VOLUME ONE

McGLAMRY'S
Foot and Ankle Surgery

FIFTH EDITION

VOLUME ONE

McGLAMRY'S
Foot and Ankle Surgery

FIFTH EDITION

BRIAN CARPENTER, DPM, FACFAS

Professor
Department of Orthopaedics
The University of North Texas Health Science Center
Fort Worth, Texas

MICHELLE L. BUTTERWORTH, DPM, FACFAS

Williamsburg Foot Center
Williamsburg Regional Hospital
Kingstree, South Carolina

WILLIAM D. FISHCO, DPM, MS, FACFAS

Faculty
The Podiatry Institute
Decatur, Georgia
Adjunct Site Director and Clinical Instructor
Creighton University PMSR/RRA
Private Practice
Anthem, Arizona

JOHN T. MARCOUX, DPM, FACFAS

Program Director, Podiatric Medicine and Surgery Residency
Department of Surgery
Steward–St. Elizabeth's Medical Center
Brighton, Massachusetts

DANIEL F. VICKERS, CAE

Executive Director
The Podiatry Institute
Decatur, Georgia

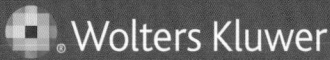 Wolters Kluwer

Philadelphia · Baltimore · New York · London
Buenos Aires · Hong Kong · Sydney · Tokyo

Executive Editor: Brian Brown
Development Editor: Stacey Sebring
Editorial Coordinator: Julie Kostelnik/Emily Buccieri
Marketing Manager: Phyllis Hitner
Production Project Manager: David Saltzberg
Design Coordinator: Stephen Druding
Manufacturing Coordinator: Beth Welsh
Prepress Vendor: SPi Global

Fifth Edition

Cataloging-in-Publication Data available on request from the Publisher

ISBN: 978-1-9751-3606-2

CONTENTS

CONTRIBUTORS

Sharif Abdelfattah, DPM, AACFAS
Foot and Ankle Surgeon
Sullivan Community Hospital
Sullivan, Indiana

Rachel H. Albright, DPM, MPH, AACFAS
Physician
Stamford Health Medical Group
Stamford, Connecticut

Dhaval K. Amin, DPM, DABPM
Staff Podiatric Foot and Ankle Surgeon
Department of Orthopaedics and
    Rehabilitation
Womack Army Medical Center
Fort Bragg, North Carolina

Robert B. Anderson, MD
Director, Foot and Ankle Service
Titletown Sports Medicine and Orthopaedics
Co-Chairman, Musculoskeletal Committee for
    the National Football League
Associate Team Physician, Green Bay Packers
Green Bay, Wisconsin

Peter J. Apel, MD, PhD
Assistant Professor
Department of Orthopaedic Surgery
Institute for Orthopaedics and Neurosciences,
    Carilion Clinic
Roanoke, Virginia

Albert V. Armstrong Jr, DPM, MS, BSRS
Professor of Radiology
Director of Advanced Medical Imaging
Former Dean
Barry University of School of Podiatric
    Medicine
Miami Shores, Florida

Christopher E. Attinger, MD
Professor, Georgetown University School of
    Medicine
Codirector, Center for Wound Healing
Department of Plastic and Reconstructive
    Surgery
MedStar Georgetown University Hospital
Washington, District of Columbia

Jayson N. Atves, DPM, AACFAS
Assistant Professor, Georgetown University
    School of Medicine
Program Director, MedStar Georgetown
    University Hospital Foot and Ankle Research
    Fellowship
Attending Physician, MedStar Health Podiatric
    Surgery Residency
Department of Plastic and Reconstructive Surgery
MedStar Georgetown University Hospital
Washington, District of Columbia

Alan S. Banks, DPM, FACFAS
Faculty
The Podiatry Institute
Decatur, Georgia
Private Practice
Tucker, Georgia

Luke C. Bates, DPM
Resident
Carilion Clinic Department of Orthopaedics
Roanoke, Virginia

Tzvi Bar-David, DPM, FACFAS
Director of Podiatric Surgery Service
Department of Orthopedic Surgery
Columbia University Medical Center
New York Presbyterian Hospital
New York, New York

Eric A. Barp, DPM, FACFAS
The Iowa Clinic-Foot and Ankle Surgery
Director of Foot and Ankle Surgery-Unity Point
    Hospital
Des Moines, Iowa

Peter A. Blume, DPM, FACFAS
Medical Director/HVC/Ambulatory Surgery
Yale New Haven Health Systems
Assistant Clinical Professor of Surgery
Anesthesia and Cardiology
Yale School of Medicine
New Haven, Connecticut

Troy J. Boffeli, DPM, FACFAS
Residency Program Director
HealthPartners Institute/Regions Hospital
Department Chair
HealthPartners Foot and Ankle Surgery
St. Paul, Minnesota

Allan M. Boike, DPM, FACFAS
Dean—CEO
Professor, Division of Foot and Ankle Surgery
Kent State University College of Podiatric
    Medicine
Independence, Ohio

Chris Bourke, DPM, AACFAS
Foot and Ankle Surgeon
Department of Orthopedics and Podiatry
Mid-Atlantic Permanente Medical Group
Kaiser Permanente
Springfield, Virginia

Aaron Bradley, MD
Private Practice
Glen Allen, Virginia

Mary R. Brandt, BA
Fourth Year Podiatric Medical Student
College of Podiatric Medicine and Surgery
Des Moines University
Des Moines, Iowa

Stephen A. Brigido, DPM, FACFAS
Section Chief, Foot and Ankle Reconstruction
Director, Foot and Ankle Fellowship
Coordinated Health at Lehigh Valley Health
    Network
Bethlehem, Pennsylvania
Clinical Professor of Surgery
The Geisinger Commonwealth
    Medical College
Scranton, Pennsylvania

Thomas A. Brosky II, DPM, FACFAS
Adjunct Faculty
Podiatric Medicine and Surgery Residency
Emory School of Medicine
Decatur, Georgia

William Brownell, DPM, MA, AACFAS
Fellow, Lower Extremity Plastic &
    Reconstructive Surgery
Division of Plastics & Reconstructive
    Surgery
Hospital of the University of
    Pennsylvania
Philadelphia, Pennsylvania

Amy E. Bruce, DPM
Chief Resident
Division of Podiatric Medicine & Surgery
University of Pennsylvania Health System–
    Penn Medicine
Philadelphia, Pennsylvania

Jennifer Buchanan, DPM, MS, FACFAS
Department of Surgery
Cambridge Health Alliance
Cambridge, Massachusetts

Michelle L. Butterworth, DPM, FACFAS
Hospital Employee
Williamsburg Foot Center
Williamsburg Regional Hospital
Kingstree, South Carolina

Jarrett D. Cain, DPM, MSc, FACFAS
Associate Professor
Department of Orthopaedics
University of Pittsburgh School of
    Medicine
University of Pittsburgh Physicians
Pittsburgh, Pennsylvania

David J. Caldarella, DPM, FACFAS
Foot and Ankle Surgery
ORTHO Rhode Island
Assistant Clinical Professor
Department of Orthopaedic Surgery
Warren Alpert School of Medicine
Brown University
Providence, Rhode Island
AO Scholar
Harborview Medical Center
Department of Orthopedic Surgery
Foot, Ankle and Amputee Service
University of Washington School of Medicine
Seattle, Washington
Alumnus, Faculty Member
The Podiatry Institute
Atlanta, Georgia

Craig A. Camasta, DPM, FACFAS, FABPS, FACSP
Private Practice
Section Chief
Department of Surgery
Emory Saint Joseph's Hospital
Atlanta, Georgia
Faculty, The Podiatry Institute
Decatur, Georgia

Steven R. Carter, DPM, FACFAS
Department of Surgery
Piedmont Hospital
Private Practice
Covington, Georgia

Andrea D. Cass, DPM, FACFAS
Faculty, The Podiatry Institute
Decatur, Georgia
Assistant Director
Atlanta Reconstructive Surgery and Limb
    Preservation Fellowship
Smyrna, Georgia

Francesca M. Castellucci-Garza, DPM, AACFAS, MS
Podiatric Surgery
Department of Orthopedics
Kaiser Permanente
Attending Surgeon
Kaiser San Francisco Bay Area Foot and Ankle
    Residency Program
Walnut Creek, California

Gage M. Caudell, DPM, FACFAS
Faculty, The Podiatry Institute
Decatur, Georgia
Fort Wayne Orthopedics
Fort Wayne, Indiana

David Chan, DPM
Private Practice
Leesburg, Virginia

Thomas J. Chang, DPM, FACFAS
Faculty, The Podiatry Institute
Decatur, Georgia
Clinical Professor and Past Chairman
Department of Podiatric Surgery
Samuel Merritt College of Podiatric Medicine,
    Formerly CCPM
Oakland, California
Redwood Orthopedic Surgery Associates
Santa Rosa, California

Jeffrey C. Christensen, DPM, FACFAS
Founder, Ankle & Foot Clinic of Everett
Past Foot & Ankle Section Chair/Attending
    Surgeon
Department of Orthopedics
Swedish Medical Center
Seattle, Washington

Robert A. Christman, DPM, EdM
Professor
College of Podiatric Medicine
Western University of Health Sciences
Pomona, California

J. Randolph Clements, DPM
Associate Professor of Orthopaedic
    Surgery
Virginia Tech Carilion School of Medicine
Roanoke, Virginia

David R. Collman, DPM, FACFAS
Site Director, Kaiser San Francisco Bay Area
    Foot and Ankle Residency Program
Assistant Chief, Podiatry/Foot and Ankle
    Surgery
Department of Orthopedics, Podiatry, Injury,
    Sports Medicine
The Permanente Medical Group, Inc.
Kaiser Foundation Hospital San Francisco
San Francisco, California

James C. Connors, DPM, FACFAS
Assistant Professor
Division of Foot and Ankle Surgery
Kent State University College of Podiatric
    Medicine
Independence, Ohio

Dustin Constant, DPM
Foot and Ankle Surgeon
Palm Beach Sports Medicine and Orthopedics
Palm Beach, Florida

Emily A. Cook, DPM, MPH, CPH, FACFAS
Assistant Professor of Surgery
Harvard Medical School
Director of Resident Education
Department of Surgery
Mount Auburn Hospital
Cambridge, Massachusetts

Jeremy J. Cook, DPM, MPH, CPH, FACFAS
Assistant Professor of Surgery
Harvard Medical School
Director of Research and Quality Assurance
Department of Surgery
Mount Auburn Hospital
Cambridge, Massachusetts

Guillaume Cordier, MD
Past President
Group of Research and Study in Minimally
    Invasive Surgery of the Foot/Minimal Invasive
    Foot Surgery
Foot and Ankle Surgeon
Clinique du Sport Bordeaux-Mérignac,
    Chirurgie du Sport–Foot and Ankle
Merignac, France

Judd Cummings, MD
Clinical Assistant Professor
Department of Orthopaedic Surgery
University of Arizona
Orthopaedic Surgical Oncology of Arizona
Scottsdale, Arizona

Miki Dalmau-Pastor, PhD, PT, DPM
Human Anatomy and Embryology Unit
Department of Pathology and Experimental
  Therapeutics
University of Barcelona
Foot and Ankle Unit
Hospital Quirón Barcelona
Barcelona, Spain

Paul Dayton, DPM, MS, FACFAS
Surgeon
Foot & Ankle Center of Iowa/Midwest Bunion
  Center
Ankeny, Iowa

Lawrence A. DiDomenico, DPM, FACFAS
Director of Residency Training
East Liverpool City Hospital
Director of Fellowship Training
NOMS (Northern Ohio Medical Specialist)
  Ankle and Foot Care Centers
Section Chief
Mercy Health St. Elizabeth Medical Center
Boardman, Ohio
Adjunct Professor
Kent State University College of Podiatric
  Medicine
Independence, Ohio

Thanh L. Dinh, DPM, FACFAS
Assistant Professor of Surgery
Harvard Medical School
Program Director
Podiatric Surgical Residency Program
Beth Israel Deaconess Medical Center
Boston, Massachusetts

Matthew B. Dobbs, MD, FACS
Director, Dobbs Clubfoot Center
Paley Orthopedic & Spine Institute
West Palm Beach, Florida
Senior Editor, Clinical Orthopaedics and
  Related Research
President, United States Bone and Joint Initiative
Secretary, Association of Bone and Joint Surgeons
Park Ridge, Illinois

Michael S. Downey, DPM, FACFAS
Chief, Division of Podiatric Surgery
Department of Surgery
Penn Presbyterian Medical Center
University of Pennsylvania Health System
Clinical Professor, Department of Surgery
Temple University School of Podiatric Medicine
Philadelphia, Pennsylvania
Private Practice
Penn Podiatry
Philadelphia, Pennsylvania and Mt. Laurel,
  New Jersey

Matthew D. Doyle, DPM, MS
Fellow
Silicon Valley Reconstructive Foot and Ankle
  Fellowship
Palo Alto Medical Foundation
Mountain View, California

Amish K. Dudeja, DPM, AACFAS
Foot and Ankle Surgical Fellow
Atlanta Reconstructive Surgery and Limb
  Preservation Fellowship
Village Podiatry Centers
Atlanta, Georgia

Karl W. Dunn, DPM, FACFAS
Compass Orthopedics
An Affiliate of Compass Rehabilitation
East Lansing, Michigan

Jordan J. Ernst, DPM, MS, AACFAS
Fellow, Foot and Ankle Deformity Correction
Fellow, Limb Lengthening and Reconstruction
Paley Orthopedic and Spine Institute
West Palm Beach, Florida

William D. Fishco, DPM, MS, FACFAS
Adjunct Site Director and Clinical Instructor
Creighton University PMSR/RRA
Private Practice
Anthem, Arizona

Adam E. Fleischer, DPM, MPH, FACFAS
Associate Professor
Dr. William M. Scholl College of Podiatric Medicine
Rosalind Franklin University of Medicine and
  Science
North Chicago, Illinois
Director of Research
Weil Foot & Ankle Institute
Mount Prospect, Illinois

Lawrence A. Ford, DPM, FACFAS
Chief of Podiatric Surgery
Department of Orthopedics
Kaiser Permanente
Attending Surgeon
Kaiser San Francisco Bay Area Foot and Ankle
  Residency Program
Oakland, California

Robert Fridman, DPM, FACFAS, CWSP
Faculty Podiatric Surgery Service
Department of Orthopedic Surgery
Columbia University Medical Center
New York Presbyterian Hospital
New York, New York

Ajay K. Ghai, DPM, AACFAS
Fellow, NOMS-Ankle and Foot Care Center
Visalia Medical Clinic
Visalia, California

David A. Goss Jr, DO
Orthopedic Foot and Ankle Surgeon
Associates of Orthopedics and Sports Medicine
Dalton, Georgia

John Grady, DPM, FFPM RCPS (G), FASPS, FAAPSM
Residency Director
Advocate Christ Medical Center
Great Lakes Foot & Ankle Institute
Oak Lawn, Illinois

David W. Gray, MD, FAAOS
Professor
Department of Surgery
Texas Christian University Medical School
Cook Children's Department of Orthopedics and
  Spine Surgery
Fort Worth, Texas

George S. Gumann Jr, DPM, FACFAS
Retired Chief, Foot and Ankle Service
Orthopedic Clinic
Martin Army Hospital
Fort Benning, Georgia

Adam L. Halverson, DO
Consultant Surgeon
Orthopedic Surgeon: Foot and Ankle
  Specialist
Bone and Joint
Wausau, Wisconsin

John C. Haight, DPM
Chief Resident
Podiatric Medicine and Surgery Residency
Emory University School of Medicine
Decatur, Georgia

Patrick B. Hall, DPM, FACFAS
Faculty, The Podiatry institute
Decatur, Georgia
Private Practice
The Bone and Joint Clinic of Baton Rouge
Baton Rouge, Louisiana

Graham Hamilton, DPM, FACFAS
Foot and Ankle Surgeon
Department of Orthopedic and Podiatric
  Surgery
Sutter Health–Palo Alto Foundation Medical
  Group
Dublin, California

Mark A. Hardy, DPM, FACFAS
Division Head, Foot and Ankle Surgery
Kent State University College of Podiatric
  Medicine
Independence, Ohio

Carl T. Hasselman, MD, FAAOS, FAOFAS
Vice Chairman of Orthopedics, UPMC St. Margaret
Clinical Associate Professor, University of
  Pittsburgh
Professor, Saint Vincent College
Pittsburgh, Pennsylvania

Daniel J. Hatch, DPM, FACFAS
Director of Surgery
North Colorado Podiatric Surgical Residency
Greeley, Colorado
Private Practice
Foot and Ankle Center of the Rockies
Denver, Colorado

Christopher R. Hood Jr, DPM
Foot and Ankle Surgery
Hunterdon Podiatric Medicine
Hunterdon Healthcare System
Flemington, New Jersey

Byron Hutchinson, DPM, FACFAS
Medical Director
CHI/Franciscan Advanced Foot & Ankle
Fellowship
Franciscan Foot & Ankle Associates: Highline
Clinic
Burien, Washington

Christopher F. Hyer, DPM, MS, FACFAS
Codirector
Foot and Ankle Reconstructive Fellowship
Orthopedic Foot and Ankle Center
Worthington, Ohio

Trusha Jariwala, DPM, AACFAS
Associate Podiatrist
Moore Foot and Ankle Specialists, PA
Asheville, North Carolina

Meagan Jennings, DPM, FACFAS
Foot and Ankle Surgeon
Department of Orthopedics and Podiatry
Sutter Health–Palo Alto Foundation Medical Group
Mountain View, California

Molly S. Judge, DPM, FACFAS
Mercy Foot & Ankle Residency Program
Cleveland, Ohio
Adjunct Faculty; Colleges of Podiatric
Medicine, USA
Faculty; Graduate Medical Education
Mercy Health Partners
Toledo, Ohio

Daniel C. Jupiter, PhD
Associate Professor
Department of Preventive Medicine and
Population Health
Department of Orthopaedic Surgery and
Rehabilitation
Assistant Dean for Recruitment
Graduate School of Biomedical Sciences
The University of Texas Medical Branch
Galveston, Texas

Andreas C. Kaikis, DPM, AACFAS
Staff Surgeon
University Hospital Health System
Augusta, Georgia

Andrew P. Kapsalis, DPM, AACFAS
Research Coordinator for Fellowship Training
Foot and Ankle Reconstructive Surgical
Services
American Health Network
Indianapolis, Indiana

Navita Khatri, DPM
Resident
Podiatric Medicine and Surgery Residency
Emory University School of Medicine
Decatur, Georgia

Michael F. Kelly, DPM, AACFAS
Foot and Ankle Surgeon
Department of Podiatry
St. Joseph Hospital–Covenant Health
Nashua, New Hampshire

Jason M. Kennedy, MD, FAAOS
Clinical Faculty, John Peter Smith Residency
Program
Clinical Faculty, Baylor University Residency
Program
Cook Children's Department of Orthopaedics
and Sports Medicine
Fort Worth, Texas

Ansab Khwaja, MD
Resident Physician
University of Arizona Orthopaedic Surgery
Residency
Tucson, Arizona

Carl Kihm, DPM, FACFAS
Attending Surgeon
Norton Audubon Hospital Residency
Program
Private Practice
Louisville, Kentucky

Christy M. King, DPM, FACFAS
Program Direction
Kaiser San Francisco Bay Area Foot and Ankle
Residency Program
Attending Physician, Kaiser Foundation
Hospital–Oakland
Department of Orthopedics and Podiatry
Oakland, California

Alex J. Kline, MD, FAAOS, FAOFAS
Clinical Associate Professor
University of Pittsburgh
Chairman
Department of Orthopedics
UPMC St. Margaret
Professor
Saint Vincent College
Pittsburgh, Pennsylvania

Bradley M. Lamm, DPM, FACFAS
Chief, Foot and Ankle Surgery
St. Mary's Medical Center & Palm Beach
Children's Hospital
Director, Foot and Ankle Deformity Center and
Fellowship
Paley Orthopedic and Spine Institute
West Palm Beach, Florida

Travis M. Langan, DPM
Fellowship Trained Foot and Ankle Surgeon
Carle Orthopedics and Sports Medicine
Champaign, Illinois

Michael S. Lee, DPM, MS-HCA, FACFAS
Foot and Ankle Surgery
Capital Orthopaedics & Sports Medicine, PC
Des Moines, Iowa

Wesley Maurice Leong, DPM
Podiatric Surgeon
Department of Foot and Ankle Surgery
Monument Health Orthopedics and Specialty
Hospital
Rapid City, South Dakota

Sara E. Lewis, DPM, AACFAS
Faculty
The Podiatry Institute
Decatur, Georgia
Health First Medical Group
Melbourne, Florida

Chandler J. Ligas, DPM
Resident
Podiatric Medicine and Surgery Residency
Emory University School of Medicine
Decatur, Georgia

George T. Liu, DPM, FACFAS
Associate Professor
Department of Orthopaedic Surgery
University of Texas Southwestern Medical Center
Dallas, Texas

Samantha A. Luer, DPM
Staff Surgeon
Department of Foot and Ankle Surgery/
Orthopedics
Avera Medical Group, St. Anthony's Hospital
O'Neill, Nebraska

**Caitlin Mahan Madden, DPM,
AACFAS**
Associate Foot and Ankle Surgeon
Podiatry Care Specialists, PC
West Chester, Pennsylvania

**Kieran T. Mahan, DPM, FACFAS,
FABFAS, FCPP**
Professor
Department of Surgery
Temple University School of Podiatric Medicine
Chair, Department of Foot and Ankle Surgery
Temple University Hospital
Philadelphia, Pennsylvania

D. Scot Malay, DPM, MSCE, FACFAS
Faculty, The Podiatry Institute
Decatur, Georgia
Staff Surgeon and Director of Podiatric
Research
Penn Presbyterian Medical Center
Philadelphia, Pennsylvania

Joshua J. Mann, DPM, FACFAS
Director
Podiatric Medicine and Surgery Residency
Emory University School of Medicine
Adjunct Assistant Professor
Department of Family and Preventive
Medicine
Emory University School of Medicine
Private Practice
Ankle and Foot Centers of Georgia
Snellville, Georgia

John T. Marcoux, DPM, FACFAS
Program Director, Podiatric Medicine and
Surgery Residency
Department of Surgery
Steward–St. Elizabeth's Medical Center
Brighton, Massachusetts

Stephen A. Mariash, DPM
Podiatric Surgeon
St. Cloud Orthopedics
Sartell, Minnesota

John A. Martucci, DPM
Resident Physician, Podiatric Medicine and
  Surgery
Division of Podiatric Surgery
Department of Surgery
Beth Israel Deaconess Medical Center
Clinical Fellow in Surgery
Harvard Medical School
Boston, Massachusetts

Stephen A. McCaughan, DO
Associate Professor
Department of Anesthesiology
Lewis Katz School of Medicine
Philadelphia, Pennsylvania

Michael C. McGlamry, DPM, FACFAS
Faculty, The Podiatry Institute
Private Practice
Cumming, Georgia

Andrew J. Meyr, DPM, FACFAS
Clinical Professor
Department of Surgery
Temple University School of Podiatric Medicine
Philadelphia, Pennsylvania

J. Michael Miller, DPM, FACFAS
Director of Fellowship Training
Foot and Ankle Reconstructive Surgical Services
American Health Network
Indianapolis, Indiana

Jason R. Miller, DPM, FACFAS
Director, Pennsylvania Intensive Lower
  Extremity Fellowship Program
Residency Director, Tower Health/Phoenixville
  Hospital PMSR/RRA
Adjunct Associate Professor
Department of Surgery
Temple University School of Podiatric Medicine
Philadelphia, Pennsylvania
Premier Orthopaedics
Malvern, Pennsylvania

Kelsey Millonig, DPM, MPH, AACFAS
Foot and Ankle Deformity Correction and
  Orthoplastics Fellow
Rubin Institute Advanced Orthopedics
International Center for Limb Lengthening
Baltimore, Maryland

Jeanne Mirbey, DPM
Physician
Emory Decatur Hospital
Decatur, Georgia

Roya Mirmiran, DPM, FACFAS
Foot and Ankle Surgeon
Sutter Medical Group
Sacramento, California

Travis A. Motley, DPM, MS, FACFAS
Professor, Department of Orthopaedic Surgery
Program Director, Podiatry Surgical Residency
Acclaim Physician Group
John Peter Smith Hospital
Fort Worth, Texas

Benjamin Meyer, DO
Resident Physician
MountainView Regional Medical Center
  Orthopaedic Surgery Residency
Las Cruces, New Mexico

Gina H. Nalbandian, DPM, AACFAS
Clinical Fellow of Surgery
Tufts University School of Medicine
Clinical Fellow of Surgery
University of California, Los Angeles
Los Angeles, California

Alan Ng, DPM, FACFAS
Foot & Ankle Surgeon, Advanced Orthopedic
  and Sports Medicine Specialists
Fellowship Director
The Rocky Mountain Reconstructive Foot &
  Ankle Fellowship at Advanced Orthopedic
Sports Medicine Specialists
Division of Orthopedic Centers of Colorado and
  Presbyterian/St. Luke's Medical Center/HCA
Residency Committee Member
Highlands-Presbyterian/St. Luke's Medical
  Center Podiatric Surgical Residency Program
Denver, Colorado

Jonathan D. Nigro, BS
Fourth Year Podiatric Medical Student
College of Podiatric Medicine and Surgery
Des Moines University
Des Moines, Iowa

Selene G. Parekh, MD, MBA, FAOA
Director of Digital Strategy & Innovation
Professor, Department of Orthopaedic Surgery
Partner, North Carolina Orthopaedic Clinic
Adjunct Faculty, Fuqua Business School
Duke University
Durham, North Carolina

Sandeep B. Patel, DPM, FACFAS
Chief of Podiatric Surgery
Department of Podiatric Surgery and Orthopedics
The Permanente Medical Group, Diablo
  Service Area
Kaiser San Francisco Bay Area Foot and Ankle
  Residency Program
Walnut Creek, California

Trevor S. Payne, DPM
Private Practice
Augusta, Georgia

Terrence M. Philbin, DO, FAOAO
Orthopedic Foot and Ankle Center
Worthington, Ohio

Alfred J. Phillips, DPM
Chief of Podiatry
St. Elizabeth Medical Center
Action, Massachusetts

Jason D. Pollard, DPM, FACFAS
Director of Research and Assistant Program
  Director
Department of Podiatric Surgery
Kaiser San Francisco Bay Area Foot and Ankle
  Residency Program
Oakland, California

Adam D. Port, DPM
Adjunct Faculty
Podiatric Medicine and Surgery Residency
Emory School of Medicine
Decatur, Georgia

Asim A. Z. Raja, DPM, FACFAS, DABPM
Director, Podiatric Medical Education (PMSR/RRA)
Department of Orthopaedics and Rehabilitation
Womack Army Medical Center
Fort Bragg, North Carolina

Nilin M. Rao, DPM, PhD, AACFAS
Fellow
Silicon Valley Reconstructive Foot and Ankle
  Fellowship
Department of Podiatric Surgery
Sutter Health–Palo Alto Medical Foundation
Mountain View, California

Rahn Ravenell, DPM, FACFAS
Assistant Professor
Medical University of South Carolina
Faculty, Podiatry Institute
Mount Pleasant, South Carolina

Christopher L. Reeves, DPM, FACFAS
Research Coordinator, Department of Podiatric
  Surgery, Advent Health System
Faculty, Advent Health East Podiatric Surgical
  Residency
Orlando Foot and Ankle Clinic/Upperline
  Health
Orlando, Florida

Rebekah Richards, DPM
Richards Orthopedic and Sports Medicine
Chambersburg, Pennsylvania

**Douglas H. Richie Jr, DPM, FACFAS,
FAAPSM**
Associate Clinical Professor
California School of Podiatric Medicine at
  Samuel Merritt University
Oakland, California

Ryan B. Rigby, DPM, FACFAS
Fellowship Trained Foot and Ankle Surgeon
Department of Orthopedics
Logan Regional Hospital
Logan Regional Orthopedics & Sports Medicine
Logan, Utah

Shayla A. Robinson, DPM
Resident
Podiatric Medicine and Surgery Residency
Emory University School of Medicine
Decatur, Georgia

Thomas S. Roukis, DPM, PhD, FACFAS
Past President (2014–2015), American College
 of Foot and Ankle Surgeons
Editor-in-Chief, Foot & Ankle Surgery:
 Techniques, Reports & Cases
Clinical Professor
Division of Foot & Ankle Surgery
Department of Orthopaedic Surgery and
 Rehabilitation
College of Medicine–Jacksonville
University of Florida
Jacksonville, Florida

Laura P. Rowe, DPM
Private Practice,
Valley Foot & Ankle Specialty Providers
Fresno, California

Shannon M. Rush, DPM, FACFAS
Tri-Valley Orthopedics Specialists, Inc
Pleasanton, California
Adjunct Professor
California College of Podiatric Medicine at
 Samuel Merritt University
Fellowship Director
Tri-Valley Foot and Ankle Reconstruction
 Fellowship
Pleasanton, California
Surgical Staff
Stanford Valley Care
Pleasanton, California

Hannah J. Sahli, DPM
Chief Resident
Advent Health East Orlando Podiatric Surgical
 Residency
Orlando, Florida

Laura E. Sansosti, DPM, AACFAS
Clinical Assistant Professor
Departments of Surgery and Biomechanics
Temple University School of Podiatric Medicine
Philadelphia, Pennsylvania

Amol Saxena, DPM, FFPM, RCPS (G), FACFAS, FAAPSM
Fellowship Director Foot and Ankle Surgery
Department of Sports Medicine
Sutter Health–Palo Alto Division
Palo Alto, California

Harry P. Schneider, DPM, FACFAS
Assistant Professor of Surgery
Harvard Medical School
Residency Program Director
Cambridge Health Alliance
Cambridge, Massachusetts

John M. Schuberth, DPM
Staff Surgeon
Dept Orthopedic Surgery, Sports Medicine &
 Podiatry
Kaiser Foundation Hospital
San Francisco, California

Josh Sebag, DPM
Chief Resident
Department of Podiatric Surgery
Advent Health East Orlando Podiatric Surgical
 Residency
Orlando, Florida

Matthew J. Seidel, MD
Surgeon Department of Orthopedic Surgery
Honor Health Hospital System
Clinical Assistant Professor of Orthopedic
 Surgery University of Arizona
Scottsdale, Arizona

Chad L. Seidenstricker, BS, DPM
Foot & Ankle Surgeon
New Mexico Orthopaedics
Albuquerque, New Mexico

Michael L. Sganga, DPM, FACFAS
Chief of Podiatry Milford Regional Medical
 Center
Foot and Ankle Surgeon
Orthopedics New England
Natick, Newton, and Hopkinton,
 Massachusetts

Amber M. Shane, DPM, FACFAS
Chair, Department of Podiatric Surgery, Advent
 Health System
Faculty, Advent Health East Podiatric Surgical
 Residency
Orlando Foot and Ankle Clinic/Upperline Health
Orlando, Florida

Eric Shi, DPM
Foot and Ankle Surgeon
Department of Podiatry
Sutter East Bay Medical Foundation
Castro Valley, California

Naohiro Shibuya, DPM, MS, FACFAS
Professor
College of Medicine
Texas A&M University
Temple, Texas

Sara Shirazi, DPM
Podiatric Surgeon
Pasadena Orthopedics, Inc.
Los Angeles, California

Louie Shou, DPM, AACFAS, FAAPSM
Reconstructive Orthopedics
Medford, New Jersey

Clay Shumway, DPM AACFAS
Fellow, Pennsylvania Intensive Lower Extremity
 Fellowship
Premier Orthopaedics & Sports Medicine
Malvern, Pennsylvania

Mickey D. Stapp, DPM, FACFAS
Private Practice
Augusta, Georgia

Jerome K. Steck, DPM
Chief of Podiatric Surgery
Carondelet Medical Group: Orthopedics
Carondelet St. Joseph's Hospital
Tucson, Arizona

John S. Steinberg, DPM, FACFAS
Professor, Georgetown University School of
 Medicine
Program Director, MedStar Health Podiatric
 Surgery Residency
Codirector, Center for Wound Healing
Department of Plastic and Reconstructive
 Surgery
MedStar Georgetown University Hospital
Washington, District of Columbia

N. Jake Summers, DPM, FACFAS
Chief of Podiatry Dartmouth-Hitchcock
 Manchester
Faculty - New England Musculoskeletal
 Institute
Dartmouth-Hitchcock
Manchester, New Hampshire

Ronald M. Talis, DPM, FACFAS
Staff Podiatric Foot and Ankle Surgeon
Department of Orthopedics and Rehabilitation
Womack Army Medical Center
Fort Bragg, North Carolina

Zach Tankersley, DPM, FACFAS
Associate Professor of Orthopaedic Surgery
Joan C. Edwards School of Medicine
Marshall University
Huntington, West Virginia

Robert P. Taylor, DPM, FACFAS
Stonebriar Foot & Ankle
Firsco, Texas

Michael H. Theodoulou, DPM, FACFAS
Chief
Division of Podiatric Surgery, Cambridge Health
 Alliance
Department of Surgery
Instructor of Surgery
Harvard Medical School
Cambridge, Massachusetts

James Thomas, DPM, FACFAS
Chief, Foot and Ankle Surgery
Professor of Orthopaedic Surgery
Joan C. Edwards School of Medicine
Marshall University
Huntington, West Virginia

Mitchell J. Thompson, DPM
Podiatric Medicine & Surgery Resident
Podiatric Medicine and Surgery
Gundersen Medical Foundation
LaCrosse, Wisconsin

Michael Van Pelt, DPM, FACFAS
Associate Professor
Department of Orthopaedic Surgery
UT Southwestern Medical Center Dallas
Dallas, Texas

Tracey C. Vlahovic, DPM, FFPM, RCPS (Glasg)
Clinical Professor
Department of Podiatric Medicine
Temple University School of Podiatric
 Medicine
Philadelphia, Pennsylvania

Mitzi L. Williams, DPM, FACFAS
Pediatric Foot and Ankle Surgery
Department of Podiatric Surgery and
 Orthopedics
Attending Surgeon
Kaiser Permanente
Oakland, California

FOREWORD

The presentation of the fifth edition of *McGlamry's Foot and Ankle Surgery* is a time to look back as well as forward. I look back to the genesis of this textbook and realize that it is one of the most satisfying chapters in my career in Podiatric Medicine and Surgery.

From 1972 to 1982, I was privileged to serve as editor of *The Journal of the American Podiatry Medical Association*. In that capacity, I made frequent visits to meet with our publisher, Williams and Wilkins Medical Publishers, in Baltimore, Maryland. This resulted in a close relationship with Norville Miller, the executive responsible for the final production and printing and distribution of the journal. Norville frequently reminded me that Podiatric Surgery was yet to produce its own textbook.

When I retired as editor of *JAPMA*, Norville called asking to meet with me in Atlanta. He was very forthright in saying that he wanted to talk about a textbook on Foot and Ankle Surgery. He also said that Williams and Wilkins (W and W) was willing to make an attractive arrangement.

Norville flew to Atlanta and met with me and two of my residents, Drs. Kieran Mahan and John Ruch. He presented the idea of doing the first medical textbook ever, with the entire book being written in computer instead of typed. The idea was to complete the book and turn over the floppy discs to W and W instead of submitting a typed manuscript. He said that W and W would purchase for us an IBM Computer, a printer, a computer desk, and most important, would purchase a support contract whereby we could call for computer instruction and technical assistance at any time of day or night. Remember, the personal computer was then new. There were no ribbons with commands at the top of the page. There was no mouse.

Dr. Mahan, Dr. Ruch, and I accepted the challenge on behalf of the relatively young Podiatry Institute. We also got a commitment from Becky McGlamry that she would serve as Author's Editor. And for the next 5 years that embryo book drove our lives and that of many of our colleagues and former residents of our program in Podiatric Surgery.

Each addition of the textbook has shown progressive maturity. This edition is no exception to that trend, and it is so written and organized as to facilitate immediate access to virtually any challenge confronting the Podiatric or Orthopedic Surgeon as they deal with foot and ankle surgery. This should provide the most accessible and in-depth information of any of the five editions, an appropriate accomplishment for the fifth edition. My personal congratulations to the editors and to the publisher, now Lippincott, Williams & Wilkins.

E. Dalton McGlamry, retired

PREFACE

We are delighted and honored to write the preface for the fifth edition of *McGlamry's Foot and Ankle Surgery*. E. Dalton McGlamry recognized the need for a complete and well-referenced textbook in foot and ankle surgery and published the first edition in 1987. Through the centuries, physicians and surgeons have been engaged in preservation of normal foot and ankle function. In ancient times, the normal functioning foot was vital to survival. Aristotle (384-322 BC) studied movement and analyzed the degeneration of muscles and the defective development of human beings, and it was believed that individuals possessing these attributes could not survive. In ancient Rome, those with disabilities were treated as objects of scorn. As early as 400 BC, Hippocrates described clubfoot and recommended nonoperative treatments using manipulation and bandaging techniques not dissimilar to the techniques utilized today.

In recent times, an abundance of medical knowledge and innovations have been unveiled and the dynamic nature of medical science continues to evolve. Professionals among the medical disciplines work collectively as interdisciplinary teams and are the cornerstone of medical organizations and health care systems representing the future of medicine. Well-trained, successful, foot and ankle surgeons exert a large influence within medicine and represent departmental chairs, current and past presidents of major medical associations, journal authors and editors, researchers, and reviewers.

This textbook is intended for use by residents in training with a focus on foot and ankle pathology as well as surgeons with interest in the foot and ankle; both nonoperative and operative techniques are described with quick reference text boxes highlighted as an educational tool for the reader.

The esteemed authors represented in this textbook were carefully selected for their educational, clinical, and surgical acumen, contributions to research and achievements in their selected subject matter. The editorial board endeavored to ensure that the information provided is accurate and current.

It is our hope and expectation that this book will provide an effective learning experience and referenced resource for all foot and ankle specialists and ultimately lead to improved patient care and outcomes.

Brian Carpenter, DPM, FACFAS
Michelle L. Butterworth, DPM, FACFAS
William D. Fishco, DPM, MS, FACFAS
John T. Marcoux, DPM, FACFAS

ACKNOWLEDGMENTS

I would like to acknowledge the authors and reviewers, Dr. Butterworth, Dr. Fishco, and Dr. Marcoux, for their dedication to this project. You have provided countless hours in bringing this to fruition and have remained steadfast friends and supportive colleagues. The world of medicine is enhanced by your contributions to academic medicine, your zeal in sharing your talent, and your ability to incentivize others by your mentorship. Your gift of time and sacrifice is immeasurable.

To the individuals with whom I have been blessed to work and serve with and those who I have had the opportunity to train and educate, I thank you for inspiring me to undertake this project. Being part of the Podiatry Institute is one of the highlights of my career being allowed to enhance the quality of life for patients with foot, ankle, and leg disorders through innovative education, research, and service is humbling. Without the experiences and support I have garnered from students, residents, and peers throughout the years, this publication would not exist.

I would be remiss if I didn't highlight those who have been instrumental in my own personal development and professional career. Physicians, nurses, and fellow residents were an integral part of my education and I am reminded of you whenever I reduce and fixate a fracture by nail or plate or when powering up a saw. I want to give special recognition and thanks to my mentors: Jeff Coen, DPM; A. Edward Mostone, DPM; Raymond Igou, MD; Michael Corbett, MD; Stephen Tubridy, DPM; Francis Wolfort, MD; and Ted Hansen, MD, who provided innumerable educational opportunities. During my training, they challenged me to never be content with my knowledge and skills. I am grateful for their stewardship and now call them friends.

Seek knowledge, serve as an ambassador for your patients, do the right thing and ultimately, your life will be blessed. I pay homage to God; without him none of this would be possible.

Brian Carpenter, DPM, FACFAS

INTRODUCTION

I am honored to have been chosen to write this introduction to the fifth edition of *McGlamry's Foot and Ankle Surgery*.

I vividly remember 30 years ago, as Dennis Martin and I began our residency at Doctors Hospital in Tucker, Georgia, the publishing of the first edition of the *McGlamry's Foot and Ankle Surgery*. No other comprehensive textbook on foot surgery had been written. The textbook included three separate volumes. The first was a text entitled the "Fundamentals of Foot Surgery" that reviewed anatomy, surgical materials, sutures, etc., and essentially provided the reader with a framework to learn the cornerstones of foot surgery. Another two volumes entitled "Comprehensive Textbook of Foot Surgery" reviewed specific pathologies of the foot and ankle and the surgical procedures associated with them. As a new resident, I looked up to the authors with reverence: E. Dalton McGlamry, John Ruch, Kieran Mahan, Gerard Yu, among others. To me, they were larger than life characters and I was humbled to be associated with them.

I remember how useful the text was as I began to learn and develop my surgical skills. In my first year, the fundamental text was invaluable to me as I learned the various biomechanical and surgical principles as well as memorizing suture materials and surgical instrumentation. The comprehensive texts were more valuable to me in my second and third years as I developed my surgical skills in the operating room and understanding complex surgical dilemmas. I am sure that my experience as an aspiring foot and ankle surgeon during this time period was not different to others in our field of expertise. The text quickly became a required text in all podiatric medical schools and remains so.

The second, third, and fourth editions built on the edition it followed. Although the editors and the authors have changed with each edition, the message and goal has been the same: to create a premier up-to-date text to teach students, residents, and attending podiatric and orthopedic surgeons foot and ankle surgery.

The fifth edition of the *McGlamry's Foot and Ankle Surgery* is a result of a collaboration of well-renowned faculty of the Podiatry Institute as well as accomplished podiatric and orthopedic foot and ankle surgeons throughout our surgical specialty. The fifth edition documents the most up-to-date information on foot and ankle surgery and does so in a unique way. As you will see, the textbook includes technique-driven color photography of surgical procedures in order to share the operative experience as well as author-specific techniques and pearls. The fifth edition also includes links in the eBook to videos illustrating surgical procedures discussed in the text, a feature not available in previous editions.

There are numerous chapters covering material that was not present in the previous texts. These include 3D imprinting, caging, cartilage replacement technology, and others.

I congratulate the editors in providing a truly new addition to the foot and ankle literature. I specifically thank Brian Carpenter, the lead editor, and the contributing editors Michelle Butterworth, William Fishco, and John Marcoux who provided endless hours reviewing and editing each chapter. I also thank Dan Vickers for his tireless work as the authors' editor. The work that they have accomplished together has provided a manuscript of supreme quality. I am certain that it will be enjoyed and treasured by all those who seek to perform foot and ankle surgery at a higher standard.

Alfred J. Phillips, DPM, FACFAS
Chairman of the Podiatry Institute 2019-2020

General Management

CHAPTER 1

Biomechanics

Douglas H. Richie, Jr.

INTRODUCTION

The human foot contains unique features enabling the primary functions of upright standing and bipedal ambulation. The goal of reconstructive foot and ankle surgery is restoration of function to the appendage that will lead to improvement of mobility for the patient. To achieve this goal, the planning of any surgical procedures requires a detailed knowledge of how the foot functions during standing and walking. More importantly, the surgeon must fully understand all of the factors that affect mobility of the foot and how they are ultimately controlled by the central nervous system. Biomechanics is a broad discipline encompassing many areas of study. This chapter will focus on certain topics that are most relevant to the foot and ankle surgeon, enabling the integration of knowledge of foot function into the planning and execution of surgical procedures.

A study of gait, focusing on the interaction of the foot with the ground as well as its interaction with proximal skeletal segments will give an introduction to moments, forces, and muscle actions. Next, a review of recent kinematic studies will give new insight into the contributions of multiple joints to overall motion of the foot, dispelling previous notions about modeling of skeletal segments of the foot during gait. Muscles and tendons, which span multiple essential joints of the foot, will be evaluated from the standpoint of power and moment arm. The physiology of sensorimotor mechanisms that control posture and lower extremity movement will be reviewed. Finally, the unique anatomic features of the human foot will be explored to elucidate how this appendage can provide compliance, stiffness, and energy storage necessary for bipedal ambulation.

Much of the insight into the function and mechanical behavior of the human foot has been gained from research contributed by several different scientific disciplines including biomechanics, movement science, neuroscience, physical medicine, and physical therapy. Terminology from these disciplines differs somewhat from common terminology used in the podiatric community. Therefore, a review of terminology is required before exploring the topics.

TERMINOLOGY

Biomechanics is a study of the mechanics of a living body, especially of the forces exerted by muscles and gravity on the skeletal structure.[1] Studies of human movement use methods of mechanical engineering studying time, mass, force, center of gravity, moments of force, and motion. The foot and ankle surgeon should be familiar with these terms and definitions as they are commonly used in publications relevant to foot and ankle surgery.

Gait studies and force plate studies utilize the millisecond as the primary unit for time. Repeated events over short periods of time are measured in frequency or hertz, abbreviated Hz. 1 Hz is one cycle per second. For example, a force plate may sample ground reaction force (GRF) at 500 Hz, which is 2-ms interval between samples.

The mass of an object is normally measured in kilograms (kg). The force acting on an object is measured in Newton. The force applied by earth's gravity on a mass of 1 kg is 9.81 N. One Newton is the force exerted by gravity on a mass of 102 g or 3 oz. Cadaver studies often apply axial load to a limb to simulate body weight. A 70-kg adult will produce a downward force from gravity of 686.7 N. Therefore, to simulate quiet standing, a cadaver model of one leg will apply axial load of ~350 N.

The center of mass is often referred to as the center of gravity in studies of human walking and standing. The center of gravity is thought to be located immediately in front of the lumbosacral junction in an upright standing human. The center of gravity can actually move away from the body depending on the movement.

The moment of force is defined as a force acting at a distance from a rotational axis. The distance is known as the lever arm or moment arm. A moment of force will cause a skeletal segment to rotate at a single joint or multiple joints. Moment of force can also be termed moment or torque. Moment of force is calculated by: $M = F \times D$, where M is the moment of force in Newton-meters (N-m), F is the force in Newton (N), and D is the distance in meters (m).

The angle of the force vector can have significant effects on the magnitude of moment of force. The above equation assumes that the force vector is aligned perpendicular to the joint axis, which applies maximal moment. If the force vector is oriented <90 degrees, a multiplier sine ℓ is used, where ℓ is the angle of the force vector relative to the axis of motion. For a force vector aligned 30 degrees from the joint axis, the formula becomes:

$$M = F \times D \times \text{sine } 30$$

which will significantly diminish the moment or power exerted on a given joint to produce rotation.

Therefore, when a tendon exerts moment of force on a joint of the foot, the overall mechanical effect is not just dependent on the length of the moment arm but also on the angle of tendon relative to the joint axis. Studies have confirmed that position of the subtalar joint will significantly affect the moment arm of the lower leg muscles. This becomes a critical issue with tendon transfers in the foot and ankle as will be discussed later in this chapter.

Stiffness is a term that is commonly used in the biomechanics literature. Stiffness is a property that describes a resistance to deformation of an elastic object or body. The term compliance is the inverse of stiffness: it describes flexibility. External forces can act on a body, which can deform and store elastic energy. This springlike behavior has been observed in various skeletal segments during gait. In the human foot, the term stiffness is frequently used to describe the behavior of the medial longitudinal arch as well as the first ray portion of the foot. However, as Latash and Zatsiorsky pointed out 25 years ago:

"The notion of stiffness has been introduced in physics to characterize properties of certain types of deformable bodies under an influence of external forces. In the absence of external forces, these bodies are supposed to maintain constant shape. Muscles are not such bodies, and joints can hardly be considered bodies at all. They are rather links between the bodies or conglomerates of bodies."[2]

Notwithstanding, the term stiffness will be used extensively in this chapter to generally describe a condition of stability or reduced range of motion. Certain structures within the foot such as tendons can function as an elastic spring system or energy storage system.

Muscle contraction can impart "stiffness" to a joint or skeletal segment. However, muscles themselves cannot store energy or have elastic recoil while tendons can. Muscles can produce active tension while shortening, which is called a concentric contraction. Alternatively, muscles can produce active tension while lengthening, which is called an eccentric contraction. A good example of stiffening and recoil due to muscular contraction is the action of the gastrocnemius and soleus during midstance and terminal stance phases of the gait cycle. These muscles contract eccentrically to restrain ankle joint dorsiflexion during the stance phase of gait. Elongation of the Achilles tendon stores elastic energy, which then recoils rapidly in preswing, providing push-off or propulsion. Push-off is not due to concentric contraction of the calf muscles but rather due to elastic recoil of the Achilles tendon.[3]

There are two types of moments that are described in the biomechanics literature. Internal moments are generated by structures within the body. Active *internal* moments are generated by muscular contraction, while passive internal moments are generated by bone and cartilage within a joint as well as ligaments surrounding a joint. The term *external* moment originates outside the body and essentially occurs from gravitational force or GRF.

To add confusion, different disciplines use the term "moment" but fail to designate whether the measurement is internal or external. An internal flexion moment at the knee is produced by the hamstrings. An external flexion moment at the knee is produced by GRFs during the loading response phase of gait. This external flexion moment causes an internal knee extension moment contributed by the quadriceps muscles, resisting knee flexion. An external knee abduction moment will cause an internal knee adduction moment contributed by the medial collateral ligament. For surgeons, appreciating internal moment of force produced by bones, cartilage, ligaments, and tendons are critical to understanding the pathomechanics of injury.

GAIT EVALUATION

Understanding normal gait and developing the skill to evaluate a patient's gait is a critical core competency for the foot and ankle surgeon. There are four basic reasons for this:

1. A cursory gait examination will allow the immediate determination of the extent of disability or impairment, which is affecting the patient's ability to ambulate.
2. A more detailed evaluation will determine if deformity or impairment proximal to the area of interest may jeopardize or impact the planned surgical procedure.
3. The etiology or pathomechanics of the condition can often be determined by gait evaluation.
4. Knowledge of the phases of gait using current terminology will allow understanding of current scientific literature, specifically those papers relevant to the pathomechanics of foot and ankle pathologies.

OLD VS NEW TERMINOLOGY DESCRIBING THE PHASES OF GAIT

Many foot and ankle surgeons were educated in "podiatric biomechanics," which has been largely based upon the theories taught by Root, Orien, and Weed.[4] Some of the foundations of these theories have been disproven, particularly the area of kinematics or observations of motions of the lower extremity during walking. The critical motions of the rearfoot in the frontal plane as proposed by Root et al. have been clarified with 2D and 3D dynamic gait studies. Originally, Root et al. proposed that the rearfoot or subtalar joint would begin supination at 30% of the stance phase of gait and would reach a neutral position by heel rise at 60% of the stance phase and continue to supinate through toe-off. Now we have learned that at 60% of the stance phase, the subtalar joint is actually at its most pronated position, averaging 5 degrees everted, during the walking cycle and never reaches its neutral position until the start of swing phase.[5-7]

PHASES OF THE GAIT CYCLE

The Root et al. divisions of the gait cycle were broken down to a stance phase and a swing phase. The stance phase had three simple divisions: contact, midstance, and propulsion. With the development of gait labs and instruments to measure all aspects of walking gait, researchers have proposed a new terminology and divisions of the gait cycle.[8]

There are eight subdivisions or gait phases that enable the limb to accomplish three tasks: weight acceptance, single limb support, and swing limb advancement (Fig. 1.1).

KEY EVENTS IN THE GAIT CYCLE

The eight phases of the gait cycle will be described focusing on the direction of GRFs, which create an external moment at various joints of the lower extremity. Traditionally, gait analysis has focused on only three joints of the lower extremity: the hip, the knee, and the ankle. Only recently have we begun to learn about the movements and forces affecting the joints of the foot itself during walking. This will be discussed later in this chapter. The external moment from GRF creates rotational moment at the joints of the lower extremity. This rotational moment is

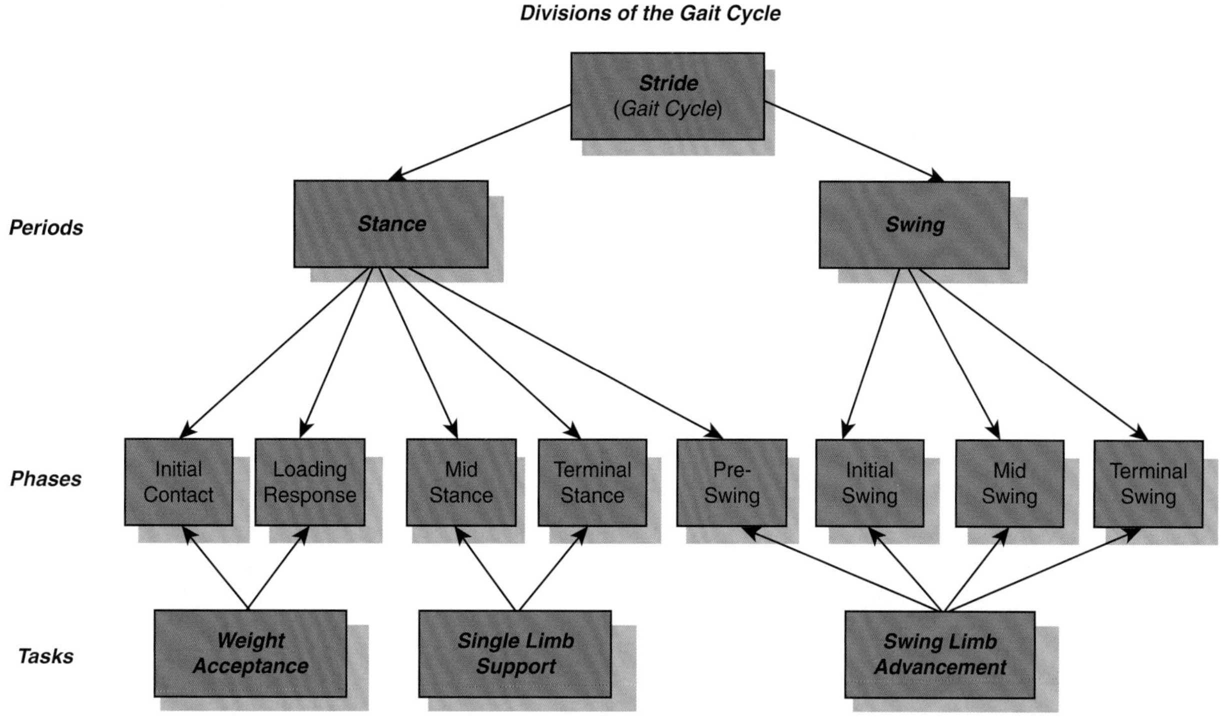

Divisions of the Gait Cycle

```
                        Stride
                      (Gait Cycle)

      Stance                              Swing

 Initial   Loading    Mid    Terminal   Pre-    Initial    Mid    Terminal
 Contact   Response  Stance   Stance    Swing   Swing     Swing    Swing


    Weight            Single Limb              Swing Limb
  Acceptance            Support               Advancement
```

Periods — Stance / Swing

Phases — Initial Contact / Loading Response / Mid Stance / Terminal Stance / Pre-Swing / Initial Swing / Mid Swing / Terminal Swing

Tasks — Weight Acceptance / Single Limb Support / Swing Limb Advancement

FIGURE 1.1 Functional division of the gait cycle. (Adapted from Perry J, Burnfield JM. *Gait Analysis: Normal and Pathological Function.* Thorofare, NJ: SLACK Incorporated; 1992.)

counteracted by muscular contraction, which provides stability to joints via controlled acceleration and deceleration.

PHASE 1: INITIAL CONTACT 0%-2% OF THE GAIT CYCLE (FIG. 1.2)

General Description

This is also known as the heel strike or "foot strike" phase of gait. Since some pathologies cause a forefoot strike only during touchdown, the term "foot strike" is preferred.

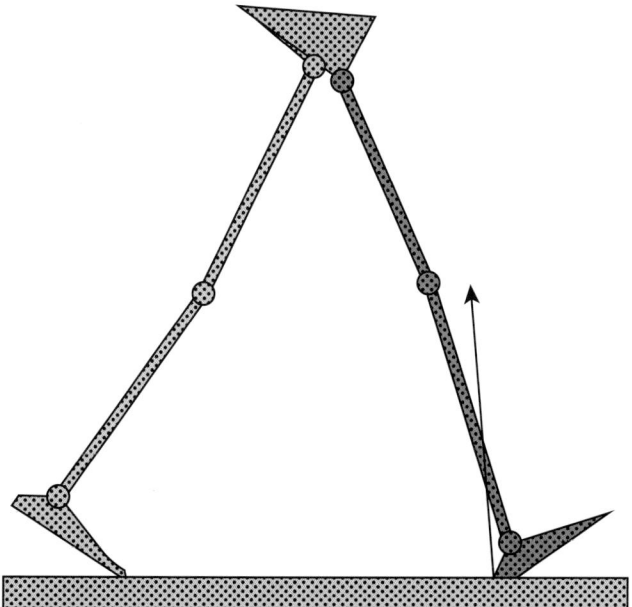

FIGURE 1.2 Phase 1: initial contact 0%-2% of the gait cycle.

Ground Reaction Forces, Moments, and Motion of the Joints: Initial Contact The hip is flexed, and the knee is straight or extended at foot strike. GRF vector is directed anterior to the hip and knee creating external extension moment. The ankle is close to a neutral or 90-degree alignment to the leg at initial contact, creating a heel strike. At this point, in the walking cycle, the presence of a tight gastrocnemius muscle can influence the attitude of the foot at touchdown. With an extended knee, the gastrocnemius is fully lengthened such that achieving a 90-degree or neutral alignment of the ankle at touchdown may not be possible if there is restriction or contracture of the gastrocnemius. As a result, initial contact might occur at the forefoot or midfoot rather than the heel.

Muscle Function and Activity During Initial Contact Anterior direction of the GRF vector places an internal extension moment on the hip generated by the gluteus maximus and the hamstrings. This continues throughout the entire stance phase of gait. The knee is held in extension at touchdown by the quadriceps, and the ankle is held at dorsiflexion by the tibialis anterior (TA).

PHASE 2: LOADING RESPONSE 2%-12% OF THE GAIT CYCLE (FIG. 1.3)

General Description

The loading response is characterized by plantar flexion of the ankle, bringing the forefoot to the supportive surface. This is also known as the "first rocker" or "heel rocker." This phase is a double support phase, which ends at the time the opposite foot leaves the ground for swing phase.

Ground Reaction Forces, Moments, and Motion of the Joints: Loading Response At heel strike, the GRF vector is posterior to the ankle joint and delivers an external plantar flexion moment to

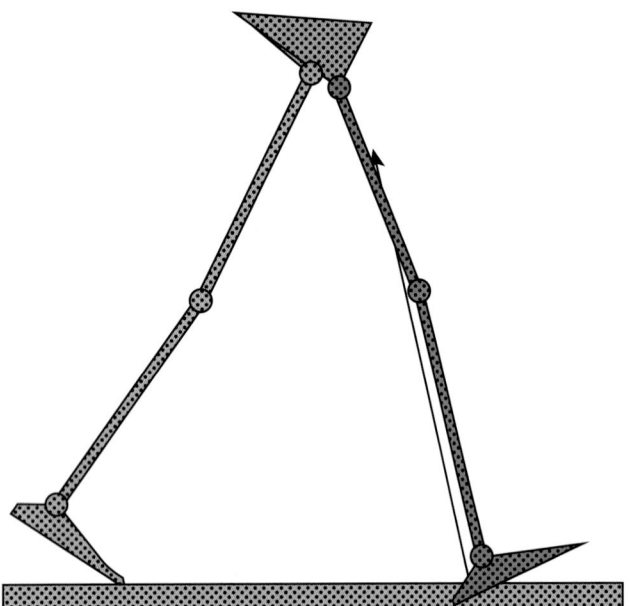

FIGURE 1.3 Phase 2: loading response 2%-12% of the gait cycle.

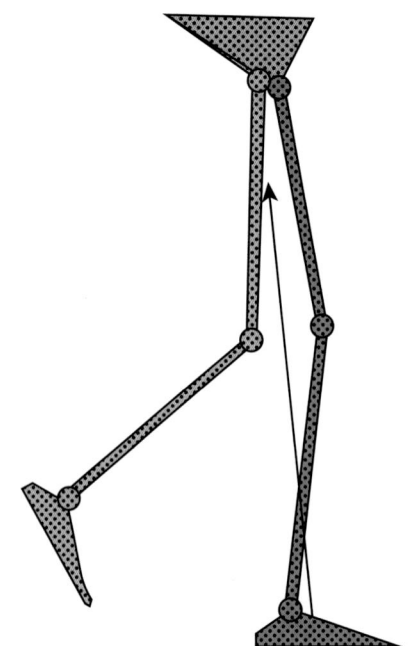

FIGURE 1.4 Phase 3: midstance 12%-31% of the gait cycle.

the ankle. At the same time, GRF vector moves posterior to the knee creating an external flexion moment. GRF vector remains anterior to the hip as it does throughout the stance phase. During this phase, momentum is generated by a forward fall. With heel strike on the rounded surface of the calcaneus, facilitating progression of the entire limb as the body falls forward. The vertical force of falling is directed forward by the unstable lever of the rounded surface of the calcaneus. During the loading response, the subtalar joint moves in the direction of pronation that is coupled to internal rotation of the tibia. This mechanism is thought to be critical to initial flexion of the knee, which occurs after foot strike.

Muscle Function and Activity: Loading Response Plantar flexion at the ankle is resisted or decelerated by the leg extensors: tibialis anterior (TA), extensor hallucis longus (EHL), and extensor digitorum longus (EDL), which all contract eccentrically as they are lengthened. Flexion of the knee is resisted by the quadriceps muscles, which also contract eccentrically. Concentric contraction of the hamstrings and gluteal muscle groups overpowers the external hip flexion moment from GRF vector, and the hip begins extending and continues to do so until just before toe-off.

PHASE 3: MIDSTANCE 12%-31% OF THE GAIT CYCLE (FIG. 1.4)

General Description

During loading response, forefoot contact on the stance limb corresponds with toe-off on the opposite limb. The end of loading response marks the end of the double support period of gait. It marks the beginning of single support and the beginning of midstance. The body is supported by one limb, rotating over the fixed foot on the ground, the so-called inverted pendulum. At the ankle, the tibia begins moving forward initiating the "second rocker" or "ankle rocker." This is the critical phase of "tibial progression," which has always thought to be due to pure sagittal plane motion at the ankle joint. However, as will be

demonstrated later in this chapter, a pure "ankle rocker" does not occur during midstance. Tibial progression occurs because multiple joints in the foot undergo dorsiflexion motion, particularly the talonavicular joint.

Ground Reaction Forces, Moments, and Motion of the Joints: Midstance At the hip, a significant external adduction moment is created by the GRF vector and loss of support of the contralateral limb, which is now off the ground. The center of gravity remains medial to the supportive limb, and the pelvis is supported only by the stance phase hip. The hip moves into extension. The knee reverses direction from flexion to extension during midstance. This is partly due to a shifting of the GRF vector anterior to the knee joint axis during midstance causing external extension moment. This change of direction occurs at about 20% of the gait cycle. The tibia appears to advance due to motion within the midfoot joints. GRF vector now passes anterior to the ankle joint creating an external dorsiflexion moment.

Muscle Function and Activity: Midstance Hip external adduction moment is resisted by contraction of the gluteus medius and the tensor fascia latae. Without this contraction, a Trendelenburg gait results demonstrating hip drop on the contralateral side. Eccentric contraction of the quadriceps converts into a concentric contraction about halfway through the midstance period as the GRF vector shifts anterior to the knee joint. Dorsiflexion of the ankle joint during midstance is resisted by the triceps surae, which contract eccentrically. This directs internal ankle plantar flexion moment, which increases plantar pressures or GRF in the forefoot. The soleus is primarily responsible for restraining tibial advancement during midstance. As tibial advancement slows, the femur catches up as it moves over the tibia, and this is the second reason that the knee moves into extension during the second half of the midstance. The ankle rocker becomes a fulcrum for tibial advancement during midstance. Proper strength and flexibility of the soleus and gastrocnemius are critical in this phase. Forward momentum causes passive dorsiflexion at the ankle joint, which is restrained by the soleus. A stable tibia allows for extension of the knee. A weak soleus will therefore keep the knee in flexion during midstance, with the patient observed to "drop down" during midstance. Conversely, a spastic or unyielding gastrocnemius-soleus complex can restrict tibial advancement and abruptly end the midstance phase prematurely with early heel-off.

PHASE 4: TERMINAL STANCE 31%-50% OF THE GAIT CYCLE (FIG. 1.5)

Key Elements

This is also known more appropriately as the *heel rise* period of the walking cycle. This phase begins when the opposite swing phase limb passes the supportive limb and continues until the opposite foot strikes the ground. During terminal stance, the heel lifts off of the ground. The rounded contour of the metatarsals serves as the third rocker or "forefoot rocker." The timing of heel rise varies among individuals depending on stability of the midfoot joints and available range of motion of the ankle joint. Timing of heel-off also varies according to walking speed. The subtalar joint begins supination just after heel rise, which is at 31% of the gait cycle and 60% of the stance phase of gait. Thus, visualization of the rearfoot would not show any inversion motion until after the swing phase limb has passed by and the heel of the supportive foot.

Ground Reaction Forces, Moments, and Motion of the Joints: Terminal Stance (Fig. 1.6) The hip has been and continues to move into extension, despite the fact that the GRF force vector is directed posterior to the joint and imposes an external hip flexion moment. Peak hip extension is achieved at the time of contact made by the opposite foot at the end of terminal stance. During heel rise, GRF vector moves forward of the knee causing an external extension moment. Heel rise does not result from ankle joint plantar flexion. In fact, the ankle does not plantarflex immediately with heel rise, and only does so late in terminal stance, at 45% of the gait cycle. Heel rise occurs from knee flexion while the ankle is maintained at maximum

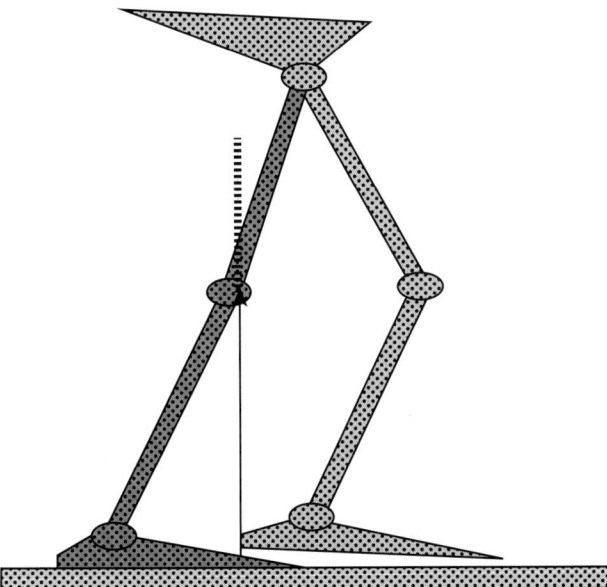

FIGURE 1.5 Phase 4: terminal stance 31%-50% of the gait cycle.

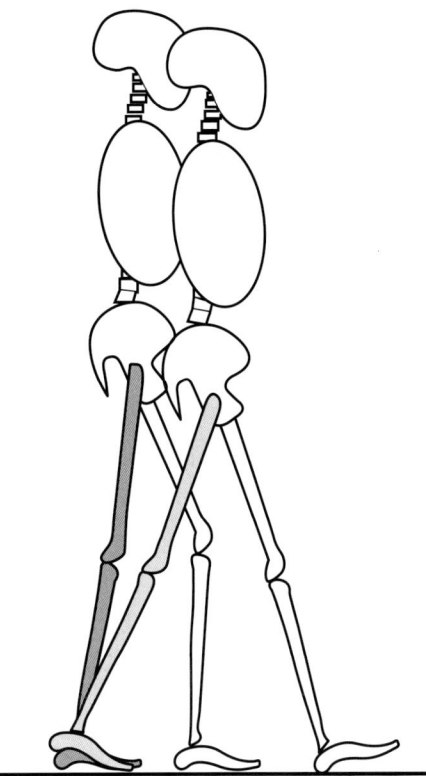

FIGURE 1.6 Terminal stance. (Adapted from Kharb A, Saini V, Jain YK, Dhiman SU. A review of gait cycle and its parameters. *Int J Comput Eng Manage.* 2011;13.)

dorsiflexion, which has already been achieved at the end of the midstance. With knee flexion, the tibia and the rearfoot are lifted off the ground. Contracture of the gastrocnemius may cause an early heel rise, but this will be due to early initiation of knee flexion, not ankle joint plantar flexion.

Muscle Function and Activity: Terminal Stance The hip abductors remain active to maintain stability of the pelvis. Despite an external extensor moment, the knee flexes due to powerful contraction of the gastrocnemius. Thus, the gastrocnemius lifts the heel off the ground by flexing the knee but not plantar flexing the ankle, which stays fixed at maximum dorsiflexion. Progression is accelerated as body weight falls forward of the area of foot support. Forward fall is controlled by the calf musculature, which develops its most powerful force during this phase. The gastrocnemius and the soleus resist ankle joint dorsiflexion at the beginning of heel rise with eccentric contraction and then both contract concentrically during later terminal stance, at 45% of the gait cycle when the ankle actually begins plantar flexion.

PHASE 5: PRESWING 50%-62% OF THE GAIT CYCLE (FIG. 1.7)

Key Elements

This starts another double support period when the opposite foot makes contact with the ground and continues through toe-off of the ipsilateral foot. The hip begins to flex, knee is already flexing, and the ankle is already plantar flexing, which started halfway through terminal stance. Accelerated limb advancement occurs at the anterior-medial margin of the forefoot.

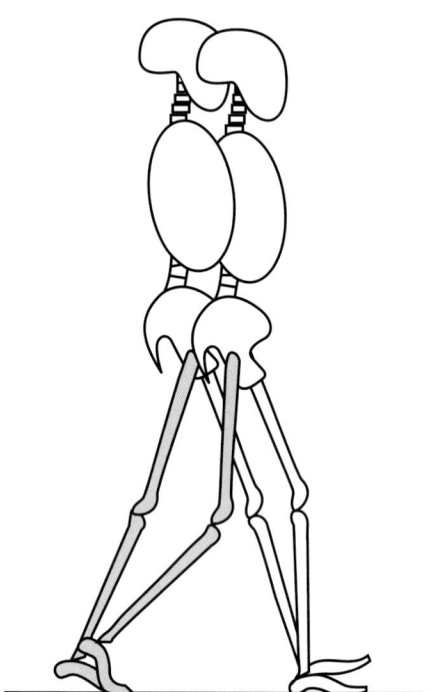

FIGURE 1.7 Phase 5: preswing 50%-62% of the gait cycle.

The fourth rocker or "toe rocker" really describes advancement over the hallux during toe-off. Supination of the rearfoot accelerates through preswing reaching maximum inversion, ~7 degrees, at the end of preswing (end of stance phase and 62% of the gait cycle).

The terminal stance and preswing phases of gait were previously combined and used to be called the "propulsive" period of gait or the "push-off" phase. This description was challenged by Jacqueline Perry who asserted that the peak of GRF at the forefoot during this period was not due to the triceps downward thrust but rather due to body position exerting increased center of pressure on the forefoot.[8] This is verified by the lack of EMG activity in the calf musculature during preswing. Perry proposes that the gastroc-soleus contractile force "locks" the ankle in terminal stance so that the limb and foot rotate on the forefoot rocker. The segment of the foot between the ankle and the metatarsal heads must be a rigid lever to support the body mass, which is now forward positioned on the foot and providing a significant dorsiflexion force across the midfoot and ankle joints. The plantar flexion force of the calf during heel rise cannot be effective if the midfoot joints are not stable during this critical phase of gait. Excessive motion across the midfoot joints will inhibit heel rise.

The calf muscles basically function to preserve the forefoot rocker. Perry states that the ankle plantar flexors restrain the body's momentum rather than propelling it forward.[8]

As the center of pressure moves forward during terminal stance, dorsiflexion increases across the MTP joints. Controlled mobility of these joints is critical to progression through the forefoot rocker. Proper functioning of the toe flexors, both extrinsic and intrinsic, as well as proper tension from the plantar aponeurosis controls or restrains dorsiflexion of the digits on the metatarsal heads.

Roll off occurs during the forefoot rocker, or terminal stance. Push-off occurs in preswing. Here, abrupt cessation of contraction of the gastroc-soleus causes elastic recoil of the

Achilles generating significant plantar flexion power across the ankle.[3] Thus, an actual propulsive event occurs. The ankle will be observed to rapidly plantarflex during preswing, at 50% of the gait cycle.

Ground Reaction Forces, Moments, and Motion of the Joints The hip reaches its maximal range of extension when the opposite foot contacts the ground, which begins the preswing phase. The GRF vector is posterior to the hip and the knee at opposite foot contact, causing a flexion moment and motion at the hip. This flexion is aided by the adductor longus. The knee continues to flex during preswing, and the rectus femoris contract eccentrically to resist excessive flexion at the knee. Flexion at the hip and knee literally "pulls" the foot off the ground during preswing.

At the ankle, despite the fact that the GRF vector is anterior to the knee joint (causing external dorsiflexion moment), the powerful concentric contraction of the triceps during terminal stance causes the ankle to continue to plantarflex during preswing. The foot rotates on the metatarsal phalangeal joints, which are moving into extension, tightening the plantar aponeurosis. This engages a "windlass mechanism" whereby the plantar aponeurosis winds around the metatarsal heads like a winch, tightening the fascia to resist bending dorsiflexion moments across the midfoot joints and metatarsals themselves. The subtalar joint continues to move in the direction of supination, which is coupled to external rotation of the tibia. The stability of the foot during this critical phase of the gait cycle is dependent upon a functioning windlass mechanism as well as a supinated position of the subtalar joint.

PHASE 6: INITIAL SWING 62%-75% OF THE GAIT CYCLE EVENTS

General Description

Also known as toe-off, this marks the end of the stance phase of gait, which occurs at 60% of the gait cycle. It also marks the beginning of the swing phase of gait.

Ground Reaction Forces, Moments, and Motion of the Joints The hip continues to flex due to contraction of the rectus femoris and the adductor magnus, which have been active during preswing. GRF has reduced to almost zero at toe-off. Hip flexion causes further knee flexion. The "ankle" reaches maximum plantar flexion, ~30 degrees at toe-off. We now know that this magnitude of plantar flexion is not solely contributed by the ankle but rather shared with multiple midfoot joints. The triceps surae stop contracting and the TA becomes the major lower leg muscle reversing ankle plantar flexion and initiating dorsiflexion that will continue through swing.

PHASE 7: MIDSWING 75%-87% OF THE GAIT CYCLE

Events

This phase begins when the swinging foot becomes adjacent to the opposite stance foot and ends when the swing limb moves forward and the tibia becomes vertical to the ground. The toes have their closest clearance to the ground when the feet are adjacent during swing.

Ground Reaction Forces, Moments, and Motion of the Joints The hip reaches 20 degrees of flexion aided by the iliopsoas contraction. There is very little muscle contraction around the knee during this phase. The knee is carried passively into flexion by hip flexion occurring more proximal. The tibia assumes a vertical alignment because the hip flexion and knee flexion magnitudes are equal. The ankle has been moving into dorsiflexion after toe-off due to contraction of the TA. The subtalar joint remains slightly supinated during swing, primarily due to the TA.

PHASE 8: TERMINAL SWING 87%-100% OF THE GAIT CYCLE

Events

The tibia moves from a vertical position to the ground to a forward position as the knee extends and the foot "reaches" forward.

Ground Reaction Forces, Moments, and Motion of the Joints The hip achieves maximum flexion as the swing phase limb reaches forward. The knee moves into extension due to inertia of the swinging shank of the lower leg. The hamstrings contract eccentrically to decelerate this motion. The TA continues to contract holding the ankle somewhere around neutral or 90-degree foot-to-leg alignment.

GAIT EVALUATION IN THE CLINICAL SETTING

Virtually every patient presenting to a clinician with a musculoskeletal pathology of the lower extremity should undergo evaluation of walking gait. A wealth of information can be obtained that can suggest etiology as well as directing appropriate treatment. Simple history taking can be very misleading in terms of determining level of impairment. Watching a patient walk can verify whether pain is causing compensation in gait and whether deformity might be either a cause or the result of another underlying pathology.

Besides detecting overall impairment, an experienced clinician can observe motion and alignment of key skeletal segments of the lower extremity during gait evaluation. Upper body posturing can suggest a neurologic deficit or a balance disorder. Limb length discrepancy can be detected by uneven pelvic alignment or asymmetrical early heel off. Congenital or acquired frontal plane deformity of the knee can have profound effects on foot posture and must be recognized before planning reconstructive foot and ankle surgery. Contracture of the gastrocnemius is attributed to be an etiology of many foot and ankle pathologies and can often be detected with a cursory gait evaluation. Traditionally, clinicians will look for an "early heel off," which would actually be an observation of heel rise occurring before the opposite limb reaches a side-by-side relationship with the stance limb. This observation, as well as most gait observations, is made from an anterior or posterior view of the walking patient.

However, many helpful and significant observations can be made from a medial/lateral or side view of the patient during gait evaluation:

1. At initial contact, a tight gastrocnemius will cause diminished ankle joint dorsiflexion and restriction of full knee extension. In the "normal" subject, the ankle should be dorsiflexed to a neutral or 90-degree position on the leg and the knee should be at full extension at heel strike.
2. Contracture of the gastrocnemius will limit tibial progression during the second rocker. This will cause an early heel off seen before the swing phase foot passes by the stance

phase foot. This heel rise is initiated by knee flexion, not ankle plantar flexion.
3. However, tibial progression can also be excessive, due to an unstable midfoot, which may undergo excessive sagittal plane motion. This will be shown as a "midfoot break" observed from a side view of the patient. There will be observed delay in heel rise as the entire tibia and rearfoot plantarflex on the forefoot. This action causes an observed "break" or flexion at the midfoot joints.
4. Heel rise begins the terminal stance phase, and this event should occur after the swing phase foot has passed by the stance phase foot. Heel rise also begins the "third rocker" as the tibia stops moving over the foot. At this point, the foot should be in its stiffest state due to tensioning of extrinsic and intrinsic muscles. This enables the tibia and foot to move together as one rigid body over the metatarsal heads and toes. Ideally, the third rocker demonstrates motion across all the toes, and most noticeably through the hallux at toe-off. In the case of functional hallux limitus, the third rocker can be observed to stop prematurely. This may be difficult to measure with direct observation. However, looking at the hip and opposite foot from a side view can help detect functional hallux limitus. Incomplete or premature ending of the third rocker will also stop full extension of the hip at the end of terminal stance. Normally, the hip continues full extension through heel rise until heel strike of the opposite foot. Functional hallux limitus will stop hip extension over the stance phase foot prematurely. When viewed from the side, the patient with functional hallux limitus will demonstrate compensation during heel rise: the midfoot may show motion in the sagittal plane while the femur stops moving backward in extension; all this occurring before heel strike of the opposite limb.
5. Preswing is the most important phase of the gait cycle in terms of generation of power and requirement for foot stability. Push-off or progression should be directed through the hallux. Dorsiflexion of the first metatarsophalangeal joint should achieve 40 degrees while engaging the windlass mechanism. Proper functioning of this mechanism should be evidenced by rearfoot supination coupled with external rotation of the tibia.

KINEMATICS OF THE FOOT AND ANKLE DURING WALKING

How do the joints move? When Root et al. proposed a model of normal and abnormal foot function, gait observations were limited to visualization of the rearfoot. A common description of motion and alignment of the "foot" often was used interchangeably with alignment of the "rearfoot" since that was the region most easily visualized when watching a patient walk in the clinical setting. Although Root et al. discussed extensively the importance of motion of other segments of the foot during walking, a general assumption in the podiatric community was that the foot primarily moved at the subtalar joint during the stance phase of gait and that the entire foot functioned as one single segment or rigid body in the direction of supination or pronation. Even today, foot and ankle surgeons will often describe a "pronated" foot posture or foot type implying a single-segment model of the foot and ignoring the significant interplay of multiple segments of the foot that may not be pronated at all.

Early kinematic studies were based upon the assumption that the foot itself could be modeled as a single rigid body and that overall position could be simply measured by comparing alignment of the calcaneus to the shank or leg. Studies of foot motion performed in the early 1990s used a single-segment model of the rearfoot and compared to motion of the shank.[9-12] These studies verified relatively small amounts of frontal plane motion of the rearfoot, which was attributed to the subtalar joint, occurring during the stance phase of gait.

However, newer insight into the importance of the talonavicular joint was discovered by Lundberg in a kinematic study of human subjects.[13] This was not a gait study but instead tracked motion of certain bones that were imbedded with metal beads. Motion of these markers was then visualized radiographically while the foot was moved passively on a platform. This investigation measured almost twice the range of motion occurring in the talonavicular joint compared to the subtalar joint.[13]

Studies of arthrodesis of the hindfoot joints further demonstrated the dominant contribution of the talonavicular joint to overall motion of the rearfoot complex. These studies showed that when the subtalar joint was fused, at least 50% residual motion was still available in the talonavicular and calcaneal-cuboid joints.[14,15] Whereas fusion of the talonavicular joint essentially eliminated all motion in the hindfoot including the subtalar joint.[14,15]

In 1999, a new approach using markers on various segments of the foot allowed measurement of motion between three segments: the leg, the rearfoot, and the forefoot.[16] In some studies, further segmentation measured motion of the hallux and the first metatarsal. Thus, began the era of three-dimensional (3D) stereophotogrammetric analysis using multisegment foot models (Fig. 1.8).

Early studies using 3D multisegment foot models demonstrated significant movement of the midfoot joints that exceeded the total motion of the subtalar joint in human subjects.[17-19] Also, studies of human subjects using (3D) multisegment foot models demonstrated that within the foot, more motion occurs in the sagittal plane than the frontal or transverse plane in gait studies of human subjects.[20,21]

At the same time, certain pathologies such as PTTD and pes planus associated with rheumatoid arthritis demonstrated a "twisting" of the forefoot on the rearfoot with significant motion in the frontal plane.[22,23] This contradicted other studies that were designed under the assumption that the forefoot functions as a rigid segment, so measurement of independent motion of the metatarsals, or joints across the midfoot was not performed.

The early multisegment foot model studies had shortcomings. There is a lack of consistency of methodology and use of segments. The plane of reference for motion in each body plane varies, and the coordinates can give misleading results. In some cases, movement of bone segments is reported relative to the supportive surface, and in other cases, relative to other bones within the foot or the tibia. For the foot and ankle surgeon, some bone realignment procedures are important relative to the supportive surface such as a medial displacement calcaneal osteotomy. In other cases, such as hallux abducto valgus hallus abductovalgus surgery, realignment of the first metatarsal is performed relative to the lesser metatarsals.

Another shortcoming of *in vivo* kinematic studies is the reliance on surface-mounted skin markers, which can have movement artifact. Also, surface markers cannot be placed on every

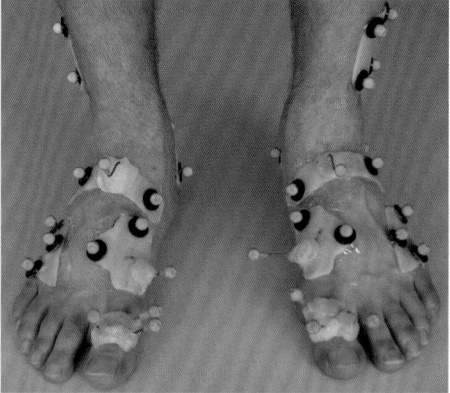
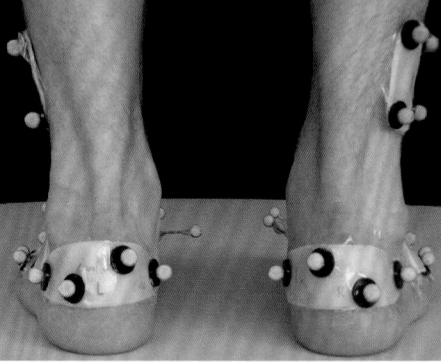

FIGURE 1.8 Marker and plate locations for the multisegment foot model. (Used with permission from Nester CJ, Jarvis HL, Jones RK, Bowden PD, Anmin L. Movement of the human foot in 100 pain free individuals aged 18–45: implications for understanding normal foot function. *J Foot Ankle Res.* 2014;7:51, Figure 1, p. 2.)

bone of the foot such as the talus, which would be critical to differentiating ankle vs subtalar joint motion.

THE BONE PIN STUDIES

Nester and co-workers, using an innovative dynamic cadaveric gait simulator, were able to place bone pin markers in multiple locations and thus were able to circumvent deficiencies of previous 3D multisegment foot model studies.[24] For the first time, measurements could be taken measuring motion of the lateral column of the foot. Nester et al. measured significant motion at the calcaneal-cuboid joint (9.8 sagittal, 7.6 frontal, 8.0 transverse), but overall motion was half that of the talonavicular joint. Both joints moved in tandem, verifying the concept of a midtarsal joint.

This was the first study measuring motion at the navicular-cuneiform as well as the metatarsal-cuneiform joints. There was considerable sagittal plane motion at the navicular-cuneiform joint in the sagittal plane, measuring 11.4 degrees, while sagittal plane motion at the first metatarsal-cuneiform joint was less than half, measuring only 5.6 degrees. The more profound finding from this study was the significant sagittal plane motion detected at the 4th and 5th metatarsal-cuboid articulation, which measured 11.5 degrees, exceeding the calcaneal-cuboid joint by 2 degrees. This compares with sagittal plane motion at metatarsals 1-3 at their respective cuneiforms, which averaged 6.1 degrees. Clearly, the metatarsals do not all move together as one rigid body segment, and the lateral metatarsals moving and the lateral metatarsals move in a greater magnitude than the medial metatarsals greater than the medial. Also, overall motion between the cuneiforms and navicular in the sagittal plane was equivalent to motion between the talus and navicular or between the calcaneus and the cuboid. In other words, the navicular-cuneiform joints contribute as much sagittal plane motion as the midtarsal joint. Surgeons should consider this finding when making decisions about joint fusion across the midfoot.

When combining sagittal plane motion across the talonavicular, navicular-cuneiform, and first metatarsal-cuneiform joints, this overall motion is equal to the net motion at the ankle and subtalar joint combined. This challenges the validity of measuring "ankle joint dorsiflexion" by dorsiflexing the entire foot and measuring alignment to the leg. At least half the motion is actually occurring in the foot, not the ankle. Furthermore, this study cast doubt on other multisegment fool model investigations, which assumed that the forefoot functions as one rigid body.

Another landmark bone pin study of foot kinematics was published by Lundgren and co-workers.[25] This study evaluated human volunteers who had bone pins implanted into multiple locations of their feet and then were evaluated with 3D stereophotogrammetric analysis. Verifying the previous observations of the cadaver bone pin study from Nester et al.[24] this in vivo study showed that the overall contribution of the joints of the medial column of the foot (talonavicular, navicular-medial cuneiform, and first metatarsal-medial cuneiform) was equivalent to the sagittal plane motion of the ankle joint. In other words, the human foot moves more during the stance phase of gait at the medial arch than at the ankle joint.

Bone pin studies allow the placement of markers on the talus, which can allow isolated measurement of the talocrural joint. Previous 3D multisegment foot model studies using skin-mounted markers could not evaluate pure frontal and transverse plane motion at the ankle, separate from the subtalar joint. Sagittal plane motion at the ankle joint verified findings from previous studies showing ~8 degrees of dorsiflexion and 8 degrees of plantar flexion.

The two bone pin studies conducted by Nester et al. and Lundgren et al. provide the most precise and reliable information about the movement of the bones of the human foot during walking gait.[24,25] Besides reaffirming previous observations about rearfoot motion during walking, new insights into the motion of the lateral column as well as the metatarsal-cuneiform joints were provided by these two studies, which dispelled previous myths and misconceptions. Furthermore, a new understanding of the complexity of ankle joint motion provides essential information for the foot and ankle surgeon. A summary of both bone pin studies showing range of motion in three body planes is provided in Table 1.1.

The two bone pin studies show motion that contradicts the "mitered hinge" perception of ankle joint motion in humans. Specifically, there is more than just pure sagittal plane motion available at the talocrural joint. Previous kinematic studies have shown surprising high amounts of transverse plane motion of transverse plane motion at the ankle joint.[26,27] This observation was verified in the two bone pin studies showing an average of 8.9 degrees of transverse motion of the talus relative to the tibia.

There is also a surprising amount of frontal plane motion in the ankle joint that averaged 8.1 degrees in the Lundgren study. This is a similar amount of frontal plane motion measured in the subtalar joint that averaged 9.8 degrees in the same study. The bone pin study from Nester et al. actually measured more frontal plane motion in the ankle compared to the subtalar

TABLE **1.1** Contribution to Motion From the Individual Joints	
Joint	**Range in Degrees**
Sagittal	
Tib-Talar	18.1[a]
Cub-5th Met	12.9
Nav-Med Cun	11.5
Talo-Nav	10.3
Calc-Cuboid	9.75
Tal-Calc	7.3
Met 1-Med Cun	5.4
Frontal	
Talo-Nav	13.6[a]
Tib-Tal	11.7
Cub-5th Met	11.6
Talo-Calc	9.8
Calc-Cub	9.45
Nav-Med Cun	9.3
Met 1-Med Cun	6.1
Transverse	
Talo-Nav	16.5[a]
Tib-Tal	8.9
Calc-Cub	8.1
Tal-Calc	7.8
Cub-5th Met	7.45
Met 1-Med Cun	5.6
Nav-Med Cun	5.3

[a]Primary joint contributor.

Data from Nester CJ, Liu AM, Ward E, et al. In vitro study of foot kinematics using a dynamic walking cadaver model. *J Biomech*. 2007;40(9):1927-1937; Lundgren P, Nester C, Liu A, et al. Invasive in vivo measurement of rear-, mid- and forefoot motion during walking. *Gait Posture*. 2008;28(1):93-100.

joint (15.3 vs 9.7 degrees).[24] It should now be recognized that frontal plane motion of the "rearfoot" observed clinically with gait analysis is actually contributed equally by both the ankle joint and the subtalar joint.

Both bone pin studies show that maximal dorsiflexion of the ankle joint (talocrural joint) occurs at 10% of the stance phase of gait, much earlier than what has been long accepted from clinical observation. The ankle joint actually moves in the direction of plantar flexion from 10% to 60% of the stance phase of gait, totally contrary to what has been reported and accepted in the medical literature.[4,8] While the talus is plantar flexing during this phase, the foot is dorsiflexing relative to the tibia. This verifies that the "dorsiflexion" motion at the ankle observed clinically during midstance through terminal stance is actually occurring at other joints of the foot, not at the ankle. Indeed, overall contribution of sagittal plane motion by the joints of the foot exceeds motion at the ankle joint by over 50%.

The bone pin studies measured greater overall motion at the talonavicular joint than motion at the talocalcaneal (subtalar) joint. In fact, the talonavicular joint has more motion in all three body planes than any of the rearfoot or midfoot joints. In comparison to the subtalar joint, the talonavicular joint moves over 40 degrees in all three body planes, while the subtalar joint moves 24 degrees. In terms of frontal plane motion, the talonavicular joint moved an average of 13.6 degrees, while the subtalar joint moved 9.8 degrees. Surprisingly, the calcaneal-cuboid joint moves 9.4 degrees in the frontal plane, which is equivalent to frontal plane motion at the subtalar joint. In fact, the calcaneal-cuboid joint moves in a larger range of motion in all three planes compared to the subtalar joint.

Motion between the navicular and the medial cuneiform is twice that of the motion occurring at the first metatarsal-medial cuneiform joint. This dispels the myth that the first metatarsal-medial cuneiform joint is the primary contributor to "hypermobility" of the first ray in many foot pathologies. In fact, the bone pin studies verify that the first metatarsal-medial cuneiform joint moves less than any other joint of the foot in all three body planes. Therefore, fusion of this joint would not be expected to have any significant effect on overall motion or function of the foot.

The cuboid 5th metatarsal joint has twice the sagittal plane motion than the first metatarsal-medial cuneiform joint. This observation, combined with the measured motion across the calcaneal-cuboid joint dispels the notion that the lateral column of the foot is relatively rigid during the stance phase of gait. In fact, the rate of nonunion with fusion of the calcaneal cuboid joint vs the first metatarsal-medial cuneiform joint might be explained by the significant difference between these joints in overall range of motion measured by the bone pin studies.

In the sagittal plane, the lateral column moves 23 degrees using combined motion at 5th metatarsal-cuboid and calcaneal-cuboid joints. Along the medial column, the combined motion of the 1st metatarsal-medial cuneiform joint, the navicular-cuneiform joint, and the talonavicular joint contribute 25 degrees. Therefore, motion in the sagittal plane is relatively equivalent when comparing the medial columns with the lateral. As with previous studies, the overall sagittal plane motion contributed by the joints of the foot exceed the motion contributed by the ankle by almost 50%. Measuring reduced foot-to-leg dorsiflexion range of motion clinically and diagnosing an ankle equinus condition is an erroneous assumption since the joints of the foot are providing most of the motion during this standard measurement technique.

HOW DO THE BONES MOVE IN A "NORMAL" FOOT?

Multisegment foot model studies have primarily focused on subjects with pathologies such as posterior tibial tendon dysfunction and rheumatoid arthritis. Most of these studies have used relatively small numbers of subjects. There has been a void in understanding "typical" or normal kinematics of the human foot. At the same time, understanding how the bones and joints move in healthy feet allows the foot and ankle surgeon to identify abnormal function and perhaps choose surgical procedures that help restore the foot to a more healthy or "normal" function.

A study performed by Nester and co-workers of 100 healthy, asymptomatic individuals provided insight into defining the kinematics of the "normal foot."[28] Unique to this study was not only the large number of healthy subjects but also the 3D multisegment model, which divided the foot into six segments: leg, calcaneus, midfoot (navicular and cuboid), medial forefoot (1st metatarsal), the lateral forefoot (4th and 5th metatarsals), and hallux. External

markers were used, rather than bone pins, but the large number of subjects gave insight, which could not be accomplished with the smaller pool of subjects in the bone pin studies.

The findings of this study verified previous studies showing overall sagittal plane motion dominates over frontal and transverse plane motion among all the joints of the foot. An important and critical finding to this study is the observation that the medial forefoot (first ray) and the lateral forefoot (4th and 5th metatarsals at the cuboid) have significant motion independent of each other and there is more frontal and transverse plane motion across the forefoot-midfoot junction than across the midtarsal joint.

Contrary to previous studies, Nester et al. found little evidence of coupling between the key segments of the foot. Furthermore, there was no evidence that the forefoot acted as a rigid body. And, as demonstrated in the bone pin studies, there was considerable motion between the forefoot and the rearfoot during terminal stance, refuting the concept of a "locking mechanism" of the midtarsal joint.

In terms of identifying predictable magnitude of "normal" or typical motion at various joints of the human foot, this study of a large number of subjects could not find any consistency. There is no pattern of motion to define a normal healthy foot. Rearfoot eversion averaged <5 degrees during the stance phase, but there was wide variation. In fact, there is wide variation of magnitude of motion among all the joints of the foot in healthy asymptomatic individuals.

At the same time, kinematic studies have verified certain patterns of motions seen in planus vs cavus foot types. These studies have measured increased frontal plane eversion of the rearfoot in pes planus foot types as well as increased transverse plane motion of the forefoot on the rearfoot in the direction of abduction.[29] Cavus feet on the other hand demonstrate a more inverted position of the rearfoot during gait.[30] However, beyond these simple and well-accepted observations of flatfooted and high-arched individuals, movement of bone segments within the foot is not predictable based upon foot type.

The variability of joint movement among healthy subjects has been a consistent finding in studies of human movement science.[31] A range of movement with variability within the range is theorized to allow the body to adapt to environmental challenges and reduce overuse of specific structures.[32] Variability in foot strike and loading of the plantar surface of the foot reduces focal repetitive loading on specific structures and thus reduces the likelihood of skin ulceration.[33] In other words, variability is a healthy finding in human locomotion.

Conversely, a reduction in variability of motion of skeletal segments can suggest a pathologic condition. Patients with chronic ankle instability (CAI) demonstrate reduced stride-to-stride variability, suggesting a more constrained neuromuscular system.[34] This reduced kinematic variability has been linked to less variability in activation of lower extremity muscles, particularly the peroneus longus (PL) and TA.[35] Reduced variability of kinematic and muscular activation during gait is thought to render patients with CAI more vulnerable to unexpected perturbation and risk of injury.[36]

Nester et al. suggested that neuromuscular mechanisms can affect direction and magnitude of joint motion within the human foot to explain the wide variation seen among healthy human subjects.[28] Joint motion during gait is largely dependent on the dynamic influence of muscle activity, which acts to resist external joint moments from GRFs. Passive restraints on joint motion are the ligamentous structures, the joint capsule, and the shape and orientation of the joint surface.

The mechanisms that contribute to neuromuscular control during standing and walking are complicated and not yet fully understood. However, this subject is worthy of study for any foot and ankle surgeon because the physiology of motor control has implications for almost all aspects of recovery from reconstructive and trauma surgery.

NEUROMUSCULAR CONTROL

Postural control is a neuromotor mechanism that functions to keep the body's center of mass within its base of support.[37] Postural control relies upon sensory input from the visual, the vestibular, and the somatosensory system. This sensory input is integrated by the sensorimotor system incorporating all the afferent, efferent, and central integration to maintain functional joint stability. The components of the sensorimotor system are depicted in Figure 1.9.

Joint stability is a major part of whole body postural control. Since loss of joint stability is a common cause of a myriad of pathologies affecting the foot and ankle, study of the sensorimotor system and neuromuscular control of the lower extremities is an important subject of interest for the foot and ankle surgeon.

Afferent input in the sensorimotor system is provided by the somatosensory system. The term proprioception refers to three perceptions: joint position sense, joint movement, and sense of resistance. The somatosensory system receives proprioceptive input from the ligaments surrounding joints as well as input from other sensors including muscle, tendon, and retinacula.[32] Pain, temperature, and tactile sensations are all part of the somatosensory system. Tactile sensation has three components: touch, pressure, and vibration (Fig. 1.10).

An essential interaction operating within the somatosensory system includes the Golgi tendon organs, the muscle spindles, and the gamma motor neuron loop.[38] These structures regulate muscle stiffness and respond to changes in length of muscle, which occur in joint movement. The muscle spindles and Golgi tendon organs are critical proprioceptors for joint position and initiate the protective reflex to activate skeletal muscles during a perturbation to prevent potential joint injury.

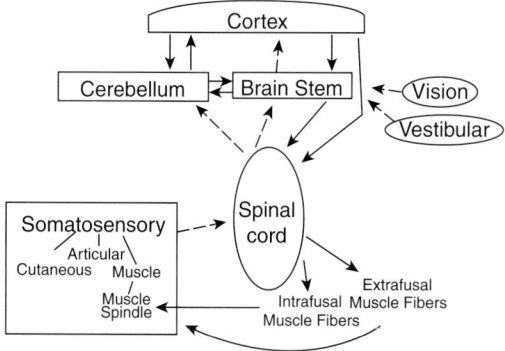

FIGURE 1.9 The sensorimotor system incorporates all the afferent, efferent, and central integration and processing components involved in maintaining functional joint stability. (Redrawn with permission from Riemann BL, Lephart SM. The sensorimotor system, part I: the physiologic basis of functional joint stability. *J Athl Train.* 2002;37(1):71–79.)

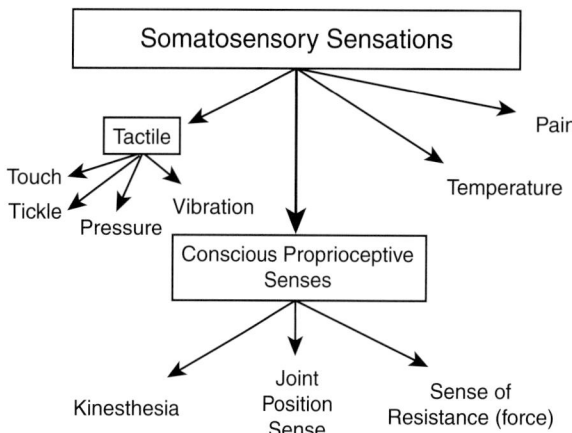

FIGURE 1.10 Sensations arising from somatosensory sources. (Redrawn with permission from Riemann BL, Lephart SM. The sensorimotor system, part I: the physiologic basis of functional joint stability. *J Athl Train.* 2002;37(1):71–79.)

Increased muscle "stiffness," which is actually increased contractile activity, enhances joint stiffness (resistance to motion), and this appears to be a benefit for functional joint stability.[39] Joint stiffness can be enhanced by co-contraction of antagonistic muscles that increases compression between articular surfaces.[40] Stiffer muscles resist sudden joint displacement more effectively.[41] This occurs when active muscles are able to recruit the muscle spindle reflex loop and shorten the reflex time needed to prevent joint subluxation and injury. In other words, the *electromechanical delay* is shortened when muscles are properly activated before a perturbation occurs, thus reducing the risk of joint injury.[42,43] This preactivation of muscles is controlled at supraspinal levels, often part of a "feed forward" mechanism.

Motor control or activation of motor neurons occurs at three primary levels of the nervous system: the spinal cord, the brainstem, and the cerebral cortex. Immediate activation occurs at the spinal cord level via reflexes, which control many of the muscular activities during gait. The brainstem modulates inhibitory muscle tone and is an essential area for postural control. The cerebral cortex regulates more fine tuned muscular activity for complex and discrete voluntary movements.

The complexity of the sensorimotor mechanism that operates in the human body explains why gait studies cannot define "normal" motion of the lower extremity skeletal segments. The timing of muscular contraction, the force of contraction, the activation of antagonist muscles, and the preactivation of muscles, all of which contribute to stiffness across joints creates multiple options for wide variation. Even when all of the elements of the sensorimotor system are functioning optimally, the ultimate effects on walking or running gait will vary significantly among healthy individuals.

When trauma disrupts key elements of the sensorimotor system, compensation or dysfunction mediated by higher (supraspinal) centers will occur. Injury to joint mechanoreceptors will disrupt neuromuscular control mechanisms. Injury can also occur to other levels of the somatosensory system, altering afferent input. Pain from injury can affect multiple levels of the sensorimotor system.

Two common orthopedic injuries have been extensively studied in terms of their effects on the sensorimotor system: the ankle sprain and anterior cruciate ligament (ACL) rupture. Subjects studied immediately after ligament disruption at the ankle show impaired proprioception and delayed lower extremity muscular activation.[44] Subjects who fail to recover from an ankle sprain develop chronic ankle instability (CAI), which is a complex disorder affecting all levels of neuromuscular control of the lower extremity.[45] Most notably, these patients demonstrate alteration in muscle activation around the ankle and in proximal joints, indicating changes at higher motor centers.[46] After ACL injury changes in muscle firing patterns are seen distally in the soleus and TA as well as proximally in the hip musculature.[47] These studies show that after orthopedic injury, alterations in motor control occur, which must be identified and treated by the treating clinician. These changes may be the result of interruption of somatosensory input or loss of integration for activation of motor response. There is significant evidence that balance training can be effective in restoring sensorimotor control after orthopedic injury.[48-51]

Ultimately, the sensorimotor system coordinates the activation of agonist and antagonist muscles to stabilize joints during locomotion. According to Perry, the each weight-bearing limb has four functions during locomotion, which are modulated by the sensorimotor system:

1. *Upright stability* is maintained despite an ever-changing posture.
2. *Progression* is generated by the interaction of selected postures, muscle force, and tendon elasticity.
3. *The shock of ground impact* at the onset of each stride is attenuated.
4. *Energy is conserved* by the optimizing coordination and minimizing muscular effort.

Not only is the timing of activation critical to this system but the eventual power and velocity of contraction of the muscle will dictate the motion at various joints. The muscles of the human body vary significantly in their physical structure, which dictates the amount of tension developed during active contraction.

Foot and ankle surgeons must consider newer insights into the influence of muscles and tendons on foot alignment and foot stability. This becomes particularly important when the foot and ankle surgeon considers a tendon transfer or considers osseous realignment procedures to off-load chronically injured tendons. When considering tendon transfer, the surgeon should evaluate the phase of activity, the strength, and excursion of the muscle itself and the moment arm or mechanical effects of a tendon acting at various joints of the foot.

PHASIC ACTIVITY

The timing and intensity of muscle activity in the lower extremities are depicted in Figures 1.11 and 1.12. In general, the extensors work in concert with each other; however, the TA is most active at initial contact, while the EHL is most active at midswing.

The ankle plantar flexors show more specialization of phasic activity. The tibialis posterior (TP) contracts immediately at initial contact to decelerate or restrain internal rotation of the tibia and subtalar joint pronation. The flexor digitorum longus (FDL) does not contract until the start of midstance and fails to provide any restraint during initial contact. This raises one of several questions about the suitability of the FDL for tendon transfer in adult acquired flatfoot (AAF) deformity.

The gastrocnemius and soleus peak activity during terminal stance or heel rise and then drop off sharply before preswing. This complete absence of muscular activity during preswing or toe-off verifies that push-off is not due to active contraction of the calf musculature.

A classic study by Silver et al. evaluated strength and excursion of the muscles of the lower extremity.[52] Excursion was determined by measuring the length of the muscle fibers. Strength was measured by taking the volume of the muscle and dividing by the fiber length. Muscle mass by itself does not determine strength. The length of the fibers of the muscle affects the strength or tension the muscle can develop. Essentially, *longer* fiber length equates to *decreased* muscle strength.

Interesting insight was gained by the Silver study, which has guided foot and ankle surgeons in decision-making for tendon transfer surgery. The ankle plantar flexors account

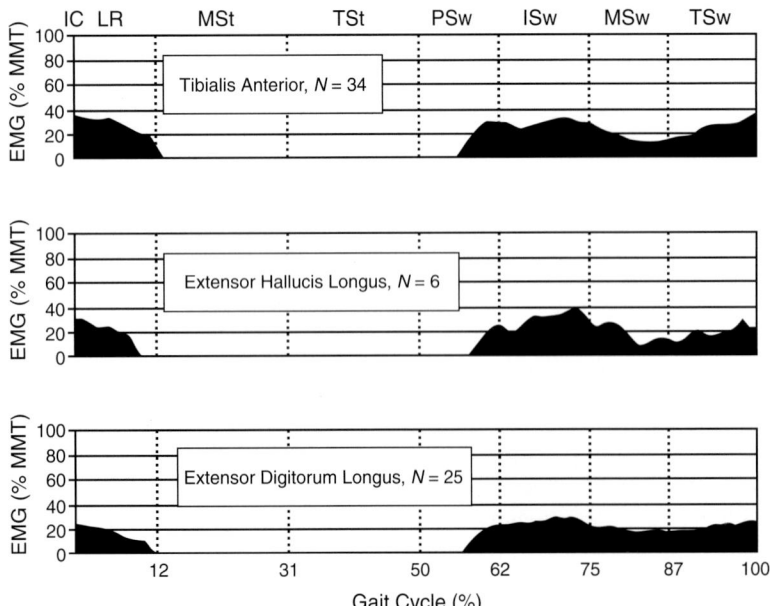

FIGURE 1.11 Ankle dorsiflexor muscles. Normal mean intensity and timing during free walking (quantified EMG). Intensity as a percent of maximum manual muscle test value (% MMT) indicated by height of *shaded area*. The *dark shading* indicates the activity pattern of the majority of subjects. *Vertical bars* designate the gait phase divisions. *N* = samples included in data. (Redrawn with permission from Jacquelin P, Burnfield JM. *Gait Analysis : Normal and Pathological Function*. 2nd ed. Thorofare, NJ: SLACK Inc.; 2010.)

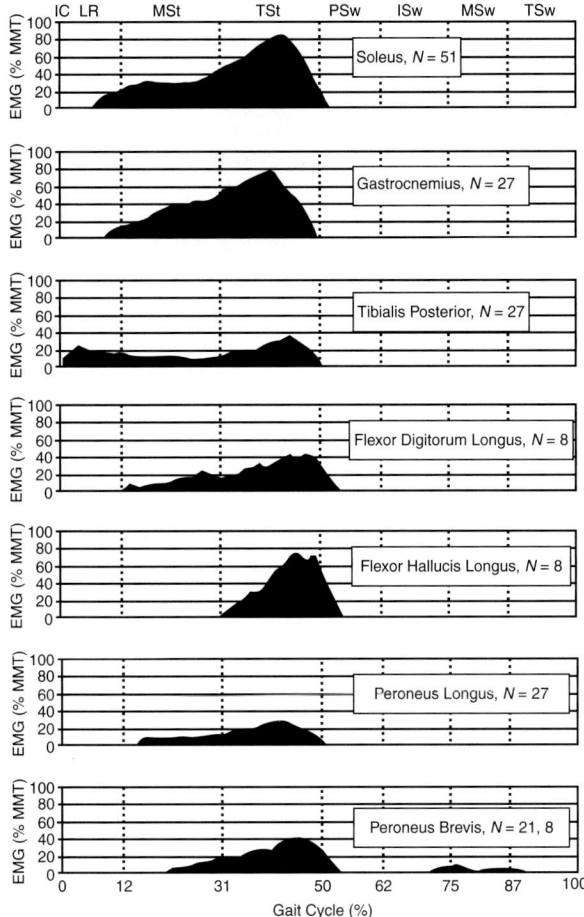

FIGURE 1.12 Ankle plantar flexor muscles including the triceps surae (soleus, gastrocnemius) and perimalleolar (TP, FDL, FHL, peroneus longus, peroneus brevis). Normal mean intensity and timing during free walking (quantified EMG). Intensity as a percent of maximum manual muscle test value (% MMT) indicated by height of *shaded area*. The *dark shading* indicates the activity pattern of the majority of subjects. *Vertical bars* designate the gait phase divisions. *N* = samples included in the data (dominant pattern, less frequent pattern if present). (Adapted from Perry J. *Gait Analysis: Normal and Pathological Function.* 2nd ed. Thorofare, NJ: SLACK Inc.; 2010, Figure 4–6, p. 59.)

for 54.5% of overall lower extremity muscle strength, while the dorsiflexors account for only 9.4%. This underscores the importance of the posterior leg musculature to control forward fall during gait. The soleus is the strongest muscle crossing the ankle joint accounting for 30% of the strength of the lower leg musculature, while the gastrocnemius provides 19.2% of overall strength. The medial head of the gastrocnemius provides 72% of the entire strength of the gastrocnemius. The primary power for dorsiflexion of the ankle comes from the TA (5.6%), which exceeds the combined power of the EHL (1.2%) and EDL (1.7%). The strength of the PL (5.5%) is more than twice that of the peroneus brevis (PB) (2.6%). The mean fiber length of the PB and the TP are identical. The strength difference between the TP (6.4%) and the FDL (1.8%) is of worthy consideration in AAF surgery.

Wickiewicz expanded on Silver's study to provide more insight in the functional differences between muscles of the lower extremity.[53] Instead of looking at gross length of the muscle fibers, microscopic measurements were taken to count the number of sarcomeres. Fiber length determines velocity of contraction with longer fibers or more sarcomeres *in series* providing higher velocity. Force or tension is determined by the number of sarcomeres *in parallel*, measured as muscle cross-sectional area. Wickiewicz evaluated lower extremity muscle performance based upon the principle that force and velocity are inversely proportional: high-velocity muscle contraction develops less tension.

The Wickiewicz study showed similar findings to Silver but showed even more contrast in strength of some of the agonist/antagonist muscles of the lower extremity. Clearly, there is no "balance" between the groups. The ankle dorsiflexors have the highest shortening velocities but develop only 15% of the tension as the plantar flexors. The EHL stands out above all the other dorsiflexors in velocity as it has three times the fiber length compared to cross-sectional area than the rest of the group. Therefore, it is the weakest of the ankle dorsiflexors. The soleus and gastrocnemius have the shortest muscle fiber length followed by the TP and the PL. Thus, these are the four top tension-producing muscles of the lower leg. Based upon muscle fiber length, the FDL is designed for higher velocity and lower tension than the TP. The PL is designed for better tension than the PB. The lateral head of the gastrocnemius is composed of fibers that are 46% longer than the medial head. Thus, the medial head of the gastrocnemius generates twice the tension compared to the lateral.

Another critical factor in muscle function of the lower extremity is the position of the tendon as it crosses key joints of the foot and ankle. Muscular contraction will produce moment or torque at a joint. Torque is a force applied over a distance that causes rotation of a joint about an axis. Moment arm is defined as the perpendicular distance from the joint's axis of rotation to the line of action of the muscle. The amount of torque generated by a muscular contraction is dependent on three variables: the strength of the contraction, the angle of application of force by the muscle-tendon unit across a joint, and the length of the moment arm or lever arm of the muscle-tendon unit. Therefore, the strength of the muscular contraction and ability to generate torque at a joint is optimized by a long moment arm, which is applied at a 90-degree angle to the axis of joint rotation.[54]

There are various methods used to measure muscle moment arms in both cadaveric (*in vitro*) and living subject (*in vivo*) studies including direct measure with radiographic imaging, load measuring, and tendon displacement measures.[55-58] Studies of moment arm of extrinsic tendons of the foot have challenges and shortcomings. The methodology of the studies differs widely. Some studies attempted to isolate movement at a specific joint by fusing other joints of the foot. Some studies manually moved the foot in one specific body plane, while other studies allowed the foot to move with 6 degrees of freedom.

Notwithstanding, consistent observations have been made from these muscle moment arm studies, which are worthy of consideration by the foot and ankle surgeon. It is important to recognize that foot position and deformity will have significant effect on the moment arms of key muscles in the lower extremity. Decision-making in reconstructive foot and ankle surgery must take into account the effects of deformity and potential correction of deformity to enhance moment arm and performance of certain muscles.

A study by Hintermann et al. showed that positioning of the ankle in dorsiflexion or plantar flexion has profound effects on moment arms of specific lower leg muscles.[57] As the ankle plantar flexes past neutral or 90 degrees, eversion moment arm of both peroneal muscles (PL and PB) significantly decreases. This verifies that the plantar flexed ankle is at risk for inversion injury not only due to change of mechanical alignment within the talocrural joint but also due to compromise in peroneal muscular efficiency for stability.

Hintermann also showed that as the ankle moves into plantar flexion, there is greater increase in plantar flexion moment arm for the gastrocnemius and soleus.[75] As the ankle moves into dorsiflexion, the moment arm of all the invertors of the ankle decreases. This study showed that as the foot moves into eversion, moment arm of the invertors, particularly the TP, decreases. In summary, the triceps surae and the TP function optimally when the ankle is plantar flexed, and the foot is in an inverted position.

A study by Lee et al. looked at the changes in moment arm of the TA, and the two heads of the gastrocnemius when the foot is inverted or everted.[59] The gastrocnemius has a small (4-mm) inversion moment arm at the rearfoot when the ankle is at 90 degrees and the subtalar joint is neutral. As the foot is moved into inversion, the inversion moment arm of the gastrocnemius increases particularly at the medial head. Eversion of the foot causes an eversion moment arm of the lateral head only, while the medial head always maintains a small inversion moment arm.[58] Eversion of the foot creates an eversion moment arm of the TA, while inversion of the foot changes this action and creates a significant inversion moment arm. This is an important consideration in flatfoot surgery. The TA can become a significant invertor of the foot provided that foot position, relative to the leg, is corrected from an everted to an inverted position.

Wang et al. performed a dynamic gait study of human subjects to measure the changes in muscle force in response to subtalar joint inversion and eversion.[60] This was not a moment arm study but rather measured joint accelerations during gait. Therefore, this study measured the effects of change of muscle force in response to foot position, which then changes the muscle moment arm. Inversion of the foot decreases the efficiency of the TA for dorsiflexion but improves the efficiency for inversion. This was verified when the researchers measured a decreased dorsiflexion acceleration in the TA when the foot was inverted. Eversion of the foot increased efficiency of the TA to dorsiflex the ankle and also increased the ability of the gastrocnemius and soleus to plantarflex the ankle and extend the knee. Therefore, inversion of the foot actually decreases efficiency of the sagittal plane stabilizers of the foot while eversion improves this efficiency. Finally, this study verified a long held belief that the triceps will further evert the subtalar joint with contractile activity if that joint is already positioned into eversion.

A comprehensive study of moment arms of the lower leg muscles was conducted by McCullough and co-workers.[61] Using a simulator that provides continuous motion in three planes, moment arms were measured in all nine extrinsic muscles of the foot in five cadaveric specimens. For the first time, moment arm was measured relative to transverse plane displacement

of the foot. In this plane, the largest moment arm for abduction (external rotation) of the foot was contributed by the PB (23 mm). For adduction (internal rotation), the FDL and the TP had similar moment arms, 22.1 mm and 21.4 mm, respectively. For eversion of the foot, the PL had the largest average moment arm of 31 mm, and for inversion of the foot, the largest moment arm was contributed by the TA (16 mm). Surprisingly, the FDL and TP had identical inversion moment arms of 10 mm, which were 30% lower than the TA. In the sagittal plane, the Achilles tendon had the largest average plantar flexion moment arm of 53 mm, while the EHL had the largest dorsiflexion moment arm of 43 mm. The peroneal tendons had surprising large moment arms for dorsiflexion with the PB contributing 16.7 mm and the PL 21.1 mm.

Evaluating moment arms alone can be misleading when considering tendon transfer surgery. For example, this study shows a surprising similarity in moment arm between the TP and the FDL, perhaps justifying the transfer of the FDL when the TP is ruptured in AAF deformity. However, several other important considerations must be made including overall muscle strength as well as change of moment arm when the tendon is transferred.

These important considerations for tendon transfer were demonstrated in a study by Hui and co-workers.[62] They measured the inversion motor arm of the intact, native FDL compared with the new inversion motor arm when the FDL tendon is transferred to the navicular, as commonly performed in AAF surgery. The hindfoot inversion moment arm of the FDL tendon in its native state averaged 19.6 mm while transfer to the navicular reduced the inversion moment arm by 45% to 10.7 mm. Furthermore, Hui factored the anticipated loss of one grade of strength with any tendon transfer, which amounts to a loss of 20% total force and then calculated overall loss of moment or torque. The native FDL produces 177 N of force, considerably less than the larger TP, which produces 727 N. Reducing the total force of the transferred FDL by 20% and then calculating moment arm, the intact FDL inversion capacity drops from 3.5 to 1.5 N-m when transferred to the navicular, a loss of over 60% inversion moment generation power.

Applying more recent knowledge about muscle moment arms as well as muscle strength measures, a hierarchy of contribution from each muscle to foot stability can be developed. While moment arms may appear similar within a group of muscles of the lower leg, factoring in the cross-sectional area or strength of the muscle with the moment arm will allow a calculation of torque capacity of the muscle.[62] The first step is to estimate the isometric force output of the muscle. Zajac calculated the peak muscle stress of skeletal muscle, assuming that all motor units would be activated simultaneously, and proposed a baseline value of 35 N cm².[54] This value can then be multiplied by the cross-sectional area of any muscle to yield an estimate of maximal isometric force expressed in Newtons.[64] By multiplying this force by the moment arm, the total moment or torque can calculated, expressed in Newton-meters. Table 1.2 lists the overall torque or moment capacity of each of the lower extremity muscles for each of six planes of motion. From this table and from studies previously cited regarding change of position of moment arms, we can summarize the major contributors of muscular control of the foot in all six body planes.

TABLE **1.2** Capacity for Moment Production in Three Planes				
Muscle	Moment Arm (mm)	Cross Section Area (cm²)	Isometric Force (N)	Moment (N-m)
Dorsiflexion				
TA	36.5	10	350	12.7[a]
EHL	43	2	70	3.0
EDL	32	5.3	175	5.6
PB	16.7	6	210	3.5
PL	21.1	12	420	8.8
Plantar flexion				
SOL	53	58	2030	107.5[a]
GAST	53	32	1120	59.3
FHL	25	5	175	4.3
FDL	12	5	175	2.1
TP	9.4	21	735	6.9
Inversion				
TP	10.2	21	735	7.5[a]
TA	16.6	10	350	5.8
Eversion				
PL	31.3	12	420	13.14[a]
PB	20.5	6	210	4.3
EDL	5	5.3	175	0.8
Internal Rotation (Adduction)				
TP	21.4	21	735	15.7[a]
FDL	22.1	5	175	3.86
External Rotation (Abduction)				
PL	16	12	420	6.72[a]
PB	23	6	210	4.83

[a]Largest moment capacity.

Data from McCullough MB, Ringleb SI, Arai K, Kitaoka HB, Kaufman KR. Moment arms of the ankle throughout the range of motion in three planes. *Foot Ankle Int.* 2011;32(3):300-306; Wickiewicz TL, Roy RR, Powell PL, Edgerton VR. Muscle architecture of the human lower limb. *Clin Orthop Relat Res.* 1983;179:317-325.

MAJOR MUSCLE CONTRIBUTORS IN SIX PLANES OF MOTION

SAGITTAL PLANE

The plantar flexion muscles provide the dominant power, exceeding the dorsiflexor power by over fivefold. As Silver has previously pointed out, there is little evidence for "balance" of power between agonist and antagonist muscles of the lower leg. Furthermore, there is no evidence that these muscles groups function in this manner as the phasic contractions do not occur together.

The significant strength advantage of the plantar flexion muscles underscores the critical requirement for the soleus and the gastrocnemius to restrain dorsiflexion and control forward fall of the body, which is the driving force of the walking gait

cycle. To further understand the importance of the plantar flexors vs the dorsiflexors, one only has to compare the impairment of an Achilles tendon rupture compared to the dropfoot condition resulting from loss of the ankle extensor muscle group. The dropfoot patient merely compensates with steppage gait, while the Achilles tendon rupture renders the patient apropulsive and incapacitated.

The soleus contributes twofold the plantar flexion moment as the medial head of the gastrocnemius. This moment increases when the ankle moves into plantar flexion and the moment arm of the Achilles moves to a perpendicular alignment to the ankle joint axis. The medial head of the gastrocnemius is a different muscle than the lateral head. The medial head has shorter muscle fibers, develops twice the ankle plantar flexion moment than the lateral, and has more inversion moment arm in all positions at the ankle compared to the lateral.

All other ankle flexors pale in comparison to the soleus and gastrocnemius: the flexor hallucis longus (FHL) provides only 5% the ankle flexion moment of the soleus. Despite a shorter moment arm, the TP is a stronger ankle plantar flexor than the FHL, which is commonly used as a transfer tendon in neglected Achilles ruptures.

The TA is the primary ankle dorsiflexor. This dorsiflexion moment of the TA weakens with foot inversion. This may contribute to dropfoot seen in patients with cavus deformity. With the longest moment arm, the minimal cross-section area of the EHL makes this muscle a negligible ankle dorsiflexor. The PL has surprising ability to dorsiflex the ankle, better than either the EHL or the EDL.

FRONTAL PLANE

The invertors and evertors are evenly balanced in muscle power indicating that walking places equal burden on the lower leg musculature in the frontal plane.

Contrary to popular belief, the TP and the TA have similar inversion moment production capacity. However, the TA becomes an evertor when the foot is everted. The TP continues to be an invertor with eversion of the foot, but moment arm for this action becomes significantly reduced with further eversion.[57] Due to favorable moment arm and larger muscle cross section, the PL is the primary everter of the foot exceeding the PB by over threefold in overall torque production capacity. This eversion power is significantly reduced with ankle joint plantar flexion.

TRANSVERSE PLANE

The internal rotators (adduction) have almost twice the moment or torque on the foot than the external rotators (abduction). Thus, walking demands significantly greater restraint of external rotation than internal rotation. The alignment of the foot relative to the leg during walking causes the foot to naturally abduct which places greater demand on the TP, which is the primary restraint to external rotation. This explains why the dominant direction of deformity assumed by the foot after posterior tibial tendon rupture is external rotation or abduction rather than frontal plane valgus deformity.[23] Furthermore, overall deformity resulting from rupture of the posterior tibial tendon is significantly more severe than what occurs in the foot after rupture of the abductors or external rotators, that is, the peroneal tendons.

The TP produces twofold greater adduction (internal rotation) moment than it does inversion moment. This muscle should be labeled primarily as an adductor in the transverse plane rather than its secondary role as an invertor. Despite the largest moment arm for abduction, the PB does not produce the greatest moment in this direction because the PL has twice the muscle cross section and still has significant moment arm to be the primary external rotator of the foot.

MUSCLE ACTIVITY/DEMAND AND FOOT TYPE

Hypertrophy of the FDL muscle has been observed with MR imaging of patients with posterior tibial tendon insufficiency.[63] Ultrasound study revealed increased cross-sectional area of the FDL and FHL muscles in patients with pes planus compared to patients with normal arch feet.[64] This verifies the role of these muscles as arch supporters, which are recruited for increased activity in pes planus.

Conversely, decreased activity of the PL and PB has been measured in patients with pes planus compared to normal-arched individuals.[65,66] Decreased cross-sectional area of the peroneal musculature has been demonstrated with ultrasound study of patients with pes planus.[64] This suggests a decrease load on the foot "pronators" in pes planus. Conversely, increased activity of the ankle inverter muscles has been shown to increase in pes planus.[65]

THE PLANTAR INTRINSIC MUSCLES

The plantar intrinsic muscles include the abductor hallucis, quadratus plantae, flexor digitorum brevis, abductor digiti minimi, flexor digiti minimi, opponens digiti minimi, adductor hallucis, dorsal and plantar interossei, and lumbricals.

The role of these muscles is just now being elucidated as key stabilizers of the foot. Understanding of the function of these muscles has been challenging due to their reduced size and depth within the foot making surface EMG studies difficult. Early studies demonstrated that the plantar intrinsics function later in the stance phase of gait to stabilize the digits during heel rise (Fig. 1.13).[67]

There was also evidence that these muscles control pronation of the subtalar joint.[68] Later studies verified the role of pronation control of the plantar intrinsics as well as an emerging concept that these muscles were important stabilizers of the medial longitudinal arch of the foot.[69,70]

Kelly and co-workers used ultrasound-guided intramuscular EMG to study the three largest plantar intrinsic muscles, specifically the abductor hallucis, flexor digitorum brevis, and quadratus plantae.[71] Significant increase of muscle activation patterns were measured with increased postural sway suggesting that the plantar intrinsic muscles play an important role in balance and postural control. This research group subsequently studied the role of the same three plantar intrinsic muscles in stabilizing or providing stiffness to the medial longitudinal arch of the foot.[72] The study measured increased stretch and activation of the plantar intrinsic muscles with increasing load deformation of the longitudinal arch of the foot. With electrical stimulation, the researchers demonstrated that the plantar intrinsic muscles act along with the plantar aponeurosis to attenuate longitudinal arch deformation during walking.

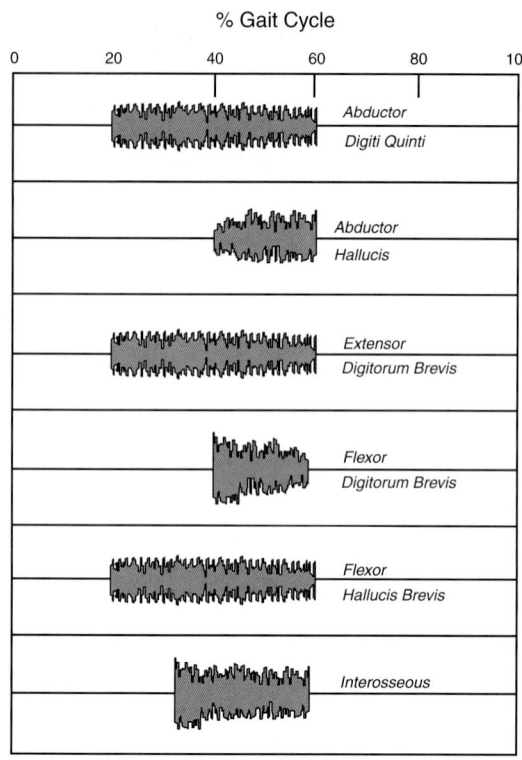

FIGURE 1.13 Intrinsic foot muscle action during stance. (Adapted from Mann R, Inman VT. Phasic activity of intrinsic muscles of the foot. *J Bone Joint Surg.* 1964:46A:469-481.)

Specific rotation of foot skeletal segments were measured depending on which muscle were stimulated. The abductor hallucis, the largest of all the plantar intrinsics, demonstrated kinematic effects in all three body planes resulting in calcaneal inversion as well as dorsiflexion (increased calcaneal inclination). The calcaneus was also observed to move into abduction with stimulation of the abductor hallucis indicating closed chain supination of the midtarsal joint. This was supported by the observation of flexion and adduction of the metatarsals with stimulation of the abductor hallucis. The flexor digitorum brevis and quadratus plantae only exerted influence in the frontal and transverse plane. The authors speculated that the more medial location of the abductor hallucis provided better moment arm to affect the sagittal plane and height of the longitudinal arch of the foot.

Other investigators have speculated that stiffness of the longitudinal arch of the foot is regulated by the active contractile elements of the plantar intrinsic muscles as well as the passive elastic elements of the plantar aponeurosis and the plantar ligaments.[73,74] The role of the passive plantar ligament structures to provide storage of energy and elastic recoil has been dubbed the "foot spring" by Ker et al.[75] They measured energy strain storage capacity in the plantar aponeurosis, the spring ligament, and the long and short plantar ligaments. It appears that the plantar intrinsics also respond to load with stretch and contraction to provide stability to the entire foot.[72]

Decreased cross-sectional area with ultrasound study of the abductor hallucis and flexor hallucis brevis has been observed in patients with pes planus compared to normal arch feet.[64,76] This contrasts with hypertrophy of other arch supporting muscles in the leg in pes planus such as the FHL and FDL.[63,65] The plantar intrinsic muscles may not have to work as hard in pes planus because the plantar fascia becomes taut in pes planus and takes over plantar flexing the toes, a so-called reverse windlass.[77]

MIDFOOT STABILITY AND THE MYTH OF "LOCKING"

The human foot is unique to all other primates containing specialized features for optimizing bipedal ambulation. These features include an enlarged calcaneal tuberosity as well as a medial and lateral longitudinal arch maintained by stable talonavicular and calcaneocuboid joints. Compared to other primates, the human foot has a well-developed spring ligament as well as long and short plantar ligaments, which stabilize these joints.[78] The critical differentiating feature of the human foot is the plantar aponeurosis, providing twice the contribution to arch stability as the spring ligament and plantar ligaments combined.[79]

During terminal stance and preswing, the human foot has been often described as a "rigid lever," which enables the powerful contraction of the triceps surae to resist dorsiflexion moment across the forefoot. This stiffness or "rigidity" facilitates heel rise due to return of elastic energy stored in the Achilles and other soft tissue structures in the plantar surface of the foot. The stretch and recoil of the Achilles tendon provides a 35% energy recovery, which is then increased to 52% recovery with stretch and recoil of the plantar aponeurosis and plantar ligaments.[3,80]

All other primates lack the stiffness of the human foot and instead demonstrate a "midfoot break" during terminal stance and preswing.[81,82] Studies demonstrate significant sagittal plane motion across all the midfoot joints of many different primate species during heel rise as well as excessive dorsiflexion of the ankle as the heel rises while the metatarsals remain on the ground.[80,81] This contrasts to significant plantar flexion of the ankle, which provides propulsion at toe-off in walking humans.

Besides the contribution of soft tissue structures to provide stiffness to the human foot, an osseous "locking mechanism" has been a long-standing accepted explanation among various disciplines explaining the conversion of the human foot from a mobile adaptor during contact phase to a rigid lever during propulsion.[4,83,84] The midtarsal joint locking mechanism was first described by Elftman who proposed that the axes of the calcaneocuboid joints and the talonavicular joints theoretically move from a parallel orientation with subtalar joint pronation to a divergent orientation when the subtalar joint was inverted.[85] Thus, the midtarsal joint was proposed to be more flexible when the subtalar joint was pronated and becomes rigid with subtalar inversion. This observation can be made when examining any human subject and pushing against the plantar surface of metatarsals 4 and 5, comparing motion with the subtalar joint held in maximum inversion and eversion.

Phillips and Phillips measured increased magnitude of eversion of the forefoot on the rearfoot as the subtalar joint was moved from neutral to a pronated position.[86] This suggested an unlocking of the midtarsal joint. Later, Gatt and co-workers used a 3D multisegment foot model to determine the change in dorsiflexion of the foot as the subtalar joint was moved from a pronated position, to a neutral position, and finally to a supinated position.[87] Although this study was intended to measure ankle joint dorsiflexion relative to subtalar joint position, the multisegment foot model detected that more sagittal plane motion was occurring between the forefoot and the rearfoot than at the ankle joint. Furthermore, moving the foot into a pronated position at the subtalar joint increased motion between the forefoot and the rearfoot. Gatt and co-workers disputed whether a midtarsal joint "locking" occurred since there was still significant motion between the forefoot and the rearfoot at both a neutral and supinated position of the subtalar joint. In both the Phillips et al. and Gatt et al. studies, the major increase in forefoot to rearfoot motion occurred when the subtalar joint moved from a neutral position to a fully pronated position. The change from subtalar neutral to supinated positioning had a mild influence on forefoot motion.

Blackwood carried out a cadaver study, which also measured greater flexibility of the forefoot in the sagittal plane when the subtalar joint was everted, and less flexibility when the subtalar joint was inverted.[88] However, this effect was only demonstrated in the sagittal plane, not the frontal plane. Blackwood et al. concluded that the stiffening of the forefoot to the rearfoot and may have involved multiple joints, not only at the midtarsal joint.

If the stiffening of the midfoot during gait was due to the establishment of divergent or conflicting joint axes at the midtarsal joint, kinematic studies would be able to demonstrate the asynchronous movement between the talonavicular and calcaneocuboid joints. However, this has not been the case. In a dynamic cadaver study, Nester et al. showed synchronous movement at the talonavicular joint and the calcaneal-cuboid joint during the stance phase of gait.[24] In a subsequent study of healthy human subjects, Nester et al. were unable to measure any consistent coupling between segments of the foot but also demonstrated that there also showed significant motion dispelling the notion of "locking" of the midtarsal joint.[28]

Okita and co-workers performed a dynamic cadaver study and also demonstrated that the midfoot joints actually become more compliant during terminal stance.[89] Interestingly, they did actually measure a divergence of joint axes in the midfoot and rearfoot, but the onset of the divergence, during the early stance phase did not correspond with increased rigidity of the foot. Instead, the foot became rigid during heel rise when the joint axes became nondivergent. The authors concluded that soft tissue structures including tendons would have to account for the stiffening of the foot during the propulsive phase of gait.

The unique ability of the human foot to stiffen in terminal stance is due to the elastic springlike performance of static and dynamic supportive structures. The dynamic influence on arch stiffness appears to be modulated by the central nervous system.[90] It does not appear to be reliant on osseous "locking" of the midfoot joints. Stiffening of the foot does occur in response to inverting the subtalar joint, as this has been clearly demonstrated in several studies.[86-88] However, this stiffening most likely is due to tensioning of key ligaments, which occurs favorably as the foot is moved from a pronated to a supinated position during terminal stance and preswing.

REFERENCES

1. The American Heritage® Stedman's Medical Dictionary Copyright © 2002, 2001, 1995 by Houghton Mifflin Company. Published by Houghton Mifflin Company.
2. Latash ML, Zatsiorsky VM. Joint stiffness: myth or reality? *Hum Mov Sci.* 1993;12:653-692.
3. Ishikawa M, Komi PV, Grey MJ, Lepola V, Bruggermann GP. Muscle-tendon interaction and elastic energy usage in human walking. *J Appl Physiol.* 2005;99(2):603-608.
4. Root ML, Orien WP, Weed JH. *Clinical Biomechanics: Normal and Abnormal Function of the Foot.* Vol. 2. Los Angeles, CA: Clinical Biomechanics Corp.; 1977:138-139.

5. Hamill J, Bates BT, Knutzen KM, Kirkpatrick GM. Relationship between selected static and dynamic lower extremity measures. *Clin Biomech (Bristol, Avon).* 1989;4:217-225.
6. McPoil TG, Cornwall MW. Relationship between neutral subtalar joint position and pattern of rearfoot motion during walking. *Foot Ankle Int.* 1994;15:141-145.
7. Mueller MJ, Norton BJ. Reliability of kinematic measurements of rear-foot motion. *Phys Ther.* 1992;72:731-737.
8. Perry J. *Gait Analysis: Normal and Pathological Function.* 2nd ed. Thorofare, NJ: SLACK Inc.; 2010.
9. Apkarian J, Naumann S, Cairns B. A three-dimensional kinematic and dynamic model of the lower limb. *J Biomech.* 1989;22(2):143.
10. Kadaba MP, Ramakrishnan HK, Wootten ME. Measurement of lower extremity kinematics during level walking. *J Orthop Res.* 1990;8(3):383-392.
11. Davis RB, Ounpuu S, Tyrburski D, Gage JR. A gait analysis data collection and reduction technique. *Hum Mov Sci.* 1991;10:575-587.
12. Siegel KL, Kepple TM, O'Connell PG, Gerber LH, Stanhope SJ. A technique to evaluate foot function during the stance phase of gait. *Foot Ankle.* 1995;16:764-770.
13. Lundberg A, Svensson OK, Bylund C, et al. Kinematics of the ankle/foot complex. Part 2: pronation and supination. *Foot Ankle.* 1989;9:248.
14. Astion DJ, Deland JT, Otis JC. Motion of the hindfoot after simulated arthrodesis. *J Bone Joint Surg Am.* 1997;79-A:241.
15. Wulker N, Stukenborg C, Savory KM, Alfke D. Hindfoot motion after isolated and combined arthrodeses: measurements in anatomic specimens. *Foot Ankle.* 2000;21:921.
16. Deschamps K, Staes F, Roosen P, Desloovere K, Bruyninckx H, Matricall G. Body of evidence supporting the clinical use of 3D multisegment foot models: a systematic review. *Gait Posture.* 2011;33(3):338-349.
17. Leardini A, Benedetti MG, Catani F, Simoncini L, Giannini S. An anatomically based protocol for the description of foot segment kinematics during gait. *Clin Biomech (Bristol, Avon).* 1999;14:528-536.
18. Cornwall MW, McPoil TG. Three-dimensional movement of the foot during the stance phase of walking. *J Am Podiatr Med Assoc.* 1999;89:56.
19. Cornwall MW, McPoil TG. Relative movement of the navicular bone during normal walking. *Foot Ankle Int.* 1999;20:507.
20. Carson MC, Harrington ME, Thompson N, O'Connor JJ, Theologis TN. Kinematic analysis of a multi-segment foot model for research and clinical applications: a repeatability analysis. *J Biomech.* 2001;34:1299-1307.
21. Hunt AE, Smith RM, Torode M, Keenan AM. Inter-segment foot motion and ground reaction forces over the stance phase of walking. *Clin Biomech (Bristol, Avon).* 2001;16:592-600.
22. Woodburn J, Nelson KM, Siegel KL, Kepple TM, Gerbber LH. Multisegment foot motion during gait: proof of concept in rheumatoid arthritis. *J Rheumatol.* 2004;31(10):1918-1927.
23. Rattanaprasert U, Smith R, Sullivan M, Gilleard W. Three-dimensional kinematics of the forefoot, rearfoot, and leg without the function of tibialis posterior in comparison with normals during stance phase of walking. *Clin Biomech (Bristol, Avon).* 1999;14:14-23.
24. Nester CJ, Liu AM, Ward E, et al. In vitro study of foot kinematics using a dynamic walking cadaver model. *J Biomech.* 2007;40(9):1927-1937.
25. Lundgren P, Nester C, Liu A, et al. Invasive in vivo measurement of rear-, mid- and forefoot motion during walking. *Gait Posture.* 2008;28(1):93-100.
26. Lundberg A, Svensson OK, Bylund C, Goldie I, Selvik G. Kinematics of the ankle/foot complex. Part 3. Influence of leg rotation. *Foot Ankle Int.* 1989;9(6):304-309.
27. Arndt A, Westblad P, Winson I, Hashimoto T, Lundberg A. Ankle and subtalar kinematics measured with intracortical pins during the stance phase of walking. *Foot Ankle Int.* 2004;25(5):357-364.
28. Nester CJ, Jarvis HL, Jones RK, Bowden PD, Anmin L. Movement of the human foot in 100 pain free individuals aged 18–45: implications for understanding normal foot function. *J Foot Ankle Res.* 2014;7:51.
29. Buldt AK, Murley GS, Butterworth P, Levinger P, Menz HB, Landorf KB. The relationship between foot posture and lower limb kinematics during walking: a systematic review. *Gait Posture.* 2013;38(3):363-372.
30. Hillstrom HJ, Song J, Kraszewski AP, et al. Foot type biomechanics part 1: structure and function of the asymptomatic foot. *Gait Posture.* 2013;37(3):445-451.
31. Lephart SM, Riemann BL, Fu FH. Introduction to the sensorimotor system. In: Lephart SM, Fu FH, eds. *Proprioception and Neuromuscular Control in Joint Stability.* Champaign, IL: Human Kinetics; 2000:37-51.
32. Riemann BL, Lephart SM. The sensorimotor system, part I: the physiologic basis of functional joint stability. *J Athl Train.* 2002;37(1):71-79.
33. Fernando M, Crowther R, Lazzarini P, et al. Biomechanical characteristics of peripheral diabetic neuropathy: a systematic review and meta-analysis of findings from the gait cycle, muscle activity and dynamic barefoot plantar pressure. *Clin Biomech (Bristol, Avon).* 2013;28:831-845.
34. Herb CC, Chinn L, Dicharry J, McKeon PO, Hart JM, Hertel J. Shank-rearfoot joint coupling with chronic ankle instability. *J Appl Biomech.* 2014;30(3):336-372.
35. Koldenhoven RM, Feger MA, Fraser JJ, Saliba S, Hertel J. Surface electromyography and plantar pressure during walking in young adults with chronic ankle instability. *Knee Surg Sports Traumatol Arthrosc.* 2016;24(4):1060-1070.
36. Koldenhoven RM, Feger MA, Fraser JJ, Hertel J. Variability in center of pressure position and muscle activation during walking with chronic ankle instability. *J Electromyogr Kinesiol.* 2018;38:155-161.
37. Richie DH. Functional instability of the ankle and the role of neuromuscular control. A comprehensive review. *J Foot Ankle Surg.* 2001;40(4):240-251.
38. Riemann BL, Lephart SM. The sensorimotor system, Part II: the role of proprioception in motor control and functional joint stability. *J Athl Train.* 2002;37(1):80-84.
39. Grillner S. The role of muscle stiffness in meeting the changing postural and locomotor requirements for force development by the ankle extensors. *Acta Physiol Scand.* 1972;86:92-108.
40. Louie JK, Mote CD Jr. Contribution of the musculature to rotatory laxity and torsional stiffness at the knee. *J Biomech.* 1987;20:281-300.
41. Sinkjaer T, Toft E, Andreassen S, Hornemann BC. Muscle stiffness in human ankle dorsiflexors: intrinsic and reflex components. *J Neurophysiol.* 1988;60:1110-1121.
42. Rack PM, Ross HF, Thilmann AF, Walters DK. Reflex responses at the human ankle: the importance of tendon compliance. *J Physiol.* 1983;344:503-524.
43. Grabiner MD. Bioelectric characteristics of the electromechanical delay preceding concentric contraction. *Med Sci Sports Exerc.* 1986;18:37-43.
44. Beckman SM, Buchanan TS. Ankle inversion injury and hypermobility: effect on hip and ankle muscle electromyography onset latency. *Arch Phys Med Rehabil.* 1995;76(12):1138-1143.
45. Munn J, Sullivan SJ, Schneiders AG. Evidence of sensorimotor deficits in functional ankle instability: a systematic review with meta-analysis. *J Sci Med Sport.* 2010;13(1):2-12.
46. Sefton JM, Hicks-Little CA, Hubbard TJ, et al. Segmental spinal reflex adaptations associated with chronic ankle instability. *Arch Phys Med Rehabil.* 2008;89(10):1991-1995.
47. Ciccotti MG, Kerlan RK, Perry J, Pink M. An electromyographic analysis of the knee during functional activities, II: the anterior cruciate ligament deficient knee and reconstructed profiles. *Am J Sports Med.* 1994;22:651-658.
48. McKeon PO, Hertel J. Systematic review of postural control and lateral ankle instability. Part 2: is balance training clinically effective? *J Athl Train.* 2008;43(3):305-315.
49. Taube W, Gruber M, Beck S, Faist M, Gollhofer A, Schubert M. Cortical and spinal adaptations induced by balance training: correlation between stance stability and corticospinal activation. *Acta Physiol (Oxf).* 2007;189:347-358.
50. Taube W, Kullmann N, Leukel C, Kurz O, Amtage F, Gollhofer A. Differential reflex adaptations following sensorimotor and strength training in young elite athletes. *Int J Sports Med.* 2007;28:999-1005.
51. Beck S, Taube W, Gruber M, Amtage F, Gollhofer A, Schubert M. Task-specific changes in motor evoked potentials of lower limb muscles after different training interventions. *Brain Res.* 2007;1179:51-60.
52. Silver RL, de la Garza J, Rang M. The myth of muscle balance. *J Bone Joint Surg.* 1985;67-B:432-437.
53. Wickiewicz TL, Roy RR, Powell PL, Edgerton VR. Muscle architecture of the human lower limb. *Clin Orthop Relat Res.* 1983;179:317-325.
54. Zajac FE. Muscle coordination of movement: a perspective. *J Biomech.* 1993;26(suppl 1):109-124.
55. Maganaris CN. In vivo measurement-based estimations of the moment arm in the human tibialis anterior muscle-tendon unit. *J Biomech.* 2000;33:375-379.
56. Klein P, Mattys S, Rooze M. Moment arm length variations of selected muscles acting on talocrural and subtalar joints during movement: an in vitro study. *J Biomech.* 1996;29:21-30.
57. Hintermann B, Nigg BM, Sommer C. Foot movement and tendon excursion: an in vitro study. *Foot Ankle Int.* 1994;15:386-395. doi: 10.1016/0021-9290(95)00025-9.
58. An KN, Takahashi K, Harrigan TP, Chao EY. Determination of muscle orientations and moment arms. *J Biomech Eng.* 1984;106:280-282.
59. Lee SM, Piazza SJ. Inversion-eversion moment arms of gastrocnemius and tibialis anterior measured in vivo. *J Biomech.* 2008;41:3366-3370.
60. Wang R, Gutierrez-Farewik EM. The effect of subtalar inversion/eversion on the dynamic function of the tibialis anterior, soleus, and gastrocnemius during the stance phase of gait. *Gait Posture.* 2011;34:29-35.
61. McCullough MB, Ringleb SI, Arai K, Kitaoka HB, Kaufman KR. Moment arms of the ankle throughout the range of motion in three planes. *Foot Ankle Int.* 2011;32(3):300-306.
62. Hui HJ, Beals TC, Brown NT. Influence of tendon transfer site on moment arms of the flexor digitorum longus muscle. *Foot Ankle Int.* 2007;28(4):441-447.
63. Wacker J, Calder JD, Engstrom CM, Saxby TS. MR morphometry of posterior tibialis muscle in adult acquired flat foot. *Foot Ankle Int.* 2003;24(4):354-357.
64. Angin S, Crofts G, Mickle KJ, Nester CJ. Ultrasound evaluation of foot muscles and plantar fascia in pes planus. *Gait Posture.* 2014;40:48-52.
65. Murley GS, Menz HB, Landorf KB. Foot posture influences the electromyographic activity of selected lower limb muscles during gait. *J Foot Ankle Res.* 2009;2(1):35.
66. Hunt AE, Smith RM. Mechanics and control of the flat versus normal foot during the stance phase of walking. *Clin Biomech (Bristol, Avon).* 2004;19(4):391-397.
67. Gray EG, Basmajian JV. Electromyography and cinematography of leg and foot ("normal" and flat) during walking. *Anat Rec.* 1968;161:1-15.
68. Mann R, Inman VT. Phasic activity of intrinsic muscles of the foot. *J Bone Joint Surg Am.* 1964;46:469-481.
69. Headlee DL, Leonard JL, Hart JM, Ingersoll CD, Hertel J. Fatigue of the plantar intrinsic foot muscles increases navicular drop. *J Electromyogr Kinesiol.* 2008;18:420-425.
70. Fiolkowski P, Brunt D, Bishop M, Woo R, Horodyski M. Intrinsic pedal musculature support of the medial longitudinal arch: an electromyographic study. *J Foot Ankle Surg.* 2003;42:327-333.
71. Kelly LA, Kuitunen S, Racinais S, Cresswell AG. Recruitment of the plantar intrinsic foot muscles with increasing postural demand. *Clin Biomech (Bristol, Avon).* 2012;27:46-51.
72. Kelly LA, Cresswell AG, Racinais S, Whiteley R, Lichtwark G. Intrinsic foot muscles have the capacity to control deformation of the longitudinal arch. *J R Soc Interface.* 2014;11:20131188.
73. Caravaggi P, Pataky T, Günther M, Savage R, Crompton R. Dynamics of longitudinal arch support in relation to walking speed: contribution of the plantar aponeurosis. *J Anat.* 2010;217:254-261.
74. Bates KT, et al. The evolution of compliance in the human lateral mid-foot. *Proc Biol Sci.* 2013;280:20131818.
75. Ker RF, Bennett MB, Bibby SR, Kester RC, Alexander RM. The spring in the arch of the human foot. *Nature.* 1987;325:147-149.
76. Angin S, Mickle KJ, Nester CJ. Contributions of foot muscles and plantar fascia morphology to foot posture. *Gait Posture.* 2018;61:238-242.

77. Aquino A, Payne C. The role of the reverse windlass mechanism in foot pathology. *J Am Podiatr Med Assoc.* 2000;34:32-34.

78. Lewis OJ. *Functional Morphology of the Evolving Hand and Foot.* Oxford: Oxford University Press; 1989.

79. Huang CK, Kitaoka HB, An KN, Chao YS. Biomechanical evaluation of longitudinal arch stability. *Foot Ankle Int.* 1993;14(6):353-357.

80. Vereecke EE, Aerts P. The mechanics of the gibbon foot and its potential for elastic energy storage during bipedalism. *J Exp Biol.* 2008;211:3661-3670.

81. Holowka NB, O'Neill MC, Thompson NE, Demes B. Chimpanzee and human midfoot motion during bipedal walking and evolution of the longitudinal arch of the foot. *J Hum Evol.* 2017;104:23-31.

82. DeSilva JM, MacLatchy LM. Revisiting the midtarsal break. *Am J Phys Anthropol.* 2008;135:S46.

83. Mann RA. Biomechanics of the foot. In: *AAOS Atlas of Orthotics: Biomechanical Principles and Application.* St. Louis, MO: C.V. Mosby Co.; 1975:257-266.

84. Donatelli RA. *The Biomechanics of the Foot and Ankle.* 2nd ed. Philadelphia, PA: F.A. Davies; 1996.

85. Elftman H. The transverse tarsal joint and its control. *Clin Orthop.* 1960;16:41-45.

86. Phillips, RD, Phillips RL. Quantitative analysis of the locking position of the midtarsal joint. *J Am Podiatry Assoc.* 1983;73(10):518-522.

87. Gatt A, Chockalingam N, Chevalier TL. Sagittal plane kinematics of the foot during passive ankle dorsiflexion. *Prosthet Orthot Int.* 2011;35:425-431.

88. Blackwood CB, Yuen TJ, Sangeorzan BJ, et al. The midtarsal joint locking mechanism. *Foot Ankle Int.* 2005;26:1074-1080.

89. Okita N, Meyers SA, Challis JH, Sharkey NA. Midtarsal joint locking: new perspectives on an old paradigm. *J Orthop Res.* 2014;32(1):110-115.

90. Kelly LA, Lichtwark G, Cresswell AG. Active regulation of longitudinal arch compression and recoil during walking and running. *J R Soc Interface.* 2015;12(102):20141076.

Imaging of the Foot and Ankle

Robert A. Christman and Albert V. Armstrong Jr

BONE AND JOINT IMAGING

Robert A. Christman

ESSENTIALS

CONSIDERATIONS WHEN ORDERING THE RADIOGRAPHIC STUDY

As the foot and ankle expert, it is in your patient's best interest to order appropriate positioning techniques for a radiographic study. Ordering radiographic views should not be routine and automatic ("dorsoplantar [DP], medial oblique, and lateral views," for example); each case should be evaluated and considered on an individual basis. First determine which radiographic view will best *isolate* or allow *visibility* of the area in question, based upon the specific, palpable location of symptomatology. The tangential surfaces concept[1] is used to select this primary positioning technique (Tables 2.1 and 2.2). For example, if focal pain or other abnormality is palpated along the superolateral aspect of the first metatarsophalangeal joint, then the first positioning technique chosen is the lateral oblique position. The resulting view will tangentially isolate the area in question. Then, additional positioning techniques are selected, based upon your provisional diagnosis, that you believe will provide additional visibility of the surrounding area. If you suspect osteoarthritis, DP and lateral projections would be included with the lateral oblique positioning technique.

The tangential surfaces concept can also be used to accurately identify the radiographic location of an unexpected lesion and correlate it to the patient clinically. For example, an exostosis is identified along the distal diaphysis of the first metatarsal in Figure 2.1. Since it is isolated in the lateral oblique view, then, based on the tangential surfaces concept, the lesion is along the inferomedial aspect of the bone. Clinically you would then palpate the patient's foot along the inferomedial aspect of the first ray.

Presentation of the talus and distal tibia and fibula may differ between the weight-bearing lateral foot and lateral ankle views. The ankle joint axis typically is not perpendicular to the x-ray image receptor in the weight-bearing lateral foot view. With the medial side of the foot placed against the image receptor, its position is such that the fibular malleolus is posterior relative to the tibial malleolus. As a result, the appearance of the ankle joint is not axial; the tibial malleolus is superimposed on the anterior portion of the talus and the fibular malleolus on the posterior portion. These presentations are especially exaggerated in a cavus and/or metatarsus adductus foot (Fig. 2.2A). In contrast, the lateral ankle view should be obtained so that the ankle joint axis is perpendicular to the image receptor (Fig. 2.2B). This is easily achieved for the non–weight-bearing ankle lateral view with the lateral side of the foot against the image receptor; however, for the weight-bearing lateral ankle view, the heel may need to be pulled away from the image receptor in order to accurately position the ankle joint axis perpendicular to the image receptor.

Other considerations: order at least two views. Ideally, two of the views should be perpendicular to each other. Bilateral studies should not be ordered routinely nor for comparison purposes; the exceptions would be for evaluating a patient with

TABLE **2.1** Selection of Primary Radiographic Positioning Technique Based Upon Tangential Surfaces Concept: Foot	
Palpable Location of Focal Symptomatology (Relative to a Specific Bone Clinically)	**Radiographic Positioning Technique**
Medial or lateral	Dorsoplantar
Superior or inferior	Lateral
Superomedial or inferolateral	Medial oblique
Superolateral or inferomedial	Lateral oblique

TABLE **2.2** Selection of Primary Radiographic Positioning Technique Based Upon Tangential Surfaces Concept: Ankle	
Palpable Location of Focal Symptomatology (Relative to a Specific Bone Clinically)	**Radiographic Positioning Technique**
Medial or lateral	Anteroposterior
Anterior or posterior	Lateral
Anteromedial or posterolateral	Medial oblique
Anterolateral or posteromedial	Lateral oblique

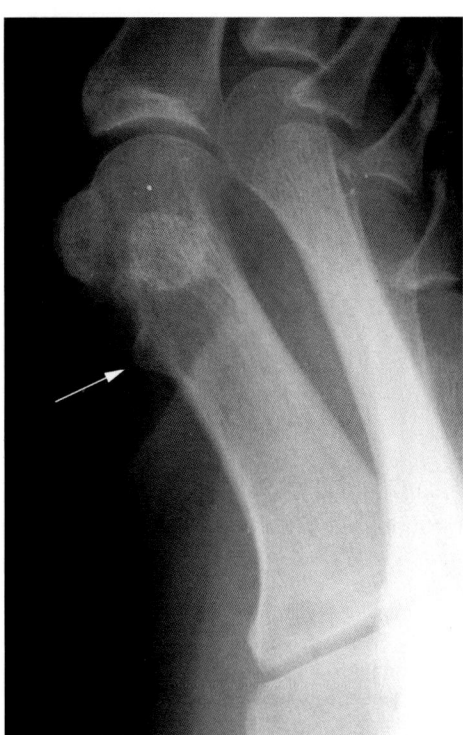

FIGURE 2.1 Lateral oblique foot view demonstrating an exostosis (*arrow*). See text for application of the tangential surfaces concept.

potential joint disease (findings and patterns of joint disease may be asymptomatic and present in the opposite foot) and, obviously, evaluating pathology of both feet. After the initial study is reviewed, then obtain additional and/or comparison views as warranted.

ANGLE AND BASE OF GAIT

When the foot is positioned for a weight-bearing radiographic study, it is recommended that the extremity be placed in its angle and base of gait. Angle and base of gait represents the attitude or relationship of the foot to the line of progression in the normal gait cycle. Radiographically, this method attempts to load the foot completely and evenly for visualizing the bony structural relationships.[2] Its purpose is to standardize the positioning technique, allowing reproducibility between patients as well as within radiographic studies of the same patient. Angle and base of gait is determined by watching the patient walk. For example, if a patient's angle of gait was determined to be 20 degrees from the line of progression, this relationship is then reproduced when positioning the foot.

What does the literature say? Bryant[3] demonstrated that positioning the feet together and straight ahead was as reliable as angle and base of gait positioning for reproducibility when measuring angles and for comparison to subsequent studies of the same patient. Though this technique is easier to perform, no study has been performed to determine whether or not radiographic findings would differ for feet with pathology. However, it has been determined that static foot placement can ensure consistency and affect measurements performed between sessions[4] and that marching in place is recommended to position a patient in angle and base.[5] Therefore, weight-bearing foot radiographs can be reliably reproduced and valid comparisons can be made over time if standardized radiographic techniques employed.

COMMON PITFALLS/ERRORS OF IMAGE INTERPRETATION

A degree of error is inevitable when interpreting radiographic studies, and it increases with fatigue and workload.[6] Search

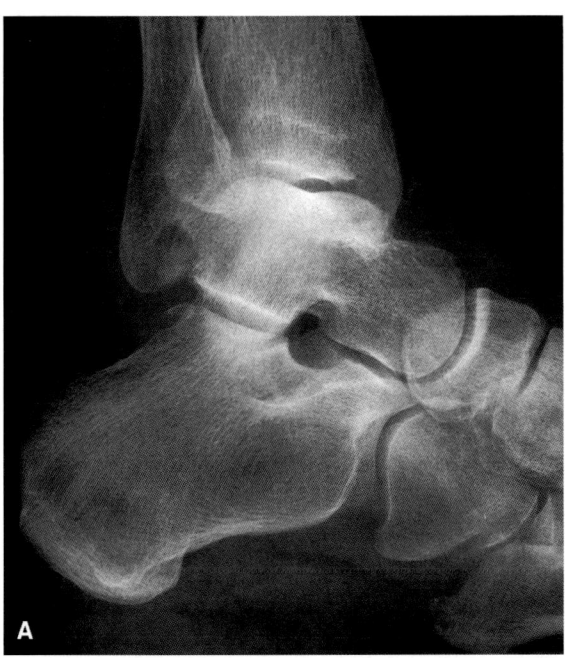

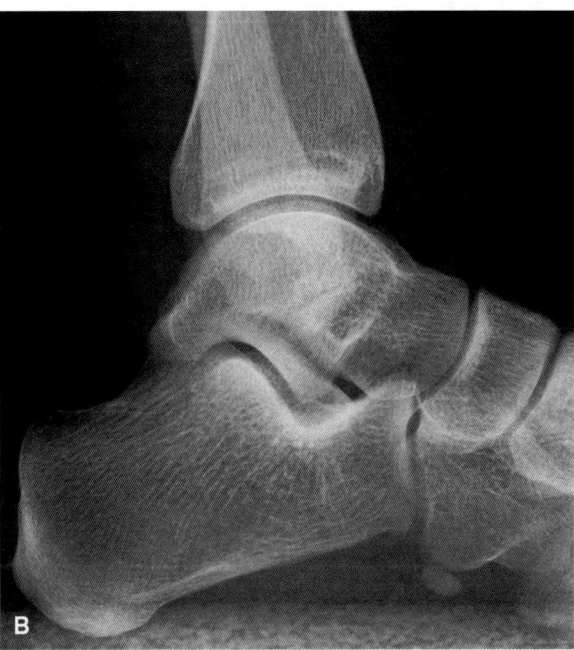

FIGURE 2.2 Lateral view. **A.** Foot (pes cavus example). Notice that the fibular malleolus is posterior to the talus, the medial and lateral shoulders of the talar dome are separated, and the ankle joint space is barely visible. **B.** Ankle; the tibial and fibular malleoli are superimposed on one another and the talar body; the ankle joint is clearly seen as the two shoulders of the talar dome are aligned.

error can result from a failure to fixate one's vision on the area of abnormality or if there is a "satisfaction of search"[7] (ie, one stops looking elsewhere). Look at all bones in all views! Recognition errors occur when an abnormality is not appreciated as abnormal[8]; this can be a result of "anatomical noise" (the lesion is superimposed on another structure), mistaking a normal finding as abnormal, or not taking into consideration how foot position (relative to the image receptor and x-ray beam) during exposure can alter form of bones and joints. Lastly, a decision-making error can occur when an abnormality is recognized but rejected as a normal variant.

A common radiographic misinterpretation of foot and ankle radiographs is interpreting normal findings as abnormal. Factors that can have a profound effect on bone form, thereby influencing the form of bones and joints, include placement of the extremity for the positioning technique, angulation of the x-ray tube head, and whether the foot is pronated vs supinated when positioned. Furthermore, if a bone is not parallel to the image receptor AND perpendicular to the x-ray beam, distortion will result,[9] which should not be ignored.[10]

The way the foot is positioned for a radiographic study can profoundly influence the appearance of bones and joints in the radiograph and may lead to misinterpretation. Therefore, when evaluating the foot and ankle radiographically, one must first determine whether or not the foot, when positioned on the orthoposer, was pronated, rectus or supinated. For example, the two DP images in Figure 2.3 are of the same person. Figure 2.3A was obtained full weight bearing after the subject externally rotated the leg, resulting in a supinated position; Figure 2.3B was obtained full weight bearing after the subject internally rotated the leg, resulting in a pronated position. LaPorta reported this effect in 1977.[11] Notice how the shapes

of bones and appearance of joints, as well as the position of bones relative to one another, has changed. For example, the navicular bone is crescent shaped in the left image, but wedge shaped on the right. The tibial sesamoid is superimposed along the medial aspect the first metatarsal head on the left, but centrally positioned on the right. The second, third, and fourth metatarsal heads appear to touch one another in the left image but are separated in the right. There appears to be only one first metatarsal-cuneiform joint in the left image, but two on the right.

THE RADIOLOGY REPORT

Payment for the radiographic study is for the description of findings, NOT the diagnosis. Insurance companies have performed random audits of patient medical records, reviewing both radiographic quality of the images and the report of radiographic findings. If unsatisfactory, the offender may be placed on a period of probation for several months. After a second review, if the reports and images are still unsatisfactory, they may stop reimbursement for this service, which results in delayed diagnosis and treatment as well as patient inconvenience to have a radiographic study performed elsewhere, not to mention the economic impact it will have on your practice.

The report of findings must be objective. State the findings in the report, and reserve diagnoses and etiologies for the conclusion. The challenge is to NOT include a diagnosis in the description of findings! And, if previous radiographic studies have been performed and are available, always compare to them and make a notation of such and any changes that may have occurred. (If prior studies had been performed but are

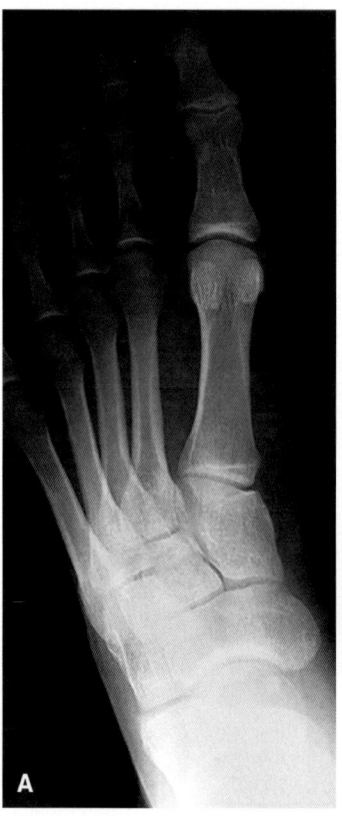
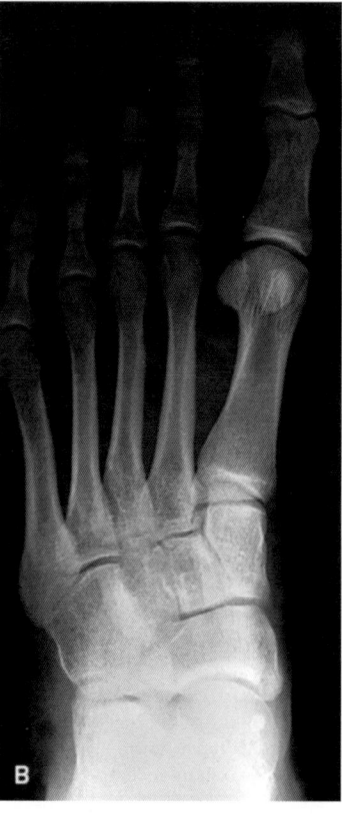

FIGURE 2.3 The effect of foot position on bone and joint form. Both images are of the same individual with the foot **(A)** supinated; **(B)** pronated. See text for further explanation.

not available, that should be documented as well.) Ideally, provide a separate report, which appears more professional than jotting a few findings in the body of your patient notes.

NORMAL RADIOGRAPHIC ANATOMY AND VARIANTS

Radiographic anatomy of the foot and ankle has recently been described in great detail elsewhere[12-16] as have the numerous skeletal variations[17] and radiographic positioning techniques.[18] The reader is encouraged to access those publications for the basic, foundational knowledge. There are, however, pertinent anatomical considerations that are sometimes overlooked or even misinterpreted; they will be discussed. Also, the variants considered here would be limited to those that may require surgical intervention or simulate pathology.

DIAPHYSEAL RIDGE OF PROXIMAL PHALANX

A bony thickening along the proximal phalangeal diaphysis of lesser toes 2, 3, and 4 is referred to as the diaphyseal ridge (Fig. 2.4). It varies in size and, when prominent, may be misinterpreted as a periosteal reaction. The extensor hood apparatus wing and fibrous flexor sheath insert along the diaphyseal ridge.[16]

BASAL TUBERCLE OF HALLUX DISTAL PHALANX

Small tubercles present along the inferomedial and inferolateral aspects of the hallux distal phalanx base. They serve as attachment for the articular collateral ligaments proximally[19]; a second "ligament" (it does not cross a joint), referred to as the interosseous ligament,[20] extends distally from each

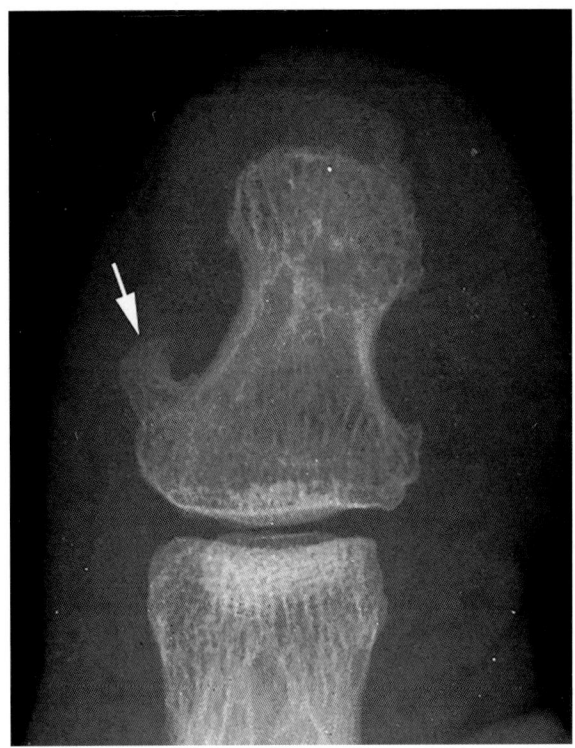

FIGURE 2.5 Large medial tubercle (*arrow*), hallux distal phalanx base. DP view.

tubercle and insert onto the ungual tuberosity.[21] The medial tubercle is larger and can range in size from negligible to large (the lateral tubercle generally is not visible radiographically) (Fig. 2.5). Lee et al.[22] reported a bony "outgrowth" just distal

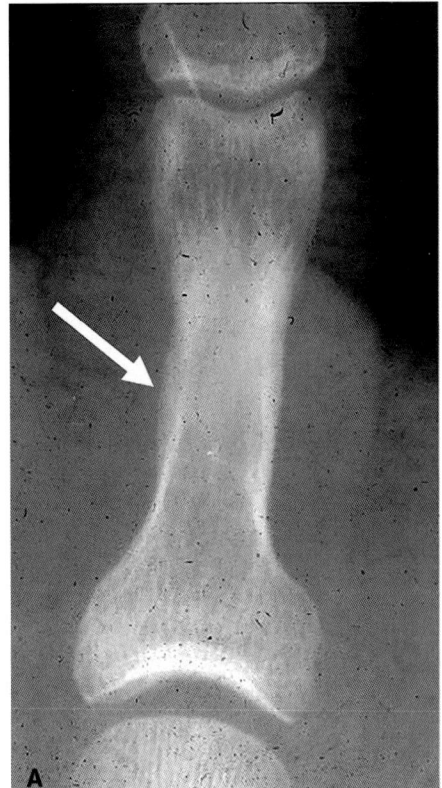

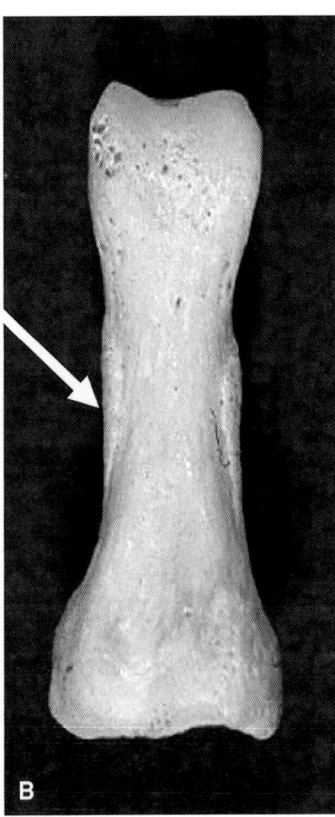

FIGURE 2.4 Diaphyseal ridge (*arrows*), lesser toe proximal phalanx. **A.** Radiograph, DP view. **B.** Bone specimen, dorsal view.

to this tubercle in 88.5% of feet and found the histologic presence of reactive bone. An elongated spur may also be seen that projects anteriorly from the medial tubercle. There has been a report of symptomatology secondary to an enlarged tubercle ("exostosis") that was excised[23]; however, any normal or variant anatomy could become symptomatic if there are faulty biomechanics. In this case, valgus rotation of the hallux causes abnormal wear and tear over the tubercle; chronic, repetitive stress may secondarily result in enlargement of the tubercle. Some patients may develop hyperkeratosis and experience discomfort. The question arises, should something that occurs in nearly 90% of patients be considered abnormal? Logic dictates that the tubercle is normal anatomy that demonstrates variable presentation and may become symptomatic under stressful conditions.

OS INTERPHALANGEUS

The os interphalangeus is found at the hallux interphalangeal joint; it is rare to see it at the interphalangeal joints of the lesser toes. The ossicle is located most commonly along the inferior aspect of the interphalangeal joint centrally and is round or oval in shape (Fig. 2.6A and B). Less commonly, it is eccentric in position (Fig. 2.6C). The eccentric os interphalangeus may be misinterpreted as fracture, though nonunion fracture may certainly be a differential diagnosis for the well-defined ossicle if there is history of prior injury. The ossicle is associated with a painful plantar hyperkeratotic lesion.[24,25] Rarely, an ossicle may be encountered along the superior aspect of an interphalangeal joint.

LATERAL EDGE OF FIRST METATARSAL HEAD

The "lateral edge" of the first metatarsal head is not "the lateral cortical surface of the metatarsal head," as portrayed by Okuda et al.[26]; it is actually the lateral edge of the trochlear articular surface for the fibular sesamoid.[15] The lateral aspect of the first metatarsal head is flat with a depression[27] and does not articulate with the hallux proximal phalanx; it appears radiographically as a linear sclerosis that is perpendicular to the anterior articular surface (Fig. 2.7). The "lateral edge" may appear continuous with the anterior articular surface sometimes in the two-dimensional radiograph, but it is not the same.

FIRST METATARSAL HEAD TRABECULATIONS AND JAGGED BIPARTITE SESAMOID MARGINS

Prominent trabeculations are normally seen in the first metatarsal head and neck (see Fig. 2.7). This finding should not be misinterpreted as osteopenia. Also, when the prominent trabeculations are superimposed on a bipartite sesamoid, the latter's apposing edges appear jagged; this should not be misinterpreted as fracture (Fig. 2.8A). Another variant bipartite presentation mistaken as fracture is when the two segments appear separated from one another (Fig. 2.8B).

PARTITE SESAMOIDS OF THE FIRST METATARSOPHALANGEAL JOINT

Partite sesamoid, tibial and/or fibular, is common and may be unilateral or bilateral (Fig. 2.9). In fact, it may be bilateral but asymmetrical. The partition may be horizontal, oblique, or vertical and may divide the sesamoid into equal halves or two unequal-sized segments. Multipartition is also possible. Well-defined margins between the two segments indicate "chronicity" and may represent a normal variant (more commonly) or an old, unhealed (nonunion) fracture. Ill-defined margins typically indicate an acute condition or

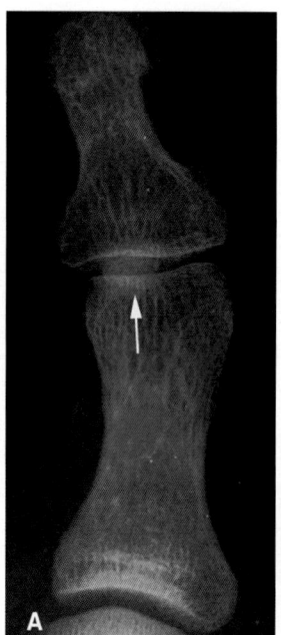
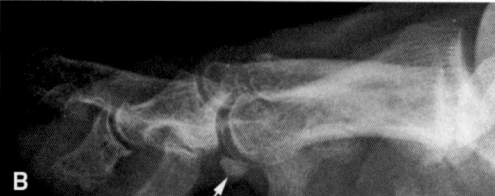
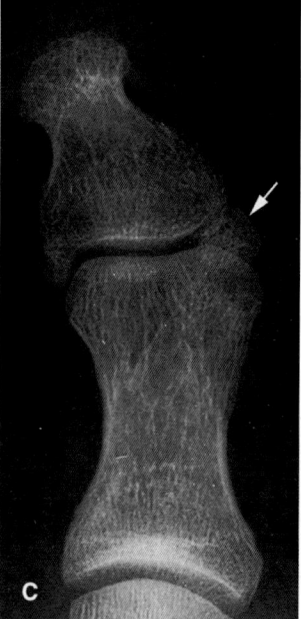

FIGURE 2.6 Os interphalangeus (*arrows*). Central location, **(A)** DP view and **(B)** lateral view. **C.** Eccentric location, DP view.

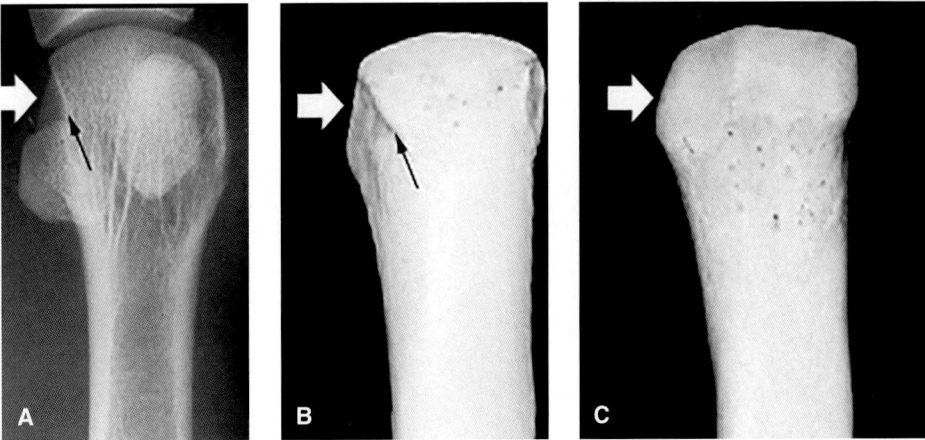

FIGURE 2.7 First metatarsal head anatomy, lateral aspect. **A.** DP view radiograph. **B.** Dorsal view bone specimen. **C.** Plantar view bone specimen. *Black arrow,* superior-lateral margin of head; *White arrow,* lateral margin of fibular sesamoid articular surface, misinterpreted as "lateral edge" or "lateral cortical surface."

fracture (Fig. 2.10A and B). It may be impossible to diagnose sesamoid fracture radiographically when it is superimposed on a metatarsal in DP and oblique views; however, the tibial sesamoid can be partially isolated in the lateral oblique view and both sesamoids isolated in the sesamoid axial view (Fig. 2.10C and D).

ACCESSORY SESAMOIDS

Accessory sesamoid bones may be encountered at any lesser metatarsophalangeal joint inferiorly (Fig. 2.11). They may occur as a single entity or in pairs, and in varying combinations, whether they are unilateral or bilateral. And, if bilateral,

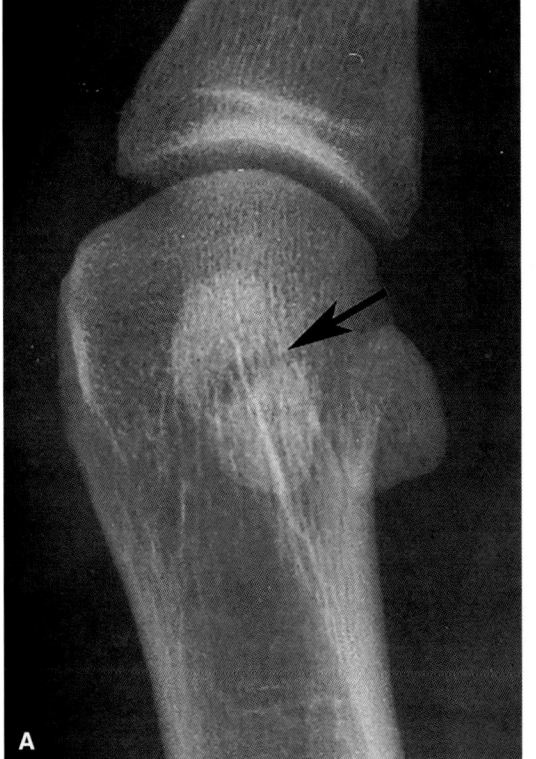

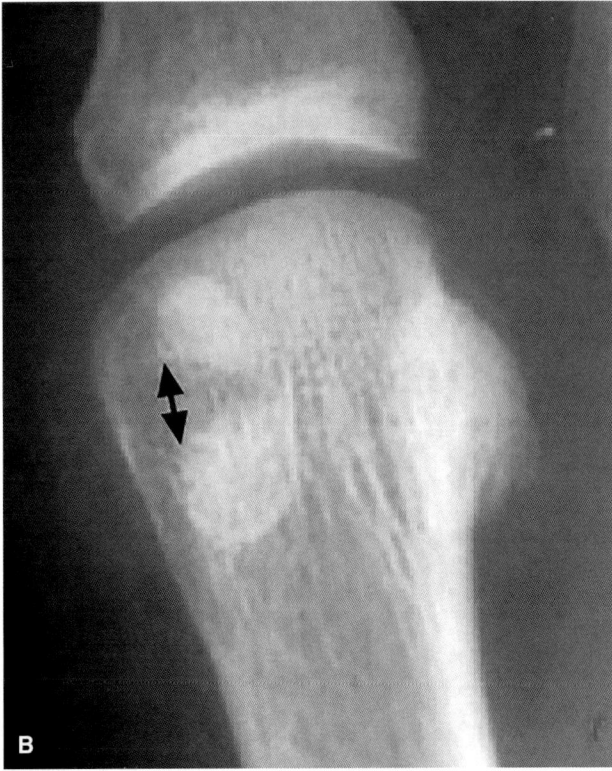

FIGURE 2.8 Simulated tibial sesamoid fracture; incidental findings with no history of trauma or pain. **A.** Jagged edges. The superimposed prominent first metatarsal head trabeculations give the partition a jagged appearance (*arrow*). **B.** Separated segments (*arrows*); this patient had no history of injury nor pain.

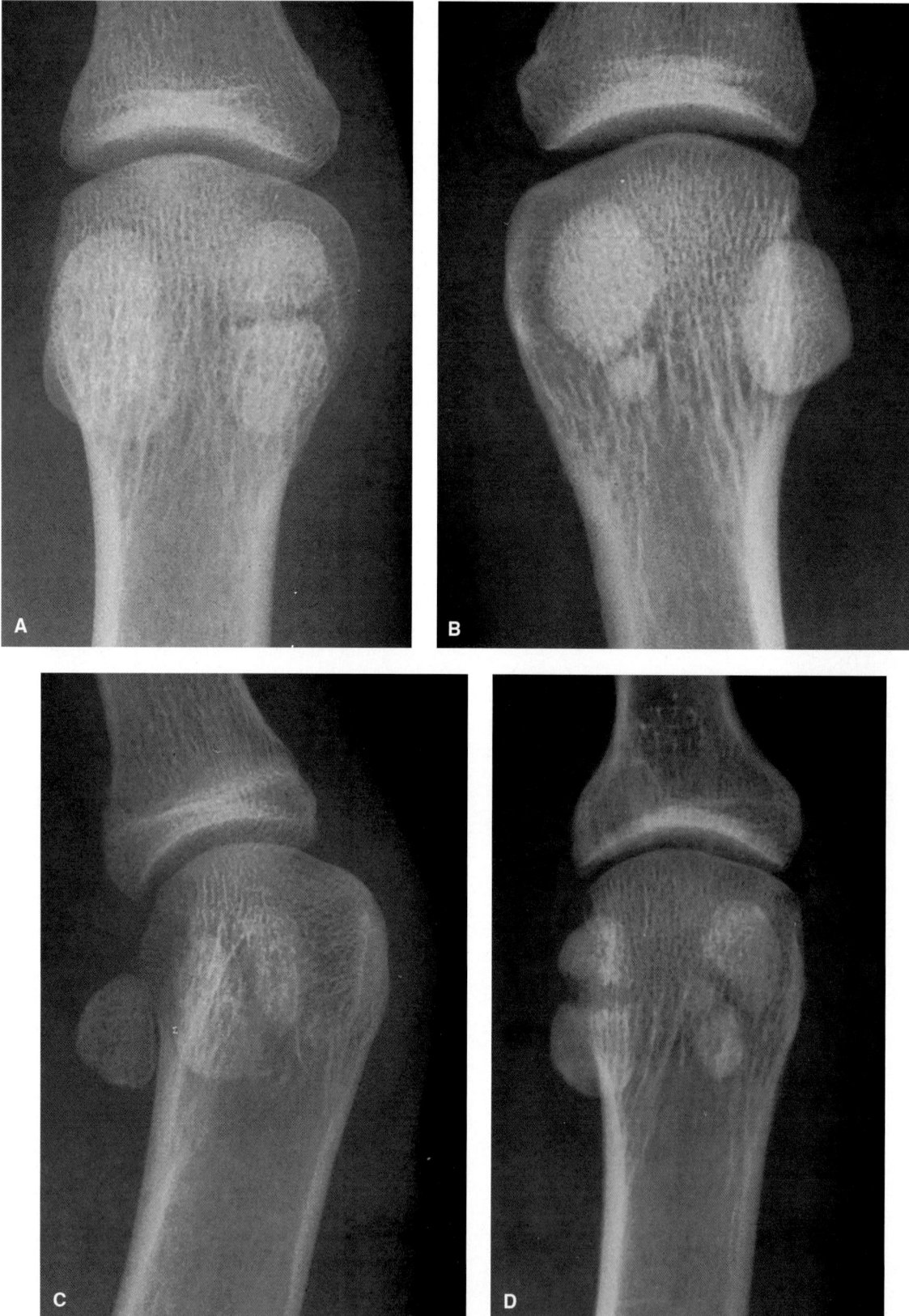

FIGURE 2.9 Partite first metatarsophalangeal joint sesamoid variations. **A.** Transverse, nearly equal halves. **B.** Extreme asymmetry in size. **C.** Oblique, nearly longitudinal partition. **D.** Tripartite tibial, bipartite fibular.

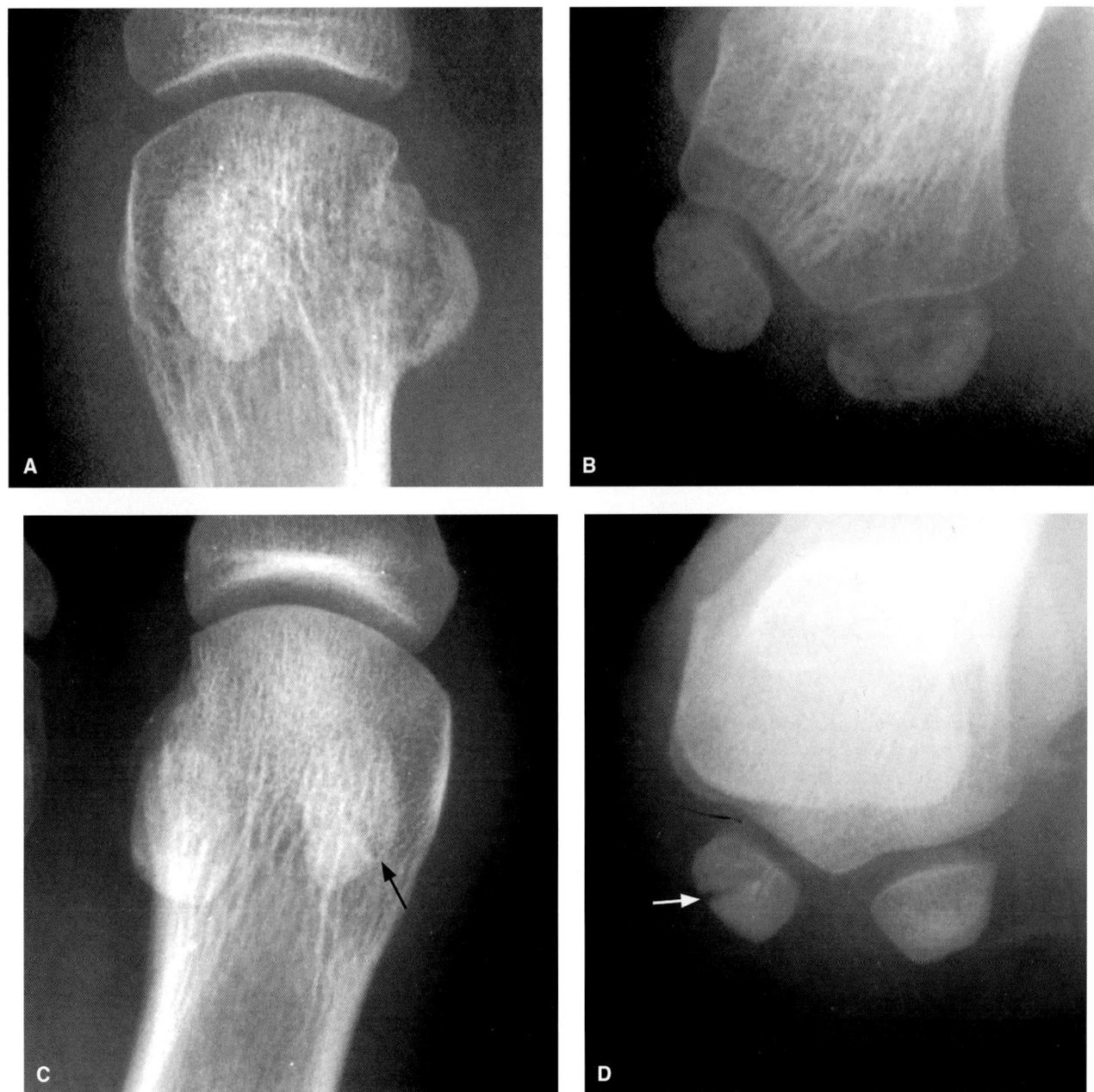

FIGURE 2.10 Sesamoid fracture. **A.** DP view; the fibular sesamoid margins are ill defined and there is fragmentation (comminution). **B.** Axial view (same patient as **A**); ill-defined fragmentation. **C.** DP view; tibial sesamoid fracture is barely perceptible (*arrow*). **D.** Axial view (same patient as **C**); fracture is identified (*arrow*).

their presence may be asymmetrically distributed. They may even be bipartite. Accessory sesamoids can be isolated in the sesamoid axial view (Fig. 2.11B). Lesions that may mimic a superimposed accessory sesamoid include bone island (Fig. 2.11C) and osteoid osteoma (when the nidus is calcified)[28]; however, they would not be seen inferior to (outside) the bone on the axial view.

BONE ISLAND (ENOSTOSIS)

The bone island, or enostosis, is a common normal variant and may be seen in any bone. It varies in size and shape but appears as a geographic, uniform increased density or sclerosis.[29] It is either seen in cancellous bone (bone island, see Fig. 2.11C) or along

the inner (endosteal) surface of the cortex (enostosis). They are not associated with symptomatology and are incidental findings.

LESSER METATARSAL CORTICAL IRREGULARITY

Variations of the girth, contour, and form of a metatarsal shaft may be encountered. One in particular is irregular thickening of the periosteal surface of the cortex. Figure 2.12 demonstrates how exuberant it may appear. Radiographically, varying degrees of periosteal new bone formation is possible, but typically it is thick and undulating (irregular). It also may be seen in the small tubular bones of the foot with tuberous sclerosis. The differential diagnosis for generalized periostitis may include venous stasis, hypertrophic osteoarthropathy, hypervitaminosis A, and thyroid acropachy.

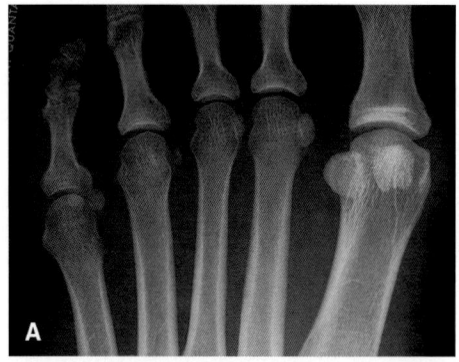

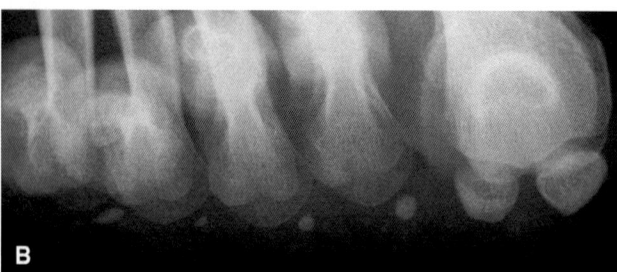

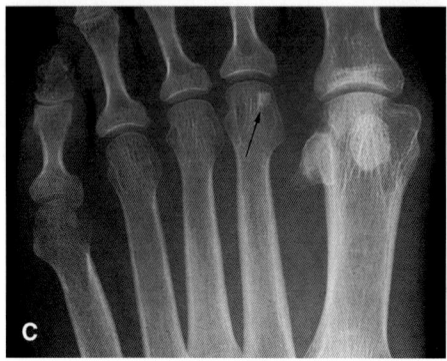

FIGURE 2.11 Accessory sesamoids **(A and B)** vs bone island.
A. DP view. **B.** Sesamoid axial view (different patient than **A**).
C. Bone island (*arrow*).

METATARSAL PARABOLA

The typical radiographic metatarsal parabola (Fig. 2.13) is as follows: the second metatarsal extends most distal; the first and third metatarsals are at the same level and slightly proximal relative to the second; and, there is a smooth steppage down from the third to the fourth and from the fourth to the fifth metatarsals.[30] Metatarsal protrusion and methods used to measure length patterns are discussed in greater detail in the "Hallux Abducto Valgus" subsection of the "Abnormalities of Position" section later in this chapter.

PERSISTENT FIFTH METATARSAL APOPHYSIS AND OS VESALIANUM

Two ossicles may be seen adjacent to the fifth metatarsal base in the adult. The persistent fifth metatarsal apophysis is more common and the os vesalianum more rare. The persistent fifth metatarsal apophysis is frequently bilateral and symmetrical but may only be found unilateral. It is an unfused apophyseal ossification center and, as such, represents a separated tuberosity (Fig. 2.14A). Its shape may vary but more commonly appears as an oval or is football shaped. It is often confused for the os

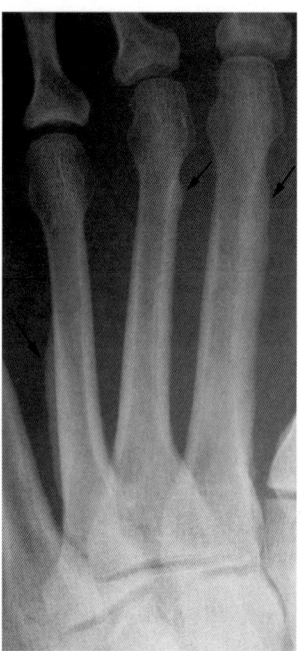

FIGURE 2.12 Undulating periosteal thickening (*arrows*), a normal variant.

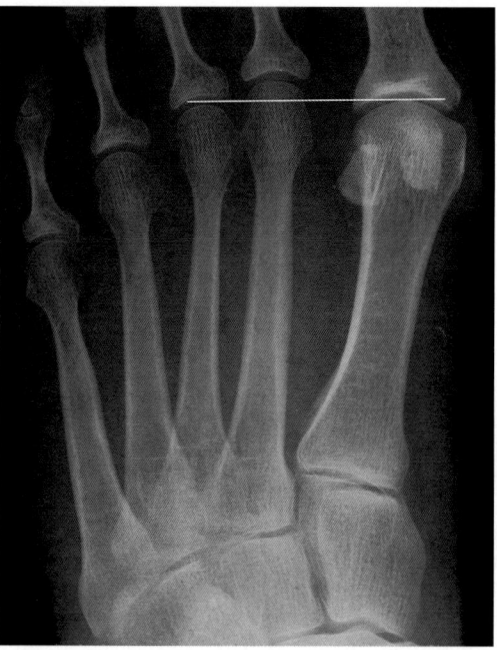

FIGURE 2.13 Normal metatarsal parabola.

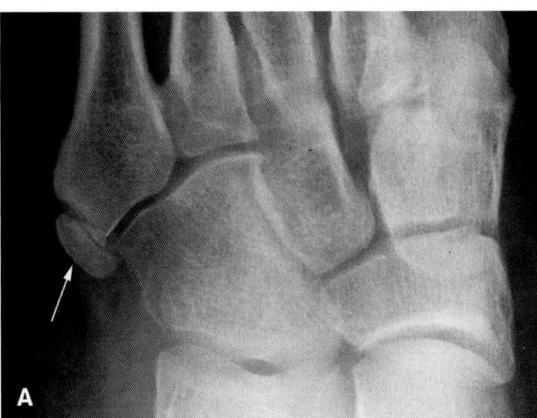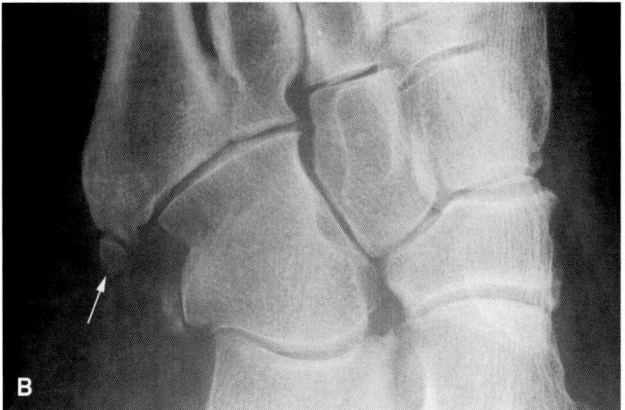

FIGURE 2.14 **A.** Persistent fifth metatarsal apophysis (*arrow*). **B.** Os vesalianum (*arrow*) (this particular case was bilateral and relatively symmetrical).

vesalianum, which presents as a small, rounded ossicle just posterior to the tip of the tuberosity (Fig. 2.14B). It is debatable whether or not the os vesalianum, in some cases, is the remnant of prior trauma.

OS INTERMETATARSEUM

The os intermetatarseum (aka os intermetatarsal I) is located between the first and second metatarsal bases superiorly (Fig. 2.15). It may be freestanding, or it may articulate or be fused with the first or second metatarsal or the medial cuneiform.[31] Its shape and size vary. The perforating branch between the dorsal and plantar metatarsal arteries may calcify and simulate the os intermetatarseum. It is infrequently associated with pain and paresthesia, related to compression of the deep peroneal nerve.[32,33]

OSSICLES MEDIAL TO FIRST METATARSAL BASE AND MEDIAL CUNEIFORM

Though extremely rare, ossicles along the medial aspect of the midfoot, if large enough, may cause pain and/or deformity.[34,35] The os cuneometatarsal 1 tibiale is located medial to the first

metatarsal-cuneiform joint; the tibialis anterior sesamoid is either medial to the medial cuneiform or the metatarsal-cuneiform joint (Fig. 2.16); the os paracuneiforme is either medial to the naviculocuneiforme 1 joint or the medial cuneiform; and the os intercuneiforme is along the posterosuperior aspect of the naviculocuneiforme 1 joint.[17]

BIPARTITE MEDIAL CUNEIFORM

The medial cuneiform is rarely divided into two segments. Unless one is specifically looking for this variation, it is easily overlooked. The overall size of the bipartite medial cuneiform tends to be larger than that of the normal medial cuneiform.[36] The partition most commonly divides it into dorsal and plantar segments; the dorsal segment is slightly smaller than the plantar (Fig. 2.17A) and tends to present bilaterally, though sometimes with asymmetry. For example, the partition may be complete in one extremity but incomplete (presenting as a cleft anteriorly, posteriorly, or both and united centrally) in the other (Fig. 2.17B). It may become symptomatic and require surgical intervention.[37] The symptomatic bipartite medial cuneiform may demonstrate bone marrow edema with magnetic resonance imaging (MRI).[38]

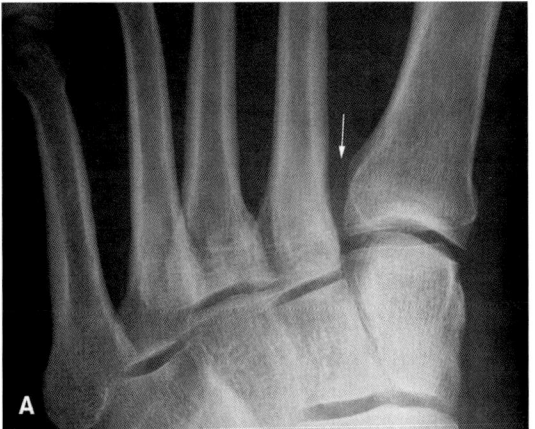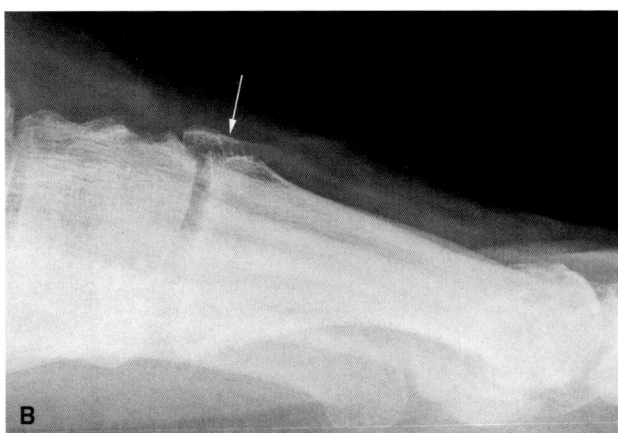

FIGURE 2.15 Large os intermetatarseum (*arrows*). **A.** DP view. **B.** Lateral view.

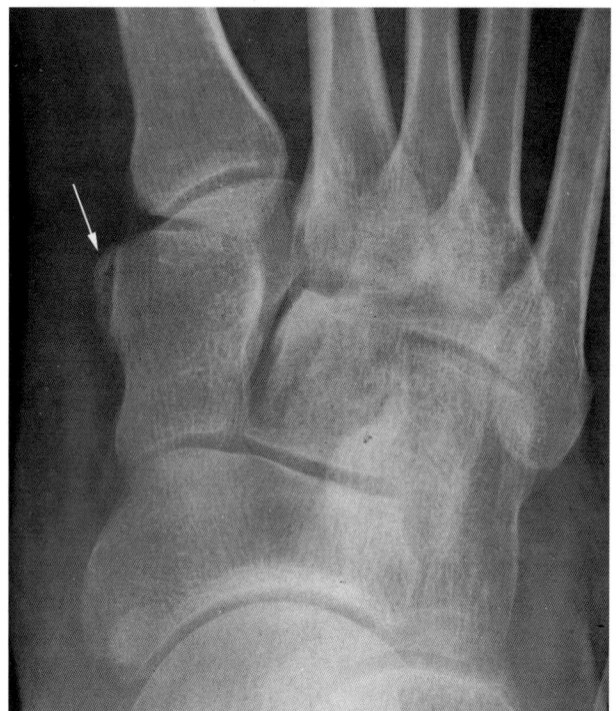

FIGURE 2.16 Tibialis anterior sesamoid (*arrow*).

BIPARTITE NAVICULAR AND MÜLLER-WEISS SYNDROME

Another rare bipartition involves the tarsal navicular. Interestingly, publications of a similar condition, Müller-Weiss syndrome, have paralleled reports of the bipartite navicular but have rarely intersected. Maceira and Rochera[39] have provided a large case cohort and detailed discussion of Müller-Weiss syndrome; five radiographic stages are presented that closely resemble the bipartite navicular. The two segments are quite asymmetrical and divided into a larger inferomedial segment and smaller superolateral segment (Fig. 2.18). In the lateral view, the smaller segment is wedge shaped, and its apex is directed inferiorly; in the DP view, the larger segment is wedge

shaped, and its apex is directed laterally.[40] Since the partitioning is superimposed and difficult to visualize radiographically, computed tomography (CT) can clearly demonstrate the morphology and help distinguish it from fracture.[41]

OS INFRANAVICULARE, OS SUPRANAVICULARE, OS SUPRATALARE, AND OS TALOTIBIALE

Two accessory ossicles may be seen along the superior aspect of the navicular in the lateral view (Fig. 2.19A). The os supranaviculare is the more frequent of the two and presents at the talonavicular joint; the os infranaviculare is located at the naviculocuneiform joint. They often are in close apposition to the parent navicular bone and appear to articulate with it. The os supranaviculare, in some cases, may demonstrate an articular surface for the talar head that is continuous with the navicular articular surface inferiorly. The ossicles are generally small and may be round, oval, or even triangular shaped. When larger, it is common to see degenerative changes, that is, spurs/osteophytes, associated with both ossicles and the navicular; this presentation suggests prior trauma and may be the result of subsequent nonunion with secondary degenerative disease. Stress fracture has been demonstrated just inferior to the os supranaviculare[42] that may subsequently result in similar findings. Also, the os supranaviculare may have a perforated attachment to the navicular bone (personal observation of a bone specimen); therefore, another scenario could be an attached ossicle that was broken off the parent bone. Avulsion fracture is typically flakelike in shape, but may, over time, remodel and look similar if a nonunion.

The os supratalare is located just posterior to the talonavicular joint, superior to the talar head/neck (Fig. 2.19B). It is best seen with the lateral view. Occasionally, it may be seen in the medial oblique view, which would indicate a superomedial position. It varies in size (small to large)[43] and shape (flat, round, oval). Occasionally, it is in direct apposition to a spur, with associated degenerative changes. It also may be seen with an os supranaviculare. Acute avulsion fracture may appear nearly identical to the accessory bone (Fig. 2.19C). CT and MRI have been used to assess a painful presentation.[44]

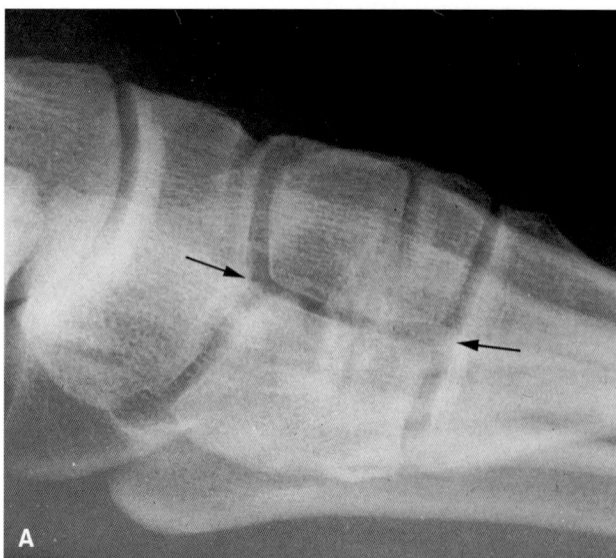
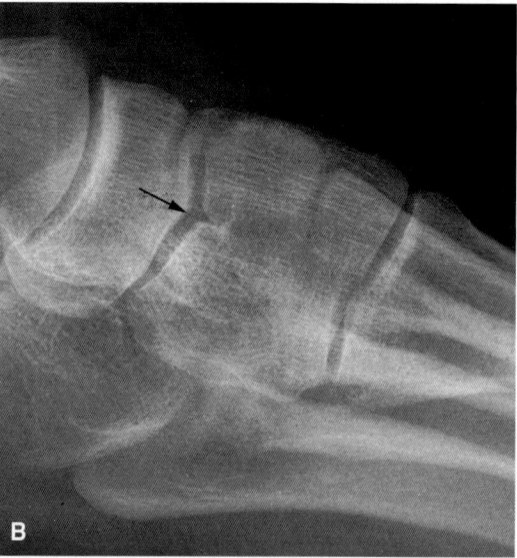

FIGURE 2.17 Bipartite medial cuneiform (*arrows*). **A.** Complete. **B.** Incomplete in opposite extremity of the same patient.

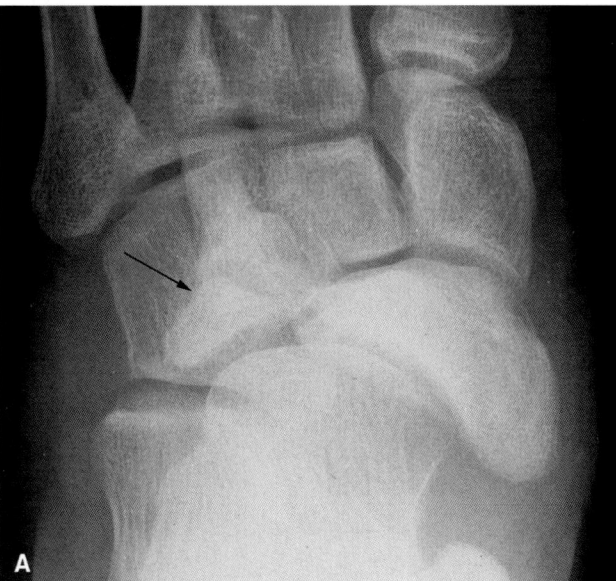
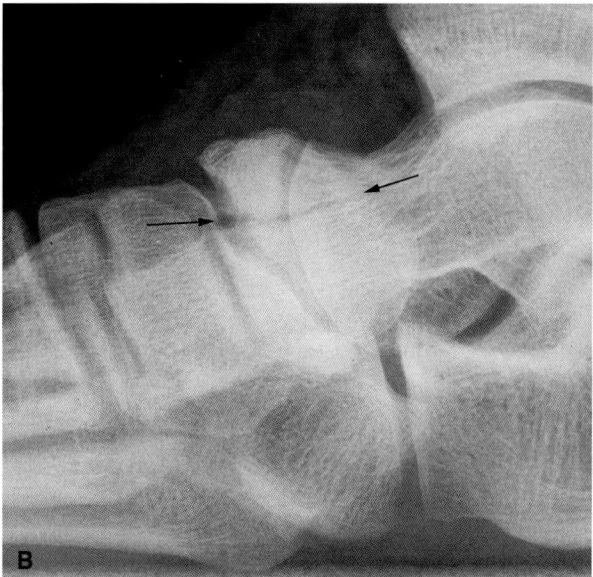

FIGURE 2.18 Bipartite navicular/Müller-Weiss syndrome (bilateral presentation in this pàtient, though somewhat asymmetric). **A.** DP view; *arrow* identifies smaller superolateral segment. **B.** Lateral view; *arrows* identify partition.

The os talotibiale is typically a small ossicle found anterior to the ankle joint, adjacent to the talar dome in the lateral view and in close apposition to the tibia (Fig. 2.19D). It may resemble a loose osseous body. One related case (not described as an os talotibiale) has been reported that is very large.[45]

ACCESSORY NAVICULAR (OS TIBIALE EXTERNUM)

Two distinct ossicles are occasionally found adjacent to the navicular tuberosity posteriorly; collectively, they are referred to as the accessory navicular. The first type is a small sesamoid bone in the posterior tibial tendon (Fig. 2.20A); it is 2-3 mm in diameter and located up to 5 mm posterior and medial to

the tuberosity.[46] This ossicle is also known as the os tibiale externum.

The second type is much larger than type 1, from 9 to 12 mm in diameter, but is located only 1-2 mm from the tuberosity posteromedially and united as a synchondrosis (Fig. 2.20B).[47] It is often triangular shaped and appears to articulate with the tuberosity. It is considered a secondary ossification center; when united as a synostosis, it is referred to as the type 3 accessory navicular (aka cornuate navicular) (Fig. 2.20C). The incidence of the type 2 accessory navicular was originally thought to be more frequent than the type 1; however, due to its small size, the latter may have been overlooked.[48] The type 2 accessory navicular has been further subdivided based upon its position

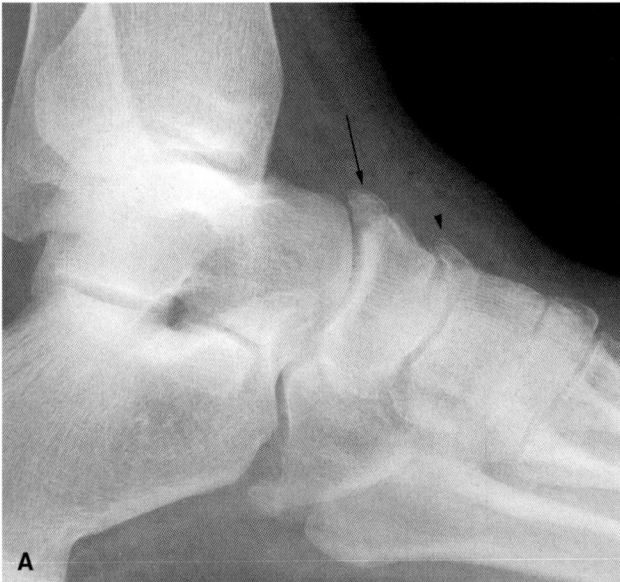
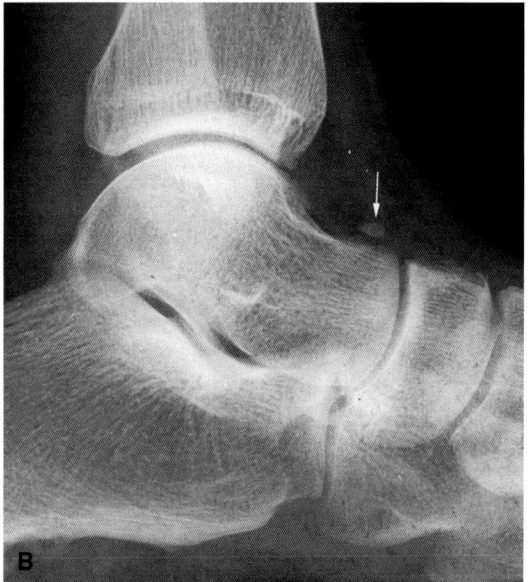

FIGURE 2.19 Ossicles superior to the tarsus. **A.** Os supranaviculare (*arrow*) and os infranaviculare (*arrowhead*). Also present is an os peroneum inferior to the cuboid. **B.** Os supratalare.

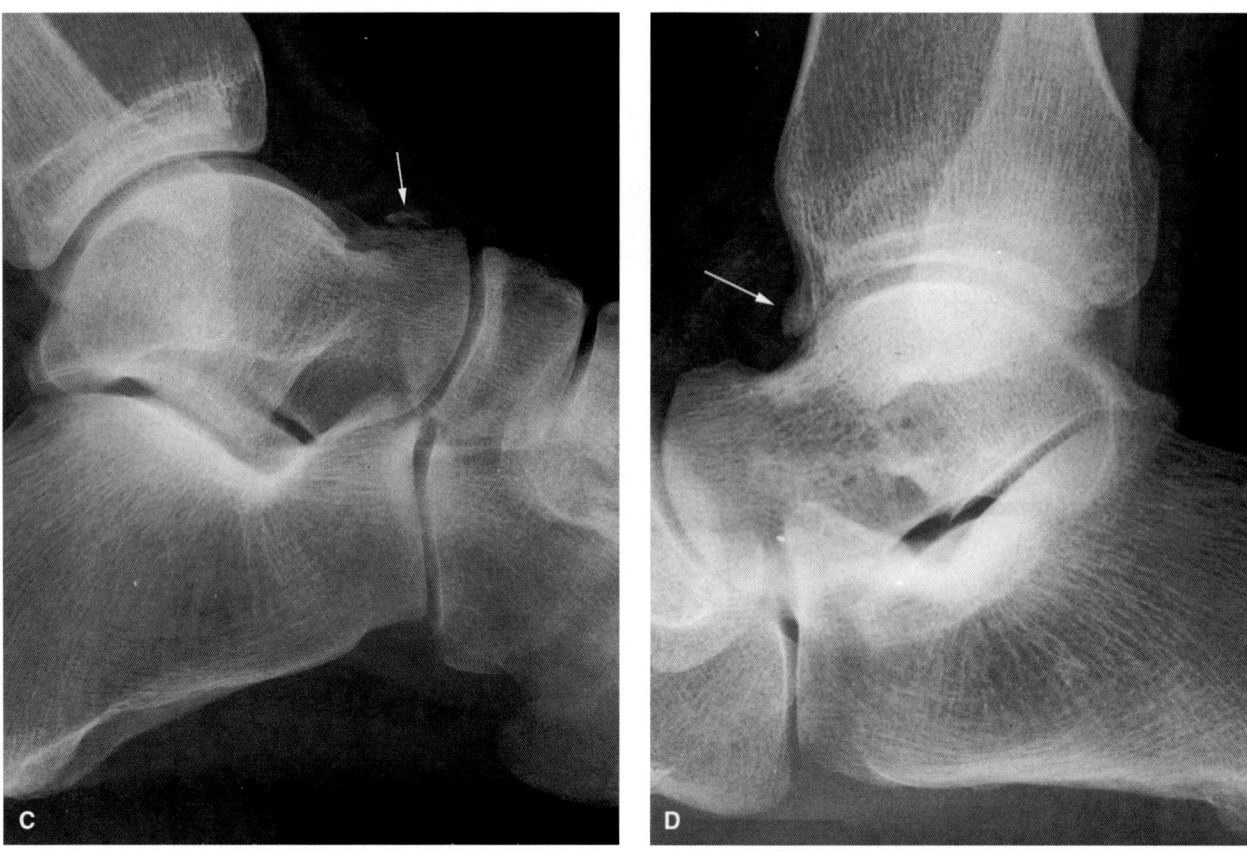

FIGURE 2.19 (*Continued*) **C.** Avulsion fracture of talar head/neck. **D.** Os talotibiale.

relative to the navicular and an angle (referred to as the synchondrosis-ossicle-talar or SOT angle) in the lateral view[49]; both types can result in symptomatology, though the investigators believed that the type 2A (which is positioned more superiorly) is more likely to become avulsed since it is subjected to tension forces (the type 2B is subjected to shear forces). Bone scintigraphy has a high negative predictive value and is useful for evaluating the symptomatic accessory navicular.[50] MRI has also been advocated to demonstrate the presence or absence of bone edema.[51]

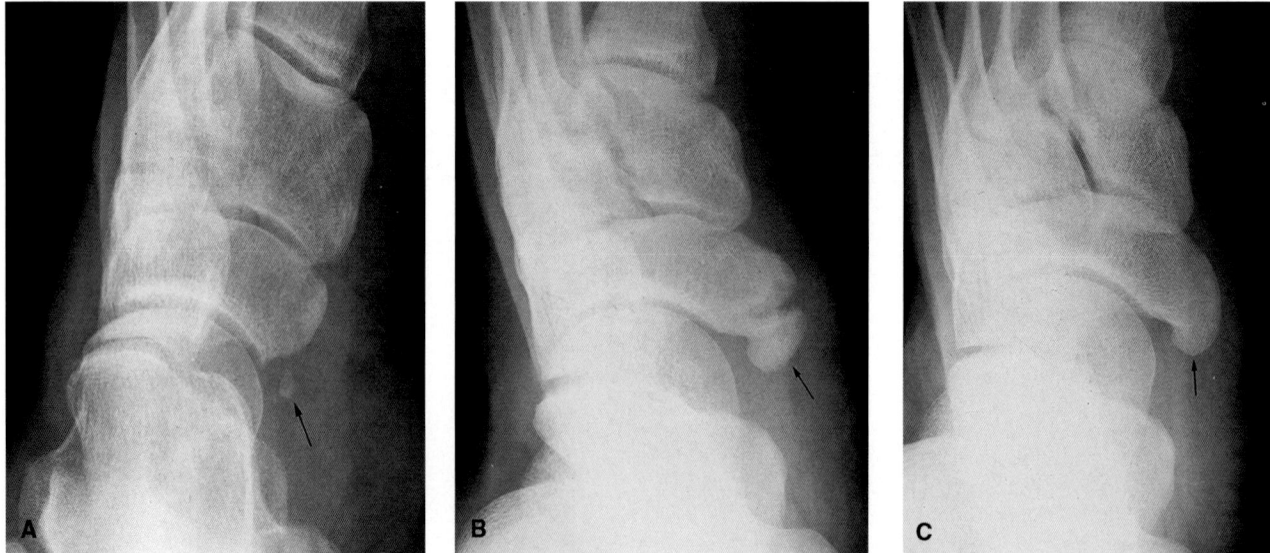

FIGURE 2.20 Accessory navicular (*arrows*). **A.** Type I (os tibiale externum). **B.** Type II (accessory ossification center). **C.** Type III (cornuate navicular).

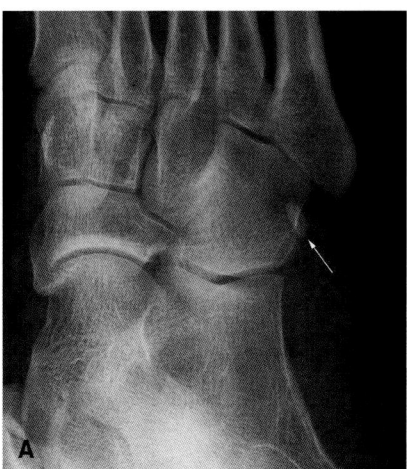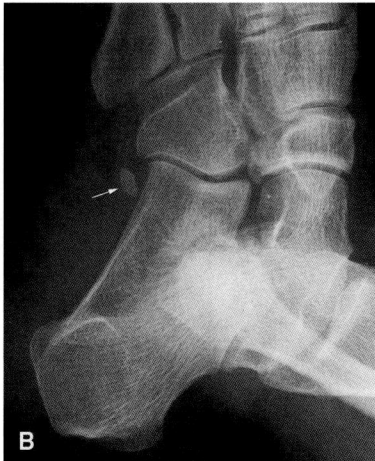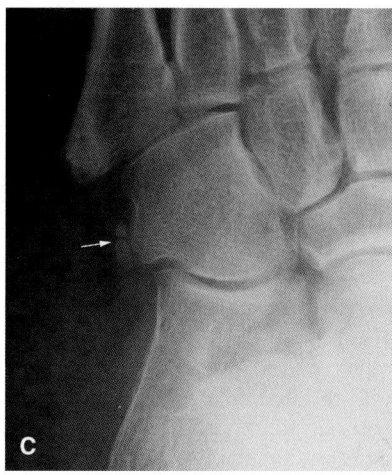

FIGURE 2.21 Os peroneum (*arrows*). **A.** Distal location. **B.** Proximal location. **C.** Central location and multipartite.

OS PERONEUM

The ossicle frequently identified adjacent to the cuboid infero-laterally is known as the os peroneum. Its size and shape vary, and it may be unilateral or bilateral, with or without symmetry. It is located in the peroneus longus tendon and is best seen in the medial oblique view; occasionally, it is isolated in the DP or lateral view (see Fig. 2.19A). Its anterior-posterior position varies; it may be superimposed anteriorly on the peroneal sulcus of the cuboid (Fig. 2.21A) or located adjacent to the calcaneus just posterior to the calcaneocuboid joint (Fig. 2.21B). The ossicle, when located adjacent to the cuboid, articulates with a facet along the antero-lateral aspect of the cuboid tuberosity,[52] and degenerative arthritis has been reported.[53] Enthesopathy-like spurring may also be

seen at its margins. Infrequently, the os peroneum may be multipartite (Fig. 2.21C). Fracture of the os peroneum and disruption of a multipartite ossicle has been reported and can be assessed additionally with ultrasound, bone scintigraphy, or MRI.[54] MRI is especially valuable when evaluating tears of the peroneus longus tendon associated with the os peroneum.[55,56]

OS CALCANEUS SECUNDARIUS

The os calcaneus secundarius is an accessory bone that is in close apposition to the calcaneus anterior process and adjacent to the talar head, navicular, and cuboid; it is isolated in the medial oblique view (Fig. 2.22). It typically is small and round or oval shaped but may be irregular or triangular in shape. (It has been

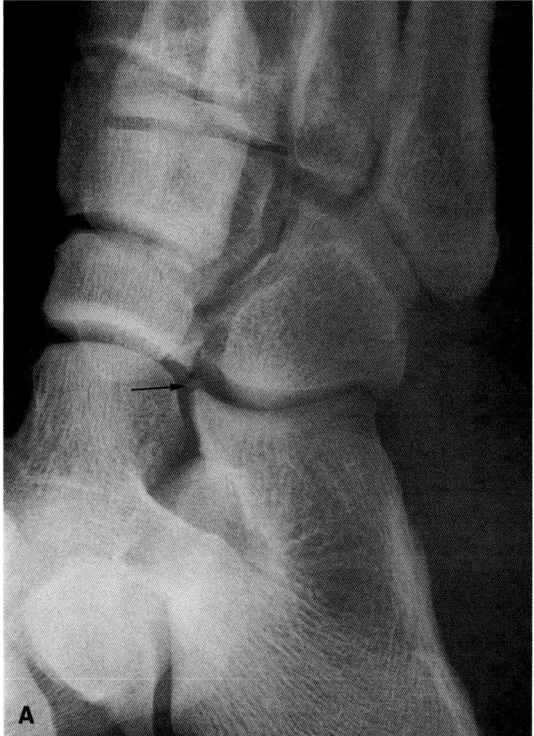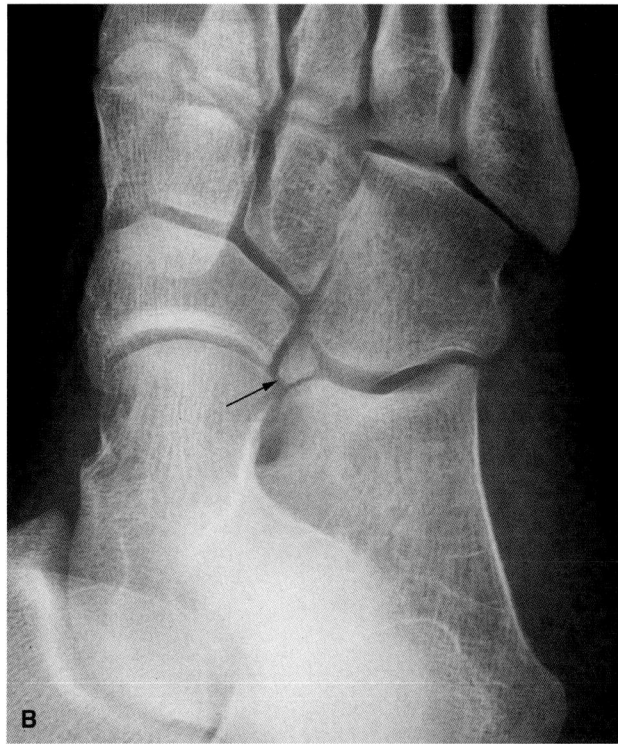

FIGURE 2.22 Os calcaneus secundarius. **A.** Small, *oval shape*. **B.** Larger, *triangular shape*.

suggested that avulsion fracture at the origin of the bifurcate ligament often is larger and triangular shaped, with ill-defined margins).[57] MRI is valuable for differentiating between fracture and accessory ossicle.[58,59] If radiographs are unremarkable but clinical suspicion is high, CT may be helpful.[60]

OS TRIGONUM AND OS ACCESSORIUM SUPRACALCANEUM

The os trigonum is located posterior to the talar posterolateral process and is visible in the lateral view (Fig. 2.23). It is reported to be round, oval, or triangular in shape[61]; however, in reality, the shape varies considerably. The ossicle usually is quite large and often appears to articulate with the talus; it may also articulate with the superior aspect of the calcaneus as an extension of the posterior talocalcaneal articular facet. Osteoarthritis may be seen, resulting in an irregular outline and/or spurring and sclerosis at the margins. Bony union with the talus is referred to as the trigonal or Stieda process.[62] The os trigonum, like the os supranaviculare, may have a perforated attachment to the posterior talus (personal observation of a bone specimen), which could break off the parent bone. The symptomatic ossicle (os trigonum syndrome) can be further assessed with a forced plantarflexion lateral view to evaluate for impingement.[63] Both CT[64] and MRI[65] are recommended for distinguishing between os trigonum vs fracture of the posterolateral talar process.

A rare ossicle, the os accessorium supracalcaneum, has been reported just posterior to where the os trigonum would be found. It may be seen with the os trigonum (Fig. 2.23C). It is independent of the talus and attached to the calcaneus.[66]

OS SUBTIBIALE AND OS SUBFIBULARE

Ossicles have been identified inferior and/or posterior to the tibial and fibular malleoli and have been collectively named as os subtibiale and os subfibulare, respectively. These ossicles may represent unfused malleolar accessory or apophyseal ossification centers, sesamoids, loose osseous bodies, or nonunion avulsion fracture fragments.

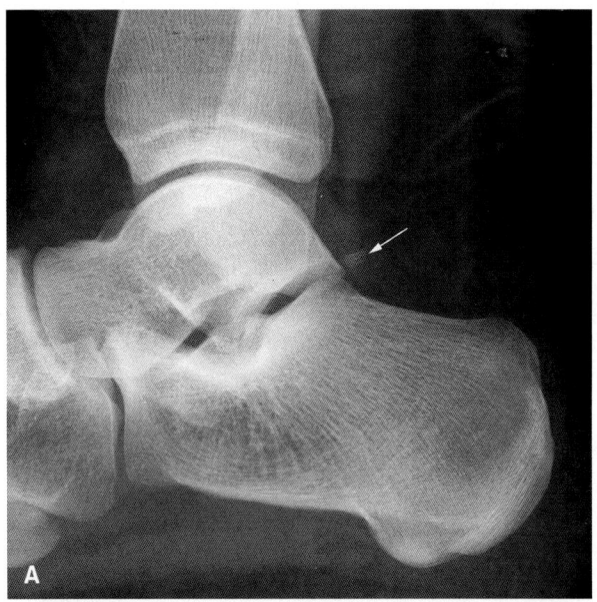

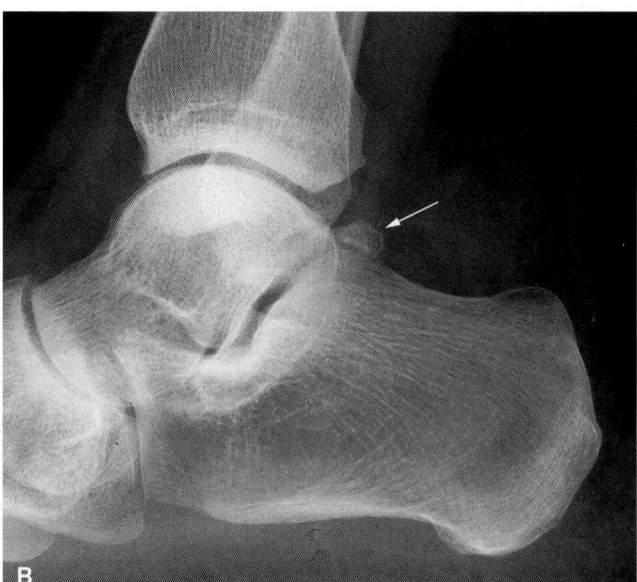

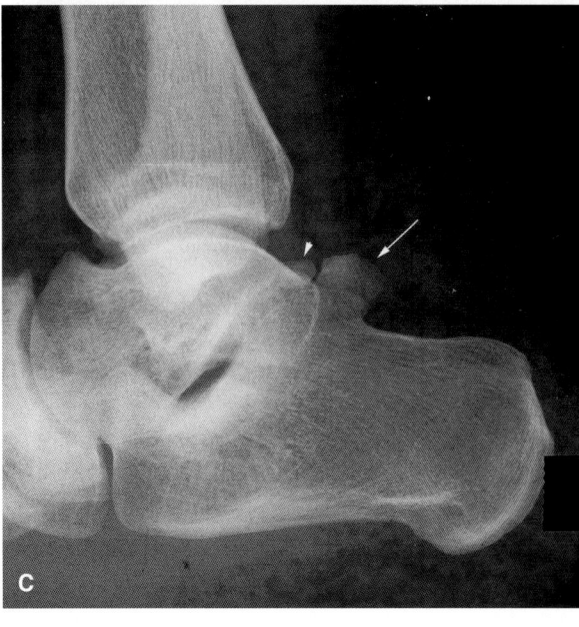

FIGURE 2.23 Os trigonum and os accessorium supracalcaneum. **A.** Small os trigonum (*arrow*). **B.** Larger os trigonum articulating with calcaneus (*arrow*). **C.** Os trigonum (*arrowhead*) and os accessorium supracalcaneum (*arrow*).

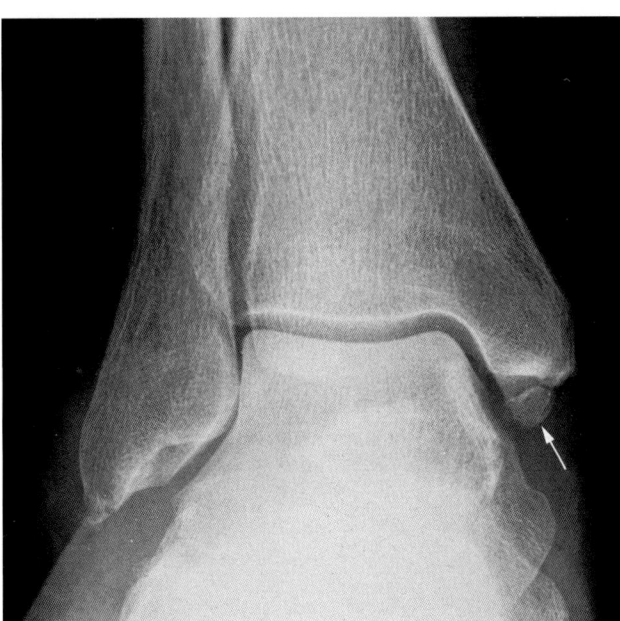

FIGURE 2.24 Os subtibiale (*arrow*).

The true os subtibiale will appear superimposed on the anterior colliculus in the AP and mortise ankle views (Fig. 2.24) and adjacent (inferior) to the posterior colliculus in the lateral view.[67] A small, rounded ossicle just inferior to the tip of the anterior colliculus may represent an unfused ossification center or avulsion (if history of trauma). Avulsion fracture may involve a larger portion of the anterior colliculus.

The true os subfibulare (Fig. 2.25) is located posterior to the tip of the fibular malleolus.[68] An unfused apophyseal ossification center is found anteriorly, and an unfused ossification center or avulsion (if history of trauma) is seen inferiorly.[69,70] Zhang et al.[71] have proposed a 9-region matrix based

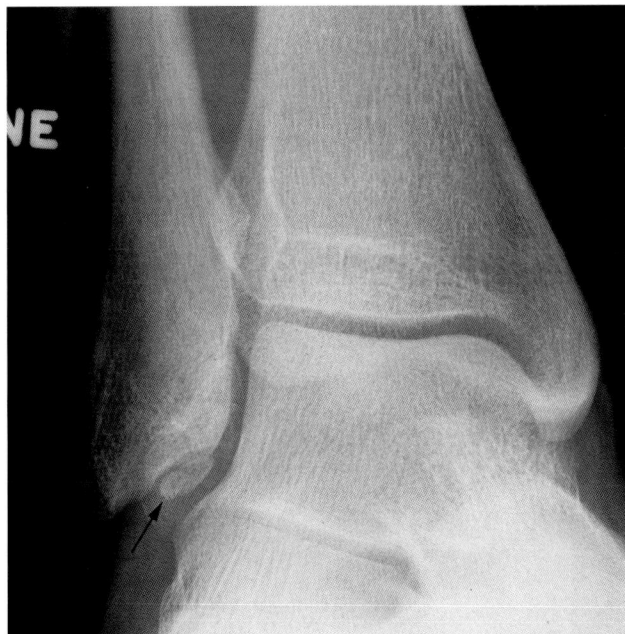

FIGURE 2.25 Os subfibulare (*arrow*). This example was located anteriorly in the lateral view, representing an unfused ossification center.

upon location and size of the ossicle in the lateral view to assist with diagnosis and treatment of symptomatic lesions. Special views have been developed to detect avulsed fragments of the anterior talofibular (ATFL) and the calcaneofibular (CFL) ligaments.[72] The ATFL view is performed with the foot posed in a 15-degree lateral oblique foot position and plantarflexed 45 degrees at the ankle joint (the image receptor is horizontal); the central ray is directed 0 degrees (from vertical) at the ankle. The CFL view is a 45-degree medial oblique position of the ankle. Another view has been devised to image avulsion fracture of the ATFL from the talus[73]; in this case, the image receptor is horizontal, the patient is seated, the heel is placed on the image receptor with the foot (ankle) plantarflexed 45 degrees and the forefoot elevated 20 degrees from the image receptor, the leg is externally rotated 30 degrees, and the central ray is directed at the dorsum of the talus at a caudal angle 20 degrees from vertical. MRI has been used for further evaluation of subfibular lesions and to assist decision management[74]; three-dimensional CT has also been advocated.[75]

COALITION (SYNOSTOSIS, SYNCHONDROSIS, AND SYNDESMOSIS)

The term coalition is used to describe an osseous (synostosis), cartilaginous (synchondrosis), or fibrous (syndesmosis) connection between two or more bones. It has also been referred to as a "bar." Coalition is often found bilaterally. Synostosis is commonly misdiagnosed due to superimposition between two bones and the apparent lack of a joint space. For example, synostosis of the proximal interphalangeal joint (PIPJ) and the third metatarsal-cuneiform joint are extremely rare; however, the PIPJ may not be seen if the toe is contracted, and the third metatarsal-cuneiform joint is frequently not visible in the DP and oblique views (a look at the lateral view will confirm the latter's presence). In any case, first attempt to trace the outline of the superimposed bone margins; if the articular end of each bone can be traced, then it is not a synostosis. Synostosis, aside from the distal interphalangeal joint and involvement of either the talus or calcaneus, is extremely rare.

INTERPHALANGEAL

Synostosis of the lesser toe distal interphalangeal joint is frequently encountered in the foot (Fig. 2.26). The fifth toe is most common, followed by the fourth, third, then second; the latter will coexist in most cases (eg, if there is synostosis of the third toe distal interphalangeal joint, there will also be synostosis of the fourth and fifth toes).

TALONAVICULAR

As obvious as it may seem, the talonavicular coalition is easily overlooked initially, having the appearance of an enlarged talar head (Fig. 2.27A and B).[76] It is often accompanied by a "ball and socket" ankle joint, as seen in the AP or mortise ankle view (Fig. 2.27C).

CALCANEONAVICULAR

The calcaneonavicular coalition is isolated and best visualized in the 45-degree medial oblique view. (If the foot is not positioned at 45 degrees but at 30 degrees, for example, there may

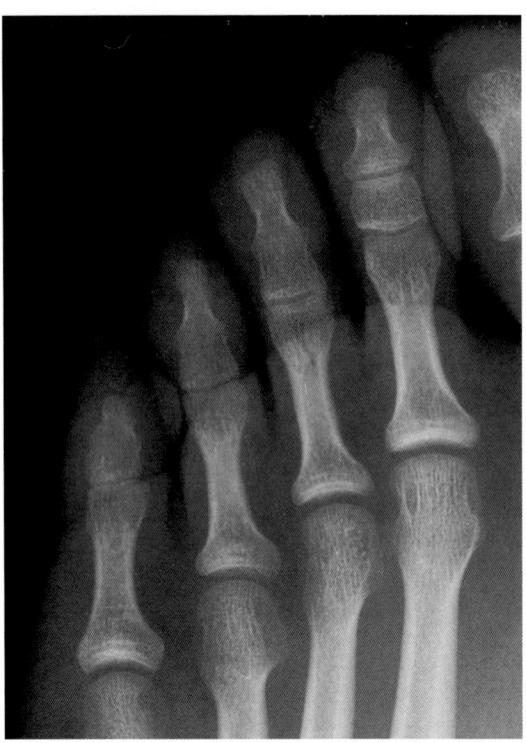

FIGURE 2.26 Distal interphalangeal synostosis of the fourth and fifth toes.

be superimposition of bony structures and the coalition will not be clearly identified.) Variable morphology may be encountered.[77] For example, there may be a slight gap between the calcaneus and navicular but with no apparent articulation (possibly a forme fruste variant or syndesmosis) (Fig. 2.28A).[78] An articulation between the two bones represents a synchondrosis; the margins of bone may appear irregular with sclerosis and spurring, mimicking an osteoarthritic joint (Fig. 2.28B). The two bones will be continuous when it is a synostosis; this presentation is the least common (Fig. 2.28C).

A prominent anterior calcaneal process, referred to as the "*anteater nose*" *sign*,[79] is seen in the lateral view (Fig. 2.28D). This finding has also been referred to as the "too long anterior process" or TLAP.[80] This sign is especially useful if an oblique view was not initially obtained. However, it may be obscured in severe pes planus or by superimposed osteoarthritis at the talonavicular joint. Occasionally, a talar beak may also be seen.

TALOCALCANEAL

Middle talocalcaneal facet and calcaneonavicular coalition are the most common tarsal joints affected; posterior talocalcaneal facet coalition is rare. Findings associated with middle talocalcaneal coalition are best demonstrated with lateral foot and Harris calcaneal axial views. CT is valuable for determining both the type (osseous vs fibrocartilaginous) as well as the facet orientation.[81] MRI may be necessary to further distinguish a fibrous coalition from cartilaginous if not detected by CT.[82]

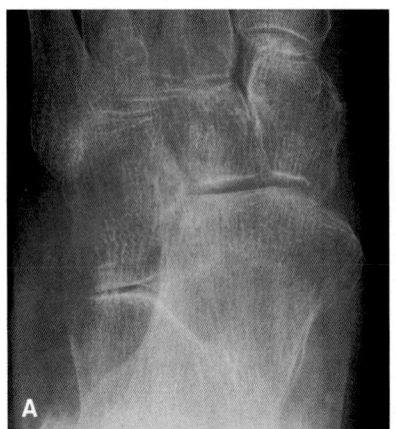
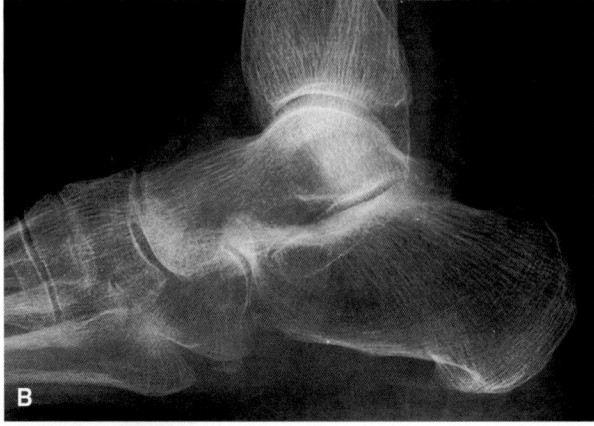
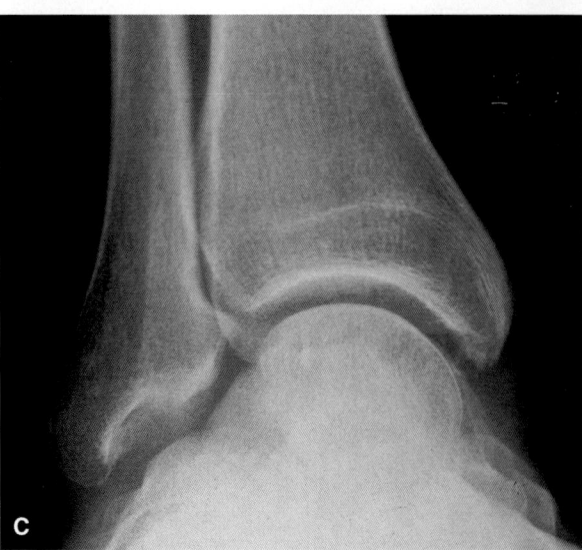

FIGURE 2.27 Talonavicular coalition. **A.** DP view. **B.** Lateral view. **C.** Mortise view: ball and socket ankle.

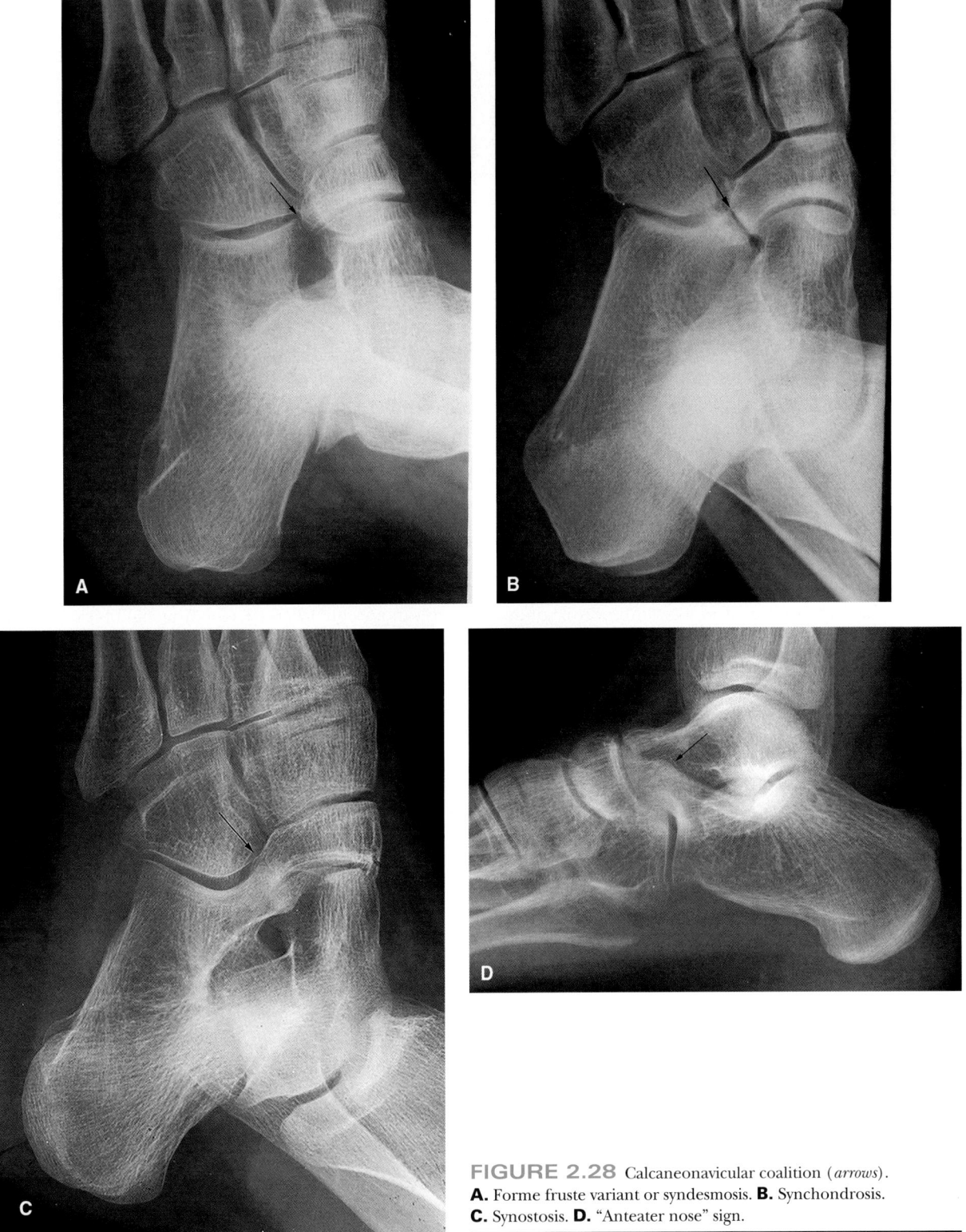

FIGURE 2.28 Calcaneonavicular coalition (*arrows*).
A. Forme fruste variant or syndesmosis. **B.** Synchondrosis.
C. Synostosis. **D.** "Anteater nose" sign.

In the lateral view, the normal sustentaculum tali is rectangular shaped and separate from the posteromedial process of the talus. With the osseous middle talocalcaneal coalition, the middle facet is not visible and the sustentaculum tali and posteromedial process of the talus are united as one landmark. The inferior margin of the sustentaculum tali continues with the inferoposterior aspect of the talar posteromedial process, which then appears to continue superiorly as the talar dome

(Fig. 2.29A); this finding has been called the "*C*" *sign*.[83] However, the "C" sign is not pathognomonic for middle talocalcaneal coalition; it has been demonstrated in some patients with flatfoot deformity but without coalition through confirmation by CT.[84] An incomplete or interrupted "C" sign will be seen with a fibrocartilaginous middle talocalcaneal coalition[85]; for example, a narrow, irregular joint (appearing osteoarthritic) may be seen between the sustentaculum tali posteriorly and the talar

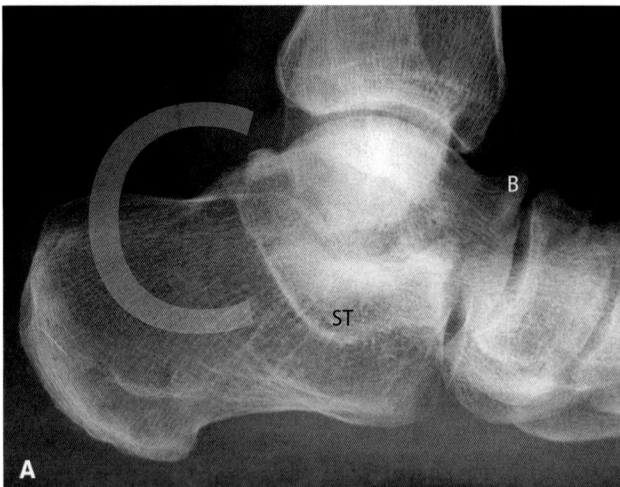
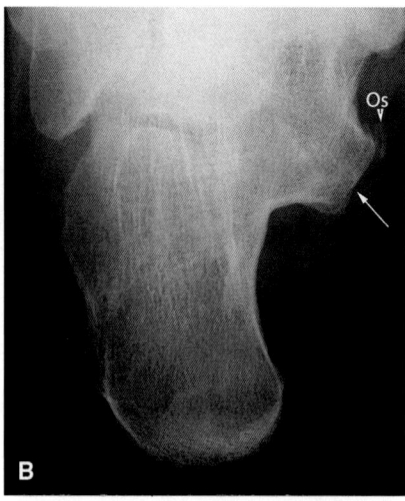

FIGURE 2.29 Osseous middle talocalcaneal coalition. **A.** Lateral view demonstrating the "C" sign, rounding of lateral talar process, dysmorphic sustentaculum tali (ST), narrowing of the posterior facet, short talar neck, and talar "beak" (B). **B.** Calcaneal axial (Harris) view. A remnant of the middle talocalcaneal joint angulates obliquely (*arrow*), and there is an os sustentaculi (Os).

posteromedial process. And, another form, the posteromedial subtalar coalition, may spare the middle facet.[86,87] Again, CT is advocated in order to confirm and detail the underlying morphology; MRI has also been used to assess fibrocartilaginous coalition in the pediatric patient.[88]

Other radiographic findings associated with some but not all talocalcaneal coalitions (Fig. 2.29A) include a *dysmorphic sustentaculum tali* (its inferior margin has a curved undersurface—it is usually flat); flattening or rounding of the lateral talar process inferiorly; narrowing of the posterior facet; a talar beak; and a short talar neck that is concave inferiorly.[89,90]

The middle and posterior talocalcaneal joints are best viewed in a calcaneal axial (Harris) projection with the tube head angulated at around 40 degrees. Normally, the two joints are horizontally oriented and nearly parallel to one another; however, the middle talocalcaneal joint or remnant of it will be oriented obliquely at ~45 degrees if there is coalition. The os sustentaculi has been associated with this anomaly (Fig. 2.29B).[91]

PEDIATRIC

Radiographic positioning techniques are the same for the child as for the adult. Weight bearing is strongly recommended for the standard DP foot/AP ankle and lateral views, whenever possible, especially for assessment of positional deformities and alignment of bones.[92] For the youngest patients who are not yet able to walk, simulated weight-bearing radiographs should be obtained; a nonpregnant parent, family member, or guardian should be instructed on how to hold and position the extremity for the study. Bilateral studies are not routinely justifiable as a comparison for unilateral trauma; however, select views of the opposite extremity may be warranted when there is a questionable finding.[93]

NORMAL DEVELOPMENT AND DEVELOPMENTAL VARIANTS

The radiographic appearance of the pediatric foot and ankle varies considerably based upon the age of the patient[94]; a variety of developmental variants may also be encountered.[95] Table 2.3 lists the major ossification centers, primary and secondary, and

their age of appearance for evaluating a patient's development pattern. Generally speaking, most ossification centers appear earlier in females than in males. Both primary and secondary ossification centers may develop from multiple ossification centers and mimic fracture (Fig. 2.30).

An *epiphysis* is a secondary ossification center, usually found at the end of a long bone. Most epiphyses distribute pressure from an adjacent bone. However, some are found at tendon insertion sites. The latter are commonly referred to as *apophyses*. Apophyses in the foot are located at the fifth metatarsal proximally and the calcaneus posteriorly. The appearance of secondary ossification centers, as well as the adjacent physis and zone of provisional calcification, can vary considerably between patients as well as within the same patient at different ages and be misinterpreted as abnormality. For example, the distal tibial physis is undulating along its anteromedial aspect (seen anteriorly in the lateral view and medially in the AP ankle view). This presentation is a feature of normal development, and since its description by Kump[96] has been referred to in the literature as the Kump hump (Fig. 2.31).[97]

The calcaneal apophysis arises from such a large ossification center that its development has been divided into six stages.[98] The normally developing calcaneal apophysis appears

TABLE 2.3	Normal Development Grouping Based on Major Ossification Centers
Age Group	**Radiographic Appearance**
Birth to 3 mo	Talus, calcaneus, cuboid
3-9 mo	Lateral cuneiform, distal tibial epiphysis
9 mo-2 y	First: distal fibular epiphysis, medial cuneiform
	Second: intermediate cuneiform, first metatarsal, proximal phalangeal basal epiphyses
2-5 y	Navicular, lesser metatarsal head epiphyses
5-9 y	Calcaneal apophysis
9-12 y	Fifth metatarsal apophysis, sesamoids

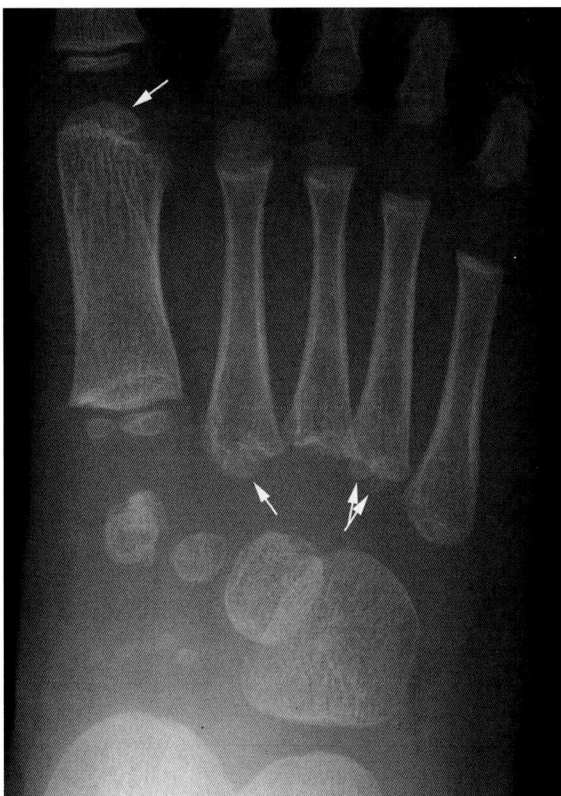

FIGURE 2.30 Multipartite primary (medial cuneiform and navicular) and secondary (first metatarsal) ossification centers. Pseudoepiphyses (*arrows*) of the first metatarsal head and lesser metatarsal bases.

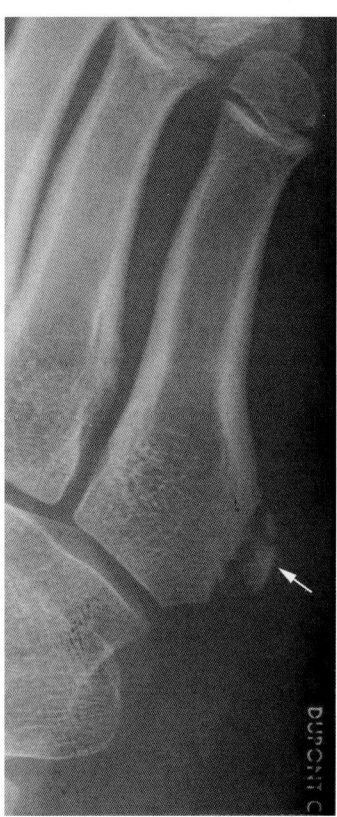

FIGURE 2.32 Fifth metatarsal apophysis. This example demonstrates multiple partitions and irregular margins (*arrow*), which were bilaterally symmetrical and asymptomatic.

sclerotic relative to the calcaneal body[99]; however, developmental variations include multipartition and a jagged adjacent metaphysis (Fig. 2.31B).

The fifth metatarsal basal apophysis may only be visible for a short period of time radiographically. And, it frequently ossifies from multiple ossification centers (Fig. 2.32). A bilateral comparison view may not be useful when fracture is a consideration; the opposite apophysis is often asymmetrical in appearance. The apophysis initially appears as a fleck of bone that is nearly parallel but slightly oblique to the fifth metatarsal diaphysis; fracture is usually more transversely oriented.[100]

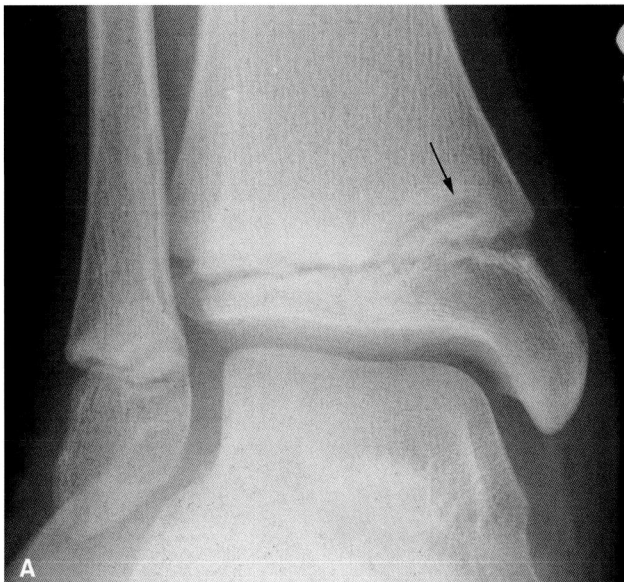

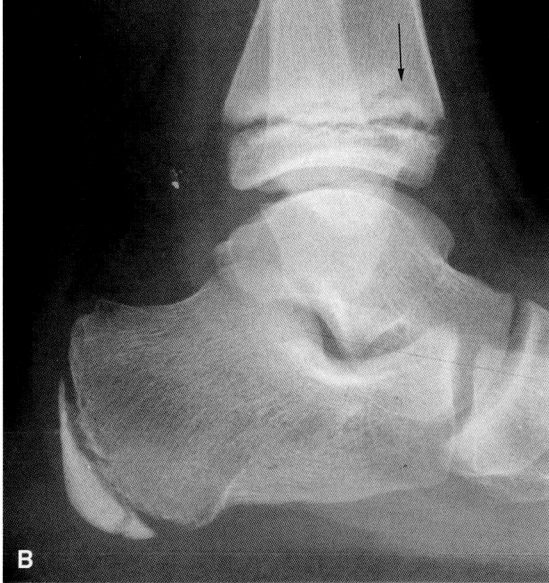

FIGURE 2.31 Kump hump (*arrows*). **A.** Mortise view. **B.** Lateral view. The normal calcaneal apophysis is sclerotic; variations include partitioning, seen inferiorly, and a jagged metaphysis. This example would be considered an osteochondrosis.

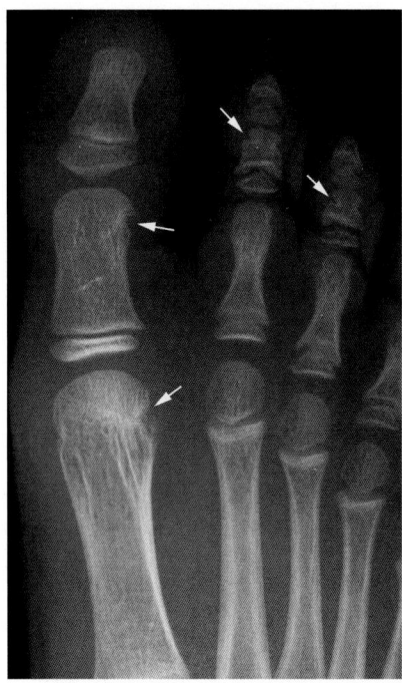

FIGURE 2.33 Variant clefts (*arrows*): pseudoepiphysis (first metatarsal head) at a later stage of development, hallux proximal phalanx head, and middle phalanx heads of the second and third toes. Also seen are variant cone-shaped epiphyses of the lesser toes.

Occasionally, the appearance of a secondary ossification center may develop at the end of a long bone that is nonepiphyseal. This frequently occurs at the head of the first metatarsal and the bases of the lesser metatarsals and is referred to as a pseudoepiphysis (see Fig. 2.30). As the first metatarsal pseudoepiphysis is closing, a cleft may be seen at the margin that may mimic an incomplete fracture; similar clefts may be seen in the heads of developing proximal and middle phalanges (Fig. 2.33).

OSTEOCHONDROSIS

Osteochondrosis is defined as fragmentation and sclerosis of an epiphysis, apophysis (see Fig. 2.31B), or epiphysoid bone (eg, the navicular).[101] The bone can also appear irregular and smaller than the expected size.[102] It may resemble fracture; however, the segmentation seen in osteochondrosis is typically well defined and the bony segments are normal density. Fracture or trauma to an epiphysis is often associated with lack of marginal definition and mixed increased and decreased densities. The diagnosis of osteochondrosis is based upon radiographic findings solely; they are named, in most cases, based upon the author first describing it in the literature (Table 2.4).

A useful categorization of osteochondrosis divides them by probable pathogenesis[102]: true osteonecrosis (Freiberg), growth disturbance with no evidence of osteonecrosis (Blount), and normal variant (Sever, Iselin). Köhler disease is unique in that it may represent either true osteonecrosis or a variation of normal.[103] Though there have been no definitive studies as to whether some osteochondroses, for example, the calcaneal and fifth metatarsal apophyses, are a result of trauma or variants of ossification, when there is pathology involving the apophysis,

TABLE 2.4 Osteochondroses	
Location	**Name**
Phalangeal base	Thiemann
Tibial sesamoid	Renander; Treves
Lesser metatarsal head (especially 2nd/3rd)	Freiberg
Fifth metatarsal basal apophysis	Iselin
Cuneiforms	Buschke
Navicular	Köhler
Calcaneal apophysis	Sever
Talar body	Diaz; Mouchet
Distal tibial epiphysis	Liffert and Arkin
Proximal tibial physis posteromedially	Blount
Tibial tubercle	Osgood-Schlatter
Capital femoral epiphysis	Legg-Calvé-Perthes

Adapted from Table 17-1, Christman RA, Marchis-Crisan C, Cohen RE. Osteonecrosis and osteochondrosis. In: Christman RA, ed. *Foot and Ankle Radiology*. 2nd ed. Philadelphia, PA: Wolters Kluwer; 2015:315.

the margins will be ill defined and osteopenic. If not, MRI may be useful for evaluation of potential bone bruising relating to underlying pathology.[104]

FRACTURE

Salter and Harris[105] published a classification for physeal fractures that is still in use today (Fig. 2.34). The type 1 fracture is separation of the physis. Type 2 partially involves the physeal plate, but the fracture then extends into the metaphysis; this latter finding results in a triangle that has been referred to as the Thurston-Holland sign. The type 3 partially involves the physeal plate, but the fracture then extends into the epiphysis. The type 4 fracture extends from the articular surface through

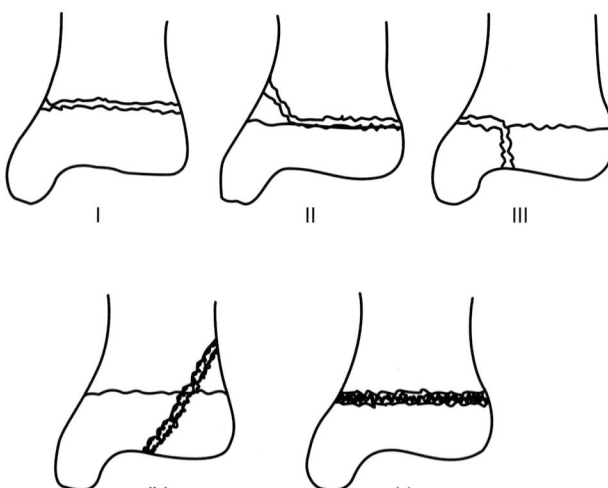

FIGURE 2.34 Salter and Harris physeal fracture classification. (From Figure 19-36 in Spinosa FA. Classification of fractures and dislocations. In: Christman RA, ed. *Foot and Ankle Radiology*. 1st ed. St. Louis, MO: Churchill Livingstone; 2003:435.)

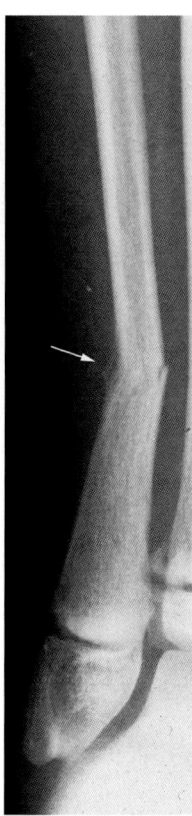

FIGURE 2.35 Pediatric diaphyseal fracture: combination greenstick and torus (*arrow*).

the epiphysis and exits through the metaphysis. The type 5 is a compression fracture of the physis, which may be hard to distinguish from the type 1 injury.

The *Salter and Harris classification* has been expanded to include fractures that do not directly involve the physis.[106] The type 6 fracture is a crushing or avulsion of only the periphery of the physis. Type 7 injury is a transepiphyseal fracture, with no physeal involvement but may be intra-articular. Metaphyseal fracture with no physeal involvement is a type 8 fracture. Selective injury to the diaphyseal periosteum is a type 9 injury.

Because bone in the developing child is still immature and not fully woven, diaphyseal fractures can have two appearances, referred to as greenstick and torus fractures. These are referred to as incomplete fractures because the fracture line usually does not extend all the way across the diaphysis. (You will not see incomplete fractures such as these in adult bones.) The *greenstick fracture* appears as convex splintering of the cortex, which is secondary to a bending force applied perpendicular to the shaft; in contrast, the *torus fracture* results in buckling along the cortex, which is secondary to an axial force applied to the shaft.[107] The phrase "lead pipe fracture" has been used to refer to a combination greenstick and torus fracture of the same bone (Fig. 2.35).[108]

OSTEOPENIA/OSTEOPOROSIS ASSESSMENT

One might think that since osteoporosis is defined as a "reduction of bone mineral density,"[109] then one would simply visually assess the radiodensity of bone to determine if radiolucency

(osteopenia) is present. The problem is determining radiolucency of bone is quite subjective and can be significantly influenced by radiographic technique (eg, in an overexposed radiograph, the bones will appear darker, ie, more radiolucent). However, bone density can objectively be assessed by examining cortical and trabecular (cancellous) bone of the second metatarsal in the DP view.

Patterns of *cortical osteopenia* in tubular bones include endosteal resorption (cortical thinning), intracortical resorption or tunneling, and periosteal resorption (the latter is only associated with hyperparathyroidism). *Cancellous osteopenia* demonstrates either prominent primary trabeculations (resorption of secondary with bone laid down on primary, which stand out in relief) or a spotty (also referred to as mottled or moth-eaten) decreased density. Occasionally, the latter is accompanied with transverse bands of decreased density. When severe, permeative decreased density may appear in both cortical and medullary bone.

Osteoporosis may either be generalized or regional. *Generalized osteoporosis* is chronic in nature, affects the entire skeleton, and primarily associated with postmenopausal women or aging men and women. Radiographically, chronic (generalized) osteoporosis demonstrates (in combination or individually) endosteal resorption (cortical thinning), intracortical tunneling, and prominent primary trabeculations (Fig. 2.36). Fleischer et al.[110] found that the presence of either diminished second metatarsal cortical thickness or intracortical tunneling correlated well with chronic osteoporosis. *Regional osteoporosis* can be chronic or acute in nature and affects an individual extremity; classic examples are immobilization (disuse) and complex regional pain syndrome (CRPS). Acute regional osteoporosis exhibits spotty, mottled, or moth-eaten decreased

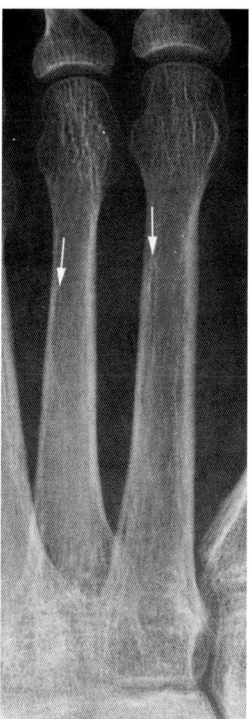

FIGURE 2.36 Chronic osteoporosis: endosteal resorption, intracortical tunneling (*arrows*), and prominent primary trabeculations.

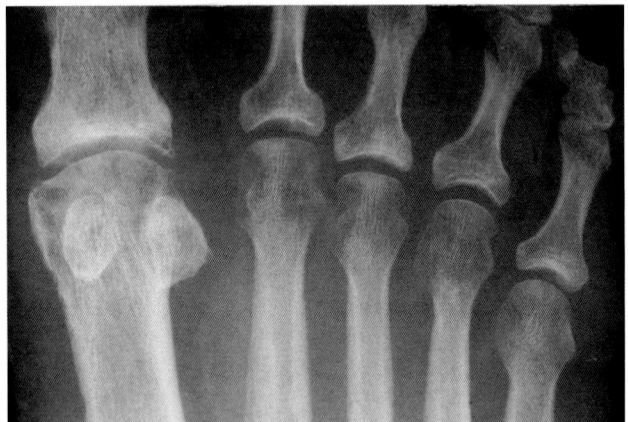

FIGURE 2.37 Acute regional osteoporosis: spotty osteopenia of all metatarsal heads.

density, with or without transverse bands of decreased density or permeative decreased density (Fig. 2.37).

Measurement of cortical thickness (also referred to as radiogrammetry) can serve as a rough guide to generalized osteoporosis in adults (but does not apply to children).[111] Although limited to the bone cortex, radiogrammetric measurements have been considered suitable for osteoporosis screening.[112] The *second metatarsal index* was found to be very useful for measuring age-appropriate bone density.[113] The second metatarsal index measures the percentage of cortical area in the DP view at the mid-diaphysis and is equal to the width of the diaphysis minus the width between the two cortices, divided by the width of the diaphysis (Fig. 2.38A). Grebing[114] found no correlation of second metatarsal hypertrophy with hypermobility of first ray that could affect the measurement. Normally, the sum of the medial and lateral cortical width should equal at least one-half the diaphyseal width (Fig. 2.38B)[115]; endosteal resorption (and, therefore, cortical thinning) has occurred if the sum is less than one-half the diaphyseal width.

Generally speaking, each second metatarsal cortex (medial and lateral) approximates 1/3 of the total width, and the medullary canal also approximates 1/3, totaling 3/3. Therefore, normally the sum of the medial and lateral cortex $(1/3 + 1/3)$ is greater than one-half. If the medullary canal appears much $>1/3$, endosteal resorption has occurred.[116]

Normally, primary trabeculations are perpendicular to the joint, running along lines of stress, and are accompanied by secondary (cross-linking, reinforcing) trabeculations that are oblique and perpendicular to the primary trabeculations. In chronic osteoporosis, as noted earlier, the secondary trabeculations are resorbed and the primary trabeculations stand out in relief. (An exception is the first metatarsal head, where the trabeculations can normally be prominent and coarse-appearing.)[117] This finding in the lesser metatarsal head was found to correlate highly with age.[113] Furthermore, new bone laid down upon the primary trabeculations makes them appear even more prominent. Also, when evaluating tubular bone for osteopenia, look for the presence of bone bars (reinforcement lines), which are prominent trabeculations running transversely across the shaft.[118]

The calcaneal trabecular pattern has been used to screen for osteoporosis. However, trabecular bone loss is difficult to recognize radiographically.[119] Jhamaria et al.[120] originally

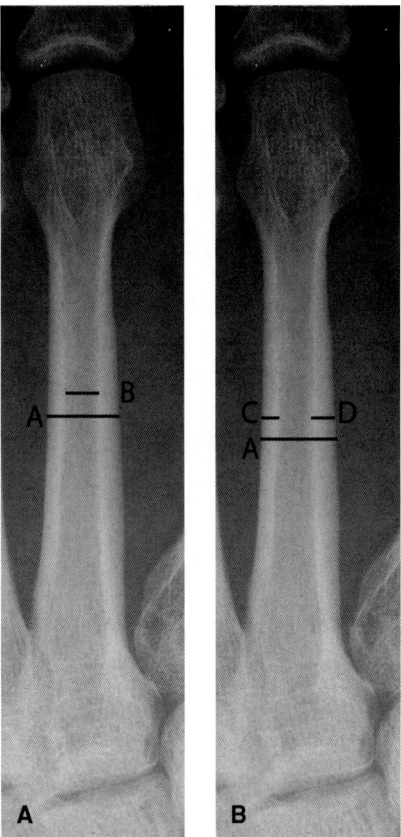

FIGURE 2.38 Cortical thickness measurement. **A.** Second metatarsal index = $(A - B) \div A$. (A, width of the diaphysis; B, width between the two cortices.) **B.** Normally, $(C + D) > (A \times 0.5)$.

proposed a 5-grade index based upon the Singh index[121] that is used with the upper end of the femur; however, there have been reports of poor correlation to bone mineral density,[122] despite its good correlation with the Singh index.[123] Pande et al. modified the calcaneal index by merging the five grades into three.[124]

ABNORMALITIES OF POSITION

RADIOGRAPHIC MEASUREMENTS AND POSITIONAL RELATIONSHIPS

The process of measuring angles radiographically inherently introduces the possibility of error. Are the measurement techniques reproducible and reliable? For example, if two people were to draw axes and measure angles on the same radiograph, would they come up with the same result (interobserver reliability)? Furthermore, if the same person was to draw axes and measure angles on the same radiograph numerous times, would the results be the same (intraobserver reliability)? The results have been mixed and vary by measurement to measurement.[125–127] Even if a technique is considered reproducible on the two-dimensional radiograph, is it accurate relative to the patient's three-dimensional foot? Lastly, a recent study questions the emphasis placed on pre- and postoperative radiographic angles used for hallux valgus surgery since they did not correlate well with patient-centered outcomes.[128]

Should you depend on these radiographic measurement tools when making clinical decisions? Despite the shortcomings listed above, radiographic measurements are not only useful to the novice learning clinical judgment for foot positional abnormalities but also provide information that is useful for patient care.[129] Static foot mechanics can be judged radiographically and are meaningful when compared to the physical examination.[130] They provide guidance and objectivity as to the severity or degree of deformity and can enhance preoperative planning. Alignment and relationships between bones and bone segments can be assessed, and the measurements are used to describe and document the deformity.

RADIOGRAPHIC BIOMECHANICAL EVALUATION: PRONATION/SUPINATION

In the world of clinical biomechanics, the terms supination and pronation refer to triplanar motion: supination indicates the combination of adduction, plantarflexion, and inversion; pronation indicates the combination of abduction, dorsiflexion, and eversion. Foot radiographs, as mentioned earlier, are static images. Therefore, the terms "pronated" and "supinated" will be used and indicate an endpoint position, not a dynamic function.

Biomechanical function of the foot is best determined by clinical examination. Radiographs are not used to determine whether or not a foot abnormally pronates or supinates and should not be used to determine foot function. The radiographic image displays whether or not the static foot is pronated or supinated when bearing weight. However, radiographs are obtained to assess foot stability, to confirm the clinical impression, and to objectively quantify the degree of deformity.[130] They are also obtained to rule out any pathology (tarsal coalition, for example) that may be contributing to abnormal biomechanical function seen clinically.

Relationships between the foot bones in the weight-bearing radiographic study vary between pronated and supinated positions.[131] Several measurement techniques (angles) are used to assess whether a foot is pronated or supinated (Table 2.5); many other positional relationships are also applied (Table 2.6). And, these angles and positional relationships are used to objectively quantify and document the many morphologic positional foot abnormalities (pes planus, pes cavus, talipes equinovarus, etc.). In order to draw and measure angles on a radiograph, though, one must first be familiar with the axes that are used for each angle and how they are placed; if

the axes are placed inaccurately, the angular measurement will be inaccurate.

In the following section, measurement techniques and other positional relationships relating to assessment of global foot deformities, such as pes planus, pes cavus, and clubfoot, will be discussed first. The remaining measurements and relationships will be included with the more specific localized abnormalities of morphologic position (eg, metatarsus adductus, hallux abducto valgus, and bunionette).

Discrepancy has existed for decades in the literature regarding use of the terms adducted/abducted and varus/valgus in the foot. For the sake of consistency, the terms adducted/abducted will be used to describe the position of a distal bone relative to a proximal bone in the transverse plane (using the body's midsagittal plane as a central reference). Therefore, if the proximal bone were lined up parallel to the midsagittal plane and the distal bone angles away from it, then the distal bone would be considered in an abducted position. Varus/valgus will be used to describe positional relationships in the coronal plane.

TRANSVERSE PLANE RELATIONSHIPS

The axes used for measuring angles in the DP view include those representing the calcaneus, talus, cuboid, and first and second metatarsal bones (Fig. 2.39).

The *calcaneal axis* is also known as the longitudinal rearfoot axis and the greater tarsus axis. Ideally, the axis would bisect the entire calcaneus, connecting the bisection point of the posterior calcaneus with a point placed at its most anterior-medial aspect. However, because only the anterior portion of the calcaneus is visible radiographically in the adult, a line is placed along the lateral aspect of the anterior calcaneus (generally speaking, this would be parallel to the calcaneal

TABLE 2.6 Other Positional Relationships Used to Assess Foot Position (Pronated or Supinated) Radiographically

DP View (Transverse Plane)	Lateral View (Sagittal Plane)
Superimposition or gap between the anterior talus and calcaneus bones	Cyma line
Talonavicular congruity (aka talar head coverage/uncoverage %)	Visibility of the sinus tarsi and middle/posterior talocalcaneal joints
Shape of the navicular bone	Cuboid visibility
Whether or not there is juxtaposition between the second through fourth metatarsal heads	Metatarsal steppage
	Height of the medial column
	Height of the lateral column
	Naviculocuboid overlap
	Navicular-cuneiform fault

TABLE 2.5 Angles Used to Assess Foot Position (Pronated or Supinated) Radiographically

DP View (Transverse Plane)	Lateral View (Sagittal Plane)
Talocalcaneal	Talar declination
Calcaneocuboid	Calcaneal inclination
Forefoot adductus	First metatarsal declination
Talus-first metatarsal	Talocalcaneal (Kite)
Talonavicular coverage	Talus-first metatarsal (Meary)

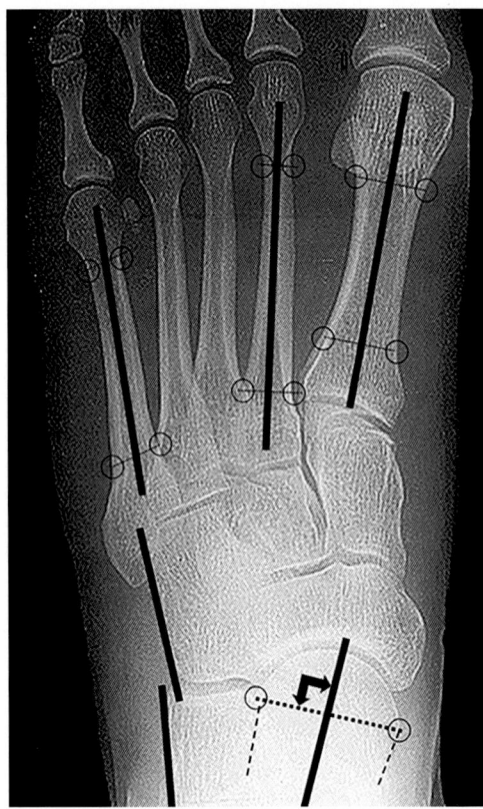

FIGURE 2.39 Dorsoplantar view axes (see text for further description).

bisection). Occasionally, the lateral surface is not flat; in that case, use the distal calcaneal trabeculations to guide axis placement.[132] In the younger child, the entire calcaneus is visible, and an axis can be drawn that bisects it longitudinally; it normally will bisect the cuboid and run through the fourth metatarsal base medial aspect[133] (being nearly parallel to the diaphysis).

The *talar axis*, also known as the longitudinal axis of the talar head and neck, is formed by first plotting points along the medial and lateral aspects of the talar neck distally at its junction with the dome-shaped articular surface. Connect these two points by a line (dotted line in the illustration) and plot the midpoint; then draw a perpendicular line at this midpoint. The perpendicular line is the talar axis (the dashed lines outline the talar neck and should run nearly parallel to the axis). (The original method for constructing the talar axis also included plotting two points at the posterior ends of the talar neck; however, because they are not consistently recognized and can result in measurement error, they probably should not be used.)

The *cuboid axis* is drawn along the lateral surface of the cuboid bone. Unfortunately, this surface is not always clearly visible and may not be flat. As with the calcaneal axis, attempt to guesstimate and flatten the surface with your line. An alternative is to plot points at the lateral aspects of the calcaneal-cuboid and fourth metatarsal-cuboid joints; connecting these two points would form an alternative cuboid axis. (The fifth metatarsal-cuboid joint is not used because it is not consistently seen in the DP view.)

The *first metatarsal axis* is formed by first selecting two points, one each along the medial and lateral cortex of the diaphysis, just proximal to the flare of the neck of the first metatarsal. Connect the two points by a straight line and mark the bisection of this line by a point on the shaft. Two additional points are selected, again, one each on the medial and lateral cortex of the diaphysis, this time just distal to the flare of the first metatarsal base. Connect the two points by a straight line and mark the bisection of this line by a point on the shaft. Connect a straight line through the bisections on the shaft of the first metatarsal. This line represents the longitudinal axis of the first metatarsal.

The *second metatarsal axis* is also known as the longitudinal axis of the forefoot or metatarsus. It is formed by first plotting two sets of points: one set along the medial and lateral aspects of the proximal shaft, just distal to the base, and the second set along the medial and lateral aspects of the distal shaft, just proximal to the neck. Connect the two distal points with a line, and the two proximal points with a line. Bisect both of these lines and connect the two bisections with another line. The resultant line is the second metatarsal axis.

The *talocalcaneal angle* is formed between the talar and calcaneal axes. Normally, the talocalcaneal angle is 19-23 degrees. In the infant, the angle is typically around 45 degrees and approaches 25 degrees in adolescence. When the foot pronates, the calcaneus abducts relative to the talus; therefore, the talocalcaneal angle will increase. When the foot supinates, the calcaneus adducts relative to the talus; therefore, the talocalcaneal angle will decrease. The talar and calcaneal axes may not cross in the DP view; in this case, move the calcaneal axis laterally such that it intersects the talar axis, such as in Figure 2.40.

The *cuboid abduction angle* is formed between the calcaneal and cuboid axes. The normal range is between 0 and 5 degrees. The angle increases when the foot is pronated. The angle is ~0 degrees in the supinated foot.

The *forefoot adductus angle* is formed between the calcaneal and second metatarsal axes. Normally, it measures between 8 and 12 degrees. The forefoot, represented by the second metatarsal axis, is abducted relative to the calcaneus in the pronated foot and results in a decreased forefoot adductus angle. In contrast, the forefoot adductus angle is increased in the supinated foot.

The *talus-first metatarsal angle* is formed by the talar and longitudinal first metatarsal axes. The talar axis normally runs collinear (0-degree angle) or lies slightly medial to the first metatarsal axis. It averages 20 degrees abducted in the infant and approaches 0 degrees in the adolescent. In the pronated foot, the first metatarsal becomes abducted relative to the talar axis and adducted in the supinated foot. (There is discrepancy in the literature as to when the talus-first metatarsal angle is positive or negative. Therefore, the terms abducted or adducted will be used when referencing the positional relationship of the first metatarsal axis to the talar axis.)

In the transverse plane radiograph, or DP view, the overpronated foot (Fig. 2.40A) is indicated by the following (relative to the rectus foot): greatly abducted position of the calcaneus relative to the talus (talocalcaneal angle); abducted position of the midfoot relative to the rearfoot (cuboid abduction angle); abducted position of the forefoot relative to the rearfoot (forefoot adductus angle); and, abducted position

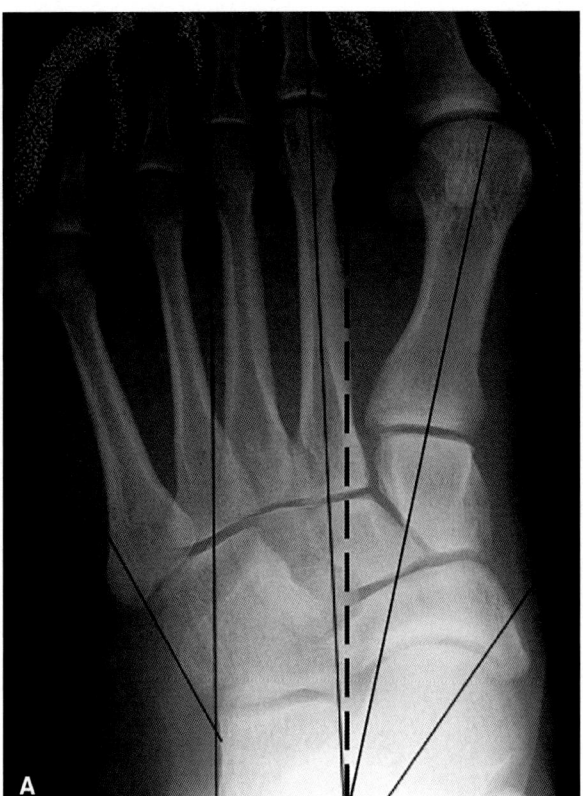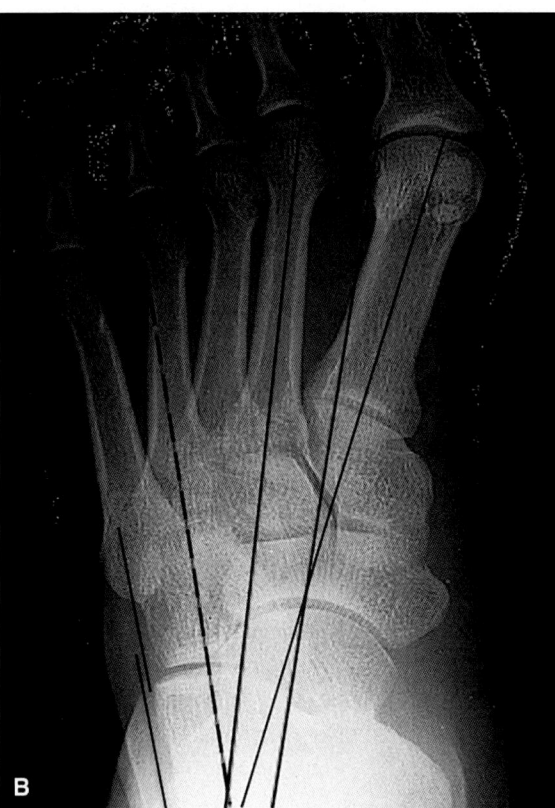

FIGURE 2.40 Examples of **(A)** overpronated and **(B)** supinated feet in the dorsoplantar view. Appreciate the differences in position between the bone axes. (The *dashed lines* represent the repositioned calcaneal axis.)

1. The calcaneal and cuboid axes are parallel to one another in the supinated foot; in contrast, notice how the cuboid axis is greatly abducted relative to the calcaneal axis in the overpronated foot.
2. In the supinated foot, the talar axis extends just lateral to the first metatarsal; however, in the overpronated foot, the talar axis is significantly directed medial to the first metatarsal.
3. The calcaneus and second metatarsal axes are nearly parallel in the overpronated foot; in the supinated foot, the second metatarsal axis is greatly adducted relative to the calcaneal axis.

of the first metatarsal axis relative to the talar axis. Generally speaking, these relationships are reversed for the supinated foot: significantly adducted position of the forefoot relative to the rearfoot (forefoot adductus angle) and adducted position of the first metatarsal axis relative to the talar axis. However, the calcaneal axis will be only mildly abducted relative to the talus, and the cuboid axis may only be parallel to the calcaneal axis (Fig. 2.40B).

Normally, the talar head lateral aspect will be slightly superimposed on the anterior calcaneus with only a small gap seen between them (Fig. 2.41). In the pronated foot, because the talus bone adducts relative to the calcaneus, a large "V"-shaped gap will be seen between the talar head and anterior calcaneus. In contrast, the talar head is superimposed upon the medial half of the anterior calcaneus in the supinated foot.

The head of the talus, in the normal foot, appears to articulate only 75% with the adjacent navicular bone (Fig. 2.42); this is because the medial portion of the talar head articulates with the spring ligament complex, which is not visible radiographically. If the head of the talus is divided into quarters, this relationship is demonstrated. Again, because the talus adducts in pronation, the talar head will appear to articulate <75% with the adjacent navicular. In contrast, the entire head of the talus may appear to articulate with the navicular in the supinated foot (except a small portion medially). This parameter estimation, referred to as talonavicular congruity,[134] has also been expressed as the talar head uncoverage percent, which would normally be 30%.[135]

Because talar head apposition with the navicular bone is somewhat subjective, the talonavicular coverage (or uncoverage)[136] angle can be used to measure this relationship (Fig. 2.43A-C). Points are plotted at both the medial and lateral margins of the talar head articular surface and the adjacent navicular articular surface. The points on each bone are connected by a line, and a perpendicular line is drawn anteriorly. The angle formed between the two perpendicular lines forms the *talonavicular coverage angle*. In the rectus foot, the talonavicular coverage angle is somewhere between 10 and 18 degrees. The angle is >18 degrees in the pronated foot, <10 degrees (and often a negative number) in the supinated foot.[137,138]

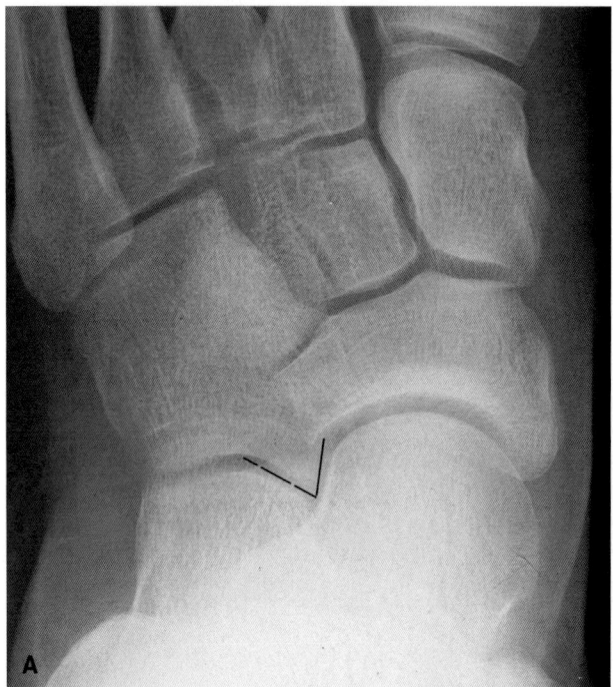

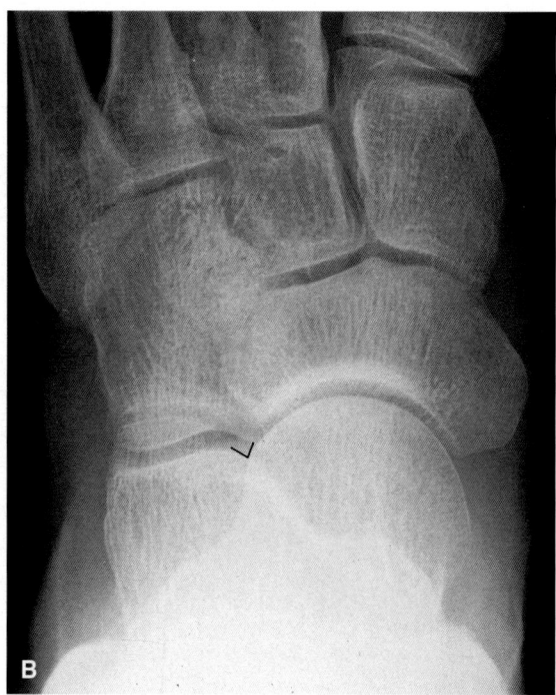

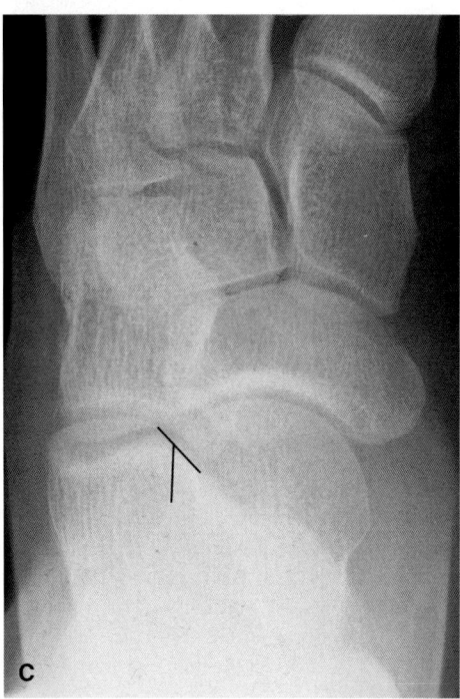

FIGURE 2.41 Gapping vs superimposition of the talar head and the calcaneus in the **(A)** pronated, **(B)** rectus, and **(C)** supinated foot. (A more objective grading system is presented in Figure 2.64.)

The *talonavicular uncoverage distance* is a simple measurement related to talar head coverage and apposition with the navicular. Points are plotted at the medial most aspect of the talar head articular surface and the navicular articular surface (Fig. 2.43D).[139] The talonavicular uncoverage distance is measured between the two points and is normally 9-12 mm.[140] It is increased in pronation, decreased in supination.

The navicular position, and therefore its shape, varies between the pronated and supinated foot. It is more wedge shaped when pronated, crescent shaped when supinated (see Fig. 2.40).

The position of the second through fourth metatarsal heads also changes between the pronated and supinated foot (Fig. 2.44). In the pronated foot, they usually are separated from one another; however, in the supinated foot, there may be superimposition. This latter picture has been described as "juxtaposed"; however, the metatarsal heads are not literally touching one another. In essence, the pronated foot in a DP view is similar to a slightly medial oblique foot position, and the supinated foot is slightly similar to a lateral oblique foot position.

Assessing the pronated vs supinated foot using nonangular relationships can also be referred to as "eyeballing" (Fig. 2.45).

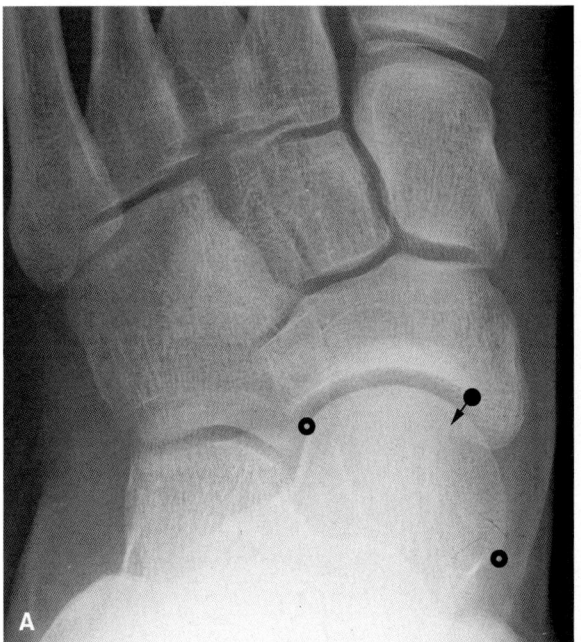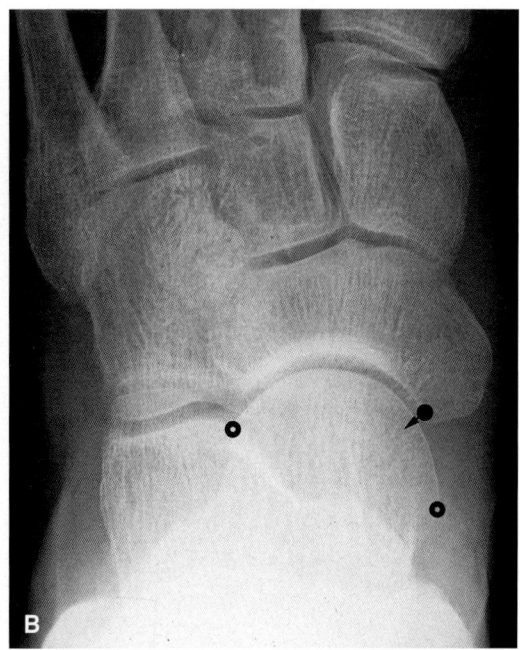

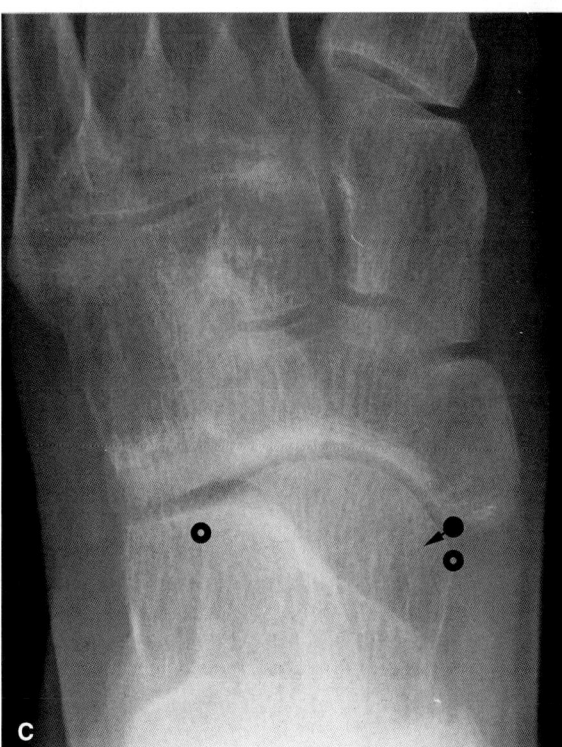

FIGURE 2.42 Talar head apposition (covering) by the navicular in the **(A)** pronated, **(B)** rectus, and **(C)** supinated foot. (Another grading system used in children is presented in Figure 2.65.)

In Figure 2.45A, there is a large gap between the talar head and anterior calcaneus; the navicular is wedge shaped and flattened medially; and, the talar head articulates ~50% with the adjacent navicular bone. Additionally, the cuboid axis is not parallel to the calcaneus axis and is abducted; the talar axis extends medial to the first metatarsal; and, the second metatarsal axis is nearly parallel to the calcaneal axis. These findings all suggest a pronated foot position.

In contrast, in Figure 2.45B, the talar head is nearly fully articular with the navicular and partially superimposed upon the anterior calcaneus, with no gapping between the talus and calcaneus bones; the navicular bone is crescent shaped and rounded medially, and the second through fourth metatarsal heads butt against each other. Additionally, the cuboid and calcaneal axes are nearly parallel to one another; the second metatarsal axis is greatly adducted relative to the calcaneal axis; and, the talar axis is directed through the first metatarsal. These findings are suggestive of a supinated foot position.

Notice that the form of the medial cuneiform grossly differs between the pronated and supinated feet. Also, the position of the tibial sesamoid varies between the two.

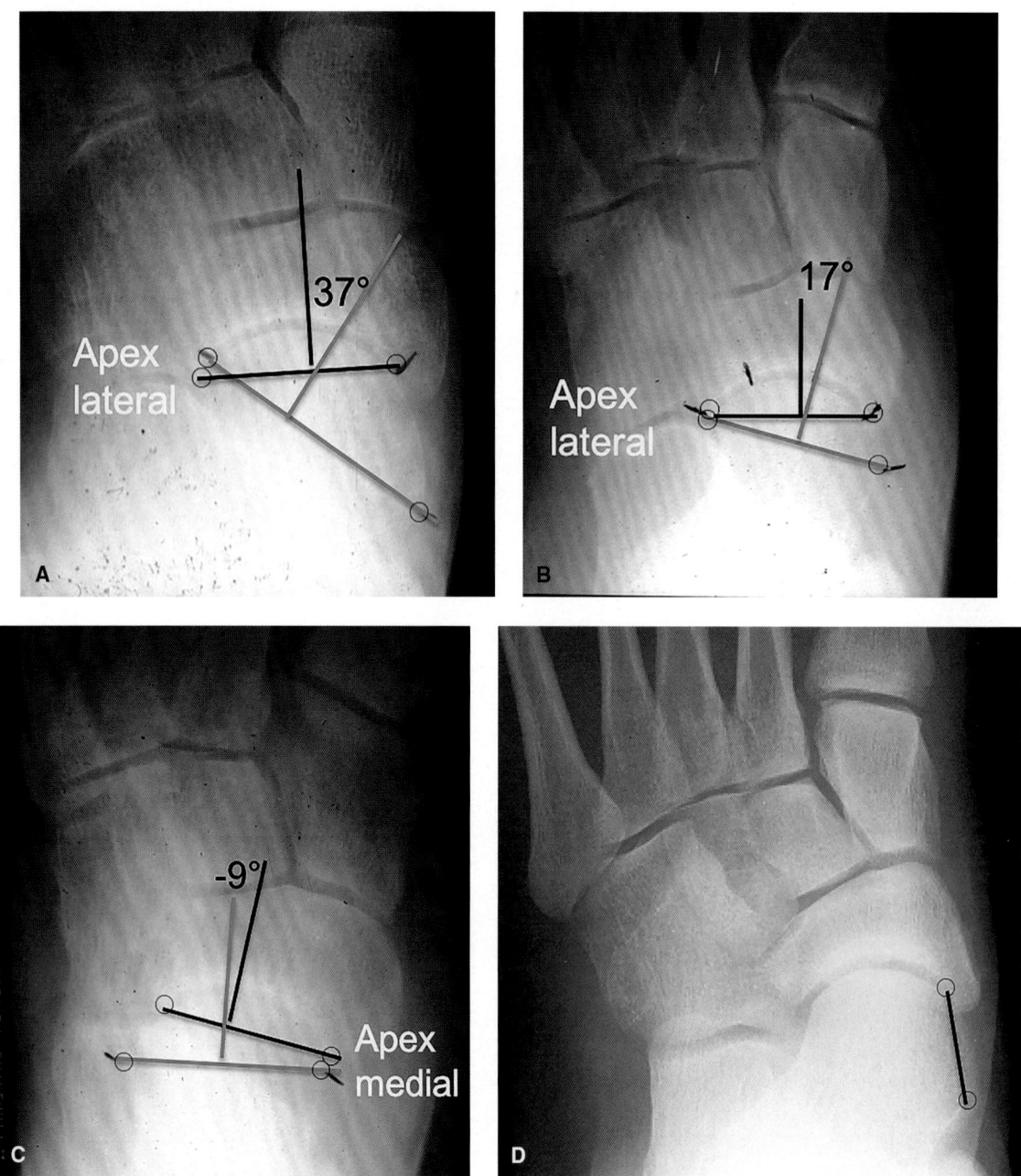

FIGURE 2.43 Talonavicular coverage/uncoverage. The talonavicular coverage angle in the **(A)** pronated, **(B)** rectus, and **(C)** supinated foot. **D.** Talonavicular uncoverage distance.

SAGITTAL PLANE RELATIONSHIPS

The axes used for measuring angles in the sagittal plane radiograph, that is, lateral view, include the talus, calcaneus, first metatarsal, and plane of support (Fig. 2.46).

For the *talar declination line*, one must first plot points along the superior and inferior aspects of the talar neck. In most circumstances, both the medial and lateral aspects of the superior talar neck are visible and superimposed. Anatomically, the lateral surface is flat, but the medial surface is concave. Since the concave medial surface is more visible, plot points at its anterior and posterior margins; the posterior margin ends where the talar dome begins. The inferior surface of the talar neck is represented by the middle talocalcaneal joint; plot points at its posterior and anterior extents. (An alternative

to plotting the anterior points uses the superior and inferior margins of the talar head articular surface for the navicular.) Connect the two posterior points and draw a bisection; connect the two anterior points and also draw a bisection. Draw a line connecting the two bisected points, which forms the talar declination line.

Connecting two points along the inferior surface of the calcaneus forms the calcaneal inclination line. The first point is plotted along the inferior aspect of the calcaneal cuboid joint; the second point is plotted along the anterior-inferior aspect of the medial tubercle. Drawing a line connecting these two points forms the calcaneal inclination line.

In order to form the *first metatarsal axis*, two sets of points must be plotted. One set of points is plotted at the distal end of the shaft where it meets the neck. The second set of points are

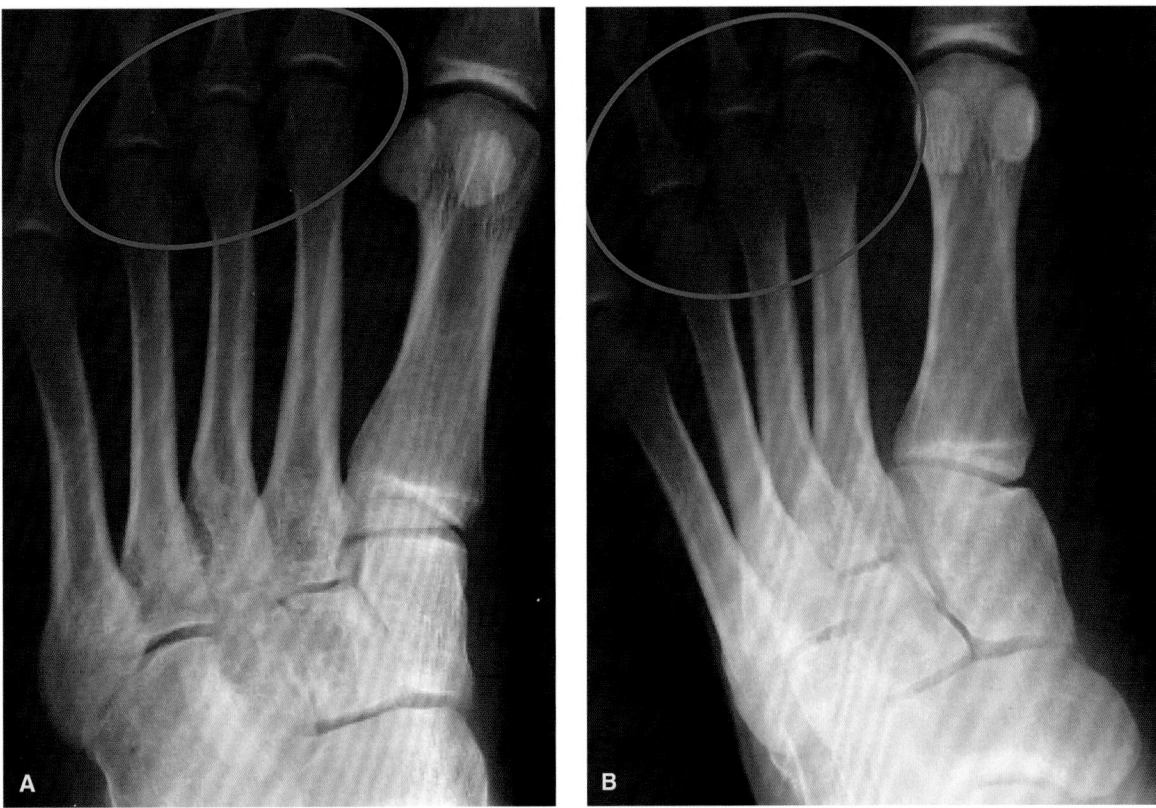

FIGURE 2.44 The position of the second through fourth metatarsal heads in the **(A)** pronated and **(B)** supinated foot.

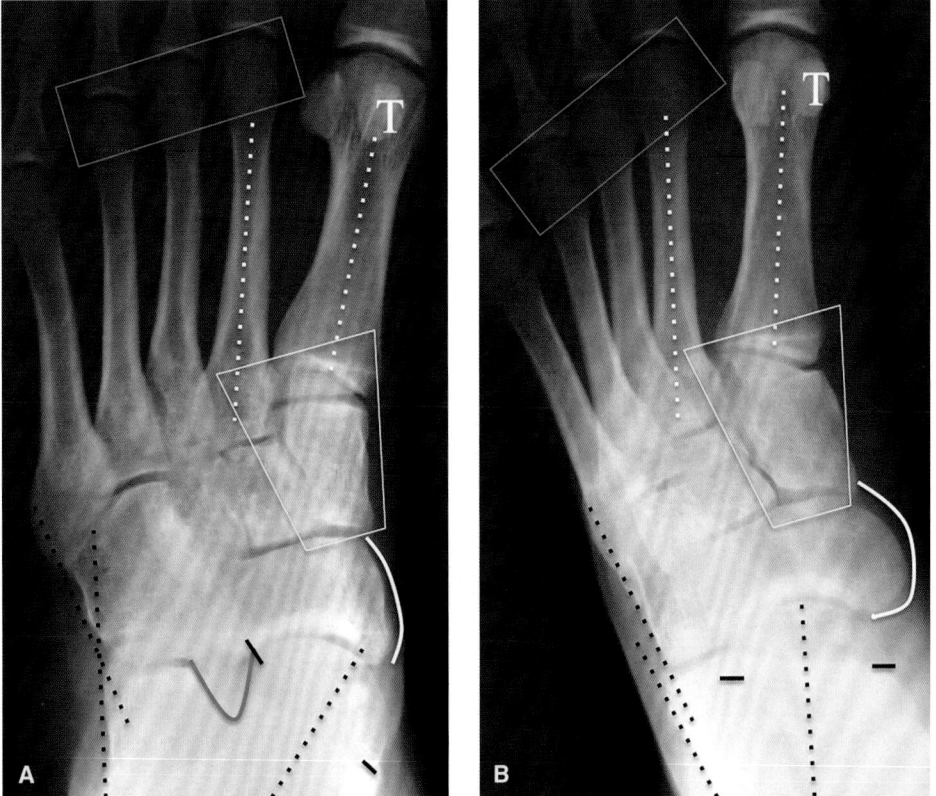

FIGURE 2.45 Eyeballing the **(A)** pronated and **(B)** supinated foot (dorsoplantar view). For further explanation, please see text.

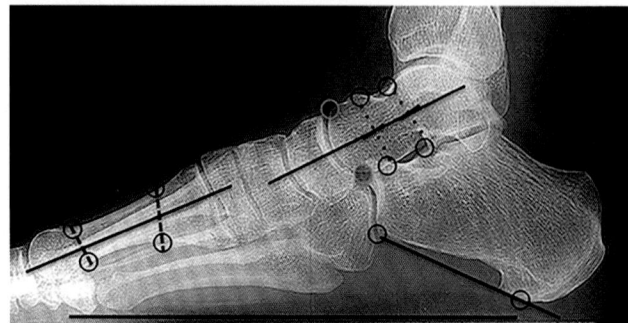

FIGURE 2.46 Lateral view axes (see text for further description).

plotted posteriorly, near the base; however, because the inferior surface extends inferiorly at the base more so than at the neck, the inferior-posterior point should be plotted somewhat more anterior to the base than the superior point. If you use the concave inferior surface of the first metatarsal as a guideline, try not to extend the posterior point any lower than the inferior point that was plotted near the neck. Next, connect the two anterior points and mark bisection, and connect the two posterior points, also marking a bisection. By connecting the two bisected points, the first metatarsal axis is formed.

The *plane of support* is simply the bottom of the image that is black. (The orthoposer that the patient stands on is lead lined, forming the plane of support.) You can also draw a line that is parallel to this so that it bisects the other axes/lines.

The *talar declination angle* is formed between the talar declination line and the plane of support. It is normally between 19 and 23 degrees. The talus plantarflexes relative to the calcaneus in the pronated foot, resulting in an increased angle with the plane of support. The angle is decreased in the supinated foot.

The *calcaneal inclination angle* (also known as the calcaneal pitch angle) is formed between the calcaneal inclination line and the plane of support. The angle is normally between 19 and 23 degrees. The calcaneus plantarflexes relative to the plane of support in the pronated foot, resulting in a decreased angle thus the angle is increased in the supinated foot. Generally speaking, however, the calcaneal inclination angle does not dramatically change in pronation or supination[141] and is less valid for discriminating between hindfoot valgus and varus deformities.[142]

The *first metatarsal declination angle* is formed between the first metatarsal axis and the plane of support. It normally measures between 19 and 23 degrees. The first metatarsal dorsiflexes relative to the plane of support in the pronated foot, resulting in a decreased angle; the angle is increased in the supinated foot.

The *lateral talocalcaneal angle* (aka Kite angle) has been used in place of the talar declination and calcaneal inclination angles. The lateral talocalcaneal angle is formed between the calcaneal inclination and talar declination lines. Normally, it measures between 35 and 40 degrees; in the child, it averages between 40 and 45 degrees. The angle increases in the pronated foot and decreases in the supinated foot.

The lateral view *talus-first metatarsal angle* is formed between the talar declination line and first metatarsal axis. The talar declination line will extend through the first metatarsal axis (collinear, 0 degrees) or very slightly inferior to it in the rectus foot. It averages from 20 degrees dorsiflexed in the infant to 5 degrees dorsiflexed in the adolescent. The lateral view talus-first metatarsal angle (aka Meary angle) demonstrates a greatly dorsiflexed angle in the pronated foot and is plantarflexed in the supinated foot. (Again, as in the DP view, there is discrepancy in the literature as to when the talus-first metatarsal angle is positive or negative; therefore, the terms dorsiflexed or plantarflexed will be used when referencing the positional relationship of the first metatarsal axis to the talar declination line.)

In the lateral view (Fig. 2.47), the overpronated foot is indicated by the following (relative to the rectus foot): significant plantarflexion of the talus relative to the plane of support (talar declination angle); mild plantarflexion of the calcaneus relative to the plane of support (calcaneal inclination angle); significant dorsiflexion of the first metatarsal relative to the plane of support (first metatarsal declination angle); and dorsiflexion of the first metatarsal axis relative to the talar declination line (lateral talus-first metatarsal angle). The talar and calcaneal axes plantarflex (talocalcaneal angle). Generally speaking, these relationships are reversed for the supinated foot: dorsiflexion of the talus relative to the plane of support (talar declination angle); mild dorsiflexion of the calcaneus relative to the plane of support (calcaneal inclination angle); plantarflexion of the first metatarsal relative to the plane of support (first metatarsal declination angle); and plantarflexion of the first metatarsal axis relative to the talar declination line (lateral view talus-first metatarsal angle). The talar and calcaneal axes dorsiflex (talocalcaneal angle).

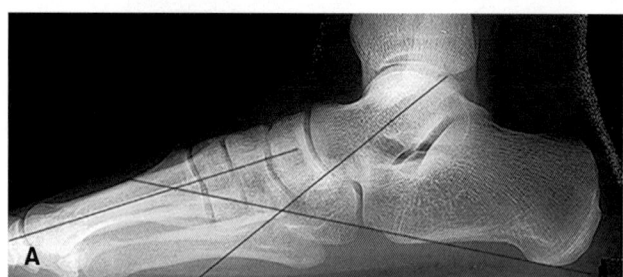
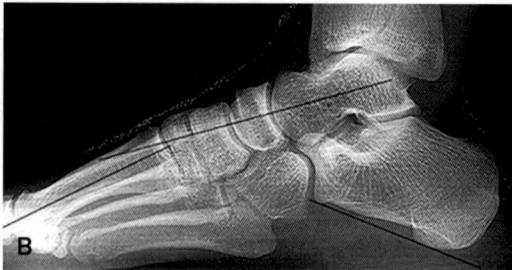

FIGURE 2.47 Examples of **(A)** overpronated and **(B)** supinated feet in the lateral view. Appreciate the differences in position between the bone axes.
1. The first metatarsal axis is dorsiflexed relative to the talar declination line in the pronated foot; in contrast, notice how the first metatarsal axis is plantarflexed relative to the talar declination line in the supinated foot.
2. In the supinated foot, the talar declination line extends just superior to the first metatarsal; however, in the pronated foot, the talar axis is significantly directed inferior to the first metatarsal.
3. Lastly, the calcaneal axis demonstrates greater inclination in the supinated foot than in the pronated foot.

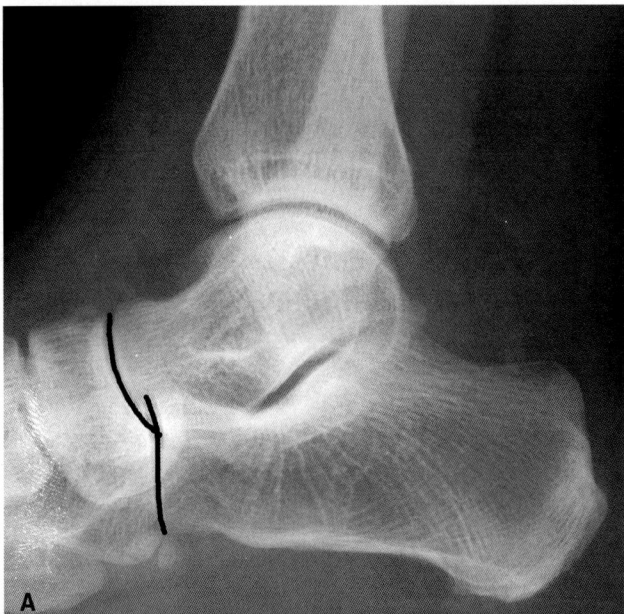

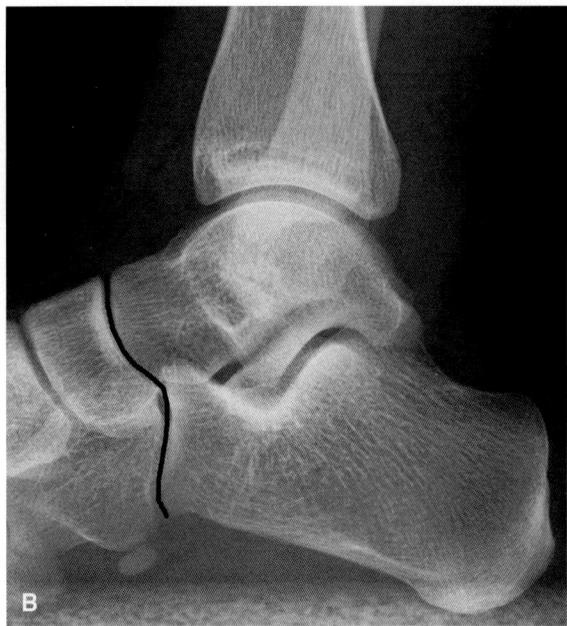

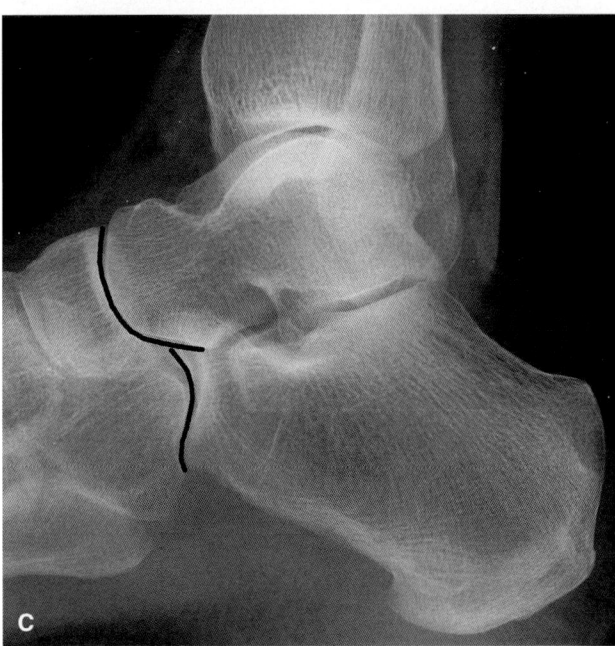

FIGURE 2.48 *Cyma line* in the **(A)** pronated, **(B)** rectus, and **(C)** supinated foot.

In the rectus foot, a continuous line running through the talonavicular and calcaneocuboid joint would appear as an "S" or cyma shape; this is referred to as the *cyma line* (Fig. 2.48). In the pronated foot, the talonavicular joint will be positioned anterior to the calcaneocuboid joint; this is referred to as an anterior break of the cyma line. This relationship is usually quite obvious in the pronated foot. In contrast, the talonavicular joint will be positioned slightly posterior relative to the calcaneocuboid joint in the supinated foot, referred to as a posterior break in the cyma line; however, the posterior break is often very subtle and not obvious.

Visibility of the talocalcaneal joints and the sinus tarsi varies between the pronated and supinated foot positions (Fig. 2.49). The middle talocalcaneal joint becomes less visible, sometimes obscured, in the pronated foot, and the posterior talocalcaneal joint becomes more visible; this latter appearance has been coined the *pseudo-sinus tarsi*. Both the middle and posterior talocalcaneal joints are visible in the rectus foot. The sinus tarsi becomes wholly visible in the supinated foot and has been referred to as the *"bullet hole" sinus tarsi.*

Because the foot rolls inward in the pronated foot, the metatarsals become more aligned with one another (Fig. 2.50A). Also, the cuboid bone becomes partially superimposed upon the navicular. In contrast, the metatarsals appear to separate from one another in a steplike fashion in the supinated foot (Fig. 2.50B). And, the cuboid nearly becomes entirely visible.

The *height of the medial column* is measured from the most inferior point of the medial cuneiform to the plane of support (Fig. 2.51). Normally, it is ~17 mm. The *height of the lateral column* is measured from the most inferior point of the cuboid to the plane of support. Normally, it is ~12 mm. They both decrease in the pronated foot, increase in the supinated foot.

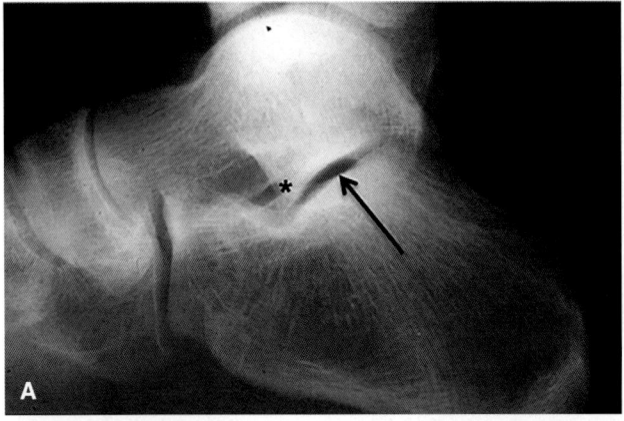

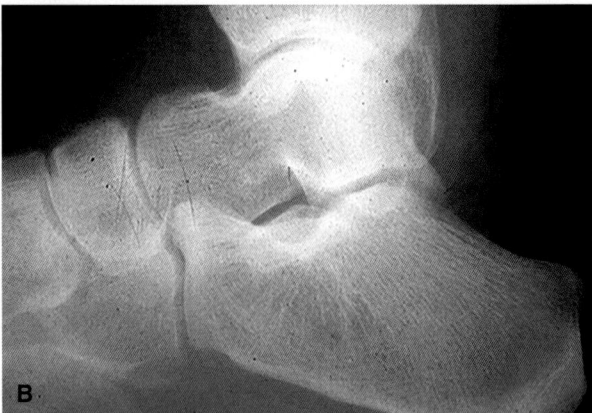

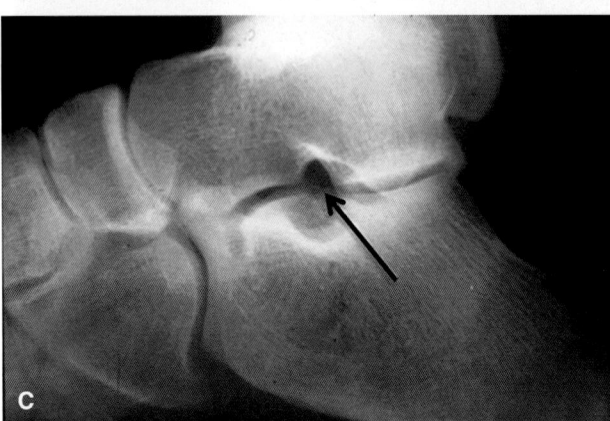

FIGURE 2.49 Visibility of the talocalcaneal joints and the sinus tarsi in the **(A)** pronated (*arrow* points to posterior talocalcaneal joint or "pseudo-sinus tarsi"), **(B)** rectus, and **(C)** supinated foot (*arrow* points to "bullet hole" sinus tarsi). (*asterisk* = lateral process of the talus, which is centered over the sinus tarsi, sometimes referred to as the "Kirby sign.") (From Green DR. Radiology and biomechanical foot types. In: *Podiatry Institute Update 1998: Chapter 48.* http://www.podiatryinstitute.com/pdfs/Update_Index.pdf. Accessed May 2, 2019.)

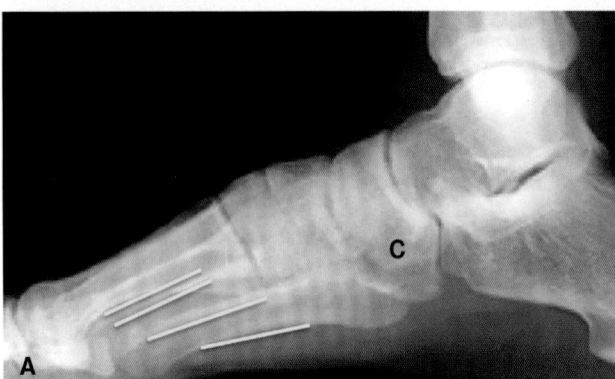

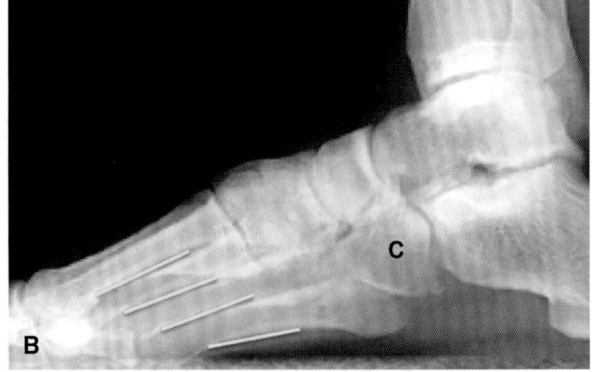

FIGURE 2.50 Metatarsal alignment and cuboid (c) visibility in the **(A)** pronated and **(B)** supinated foot.

FIGURE 2.51 Height of the medial (*solid line*) and lateral (*dashed line*) columns.

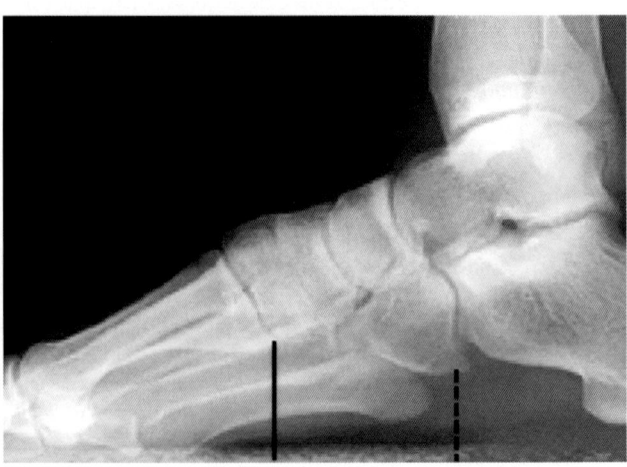

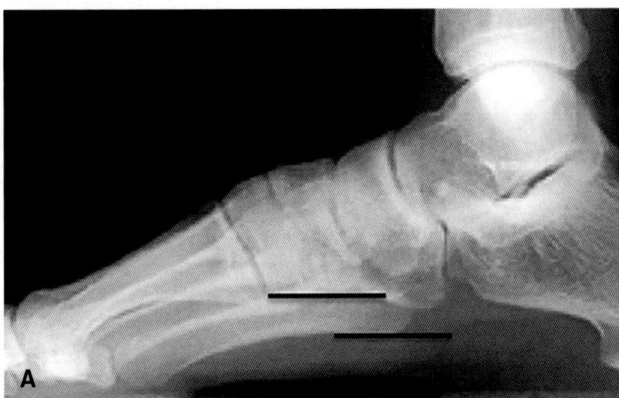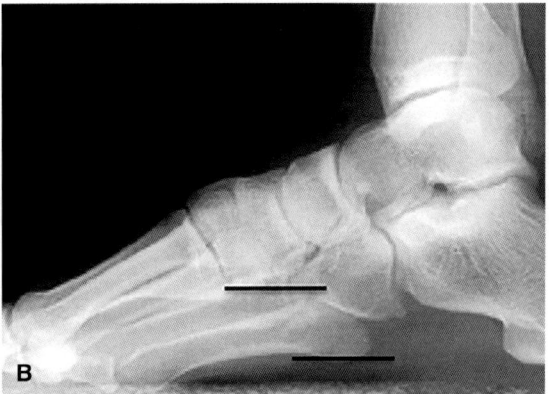

FIGURE 2.52 Medial cuneiform-fifth metatarsal height (measured between solid bars) in the **(A)** pronated and **(B)** supinated foot.

The *medial cuneiform-fifth metatarsal height* (Fig. 2.52) is determined by measuring the distance between the most plantar aspects of the medial cuneiform and fifth metatarsal base, averaging 17.5 mm.[140,143] The distance decreases in the pronated foot, increases in the supinated foot. The measured value is considered a negative number when the inferior aspect of the medial cuneiform is inferior to that of the fifth metatarsal base.

Naviculocuboid overlap is the overlapped portion of the navicular and cuboid divided by the vertical height of the cuboid (Fig. 2.53). Normally ~30% overlapped, it increases to ~70% in the pronated foot, and decreases to 7% in the supinated foot. A useful technique, but it does not reflect the degree of the deformity in severe varus or valgus feet.[142]

A *"fault," "sag," "breach," or "break"* due to excess dorsiflexion may occur at the talonavicular, naviculocuneiform, and calcaneocuboid joints.[144] Radiographically, the superior aspect of the joint appears compressed and the inferior aspect separated. The navicular-cuneiform fault refers to an apparent lack of linearity between the superior surfaces of the navicular and cuneiform bones (Fig. 2.54). However, the posterior half of the medial cuneiform bone's superior surface normally slants inferiorly and is often misinterpreted as faulty alignment.

"Eyeballing" the pronated vs supinated foot in the lateral view is illustrated in Figure 2.55A and demonstrates the following: the talar dome is rounded; the posterior talocalcaneal joint is somewhat more visible than the middle talocalcaneal joint; the cyma line is broken anteriorly; the cuboid bone is barely

visible and superimposed on the navicular; and, the metatarsals are closer to one another. Additionally, the talar declination line is greatly plantarflexed relative to the first metatarsal bone, and the calcaneal declination line is becoming closer to parallel with the plane of support. These findings all suggest a pronated foot position.

In contrast, in Figure 2.55B, a bullet-hole sinus tarsi is visible, the cuboid bone is almost entirely visible, the cyma line is slightly broken posteriorly, and the inferior margins of the metatarsals are separated in a steplike fashion. Additionally, the calcaneal declination line is greatly dorsiflexed relative to the plane of support, the talar declination line runs through the first metatarsal (it often is superior to it), the medial cuneiform is prominent superiorly and presents as a hump, and the talar dome is flattened. These findings are suggestive of a supinated foot position.

PES PLANUS, PLANOVALGUS, AND VERTICAL TALUS

Measurements used to assess pes planus in the DP, lateral, and calcaneal axial (hindfoot alignment) views are listed in Table 2.7. Generally speaking, the findings in the adult mimic those seen in the classic pronated foot, discussed above (see Figs. 2.40A, 2.45A, 2.47A, and 2.55A). Younger et al.[140] compared the symptomatic flatfoot to a normal control group (asymptomatic flatfoot was not studied). They found that the talar head uncoverage distance was the most

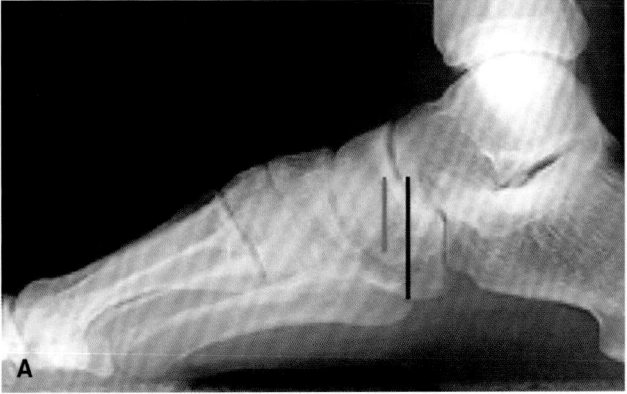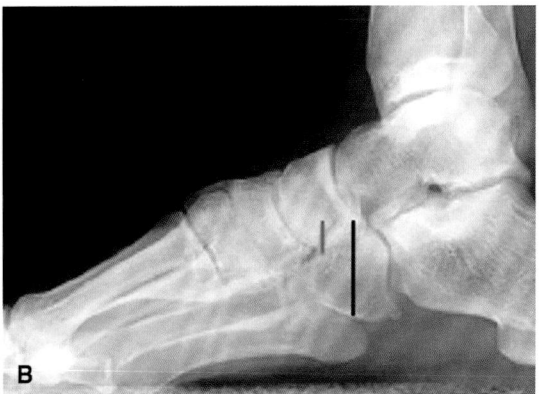

FIGURE 2.53 Naviculocuboid overlap in the **(A)** pronated and **(B)** supinated foot. (Black bar = vertical height of cuboid; blue bar = overlap of cuboid on navicular.)

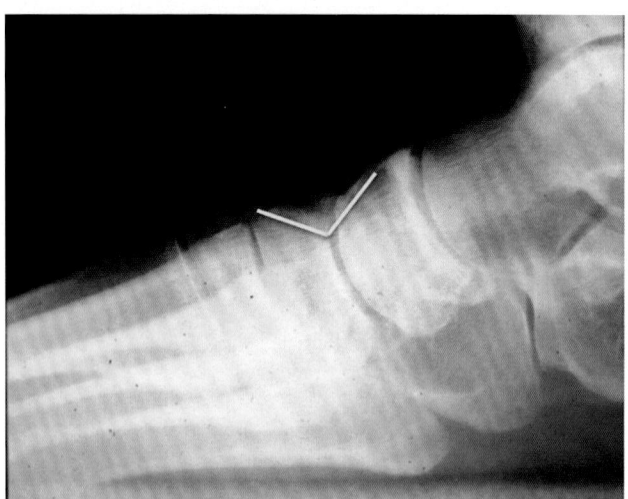

FIGURE 2.54 Navicular-cuneiform fault.

statistically significant value on the DP view, despite low inter- and intraobserver reliability. In the lateral radiograph, they found that the talus-first metatarsal angle was the most discriminating radiographic parameter and most consistently accurate radiographic parameter of flatfoot; however, Sensiba et al.[145] found poor interobserver reliability. Additionally, there were significantly different values compared to controls (lateral view) with the talar-first metatarsal angle, calcaneal pitch angle, and medial cuneiform-fifth metatarsal height; Sensiba et al.[145] found the latter two measurements most reliable in their study.

Specialized radiographic techniques have been devised to assess the rearfoot in the coronal plane: the long leg calcaneal axial view, and the hindfoot alignment view. The *long leg calcaneal axial view* can be performed with standard weight-bearing lower extremity radiography equipment; however, a 14 × 17-in cassette is preferable in order to see more of the tibia to draw its axis. This positioning technique is performed the same as a weight-bearing Harris and Beath calcaneal axial study with the tube head angled at 45 degrees.[91] In contrast, the *hindfoot alignment view* requires the construction of a specialized radiolucent platform with a 20-degree angled slot from vertical for a 11 × 14- or 14 × 17-in image receptor; the tube head is angled at 20 degrees from horizontal such that the x-ray beam is perpendicular to the image receptor.[146,147] Both techniques are well illustrated by Mendicino et al.,[148] although they use a 15-degree angulation of tube head (from horizontal)

TABLE 2.7	Pes Planus Measurement Considerations	
DP View	**Lateral View**	**Calcaneal Axial (Hindfoot Alignment) View**
Increased talocalcaneal angle	Increased talar declination angle	Valgus tibiocalcaneal (hindfoot alignment) angle
Increased cuboid abduction angle	Decreased calcaneal inclination (pitch) angle	Increased tibial/calcaneal displacement
Decreased forefoot adductus angle	Decreased first metatarsal declination angle	
Talar-first metatarsal angle (abducted metatarsal)	Talar-first metatarsal (Meary) angle (dorsiflexed metatarsal)	
Decreased talonavicular joint "congruency" (aka talar head coverage/uncoverage %)	Increased talocalcaneal (Kite) angle	
Increased talonavicular coverage angle	Anterior break in the cyma line	
Increased talonavicular uncoverage distance	Decreased medial column height	
	Decreased lateral column height	
	Decreased medial cuneiform-fifth metatarsal height	
	Increased naviculocuboid overlap	
	Naviculocuneiform "fault"	

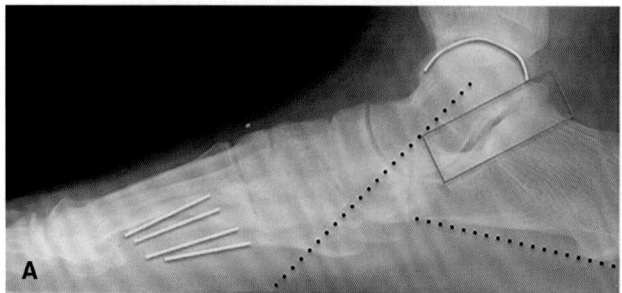
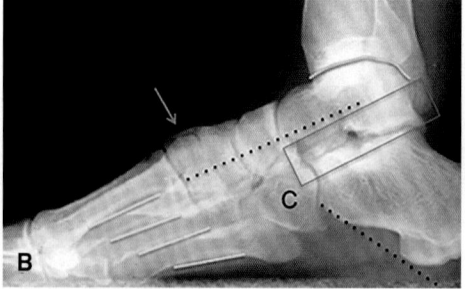

FIGURE 2.55 Eyeballing the **(A)** pronated and **(B)** supinated foot (lateral view). For further explanation, please see text C, cuboid bone. The *arrow points* to the prominent medial cuneiform.

Chapter 2 **Imaging of the Foot and Ankle** **57**

and image receptor (from vertical). Reilingh et al.[149] found that the long leg axial view had better intra- and inter-rater reliability and recommended performing the study as a single bilateral weight-bearing stance as opposed to unilateral. The hindfoot alignment view was subsequently modified such that the image receptor is vertical (perpendicular to the floor); however, the tube head remains angled at 20 degrees from horizontal.[150,151] A modified radiolucent, elevated platform is still necessary.

Angles and measurements relating to the coronal/frontal plane include the tibiocalcaneal (or hindfoot alignment) angle, tibial/calcaneal displacement (or alignment, distance), and lateral distal tibial angle. The following axes are used: anatomic tibial axis, ankle joint orientation line, and calcaneal axis.

The anatomic tibial axis is represented by a parallel line running through the mid-diaphysis (Figs. 2.56 and 2.57A). The axis can be determined by plotting points at the proximal and distal aspects of the middle one-third diaphysis medially and laterally, connecting the respective points, and then connecting the two bisecting points. In the AP ankle view, it runs slightly medial to the talus midline.[152]

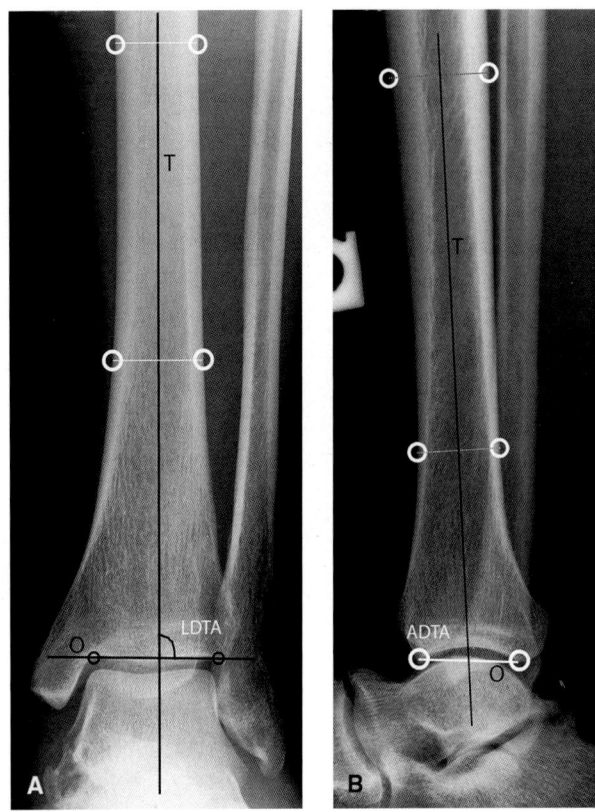

FIGURE 2.57 Distal tibial (articular) angles. **(A)** AP ankle view, **(B)** lateral ankle view. O, tibial ankle joint orientation line; T, anatomic tibial axis; LDTA, lateral distal tibial angle; ADTA, anterior distal tibial angle.

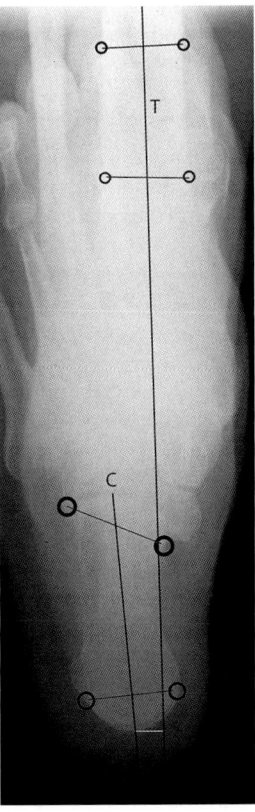

FIGURE 2.56 Coronal/frontal plane angles and measurements, long leg calcaneal axial view. T, anatomic tibial axis; C, calcaneal axis; *white line*, tibial/calcaneal displacement. Points for calcaneal axis determination are placed at the lateral aspect of the posterior talocalcaneal joint, the inferior aspect of the base of the sustentaculum tali, and along the medial and lateral aspects of the posterior process of the calcaneus. (Buck P, Morrey BF, Chao EY. The optimum position of arthrodesis of the ankle. A gait study of the knee and ankle. *J Bone Joint Surg.* 1987;69(7):1052-1062.)

The tibial ankle joint orientation line represents the distal tibial articular surface.[153] It is drawn across the flat distal tibial plafond in the AP and mortise ankle views (Fig. 2.57A).[154]

Several methods have been described for drawing the calcaneal axis. The simplest method is to draw a line through the center of the calcaneus that is parallel to its lateral surface.[145] Other methods entail the following: plotting points at varying aspects of the posterior calcaneus and connecting bisections (Fig. 2.56)[150,155]; using skin markers[156]; overlaying an egg-shaped elliptical[151]; and using a 60:40 ratio as a bisector to compensate for asymmetrical width of the posterior calcaneus relative to the distal calcaneus.[149]

The tibiocalcaneal (or hindfoot alignment) angle is measured between the anatomic tibial and calcaneal axes on either the long leg calcaneal axial or hindfoot alignment view. Normally, the two axes are parallel (0-degree angulation).[149]

Tibial/calcaneal displacement, alignment, or distance is determined by measuring the horizontal distance between the weight-bearing axis of the tibia and the most inferior aspect of the calcaneus (ie, closest to "floor") (see Fig. 2.56).[147,157] Normally, the calcaneal lowest point is 5-10 mm lateral to the tibial mid-diaphyseal axis.[149] (The measured numerical value is considered negative if the tibial axis is lateral to the lowest point of the calcaneus.[147]) Sometimes, the anatomic axis of the calcaneus is used instead of the lowest calcaneal point to determine the distance relative to the tibial axis.[158] In this case, the normal range would be between 1 and 20 mm.[159]

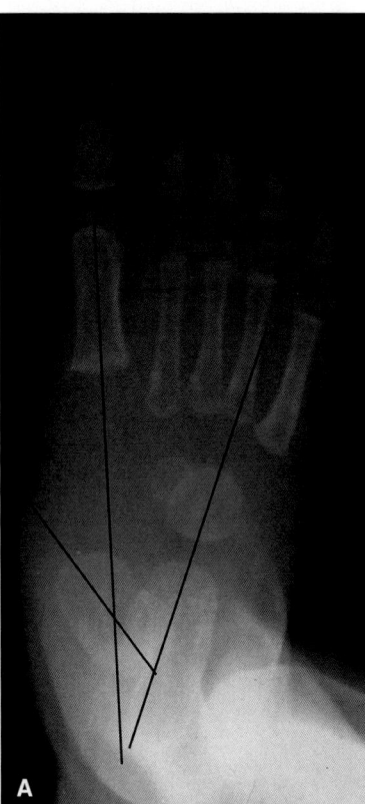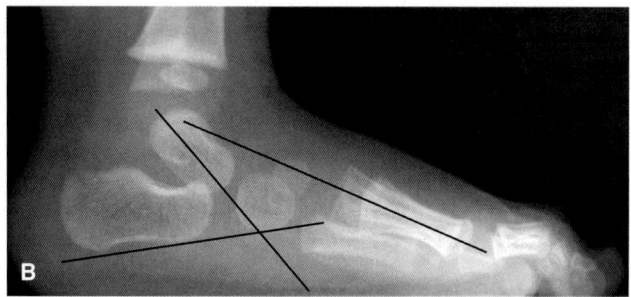

FIGURE 2.58 Pediatric pes planus. **(A)** DP view, **(B)** lateral view.

The lateral distal tibial (articular) angle has been measured on the AP ankle, mortise, and hindfoot alignment views. The angle is measured between the anatomic tibial axis and the tibial ankle joint orientation line (Fig. 2.57A). The normal lateral distal tibial angle averages 89 degrees.[160]

The anterior distal tibial (articular) angle (sagittal plane) has also been measured in the lateral ankle view (Fig. 2.57B). Points for the tibial ankle joint orientation line are plotted at the anterior and posterior margins of the distal tibial plafond and connected by a line.[161] The anatomic tibial axis can be determined by plotting points at the proximal and distal aspects of the middle one-third diaphysis anteriorly and posteriorly, connecting the respective points, and then connecting the two bisecting points. The anatomic tibial axis will normally pass through the lateral talar process.[152] The anterior distal tibial angle in the lateral ankle view averages 80 degrees.[160]

In the younger pediatric foot, radiographic analysis is limited, especially if weight-bearing radiographs are not possible. Pes planus is very common in this group and presents with the following radiographic findings (Fig. 2.58): increased talocalcaneal angles (DP and lateral views); the calcaneal axis is relatively parallel to the fourth metatarsal (DP view); the cuboid is bisected by the calcaneal (mid-body) axis (DP view); and the talus-first metatarsal angle is abducted (DP view) and dorsiflexed (lateral view).

A more severe deformity, *convex pes planus* (also known as pes planovalgus or simply pes valgus), demonstrates the same presentation as pes planus; however, the fourth metatarsal is abducted relative to the calcaneal axis (Fig. 2.59A). Also, when the forefoot is abducted, the lesser metatarsals will appear parallel to one another in the DP view.[162]

Congenital *vertical talus* (also known as talipes convex pes valgus) is a condition where the talus and navicular bones demonstrate no apposition, and the navicular "articulates," so to speak, with the dorsal surface of the talar neck. This is best demonstrated in the lateral view. The resulting picture has also been referred to as a "rocker bottom foot" (plantarflexed rearfoot and dorsiflexed forefoot), a reversal of the normal longitudinal arch; the calcaneus-fifth metatarsal angle is >180 degrees (Fig. 2.59B).[163] Congenital vertical talus is obvious to see radiographically when the navicular is ossified and visible. The calcaneus demonstrates an equinus (plantarflexed) position in the lateral view, and the tibiotalar angle can reach 180 degrees.[164] In the DP view, the talocalcaneal angle will be greatly increased and there is significant forefoot abduction, as demonstrated in severe pes planovalgus.

Vertical talus is difficult to diagnose when the navicular has not yet ossified. It can be inferred by the position of the talus relative to the lateral cuneiform, assuming that the navicular will lay directly posterior to the latter (see Fig. 2.59B).[162] A lateral (forced, maximum) plantar flexion stress view can be obtained in an attempt to reduce the deformity (Fig. 2.59C).[165] In this view, the first metatarsal axis normally is plantar to the talar axis; in vertical talus, the first metatarsal axis runs dorsal to the talar axis (which is locked in plantarflexion).[166] The talar axis will also point below the cuboid.[167] Drennan[168] also recommends performing the lateral view in forced (maximum) dorsiflexion and measures the tibiocalcaneal angle to determine if the equinus deformity is fixed.

Oblique talus may simulate vertical talus, where the partially ossified navicular appears dorsal to the talar head. In this case, there is partial articulation (subluxation) with the navicular in the lateral view. Upon performance of a maximum plantarflexion lateral view, the navicular will come to lie anterior to the talar head and the talar axis will intersect the metatarsals, unlike congenital vertical talus.[169]

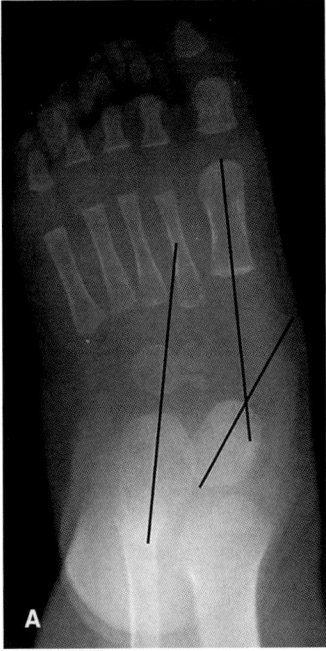
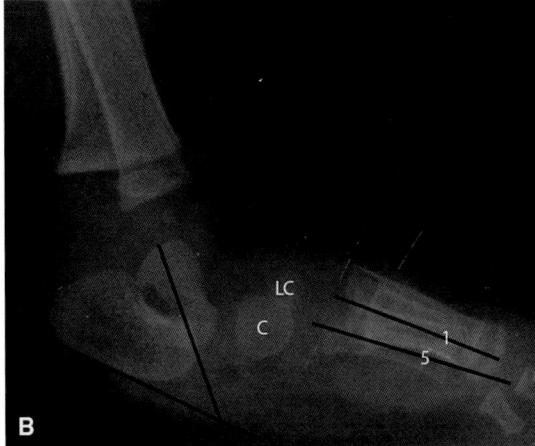
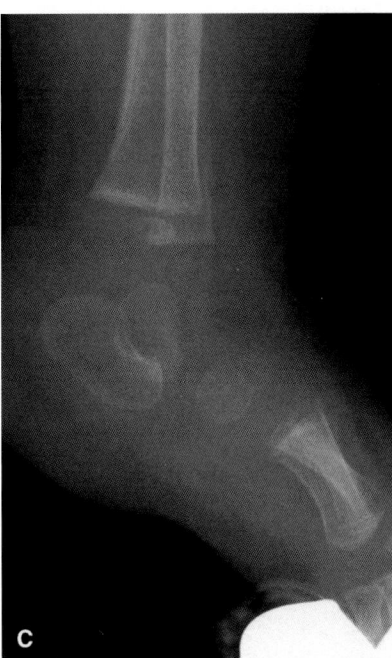

FIGURE 2.59 Vertical talus. **A.** DP view. The fourth metatarsal is abducted relative to the calcaneal axis in the DP view, a finding differentiating pes planovalgus from pes planus. **B.** Lateral view. **C.** Forced plantarflexion lateral view (no reduction of deformity demonstrated). LC, lateral cuneiform; C, cuboid; 5, fifth metatarsal axis; 1, first metatarsal axis.

PES CAVUS

Pes cavus can demonstrate deformity in three planes: sagittal (the primary deformity), coronal, and transversal. Cavus deformity may also be referred to as cavovarus and calcaneocavus, depending on location of the deformity. High medial arch is the primary feature seen in the sagittal plane. It may be characterized by plantarflexed metatarsals and digital contractures (anterior cavus, more common), a vertical position of the calcaneus (posterior cavus), or a combination of the two.[170] Varus (sometimes valgus) calcaneus is seen in the coronal plane, and metatarsus adductus is seen in the transverse plane. Measurements used to assess pes cavus in the DP and lateral views are listed in Table 2.8.

The cavus foot in the DP radiograph appears severely supinated (see Figs. 2.40B and 2.45B). The talocalcaneal angle is decreased, and the cuboid abduction angle is normal or decreased (especially with severe deformity). The forefoot adductus and metatarsus adductus angles are increased, and the talus-first metatarsal angle is adducted. Perera et al.[171] state that hindfoot varus causes the metatarsus adductus to look worse than it really is, so they recommend subtracting the tibio-calcaneal angle (in the hindfoot view) from the talus-first metatarsal angle to achieve a "true" measurement.

Pes cavus is best assessed in the lateral view (see Figs. 2.47B and 2.55B). Radiographically, the talus-first metatarsal angle (Meary angle) is abnormal such that the first metatarsal is severely plantarflexed relative to the talus. The talocalcaneal angle is decreased. The calcaneal inclination angle is increased and >30 degrees in posterior cavus, near normal in anterior cavus. The calcaneus-first metatarsal Hibbs[172] angle has also been used to assess cavus deformity; the angle is measured anteriorly between the calcaneal and first metatarsal axes

(Fig. 2.60).[173] It is typically <45 degrees in the normal foot, sometimes reaching 90 degrees in the cavus foot.[174] Jahss[175] also evaluates the tibioplantar angle (anatomic tibial axis relative to the weight-bearing surface, normally 90 degrees) to determine how much bone resection is needed; for example, a distal wedge procedure may not be adequate if the tibioplantar angle is >120 degrees.

The anterior pes cavus deformity can be subdivided based upon the apex of the deformity in the sagittal plane.[176] This may be accomplished by determining where the talar and first metatarsal axes cross in the lateral view (Fig. 2.61)[177]: if the axes cross at Lisfranc joint, it is called metatarsal cavus; if the apex is at the region of the naviculocuneiform joints, it is named lesser tarsal cavus; and, lastly, if the apex is at Chopart joint, it is considered a forefoot cavus.[178] A combined anterior cavus occurs at more than one location and is generalized to the lesser tarsus.[179] Evaluation of the first metatarsal/calcaneus and calcaneus/fifth metatarsal relationships has also been recommended for determining cavus in the lateral view.[180] The calcaneus-fifth metatarsal angle is measured plantarly and will decrease below 150 degrees in the cavus foot (see Fig. 2.60).[181]

External rotation of the ankle in the lateral positioning technique causes several findings to occur radiographically (see Fig. 2.60). The fibular malleolus is positioned posteriorly relative to the tibial malleolus and talus, which has been coined "sagittal breech."[182] The talar dome demonstrates a "double shadow" since the medial and lateral trochlear shoulders are no longer superimposed on one another. The sinus tarsi may appear widened,[183] or as Coleman and Chesnut[184] describe it, "the through and through view of the subtalar joint." The navicular will be positioned much more superiorly to the cuboid than normal. Also, a posterior break of the cyma line may be evident. One may want to reposition the foot, after obtaining

TABLE **2.8** **Pes Cavus Measurement Considerations**

DP View	Lateral View	Calcaneal Axial (Hindfoot Alignment) View
Decreased talocalcaneal angle	Decreased talar declination angle	Varus tibiocalcaneal (hindfoot alignment) angle
Normal or decreased cuboid abduction angle	Normal or increased calcaneal inclination (pitch) angle	
Increased forefoot adductus angle	Increased first metatarsal declination angle	
Increased metatarsus adductus angle	Talar-first metatarsal (Meary) angle (plantarflexed metatarsal)	
Talar-first metatarsal angle (adducted metatarsal)	Increased calcaneus-first metatarsal (Hibbs) angle	
Metatarsal "stacking"	Decreased talocalcaneal (Kite) angle	
	Increased tibioplantar angle	
	Posterior position of fibula (aka "sagittal breech")	
	"Double shadow" of talar dome	
	"Widened" sinus tarsi or "through and through view of subtalar joint"	
	Posterior break in the cyma line	
	Decreased naviculocuboid overlap	

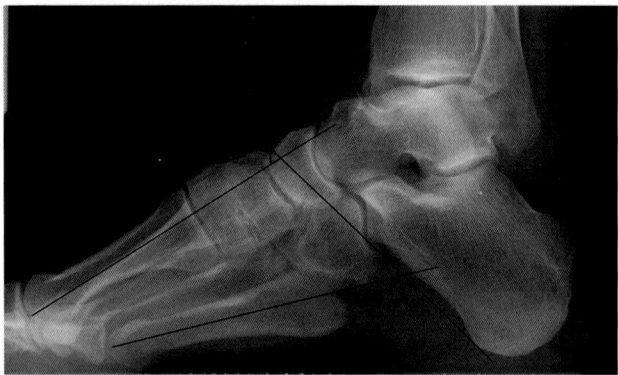

FIGURE 2.60 Posterior cavus. Hibbs angle is 75 degrees, the calcaneal inclination angle is 43 degrees, and the calcaneus-fifth metatarsal angle is 125 degrees.

the standard lateral view, by positioning the ankle joint axis so that it is perpendicular to the image receptor to assess true radiographic anatomy, especially of the talus.

In the cavus foot, the talar dome may appear flat in the lateral view, referred to as a *"flat-topped" talus* (see Fig. 2.60). This illusion occurs because when the cavus foot is placed against the x-ray image receptor, the rearfoot is anatomically rotated away from the receptor relative to the forefoot. One must adjust the positioning technique for the cavus foot by pulling the heel away from the image receptor so that the ankle joint axis is perpendicular to the image receptor.

Coleman and Chesnut[184] recommend additionally performing the DP and lateral foot views with a 1-in radiolucent block under the heel and lateral border of the foot. These images can be used to determine and "document" whether the deformity is a fixed or flexible.

The long leg calcaneal axial or hindfoot alignment views (discussed in the Pes Planus section) can be used to determine if a varus attitude is present in the rear foot.

Associated abnormalities are assessed in the ankle AP view. Talar tilting (varus) implies an incompetent lateral ligament complex and a tight deltoid ligament; ankle stress radiographs may be necessary to better assess the ligaments. Tibial varus can be evaluated by determining whether or not the tibial axis is perpendicular to the tibial plafond (lateral distal tibia angle, described in the Pes Planus section).[185] AP and lateral ankle radiographs are obtained to assess whether or not there is any joint disease.

Pes cavus, in the younger pediatric patient, is best demonstrated radiographically by abnormal talus-first metatarsal relationships, adducted and plantarflexed, in both the DP and lateral views, respectively. The talocalcaneal angles are decreased as well. In the lateral view, the calcaneus is greatly dorsiflexed and the metatarsals plantarflexed.

Fluoroscopy, MRI, and CT, in addition to radiography, have been used to assess the cavus foot. Radiography is the primary study and provides the ability to determine the severity of deformity such that an appropriate surgical procedure or procedures can be selected. Fluoroscopy may be useful for evaluating the ankle integrity via stress and for intraoperative review of the procedure being performed. MRI is valuable for assessing the peroneal tendons, if symptomatic. CT is useful for evaluating the existence of osteoarthritis, coalition, and misalignment (relative to the talar dome) of the tarsal joints.

CLUBFOOT (CONGENITAL TALIPES EQUINOVARUS, TEV)

The radiographic technique used to image the patient with clubfoot is especially important due to the severe deformity and its presence in the newborn. DP and lateral foot radiographs should be obtained weight bearing or, if not possible, as simulated weight bearing. The two feet should not be positioned in the "frog-leg" position for lateral views but imaged individually.[181]

Simons[186] strongly recommends performing the DP image with the foot placed in its "maximally corrected position" (ie, manually pushing against the medially deviated forefoot, if flexible). He also advises that the foot be adequately dorsiflexed at the ankle, unless prevented by significant equinus; visibility of the tibial and fibular shafts in the DP view would indicate inadequate ankle dorsiflexion. And, avoid positioning the foot inverted, which would cause the metatarsals to overlap one another.

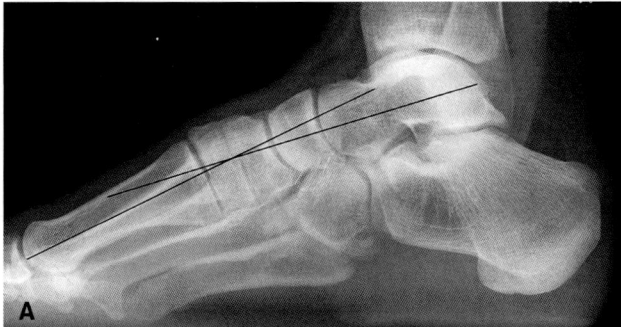
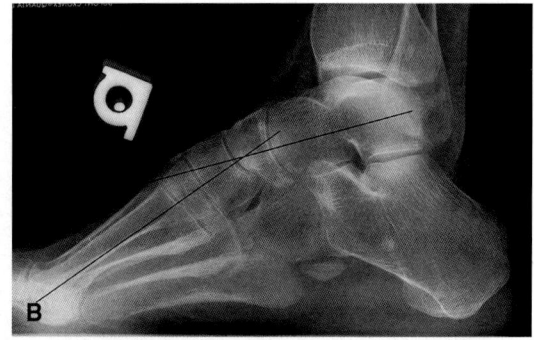
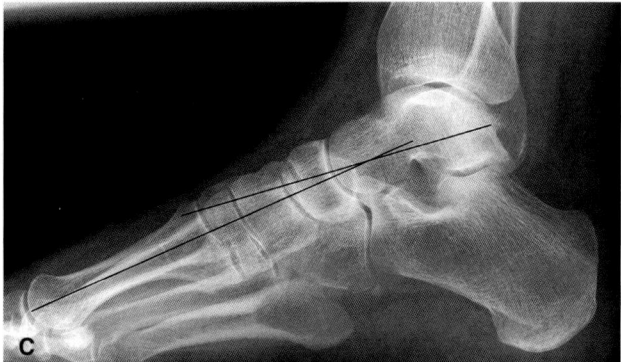

FIGURE 2.61 Anterior pes cavus subtypes based upon the deformity apex, lateral view. **A.** Metatarsal cavus. **B.** Lesser tarsal cavus. **C.** Forefoot cavus.

For the lateral view, Simons[186] recommends maximally dorsiflexing the foot at the ankle without raising the heel off the floor (for an accurate depiction of the talocalcaneal relationship) and positioning the medial aspect of the rearfoot parallel to the image receptor (which requires pulling the rearfoot away from it; if not, the rearfoot foot will be externally rotated relative to the image receptor). This lateral position can also be determined by lining up the malleolar axis such that it is perpendicular to the image receptor. An alternative is to position the lateral aspect of the rearfoot against the image receptor.[187] Observe the position of the fibular malleolus in the lateral view; if it is positioned posterior to the tibial malleolus and not superimposed upon it, then there was external rotation of the extremity. Also, improper inversion positioning of the foot will cause the metatarsals to become stacked, that is, lose their overlapping appearance.[186]

Measurements used to assess clubfoot in the DP and lateral views are listed in Table 2.9. Clubfoot demonstrates very decreased talocalcaneal angles, which are usually <20 degrees in both the DP and lateral views (Fig. 2.62). The talus and calcaneus become more parallel to one another. Furthermore, the talus-first metatarsal relationships are severely abnormal (adducted in the DP view and plantarflexed in the lateral view).

The calcaneal axis, in clubfoot, runs lateral to the cuboid center in the DP view; LeNoir[188] referred to this finding, along with the cuboid center positioned inferior to the calcaneal axis in the lateral view, as the "inverted cuboid sign." Simons[189] grades the severity of this relationship as illustrated in Figure 2.63. Talocalcaneal divergence (Fig. 2.64) and navicular position (Fig. 2.65) are also abnormal.[190]

In most cases, three of the four primary deformities can be assessed radiographically: the adducted forefoot, varus

rearfoot, and hindfoot equinus.[191] However, because the navicular is not yet ossified in the younger child, talonavicular joint subluxation is not obvious. In this case, the "15-degree rule" can be applied: talonavicular subluxation exists if the talocalcaneal angle is <15 degrees and the talus-first metatarsal angle is >15 degrees adducted (an exception is when there is severe forefoot adduction along with hindfoot equinus and varus).[192] Thometz and Simon[193] found that, if the calcaneocuboid joint is subluxated substantially, then there is severe subluxation of the talonavicular joint.

In the lateral view, the calcaneus is in equinus position (plantarflexed) and nearly parallel to the talus. The tibiocalcaneal angle (normally 42-68 degrees) has been used to document the amount of equinus (the angle decreases in clubfoot).[194] The normal tibiocalcaneal angle is reported between 25 and 60 degrees.[186] The metatarsals have a "stair-step" appearance, and the first metatarsal is greatly plantarflexed (see Fig. 2.62B).

TABLE 2.9 Clubfoot Measurement Considerations	
DP View	**Lateral View**
Decreased talocalcaneal angle	Decreased talocalcaneal angle
Talo-first metatarsal angle (adducted metatarsal)	Talo-first metatarsal (Meary) angle (plantarflexed metatarsal)
Cuboid medial to calcaneal bisection axis	Metatarsal "stair-step" appearance
Abnormal navicular position	Abnormal navicular position
Abnormal talocalcaneal divergence	Increased tibiocalcaneal angle

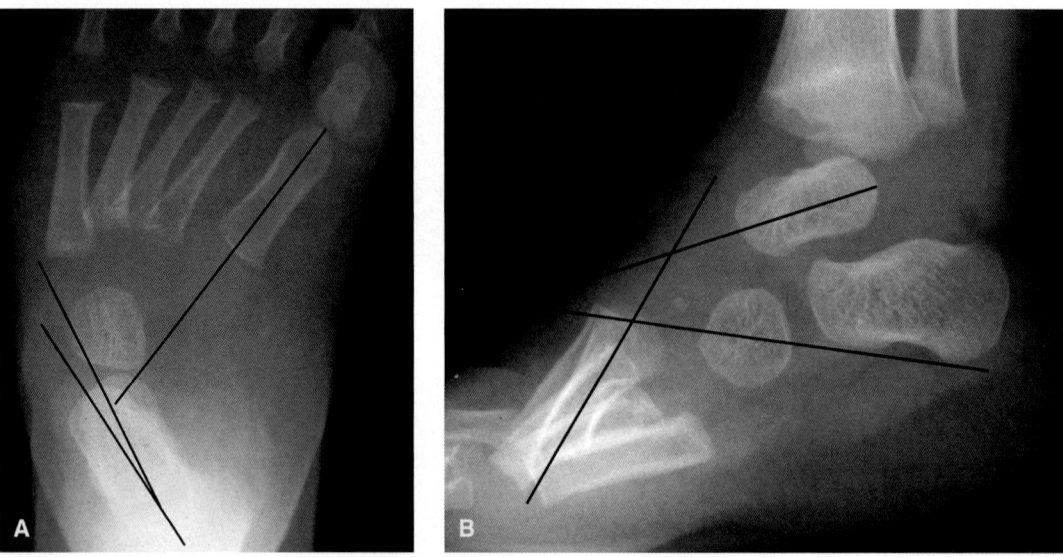

FIGURE 2.62 Clubfoot. **(A)** DP view, **(B)** lateral view.

A maximum dorsiflexion lateral view is sometimes obtained to better assess the talocalcaneal relationship (the maximum dorsiflexion talocalcaneal angle is normally 40-45 degrees and is decreased in clubfoot). It has also been used with a stress plantarflexion lateral view to determine flexibility.[195,196] The tibiotalar angle can be used to measure ankle range of motion; it is considered unsatisfactory if >110 degrees with dorsiflexion and <110 degrees in plantarflexion.[190]

Flattening of the talar dome is a radiographic hallmark associated with clubfoot. It appears to be related to cast treatment, but the etiology is undetermined.[197,198] Since talar dome flattening may influence ankle motion, a measurement has been developed and is advocated to assess talar distortion, referred to as the R/L (radius/length) ratio.[199-201] "R" is the radius of the talar dome trochlear curvature, and "L" is the length of the talus between the head distally (at the articular surface) to the most posterior aspect of the talar process. The normal R/L ratio is 0.365 mm.[199]

METATARSUS ADDUCTUS

Metatarsus adductus is a deformity in the transverse plane occurring at the tarsal-metatarsal, or Lisfranc, joint.[202] There is a greater than normal deviation of the forefoot (metatarsals)

toward the body's midline. The relationship is classically measured between the second metatarsal and lesser tarsal axes. However, there have been some variation of this technique in the adult and alternate methods in the young child.

The metatarsus adductus angle, generally speaking, is not influenced by pronation or supination.[144] Abnormality of this angle, therefore, is considered to represent a structural, not a functional, abnormality.[203] However, the angle does change depending on whether the foot is supinated or pronated, though not as extreme as other angular relationships.[11,131] (The idea that the metatarsus adductus angle is structural and not functional has not been questioned, despite the discrepancy.) Several methods have been used to measure this angle. However, the two methods used more commonly are the classic method and a simplified method, also known as the Engel angle.

The *classic metatarsus adductus angle* is measured between the second metatarsal and the lesser tarsus longitudinal axis (Fig. 2.66A). The lesser tarsus axis is created in the following manner: (1) Points are plotted at the most medial aspect of the first metatarsal-medial cuneiform articulation and the most medial aspect of the talonavicular articulation. The two points are connected by a straight line, which is then bisected with another plotted point. (2) Points are plotted at the most lateral

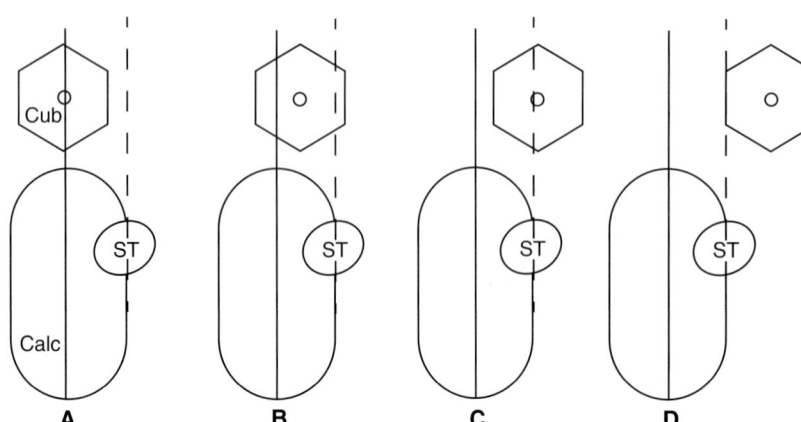

FIGURE 2.63 The "cuboid sign" (relationship between calcaneal axis and medial tangent with cuboid in DP view). **A.** Normal alignment. **B.** +1 grade. **C.** +2 grade. **D.** +3 grade. Calc, calcaneus; Cub, cuboid; ST, sustentaculum tali; *dashed line*, medial tangent to calcaneus.

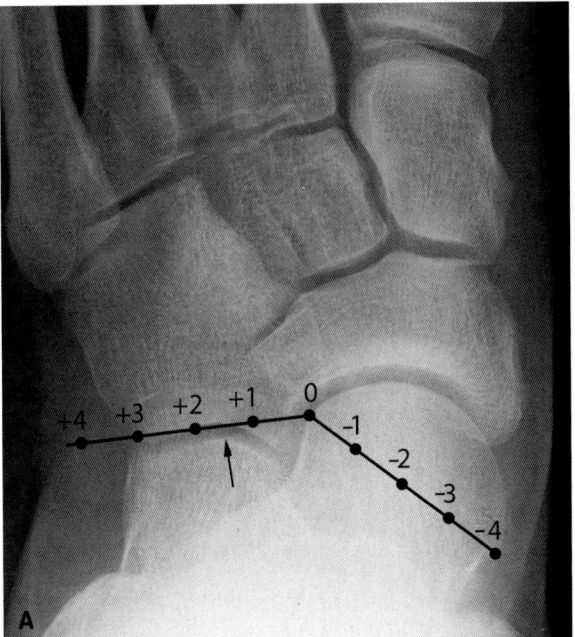

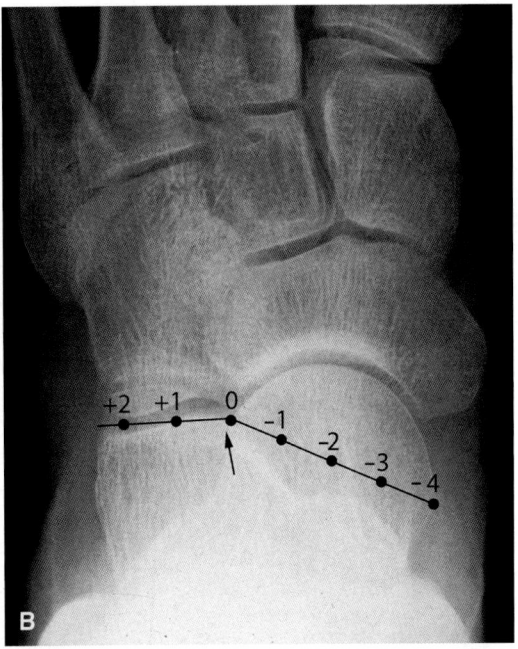

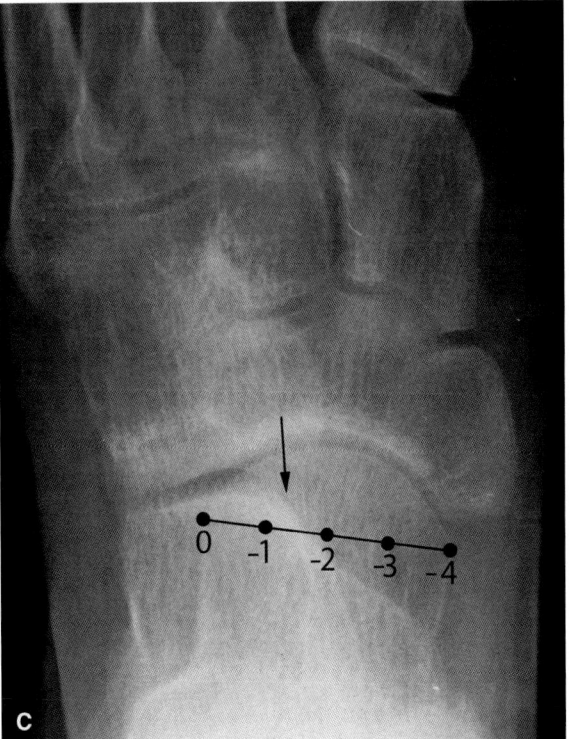

FIGURE 2.64 Talocalcaneal divergence. **A.** Separation or divergence between the anterior ends of the talus and calcaneus designated as +1.5 (pronated foot). **B.** Minimal to no separation or overlap or 0 (normal foot). **C.** Overlap designated as −1.5 (supinated foot). (*Arrow* indicates medial edge of anterior calcaneus.) (This grading system is more objective than that presented in Figure 2.41.)

FIGURE 2.65 Navicular position (when visible), based upon the amount of talar head articulating with the adjacent navicular (dashed lines = talar axis). **(A)** Pronated (half of the talar head is covered laterally; therefore, this is a grade +2), **(B)** rectus (grade 0), and **(C)** supinated (half of the talar head is covered medially; therefore, this is a grade −2) foot. Grade 4 is used if there is total displacement medially or laterally. If the navicular is not ossified, the first metatarsal is used in its place.

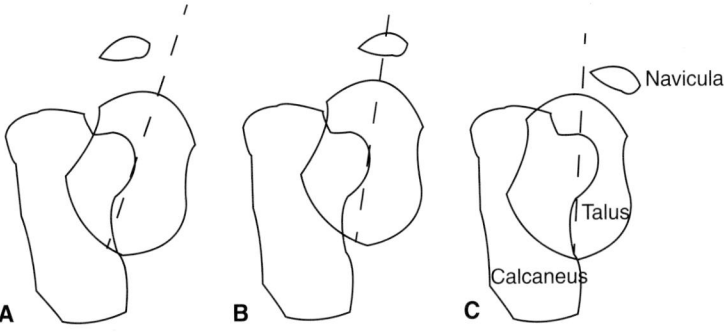

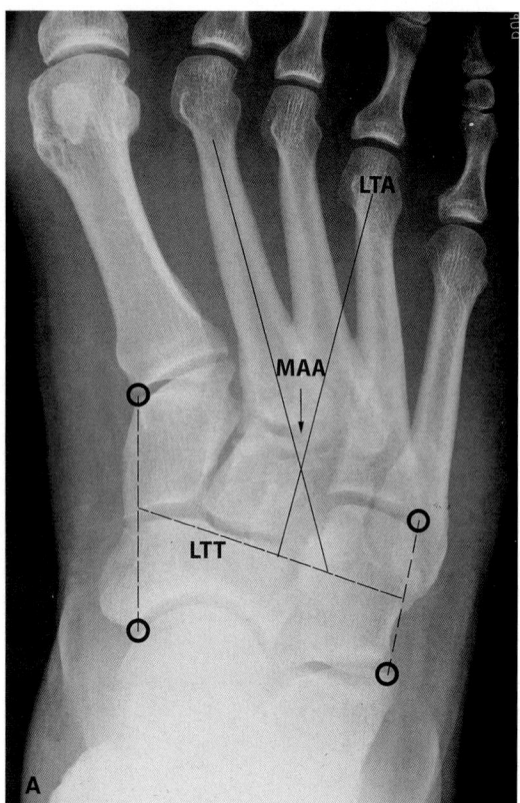
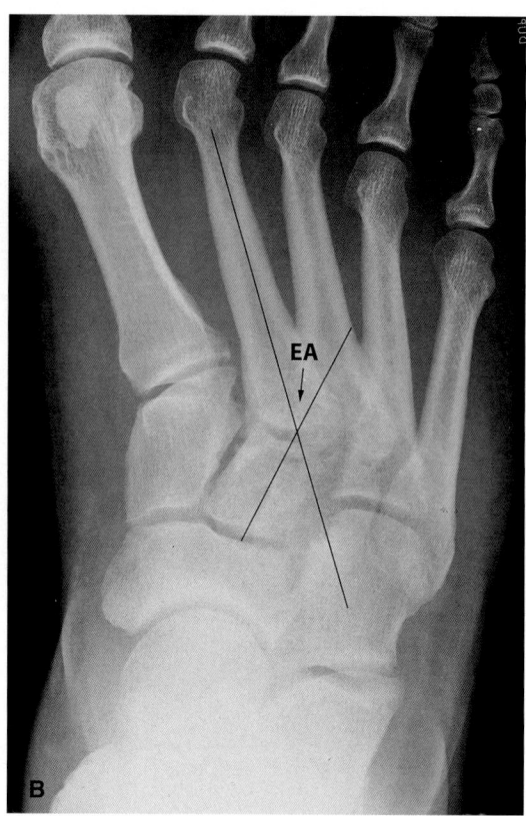

FIGURE 2.66 Metatarsus adductus angle, **(A)** classic method using the fourth metatarsal-cuboid joint, and **(B)** simplified method. LTA, lesser tarsus axis; MAA, metatarsus adductus angle; LTT, lesser tarsus transection; EA, Engel angle.

aspect of the fourth (preferred) or fifth metatarsal-cuboid articulation and the most lateral aspect of the calcaneocuboid articulation. The two points are connected by a straight line, which is then bisected with another plotted point. (3) Draw a line connecting the two bisection points. This line is the lesser tarsus transection. (4) Draw a perpendicular to lesser tarsus transection to obtain the lesser tarsus longitudinal axis.

Kilmartin and Wallace[204] measured the angle formed between the second metatarsal and the lesser tarsus transection (using the fifth metatarsal-cuboid articulation point). This angle, subtracted from 90 degrees, is the same as the metatarsus adductus angle formed by the classic method.

Varying normal ranges have been published, differing between the method used and also between men and women.[205-208] Generally speaking, the classic metatarsus adductus angle using the fourth metatarsal-cuboid articulation point is considered normal if <14 degrees, high normal/borderline between 15 and 20 degrees, and abnormal if over 20 degrees. (Add 3 degrees to those numbers if using the classic metatarsus adductus angle using the fifth metatarsal-cuboid articulation point.)[209]

The simplified method for the metatarsus adductus angle is formed between the longitudinal axes of the second metatarsal and intermediate cuneiform (Fig. 2.66B). This method, originally described by Engel et al.,[210] is easier to perform. The ranges for normal and abnormal were determined to be 3 degrees greater than those for the classic method using the fifth metatarsal-cuboid articulation point. Therefore, the normal range is up to 20 degrees, and the angle is considered pathologic if over 23 degrees. (However, according to the results obtained

by Crawford and Green,[209] one may want to consider pathologic as over 29 degrees using the simplified method.) Thomas et al.[211] further modified the Engel angle; instead of bisecting the intermediate cuneiform to create its axis, they formed the axis as a perpendicular to a line drawn across the proximal articular surface.

Dawoodi et al.[212] concluded that, of the several techniques used to measure the metatarsus adductus angle, the classic method using the fourth metatarsal-cuboid articulation point should be considered the standard method because it demonstrated: (1) the highest inter- and intraobserver reliability and (2) a significant positive correlation between the hallux abductus and metatarsus adductus angles. Furthermore, Crawford and Green[209] agreed that the classic method using the fourth metatarsal-cuboid articulation point (which is more easily identified than the fifth) is the most ideal and warned against using the Engel angle due to, when compared to the classic method, a wide range of difference and poor correlation.

Many of the lesser tarsal bones are either not yet ossified or, if ossified, rudimentary in appearance in the young child and infant. Alternative means of assessing metatarsus adductus in this age group have, therefore, been proposed since the methods used in the adult do not suffice. The following angular relationships have been used in the DP view: calcaneus-fifth metatarsal (normal value is 5 degrees, abnormal is >10 degrees), calcaneus-second metatarsal (normal value is <22 degrees), first-fifth metatarsal (normal is 22 degrees, abnormal is >27 degrees), and talus-first metatarsal (Fig. 2.67).[206,213] Of these methods, the angle measured between the first metatarsal axis relative to the talar axis is most commonly used.

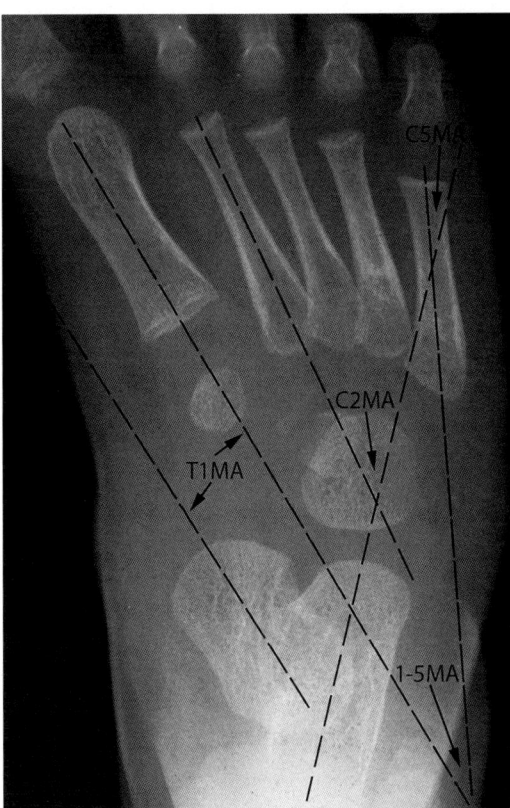

FIGURE 2.67 Angles used to assess metatarsus adductus in the young child and infant. C5MA, calcaneus-fifth metatarsal angle; C2MA, calcaneus-second metatarsal angle; 1-5MA, first-fifth metatarsal angle; T1MA, talus-first metatarsal angle.

The talus-first metatarsal angle has a normal range between 0 and 20 degrees (ie, the first metatarsal is parallel or abducted relative to the talus); metatarsus adductus is associated with a first metatarsal axis adducted relative to the talar axis. (However, La Reaux[206] cautions that a false positive may result if rearfoot supination is present.) According to French et al.,[214] an abnormality of two of the three angles (calcaneus-fifth metatarsal, first-fifth metatarsal, and talus-first metatarsal) supported a diagnosis of metatarsus adductus; they also noted that the first and fifth metatarsal axes converged laterally outside the rearfoot in the metatarsus adductus foot. Generally speaking, the metatarsal bases converge posteriorly, more than normal.

Lepow et al.[215] developed a novel pediatric metatarsus adductus angle. It requires the use of a compass in order to plot points and subsequently construct lines, which is probably why it has rarely been cited in the literature.[216]

Berg[217] described four types of metatarsus adductus, depending upon the talocalcaneal angle (normal or increased) and the cuboid position relative to the calcaneal axis. All four types demonstrate an abnormal talus-first metatarsal angle (adducted metatarsal); however, it is the varying combinations of talocalcaneal angle and the cuboid position relative to the calcaneal axis that distinguish between them (Fig. 2.68). *Common metatarsus adductus* demonstrates a normal talocalcaneal angle and the calcaneal axis roughly bisects the cuboid. *Complex metatarsus adductus* (also known as metatarsus adductovarus and cavometatarsus adductus) demonstrates a normal talocalcaneal angle but the calcaneal axis falls medial to the cuboid bisection. *Skewfoot* (also referred to as metatarsus varus)[218] demonstrates an increased talocalcaneal angle, but the calcaneal axis roughly bisects the cuboid. *Complex skewfoot* (also known as the serpentine foot) demonstrates both an increased talocalcaneal

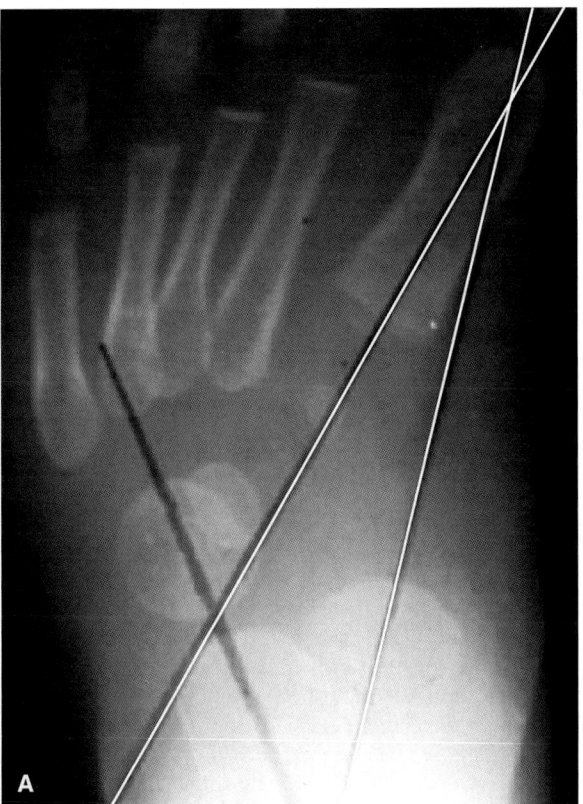

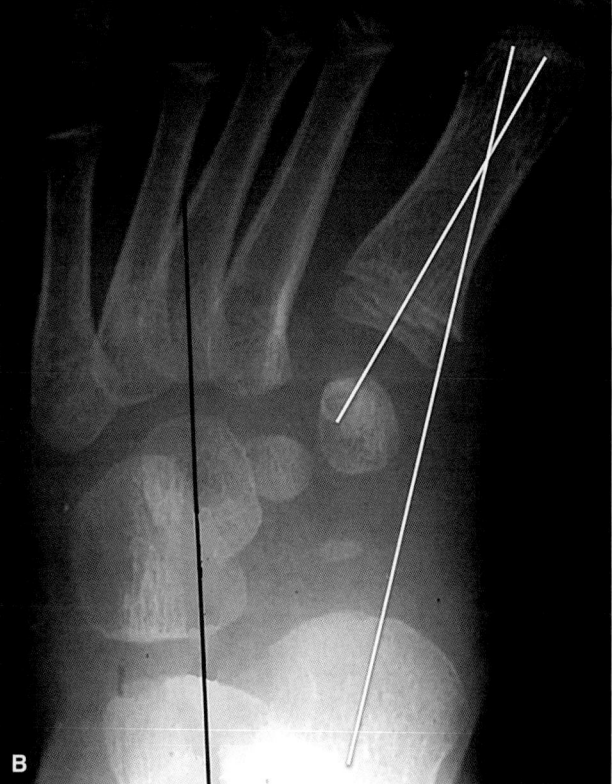

FIGURE 2.68 Four types of metatarsus adductus according to Berg.[217] **A.** Common metatarsus adductus. **B.** Complex metatarsus adductus.

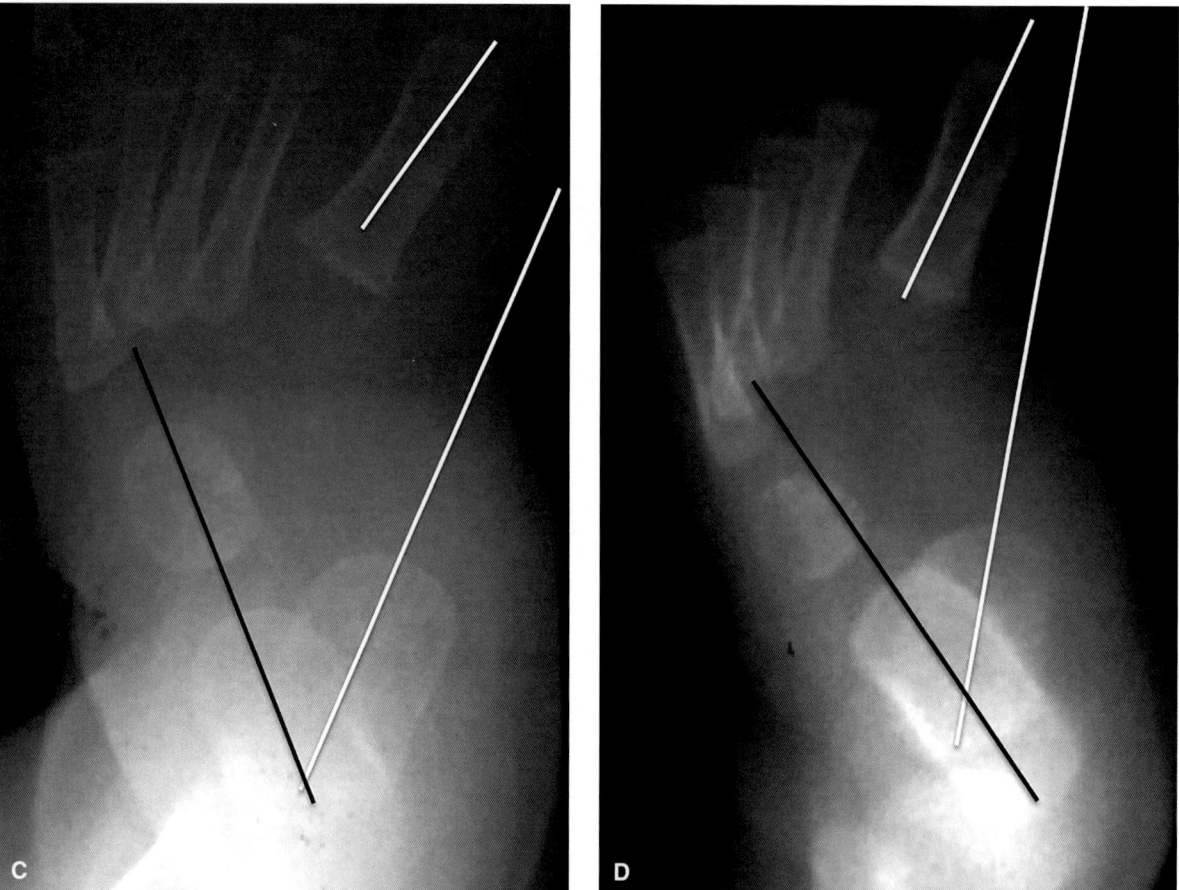

FIGURE 2.68 (*Continued*) **C.** Skewfoot. **D.** Complex skewfoot.

angle and the calcaneal axis falls medial to the cuboid bisection. Unfortunately, due to irregularity of the tarsal ossification centers, changes in shape during ossification, and foot positioning variability, the talocalcaneal angles in particular can be measured inconsistently, making this classification unreliable.[219]

Ultrasound may prove to be valuable for assessing the pediatric foot deformity when ossification centers are either not visible or only partially ossified. Miron and Grimard[220] have described ultrasound findings for clubfoot, metatarsus adductus (including skewfoot), and oblique and vertical talus; a specific imaging protocol is proposed for each deformity.

HALLUX ABDUCTO VALGUS

Radiographic preoperative assessment of hallux abducto valgus deformity should include at least the following three views: DP, lateral, and sesamoid axial. The sesamoid axial (tangential) view is required in order to assess coronal position of the first metatarsal and to assess integrity of the sesamoid-metatarsal joints. Oblique views may be included, if warranted. For example, first metatarsophalangeal osteophytes tend to occur dorsolaterally; therefore, if spurs are palpated in this area clinically, a lateral oblique view should also be included.

Criteria used to preoperatively assess hallux abducto valgus deformity consist of numerous positional relationships, many of them angles; several nonpositional criteria are also used. Table 2.10 lists some of the more common criteria. Almost all parameters are assessed in the DP view. Recently, there has

been a renewed interest regarding the influence and evaluation of coronal (frontal) plane parameters.[221] And with the advent of weight-bearing extremity CT, the accurate assessment of coronal plane bone position may become possible.[222,223]

Many of the axes for the angles mentioned below are described in the "Transverse" or "Sagittal Plane Relationships" sections above. Otherwise, axes will be described when appropriate.

First Intermetatarsal Angle

The first intermetatarsal (or, intermetatarsal 1) angle is formed between the first and second metatarsal longitudinal axes (Fig. 2.69). In the normal foot, it measures ≤8 degrees. When the angle is >8 degrees, the deformity is referred to as metatarsus primus adductus.

Metatarsus Adductus Angle

Metatarsus adductus deformity, discussed previously, may exaggerate the true intermetatarsal angle. In this case, the true intermetatarsal angle (aka total adductus angle)[224] is determined by adding the measured intermetatarsal angle to the metatarsus adductus angle and subtracting 15 (which would be the normally expected metatarsus adductus angle). Or, another way of looking at this, the total adductus angle (intermetatarsal angle plus the metatarsus adductus angle) should normally be 20 degrees or less.[225]

TABLE 2.10	Radiographic Parameters Frequently Used to Assess Hallux Abducto Valgus. (Unless Otherwise Indicated, All Parameters Are Assessed in the DP View)		
Angular Relationships	**Other Positional Relationships**	**Nonpositional Criteria**
Intermetatarsal 1	Metatarsal-sesamoid position (DP view)	First metatarsal head "shape"
Hallux abductus	Axial sesamoid position (sesamoid axial view)	Width of the medial eminence
Hallux interphalangeus	Joint "status" (congruous, deviated, subluxated)	First metatarsophalangeal joint space
Proximal articular set	Structural vs positional deformity	Presence or absence of osteophytes, loose bodies, subchondral sclerosis, or geodes
Distal articular set	First metatarsal length (metatarsal protrusion distance)	Presence or absence of osteopenia
Metatarsus adductus	First metatarsal head "movement"	Medial cuneiform-first metatarsal joint shape
Tangential angle to the second axis	Metatarsus primus elevatus (lateral view)	
First metatarsal declination (lateral view)		
First metatarsal pronation (sesamoid axial view)		

Hallux Abductus Angle

The hallux abductus angle measures the amount of hallux lateral deviation relative to the first metatarsal. It is formed between the longitudinal axes of the first metatarsal and hallux proximal phalanx (see Fig. 2.69). The phalangeal longitudinal axis is formed in the following manner: (1) Points are plotted on the medial and lateral cortex of the diaphysis, just proximal to the flare of the phalanx neck and connected by a straight line; the bisection of this line is marked by a point on the shaft. (2) Two more points are plotted on the medial and lateral cortex of the diaphysis, this time just distal to the flare of the phalanx base, connecting them by a straight line and marking the bisection of this line by a second point on the shaft. (3) Connect a straight line through the two bisections on the shaft of the phalanx; this line represents the longitudinal axis of the phalanx.

The hallux abductus angle is normally ≤15 degrees. If the angle measures >15 degrees, the deformity is referred to as hallux abductus. If the angle is a negative number, the deformity is referred to as hallux adductus.

Hallux Interphalangeus Angle

The hallux interphalangeus angle is formed between the longitudinal axes of the hallux proximal (described above) and distal phalanges (see Fig. 2.69). Four methods have been described for drawing the distal phalanx axis: Strydom et al.[226] plotted points that were 5 mm distal to the basal articular surface and were 5 mm proximal to the anterior tip of the ungual tuberosity; Coughlin and Shurnas[227] plotted points at the center of the basal articular surface and the distal tip of the ungual tuberosity. Barnett[228] and Sorto et al.[229] drew lines tangential to the medial and lateral aspects of the distal phalanx, which crossed distally; the axis was formed by bisecting the resultant "triangle." Whitney[230] bisected the diaphysis in a fashion similar to that of the proximal phalanx. The hallux interphalangeus angle is considered pathologic when it measures >10 degrees. However, the angle is often underestimated due to coronal plane rotation of the first ray.[231]

Total Valgus Deformity of the Hallux

The total "valgus" deformity of the hallux (TVDH) is equivalent to the sum of the hallux abductus and hallux interphalangeus angles. It normally measures <25 degrees.[226]

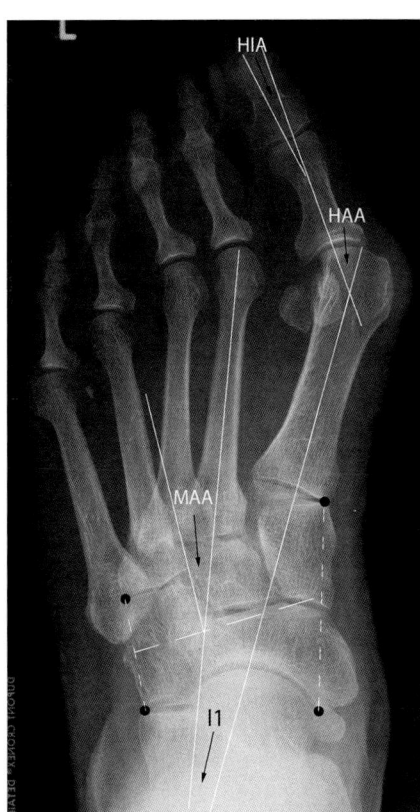

FIGURE 2.69 Hallux abductus measurements.
I1, intermetatarsal 1 angle; MAA, metatarsus adductus angle; HAA, hallux abductus angle; HIA, hallux interphalangeus angle.

Proximal Articular Set Angle

The proximal articular set angle, or PASA, determines whether or not the effective articular surface of the first metatarsal head is perpendicular to the shaft. It has also been referred to as the distal metatarsal articular angle, or DMAA.[232] It is formed between the first metatarsal longitudinal axis and the proximal articular set axis (Fig. 2.70). The latter axis is formed as follows: (1) Connect the following two points by a straight line: (a) the most medial aspect on the effective articular surface near the cortex of the first metatarsal head (sometimes denoted by a "sagittal groove") and (b) the most lateral aspect on the effective articular surface near the superior-lateral margin of the first metatarsal head. This line represents the proximal articular set line. (2) Draw a line perpendicular to the proximal articular set line; this is the proximal articular set axis.

The PASA normally measures ≤8 degrees. Unfortunately, the radiographic measurement does not correlate well with the intraoperative evaluation of the articular surface, especially if lateral adaptation of the cartilage has occurred.[233] Also, the measurement's accuracy and validity have been questionable, owing primarily to inter-rater reliability (relating to point selection for the proximal articular set axis) and the effect of varus rotation (pronation) of the metatarsal.[234,235] However, reliability can become more consistent by (1) selecting the lateral point based upon the identifiable superior-lateral margin of the first metatarsal head,[15] which appears radiographically as a linear sclerosis that is perpendicular to the anterior articular surface (Fig. 2.7), and (2) knowing that the PASA is dependent upon rotational deformity and will increase with increasing

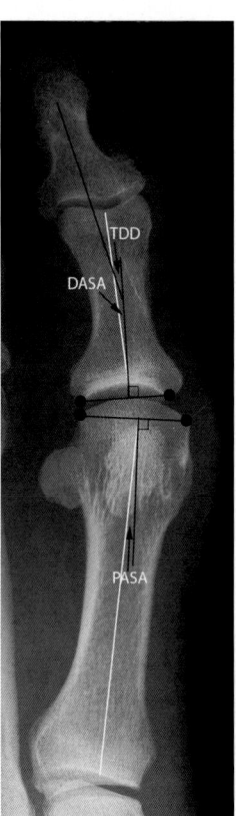

FIGURE 2.70 Hallux abductus measurements. PASA, proximal articular set angle; DASA, distal articular set angle; TDD, total distal deformity.

pronation of the first metatarsal.[236] Articular surface deformity relating to PASA is recognized accurately upon visualizing the articular cartilage intraoperatively.[233,237]

Distal Articular Set Angle

The distal articular set angle, or DASA, measures internal deviation of the proximal phalanx shaft relative to its base. (This measurement has also been referred to as the proximal phalangeal articular angle, or PPAA.)[238] It is formed between the longitudinal axis of the proximal phalanx and the distal articular set axis (see Fig. 2.70). The latter axis is formed as follows: (1) Plot points at the most medial and lateral aspects of the effective articular surface of the hallux proximal phalanx base and connect them by a straight line. This line represents the distal articular set line. (2) Draw a line perpendicular to the distal articular set line; this is the distal articular set axis.

Like the PASA, the DASA normally measures ≤8 degrees. However, it has been demonstrated that coronal plane rotation of the hallux significantly changes the proximal phalanx morphology and results in significantly different DASA measurements in the transverse plane.[239]

Total Deformity Distal to the First Metatarsophalangeal Joint

Spinner et al.[240] take into consideration the entire hallux deformity in the transverse plane distal to the first metatarsophalangeal joint. The angle, named total hallucal deviation (THD), is measured between the distal articular set axis and the distal phalanx axis (the bisection method was not specified) (see Fig. 2.70). The mean value was 8.6 degrees; a value >12 degrees was considered to be a significant deformity.

Elliot and Saxby[241] reinvented this measurement method and referred to it as the total distal deformity. They used the Coughlin and Shurnas[227] method to draw the distal phalanx axis, described above in the "Hallux Interphalangeus Angle" section. Elliot and Saxby found an average total distal deformity angle of 20 degrees in their hallux "valgus" cohort (the hallux interphalangeal angle average was 11 degrees) but did not state a normal value; since the angle incorporates the DASA (pathologic >8 degrees) and hallux interphalangeal angles (pathologic >10 degrees), the total distal deformity should measure no >18 degrees. However, as with most transverse plane measurements, first ray pronation can influence the actual value, which is also the case with the total distal deformity angle.[238]

Tangential Angle to the Second Metatarsal Axis

The tangential angle to the second metatarsal axis, aka TASA, assesses the position of the first metatarsal head articular surface relative to the second metatarsal.[242] The angle is formed between a perpendicular to the second metatarsal axis and the proximal articular set line; the normal value is −5 to 5 degrees. The measurement should equal the intermetatarsal 1 angle minus the PASA. Since TASA focuses on the direction of the distal articular surface, it is proposed to be useful for determining the angulation for an Austin-type bunionectomy/osteotomy procedure, especially when the intermetatarsal 1 angle is normal.

This angle has rarely been assessed in the literature. In one publication,[243] TASA was used to assess outcomes after Lapidus arthrodesis; however, large individual differences in TASA values were found, and the measurement was not recommended.

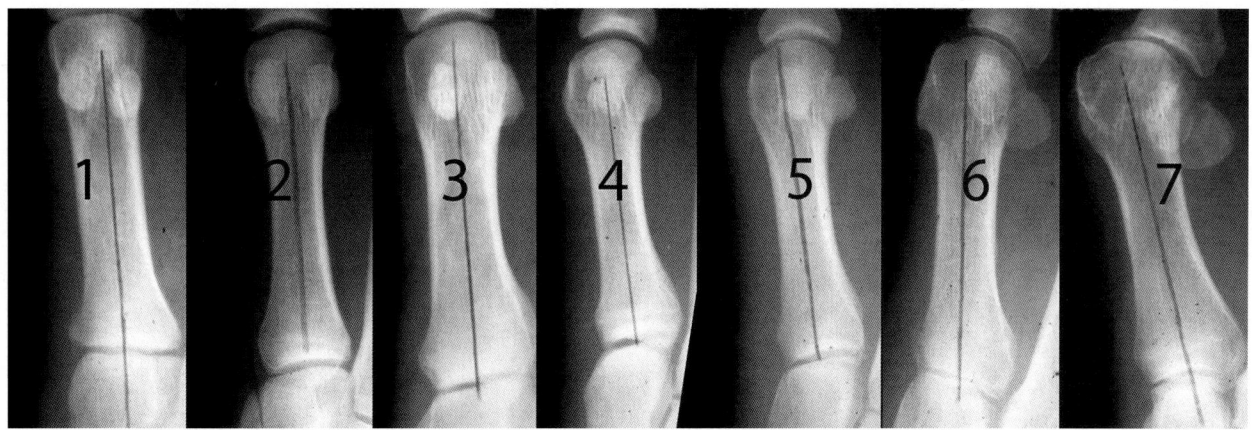

FIGURE 2.71 Tibial sesamoid position using the 7-position system.

Metatarsal-Sesamoid Position (DP View)

The first metatarsophalangeal joint sesamoids do not move relative to the first metatarsal; they maintain their relationship with the second metatarsal.[244] The metatarsal-sesamoid position describes the position of the first metatarsal relative to either the tibial or fibular sesamoid. Each method was originally described using a 7-position system.

The tibial sesamoid method describes the position of the tibial sesamoid relative to the first metatarsal longitudinal axis.[245] Radiographic examples for the seven tibial sesamoid positions are presented in Figure 2.71. Position 4 out of 7 could be considered a "tipping point" regarding deformity progression and may represent an acceptable upper limit when considering surgical correction.[246] An abnormal (4+) sesamoid position may be perceived as subluxation with the metatarsal head; however, one must correlate this finding with the axial sesamoid position. Coronal plane rotation of the metatarsal may demonstrate normal positioning of the sesamoid relative to the crista in the axial view despite an abnormal sesamoid position in the DP view.[221,247]

The fibular sesamoid method describes the position of the fibular sesamoid relative to the lateral border of the first metatarsal head flare.[248] The bone's lateral margin bisects the fibular sesamoid in position 4.

Smith et al.[249] recommended a 4-grade sesamoid position for either method in that it is easier to use and provides adequate distribution of data: 0, completely medial, no overlap or displacement; 1, <50% overlap; 2, > 50% overlap; and, 3, completely lateral, complete displacement. The 4-grade fibular (lateral) sesamoid position has been addressed in recent literature, noting significant correlation with the intermetatarsal and hallux abductus angles as well as high inter- and intraobserver reliability.[250,251]

Congruency of the First Metatarsophalangeal Joint

Coughlin[252] described the concept of joint congruency, where the medial and lateral margins of the proximal phalanx basal articular surface match the first metatarsal head articular surface. A measurement quantifying this variable plots points at the middle of the proximal phalanx articular surface and the distal end of the first metatarsal head at its intersection with the first metatarsal mechanical axis.[253] Normally, in the DP view,

the center of the first metatarsal head articular surface should directly appose the center of the proximal phalanx base articular surface (a distance of 0 mm). If they do not, the distance in millimeters can be measured between these two central points (Fig. 2.72). This distance can be used to determine the amount of intermetatarsal angle correction required to reduce the deformity, which should correlate with the distance measured in the sesamoid axial view between the first metatarsal head crista and a point centered between the two sesamoids.[254]

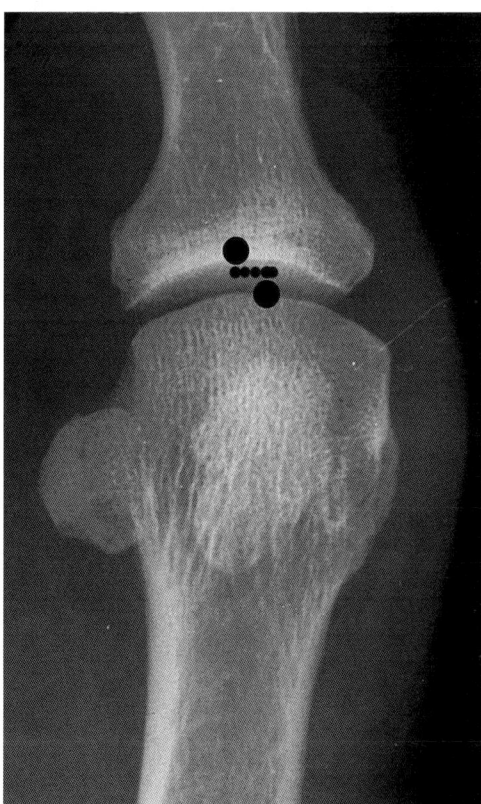

FIGURE 2.72 First metatarsophalangeal joint congruency. The two central points should be directly opposite one another; since they are not in this case, the distance between the two points (*dotted line*) can be measured.

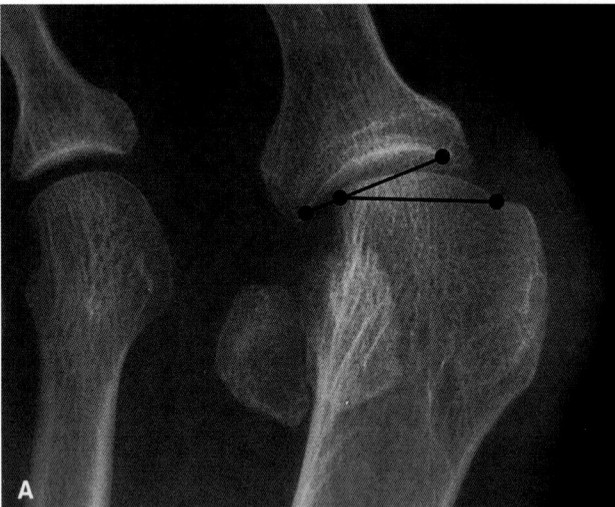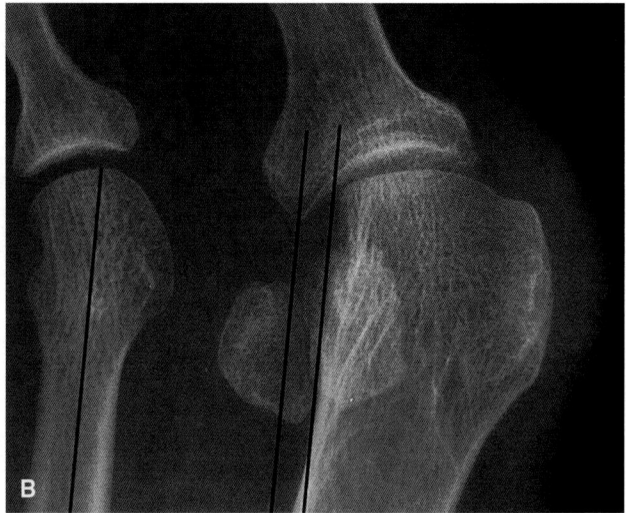

FIGURE 2.73 Joint status. **A.** The distal and proximal articular set lines should be parallel to one another; since they cross with the joint, the joint status is considered subluxated. Figure 2.70 is an example of deviated, since the two lines, if extended laterally, will cross outside the joint. **B.** *Parallel lines* to the second metatarsal demonstrate separation between the first metatarsal and hallux proximal phalangeal articular surfaces laterally; >2 mm separation is grade 2 in the 3-grade system.

Joint Status

Assessing the position of the articular surfaces relative to one another aids in establishing whether the deformity is related to anatomic variation or phalangeal displacement (positional deviation).[255] The first metatarsophalangeal joint status is determined by comparing the position of the proximal and distal particular set lines. Figure 2.73A illustrates joint status: if the two lines are parallel to one another, the joint is considered to be congruous; if the two lines cross outside the joint, the joint is said to be deviated; finally, if the lines cross within the joint, the joint is subluxated.

Smith et al.[249] use a 3-grade system and determine the joint status in the following manner: after drawing the second metatarsal longitudinal axis, parallel lines are drawn at the lateral edge of both the first metatarsal and hallux proximal phalangeal articular surfaces; the distance (if any) is measure between the two parallel lines. If there is no separation between the lines (superimposition), there is no subluxation (grade 0); if the distance of subluxation is 2 mm or less, it is grade 1, and grade 2 if the subluxation distance is >2 mm (Fig. 2.73B).

Structural, Positional, or Combined Deformity (Table 2.11)

Hallux abducto valgus can either be a structural or positional abnormality. A more detailed way to determine this is to correlate the PASA and DASA to the hallux abductus angle and relating it to the joint status described above (congruous, deviated, or subluxated).[256] If the sum of the proximal and the DASA equals the hallux abductus angle, and the proximal and/or DASA are abnormal, but the joint is congruous, then the deformity is considered to be structural. However, if the sum of the proximal and DASA is less than the hallux abductus angle, the proximal and DASA are both normal, and the joint is either deviated or subluxated, then the deformity is considered to be positional. A combined deformity is accompanied by a hallux abductus angle greater than the sum of the proximal and the

DASA, the proximal and/or DASA are abnormal, and the joint is either deviated or subluxated.

Metatarsal Protrusion

Numerous methods have been described in an attempt to measure the length of the first metatarsal relative to the second. This difference in length has been referred to as the metatarsal protrusion distance (MPD), metatarsal protrusion index, and relative metatarsal protrusion.

Nilsonne,[257] in 1930, drew a line perpendicular to the second metatarsal longitudinal axis at the head's most distal point; a second perpendicular line, parallel to the first, was drawn from the second metatarsal axis to the most distal point of the first metatarsal head. The metatarsal protrusion index is the distance between the two lines. A positive value was given when the first metatarsal was longer than the second metatarsal, a negative value when shorter.

TABLE 2.11	Criteria for Determining If a Hallux Abducto Valgus Deformity Is Structural, Positional, or Combined
Deformity	**Criteria**
Structural	PASA + DASA = HAA
	PASA and/or DASA abnormal
	Congruous joint
Positional	PASA + DASA < HAA
	PASA and DASA normal
	Deviated or subluxated joint
Combined	PASA + DASA < HAA
	PASA and/or DASA abnormal
	Deviated or subluxated joint

Harris and Beath[258] drew two lines from the distal ends of the first and second metatarsal heads to a single point along the most posterior aspect of the calcaneus (the view used was a combination of the DP foot and calcaneal axial projections). They found the most common length to be equal.

Hardy and Clapham[245] created a transverse reference line by connecting two points: one at the lateral aspect of the calcaneocuboid joint and the second at the medial aspect of the talonavicular joint. The longitudinal axis of the second metatarsal is drawn, placing a point where it intersects the transverse reference line; this point serves as the rotation point for measurement. Two arcs are drawn with a compass, one at the distal aspect of the first metatarsal distal articular surface and one at the distal aspect of the second metatarsal articular surface (Fig. 2.74). A perpendicular line is then drawn between the two arcs. The MPD is measured in mm between the two arcs. A positive value is used when the first metatarsal is longer that the second; a negative value is used when the first metatarsal is shorter than the second metatarsal. This method was preferred by the American Orthopaedic Foot and Ankle Society (AOFAS).[249] Measurements between −1 and 1 mm were considered equal.[227] A first metatarsal head that protrudes longer than the second metatarsal head has been associated with hallux abducto valgus; if true, then the slight shortening that occurs with metatarsal osteotomies may be acceptable.[232]

Lundberg and Sulja[259] developed a measurement method that they believed corrected for metatarsus primus adductus. The axes for the first and second metatarsals are drawn. The compass point is placed where the first metatarsal axis intersects its base; an arc is drawn at the most distal end of the first

metatarsal. A "new" first metatarsal axis is drawn, originating at the base of the first metatarsal at its intersection with its axis and parallel to the second metatarsal axis. A perpendicular line is drawn from the distal end of the second metatarsal head at its axis to the "new" first metatarsal axis. At this point, the distance is measured to the end of the first metatarsal, referred to as the relative metatarsal protrusion.

Ideally, the creation of arcs as suggested by Hardy and Clapham[245] should be performed using the intersection of the first and second metatarsal longitudinal axes for compass placement.[259] This technique is commonly used; the distance measured between the two arcs is the metatarsal protrusion, which is normally between +2 and −2 mm.[260] However, the intersection may form off the image, which occurs with smaller intermetatarsal angles; Osher et al.[261] solved this problem mathematically by creating a "virtual" isosceles triangle (and, a compass is not required).

Maestro et al.[262] developed a measurement technique useful for evaluating metatarsal lengths relative to one another. They found a geometrical progression of the "normal" lesser metatarsal head position that approximated a factor of 2; for example, the distance from the tip of one lesser metatarsal head to the next might be 3 to 6-12 mm (a transmetatarsal line, constructed between the center of the fibular sesamoid and perpendicular to the second metatarsal longitudinal axis, was used as a reference). Also, this transmetatarsal axis would normally, when extended laterally, cross through the middle one-third of the fourth metatarsal head. It appears that they found this same geographic progression with the distances measured between the distal tip of each lesser metatarsal head and transmetatarsal line. Ali et al.[263] found the technique to be reproducible and reliable statistically.

Metatarsal Break Angle

The metatarsal break angle has also been referred to as the metatarsal parabolic angle and the metatarsal length pattern.[264] Three points are plotted, one each at the end of the first, second, and fifth metatarsals. The first and second metatarsals points are connected by a line, and the second and fifth metatarsals are connected by a line (Fig. 2.75). The angle formed between these two lines has a mean of 142.5 degrees.[265] An angle <135 degrees indicates a short first metatarsal. The value of this measurement is questionable.[261]

First Metatarsal Head Shape

The first metatarsal head has been described as having one of three shapes (Fig. 2.76): round (or curved, convex, oval); flat (or square); and oblique (or square with ridge, chevron). It is believed that a flat metatarsal head shape resists deforming forces (due to greater stability in the transverse plane), while a round shape is more prone to hallux abductus development.[266] The flat head with ridge is more commonly associated with hallux limitus.[207]

It is erroneous to use the measurement system for metatarsal head shape devised by Okuda et al.[267] (explained earlier in the Radiographic Anatomy section). Hatch et al.[221] have referred to this as the "round sign" and relate it to frontal plane rotation of the metatarsal; yes, position can definitely influence the visibility of the "lateral edge."[268] Just keep in mind that the "rounding" is actually visibility of the fibular sesamoid articular margin

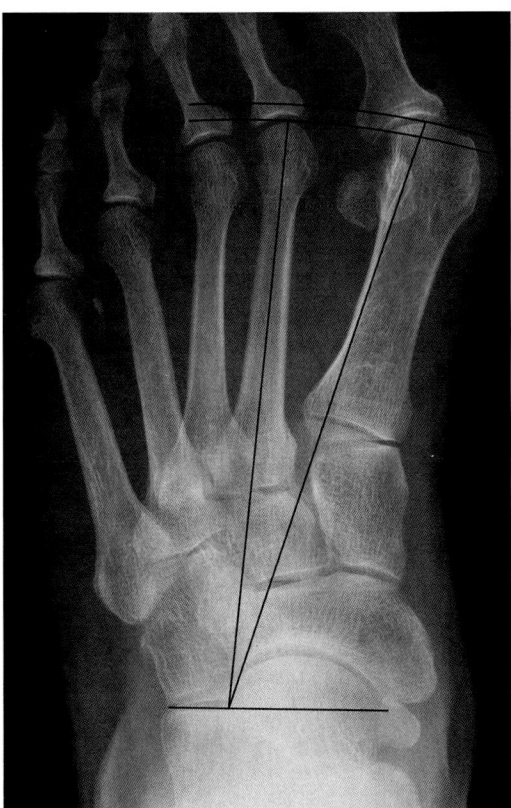

FIGURE 2.74 Metatarsal protrusion, Hardy and Clapham method.

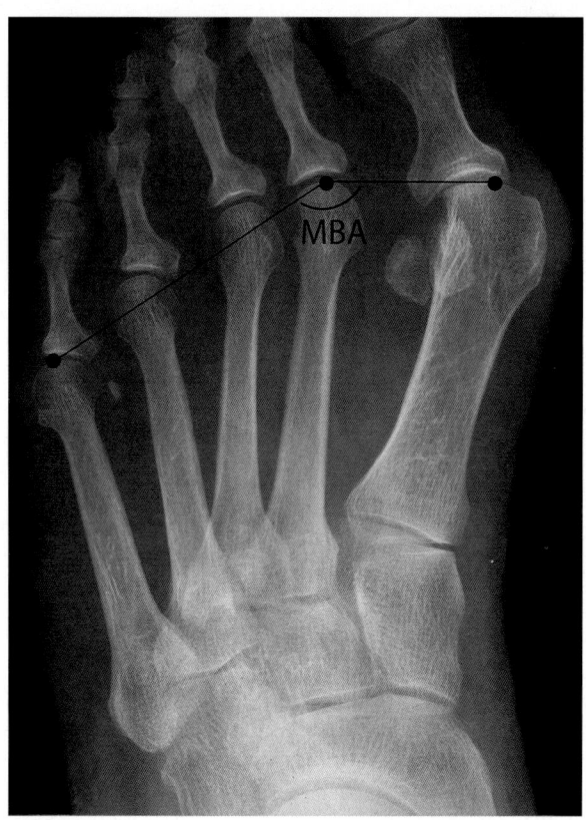

FIGURE 2.75 Metatarsal break angle (MBA).

appearing colinear with the proximal phalanx articular surface. Its visibility, however, associated with a high tibial sesamoid position do correlate with a metatarsal head rotated in the coronal plane.[269]

Width of Medial Eminence

First, a line is drawn along (tangent to) the medial aspect of the first metatarsal diaphysis; it is extended distally to the joint. Plot a point at the most medial aspect of the medial eminence (the widest point). Draw a perpendicular line from the medial diaphyseal line that connects to the medial eminence point; measure the distance in mm, which represents the size of the medial eminence (Fig. 2.77).[232,270]

First Metatarsal Declination Angle

The first metatarsal declination angle is formed between the first metatarsal longitudinal axis and the plane of support in the lateral view. A line tangent to the dorsal surface of the first metatarsal shaft also has been used in place of the longitudinal axis bisection (Fig. 2.78). It normally measures between 19 and 23 degrees. A decreased angle is associated with metatarsus primus elevatus; an increased angle suggests a plantarflexed first ray.

Second Metatarsal Declination Angle

The second metatarsal declination angle is formed between the second metatarsal axis and the plane of support in the lateral view. Since the second metatarsal is fully superimposed and not

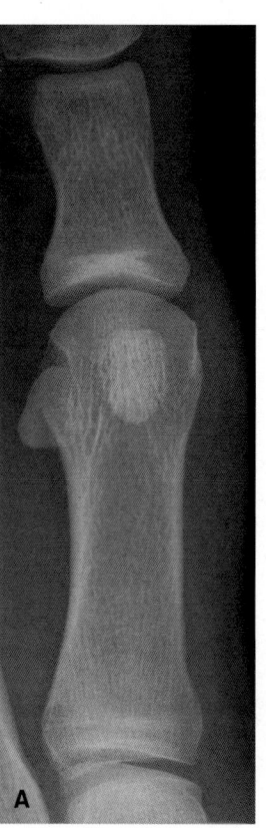
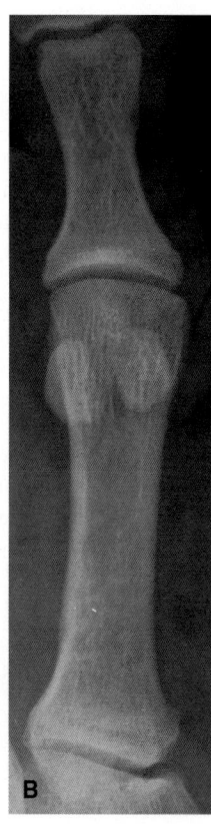
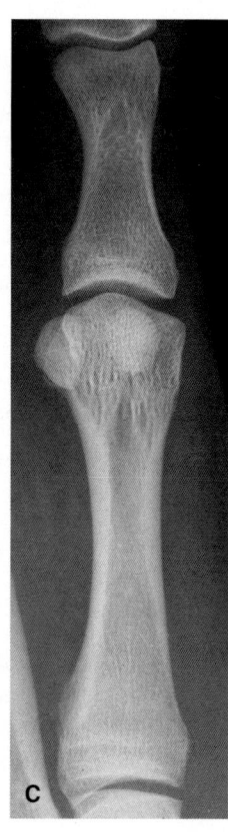

FIGURE 2.76 First metatarsal head shape. **(A)** Round, **(B)**, flat, **(C)** oblique.

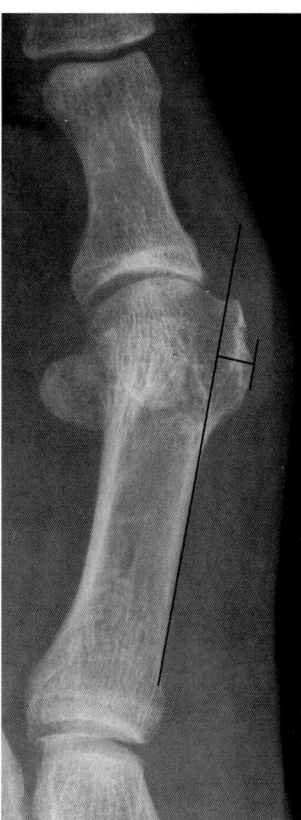

FIGURE 2.77 Width of the medial eminence.

clearly visible, a tangent line is drawn along the dorsal surface of its diaphysis to form its axis (see Fig. 2.78).[271] This angle has been used with the first metatarsal declination angle to assess metatarsus primus elevatus.

Metatarsus Primus Elevatus

Metatarsus primus elevatus, generally speaking, refers to elevation of the first metatarsal relative to the second metatarsal, an extrinsic relationship, in the weight-bearing lateral foot view. (Intrinsically, the first metatarsal may be deformed, where the diaphysis is not perpendicular to the base.) Normally, there is no plantar declination nor dorsal angulation of the first metatarsal relative to the second.[272] The dorsal cortical surfaces of the two metatarsals should be parallel to one another, which is

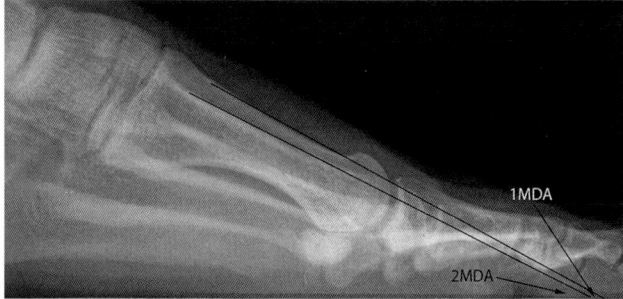

FIGURE 2.78 Metatarsal declination angles using lines tangent to the metatarsal diaphyseal dorsal surface. 1MDA, first metatarsal declination angle; 2MDA, second metatarsal declination angle.

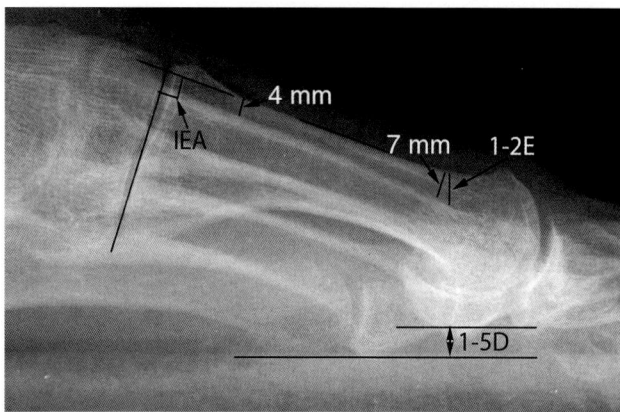

FIGURE 2.79 Metatarsus primus elevatus. The dorsal cortices of the first and second metatarsals are parallel to one another in this example; therefore, the sagittal intermetatarsal angle would be 0 degrees. Using the Seiberg index, the displacement value is 3 mm (7 minus 4). 1-2E, first to second metatarsal head elevation; 1-5D, first to fifth metatarsal head distance; IEA, intrinsic elevation angle of the first metatarsal; *dashed line*, tangent to dorsal surface of first metatarsal diaphysis.

not affected by x-ray tube head position or angulation.[273] Several methods have been used to assess extrinsic elevation of the first metatarsal. They include first to second metatarsal head elevation, the Seiberg index, the sagittal intermetatarsal angle, and the first to fifth metatarsal head distance (Fig. 2.79).

First to second metatarsal head elevation is determined by measuring the vertical distance between the superior aspects of the distal metaphyseal flare of the first metatarsal and the second metatarsal; the measurement is performed perpendicular to the ground.[274,275] A normal value is considered to be equal to or less than 8 mm, and a negative value when the first metatarsal point is positioned inferior to the second metatarsal point. Bouaicha et al.[276] modified this measurement technique using a method that provided a different measurement point along the dorsum of the distal metatarsal. However, Christman et al.[277] demonstrated that slight changes in x-ray tube head position can influence the measurement of first to second metatarsal head elevation.

The *Seiberg index* uses two reference points plotted along the dorsum of the first metatarsal: one distal at the distal metaphyseal flare just posterior to the head convexity, and the second 1.5 cm anterior to the first metatarsal-cuneiform joint.[278] Lines perpendicular to the first metatarsal longitudinal axis were made from each point and drawn to the top of the second metatarsal cortex. A negative value is assigned when the first metatarsal point is positioned inferior to the second metatarsal point. The value of the proximal point is then compared to that of the distal point. (The second proximal point was used to account for positional variations that may occur by just using the distal point.) The index value was attained by subtracting the proximal point value from the distal point value.

The *sagittal intermetatarsal angle* is formed between the first and second metatarsal axes in the lateral view; lines tangent to the dorsal surfaces of the two metatarsals are used as the axes as opposed to their longitudinal axes formed by bisections.[279] This technique simplifies the method of subtracting the second metatarsal declination angle from the first metatarsal declination angle used by Schuberth.[271] The normal angle should be nearly 0 degrees, since the two metatarsals are considered normal when the dorsal surfaces of their diaphyses are parallel. The angle is considered a negative value when the first metatarsal is plantarflexed relative to the second metatarsal.

First to fifth metatarsal head distance is measured between the two rays in the lateral view. Lines are drawn tangent to the plantar aspects of the tibial sesamoid and the fifth metatarsal head that are parallel to the plane of support. The perpendicular distance is measured; a value of 5 mm or less was considered normal.[280]

Intrinsic elevation of the first metatarsal can be determined by measuring the angle formed between the tangent to the dorsal diaphyseal surface of the first metatarsal and a tangent line along the cuneiform articular surface of the first metatarsal base, which is normally 90 degrees (Fig. 2.79). Abnormality of this intrinsic relationship is often associated with postoperative metatarsal osteotomy malunion.[281]

Camasta[282] demonstrated that true or primary metatarsus primus elevatus (structural) could be distinguished from secondary (positional) elevatus by repeating the lateral view with the entire foot, from heel to the metatarsophalangeal joints (excluding the toes), under a 1- to 2-in block. The position of the first metatarsal relative to the second metatarsal will remain unchanged with a true metatarsus primus elevatus; however, if the elevatus is positional, for example, related to flexible flatfoot and hallux limitus/rigidus, then the first metatarsal will demonstrate a normal position relative to the second metatarsal.

Axial Sesamoid Position

The position of the tibial sesamoid relative to the first metatarsal head crista (or, intersesamoid ridge) is observed in the sesamoid axial (tangential) view. The traditional method uses 5 positions graded 1-5 (Fig. 2.80); in position 1, the sesamoid

is entirely medial to the crista; in position 3, the sesamoid lays directly under the crista of the first metatarsal head; and in position 5, the sesamoid is entirely lateral to the crista. It has been demonstrated that the amount of dorsiflexion at the first metatarsophalangeal joint can influence this relationship[283]; this stresses the importance of using a weight-bearing sesamoid axial poser for consistency.

First Metatarsal Pronation Angle

Surgical planning for hallux abducto valgus deformity relies heavily on transverse plane radiographs (DP view). However, not taking into consideration, the coronal plane rotation of the first metatarsal can produce disappointing results.[284] Assessing coronal plane rotation is necessary to understand and interpret transverse plane variables. Generally speaking, the terms "external rotation," "valgus," "eversion," and "pronation" are equivalent when referring to coronal plane rotation of the first metatarsal.[285]

Scranton and Rutkowski[286] obtained non–weight-bearing sesamoid axial views on cadavers and measured the angle between two lines drawn as follows: (1) connect points plotted at the center of the first and fifth metatarsal heads and (2) connect points plotted along the inferior aspects of the first metatarsal articular condyles. They found that the angle averaged 3.1 degrees in "normal feet" and 14.5 degrees in feet with "degenerative changes." Unfortunately, application of this method to the weight-bearing sesamoid axial view is difficult because the centers of the first and fifth metatarsal heads are superimposed by their respective phalanges, impairing visibility; possibly using the most inferior points of the fifth metatarsal head and the first metatarsal crista would be an alternative (Fig. 2.81A).

Saltzman reported a method for determining the amount of metatarsal pronation in a weight-bearing sesamoid axial (tangential) view.[287] A line is drawn across the inferior aspect of the

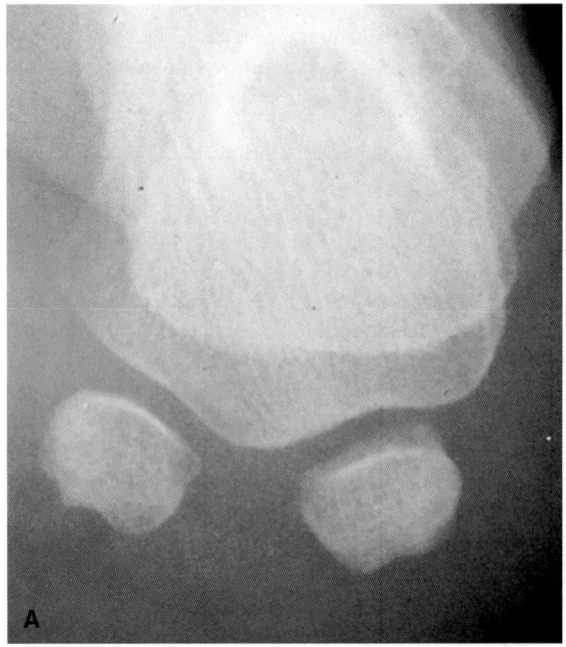
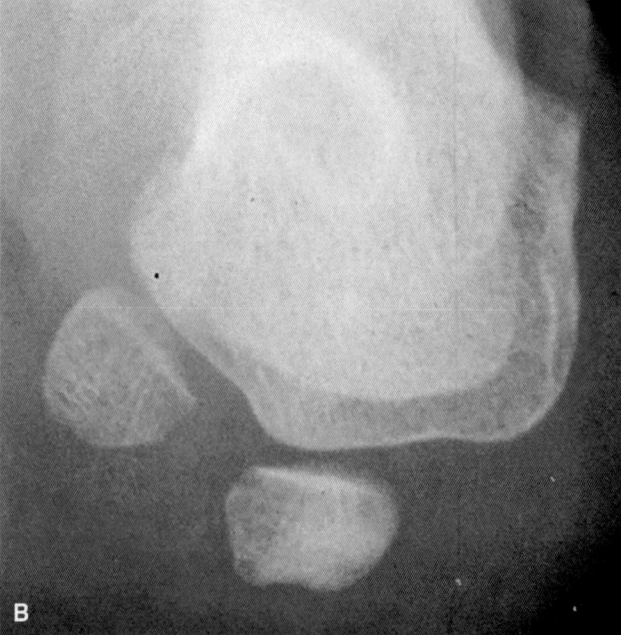

FIGURE 2.80 Axial sesamoid position, 5-grade system. **(A)** Grade 1, **(B)** grade 2, **(C)** grade 3, **(D)** grade 4, **(E)** grade 5.

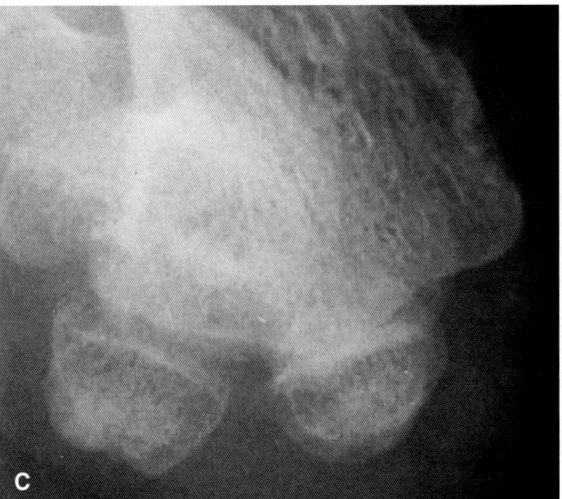

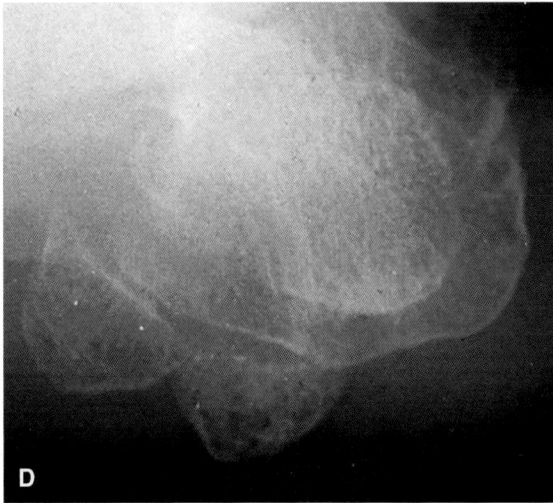

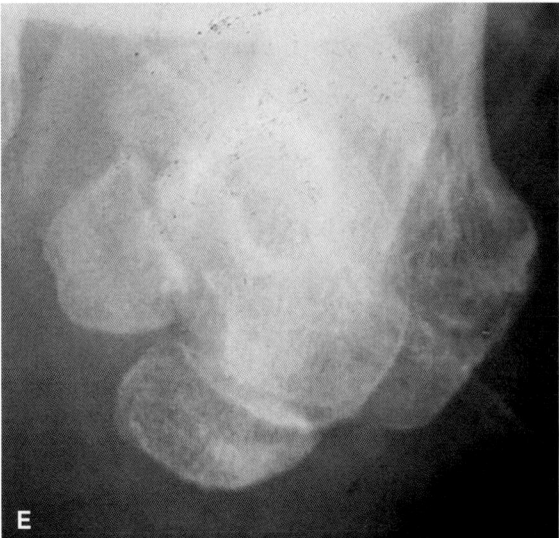

FIGURE 2.80 (*Continued*)

metatarsal head by connecting the following two points: one at the inferolateral aspect of the lateral sulcus and the second at the inferomedial aspect of the medial sulcus (Fig. 2.81B). The rotation angle is measured between this line and the plane of support; the mean metatarsal rotation value was 1.6 degrees for the control group. Ideally, both feet would be positioned in a weight-bearing sesamoid positioning device with equal weight on both feet while performing the radiographic study for each foot.

Eustace et al.[288] described a method to assess metatarsal pronation using the DP view. The position of the posterior apex of the first metatarsal basal tuberosity (inferiorly) was located relative to the first metatarsal axis in the DP view to determine the amount of first metatarsal pronation. They determined that the

tuberosity lined up with the metatarsal axis in its neutral position; the lateral half of the base was then divided into thirds representing 10, 20, and 30 degrees of metatarsal pronation at each one-third position. These categories were then used to classify the amount of metatarsal pronation in weight-bearing DP radiographs (Fig. 2.82).

Hallucal Rotation Angle

There is little attention in the literature regarding coronal plane rotation of the hallux. Talbot and Saltzman[289] developed a radiographic technique for measuring hallucal rotation in the weight-bearing sesamoid axial view. Beadlets (small BBs) are placed on

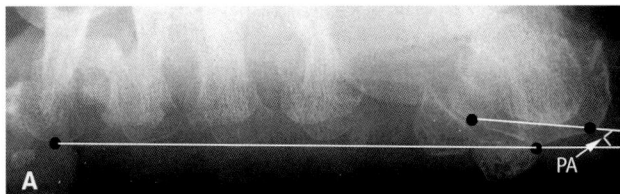

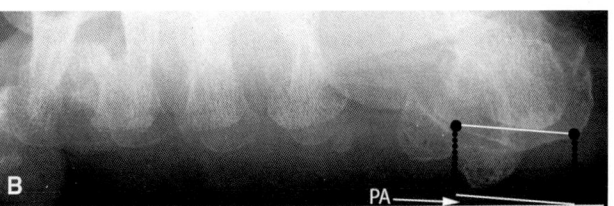

FIGURE 2.81 First metatarsal pronation angle. **A.** Scranton and Rutkowski method. **B.** Saltzman et al. method.

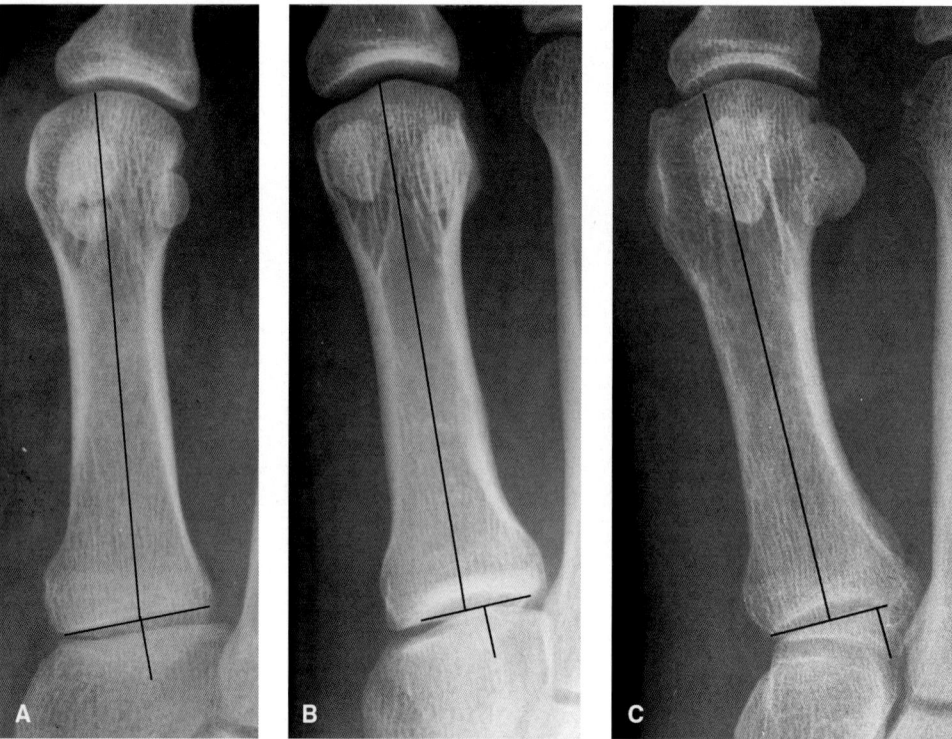

FIGURE 2.82 First metatarsal pronation evaluated by the DP view (Eustace et al. method). **(A)** 0-degree rotation, **(B)** 10-degree rotation, and **(C)** 20-degree rotation.

the medial and lateral aspects of the toenail lunula; these two markers are connected by a line in the resultant radiograph, and the angle is measured between it and the plane of support. The mean hallucal rotation measurement was 7 degrees for the control group and 19 degrees for the bunion group.

Sesamoid Rotation Angle

Kuwano et al.[290] developed the sesamoid rotation angle in order to assess the rotational position of the hallucal sesamoids in the weight-bearing sesamoid axial view. Points were plotted along the most inferior aspects of the tibial and fibular sesamoids; the angle created between a line connecting these points and the plane of support represents the sesamoid rotation angle (Fig. 2.83). The mean angular value for the control group was 7 degrees and 29 degrees for the hallux valgus group.

Medial Cuneiform-First Metatarsal Joint Considerations

The first metatarsal-cuneiform joint has been implicated as an etiology of metatarsus primus varus (or metatarsus adducto valgus), the triplanar term suggested by Dayton et al.,[291] which is

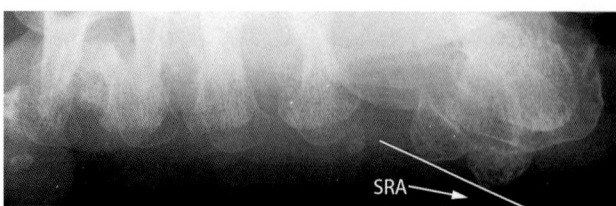

FIGURE 2.83 Sesamoid rotation angle (SRA).

considered to be a major factor in the development of hallux abducto valgus.[253] As a result, many variables have been investigated relating to the shape (square or flat vs round or curve) and orientation (transverse vs oblique or atavism) of the medial cuneiform and its distal articular surface.[256,266]

Obliquity of the medial cuneiform articular surface for the first metatarsal has been assessed using several methods in the DP view (Fig. 2.84). The relationship should normally approximate 90 degrees. The *first metatarsal-medial cuneiform angle* is formed between the first metatarsal bisection and a tangent to the medial cuneiform distal articular surface.[292] The *angle of inclination of the proximal articular surface of the first metatarsal* was formed between a perpendicular to the second metatarsal axis and the first metatarsal proximal articular surface (the latter was considered more precisely drawn than the medial cuneiform distal articular surface).[293] The *obliquity_1 angle* (similar to the angle of inclination of the proximal articular surface of the first metatarsal) is formed between a line parallel to the medial cuneiform-first metatarsal joint and a perpendicular line to the second metatarsal bisection longitudinal axis; the mean value was 17 degrees.[294] The *medial inclination angle* is formed between the transverse tarsal line and the medial cuneiform distal articular surface; the normal mean angle was measured to be 11 degrees in a 10-degree tube head angulation DP view and −6 degrees in a 20-degree DP view.[295] The *first metatarsal proximal obliquity angle* is measured between the first metatarsal longitudinal axis and its basal articular surface; the overall mean angle was 3.42 degrees (measured on bone specimens).[296] The *proximal obliquity angle* was 2.92 degrees when no intermetatarsal facet was present and 4.63 degrees when present.[297] (The presence or absence of a lateral articular facet for the second metatarsal has been investigated as another factor.)[298] The *medial cuneiform joint angle* is

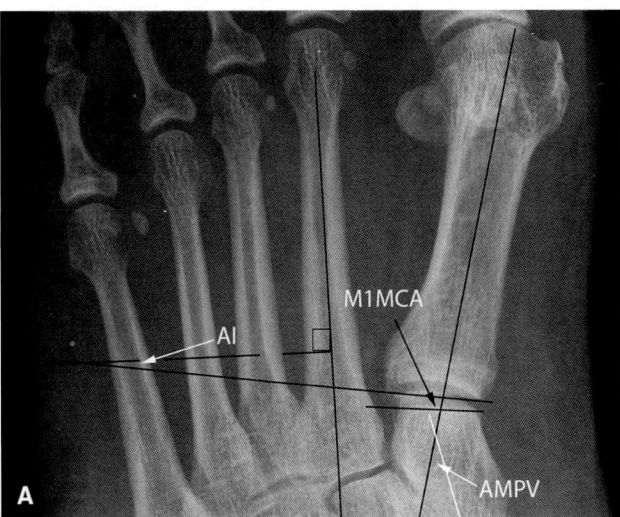
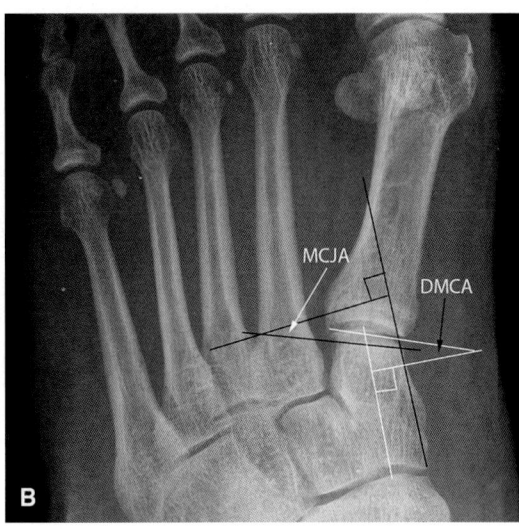

FIGURE 2.84 Medial cuneiform-first metatarsal joint considerations. **A.** First metatarsal-medial cuneiform angle (M1MCA), the angle of inclination of the proximal articular surface of the first metatarsal (AI), and the angle of metatarsus primus varus (AMPV). **B.** Medial cuneiform joint angle (MCJA) and distal medial cuneiform angle (DMCA).

formed between a line perpendicular to a tangent to the medial border of medial cuneiform and a line tangent to the distal articular surface for the first metatarsal; up to 8 degrees medial angulation was considered normal.[299] In a similar fashion, the *distal medial cuneiform angle* is measured between a line through the medial cuneiform-first metatarsal joint and a perpendicular to the medial cuneiform mechanical axis.[300]

The *angle of metatarsus primus varus* is formed between the longitudinal axes of the first metatarsal and medial cuneiform in the DP view (Fig. 2.84A); the angle averaged 18 degrees in the control group.[301] Tanaka[293] found a normal average of 15 degrees. Though controversial, it has been suggested that the metatarsus primus varus deformity is secondary to hallux abducto valgus, since distal surgical correction of the latter reduces the metatarsus primus varus angle.[302]

Plantar gapping (or wedging) of the first metatarsal-medial cuneiform joint and first ray hypermobility has also been investigated.[303] King and Toolan[304] devised two parameters to assess this in the lateral view (Fig. 2.85): the first metatarsal-medial

cuneiform angle is formed between lines drawn tangent to the articular surfaces (normally should be parallel or 0 degrees); the first metatarsal lift measures the distance (perpendicular) between the inferior surface of the first metatarsal base and a line tangent to the inferior surface of the medial cuneiform (normally the two lines should be colinear and, therefore, no measurable distance between them).

The bad news: Sanicola et al.[305] reported that the shape of the joint, medial cuneiform, and base gapping can be changed by foot position during the radiograph exposure, thus causing obliquity of the bone and joint. Differing x-ray beam orientations and changes in foot position can also influence the resulting measurements.[295,299,306] And, in most instances, no statistical significance was found between metatarsal-cuneiform joint obliquity and other hallux abducto valgus parameters. Anatomically, variant obliquity of the joint surface has been described[296,307]; however, how can it be distinguished from positional variation radiographically?

Assessment of Joint Disease and Osteopenia

Preoperative assessment for hallux abducto valgus requires evaluating the first metatarsophalangeal joint for any evidence of joint disease. For example, is the joint space abnormal? Are there any primary joint abnormal findings, such as osteophytes or erosions? Are there any secondary joint abnormalities, such as subchondral sclerosis or geodes? Osteoarthritis is the most common joint disease affecting the first metatarsophalangeal joint and its presence could alter the treatment plan. Hallux limitus and rigidus are discussed later in the "Arthritis" section of this chapter.

The presence or absence of osteopenia is also important to consider preoperatively. This was discussed earlier in this chapter in the section titled "Osteopenia/Osteoporosis Assessment."

BUNIONETTE (TAILOR BUNION)

The literature has discussed numerous methods for radiographic evaluation of tailor bunion; most are performed on

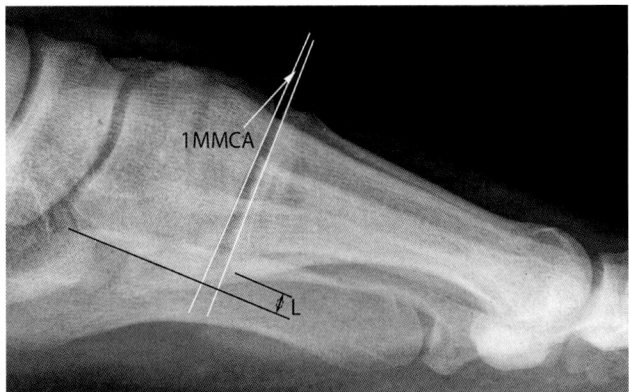

FIGURE 2.85 Plantar gapping of the first metatarsal-medial cuneiform joint. L, lift; 1MMCA, first metatarsal-medial cuneiform angle.

the DP view. The more common measurements/criteria used include the fourth intermetatarsal angle (sometimes referred to as the mini intermetatarsal) angle, the lateral deviation angle, and the size and shape of the fifth metatarsal head. Occasionally, the fifth metatarsophalangeal angle is used as well. Of the angles listed above, only the lateral deviation angle was found to be both poorly reliable and reproducible.[308]

The *fourth intermetatarsal angle* measures divergence between the fourth and fifth metatarsals (Fig. 2.86). The "classic" method uses the longitudinal axes of both metatarsals, which are formed by bisecting the medial and lateral margins of both the proximal and distal metaphyses. The reported range for normal and abnormal varies; however, an angle equal to or greater than 9 degrees has been considered as abnormal and is often associated with symptomatology.[309,310] The angle varies 3 degrees between supination and pronation.[310] The distance between the fourth and fifth metatarsal heads is normally <3 mm.[311]

An alternate method for measuring the fourth intermetatarsal angle was proposed by Fallat and Buckholz[310] to account for anatomical variation of the fifth metatarsal diaphysis, in particular, lateral bowing distally and a wide base proximally. The fifth metatarsal axis is formed by a line adjacent and parallel to the medial surface of the diaphysis proximal half. The angle is formed between this modified axis and the fourth metatarsal longitudinal axis (see Fig. 2.86). Fallat and Buckholz[310] found that, in the normal population, the alternate fourth intermetatarsal angle is 6.47 degrees; a foot with bunionette deformity averaged 8.7 degrees.

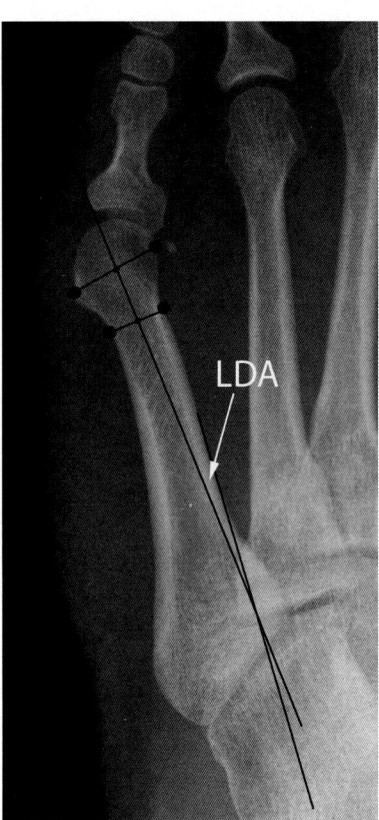

FIGURE 2.87 Lateral deviation angle (LDA). The larger points plotted to determine the head and neck bisections can also be used to measure head and neck widths.

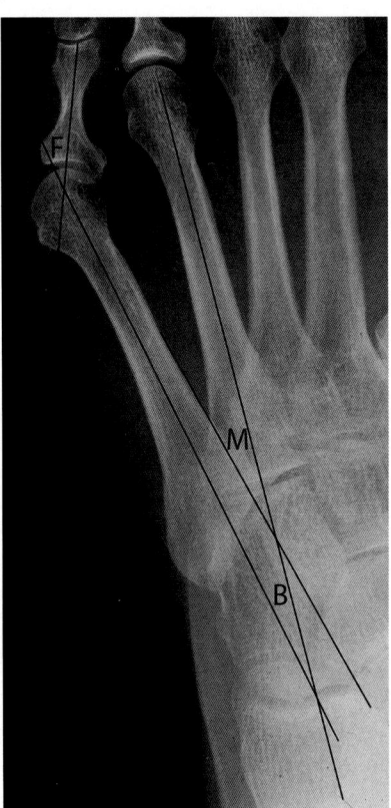

FIGURE 2.86 Fourth intermetatarsal angle. B, angle using bisection of fifth metatarsal; M, angle using medial surface of proximal one-half fifth metatarsal; F, fifth metatarsophalangeal angle.

The *lateral deviation angle* is used to evaluate lateral bowing or curving of the fifth metatarsal shaft distally. The angle was developed to distinguish between fifth metatarsal splaying from the fourth metatarsal (fourth intermetatarsal angle) and distal lateral curving of the fifth metatarsal head on the proximal metatarsal.[310] Although lateral bowing is not commonly associated with bunionette,[312] excessive bowing is believed to contribute to the development of a painful lateral condyle prominence.[309] The lateral deviation angle is formed between the longitudinal bisection of the fifth metatarsal head and neck and a line drawn parallel to the proximal-medial border of the fifth metatarsal diaphysis (Fig. 2.87). Fallat and Buckholz[310] found a significant difference between symptomatic and normal feet; the average angle was 8.05 degrees in symptomatic feet (range 0-16 degrees) compared to 2.64 degrees in "normal" feet (range 0-7 degrees). Pronation of the foot does not change this structural angle. Nestor et al.,[312] however, did not find any significant difference in lateral bowing between symptomatic feet and controls, which averaged 2.4 degrees for each.

The *fifth metatarsophalangeal angle* demonstrates the degree of medial deviation of the fifth toe relative to the fifth metatarsal shaft. The axes used to measure this angle are the bisections of the fifth metatarsal and proximal phalangeal shafts (see Fig. 2.86). The average angle in normal feet is 10 degrees.[313] Patients with bunionette deformity averaged a 16-degree angle, with a range of −5 to +30 degrees.[309] Nestor et al.[312] found a significant difference between symptomatic feet and controls: 16.6 degrees vs 10.2 degrees, respectively.

Several other measurements have been mentioned in the literature relating to bunionette assessment. *Prominence of the fifth*

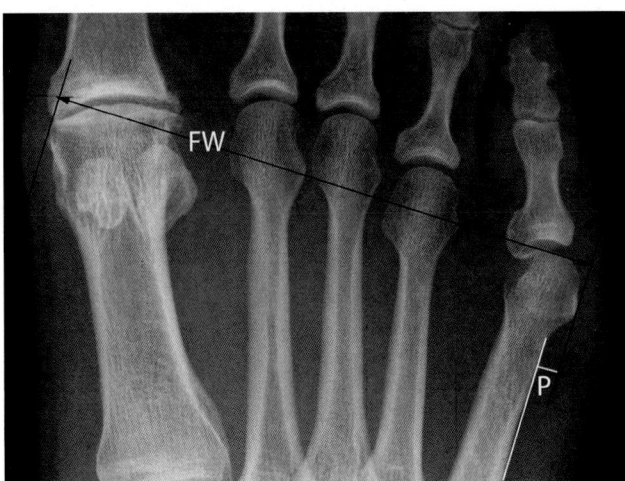

FIGURE 2.88 Prominence of the fifth metatarsal head (P) and forefoot width (FW) measurements.

metatarsal head is measured between the following two lines: (1) a line parallel to the lateral aspect of the fifth metatarsal diaphysis and (2) a line parallel to the first line that is tangent to the most lateral aspect of the prominent fifth metatarsal head (Fig. 2.88); the average distance is 4 mm with a range of 2-9 mm.[314]

Nestor et al.[312] studied the *widths of the fifth metatarsal head and neck* (see Fig. 2.87) in patients with and without Tailor bunion. The fifth metatarsal head width was significantly greater in the symptomatic foot vs the control, 14.2 mm vs 13.2 mm, respectively. They also found that the fifth metatarsal neck width was significantly greater in the symptomatic foot vs the control, 7.5 mm vs 7.0 mm, respectively. However, there was no significant difference in the fifth metatarsal head-neck ratio.

Nestor et al.[312] also advocated analyzing foot width, pre- and postoperatively, as a means to evaluate bunionette deformity and correction. They measured *forefoot width* as the distance between parallel lines that were tangent to the first metatarsal head distal-medially and fifth metatarsal head laterally (Fig. 2.88) and found that forefoot width was significantly greater in patients with bunionette deformity vs the control group (92.5 mm vs 86.8 mm, respectively). Postoperatively, the average foot width was reduced by 6 mm (range, 2-15 mm). However, this technique could be unreliable if patients had prior hallux abducto valgus surgery.[309] Nestor et al.[312] also found that the forefoot width-to-length ratio was significantly greater than the control (second metatarsal length was arbitrarily chosen as the forefoot length).

Bunionette deformity has been classified as four types based upon radiographic findings in the weight-bearing DP radiograph (Fig. 2.89).[315] The *type I bunionette* is an enlarged lateral aspect of the fifth metatarsal head; enlargement may be due to a prominent or hypertrophied lateral tubercle, head rotation secondary to pronation, or a round or dumbbell-shape. However, there is no fifth metatarsal bowing and the fourth intermetatarsal angle is normal. The *type II bunionette* demonstrates lateral bowing of the metatarsal, but the fourth intermetatarsal angle is normal and there is no enlargement of the metatarsal head. The *type III bunionette* exhibits an increased intermetatarsal angle, but there is no metatarsal bowing and no head enlargement. The *type IV bunionette* is a combination of two or more of types of those just described; it has been associated with rheumatoid arthritis.

LESSER TOE DEFORMITY

Positional abnormality of the lesser toe is common and has several appearances. Examples include hammertoe, mallet toe,

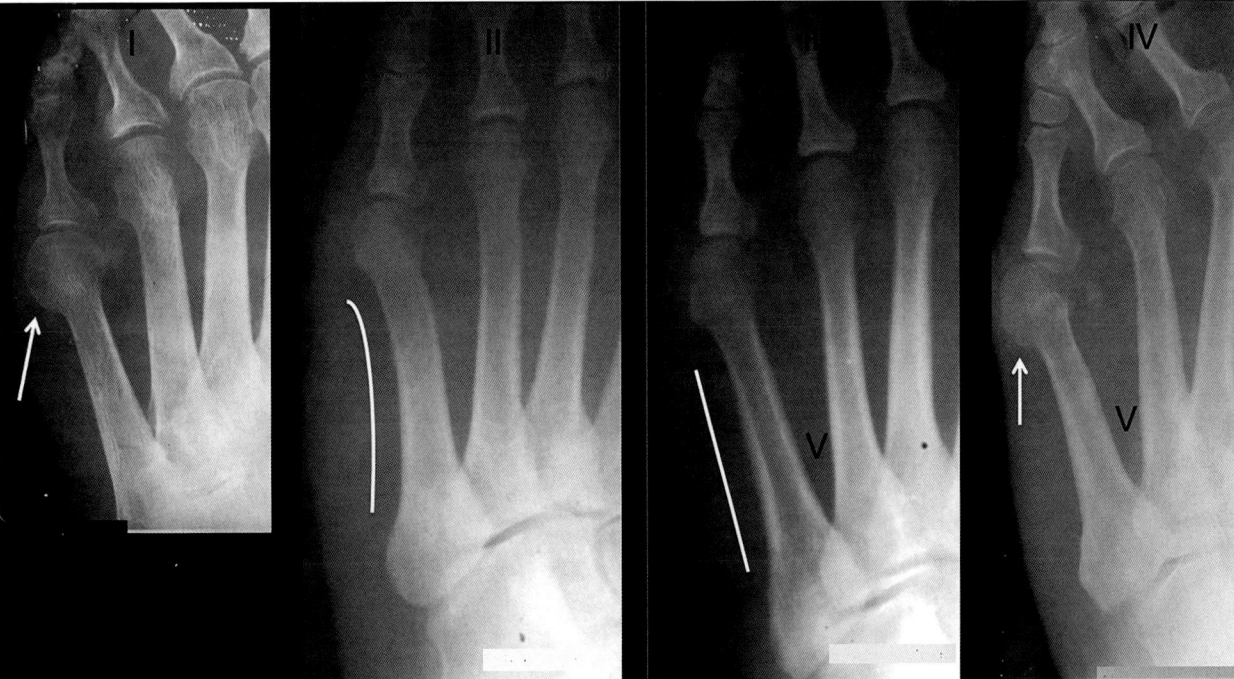

FIGURE 2.89 Bunionette classification, four types (see text for further description). *Arrow*, enlarged head; V, increased intermetatarsal angle; *curved line*, bowing.

adductovarus toe, crossover toe, and divergent toe. The abnormality may be seen in the DP or lateral view, depending upon the plane of the deformity.

The interphalangeal joints are not clearly visible in the DP view when there is sagittal plane deformity due to superimposition of the phalanx base on the adjacent phalanx head; in this case, the deformity is assessed in the lateral view, though superimposition on adjacent toes impairs clear visibility. *Hammertoe* deformity has PIPJ flexion contracture and distal interphalangeal joint hyperextension; the metatarsophalangeal joint is either neutral or extended (Fig. 2.90A). *Claw toe* consists of flexion contractures at the interphalangeal joints of the digit, and most characteristically, extension deformity at the metatarsophalangeal joint (Fig. 2.90B).[316] *Mallet toe* is a plantarflexion deformity of the distal interphalangeal joint; there is minimal to no deformity at the PIPJ or metatarsophalangeal joint (Fig. 2.90C).[317]

The *adductovarus toe* is also referred to as the curly toe. The fifth toe is commonly affected, the fourth and third toes to a lesser degree. There is flexion of the distal and PIPJs, but either flexion or neutral position of the metatarsophalangeal joint. Additionally, there is varus rotation of the toe, which will appear oblique in the DP view (Fig. 2.90D). Therefore, positioning the foot for a medial oblique view will derotate the toe so that it is viewed straight-on. The lateral oblique view will position the adductovarus toe such that it is in a lateral position.

The *crossover toe* demonstrates medial or lateral deviation at the metatarsophalangeal joint. The PIPJ may be neutral or flexed; the distal interphalangeal joint may be neutral, flexed, or extended.[317] It is best appreciated with the DP view (Fig. 2.90E). Crossover toe is frequently associated with severe hallux abducto valgus; the second toe typically deviates medially and dorsally over the hallux.[318] Or, the hallux may push and displace the second toe laterally and dorsally over the third toe. They both may be associated with second metatarsophalangeal joint subluxation. Crossover toe is also associated with first metatarsophalangeal joint osteoarthritis.[319]

Divergent toe exhibits splaying of one digit away from an adjacent digit; depending upon the direction of divergence,

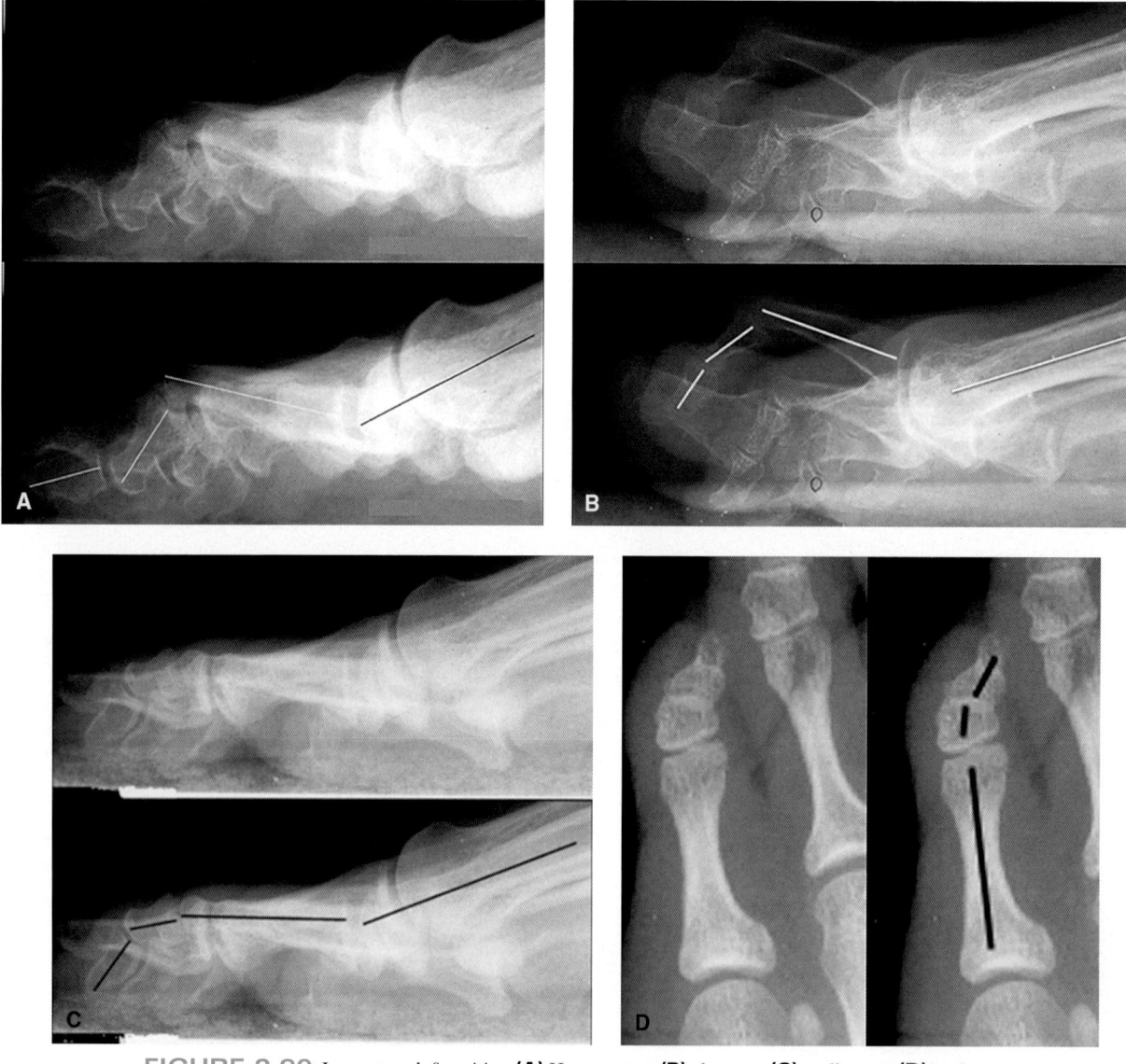

FIGURE 2.90 Lesser toe deformities. **(A)** Hammertoe, **(B)** claw toe, **(C)** mallet toe, **(D)** curly toe, **(E)** crossover toe, and **(F)** divergent toe (*arrow,* uncovering of metatarsal head).

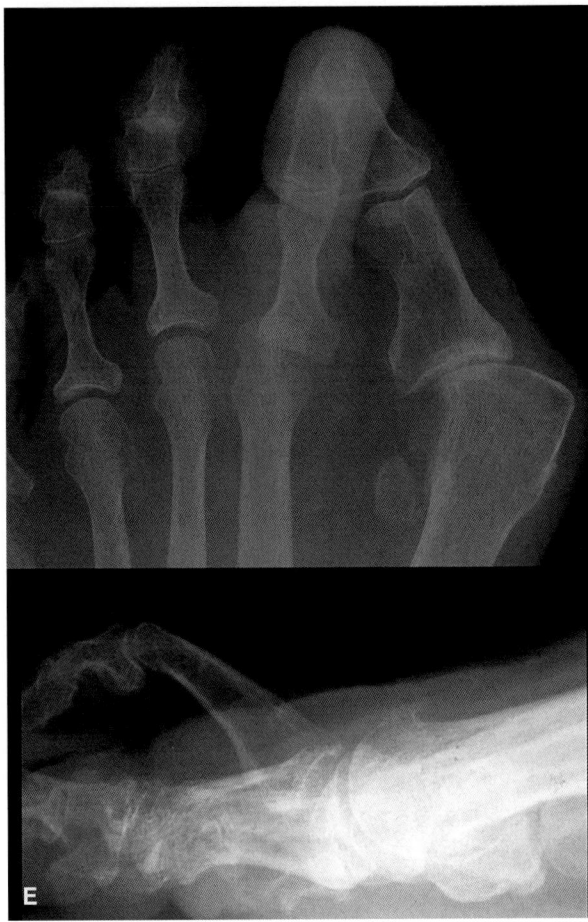

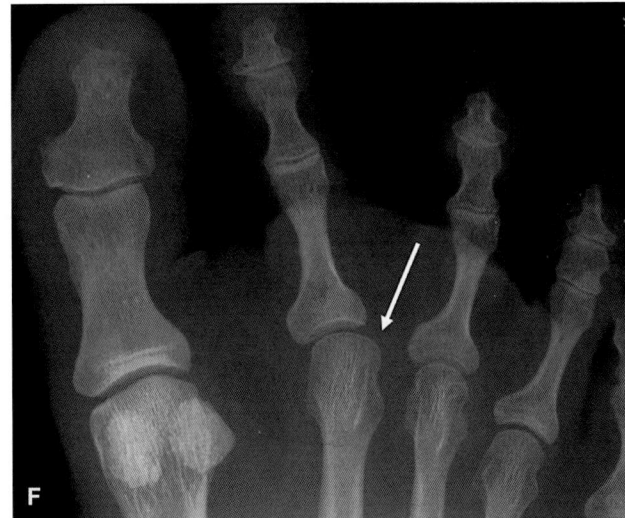

FIGURE 2.90 (*Continued*)

it may be referred to as either digitus adductus or abductus.[320] Uncovering of the metatarsal head may occur (Fig. 2.90F), which is suggestive of plantar plate degeneration or tear in the proper clinical setting. Plantar plate degeneration or tear can also be evaluated by arthrography, ultrasound, and MRI.

PREDISLOCATION SYNDROME

A condition that results in progressive subluxation or dislocation of the lesser metatarsophalangeal joint has been referred to as predislocation syndrome. It typically involves the second metatarsophalangeal joint and is related to plantar plate pathology (degeneration, tearing). The second toe drifts into varus, eventually crossing over the hallux. Radiographically, DP, lateral, and sesamoid axial views are recommended. Findings may include splaying between the second and third toes and uncovering of the second metatarsal head laterally (Fig. 2.90F) that progresses to subluxation and, ultimately, dislocation if left untreated. Since it is progressive, its presentation radiographically may vary depending upon the severity. It has been associated with a long second metatarsal, which is considered a risk factor; the best method to assess this was by Nilsonne metatarsal protrusion index (described earlier in the "Hallux Abducto Valgus" section).[321] The condition is further assessed and confirmed by musculoskeletal ultrasound or MRI (or arthrography, less commonly).

TRAUMA

GENERAL CONSIDERATIONS

Radiography should not be performed on every patient presenting with a history of trauma. Nor should they be ordered prior to performing an appropriate history and physical examination. Criteria are available for the acutely injured ankle and foot, known as the *Ottawa Ankle Rules* (OAR), which were designed to minimize false-negative results. They have been reproduced and validated in different types of medical settings and boast a nearly 100% sensitivity.[322] The need for radiographs associated with acute ankle injury, especially in the emergency department, has the potential to be reduced by at least 30%, reducing the cost of treating ankle injuries.[323] Ankle radiographs are indicated if there is tenderness upon palpation of either malleolus inferiorly or posteriorly or along the distal 6 cm posterior edge of the tibia/fibula. The inability to bear weight both immediately following the injury and upon evaluation for four steps independently, even if limping, is an indication for radiography. A modification of the OAR, referred to as the "Buffalo Rule," includes tenderness over the crest or midportion of the tibial or fibula, between the tip of the malleolus up to 6 cm proximally.[324] The OAR has been refined to include the midfoot: radiography is indicated if there is tenderness at the fifth metatarsal base or navicular bone following injury.[325] The OAR can also be applied to children older than 5 years of age.[326]

The *Low Risk Ankle Rule* is a decision rule used for children with acute ankle injury. It states that radiography may not be indicated if swelling and/or tenderness are isolated to the lateral ligaments distal to the tibial plafond and/or the distal fibula. This rule also boasts 100% sensitivity for "clinically important" fractures of the distal fibula and has the potential to reduce radiographic studies by nearly 60%.[327]

Despite these guidelines, not all patients with acute injury meet the inclusion criteria. For example, the OAR should not be used if the patient is a diabetic with peripheral neuropathy,[328] there is any skin wound or evidence of penetrating trauma, other bone pathology exists, or the injury occurred at least 10 days ago and the patient is experiencing persistent pain.[329] Radiographs should be ordered if there is the potential for a midfoot/Lisfranc injury, since they are frequently overlooked.[330] Toes and metatarsal heads are not included in these criteria.

Radiography is considered the initial study of choice when appropriate; if radiographs are not conclusive, then further study with CT, MRI, or bone scintigraphy may be indicated. A minimum of two views are required, preferably planar and orthogonal (DP and lateral foot; AP and lateral ankle); however, three views are often recommended, including the medial oblique (foot) and mortise (ankle). Choose views intelligently; do not just choose routine views. For example, pain on palpation of the superolateral aspect of the calcaneocuboid joint region is best isolated with the lateral oblique foot view, not the medial oblique (see "Considerations When Ordering the Radiographic Study" at the beginning of this chapter). If there is suspicion of abnormality, consider obtaining additional views. And, do not dismiss specialty views; Broden views are valuable for assessing intra-articular calcaneal fractures.[331] Repeat the radiographic study in 10 days if the initial study is unremarkable but fracture is suspected and symptoms persist.

Radiographs should be obtained following the initial study after ~6-8 weeks to assess the presence of healing. One may be tempted to order radiographs more frequently, especially postoperatively. However, if clinically the patient is doing well and there have been no setbacks (reinjury, unexpected pain or swelling, etc.), then radiographs will more than likely show no significant changes or evidence of healing for at least 4 weeks. A radiographic study should also be performed postfracture reduction and postimmobilization, as well as after each cast or traction change and before final discharge of the patient from your care. Any radiographic changes in fracture position should be reassessed 1 or 2 weeks later.

Accessory ossicles are occasionally misinterpreted as fracture. Examples are presented in the "Normal Radiographic Anatomy and Variants" section of this chapter.

FRACTURE TERMINOLOGY

The term fracture refers to a break in the bone's continuity. A complete fracture involves the entire circumference or both cortical surfaces of a bone; an incomplete fracture does not. Incomplete fractures (greenstick, torus) occur in children and were discussed earlier in this chapter in the section "Pediatrics."

A *comminuted fracture* is defined as having at least two fracture lines that result in at least three or more fracture segments. A small triangular or wedge-shaped fragment off the cortex of a tubular bone is referred to as a "butterfly" fragment. The term segmental is used when an intact segment of diaphyseal bone is located between two fracture lines.

A *pathologic fracture* is a break through existing abnormal bone (such as a bone tumor). An avulsion fracture occurs at the insertion of a tendon or ligament. An *intra-articular fracture* extends into the subchondral bone plate and enters the joint. A *malunion fracture* results after the healing of two bone segments that are significantly malaligned and/or displaced; there typically is significant angulation and/or displacement between the two segments with compensatory remodeling.

An *impaction (depression) fracture* typically results from a portion of harder bone jamming into softer adjacent bone; it can be very subtle, resulting in only minimal deformity, including bone shortening. A double cortical contour may be the only finding.[332]

Osteochondritis dissecans (osteochondrosis dissecans) is an osteochondral fracture, with complete or incomplete separation of a portion of joint cartilage and underlying bone. The fragment may appear as a loose body of bone in the joint.

Osteonecrosis results from bone ischemia; trauma is probably the most common etiology of osteonecrosis in the foot. Initially, bone appears normal radiographically; therefore, acute posttraumatic osteonecrosis is difficult to diagnose with radiographs. The "classic" radiographic picture of osteonecrosis in bones such as the talus or navicular is sclerosis, which represents an old, healed process after bone remodeling has occurred months or years later. The presence of a curvilinear decreased density that parallels the subchondral bone plate, such as along the talar dome (Hawkins sign), indicates an intact vascular supply to the talar body.

Repetitive stress to normal or abnormal bone can result in a *stress fracture*. An insufficiency stress fracture results from normal stress on weakened bone (such as in osteoporosis), a type of pathologic fracture. A fatigue stress fracture results from abnormal stress to normal bone. The radiographic findings vary and depend on whether the stress fracture involves cortical or cancellous bone. Cortical bone stress fracture, such as that seen in the lesser metatarsal diaphysis, demonstrates a small cortical discontinuity and/or periosteal reaction after ~10-14 days (Fig. 2.91A). The longer the delay in imaging and treatment, the more exuberant the periosteal reaction. If the patient continues to walk on the injured bone, it may proceed to become a complete fracture. In contrast, cancellous bone stress fracture, affecting the tarsal bones or the metatarsal base or head, will demonstrate an ill-defined increased density within the bone, a finding not visible radiographically until 4-8 weeks later (Fig. 2.91B). Bone scintigraphy or MRI can be used for earlier diagnosis.

JOINT AND SOFT TISSUE

Normally, the articular surfaces of two bones appose each other 100%. Partial apposition (1%-99%) between two bones at a joint is referred to as *subluxation*; 0% apposition is known as *luxation* or *dislocation*. Terminology used to describe positioning of the distal bone relative to the proximal are the same that are used to describe the position of fracture fragments.

Dislocation of a metatarsophalangeal or interphalangeal joint may be difficult to appreciate radiographically. The dorsally dislocated phalanx is often superimposed on the metatarsal head in the DP view, as one might see in joint contracture. Though there is superimposition of multiple bones in the lateral view, it is the only image demonstrating displacement that

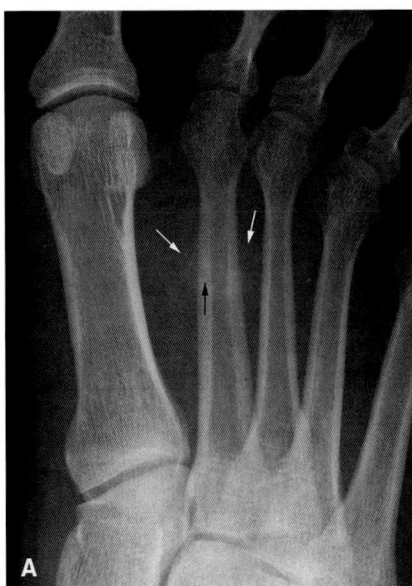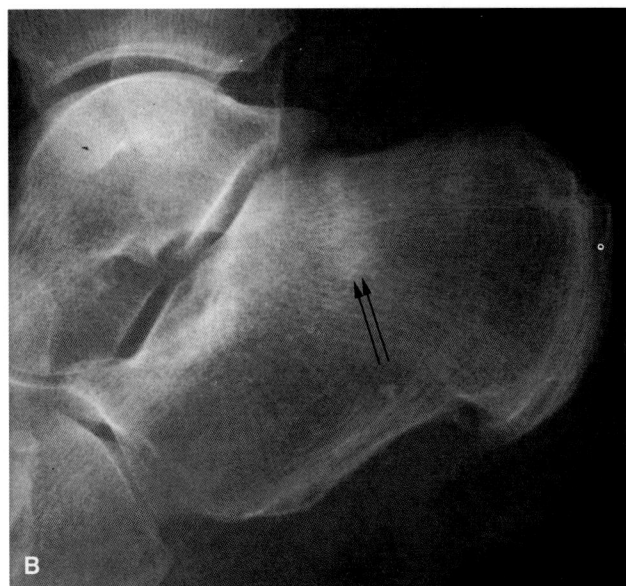

FIGURE 2.91 Stress fracture of **(A)** cortical bone and **(B)** cancellous bone. *White arrows,* periosteal reaction; *single black arrow,* hairline cortical discontinuity; *double black arrows,* ill-defined increased density.

occurs in the sagittal plane. Oblique views are helpful but not necessarily definitive.

Diastasis refers to separation or widening between two normally attached bones where there is no true joint.[109] The best example in the lower extremity is the syndesmosis between the distal tibia and fibula.

The ankle joint capsule is redundant anteriorly and posteriorly to allow for ankle dorsiflexion and plantarflexion. When inflammatory fluid accumulates following trauma, it appears radiographically as increased soft tissue density and can be diagnosed as *joint effusion* (Fig. 2.92). Increased soft tissue density

seen anteriorly in the lateral ankle view, whether it be related to trauma, arthritis, or infection, etc., may have a distinct shape that has been referred to as the teardrop sign.[333] It has been reported that 5 mL of fluid is necessary for ankle effusion to be visualized in a lateral radiograph; smaller amounts may be detected with MRI and sonography.[334]

FRACTURE DESCRIPTION

Terminology should be used to fully describe the fracture configuration, location, alignment, and amount of apposition; other terms, such as intra-articular, are used when appropriate. The term "fracture," the diagnosis, should not be used in the interpretation of findings; descriptive terms may include cortical or focal discontinuity, linear decreased density, etc. Eponyms and/or classifications should not be used alone, which are sometimes confusing or may be archaic; also, some fractures may not always fit into a category.[335] At a minimum, describe the fracture in a fashion such that it resembles the radiographic picture.[336] If prior diagnostic images are available, compare them to the latest study and document any changes.

Fracture configuration refers to the orientation or geometry of the fracture line. In a tubular bone, it may be transverse (perpendicular to the diaphysis), oblique (diagonal to the diaphysis), or spiral (wrapping around the diaphysis).[337] The edges of the spiral fracture bone fragments may appear sharp and pointed; the fracture line itself may not be clearly visible.[338] The term "oblique-transverse" is sometimes used to describe a fracture line that is <30 degrees angulated to the diaphysis.

A tubular bone diaphysis can be divided into thirds, and the fracture location is then described based on this location "grid," if possible. In Figure 2.93, for example, the second metatarsal fracture is transverse/slightly oblique and located in the distal one-third of the diaphysis. If the fracture were in between the distal and middle one-third of the diaphysis, one would state that it is located at the junction between the distal and middle thirds shaft. Anatomic landmarks may be referenced, when

FIGURE 2.92 Ankle joint effusion (*arrows*).

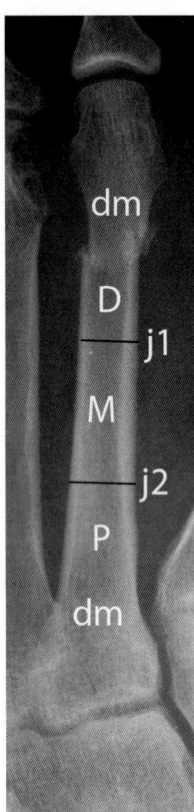

FIGURE 2.93 Tubular bone "grid" for describing fracture location. D, distal one-third diaphysis; M, middle one-third diaphysis; P, proximal one-third diaphysis; j1, junction between the distal and middle thirds shaft; j2, junction between the middle and proximal thirds shaft; dm, diametaphysis.

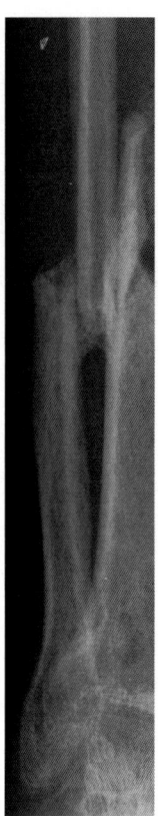

FIGURE 2.94 Bayonet position of the distal fibula lateral to the proximal segment.

appropriate. Otherwise, be very descriptive as to its location (distal or proximal diametaphysis, distal or proximal metaphysis, etc.).

Fracture assessment includes a description of the position of one fragment's longitudinal axis relative to another; the convention is to describe the position of the distal segment relative to the proximal segment.[339] More specifically, displacement (translation) and angulation (alignment) are described, including the direction and amount (a percentage or angle). The position in two planar views at 90 degrees should be described together. There may be displacement with or without angulation, and vice versa. (This same terminology is used to describe position abnormality associated with joint subluxation and dislocation.) It is very difficult to determine if there is rotation of a fracture segment but report it if obvious.

Fracture *displacement*, or translation, refers to the amount of apposition between the two segments. No displacement demonstrates 100% apposition. Attempt to specify the amount of apposition in addition to the displaced direction of the distal segment relative to the proximal when present; for example, in Figure 2.93, the distal fracture segment is displaced medially ~20% (or, with 80% apposition between the two segments). Rarely, the distal segment may be fully displaced, retracted (resulting in shortening), and positioned longitudinally alongside the proximal segment; this is referred to as bayonet position (Fig. 2.94). Any separation or gap between the two fragments, that is, distraction, should be mentioned as well.

Angulation refers to when two fracture segments are not aligned, that is, they are angled. The term alignment indicates an arrangement between the two fragments that are in a straight or parallel line; there is no angulation. The direction of angulation can be described in two manners: (1) by the distal segment axis direction relative to the proximal segment axis and (2) by the direction of the vertex formed between longitudinal axes of the two segments. The latter method is the opposite direction of the former and one should specify that it is the vertex direction; if this method is used, it is preferable to mention both so as to avoid confusion.[339] The direction of the distal segment relative to the proximal can also be determined by drawing lines along the ends of the two fracture surfaces; the vertex formed between these two lines corresponds to the fracture direction (Fig. 2.95).

Unless the true angular deformity is in a reference plane (DP view-transverse plane and lateral view-sagittal plane for the foot, AP view-coronal plane and lateral view-sagittal plane for the ankle), which is infrequent, the true angular deformity in an image will always be underestimated as a translational deformity.[9] Correlating the fracture position in both 45-degree oblique views improves precision. This principle applies to both long bone fractures and osteotomies.

Calcaneal joint depression fracture may be subtle and overlooked; two angles measured in the lateral view have been used to assess this fracture: Böhler angle and the critical angle of Gissane.

Böhler (or tuber joint) angle is formed by plotting three points: one at the highest point of the anterior calcaneal process, a second at the highest point of the posterior articular surface, and the third at the most superior point of the bursal projection

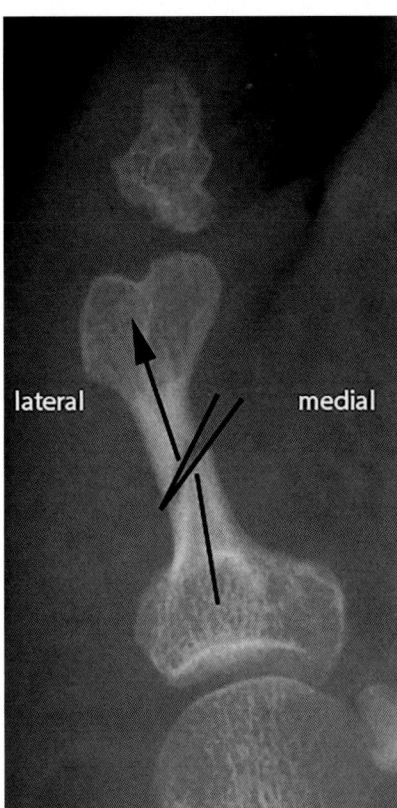

FIGURE 2.95 Fracture angulation. The distal segment axis (*arrow*) is angulated (*points*) laterally relative to the proximal segment. The *two horizontal lines* are tangent to the fracture segment ends; since the apex points laterally, this confirms the initial assessment using the axes.

(Fig. 2.96). By connecting these three points, two lines will form, and the normal angle between them has been reported as ranging anywhere between 10 and 40 degrees,[340] though Böhler[341] originally described it as being between 30 and 35 degrees. Böhler angle will decrease with joint depression fractures; the two lines may even appear to be parallel to one another.

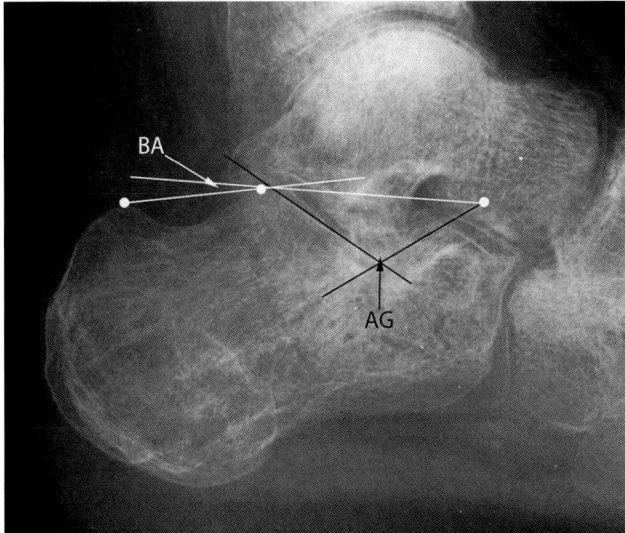

FIGURE 2.96 Böhler angle (BA) and critical angle of Gissane (AG).

The *critical or crucial angle of Gissane* is formed by two lines that have not been clearly defined in the literature. One line is formed along the articular surface of the posterior calcaneal facet, and the second line extends from the highest point of the anterior calcaneal process to the calcaneal sulcus (or fossa) of the sinus tarsi (see Fig. 2.96); generally speaking, the lines parallel the margins of the lateral talar process. The normal range was established to be between 120 and 145 degrees.[342] However, the angle was found to have poor inter-rater reliability and was not useful for diagnosing calcaneal fractures in an emergency department setting.[343] Of interest, the original source referenced for this angle in the literature has no mention of the measurement; in fact, the reference is to the minutes ("news notes") of a British Orthopaedic Association meeting, and one sentence refers to Mr. Gissane.[344] Furthermore, the measurement range was established 35 years later! The critical angle may be crucial but apparently was a reference to an anatomical landmark, not a measured angle.[345]

FRACTURE HEALING

The earlier radiographic features of secondary fracture healing in a tubular bone include increased soft tissue density and volume, localized osteopenia, bone resorption at the fracture margins, and ill-defined periosteal reaction, followed by diffuse sclerosis, well-defined periosteal reaction and bone remodeling. The findings just described occur in the sequence listed, for the most part; however, there is significant overlap, especially with the earlier findings. And, mixed osteopenia and increased density (sclerosis) may be seen together. The time frame can also vary considerably and is dependent upon the fracture configuration and type, patient age, immobilization (or lack of), whether or not there is intra-articular extension or comminution, etc. Remodeling at the fracture site, depending upon the amount of malposition, may occur over the course of months or even years. Due to superimposition of the latter findings (diffuse sclerosis, well-defined periosteal reaction) on the fracture line, the fracture may appear united; these findings must be correlated with the clinical picture and can be confirmed with fluoroscopy or CT, if indicated. Bone scintigraphy, ultrasound, and MRI also have been used, with mixed results.[346]

Nontubular bone fracture healing may only exhibit ill-defined increased density that progresses to well-defined sclerosis.

Though there is no uniform consensus regarding the definition of fracture union, the following criteria have commonly been used: callus or trabeculae bridging the fracture line; callus that bridges in at least 3 of the 4 cortices in radiographs taken in 2 planes; and cortical continuity with no visible fracture line.[347] However, radiographs alone should not be used to decide if the fracture is healed; clinical criteria should be considered as well. There is no uniformly accepted definition of delayed union; it is based upon clinical appraisal.

There are no standard criteria for diagnosing nonunion fracture.[346] In general, a fracture is said to be a nonunion if it has failed to heal in a 9-month period of time and there has been no radiographic evidence of progression over a 3-month time frame.[348] The radiographic appearance of nonunion varies and has been classified based upon four types: hypertrophic "elephant foot," hypertrophic "horse foot," oligotrophic, and atrophic.[349] *Hypertrophic "elephant foot"* nonunion demonstrates significant sclerosis at the fracture margins and an overabundance of well-defined periosteal reaction that does

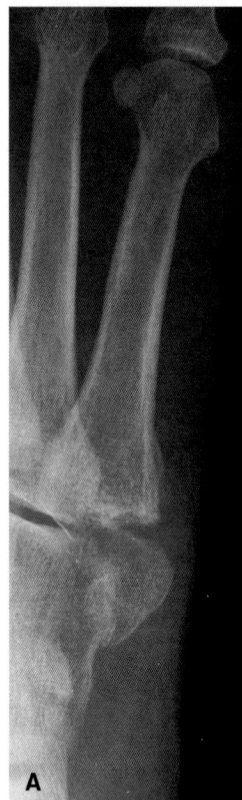

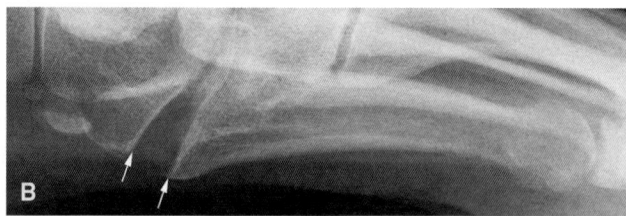

FIGURE 2.97 Oligotrophic nonunion. **(A)** DP view, **(B)** lateral view. *Arrows* identify thin, well-defined sclerotic margins.

not bridge the fracture line. *Hypertrophic "horse foot" nonunion* demonstrates sclerosis at the fracture margins and a smaller amount of well-defined periosteal reaction. The *oligotrophic nonunion* has sclerotic margins with no evidence of well-defined periosteal reaction (Fig. 2.97). The *atrophic nonunion* type has minimal or no sclerosis at the fracture margins and no evidence of well-defined periosteal reaction; there may even be osteopenia at the fracture margins. *Pseudarthrosis* is a term used for an end-stage nonunion that develops a synovial-like joint.

ARTHRITIS

The primary joint disorders affecting the foot and ankle include osteoarthritis, rheumatoid arthritis, seronegative arthritis, gouty arthritis, Charcot neuropathic osteoarthropathy, and septic arthritis. A radiologic classification of these joint disorders is based on primary radiographic findings, which include the following: osteophyte, osseous erosion, subchondral resorption, and arthritis mutilans.[350] Table 2.12 lists joint disorders associated with these findings; note that two joint disorders, Charcot neuropathic osteoarthropathy and psoriatic arthritis, may present with one of two primary findings.

PRIMARY FINDINGS

An *osteophyte* is a bony outgrowth at the marginal or central region of a joint.[351] To further define the osteophyte, it can be differentiated from two other terms, spur and exostosis (Fig. 2.98). A spur, or *enthesophyte*, forms at an enthesis (attachment site for joint capsule, ligament, or tendon), that is, where soft tissue attaches to bone; the diagnosis is referred to as enthesopathy.[352]

In contrast, an exostosis is not found at an enthesis; exostoses are typically found along the outer surface of the diaphysis (examples include the posttraumatic exostosis and osteochondroma).

An osteophyte can have many different presentations, and figurative terms have been used to describe them. The more common figurative terms include "flagging," such as seen along the dorsal aspect of the first metatarsal head, and "lipping," seen along the dorsal aspect of the talonavicular joint. The term talar "beak," associated with tarsal coalition, probably represents a spur; this bony outgrowth is found proximal to the articular edge at the talar neck ridge, an enthesis for talonavicular and ankle joint capsule and ligaments.[353]

TABLE 2.12	Radiologic Classification of Primary Joint Disorders in the Foot and Ankle Categorized by Primary Radiographic Findings
Primary Radiographic Finding	**Joint Disorder**
Osteophyte	Osteoarthritis
Erosion (osseous)	Rheumatoid arthritis, seronegative arthritis (psoriatic arthritis, reactive arthritis, and ankylosing spondylitis), gouty arthritis
Subchondral resorption	Charcot neuropathic osteoarthropathy, septic arthritis
Arthritis mutilans	Charcot neuropathic osteoarthropathy, psoriatic arthritis, rheumatoid arthritis (fifth MPJ only)

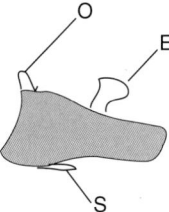

FIGURE 2.98 Examples of "bony outgrowth." Spur (S), osteophyte (O), and exostosis (E). (Figure 11-10 from Marchis-Crisan C, Christman RA. Joint disease. In: Christman RA, ed. *Foot and Ankle Radiology*. 2nd ed. Philadelphia, PA: Wolters Kluwer; 2015:345-380.)

Osseous erosion, in contrast to cartilaginous erosion that cannot be directly seen radiographically, is typically found along the margin of a joint (medial and/or lateral margin in a DP view). Its location may be intra-articular (within the joint capsule) or extra-articular. When intra-articular, it is important to note whether the erosion is located along the medial, lateral, or both sides of the joint; rheumatoid arthritis, for example, rarely affects the lateral side of the second, third, or fourth metatarsal heads. (Be aware that the normal concavity along the lateral aspect of the lesser metatarsal head in the DP view is often misinterpreted as an erosion, as in Fig. 2.99.) Also, erosion along both the medial and lateral aspects of a joint may lead to arthritis mutilans. The margin of an erosion may either be ill defined or well defined; the latter may or may not be accompanied by a sclerotic margin. An ill-defined erosion indicates an acute process, a well-defined erosion a chronic one. Erosion may or may not be accompanied with joint space narrowing. Furthermore,

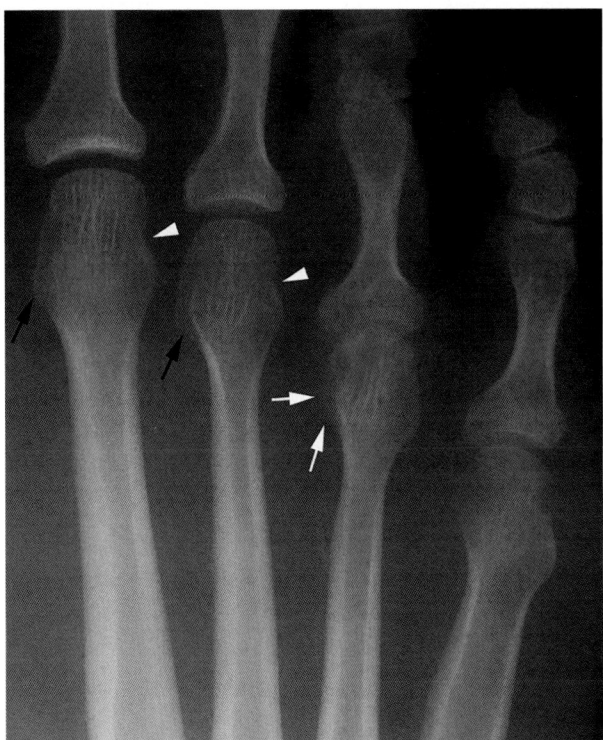

FIGURE 2.99 Pre-erosion, fourth metatarsal head medial aspect. *White arrowheads,* normal concavity sometimes misinterpreted as erosion; *black arrows,* normal subchondral bone plate; *white arrows,* absent subchondral bone plate (pre-erosion).

erosion may or may not be associated with new bone production. The presence or absence of secondary findings (discussed next) will help to narrow down the differential diagnosis.

The subchondral bone plate presents as a thin, well-defined increased density along the cartilaginous margin of a joint; it should be continuous from one side of the joint to the other. A pre-erosion becomes evident when a portion of that subchondral bone plate is absent (see Fig. 2.99). If you were to trace the subchondral bone plate at an affected joint, you may notice a "skip" in the bone plate; if there is more than one "skip," this may give a "dot-dash" appearance.

Subchondral resorption, which occurs centrally in a joint, may have one or a combination of the following three presentations: (1) disappearance of the subchondral bone plate centrally; (2) the subchondral bone plate may be visible, but there is rarefaction (decreased density) immediately adjacent to it; or (3) there may be loss of the subchondral bone plate centrally and adjacent rarefaction, which usually presents as osteolysis.

Arthritis mutilans is a combination of marginal erosion and central subchondral resorption.

At a metatarsophalangeal joint, the combination of medial and lateral erosion of the metatarsal head and central subchondral resorption of the adjacent phalanx base results in a picture that has been figuratively described as "pencil-in-cup," "mortar-in-pestle," "whittling," and "sucked candy." At an interphalangeal joint, arthritis mutilans usually appears as absence (resorption) of a phalangeal head and the adjacent phalanx base. Severe cases of arthritis mutilans demonstrate gross disappearance of bones.

SECONDARY FINDINGS

The secondary findings associated with joint disease help one narrow the differential diagnosis. These may include one or more of the following: bone production; alteration of joint space; soft tissue abnormality; detritus; and geode.

Bone production examples include periostitis, whiskering, ivory phalanx, sclerosis (diffuse or subchondral), and an overhanging margin of bone over an erosion (Martel sign). It is unusual for any bone production listed above to be associated with rheumatoid arthritis. Periostitis adjacent to affected joints may be seen in seronegative arthritis. Whiskering and the ivory phalanx, targeting the hallux distal phalanx, are associated with psoriatic arthritis. A C-shaped erosion with an overhanging margin of bone is a characteristic feature of long-standing gouty arthritis. Diffuse sclerosis is seen in the midfoot as Charcot neuropathic osteoarthropathy remodels. Subchondral sclerosis may be seen with osteoarthritis.

Joint space alterations include narrowing (uneven or even), widening, and loss of 100% apposition between the two bones. Since erosion in gouty arthritis is often extra articular, there is sparing of the joint space; in contrast, the joint space narrows early in inflammatory arthritis, such as rheumatoid or seronegative arthritis. Joint space narrowing is evenly (uniformly) distributed in rheumatoid arthritis, uneven in osteoarthritis. Subchondral resorption at both ends of the joint will give the appearance of joint space widening.[354] Loss of 100% joint apposition occurs in rheumatoid arthritis.

Soft tissue abnormalities include increased volume and density, "sausage toe," "lumpy-bumpy" and fusiform-shaped masses, and calcification. The presence of a "lumpy-bumpy" mass with calcification adjacent to a joint occurs in gouty arthritis.

A fusiform soft tissue mass may represent a rheumatoid nodule, and edema involving an entire digit ("sausage toe") is seen with psoriatic and reactive arthritis.

Detritus refers to bony fragmentation and the presence of a loose body in a joint (sometimes referred to as a "joint mouse"). Fragmentation is associated with Charcot neuropathic osteoarthropathy and septic arthritis, and loose bodies with osteoarthritis.

A *geode*, commonly referred to as a bone "cyst," may or may not have a sclerotic margin. It is typically subchondral in location and frequently associated with osteoarthritis but may also be seen in rheumatoid arthritis, usually without the sclerotic margin.

ENTHESOPATHY

Several joint disorders may demonstrate abnormal findings in the lateral foot view at the calcaneal entheses. Enthesopathy, defined as an alteration at an enthesis,[355] may present as either bone production, resorption, or a combination (Fig. 2.100A). Spurs (enthesophytes) are the most common example of bone production and may be well or ill defined. Well-defined spurs are a feature of the common degenerative joint disease; inferior calcaneal spurs classically are hooked and pointed but may appear blunt and straight. Another rheumatic disorder, DISH (diffuse idiopathic skeletal hyperostosis) is associated with unusually large spurs.

Inferior calcaneal spurring is also associated with inflammatory joint disease (rheumatoid and seronegative arthritis); though these spurs, when well formed, may not be distinguishable from degenerative spurs, they may appear irregular and/or ill defined if encountered early in the disease process.[356] They also may be accompanied by ill-defined increased density in the adjacent tubercle and mixed with ill-defined osteopenia or even erosion in seronegative arthritis. It has been reported that 50% of patients have a bursa inferior to the calcaneal tuberosity[357]; this may account for erosion associated with inflammatory joint disease. Inferior calcaneal erosion may also be seen with gouty arthritis. A similar finding, referred to as the "saddle sign," has been reported in patients with painful heel but no evidence of joint disease (Fig. 2.100B).[358]

Spurs are frequently encountered along the posterior calcaneus at the Achilles tendon insertion. Different aspects of these spurs, which may run transversely across the entire Achilles enthesis, can be seen in the oblique foot views as well as the lateral view. Achilles tendon spurring associated with Haglund syndrome has also been referred to as the posterior calcaneal step spur (Fig. 2.100C).[359]

In addition to degenerative and rheumatic inflammatory processes, enthesopathy has also been associated with trauma, crystal deposition diseases (hydroxyapatite and calcium pyrophosphate dihydrate), and metabolic disorders, including diabetes mellitus and acromegaly.[360]

OTHER CONSIDERATIONS

The retrocalcaneal bursa lays over the posterosuperior portion of the calcaneus; the latter is referred to as the bursal projection.

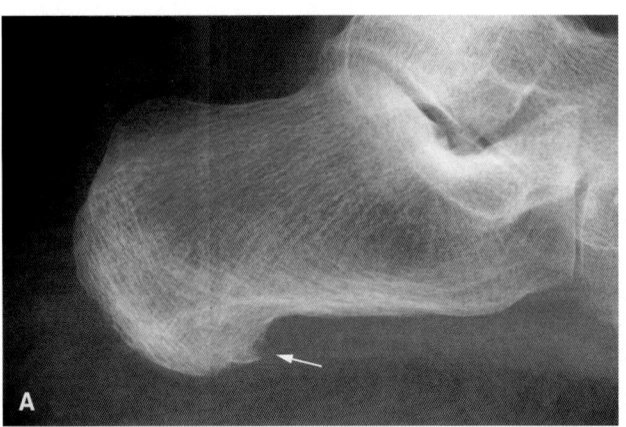

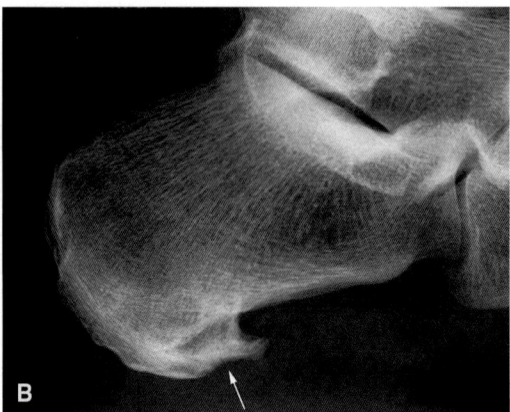

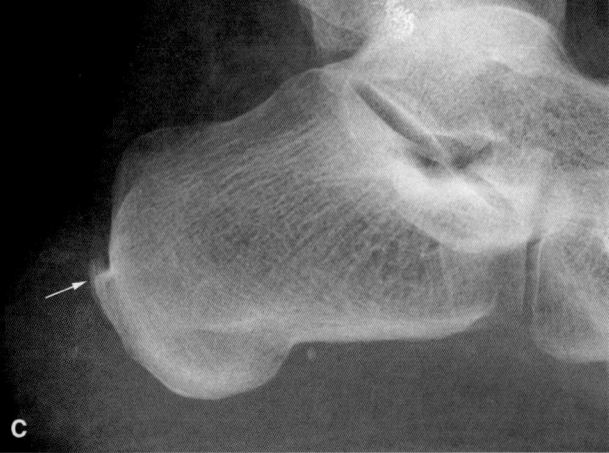

FIGURE 2.100 Calcaneal enthesopathy. **(A)** A combination of bone production and erosion (*arrow*), **(B)** a well-defined spur and "saddle sign" (*arrow*), and **(C)** a posterior calcaneal step spur (*arrow*).

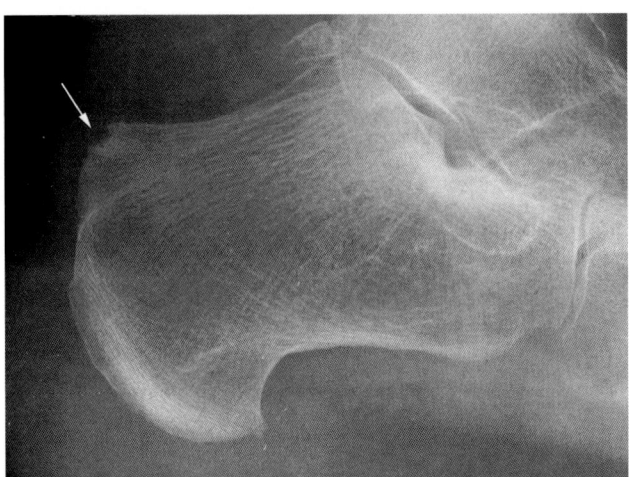

FIGURE 2.101 Erosion along calcaneal bursal projection (*arrow*) in a patient with rheumatoid arthritis.

Inflammation of the bursa has been associated with inflammatory arthritis, especially rheumatoid arthritis, and results in erosion (Fig. 2.101).[361]

Ankylosis (union between two bones) is an end-stage finding of some joint disorders and may be fibrous (rheumatoid arthritis) or osseous (seronegative arthritis).[362] Ankylosis is not seen in osteoarthritis or gouty arthritis.

Most joint disorders target specific joints in the foot; they will be identified subsequently with descriptions for each joint disorder. However, joints may be affected that are clinically asymptomatic, and there frequently is bilateral distribution. For this reason, it is strongly recommended that bilateral foot studies be obtained when evaluating a patient for joint disease, and that all joints and the calcanei be assessed routinely.[363]

OSTEOARTHRITIS (INCLUDING HALLUX LIMITUS AND RIGIDUS)

The primary finding in osteoarthritis (Fig. 2.102) is the osteophyte; its appearance will vary at different joints. Secondary findings, that may be found individually or in combination, include uneven (nonuniform) joint space narrowing, subchondral sclerosis (eburnation), geode (subchondral "cyst") with sclerotic margin, and detritus (sometimes referred to as a loose body or "joint mouse"). Detritus is usually posttraumatic in origin and may have been an osteophyte that broke off.

Osteoarthritis targets joints along the medial column of the foot, including the first metatarsophalangeal, hallux interphalangeal, second metatarsal-cuneiform (and less commonly the first metatarsal-cuneiform), and talonavicular joints. It may be monoarticular or polyarticular, unilateral or bilateral, and symmetrical or asymmetrical. However, any joint can develop osteoarthritis following trauma, especially the ankle.[364]

When is it NOT osteoarthritis? Erosion is not seen in osteoarthritis. (There is a rare form known as erosive osteoarthritis; however, this is primarily seen in the fingers, not the toes.)[365] The presence of erosion suggests another joint disorder, such as rheumatoid, seronegative, gouty, and septic arthritis. Subchondral resorption at multiple joints, such as Lisfranc, suggests Charcot neuropathic osteoarthropathy.

Radiographic grading systems for osteoarthritis have been developed for the entire body[366]; however, there has not been as much attention to the foot.[367,368] Osteoarthritis at the first metatarsophalangeal joint causing limited or loss of range of motion has been referred to as hallux limitus and rigidus, respectively.

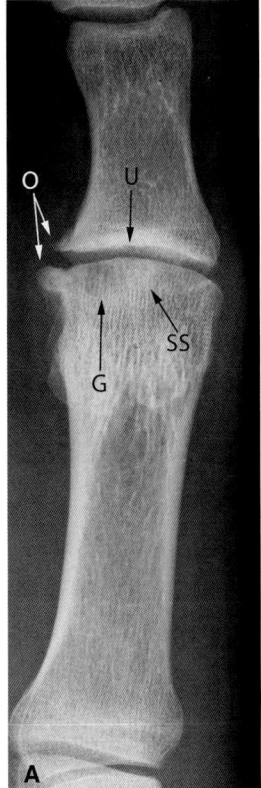

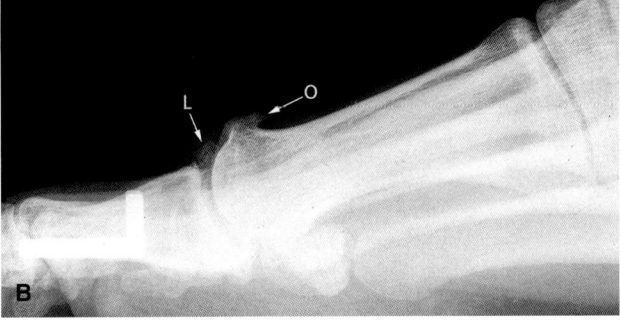

FIGURE 2.102 Osteoarthritis, first metatarsophalangeal joint. **(A)** DP view, **(B)** lateral view. G, geode; L, loose body; O, osteophyte; SS, subchondral sclerosis; U, uneven joint space narrowing.

A few radiographic grading systems have been proposed, some with clinical correlation, some without.[227,369-373] Generally speaking, there are three categories, corresponding to the severity of osteophyte formation, joint space narrowing, and subchondral sclerosis. Category 1 presents with mild osteophyte formation, and minimal or no joint space narrowing or subchondral sclerosis. Category 2 demonstrates larger and/or more osteophytes, with mild to moderate joint space narrowing and subchondral sclerosis. Category 3 involves the entire joint with a combination of significant osteophyte proliferation, joint space narrowing, and subchondral sclerosis; loose bodies and geodes may also be present, as well as involvement of the sesamoid-metatarsal joints.

Maximum dorsiflexion range of motion of the first metatarsophalangeal joint can be documented with the stress lateral dorsiflexion view.[374,375] The foot is positioned as a lateral weight-bearing radiograph; however, prior to exposure, the patient is instructed to raise their heel while leaving the ball of the forefoot firmly on the orthoposer, such that the hallux is maximally dorsiflexed. The central x-ray beam is directed at the first metatarsophalangeal joint. The angle of maximum forced dorsiflexion is measured between the longitudinal axes of the first metatarsal and hallux proximal phalanx. The normal value decreases with age; the normal mean has been reported between 63 and 77 degrees,[376] and the normal average between 65 and 95 degrees.[377]

GOUTY ARTHRITIS

The primary radiographic finding in gouty arthritis (Fig. 2.103) is erosion. Gouty erosions are often periarticular (extra-articular) and, as a result, spare the joint space. They frequently are well defined and "C" shaped. Though not seen in all cases,

new bone production in the form of an overhanging margin adjacent to an erosion (Martel sign) is strongly suggestive of gouty arthritis.[378] Secondary findings may include a "lumpy-bumpy" soft tissue mass and calcification. The joint space often appears normal despite the appearance of significant periarticular erosion,[379] unless tophi and erosions become intra-articular. Gouty arthritis targets the first metatarsophalangeal and hallux interphalangeal joints; however, erosion may be encountered at any foot joint. Distribution in the foot may be unilateral or bilateral, asymmetric or symmetric, and monoarticular or polyarticular.

RHEUMATOID ARTHRITIS

The primary radiographic finding of rheumatoid arthritis (Fig. 2.104) is erosion. The classic picture demonstrates medial erosion at all metatarsal heads and lateral erosion of the fifth metatarsal head[380]; the latter may result in arthritis mutilans. Secondary findings include even joint space narrowing, fibular deviation of all digits except the fifth bilaterally, loss of 100% joint apposition resulting in subluxation and/or dislocation, and geodes (sometimes referred to as pseudocysts). Periarticular osteopenia may also be seen. There is rarely involvement of lesser toe interphalangeal joints. Rheumatoid arthritis targets the metatarsophalangeal and hallux interphalangeal joints; tarsal involvement is infrequent, and erosion of the calcaneal bursal projection may occur. Foot distribution classically is bilateral and symmetrical; however, it appears monoarticular initially (notably at the fifth metatarsophalangeal joint), then becomes polyarticular.[381] Erosion of the distal fibula, seen in the ankle mortise view adjacent to the triangular lateral surface of the distal tibia, has been associated with rheumatoid arthritis.[382]

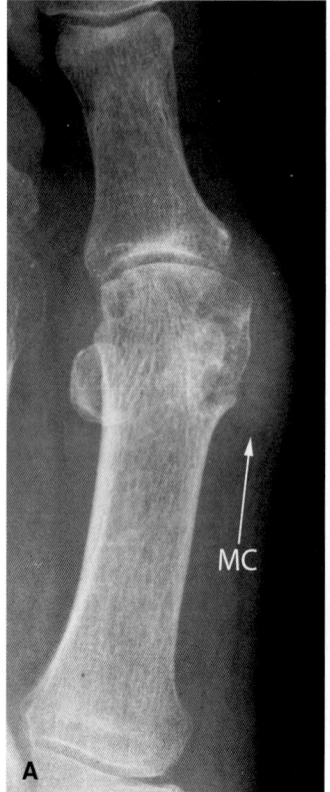
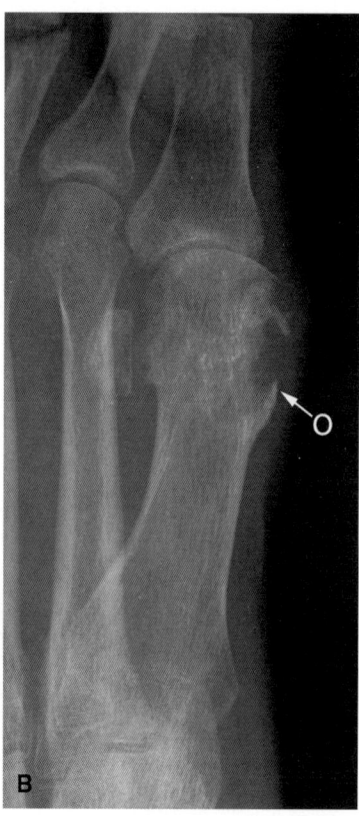

FIGURE 2.103 Gouty arthritis, first metatarsophalangeal joint. **(A)** DP view, **(B)** medial oblique view. There is a large, extra-articular C-shaped erosion; note the relative sparing of the joint space. MC, lumpy-bumpy soft tissue mass with calcification; O, overhanging margin.

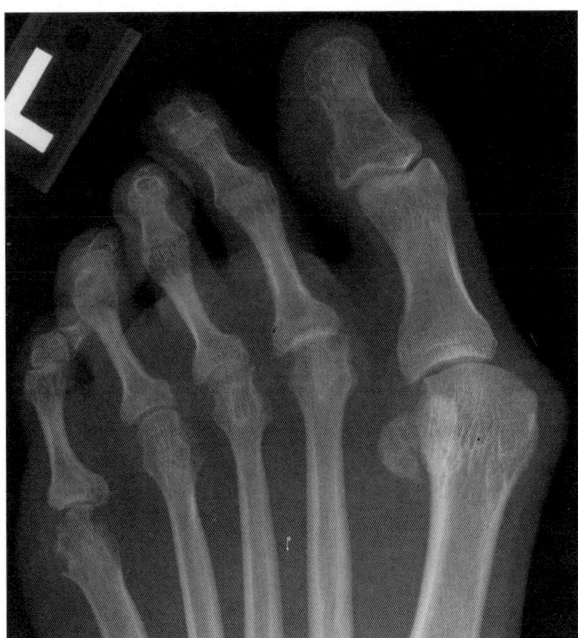

FIGURE 2.104 Rheumatoid arthritis. There is involvement of all lesser metatarsophalangeal joints accompanied by even joint space narrowing: erosion along the medial aspects of the second and third, pre-erosion medially at the fourth, and erosions along the medial and lateral aspects of the fifth.

PSORIATIC ARTHRITIS

Erosion is the primary radiographic finding of psoriatic arthritis (Fig. 2.105). Unlike rheumatoid arthritis, the erosions occur along the medial and/or lateral sides of affected joints and may result in arthritis mutilans. Secondary findings vary and may include joint space narrowing or widening, periostitis adjacent

to an affected joint, whiskering and/or ivory phalanx involving the hallux distal phalanx, and edema of a single digit referred to as sausage toe. Calcaneal enthesopathy, including erosion and bone proliferation, may also occur.[383]

Psoriatic arthritis has several different presentations in the foot, which may occur individually (more likely) or in combination. (1) More commonly, there is bilateral but asymmetrical metatarsophalangeal involvement, unlike rheumatoid arthritis (which is classically symmetrical). (2) Psoriatic arthritis may target the lesser toe distal interphalangeal joint, which would not be seen in rheumatoid arthritis. (3) Ray distribution is another presentation where all joints of one ray are involved (eg, the distal and PIPJs as well as the metatarsophalangeal joint of the second ray). (4) A hallux distal phalanx presentation consists of the ivory phalanx (increased density) and/or whiskering (bony proliferation adjacent to superficial bony erosion); there also may be erosion of the ungual tuberosity. (5) A less common presentation mimics rheumatoid arthritis, demonstrating bilateral, symmetrical metatarsophalangeal joint involvement.

REACTIVE ARTHRITIS AND ANKYLOSING SPONDYLITIS

Both reactive arthritis and ankylosing spondylitis resemble psoriatic arthritis; the primary radiographic finding is erosion of medial and/or lateral sides of affected joints. The secondary findings, however, are not as diverse and include joint space narrowing or widening, periostitis adjacent to affected joints, and sausage toe (reactive arthritis). The clinical history and type of sacroiliac involvement help to distinguish between reactive arthritis and ankylosing spondylitis, respectively. Target joints include the metatarsophalangeal joints, and there may also be calcaneal enthesopathy; additionally, reactive arthritis targets the lesser toe interphalangeal joints and ankylosing spondylitis the hallux interphalangeal joint.[384] The foot distribution is bilateral and polyarticular; ankylosing spondylitis may be symmetrical or asymmetrical, but classic reactive arthritis is asymmetrical.[385]

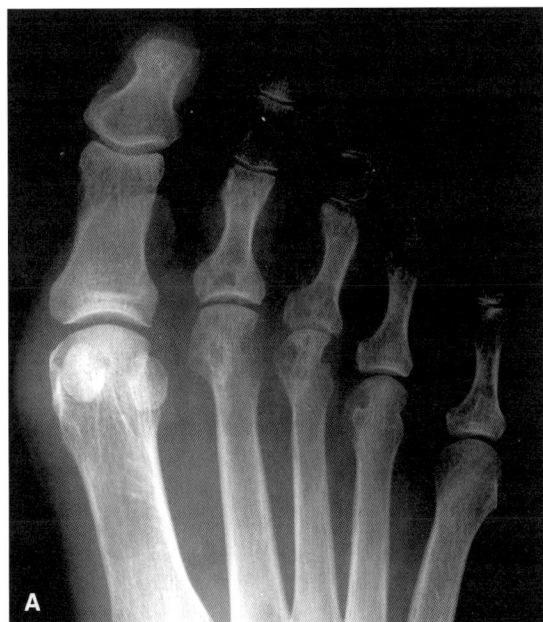
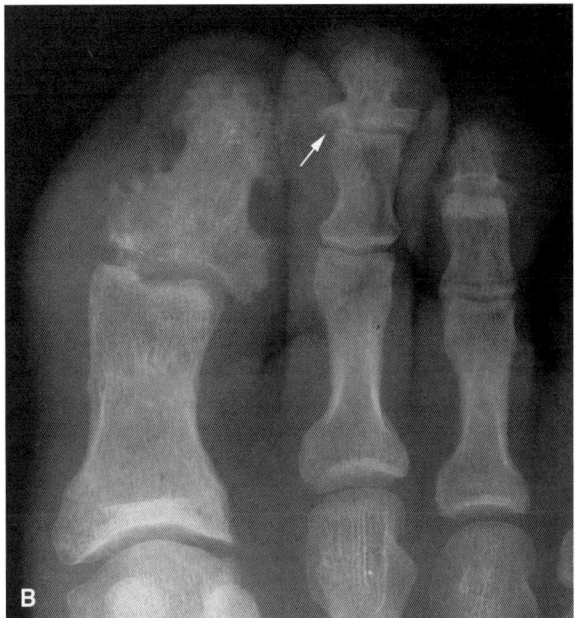

FIGURE 2.105 Psoriatic arthritis. **A.** Erosion along medial and lateral aspects of the second and third metatarsophalangeal joints. **B.** Whiskering of hallux distal phalanx margins and erosion along medial aspect of the second toe distal interphalangeal joint (*arrow*).

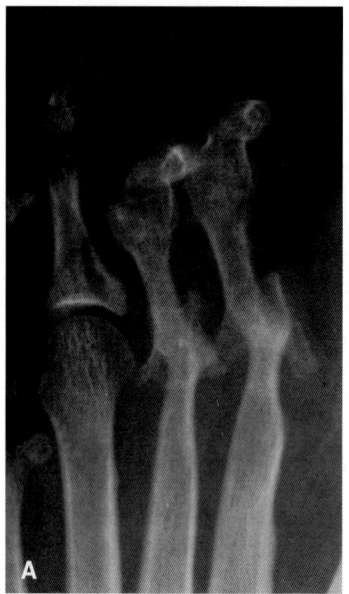 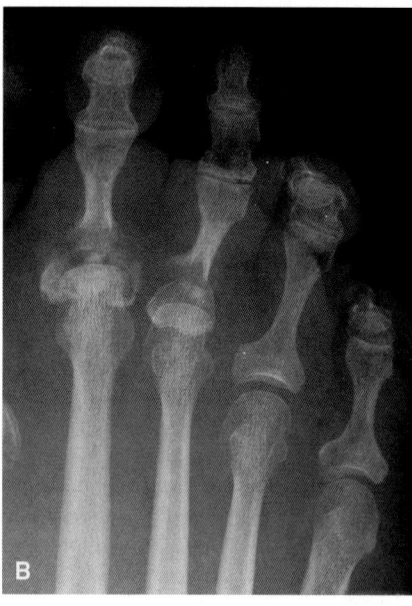 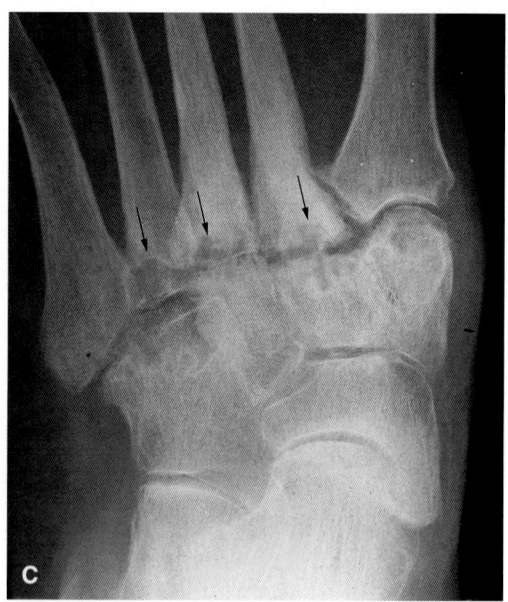

FIGURE 2.106 Charcot neuropathic osteoarthropathy. **A.** Forefoot: arthritis mutilans, second and third metatarsophalangeal joints. **B.** Forefoot: early findings include subchondral resorption and detritus (osteolysis), second metatarsophalangeal joint. **C.** Lisfranc joint: subchondral resorption (*arrows*) accompanied with sclerosis.

CHARCOT NEUROPATHIC OSTEOARTHROPATHY

Charcot neuropathic osteoarthropathy, or Charcot foot, is a grossly destructive arthritis associated with diabetes. It tends to focus on one of the following five distinct locations: the forefoot; the tarsometatarsal (Lisfranc) joint; the naviculocuneiform, talonavicular, and calcaneocuboid joints; the ankle and subtalar joints; or, the posterior calcaneus.[386] Foot distribution is typically unilateral and may be monoarticular but is often polyarticular.

The primary radiographic finding of forefoot Charcot foot is subchondral resorption that ultimately results in arthritis mutilans (Fig. 2.106A). Secondary findings are osteolysis and periostitis; loss of joint apposition and fragmentation (detritus) may also be seen (Fig. 2.106B). Sclerosis is relatively absent in the forefoot form.

The primary radiographic finding of tarsal Charcot foot is subchondral resorption (Fig. 2.106C). Secondary findings include loss of 100% apposition between bones (subluxation/dislocation), fragmentation (detritus), and, diffuse sclerosis. The loss of apposition may not be discernable in the DP and medial oblique views, but it is obvious in the lateral view. Increased soft tissue density and volume is significant. Posttraumatic osteoarthritis at the tarsometatarsal joints has been misdiagnosed as Charcot foot in patients that are diabetic. Posttraumatic osteoarthritis will demonstrate osteophytes and subchondral sclerosis; however, there is no subchondral resorption.

Eichenholtz[387] described the radiographic "evolution of a Charcot joint," which distinguishes in three stages whether or not the underlying pathologic process appears acute or chronic. Stage 1, development, consists of bony debris, fragmentation of subchondral bone, periarticular fracture, and subluxation and/or dislocation. Stage 2, coalescence, demonstrates resorption of the fine debris, larger fragment union with joint ankylosis, and sclerosis of bone ends. Stage 3, remodeling, exhibits rounding of bone margins and decreased sclerosis.

Stage 0 was later added to the system to account for the affected joint or joints that have not yet demonstrated significant abnormality; radiographic findings are minimal or absent.[388] Thus, the importance is placed upon early detection, prior to radiographic visibility of pathology, in an attempt to arrest the acute process and to prevent the development of fracture, dislocation, etc.[389] Special imaging studies (MRI or, if contraindicated or not available, bone scintigraphy) have been and can be used when Charcot neuropathic osteoarthropathy is suspected clinically yet radiographs are normal.[390]

A bone fleck, seen along the superior aspect of the midfoot in the lateral view, was reported in one case as a potential early finding associated with tarsal Charcot foot. Stage 0 is unremarkable radiographically, but a small fleck of bone may be commonly overlooked and could indicate an overall foot alignment change.[391]

SEPTIC ARTHRITIS

Subchondral resorption is the primary radiographic finding for pyogenic septic arthritis (Fig. 2.107). Secondary findings include osteolysis and increased soft tissue density and volume. Septic arthritis can target any joint, and its distribution is monoarticular.

OSTEOMYELITIS

SOFT TISSUE

Soft tissue infection appears as increased soft tissue density and volume. This is nonspecific, since increased soft tissue density and volume may be seen with other inflammation pathology. A tractlike soft tissue decreased density that runs between bone and the skin surface is referred to as a *sinus*; however, sinuses are not clearly seen in a radiograph without the addition of a

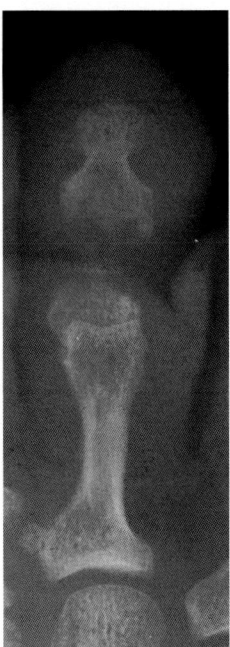

FIGURE 2.107 Septic arthritis, third toe distal interphalangeal joint. Subchondral resorption of the middle phalanx head and distal phalanx base resulted in a large "space" between the two bones.

contrast agent (known as sinography). The term *abscess* refers to a focal collection of pus, and *cellulitis* is a localized or diffuse inflammation of connective tissue involving the dermal and subcutaneous layers of skin. MRI is considered the modality of choice for soft tissue infection.[392]

The presence of one or multiple geographic airlike decreased densities in the soft tissue may be secondary to a gas-forming bacterial infection; the finding is described as *soft tissue emphysema*, and the diagnosis is gas gangrene (Fig. 2.108). An ulcer, depending upon its size, will be seen as a soft tissue defect if it is tangent to the x-ray beam; however, if viewed *en face*, the ulcer may appear as a geographic decreased density and be mis-diagnosed as gas gangrene. In this case, it is important to correlate the radiograph with the clinical picture.

JOINT

The primary finding of pyogenic septic arthritis is subchondral resorption. Septic arthritis is monoarticular and, when full-blown, appears as "osteolysis," the primary finding being

subchondral resorption (see Fig. 2.107). Secondary findings may include periostitis, rarefaction, and erosion. The adjacent soft tissue will demonstrate increased density and volume. The differential diagnosis for subchondral resorption is Charcot neuropathic osteoarthropathy, which may be polyarticular. Gout is primarily a clinical differential diagnosis; you should not see any osseous abnormality in acute, early gout. Rarefaction (a secondary finding) may occur prior to subchondral resorption and be the earliest finding. The remaining radiographic features of septic arthritis, loss of joint apposition (joint space widening), periostitis, rarefaction, and fragmentation are considered secondary findings.

BONE

Osteomyelitis is defined as infection of the bone and marrow. However, there may be times that the infectious process does not involve the marrow and may only be under the periosteum, known as *infective periostitis* (Fig. 2.109), or may involve only the periosteum and underlying cortex, referred to as *infective osteitis*.[393]

Osteomyelitis may be classified as either hematogenous (blood borne) or as secondary to a contiguous source of infection, also referred to as direct extension; the route of contamination can affect its radiographic appearance. Infective periostitis or osteitis may result from direct extension; once the marrow is involved, it is then osteomyelitis. Infection may also result from direct implantation or via surgery.[394]

Hematogenous osteomyelitis will have a different presentation in three age groups due to the vascular pattern at these times of development.[395] Since the metaphyseal blood vessels communicate with the epiphysis in the infant, hematogenous osteomyelitis will involve both the metaphysis and epiphysis. However, metaphyseal blood vessels do not cross the physis in the child (~1-16 years of age), and hematogenous osteomyelitis will be isolated to the metaphysis. Because the physis is closed in the adult, hematogenous osteomyelitis can be seen at the end of a long bone.

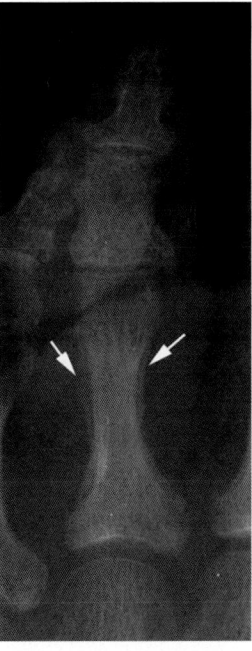

FIGURE 2.109 Infective periostitis (*arrows*).

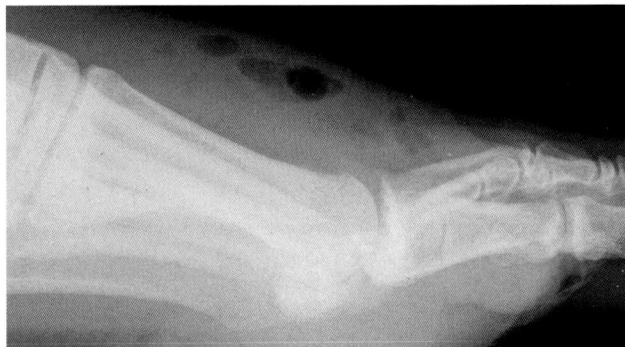

FIGURE 2.108 Soft tissue emphysema. Large, geographic decreased densities are seen in the dorsum of the foot.

Osteomyelitis can clinically be categorized into three stages: acute, subacute, or chronic.[396] Acute refers to an abrupt, initial infection. Subacute is usually reserved for bone abscess and Garre sclerosing osteomyelitis, which could also be considered chronic. Chronic indicates an infection that has never resolved and remains indefinitely. Chronic osteomyelitis may be active or inactive, and there are specific terms used to describe associated findings, including sequestrum, involucrum, and cloaca.

Radiographic findings associated with acute bone infection (in particular, direct extension) include periostitis, rarefaction, erosion, and osteolysis, which may appear collectively or individually (Fig. 2.110). These findings are not necessarily specific for osteomyelitis as they may be associated with Charcot neuropathic osteoarthropathy as well. If pus gets underneath the periosteum, a periosteal reaction (aka periostitis) will eventually be seen, presenting as an ill-defined increased density along the

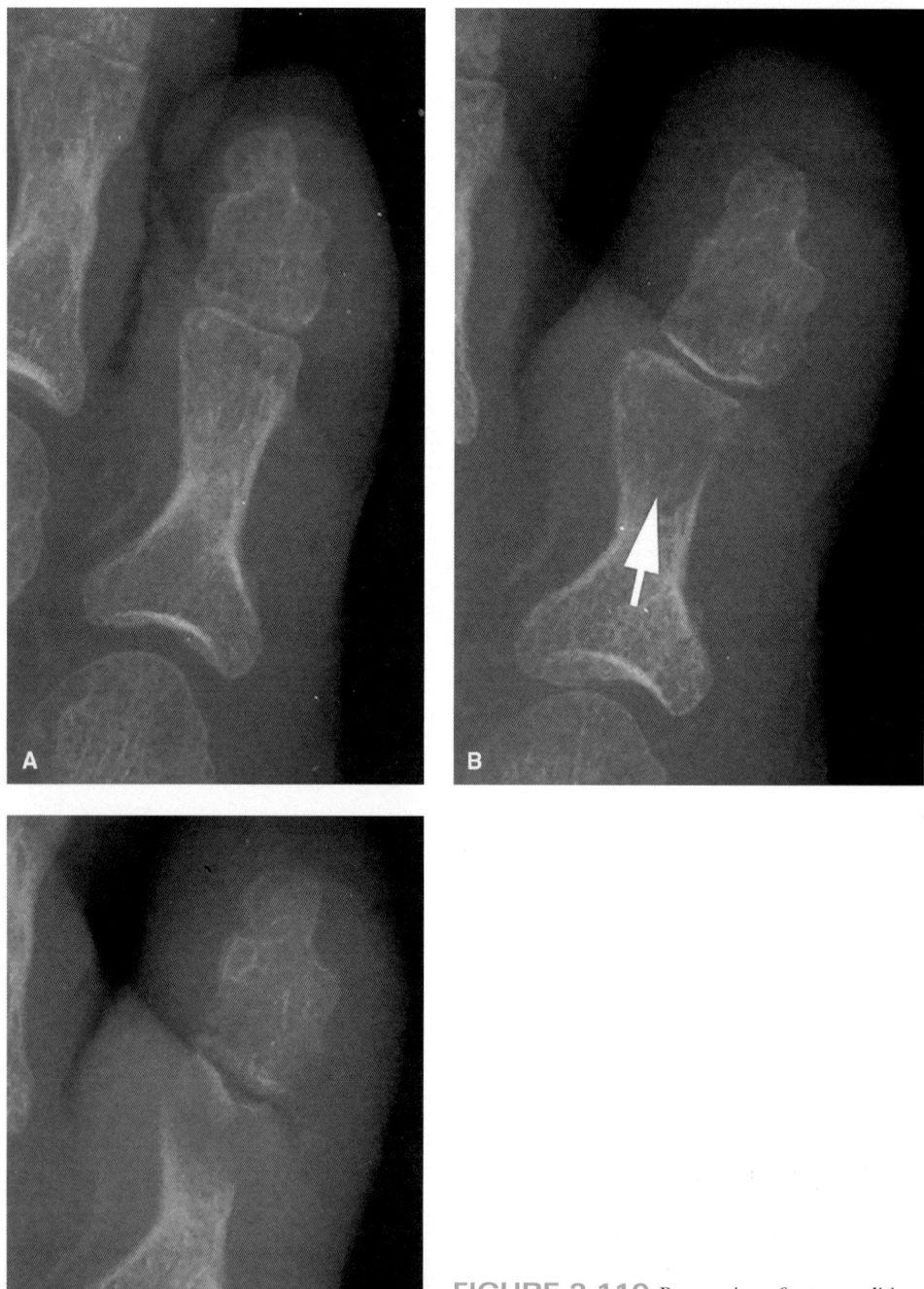

FIGURE 2.110 Progression of osteomyelitis, fifth toe proximal phalanx. **A.** Increased soft tissue volume and density. **B.** Rarefaction (*arrow*). **C.** Osteolysis. (Figure 18-8 from Williams M, Christman RA. Bone infection. In: Christman RA, ed. *Foot and Ankle Radiology*. 2nd ed. Philadelphia, PA: Lippincott Williams & Wilkins; 2015:331-344.)

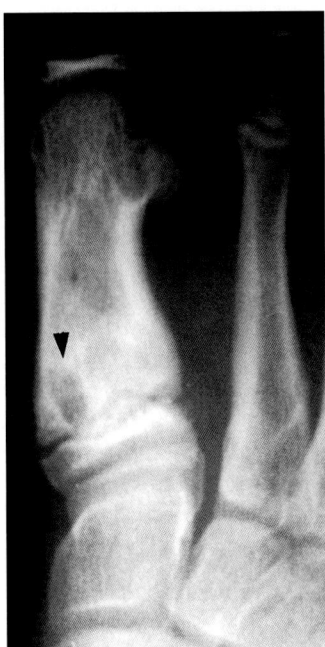

FIGURE 2.111 Bone abscess (*arrowhead*). (Figure 18-9 from Williams M, Christman RA. Bone infection. In: Christman RA, ed. *Foot and Ankle Radiology*. 2nd ed. Philadelphia, PA: Lippincott Williams & Wilkins; 2015:331-344.)

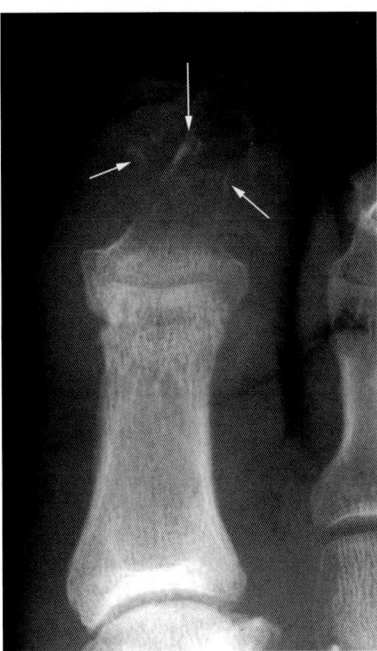

FIGURE 2.112 Sequestra (*arrows*), acute osteomyelitis.

outer surface of the cortex. Rarefaction is a synonym for localized decreased bone density within bone. Erosion occurs along the outer margin of a bone and results in a segment of the bone border to be absent. The term *osteolysis* refers to fragmentation, rarefaction, and ill-defined bone resorption that result in a loss of the bone's form (Fig. 2.110C).

Bone abscess is a geographic decreased density with a diffuse surrounding sclerosis. The bone abscess, also known as Brodie abscess, is the result of hematogenous spread to bone and is almost exclusive to adults.[397] Its characteristic features are a geographic decreased density surrounded by diffuse sclerosis (Fig. 2.111). This lesion does not occur abruptly but takes time to develop, hence its classification as "subacute" or chronic. For "subacute" osteomyelitis, consider a pot of sauce simmering on the stove; still contained, but ready to overflow.

Garre sclerosing osteomyelitis is rare in the foot and represents a nonpurulent form of osteomyelitis, hence its classification as "subacute." Marked periosteal bone deposition is seen, resulting in a very sclerotic appearance. It may be either subacute or chronic and targets the anterior tibia and mandible.[398]

The terms sequestrum, involucrum, and cloaca are only used in known cases of osteomyelitis. *Sequestrum* is dead bone separated by living bone by granulation tissue; in other words, the bone fragment is floating in a sea of pus (Fig. 2.112). It is seen in acute osteomyelitis, and when present in chronic osteomyelitis, the infection is active.[399] It is especially associated with hematogenous origin. Sequestrum can harbor living organisms and evoke acute flare-ups. In the adult, involucrum and cloaca are only seen in chronic osteomyelitis. *Involucrum* represents a layer or collar of new bone that has formed around the necrotic, infected bone (Fig. 2.113). It represents the body's attempt to wall off the infection and keep it contained.[400] (Involucrum is also seen in infants and children, but not necessarily in chronic osteomyelitis, since the periosteum

is less adhered to the cortex.) Holes or openings may be present in the involucrum, which allow pus, with or without sequestrum, to escape; this opening or tract through the involucrum is referred to as a *cloaca*.[401]

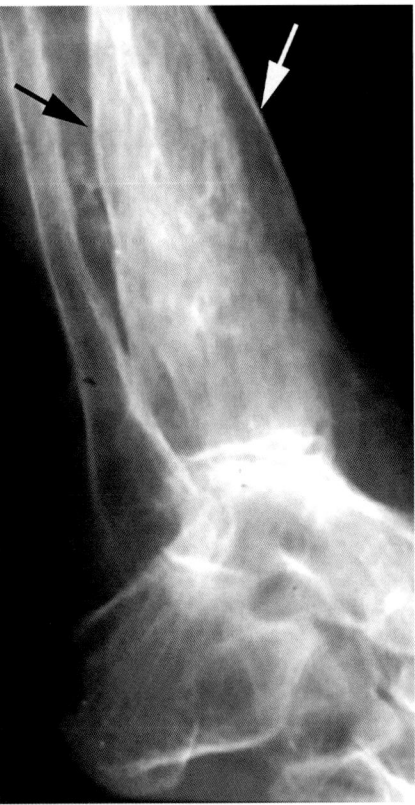

FIGURE 2.113 Involucrum (*arrows*), chronic osteomyelitis. (Figure 18-10 from Williams M, Christman RA. Bone infection. In: Christman RA, ed. *Foot and Ankle Radiology*. 2nd ed. Philadelphia, PA: Lippincott Williams & Wilkins; 2015:331-344.)

BONE IMAGING ALGORITHM

Radiographic evidence of bone abnormality may take 10-14 days before visible to the naked eye; this is because radiographs are insensitive to changes in bone calcium content until ~30%-60% of bone has been resorbed or added.[402] As a result, numerous days or weeks may pass before bone resorption, the primary finding of septic arthritis or osteomyelitis is visible on a radiograph. And, one certainly does not want to wait 2 weeks in order to make the diagnosis of bone or joint infection and delay treatment. This is where adjunctive imaging studies come in to play.[403]

When infection is suspected clinically, radiographs will be ordered first. If the radiographs reveal obvious findings associated with osteomyelitis, such as osteolysis, then the diagnosis is confirmed, and no further studies are necessary. If, however, the radiographs are entirely normal, then either MRI or bone scintigraphy (if MRI is contraindicated or unavailable) would be requested. MRI can be ordered with gadolinium to enhance the images; some imaging centers include it as normal protocol for suspected infection. MRI will demonstrate high signal intensity in areas of concern on T2, STIR, and fat-suppressed T1 images (with gadolinium) if infection is present. If all three phases of the bone scintigram demonstrate focal uptake in the area of concern, this would also be consistent with osteomyelitis.

If, however, the initial radiographic study reveals a superimposed or co-existing pathology or process, such as Charcot neuropathic osteoarthropathy, osteoarthritis, or prior surgery, then differentiation of osteomyelitis becomes much more challenging. In this case, one could follow several different paths: MRI; a third phase bone scintigram + gallium; a third phase bone scintigram + indium; a technetium HMPAO scan; an FDG-PET (positron emission tomography) study; or a SPECT (single photon emission computed tomography)/CT study. The latter two are newer modalities that may not be readily available. (Also, Tc-99m sulfur colloid marrow imaging has been used with In-111 to improve its sensitivity, specificity, and accuracy.) In any case, if surgery is being planned, an MRI would be obtained for preoperative planning, which is one reason why this study is preferred over all the others.

BONE TUMOR

There are two caveats regarding bone tumors and tumorlike lesions. First, most bone tumors cannot be diagnosed by radiographic appearance alone; however, lesion growth rate can be estimated and appropriate differential diagnoses can be determined based upon specific radiographic findings. Second, other conditions may mimic bone tumor; examples include fibrous dysplasia, osteomyelitis, and eosinophilic granuloma. Therefore, the goal is to recognize and describe the radiographic findings of a solitary bone lesion, determine its growth rate, and list differential diagnoses.[404] Special imaging studies may be useful after analyzing the radiographic presentation; however, radiography provides the most useful information about a lesion and remains the gold standard for formulating differential diagnoses for tumorlike lesions of bone.[405]

Radiographic findings useful for determining the growth rate of a bone lesion include its destructive (lytic) pattern, the level of cortical involvement, presence of a soft tissue component, type of periosteal reaction (if present), and the size, shape, and number of lesions. Other factors that can additionally be helpful in developing a differential diagnosis but do not provide information as to the lesion's growth rate include the tumor's position in a tubular bone, the tumor's location (some tumors have a predilection for a specific bone), the presence or absence of trabeculations, whether or not the tumor demonstrates a visible matrix, and the patient's age. The tumor's position in a tubular bone and the patient's age are the most important clues for narrowing the differential diagnosis.[406]

DESTRUCTIVE (LYTIC) PATTERN

The destructive or lytic pattern of a lesion will either be geographic, moth-eaten, or permeative.[407] Geographic lesions (Fig. 2.114A) typically are slower growing, or, less aggressive, than lesions demonstrating moth-eaten or permeative destruction. And, likewise, slow growing lesions will generally demonstrate well-defined margins that have a sharp, narrow zone of transition between the lesion and surrounding normal bone. In comparison, it is difficult to see where an aggressive lesion begins or ends (Fig. 2.114B).

A geographic destructive lesion also can demonstrate features that infer varying degrees of aggressiveness. The presence of a well-defined sclerotic margin indicates slow growth compared to the geographic lesion with no sclerotic margin and/or an ill-defined margin (Fig. 2.114C). If, over time, a lesion's destructive pattern changes and becomes less defined, one should consider an increase in lesion activity, for example, malignant transformation of a benign lesion. A potential complication of any destructive lesion is fracture, referred to as a pathologic fracture since it occurs through abnormal bone.

Moth-eaten destruction may occur in either cancellous or cortical bone or both; the individual decreased densities are usually well defined. In contrast, permeative destruction is ill defined and permeates through cortical and cancellous bone. Moth-eaten and permeative destruction demonstrate an ill-defined margin with a wide transition zone and indicate very aggressive processes (see Fig. 2.114B).

The majority of tumors that exhibit geographic destruction are benign processes. Lesions demonstrating moth-eaten and permeative destruction are usually malignant. Notice, however, that some malignant tumors, most notably chondrosarcoma and fibrosarcoma, may demonstrate geographic destruction and slow growth rate, especially early on.[407]

CORTICAL INVOLVEMENT

Another consideration when assessing the lesion and its growth rate is whether or not, if located in the medullary canal of a long bone, there is any cortical involvement. Four scenarios may be encountered: no cortical involvement; scalloping of the cortex; "expansion" of the cortex; and break through the cortex.

A lesion that is geographic and elongated in shape, following the contour of the medullary canal and not causing any adjacent cortical erosion, is likely very slow growing. The lesion is simply following the path of least resistance and is probably not aggressive. If there is erosion along the endosteal (or inner) surface of the cortex, also referred to as scalloping, a more active lesion is usually indicated, although it may slowly form over a prolonged time period. An "expanded" cortex results when there is endosteal erosion that continues over a long period of time, usually months or years. Since the lesion is slow growing, the body reacts by trying to contain it, and periosteal new bone is formed along the outside of the cortex, referred to as a shell periosteal reaction (Fig. 2.115). Cortical expansion

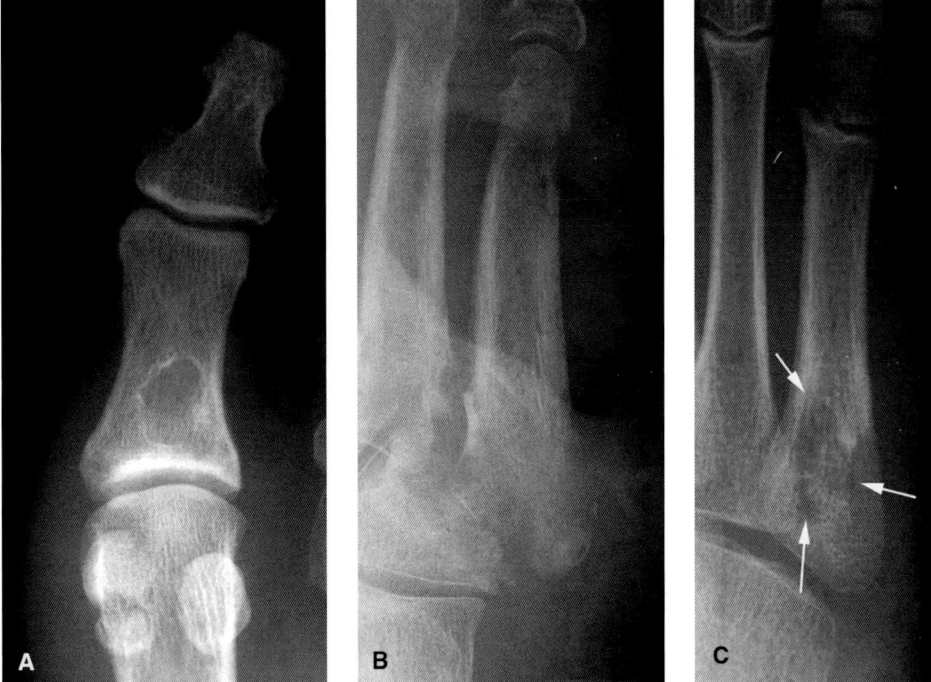

FIGURE 2.114 Destructive pattern. **A.** Geographic lesion with sclerotic margin. **B.** Mixed moth-eaten and permeative destruction involving the entire fifth metatarsal. **C.** A "geographic" lesion with ill-defined margins (*arrows*).

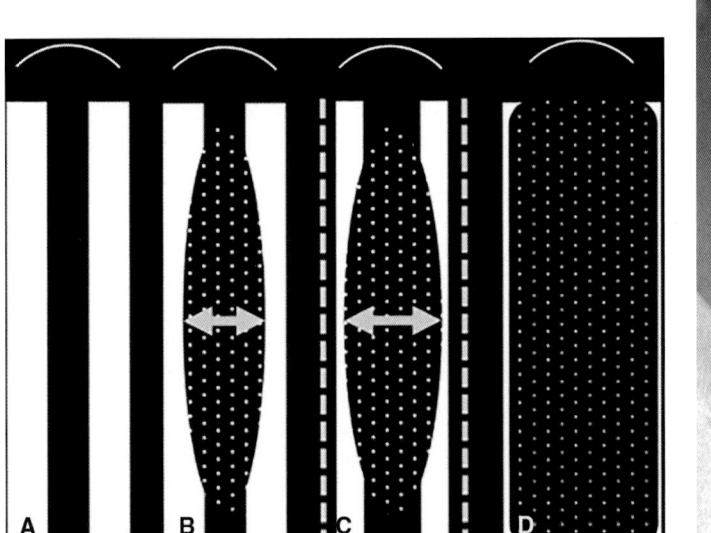
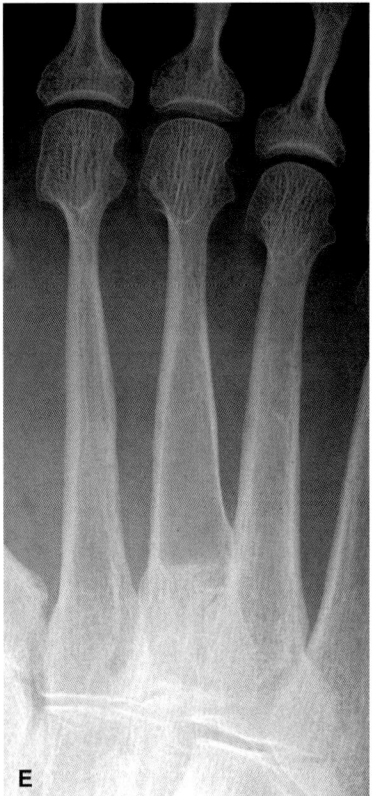

FIGURE 2.115 Formation of the "expanded" cortex. **A.** Normal cortical thickness of a shaft. **B.** Endosteal scalloping due to pressure atrophy; a central lesion is pressing against the inner (endosteal) margins of each cortex. **C.** As the lesion enlarges, pressure atrophy continues (the original cortices become thinner), and periosteal reaction (*dashed lines*) form to contain the lesion as it slowly enlarges. **D.** Lastly, after the original cortices are resorbed, a thin periosteal shell remains. **E.** Example of an "expanded" cortex, that is, shell periosteal reaction.

also indicates a slow-growing process; if the lesion were aggressive, it would simply break through the thin cortical shell. A lesion that breaks through the cortex indicates an aggressive process that very well may be malignant. Cortical destruction associated with "onion skin," "sunburst," or Codman angle periosteal reactions indicate aggressive, usually malignant (or infectious) processes.[408]

SOFT TISSUE COMPONENT

A primary bone tumor that breaks through the cortex and invades the soft tissues more than likely represents a malignant process, such as osteosarcoma; the adjacent bone destructive pattern likely is moth-eaten or permeative. However, a primary soft tissue mass may "invade" bone and mimic malignancy; enlargement of a primary soft tissue mass, which typically is a slow process, causes pressure against adjacent bone. The bone, due to pressure atrophy, resorbs in an attempt to allow room for the soft tissue mass. (A similar process can cause the C-shaped erosion associated with adjacent tophi in gouty arthritis.) As a result, the bone destructive pattern is geographic and well defined, sometimes with a thin sclerotic margin (Fig. 2.116).

PERIOSTEAL REACTION

Occasionally, a periosteal reaction may be seen with a destructive lesion. Generally speaking, periosteal reactions are either continuous (with or without the underlying original cortex), interrupted, or complex.[409] There is a relationship of a tumor's growth rate to the type of periosteal reaction.

Continuous periosteal reactions with no underlying original cortex include lesions with slow growth (relatively speaking) but aggressive enough to cause the cortex to be totally resorbed and replaced by new bone. These are referred to as shell periosteal reactions (aka "expanded" cortex) and may be smooth, lobulated, or ridged. Lobulations are usually related to cartilage tumors (that typically are lobular), and ridges are related to adjacent trabeculations formed by the tumor. The shell periosteal reaction is the result of endosteal bone resorption and periosteal apposition of new bone that occurs over a long period of time (months, years), indicating a slow, nonaggressive process (see Fig. 2.115).

A continuous periosteal reaction with an intact original cortex may be solid, a single lamella (or layer), multiple lamellated (aka "onion skin" appearance, like the layers of an onion peeling apart), or parallel spiculated (perpendicular to the cortex, also referred to as "hair on end" appearance). Lesions with solid and single lamella periosteal reactions are typically slow growing, allowing the periosteum to enclose the lesion (Fig. 2.117). However, a multiple lamellated periosteal reaction suggests an aggressive process that is intermediate, and parallel spiculated a process that may be very aggressive.

A continuous periosteal reaction may become interrupted by the underlying lesion. The buttress is the result of a solid, continuous periosteal reaction that was interrupted (Fig. 2.118); the Codman angle is the result of a single lamella periosteal reaction that was interrupted; the interrupted multiple lamellated is the result of a multiple lamellated periosteal reaction that was interrupted; and the interrupted spiculated is the result of a spiculated

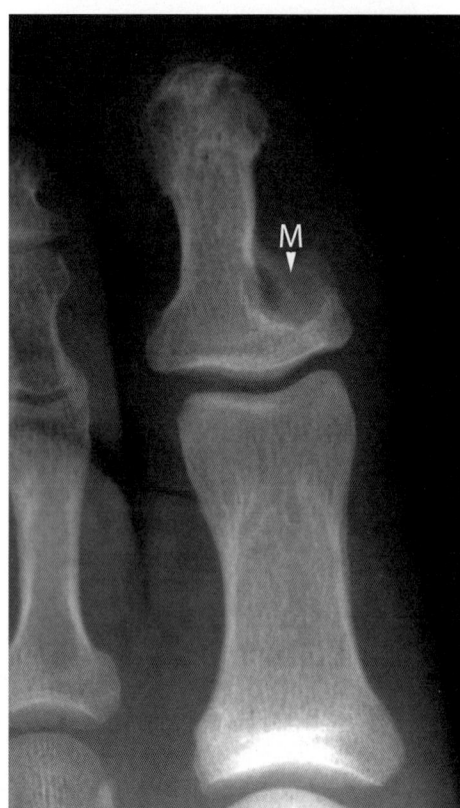

FIGURE 2.116 Soft tissue mass (M) causing pressure atrophy (*arrowhead*) of adjacent bone.

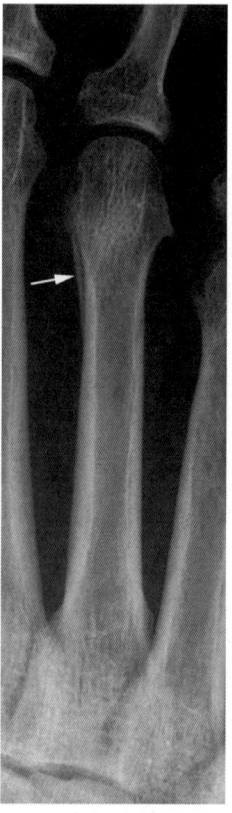

FIGURE 2.117 Single lamella periosteal reaction (*arrow*).

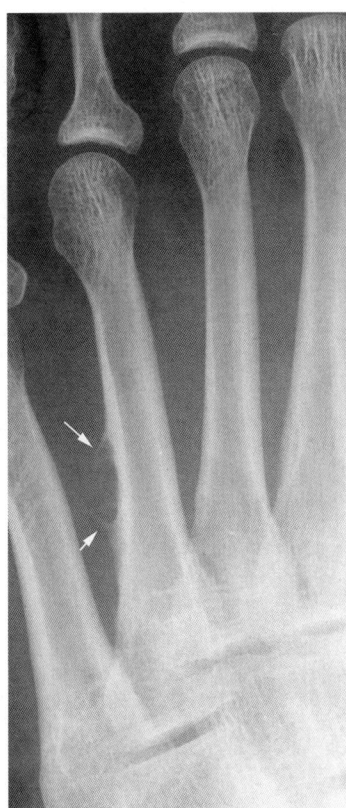

FIGURE 2.118 Buttress periosteal reactions (*arrows*). (Figure 20-30 from Osher L, Petrozzi R, Christman RC. Tumors and tumor-like lesions. In: Christman RA, ed. *Foot and Ankle Radiology.* 2nd ed. Philadelphia, PA: Wolters Kluwer; 2015:381-427.)

periosteal reaction that was interrupted. The presence of an interrupted periosteal reaction strongly suggests that the underlying lesion has broken through the cortex and is an aggressive process.

Complex periosteal reactions include those with exaggerated appearances, such as sunburst and radiating periosteal reactions, as well as a combination of multiple types of periosteal reactions. These presentations are associated with extremely aggressive processes.

SIZE, SHAPE, AND NUMBER

Larger lesions can indicate that a lesion is more aggressive, unless its margins are well defined and/or there is a shell-type periosteal reaction, which would indicate an intermediate growth rate or a long-standing, slowly progressive process. The presence of multiple lesions can indicate metastasis or multiple myeloma, which are malignant processes; however, differential diagnoses may include potentially benign processes, including histiocytic lesions, fibrous dysplasia, and enchondromatosis.

POSITION IN A TUBULAR BONE

Many tumors have a predilection for a certain position in the long bone. What is the tumor's transverse position in a long bone? The midpoint of the lesion may be found in the central aspect of the bone, off-center or eccentric, in the cortex, or along the outer surface of the periosteum, also referred to as parosteal. Enchondroma, simple bone cyst, and fibrous dysplasia are commonly centrally positioned; osteosarcoma and chondromyxoid fibroma are frequently eccentric; fibrocortical defect is centered in the cortex; and osteoid osteoma has a predilection for a parosteal position.

Longitudinally, is the lesion centered in the epiphysis, metaphysis, or diaphysis? For example, fibrous dysplasia and round cell tumors, which include reticulum cell sarcoma, Ewing sarcoma, and multiple myeloma, have a predilection for the diaphysis. Chondroblastoma, clear cell chondrosarcoma, and giant cell tumor have a predilection for the epiphysis and distal metaphysis, depending on whether in a child or adult, respectively. However, the majority of bone tumors are found in the metaphysis and may extend into either the diaphysis or epiphysis. The small bones of the midfoot may be considered as an "epiphyseal" equivalent position.[410]

LOCATION (BONE PREDILECTION)

A few tumors have predilection for a specific bone or bones in the body. For example, enchondroma is commonly found in phalanges of the fingers and toes. The simple bone cyst and intraosseous lipoma have a predilection for the neutral triangle of the calcaneus. Osteoid osteoma has a predilection for the talar neck. And, metaphyseal fibrous defect is commonly found in the distal tibia.

TRABECULATIONS

A handful of tumors may demonstrate trabeculations (sometimes referred to as a "soap bubbles," "multiloculated," "honeycomb," or "bundle of grapes" appearance). The nature of the tumor may be predicted based upon the type of trabeculations.[410] Giant cell tumor and aneurysmal bone cyst both demonstrate fine, delicate trabeculations (Fig. 2.119); occasionally, the trabeculations are horizontally oriented in aneurysmal bone cyst due to fluid-air levels. The trabeculations associated with fibrocortical defect (and nonossifying fibroma, which is the same tumor but larger in size) may appear lobulated. Chondromyxoid fibroma typically demonstrates coarse, thick trabeculations. Hemangiomas may demonstrate striated, radiating, or sunburst trabeculations.

VISIBLE TUMOR MATRIX

Another feature of tumors, though infrequent, is the presence of a visible tumor matrix.[411] When osteogenic tumors, such as enostosis (or bone island), osteoma, osteoid osteoma, osteoblastoma, and osteosarcoma, produce a visible matrix, it typically appears solid, cloudlike, or ivorylike. In contrast, the visible matrix of chondrogenic tumors such as osteochondroma, chondroblastoma, chondromyxoid fibroma, enchondroma, and chondrosarcoma has been described as punctate, stippled, flocculent, comma shaped, or rings and arcs (Fig. 2.120); they have also been referred to as "pebbles" or "popcorn shaped." Lastly, the visible tumor matrix of fibrogenic lesions such as fibrous dysplasia will appear as ground glass or have a "smudgy" or "milky" appearance.

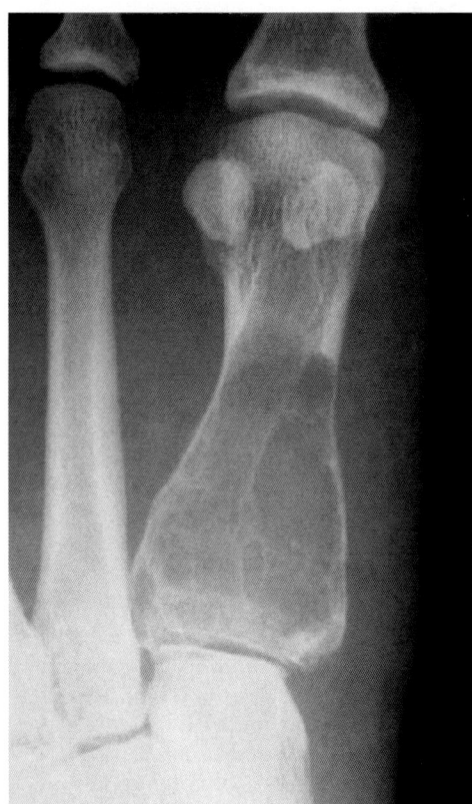

FIGURE 2.119 Lesion demonstrating trabeculations. Also note the shell periosteal reaction. (Figure 20-7 from Osher L, Petrozzi R, Christman RC. Tumors and tumor-like lesions. In: Christman RA, ed. *Foot and Ankle Radiology.* 2nd ed. Philadelphia, PA: Wolters Kluwer; 2015:381-427.)

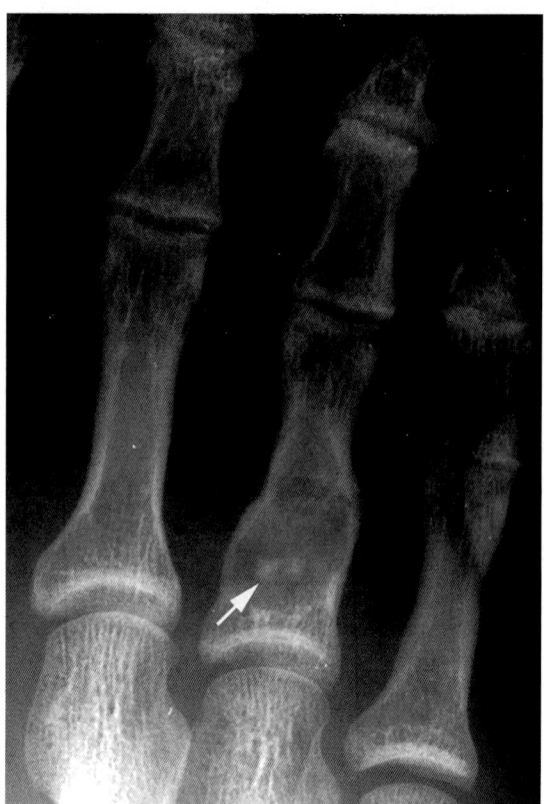

FIGURE 2.120 Visible tumor matrix in the form of flocculent calcifications (*arrows*).

PATIENT AGE

A final diagnostic, nonradiographic clue that is valuable when determining differential diagnoses is the age of the patient.[412] Some tumors have a predilection for those under the age of 20. Examples include fibrocortical defect and Ewing sarcoma. Tumors seen from adolescence to young adult include osteogenic osteosarcoma and aneurysmal bone cyst. Giant cell tumors are frequently seen in the 20-40 age group. Some tumors cross over and may be seen between 10 and 40 years of age, such as osteoid osteoma, enchondroma, and primary osteosarcoma. Multiple myeloma and metastasis frequent the over 40 age group.

MALIGNANT BONE TUMORS

Metastatic carcinoma is the most frequent malignant tumor of bone. The five most common metastatic lesions to bone are breast, lungs, thyroid, kidney, and prostate; however, the gastrointestinal and genitourinary tract may be common sources for the foot.[413,414] Malignant neoplasms of hematopoietic histologic type (including multiple myeloma, lymphoma, and leukemia) represent the most common primary malignancy of bone, followed by sarcoma (osteosarcoma, Ewing).

As a rule, malignant tumors with rapid growth do not expand bone but cause permeative destruction and soft tissue extension. Sometimes, the metastasis is so aggressive that

the bone literally disappears; however, metastasis to bone may also radiographically appear sclerotic, or as mixed lysis and sclerosis.[415]

ADJUNCTIVE IMAGING STUDIES

Special imaging studies may prove useful for further evaluation of tumors that require additional anatomical information or if surgery is being considered. In most cases, MRI or CT is most appropriate for further characterization and preoperative assessment of primary bone tumors.[416]

CT has been used to identify matrix mineralization and is especially good at differentiating between chondrogenic and osteogenic tumor matrix, which may be difficult to perceive on radiographs.[417] CT can accurately detect the central nidus of an osteoid osteoma, which may not be visible on the radiograph, and is superior at delineating the integrity of the cortex[418]; in other words, is the thin shell of a cystic or aneurysmal lesion intact, or has it been broken through by the tumor, which then extends into the soft tissue? The latter case would strongly suggest malignancy. CT can also provide information as to the composition of a tumor or tumorlike lesion via the Hounsfield units measured in it. CT can also be used to guide the biopsy of a lesion.

Compared to CT, MRI demonstrates superior soft tissue contrast and is, therefore, better at assessing the soft tissue extent of malignant lesions in particular. This assists the surgeon for determining the stage of the tumor and planning surgical excision.[419] MRI is also useful for evaluating the extent of bone marrow involvement.[420] The use of gadolinium as a contrast agent helps distinguish between viable tumor and reactive edema; it can also demonstrate areas of increased blood flow and vascular permeability.

Bone scintigraphy is valuable when looking for metastasis in the entire skeleton.[421] Metastatic lesions usually will appear as increased uptake (or, "hot spots") on the image. One would then order radiographs of that particular skeletal location or locations. Bone scintigraphy has also been used to identify occult lesions.

The activity of a lesion may be assessed using bone scintigraphy.[422] For example, a bone island should appear as normal in a bone scintigram vs an osteoid osteoma, which will demonstrate increase uptake. Malignant lesions will typically demonstrate greater activity than a benign lesion. Indolent or inactive lesions will demonstrate minimal skeletal uptake and generally rules out malignancy. Examples of tumors demonstrating indolent activity are nonossifying fibroma, enchondroma, and fibrous dysplasia. However, a lesion that was once indolent and later demonstrates increased activity should be suspected as malignant transformation.

Positron emission tomography or PET is a newer functional imaging technique. It enables evaluation of tissue metabolism and physiology *in vivo*.[423] PET can be further enhanced by adding CT. PET has high sensitivity, which allows detection of small lesions. It also provides accurate evaluation of a tumor's local extension. However, PET has a relatively low specificity, similar to bone scintigraphy. PET is superior to bone scintigraphy in that it can detect metastatic lesions earlier and more precisely.[424] PET also can identify osteolytic or mixed lytic/blastic osseous metastases better as well as metastases of multiple myeloma and Ewing sarcoma.

HAGLUND DEFORMITY

Haglund deformity has been defined as a "distortion of the posterosuperior and lateral portion of the calcaneus."[425] Prominence of this location, also referred to as the bursal projection, has been evaluated by using several radiographic measurement techniques, including the Fowler-Philip angle,

Steffensen and Evensen angle, total angle of Ruch, parallel pitch lines, Chauveaux-Liet (CL) angle, and the X/Y ratio. All measurements are performed on the weight-bearing lateral foot view.

The Fowler-Philip angle is formed between the inferior calcaneal axis and an axis tangent to the upper one-third posterior calcaneal surface (Fig. 2.121A).[426] The normal range is between 44 and 69 degrees and is considered abnormal when >75 degrees.

The Steffensen and Evensen angle is formed between a longitudinal calcaneal axis and a line tangent to the upper two-thirds posterior calcaneal surface (Fig. 2.121B).[427] The longitudinal calcaneal axis is drawn between two points: the most superior aspect of the posterior calcaneus at the Achilles enthesis, which corresponds to the inferior aspect of the posterior one-third surface, and the most anterior aspect of the posterior articular surface for the talus. The posterior tangent line is formed by connecting the following two points: the superior aspect of the bursal projection and the posterior point of the calcaneus drawn for the longitudinal axis. A normal value averaged 60 degrees, and abnormal was considered >63-65 degrees.

Ruch[428] proposed adding the Fowler-Philip angle measurement to the calcaneal inclination angle, since the latter, when increased, can influence prominence of the bursal projection. A few years later, Vega et al.[429] expanded Ruch's suggestion and introduced the "total angle," which is formed between the line along the upper one-third posterior calcaneus and the plane of support (which is just a simpler way to measure the sum of the calcaneal inclination and Fowler-Philip angles) (Fig. 2.121C). It has since been referenced to as the "total angle of Ruch"; the normal range is between 64 and 89 degrees, and an angle ≥90 degrees is considered abnormal.

Pavlov et al. developed a novel approach that looked at the position of the bursal projection relative to the calcaneal pitch, referred to as the parallel pitch lines (Fig. 2.121D).[430] Firstly, the inferior calcaneal inclination axis is drawn. After plotting a point at the most posterior aspect of the posterior talocalcaneal joint, a line is drawn from this point that is perpendicular

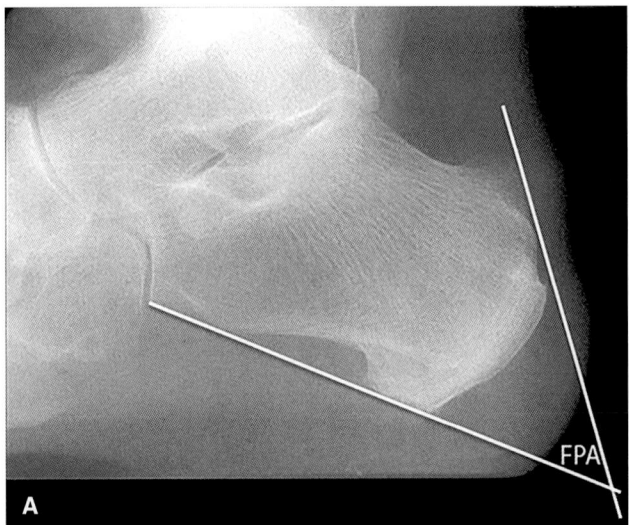

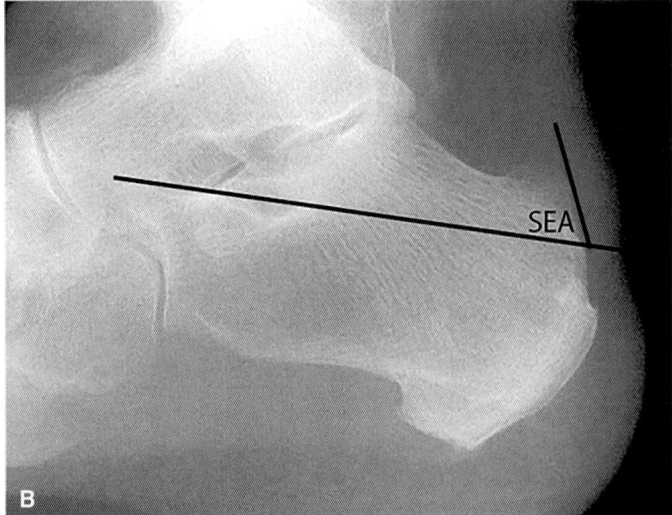

FIGURE 2.121 Haglund deformity measurement techniques. **A.** Fowler-Philip angle (FPA). **B.** Steffensen and Evensen angle (SEA).

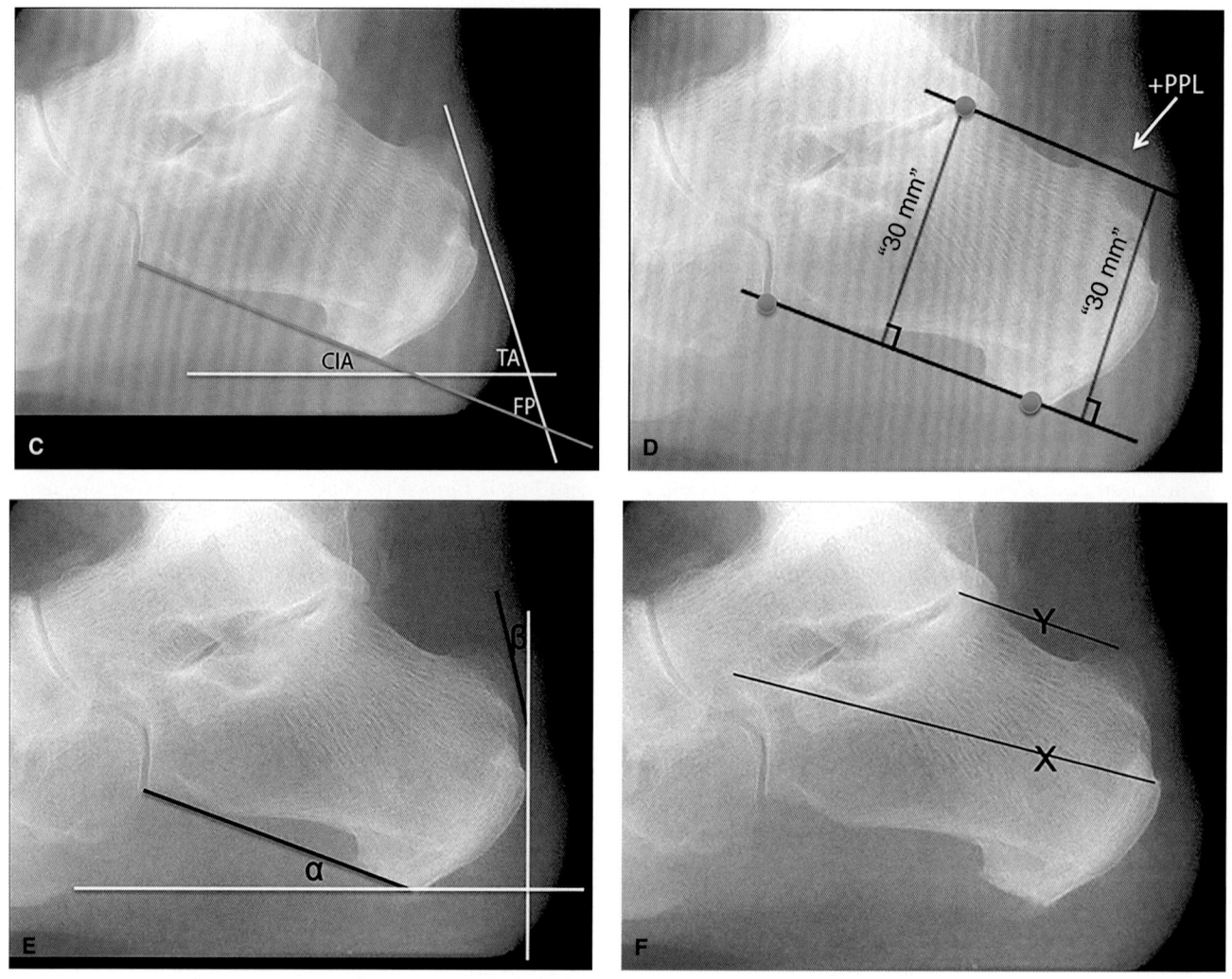

FIGURE 2.121 (*Continued*) **C.** Total angle (TA). CIA, calcaneal inclination angle; FP, Fowler-Philip angle. **D.** Parallel pitch lines (PPL). **E.** Chauveaux-Liet angle = α − β. **F.** X/Y calcaneal ratio.

to the calcaneal axis. After measuring the length of this line, another line is drawn at that length near the bursal projection and a point plotted at its top. The two plotted points are connected by a fourth line (which should be parallel to the inferior calcaneal inclination axis). Normally, the bursal projection is below the parallel pitch line or PPL, which is referred to as a negative PPL. If the bursal projection extends above this line, it is a positive PPL.

The CL angle (Fig. 2.121E) measures the difference between the calcaneal inclination (pitch) angle, α, and the morphologic angle, β (ie, the CL angle = α − β).[431] The morphologic angle (β) is formed between the following and measured superiorly: (1) a line that is perpendicular to the plane of support and tangent to the Achilles tendon enthesis and (2) a line drawn along the posterior aspect of the upper one-third calcaneal posterior surface. An angle >12 degrees is considered abnormal.

The X/Y calcaneal ratio (Fig. 2.121F) assesses total calcaneal length (X) relative to length of the greater tuberosity (Y).[432] X is measured from most anterior point of the anterior process to the most posterior point of the calcaneus (the Achilles tendon

enthesis, at the inferior aspect of the middle one-third surface); Y is measured from the most posterior point of the posterior talocalcaneal joint to the summit of the bursal projection. A normal ratio is >2.5; abnormal is considered <2.5, which considers the calcaneus as "long" and causing posterior impingement and tension with posterior soft tissues. The X/Y calcaneal ratio was compared to the Fowler-Philip angle, total angle of Ruch, parallel pitch lines, and CL angle.

Fiamengo et al.[359] discovered no statistically significant difference between the Fowler-Philip angle and symptomatology. Pavlov et al.[430] determined that the parallel pitch lines were a more valid measurement technique than the Fowler-Philip angle. Mishra et al.[433] did not find the Fowler-Philip angle or parallel pitch lines to be reliable indicators to assess the bursal projection. Lu et al.[434] found the Fowler-Philip angle and parallel pitch lines were not reliable enough to make a surgical decision. Singh et al.[435] concluded that the CL angle and parallel pitch lines were reliable diagnostic indicators of calcaneal abnormality. And, Tourne et al.[432] found the X/Y ratio's specificity and sensitivity to be more reliable and reproducible than the other measurements.

Albert V. Armstrong, Jr

SOFT TISSUE IMAGING

SOFT TISSUE INFECTION

The physician needs to remember that Patient history and physical examination are the most important aspects to consider when ordering and evaluating any imaging study. Soft tissue infections most commonly seen in the foot and ankle are cellulitis and abscess formation.[436] Less commonly seen, are septic tenosynovitis, necrotizing fasciitis, and infectious myositis. After plain film radiography, MRI would be the advanced imaging method of choice for these conditions.[437] One should remember to give the radiologist as much information as possible regarding the patient history and clinical findings. Soft tissue infection is usually the result of direct contamination by a penetrating injury, spread from adjacent osteomyelitis or hematogenous seeding.[438] What one looks for on plain radiographs are swelling, blurring of soft tissue planes, and gas in the tissues (Fig. 2.122).

FOREIGN BODIES

One should also consider the possibility of a foreign body, especially in the diabetic neuropathic patient. In this case, plain radiographs should be done first. One should always be sure to get a minimum of two views when imaging for foreign bodies: an AP (or DP) and a lateral. Radiopaque foreign bodies may be easily seen on a radiograph, but other foreign bodies such as glass, wood, palm fronds, or stingers from aquatic animals may not be apparent. Ultrasound has become an important adjunct imaging modality for the detection and removal of soft tissue foreign bodies.[439] What one looks for

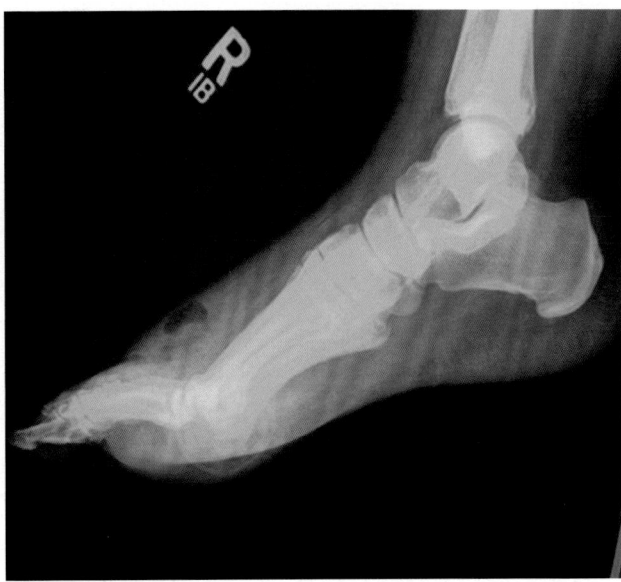

FIGURE 2.122 Soft tissue infection. Lateral radiograph of the foot in a diabetic patient with a medial wound near the first metatarsal head. One can see radiolucencies in the dorsal soft tissues, confirming the clinical diagnosis of soft tissue infection.

is an echogenic focus, with an echolucent halo, indicating a granuloma around the foreign body. Another indication one should look for is an acoustic shadow, which will virtually point to the retained foreign body (Fig. 2.123). For abscess formation, MRI would be the imaging method of choice after plain film radiography.

SOFT TISSUE ULCER

Medical imaging is somewhat limited when evaluating soft tissue foot and ankle wounds. One may see the soft tissue

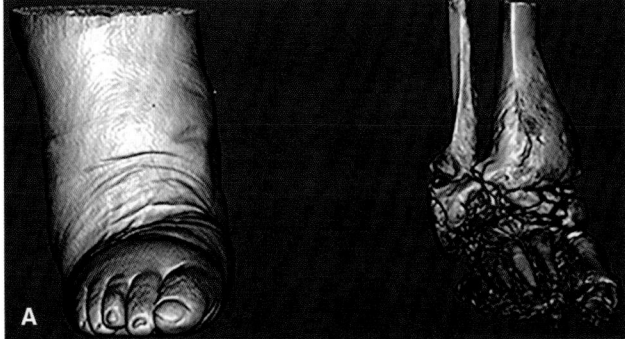
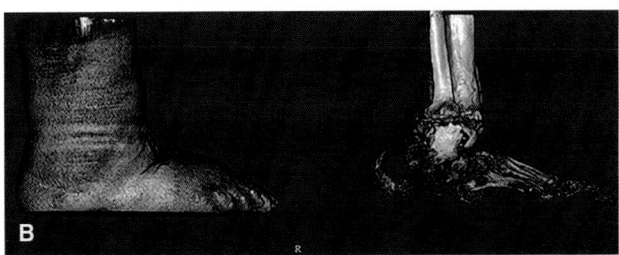

FIGURE 2.123 **A.** Charcot foot with plantar ulcer. 3D CT, AP image with soft tissue and without soft tissue. **B.** Same patient as above, 3D lateral image with and without soft tissue. Note how the cuboid is angled plantarly.

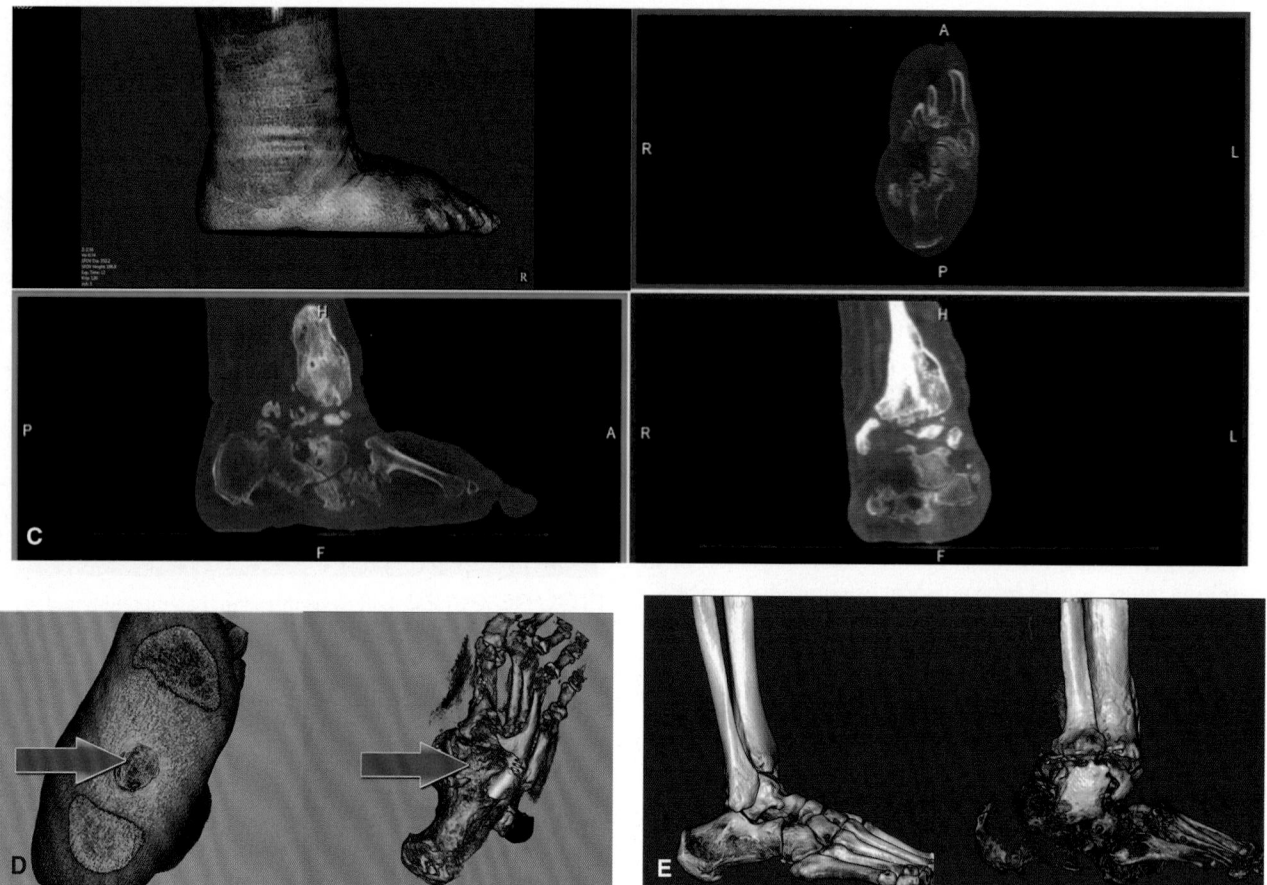

FIGURE 2.123 (*Continued*) **C.** Included with the 3D image are now the 2D sagittal, axial, and coronal slices, again showing how the cuboid is angled plantarly. **D.** Plantar ulcer (*red arrow*) with and without soft tissue, showing evidence that the displaced cuboid is the bone causing the ulcer. (Images courtesy of CurveBeam 3D Extremity Imaging, 2800 Bronze Drive, Suite 110, Hatfield PA 19440.)

defect on plain film radiography or ultrasound. One may also see a soft tissue defect on CT, especially with the newer generations. The new 3D weight-bearing CT has the capability to image the skin and then strip away the soft tissue to see the bones underneath. This is important with plantar pressure ulcers, especially those patients with the Charcot foot. One can actually remove the soft tissue and see exactly which bone is causing the ulcer. With CT, one can also see the decreased bone density also associated with the Charcot foot (Fig. 2.123A-E).

COMPLEX REGIONAL PAIN SYNDROME

CRPS is also known as reflex sympathetic dystrophy, causalgia, and Sudeck atrophy. The cause is unknown, but the condition is associated with injury. The pain may be severe, often disproportionate to the initial injury. It can also be associated with a surgical procedure. Although the pain of CRPS may

be limited to one extremity, the contralateral limb can also show swelling, and hyperemia, though to a lesser extent.[2,3] If CRPS is suspected, one should begin with plain radiographs. The radiographs will appear normal early in the course of the condition, but later radiographic findings include patchy osteoporosis, intracortical tunneling, and bone resorption (it should be noted that these findings are radiographically indistinguishable from disuse osteoporosis.[436] These findings will also be seen with CT (Fig. 2.124). A TC99MDP triple phase bone scan will show increased uptake in all three phases. Uptake will be centered around the joints in the third or delayed phase (Fig. 2.125).

SYNDESMOTIC AND LIGAMENTOUS INJURIES

The syndesmotic ligaments consist of four ligaments. From above downward, they consist of the interosseous ligament, the anterior tibiofibular ligament, the posterior tibiofibular

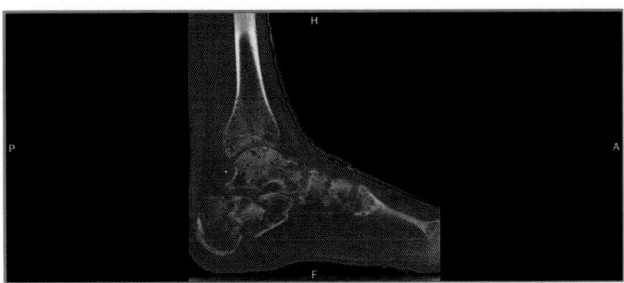

FIGURE 2.124 Complex regional pain syndrome (CRPS). This patient was injured at work and went to a nearby hospital emergency department for treatment. Radiographs were read as negative, and the patient was diagnosed with an ankle sprain. The patient was without health insurance and remained in an ace wrap and with crutches for 2 months. After seeing a podiatrist, the above CT scan was ordered. Shown are intra-articular calcaneal fractures. Also seen is patchy osteoporosis. The diagnosis of complex regional pain syndrome (CRPS) was made in addition to the calcaneal fractures.

ligament, and the transverse tibiofibular ligament. The interosseous ligament represents the lowermost portion of the crural interosseous membrane. The anterior inferior tibiofibular ligament is the weakest of the four. The transverse tibiofibular ligament is the lowermost portion of the posterior inferior

tibiofibular ligament.[437] If the patient presents with an injury to the ankle, and there is a concern of a high ankle sprain, plain radiographs of the ankle should be done first: AP, mortise, and lateral. On the AP radiograph, the tibiofibular clear space should be <6 mm. The tibiofibular overlap should be >6 mm. On the ankle mortise, the medial clear space should be ≤4 mm (Fig. 2.126A and B).[442] According to the Lauge-Hansen fracture classification system, if a Volkman (posterior malleolar) fracture is seen, there must be a fracture of the fibula somewhere.[440-442] Therefore, one should obtain AP and lateral lower leg radiographs to include the knee joint, in order to determine if there is a more proximal fibular fracture than would be seen on an ankle series. A proximal fibular fracture, according to Danis-Weber, indicates a syndesmotic rupture, a poor prognostic indicator.[443] Another indicator of a syndesmotic injury is an avulsion fracture. Neither the Lauge-Hansen nor the Danis-Weber are perfect fracture classification systems. Therefore, the physician should do comparison studies. This can be done with podiatric medical imaging equipment if necessary. It must be emphasized, however, that stress studies for syndesmotic injuries may be appropriate for initial evaluation. Advance imaging is necessary for more precise evaluation. According to Kellett et al., even intraoperative stress radiography failed to detect approximately half of instability injuries confirmed at arthroscopy.[444] CT is valuable for

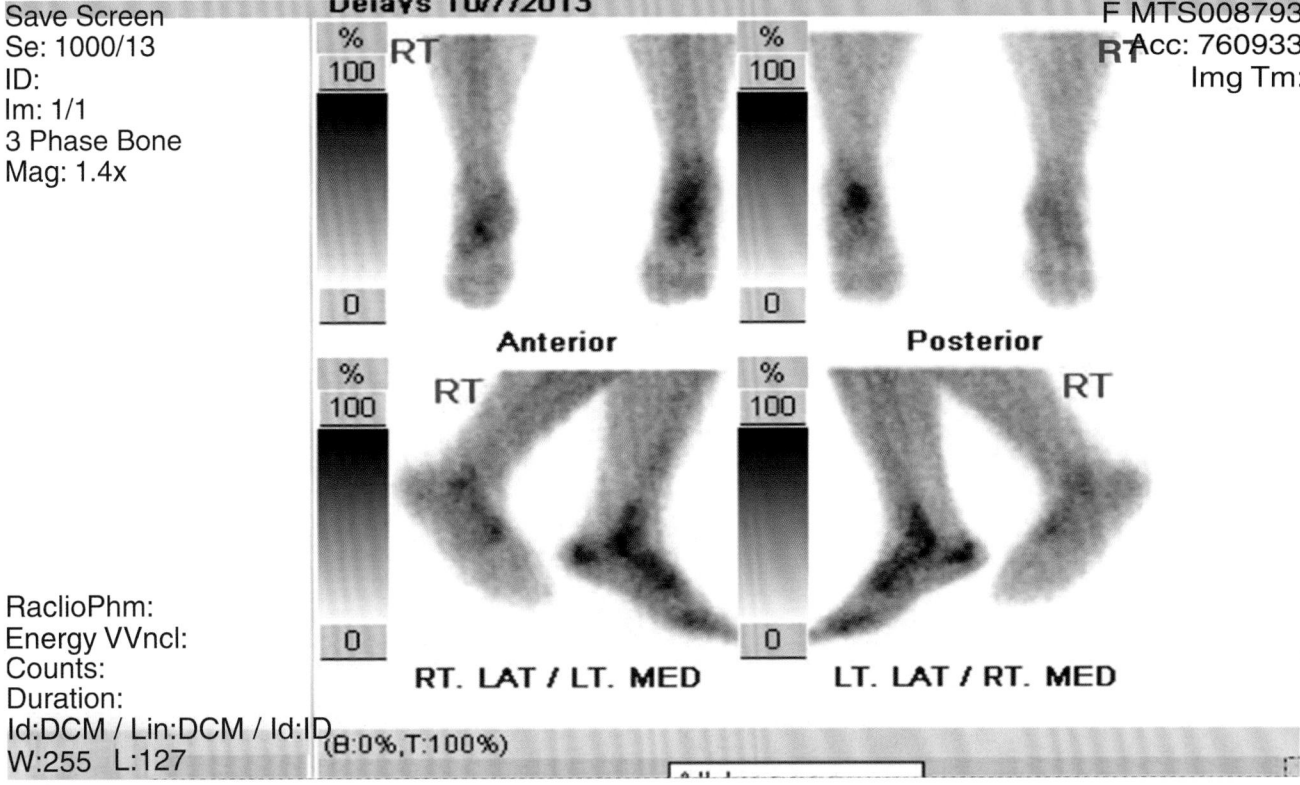

FIGURE 2.125 Complex regional pain syndrome. The delayed phase of this triple phase bone scan shows increased uptake in the joints of the left foot. The patient had complained of severe pain and swelling in her left lower leg for months after a minor injury at work. Her history, physical examination, and this bone scan helped to confirm the diagnosis.

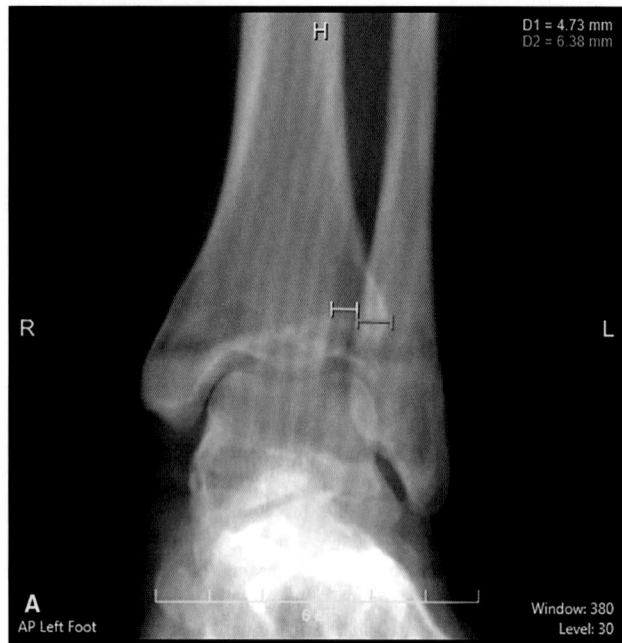
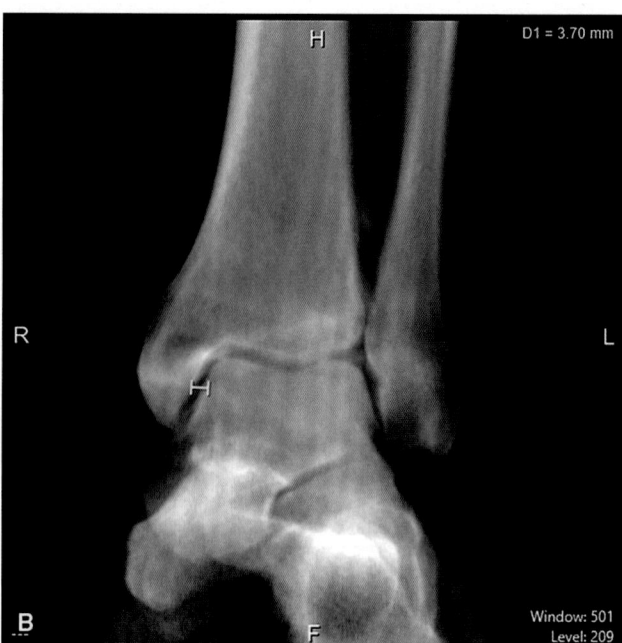

FIGURE 2.126 A. Normal AP radiograph of the left ankle. *Blue measurement*: tibiofibular clear space, which measures 4.73 mm. Normal should be <6 mm on both the AP and mortise views. *Orange measurement*: tibiofibular overlap, which measures 6.38 mm. Normal should be >6 mm on the AP view. **B.** Normal mortise of the left ankle. *Blue measurement*: medial clear space, which should be ≤4 mm. Images reconstructed, and measurements obtained from 3D weight-bearing CT software.

the detection of syndesmotic avulsion fractures (Fig. 2.127). If weight-bearing CT is available, one should do a bilateral scan for comparison.[445] However, the imaging methods of choice for syndesmotic ankle injury and instability is high powered MRI (3T) or arthroscopic viewing with stress examination.[444] Stress radiography can be used to evaluate ligamentous integrity. The three stress examinations in radiography to evaluate ankle ligaments are the inversion stress (ATF and CF ligaments), anterior drawer (ATF), and eversion stress (deltoid). For inversion stress, AP radiograph, the inferior surface of the tibia, and superior surface of the talus should be nearly parallel. A talar tilt angle >10 degrees or 5 degrees more than the normal ankle is considered abnormal.[442] A positive anterior drawer is a distance of >10 mm between the tibial articular surface posteriorly and adjacent talus[442] (Fig. 2.128A-D). In the doctor's office, diagnostic ultrasound is another fast and affordable method to evaluate ligamentous injury (Fig. 2.129A and B).[442,446,447]

SOFT TISSUE TUMORS

There are several bone and soft tissue tumors that have a predilection for the lower extremity.[448] Diagnostic imaging is much more limited for the diagnosis of soft tissue tumors than with bone tumors.[436] As with bone tumors, one should always start with plain film radiography, which may show blurring of soft tissue planes, calcifications, phleboliths, or splaying of bones. With bone tumors, advanced imaging should be CT after plain radiographs, because CT is better than MRI at imaging cortical bone. However, with a soft tissue tumor, one should order an MRI with contrast after plain radiography. MRI is superior

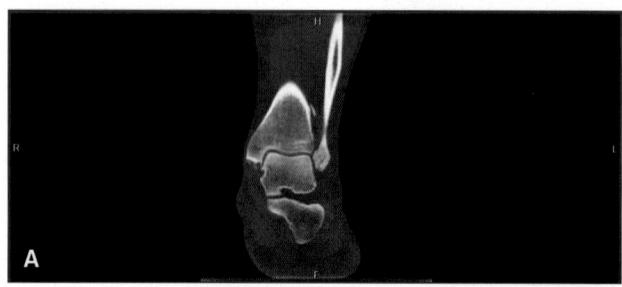
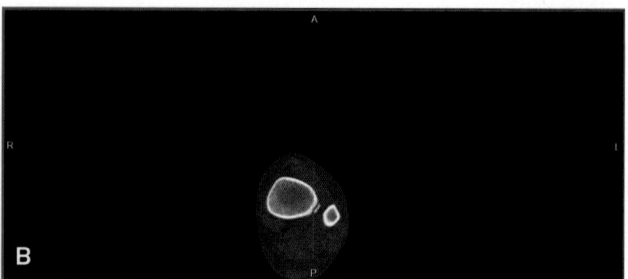

FIGURE 2.127 Syndesmotic injury. **A.** Weight-bearing CT, coronal slice of a patient with a history of high ankle sprain. Avulsion fracture seen from the lateral aspect of the distal tibia, indicative of an interosseous membrane sprain. Also note the arthritic changes in the medial ankle, which can result from an old high ankle sprain. **B.** Axial slice. Avulsion fracture is seen, posterior-lateral.

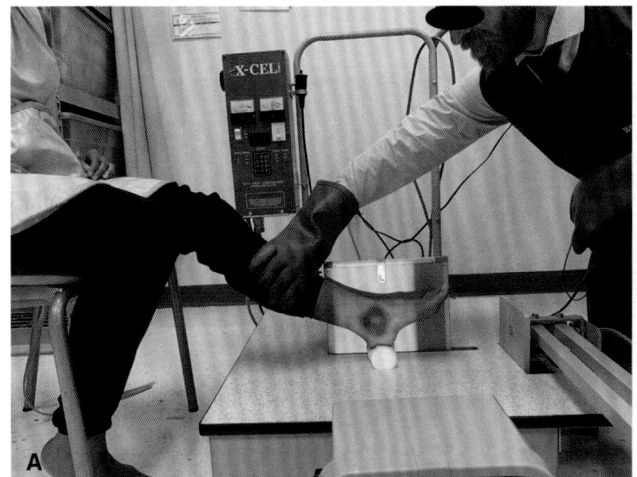
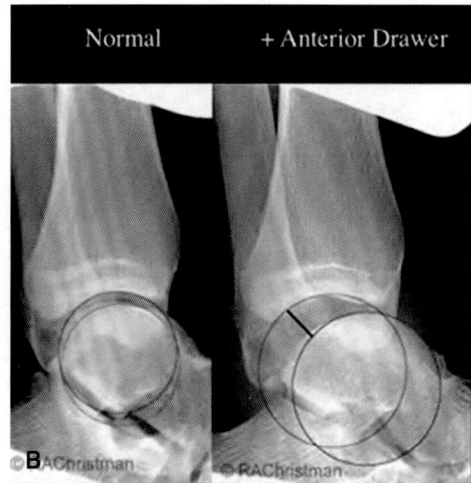
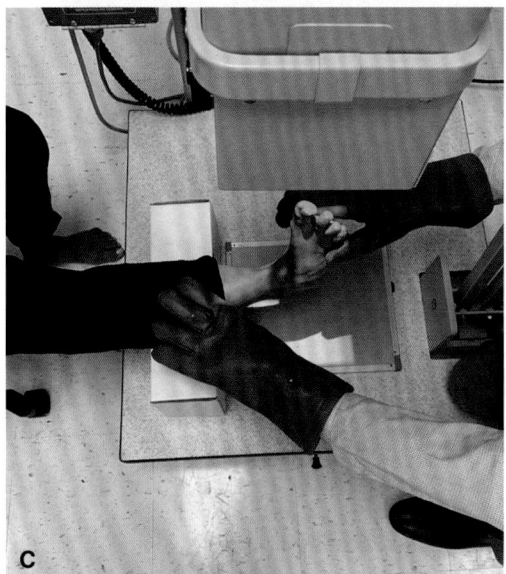
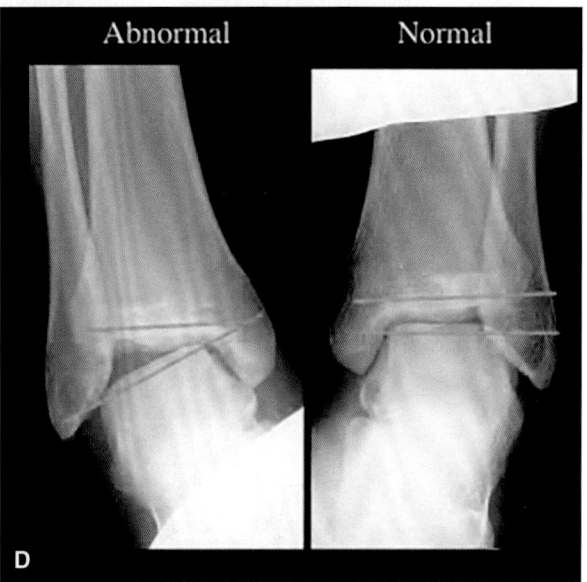

FIGURE 2.128 **A.** Anterior drawer method using a standard foot and ankle radiographic unit. **B.** Anterior drawer sign. Stress radiographs. *Left*: negative anterior drawer (normal). *Right*: positive anterior drawer: a distance of >10 mm between the tibial articular surface posteriorly and adjacent talus. **C.** Talar tilt using a standard foot and ankle radiographic unit. **D.** Talar tilt stress radiographs. *Left*: abnormal; the angle >10 degrees indicating a rupture of the calcaneofibular ligament. *Right*: normal; the two lines are nearly parallel. (Radiographs courtesy of Dr. Robert A. Christman.)

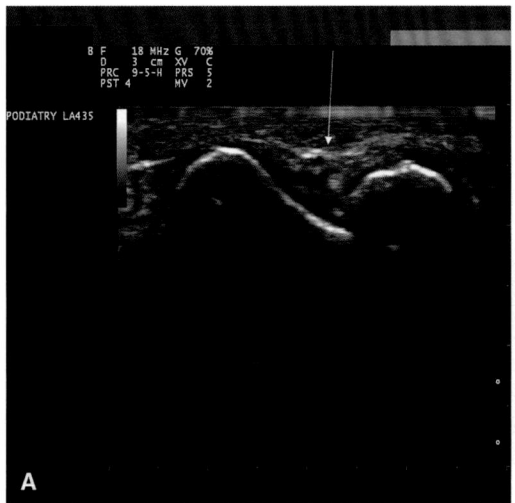
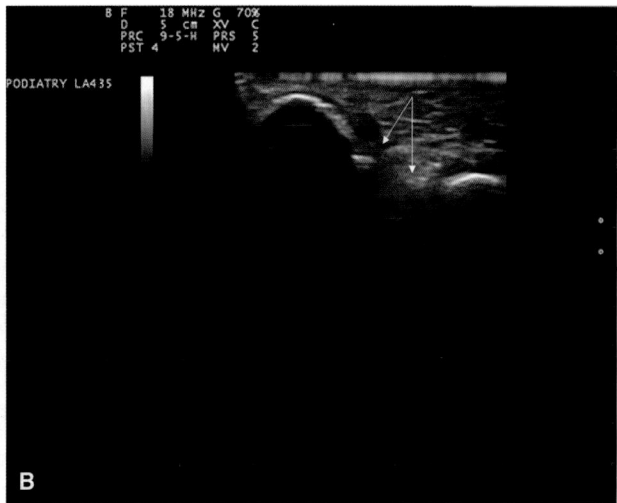

FIGURE 2.129 **A.** Intact anterior talofibular ligament (*arrow*), long axis with ultrasound. **B.** Ruptured anterior talofibular ligament (*arrows*).

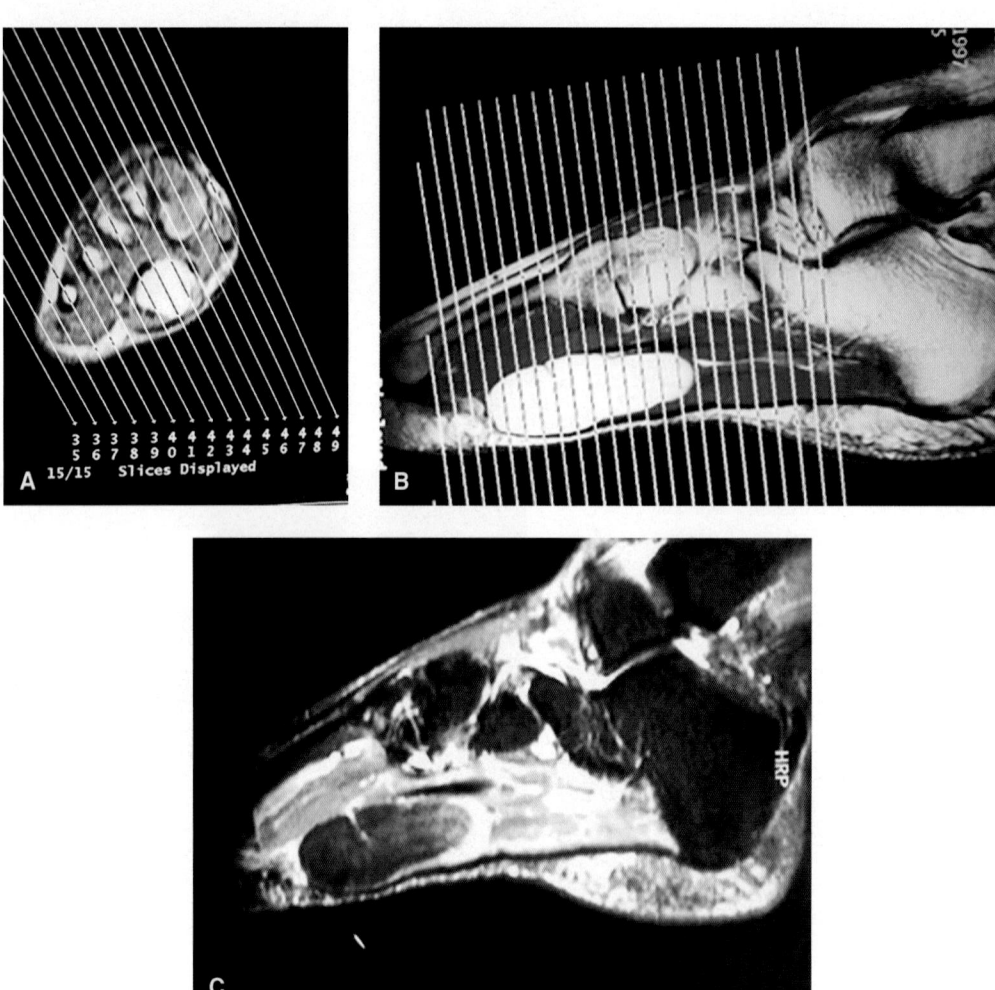

FIGURE 2.130 Lipoma. **A.** MRI, coronal slice, T1 weighted. One can see the circular high signal lesion at the plantar aspect of the foot. **B.** Sagittal slice, also T1 weighted. One can again see the now oval-shaped high signal lesion in the plantar aspect of the foot. **C.** Sagittal slice, the weighting is balanced, with fat suppression. The lipoma is now low signal, consistent with a fat suppressed image.

to CT at imaging soft tissue, and contrast should be ordered to evaluate if there is a blood supply to the tumor. There are numerous soft tissue tumors that can be imaged with MRI.[437] This chapter focuses on a few of those. There are some benign tumors that have a distinctive appearance on MRI. A lipoma, of course, is going to appear as a homogeneous high signal lesion on a T1-weighted image (Fig. 2.130A-C). Synovial and

ganglion cysts will appear as a homogeneous high signal lesion on a T2-weighted image due to its fluid content (Fig. 2.131). Hemangiomas are not well defined and have a heterogeneous appearance on MRI.[436] Morton neuroma is actually a misnomer. It is not a true nerve tumor, but rather a peripheral nerve entrapment, with fibrotic response in and around the nerve.[2,446,447] Plain radiography can demonstrate splaying of the

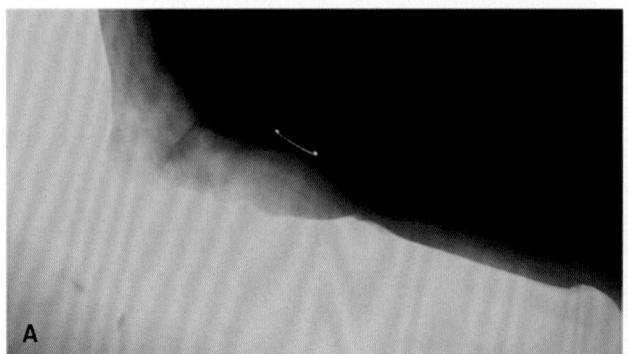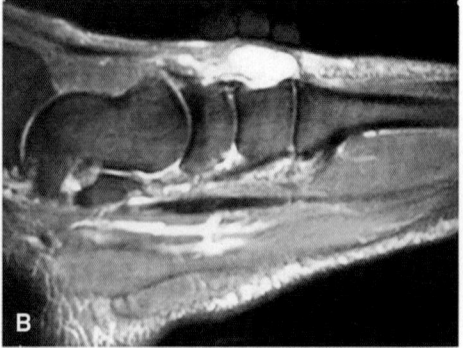

FIGURE 2.131 Ganglion cyst. **A.** Lateral radiograph of the foot with a lesion marker on the soft tissue mass. **B.** T2 weighted MRI (also with a lesion marker) showing the homogeneous, high signal lesion, consistent with a fluid-filled ganglion cyst.

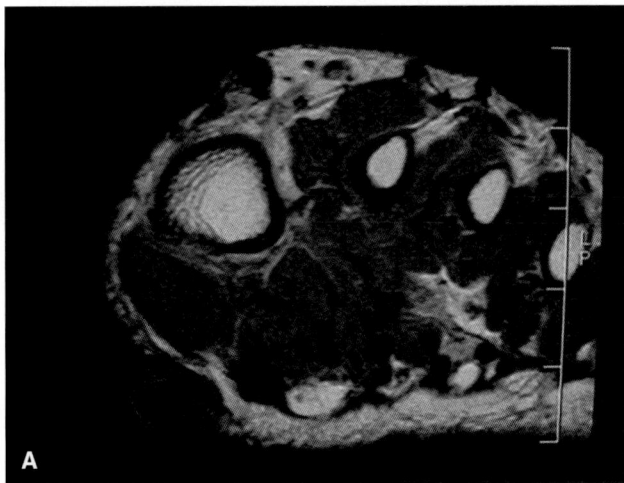

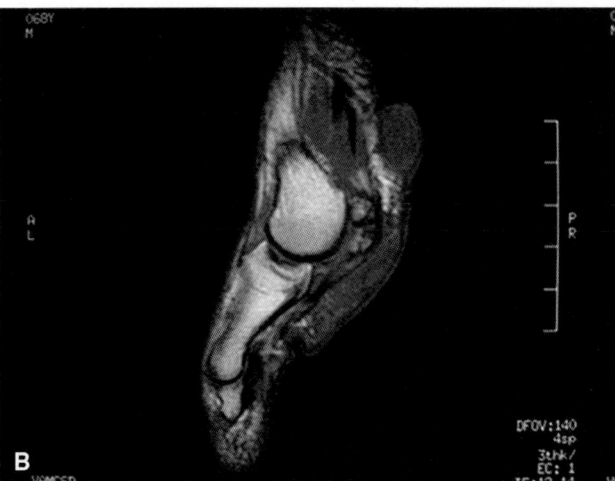

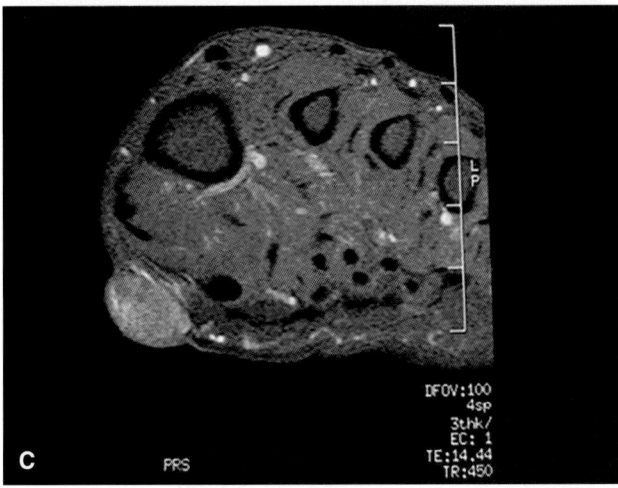

FIGURE 2.132 Dermatofibroma. **A.** Coronal slice, T1-weighted MRI, shows a low signal intensity lesion on the plantar-medial aspect of the foot, inferior to the first metatarsal shaft. **B.** Sagittal slice, also T1 weighted, also shows the low signal lesion on the plantar aspect of the foot. **C.** The lesion shows enhancement with gadolinium. (Images courtesy of Dr. Sandra Garcia-Ortiz.)

digits affected by the neuroma. Plantar fibromatosis, a nodular proliferation of the plantar fascia, will usually have a low signal intensity on MRI. A dermatofibroma will appear as low signal on both T1- and T2-weighted images and will show enhancement with gadolinium (Fig. 2.132A-C). Synovial sarcoma is a malignant tumor, ninety percent of which occur in the extremities. On MRI, they have a lobulated, low signal appearance on T1 and high signal on T2 (or STIR proton density) (Fig. 2.133A and B).

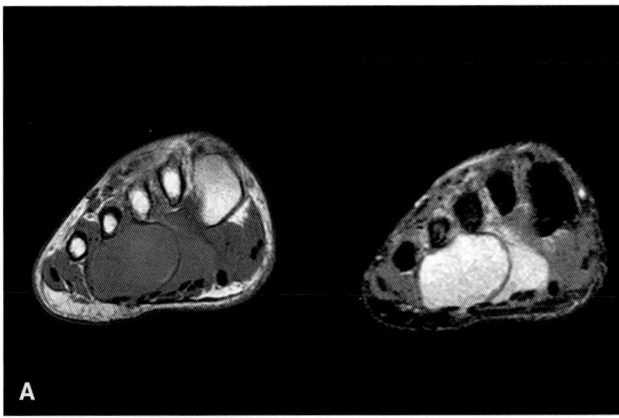

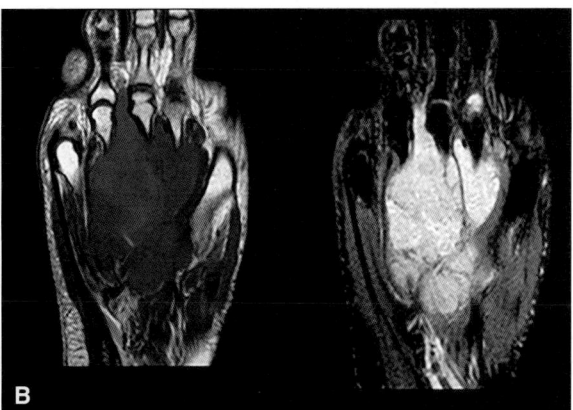

FIGURE 2.133 Synovial sarcoma, MRI. **A.** Coronal images show the soft tissue mass low signal on the T1-weighted image (*left*) and high signal on the STIR image (*right*). **B.** Axial slices also show the soft tissue mass low signal on the T1-weighted image (*left*) and high signal on the STIR image (*right*).

TENDONS

Can be imaged with MRI or ultrasound. Tendons, if they are normal will appear black on MRI, whether the image is T1, T2, or balanced (proton density). When pathology is suspected, one should look for increased signal intensity in the tendon or an abnormal shape of the tendon. With ultrasound, tendons appear as slightly echogenic and will look like cables in long axis. Pathology of a tendon will show decreased echogenicity and/or abnormal shape. The Achilles tendon can be imaged initially with plain radiography. One can see the shadow of this tendon, as the posterior border of Kager triangle. If rupture or pathology is suspected, one looks for distortion or obliteration of Kager triangle (Fig. 2.134). On MRI, especially on the T2-weighted image, Achilles tendon rupture will show stranding of the tendon, with areas of high signal intensity indicating hemorrhage (Fig. 2.135).[442] The plantar fascia is basically a continuation of the Achilles tendon. Therefore, like tendon, the normal plantar aponeurosis should appear black on MRI. When considering pathology, one should look for the same abnormalities seen with tendon, that is, increased signal intensity, or abnormal shape on MRI, or decreased echogenicity and abnormal shape on ultrasound (Fig. 2.136).

BONE MARROW

Bone marrow can be imaged with MRI and will appear high signal on T1, and low signal on T2, or with fat suppression. Bone marrow edema will appear high signal on T2, and MRI is the imaging method of choice for acute osteomyelitis. However, impacted bone marrow due to trauma or surgery can also appear as high signal on a T2 weighted image. Bone marrow imaging with nuclear medicine can help with this dilemma.[449] A marrow scan is usually done to supplement a labeled white blood cell scan when looking for infection in bones and joints. The scan is performed with an intravenous injection of Tc-99m sulfur colloid. This increases the diagnostic accuracy of the white blood cell scan by making it far more specific for the detection of infection. Generally speaking, if both the white blood cell scan and the sulfur colloid scan show increased uptake in the area of concern, there is no infection, and the uptake is due to impacted bone. However, if there is increased uptake with the white blood cell scan, and normal uptake with the sulfur colloid scan, infection would be suspected (Fig. 2.137).

Stressed again here is the importance of the patient history, physical examination, and clinical diagnosis when ordering and evaluating any imaging study. The more precise information the radiologist can be given, the better he or she is able to confirm or exclude a diagnosis or suggest additional imaging if necessary.

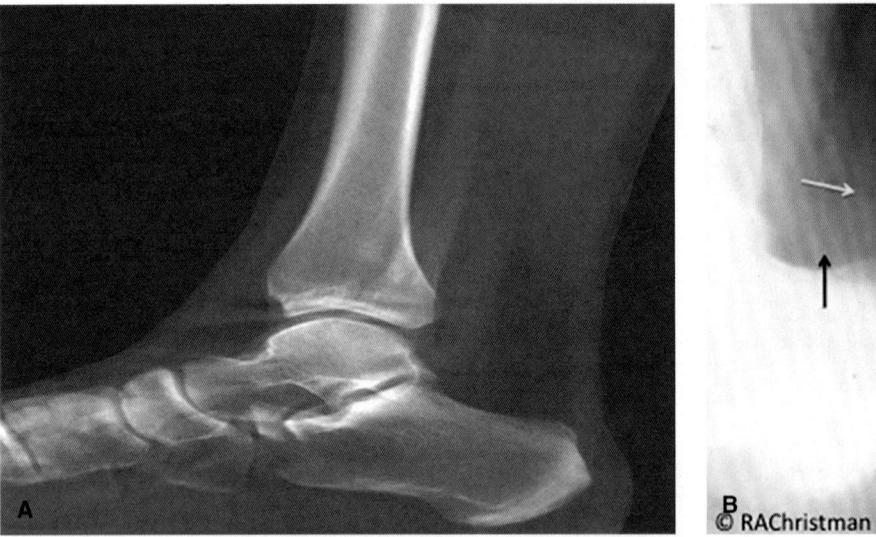
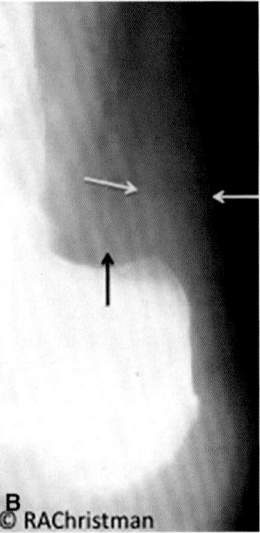

FIGURE 2.134 Kager triangle. **A.** Normal Kager triangle. **B.** Achilles tendonitis, (*arrows*) showing obliteration of Kager triangle. (**Part B** image courtesy of Dr. Robert A. Christman.)

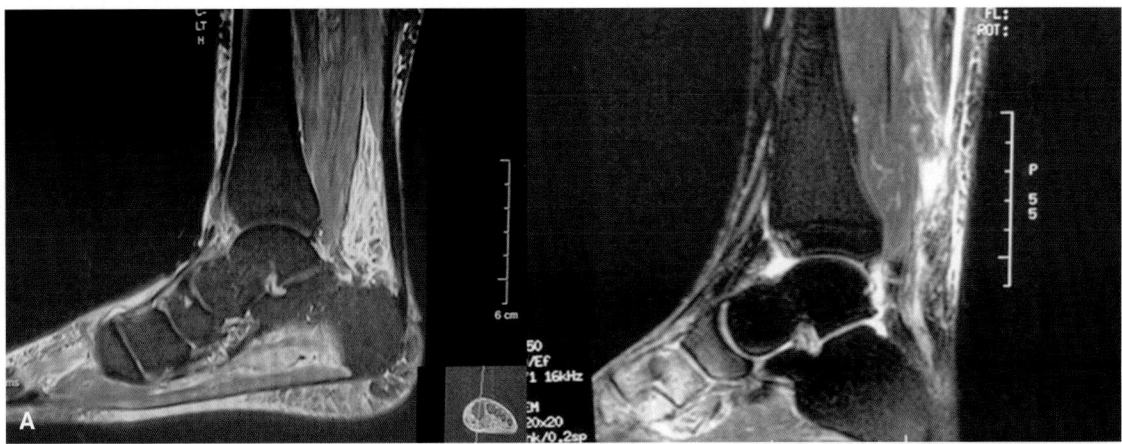

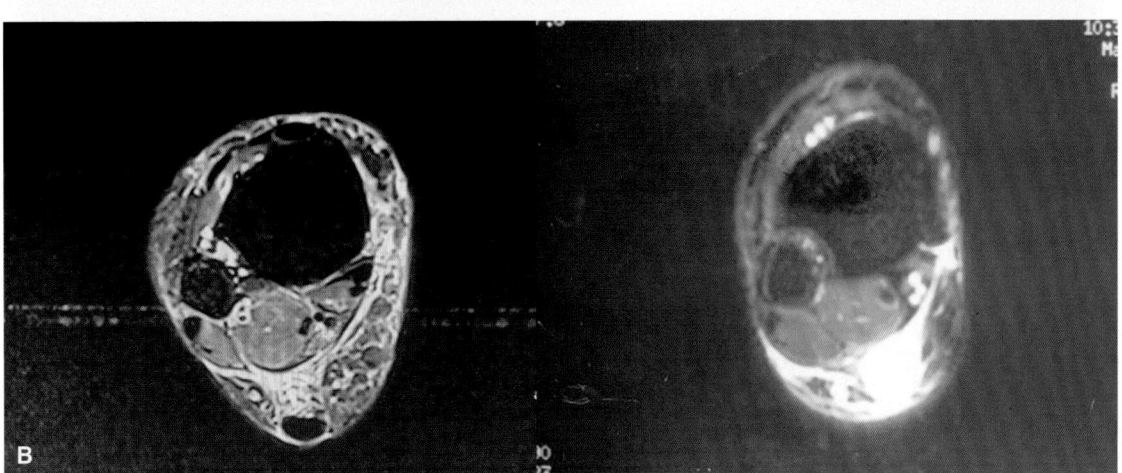

FIGURE 2.135 Achilles tendon rupture. **A.** T2-weighted sagittal slices through the ankle. The *left* image shows a normal Achilles tendon, which appears as a black strip in the posterior ankle as it should. On the *right*, one can see stranding of the tendon, and the high signal intensity hemorrhage in place of the normally black tendon. **B.** T2-weighted axial slices through the ankle. The *left* image shows a normal Achilles tendon in short axis, which is *black* and *oval* in shape. On the *right*, there is disappearance of the tendon, which is replaced with high signal hemorrhage, consistent with an Achilles tendon rupture.

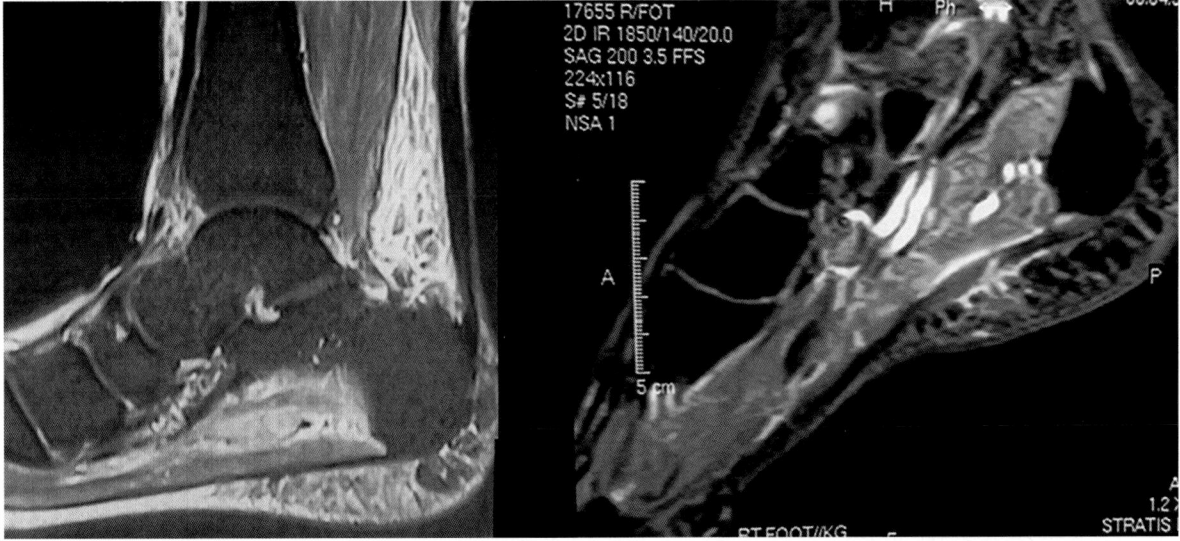

FIGURE 2.136 MRI, partial rupture, plantar aponeurosis. On the *left* is the normal appearance of the plantar aponeurosis on MRI, T2 weighted. On the *right*, also T2 weighted, one can see the increase signal intensity, and abnormal shape of the plantar aponeurosis, consistent with a partial rupture.

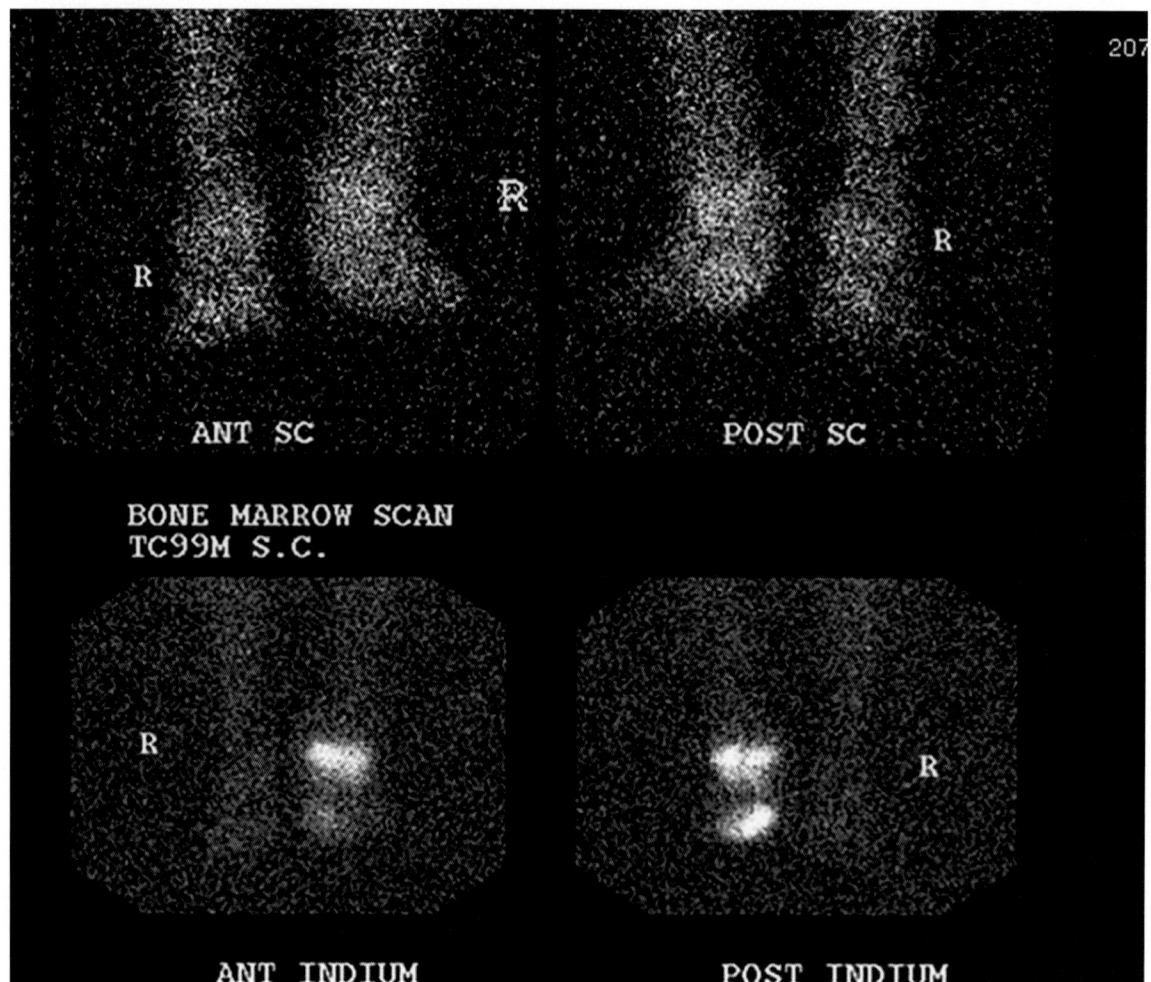

FIGURE 2.137 Bone marrow scan of a patient with recent ankle surgery and a heel ulcer on the *left*. The two *top* images are the sulfur colloid images. One does not see intense increased uptake in the left foot. The *bottom* two images are indium 111 white blood cell labelled images. These images show increased uptake in the ankle and the heel, which helped confirm the diagnosis of osteomyelitis.

REFERENCES

1. Christman RA. View selection for the radiographic study. In: Christman RA, ed. *Foot and Ankle Radiology*. 2nd ed. Philadelphia, PA: Wolters Kluwer; 2015:167-178.
2. Ruch JA. Significance and use of radiographs in the angle and base of gait. *PAL Perspectives in Podiatry*. 1980;1(2):1-4 (Podiatry Arts Lab).
3. Bryant JA. A comparison of radiographic foot measurements taken in two different positions. *J Am Podiatr Med Assoc*. 2001;91(5):234.
4. McPoil TG, Carrell D, Ehlers D, et al. Does foot placement affect the reliability of static foot posture measurements? *J Am Podiatr Med Assoc*. 2014;104(1):34-42.
5. McPoil TG, Cornwall MW, Taylor O, et al. The consistency of individual-selected versus rater-determined angle and base of gait. *J Am Podiatr Med Assoc*. 2014;104(3):247-252.
6. Waite S, Scott J, Gale B, et al. Interpretive error in radiology. *AJR Am J Roentgenol*. 2017;208:739-749.
7. Eastman GW, Wald C, Crossin J. Phenomena in imaging and perception. In: Eastman GW, Wald C, Crossin J, eds. *Getting Started in Clinical Radiology: From Image to Diagnosis*. New York, NY: Thieme; 2006:18-26.
8. Gunderman RB. Introduction to radiology. In: Gunderman RB, ed. *Essential Radiology*. 2nd ed. New York, NY: Thieme; 2006:1-38.
9. Green SA, Green HD. The influence of radiographic projection on the appearance of deformities. *Orthop Clin North Am*. 1994;25(3):467-475.
10. Weijers R, Kemerink G, van Mameren H, et al. The intermetatarsal and metatarsal declination angles: Geometry as a source of error. *Foot Ankle Int*. 2005;26(5):387-393.
11. LaPorta GA, Scarlet J. Radiographic changes in the pronated and supinated foot. *J Am Podiatry Assoc*. 1977;67(5):334.
12. Christman RA. Radiographic anatomy of the foot and ankle. Part 1: the distal leg. *J Am Podiatr Med Assoc*. 2014;104(4):402.
13. Christman RA. Radiographic anatomy of the foot and ankle. Part 2: the greater tarsus. *J Am Podiatr Med Assoc*. 2014;104(5):493.
14. Christman RA. Radiographic anatomy of the foot and ankle. Part 3: the lesser tarsus. *J Am Podiatr Med Assoc*. 2014;104(6):633.
15. Christman RA. Radiographic anatomy of the foot and ankle. Part 4: the metatarsals. *J Am Podiatr Med Assoc*. 2015;105(1):51.
16. Christman RA. Radiographic anatomy of the foot and ankle. Part 5: the toes. *J Am Podiatr Med Assoc*. 2015;105(2):141.
17. Christman RA. Normal variants and anomalies. In: Christman RA, ed. *Foot and Ankle Radiology*. 2nd ed. Philadelphia, PA: Wolters Kluwer; 2015:79-119.
18. Baron RL, Strugielski CF, Christman RA. Positioning techniques and terminology. In: Christman RA, ed. *Foot and Ankle Radiology*. 2nd ed. Philadelphia, PA: Wolters Kluwer; 2015:43-62.
19. Draves DJ. *Anatomy of the Lower Extremity*. Baltimore, MD: Williams and Wilkins; 1986: 135-136.
20. Shrewsbury M, Johnson RK. The fascia of the distal phalanx. *J Bone Joint Surg Am*. 1975; 57-A(6):784-788.
21. Wilkinson JL. The terminal phalanx of the great toe. *J Anat*. 1954;88:537-541.
22. Lee M, Hodler J, Haghighi P, et al. Bone excrescence at the medial base of the distal phalanx of the first toe: normal variant, reactive change, or neoplasia? *Skeletal Radiol*. 1992;21:161-165.
23. Chinn S, Jenkin W. Proximal nail groove pain associated with an exostosis. *J Am Podiatr Med Assoc*. 1986;76(9):506-508.
24. Roukis TS, Hurless JS. The hallucal interphalangeal sesamoid. *J Foot Ankle Surg*. 1996;35(4):303-308.
25. Sharon SM. Interphalangeal joint hallux ossicle. *J Foot Surg*. 1977;16(2):69-72.
26. Okuda R. Proximal supination osteotomy of the first metatarsal for hallux valgus. *Foot Ankle Clin*. 2018;23:257-269.
27. Christman RA, Ly P. Radiographic anatomy of the first metatarsal. *J Am Podiatr Med Assoc*. 1990;80(4):177-203.
28. Spencer EE, Beirman JS, Femino JE. Osteoid osteoma of the fifth metatarsal: a case report and literature review. *Foot Ankle Surg*. 2002;8:71-78.
29. Resnick D, Kransdorf MJ. Enostosis, hyperostosis, and periostitis. In: Resnick D, Kransdorf MJ, eds. *Bone and Joint Imaging*. 3rd ed. Philadelphia, PA: Elsevier Saunders; 2005:1424-1446.
30. Gamble FO, Yale I. Normal foot structure. In: Gamble FO, Yale I, eds. *Clinical Foot Roentgenology*. 2nd ed. Huntington, NY: Krieger Publishing; 1975:186-208.
31. Case DT, Ossenburg NS, Burnett SE. Os intermetatarseum. *Am J Phys Anthropol*. 1998;107:199-209.
32. Nakasa T, Fukuhara K, Adachi N, et al. Painful os intermetatarseum in athletes: report of four cases and review of the literature. *Arch Orthop Trauma Surg*. 2007;127(4):261-264.
33. Knackfuss IG, Giordano V, Nogueira M, et al. Compression of the medial branch of the deep peroneal nerve, relieved by excision of an os intermetatarseum: a case report. *Acta Orthop Belg*. 2003;69:568.
34. Haliburton RA, Butt EG, Barber JR. The tibialis anterior sesamoid. *Can J Surg*. 1961;4:480.
35. Morrison AB. The os paracuneiforme. Some observations on an example removed at operation. *J Bone Joint Surg Am*. 1953;35B(2):254.
36. Burnett SE, Case DT. Bipartite medial cuneiform: new frequencies from skeletal collections and a meta-analysis of previous cases. *HOMO*. 2011;62:109-125.
37. Steen EF, Brancheau SP, Nguyen T, et al. Symptomatic bipartite medial cuneiform. Report of five cases and review of the literature. *Foot Ankle Spec*. 2016;9(1):69-78.
38. Elias I, Dheer S, Zoga AC, et al. Magnetic resonance imaging findings in bipartite medial cuneiform—a potential pitfall in diagnosis of midfoot injuries: a case series. *J Med Case Reports*. 2008;2:272.
39. Maceira E, Rochera R. Muller-Weiss disease: clinical and biomechanical features. *Foot Ankle Clin*. 2004;9:105-125.
40. Sizensky JA, Marks RM. Imaging of the navicular. *Foot Ankle Clin*. 2004;9:181-209.
41. Dionisio P, Lomasney LM, Demos TC, et al. Bipartite navicular. *Orthopedics*. 2009;32(11):856-858.
42. Ingalls J, Wissman R. The os supranaviculare and navicular stress fractures. *Skeletal Radiol*. 2011;40:937-941.
43. Henriques M. Os supratalare. *Acta Med Port*. 2018;31(5):280.
44. Kim SJ, Kim O. Imaging findings of CT and MRI of Os supratalare: a case report. *J Korean Soc Radiol*. 2013;69(4):317-320.
45. Salekzamani Y, Shakeri-Bavil A, Nezami N, et al. Ankle patella: a report of a large accessory bone in the ankle: a case report. *Cases J*. 2009;2:8512.
46. Lawson JP, Ogden JA, Sella E, et al. The painful accessory navicular. *Skeletal Radiol*. 1984;12:250-262.
47. Lawson JP. International Skeletal Society Lecture in honor of Howard D. Dorfman. Clinically significant radiologic anatomic variants of the skeleton. *Am J Roentgenol*. 1994;163:249-255.
48. Perdikakis E, Grigoraki E, Karantanas A. Os naviculare: the multi-ossicle configuration of a normal variant. *Skeletal Radiol*. 2011;40:85-88.
49. Sella EJ, Lawson JP. Biomechanics of the accessory navicular synchondrosis. *Foot Ankle*. 1987;8:156-163.
50. Chong A, Ha JM, Lee JY. Clinical meaning of hot uptake on bone scan in symptomatic accessory navicular bones. *Nucl Med Mol Imaging*. 2016;50:322-328.
51. Bernaerts A, Vanhoenacker FM, Van de Perre S, et al. Accessory navicular bone: not such a normal variant. *JBR-BTR*. 2004;87:250-252.
52. Kelikian AS. *Sarrafian's Anatomy of the Foot and Ankle*. 3rd ed. Philadelphia, PA: Lippincott Williams & Wilkins; 2011:72.
53. Burton SK, Altman MI. Degenerative arthritis of the os peroneum: a case report. *J Am Podiatr Med Assoc*. 1986;76(6):343-345.
54. Corey SV. Management of pathology associated with the presence of an os peroneum. *Podiatry Institute Update*. 2012;46:233-235.
55. Bianchi S, Bortolotti C, Draghi F. Os peroneum imaging: normal appearance and pathological findings. *Insights Imaging*. 2017;8:59-68.
56. Stockton KG, Brodsky JW. Peroneus longus tears associated with pathology of the os peroneum. *Foot Ankle Int*. 2014;35(4):346-352.
57. Degan TJ, Morrey BF, Braun DP. Surgical excision for anterior-process fractures of the calcaneus. *J Bone Joint Surg Am*. 1982;64:519-524.
58. Ouellette H, Salamipour H, Thomas BJ, et al. Incidence and MR imaging features of fractures of the anterior process of calcaneus in a consecutive patient population with ankle and foot symptoms. *Skeletal Radiol*. 2006;35(11):833-837.
59. Kürklü M, Köse Õ, Yurttas Y, et al. Anterosuperior calcaneal process fracture or os calcaneus secundarius? *Am J Phys Med Rehabil*. 2010;89(6):522.
60. Fadl SA, Ramzan MM, Sandstrom CK. Core curriculum illustration: anterior process fracture of the calcaneus. *Emerg Radiol*. 2018;25:205-207.
61. Nwawka OK, Hayashi D, Diaz LE, et al. Sesamoids and accessory ossicles of the foot: anatomical variability and related pathology. *Insights Imaging*. 2013;4:581-593.
62. Mellado JM, Ramos A, Salvado E, et al. Accessory ossicles and sesamoid bones of the ankle and foot: imaging findings, clinical significance and differential diagnosis. *Eur Radiol*. 2003;13:L164-L177.
63. Nault ML, Kocher MS, Micheli LJ. Os trigonum syndrome. *J Am Acad Orthop Surg*. 2014;22:545-553.
64. Kose O. The accessory ossicles of the foot and ankle; a Diagnostic Pitfall in Emergency Department in Context of Foot and Ankle Trauma. *JAEM*. 2012;11:106-114.
65. Berkowitz MJ, Kim DH. Process and tubercle fractures of the hindfoot. *J Am Acad Orthop Surg*. 2005;13:492-502.
66. Milgrom C, Kaplan L, Lax E. Case report 341: Os accessorium supracalcaneum of the left hind foot (also present, but to a lesser extent, on the right). *Skeletal Radiol*. 1986;15:150-153.
67. Coral A. The radiology of skeletal elements in the subtibial region: incidence and significance. *Skeletal Radiol*. 1987;16:298-303.
68. Coughlin MJ. Sesamoids and accessory bones of the foot. In: Coughlin MJ, Mann RA, Saltzman CA, eds. *Surgery of the Foot & Ankle*. 8th ed. St. Louis, MO: Mosby; 2006:531-610.
69. Berg EE. The symptomatic os subfibulare. Avulsion fracture of the fibula associated with recurrent instability of the ankle. *J Bone Joint Surg Am*. 1991;73(8):1251.
70. Kono T, Ochi M, Takao M, et al. Symptomatic os subfibulare caused by accessory ossification: a case report. *Clin Orthop Relat Res*. 2002;399:197.
71. Zhang C, Wang X, Ma X, et al. A novel 9-region systematic assessment tool for separated ossicles at the fibular top effects on lateral ankle ligament complex integrity: a cadaveric study. *Surg Radiol Anat*. 2014;36:281-288.
72. Haraguchi N, Kato F, Hayashi H. New radiographic projections for avulsion fracture of the lateral malleolus. *J Bone Joint Surg Br*. 1998;80:684-688.
73. Miyamoto W, Takao M, Nishiguchi K, et al. Technique tip: a radiographic projection for an avulsion fracture of the talar attachment of the anterior talofibular ligament. *Foot Ankle Int*. 2008;29:435-437.
74. Sugi MT, Tileston K, Krygier JE, et al. Transepiphyseal (Type VII) ankle fracture versus os subfibulare in pediatric ankle injuries. *J Pediatr Orthop*. 2018;38:e593-e596.
75. Nakasa T, Fukuhara K, Adachi N, et al. Evaluation of anterior talofibular ligament lesion using 3-dimensional computed tomography. *J Comput Assist Tomogr*. 2006;30(3):543-547.
76. Kernbach KJ. Tarsal coalitions: etiology, diagnosis, imaging, and stigmata. *Clin Podiatr Med Surg*. 2010;27:105-117.
77. Lysack JT, Fenton PV. Variations in Calcaneonavicular morphology demonstrated with radiography. *Radiology*. 2004;230:493-497.

78. Upasani VV, Chambers RC, Mabarak SJ. Analysis of calcaneonavicular coalitions using multi-planar three-dimensional computed tomography. *J Child Orthop.* 2008;2:301-307.

79. Oestreich AE, Mize WA, Crawford AH, et al. The "anteater nose": a direct sign of calcaneonavicular coalition on the lateral radiograph. *J Pediatr Orthop.* 1987;7:709-711.

80. Pouliquen JC, Duranthon LD, Glorion CH, et al. The too long anterior process calcaneus: a report of 39 cases in 25 children and adolescents. *J Pediatr Orthop.* 1998;18:333-336.

81. Rozansky A, Varley E, Moor M, et al. A radiologic classification of talocalcaneal coalitions based on 3D reconstruction. *J Child Orthop.* 2010;4:129-135.

82. Linklater J, Hayter CL, Vu D, et al. Anatomy of the subtalar joint and imaging of talocalcaneal coalition. *Skeletal Radiol.* 2009;38:437-449.

83. Lateur LM, Van Hoe LR, Van Ghillewe KV, et al. Subtalar coalition: diagnosis with the C sign on lateral radiograph of the ankle. *Radiology.* 1994;193:847-851.

84. Brown RR, Rosenberg ZS, Thornhill BA. The C sign: more specific for flatfoot deformity than subtalar coalition. *Skeletal Radiol.* 2001;30:84-87.

85. Moraleda L, Gantsoudes GD, Mubarak SJ. C Sign: talocalcaneal coalition or flat foot deformity? *J Pediatr Orthop.* 2014;34:814-819.

86. Mahan ST, Prete VI, Spencer SA, et al. Subtalar coalitions: does the morphology of the subtalar joint involvement influence outcomes after coalition excision? *J Foot Ankle Surg.* 2017;56:797-801.

87. Bixby SD, Jarrett DY, Johnston P, et al. Posteromedial subtalar coalitions: prevalence and associated morphological alterations of the sustentaculum tali. *Pediatr Radiol.* 2016;46:1-8.

88. Exner GU, Jacob HAC, Maquiera GJ. Fibulocalcaneal impingement in a growing child with otherwise asymptomatic talocalcaneal coalition. *J Foot Ankle Surg.* 2017;56:1323-1327.

89. Beckly DE, Anderson PW, Pedegana LR. The radiology of the subtalar joint with special reference to talo-calcaneal coalition. *Clin Radiol.* 1975;26:333-341.

90. Crim J, Kjeldsberg K. Radiographic diagnosis of tarsal coalition. *Am J Roentgenol.* 2004;18:323-328.

91. Harris RI, Beath T. Etiology of peroneal spastic flat foot. *J Bone Joint Surg Br.* 1948;30B(4):624-634.

92. Oestreich AE. Radiology. In: Drennan JC, ed. *The Child's Foot and Ankle.* New York, NY: Raven Press; 1992.

93. Don S, Slovis TL. Musculoskeletal imaging strategies and controlling radiation esposure. In: Stein-Wexler R, Wooten-Gorges SL, Ozonoff MB, eds. *Pediatric Orthopedic Imaging.* New York, NY: Springer Verlag Berlin Heidelberg; 2015.

94. Christman RA, Truong J. Normal development. In: Christman RA, ed. *Foot and Ankle Radiology.* 2nd ed. Philadelphia, PA: Wolters Kluwer; 2015:121-143.

95. Christman RA, Truong J. Developmental variants. In: Christman RA, ed. *Foot and Ankle Radiology.* 2nd ed. Philadelphia, PA: Wolters Kluwer; 2015:145-158.

96. Kump WL. Vertical fractures of the distal tibial epiphysis. *Am J Roentgenol Radium Ther Nucl Med.* 1966;97(3):676-681.

97. Keats TE, Anderson MW. *Atlas of Normal Roentgen Variants That May Simulate Disease.* 9th ed. Philadelphia, PA: Saunders; 2013.

98. Nicholson AD, Liu RW, Sanders JO, et al. Relationship of calcaneal and iliac apophyseal ossification to peak height velocity timing in children. *J Bone Joint Surg Am.* 2015;97:147-154.

99. Shopfner CE, Coin CG. Effect of weight-bearing on the appearance and development of the secondary calcaneal epiphysis. *Radiology.* 1966;86:201.

100. Frush TJ, Lindenfeld TN. Peri-epiphyseal and overuse injuries in adolescent athletes. *Sports Health.* 2009;1:201-211.

101. Resnick D, Kransdorff MJ. Osteochondroses. In: Resnick D, Kransdorff MJ, eds. *Bone and Joint Imaging.* 3rd ed. Philadelphia, PA: Elsevier Saunders; 2005:1089-1107.

102. Brower AC. The osteochondroses. *Orthop Clin North Am.* 1983;14:99-117.

103. Ferguson AB, Gingrich RM. The normal and the abnormal calcaneal apophysis and tarsal navicular. *Clin Orthop.* 1957;10:87-95.

104. Ogden JA, Ganey TM, Hill JD, et al. Sever's injury: a stress fracture of the immature calcaneal metaphysis. *J Pediatr Orthop.* 2004;24:488.

105. Salter RB, Harris R. Injuries involving the epiphyseal plate. *J Bone Joint Surg Am.* 1963;45:587-622.

106. Ogden JA. Skeletal growth mechanism injury patterns. *J Pediatr Orthop.* 1982;2(4):371-377.

107. Lee P, Hunter TB, Taljanovic M. Musculoskeletal colloquialisms: how did we come up with these names? *Radiographics.* 2004;24(4):1009-1027.

108. http://learningradiology.com/radsigns/radsignspages/L-radsigns.htm. Accessed April 23, 2019.

109. Dorland WAN. *Dorland's Illustrated Medical Dictionary.* 31st ed. Philadelphia, PA: Saunders; 2007.

110. Fleischer A, Amidi A, Kelly M, et al. Look Before You Cut: Risk Factors for Skeletal Osteoporosis on Foot X-rays. Poster presentation at 2017 ACFAS Annual Scientific Conference; February 27, 2017; Las Vegas, NV. Poster presentation at APMA Annual Scientific Meeting; July 13, 2017; Nashville, TN. Oral presentation also at American Academy of Orthopaedic Surgeons/American 14 Association of Orthopaedic Surgeons (AAOS) 2018 Annual Meeting; March 7, 2018; New Orleans, LA.

111. Manaster BJ, May DA, Disler DG. Osteoporosis. In: Manaster BJ, May DA, Disler DG, eds. *Musculoskeletal Imaging.* 4th ed. Philadelphia, PA: Elsevier; 2013.

112. Meema HE, Meema S. Postmenopausal osteoporosis: simple screening method for diagnosis before structural failure. *Radiology.* 1987;164:405-410.

113. Fleischer AE, Baron R, Scholl D, et al. Age-appropriate bone density on foot X-rays is best evaluated by the 2nd metatarsal index. Poster presentation at the APMA Annual Scientific Meeting; July 23, 2013; Las Vegas, NV.

114. Grebing BR, Coughlin MJ. Evaluation of Morton's theory of second metatarsal hypertrophy. *J Bone Joint Surg Am.* 2004;86A(7):1375-1386.

115. Kaplan FS. Osteoporosis. *Clin Symp.* 1983;35(5):2-32.

116. Baron RL, Gianfortune PJ, Evans DP, et al. Imaging/Radiology. In: Edwards AA, Walter Jr. JH, Goss LR, eds. *Review Text in Podiatric Orthopedics & Primary Medicine.* 2nd ed. Bethesda, MD: American College of Foot & Ankle Orthopedics & Medicine; 2004:36.

117. Christman RA. Normal variants and anomalies. In: Christman RA, ed. *Foot and Ankle Radiology.* 2nd ed. Philadelphia, PA: Wolters Kluwer; 2015:102.

118. Pitt MJ, Morgan SL, Lopez-Ben R, et al. Association of the presence of bone bars on radiographs and low bone mineral density. *Skeletal Radiol.* 2011;40:905-911.

119. Meema HE. Recognition of cortical bone resorption in metabolic bone disease in vivo. *Skeletal Radiol.* 1977;2:11-19.

120. Jhamaria NL, Lal KB, Udawat M, et al. The trabecular pattern of the calcaneum an index of osteoporosis. *J Bone Joint Surg Br.* 1983;65;195-198.

121. Singh M, Nagrath AR, Maini PS. Changes in trabecular pattern of the upper end of the femur as an index of osteoporosis. *J Bone Joint Surg Am.* 1970;52:457-467.

122. Cockshott WP, Occleshaw CJ, Webber C, et al. Can a calcaneal morphologic index determine the degree of osteoporosis? *Skeletal Radiol.* 1984;12:119-122.

123. Aggarwal ND, Singh GD, Aggarwal R, et al. A survey of osteoporosis using the calcaneum as an index. *Int Orthop.* 1986;10:147-153.

124. Pande KC, Pande SK, Takats DD, et al. Modified calcaneal index: a new screening tool for osteoporosis based on plain radiographs of the calcaneum. *J Orthop Surg (Hong Kong).* 2005;13:27-33.

125. Saltzman CL, Brandser EA, Berbaum KS, et al. Reliability of standard foot radiographic measurements. *Foot Ankle Int.* 1994;15(12):661-665.

126. Brage ME, Bennett CR, Whitehurst JB, et al. Observer reliability in ankle radiographic measurements. *Foot Ankle Int.* 1997;18(6):324-329.

127. Condon F, Kaliszer M, Conhyea D, et al. The first intermetatarsal angle in hallux valgus: an analysis of measurement reliability and the error involved. *Foot Ankle Int.* 2002;22(8):717-721.

128. Matthews M, Klein E, Youssef A, et al. Correlation of radiographic measurements with patient-centered outcomes in hallux valgus surgery. *Foot Ankle Int.* 2018;39(12):1416-1422.

129. Oestrich AE. *How to Measure Angles from Foot Radiographs. A Primer.* New York: Springer-Verlag; 1990.

130. Sanner WH. Principles of biomechanical radiographic analysis of the foot. In: Christman RA, ed. *Foot and Ankle Radiology.* 2nd ed. Philadelphia, PA: Wolters Kluwer; 2015:199-207.

131. Hlavac HF. Differences in x-ray findings with varied positioning of the foot. *J Am Podiatry Assoc.* 1967;57(10):465-471.

132. Weissman SD. Biomechanically acquired foot types. In: Weissman SD, ed. *Radiology of the Foot.* 2nd ed. Baltimore, MD: Williams & Wilkins, 1989:66-90.

133. Templeton AW, McAlister WH, Zim ID. Standardization of terminology and evaluation of osseous relationships in congenitally abnormal feet. *Am J Roentgenol.* 1965;93:374-381.

134. Green DR. Radiology and biomechanical foot types. In: *Podiatry Institute Update 1998: Chapter 48.* http://www.podiatryinstitute.com/pdfs/Update_Index.pdf. Accessed May 2, 2019.

135. Ellis SJ, Yu JC, Williams BR, et al. New radiographic parameters assessing forefoot abduction in the adult acquired flatfoot deformity. *Foot Ankle Int.* 2009;30:1168-1176.

136. Kang S, Charlton TP, Thordarson DB. Lateral column length in adult flatfoot deformity. *Foot Ankle Int.* 2013;34:392-397.

137. Sangeorzan BJ. Effect of calcaneal lengthening on relationships among the hindfoot, midfoot, and forefoot. *Foot Ankle.* 1993;14(3):136.

138. Scharfbillig R, Evans AM, Copper AW, et al. Criterion validation of four criteria of the foot posture index. *J Am Podiatr Med Assoc.* 2004;94(1):31.

139. Chadha H, Pomeroy G, Manoli A. Radiologic signs of unilateral pes planus. *Foot Ankle Int.* 1997;18:603-604.

140. Younger AS, Sawatzky B, Dryden P. Radiographic assessment of adult flatfoot. *Foot Ankle Int.* 2005;26(10):820-825.

141. DiGiovanni JE, Smith SD. Normal biomechanics of the adult rearfoot: A radiographic analysis. *J Am Podiatry Assoc.* 1976;66(11):812-824.

142. Lee KM, Chung CY, Park MS, et al. Reliability and validity of radiographic measurements in hindfoot varus and valgus. *J Bone Joint Surg Am.* 2010;92-A(13):2319-2327.

143. Faciszewski T, Burks RT, Manaster BJ. Subtle injuries of the Lisfranc joint. *J Bone Joint Surg.* 1990;72A(10):1519-1522.

144. Sanner WH. Foot segmental relationships and bone morphology. In: Christman RA, ed. *Foot and Ankle Radiology.* 2nd ed. Philadelphia, PA: Wolters Kluwer; 2015:209-234.

145. Sensiba PR, Coffey MJ, Williams NE, et al. Inter- and intraobserver reliability in the radiographic evaluation of adult flatfoot deformity. *Foot Ankle Int.* 2010;31(2):141-145.

146. Cobey JC. Posterior roentgenogram of the foot. *Clin Orthop.* 1976;118:202-207.

147. Saltzman CL, El-Khoury GY. The hindfoot alignment view. *Foot Ankle Int.* 1995;16:572-576.

148. Mendicino RW, Catanzariti AR, John S, et al. Long leg calcaneal axial and hindfoot alignment radiographic views for frontal plane assessment. *J Am Podiatr Med Assoc.* 2008;98:75-81.

149. Reilingh ML, Beimers L, Tuijthof GJ, et al. Measuring hindfoot alignment radiographically: the long axial view is more reliable than the hindfoot alignment view. *Skeletal Radiol.* 2010;39(11):1103-1108.

150. Buck P, Morrey BF, Chao EY. The optimum position of arthrodesis of the ankle. A gait study of the knee and ankle. *J Bone Joint Surg Am.* 1987;69(7):1052-1062.

151. Johnson JE, Lamdan R, Granberry WF, et al. Hindfoot coronal alignment: a modified radiographic method. *Foot Ankle Int.* 1999;20(12):818-825.

152. Lamm BM, Paley D. Deformity correction planning for hindfoot, ankle, and lower limb. *Clin Podiatr Med Surg.* 2004;21:305-326.

153. Mendicino RW, Catanzariti AR, Reeves CL, et al. A systematic approach to evaluation of the rearfoot, ankle, and leg in reconstructive surgery. *J Am Podiatr Med Assoc.* 2005;95(1):2-12.

154. Paley D. Ankle and foot considerations. In: Herzenberg JE, ed. *Principles of Deformity Correction.* New York, NY: Springer; 2002:571-645.

155. Williamson ERC, Chan JY, Burket JC, et al. New radiographic parameter assessing hindfoot alignment in stage II adult-acquired flatfoot deformity. *Foot Ankle Int.* 2015;36(4):417-423.

156. Robinson I, Dyson R, Halson-Brown S. Reliability of clinical and radiographic measurement of rearfoot alignment in a patient population. *The Foot.* 2001;11:2-9.

157. Aebi J, Horisberger M, Frigg A. Radiographic study of pes planovarus. *Foot Ankle Int.* 2017;38(5):526-531.

158. Labovitz JM. The Algorithmic approach to pediatric flexible pes planovalgus. *Clin Podiatr Med Surg.* 2006;23:57-76.

159. Lamm BM, Stasko PA, Gesheff MG, et al. Normal foot and ankle radiographic angles, measurements, and reference points. *J Foot Ankle Surg.* 2016;55:991-998.

160. Lamm BM, Mendicino RW, Catanzariti AR, et al. Static rearfoot alignment: a comparison of clinical and radiographic measures. *J Am Podiatr Med Assoc.* 2005;95:26-33.

161. Magerkurth O, Knupp M, Ledermann H, et al. Evaluation of hindfoot dimensions: a radiological study. *Foot Ankle Int.* 2006;27:612-616.

162. Ozonoff MB. The foot. In: Ozonoff MB, ed. *Pediatric Orthopedic Radiology.* Philadelphia, PA: WB Saunders Co.; 1992:397-460.

163. Berquist TH, Bancroft LW, Merinbaum DJ. Pediatric foot and ankle disorders. In: Berquist TH, ed. *Imaging of the Foot and Ankle.* 3rd ed. Philadelphia, PA: Lippincott Williams & Wilkins; 2011:528-558.

164. McKie J, Radomisli T. Congenital vertical talus: a review. *Clin Podiatr Med Surg.* 2010;27(1):145-156.

165. Greenspan A, Beltran J. Anomalies of the upper and lower limbs. In: Greenspan A, Beltran J, eds. *Orthopedic Imaging: A Practical Approach.* 6th ed. New York, NY: Wolters Kluwer Health; 2015:1057-1099.

166. Haendlmayer KT, Harris NJ. Flatfoot deformity: an overview. *Orthop Trauma.* 2009;23(6):395-403.

167. Oestreich AE, Crawford AH. The lower extremity. In: Oestreich AE, ed. *Atlas of Pediatric Orthopedic Radiology.* New York, NY: Thieme Inc.; 1985:173-266.

168. Drennan JC. Congenital vertical talus. *J Bone Joint Surg Am.* 1995;77A(12):1916-1923.

169. Jacobsen ST, Crawford AH. Congenital vertical talus. *J Pediatr Orthop.* 1983;3(3):306-310.

170. Japas LM. Surgical treatment of pes cavus by V-osteotomy: preliminary report. *J Bone Joint Surg Am.* 1968;50(5):927-944.

171. Perera A, Guha A. Clinical and radiographic evaluation of the cavus foot: surgical implications. *Foot Ankle Clin.* 2013;18(4):619-628.

172. Hibbs RA. An operation for claw foot. *JAMA.* 1919;73:1583-1585.

173. Lin CS, Wu TY, Wang TM, et al. A new technique to increase reliability in measuring the axis of bone. *J Foot Ankle Surg.* 2016;55:106-111.

174. Marks RM. Midfoot and forefoot issues cavovarus foot: Assessment and treatment issues. *Foot Ankle Clin.* 2008;13:229-241.

175. Jahss MH. Evaluation of the cavus foot for orthopedic treatment. *Clin Orthop.* 1983;181:52-63.

176. Whitney AK, Green DR. Pseudoequinus. *J Am Podiatry Assoc.* 1982;72:365-371.

177. Leal LO, Bosta SO, Feller DP. Anterior tarsal resection (Cole osteotomy). *J Foot Surg.* 1988;27:259-263.

178. Smith TF, Green DR. Pes cavus. In: Banks AS, Downey MS, Martin DE, Miller SJ, eds. *McGlamry's Comprehensive Textbook of Foot and Ankle Surgery.* 3rd ed. Philadelphia, PA: Lippincott Williams and Wilkins; 2001:761-798.

179. Green DR, Smith TF. Pes cavus classification: a simplified approach. In: Camasta CA, Vickers NS, Ruch JA, eds. *Reconstructive Surgery of the Foot and Leg: Update '94.* Tucker, GA: The Podiatry Institute; 1994:197-200.

180. Oestreich AE. The lateral foot. In: Oestreich AE, ed. *How to Measure Angles from Foot Radiographs. A Primer.* New York, NY: Springer-Verlag; 1990:31-41.

181. Templeton AW, McAlister WH, Zim ID. Standardization of terminology and evaluation of osseous relationships in congenitally abnormal feet. *AJR Am J Roentgenol.* 1965;93:374-381.

182. Lloyd-Roberts GC, Swann M, Catterall A. Medial rotation osteotomy for severe residual deformity in clubfoot. A preliminary report on a new method of treatment. *J Bone Joint Surg.* 1974;56B:37-43.

183. Apostle KL, Sangeorzan BJ. Anatomy of the varus foot and ankle. *Foot Ankle Clin.* 2012;17:1-11.

184. Coleman SS, Chesnut WJ. A simple test for hindfoot flexibility in the cavovarus foot. *Clin Orthop Relat Res.* 1977;123:60-62.

185. Paley D, Herzenberg JE, Tetsworth K, et al. Deformity planning for frontal and sagittal plane corrective osteotomies. *Orthop Clin North Am.* 1994;25:425-465.

186. Simons OW. A standardized method for the radiographic evaluation of club feet. *Clin Orthop.* 1978;135:107-118.

187. Cummings RJ, Davidson RS, Armstrong PF, et al. Congenital clubfoot. *J Bone Joint Surg Am.* 2002;84-A(2):290-308.

188. LeNoir JL. A perspective focus on the indicated surgical treatment of persistent club feet in the infant. *South Med J.* 1976;69:837-843.

189. Simons GW. Calcaneocuboid joint deformity in talipes equinovarus: an overview and update. *J Pediatr Orthop B.* 1995;4:25-35.

190. Simons GW. Complete subtalar release in club feet. Part II—Comparison with less extensive procedures. *J Bone Joint Surg Am.* 1985;67(7):1056-1065.

191. Simons GW. Analytical radiography of club feet. *J Bone Joint Surg Br.* 1977;59:485-489.

192. Simons GW. The diagnosis and treatment of deformity combinations in clubfeet. *Clin Orthop Relat Res.* 1980;150:229-244.

193. Thometz JG, Simons GW. Deformity of the calcaneocuboid joint in patients who have talipes equinovarus. *J Bone Joint Surg Am.* 1993;75:190-195.

194. Prasad P, Sen RK, Gill SS, et al. Clinico-radiological assessment and their correlation in clubfeet treated with postero-medial soft-tissue release. *Int Orthop.* 2009;33:225-229.

195. Heywood AWB. The mechanics of the hindfoot in clubfoot as demonstrated radiographically. *J Bone Joint Surg Br.* 1964;46B(1):102-107.

196. Joseph B, Bhatia M, Nair NS. Talo-calcaneal relationship in clubfoot. *J Pediatr Orthop.* 2001;21:60-64.

197. Dunn HK, Samuelson KM. Flat-top talus. A long-term report of twenty club feet. *J Bone Joint Surg Am.* 1975;56(1):57-62.

198. Burger D, Aiyer A, Myerson MS. Evaluation and surgical management of the overcorrected clubfoot deformity in the adult patient. *Foot Ankle Clin.* 2015;20:587-599.

199. Hjelmstedt A, Sahlstedt B. Arthrography as a guide in the treatment of congenital clubfoot: findings and treatment results in a consecutive series. *Acta Orthop Scand.* 1980:51:321-334.

200. Hutchins PM, Foster BK, Paterson DC, et al. Long-term results of early surgical release in clubfeet. *J Bone Joint Surg Br.* 1985;67:791-799.

201. Bach CM, Wachter R, Stockl B, et al. Significance of talar distortion for ankle mobility in idiopathic clubfoot. *Clin Orthop Relat Res.* 2002;398:196-202.

202. Dawoodi A, Perera A. Radiological assessment of metatarsus adductus. *Foot Ankle Surg.* 2012;18:1-8.

203. Weissman SD. Biomechanically acquired foot types. In: Weissman SD, ed. *Radiology of the Foot.* 2nd ed. Baltimore, MD: Williams & Wilkins; 1983:66-90.

204. Kilmartin TE, Barrington RL, Wallace WA. Metatarsus primus varus. A statistical study. *J Bone Joint Surg Br.* 1991;73:937-940.

205. Ferrari J, Malone-Lee J. A radiographic study of the relationship between metatarsus adductus and hallux valgus. *J Foot Ankle Surg.* 2003;42:9-14.

206. La Reaux RL, Lee BR. Metatarsus adductus and hallux abducto valgus: their correlation. *J Foot Surg.* 1987;26:304-308.

207. Martin DE, Pontious J. Introduction and evaluation of hallux abducto valgus. In: Banks AS, Downey MS, Martin DE, eds. *McGlamry's Comprehensive Textbook of Foot and Ankle Surgery.* Vol 1. 3rd ed. Philadelphia, PA: Lippincott Williams & Wilkins; 2001:481.

208. Domínguez G, Munuera PV. Metatarsus adductus angle in male and female feet: normal values with two measurement techniques. *J Am Podiatr Med Assoc.* 2008;98:364-369.

209. Crawford M, Green D. Metatarsus adductus: Radiographic and pathomechanical analysis. In: *Podiatry Institute Update, 2014: Chapter 5.* http://www.podiatryinstitute.com/pdfs/Update_Index.pdf. Accessed May 29, 2019.

210. Engel E, Erlick N, Krems I. A simplified metatarsus adductus angle. *J Am Podiatry Assoc.* 1983;73:620-628.

211. Thomas JL, Kunkel MW, Lopez R, et al. Radiographic values of the adult foot in a standardized population. *J Foot Ankle Surg.* 2006;45:3-12.

212. Dawoodi A, Perera A. Reliability of metatarsus adductus angle and correlation with hallux valgus. *Foot Ankle Surg.* 2012;18:180-186.

213. Bresnahan PJ. Congenital and developmental pediatric abnormalities. In: Christman RA, ed. *Foot and Ankle Radiology.* 2nd ed. Philadelphia, PA: Wolters Kluwer; 2015:235-246.

214. French S, Niespodziany J, Wysong D, et al. A radiographic study of infant metatarsus adductus treatment by serial casting. *J Foot Surg.* 1985;24(3):222-229.

215. Lepow GM, Lepow RS, Lepow RM, et al. Pediatric metatarsus adductus angle. *J Am Podiatr Med Assoc.* 1987;77(10):529-532.

216. Marshall N, Ward E, Williams CM. The identification and appraisal of assessment tools used to evaluate metatarsus adductus: a systematic review of their measurement properties. *J Foot Ankle Res.* 2018;11:25.

217. Berg EE. A reappraisal of metatarsus adductus and skewfoot. *J Bone Joint Surg.* 1986;68-A:1185-1196.

218. Thompson GH, Abaza H. Metatarsus adductus and metatarsus varus. In: McCarthy JJ, Drennan JC, eds. *Drennan's The Child's Foot and Ankle.* 2nd ed. Philadelphia, PA: Lippincott Williams and Wilkins; 2010:117-125.

219. Cook DA, Breed AL, Cook T, et al. Observer variability in the radiographic measurement and classification of metatarsus adductus. *J Pediatr Orthop.* 1992;12:86-89.

220. Miron MC, Grimard G. Ultrasound evaluation of foot deformities in infants. *Pediatr Radiol.* 2016;46:193-209.

221. Hatch DJ, Santrock RD, Smith B, et al. Triplane hallux abducto valgus classification. *J Foot Ankle Surg.* 2018;57:972-981.

222. Collan L, Kankare JA, Mattila K. The biomechanics of the first metatarsal bone in hallux valgus: a preliminary study utilizing a weight bearing extremity CT. *Foot Ankle Surg.* 2013;19:155-161.

223. Kim Y, Kim JS, Young KW, et al. A new measure of tibial sesamoid position in hallux valgus in relation to the coronal rotation of the first metatarsal in CT scans. *Foot Ankle Int.* 2015;36:944-952.

224. Palladino SJ. Preoperative evaluation of the bunion patient. In: Gerbert J, ed. *Textbook of Bunion Surgery.* 3rd ed. Philadelphia, PA: W.B. Saunders Company; 2001:3-71.

225. Gerbert J, Palladino SJ. Preoperative evaluation of the bunion patient. In: Gerbert J, ed. *Textbook of Bunion Surgery.* 4th ed. Brooklandville, MD: Data Trace Publ Co.; 2012:1-46.

226. Strydom A, Saragas NP, Ferrao PNF. A radiographic analysis of the contribution of hallux valgus interphalangeus to the total valgus deformity of the hallux. *Foot Ankle Surg.* 2017;23:27-31.

227. Coughlin MJ, Shurnas PS. Hallux rigidus: demographics, etiology, and radiographic assessment. *Foot Ankle Int.* 2003;24:731-743.

228. Barnett CH. Valgus deviation of the distal phalanx of the great toe. *J Anat.* 1962;96(2):171-177.

229. Sorto L, Balding M, Weil L, et al. Hallux abductus interphalangeus: etiology, x-ray evaluation and treatment. *J Am Podiatry Assoc.* 1976;66(6):384-396.

230. Whitney AK. *Radiographic Charting Technic.* Philadelphia, PA: Pennsylvania College of Podiatric Medicine; 1978.

231. Park JY, Jung HG, Kim TH, et al. Intraoperative incidence of hallux valgus interphalangeus following basilar first metatarsal osteotomy and distal soft tissue realignment. *Foot Ankle Int.* 2011;32(11):1058-1062.

232. Coughlin MJ, Jones CP. Hallux valgus: demographics, etiology, and radiographic assessment. *Foot Ankle Int.* 2007;28(7):759-777.

233. Martin DE. Pre-operative radiographic evaluation in HAV surgery: a critical analysis of PASA and other soft tissue adaptations. In: Camasta CA, Vickers NS, Ruch JA. *Reconstructive Surgery of the Foot and Leg: Update '93.* Tucker, GA: The Podiatry Institute; 1993:338-341.

234. Sullivan BT, Robinson JB, Palladino SJ. Interevaluator variability in the measurement of proximal articular set angle. *J Foot Surg.* 1988;27(5):466-468.

235. Vittetoe D, Saltzman C, Krieg J, et al. Reliability and validity of distal metatarsal articular angle. *Foot Ankle Int.* 1994;15:541-547.

236. Cakmak G, Kanatli U, Kilinc B, et al. The effect of pronation and inclination on the measurement of the hallucal distal metatarsal articular set angle. *Acta Orthop Traumatol Turc.* 2013;47(5):354-358.

237. Amarnek DL, Mollica A, Jacobs AM, et al. A statistical analysis on the reliability of the proximal articular set angle. *J Foot Surg.* 1986;25:39-43.

238. Dixon A, Lee L, Charlton T, et al. Increased incidence and severity of postoperative radiographic hallux valgus interphalangeus with surgical correction of hallux valgus. *Foot Ankle Int.* 2015;36:961-968.

239. Christman RA. Radiographic evaluation of the distal articular set angle. *J Am Podiatr Med Assoc.* 1988;78(7):352-354.

240. Spinner SM, Lipsman S, Spector F. Radiographic criteria in the assessment of hallux abductus deformities. *J Foot Surg.* 1984;23:25-30.

241. Elliot RR, Saxby TS. A new method for measuring deformity distal to the hallux metatarsophalangeal joint. *Foot Ankle Int.* 2010;31(7):609-611.

242. Shechter DZ, Doll PJ. Tangential angle to the second axis. A new angle with implications for bunion surgery. *J Am Podiatr Med Assoc.* 1985;75:505.

243. Klouda J, Hromádka R, Šoffová S, et al. The change of first metatarsal head articular surface position after Lapidus arthrodesis. *BMC Musculoskelet Disord.* 2018;19:347.

244. Geng X, Zhang C, Ma X, et al. Lateral sesamoid position relative to the second metatarsal in feet with and without hallux valgus: a prospective study. *J Foot Ankle Surg.* 2016;55:136-139.

245. Hardy RH, Clapham JCR. Observations on hallux valgus. Based on a Controlled Series. *J Bone Joint Surg Br.* 1951;133-B(3):376-391.

246. Meyr AJ, Myers A, Pontious J. Descriptive quantitative analysis of hallux abductovalgus transverse plane radiographic parameters. *J Foot Ankle Surg.* 2014;53:397-404.

247. Talbot KD, Saltzman CL. Assessing sesamoid subluxation: How good is the AP radiograph? *Foot Ankle Int.* 1998;19:547-554.

248. Swanson AB, Lumsden RM, Swanson GD. Silicone implant arthroplasty of the great toe. A review of single stem and flexible hinge implants. *Clin Orthop Relat Res.* 1979;142:30-43.

249. Smith RW, Reynolds JC, Stewart NJ. Hallux valgus assessment: report of research committee of American Orthopaedic Foot and Ankle Society. *Foot Ankle.* 1984;5:92-103.

250. Agrawal Y, Desai A, Mehta J. Lateral sesamoid position in hallux valgus: Correlation with the conventional radiological assessment. *Foot Ankle Surg.* 2011;17:308-311.

251. Panchani S, Reading J, Mehta J. Inter and intra-observer reliability in assessment of the position of the lateral sesamoid in determining the severity of hallux valgus. *The Foot.* 2016;27:59-61.

252. Coughlin MJ. Juvenile hallux valgus. Etiology and treatment. *Foot Ankle Int.* 1995;16:682-697.

253. Tanaka Y, Takakura Y, Sugimoto K, et al. Precise anatomic configuration changes in the first ray of the hallux valgus foot. *Foot Ankle Int.* 2000;21(8):651-656.

254. Boberg JS. Evaluation and procedural selection in hallux valgus surgery. In: Southerland JT, Boberg JS, Downey MS, et al., eds. *McGlamry's Comprehensive Textbook of Foot and Ankle Surgery.* 4th ed. Philadelphia, PA: Lippincott Williams & Wilkins; 2014:245-249.

255. Piggott H. The natural history of hallux valgus in adolescence and early adult life. *J Bone Joint Surg.* 1960;42-B(4):749-760.

256. LaPorta G, Melillo T, Olinsky D. X-ray evaluation of hallux abducto valgus deformity. *J Am Podiatry Assoc.* 1974;64:544-566.

257. Nilsonne H. Hallux rigidus and its treatment. *Acta Orthop.* 1930;1(1-4):295-303.

258. Harris R, Beath T. The short first metatarsal. Its incidence and clinical significance. *J Bone Joint Surg.* 1949;31A:553-565.

259. Lundberg BJ, Sulja T. Skeletal parameters in the hallux valgus foot. *Acta Orthop Scand.* 1972;43:576-582.

260. LaPorta DM, Melillo TV, Hetherington VJ. Preoperative assessment in hallux valgus. In: Hetherington VJ, ed. *Hallux Valgus and Forefoot Surgery.* St. Louis, MO: Churchill Livingstone; 1994:107-123.

261. Osher L, Blazer MM, Buck S, et al. Accurate determination of relative metatarsal protrusion with a small intermetatarsal angle- a novel simplified method. *J Foot Ankle Surg.* 2014;53:548-556.

262. Maestro M, Besse JL, Ragusa M, et al. Forefoot morphotype study and planning method for forefoot osteotomy. *Foot Ankle Clin.* 2003;8(4):695-710.

263. Ali Z, Karim H, Wali N, et al. The inter- and intra-rater reliability of the Maestro and Barroco metatarsal length measurement techniques. *J Foot Ankle Res.* 2018;11:47.

264. Meshan I. Radiology of the normal foot. *Semin Roentgenol.* 1970;5(4):327-340.

265. Gamble FO, Yale I. Normal foot structure. In: Gamble FO, Yale I, eds. *Clinical Foot Roentgenology.* Baltimore, MD: Williams & Wilkins Co.; 1966:145-162.

266. Mann RA, Coughlin MJ. Hallux valgus—etiology, anatomy, treatment and surgical considerations. *Clin Orthop.* 1981;157:31-41.

267. Okuda R, Kinoshita M, Toshito Y, et al. The shape of the lateral edge of the first metatarsal head as a risk factor for recurrence of hallux valgus. *J Bone Joint Surg Am.* 2007;89:2163-2172.

268. Wagner P, Wagner E. Is the rotational deformity important in our decision-making process for correction of hallux valgus deformity? *Foot Ankle Clin.* 2018;23205-23217.

269. Dayton P, Feilmeier M. Comparison of tibial sesamoid position on anteroposterior and axial radiographs before and after triplane tarsal metatarsal joint arthrodesis. *J Foot Ankle Surg.* 2017;56:1041-1046.

270. Thordarson DB, Krewer P. Medial eminence thickness with and without hallux valgus. *Foot Ankle Int.* 2002;23(1):48-50.

271. Schuberth JM, Reilly CH, Gudas CJ. The closing wedge osteotomy: a critical analysis of first metatarsal elevation. *J Am Podiatry Assoc.* 1984;74:13-20.

272. Roukis TS. Metatarsus primus elevatus in hallux rigidus: fact or fiction? *J Am Podiatr Med Assoc.* 2005;95:221-228.

273. Camasta CA. Radiographic evaluation and classification of metatarsus primus elevatus. In: Camasta CA, Vickers NS, Ruch JA, eds. *Reconstructive Surgery of the Foot and Leg: Update '94.* Tucker, GA: The Podiatry Institute; 1994:122-127.

274. Meyer JO, Nishon LR, Weiss L, et al. Metatarsus primus elevatus and the etiology of hallux rigidus. *J Foot Surg.* 1987;26:237-241.

275. Horton GA, Park YW, Myerson MS. Role of metatarsus primus elevatus in the pathogenesis of hallux rigidus. *Foot Ankle Int.* 1999;20:777-780.

276. Bouaicha S, Ehrmann C, Moor BK, et al. Radiographic analysis of metatarsus primus elevatus and hallux rigidus. *Foot Ankle Int.* 2010;31:807-814.

277. Christman RA, Flanigan KP, Sorrento, DL, et al. Radiographic analysis of metatarsus primus elevatus: a preliminary study. *J Am Podiatr Med Assoc.* 2001;91(6):294-299.

278. Seiberg M, Felson S, Colson JP, et al. Closing base wedge versus Austin bunionectomies for metatarsus primus adductus. *J Am Podiatr Med Assoc.* 1994;84:548-563.

279. Bryant A, Mahoney B, Tinley P. Lateral intermetatarsal angle: a useful measurement of metatarsus primus elevatus? *J Am Podiatr Med Assoc.* 2001;91:251-254.

280. Meyer JM, Tomeno B, Burdet A. Metatarsalgia due to insufficient support by the first ray. *Int Orthop.* 1981;5:193-201.

281. Cicchinelli LD, Camasta CA, McGlamry ED. Iatrogenic metatarsus primus elevatus: etiology, evaluation, and surgical management. *J Am Podiatr Med Assoc.* 1997;87:165-177.

282. Camasta CA. Hallux limitus and hallux rigidus: clinical examination, radiographic findings, and natural history. *Clin Podiatr Med Surg.* 1996;3:423-448.

283. Yildirim Y, Cabukoglu CE, Erol B, et al. Effect of metatarsophalangeal joint position on the reliability of the tangential sesamoid view in determining sesamoid position. *Foot Ankle Int.* 2005;26(3):247-250.

284. Kay DB, Njus G, Parrish W, et al. Basilar crescentic osteotomy. A three-dimensional computer simulation. *Orthop Clin North Am.* 1989;20(4):571-582.

285. Dayton P, Merrell K, Feilmeier M. Is our current paradigm for evaluation and management of the bunion deformity flawed? A discussion of procedure philosophy relative to anatomy. *J Foot Ankle Surg.* 2015;54:102-111.

286. Scranton PE, Rutkowski R. Anatomic variations in the first ray: part 1. Anatomic aspects related to bunion surgery. *Clin Orthop Relat Res.* 1980;151:244-255.

287. Saltzman CL, Brandser EA, Anderson C, et al. Coronal plane rotation of the first metatarsal. *Foot Ankle Int.* 1996;17:157-161.

288. Eustace S, O'Byrne J, Stack J, et al. Radiographic features that enable assessment of first metatarsal rotation: the role of pronation in hallux valgus. *Skeletal Radiol.* 1993;22:153-156.

289. Talbot KD, Saltzman CL. Hallucal rotation: a method of measurement and relationship to bunion deformity. *Foot Ankle Int.* 1997;18(9):550-556.

290. Kuwano T, Nagamine R, Sakaki K, et al. New radiographic analysis of sesamoid rotation in hallux valgus comparison with conventional evaluation methods. *Foot Ankle Int.* 2002;23:811-817.

291. Dayton P, Kauwe M, Feilmeier M. Clarification of the anatomic definition of the bunion deformity. *J Foot Ankle Surg.* 2014;53:160-163.

292. Saragas NP, Becker PJ. Comparative radiographic analysis of parameters in feet with and without hallux valgus. *Foot Ankle Int.* 1995;16(3):139-143.

293. Tanaka Y, Takakura Y, Kumai T, et al. Radiographic analysis of hallux valgus: A two-dimensional coordinate system. *J Bone Joint Surg Am.* 1995;77-A(2):205-213.

294. Patel K, Hasenstein T, Meyr AJ. Quantitative assessment of the obliquity of the first metatarsal-medial cuneiform articulation. *J Foot Ankle Surg.* 2019;58(4):679-686. doi:10.1053/j.jfas.2018.11.017.

295. Doty JF, Coughlin MJ, Hirose C, et al. First metatarsocuneiform joint mobility: radiographic, anatomic, and clinical characteristics of the articular surface. *Foot Ankle Int.* 2014;35:504-511.

296. Hyer CF, Philbin TM, Berlet GC, et al. The obliquity of the first metatarsal base. *Foot Ankle Int.* 2004;25:728-732.

297. Hyer CF, Philbin TM, Berlet GC, et al. The incidence of the intermetatarsal facet of the first metatarsal and its relationship to metatarsus primus varus: a cadaveric study. *J Foot Ankle Surg.* 2005;44:200-202.

298. Romash MM, Fugate D, Yanklowit B. Passive motion of the first metatarsal cuneiform joint: preoperative assessment. *Foot Ankle.* 1990;10(6):293-298.

299. Brage ME, Holmes JR, Sangeorzan BJ. The influence of x-ray orientation on the first metatarsocuneiform joint angle. *Foot Ankle Int.* 1994;15:495-497.

300. Hatch DJ, Smith A, Fowler T. Radiographic relevance of the distal medial cuneiform angle in hallux valgus assessment. *J Foot Ankle Surg.* 2016;55:85-89.

301. Houghton GR, Dickson RA. Hallux valgus in the younger patient. The structural abnormality. *J Bone Joint Surg Br.* 1979;61-B(2):176-177.

302. Antrobus JN. The primary deformity in hallux valgus and metatarsus primus varus. *Clin Orthop.* 1984;184:51-255.

303. Myerson M. *Foot and ankle disorders, hallux valgus.* Philadelphia, PA: WB Sanders Co.; 1999:213-289.

304. King DM, Toolan BC. Associated deformities and hypermobility in hallux valgus: an investigation with weightbearing radiographs. *Foot Ankle Int.* 2004;25:251-255.

305. Sanicola SM, Arnold TB, Osher L. Is the radiographic appearance of the hallucal tarso-metatarsal joint representative of its true anatomical structure? *J Am Podiatr Med Assoc.* 2002;92:491-498.

306. Dayton P, Kauwe M, Kauwe JS, et al. Observed changes in first metatarsal and medial cuneiform positions after first metatarsophalangeal joint arthrodesis. *J Foot Ankle Surg.* 2014;53:32-35.

307. Haines W, Mcdougall A. The anatomy of hallux valgus. *J Bone Joint Surg Br.* 1954;36:272-293.

308. Shofler D, McKenna B, Huang J, et al. Reproducibility and reliability of the radiographic angles used to assess tailor's bunions. *J Am Podiatr Med Assoc.* 2018;108(3):205-209.

309. Coughlin MJ. Treatment of bunionette deformity with longitudinal diaphyseal osteotomy with distal soft tissue repair. *Foot Ankle.* 1991;11:195-203.

310. Fallat LM, Buckholz J. An analysis of the tailor's bunion by radiographic and anatomical display. *J Am Podiatry Assoc.* 1980;70:597-603.

311. Schabler JA, Toney M, Hanft JR, et al. Oblique metaphyseal osteotomy for the correction of tailor's bunions: a 3-year review. *J Foot Surg.* 1992;31(1):79-84.

312. Nestor BJ, Kitaoka HB, Ilstrup DM, et al. Radiologic anatomy of the painful bunionette. *Foot Ankle.* 1990;11(1):6-11.

313. Steel MW, Johnson KA, DeWitz MA, et al. Radiographic measurements of the normal adult foot. *Foot Ankle.* 1980;1:151-158.

314. Steinke MS, Boll KL. Holmann-Thomasen metatarsal osteotomy for tailor's bunion (bunionette). *J Bone Joint Surg.* 1989;71A:423-426.

315. Fallat LM. Pathology of the fifth ray. *Clin Podiatr Med Surg.* 1990;7:689-715.

316. Schrier JCM, Verheyen CCPM, Louwerens JW. Definitions of hammer toe and claw toe: an evaluation of the literature. *J Am Podiatr Med Assoc.* 2009;99(3):194-197.

317. Shirzad K, Kiesau CD, DeOrio JK, et al. Lesser toe deformities. *J Am Acad Orthop Surg.* 2011;19:505-514.

318. Coughlin MJ. Crossover second toe deformity. *Foot Ankle.* 1987;8:29-39.

319. Kaz AJ, Coughlin MJ. Crossover second toe: Demographics, etiology, and radiographic assessment. *Foot Ankle Int.* 2007;28(12):1223-1237.

320. McGlamry ED, Jimenez AL, Green DR. Deformities of the intermediate digits and the metatarsophalangeal joint. In: Banks A, Downey MS, Martin DE, Miller SJ, eds. *McGlamry's Comprehensive Textbook of Foot and Ankle Surgery.* 3rd ed. Philadelphia, PA: Lippincott Williams & Wilkins; 2001:253-304.

321. Fleischer AE, Klein EE, Ahmad M, et al. Association of abnormal metatarsal parabola with second metatarsophalangeal joint plantar plate pathology. *Foot Ankle Int.* 2017;38(3):289-297.

322. Stiell IG, Greenberg GH, McKnight RD, et al. Decision rules for the use of radiography in acute ankle injuries: Refinement and prospective validation. *JAMA.* 1993;269:1127-1132.

323. Stiell IG, McKnight RD, Greenberg GH, et al. Implementation of the Ottawa ankle rules. *JAMA.* 1994;271:827-832.

324. Leddy JL, Smolinski RJ, Lawrence J, et al. Prospective evaluation of the Ottawa ankle rules in a University Sports Medicine Center. With a modification to increase specificity for identifying malleolar fractures. *Am J Sports Med.* 1998;26:158-165.

325. Pigman EC, Klug RK, Sanford S, et al. Evaluation of the Ottawa clinical decision rules for the use of radiography in acute ankle and midfoot injuries in the emergency department. *Ann Emerg Med.* 1994;24:41-45.

326. Dowling S, Spooner CH, Liang Y, et al. Accuracy of Ottawa Ankle Rules to exclude fractures of the ankle and midfoot in children: a meta-analysis. *Acad Emerg Med.* 2009;16(4):277-287.

327. Boutis K, Grootendorst P, Willan A, et al. Effect of the low risk ankle rule on the frequency of radiography in children with ankle injuries. *CMAJ.* 2013;185(15):E731-E738.

328. McLaughlin SA, Binder DS, Sklar DP. Ottawa ankle rules and the diabetic foot. *Ann Emerg Med.* 1998;32(4):518.

329. ACR Appropriateness Criteria, Acute trauma to the foot. https://www.acr.org/Clinical-Resources/ACR-Appropriateness-Criteria. Accessed June 26, 2019.

330. Sands AK, Grose A. Lisfranc injury. *Injury.* 2004;35:S-B71-S-B76.

331. Looijen RC, Misselyn D, Backes M, et al. Identification of postoperative step-offs and gaps with Broden's view following open reduction and internal fixation of calcaneal fractures. *Foot Ankle Int.* 2019;40(7):797-802.

332. Greenspan A, Beltran J. Radiologic evaluation of trauma. In: Greenspan A, Beltran J, eds. *Orthopedic Imaging, A Practical Approach.* 6th ed. Philadelphia, PA: Wolters Kluwer Health; 2015:55-106.

333. Towbin R, Dunbar JS, Towbin J, et al. Teardrop sign: plain film recognition of ankle effusion. *AJR Am J Roentgenol.* 1980;134:985-990.

334. Jacobson JA, Andresen R, Jaovisidha S, et al. Detection of ankle effusions: comparison study in cadavers using radiography, sonography, and MR imaging. *AJR Am J Roentgenol.* 1998;170:1231-1238.

335. McRae R, Esser M. *Practical Fracture Treatment.* 5th ed. St. Louis, MO: Churchill Livingstone; 2008:22.

336. Martin RE. Initial assessment and management of common fractures. *Prim Care.* 1996;23(2):405-409.

337. Scherl SA, Templeton K. Fracture. In: Bernstein J, ed. *Musculoskeletal Medicine.* Rosemont, IL: American Academy of Orthopedic Surgeons; 2003:161-174.

338. Weissman BNW, Sledge CB. General principles. In: Weissman BNW, Sledge CB, eds. *Orthopedic Radiology.* Philadelphia, PA: WB Saunders Co.; 1986:1-69.

339. Reinus WR. Imaging approach to musculoskeletal trauma. In: Bonakdarpour A, Reinus WR, Khurana JS, eds. *Diagnostic Imaging of Musculoskeletal Diseases, A Systematic Approach.* New York, NY: Springer; 2010:125-201.

340. Palmer I. The mechanism and treatment of fractures of the calcaneus. Open reduction with the use of cancellous grafts. *J Bone Joint Surg.* 1948;30A:2-8.

341. Böhler L. Diagnosis, pathology, and treatment of fractures of the os calcis. *J Bone Joint Surg.* 1931;13:75-89.

342. Stephenson JR. Displaced fractures of the os calcis involving the subtalar joint: the key role of the superomedial fragment. *Foot Ankle.* 1983;4(2):91-101.

343. Knight JR, Gross EA, Bradley GH, et al. Boehler's angle and the critical angle of Gissane are of limited use in diagnosing calcaneus fractures in the ED. *Am J Emerg Med.* 2006;24(4):423-427.

344. Gissane W. Proceedings of the British Orthopedic Association. *J Bone Joint Surg Br.* 1947;29:254-255.

345. Essex-Lopresti P. The mechanism, reduction technique and results in fractures of the as calcis. *Br J Surg.* 1952;39:395-419.

346. Bishop JA, Palanca AA, Bellino MJ, et al. Assessment of compromised fracture healing. *J Am Acad Orthop Surg.* 2012;20:273-282.

347. Corrales LA, Morshed S, Bhandari M, et al. Variability in the assessment of fracture-healing in orthopaedic trauma studies. *J Bone Joint Surg Am.* 2008;90:1862-1868.

348. United States Food and Drug Administration (USFDA), Office of Device Evaluation. *Guidance Document for Industry and CDRH Staff for the Preparation of Investigational Device Exemptions and Premarket Approval Application for Bone Growth Stimulator Devices.* 1988.

349. Frolke JPM, Patka P. Definition and classification of fracture non-unions. *Injury.* 2007;38S:S19-S22.

350. Marchis-Crisan C, Christman RA. Joint disease. In: Christman RA, ed. *Foot and Ankle Radiology.* 2nd ed. Philadelphia, PA: Wolters Kluwer; 2015:345-380.

351. Hayeri MR, Trudell DJ, Resnick D. Anterior ankle impingement and talar bony outgrowths: osteophyte or enthesophyte? Paleopathologic and cadaveric study with imaging correlation. *AJR Am J Roentgenol.* 2009;193:W334-W338.

352. Esposito A, Souto SC, Catalano OA, et al. Pattern of osteophytes and enthesophytes in the proximal ulna: an anatomic, paleopathologic, and radiologic study. *Skeletal Radiol.* 2007;35:847-856.

353. Resnick D. Talar ridges, osteophytes, and beaks: a radiologic commentary. *Radiology.* 1984;151(2):329-332.

354. Forrester DM, Brown JC. *The Radiology of Joint Disease.* 3rd ed. Philadelphia, PA: WB Saunders; 1987.

355. Resnick D, Niwayama G. Entheses and enthesopathy. *Radiology.* 1983;146:1-9.

356. Resnick D, Feingold ML, Curd J, et al. Calcaneal abnormalities in articular disorders. *Radiology.* 1977;125:355-366.

357. Sarrafian SK, Kelikian AS. Tendon sheaths and bursae. In: Kelikian AS, ed. *Sarrafian's Anatomy of the Foot and Ankle.* Philadelphia, PA: Lippincott Williams & Wilkins; 2011:292-301.

358. Amis J, Jennings L, Graham D, et al. Painful heel syndrome: radiographic and treatment assessment. *Foot Ankle.* 1988;9(2):91-95.

359. Fiamengo SA, Warren RF, Marshall JL. Posterior heel pain associated with a calcaneal step and Achilles tendon calcification. *Clin Orthop.* 1982;167:203-211.

360. Slobodin G, Rimar D, Boulman N, et al. Entheseal involvement in systemic disorders. *Clin Rheumatol.* 2015;34:2001-2010.

361. Bywaters EGL. Heel lesions of rheumatoid arthritis. *Ann Rheum Dis.* 1954;13:42-51.

362. Resnick D, Niwayama G. Rheumatoid arthritis and the seronegative spondyloarthropathies: radiographic and pathologic concepts. In: Resnick D, Niwayma G, eds. *Diagnosis of Bone and Joint Disorders.* 2nd ed. Philadelphia, PA: WB Saunders Co.; 1988:895-953.

363. Christman RA. A systematic approach for radiographically evaluating joint disease in the foot. *J Am Podiatr Med Assoc.* 1991;81(4):174-180.

364. Saltzman CL, Salamon ML, Blanchard GM, et al. Epidemiology of ankle arthritis: report of a consecutive series of 639 patients from a tertiary orthopaedic center. *Iowa Orthop J.* 2005;25:44-46.

365. Belhorn LR, Hess EV. Erosive osteoarthritis. *Semin Arthritis Rheum.* 1993;22:298-306.

366. Kellgren JH, Lawrence JS. Radiological assessment of osteoarthrosis. *Ann Rheum Dis.* 1957;16(4):494-502.

367. Menz HB, Munteanu SE, Landorf KB, et al. Radiographic classification of osteoarthritis in commonly affected joints of the foot. *Osteoarthritis Cartilage.* 2007;15:1333-1338.

368. Trivedi B, Marshall M, Belcher J, et al. A systematic review of radiographic definitions of foot osteoarthritis in population-based studies. *Osteoarthr Cartil.* 2010;18:1027-1035.

369. Roukis TS, Jacobs PM, Dawson DM, et al. A prospective comparison of clinical, radiographic, intraoperative features of hallux rigidus. *Foot Ankle Surg.* 2002;41:76-95.

370. Hanft JR, Mason ET, Landsman AS, et al. A new radiographic classification for hallux limitus. *J Foot Ankle Surg.* 1993;32:397-404.

371. Hattrup SJ, Johnson KA. Subjective results of hallux rigidus following treatment with cheilectomy. *Clin Orthop.* 1988;226:182-191.

372. Regnauld B. Disorders of the great toe. In: Elson R, ed. *The Foot: Pathology, Aetiology, Seminology, Clinical Investigation and Treatment.* New York, NY: Springer-Verlag; 1986:269-281, 344-349.

373. Drago JJ, Oloff L, Jacobs AM. A comprehensive review of hallux limitus. *J Foot Surg.* 1984;23:213-220.

374. Samimi R, Green DR, Malay DS. Evaluation of first metatarsophalangeal range of motion pre and post bunion surgery: A clinical and radiographic correlation with stress lateral dorsiflexion views; A retrospective approach. In: *Podiatry Institute Update, 2009: Chapter 16:97-114.* http://www.podiatryinstitute.com/pdfs/Update_Index.pdf. Accessed July 08, 2019.

375. Boffeli TJ, Collier RC. Lateral stress dorsiflexion view: a case series demonstrating clinical utility in midterm hallux limitus. *J Foot Ankle Surg.* 2015;54:739-746.

376. Joseph J. Range of movement of the great toe in men. *J Bone Joint Surg Br.* 1954;36B(3):450-457.

377. Buell T, Green D, Risser J. Measurement of the first metatarsophalangeal joint range of motion. *J Am Podiatr Med Assoc.* 1988;78(9):439-449.

378. Martel W. The overhanging margin of bone: a roentgenologic manifestation of gout. *Radiology.* 1968;91:755-756.

379. Resnick D. The radiographic manifestations of gouty arthritis. *CRC Crit Rev Diagn Imaging.* 1977;9:265-335.

380. MacKenzie JD, Karasick D. Imaging of rheumatoid arthritis. In: Weissman BN, ed. *Imaging of Arthritis and Metabolic Bone Disease.* Philadelphia, PA: Saunders; 2009:340-364.

381. Brower AC, Flemming DJ. Approach to the foot. In: Brower AC, Flemming DJ, eds. *Arthritis in Black & White.* 3rd ed. Philadelphia, PA: Saunders; 2012:62-92.

382. Karasick D, Schweitzer ME, O'Hara BJ. Distal fibular notch: a frequent manifestation of the rheumatoid ankle. *Skeletal Radiol.* 1997;26:529-532.

383. Resnick D, Kransdorf MJ. Psoriatic arthritis. In: Resnick D, Kransdorf MJ, eds. *Bone and Joint Imaging.* 3rd ed. Philadelphia, PA: Elsevier Saunders; 2005:288-297.

384. Resnick D, Kransdorf MJ. Ankylosing spondylitis. In: Resnick D, Kransdorf MJ, eds. *Bone and Joint Imaging.* 3rd ed. Philadelphia, PA: Elsevier Saunders; 2005:267-287.

385. Resnick D, Kransdorf MJ. Reiter's syndrome. In: Resnick D, Kransdorf MJ, eds. *Bone and Joint Imaging.* 3rd ed. Philadelphia, PA: Elsevier Saunders; 2005:298-305.

386. Frykberg RG, Mendeszoon E. Management of the diabetic Charcot foot. *Diabetes Metab Res Rev.* 2000;16(suppl 1):S59-S66.

387. Eichenholtz SN. General considerations. In: Eichenholtz SN, ed. *Charcot Joints.* Springfield, IL: Charles C. Thomas; 1966:1-20.

388. Shibata T, Tada K, Hashizume C. The results of arthrodesis of the ankle for leprotic neuroarthropathy. *J Bone Joint Surg Am.* 1990;72:749-756.

389. Frykberg RG, Eneroth M. Principles of conservative management. In: Frykberg RG, ed. *The Diabetic Charcot Foot: Principles and Management.* Brooklandville, MD: Data Trace Publishing Company; 2010:93-116.

390. Wukich DK, Sung W. Charcot arthropathy of the foot and ankle: modern concepts and management review. *J Diabetes Complications.* 2009;23:409-426.

391. Yu GV, Hudson JR. Evaluation and treatment of stage 0 Charcot's neuroarthropathy of the foot and ankle. *J Am Podiatr Med Assoc.* 2002;92(4):210-220.

392. Turecki MB, Taljanovic MS, Stubbs AY, et al. Imaging of musculoskeletal soft tissue infections. *Skeletal Radiol.* 2010;39:957-971.

393. Resnick D, Kransdorf MJ. Osteomyelitis, septic arthritis, and soft tissue infection: mechanisms and situations. In: Resnick D, Kransdorf MJ, eds. *Bone and Joint Imaging.* 3rd ed. Philadelphia, PA: Elsevier Saunders; 2005:713-742.

394. Rowe LJ, Yochum TR. Infection. In: Yochum TR, Rowe LJ, eds. *Essential of Skeletal Radiology.* 3rd ed. Philadelphia, PA: Lippincott Williams & Wilkins; 2005:1373-1426.

395. Greenspan A, Beltran J. Radiologic evaluation of musculoskeletal infections. In: Greenspan A, Beltran J, eds. *Orthopedic Imaging: A Practical Approach.* 6th ed. New York, NY: Wolters Kluwer Health; 2015:933-944.

396. Greenspan A, Beltran J. Osteomyelitis, infectious arthritis, and soft tissue infections. In: Greenspan A, Beltran J, eds. *Orthopedic Imaging: A Practical Approach.* 6th ed. New York, NY: Wolters Kluwer Health; 2015:945-972.

397. Bohndorf K, Anderson M, Davies M, et al. Infections of the bones, joints, and soft tissues. In: Bohndorf K, Anderson M, Davies M, et al., eds. *Imaging of Bones and Joints.* New York, NY: Thieme; 2008:228-254.

398. Reinus WR. Imaging approach to musculoskeletal infections. In: Bonakdarpour A, Reinus WR, Khurana JS, eds. *Diagnostic Imaging of Musculoskeletal Diseases, A Systematic Approach.* New York, NY: Springer, 2010:363-405.

399. Lecomte AR, Ossiani M, Aliabadi P. Imaging of infection. In: Weissman BN, ed. *Imaging of Arthritis and Metabolic Bone Disease.* Philadelphia, PA: Saunders; 2009:314-339.

400. Manaster BJ, Roberts CC, Petersilge CA, et al. Osteomyelitis. In: Manaster BJ, ed. *Diagnostic Imaging. Musculoskeletal: Non-Traumatic Disease.* Vol 8. Canada: Amirsys; 2012:2-21.

401. Chew FS. Infection and marrow disease. In: Chew FS, ed. *Skeletal Radiology: The Bare Bones.* 3rd ed. Philadelphia, PA: Lippincott Williams & Wilkins; 2010:297-314.

402. Christman RA. The radiographic presentation of osteomyelitis in the foot. *Clin Podiatr Med Surg.* 1990;7(3):433-448.

403. Williams M, Christman RA. Bone infection. In: Christman RA, ed. *Foot and Ankle Radiology.* 2nd ed. Philadelphia, PA: Lippincott Williams & Wilkins; 2015:331-344.

404. Osher L, Petrozzi R, Christman RC. Tumors and tumor-like lesions. In: Christman RA, ed. *Foot and Ankle Radiology.* 2nd ed. Philadelphia, PA: Wolters Kluwer; 2015:381-427.

405. Unni KK, Inwards CY. *Dahlin's Bone Tumors.* 6th ed. Philadelphia, PA: Lippincott Williams & Wilkins; 2010.

406. Miller TT. Bone tumors and tumorlike conditions: analysis with conventional radiography. *Radiology.* 2008;246(3):662-674.

407. Madewell JE, Ragsdale BD, Sweet DE. Radiologic and pathologic analysis of solitary bone lesions. Part I. Internal margins. *Radiol Clin North Am.* 1981;19(4):715-748.

408. Kang HS, Ahn JM, Kang Y. *Oncologic Imaging: Bone Tumors.* Singapore: Springer; 2017.

409. Ragsdale BD, Madewell JE, Sweet DE. Radiologic and pathologic analysis of solitary bone lesions. Part II. Periosteal reactions. *Radiol Clin North Am.* 1981;19(4):749-783.

410. Resnick D, Kransdorff MJ. Tumors and tumor-like lesions of bone: radiographic principles. In: *Bone and Joint Imaging.* 3rd ed. Philadelphia, PA: Elsevier Saunders; 2005:1109-1119.

411. Sweet DE, Madewell JE, Ragsdale BD. Radiologic and pathologic analysis of solitary bone lesions. Part III. Matrix patterns. *Radiol Clin North Am.* 1981;19(4):785-814.

412. Wilner D. *Radiology of Bone Tumors and Allied Disorders.* Philadelphia, PA: WB Saunders Co.; 1982.

413. Libson E, Bloom R, Husband J, et al. Metastatic tumors of bones of the hand and foot: a comparative review and report of 43 additional cases. *Skeletal Radiol.* 1987;16:387-392.

414. Bakotic B, Huvos A. Tumors of the foot: a review of 150 cases. *J Foot Ankle Surg.* 2001;405:277-286.

415. El Ghazaly SA, DeGroot H. Metastases to bones of the foot: a case series, review of the literature, and a systematic approach to diagnosis. *Foot Ankle Spec.* 2008;1(6):338-343.

416. American College of Radiology. *ACR appropriateness criteria. Musculoskeletal: Primary bone tumors.* 2013. https://acsearch.acr.org/list/) (https://acsearch.acr.org/docs/69421/Narrative/. Accessed July 11, 2019.

417. Kransdorf MJ, Murphey MD. Adult bone and soft tissue tumors: fundamental concepts. In: Hodler J, Kubik-Huch RA, von Schulthess GK, eds. *Musculoskeletal Diseases 2017-2020.* New York, NY: Springer; 2017:3-16.

418. Toepfer A. Tumors of the foot and ankle—A review of the principles of diagnostics and treatment. *Fuß Sprunggelenk.* 2017;15:82-96.

419. Manaster BJ, May DA, Disler DG. Introduction to musculoskeletal tumor imaging. In: Manaster BJ, May DA, Disler DG, eds. *Musculoskeletal Imaging.* 4th ed. Philadelphia, PA: Saunders; 2013:355-364.

420. Aisen AM, Martel W, Braunstein EM, et al. MRI and CT evaluation of primary bone and soft-tissue tumors. *AJR Am J Roentgenol.* 1986;146:749-756.

421. Gunderman RB. The musculoskeletal system. In: Gunderman RB, ed. *Essential Radiology: Clinical Presentation, Pathophysiology, Imaging.* 2nd ed. New York, NY: Thieme; 2006:220-256.

422. Wu JS, Hochman MG. *Bone Tumors.* New York, NY: Springer; 2012.

423. Lakkaraju A, Patel CN, Bradley KM, et al. PET/CT in primary musculoskeletal tumours: a step forward. *Eur Radiol.* 2010;20:2959-2972.

424. Peterson JJ. F-18 FDG-PET for detection of osseous metastatic disease and staging, restaging, and monitoring response to therapy of musculoskeletal tumors. *Semin Musculoskelet Radiol.* 2007;11:246-260.

425. Sella EJ, Caminear DS, McLarney EA. Haglund's syndrome. *J Foot Ankle Surg.* 1998;37(2):110-114.

426. Fowler A, Philip JF. Abnormalities of the calcaneus as a cause of painful heel: its diagnosis and operative treatment. *Br J Surg.* 1945;32:494-498.

427. Steffensen JCA, Evensen A. Bursitis retrocalcanea Achilli. *Acta Orthop Scand.* 1958;27:228-236.

428. Ruch JA. Haglund's disease. *J Am Podiatry Assoc.* 1974;64:1000-1003.

429. Vega MR, Cardo DJ, Green RM, et al. Haglund's deformity. *J Am Podiatry Assoc.* 1984;74:129-135.

430. Pavlov H, Heneghan MA, Hersh A, et al. The Haglund's syndrome: initial and differential diagnosis. *Radiology.* 1982;144(1):83-88.

431. Chauveaux D, Liet P, Le Huec JC, et al. A new radiologic measurement for the diagnosis of Haglund's deformity. *Surg Radiol Anat.* 1991;13:39-44.

432. Tourne Y, Baray AL, Barthelemy R, et al. Contribution of a new radiologic calcaneal measurement to the treatment decision tree in Haglund syndrome. *Orthop Traumatol Surg Res.* 2018;104:1215-1219.

433. Mishra DK, Kurup HV, Musthyala S, et al. Role of calcaneus in heel pain: radiological assessment. *Foot Ankle Surg.* 2006;12:127-131.

434. Lu CC, Cheng YM, Fu YC, et al. Angle analysis of Haglund syndrome and its relationship with osseous variations and Achilles tendon calcification. *Foot Ankle Int.* 2007;28:181-185.

435. Singh R, Rohilla R, Siwach RC, et al. Diagnostic significance of radiologic measurements in posterior heel pain. *The Foot.* 2008;18:91-98.

436. Crim JR. *Imaging of the Foot and Ankle.* London, England: Lippincott-Raven; 1996.

437. Resnick D, Kransdorf M. *Bone and Joint Imaging.* 3rd ed. Philadelphia, PA: Elsevier Saunders; 2004.

438. Manaster BJ, May DA, Disler DG. *Musculoskeletal Imaging: The Requisites.* 3rd ed. Philadelphia, PA: Mosby. 2007;200(445):253-255.

439. Adler R, Sofka C, Positano R. *Atlas of Foot and Ankle Sonography.* Philadelphia, PA: Lippincott Williams & Wilkins; 2004.

440. Okanobo H, Khurana B, Sheehan S, Duran-Mendicuti A, Arianjam A, Ledbetter S. Simplified diagnostic algorithm for Lauge-Hansen classification of ankle injuries. *Radiographics.* 2012;32(2):E71-E84.

441. Tartaglione J, Rosenbaum A, Abousayed M, Dipreta J. Classifications in brief: Lauge-Hansen classification of ankle fractures. *Clin Orthop Relat Res.* 2015;473(10):3323-3328.

442. Christman R. *Foot and Ankle Radiology*. 2nd ed. Philadelphia, PA: Wolters Kluwer; 2015.

443. Mcrae R, Esser M. *Practical Fracture Treatment*. 5th ed. 2008.

444. Kellett JJ, Lovell GA, Eriksen DA, Sampson MJ. Diagnostic imaging of ankle syndesmosis injuries: a general review. *J Med Imaging Radiat Oncol*. 2018;62(2):159-168.

445. Guss D. https://www.curvebeam.com/blog/evaluating-the-ankle-syndesmosis-injury-vs-instability/. 2019.

446. Schwartz N. *Ultrasound of the Foot and Ankle*. New York, NY: McGraw-Hill; 2016.

447. Tassone J Jr, Barrett S. *Diagnostic Ultrasound of the Foot and Ankle*. Brooklandville, MD: Data Trace Publishing Company; 2013.

448. Armstrong A, Aedo A, Phelps S. Synovial sarcoma: a case report. *Clin Podiatr Med Surg*. 2008;25:167-181.

449. Palestro C, Love C, Tronco G, et al. Combined labeled leukocyte and Technetium 99m sulfur colloid bone marrow imaging for diagnosing musculoskeletal infection. *RadioGraphics*. 2006;26(3).

Perioperative Management

CHAPTER 3

Perioperative Evaluation

Andrea D. Cass and Roya Mirmiran

INTRODUCTION

Perioperative evaluation includes initial patient assessment as well as planning for any pertinent preoperative labs, imaging, and referrals. The evaluation does not end with the planned surgery, as intraoperative concerns and potential immediate postoperative issues still need to be considered. This chapter discusses elements of a history and physical as well as pre-, intra-, and postoperative considerations for patients undergoing foot and ankle surgery. Although it is impossible to discuss all elements of perioperative management, an attempt was made to not only highlight the significant topics but also present areas of controversy in perioperative management of patients.

PATIENT ASSESSMENT

With increase in life expectancy and upsurge incidence of illnesses such as diabetes mellitus and hypertension, obtaining a thorough history and physical becomes even more crucial in achieving a successful surgical outcome.[1] The main goal of a history and physical is to provide means for risk mitigation. The financial implications of risk stratification cannot be ignored, and the need for thorough and efficient perioperative risk evaluation is warranted.

The podiatric surgeon, internist, and anesthesiologist are key players in determining perioperative risk for each patient prior to surgery. In addition to the patient's list of illnesses, there are other factors that can play a significant role on the final outcome of a surgery. Nutritional status, psychosocial history, social habits, and patient compliance may even have a higher impact on the procedure selection, length of recovery, and overall outcome. A thorough perioperative medical assessment can decrease the length of hospital stay as well as minimize postponed or cancelled surgeries.[2]

GUIDELINES ON PREOPERATIVE EVALUATIONS

The risk of perioperative morbidity and mortality is strongly related to physiologic stress induced by surgery. Foot and ankle surgery are considered at low to intermediate risk by the American College of Cardiology (ACC).[2] Current guidelines for preoperative evaluations are less complicated, but the focus remains on cardiac and pulmonary risk stratification. One of the most commonly used surgical risk stratification method is the American College of Surgeon's National Surgical Quality

Improvement Program (NSQIP) questionnaire. This risk assessment weighs in the type of surgery along with common risk factors. The physician enters the Common Procedural Terminology (CPT) code for the procedure along with patient's medical history to calculate the postoperative risks associated with the particular procedure. The calculated postoperative risks include probabilities for serious complication, cardiac complications, renal failure, urinary tract infection, pneumonia, venous thrombosis, readmission, and return to the operating room (OR). This risk calculator can be accessed via https://riskcalculator.facs.org/RiskCalculator/PatientInfo.jsp. Not all foot and ankle surgery Current Procedural Terminology (CPT) codes are listed, but one can find a closely related CPT code to achieve an approximate risk stratification.

In addition to cardiac and pulmonary risk factors, other risk factors such as nutrition (ie, vitamin D deficiency, low protein and albumin levels), social habits (such as tobacco and alcohol use), psychiatric history (eg, depression and anxiety), socioeconomic and work issues, medical illnesses (such as diabetes and rheumatoid arthritis), and patient compliance can play an even stronger role in surgical outcome.

PHYSIOLOGIC EFFECT OF SURGERY

Epinephrine, norepinephrine, and cortisol levels increase during surgery and remain elevated for 24-72 hours.[3] Serum antidiuretic hormone levels may be elevated for up to 1 week postoperatively, leading to nausea and vomiting. There is evidence that anesthesia and surgery may be associated with a relative hypercoagulable and inflammatory state mediated by increases in plasminogen activator-1, factor VIII, and platelet reactivity, and increased levels of tumor necrosis factor, interleukins 1 and 6, and C-reactive protein.[3] The body attempts to stabilize itself and restore hemostasis after surgery. For those patients with medical comorbidities and inability to fully recuperate, the recovery can be associated with significant postoperative complications. As physicians, it is our duty to recognize and understand the medical condition of a patient in the preoperative phase to avoid or reduce occurrence of any postoperative complication.

PREOPERATIVE ASSESSMENT

Preoperative assessment for elective surgery is typically performed days before surgery. Per Centers for Medicare and Medicaid Services (CMS), a medical history and examination should be performed within 30 days of the planned surgery.[4] Furthermore, CMS Conditions of Participation requires an update to an H&P. "*When the H&P is conducted within 30 days before admission or registration, an update must be completed and documented by a licensed practitioner who is credentialed and privileged by the hospital's medical staff to perform an H&P. (71 FR 68675).*"[4] Per the Joint Commission (TJC) requirement, this update must be completed within 24 hours of patient's registration to the hospital but prior to surgery or a procedure requiring anesthesia.[5]

A complete H&P includes patient's chief complaint, thorough review of patient's current and past medical history, drug history, surgical, anesthetic and psychiatric history, alcohol and tobacco use, allergies, bleeding history, functional class, as well as a thorough physical examination.

History

The history includes a chief complaint along with any information about the condition for which the surgery is planned, any past surgical procedures, patient's experience with anesthesia, and current and chronic medical conditions, particularly of the heart and lungs. In children, the history includes birth history, focusing on risk factors such as prematurity at birth, perinatal complications, congenital chromosomal or anatomic malformations, and history of recent infections, particularly upper respiratory infections or pneumonia. Socioeconomic and a psychiatric history can help the surgeon with appropriate postoperative planning to assure a safe and smooth recovery.

Social history such as smoking, alcohol, and drug use history are important considerations when assessing potential perioperative pulmonary and cardiac complications.[6] Smoking has known detrimental effect on healing bone and tissue. In a small study of patients undergoing first metatarsal osteotomy, a 42% increase in time to bone healing was noted among smokers. The delay in bone healing correlated to increased urine cotinine level.[7] Cotinine is a metabolite formed in the body after exposure to nicotine. Cotinine levels can be elevated for 3 or more weeks after exposure to nicotine. Nicotine has shown to cause delay in tendon-to-bone healing in animal models.[8] Higher rates of infection, pain, delayed osseous union, and wound healing issues in smokers have been reported in several foot and ankle studies.[9-11] The patient should quit smoking 8 or more weeks before surgery to minimize surgical wound complications associated with smoking.[12,13] If a physician is concerned about nicotine use or compliance prior to surgery, checking cotinine levels can be helpful.

Both acute intoxication and chronic abuse of alcohol and recreational drugs can present challenges for anesthetic management and postoperative complications. Alcohol consumption is associated with increased postoperative complications such as infections, cardiopulmonary complications, and bleeding episodes. Excessive alcohol consumption affects many organs such as liver, pancreas, and nervous system. There is reported fivefold increase in probability of cardiac arrest among patients with history of heavy drinking.[14] Cessation of alcohol prior to surgery may help normalize the affected organ systems and lower liver enzymes to some degrees. However, a 2018 Cochrane data base study could not find any supportive evidence that alcohol cessation would have any impact in improving postoperative outcome.[15] We recommend against performing elective foot and ankle surgery on a patient with acute drug intoxication. Urgent and emergent surgeries in acutely intoxicated patients should be postponed or performed only after weighing in associated risks vs benefits.

There are no specific guidelines on timing of surgery in cocaine positive patients. It is unclear if history of substance abuse, such as use of cocaine, increases intra- or postoperative mortality or morbidity. A significantly higher incidence of pneumonia was found among cocaine positive patients, posttrauma surgery.[16] Surgery should be considered carefully among patients with history of marijuana use. Hepatomegaly and splenomegaly have been reported among 57.7% and 73.1% of patient with history of marijuana use, respectively.[17]

Medications

Medications (with dosages), including over-the-counter medications, vitamins, and herbal medicines, are reviewed and documented. Drug dosages may need to be adjusted in the perioperative period. Table 3.1 lists preoperative recommendations for the most common cardiovascular, pulmonary, diabetes, and other medications.[18] Adjusting preoperative medications should be patient and/or procedure specific as times risks of withholding a medication may outweigh its benefit. As such, a patient's primary care physician or cardiologist may need to be consulted. Immunization status can be documented, and vaccines can be updated if necessary.

Allergies

Latex allergy is increasingly becoming more common and occurs in 5%-10% of the population.[1] Patients with a history of chronic urologic problems, spina bifida, and atopic dermatitis are considered at high risk for latex allergy.[19-23] The latest data show average prevalence of latex allergy worldwide to be at 9.7%, 7.2%, and 4.3% among health care workers, susceptible patients, and general population, respectively.[19] Due to increased incidence of latex allergy in health care workers and general population, there has been a highlighted movement in providing a latex-free environment within the clinics and ORs.

Although it is suggested that patients with shellfish allergies may have hypersensitivity to use of betadine prep materials, such statement is not well supported in literature.[24] In matter of fact, research has shown lack of evidence for allergic reaction to intravenous iodine-based contrast among patients with shellfish allergy.[25] An allergy to antibiotics, pain medications, metal, and adhesive tapes are common. As some of the patient's self-reported adverse reaction to medications may not be true allergy (IgE mediated), it is important to obtain detail information about the type of reaction the patient experienced with the specific allergen.

Laboratory Testing

Preoperative laboratory testing should be selective and not routine. Current recommendations are for considering laboratory tests based on a specific sign, symptoms, and diagnosis.[26] Normal laboratory test results obtained 4-6 months before surgery may be used as preoperative tests, provided there are no changes in the clinical status of the patient. MacPherson et al. found that <2% of test results conducted 4 months before surgery had changed at the time of clinical evaluation.[27]

Preoperative laboratory studies may include a complete blood count, extensive blood chemistry profile, coagulation

TABLE 3.1	Pharmacologic Categories and Their Recommendations
Adjusting preoperative medications should be patient and/or procedure specific as times risks of withholding a medication may outweigh its benefit	
Frequently used medications	
Acetaminophen	CONTINUE use
Aspirin	HOLD 7-10 d prior to surgery - due to irreversible inhibitor activity of platelet cyclooxygenase
NSAID	HOLD 3 d prior to surgery - due to reversible inhibitor activity of platelet cyclooxygenase
Clopidogrel	HOLD 7-10 d prior to surgery - due to its irreversible antiplatelet effect
Cardiovascular medications	
Digoxin Clonidine Beta-blockers Ca channel blockers	CONTINUE up to and including day of surgery
Diuretics ACE inhibitors Angiotensin II receptor blocker	HOLD on the morning of surgery - especially if indication is CHF because there is an increased risk of hypotension during surgery
Cholesterol-lowering drugs	HOLD 1 d prior to surgery - carry risk of rhabdomyolysis and myositis
Pulmonary medications	
Inhaled beta-agonist Inhaled ipratropium Inhaled corticosteroid	CONTINUE up to and including day of surgery
Diabetes medications	
Insulin	Give long-acting insulin at ½ the normal dose, hold short-acting morning of surgery
Metformin	HOLD 2 d prior to surgery - due to risk of lactic acidosis if patient has renal problems preoperatively
Sulfonylureas Thiazolidinediones Alpha-glucosidase inhibitors	HOLD on the morning of surgery
Vitamins	
Vitamin E supplements	HOLD 7-10 d prior to surgery - due to a risk of bleeding

profile, urinalysis, electrocardiogram (ECG), and chest radiographs. Indications for specific tests are as follows:

1. Urine pregnancy test should be considered for women of childbearing age.
2. Chemistry profile should be performed in patients with a history of hypertension, diuretic use, chronic obstructive pulmonary disease (COPD) or obstructive sleep apnea, diabetes, renal disease, or chemotherapy.

3. Complete blood count should be performed in patients with a history of fatigue, dyspnea on exertion, liver disease, blood loss, signs of coagulopathy, diabetes, or tachycardia.
4. Coagulation profile is indicated if the patient is receiving anticoagulant therapy, has a family or personal history that suggests a bleeding disorder, or has evidence of liver disease.
5. Renal and hepatic function tests are indicated for patients who have a medical condition such as history of liver disease, alcoholism, severe hypertension, lupus, diabetes, colon cancer, and medication use (ie, NSAIDs, hydrochlorothiazide use, etc.) that would serve as indications for these tests.
6. ECG is generally recommended in men over the age of 40 years, and in women older than 50 years, and in those with known underlying cardiovascular disease. Per 2014 ACC/American Heart Association (AHA) guidelines,[28] if patient has a low risk (<1%) for major adverse cardiac event (MACE), then no ECG is needed and one can proceed with surgery. If the patient is at elevated risk of MACE, then one needs to measure patient's functional capacity. If patient has moderate to excellent functional capacity (≥ 4 METs), then surgery can be done without any further testing. If patient has unknown or poor functional capacity (<4 METs), further testing such as ECG and stress testing is recommended. Routine 12-lead ECG is not usually recommended in asymptomatic patients undergoing low-risk surgical procedures.[28]
7. Chest radiographs should be obtained if there are signs of pulmonary disease.

PERIOPERATIVE ANESTHESIA ASSESSMENT

The American Society of Anesthesiologists (ASA) in 1987 adopted basic standards for the evaluation of patients prior to surgery. The ASA classification was designed to estimate overall mortality risk in patients undergoing surgery, but a number of studies have shown that it also predicts cardiovascular and pulmonary complications. Patients who are graded higher than class II in the 5-class ASA system have a 2- to 3-fold increased risk of postoperative pulmonary complications compared with those graded class II or lower. Although subjective, a score of II-V indicates an increased level of severity and increased postoperative morbidity (Table 3.2).[29]

Anesthesia and surgery are coupled with physiologic response to preserve homeostasis. Homeostasis is carefully monitored through the perioperative period. Inhaled, intravenous, and local anesthesia cause diverse effects on the nervous, cardiovascular, and respiratory systems. Inhalational anesthetic agents have predictable physiologic effects. All inhalational anesthetic agents are myocardial depressants. While not clinically significant in healthy patients, this effect leads to a dependence on cardiac preload that may cause an accentuated response to the induction of anesthesia in patients who are volume depleted due to illness or over diuresis or who have left ventricular dysfunction. Anesthesia leads to a decrease in lung volumes, which may lead to atelectasis and is a principal factor leading to the development of postoperative pulmonary complications.[3]

Controversy exists regarding the relative safety of general vs spinal or epidural anesthesia in patients at risk for postoperative cardiac or pulmonary complications. In a recent large meta-analysis of randomized controlled trials of anesthetic

TABLE **3.2** **Preoperative Anesthesia Assessment: American Society of Anesthesiology (ASA) Classification**

Class I	A normal, healthy patient Eg: healthy with good exercise tolerance
Class II	A patient with mild systemic disease Eg: controlled hypertension or controlled diabetes without systemic effects, cigarette smoking without COPD, anemia, mild obesity, age younger than 1 y or older than 70 y, pregnancy
Class III	A patient with severe systemic disease Eg: controlled congestive heart failure (CHF), stable angina, old myocardial infarction, poorly controlled hypertension, morbid obesity, bronchospastic disease with intermittent symptoms, chronic renal failure
Class IV	A patient with severe systemic disease that is a constant threat to life Eg: unstable angina, symptomatic COPD, symptomatic CHF, hepatorenal failure
Class V	A patient with a critical medical condition with little change of survival with or without the surgical procedure Eg: multiorgan failure, sepsis syndrome with hemodynamic instability hypothermia, poorly controlled coagulopathy
Class VI	A declared brain-dead patient who is undergoing anesthesia care for the purposes of organ donation
E	If the procedure is an emergency, the physical status is followed by "E" (eg, "2E")

Based on ASA Physical Status Classification System. A copy of the full text can be obtained from ASA, 1061 American Lane, Schaumburg, IL 60173. https://www.asahq.org/standards-and-guidelines/asa-physical-status-classification-system. Last Amended December 13, 2020.

technique, patients who were randomized to receive spinal or epidural anesthesia as a component of their anesthesia had significantly lower rates of venous thromboembolism, pneumonia, respiratory depression, myocardial infarction (MI), or death than patients receiving general anesthesia exclusively.[30,31] In some cases, patients undergoing foot and ankle surgery are considered for local with monitored anesthesia care (MAC). Such patients are noted to experience less postoperative pain and have significantly lower levels of anxiety postoperatively in comparison to patients receiving general anesthesia.[32] In general, the choice of anesthetic technique or agent, the decision to use invasive hemodynamic monitoring, and the regulation of body temperature should be left to the anesthesiologist.

PERIOPERATIVE CARDIAC ASSESSMENT

Cardiac complications create one of the most significant risks to patients undergoing noncardiac surgery. A cohort study of 7508 patients, published in 2017, reported an overall mortality rate of 2.8% for patients who developed postoperative complications after elective surgery. A total of 43.9% of these patients died from cardiac arrest.[33] Therefore, understanding a patient's cardiovascular status is essential in order to help reduce these sometimes-fatal complications.

Cardiac risk stratification prior to noncardiac surgery serves a number of goals.[34] First, it determines the patient's current health status, followed by the establishment of a surgical risk profile. It will also help to determine whether further cardiac testing is indicated and to identify the actions that might reduce the patient's perioperative risk. For instance, history of diabetes and peripheral vascular disease, which is often encountered in foot and ankle surgery, places a patient at higher risk for cardiac complication. It is important to identify, recognize, and refer patients at risk for cardiac disease for the needed workup and assessment in order to reduce potential perioperative cardiac adverse events.[35] Over the years, there have been multiple indices introduced to help surgeons better understand the cardiac risk of a patient undergoing noncardiac surgery. The most widely accepted index was developed in 2002 (and later revised in 2014) by the ACC/AHA.[28] The ACC/AHA guidelines summarized clinical predictors for increased perioperative risk of a MI, heart failure (HF), and cardiac death based on history, physical examination, and resting ECG. These predictors are divided into major, intermediate, and minor predictors. Major predictors require intensive management, which may cause a delay or cancellation of surgery. These include recent MI (within 6 months), severe angina, recent percutaneous coronary intervention, and significant arrhythmias. Intermediate predictors may necessitate further noninvasive workup and include mild angina, prior MI by history of ECG, rhythm other than sinus, decompensated HF, diabetes mellitus, and renal insufficiency. Minor predictors are recognized markers for cardiovascular disease but have not been proven to increase perioperative risk. These include advanced age, abnormal ECG, rhythm other than sinus, low functional status, history of stroke, and uncontrolled systolic hypertension.

A thorough medical history is important in order to obtain pertinent information of a patient's cardiovascular status including a history of MI, congestive heart failure, arrhythmias, or valvular disease. It is also important to be aware of any diagnostic or therapeutic procedures the patient has undergone for such conditions, when they were performed, and the specific results/outcome.[36] Such detailed history will also give insight on the patient's functional capacity. Functional capacity is expressed in metabolic equivalents (METs) (1 MET equals 3.5 mL oxygen uptake/kilogram/minute, or the resting oxygen uptake in a sitting position). Patients who are able to walk up a flight of steps without suffering from shortness of breath or chest pain are said to have a 4 MET functional capacity. Those who are unable to meet a functional capacity of 4 METs are associated with an increased risk of postoperative cardiopulmonary complications after major noncardiac surgery.[28] Specific questions should be asked of the patient regarding how many blocks they can walk or how many flights of stairs they can climb before having to stop.

The physical examination, such as assessment of vital signs, murmurs, a third heart sound, jugular venous distention, and rales, is also important, which will further confirm what may already be known based on the history.[36] An ECG is often ordered prior to surgery. Although, ECG is generally recommended in men older than 40 years of age, women older than 50 years, and those with known underlying cardiovascular disease, the most up-to-date ACC-AHA guidelines rely on patient's risk factors in determining the need for an EKG.[28]

Patients with automatic implantable cardioverter defibrillators (AICDs), or pacemakers, may also present a challenge in the perioperative setting. Preoperative management of these patients includes evaluation and optimization of coexisting diseases. No special laboratory tests or radiographs are needed for the patient with a conventional pacemaker.[18] Certain devices may require a standard chest radiograph to document the position of the coronary sinus lead. Important information for current pacemakers, such as battery voltage, battery impedance, lead performance, and adequacy of current setting, may be obtained with a device interrogation with a programmer. Reprogramming is the safest way to avoid intraoperative problems, especially if monopolar electrocautery is to be used.[18] The type of the pacemaker must be known prior to surgery or the patient should carry information about the pacemaker. In certain cases, a magnet must be available or a company representative may need to be notified prior to surgery. The representative will be able to further inform the physician of the steps that need to be taken in the perioperative setting.

Another important issue includes a thorough understanding of which cardiac medications should be, and more importantly should not be, taken perioperatively. Based on the type of foot or ankle procedure, anticoagulants are often discontinued before surgery to reduce bleeding risks. Aspirin and Plavix are discontinued 7-10 days prior to surgery. Coumadin can be stopped 5 days before surgery, and an INR should be performed on the day of surgery. Pradaxa (dabigatran) should be stopped 3 days prior to surgery; Eliquis (apixaban) stopped 48 hours prior to surgery; and Xarelto (rivaroxaban) stopped 24 hours before surgery. Most of these can be restarted the day following the procedure. Preoperative management of anticoagulation medications should be discussed with the patient's cardiologist or internist.

Drugs that should be taken up to and including the day of surgery are beta-blockers, clonidine, antiarrhythmics, calcium channel blockers, nitrates, and digoxin. Statins should also be continued in the perioperative period as they have been shown to prevent cardiovascular events.[37] Medications such as diuretics, ACE inhibitors, and angiotensin II receptor blockers result in electrolyte imbalance and should be held on the day of surgery especially if their main indication is for management of hypertension and the patient's blood pressure is well controlled. Drugs such as niacin, fibric acid derivatives, cholestyramine, and colestipol should be held at least 1 day before surgery.[37]

PERIOPERATIVE PULMONARY ASSESSMENT

Postoperative pulmonary complications are as prevalent as cardiac complications and contribute equally to morbidity, mortality, and length of hospital stay. In a study of 3790 patients undergoing major noncardiac surgery, the rates of pulmonary complications were respiratory failure 2% and bacterial pneumonia 1%. Cardiac complications occurred with an overall frequency of 2%.[38] Therefore, estimation of the risk of pulmonary complications is a necessary part of the preoperative evaluation. Important postoperative pulmonary complications include pneumonia, respiratory failure with prolonged mechanical ventilation, atelectasis, bronchospasm, and exacerbation of underlying COPD.[39]

A history of asthma, prior or current tobacco use, exercise intolerance, chronic cough, sleep apnea, or unexplained dyspnea should be obtained. The physical examination may identify findings suggestive of unrecognized pulmonary disease such as decreased breath sounds, dullness to percussion, wheezes, rhonchi, and a prolonged expiratory phase that predicts an increase in the risk of pulmonary complications.[39]

The ASA classification and the Goldman cardiac risk class can help predict the risk of postoperative pulmonary complications. Although the primary objective of the ASA classification is to determine overall perioperative mortality, this index is also a useful tool to determine pulmonary risk. Patients with ASA class greater than II (on a scale of I-V) have a 1.5-3.2-fold increased risk of pulmonary complications.[39] Other patient-related risk factors known to increase the risk for perioperative pulmonary dysfunction include advanced age, low functional capacity, history of COPD, and CHF (Table 3.3). Procedure-related risk factors include use of general anesthesia, emergency, and/or prolonged surgery.[40] One of the suggested laboratory testing used to stratify pulmonary complication risk is level of serum albumin. Serum albumin level <35 g/L is noted to be a good predictor of potential perioperative pulmonary complication.[39,40]

A useful method (Table 3.3) for calculation of perioperative pulmonary risk factors is the Assess Respiratory Risk in Surgical Patients in Catalonia (ARISCAT) risk index[41] that can be found using the following link: https://www.mdcalc.com/ariscat-score-postoperative-pulmonary-complications.

Patients with a history of asthma are considered to have increased risk of postoperative pulmonary complication only if the patient is actively wheezing. However, in patients with well-controlled asthma, there is no added risk of pulmonary complications. In a large study of 706 patients with asthma undergoing surgery, the incidence of perioperative bronchospasm was 1.7%. There was one episode of postoperative respiratory failure, and no episodes of pneumonia or postoperative death.[12] In patients with a history of controlled asthma or COPD, pulmonary complications may be prevented by providing patients with instructions on how to perform incentive spirometry and deep-breathing exercises preoperatively. In uncontrolled

TABLE 3.3 ARISCAT Risk Index
Risk factors: perioperative pulmonary complication risk factors by patient factors
Current tobacco use ASA class II or higher CHF COPD Age over 60 years old Serum albumin <3.5 mg/dL Sleep apnea
Risk factors: perioperative pulmonary complication risk factors by surgery
Aortic aneurysm repair Thoracic surgery Abdominal surgery Neurosurgery Emergency surgery General anesthesia Prolonged surgery > 3 h Unplanned postoperative intubation Head and neck surgery Vascular surgery

asthmatic or COPD patients, a combination of inhaled bron-chodilators, systemic corticosteroids, and in some cases, chest physical therapy are suggested.[42] Deep-breathing exercises and incentive spirometry in the postoperative period may be particularly beneficial in obese patients or patients with lung disease.

Smoking is a risk factor for postoperative pulmonary complications among patients with and without COPD. Tobacco use affects the respiratory tract and has direct impact on cardiovascular function as well as the blood clot cascade. Studies have shown current cigarette smokers have a 1.4- to 5-fold increase of postoperative complications.[39,43] It is suggested that a minimum of 3-4 weeks of tobacco cessation is required to achieve significantly reduced respiratory-associated postsurgical complication. A decrease in airway secretions and an improvement in mucocillary transport is noted with cessation of smoking within 2-4 weeks of surgery.[44,45]

Poor exercise tolerance is a risk factor for postoperative pulmonary complications. In a questionnaire study of 600 patients undergoing major noncardiac surgery, patients who were unable to walk four blocks or climb two flights of stairs had a modest increase in the rate of pulmonary complications when compared with those with good self-reported exercise capacity (9.0% vs 6.3%).[46]

Although contrary to traditional assumption, multiple studies have shown no increased risk of postoperative pulmonary complications in obese patients.[39] Adequate maintenance of comorbid conditions is essential to reducing pulmonary risks. Finally, adequate control of pain in the postoperative period is paramount in reduction of postoperative pulmonary complications. A systematic review and meta-analysis of randomized trials found that regional anesthetic techniques such as postoperative epidural analgesia and paravertebral nerve blocks provide more effective pain relief than parenteral opiates.[47]

PERIOPERATIVE ENDOCRINE ASSESSMENT

Increased mortality is noted among patients with tight control than a less strict target.[48] It is suggested that tight glucose control may be more practical in surgical rather than nonsurgical intensive care unit (ICU) patients. However, tight glucose control may not be beneficial for all surgical patients. A tight control seems to be even more effective in nondiabetic patients who have pre-/perioperative hyperglycemia, whereas a moderate control is more practical in patients with preexisting diabetes.[49] One of the main concerns regarding perioperative hyperglycemia is the increased risk for skin and soft tissue infections (SSIs). As such, previous recommendations have been to address glucose levels above 200 mg/dL. There is insufficient evidence to support strict glycemic control for the prevention of SSIs.[50] Having said that, glucose level above 200 mg/dL as well as elevated A1C levels >6.5 percent are reported to be significantly associated with increased rates of dehiscence and reoperation in foot and ankle surgery.[51] It is important to be careful in achieving a tight glycemic control since hypoglycemia is commonly seen when trying to rapidly or tightly lower the glucose down to 80-110 mg/dL.[52,53] Therefore, frequent monitoring and measurement is required to watch for hypoglycemia. The data may suggest controlling hyperglycemia in surgical patients to a glucose level of <200 mg/dL; however, an absolute target range remains unknown.[52]

In 2003, the World Health Organization (WHO) and the American Diabetes Association (ADA) introduced a new classification for diabetes.[54] Type I diabetes is characterized as immune mediated or idiopathic while type II ranges from insulin resistance with relative insulin deficiency to a secretory defect with insulin resistance. In the perioperative state, a clear distinction is necessary between the insulin-dependent patient and those on oral antidiabetic drugs. In the latter group, oral hypoglycemic medications are generally withheld on the day of surgery and resumed when a normal diet is restarted. Metformin, which may alter renal function and increase risk for ketoacidosis, is commonly stopped for 48 hours preoperatively. Metformin is continued once normal renal function is confirmed 48-72 hours postoperatively. Type II diabetics treated with insulin often only require supplemental short-acting sliding scale insulin and may resume their normal regimen when dietary intake is normal.

The insulin-dependent patient often requires more elaborate management. Ideally subcutaneous insulin is replaced by continuous intravenous insulin in combination of intravenous dextrose, especially is patients undergoing general anesthesia. When this is not an option, glycemic control can be established by using reduced doses of subcutaneous insulin as a combination of intermediate and short acting. Patients taking long-acting insulin should take half to two-thirds of their bedtime dose the evening before surgery and one-half of their morning dose on the morning of surgery.[55] A common mistake made preoperatively is stopping a patient's basal insulin when they are receiving nothing by mouth prior to surgery (NPO). This results in difficult intraoperative and postoperative glucose control. If the patient is using an insulin pump, basal rate should be continued. As noted previously, intensive glucose control and hypoglycemia is more harmful than a moderately elevated serum glucose level on the day of the surgery in diabetic patients.[56-58]

Postoperatively, diabetic regimens may be resumed once the patient resumes their diet. If a patient undergoing outpatient surgery suffers from adverse gastrointestinal affects of surgery, it is important that they do not resume their insulin or oral hypoglycemic regimen until they are tolerating food or liquid. In the inpatient setting, intravenous dextrose may be necessary until the patient is able to resume a normal diet.

Other than blood glucose control, a thorough evaluation of the comorbidities of the patient with diabetes is also important. Many patients with diabetes have concomitant cardiac, pulmonary, or renal problems that should be addressed preoperatively. Other complications of diabetes that may exist include microvascular, macrovascular, and neuropathic manifestations, all of which increase the risk of morbidity and mortality in the perioperative setting.[59] A cardiac risk assessment should assume high priority in the preoperative examination of the patient with diabetes, since coronary heart disease (CHD) is increased 2-fold in this population, especially in those patients who do not commonly present with the "characteristic" symptoms of CHD.[55] A patient with diabetes and a history of MI and/or unstable angina, autonomic neuropathy, gastroparesis, or orthostatic hypotension should have a thorough cardiovascular evaluation before surgery.

PERIOPERATIVE RENAL ASSESSMENT

Understanding the risk of acute renal failure (ARF) in patients with renal insufficiency is another important topic, since it is associated with a considerably high mortality rate perioperatively. One-half of patients who develop ARF postoperatively will die, and only 15% that survive will ever fully recover their baseline kidney function.[60] It has been shown that the most critical determinants of risks for a postoperative renal failure include preoperative renal function, maintenance of appropriate intravascular volume, and degree of myocardial function.[61]

Postoperative ARF is associated with many acute and chronic risk factors that should be assessed preoperatively. Acute risk factors include volume depletion, use of aminoglycosides, contrast dye exposure, use of NSAIDs, septic shock, and pigmenturia. The podiatric physician should pay special attention to the chronic risk factors as these may be more pertinent in an elective outpatient surgical setting. These chronic risk factors include preexisting renal disease, hypertension, congestive heart failure, diabetes mellitus, peripheral vascular disease, advanced age, and cirrhosis of the liver.[61] It has been shown that a preoperative creatinine level of 2.0 mg/dL or higher is an independent risk factor for postoperative cardiac complications.[62] Females with underlying renal insufficiency are also more likely than their male counterparts to develop ARF postoperatively.[60] Identification of coexisting cardiovascular, circulatory, hematologic, and metabolic derangements secondary to renal dysfunction are the goals of preoperative evaluation.[62] A thorough history and physical in patients with known renal insufficiency with specific focus on symptoms of ischemic heart disease is helpful. A patient's functional status and exercise tolerance should be elicited.

Diagnostic testing should include ECG, complete blood count, and serum chemistry panel in patients with renal dysfunction.[62] Urinalysis and urinary electrolyte studies are generally not helpful in those with established renal disease but may be diagnostic in those with new-onset renal insufficiency. Perioperative antibiotics and postoperative pain medications such as NSAIDs may require further adjustments in patients with known renal failure. One way to minimize the risk of postsurgical renal failure is to calculate the glomerular filtration rate (GFR) and adjust the dose and/or frequency of the medications accordingly. Those with end-stage renal disease and/or on dialysis frequently require treatment perioperatively for hyperkalemia, hypocalcemia, or hyperphosphatemia. A discussion with a nephrologist may be beneficial to assist in enhancing renal function and optimization of the patient preoperatively. In patients with end-stage renal disease, uremia can cause platelet dysfunction, which can then result in increased perioperative bleeding. Such patients should undergo dialysis before surgery to reduce risk of intra- or postoperative bleeding. In most cases, dialysis is performed 1 day prior to surgery and avoided on the day of surgery unless the situation is emergent. Heparin is commonly used with dialysis. Unless heparin-free dialysis is used, it is best to hold off on an elective surgery for least 12 hours after the last hemodialysis with heparin.

PERIOPERATIVE VASCULAR ASSESSMENT

Peripheral arterial disease (PAD) is the most common manifestation of atherosclerosis, and ~50% of such patients are symptomatic. Many of these patients have coexisting coronary and cerebrovascular atherosclerosis, putting their risk of death secondary to cardiovascular disease at a sixfold increase compared to patients without PAD.[63] In obtaining a vascular history of a patient, the physician should aim to determine if risk factors for atherosclerosis, such as diabetes mellitus, dyslipidemia, hypertension, family history of cardiovascular disease, and cigarette

smoking, exists. A prior history of CHD, including prior MI, stroke, angina, or prior revascularization procedure, should also be documented.[63] Identifying the patient's risk factors for PAD, as well as the patient's current symptoms will assist in minimizing perioperative complications. A comprehensive vascular examination should be performed preoperatively on all patients. Vital signs are an important part of the examination and should be recorded. The dorsalis pedis and posterior tibial pulses should be palpated. Bounding pulses or absent of pulses should be documented. Other associated findings such as changes in skin color, poor hair growth, presence of cyanosis or clubbing of the fingers, and a decrease in temperature of the lower extremities must be evaluated.[64]

If the pedal pulses are nonpalpable, an arterial Doppler examination should be performed prior to the planned procedure. An ankle brachial index (ABI) is a simple test that can be performed in the office. An ABI <0.9 is strongly associated with limitations in lower extremity function and tolerance of physical activity.[65] Other noninvasive testing includes segmental Doppler pressures, pulse volume recordings, and transcutaneous oximetry.

One of the most specific symptoms of PAD is intermittent claudication. This occurs as a result of skeletal muscle ischemia that is produced with exertion, as the muscle energy requirements are not served by sufficient augmentation in blood supply.[63] As a result, patients describe discomfort in the affected limb as aching, burning, cramping, and/or tightness. Peripheral arterial stenosis may not compromise muscular function at rest, resulting in the intermittent symptoms. These symptoms may occur in any portion of the limb, from the buttock, hip, thigh, calf or foot, and this is a reflection of the arterial segment that an arterial stenosis may exist. Critical limb ischemia occurs when limb blood flow is inadequate to meet of metabolic demands of the tissues at rest. Patients may describe persistent pain, especially in the toes, ball of the foot, or heel. Sensitivity to cold, joint stiffness, and hypesthesia may also exist.[63] The pain is often increased with elevation of the limb and is relieved with limb dependency.

Arterial embolism or thrombosis may produce acute limb ischemia with symptoms ranging from an asymptomatic loss of a pulse to a sudden onset of severe pain at rest. Pain, pallor, poikilothermia, paresthesia, and paralysis characterize the findings of acute limb ischemia. Atheroembolism may also occur from atherosclerotic debris, compromising distal arteries of the lower extremities. This leads to occlusion of small arterioles, and patients present with calf, foot, or toe pain. Violaceous discoloration or cyanosis may occur in the toes, followed by ulceration of the digit.[63]

There also exist numerous uncommon diseases of peripheral arteries that should be considered as differential diagnoses in patients with claudication or evidence of ischemia. Takayasu arteritis is a condition that occurs in people between the age of 20 and 40 years. In addition to vascular symptoms, such as muscle pain and a diminished pulse and claudication of an upper extremity, patients may also have constitutional symptoms, including fevers, arthralgias, fatigue, and weight loss. Thromboangiitis obliterans (TAO), or Buerger disease, affects the distal vessels of the arms and legs in people under the age of 40 who smoke cigarettes. It is more common in men than in women. The classic triad of TAO is claudication, Raynaud's phenomenon, and superficial thrombophlebitis.[63] This disease may also result in ulcerations of the digits.

Raynaud's phenomenon is another important vascular entity in which the podiatric physician should have a thorough understanding, since it is the most common vasospastic disorder. Classic signs include pale or cyanotic changes of the digits during cold exposure. Although the fingers are most commonly affected, the toes may develop symptoms in 40% of patients.[63] Patients may also develop pain or paresthesia in the digits. Increased erythema is generally seen in rewarming of the digits from the release of the vasospasm. Two forms of Raynaud's exist. The first, primary Raynaud disease or idiopathic episodic digital vasospasm, is characterized by intermittent attacks of ischemic discoloration of the extremities that generally occurs in bilateral distribution.[64] Trophic changes of the skin may also be present. It is the most common type of Raynaud's phenomenon and occurs five times more often in females. The other form is Secondary Raynaud's that is a result of another condition such as connective tissue disorders (ie; lupus), arterial occlusive disease, blood dyscrasias, trauma and certain drugs such as birth control pills. The use of epinephrine as a homeostatic agent should be avoided in these patients, especially in the digits, as this may result in irreversible vasospasm. Some physicians also recommend that ice be avoided postoperatively. Smoking cessation should be strongly discussed in patients with vascular compromise. Proper referral for patients with symptoms or clinical findings of arterial disease may be necessary before elective surgery is considered.

Presence of lower extremity edema should also be evaluated, including location and symmetry. Edema should be graded, as well as assessed for pitting. Unilateral edema may indicate deep venous thrombosis, lymphedema, or cellulitis. Bilateral edema may be a sign of chronic venous insufficiency or congestive heart failure.[65] Patients with chronic venous stasis and superficial venous disease are at higher risk for a postoperative deep venous thrombosis (DVT). Although the routine use of chemical venous thrombosis prophylaxis is not justified, nor supported in foot and ankle surgery, chemical prophylaxis should be considered in patients at high risk for DVT or pulmonary embolism (PE). Such risks include a family or personal history of venous thromboembolism and/or a hypercoagulable state, hormonal or birth control pill use, history of cancer, advanced age, obesity, smoking, and need for prolonged lower extremity immobilization. If feasible, hormonal therapy should be placed on hold in anticipation of an elective foot and ankle surgery. The 2012 American College of Chest Physicians (ACCP) guideline does not recommend any pharmacologic prophylaxis in patients with isolated lower extremity injuries requiring immobilization.[66] However, patient education and identifying potential risk factors are essential during a preoperative examination.

PERIOPERATIVE RHEUMATOLOGY ASSESSMENT

Both inflammatory and noninflammatory types of arthritis can lead to significant deformities and joint destruction in the foot and ankle requiring reconstructive surgery. This patient population, especially those with inflammatory arthritis, can be difficult to manage because of other systemic manifestations of the disease, as well as the use of immunosuppressive medications that may complicate the postoperative healing.

The majority of patients with arthritis take aspirin or nonsteroidal anti-inflammatory drugs (NSAIDs) that may produce difficulties with intraoperative and postoperative bleeding. Aspirin should be discontinued 7-10 days prior to surgery, and NSAIDs should be stopped 3 days prior. Many patients are also

receiving glucocorticoids before surgery. Ideally, the dosage of steroids should be reduced to the lowest possible maintenance dose in the perioperative setting to reduce the risk of postoperative infection and wound healing complications. Supplemental glucocorticoids in the perioperative setting should be considered in patients who are on chronic corticosteroids for more than a few weeks in the last year.[67] Physiologic cortisol secretion in response to major surgery is 75-150 mg/day and returns to baseline in 48-72 hours. At our institution, 100 mg of methyl prednisone is utilized preoperatively, which is sufficient in most podiatric surgical situations. If the patient's disease is severe or a more extensive procedure is performed, the methyl prednisone may be continued postoperatively at a dose of 25-50 mg every 8 hours for 48-72 hours.[67] Recent data suggest that patients on chronic oral steroid use may not need supplemental therapy before surgery. It is recommended to maintain the patients on their usual preoperative dose and only treat if refractory hypotension presents in the perioperative period.[68-70] Moreover, it is recommended that one considers and assesses anticipated degree of surgically induced stress to determine the need or the appropriate perioperative corticosteroid stress dose.[71] The 2016 Endocrine Society Clinical Practice Guideline[72] suggests use of supplemental steroids perioperatively in patients with primary adrenal insufficiency. For minor or moderate surgery-related stress, the recommend supplement is hydrocortisone 25-75 mg/24 hours (usually 1-2 days). For major surgery with general anesthesia, trauma, or situations that require intensive care, the recommended dose is hydrocortisone 100 mg IV injection followed by continuous IV infusion of 200-mg hydrocortisone/24 hours (alternatively 50 mg every 6 hours IV or IM).[72] This should be discussed with the patient's rheumatologist since maintenance doses vary widely from patient to patient. Methotrexate (MTX) has been shown in some studies to increase susceptibility to postoperative infections and should be discontinued 2 weeks before surgery and not reinstituted until wound healing is ensured. MTX should not be resumed immediately postsurgery, as it may cause subtle reductions in renal function leading to precipitation of the drug in the renal tubules and subsequent toxicity.[73] There is additional concern that penicillamine, indomethacin, cyclosporin, hydroxychloroquine, chloroquine, and prednisolone may significantly increase the risk of infection and postoperative complications.[73] It is essential to communicate with the physician managing the patient's condition and medications so that they fully understand the extent of the planned surgery and can subsequently manage the patient's medications appropriately.

Another concern especially in patient with RA is presence of poor bone quality. These patients may require more fixation or longer periods of non–weight bearing in certain circumstances. Patients with arthritis should also be adequately assessed for problems with the neck and jaw, which could interfere with intubation. Flexion radiographs of the neck may show atlantoaxial subluxation, especially in patients with RA and ankylosing spondylitis.[74]

Most patients with chronic inflammatory arthritis have some degree of anemia. Many of the medications used to control the disease also have a hematologic effect of some kind. A thorough hematologic laboratory assessment should be performed on all patients with inflammatory arthritis. If abnormalities are discovered, patients should undergo the proper treatment prior to surgery. For example, it may be advantageous for patients with low hemoglobin levels to receive erythropoietin preoperatively.[75]

Finally, it is important to thoroughly assess the overall physical status of the patient before surgery. Preoperative evaluation by physical and occupational therapists may be helpful. For example, patients with RA may not be able to ambulate with a walker or crutches postoperatively due to deformities of hands and upper extremities. It may be difficult, if not impossible, for many of these patients to be non–weight bearing for extended periods of time. Also, an understanding of the patient's support system at home will be helpful in determining what is realistic postoperatively for the patient. The physician needs to have extensive conversations with the patient about the increased risks of surgery in this population as well as what the realistic expectations are postoperatively.

Another arthritic disease that should be mentioned is gout. Most patients with chronic gout, if managed adequately, do not need supplemental medication in the perioperative setting. These patients should continue their prescribed medication throughout the perioperative period. Since surgical insult may precipitate an attack of acute gouty arthritis, patients with recent history of a gout attack may benefit from one week of an anti-inflammatory medication such as indomethacin post-surgery to reduce the possibility of a gout attack. Alternatively, such patients can be placed on indomethacin for 1 week after surgery to reduce the possibility of a gout attack.

PERIOPERATIVE NUTRITION ASSESSMENT

Perioperative evaluation includes an assessment of risk factors of malnutrition. Malnutrition refers the surgical patient that is overweight or underweight based on the body mass index (BMI). Malnutrition has implications on impaired wound healing, immune system compromise, diminished cardiac and respiratory function, and a host of other complications that can lead to longer hospitalizations and higher mortality rates. Malnourished patients experience increased surgical morbidity and mortality. Social isolation, limited financial resources, poor dentition, weight loss, and chronic disorders such as pulmonary disease, congestive heart failure, depression, diarrhea, and constipation are commonly associated with malnutrition.[76] Weight loss of more than 5% in 1 month or of 10% or more over 6 months, a serum albumin of <3.2 g/dL, and a total lymphocyte count of <3000 cells/m^3 signify an increased risk of postoperative complications.[77]

The most optimal means of defining a patient's nutritional status has not been established. Measurement of any of the visceral proteins—albumin, transferrin, or prealbumin—can be used to determine the degree of protein malnutrition. Malnutrition, as manifested by decreased serum albumin levels, is a powerful predictor of higher perioperative morbidity. If concerns exist about a patient's nutritional status preoperatively, this should be addressed by the patient's internist or a nutritional specialist in order to minimize postoperative complications.

PERIOPERATIVE DEEP VEIN THROMBOSIS

Deep vein thrombosis (DVT), also known as venous thromboembolism (VTE), is a potential postoperative complication seen in a patient undergoing any surgery. A lower leg venous thrombotic event may result in a PE and subsequent death. The incidence of DVT and PE is low among patients who undergo foot and ankle surgery. However, due to its possible associated mortality risk, it is important that a surgeon is able to identify patients at potential risk, and recognize signs and symptoms of DVT. Patient education on signs and symptoms of DVT/PE is of most importance during any preoperative visit. The mechanism for developing a DVT is well described as Virchow triad that includes presence of a hypercoagulable state, damage to endothelial venous wall, and venous stasis.[78] Injury to the venous endothelium during surgery may promote platelet and fibrin adherence and activates the clotting cascades.[79] Signs and symptoms of DVT include possible calf tenderness/tightness, edema, localized increase in temperature, and pain with passive dorsiflexion of the ankle. However, at times a VTE may go undiagnosed due to absence of classical signs and symptoms.[80]

INCIDENCE IN FOOT AND ANKLE SURGERY

The incidence of DVT post foot and ankle surgery ranges from 0.22% to 3.5%. The incidence for PE, subsequent to a foot or ankle surgery, remains low at about 0.15%-0.3%. A study by Solis and Saxby[81] involving 201 patients, who underwent foot and ankle surgery, found a 3.5% incidence of DVT. In their study, the authors noted rearfoot surgery (without regard to immobilization), increasing age, and tourniquet time to be a risk factor for a postoperative DVT. In a prospective multicenter study of 2733 patients, Mizel et al. reported 0.22% incidence of DVT with 0.15% occurrence for a nonfatal pulmonary embolus (PE) in patients post foot or ankle surgery.[82] In a different study, incidence of DVT was 0.4%, whereas 0.3% of population had a nonfatal PE after foot and ankle surgery among 1000 patients.[83] A retrospective review of 1821 patients showed a 0.5% and 0.16% incidence rates for DVT and nonfatal PE, respectively.[79]

Consensus statement papers by the American College of Foot and Ankle Surgeons in 2015[84] and again in 2017[85] concluded that routine use of chemical prophylaxis is not necessary after foot and ankle surgery. However, the authors of both papers note that the use of chemical prophylaxis should be considered in patients at high risk for venous thromboembolic event.[84,85] Moreover, in 2012, the ACCP suggested that there was no need for pharmacologic prophylaxis in patients with isolated lower extremity injuries requiring immobilization.[86]

WHO IS AT RISK?

Patients with family history of VTE, end-stage renal failure, platelet dysfunction, factor V deficiency, pregnancy, hormone therapy (ie, birth control pills), and cancer carry a higher risk for developing VTE posttrauma or surgery. In addition, if a patient has had prior incident of DVT, he/she remains at higher risk for recurrent venous thrombosis. In a retrospective study of 259 231 patients who had undergone an outpatient surgery, the highest incidence for a postoperative DVT/PE was in patients undergoing vascular surgery, lymphatic surgery with musculoskeletal surgeries taking the third highest rank. Identified risk factors for DVT/PE were current pregnancy, active cancer, age $\geq$ 60, BMI $\geq$ 40, and operative time $\geq$120 minutes. Although, a patient can be at risk for a venous thrombosis for up to 3 months postoperatively, the authors noted a median time for a VTE event to be at 8 days postoperatively.[87] It is prudent that patients undergoing any foot and ankle surgery are screened at the time of their preoperative visit or admission to the hospital/surgery center. Preventive measures can be instituted intraoperatively and/or immediately postoperatively.

PREVENTIVE MEASURES

Venous thrombosis is recognized to be one of the most preventable cause of hospital deaths. This section focuses on prophylactic aspect of DVT/PE, rather than postevent treatment options. Venous thrombosis prophylaxis may be achieved by use of mechanical and/or pharmacological measures. Intraoperatively, patient may be considered for use of graduated compression stockings or intermittent pneumatic compression pumps. It is difficult to utilize compression devices or stockings if surgery is being performed on both feet/ankles. Caution must be taken when using compression devices or stockings in patients with advanced occlusive peripheral vascular disease, septic phlebitis, congestive heart failure, infection, and gangrene. Although compression devices and stockings are often used in surgery, their true effectiveness in preventing a venous thrombotic event is not well proven.[88]

Pharmacological measures are often used in patients at high risk for a postoperative venous thrombosis. Recommended pharmacological therapy for DVT prophylaxis includes aspirin, unfractionated heparin, low molecular weight heparin (LMWH), adjusted dose vitamin K antagonists, synthetic pentasaccharide factor Xa inhibitor (fondaparinux), and newer oral anticoagulants. There are possible contraindications to the use of anticoagulants in DVT prophylaxis. Relative contraindications include previous cerebral hemorrhage, stroke or history of intestinal/gastric bleed in past 6 months, known history of coagulopathy, thrombocytopenia, active intracranial lesions or neoplasms, and proliferative retinopathy. Absolute contraindications include active wound or lesion hemorrhage, history of heparin-induced thrombocytopenia and thrombosis, warfarin use in pregnancy, severe trauma to the head, spinal cord, or extremities with hemorrhage in the past 4 weeks. Spinal or epidural anesthesia should not be performed if patient is on anticoagulation therapy.[89] When choosing an anticoagulation therapy, one must consider the associated risk for major internal bleeding, hematoma formation at the surgical site, thrombocytopenia, and possible potential drug interactions. For instance, the use of warfarin should be closely monitored if patient is on oral antibiotics. In older patients, additional caution should be taken as such patients are at higher risk for fall and easy bleeding. In such situations, the benefits of anticoagulation therapy must outweigh the associated risks. A thorough evaluation of the patient, the proposed surgery, postoperative recovery course, and all associated risk factors is recommended to assist with this decision.

There is ongoing controversy on use of aspirin and its effectiveness in reducing a thrombotic event. In the past, heparin was used frequently for DVT prophylaxis, but its use has diminished after newer medications were introduced into the market. Heparin if used for DVT prophylaxis is dosed at 5000 units, injected subcutaneously, every 8-12 hours. This low-dose regimen is found to reduce the risk for DVT and PE for up to 60%-70% when compared with placebo.[90] Heparin remains a good alternative anticoagulation therapy for inpatients with renal disease who are unable to receive LMWH.

LMWH is a smaller chain pentasaccharide and has less anti-IIa activity. LMWH inhibits factor Xa and activates antithrombin. There is less incidence of postoperative hematoma formation with LMWH and monitoring is unnecessary. The main disadvantage is that since LMWH is cleared renally, it should not be used in patients with renal failure. LMWH should be continued for 7-14 days postoperatively if used for DVT prophylaxis. LMWH are as effective as heparin in reducing risks of DVT/PE and can be used easily in outpatient settings.[91]

Fondaparinux, a synthetic analog of heparin and LMWH, indirectly inhibits factor Xa by binding to antithrombin (AT III). Fondaparinux similar to LMWH is injected subcutaneously when used in DVT prophylaxis. A newer oral anticoagulation therapy, rivaroxaban, is a highly selective and direct factor Xa inhibitor, which inhibits both free factor Xa and bound factor Xa. Unlike heparin, none of these medications have a direct effect on platelets.

Warfarin was commonly prescribed as an oral agent for DVT/PE prophylaxis. Warfarin inhibits the binding of vitamin K to coagulation factors II, VII, XI, X, and proteins C and S. With introduction of newer oral anticoagulation therapy, warfarin plays a greater role in chronic, long-term anticoagulation therapy. It usually takes 36-72 hours after initiation of therapy for the peak effect to occur.

Having said that, the best prophylactic treatment remains early mobility and ambulation, once it is otherwise medically safe for the postsurgical patient.

PERIOPERATIVE ANTIBIOTIC THERAPY

Surgical wounds are classified as clean, clean-contaminated, contaminated, and dirty/infected.[92] The overall risk for postoperative infection can be estimated utilizing this wound classification (Table 3.4). The postoperative infection rate for clean, elective procedures is generally <2%. Currently, the literature lacks strong evidence to support the need for antibiotic prophylaxis prior to an elective foot and ankle surgery. Having said that each institution or medical community may have its own established protocol or an acceptable common practice in using preoperative antibiotic therapy.

The risk of surgical site infection is significantly increased if site contamination with >10^5 microorganisms per gram of tissue are present. Infection may ensue with concentrations of <100 microorganisms per gram of tissue when foreign material is present at the site, that is, foreign body, implants, or sutures.[94] Patient factors such as age, poor nutritional status, immunosuppression, and obesity may have a greater impact in increasing risk for a postoperative infection[92-94] (Table 3.5). Other factors such as preoperative skin preparation, careful anatomic dissection, appropriate tissue handling, and layered closure may also have an influence in reducing risks for a postoperative infection. Drains should be used when indicated.

A retrospective review of 555 elective foot and ankle surgical procedures showed an overall infection rate of 1.6% among 306 patients who were given preoperative antibiotics. In comparison, there was 1.4% incidence of infection in remainder of patients ($n = 249$) who were not prophylaxed. The authors conclude that routine intervenors antibiotic prophylaxis is not warranted in elective foot and ankle surgery.[95] Although, the literature lacks sufficient studies to support use of antibiotics prior to a foot or ankle surgery, the following is some general guideline on appropriate use of preoperative antibiotic therapy.

1. Prophylactic intravenous (IV) antibiotics may not provide any additional benefits when used in clean elective cases where no prosthetic material is being placed unless the patient meets certain high-risk criteria.

TABLE 3.4		Wound Classification Scheme as a Predictor of Infection Risk[92,93]		
Class	**Type**	**Description**	**Infection Risk**
I	Clean	Nontraumatic wound, noninflammatory in nature, no breaks in technique, accounts for 75% of all surgical procedures	<5%
II	Clean-contaminated	Minor technique break, procedure requires entry into the oropharynx, gastrointestinal, or genitourinary tracts, 15% of all cases	10%
III	Contaminated	Major breaks in sterile technique, a fresh traumatic wound, open fractures	20%-40%
IV	Dirty	Infected, acute bacterial inflammation occurs because of devitalized tissue, foreign bodies, fecal contamination, trauma from a dirty source, delayed treatment or the presence of frank purulence	>40%

Adapted from Woods RK, Dellinger EP. Current guidelines for antibiotic prophylaxis of surgical wounds. *Am Fam Physician.* 1998;57:1-12; Mader JT, Cierny G. The principles and use of preventive antibiotics. *Clin Orthop Relat Res.* 1984;190:75-82.

2. Prophylaxis may be beneficial in cases where the wound is classified as clean-contaminated, contaminated, or dirty.[92]
3. IV antibiotics may have a greater impact in reducing postoperative infection in cases of prolonged surgery time (ie, more than 2 hours) or in cases where an internal hardware is used to discourage formation of bacterial "slime" layer on surface of the implant.
4. Prophylaxis against bacterial endocarditis is not warranted in clean orthopedic procedures, but is indicated in incision and drainage of severe foot infections when sepsis is of concern. In these patients, intubation increases the risk of introduction of infectious organisms into the retropharyngeal space[96] and may result in endocarditis.
5. Routine prophylaxis preceding dental work is not warranted in patients with retained orthopedic implants unless they are at high risk, are severely immunocompromised, and have a history of repeated systemic infections. To date, there are no clinical data to justify routine administration of antibiotics prior to dental work.[97]
6. In cases of open fractures, intravenous antibiotics should be initiated immediately upon presentation of patient to the emergency room. Studies have shown that immediate use of intravenous antibiotics along with irrigation and debridement is vital in reducing infection rates when treating lower extremity open fractures. Most studies recommend that the antibiotic therapy should be continued for 48-72 hours posteventual wound closure.[98-103]
7. When possible and medically safe, it is generally recommended to withhold preoperative antibiotics in surgical cases where the goal of surgery is to obtain a tissue or bone biopsy, as part of an infection workup.
8. Prophylaxis is always indicated when the risk of postoperative infection would be devastating to the outcome and overshadows the risks of antibiotic therapy.[94]

ANTIBIOTIC SELECTION

The chosen antibiotic should be active against the most commonly expected microorganisms, pose minimal risk to the patient, and be reasonably inexpensive.[94] *Staphylococcus* and *Streptococcus* species are the most commonly encountered organisms in foot and ankle infection. Exceptions include diabetic/vascular foot infections, open fractures, penetrating trauma, and severely immunocompromised patients, where polymicrobial coverage with broad-spectrum agents is warranted. Ideally, the IV dose should be given within 60 minutes of the procedure and completed just prior to the skin incision and/or before inflating the tourniquet. The half-life of the chosen antibiotic should be long enough to provide therapeutic levels through the entire operation and early postoperative period.

Cefazolin is by far the most common agent used in routine prophylaxis. It is inexpensive and highly effective against *Staphylococcus* and *Streptococcus* species. It has the longest half-life of the first-generation cephalosporins at 1.8-2 hours. Cefazolin should be administered as a single 1-g IV dose preoperatively. A 2-gm dose should be given in all patients weighing >175 lb to ensure adequate serum tissue levels.[104]

Clindamycin or vancomycin may be safely administered in patients with known penicillin allergy. Among the two, clindamycin is a preferred alternative to cefazolin. Clindamycin penetrates the glycocalyx around prosthetic implants. Clindamycin is generally given as a single dose of 600-mg IV preoperatively and has a serum half-life of 2.4 hours. Redosing during podiatric procedures is generally not necessary. Unlike vancomycin, clindamycin is preferred in patients with renal insufficiency or at high risk for renal disease since renal dosage adjustment is not necessary.

TABLE 3.5	Patient Systemic and Local Factors Contributing to the Development of Surgical Site Infection	
Systemic Factors	**Local Factors**
■ Diabetes ■ Corticosteroid use ■ Obesity ■ Smoking history ■ Extremes of age ■ Malnutrition ■ Recent surgery ■ Infection at a remote body site ■ Length of preoperative stay ■ Massive transfusion ■ Multiple (>3) preoperative comorbid conditions ■ ASA classes III, IV, V	■ Foreign body ■ Electrocautery ■ Duration of surgical scrub ■ Preoperative skin prep ■ OR ventilation ■ Injection with epinephrine ■ Wound drains ■ Hair removal with razor ■ Previous irradiation of site

Adapted from Woods RK, Dellinger EP. Current guidelines for antibiotic prophylaxis of surgical wounds. *Am Fam Physician.* 1998;57:1-12; Mangram AJ, Horan TC, Pearson ML, Silver LC, Jarvis WR. Guideline for prevention of surgical site infection, 1999. *Infect Control Hosp Epidemiol.* 1999;20:247-278.

Vancomycin offers an extended half-life of 6 hours and as such a one-time dosing regimen of 1 g infused intravenously, slowly over 1 hour, prior to tourniquet application or surgical cut will be sufficient. Vancomycin should not be used routinely to avoid development of highly resistant strains. The best indication for use of vancomycin is in patients with prior known history of methicillin-resistant *Staphylococcus aureus* (MRSA), resistant MRSA, or a prolonged preoperative hospital stay.

Nasal carriers of *Staphylococcus* species are 2 to 9 times more likely to develop a postoperative surgical site infection and also more likely to develop nosocomial infection while hospitalized.[105] The use of preoperative nasal mupirocin has been demonstrated to reduce MRSA infection in cardiac, spinal, and total joint replacement procedures but remains controversial due to the necessity of proven preoperative colonization prior to instituting therapy.[106] It has been reported that nasal mupirocin may reduce the risk of staphylococcal surgical site infection in MRSA or SA carrier patients; however, this beneficial effect has not shown to be statistically or clinically significant.[107] The challenge in treating patients with nasal mupirocin is lack of a universal decontamination protocol. There are numerous protocols described and studied in current literature.[107-114]

LENGTH OF THERAPY

There is no additional benefit in continuing antibiotic therapy beyond the operative day, in clean elective procedures, with or without internal fixation. One properly delivered preoperative dose guarantees adequate prophylaxis.[115,116]

ADVERSE EFFECT OF PROPHYLAXIS

Overuse of antibiotics can be of a great concern due to emergence of multidrug-resistant organisms. Prolonged and inappropriate use of IV antibiotics may increase the risk of developing resistant organisms, result in adverse drug reactions, and may mask anatomically unrelated infections.[93] Moreover, late infections, or "superinfections," are becoming more prevalent. In recent years, *Clostridium difficile* colitis has reached epidemic heights and is often associated with prolonged antibiotic use.[117]

Unnecessary prophylaxis also results in increased cost of drugs and drug administration and millions of wasted dollars every year. The careful selection and planned duration of antibiotic prophylaxis should focus on minimizing risk to the patient while reflecting current trends in hospital microbiology,[103] local flora, and sensitivity patterns.[93] Careful measures, along with appropriate antibiotic prophylaxis, significantly reduce the risk of postoperative infection as well as the length of hospital stay and associated costs.

LOCAL/REGIONAL ANESTHESIA

The use of local anesthetics in foot and ankle surgery is a topic of great importance. Not only does local anesthesia interrupt transmission of the autonomic, sensory, and motor neural impulses but the usage of local agents also decreases a patient's requirement for both inhaled anesthesia and intravenous medications. This can only assist patients with an expedited return to physiologic function and further pain control. When placed in proximity to nerve membranes, a reversible blockade is produced.[118] Subsequently, recovery from the effects of

local anesthetics is spontaneous with rare nerve fiber damage. With an understanding of anatomy, anesthetic agents, and technique, local anesthesia benefits patients in both surgical and clinical setting.

STRUCTURE

Two broad groups exist for classifying local anesthetic agents. The basis for classification depends on the local anesthetic's structure. Local anesthetics consist of a lipophilic unsaturated benzene ring, hydrophilic tertiary amine, and proton acceptor. These constructs are separated by a hydrocarbon chain. This hydrocarbon chain is linked to the lipophilic portion by either an ester (-CO-) or amide (-HNC-) bond.[119,120] Esters, such as procaine ($C_{13}H_{20}N_2O_2$), undergo hydrolysis by plasma esterases in the blood. The incidence of an allergic reaction is rare yet a greater potential for an allergic response exists for this group. Procaine has a half-life of 40-80 seconds and is excreted via the renal system. Procaine has the advantage of constricting blood vessels as does cocaine. Still, procaine does not produce the euphoric and addictive qualities of cocaine.

Hypoallergenic alternatives such as lidocaine are used more frequently today. Amides, in general, are metabolized by the liver and most commonly excreted by the renal system. Lidocaine ($C_{14}H_{22}N_2O$) is fast acting and has a half-life of 1.5-2 hours. Bupivacaine ($C_{18}H_{28}N_2O$), on the other hand, is longer acting with a half-life of 3.5 hours in adults and 8.1 hours in neonates. Amides are not risk free as they can lead to toxicity. Care should be taken with patients who have hepatic impairment or congestive heart failure. Most adverse drug reactions result from improper administration technique resulting in systemic exposure. It is important that one is aware of differences in onset, duration, and allowed dosage for each anesthetic (Tables 3.6-3.8).

Lidocaine and Marcaine are commonly used in foot and ankle surgery. Lidocaine serves as an excellent clinical and preoperative agent due to its rapid onset of action and moderate duration of action. The toxic dose of lidocaine should not exceed 4 mg/kg or 300 mg. If epinephrine is added, the toxic dose increases to 7 mg/kg or 500 mg. On the other hand, Marcaine is two to three times more toxic. Marcaine has a longer onset of action of 10-20 minutes and has a longer duration of action of 400 minutes. A mixture of the two agents is often utilized. The toxic dose of Marcaine is 175 mg. If epinephrine is used, the toxic dose increases to 225 mg.[119]

TABLE 3.6 Comparative Pharmacology

Classification	Onset	Duration After Infiltration (min)	Maximum Single Dose for Infiltration (mg)
Procaine	Rapid	45-60	500
Chloroprocaine	Rapid	30-45	600
Lidocaine	Rapid	60-120	300
Tetracaine	Slow	60-180	100
Mepivacaine	Slow	90-180	300
Prilocaine	Slow	60-120	400
Bupivacaine	Slow	240-480	175
Ropivacaine	Slow	240-480	200

TABLE 3.7 Dose per Kilogram

Local Anesthetic	mg/kg dose
Lidocaine	3-4.5 mg/kg
Lidocaine with epinephrine	7 mg/kg
Bupivacaine	2-2.5 mg/kg

Epinephrine or sodium chloride can be added to local anesthetics. Epinephrine can be added to lidocaine to produce a 1:200 000 dilution. Epinephrine retards anesthesia absorption and, therefore, increases duration of action.[120] Epinephrine causes temporary vasoconstriction and can decrease the need for tourniquet use. Although some literature recommends against epinephrine containing local anesthetics in digital surgery, this warning appears to be based on anecdotal evidence vs research. Surveys and studies have documented that epinephrine is safe to use with local anesthetics when administered cautiously.[121-123] Epinephrine shortens the onset of anesthesia, prolongs the effect, and produces vasoconstriction.[120] Vasoconstriction not only decreases bleeding but also slows the rate of absorption of anesthetic. This allows more time to metabolize the anesthetic and further prolongs its action. Therefore, larger doses of local anesthesia with epinephrine can be used as compared to anesthesia without epinephrine. Epinephrine in concentrations of 1:100 000 and 1:200 000 works well and safely for surgery. The most common side effect is transient tachycardia after inadvertent intravascular injection.

The maximum dose of epinephrine is 1 mg or 100 mL of a 1:100 000 solution. The maximum dose should be decreased in patients with heart disease to 0.2 mg or 20 mL of a 1:100 000 solution. Epinephrine is contraindicated in patients with pheochromocytoma, hyperthyroidism, severe hypertension, or severe peripheral vascular disease. Relative contraindications include pregnancy and psychological instability.[124]

SIDE EFFECTS OF LOCAL ANESTHESIA

Local and systemic side effects can result from use of local anesthetics. The majority of local side effects can be attributed to injection technique, infiltration rate, and volume of anesthetic utilized. To minimize complications, physicians must be equally critical of these parameters prior to the start of a procedure.

TABLE 3.8 Maximum Allowed Doses

Local Anesthetic	mg/mL	Maximum (mg)	Maximum (mL)
1% Lidocaine plain	10	300	30
2% Lidocaine plain	20	300	15
1% Lidocaine w/epinephrine	10	500	50
2% Lidocaine w/epinephrine	20	500	25
1% Carbocaine	10	300	30
2% Carbocaine	20	300	15
0.5% Marcaine plain	5	175	35
0.5% Marcaine w/epinephrine	5	225	45

Common side effects are pain, ecchymosis, hematoma formation, infection, nerve laceration, and tissue irritation. In general, quick penetration and slow infiltration are essential. Both concepts not only produce less pain and tissue irritation but also decrease trauma and distortion of surrounding tissue. A small gauge needle (27G or 30G) should be utilized with slow infiltration. Tissue irritation, secondary to the acidity of the local agent, can also be minimized by a slow infiltration rate. Aggressive treatment is recommended if true infection does occur. Nerve laceration, although rare, can occur secondary to regional nerve blocks. Common signs of nerve laceration are paresthesia, sharp shooting pain, and excessive pain with needle insertion.

Systemic side effects are most commonly associated with inappropriate administration technique. Inaccurate technique or exceeding maximum doses can place the patient at great risk of systemic complications. Systemic side effects manifest in both the central nervous system and cardiovascular system. Furthermore, patients may show signs of allergic reactions, methemoglobinemia, or toxicity. Local anesthetics can alter the central nervous system via selective depression of inhibitory neurons. This leads to cerebral excitation and further generalized convulsions. Other side effects include coma, respiratory arrest, and death. These side effects are most commonly the result of an increase in plasma levels postintravenous administration, toxic dose, or direct exposure of CNS.

The conductive system of the heart is highly sensitive to local anesthesia. Lidocaine, for example, is an antiarrhythmic agent, which blocks sodium channels. This can produce a slower conduction of impulses leading to either tachyarrhythmia or bradycardia. Higher plasma levels of lidocaine can also produce AV blockage, coma, or death.

Toxicity and allergic reactions are also rare side effects. Toxicity is a risk, which is highly associated with inaccurate dose and route. Over dose of bupivacaine has been associated with cardiotoxicity. This can be reversed with an intravenous lipid emulsion otherwise known as lipid rescue. Allergies are also rare. Still adverse drug reactions are not infrequent. The majority of allergic reactions are not from the local anesthetic agent but are from its preservative: paraben. Methemoglobinemia is defined as a reduction of hemoglobin available for oxygen transport. This side effect has been associated with exceeding the maximum dose for prilocaine. Although systemic toxicity of prilocaine is rare, its metabolite o-toluidine is associated with methemoglobinemia.[118,125,126]

Sciatic Nerve Block (L4, L5, S1-S3)

There is only one nerve that innervates the foot that is not an extension of the sciatic nerve. This is known at the saphenous nerve. Otherwise, the remainder of the foot is innervated by nerve branches from the sciatic nerve. A sciatic nerve block provides extended pain relief and decreases the patient's requirement for general anesthesia.[127]

Anatomy The sciatic nerve courses through the greater sciatic foramen and deep to the piriformis muscle. It then travels across the posterior border of the hip joint capsule where it is protected by the gluteus maximus muscle belly. The nerve then courses over the quadratus femoris muscle belly and deep to the biceps femoris muscle. Deep to the biceps femoris muscle, the sciatic nerve descends into the popliteal fossa and divides into the common peroneal nerve and tibial nerve branches.

Technique The patient is placed into the prone or lateral decubitus position. The buttock is then visibly divided into four distinct quadrants. The nerve is easily encountered just medial to the ischial tuberosity and near the intersection of lines. The needle is advanced until paresthesia is experienced. Care is taken to aspirate to avoid intravascular injection. Likewise, the needle is withdrawn 2.5 mm to avoid intraneural injection. The anesthetic of choice is then administered. This is usually a block requiring a longer-acting anesthetic agent.

Tibial Nerve (Popliteal) Block (L4, L5, S1-S3)

The tibial nerve innervates the posterior aspect of the leg as well as the sole of the foot. The nerve is accessible at the level of the popliteal fossa and is an excellent block for the following procedures: tendo Achilles lengthening, gastrocnemius recession, repair of tendo Achilles rupture, extensive clubfoot releases, and pediatric pain management.

Anatomy The diamond-shaped popliteal fossa is defined inferiorly by the medial and lateral heads of the gastrocnemius, superolaterally by the long head of the biceps femoris muscle, and superomedially by the tendons of both semitendinosus and semimembranosus muscles. As the common peroneal branch of the sciatic nerve diverges laterally, the tibial nerve branch continues in the same direction as the sciatic nerve through the popliteal fossa. The tibial nerve branch can be found 0.5-1 cm lateral to the midline of the popliteal fossa. The tibial nerve branch is ~1.5-2 cm deep to the skin.

Technique There are two positions available to approach this nerve block. The adult patient is placed in the prone position with the knee flexed 30 degrees. This provides the bordering structures of the popliteal fossa to be easily visible. The pediatric patient can be placed into the supine position if assistance is available. The assistant holds the leg in the vertical upright position so the block can be administered. An intradermal wheal of local anesthesia is administered 5-7 cm proximal to the skin crease and 0.5-1 cm lateral to the midline of the popliteal fossa. The needle is advanced until paresthesia is obtained and then withdrawn 1.5 mm. Care must be taken to minimize intraneural trauma via injection. The local anesthetic of choice is administered. Often a peripheral nerve stimulator can be used to assist with tibial nerve location. Location is confirmed by a visible twitch in the direction of inversion and plantarflexion.[128] This is an excellent modality for postoperative pain management and the pediatric patient. This block is often approached by either the surgeon or anesthesiologist.

Common Peroneal Nerve Block (L4, L5, S1-S2)

The common peroneal nerve innervates the muscles on both the lateral and anterior aspects of the lower leg. This nerve also supplies the dorsum of the foot. The common peroneal nerve block is useful in the following procedures: ankle stress radiographs, peroneal spastic flatfoot, and when it is not safe to perform a more distal block.[129]

Anatomy The common peroneal nerve branches from the sciatic nerve to course laterally across the popliteal fossa. The nerve then travels around the neck of the fibula proximally and further divides into its terminal branches: the deep peroneal nerve and superficial peroneal nerve. This division occurs near the proximal fibers of the peroneus longus muscle belly. The common peroneal nerve is palpable at the posterior aspect of the fibular neck.

Technique The common peroneal nerve is best palpable posterior to the fibular neck. At this location, an intradermal wheal is raised 2.5 cm distal to the fibular head.[129] The nerve is not deep. Hence, at a depth of 1-1.5 cm paresthesia should be accomplished. Care must be taken to avoid intravascular or intraneural injection. One should always aspirate prior to injection of local anesthesia.

Superficial Peroneal Nerve Block (L4, L5, S1)

Cutaneous sensation to the lower anterior leg and dorsum of the foot is supplied by the superficial peroneal nerve branches. Both the medial dorsal cutaneous nerve and intermediate dorsal cutaneous nerve are terminal branches of the superficial peroneal nerve. The medial dorsal cutaneous nerve provides cutaneous sensation to the hallux, second digit, and medial aspect of the third digit. The intermediate dorsal cutaneous nerve supplies sensory innervation to the lateral aspect of the third digit, fourth digit, and medial aspect of the fifth digit.

Anatomy The superficial peroneal nerve trunk is found subcutaneously along the anterior border of the fibula about 10.5 cm above the lateral malleolus.[129] The nerve is located at this level in the groove between the peroneal group of muscles and the extensor digitorum longus. The superficial peroneal nerve divides into its two terminal branches at 6.5 cm proximal to the lateral malleolar tip.

The intermediate dorsal cutaneous nerve is easily palpated through the skin. With inversion, the nerve becomes taut and visible. This nerve courses along the tibiofibular syndesmosis, over the inferior extensor retinaculum, and obliquely across the lateral extensor digitorum longus tendons. The intermediate dorsal cutaneous nerve divides into a dorsal lateral and dorsal medial branch. The intermediate dorsal cutaneous nerve supplies sensory innervation to the lateral aspect of the third digit, fourth digit, and medial aspect of the fifth digit.

The medial dorsal cutaneous nerve overlies the extensor digitorum longus tendon, courses parallel to the extensor hallucis longus tendon, and crosses superficially over the inferior extensor retinaculum. The medial dorsal cutaneous nerve divides into three branches and provides cutaneous sensation to the hallux, second digit, and medial aspect of the third digit. Care must be taken to protect these nerves in the following procedures: ankle arthroscopy (anterolateral portal), triple arthrodesis, tarsometatarsal surgery, central metatarsal surgery, and bunion surgery.

Technique The medial dorsal cutaneous nerve is noted lateral to the extensor hallucis longus tendon, 1 cm proximal to the medial malleolar base, while the intermediate dorsal cutaneous nerve is palpated 1-1.5 cm anterior to the lateral malleolus. One can easily locate the intermediate dorsal cutaneous nerve by inverting and plantarflexing the foot.[128] Once each nerve is identified, 0.5-1 mL of local anesthetic can be infiltrated. The infiltration takes place directly adjacent to these nerves.

Deep Peroneal Nerve Block

The deep peroneal nerve provides cutaneous sensation to the first dorsal interspace. It also provides motor branches to the anterior lower leg. The lateral terminal branch of the deep peroneal nerve innervates the extensor digitorum brevis.

Anatomy The anterior tibial nerve pierces the extensor digitorum longus in the upper one-third of the lower leg. Here, it travels with the anterior tibial artery. In the upper one-third of the lower leg, the nerve is located between the tibialis anterior and extensor digitorum longus. In the middle one-third of the lower leg, the nerve is isolated between the tibialis anterior and extensor hallucis longus. In the lower one-third of the leg, ~2.5-5 cm proximal to the ankle, the nerve travels deep to the extensor hallucis longus to finally be located between the extensor hallucis longus and extensor digitorum longus.[129] At this location, the nerve is accurately named the deep peroneal nerve.

The deep peroneal nerve is usually found lateral to the anterior tibial artery. Horwitz found in 98% of cases the deep peroneal nerve divided into its terminal branches 1.3 cm proximal to the ankle joint.[130] The medial terminal branch of the deep peroneal nerve courses medial to the dorsalis pedis artery.

Technique The nerve is located between the extensor hallucis longus and extensor digitorum longus about 2.5 cm proximal to the ankle joint. The needle is placed just lateral to the arterial pulse. Approximately 1-2 mL of local anesthesia is needed as the average diameter of the nerve is 1-3 mm.[129] One should always aspirate to avoid intravascular infiltration.

Posterior Tibial Nerve Block

The posterior tibial nerve supplies cutaneous innervation to the medial posterior heel and plantar foot. The posterior tibial nerve also provides motor innervation to the posterior lower leg and majority of intrinsic muscles of the foot via its division into the medial and lateral plantar nerves. This is a common nerve block in foot and ankle surgery. This can also provide sympathetic blockade in the treatment of complex regional pain syndrome (CRPS). CRPS is an uncommon chronic condition that usually affects extremities. Type 1, previously known as regional sympathetic dystrophy (RSD), occurs after an illness or injury that did not directly damage the nerves in the affected limb. On the other hand, type 2 follows a distinct nerve injury. CRPS was first described during the civil war when soldiers continued to report excessive pain after wounds had healed. More detail information on CRPS, including its etiology, diagnosis, and treatment, is provided elsewhere in this book.

Anatomy The posterior tibial nerve is usually located ~7.5 cm proximal to the medial malleolus tip and parallel to the medial border of the Achilles tendon.[129] The posterior tibial nerve is posterior to the posterior tibial artery. The nerve divides into its terminal branches just proximal to the porta pedis. The medial calcaneal branch bifurcates higher than the remaining branches. Dellon found that the medial calcaneal nerve originates from the posterior tibial nerve in 90% of cases.[129] In 10% of cases, the medial calcaneal nerve is found to be a branch of the lateral plantar nerve. The medial and lateral plantar nerves innervate the majority of the foot. The medial plantar nerve

innervates the medial three digits and the medial aspect of the fourth digit. The lateral plantar nerve innervates the fifth digit and lateral aspect of the fourth digit.

Technique The posterior tibial artery is palpated posterior to the medial malleolus. After aspiration, the local anesthetic agent is infiltrated 0.5-1 cm superior to the reference mark. The nerve is usually located 1.5-2 cm in depth. For most injections, quick penetration and slow infiltration minimizes discomfort. If intravascular placement occurs, the needle should be redirected and re-aspirated. Infiltration of 3-5 mL of local anesthetic agent is usually adequate.

Sural Nerve Block

The sural nerve provides cutaneous innervation to the lateral lower leg and lateral aspect of the foot. The sural nerve block is a useful nerve block in foot and ankle surgery.

Anatomy The sural nerve is formed by the medial sural nerve (branch of tibial nerve) and an anastomotic peroneal communicating branch from the lateral sural nerve or common peroneal nerve. The sural nerve courses along the lateral border of the Achilles tendon to remain anterolateral to the small saphenous vein. The sural nerve proceeds to course 1-1.5 cm distal to the lateral malleolus. The peroneal tendons separate the nerve from the lateral malleolus. The sural nerve terminates as the lateral dorsal cutaneous nerve. Prior to its termination, the nerve provides lateral calcaneal branches.

Technique The nerve can be blocked just inferior or superior to the lateral malleolus. The most common location for the sural nerve is 10 cm above the tip of the lateral malleolus just at the lateral border of the Achilles tendon.

Saphenous Nerve Block (L3, L4)

The saphenous nerve is the only nerve to innervate the foot, which is not a branch of the sciatic nerve. The saphenous nerve, a branch of the femoral nerve, is commonly blocked for foot and ankle surgery.

Anatomy The saphenous nerve is located anterior to the medial malleolus and posterior medial to the great saphenous vein. The nerve courses along the medial aspect of the foot to terminate near the first metatarsal phalangeal joint.

Technique The saphenous nerve is blocked near the saphenous vein. The nerve crosses the ankle joint just lateral to the vein. Often the saphenous nerve is palpable. The nerve can be blocked with 0.5-1 mL of local anesthetic.

Ankle Block

An ankle block is an excellent approach to regional anesthesia of the foot and ankle. During an ankle block, one applies anesthesia to the following nerves: tibial, saphenous, deep peroneal, superficial peroneal, and sural. With an understanding of anatomy, one can target the individual nerves with minimal anesthesia. Many of these nerves are superficially located. These specific nerve blocks allow the anesthesiologist to carry the patient on a lighter plane of anesthesia.[129]

Mayo Block

The Mayo block is a type of field block, which provides anesthesia proximal to the surgical site. This preserves the surgical tissue planes. The Mayo block targets the saphenous nerve, deep peroneal nerve, medial plantar nerve, and medial dorsal cutaneous nerve. This is a common technique prior first metatarsophalangeal joint surgery. A wheal is raised proximally in the first interspace. The needle is advanced from dorsal to plantar to anesthetize the deep peroneal nerve. The needle is withdrawn and redirected medially where a second wheal is formed to block the saphenous and medial dorsal cutaneous branch. The anesthetic agent is infiltrated medial to plantar. The needle is then reintroduced in a medial to lateral direction, deep to the first metatarsal. This provides anesthesia to the deep and superficial branches of the medial plantar nerves. Additional local anesthetic is administered to the distal first interspace, if needed.

Digital Nerve Block

The two-point digital block provides local anesthesia to a digit. This block is often used in a clinical setting or surgical setting. Each digit is supplied by two dorsal digital nerves and two plantar digital nerves. As such, two wheals are raised on the dorsomedial and dorsolateral aspects of the digit. The needle is advanced until noted plantarly.

ANESTHESIA

IV CONSCIOUS SEDATION

This form of anesthesia can be described as a drug-induced depression of consciousness, during which patients continue to respond to physical and verbal stimuli. The goal of conscious sedation (CS) is to relieve anxiety and relax the patient without depressing the level of consciousness to a degree that the airway is compromised. Commonly used in surgery centers, minor procedure rooms, and in the emergency department, physicians typically administer an intravenous sedative along with an analgesic or amnestic, which allows for patient relaxation and ease of surgery. Typical dosing (2 mg IV midazolam, 2 mg IV morphine) allows patients to maintain their own airway.[131]

Since in most cases an anesthesia team may not be present, these patients must be carefully monitored by the OR staff. CS should be limited to settings where there is appropriate equipment for monitoring and resuscitation. It is imperative that a blood pressure monitor, pulse oximeter, cardiac monitor, airway maintenance devices, oxygen source and delivery devices, IV drugs, defibrillator, and a crash cart are readily available.[131] Each facility will have their own specific guidelines but most require the patient meet certain postprocedural criteria prior to being discharged home. Overall, with the help of a qualified assistant, CS can safely allow surgeons to perform minor procedures on relaxed patients, without the need for an anesthesia team.

MONITORED ANESTHESIA CARE

MAC is similar to IV CS except that patients may be taken to deeper levels of sedation in which they cannot be easily aroused but still respond purposefully to repeated or painful stimulation.[132] The anesthesia team is in attendance to monitor vital signs, administer oxygen, and deal with potential respiratory depression. More complex surgical procedures can be performed under MAC, as the level of sedation may be deeper, with the anesthesia team managing the patient's vital functions. MAC is ideal for the majority of forefoot and certain midfoot procedures. Lengthier or involved procedures, such as reconstructive surgery, are probably best reserved for general or regional anesthesia.

During MAC, the patient is often taken briefly to a deeper level of sedation, which allows the surgeon to administer local anesthesia into the operative site without patient discomfort. As the local anesthetic provides analgesia at the surgical site, anesthesiologists are able to gradually reduce the amount of patient sedation for the remainder of the procedure. Patients are kept comfortable, the airway is maintained, and vital signs are continuously monitored. Though many patients fall asleep during MAC, they should be able to quickly arouse and respond to verbal stimuli. MAC is typically a pleasant outpatient surgical experience for the patients since recovery times are short and the incidence of nausea is reduced.

GENERAL ANESTHESIA

General anesthesia, as defined by the ASA, is when a patient "loses consciousness and the ability to respond purposefully."[132] General anesthesia may be said to consist of the following five components:

- Loss of consciousness
- Blocking of pain sensation (analgesia)
- Loss of memory (amnesia)
- Muscle relaxation/lack of movement
- Blunting of autonomic reflexes (eg, hypertension, tachycardia)

General anesthesia is typically accomplished with a combination of IV and inhalational agents, although purely IV or inhalational techniques may be used as well. In addition to managing hemodynamics and cardiac rhythm, the anesthesia care team is responsible for protecting and ensuring a competent airway and ventilation, oxygenation and CO_2 regulation, acid/base balance, IV fluid balance, blood loss and blood product replacement, temperature, urine output, patient positioning, and movement.

General anesthesia consists of induction, maintenance, and emergence phases. Induction is taking the patient from being alert and awake to unconsciousness. Respirations and ventilation are usually depressed during this phase. The airway is also commonly compromised, and care must be taken to ensure an adequate airway and ventilation. The most common induction agent used today is propofol, administered IV. For the duration of surgery, general anesthesia is most often maintained with inhalation agents such as isoflurane or sevoflurane with or without nitrous oxide. Discontinuation of inhaled anesthetics leads to patient awakening, that is, emergence.

Airway Management

Airway management is an important part of every anesthetic since loss of consciousness and resulting loss of airway is always a possibility even in regional or local anesthetics with sedation.

Nasal cannulas can be utilized to deliver supplemental oxygen to spontaneously ventilating patients. One end of the tubing rests loosely in the nares, while the other end is connected to the oxygen source. One can deliver 24%-44% oxygen with flow rates of 1-6 L/min, respectively. Nasal cannulas work by using the nasopharynx as a reservoir and are effective whether the patient is a nose breather or mouth breather. Technically easy and cost effective, nasal cannulas are often the first line in maintaining oxygenation.

Variant methods of oxygen delivery in the spontaneously breathing patient include the addition of simple facemasks and partial rebreather or nonrebreather face masks. These can deliver up to 70% oxygen.

It is common to have a degree of airway obstruction when patients lose consciousness, as muscle tone is lost and soft tissue structures (soft palate, epiglottis, tongue) fall back and obstruct the upper airway. The head-tilt/chin-lift maneuver (head extension/jaw thrust) can help relieve the obstruction. If this maneuver fails to relieve the obstruction, then inserting oropharyngeal or nasopharyngeal airways will often succeed. Continuous positive airway pressure (CPAP) may also be utilized in a variety of settings.

Laryngeal mask airway (LMA) is a frequently employed airway device in general anesthesia. The basic skills for inserting and using an LMA are considered easier to acquire than those required for facemask ventilation or endotracheal insertion. LMAs may also be used as rescue devices when facemask ventilation or intubation is not possible in both planned and emergency situations. The classic LMA consists of an inflatable laryngeal mask, airway tube, and inflation line, while newer versions of the LMA consist of a noninflatable gel-filled laryngeal mask and airway tube. The basic premise is the same: proper functioning is based on obtaining an airtight seal around the larynx. It is important to note that the LMA does not protect the trachea and lungs from aspiration of stomach contents nor may one use positive pressure mechanical ventilation as with an endotracheal tube. While the airway tube of the LMA resembles an endotracheal tube, it is important to remember that the LMA is much more like a facemask than an endotracheal tube.

Tracheal intubation is the passing of an endotracheal tube through the larynx (vocal cords) into the trachea. The tube is made with a high volume-low pressure cuff at the distal end, which is inflated to provide a seal below the larynx. Tracheal intubation is a highly skilled procedure in which the operator must overcome several natural barriers while entering the trachea such as the epiglottis while managing possible airway reactivity (gagging) in awake and semi-awake patients. Most commonly, tracheal intubation is achieved by laryngoscopy after blunting airway reflexes through the use of local anesthetics in awake patients or the induction of general anesthesia along with neuromuscular blockade. There are multiple devices for laryngoscopy currently available: traditional laryngoscopes (straight and curved) for direct laryngoscopy, flexible fiberoptic laryngoscopes, rigid indirect laryngoscopes, and optical stylets. In addition, there are multiple modes of tracheal intubation utilizing LMAs and other devices, which can be performed "blind" or with visualization of the larynx. Correct tracheal tube placement is best confirmed by multiple modalities including auscultation of the chest, capnography, and chest radiography. Tracheal intubation provides a secure airway, protects the lungs from accidental aspiration of stomach contents or other foreign bodies, and allows for mechanical ventilation with various ventilatory modes. It allows for the delivery of positive end-expiratory pressure (PEEP) and CPAP as needed for patients with impaired gas exchange and oxygenation problems.

POSTANESTHESIA CARE UNIT

The postanesthesia care unit (PACU) receives patients directly from the OR and is designed to closely monitor patients' level of consciousness, breathing, and cardiovascular status. Patient transfer from the OR to the PACU is usually uneventful in the majority of cases. In a prospective study of over 18 000 patients admitted to the PACU, 24% had postoperative complications, including nausea and vomiting (9.8%), the need for upper airway support (6.8%), and hypotension (2.7%) (ASA). Another common complication seen postoperatively is urinary retention. Other concerns in the PACU are fluid management, pain control, and neurovascular status of the digits.

Recognition of complications and pending complications is the responsibility of the PACU team. Quick assessment and adequate knowledge of multiple organ system physiology will allow PACU members to effectively reduce risk for or treat any potential complications that may result.

POSTOPERATIVE NAUSEA AND VOMITING

Postoperative nausea and vomiting (PONV) are common problems that can delay discharge from the PACU or lead to an unplanned admission. Some facilities assign patients to low, moderate, and high PONV risk stratification groups, taking into account age, sex, previous history of nausea and vomiting, and anticipated opioid usage. Following a trial of six separate combinations of antiemetics in 5199 patients, similar reduction in PONV were seen when ondansetron, dexamethasone, and droperidol were used with an approximate reduction rate of 26%.[133] They concluded that because of the similar nature of the reduction in each combination, the safest and least expensive should be used first and that prophylaxis was rarely needed in low-risk patients.

A number of pharmacologic agents are available to treat PONV with each agent working on a specific receptor involved in nausea and the vomiting reflex. They can be thus classified by their site of action. Treatment is often based on clinical experience, etiology, and route of administration.

Scopolamine, an anticholinergic, can be administered by transdermal patch administration for PONV prophylaxis. To achieve maximal benefit, it needs to be placed at least 8 hours preoperatively. The patch will continue to release medication for up to 72 hours. Promethazine is a commonly used phenothiazine, which is utilized for its antiemetic effects rather than its antipsychotic effects. Among the dopamine receptor antagonists, metoclopramide has antiemetic properties but can also be associated with extrapyramidal side effects. The use of ondansetron and other serotonin antagonists, once reserved for chemotherapy-induced nausea, is becoming ever more widespread in the perioperative treatment of nausea. Corticosteroids such as dexamethasone have also been shown to help reduce PONV.

POSTOPERATIVE URINARY RETENTION

A multitude of studies report on incidence of postoperative urinary retention (POUR) ranging from 5% to 70%, with a slightly higher percentage occurring in men compared to women. Diagnosis is made clinically at bedside but can also be confirmed with ultrasound. POUR has been defined as the inability to void in the presence of a full bladder.[31] In addition, the patient will complain of a straining sensation with an urge to urinate, as well as the presence of a distended and painful bladder.

Certain medications, such as anticholinergic drugs and opioids, may cause POUR. While comorbidities such as neurological diseases, medications, type and length of surgery, as well as type of anesthesia are all factors that should be taken into account, they are not considered independent variables. However, age, amount of intraoperative fluids, and bladder volume (over 270 mL urine) at the time of arrival to the PACU are reported to be independent predictive factors for POUR.[34]

When managing POUR, both medication and catheterization may be utilized. Bethanechol is an agonist of the parasympathetic system and helps to increase bladder muscle tone and contractility. The role of bladder catheterization is a simple therapy that can be utilized with the caveat that catheterization increases the chance of urinary tract infections; so caution should be taken. The decision to catheterize should be based on the functional capacity of the bladder and the ability to void. If the sensation to void is not present and the patient is of a low risk category, the patient could be discharged to home.

POSTOPERATIVE FLUID MANAGEMENT

Fluid management consists of two types of therapy: maintenance and replacement therapy. Maintenance therapy is initiated when the patient is not expected to eat or drink for a certain amount of time, that is, perioperatively. Replacement therapy is aimed at replenishing any additional water and electrolyte deficits, including bleeding, evaporative losses, profuse sweating, and other gastrointestinal losses. The aim of both is to preserve the water and electrolyte balance that is normally lost throughout the day. For a 70-kg adult, these losses account for 30-35 mL/kg/d (~2100-2500 mL/day) and should be replenished according to the 4-2-1 rule.[134] The 4-2-1 rule allocates 4 mL/kg/h for the first 10 kg of weight, followed by 2 mL/kg/h for the second 10 kg of weight, followed by 1 mL/kg/h for every kg thereafter.

Fluid selection is made largely by physician preference. Crystalloid solutions are most frequently used and include normal saline (NS) and lactated Ringer's (LR). Crystalloids are essentially a solution of sterile water with added electrolytes to approximate the content of human plasma.[134] The most common 0.9% NS consists of a pH of 5.0, 154 mEq/L sodium, 154 mEq/L chloride, with an osmolality of 308 mEq/L. LR more closely mimics human plasma with a pH of 6.5, 130 mEq/L sodium, 109 mEq/L chloride, 4 mEq/L potassium, 3 mEq/L calcium, 28 mEq/L lactate, with an osmolality of 275 mEq/L. However, care should be taken when using LR in diabetic patients, as lactate can be converted to glucose. Crystalloids are at a disadvantage in that they have limited ability to remain in the intravascular space (25% after 1 hour of administration) and must be given in large volumes.[134] Colloids are based on crystalloid solutions but have an added component of a colloidal substance that does not freely diffuse across a semipermeable membrane. They may have a greater capacity to remain within the intravascular space and may restore plasma volume more efficiently.[134]

CONCLUSION

This chapter serves as a mere guideline to help podiatric physicians individualize each patient based on medical comorbidities. Numerous other medical conditions exist that are not addressed here and these should not be considered less significant. The authors chose to focus on the conditions that are responsible for the majority of perioperative complications that may be encountered in patients undergoing foot and ankle surgery. Although the podiatric surgeon is not often directly involved in the diagnosis or treatment of medical conditions, a multidisciplinary approach will help maximize surgical outcomes. Perioperative management of patients requires a careful history and examination to help in assessing the need and to select the most appropriate means of preventing postoperative complications such as infection and DVT. Perioperative pain management also plays a part in overall outcome of the procedure. Future research will aid in predicting which testing and management interventions have evidence-based proof of their role in reducing complications and length of hospital stay, while still maintaining cost efficiency.

REFERENCES

1. Perioperative medicine summit: using evidence to improve quality, safety and patient outcomes. *Cleve Clin J Med.* 2006;73(suppl 1):1-120.
2. Kloehn GC, O'Rourke RA. Perioperative risk stratification in patients undergoing noncardiac surgery. *J Intensive Care Med.* 1999;14(2):95-108.
3. Dennis L, Kasper DL, Braunwald E, Fauci A, et al. Harrison's Principles of Internal Medicine, 16th edition. In: Smetana GW, ed. *Introduction to Clinical Medicine: Chapter 7. Medical Evaluation of the Surgical Patient.* Philadelphia, PA: McGraw-Hill; 2004.
4. https://www.cms.gov/Medicare/Provider-Enrollment-and-Certification/SurveyCertificationGenInfo/downloads/SCLetter08 12.pdf
5. https://www.jointcommission.org/standards_information/jcfaqdetails.aspx?StandardsFAQId=1445
6. Moller, AM, Pedersen T, Villebro N. Effect of smoking on early complications after elective orthopaedic surgery. *J Bone Joint Surg Am.* 2003;85-B:178-181.
7. Krannitz KW, Fong HW, Fallat LM, Kish J. The effect of cigarette smoking on radiographic bone healing after elective foot surgery. *J Foot Ankle Surg.* 2009;48(5):525-527.
8. Galatz LM, Silva MJ, Rothermich SY, Zaegel MA, Havlioglu N, Thomopoulos S. Nicotine delays tendon-to-bone healing in a rat shoulder model. *J Bone Joint Surg Am.* 2006;88-A:2027-2034.
9. Nasell H, Ottosson C, Tornqvist H, Linde J, Ponzer J. The impact of smoking on complications after operatively treated ankle fractures-a follow-up study of 906 patients. *J Orthop Trauma.* 2011;25(12):748-755.
10. Ding L, He Z, Xiao H, Chai L, Xue F. Risk factors for postoperative wound complications of calcaneal fractures following plate fixation. *Foot Ankle Int.* 2013;34(9):1238-1244.
11. Bettin CC, Gower K, McCormick K, et al. Cigarette smoking increases complication rate in forefoot surgery. *Foot Ankle Int.* 2015;36(5):488-493.
12. Warner DO, Warner MA, Barnes RD, et al. Perioperative respiratory complications in patients with asthma. *Anesthesiology.* 1996;85:460-467.
13. Moller AM, Villebro N, Pedersen T, Tønnesen H. Effect of preoperative smoking intervention on postoperative complications: a randomised clinical trial. *Lancet.* 2002;359(9301):114-117.
14. Siriphuwanun V, Punjasawadwong Y, Saengyo S, Rerkasem K. Incidences and factors associated with perioperative cardiac arrest in trauma patients receiving anesthesia. *Risk Manag Healthc Policy.* 2018;11:177-187.
15. Egholm JW, Pedersen B, Moller AM, Adami J, Juhl CB, Tonnesen H. Perioperative alcohol cessation intervention for postoperative complications. *Cochrane Database Syst Rev.* 2018;8:11.
16. Hadhizacharia P, Green DJ, Plurad D, et al. Cocaine use in trauma: effect on injuries and outcomes. *J Trauma.* 2009;66(2):491-494.
17. Borini P, Guimaraes RC, Borini SB. Possible hepatotoxicity of chronic marijuana usage. *Sao Paulo Med J.* 2004;122(3):110-116.
18. Saber W. Perioperative medication management: a case-based review of general principles. *Cleve Clin J Med.* 2006;73(1):S82-S87.
19. Wu M, McIntosh J, Liu J. Current prevalence rate of latex allergy: Why it remains a problem? *J Occup Health.* 2016;58(2):138-144.
20. Bueno de Sa A, Camilo Araujo RF, et al. Profile of latex sensitization and allergies in children and adolescents with myelomeningocele in Sao Paulo, Brazil. *J Investig Allergol Clin Immunol.* 2013;23:43-49.
21. Mertes PM, Alla F, Trechot P, Auroy Y, Jougla E. Anaphylaxis during anesthesia in France: an 8-year national survey. *J Allergy Clin Immunol.* 2011;128(2):366-373.

22. Mota AN, Turrini RN. Perioperative latex hypersensitivity reactions: an integrative literature review. *Rev Lat Am Enfermagem.* 2012;20:411-420.

23. Sussman GL, Lem D, Liss G, Beezhold D. Latex allergy in housekeeping personnel. *Ann Allergy Asthma Immunol.* 1995;74:415-418.

24. Dewachter P, Mouton-Faivre C, Castells MC, Hepner DL. Anesthesia in the patient with multiple drug allergies: are all allergies the same? *Curr Opin Anaesthesiol.* 2011;24(3):320-325.

25. Baig M, Farag A, Sajid J, Potluri R, Irwin RB, Khalid HM. Shellfish allergy and relation to iodinated contrast media: United Kingdom survey. *World J Cardiol.* 2014;6(3):107-111.

26. Marcello PW, Roberts PL. "Routine" preoperative studies: which studies in which patients. *Surg Clin North Am.* 1996;76:11-23.

27. Macpherson DS, Snow R, Lofgren RP. Preop screening: value of previous testing. *Ann Intern Med.* 1990;113: 969-973.

28. Fleisher LA, Fleischmann KE, Auerbach AD, et al. 2014 ACC/AHA guideline on perioperative cardiovascular evaluation and management of patients undergoing noncardiac surgery: executive summary: a report of the American College of Cardiology/American Heart Association Task Force on practice guidelines. Developed in collaboration with the American College of Surgeons, American Society of Anesthesiologists, American Society of Echocardiography, American Society of Nuclear Cardiology, Heart Rhythm Society, Society for Cardiovascular Angiography and Interventions, Society of Cardiovascular Anesthesiologists, and Society of Vascular Medicine Endorsed by the Society of Hospital Medicine. *J Nucl Cardiol.* 2015;22(1):162-215.

29. American Society of Anesthesiologists approved by the House of Delegates on October 14, 1987.

30. Tuman KJ, McCarthy RJ, March RJ, DeLaria GA, Patel RV, Ivankovich AD. Effects of epidural anesthesia and analgesia on coagulation and outcome after major vascular surgery. *Anesth Analg.* 1991;73:696-704.

31. Yeager MP, Glass DD, Neff RK, Brinck-Johnsen T. Epidural anesthesia and analgesia in high-risk surgical patients. *Anesthesiology.* 1987;66:729-736.

32. Wright J, MacNeill AL, Mayich DJ. A prospective comparison of wide-awake local anesthesia and general anesthesia for forefoot surgery. *Foot Ankle Surg.* 2019;25(2):211-214.

33. Pearse RM, Beattie S, Clavien PA, et al. Global patient outcomes after elective surgery: prospective cohort study in 27 low-, middle- and high-income countries. *Br J Anaesth.* 2016;117(5):601-609.

34. Goldman L, Caldera D, Nussbaum S, et al. Multifactorial index of cardiac risk in noncardiac surgical procedures. *N Engl J Med.* 1977;297:845.

35. Cohn SL. Cardiac risk stratification before noncardiac surgery. *Cleve Clin J Med.* 2006;73(1):S18-S24.

36. Sayyed R, Alam MB. Perioperative cardiac considerations in the surgical patient. *Clin Podiatr Med Surg.* 2019;36(1):103-113.

37. Salerno S, Carlson D, Soh E, et al. Impact of perioperative cardiac assessment guidelines on management of orthopedic surgery patients. *Am J Med.* 2007;120:185.e1-e6.

38. Fleischmann KE, Goldman L, Young B, Lee TH. Association between cardiac and noncardiac complications in patients undergoing noncardiac surgery: outcomes and effects on length of stay. *Am J Med.* 2003;115:515-520.

39. Smetana GW, Lawrence VA, Cornell JE. Preoperative pulmonary risk stratification for noncardiothoracic surgery: systematic review for the American College of Physicians. *Ann Intern Med.* 2006;144(8):581-595.

40. Diaz-Fuentes G, Hashmi HR, Venkatram S. Perioperative evaluation of patients with pulmonary conditions undergoing non-cardiothoracic surgery. *Health Serv Insights.* 2016;9(suppl 1):9-23.

41. Langren O, Carreira S, Le Sache F, Raux M. Postoperative pulmonary complications updating. *Ann Fr Anesth Reanim.* 2014;33(7-8):480-483.

42. Tarhan S, Moffitt EA, Sessler AD, Douglas WW, Taylor WF. Risk of anesthesia and surgery in patients with chronic bronchitis and chronic obstructive pulmonary disease. *Surgery.* 1973;74:720-726.

43. Bluman LG, Mosca L, Newman N, Simon DG. Preoperative smoking habits and postoperative pulmonary complications. *Chest.* 1998;113:883-889.

44. Myers K, Hajek P, Hinds C, McRobbie H. Stopping smoking shortly before surgery and postoperative complications: a systematic review and meta-analysis. *Arch Intern Med.* 2011;171(11):983-989.

45. Wong J, Lam DP, Abrishami A, Chan MT, Chung F. Short-term preoperative smoking cessation and postoperative complications: a systematic review and meta-analysis. *Can J Anaesth.* 2012;59(3):268-279.

46. Reilly DF, McNeely MJ, Doerner D, et al. Self-reported exercise tolerance and the risk of serious perioperative complications. *Arch Intern Med.* 1999;159:2185-2192.

47. Block BM, Liu SS, Rowlingson AJ, Cowan AR, Cowan JA Jr, Wu CL. Efficacy of postoperative epidural analgesia: a meta-analysis. *JAMA.* 2003;290:2455-2463.

48. Abdelmalak BB, Lansang MC. Revisiting tight glycemic control in perioperative and critically ill patients: when one size may not fit all. *J Clin Anesth.* 2013;25(6):499-507.

49. Navaratnarajah M, Rea R, Evans R, et al. Effect of glycaemic control on complications following cardiac surgery: literature review. *J Cardiothorac Surg.* 2018;13(1):10.

50. Kao LS, Meeks D, Moyer VA, Lally KP. Peri-operative glycaemic control regimens for preventing surgical site infections in adults. *Cochrane Database Syst Rev.* 2009;(3):CD006806. doi: 10.1002/14651858.CD006806.pub2.

51. Endara M, Masden D, Goldstein J, Gondek S, Steinberg J, Attinger C. The role of chronic and perioperative glucose management in high-risk surgical closures: a case for tighter glycemic control. *Plast Reconstr Surg.* 2013;132(4):996-1004.

52. May AK, Kauffmann RM, Collier BR. The place for glycemic control in the surgical patient. *Surg Infect (Larchmt).* 2011;12(5):405-418.

53. Buchleitner AM, Martinez-Alonso M, Hernandez M, Sola I, Mauricio D. Perioperative glycaemic control for diabetic patients undergoing surgery. *Cochrane Database Syst Rev.* 2012;(9):CD007315. doi: 10.1002/14651858.CD007315.pub2.

54. Borg H, Arnqvist HJ, Bjork E, et al. Evaluation of the new ADA and WHO criteria for classification of diabetes mellitus in young adult people (15-34 yrs) in the Diabetes Incidence Study in Sweden (DISS). *Diabetologia.* 2003;46(2):173-181.

55. Hoogwerf B. Perioperative management of diabetes mellitus: How should we act on the limited evidence? *Cleve Clin J Med.* 2005;73(1):S95-S99.

56. Duncan AE. Hyperglycemia and perioperative glucose management. *Curr Pharm Des.* 2012;18(38):6195-6203.

57. Sheehy AM, Gabbay RA. An overview of preoperative glucose evaluation, management, and perioperative impact. *J Diabetes Sci Technol.* 2009;3(6):1261-1269.

58. Drews HL III, Castiglione AL, Brentin SN, et al. Perioperative hypoglycemia in patients with diabetes: incidence after low normal fasting preoperative blood glucose versus after hyperglycemia treated with insulin. *AANA J.* 2012;80(4 suppl):S17-S24.

59. Turnia M, Christ-Crain M, Polk H. Impact of diabetes mellitus and metabolic disorders. *Surg Clin North Am.* 2005;85:1153-1161.

60. Schreiber M. Minimizing perioperative complications in patients with renal insufficiency. *Cleve Clin J Med.* 2006;73(1):S116-S120.

61. Neumayer L and Vargo D. Principles of Preoperative and Operative Surgery. In: Townsend CM, Beauchamp RD, Evers BM, eds. *Sabiston Textbook of Surgery: The Biological Basis of Modern Surgical Practice.* 18th ed. St. Louis: Saunders Elsevier; 2008:251-279.

62. Liu K, Stafford-Smith M, Shaw A. Renal Function Monitoring. In: Miller RD, Cohen NE, Eriksson LI, Fleischer LA, Wiener-Kronish JP, Young WL. eds. *Miller's Anesthesia.* 8th ed. Philadelphia, PA: Saunders Elsevier; 2015:1580-1603.

63. Beckman JA, Creager MA. The History and Physical Examination. In: Creager MA, Dzau VJ, Loscalzo J, eds. *Vascular Medicine.* Philadelphia, PA: Saunders Elsevier; 2006:135-145.

64. Creager MA, Halperin JL, Coffman JD. Raynaud's Phenomenon. In: Creager MA, Dzau VJ, Loscalzo J, eds. *Vascular Medicine.* Philadelphia, PA: Saunders Elsevier; 2006:689-706.

65. Gerhard-Herman M, Gardin JM, Jaff M, et al.; American Society of Echocardiography; Society of Vascular Medicine and Biology. Guidelines for noninvasive vascular laboratory testing: a report from the American Society of Echocardiography and the Society of Vascular Medicine and Biology. *J Am Soc Echocardiogr.* 2006;19(8):955-972.

66. Kearon C, Akl EA, Comerota AJ, et al. Antithrombotic therapy for VTE disease: Antithrombotic therapy and prevention of thrombosis, 9th ed: American College of Chest Physicians Evidence-Based Clinical Practice Guidelines. *Chest.* 2012;141(2 suppl):e419S-e496S.

67. Stein CM, Pincus T. Glucosteroids. In: Ruddy S, Harris ED, Sledge CB, eds. *Kelley's Textbook of Rheumatology.* 6th ed. Philadelphia, PA: WB Saunders Company; 2001:823-840.

68. Kelly KN, Domajnko B. Perioperative stress-dose steroids. *Clin Colon Rectal Surg.* 2013;26:163-167.

69. de Lange DW, Kars M. Perioperative glucocorticosteroid supplementation is not supported by evidence. *Eur J Intern Med.* 2008;19:461-467.

70. Brown CJ, Buie WD. Perioperative stress dose steroids: Do they make a difference? *J Am Coll Surg.* 2001;193:678-686.

71. Liu MM, Reidy AB, Saatee S, Collard CD. Perioperative steroid management: approaches based on current evidence. *Anesthesiology.* 2017;127(1):166-172.

72. Bornstein SR, Allolio B, Arlt W, et al. Diagnosis and treatment of primary adrenal insufficiency: An Endocrine Society Clinical Practice Guideline. *J Clin Endocrinol Metab.* 2016;101:364-389.

73. Weinblatt ME. Methotrexate. In: Ruddy S, Harris ED, Sledge CB, eds. *Kelley's Textbook of Rheumatology.* 6th ed. Philadelphia, PA: WB Saunders Company; 2001:841-852.

74. Weismann BN, Resnick D, Kaushik S, Sem AW, Yu JS. Imaging. In: Ruddy S, Harris ED, Sledge CB, eds. *Kelley's Textbook of Rheumatology.* 6th ed. Philadelphia, PA: WB Saunders Company; 2001:621-683.

75. Sledge CB. Introduction to surgical management of patients with arthritis. In: Ruddy S, Harris ED, Sledge CB, eds. *Kelley's Textbook of Rheumatology.* 6th ed. Philadelphia, PA: WB Saunders Company; 2001:1691-1697.

76. Seidner DL. Nutritional issues in the surgical patient. *Cleve Clin J Med.* 2006;73(1):S77-S81.

77. Gibbs J, Cull W, Henderson W, Daley J, Hur K, Khuri SF. Preoperative serum albumin level as a predictor of operative mortality and morbidity: results from the National VA Surgical Risk Study. *Arch Surg.* 1999;134:36-42.

78. Virchow R. Neuer fall von todlicher. Embolie der lungenarterien. *Arch Anat Cytol Pathol.* 1856;10:225.

79. Slaybaugh RS, Beasley BD, Massa EG. Deep venous thrombosis risk assessment, incidence, and prophylaxis in foot and ankle surgery. *Clin Podiatr Med Surg.* 2003;20:269-289.

80. Judge MS, Budny AM, Shibuya N, et al. Current concepts in deep venous thrombosis prophylaxis. In: *The Proceedings of the Annual Meeting of the Podiatry Institute–Update 2006.* Tucker, GA: Podiatry Institute; 2006:266-272.

81. Solis G, Saxby T. Incidence of DVT following foot and ankle surgery. *Foot Ankle Int.* 2002;23:411-414.

82. Mizel MS, Temple HT, Michelson JD, et al. Thromboembolism after foot and ankle surgery: a multicenter study. *Clin Orthop Relat Res.* 1998;348;180-185.

83. Wukich D, Waters DH. Thromboembolism following foot and ankle surgery: a case series and literature review. *J Foot Ankle Surg.* 2008;47:243-249.

84. Fleischer AE, Abicht BP, Baker JR, Boffeli TJ, Jupiter DC, Schade VL. American College of Foot and Ankle Surgeons' clinical consensus statement: risk, prevention, and diagnosis of venous thromboembolism disease in foot and ankle surgery and injuries requiring immobilization. *J Foot Ankle Surg.* 2015;54:497-507.

85. Meyr AJ, Mirmiran R, Naldo J, Sachs BD, Shibuya N. American College of Foot and Ankle surgeon's clinical consensus statement: perioperative management. *J Foot Ankle Surg.* 2017;56(2):336-356.

86. Douketis JD, Spyropoulos AC, Spencer FA, et al.; American College of Chest Physicians. Perioperative management of antithrombotic therapy: antithrombotic therapy and prevention of thrombosis, 9th ed: American College of Chest Physicians Evidence-Based Clinical Practice Guidelines. *Chest.* 2012;141(2 suppl):e326S-e350S.

87. Pannucci CJ, Shanks A, Moote MJ, et al. Identifying patients at high risk for venous thromboembolism requiring treatment after outpatient surgery. *Ann Surg.* 2012;255(6):1093-1099.

88. Geerts WH, Pineo GF, Heit JA, et al. Prevention of venous thromboembolism: the Seventh ACCP Conference on Antithrombotic and Thrombolytic Therapy. *Chest.* 2004;126(suppl):338S-400S.

89. Muntz JE. Deep vein thrombosis and pulmonary embolism in the perioperative patient. *Am J Manag Care.* 2000;6:1045-1052.
90. Deep venous thrombosis: prevention. In: Browse NL, Burnand KA, Thomas ML, eds. *Diseases of the Veins.* London, England: Edward Arnold; 1988.
91. Turpie AG. Efficacy of a postoperative regimen of enoxaparin in deep vein thrombosis prophylaxis. *Am J Surg.* 1991;161:532.
92. Woods RK, Dellinger EP. Current guidelines for antibiotic prophylaxis of surgical wounds. *Am Fam Physician.* 1998;57:1-12.
93. Mader JT, Cierny G. The principles and use of preventive antibiotics. *Clin Orthop Relat Res.* 1984;190:75-82.
94. Mangram AJ, Horan TC, Pearson ML, Silver LC, Jarvis WR. Guideline for prevention of surgical site infection, 1999. *Infect Control Hosp Epidemiol.* 1999;20:247-278.
95. Zgonis T, Jolly GP, Garbalosa JC. The efficacy of prophylactic intravenous antibiotics in elective foot and ankle surgery. *J Foot Ankle Surg.* 2004;43:97-102.
96. Joseph WS. *Handbook of Lower Extremity Infections.* St. Louis, MO: Churchill Livingstone; 2003.
97. American Dental Association; American Academy of Orthopedic Surgeons. Antibiotic prophylaxis for dental patients with total joint replacements. *J Am Dent Assoc.* 2003;134:895-898.
98. Patzakis MJ, Wilkins J, Moore TM. Use of antibiotics in open tibial fractures. *Clin Orthop Relat Res.* 1983;178:31-35.
99. Malhotra AK, Goldberg S, Graham J, et al. Open extremity fractures: impact of delay in operative debridement and irrigation. *J Trauma Acute Care Surg.* 2014;76:1201-1207.
100. Ovaska MT, Madanat R, Honkamaa M, Makinen TJ. Contemporary demographics and complications of patients treated for open ankle fractures. *Injury.* 2015;46:1650-1655.
101. Dellinger EP, Caplan ES, Weaver LD, et al. Duration of preventive antibiotic administration for open extremity fractures. *Arch Surg.* 1988;123:333-339.
102. Henley MB, Chapman JR, Agel J, Harvey EJ, Whorton AM, Swiontkowski MF. Treatment of type II, IIIA and III B open fractures of the tibial shaft: a prospective comparison of unreamed interlocking intramedullary nails and half-pin external fixators. *J Orthop Trauma.* 1998;12:1-7.
103. Hohmann E, Tetsworth K, Radziejowski MJ, Wiesniewski TF. Comparison of delayed and primary wound closure in the treatment of open tibial fractures. *Arch Orthop Trauma Surg.* 2007;127:131-136.
104. Bratzler DW, Houck PM. Antimicrobial prophylaxis for surgery: an advisory statement from the national surgical infection prevention project. *Clin Infect Dis.* 2004;38:1706-1715.
105. Perl T. Prevention of staphylococcus aureus infections among surgical patients: beyond traditional prophylaxis. *Surgery.* 2003;134:s10-s17.
106. Pavel A, Smith RL, Ballard A, Larsen AJ. Prophylactic antibiotics in clean orthopaedic surgery. *J Bone Joint Surg.* 1974;56:777-782.
107. Kallen AJ, Wilson CT, Larson RJ. Perioperative intranasal mupirocin for the prevention of surgical site infections: systematic review of the literature and meta-analysis. *Infect Control Hosp Epidemiol.* 2005;26:916-922.
108. Kim DH, Spencer M, Davidson SM, et al. Institutional prescreening for detection and eradication of methicillin-resistant *Staphylococcus aureus* in patients undergoing elective orthopedic surgery. *J Bone Joint Surg Am.* 2010;92:1820-1826.
109. Schweizer ML, Chiang HY, Septimus E, et al. Association of a bundled intervention with surgical site infections among patients undergoing cardiac, hip or knee surgery. *JAMA.* 2015;313:2162-2171.
110. Chen AF, Heyl AE, Xu PZ, Rao N, Klatt BA. Preoperative decolonization effective at reducing staphylococcal colonization in total joint arthroplasty patients. *J Arthroplasty.* 2013;28(8 suppl):18-20.
111. Chen AF, Wessel CB, Rao N. Staphylococcus aureus screening and decolonization in orthopedic surgery and reduction of surgical site infection. *Clin Orthop Relat Res.* 2013;471:2383-2399.
112. Kalmeijer MD, van Nieuwland-Bollen E, Bogaers-Hofman D, de Baere GA. Nasal carriage of *Staphylococcus aureus* is a major risk factor for surgical site infections in orthopedic surgery. *Infect Control Hosp Epidemiol.* 2000;21:319-323.
113. Rao N, Cannella B, Crossett LS, Yates AJ Jr, McGough R III. A preoperative decolonization protocol for Staphylococcus aureus prevents orthopedic infections. *Clin Orthop Relat Res.* 2008;466:1343-1348.
114. Economedes DM, Deirmengian GK, Deirmengian CA. *Staphylococcus aureus* colonization among arthroplasty patients previously treated by a decolonization protocol: a pilot study. *Clin Orthop Relat Res.* 2012;471:3128-3132.
115. DeLalla F. Perioperative antibiotic prophylaxis: a critical review. *Surg Infect (Larchmt).* 2006;7(suppl 2):s37-s39.
116. Ali M, Raza A. Role of single dose antibiotic prophylaxis in clean orthopedic surgery. *J Coll Physicians Surg Pak.* 2006;16:45-48.
117. Kanter G, Connelly NR, Fitzgerald J. A system and process redesign to improve perioperative antibiotic administration. *Anesth Analg.* 2006;103:1517-1521.
118. Stoelting R, Miller R. *Basics of Anesthesia.* Philadelphia, PA: Churchill Livingstone; 2000.
119. Roth RD. Utilization of epinephrine containing anesthetic solution in the toes. *J Am Podiatr Med Assoc.* 1981;71:189-199.
120. Myerson M, Ruland C, Allon S. Regional anesthesia for foot and ankle surgery. *Foot Ankle Int.* 1992;13:282-288.
121. Tipton PE, Gudas CJ. The effects of a local anesthetic on digital circulation. *J Am Podiatr Med Assoc.* 1980;70:142-146.
122. Green D, Walter J, Heden R, et al. The effects of local anesthesia containing epinephrine on digital blood perfusion. *J Am Podiatr Med Assoc.* 1979;69:397-409.
123. Kaplan EG, Kashuk K. Disclaiming the myth of epinephrine local anesthesia in feet. *J Am Podiatr Med Assoc.* 1971;61:335-340.
124. Crawford ME, Dockery GD. Anesthesia. In: *Lower Extremity Soft Tissue and Cutaneous Plastic Surgery.* 2nd Ed. Edinburgh. Saunders Elsevier; 2012:45-52.
125. Scarlet J, Walter J, Bachman R. Digital perfusion following injection of plain lidocaine and lidocaine with epinephrine: a comparison. *J Am Podiatr Med Assoc.* 1978;68:339-346.
126. Steinberg MV, Block P. The use and abuse of epinephrine in local anesthetics. *J Am Podiatr Med Assoc.* 1971;61:341-343.
127. Carron H, Giorgio A, Kepes E. Nerve block. *Aches Pains.* 1983;4:41-46.
128. Lemont H. A simplified nerve block to control postoperative pain. *J Am Podiatry Assoc.* 1978;68:193.
129. Sarrafian SK, Ibrahim IN, Breihan JH. Ankle–foot peripheral nerve block for mid- and forefoot surgery. *Foot Ankle.* 1983;4:86-90.
130. Horwitz MT. Normal anatomy and variations of the peripheral nerves of the leg and foot. *Arch Surg.* 1938;36:626.
131. Smith DF. Conscious Sedation, Anesthesia and the JCAHO. In. *The JACHO's Anesthesia Related Standards.* Marblehead, MA: Opus Communication Inc; 1999:59-122.
132. Phillip BK. Sedation with Propofol: A New ASA Statement. *ASA Monitor.* 2005;69(2):29-30.
133. Apfel CC, Korttila K, Abdalla M, et al. A factorial trial of six interventions for prevention of postoperative nausea and vomiting. *N Engl J Med.* 2004;350:2441.
134. Schneider TW, Minto CF, Shafer SL, et al. The influence of age on propofol pharmacodynamics. *Anesthesiology.* 1999;6:1502-1516.

CHAPTER 4

Perioperative Pain Management

Andrew J. Meyr and Stephen A. McCaughan

INTRODUCTION

Although much has changed concerning the topic of perioperative pain management since the previous edition of this text was published, one might broadly consider that this has primarily been a change of awareness and perspective, and not of the basic science that underlies the topic. This contemporary perspective has certainly affected physicians with respect to regulations on the prescribing practices of controlled substances, but most importantly, it has affected our patients, many of whom have truly suffered, in part, as a result of years of relatively imprecise practice standards. Any number of troubling statistics from the US Center for Disease Control paint the troubling picture: more than 4 million Americans report engaging in the nonmedical use of prescription opioids on a monthly basis, in 2013 enough prescriptions were filled so that every US adult could have a bottle of opioids, and more than 40 people die each day as a result of overdoses involving prescription opioids.[1] The total annual number of US overdose deaths involving prescription opioids (including methadone) rose dramatically from 3442 in 1999 to 17 029 in 2017.[2] Public awareness of this situation likely peaked in October of 2018 as the SUPPORT for Patients and Communities Act was signed into US law to assist in combating the opioid crisis.[3]

Why, when, and how did this occur? Although this is a challenging question that extends beyond the scope of this specific chapter, it is interesting to consider that Dr. John J. Bonica (1917–1994), considered the founder of the contemporary multidisciplinary, multimodal approach to pain management, likely would have argued that the writing had been on the wall for years so to speak. He argued that physicians had relatively "passive" attitudes toward pain management because the source of postoperative pain is usually easy to deduce, the conditions are often self-limiting, and treatments are generally very effective.[4] This last point is perhaps the most critical. Following publication of reports on the safety and efficacy of opioids prescribed to small numbers of patients with chronic nonmalignant pain, and the publication of a seminal article entitled "The tragedy of needless pain," the use of opioids to treat chronic nonmalignant pain became more widely practiced and incorporated into clinical guidelines.[5,6] Secondary to a confluence of factors, including but not limited to increased emphasis on in-hospital pain documentation as the so-called "5th vital sign" and increasing patient expectations with respect to treatment, physicians in the United States simply began prescribing more opioids at higher quantities and stronger dosages. This activity

might have been further initiated by the landmark 1996 consensus statement that "<1% of opioid users become addicted," from both the American Pain Society and the American Academy of Pain Management.[7] Several studies on national prescribing patterns have indicated that although patients generally present with roughly the same complaints in the same intensity as they did decades ago, physicians simply became more likely to prescribe an opioid for these same complaints moving into the 21st century.[8-10]

Dr. Bonica often included on the cover of his *Management of Pain* textbooks a picture of a sculpture of the mythological Herculus fighting the multiheaded hydra, and a painting by American artist John Singer Sargent with a similar theme also enforces this illustration as it relates to physicians and pain management (Fig. 4.1).[11] In this example, physicians represent Hercules doing battle with a formidable opponent

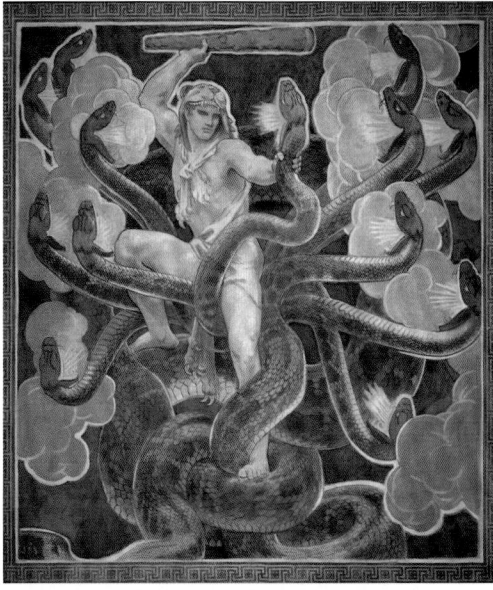

FIGURE 4.1 Multimodal Pain Management. This painting entitled Hercules by John Singer Sargent is on display on the ceiling of the Boston Museum of Fine Arts (1921). Postoperative pain management has been compared to fighting a multiheaded hydra. The use of unimodal therapy is like focusing on only one the hydra's heads, but an active multimodal approach with maximization of adjuvant therapy enables the surgeon to attack multiple pain mechanisms simultaneously.

(pain management represented as the hydra). For too long, physicians have been entirely too focused on only a single head of the hydra (opioids), while completely ignoring all the other heads that continue to attack Hercules unabated. Considering the recent history of pain management in the United States, frankly the hydra had won because of the overreliance on opioids and sequela therein. *Better* pain management in actuality means more *efficient* pain management through a multimodal approach, not simply prescribing higher quantities and stronger dosages of the same class of medications. Moving forward, physicians should have a broader focus on each of the heads of the hydra (representing a multimodal approach), and not simply passively attack one head with a primary focus.

HISTORY

Although it has certainly received increased contemporary attention, in fact the management of pain has served as the focus and foundation of the science of medicine since the beginnings of recorded history. This is because pain is not only the primary reason that people seek medical care, but it is also an expected sequela of surgical intervention.[12-15] Because of this, one might argue that it is the responsibility of all surgeons to appreciate the management of this most basic of human complaints and to understand how to implement appropriate interventions for the benefit of their patients.

The act of surgery provides unique perspective on how modern medicine approaches concepts of pain. Despite pain relief acting as the driving force of medical interventions for thousands of years, perioperative anesthetic techniques were not consistently utilized until the middle of the 19th century. Historical physicians such as Hippocrates (460–377 BC) and Ambrose Paré (1520–1590) were known to use carotid compression in the perioperative setting, but it was a dentist in 1846 who is recognized with pioneering modern anesthesia. William Morton (1819–1868) first led a surgical demonstration of a tumor excision from the jaw of a patient preoperatively anesthetized with ether before an astonished crowd at the Massachusetts General Hospital in Boston.[16,17] Interestingly, the medical community and general public needed to be convinced that this form of intervention to prevent pain during surgery was necessary or even socially acceptable. Generations of public conception viewing pain as its Latin root *poena*, or "punishment," relatively spurned medical advances to treat and prevent pain in elective situations.[18] It was not until the later part of the century when Queen Victoria was anesthetized during labor, and Pope Pius XII declared approval for anesthetic techniques, that the public grew to accept it.[16-18] Physicians were also initially skeptical. Surgeons often took pride in the ability to perform painful surgery on sensate patients, and some even considered it a rite of passage for younger surgeons.[19,20] A history of surgery with this hindsight perspective reveals the almost barbaric nature of the practice.

Although it is now generally considered unacceptable to operate on sensate patients without any anesthesia, we likely continue to allow some unnecessary pain in the postoperative recovery period. Many patients report experiencing moderate to severe pain within the first 48 hours of outpatient ambulatory surgery, while patient satisfaction levels are lower than might be expected.[21-29] In studies specifically examining lower extremity

orthopedic procedures, a majority of patients admitted experiencing episodes of moderate to severe pain that resulted in the loss of sleep and impairment of activities of daily living.[24,25]

Additionally, pain as a negative surgical sequela has the potential to contribute to other short and long-term complications. Uncontrolled postoperative pain leads to increased levels of patient dissatisfaction, longer hospital stays and higher health care costs.[30-35] Acute postoperative pain also activates the postinjury stress response and systemic effects extending beyond the operative site.[31] Increased circulating catecholamines, vasoconstriction, platelet aggregation, peripheral thrombosis, hyperglycemia, and a decreased immune response with increased infection rates might all be associated with uncontrolled postoperative pain.[31,36-38]

CLINICAL POINTS OF EMPHASIS

All surgeons should take an active approach to postoperative pain management. This chapter will highlight how the known physiologic and pathophysiologic mechanisms contributing to operative pain can be used in treatment interventions throughout the perioperative period. Specific consideration will be given to preemptive analgesia, a multimodal analgesic approach, and the perioperative management of the chronic pain patient.

PHYSIOLOGY OF OPERATIVE PAIN

"ATTACK POINTS" OF PAIN PROCESSING

An evidence-based approach requires that medical interventions are based on known mechanisms. A thorough understanding of the underlying physiology allows physicians to actively attack the source of a patient complaint, instead of passively covering up the symptoms. Particularly in the acute pain setting, such as surgery, these mechanisms are well understood and medical interventions that directly interrupt pain processing pathways are readily available.

In many ways, acute pain can be viewed as a "healthy" or "normal" physiologic response. Following the initiation of a noxious stimulus in the form of tissue damage, the body activates pathways alerting the organism that homeostasis has been disrupted and that a change in behavior is necessary to prevent further injury. In fact, the spinal reflexes that respond to acute pain form the most basic components of the peripheral and central nervous systems.[4,39,40] While operative pain is best described by the mechanism of acute peripheral pain physiology, it serves no biologic function. The "normal" physiology of this type of pain can only lead to complications.[36]

For a basic understanding of acute pain physiology, the process is viewed as a serial bottom-up system in which an external stimulus leads to a series of staged reactions within the peripheral and central nervous systems.[41] The following model emphasizes clinical diagnosis and treatment presented in terms of four "attack points" where active intervention is possible to address the source and interrupt the physiology of pain.[42]

STIMULUS

The initiation of the acute pain pathway comes in the form of a noxious stimulus. Interestingly, there is no quantitative or objective definition that separates a noxious stimulus from a non-noxious stimulus. Put most simply, a stimulus is considered noxious if it leads to *transduction* or activation of specialized peripheral nociceptors.[41-44] These free nerve endings are located in skin, viscera, muscle, fascia, blood vessels, and joint capsules.[45] Three general forms of peripheral nociceptors are likely to be activated during a surgical procedure: chemical, mechanical, and thermal.[41,46]

Chemical Nociceptors

Chemical nociceptors undergo transduction when the free nerve endings are exposed to specific ions and cytokines within the surrounding extracellular matrix. These substances are released either directly as a result of cellular damage or indirectly through the normal inflammatory processes that accompany tissue damage and wound healing. Additionally, these substrates can either directly activate the nociceptor or sensitize the nerve endings making transduction more likely to occur.[39,41-44,46-48]

Direct cellular damage primarily occurs during dissection to the surgical target tissue and during the definitive procedure as intracellular components are spilled into the extracellular environment. The degree of tissue damage will determine the quantity and quality of the postoperative inflammatory response, particularly in the superficial layers.[49] Uncontrolled hemostasis can also lead to direct and indirect activation of peripheral chemical nociceptors through the action of platelets.[50] And although damage to any type of cell will result in the release of inflammatory cytokines, direct nerve damage additionally amplifies the noxious signal through the processes of ectopic discharge, peripheral sensitization, and central sensitization.[41,51-53]

Mechanical Nociceptors

Transduction of mechanical nociceptors occurs when a physical stretch deforms unique transmembrane channels on free nerve endings. The resultant distortion of the channel allows for the influx of extracellular ions (Na+, K+ and Cl−), and nociceptor depolarization occurs.[41] Most mechanical noxious stimuli result in plastic deformation of the channel, but excessive stimuli can result in permanent damage.[39] Activation of mechanical nociceptors is likely during an elective procedure with both retraction[55-57] and tourniquet use.[58,59]

Thermal Nociceptors

Thermal nociceptors are activated by both heat and cold stimuli, although most in the lower extremities are activated by heat between 42°C and 45°C.[47,60] These temperatures are routinely generated during orthopedic procedures, with the secondary sequela of thermal necrosis, from the use of power instrumentation and electrocautery devices.[61-65]

TRANSMISSION

The transmission phase of the acute pain pathway involves peripheral afferent nerve fibers carrying the action potential generated by the noxious stimulus from the local site of tissue injury to the dorsal horn of the spinal cord.[41-44] Two unique types of afferent nerve fibers are responsible for this

conduction in the acute operative pain setting: the alpha-delta (A-δ) fiber and the C fiber.

The speed of transmission is directly correlated to the diameter of the axons of sensory neurons and whether or not they are myelinated.[66] Nociceptive fibers have been classified on the basis of their conduction velocity, sensitivity, and threshold to noxious mechanical, heat, and cold stimuli.[66] A-δ fibers are thinly myelinated nociceptors that are activated by both mechanical and thermal but rarely chemical, stimulation. Some describe the A-δ fibers as giving rise to *first pain* because of the rapid nature of their transmission, nearly 10-25 times the speed of the unmyelinated C-fibers.[22] This pain is described as brief, localized, and sharp in nature. It is theorized that it provides the central nervous system with rapid information regarding intensity, location, and duration of the noxious stimulus.[31,36,41,43,67]

C fibers are unmyelinated nociceptors that are activated by chemical, mechanical, and thermal stimulation. They are thought to play a significant role in the development of pain associated with the inflammatory process because of their ability to respond to chemical stimulation. These unmyelinated fibers are inherently slower, giving rise to *second pain*. This is described as burning, throbbing, and aching in nature and may provide the central nervous system with information regarding the extent or severity of the injury.[31,36,41,43]

MODULATION

At the most basic level, the modulation phase represents the synapse between the primary sensory afferent of the periphery and the second-order neuron of the central nervous system. This site, however, at the dorsal horn of the spinal cord, is actually a complex interaction of excitatory and inhibitory signals from both ascending and descending pathways (Fig. 4.2).

A simplified explanation that provides a basic visual model of this stage was proposed by Wall and Melzack in the middle of the 20th century.[68] The *gate control theory* depicts the dorsal horn of the spinal cord as a single gate that is either opened (leading to propagation of the noxious stimuli into the central nervous system) or closed (blocking the peripheral noxious stimuli from being processed by the central nervous system). The status of the "gate" is determined by the interaction of various inhibitory and excitatory signals from peripheral and central sources in a constant balance. If the cumulative inhibitory signal is stronger than the net excitatory signal, then the gate remains closed. But if the cumulative excitatory signal is stronger than the net inhibitory signal, then the gate is opened and the signal is transmitted on.[44,68-70]

While it is now known that the mechanisms of modulation are more complex than the status of a single gate being either opened or closed, the fundamental principles of the gate control theory likely remain conceptually accurate. The term modulation was specifically chosen to describe this stage because of the modification of the peripheral noxious signal that occurs. For each A-δ and C fiber that has been stimulated and is transmitting a noxious signal, there are thousands of peripheral nociceptors in the extremity that are not. For example, A-beta (Aβ) fibers are large diameter myelinated nociceptors that do not normally transmit the sensation of pain when activated, but rather of light touch, pressure, and hair movement.[67,71] In the same way, there are descending pathways from higher brain centers sending a constant stream of excitatory and inhibitory signals

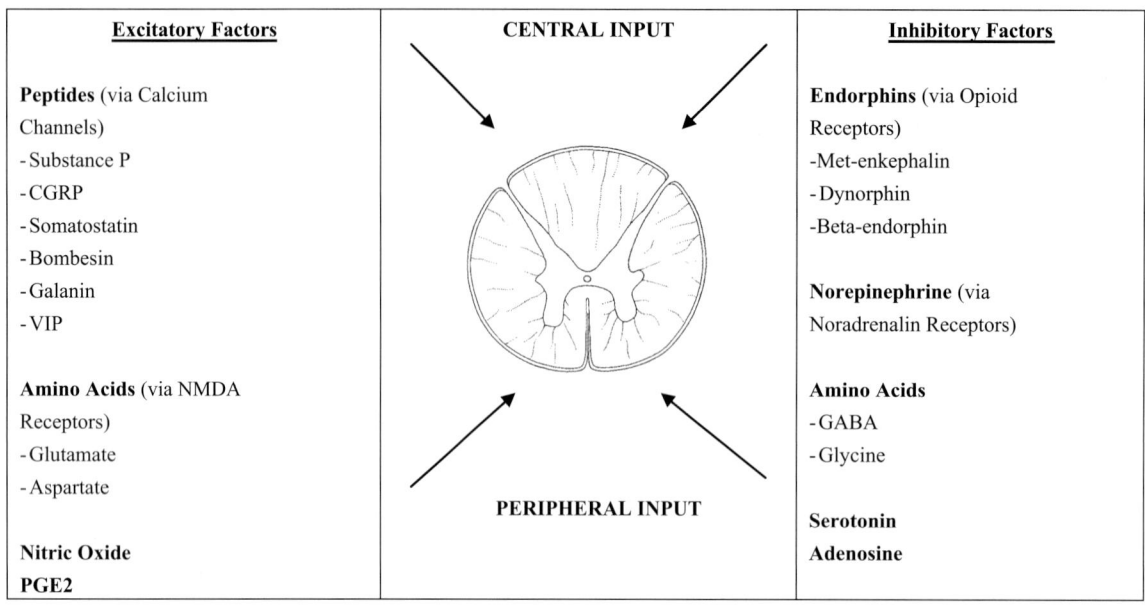

FIGURE 4.2 The Modulation Attack Point. The influence of a noxious stimulus transmitted to the dorsal horn of the spinal cord is dependent on the complex interaction of central and peripheral, excitatory and inhibitory factors. (Reproduced with permission from Meyr AJ, Steinberg JS. The physiology of the acute pain pathway. *Clin Podiatr Med Surg.* 2008;25(3):305-326.)

to the dorsal horn. Through these mechanisms, the dorsal horn synapse represents a balance of excitatory and inhibitory signals that has been triggered by the initial noxious stimulus.

PERCEPTION

In many ways, perception represents the qualitative and psychological aspects of pain physiology. The previous attack points have emphasized concrete physiologic mechanisms and changes that occur in response to a noxious stimulus. While perception does involve the paleospinothalamic and neospinothalamic tracts terminating the noxious signal in the higher brain centers of the limbic system, frontal cortex and somatosensory cortex, pain cannot be fully described in terms of a physiologic mechanism.[36,43,44] Pain is not tissue damage, it is not an action potential, and it is not the influx of calcium ions within synapses of the spinal cord. It is a biologic and psychologic *experience* influenced by previous history, culture, religious beliefs, mood, and even the time of day or number of people in the room.[72-78] Perception is the process of transforming an objective physiologic mechanism into a subjective patient complaint.

PATHOPHYSIOLOGY OF OPERATIVE PAIN

The physiology of acute operative pain can be thought of as a distinct pathway beginning with the noxious stimulus and ending with perception. In the absence of sustained stimulation, the consequent physiology leading to perception is not expected to occur. In more basic terms, the pain stops when the stimulus is removed. However, through both peripheral and central sensitization, this normally linear pathway can be transformed into a chronic cycle without a beginning or endpoint. In this situation, the perception of pain continues even in the absence of noxious stimulation. Although many of the

molecules, synapses, and mechanisms used in these processes are the same, they are functioning in different ways. It is the pathophysiology of these systems that initiates chronic pain.[79-82]

PERIPHERAL SENSITIZATION

Localized, peripheral inflammation is a normal consequence of tissue damage and represents an important initial phase of the healing process.[41] However, peripheral sensitization is an imbalance of this inflammation leading to the transmission of painful signals to the central nervous system out of proportion to or in the absence of a noxious stimulus. It is a pathophysiologic process using the normal physiology of stimulus and transmission phases.

Inflammatory cytokines can either directly activate chemical nociceptors or sensitize nociceptors making them more susceptible to transduction. This nociceptor sensitization is a relatively unique concept in human physiology in that constant stimulation leads to a greater reaction and not functional adaptation with a decreased response.[36,41,50] In the presence of peripheral sensitization, quantitatively more nociceptors are available for activation, and transduction occurs at lower thresholds.[39,44,70,79-91] This results in an amplification of the noxious signal because a given stimulus leads to a relatively greater degree of transduction and transmission.

CENTRAL SENSITIZATION

In a similar way, central sensitization can be thought of as an imbalance of the modulation phase. There is a disproportionate excitatory signal from peripheral and central sources "opening the gate" and leading to noxious processing. Centrally at the dorsal horn, excitatory signals from C fibers displace magnesium ions from NMDA receptors and open calcium channels at other excitatory synapses. A "wind-up" phase results in the postsynaptic neurons as excitatory neuropeptides and amino acids accumulate within the synapse.[39,41,81,87,92-95]

Central sensitization is driven by peripheral excitatory signals (particularly from the C fibers), and it cycles to increase peripheral effects. Axonal reflexes lead to a *secondary hyperalgesia* where the perceived physical area of pain increases. A reflex arc develops within the activated peripheral nerve and spinal cord to cause activation and sensitization along the entire distal extent of that peripheral nerve, not just the branches of the injured tissue. Through this mechanism, nociceptors in the surrounding area of the injured tissue become activated.[39,41,96-98] *Allodynia* also develops in the periphery when non-noxious stimuli are perceived to be painful. In the setting of central sensitization and displaced magnesium ions, A-β peripheral afferents that are activated by light touch are registered as a noxious signal by NMDA receptors at the dorsal horn.[36,41,81,92,99-101]

Peripheral and central sensitization have been described as a more efficient pain signal where amplification of the noxious stimulus creates a cycle of inflammation and further sensitization. If noxious stimuli or peripheral sensitization are maintained, then central sensitization can be sustained indefinitely. In contrast, when the peripheral signal is removed, there is evidence that central sensitization can resolve within minutes.[39,41,81]

The noxious stimuli produced by the physical act of surgery are sufficient enough to generate peripheral and central sensitization pathophysiology in addition to the physiology of the acute pain pathway.[11] An active approach to perioperative pain management takes into account and intervenes into both the physiology and pathophysiology of these mechanisms.

MULTIMODAL MANAGEMENT OF PERIOPERATIVE PAIN

The goals of pain management in the perioperative setting can be viewed in several ways. *Physiologically*, interventions should interrupt the known acute and chronic pain mechanisms to limit, in an attempt to prevent, peripheral sensitization, central sensitization, and the perception of pain. Put more broadly, the physiologic goal is to reach a resolution of the acute pain pathway without the development of a pathophysiologic chronic pain cycle. *Objectively*, the goals of pain management include quantifiable outcome measures such as increased time to the first perception of pain and a decreased total opioid usage, total duration of pain, need for rescue analgesia, average pain intensity score, maximum pain intensity score, length of hospital stay, and pain/medication side effects. Finally, *subjectively* high levels of patient satisfaction with regard to pain management are sought. Although multifactorial, patient satisfaction involves an effective physician-patient relationship with respect to communication and the development of mutual expected outcomes. These goals are all likely best achieved with a multimodal approach.[11,32-37,82,102,103]

PREOPERATIVE CONSIDERATIONS

The idea of *preemptive analgesia* employs acute pain physiology intervention before the actual noxious stimulus or the first perception of pain. Surgery is a situation in which the anticipated tissue damage will activate peripheral nociceptors leading to pain perception and sensitization. Taking action prior to the development of this physiology might accomplish some

of the goals of pain management including the prevention of peripheral and central sensitization, increasing the time until the first perception of pain, and decreasing total opioid usage and pain scores.[11,35,102-106]

Surgeons should appreciate several thoughts with respect to the topic of preemptive analgesia. First, some of these principles are likely already incorporated in their existing perioperative protocols. For example, the use of general anesthesia is considered preemptive in that it blocks nociceptive input at the modulation stage prior to the surgical procedure. Additionally, preoperative local anesthetic peripheral blockades interrupt the physiology of the transmission phase[31,36,41,44,107] and have been demonstrated to be one of the most effective preemptive analgesic strategies.[105,106] Another consideration is that while many of these techniques have been found effective in clinical trials, no rigid protocols or recommendations exist for their use. Surgeons are encouraged to actively examine their own clinical practices, stay current on the medical literature, and decide if any of these techniques may be used to improve patient care in their respective practices.

Anxiolysis

Preoperative anxiety activates excitatory descending pathways from higher brain centers at the modulation and perception phases and might have a detrimental effect on postoperative pain and patient satisfaction.[12,108,109] Anxiolysis can often be accomplished through proper patient education in the preoperative phase. Studies have demonstrated that a reduction in preoperative anxiety scores is possible through counseling and education, and that this intervention leads to lower levels of postoperative pain.[110-114] Reduction of anxiety levels with preoperative pharmaceuticals has also been shown to significantly reduce postoperative pain. Although this form of intervention might usually be unnecessary, the use of benzodiazepines might be considered in some situations.[114,115]

Preoperative patient education with respect to lower extremity orthopedic procedures involves several considerations. Most importantly, the physician and the patient should have effective communication and a mutual understanding of the expected outcomes of the surgical procedure. The patient should be aware of the criteria that the surgeon will use to judge a successful outcome, just as the surgeon should fully appreciate the patient's complaint and expected results. The patient should also understand what to expect in the immediate postoperative period in terms of pain (onset, duration, intensity, quality, normal and abnormal sensations, etc.), physical constraints (dressings, immobilization devices, activities of daily living, driving, bathing, etc.), physical deformity (extent of incisions, expected scar formation, permanent or temporary fixation, etc.), and potential complications. Patients should also be made aware that the complete relief of pain is an unrealistic expectation. Instead, some controlled pain should be expected postoperatively.

Opioids

Opioids are still considered the gold standard for postoperative pain control[116] but might also be used preoperatively.[105,106,117-119] They act at both the modulation and perception stages, specifically by increasing the inhibitory signal at the dorsal horn of the spinal cord. Pharmaceutical opioids mimic the mechanism of action of endogenous opioids by binding inhibitory receptors and preventing the release of excitatory neurotransmitters. They also have an effect on higher brain centers within the limbic system to control the emotional response to pain.[120-122]

The use of opioids as a frontline treatment in the management of acute pain remains unquestioned. They form the basis of the World Health Organization (WHO) "three step" analgesic ladder for cancer treatment and have been additionally validated in perioperative pain management studies.[116,123-127] However, there is obviously appropriate concern for their overuse and an over reliance on these agents because of their efficacy and ease of administration.[8-10] This is particularly true when they represent the solitary form of analgesia. Opioids have a significant side effect profile including nausea, constipation, sedation, seizures, allodynia, opioid-induced hyperalgesia, and dependence.[31-33,128,129] These adverse effects can be reduced while improving overall patient outcomes with the proper use of adjuvants within a multimodal approach.

Anti-inflammatories

One of the goals of perioperative pain management is to maintain a balance between the physiologic inflammation associated with wound healing, and the pathophysiologic processes of peripheral sensitization at the stimulus stage. Despite the concept that central sensitization might be maintained indefinitely in the setting of peripheral sensitization, relatively few of the pharmaceutical interventions most commonly used for perioperative pain control have effects at the local area of tissue damage and chemical nociceptor transduction.[39,41,81] Anti-inflammatory medications, particularly the nonsteroidal anti-inflammatory drugs (NSAIDs), have local effects and show durable results when used in the perioperative period for pain control.[104,106,115,130-134] All NSAIDs have antipyretic, analgesic, and anti-inflammatory action secondary to prostaglandin synthesis inhibition; however, cyclooxygenase-2 (COX-2) agents might be preferred in the perioperative setting because they maintain platelet function while sparing gastrointestinal side effects.[115,130-132]

The use of these drugs should be assumed with some caution, however. The goal is to create a balance where the uncontrolled local inflammatory processes of peripheral sensitization are blunted, but the normal inflammation associated with wound healing is maintained. Although the use of NSAIDs at high dosages and for extended durations might have detrimental effects on wound and bone healing, this is likely not as much of a concern with single preoperative doses (to diminish the initial inflammatory response) or in the immediate postoperative inflammatory phase of wound healing at recommended dosages (2-5 days).[135-142]

Calcium Channel Blockers

The calcium channels at the dorsal horn of the spinal cord play an important role in the physiology of the modulation attack point, in addition to the pathophysiology of central sensitization. Unlike opioid receptors that are inhibitory in nature, the calcium channels are directly excitatory (Fig. 4.2). Their activation tips the modulation balance in the direction of an "open gate" when influenced by stimulated C fibers and excitatory peptides. Blocking the calcium channel directly inhibits the excitatory signal and might stop the mechanisms of pain processing.[143-145]

The use of calcium channel blockers as an adjuvant therapy should be considered in both acute and chronic pain situations. Although originally designed as an anticonvulsant, gabapentin has also shown analgesic properties through an affinity for and an inhibitory action on calcium channel subunits.[146,147] Its use in chronic pain states and preoperatively for pain management is well documented with encouraging results.[148-154]

Acetaminophen

Acetaminophen has experienced a recent resurgence as being a popular choice for managing mild to moderate surgical pain and is an effective and well-tolerated analgesic with an excellent safety profile within the therapeutic dose ranges. The acetaminophen mechanism of action remains poorly defined. It has been shown to act with modest efficacy against cyclooxygenase (prostacyclin endoperoxidase H2 synthase) *in vitro* prompting its loose affiliation with NSAIDs.[155,156] At the spinal cord level, it has been shown to antagonize neurotransmission by NMDA, substance P, and nitric oxide pathways.[157] It does seem that acetaminophen exerts simultaneous antinociception effects at spinal and supraspinal sites and shows self-synergy between these two routes of activity.[158] Intravenous acetaminophen produces a much higher plasma concentration, which then leads to higher levels in the cerebrospinal fluid. The safety profile and relative lack of systemic adverse reactions make this an attractive analgesic for a wide variety of surgical patients.[159]

N-Methyl D-aspartate (NMDA)-receptor Antagonists

Like the calcium channel, the NMDA receptor is directly excitatory in acute pain states at the modulation attack point through the mechanisms of the excitatory amino acids glutamate and aspartate. This receptor is also involved in chronic pain states through the process of allodynia as discussed with central sensitization.[85,160,161] The use of NMDA-receptor antagonists is most easily accomplished immediately perioperatively because of intravenous, intramuscular, or subcutaneous administration. Preoperative dosing of ketamine may improve postoperative outcomes and prevent the development of central sensitization.[162-165] Intravenous ketamine infusions appear to particularly improve pain control when used with epidural analgesia or IV patient-controlled analgesia, with opioid-tolerant patients, or for surgeries known to have higher incidences of chronic postsurgical pain.[166]

INTRAOPERATIVE CONSIDERATIONS

Anesthesia

A number of interventions that take place within the operating room will likely have an effect on postoperative pain management. Certainly, one of these considerations is the form of delivered anesthesia, whether it is general anesthesia, spinal/epidural anesthesia, or monitored anesthesia care (intravenous sedation). Conscious awareness of noxious stimulation is not required for pain processing to occur.[11] In other words, the development of central sensitization pathophysiology at the modulation attack point will occur if a noxious stimulus reaches the spinal cord regardless of whether or not the patient consciously perceives it. The ideal care offered by the anesthesiology team should complement the surgeon's own analgesic practices. The anesthetic should help block noxious processing at the spinal level and the modulation/perception attack points. The different forms of anesthesia intervention are not uniform in their ability to accomplish this. For example, epidural anesthesia is very effective at blunting the postinjury stress response[11,49,167,168] and might be more effective at maintaining postoperative pain control.[126,169,170]

Local Anesthesia

The use of local anesthetics for peripheral nerve blockade in the perioperative period warrants additional emphasis. It represents the surgeon's primary intervention into the transmission attack point, and its importance cannot be overstated as a complete peripheral blockade with local anesthesia effectively prevents the conduction of the noxious stimulus from reaching the spinal cord.[36,41,44,107,171] Modulation and central sensitization will not occur if the signal does not reach the dorsal horn from the periphery. Two goals of perioperative pain management, increasing the time until the first perception of pain and the prevention of central sensitization, are directly influenced by the quality of the peripheral nerve blockade.

Several variables affect the impact of the regional block on postoperative pain management outcome measures. The first consideration is the timing of the block. Although not overwhelming, theory and some of the medical literature support preoperative infiltration.[105,106] Central sensitization develops in response to the surgical noxious stimuli even in the absence of conscious awareness,[11] so modulation pathophysiology occurs during the course of an operation even if general anesthetic measures temporarily mask it. If possible, all noxious stimuli should be prevented from reaching the central nervous system, not just when the patient has the ability to perceive it. Another consideration is the specific anesthetic agent utilized. The onset and duration of action should be considered, as well as the fact that the quality of the block may be related to the quantity of the drug injected. Longer-acting agents, such as bupivacaine, are better able to increase the time until the first perception of pain. The use of adjuvants including ketamine, ketorolac, clonidine, magnesium, and opioids in addition to local anesthetic agents in the injection have also been described, although the contemporary evidence is relatively limited.[172-175]

A final consideration is the location of the block. Several localized, ring-type blockades are available to the foot and ankle surgeon based on the specific target tissue of the operative intervention.[176-178] These blocks focus attention on the peripheral nerves supplying the dermatomes of the surgical site. However, dermatomes only describe the sensory innervation of the skin and superficial fascia and often do not correspond to the sensory innervation of the structures below the level of the deep fascia. The innervation of these structures, including bone and musculotendinous elements that are often the surgical target tissue, is better described by separate sensory maps, specifically sclerotomes and myotomes.[4,36,179-182] Only rudimentary maps of the sensory innervation of the deep somatic structures of the lower extremity have been derived, but it is clear that a degree of depth should be appreciated when considering the innervation of a given anatomic area.[4,42,181,182] This concept might lead the surgeon to consider a more proximal blockade to ensure complete paresthesia of the operative site. A popliteal nerve block with supplemental saphenous nerve blockade provides complete paresthesia of the lower extremity, has been shown

to be effective and superior in postoperative pain management outcomes, and represents the block of choice for many foot and ankle surgeons.[183-187]

Surgical Technique

Meticulous anatomic dissection technique and strict maintenance of hemostasis in the surgical field should have a positive impact on the postoperative pain course. The quality of the postoperative local inflammatory response is dependant on the quantity of the released cytokines and mediators.[49] Tissue damage should be minimized to diminish this release, particularly in the superficial surgical layers of dissection away from the deeper operative target tissue. Additionally, platelets store and release local inflammatory factors leading to direct and indirect transduction of peripheral chemical nociceptors including serotonin, histamine, thromboxane A2, and platelet factors.[50] This underscores the importance of hemostatic control in the surgical field. Furthermore, unnecessary retraction and tourniquet use, specifically with regard to total time and maximum pressure, should be minimized as both significantly contribute to postoperative pain and patient dissatisfaction.[55-59]

POSTOPERATIVE CONSIDERATIONS

Multimodal Analgesia

Postoperative pain management should be considered an extension of pre- and intraoperative therapies within the multimodal analgesic model. Although there are no standardized postoperative pain management protocols, an individual strategy should work toward the physiologic, objective, and subjective goals outlined earlier in this chapter. The rationale of a multimodal approach is to achieve effective analgesia with the cumulative effects of different interventions at multiple attack points, in order to reduce the dosing and adverse effects of each individual therapy (Table 4.1).[82] A multimodal plan must include consideration of the intensity of the noxious stimuli, the ideal route of administration, and the unique requirements of the individual patient.[188,189]

Adjuvants

Maximization of adjuvant therapy should be utilized before progression to a stronger dosage or class of opioids. The majority of the potential adjunctive therapies have already been described in this chapter including anti-inflammatories, anxiolytics, calcium channel blockers, NMDA-receptor antagonists, and local anesthetics. Muscle relaxants may also be considered an adjuvant therapy, specifically in the setting of muscle spasm and cramping.[190,191] All adjunctive therapies aim to decrease overall pain perception, but the specific mechanisms of action should be considered prior to use. For example, anti-inflammatories and local anesthetics might have the greatest effect in the setting of peripheral sensitization, while calcium channel blockers and NMDA-receptor antagonists might be better served in clinical situations consistent with central sensitization.

Nonpharmacologic Intervention

Not all postoperative pain management interventions are pharmacologic. One of the primary physiologic goals of perioperative pain management is to reach a resolution of the acute pain

TABLE 4.1	An Active Approach to Multimodal Analgesia
Attack Point	**Potential Interventions**
Stimulus	Minimize tissue damage/noxious stimulation ■ Meticulous anatomic dissection ■ Hemostatic control ■ Minimize tourniquet use ■ Minimize retraction ■ Minimize thermal necrosis Physical therapeutics ■ Protection ■ Immobilization ■ Cryotherapy ■ Compression ■ Elevation ■ Minimize secondary reaggravation Pharmacology ■ Anti-inflammatories ■ Nonopioid analgesics ■ Muscle relaxants
Transmission	Pharmacology ■ Local anesthetics
Modulation	Pharmacology ■ Opioids ■ Calcium channel blockers ■ NMDA-receptor antagonists ■ Anti-inflammatories ■ Nonopioid analgesics ■ Alpha-2 agonists
Perception	Patient Education Pharmacology ■ Anxiolytics ■ Antidepressants

The rationale of a multimodal approach is to achieve effective analgesia with the cumulative effects of different interventions at multiple attack points throughout all phases of the perioperative period.

pathway without the development of a chronic pain cycle. This is best accomplished by removing the noxious stimulus, in this case the tissue damage caused by the surgical procedure. While the transduction portion of the stimulus attack point may continue through the processes of local inflammation, additional noxious stimulation through tissue damage should no longer occur. Physicians are encouraged to maximize nonpharmacologic interventions to avoid secondary reaggravation of the damaged tissue and reduce the local effects of sensitization.[42]

In addition to providing a direct analgesic effect, cryotherapy, immobilization, compression, and elevation are the primary physical therapeutics that contribute to the prevention of peripheral sensitization in the postoperative setting.[192-195] Although these techniques are generally not the focus of research trials because of a relative lack of quantifiable variables, they should form the foundation of any postoperative pain management protocol. These therapies have been a constant point of emphasis throughout the history of pain management underscoring the importance of nonpharmacologic physical measures in the interruption of the physiology of pain processing.

CHRONIC PAIN IN THE PERIOPERATIVE SETTING

There are two distinct topics when considering chronic pain in the perioperative setting. The first is that chronic pain

represents a potential complication following any form of surgical intervention, even if a multimodal approach is utilized to prevent it.[102] Surgeons do not hesitate to immediately intervene when signs or symptoms of infection are present in the postoperative phase. The development of chronic pain can be just as significant as an infection, and it should be recognized and treated just as aggressively. By one estimate, 20% of patients presenting to a chronic pain clinic listed an elective surgical procedure as the initiating event of their complaint.[102] An immediate second opinion from a multidisciplinary pain clinic is strongly recommended for patients who develop persistent postoperative pain that only appears to respond to opioid use.[196,197]

A second concern is the perioperative management of an established chronic pain, opioid tolerant or addicted patient. Regardless of the patient's preoperative history, the physician needs to appreciate that surgical intervention will result in the development of acute pain physiology likely requiring additional treatment. These patients have the right to be afforded the same opportunities for pain relief as any other patient to avoid the sequelae of undertreatment. A multimodal approach with maximization of adjuvant pharmacologic and nonpharmacologic therapy should be immediately implemented in these situations, although supplemental opioid therapy is usually required for the appropriate management of these patients.[198-205]

OTHER PERIOPERATIVE PAIN MANAGEMENT CONSIDERATIONS

DOCUMENTATION

Appropriate documentation with respect to controlled substance prescription should be maintained throughout the perioperative period. The model policy established by the Federation of State Medical Boards of the United States and acknowledged by the Drug Enforcement Agency outlines six domains of appropriate documentation when controlled opioids are prescribed.[206,207] These are areas of assessment that should be documented with each patient encounter, including the operative note. The first criteria is an evaluation of the patient to include the nature and intensity of the pain, current and past treatments for pain, underlying diseases or conditions, the effect of pain on physical and psychological function, any history of substance abuse, and one or more recognized indications for the use of a controlled substance. The second criterion is a written treatment plan including clear objectives that will be used to establish the success or failure of the intervention. The third criterion is documentation of obtained informed consent detailing the alternatives, risks, and complications associated with the use of controlled substances. Fourth, periodic review should be performed incorporating objective evidence of improved or diminished function in response to continued or modified treatment. Further, the physician should be willing to obtain consultation for additional evaluation in order to achieve treatment outcomes if necessary. Finally, accurate and complete records should be maintained to demonstrate compliance with state and federal laws and regulations with respect to the use of controlled substances.

PRESCRIPTION DRUG MONITORING PROGRAMS

Although currently not available on a national basis, individual state and interstate prescription drug monitoring programs allow (and often require) physicians to query a specific patient's prescription history prior to dispensing a new prescription for a controlled substance.[208-212] This primarily allows physicians to ensure that an individual patient is not receiving multiple prescriptions from multiple providers, calculate the total amount of opioids prescribed per day (in MME/day), and identify patients who are being prescribed other substances that may increase risk of opioids—such as benzodiazepines.[212] These programs have been demonstrated to be effective in decreasing the quantity of opioid dispensements.

PREOPERATIVE OPIOID CONTRACTS

A so-called opioid contract might also be employed in the perioperative setting to establish responsibilities with respect to the prescription of controlled substances. This not only includes responsibilities of patients (they should only receive prescriptions from one provider, utilize only one pharmacy, never share, distribute, or sell prescriptions, play an active role in their therapy and consent to random drug testing) but also physicians (they should never prescribe a controlled substance without a complete evaluation, observe the patient at regular intervals, actively change medications based on patient complaints, consider a second opinion, and evaluate the patient for adverse effects).[213-215]

INSURANCE RESTRICTIONS AND OPIOID CLIFFS

A final concept is potential restrictions placed on prescribing providers by third parties including state laws, insurance companies, and pharmacies. These might dictate the quantity, duration, and specific substances that might be prescribed including the need for pre-authorization in many cases. As specific restrictions vary, physicians are encouraged to utilize resources detailing individual state laws and requirements.[216-218]

CONCLUSION

An active approach to pain management utilizes the physiologic and pathophysiologic mechanisms leading to the development of surgical pain in treatments throughout all phases of the perioperative period. Unnecessary sequelae of this expected surgical complication can be mitigated through active physician intervention. All practicing physicians and surgeons should be aware of both the ability and the obligation to utilize modern pain management approaches in the perioperative setting.

REFERENCES

1. CDC Guideline for prescribing opioids for chronic pain. https://www.cdc.gov/drugoverdose/pdf/guidelines_at-a-glance-a.pdf. Accessed March 12, 2019.
2. National Institute on Drug Abuse overdose death rates. https://www.drugabuse.gov/related-topics/trends-statistics/overdose-death-rates. Accessed March 12, 2019.
3. H.R.6—SUPPORT for Patients and Communities Act. https://www.congress.gov/bill/115th-congress/house-bill/6. Accessed March 12, 2019.
4. Bonica JJ, Loeser JD. Applied anatomy relevant to pain. In: Loeser JD, ed. *Bonica's Management of Pain*. 3rd ed. Philadelphia, PA: Lippincott Williams & Wilkins; 2001:196-221.
5. Portenoy RK, Foley KM. Chronic use of opioid analgesics in non-malignant pain: report of 38 cases. *Pain*. 1986;25(2):171-186.
6. Melzack R. The tragedy of needless pain. *Sci Am*. 1990;262(2):27-33.
7. Flansbaum B. Less than one percent of pain sufferers become addicted. https://thehospitalleader.org/less-than-one-percent-of-pain-sufferers-become-addicted. Accessed March 12, 2019.
8. Caudill-Slosbery MA, Schwartz LM, Woloshin S. Office visits and analgesic prescriptions for musculoskeletal pain in US: 1980 vs. 2000. *Pain*. 2004;109(3):514-519.
9. Olfson M, Wang S, Iza M, et al. National trends in the office-based prescription of schedule II opioids. *J Clin Psychiatry*. 2013;74(9):932-939.
10. Olsen Y, Daumit GL, Ford DE. Opioid prescriptions by U.S. primary care physicians from 1992 to 2001. *J Pain*. 2006;7(4):225-235.
11. Niv D, Devor M. Preemptive analgesia: can it prevent subacute postoperative pain? In: Raj PP, ed. *Practical Management of Pain*. 3rd ed. St. Louis, MO: Mosby; 2000:986-1000.
12. Gatchel RJ. A biopsychosocial overview of pretreatment screening of patients with pain. *Clin J Pain*. 2001;17(3):192-199.
13. Hing E, Cherry DK, Woodwell DA. National Ambulatory Medical Care Survey: 2004 summary. *Adv Data*. 2006;(374):1-33.
14. Loeser JD, Melzack R. Pain: an overview. *Lancet*. 1999;353(9164):1607-1609.
15. Helfand AE. Foot problems in older patients. A focused podogeriatric assessment study in ambulatory care. *J Am Podiatr Med Assoc*. 2004;94(3):293-304.
16. Kucharski A, Todd EM. Pain: historical perspectives. In: Warfield CA, Bajwa ZH, eds. *Principles and Practice of Pain Medicine*. 2nd ed. New York: McGraw-Hill; 2004:1-10.
17. Bonica JJ, Loeser JD. History of pain concepts and therapies. In: Loeser JD, ed. *Bonica's Management of Pain*. 3rd ed. Philadelphia, PA: Lippincott Williams & Wilkins; 2001:3-16.
18. Parris WCV. The history of pain medicine. In: Raj PP, ed. *Practical Management of Pain*. 3rd ed. St. Louis, MO: Mosby; 2000:3-9.
19. Magner LN. *A History of Medicine*. 2nd ed. Boca Raton, FL: Taylor & Francis; 2005:461-493.
20. Denney RE. *Civil War Medicine Care and Comfort of the Wounded*. New York: Sterling Publishing Co; 1994:1-400.
21. Kuusniemi K, Poyhia R. Present-day challenges and future solutions in postoperative pain management: results from PainForum 2014. *J Pain Res*. 2016;9:25-36.
22. Dexter F, Candiotti KA. Multicenter assessment of the Iowa Satisfaction with Anesthesia Scale, an instrument that measures patient satisfaction with monitored anesthesia care. *Anesth Analg*. 2011;113(2):364-368.
23. Beauregard L, Pomp A, Choiniere M. Severity and impact of pain after day-surgery. *Can J Anaesth*. 1998;45:304.
24. Strassels SA, Chen C, Carr DB. Postoperative analgesia: economics, resource use, and patient satisfaction in an urban teaching hospital. *Anesth Analg*. 2002;94:130-137.
25. Pavlin DJ, Chen C, Penaloza DA, Buckley FP. A survey of pain and other symptoms that affect the recovery process after discharge from an ambulatory surgical unit. *J Clin Anesth*. 2004;16(3):200-206.
26. Rawal N, Hylander J, Nydahl PA, et al. Survey of postoperative analgesia following ambulatory surgery. *Acta Anaesthesiol Scand*. 1997;41(8):1017-1022.
27. Gramke HF, de Rijke JM, van Kleef M, et al. The prevalence of postoperative pain in a cross-sectional group of patients after day-case surgery in a university hospital. *Clin J Pain*. 2007;23(6):543-548.
28. Apfelbaum JL, Chen C, Mehta SS, Gan TJ. Postoperative pain experience: results from a national survey suggest postoperative pain continues to be undermanaged. *Anesth Analg*. 2003;97(2):534-540.
29. Sommer M, de Rijke JM, van Kleef M, et al. Predictors of acute postoperative pain after elective surgery. *Clin J Pain*. 2010;26(2):87-94.
30. Chung F, Ritchie E, Su J. Postoperative pain in ambulatory surgery. *Anesth Analg*. 1997;85(4):808-816.
31. Crews JC. Acute pain syndromes. In: Raj PP, ed. *Practical Management of Pain*. 3rd ed. St. Louis, MO: Mosby; 2000:169-195.
32. Raj PP. The problem of postoperative pain: an epidemiologic perspective. In: Ferrante FM, VadeBoncouer TR, eds. *Postoperative Pain Management*. New York: Churchill Livingstone; 1993:1-15.
33. Engoren M. Cost-effectiveness of different postoperative analgesic treatments. *Expert Opin Pharmacother*. 2003;4(9):1507-1519.
34. Lie SS, Wu CL. The effect of analgesic technique on postoperative patient-reported outcomes including analgesia: a systematic review. *Anesth Analg*. 2007;105(3):789-808.
35. Joshi GP. Multimodal analgesia techniques and postoperative rehabilitation. *Anesthesiol Clin North America*. 2005;23(1):185-202.
36. Coda BA, Bonica JJ. General considerations of acute pain. In: Loeser JD, ed. *Bonica's Management of Pain*. 3rd ed. Philadelphia, PA: Lippincott Williams & Wilkins; 2001:222-240.
37. Joshi GP, Ogunnaike OB. Consequences of inadequate postoperative pain relief and chronic persistent postoperative pain. *Anesthesiol Clin North America*. 2005;23(1):21-36.
38. Hallivis R, Derksen TA, Meyr AJ. Peri-operative pain management. *Clin Podiatr Med Surg*. 2008;25(3):443-463.
39. Byers MR, Bonica JJ. Peripheral pain mechanisms and nociceptor plasticity. In: Loeser JD, ed. *Bonica's Management of Pain*. 3rd ed. Philadelphia, PA: Lippincott Williams & Wilkins; 2001:26-72.
40. Le Bars D, Gozariu M, Cadden SW. Animal models of nociception. *Pharmacol Rev*. 2001;53(4):597-652.
41. Devor M. Neurobiology of normal and pathophysiologic pain. In: Aranoff GM, ed. *Evaluation and Treatment of Chronic Pain*. 3rd ed. Philadelphia, PA: Lippincott Williams & Wilkins; 1999:11-25.
42. Meyr AJ, Steinberg JS. The physiology of the acute pain pathway. *Clin Podiatr Med Surg*. 2008;25(3):305-326.
43. Katz N, Ferrante FM. Nociception. In: Ferrante FM, VadeBoncouer TR, eds. *Postoperative Pain Management*. New York: Churchill Livingstone; 1993:17-67.
44. Suchdev PK. Pathophysiology of pain. In: Warfield CA, Fausett HJ, eds. *Manual of Pain Management*. Philadelphia, PA: Lippincott Williams & Wilkins; 2002:6-12.
45. Dickinson B, Altman R, Neilsen N, Williams M. Use of opioids to treat chronic, non cancer pain. *West J Med*. 2000;172(2):107-115.
46. Yaksh TL. Anatomy of the pain-processing system. In: Waldman SD, ed. *Interventional Pain Management*. 2nd ed. Philadelphia, PA: W.B. Saunders Company; 2001:11-20.
47. Fausett HJ. Anatomy and physiology of pain. In: Warfield CA, Bajwa ZH, eds. *Principles and Practice of Pain Medicine*. 2nd ed. New York: McGraw-Hill; 2004:28-34.
48. Aimone LD. Neurochemistry and modulation of pain. In: Sinastra RS, Hord AH, Ginsberg B, Preble LM, eds. *Acute Pain: Mechanisms and Management*. St. Louis, MO: Mosby Year Book; 1992:29-43.

49. Lie SS, Benzon HT. Outcomes and complications of acute pain management. In: Abrams BM, Benzon HT, Hahn MB, et al., eds. *Practical Management of Pain*. 3rd ed. St. Louis, MO: Mosby, Inc; 2000:871-889.

50. Handwerker HO, Ringkamp M, Schmelz M. Neurophysiological basis for chemogenic pain and itch. In: Boivie J, Hansson P, Lindblom U, eds. *Touch, Temperature, and Pain in Health and Disease: Mechanisms and Assessments*. Seattle, WA: IASP Press; 1994:195-206.

51. Sun Q, Tu H, Xing GG, et al. Ectopic discharges from injured nerve fibers are highly correlated with tactile allodynia only in early, but not late, stage in rates with spinal nerve ligation. *Exp Neurol*. 2005;191(1):128-136.

52. Schwartzman RJ, Grothusen J, Kiefer TR, Rohr P. Neuropathic central pain: epidemiology, etiology, and treatment options. *Arch Neurol*. 2001;58(10):1547-1550.

53. Chen Y, Devor M. Ectopic mechanosensitivity in injured sensory axons arises from the site of spontaneous. *Eur J Pain*. 1998;2(2):165-178.

54. Lisney SJ, Devor M. Afterdischarge and interactions among fibers in damaged peripheral nerve in the rat. *Brain Res*. 1987;415(1):122-136.

55. Flatters SJ. Characterization of a model of persistent postoperative pain evoked by skin/muscle incision and retraction (SMIR). *Pain*. 2008;135(1–2):119-130.

56. Bolotin G, Buckner GD, Jardine NJ, et al. A novel instrumented retractor to monitor tissue-disruptive forces during lateral thoracotomy. *J Thorac Cardiovasc Surg*. 2007;133(4):949-954.

57. Pitcher GM, Henry JL. Nociceptive response to innocuous mechanical stimulation is mediated via myelinated afferents and NK-1 activation in a rat model of neuropathic pain. *Exp Neurol*. 2004;186(2):173-197.

58. Konrad G, Markmiller M, Lenich A, et al. Tourniquets may increase postoperative swelling and pain after internal fixation of ankle fractures. *Clin Orthop Relat Res*. 2005;433:189-194.

59. Ömeroğlu H, Ucaner A, Tabak AY, et al. The relationship between the use of tourniquet and the intensity of postoperative pain in surgically treated malleolar fractures. *Foot Ankle Int*. 1997;18(12):798-802.

60. Jones SL. Anatomy of pain. In: Sinastra RS, Hord AH, Ginsberg B, Preble LM, eds. *Acute Pain: Mechanisms and Management*. St. Louis, MO: Mosby Year Book; 1992:8-28.

61. Krause WR, Bradbury DW, Kelly JE, Lunceford EM. Temperature elevations in orthopaedic cutting operations. *J Biomech*. 1982;15(4):267-275.

62. Li S, Chien S, Brånemark PI. Heat shock-induced necrosis and apoptosis in osteoblasts. *J Orthop Res*. 1999;17(6):891-899.

63. Toksvig-Larsen S, Ryd L, Lindstrand A. Temperature influence in different orthopedic saw blades. *J Arthroplasty*. 1992;7(1):21-24.

64. Piska M, Yang L, Reed M, Saleh M. Drilling efficiency and temperature elevation of three types of kirschner-wire point. *J Bone Joint Surg Br*. 2002;84(1):137-140.

65. Brisman DL. The effect of speed, pressure, and time on bone temperature during the drilling of implant sites. *Int J Oral Maxillofac Implants*. 1996;11(1):35-37.

66. Dubin A, Patpoutain A. Nociceptors: the sensors of the pain pathway. *J Clin Invest*. 2010;120(11):3760-3772.

67. Benzon H, Raja S, Molloy R, Liu S, Fishman S. *Essentials of Pain Medicine and Regional Anesthesia*. 2nd ed. Philadelphia, PA: Elsevier; 2005:1-5.

68. Wall PD, Melzack R. *Textbook of Pain*. Edinburgh, Scotland: Churchill Livingstone; 1994.

69. Melzack R, Wall PD. Evolution of pain theories. *Int Anesthesiol Clin*. 1970;8(1):3-34.

70. Deleo JA. Basic science of pain. *J Bone Joint Surg Am*. 2006;88(suppl 2):58-62.

71. Woolf CJ, Doubell TP. The pathophysiology of chronic pain—increased sensitivity to low threshold A beta-fibre inputs. *Curr Opin Neurobiol*. 1994;4(4):525-534.

72. Jensen MP, Karoly P. Self-report scales and procedures for assessing pain in adults. In: Turk DC, Melzack R, eds. *Handbook of Pain Assessment*. 2nd ed. New York: The Guilford Press; 2001:15-29.

73. Jackson T, Iezzi T, Chen H, et al. Gender, interpersonal transactions, and the perception of pain: an experimental analysis. *J Pain*. 2005;6(4):228-236.

74. Kállai I, Barke A, Voss U. The effects of experimenter characteristics on pain reports in women and men. *Pain*. 2004;112(1–2):142-147.

75. Levine FM, De Simone LL. The effects of experimenter gender on pain report in male and female subjects. *Pain*. 1991;44(1):69-72.

76. Unruh AM. Spirituality, religion, and pain. *Can J Nurs Res*. 2007;39(2):66-86.

77. Chen AC, Dworkin SF, Haug J, Gehrig J. Human pain responsivity in a tonic pain model: psychological determinants. *Pain*. 1989;37(2):143-160.

78. Folkard S, Glynn CJ, Lloyd JW. Diurnal variation and individual differences in the perception of intractable pain. *J Psychosom Res*. 1976;20(4):289-301.

79. Meyr AJ, Saffran B. The pathophysiology of the chronic pain cycle. *Clin Podiatr Med Surg*. 2008;25(3):327-346.

80. Jacobson L, Mariano AJ. General considerations of chronic pain. In: Loeser JD, ed. *Bonica's Management of Pain*. 3rd ed. Philadelphia, PA: Lippincott Williams & Wilkins; 2001:241-254.

81. Niv D, Devor M. Transition from acute to chronic pain. In: Aronoff GM, ed. *Evaluation and Treatment of Chronic Pain*. 3rd ed. Philadelphia, PA: Lippincott Williams & Wilkins; 1998:27-45.

82. Reuben SS, Buvanendran A. Preventing the development of chronic pain after orthopedic surgery with preventative multimodal analgesic techniques. *J Bone Joint Surg Am*. 2007;89:1343-1358.

83. Wilder-Smith OH. Changes in sensory processing after surgical nociception. *Curr Rev Pain*. 2000;4(3):234-241.

84. Graven-Nielsen T, Mense S. The peripheral apparatus of muscle pain: evidence from animal and human studies. *Clin J Pain*. 2001;17(1):2-10.

85. Bolay H, Moskowitz MA. Mechanisms of pain modulation in chronic syndromes. *Neurology*. 2002;59(5 suppl 2):S2-S7.

86. Bhave G, Gereau RW. Posttranslational mechanisms of peripheral sensitization. *J Neurobiol*. 2004;61(1):88-106.

87. Katz WA, Rothenberg R. Section 3: the nature of pain: pathophysiology. *J Clin Rheumatol*. 2005;11(2 suppl):S11-S15.

88. Omoigui S. The biochemical origin of pain: the origin of all pain is inflammation and the inflammatory response. Part 1 of 3—a unifying law of pain. *Med Hypotheses*. 2007;69(1):70-82.

89. Omoigui S. The biochemical origin of pain: the origin of all pain is inflammation and the inflammatory response. Part 2 of 3—inflammatory profile of pain syndromes. *Med Hypotheses*. 2007;69(6):1169-1178.

90. Katz EJ, Gold MS. Inflammatory hyperalgesia: a role for the C-fiber sensory neuron cell body? *J Pain*. 2006;7(3):170-178.

91. Jensen TS, Finnerup NB. Allodynia and hyperalgesia in neuropathic pain: clinical manifestations and mechanisms. *Lancet Neurol*. 2014;13(9):924-935.

92. Cohen SA. Pathophysiology of pain. In: Raj PP, ed. *Practical Management of Pain*. 3rd ed. St. Louis, MO: Mosby; 2000:35-48.

93. Vikman KS, Kristensson K, Hill RH. Sensitization of dorsal horn neurons in a two-compartment cell culture model: wind-up and long-term potentiation-like responses. *J Neurosci*. 2001;21(19):RC169.

94. Eide PK. Wind-up and the NMDA receptor complex from a clinical perspective. *Eur J Pain*. 2000;4(1):5-15.

95. Traub RJ. Spinal modulation of the induction of central sensitization. *Brain Res*. 1997;778(1):34-42.

96. Klede M, Handwerker HO, Schmelz M. Central origin of secondary mechanical hyperalgesia. *J Neurophysiol*. 2003;90(1):353-359.

97. Blunk J, Osiander G, Nischik M, Schmelz M. Pain and inflammatory hyperalgesia induced by intradermal injections of human platelets and leukocytes. *Eur J Pain*. 1999;3(3):247-259.

98. Kawamata M, Watanabe H, Nishikawa K, et al. Different mechanisms of development and maintenance of experimental incision-induced hyperalgesia in human skin. *Anesthesiology*. 2002;97(3):550-559.

99. Li X, Conkin D, Ma W, et al. Spinal noradrenergic activation mediates allodynia reduction from an allosteric adenosine modulator in a rat model of neuropathic pain. *Pain*. 2002;97(1–2):117-125.

100. Minami T, Matsumura S, Okuda-Ashitaka E, et al. Characterization of the glutamatergic system for induction and maintenance of allodynia. *Brain Res*. 2001;895(1–2):178-185.

101. Gottrup H, Nielsen J, Arendt-Nielsen L, Jensen TS. The relationship between sensory thresholds and mechanical hyperalgesia in nerve injury. *Pain*. 1998;75(2–3):321-329.

102. Macrae WA, Davies HTO. Chronic postsurgical pain. In: Crombie IK, Croft PR, Linton SJ, LeResche L, Von Korff M, eds. *Epidemiology of Pain*. Seattle, WA: IASP Press; 1999:125-142.

103. Manchikanti L. Evidence-based medicine, systemic reviews and guidelines in interventional pain management, part 1: introduction and general considerations. *Pain Physician*. 2008;11(2):161-186.

104. Kissin I. Preemptive analgesia. *Anesthesiology*. 2000;93:1138-1143.

105. Moiniche S, Kehlet H, Dahl JB. A qualitative and quantitative systematic review of preemptive analgesia for postoperative pain relief: the role of timing of analgesia. *Anesthesiology*. 2002;96:725-741.

106. Ong CK, Lirk P, Seymour RA, Jenkins BJ. The efficacy of preemptive analgesia for acute postoperative pain management: a meta-analysis. *Anesth Analg*. 2005;100:757-773.

107. Breivik H. Local anaesthetic blocks and epidurals. In: McMahon SB, Koltzenburg M, eds. *Wall and Melzack's Textbook of Pain*. 5th ed. Philadelphia, PA: Elsevier Churchill Livingstone; 2006:507-519.

108. Turk DC, Melzack R. The measurement of pain and assessment of people experiencing pain. In: Turk DC, Melzack R, eds. *Handbook of Pain Assessment*. 2nd ed. New York: The Guildford Press; 2001:3-11.

109. Marcus DA. Pathogenesis of chronic pain. In: Marcus DA, ed. *Chronic Pain: A Primary Care Guide to Practical Management*. Totowa, NJ: Humana Press; 2005:17-28.

110. Pour AE, Parvizi J, Sharkey PF, et al. Minimally invasive hip arthroplasty: what role does patient preconditioning play? *J Bone Joint Surg Am*. 2007;89(9):1920-1927.

111. McDonald S, Hetrick S, Green S. Pre-operative education for hip or knee replacement. *Cochrane Database Syst Rev*. 2004;(1):CD003526.

112. Bondy LR, Sims N, Schroeder DR, et al. The effect of anesthetic patient education on preoperative patient anxiety. *Reg Anesth Pain Med*. 1999;24(2):158-164.

113. Gocen Z, Sen A, Unver B, et al. The effect of preoperative physiotherapy and education on the outcome of total hip replacement: a prospective randomized controlled trial. *Clin Rehabil*. 2004;18(4):353-358.

114. Ciccozzi A, Marinangeli F, Colangeli A, et al. Anxiolysis and postoperative pain in patients undergoing spinal anesthesia for abdominal hysterectomy. *Minerva Anestesiol*. 2007;73(7–8):387-393.

115. Phero JC, Becker DE, Dionne RA. Contemporary trends in acute pain management. *Curr Opin Otolaryngol Head Neck Surg*. 2004;12:209-216.

116. Sinatra RS, Torres J, Bustos AM. Pain management after major orthopedic surgery: current strategies and new concepts. *J Am Acad Orthop Surg*. 2002;10(2):117-129.

117. Reuben SS, Steinberg RB, Maciolek H, Joshi W. Preoperative administration of controlled-release oxycodone for the management of pain after ambulatory laparoscopic tubal ligation surgery. *J Clin Anesth*. 2002;14(3):223-227.

118. Woolf CJ, Chong MS. Preemptive analgesia—treating postoperative pain by preventing the establishment of central sensitization. *Anesth Analg*. 1993;77(2):362-379.

119. McQuay HJ, Carroll D, Moore RA. Postoperative orthopaedic pain—the effect of opiate premedication and local anaesthetic blocks. *Pain*. 1988;33(3):291-295.

120. Stein C. The control of pain in peripheral tissue by opioids. *N Engl J Med*. 1995;332(25):1685-1690.

121. Somogyi AA, Barratt DT, Coller JK. Pharmacogenetics of opioids. *Clin Pharmacol Ther*. 2007;81(3):429-444.

122. Sawynok J. Topical and peripherally acting analgesics. *Pharmacol Rev*. 2003;55(1):1-20.

123. Ventafridda V, Saita L, Ripamonti C, De Conno F. WHO guidelines for the use of analgesics in cancer pain. *Int J Tissue React*. 1985;7(1):93-96.

124. World Health Organization. Pain relief ladder. https://www.who.int/cancer/palliative/painladder/en/. Accessed March 12, 2019.

125. Bourne MH. Analgesics for orthopedic postoperative pain. *Am J Orthop.* 2004;33(3):1128-1135.
126. Viscusi ER. Emerging techniques for postoperative analgesia in orthopedic surgery. *Am J Orthop.* 2004;33(5 suppl):13-16.
127. Montane E, Vallano A, Aguilera C, et al. Analgesics for pain after traumatic or orthopedic surgery: what is the evidence—a systematic review. *Eur J Clin Pharmacol.* 2006;62(11):971-988.
128. Quigley C, Wiffen P. A systematic review of hydromorphone in acute and chronic pain. *J Pain Symptom Manage.* 2003;25(2):169-178.
129. Schnitzer TJ. Update on guidelines for the treatment of chronic musculoskeletal pain. *Clin Rheumatol.* 2006;25(suppl 1):S22-S29.
130. Ekman EF, Koman LA. Acute pain following musculoskeletal injuries and orthopaedic surgery: mechanisms and management. *J Bone Joint Surg Am.* 2004;86:1316-1327.
131. Reuben SS, Ekman EF, Raghunathan K, et al. The effect of cyclooxygenase-2 inhibition on acute and chronic donor-site pain after spinal-fusion surgery. *Reg Anesth Pain Med.* 2006;31(1):6-13.
132. Buvanendran A, Kroin JS, Tuman KJ, et al. Effects of perioperative administration of a selective cyclooxygenase 2 inhibitor on pain management and recovery of function after knee replacement: a randomized controlled trial. *JAMA.* 2003;290(18):2411-2418.
133. Desjardins PJ, Black PM, Daneils S, et al. A randomized controlled study comparing rofecoxib, diclofenac sodium, and placebo in post-bunionectomy pain. *Curr Med Res Opin.* 2004;20(10):1523-1537.
134. Desjardins PJ, Traylor L, Hubbard RC. Analgesic efficacy of preoperative parecoxib sodium in an orthopedic pain model. *J Am Podiatr Med Assoc.* 2004;94(3):305-314.
135. Reuben SS, Ekman EF. The effect of cyclooxygenase-2 inhibition on analgesia and spinal fusion. *J Bone Joint Surg Am.* 2005;87(3):536-542.
136. Endo K, Sairyo K, Komatsubara S, et al. Cyclooxygenase-2 inhibitor delays fracture healing in rats. *Acta Orthop.* 2005;76(4):470-474.
137. Keller J, Bunger C, Andreassen TT, et al. Bone repair inhibited by indomethacin: effects on bone metabolism and strength of rabbit osteotomies. *Acta Orthop Scand.* 1987;58(4):379-383.
138. Dahners LE, Mullis BH. Effects of nonsteroidal anti-inflammatory drugs on bone formation and soft-tissue healing. *J Am Acad Orthop Surg.* 2004;12(3):139-143.
139. Bo J, Sudmann E, Marton PF. Effect of indomethacin on fracture healing in rats. *Acta Orthop Scand.* 1976;47(6):588-599.
140. Harder AT, An YH. The mechanisms of the inhibitory effects of nonsteroidal anti-inflammatory drugs on bone healing: a concise review. *J Clin Pharmacol.* 2003;43(8):807-815.
141. Wheatley BM, Nappo KE, Christensen DL, et al. Effect of NSAIDs on bone healing rates: a meta-analysis. *J Am Acad Orthop Surg.* 2019;27:e330-e336.
142. Dodwell ER, Latorre JG, Parisini E, et al. NSAID exposure and risk of nonunion: a meta-analysis of case–control and cohort studies. *Calcif Tissue Int.* 2010;87(3):193-202.
143. Wallace MS. Calcium and sodium channel antagonists for the treatment of pain. *Clin J Pain.* 2000;16(2 suppl):S80-S85.
144. Yaksh TL. Calcium channels as therapeutic targets in neuropathic pain. *J Pain.* 2006;7(1 suppl 1):S13-S30.
145. Nelson MT, Todorovic SM. Is there a role for T-type calcium channels in peripheral and central sensitization? *Mol Neurobiol.* 2006;34(3):243-248.
146. Dahl JB, Mathiesen O, Moiniche S. 'Protective premedication': an option with gabapentin and related drugs? A review of gabapentin and pregabalin in the treatment of post-operative pain. *Acta Anaesthesiol Scand.* 2004;48(9):1130-1136.
147. Luo ZD, Chaplan SR, Higuera ES, et al. Upregulation of dorsal root ganglion (alpha)2(delta) calcium channel subunit and its correlation with allodynia in spinal nerve-injured rats. *J Neurosci.* 2001;21(6):1868-1875.
148. Hurley RW, Cohen SP, Williams KA, et al. The analgesic effects of perioperative gabapentin on postoperative pain: a meta-analysis. *Reg Anesth Pain Med.* 2006;31(3):237-247.
149. Gilron I. Gabapentin and pregabalin for chronic neuropathic and early postsurgical pain: current evidence and future directions. *Curr Opin Anaesthesiol.* 2007;20(5):456-472.
150. Pandey CK, Navkar DV, Giri PJ, et al. Evaluation of the optimal preemptive dose of gabapetin for postoperative pain relief after lumbar diskectomy: a randomized double-blind, placebo-controlled study. *J Neurosurg Anesthesiol.* 2005;17(2):65-68.
151. Montazeri K, Kashefi P, Honarmand A. Pre-emptive gabapentin significantly reduces postoperative pain and morphine demand following lower extremity orthopaedic surgery. *Singapore Med J.* 2007;48(8):748-751.
152. Li F, Ma J, Kuang M, et al. The efficacy of pregabalin for the management of postoperative pain in primarily total knee and hip arthroplasty: a meta-analysis. *J Orthop Surg Res.* 2017;12(1):49.
153. Lam DM, Choi SW, Wong SS, et al. Efficacy of pregabalin in acute postoperative pain under different surgical categories: a meta-analysis. *Medicine (Baltimore).* 2015;94(46):e1944.
154. Yadeau JT, Paroli L, Kahn RL, et al. Addition of pregabalin to mutlimodal analgesic therapy following ankle surgery: a randomized double-blind, placebo-controlled trial. *Reg Anesth Pain Med.* 2012;37(3):302-307.
155. Lucas R, Warner TD, Vojnovic I, Mitchell JA. Cellular mechanisms of acetaminophen: role of cyclo-oxygenase. *Faseb J.* 2005;19:635-637.
156. Mitchell JA, Akarasereenont P, Thiemermann C, et al. Selectivity of nonsteroidal antiinflammatory drugs as inhibitors of constitutive and inducible cyclooxygenase. *Proc Natl Acad Sci.* 1993;90:11693-11697.
157. Vadivelu N, Sukanya M, Narayan, D. Recent advances in postoperative pain management. *Yale J Biol Med.* 2010;83(1):11-25.
158. Pickering G, Loriot MA, Libert F, et al. Analgesic effect of acetaminophen in humans: first evidence of a central serotonergic mechanism. *Clin Pharmacol Ther.* 2006;79:371-378.
159. Lachiewicz P. The role of intravenous acetaminophen in multimodal pain protocol for perioperative orthopedic patients. *Orthopedics.* 2013;36(2):15-19.
160. Woolf CJ. The pathophysiology of peripheral neuropathic pain-abnormal peripheral input and abnormal central processing. *Acta Neurochir Suppl.* 1993;58:125-130.
161. Persson J, Axelsson G, Hallin RG, Gustafsson LL. Beneficial effects of ketamine in a chronic pain state with allodynia, possibly due to central sensitization. *Pain.* 1995;60(2):217-222.
162. Schmid RL, Sandler AN, Katz J. Use and efficacy of low-dose ketamine in the management of acute postoperative pain: a review of current techniques and outcomes. *Pain.* 1999;82(2):111-125.
163. Subramaniam K, Subramaniam B, Steinbrook RA. Ketamine as adjuvant analgesic to opioids: a quantitative and qualitative systematic review. *Anesth Analg.* 2004;99(2):482-495.
164. Tverskoy M, Oren M, Vaskovich M, et al. Ketamine enhances local anesthetic and analgesic effects of bupivacaine by peripheral mechanism: a study in postoperative patients. *Neurosci Lett.* 1996;215(1):5-8.
165. Wang X, Xie H, Wang G. Improved postoperative analgesia with coadministration of preoperative epidural ketamine and midazolam. *J Clin Anesth.* 2006;18(8):563-569.
166. Benzon H, Shah R, Benzon HT. Perioperative nonopioid infusions for postoperative pain management. In: Benzon HT, Raja SN, Fishman SM, Liu SS, Cohen SP, eds. *Essentials of Pain Medicine.* 4th ed. Philadelphia, PA: Elsevier; 2018:111-116.
167. Adams HA, Saatweber P, Schmitz CS, Hecker H. Postoperative pain management in orthopaedic patients: no differences in pain score, but improved stress control by epidural anaesthesia. *Eur J Anaesthesiol.* 2002;19:658-665.
168. Peeters-Asdourian C. Acute pain. In: Warfield CA, Fausett HJ, eds. *Manual of Pain Management.* 2nd ed. Philadelphia, PA: Lippincott Williams and Wilkins; 2002:215-222.
169. Capdevila X, Barthelet Y, Biboulet P, et al. Effects of perioperative analgesic technique on the surgical outcome and duration of rehabilitation after major knee surgery. *Anesthesiology.* 1999;91(1):8-15.
170. Slowikowski RD, Flaherty SA. Epidural analgesia for postoperative orthopaedic pain. *Orthop Nurs.* 2000;19(1):23-31.
171. Chelly JE, Ben-David B, Williams BA, Kentor ML. Anesthesia and postoperative analgesia: outcomes following orthopedic surgery. *Orthopedics.* 2003;26(8 suppl):S865-S871.
172. Reinhart DJ, Stagg KS, Walker KG, et al. Postoperative analgesia after peripheral nerve block for podiatric surgery: clinical efficacy and chemical stability of lidocaine along versus lidocaine plus ketorolac. *Reg Anesth Pain Med.* 2000;25(5):506-513.
173. Gentili M, Bernard JM, Bonnet F. Adding clonidine to lidocaine for intravenous regional anesthesia prevents tourniquet pain. *Anesth Analg.* 1999;88(6):1327-1330.
174. Gorgias NK, Maidatsi PG, Kyriakidis AM, et al. Clonidine versus ketamine to prevent tourniquet pain during intravenous regional anesthesia with lidocaine. *Reg Anesth Pain Med.* 2001;26(6):512-517.
175. Lysakowski C, Dumont L, Czarnetzki C, Tramèr MR. Magnesium as an adjuvant to postoperative analgesia: a systemic review of randomized trials. *Anesth Analg.* 2007;104(6):1532-1539.
176. Reilley TE, Gerhardt MA. Anesthesia for foot and ankle surgery. *Clin Podiatr Med Surg.* 2002;19(1):125-147.
177. Enneking FK, Chan V, Greger J, et al. Lower-extremity peripheral nerve blockade: essentials of our current understanding. *Reg Anesth Pain Med.* 2005;30(1):4-35.
178. Klein SM, Evans H, Nielsen KC, et al. Peripheral nerve block techniques for ambulatory surgery. *Anesth Analg.* 2005;101(6):1663-1676.
179. Ivanusic JJ. The evidence for the spinal segmental innervation of bone. *Clin Anat.* 2007;20(8):956-960.
180. Kellgren JH. Deep pain sensibility. *Lancet.* 1949;1(23):943-949.
181. Inman VT, Saunders JB. Anatomicophysiological aspects of injuries to the intervertebral disc. *J Bone Joint Surg Am.* 1947;29:461-534.
182. Bonica JJ, Cailliet R, Loeser JD. General considerations of pain in the neck and upper limb. In: Loeser JD, Butler SH, Chapman CR, Turk DC, eds. *Bonica's Management of Pain.* 3rd ed. Philadelphia, PA: Lippincott Williams & Wilkins; 2001:983-1002.
183. Goss K. Lower extremity regional anesthesia with the low sciatic nerve block. *Clin Podiatr Med Surg.* 2008;25(3):431-441.
184. Migues A, Slullitel G, Vescovo A, et al. Peripheral foot blockade versus popliteal fossa nerve block: a prospective randomized trial in 51 patients. *J Foot Ankle Surg.* 2005;44(5):354-357.
185. Provenzano DA, Viscusi ER, Adams SB Jr, et al. Safety and efficacy of the popliteal fossa nerve block when utilized for foot and ankle surgery. *Foot Ankle Int.* 2002;23(5):394-399.
186. Zaric D, Boysen K, Christiansen J, et al. Continuous popliteal sciatic nerve block for outpatient foot surgery-a randomized, controlled trial. *Acta Anaesthesiol Scand.* 2004;48(3):337-341.
187. McLeod DH, Wong DH, Vaghadia H, et al. Lateral popliteal sciatic nerve block compared with ankle block for analgesia following foot surgery. *Can J Anaesth.* 1995;42(9):765-769.
188. Chou R, Gordon DB, de Leon-Casasola PA, et al. Management of postoperative pain: a clinical practice guidelines from the American Pain Society of Regional Anesthesia and Pain Medicine, and the American Society of Anesthesiologists' Committee on Regional Anesthesia, Executive Committee, and Administrative Council. *J Pain.* 2016;17(2):131-157.
189. American Society of Anesthesiologists Task Force on Acute Pain Management. Practice guidelines for acute pain management in the perioperative setting: an updated report by the American Society of Anesthesiologists Task Force on Acute Pain Management. *Anesthesiology.* 2012;116(2):248-273.
190. See S, Ginzburg R. Skeletal muscle relaxants. *Pharmacotherapy.* 2008;28(2):207-213.
191. Sullivan WJ, Panagos A, Foye PM, et al. Industrial medicine and acute musculoskeletal rehabilitation: medications for the treatment of acute musculoskeletal pain. *Arch Phys Med Rehabil.* 2007;88(3 suppl 1):S10-S13.
192. Adams ML, Arminio GJ. Non-pharmacologic pain management intervention. *Clin Podiatr Med Surg.* 2008;25(3):409-429.
193. Waldman SD, Waldman KA, Waldman HJ. Therapeutic heat and cold in the management of pain. In: Waldman SD, ed. *Pain Management,* Volume 2. Philadelphia, PA: Saunders Elsevier; 2007:1033-1042.
194. Wright A, Sluka KA. Nonpharmacological treatment for musculoskeletal pain. *Clin J Pain.* 2001;17(1):33-46.

195. Helfand AE. Physical modalities in the management of mild to moderate foot pain. *Clin Podiatr Med Surg.* 1994;11(1):107-123.

196. Sherlekar S. Pain management clinics. *Clin Podiatr Med Surg.* 2008;25(3):477-491.

197. Nicholas MK. When to refer to a pain clinic. *Best Pract Res Clin Rheumatol.* 2004;18(4):613-629.

198. Althari HK, Keplinger M, Bobbitt KL. Understanding addiction: the orthopedic surgical perspective to a significant problem. *Clin Podiatr Med Surg.* 2008;25(3):493-515.

199. Tucker C. Acute pain and substance abuse in surgical patients. *J Neurosci Nurs.* 1990;22(6):339-349.

200. Gilson AM, Joranson DE. U.S. policies relevant to the prescribing of opioid analgesics for the treatment of pain in patients with addictive disease. *Clin J Pain.* 2002;18(4 suppl):S91-S98.

201. Wesson DR, Ling W, Smith DE. Prescription of opioids for treatment of pain in patients with addictive disease. *J Pain Symptom Manage.* 1993;8(5):289-296.

202. Peng PW, Tumber PS, Gourlay D. Review article: perioperative pain management of patients on methadone therapy. *Can J Anesth.* 2005;52(5):513-523.

203. Schultz JE. The integration of medical management with recovery. *J Psychoactive Drugs.* 1997;29(3):233-237.

204. Alford DP, Compton P, Samet JH. Acute pain management for patients receiving maintenance methadone or buprenorphine therapy. *Ann Intern Med.* 2006;144(2):127-134.

205. Passik SD, Kirsh KL. Opioid therapy in patients with a history of substance abuse. *CNS Drugs.* 2004;18(1):13-25.

206. Federation of State Medical Boards of the United States. Model guidelines for the use of controlled substances for the treatment of pain. May 1998. https://www.ihs.gov/pain-management/includes/themes/newihstheme/display_objects/documents/modelpolicytreatmentpain.pdf. Accessed March 12, 2019.

207. Passik SD, Kirsh KL. Protecting your practice: appropriate documentation for pain management. In: McCarberg B, Passik SD, eds. *Expert Guide to Pain Management.* Philadelphia, PA: American College of Physicians; 2005:299-308.

208. Soelberg CD, Brown RE Jr, Du Vivier D, et al. The US opioid crisis: current federal and state legal issues. *Anesth Analg.* 2017;125(5):1675-1681.

209. Winstanley EL, Zhang Y, Mashni R, et al. Mandatory review of a prescription drug monitoring program and impact on opioid and benzodiazepine dispensing. *Drug Alcohol Depend.* 2018;188:169-174.

210. Davis CS, Johnston JE, Pierce MW. Overdose epidemic, prescription monitoring programs, and public health: a review of state laws. *Am J Public Health.* 2015;105(11):e9-e11.

211. Moyo P, Simoni-Wastila L, Griffin BA, et al. Impact of prescription drug monitoring programs (PDMPs) on opioid utilization among Medicare beneficiaries in 10 US states. *Addiction.* 2017;112(10):1784-1796.

212. Centers for Disease Control and Prevention. Prescription Drug Monitoring Programs. https://www.cdc.gov/drugoverdose/pdf/pdmp_factsheet-a.pdf. Accessed March 12, 2019.

213. Fishman SM, Kreis PG. The opioid contract. *Clin J Pain.* 2002;18(4 suppl):S70-S75.

214. Vadivelu N, Kai AM, Kodumudi V, et al. Pain management of patients with substance abuse in the ambulatory setting. *Curr Pain Headache Rep.* 2017;21(2):9.

215. Meyr AJ, Steinberg JS. Legal aspects of podiatric pain management. *J Am Podiatr Med Assoc.* 2010;100(6):511-517.

216. Center for Disease Control Public Health Law Program Prescription Drugs module. https://www.cdc.gov/phlp/publications/topic/prescription.html. Accessed March 12, 2019.

217. Center for Disease Control Public Health Law Program Prescription Drug Time and Dosage Limit Laws. https://www.cdc.gov/phlp/docs/menu_prescriptionlimits.pdf. Accessed March 12, 2019.

218. American Podiatric Medical Association Opioid Use and Abuse Prevention Resources. https://www.apma.org/PracticingDPMs/content.cfm?ItemNumber=26349. Accessed March 12, 2019.

CHAPTER 5

Complex Regional Pain Syndrome

Naohiro Shibuya and Daniel C. Jupiter

DEFINITION

Complex regional pain syndrome (CRPS) "describes an array of painful conditions that are characterized by a continuing (spontaneous and/or evoked) regional pain that is seemingly disproportionate in time or degree to the usual course of any known trauma or other lesion. The pain is regional (not in a specific nerve territory or dermatome) and usually has a distal predominance of abnormal sensory, motor, sudomotor, vasomotor, and/or trophic findings."[1] This general definition was created by an international consensus panel that met in Budapest, Hungary in 2003. The definition was evolved from their original criteria developed in 1994.[2] Since then, a workshop conducted by experts was conducted in Budapest to establish new clinical criteria, which were turned in to the International Association for the Study of Pain (IASP) to be published by the IASP press.[3] Since then, the criteria have gone through a series of validation processes. In the past, the condition has been referred to as regional sympathetic dystrophy, causalgia, Sudeck atrophy/dystrophy, shoulder/hand syndrome, algodystrophy, transient osteoporosis, and/or posttraumatic dystrophy. These terms are often used interchangeably; however, each describes a different subtype, stage, and clinical finding of CRPS.

In foot and ankle, CRPS is common after injuries and surgeries, and it can result in devastating and debilitating condition.[4] It causes diffuse pain beyond the area of injury or surgery. The condition usually initiates from some form of traumatic stimuli, including injury and surgical intervention.[5,6] Patients with this condition also often complain of edema, erythema, sudomotor, and motor dysfunctions.[5,7,8] Prognosis of this condition is fair when treated early but becomes poor when it becomes chronic.[4,9-11] It has been shown that the high percentage of cases of this condition can involve lawsuits and worker's compensation cases.[12]

Although epidemiology of this condition is not well understood, a few population studies have reported that the condition can present in 5.5-26 per 100 000 persons per year in the general population.[5,13] Bruehl translated these results to the U.S. population and estimated that the incidence of CRPS in the United States is ~50 000 new cases annually.[14] Within the populations studied, female gender of postmenopausal ages has been shown to have higher incidence of this condition. Fractures and sprains are the most common inciting events resulting in CRPS.

Who Is At Risk?

- Postmenopausal female
- Patient with history of CRPS
- Patient after trauma (ie, fracture and sprain)
- Patient with chronic pain
- Patient under stress/anxiety
- Patient undergoing surgery

Foot and ankle surgeons encounter many patients with musculoskeletal and neuropathic pain every day; therefore, identification of CRPS among all of these patients with similar symptoms can be difficult. Yet, delay in diagnosis of this condition can result in worse prognosis; therefore, understanding clinical criteria and classification of the condition are essential to effective treatments. In addition, prevention of this condition in elective surgical patients as well as effective systematic treatment for this condition are critical skills that the foot and ankle surgeon should possess for providing comprehensive foot and ankle care.

CLASSIFICATION

The condition has been traditionally classified in terms of types and staging. Types are based on integrity of the nerve. When there is no major nerve damage, it is considered type 1 CRPS, often referred to as reflex sympathetic dystrophy (RSD). When there is evidence for major nerve damage, it is classified as type 2 CRPS, often referred as causalgia. When patients who do not belong to either of these types, they are placed into the "not otherwise specified (NOS)" group. While popular, this classification is based on subjective assessment of condition of the nerve, and often this distinction does not provide any clinically significant information, including treatment regimen. Also, the definition of "major nerve damage" is not well documented.

The other classification system depicts different stages of the CRPS process. Historically, it was suggested that the condition progresses to different stages as duration of the condition increases. In the acute phase, it was believed that the condition was inflammatory, often accompanied with edema and redness. In this stage, it was thought that the prognosis was better than that of more chronic stages. It was believed that CRPS in the acute phase progressed to the dystrophic phase, where the inflammation subsided and patients lost mobility. This led to the final, dystrophic stage, where the foot or ankle became cold and mottled. The prognosis was believed to be guarded at this stage.

Despite this classic belief, more recent population studies have shown that this sequential staging is not well established. Bruehl et al. studied 113 CRPS patients, diagnosed with the IASP criteria, and found three distinctive subtypes in the cohort: vasomotor predominating, neurological predominating, and "classic RSD."[15] The "classic RSD" group had the most trophic and motor changes, with the lowest bone density. However, duration of pain was similar between all the subgroups, suggesting that the sequential staging may not be fully supported. On the other hand, progression of "hot" CRPS to "cold" CRPS is common,[16] though duration of each phase may vary between patients.[3] Therefore, while the progression of CRPS may still exist, some CRPS may not follow the exact sequence, and certainly the duration of each stage can vary significantly.

CLASSIFICATION BY CONDITION OF THE NERVE

- Type 1: RSD—No sign of nerve damage
- Type 2: Causalgia—Evidence of nerve damage
- NOS: Not otherwise specified

CLASSIFICATION BY SEQUENTIAL STAGING

- Acute
- Dystrophic
- Atrophic

CLASSIFICATION BY CLUSTERING

- Vasomotor predominating
- Neuropathic pain/sensory abnormality predominating
- "Classic RSD"

PHYSICAL EXAMINATION

Original International Association for the Study of Pain Criteria[17]

- The presence of an initiating noxious event or a cause of immobilization.
- Continuing pain, allodynia or hyperalgesia with which the pain is disproportionate to any inciting event.
- Evidence at some time of edema, changes in skin blood flow, or abnormal sudomotor activity in the region of pain.
- This diagnosis is excluded by the existence of conditions that would otherwise account for the degree of pain and dysfunction.

Budapest Criteria

- Continuing pain, which is disproportionate to any inciting event
- Must report at least one symptom in three of the four following categories:
  - Sensory: Reports of hyperalgesia and/or allodynia
  - Vasomotor: Reports of temperature asymmetry and/or skin color changes and/or skin color asymmetry
  - Sudomotor/edema: Reports of edema and/or sweating changes and/or sweating asymmetry
  - Motor/trophic: Reports of decreased range of motion and/or motor dysfunction (weakness, tremor, dystonia)
- Must display at least one sign at time of evaluation in two or more of the following categories
  - Sensory: Evidence of hyperalgesia (to pinprick) and/or allodynia (to light touch and/or deep somatic pressure and/or joint movement)
  - Vasomotor: Evidence of temperature asymmetry (>1°C) and/or skin color changes and/or asymmetry
  - Sudomotor/edema: Evidence of edema and/or sweating changes and/or sweating asymmetry
  - Motor/trophic: Evidence of decreased range of motion and/or motor dysfunction (weakness, tremor, dystonia) and/or trophic changes (hair, nail, skin)
- There is no other diagnosis that better explains the sign and symptoms.

Veldeman Criteria

1. Four or five of
   - Unexplained or diffuse pain
   - Difference in skin color relative to other limb
   - Diffuse edema
   - Difference in skin temperature relative to other limb
   - Limited active range of motion
2. Occurrence or increase of above signs and symptoms after use
3. Above signs and symptoms present in an area larger than the area of primary injury or operation and including the area distal to the primary injury

The diagnosis of CRPS is mainly made by clinical examination. There are several physical factors that foot and ankle surgeons should be looking for in patients for diagnosing CRPS. Again, early detection of the condition is needed for better prognosis.

To assist in diagnosing this condition, surgeons should use well-validated clinical criteria. There are several useful clinical criteria available. These criteria have evolved over years to guide physicians to diagnose CRPS with higher accuracy. Many population studies with effort to cluster and categorize patients into subtypes helped identify specific clinical signs to be included in the criteria, to improve both sensitivity and specificity. Major guidelines such as American Academy of Pain Medicine,[3] Netherlands guideline on CRPS-1,[18] and British guidelines by the Royal College of Physicians[19] all list useful clinical diagnosis criteria, which can be used in a clinical practice. The Netherland's guideline advocates the use of Veldeman criteria, while many others list the Budapest criteria, which evolved from their original International Association of Study of Pain criteria.

While they differ from each other, these criteria have similar key physical features that should be identified by a surgeon in order to diagnose CRPS. Across all the criteria, they describe neurological findings, trophic changes, motor abnormalities, and vasomotor dysfunction to be key findings for this condition. Identifying some or all of these key features is required to detect this condition. While some criteria are stricter, some are less so, in order to make sure that the condition is not underdiagnosed. While stricter criteria (which require more matching physical findings to diagnose CRPS) can provide better specificity, they can potentially miss some patients with CRPS. Therefore, many criteria are made less strict to maximize their sensitivity to avoid potential delay in treatment. On the other hand, stricter criteria are useful for the purpose of research, where underdiagnosing is not as critical, but overdiagnosing can result in selection bias for the study. The Budapest criteria have both more sensitive and specific versions to be used for clinical and research purposes, respectively, by adjusting the number of physical findings needed to diagnose CRPS.

CHARACTERISTICS OF PAIN IN CRPS

In CRPS, description of pain is often characterized as continuous, disproportionate, or diffused. As noted in the original IASP criteria, CRPS provides "spontaneous pain, allodynia or hyperalgesia, which is not limited to the territory of a single peripheral nerve and is disproportionate to the inciting event."[2] This characteristic of pain needs to be distinguished from postoperative, posttraumatic pain, or other neuropathic pain. To distinguish from postoperative or posttraumatic pain, a key feature that should be closely examined is the characteristics of the diffuse pain. Foot and ankle surgeon should be suspicious of pain in an area that is away from the operative site. Similarly, after thorough clinical and radiographic examinations, a clinician should be aware of pain that is not in the area of injury in a case of trauma. If the pain the patient is complaining of is diffused beyond the area of surgery or injury, then one should be suspicious about the pain being of neurologic origin. For example, if a patient underwent a hallux valgus correction, then the postsurgical pain should not extend beyond the area of the surgical site over the first ray generally. In CRPS, the patient can have pain not only over the first ray but also diffused over to lateral side of the foot. A surgeon should, however, remember that global edema stemming from postoperative or posttraumatic inflammation can mimic the symptoms of diffused neurological pain. Tight bandages, or excessive use of ice can also provide similar pain characteristics to those of pain of neurologic origin.

Other characteristics of pain such as pain "which is disproportionate to any inciting event" are useful in distinguishing CRPS from other sources of pain. Light touch examination with a finger, or pinprick examination with some sharp instrument in the area away from the site of injury can produce "disproportionate" pain in CRPS. However, it should be noted that involuntary guarding mechanism of patients after injury can also mimic disproportionate response to such stimuli.

CHARACTERISTICS OF AUTONOMIC DISORDERS IN CRPS

Examination of the pain and its characteristics, alone does not qualify to diagnose CRPS, according to commonly accepted clinical criteria. Criteria require other findings such as vasomotor, sudomotor, motor, and trophic changes and abnormalities. Many of the vasomotor and sudomotor abnormalities are indication of autonomic disorders resulting from CRPS. Edema, skin color and temperature changes, and excessive sweating/dryness can be the result of this condition.

Edema is a common finding after foot and ankle surgery or injury. Therefore, distinguishing the surgical or traumatic edema from edema caused by CRPS's autonomic dysfunction is challenging. An examiner can, however, notice atypical pattern

to the edema in postoperative or posttraumatic patients. During the acute phase of healing, edema is a normal finding; however, as the healing process progresses beyond the acute phase, the edema should naturally subside. During this period, an examiner may notice abnormal edema that is distinguishable from the edema due to normal healing process.

Skin color changes are more unique to those with CRPS among postoperative or posttraumatic patients. Redness, often with dark hue, is not as common in patients undergoing a normal postoperative or posttraumatic course (Fig. 5.1). A clinician, however, should be able to rule out other differential diagnoses such as infection, dermatitis, and/or deep or superficial vein thrombosis. Infectious process, especially with *Streptococcus*, can mimic the typical color changes created by CRPS (Fig. 5.2). Ruling out this condition, however, is not difficult for average clinicians during the postoperative period. The color change surrounds the area of infection or surgical site in an infectious case. A patient may also have constitutional symptoms and abnormal laboratory results, indicative of infection. Dermatitis from a bandage can also mimic the color changes in CRPS; however, there is usually no pain associated with the condition unless the bandage is too tight (Fig. 5.3). Loosening of the bandage should relieve most of the pain if there is no underlying CRPS. A tight bandage, however, often causes chronic neurological problems especially in the anterior aspect of the ankle. This is usually accompanied with bruising and decubitus ulceration in the area of the pain. Venous thrombosis when symptomatic has an acute onset, and the description of pain is not consistent with that of CRPS.

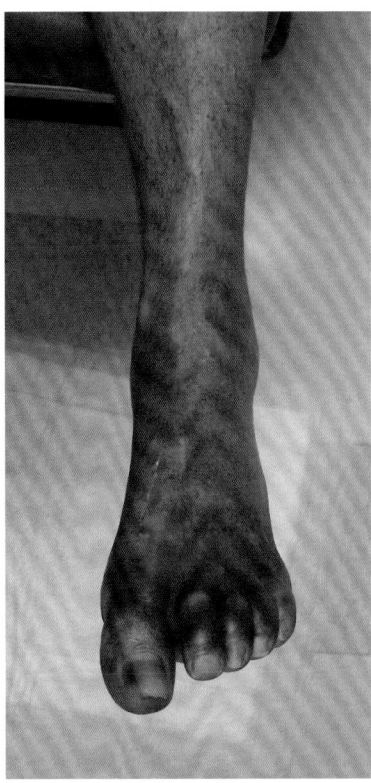

FIGURE 5.1 Skin color change noted in a patient with complex regional pain syndrome. The patient had a midfoot fusion 3 months prior to this presentation.

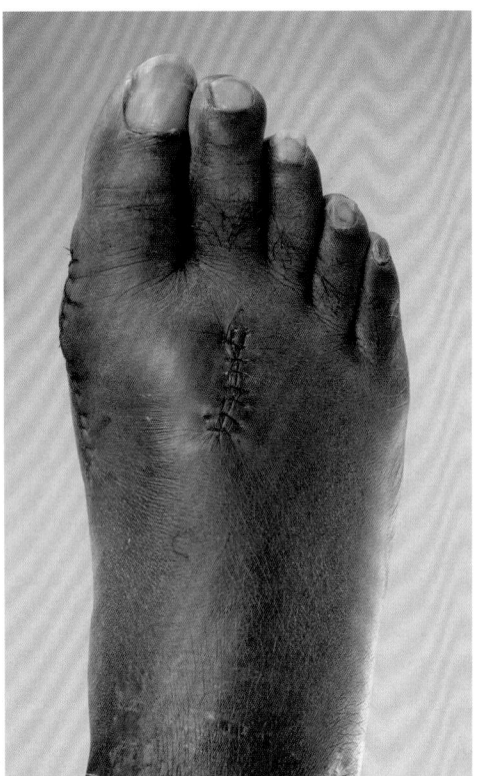

FIGURE 5.2 Skin color change due to underlying infection.

Sudomotor dysfunction, or abnormality in perspiration, unlike edema and color changes that can happen in an acute inflammatory phase, is unique to neurological disorders such as CRPS. It is a sign of abnormality in the sympathetic nervous system controlling mainly the sweat glands. In some cases, moisture on the skin is easily felt over the dorsum of a foot especially when compared with the contralateral foot. However, lack of this finding does not itself preclude from diagnosing CRPS (see criteria).

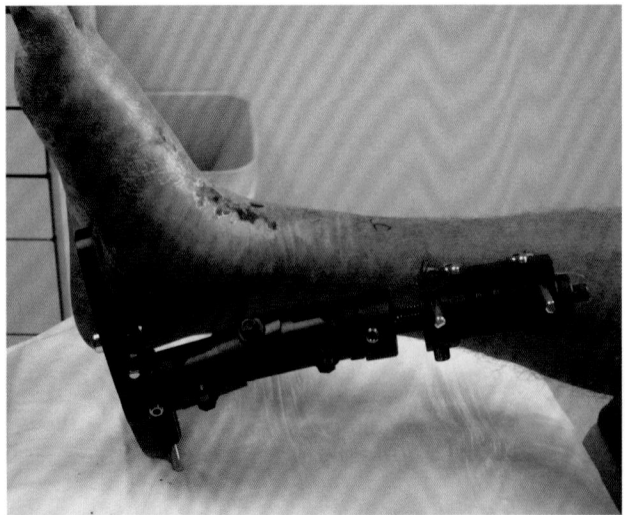

FIGURE 5.3 Skin color change due to bandage irritation and dermatitis.

TROPHIC CHANGES IN CRPS

Trophic changes not only include presence of thin shiny skin, but also result in decreased density of the pedal bones noted in x-rays (often referred as Sudeck atrophy), and fibrosis or stiffening of the supple foot, or ankle and hair/nail growth abnormality. These findings provide the classic "RSD" appearance. These changes were believed to present in the late stage of the condition. However, the actual time frame which it takes to get to the stage varies significantly between patients, and some may not go through the classic sequential staging before reaching this level. It has been noted that duration of the pain due to CRPS was not necessarily longer in patients with trophic changes when compared to those without.[15]

"Mottled" skin is a sign of fibrosis, and this can result in physical limitation in range of motion in the pedal joints. Shiny, thin skin appears similar to those with vascular abnormalities, which are often seen in elder patients. Decrease in bone density is often noted in radiographic examination during the postoperative period; therefore, this finding alone does not have good sensitivity or specificity to detect CRPS, especially when the surgery requires patients to be inactive. The decrease of bone density in CRPS can originate from actual increase in osteoclastic activity mediated by proinflammatory cytokines such as Substance P and TNF-alpha,[20] but may also be due to disuse from fear of movement (kinesiophobia) or weight bearing in these patients experiencing severe pain.

Motor abnormality, therefore, can be common in the CRPS patients due to the kinesiophobia from pain, but CRPS can also directly cause tremor, dystonia, and weakness. Posttraumatic patients often present to a specialist weeks or months after the injury, complaining of lack of improvement in pain, but also for weakness, often accompanied by tremor. For example, a patient with grade I or II ankle sprain treated with immobilization for several weeks comes in with worsened to see a foot and ankle specialist. The patient may still have pain over the lateral collateral ligaments, but the chief complaint now can be a neurological pain diffused throughout the foot and ankle. The area of diffused pain can vary between patients, but the pain is not confined to the lateral ankle. Such patients often present with spontaneous tremor, weakness, and loss of motion.

Knowing these clinical characteristics of CRPS and distinguishing them from other postoperative and posttraumatic findings is crucial for early detection and to obtain better prognosis. It should, however, be noted that not all findings are needed to diagnose CRPS or to initiate treatment in these patients. For example, while the Budapest criteria have four categories, within the second category, only 3 out of 4 symptoms, and within the third category, only 2 out of 4 physical findings need to be met to diagnose CRPS. The number of measure needed increase the sensitivity of the criteria, as underdiagnosing the problem can cause a delay in treatment for some patients, and is problematic in the clinical setting. Similarly, in Veldeman criteria, only 3 out of 4 clinical signs have to be met in their first category in order to diagnose.

PATHOGENESIS

Pathophysiology of CRPS is complex and multifactorial. It involves both central and peripheral nervous systems.[21] While understanding the pathophysiology may not affect daily clinical practice for the most surgeons, it will help develop more accurate diagnosis and effective, targeted treatment for this condition. In the past, it was believed that CRPS is a disorder of the sympathetic nervous system (hence, the name, RSD); however, more recent studies show involvement of multiple systems, including the central nervous system.

Though the exact mechanism has not been identified, it has been suggested that the condition is initiated by minor local nerve damage after an injury or surgery.[22] The normal resultant inflammatory response produces and releases inflammatory cytokines and neuropeptides. However, with potential predisposition due to underlying genetic factors,[23,24] psychological factors[25] and/or even preexisting chronic pain,[26] the inflammatory response can be uncontrollably up-regulated in patients, resulting in peripheral sensitization. The sympathetic nervous system function is also known to be impaired initially in this population. Specifically, recent findings suggest that the SNS is down-regulated rather than up-regulated, despite the past beliefs.[27,28]

When the sympathetic nervous system outflow is reduced, vasodilatation can occur; hence, vasomotor responses, such as edema and skin color changes, can be apparent in the acute phase. To compensate for this reduced outflow, adrenergic receptors are up-regulated. This results in excessive vasoconstriction in the later stage of CRPS. In addition, excessive catecholamine response in CRPS patients from physical and psychological stresses on top of the overexpressed adrenergic receptors, further activates the adrenergic response and vasoconstriction, leading to more trophic changes. This series of events can also result in central sensitization at spinal and brain levels that alter nociceptive response to stimuli, resulting in allodynia (pain following normally nonpainful stimuli) and hyperalgesia (increased sensitivity).

IMAGING AND DIAGNOSTIC STUDIES

Most of the major guidelines on CRPS do not advocate the routine use of radiographic studies or diagnostic tests for diagnosing this condition. Plain x-rays can show patchy demineralization in some subjects.

In the bone or Sudeck atrophy (Fig. 5.4), it has been shown that this finding is not sensitive enough to detect CRPS, as demineralization can be due to osteoclastic activity often seen in neurological conditions such as CRPS. This can be seen as well in other neurological disorders such as Charcot arthropathy or disuse conditions in many postsurgical or posttraumatic patients.

Similarly, while nuclear imaging, such as triphase bone scan, can show hyperperfusion and periarticular uptake in early CRPS (Fig. 5.5), the detection of this condition is dependent

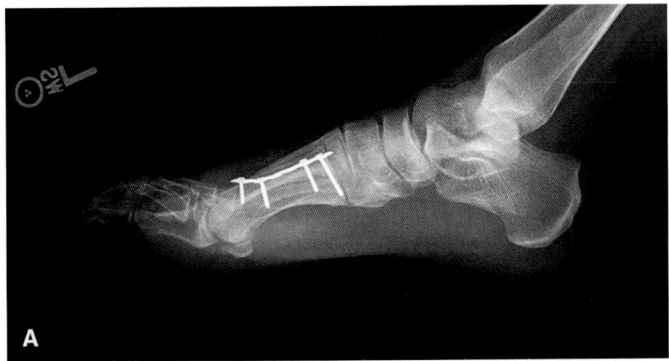

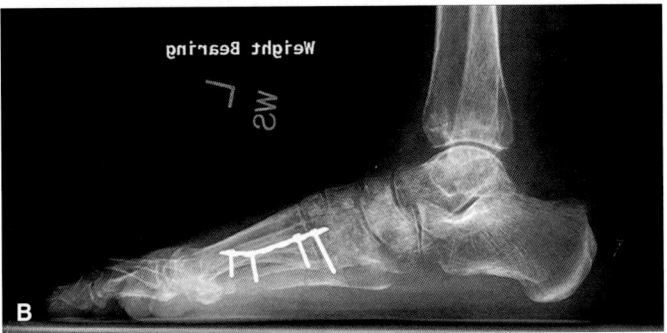

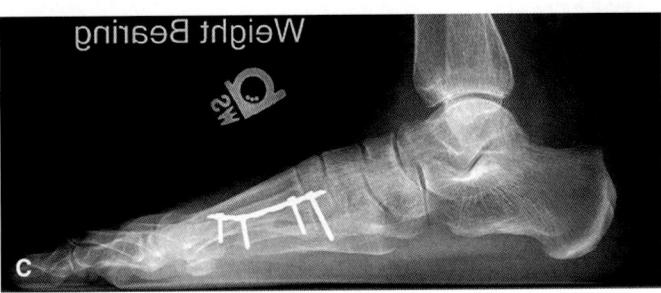

FIGURE 5.4 A. The patient with normal bone density goes through open reduction of the metatarsal. **B.** The patient subsequently develops CRPS and patchy demineralization (Sudeck atrophy) is evident in the x-ray. **C.** After functional restoration and improvement of CRPS, the bone density is restored.

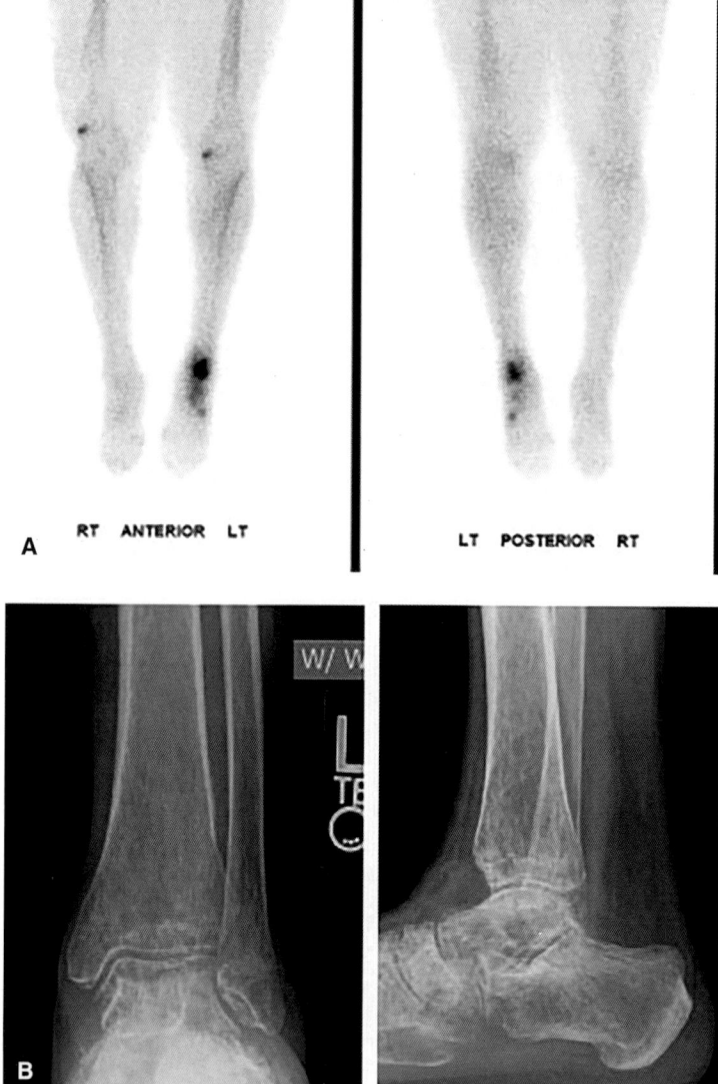

A   RT ANTERIOR LT   LT POSTERIOR RT

B

FIGURE 5.5 A. Hyperperfusion and bone uptake are noted in the ankle area in this delay phase of the technetium bone scan. **B.** The area of the hyperperfusion and bone uptake corresponds to demineralization noted in the plain x-rays in the same patient with CRPS.

on subtypes/stages at the time of examination; therefore, the use of this modality for general diagnosis of CRPS is not recommended. The modality is not sensitive enough and, therefore, can result in underdiagnosing of the condition. However, this modality may be useful for monitoring the course of CRPS during treatment.[29]

EMG/NCV studies are not useful in detecting CRPS unless one is looking for a "major" nerve damage in the case of type II CRPS or causalgia. While this may be useful in distinguishing types within CRPS patients, a negative finding does not rule out the presence of CRPS. In addition, distinction of these types may not have significant clinical implications, and the test itself can provide unnecessary pain, which can exacerbate the condition. Invasive tests such as sympathetic block or somatosensory evoked potential (SSEP) can also provide more risks than benefits.

Temperature measurements, such as resting skin temperature measurement or thermography, are nonspecific, especially in posttrauma or postsurgical patients who often have inflamed foot or ankle. It is also dependent on subtypes and stages of CRPS.

Modalities to test for sudomotor dysfunction, such as a quantitative sudomotor axon reflex test (QSART), or resting sweat output (RSO), can be specific, but availability of these tests may be limited to larger institutions. A negative result from these tests again will not rule out CRPS.

It should be noted that diagnosis of CRPS is mainly made by clinical examination. Accepted criteria set forth by major organizations and expert panels are standard for diagnosing this pathology. Relaying on a single diagnostic test or imaging is not recommended.

TREATMENT

Prevention is one of the most important aspects of this condition. Being aware of risk factors for this condition is essential in avoiding CRPS in elective surgical cases. It has been shown that female patients, especially postmenopausal females, are more likely to suffer this condition as compared to male counterparts.[13] Also, those patients who have been suffering from chronic pain are predisposed to CRPS. While postoperative pain management is key to avoiding central sensitization, those with chronic pain who are dependent on pain medication are difficult patients to manage postoperatively. Pain management consultation prior to an elective surgery in these high-risk patients may be warranted. In addition, patients with history of CRPS are more likely to have CRPS compared to those who have never had CRPS.[28] It has also been suggested that underlying stress may be associated with development of CRPS.[30] Therefore, it is as important for a surgeon to evaluate psychological and socioeconomic status of these patients along with musculoskeletal issues. It is imperative to distinguish musculoskeletal pain from other neurological chronic pain in these patients.

It has been shown that administration of high-dose vitamin C is effective in reducing occurrence of CRPS after trauma or surgery. Shibuya et al., in their systematic review and meta-analysis, demonstrated that the potential reduction of CRPS with this regimen was five folds.[31] However, a subsequent study in contrary showed no difference between those who consumed high-dose vitamin C versus those did not.[32] The risk and cost of high-dose vitamin C is minimal; therefore, routine use of this regimen may be warranted. The Dutch guidelines advocate the use of vitamin C in prevention of CRPS.[18] Typically, daily 500-1000 mg of oral vitamin C is utilized. High-dose vitamin C is readily available over the counter.

Once a patient develops CRPS, early initiation of multidisciplinary treatments is warranted. To provide effective treatments, foot and ankle surgeons should be reminded that CRPS not only causes pain but also results in functional disability and psychological distress. Addressing all of these aspects is, therefore, important in comprehensive management of the patient with CRPS: pain management, functional restoration, and psychological care should all be considered.

The fourth edition of the practical diagnostic and treatment guidelines, sponsored by the RSD Association, which was published in 2013, recommends prioritizing functional restoration over pharmacological and psychological treatment.[3] The Dutch guidelines list drug treatment, invasive treatment, physical therapy (PT), occupational therapy (OT), rehabilitation medicine, and psychological treatment methods separately, and discuss evidence behind each approach and their recommendation.[18] Categorically, both guidelines focus on functional rehabilitation, pharmacological treatment, and psychological treatment for these patients.

Three Major Categories in Management of CRPS

PSYCHOLOGICAL MANAGEMENT
- Relaxation, behavioral training

FUNCTIONAL RESTORATION
- Physical, occupational, recreational, vocational therapy

PHARMACOLOGICAL MANAGEMENT
- Oral, topical, and interventional administration of pharmacological agents

---

PSYCHOLOGICAL MANAGEMENT

While evidence for psychological treatment for CRPS and/or any neuropathic pain is scarce, it is a modality recommended by practice guidelines.[3,33] It is known that emotional stress can lead to a physiological catecholamine release, which can further activate the already up-regulated catecholamine receptors (due to

decreased sympathetic outflow: see mechanism) in CRPS patients, and result in further vasoconstriction and trophic changes. Therefore, it is beneficial to consider psychological management in CRPS patients, especially as the risks and cost of this modality are relatively low. While not specific to CRPS, psychological management has been shown to be effective in patients with chronic pain, by multiple randomized clinical trials.[34,35]

Psychological management starts with informing the patient about the condition, prognosis, and short/long-term management plans. Providing written information regarding this condition is helpful, as many patients may not register every detail of what has been explained during the office/clinic visit. While information regarding CRPS is readily available on the Internet, it is important to direct patients to reliable sources. For example, www.rsds.org, which is run by a nonprofit organization in the United States, provides comprehensive and reliable information needed for a patient to understand CRPS. It also provides references patients can use to get further information on any specific topic. It is advisable to visit the Web site prior to providing the address to avoid discrepancy in information provided to the patient. The patients may also benefit from reading blogs written by other patients with the same condition. However, patients should be warned before visiting these blogs that some information presented in the blog can be inaccurate, and CRPS can manifest differently in each individual.

After informing the patient about the condition, psychology consultation may be warranted. It should be noted that some patients may perceive this as offensive, as they may think that the surgeon feels that the pain is psychological. It is, therefore, important to inform the patient that it is not the case. It may be beneficial not to use the term "psychological" during the conversation. Rather, a surgeon can describe the psychotherapies by what actually takes place and how each modality can help physiologically with the patient's chronic pain. The psychological interventions can include, but are not limited to, relaxation/autogenic training, behavioral therapy, and biofeedback training.

It is also important to observe patients' socioeconomic status and the mood of people surrounding the patient. Financial struggle, job insecurity, health issues/death in family, and negative remarks from the patient's own family member/friends can all contribute to the negative feedback mechanism in this condition. Getting appropriate assistance for life struggles and education of people around the patient may be necessary. Recreational therapy and vocational therapy can also help patients improve their life situation and minimize the negative feedback that is detrimental to the chronic pain.

FUNCTIONAL RESTORATION

Functional restoration is considered the most important aspect of CRPS management. Returning patients to their original activity level should be the main goal in treatment of CRPS. Functional restoration modalities reduce pain, avert disuse, and prevent fear of movement. They are achieved by multiple disciplines including, but not limited to, PT, OT, recreational therapy, and vocational rehabilitation.[3]

PT/OT is recommended almost universally by practice guidelines. Modalities used by these disciplines attempt to reduce edema, desensitize the area of pain, restore a range of motion, and reestablish relationship between sensory input and motor output. To most surgeons, this entails timely referral to PT/OT for modalities utilized for this condition. Surgeons should also remind the patient that they should avoid inactivity, though the surgical site is reasonably protected. Also, if a patient is using ice for postoperative edema and pain control, it should be discontinued immediately: icing may accelerate trophic changes and decrease mobility in CRPS patients. On the other hand, aggressive attempt at desensitization and mobilization can also exacerbate CRPS; rather, gradual improvement from the periphery of the pain is preferred. Desensitization typically starts out with a softer, more tolerable material with less friction brushing across the skin before progressing into more coarse and stimulating material.

It is recommended for surgeons to have some understanding of what actually takes place when patients are refereed to PT/OT. Modalities include, but are not limited to, mirror therapy, desensitization, mild compression, movement therapy, gait training with gradual increase in weight, aquatic/pool therapy, light therapy, range of motion exercises, massage, and stretching. Because most of the patients during postoperative or posttraumatic period are restricted in certain motions or weight bearing, communication between a surgeon and therapist is essential. It should also be noted that some PT/OT providers are not specialized in this condition and are not familiar with modalities utilized specifically for different types or stages of this condition.

Because inactivity is detrimental to patients with CRPS, recreational therapy is often utilized to make movement more enjoyable and less fear inducing for a patient. On the other hand, returning to work can be one of the most difficult tasks that patients with CRPS can experience. Constant communications with their employer may be required to avoid premature return to work or excessive disability and inactivity. A conditional return to work may help patients remain active while avoiding exacerbation. Vocational rehabilitation may be necessary in those who are out of work for a long time.

PHARMACOLOGICAL MANAGEMENT

While pharmacological management addresses mainly pain, it can also manage other symptoms of CRPS such as edema, dystonia, and other associated conditions resulting from CRPS. Some pharmacotherapies can be initiated by a foot and ankle surgeon, but appropriate referrals are necessary to initiate other agents especially those require an intervention. Understanding pharmacological options available for this condition is useful in having conversations with a patient and initiating an appropriate referral.

Anti-inflammatory Drugs

Anti-inflammatory drugs may be useful in reducing pain and edema. While NSAIDs may not reduce neurogenic inflammation, they help with musculoskeletal pain that the patient may be simultaneously experiencing due to the operation or trauma. However, evidence for anti-inflammatory medications in CRPS is limited.

Oral corticosteroids have been tested in treatment of CRPS. Christensen et al. showed efficacy of oral prednisone used mostly for acute CRPS.[36] They used 10 mg of prednisone for up to 12 weeks in 13 patients, and found significant clinical improvement compared to placebo. Proper dosing and effectiveness of corticosteroids in chronic CRPS are still not clear.

Opioids

There is insufficient evidence for opioids to be used in CRPS. Not only is the efficacy of this group of medication questionable, it can also lead to many side effects, such as dependency and exacerbation of hyperalgesia and allodynia. A randomized clinical trial tested the efficacy of oral sustained-release morphine (taken 90 mg daily for 8 days) and showed no detectible difference compared to placebo.[37]

Due to the recent opioid crisis, narcotic use in a postoperative setting is highly regulated. Surgeons should be mindful of opioid overdose, especially in those with history of chronic pain. Some patients may have a pain contract with other specialists; therefore, no pain medication should be prescribed by a surgeon without modification of the contract. Many states require physicians to check patients' prescription records prior to prescribing new narcotics.

Efficacy of opioid use as a rescue medicine or for breakthrough pain is controversial. A proper pain management consult may be warranted.

Anticonvulsants/Antidepressants

The efficacy of both anticonvulsants and antidepressants in neuropathic pain is well documented.[38-44] Administration of these drugs, therefore, may be beneficial for patients with CRPS. Antidepressants may help those with chronic CRPS, also by managing depression, which is often associated with chronic pain.

While the efficacy of antidepressants specifically for CRPS patients has not been evaluated in clinical trials, Van de Vusse et al. studied the efficacy of anticonvulsant (gabapentin) in patients with chronic CRPS.[45] They found that daily administration of gabapentin 600-1800 mg led to a significant improvement in pain and sensory deficit. By design, they started the pharmacotherapy with a daily dose of 600 mg, and the dose was titrated to 1800 mg over the course of 5 days. The course of treatment in the study was 21 days.

Bisphosphonates and Calcitonin

Foot and ankle surgeons may be familiar with bisphosphonates and calcitonin due to their off-label use in treatment of Charcot arthropathy. They not only inhibit osteoclastic activity resulting from neuropathic osteolysis but also have been shown to decrease temperature and symptoms such as pain.[46,47]

This class of drugs is also studied in CRPS patients. Overall, the efficacy of bisphosphonates, especially in pain reduction, is favorable. There are multiple randomized clinical trials with similar results. Varrena et al. tested 10-day administration of intravenous daily clodronate of 300 mg and found that the bisphosphonate reduced pain and symptoms of CRPS more than placebo.[48] Similarly, Varrena et al. tested 100 mg of neridronate infused intravenously a total of four times, and found that it too reduced pain and symptoms of CRPS.[49] Adami et al. evaluated daily intravenous alendronate 7.5 mg for 3 days against placebo and found it improved pain, edema, and range of motion.

The results of clinical trials testing calcitonin for treatment of CRPS are, however, conflicting. Gobelet et al. showed that nasal salmon calcitonin of 100 IU, given three times a day, improved pain, range of motion, and ability to work in CRPS patients, more than placebo.[50] On the other hand, Bickerstaff and Kanis found that such a difference was not detectable when 200 IU of the nasal spray was used twice daily.

Muscle Relaxants

While most of the clinical studies concern intrathecal administration of baclofen, oral muscle relaxants may improve the symptom of CRPS-induced dystonia.[3,18,33] There is insufficient evidence on botulinum toxin injections in CRPS patients. They are generally not recommended by major guidelines.[3,18]

Antihypertensive Drugs

The rationale behind the use of antihypertensive drugs is to improve peripheral blood circulation. Muizelaar et al. tested both a calcium channel (nifedipine) and alpha blockers (phenoxybenzamine) for efficacy in treating both acute and chronic CRPS.[51] They reviewed the cases of patients who had an 8-12 week course of these medications and found overall cure rates of 92% and 40% in acute (n = 12) and chronic (n = 47) CRPS, respectively. The side effects experienced during the course of treatment included orthostatic hypotension, impotence in men, headache, and lightheadedness. The Dutch guidelines recommend that a calcium channel blocker can be indicated in a cold type 1 CRPS but should be discontinued if no effect is seen within a week.[18]

Topical Medications

There is no sufficient evidence on low-concentration capsaicin (which is readily available over the counter) in treating neuropathic pain. On the other hand, high-concentration (>8%) topical capsaicin in neuropathic patients has been shown effective in multiple studies.[52] However, such evidence does not exist for neuropathic pain caused specifically by CRPS. Indeed, the topical agent is usually not well tolerated in CRPS patients as it causes a severe burning sensation in the area of application. The Dutch guidelines recommend against the use of capsaicin in patients with CRPS.[18]

Lidocaine, when applied in high concentration, has been shown efficacious in neuropathic pain as well.[53] Specifically to CRPS patients, Calderón et al. observed 10 patients, who were administered 5% lidocaine-medicated plaster, and showed that 7 patients had at least 50% pain relief[54] though this was not tested against placebo. It should be noted that each over-the-counter topical lidocaine has different concentration, formula, and absorption properties, so should be used with caution.[55] Higher concentration patches can be expensive, especially for long-term use. Often patients with severe hyperalgesia are unable to tolerate any topical medication; therefore, it has to be initiated with application in the periphery, rather than in the center of the pain. There is no sufficient evidence for use of compound topical pain medications. Topical amitriptyline is not effective in treatment of neuropathic pain.[56]

A free radical scavenging agent such as dimethylsuphoxide (DMSO) cream has been tested and shown to be beneficial for CRPS patients.[57,58] A randomized controlled study conducted by Perez et al. found that a 50% DMSO cream applied five times a day to the affected area improved function compared to placebo, especially in hot CRPS.[57] The cream of an equal or greater concentration is readily available over the counter in the United States.

INTERVENTIONAL TREATMENTS

While foot and ankle surgeons are not the primary provider for these interventional treatments, having basic understanding of efficacy and safety of some of the most common modalities is useful in having conversation with the patients.

Intravenous Regional Sympathetic Block

A regional sympathetic blocking agent is introduced intravenously in an extremity isolated from rest of the body via a tourniquet. Multiple agents, such as guanethidine, atropine, bretylium, droperidol, and ketanserin, have been tested in CRPS patients; however, they mostly show no added benefit in pain reduction when compared to placebo.[59,60] The Dutch guidelines suggest that intravenous sympathetic blockade has no place in the treatment of CRPS.[18]

Local (Percutaneous) Sympathetic Block

The nerve block is often performed by interventional radiologist, anesthesiologist, neurologist, or a spine surgeon at the cervical, thoracic, or lumber level for CRPS manifesting in an upper or lower extremity, respectively. This classic procedure is still commonly used in patients with CRPS and often found in part of treatment algorithms. There is some evidence that shows that the regional sympathetic block is effective in CRPS patients.[19] Studies have not only shown its effectiveness in pain reduction but also in improving blood flow and temperature of extremities.[61] However, routine use is not recommended, and the success rate may be low.[18,62]

Spinal Infusion

Epidural and intrathecal infusion of various agents have been shown to benefit patients with CRPS.[63-69] However, due to its potential complications such as infection, it is generally reserved for those who have failed percutaneous blocks.[3]

Implantable Neurostimulation

An implantable electrode is placed in the epidural space or dorsal root ganglion to induce paresthesia. Pain control specifically for CRPS patients has been documented by recent studies.[70-72] Guidelines advocate the procedure in carefully selected patients when other less invasive measures fail.[3,18] The procedure may not directly improve function, but it can assist patients with severe pain become tolerant of various functional restoration modalities.

Amputation

Amputation may not be avoidable in patients who have exhausted all the other measures and still have intractable pain. However, it should be noted that risk of persistent or recurrent pain even after amputation is high. Dielissen et al. found that only 2 out of 28 amputees with CRPS had relief of pain.[73] Krans-Schreuder et al. showed recurrence of CRPS in 24% (5/22) of their CRPS patients who underwent a limb amputation.[74] The patient should be aware that an amputation can result in phantom pain, recurrence of CRPS, and development of new CRPS in different locations.

Despite these possible risks and complications associated with the amputation, it may help improve function and quality of life in many. The satisfaction rates, despite persistent pain, were high in patients in the above studies. Midbari et al. compared those who had and did not have amputation in a population of intractable CRPS pain.[75] Those patients who underwent amputation had better pain, quality of life, and psychological scores in the study.

Before proceeding with amputation, a surgeon should make sure that the patient is well aware of prognosis, has reasonable expectations, is psychologically stable, and has tried and exhausted a reasonable amount of other treatment modalities.

Elective Foot and Ankle Surgery on Patients With CRPS

Elective surgery unrelated to CRPS should be avoided in most cases until the symptoms of CRPS are resolved, as the surgery can exacerbate the condition. If a unique circumstance arises where an unrelated musculoskeletal pathology can be addressed and potentially improves the function of a patient, the procedure should be carefully planned and executed by an experienced surgeon with consultation of anesthesia and pain management.

It should, however, be noted that recurrence of CRPS is common.[76,77] Surgical neurolysis to treat CRPS is not indicated unless there is a clearly identifiable nerve damage and the benefit of the procedure overweighs the risk of exacerbation.[19]

CONCLUSION

The condition is common and frequently seen by foot and ankle surgeons. When becoming chronic, prognosis of this condition worsens. It is imperative to detect and diagnose this condition for early, effective treatments. While laboratory and radiographic examinations are sometimes useful in monitoring the progress of the condition, the diagnosis is made with clinical examination. Well-established clinical criteria assist surgeons to accurately diagnose this condition. The broad categories of treatments include functional restoration, pharmacological treatment, and psychological management. Managing all of these aspects will require multiple consultations to appropriate disciplines.

REFERENCES

1. Harden RN, Bruehl S, Stanton-Hicks M, Wilson PR. Proposed new diagnostic criteria for complex regional pain syndrome. *Pain Med.* 2007;8:326-331.
2. Stanton-Hicks M, Janig W, Hassenbusch S, Haddox JD, Boas R, Wilson P. Reflex sympathetic dystrophy: changing concepts and taxonomy. *Pain.* 1995;63:127-133.
3. Harden RN, Oaklander AL, Burton AW, et al. Complex regional pain syndrome: practical diagnostic and treatment guidelines, 4th edition. *Pain Med.* 2013;14:180-229.
4. Anderson DJ, Fallat LM. Complex regional pain syndrome of the lower extremity: a retrospective study of 33 patients. *J Foot Ankle Surg.* 1999;38:381-387.
5. Sandroni P, Benrud-Larson LM, McClelland RL, Low PA. Complex regional pain syndrome type I: incidence and prevalence in Olmsted County, a population-based study. *Pain.* 2003;103:199-207.
6. Perez RS, Collins S, Marinus J, Zuurmond WW, de Lange JJ. Diagnostic criteria for CRPS I: differences between patient profiles using three different diagnostic sets. *Eur J Pain.* 2007;11:895-902.
7. Veldman PH, Reynen HM, Arntz IE, Goris RJ. Signs and symptoms of reflex sympathetic dystrophy: prospective study of 829 patients. *Lancet.* 1993;342:1012-1016.
8. Vogel T, Gradl G, Ockert B, Pellengahr CS, Schurmann M. Sympathetic dysfunction in long-term complex regional pain syndrome. *Clin J Pain.* 2010;26:128-131.
9. Lee KJ, Kirchner JS. Complex regional pain syndrome and chronic pain management in the lower extremity. *Foot Ankle Clin.* 2002;7:409-419.
10. Harris J, Fallat L, Schwartz S. Characteristic trends of lower-extremity complex regional pain syndrome. *J Foot Ankle Surg.* 2004;43:296-301.
11. Perez RS, Kwakkel G, Zuurmond WW, de Lange JJ. Treatment of reflex sympathetic dystrophy (CRPS type 1): a research synthesis of 21 randomized clinical trials. *J Pain Symptom Manage.* 2001;21:511-526.
12. Allen G, Galer BS, Schwartz L. Epidemiology of complex regional pain syndrome: a retrospective chart review of 134 patients. *Pain.* 1999;80:539-544.
13. de Mos M, de Bruijn AG, Huygen FJ, Dieleman JP, Stricker BH, Sturkenboom MC. The incidence of complex regional pain syndrome: a population-based study. *Pain.* 2007;129:12-20.
14. Bruehl S, Chung OY. How common is complex regional pain syndrome-Type I? *Pain.* 2007;129:1-2.
15. Bruehl S, Harden RN, Galer BS, Saltz S, Backonja M, Stanton-Hicks M. Complex regional pain syndrome: are there distinct subtypes and sequential stages of the syndrome? *Pain.* 2002;95:119-124.
16. Wasner G, Schattschneider J, Heckmann K, Maier C, Baron R. Vascular abnormalities in reflex sympathetic dystrophy (CRPS I): mechanisms and diagnostic value. *Brain.* 2001;124:587-599.
17. Merskey H, Bogduk N. *Classification of Chronic Pain: Descriptions of Chronic Pain Syndromes and Definitions of Pain Terms* [press release]. Seattle, WA: IASP Press; 1994.
18. Geertzen J, Perez R, Dijkstra P, Kemler M, Rosenbrand C. *Complex Regional Pain Syndrome Type I Guidelines.* Alphen aan den Rijn: Van Zuiden Communications B.V.; 2006.
19. Goebel A, Barker C, Turner-Stokes L, Atkins R, Cameron H, Cossins L. *Complex Regional Pain Syndrome in Adults: UK Guidelines for Diagnosis, Referral and Management in Primary and Secondary Care.* London, England: The Royal College of Physicians (RCP); 2012:2012.
20. Birklein F, Schmelz M. Neuropeptides, neurogenic inflammation and complex regional pain syndrome (CRPS). *Neurosci Lett.* 2008;437:199-202.
21. Bruehl S. An update on the pathophysiology of complex regional pain syndrome. *Anesthesiology.* 2010;113:713-725.
22. Oaklander AL, Rissmiller JG, Gelman LB, Zheng L, Chang Y, Gott R. Evidence of focal small-fiber axonal degeneration in complex regional pain syndrome-I (reflex sympathetic dystrophy). *Pain.* 2006;120:235-243.
23. de Rooij AM, de Mos M, Sturkenboom MC, et al. Familial occurrence of complex regional pain syndrome. *Eur J Pain.* 2009;13:171-177.
24. de Rooij AM, de Mos M, van Hilten JJ, et al. Increased risk of complex regional pain syndrome in siblings of patients? *J Pain.* 2009;10:1250-1255.
25. Bruehl S, Chung OY, Burns JW. Differential effects of expressive anger regulation on chronic pain intensity in CRPS and non-CRPS limb pain patients. *Pain.* 2003;104:647-654.
26. Harden RN, Bruehl S, Stanos S, et al. Prospective examination of pain-related and psychological predictors of CRPS-like phenomena following total knee arthroplasty: a preliminary study. *Pain.* 2003;106:393-400.
27. Schurmann M, Gradl G, Zaspel J, Kayser M, Lohr P, Andress HJ. Peripheral sympathetic function as a predictor of complex regional pain syndrome type I (CRPS I) in patients with radial fracture. *Auton Neurosci.* 2000;86:127-134.
28. Ackerman WE III, Ahmad M. Recurrent postoperative CRPS I in patients with abnormal preoperative sympathetic function. *J Hand Surg Am.* 2008;33:217-222.
29. Howard BA, Roy L, Kaye AD, Pyati S. Utility of radionuclide bone scintigraphy in complex regional pain syndrome. *Curr Pain Headache Rep.* 2018;22:7.
30. Geertzen JH, de Bruijn-Kofman AT, de Bruijn HP, van de Wiel HB, Dijkstra PU. Stressful life events and psychological dysfunction in Complex Regional Pain Syndrome type I. *Clin J Pain.* 1998;14:143-147.
31. Shibuya N, Humphers JM, Agarwal MR, Jupiter DC. Efficacy and safety of high-dose vitamin C on complex regional pain syndrome in extremity trauma and surgery—systematic review and meta-analysis. *J Foot Ankle Surg.* 2013;52:62-66.
32. Ekrol I, Duckworth AD, Ralston SH, Court-Brown CM, McQueen MM. The influence of vitamin C on the outcome of distal radial fractures: a double-blind, randomized controlled trial. *J Bone Joint Surg Am.* 2014;96:1451-1459.
33. Perez RS, Zollinger PE, Dijkstra PU, et al. Evidence based guidelines for complex regional pain syndrome type 1. *BMC Neurol.* 2010;10:20.
34. Malone MD, Strube MJ, Scogin FR. Meta-analysis of non-medical treatments for chronic pain. *Pain.* 1988;34:231-244.
35. Eccleston C, Williams AC, Morley S. Psychological therapies for the management of chronic pain (excluding headache) in adults. *Cochrane Database Syst Rev.* 2009;(2):CD007407.
36. Christensen K, Jensen EM, Noer I. The reflex dystrophy syndrome response to treatment with systemic corticosteroids. *Acta Chir Scand.* 1982;148:653-655.
37. Harke H, Gretenkort P, Ladleif HU, Rahman S, Harke O. The response of neuropathic pain and pain in complex regional pain syndrome I to carbamazepine and sustained-release morphine in patients pretreated with spinal cord stimulation: a double-blinded randomized study. *Anesth Analg.* 2001;92:488-495.
38. Serpell MG; Neuropathic Pain Study Group. Gabapentin in neuropathic pain syndromes: a randomised, double-blind, placebo-controlled trial. *Pain.* 2002;99:557-566.
39. Yasuda H, Hotta N, Kasuga M, et al. Efficacy and safety of 40 mg or 60 mg duloxetine in Japanese adults with diabetic neuropathic pain: Results from a randomized, 52-week, open-label study. *J Diabetes Investig.* 2016;7:100-108.
40. Gao Y, Guo X, Han P, et al. Treatment of patients with diabetic peripheral neuropathic pain in China: a double-blind randomised trial of duloxetine vs. placebo. *Int J Clin Pract.* 2015;69:957-966.
41. Irving G, Tanenberg RJ, Raskin J, Risser RC, Malcolm S. Comparative safety and tolerability of duloxetine vs. pregabalin vs. duloxetine plus gabapentin in patients with diabetic peripheral neuropathic pain. *Int J Clin Pract.* 2014;68:1130-1140.
42. Tanenberg RJ, Clemow DB, Giaconia JM, Risser RC. Duloxetine compared with pregabalin for diabetic peripheral neuropathic pain management in patients with suboptimal

pain response to gabapentin and treated with or without antidepressants: A post Hoc analysis. *Pain Pract.* 2014;14:640-648.

43. Boyle J, Eriksson ME, Gribble L, et al. Randomized, placebo-controlled comparison of amitriptyline, duloxetine, and pregabalin in patients with chronic diabetic peripheral neuropathic pain: impact on pain, polysomnographic sleep, daytime functioning, and quality of life. *Diabetes Care.* 2012;35:2451-2458.

44. Raskin J, Pritchett YL, Wang F, et al. A double-blind, randomized multicenter trial comparing duloxetine with placebo in the management of diabetic peripheral neuropathic pain. *Pain Med.* 2005;6:346-356.

45. van de Vusse AC, Stomp-van den Berg SG, Kessels AH, Weber WE. Randomised controlled trial of gabapentin in Complex Regional Pain Syndrome type 1 [ISRCTN84121379]. *BMC Neurol.* 2004;4:13.

46. Jude EB, Selby PL, Burgess J, et al. Bisphosphonates in the treatment of Charcot neuroarthropathy: a double-blind randomised controlled trial. *Diabetologia.* 2001;44:2032-2037.

47. Anderson JJ, Woelffer KE, Holtzman JJ, Jacobs AM. Bisphosphonates for the treatment of Charcot neuroarthropathy. *J Foot Ankle Surg.* 2004;43:285-289.

48. Varenna M, Zucchi F, Ghiringhelli D, et al. Intravenous clodronate in the treatment of reflex sympathetic dystrophy syndrome. A randomized, double blind, placebo controlled study. *J Rheumatol.* 2000;27:1477-1483.

49. Varenna M, Adami S, Rossini M, et al. Treatment of complex regional pain syndrome type I with neridronate: a randomized, double-blind, placebo-controlled study. *Rheumatology (Oxford).* 2013;52:534-542.

50. Gobelet C, Waldburger M, Meier JL. The effect of adding calcitonin to physical treatment on reflex sympathetic dystrophy. *Pain.* 1992;48:171-175.

51. Muizelaar JP, Kleyer M, Hertogs IA, DeLange DC. Complex regional pain syndrome (reflex sympathetic dystrophy and causalgia): management with the calcium channel blocker nifedipine and/or the alpha-sympathetic blocker phenoxybenzamine in 59 patients. *Clin Neurol Neurosurg.* 1997;99:26-30.

52. Derry S, Rice AS, Cole P, Tan T, Moore RA. Topical capsaicin (high concentration) for chronic neuropathic pain in adults. *Cochrane Database Syst Rev.* 2017;(1):CD007393.

53. Baron R, Mayoral V, Leijon G, Binder A, Steigerwald I, Serpell M. 5% lidocaine medicated plaster versus pregabalin in post-herpetic neuralgia and diabetic polyneuropathy: an open-label, non-inferiority two-stage RCT study. *Curr Med Res Opin.* 2009;25:1663-1676.

54. Calderon E, Calderon-Seoane ME, Garcia-Hernandez R, Torres LM. 5% Lidocaine-medicated plaster for the treatment of chronic peripheral neuropathic pain: complex regional pain syndrome and other neuropathic conditions. *J Pain Res.* 2016;9:763-770.

55. Oni G, Brown S, Kenkel J. Comparison of five commonly-available, lidocaine-containing topical anesthetics and their effect on serum levels of lidocaine and its metabolite mono-ethylglycinexylidide (MEGX). *Aesthet Surg J.* 2012;32:495-503.

56. Ho KY, Huh BK, White WD, Yeh CC, Miller EJ. Topical amitriptyline versus lidocaine in the treatment of neuropathic pain. *Clin J Pain.* 2008;24:51-55.

57. Perez RS, Zuurmond WW, Bezemer PD, et al. The treatment of complex regional pain syndrome type I with free radical scavengers: a randomized controlled study. *Pain.* 2003;102:297-307.

58. Zuurmond WW, Langendijk PN, Bezemer PD, Brink HE, de Lange JJ, van loenen AC. Treatment of acute reflex sympathetic dystrophy with DMSO 50% in a fatty cream. *Acta Anaesthesiol Scand.* 1996;40:364-367.

59. Forouzanfar T, Koke AJ, van Kleef M, Weber WE. Treatment of complex regional pain syndrome type I. *Eur J Pain.* 2002;6:105-122.

60. Jadad AR, Carroll D, Glynn CJ, McQuay HJ. Intravenous regional sympathetic blockade for pain relief in reflex sympathetic dystrophy: a systematic review and a randomized, double-blind crossover study. *J Pain Symptom Manage.* 1995;10:13-20.

61. Malmqvist EL, Bengtsson M, Sorensen J. Efficacy of stellate ganglion block: a clinical study with bupivacaine. *Reg Anesth.* 1992;17:340-347.

62. Cepeda MS, Carr DB, Lau J. Local anesthetic sympathetic blockade for complex regional pain syndrome. *Cochrane Database Syst Rev.* 2005;(4):CD004598.

63. Rauck RL, Eisenach JC, Jackson K, Young LD, Southern J. Epidural clonidine treatment for refractory reflex sympathetic dystrophy. *Anesthesiology.* 1993;79:1163-1169; discussion 27A.

64. Goto S, Taira T, Horisawa S, Yokote A, Sasaki T, Okada Y. Spinal cord stimulation and intrathecal baclofen therapy: combined neuromodulation for treatment of advanced complex regional pain syndrome. *Stereotact Funct Neurosurg.* 2013;91:386-391.

65. van der Plas AA, van Rijn MA, Marinus J, Putter H, van Hilten JJ. Efficacy of intrathecal baclofen on different pain qualities in complex regional pain syndrome. *Anesth Analg.* 2013;116:211-215.

66. van Rijn MA, Munts AG, Marinus J, et al. Intrathecal baclofen for dystonia of complex regional pain syndrome. *Pain.* 2009;143:41-47.

67. Cooper DE, DeLee JC, Ramamurthy S. Reflex sympathetic dystrophy of the knee. Treatment using continuous epidural anesthesia. *J Bone Joint Surg Am.* 1989;71:365-369.

68. Munts AG, van der Plas AA, Voormolen JH, et al. Intrathecal glycine for pain and dystonia in complex regional pain syndrome. *Pain.* 2009;146:199-204.

69. Kemler MA, de Vet HC, Barendse GA, van den Wildenberg FA, van Kleef M. Effect of spinal cord stimulation for chronic complex regional pain syndrome Type I: five-year final follow-up of patients in a randomized controlled trial. *J Neurosurg.* 2008;108:292-298.

70. Deer TR, Levy RM, Kramer J, et al. Dorsal root ganglion stimulation yielded higher treatment success rate for complex regional pain syndrome and causalgia at 3 and 12 months: a randomized comparative trial. *Pain.* 2017;158:669-681.

71. Yang A, Hunter CW. Dorsal root ganglion stimulation as a salvage treatment for complex regional pain syndrome refractory to dorsal column spinal cord stimulation: a case series. *Neuromodulation.* 2017;20:703-707.

72. Skaribas IM, Peccora C, Skaribas E. Single S1 dorsal root ganglia stimulation for intractable complex regional pain syndrome foot pain after lumbar spine surgery: a case series. *Neuromodulation.* 2019;22:101-107.

73. Dielissen PW, Claassen AT, Veldman PH, Goris RJ. Amputation for reflex sympathetic dystrophy. *J Bone Joint Surg Br.* 1995;77:270-273.

74. Krans-Schreuder HK, Bodde MI, Schrier E, et al. Amputation for long-standing, therapy-resistant type-I complex regional pain syndrome. *J Bone Joint Surg Am.* 2012;94:2263-2268.

75. Midbari A, Suzan E, Adler T, et al. Amputation in patients with complex regional pain syndrome: a comparative study between amputees and non-amputees with intractable disease. *Bone Joint J.* 2016;98-B:548-554.

76. Katz MM, Hungerford DS. Reflex sympathetic dystrophy affecting the knee. *J Bone Joint Surg Br.* 1987;69:797-803.

77. Veldman PH, Goris RJ. Surgery on extremities with reflex sympathetic dystrophy. *Unfallchirurg.* 1995;98:45-48.

Forefoot Surgery

CHAPTER 6

Hallux Surgery

Allan M. Boike and James C. Connors

DEFINITION

The goal of hallux surgery is to remove the osseous deformity created by an angular deformity of the hallux interphalangeal joint (HIPJ) which leads to altered joint mechanics as well as adjacent toe soft tissue irritation. Located at the most distal great toe joint, hallux interphalangeus is defined as lateral deviation of the distal phalanx with ~10 degrees or greater being considered pathologic.[1] This pathologic condition presents either as a primary abnormality or in combination with the more proximal hallux valgus deformity as well as hallux rigidus. Several surgical options exist focusing on the proximal phalanx of the hallux depending on the apex of the deformity. The Akin osteotomy is a closing wedge osteotomy on the medial aspect of the proximal phalanx with a lateral apex for correction of the hallux interphalangeal deformity.[2] This procedure serves as the most common type of correction, but other options must be considered with atypical presentations. The Moberg osteotomy, a dorsiflexory closing wedge type osteotomy of the proximal phalanx is an effective joint sparing procedure in combination with a simple cheilectomy for treatment of early stage of hallux rigidus.[3,4] An obliquely oriented osteotomy of the proximal phalanx, commonly referred to as a "Miami Osteotomy" provides a potential alternative for transverse plane HIPJ deformity as well as sagittal plane correction in the setting of hallux limitus.[5] In cases of degenerative joint disease at the HIPJ, procedural options include arthrodesis or arthroplasty depending on ambulatory demand as well as co-impacting factors.[6] The use of an isolated HIPJ arthroplasty as a treatment for a plantar medial soft tissue ulceration offers a method for internal joint offloading when local wound care and shoe modifications fail.[7]

INDICATIONS AND PITFALLS

The Akin osteotomy provides true transverse plane correction in the setting of hallux interphalangeal deviation or as a versatile adjunctive procedure for hallux valgus correction.[8,9] The proximal phalanx osteotomy affords finer tuned correction to lessen the need for overly aggressive medial eminence resection and extensive sagittal groove violation which potentially leads to hallux varus complications.[10] The Akin osteotomy limits the need for disproportionate lateral soft tissue release in combination with distal or shaft metatarsal osteotomies.[11,12] The adjunctive Akin decreases the need for over displacement of the distal first metatarsal osteotomy capital fragment.

The lateral aspect of the osteotomy requires gradual completion to avoid fracture of the lateral hinge. The intact lateral cortex provides inherent stability to the osteotomy and allows for single axis fixation. Hinge fracture greatly increases the occurrence of nonunion and hardware failure.[13] Avoid excessive shortening of the proximal phalanx by limiting the osseous resection to the minimal amount required for deformity correction.

In greater intermetatarsal (IM) angle deformity, the best utilization of the Akin is as a secondary procedure to provide additional, augmented correction.[8,9] The Akin has limited capability for larger deformity correction due to the constrained length of the proximal phalanx. Studies demonstrate a correction of the Hallux abductus interphalangeal of 10 degrees requires a 3 mm osteotomy thus increasing the potential for shortening.[14] The potential for under-correction exists if the majority of the deformity correction is dependent on the proximal phalanx procedure.[10,15] The proximal Akin osteotomy is contraindicated in the skeletally immature patient.

The Moberg osteotomy imparts only sagittal plane correction of the proximal phalanx. The dorsal wedge osteotomy establishes a dorsiflexed proximal phalanx and decreases the contact pressure at the 1st metatarsal phalangeal joint (MTPJ).[3,4] The Moberg osteotomy is commonly performed as an adjunctive procedure for hallux rigidus and helps to decompress the joint. The limited motion at the MTP can result in hallux jamming with ambulation. The hallux osteotomy is performed in conjunction with a cheilectomy procedure to remove osseous prominence at the dorsal aspect of the proximal phalanx base as well as the 1st metatarsal head.

In contrast to an Akin, a plantar hinge is created to provide stability to the osteotomy and allow for singe staple or combined staple/plate fixation.[4] This procedure does not provide correction for hallux interphalangeus and is limited to only sagittal plane correction. Caution must be taken to verify adequate plantarflexion deformity preoperatively to provide adequate hallux ground purchase following the procedure. The potential for a progressive hallux malleus and degeneration of the HIPJ is present if plantarflexion is limited at the MTP joint due to distal compensation.

The "Miami Osteotomy" provides combined transverse plane correction as well as minor sagittal plane correction with one simple osteotomy.[5] This oblique osteotomy is performed at the base of the proximal phalanx and is oriented dorsal proximal to plantar distal. A complete osteotomy eliminates the need for a cortical hinge and allows for the ability to swivel the proximal phalanx for mild to moderate correction of hallux interphalangeus.

However, the "Miami Osteotomy" is unstable and requires two points of fixation to prevent axial rotation around a single screw.

Arthrodesis of the HIPJ is an excellent procedure for consideration in degenerative joint disease of the HIPJ. This is a joint destructive procedure and must be reserved for end stage joint degeneration. The cartilage is removed on both sides of the joint typically by sagittal saw, power rasp or hand instrumentation. Two parallel osseous surfaces are created and fixated in close opposition.

When considering a HIPJ fusion, the surgeon must evaluate the adjacent 1st MTPJ for pre-existing arthritic changes. If present, adjunctive procedures may be necessary to preserve proximal joint function. Adjunctive procedures are necessary to prevent accelerative damage at the 1st MTP due to creating a longer rigid lever arm at push off.[6]

There are many fixation options for the HIPJ fusion. Due to the potential for axial rotation, two points of fixation provide the most stable construct.

Arthroplasty of the HIPJ has a smaller window for procedural consideration. This is a joint destructive procedure that resects the head of the hallux proximal phalanx just distal to the condyles. This procedure provides immediate internal offloading to heal chronic plantar/medial hallux ulcerations as well as correction of rigid hallux malleus in the neuropathic patient. Increased motion at the HIPJ in dorsiflexion is observed on the operating room table. The shear force and friction that was present before surgery is now permitted to dissipate through the improved range of motion of the joint. The joint however is not intended to fuse so this procedure is best reserved for patients who have failed conservative care.

INDICATIONS

- Isolated hallux interphalangeus angular deformity
- Adjunctive procedure for improved correction of hallux valgus deformity
- Painful joint restriction at the hallux interphalangeal joint
- Nonhealing ulceration of the hallux soft tissue

ANATOMIC FEATURES

The proximal phalanx is a cylindrical long bone with an abrupt diaphysis. The proximal phalanx is the central component of the hallux lever arm. A truncated lateral metaphyseal diaphyseal junction causes distal angulation deformity at the HIPJ. Conversely, a function deformity is created at the HIPJ due to the soft tissue imbalance in the setting of hallux valgus. The presence of an intra-capsular accessory sesamoid have been observed. The sesamoid may potentially restrict motion in the setting of altered joint mechanics.

FUNCTIONAL ANALYSIS OF THE ANATOMY

The joint functions in dorsiflexion and plantarflexion. The distal phalanx is the final anatomic weightbearing structure

before push-off in the gait cycle. The hallux generates the final component of the necessary force to completely propel the full body weight off the ground. Limitation or joint deviation at the MTP leads to a lateralizing force to the HIPJ and alters the mechanical lever arm of the hallux. The abnormal force weakens soft tissue stabilizing structures and worsen or increases the tendon imbalance present with proximal deformities. Proximal procedures allow functional return of length to the first metatarsal, which creates a bowstring effect on the extensor halluces longus (EHL). The proximal phalanx osteotomy reduces the tendon lever arm and realigns the soft tissue balance across the first metatarsophalangeal joint. This potentially prevents recurrence and hallux drift.[16]

PHYSICAL EXAMINATION

The initial complaint routinely accompanies concomitant bunion pain. Irritation at the second digit is commonly noted. Subluxation or dislocation is a likely consequence of the progressive deformity. The deformity typically presents independent of shoe gear and is resistant to padding as well as spacers. The hallux IPJ range of motion must be evaluated for restriction. The joint limitations may proceed to rigidity without intervention. The distal phalanx appears plantarflexed in a mallet contracture in advanced presentations. Early identification of HIPJ space narrowing both radiographically and clinically allows for joint sparing procedures to remain in consideration.

PATHOGENESIS

Hallux valgus deformity centered at the HIPJ requires correction at the apex of the deformity. This subset of the deformity is driven by a soft tissue imbalance extenuated by imperfect inherent osseous abnormalities. Hallux interphalangeus or an isolated obliquity of the hallux interphalangeal angle is responsible for the hallux misalignment in the centered hallux valgus deformity.[5] In the setting of a relatively maintained IM 1-2 angle and proper first metatarsal alignment, a lateral cortical length disparity sets the stage for long tendon imbalance and distal bunion pathology. The distal instability causes proximal altered mechanics and first metatarsophalangeal joint deviation.

IMAGING AND DIAGNOSTIC STUDIES

Weight bearing radiographs in the anterior posterior views to assess for:

- Hallux abductus interphalangeal HAI angle. Normal 0-10 degrees
- Lateral and medial proximal phalanx cortex disparity
- Distal Articular Set Angle
- HIPJ sesamoid

Weight bearing radiographs in the lateral view to assess for:

- Hallux sagittal malalignment
- HIPJ sesamoid

TREATMENT

NONOPERATIVE

Splints and toe spacers offer temporary stability without lasting deformity correction. Rigid carbon fiber inserts may provide external stability and reduce motion in the setting of degenerative joint disease.

OPERATIVE TREATMENT

Indicated after failure of conservative care.

> *positioning* PEARLS
> - Patient positioned supine on the operating table with an ipsilateral hip bump to maintain the foot rectus

Akin Osteotomy

Surgical Procedures and Techniques

The incision placement is dorsal linear, directed just medial to the EHL tendon extending from the HIPJ to the 1st MTPJ. This incision can also be incorporated into the primary procedure by extending the incision placement distally. The dissection is carried to the medial aspect of the EHL, which is isolated and retracted laterally while maintaining the distal attachment. The periosteum is reflected sharply off the base of the proximal phalanx.

For the proximal Akin, the transverse osteotomy is performed ~5-7 mm from the metatarsophalangeal joint at the proximal metaphyseal diaphyseal junction of the proximal phalanx. The proximal transverse osteotomy provides ease of access due to the minor incision extension and anatomic dissection needed for access. For the distal Akin, the transverse osteotomy is made ~5-7 mm from the HIPJ at the distal metaphyseal diaphyseal junction of the proximal phalanx.

A 0.045-in Kirschner wire (K-wire) is utilized as an apex guide and is inserted into the lateral aspect of the proximal phalanx either proximal or distal depending on the osteotomy site. The wire is placed into the proximal phalanx at the lateral edge with caution to place the wire in the widest portion of the phalanx at the metaphyseal diaphyseal junction. Verify that the guidewire is placed perpendicular to the long axis of the proximal phalanx.

The osteotomy can be marked out before making the individual cuts to visualize the degree of correction needed. Draw the osteotomy by surgical marker or the cuts can be lightly scored by the sagittal saw. The distal cut is made first to the degree of correction due to the anatomic stability while the proximal cut is then produced second parallel to the joint due to the retained anatomic stability. Complete the osteotomy superiorly and inferiorly with thorough removal of the osseous wedge. The apex of the osteotomy is then "feathered" by sagittal saw until the osteotomy is manually reduced and held in place by clamp or guidewire. The feathering technique gradually removes a portion of cortical bone until the osteotomy is reducible while maintain the cortical hinge. First the osteotomy is extended plantary while hold slight compression force distally. If the osteotomy remains nonreducible then the osteotomy is extended gradually at the dorsal aspect. This technique is repeated in increments until the osteotomy is reducible and able to be held in compression manually.

The oblique wedge osteotomy provides powerful correction while allowing for screw fixation in the preferred perpendicular direction. The osteotomy is directed distal medial to proximal lateral within the phalanx shaft (Figs. 6.1 through 6.4). A transversely oriented osteotomy may also be considered. Both directions are amendable to single screw fixation if the cortical hinge is maintained.

> PEARLS
> - Plantarflex the hallux at the interphalangeal joint to allow slack in the flexor hallucis longus tendon and minimizes iatrogenic injury risk.
> - Dental pick to remove osseous fragment.
> - Feather the superior and inferior aspect individually in a gradual manner.
> - Lightly compress at the osteotomy until closure is noted.

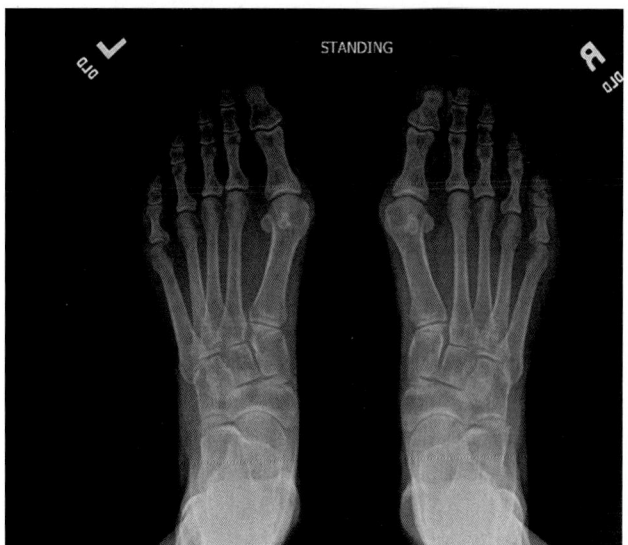

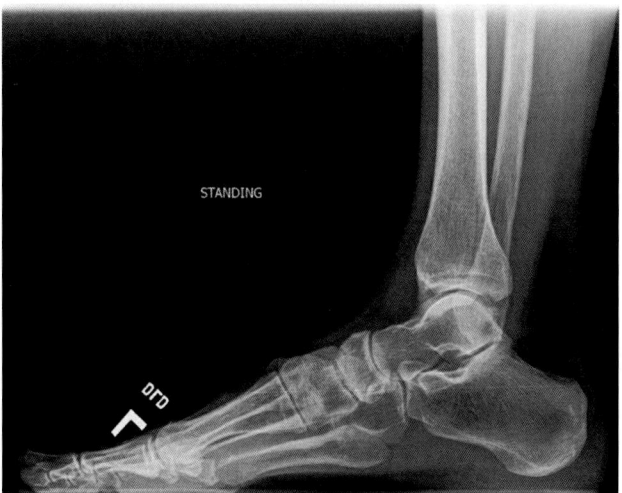

FIGURE 6.1 Preoperative radiographs of a 62-year-old female with a chief compliant of painful hallux valgus.

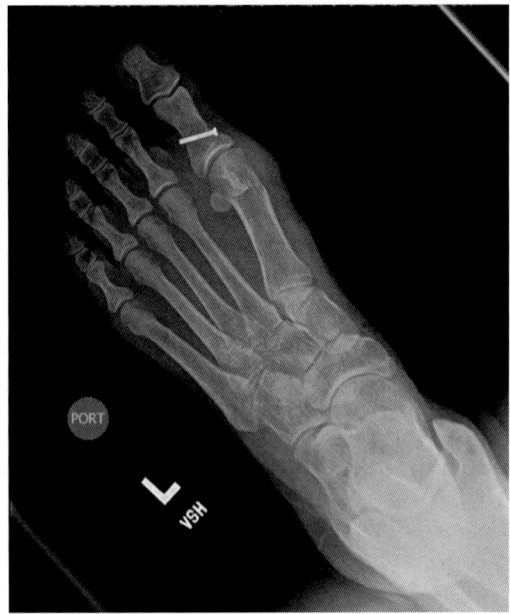

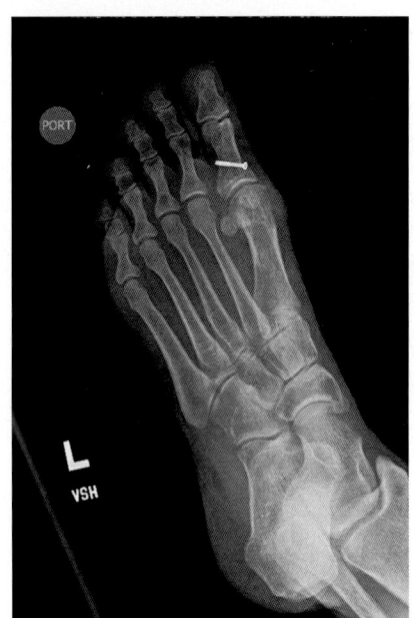

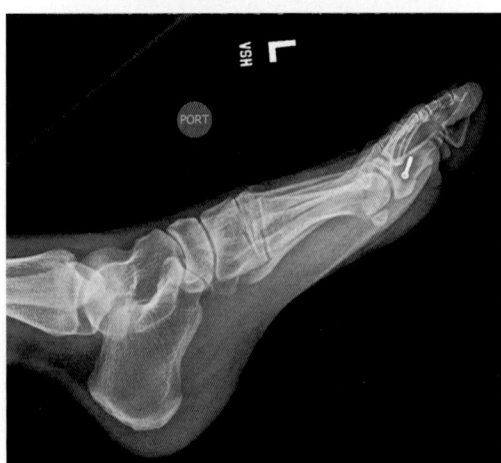

FIGURE 6.2 Three postoperative radiographs of a bunionectomy combined with an oblique Akin with single screw fixation.

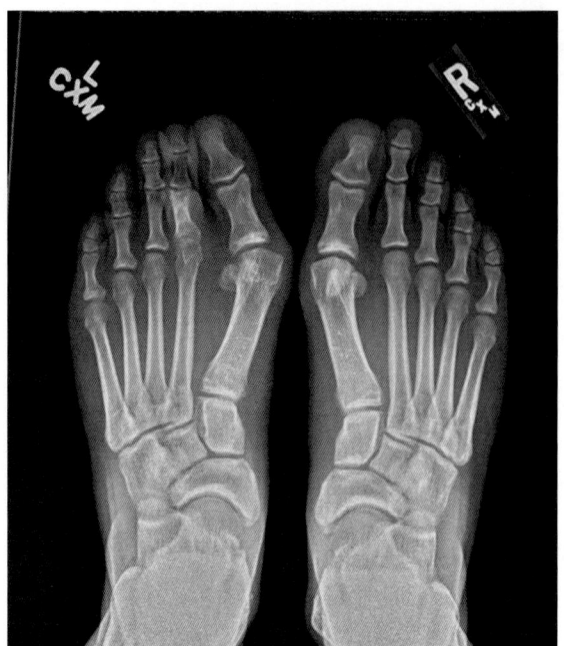

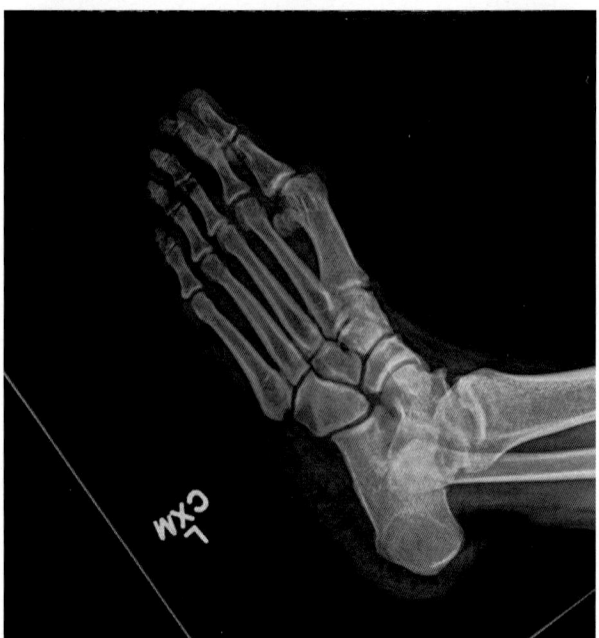

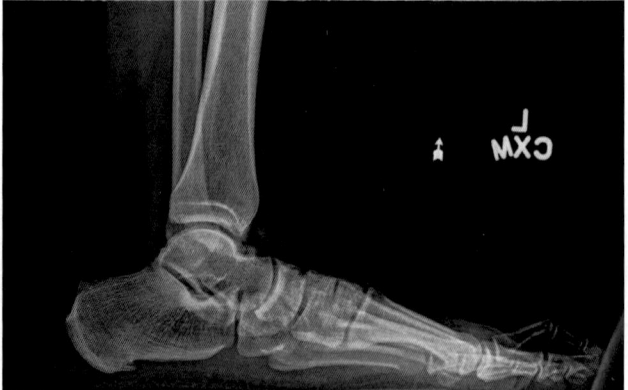

FIGURE 6.3 Preoperative radiographs of a 65-year-old female with a chief compliant of painful hallux valgus and 2nd digit hammer toe.

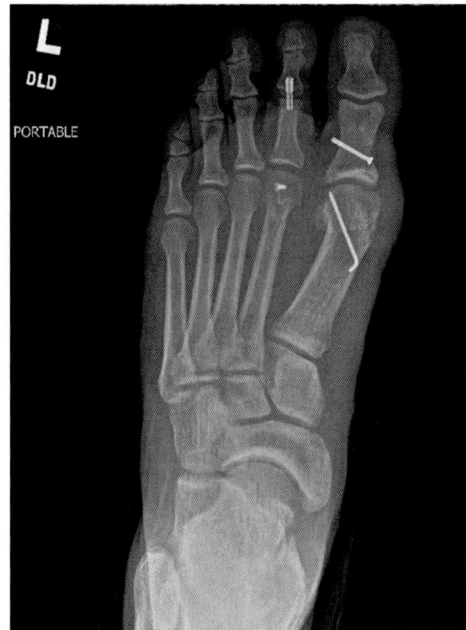

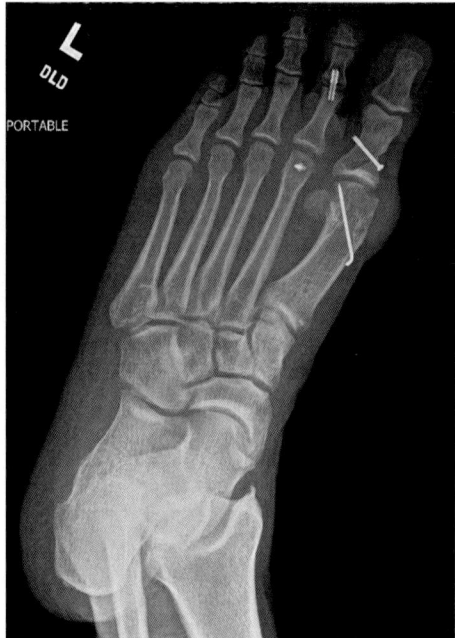

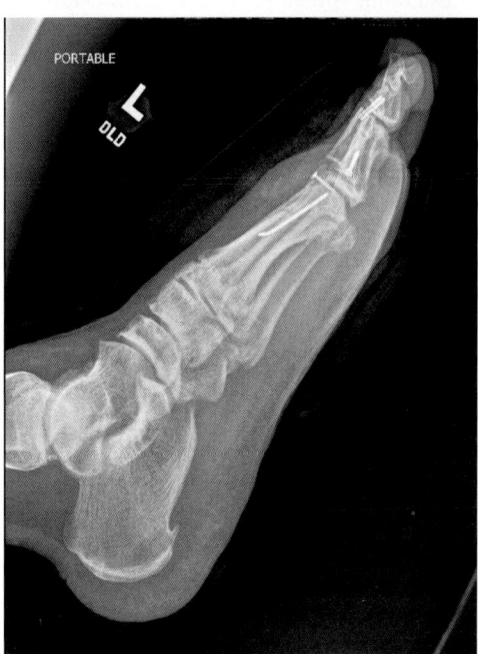

FIGURE 6.4 Postoperative radiographs of a distal metatarsal chevron osteotomy combined with an oblique Akin osteotomy with screw fixation.

Several fixation options are available for the Akin osteotomy. The intact lateral hinge imparts inherent stability to the osteotomy and is thus amendable to single axis fixation.[17] Historically the osteotomy was secured by monofilament wire. For the proximal Akin, a single headless compression screw placed at the proximal medial condyle of the proximal phalanx provides reliable fixation with minimal soft tissue prominence. The screw should exit the lateral cortex within the concave portion of the diaphysis. For the distal Akin, the technique is reversed, and a single screw is placed in the distal medial condyle with the screw directed to exit the bone at lateral diaphysis. Staples are easily inserted perpendicular to the osteotomy. Ensure pilot hole drilling for staple placement is done parallel to the osteotomy. This may be accomplished by placing one of the drill guide arms slightly off of the bone. Failure to do so may lead to one of the arms of the staple off kilter in the osteotomy or within the adjacent joint.

The osteotomy at the distal aspect of the proximal phalanx allows correction closer to the apex of the hallux interphalangeus deformity. This approach requires the incision to be extended further distally overlying the HIPJ. The EHL attachment must be restored to avoid a functionally plantarflexed hallux. The wedge osteotomy is placed at the medial cortex with the apex placed laterally just proximal to the distal condyle. Fixation is oriented in the opposite direction from distal medial to proximal lateral.

The Moberg Osteotomy

Surgical Procedures and Techniques

The incision placement is dorsal linear directed just medial to the EHL tendon extending from the HIPJ to the 1st MTPJ. This incision can also be incorporated into the adjunctive 1st MTP procedure by extending the incision placement distally. The dissection is carried to the EHL, which is isolated and retracted laterally while maintaining the distal attachment. The periosteum is reflected sharply off the base of the proximal phalanx. A 0.045-in K-wire is utilized to protect erroneous entry into the 1st MTP. The wire is inserted in a medial to lateral orientation with care to provide adequate area for fixation to the base of the proximal phalanx.

The proximal osteotomy is performed first in the superior to inferior direction perpendicular to the proximal phalanx and not to the weightbearing surface. The cut is made distal to the MTPJ (metatarsophalangeal joint) ~5 mm from the cartilaginous surface of the proximal phalanx based with care taken to not violate the metatarsophalangeal joint. The osteotomy is stopped before the plantar cortex to maintain the plantar hinge as well as protect the FHL from iatrogenic laceration. The second osteotomy is made ~2-4 mm distal to the first osteotomy and is oriented in a dorsal wedge to be completed at the inferior aspect of the first cut.[4] The two cuts must be parallel at the dorsal starting point with the equal removal of bone at the medial and lateral aspect of the wedge to prevent added hallux interphalangeus deformity.

The dorsal wedge osteotomy provides hallux dorsiflexion while the plantar hinge provides added stability. This osteotomy requires gradually extension of the osteotomy in closer proximity to the hinge by sagittal saw, also known as "feathering." As describe in the Akin section, this technique carefully extends the bone cut closer to the hinge to allow for manual compression of osteotomy site utilizing the modules of elasticity of bone while maintaining the cortical hinge. The reduced position is held in place by temporary K-wire or clamp. Staple fixation is considered adequate if performed perpendicular to the osteotomy after manual compression either dorsally or medially.

> ## PEARLS
> - Carefully anatomic preservation of the EHL maintains physiologic resting tension which provides an additional soft tissue tether to oppose plantarflexion and decrease potential for malunion/nonunion.

The "Miami Osteotomy"

Surgical Procedures and Techniques

The incision placement is dorsal linear directed just medial to the EHL tendon extending from the HIPJ to the 1st MTPJ. This incision can also be incorporated into the primary 1st MTPJ procedure by extending the incision placement distally. The dissection is carried to the EHL, which is isolated and retracted laterally while maintaining the distal attachment. The periosteum is reflected sharply off the base of the proximal phalanx.

The proximal oblique osteotomy is performed just superior to the cartilaginous surface at the dorsal aspect of the proximal phalanx base. The osteotomy is directed ~25-30 degrees to the longitudinal bisection of the proximal phalanx base.[5] The saw is oriented dorsal proximal to plantar distal and is a complete through and through cut without maintaining a plantar hinge. The hallux distal phalanx must be held in a plantarflexed position at the HIPJ to reduce tension on the FHL.

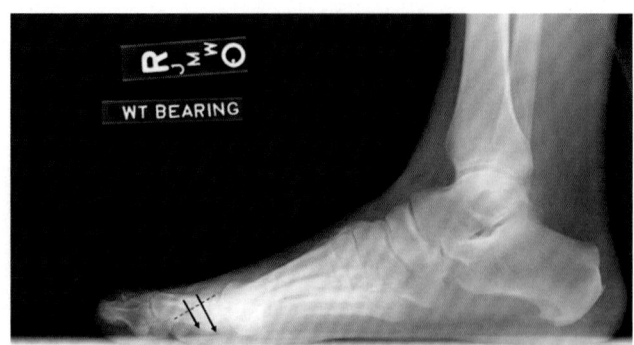

FIGURE 6.5 The Miami osteotomy (*red dashed line*) is oriented dorsal proximal to plantar distal and is a complete through and through cut. Two screws (*black arrows*) are oriented perpendicular to the osteotomy. Care must be taken to leave enough of an osseous shelf both dorsal and plantar to aid in screw purchase and compression of the osteotomy. Apply plantar pressure to maintain osseous apposition during screw insertion.

The oblique proximal phalanx osteotomy provides powerful correction in the transverse plane while allowing an adequate shelf for two screw fixation in the preferred perpendicular direction. Temporary fixation of the osteotomy is achieved by screw guidewire placement or 0.045 K-wire insertion once the corrected position is attained. The guidewires for small cannulated partially threaded screws, preferably 2.7 mm or smaller depending on the proximal phalanx dimensions, are placed using intraoperative fluoroscopy to verify the correct obliquity needed for perpendicular fixation. Due to the oblique angulation of the osteotomy the distal screw is placed first while the proximal guidewire maintains a second point of temporary fixation. The second screw is placed under the same technique. Similar to a Weil osteotomy for a lesser metatarsal, the ideal screw configuration for the Miami osteotomy is spaced adequately apart to accommodate the individual screw land while maintaining an intact osseous shelf for screw purchase and compression (Fig. 6.5).

Care must be taken to avoid placing the screws too close to the ends of the osteotomy arms as the thin cortex is susceptible to cracking during screw placement resulting in loss of purchase.

> ## PEARLS
> - Verify guidewire placement prior to screw insertion to assess adequate cortical thickness for screw purchase.
> - Place manually plantar force underneath the osteotomy to decrease likelihood of gapping at the osteotomy during screw placement.

Arthrodesis of the HIPJ

Surgical Procedures and Techniques

The incision placement is dorsal linear, directed just medial to the EHL tendon with two perpendicular arms one medial and one lateral placed over the HIPJ. An extension of a linear incision can also be incorporated into the adjunctive 1st MTP procedure by extending the incision placement distally. The dissection is carried to the EHL, which is isolated and transected proximally to the distal attachment. The tendon is reflected proximally and protected throughout the procedure. Maintain adequate distal tendon for later reattachment. The HIPJ is sharply incised transversely and the collateral ligaments are released both medial and lateral. Dissection should be limited to adequate joint exposure without unnecessary periosteal stripping of adjacent osseous surfaces. Inspection of the plantar aspect of the joint to allow for removal of a HIPJ sesamoid if present.

Both the distal and proximal cartilaginous surfaces of the joint are resected by sagittal saw or hand instrumentation per surgeon preference. Joint preparation is planar where the cuts must be oriented parallel to each other to allow for complete opposition of the osseous surfaces. Depending on concurrent interphalangeal deformity joint resection can incorporate a wedge cut to provide proper hallux alignment. A 0.045-in K-wire may be used as a cutting orientation guide to verify the joint is resected perpendicular to osseous surface opposed to the weightbearing surface. The guidewire also provides a means to confirm equal and adequate deformity correction in the setting of hallux interphalangeus. The adjacent joint surfaces are prepared for fusion by removing all remaining cartilage and soft tissue. Intramedullary drilling of the head of the proximal phalanx is performed with caution but it is not recommended for the distal phalanx due to the potential for iatrogenic fracture. Aggressive fish scaling should be avoided.

The alignment of the HIPJ during fixation is the key to providing the patient with the proper deformity correction without significantly altering the mechanics proximally at the 1st MTP. Fusion of the HIPJ creates a rigid lever arm that may accelerate joint degeneration due to poor position.

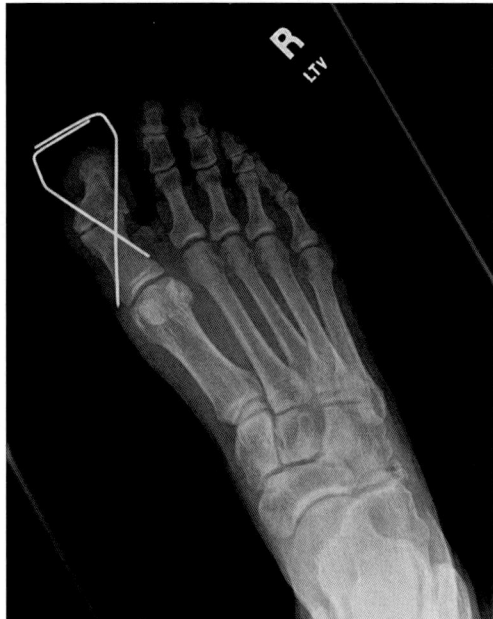

> ### PEARLS
> - Utilizing K-wires as cut guides reduces angulation at the osseous surface of the fusion sites.
> - Verify the removal of cartilage and soft tissue between the opposing osseous surfaces prior to fixation.
> - Avoid excessive shortening by performing cautious joint resection.

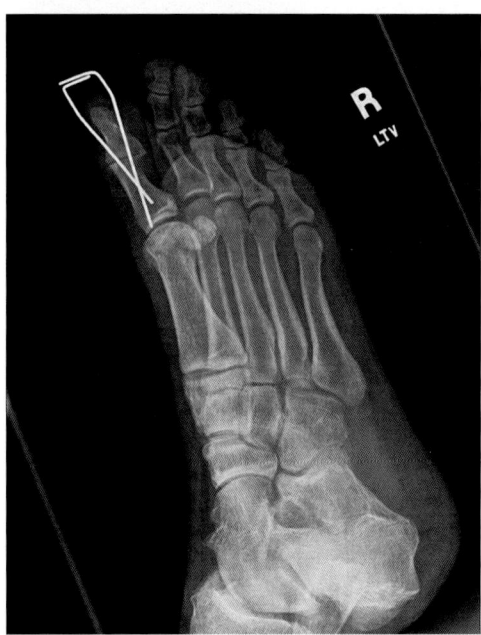

Several fixation options are available for the HIPJ arthrodesis procedure.

Permanent fixation is recommended but not absolutely required for joint fusion. The joint may be temporarily stabilized by either one or two 0.062 K-wire placed in retrograde or anterograde fashion.

For retrograde single K-wire fixation: the distal phalanx is held while the K-wire is driven from within the joint out through the tip of the toe. Care must be taken not to violate the nail plate. In cases of nail disruption, the K-wire should be completely driven through the exit point and discarded. Resist pulling the K-wire back and redirecting due to possible contamination of the wire from the undersurface of the nail.

For retrograde double K-wire fixation: the distal phalanx is held while the K-wire is driven from within the joint out through the tip of the toe. The wires should cross in the proximal phalanx away from the joint. The distal ends of the wires are then bent and taped together to resemble a "bucket handle" (Fig. 6.6). This technique allows the 2 K-wires to work as a unit which prevents accidental pull out and more stable fixation.

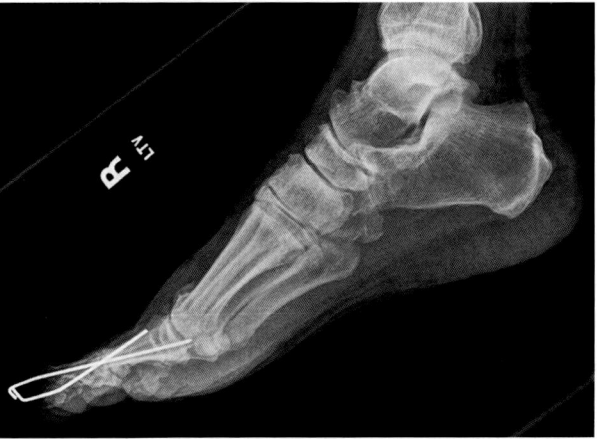

FIGURE 6.6 Hallux interphalangeal joint arthrodesis by crossed Kirschner wires in the "bucket handle" configuration.

Either single or double K-wire fixation can be performed in anterograde fashion. The distal phalanx is held while the K-wire is driven from the distal tip of the toe. The wires should cross with in the proximal phalanx.

Screw fixation provides a permanent fixation option for joint fusion. Two crossing screws provide a strong construct that resists axial rotation at the fusion site. Dependent on an individual patient's anatomy, the distal phalanx has a limited osseous structure that possibly prevents two screw configuration. The necessary angle to accomplish two screw fixation poses a challenge that is mitigated by using cannulated screws. The distal phalanx is at risk of iatrogenic fracture with multiple redirected fixation attempts. A simpler screw fixation technique entails the use of a single solid fully threaded screw placed under modified cannulated technique. The joint is prepared and the guidewire for a 2.7, 3.5 or 4.0 mm is placed retrograde from the center of the distal phalanx out through the tip of the hallux inferior to the nail plate. Standard AO technique of overdrill, underdrill and careful countersinking are performed after insuring proper pin placement and alignment with intraoperative fluoroscopy. Next the guidewire is advanced into the predetermined site of the proximal phalanx. Now both the under and over drill is performed with the assistance of the guidewire using cannulated technique to provide lag by technique. The solid screw is inserted and the joint is compressed evenly (Fig. 6.7). Single screw fixation has the potential for axial rotation. Once the fixation and position are noted to be well aligned, the EHL is reapproximated by 4-0 vicryl. Careful reapproximation of the EHL tendon provides a minor soft tissue restraint to motion.

PEARLS

- The retrograde approach allows direct visualization of the fixation within the HIPJ and is the preferred method.
- Flush apposition of joint resection is required for arthrodesis.
- Perform co-axial drilling over a wire. Do not free-hand drill distal and proximal phalanx separately which may result in reduced surface contact area or gapping.
- Use of a fully threaded screw is preferred over a partially threaded screw to avoid loss of thread purchase in the medullary canal of the proximal phalanx.

Arthroplasty of the HIPJ

Surgical Procedures and Techniques
The incision placement is dorsal linear, directed just medial to the EHL tendon with two perpendicular arms one medial and one lateral placed over the HIPJ. The dissection is carried to the EHL, which is isolated and transected proximally to the distal attachment. The tendon is reflected proximally and protected throughout the procedure. Maintain adequate distal tendon for later reattachment. The HIPJ is sharply incised transversely and the collateral ligaments are released both medial and lateral. Dissection should be

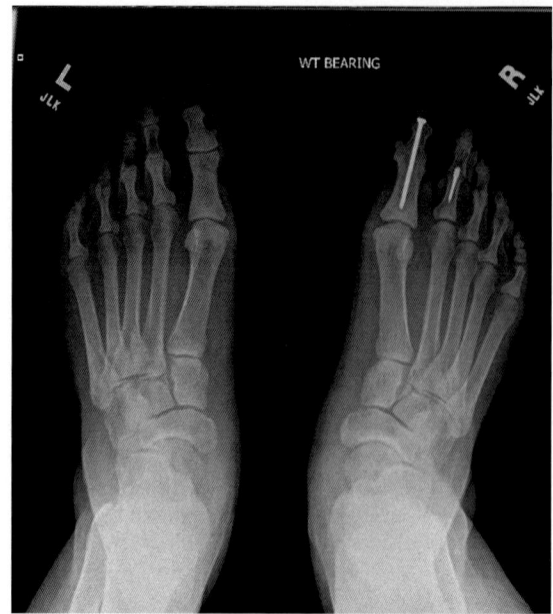

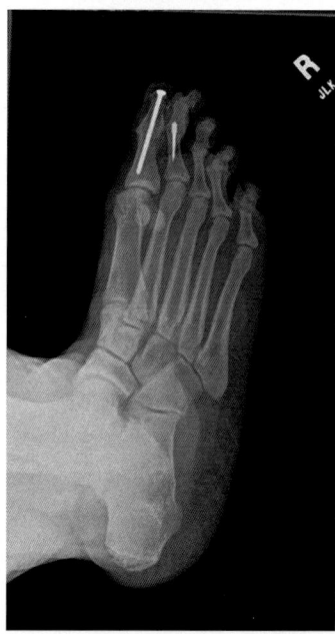

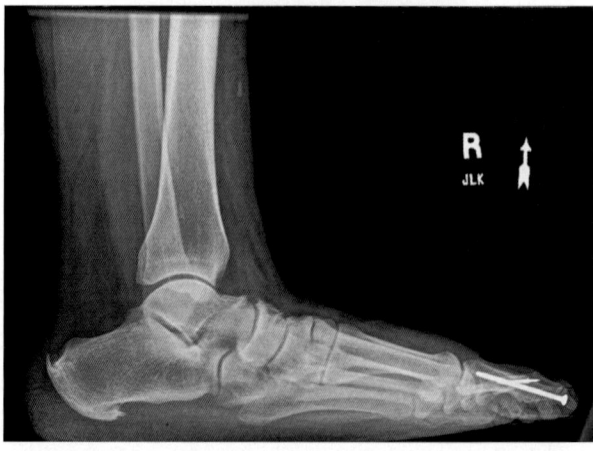

FIGURE 6.7 Hallux interphalangeal joint arthrodesis performed by single screw fixation.

limited to adequate joint exposure without unnecessary periosteal stripping of adjacent osseous surfaces. Inspection of the plantar aspect of the joint to allow for removal of a HIPJ sesamoid if present.

Only the head of the proximal phalanx is resected by sagittal saw. Orient the placement of the cut just proximal to the condyles of the proximal phalanx. The cut is directed perpendicular to the long axis of the proximal phalanx. A 0.045-in K-wire may be used as a cutting orientation guide to verify the head of the proximal phalanx is resected perpendicular to osseous surface opposed to the weightbearing surface. The guidewire also provides a means to confirm equal and adequate deformity correction in the setting of hallux interphalangeus.

Upon completion of the arthroplasty the EHL is reapproximated by absorbable suture, preferable 4-0 vicryl.

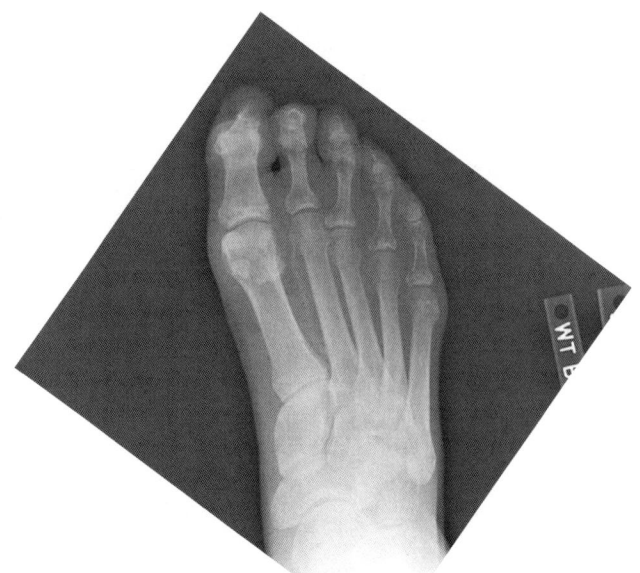

PEARLS

- Plantarflex the hallux at the interphalangeal joint to allow slack in the flexor hallucis longus tendon and minimizes iatrogenic injury risk.

No permanent fixation is required. The joint may be temporarily stabilized by either one or two 0.062 K-wire placed in retrograde or anterograde fashion. The wire prevents excess motion and allows the incision to heal without delays. The wires can easily be removed in the clinic setting using a pair of pliers. Plain film radiographs can be taken before removal to verify the wire has not shifted or bent during the postoperative period. Wire removal is typically performed 3-4 weeks after surgery.

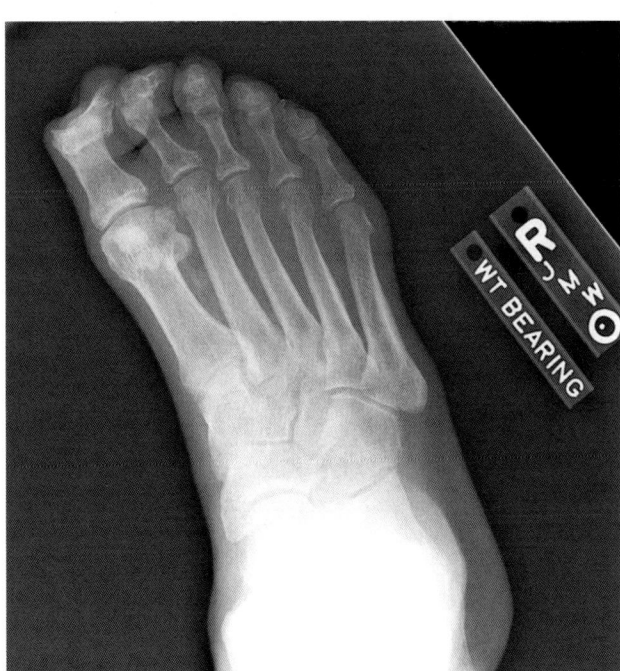

PEARLS

- In cases of nail disruption, the K-wire should be completely driven through the exit point and discarded. Resist pulling the K-wire back and redirecting due to possible contamination of the wire from the undersurface of the nail (Figs. 6.8 through 6.11).
- In the setting of open ulceration, no fixation is preferred.

AUTHORS PREFERRED TREATMENT

The authors recommend the Akin proximal phalanx osteotomy for enhanced correction of large IM angle hallux valgus deformity in conjunction with a primary procedure (Fig. 6.12). Osteotomy orientation either transverse or oblique at the proximal base provides the ability to dial in the necessary correction. This technique provides slightly more protection of the lateral hinge due to the apex being easily placed at the metaphyseal diaphyseal junction. Complete the primary hallux abductovalgus corrective procedure first then assess additional need for proximal phalanx correction (Fig. 6.13).

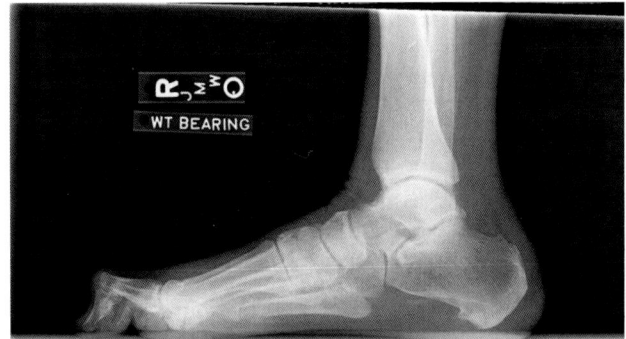

FIGURE 6.8 Preoperative radiographs of a 73-year-old patient with a severe mallet toe deformity that was rigid in nature.

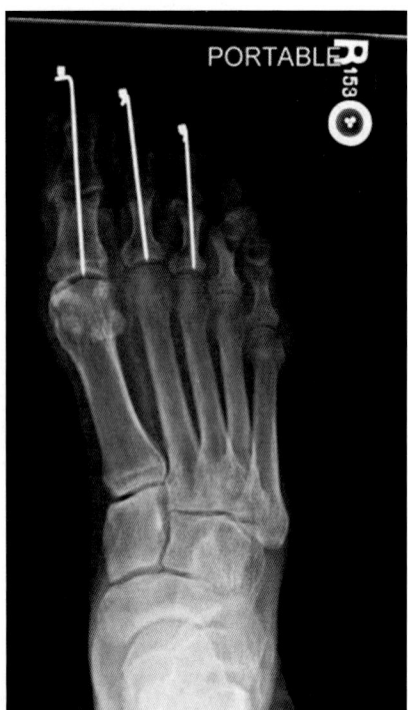

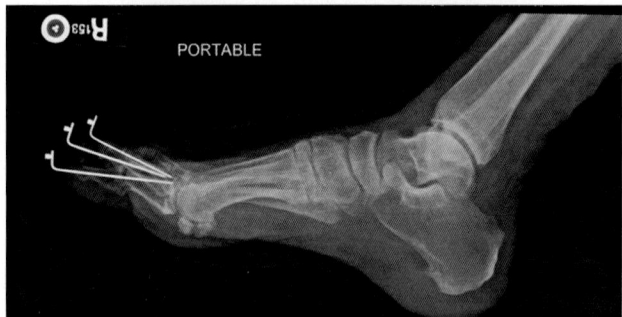

FIGURE 6.9 Postoperative radiographs of the hallux interphalangeal joint arthroplasty with Kirschner wire temporary stabilization.

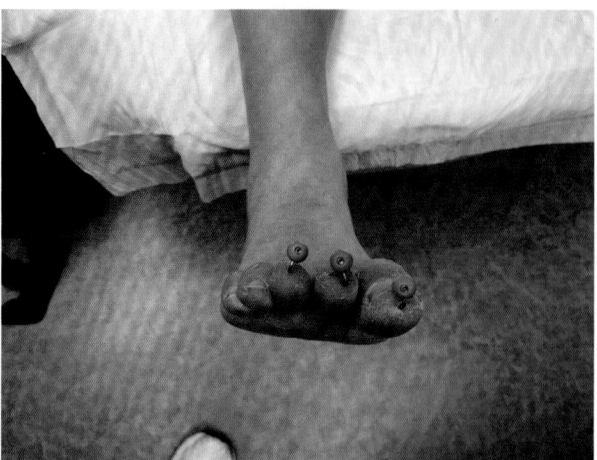

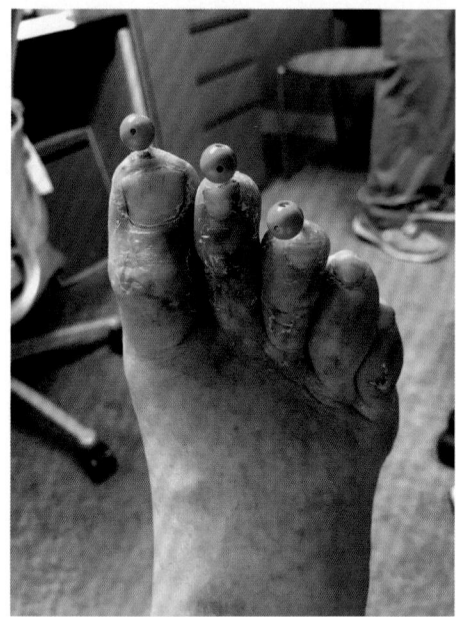

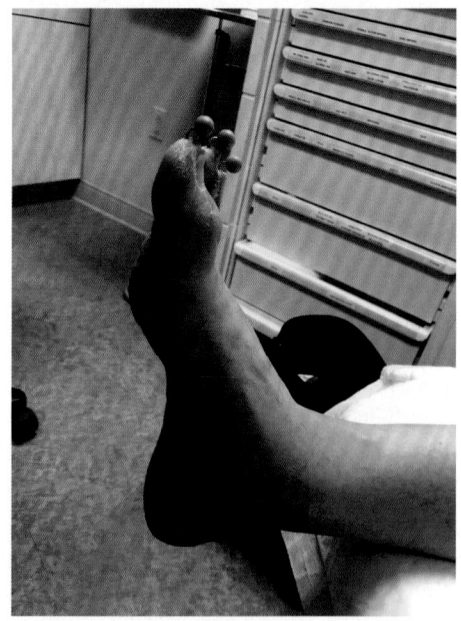

FIGURE 6.10 Clinical pictures with the K-wires intact.

The K-wire axis guide is essential and helps prevent sagittal malalignment of the osteotomy orientation (Fig. 6.14). The osteotomy is completed first distally then the proximal portion. The osseous fragment is then removed by dental pick (Fig. 6.15). The osteotomy lateral apex is feathered by sagittal saw while gentle compression is applied. Once osteotomy closure is complete, a single 2.5-3.0 mm headless compression screw is placed across the osteotomy. The screw is oriented medial to lateral and started in the medial condyle of the proximal phalanx. A small percutaneous incision may be utilized to allow for deeper screw application and reduce the risk of stress riser fracture of the dorsal shelf of the osteotomy. Verify guidewire placement on intra-op fluoroscopy to verify appropriate far cortex exit and drill utilizing cannulated technique (Fig. 6.16). It is recommended to drill completely through the far cortex to allow for easy screw insertion and to avoid excessive torque on the lateral hinge. Verify even appearance of both medial and lateral cortices as well as reduction of the

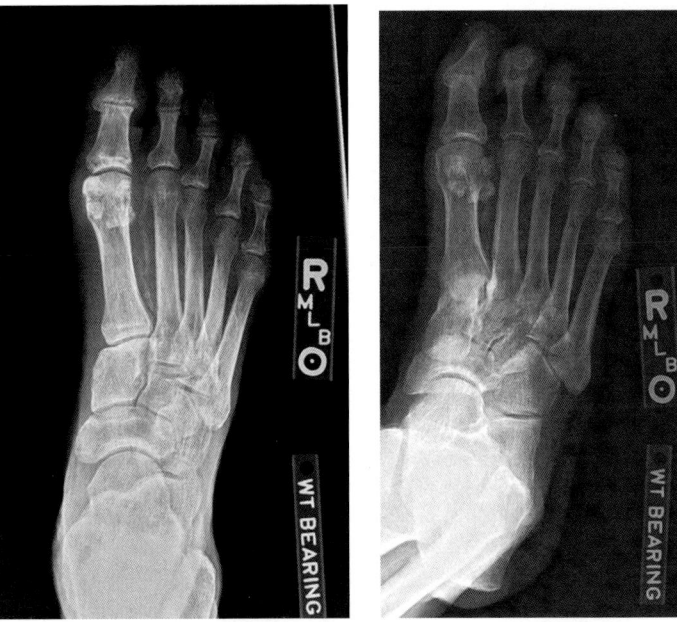

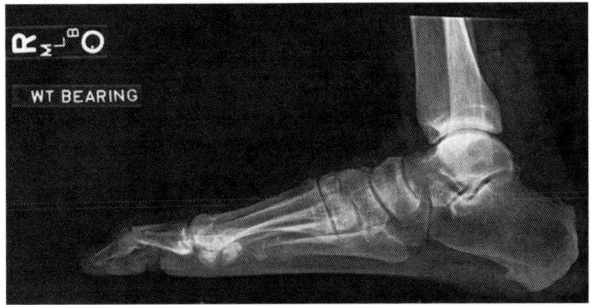

FIGURE 6.11 Postoperative radiographs showing deformity correction after K-wire removal.

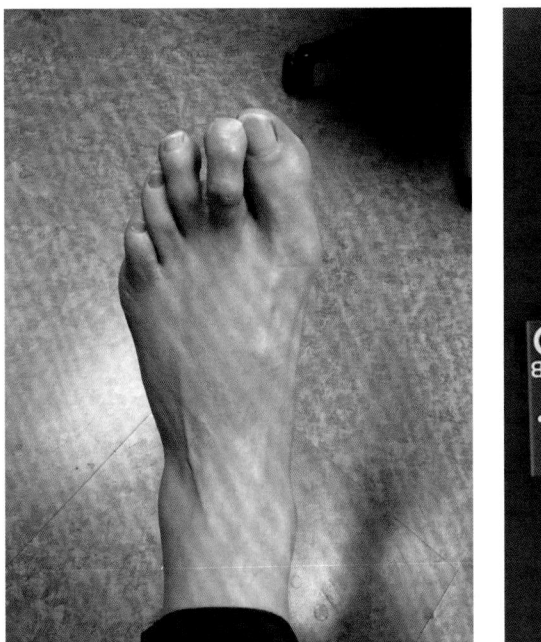

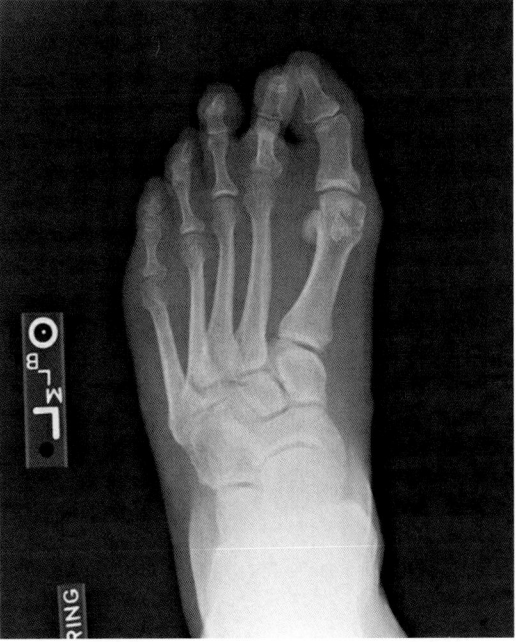

FIGURE 6.12 Clinical and radiographic images of a 52-year-old male patient with a painful hallux valgus deformity as well as a second digit hammer toe deformity.

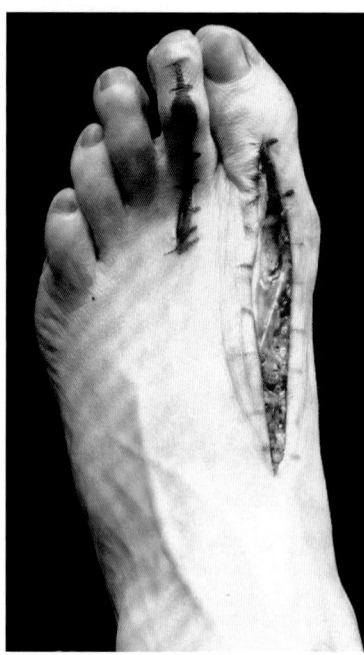

FIGURE 6.13 Intraoperative image of the hallux position following Lapidus correction with lateral deviation of the hallux still apparent.

POSTOPERATIVE CARE

Well-padded soft compressive dressing with heel weight bearing in a stiff sole surgical shoe to avoid propulsion at the operative digit. If K-wires are present, the pin sites should be inspected on a regular basis. The insertion sites are kept dry and dressed with nonadherent dressing with bacitracin or betadine. In the postoperative period the K-wires can be removed typically 3-4 weeks after surgery. Plain film radiographs are useful to verify the wires have not bent or shifted postoperatively. The tip of the wire is grasp just distal to the skin and the wire is pulled straight back while maintaining a side to side twisting motion of the hand. The sites are then dressed and monitored until closure is completed.

REHABILITATION

Activity limitation until radiographic healing of the osteotomy is noted. The patient can progress to passive range of motion at the first metatarsophalangeal joint and interphalangeal joint depending on the procedure selected.

hallux interphalangeus angle (Figs. 6.17 and 6.18). Obtain regular postoperative radiographs to verify proper healing of the osteotomy without displacement of the fixation and maintenance of the correction (Fig. 6.19).

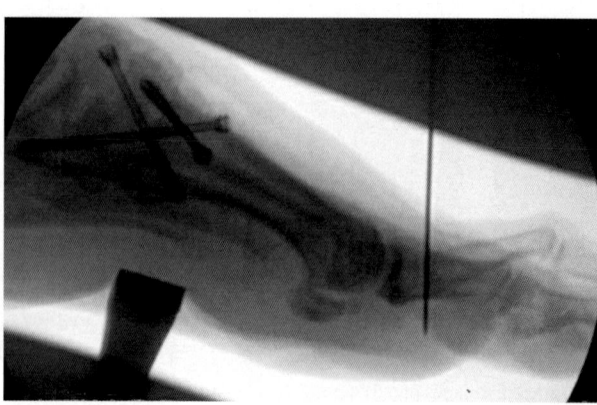
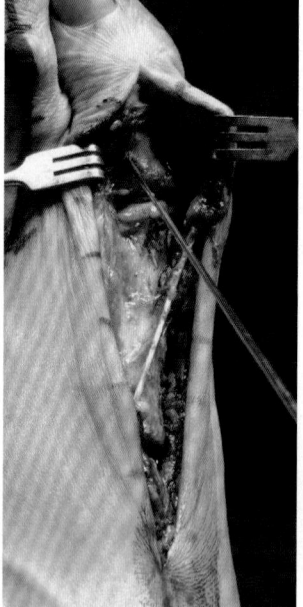

FIGURE 6.14 Placement of the osteotomy apex guidewire in the lateral aspect of the proximal phalanx.

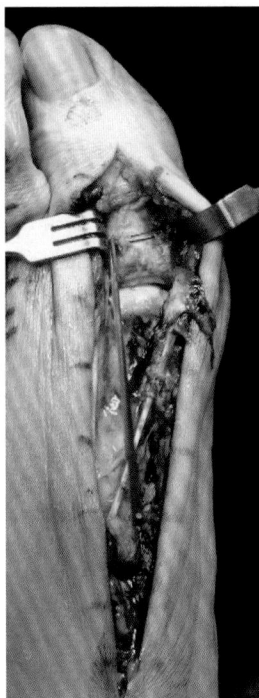
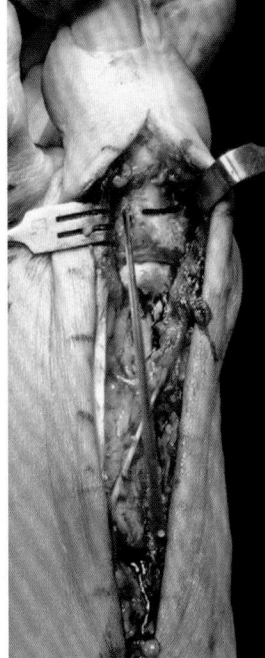
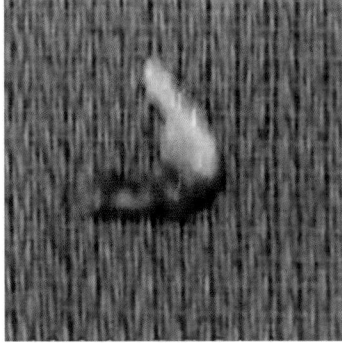

FIGURE 6.15 Intraoperative image following osteotomy complete and then removal osseous fragment.

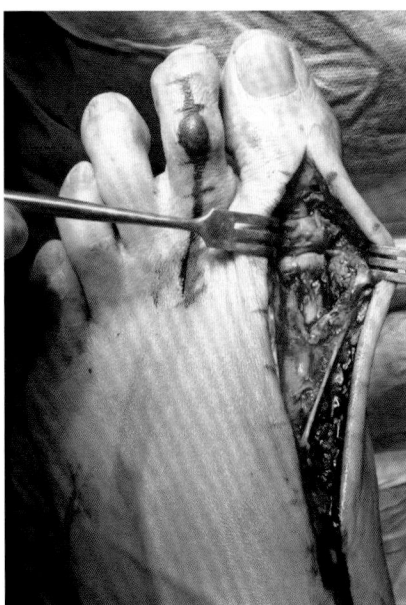
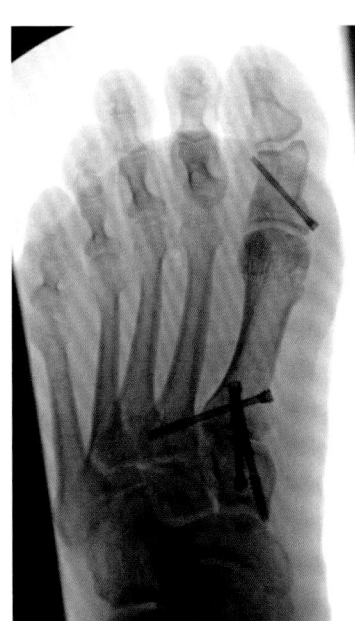
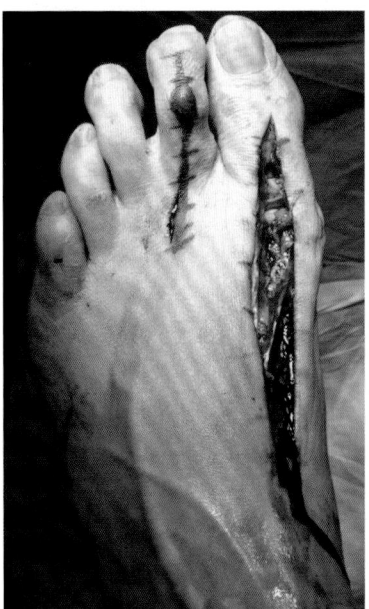

FIGURE 6.16 Intraoperative and fluoroscopic images of the osteotomy closure and singe 2.5 mm headless compression screw fixation.

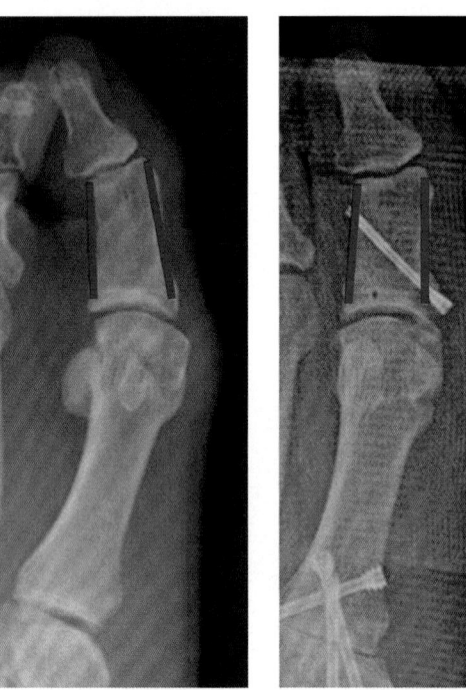

FIGURE 6.17 Preoperative and immediate postoperative demonstration of medial and lateral cortical length.

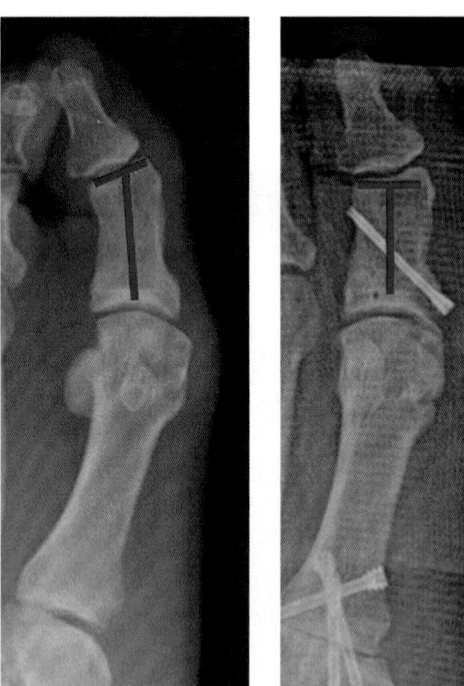

FIGURE 6.18 Preoperative and immediate postoperative demonstration of hallux interphalangeus angle reduction.

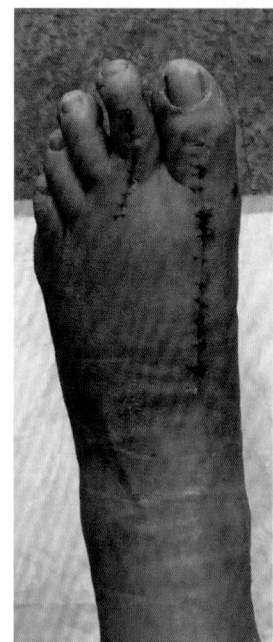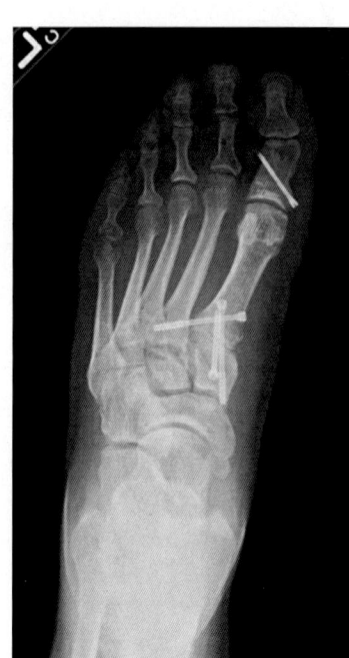

FIGURE 6.19 Clinical and radiographic images of the Lapidus with adjunctive Akin osteotomy postoperative 4 weeks.

REFERENCES

1. Daw SW. An unusual type of hallux valgus (two cases). *Br Med J.* 1935;2:580.
2. Akin OF. The treatment of hallux valgus: a new operative procedure and its results. *Med Sentinel.* 1925;33:678-679.
3. Moberg E. A simple operation for hallux rigidus. *Clin Orthop Relat Res.* 1979;(142):55-56.
4. Warganich T, Harris T. Moberg osteotomy for hallux rigidus. *Foot Ankle Clin.* 2015;20(3):433-450.
5. Cohen M. The oblique proximal phalangeal osteotomy in the correction of hallux valgus. *J Foot Ankle Surg.* 2003;42:282-289.
6. Derner R, Meyr AJ. Hallux interphalangeal joint arthrodesis. *J Foot Ankle Surg.* 2009;48:408-410.
7. Lew E, Nicolosi N, McKee PJ. Evaluation of hallux interphalangeal joint arthroplasty compared with nonoperative treatment of recalcitrant hallux ulceration. *J Foot Ankle Surg.* 2015;54(4):541-548.
8. Frey C, Jahss M, Kummer F. The Akin procedure an analysis of results. *Foot Ankle.* 1991;12:1-6.
9. Rettedal D, Lowery NJ. Proximal phalangeal osteotomies for hallux abductovalgus deformity. *Clin Podiatr Med Surg.* 2014;31(2):213-220.
10. Shibuya N, Thorud JC, Martin LR, Plemmons BS, Jupiter DC. Evaluation of hallux valgus correction with versus without akin proximal phalanx osteotomy. *J Foot Ankle Surg.* 2016;55(5):910-914.
11. Kerr HL, Jackson R, Kothari P. Scarf-Akin osteotomy correction for hallux valgus: short-term results from a district general hospital. *J Foot Ankle Surg.* 2010;49:16-19.
12. Pinney SJ, Song KR, Chou LB. Surgical treatment of severe hallux valgus: the state of practice among academic foot and ankle surgeons. *Foot Ankle Int.* 2006;27:1024-1029.
13. Douthett SM, Plaskey NK, Fallat LM, Kish J. Retrospective analysis of the akin osteotomy. *J Foot Ankle Surg.* 2018;57:38-43.
14. Shannak O, Sehat K, Dhar S. Analysis of the proximal phalanx size as a guide for an akin closing wedge osteotomy. *Foot Ankle Int.* 2011;32(4):419-421.
15. Dixon AE, Lee LC, Charlton TP, Thordarson DB. Increased incidence and severity of postoperative radiographic hallux valgus interphalangeus with surgical correction of hallux valgus. *Foot Ankle Int.* 2015;36:961-968.
16. Park JY, Jung HG, Kim TH, Kang MS. Intraoperative incidence of hallux valgus interphalangeus following basilar first metatarsal osteotomy and distal soft tissue realignment. *Foot Ankle Int.* 2011;32(11):1058-1062.
17. Christensen JC, Gusman DN, Tencer AF. Stiffness of screw fixation and role of cortical hinge in the first metatarsal base osteotomy. *J Am Podiatr Med Assoc.* 1995;85:73-82.

CHAPTER 7

Second Metatarsophalangeal Joint

Amber M. Shane, Christopher L. Reeves, Hannah J. Sahli, and Josh Sebag

DEFINITION

Pathology of the second metatarsal phalangeal joint, namely metatarsalgia, is a comprehensive term comprised of several differential diagnoses that encompass the lesser rays and forefoot. It is a common, often misunderstood, and painful condition seen by foot and ankle specialists. Often, crossover toe and plantar plate dysfunction come to mind as pain generators and causes of metatarsalgia. This term may also include predislocation syndrome, capsulitis, Freiberg's, or synovitis.[1,2] Many of these differentials involve similar treatment modalities that have been addressed and classified.[1,3] Inflammatory, noninflammatory, and crystalline arthropathies may also lead to forefoot pathologies that can be difficult to diagnose due to similar clinical presentation.[4] Second metatarsophalangeal joint (MTPJ) deformities, specifically, have long plagued the foot and ankle surgeon due to their complexity. Anatomic and biomechanical complexities exist about the weight-bearing forefoot with the longest ray, most commonly the second, often affected.[5] Many nonoperative and operative treatment modalities exist with an aim to treat the region. However, a single surgical procedure that consistently provides a rectus pain free toe is not typical. The literature frequently demonstrates that surgery about the forefoot is not without issue. Metatarsal osteotomies may lead to floating toe, flexor tendon transfers may lead to digital stiffness, and joint destructive procedures may greatly alter biomechanics of the foot and thus should be reserved for severe cases recalcitrant to conservative care.[6] The modern era of orthopedic fixation devices has acted to influence medicine, advance surgical techniques, and accelerate postoperative protocols. Cruveilhier, in 1844, was credited with the first description of the plantar plate. This complex anatomic connective tissue structure is still known for its challenges in diagnosis and treatment.[7] In this chapter, we will focus on lesser MTPJ instability, including the plantar plate, and discuss common nonsurgical and surgical modalities. Recreation of a well-aligned metatarsal parabola and technical detail in plantar plate reconstruction to achieve anatomical and functional balance of the forefoot will be described. In addition, we will also discuss avascular necrosis (AVN) of the lesser MTPJ, Freiberg infraction, briefly as this diagnosis and treatment warrants focused discussion.

CLASSIFICATION

Multiple classification systems have been described for clinical and anatomic plantar plate dysfunction as well as Freiberg infraction. Yu and Coughlin have both described clinical and anatomic staging based upon physical appearance and plantar plate integrity. Table 7.1 depicts the classification systems. Smillie classified a staging system for Freiberg infraction that is based upon progression of second metatarsal head deterioration; Table 7.2 depicts this classification system.

CLASSIFICATION

- Plantar plate dysfunction clinical staging
  - Grade 0—Plantar plate or capsular attenuation
  - Grade 1—Transverse distal midsubstance tear, <50%
  - Grade 2—Transverse distal or midsubstance tear, >50%
  - Grade 3—Longitudinal tear with or without transverse tear
  - Grade 4—Extensive stellate tear with dislocation/degeneration
- Smillie staging system for Freiberg infraction
  - Fissure fracture in ischemic epiphysis
  - Changes to articular surface with absorption of cancellous bone, central portion begins to collapse into metatarsal head. Plantar hinge intact
  - Articular surface sinks well into the head, leaving sizable projections on either side
  - Plantar hinge fails and projections on either side fracture, creating loose bodies
  - Arthrosis with marked flattening and deformity of the metatarsal head

ANATOMIC FEATURES

Before we can understand the abnormal second MTPJ, we must discuss normal second MTPJ anatomy. The second MTPJ is an ellipsoidal, ginglymus, synovial joint with ~40 degrees of flexion and extension.[9] Many intrinsic and extrinsic structures

TABLE 7.1	Anatomic and Clinical Staging for Plantar Plate Dysfunction	
	Yu Anatomic Staging[1,2]	**Coughlin Clinical Staging[3]**
Grade 0		Plantar plate or capsular attenuation
Grade 1	Subtle edema to dorsal and plantar lesser MTPJ, alignment of the digit unchanged	Transverse distal midsubstance tear, <50%
Grade 2	Mild edema with noticeable deviation of the digit Loss of toe purchase with weight bearing	Transverse distal or midsubstance tear, >50%
Grade 3	Moderate edema around the entire joint and toe More pronounced deviation and possible subluxation present End result of crossover second-toe deformity	Longitudinal tear +/− transverse tear
Grade 4		Extensive stellate tear with "button hole" dislocation/degeneration

cross the joint and thus each play a role in biomechanical function and stability. The lesser MTPJs are crossed dorsally by two extensor tendons, the extensor digitorum longus and brevis. The extensor digitorum longus divides into three slips over the lesser digit. The middle slip inserts on the base of the middle phalanx, while the two lateral slips extend over the dorsolateral aspects of the middle phalanx and converge with the extensor digitorum brevis (EDB) to insert at the base of the distal phalanx.[10] The tendons act to dorsiflex the digits during the swing phase of gait and stabilize the digits during propulsion.[11] Proximally, at the level of the MTPJ, the sheath of the extensor tendons blend with the capsule of the MTPJ (Fig. 7.1), which subsequently attaches to the plantar plate and deep transverse intermetatarsal ligament connecting one MTPJ to the adjacent. This anatomic configuration allows for a strong dorsiflexory function of the proximal phalanx. In contrast, the flexor digitorum longus and brevis tendons function as the primary flexors of the interphalangeal joints, with a passive plantarflexory force across the MTPJ. Unlike the lateral lesser joints, the flexor tendon runs beneath the second metatarsal head in a groove immediately plantar to the plantar plate.[12] If abnormal bony architecture, gait, or other mechanical demands are present, this system may become pathologic.[13]

In addition to extrinsic forces, there are intrinsic attachments about the second MTPJ as well. Unlike the remaining lesser rays, this joint has two dorsal interosseous muscles crossing the joint. These interossei muscles serve to stabilize the MTPJ in the transverse plane. The lumbricals of the foot originate from the long flexor tendons and attach on the medial aspect of the MTPJ capsule.[10] This allows an unopposed adductory force across the MTPJ. However, with an intact lateral capsule, plantar plate, and lateral collateral ligaments, this adductory force is easily balanced.[14]

Another major structure of the second MTPJ is the plantar, or flexor, plate and collateral ligaments. The plantar plate is a dense trapezoidal fibrocartilaginous structure, composed of 75% type I collagen, 21% type 2 collagen, and the remaining from blended connective tissue elements from its attachments. The dorsal two-thirds of the plantar plate have longitudinal fibers while the planter third has transverse fibers. The average length of the plate is 19 mm with an average width of 11 mm. The additional attachments to the plantar plate are extensive and include the deep transverse intermetatarsal ligament, plantar fascia, capsular tissues, interossei tendons, and flexor sheath. The plantar plate has a firm attachment to the base of the proximal phalanx, the collateral ligaments, and plantar fascia; however, it has a thin synovial tissue attachment to the

TABLE 7.2	Staging System for Freiberg Infraction by Smillie
Stage 1	Fissure fracture in ischemic epiphysis
Stage 2	Changes in articular surface. Absorption of cancellous bone, central portion begins to collapse into the metatarsal head Leaves an intact plantar hinge
Stage 3	Articular surface sinks well into the head, leaving sizable projections on either side
Stage 4	Plantar hinge fails and projections on either side fracture, creating loose bodies
Stage 5	State of arthrosis with marked flattening and deformity of the metatarsal head

Smillie IS. Treatment of Freiberg's infraction. *Proc R Soc Med*. 1967;60:29-31. Ref.[8]

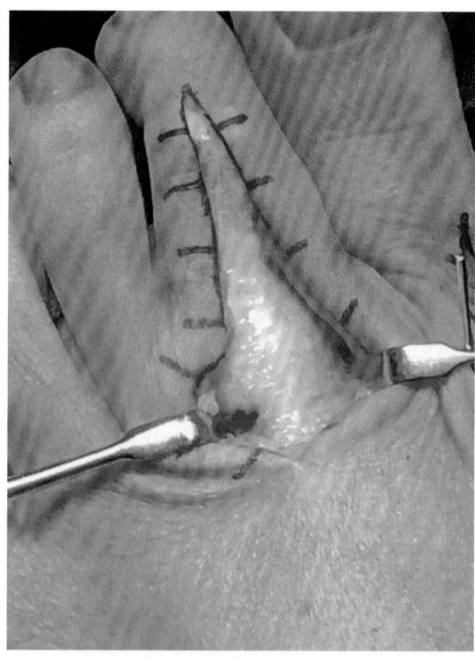

FIGURE 7.1 Healthy appearing second MTPJ, note the transversely oriented fibers of the extensor hood apparatus in relation to the long axis of the ray.

metatarsal neck.[11] The inherent stability of a normal plantar plate apparatus has been discussed by many authors. It is considered the most dynamic stabilizing element of the lesser MTPJ. Ford et al, in a cadaveric study evaluating stabilization of the second MTPJ, found that a transected plantar plate markedly increased dorsal displacement of the digit by 74%.[15] In addition to the plantar plate, the collateral ligaments aid in positioning and stabilization of the MTPJ. These are composed of two main structures; the phalangeal collateral ligament (PCL), which inserts at the base of the proximal phalanx, as well as the accessory collateral ligament (ACL) that inserts into the plantar plate.[11] With these structures intact, the plantar plate has three main functions; serve as a cushion to offload compressive loads transferred to the forefoot, assist with MTPJ stability, and provide support to the windlass mechanism with direct insertion on the plantar fascia.

In addition to the extensive soft tissue complex about the second MTPJ, it is important to review the vascular supply. In 2002, Peterson and Lankes performed a cadaver study to map the arterial supply of the lesser metatarsals and found each metatarsal head has two arterial sources: the dorsal metatarsal arteries, which arise from the dorsalis pedis artery, and the plantar metatarsal arteries, which are branches of the posterior tibial artery. These two vessels typically anastomose about the metatarsal head forming a vascular ring that acts to perfuse the region. The nutrient arteries traverse the cortex of the metaphysis close to the capsular and ligamentous insertions to provide multiple branches for the supply of the subchondral bone. They also found variations in normal anatomy in which some cadavers were missing one or both of the main arterial supplies and were left with just collateral circulation leaving some predisposed for vascular compromise.[15] Due to the extensive vascular and soft tissue network about the second MTPJ, there are multiple opportunities for pathology, including AVN, or Freiberg infraction.

PHYSICAL EXAMINATION

Depending on the stage of the deformity at initial presentation, multiple clinical and radiographic signs are examined and used for diagnosis. As originally described by Yu, "predislocation syndrome" often presents as a rectus digit with isolated plantar sulcus pain. Pain is typically distal to the plantar aspect of the metatarsal head as this is consistent with the anatomic location of the insertion of the plantar plate, to the proximal phalangeal base.[1,2] Local edema isolated to the joint as well as joint line tenderness may be particularly helpful when distinguishing plantar plate irregularities vs other forefoot abnormalities such as neuromas, stress fracture, and MTPJ synovitis. In 2002, Yu went on to outline multiple ways to help the practitioner differentiate plantar plate dysfunction from other common ailments.[1]

Stress fractures may be differentiated from other MTPJ pathology with pain on direct palpation on the midshaft of a metatarsal or by using a tuning fork, which is classically positive for tenderness, mostly dorsal, in cases of stress fracture. This may be particularly helpful when the patient presents during the early period of time in which radiographs may not depict callus formation. Additionally, differentiating plantar plate pathology from a neuroma is of importance. A neuroma is most commonly seen at the third interspace and occasionally at the second. A positive Mulder click may be present when there is a

significant soft tissue mass. This is unlike plantar plate pathology that is frequently seen at the second MTPJ rather than the innerspace. Further, in cases of neuroma, edema is infrequent, however, quite common in plantar plate dysfunction, and with musculoskeletal disease.

Predislocation syndrome may insidiously develop toward MTPJ subluxation as the deformity is progressive in nature. Mendicino and others have described a prodromal period prior to subluxation.[12] This is often characterized by pain and swelling, isolated to the lesser MTPJ. Patients may present initially with vague symptoms including discomfort to the digits, metatarsals, and intermetatarsal space. Umans, in 2014, evaluated skeletal radiology and found that 67% of plantar plate tears were associated with coexistent non-neuroma interspace lesions, namely pericapsular fibrosis.[16] In subtle cases, this clinical presentation may create challenges in diagnosis to the clinician. As the deformity progresses, subluxation about the joint, both in weight bearing and in static assessment, may be seen as digital contracture.[13,17] Due to this, hyperkeratotic lesions are frequently seen at areas of high pressure such as the plantar second metatarsal head and the dorsal aspect of the proximal interphalangeal joint (PIPJ) due to irritation with shoe gear. Rigidity and hyperkeratotic lesions may indicate chronicity of the deformity.

A thorough non–weight-bearing examination must be performed to help assist with the diagnosis of plantar plate disruption. The vertical drawer, or Lachman examination, should be used to test the local soft tissues for sagittal plane insufficiency.[1,2] This is the most useful clinical examination to isolate and assess the integrity of the plantar plate and associated collateral and suspensory ligaments. This examination may be painful, and a local anesthetic block may be considered to fully appreciate potential subluxation. Additionally, an anesthetic block may be helpful to distinguish pain associated with an interdigital neuroma vs an unstable lesser MTPJ.[18] Injections in this fashion are both diagnostic and therapeutic when used appropriately. To perform the Lachman examination, the digit is dorsiflexed ~20-25 degrees at the MTPJ and a vertical stress is performed upon the digit while the clinicians other hand stabilizes the forefoot and immediately adjacent metatarsal heads from motion (Fig. 7.2).[19] If the toe is not dorsiflexed prior to vertical translation, the plantar portion of the phalangeal base may abut the metatarsal head leading to a false negative. The vertical stress test is defined as positive if 5-mm dorsal translation of the joint is noted.[5] This alone is thought by many to be pathognomonic for plantar plate insufficiency. In more advanced cases of instability, frank subluxation is present without elicitation of the vertical stress test, as complete attenuation has already led to dorsal subluxation of the digit. In the setting of long-standing dorsal dislocation, concurrent degenerative joint changes are not uncommon.[5] In this scenario, treatment options may be more limited or require more significant interventions vs isolated plantar plate reconstruction as multiple architectural factors are likely correlated. Reasonable patient expectations should be discussed at length prior to any surgical intervention. The Kelikian push up test, another non–weight-bearing examination, may help assess flexible vs rigid lesser digital deformities and may also be helpful when assessing the competence of the plantar plate. The practitioner applies a dorsally directed force to the plantar surface of the metatarsal head. In a flexible deformity, one will notice the digit and MTPJ to reduce. This test has been well described and may be helpful in surgical

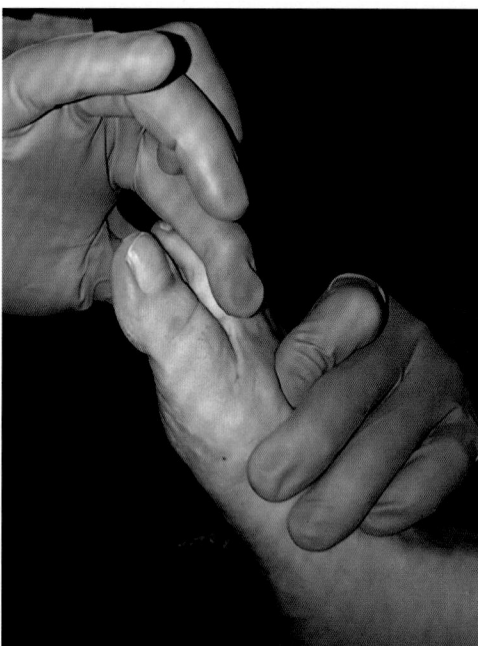

FIGURE 7.2 Lachman examination is a vertical stress on the second metatarsophalangeal joint to test the integrity of the plantar plate. Image shows a positive examination with a torn plantar plate.

decision-making intraoperatively.[20] In a rigid scenario, the digit will not reduce and a positive plantar plate tear may be suspected if the test demonstrates medial digital deviation.

Another, less sensitive yet effective examination, described by Bouche, is the paper pull out test.[21] While the patient is weight bearing, the affected digit is tested for toe purchase and strength by placing and pulling a strip of paper from beneath the toe pulp (Fig. 7.3). In an unaffected second MTPJ, the

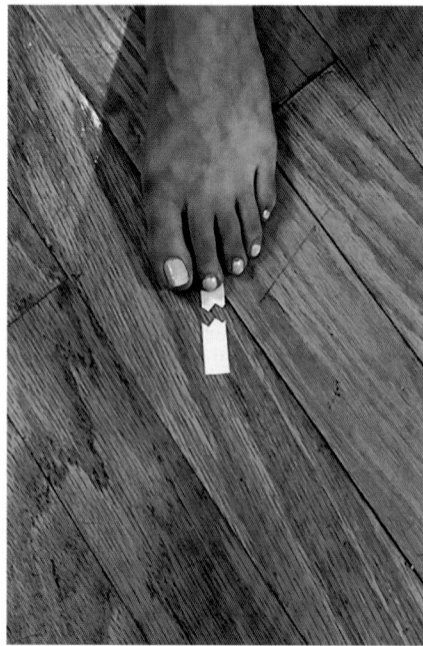

FIGURE 7.3 Bouche paper pull out test is a weight-bearing examination used to test plantar flexion strength about the lesser MTPJ.

patient is able to engage the second digit into the paper via the flexors and prevent pull out of the test strip. In the setting of plantar plate disruption, digital purchase and strength may be lost, and the paper may easily be removed. The toe may rest abnormally high and lack the ability to adequately make contact with the paper despite instruction to flex the digit. If the patient is unable to prevent the paper from being pulled out, this is considered a positive test. This is further suggestive of plantar plate instability, attenuation, and disruption. Lastly, evaluation of the plantar forefoot may reveal fat pad atrophy, whether from previous injections or anatomic variation. This is not to be overlooked as this may decrease the buffer between the plantar metatarsal head, plantar plate apparatus, and the ground reactive forces.

In our experience, intraoperative findings correlate with physical examination findings seen with the Lachman, Kelikian, and Bouche paper pull out examinations. After obtaining subjective and objective clinical findings, consider that 95% of patients with plantar second metatarsal head pain, localized edema, positive Lachman examination, and pain that has been present for more than 6 months have a true plantar plate disruption.[22] When a patient presents with localized pain and edema to the second MTPJ with a negative Lachman and Bouche paper examination, other sources of pathology must be considered. Freiberg disease as well as capsulitis, synovitis, neuroma, or other biomechanical imbalance may present with similar initial patient complaints. Further examination including advanced imaging may be warranted to assist in differentiating the diagnosis.

PATHOGENESIS

Etiology of second MTPJ pathology is vast and often affects the biomechanical function of the foot and ankle. This impacts >2 million patients annually in the United States leading to more than 350 000 MTPJ and 500 000 PIPJ procedures each year.[23] There have been many causes suggested for the development of predislocation syndrome. These include hallux valgus deformity, hypermobile first ray, abnormal metatarsal protrusion, trauma, neuromuscular, anomalous muscle, and other anatomic abnormalities.[24] Each of these causes hold merit on the development of the deformity; however, congenital predilection, combined with the aging process, female gender, and chronic ill-fitting shoe gear, may be among the most likely cause.[25] Yu and colleagues postulated that common anatomic and biomechanical variants were the fundamental causes of predislocation syndrome. They suggested that the long second metatarsal and pronated pedal architectures created an increased plantar pressure to the second MTPJ, causing both initiation and progression of the disease. Further, gait analysis studies reveal that during the heel-off phase, the forefoot can experience up to 120% of the total body load.[26] Additionally, the role of equinus and its contribution to increased forefoot pressures must be considered. Several investigators suggest that external patient factors should be considered as well. Individual activity level, the use of high-heeled shoes, and tight toe boxes increase the forefoot pressure that may predispose individuals to lesser metatarsalgia.[25]

As mentioned previously, women appear to be more at risk of developing the deformity. This is likely because of the aforementioned forefoot loading and shoe gear that tends to be associated with the syndrome. In a series of patients by Kaz and Coughlin, they found that 86% of their patients were women. This is similar to other reports in which most 70%-100% of subjects with symptoms were women.[5] Acute and chronic trauma may also lead to the progression of second MTPJ instability. These events can include activities such as running, weight lifting, baseball, gymnastics, or even daily activities like using the stairs.[27] All of the causes previously mentioned act to test the competence of and potentially negatively influence capsular, collateral ligament, and plantar plate structure. As previously discussed, the aforementioned play important roles in actively stabilizing the digit in gait and maintaining a rectus digit at rest. It has been shown in cadaveric studies that rupture of the plantar plate can increase dorsal MTPJ instability by 74% and sagittal plane instability by 33%.[28,29] Prior to any dislocation, nonspecific localized edema and pain may occur, typified as the classic predislocation syndrome. The patient may work through a subacute and acute phase leading to dorsal subluxation at the PIPJ and MTPJ. This is followed by a varus and often medial malalignment about the digit, if conservative treatment measures to mitigate the progression are not employed. Much discussion exists on the position of the second digit and its unique orientation in crossover toe deformities. We believe that various contributing force vectors allow its position. The lumbrical insertion into the medial extensor hood apparatus is a medial deforming force that may tether beneath the deep transverse intermetatarsal ligament. The more prominent lateral metatarsal condyle has also been suggested as a predisposing factor to more lateral collateral ligamentous attenuation. Further, in cases of plate dysfunction, the flexor tendons may become unbound and displace medially acting to change directional pulling forces. This coupled with a nonaxial pull of the extrinsic extensor tendons and an often space occupying hallux valgus contribute to consequent adductovarus digital malposition.

Another concept to consider is the idea of a second MTPJ bunion. This largely theoretical biomechanical theory has been demonstrated by Beren, with subsequent bunion like treatments suggested.[30] Here, given the anatomic similarities to the first ray, one may correlate the lesser MTPJ plantar plate apparatus similar to that of the first MTPJ sesamoid complex. Further, the flexor tendons of the first MTPJ correlate with that of the lesser MTPJs. Effects of a long first metatarsal and its relationship to hallux limitus may be extrapolated to the long second metatarsal and its contribution to predislocation syndrome. This interesting take on lesser MTPJ pathology and treatment has been discussed in the literature by various authors. Given the vast treatment algorithms for the first MTPJ to include cheilectomy, osteotomy, and arthrodesis, Beren has discussed cartilaginous transposition osteotomy similar to that of a Reverdin, used for the lesser ray.[30] A number of authors have also discussed lesser MTPJ fusion as a viable option in advanced cases. In 2019, Hollawell et al. demonstrated resolution of symptoms with arthrodesis of the lesser MTPJ, in a small cohort, achieving radiographic fusion on average at 16.4 weeks.[31] However, Sigvard Hansen, in his book, has outlined what he deemed essential joints of the foot and ankle.[32] These are determined as such by the nature of their biomechanical requirement and subsequent importance in normal foot motion. The first MTPJ, although useful, is described as a nonessential joint, which may be fused with impunity. This is unlike the lesser MTPJ as they have a role in push off in the late stance phase of gait that should not be compromised. This largely dispels the notion of

lesser MTPJ being treated with bunion-type methods. This further suggests the need for a deeper understanding of the plantar plate and surrounding structures. The theory of essential vs nonessential joints, the implications of a load bearing nonessential joint (first MTPJ) immediately adjacent to that of a load bearing essential joint (second MTPJ) may play a role on one another. We believe that this coupled with the compact nature of the anatomy in this region of the foot often complicates treatment. This theory is quite simplistic, essentially suggesting that acceptable semiconstrained motions, like that of the first MTPJ, are liable to create unintended motions, shear, and thereby pathology, deformity, and pain of an adjacent joint should they go unchecked. The authors believe that this theory plays a role in lesser MTPJ pain. This is further demonstrated by the frequency of first MTPJ pathology seen in symptomatic patients with lesser MTPJ complaints as the two are not mutually exclusive.

The etiology of Freiberg's, or AVN, is different than that of plantar plate injuries. AVN of the second metatarsal head is the fourth most common AVN in the body. The second metatarsal is the longest and most constricted metatarsal and can increase the stress on the metatarsal head. This theory correlates with a study done by Stanley et al.[33] who found that the longest metatarsal is affected by AVN in 85% of cases when comparing it to other lesser metatarsals. This may be further supported by the fact the second metatarsal is most likely to incur a stress fracture and associated potential vascular compromise. The cause is thought to be vascular or traumatic and is most likely a combination of both. One theory is that Freiberg's is due to disruption of vascular supply to the epiphysis of the metatarsal head. The epiphysis of the second metatarsal is supplied by branches of the medial deep plantar artery and the dorsal metatarsal artery as well as the nutrient and periosteal arteries. Peterson and Lankes performed a cadaveric study to map the arterial supply of the lesser metatarsals and found the two vessels mentioned above typically join at two sites about the metatarsal head, forming a vascular ring. This provides an extensive extraosseous arterial network around the metatarsal head. Small arterial branches from this complex network run distally on the metatarsal cortex to enter the bone at the level of the metatarsal head. The nutrient artery also traverses the cortex of the metaphysis close to the capsular and ligamentous insertions to provide multiple branches to supply the subchondral bone. The study found that limited periosteal stripping and care not to over penetrate the plantar cortex aids in avoiding the risk of AVN with metatarsal osteotomies. Also, some believe the angle of common bone cuts at this location may attribute to the very low rate of AVN seen with a Weil osteotomy.[28] Wiley and Thurston also conducted a cadaver study and found variations in normal anatomy in which some cadavers were missing one or both of the main arterial supplies and were left with just collateral circulation.[34] Therefore, anatomic variation plays a role. The other theory is a traumatic theory. Here, it is thought that trauma to the metatarsal head is the source of degenerative changes. In Freiberg original study, several patients reported previously stubbing their toes, he also postulated biomechanical factors such as long second metatarsals, hallux valgus, and hallux rigidus, which can cause chronic microtrauma, or second ray overload related to causation, but that a single trauma was unlikely to be a cause.[35] Systemic disease must also be considered. Diseases, such as systemic lupus erythematosus, and any disease that may cause a hypercoagulable state, may lead to Freiberg disease.[5] We believe that the true etiology is likely a combination of many factors without individual causation. Early recognition, although difficult to diagnose in many instances, can lead to less aggressive treatment and favorable outcomes, as the early stages usually respond to conservative treatment more effectively.

IMAGING AND DIAGNOSTIC STUDIES

Plain film weight-bearing radiographs are often the first imaging of choice when assessing second MTPJ pathology. Radiographs may help determine the length of the metatarsal and to evaluate concurrent foot and ankle abnormalities. This allows for evaluation of joint congruity, generalized bone structure, and bone stock. There are several findings to take note of with a few key nuances that may be prognostic for plantar plate tears.[13]

On the AP projection, we can assess digital splay, metatarsal protrusion distance, and intermetatarsal angles as it is helpful in assessing transverse plane deformity. We can also asses the clear space of the MTPJ in evaluating for degenerative joint disease. In normal anatomy, we expect to see 2-3 mm of clear space. As the digit becomes dorsally subluxed on the metatarsal head, the apparent joint space decreases. While the digit rides dorsally it moves proximally, a classic gun barrel sign may be seen.[13] Klein et al. eloquently discussed the importance of foot architecture noted on radiographs and their correlation with forefoot pathology. They radiographically evaluated 106 ft that underwent surgical repair of suspected plantar plate tears, 97

of which had intraoperative findings positive for plantar plate tear. The radiographic data revealed that patients with an intermetatarsal angle larger than 12, medial deviation of the second digit, and splaying of the digits were most commonly correlated to intraoperative plantar plate tears.[22] Although weight-bearing radiographs by themselves are somewhat nonspecific, understanding architectural normal vs abnormal may help with diagnosis in the absence of other foot pathology. These findings may also suggest that the long-term health of the forefoot may be correlated to parabolic normal. Therefore, the parabola should be corrected to help with avoidance of plantar plate pathology (Fig. 7.4).[22] There are at least three methods that may be used to evaluate metatarsal protrusion distances. The Coughlin method, which may be the simplest to employ quickly, measures the distance from the apex of the second metatarsal to a line from the apex of the first and third metatarsals.[14] This is the author's preferred method and addresses the second metatarsal independent of hallux valgus deformity in terms of length. The second method is Maestro's; this utilizes a transmetatarsal line centered from the lateral border of the tibial sesamoid and perpendicular to the medial border of the second metatarsal with distance to the apex of each metatarsal measured independently. The third and final method is used widely among foot and ankle surgeons. Here, a dual arc method measuring the metatarsal parabola and assessing metatarsal protrusion is done. For completeness sake, the intermetatarsal angle between the first and second metatarsals as well as signs of metadductus need to be evaluated.

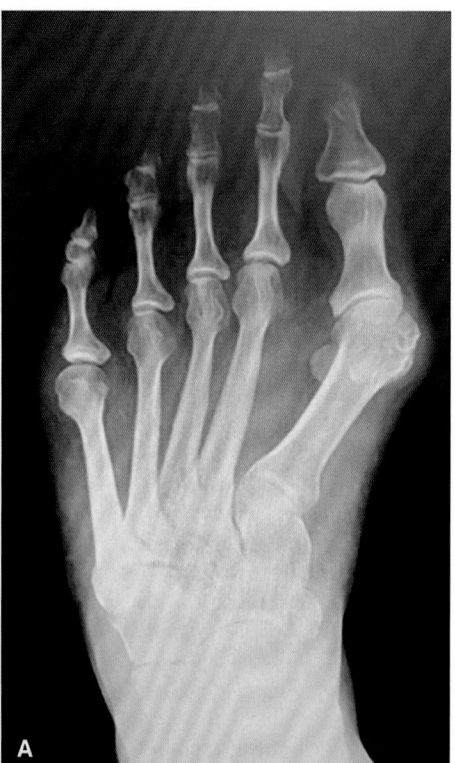
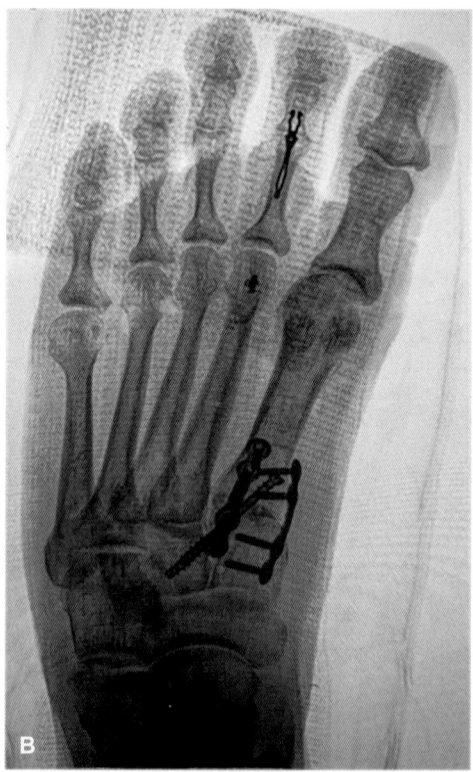

FIGURE 7.4 A. AP radiograph of abnormal parabola showing elongated second metatarsal. Additionally, clinically relevant metatarsus adductus and HAV. **B.** AP postoperative radiograph of a surgically corrected bunion via a Lapidus bunionectomy, second metatarsal Weil-type osteotomy with FDL transfer, intramedullary IPJ implant, and radiolucent staple fixation for a proximal akin osteotomy.

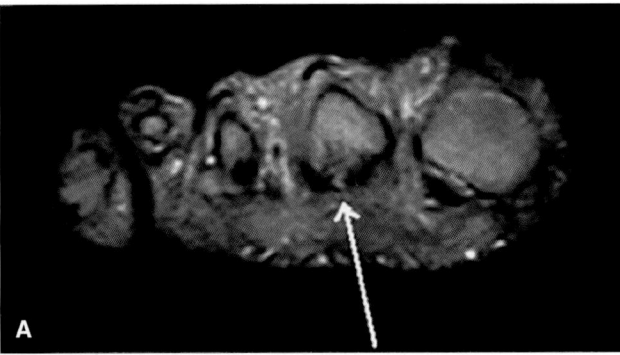 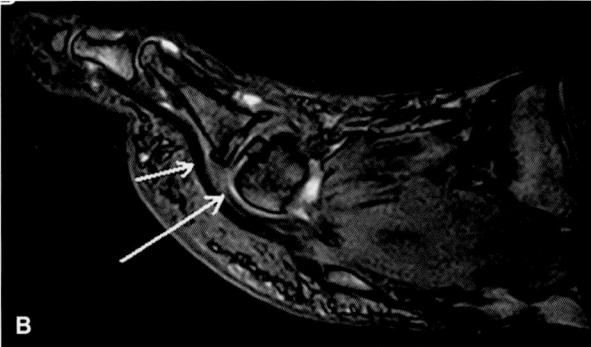

FIGURE 7.5 A, B. Magnetic resonance imaging of the second plantar plate. Arrows depict linear signal hyperintensity along the plantar plate.

Should any concurrent hallux valgus or metadductus be identified, this too should be documented and if needed, corrected. These measurements together can give insight to the relative length of the second metatarsal in comparison to the first as this impacts the stability of the lesser MTPJs. Lastly, the AP view may provide the clinician a quick evaluation of the bone stock. Osteopenic bone is more easily appreciated on this view. The authors often make decisions regarding hardware specifics using this view in order to help avoid periprosthetic fracture. If any doubt, further studies including DEXA scans and various laboratory tests to include vitamin D, PTH, Ca++, to name a few, may be helpful markers to assess overall bone health.[36]

On the lateral projection, the sagittal plane deformity may be more specifically evaluated. It is important to remember the quality of the plantar plate may not be directly appreciated since soft tissues are poorly seen on plain film radiographs. However, we can appreciate any digital subluxation or hyperextension from this view. The thickness of the plantar fat pad or lack thereof may also be noted beneath the metatarsal heads on this view.

There is a 2-5 times increase risk for plantar plate rupture if the following findings are observed on AP and lateral radiographs: intermetatarsal angle >12 degrees, medial deviation of the second digit, and an elongated second metatarsal.[37]

Given the relative simplicity, ease of access, low cost, and examination benefits of ultrasound, continued interest remains among physicians in the diagnosis of musculoskeletal pathologies. Klein et al. evaluated ultrasound in the diagnosis of plantar plate tears unilaterally using the unaffected limb as a control on fifty consecutive patients with suspected plantar plate dysfunction. Images were then graded as "torn" or "intact." Results of the ultrasound were then compared with intraoperative evaluation, comparing both longitudinal and transverse ultrasound for accuracy in identifying tears. Forty-five plantar plate tears were identified intraoperatively with longitudinal ultrasound correctly identifying 40 of them. Transverse ultrasound, however, identified 36 plantar plate tears, with only 19 seen intraoperatively. At best, sensitivity was found to be upward of 91%; however, specificity remained low at 25%. Ultrasound use and reliability is often technician dependent for this type of pathology. Therefore, the authors surmise that ultrasound as an advanced imaging technique for the diagnosis of plantar plate dysfunction may not be as useful as magnetic resonance imaging.[38]

Magnetic resonance imaging (MRI) can be useful in obtaining a final diagnosis for second MTPJ pathology. MRI has been shown to be 95% sensitive and 100% specific. This modality can assess the continuity and micro attenuation of the plantar plate prior to visual clinical deformity. Plantar plate tears identified on MRI are typically lateral full-thickness tears at the proximal phalanx insertion point (Fig. 7.5).[39]

MRI may also be useful in assessing joint effusion and synovitis. Increased thickness of the plate may be noted due to longstanding inflammation. Consider stress dorsiflexion during MRI to reduce false-negative findings that may be seen by the tear reapproximating in a relaxed position should the digit become plantarflexed.[35] Given the small area of the plantar plate and its focal attachments (see Fig. 7.5), a T3 MRI should be obtained, if available. T3 strength MRI may help delineate small structures down to the micron level. A standard 1.5T MRI provides very few "imaging cuts" through the second MTPJ. This could result in poor clarity. Most MRIs cannot obtain images smaller than 3 mm. The plantar plate averages 19 × 11 mm without pathology.[40] Due to the size constraints, a standard MRI would need perfect cuts to give the results needed for diagnosis and operative planning. T3 imaging provides increased clarity in the small detail needed to identify tearing in the thin plantar plate.[41] It should be noted that not every patient benefits from MRI for diagnostic use. It may be most beneficial in patients with early disease or with multiple factors affecting the MTPJ. Additionally, in scenarios where other focal pathology may be suspected and not ruled out, like that of Freiberg infraction, or metatarsal stress fracture, an MRI will provide added information.

While weight-bearing radiographs, ultrasound, and MRI are common, there is, however, some evidence suggesting the benefit of arthrography. Arthrography may provide verification of a capsular tear or instability; however, it can be unreliable. Dye seen to leak into the tendon sheath will indicate a plantar plate rupture.[42]

Computed tomography (CT) is uncommonly used for this pathology due to requirements for increased exposure to radiation without increased soft tissue visualization. This study is primarily reserved for evaluating the bony structures in more detail inconsistent with the goals of pathologic plantar plate evaluation. However, recent technology has brought forth office-sized weight-bearing CT machines, which are gaining in popularity. These offer the clinician immediate full weight-bearing CT scans, in office, to be used for diagnosis and treatment and appear to have minimal radiation exposure while providing high-resolution images. Cost, availability, and overall effectiveness in comparison to standard x-rays are being studied.

TREATMENT

NONOPERATIVE

First-line treatment for all second MTPJ pathology includes conservative care modalities aimed at slowing, or stopping, the progression of the disease as well as pain relief. Shoe modification is often the easiest and most effective change to make during an initial consultation where second MTPJ symptomatology is to be treated. Advise patients to find shoes with a wider toe box, reduced heel height, and a rocker bottom-type sole to alleviate forefoot pressures during the gait cycle. Plantarflexed toe splinting may also be therapeutic. This is called a bunion splint (Fig. 7.6) and is based upon Davis law of soft tissue remodeling; soft tissues heal according to the manner in which they are mechanically stressed.[43] Metatarsal padding may also help offload, stabilize, and support the second metatarsal head and joint. If the patient has severe pain with weight bearing, one can consider these splints, taping, and padding within an offloading shoe or boot. In addition to these external factors, corticosteroids and topical or oral NSAIDs may provide relief. While tapered oral corticosteroids can be beneficial, the same cannot be guaranteed for repetitive intra-articular steroid injections. Instability and dislocation at the metatarsal phalangeal joint following repeat injections have been documented in the literature as unintended sequelae.[44] Intra-articular injections can weaken an already compromised plantar plate and ligamentous structure. It has been shown that methylprednisolone decreases the tensile strength of surrounding structures for up to 1 year.[45] Despite possible risks, if the decision is made to inject the lesser MTPJ, one should perform plantar flexion taping postinjection to protect excess strain on the soft tissues. Given the possibility of misdiagnosis for interdigital neuroma, where steroid injections are considered by many as the cornerstone of nonoperative treatment, the potential for lesser MTPJ harm and flexor plate damage with repeat injections to an already attenuated soft tissue structure is real. Oral steroid regimens have, therefore, been touted by some as a potentially joint sparing method for treatment in certain cases. This typifies the importance of the physical examination and the benefits of advanced imaging in uncertain etiology situations.

Nonoperative care for Freiberg's is similar to that of plantar plate injuries. The primary focus is on resolution of forefoot symptoms. In this disease, conservative care is most effective in the early stages. When an early diagnosis is made, patient outcomes are best with limited weight bearing and immobilization in cast or walking boot. The patient may then gradually return to activity in supportive shoe gear. It is recommended that the metatarsal head is still off-loaded through orthotics or metatarsal pads until there is radiographic evidence of healing, this may be two or more years.[35] When the disease continues to progress for both plantar plate injuries and Freiberg disease, and exhaustive efforts for nonoperative treatments have been completed, surgical treatment options should be discussed with patients.

INDICATIONS

- Recalcitrant pain at metatarsal head plantarly and/or within the joint
- Abnormal metatarsal parabola
- MRI evidence of plantar plate insufficiency
- Radiographic evidence of Freiberg infraction
- Clinical changes in positioning of the second digit

OPERATIVE

Surgical treatment options for both plantar plate insufficiency and Freiberg disease are numerous. In dealing specifically with plantar plate dysfunction, the severity and rigidity of the deformity often dictates treatment options. The goals of surgical correction at the second MTPJ are to recreate normal biomechanical function in this essential joint, regain stability, and prevent painful or abnormal movement. We prefer to follow an algorithm shared by multiple other leading specialists in the field whereby clinical, radiographic, and advanced imaging modalities

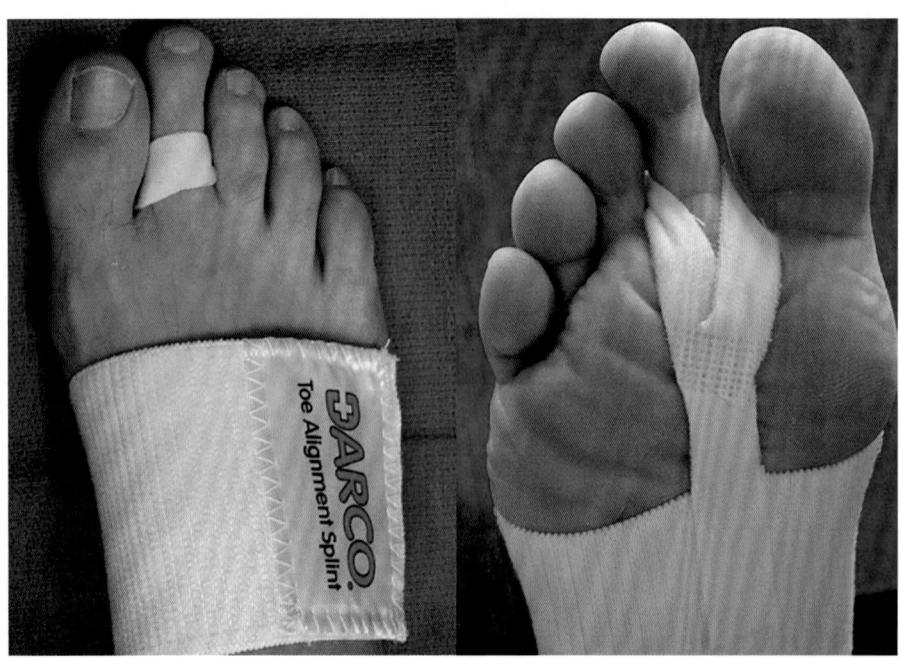

FIGURE 7.6 Plantarflexion splint for conservative care about the second metatarsophalangeal joint to alleviate strain on the plantar plate. Used with permission from DARCO International.

are used collectively to aid in treatment. The authors feel MTPJ reconstruction can be likened to that of a Broström procedure, through which the primary stabilizing structure of a joint undergoes repair, the entire joint and its function become more stable. Additionally, in line with Pauwels theory of causal histogenesis, collagen fibrils are always oriented in the direction of greatest tension.[43] One can choose to repair the plantar plate directly, indirectly, or not at all. Often, the decision can be made to leave a subjective plantar plate tear and address the joint through metatarsal osteotomies and capsular balancing as this may alone provide relief. As for Freiberg infraction, treatment options can range from debridement of the joint, to osteotomies, and even joint replacement or fusion. Moving forward we will discuss the vast array of surgical procedures for second MTPJ pathology, namely plantar plate dysfunction. Additionally, we will also discuss the operative treatment of Freiberg infraction in more detail.

PLANTAR PLATE TREATMENTS

Arthroscopy

Nery and colleagues discussed using small joint arthroscopy techniques via two portals at the dorsomedial and dorsolateral aspects of the lesser MTPJ to evaluate and treat the lesser MTPJ. This has been shown to be a good method to identify diseased tissue prior to committing to more invasive methods. They noted a healthy plantar plate to have a shine.[46] Shiny platelike tissue may be not be easily assessed intraoperatively with open procedures or in cases where hemostasis is not well maintained. In addition, arthroscopy may also be beneficial in shrinking the capsule with radio ablative wands. This technique is most effective in a grade 0 and grade 1 plantar plate disease.[47] Arthroscopy of the second MTPJ may also be beneficial in debridement of inflammatory and synovitic tissue.[48]

Tendon Transfers

Tendon transfers are a commonly used procedure about the lesser MTPJs. These can be used in isolation or as an adjunct to other procedures to regain stability and alignment about the MTPJ. Bouche et al., in 2008, evaluated the combined plantar plate repair with direct flexor digitorum longus tendon transfer in 17 ft.[21] This study was able to display 37-month AOFAS scores of 83 overall and demonstrated that direct plantar plate approach with the addition of a supplemental tendon transfer is a viable alternative in the surgical treatment and repair of plantar plate tears.[21] It has been shown that when combined with a plantar plate repair, the plantar plate will provide static stabilization of the joint while the flexor tendon transfer provides a dynamic tether (Fig. 7.7).[21]

Additionally, Lui in 2019 looked at using the short flexor tendon in a minimally invasive approach to alleviate second MTPJ pathology from a dorsal approach.[49] In the crossover deformity specifically, one will notice primarily sagittal and transverse plane components to the digits position. The EDB transfer in this cohort was able to address both the dorsal and medial malposition of the digit. Flexor plate tenodesis and EDB transfer

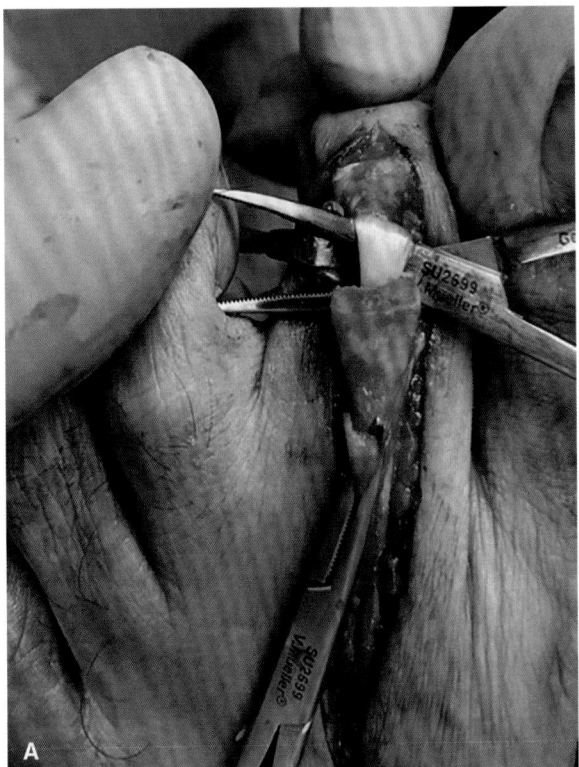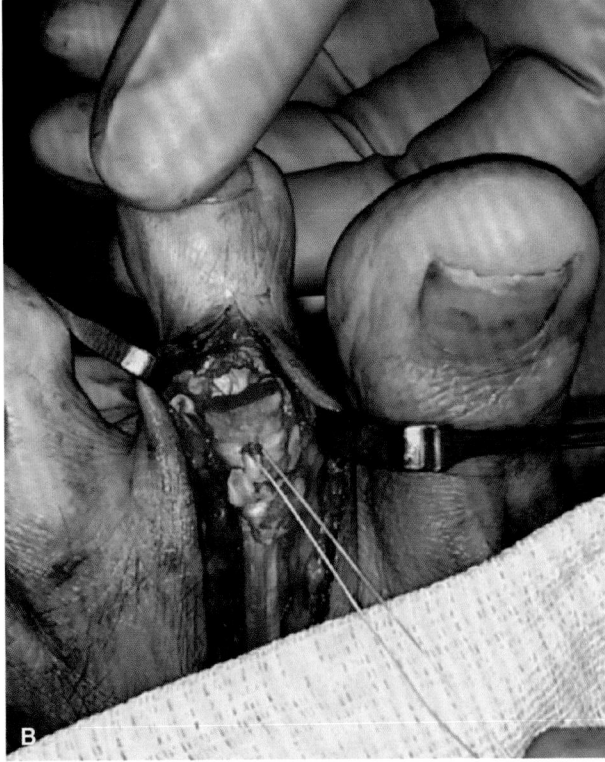

FIGURE 7.7 A, B. FDL transfer. The capital phalangeal fragment is osteotomized allowing for ease of access to the flexor tendons. The FDL is harvested as far distal as possible, split longitudinally, and brought up on either side of the phalanx. The two tendon ends are then tied with a nonabsorbable suture, usually a 3-0 polyethylene, on the dorsal aspect of the bone.

is, therefore, another reasonable surgical option, as the dual EDB tendon slips lend themselves to this application. In general, various opinions exist whether flexor transfer should be performed alone or in conjunction with a plantar plate repair. Coughlin recommends flexor tendon transfer in addition to a Weil osteotomy and possible plantar plate repair with grade 4 plantar plate tears (Table 1).[47] We believe the flexor tendon transfer is a powerful procedure that should be reserved in cases of revision and late stage or neglected plantar plate rupture as it may lead to joint stiffness due to its dynamic nature.

Plantar Approach Plantar Plate Repair

The greater soft tissue structures that intertwine and envelope one another about the second MTPJ in many instances have an intimate relationship with that of the capsule and fascial attachments. Additionally, a more global approach is being taken by many surgeons who wish to attempt rebalancing the soft tissue structures vs remote plantar plate repair as a standalone procedure in cases of instability. Nery et al., in 2012, performed a prospective study evaluating indirect plantar plate repairs and capsular insufficiency.[50] Forty MTPJs with instability were followed for 17 months. They then designed a treatment algorithm. In summary, grade 1 and 2 lesions using the Coughlin classification demonstrated the best AOFAS scores 95 and 96, respectively. Grade 3 lesions were noted to be the most common and showed the greatest net improvement.[50] In early stages, 0 and 1, those authors advocated for Weil osteotomy and radiofrequency capsular shrinkage techniques. In grades 2 and 3, the Weil osteotomy is performed with direct repair of the plantar plate. In more advanced stages, these authors suggest adding the flexor tendon transfer to the aforementioned list of procedures to further stabilize the markedly unstable joint. Moreover, the study established some closing points suggesting that both osseous and soft tissue work in combination were best. Specifically, a dorsal approach, Weil osteotomy, lateral soft tissue capsular, and collateral ligament reefing in conjunction with appropriate postoperative guidelines are important.

Dorsal Approach Plantar Plate Repair

Dorsal approaches to plantar plate repair, described as an indirect approach, may be limited by accessibility to the plantar plate. Recently, complex instrumentation has been developed to aid in this approach; there is a learning curve to achieve a reproducible result. Additionally, this approach may limit the surgeon in visualization of the pertinent structures. Therefore, the plantar plate repair may also be addressed from a direct, plantar approach. The primary benefit of the direct approach is complete exposure of the plantar plate with no requirement for metatarsal osteotomy. Potential disadvantages to the plantar approach include incisional placement, scar formation, and potential need for secondary incision for concurrent metatarsal osteotomy if necessary. Both approaches have been extensively studied. Jastifer and Coughlin dissected multiple second MTPJs to evaluate exposure of the plantar plate from a dorsal approach. They found that after a capsulotomy was performed, 1.1 mm of exposure to the plantar plate was gained. Release of the collateral ligaments achieved 2.5 mm, and the use of a McGlamry elevator achieved 4.1 mm of visualization within the joint space. This shows that successful plantar plate repair can be done dorsally with sufficient access after sequential release

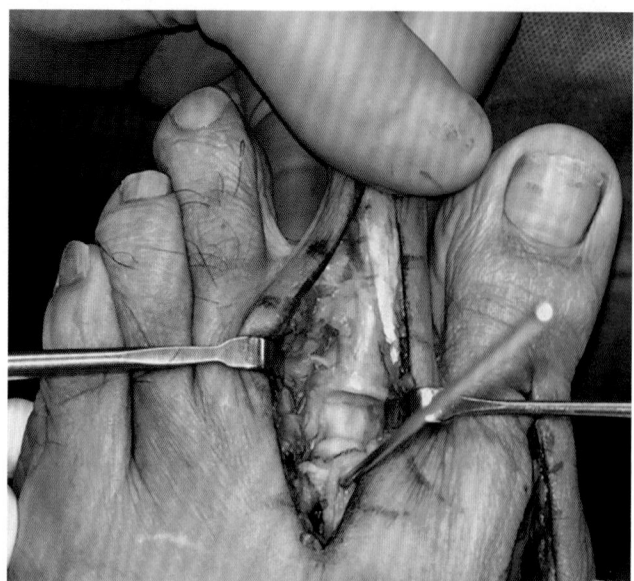

FIGURE 7.8 Through a dorsal exposure, following metatarsal osteotomy, the vast majority of the plantar plate and its attachments may be evaluated. Take note of the strong ligamentous plantar bonds maintaining the plantar plate apparatus.

of soft tissue structures.[47] Figure 7.8 shows anatomic dissection and plantar plate access via a dorsal approach after a metatarsal osteotomy has been performed. Weil et al. have also evaluated indirect plantar plate repairs with concomitant Weil osteotomy. In their cohort of 13 patients with a 22-month follow-up, they found 85% to have improved function. The authors concluded that the plantar plate can be visualized through a dorsal incision, repaired anatomically, and advanced appropriately after the Weil osteotomy is performed.[51] However, given the anatomic constraints of a dorsal approach, a direct repair has also been studied. McAlister et al. published on the plantar approaches finding this method beneficial to obtain precise correction of the plantar plate and potentially avoid requirements for metatarsal osteotomy, especially helpful in cases of parabolic normals.[52]

The author's preferred technique is a direct approach in repairing the plantar plate with a separate dorsal incision for metatarsal osteotomy if necessary.

The Weil osteotomy, a classic dorsal distal to plantar proximal oriented osteotomy, has by many been considered the core procedure of lesser ray pathology due to high patient satisfaction and a myriad of research demonstrating successful outcomes when performed appropriately (Fig. 7.9). Klein et al. described the underlying osseous contributions associated with lesser MTPJ pathology. Here, the authors identified a double risk for patients with a first intermetatarsal angle >12 degrees, a long second metatarsal, and medial deviation of the second digit as pathoanatomical contributors.[22] A lesser metatarsal osteotomy should be considered when actively treating the second MTPJ.

Through the years, this osteotomy has evolved from its initial description to various modifications addressing the specifics of anatomic regions and its inherent difficulties. Typically, from the dorsal approach, a metatarsal osteotomy must be performed in order to access and adequately visualize the plantar plate structures. As discussed above, the plantar plate can be visualized without an osteotomy, however.[47] Despite their findings, at our institution, we routinely utilize and recommend

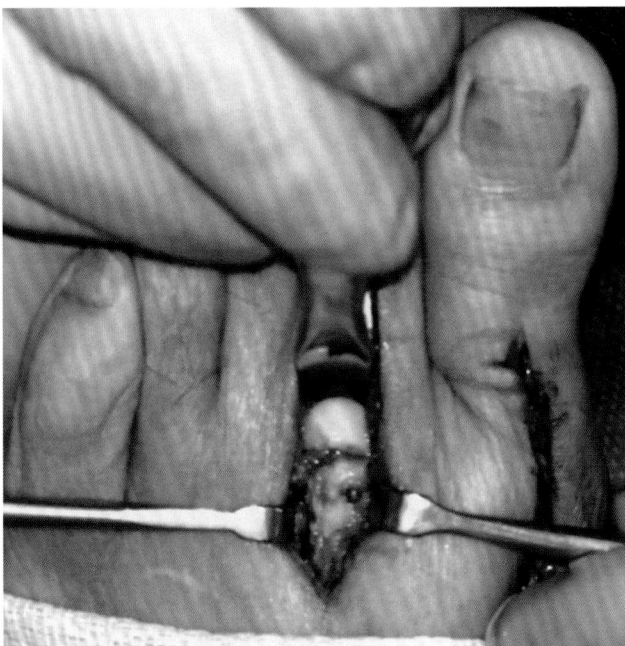

FIGURE 7.9 Weil osteotomy pictured with the usage of a McGlamry elevator to stabilize the capital fragment, fixation may be placed, and the overhanging portion of cartilage resected.

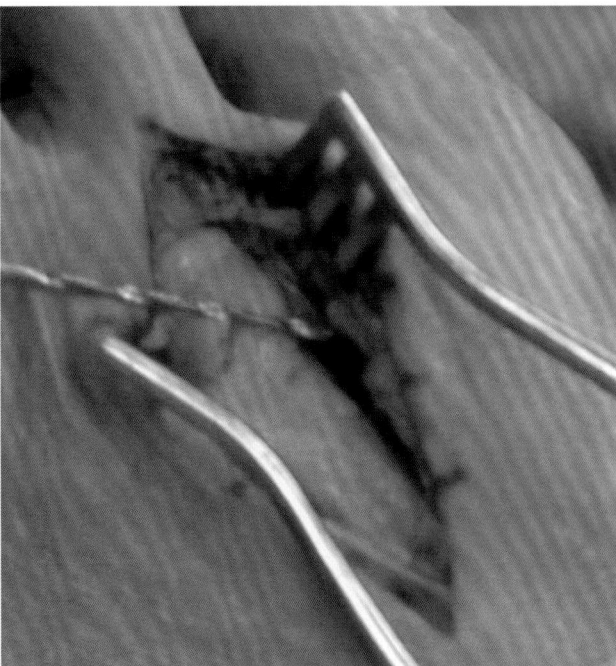

FIGURE 7.10 Oblique drill orientation indicating the direction of screw placement for fixation of an oblique Weil-type osteotomy. Specifically indicated to translate the capital fragment in the direction of the digital deformity.

considering preparing for a Weil-type osteotomy in order to adequately decompress the joint capsule and allow ease of repair. A successful Weil osteotomy can provide many benefits; it decompresses the lesser MTPJ as well as the plantar plate. It can also be used to stabilize intra-articular structures through scarring.

In certain cases where digital excursion is limited, or when somewhat trackbound, a McGlamry elevator is used to help free any plantar adhesions and to aid in mobilization of the joint in preparation for repair. In our experience, this by itself typically allows for a significant increase in motion. Medial deviation of the digit can be addressed with the metatarsal osteotomy as well. An obliquely oriented osteotomy technique is gaining in popularity. Here, the metatarsal head is allowed to transpose in the direction of the digital deformity, this may be particularly helpful in cases of crossover toe and enlarged intermetatarsal angles (Fig. 7.10). By shifting the metatarsal head in the direction in which the toe is moving allows for a more congruous MTPJ and also acts to mitigate forces upon the medial or lateral soft tissue repairs. Regardless of which osteotomy technique is chosen, stability of construct is of utmost importance.

AUTHOR'S PREFERRED TREATMENT

With a painful second MTPJ, and metatarsal protrusion >4 mm, in addition to evidence of plantar plate pathology identified on advanced imaging, the authors will typically utilize a dorsal approach for the metatarsal osteotomy and concomitant direct plantar approach for repair of the plantar plate. We believe that greater overall MTPJ control may be obtained with metatarsal osteotomy coupled with direct plantar plate repair. We have found that this conjoined incisional technique allows us for the most reproducible and dramatic repair. Additionally, we have found the direct plantar plate repair to have virtually eliminated the feared floating toe postoperatively.

positioning PEARLS

- Supine position with heels at the end of the bed
- Ipsilateral hip bump to rotate foot into rectus position

The patient is placed in a supine position; an ipsilateral hip bump is added to internally rotate the foot to rectus position. A calf tourniquet is then placed to the operative extremity. Following administration of local anesthetic, the foot is scrubbed, prepped, and draped in normal aseptic technique and the surgical foot is elevated, exsanguinated, and the tourniquet inflated to obtain hemostasis. We find it helpful to use a K-wire through the MTPJ as a radiographic marker on the skin to identify the location of the plantar plate and then mark this location on the skin with a marker. This may help to identify target structures during dissection. The metatarsal osteotomy, if needed, starts with a 2-cm linear incision centrally over the second metatarsal head. Dissection in a layered fashion is performed. The extensor tendons are carefully retracted allowing for visualization of the dorsal capsule. Make a linear capsulotomy and assess the medial and lateral collateral ligaments. If necessary, the collateral ligaments are freed. The McGlamry elevator is placed into the joint with care taken not to violate the cartilaginous surface. At this stage, and with the McGlamry elevator in place with soft tissue structures retracted, an oscillating saw is used to make a Weil-type osteotomy of the metatarsal. Start this osteotomy 2 mm inside the dorsal cartilage flare. The saw is oriented dorsal distal to plantar proximal, as well as parallel with the weightbearing surface. This is a true through and through osteotomy. The McGlamry is retrieved and the metatarsal head is then transposed proximally. The osteotomy is then provisionally fixated with a 0.45 K-wire and definitively fixated with one or two

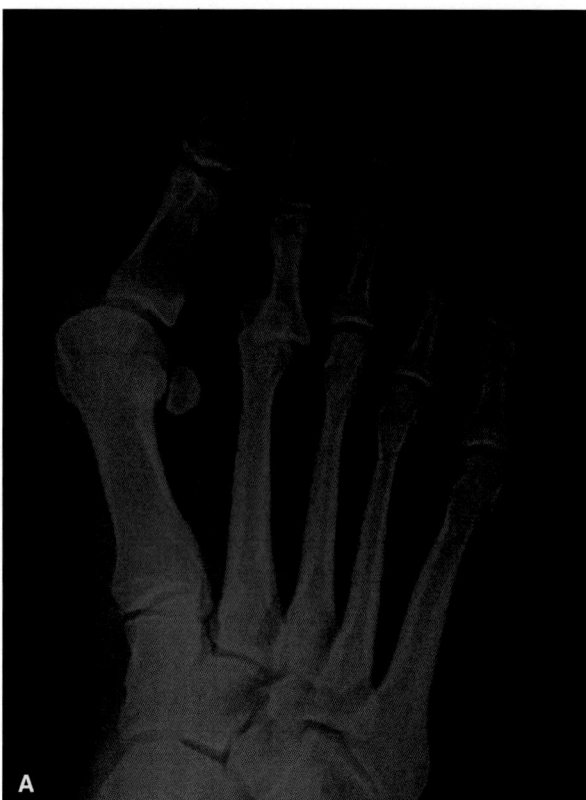
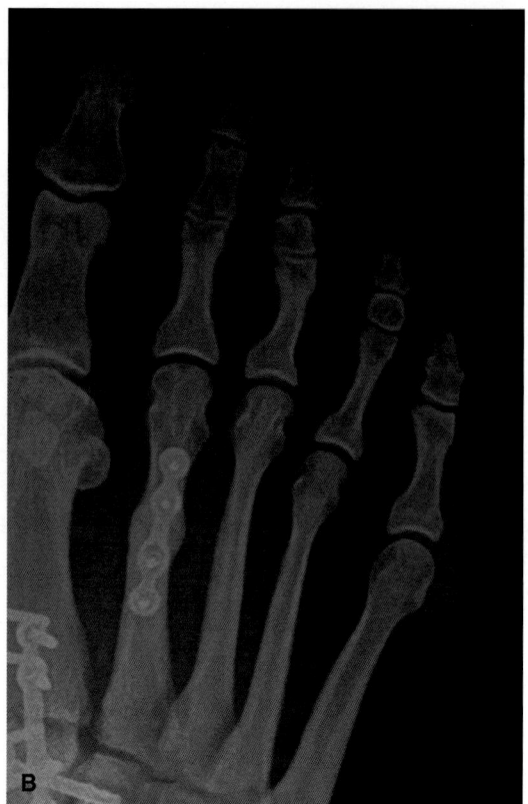

FIGURE 7.11 A. Preoperative AP radiograph revealing hallux valgus, a significantly elongated second metatarsal as well as a dorsally dislocation second digit. **B.** A postoperative AP radiograph status postbunion correction with a metadiaphyseal shortening osteotomy of the second metatarsal. This is ideal for patients with a significantly elongated second metatarsal.

screws depending on size of the metatarsal once radiographs have demonstrated appropriate parabola realignment.

In situations where we encounter excessive length discrepancies or with insufficient bone stock to accept screw fixation, we will employ segmental shortening or decompression osteotomies with low profile locking plate fixation. The dissection is largely the same as with the Weil-type osteotomy, however, will usually require a longer incision to accommodate plate fixation. Due to vascular concerns, metaphyseal and metadiaphyseal junction segmental shortening osteotomies are preferred over pure diaphyseal bone cuts. Additionally, subperiosteal plating at the central portion of the metatarsal is not required. To increase stability of the metatarsal, we recommend making two modified chevron-type osteotomies starting with the distal most osteotomy first to aid in stability of the bone cut. The segmental v-shaped piece of bone is removed. A pure dorsal to plantar osteotomy perpendicular to the long axis of the metatarsal (Fig. 7.11) is also acceptable, however, somewhat more unstable until fixated. Should any dorsal translation be necessary this can be addressed at this time due to the inherent stability of the chevron bone cut. We then loosely place screws into the distal fragment first of the plate. This helps drive the segment with relation to the proximal stable metatarsal segment. Once positioned appropriately, we lock the proximal screw holes and finalize the distal locking screws. T plates or straight plates are particularly useful in this application. Herzog et al. in 2014 reported on 30 consecutive patients utilizing a similar technique for the treatment of pathologic central ray metatarsalgia recalcitrant to conservative care.[53] On average, 2.7 mm

of shortening was documented, and no incidence of malunion or AVN reported. Good or excellent results were rated in 72% of this patient cohort.[53] We have found similar results in our patient population and feel segmental shortening is a viable option should surgeon preference and patient factors lend themselves toward more than 2 mm of shortening.

After the completion of the metatarsal osteotomy, in cases of plantar plate disruptions, we utilize K-wire fixation and use this to cross the MTPJ with the toe in slight plantar flexion to reduce the stress on the plantar plate repair. The digital procedure is performed last.

In the plantar approach, a curvolinear incision of ~3-5 cm is carried out about the web space directly adjacent to the weight-bearing portion of the ray, taking care to avoid direct metatarsal head incisional approaches (Fig. 7.12). Given the change in thickness of the skin at this anatomic level of the foot, ensuring a perpendicular approach with the blade is of extreme importance as skiving is more likely to occur. Sharp dissection is preferred through the fascial and subcutaneous layer to assist reduction of scar tissue formation.[54] A self-retaining retractor may be helpful to maintain visualization when working in the setting without assistance or residents. The distal digital nerves are identified and retracted exposing the flexor sheath. Care is taken to avoid neurovascular structures. The flexor tendon sheath is then incised parallel to the tendon. The interval of the short and long extensor tendons are identified and the tendons are then retracted (Fig. 7.13). This critical juncture exposes the plantar plate as the tendons lie directly inferior to it. In treatment of direct linear tears, a small wedge of plantar plate, often

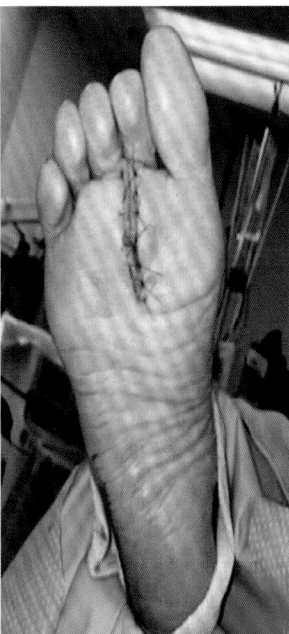

FIGURE 7.12 Incision placement for direct plantar plate repair.

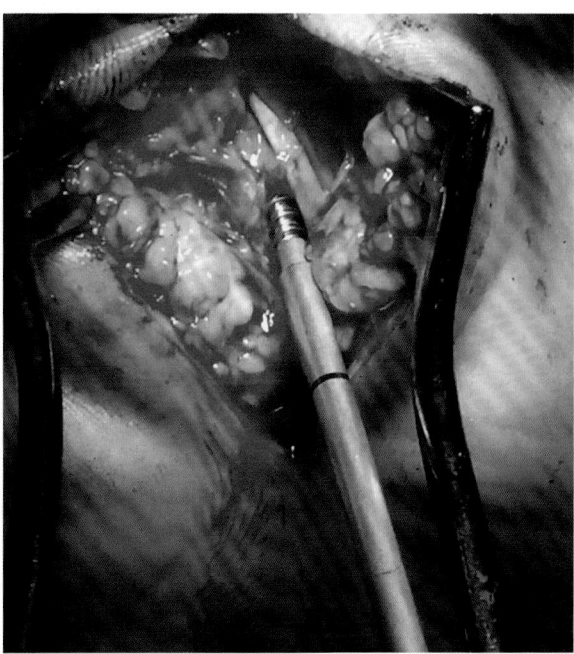

FIGURE 7.14 Suture anchor inserted into the plantar proximal aspect of the base of the proximal phalanx.

no more than a few millimeters, is removed from the plantar plate taking care to avoid skiving the articular surfaces directly deep to the plate nor creating vascular insult to the metatarsal head. Next, a no. 0 or no. 2-0 nonabsorbable suture on a tapered needle may be used for direct repair of the plantar plate, proximal to distal. At least two independent stitches are recommended. In some cases, we have also found it helpful to have small suture anchors available as they may be used to supplement repair and assist in (Fig. 7.14). The use of an anchor may aid in a stronger repair as the distal tissues are often weaker

and difficult to grasp. The anchor is placed plantar to dorsal through the base of the proximal phalanx. The nonabsorbable suture from the anchor is then passed through the proximal portion of the plantar plate (Fig. 7.15). At this time, if a digital contraction is noted at the proximal or distal interphalangeal joints, this is now corrected. This can be corrected with arthroplasty or arthrodesis procedures. When a concomitant hammertoe deformity is present, we prefer a proximal interphalangeal arthrodesis fixated with 0.045-in Kirschner wire, or an implant that allows for wire fixation of the PIPJ, DIPJ, or both. Once the digit is corrected, the wire is then passed across

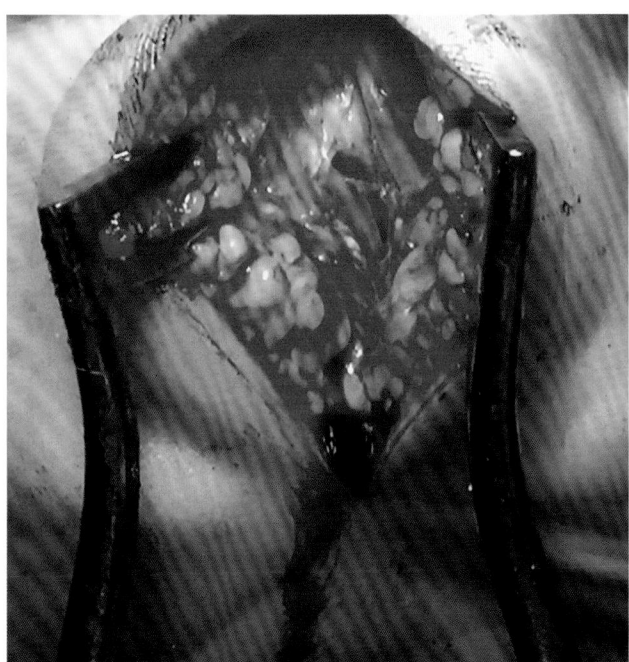

FIGURE 7.13 Visualization of the plantar plate with flexor tendons retracted.

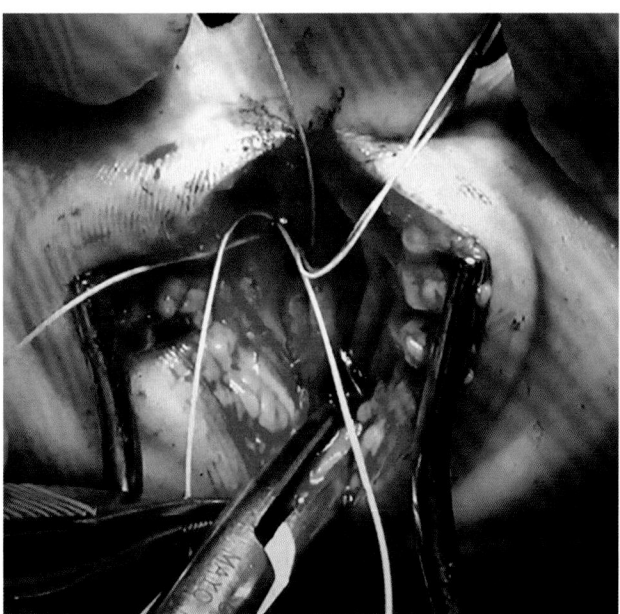

FIGURE 7.15 Suture from the anchor is then passed through the proximal portion of the plantar plate.

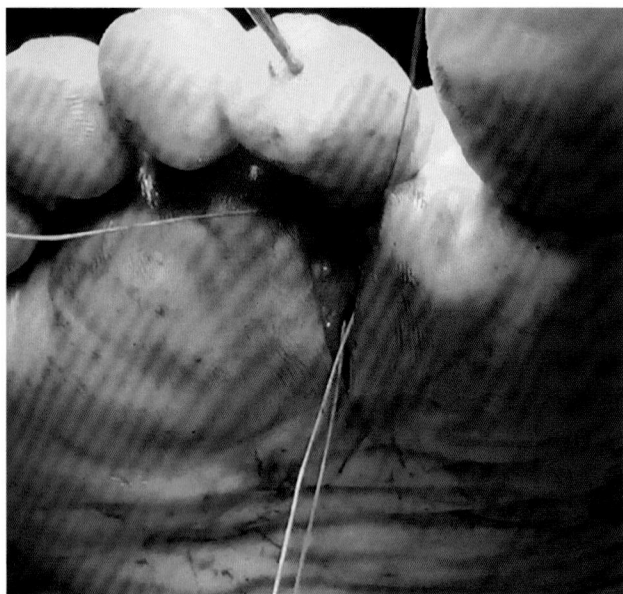

FIGURE 7.16 The sutures are then hand tied with the toe in pinned in slight plantar flexion.

the MTPJ and into the metatarsal head in slight plantar flexion. With the toe pinned in its relaxed position, the suture is hand tied into place (Fig. 7.16). Should higher-grade tears be noted, various oblique wedge resection and reefing techniques might be used; however, ultimately, the capsulorrhaphy should be measured to allow the native tissues to be coapted under anatomic tension. The flexor tendon sheath is not repaired unless markedly bowstrung and the tendons are allowed to glide back into their native position unbound.

PEARLS

- If utilizing a plantar approach, passing a K-wire through the joint from dorsal to plantar can help identify plantar location of the joint.
- Segmental shortening with a dorsal plate may be used when the metatarsal needs to be shortened more than 2 mm.
- When end to end repair of the plantar plate cannot be achieved, a small suture anchor into the plantar base of proximal phalanx can provide a fixed insertion for the proximal portion of the plantar plate.
- When other procedures are combined with a plantar plate repair from a plantar approach, tie the plantar plate suture last.

POSTOPERATIVE

The postoperative period is critical regardless of procedure as this is may dictate ultimate outcome. Additionally, our protocols do not change for patients who receive the dual incisional approach, single incisional approach, or isolated direct vs indirect plantar plate repair. In our experience, we find it helpful when treating postsurgical plantar plate repairs to maintain our surgical extremity in a well-padded, non–weight-bearing splint for 10 days. We then transition our patients to a removable boot that they may weight bear in. Between 6 and 8 weeks, the pin is

pulled from the toe in office and the patient may transition to a supportive tennis shoe. The patient is to tape the toe plantar grade for the following 2 months while walking to help mitigate recurrence.

FREIBERG TREATMENT

When conservative care for Freiberg's has failed, there are many surgical options available. One of the least invasive is arthroscopic debridement of the joint. As discussed above, arthroscopy of the second MTPJ can be performed through dorsomedial and dorsolateral portals. The use of small joint arthroscopy can be used in early stages for debridement and synovectomy. Carro et al. also noted excellent results with arthroscopic excision of the base of the proximal phalanx in late stages.[55] Whether open, or arthroscopic, debridement of the joint with microfracture of the metatarsal head can be a successful procedure in stages 1, 2, and 3 of Freiberg infraction.[56] Debridement must include removal of all osteophytes and loose bodies, hypertrophic synovium, and areas of denuded cartilage. Some of the most common procedures to treat Freiberg's include dorsiflexory osteotomies, osteochondral autograft transposition (OAT), and interpositional arthroplasty. Dorsiflexory osteotomies are recommended for Smillie stages 1-4.[57] This procedure was originally described by Gautheir and Elbaz in 1974. It allows for removal of the dorsally located necrotic bone and transposition of the healthy plantar cartilage into a highly articular area. Since the 1970s, this procedure has continued to be utilized with a 93% success rate.[57] Lee et al. found that shortening of the metatarsal as well as dorsiflexion of the head allowed for nearly 3 mm of shortening without complaints of transfer metatarsalgia. This allows for better fixation options, correction of a typically elongated metatarsal, decompression of the MTPJ, as well as transfer of healthy cartilage.[58] The OAT procedure is typically recommended for stages 3 and 4. Devries and colleagues as well as Tsuda and colleagues performed OAT procedures on adolescent athletes in which the harvest was taken from the lateral femoral condyle. It is not uncommon to harvest a cartilaginous plug from a nonarticular portion of the talus in certain cases. Although among smaller cohorts, in each study, the authors reported excellent results. Postoperative imaging was obtained acting to help reveal incorporation status of the grafts.[5] The current literature supports this as a reasonable surgical solution. Interpositional arthroplasty is most often performed with the EDB tendon. This procedure can be used in all stages of Freiberg's. In this technique, a dorsal incision is made over the MTPJ, the EDB tendon to the second digit is identified, isolated, and transected. The joint is then debrided, removing all osteophytes, and the joint margins are remodeled. Next, the harvested EDB tendon is spun into a sphere and placed within the joint. The capsule is then repaired around the joint.[59,60] Interpositional arthroplasty may also be accomplished successfully with acellular dermal allograft. The literature is limited on this, however. It may help preserve anatomic structures and joint function in even late stage disease.[61] Given the advancement and availability of dermal allograft at our institution, we have found this to be useful vs tendon harvest when employing interpositional arthroplasty in late stage cases of Freiberg's. When the disease has progressed toward end stages, surgical options are limited to joint destructive procedures.

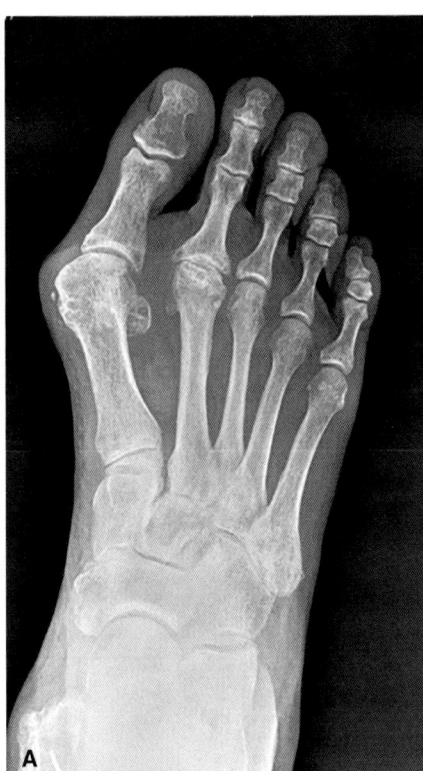 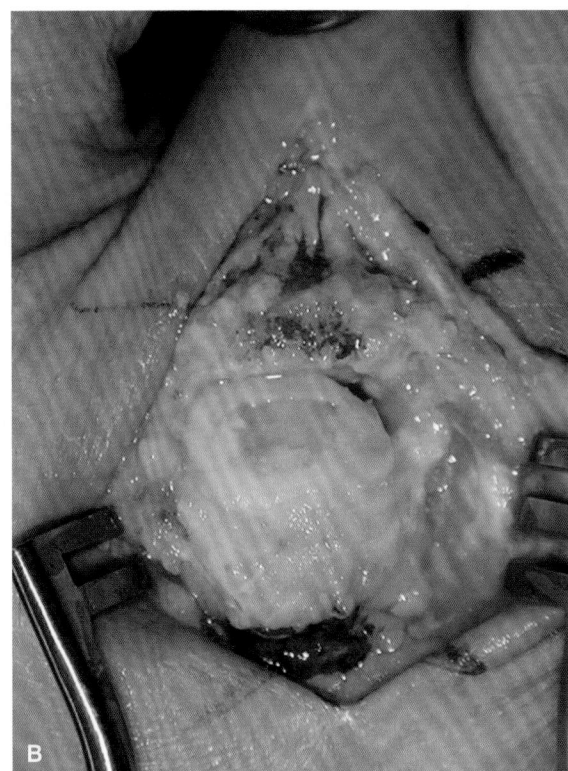

FIGURE 7.17 A stage 4 Freiberg infraction seen at the second metatarsal head both radiographically **(A)** and clinically **(B)**.

Multiple total and hemi-implants are available to the surgeon. Unfortunately, the short-term results have mixed outcomes and long-term results consistently show high failure rates. Multiple complications exist including implant loosening, synovitis, osteolysis, infection, and transfer metatarsalgia.[61] In severe cases of joint arthrosis (Fig. 7.17), when joint salvage is unreasonable or the patient is unwilling, lesser MTPJ resection and arthrodesis has been proposed.[31] Hollawell et al. have discussed fusion of the second and third MTPJs joint with successful results in a short series of patients with severe recalcitrant deformity (Fig. 7.18). The authors believe that arthrodesis of the joint may be a viable salvage procedure.[31]

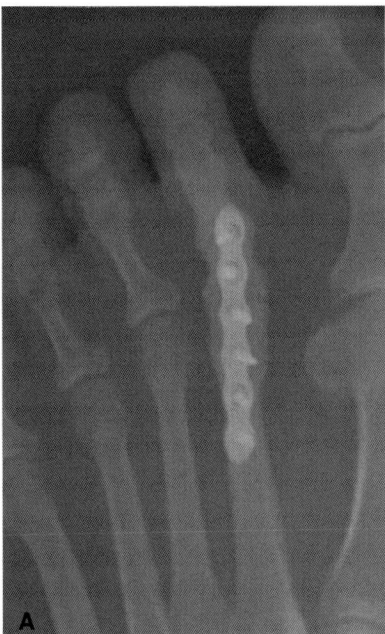 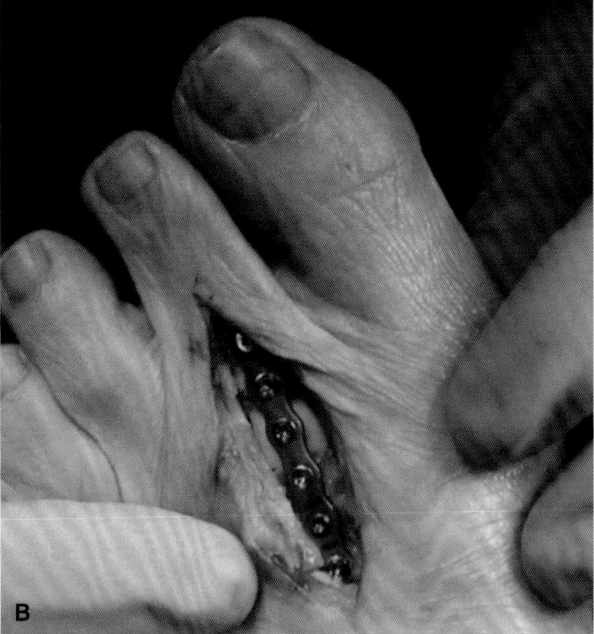

FIGURE 7.18 A, B. Second MTPJ arthrodesis with plate and screw construct in a case of recurrent lesser MTPJ dysfunction despite previous surgical intervention.

AUTHOR'S PREFERRED TECHNIQUE

The author's preferred technique for stages 1-4 of Freiberg infraction is a dorsiflexory modification of a Weil osteotomy. Incision is made directly over the second metatarsal ~3-4 cm in length. Dissection is carefully taken in layers to the level of capsule. A capsular and periosteal incision is made and the structures are freed from the dorsal aspect of the metatarsal head. The second metatarsal head is inspected to assess the level of damage to the cartilage. Next, osteophytes and necrotic bone are removed and the metatarsal head is remodeled. Following this, an oblique distal to proximal osteotomy parallel to the weight-bearing surface is performed in the metatarsal head at the dorsal most level of viable cartilage. A second distal to proximal oblique osteotomy is then performed at the metatarsal neck removing a wedge of avascular bone.[58] Due to the oblique nature of the cuts, the head of the metatarsal will dorsiflex as well as shorten. This osteotomy is then temporarily fixed with a K-wire. The MTPJ is then passed through range of motion to ensure improvement in anatomic function. The osteotomy is then fixated with one small screw, much like our standard Weil osteotomy.

For early stages not amenable to conservative care, we employ subchondral fenestration techniques. Our incision and dissection remains the same. We then use a 0.045 K-wire to drill the subchondral plate 1 mm apart from each other. The dorsal tissues are then irrigated and closed in anatomic layers.

COMPLICATIONS

Although not ideal, complications are part of every surgical procedure. Some common complications when working at the second MTPJ include pain, swelling, numbness to the digit, weakness, loss of purchase, persistent or recurrent deformity, stiffness about the joint, wound dehiscence, and infection. Most of which may be mitigated with appropriate technique and patient selection.

PEARLS

- Mildly overcorrect in a plantar position, bandage splintage alone is insufficient, always use a K-wire and maintain position for at least 4 weeks.
- Perform all ancillary procedure prior to repairing the plantar plate.
- Interdigital neuromas generally are not the cause of edema, nor the cause of pain at the MTPJ. Use caution when making a diagnosis.
- Compare the Lachman examination to the contralateral side in order to make a diagnosis.
- In repairing the plantar plate, pay attention to decorticate the phalangeal base, ensuring capsulodesis and near anatomic repair.
- Plantar forefoot calluses indicate chronicity and sub two pain should be addressed.
- Avoid intra-articular steroid injections as they selectively atrophy collagen.
- When transverse plane deformity exists at the lesser MTPJ, consider displacement osteotomies in the direction of the digital deformity to mitigate forces.

PERILS and PITFALLS

- Mildly overcorrect in a plantar position, bandage splintage alone is insufficient, always use a K-wire and maintain position for at least 4 weeks.
- Perform all ancillary procedures prior to repairing the plantar plate.
- Interdigital neuromas generally are not the cause of edema, nor the cause of pain at the MTPJ. Use caution when making a diagnosis.
- Compare the Lachman examination to the contralateral side in order to make a diagnosis.
- In repairing the plantar plate, pay attention to decorticate the phalangeal base, ensuring capsulodesis and near anatomic repair.
- Plantar forefoot calluses indicate chronicity and sub two pain should be addressed.
- Avoid intra-articular steroid injections as they selectively atrophy collagen.
- When transverse plane deformity exists at the lesser MTPJ, consider displacement osteotomies in the direction of the digital deformity to mitigate forces.

CONCLUSION

Many medical practitioners across disciplines have identified the plantar plate as a source of pathology that accompanies metatarsalgia and other progressive forefoot deformity. Pathology of the second MTPJ is a broad term that can include predislocation syndrome, capsulitis, Freiberg's, or synovitis. The importance of a thorough clinical examination cannot be overstated as many of these conditions present with similar findings. Plain film radiographs and MRI, coupled with physical findings, may be the most beneficial examinations for diagnosis. A growing list of surgical procedures exist to tackle lesser MTPJ pathology, ranging from tendon transfers, osteotomies, soft tissue balancing, and even arthrodesis. Rarely is a plantar plate repair done as an isolated procedure, as each foot has a different complex of symptoms and findings. Primary repair of the ruptured or attenuated plantar plate through a dorsal or plantar approach has proven to be a safe and effective surgical option in the management of one of the most difficult conditions of the lower extremity. Patient education is crucial, and it may be necessary to discuss that complete resolution may be unreasonable in severe cases. When it comes to treatment, regardless of the diagnosis, off-loading and stabilization of the joint are first-line treatments along with physical therapy. The addition of oral or intra-articular anti-inflammatory modalities may provide relief as well. When conservative care and shoe gear modification have failed and the condition is recalcitrant to nonoperative treatment, there are many surgical procedures to consider which when performed appropriately may be effective.

REFERENCES

1. Yu GV, Judge MS, Hudson JR, et al. Predislocation syndrome-progressive subluxation/dislocation of the lesser metatarsophalangeal joint. *J Am Podiatr Med Assoc.* 2002;92(4):192-199.
2. Yu GV, Judge MS. Predislocation syndrome of the lesser metatarsophalangeal joint: a distinct clinical entity. In: Camasta CA, Vickers NS, Carter SR, eds. *Reconstructive Surgery of the Foot and Leg: Update '95.* Tucker, GA: The Podiatry Institute; 1995:109.
3. Caio N, et al. "Prospective evaluation of protocol for surgical treatment of lesser MTP joint plantar plate tears." *Foot Ankle Int.* 2014;35(9):876-885. doi: 10.1177/1071100714539659.

4. Brooks F, Hariharan K. The rheumatoid forefoot. *Curr Rev Musculoskelet Med.* 2013;6:320.
5. Shane A, Reeves C, Wobst G, Thurston P. Second metatarsophalangeal joint pathology and Freiberg disease. *Clin Podiatr Med Surg.* 2013;30(3):313-325. doi: 10.1016/j.cpm.2013.04.009.
6. Trnka H-J, Nyska M, Parks BG, et al. Dorsiflexion contracture after the Weil osteotomy; results of cadaver study and three-dimensional analysis. *Foot Ankle Int.* 2001;22(1):47-50.
7. Cruveilhier J. *The Anatomy of the Human Body.* New York, NY: Harper & Bros; 1844:176.
8. Smillie IS. Treatment of Freiberg's infraction. *Proc R Soc Med.* 1967;60:29-31.
9. Norkin CC, White DJ. Techniques and procedures. In: Norkin CC, White DJ, eds. *Measurement of Joint Motion: A Guide to Goniometry.* Philadelphia, PA: FA Davis; 1988:9-24.
10. Sarrafian SK, Topouzian LK. Anatomy and physiology of the extensor apparatus of the toes. *J Bone Joint Surg Am.* 1969;51:669-679.
11. Deland JT, Lee KT, Sobel M, et al. Anatomy of the plantar plate and its attachments in the lesser metatarsal phalangeal joint. *Foot Ankle Int.* 1995;16:480-486.
12. Medicino RW, Statler TK, Saltrick KR, et al. Predislocation syndrome: a review and retrospective analysis of eight patients. *J Foot Ankle Surg.* 2001;40(1):214-224.
13. Coughlin MJ. Crossover second toe deformity. *Foot Ankle.* 1987;8:29-39.
14. Coughlin MJ. Subluxation and dislocation of the second metatarsophalangeal joint. *Orthop Clin North Am.* 1989;20:535-551.
15. Ford LA, Collins KB, Christensen JC. Stabilization of the subluxed second metatarsophalangeal joint: flexor tendon transfer versus primary repair of the plantar plate. *J Foot Ankle Surg.* 1998;37(3):217-222. doi: 10.1016/s1067-2516(98)80114-2.
16. Umans H, Srinivasan R, Elsinger E, Wilde GE. MRI of lesser metatarsophalangeal joint plantar plate tears and associated adjacent interspace lesions. *Skeletal Radiol.* 2014;43(10):1361-1368.
17. Coughlin MJ. When to suspect crossover second toe deformity. *J Musculoskel Med.* 1987;4:29-48.
18. Miller SD. Technique tip: forefoot pain: diagnosing metatarsophalangeal joint synovitis from interdigital neuroma. *Foot Ankle Int.* 2001;22:914-915.
19. Coughlin MJ. Common causes of pain in the forefoot in adults. *J Bone Joint Surg Br.* 2000;82:781-790.
20. How to Reduce Complication Risk in Hammertoe Surgery. 2013. https://www.podiatry-today.com/how-reduce-complication-risk-hammertoe-surgery
21. Bouche RT, Heit EJ. Combined plantar plate and hammertoe repair with flexor digitorum longus tendon transfer for chronic, severe sagittal plane instability of the lesser metatarsophalangeal joints: preliminary observations. *J Foot Ankle Surg.* 2008;47(2):125-137.
22. Klein EE, Weil L Jr, Weil LS Sr, Knight J. The underlying osseous deformity in plantar plate tears: a radiographic analysis. *Foot Ankle Spec.* 2013;6:108-118.
23. McGlamry ED, Southerland JT. Chapter 19. Plantar plate repair of the second metatarsophalangeal joint. In: *McGlamry's Comprehensive Textbook of Foot and Ankle Surgery.* Philadelphia, PA: Wolters Kluwer Health/Lippincott Williams & Wilkins; 2013.
24. Sferra J, Arndt S. The crossover toe and valgus toe deformity. *Foot Ankle Clin.* 2011;16:609-620.
25. Kaz MD, Coughlin MJ. Crossover second toe: demographics, etiology, and radiographic assessment. *Foot Ankle Int.* 2007;28(12):1223-1237.
26. Stokes IA, Hutton WC, Stott JR. Forces acting on the metatarsals during normal walking. *J Anat.* 1979;129:579-590.
27. Coughlin MJ. Second metatarsophalangeal joint instability in the athlete. *Foot Ankle.* 1993;14:309-319.
28. Petersen WJ, Lankes JM, Paulsen F, Hassenpflug J. The arterial supply of the lesser metatarsal heads: a vascular injection study in human cadavers. *Foot Ankle Int.* 2002;23(6):491-495.
29. Chalayon O, Chertman C, Guss AD, et al. Role of plantar plate and surgical reconstruction techniques on static stability of lesser metatarsophalangeal joints: a biomechanical study. *Foot Ankle Int.* 2013;34:1436-1442.
30. Berens TA. Laterally closing metatarsal head osteotomy in the correction of a medially overlapping digit. *Clin Podiatr Med Surg.* 1996;13(2):293-307.
31. Hollawell SM, Kane BJ, Paternina JP, Santamaria GJ, Heisey CM. Lesser metatarsophalangeal joint pathology addressed with arthrodesis: a case series. *J Foot Ankle Surg.* 2019;58(2):387-391. doi: 10.1053/j.jfas.2018.08.039.
32. Hansen ST. *Functional Reconstruction of the Foot and Ankle.* Philadelphia, PA: Lippincott Williams & Wilkins; 2000.
33. Stanley D, Betts RP, Rowley DI, et al. Assessment of etiologic factors in the development of Freiberg's disease. *J Foot Surg.* 1990;29:444-447.
34. Wiley J, Thurston P. Freiberg's disease. *J Bone Joint Surg.* 1981;63B:459-463.
35. McGlamry ED, Southerland JT. Chapter 54. Osteochondroses of the foot and ankle. In: Southerland JT, ed. *McGlamry's Comprehensive Textbook of Foot and Ankle Surgery.* Philadelphia, PA: Wolters Kluwer Health/Lippincott Williams & Wilkins; 2013.
36. Farmer RP, Herbert B, Cuellar DO, et al. Osteoporosis and the orthopaedic surgeon: Basic concepts for successful co-management of patients' bone health. *Int Orthop.* 2014;38(8):1731-1738. doi: 10.1007/s00264-014-2317-y.
37. Barca F, Acciaro AL. Surgical correction of crossover deformity of the second toe: a technique for tenodesis. *Foot Ankle Int.* 2004;25:620-624.
38. Klein EE, Weil L Jr, Weil LS Sr, Knight J. Musculoskeletal ultrasound for preoperative imaging of the plantar plate: a prospective analysis. *Foot Ankle Spec.* 2013;6(3):196-200.
39. Dinoa V, von Ranke F, Costa F, et al. Evaluation of lesser metatarsophalangeal joint plantar plate tears with contrast-enhanced and fat-suppressed MRI. *Skeletal Radiol.* 2016;45:635-644.
40. Maas NMG, Van Der Grinten M, Bramer WM, Kleinrensink G-J. Metatarsophalangeal joint stability: a systematic review on the plantar plate of the lesser toes. *J Foot Ankle Res.* 2016;9:32.
41. Yao L, Cracchiolo A, Farahani K, Seeger LL. Magnetic resonance imaging of plantar plate rupture. *Foot Ankle Int.* 1996;17(1):33-36. doi: 10.1177/107110079601700107.
42. Karpman RR, MacCollum MS III. Arthrography of the metatarsophalangeal joint. *Foot Ankle.* 1988;9:125-129.
43. Ellenbecker TS, De Carlo M, DeRosa C. *Effective Functional Progressions in Sport Rehabilitation.* Human Kinetics; 2009.
44. Reis ND, Karkabi S, Zinman C. Metatarsophalangeal joint dislocation after local steroid injection. *J Bone Joint Surg Br.* 1989;71:864.
45. Noyes FR, Nussbaum NS, Delucas JL, et al. Biomechanical and ultrastructural changes in ligaments and tendons after corticosteroid injection. *J Bone Joint Surg Am.* 1975;57:876.
46. Nery C, Coughlin MJ, Baumfeld D, et al. Lesser metatarsal phalangeal joint arthroscopy: anatomic description and comparative dissection. *Arthroscopy.* 2014;30(8):971-979.
47. Jastifer JR, Coughlin MJ. Exposure via sequential release of the metatarsophalangeal joint for plantar plate repair through a dorsal approach without an intra articular osteotomy. *Foot Ankle Int.* 2014;36(3):335-338. doi: 10.1177/1071100714553791.
48. Reeves CL, Shane AM, Payne T, Cavins Z. Small joint arthroscopy in the foot. *Clin Podiatr Med Surg.* 2016;33(4):565-580.
49. Lui TH. Correction of crossover deformity of second toe by combined plantar plate tenodesis and extensor digitorum brevis transfer: a minimally invasive approach. *Arch Orthop Trauma Surg.* 2011;131(9):1247-1252. doi: 10.1007/s00402-011-1293-6.
50. Nery C, Coughlin MJ, Baumfeld D, Mann TS. Lesser metatarsophalangeal joint instability: prospective evaluation and repair of plantar plate and capsular insufficiency. *Foot Ankle Int.* 2012;33(4):301-311. doi: 10.3113/fai.2012.0301.
51. Weil L, et al. Anatomic plantar plate repair using the Weil metatarsal osteotomy approach. *Foot Ankle Spec.* 2011;4(3):145-150. doi: 10.1177/1938640010397342.
52. Mcalister JE, Hyer CF. The direct plantar plate repair technique. *Foot Ankle Spec.* 2013;6(6):446-451. doi: 10.1177/1938640013502723.
53. Herzog JL, Goforth WD, Stone PA, Paden MH. A modified fixation technique for a decompressional shortening osteotomy: a retrospective analysis. *J Foot Ankle Surg.* 2014;53(2):131-136. doi: 10.1053/j.jfas.2013.12.018.
54. Blitz NM, Ford LA, Christensen JC, Plantar plate repair of the second metatarsophalangeal joint: technique and tips. *J Foot Ankle Surg.* 2004;43:266-270.
55. Carro LP, Golano P, Farinas O, Cerezal L, Abad J. Arthroscopic Keller technique for Freiberg disease. *Arthroscopy.* 2004;20(suppl 2):60-63.
56. Mareca G, Adriani E, Fale F, et al. Arthroscopic treatment of Freiberg's infraction. *Arthroscopy.* 1996;12:103-108.
57. Helix-Gioranino M, Randier E, Frey S, Picket B. Treatment of Freiberg's disease by Gauthier's dorsal cuneiform osteotomy: retrospective study of 30 cases. *Orthop Traumatol Surg Res.* 2015;101(6):221-225.
58. Lee H-S, Kim Y-C, Choi J-H, Chung J-W. Weil and dorsal closing wedge osteotomy for Freiberg's disease. *J Am Podiatr Med Assoc.* 2016;106(2):100-108. doi: 10.7547/14-065.
59. Zgonis T, Jolly GP, Kanuck DM. Interpositional free tendon graft for lesser metatarsophalangeal joint arthropathy. *J Foot Ankle Surg.* 2005;44(6):490-492. doi: 10.1053/j.jfas.2005.08.005.
60. Özkan Y, Öztürk A, Özdemir R, Aykut S, Yalşin N. Interpositional arthroplasty with extensor digitorum brevis tendon in Freiberg's disease: a new surgical technique. *Foot Ankle Int.* 2008;29(5):488-492. doi: 10.3113/fai.2008.0488.
61. Seybold JD, Zide JR. Treatment of Freiberg disease. *Foot Ankle Clin.* 2018;23:157–169.

CHAPTER 8

Digital Surgery

Jarrett D. Cain, Rahn Ravenell, Miki Dalmau-Pastor, Guillaume Cordier, and Amy E. Bruce

DEFINITION AND CLASSIFICATION

Digital deformities are commonplace conditions seen by the foot and ankle specialist. While the condition is commonly seen in the sagittal plane; abnormalities can also exist in the transverse and frontal planes and in any combination of these.[1] This condition involves ligamentous, tendon as well osseous pathologies of the digit that can occur at the metatarsophalangeal joint, the proximal interphalangeal joint (PIPJ) and/or distal interphalangeal joint.[2] While the etiology is multifactorial, digital pathologies are a result of imbalances between the anatomic structures during weight-bearing and lead to chronic structural abnormalities.[3]

A hammertoe deformity is defined as a disorder resulting in plantarflexion at the PIPJ with dorsiflexion at both the metatarsophalangeal joint and the distal interphalangeal joint (Fig. 8.1A). When dorsiflexion is present at the metatarsophalangeal joint with plantarflexion at both the PIPJ and the distal interphalangeal joint, a claw toe deformity is present (Fig. 8.1B). A mallet toe is present when there is plantarflexion isolated to only the distal interphalangeal joint.

ANATOMY

EXTENSOR APPARATUS

When the tendons of the extensor digitorum longus (EDL) and extensor digitorum brevis (EDB) arrive to join the interossei and lumbrical muscles at the metatarsophalangeal joint of each of the lesser toes, they form a tendinofibroaponeurotic structure known as the extensor apparatus. This complex structure can be divided between an extrinsic contribution (EDL), an intrinsic contribution (EDL, interossei and lumbrical muscles), and stabilizing ligaments (extensor sling, extensor wing, and triangular lamina).[4,5]

The EDL is a muscle in the anterior compartment of the leg. It provides 4 tendons for the 2nd through 5th toes. The EDB is the only intrinsic muscle in the dorsum of the foot, and it provides 4 tendons for the 1st through 4th toes. Thus, the extensor apparatus is a structure mainly developed in the 2nd, 3rd, and 4th toes.

The extensor tendons are attached to the digital axis through a fibroaponeurotic structure known as the extensor sling, which is a stabilizing ligament located at the metatarsophalangeal joint. In this location, the EDL tendon divides into three tendinous components (Fig. 8.2): The middle component inserts in the dorsum of the middle phalanx, while the medial and lateral components receive contribution from the intrinsic muscles (lumbrical muscles medially, EDB laterally) and insert into the distal phalanx and are maintained in position by an aponeurotic structure known as the triangular lamina. The interossei muscles insert at the proximal area of the proximal phalanx and plantar plate, covered by the extensor sling.

The extensor hood, which consist of the sling portion proximally and the wing portion distally, is an important structure in digital surgery (Fig. 8.3). When an extensor tenotomy is performed at this level, it prevents proximal displacement of the tendon ends. It should be noted that in lesser digital deformities, the EDB acquires a more lateral position than usual at the metatarsophalangeal joint. This is a key aspect to remember, as failure in releasing the EDB could lead to incomplete reduction of the deformity.

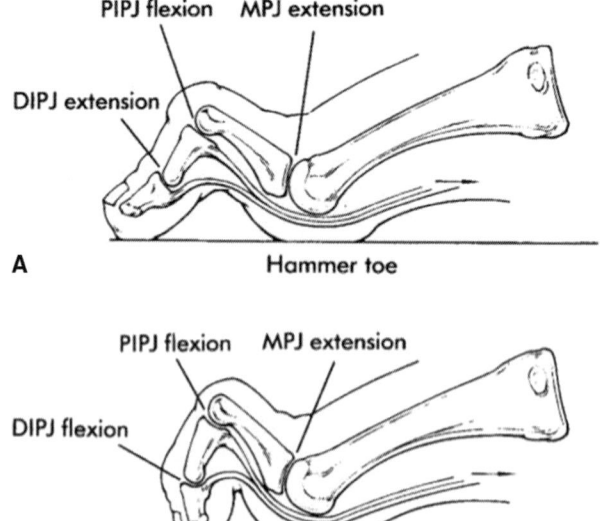

FIGURE 8.1 Digital deformities. **A.** Hammertoe deformity with dorsiflexion at the metatarsophalangeal joint, plantarflexion at the proximal interphalangeal joint and hyperextension at distal interphalangeal joint. **B.** Claw toe deformity with dorsiflexion at the metatarsophalangeal joint, plantarflexion at the proximal interphalangeal joint and distal interphalangeal joint.

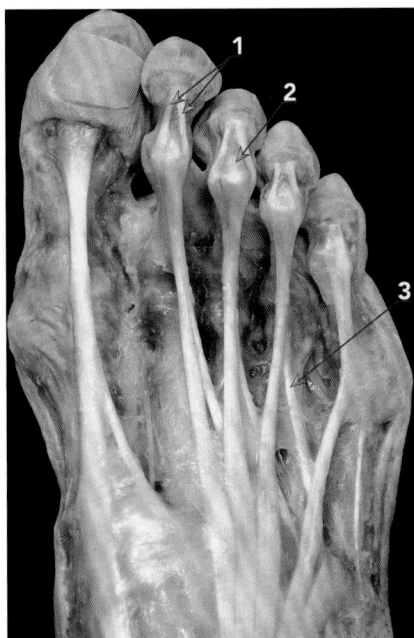

FIGURE 8.2 General view extensor apparatus: dorsal view of a dissection of the extensor apparatus. *1.* Lateral and medial slips of the extensor apparatus. *2.* Central slip of the extensor apparatus. *3.* Extensor digitorum brevis tendon, that incorporates laterally to the extensor digitorum longus.

FLEXOR APPARATUS

The flexor apparatus of the toes is a system formed by the flexor digitorum longus (FDL) and flexor digitorum brevis (FDB) tendons, the quadratus plantae and the synovial sheaths and pulleys that accompany the tendons at the level of the toes.

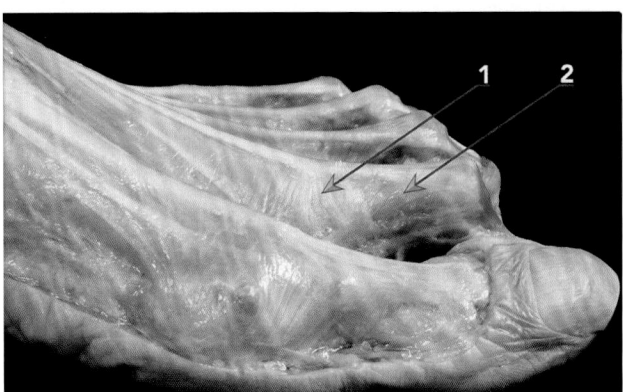

FIGURE 8.3 Extensor hood (sling/wing): medial view of the extensor apparatus demonstrating the stabilizing structures. *1,* Extensor sling. *2,* Extensor wing.

When both the FDL and FDB tendons direct to the four toes, each pair of tendons travels through a fibro-osseous tunnel. In this tunnel, at the level of the proximal phalanx, the FDB tendon divides to allow the FDL to pass between its two slips on its way to insert into the base of the distal phalanx. The fibers of the FDB tendon decussate after the passage of the FDL tendon, and the two-slip configuration is maintained until its insertion into the sides of the middle phalanx (Fig. 8.4).

The flexor tendons of the toes are embedded in a synovial sheath that starts over the metatarsal head and finishes at the distal interphalangeal joint. Inside this synovial sheath, the tendons of FDB and FDL receive nerves and vessels, which pass to the tendons through mesotendinous structures called "vincula tendinum".[6] The vinculae tendinum are subdivided into two sets: vincula longus and vincula brevis. The vincula longus is a triangular structure with a free concave border,

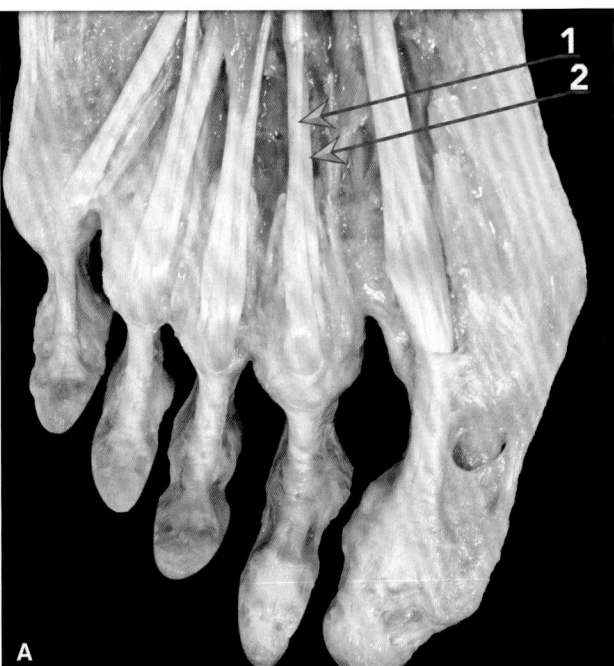

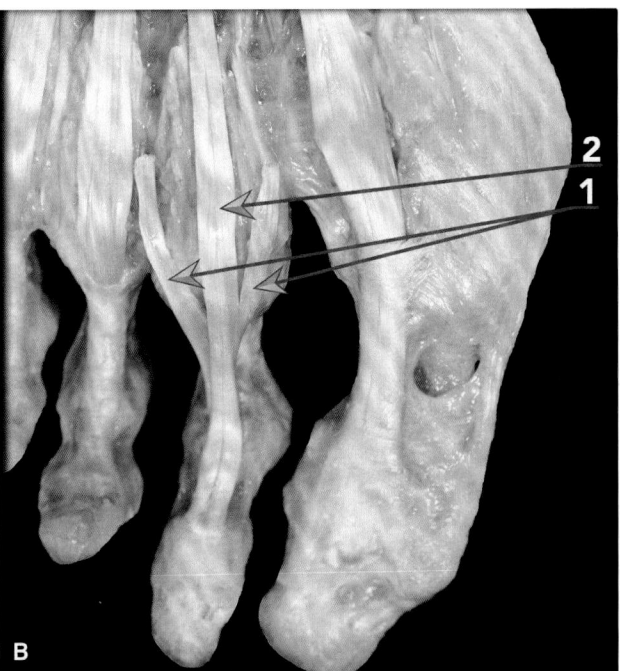

FIGURE 8.4 General flexor apparatus. **A.** General view of the flexor apparatus of the toes. **B.** Macroscopic view where flexor digitorum brevis (*1*) slips have been cut and their insertion in the middle phalanx can be observed, while flexor digitorum longus (*2*) inserts in the distal phalanx.

present at the insertion of the tendons of both the FDB and FDL tendons. The vincula brevis is a cord-like structure that is situated between the tendons of FDB and FDL tendons. There are instances where an extra vincula longus is present at the level of proximal third of the proximal phalanx.

Focal thickened areas of the flexor tendon sheath function to hold the tendons in the right position, forming the flexor pulley system.[7,8] Four annular pulleys and two cruciform pulleys are present in each toe:

A1: the first annular pulley is located at the metatarsophalangeal joint. It has its origin at the plantar plate, so it leaves the flexor tendons in a tunnel formed by the plantar plate and the A1 pulley.

A2: the second annular pulley is located at the middle of the diaphysis of the proximal phalanx. It has an osseous origin, and it is the longest and strongest of all the toe pulleys.

A3: the third annular pulley is located at the PIPJ. It covers the insertion of the FDB tendon into the base of the middle phalanx. It is continuous with the extensor apparatus.

A4: the fourth annular pulley is the smallest of the pulleys, located at the distal interphalangeal joint. It does not cover the insertion of the FDL tendon, because the pulley and also the sheath finish just proximal of this point.

C1: the first cruciform pulley is located distally to the A1 pulley. It is formed by an expansion of the interosseous muscle that, after inserting into the base of the proximal phalanx gives a slip that covers the synovial sheath of the flexor tendons.

C2: the second cruciform pulley is located between the A2 and A3 pulleys, at the head of the proximal phalanx.

Due to the disposition of the flexor tendons, a tenotomy performed at the base of the proximal phalanx will most likely release both the FDL and FDB tendons, while a tenotomy performed at the head of the proximal phalanx can release only the FDB tendon.

NEUROVASCULAR

Five nerves are in charge of the innervation of the foot: the saphenous, tibial, sural, deep, and superficial peroneal nerves.

The saphenous nerve passes anterior to the medial malleolus with distribution over the medial side of the foot, rarely extending to the 1st metatarsophalangeal joint.

The tibial nerve divides into the medial and lateral plantar nerves and innervate the sole of the foot and the dorsum of the distal phalanx of each toe.

Finally, three nerves supply the innervation of the dorsum of the foot: the sural nerve, superficial, and deep peroneal nerves.

Innervation pattern to the digits are quite variable.[9] When performing digital surgery, it is important to remember that regardless of the nerve providing the branch, four nerves innervate each toe: the dorsomedial, dorsolateral, plantarmedial, and plantarlateral branches (Fig. 8.5).

EXAMINATION

Clinical examination of digital deformities should commence with a thorough understanding of the past medical history, particularly noting history of trauma, metabolic disorders, inflammatory arthritis, and neuromuscular disorders.

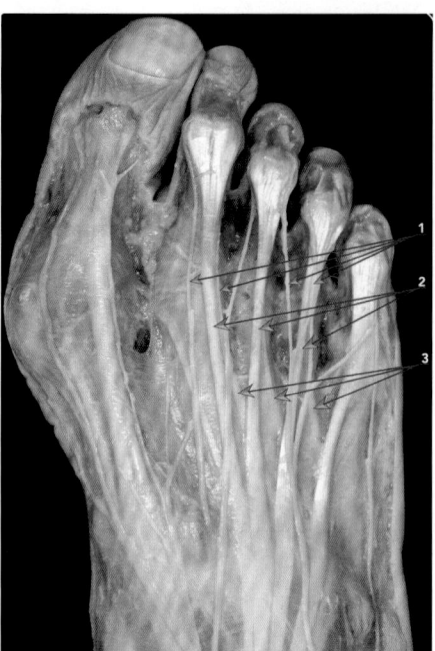

FIGURE 8.5 Dorsal nerves: dorsal view of the nerves of the dorsum of the foot demonstrating the pattern of innervation (one dorsomedial and one dorsolateral nerve for each toe). *1*, Digital nerves. *2*, Extensor digitorum longus tendons. *3*, Extensor digitorum brevis tendons.

A comprehensive biomechanical evaluation of the foot in stance and gait should ensue to assess the functional significance of the deformity. Once the biomechanical pathology is identified, focus should shift to the interphalangeal and metatarsophalangeal joint level. Typically, patients will report pain and tenderness to the dorsal PIPJ where a dorsal callosity might be noted. Occasionally significant plantar calluses under the metatarsal head are present due to significant points of pressure from the retrograde force of the flexion deformity. The reducibility of the deformity, and whether it is deemed flexible or rigid, range of motion, and the plane of the deformity should be noted. The Kelikian push up test reproduces weight-bearing by eliciting a plantar loading force on the lesser metatarsal head. This force will tension the plantar fascia, and if this mechanism is intact and the deformity is flexible, it will recreate the rectus alignment of the digit allowing the PIPJ to extend.[10] A rigid deformity will maintain the flexion deformity with this maneuver, and a semirigid deformity is noted to only partially reduce (Fig. 8.6).

PATHOGENESIS

Digital deformities can occur due to a multitude of factors that disrupt the delicate balance between static stabilizers and dynamic stabilizers. Nonmechanical etiologies are posttraumatic, inflammatory, neurologic, metabolic, congenital, or postsurgical in nature. However, the majority of digital deformities are due to biomechanical dysfunction. McGlamry et al. described three main etiologies of digital deformities due to failure of the intricate balance of the intrinsic/extrinsic musculature that stabilizes metatarsophalangeal joint and the digit.[11] These include flexor stabilization, flexor substitution, and extensor substitution.

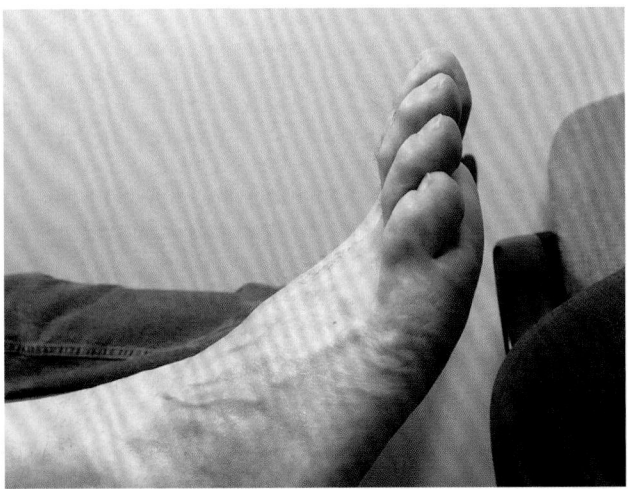

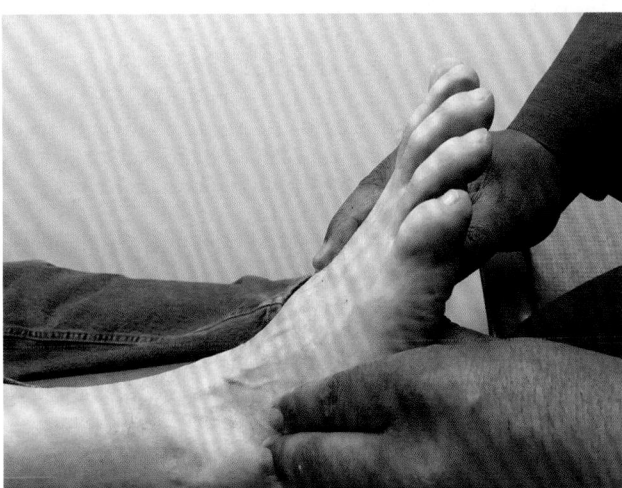

FIGURE 8.6 Kelikian push up. Flexible digital deformity.

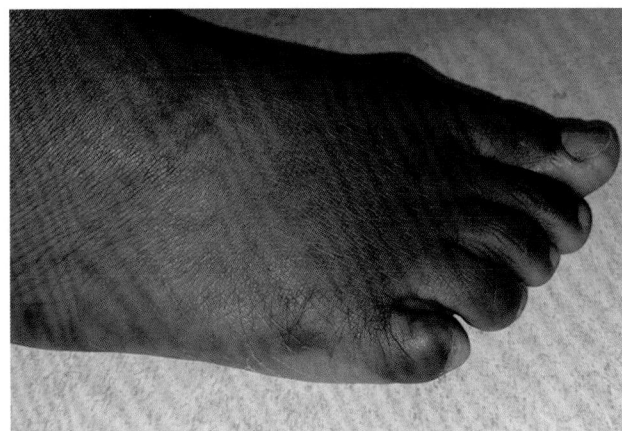

FIGURE 8.7 Flexor stabilization with adductovarus deformity.

FLEXOR STABILIZATION

Flexor stabilization is the most common mechanism leading to digital deformities, typically seen in a pronated foot during the late stance phase of gait. During gait, the long flexors are supinators of the subtalar and midtarsal joint.[12] With excessive pronation, the long flexor tendons fire earlier and longer in the gait cycle during stance. The long flexor tendons gain mechanical advantage and overpower the interossei causing fatigue and failure. The interossei lose the ability to stabilize the proximal phalanx on the weight-bearing surface, leading to mild hyperextension deformity at the metatarsophalangeal joint. As the intrinsic muscles continue to weaken, the short flexor will fail to stabilize the middle phalanx on the weight-bearing surface leading to the long flexors overpowering, creating a recognizable claw toe or hammertoe deformity during stance (Fig. 8.7). Quadratus plantae loses its mechanical advantage and therefore loses its lateralizing pull on the FDL, leading to adductovarus deformity of the fourth and fifth digits.[11-14]

FLEXOR SUBSTITUTION

Flexor substitution is the least common of the three mechanisms attributing to digital deformities occurring typically during stance in a supinated foot. During gait, the deep posterior

and peroneal muscles will function and gain advantage as major plantar flexors to aid in heel off when there is weakness in the triceps surae.[11] This can occur in situations of an overlengthened Achilles tendon with calcaneal gait or neuromuscular pathologies with a high arched foot. While these deep posterior and lateral muscles pass posterior to the ankle joint axis, the plantarflexory lever arm is short and therefore not as effective at eliciting heel lift.[11] Due to the overuse of these flexor tendons, they over power the extensors and claw-type deformities will develop.

EXTENSOR SUBSTITUTION

Extensor substitution occurs during the swing phase in the pes cavus foot or in neuromuscular disorders such as Charcot Marie Tooth that manifest with a cavus deformity. In the cavus foot, equinus of the foot and ankle can be present with the forefoot plantar in orientation relative to the rearfoot.[15] During gait, in order for the forefoot to clear the weight-bearing surface during swing phase, the EDL fires early and forcefully gains a mechanical advantage over the stabilizing effects of the lumbricals, leading to severe hyperextension at the metatarsophalangeal joint.[11-14] This deformity in the early stages is flexible, occurring during the swing phase and reducing during stance. On examination, the digits will be hyperextended at the metatarsophalangeal joint, a common site of pain plantarly at the metatarsal heads, and notable bowstringing of the long extensor tendons, along with clawing or flexion of the digits purely in the sagittal plane (Fig. 8.8). Over time, this flexible deformity will become rigid in nature with fixed metatarsalphalangeal joint (MTPJ) subluxation from progressive and chronic contraction of the extensor tendons.

IMAGING AND DIAGNOSTIC STUDIES

Standard weight-bearing dorsoplantar, medial oblique, and lateral radiographs are used in evaluating digital deformities. Assessment of joint congruity, arthritic changes, angular deformities, and the metatarsal parabola can be evaluated.[11] Associated deformities such as hallux valgus and other contributing pathology that might need to be addressed such as cavus foot or metatarsus adductus should also be evaluated.

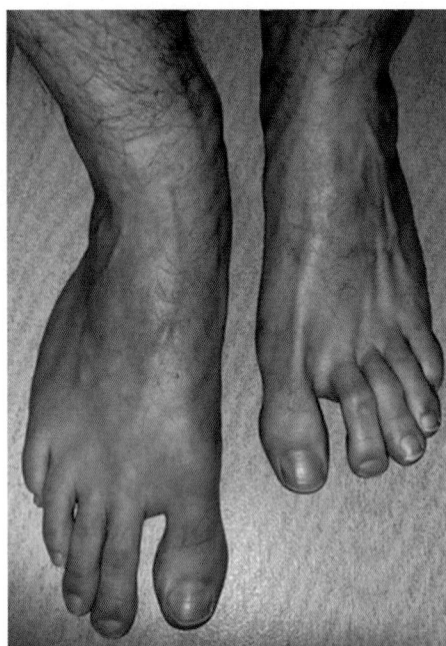

FIGURE 8.8 Extensor substitution during stance and swing with bowstringing tendons.

On the dorsoplantar view in the presence of the severe digital deformity, the typical positive "gun barrel sign" is readily apparent (Fig. 8.9A). On the lateral radiograph, the degree of hyperextension or dorsal dislocation of the digit can be observed (Fig. 8.9B).

The use of magnetic resonance imaging (MRI) while not essential in the diagnosis of digital deformities has been reported to have high sensitivity and specificity for detecting plantar plate tears, a concomitant finding in some digital deformities with predislocation syndrome.[15-17] While, plantar plate tears are a clinical diagnosis, MRI is useful for diagnosing injuries of the plantar plate in cases where the physical examination is equivocal. Ultrasonography is a low-cost imaging modality that offers a dynamic assessment of the plantar plate integrity, detecting partial and complete tears with high sensitivity and noting the adjacent joint structure pathology[16,18,19] While useful, ultrasound may be limited by the experience of the technologist. Arthrography while not frequently utilized can also aid in detecting tears of the plantar plate and metatarsophalangeal joint capsule.[20]

NONSURGICAL TREATMENT

Nonsurgical measures should always be initiated as the first line of treatment, with the goal of relieving local pain and aiding in normal ambulation. The mainstay of treatment involves foot wear modification: utilizing wider shoes, larger toe box, and lower heels.[21] A rocker-bottom sole may diminish pain and relieve dorsiflexion stress to the forefoot. Adding a cushioned insole or a metatarsal pad can offload and reduce plantar forefoot pressure. Pressure areas over the PIPJ may be relieved with toe cushions or sleeves to alleviate impingement of the digits. In cases of plantar plate tear or dysfunction with flexible MTPJ subluxation, tapping or the use of a splint that positions the affected digit in a plantarward direction can eliminate symptoms and facilitate scarring in this new plantar position. Although nonsurgical treatment of an unstable MTP joint deformity may temporarily relieve pain or slow progression, it cannot be expected to permanently correct the malalignment. In a report on the conservative treatment of patients with a crossover toe deformity, Coughlin observed that digital taping slowed progression of the deformity, but the patients continued to have pain long term, necessitating surgical intervention.[22,23]

Nonsteroidal anti-inflammatory drugs (NSAIDs) can be utilized to manage discomfort but should be used cautiously and only after thorough review of patient's medical comorbidities.

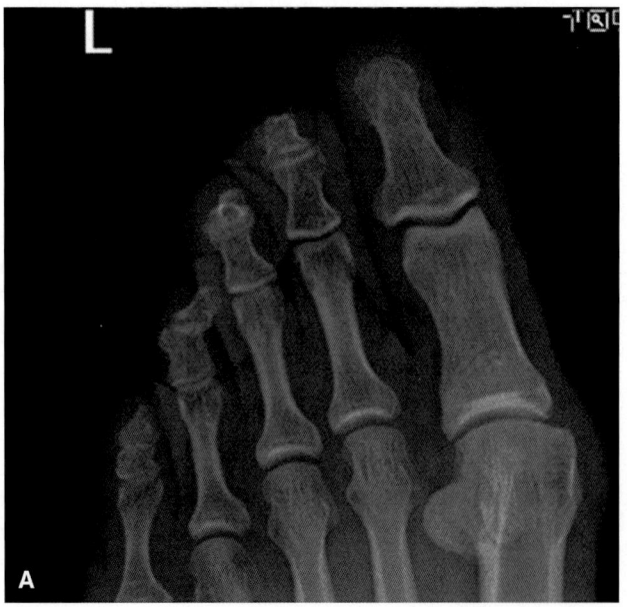

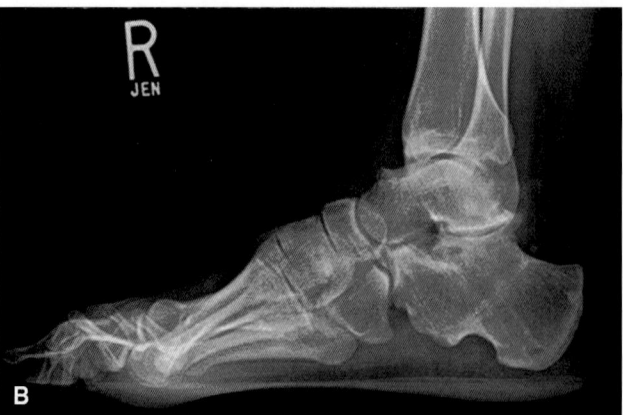

FIGURE 8.9 Weight-bearing radiographs: **(A)** AP "gun barrel sign," **(B)** lateral severe hyperextension/flexion deformity.

Selective corticosteroid injections can be diagnostic and therapeutic, but should be used with extreme caution when a plantar plate tear is suspected as they can potentially disguise symptoms, potentiate further capsular and plantar plate degeneration and result in further joint subluxation or dislocation requiring surgical intervention.

SURGICAL TREATMENT

Once conservative treatment has failed, surgical correction of the condition is warranted to relieve symptoms of digital deformities. The patient should have symptoms with shoe gear and activity that interfere with their daily activities. While relief of pain and symptoms are the goal, it is important to address the deformity at the level of the pathology of the digit.[24] This reduces the chances of reoccurrence of the condition along with pain-free activity. It is important that the patient has realistic expectations when approaching surgical correction of the condition.

positioning PEARLS

- The patient is placed in a supine position on the operating table.
- The lower extremity is internally rotated with the use of a bump underneath the ipsilateral hip to keep the foot in a neutral position.
- A nerve block is performed at the level of the digit to provide anesthesia to the medial and lateral nerves along the digit.
- Once the toe has been prepped and appropriately draped, attention is directed to the pathological digit.
- An ankle tourniquet is utilized for hemostasis.
- Intraoperative Mini C-arm is essential for digital procedures and fixation.

ARTHROPLASTY

This procedure is performed at the level of the PIPJ. It is indicated for flexible and semi-rigid deformities, which are commonly caused by overpowering of the flexor tendons that are correctable on clinical examination. Also, the procedure can be employed on structurally long digits that fail conservative treatment.

The arthroplasty procedure allows for shortening of the digit to reduce the contraction by removing a portion of the proximal or middle phalanx depending on the level of the deformity.[25] This weakens the function of the flexor tendons at the insertion that contribute to the condition for flexor hammertoe deformities.[26]

Technique

An incision can be made either horizontally or longitudinally (Fig. 8.10). A horizontal incision at the level of the PIPJ is preferred when the deformity is isolated at the level of the PIPJ only. A longitudinal incision is preferred when correction of the deformity is needed at the level of both the metatarsophalangeal joint and the PIPJ. Proper soft tissue release in a stepwise fashion at the metatarsophalangeal

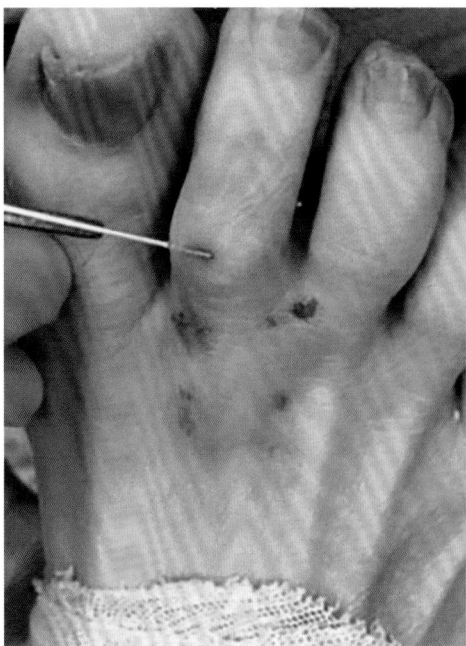

FIGURE 8.10 Horizontal incision utilized for arthroplasty procedure.

joint to reduce the deformity is performed when needed before proceeding to the PIPJ.

After skin incision, the subcutaneous tissues are reflected to reveal the extensor tendon. A transverse tenotomy is then performed or an extensor tendon lengthening can be performed if necessary. The medial and lateral collateral ligaments are then incised at the level of the PIPJ to expose the head of the proximal phalanx. Care is taken to avoid the FDL tendon (Figs. 8.11 through 8.14). Once exposed, the distal aspect of

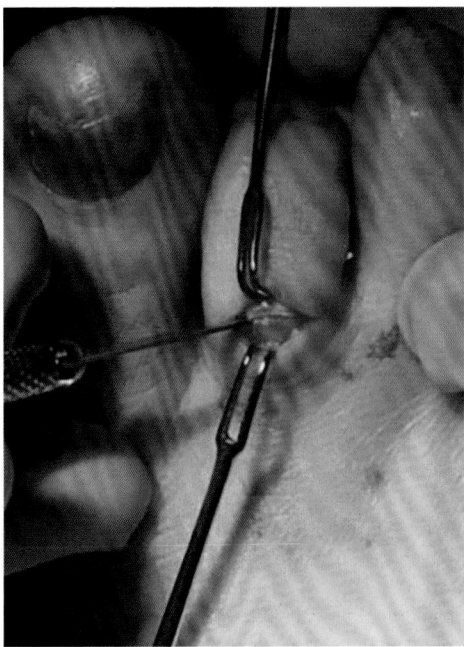

FIGURE 8.11 Extensor tendon is identified and released through a horizontal incision.

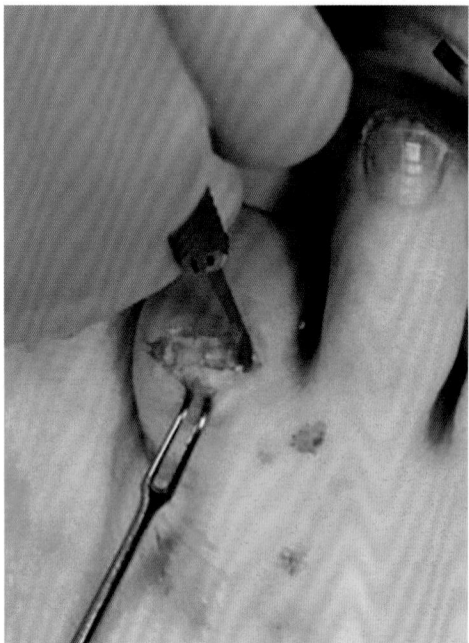

FIGURE 8.12 Release of the lateral collateral ligaments to allow for exposure of the distal aspect of the proximal phalanx.

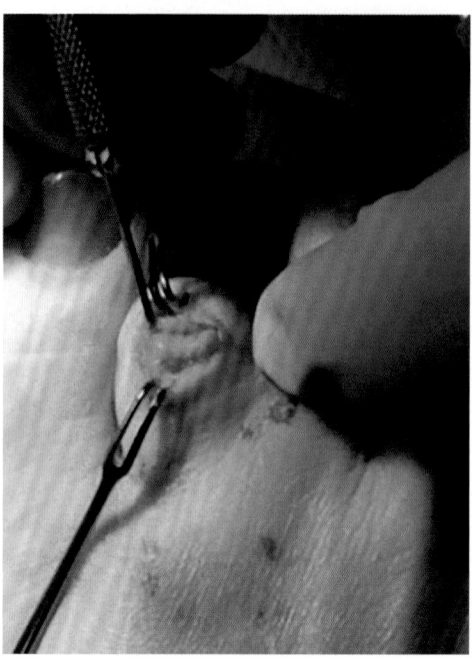

FIGURE 8.13 Release of the medial collateral ligaments to allow for exposure of the distal aspect of the proximal phalanx.

the proximal phalanx is removed making sure to resect just proximal to the condyles (Figs. 8.15 and 8.16). After osseous resection, the extensor tendon is reapproximated followed by the appropriate skin closure (Figs. 8.17 through 8.19).

Multiple arthroplasty procedures performed on adjacent digits should be avoided as this can create destabilization of the foot during the late stance phase of gait.

ARTHRODESIS

Arthrodesis is commonly performed at the proximal phalangeal joint for correction of rigid or semi-rigid hammertoe deformities.[27] This procedure is done when contraction is present at the metatarsophalangeal joint and the PIPJ, and it is unable to be reduced based on clinical examination. While the deformity is commonly corrected in the sagittal plane, it can be useful for correction in the transverse plane as well.[28]

SURGICAL PEARLS OF ARTHROPLASTY PROCEDURE

- Success of this procedure depends on adequate bone resection to correct the deformity. Excessive resection of the proximal phalanx should be avoided. Resection of more than condyles of the proximal phalanx can lead to a short digit, destabilized digit, or more commonly a flail digit.
- Resection of the condyles can be performed with either a micro sagittal saw or a bone cutting forceps. With the use of bone forceps, the surgeon maintains control of the amount of bone resection; however, with the microsagittal saw, there exists a greater risk of thermal necrosis of the bone along with a greater chance of excessive bone resection during the procedure.
- Regardless of the type of instrument utilized for bone resection; it is important to protect the adjacent skin and neurovascular structures as well as the flexor tendons plantarly.
- If correction of the condition at the proximal interphalangeal joint is performed, the distal interphalangeal joint may still be in a contracted position as in a mallet toe.

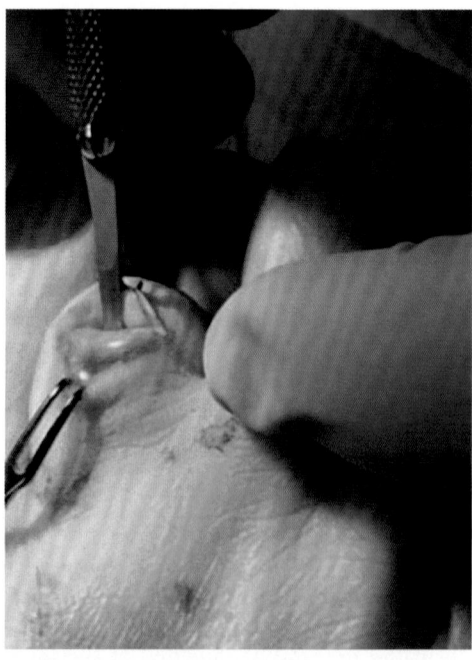

FIGURE 8.14 Release of the flexor tendons to allow for greater exposure of the proximal phalanx.

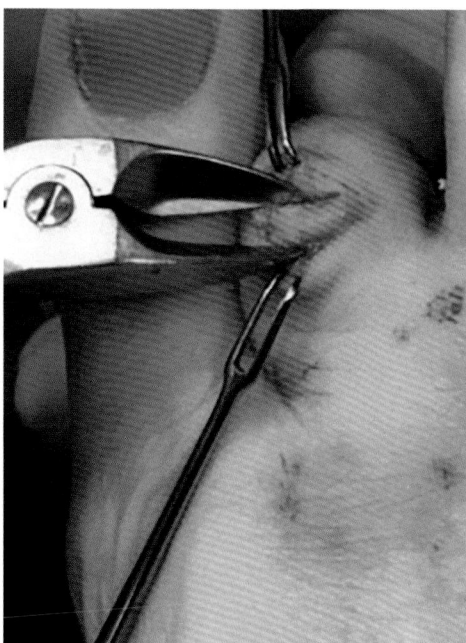

FIGURE 8.15 Bone forceps are used to remove the condyles of the proximal phalanx.

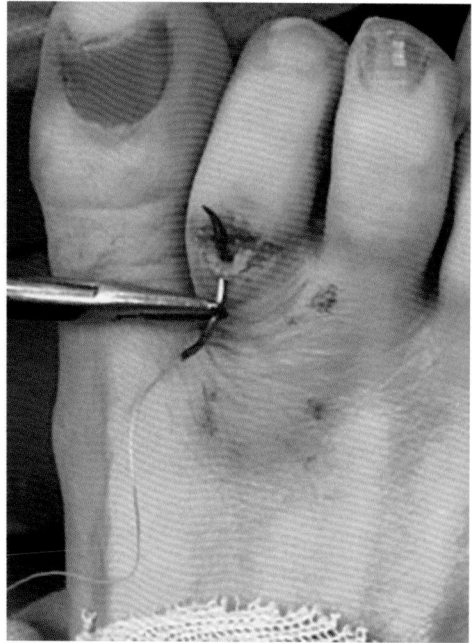

FIGURE 8.17 Reapproximation of the extensor tendon once the arthroplasty is complete.

Technique

A longitudinal incision is used to correct the deformity at the level of the metatarsophalangeal joint and the PIPJ. Incision placement is important to preserve the neurovascular structures during the incision (Fig. 8.20). As blunt dissection is done through the subcutaneous layer, then attention is directed to the metatarsophalangeal joint. A soft tissue release

in a stepwise fashion is then performed to reduce the deformity as needed.

Attention is then directed to the PIPJ. A transverse tenotomy or an extensor tendon lengthening is then performed and the medial and lateral collateral ligaments are incised to expose the proximal aspect of the middle phalanx and the condyles of the distal aspect of the proximal phalanx (Fig. 8.21A and B).

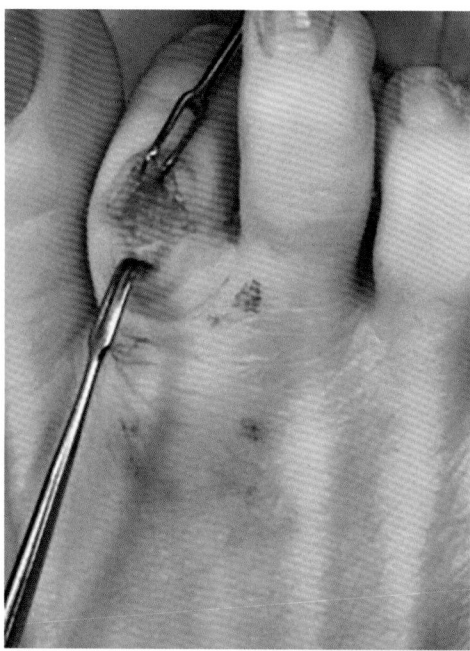

FIGURE 8.16 Proximal phalanx after the condyles have been removed from the proximal phalanx.

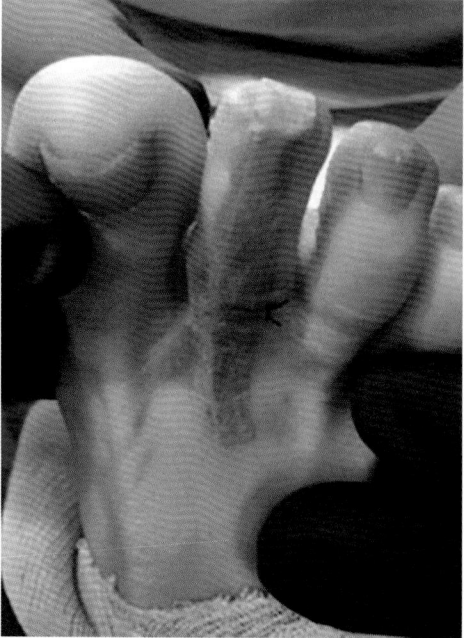

FIGURE 8.18 Correction of the deformity is maintained with steri-strips bandages.

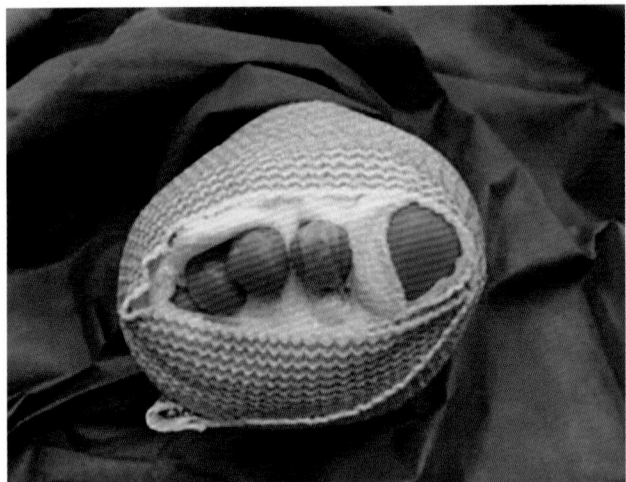

FIGURE 8.19 Full bandage to maintain correction of the arthroplasty procedure.

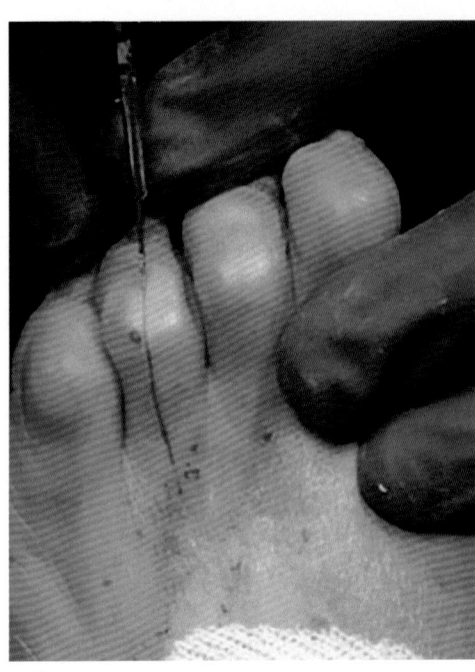

FIGURE 8.20 A longitudinal incision to allow exposure of the proximal interphalangeal joint with the metatarsophalangeal joint.

Once the PIPJ is exposed, osseous resection is performed to remove the articular cartilage with subchondral bone, the condyles of the proximal phalanx, and the base of the middle phalanx (Fig. 8.22A and B). The osseous resection to correct the deformity can be performed with microsagittal saw or bone forceps.

Once the joint is resected, an intraoperative push up test is performed to evaluate further contraction that may be present at the metatarsophalangeal joint. This is commonly seen in rigid hammertoe deformities and can lead to reoccurrence of the condition if not properly addressed. An incision is made medial to the EDL tendon through the extensor hood apparatus from the proximal aspect of the metatarsophalangeal

joint. The extensor tendon is identified and once exposed, a Z-plasty of the extensor tendon lengthening is performed with 2 horizontal and 1 longitudinal incisions. One horizontal incision is made medial to the EDL tendon at the distal one-fourth of the metatarsal followed by a longitudinal incision between the EDL and EDB tendons (Fig. 8.23A-C). A horizontal incision lateral to the extensor tendon at the level of the extensor apparatus completes the tendon lengthening.

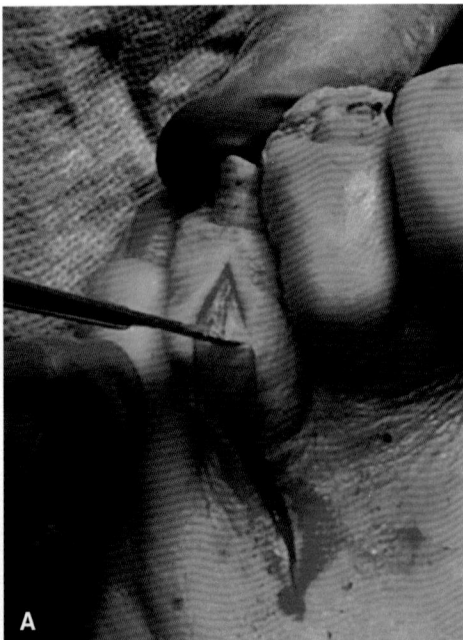
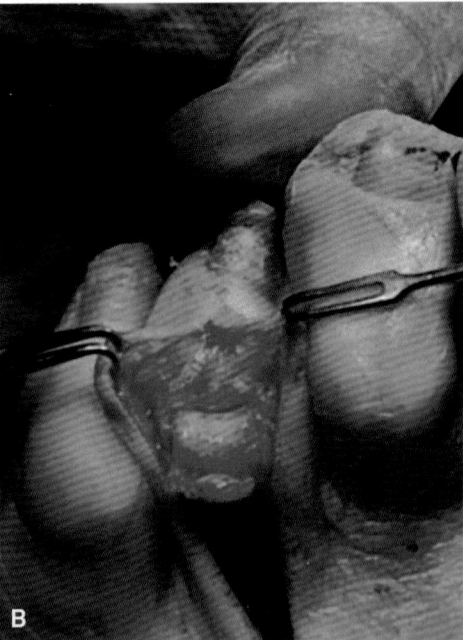

FIGURE 8.21 **A.** Release of the extensor tendon along with the medial and lateral collateral ligaments. **B.** Exposed proximal interphalangeal joint after soft tissue release.

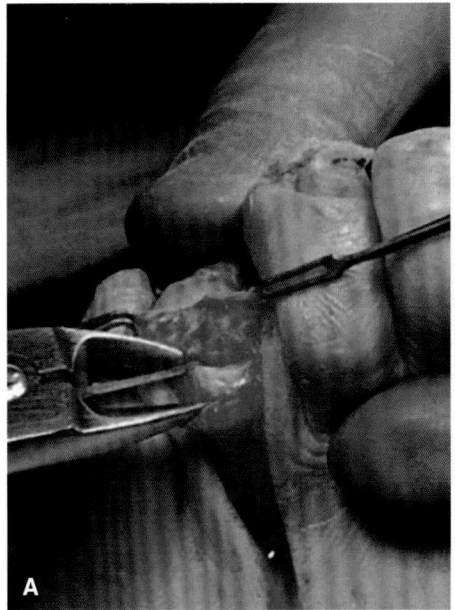
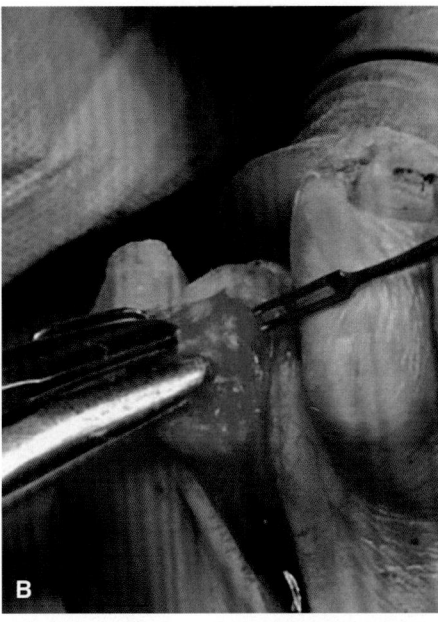

FIGURE 8.22 **A.** Removal of condyles with bone forceps at the distal aspect of the proximal phalanx. **B.** Utilizing a curette, removal of cartilage with subchondral bone at the distal aspect of the middle phalanx.

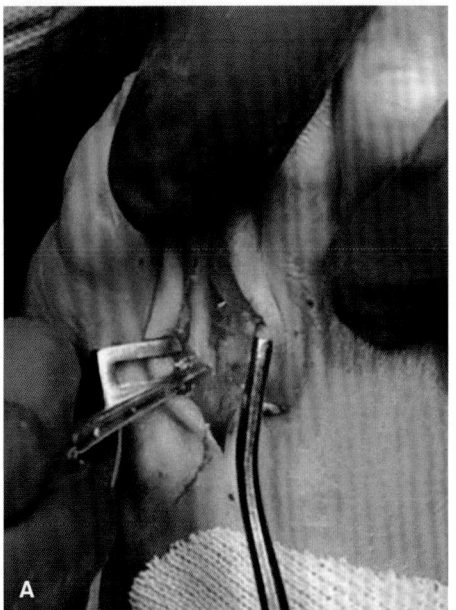
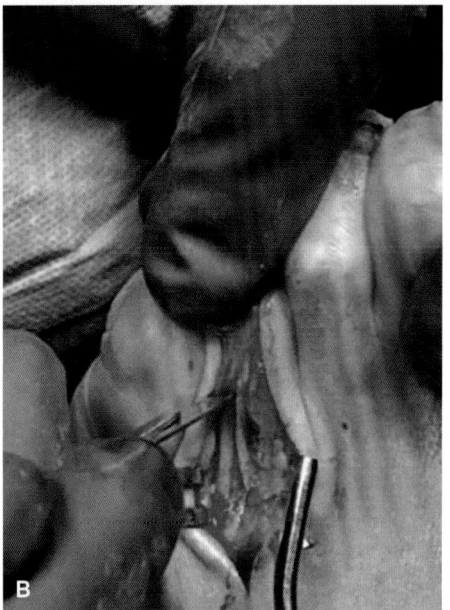
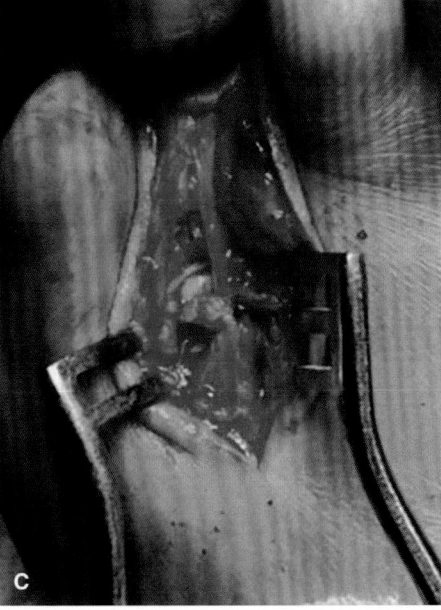

FIGURE 8.23 **A.** Horizontal cut for a Z-plasty tendon lengthening of the extensor tendon. **B.** Distal horizontal incision for Z-plasty extensor tendon lengthening. **C.** Corrected position after Z-plasty extensor tendon lengthening.

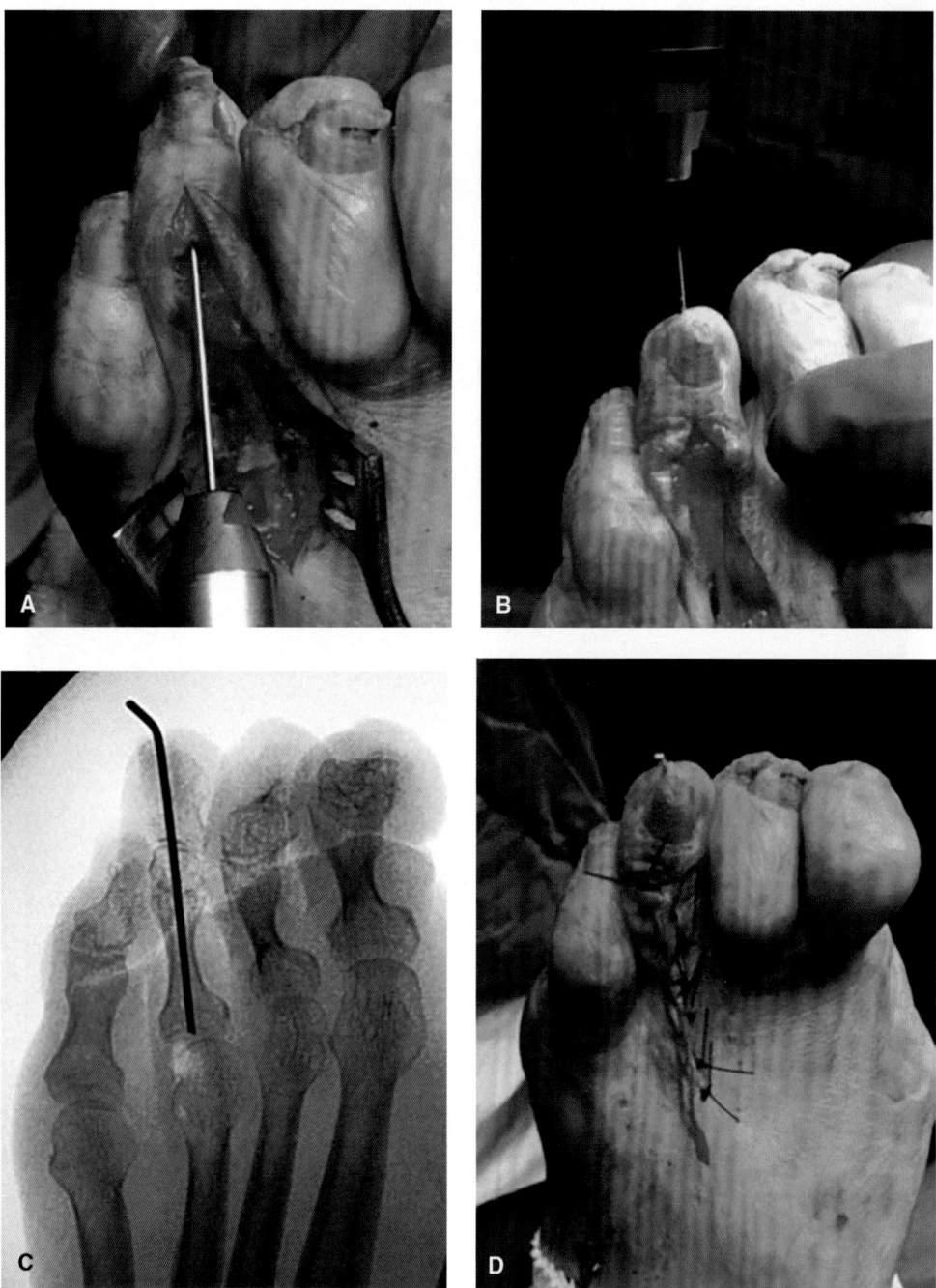

FIGURE 8.24 A. Drilling of the middle phalanx for Kirschner wire (K-wire) for fixation of arthrodesis for the proximal phalanx. **B.** Retrograde drilling through the proximal interphalangeal joint for arthrodesis of the proximal interphalangeal joint. **C.** Radiograph of K-wire fixation for arthrodesis of the proximal interphalangeal joint. **D.** Postoperative correction with external K-wire fixation.

Once the digit is placed in the appropriate position to reduce the deformity, the extensor tendon is reapproximated at this appropriate length.

Once the soft tissue contraction has been reduced, fixation of the PIPJ is performed. Kirschner wires (K-wires), in the size of 0.045, 0.054, or 0.062, have been commonly utilized for fixation for digital arthrodesis[29,30] Once the appropriate size K-wire is selected, the proximal phalanx is predrilled then the K-wire is placed into the base of the middle phalanx and run distally out the end of the toe. It is then retrograded back across the PIPJ into the proximal phalanx (Fig. 8.24A-D).

While K-wires provide a level of convenience and versatility with ease of use, patients still experience complications such as exposed hardware that increase risk of infection as well as instability of fixation that leads to delayed and nonunion.[31] With the advent of new technology, multiple options for intramedullary fixation now exist that allow for reduced postoperative complications from external K-wires (Fig. 8.25). These include but are not limited to bioabsorbable pins, metallic intramedullary implants, thermal activated metallic fixation, allogenic bone implant, Polyetheretherketone fixation, and cannulated screws.[32-39]

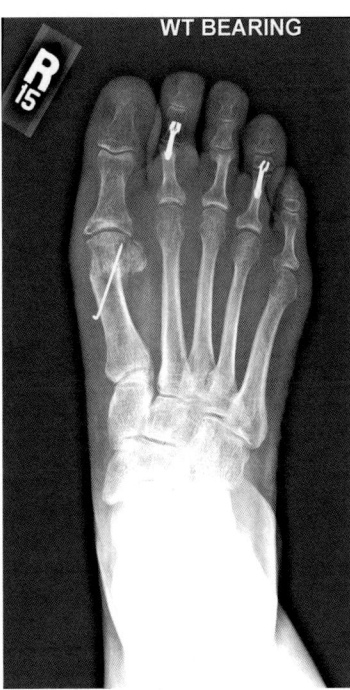

FIGURE 8.25 Metallic intramedullary internal fixation for arthrodesis of the PIP joint.

SURGICAL PEARLS OF ARTHRODESIS PROCEDURE

- When performing arthrodesis of the digit, it is important that the digit is placed in a plantarflexed position. By performing the fusion in mild plantarflexion, it provides for function of the flexor tendons during the stance phase of gait to allow the digit to purchase the ground.
- When utilizing a K-wire for fixation, it is important that the digit be in slight plantarflexion and the fixation remains at the center of the arthrodesis site of the digit. If the K-wire

is too plantar, not only will it not cross the arthrodesis site, but it will cause pain, hardware failure, migration, and possible infection.
- Proximal correction at the metatarsophalangeal joint is performed prior to the proximal interphalangeal joint arthrodesis. If not properly performed, the lack of correction would be heightened further at the metatarsophalangeal joint in the sagittal and possibly transverse planes, respectively.
- External fixation of the proximal interphalangeal joint must not cross the metatarsophalangeal joint as it can lead to early arthritic changes.
- With this procedure, lack of purchase of the digits during gait is a common postoperative complication.

FLEXOR DIGITORUM LONGUS TENDON TRANSFER

The transfer of the flexor tendon is a very useful and powerful procedure in the correction of many digital deformities. It is most effective for sagittal plane deformities in which there is a dorsal contracture of the metatarsal phalangeal joint of the lesser toes. However, the procedure can be modified or used in combination with other procedures to correct transverse and frontal plane deformities.[40] While this procedure can be combined with digital arthroplasty or arthrodesis in nonreducible hammertoe deformities, it has also been shown to be an effective isolated procedure.

Surgical Technique

The patient is positioned on the operating table in the supine position. Typically, a sequential release of the dorsal contracted structures is performed. This includes Z-lengthening of the EDL tendon and appropriate capsulotomy at the metatarsal phalangeal joint—dorsal, medial and lateral capsulotomy as necessary to correct any angular deformity present (Fig. 8.26A-C). If extensor deformity is still present despite

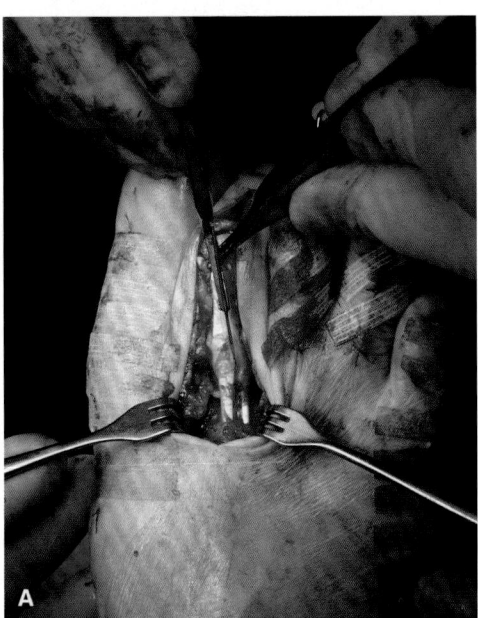
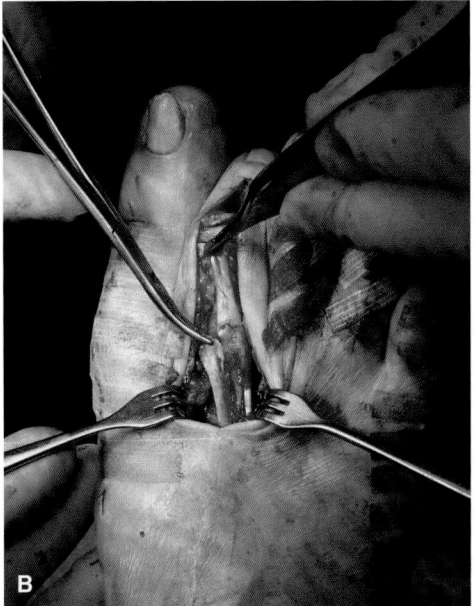

FIGURE 8.26 A. Longitudinal incision between extensor digitorium longus tendon medially and extensor digitorium brevis laterally. **B.** The extensor digitorium longus tendon is identified and transected distally.

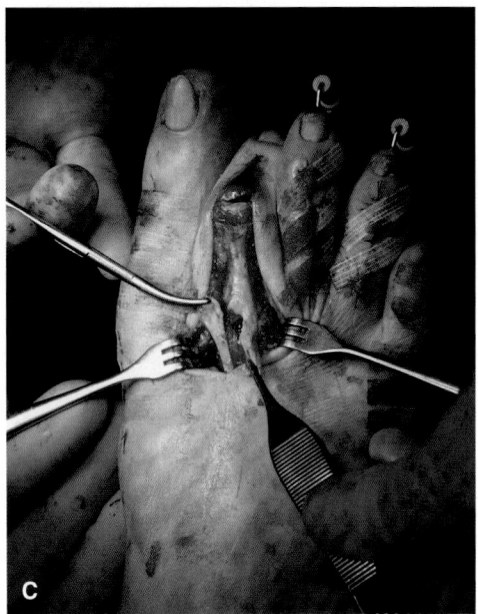

FIGURE 8.26 (*Continued*) **C.** To complete the Z-plasty lenghteinging, the extensor digitorium longus is transected proximally.

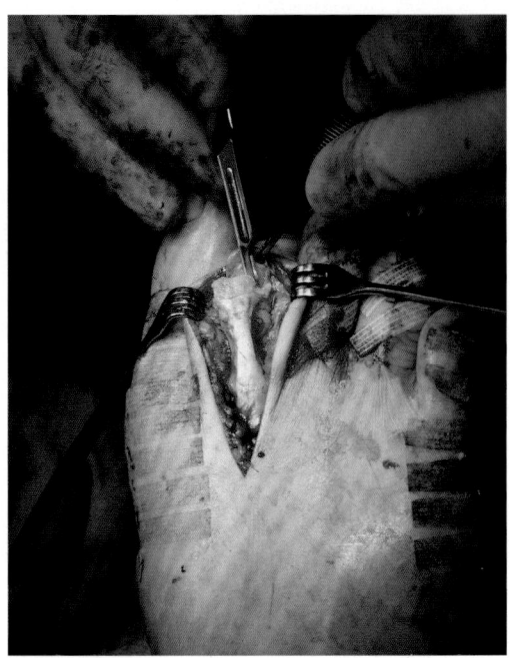

FIGURE 8.27 Proximal interphalangeal joint disarticulation.

sequential release dorsally, and the toe does not purchase the weight-bearing surface during simulated weight bearing (Kelikian push-up test), a FDL tendon transfer is indicated, and proceeds as follows.

1. Attention is directed to the PIPJ where the medial and lateral collateral ligaments are transected. Care is taken to preserve the ligament for use in final closure (Fig. 8.27).
2. Periosteal dissection along the plantar aspect of the proximal phalanx is performed to allow dorsal traction to be

placed on the bone to expose the digital flexor apparatus (Fig. 8.28A and B).
3. The PIPJ is distracted, and the plantar capsular thickening (plantar plate) of the IPJ is identified. This thickened capsule is carefully transected to expose the flexor tendons (Fig. 8.29A and B). Care is taken to not cut through the flexor tendons during capsular transection.
4. The flexor tendons are identified (Fig. 8.30). Three tendons should be visualized. The medial and lateral tendons are the

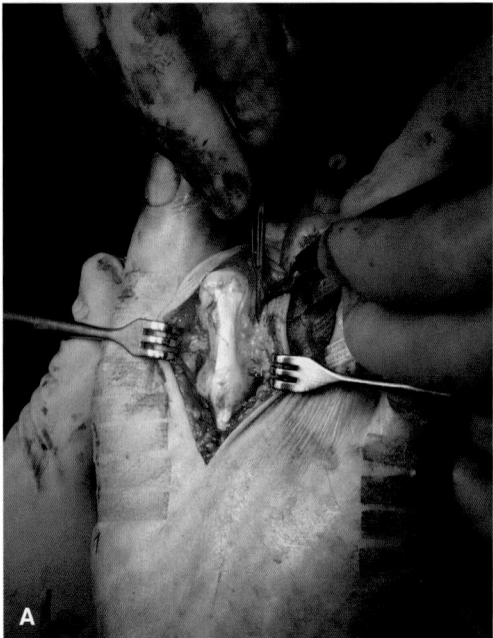

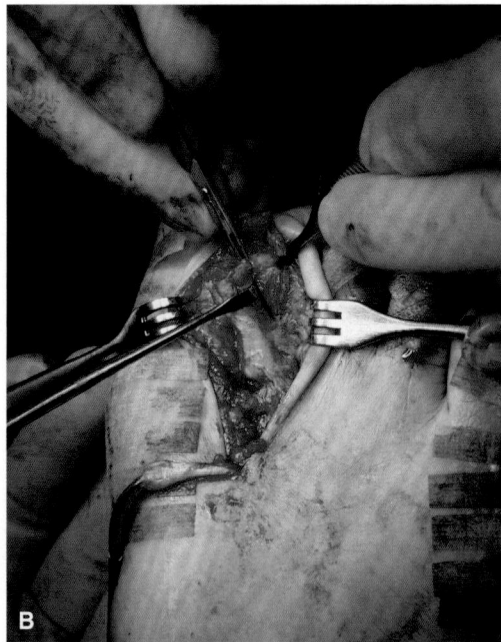

FIGURE 8.28 **A.** Plantar disarticulation. **B.** Plantar dissection to expose flexor plate.

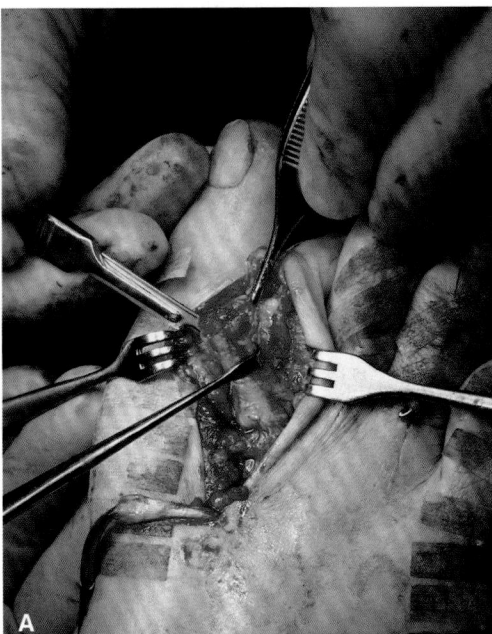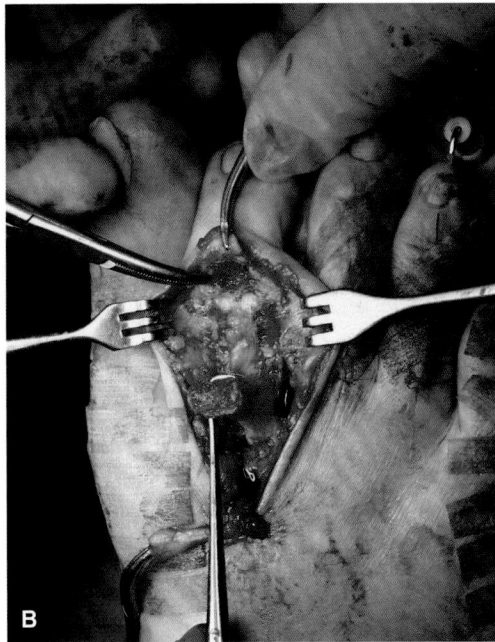

FIGURE 8.29 **A.** Dissection to identify the flexor tendon. **B.** Capsule of the flexor tendon identified.

bifurcation of the FDB tendon and are inserting on the shaft of the middle phalanx. These are preserved. The FDL tendon is the central tendon and should be sitting dorsal to the brevis tendons. A curved mosquito hemostat is placed beneath the long tendon and the jaws are spread (Fig. 8.31).

5. With the jaws of the hemostat spread, one is able to appreciate the longitudinal fibers of the tendon. A no. 15 blade is then utilized to make a stab incision centrally within the

tendon. Care is taken to create equal medial and lateral sections of the tendon.

6. A second hemostat is then used to gently grasp the medial half of the tendon. The original hemostat is now used to grasp the lateral half of the tendon. Once both halves of the tendon are secured, a no. 15 blade is used to incise the tendons as distally as possible to ensure adequate length of tendon for transfer (Fig. 8.32).

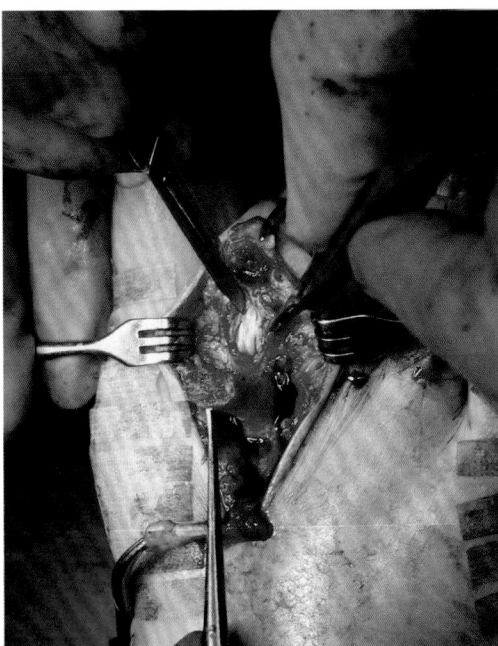

FIGURE 8.30 Flexor tendon identified.

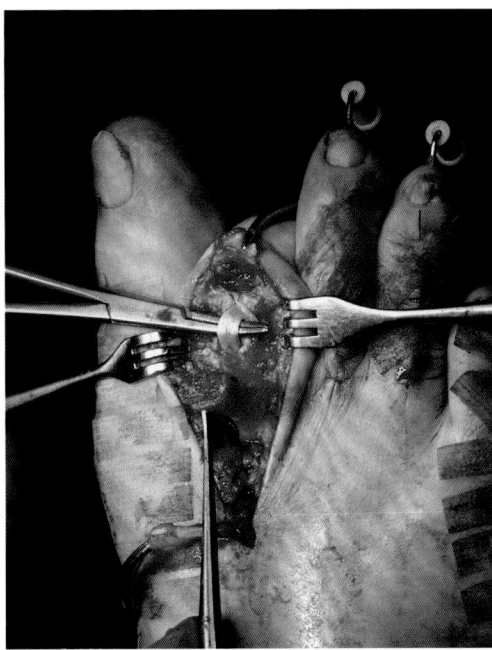

FIGURE 8.31 Flexor tendon isolated prior to release.

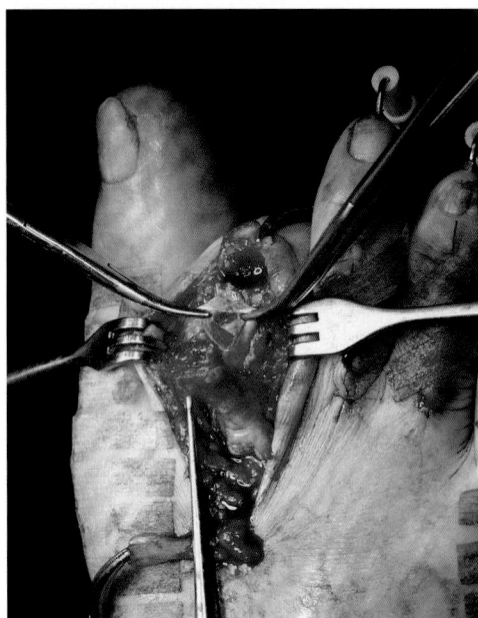

FIGURE 8.32 Flexor tendon incised into halves.

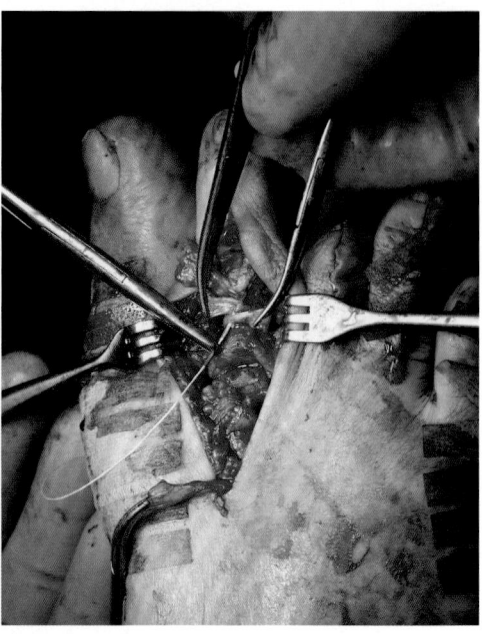

FIGURE 8.34 Securing of dorsal tied flexor tendon.

7. Because of the longitudinal direction of the fibers, no further sharp dissection is needed, and the tendon is easily split into a medial and lateral half with moderate, but gentle medial and lateral traction (Fig. 8.33).

8. The proximal phalanx is then plantar flexed, and the medial and lateral halves of the tendon are passed from plantar to dorsal around the medial and lateral shaft of the phalanx, respectively.

9. Once the tendons are on the dorsal side of the bone, they are secured under appropriate tension to one another with the surgeon's desired suture (Fig. 8.34).

SURGICAL PEARLS OF FLEXOR DIGITORUM LONGUS TENDON TRANSFER

- After plantar dissection to expose the flexor tendons, a Ragnell retractor is useful to keep the proximal phalanx dorsally retracted. Be sure to dissect far enough proximally to adequately expose the tendons.

- If a proximal interphalangeal joint arthrodesis is performed, one should pin this joint prior to final suturing of the tendons. Additionally, temporarily pinning across the metatarsal phalangeal joint, slightly over correcting for the present deformity, will assist in maintaining correction, while the tendons are sutured in their transferred position (Fig. 8.35).

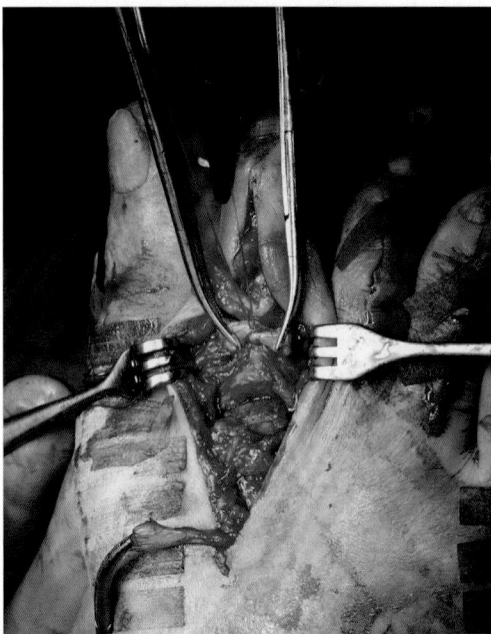

FIGURE 8.33 Flexor tendon transferred dorsal and tied to proximal phalanx.

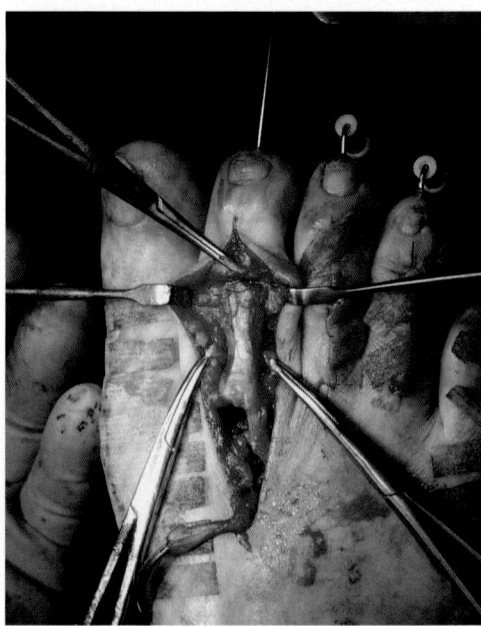

FIGURE 8.35 Arthrodesis of the proximal phalangeal joint after flexor tendon transfer.

POSTOPERATIVE COURSE

A moist to dry sterile compressive dressing is applied. Steri strips are often used to "splint" toe in its corrected position. This dressing is left in place for 5-7 days and then changed. If nonabsorbable sutures are used for skin closure, these are removed 14 days after procedure. At 4 weeks postoperation, the pin is backed out of the metatarsal phalangeal joint but remains across the PIPJ for an additional 2 weeks. The pin is completely removed from the digit at the 6-week mark. The patient is allowed protected weight bearing in a stiff soled postoperative shoe for 6 weeks and then transitions to a stable athletic shoe thereafter.

FIFTH DIGIT DEFORMITIES

Pathology of the fifth digit can be some of the most difficult and challenging deformities a foot and ankle surgeon may encounter. Patients may complain of pain associated with irritation and corn formation due to rubbing of the shoe or adjacent fourth digit. This, coupled with the potential multiplane deformity of the toe, makes surgical intervention complex in some situations. Hyperkeratosis (hard corn), usually seen dorsal-lateral on the fifth toe, or interdigital keratosis (soft corn), arise primarily due to the plane(s) of deformity. One or more planes may be involved in the deformity and would need to be addressed either conservatively or surgically to alleviate patient complaints.

Lesion Patterns and Types

Several lesion patterns may develop on the fifth digit, and particular patterns are due to the planes of deformity coupled with the flexibility or rigidity of the deformity. These lesions may occur in isolation, or in combination with one another.

1. A nucleated lesion present on the distal aspect of the fifth digit beneath the border of the toenail is typically due to an adductovarus deformity, prominent epicondyle of the distal phalanx, or ankylosis of the interphalangeal joint commonly known as symphalangism.[42] This lesion pattern, original described as Durlacher or Lister's Corn,[43,44] is commonly seen on the lateral border of the toe but can also present medially. Clinically, the toenail may present thickened due to fungal infection, ingrown, dystrophic due to constant irritation from the position of the digit. As a result, it may require debridement in order to expose the nucleated skin lesion to relieve the significant source of pain.

2. A hyperkeratotic lesion on the distal medial tuft of the fifth digit due to friction between the head of the fifth distal phalanx and the head of the fourth proximal phalanx has been described as a heloma molle.[45] While the lesion may clinically present on both sides of the distal or PIPJs, it varies in location depending on the pathomechanics of the digits. Patient with the heloma molle commonly present with varus rotation of the fifth toe where there is slight underlapping of the fourth digit. As a result, the head of the proximal phalanx at the PIPJ of the fifth digit is compressed against the lateral condyle at the base of the proximal phalanx of the fourth digit.

3. Hyperkeratotic lesion present over the dorsal-lateral aspect of the fifth digit are commonly seen with flexion contracture, varus rotation, or a combination of both pathologies. These lesions are present on the dorsolateral aspect of the middle or proximal phalanx and is one of the more common lesion patterns seen involving the fifth digit.

4. Hyperkeratotic lesions present in the fourth interdigital space keratosis are commonly known as "kissing lesions," or soft corns. These lesions may be seen on the medial aspect of the proximal phalanx of the fifth digit and the lateral aspect of the proximal phalanx of the fourth digit. Clinically, these lesions are macerated in appearance.[46]

Surgical Procedures

The goals of surgical intervention to the fifth digit are to correct all planes of deformity, obtain near or complete anatomic alignment, alleviate pain, and maintain function of the toe when possible. A thorough preoperative assessment is paramount to ensure proper procedure selection. One must observe the clinical presentation of the toe, lesion patterns, and involved anatomic planes.

MEDIAL OR LATERAL DISTAL INTERPHALANGEAL CONDYLECTOMY

Painful and well-localized hyperkeratosis can occur on the fifth toe either within the lateral nail groove laterally or medially near the base of the proximal nail fold. These lesions typically overlie the prominent medial or lateral margins of the fifth distal interphalangeal joint or distal interphalangeal joint synostosis site. The lateral lesion, or Lister's corn, is often confused by patients as an ingrowing lateral fifth digital nail margin or a second fifth digital nail. Isolated exostoses, whether medial or lateral, in the absence of a digital deformity, can be resected through an incision that also excises the painful deep-seated hyperkeratosis. Any significant associated frontal plane varus rotational deformity of the fifth toe should be considered for correction by skin plasty combined with the exostosis resection. Lack of correction of any frontal plane varus rotation of the fifth toe can leave the surgical site and scar weight-bearing and potentially as painful postoperatively as the exostosis and pressure hyperkeratosis were preoperatively.

DISTAL PHALANGECTOMY

Painful pressure hyperkeratosis located medial and lateral over the margins of the fifth distal interphalangeal joint can be aggravated by a painful and dystrophic fifth digital nail. If the nail and pressure hyperkeratosis are symptomatic or if there is recurrence from previously failed fifth distal interphalangeal joint medial or lateral condylectomy, then distal phalangectomy of the fifth toe is a consideration. Fifth toe distal phalangectomy involves not only resection of the fifth distal phalanx through disarticulation at the distal interphalangeal joint or transection through the synostosis but also excision of the fifth digital nail and nail matrix. Any associated fifth digital nail problems or complaints can thus be surgically addressed simultaneously. Through this distal incision approach, the medial and lateral condyles on the distal aspect of the fifth middle phalanx can be reached and resected.

SUPPLEMENTAL SURGICAL PROCEDURES

DEROTATIONAL SKIN PLASTY

Frontal plane varus rotation can be addressed surgically by relaxation of soft tissues either through bone resection of the head of the fifth proximal phalanx or occasionally by excision of a wedge-shaped middle phalanx. Further reduction of the varus fifth toe positioning can be aided and reinforced by derotational skin plasty. Two converging semielliptical incisions are employed over the area of bone resection oriented on an axis to derotate the fifth toe in the plane desired with closure of the incisions. The skin can actually be gently pinched with forceps preoperatively to test various orientations for the wedge to aid placement. The axis of orientation of the incisions on the fifth toe is typically from proximal lateral to distal medial centered over the PIPJ dorsally to allow access for the bone resection. The more vertical the orientation of the two converging semielliptical incisions, the greater degree of abduction is possible on the transverse plane. The more horizontal the orientation of the incisions, the greater the degree of varus derotation is possible on the frontal plane. The incisions can be of a length as needed to effect correction and aid surgical access to deeper tissues. The skin wedge should not be more than 3-4 mm at the widest point. The excision of a skin wedge that is too wide may result in a toe that appears misshapen and constricted. Too small of a skin wedge may result in ineffective correction. The skin wedge is of controlled depth to the superficial fascia only. Deeper dissection through the superficial fascia is linear and respects neurovascular structures. Closure of all layers including skin is affected with the toe held in corrected position.

PLANTAR SKIN PLASTY

Few surgical techniques are available to aid plantarflexory alignment of the fifth toe. Resection of the head of the proximal phalanx is intended to weaken flexor contracture and can result in weakened purchase of the fifth toe to the floor. PIPJ arthrodesis of the fifth toe is typically avoided to maintain flexibility and aid comfort with shoe wear. Plantar skin plasty is an effective adjunctive procedure to aid fifth toe plantarflexory positioning. Unlike the remaining lesser toes, the fifth toe is suitable for this procedure due to the proximity of the pulp of the toe to the plantar forefoot. The skin of the plantar sulcus of the fifth toe is excised to include all contiguous skin from the pulp of the toe to the forefoot. The distal fifth toe skin incision can be drawn with a skin pencil then opposed and pressed into a corrected position leaving a mirror image mark proximally on the plantar forefoot. The entire wedge of skin thus marked is excised to the level of the superficial fascia much like taking a full thickness skin graft or syndactyly. Closure may be affected with horizontal mattress-type sutures to aid eversion of the skin margins laying all in place first then tying to allow ease of insertion. This procedure can be combined with other dorsal approach fifth toe surgeries as there is limited deep dissection to impact the plantar neurovascular structures of the toe.

SYNDACTYLY

Reconstructive procedures to stabilize the small joints of the fifth toe may be impractical. If the fourth toe is functional and stable, syndactyly can help transfer the stability of the fourth toe to the fifth toe. Syndactyly can be employed for painful proximal or distal fourth and fifth toe interdigital keratoses. The procedure involves excision of the interdigital fourth and fifth toe skin to the level of the superficial fascia. The dorsal incision is linear to the dorsal aspect of the toes, and the plantar incision is relatively angled to the first incision, respecting the curvature to the underside of the toes. The syndactyly incision extends proximally from the interdigital space to end distally limited by the length of the fifth toe. If the incision is ended short on the fifth toe, the contiguous skin at the tip of the toes can become macerated and difficult to clean.

1. The incision is drawn with a skin pencil on the fifth toe. The fourth and fifth digits are then compressed leaving a shadow mark on the fourth toe.
2. The skin wedge is excised to the level of the superficial fascia.
3. Closure is facilitated by placing all the sutures first then tying them once all are placed.

Z PLASTY AND V-Y SKIN PLASTY

Either a Z-plasty or a V-Y plasty can be employed to lengthen any associated dorsal skin contracture for the fifth toe. The skin plasty incisions are placed on the distal forefoot at the base of the fifth toe. The Z-plasty flaps are dissected full thickness to the deep fascia to preserve their blood supply. The Z-plasty is first drawn with the central arm of the incision along the line of contracture. The length of the central arm is determined not only by the amount of corrective length needed but also by the anticipated location of the proximal and distal arms of the Z. The length of the proximal and distal arms must be of the same length as the central arm just as the two connecting angles must be of the same degree. The longitudinal length of the Z-plasty increases with interposition of the flaps, at the expense of the transverse width decreasing. This associated constriction can be a problem impacting closure due to the limited mobility of tissues over the dorsal distal fifth metatarsal and fifth metatarsophalangeal joint area. The amount of length gained may or may not be sufficient. Once the incisions are placed, the degree of lengthening is fixed and cannot be adjusted for greater or lesser corrections. The exact amount of skin lengthening needed relative to the size of the Z-plasty is nearly impossible to determine preoperatively.

The V-Y plasty is a more versatile and easily applied procedure for release of fifth toe extensor contracture than Z-plasty. The initial V portion of the skin plasty is typically placed with the apex proximally and the legs ending medially and laterally toward the base of the fifth toe. The apex may be placed distally; however, the arms would need to end at the fifth metatarsophalangeal joint with the apex on the fifth toe itself making closure difficult with associated constriction of the toe. The triangular flap of skin is dissected full thickness to the deep fascia. Release of the extensor tendon and joint contracture can be affected through the V flap incision. With flexion of the fifth toe, the V flap should move with the toe and displace distally creating the proximal arm of the Y. Lengthening linearly of the skin occurs in a V-Y plasty just as a Z-plasty at the expense of transverse skin narrowing. The potential must exist for the skin to narrow to permit the skin to lengthen and the incision to close. Scarring or local anatomy considerations at the dorsal base of the fifth toe can prevent this skin movement from occurring obviating the desired effect of the skin plasty. Unlike a Z-plasty, the amount of correction can be adjusted in the V-Y plasty as needed.

MINIMAL INVASIVE SURGERY

Minimal invasive surgery, MIS, practice has increased in the use in its indications for foot surgery, especially to treat digital deformities (Fig. 8.36). These techniques offer a substitute to open procedures; however, it requires dedicated anatomical knowledge and instrumentation to reduce the learning curve and avoid failure.

EXTENSOR TENOTOMY

The procedure is performed at the level of the metatarsophalangeal joint where the EDL and brevis are separate tendons within the extensor hood. The portal to introduce the beaver blade is dorsal, at the level of the MTP joint; the percutaneous incision is parallel to the tendon to avoid soft tissue damages to the nerve and vessels (Fig. 8.37A). The beaver blade is then rotated 90 degrees (Fig. 8.37B) in order to perform the sectioning of the tendons (Fig. 8.37C). The surgeon should drive the toe into plantarflexion to feel and confirm the full tendon section (Fig. 8.38A and B). The procedure is confirmed by plantarflexion of the joint and if it is deemed insufficient for correction of the deformity, a dorsal transverse capsulotomy of the metatarsophalangeal joint can be added once confirmed by fluoroscopy with manual traction to distract the joint. It is preferred to maintain integrity of one of the extensor tendon to avoid poor functioning of the extensor mechanism.[47]

FLEXOR BREVIS AND LONGUS TENOTOMIES

Flexor tenotomies are performed for sagittal plane deformities at the middle and distal interphalangeal joint. The percutaneous stab incision is located on the plantar side,

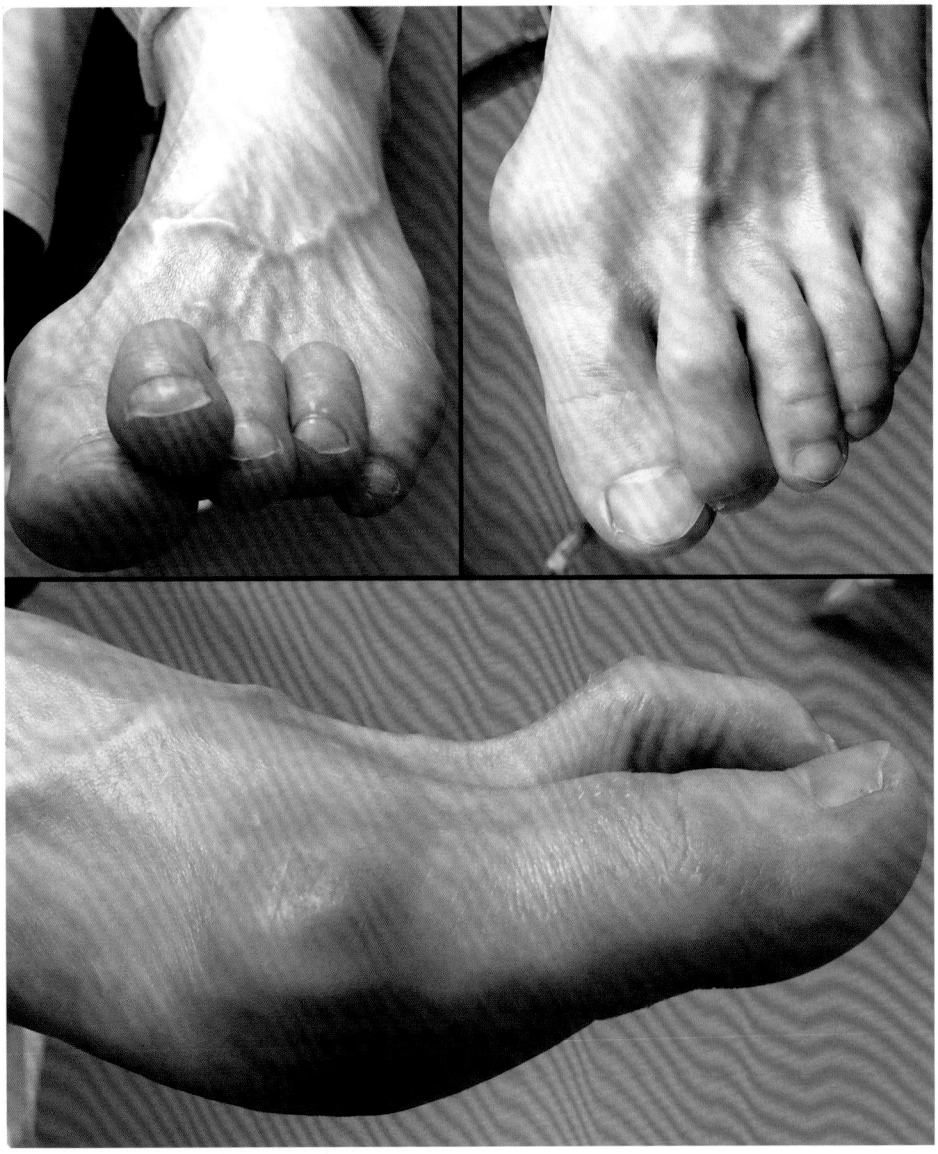

FIGURE 8.36 Multiplanar digital deformities.

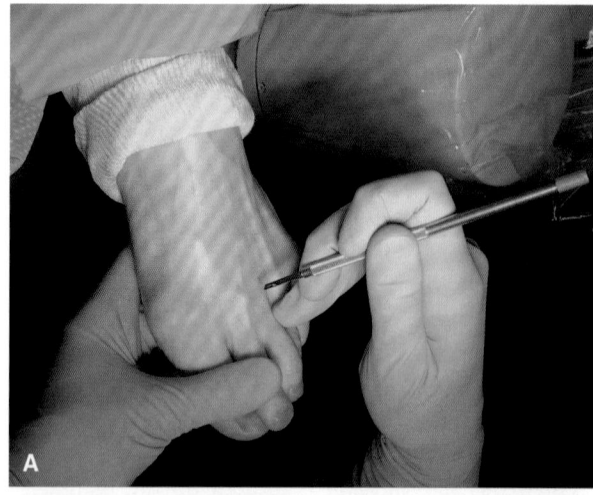

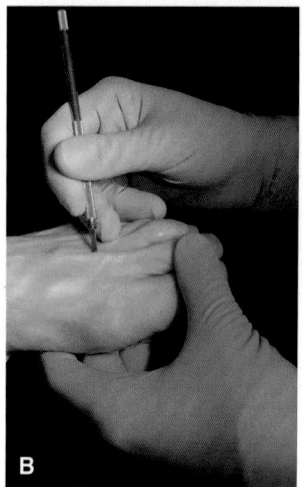
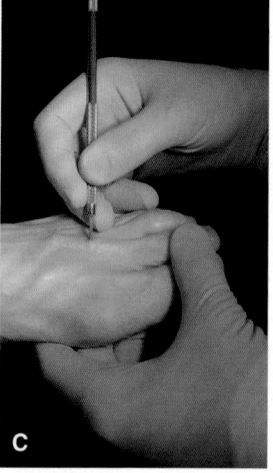

FIGURE 8.37 Stepwise approach to extensor tenotomy.
A. An incision parallel to the extensor tendon. **B.** Rotation of the beaver blade 90 degrees to the extensor tendon. **C.** Sectioning of the extensor tendon.

1 cm distal to metatarsophalangeal joint. The beaver blade is introduced parallel to the tendon (Fig. 8.39A) and rotated 90 degrees (Fig. 8.39B) as both of the tendons are sectioned by means of a lateral movement. Care is taken to avoid the neurovascular structures with the careful release of the tendons. It is helpful to drive the toe into dorsiflexion to put tension on the tendons, feel the cut, and check if both tendons are fully sectioned; however, it is important the toe is not forced in an erect position while performing the release to protect the neurovascular structures against traumatic injury.

FLEXOR DIGITORUM BREVIS TENOTOMY

The procedure is initiated at the level of the PIPJ of the digit. The beaver blade is introduced directly to the bone either on the medial or lateral aspect of the digit (Fig. 8.40A). This is done to protect the neurovascular bundle of the digit. With the toe in a plantarflexed position, a capsulotomy is done at the distal aspect of the proximal phalanx by rotating the blade 90 degrees (Fig. 8.40B). Once the capsulotomy is performed, the FDB is released from its insertion on the middle phalanx (Fig. 8.40C). The procedure may require small advancement of the beaver blade on the plantar surface of the middle phalanx to release any tendon attachments that maybe present. Once the FDB tenotomy is complete, the digit is dorsiflexed to confirm the entire release of the FDB tendon (Fig. 8.40D). The advantage of the FDB tenotomy, with or without a phalangeal osteotomy,[48] is to preserve passive and active plantar flexion while avoiding floating toe syndrome.

FLEXOR DIGITORUM LONGUS TENOTOMY

A selective flexor digitorum tenotomy can be performed by a distal plantar approach at the level of distal interphalangeal joint. The procedure can be utilized for flexible deformities at the distal interphalangeal joint. A beaver blade is

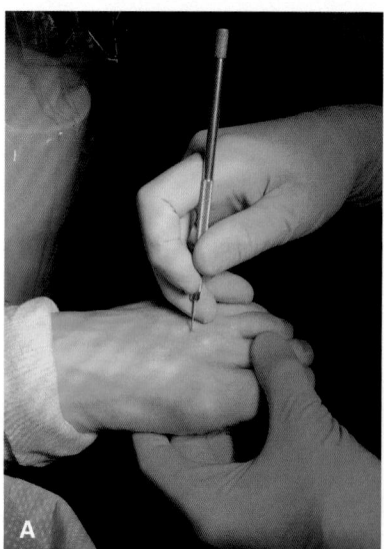
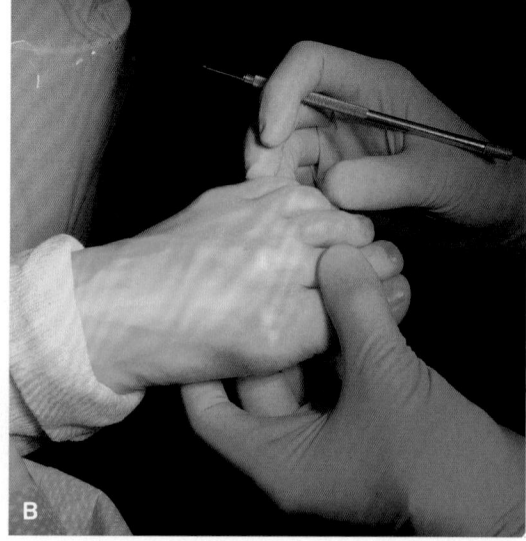

FIGURE 8.38 A. Sectioning of the extensor tendon with plantarflexion of the digit. **B.** Further plantarflexion of the digit to confirm release of the extensor tendon.

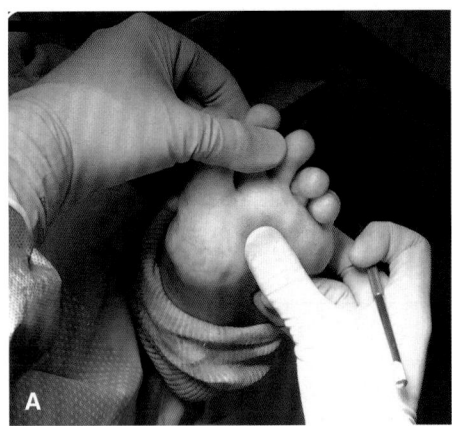
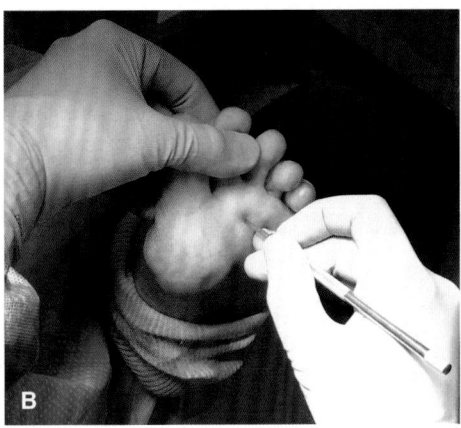

FIGURE 8.39 A. Identification of flexor tendons on dorsiflexion of the digit. **B.** Once the location is identified, a beaver blade is introduced parallel to the tendons and rotated 90 degrees as both of the tendons are sectioned by lateral movement of the tendon.

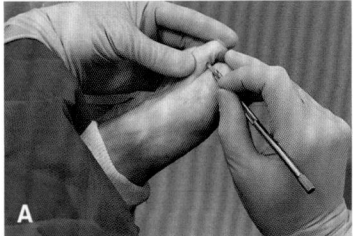
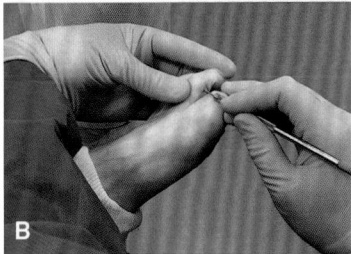
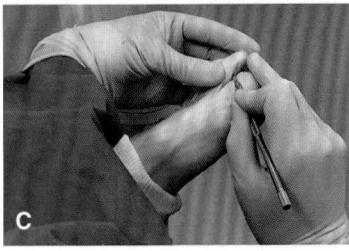
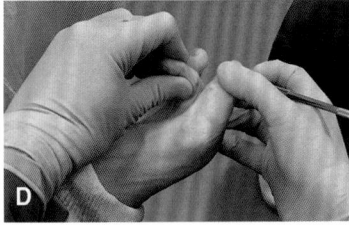

FIGURE 8.40 Stepwise approach for a flexor digitorum brevis tenotomy. **A.** Proximal interphalangeal joint capsulotomy is performed at the distal aspect of the proximal phalanx. **B.** Rotating the blade 90 degrees, the insertion of the flexor digitorum brevis is released from the base of the middle phalanx. **C.** Small advancement of the beaver blade on the plantar surface of the middle phalanx is performed for additional tendon release that may be present more distally. **D.** Once the flexor digitorum brevis tenotomy is complete, the procedure is confirmed by dorsiflexion of the digit.

introduced to the plantar aspect of the distal interphalangeal joint through a small stab incision. Once this is done, the beaver blade is rotated 90 degrees both medially and laterally to release the FDL tendon, while distal phalanx is dorsiflexion position. The success of the procedure is confirmed by dorsiflexion of the distal phalanx at the distal interphalangeal joint and can be maintained by steri-strips postoperatively.

PHALANGEAL OSTEOTOMY

Phalangeal osteotomies can be performed for multiple digital deformities, which soft tissue correction procedures are inadequate.

Historically, the portal for a proximal phalangeal osteotomy was the same as for the FDL tenotomy, distal to the plantar aspect of the metatarsophalangeal joint (Fig. 8.41A). A dedicated percutaneous burr (2 × 8 mm) is utilized and placed perpendicular to the proximal metaphysis-diaphysis junction of the proximal phalanx (Fig. 8.41B). It is important that the burr is placed medial or lateral to the flexor sheath so that it lies directly against the bone. Once this is confirmed under fluoroscopy, an osteotomy is performed on the plantar aspect of the proximal phalanx by rotating the burr from medial to lateral or vice versa. It is important when performing the osteotomy; the burr is kept at a low speed to prevent iatrogenic trauma to the skin, neurovascular structures, and/or tendon. A partial osteotomy can be performed by leaving the dorsal cortex intact or a complete osteotomy can be performed depending on the correction needed with plantarflexion of the osteotomy (Fig. 8.41D). Alternatively, the procedure can be performed with a dorsal incision for varus and valgus deformity of the proximal phalanx. Once the proximal metaphyseal-diaphyseal junction of the proximal phalanx has been identified under fluoroscopy, the burr can be used to create an osteotomy in the direction (medial or lateral) necessary to correct the deformity with the opposite cortex left intact.

While technically more challenging, the same principles can also be applied for middle phalangeal osteotomies. Other less frequently used procedures can also be performed like arthrolysis, condylectomy, arthrodesis, and arthroplasty through the same portal.

The postoperative bandaging is an important part of the surgical procedure and is confirmed under fluoroscopy, to maintain correction obtained from the operation.

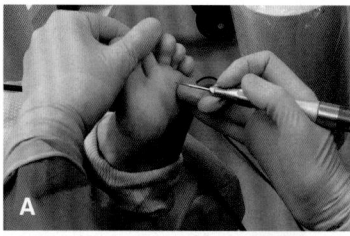
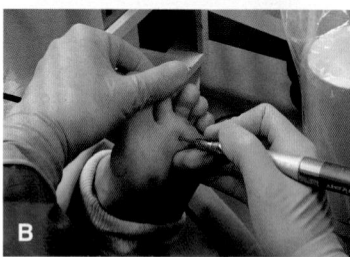
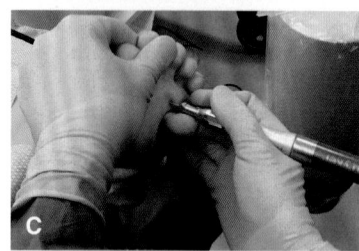
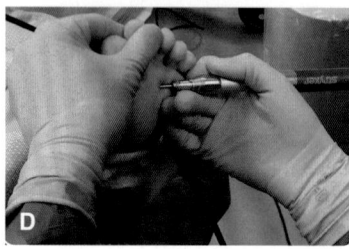

FIGURE 8.41 Stepwise approach to a proximal phalanx osteotomy. **A.** Plantar aspect of the proximal phalanx is identified. **B.** Percutaneous burr is perpendicular to the proximal metaphysis-diaphysis junction of proximal phalanx. **C.** With burr at low speed, an osteotomy is performed. **D.** After osteotomy is performed, dorsiflexion of the phalanx is performed for correction of the deformity.

SURGICAL PEARLS OF MINIMAL INVASIVE SURGERY

- MIS procedures require respect for anatomy and special instrumentation.
- An extensor tenotomy should be done with the digit in plantarflexion to feel and confirm the full tendon section. Performing the procedure at the metatarsophalangeal joint will maintain the extensor hood connection to the proximal part of the tendon allowing for some dorsiflexion function to be preserved.
- When performing flexor tenotomies, the toe should be in a dorsiflexed position to put tension on the flexor tendons.
- One disadvantage of a flexor digitorum longus/brevis tenotomy is that it can lead to loss of purchase of the digit postoperatively.
- Phalangeal osteotomies can be performed through medial, lateral, or plantar approaches.
- Phalangeal osteotomies can be partial or complete.

COMPLICATIONS

Digital surgery can be very challenging procedures that can lead to long-term edema of the toe along with reoccurrence of the condition. Loss of a digit can also occur secondary to vascular compromise during the procedure. The patient can also have stiffness of the digits after an arthroplasty procedure or a fibrous nonunion after an arthrodesis procedure which can lead to a prolonged recovery

PERILS and PITFALLS

- Prolonged digital edema
- Reoccurrence of the deformity
- Loss of a digit secondary to vascular compromise during the procedure
- Stiffness of the digits after an arthroplasty procedure
- Fibrous nonunion after an arthrodesis procedure
- Recurrence of condition due to inadequate correction of the deformity

REFERENCES

1. McGlamry ED, Jimenez AL, Green DR. Lesser ray deformities. In: Banks AS, Downey MS, Martin DE, et al., eds. *McGlamry's Comprehensive Textbook of Foot and Ankle Surgery.* 3rd ed. Philadelphia, PA: Lippincott Williams & Wilkins; 2001:253-304.
2. Morris JL. Biomechanical implications of hammertoe deformities. *Clin Podiatr Med Surg.* 1986;3:339-346.
3. Shirzad K, Kiesau CD, DeOrio JK, Parekh SG. Lesser toe deformities. *J Acad Orthop Surg.* 2011;19:505-514.
4. Dalmau-Pastor M, Fargues B, Alcolea E, et al. Extensor apparatus of the lesser toes: anatomy with clinical implications—topical review. *Foot Ankle Int.* 2014;35(10):957-969.
5. Sarrafian SK, Topouzian LK. Anatomy and physiology of the extensor apparatus of the toes. *J Bone Joint Surg Am.* 1969;51(4):669-679.
6. Haynes Lovell AG, Tanner HH. Synovial membranes, with special reference to those related to the tendons of the foot and ankle. *J Anat Physiol.* 1908;42(Pt 4):415-432.
7. Doyle JR. Anatomy of the finger flexor tendon sheath and pulley system. *J Hand Surg Am.* 1988;13(4):473-484.
8. Martin MG, Masear VR. Triggering of the lesser toes at a previously undescribed distal pulley system. *Foot Ankle Int.* 1998;19(2):113-117.
9. Kosinski C. The course, mutual relations and distribution of the cutaneous nerves of the metazonal region of leg and foot. *J Anat.* 1926;60(Pt 3):274-297.
10. Kelikian H. Deformities of the lesser toes. In: *Hallux Valgus, Allied Deformities of the Forefoot and Metatarsalgia.* Philadelphia, PA: W.B. Saunders Co; 1965:282–336.
11. McGlamry ED, Jimenez AL, Green DR. Deformities of the intermediate digits and the metatarsophalangeal joint. In: *McGlamry's Comprehensive Textbook of Foot and Ankle Surgery.* 3rd ed. Philadelphia, PA: Lippincott Williams & Wilkins; 2001;1:253-304.
12. Mann R, Inman VT. Phasic activity of intrinsic muscles of the foot. *J Bone Joint Surg Am.* 1964;46(3):469-481.
13. Root MC, Orien WP, Weed JH. *Normal and Abnormal Function of the Foot: Clinical Biomechanics.* Vol. 2. Los Angeles, CA: Clinical Biomechanics Corp.; 1977.
14. Jarret BA, Manzi JA, Green DR. Interossei and lumbrical muscles of the foot an anatomical and functional study. *J Am Podiatry Assoc.* 1980;70:143.
15. Whitney AK, Green DR. Pseudoequinus. *J Am Podiatry Assoc.* 1982;72:365-371.
16. Sung W, Weil L Jr, Weil LS Sr, et al. Diagnosis of plantar plate injury by magnetic resonance imaging with reference to intraoperative findings. *J Foot Ankle Surg.* 2012;51:570-574.
17. Yu GV, et al. Predislocation syndrome. Progressive subluxation/dislocation of the lesser metatarsophalangeal joint. *J Am Podiatr Med Assoc.* 2002;92(4):182-199.
18. Gregg JM, Schneider T, Marks P. MR imaging and ultrasound of metatarsalgia-the lesser metatarsals. *Radiol Clin North Am.* 2008;46:1061-1078.
19. Carlson RM, Dux K, Stuck RM. Ultrasound imaging for diagnosis of plantar plate ruptures of the lesser metatarsophalangeal joints: a retrospective case series. *J Foot Ankle Surg.* 2013;52:786-788.
20. Kier R, et al. MR arthrography of the second and third metatarsophalangeal joints for the detection of tears of the plantar plate and joint capsule. *Am J Roentgenol.* 2010;194(4):1079-1081.
21. Trepman E, Yeo SJ. Nonoperative treatment of metatarsophalangeal joint synovitis. *Foot Ankle Int.* 1995;16(12):771-777.
22. Coughlin MJ. Crossover second toe deformity. *Foot Ankle.* 1987;8(1):29-39.
23. Coughlin MJ. Second metatarsophalangeal joint instability in the athlete. *Foot Ankle.* 1993;14(6):309-319.
24. Jimenez AL, McGlamry ED, Green DR. Lesser ray deformities. In: McGlamry ED, ed. *Comprehensive Textbook of Foot Surgery.* 1st ed. Baltimore, MD: Lippincott Williams & Wilkins; 1987:71-73.
25. Boberg J, Willis JL. Digital deformities: etiology, procedural selection and arthroplasty (Chap. 13). In: Banks AS, Downey MS, Martin DE, eds. *McGlamry's Forefoot Surgery.* Philadelphia, PA: Wolters Kluwer Health; 2015.

26. Malay DS, Hillstrom H, Stanifer EG, Lefkowitz, LR. The influence of digital stabilization on lesser metatarsalgia. DiNapoli DR. ed. In: *Reconstructive Surgery of The Foot And Leg, Update 1990*. Doctors Hospital Podiatric Education and Research Institute; 1990:50-51.

27. McGlamry ED, Jimenez AL, Green DR. Lesser ray deformities. Part I: deformities of the intermediate digits and the metatarsophalangeal joint. In: Banks AS, Downey MS, Martin DE, Miller SJ, eds. *McGlamry's Comprehensive Textbook of Foot and Ankle Surgery*. 3rd ed. Philadelphia, PA: Lippincott Williams & Wilkins; 2001:253-304.

28. Angirasa AK, Augoyard M, Coughlin MJ, Fridman R, Ruch J, Weil L Jr. Hammer toe, mallet toe, and claw toe (roundtable discussion). *Foot Ankle Spec*. 2011;4(3):182-187.

29. Hofbauer MH, Shane AM. Lesser digital surgery: arthroplasty, arthrodesis, and flexor tendon transfer. In: Chang TJ, ed. *Master Techniques in Podiatric Surgery: The Foot and Ankle*. Philadelphia, PA: Lippincott Williams & Wilkins; 2005:35-47.

30. Butterworth M. Proximal interphalangeal joint arthrodesis via Kirschner wire fixation. In: Cook EA, Cook JJ, eds. *Hammertoes: A Case Based Approach*. Switzerland: Springer Nature Switzerland AG; 2019:85-101.

31. Ellington K, Anderson RB, Davis WH, Cohen BE, Jones CP. Radiographic analysis of proximal interphalangeal joint arthrodesis with an intramedullary fusion device for lesser toe deformities. *Foot Ankle Int*. 2010;31(5):372-376.

32. Cook JJ, Cook EA. Proximal interphalangeal joint (PIPJ) arthrodesis with a polyetheretherketone (PEEK) implant. In: Cook E, Cook J, eds. *Hammertoes: A Case Based Approach*. Springer Nature Switzerland AG. 2019:141-148.

33. Konkel KF, Menger AG, Retzlaff SA. Hammer toe correction using an absorbable intramedullary pin. *Foot Ankle Int*. 2007;28(8):916-920.

34. Pietrzak WS, Lessek TP, Perns SV. A bioabsorbable fixation implant for use in proximal interphalangeal joint (hammer toe) arthrodesis: biomechanical testing in a synthetic bone substrate. *J Foot Ankle Surg*. 2006;45(5):288-294.

35. Shaw AH, Alvarez G. The use of digital implants for the correction of hammer toe deformity and their potential complications and management. *J Foot Surg*. 1992;31(1):63-74.

36. Rivera MA, Chang TJ. PIPJ arthrodesis with a thermal-activated metallic implant. In: Cook E, Cook J, eds. *Hammertoes: A Case Based Approach*. Springer Nature Switzerland AG. 2019:115-128.

37. Miller SJ. Hammer toe correction by arthrodesis of the proximal interphalangeal joint using a cortical bone allograft pin. *J Am Podiatr Med Assoc*. 2002;92:563-569.

38. Konkel KF, et al. Hammertoe correction using an absorbable pin. *Foot Ankle Int*. 2011;32(10):973-978.

39. Caterini R, Farsetti P, Tarantino U, Potenza V, Ippolito E. Arthrodesis of the toe joints with an intramedullary cannulated screw for correction of hammertoe deformity. *Foot Ankle Int*. 2004;25(4):256-261.

40. Isham S, Nunez O. Isham hammertoe procedures for the correction of lesser digital deformities. In: Maffuli N, Easly M, eds. *Minimally Invasive Surgery of the Foot and Ankle*. London/Dordrecht/Heidelberg/New York: Springer; 2011:171-183.

41. Kearney TP, Hunt NA, Lavery LA. Safety and effectiveness of flexor tenotomies to heal toe ulcers in persons with diabetes. *Diabetes Res Clin Pract*. 2010;89:224-226.

42. Thompson FM, Change UK. The two-boned fifth toe: clinical implications. *Foot Ankle Int*. 1995;16:34-36.

43. Durlacher L. *A Treatise on Corns, Bunions, the Diseases of Nails, and the General Management of the Feet*. London: Simpkin, Marshall and Co; 1845:196.

44. Alder DC, Fishco WD, Ruch JA. Surgical treatment of Lister's corn. A case illustration. *J Am Podiatr Med Assoc*. 1998;88(1):30-33.

45. Gillett HG, du P. Webbing corn incidence and etiology. *Chiropodist*. 1971;26:403-418.

46. Coughlin MJ, Kennedy MP. Operative repair of fourth and fifth toe corns. *Foot Ankle Int*. 2003;24(2):147-157.

47. Redfern DJ, Vernois J. Percutaneous surgery for metatarsalgia and the lesser toes. *Foot Ankle Clin*. 2016;21:527-550.

48. Frey S, Hélix-Giordanino M, Piclet-Legré B. Percutaneous correction of second toe proximal deformity: proximal interphalangeal release, flexor digitorum brevis tenotomy and proximal phalanx osteotomy. *Orthop Traumatol Surg Res*. 2015;101(6):753-758.

CHAPTER 9

Lesser Rays

William D. Fishco

DEFINITION

Metatarsalgia is an all inclusive diagnostic term for pain in the submetatarsal region of the foot.[1] For the purposes of this chapter, the focus will be for the condition of pain under the metatarsal head(s) due to plantar pressures and to address tailor's bunion deformity. Lesser metatarsal surgery is typically performed to address metatarsalgia related to high plantar pressures when nonoperative treatments fail to adequately resolve pain.

ANATOMIC FEATURES AND FUNCTIONAL ANALYSIS

Central metatarsal surgery is typically performed to "adjust" the height or length of a metatarsal head that is causing pain due to pressure overload. It is important to remember that the central metatarsal conditions have mechanical influences that contribute to pathology such as ankle equinus, instability of the medial column, hallux valgus, and hammer toes. The 5th metatarsal is generally associated with more of a structural problem of the metatarsal bone. A tailor's bunion typically has lateral bowing or a wide metatarsal head leading to a lateral and/or plantar lateral prominence of bone. Typically, a higher arched foot or one that oversupinates has trouble under the 5th metatarsal head.

PHYSICAL EXAMINATION

History and physical examination can determine the etiology of the pain and treatment can be initiated based upon those findings. When a patient presents with "pain in the ball of the foot," the physical examination includes a complete radiographic examination, palpation and range of motion examination of the metatarsophalangeal joints, anterior drawer test of the metatarsophalangeal joints, palpation/squeeze test into the intermetatarsal spaces, and a dermatologic examination to assess for associated keratoses. In the elderly, diminished plantar fat pad under the metatarsals may be a factor.

The common clinical findings associated with metatarsalgia that should be evaluated for include ankle equinus and hammer toes,[2] hallux valgus deformity with first ray insufficiency,[3-5] and acute inflammatory joints.

When there is pain and/or crepitation with range of motion to a lesser metatarsophalangeal joint, then an inflammatory or degenerative joint condition such as rheumatoid arthritis, Freiberg infraction, or an acute synovitis/capsulitis should be considered. Pain with plantar flexion of the digit and pain with palpation of the plantar plate is consistent with an acute synovitis/capsulitis, which can lead to hammer toe or dislocation deformity. This condition has also been referred to as predislocation syndrome.[6] Morton neuroma should be considered when there is pain and clicking noted with palpation and squeezing into the interspace between the metatarsals.

DIAGNOSTIC IMAGING

The commonly accepted "normal" metatarsal length pattern or parabola is $II \geq I > III > IV > V$.[7] Just how much metatarsal length variation is acceptable and what the length pattern should be is still very much a debate.[8] A relatively long 2nd metatarsal is still considered to be a leading causation of metatarsalgia and hammer toe development of the 2nd toe.[9] A complete set of radiographs is necessary to determine whether there is any structural deformity. An anteroposterior radiograph is helpful in determining the metatarsal parabola. An oblique view will assess sagittal plane abnormalities of the central metatarsals and lateral bowing of the 5th metatarsal (Fig. 9.1). The lateral view and sesamoid axial view will allow visualization of sagittal plane positions of the metatarsal heads (Fig. 9.2). Radiographs will also rule out arthritic conditions.

TREATMENT

Treatment

- Designed to resolve high peak pressures causing pain under the metatarsal head

Nonsurgical treatment includes wearing stiff soled shoes with orthotics to reduce high peak plantar pressures to the painful metatarsal head(s). Debridement of any associated hyperkeratotic lesions help reduce pressure. In older patients with fat pad atrophy, cushioned liners with shock absorbing properties can be used.

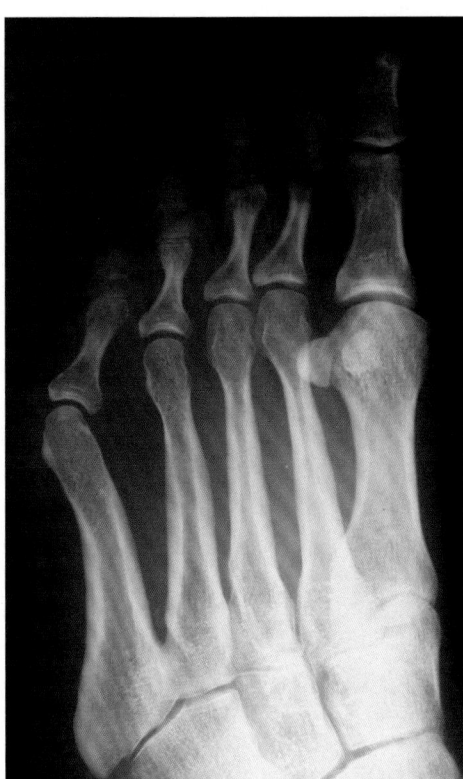

FIGURE 9.1 Oblique view illustrating lateral bowing of the 5th metatarsal.

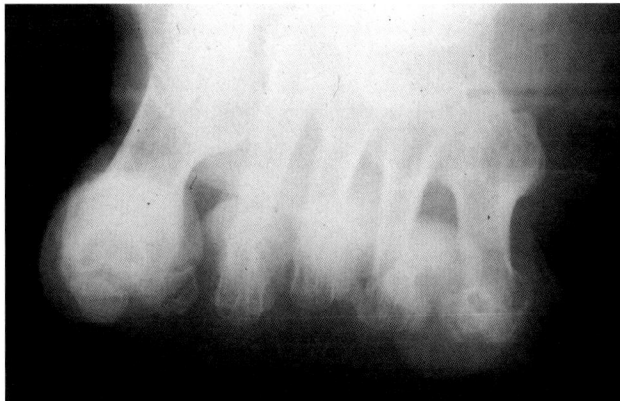

FIGURE 9.2 Sagittal plane abnormalities can be seen on and axial view. Note elevated 3rd metatarsal.

When surgery is performed to address metatarsalgia, the end goal is to resolve high peak plantar pressure areas, which would lead to pain and dysfunction. There is a combination of four surgical approaches that are typically used, which includes removal of bone, which can be done with a plantar condylectomy or partial/complete metatarsal head resection, shortening/lengthening a metatarsal, raising/lowering a metatarsal head (sagittal plane correction), or medial/lateral translocation (transverse plane correction), which is typically performed when repairing a concomitant transverse plane hammer toe deformity or tailor's bunion deformity.

Surgery of the 5th metatarsal is typically performed for a tailor's bunion. The techniques used typically involve shaving of the lateral bony prominence (exostectomy) and/or osteotomy to move the metatarsal medially and/or dorsally depending on the location of pain.

Metatarsal osteotomies can be performed in the neck, midshaft, or base of the bone. The majority of surgery is performed at the metatarsal neck due to the typical need of minor adjustments of height and/or length, ease of dissection/osteotomy/fixation, and proximity to the digit (which often times is also addressed). Moreover, healing potential is greatest in metaphyseal bone (Figs. 9.3 through 9.5). When larger amounts of correction are needed, then a midshaft osteotomy or base osteotomy is recommended. A midshaft sagittal Z osteotomy is ideal for metatarsals requiring greater amounts of shortening that can be obtained with a distal metatarsal osteotomy or if lengthening of the bone is required (Fig. 9.6A and B). For large amounts of sagittal plane correction, a dorsiflexion or plantarflexion osteotomy of the metatarsal base is recommended as the proximal location leads to greater correction with minimal bone wedging (Fig. 9.7A and B). Osteotomies placed in the metatarsal base have a longer radius arm. The more proximal the osteotomy, the longer the lever arm will be and thus allow for larger amounts of correction. In the cavus foot, for example, a dorsiflexory base osteotomy is often used.

The most common metatarsal osteotomies of the metatarsal head/neck include the Weil osteotomy, a "V" osteotomy, and an oblique osteotomy that can be used as a "tilt-up" or through and through osteotomy with a single or double cut (Figs. 9.8 through 9.10). Certainly any osteotomy that can afford repositioning of bone to the desired location that is amenable for

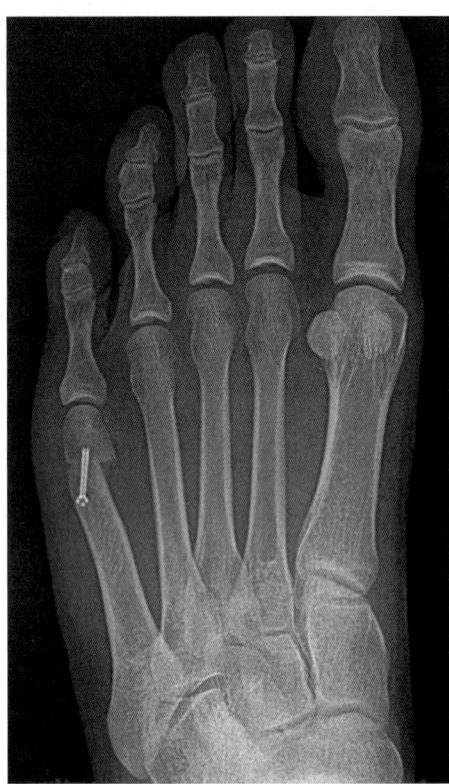

FIGURE 9.3 Traditional chevron osteotomy.

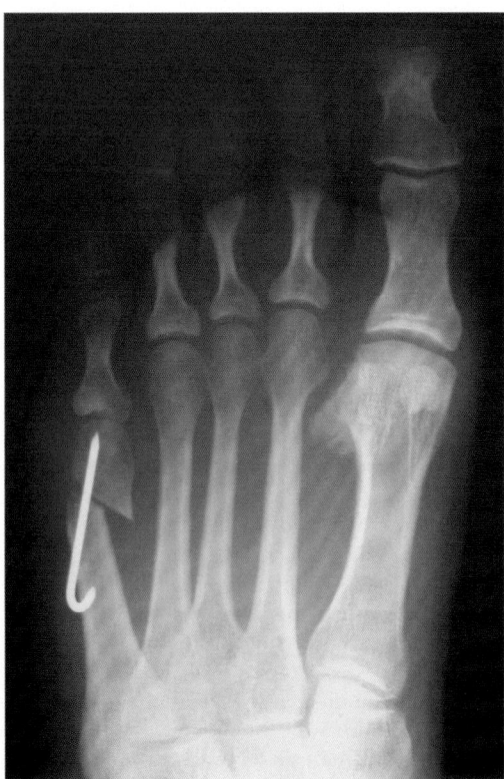

FIGURE 9.4 Oblique osteotomy is simple and effective in reducing the deformity.

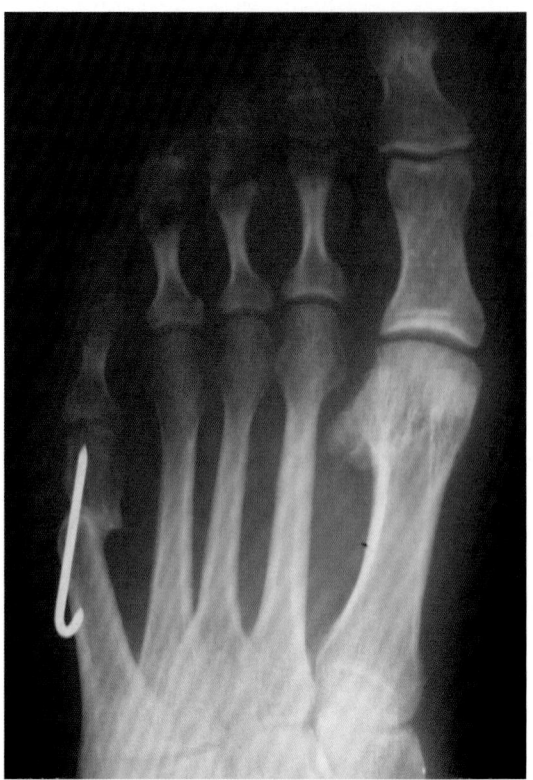

FIGURE 9.5 Healed osteotomy

internal fixation is acceptable. Fixation of a "V" osteotomy can be difficult and as a result has fallen out of favor. One can modify the osteotomy with unequal arms of the chevron to make it easier to fixate (Fig. 9.11). In addition, small plates and screws can be used for traditional chevron osteotomies.[10] With the advent of small superelastic memory staples, a transverse osteotomy can be simple and easy to fixate (Fig. 9.12).

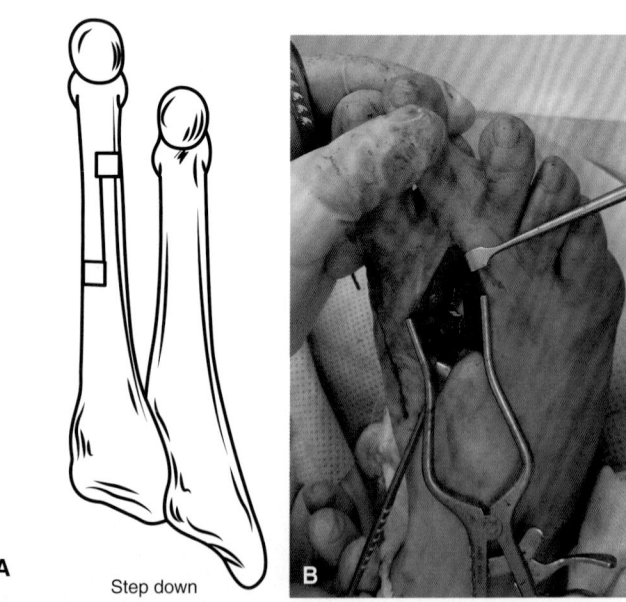

FIGURE 9.6 A. Diagram illustrating a "step-down" sagittal Z osteotomy. **B.** Intraoperative view of a sagittal Z osteotomy in a patient with iatrogenic deformities requiring more shortening than could be obtained with a distal metatarsal osteotomy.

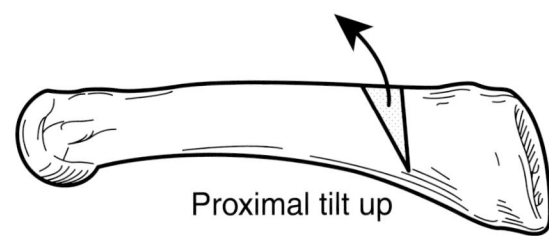

Proximal tilt up

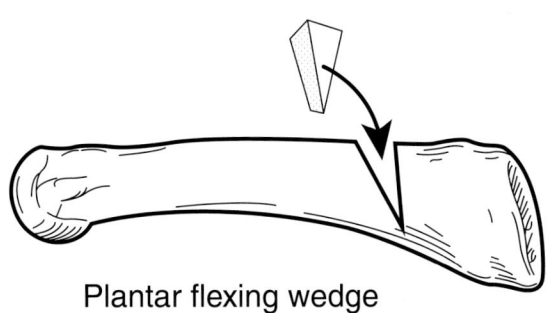

Plantar flexing wedge

FIGURE 9.7 A. Diagram illustrating a dorsiflexing base wedge osteotomy. **B.** Diagram illustrating a plantarflexing base wedge osteotomy using a bone graft.

DISSECTION TECHNIQUE

Surgical exposure for lesser metatarsal surgery includes a mid-line linear skin incision over the affected ray from the base of the phalanx to the metatarsal neck and shaft. Depending on which procedure is being performed will dictate how long the incision should be and whether the metatarsopha-

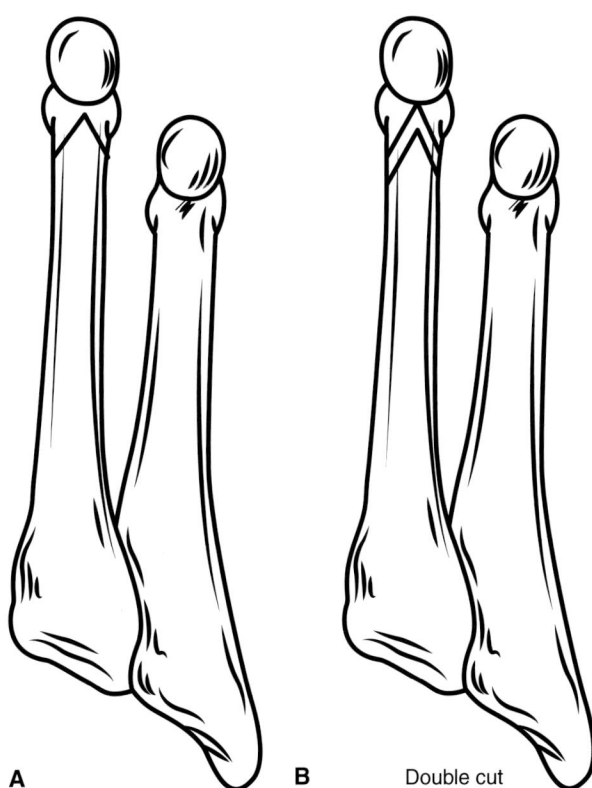

A   B   Double cut

FIGURE 9.8 A, B. Diagram illustrating a chevron osteotomy to adjust the height of a metatarsal or a double cut for more shortening.

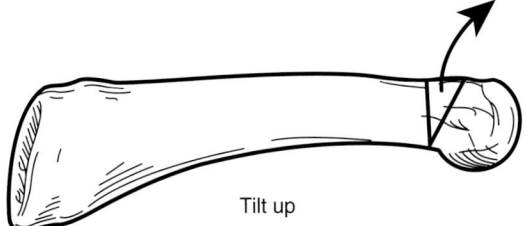

Tilt up

FIGURE 9.9 Diagram illustrating a "tilt up" oblique osteotomy.

langeal joint needs to be opened. When performing a condylectomy, the dissection starts more distally on the toe and ends just proximal to the metatarsophalangeal joint. For extra-articular distal metatarsal osteotomies, the dissection can start just proximal to the metatarsophalangeal joint. If an intra-articular osteotomy, such as a Weil osteotomy is going to be performed, then the incision will need to encompass the base of the toe and extend to the metatarsal neck. Once the skin incision is made, the subcutaneous tissues are dissected and separated from the long extensor tendon. A moist gauze sponge is useful in clearing away the fatty tissue off of the extensor tendon apparatus. The tendon can be reflected by releasing the hood fibers on lateral side and retracting the tendon medially or vice versa. This will expose the joint capsule and periosteum. A transverse capsulotomy of the metatarsophalangeal joint is performed followed by a linear incision on the periosteum of the metatarsal neck. This will have the appearance of a "T." The periosteum is reflected medially and laterally for exposure of the bone and is now ready for the osteotomy. Use intraoperative fluoroscopy to ensure proper amount of correction is obtained (Fig. 9.13). Alternative approaches for the tendon include splitting the tendon in the midline and retract medially and laterally, or finally one can do a z-plasty of the tendon and repair after the bone work is done. For basilar osteotomies, the dissection starts more proximal in midshaft area of the metatarsal and carried toward the base of the bone.

Plantar condylectomies are considered when there is not a significant deformity of the metatarsal, yet there is chronic pain, keratosis, and/or skin breakdown under the metatarsal head (Fig. 9.14). Condylectomies are ideal for patients with osteopenic bone or if they are not good candidates for an osteotomy and internal fixation.

PEARLS

CENTRAL METATARSAL OSTEOTOMIES
- Use flouroscopy to confirm metatarsal positioning to avoid over shortening.
- Aggressive postoperative ROM of toes helps prevent stiff joints.
- Bandaging toes in excessive plantarflexion and splinting in this position for the first few weeks help prevent floating toes.
- Consider concomitant hammer toe repair when shortening a metatarsal as a digital deformity may worsen or develop due to loss of intrinsic stability of the toe.

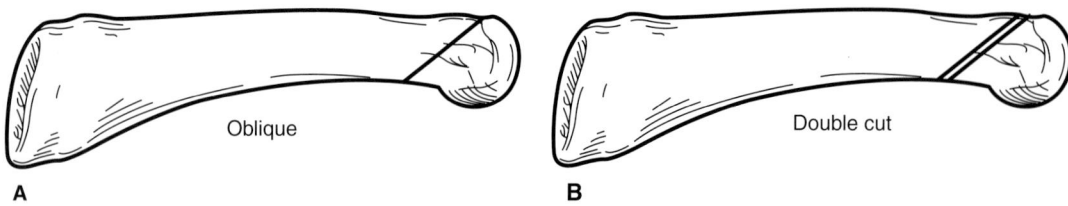

FIGURE 9.10 A, B. Diagram illustrating a single cut oblique osteotomy and a double cut for more shortening.

TAILOR'S BUNION

Tailor's bunion, also known as a bunionette, is a common cause of pain to the lateral or plantar lateral 5th metatarsal head. Radiographic findings associated with tailor's bunions include a large intermetatarsal angle between the 4th and 5th metatarsals, lateral bowing of the 5th metatarsal, and/or a large dumbbell-shaped metatarsal head[11] (Fig. 9.15).

Surgical techniques to address a tailor's bunion include lateral condylectomy, distal neck, midshaft, basilar osteotomies, and on rare occasions a 5th metatarsal head resection.

Lateral condylectomies are selected when there is pain to the lateral aspect of the 5th metatarsal head without any significant radiographic evidence of intermetatarsal splaying or lateral bowing. There may be a wide metatarsal head or prominent lateral condyle. Approximately ⅓ of the lateral metatarsal can be resected with a power saw or osteotome.

Fifth metatarsal head resections are rarely performed due to inherent complications. The notable exceptions may be in geriatric patients with osteoporosis, a very large deformity, or in a patient with a neurotrophic ulceration on the lateral or plantar aspect of the 5th metatarsal head. Potential problems that occur with a metatarsal head resection include a retracted/flail 5th toe, transfer metatarsalgia, and in rare cases can trigger Charcot arthropathy in neuropathic patients.[12]

Distal metatarsal osteotomies are most commonly performed for tailor's bunion correction just as in central metatarsal osteotomies for same reasons. Various osteotomy designs have been described and used without a clear advantage of one over another. A chevron osteotomy with or without a long dorsal or plantar arm, oblique osteotomies, closing wedge osteotomies, and transverse osteotomies are used (Fig. 9.16). After the osteotomy is complete, a shift of no more than half of the width of the metatarsal head should be performed to avoid instability.

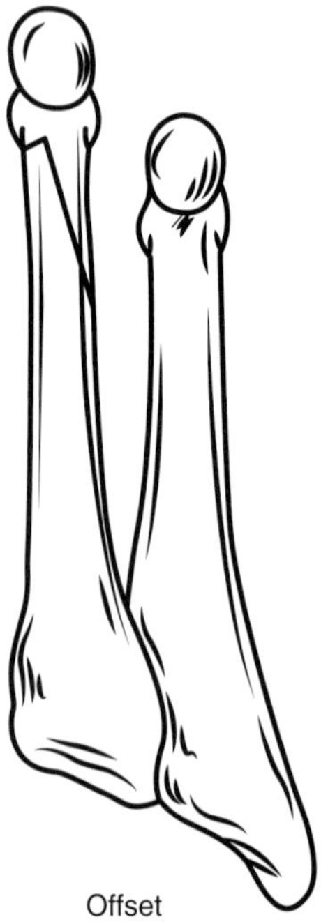

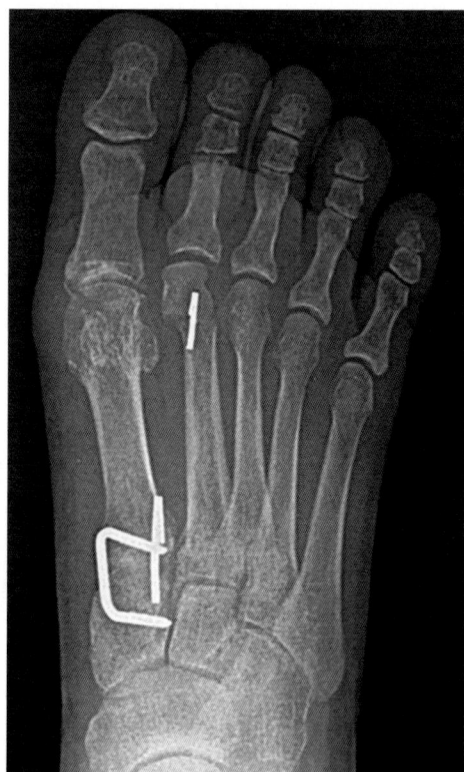

FIGURE 9.12 A transverse osteotomy with superelastic staple may be ideal for minimal shortening and transverse plane correction. This patient had a large hallux valgus deformity with a medially deviated 2nd toe.

FIGURE 9.11 Diagram illustrating an offset chevron osteotomy, which may be easier to fixate than a traditional chevron osteotomy.

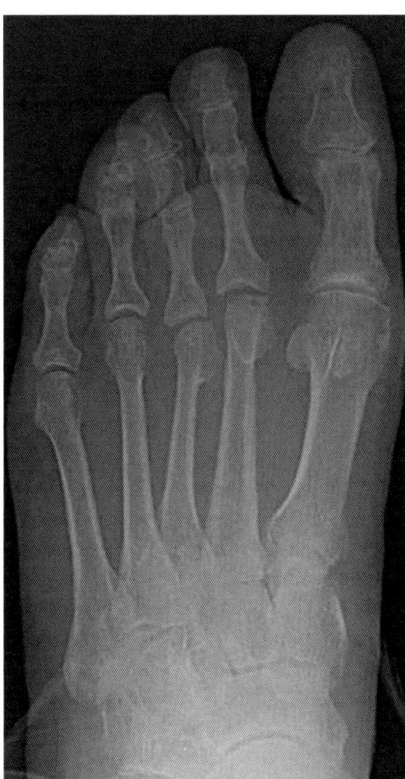

FIGURE 9.13 Over shortening of the 3rd metatarsal could have been avoided with the use of intraoperative fluoroscopy.

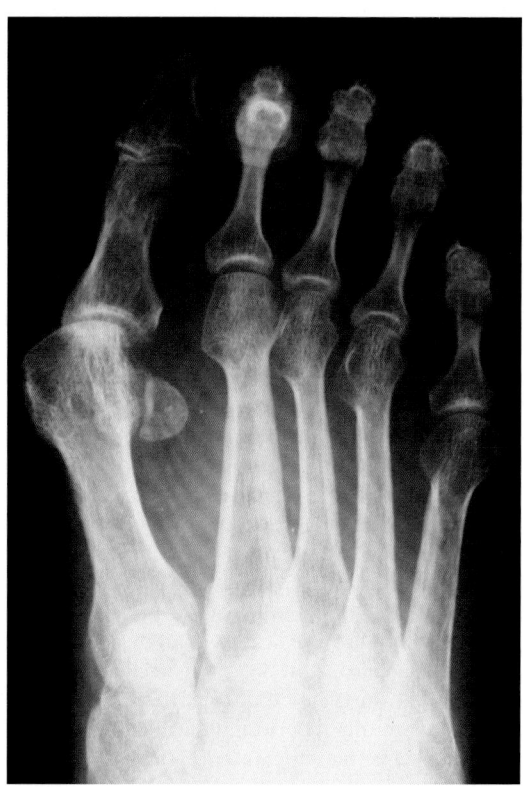

FIGURE 9.15 Note dumbbell-shaped 5th metatarsal in a patient with a bunion and tailor's bunion.

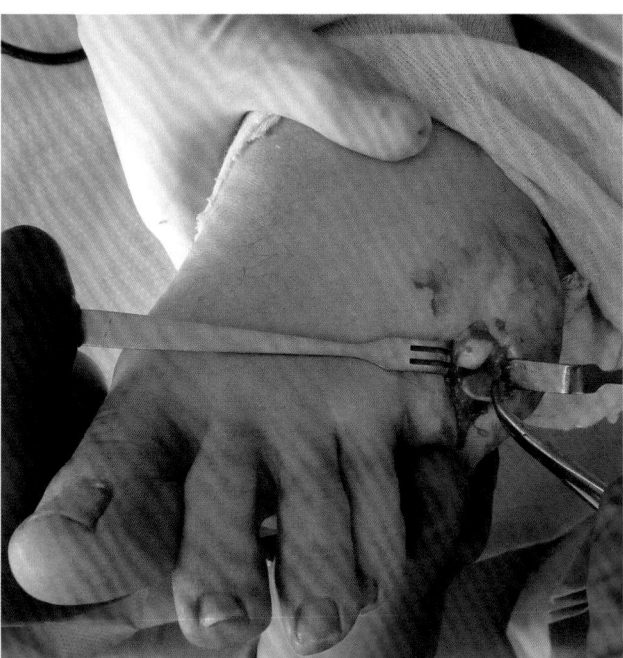

FIGURE 9.14 Intraoperative view of a condylectomy of the 5th metatarsal for a patient having sub 5 pain without any significant metatarsal deformity.

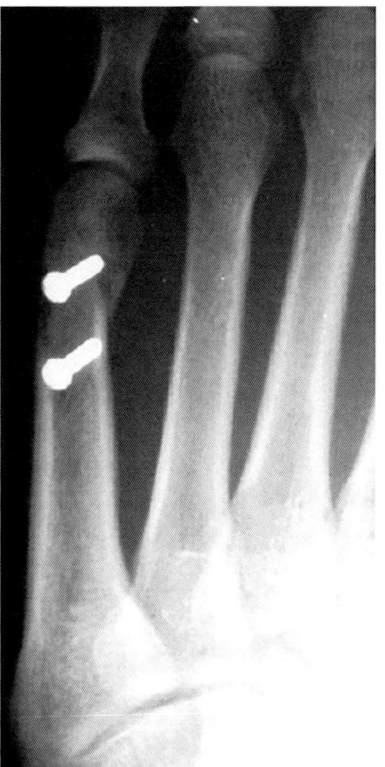

FIGURE 9.16 Postoperative x-ray of a tailor's bunion repaired with a chevron osteotomy with a long plantar arm fixated with 2.0-mm cortical screws. This is a very stable construct.

For large deformities or in cases where there has already been surgery such as a lateral condylectomy, midshaft or proximal osteotomy is considered. The most common midshaft osteotomy is a SCARF design. Basilar osteotomies typically include a closing wedge osteotomy with a lateral apex and hinge.

SURGICAL TECHNIQUE

A skin incision is made overlying the 5th metatarsal and extended to the base of the 5th toe. The incision should be just lateral to the extensor tendon. The subcutaneous tissues are reflected away from the extensor tendon and hood apparatus. The periosteum of the 5th metatarsal is incised. Use forceps to palpate the bone, this will avoid slipping off the side of the bone where there is intrinsic muscle. As the periosteum is incised lateral to the extensor tendon, it is extended to the base of the proximal phalanx. Now the joint is visualized. The 5th toe can be distracted and that will lead to puckering of the lateral capsule, which will leave a pouch to the lateral side of the joint where the scalpel blade can be inserted to detach the capsule from the lateral aspect of the metatarsal head. Depending on the type of osteotomy to be performed will determine how much periosteum will need to be reflected for bone access. The lateral eminence can be removed with a sagittal saw or osteotome. Avoid removing too much bone as you will only be able to move the metatarsal head ⅓ to ½ of the width of the head. The desired osteotomy can now be performed (Fig. 9.17A–E). An alternative method involves removing the eminence and overhang of bone after the osteotomy is made and fixated so that there is more metatarsal head available for shifting.

PEARLS

TAILOR'S BUNIONECTOMY

- A traditional chevron osteotomy can be difficult to fixate. Modifying the osteotomy with a long plantar arm allows for easier and more stable fixation with two 2.0-mm cortical screws.
- Do not medially translocate the metatarsal head more than half the width of the metatarsal head.
- When performing a distal metatarsal osteotomy, do not remove too much of the lateral eminence so that you have greater ability to shift the head.
- Avoid plantar and lateral condylectomy as this will weaken the bone.
- Avoid basilar osteotomies unless the deformity cannot be fixed with a distal osteotomy.
- Use caution with 5th metatarsal head resections. In the cavovarus foot type, a new lesion will occur at the stump of the metatarsal. In neuropathic patients, it may trigger a Charcot event.

POSTOPERATIVE CARE

Distal metatarsal osteotomies can be managed with weight bearing to tolerance in a fracture boot or surgical shoe. Base wedge osteotomies will require 4-6 weeks of non–weight bearing followed by protected weight bearing in a fracture boot for an additional 2-4 weeks based upon radiographic signs of bone healing. Stiff and floating toes are common with these procedures; therefore, aggressive range of motion exercises of toes, bandaging toes in plantar flexion, and the use of splints after surgery can help mitigate those problems.

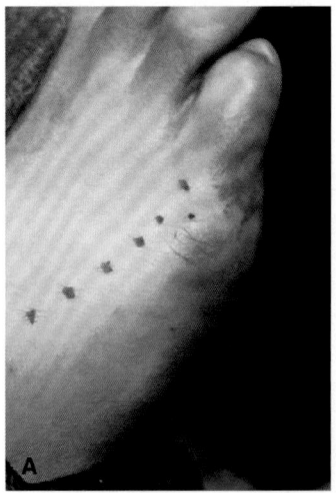
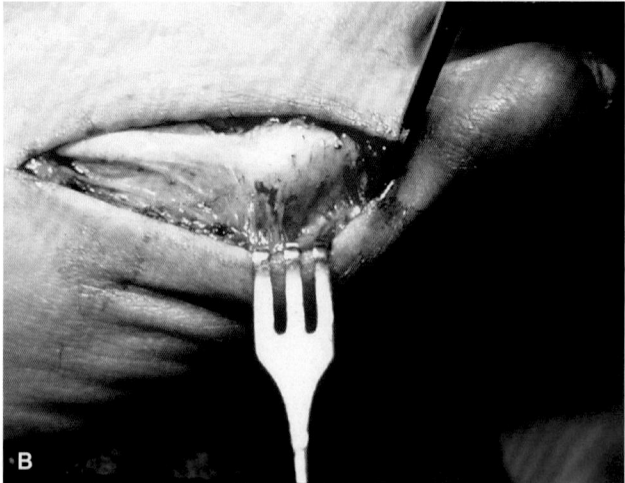

FIGURE 9.17 A. Skin incision is dorsolateral from the base of the 5th toe to the metatarsal shaft. **B.** The subcutaneous tissues are dissected off of the joint capsule and extensor tendon apparatus.

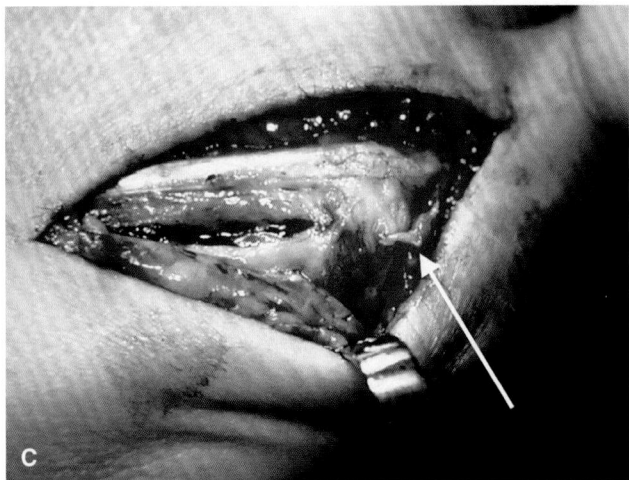

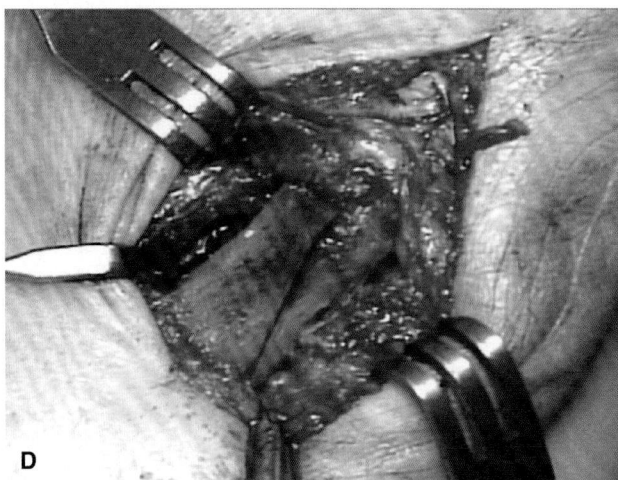

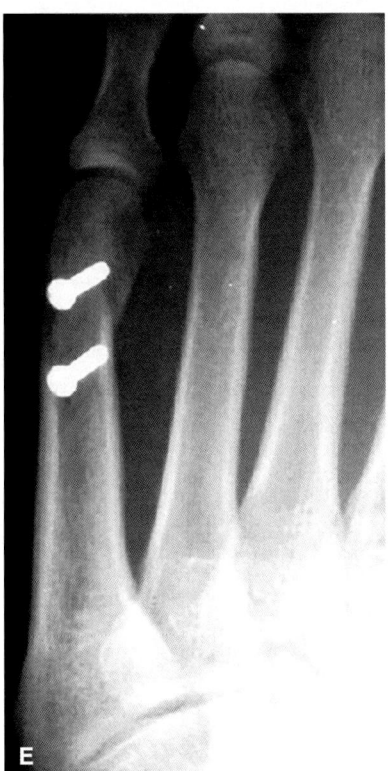

FIGURE 9.17 (*Continued*) **C.** The periosteum is incised from the metatarsal shaft and then the capsule is incised to visualize the joint. When the 5th toe is pulled/distracted, the lateral capsule will pucker and a scalpel can be inserted in the pocket to detach the lateral capsule (*arrow*). **D.** A long plantar arm osteotomy. **E.** Healed osteotomy with cortical screws.

REFERENCES

1. Schuh R, Trnka HJ. Metatarsalgia: distal metatarsal osteotomies. *Foot Ankle Clin.* 2011;16(4):583-595.
2. Searle A, Spink MJ, Ho A, et al. Association between ankle equinus and plantar pressures in people with diabetes. A systematic review and meta-analysis. *Clin Biomech (Bristol, Avon).* 2017;43:8-14.
3. Greisberg J, Prince D, Sperber L. First ray mobility increase in patients with metatarsalgia. *Foot Ankle Int.* 2010;31(11):954-958.
4. Walker AK, Harris TG. The role of first ray insufficiency in the development of metatarsalgia. *Foot Ankle Clin.* 2019;24(4):641-648.
5. Lopez V, Slullitel G. Metatarsalgia: assessment algorithm and decision making. *Foot Ankle Clin.* 2019;24(4):561-569.
6. Yu GV, Judge MS, Hudson JR, et al. Predislocation syndrome. Progressive subluxation/dislocation of the lesser metatarsophalangeal joint. *J Am Podiatr Med Assoc.* 2002;92(4):182-199.
7. Barrôco R, Nery C, Favero G, et al. Evaluation of metatarsal relationships in the biomechanics of 332 normal feet using the method of measuring relative lengths. *Rev Bras Ortop.* 2011;46(4):431-438.
8. Stoupine A, Singh BN. A cadaveric study of metatarsal length and its function in the metatarsal formula and forefoot pathology. *J Am Podiatr Med Assoc.* 2018;108(3):194-199.
9. Fleischer AE, Hshieh S, Crews RT, et al. Association between second metatarsal length and forefoot loading under the second metatarsophalangeal joint. *Foot Ankle Int.* 2018;39(5):560-567.
10. Herzog JL, Goforth WD, Paden MH. A modified fixation technique for a decompressional shortening osteotomy: a retrospective analysis. *J Foot Ankle Surg.* 2014;53(2):131-136.
11. Coughlin MJ. Treatment of bunionette deformity with longitudinal diaphyseal osteotomy with distal soft tissue repair. *Foot Ankle.* 1991;11(4):195-203.
12. Fishco WD. Surgically induced Charcot's foot. *J Am Podiatr Med Assoc.* 2001;91(8):388-393.

CHAPTER 10

Distal Metatarsal Osteotomies in Hallux Abducto Valgus Surgery

Navita Khatri, Chandler J. Ligas, Shayla A. Robinson, Joshua J. Mann, Thomas A. Brosky II, and Patrick B. Hall

INTRODUCTION

Hallux abducto valgus deformity (HAV), a bunion, is one of the most common surgical problems encountered by foot and ankle surgeons. The first metatarsal deviates medially and the hallux deviates laterally into a pronated position. The cause of them are multifactorial but can be attributed to both extrinsic and intrinsic factors including genetic predisposition, footwear, and biomechanics. Incidence has been reported between 23.0% and 35.7%.[1] HAV can be mild, moderate, or severe and cause an array of symptoms (Figs. 10.1 and 10.2). Over 100 procedures have been described to correct HAV deformities, each patient needs to be considered individually to determine the appropriate procedure. The goal of any HAV procedure is to restore the correct alignment of the hallux and the congruity of the first metatarsophalangeal joint.

INDICATIONS

Distal metatarsal osteotomies (DMOs), when performed under the right indications, are very successful in treating HAV deformities. There are several factors to consider when evaluating a patient with HAV deformity both clinically and radiographically. Both non–weight-bearing and weight-bearing examinations should be performed. The range of motion of the first metatarsophalangeal and first metatarsocuneiform joints should be assessed to determine the flexibility and severity of the deformity. Other foot deformities should also be noted and addressed as necessary. Radiographically, the intermetatarsal angle (IMA) is one factor to help determine the appropriate surgical procedure. DMOs have been indicated for mild to moderate HAV deformities with an IMA of up to 15 degrees. However, reports have shown that distal procedures can correct larger angular deformities, and distal osteotomies can provide multiplanar correction depending on the type of osteotomy performed. Sesamoid alignment and first metatarsophalangeal joint congruity also need to be assessed on preoperative radiographs.

There are several details to be considered when performing distal metaphyseal osteotomies in HAV that will lead to surgical success. These details will be covered in this chapter. Percutaneous, or minimally invasive bunion techniques are currently evolving, so the focus of this chapter will be to discuss the most commonly performed open distal metaphyseal osteotomies for the correction of HAV deformities.

SURGICAL PROCEDURES AND TECHNIQUES

Positioning PEARLS

- Patient to be positioned in a supine position on a radiolucent table.
- A well-padded tourniquet can be applied to the ankle or mid-calf according to surgeon's preference. The author prefers to perform the procedure without tourniquet and utilize local anesthetic with epinephrine (unless contraindicated).
- Place a bump under the ipsilateral hip to decrease external rotation of the limb.
- Surgical assistant is on the side of the operative foot, and surgeon is at the foot of the bed with the surgical table placed in slight reverse trendelenburg.

APICAL AXIS GUIDE

When performing a distal metaphyseal osteotomy of the first metatarsal to correct a hallux valgus deformity, the axis guide is critical in performing a quality and reproducible osteotomy. An apical axis guide is a technique, which uses a Kirschner wire (K-wire) to allow for visualization and provide directional control of the osteotomy. The placement of this K-wire can help to correct the deformity in the sagittal plane and transverse plane and to allow for any shortening/lengthening that is needed (Fig. 10.3A and B). The principles of placing the guide needs to be understood to help achieve the proper correction. Plantarflexion of the capital fragment is commonly performed and can effectively restore the weight-bearing function of the first metatarsal. In addition, it can cause relaxation of the periarticular soft tissues.[2]

Typically, a 0.045-in smooth K-wire is used as the axis guide. Once the axis guide is inserted, the saw blade is aligned parallel to the guide in order to execute a well-fitting, stable osteotomy.

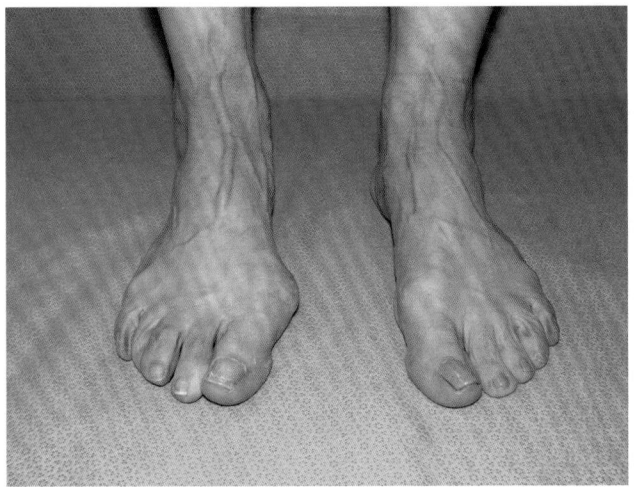

FIGURE 10.1 Clinical weight-bearing photograph showing mild HAV deformity.

Deviation from the axis guide may result in an incomplete osteotomy, converging bone cuts that impede lateral translation, or stress risers that result in fracture of the osteotomy.

AUSTIN (CHEVRON) BUNIONECTOMY

Traditional Austin

The Austin or distal chevron bunionectomy was first performed in 1962. It was a horizontally directed "V" displacement osteotomy.[3] In 1981, Austin and Leventen published their description of the distal V-shaped osteotomy in the distal head of the first metatarsal.[4] The goal of this osteotomy was to restore the alignment of the first MPJ, correct the hallux valgus, and correct the metatarsus primus varus while maintaining osteotomy stability and allowing early ambulation.[3] Since then, there have

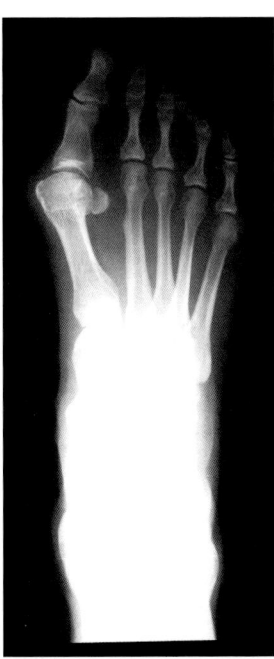

FIGURE 10.2 DP view of a mild, moderate, and severe HAV deformity.

been many modifications to this osteotomy. The Austin remains a popular choice because of its stability and relative ease of performance. In 2001, Shaw and colleagues published their study in which they compared the mechanical strength between the offset V, inverted Z, Mau, and Ludloff osteotomy groups.[5] They concluded that one could expect a safer, immediate return to weight-bearing postoperatively with the offset V osteotomy when compared with other osteotomies. In 2016, Choi and colleagues compared the modified McBride procedure and the distal chevron osteotomy for treatment of moderate hallux valgus.[6] They concluded that the chevron group experienced significantly greater correction in hallux valgus and IMA, had improvement in AOFAS scores, and had a lower incidence of recurrence.

OSTEOTOMY SITE PREPARATION

The resection of the prominent dorsomedial eminence of the first metatarsal head will be performed after a sufficient lateral release of the contracted soft tissues of the first metatarsophalangeal joint and first metatarsophalangeal joint capsulotomy is completed.

It is important to maintain the dorsal and plantar synovial folds of the first metatarsophalangeal joint capsule. A freer or elevator is very useful to reflect the periosteum of the first metatarsal head. The resection of the prominent dorsomedial eminence can be accomplished utilizing a power saw or osteotome, and initially is performed to create a flat surface for the osteotomy (Fig. 10.4). It is important to maintain the sagittal groove of the first metatarsal head, a further contouring of the first metatarsal head will be performed after the osteotomy is performed and the correction is achieved. The apical axis guide is then inserted. Traditionally, this was placed centrally in the metatarsal head. However, placing the axis guide slightly superior to the midpoint of the head will increase the surface and strength of the weight-bearing portion and provide a greater area for fixation of the osteotomy (Figs. 10.5 and 10.6). Placement of the axis guide too proximal will place the osteotomy in diaphyseal bone, and placement too distal may result in an intra-articular fracture. Satisfactory dissection of capsular tissues and good retraction are critical to enable accurate evaluation of this surface for axis guide placement. Retractors will be placed dorsal lateral and plantar medial to provide visualization for the osteotomy and protect the soft tissues. The exit site for the plantar arm of the osteotomy is determined by the proximal extent of the synovial fold.[7]

OSTEOTOMY AND FIXATION TECHNIQUE

The osteotomy may be performed with either a sagittal or oscillating saw, and the saw blade needs to be in perfect alignment with the guide wire. It is also important to consider the orientation of fixation to be used prior to making the osteotomy, and the angle between the dorsal and plantar segments is ~60 degrees (Fig. 10.7). The plantar arm must avoid the sesamoid articulation.

Following completion of the osteotomy, the hallux is distracted distally, and a lateral force is then applied on the capital fragment to place it in the corrected position (Fig. 10.8). Once adequate correction is achieved, a slight impaction of the capital fragment will seat the osteotomy. Temporary fixation with a 0.045-in smooth K-wire is then placed. The temporary K-wire is

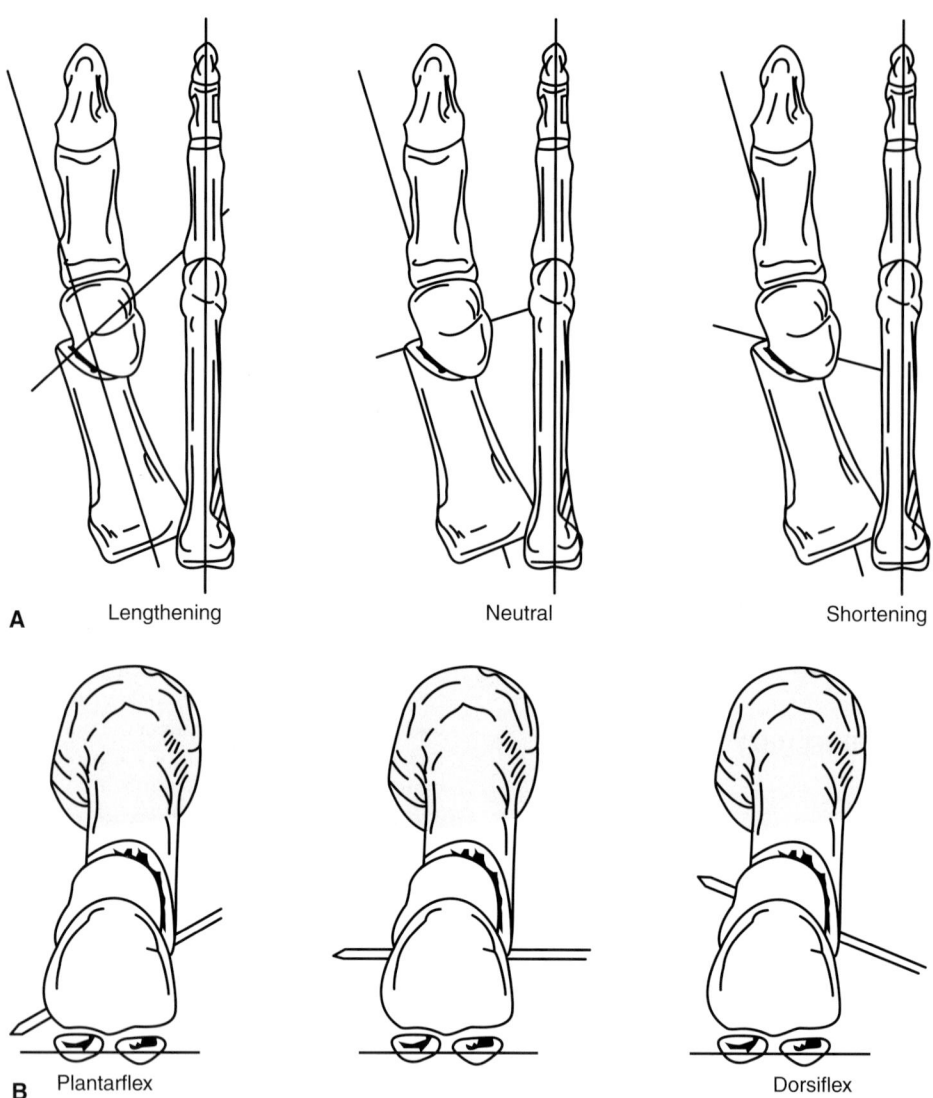

A   Lengthening   Neutral   Shortening

B   Plantarflex   Dorsiflex

FIGURE 10.3 A. Transverse plane orientation of the K-wire as an apical axis guide. When the wire is directed proximally, the capital fragment will shorten. If maintenance of length is desired, then the wire is directed perpendicular to the long axis of the 1st metatarsal. And when the wire is directed distally, it will lengthen. **B.** Frontal plane orientation demonstrates the ability of the axis guide to direct dorsiflexion, plantarflexion, or maintenance of position.

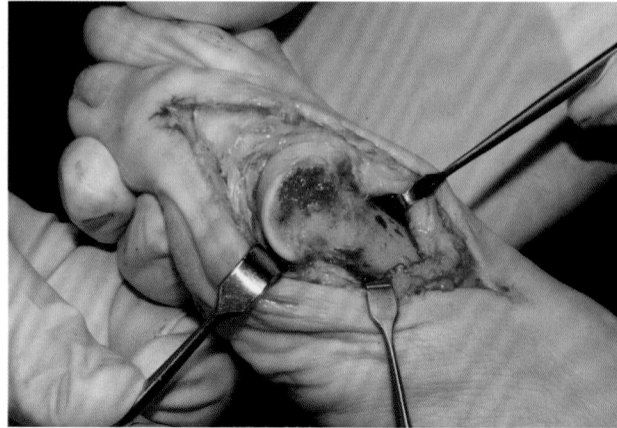

FIGURE 10.4 Intraoperative image of the 1st metatarsal head following resection of medial eminence tissue.

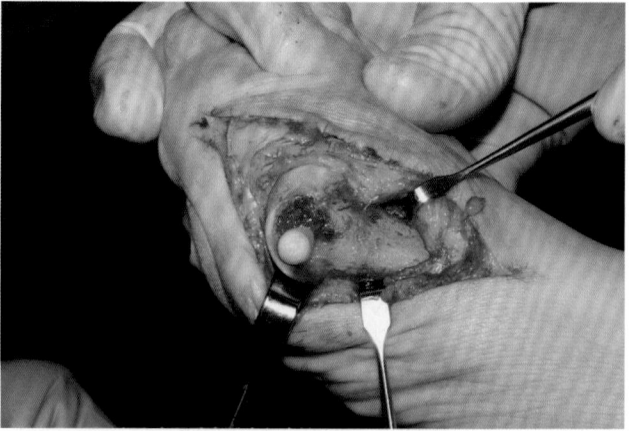

FIGURE 10.5 Position of the axis guide from a medial view. Notice: the wire is centered from proximal to distal and slightly superior to midline from dorsal to plantar.

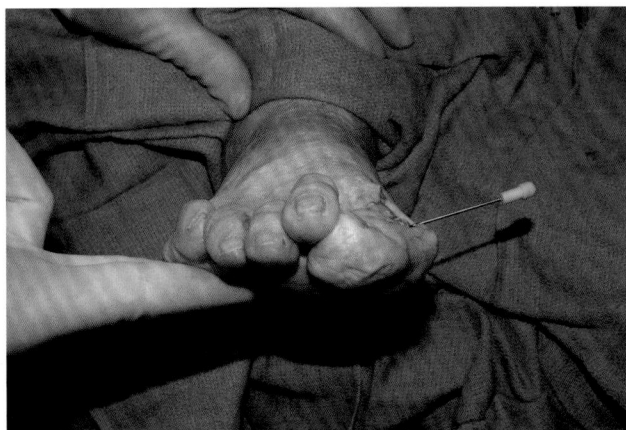

FIGURE 10.6 Position of the axis guide from an anterior to posterior view. Notice: slight plantarflexion of the capital fragment will be achieved.

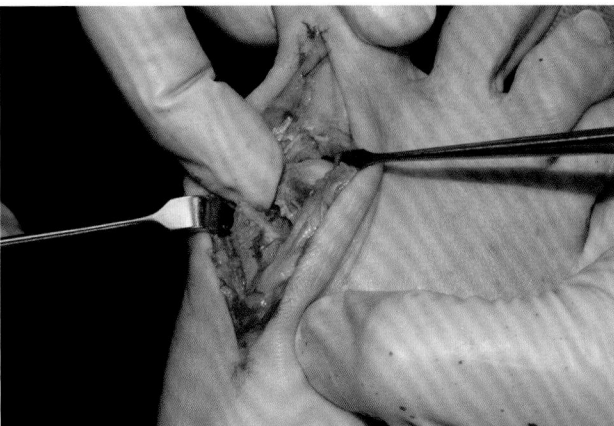

FIGURE 10.8 A gentle distraction force on the hallux will allow easy lateral translocation of the capital fragment.

placed with consideration for avoiding the permanent fixative device (Fig. 10.9). To confirm appropriate positioning of the osteotomy, intraoperative fluoroscopy is utilized to visualize the sesamoid position and first metatarsophalangeal joint congruity. The first metatarsophalangeal joint range of motion is also assessed.

FIXATION OPTIONS

The original Austin did not use fixation. Though the osteotomy is intrinsically stable, there can still be rotation and/or displacement of the capital fragment, which is why fixation is used today. There are a number of fixation options for the Austin osteotomy. These include smooth K-wires in a "locked" fashion (Fig. 10.10A and B), threaded K-wires, cortical and cancellous screws ranging from 2.0- to 4.0-mm (Fig. 10.11), both cannulated and noncannulated screws, as well as traditional and headless designs (Fig. 10.12). Screw fixation has shown the greatest strength of construct experimentally.[7] An axial loading screw in conjunction with a dorsally placed compression screw can also be used.[8] T plate fixation has also been described for decompression, shortening metatarsal osteotomies.[9] One study by Andrews and colleagues compared screw vs plate fixation for the osteotomy.[10] Neither fixation proved to be "better" than

the other, but perhaps a locking plate with an interfragmentary screw can be considered an option for patients with osteoporotic and cystic bone. Ultimately choice of fixation is dependent on the bone quality, surgeon preference, and patient allergies.

Placement of Screw Fixation

A 0.062-in smooth K-wire is first inserted as a predrill. The orientation of the K-wire should be perpendicular to the plantar arm of the osteotomy, and it will be aimed toward the cristae between the sesamoid articular surfaces. The direction of the K-wire is from proximal-dorsal-medial to distal-plantar-lateral (Fig. 10.13). After insertion of the guide, the position and exit site should be inspected, to ensure adequate purchase of the plantar segment (Fig. 10.14).

After this, the pilot hole is then created with the "under" drill. The size of this drill bit is dependent upon the screw size and manufacturer being used. Its diameter corresponds to the core diameter of the screw (Fig. 10.15). The countersink is then used to help seat the screw head and prevent stress risers (Fig. 10.16).[11] When using a fully-threaded screw, the "lag by technique" principle can be applied. This is accomplished by

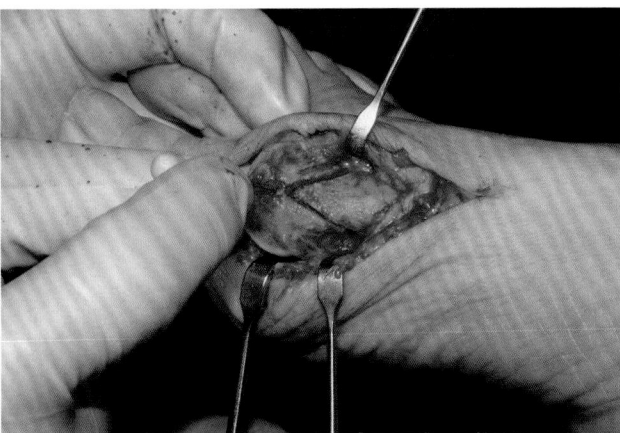

FIGURE 10.7 Completed Austin osteotomy, with the angle being ~60 degrees.

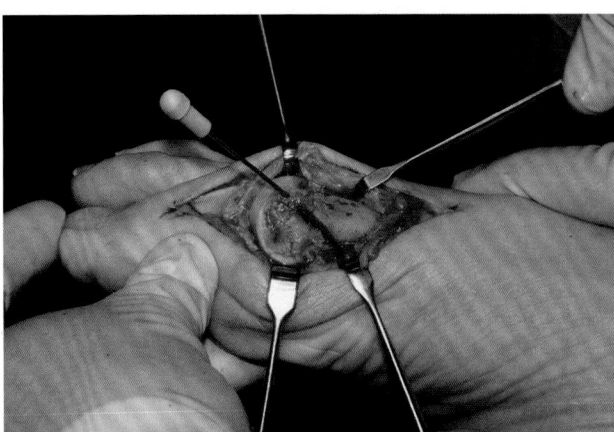

FIGURE 10.9 Temporary fixation of the osteotomy with a 0.045-in K-wire maintains the position of translocation, allowing the surgeon to focus on the permanent fixative without losing correction. Care should be taken to place the temporary wire away from the designated path of the permanent device.

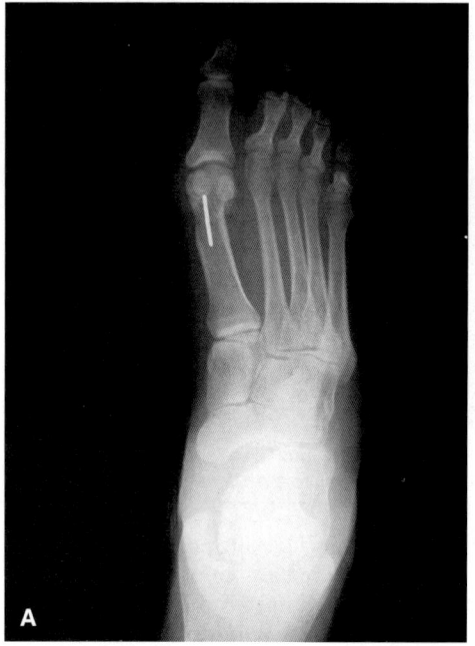
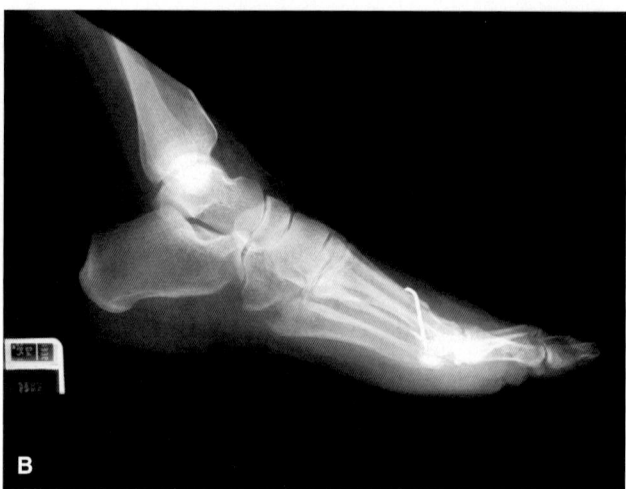

FIGURE 10.10 A. Dorsoplantar view of a smooth K-wire used in a "locked" fashion. **B.** Lateral views of a smooth K-wire used in a "locked" fashion.

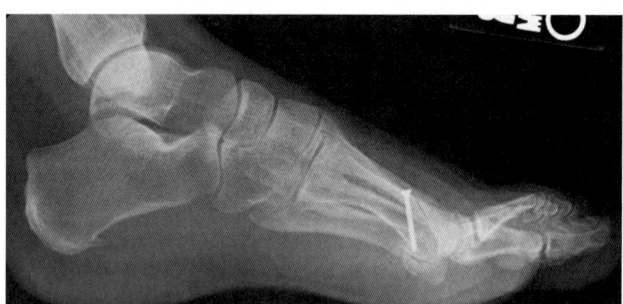

FIGURE 10.11 Lateral view of a cortical screw for fixation.

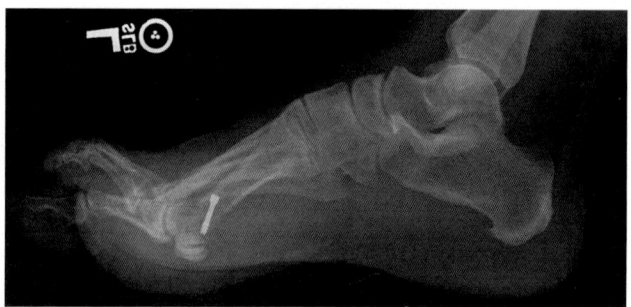

FIGURE 10.12 Fixation with a 3.0-mm partially threaded, headless screw.

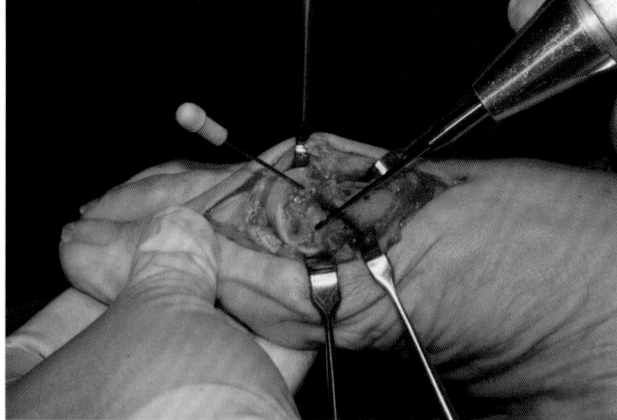

FIGURE 10.13 The initial path of the screw is accomplished with a 0.062-in smooth K-wire. This allows penetration of both proximal and distal cortices in an accurate and deliberate manner without the risk of having the drill bit skive or slide along one of the two cortices. The direction of the K-wire should be perpendicular to the plantar arm of the osteotomy on the lateral view and aimed toward the cristae between the sesamoid articular surfaces in the dorsoplantar orientation. This should be directed from proximal-dorsal to distal-plantar.

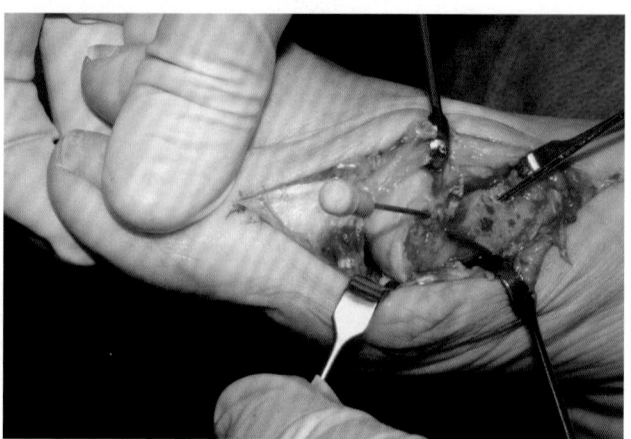

FIGURE 10.14 Evaluation of the exit point of the K-wire, demonstrating sufficient purchase of the plantar segment.

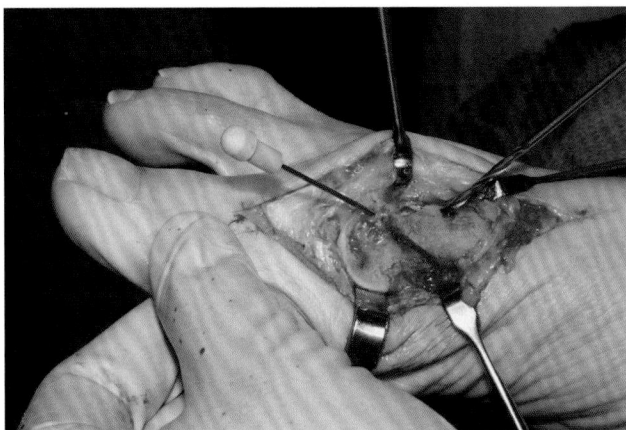

FIGURE 10.15 Having established the initial path for screw placement, the pilot hole is then established with the "under" drill or lesser drill bit.

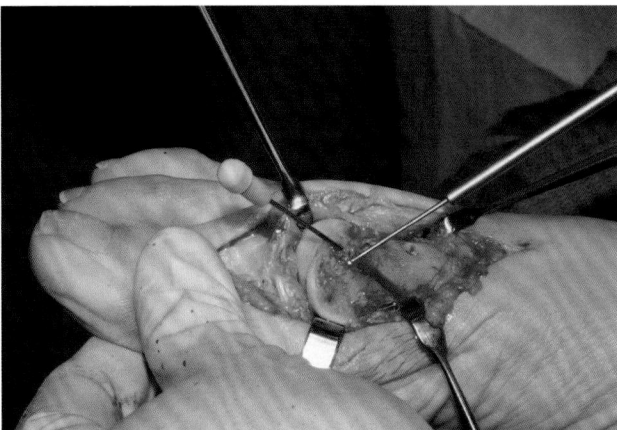

FIGURE 10.17 A depth gauge is inserted to measure the screw length. In the instance of this orientation, one does not want to use a longer screw than measured, as it would enter the joint and likely irritate the sesamoids.

using an "over" drill on the near cortex only, whose diameter corresponds with the screw's thread diameter.

The depth gauge is then inserted to measure the screw length (Fig. 10.17). Care should be taken to accurately measure the screw length as using too long a screw would enter the joint and likely irritate the sesamoids (Fig. 10.18). This can be assessed intraoperatively by checking where the depth gauge is exiting the first metatarsal head plantarly. The screw is then inserted, in the same orientation as the drill holes. Next, temporary fixation is removed and the screw is further tightened. The medial overhanging bone is resected and further contoured with power instrumentation (Figs. 10.19-10.25). Intraoperative fluoroscopy can be utilized to assess the correction of the deformity, fixation position, and osteotomy apposition. Postoperative radiographs should also be performed. These radiographs will show a decreased IM angle, show congruity of the first metatarsophalangeal joint, and verify appropriate screw length and apposition of the osteotomy (Fig. 10.26A and B).

LONG DORSAL ARM MODIFICATION

The long dorsal arm modification has been utilized frequently in foot and ankle surgery for the correction of mild to moderate bunions. The original idea of the long dorsal arm was fashioned to address the limitations of the standard chevron osteotomy. These included displacement and malposition of the capital fragment, delayed or nonunion, difficulties with fixation, and limited postoperative first metatarsophalangeal joint range of motion.[12] The long dorsal cut changes the acuity of the osteotomy, which in turn preserves the nutrient artery to the capital fragment.[13] This specific osteotomy is performed with the apical guide wire just plantar to midline. The angle of the dorsal and plantar osteotomy cuts is created at a more acute 55-degree angle. This allows for the dorsal cut to be longer than the plantar cut. Because the dorsal arm determines the orientation of the fixation, it is preferred to execute the dorsal osteotomy first followed by the plantar arm. Once the capital fragment is freed and transposed laterally to correct the deformity, two screw fixation can be utilized. It is important here to position the screws so that they do not create stress risers in the dorsal cortex. Therefore, there should be enough

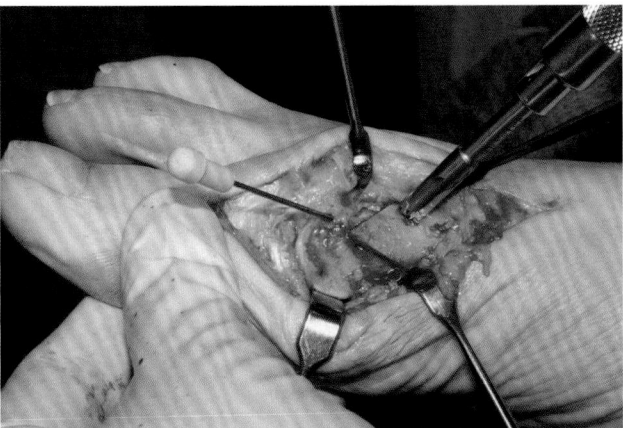

FIGURE 10.16 The countersink is then utilized to create a space for seating the land of the screw head. Even with headless screws, a small amount of countersinking will weaken the dorsal cortex preventing stress riser formation and increasing the compressive surface area for the screw upon engagement.

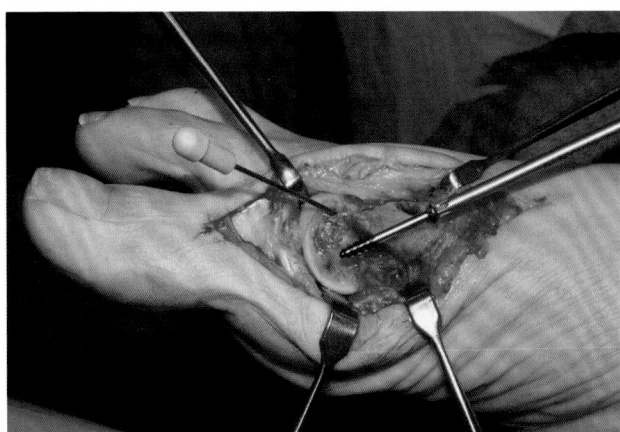

FIGURE 10.18 If screw length is in doubt, it may be superimposed medial to the metatarsal head to allow further inspection of the length desired.

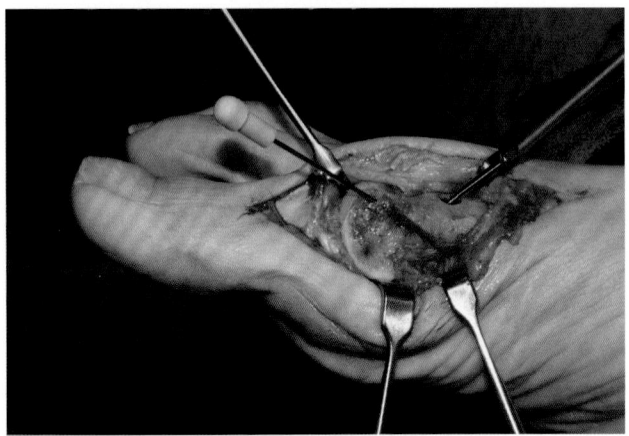

FIGURE 10.19 The screw is then inserted and temporary fixation is removed.

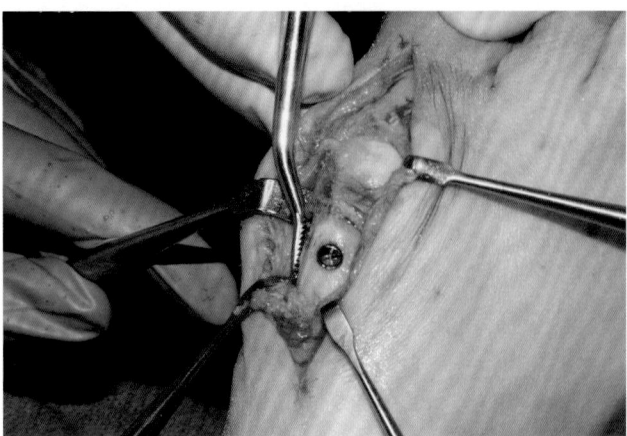

FIGURE 10.22 A power burr can easily bury itself within metaphyseal bone creating a defect, or even loosening and disrupting the fixation. For this reason, sharp prominences are best contoured with a small hand rasp.

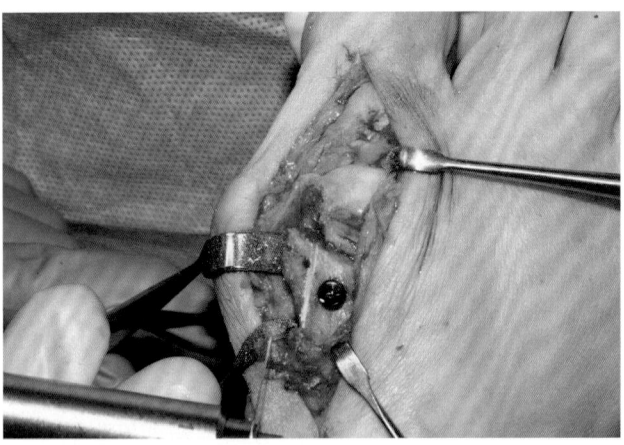

FIGURE 10.20 Overhanging medial osseous tissue is scored.

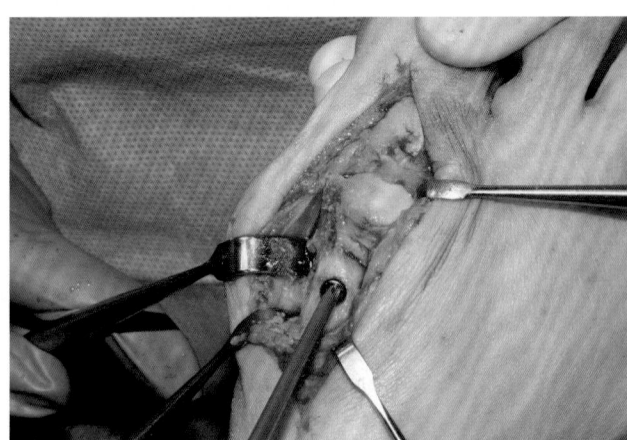

FIGURE 10.23 Final screw tightening is then performed.

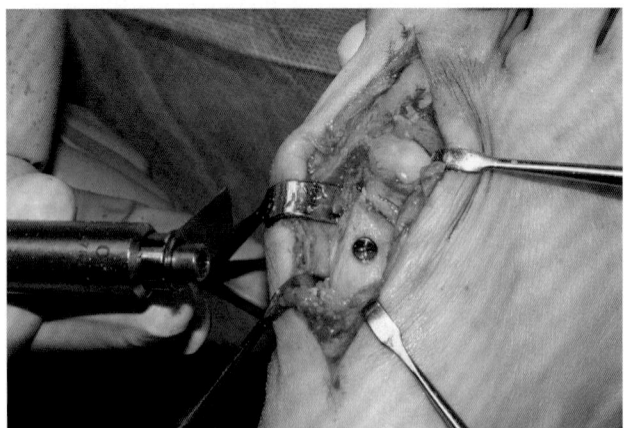

FIGURE 10.21 Overhanging medial osseous tissue is excised.

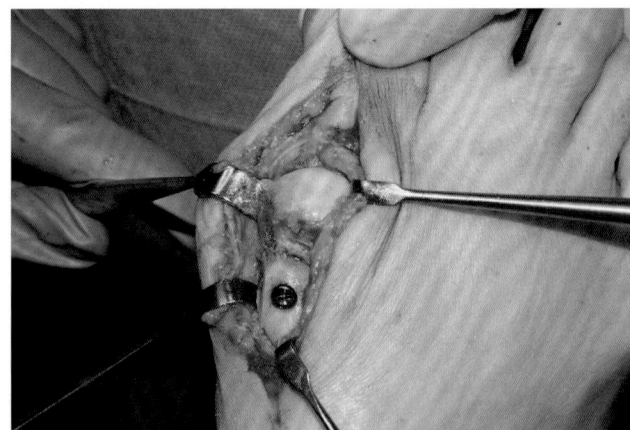

FIGURE 10.24 Final appearance of fixated osteotomy from dorsoplantar view.

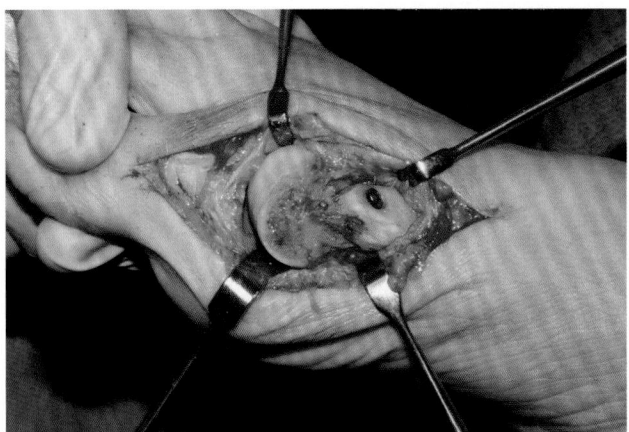

FIGURE 10.25 Final appearance of fixated osteotomy from medial view.

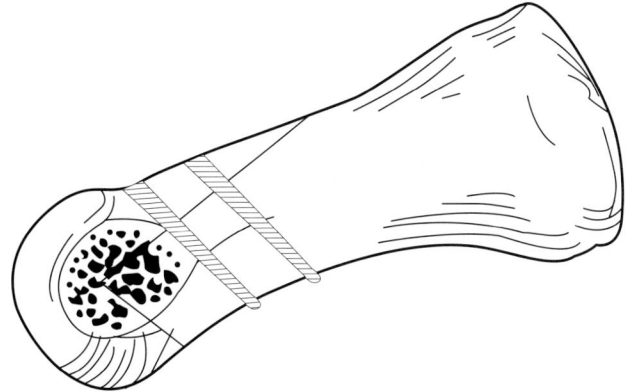

FIGURE 10.27 Artistic rendering of a long dorsal arm Austin fixated with two cortical screws, medial to lateral view. Notice: exact screw length is less critical because extra threads rest in soft tissue.

distance between the screws to allow for proper countersinking of each screw and ensure proper compression through the entire osteotomy site. Some authors have found that the proximal aspect of the osteotomy can create some callus formation due to its friability and have recommended resection of this part with the use of bone cutting forceps.[14] Orientation of the screws is perpendicular to the dorsal osteotomy cut, and thread purchase in the plantar cortex is imperative to osteotomy stability (Fig. 10.27). Screw length is important to consider, but the surgeon can afford a couple of threads through the plantar cortex because the screw tip will rest in the plantar soft tissues. With correction of the deformity, utilizing two screws will aid in compressive benefits and the resistance against rotation during the postoperative period.

LONG PLANTAR ARM MODIFICATION

The long plantar arm modification has gained some popularity over the years. It was originally investigated because some surgeons believe that the long dorsal osteotomy has inherent

failure occurring at one or both of the screw holes, between screws, and within the metatarsal proximal to fixation.[15] This, in combination with the possibility that patients may excessively bear weight before the osteotomy has healed, led to the long plantar arm modification. The angle in this modification is wider, and the plantar arm is longer than the dorsal arm. This modification has been investigated and found to have the greatest load to failure when comparing different osteotomies with similar fixation. The strength of this osteotomy is due to its plantar cortex fixation, as well as due to the increased plantar surface area for fixation (Fig. 10.28). The entire construct will be compressed with early weight bearing.[7,16] It is the authors' preference for this osteotomy to be used in patients with mild to moderate bunion deformities whom also have a larger body mass index and will have difficulty with off-loading during the postoperative period.

The osteotomy is performed with the apical guide oriented just superior to the midline of the halfway point between articular cartilages at the first metatarsal head. The plantar osteotomy will be performed first due to it determining the fixation.

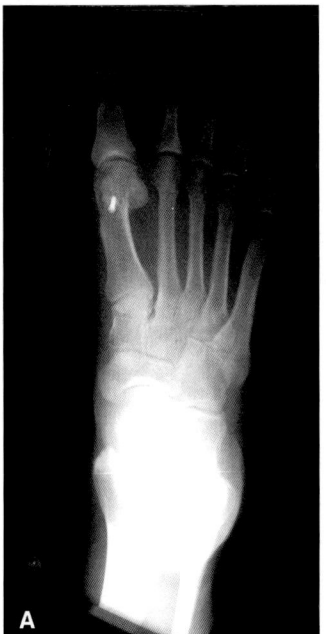

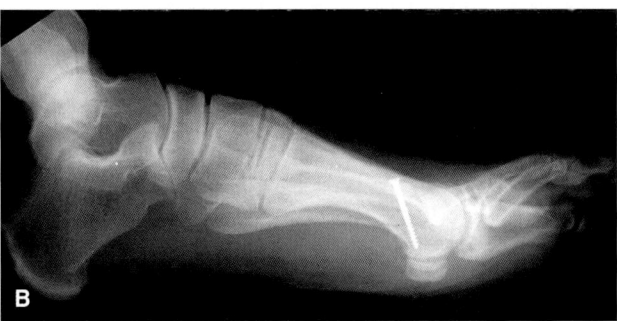

FIGURE 10.26 **A.** AP postoperative x-ray of Austin osteotomy fixated with a 3.0-mm partially threaded screw. **B.** Lateral postoperative x-rays of Austin fixated with a 3.0-mm partially threaded screw.

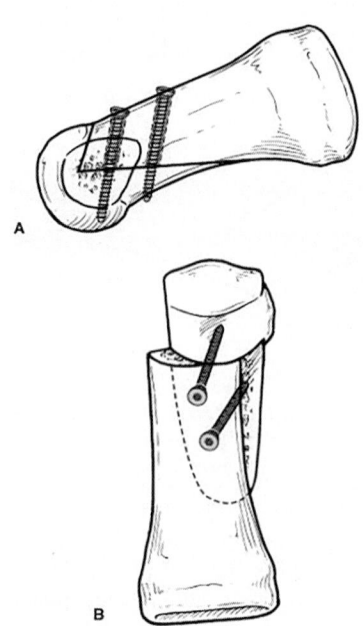

FIGURE 10.28 **(A)** DP and **(B)** lateral artistic rendering of a long plantar arm Austin fixated with two cortical screws.

Fixation options vary and depends on the surgeon preference. Typically, the author will use a single 2.4-mm screw (Fig. 10.29A and B).

REVERDIN BUNIONECTOMY

Traditional Reverdin

The Reverdin was first described in 1881 by Swiss Genevian physician, Jacques-Louis Reverdin to correct bunion deformities by partially resecting the medial bony eminence of the metatarsal combined with a wedge resection with a laterally based hinge (Fig. 10.30). The resection was designed to correct inherent metatarsal head and articular surface changes, also known as the proximal articular set angle (PASA). The IMA will then correct up to 3.5 degrees through a process called reverse buckling in flexible deformities described by McGlamry and Fenton.[17] The soft tissue balance between the muscle, soft tissue, and capsule will be shifted medially, as long as the wedge resection corrects the PASA to neutral or negative. It cannot be corrected if the metatarsal is rigid and plantarflexed.[18] The dorsal cuts are made approximately one-eighth to one inch from the articular surface with the distal osteotomy made parallel to the cartilage. The proximal cut is created perpendicular to the long axis of the bone. The cuts should be connected, but care must be taken to keep the lateral cortex intact. The hinge provides additional stability to the osteotomy site. The proximal cut can be adjusted to determine the amount of wedge needed to correct the deformity. A dorsal to plantar apical guide can be used to ensure the lateral cortex remains intact with its placement being slightly medial to the lateral cortex. Fixation is not required due to the hinge stability, but K-wires and monofilament wires can be used.[18,19] Several modifications of the osteotomy have been made over the years designed to correct different types of deforming forces that cause the HAV.

Reverdin-Green

Green modified Reverdin's procedure by describing an additional oblique plantar osteotomy in 1977. The osteotomy is a through and through cut parallel to the weight-bearing surface of the head of the first metatarsal. The cut can provide more stability for screw fixation (Fig. 10.31),[18,19] and the plantar cut allows for prevention of disturbing the sesamoid apparatus.[19] Indications for the procedure are the same as the Reverdin, which are correcting PASA with the added benefit of stability and maintaining sesamoid integrity.

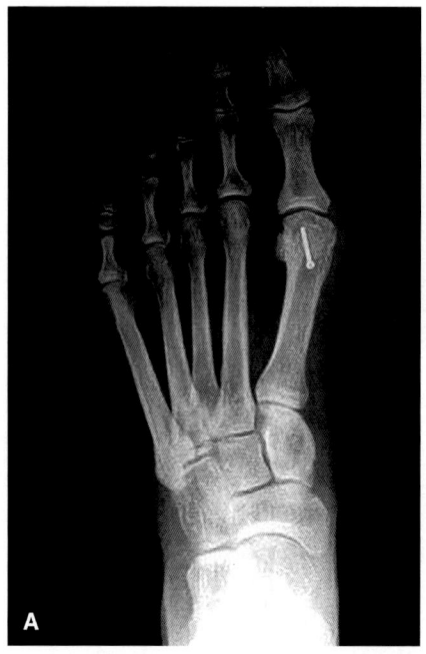

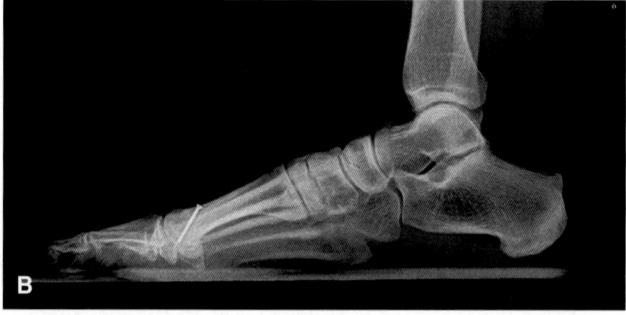

FIGURE 10.29 **A.** AP postoperative x-ray of long plantar arm chevron with 2.4 mm screw. **B.** Lateral postoperative x-ray of long plantar arm chevron osteotomy with 2.4 mm screw.

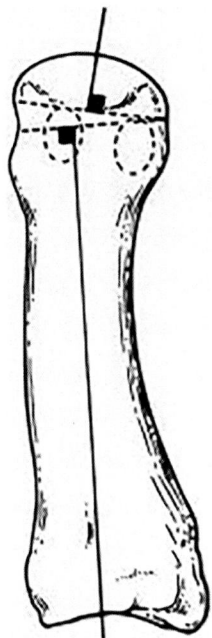

FIGURE 10.30 Reverdin osteotomy. The distal segment is oriented parallel to the articular surface of the 1st metatarsal head. The proximal segment is oriented perpendicular to the long axis of the 1st metatarsal.

Reverdin-Laird

The Reverdin-Laird is another commonly used modification. The dorsal osteotomies are completed with no preservation of the lateral hinge. This technique provides the ability to correct not only PASA but also the IMA, by allowing the shifting of the capital fragment (Fig. 10.32A and B).[19,20] The Reverdin-Laird differs from the chevron bunionectomy in that the apex of the deformity is more distal and plantar. The angle of the osteotomy is 90 degrees compared to 60 degrees, which reduces impaction and troughing (Fig 10.33). The Reverdin and its modifications can be combined with base and shaft osteotomies to increase correction.

When considering the Reverdin or its modifications, several considerations must be made, including quality of the bone stock. Wedge resection or even transposition of the capital fragment can be difficult in osteopenic patients and greatly reduces stability and fixation options. Care must be taken when determining fixation options as the articular cartilage must be preserved, however stable fixation is critical.

PERILS and PITFALLS

- Avoid excessive dissection of the soft tissue from the first metatarsal head. It is important to maintain the dorsal and plantar synovial folds of the first metatarsophalangeal joint capsule.
- Avoid the sesamoids with the osteotomy and fixation to prevent irritation and long-term complications.
- Avoid over or under correction by maintaining the sagittal groove of the first metatarsal head and not staking the head. Assessing the congruity of the first metatarsophalangeal joint and sesamoid positioning using intraoperative fluoroscopy.

POSTOPERATIVE CARE AND REHABILITATION

The postoperative care for distal metaphyseal osteotomies is determined by the inherent stability of the osteotomy performed and surgeon preference. Postoperative radiographs are taken after surgery to evaluate correction of the deformity, apposition of the osteotomy, and fixation position. Weight-bearing status is dictated by intraoperative findings including the quality of bone stock and stability of the osteotomy.

Postoperatively the hallux is bandaged in a rectus alignment with a kling dressing over a well-padded compression dressing. Typically, the patient will be partial weight bearing as tolerated immediately postoperatively with use of a postoperative shoe or cam boot and crutches. Passive range of motion exercises of the hallux are encouraged starting on the third postoperative day. The amount of walking or dependency is restricted for the first 2 weeks to assist in control of edema. Patients return to clinic

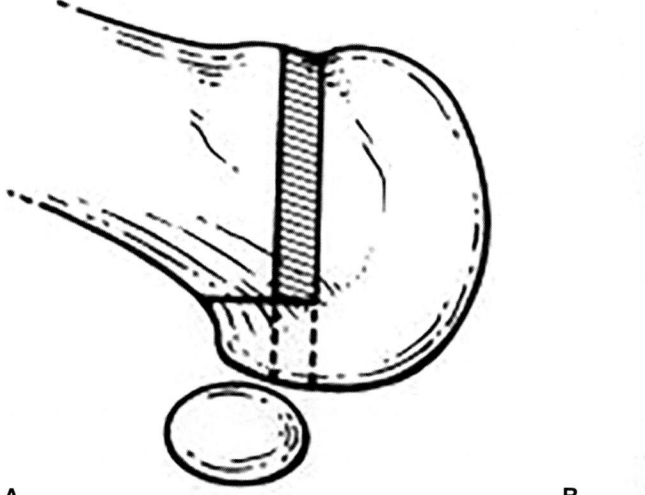

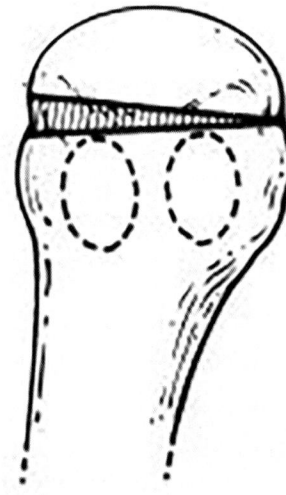

A   B

FIGURE 10.31 **A, B.** Green modification to the Reverdin osteotomy. This entails an oblique plantar osteotomy similar to that of an Austin. This preserves the sesamoids articular surface and increases the weight-bearing stability.

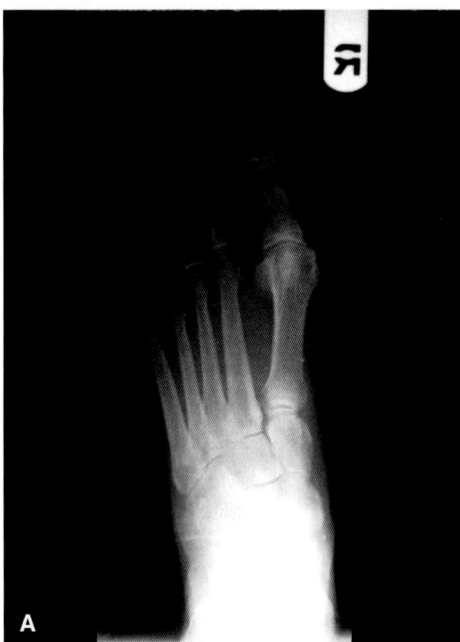
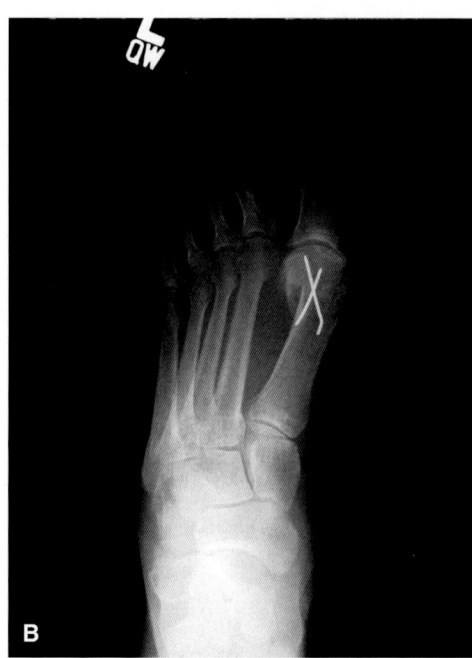

FIGURE 10.32 A. DP preoperative radiographs of a Reverdin-Laird. Subtle cystic changes can be appreciated at the medial aspect of the 1st metatarsal head on the preoperative image. **B.** DP postoperative radiographs of a Reverdin-Laird.

at 1 and 2 weeks for bandage changes, and a toe spacer can be used between the hallux and second toe as a retainer (provided the second toe has not undergone surgery). Patients will wear an elastic bandage to help control edema for an additional 4 weeks, and patients can expect edema to remain up to 6-12 months following surgery.

Postoperative x-rays are taken immediately following surgery and at desired intervals, typically 2 and 6 weeks, to evaluate the osteotomy stability and healing. Patients are transitioned to tennis shoes once adequate bone healing and swelling control is noted around the 6- to 8-week period. Formal physical therapy can be utilized as needed. The patient should gradually return to their normal activities, and it can take 4-6 months for the patient to return to all activities as tolerated.

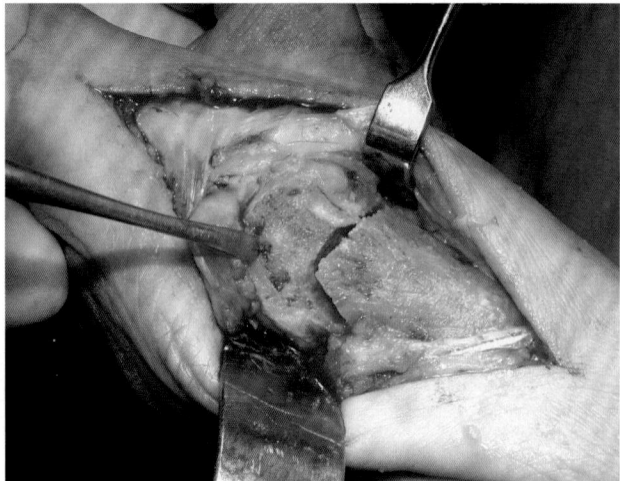

FIGURE 10.33 Completed Reverdin Laird osteotomy. Note the apex of the deformity is more distal and plantar and 90 degrees.

REFERENCES

1. Smyth NA, Aiyer AA. Introduction: why are there so many different surgeries for hallux valgus? *Foot Ankle Clin.* 2018;23(2):171-182. doi: 10.1016/j.fcl.2018.01.001.
2. Cain T, Boyd D. Defining the limits of the modified Austin bunionectomy. In: DiNapoli D, ed. *Reconstructive Surgery of the Foot and Leg: Update '90.* Tucker, GA: Podiatry Institute; 1990:129-134.
3. Chandler LM. First metatarsal head osteotomies for the correction of hallux abducto valgus. *Clin Podiatr Med Surg.* 2014;31(2):221-231. doi: 10.1016/j.cpm.2013.12.004.
4. Austin DW, Leventen EO. A new osteotomy for hallux valgus: a horizontally directed "V" displacement osteotomy of the metatarsal head for hallux valgus and primus varus. *Clin Orthop Relat Res.* 1981;(157):25-30.
5. Shaw N, Wertheimer S, Krueger J, et al. A mechanical comparison of first metatarsal diaphyseal osteotomies for the correction of hallux abducto valgus. *J Foot Ankle Surg.* 2001;40(5):271-276. doi: 10.1016/s1067-2516(01)80062-4.
6. Choi GW, Kim HJ, Kim TS, et al. Comparison of the modified McBride procedure and the distal Chevron osteotomy for mild to moderate hallux valgus. *J Foot Ankle Surg.* 2016;55(4):808-811. doi: 10.1053/j.jfas.2016.02.014.
7. Chang TJ, Landsman AS, Ruch JA. Relative strengths of internal fixation in osteotomies and arthrodesis of the first metatarsal. In: Miller S, Mahan K, Camasta CA, Ruch JR, eds. *Reconstructive Surgery of the Foot and Leg: Update 1996.* Tucker, GA: Podiatry Institute Publishing; 1996.
8. Rigby RB, Fallat LM, Kish JP. Axial loading cross screw fixation for the Austin bunionectomy. *J Foot Ankle Surg.* 2011;50(5):537-540. doi: 10.1053/j.jfas.2011.04.024.
9. Herzog JL, Goforth WD, Stone PA, et al. A modified fixation technique for a decompressional shortening osteotomy: a retrospective analysis. *J Foot Ankle Surg.* 2014;53(2):131-136. doi: 10.1053/j.jfas.2013.12.018.
10. Andrews BJ, Fallat LM, Kish JP. Screw versus plate fixation for chevron osteotomy: a retrospective study. *J Foot Ankle Surg.* 2016;55(1):81-84. doi: 10.1053/j.jfas.2015.06.024.
11. Brosky T II, Hall P. Distal metaphyseal osteotomies in hallux abducto valgus surgery. In: *McGlamry's Comprehensive Textbook of Foot and Ankle Surgery.* Vol 1. 4th ed. Philadelphia, PA: Lippincott Williams & Wilkins; 2012:1510-1552.
12. Kalish SR, Bernbach MR. Modification of the Austin bunionectomy. In: McGlamry ED. *Reconstructive Surgery of the Foot and Leg, Update '87.* Tucker, GA: Podiatry Institute; 1987:86-89.
13. Weinraub GM, Steinberg J. Vascular perfusion of the long dorsal arm versus Chevron osteotomy: a Cadaveric injection study. *J Foot Ankle Surg.* 2004;43(4):221-224. doi: 10.1053/j.jfas.2004.05.008.
14. Dairman MC, Hatch DJ. Modified Kalish osteotomy: a simple approach to minimizing proximal dorsal stress risers. *J Foot Ankle Surg.* 2003;42(2):108-110. doi: 10.1016/s1067-2516(03)70011-8.
15. Dalton SK, Bauer GR, Lamm BR, et al. Stability of the offset V osteotomy: effects of fixation, orientation, and surgical translocation in polyurethane foam models and preserved cadaveric specimens. *J Foot Ankle Surg.* 2003;42(2):53-62.
16. Ravenell RA, Kihm CA, Lin AS, et al. The offset V osteotomy versus the modified Austin with a longer plantar arm: a comparison of mechanical stability. *J Foot Ankle Surg.* 2011;50(2):201-206. doi: 10.1053/J.JFAS.2010.12.012.

17. Fenton CF III, McGlamry ED. Reverse buckling to reduce metatarsus primus varus: a preliminary investigation. *J Am Podiatry Assoc.* 1982;72(7):342-346.

18. McGlamry D, Banks A. Reverdin hallux valgus correction. In: *The Proceedings of the Annual Meeting of the Podiatry Institute.* Tucker, GA: Podiatry Institute, Inc.; 1992:227-230.

19. Todd W, Randall T. Reverdin procedure and its modifications. In: *Hallux Valgus and Forefoot Surgery.* Churchill Livingstone. 1994:203-213.

20. Banks A. The Reverdin Laird osteotomy. In: *The Proceedings of the Annual Meeting of the Podiatry Institute.* Tucker, GA: Podiatry Institute, Inc.; 2004:282-284.

CHAPTER 11

Proximal First Metatarsal Osteotomy

Molly S. Judge

CLOSING BASE WEDGE OSTEOTOMY

DEFINITION

The long oblique wedge osteotomy is designed to affect reduction of high intermetatarsal angle (IMA) hallux abducto valgus (HAV) deformity with excision of a wedge of bone.

This osteotomy is cut from proximal medial to distal lateral excising ample bone to reduce a high IMA. It is designed for support by two points of internal fixation. Optimal stabilization of the construct is achieved with two interfragmentary compression screws and prolonged non–weight bearing. The learning curve for this technique is steep and should not be underestimated.

The closing base wedge osteotomy (CBWO) was described in the early 1900s for the correction of severe HAV deformity. At that time, the critical deformity of metatarsus primus adductus was addressed at its apex using a short transverse plane osteotomy.[1,2] Juvara studied the limitations of this short oblique osteotomy suggesting the use of two long oblique cuts extending into the diaphyseal-metaphyseal junction creating a more stable construct.[3-5] With the advent of internal fixation technique a modification of the CBWO, the Podiatry Institute described the long oblique CBWO in 1977.[6] This modification provided a lengthened radius arm for enhanced reduction of deformity. This also increases the surface area of the osteotomy providing room for two screws for enhanced fixation of the parts.[7-9]

To that end, Fillinger et al. demonstrated double screw fixation to be more stable than single screw fixation in comparing proximal crescentic and oblique wedge osteotomies.[10] The oblique CBWO is challenging and requires practice to master the intricacies of the technique. Proficiency using saw bones or cadaver specimens is encouraged and the mechanics of the CBWO were described in detail for this purpose.[11]

INDICATIONS AND PITFALLS

Designed for metatarsus primus adductus with a high intermetatarsal angle (IMA ≥ 15-degrees), the base wedge osteotomy is a powerful procedure for reducing severe multiplanar deformity of the first ray segment. The technique has withstood the test of time and is likely underutilized due to the history of reported complications. The technique is predictable, reproducible and proves to be very effective when performed accurately. It should be clarified that the complications reported in the literature are resultant of technical failures not flaws inherent to the technique.[12]

The procedure has been criticized for excessive shortening of the metatarsal segment. With closer study, this shortening was often found to be the result of first ray elevation. With time and experience, an appreciation for hinge mechanics would serve to reduce the risk of this complication.[6] When the axis guide is designed accurately, the metatarsal is translocated purely in the transverse plane, shortening is minimized as noted in multiple retrospective studies.[13-16] The greatest shortening of those articles reporting an average 3.18-mm shortening in long-term review of 159 cases.[13] Banks et al. demonstrated mathematically using geometric analysis that the shortening due to a CBWO was in fact due to metatarsal elevation and correlated that with the width of the metatarsal segment.[16] Metatarsus elevatus was also noted to occur due to malunion in the face of premature weight bearing after CBWO. Strict non–weight-bearing measures are enforced postoperatively to ensure optimal outcome. Alternative proximal osteotomies have been designed in an attempt to avoid these complications such as the proximal crescentic and Chevron (aka Austin) osteotomies. In a cadaveric study, the base wedge osteotomy using the two-screw technique proved to be 82% stronger than the crescentic customarily using a single screw.[17]

INDICATIONS LONG OBLIQUE CLOSING BASE WEDGE OSTEOTOMY

- **High intermetatarsal angle:** The long radius arm of the CBWO can reduce high IMAs predictably while allowing for two points of internal fixation.
- **Rigid first ray:** When the deformity is nonreducible in the transverse plane, a proximal CBWO will more effectively correct deformity and reduce the risk of recurrence vs a distal osteotomy.
- **Elevated first metatarsal (elevatus):** The CBWO can be modified to affect change in the sagittal plane reproducibly with strict attention to the details of the technique.
- **Juvenile hallux abductovalgus deformity:** Not uncommonly HAV deformity in the juvenile is associated with a flexible deformity and residual metatarsus adductus. Often there is a mismatch between the radiographs and the clinical findings where the clinical deformity appears dramatic and yet the residual metatarsus adductus masks the significance of the IMA on the radiograph. In this event, measurement of the true IMA is critical in determining the size of wedge to be resected for realignment.

(Continued)

■ **Iatrogenic deformity:** When a distal osteotomy has failed and recurrence is evident, often the residual bone stock at the head of the metatarsal is insufficient for revision. The head and neck may have been narrowed, the quality and cubic content of bone may be diminished once retained fixation devices are removed, or residual degenerative defects may increase the risk of nonunion should a distal procedure be performed. In these cases, a proximal osteotomy may reduce the risk of technical complications and provide long-standing correction of deformity.

ANATOMIC FEATURES

1. Consider the *crescentic shape* of the first metatarsal base as the lateral flare rides beneath the proximal medial border of the second metatarsal at times obscuring the intermetatarsal joint on the plain film. This anatomy is important especially when determining the level for the bone cut for the crescentic osteotomy. The first metatarsal base flare has *two discrete facets;* one articulates with the medial base of the second while the other provides articulation with the cartilage of the inferior surface of the first (medial) cuneiform (Fig. 11.1). This lateral flare rests much more plantar than the medial flare and so is deeper within the intermetatarsal vault (Fig. 11.20). When running the compression screw, this flare provides bone volume to facilitate screw thread capture and compression of the base while allowing ingrowth about the screw during primary bone healing.

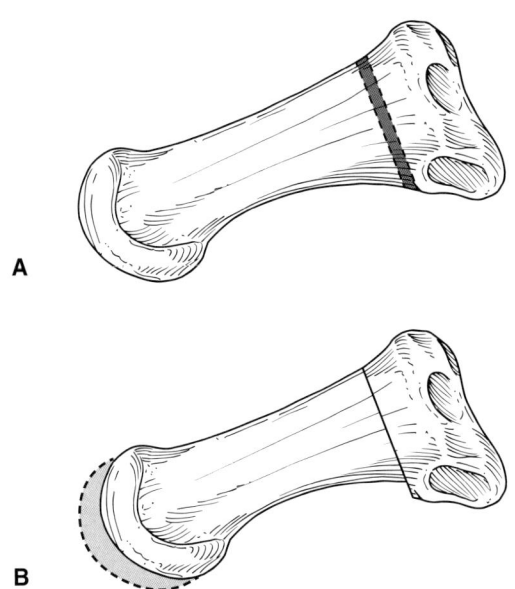

FIGURE 11.1 **A.** Illustration right lateral metatarsal. This later flare rests much more plantar than the medial flare and so is deeper within the vault. This flare has two discrete facets for articulation laterally; one with the medical base of the second metatarsal the other articulates with the cartilage of the inferior surface of the first medial cuneiform. **B.** After osteotomy demonstrating shortening and a virtual dorsiflexion of the metatarsal. For every millimeter of bone excised a degree of elevation results. Fig 11.1a. A wedge resection of bone (two passes of a 1 mm thick sagittal saw blade) results in a minimum of 2mm shortening. Fig 11.1b. The shortened metatarsal segment will rest higher in the sagittal plane (off the weight bearing surface) as seen here. This shortening results in a virtual dorsiflexion of the metatarsal segment as seen in lateral radiographs.

2. Consider the declination of the first metatarsal from the lateral view (Fig. 11.1). For every millimeter of metatarsal, bone excised simply from the excursion of the saw blade elevation will result. The residual metatarsal segment being shorter rests more dorsal in the sagittal plane (Fig. 11.1). When resecting a wedge of bone from the metatarsal, the degree of shortening is predictable and has been determined specifically to be 1.1 mm for every 5-degree wedge of bone resected and 2.5-mm shortening for every 15-degree wedge resected.[16]

3. The periosteum of bone is a major source of perfusion facilitating primary bone healing. Over time there has been debate over the impact of periosteal reflection, so called stripping, and the suspected adverse effect that has on bone healing.

In a study by Whiteside et al., the notion that periosteal stripping would significantly decrease perfusion to bone was refuted.[18] In fact, Zucmans' study demonstrated that periosteal stripping results in dilatation of periosteal vessels increasing perfusion and yields a positive impact on primary bone healing.[19]

FUNCTIONAL ANALYSIS

See chapter on HAV evaluation & management.

PATHOGENESIS

The overall position and alignment of the foot and ankle are genetically determined. The position and alignment of the metatarsal bones and the integrity of the capsular and ligamentous structures are realized as the patient begins to weight bear and adapt to their environment. With maturity the rear foot and ankle adapt to activity, terrain and weight-bearing function and the medial arch assumes a posture in response to physical demands and the strength and stability of the limbs. As hallux valgus progresses, the lateral capsular and ligamentous structures contract drawing the hallux toward the second ray and ultimately can rotate the hallux into valgus. When pronatory changes occur in the ankle and rear foot increased demand is placed along the medial column and first ray segment. With increasing pronatory forces, weight-bearing function of the first ray diminishes and load is transferred onto the 2nd ray, specifically the second metatarsal phalangeal joint (MTPJ). With progressive pronatory force first ray instability increases, lateral joint contractures progress and medial joint structures fatigue and attenuate allowing for a drift and lateral rotation of the sesamoid apparatus. As the first metatarsal splays toward the midline, the medial eminence of the metatarsal head becomes prominent. In the earliest stage of deformity, this prominence represents normal bone in an abnormal position. With time and progression of deformity, the medial eminence is often exposed to mechanical irritation within shoe gear and a fibrocartilaginous overgrowth develops. This hypertrophic overgrowth may or may not be associated with a fluid-filled shock absorbing sac (aka bursal projection). It is this fibrocartilaginous overgrowth that often yields a mismatch between the clinical appearance of a grossly inflamed and enlarged bunion deformity and the radiographic appearance. With significant hypertrophic fibrocartilaginous over growth, the clinical presentation can be profound often with soft tissue inflammation, erythema, and tenderness; however, if the intermetatarsal metatarsal angle is low to moderate (8-12 degrees), radiographic findings may not be impressive. The apex of the first metatarsal deviation is believed to be within the first MTPJ when the hallux deviates and prompts retrograde forces upon the metatarsal head increasing the IMA beyond normal limits beyond 8 degrees.[20] When instability is noted within the metatarsal cuneiform joint (MCJ), the apex of deformity is proximal in first ray and splaying of the metatarsal commonly results in higher IMAs, often >15 degrees. The incidence, etiology, predisposing factors, clinical, and radiographic evaluation of the bunion deformity have been discussed in great detail.[21-23]

PHYSICAL EXAMINATION

Stance

Evaluation in relaxed stance and base of gait will reveal concomitant deformity such as spine, shoulder, and or hip malalignment that contributes to imbalance and dynamic deformity in both stance and gait. Frontal plane malalignment of the knee (genu valgus or varus) contributes to weight-bearing imbalances stressing the medial or lateral foot, respectively. Genu recurvatum, convexity of the posterior knee resultant of knee hyperextension, is evident when limitation of ankle joint is present and should be taken into consideration prior to foot and ankle surgery. In the face of subtalar joint (STJ) and midtarsal joint (MTJ), pronation subluxation of the talus within the navicular mortise may be appreciated in all three planes of motion. Talar ptosis and medial column insufficiency translates into higher mid foot and fore foot pressure for a longer duration during the gait cycle. In the face of flexible deformity, position and alignment can be reduced to normal with manual manipulation and deliberate posturing of the foot and ankle (see also neutral position foot films under radiographic evaluation).

Frontal View

It is easy to appreciate that the medial arch in this case is full weight bearing and the midfoot is abducted with prominence of the styloid process of the fifth ray. STJ and MTJ prolapse can be evidenced by peri talar subluxation (PTS) in the frontal plane and exacerbates fore foot deformity such as hallux abduction and metatarsus primus adductus, flexor stabilization of the lateral digits, and crossover second toe deformities (Fig. 11.1 and 11.2). The summation of these deformities results in an increased girth of the fore foot while the rearfoot and heel remain relatively narrow resulting in heel slippage from the shoe in gait and makes shoe fitting troublesome. In (Fig 11.2), the right foot was corrected with the benefit of the CBWO, sequential reduction, and arthrodesis of the second toe years prior. The nature and extent of deformity in the left foot documents the preoperative deformity addressed with a CBWO on the right. The enlarged medial eminence of the first ray exaggerated by metatarsus primus adductus is associated with hallux abduction that underlaps the second digit. With overloading of the second MTPJ instability results in digital subluxation progressing into elevation and adduction at the MTPJ and flexion at the proximal interphalangeal joint (PIPJ).

Range of Motion

Flexibility of the first ray and metatarsophalangeal joint (MTPJ) should be assessed with the foot in neutral position while the metatarsal is stabilized, and the hallux is moved in

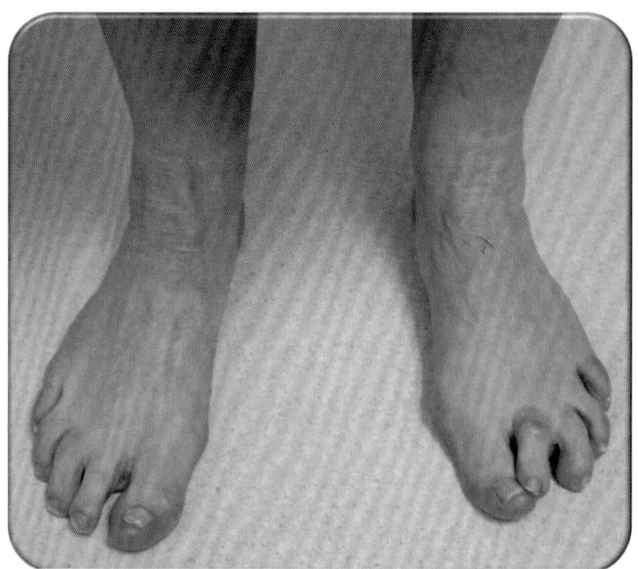

FIGURE 11.2 In this clinical photo, the right foot was corrected with the benefit of the CBWO, sequential reduction, and arthrodesis of the second toe 6 years prior. The nature and extent of deformity was nearly identical preoperatively and the left foot documents the preoperative deformity. The overall change in foot girth and first ray congruity is markedly improved and weight-bearing function of the first MTPJ has been restored.

the sagittal plane. If the range of motion is limited with the hallux in neutral position, angular deformity or arthritic disease is suspected. Osteoarthritis of the MTPJ may present as hallux limitus due to a dorsal rather than medial eminence and transverse plane deformity of the hallux may be absent in that case. Attention should be directed to the MCJ to determine if that joint is stable or hypermobile. Testing for MCJ instability is performed by holding the first and second MCJs in neutral position. The first ray is then translated dorsally in the sagittal plane; this is the wrong one when the metatarsal base is able to be shifted 5 mm above, the second instability is confirmed and an alternate procedure should be entertained. Details regarding evaluation and assessment of first MCJ stability have been discussed in detail within the literature.[24-28]

Flexibility of the First Ray

In the face of a nonflexible (rigid or semi rigid) first ray, a proximal procedure can predictably reduce the IMA. When a nonreducible transverse plane deformity is present, a distal procedure may be met with recurrent deformity.

The capsular repair and soft tissue balancing cannot predictably prevent recurrence when the ray is rigid with a moderate or high IMA. Conversely, in the face of excess flexibility or hypermobility of the first MCJ, an alternate procedure should be considered, for example, arthrodesis of the first MCJ and is detailed in an alternate chapter.

Metatarsus Primus Elevatus

Often evidenced by keratosis beneath the second metatarsal head, an elevated first ray can be the result of congenital deformity, trauma, or iatrogenic defect. Keratotic transfer lesions are often an indicator of MTPJ instability and lateral overloading in weight bearing. Off weight bearing with the STJ and MTJs placed in neutral position, the forefoot alignment can be evaluated. With the foot in neutral position loading, the fifth ray and comparing the metatarsal parabola from medial to lateral the forefoot alignment can be assessed. The plantar level of the first metatarsal can be seen as dorsal to the second when metatarsus primus elevatus (MPE) is present. When present, an uncompensated fore foot varus deformity is associated with a keratotic lesion beneath the fifth metatarsal head and partially compensated deformity is associated with a keratotic lesions beneath the first and the first metatarsal heads. Fully compensated varus deformity results in a focal lesion beneath the fifth metatarsal head and increases the risk for preulceration. The various etiologies for MPE include an abnormal length pattern of the first metatarsal, a short proximal phalanx of the hallux, and a hypermobile medial column or first metatarsal can also lead to MPE. Structural abnormalities of the fore foot include uncompensated or partially compensated forefoot varus (fore foot) supinatus, rearfoot, or ankle varus and can prevent weight-bearing function of the first metatarsal. Loss of integrity of the load-bearing medial column of the foot can lead to an acquired elevatus. This can be resultant of degenerative arthritis, compensatory gait due to pain or neuropathic arthropathy. Iatrogenic elevatus can be a debilitating sequela of first ray surgery and so specific modifications to first ray osteotomies or other procedures should be made to avoid residual MPE.

Forefoot Valgus

A reducible forefoot valgus is often associated with a pronated foot type and bunion deformity. Commonly such angular deformity can be identified by characteristic patterns of plantar keratosis. When uncompensated deformity is present, keratosis beneath the first metatarsal head is apparent and combination lesions beneath the first and the fifth metatarsal heads manifest when partially compensated. Fully compensated deformity is associated with keratotic lesions beneath the 5th metatarsal head and may pose a threat of ulceration if not appropriately accommodated.

RADIOGRAPHIC EVALUATION

Position and alignment in multiple orthogonal planes, quality of bone, joint alignment, and presence of intra-articular degenerative changes are key parameters to assess in a step-wise progression when assessing plain films of the foot and ankle. Beginning with the dorsoplantar view position and alignment of the larger complexes of the foot can be assessed: STJ, MTJ, and Lis Franc joint complexes. Deformities of the metatarsal parabola and digital rays are assessed next. The most common radiographic parameters to assess the first ray in cases of HAV deformity are the hallux abductus angle (HAA), intermetatarsal angle (IMA), metatarsus adductus angle (MA), true IMA, metatarsal primus elevatus (MPE), Meary angle or lateral talo-first metatarsal angle, and fore foot axial (FFA).

In the dorsal plantar (DP) view of the severe bunion deformity, a high IMA, HAA, and deviated sesamoid apparatus are often associated with malalignment of the lesser rays and a cross-over second toe (Fig. 11.3). A diastasis between the first and second rays can be an indicator of available motion between the parts. A measurable space between the metatarsal bases is an indicator of increased flexibility and often instability that can exacerbate the HAV deformity (Fig. 11.4). Conversely, the presence of an enlarged articular facet, a very tight or restrictive

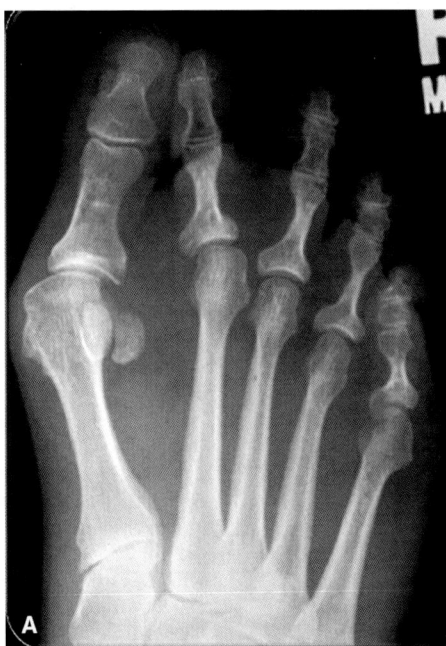 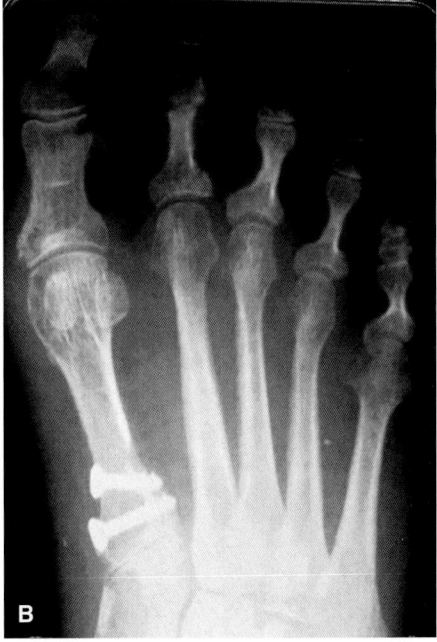

FIGURE 11.3 A. Preoperative radiograph demonstrates a high IMA, deviated hallux, and sesamoid apparatus and at a glance it seems there is a diastasis between metatarsal bases 1-2. Seen here the 2nd metatarsal base is deeply recessed along the lateral aspect of the medial cuneiform. **B.** The base of the metatarsal remains congruent with the chondral surface of the cuneiform and was stable.

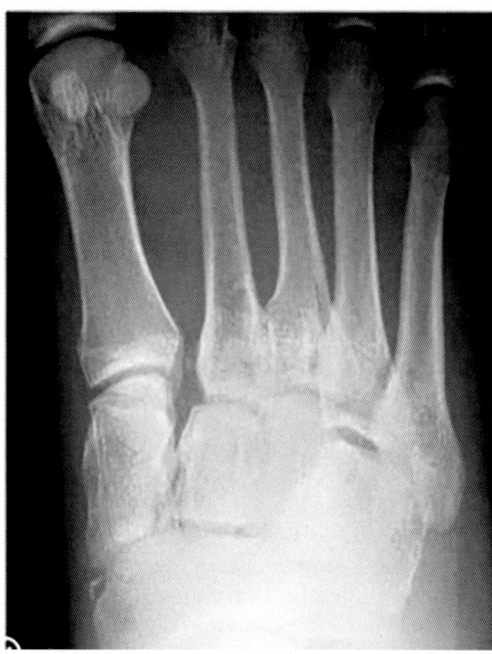

FIGURE 11.4 As seen in this plain film x-ray, a true diastasis between the metatarsal bases is noted. When present this incongruity is an indicator of available motion and is often associated with instability between the rays. When present in the face of chronic bunion deformity an alternative to the CBWO procedure should be considered. In this case, a Lis Franc injury is the culprit for this instability and this hallmark radiographic change.

articulation of the associated rays or the presence of an os intermetatarsia,[29] is more suggestive of limited motion of the first ray and is favorable when considering a CBWO (Fig. 11.5). Osteoarthritis and dorsal bossing about the MTPJ can cause irritation of the medial dorsal cutaneous nerve and may be associated with HAV deformity clinically and radiographically.[30,31] HAV complicated by residual metatarsus adductus should take into consideration the calculation of the true IMA and often supports the

use of a proximal metatarsal osteotomy. Further, a more recent discussion analyzed the change in proximal intermetatarsal divergence angle *after distal metatarsal osteotomy* underlining an increased metatarsal divergence and increased maximum intermetatarsal distance in low-angle IMA deformity.[32] This *postoperative finding* may be an indication for candidates that would benefit from a proximal arthrodesis when revision is considered.

In the lateral (Lat) view of the foot, sagittal plane deformity of the first metatarsal can be identified. MPE is a clinical diagnosis resultant of either structural or functional abnormality that can be assessed radiographically. Determining the etiology of MPE is important to a successful HAV correction and will allow selection of adjunctive procedures that will optimize postoperative function.

It is important to determine whether deformity is within the metatarsal bone itself (intrinsic) or is the result of dynamic abnormalities outside the bone itself (extrinsic). When comparing the dorsal cortex of the first and second metatarsal diaphysis, divergence of the cortices supports the presence of elevatus while a parallel alignment supports a more neutral sagittal plane configuration (Fig. 11.6A). Correction of MPE depends on the nature of the condition; whether MPE is a structural or dynamic deformity. To study this concept, the physician must determine whether the deformity is intrinsic or extrinsic to the metatarsal bone (Fig. 11.6B).[33] Camasta underlined that a proper imaging technique is integral to an accurate assessment of first ray position and alignment. If the x-ray tube head is angled 10 degrees cephalad (upward aiming toward the head), the lateral radiograph will give the appearance of first ray elevation; however, the dorsal cortices remain in a parallel arrangement when a neutral ray position is present (Fig. 11.7).

Neutral Radiographs

Dorsal plantar (DP), lateral (LAT), AP ankle (AP AJ), and calcaneal axial views can be obtained in a mechanically neutral position to determine the degree of reducibility of deformity within the ankle, rearfoot, and forefoot. Often this information

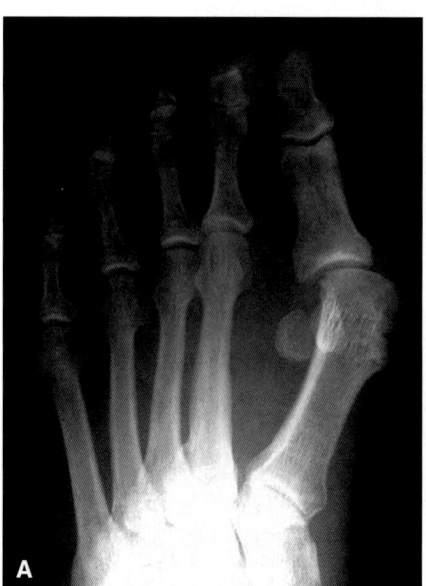

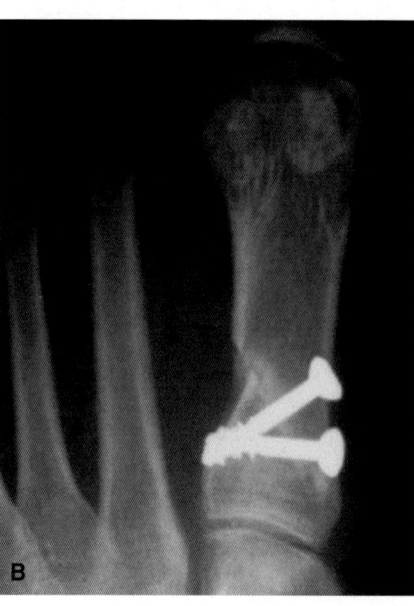

FIGURE 11.5 A. Preoperative radiograph demonstrates a high IMA, deviated hallux and sesamoid apparatus and at a glance there is a noticeable diastasis between metatarsal bases 1-2. Seen here the 2nd metatarsal base is deeply recessed along the lateral aspect of the medial cuneiform. The base of the metatarsal remains congruent with the chondral surface of the cuneiform and was stable. **B.** At midterm follow up the CBWO has maintained alignment and correction of deformity unchanged at 6-years post op. Notice the narrow width of the metatarsal base as compared to the large caliber of the 4.0mm cancellous screws. Given the girth of this bone segment smaller screws could have been used as an alternative in this case had they been available. These radiographs correspond to the clinical photo seen in Fig 11.2.

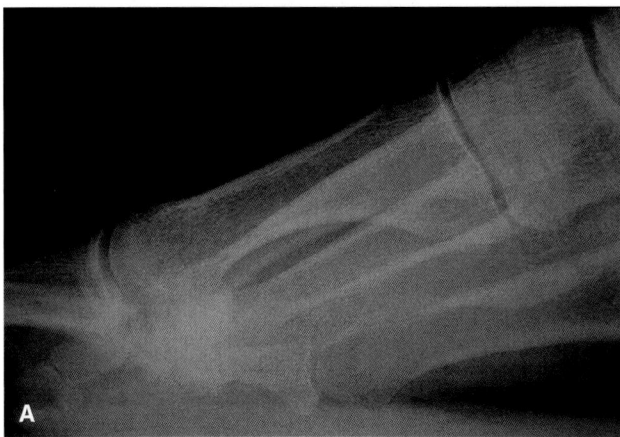
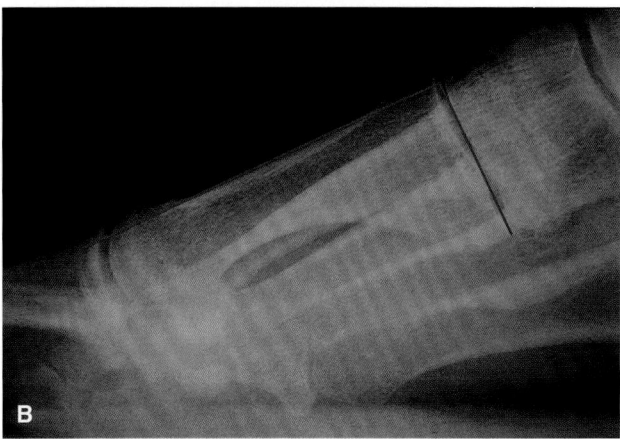

FIGURE 11.6 **A.** From the lateral radiograph, first metatarsal elevatus can be assessed by comparing the cortical margins of metatarsals one and two. A divergent configuration as seen here indicates an elevated metatarsal position. **B.** When comparing the angle created by the articular surface of the 1st metatarsal base and the cortical margin the etiology of the metatarsal elevation can be surmised. Seen here a 90-degree relationship indicates that the elevation is not inherent to the bone but rather is extrinsic to the metatarsal and is positional in nature.

will assist in determining primary and adjunctive surgical procedures as they may reveal compensatory mechanics not obviated during the clinical evaluation. The ability for the ankle, subtalar, midtarsal, and medial column to achieve a neutral position is important to a successful rebalancing procedure. When performing the Heubscher maneuver in the LAT and DP foot views faulting within the medial column, mid foot or rear foot may indicate an inability to compensate when the first ray is realigned (Fig. 11.8). Such radiographic findings should be discussed with the patient and the potential need for adjunctive procedures should be considered.

TREATMENT

Conservative therapy can include insole modifications or more predictably prescription orthotic devices can be prepared to rebalance the forefoot as an alternative to surgical intervention. When an elevatus is present, the prescription should provide

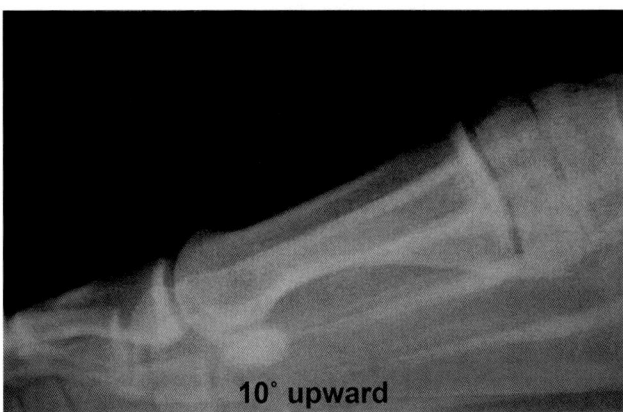

10° upward

FIGURE 11.7 Camasta underlined that proper imaging technique is integral to an accurate assessment of the position and alignment of the first ray segment. Here it was demonstrated that deviation of the x-ray tube head during weight bearing lateral plain film x-rays can mimic a metatarsal elevation. (Reproduced with permission from Camasta CA. *Radiographic Evaluation and Classification of Metatarsus Primus Elevatus.* The Podiatry Institute; 1994;123-127.)

relief beneath the 5th metatarsal head with a partial fill beneath the first metatarsal. Options in orthotic materials include semiflexible polypropylene, copolymers, poly-laminates, or cork-based prescriptions. Accommodation of the rigid first ray can be achieved using a medial forefoot wedge. Alternatively, for the most aggressive orthotic prescription, a University of California Biomechanics Laboratory (UCBL) custom molded orthotic can provide control of the rear foot that can derotate malalignment of the heel, provide firm buttressing of the medial arch, provide a lateral flange to counter midfoot abduction, and improve fore foot balance. As with any orthotic device, custom fabrication is reliant on a detailed and thoughtful prescription. Final customizing of an orthotic prescription cannot be overstated as this serves to ensure proper fit, function, and comfort especially when taking into consideration heavy weight-bearing demands. While precise orthotic fabrication is key to success, patient education regarding appropriate shoe gear for desired function is also critical for success. Should orthotic therapy fail the proximal first metatarsal osteotomy can provide predictable and reproducible results with strict attention to the details of the technique. Postoperatively orthotic therapy to support the arch and reduce weight-bearing imbalance may optimize long-term function.

AUTHORS PREFERRED TREATMENT

Technique Tip 1

Principals of the hinge axis should be studied in advance by practicing this technique in the laboratory using bone models or cadaver specimens. Once mastered in the lab, the technique can be employed reliably with predictable reduction of deformity. Refer to Mcglamry's Comprehensive Textbook of Foot Surgery for further details of mechanical and surgical principals associated with this technique.[34]

The procedure begins with an extensile dorsolinear incision medial to the extensor hallucis longus (EHL) tendon beginning just proximal to the MCJ and extending over the proximal phalanx (Fig. 11.9A and B). After the first interspace release (release of the deep transverse intermetatarsal

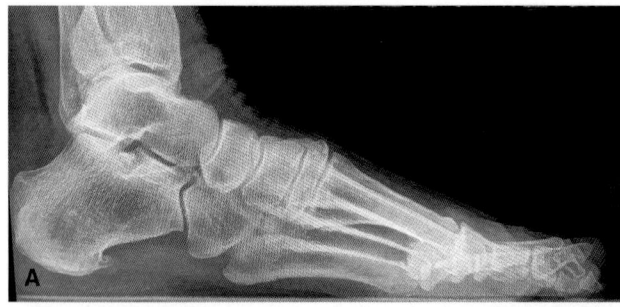

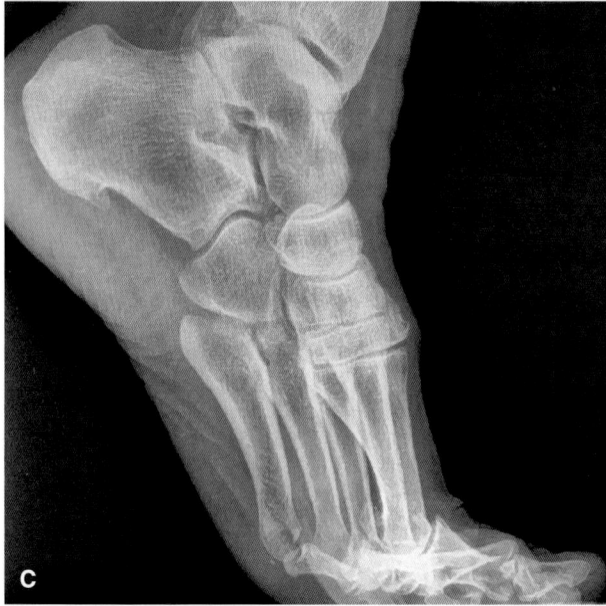

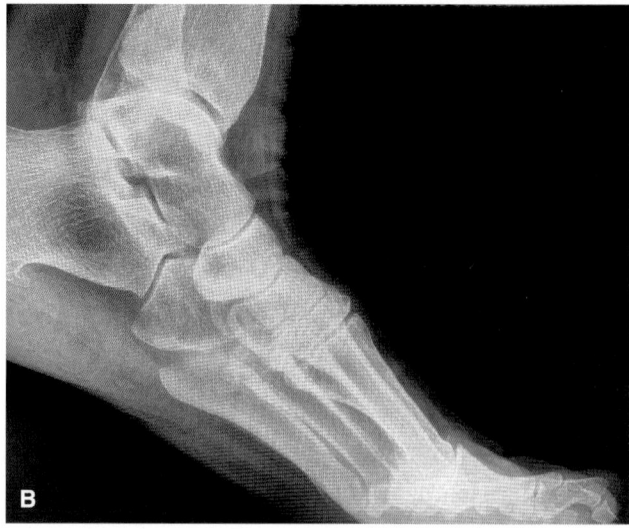

FIGURE 11.8 When irregularity is noted at the dorsum of the 1st metatarsal cuneiform joint dysfunction and instability is suspected at the MCJ. If instability is present, then the CBWO is not the preferred procedure and an arthrodesis of the MCJ may be most appropriate. **A. Lateral view:** Dysfunction and joint instability is suspected given the exuberant bone formation at the distal aspect of the cuneiform in an otherwise congruous joint. It is prudent in this case to stress the joint to ensure that there is no evidence of joint insufficiency or laxity that may preclude the use of a CBWO. **B. Stress lateral view 45-degree angle:** Reveals maintenance of joint congruency. **C. High angle stress lateral:** Fails to reveal faulting at the MCJ and the CBWO can be considered in correction of the HAV deformity in this instance.

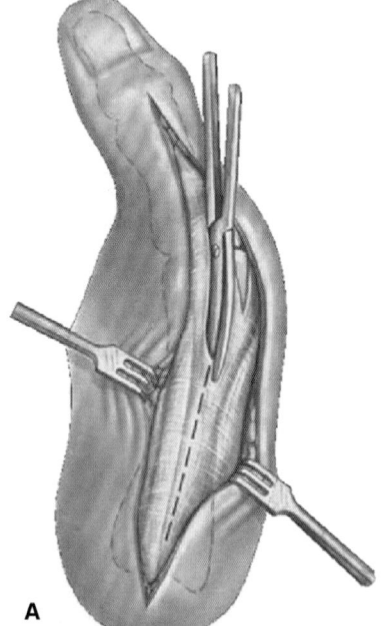

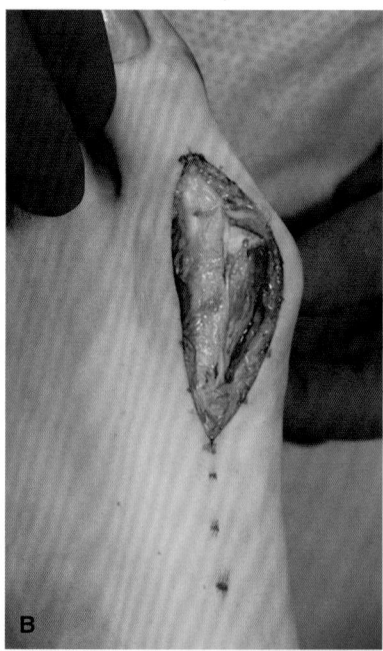

FIGURE 11.9 A. Illustration of the distal skin and deep fascial incision facilitating the interspace release. Use of a Metzenbaum scissor allows precise incision of the deep fascia and exposure of the EHL tendon. (Courtesy of John A. Ruch, DPM.) **B.** Intraoperative photo. With the EHL exposed, the tendon can be inspected for attenuation, contracture, or chronic tendinosis, and the need for adjunctive procedures can be considered at this time.

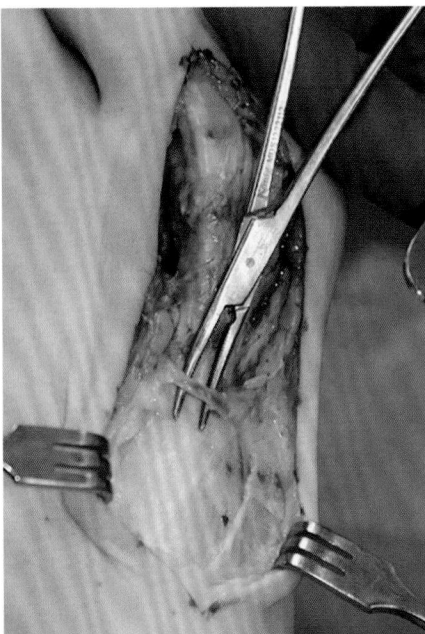

FIGURE 11.10 Intraoperative photo of the nature and location of the medial marginal vein to be identified, isolated, and ligated.

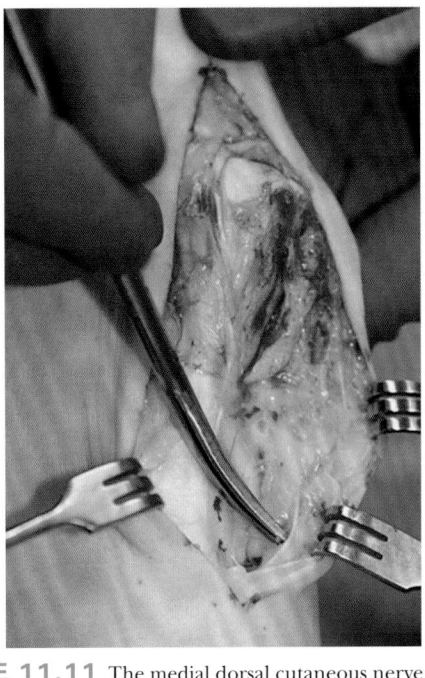

FIGURE 11.11 The medial dorsal cutaneous nerve or its branches are encountered, isolated, and retracted medially.

ligament, lateral capsular contractures, and fibular sesamoi-dal ligament), the medial eminence is resected and blunt dissection is continued proximally. The medial marginal vein (Fig. 11.10) and the medial dorsal cutaneous nerve (Fig. 11.11) or its branches are encountered and retracted medially. Once subcutaneous tissues have been reflected proximally, an incision into the deep fascia is made medial to the EHL tendon to afford lateral retraction of the tendon (Fig. 11.12A and B). This exposure allows best visualization of the metatarsal base, shaft, and the MCJ.

Technique Tip 2

The first ray should be manipulated to identify the MCJ capsule. An 18G hypodermic needle can be placed in the MCJ as a marker to prevent placing the axis guide too close to the joint (Fig. 11.13). The freer elevator in this figure indicates the desired location of the axis guide ~1 cm distal to the MCJ. In the case of juvenile HAV, it is vastly important to recheck your anatomic landmarks to ensure that the growth plate within the base of the first metatarsal is not violated during the procedure. In the event that an interspace release is not required, the deep fascial incision can be designed for limited

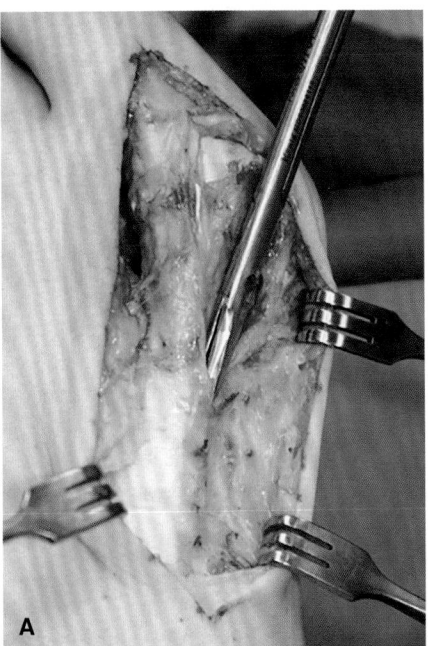

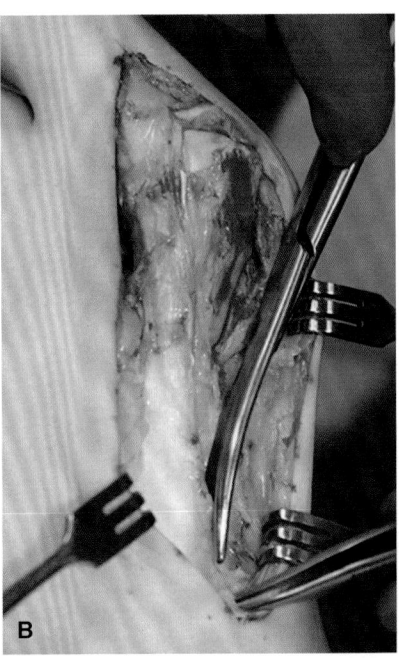

FIGURE 11.12 A, B. Continuing within the first ray dissection, the deep fascial incision is extended proximally and the EHL tendon can then be retracted laterally.

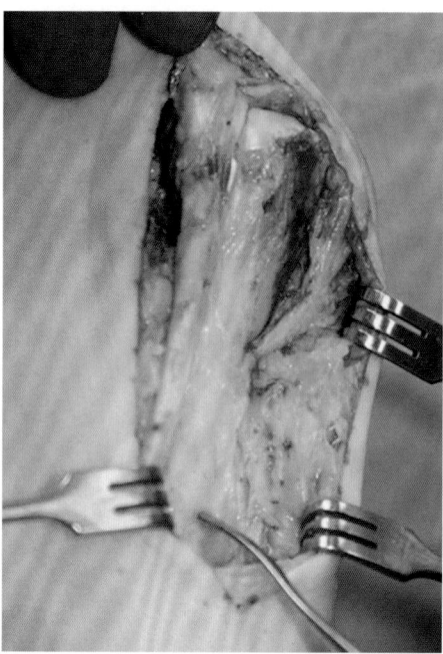

FIGURE 11.13 Intraoperative photo: The freer elevator illustrates the location of the most proximal metatarsal ~1 cm distal to the MCJ, Technique Tip 7. This landmark facilitates localization for the axis guide of the base wedge osteotomy. Preparing the axis guide in this location reduces the risk of untoward violation of the joint, see Technique Tip 4.

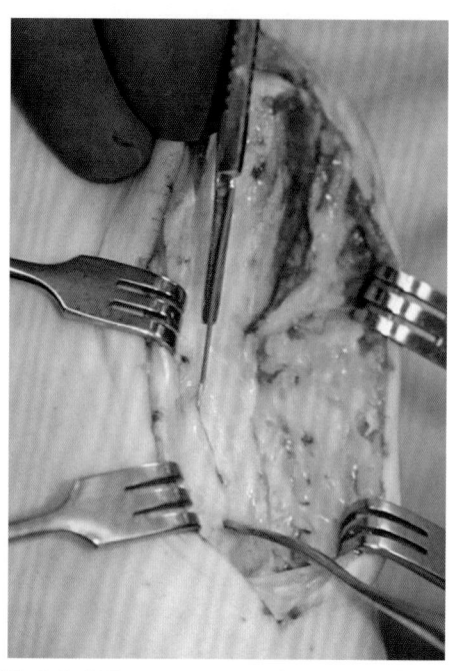

FIGURE 11.15 The periosteal incision begins 1 cm distal to the MCJ on the medial metatarsal base and runs from proximal medial to central lateral within the central metatarsal shaft and is completed distally on the shaft as seen in Figure 11.16.

exposure of the proximal metatarsal and the distal medial eminence (Fig. 11.14). The periosteal incision is begun with a stab incision medially at the proximal base of the first metatarsal ~1 cm distal to the MCJ. This incision runs obliquely from

proximal medial to distal lateral across the metatarsal base (Fig. 11.15). This incision extends distally along the central metatarsal shaft providing ample exposure for the osteotomy and internal fixation (Fig 11.16). The periosteum is incised and reflected using the freer elevator (Fig. 11.17).

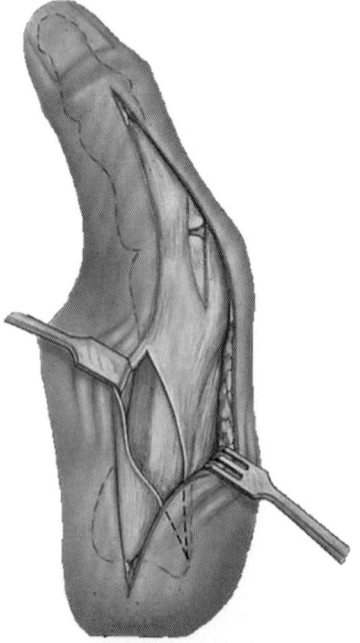

FIGURE 11.14 The deep fascial incision can be completed in two parts lending exposure for the distal interspace soft tissue release and proximally to provide exposure for osteotomy cuts and internal fixation. (Courtesy of John A. Ruch, DPM.)

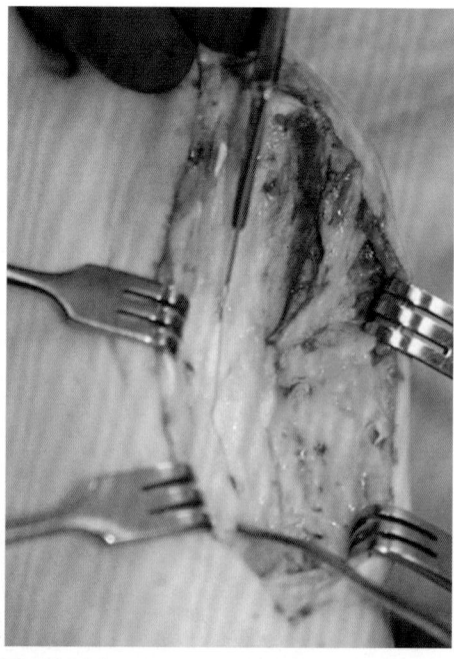

FIGURE 11.16 The periosteum is incised and reflected using the freer elevator

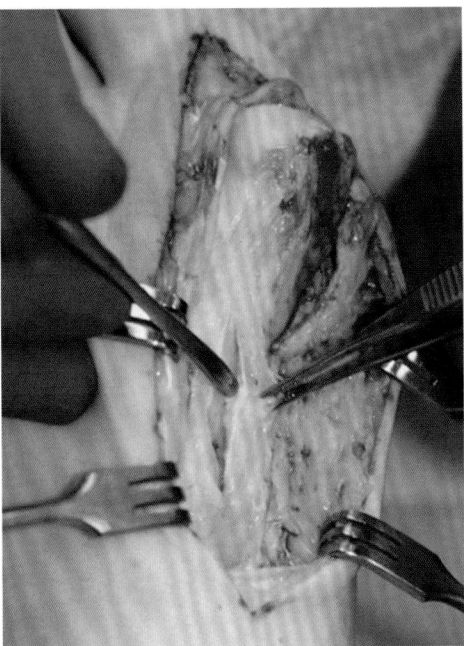

FIGURE 11.17 Use of the sharp end of the freer elevator facilitates reflection of the periosteum in a single tissue layer in preparation for later closure, see Technique Tip 8.

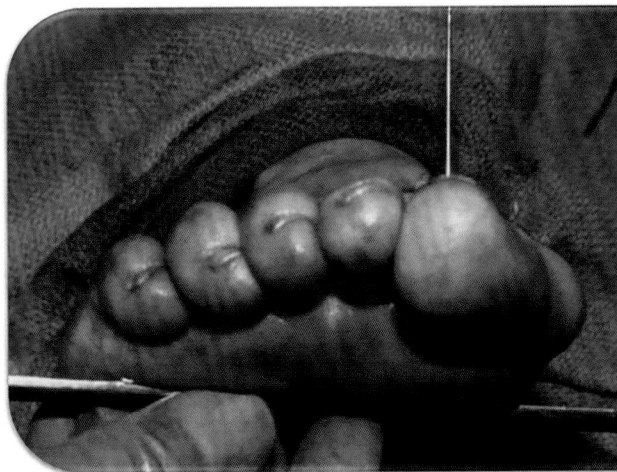

FIGURE 11.18 Intraoperative view with the fore foot loaded in neutral position using an osteotome. This maneuver confirms the osteotomy axis guide is perpendicular to the weight-bearing surface, see Technique Tip 5.

See Technique Tip 3

The periosteum can be tagged and retracted with nonabsorbable suture for later closure. This suture retraction technique facilitates exposure of the metatarsal base while preserving the tissue layer for later closure. *Notice that the periosteum is not reflected from the medial base of the osteotomy site.* This periosteal attachment provides enhanced support for the hinge after the osteotomy has been cut and fixated and is in essence a third point of fixation. Definitive mechanical stress testing experiments have demonstrated that the medial cortical hinge of the CBWO is the primary stabilizing force of this construct.[6] The periosteum is an important component of perfusion for the metatarsal base and so is preserved by meticulous delicate handling.[18,19] In a 3-year prospective study of 65 CBWO procedures, cases with periosteal reflection vs no periosteal reflection (stripping vs no stripping) were compared revealing reduced incidence of displacement and delayed union in the nonstripped group.[35]

Axis Guide Placement

It is important to simulate weight bearing of the foot before driving the K-wire into place. The **K-wire axis is to be perpendicular to the weight-bearing surface** (NOT perpendicular to the metatarsal) as this allows pure transverse plane rotation of the osteotomy (see Fig. 11.18) **and Technique Tip #1**. Note that an osteotome simulates the weight-bearing surface and creates a neutral forefoot to better assess the position of the K-wire. The axis guide uses either a 0.035 or 0.045 K-wire depending on the girth of the metatarsal base. This is placed ~1 cm distal to the MCJ on the medial shoulder of the metatarsal base. This allows ample space for reciprocal planning of the osteotomy once the axis guide is removed. Finally inspect the axis placement in both the sagittal and frontal plane to ensure the design will affect accurate correction of the given deformity (Figs. 11.18 and 11.19). When driving the axis guide wire tilting the hand laterally will

plantarflex the metatarsal and tilting medially will dorsiflex the metatarsal once the osteotomy is closed (Fig. 11.20). If the position of the axis guide is unacceptable, the K-wire can be removed and driven to optimize its position when necessary. When satisfied with the position and alignment of the axis guide in both planes, the K-wire is then cut and capped leaving a short wire segment for aligning the saw blade.

BONE CUTS

See Technique Tips 4 and 5. The design of the osteotomy is scored into the bone using a sagittal saw or osteotome. These markings run from the K-wire axis toward the cortical margin. It is important to understand that *the angle of the most proximal bone cut determines the length of the final osteotomy plane.* Designing these bone markings accurately begins with scoring the proximal cut no >45 degrees from the long axis of the distal metatarsal segment (Fig. 11.21A-C). This cut is performed first as this proximal cut determines the plane of the osteotomy and dictates the surface

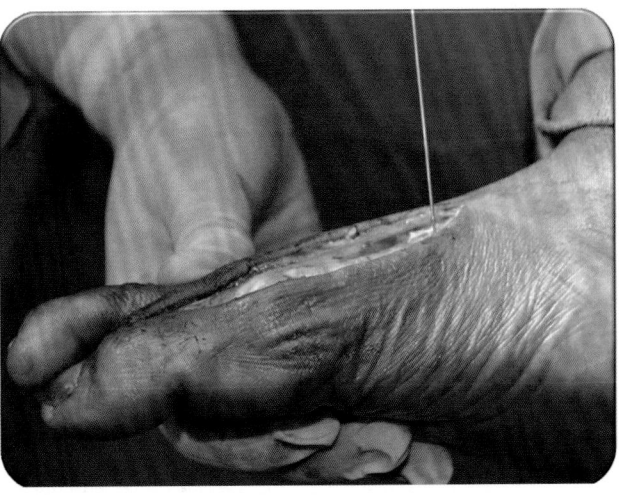

FIGURE 11.19 Confirmation of sagittal plane alignment of the axis guide with the fore foot loaded, see Technique Tip 5.

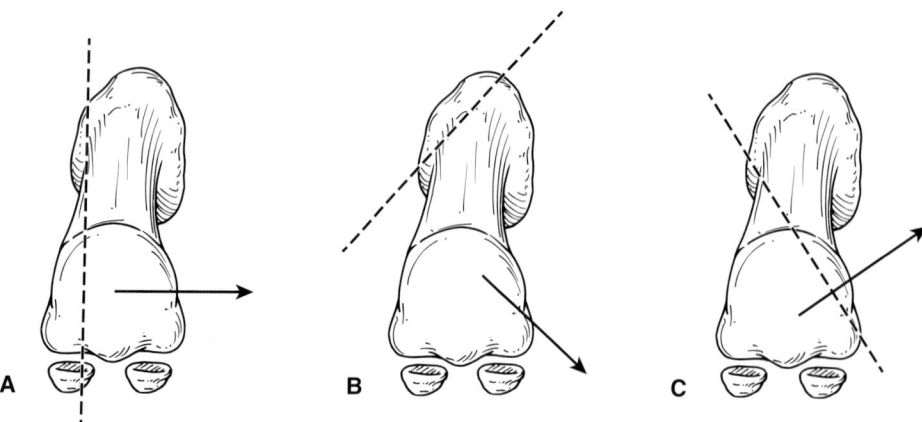

FIGURE 11.20 A. The frontal view of the 1st metatarsal left foot. Notice the lateral flare is much larger and extends more plantarly than the medial flare of the metatarsal base. The axis guide placement determines the orientation of the osteotomy and therefore determines the final position of the distal metatarsal. When pure transverse plane motion is desired, the axis guide is driven perpendicular to the weight-bearing surface. **B.** When plantarflexion is desired, the axis guide is tilted laterally creating a dorsomedial hinge that plantarflexes as it is closes. **C.** When elevation of the metatarsal is desired, tilting the axis guide medially a plantar medial hinge is created and dorsiflexion of the distal metatarsal results in elevation of the part.

available for fixation. The long arm is scored at an angle that will best achieve reduction of the IMA keeping in mind the relationship between the size of the wedge removed and resultant shortening of the metatarsal.[16] Once satisfied with the scoring of the cuts, the sagittal saw is used to cut the osteotomy. The deep soft tissues (not just the skin) should be retracted at the distal lateral edge of the intended osteotomy. It is customary to make

the proximal cut in the metatarsal first as that solid bone is stable to work with. The lateral cortex is penetrated first opening the cortical bone with an oscillating saw (Fig. 11.22). Normal saline is applied to the oscillating saw blade during the osteotomy cut to prevent overheating and thermal necrosis of bone. Irrigation is prudent as it serves to preserve bone quality and promotes primary bone healing. Upon entering the marrow

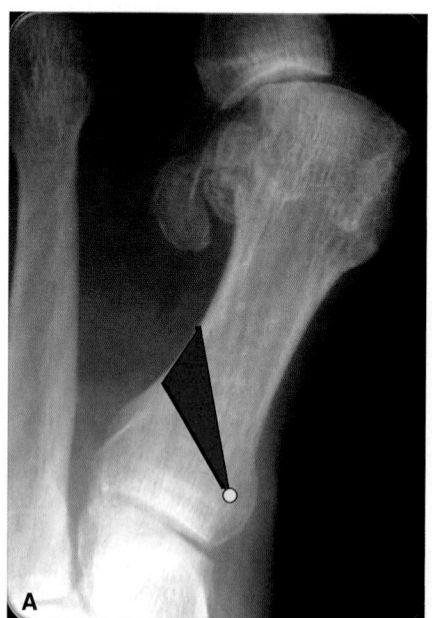
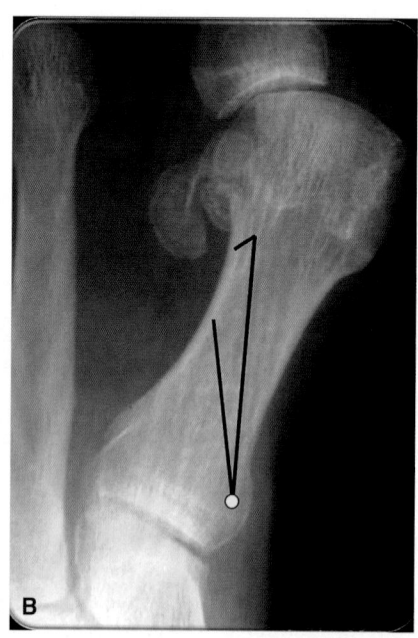
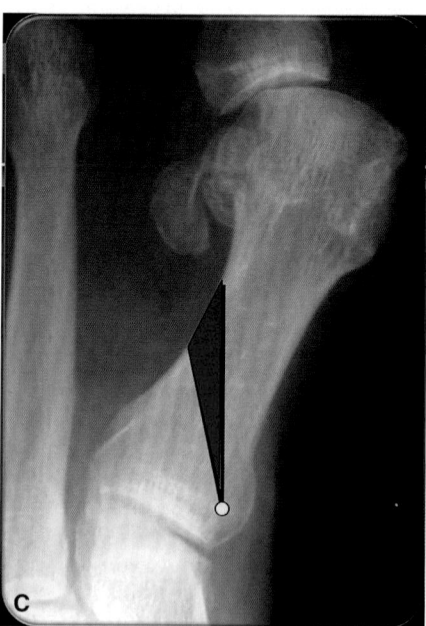

FIGURE 11.21 A. Considerations in designing the base wedge osteotomy. If the first bone cut is angulated too acutely in the transverse plane, a short transverse osteotomy will be created, which cannot facilitate two points of fixation. **B.** If the first bone cut is angulated obtusely, a very long osteotomy will result in bone cuts that can approach or interfere with the sesamoid apparatus. **C.** When the first bone cut is made ~45 degrees to the base of the metatarsal, the cut will exit the lateral cortex within the proximal diaphysis allowing for a second cut to create a long oblique osteotomy that can accommodate two points of fixation.

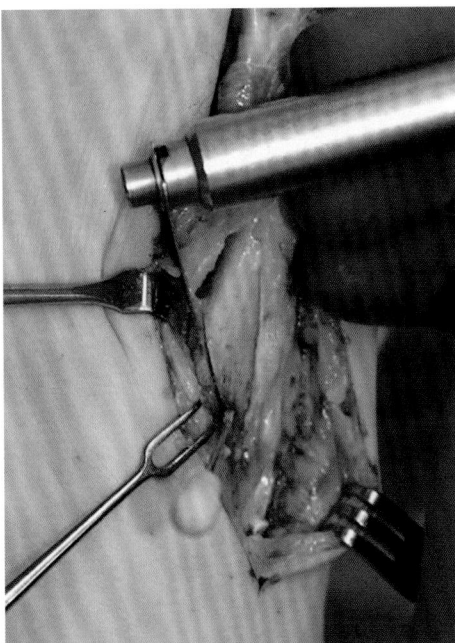

FIGURE 11.22 The first cut of the osteotomy is the proximal cut where the oscillating saw is applied to the lateral margin of the proximal metatarsal base and is oriented parallel to the axis guide. The blade is manipulated from dorsal to plantar cutting the full thickness of the bone as the cut is made up to but not against the axis guide, see Technique Tips 9 and 10.

cavity, the blade will achieve full excursion as it works its way into the marrow to begin the cut. This first bone cut ends immediately distal to the K-wire allowing room for later feathering (Fig. 11.23). The second cut is made in the distal segment converging with the first cut just before the pin (Fig. 11.24). Notice these bone cuts converge distal to the pin NOT on the pin.

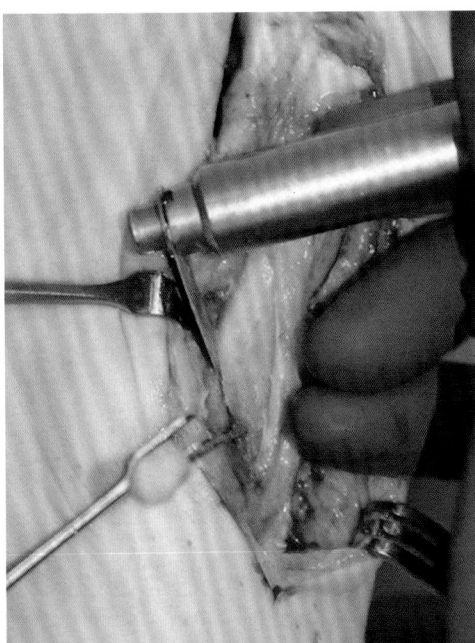

FIGURE 11.23 The second cut of the osteotomy is made distally and the blade is oriented parallel to the axis guide as the cut is made from distal to proximal cutting up to but not against the axis guide.

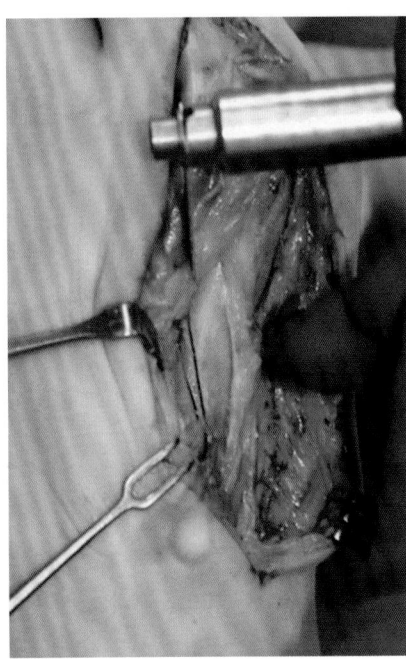

FIGURE 11.24 The osteotomy cuts converge near but not onto the axis guide. This will allow for feathering the cuts when necessary for closing the osteotomy.

This will allow reciprocal planning (*feathering*) of bone after the K-wire is removed. Bone wedge has been removed from the base wedge osteotomy. Notice with meticulous handling the wedge is removed entoto and is seen here distal to the osteotomy void held in hemostat. Removal of the bone wedge from deep within the lateral margin of the metatarsal base is best facilitated by a dental hook as residual fragments here may impede osteotomy closure. This *feathering* of bone creates a malleable hinge that can be coapted and fixated without fracturing. If both cuts are made *onto* the pin, the axis will appear squared off once the pin is removed and the segment will be

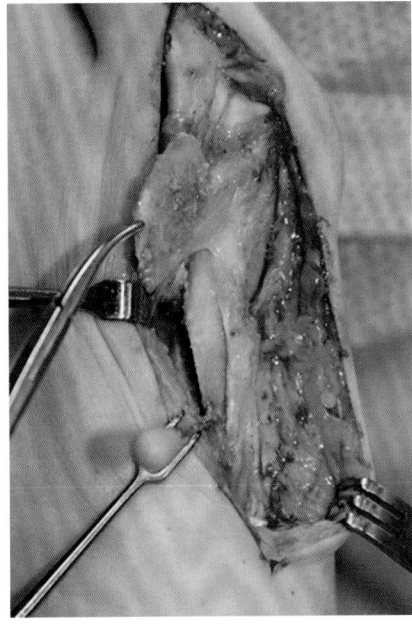

FIGURE 11.25 Bone wedge has been removed from the osteotomy.

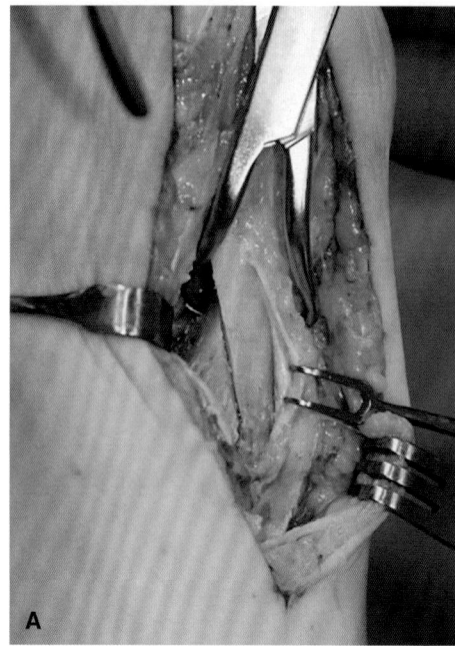
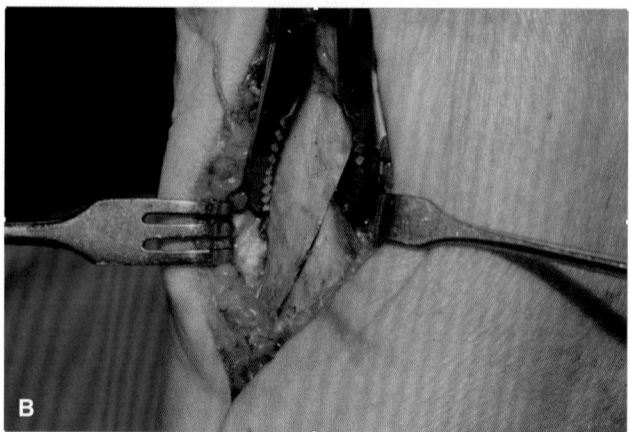

FIGURE 11.26 A. Double sharp bone clamp can be used to reduce the osteotomy when good bone stock is evident. **B.** In osteoporotic bone, an atraumatic style clamp may be preferred.

less pliable and at greater risk for fracture upon closure. When the cuts are made accurately, a small wedge of bone can be removed in to using a dental hook (Fig. 11.25). The axis guide is then removed and reciprocal planning of the osteotomy at its apex is completed. An atraumatic bone clamp is positioned out of the lines intended for fixation. Approaching the osteotomy from distal to proximal with the clamp allows closure of the parts while leaving the handles of the clamp distal on the first ray (Fig. 11.26). Caution is required if a double sharp tip bone clamp is used as it may overpenetrate in osteopenic or osteoporotic bone. Inadvertent overpenetration may well compromise fixation. Intraoperative fluoroscopy should be obtained in addition to clinical assessment of the IMA reduction, position, and alignment of the first ray segment. If greater reduction is needed further, reciprocal planning can be completed at this time.

INTERNAL FIXATION OBLIQUE CLOSING BASE WEDGE OSTEOTOMY

The angulation of the compression screws is dependent on the orientation of the osteotomy plane and the surface area available for fixation devices. A short oblique osteotomy will only facilitate a single screw and so mechanics of screw placement will be different from that of a long oblique osteotomy that has ample surface area to afford two points of fixation, **see Technique Tip #6.** The author prefers the long oblique osteotomy using a two-screw fixation technique; one as an anchor screw and the other as a compression screw. The size of the screw is selected based upon the width of the metatarsal and quality of bone. Alternatively, two 3.5-mm or 2.7-mm fully threaded cortical screws or a combination of these are alternatives. Partially threaded cancellous screws are preferred as the osteotomy plane lies predominantly in metaphyseal bone. **See anatomic considerations first metatarsal bone in this chapter.** In the case of a more narrowed metatarsal width, a smaller core diameter will be better suited

and will afford more threads for bone ingrowth, for example, 2.7-mm or 2.0-mm cortical screws, **see Technique Tip 7.**

1ˢᵗ Screw = Anchor Screw (Fig. 11.27A and B): This screw is placed in the most dorsal-proximal aspect of the medial metatarsal base and runs perpendicular to the long axis of the bone. *Predrill* using 1.6-mm K-wire checking that the angulation is accurate (Fig. 11.28). Create a *thread hole* using 2.5-mm drill (Fig. 11.29) followed by counter sinking in line with the thread hole (Fig. 11.30A), **see Technique Tip #8.**

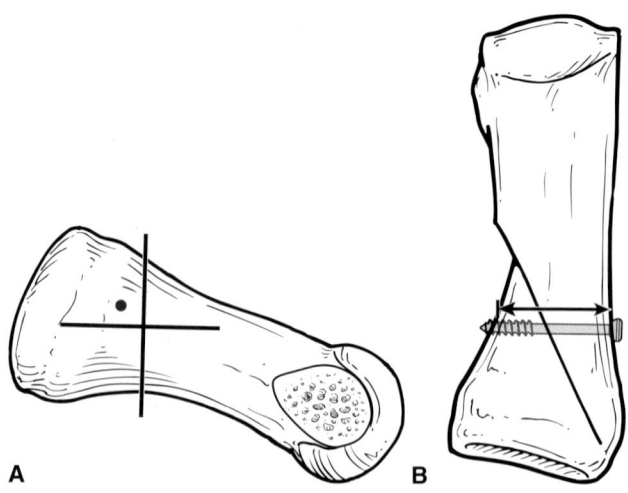

FIGURE 11.27 Diagrams for anchor screw placement. **A.** The metatarsal base is divided into quadrants where the anchor screw guide wire will be placed within the dorsal proximal quadrant. **B.** The screw will be oriented *perpendicular to the medial cortex* (not the osteotomy) to stabilize or anchor the proximal osteotomy hence the term "anchor screw." Notice that the bone in this region is purely metaphyseal and is >1 cm from the articulation.

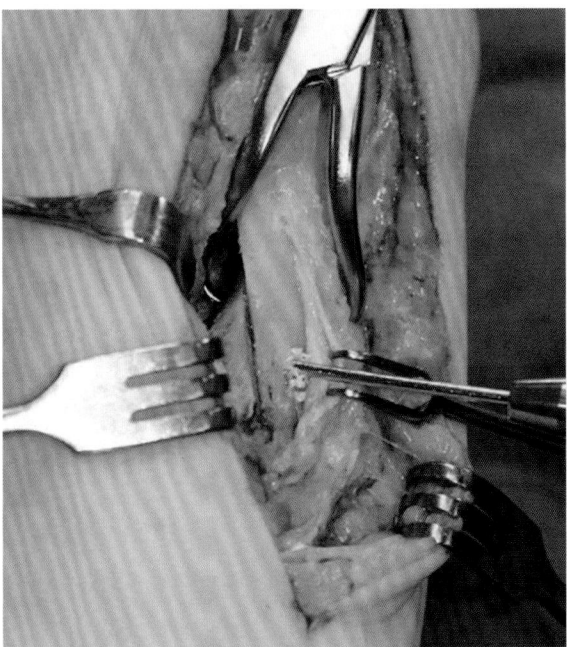

FIGURE 11.28 Notice that pre drilling is performed perpendicular to the medial cortex; the long axis of the metatarsal NOT perpendicular to the osteotomy. With adequate exposure, the guide wire will be seen as it exits the lateral cortex near to or within the proximal metaphyseal flare.

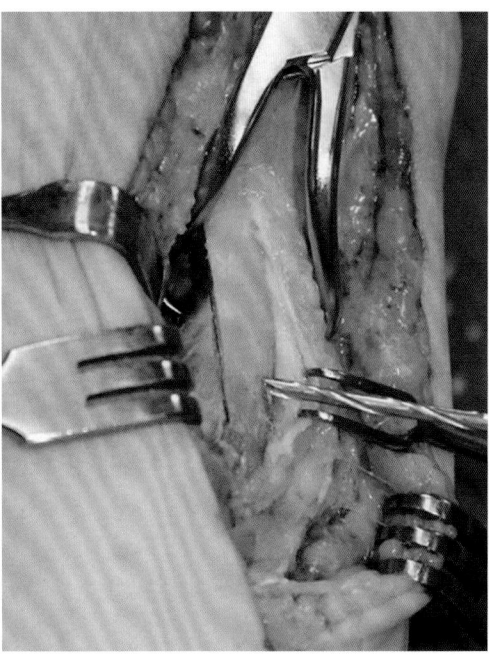

FIGURE 11.29 Application of the drill coaxial with the guide hole to ensure proper alignment of the screw.

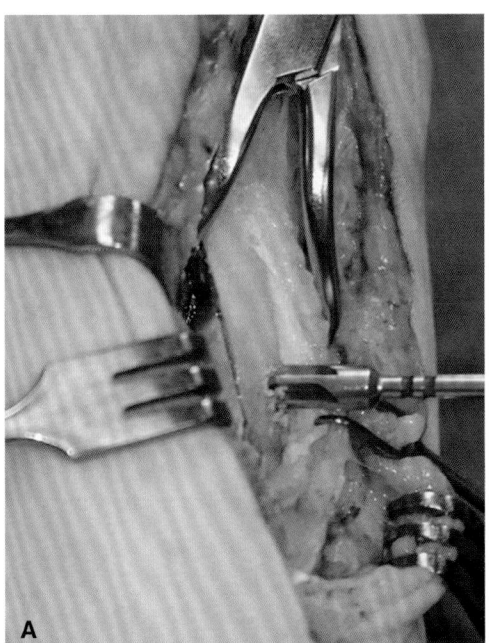

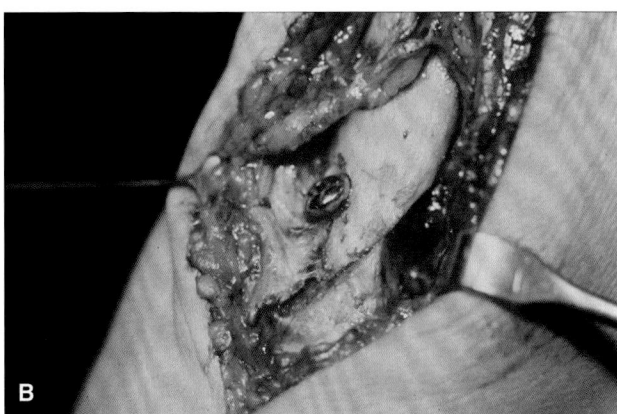

FIGURE 11.30 **A.** It is vastly important to countersink coaxial to the drill hole. When the countersink is offset, the land of the screw will not seat flush with the cortex. **B.** When the screw head is not seated flush to bone a stress riser will develop breeching the cortex and disrupts the stability of the screw. In this intraoperative photo, note the proximal migration of the distal bone segment as it ruptured the medial cortical and rotated the compression screw distracting the parts.

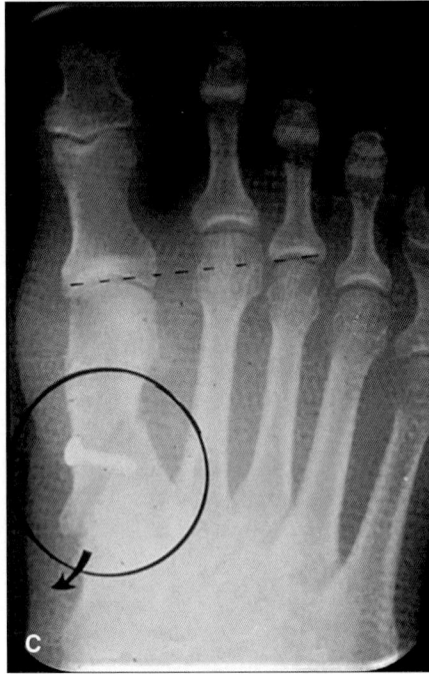

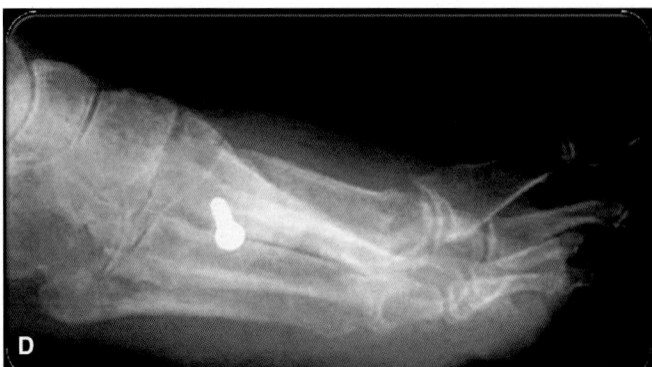

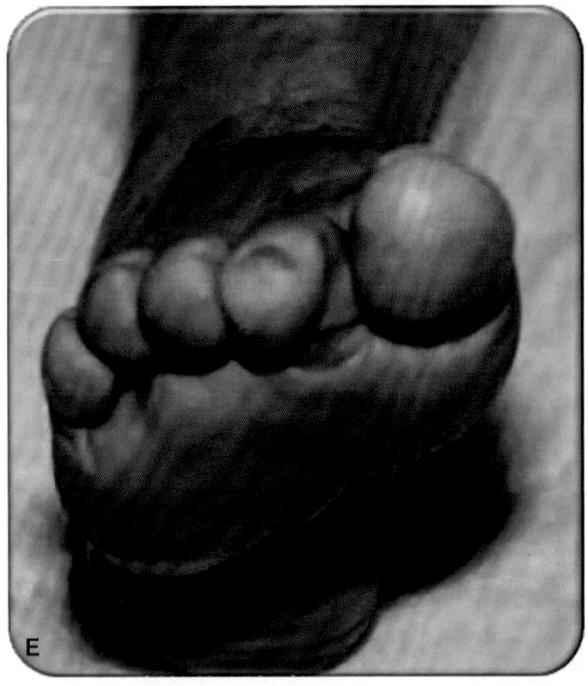

FIGURE 11.30 (*Continued*) **C.** Plain film radiograph documents hinge failure and the telescoping that creates a cortical breech resulting in shortening of the ray. In this instance, application of an anchor screw may have prevented this complication. Radiographically, the shortening of the metatarsal is significant and can be measured on the dorsal plantar view. **D.** The lateral radiograph depicts the severity of the sagittal plane malalignment. **E.** When plastic deformations occur at the hinge, the resultant damage and deformity is not compatible with weight-bearing function.

Visualize the *depth gauge* as it captures the most *proximal* lateral cortex to ensure proper screw length. If the distal lateral cortex is captured, the measure will be shorter than optimal and fixation will be less secure. Measurement of screw length is followed by use of a 4.0-mm *cancellous tap* (Fig. 11.31) **(Fig. 20.26 from 2nd ed Chapter 20 p. 514), see Technique Tip #9.** Finally, insertion of the 4.0-mm partially threaded screw is completed taking care not to over tighten (Fig. 11.32A and B). As the osteotomy is compressed, watch the hinge for evidence of

telescoping to prevent rupture. Overtightening increases the risk of hinge fracture. Definitive tightening of the anchor screw will be completed *after* insertion and final tightening of the compression screw.

2ⁿᵈ Screw = Compression Screw: (Fig. 11.33A and B): The instrumentation for this screw will be run oblique to the osteotomy and so penetration of the cortical margin can prove challenging. To facilitate this process, create the pre-drill hole perpendicular to the medial cortex then withdraw

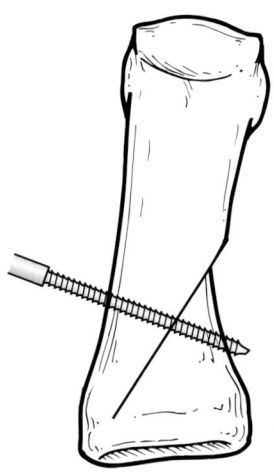

FIGURE 11.31 Using the 4.0-mm *cancellous tap*, a forward-reverse technique is used where the instrument is advanced three turns and is then reversed for one turn alternating to empty the flutes of bone with each reversal of the device.

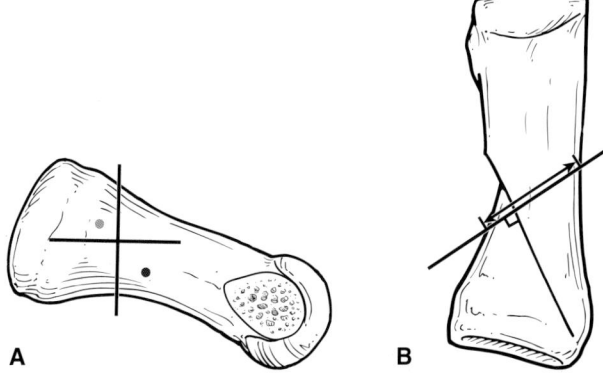

FIGURE 11.33 Diagram for compression screw placement. **A.** Notice the compression screw is applied within the distal plantar quadrant of the proximal metatarsal and is oriented obliquely to the bone. **B.** It is important to note that the screw hole is to be prepared perpendicular to the osteotomy to provide effective compression of the parts.

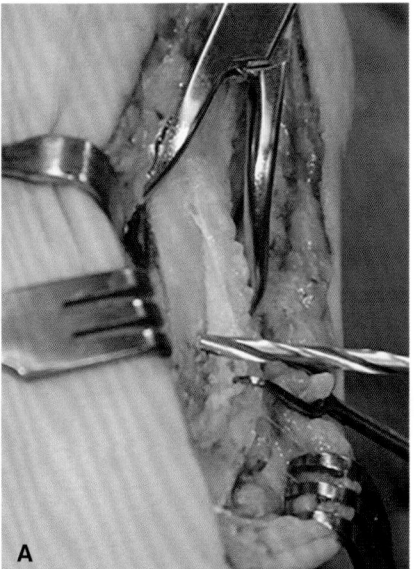

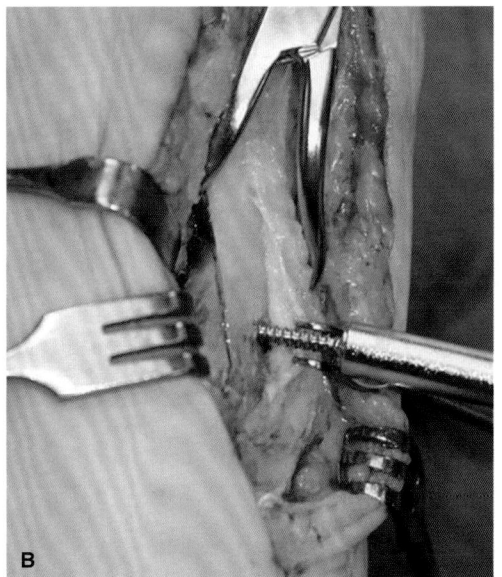

FIGURE 11.32 **A.** Drilling for anchor screw. **B.** When the anchor screw is inserted coaxial to the drill hole, this partially threaded cancellous screw will draw the lateral cortex medially compressing the parts with insertion. **C.** As the osteotomy is compressed and the screw head is seated flush to the cortex coaptation of the parts has now anchored the osteotomy in place without angulation of the screw head or gapping at the osteotomy site.

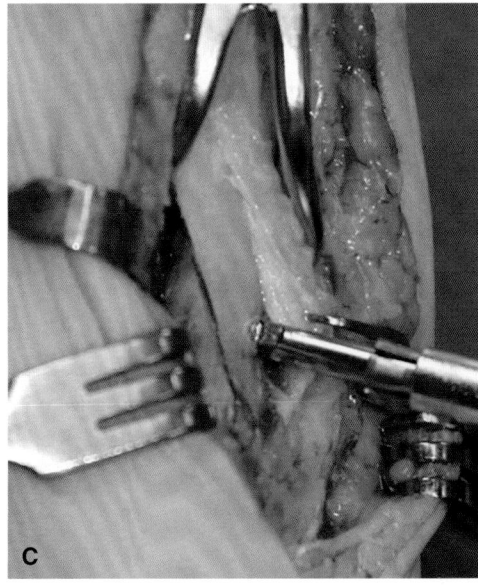

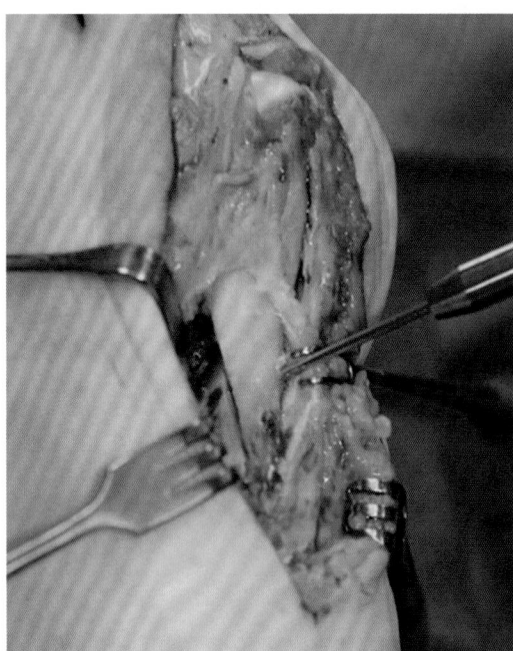

FIGURE 11.34 Notice that the predrill for the compression screw is angulated as it enters the medial cortex and penetrates perpendicular to the osteotomy site. This orientation best facilitates compression of the parts identical to fracture reduction principals.

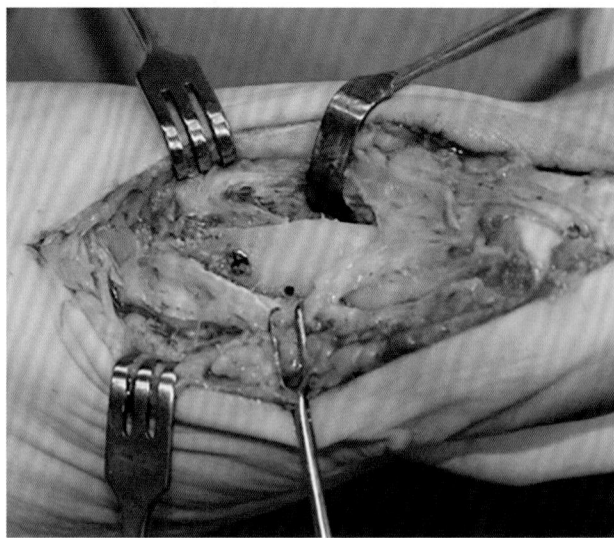

FIGURE 11.35 Seen here is the predrill holes for the anchor screw (dorsal proximal quadrant) and the compression screw (distal plantar quadrant). Notice that there is ample distal between these holes to assure seating of the screw heads without overlap or stress riser.

and redirect the wire to run perpendicular to the osteotomy (Fig. 11.34). This screw is placed in the distal-plantar quadrant of the medial metatarsal base oriented perpendicular to the osteotomy using the same technique as for the anchor screw described above (Fig. 11.35). Just as in tapping, it is important to maintain the appropriate orientation of the screw with insertion. With malalignment, the screw may glide along the inner lateral cortex and miss the intended thread hole. The compression screw is secured to *two finger tightness* followed by retightening the anchor screw (Fig. 11.36A and B). Final seating of the screws gently to two finger tightness will result in rigid coaptation of the parts without fracturing the hinge. The head of the screw should rest flush to bone and at least 1-2 full screw thread should be visualized penetrating the proximal lateral cortex. The bone clamp is removed and final radiographs can be obtained (Fig. 11.37A and B).

Closure of the periosteum is completed with undyed 3.0 absorbable suture. The periosteum is an important component of perfusion for the metatarsal base and so must be handled meticulously and delicately closed as a single layer covering the screw heads and the hinge at the conclusion of the procedure. The subcutaneous tissues and skin as separate layers after excellent hemostasis has been confirmed. Neurovascular status is rechecked prior to application of the dressing. A sterile bulky gauze dressing is applied to the foot positioned at 90 degrees to the leg and a modified Jones compression dressing is applied from the distal forefoot to the pretibial region. Finally, an eggshell fiberglass cast can be applied or alternatively a posterior splint of plaster or fiberglass or prefabricated non–weight-bearing boot may be applied to further encourage non–weight bearing postoperatively.

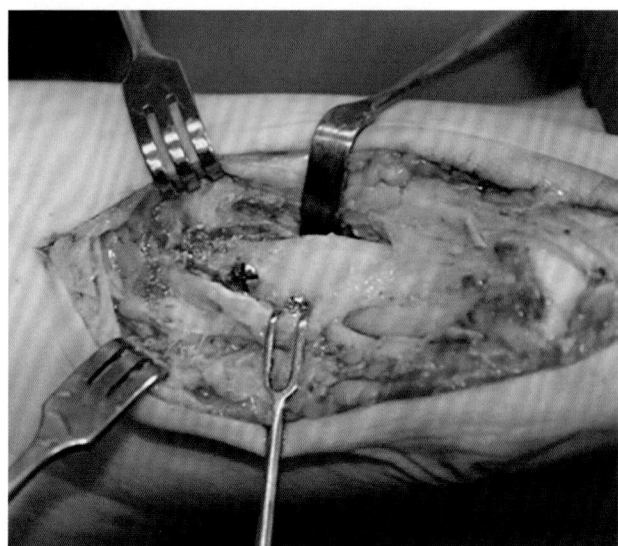

FIGURE 11.36 Final seating of the screw demonstrating sufficient spacing to allow compression of the parts with flush seating of the screw heads.

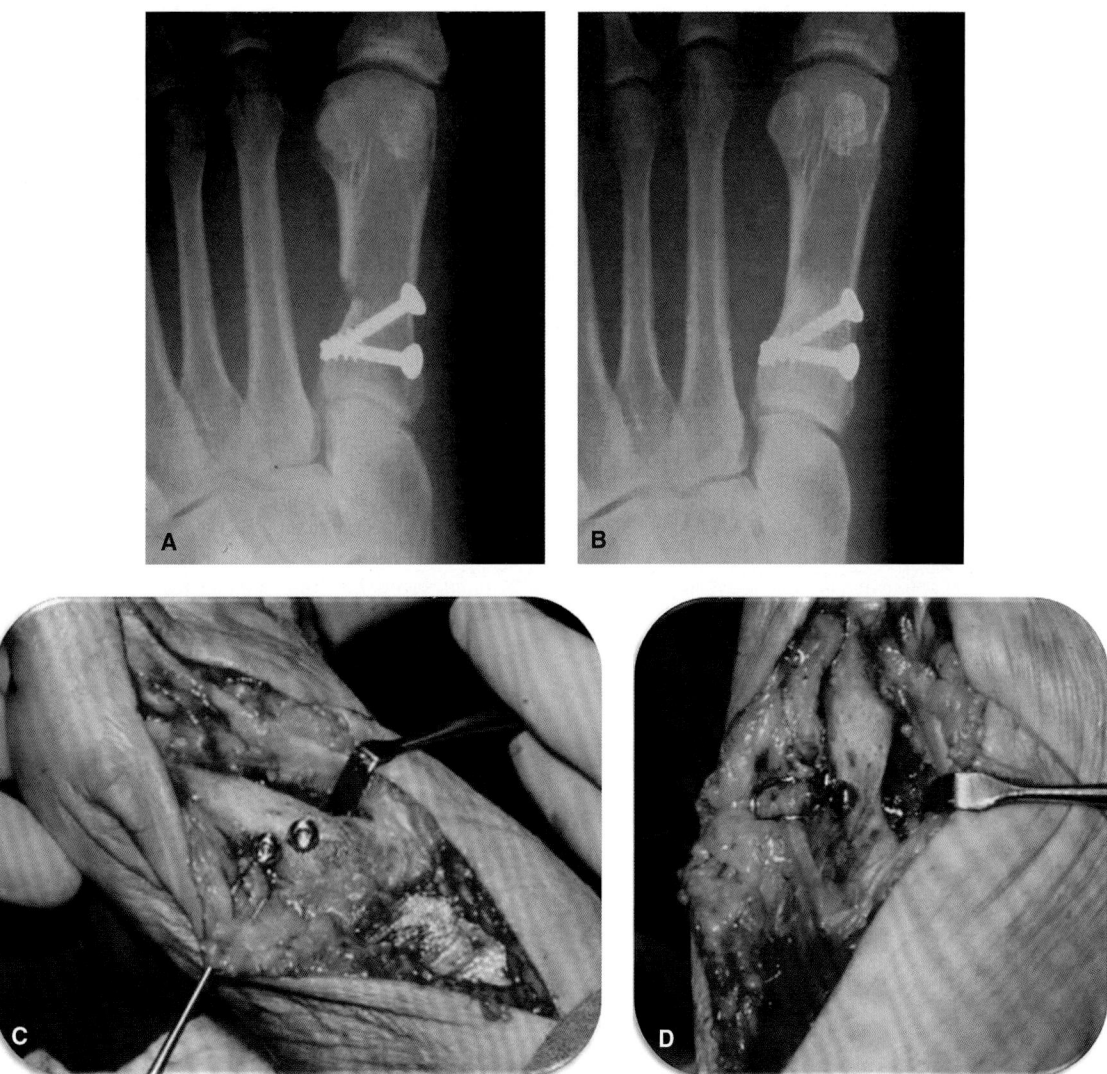

FIGURE 11.37 Plain film radiographs reveal position and alignment of the osteotomy and internal fixation devices immediate postoperative films **(A)** and long-term follow-up **(B)**. Recall that the screws are stacked in different planes; the anchor screw running dorsal within the transverse plane and the compression screw running obliquely through the sagittal plane **(C and D)**. This gives a false appearance of the screws colliding within the lateral margin of the osteotomy.

TECHNIQUE TIPS & ANATOMICAL CONSIDERATIONS

1. **Principals of the hinge axis in CBWO:** This concept should be studied in advance of practicing this technique in the laboratory using bone models or cadaver specimens. Once mastered in the lab, the technique can be employed reliably with predictable reduction of deformity (Fig. 11.20A-C). This information has been detailed thoroughly *refer to the 2nd edition McGlamry Comprehensive Textbook of Foot Surgery.*[34]
2. **Axis Guide:** The long oblique osteotomy is designed using an axis in the metatarsal base, the farther the axis is from the distal metatarsal ensures the longest radius arm for the base wedge. The longer the radius arm, the greater the reduction of the IMA. The larger the wedge, the greater the metatarsal heads arc of rotation as the osteotomy is closed.
3. Consider the anatomy of the first metatarsal base in preparing the osteotomy axis guide. The base of the metatarsal has a large cubic content of medullary bone providing for a flexible hinge. If the axis is placed too far distal into diaphyseal bone, the hinge will be rigid. This increases resistance to closure and risk of fracturing the hinge.
4. The axis guide is placed ~1 cm distal to the MCJ on the medial shoulder of the metatarsal base. The shape of the medial most base of the metatarsal is convex making placement of the axis guide challenging. Use of a spiked drill sleeve grips stabilizes the metatarsal bone at the medial summit of the metatarsal base allowing the K-wire to be driven perpendicular to the weight-bearing surface.
5. When the K-wire axis is run perpendicular to the weight-bearing surface, closure of the wedge will produce purely transverse plane reduction of the parts. If the K-wire is INADVERTENTLY run perpendicular to the bone dorsiflexion

(Continued)

TECHNIQUE TIPS & ANATOMICAL CONSIDERATIONS (*Continued*)

results with shortening, the metatarsal as the wedge is closed and the IMA is reduced. If the superior pole of the K-wire axis is tilted medially, closure of the wedge results in dorsiflexion of the parts. Alternatively, when the superior pole axis is tilted laterally, plantarflexion of the parts will result (Fig. 11.20A-C).

6. **(Refer to video 2019 CBWO hinge axis audio)**

7. **The first ray should be manipulated to identify the MCJ capsule.** An 18G hypodermic needle can be placed in the MCJ as a marker to prevent placing the axis guide too close to the joint. In the case of juvenile HAV, it is vastly important to check and recheck your anatomic landmarks to ensure that the growth plate within the base of the first metatarsal is not violated during the procedure.

8. **Reflection of the periosteum:** It often goes unnoticed that the two ends of a freer elevator are functionally distinct having both sharp and blunt ends. When the periosteum is thick and easily reflected from the bone, the blunt end can be used safely without buttonholing the periosteum. When the periosteum is thin and adhered to the bone, the sharp end will best facilitate reflection of the tissue. The importance of periosteal reflection, so called stripping, was reviewed and the notion that periosteal stripping would significantly decrease perfusion to bone was refuted.[18] In fact it was demonstrated that periosteal stripping results in dilatation of periosteal vessels increasing perfusion and yields a positive impact on primary bone healing.[19]

9. **Bone cuts;** *Measure Twice Cut Once:* The proximal bone cut determines the angulation of the osteotomy and ultimately dictates whether the osteotomy is transverse or oblique in nature. An error in performing the proximal cut of the osteotomy will negatively impact the procedure. To avoid error, the plan for these bone cuts should be scored in the dorsal cortex using a sagittal saw or osteotome. This serves as a litmus test for determining the size and shape of the osteotomy. Once the osteotomy has been scored in the dorsal cortex and appropriate size and shape of the osteotomy is confirmed, then the bone cuts can be made with confidence.

    Proper angulation of the proximal arm of the osteotomy is critical to the internal fixation plan. If the proximal arm is cut too acutely (more than 45 degrees from the long axis of the metatarsal), the osteotomy will be more transverse and the final osteotomy plane will be shortened reducing the surface area for fixation. The distal cut is angulated to achieve an appropriate degree of IMA reduction (Fig. 11.21A-C).

10. **Bone cuts; Which arm of the osteotomy do you cut first?:** When scoring the bone, the proximal line is scored first as this will determine the plane of the osteotomy and predetermines the space available for fixation. The most proximal bone cut is performed first for this same reason. The proximal metatarsal is stabilized by the metatarsal cuneiform ligaments and remains stable as the proximal bone cut is completed.

11. **Closure of the osteotomy:** A bone clamp is used to facilitate and maintain closure of the osteotomy. When there is resistance to closure, the apex of the osteotomy may feel stiff creating tension at the medial hinge. If this occurs, *feathering* or further planing of the osteotomy is required. In this event, the saw blade is passed within the osteotomy removing a very small amount of bone nearing the site of the axis guide. When sufficient bone has been removed, the hinge will become more malleable and the osteotomy will close

without tension. This feathering maneuver takes finesse to master. Practice using bone models or cadaver specimens is most prudent.

12. **Orientations in two lag screw technique:**
    1st Screw = Anchor Screw: This screw is placed in the most dorsal-proximal quadrant of the medial metatarsal base and runs perpendicular to the long axis of the bone. In the event of hinge failure, any proximal shift or telescoping of the distal fragment would be countered by the presence of the first screw, hence the term *anchor screw*. Note the proximal migration of the distal segment as it ruptured the medial cortical and rotated the compression screw distracting the parts. The shortening of the metatarsal is significant in this event (Fig. 11.27A and B).

    2nd Screw = Compression Screw: This screw is placed in the distal-plantar quadrant of the medial metatarsal base running perpendicular to the osteotomy (Fig. 11.33A and B). With the screw-oriented perpendicular to the osteotomy, it provides compression of the parts without stressing the medial hinge. Notice from the diagram (Fig. 11.33A), these screws are stacked in separate planes and will not collide when strict attention is given to the application technique.

13. **Counter Sinking:** Countersinking is designed to allow seating of the *land* of the screw head flush into the cortical margin during screw insertion. If countersinking is not deep enough to seat the head or is misaligned, then the distal edge of the screw head will contact the bone first and will shift the shaft of the screw proximally compromising the medial cortical hinge and fixation of the parts (Fig. 11.30B and C).

14. **Tap:** Use of the tap sleeve will protect soft tissues from entanglement. When using the tap, a *forward-reverse* technique (3-turns forward then 2-turns in reverse to clear the flutes) will allow bone removal from the flutes as the instrument progresses toward the opposite cortex. As with using the depth gauge, it is important to visualize the tap to ensure that it exits the lateral cortex and does not advance into the second ray. If the tap overpenetrates the lateral cortex, it may strip the medial threads destabilizing the screw.

15. **Cortical screws used as lag screws:** In smaller or more narrow bone, a cortical screw can be used to achieve compression by modifying the technique. Recall that *the core diameter of the 3.5-mm cortical screw and the 4.0-mm cancellous screw are the same (2.5 mm); however, the pitch of their threads is decidedly different 1.25 and 1.75 mm, respectively.* To achieve compression with a 3.5-mm fully threaded cortical screw, it requires the use of a 2.5-mm thread hole and appropriate countersink. Next prepare a 3.5-mm glide hole in the *near cortex only* (medial cortex). This drill hole is larger than that of the larger cancellous screw (3.2 mm). *This should be considered as it may reduce the strength of the medial cortex.* The combination of a small cortical screw (3.5 or 2.7) with a larger 4.0-mm cancellous screw can be entertained as an alternative. Measurement for the screw is always done before tapping to avoid damaging the cut of the threads with the depth gauge. Use the 3.5-mm *cortical tap* (remember the pitch of the threads are smaller; 1.25 mm) to cut the thread. The 3.5-mm cortical screw of appropriate measure is applied in line with the threads ensuring capture of the lateral cortex with 1-2 threads exposed upon seating the screw head. As the screw is driven compression across the osteotomy is

TECHNIQUE TIPS & ANATOMICAL CONSIDERATIONS (*Continued*)

appreciated. When cortical screws are used and *the hinge fails, the distal bone telescopes proximally causing the cortical screw to rotate and distract the parts further compromising the osteotomy.* Cortical screws have some advantages over cancellous screws. The cortical screw can be replaced with a larger screw if the technique should fail. Because they are fully threaded, cortical screws cut their way out of cortical bone as they are removed. Smaller cortical screws are preferable in dense bone typical of adolescents or young adults.

16. **Supplemental Fixation:** This technique of cerclage wire enhancement, popularized by John Ruch, DPM of the Podiatry

Institute, Georgia, should be considered as an addition to the CBWO procedure to enhance stability and long-term performance of the construct. In the untoward event of hinge, fracture or other failure in technique that may compromise stability supplemental fixation should be considered. Using monofilament wire, a cerclage wire is secured between the 2 compression screws of the CBWO. This serves to protect the construct against untoward weight bearing that could cause a retrograde translation of force against the hinge of the CBWO. Figure 11.38A-C illustrates the technique and diagrams stress as applied along a supplemental cerclage wire in the CBWO.

INDICATIONS AND PITFALLS

- **HAV with high IMA:** The long radius arm (the distance between the proximal axis and the distal metatarsal) allows for greater correction of the deformity while preventing overcorrection (prevents negative IMA). The metatarsal will only close down until parallel to the 2nd metatarsal. In a distal osteotomy, extreme lateral translocation of the head can create a negative IMA and increase the risk of residual varus deformity.

- **Juvenile hallux abductovalgus deformity:** Not uncommonly HAV deformity in the juvenile is associated with a flexible deformity and residual metatarsus adductus, which can result in a mismatch between clinical findings and radiographic appearance of the deformity. Often the radiographs are far less impressive than the clinical condition. Short-term failure of distal osteotomy procedures in these cases is the result of insufficient reduction of transverse plane deformity, residual metatarsus adductus in the face of continued bone growth, and change in habitus with time.

- **Metatarsus primus elevatus (MPE):** By tilting the axis guide and resecting a small wedge of bone at the metatarsal base, the metatarsal segment can be shifted plantarly eliminating elevatus while restoring stability to the MTPJ. If a distal osteotomy was modified to achieve a similar degree of plantarflexion, the abrupt change in the vectors of the extensor and flexor tendons as they cross the MTPJ could shift the muscle tendon balance toward extension resulting in hallux extensus and a nonpurchasing or cock-up deformity. A CBWO can be modified to correct a plantarflexed first ray segment by modifying the placement of the axis guide.

- **Radiographic evaluation of MPE (lateral view):** Care must be taken to obtain weight-bearing radiographs *reproducibly* in weight-bearing angle and gait with the tube head parallel to the weight-bearing surface. It has been demonstrated that when the tube head is angled 10 degrees upward (for the lateral view), the ray will appear dorsiflexed. Note the amount of separation of the first and second metatarsals, while the angular relationship between these two bones remains constant. Conversely, when the tube head is angled downward by 10 degrees, the ray will appear plantarflexed.[33]

- **Plastic deformation causing metatarsus primus elevatus (MPE):** Premature weight bearing can cause plastic deformation of bone and/or rupture of the medial hinge resulting in elevation of the distal metatarsal (Fig. 11.30D).[36]

- **Rigid deformity:** An isolated intermetatarsal release and capsular reefing is unlikely to affect the final position of the ray in rigid deformities and is unable to counteract the pronatory forces of weight bearing and hallux abduction at the MTPJ.

- **Proximal articular set angle:** In rare events, deviation of the articular cartilage may contribute to hallux deviation and requires a distal realignment procedure such as a Reverdin or Austin.

- **Patient selection:** Patient selection is not based upon deformity alone. The patient profile; personality, health, physique, and profession will also influence the outcome in surgery. In patient selection also consider the flexibility of the deformity, the sagittal plane position of the metatarsal, the patients age, ability to remain non–weight bearing, the patients activity goals, required activities, concomitant foot and ankle deformities, as well as more proximal musculoskeletal deformities affecting base and gait.

- **Metatarsus primus elevatus (MPV):** When metatarsal primus elevatus exists, a CBWO osteotomy can produce plantar deflection of the metatarsal based upon the hinge-axis principal. Strict attention to detail in modifying the axis of rotation of the osteotomy will allow for plantarflexion.

- **Premature weight bearing:** Despite advances in A-O (Arbeitsgemeinschaft für Osteosynthesefragen) technique, no internal fixation devices are expected to counter the unsupported stresses of weight bearing especially in the case of a proximal metatarsal osteotomy. Dorsiflexion and distraction of the parts are often the result of premature and untoward weight bearing resulting in malunion, delayed, or nonunion of bone and dysfunction.

- **Insufficient internal fixation:** Failure to use strict A-O technique when applying the anchor and compression screws may result in available motion about the osteotomy disrupting primary bone healing. This sets the stage then for secondary bone healing (healing by callus formation) setting the stage for malunion, delayed, or nonunion of bone.

(*Continued*)

INDICATIONS AND PITFALLS (*Continued*)

- **Inherent metatarsal shortening:** Since there is bone loss with every pass of the sagittal saw, it is often beneficial to slightly plantarflex the osteotomy to counteract the small amount of shortening that is inherent to the bone cuts. Given the declination of the first metatarsal, every millimeter excised results in dorsiflexion (elevation) of the part. The residual metatarsal segment being shorter rests more dorsal in the sagittal plane (Fig. 11.1). When considering the shortening associated with removal of a wedge of bone, there are specific geometric considerations. The mathematics behind this have been thoroughly discussed and generally it is accepted that with removal of a 5-degree wedge of bone, there is 1.1-mm shortening. If a much larger segment is removed 15-degree wedge, there is a predictable 2.5 mm of shortening.[16]

- **Increased metatarsal shortening:** This risk is increased when there is a breech in the technique. There are many steps integral to the success of this technique as mentioned in the Technique Tips. Among those affecting the final metatarsal length are improper placement of the axis guide, errors in cutting the bone resulting in weakness, excess rigidity or fracture of the hinge, errors in executing screw preparation and insertion, over aggressive counter sinking weakening the medial cortical margin of bone affecting the hinge, and premature weight bearing just to name a few. All of these untoward events may lead to increased dorsiflexion of the metatarsal,

distraction of the osteotomy, failure of internal fixation devices (the hinge among them), and resultant shortening, malunion of bone, and dysfunction at the MTPJ.

- **Complications of the CBWO:** As with all osteotomy procedures, there is a risk of infection of soft tissue or bone, malunion, delayed union, and nonunion of bone. Soft tissue complications may include dehiscence, painful or unsightly scar, neuritis, and nerve entrapment among others. While shortening and metatarsus primus elevatus are most commonly associated with the CBWO, Lagaay et al. compared the complication rates between the Austin, CBWO, and Lapidus and found no statistically significant difference between them.[37]

- **Overcorrection of deformity** (large negative IMA): If wedge of bone resected is excessively large, overcorrection of the first ray position will be evidenced by a negative IMA. In this event, a bone graft may be required to achieve the desired correction.[36] If the wedge of bone removed was preserved that autogenous bone could be planed and reinserted to reduce overcorrection.

- **Undercorrection of deformity:** When the wedge osteotomy is cut too small, the metatarsal will fail to reduce in the transverse plane. This will require replanning of the distal cut of the osteotomy. Caution in manipulating the metatarsal to achieve this effect as over manipulation can result in rupture of the hinge and will complicate fixation.

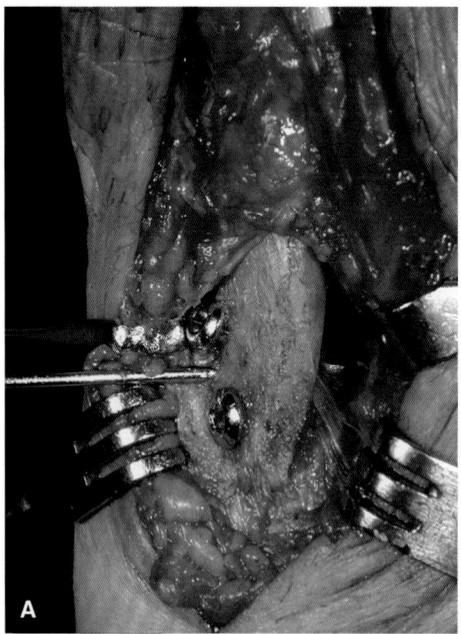 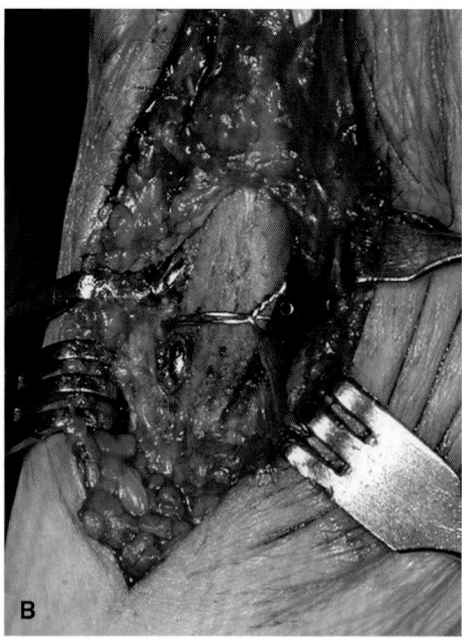 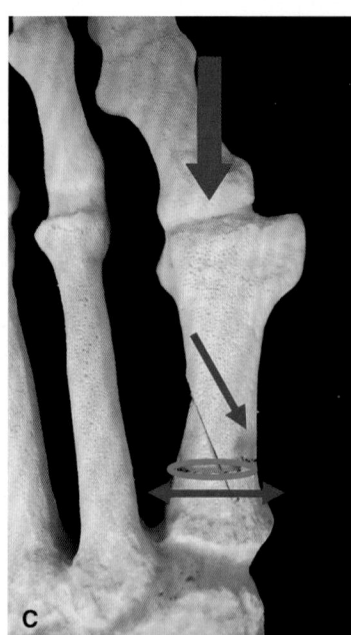

FIGURE 11.38 **A.** The principles in applying a supplemental cerclage wire. When the cerclage wire is secured through the transverse plane, it stabilizes the hinge supplementing the anchor screw. The wire is secured perpendicular to the bisection of the metatarsal once the osteotomy is closed. Intraoperative photo of drilling for the cerclage wire. **B.** Shown here is a double banding of the wire through the proximal metatarsal. Using a compromised technique (the osteotomy is already compressed), tensioning the wire and burying the free end completes the process. **C.** With an axial force, the stress is translated medially challenging the hinge. The cerclage wire will resist stress as it reinforces the medial hinge.

POSTOPERATIVE CARE

Regardless of the technique used, fixation of the CBWO is not designed to withstand weight bearing, **see Technique Tip #15: Supplemental fixation**. Non–weight bearing should be maintained for a minimum of 6 weeks with sufficient evidence of bone healing evident in serial radiographs simulating weight-bearing conditions. The use of antithrombotics during this period is dependent upon the individuals' risk factors. In general, recommendations for passive range of motion exercises for the MTPJ and active exercises for muscle contractions in the thigh and calf are of benefit. Removable posterior splints, bivalved casts, and removable non–weight-bearing braces will facilitate this process. Options for use during the non–weight-bearing period include crutches, knee roller, and modified walkers with knee stands among others. Integral to a successful postoperative course is appropriate selection of the assistive device and this is dependent on the patient's baseline balance, coordination, upper body strength, strength of the contralateral limb, and competence in understanding the purpose and importance of the non–weight-bearing plan. If erythema, calor, swelling, tenderness, or a combination of these are present, then non–weight bearing should continue until these outward signs are resolved. Erythema and calor beyond the time of primary wound healing are most suspicious of infection and or symptomatic nonunion of bone. When this occurs, instability of fixation or premature weight bearing may be suspected. Serial radiographs and a keen clinical acumen are essential when determining sufficient bone healing to begin advancement of the weight-bearing process.

REHABILITATION

Range of motion exercises, passive and active, can be encouraged for the first MTPJ in a non–weight-bearing attitude once wound healing has been completed. In general, recommendations for passive range of motion exercises for the MTPJ and active exercises for muscle contractions in the thigh and calf are of benefit. Removable posterior splints, bivalved casts, and removable non–weight-bearing braces will facilitate this process.

In conclusion, the base wedge osteotomy is a powerful procedure that has an important role in the treatment of moderate to high angle bunion deformity in appropriate patients. The procedure is technically challenging as it requires a deep mechanical understanding of the hinge axis concept and A-O technique as well as manual dexterity and finesse. Mastery of this technique requires practice to meet the challenges of the steep learning curve.

Video: Mechanics of the hinge axis concept and fundamental screw placement.

CRESCENTIC OSTEOTOMY

DEFINITION

Popularized in the 1990s, the crescentic technique is a proximal osteotomy requiring a special blade to create a concavity in the base of the metatarsal allowing triplanal rotation of the entire distal metatarsal to reduce deformity.[38] These pestle in mortar shapes allow for triplane motion when re-establishing the position of the metatarsal segment; however, reduction and stabilization of the parts proves challenging as many authors can attest 1-4. Consequently, the osteotomy design has been modified overtime to enhance stability and reduce the risk of stress risers with fixation of the construct.

The great liberty that the osteotomy allows in transverse plane motion is countered by instability and poor reproducibility in sagittal plane positioning. Brodsky reported this downfall when prospectively studying plantar pressures in 43 procedures over an average of 29 months follow-up. Despite surgical expertise, a 20% incidence of increased pressure beneath the second metatarsal head was reported.[39] Primary complications associated with the crescentic osteotomy have been reported with an incidence as high as 40% and include shortening, delayed union, malunion, or difficulty in fixation causing metatarsal elevatus among others.[38,40] In an attempt to improve the stability of the osteotomy and minimize the risk of complications, modifications to the crescentic osteotomy have been made. These include the addition of a plantar shelf and reversing the orientation of the crescentic cut. Using a plantar shelf, the osteotomy is stabilized and the surface area for internal fixation has been optimized. By reversing the direction of the ball and socket (socket distal), the direction of the force in translocating the osteotomy is changed from medial to lateral along the first ray.[41-44] The lateral border of the first ray being more stable as it is buttressed by the second ray.

INDICATIONS

- High angle IMA deformity including triplane deformity of the first metatarsal associated with HAV, metatarsus primus elevatus congenital or iatrogenic, and rigid or semi rigid plantarflexed first metatarsal.
- Absence of osteoarthritis within the first MTPJ and TMTJ.
- Hypermobility at the MCJ has historically been an indicator for arthrodesis of that joint; however, it has been demonstrated that this hypermobility can be reduced after the benefit of a proximal first metatarsal osteotomy.[45]

ANATOMIC FEATURES

1. Consider the *crescentic shape* of the first metatarsal base as the lateral flare rides beneath the proximal medial border of the second metatarsal that at times obscuring the intermetatarsal joint on the plain film. This anatomy is important especially when determining the level for the bone cut for the crescentic osteotomy. The first metatarsal base flare has *two discrete facets*; one articulates with the medial base of the second while the other provides articulation with the cartilage of the inferior surface of the first (medial) cuneiform (Fig. 11.1). This lateral flare rests much more plantar than the medial flare and so is deeper within the intermetatarsal vault (Fig. 11.20). When running the compression screw, this flare provides bone volume to facilitate screw thread capture and compression of the base while providing bone for ingrowth about the screw during primary bone healing.

2. Consider the declination of the first metatarsal from the lateral view. For every millimeter of metatarsal bone excised from the excursion of the saw blade elevation results (Fig. 11.1).

3. Consider the total girth of the distal aspect of the proximal one-third of the metatarsal bone. If the concavity of the proximal cut is narrow due to the size of the crescentic blade, the total lateral excursion available to the distal segment is limited. If, however, a crescentic blade wider than the metatarsal base is used, then a greater degree of lateral excursion is available when the bone is rotated lateralward[46] **Technical Tip #4.**

FUNCTIONAL ANALYSIS OF THE ANATOMY

Consider the *dorsal proximal cut of the crescentic osteotomy* in the base of the first metatarsal bone. If the crescentic blade is oriented to cut a *concavity in the proximal metatarsal base*, it creates a ball in cup morphology from distal to proximal. When the distal metatarsal (ball) is rotated lateralward, a retrograde line of pressure is created within the medial aspect of the proximal osteotomy (the ball rotates within the cup creating maximal stress at the medial border of the cup). This force creates a line of stress, potentially a stress riser, that can destabilize the proximal medial aspect of the construct (Fig. 11.39A). A similar relationship is noted when considering the ball and cup articulation of the talonavicular joint (TNJ). The articulation is more stable in a cavus foot where the talus rests lateralward within the navicular cup. The lateral structures of the midfoot are a buttress to the TNJ. As opposed to the hyperpronated foot where there are no adjacent osseous structures to stabilize the talar head as it rotates medially out of the navicular mortise.

Alternatively, if the crescentic blade is oriented to cut a *convexity in the proximal metatarsal base*, it creates a ball in cup morphology from proximal to distal. When the distal metatarsal is rotated lateralward, a retrograde line of pressure along the lateral aspect of the proximal osteotomy (the cup is rotated lateral ward on the ball) is countered (stabilized) by the adjacent second metatarsal base[44] (Fig. 11.39B).

PHYSICAL EXAMINATION

Described earlier in the chapter under CBWO.

TREATMENT

Nonoperative Treatment

Conservative therapy can include insole modifications or, more predictably, prescription orthotic devices can be prepared to rebalance the forefoot as an alternative to surgical intervention. When an elevatus is present, the prescription should provide relief beneath the 5th metatarsal head with a partial fill beneath the first metatarsal. Options in orthotic materials include semiflexible polypropylene, copolymers, poly-laminates, or cork-based prescriptions. Accommodation of the rigid first ray can be achieved using a medial forefoot wedge. Should orthotic therapy fail the proximal first metatarsal osteotomy can provide predictable and reproducible results with strict attention to the details of the technique. Postoperatively, orthotic therapy to support the arch and reduce weight bearing imbalance can optimize long-term function.

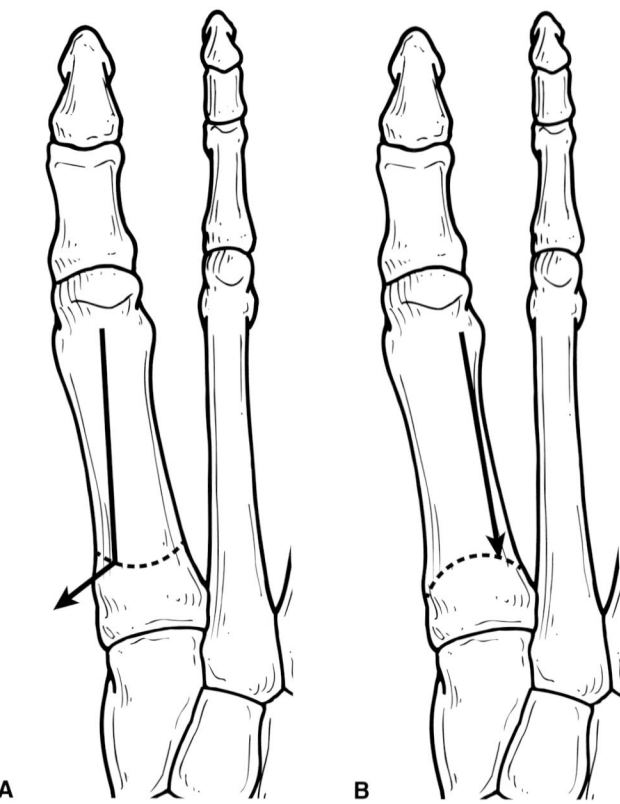

FIGURE 11.39 Considerations in performing the crescentic osteotomy; creating a convexity or concavity at the metatarsal shaft determines the contact area for aligning the osteotomy and impacts stability and axial loading of the ray. **A.** When a convexity is made in the proximal shaft, an axial load will propagate stress along the medial ray and out the proximal medial aspect of the contact area; the less stable side of the ray. **B.** As an alternative, creating a concavity in the proximal metatarsal shaft increases the surface area of contact and improves the cubic content of bone available for fixation. With axial loading, the stress propagates along the lateral more stable border of the osteotomy and is buttressed by the second metatarsal.

AUTHORS PREFERRED TREATMENT

The authors preferred technique is a modified crescentic shelf osteotomy described by numerous authors to enhance stability and reduce the risk of elevatus upon return to weight bearing.[41-44] The plantar shelf is made within the proximal metaphysis creating a surface area to stabilize the osteotomy against elevation and enhance fixation (Fig. 11.40).

The crescentic osteotomy requires a special crescentic blade to create a convexity in the base of the metatarsal allowing triplanar rotation of the entire distal metatarsal to reduce deformity. The convexity being proximal allows for a long distal segment that provides ample excursion as the osteotomy is rotated. In making a convex cut within the proximal metatarsal base, a matching concavity is created for the distal (free) segment. Given this ball-in-cup configuration, the distal segment can be manipulated like a joystick on the base. Given the saw blade width, there is minimal yet predictable shortening typically 1-2 mm. This procedure requires rigid internal fixation that should be protected with absolute non–weight bearing to achieve primary bone healing. The literature will suggest

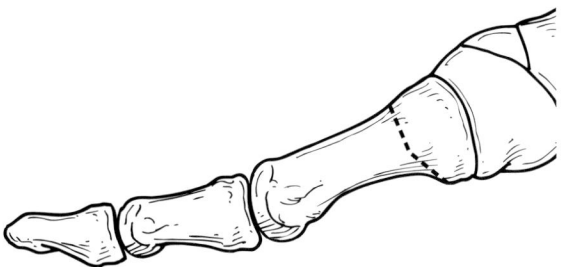

FIGURE 11.40 The plantar shelf is made within the proximal metaphysis creating a surface area to stabilize the osteotomy against elevation and enhance fixation. The dotted line indicates the plantar shelf for a crescentic osteotomy as modified by Carpenter et al. Similar to alternative constructs where the shelf extends distally within cortical bone of the metatarsal shaft (see Fig. 11.47A and B), this shelf is located more proximally creating a more stout and stable shelf in metaphyseal bone.

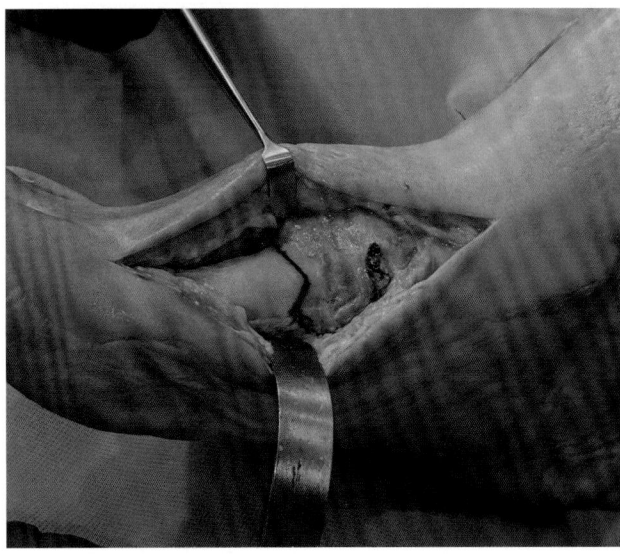

FIGURE 11.41 The angulation of the plantar cut can be seen in this cadaveric model.

good benefit from the procedure and further reveals the steep learning curve associated with it.[42,47-58]

It is the surgeon's preference when and if to perform an intermetatarsal release. The skin incision and dissection required to perform an intermetatarsal space release are described in the section on hallux abducto valgus deformity and the distal metatarsal osteotomy.

In preparation for the proximal crescentic osteotomy, a dorsal linear incision is begun 1 cm proximal to the MCJ and extends ~3-5 cm distally to expose the metatarsal base allowing for wide exposure and ease of soft tissue retraction. The incision length will vary with the size of the anatomy and the girth of the soft tissues. When the soft tissue envelop is thick, a longer incision may be required to facilitate exposure. A linear periosteal incision completes exposure of the metatarsal base. Use a freer elevator to bluntly reflect the periosteum. The periosteum of bone is a major source of perfusion facilitating primary bone healing and so is handled meticulously and is tagged for later closure, see **Technique Tip #1.**

Periosteal Incision

Before the osteotomy is prepared, a plantar shelf is created from a medial to lateral direction and is made as close to parallel as possible to the weight-bearing surface with a sagittal saw (Fig. 11.41), **see Technique Tip #2.** This plantar shelf exits the metatarsal proximal to the planned placement of the crescentic osteotomy and distal to the first MCJ. After this shelf is completed, the crescentic blade is used to create the osteotomy in the superior two-thirds of the metatarsal.

The osteotomy is scored using the crescentic blade 1.5-2 cm distal to the MCJ to afford the longest radius arm of the osteotomy. Contrary to the original description of this technique, the author prefers to orient the blade to create a convexity within the metatarsal base (ball in the metatarsal base) (Fig. 11.42A and B), **see Technique Tip #3.**

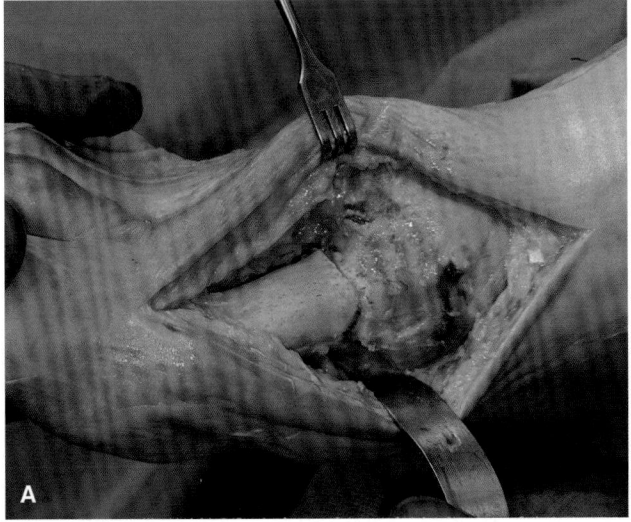
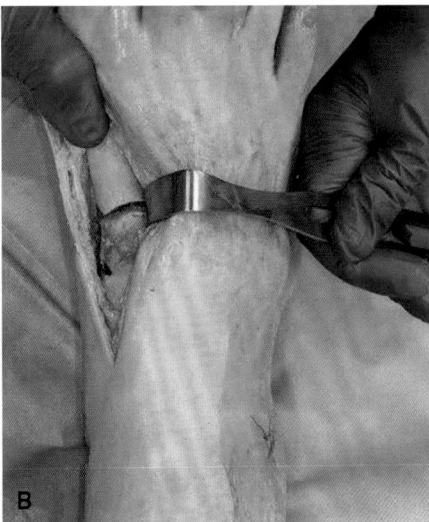

FIGURE 11.42 Contrary to the original description of this technique, the author prefers to orient the blade to create a convexity within the metatarsal base (ball in the metatarsal base) shown in **(A)** medial and **(B)** dorsal plantar perspectives.

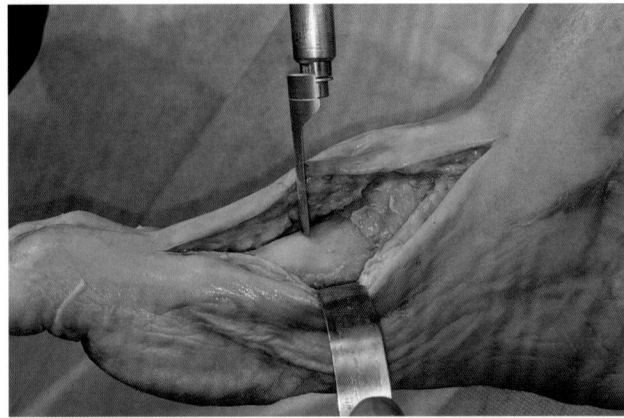

FIGURE 11.43 The blade is tilted slightly toward the sesamoids to create a slight plantar tilt to prevent an iatrogenic elevatus as seen in this cadaveric model.

A *specialized oscillating blade* is selected as appropriate for the size of the metatarsal base, **see Technique Tip #4: Preparation of the bone cut.** The oscillating saw blade is first positioned perpendicular to the weight-bearing surface. *The hand is tilted slightly lateral and the tip of the blade angled slightly toward the sesamoid apparatus to affect slight plantarflexion* countering the shortening effect inherent to the bone cut (Fig. 11.43).[46] Normal saline is applied to the oscillating saw blade during the osteotomy cut to prevent overheating and thermal necrosis of bone. Continuous irrigation during the cuts is prudent as it preserves bone quality and promotes primary bone healing. With liberation of the parts, the metatarsal can be rotated like a pestle in mortar or "joystick." The proximal metatarsal can be medialized using a dental hook while the distal metatarsal is manually translocated lateralward until parallel with the second metatarsal. Slight plantarflexion is typically desired.[58] Provisional stabilization with a 0.062 K-wire is completed running from dorsal proximal to plantar distal within the central metatarsal base and across the osteotomy (Fig. 11.44). A second 0.062 K-wire

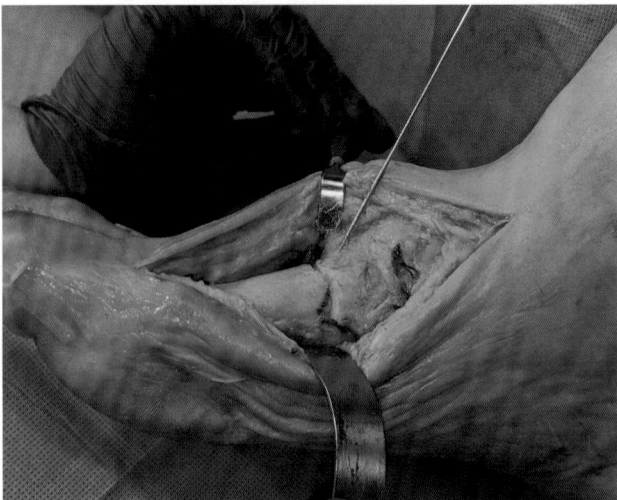

FIGURE 11.44 Provisional stabilization with a 0.062 K-wire is completed running from dorsal proximal to plantar distal within the central metatarsal base and across the osteotomy. Notice the plantar shelf coapted at the inferior surface of the crescentic cut.

is placed distal to the osteotomy running from the medial shaft of the first metatarsal into the shaft of the second metatarsal stabilizing the segment for definitive fixation, **see Technique Tip #5: Provisional fixation.** Intraoperative fluoroscopy is used to confirm position and alignment in multiple orthogonal planes prior to applying definitive fixation. *Applying the screw from proximal to distal is preferred* given the inherent stability of the proximal aspect of the metatarsal as it remains anchored by the MCJ.

Once the distal segment stability is confirmed, the proximal wire is removed and replaced with a fully threaded 3.5-mm cortical screw using standard A-O technique (Fig. 11.45A and B). The importance of countersinking cannot be underestimated and is essential to prevent screw head prominence and subsequent nerve and soft tissue irritation given the location of the screw (Fig. 11.46). Definitive seating of the screw without overpenetration of the cortex is facilitated by precise

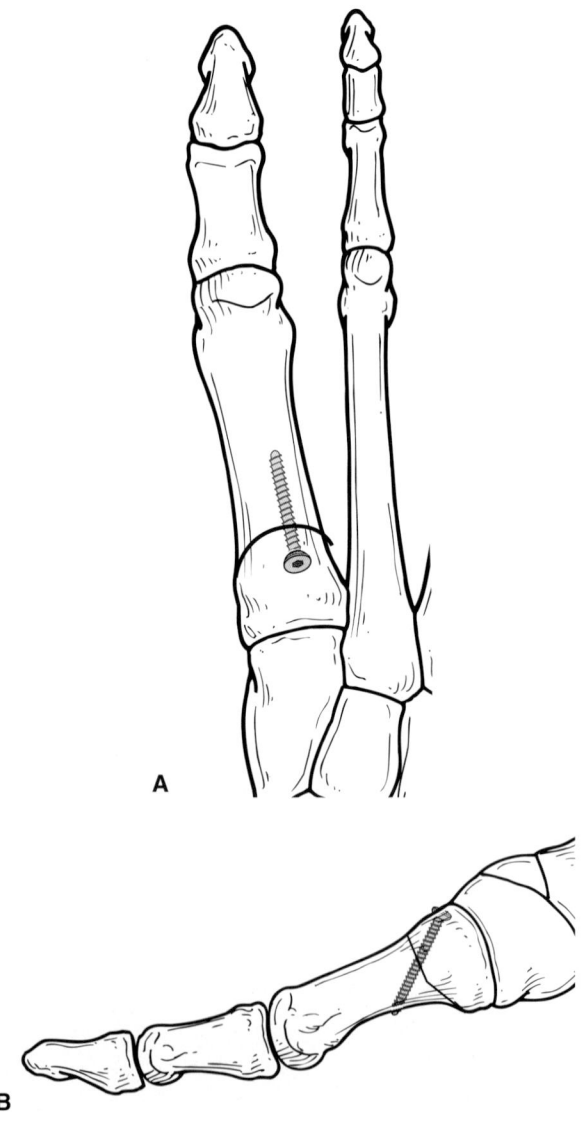

FIGURE 11.45 A, B. Internal fixation in the crescentic-plantar shelf osteotomy. The cortical screw is oriented proximal to distal **(A)** dorsal and **(B)** lateral view.

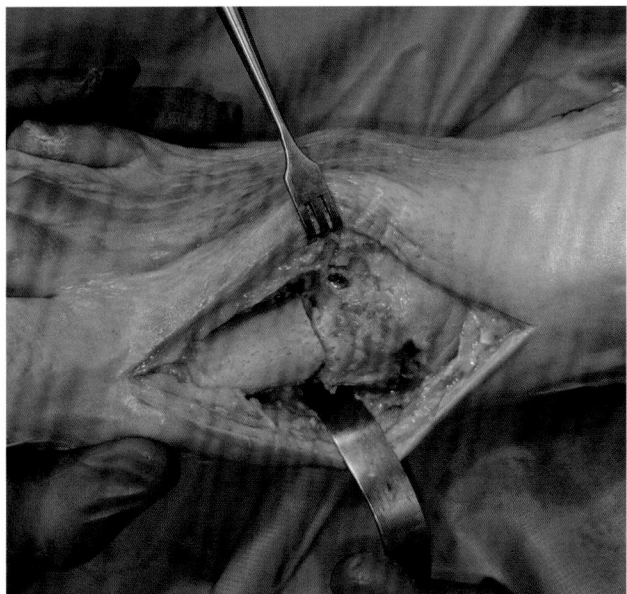

FIGURE 11.46 The importance of countersinking the screw head cannot be overstated. Despite the fact that the screw is drive on an angle, the screw head is seated flush within bone. The risks associated with a prominent screw head include nerve irritation, development of bursal projection, wound dehiscence, and shoe gear irritation among others. Notice the screw is implanted at least 1 cm proximal to the joint.

countersinking, **see Technique Tip #6: Seating the screw**. Overpenetration of the screw head will result in a loss of compression and instability of the osteotomy. Alternative screw size and two-point fixation is selected based upon the size of the bone and surgeon's preference as various orientations using a variety of fixation devices have been described including use of a 3.5-mm cortical screw,[39] crossing 3.0-mm cannulated screws,[59] crossing K-wires, multiple staples,[57] 4.0-mm cancellous screws, and 5/8 Steinman pins[38] each described with good success.

With final confirmation of anatomic reduction of the osteotomy and correction of the deformity, the wound can be irrigated and prepared for closure. Closure of the periosteum should be meticulous to provide coverage of the fixation device(s) as it is a major source of perfusion to bone. A layered closure and sterile compressive dressing is completed identical to that used in the CBWO technique.

A modified Jones compression dressing with an egg shell fiberglass cast can be maintained for the first 2 weeks of non–weight bearing. Once sufficient wound healing has been completed, the use of a short leg fiber glass cast can be employed until sufficient clinical and radiographic evidence of bone healing typically 6-8 weeks. This clinical case (Fig. 11.47A) provides short- and long-term follow-up weight-bearing radiographs status post modified plantar shelf crescent osteotomy (Fig. 11.47B and C) confirming reduction of IMA and maintenance of internal fixation position and alignment.

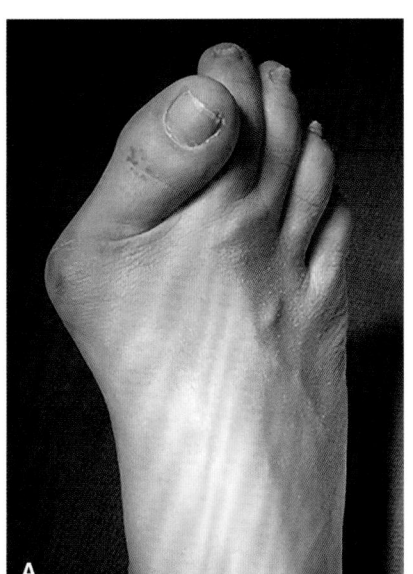
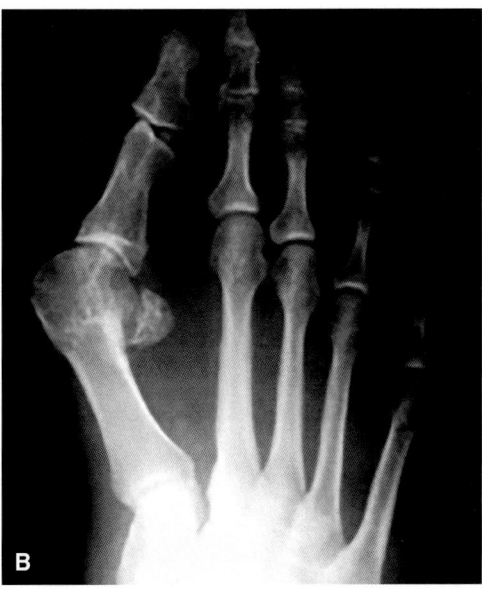
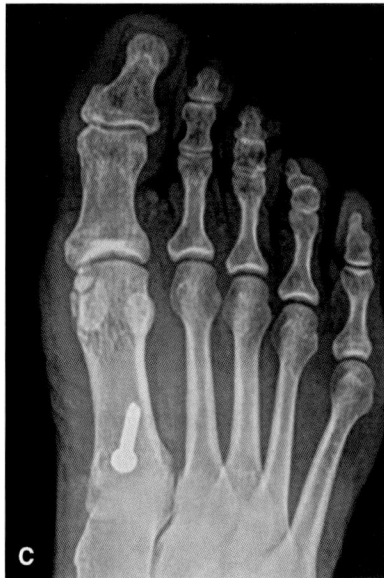

FIGURE 11.47 A, B. Clinical photograph and **(B)** preop x-ray demonstrating the high angle IMA and valgus hallux rotation associated with a cross over hallux deformity. Notice the rotation of the HIPJ nearly dislocates the joint in this end stage deformity. **C.** Postop x-ray of the same patient illustrates the power of this osteotomy as it reduces the IMA to zero and virtually lengthens the first ray restoring a congruous MTPJ and normalizes the metatarsal parabola. The internal fixation remains stable and there are no residual markings of the osteotomy cuts in this long-term follow-up film. (Illustrations compliments of Brian Carpenter, DPM.)

TECHNIQUE TIPS AND PITFALLS

Technique Tip #1: Periosteal incision: The periosteum of bone is a major source of perfusion facilitating primary bone healing and is to be handled meticulously. Over time, there has been debate over the impact of periosteal reflection, so-called stripping, and the suspected adverse effect that has on bone healing. In Whiteside et al., the notion that periosteal stripping would significantly decrease perfusion to bone was *refuted* in an anatomical study.[18] In fact, Zucmans' study demonstrated that *periosteal stripping results in dilatation of periosteal vessels* increasing perfusion and yields a positive impact on primary bone healing.[19] Directly related to proximal metatarsal osteotomy in a 3-year prospective study of sixty-five CBWO procedures, cases with periosteal reflection vs no periosteal reflection (stripping vs no stripping) were compared to determine the impact on bone healing. Although no significant difference was noted between the two groups, the authors found increased rates of osteotomy displacement and delayed bone healing in the groups *without* periosteal reflection and suspected periosteal injury as the culprit.

Technique Tip #2: Modification to add stability; plantar shelf: After making the crescentic bone cut, an unstable distal segment is created that is difficult to stabilize for fixation.[60] With a plantar shelf, the osteotomy may be easier to fixate and prevent untoward sagittal plane deviation with transverse plane reduction of the parts.[41-44,61] Gocke performed a bench analysis of the crescentic osteotomy comparing the long arm and short arm shelf osteotomies where the short arm modification outperformed the long arm in each of three elements; moment to failure, stiffness, and failure load[62] (Fig. 11.48A and B).

Technique Tip #3: When implementing the traditional crescentic osteotomy, ball and cup oriented distal to proximal, the benefit of triplane motion is countered by inherent instability. Modifications to *counter this instability* can be made effectively by reversing the orientation of the ball and cup by 180 degrees *creating a proximal to distal ball and cup configuration* (*Fig. 11.42A and B*). In addition, preparing a plantar shelf in the metatarsal base will stabilize the osteotomy countering the ground reactive forces that can lead to elevation and enhances internal fixation of the final construct (Fig. 11.42B).

Technique Tip #4: Preparation for the crescentic bone cut
a. **Orientation of blade:** After the plantar shelf is cut, the appropriate crescentic blade is selected for the girth of the metatarsal. The crescentic saw blade is first *oriented on an axis perpendicular to the weight-bearing surface* in the *metaphyseal-diaphyseal junction then the blade is tilted slightly toward the sesamoids to create a convexity within the proximal metatarsal base and a concavity within the distal segment* (*Fig. 11.43*). With the ball and socket configurated in this fashion, the osteotomy is tilted slightly plantar and is easier to manipulate, and retrograde forces are lateralized within the more stable side of the first ray. Avoid cutting the osteotomy too far proximal within the metaphyseal bone. If the cut is made too far proximal, it will be difficult to complete the bone cut given the depth of the lateral flare of the first metatarsal base. Furthermore, *the blade should be tilted slightly lateral* and the distal tip of the saw blade should be *angled slightly toward the sesamoids* to ensure reduction of the IMA with slight plantarflexion and external rotation as the metatarsal is translocated parallel to the 2nd metatarsal.[46]
b. **Crescentic blade:** Crescentic blades have variable sizes. If the width of the crescentic blade is small, the concavity in the distal bone is narrow and the total lateral excursion available will be limited. If, however, a crescentic blade wider than the metatarsal base is used, then a greater degree of lateral excursion will be available when the bone is rotated lateralward affording greater reduction of the IMA.[46]
c. **Anatomy metatarsal base:** The first metatarsal base lateral flare rests much more plantar than the medial flare and so is deeper within the vault of the intermetatarsal region. If the crescentic blade is positioned too far proximal, it may be difficult to complete the bone cut given the extreme plantar and lateral extension of the metatarsal base.
d. **Plantarflex the osteotomy:** As in the CBWO, it is often beneficial to slightly plantarflex the osteotomy to counteract the small amount of shortening that is inherent to the bone cuts. Given the declination of the first metatarsal, every millimeter excised results in dorsiflexion (elevation) of the part.
e. **Metatarsal shortening:** As in every osteotomy, there is bone loss with every pass of the saw and so it is beneficial to slightly plantarflex the osteotomy to counteract the small amount of shortening that is inherent to the bone cuts. Given the declination of the first metatarsal, every millimeter excised 1 mm of shortening results that yields a virtual dorsiflexion (elevation) of the part. The residual metatarsal segment being shorter rests more dorsal in the sagittal plane (Fig. 11.1).

Technique Tip #5: Provisional stabilization: A variation in technique described transfixes the first and second metatarsal heads after transposition of the metatarsal using a smooth K-wire in advance of definitive fixation that is stabilizing for application of either a 4.0-mm cancellous screw, staples or parallel K-wires.[57]

Technique Tip #6: Definitive seating of the screw head: Not a minor detail since the orientation of the screw is at an angle to the dorsal cortex. If the screw head overpenetrates the cortical margin, then the screw loses purchase destabilizing the construct. With appropriate position and alignment of the countersink, the land of the screw head will seat flush within that space reducing the incidence of stress riser. Completing screw placement with two-finger tightness will seat the screw head firmly without rupturing the cortical bone.

Primary pitfalls: Widely published down falls associated with this technique are sagittal plane instability resulting in residual metatarsal elevatus and difficulty in establishing rigid internal fixation. An average dorsiflexion of 6.2 degrees was noted in 33 cases in a short-term follow-up study where the greatest deformity was associated with the use of staple fixation.[57] The incidence of residual metatarsal dorsiflexion specific to the crescentic osteotomy has been reported as high as 28%[38] while others have noted dorsiflexion to various degrees in *all* basilar osteotomies.[10]

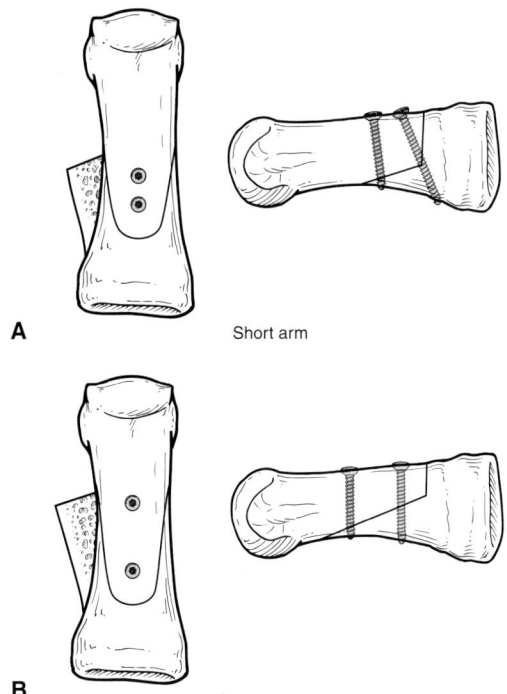

FIGURE 11.48 A, B. Crescentic osteotomy with the convex cut within the proximal metatarsal shaft. Shown here is the short and long arm shelf modifications. While this configuration is conducive to two points of fixation, the distal shelf is relatively thin with a smaller surface area for screw purchase.

POSTOPERATIVE CARE AND REHABILITATION

Regardless of the technique used, fixation of the crescentic is not designed to withstand weight bearing. Non–weight bearing should be maintained for a minimum of 6 weeks with sufficient evidence of bone healing evident upon serial radiographs in simulated weight-bearing condition. The use of antithrombotics during this period is dependent upon the individuals' risk factors. In general, recommendations for passive range of motion exercises for the MTPJ and active exercises for muscle contractions in the thigh and calf are of benefit. Options for use during the non–weight-bearing period include an ortho wedge shoe, crutches, knee roller, and modified walkers with knee stands among others. Integral to a successful postoperative course is appropriate selection of the assistive device and this is dependent on the patient's baseline balance, coordination, upper body strength, strength of the contralateral limb, and competence in understanding the purpose and importance of the non–weight-bearing plan.

If erythema, calor, swelling, tenderness, or a combination of these are present, then non–weight bearing should continue until these outward signs are resolved. Erythema and calor beyond the time of primary wound healing are most suspicious of infection and or symptomatic nonunion of bone. When this occurs, instability of fixation or premature weight bearing may be suspected. Serial radiographs and a keen clinical acumen are essential when determining sufficient bone healing to begin advancement of the weight-bearing process (Fig. 11.49A and B).

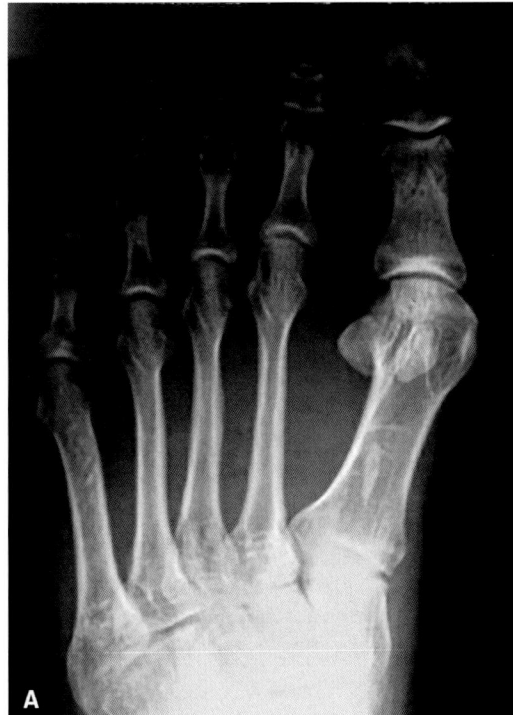
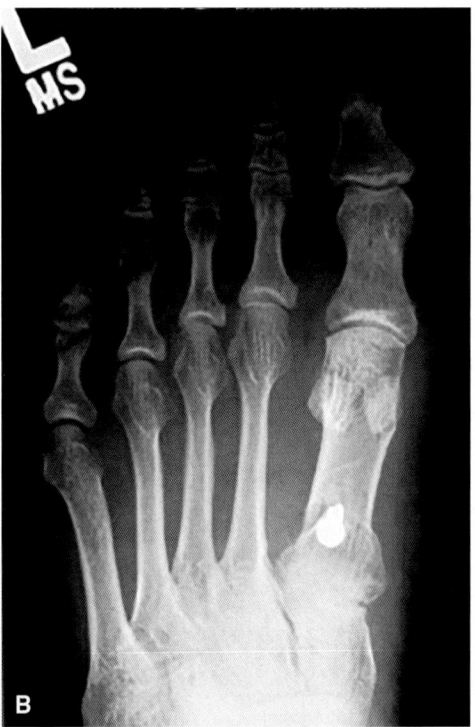

FIGURE 11.49 A, B. Pre and post x-ray comparison in weight-bearing dorsal plantar films showing dramatic reduction of the IMA and congruity of the MTPJ.

REHABILITATION

Range of motion exercises, passive and active, can be encouraged for the first MTPJ in a non–weight-bearing attitude once wound healing has been completed. Removable posterior splints, bivalved casts, and removable non–weight-bearing braces will facilitate this process. In general, recommendations for passive range of motion exercises for the MTPJ and active exercises for muscle contractions in the thigh and calf are of benefit.

CONCLUSION

The proximal crescentic osteotomy is a powerful procedure that has its primary strength in addressing high angle multiplanar bunion deformity in appropriate patients. When implementing this technique, the benefit of triplane motion is countered by a lack of inherent stability. The procedure is technically challenging as it requires a deep understanding of the mechanics of creating and manipulating a ball and socket configuration of bone. As with any procedure, strict attention to details of the technique and finesse in bone and soft tissue manipulation is required for accurate reduction of the deformity. Understanding fundamental A-O principals as well as having manual dexterity are important components to a successful procedure. Rigid internal fixation is protected with the benefit of absolute non–weight bearing to encourage primary bone healing. Mastery of the proximal crescentic osteotomy requires practice to meet the challenges of the steep learning curve.

PROXIMAL CHEVRON (AUSTIN) OSTEOTOMY

DEFINITION

The proximal Chevron aka Austin osteotomy is a "V" osteotomy that is cut through the transverse plane in the first metatarsal from medial to lateral. The technique uses a K-wire as an axis

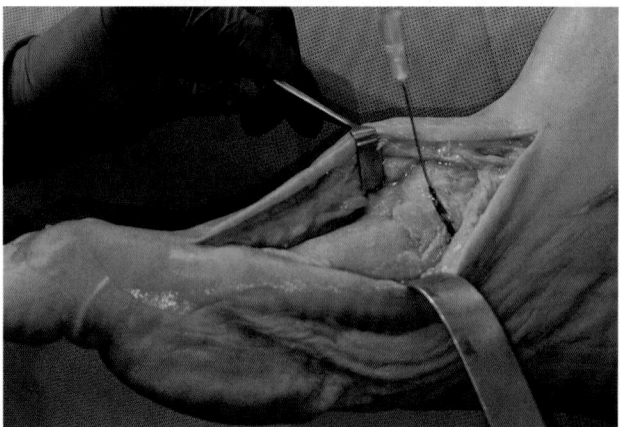

FIGURE 11.50 The enthesis of tibialis anterior is seen superior to the ribbon retracted within the plantar soft tissue sleeve. Care is taken to identify, isolate, and preserve the enthesis during this procedure.

guide identical to that used for the distal version of this technique. While the angle of the cuts are similar in both versions, 60-70 degrees, the orientation of the apex in the proximal "V" is 180 degrees opposite and lies 1 cm or more distal to the MCJ with the arms of the "V" cut extending distally into the metatarsal shaft[63] (Fig. 11.50). Alternatively, the technique can be modified using a distal apex cutting the arms of the "V" proximally.[64] The mechanical advantages of performing the osteotomy using the arms cut distally vs proximally has not been noted in the literature to date.

The proximal Chevron aka Austin osteotomy is an option when correcting high IMA bunion deformities, however, is not frequently discussed.[36,56,65,66] Interestingly, a prospective controlled study comparing the proximal and distal Chevron for correcting moderate to severe bunion deformity revealed both procedures were effective with radiographic and clinical outcomes being comparable.[67] Unique to this study is the fact that each patient had simultaneous bilateral surgery with a distal Chevron performed on one foot and a proximal Chevron on the opposite foot. Since both procedures were performed in each patient, the variability introduced by differences in age, gender, body mass index, comorbidity, bone quality, and activity level were equalized. While the proximal osteotomy affords greater correction of deformity both procedures performed side by side produced comparable radiographic and clinical outcomes in an average follow-up of 40.2 months. Another study comparing distal and proximal osteotomy in the treatment of HAV pain with moderate to high IMA reported both (distal Chevron and Mau osteotomy) procedures provided pain-relief in functional scores; however, less radiographic improvement was noted in the distal osteotomy group.[68] Given that proximal wedge osteotomies rely on a hinge for maintenance of stability, failure of the hinge often results in shortening, elevation of the ray, malunion, and MTPJ dysfunction.[69,70] Given the learning curve associated with the CBWO, this downfall leaves the surgeon to consider alternatives in approaching the high IMA bunion deformity. Duke considered the alternatives to the CBWO and delineated the seven characteristics that should be considered when entertaining an alternative technique: (1) proximal apex of correction; (2) resist stresses of weight bearing; (3) simple to perform; (4) simply and effectively fixated; (5) easily adjustable; (6) versatile in correction; and (7) minimal surgical trauma.[71]

> **Indications:** Moderate to severe hallux abducto valgus deformity including 18-20 degrees intermetatarsal angles (IMAs). Some authors find the proximal Chevron (Austin) osteotomy superior to others such as the crescentic sighting improved stability with internal fixation demonstrated in a head to head comparison in one publication.[56] For larger IMAs, >18 degrees, a transverse plane swivel of the osteotomy is required, **see Technique Tip: Swivel technique.**
>
> **Pitfall:** Larger IMA deformities (>20 degrees) are not included here as the modifications needed to accommodate higher IMA are believed to decrease the stability of the osteotomy.[36,56,65]

ANATOMIC FEATURES

Recall that the tibialis anterior tendon along the medial cuneiform and has a point of insertion on the most medial aspect of the first metatarsal base. This tendon should be identified, isolated, and preserved in dissecting and preparing the osteotomy in this area (Fig. 11.50). Seen in this figure the tibialis anterior enthesis is just superior to the ribbon retractor. An ink line marks the level of the MCJ and a shorter hypodermic needle can be inserted there to serve as a landmark to prevent violating the joint surface.

TREATMENT

Conservative therapy can include insole modifications or more predictably prescription orthotic devices can be prepared to rebalance the forefoot as an alternative to surgical intervention. When an elevatus is present, the prescription should provide relief beneath the 5th metatarsal head with a partial fill beneath the first metatarsal. Options in orthotic materials include semiflexible polypropylene, copolymers, poly-laminates, or cork-based prescriptions. Accommodation of the rigid first ray can be achieved using a medial forefoot wedge. Should orthotic therapy fail the proximal first metatarsal osteotomy can provide predictable and reproducible results with strict attention to the details of the technique. Postoperatively, orthotic therapy to support the arch and reduce weight-bearing imbalance may optimize long-term function.

AUTHORS PREFERRED TREATMENT

The procedure begins with an extensile dorsal linear incision medial to the EHL tendon beginning proximal to the MCJ and extending distally over the proximal phalanx. After the first interspace release (release of the deep transverse intermetatarsal ligament, lateral capsular contractures, and fibular sesamoid ligament), the medial eminence is resected and recontoured taking care not to violate diaphyseal bone in the process. Then blunt dissection is continued proximally. The medial dorsal cutaneous nerve or its branches are encountered and retracted medially. Once subcutaneous tissues have been reflected proximally, an incision into the deep fascia is made medial to the EHL tendon to afford lateral retraction of the tendon. This exposure allows best visualization of the metatarsal base, shaft, and the MCJ. The first ray should be manipulated to identify the MCJ capsule. An 18G hypodermic needle can be placed in the MCJ as a marker to prevent inadvertent violation of the joint (Fig. 11.50). Care is taken in reflecting the deep fascia and periosteum as the tibialis anterior tendon inserts along the plantar aspect of the first metatarsal and the medial cuneiform. This enthesis identified, isolated, and preserved during proximal exposure of the first metatarsal base, see **Technique Tip #1: Periosteal incision CBWO**. With the deep fascia retracted, the apical axis guide is placed across the transverse plane using a 0.045 K-wire run perpendicular to the second ray (Fig. 11.51), see **Technique Tip #1: Apical axis guide**. The "V" osteotomy is scored within the proximal metatarsal using a #10 osteotome and mallet or sagittal saw (Fig. 11.52), see **Technique Tip #2: Preparing the osteotomy.** The plantar arm is designed to be longer than the dorsal arm as this will facilitate fixation and stability of the construct. The arms of the "V" are oriented distal to the apex and are prepared at approximately a 60-degree angle in the same manner as a distal "V" osteotomy. Once the osteotomy has been scored,

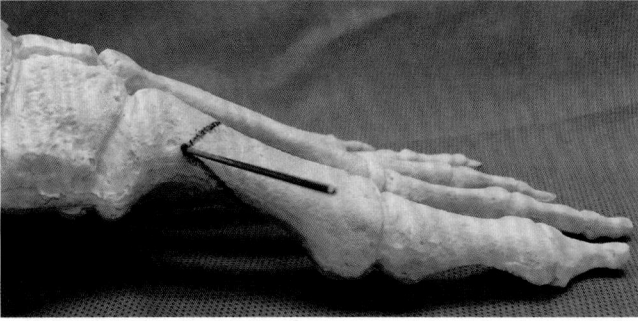

FIGURE 11.51 The axis guide is used as a reference for the proximal Chevron "V".

the arms of the "V" cut are reassessed. The sagittal saw is used to make the cuts. With the blade parallel to the axis guide, use the saw to penetrate the cortex and run the blade from distal (through the thinnest margin) to proximal toward the axis guide. It is important to keep the axis guide in place for the plantar cut. The cuts should both run up to the pin. If the apical axis guide K-wire inadvertently vibrates out, it should be replaced to ensure a precise plantar cut of the osteotomy. (In this event, the blunt end is reintroduced to the hole to prevent cutting a new hole.) Once both cuts are completed through to the wire, the guide wire can be removed. The osteotomy can then be shifted laterally taking care not to impinge the lateral border of the osteotomy into the 2nd metatarsal. A clean cut of the osteotomy will result in a press fit as desired. In cases of more severe deformity, the osteotomy will be lateralized maximally and the lateral border of the proximal osteotomy may need to be reduced using power instrumentation. If greater correction of the deformity is required, the osteotomy can be rotated to reduce the IMA further. The proximal osteotomy shaft can be rotated medialward shifting the distal portion of the metatarsal toward the second

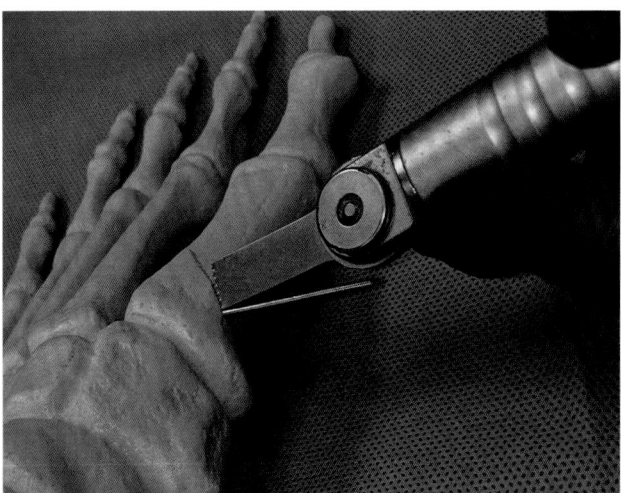

FIGURE 11.52 Once the cuts are scored onto the bone, the position and alignment of the dorsal and plantar arms can be reassessed before definitive bone cuts are made.

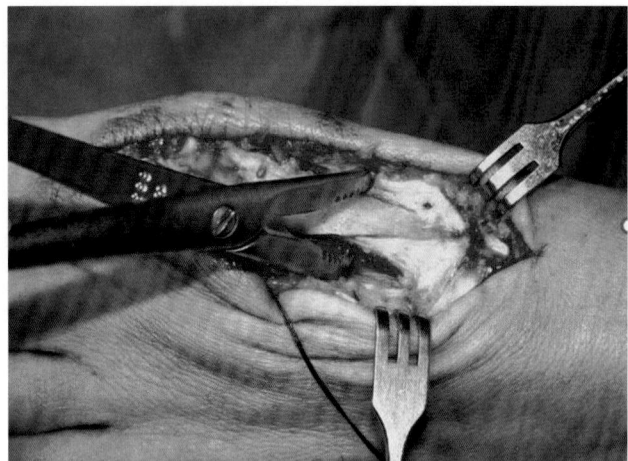

FIGURE 11.53 Intraoperative view of the proximal "V" osteotomy with a long plantar arm stabilized with a bone clamp preparing for internal fixation.

metatarsal. As the proximal metatarsal pivots within the apical cut, the distal metatarsal will further reduce the IMA as it approaches the second metatarsal, see **Technique Tip #3: Modification for severe deformity**. A bone clamp should be applied to compress and stabilize the parts without interfering with fixation placement (Fig. 11.53). The osteotomy is stabilized using 0.062 K-wires run obliquely in a parallel pattern. The first point of fixation runs obliquely from distal to proximal through the sagittal plane capturing of the plantar shelf of the first metatarsal base. The next wire is driven proximal to the first taking care to space the wires by 1.5-2 cm as this will accommodate the size and seating of the screw heads (Figs. 11.54 and 11.55). Allowing for ample space between the screw heads will reduce the risk of stress fracture within the dorsal cortex. Application of two parallel 3.5-mm cortical lag screws is completed using strict A-O technique. Use the 2.5-mm drill bit to create a thread hole matching the core of the 3.5-mm screw (Fig. 11.56). Countersinking is important as it allows seating of the screw head at an angle without causing undue stress or fracture of the dorsal cortex (Fig. 11.57). Measure the length of the screw by seating the depth gauge flush within the countersink and capture the most proximal

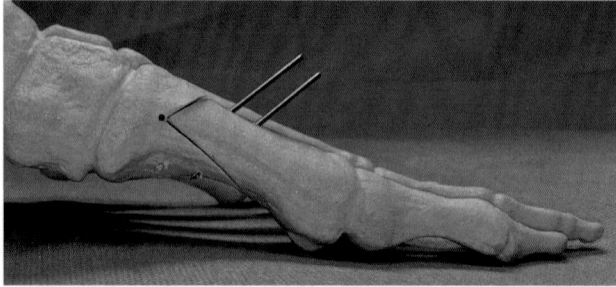

FIGURE 11.54 Medial view provisional fixation in proximal "V" osteotomy with long plantar arm using parallel K-wire stabilization. Take care to space the wires by 1.5-2 cm as this will accommodate the size and seating of the screw heads.

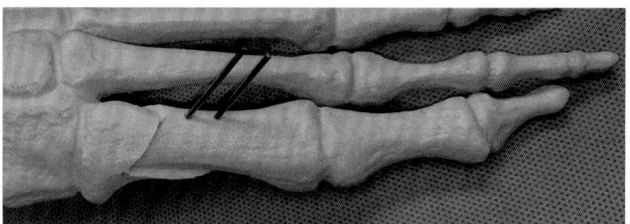

FIGURE 11.55 Dorsal view provisional fixation in proximal "V" osteotomy with short dorsal arm using parallel K-wire stabilization. K-wires are run parallel from dorsal lateral to plantar and slightly medial to capture the plantar arm taking care to space the wires by 1.5-2 cm to accommodate the size and seating of the screw heads.

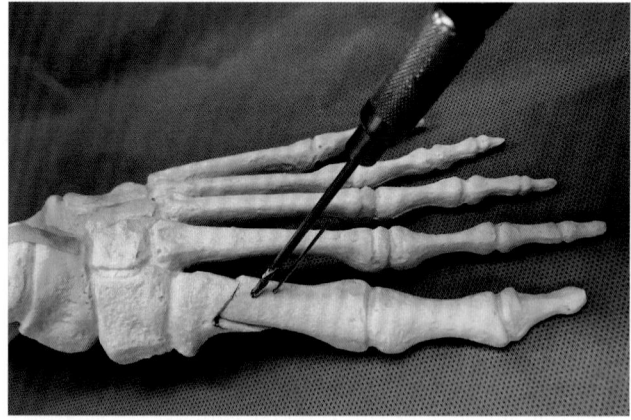

FIGURE 11.56 The most proximal screw is prepared 1 cm distal to the dorsal osteotomy cut using a 2.5-mm drill to match the core of the screw.

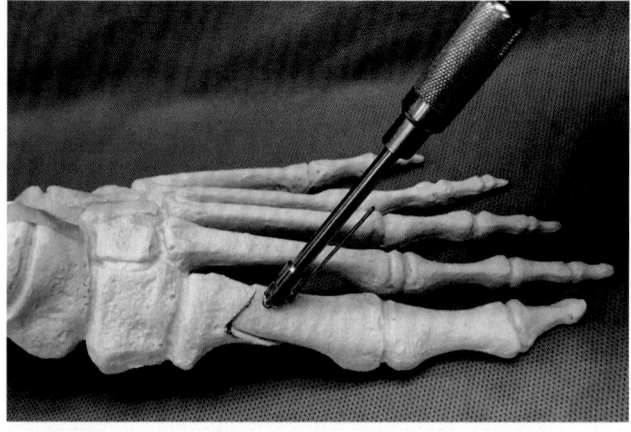

FIGURE 11.57 Notice the countersink is oriented perfectly coaxial to the thread hole; this allows seating of the screw head at an angle without causing undue stress or fracture of the dorsal cortex while leaving ample space between the two screw heads.

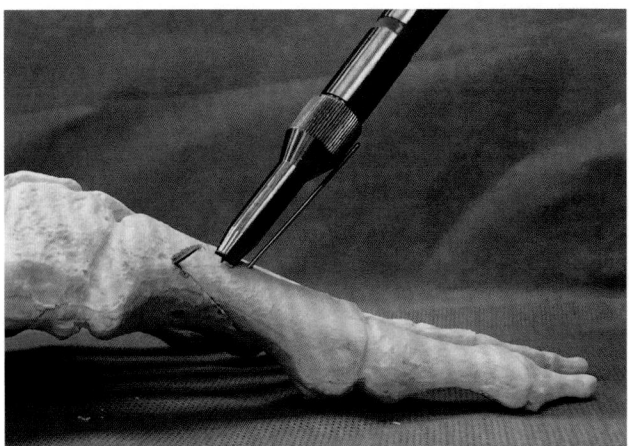

FIGURE 11.58 Measure the length of the screw by seating the depth gauge flush within the countersink coaxial with the thread hole. Be certain to capture the most proximal plantar shelf to ensure the greatest measure.

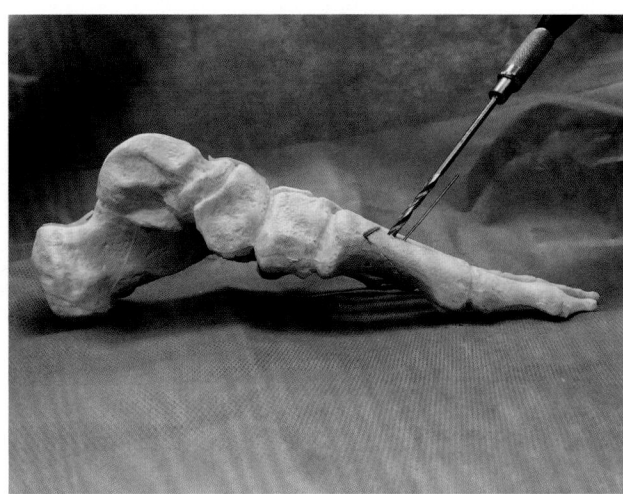

FIGURE 11.60 The *near cortex* is overdrilled using a 3.5-mm drill bit to provide a glide hole for the compression screw.

plantar shelf to ensure the greatest measure (Fig. 11.58). The measure should provide length for 2-3 threads beyond the plantar cortex for purchase and compression of the parts. The 3.5-mm cortical tap is used employing the three turns forward followed by one turn in reverse to clear the flutes of the tap (Fig. 11.59). Once tapping is complete, the *near cortex* is overdrilled using a 3.5-mm drill bit (Fig. 11.60). The screw is then inserted until the screw head compresses the parts (Fig. 11.61). Definitive tightening of the first screw is not completed until the second, more proximal screw is applied. Then the screws are each secured to two finger tightness in this same sequence (Fig. 11.62A and B). Final evaluation of the construct and radiographic evaluation is followed by copious irrigation.

Closure of the periosteum is completed with undyed 3.0—absorbable suture. The periosteum is an important component of perfusion for the metatarsal base and so must be handled meticulously and delicately closed as a single layer covering the screw heads and the hinge at the conclusion of the procedure. The subcutaneous tissues and skin are closed as separate layers after hemostasis have been confirmed. Neurovascular status is rechecked prior to application of the dressing. A sterile bulky gauze dressing is applied to the foot positioned at 90 degrees to the leg and a modified Jones compression dressing is applied from the distal forefoot to the pretibial region. Finally, an egg shell fiberglass cast can be applied or alternatively a posterior splint of plaster or fiberglass or prefabricated non–weight-bearing boot may be applied to further encourage non–weight bearing postoperatively.

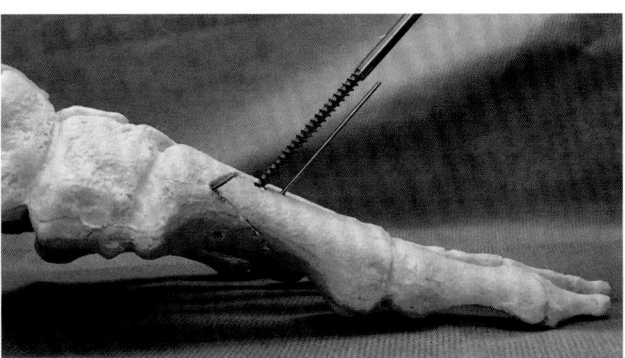

FIGURE 11.59 The 3.5-mm cortical tap is used employing the three turns forward followed by one turn in reverse to clear bone from the flutes of the tap.

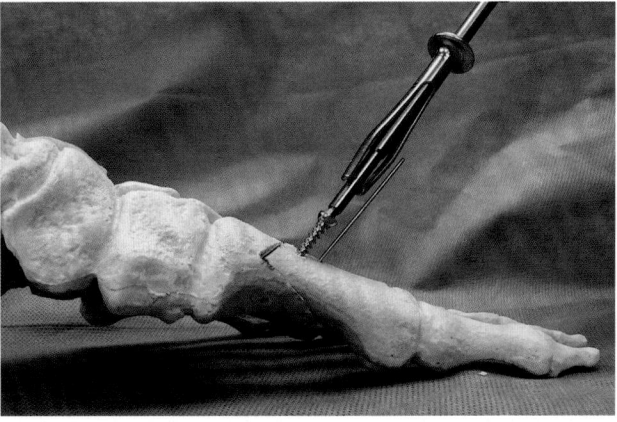

FIGURE 11.61 With the 3.5-mm screw inserted, the osteotomy is compressed and preparation of the distal screw can be completed prior to definitive tightening of the proximal screw.

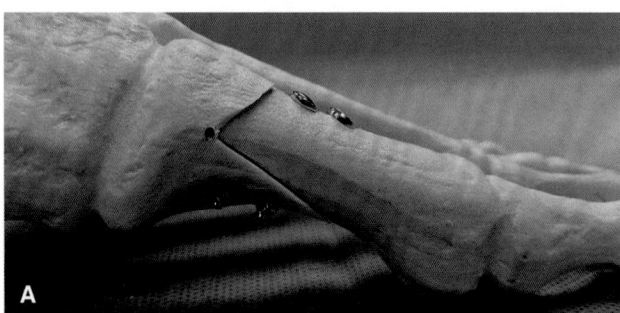
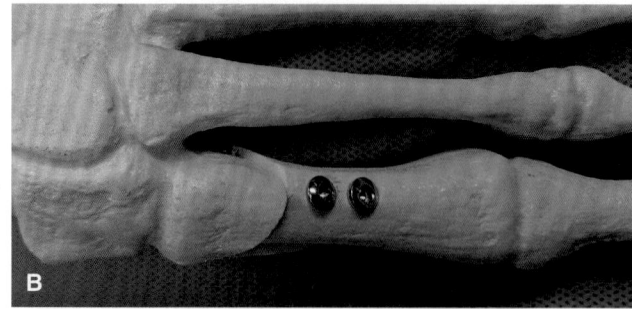

FIGURE 11.62 Rigid internal fixation of the proximal "V" osteotomy with long plantar arm with application of parallel 3.5-mm cortical screws using lag technique. The choice of either 2.7- or 3.5-mm screws will vary with the size of the metatarsal. Screw selection depends on the size and quality of the bone. **(A)** Medial projection and **(B)** dorsal projection of the 3.5-mm lag screw technique.

TECHNIQUE TIPS

1. **Apical axis guide:** The apex of the proximal basilar osteotomy is prepared by identifying the distal portion of the medial metaphysis and placing the wire within its bisection. A 0.045 K-wire is used as the axis guide and is run through the transverse plane ~1.0-1.5 cm distal to the MCJ. This location varies based upon the length of the metatarsal base. The apex should rest within medullary bone in an identical manner as in a distal "V" osteotomy.

2. **Preparing the osteotomy: Length of the dorsal osteotomy cut:** Conventional wisdom suggests that the dorsal arm be shorter than the plantar arm to reduce the risk of creating a stress riser when placing the screw (Fig. 11.51). If the dorsal arm of the osteotomy cut is too long, the risk of stress riser and fracture increases.[36] When a long dorsal arm is prepared, the screw head generates shear as it encounters the thin distal cortical margin. As the screw head seats into the bone at an angle, it can rupture that arm of the osteotomy destabilizing fixation. When the dorsal arm is fractured, instability and healing complications have been reported (Fig. 11.52). Use of a long plantar arm and short dorsal arm provides geometry that enhances stability without increased risk of stress riser formation.

3. **Score the osteotomy:** With the apical axis guide in place, score the diagram of the "V" cuts precisely. This ensures that the location and length of the cuts will be effective. Use a no. 10 osteotome and small mallet to score the "V" pattern. Reassess the scored cuts checking the relationship of the arms of the osteotomy; plantar longer than dorsal to facilitate the fixation plan. If the appearance is not accurate at this point, you have NOT gone too far and can "redraw" your intentions for the cuts optimally.

4. **Cutting the osteotomy:** Cutting of bone begins with the blade penetrating the distal arm of the dorsal cortex and continues proximally up to the apical guide wire. Irrigation to prevent thermal necrosis is important to reduce risk of bone healing complications. If the K-wire vibrates out of the bone, it should be replaced to ensure precision in preparing the plantar arm of the osteotomy. When the cuts are made clean to the wire is removed easily. If the cuts remain short of the wire, the pin will be difficult to remove. Keeping the axis guide intact when cutting the osteotomy prevents cross cutting at the apex or

otherwise creating irregular cuts that prevent a smooth press fit of the parts. If the osteotomy is difficult to move, then the cuts may not be completely through the deep portion of the lateral cortex. In this event, a fine instrument such as a *flat bovie tip* can be used to clear the osteotomy cuts ensuring full mobility of the parts.

5. **Modification for severe deformity:** The osteotomy can be lateralized maximally in some cases and the lateral border of the proximal osteotomy may need to be reduced using power instrumentation. If *even greater correction* of the deformity is required, the osteotomy can be rotated to reduce the IMA further. The proximal osteotomy shaft can be rotated lateralward. As the proximal metatarsal pivots within the apical cut, the distal metatarsal will further reduce the IMA as it approaches the second metatarsal.

6. **Anatomy metatarsal base:** The first metatarsal base lateral flare rests much more plantar than the medial flare and so is deeper within the vault of the intermetatarsal region. When making the "V" cuts, the increased depth of bone is appreciated proximally.

7. **Internal fixation:** Considerations in fixation techniques for the proximal Chevron are born from the query as to which configuration of the osteotomy and fixation devices can withstand the most weight-bearing load.[72]

    Multiple variations in fixation techniques have been described over time. Most authors describe the use of one or more points of fixation to enhance stabilization of the construct in preparation for weight-bearing activity. It is preferred to apply parallel screws inserted in tandem along the sagittal plane of the metatarsal dorsally. Alternatively, a cross screw technique can be used where the screws are inserted dorsomedial and dorsolateral aiming proximally to capture the plantar cuts of the osteotomy. Instron testing in saw bone models demonstrated the parallel configuration to be twice as strong as the crossing screw technique. (Personal communication Alan Mlodzienski, DPM.) There remain a few basic tenents in fixation techniques regardless of where you apply them in the proximal metatarsal segment. (1) When possible, fixating bone perpendicular to the osteotomy is preferred; hence, parallel screws running through the sagittal plane should be stronger than a cross

TECHNIQUE TIPS (*Continued*)

screw technique. (2) Two points of fixation are more stable than one in addressing osteotomies made along the natural declination of the first metatarsal bone. (3) The increased stress in weight bearing and the retrograde forces generated up stream along the metatarsal segment merit stout devices and precise application to ensure optimal long-term apposition of the parts. There are several biomechanical studies on the fixation of saw bones or cadaveric feet. Lian et al. and Bozkurt et al. reported screw fixation to be significantly stronger than K-wires or staples.[17,73]

Fillinger et al. demonstrated a double screw fixation to be more stable compared to single screw fixation in comparing proximal crescentic and oblique wedge osteotomies.[73] Varner et al. reported greater stability of plate fixation compared to single screw fixation for metatarsal crescentic

osteotomy.[10] In a recent biomechanical study of the proximal Chevron, aka "V" osteotomy, parallel screw fixation out performed both locking plate/screw and parallel K-wire techniques. In that bench study, the parallel K-wires did not withstand the walking fatigue challenge. The parallel headless screws were superior in resistance to bending forces and smaller dorsal angulation than the locking plate system.[74] Interestingly, others support the use of a single screw stabilization and immediate weight bearing with satisfactory results.[72]

8. **Screw spacing:** When placing multiple screws in series, it is important to space the screws sufficiently apart to reduce the risk of stress fracture. A rule of thumb is to allow *at least the measure of a single screw head* between the implants that are inserted (Fig. 11.55).

PERILS and PITFALLS

While a bench study can validate the technique of proximal first metatarsal osteotomies, it cannot attest to how the osteotomy will hold up in real life weight bearing or how it will fair with the test of time.[75] In moderate to severe HAV deformity, the proximal osteotomy should be used with caution as some authors report long-term complications. Strict attention to patient selection will improve compliance postoperatively. Often patients believe that they can be compliant with non–weight bearing; however, their life circumstances will not allow it. Caution is suggested when considering appropriate patients for proximal metatarsal osteotomies.[76,77]

Regarding long-term complications, shortening and elevation seem to be among the most prevalent.[49,73,78]

POSTOPERATIVE CARE AND REHABILITATION

Regardless of the technique used, fixation of the proximal Chevron osteotomy aka proximal Austin or "V" osteotomy is not designed to withstand weight bearing. Non–weight bearing should be maintained for a minimum of 6 weeks with sufficient evidence of bone healing evident upon serial radiographs in simulated weight-bearing condition. The use of antithrombotics during this period is dependent upon the individuals' risk factors. In general, recommendations for passive range of motion exercises for the MTPJ and active exercises for muscle contractions in the thigh and calf are of benefit. Options for use during the non–weight-bearing period include an ortho wedge shoe, crutches, knee roller, and modified walkers with knee stands among others. Integral to a successful postoperative course is appropriate selection of the assistive device and this is dependent on the patients' baseline balance, coordination, upper body strength, strength of the contralateral limb, and competence in understanding the purpose and importance of the non–weight-bearing plan.

REHABILITATION

Range of motion exercises, passive and active, can be encouraged for the first MTPJ in a non–weight-bearing attitude once

wound healing has been completed. Removable posterior splints, bivalved casts, and removable non–weight-bearing braces will facilitate this process. If erythema, calor, swelling, tenderness, or a combination of these are present, then non–weight bearing should continue until these outward signs are resolved. Erythema and calor beyond the time of primary wound healing are most suspicious of infection and or symptomatic nonunion of bone. When this occurs, instability of fixation or premature weight bearing may be suspected. Serial radiographs and a keen clinical acumen are essential when determining sufficient bone healing to begin advancement of the weight-bearing process.

COMPLICATIONS

Potential complications reported in using the proximal Chevron aka proximal "V" osteotomy include a myriad of problems associated with premature weight bearing. Disruption of fixation potentially results in malunion, delayed union, or nonunion of bone. In these events, the need for further surgery is possible. Wound healing complications, nerve irritation, the development of a thickened unsightly or even painful scar may arise from prominent fixation devices. Undercorrection may lead to recurrence while overcorrection may result in hallux varus deformity. Late complications have been reported and include MPE and symptomatic metatarsal shortening.

CONCLUSION

The proximal Chevron aka proximal "V" osteotomy is a powerful procedure that has its primary strength in addressing high angle bunion deformity in appropriate patients. As with any procedure, strict attention to details, finesse in making bone cuts, and manipulation of the parts are required for accurate reduction of the deformity. Understanding fundamental A-O principals and good manual dexterity are important components to a successful procedure. Rigid internal fixation is protected with the benefit of absolute non–weight bearing to encourage primary bone healing. Serial radiographs and a keen clinical acumen are essential when determining sufficient bone healing to begin advancement of the weight-bearing process. Mastery of this technique requires practice to meet the challenges of the learning curve.

ACKNOWLEDGMENTS

Closing Base Wedge Osteotomy

A debt of gratitude to *John Ruch, DPM* for taking upon himself the onus of detailing the clinical, surgical, and mechanical principals of the closing base wedge osteotomy and hallux abducto valgus surgery. These efforts benefit surgeons across the globe. His depth of thought in producing illustrations, textbook chapters, and journal articles has set the bar exceedingly high for the next generation in foot and ankle surgery.

Special appreciation to *Jack Schuberth, DPM* for his exacting thoughts in the original description of the hinge axis concept that has served a wealth of physicians, residents, and medical students since the early 1980s.

Special thanks to Thomas Smith, DPM for his drive to publish the original discussion of the hinge axis concept. His shear intelligence was exceeded only by his chivalry.

In memory of *Gerard V. Yu, DPM* whose zest for life and insatiable intrigue for the details of foot and ankle surgery has touched the lives of patients and surgeons too numerous to count. His enthusiasm, specifically for the closing base wedge osteotomy, and his ability to project that from the podium was epic.

Special thanks for the exemplary efforts of Lisa Nichols and the medical library staff at St. Vincent Mercy Health Partners of Toledo, Ohio for their assistance in research and acquisition of articles required for this publication.

Proximal Crescentic Osteotomy

Special thanks to Brian Carpenter, DPM for his input, contributions to illustrations, and willingness to share personal experience in using the proximal crescentic osteotomy. Many thanks to a team of residents and medical students who entrenched themselves into the task of dissecting and preparing bone models to benefit the reader. This team includes Adam D. Port, DPM, PGY-III, Charles B. Penvose, DPM, PGY-II, and Jeanne M. Mirbey, DPM PGY-I of Emory Decatur Podiatry Residency Program 2701 North Decatur Road, Decatur, Georgia, 30033.

As well as Medical students: Rupinder K. Boora, MS-4 and Marisa Giustiniano MS-4 of The New York College of Podiatric Medicine, 53 East 124th Street, New York, New York, 10035.

Special thanks for the exemplary efforts of Lisa Nichols and the medical library staff at St. Vincent Mercy Health Partners of Toledo, Ohio for their assistance in research and acquisition of articles required for this publication.

Crescentic Osteotomy

Special thanks to Dennis Martin, DPM and Alan Mlodzienski, DPM for their input, contributions to illustrations, and willingness to share their personal experience in using this technique

Many thanks to a team of residents and medical students who entrenched themselves into the task of dissecting and preparing bone models to benefit the reader. This team includes: Adam D. Port, DPM, PGY-III, Charles B. Penvose, DPM, PGY-II, and Jeanne M. Mirbey, DPM PGY-I of Emory Decatur Podiatry Residency Program 2701 North Decatur Road, Decatur, Georgia, 30033.

As well as Medical students: Rupinder K. Boora, MS-4 and Marisa Giustiniano MS-4 of The New York College of Podiatric Medicine, 53 East 124th Street, New York, New York, 10035.

Special thanks for the exemplary efforts of Lisa Nichols and the medical library staff at St. Vincent Mercy Health Partners of Toledo, Ohio for their assistance in research and acquisition of articles required for this publication.[35,79]

REFERENCES

1. Loison M. Note sur le traitement chirugical de l'hallux valgus d'apres l'etude radiographic de la deformation. *Bull Mem Soc Chir Paris.* 1901;27:528-531.
2. Balacescu J. Un cas de hallux valgus simetric. *Rev Chir Orthop.* 1903;7:128-135.
3. Juvara E. Nouveau procedure por-la cure radicale du hallux valgus. *Nouv Presse Med.* 1919;40:395.
4. Juvara E. Cure Radicale de l'hallux-valgus per la resection cuneiform de la portion moyenne de la diaphyse du metatarsien, suivie de l'osteosynthese des fragments. *Lyon Chir.* 1926;23:429.
5. Juvara E. L'hallux-valgus; son traitement operatoire. *Rev Chir.* 1932;5:321.
6. Vickers NS, Ruch JA. Current use of the oblique base wedge osteotomy in hallux abducto valgus surgery. In: *Reconstructive Surgery of the Foot and Leg Update 1994.* Tucker, GA: Podiatry Institute Publishing Co.; 1994:128-132.
7. Laporta GA, Richter KP, Jolly GP. Pressure osteosynthesis for internal fixation of metatarsal angulational osteotomies. *J Am Podiatry Assoc.* 1976;66:173-180.
8. Schlicke LH, Panjabi M, White A. Optimal orientation of transfixation screws across oblique fracture lines. *Clin Orthop Relat Res.* 1979;143:271.
9. Christensen JC, Gusman DN, Tencer AF. Stiffness of screw fixation and role of cortical hinge in the first metatarsal base osteotomy. *J Podiatr Med Assoc.* 1995;85(2):73-82.
10. Fillinger EB, McGuire JW, Hesse DF, Solomon MG. Inherent stability of proximal first metatarsal osteotomies: a comparative analysis. *J Foot Ankle Surg.* 1998;37(4):292-302.
11. Schuberth JM, Reilly CH, Gudas CJ. Closing abductory base wedge osteotomies: a comprehensive analysis of first metatarsal elevation. Presented at American Podiatry Association Meeting, Chicago, Illinois, August 1982.
12. Denton J, Kuwada G. Retrospective study of closing wedge osteotomy complications at the base of the first metatarsal with bone screw fixation. *J Foot Surg.* 1983;22(4):314-319.
13. Schuberth JM, Reilly CH, Gudas CJ. The closing base wedge osteotomy. *J Am Podiatr Med Assoc.* 1984;74:13-24.
14. Jeremins PJ, DeVincentis A, Goller W. Closing base wedge osteotomy: an evaluation of 24 cases. *J Foot Surg.* 1982;21:316-323.
15. Zlotoff H. Shortening of the first metatarsal following osteotomy and its clinical significance. *J Am Podiatry Assoc.* 1977;67:412-426.
16. Banks AS, Cargill RS, Carter S, Ruch JR. Shortening of the first metatarsal following closing base wedge osteotomy. *J Am Podiatr Med Assoc.* 1997;87:199-208.
17. Lian GJ, Markolf K, Cracchiolo A. Strength of fixation constructs for basilar osteotomies. *Foot Ankle.* 1992;13:509-514.
18. Whiteside LA, Ogata K, Lesker P, Reynolds FC. The acute effects of periosteal stripping and medullary reaming on regional blood flow. *Clin Orthop.* 1978;131:266.
19. Zucman J. Studies on the vascular connections between periosteum, bone and muscle. *Br J Surg.* 1960;48:324-328.
20. Sanders AP, Snijders CJ, Linge BV. Medial deviation of the first metatarsal head as a result of flexion forces in hallux valgus. *Foot Ankle.* 1992;13:515-522.
21. Martin D, Pontius J. Anatomical Dissection of the First Metatarsal Phalangeal Joint. In: Banks AS, Downey MS, Martin DE, Miller SJ, eds. *Comprehensive Textbook of Foot Surgery.* 3rd ed. Philadelphia, PA: Lippincott Williams & Wilkins; 2001:481-491.
22. Landers P. Introduction and Evaluation of Hallux Abducto Valgus. In: McGlamry ED, Banks AS, Downey MS, eds. *Comprehensive Textbook of Foot Surgery.* 2nd ed. Baltimore, MD: Lippincott Williams & Wilkins; 1992:459-466.
23. Lynch FR. Juvenile Hallux Abducto Valgus. In: McGlamry ED, Banks AS, Downey MS, eds. *Comprehensive Textbook of Foot Surgery.* 2nd ed. Baltimore, MD: Lippincott Williams & Wilkins; 1992:566-570.
24. DiDomenico LA, Wargo-Dorsey M. Lapidus Bunionectomy: First Metatarsal- Cuneiform Arthrodesis. In: Southerland JT, ed. *Comprehensive Textbook of Foot Surgery.* 4th ed. Philadelphia, PA: Wolters Kluwer/Lippincott Williams & Wilkins; 2013:322.
25. Roukis TS, Landsman AS. Hypermobility of the first ray: a critical review of the literature. *J Foot Ankle Surg.* 2003;6:377-390.
26. Bednarz PA, Manoli A. Modified Lapidus procedure for the treatment of hypermobile hallux valgus. *Foot Ankle Int.* 2000;10:816-821.
27. Root MI, Orien WP, Weed JH. Muscle function of the foot during locomotion. In: Root ML, O'Rien WOP, Weed JH, eds. *Clinical Biomechanics,* Vol. 2. Los Angeles, CA: Clinical Biomechanics Corporation; 1977.
28. Root MI, Orien WP, Weed JH, et al. Technique for the examination of the first ray. In: *Biomechanical Examination of the Foot.* Vol. 1. Los Angeles, CA: Clinical Biomechanics; 1971:80-87.
29. Tobin R, Krych S, Harkless LB. First metatarsal-cuneiform dorsal exostosis: its anatomical relation with the medial dorsal cutaneous nerve. *J Foot Surg.* 1989;28(5):442-444.
30. Marcinko DE, McGlamry ED. The first cuneometatarsal exostosis. *J Am Podiatry Assoc.* 1985;75:401.
31. Schuster O. *Foot Orthopedics.* New York: J.B. Lyon; 1939.
32. Akpinar E, Buyuk AF, Cetinkaya E, Gursu S, Ucpunar H, Albayrak A. Proximal intermetatarsal divergence in distal chevron osteotomy for hallux valgus: an overlooked finding. *J Foot Ankle Surg.* 2016;55:504-508.
33. Camasta C. Evaluation and classification of metatarsus Primus Elevatus, In: *Reconstructive Surgery of the Foot and Leg Update 1994.* Tucker, GA: Podiatry Institute Publishing Co.; 1994:123-127.
34. Ruch J. In: McGlamry ED, Banks AS, Downey MS, eds. *Comprehensive Textbook of Foot Surgery.* 2nd ed. Baltimore, MD: Lippincott Williams & Wilkins; 1992:504-507.

35. Christenson C, Jones RO, Basque M, Mollohan E. Comparison of oblique closing base wedge osteotomies of the first metatarsal: stripping versus non-stripping of the periosteum. *J Foot Surg.* 1991;40(30):107-113.

36. Martin DE, Blitch EL. Alternatives to the closing base wedge osteotomy. *Clin Podiatr Med Surg.* 1996;13(3):515-531.

37. Lagaay PM, Hamilton GA, Ford LA, Williams ME, Rush SM, Schuberth JM. Rates of revision surgery using chevron- Austin osteotomy, Lapidus arthrodesis, and closing base wedge osteotomy for correction of hallux valgus deformity. *J Foot Ankle Surg.* 2008;47(4):267-272.

38. Mann R, Rudicel S, Graves S. Repair of hallux valgus with a distal soft-tissue procedure and proximal metatarsal osteotomy. *J Bone Joint Surg.* 1992;74:124-129.

39. Brodsky JW, Beischer AD, Robinson AHN, Westra S, Negrine JP, Shabat S. Surgery for hallux valgus with proximal crescentic osteotomy causes variable postoperative pressure patterns. *Clin Orthop Relat Res.* 2006;443:280-286.

40. Coughlin M, Mann R. Hallux valgus. In: Coughlin M, Mann R, Saltzman C, eds. *Surgery of the Foot and Ankle.* 8th ed. Philadelphia, PA: Mosby; 2007:259-260.

41. Jimenez L. The wedge shelf osteotomy. In: *Update 1994: Reconstructive Surgery of the Foot and Leg.* Tucker, GA: Podiatry Institute Publishing; 1994:135.

42. Cohen M, Roman A, Ayres M, et al. The crescentic shelf osteotomy. *J Foot Ankle Surg.* 1993;32:204-226.

43. Fabrikant JM, Colarco J. A study of the proximal wedge shelf osteotomy for correction of large IM angle HAV deformity. *Foot Ankle Spec.* 2012;5(1):23-30.

44. Carpenter B, Motley T. Adding stability to the crescentic basilar first metatarsal osteotomy. *J Am Podiatr Med Assoc.* 2004;94:502-504.

45. Coughlin MJ, Jones CP. Hallux valgus: demographics, etiology, and radiographic assessment. *Foot Ankle Int.* 2007;28:759-777.

46. Lippert FG III, McDermott JE. Crescentic osteotomy for hallux valgus: a biomechanical study of variables affecting the final position of the first metatarsal. *Foot Ankle.* l991;11:204-207.

47. Pehlivan O, Akmaz I, Solakoglu C, Kiral A, Kaplan H. Proximal oblique crescentic osteotomy in hallux valgus. *J Am Podiatr Med Assoc.* 2004;94:43-46.

48. Thordarson DB, Rudicel SA, Ebramzadeh E, Gill LH. Outcome study of hallux valgus surgery: an AOFAS multi-center study. *Foot Ankle Int.* 2001;22:956-959.

49. Veri JP, Pirani SP, Claridge R. Crescentic proximal metatarsal osteotomy for moderate to severe hallux valgus: a mean 12.2 year follow-up study. *Foot Ankle Int.* 2001;22:817-822.

50. Trnka HJ, Parks BG, Ivanic G, et al. Six first metatarsal shaft osteotomies: mechanical and immobilization comparisons. *Clin Orthop Relat Res.* 2000;381:256-265.

51. Zettl R, Trnka HJ, Easley M, Salzer M, Ritschl P. Moderate to severe hallux valgus deformity: correction with proximal crescentic osteotomy and distal soft-tissue release. *Arch Orthop Trauma Surg.* 2000;120:397-402.

52. Kitaoka HB, Patzer GL. Salvage treatment of failed hallux valgus operations with proximal first metatarsal osteotomy and distal soft-tissue reconstruction. *Foot Ankle Int.* 1998;19(3):127-131.

53. Fox IM, Caffiero L, Pappas E. The crescentic first metatarsal basilar osteotomy for correction of metatarsus primus varus. *J Foot Ankle Surg.* 1998;38:203-207.

54. Markbreiter LA, Thompson FM. Proximal metatarsal osteotomy in hallux valgus correction: a comparison of crescentic and chevron procedures. *Foot Ankle.* 1997;18:71-76.

55. Easley ME, Kiebzak GM, Davis WH, Andersen RB. Prospective, randomized comparison of proximal crescentic and chevron osteotomies for correction of hallux valgus deformity. *Foot Ankle.* 1996;17:307-316.

56. McCluskey LC, Johnseon JE, Wynarsky GT, Harris GF. Comparison of stability of proximal crescentic metatarsal osteotomy and proximal horizontal "V" osteotomy. *Foot Ankle Int.* 1994;15:263-270.

57. Thordarson DB, Leventen EO. Hallux valgus correction with proximal metatarsal osteotomy: two - year follow up. *Foot Ankle.* 1992;13(6):321-326.

58. Nyska M, Liberson A, McCabe C, Linge K, Klenerman L. Plantar foot pressure distribution in patients with hallux valgus treated by distal soft tissue procedure and proximal metatarsal osteotomy. *Foot Ankle Surg.* 1998;4:35-41.

59. Fox IM, Caffiero L. The crescentic first metatarsal basilar osteotomy for correction of metatarsus primus varus. *J Foot Ankle Surg.* 1999;38(3):203-207.

60. Hyer CF, Glover JP, Berlet GC, Philbin TM, Lee TH. A comparison of the crescentic and mau osteotomies for correction of hallux valgus. *J Foot Ankle Surg.* 2008;47(2):103-111.

61. Earl M, Wayne J, Caldwell P, et al. Comparison of two proximal osteotomies for the treatment of hallux valgus. *Foot Ankle Int.* 1998;19:425-429.

62. Gocke SP, Rottier FJ, Havey RM, et al. Quantitative analysis of long and short arm crescentic shelf bunionectomy osteotomies in fresh cadaveric matched pair specimens. *J Foot Ankle Surg.* 2011;50(2):158-164.

63. Sammarco GJ, Brainard BJ, Sammarco V. Bunion correction using proximal chevron osteotomy. *Foot Ankle.* 1993;l4:8-l4.

64. Abidi NA, Conti SF. Hallux valgus: indications and technique of proximal chevron osteotomy combined with distal soft tissue release. *Operat Tech Orthop.* 1999;9(1):8-14.

65. Easely M, Kiebzak GM, Davis WH, Anderson RB. Prospective randomized comparison of proximal crescentic and proximal chevron osteotomies for hallux valgus deformity. *Foot Ankle Int.* 1996;17:307-316.

66. Markbreiter LA, Thompson F. Proximal metatarsal osteotomy in hallux valgus correction: a comparison of crescentic and chevron procedures. *Foot Ankle Int.* 1997;18:71-76.

67. Lee KB, Cho NY, Park HW, Seon JK, Lee SH. A comparison of proximal and distal Chevron osteotomy, both with lateral soft-tissue release, for moderate to severe hallux valgus in patients undergoing simultaneous bilateral correction. A prospective randomized controlled trial. *Bone Joint J.* 2015;97-B(2):202-207.

68. Chuckpaiwong B. Comparing proximal and distal metatarsal osteotomy for moderate to severe hallux valgus. *Int Orthop.* 2012;36:2275-2278.

69. Cedel CA, Astrom M. Proximal metatarsal osteotomy in hallux valgus. *Acta Orthop Scand.* 1982;53:1013-1018.

70. Landsman AS, Vogler HW. As assessment of oblique base wedge osteotomy stability in the first metatarsal using different modes of internal fixation. *Foot Ankle Surg.* 1992;31: 211-218.

71. Duke H. Rotational SCARF (Z) osteotomy bunionectomy for correction of high intermetatarsal angles. *J Am Podiatr Med Assoc.* 1992;82:352.

72. Kim JS, Cho HK, Young KW, Kin JS, Lee KT. Biomechanical comparison study of three fixation methods for proximal chevron osteotomy of the first metatarsal in hallux valgus. *Clin Orthop Surg.* 2017;9:514-520.

73. Bozkurt M, Tigaran C, Dalstra M, Jensen NC, Linde F. Stability of a cannulated screw versus a Kirschner wire for the proximal crescentic osteotomy of the first metatarsal: a biomechanical study. *J Foot Ankle Surg.* 2004;43(3):138-143.

74. Varner KE, Matt V, Alexander JW, et al. Screw versus plate fixation of proximal first metatarsal crescentic osteotomy. *Foot Ankle Int.* 2009;30(2):142-149.

75. Mittag F, Leichtle U, Meisner C, Ipach I, Wulker N, Wunschel M. Proximal metatarsal osteotomy for hallux valgus: an audit of radiologic outcome after single screw fixation and full postoperative weightbearing. *J Foot Ankle Res.* 2013;6:22.

76. Costa MT, de Almeida Pinto RZ, Ferreira RC, Sakata MA, Frizzo GG, Santin RA. Osteotomy of the first metatarsal base on the treatment of moderate to severe hallux valgus results after a mean follow-up time of eight years. *Rev Bras Orthop.* 2009;44(3):247-253.

77. Okuda R, Kinoshita M, Morikawa J, Jotoku T, Abe M. Proximal metatarsal osteotomy: relation between 1-to greater than 3-years results. *Clin Orthop Relat Res.* 2005;(435):435-436.

78. Trnka HJ, Mühlbauer M, Zembsch A, Hungerford M, Ritschl P, Salzer M. Basal closing wedge osteotomy for correction of hallux valgus and metatarsus primus varus: 10- to 22-year follow-up. *Foot Ankle Int.* 1999;20(3):171-177.

79. Nyska M, Trnka HJ, Parks BG, Myerson MS. Proximal metatarsal osteotomies: a comparative geometric analysis conducted on saw bone models. *Foot Ankle Int.* 2002;23(10):938-945.

CHAPTER 12

Proximal Midshaft Osteotomies of the First Metatarsal–The Mau, Ludloff, and Scarf Procedures

Tzvi Bar-David and Robert Fridman

INTRODUCTION

In this chapter, we will focus on three popular midshaft osteotomies: the Mau osteotomy as a standalone procedure or combined with a Reverdin-Laird osteotomy, the Ludloff osteotomy, and separately, the Scarf osteotomy.

DEFINITION

Midshaft osteotomies are mostly centered in the hard cortical bone of the shaft of the first metatarsal. Ludloff in 1913 and 1918 was the first to describe an oblique first metatarsal osteotomy oriented from dorsal proximal to plantar distal.[1] Mau challenged the inherent instability of the Ludloff procedure and described the reverse osteotomy oriented from dorsal distal to proximal plantar, producing an inherent stable and rigid dorsal shelf to resist the ground reactive forces[2] (Fig. 12.1). As originally published, both of these procedures were not fixated and thus lacked stability. Furthermore, their location within hard cortical mid-diaphyseal bone was a cause for concern for more healing difficulties. These procedures were not popular until the mid-1990s when several authors described modifications of lengthening these osteotomies into the more proximal cancellous region of the metatarsal. This created a more proximal center of rotation and, together with rigid internal fixation, increased stability and ease of healing.[3-6] The Mau and Ludloff osteotomies regained favor since they are easily performed involving only a single cut and are reliably reproducible.

RELEVANT ANATOMIC CONSIDERATIONS FOR MAU AND LUDLOFF

The anatomic topography of the first metatarsal becomes important with shaft osteotomies. The shaft of the first metatarsal is concave plantarly and becomes triangular as it approaches the base of the metatarsal at its articulation with the medial cuneiform. The medial surface is narrow and short, and the lateral surface is longer and flatter. The nutrient foramen is usually found on the lateral surface.[7,8] The head of the first metatarsal derives its circulation from the first intermetatarsal artery and medial plantar artery.

Another important anatomic note is the insertion of the peroneus longus tendon on a tubercle on the inferolateral aspect of the base.[7,8]

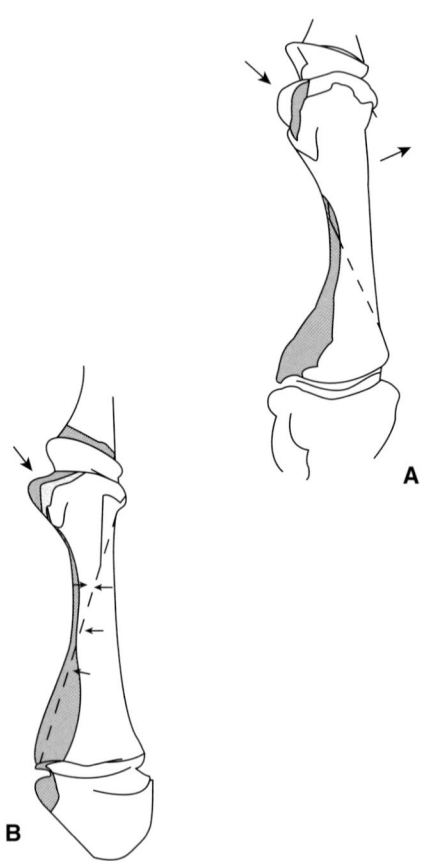

FIGURE 12.1 **A.** Ludloff osteotomy. Ground reactive forces will distract the dorsal fragment containing the head of the metatarsal. **B.** Mau osteotomy. Ground reactive force will not allow distraction of the plantar fragment containing the head of the metatarsal as the dorsal shelf will block the motion.

SURGICAL PEARLS FOR MAU AND LUDLOFF OSTEOTOMIES RELATED TO ANATOMY OF THE FIRST METATARSAL

- Because of the triangular undersurface of the first metatarsal, when fixating these osteotomies, the orientation of the screws should be directed slightly medially and not directly plantarly through the center of the plantar triangular surface. Doing so may split the plantar bone and cause a stress fracture along the length of the plantar cut, which will compromise fixation and stability (Fig. 122.2).
- Midshaft osteotomies are always made on the medial surface along the length of the metatarsal and extend to the lateral surface. Care must be taken not to make the dorsal or plantar surface too thin, or this may also cause an increased chance for stress fractures or failed fixation.
- The Mau osteotomy exits in the area of the peroneus longus insertion at the base of the first metatarsal. Therefore, care should be taken to avoid severing the peroneus longus tendon insertion.[7,8] We recommend not completing the full plantar cut with an oscillating saw. Rather, we start the cut with a saw, and we complete it with an osteotome by distracting the dorsal and plantar fragments from each other. When performing the Mau, we routinely enter the very endpoint of the plantar base to provide the most proximal hinge for axis of rotation, as will be described in the Mau osteotomy technique section later in the chapter.
- Caution should also be used when performing these procedures on a narrow metatarsal, as this may complicate fixation when translated or rotated.

PEARLS FOR THE MAU OSTEOTOMY

- Make a long osteotomy parallel to the weight-bearing surface.
- Position the foot laterally on the operative table when making the osteotomy.
- Most stable construct recommended by the author is with screw and plate fixation.
- First, fixate with a 3.5-mm cortical screw at the point of rotation replacing the K-wire. Follow this with application of 5-6 holes thin compression plate with 2.4-mm locking screws. Insert first two screws proximally at the osteotomy and then apply the screws distal to the osteotomy securing the plate on the metatarsal. Leave the plate hole over the dorsal exit site of the osteotomy open. If have room, add last screw placement to insert again proximally over osteotomy.
- If adding Reverdin-Laird osteotomy, it is fixed with a 3.0-mm headless double-threaded screw. Oriented from medial dorsal shaft to lateral plantar into the metatarsal head.

AXIS AND PLANE OF MOTION AS IT RELATES TO MIDSHAFT OSTEOTOMIES

In wedge osteotomies, the axis of motion is influenced by the orientation of the hinge. For example, in a closing base wedge procedure, the metatarsal may plantar flex or dorsiflex with closure of the wedge depending on the orientation of the hinge axis.

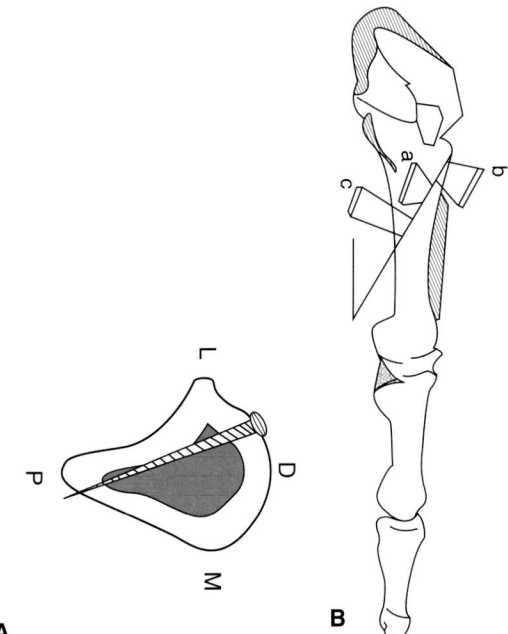

FIGURE 12.2 A. Orientation of the screws should be directed slightly medially and not directly plantarly through the center of plantar triangular surface, which can cause a stress fracture along the length of the plantar cut compromising fixation and stability. **B.** In plane-of-motion osteotomies such as Mau and Ludloff. The orientation of the hand and saw will influence the direction of motion. Example of Ludloff osteotomy with (a) hand neutral, (b) saw tilted down metatarsal head will declinate—plantar flex, and (c) saw tilted up metatarsal head will elevate—dorsiflex. (Adapted with permission from Nyska M, Trnka H-J, Parks BJ, Myerson MS. The Ludloff metatarsal osteotomy: guidelines for optimal correction based on geometric analysis conducted on a sawbone model. *Foot Ankle Int.* 2003;24(1):34-39.)

In contrast, The Mau, Ludloff, and Scarf are "plane-of-motion" osteotomies, where the orientation of the cut itself will influence the direction of motion. For example, the metatarsal may plantar flex or dorsiflex depending on the position of the saw as the cut is made (see Fig. 12.2). Therefore, care must be taken when creating the osteotomy to have the hand positioned properly so as not to cause an undesired elevation or declination of the metatarsal.

Plane-of-motion osteotomies can be categorized into two types:

1. *Translational*: one segment of bone is slid or transposed over another. The scarf is primarily a transpositional osteotomy but may allow for minimal rotation and some proximal articular set angle (PASA) correction as will be discussed later in the Scarf historical review section.

2. *Rotational*: one segment of bone is rotated over another. Both the Ludloff and Mau are primarily rotational osteotomies. However, they can allow for some transposition as will be described later in the chapter. Care must be taken when translating the bone so not to overtranslate more than 5 mm as this may compromise stability and fixation.[9] Furthermore, as rotation increases, the first metatarsophalangeal (MTP) joint becomes incongruent, increasing the chance for arthritis. This maneuver also increases the PASA and chance of recurrent bunion deformity[10-12]

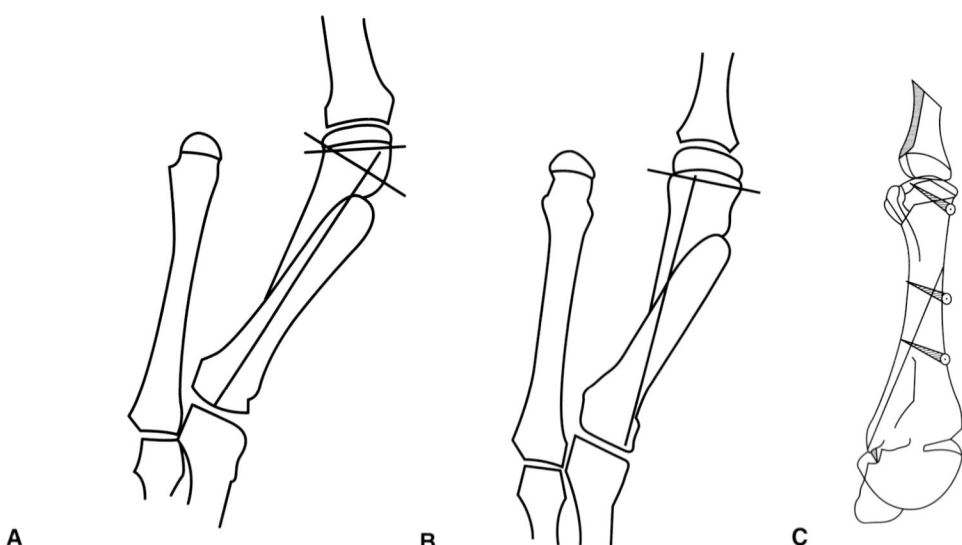

FIGURE 12.3 A. As rotation increases, the congruity of the joint is compromised increasing the proximal articular set angle (PASA) and making the joint incongruent. **B.** The Mau as shown or Ludloff can be combined with a Reverdin-Laird osteotomy, which can correct for the increased PASA at the capital fragment. It can also correct some for additional increased intermetatarsal angle by translating the capital fragment laterally after realignment of the PASA. **C.** Mau-Reverdin shown after fixation. (Adapted from Neese DJ, Zelent ME. The modified Mau-Reverdin double osteotomy for correction of hallux valgus: a retrospective study. *J Foot Ankle Surg.* 2009;48(1):22-29.)

(Fig. 12.3A). The Mau and Ludloff can be combined with a distal head osteotomy, such as a Reverdin-Laird,[13] which can correct for the increased PASA at the capital fragment. It can also correct some for additional increased intermetatarsal angle by translating the capital fragment laterally after realignment of the PASA[3,9,11,14,15] (Fig. 12.3B and C). This will be discussed in more detail at the end of the fixation section.

INDICATIONS

The Mau, Ludloff, and Scarf midshaft osteotomies are mostly reserved for when distal, capital head procedures are not sufficient to reduce a high intermetatarsal angle. The goal of midshaft osteotomies is to adequately correct a large intermetatarsal angle without the need for a wedge osteotomy and to avoid invasion of the first metatarsal-cuneiform joint.

Midshaft osteotomies are primarily indicated for moderate hallux valgus deformities. The overall radiographic criteria range would be an intermetatarsal (IM) angle of 12-20 degrees and a hallux abductus (HA) angle > 30 degrees.[12] Average IM correction of 9 degrees and HA correction of 22

degrees is relatively similar with the Ludloff[12,16-19] and Mau osteotomies.[11,14,15,20-22] Ideally, there should be no arthritis of the first MTP joint. The PASA should not be excessively elevated as this may become worsened with rotation and translation as described above.

SURGICAL TECHNIQUE FOR MAU AND LUDLOFF

CONTRAINDICATIONS

- Arthrosis of first MTP joint
- Poor bone quality

ADVANTAGES OF MAU/LUDLOFF OSTEOTOMIES

- Correction of advanced bunion deformities
- Stable construct maintaining intrinsic stability of the first metatarsal
- Minimal or no shortening of the first metatarsal

SKIN INCISION AND SOFT TISSUE RELEASE

The author's (TBD) midshaft procedure of choice is the Mau osteotomy and is most often combined with a distal Reverdin-Laird procedure for realignment of the PASA and additional IM correction if needed.

The initial incision and release are the same for both the Mau and Ludloff osteotomies. A dorsolinear and slightly medially based skin incision is made over the first MTP joint medial and parallel to the extensor hallucis longus tendon. It extends prox-

INDICATIONS FOR MAU/LUDLOFF OSTEOTOMIES

- IM angle 12-20 degrees
- HA angle >30 degrees
- Short metatarsal
- Desire not to fuse first metatarsal-cuneiform joint

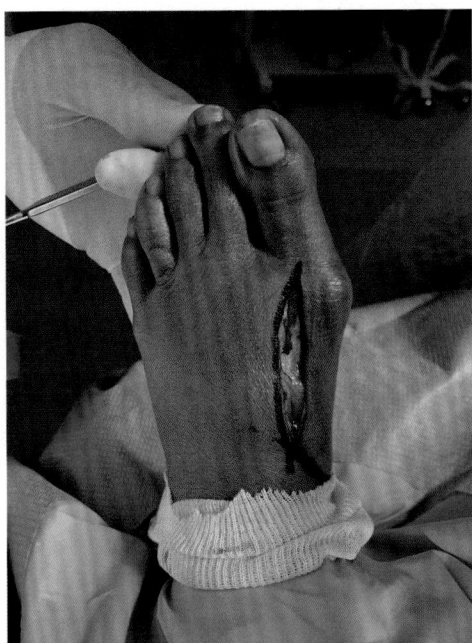

FIGURE 12.4 Skin incision dorsal linear and slightly medial over the first MTP joint medial and parallel to the extensor hallucis longus tendon extending proximally to the base of the first metatarsal just at the cuneiform joint.

imally to the base of the first metatarsal at the cuneiform joint (Fig. 12.4). The incision is deepened to the periosteum and capsule, where an inverted-L capsulotomy is made at the head of the metatarsal with the long arm ending at the proximal edge of the incision. The first MTP joint is then inspected for any

increased PASA (Fig. 12.5A). Next, the medial metatarsal exostoses at the head are resected with a sagittal saw. The capsule and full-thickness periosteum are reflected dorsally and plantarly, exposing the plantar surface of the metatarsal down to the base, where the apex of the triangular base or "flare" will be palpable and visualized (Fig. 12.5B). A soft tissue release of the first interspace is performed by cutting the conjoined adductor hallucis tendon and release of the fibular sesamoid metatarsal suspensory ligament (Fig. 12.6). The hallux is then manipulated in the direction of maximum allowable adduction to release any further adhesions or scarring within the first metatarsal interspace, which may be still maintaining the toe in the abducted position. The fibular sesamoid is palpated to ensure it can be realigned under the metatarsal as the hallux is repositioned medially.

OSTEOTOMY TECHNIQUE

Mau Osteotomy

The foot is repositioned on the table with the lateral aspect against the operative table and the dorsal, medial, and plantar aspect of the first metatarsal exposed and facing dorsally. We minimize lateral and dorsal dissection of the soft tissues surrounding the metatarsal head, thus protecting the blood flow to the head. Adequate protection of the dorsal and plantar soft tissue and neurovascular structures is achieved with Hohmann, malleable, and Senn retractors.

A sagittal saw is then used to create the Mau osteotomy with a single cut starting distally and dorsally and ending proximally and plantarly. The osteotomy is made as close to parallel to the weight-bearing surface as possible. The osteotomy begins approximately 1.5-2.0 cm proximal to the first MTP

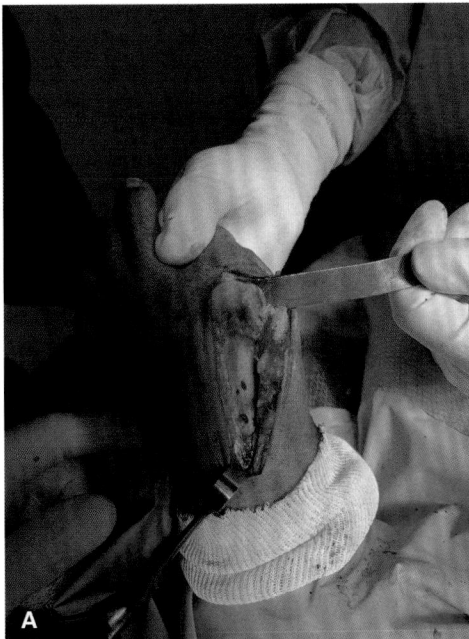
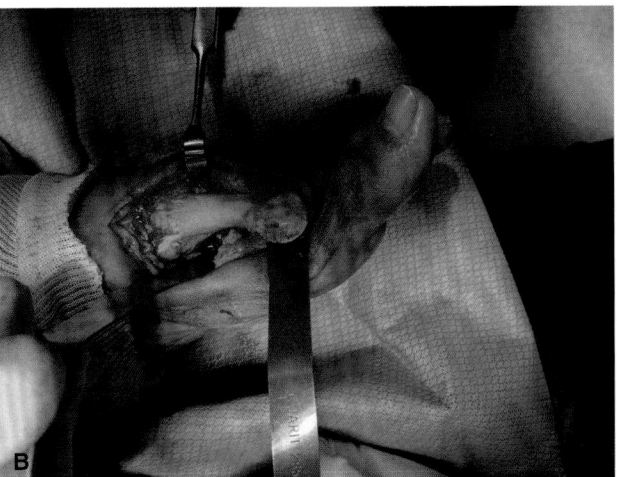

FIGURE 12.5 A. The first MTP joint is then inspected for any increased PASA. **B.** Capsule and full-thickness periosteum are reflected dorsally and plantarly with exposed plantar surface of the metatarsal down to the base, where the apex of the triangular base or "flare" is palpable and visualized. The medial metatarsal exostoses at the head have been resected with a sagittal saw.

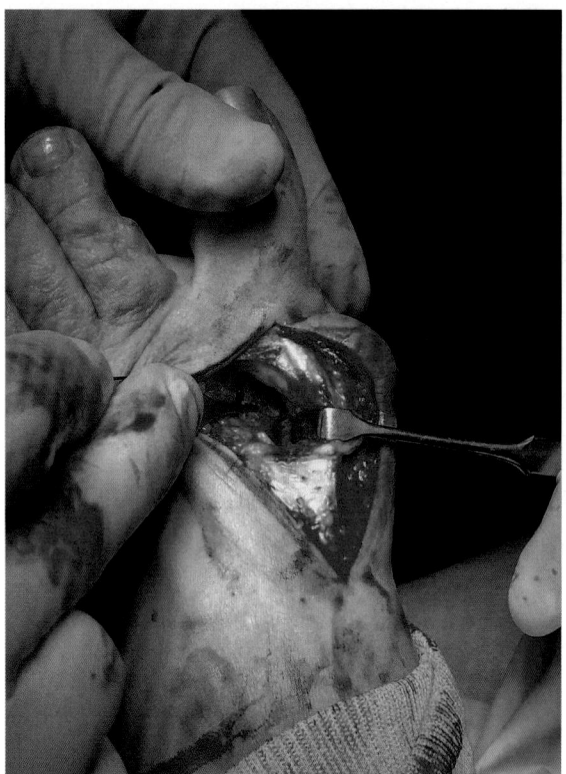

FIGURE 12.6 The first interspace soft tissue release is achieved by releasing of the conjoined adductor hallucis tendon and release of the fibular sesamoid metatarsal suspensory ligament. Note forceps pointing to the dorsal articular surface of the fibular sesamoid visualized in the interspace.

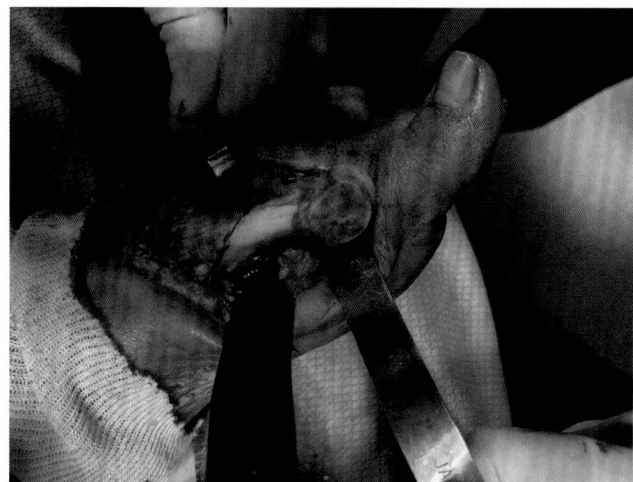

FIGURE 12.7 Outline of the Mau osteotomy. Note the cut is made as close to parallel to the weight-bearing surface as possible. The osteotomy begins approximately 1.5-2.0 cm proximal to the first MTP joint, extending into the shaft, and ending distally just shy of the first metatarsal-cuneiform joint. It can extend into the metatarsal base at its flare at the edge of the medial cuneiform joint.

joint, extending into the shaft, and ending approximately 1.0 cm distal to the first metatarsal-cuneiform joint. The cut should be sufficiently long enough to allow for appropriate fixation, and it can extend into the metatarsal base at its flare and, if necessary, to the metatarsal at the edge of the medial cuneiform joint (Fig. 12.7). In both the Mau and Ludloff procedures, rotation of the metatarsal osteotomy occurs around a single axis point. The further proximal the rotational axis point is (ie, the closer the axis of rotation is to the tarsometatarsal joint), the less the angular correction will be distally within the metatarsal itself.[23] When reducing a high IM angle, if the axis is too far distal, the metatarsal will have a "banana-shape" from increased acuity and create an increased PASA and incongruent joint. Sammarco[9] described modifying the Mau with a second cut made with a smaller, 5-mm blade transversely through the plantar metaphyseal cortex. This allows for extension of the osteotomy more proximally to gain more significant correction, since the axis of rotation will be more proximal. Our experience has not led us to see the need for this second cut. We always enter the proximal cortex and create the rotational axis point close to the metatarsal-cuneiform joint at the apex of the plantar triangular portion of the proximal metatarsal and have not seen complications from this (Fig. 12.8). Hence, at times, the osteotomy ends at the metatarsal-cuneiform joint at the end point of the apex of the plantar flare. Recognizing that we are in the area of the peroneus longus insertion at the metatarsal base, the cut is not completed proximally with the saw, but rather a

thin osteotome, which is inserted at the proximal ¼ of the metatarsal. The osteotome is extended dorsally and plantarly between the fragments, separating them and completing the cut. This protects the peroneal longus tendon insertion point at the base of the first metatarsal. It also creates a fixed, thick dorsal shelf and a plantar segment that includes the metatarsal head (Fig. 12.9). The head of the first metatarsal should be parallel to the weight-bearing surface. Maintaining this position, the osteotomy is stabilized with a bone clamp, and the foot is then repositioned to face dorsally on the opera-

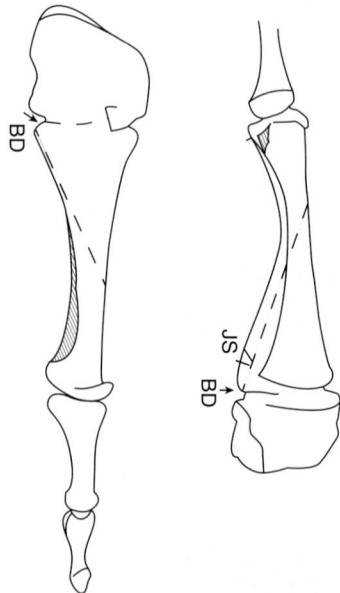

FIGURE 12.8 **A.** Sammarco[9] described modifying the Mau with a second cut made with a smaller, 5-mm blade transversely through the plantar metaphyseal cortex **B.** The author's (TBD) preferred osteotomy enters the proximal cortex close to the metatarsal-cuneiform joint at the apex of the plantar triangular portion of the proximal metatarsal.

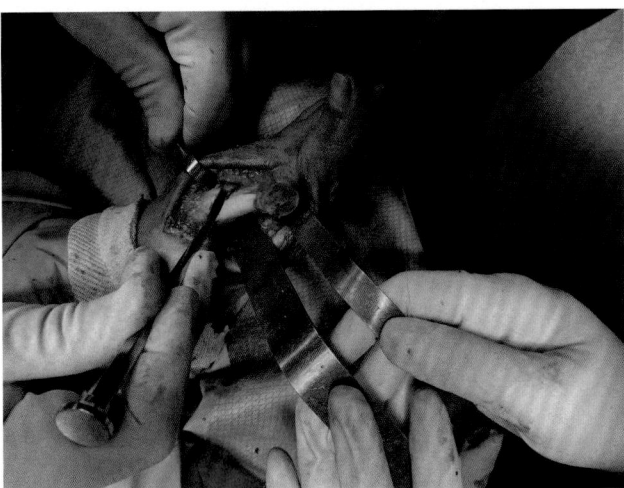

FIGURE 12.9 The cut is completed proximally with a thin osteotome inserted at the proximal quarter and the hand extended dorsally and plantarly between the fragments, thus separating the fragments and completing the cut while protecting the peroneal longus tendon insertion at the base of the first metatarsal. Note the thick dorsal shelf and plantar fragment that includes the metatarsal head.

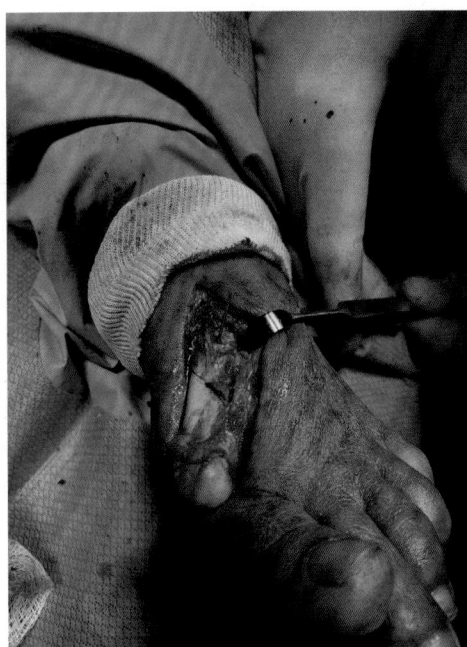

FIGURE 12.11 A 0.45 K-wire, or guidewire if fixating with cannulated screw, is drilled at the proximal aspect, perpendicular to the osteotomy from dorsal to plantar, providing stabilization and a rotational axis point.

tive table (Fig. 12.10). A 0.045 K-wire (or a guidewire if using cannulated screws) is inserted at the proximal aspect, perpendicular to the osteotomy from dorsal to plantar, to provide stabilization and a rotational axis (Fig. 12.11). When placing the wire, it is important to maintain the original length of the first metatarsal unless there is a specific need to shorten or lengthen it. The clamp is removed and the plantar shelf, which contains the metatarsal head, is rotated laterally and under the stable dorsal shelf to reduce the IM angle (Fig. 12.12). This is achieved by pulling the plantar fragment medially with a towel or bone clamp and rotating the dorsal shelf either with a bone clamp or with thumb pressure. When necessary, the metatarsal can be slightly lengthened or shortened by sliding the plantar segment on the distal segment prior to inserting the stabilizing axis wire. Using a bone

clamp, the osteotomy is compressed to stabilize the metatarsal in its corrected position, and a secondary K-wire or guidewire can be inserted to help maintain this corrected position while fixating the osteotomy (Fig. 12.13).

A fluoroscope is used intraoperatively to visualize the correction. If additional IM correction is necessary, it can be

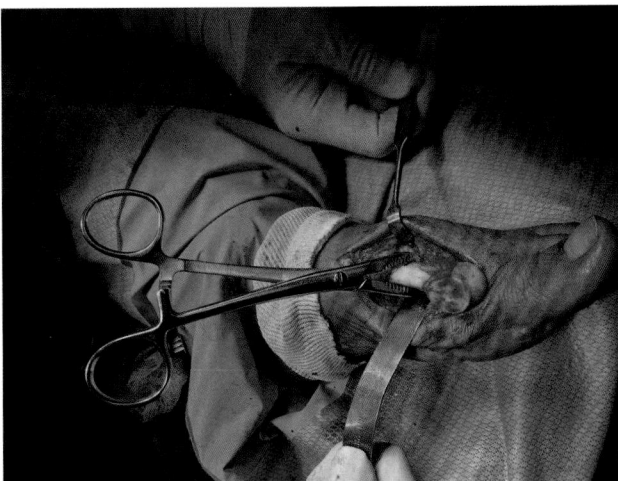

FIGURE 12.10 The osteotomy is stabilized with a bone clamp, and the foot is then repositioned to face dorsally on the table.

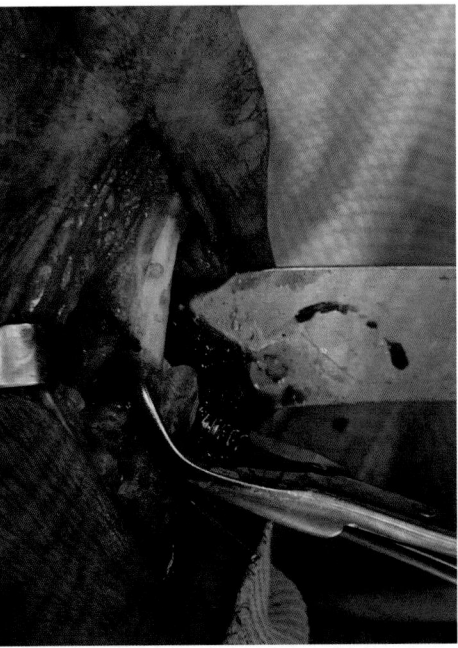

FIGURE 12.12 The plantar shelf, which contains the metatarsal head, is rotated laterally and under the stable dorsal shelf to reduce the IM angle and then clamped in the fixed position.

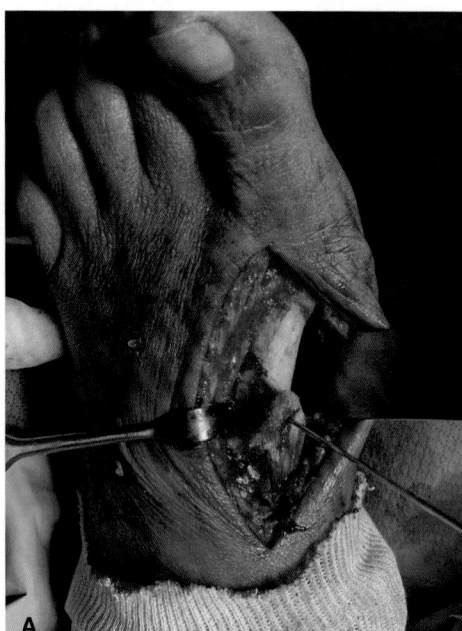
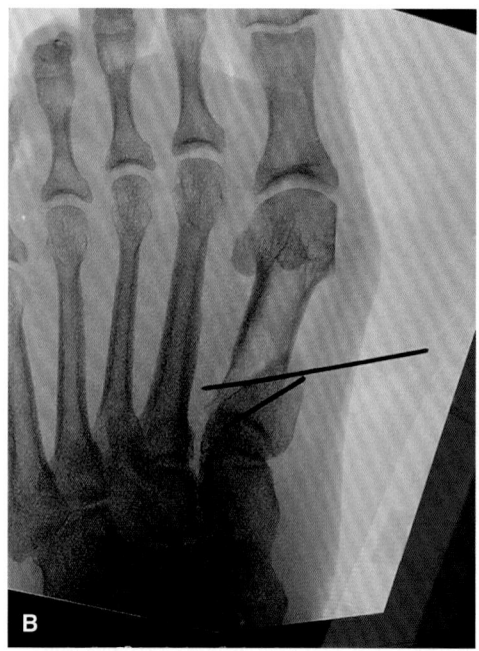

FIGURE 12.13 A. A secondary K-wire can be inserted to help maintain the corrected position while fixating the osteotomy. **B.** Intraoperative fluoroscope. Correction of IM deformity with the 0.45 K-wire rotational axis point proximal and secondary distal 0.45 K-wire stabilizing the bone.

achieved by initially sliding the plantar segment on the dorsal segment laterally to a limit of 5 mm before the axis wire is placed and rotational correction achieved.[9] As explained above, excessive translation of the plantar fragment may compromise stability and fixation. In cases where a distal Reverdin-Laird osteotomy will be required, the distal capital fragment can be translated laterally for additional IM angle correction.

Ludloff Osteotomy

Beischer et al.,[24] using three-dimensional computer modeling, found the optimal geometric parameters for the Ludloff osteotomy started at the dorsum of the first metatarsal base just at the joint and extended distally and plantarly to a point just proximal to the sesamoid articulation. Furthermore, a tilt of 10 degrees in the coronal plane of the osteotomy (ie, saw tilted down) was necessary to limit first metatarsal head elevation.[24,25] The best axis of rotation was within 5 mm of the proximal end of the osteotomy. The most common configuration of the Ludloff osteotomy is an oblique cut starting approximately 5-8 mm anterior to the metatarsal cuneiform joint and continuing toward the plantar-distal diaphysis with about 30 degrees of inclination (Fig. 12.14). This construct permits a broad area of bony contact involving some metaphyseal bone for better stability and healing, and allows for greater IM angle correction by being closer to the apex of the deformity. It is important to place retractors, such as Hohmann or malleable-type retractors, dorsal proximal to protect the extensor hallucis longus tendon and plantar-distal to protect the plantar artery to the metatarsal head.[23] Initially, the dorsal two-thirds of the osteotomy is carried out without completion of the plantar cortex distally.[17,18,23] A proximal screw, most commonly through a guidewire, is inserted and directed from dorsal to plantar.

This will act as the center of rotation. As stated with the Mau above, the further proximal the osteotomy is performed (ie, the closer the axis of rotation is to the tarsometatarsal joint), the less the angular correction is distally.[23] The osteotomy is then completed, and the distal fragment is rotated around the proximal screw. The second screw is placed about 1 cm distal to the first one to complete the fixation.[12] To rotate the osteotomy, pull the plantar fragment medially either with an instrument and rotate the dorsal fragment laterally either with a bone clamp or by the use of thumb pressure on the shaft or head. The first screw is fully tightened to hold the correction. The second screw is then inserted either from dorsal to plantar or as recommended by some[12,18,26] from plantar to dorsal, across the distal aspect of the osteotomy and approximately 1 cm distal to the first screw as described below in the fixation technique section.

FIXATION TECHNIQUES

Mau and Ludloff Osteotomies

The Mau and Ludloff midshaft osteotomies are commonly fixated with compression screws. The alignment of the screws is as close to perpendicular to the osteotomy as possible, with supplemental K-wire or plate fixation. Sometimes, correction can be lost when orienting the screws perpendicular due to tension across the osteotomy. In this case, orient the screws in a position that will maintain the greatest correction. Additionally, the screws are placed slightly medial to capture the opposing cortex and not oriented directly plantar. This avoids the screws exiting through the center of the plantar triangular surface and potentially splitting the plantar bone creating a fracture along the length of the plantar cut (Fig. 12.15). When fixating the Mau, multiple screws can be used. The first screw to be inserted

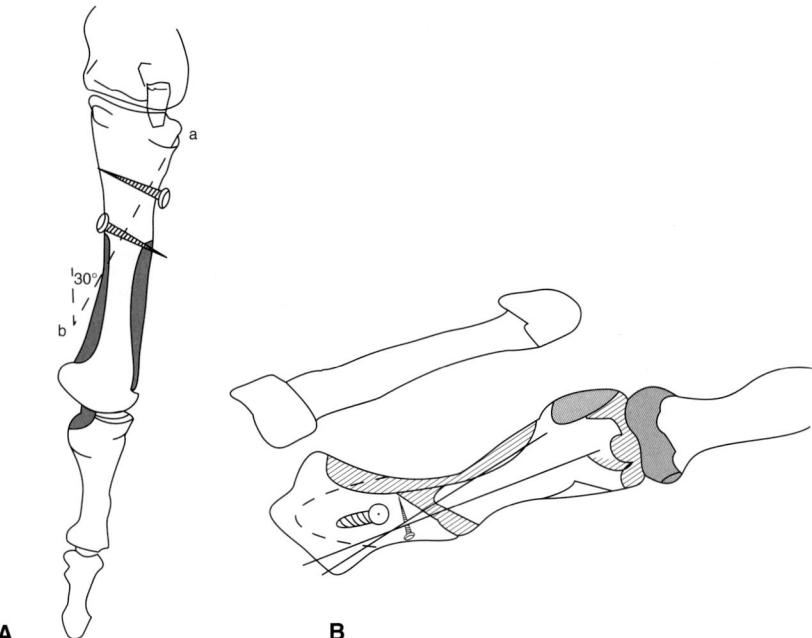

FIGURE 12.14 A. The most common configuration of the Ludloff osteotomy is an oblique cut starting dorsally approximately 5-8 mm anterior to the metatarsal cuneiform joint and continuing toward the plantar-distal diaphysis with about 30 degrees of inclination. (*Adapted* from Bae SY, Schon L. Surgical strategies: Ludloff first metatarsal osteotomy. *Foot Ankle Int.* 2007;28(1):137-144; Schon LC, Dom KJ, Jung H-G. Clinical tip: stabilization of the proximal Ludloff osteotomy. *Foot Ankle Int.* 2005;26(7):579-580.) **B.** Some authors recommend that the second distally oriented screw in the Ludloff be inserted from plantar to dorsal across the distal aspect of the osteotomy and approximately 1 cm distal to the first screw. Two K-wires for supplemental reinforcement for the Ludloff. The wires are oriented from proximal medial and driven distal into the metatarsal head or shaft and oriented parallel to the cut.

is at the proximal axis point. Fixation is then carried distally with one or two more screws inserted distal to the initial screw. Sizes range from 2.7 to 4.0 mm at the proximal apex and as small as 2.0 mm at the distal aspect of the osteotomy. We recommend using headed screws. Robinson et al.[17] compared Scarf and Ludloff osteotomies and determined that headless screws are insufficient to hold the Ludloff osteotomy and may attribute to delayed union and malunion. Countersinking the screws, especially the proximal one, is important to reduce the risk of fracture of the dorsal metatarsal cortex.[18,23] This is true for both the Mau and Ludloff. Some authors[12,18,26] recom-

mend that the second distally oriented screw in the Ludloff be inserted from plantar to dorsal across the distal aspect of the osteotomy and approximately 1 cm distal to the first screw (see Fig. 12.14). There is no literature to support inserting the distal screws from plantar to dorsal in the Mau, although this may be beneficial. Schon[26] does not use a lag screw here with the Ludloff, as he feels the screw will not be perpendicular when the bones are in the corrected position. Attempting a lag screw in this case may cause loss of correction through tension across the osteotomy.

> **PERILS and PITFALLS**
> - "Banana" metatarsal by making a short osteotomy or overrotation of the first metatarsal.
> - Beware of compromised peroneal longus tendon insertion.
> - Do not translate more than 5 mm if at all. Mau and Ludloff are primarily rotational osteotomies.

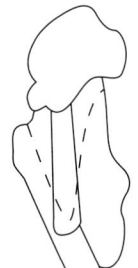 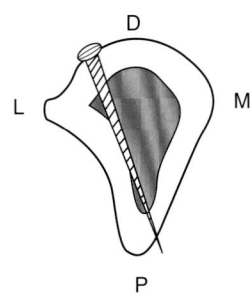

FIGURE 12.15 When fixating the Mau and Ludloff, the screws are oriented slightly medial to capture the opposing cortex and not directly plantar thereby avoiding the center of the plantar triangular surface and a potential stress fracture along the length of the plantar cut compromising fixation and stability. L, lateral; D, dorsal; M, medial; P, plantar.

To bolster stability in the Ludloff, Bae, and Schon, insert two K-wires for supplemental reinforcement.[12] This is especially helpful when encountering osteoporotic bone. The wires are oriented from proximal medial and driven distal into the metatarsal head or shaft and oriented parallel to the cut. Choi et al.[27] showed that insertion of a supplementary K-wire in the Ludloff also reduces the loss of IM correction, which can occur with these osteotomies at the time of immediate fixation or up to 1year from the surgery[17] (see Fig. 12.14).

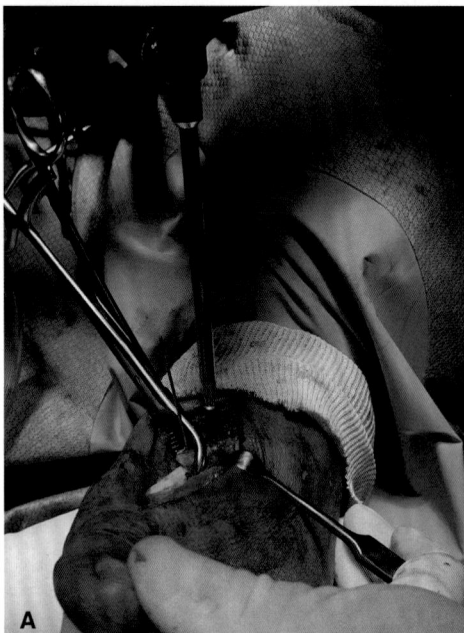 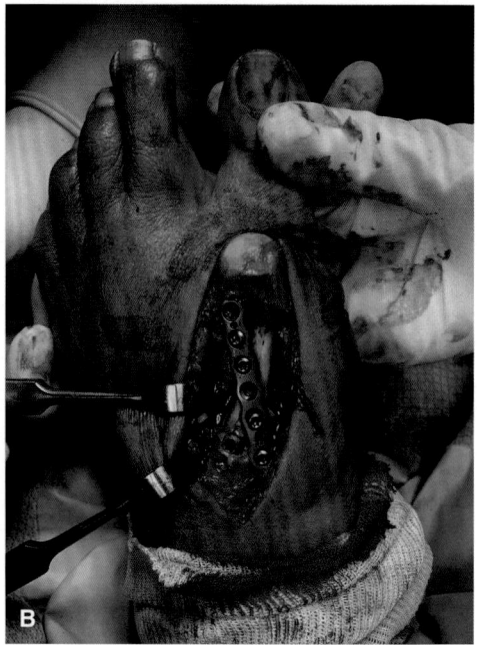

FIGURE 12.16 A. Mau osteotomy fixated with screw and plate construct. Note the proximal 3.5-mm solid cortical compression screw (Stryker Corp) replaced the proximal 0.45 K-wire. **B.** Following this, a plate is aligned medial to the screw and extends dorsal and lateral over the osteotomy. Note 5-6 hole slim compression plate with 2.4-mm locking screws (Stryker Corp). Authors preferred construct includes 2-3 screws proximal and crossing the osteotomy, thus providing additional fixation to the osteotomy through the plate. The dorsal edge of the osteotomy is aligned with an empty plate hole. Distal to the osteotomy 2 compression screws secure the plate on the bone. Image reprinted with permission from Stryker Corporation. © [2021] Stryker Corporation. All rights reserved.

More recently, there has been a push for fixation utilizing locking plates to add more stability, resistance to fatigue, and loss of fixation.[23,28-30] Saxena found that fixation of the Ludloff with a locking plate provided superior stabilization to two lag screws.[24] A locking plate may also minimize loss of correction.

Reports of supplemental K-wires or using locking plates have not as of now been documented in the literature with the Mau.[11] However, we have started to employ plating techniques for the Mau osteotomy. When fixating the Mau with a plate, we recommend fixating the osteotomy proximally with an independent compression screw and then applying the plate distal to this screw. A second screw is placed through the plate (either standard technique or locking) fixating the osteotomy at a second point. The rest of the screws crossing the plate will stabilize the dorsal and plantar fragments against load and shearing forces (Fig. 12.16).

Once full fixation is complete, the osteotomy is tested for stability by attempting to place a slight bending force at the head with one's fingers and observing for distraction of the osteotomy.

When complete, the Mau and Ludloff will have a redundant medial shelf of bone, which is smoothed with a power bur.

At this point, if articular deviation is present or additional IM correction is warranted, a Reverdin-Laird osteotomy[13] is performed. The authors preferred method of fixating this osteotomy is with a single cannulated headless 3.0-mm-diameter screw oriented from dorsal proximal to distal plantar and directed into the head with avoidance of the articular cartilage of the distal metatarsal (Fig. 12.17A-C).

Alternative fixation techniques include staples or a K-wire (Figs. 12.18A-C and 12.19A-C).

POSTOPERATIVE PROTOCOLS FOR MAU AND LUDLOFF OSTEOTOMIES

The literature does not have a consensus on postoperative protocols for the Mau and Ludloff procedures. There is a wide variation ranging from immediate heel weight bearing in a rigid post-op shoe with an assistive device, immediate walking with a CAM boot walker, to immobilization with a cast for 1-6 weeks prior to full weight bearing.[11,15,17,18,20-23,27,29,30] Constructs with more rigid fixation, such as locking plates and the presence of better bone quality, may allow for earlier weight bearing.[29] Neufeld found that locking plates used with the Ludloff provided ability for immediate weight bearing with no increased recurrence rates compared to other protocols.[29] When fixating the Mau with only screws, we recommend 4 weeks of non–weight bearing. With plate fixation, the osteotomy appears much more stable and resistant to shear and distraction; therefore, we are more liberal. In this case, we use a forefoot splint with partial weight bearing on the heel for 3 weeks in a post-op shoe before returning to partial weight bearing in a sneaker. Serial radiographs are taken to ensure healing of the osteotomy before allowing for full weight bearing in a supportive sneaker shoe. Most patients are able to wear casual shoes between 8 and 12 weeks, while full recovery is typically not achieved for 6-9 months.

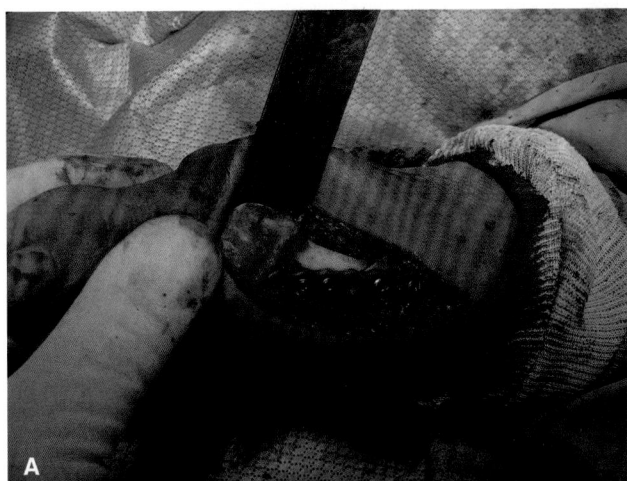

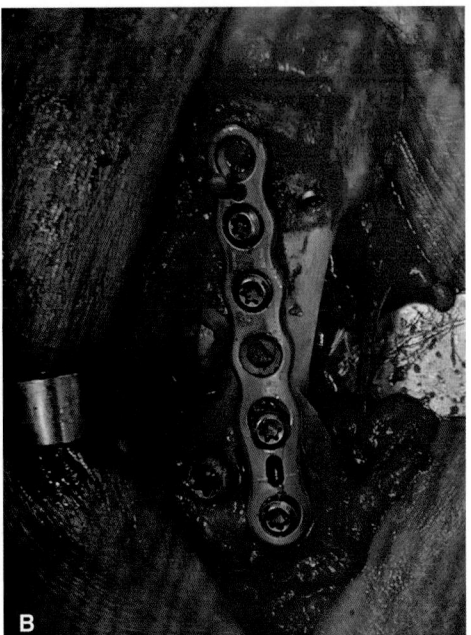

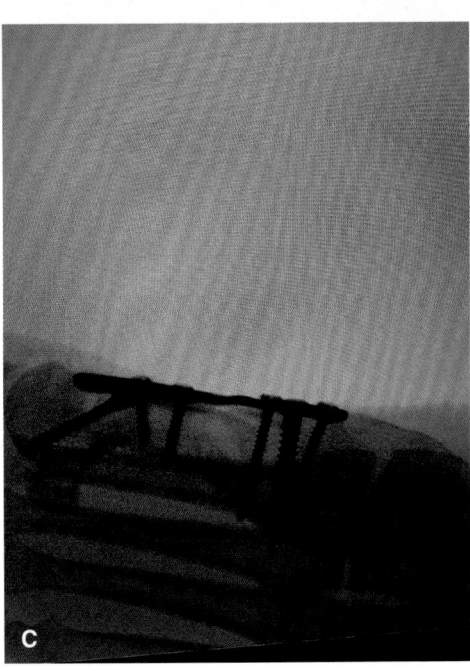

FIGURE 12.17 Fixating the Reverdin-Laird osteotomy with a single 3.0-mm cannulated headless double-threaded screw (Stryker Corp) oriented from dorsal proximal medial to plantar distal lateral and directed into the head with care not to penetrate the articular cartilage of the distal metatarsal. Image reprinted with permission from Stryker Corporation. © [2021] Stryker Corporation. All rights reserved.

COMPLICATIONS OF MAU AND LUDLOFF OSTEOTOMIES

Ludloff osteotomies have been associated with a delayed union rate of 2%-7%, metatarsal shortening, loss of IM correction with recurrent deformity, and a malunion revision rate of 1.5%-5%.[28] Delayed union in the Ludloff osteotomy may further lead to dorsiflexory malunion with subsequent elevation and metatarsalgia. Malunion with dorsiflexion of the osteotomy is most common with the Ludloff and least with the Mau osteotomy.[9,11] Comparing the Scarf and Ludloff procedures, Robinson et al.[17] found the Scarf to have superior outcomes in clinical and radiologic outcomes. Of 57 patients, 5%

of patients had a delayed union with the Ludloff, which may have been attributed to the use of headless screws. Two of the three nonunions in that series went on to develop a dorsiflexory nonunion.[17]

In the Ludloff, the load is transferred from the distal fragment to the proximal fragment through the fixation device.[28] This can lead to an irritation callus at the osteotomy site with a reported incidence of 16%-27%.[28] Gapping and load failure can also occur with the Ludloff as the osteotomy will distract and usually fracture at the proximal screw on the dorsal aspect of the metatarsal.[31,32] Mechanical cadaveric studies by Trnka[33] and saw bone studies by Acevedo[31] showed the Mau osteotomy to be more stable than the Ludloff and Scarf

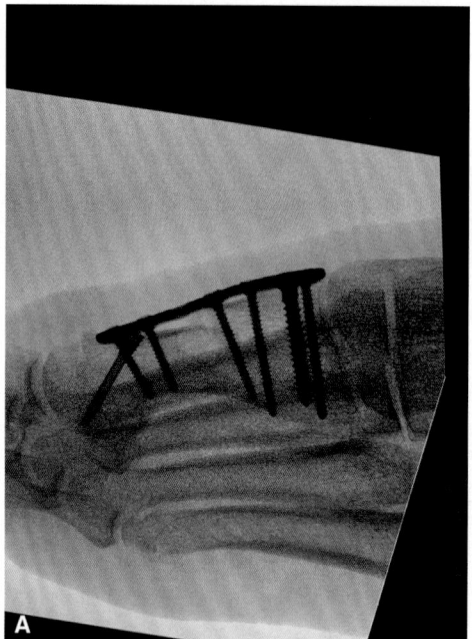

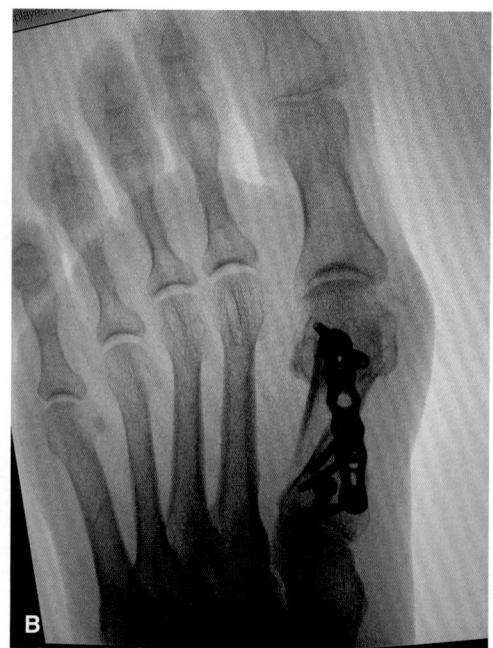

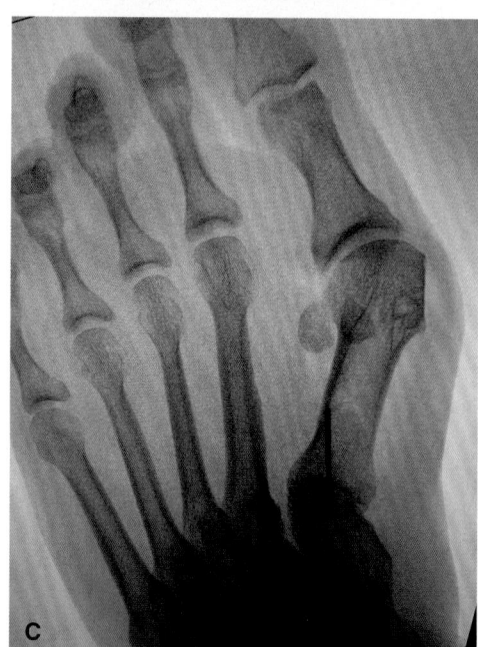

FIGURE 12.18 Preoperative and postprocedure intraoperative fluoroscope of Mau-Reverdin osteotomy fixed with plate and screws. Note the apex screw proximally is out of the plate. The distal Reverdin screw does not penetrate the articular cartilage at the head. The second proximal screw through the plate is also compressing the osteotomy. The rest of the screws are stabilizing the dorsal and plantar fragments against load and shearing forces.

osteotomies. Saw bone studies by Meric demonstrated failure in the distal screw region with the Ludloff, in the proximal screw region in the Mau, and between the screws with the Scarf.[34] Many studies demonstrated failure with the Ludloff in the proximal screw region.[12,33,35,36] Gapping has not been reported with failure in the Mau due to the inherent strong dorsal shelf. Loss of the intraoperative IM correction can occur with both Mau and Ludloff procedures, which can be minimized by orienting the screws perpendicular to the osteotomy whenever possible.

As with any capital osteotomy, when adding a Reverdin-Laird osteotomy to the Mau, there is low risk of avascular necrosis of the head. The incidence does not seem to be increased with the added osteotomy through the midshaft.[11,15]

HISTORICAL REVIEW

SCARF OSTEOTOMY

The midshaft Z-osteotomy was initially described by Burutaran[37] and Zygmunt and Gudas.[38] The "scarf osteotomy" was first coined by Weil Sr. in 1984[39,40] and describes a carpentry term whereby the two ends of a piece of wood are beveled and secured together so that they create one longer uninterrupted beam[41] (Fig. 11.20). Due to its stability, the scarf construct withstands tension and compression forces along the osteotomy.[42] Barouk popularized its usage in Europe, supported by the Scarf osteotomy's inherent stability, versatility, and ease of internal fixation, which allows for early weight bearing.[43] Barouk also

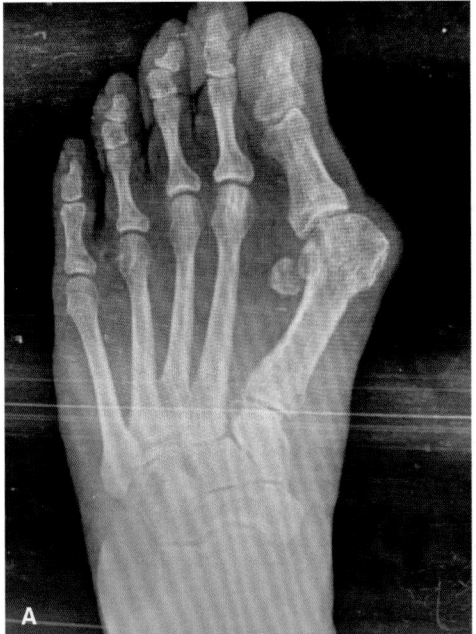

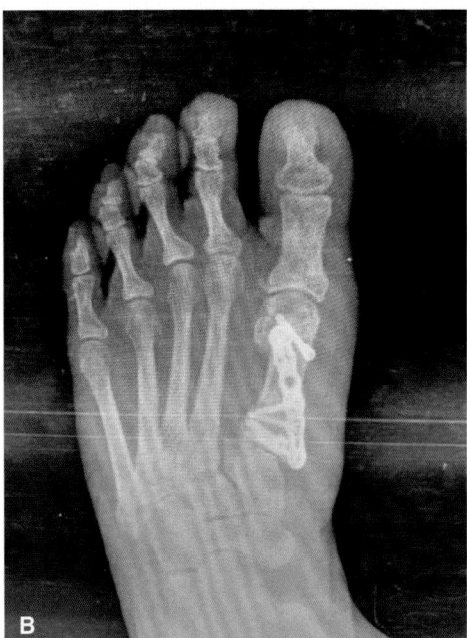

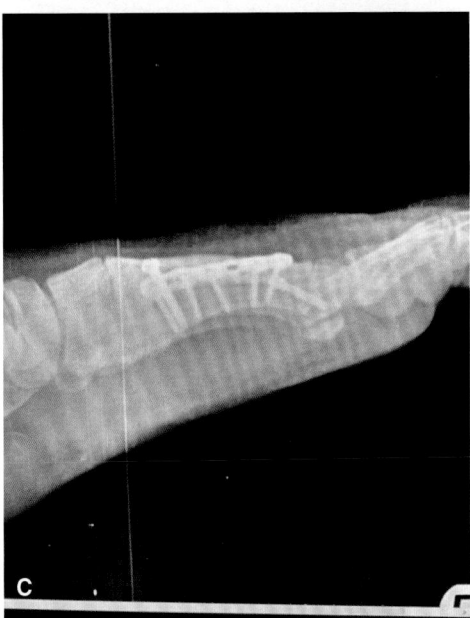

FIGURE 12.19 Preoperative and postoperative x-rays of the Mau-Reverdin osteotomy fixed with compression screw, plate, and distal headless screw.

reported that the Scarf osteotomy does not violate the blood supply to the first metatarsal, which is mainly from a plantar origin,[44] as can be the rare case with distal metatarsal head osteotomies, such as the Chevron (Fig. 12.21).[45]

INDICATIONS FOR SCARF OSTEOTOMY

The indications for a Scarf osteotomy are a moderate to severe hallux valgus deformity with intermetatarsal angles ranging from 12 to 23 degrees.[42] Proximal articular set angle (PASA) of up to 10 degrees can also be addressed with the osteotomy.[40] The technique can also be performed safely, simultaneously, bilaterally with early return to full weight bearing in shoes.[46] Contraindications to the procedure are moderate to severe first MTP joint arthritis, osteoporosis, extremely large intermetatarsal angles >25 degrees, and frank hypermobility of the first ray.[47]

INDICATIONS

- IM angle 12-23 degrees
- Can address elevated first metatarsal with modifications
- Can address increased PASA with modifications
- Can be performed bilaterally simultaneously
- Patients can start protective weight bearing immediately following surgery

CONTRAINDICATIONS

- Arthrosis of first MTP joint
- Poor bone quality

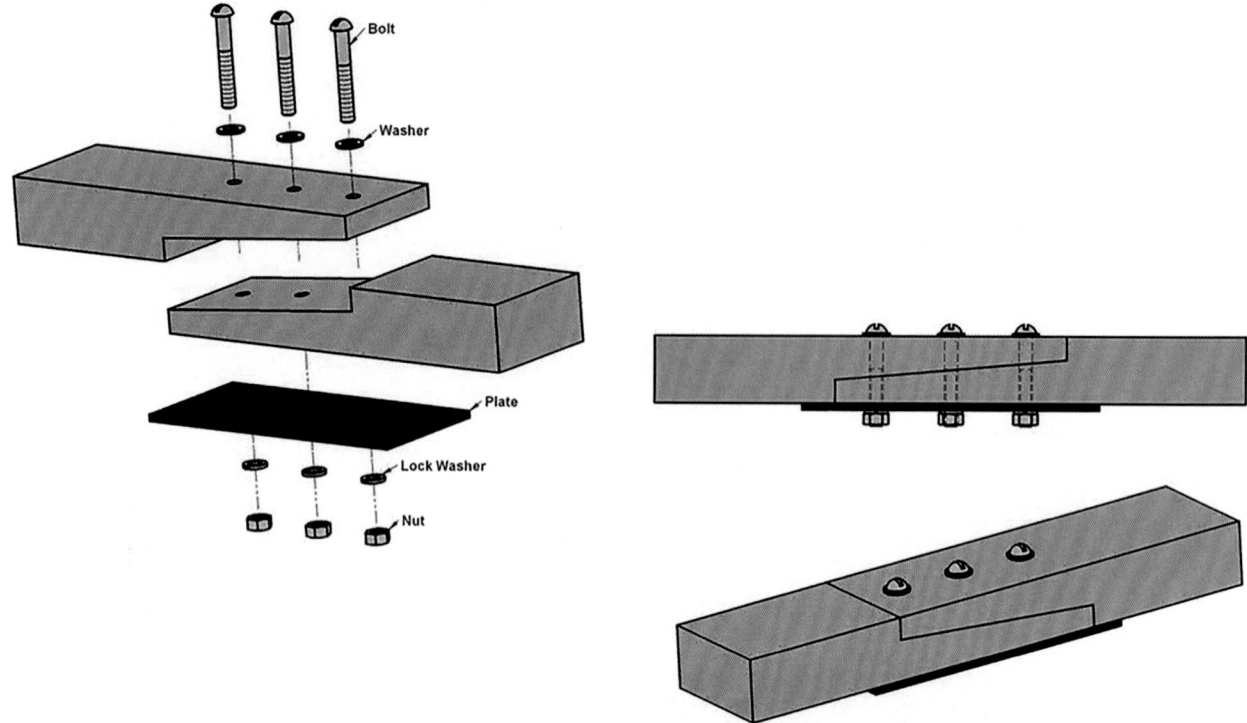

FIGURE 12.20 Illustration of a Scarf carpentry joint. With permission from Barouk LS. *Forefoot Reconstruction.* 2nd ed. Paris, France: Springer-Verlag; 2005.

SURGICAL TECHNIQUE

INCISION

Surgery is performed with the patient in a supine position with a combination of monitored sedation and a local Mayo block[48] using 15-18 cc bupivacaine 0.5% plain. If bilateral simultaneous surgery is being performed, a mixture of 0.5% bupivacaine plain and 1% lidocaine plain in a 1:1 ratio is used to avoid a potential toxic dose of local anesthetic.[49] An Esmarch bandage is used to exsanguinate the foot. An ankle tourniquet set at 250 mm Hg is employed, as it facilitates hemostasis and visibility of the surgical field. The author (RF) prefers to use a medial incision of the first metatarsal as it avoids the dorsomedial neurovascular bundle, allows for better visibility of the osteotomies and fixation, and gives a more cosmetic scar (Fig. 12.22).[40] The incision measures approximately 5-7 cm and is made just above the junction of the glabrous plantar skin and dorsal skin, from the base of the proximal phalanx to the midshaft of the metatarsal. The incision is deepened to subcutaneous tissue to the level of the joint, and any bleeding veins are ligated or cauterized. At this point, a Metzenbaum scissor is used to free up any attachments at the plantar portion of the incision. In addition, a soft tissue flap inferior to the neurovascular bundle is made dorsally, which envelopes the structures and enables them

FIGURE 12.21 Blood supply to first metatarsal in relation to Scarf osteotomy. 1. Dorsalis pedis artery; 2. Nutrient artery (variable); 3. Metaphyseal capital dorsal branch; 4. Medial plantar artery; 5. Medial plantar metaphyseal capital branch; 6. First intermetatarsal artery (main artery to the first metatarsal head); and 7. Lateral plantar metaphyseal capital branch. (With permission from Barouk LS. *Forefoot Reconstruction.* 2nd ed. Paris, France: Springer-Verlag; 2005.)

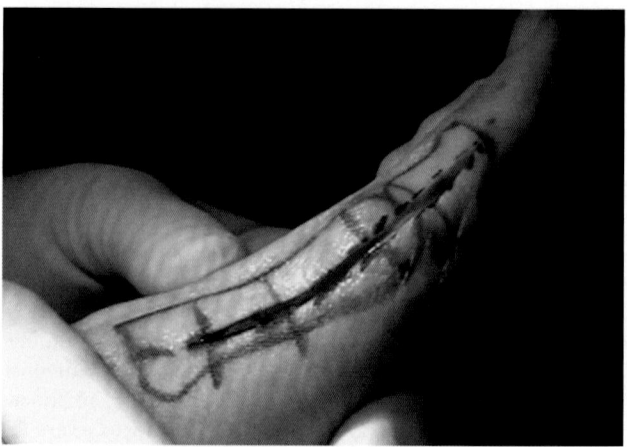

FIGURE 12.22 Skin incision.

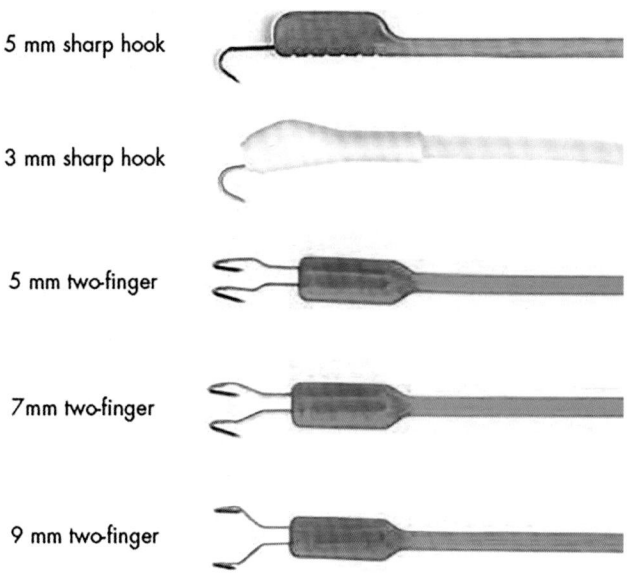

5 mm sharp hook

3 mm sharp hook

5 mm two-finger

7mm two-finger

9 mm two-finger

FIGURE 12.23 Flexible skin hooks. (Image provided courtesy of CooperSurgical Inc.)

to be carefully retracted out of the field. Flexible abdominal skin hooks aid in retraction and keep the operative field free of handheld instruments, allowing the procedure to be performed unassisted (Fig. 12.23).

PEARLS

- Use fluoroscopy.
- Use "one-third to two-third" relationship of the metatarsal when planning the osteotomy.
- Make head osteotomy in cancellous metaphyseal bone 4-5 mm proximal to articular cartilage to prevent troughing.
- Use an osteotomy guide to make accurate cuts.
- Make a long osteotomy.
- Use threaded head screws for fixation to provide stability and compression of fragments.

PITFALLS

- Troughing from making osteotomy in cortical bone or having inaccurate cuts
- Stress fracture or fracture from making a short osteotomy
- Malunion
- Metatarsalgia from shortening or elevation

CAPSULOTOMY AND LATERAL RELEASE

Two semielliptical converging incisions are made at the joint, which act as both a capsulotomy and subsequent capsulorrhaphy once the redundant tissue is excised. This gives excellent visualization of the medial aspect of the joint. Blunt dissection of the plantar tissue is achieved using the end of the scalpel handle and is extended distally to the plantar flare of the metatarsal. The dorsal joint tissue and periosteum are reflected sharply off the metatarsal head and shaft, and the skin hooks are reappropriated to encompass the deeper tissues. Through

the same medial incision, a McGlamry elevator is used to free up any adhesions of the lateral joint capsule and to mobilize the sesamoids with care being taken to avoid the plantar blood supply to the sesamoids. A Weitlaner smooth self-retaining retractor is then positioned and expanded between the plantar joint capsule and metatarsal head. This allows intracapsular release of the lateral sesamoid suspensory ligament using a Beaver 6400 blade. Ergonomically, for the right-handed surgeon, the technique is best performed from the base of the operating table on the right foot and overarching the left foot to the surgical area from the lateral aspect. This is the opposite for the left-handed surgeon. The hallux is then extended into a varus position to further relax the lateral joint structures.

OSTEOTOMY

The Scarf osteotomies create a "z-cut," which is inherently stable and is fixated using rigid internal fixation. Minimal removal of the dorsomedial bump is performed with an oscillating saw to give a flat surface for the osteotomy. As described by Weil Jr. and Bowen, a 0.045 smooth K-wire is placed at the dorsal one-third of the first metatarsal head and driven laterally. The guidewire can be positioned to maintain length, shorten or lengthen the metatarsal, as well as for plantar or dorsal displacement based on axis guide principles.[40,50,51] In most cases, slight shortening and plantar displacement are desired, so the guidewire is directed approximately 25-30 degrees dorsal-to-plantar with slight shortening by aiming the wire toward the fourth metatarsal head. Slight plantar displacement of the first metatarsal osteotomy decreases the risk of second metatarsal overload.[47] A Reese osteotomy guide is then placed over the guidewire in order to make predictable and reproducible cuts. It is the authors' opinion and others[40,47] that this is one of the most important components in the success of the Scarf osteotomy. A marker is used to draw out the cuts on the bone in preparation for the osteotomy. The dorsal portion of the z-cut is made first. It is angled approximately 60-70 degrees and exits 4-5 mm proximal to the articular cartilage of the first metatarsal head. This cut must be made in the cancellous metaphyseal bone of the metatarsal head to prevent troughing during translation of the osteotomy. Next, the transverse cut is made. A "one-third, two-third" concept is used to orient this portion of the osteotomy; at the distal end, there should be one-third of the bone dorsal to the osteotomy, and two-thirds below the osteotomy. This is reversed at the proximal end where one-third is plantar and two-thirds is dorsal to the cut. The cut is angled toward the base of the first metatarsal near its anatomic flare. The K-wire in the head and guide is then removed, and the plantar proximal cut is made free-handed with the edge of the blade, corresponding to the same angle as the dorsal distal cut (Fig. 12.24). An axis guide is usually not needed for the proximal plantar cut but can be placed if so desired. It is important that this cut be parallel to the dorsal cut so that there is an easily translatable osteotomy. Distal traction on the hallux can help with completing this portion of the cut.

Once the osteotomy is completed and mobilized, it is translated laterally using a push-pull technique (Fig. 12.25).[47] A small phalangeal clamp attached at the corner of the capital fragment and is used to pull the dorsal fragment medially, while the plantar portion is pushed laterally with a blunt instrument or thumb to close down the intermetatarsal angle.

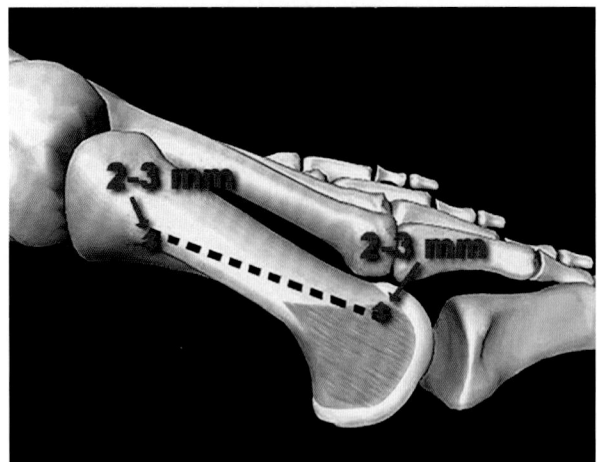

FIGURE 12.24 Scarf osteotomy placement. (With permission from Barouk LS. *Forefoot Reconstruction.* 2nd ed. Paris, France: Springer-Verlag; 2005.)

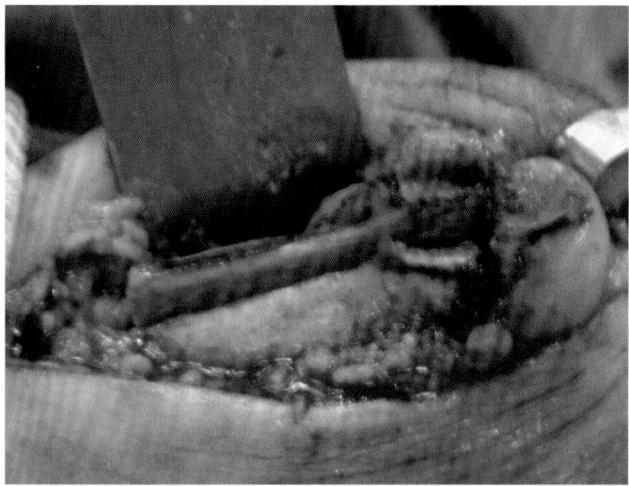

FIGURE 12.25 Scarf translation.

Some authors extend the limits of translation to 75% of the width of the metatarsal shaft,[12] but rarely does it go more than 50%. A specialized Scarf clamp is used to hold the osteotomy in place (Fig. 12.26A-C).

The Scarf is primarily a transpositional osteotomy. It prevents rotation since the proximal plantar cut will be blocked by the shelf of bone behind it. The Scarf can be modified to correct for increases in PASA/DMAA of up to 20 degrees. Small increased can be managed by rotating the capital fragment

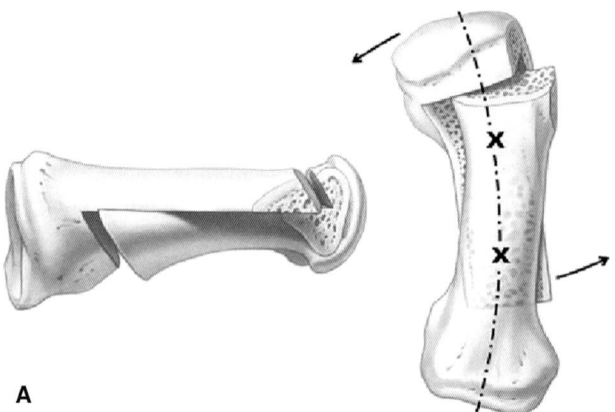

A

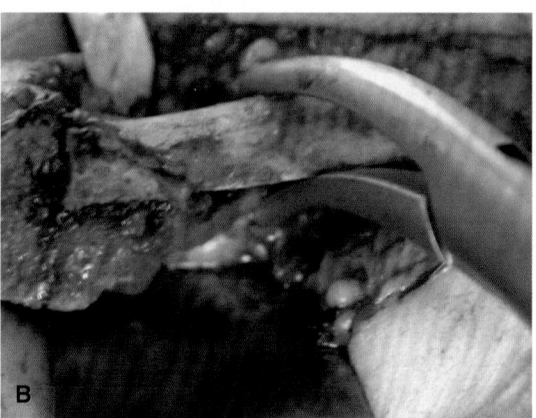

B

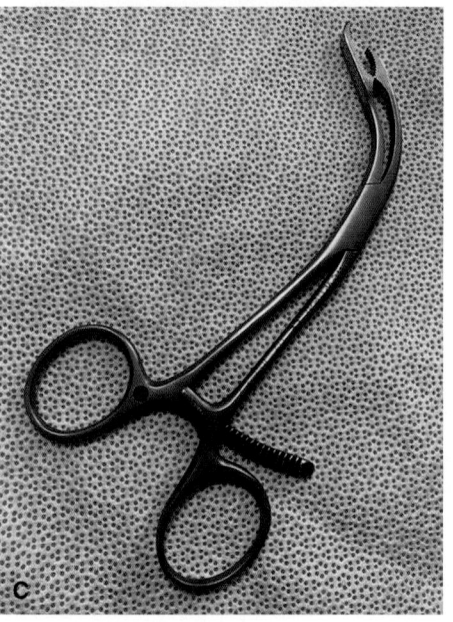

C

FIGURE 12.26 Scarf stabilization using specialized scarf clamp.

to make the joint congruent. Larger PASA/DMAA correction can be achieved by removing a small mirror-image wedge at the dorsal distal cut and proximal plantar cut, which will now allow for additional rotation to occur (see Fig. 12.26A). However, intermetatarsal angular correction is achieved only by translation.

FIXATION

Fixation is achieved using two cannulated threaded-head compression screws, usually 2.5-3.0 mm in size. Two provisional K-wires are placed to guide the cannulated screws. The first screw is unicortical and is positioned distal and plantar toward the crista of the first metatarsal head (Fig. 12.27A). Care is taken to avoid hitting the sesamoids when advancing the wire. This can be done via visual inspection or with the help of intraoperative fluoroscopy. When using compression screws, a good rule of thumb is to subtract about 4 mm from the length of the wire to get the correct screw size. This will allow appropriate countersinking of the head of the screw without violating the plantar joint space from using an inappropriately long screw. The proximal screw is bicortical and is directed from dorsal medial to plantar lateral to capture the cortex of the plantar shelf (Fig. 12.27B). Once screw fixation is obtained, the Scarf clamp is removed, the screws are finger tightened, and the remaining overhanging bone shelf at the dorsomedial head is resected with a saw. At this point, a fluoroscopic image in multiple planes is performed to ensure maintained correction and appropriate screw length and placement. An assessment for any adjunctive first ray procedures, such as an Akin phalangeal osteotomy, is then made.

TROUGHING

A rare complication of the Scarf osteotomy is troughing, which occurs during translation of the osteotomy.[40,52] The medial portion of the dorsal shelf falls into the soft medullary canal of the plantar bone and essentially creates a dorsiflexion of the first ray with loss of metatarsal height (Fig. 12.28). The risk may occur with osteopenic bone, multiple passes of the saw blade, and exceeding the recommended amount of lateral translation of the osteotomy.[53] Meticulous surgical technique is important to help prevent troughing. By making the proximal and distal cuts in strong cancellous bone, this limits the effect. Using an osteotomy guide eliminates the need for multiple passes of the saw blade. If troughing is encountered intraoperatively, Lee et al advocates inserting a free oscillating saw blade in the longitudinal cut, clamping the bone, inserting the screws, and then removing the saw blade.[54] A similar technique was described by Saragas using the flat end of the McDonald dissector.[55] Others have used the resected medial eminence as bone graft to resist troughing.[56]

CLOSURE

The toe is held in a corrected position, and the joint capsule is closed with 2-0 absorbable suture in a running fashion. The closure starts with a pulley suture directed from plantar capsule to dorsal capsule, which help maintain joint alignment. The subcutaneous closure and skin closure are performed as per surgeon's preference. A multilayer compression dressing is used to maintain the correction.

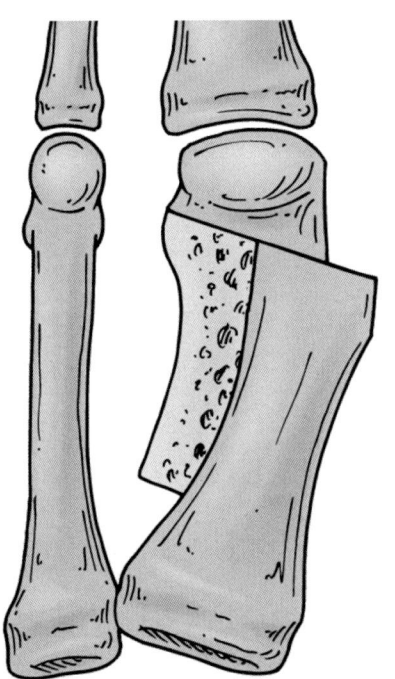 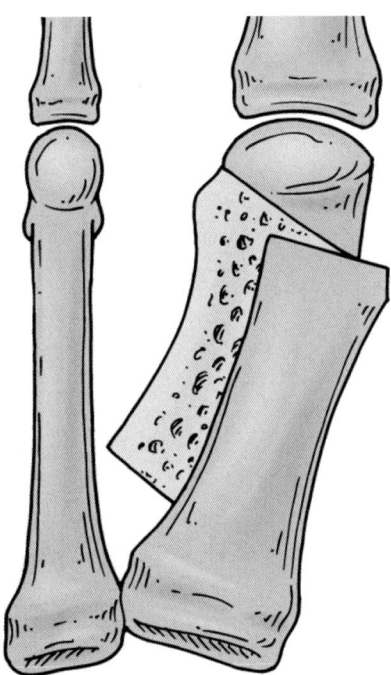

FIGURE 12.27 Scarf correction for PASA/DMAA. On the left, is normal translation without any correction of the cartilage deviation. On the right, the capital fragment is rotated to allow for PASA/DMAA correction. Larger angles are addressed by removing a small, mirroring bone wedges from the dorsal distal metatarsal and the proximal plantar fragment. (Courtesy of the Podiatry Institute.)

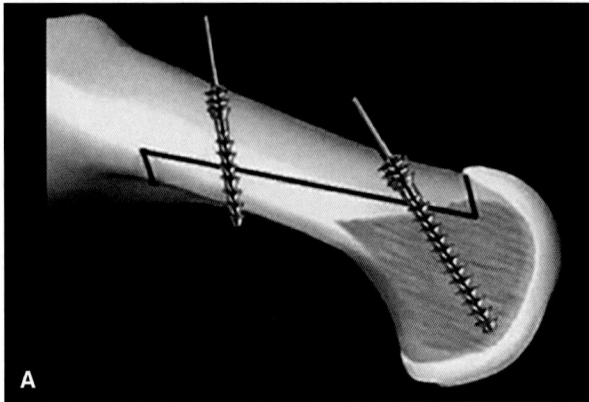

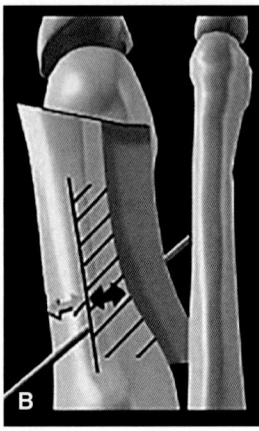

FIGURE 12.28 Scarf screw placement. **A.** Note that placement of the distal screw is in the head of the first metatarsal and avoids violating the joint. **B.** Note the placement of the guidewire goes from dorsal proximal medial to plantar distal lateral in order to catch the plantar cortex with the screw. (With permission from Barouk LS. *Forefoot Reconstruction.* 2nd ed. Paris, France: Springer-Verlag; 2005.)

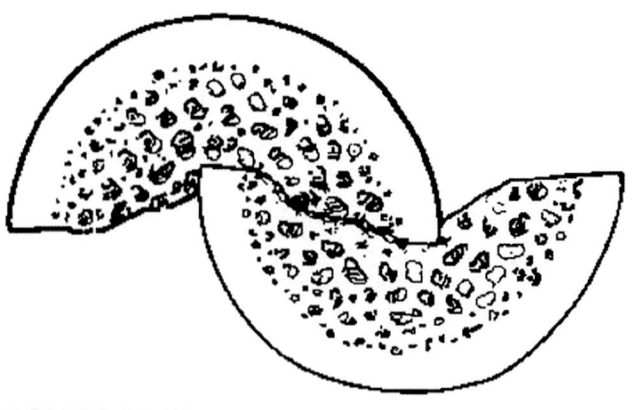

FIGURE 12.29 Troughing.

POSTOPERATIVE PROTOCOL

Guarded weight bearing in a postoperative shoe or CAM walker is started immediately. Advancement to a stable running shoe occurs between 10 and 21 days, depending on the patient's activity level and type of work they perform.[46] Physical therapy range-of-motion exercises are started at 7-10 days post-op, as evidence has shown that early adoption of therapy increases function and decreases pain after bunion surgery.[57,58] If appropriate healing is clinically and radiographically apparent at 6 weeks, transition to any type of footwear is allowed, and low-impact exercises, such as elliptical machine and walking, can be started. Full-impact activity, such as running, is permitted at 3 months (Figs. 12.29 and 12.30).

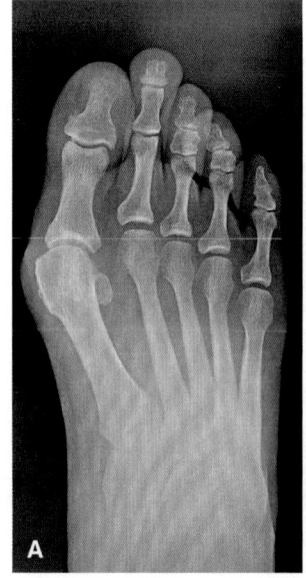

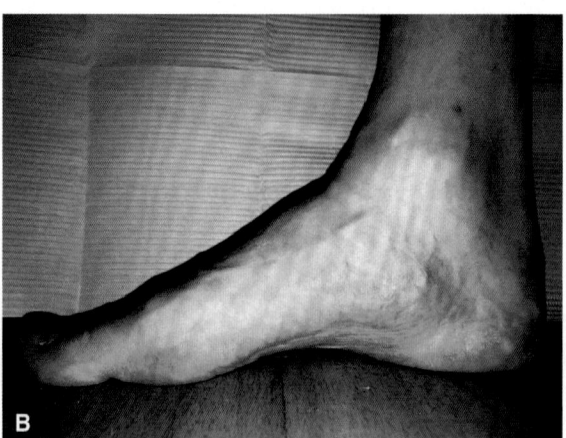

FIGURE 12.30 **A,B.** Pre-operative radiographic and clinical image of foot prior to Scarf bunionectomy. **C,D,E.** 10-year post-operative Scarf bunionectomy clinical and radiographic images.

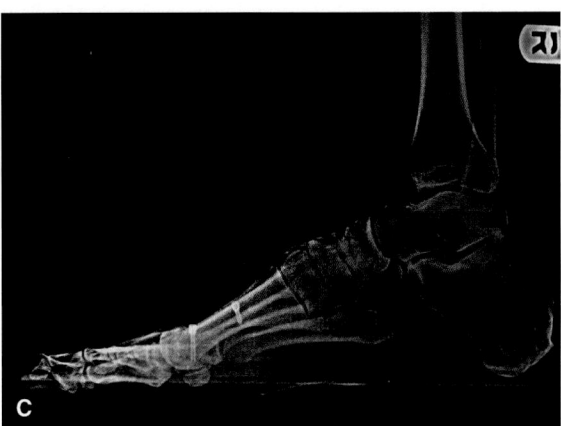

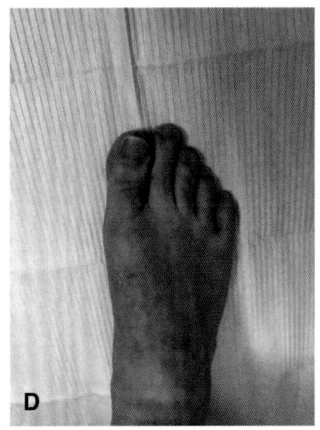

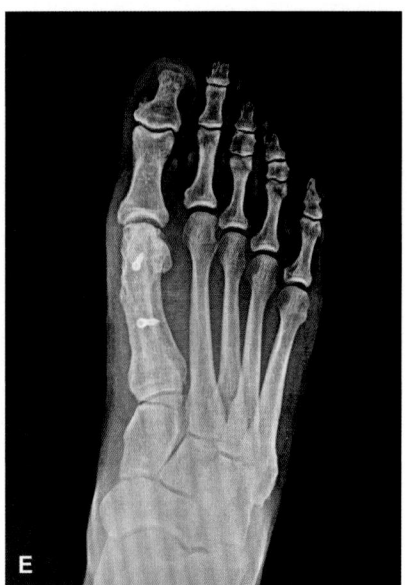

FIGURE 12.30 (*Continued*)

REFERENCES

1. Ludloff K. Die beseitigung des hallux valgus durch die schrage planta-dorsale osteotomie des metatarsus I. *Arch Klin Chir.* 1918;365.
2. Mau C, Lauber HT. Die operative behalung des hallux valgus (Nochunt Suchungen). *Dtsch Z Chir.* 1926;197:361.
3. Neese D, Zelichowski J, Patton G. Mau osteotomy: an alternative procedure to the closing abductory base wedge. *J Foot Surg.* 1989;28(4):352-362.
4. Vogler HW. Shaft osteotomies in hallux valgus. *Clin Podiatr Med Surg.* 1989;6:47-69.
5. Martin DE, Blitch EL. Alternatives to the closing base wedge osteotomy. *Clin Podiatr Med Surg.* 1996;13:515-531.
6. Saxena A, McCammon D. The Ludloff osteotomy: a critical analysis. *J Foot Ankle Surg.* 1997;36(2):100-105.
7. Draves DJ. *Anatomy of the Lower Extremity.* Philadelphia, PA: Williams & Wilkins; 1986: 127-128.
8. Sarrafian SK. *Anatomy of the Foot and Ankle.* Philadelphia, PA: J. B. Lippincott; 1983:78-79.
9. Sammarco VJ. Surgical strategies: Mau osteotomy for correction of moderate and severe hallux valgus deformity. *Foot Ankle Int.* 2007;28(7):857-864.
10. Ferraro PN, Saragas NP. Rotational and opening wedge basal osteotomies. *Foot Ankle Clin.* 2014;19(2):203-221.
11. Arcuri N, Bar-David T. The Mau-Reverdin osteotomy: a short term retrospective analysis. *J Foot Ankle Surg.* 2016;55:794-798.
12. Bae SY, Schon L. Surgical strategies: Ludloff first metatarsal osteotomy. *Foot Ankle Int.* 2007;28(1):137-144.
13. Beck E. Modified Reverdin technique for hallux abducto valgus (with increased proximal articular set angle of the first metatarsal phalangeal joint). *J Am Podiatry Assoc.* 1974;64:662-667.
14. Bar-David T, Greenberg P. Retrospective analysis of the Mau osteotomy and effect of a fibular sesamoidectomy. *J Foot Ankle Surg.* 1998;37(3):212-216.
15. Neese DJ, Zelent ME. The modified Mau-Reverdin double osteotomy for correction of hallux valgus: a retrospective study. *J Foot Ankle Surg.* 2009;48(1):22-29.
16. Schuh R, Willegger M, Holinka J, Ristl R, Windhager R, Wanivenhaus AH. Angular correction and complications of proximal first metatarsal osteotomies for hallux valgus deformity. *Int Orthop (SICOT).* 2013;37:1771-1780.
17. Robinson A, Bhatia M. Prospective comparative study of the scarf and Ludloff osteotomies in the treatment of hallux valgus. *Foot Ankle Int.* 2009;30(10):955-963.
18. Trnka HJ, Hofstaetter MD, Easley ME. Intermediate term results of the Ludloff osteotomy in one hundred and eleven feet. *J Bone Joint Surg Am.* 2009;91 (Suppl 2; part 1): 156-168.
19. Chiodo C, Schon L, Myerson M. Clinical results with the Ludloff osteotomy for correction of adult hallux valgus. *Foot Ankle Int.* 2004;25(8):532-536.
20. Thangarajah T, Ahmed U, Shahbaz M, Tilu A. The early functional outcome of Mau osteotomy for the correction of moderate-severe hallux valgus. *Orthop Rev.* 2013;5(e37): 159-161.
21. Hyer CF, Glover JP, Berlet GC, Philbin TM, Lee TH. A comparison of the crescentic and Mau osteotomies for correction of hallux valgus. *J Foot Ankle Surg.* 2008;47(2):103-111.
22. Glover JP, Hyer CF, Berlet GC, Lee TLJ. Early results of the Mau osteotomy for correction of moderate to severe hallux valgus: a review of 24 cases. *J Foot Ankle Surg.* 2008;47(3): 237-242.
23. Castaneda DA, Myerson MS, Neufeld SK. The Ludloff osteotomy: a review of current concepts. *Int Orthop (SICOT).* 2013;37:1661-1668.
24. Beischer AD, Ammon P, Corniou A, Myerson M. Three-dimensional computer analysis of the modified Ludloff osteotomy. *Foot Ankle Int.* 2005;26(8):627-632.
25. Nyska M, Trnka H-J, Parks BJ, Myerson MS. The Ludloff metatarsal osteotomy: guidelines for optimal correction based on geometric analysis conducted on a sawbone model. *Foot Ankle Int.* 2003;24(1):34-39.
26. Schon LC, Dom KJ, Jung HG. Clinical tip: stabilization of the proximal Ludloff osteotomy. *Foot Ankle Int.* 2005;26(7):579-580.
27. Choi GW, Choi WJ, Yoon HS, Lee JW. Additional surgical factors affecting the recurrence of hallux valgus after Ludloff osteotomy. *Bone Joint J.* 2013;95B(6):803-808.
28. Chatzistergos PE, Karaoglanis GC, Kourkoulis SK, Tyllianakis M. Supplementary medial locking plate fixation of Ludloff osteotomy versus sole lag screw fixation: a biomechanical evaluation. *Clin Biomech.* 2017;47:66-72.
29. Neufeld SK, Marcel JJ, Campbell M. Immediate weight bearing after hallux valgus correction using locking plate fixation of the Ludloff osteotomy. *Foot Ankle Spec.* 2018;11(2):148-155.
30. Saxena A, St. Louis M. Medial locking plate versus screw fixation for fixation of the Ludloff osteotomy. *J Foot Ankle Surg.* 2013;52:153-157.
31. Acevedo JI, Sammarco J, Boucher HR, Parks BG, Schon L, Myerson MS. Mechanical comparison of cyclic loading in five different first metatarsal shaft osteotomies. *Foot Ankle Int.* 2002;23(8):711-716.
32. Scott AT, DeOrio JK, Montijo HE, Glisson RR. Biomechanical comparison of hallux valgus correction using the proximal chevron osteotomy with a medial locking plate and the Ludloff osteotomy fixed with two screws. *Clin Biomech.* 2010;25:271-276.
33. Trnka HJ, Parks BG, Ivanic G, Chu IT, Easley ME, Schon LC, et al. Six metatarsal shaft osteotomies mechanical and immobilization comparisons. *Clin Orthop Relat Res.* 2000;381:256-265.
34. Unal A, Baran O, Uzun B, Turan AC. Comparison of screw stabilities of first metatarsal shaft osteotomies: a biomechanical study. *Acta Orthop Traumatol Turc.* 2010;44(1):70-75.
35. Rockett MS, Goss LR. Midshaft first ray osteotomies for hallux valgus. *Clin Podiatr Med Surg.* 2005;22:169-195.
36. Trnka HJ. Osteotomies for hallux valgus correction. *Foot Ankle Clin.* 2005;10:15-33.
37. Burutaran JM. Hallux valgus y cortedad anatomica del primer metatarsiano (correction quirurgica). *Actual Méd Chir Pied* 1976;XIII:261-266.
38. Zygmunt KH. Z-bunionectomy with internal screw fixation. *J Am Podiatr Med Assoc.* 1989;79(7):322-329.
39. Weil LS, Borelli AH. Modified Scarf bunionectomy: our experience in more than 1000 cases. *J Foot Surg.* 1991;30:609-622.
40. Weil LS. Scarf osteotomy for correction of hallux valgus. Historical perspective, surgical technique, and results. *Foot Ankle Clin.* 2000;5:559-580.
41. Molloy A. Scarf osteotomy. *Foot Ankle Clin.* 2014;19(2):165-180.
42. Weil LJ. Scarf osteotomy for correction of hallux abducto valgus deformity. *Clin Podiatr Med Surg.* 2014;31(2):233-246.
43. Barouk LS. Scarf osteotomy of the first metatarsal in the treatment of hallux valgus. *Foot Dis II.* 1991;1:35-48.
44. Barouk LS. Scarf osteotomy for hallux valgus correction, local anatomy, surgical technique, and combination with other forefoot procedures. *Foot Ankle Clin.* 2000;5(3):525-558.
45. Easley ME. Avascular necrosis of the hallux metatarsal head. *Foot Ankle Clin.* 2000;5(3):591-608.
46. Fridman R, Cain JD, Weil LJ, et al. Unilateral versus bilateral first ray surgery: a prospective study of 186 consecutive cases—patient satisfaction, cost to society, and complications. *Foot Ankle Spec.* 2009;2:123-129.
47. Weil LS. Scarf bunionectomy. In: Chang TJ, ed. *Master Techniques in Podiatric Surgery: The Foot and Ankle.* Philadelphia, PA: Lippincott Williams & Wilkins; 2005:149-159.

48. Worrell JB, Barbour G. The Mayo block: an efficacious block for hallux and first metatarsal surgery. *AANA J.* 1996;64:146-152.

49. Williams DJ, Walker JD. A nomogram for calculating the maximum dose of local anaesthetic. *Anaesthesia.* 2014;69:847-853.

50. Chang TJ. Distal metaphyseal osteotomies in hallux abducto valgus surgery. In: Banks AS, et al., eds. *McGlamry's Comprehensive Textbook of Foot and Ankle Surgery.* 3rd ed. Philadelphia, PA: Lippincott Williams & Wilkins; 2001:505-527.

51. Cain TD. Distal metaphyseal osteotomies in hallux abducto valgus surgery. In: Banks AS, et al., eds. *McGlamry's Comprehensive Textbook of Foot and Ankle Surgery.* 2nd ed. Baltimore, MD: Williams & Wilkins; 1992:493-505.

52. Coetzee JC. Scarf osteotomy for hallux valgus repair: the dark side. *Foot Ankle Int.* 2003;24(1):29-33.

53. Schoen NS, Zygmunt K, Gudas C. Z-bunionectomy: retrospective long-term study. *J Foot Ankle Surg.* 1996;35(4):312-317.

54. Lee SC, Hwang SH, Nam CH, Baek JH, Yoo SY, Ahn HS. Technique for preventing troughing in Scarf osteotomy. *J Foot Ankle Surg.* 2017;56(4):822-823.

55. Saragas NP. Technique tip: preventing "troughing" with the scarf osteotomy. *Foot Ankle Int.* 2005;26(9):779-780.

56. Duke HF. Rotational scarf (Z) osteotomy bunionectomy for correction of high intermetatarsal angles. *J Am Podiatr Med Assoc.* 1992;82(7):352-360.

57. Hawson ST. Physical therapy post-hallux abducto valgus correction. *Clin Podiatr Med Surg.* 2014;31(2):309-322.

58. Schuh R, Hofstaetter SG, Adams SB Jr, Pichler F, Kristen KH, Trnka HJ. Rehabilitation after hallux valgus surgery: importance of physical therapy to restore weight bearing of the first ray during the stance phase. *Phys Ther.* 2009;89(9):934-945.

59. Shaw N, Wertheimer S, Kruger J, Haut R. A mechanical comparison of first metatarsal diaphyseal osteotomies for the correction of hallux abducto valgus. *J Foot Ankle Surg.* 2001;40(5):271-276.

60. Nyska M, Trnka H-J, Parks BG, Myerson MS. Proximal metatarsal osteotomies: a comparative geometric analysis conducted on sawbone models. *Foot Ankle Int.* 2002;23(10):938-945.

61. Bar-David T, Greenberg P. *McGlamry's Comprehensive Textbook of Foot and Ankle Surgery.* Volume I. Lippincott Williams & Wilkins; 2001:572-579.

CHAPTER 13

Lapidus Bunionectomy

Paul Dayton and Daniel J. Hatch

DEFINITION

HISTORY

The Lapidus bunionectomy has evolved over the years and has become increasingly popular with foot and ankle surgeons. Our re-discovery that the first tarsometatarsal joint (1st TMT) is the anatomic apex of the deformity, a concept originally associated with the procedure indications, is driving new discussions on the utility of this procedure. Albrecht first described 1st TMT arthrodesis in 1911.[1] Truslow coined the term metatarsus primus varus in 1925.[2] This was in reference to the adduction deformity in the transverse plane and not varus as we understand it now in the frontal plane. In 1934, Lapidus stated "the only mechanically sound osteotomy for metatarsus primus varus should be at the metatarsocuneiform joint which is at the apex of the angulation between the first metatarsal and cuneiform joint."[3] A true Lapidus procedure involves arthrodesis of the first tarsometatarsal joint and the bases of the first and second metatarsals. Modifications are commonly performed by either only fusing the first tarsometatarsal joint or employing screw stabilization or arthrodesis between the first and second rays if instability is observed in either the sagittal or transverse plane.

Although Dr. Lapidus' name is still ascribed to 1st TMT arthrodesis for correction of hallux valgus, the procedure as well as the indications have evolved. For the past two decades, we have seen dramatic improvement in fixation and bone healing and a new understanding of surgical anatomy. These factors have put aside some of the traditional fears of the 1st TMT arthrodesis such as healing problems and prolonged convalescence with earlier iterations of the procedure. We now know that the 1st TMT is a powerful site to correct not only the intermetatarsal (IM) angle but also the other triplane components of the deformity.[4] We no longer see this as a procedure reserved for the most severe deformities or only for those needing first ray stabilization. In fact, there are many surgeons that use the 1st TMT corrective arthrodesis as their priority procedure for correction of hallux abducto valgus (HAV).

HISTORICAL INDICATIONS

Traditional indications for the Lapidus bunionectomy have been based upon severity-based algorithms. In the past, and to a large extent today, the procedure fits in the spectrum of severity only for the most severe deformities of the IM angle.

Other indications are the presence of osteoarthritis of the first tarsometatarsal joint, which is not a common component of hallux valgus deformity, and significant elevation of the first ray. Condon et al. in 2002 described a severity-based algorithm for hallux valgus repair in which a severe deformity was classified as an IM angle of 16 degrees or greater.[5] This also was supported by Coughlin and Jones in 2007.[6] Traditionally, it has been in this severe class that the Lapidus procedure would be performed. Additionally, hypermobility of the first ray has also been a criterion for the Lapidus procedure. While still a clinical enigma, many descriptions of hypermobility have been attempted. Due to the difficulty of definition, many now prefer to call this first ray insufficiency or functional instability. Many authors believe that hypermobility of the first ray unlocks the forefoot predisposing it to HAV deformity.[3,7,8] D'Amico wrote a review of first ray mechanics in 2016.[9] In that article he stated "hypermobility of the first ray ... occurs primarily at the medial cuneiform-navicular articulation caused by subtalar and midtarsal joint pronation as a result of inherently induced phylogenetic and ontogenic induced imperfections." Kimura et al. in 2017 stated that hypermobility occurs along the entire first ray and is not limited to or predominated by range of motion at the 1st TMT.[10]

Most commonly those that have studied and discussed first ray range of motion discuss hypermobility in the sagittal plane. Root et al. in 1977 defined hypermobility as motion in excess of equal amounts of dorsal and plantar displacement of the first ray compared to the second ray.[11] Roukis and Landsman described a dynamic Hick test in their review of the literature in 2003.[12] In this case, the windlass mechanism would be engaged while evaluating the disbursement of the first ray. The power of the windlass mechanism was detailed in Rush et al. article in 2000.[13] They found that there was significant loss of the windlass with hallux valgus deformity. Additionally, realignment of the first ray and sesamoids provides successful engagement of the windlass. Shibuya et al. found in their systematic review that there was 3.62-mm displacement in the sagittal plane in the hallux valgus group.[14] Radiographic signs of sagittal plane instability include second ray overload with stress fractures and plantar gapping of the 1st TMT (Fig. 13.1).

Descriptions of transverse instability or splay are less common in the literature. Weber et al. described a "splay test" that represented transverse plane instability especially in a Romash 1 foot type.[15] This was later reinforced by a study from Flemming et al. finding that in patients with hallux valgus, 73.8% had transverse plane instability.[16]

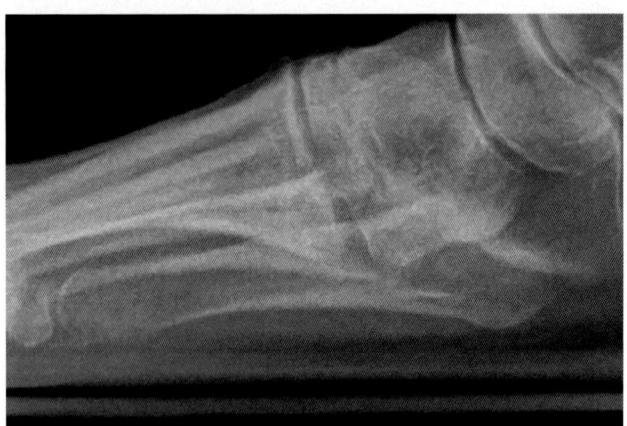

FIGURE 13.1 Sagittal plane instability with plantar gap at the first TMTJ. (From Hatch DJ, Santrock RD, Smith B, Dayton P, Weil L. Triplane Hallux Abducto Valgus Classification. *J Foot Ankle Surg.* 2018;57(5):972-981.)

Hypermobility not only influences the HAV deformity but it increases the chance of recurrence and overload to the second rays as pointed out by Feilmeier et al.[17] As with sagittal plane instability, transverse plane movement and potential functional instability occurs at multiple first ray joints including the 1st TMT. Traditional thought is that fusing the 1st TMT as part of the Lapidus procedure will eliminate recurrence of the deformity. Because the motion comes from multiple joints, recurrence of HAV is certainly possible even when the 1st TMT is solidly fused. This especially may occur if the IM angle is not reduced enough. Lapidus in his original description included fusion of the first and second metatarsal bases, possibly because he recognized this. Fusion of metatarsals 1-2 at the bases certainly reduces the chances of recurrence but may limit the desirable windlass function of the first ray. As we will discuss later in this chapter, a more modern approach to 1st TMT fusion for HAV is a triplanar correction philosophy.

MODERN INDICATIONS

Current indications for Lapidus originate from improved understanding of three-dimensional (3-D) anatomy of the first ray. This triplanar anatomic-based approach has been discussed by Hatch et al.[18] (Table 13.1). Understanding of the frontal plane component of the first ray as a component of HAV and adherence to the principle that the 1st TMT is the anatomic apex of the deformity changes our thought process from the 1st TMT fusion being an occasionally performed procedure, to one that is indicated for most HAV deformities. Comprehension of the 3-D aspects of the first ray has evolved since Mizuno first described this in 1956.[19] Scranton and Rutkowski in their 1980 study found that patients with HAV had 14.5 degrees of valgus rotation of the first ray vs 3.1 degrees in the normal population.[20] Eustace in 1994 described a valgus rotation of the first metatarsal with bunion deformity.[21] Talbot and Saltzman found that pronation of the first metatarsal changed the apparent position of the sesamoids on the AP radiographic view.[22] Okuda et al. described a lateral rounding of the first metatarsal in his HAV group indicating a rotation in the frontal plane.[23] This was also substantiated by Yamaguchi et al. in 2015.[24] Mortier in 2012 found that the first ray was pronated in the HAV group by an average of 12.7 degrees.[25] Dayton et al. pointed out that our traditional evaluations of the bunion deformity may be flawed if the frontal plane is not considered and also found significant valgus rotation of the first ray in HAV patients.[26] With improved imaging provided by three-dimensional computerized tomography (CT), it has become clear that a majority of patients with hallux valgus possess a valgus rotation of the first ray. This may be intrinsic as described by Ota et al.[27] or extrinsically rotated in valgus as elucidated by many recent authors. Unless the valgus rotation is addressed surgically, recurrences can be expected due to malalignment of the sesamoid complex.[28]

TABLE 13.1	Triplane Classification of HAV		
Triplane Hallux Valgus Classification and Treatment Algorithm			
Class	**Anatomic Findings**	**MTP Joint Status**	**Treatment Recommendation**
1	Increased HVA and IMA **No first metatarsal pronation evident on AP and sesamoid axial radiograph** Sesamoids may be subluxed	No clinical or radiographic evidence of DJD	Metatarsal osteotomy or TMT correction. Sesamoid release to help realign complex
2A	Increased HVA and IMA **First metatarsal pronation evident on AP and sesamoid axial radiograph** No sesamoid subluxation on axial	No clinical or radiographic evidence of DJD	Triplane correction including first metatarsal inversion
2B	Increased HVA and IMA **First metatarsal pronation evident on AP and sesamoid axial radiograph** With sesamoid subluxation on axial	No clinical or radiographic evidence of DJD	Triplane correction including first metatarsal inversion Lateral capsular/sesamoidal release prior to correction
3	Increased HVA and IMA >20 degrees MTA	No clinical or radiographic evidence of DJD	Metatarsal 2 and 3 transverse plane correction Metatarsal osteotomy or TMT correction per class 1 and 2 recommendations
4	Increased HVA and IMA ± first metatarsal pronation	**Clinical and/or radiographic evidence of DJD**	First MTP arthrodesis preferred Resectional/implant arthroplasty may also be utilized

The center of rotation and angulation (CORA) is defined by Paley as either mechanical or anatomic and is a vital concept for deformity mapping and choosing the most appropriate site for correction.[29] The 1st TMT is the most advantageous site to address the triplane components of HAV because it represents the anatomic apex of the deformity between the medial cuneiform and the first metatarsal.[26,30,31] The mechanical axis of the first ray has been discussed by LaPorta et al. in 2016 as more proximal in the midfoot.[32] Indeed the majority of motion within the first ray is at the navicular-medial cuneiform joint.[9] With traditional severity-based algorithms, we measure and address the transverse plane variables (two-dimensional approach) and chose from a variety of metatarsal osteotomies. Because metatarsal osteotomy does not move the segment at the anatomic apex and can provide only limited 3-D correction, we are left with less than desirable alignment in many instances. This is highlighted by the fact that the overall foot width following osteotomy is not reduced after osteotomy as described by Tenenbaum.[33] When correcting the deformity at the anatomic apex, a true correction can be obtained with consistent reduction in the width of the forefoot. We measured a consistent width reduction in 109 1st TMT arthrodesis procedures along with true IM angle correction and consistent decrease in forefoot width (Dayton, unpublished results, 2019). Central concepts that have changed our thinking regarding the indications for 1st TMT arthrodesis are the concept of anatomic apex, the need for multiplane correction, which is most surgically amenable at the 1st TMT, and ease of addressing first and second ray instability at that site when it exists.

INDICATIONS

- No longer severity based. It is anatomic based with anatomic CORA at the 1st TMT.
- Based upon HAV and any increased IM angle.
- Presence of frontal plane rotation.

RADIOGRAPHIC EVALUATION

Both clinical and radiographic preoperative planning is essential to set the stage for adequate deformity correction. The weight-bearing AP projection is used to evaluate the IM angle and the hallux valgus angles (HVA). Good intra- and inter-rater reproducibility of these angles has been studied and published. The distal metatarsal articular angle (DMAA), also known as the proximal articular set angle (PASA), has proven to be less reliable.[6,34,35] The possibility that DMAA is a radiographic artifact has been raised by several researchers who have noted the articular surface alignment to change substantially with repositioning of the first metatarsal without osteotomy.[4,36] Tibial sesamoid position (TSP) is also assessed on the AP radiographic projection and is thought to be an important indicator of both severity of deformity and a marker of adequate correction. Recent findings have confirmed that dramatic changes in the apparent AP TSP can be affected by frontal plane rotation of the first ray.[37,38] The sesamoids may appear subluxed on the AP projection when in fact they are in their normal location medial and lateral to the median crista. Axial sesamoid views or weight-bearing CT scans are needed to assess the true positions of the sesamoids, and the AP radiograph should not be relied

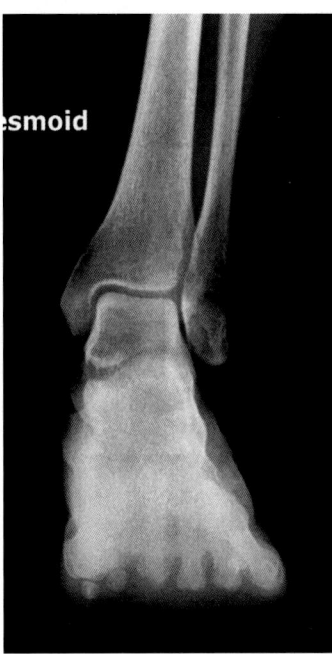

FIGURE 13.2 Axial sesamoid view demonstrating eversion of the first ray.

upon exclusively preoperative, intraoperative, or postoperative. There is a renewed importance of the weight-bearing axial sesamoid view since Kim et al. demonstrated frontal plane rotation via 3-D CT analysis.[39] The axial view will evaluate the amount of eversion of the metatarsal when it exists and the degree if any of sesamoid subluxation (Fig. 13.2). When sesamoid subluxation occurs, a first MTPJ lateral release should be performed to properly align the sesamoid complex upon realignment of the metatarsal. The weight-bearing lateral projection is utilized to mainly assess the Meary angle and Seiberg index. If elevation of the first ray is observed, then it should also be addressed at the time of surgery.

As discussed previously using a more modern approach, the angular severity measurements are not as important as the 3-D relationship of the first ray to the remainder of the foot. We do not ascribe to an absolute minimum or maximum value for IMA, HAV, or TSP in the selection of 1st TMT arthrodesis correction. Instead we observe the entire three-dimensional relationship and design the correction based on these findings.

ANATOMY AND SURGICAL BIOMECHANICS

It has long been thought that the obliquity of the medial cuneiform was a primary etiological factor in hallux valgus. Tuslow in 1925 coined the term "metatarsus primus varus" with his understanding of the deviation of the first metatarsal cuneiform joint in the transverse plane even though we understand varus to be a component of the frontal plane.[2] D.J. Morton described metatarsus atavicus in 1927.[7] Lapidus described the "atavistic" foot in 1934 as an etiological factor in hallux valgus.[3] However, more recent studies show that the obliquity of this joint does not correlate with HAV deformity.[40-43] Vyas specifically found that the morphology of the medial cuneiform was not involved in HAV deformity.[40] Others have observed change in the perceived obliquity after rotation without manipulations at the 1st TMT, indication that the AP representation of the cuneiform angle may not be an accurate representation.[4] Doty et al. gave a comprehensive description of the first metatarsal cuneiform joint.[41] Their cadaveric study revealed an average depth of 28.3 mm and width of 13.1 mm. The joint is typically continuous (59%) vs bi-lobed (38%). The lateral inclination angle averages 26.5 degrees. The first ray is inherently unstable and as such there are stabilizers of the first ray that should be appreciated. There are static and dynamic stabilizers of the first ray. Static stabilizers are the articulations of the 1st TMT: intercuneiform joint and the medial cuneiform and second metatarsal base.[11,44,45] Additionally, the plantar first metatarsal medial cuneiform ligament is a static force.[46] Dynamic stabilizers include the plantar aponeurosis and the peroneus longus. The effects of the plantar aponeurosis on stabilization of the first ray have been described by Rush et al.[13] Later Coughlin et al. also noted this effect.[47] The peroneus longus will lock the first ray in eversion.[48-50] This action is inhibited by significant equinus and pronation of the subtalar and midtarsal joints.[9,51] Bierman et al. discussed the effects of the Lapidus on peroneal longus function.[52] They found increased efficiency of the longus in stabilizing the first ray after the Lapidus procedure. It also everts the medial cuneiform and elevates the talus. Lastly, as previously stated, the windlass mechanism is now more functionally employed.[13,51]

SURGICAL CONSIDERATIONS

There are many variations of this surgical technique with the common denominator being fusion of the 1st TMT. Incisional exposure is based upon surgeon preference and may be a long dorsal incision or a smaller dorsal at the base of the 1st TMT and an additional medial incision if needed over the first MTPJ. Medial-based incisions over the TMT have also been described and have the cosmetic benefit that the scar is more hidden from the patient's sight. Because the 3-D alignment is complicated to observe intraoperatively, we find the dorsal incision to be more advantageous to visualize the angular and rotational positions of each segment simultaneously.

Research has supported the importance of proper sesamoid alignment postoperatively to prevent recurrence of the HAV deformity.[28,53] Understanding of the sesamoid-metatarsal complex has evolved through current 3-D CT that the deformity is indeed a triplanar condition. Hatch et al. have developed a new classification scheme that is based upon this 3-D anatomy (Table 13.1).[18] In that system, the sesamoids may be rotated with the metatarsal and or displaced. When displaced, especially in longstanding conditions, the sesamoid complex must be released in order to be properly realigned (Fig. 13.3). When the sesamoids are deviated in the AP projection but aligned in the axial, that is a sign of net first ray rotation that must be addressed at the time of surgery (Fig. 13.4). Adjacent ray fusion is employed when transverse or sagittal plane instability is observed or noted.[15,16] This later technique may fuse the medial cuneiform to second metatarsal base or intercuneiform joints (Fig. 13.5).

Unlike the traditional Lapidus procedure that prioritized transverse plane correction, we approach the procedure with a multiplanar mindset. Regardless of the degree of IMA, sagittal deviation, and frontal plane rotation, the procedure is approached in the same manner. All three components are

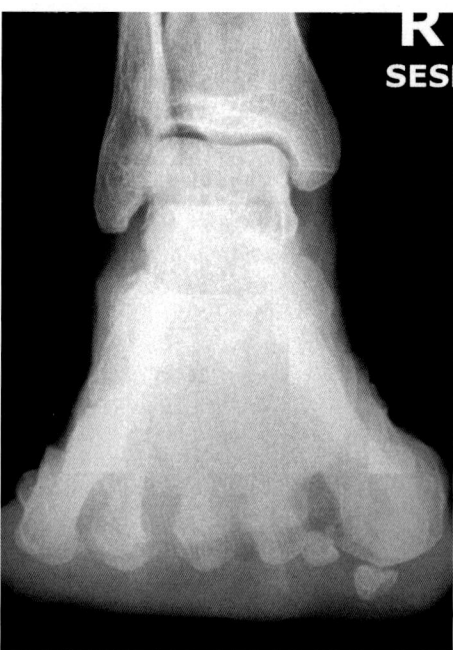

FIGURE 13.3 Displaced sesamoid complex that should be surgically released.

corrected to the amount necessary concurrently, not individually. Correction is assessed clinically and fluoroscopically in real time using anatomic landmarks rather that arbitrary and inaccurate measurements. That is, the first metatarsal is angulated in the transverse and sagittal planes and rotated in the frontal plane until the IMA, HVA, TSP, and lateral round sign are normal (Fig. 13.6). Using this multiplanar approach, the degree of each planar deformity does not matter preoperatively, as all patients receive the same three plane realignment. Three-dimensional correction can be made easier with a joystick pin in the first metatarsal and with specialized guides and jigs. It must be emphasized that the 1st TMT must be fully mobilized and any lateral ankylosis at the metatarsophalangeal joint released to allow for three plane correction. We have found that attempts to correct one planar component at a time are frustrating and do not result in satisfying alignment.

SURGICAL PEARLS
- Correct the deformity, then make precise cuts utilizing a cutting jig (preferred by authors).
- Release sesamoids if subluxed on axial views.
- Pay attention to all three planes when correcting deformity.
- Employ fixation that is amenable to early weight bearing.

As with any fusion procedure, healing is dependent on many factors. Patient health concerns such as smoking, diabetes, metabolic bone disease, and other factors must be identified and controlled. Surgical dissection should be minimally invasive and avoidance of excessive tissue plane separation is priority. We prefer intracapsular and subperiosteal dissection at both the 1st TMT and the first MTP to maintain all blood supply in full-thickness flaps (Fig. 13.7). Bone preparation

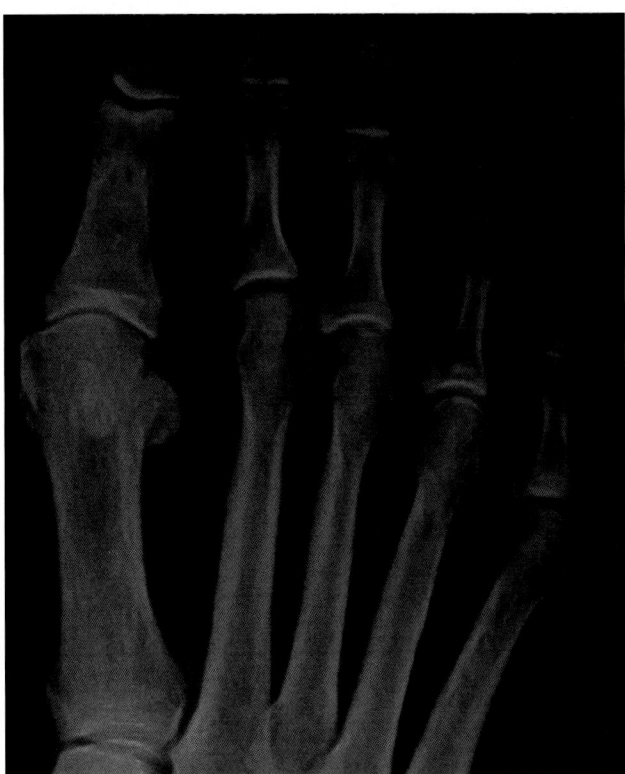

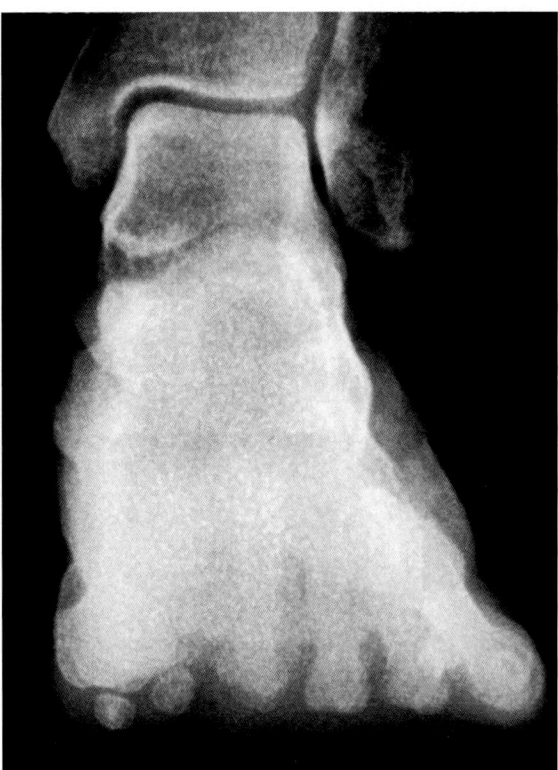

FIGURE 13.4 AP—apparent subluxation of sesamoids; and axial—normal alignment— illustrative of rotation.

must also be carried out appropriately to foster rapid healing. Curettage of the cartilage is a common method of fusion site preparation. Although curettage may have some advantage of reducing bone removal and limiting first ray shortening, studies have suggested that up to 50% of the surfaces prepared

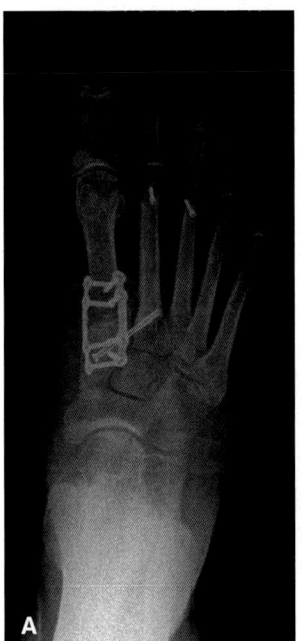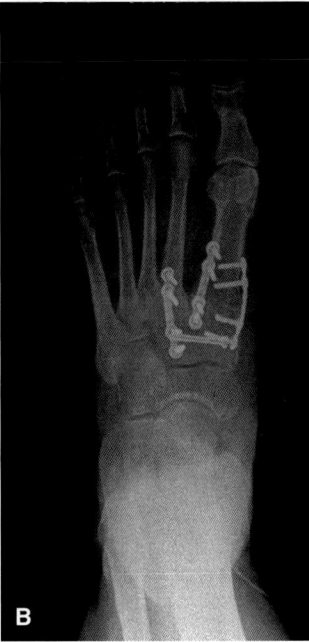

FIGURE 13.5 Arthrodesis between first and second rays to prevent transverse plane instability. **A.** Between medial cuneiform and second metatarsal base. **B.** Between cuneiform 1 and 2.

with curettage maintain calcified cartilage, which theoretically reduces the surface area for healing.[54] We prefer complete removal of all cartilage and subchondral plate using low heat generating saws. Additionally, we find benefit in fenestration of the fusion surfaces with a fluted drill bit. Unlike a wire, when a drill is used for fenestration less heat is generated and bone fragments are pulled into the fusion site acting as autogenous graft. The fragments are left in the site and not irrigated (Fig. 13.8). Shortening is limited by careful execution of bone cuts and alignment of the surfaces before the cuts are made. We generally find 3 mm or less shortening is possible with careful execution. Allograft products and other proprietary products are sometimes recommended as potential adjuvants to fusion healing. We find no need for addition of graft products and feel these products can interfere with the natural healing characteristics of a properly prepared and fixated fusion site. Most products require a separate biologic process and may compete with the body's healing resources, despite our hopes for augmentation. Another factor that is not often discussed is maximizing fusion surface area by reducing the amount of hardware crossing the surfaces. The 1st TMT has a relatively small surface area for healing, and any reduction of bone surface by intraosseous hardware represents a relative reduction in bone contact. We prefer multiplane locking plates because there is not intra-arthrodesis reduction in bone surface area taken up by screws or other devices.

Fixation constructs have evolved over time with the quest for earlier weight bearing postoperatively. The priorities are to both set the stage for consistent healing of the arthrodesis and allow the patient to maintain active range of motion and protected weight bearing throughout the entire recovery. This prevents or reduces the incidence of stiffness, weakness, and

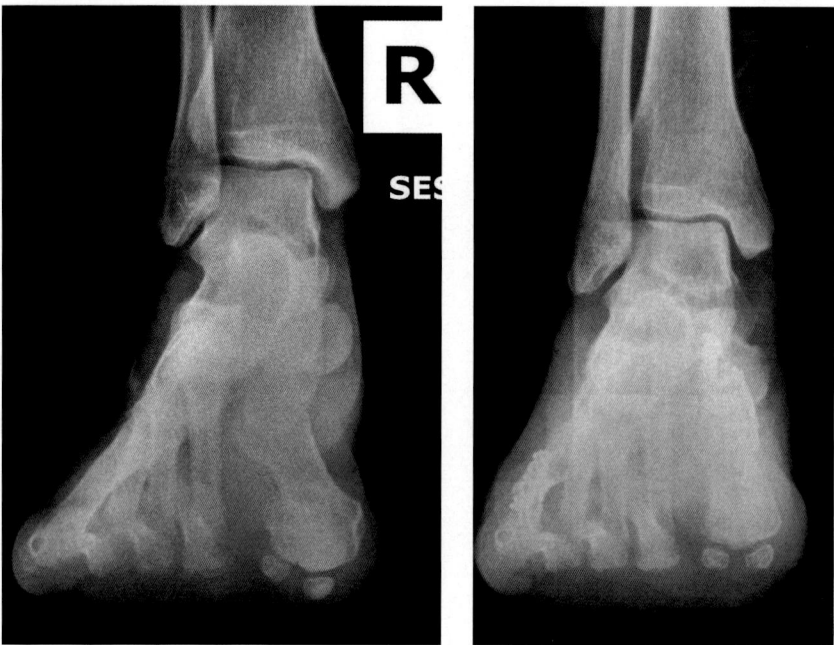

FIGURE 13.6 Pre- and postop axial view demonstrating rotational correction of the first metatarsal and sesamoid complex.

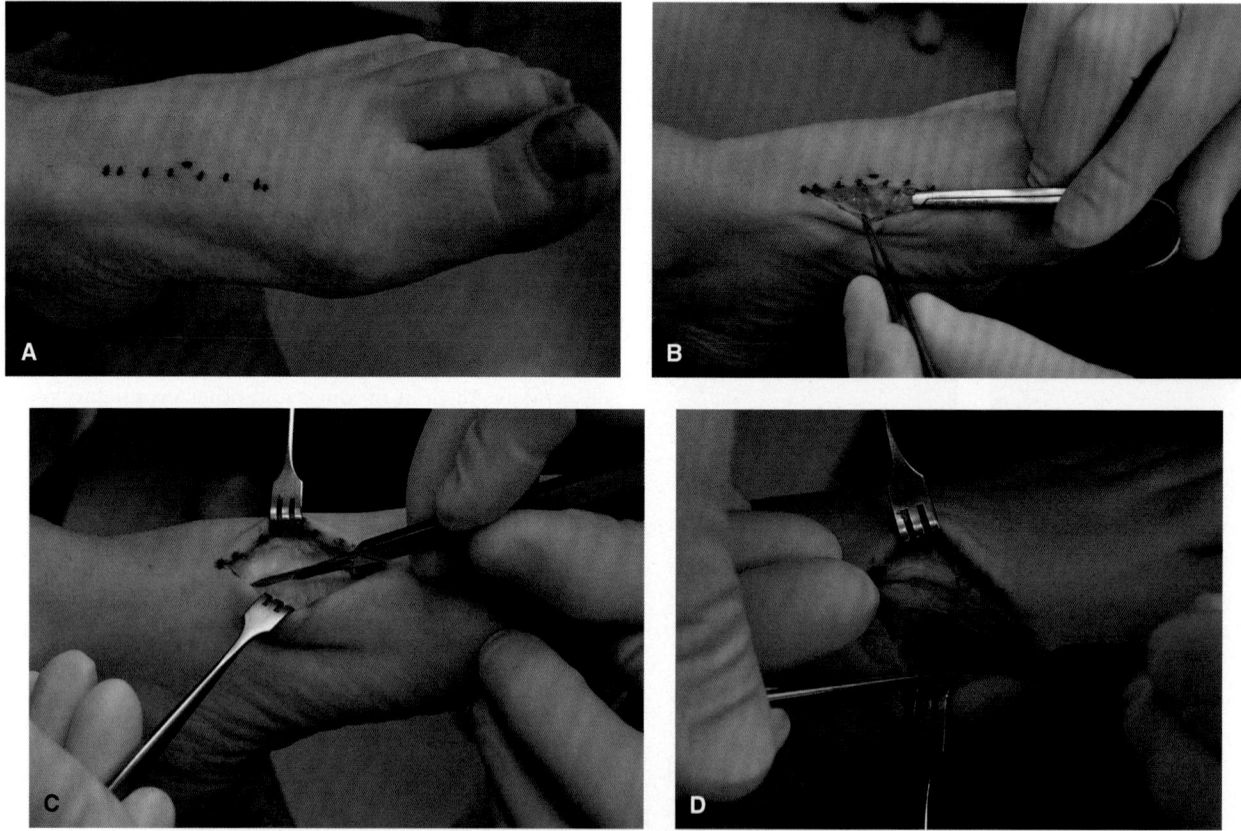

FIGURE 13.7 Photographs illustrating minimal dissection technique: **A.** Incision is medial to EHL from midshaft first metatarsal to proximal of medial cuneiform. **B.** No subcutaneous undermining. **C.** Capsule and periosteal incision is medial to EHL. **D.** Expose medial ridge of first metatarsal then dissect proximally.

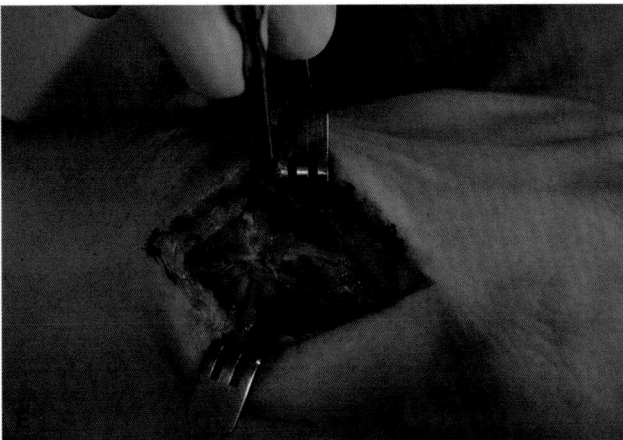
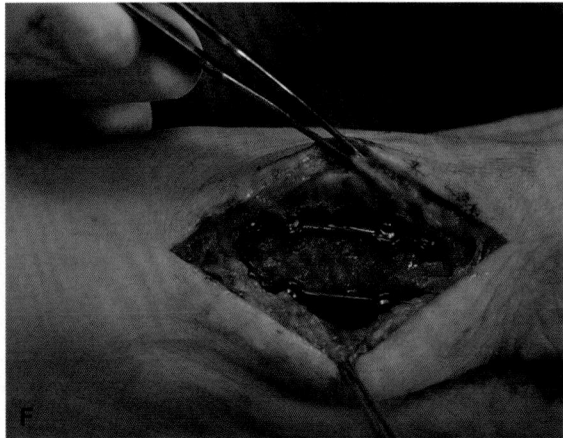

FIGURE 13.7 (*Continued*) **E.** Create a pocket for the fulcrum. **F.** Final construct after cuts are made using a jig. Flap remains full thickness.

DVT seen with casting and non–weight bearing. Commonly, a 2-3 screw construct is employed using the principles of friction-based rigidity produced with compression screws. Hansen realized that precompressing a joint and allowing the patient to weight bear created sheer at the fusion site due to the angular loading of the compressed surfaces can impairing healing.[55] Hence, he developed a shear strain relieved bone graft to mitigate this effect. This has been supported by a level four study by Mani et al. study in 2015.[56] Commonly, screw constructs include 6 weeks of NWB with or without casting, followed by 6 weeks of protected weight bearing in a CAM boot. King reported results with a screw construct and early partial WB at 12 days and full at 4 weeks.[57] Patient acceptance of these parameters was low and hence a strive for earlier weight bearing and newer surgical constructs. Several recent studies have advocated early weight bearing with conventional screw constructs.[57,58] Plate and screw combinations have evolved earlier weight bearing.[59] Newer biplanar construct takes into account the concept of "biologic healing" and advocated by Perren in 2002.[60] Micromotion at the arthrodesis site allows for callus formation yielding a faster and stronger arthrodesis. Consistent healing in a series of 195 first ray fusions using a biplane locked plate construct and protected weight bearing in a cam boot within the first postoperative week was published in 2018.[61] Using stable multiplanar fixation fosters callus healing, which is known to achieve intrinsic stability quicker than primary healing seen in compression screw fixation. While at the same time we can encourage protected weight bearing when multiplane stability is provided. A large level III study was done by Prissel et al. 2016 comparing early vs delayed weight bearing and found no differences in

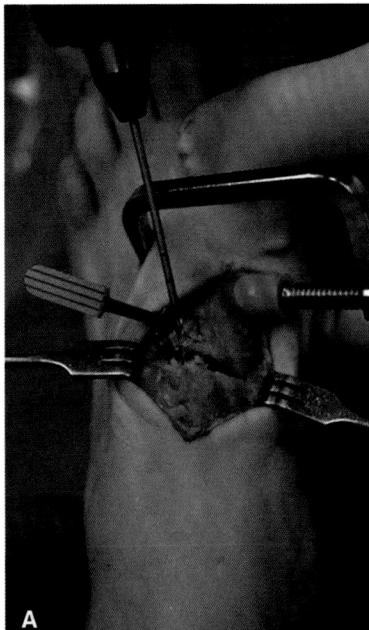
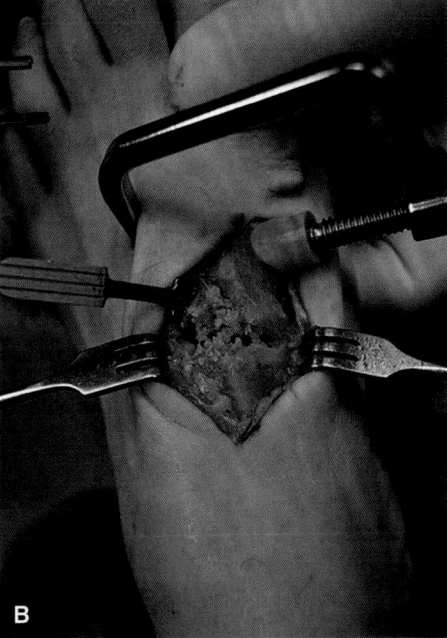

FIGURE 13.8 **A.** Joint preparation technique with drill bit. **B.** Note fenestrations and bone debris in arthrodesis site.

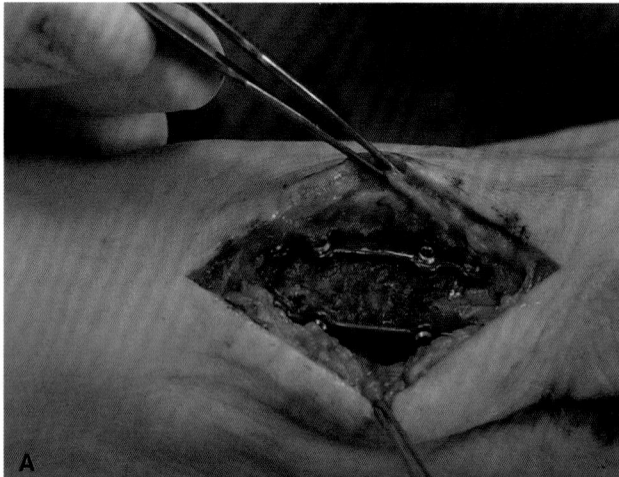
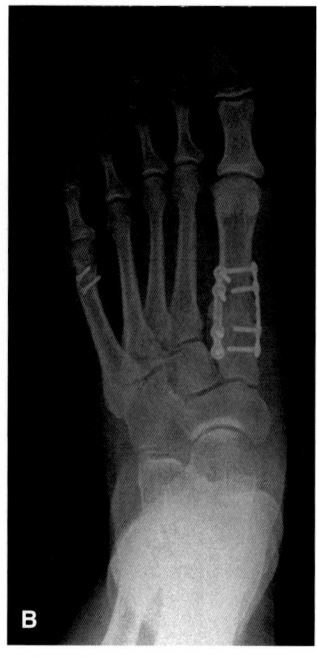
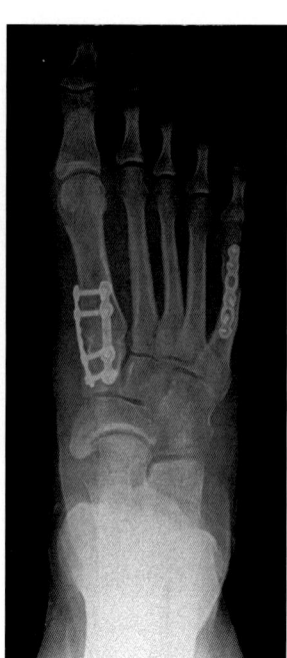

FIGURE 13.9 Biplanar construct **(A)** clinically and **(B)** radiographically.

union rates when appropriate stability was provided.[62] Newer constructs may allow for weight bearing from immediate to early (2 weeks) (Fig. 13.9).

COMPLICATIONS

The complications of the Lapidus bunionectomy are not different from other types of bunion procedures. These would include shortening, elevation, nonunion, and recurrence of deformity. Shortening is minimized by paying attention to minimal joint resection. Elevation of the first metatarsal is avoided by proper technique and checking during the surgical procedure with intraoperative fluoroscopy. Reports of nonunion have ranged from 5% to 10%.[57] Barp et al. reported nonunion rates of 6.7% in 147 procedures.[63] Even more encouraging was Mani et al. study in 2015 reporting a 2.7% nonunion rate if meticulous joint preparation, internal fixation, and a shear-strain bone graft is utilized.[56] The shear strain relieved bone graft was advocated by Hansen in 2000.[55] Since the foot is loaded tangentially to the long axis of the bone, shear forces are created with weight bearing and joint compression with standard rigid internal fixation. The bone graft allows micromotion and secondary bone healing, which has shown to be quicker and stronger by Perren's studies.[60] Recurrences are due to lack of sesamoid alignment[28,64] and undercorrection of the first metatarsal second metatarsal angle.[65] Achieving a collinear alignment of the first ray will optimize the direct pull of the tendons inserting into the hallux. With a dorsal incision, there may be compromise or irritation to the cutaneous nerve branch of the medial dorsal cutaneous nerve.

PERILS and PITFALLS

- Imperative to analyze correction in all three planes
- Ensure first metatarsal is neutrally aligned in the sagittal plane
- Must strive to reduce IM deformity to 4 degrees or less
- Must check instability of the first and second rays

SUMMARY

The Lapidus bunionectomy is a dependable procedure that helps minimize chances of recurrences while providing a surgically amenable site to address the triplane deformity of the first ray. The 1st TMT site is considered the anatomic apex of the deformity. That is not discounting that more proximal motions are pathologic for this condition. This especially involves motion at the intercuneiform joint and navicular cuneiform joint. When excessive motion occurs at those joints stabilization may be achieved by intercuneiform or medial cuneiform-second metatarsal base arthrodesis. The triplane deformity of the first ray may be easily addressed at the 1st TMT, and by arthrodesis at that site, the effects of the peroneus longus and windlass mechanisms are enhanced to stabilize the first ray.

REFERENCES

1. Albrecht GH. The pathology and treatment of hallux valgus. *Russ Vrach.* 1911;10(14): 14-19.
2. Truslow W. Metatarsus primus varus or hallux valgus. *J Bone Joint Surg Br.* 1925;7:98.
3. Lapidus P. Operative correction of the metatarsal varus primus in hallux valgus. *Surg Gynecol Obstet.* 1934;58:183-191.
4. Dayton P, Feilmeier M, Kauwe M, Hirschi J. Relationship of frontal plane rotation of first metatarsal to proximal articular set angle and hallux alignment in patients undergoing tarsometatarsal arthrodesis for hallux abducto valgus: a case series and critical review of the literature. *J Foot Ankle Surg.* 2013;52(3):348-354.
5. Condon F, Kaliszer M, Conhyea D, O' Donnell T, Shaju A, Masterson E. The first intermetatarsal angle in hallux valgus: an analysis of measurement reliability and the error involved. *Foot Ankle Int.* 2002;23(8):717-721.
6. Coughlin MJ, Jones CP. Hallux valgus: demographics, etiology, and radiographic assessment. *Foot Ankle Int.* 2007;28(7):759-777.
7. Morton DJ. Metatarsus atavicus. *J Bone Joint Surg Br.* 1927;9:531-534.
8. Hansen ST Jr. Introduction: the first metatarsal: it's importance in the human foot. *Clin Podiatr Med Surg.* 2009;26(3):351-354, Table of Contents.
9. D'Amico JC. Understanding the first ray. *Podiatr Manag.* 2016:109-120.
10. Kimura T, Kubota M, Taguchi T, Suzuki N, Hattori A, Marumo K. Evaluation of first-ray mobility in patients with hallux valgus using weight-bearing CT and a 3-D analysis system: a comparison with normal feet. *J Bone Joint Surg Am.* 2017;99(3):247-255.
11. Root ML, Orien WP, Weed JH. Normal and abnormal function of the foot. *Clin Biomech.* 1977;2. https://ci.nii.ac.jp/naid/10031091761/. Accessed July 25, 2018.
12. Roukis TS, Landsman AS. Hypermobility of the first ray: a critical review of the literature. *J Foot Ankle Surg.* 2003;42(6):377-390.

13. Rush SM, Christiansen JC, Johnson CH. Biomechanics of the first ray. Part II: Metatarsus primus varus as a cause of hypermobility. A three dimensional kinematic analysis in a cadaver model. *J Foot Ankle Surg.* 2000;39(2):68-77.

14. Shibuya N, Roukis T, Jupiter DC. Mobility of the first ray in patients with or without hallux valgus deformity: systematic review and meta-analysis. *J Foot Ankle Surg.* 2017;56(5):1070-1075.

15. Weber AK, Hatch DJ, Jensen JL. Use of the first ray splay test to assess transverse plane instability before first metatarsocuneiform fusion. *J Foot Ankle Surg.* 2006;45(4):278-282.

16. Fleming JJ, Kwaadu KY, Brinkley JC, Ozuzu Y. Intraoperative evaluation of medial intercuneiform instability after Lapidus arthrodesis: intercuneiform hook test. *J Foot Ankle Surg.* 2015;54(3):464-472.

17. Feilmeier M, Dayton P, Wienke JC Jr. Reduction of intermetatarsal angle after first metatarsophalangeal joint arthrodesis in patients with hallux valgus. *J Foot Ankle Surg.* 2014;53(1):29-31.

18. Hatch DJ, Santrock RD, Smith B, Dayton P, Weil L. Triplane hallux abducto valgus classification. *J Foot Ankle Surg.* 2018;57:972-981.

19. Mizuno S, Sima Y, Yamazaki K. Detorsion osteotomy of the first metatarsal bone in hallux valgus. *J Jpn Orthop Assoc.* 1956;30:813-819.

20. Scranton PE Jr, Rutkowski R. Anatomic variations in the first ray: part I. Anatomic aspects related to bunion surgery. *Clin Orthop Relat Res.* 1980;151:244-255.

21. Eustace S, Byrne JO, Beausang O, Codd M, Stack J, Stephens MM. Hallux valgus, first metatarsal pronation and collapse of the medial longitudinal arch—a radiological correlation. *Skeletal Radiol.* 1994;23(3):191-194.

22. Talbot KD, Saltzman CL. Assessing sesamoid subluxation: how good is the AP radiograph? *Foot Ankle Int.* 1998;19(8):547-554.

23. Okuda R, Kinoshita M, Yasuda T, Jotoku T, Kitano N, Shima H. The shape of the lateral edge of the first metatarsal as a risk factor for recurrence of hallux valgus. *J Bone Joint Surg Br.* 2007;89(10):2161-2172.

24. Yamaguchi S, Sasho T, Endo J, et al. Shape of the lateral edge of the first metatarsal head changes depending on the rotation and inclination of the first metatarsal: a study using digitally reconstructed radiographs. *J Orthop Sci.* 2015;20(5):868-874.

25. Mortier JP, Bernard JL, Maestro M. Axial rotation of the first metatarsal head in a normal population and hallux valgus patients. *Orthop Traumatol Surg Res.* 2012;98(6):677-683.

26. Dayton P, Kauwe M, Feilmeier M. Is our current paradigm for evaluation and management of the bunion deformity flawed? A discussion of procedure philosophy relative to anatomy. *J Foot Ankle Surg.* 2015;54(1):102-111.

27. Ota T, Nagura T, Kokubo T, et al. Etiological factors in hallux valgus, a three-dimensional analysis of the first metatarsal. *J Foot Ankle Res.* 2017;10:43.

28. Shibuya N, Kyprios EM, Panchani PN, Martin LR, Thorud JC, Jupiter DC. Factors associated with early loss of hallux valgus correction. *J Foot Ankle Surg.* 2018;57(2):236-240.

29. Paley D. *Principles of Deformity Correction.* Berlin, Heidelberg: Springer Berlin Heidelberg; 2002.

30. Tanaka Y, Takakura Y, Kumai T, Samoto N, Tamai S. Radiographic analysis of hallux valgus. *J Bone Joint Surg Br.* 1995;77A(2):205-213.

31. Paley D, Correction D. Principles of foot deformity correction: Ilizarov technique. In: Gould JS, ed. *Operative Foot Surgery.* Philadelphia, PA: WB Saunders; 1994:476-514.

32. LaPorta GA, Nasser EM, Mulhern JL, Malay DS. The mechanical axis of the first ray: a radiographic assessment in hallux abducto valgus evaluation. *J Foot Ankle Surg.* 2016;55(1):28-34.

33. Tenenbaum SA, Herman A, Bruck N, Bariteau JT, Thein R, Coifman O. Foot width changes following hallux valgus surgery. *Foot Ankle Int.* 2018;39(11):1272-1277.

34. Coughlin MJ, Freund E. The reliability of angular measurements in hallux valgus deformities. *Foot Ankle Int.* 2001;22(5):369-379.

35. Lee KM, Chung CY, Park MS, Lee SH, Cho JH, Choi IH. Reliability and validity of radiographic measurements in hindfoot varus and valgus. *J Bone Joint Surg Am.* 2010;92(13):2319-2327.

36. Chi TD, Davitt J, Younger A, Holt S, Sangeorzan BJ. Intra- and inter-observer reliability of the distal metatarsal articular angle in adult hallux valgus. *Foot Ankle Int.* 2002;23(8):722-726.

37. Okuda R, Kinoshita M, Yasuda T, Jotoku T, Kitano N, Shima H. Postoperative incomplete reduction of the sesamoids as a risk factor for recurrence of hallux valgus. *J Bone Joint Surg Am.* 2009;91(7):1637-1645.

38. Dayton P, Feilmeier M. Comparison of tibial sesamoid position on anteroposterior and axial radiographs before and after triplane tarsal metatarsal joint arthrodesis. *J Foot Ankle Surg.* 2017;56(5):1041-1046.

39. Kim Y, Kim JS, Young KW, Naraghi R, Cho HK, Lee SY. A new measure of tibial sesamoid position in hallux valgus in relation to the coronal rotation of the first metatarsal in CT scans. *Foot Ankle Int.* 2015;36(8):944-952.

40. Vyas S, Conduah A, Vyas N, Otsuka NY. The role of the first metatarsocuneiform joint in juvenile hallux valgus. *J Pediatr Orthop B.* 2010;19(5):399-402.

41. Doty JF, Coughlin MJ, Hirose C, et al. First metatarsocuneiform joint mobility: radiographic, anatomic, and clinical characteristics of the articular surface. *Foot Ankle Int.* 2014;35(5):504-511.

42. Hatch DJ, Smith A, Fowler T. Radiographic relevance of the distal medial cuneiform angle in hallux valgus assessment. *J Foot Ankle Surg.* 2016;55(1):85-89.

43. Houghton GR, Dickson JR. Hallux valgus in the younger patient. *J Bone Joint Surg Br.* 1979;61(2):176-177.

44. Hicks JH. The mechanics of the foot. *J Anat.* 1954;88(Pt 1):25-30.1.

45. Dykyj D, Ateshian GA, Trepal MJ, MacDonald LR. Articular geometry of the medial TMTJ comparison of metatarsus primus adductus and metatarsus primus rectus. *J Foot Ankle Surg.* 2001;40(6):357-365.

46. Mizel MS. The role of the plantar first metatarsal first cuneiform ligament in weightbearing on the first metatarsal. *Foot Ankle.* 1993;14(2):82-84.

47. Coughlin MJ, Jones CP, Viladot R, et al. Hallux valgus and first ray mobility: a cadaveric study. *Foot Ankle Int.* 2004;25(8):537-544.

48. Johnson CH, Christensen JC. Biomechanics of the first ray part I. The effects of peroneus longus function: a three-dimensional kinematic study on a cadaver model. *J Foot Ankle Surg.* 1999;38(5):313-321.

49. Dullaert K, Hagen J, Klos K, et al. The influence of the peroneus longus muscle on the foot under axial loading: a CT evaluated dynamic cadaveric model study. *Clin Biomech.* 2016;34:7-11.

50. Klemola T, Leppilahti J, Laine V, et al. Effect of first tarsometatarsal joint derotational arthrodesis on first ray dynamic stability compared to distal Chevron osteotomy. *Foot Ankle Int.* 2017;38(8):847-854.

51. Faber F, Mulder P, Verhaarr J. Role of first ray hypermobility in the outcome of the Hohmann and the Lapidus procedure. *J Bone Joint Surg Br.* 2004;86A(3):486-495.

52. Bierman RA, Christensen JC, Johnson CH. Biomechanics of the first ray. Part III. Consequences of Lapidus arthrodesis on peroneus longus function: a three-dimensional kinematic analysis in a cadaver model. *J Foot Ankle Surg.* 2001;40(3):125-131.

53. Chen JY, Rikhraj K, Gatot C, Lee JYY, Singh Rikhraj I. Tibial sesamoid position influence on functional outcome and satisfaction after hallux valgus surgery. *Foot Ankle Int.* 2016;37(11):1178-1182.

54. Johnson JT, Schuberth JM, Thornton SD, Christensen JC. Joint curettage arthrodesis technique in the foot: a histological analysis. *J Foot Ankle Surg.* 2009;48(5):558-564.

55. Hansen ST. *Functional Reconstruction of the Foot and Ankle.* Philadelphia, PA: Lippincott Williams & Wilkins; 2000.

56. Mani SB, Lloyd EW, MacMahon A, Roberts MM, Levine DS, Ellis SJ. Modified Lapidus procedure with joint compression, meticulous surface preparation, and shear-strain-relieved bone graft yields low nonunion rate. *HSS J.* 2015;11(3):243-248.

57. King CM, Richey J, Patel S, Collman DR. Modified Lapidus arthrodesis with crossed screw fixation: early weightbearing in 136 patients. *J Foot Ankle Surg.* 2015;54(1):69-75.

58. Basile P, Cook EA, Cook JJ. Immediate weight bearing following modified Lapidus arthrodesis. *J Foot Ankle Surg.* 2010;49(5):459-464.

59. Cottom JM, Vora AM. Fixation of Lapidus arthrodesis with a plantar interfragmentary screw and medial locking plate: a report of 88 cases. *J Foot Ankle Surg.* 2013;52(4):465-469.

60. Perren SM. Evolution of the internal fixation of long bone fractures. *J Bone Joint Surg.* 2002;84-B:1093-1110.

61. Dayton P, Hatch D, Santrock R, Smith B. Biomechanical characteristics of biplane multiplanar tension-side fixation for Lapidus fusion. *J Foot Ankle Surg.* 57(4):766-770.

62. Prissel MA, Hyer CF, Grambart ST, et al. A multicenter, retrospective study of early weightbearing for modified Lapidus arthrodesis. *J Foot Ankle Surg.* 2016;55(2):226-229.

63. Barp EA, Erickson JG, Smith HL, Almeida K, Millonig K. Evaluation of fixation techniques for metatarsocuneiform arthrodesis. *J Foot Ankle Surg.* 2017;56(3):468-473.

64. Park CH, Lee WC. Recurrence of hallux valgus can be predicted from immediate postoperative non-weight-bearing radiographs. *J Bone Joint Surg Am.* 2017;99(14):1190-1197.

65. Raikin SM, Miller AG, Daniel J. Recurrence of hallux valgus: a review. *Foot Ankle Clin.* 2014;19(2):259-274.

CHAPTER 14

Hallux Limitus

Mitchell J. Thompson and Thomas S. Roukis

DEFINITION

Hallux limitus is a widespread condition affecting ~1 out of 40 people over the age of 50 and is the second most common foot ailment, behind hallux valgus.[1,2] Arthrosis of the first metatarsophalangeal joint (MPJ) was first described in 1881 by Nicoladoni[3] and later popularized by Davis-Colley in 1887; the term hallux rigidus was not coined until 1887 by Cotterill.[3] The term hallux limitus was not invented until a mere 40 years later when in 1931 hallux limitus was described by Hiss.[3] The condition described in those texts is defined as degenerative arthrosis of the first MPJ. Arthrosis of the joint leads to limited range of motion (ROM), often accompanied by pain. Today, the term hallux limitus is widely used in foot and ankle clinics for conditions with limited ROM of the first MPJ. When motion is virtually nonexistent at the first MPJ, the term hallux rigidus is often applied.

Multiple etiologies have been described through history, though there are little data and much debate about the main cause of hallux limitus.[6] Most common etiologies encompass a combination of foot structure and biomechanical imbalances, which limit motion at the first MPJ and cause excess stress leading to arthrosis. Examples of these etiologies would be excessive first metatarsal elevation, flatfoot deformity, and gastrocnemius equinus.[4,5] Other possible etiologies include systemic arthropathies, acute trauma, neuromuscular disorders, and iatrogenic causes.[6-9]

The total amount of treatment options for hallux limitus are just as wide spread as the possible etiologies of the condition. A myriad of options exist ranging from initial nonoperative treatments to surgical reconstruction of the MPJ.[10,11] The aim of this chapter is to provide a synopsis of the anatomical and pathological concepts of hallux limitus along with a detailed overview of surgical and nonsurgical treatment options.

CLASSIFICATION

Multiple classifications have been produced throughout the years regarding hallux limitus. The main focus of these classifications has been based on findings of the radiographic assessment. Roukis et al. in 2002 developed a classification based off of radiographic assessment and clinical findings[12] (Table 14.1). This classification is unique in that it can predict articular erosions when additional clinical findings are included, setting it apart from other classifications. In 2003, Coughlin and Shurnas developed a modification of the Hattrup and Johnson grading system, which took into account both radiographic and clinical assessment of the first ray[13,14] (Table 14.2). Both classifications systems are similar in that they both grade end-stage hallux rigidus as a grade 4. The Coughlin classification consists of a grade 0, which is completely subjective stiffness and no radiographic findings. Roukis and colleagues begin their classification scale at 1, when radiographic findings are first evident.

INDICATIONS

- Pain to first MPJ with activity.
- Arthritic spurring causes osseous prominence leading to decreased range of motion (ROM) and irritation.
- Transfer lesion to plantar hallux interphalangeal joint due to mechanical stress caused by decreased first MPJ motion.

TABLE 14.1	Hybrid Radiographic Grading System for Hallux Rigidus
Grade	**Criteria**
Grade 1	Metatarsus primus elevatus with hallux equinus Periarticular subchondral sclerosis Minimal dorsal exostosis (first metatarsal head and base of proximal phalanx) Minimal flattening of first metatarsal head
Grade 2	Moderate dorsal exostosis (first metatarsal head and base of proximal phalanx) Moderate flattening of the first metatarsal head Minimal joint space narrowing Lateral first metatarsal head erosion and/or joint flare/exostosis Sesamoid hypertrophy Subchondral cyst formation/loose body formation
Grade 3	Severe dorsal exostosis (first metatarsal head and base of proximal phalanx) Irregular joint space narrowing Traction enthesopathic sesamoid hypertrophy with immobilization-induced osteopenia Definite subchondral cyst formation and presence of loose bodies
Grade 4	Excessive exostosis proliferation with trumpeting of the first metatarsal head, base of the proximal phalanx, and sesamoid apparatus Minimal or absent joint space Sesamoid fusion Hallucal interphalangeal and/or first metatarsal-medial cuneiform osteoarthritic changes

TABLE 14.2	Hallux Rigidus Classification Developed by Coughlin and Shurnas in 2003
Grade	**Criteria**
Grade 0	*ROM*: Dorsiflexion 40-60 degrees and/or 10%-20% loss compared with normal side *Radiographic*: Normal or minimal findings *Clinical*: No subjective pain, only stiffness, loss of passive motion on examination
Grade 1	*ROM*: Dorsiflexion 30-40 degrees and/or 20%-50% loss compared with normal side *Radiographic*: Dorsal spur is main finding, minimal joint narrowing, minimal periarticular sclerosis, minimal flattening of metatarsal head *Clinical*: Mild or occasional subjective pain and stiffness, pain at extremes of dorsiflexion and/or plantar flexion on examination
Grade 2	*ROM*: Dorsiflexion 10-30 degrees and/or 50%-75% loss compared to normal side *Radiograph*: Dorsal, lateral, and possibly medial osteophytes give flattened appearance to metatarsal head, no more than one-fourth of dorsal joint space involvement on lateral radiograph, mild to moderate joint narrowing and sclerosis, sesamoids not usually involved but may be irregular in appearance *Clinical*: Moderate to severe subjective pain and stiffness that may be constant, pain just before maximal dorsiflexion, and/or plantar flexion on examination
Grade 3	*ROM*: Dorsiflexion of 10 degrees or less and/or 75%-100% loss compared with normal side and notable loss of plantar flexion *Radiographic*: As in grade 2 but with substantial narrowing, possibly periarticular cystic changes, more than one-fourth dorsal joint may be involved on lateral, sesamoids (enlarged and/or cystic and/or irregular) *Clinical*: Nearly constant subjective pain and substantial stiffness, pain throughout ROM on examination (but not at midrange)
Grade 4	Same criteria and findings as grade 3, but definite pain at mid-ROM on examination

ANATOMIC FEATURES

The first MPJ consists of four bones, multiple ligaments, and is traversed by six tendons (flexor hallucis longus [FHL], flexor hallucis brevis [FHB], abductor hallucis [ABH], adductor hallucis [ADH], extensor hallucis longus [EHL], and extensor hallucis brevis). The first metatarsal head has a sinusoidal shape, which aligns with the ellipsoid shape of the proximal phalanx creating a biaxial condylar articulation.[15] The first metatarsal head also shares an articulation with two sesamoid bones that lie directly plantar to the metatarsal head within the flexor hallucis brevis tendon. The sesamoids are separated by the crista, which is located on the plantar first metatarsal head surface. Multiple ligaments hold these four bones in the first MPJ complex. There is an intersesamoid ligament connecting the two sesamoid bones and then off each sesamoid is a sesamoid-phalangeal ligament and an accessory sesamoid ligament attaches to the metatarsal. Collateral ligaments are then seen connecting the first

metatarsal head to the proximal phalanx both medially and laterally. The FHB, which has two heads, each inserting onto to the base of the proximal phalanx, encompasses the sesamoid bones. The FHL tendon extends to the distal phalanx and lies in between the medial and lateral heads of the FHB. Dorsally, the extensor hallucis longus traverses the first MPJ, and the extensor hallucis brevis is seen laterally inserting on the base of the proximal phalanx.[16,17] The abductor hallucis tendon traverses along the medial aspect of the first MPJ to insert on the medial aspect of the base of the proximal phalanx. The adductor hallucis muscle produces two tendons, and oblique and transverse head, both of which have a common insertion on the lateral aspect of the base of the proximal phalanx.

FUNCTIONAL ANALYSIS

The functional sequence of events of the first MPJ during every day walking is quite complex in comparison to many other joints in the foot and ankle when considering all the moving anatomy described above. During the propulsive phase of gait as the weight of the body moves forward to the forefoot, there is natural plantar flexion of the first metatarsal. This plantar flexion in a normal joint causes the metatarsal head to slide proximal off the sesamoid apparatus allowing dorsiflexion of the proximal phalanx and hallux, on the metatarsal head.[18] Subsequently, this action pulls the sesamoid apparatus slightly distal within the FHB tendon as the windlass mechanism engages. A normal first MPJ allows approximately at least 65 degrees of hallux dorsiflexion and 20 degrees of plantar flexion.[19]

The analysis of the ROM and ultimately the diagnosis of hallux limitus can be divided into either functional or structural hallux limitus. Functional hallux limitus occurs when the ROM of the hallux is limited with the foot loaded, simulating weight bearing, but normal ROM is present at the first MPJ when the foot is non–weight bearing. Functional assessment by loading the foot is most representative of normal gait, although some studies have eluded that motion of the hallux may be different between static weight bearing and during normal phases of gait.[20] The discovery of functional hallux limitus is most indicative of a functional deficiency between the complete working complex of the first MPJ. Functional hallux limitus is typically seen first in the progression of this disease. Structural hallux limitus is defined as limited ROM due to the static structural nature of the foot.[21] For instance, narrow joint space caused by arthritic changes, dorsiflexed first metatarsal, or overly tight ligamentous complex may not allow the first MPJ to go through full arc of motion regardless of the foot is loaded or not. Structural hallux limitus is typically seen in later stages of the disease.

PHYSICAL EXAMINATION

After gaining a proper history, the physical examination will be the next most important step to diagnosing hallux limitus. As with all foot and ankle examinations, vascular status, especially capillary refill to the hallux, should be checked. Next, it is important to note the overall structure of the foot. A cavus foot may be accompanied by a plantar flexed first metatarsal and overall plantar flexed forefoot in regard to the rearfoot, which has been linked to hallux limitus. A pes planus foot structure is more likely to produce a dorsiflexed first metatarsal, especially in regard to the second metatarsal, which would naturally cause impingement with dorsiflexion of the hallux.[22] Any form of valgus forefoot, compensatory or not, may also cause increased loading to the first ray and possible elevation leading to hallux limitus. After recognizing the structure of the foot in your initial survey, a simple glance to the first MPJ can elude to any trauma, dorsal bump from osteophytes, or any possible irritation to the skin noted from shoe gear.[23] At this time, attention is turned to a hands-on examination of the first ray. It is important to assess the stability of the entire first ray from the navicular cuneiform joint down to the interphalangeal joint of the hallux. The reason for this is to assess the excursion in the sagittal plane the first ray will go through during the phases of gait. If upon weight bearing, the first metatarsal becomes too far elevated; this can lead to limited ability of the hallux to dorsiflex. In a study done by Roukis et al., elevating the first ray 4 mm from normal resting position decreased the first MPJ dorsiflexion by 19% from 22.7 to 18.4 degrees.[6] Elevating the first ray 8 mm from normal resting stance decreased first MPJ dorsiflexion by 34.7% from 22.7 degrees of dorsiflexion to 14.8 degrees. Excursion of the first ray in the sagittal plane should not exceed 5 mm.[6] Focusing now on the first MPJ, it is important to assess the ROM again with the foot in both open and closed kinetic chain to better assess the etiology as explained above. Palpation to an inflamed and irritated joint may very well cause the patient discomfort and should be kept in mind during the examination. The dorsal osteophytes will be palpable at this time. The patient may also feel discomfort both with dorsiflexion and with plantar flexion of the MPJ. Pain with dorsiflexion is due to the impingement of the proximal phalanx base on the head of the first metatarsal. Early on in the disease, pain is most commonly noted at end-stage dorsiflexion only, whereas later in the disease, any amount of dorsiflexion may cause pain as the arthritis progresses. Discomfort is seen with plantar flexion, as well, due to the stretching of the joint capsule over the osteophytes that have formed over time on the dorsal first metatarsal head. Finally, moving distally, the hallux may be in slight hyperextension due to compensation from limited motion at the MPJ, and now, the dorsiflexion of the hallux is being transferred through the IPJ causing a hallux extensus. Gait analysis can also be helpful when evaluating for hallux limitus, most commonly the patient will have a compensatory gait, transferring weight to the lateral aspect of the foot. Limited motion at the first MPJ will also be seen with walking, and if this is combined with a pes planus foot structure and dorsiflexed first ray, late heel off may also be noted on gait analysis.

Hallux limitus can also have dermatologic and neurologic manifestations in the foot. First as previously mentioned, there may be redness and irritation noted to the skin overlying any osteophyte seen at the level of the dorsal MPJ due to the arthritic changes. This irritation is likely due to shoe gear and is especially noted in colder climates where closed-toed shoes are a must. Transfer lesions may be noted on the plantar aspect of the hallux IPJ due to the increased stressed placed on this joint when there is limited motion at the IPJ. Neuropraxias can be seen with positive Tinel sign, as the medial dorsal cutaneous nerve branch is impinged as it traverses over the osteophytes to supply the great toe.

PATHOGENESIS

The pathogenesis of hallux limitus and ultimately hallux rigidus is the consistent trauma of the dorsal proximal aspect of the base of the proximal phalanx impinging against the dorsal aspect of the articular surface of the first metatarsal head during ROM, specifically propulsion phase of gait.[7] During heel lift, the windlass mechanism engages as the metatarsal head plantar flexes and the proximal phalanx dorsiflexes on the metatarsal head; in hallux limitus, the dorsal proximal base of the proximal phalanx impinges on the metatarsal head due to a variety of reasons discussed earlier. This repeated trauma causes destruction of the hyaline cartilage, more so on the metatarsal head but also on the proximal phalanx.[24] This trauma also causes formation of osteophytes as the body attempts to protect itself by laying down new bone. As these osteophytes continue to enlarge, along with the repeated trauma, the first metatarsal head begins to take a squared shape and the joint space continues to narrow.[25] Clinically, as the joint space narrows, the ROM continues to decrease and pain increases.[24]

IMAGING

Initial imaging should consist of the typical three views of the foot including anterior posterior (AP), medial oblique (MO), and lateral (L). All imaging should be taken with the patient weight bearing to best simulate the osseous structures during gait. The AP radiograph is best used to assess the joint space of the first MPJ. In hallux limitus, the joint space will be narrowed and flattening of the metatarsal head will be seen in later stages. The AP view is also where the medial and lateral spurring off both, the metatarsal head and proximal phalanx base, can best be appreciated. The lateral view best shows the dorsal spurring on the metatarsal head. This dorsal spurring is one of the first radiographic signs noted in hallux limitus and is seen beginning in a stage 2. The lateral view can also help evaluate for an elevated first metatarsal when weight bearing as a possible etiology for the hallux limitus. In late stages, where compensatory hallux extensus has developed, this may also be visualized on a lateral weight-bearing radiograph. The MO view provides another point of view to evaluate the first MPJ and can express the narrowed joint space and spurring associated with hallux limitus. All three views can be used to assess for any subchondral cyst formation or sclerosis of the bone seen in later stages of hallux limitus. In some cases, a lateral view with forced hallux extension can be helpful to visualize the exact area of impingement on the metatarsal head or if the sesamoids are fused to the metatarsal head, but rarely is this view needed. Roukis et al. developed a radiographic classification system in 2002 taking into consideration all of these possible findings.[12]

Rarely is advanced imaging indicated in hallux limitus. A magnetic resonance image (MRI) may be helpful if concerned about soft tissue disruption/impingement, synovitis, or to evaluate cyst formation. A computed tomography (CT) scan may also be helpful in evaluating osseous cysts, especially if surgery is going to be pursued.

NONOPERATIVE TREATMENT

Initial treatment of hallux limitus should focus on nonoperative techniques. Studies have shown that upward of 50% of hallux limitus can be met with satisfactory results when using conservative cares.[26] When discussing these options with patients, it is important to be clear that the nonoperative treatments are to decrease symptoms but would not cure their hallux limitus. Multiple treatments have been discussed with decreased symptoms, but overall poor evidence exists to support these results.[27] Nonoperative treatments are best tailored after understanding the individual cause for the hallux limitus, but initial rest, use of nonsteroidal anti-inflammatories (oral or topical), and heat or ice may be helpful. The next and most commonly used treatment option is to modify the patients shoe gear. A stiff-soled shoe and a shoe with a rocker bottom both can be helpful to reduce stress across the first MPJ by negating the need for full ROM of the MPJ to maintain a normal gait pattern. If a majority of the discomfort is due to irritation on the skin over the first MPJ, the toe box of the shoe can be stretched to accommodate any dorsal prominence or spurring of the MPJ.

Customized inserts or orthotics can be utilized should initial shoe gear modification not be met with satisfactory results. Morton extension modification to an insert can be used to limit motion at the first MPJ. The Morton extension also disperses the ground forces during propulsion to MPJ's 2-5 during gait. This modification can also be incorporated into a custom orthotic, which may supply arch support in patients with pes planus foot structure to decrease pronation and alleviate the elevated first ray allowing increased dorsiflexion of the hallux.

Corticosteroid injections are often used as a last resort prior to surgery for symptom relief. It is important to make sure patients are aware that these injections will not cure their hallux limitus but simply reduce the inflammation in attempt to decrease discomfort. These injections are given intra-articular, therefore within the first MPJ capsule. Due to the intra-articular nature, it is best to use a phosphate-based steroid to prevent further damage of the articulating cartilage. Mixing local anesthetic in with the steroid is a common practice, this way depending on total time of symptom relief this injection can be used both as a diagnostic and therapeutic injection. Relief of symptoms can last upward and possibly even beyond the 3-month mark.[28]

OPERATIVE TREATMENT

Operative treatments should be considered only after the patient has failed nonoperative treatments with continued pain and decreased functionality to the first MPJ. Multiple surgical options exist to correct for hallux limitus and can partially be indicated depending on the progression of the disease and clinical/radiographic findings.[29-32] Surgical treatments are best broken down into two distinct categories, joint sparing and joint destructive. Joint-sparing procedures aim to maintain the integrity of the joint and limit any destruction to the articular cartilage. Joint-sparing procedures consist of cheilectomy, proximal phalanx osteotomies, first metatarsal osteotomies, and joint distraction techniques. These procedures are typically used when the articular cartilage is without or very little damage and there is adequate joint space to allow motion after removal of the spurs. Therefore, these procedures are typically indicated in grade 2 or less. Joint destructive procedures, much as the name would suggest, entails reconstruction, replacement, or removal of the articulating aspect of the first MPJ. Procedures in the joint destructive category consist of first MPJ arthrodesis, arthroplasty, interpositional arthroplasty, or implant placement. Joint destructive procedures are indicated in grade 3 and 4 hallux limitus.

EXPOSURE

The typical approach is a dorsal medial incision just medial to the long extensor tendon (Fig. 14.1). The extensor hallucis longus tendon is then retracted laterally. Careful dissection is carried out within the incision down to the first MPJ capsule, being careful to identify and retract the medial dorsal cutaneous nerve if this is encountered. All veins should be

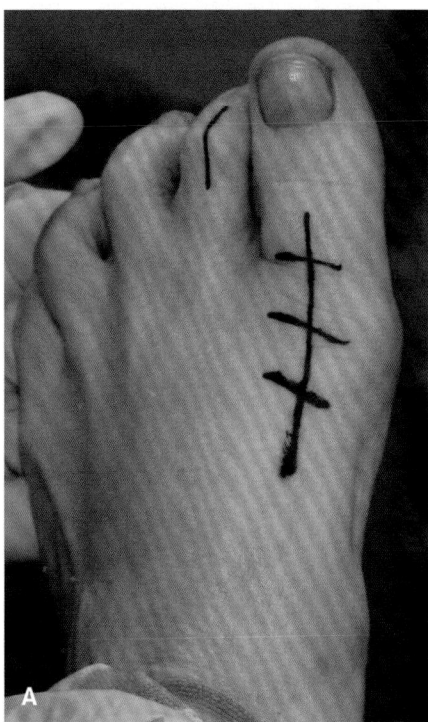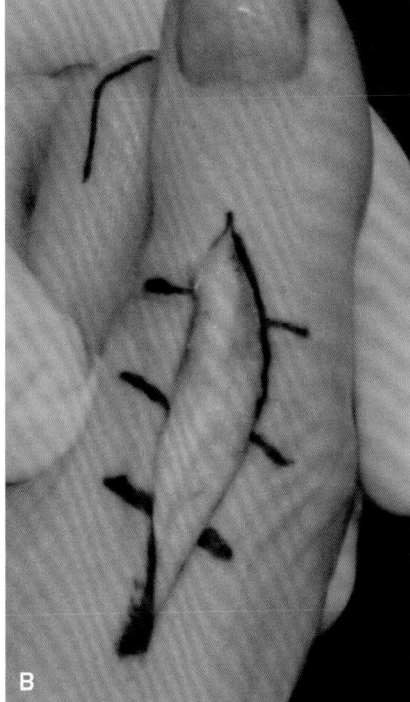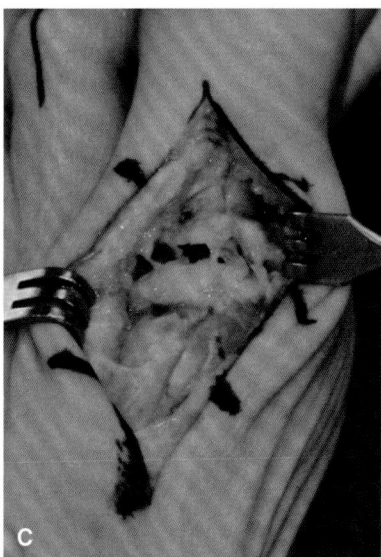

FIGURE 14.1 **A.** Incision for exposure to the first MPJ drawn over the dorsal aspect of the joint just medial to the extensor tendon. **B.** Extensor tendon and capsular tissue encountered after excision through the skin. **C.** Longitudinal capsulotomy the full length of the skin incision exposing the first MPJ.

cauterized or tied off to ensure hemostasis after the procedure. The extensor hallucis capsularis may be encountered overlying the capsule and may be incised when performing the capsulotomy. A capsular incision is made down to bone and, in line with and the full length, of the skin incision. The capsular tissue is then reflected off the head of the metatarsal and base of the proximal phalanx. When reflecting the periosteum off of the metatarsal, it is important to not disrupt the nutrient artery inserting plantarly on the metatarsal neck. Any capsular work should be reserved until the end of the procedure to ensure proper repair.

JOINT SPARING

Cheilectomy

The cheilectomy was first described by Duvries in 1959 as a joint-sparing procedure typically indicated in early-onset disease (grade 2).[33] Cheilectomy is indicated when adequate joint space is present, though spurring exists to limit the first MPJ ROM, grades 1-2. The purpose of a cheilectomy is to remove any spurring and restore normal anatomy to the first MPJ. The cheilectomy has been proven to be a great first-line treatment with published data supporting only an 8.8% revision rate after isolated cheilectomies at >12-year follow-up.[34]

Technique

The typical dorsal medial incisional approach over the first MPJ is performed with dissection down to the first MPJ. It is important to expose the metatarsal head including medial and lateral aspects (Fig. 14.2). It is also important to expose the base of the proximal phalanx, as spurring may be evident here as well, which can affect the motion of the first MPJ. Plantar soft tissue adhesions are released from the plantar metatarsal head utilizing a McGlamry or freer elevator. Once the entire MPJ is exposed, run the joint through full ROM to assess the exact areas of impingement that limit the dorsiflexion. The authors do advocate to distract the joint and to inspect the articulating cartilage on both the metatarsal head and proximal phalanx, as mentioned; since the cheilectomy is performed on grade 2 or less hallux limitus, the damage cartilage will be limited to the dorsal aspect of the joint. The traditional cheilectomy involves resection of the dorsal one-third of the metatarsal head with a sagittal saw to ensure removal of osteophytes and any damaged cartilage[33] (Fig. 14.2). Next, the medial and lateral spurring of the metatarsal head can be removed with the sagittal saw, rotatory bur, or rongeur. It is recommended that a bone rasp be used to ensure smooth osseous contours of the metatarsal head, ensuring to rasp away from the articulating cartilage not to damage the cartilage. Attention can then be directed to the proximal phalanx base where any spurring, whether dorsal,

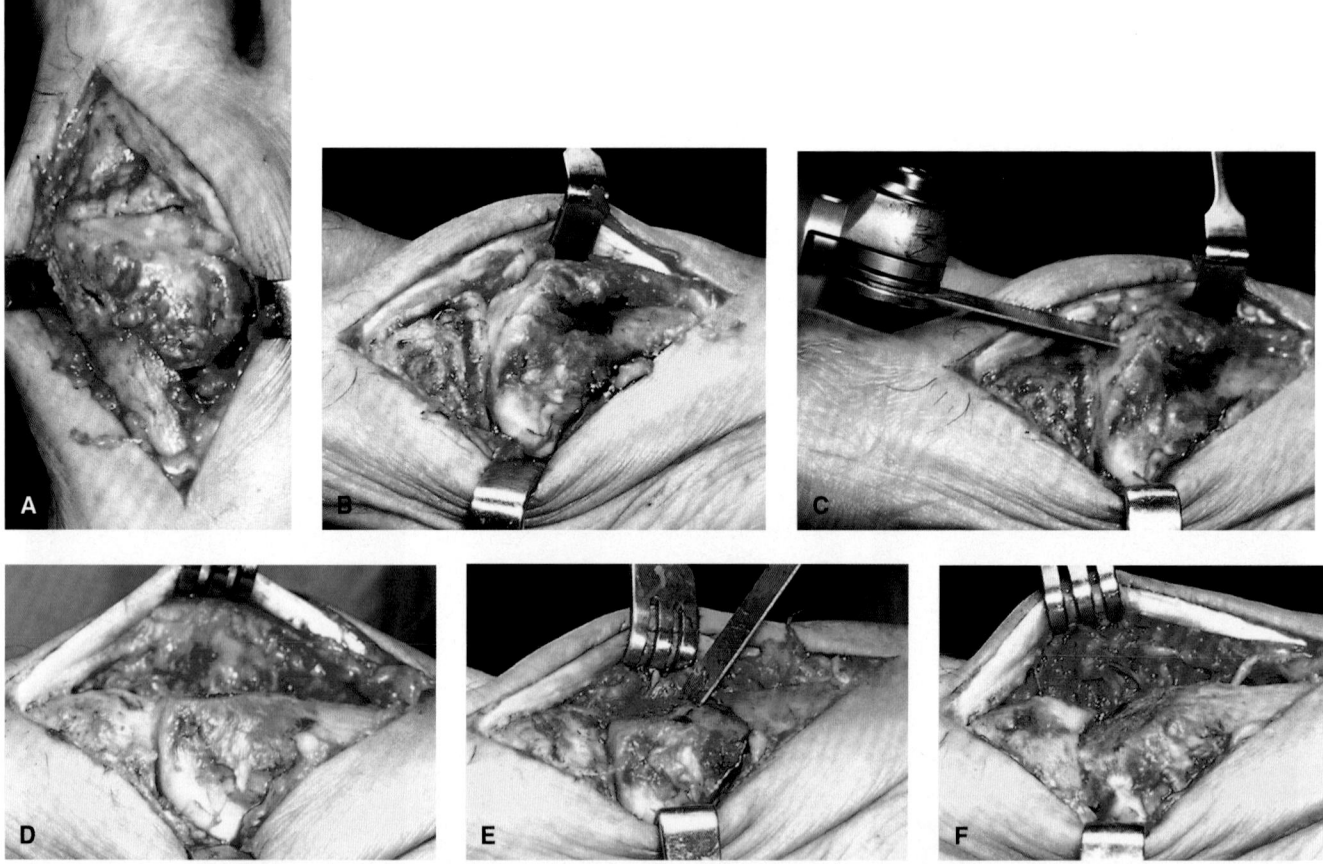

FIGURE 14.2 A. Dorsal view of the first MPJ showing narrowed joint space. **B.** Lateral view of the first MPJ in which dorsal spurring of the metatarsal head is evident. **C.** Sagittal saw being used to remove the dorsal spurring, aligning the saw blade with the dorsal cortex of the metatarsal. **D.** Removal of the dorsal spurring. **E.** Placement of saw to remove the dorsal one-third of the articular cartilage. **F.** Completed cheilectomy with removal of entire dorsal one-third of the metatarsal head.

lateral, or medial should be removed with the use of a rongeur (see Fig. 14.2). At this time, the first MPJ should be run through the full arch of motion to assess dorsiflexion, which should be ~65 degrees.[19] Once proper ROM is obtained, the surgical site should be irrigated, and then, capsular closure can be performed with absorbable suture, followed by skin closure.

Waterman

The Waterman osteotomy first described in 1927 by Waterman[35] is a joint-sparing osteotomy performed within the head of the first metatarsal. The Waterman is a dorsal-based wedge osteotomy that aims to bring the intact plantar cartilage dorsally (Fig. 14.3). This osteotomy is indicated in grade 2 hallux limitus.

Technique

Exposure to the first metatarsal head is gained, and any spurring off of the metatarsal head is removed via hand instruments. The medial eminence may be removed off of the metatarsal head should there be one. Next, the osteotomy cuts are drawn. A dorsal-based wedge osteotomy angles are drawn such that a trapezoidal wedge will be resected (see Fig. 14.3). The proximal cut is drawn perpendicular to the weight-bearing surface, and the distal cut is angled roughly 30 degrees (see Fig. 14.3). The size of the wedge determines the amount of dorsiflexion needed. The cuts are made with the sagittal saw and are through and through cuts, but it is important not to disrupt the sesamoid apparatus when cutting through the plantar cortex. The wedge of bone is then removed, and the metatarsal head is rotated dorsally onto the metatarsal. The metatarsal head is then temporarily fixated with a Kirschner wire (K-wire). A single 2.7-mm screw is then used for permanent fixation in a dorsal proximal to distal plantar direction from the metatarsal neck into the capital fragment ensuring not to violate the joint.

Modified Oblique Waterman

A modification to the Waterman osteotomy can also be made is unique circumstances. In the late 1980s M. P. Jacobs developed a modified oblique Waterman osteotomy. There are only specific indications in which Jacobs states this procedure is to be used. The indications are low-grade hallux limitus in which the first metatarsal is already short and cannot afford any further shortening and contraindicated in long or elevated first metatarsals. This technique is used in grade 1-2 hallux limitus.

Technique

The typical exposure to the first MPJ is performed along with removal of all osteophytes off of the first metatarsal head. Any medial eminence of the metatarsal head may also be removed. A cheilectomy is also performed to remove and dorsal spurring or denuded dorsal cartilage. Next, the osteotomy cuts are to be drawn. The apex of the osteotomy is on the distal plantar aspect of the metatarsal head, distal to the sesamoids. The plantar arm of the osteotomy is drawn proximally in an oblique fashion to the metatarsal neck. The angle of the dorsal arm is determined by the amount of wedge needing to be removed but is also drawn proximally in an oblique fashion. The cuts are made with a sagittal saw and care is taken to leave the plantar hinge intact. The wedge of bone is then removed, and the capital fragment is dorsiflexed back onto the metatarsal. Temporary fixation may be performed with a K-wire. The hallux and first MPJ is ran through ROM to ensure no impingement remains. Final fixation is performed with two parallel 2.7 screws from dorsal distal to plantar proximal. The screws are to be bicortical and will exit proximal to the sesamoid apparatus.

Waterman-Green

The Waterman-Green osteotomy is another joint-sparing surgical procedure for the treatment of hallux limitus, specifically grade 2. The Green modification was added in 1987 by Bernbach[36] as a way to protect the sesamoids from any possible disruption during the osteotomy cuts. The Waterman-Green osteotomy also allows for plantar translation of the metatarsal head along with decompression of the first MPJ (Fig. 14.4).

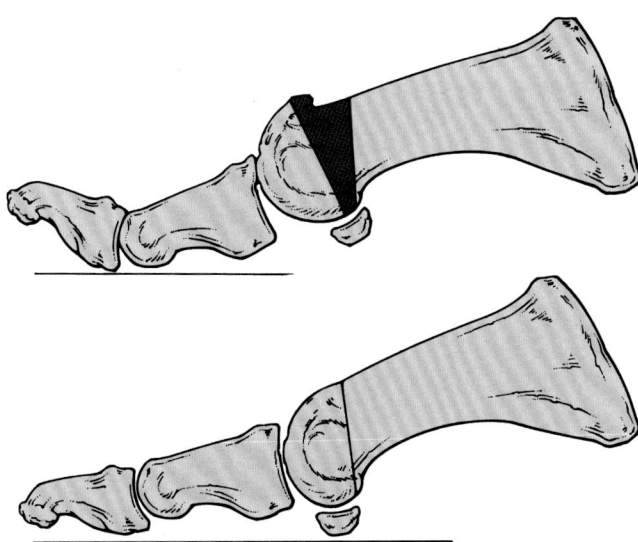

FIGURE 14.3 Dorsal based wedge to be removed allowing dorsal translation of the cartilage and decompression of the joint upon implantation of the metatarsal head on the metatarsal.

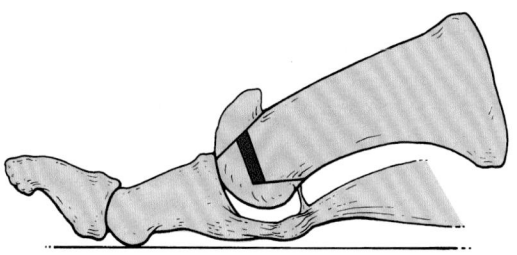

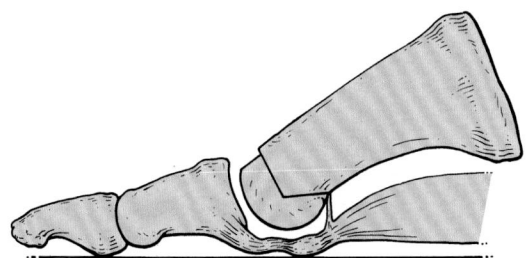

FIGURE 14.4 Waterman osteotomy with Green modification showing plantar shelf extent out the neck of the metatarsal proximal to the sesamoids. Both plantar flexion and decompression of the joint is achieved upon implantation.

Technique

The dorsal medial incisional approach is again used to gain access to the first MPJ. Dorsal spurring of the first metatarsal head is typically removed first with a rongeur, rotary bur, or sagittal saw. Next, any medial eminence of the first metatarsal head may be removed to allow a flat surface to perform the osteotomy cuts (Fig. 14.5). The apex of the osteotomy is marked one-third to one-half of the distance from the dorsal proximal

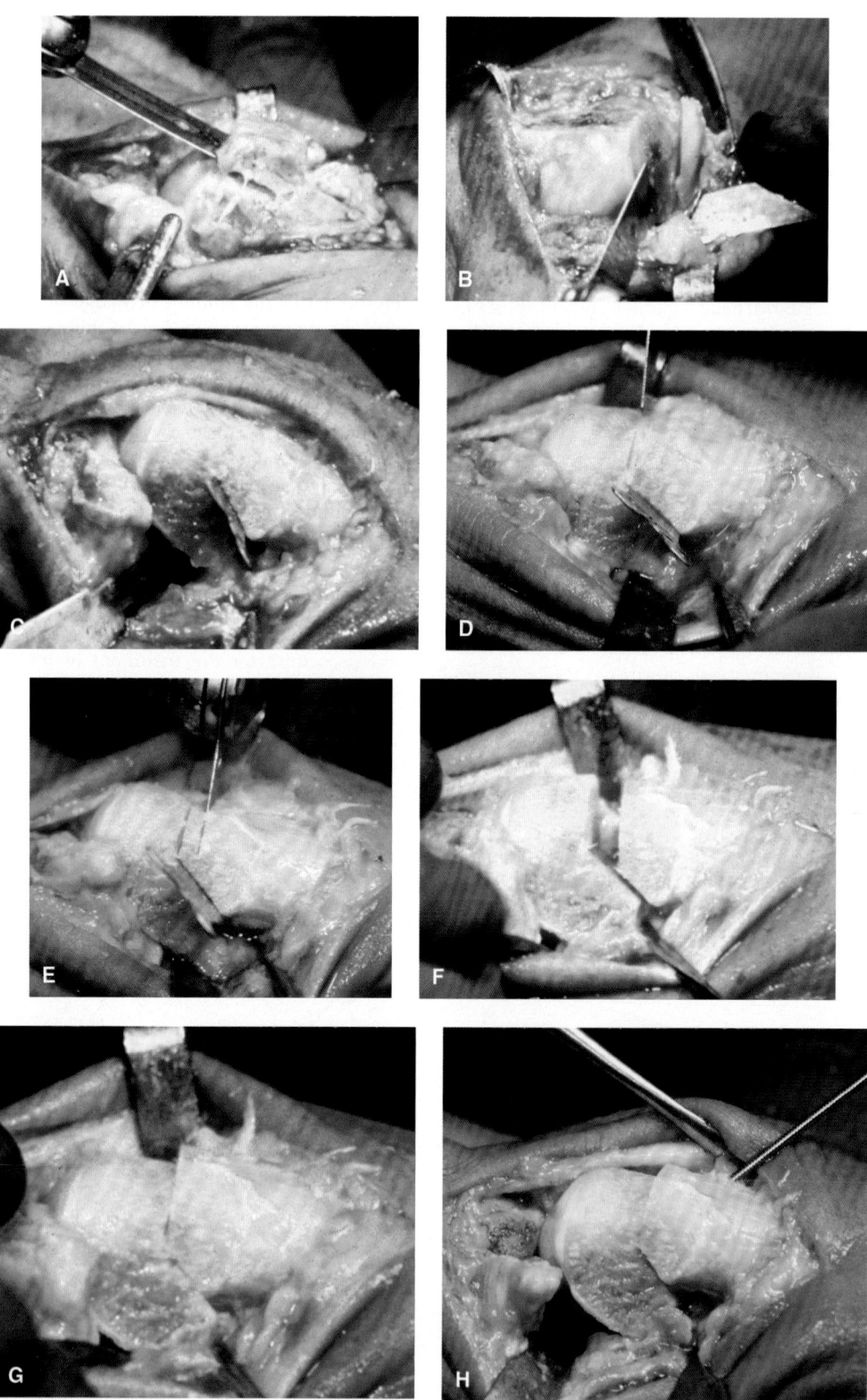

FIGURE 14.5 A, B. Removal of spurring off of the metatarsal head. **C, D.** Showing the plantar and dorsal arms of the osteotomy with apex central to slightly dorsal. **E.** Proximal dorsal cut being made parallel to the first dorsal cut. **F.** Removal of the dorsal wedge of bone. **G, H.** Reduction of osteotomy showing plantar flexion and shortening of the metatarsal head. (Courtesy of Donald R. Green, DPM.)

extent of the cartilage to the proximal plantar extent of the articulating cartilage (see Fig. 14.5). Next, using a marking pen, the dorsal and plantar arms of the osteotomy can be drawn. The plantar arm extends from the apex drawn just proximally to the metatarsal neck, ensuring to be proximal to the sesamoids. The dorsal arm is then drawn slightly proximal and dorsally. The more acute the angle of the osteotomy is, the more shortening that will be achieved, and the more vertical the osteotomy cuts the greater plantar flexion that will be achieved.[37] The dorsal and plantar cuts are both made perpendicular to the long axis of the metatarsal in the transverse plane. Next, there is a proximal cut taken off of the dorsal aspect of the metatarsal (see Fig. 14.5). This cut is parallel to the dorsal distal cut already made and exits through the plantar cut, effectively lowering the apex. The width of the wedge needing to be taken out is measured preoperatively to give proper decompression of the first MPJ. The wedge of bone is then removed. The capital fragment is then compressed onto the metatarsal and plantarly displaced (see Fig. 14.5). The capital fragment can be temporarily fixated with a single K-wire and the first MPJ put through full arch of motion to ensure no impingement exists (Fig. 14.5). Once full ROM is noted, a single 2.7-mm screw using AO technique can be placed from the metatarsal neck into the metatarsal head from dorsal proximal to plantar distal. The surgical site is then irrigated, and capsular closure can be ensued followed by skin closure.

Austin-Youngswick

The Austin osteotomy with Youngswick modification is another distal metatarsal osteotomy used for hallux limitus (Fig. 14.6). Many similarities exist between this osteotomy and the Waterman-Green procedure. The Austin-Youngswick is a traditional Austin with a dorsal wedge of bone resected (see Fig. 14.6). In theory, the shortening effects of this osteotomy will be offset by the plantar displacement of the head to allow for proper mechanics of the medial column, but recent studies have indicated this not to be the case.[38] Although patients do have the potential to do well after the Austin-Youngswick procedure,

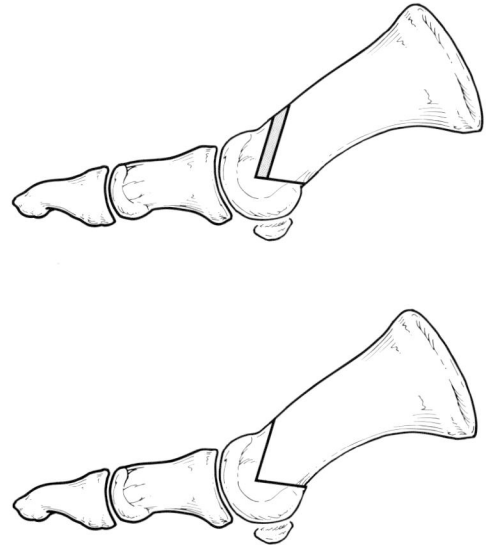

FIGURE 14.6 Standard Austin osteotomy with dorsal wedge removed.

Roukis has shown roughly a quarter of these osteotomies need revision.[39] The Austin osteotomy with Youngswick modification is indicated in grade 2 and 3 hallux limitus.

Technique

Once the metatarsal head is exposed, any spurring should be removed with a sagittal saw, rotary bur, or bone rongeur. The medial eminence, if there is one, may be removed allowing for a flat surface to perform the osteotomy cuts. The center of the metatarsal head is then found and used as the apex for the osteotomy cut (Fig. 14.7). The typical Austin cuts are made 60 degrees from each other. The angle of your Austin cut can be made more acute to allow greater shortening of the metatarsal or the cuts can be made at a larger angle to have more plantar flexion of the metatarsal head. Gerbert showed that keeping the dorsal arm at 60 degrees from the long axis and angling the plantar cut at 45 degrees will allow for 1.5 mm of both shortening and plantar displacement of the metatarsal head. He also showed that if the plantar arm is kept at 30 degrees and the dorsal arm is cut anywhere from 45 to 90 degrees, there is a consistent 2 mm of shortening and 1 mm of plantar displacement.[40] Next, the second dorsal cut is made in a parallel fashion and just proximal to the first dorsal cut (see Fig. 14.7). The width of the wedge removed depends on the amount of space needed to properly decompress the joint space. Once the proximal dorsal cut is performed, the wedge of bone is removed and the metatarsal head is impacted onto the metatarsal. Temporary fixation is performed with a K-wire, and adequate ROM, absent of any impingement, should be noted. Next, the osteotomy is fixated with a single 2.7-mm screw from the dorsal metatarsal direct plantar and distal into the metatarsal head (see Fig. 14.7).

Plantarflexory First Metatarsal Osteotomy (Lambrinudi)

The plantarflexory osteotomy described by Lambrinudi in 1938[41] is used in cases where metatarsus primus elevatus is thought to be the primary contributing etiology for the hallux limitus. As the name suggest, this osteotomy plantar flexes the metatarsal head to allow dorsiflexion of the hallux without impingement (Fig. 14.8). The plantarflexory osteotomy is indicated in grade 2-3 hallux limitus.

Technique

Exposure is much more extensive for the plantarflexory osteotomy; the incision will need to be extended proximally to the base of the first metatarsal. The periosteum will need to be elevated to expose the diaphyseal portion of the metatarsal. Once proper exposure is achieved, any osteophytes on the metatarsal head should be removed with a sagittal saw, rotary bur, or bone rongeur. Next, the osteotomy can be drawn out on the medial aspect of the middiaphyseal metatarsal. The apex of the osteotomy will be dorsally and ~1 cm from the metatarsal cuneiform joint. The apex hinge will consist of the dorsal cortex of the metatarsal; therefore, the apex should be drawn just inferior. Next, the two arms of the osteotomy are drawn in a wedge type fashion, distally and obliquely with the base being plantarly on the diaphyseal bone of the metatarsal (see Fig. 14.8). The proximal wedge cut should be angled 45 degrees from the first metatarsal cuneiform joint line. The distal wedge cut will be determined by the size of the bone wedge needed to be removed. These cuts will go through the plantar cortex. The larger the wedge that is resected, the more plantar flexion that

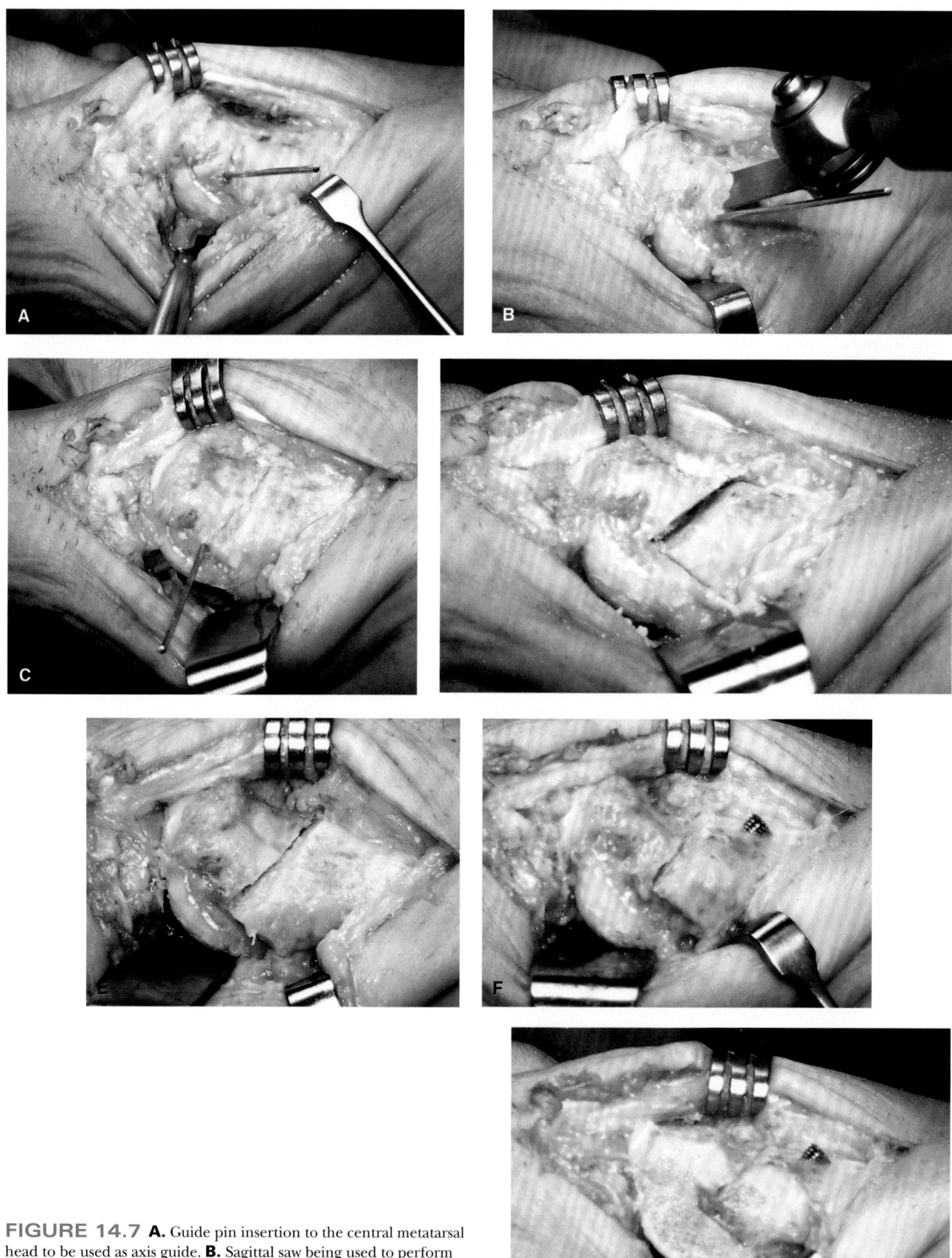

FIGURE 14.7 A. Guide pin insertion to the central metatarsal head to be used as axis guide. **B.** Sagittal saw being used to perform the dorsal distal cut. **C.** After completion of plantar cut. **D.** Removal of dorsal wedge of bone after a proximal dorsal cut has been made. **E-G.** Reduction and fixation of the osteotomy.

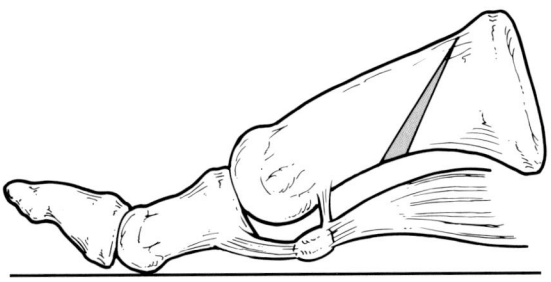

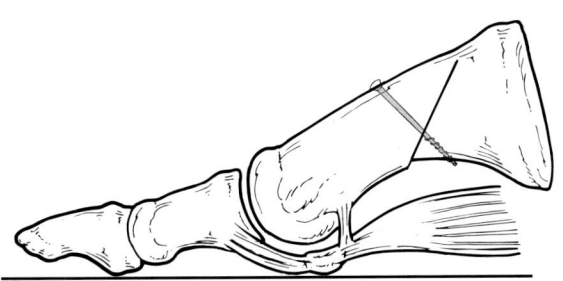

FIGURE 14.8 Plantarflexory osteotomy (Lambrinudi), which is a slightly oblique closing-based wedge in the diaphyseal of the first metatarsal.

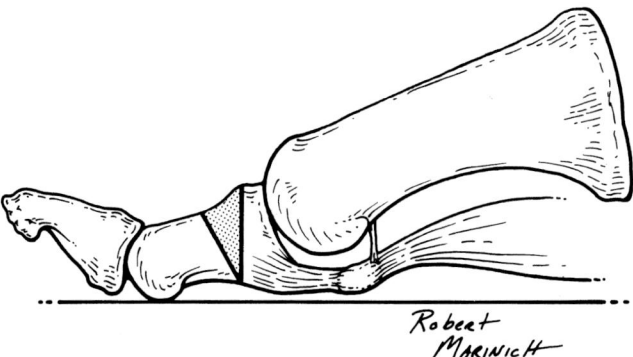

Robert
MARINICH

FIGURE 14.9 Illustration indicating the dorsal closing-based wedge within the proximal phalanx.

dorsally based wedge with the plantar apex being left intact as a hinge and point of fixation (Fig. 14.9). The width of the base of the wedge will determine the total amount of dorsiflexion of the hallux. The wider the base, the more dorsiflexion that is achieved and vice versa. Next, the osteotomy cuts are made with a sagittal saw; cuts can be made dorsal to plantar or medial to lateral depending on the surgeon's comfort level. The important factor to note is that the cuts must be perpendicular to the long axis of the proximal phalanx to ensure no transverse plane deformities upon closing of the wedge. Once the cuts are complete, the distal aspect of the proximal phalanx is dorsiflexed in attempt to close the wedge, feathering with the saw may be indicated to accomplish complete closure. Once the wedge is closed and good osseous contact is seen at the osteotomy site, fixation can be performed. Fixation is usually accomplished with a dorsally placed staple. A screw placed from proximal and medial oriented distal and lateral across the osteotomy using AO technique may also be used.

Valenti

The Valenti procedure was originally described in 1976 by Valenti, an Italian surgeon, and has many similarities to a cheilectomy.[45] The Valenti procedure consists of an aggressive cheilectomy type resection of one-third to one-half of both the metatarsal head and base of the proximal phalanx in order to alleviate all possible impingement of the dorsal first MPJ. Studies have proven that the Valenti procedure as a reliable procedure with positive outcomes and a revision rate of only 4.6% at >12-month follow-up.[46] This procedure is indicated in grade 2-3 hallux limitus.

Technique

The first order of business is to remove all dorsal spurring off of the metatarsal head and base of the proximal phalanx. This allows for complete visualization of the joint. Next, using a sagittal saw, the dorsal one-third to one-half of the articular cartilage of the metatarsal head is resected in a distal plantar to proximal dorsal manner. Next, the dorsal one-half of the proximal phalanx articulating cartilage is removed off of the base. The saw is oriented in a distal dorsal to proximal plantar position. Careful control is needed when cutting in this direction to not affect the cartilage on the metatarsal head. (Pearl is to place a Seeberger retractor in the first MPJ to act as protector.) Once the cut is made, the dorsal piece of bone is removed. Upon completion of the cuts, there is approximately a 90-degree angle between the cuts. Any and all sharp edges can be smoothed down with

will be achieved. Using a sagittal saw, the osteotomy cuts are now made from medial to lateral starting with the distal cut first. It is important to note that once the lateral cortex is penetrated, not to continue due to the dorsalis pedis artery and deep peroneal nerve being within the interspace. Once both cuts have been made, the wedge is taken out and the distal metatarsal is plantar flexed on the dorsal hinge that is now created. If the osteotomy does not close down, the sagittal saw is used to "feather" the osteotomy apex until the hinge is susceptible to closing down. Once the metatarsal is plantar flexed, temporary fixation is achieved with a K-wire. Once adequate ROM of the first MPJ is achieved due to the now plantar flexed first metatarsal head, permanent fixation can be performed with a dorsal distal to plantar proximal or a medial distal to lateral proximal 3.5 screw using AO technique (see Fig. 14.8). Fixation may also be achieved with a medial-based plate or staple.

Kessel-Bonney

This procedure was first described in 1952 by Kessel[42] as a way to fixate the hallux in an extended position, lessening the need for dorsiflexion at the first MPJ during gait. This technique was initially described as a procedure for adolescents.[42] This procedure can be performed independently or with a first metatarsal procedure such as a cheilectomy. Moberg described a similar type dorsiflexory phalangeal osteotomy in adults calling it the Moberg osteotomy.[43] Studies have shown a Moberg osteotomy combined with a cheilectomy can improve symptoms in 89% of patients and increase the dorsiflexion of the hallux to 9 degrees.[44] The Kessel-Bonney and Moberg osteotomies are indicated in grade 2-3 hallux limitus.

Technique

The first MPJ exposure is carried out, and the initial incision is extending slightly distal to the interphalangeal joint of the hallux. After full exposure of the proximal phalanx diaphyseal bone, the osteotomy can be drawn out. The osteotomy is a a bone rongeur or bone rasp. The hallux is then dorsiflexed to assess for any catching or impingement.

Distraction Arthrodiastasis

Arthrodiastasis has been a well-documented procedure to reduce stiffness in many joints throughout the body.[47] Arthrodiastasis of the first MPJ is typically reserved for grade 2-3 hallux limitus in patients who are particularly active and wish to preserve motion at the first MPJ. The goal of arthrodiastasis is to stretch the soft tissues structures surrounding the joint as well as to alleviate any pressure on the articular cartilage.[47] Therefore, arthrodiastasis may allow for more ROM and decrease the pain caused by the impinging joint.

Technique

The first step to this procedure is removing any exostosis present at the first MPJ utilizing the usual exposure. If the joint is opened to remove spurring, the cartilage can be assessed at this time, and if subchondral drilling is indicated, it can be done at this time. The next step would be to apply the external fixator device. Typically, a MiniRail fixator device is utilized and applied medially to avoid disrupting the tendinous structures (Fig. 14.10). The external device is held parallel to the first metatarsal such that the distraction portion of the device faces distally. The screw clamps should be on either side of the first MPJ, and the distal screw clamp should be position as far proximal as possible to allow for maximal distraction upon application (see Fig. 14.10).

The first metatarsal screw may now be placed through the proximal seat of the proximal clamp on the external fixator and into the central shaft of the metatarsal, perpendicular to the long axis. It is important to note that all screws should be bicortical to ensure stability. Next, the hallux is held in neutral position and in line with the external fixator, and the first hallux screw is placed into the proximal seat of the distal clamp and into the proximal phalanx. Proper alignment of the joint and bicortical insertion of the screws may now be verified using intraoperative radiographs. After confirmation of proper placement, the second metatarsal and hallux screws may be placed. The external fixator device should be placed at least 5 mm off of the soft tissues to allow for swelling (see Fig. 14.10). The first MPJ may now be distracted up to 5 mm intraoperatively prior to closure of the incision. It is recommended that the distraction is checked under fluoroscopy to ensure proper distraction and alignment of the joint before closure (Fig. 14.11).

The postoperative protocol for proper distraction of the first MPJ follows the standard external fixator distraction template. In the first week, there is no distraction to allow for the soft tissues to accommodate the distraction performed prior to closure. Beginning the 2nd postoperative week, distraction may proceed. Distraction is typically done at 0.5 mm/day. This can be done by the patient and can be performed by a single 0.5 mm increase once daily or by two 0.25 mm increases per day. One full turn of the screw by the patient is 1 mm, so this would relate to one-half turn daily or two-quarter turns daily, respectively. Distraction is carried out for 14 days, allowing an additional 7 mm of distraction, making a total of 12 mm of distraction. During weeks 4 and 5 postoperative, no distraction is carried out to allow the soft tissues to again adapt to the increased length and tension on the joint. After week 5, if adequate distraction has been achieved, the external fixator may be removed with patient beginning a rehabilitation program to assist is first MPJ ROM.

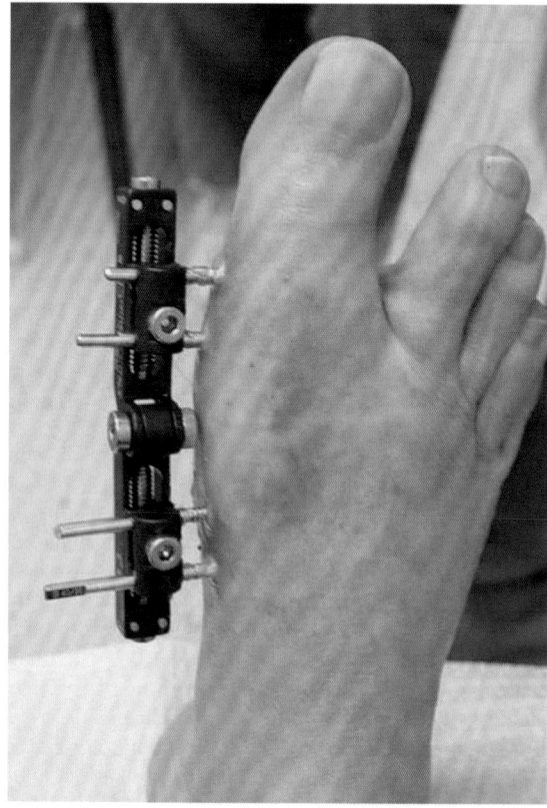

FIGURE 14.10 Application of external fixator device to the first rat. (Courtesy of George Vito, DPM.)

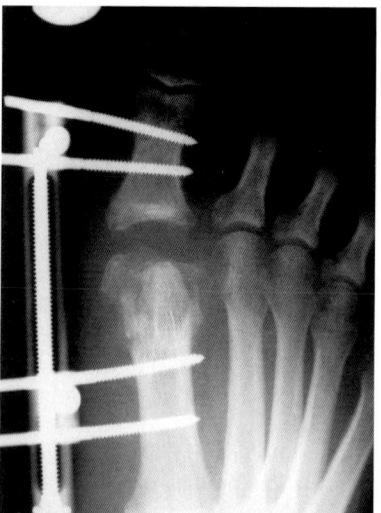

FIGURE 14.11 Radiographs showing distraction of the first MPJ and proper alignment of the pins into the first metatarsal and proximal phalanx. All pins are noted to be bi-cortical. (Courtesy of George Vito, DPM.)

JOINT DESTRUCTIVE

Osteochondral Grafting

Osteochondritis dissecans can be a common finding in hallux limitus, especially when the etiology is due to trauma.[48] Osteochondral defects may allow for acceleration of the arthritic process within the first MPJ and cause progressively worse hallux limitus. The aim of osteochondral grafting is to repair the chondral defect with either allo- or autograft hyaline cartilage to deter further destruction.

Technique

Exposure of the first MPJ occurs in the standard manner. Once the joint is exposed, all spurring may be removed utilizing a rongeur and/or a burr. Next, the first metatarsal is inspected for the chondral defect (confirmed on MRI prior to surgery). The damaged cartilage is excised to healthy cartilage margins. The defect circumference is then measured. Next, the proper allograft or autograft is obtained. Possible donor sites include the talus, knee, or even the dorsal aspect of the metatarsal head if the lesion is isolated centrally.[49] Newer synthetic grafts are also now available, although short to midterm outcomes with these synthetic grafts are promising, longer-term studies need to be performed.[50] A special harvesting tool is utilized to harvest the hyaline cartilage plug, which is ~1 mm larger in circumference than the defect measured and ~12 mm in length.[49] Once the graft is harvested, the same type of instrument, but smaller circumference, is used to remove the damaged lesion. The depth when removing the lesion is typically 1-2 mm shorter than the actual graft. Next, the graft is placed in the defect; this will be a snug fit as the graft circumference is wider than what was removed. The hyaline graft will also sit proud on the metatarsal head after impaction as well; this is to account for any possible absorption of the graft as it incorporates into the metatarsal head. Compression of the joint is performed via axial loading of the proximal phalanx on the metatarsal head.[49] If the graft was harvested from the dorsal cartilage, then a dorsal cheilectomy is now performed; otherwise, once proper ROM is achieved, closure may ensue.

Arthroplasty

The arthroplasty procedure has long been a reliable procedure for hallux rigidus, and now, arthroplasty with implants are gaining popularity in the treatment of hallux rigidus.[51] Arthroplasties are often indicated in patients with severe joint space narrowing and destruction of joint space due to arthritic changes. Many times, upon evaluation of the articulating surfaces, the cartilage is absent or fibrocartilage has replaced the native hyaline cartilage. Excisional arthroplasties are often indicated in instances where the joint is destroyed from arthritic changes, but the bone stock is also poor, likely from systemic disease, making implantation of prosthetic devices very difficult. Arthroplasty with implant placement is used in end-stage hallux rigidus where maintenance of joint motion is of high priority.

Mayo

The Mayo arthroplasty was originally described for hallux valgus deformity in 1908 but now is also indicated in end-stage hallux rigidus typically seen in patients with systemic arteriopathies such as rheumatoid arthritis.[52] Mayo arthroplasty is performed at the head of the first metatarsal. The Mayo arthroplasty is indicated in stages 3-4 hallux rigidus and is also routinely used as a salvage-type procedure.

Technique

The first metatarsal head is exposed per usual fashion. It is important to remove all metatarsal head spurring to ensure adequate visualization of the joint space. This can be done with a bone rongeur or a sagittal saw. At this time, the transverse arthroplasty cut is drawn on the metatarsal head. It is important to make the transverse cut so that all articulating cartilage is removed. The amount of resection can be determined by preoperative measurements on radiographs or an intraoperative decision, but typically, 0.5-1 cm of bone is resected. The bone cuts are typically made dorsal to plantar, but care is taken when going through the plantar cortex to not disturb the flexor tendons. Care is also taken to ensure that the transverse cut is made perpendicular to the long axis of the first metatarsal. Next, the distal first metatarsal bone is dissected out and free of all soft tissue attachments. At this point, any sharp edges of the metatarsal are removed with a bone rongeur or the sagittal saw. Rough edges can also be smoothed down with a bone rasp. The hallux is then ran through the arc of motion to ensure that adequate amount of bone was removed and no impingement is seen. It is at this time, the stability of the joint after resection is assessed; if the joint appears unstable or appears to sit in a nonrectus position, retrograde pinning of the first MPJ can be achieved with a 0.62-in K-wire to the desired position. This pin will remain in the foot be pulled around the 4-week mark. The joint space is left open to fill in with hematoma and scar tissue. Capsular and skin closure is then ensued.

Keller

The Keller excisional arthroplasty was first described in 1904 and parallels the Mayo osteotomy except it is performed on the base of the proximal phalanx and not the metatarsal.[53] Often times, the Keller arthroplasty may also be used in conjunction with the Mayo arthroplasty for severely damaged first MPJs. The Keller arthroplasty is indicated in grade 3-4 hallux limitus.

Technique

The proximal phalanx is exposed through the dorsal incision. Any osteophytes off of the metatarsal head or proximal phalangeal base should be removed to allow visualization of the joint. The transverse osteotomy is then made with a sagittal saw resecting approximately the proximal one-third of the proximal phalanx, staying perpendicular to the long axis. Again, it is important to ensure that the transverse cut is perpendicular to the long axis of the proximal phalanx. Care is taken when cutting through the plantar cortex to ensure not to violate the flexor tendons. The proximal phalanx base is now removed in total. The hallux is ran through the arch of motion to ensure that adequate excision of bone was performed. Next, the hallux is pinned in proper rectus position with a 1-cm joint space utilizing an 0.62-in K-wire inserted in a retrograde fashion through the hallux and then into the first metatarsal. Through the osteotomy site any possible flexor tenotomy may be performed if indicated to have the hallux rest in a rectus position. Modifications can be made to the Keller bone cuts in order to preserve plantar soft tissue attachments at the base of the proximal phalanx. The transverse cut is still perpendicular to the longitudinal axis in the transverse plane but is angled slightly in the sagittal plane to resect more dorsally than plantarly on the proximal phalanx base. The cut is oriented dorsal distal to proximal plantar and also maintenance of vital soft tissue attachments at the plantar base of the proximal phalanx.

Interposition Arthroplasty

The interpositional arthroplasty is indicated in destructive joints in which motion is imperative to the patient. Specifically, younger and more active patients are the typical candidates for the interpositional arthroplasty. This procedure is indicated in grade 2-4 hallux limitus. Studies have shown with autogenous soft tissue interposition arthroplasty, patients do quite well and have an overall low incidence of complications. In the same

study, these improved patient outcomes were consistent at >12 months postoperative.[54] Using the technique detailed below, dorsiflexion of the hallux on average has increased 52% postoperatively.[55]

Technique
Roukis

The initial dorsal medial incision and dissection to capsule follows the technique listed previously, but once down to the capsule, the exposure technique deviates. Approximately 4.0 cm proximal to the MPJ, a transverse full-thickness capsular incision is made. Extending from the medial and lateral aspects of the transverse incision, and made distally in a longitudinal fashion, two full-thickness capsular incisions are made extending distally to the first MPJ (Fig. 14.12). Starting proximally where the transverse incision was made, the dorsal capsular and periosteal flap is dissected off of the metatarsal.

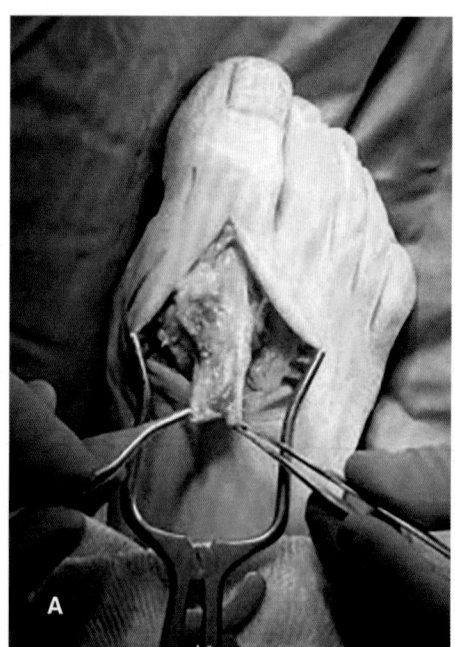
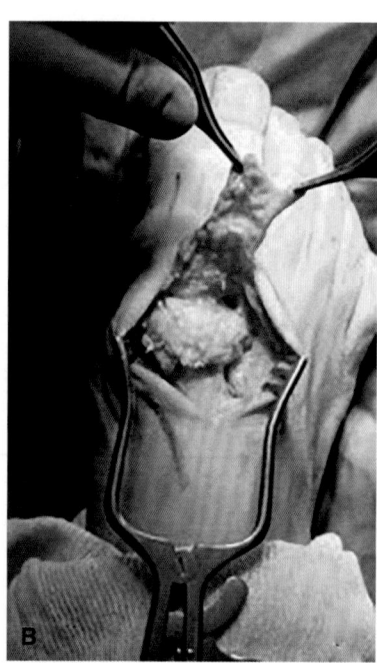
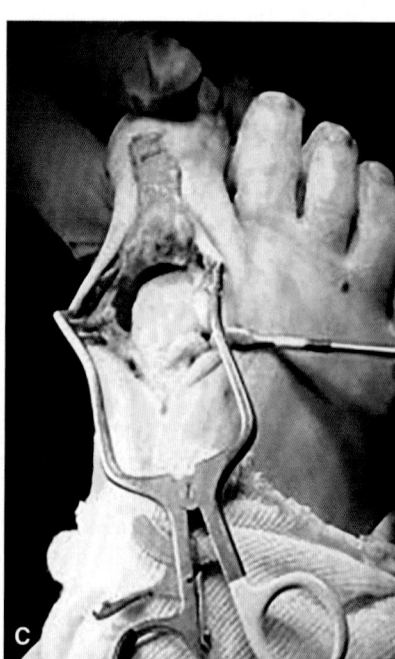
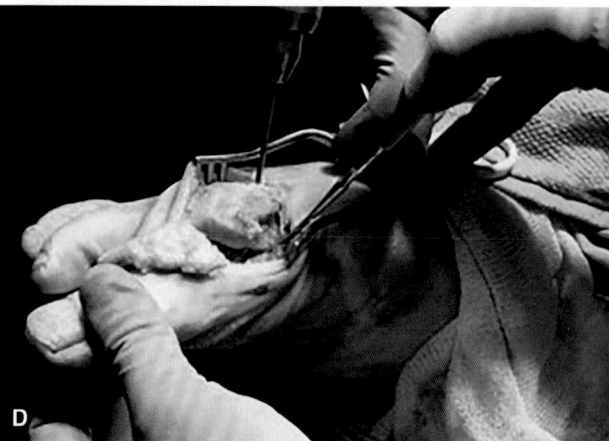
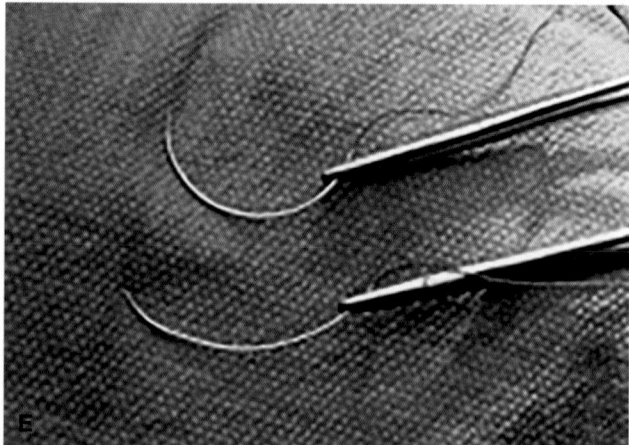

FIGURE 14.12 A. Capsule and periosteum flap created off of the dorsal first MPJ. **B.** Reflection of the flap showing the remaining attachment to the proximal phalangeal base. **C.** A debrided first metatarsal head to normal anatomic shape with the flap maintained. **D.** Dorsal to plantar drill placement, which will be used to secure the flap with suture. **E.** The superior needle is a ½ circular needle that comes standard with suture. The inferior needle has been carefully bent to enlarge the curvature, making it easier to pass through the drill holes.

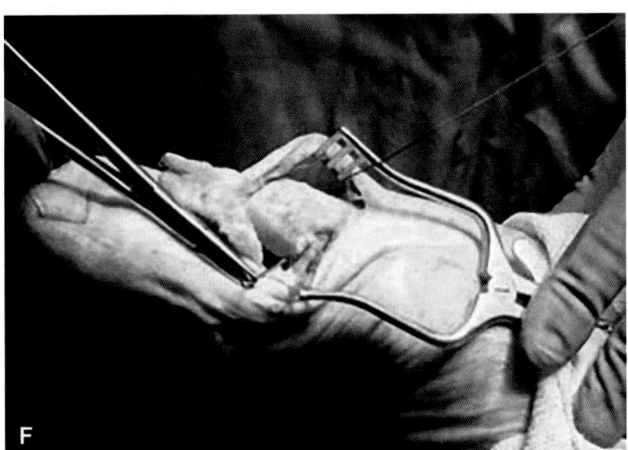

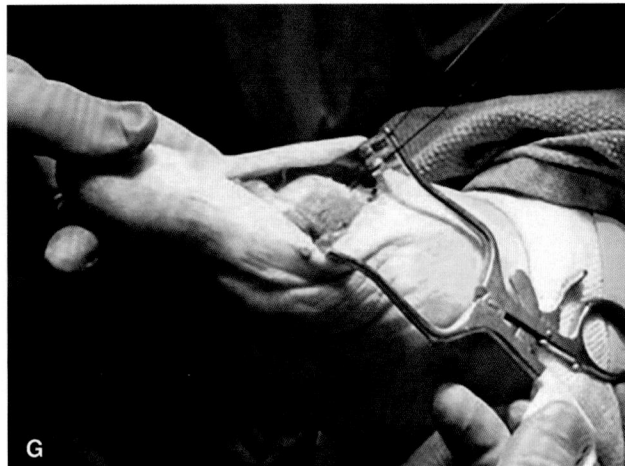

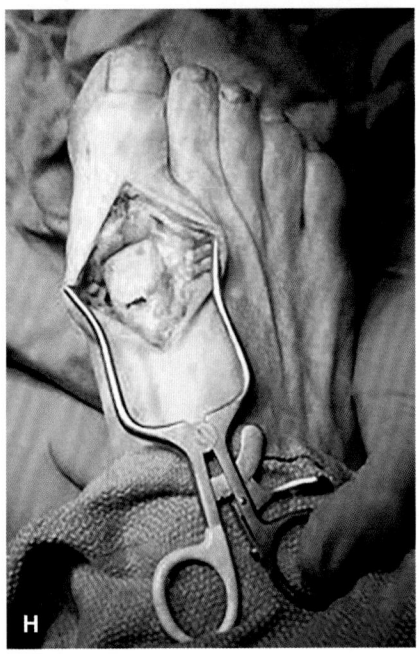

FIGURE 14.12 (*Continued*) **F.** Passing of the needle and suture through the drill hole. **G.** The capsule periosteum flap placed into the first MPJ with tension on the sutures to secure flap in place. **H.** The capsule periosteum flap seated into the first MPJ and tightly secured by a tied suture on the dorsal aspect of the metatarsal. (Courtesy Thomas Roukis, DPM, PhD.)

The dissection is carried distally, and 2-3 mm is also dissected off of the base of the proximal phalanx (see Fig. 14.12). The extensor hallucis brevis tendon is transected during this dissection and remains within the flap to provide bulk and support to the flap. The articulating cartilage is then inspected for any denuded cartilage. The first metatarsal head will undergo an aggressive cheilectomy removing the dorsal one-half of the articulating cartilage. The medial and lateral spurring of the metatarsal head is then removed, and the head is recontoured with rotatory bur or bone rasp. The plantar distal aspect of the first metatarsal head is assessed for any spurring or arthrofibrosis to underlying structures. If spurring is present, osteophytes are removed to leave a smooth surface. It is important to resect as little bone as possible in this area, as to preserve the weight-bearing surface of the metatarsal head. Fibrosis of the metatarsal head to underlying structures may be freed using a McGlamry or freer elevator; caution should be used to strip as little periosteum as possible to preserve blood supply. As for the proximal phalanx, if the hallux is long in comparison to the second digit, a 2- to 3-mm resection of the base of the proximal phalanx may be performed. If the hallux sits in a corrected position, subchondral drilling may then be performed wherever denuded cartilage is seen.

Once all resection has occurred, the hallux should be ran through the arc of motion to ensure no impingement, catching, or clicking exists. Next, a 2.0-mm drill is used to drill two holes from dorsal to plantar, one medial and one lateral. These holes are to be drilled just proximal to the proximal extent of the tibial and fibular sesamoids (see Fig. 14.12). Absorbable suture of the surgeon's preference (the authors advise a 3-0) on a needle, the needle curve is first bent for easier passage through the hole, then passed from dorsal to plantar through the lateral drill hole first (see Fig. 14.12). A Kessler-Kleinert (ie, locking Kessler) stitch is performed in the capsular flap extending ~3.0 mm from the distal end of the flap. Once the stitch has been placed, the needle is then brought plantar to dorsal in the medial drill hole (see Fig. 14.12). The capsular flap should now be positioned overlying the proximal phalanx base and diving plantar in between the first metatarsal head and proximal phalanx. The proximal extend of the flap should be positioned between the plantar first metatarsal head and sesamoid bones. Once the flap is properly positioned, the medial and lateral suture ends on the dorsal aspect of the metatarsal may be tied down together (see Fig. 14.12). The medial and lateral aspects of the capsuleperiosteum flap may be reinforced and sutured to surrounding capsule with absorbable suture and skin closure is ensued.

Technique

McGlamry

Full exposure of the first MPJ is obtained, and then, cheilectomy is performed to remove all osteophytes off of both the metatarsal head and base of the proximal phalanx. Keller arthroplasty is performed as noted above and often the modified Keller cut is preferred to preserve the attachment of the plantar soft tissues, specifically the flexor hallucis brevis, in these patients. Next, it is important to free the metatarsal head from the underlying sesamoid bones as this will be important for the interpositional graft placement. Typically, a McGlamry elevator can be used to release the sesamoids from the metatarsal head; however, an alternative method would be to use a curved osteotomy or freer elevator. It is important to not strip the metatarsal head of nutrient vessels and vital blood supply while releasing the sesamoids. The next steps can vary depending on if using the capsule for the interpositional aspect or using an allograft. If using the capsule, once the joint is contoured and clean of any osteophytes, the medial capsule is incised parallel to the joint. The dorsal medial capsule can be transposed into the joint over the metatarsal head and sutured to the underlying plantar plate using 4-0 absorbable suture.

Own Allograft Technique

If the surgeon's preference is to use an allograft, the steps deviate from the above technique. After dissection down to the first MPJ and removal of all spurring, four holes are now made within the distal metatarsal, which will serve as anchoring points for the graft. The holes are made using a 0.045-in K-wire. The four holes are made in the metaphyseal bone of the distal metatarsal just proximal to sesamoid apparatus. Dorsal holes are made, one medial and one lateral, starting on the dorsal aspect and at a 45-degree angle out the medial and lateral sides of the bone. Similar types of holes are made plantarly, but this time, the K-wire is started on the plantar one-third of the medial and lateral metatarsal metaphyseal and aimed at a 45-degree angle through the plantar cortex more centrally on the bone. The reason four holes are made instead of just two straight dorsal to plantar on the medial and lateral aspect of the metatarsal is that the authors find it easier to feed the suture through and easier to contour the free allograft to each of the individual holes. Next, the interpositional graft is prepared. The authors typically use a freeze-dried allograft. The use of allograft requires

soaking in gentamicin (360 mg in solution) for 5 minutes prior to use; this also makes the graft more malleable for use. The graft is typically a 1 × 4-in piece, and the graft is folded over on itself two times to make a 2 × 1-in piece with one-half of the graft being three layers thick. The thicker end is the end that will be between the metatarsal and phalanx, while the single layer end will be placed between the plantar metatarsal head and sesamoid bones. Each of the four corners of the graft are now tagged with 4-0 absorbable suture. The graft is then placed as noted above, and the suture needles are passed through the respective holes, and the graft is sutured in place. The hallux is then ran through arch of motion to ensure proper motion with the graft present. Capsular closure is then performed followed by skin.

Implant Arthroplasty

Implant arthroplasty is a joint destructive procedure, which aims to recreate the joint through a prosthetic implant. This procedure is usually offered to patients who are older and still would like to maintain motion at their great toe joint but are of only moderate activity level. These implants typically are not indicated in highly active patients for fear of failure. It is important to counsel patients on the fact that these implants may only last a few years and may need to be replaced.[56] Multiple different joint implants exist including hemi-implants, hinged implants, total joint implants, and even newer technologies. Most of the implants are made out of a metallic metal or titanium or a silicone type material. Implant arthroplasty is indicated in grade 3-4 hallux limitus.

Technique

The first MPJ is exposed in the usual fashion as described in this text. Initial treatment should be focused on removal of all spurring noted on the metatarsal head and base of the proximal phalanx to appropriately contour the joint and gain complete visibility of the anatomical first MPJ. Depending on the type of implant that is going to be placed, a Mayo, Keller, or both arthroplasties may be performed.

Hemi-implant

The hemi-implant comes in many different varieties and will be placed on the proximal phalanx (Fig. 14.13). First a cheilectomy with removal of all osteophytes is performed upon exposure of the joint to allow proper visualization of the joint space (Fig. 14.14). Next, the base of the proximal phalanx is removed using a sagittal saw, the cut is perpendicular to the longitudinal axis of the phalanx (Fig. 14.15). The trial sized implants will be used to estimate the amount of bone to resect (2-3 mm). The transverse cut is to be perpendicular to the long axis of the proximal phalanx. Upon sawing through the plantar cortex, it is important to not violate the flexor tendons. Next, a hole is drilled down the central axis of the proximal phalanx for the trial implant, this hole is guided by the sizing guide. The trial implants are then placed on the proximal phalanx (Fig. 14.16). The implant should extend to the outer aspects of the proximal phalanx base and allow for proper dorsiflexion of the hallux. Error should be on the larger sized implant to deter any osseous overgrowth that would affect the implant. Once satisfied with the implant and motion of the hallux, the trial implant is removed and a broach is placed, centered on the trial pin

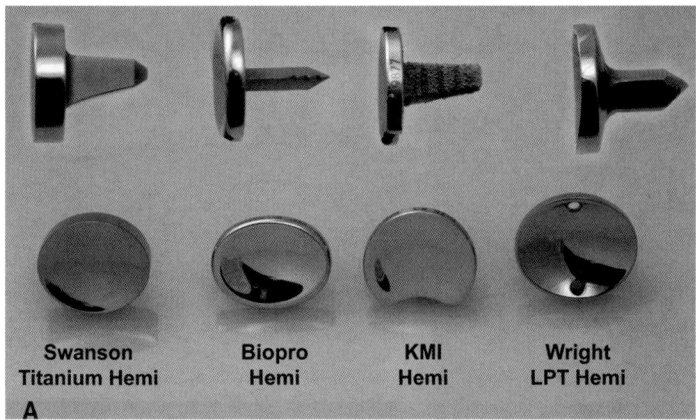
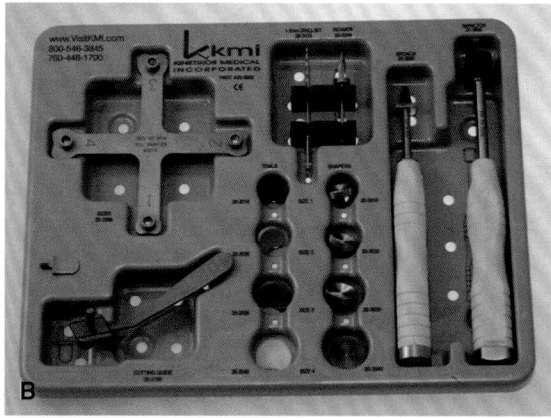

FIGURE 14.13 **A.** Picturing four hemi-implants for the first MPJ. From left to right: Swanson great toe implant BioPro hemi-implant, KMI hemi-implant, Wright LPT hemi-implant. **B.** Instrumentation set utilized for implantation of the KMI hemi-phalanx implant.

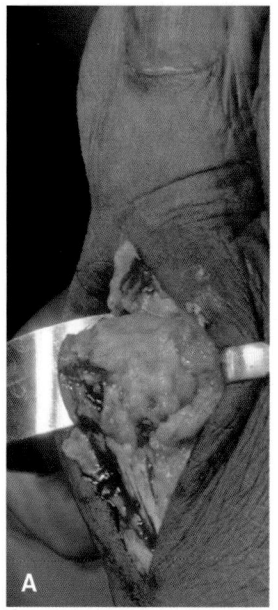
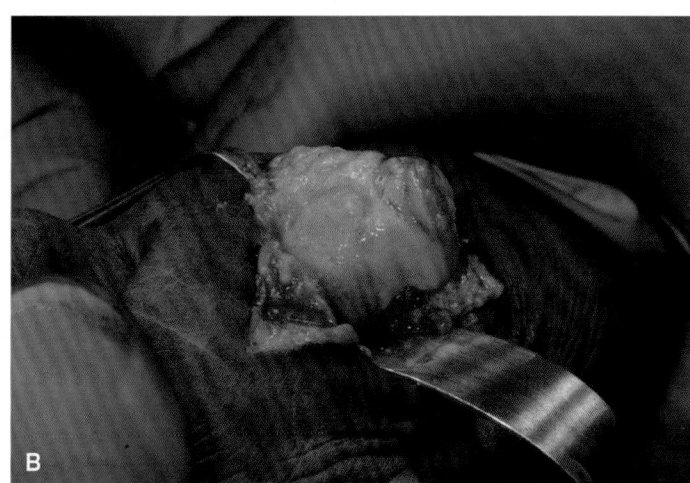
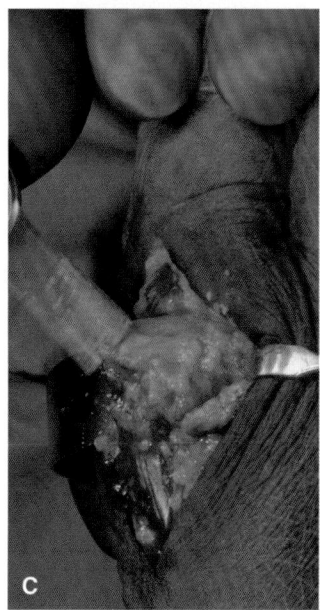
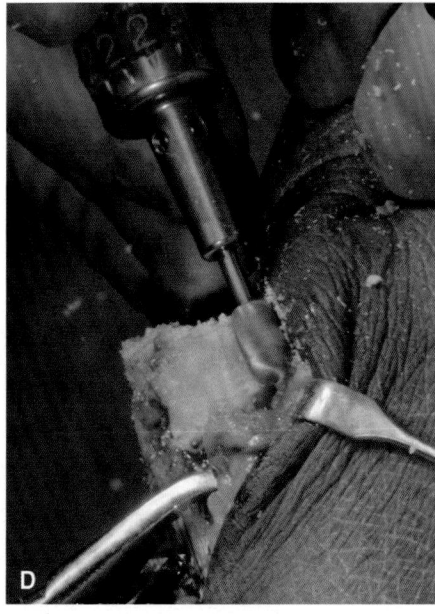

FIGURE 14.14 **A.** Exposure of the first MPJ. **B.** Denuded articular cartilage on the metatarsal head. **C, D.** Removal of osteophytes off of the metatarsal head with smoothing of the bone.

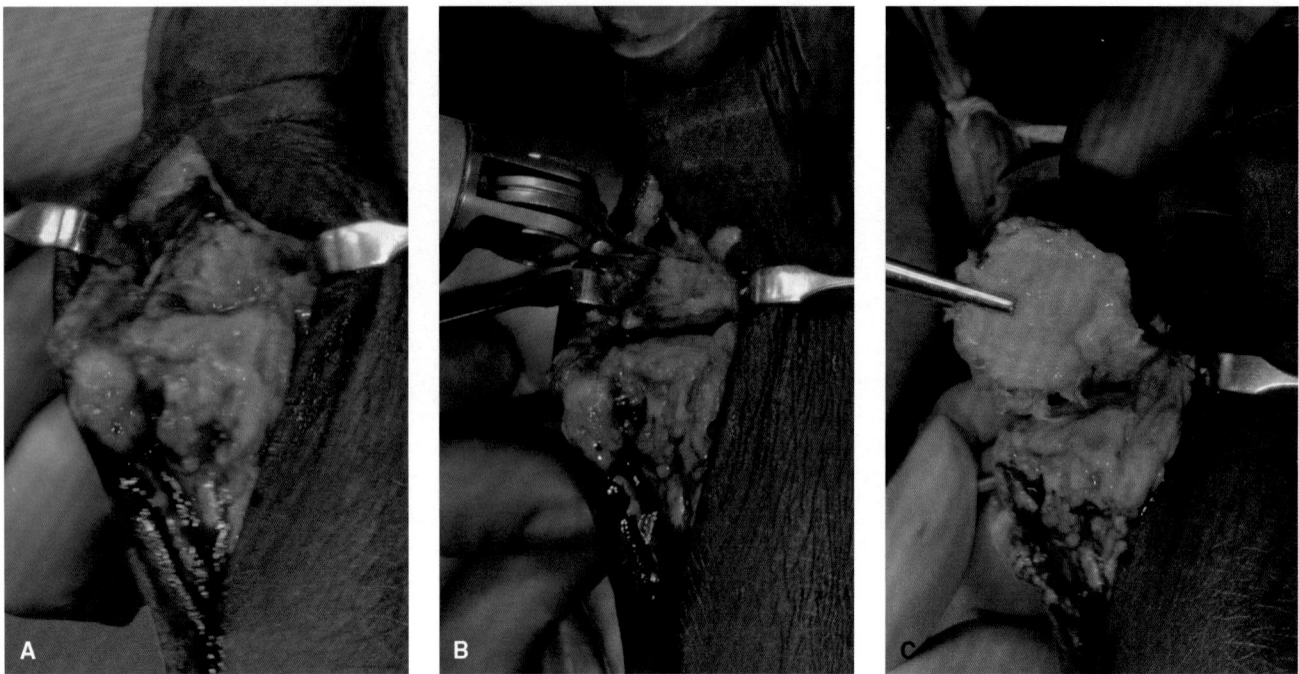

FIGURE 14.15 A. Exposure of the proximal phalanx base. **B.** Sagittal being used to remove the proximal one-third of the phalanx perpendicular to longitudinal axis. **C.** Removal of the proximal phalanx base.

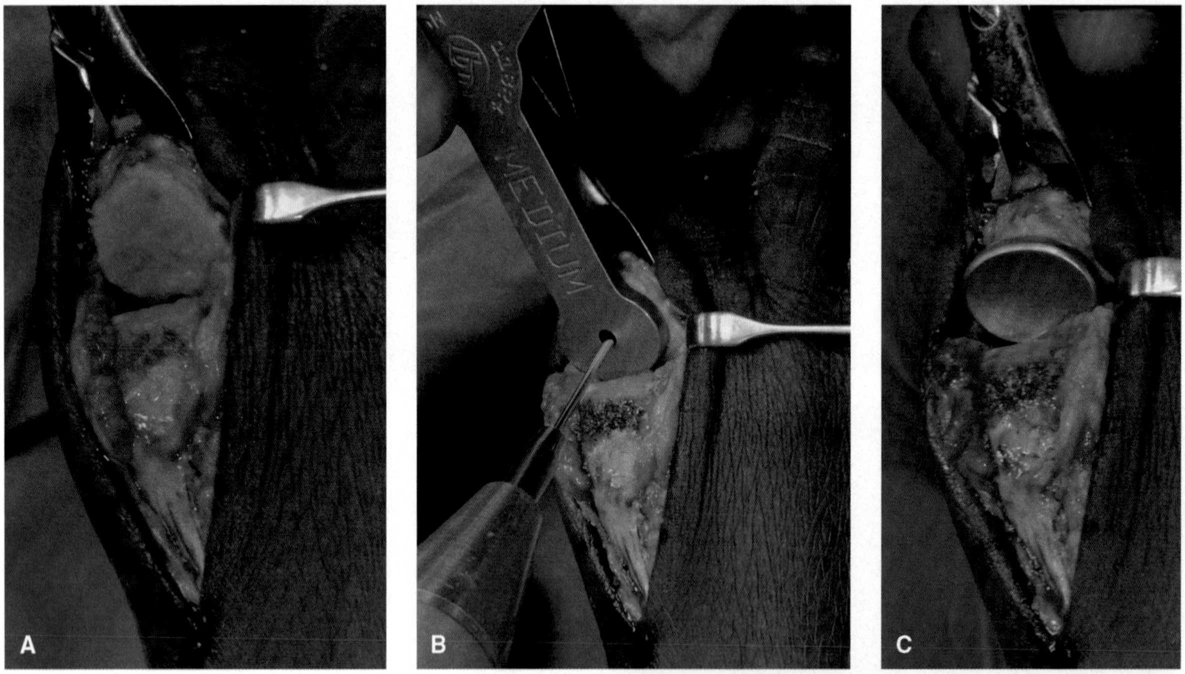

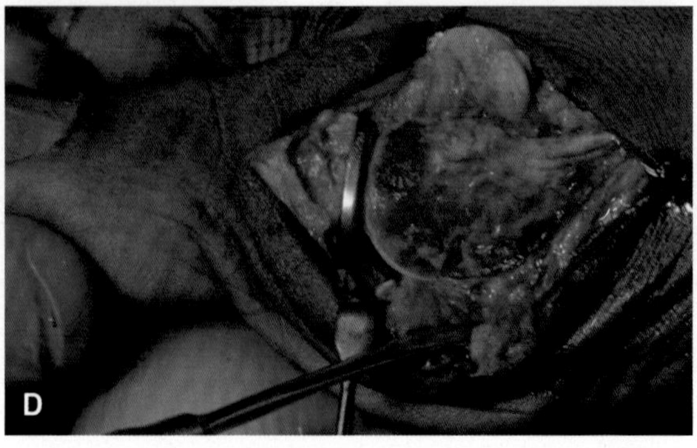

FIGURE 14.16 A. Flat surface of the proximal phalanx base for implant. **B.** Sizing guide placed on the base of proximal phalanx used to guide central drill hole. **C.** Trial implant inserted with stem inserting into the drill hole. **D.** Proper fitting of trial implant.

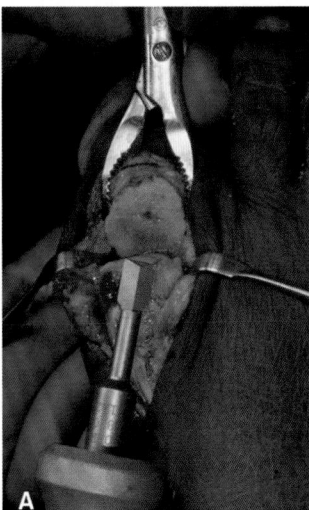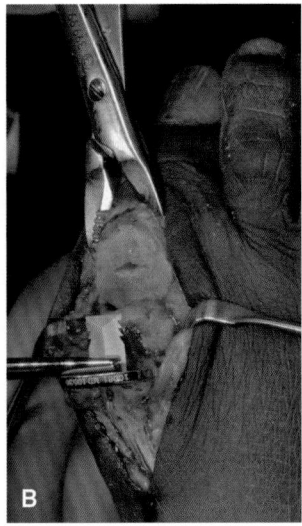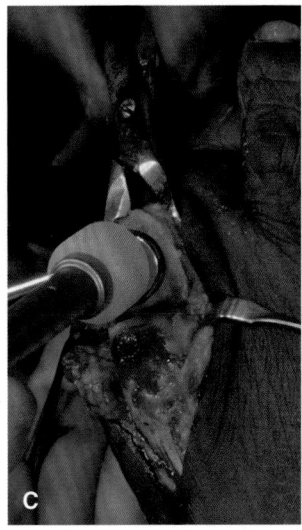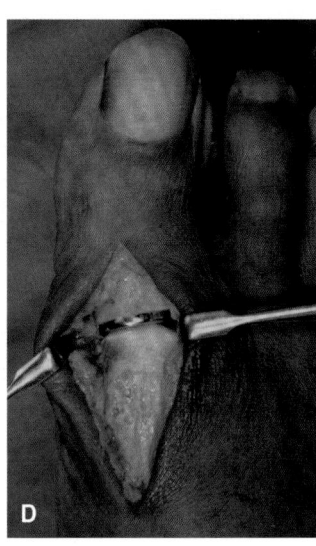

FIGURE 14.17 A. Broached used to prepare the canal of the phalanx. **B.** Implant insertion using no-hands technique. **C.** Impaction of implant onto the phalanx. **D.** Proper fitting hemi-implant.

hole already drilled. The broach is manually inserted and typically has a laser line or stopping mark to indicate when the broach has been inserted the proper distance for the implant (Fig. 14.17). The proper sized implant is then opened, and using a no touch technique, if possible, the implant is grasped with forceps and the stem is placed into the proximal phalanx. Next, the impactor that comes with the implant hardware is used to impact the implant onto the proximal phalanx until flush apposition between implant and bone stalk is noted (see Fig. 14.17). The hallux is again ran through the full arc of motion to ensure no impingement. If the joint is stiff or limited ROM noted, often more bone resection is needed. Implant position is often verified with intraoperative radiographs, and after verifying proper position, closure is ensued (Fig. 14.18).

Metatarsal Head Resurfacing

Similar to the technique described above, metatarsal head resurfacing is a hemi-implant that is inserted onto the metatarsal head. Although this resurfacing technique has been described in other joints in the body such as the knee and the hip, it was first described for the first metatarsal head in 2008.[57] This procedure has gained popularity over recent years for multiple reasons. Carpenter and colleagues have shown an increase in patient satisfaction after undergoing the procedure over a 10-year period.[58] Also, the literature supports a significant increase, as much as 50 degrees, in dorsiflexion at the first MPJ.[59] Metatarsal head resurfacing is indicated in grade 2-3 hallux limitus.

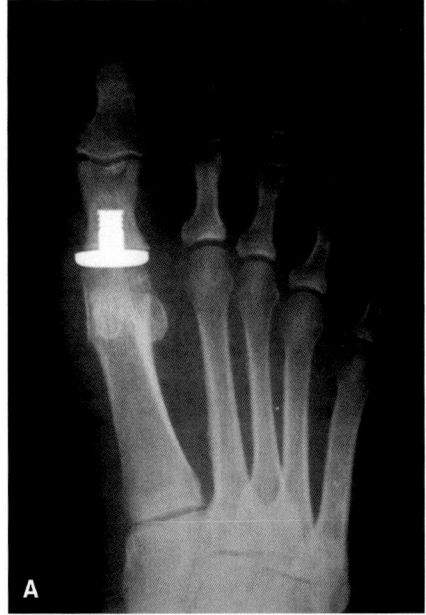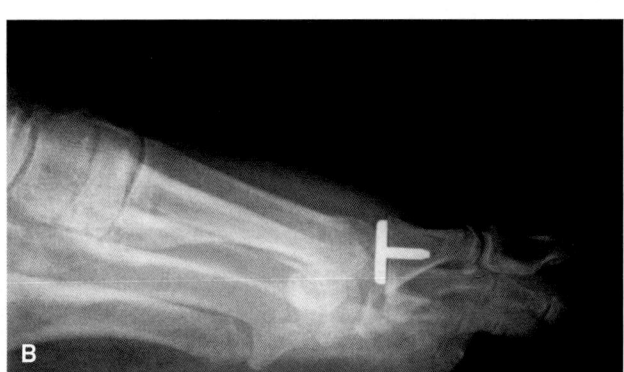

FIGURE 14.18 A. An AP depicting proper size and placement of hemi-implant into the proximal phalanx. **B.** Lateral radiograph showing proper placement of hemi-implant.

Technique

The first metatarsal head is exposed through the dorsal medial incision as described. It is important to release the soft tissue from the entire metatarsal head in order to expose both medial and lateral aspects. Next, removal of the medial eminence can be performed if indicated. All spurring should be removed until normal anatomic metatarsal head is appreciated. It is important to remove all soft tissue attachments to the metatarsal head as well as releasing the sesamoids to gain the most motion. A freer or McGlamry elevator may be sued to release the sesamoids. Next, a K-wire is placed centrally in the metatarsal head and inserted down the longitudinal axis, a drill guide that comes with the hardware is used to find the proper placement of the K-wire (Fig. 14.19). The over drill is then used to drill over the guidewire until the drill stop reaches the metatarsal head (see Fig. 14.19). A tap is then placed over the guide pin and used to tap the hole that was just drilled. Once the central metatarsal is properly tapped, the taper post is then inserted over the guidewire using a power drill until the taper post is flush with the metatarsal head. The guide pin is then removed, and the trial sizes for the implant are inserted. The trial device must be flush with the existing articular surface. Your hardware set should also come with a measuring device to measure the distance both dorsal to plantar and medial to lateral from the central aspect of the metatarsal head and then use these measurements in relation to a sizing chart to pick the proper implant size. Once proper implant size is determined, the metatarsal head is reamed of all cartilage down to subchondral bone and your reamer will be stopped by the taper post previously placed, ensuring the proper distance of reaming (see Fig. 14.19). Next, all unessential remaining cartilage can be removed from the metatarsal head with a rongeur, but be mindful not to interfere with the sesamoid apparatus plantarly.

The angled reamer for the dorsal aspect of the metatarsal head is used next (see Fig. 14.19). The guide pin of the reaming device is placed into the taper post within the metatarsal

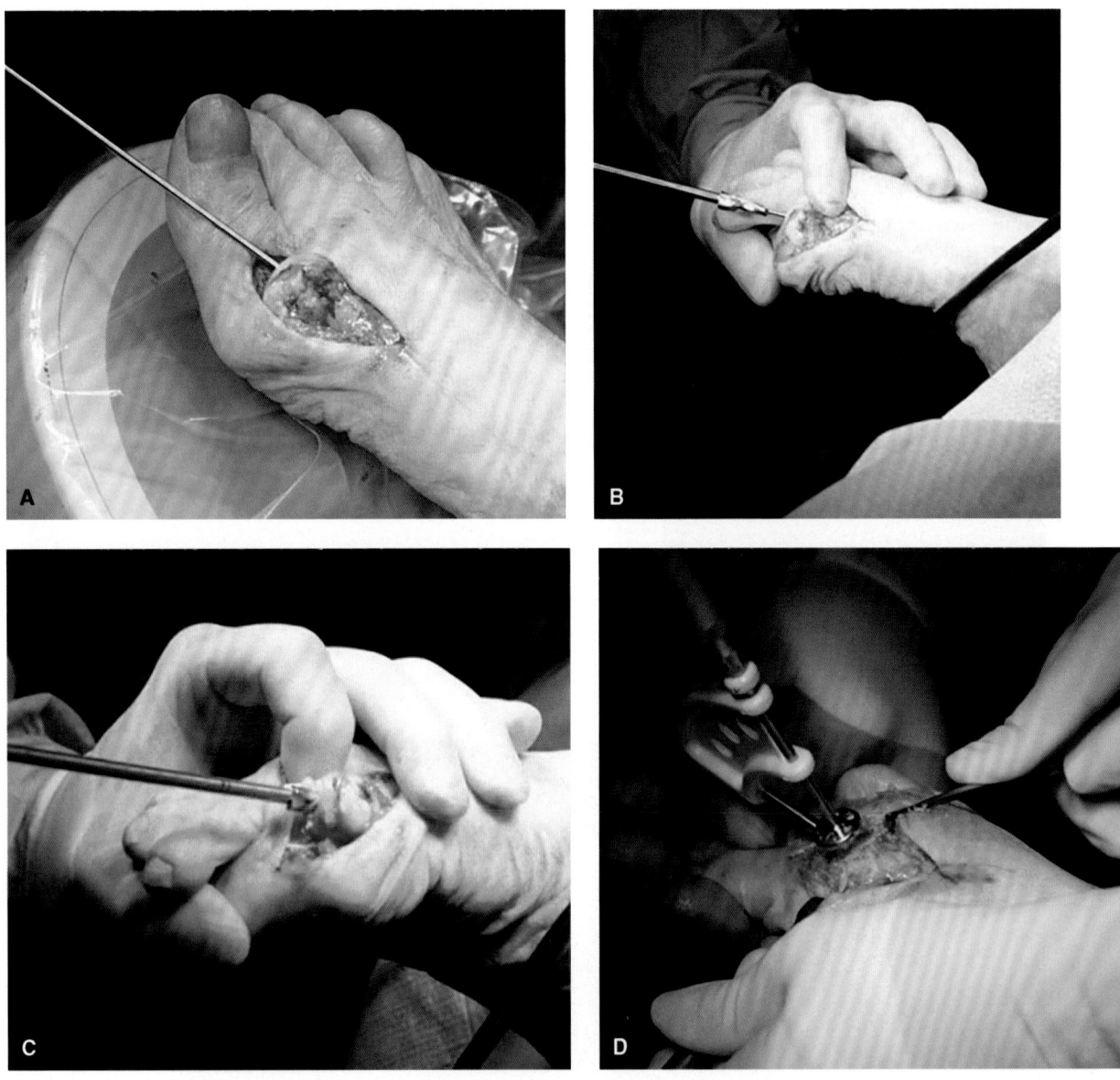

FIGURE 14.19 A. Initial guidewire placement into the first metatarsal. **B, C.** Initial reaming for taper post over the guidewire. **D.** Reaming guide to properly ream the dorsal aspect of the metatarsal head. (Courtesy of Brian Carpenter, DPM.)

head and the drill is then placed onto the reamer. The entire reaming apparatus should be in line in the sagittal plane with the cristae to ensure proper placement of the reamer, as it is not to be offset medial or lateral. Reaming is then carried out until the reamer bottoms out. Next, the trial sized implants are inserted to ensure proper sizing (Fig. 14.20). The hallux is ran through dorsiflexion with the trial implant in place to ensure adequate ROM. If dorsiflexion appears limited, further plantar soft tissue release may need to be performed. Once proper size is known, the implant is inserted into the taper post and compressed into placed with the tamp (see Fig. 14.20). Once in place, increased dorsiflexion at the first MPJ should be noted. Soft tissues are then closed. Final alignment may also be checked with intraoperative imaging as well (see Fig. 14.20).

PEARLS

- Aggressive soft tissue release of sesamoids if you want to regain motion
- Decompress joint as needed to regain metatarsal parabola with reaming to regain motion
- Smooth any plantar ridge from cristae to implant so sesamoids will articulate with implant at maximum dorsiflexion
- Resect dorsal lip/exostosis of proximal phalanx base
- Immediate ROM postoperatively and PT if patient not maintaining over 40 degrees of dorsiflexion at 2 weeks
- Immediate WB in surgical shoe and without shoe at home
- Normal shoe gear when skin is healed

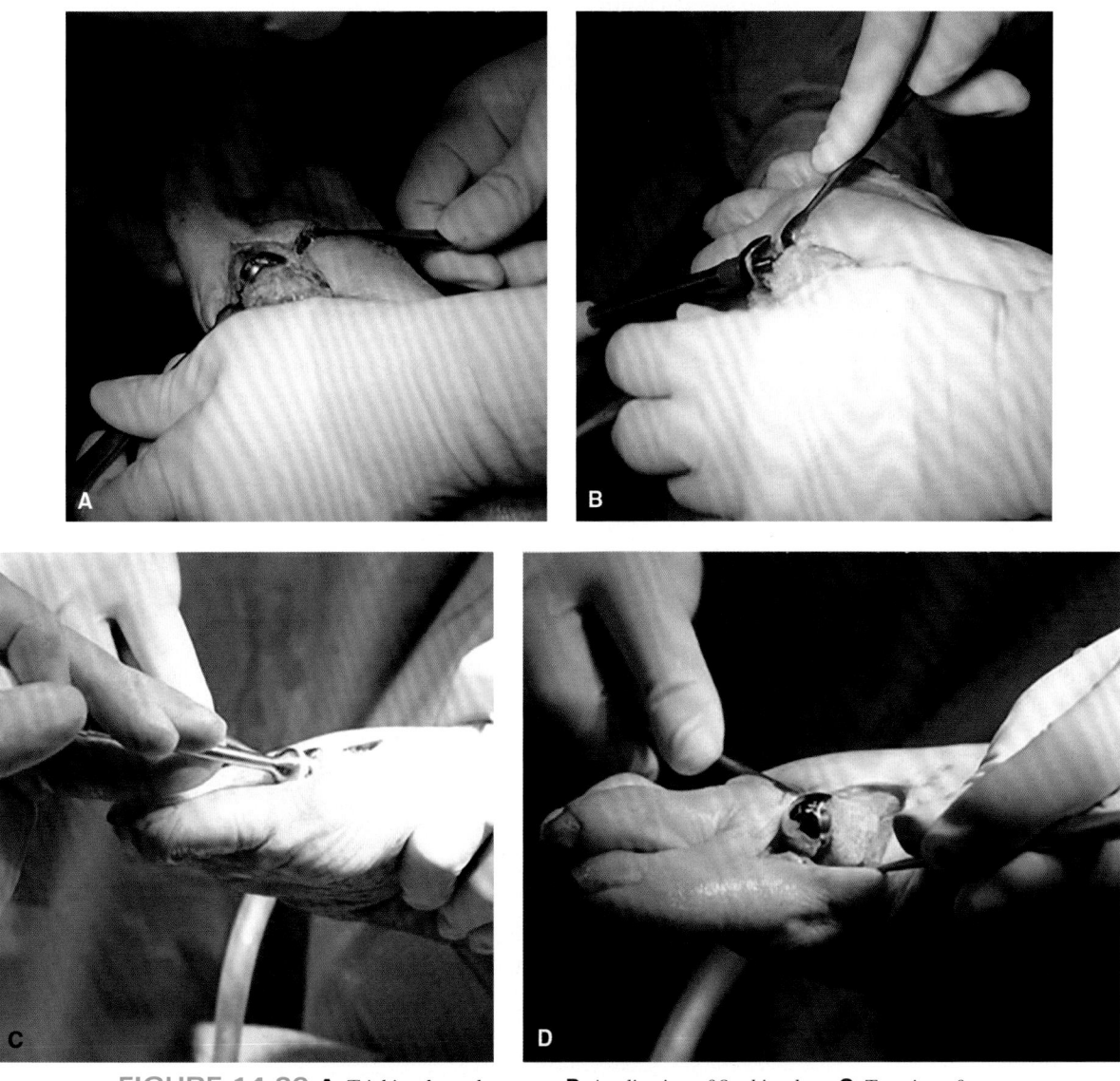

FIGURE 14.20 A. Trial implant placement. **B.** Application of final implant. **C.** Tamping of implant into the taper post. **D.** Implant securely in the first metatarsal head.

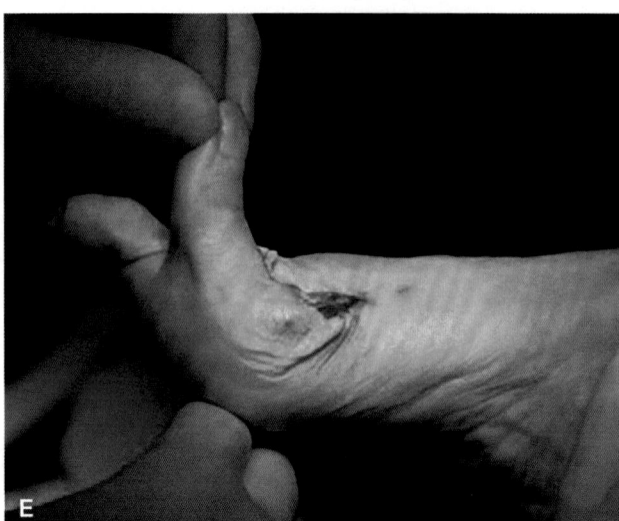
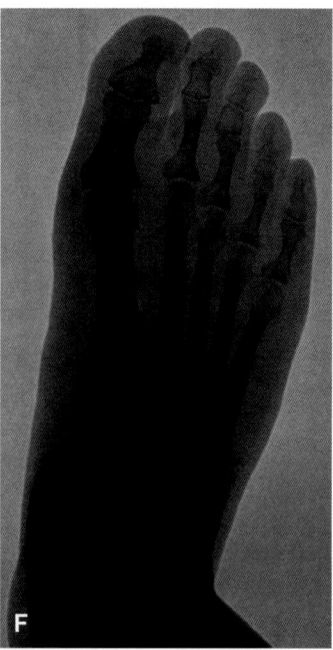

FIGURE 14.20 (*Continued*) **E.** Increased range of motion after implant placement and release of soft tissue adhesions. **F.** AP radiograph showing proper implant placement. (Courtesy of Brian Carpenter, DPM.)

Total Joint

Total joint implant arthroplasty is used for end-stage grade 3-4 hallux rigidus as a primary procedure and can even be used as a salvage procedure from previous implant failure. End-stage hallux rigidus has severe destruction of the articulating surface of the metatarsal head; therefore, a total joint implant and not a hemi-implant is indicated. The total joint implant is two components with the phalanx component being flatter and having the plastic spacer attached and the metatarsal component taking on a more rounded shape to best imitate an anatomic joint (Fig. 14.21).

Technique

The typical dorsal medial exposure is used to gain access to the first MPJ. The joint is then contoured to an anatomic structure by removing all osteophytes and exostosis off of the metatarsal head and proximal phalanx base. This can be done with bone rongeur, sagittal saw, or rotary burr. Once the normal joint anatomy can be appreciated, resection arthroplasty can be performed. The osteotomy cuts are guided by the particular guide provided with the implant hardware. The guide is inserted into the first MPJ with the concave side butting against the curved anatomy of the metatarsal head and the flattened portion of the guide aligns with the base of the proximal phalanx (Fig. 14.22). The arthroplasty cuts are then performed as directed by the guide using a sagittal saw. The cut on the proximal phalanx is perpendicular to the longitudinal axis of the proximal phalanx. The cut on the metatarsal head is typically angled dorsal proximal to distal plantar to preserve the plantar cortex and sesamoid articulation (see Fig. 14.22). The cuts are initiated with the guide in place for the first 50% of the cut and then the guide is removed to allow completion of the cuts. The osseous pieces are removed, and the bones are ready for medullary canal preparation and implant sizing.

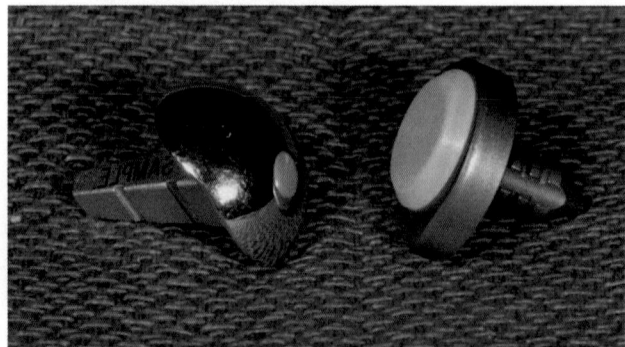

FIGURE 14.21 Two component total joint implants with the plastic spacer on the phalangeal implant. KGTI Kinetik Great Toe Implant.

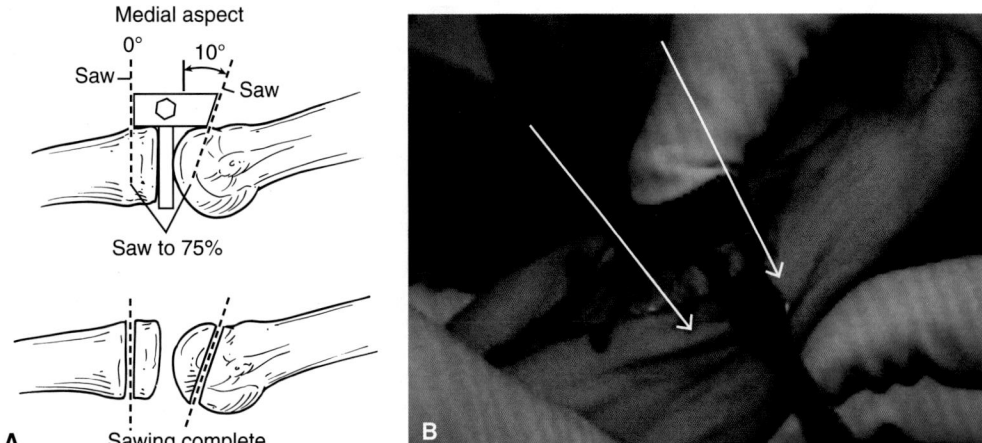

FIGURE 14.22 **A.** Illustration indicating proper placement of the cutting guide properly inserted into the first MPJ. Note the white arrows designate the proper path of the osteotomies to resect the first MPJ surfaces. **B.** Intraoperative photo of the cutting guide properly inserted into the first MPJ.

The implant sizer will come with the implant hardware set and typically includes the drilling guide as well. The implant sizer is placed flush onto the distal aspect of the metatarsal head (Fig. 14.23). It is important to ensure that the sizer/drill guide is properly aligned and not displaced in any of the three planes. Once proper placement is achieved, the sizer/drill guide is held in place with two K-wires. The metatarsal head is then reamed according to the implant's technique guide (see Fig. 14.23). After the canal has been reamed, the metatarsal canal is ready to be broached. Broaching the canal is important to mold the canal to accept the stem of the implant. The broach guide is attached to the metatarsal head with two K-wires in a similar fashion as the drill guide. The handled broach is then manually inserted, there will be a notch or laser line on the broach handle that will ensure proper orientation upon insertion (Fig. 14.24). There is also a stop on the broach handle, which will abut against the guide when the broach has been inserted the proper distance. Attention is then directed to the proximal phalanx, which has

its canals prepared in a similar fashion (Fig. 14.25). The proximal phalanx preparation may or may not include broaching depending on the technique of the implant guide, in that case the reamer will provide the proper canal preparation to accept the implant stem.

The trial implants for both the metatarsal and proximal phalanx are now inserted (Fig. 14.26). The correct implant size will abut flush against the bone and allow full ROM to the first MPJ without catching or clicking. If the joint is stiff and too tight, more bone may need to be resected followed by repeating the reaming and broaching steps. If the joint appears unstable, then possibly a larger size implant is indicated. Once the correct size has been decided, the implants are inserted into their respective bones and tamped into placed with gentle taps via a mallet until tight flush apposition of the implant on the bone surface is achieved (see Figs. 14.26 and 14.27). Proper placement and alignment is then verified with intraoperative radiographs (Fig. 14.28). At this time, the capsule can be sutured together, followed by skin closure.

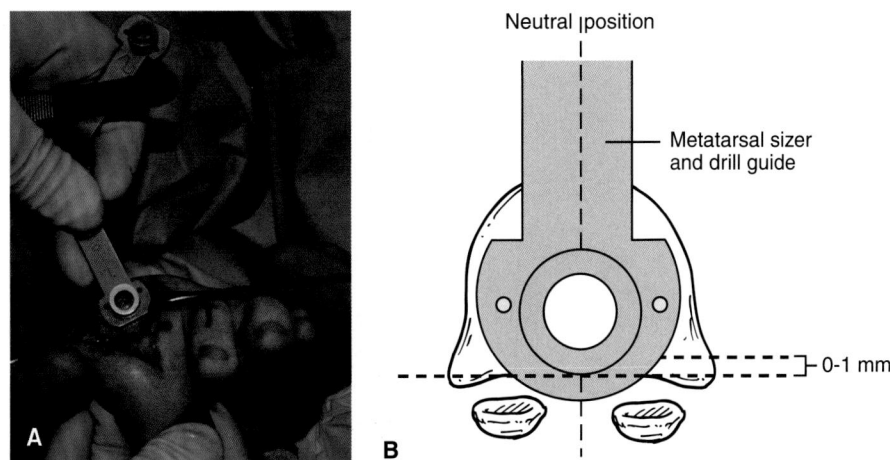

FIGURE 14.23 **A.** Placement of the sizer/drill guide onto the first metatarsal head. **B.** Illustrates the correct alignment of the sizer/drill guide onto the metatarsal head in neutral position.

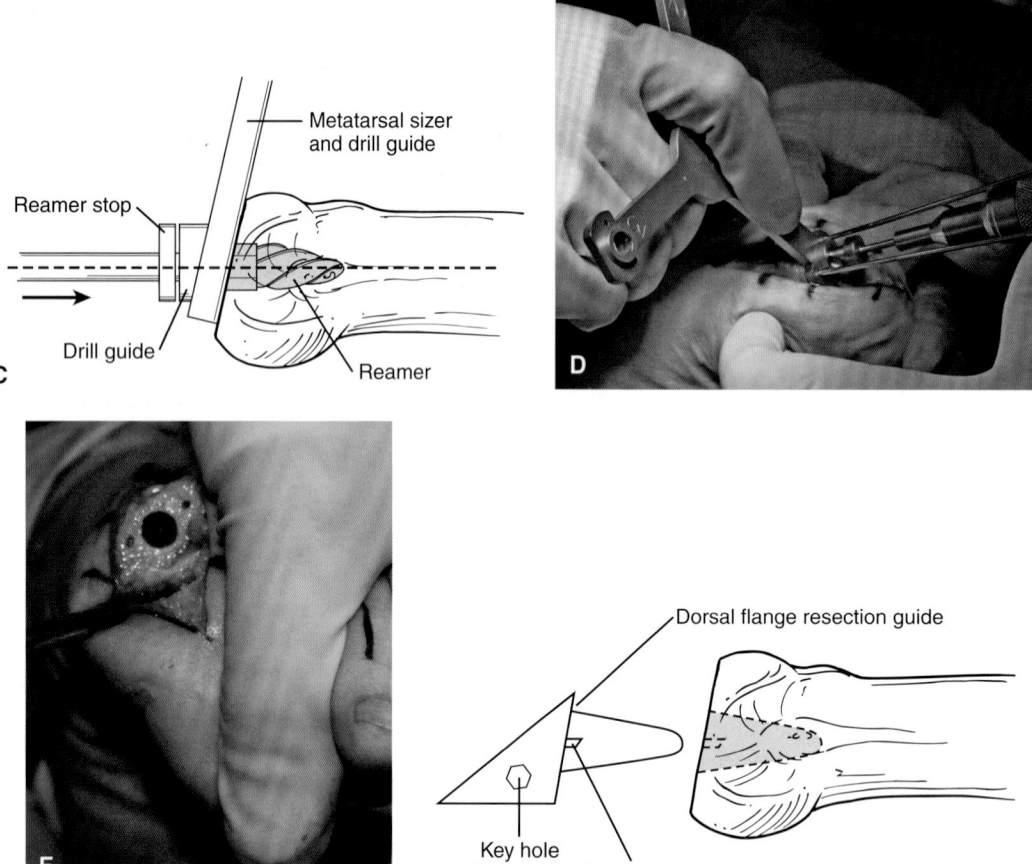

FIGURE 14.23 (*Continued*) **C.** Lateral view illustration showing the sizer/drill guide placement along with the reaming of the first metatarsal head centrally along the longitudinal axis. Note the reamer stop to indicate when the reamer has been inserted the proper distance. **D.** Intraoperative photo depicting the reaming process. **E.** Frontal view of the metatarsal head showing the central canal after being reamed along with the two K-wire holes, medial and lateral, used to hold the drill guide in place. **F.** Resection guide inserted into the metatarsal head to guide resection of dorsal osteophytes; this step may or may not be performed.

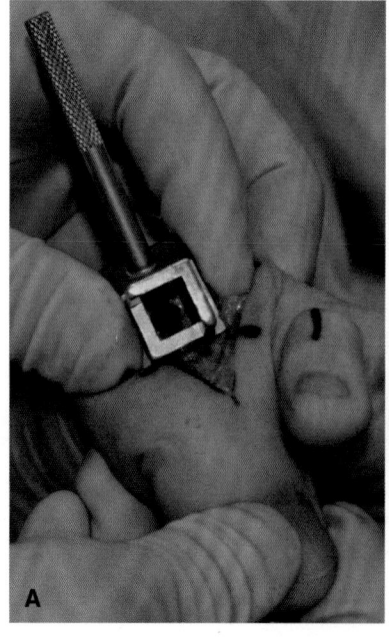

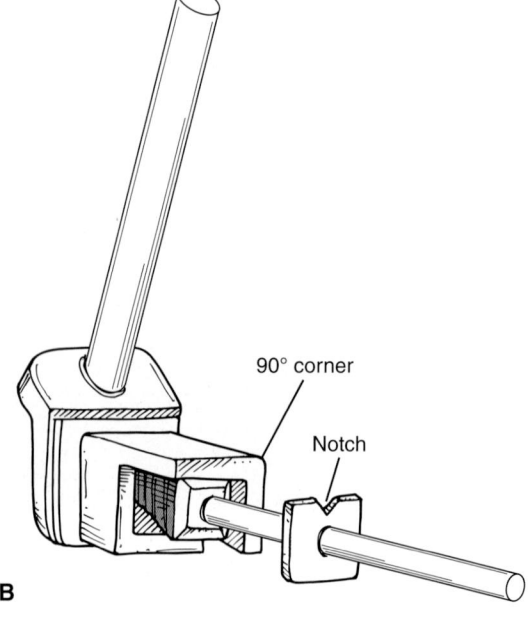

FIGURE 14.24 **A.** Placement of the broach guide onto the first metatarsal. **B.** Illustration depicting the insertion of the broach into the guide.

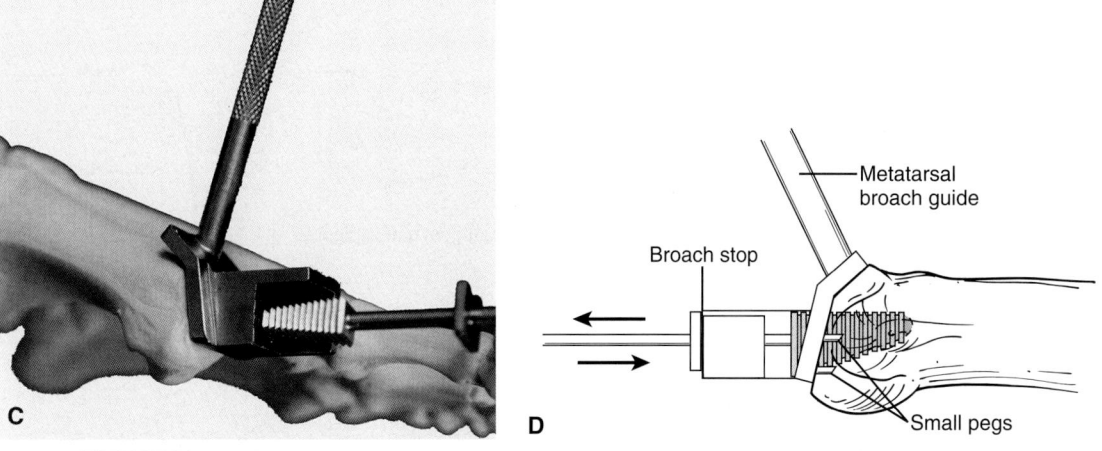

C

D — Metatarsal broach guide — Broach stop — Small pegs

FIGURE 14.24 (*Continued*) **C, D.** Showing proper insertion of the broach into the first metatarsal head.

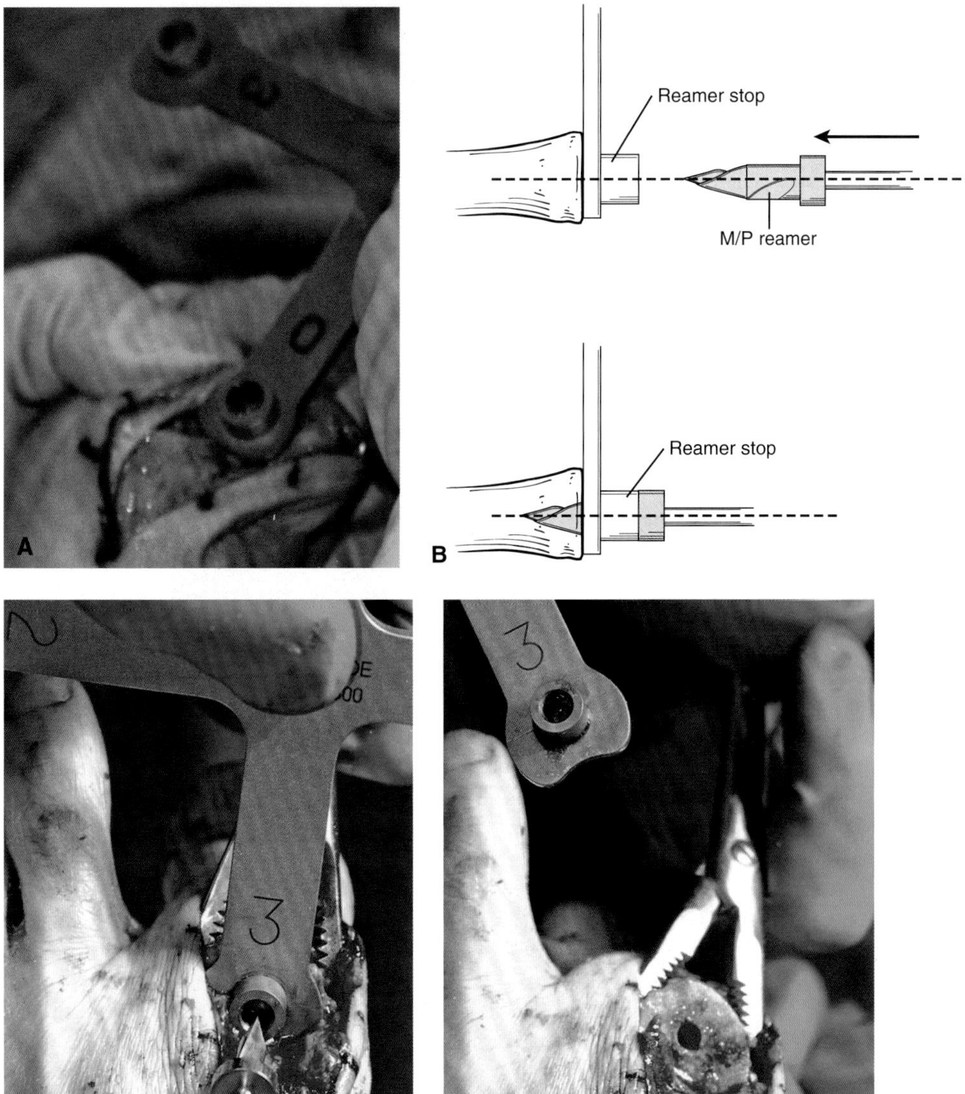

A

B — Reamer stop — M/P reamer — Reamer stop

C

D

FIGURE 14.25 A. Sizer now placed onto the base of the proximal phalanx. **B.** Illustration depicting proper reaming of the phalangeal canal. **C, D.** Reaming of the proximal phalanx.

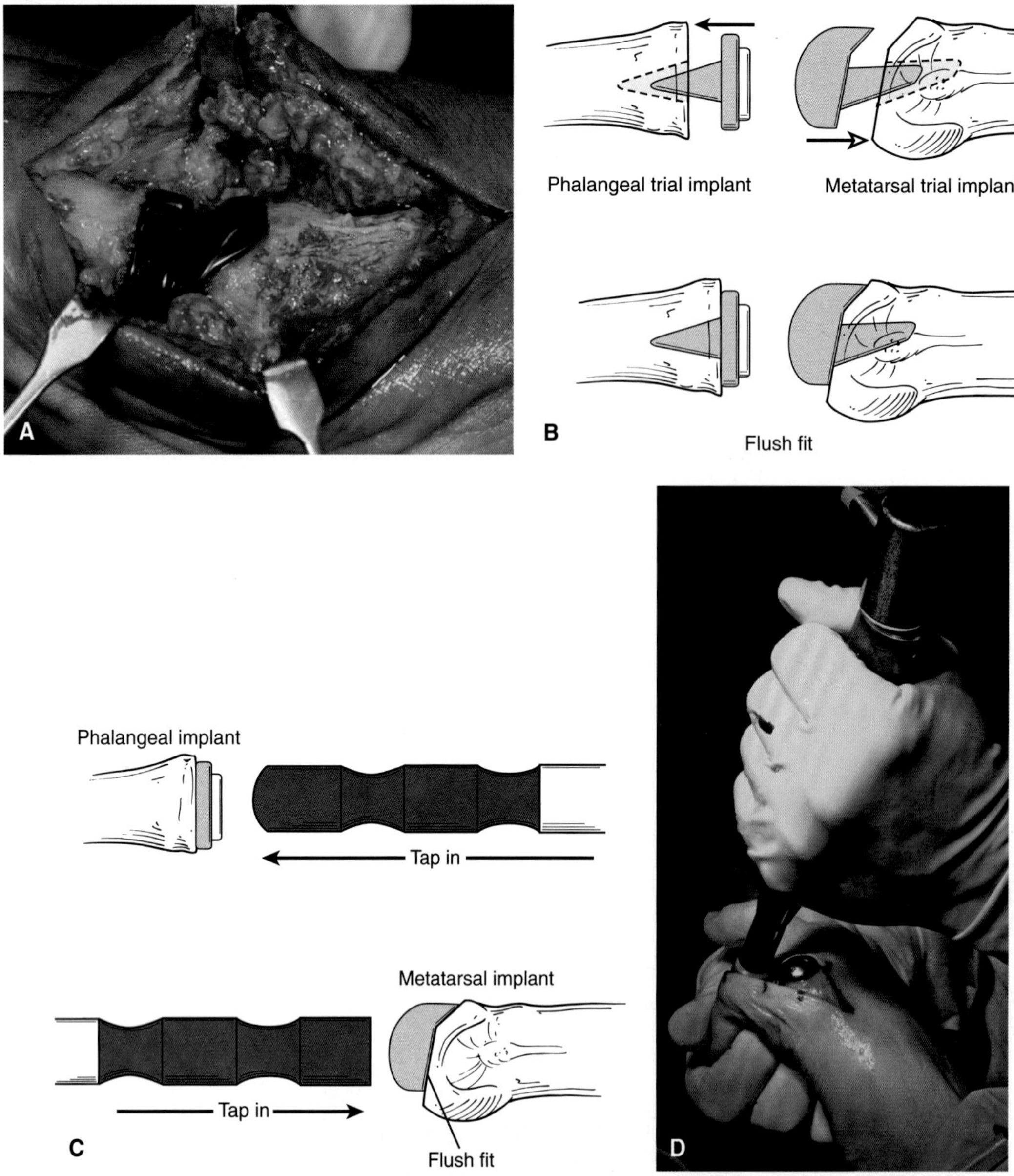

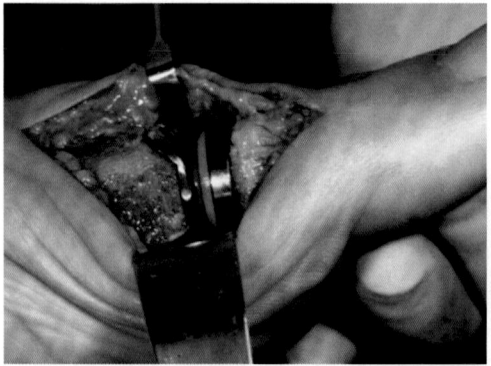

FIGURE 14.26 **A.** Trial implant inserted into the MPJ. **B.** Illustrating showing proper insertion and alignment of implants. **C.** Illustration depicting proper tapping and insertion of the implants with proper instruments. **D.** Intraoperative photo of tapping in the implant into the proximal phalanx.

FIGURE 14.27 Proper implantation of two component total joint implant with proper alignment.

Hinged

The typical hinged implant most commonly used is a silicone implant of the Swanson design (Fig. 14.29). After exposure to the first MPJ is obtained, resection of all osteophytes should be removed off of both the proximal phalanx base and metatarsal head to allow exposure and visualization of the joint. Next, variations of the Keller and Mayo arthroplasties are performed. The amount of resection depends on the exact implant used. It is important that enough bone is removed to allow proper ROM of the first MPJ after implant is placed. The proximal phalanx arthroplasty is typically performed first (Fig. 14.30). The amount of proximal phalanx resection again depends on the size of the implant and any technique guide specific to the implant, but typically, ¼ to ⅓ of the proximal phalanx base is resected. The osteotomy is made transverse

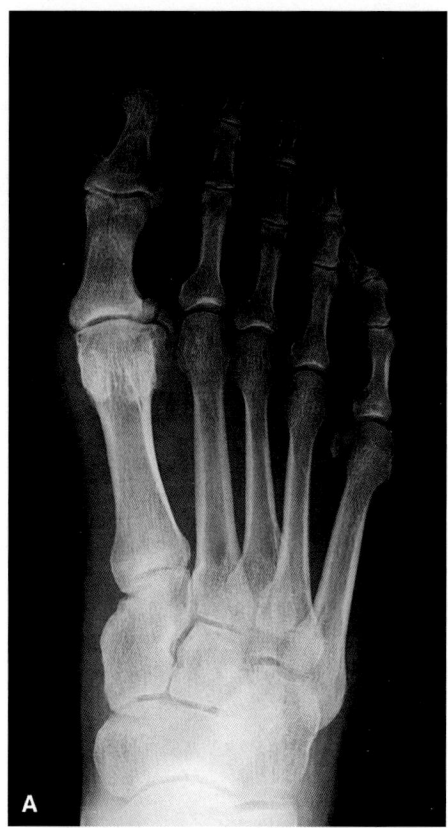

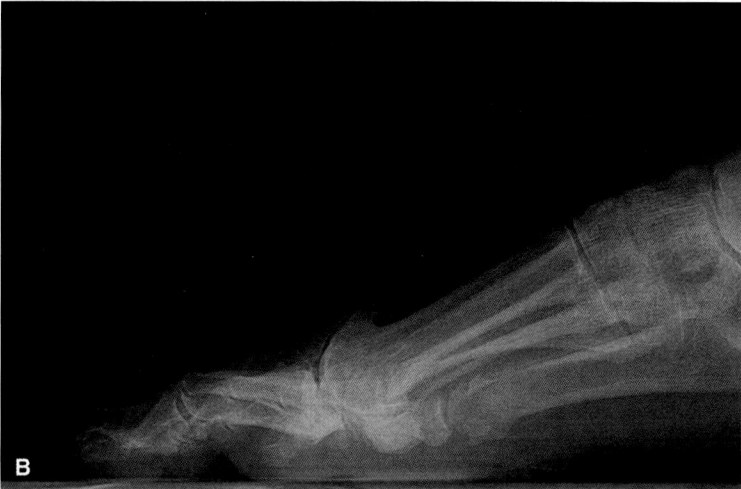

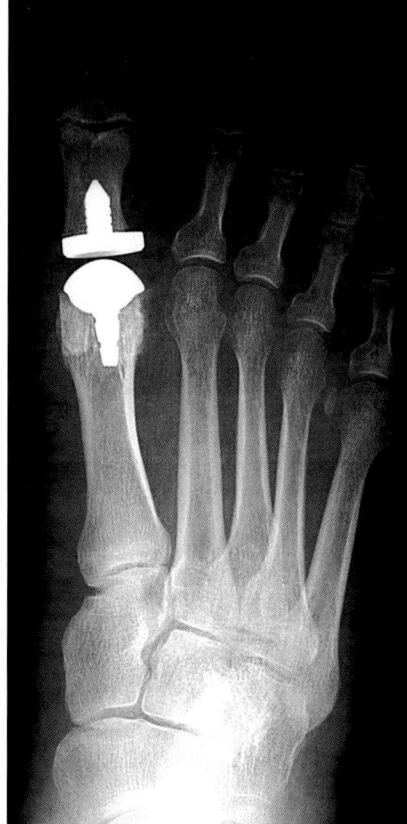

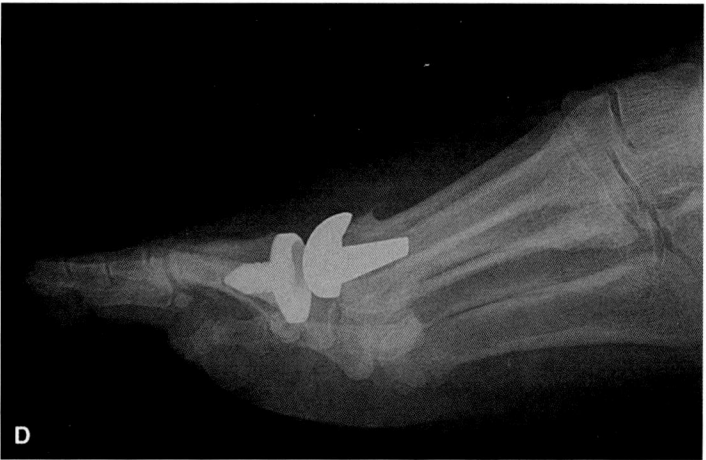

FIGURE 14.28 **A.** AP radiograph of grade 3 hallux limitus preoperatively. **B.** Lateral radiograph of grade 3 hallux limitus preoperatively. **C.** AP radiograph depicting two component total joint implant properly inserted. **D.** Lateral radiograph showing rectus alignment of the first MPJ after total joint implantation.

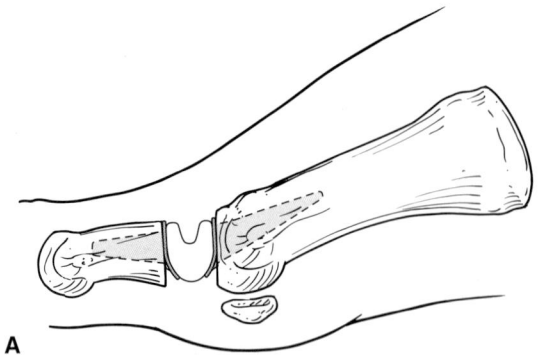

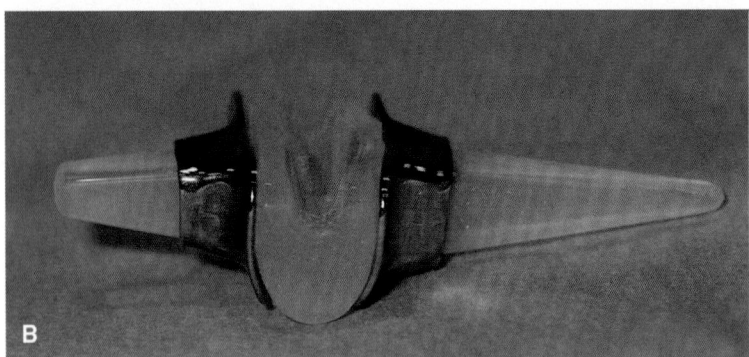

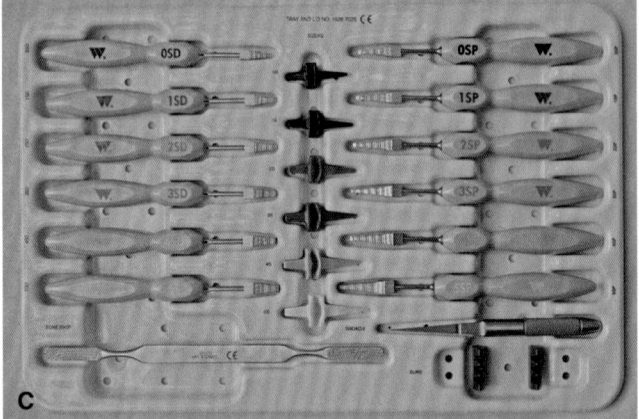

FIGURE 14.29 A. Illustration showing hinged silicone implant placement into the first MPJ. **B.** Swanson silicone hinged implant with grommet placement (Wright Medical, Arlington, TN). Note the longer tapered end for the metatarsal and the stubbier rectangular end for the proximal phalanx. **C.** Broaches and sizing set for hinged implant.

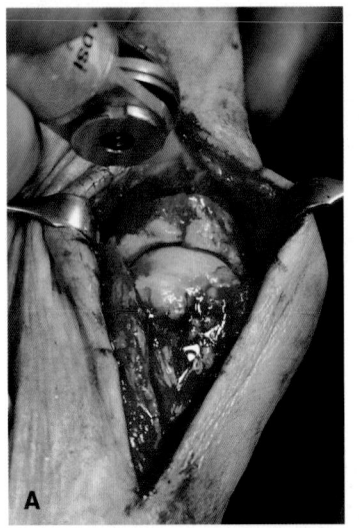

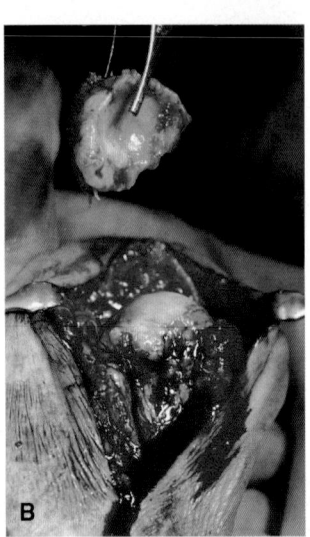

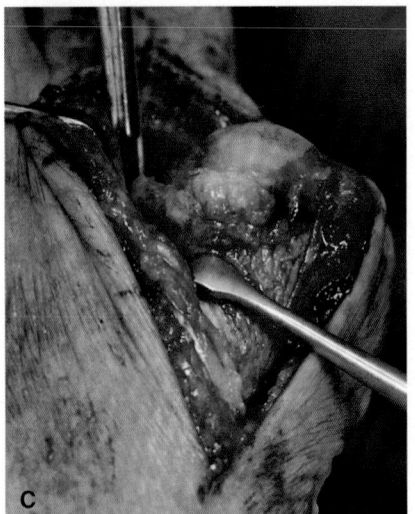

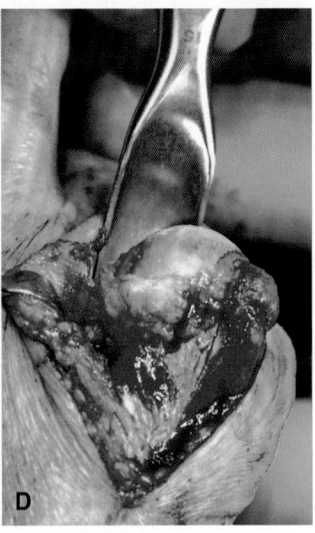

FIGURE 14.30 A, B. Resection of the proximal phalanx base via use of a sagittal saw cutting perpendicular to the long axis of the phalanx. **C, D.** Removal of all soft tissue attachment's to the metatarsal head.

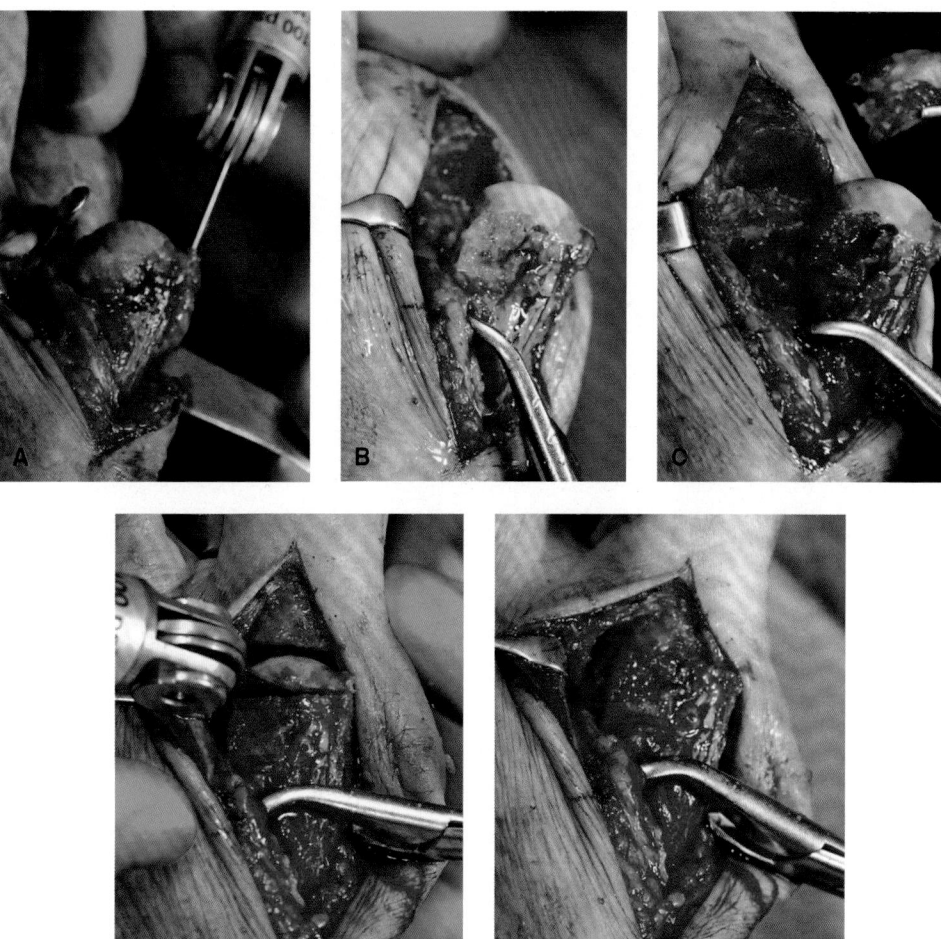

FIGURE 14.31 A-C. Removal of osteophytes and medial eminence off of the metatarsal head. **D, E.** Resection of the articulating cartilage off of the metatarsal head perpendicular to the long axis of the metatarsal.

and perpendicular to the long axis of the proximal phalanx. Resection of the first metatarsal head is performed next. Prior to resection, any adhesions to the plantar metatarsal head may need to be released (Fig. 14.31). Resection on the first metatarsal is limited to the distal metatarsal articular surface only, as to limit the effect on the weight-bearing surface of the metatarsal and not disrupt the biomechanics of the first metatarsal/sesamoid apparatus (see Fig. 14.31). Resection of the metatarsal articular surface is a transverse cut and is made perpendicular to weight-bearing surface. This cut alignment leaves the plantar cortex and cristae intact to again aid in preservation of the sesamoid articulation. Once removal of bone is accomplished, a trial implant may be placed alongside the joint space to gain rough estimate if enough bone has been resected.

The medullary canals of both the proximal phalanx and the metatarsal must be prepared next, typically starting with the metatarsal. Although resection arthroplasties have been performed, if access to the canals is not readily available, a straight hemostat or rotary burr may be used to gain access to the canals (Fig. 14.32). Beginning with the metatarsal, broaches are used to ream the canals in preparation for the implant stem. The broaches are specific to the implant used, and reaming technique depends on the particular implant technique

guide, but typically, the smallest broach is used first working up to larger sizes that fill the medullary canal. Final broach size is determined by the implant size expected to be used. The proximal phalanx medullary canal is prepared in a similar fashion (Fig. 14.33).

Trial implants are now inserted into the first MPJ with each stem going into its respected canal (see Fig. 14.33). Proper fit will allow from abutment of the hinge with the bone of both the metatarsal and phalanx. It is important to ensure that the hallux is sitting in neutral position without deviation in the transverse, sagittal, or frontal planes. Finally, the correct size will allow for controlled full ROM without impingement, laxity, or resistance. If the MPJ feels stiff to movement and sits in an incorrect position, additional bone resection or decrease in implant size may be needed. If the implant is loose within the joint, a larger size is often indicated. Once the proper implant size is determined, grommets are to be placed. Each size of implant will have a corresponding grommet pair to be inserted in the phalanx and metatarsal medullary canals. The grommets are titanium implants used to provide an interface between the silicone implant and bone. Importance of these grommets are to avoid osseous overgrowth, which could potentially cause damage to the silicone implant over time. The grommets are placed into the canals prior to implant placement (Fig. 14.34).

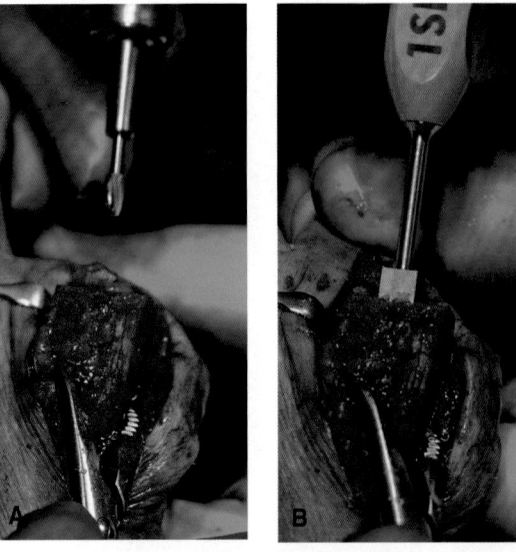
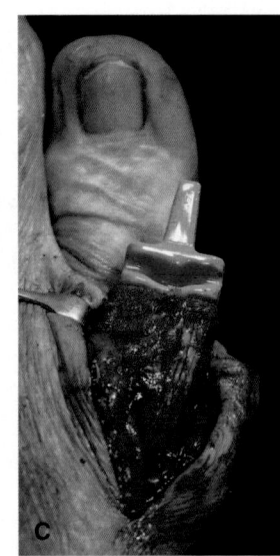
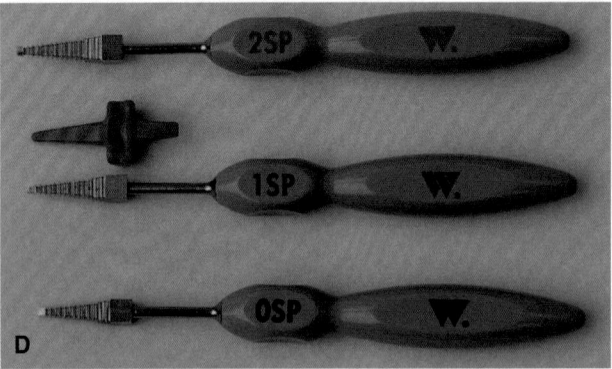

FIGURE 14.32 **A.** Rotary bur being used to gain access to medullary canal. **B.** Insertion of the broach. **C.** Trial hinged implant fitting flush into the first metatarsal. **D.** Photo of the different broach sizes along with trial implant. Note they are color coordinated.

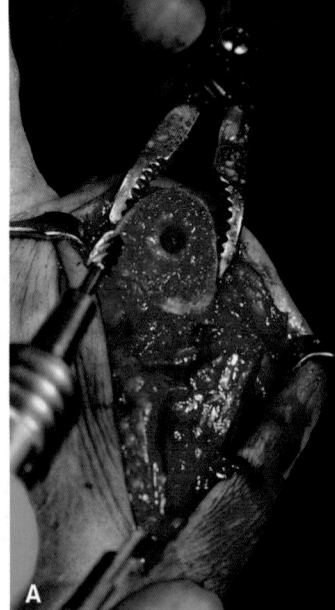
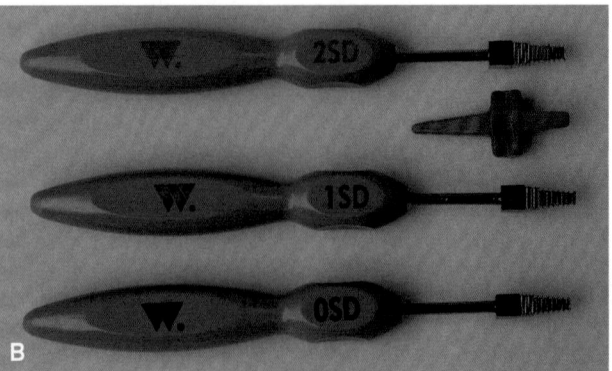

FIGURE 14.33 **A.** Rotary bur being used to gain access to proximal phalanx medullary canal. **B.** The proximal phalanx broaches and trial implant, also color coordinated.

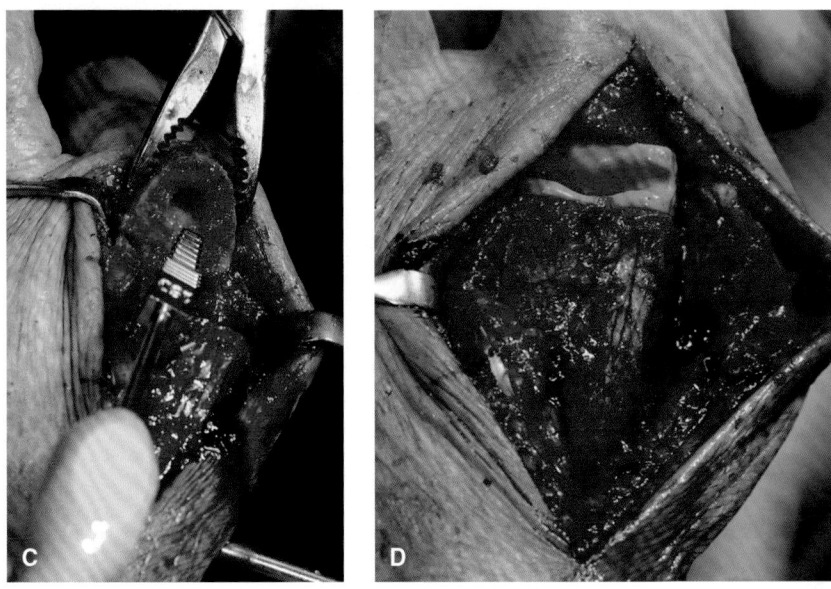

FIGURE 14.33 (*Continued*) **C.** Broach insertion into the phalanx. **D.** Trial implant properly seated into the first MPJ.

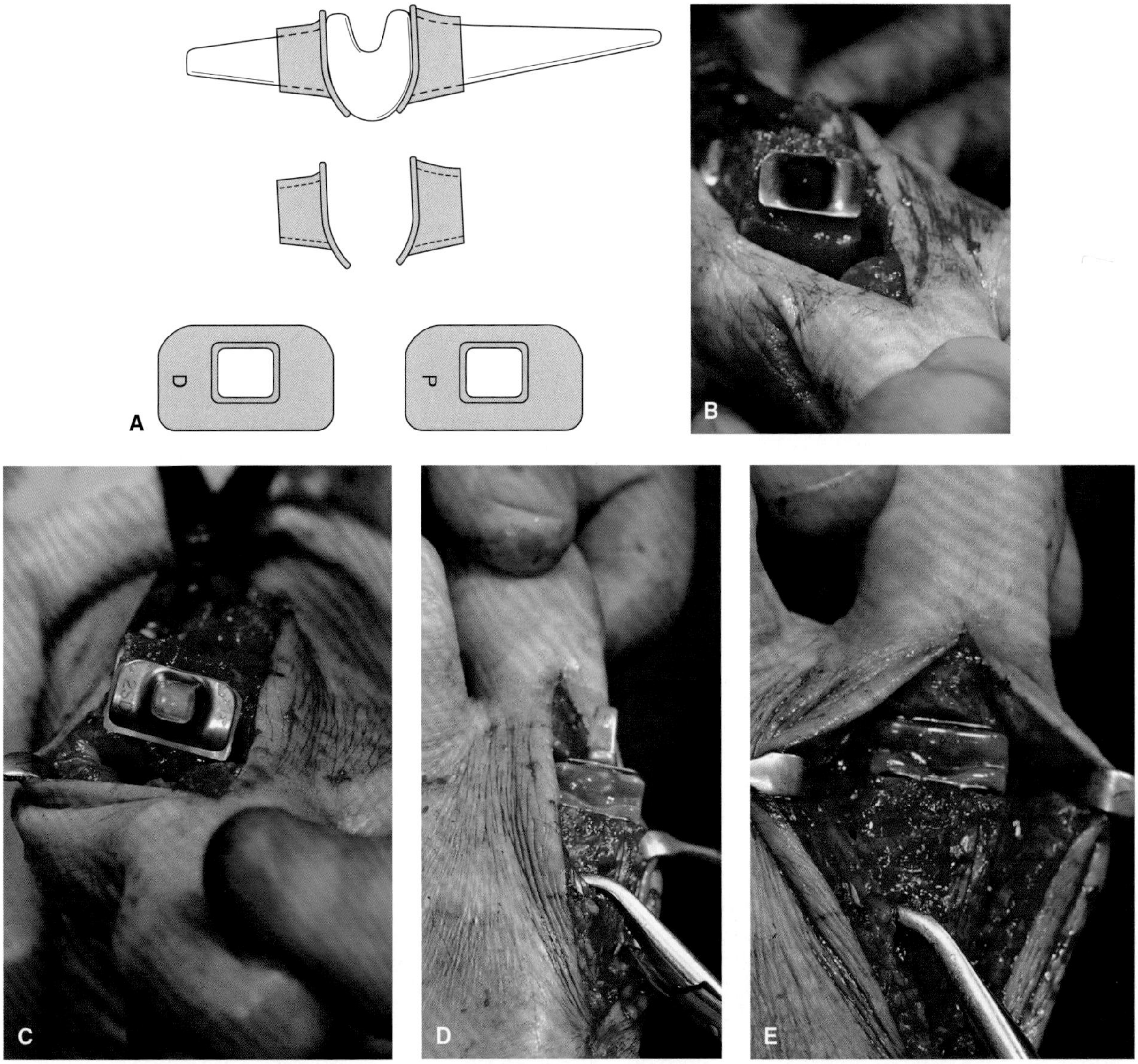

FIGURE 14.34 A. Illustration depicting how the grommets fit onto the implant and how they are specifically contoured to the hinge of the implant. **B.** Grommet insertion into the metatarsal canal. **C, D.** Grommet placement onto the phalanx stem of the implant. **E.** Silicone hinged implant with grommets inserted into the first MPJ.

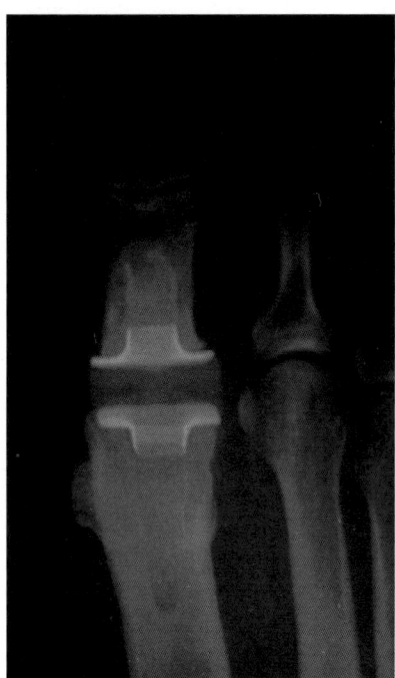

FIGURE 14.35 AP radiograph showing proper placement of hinged silicone implant with grommets into the first MPJ.

The implant is opened once proper size is determined, and a no-hands technique is used for insertion, typically with forceps. The stem into the metatarsal is inserted first followed by insertion into the phalanx. Attempts should be made to ensure that the implants does not touch any other structures or soft tissue that could cause contamination to the implant. Distraction along with plantar flexion of the hallux will aid in insertion of the stem into the proximal phalanx. After insertion, it is important to reassess both the static resting position of the hallux and the full ROM of the hallux. Proper alignment is also then checked under fluoroscopy to ensure proper placement of grommets and implant (Fig. 14.35). Capsular repair is then ensued followed by skin closure.

First Metatarsal Phalangeal Joint Arthrodesis

First MPJ arthrodesis is covered in other sections of this text, but we will also mention it here, as it is a common procedure performed for end stage hallux limitus. First MPJ arthrodesis is indicated in patients with severe arthritic changes and narrowed joint space and can also be used as a salvage option for previously failed hallux limitus surgeries. Many times, these joints will have already begun to auto-fuse or have virtually no motion, but there is concurrent pain. Patients initially will be hesitant to fuse their great toe joint, but studies have shown that with first MPJ fusion, patients return to activity with satisfactory results and great pain relief.[60,61] This procedure is indicated in grade 3-4 hallux limitus.

Technique

The first MPJ is exposed in the usual manner described. Again, it is important to remove all spurring off of the metatarsal head and base of the proximal phalanx. Next, the cartilage is inspected and resection of the cartilage off of the metatarsal head and base of the proximal phalanx is ensued. There are multiple ways in which the cartilage can be resected, but keep in mind, in most cases, it is important to shorten the first ray as little as possible during this procedure to not introduce iatrogenic problems such as transfer lesions. The three main options for removal of cartilage down to subchondral bone are with hand instruments (ie, curettes, rongeur, osteotome), cup and cone drilling method, and planar cuts with a saw. Planar cuts using a sagittal saw are also an option for prepping the joint surfaces but do have the potential to cause the most shortening of the first ray. It is important that these transverse cuts are perpendicular to the long axis of the metatarsal and proximal phalanx and to resect only the cartilage (Fig. 14.36). The cup and cone method of joint preparation involves placing a K-wire longitudinally down the central axis of the metatarsal head. The cup-shaped reamer is then placed onto the K-wire and down to the metatarsal head. These reamers can be ran by hand or the power drill. Similar steps are used on the base of the proximal phalanx where a K-wire is placed longitudinally down the center of the metatarsal starting at the base, and this

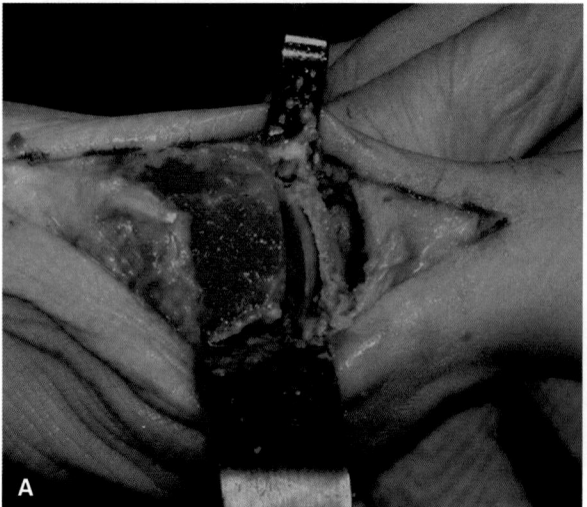 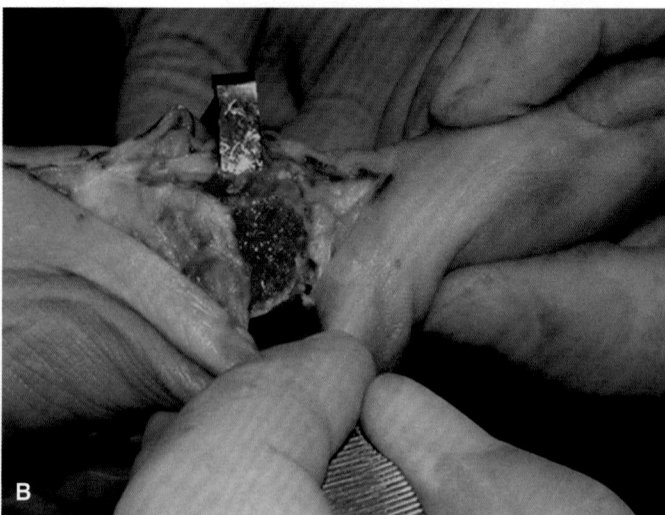

FIGURE 14.36 A. First MPJ after removal of all osteophytes and plantar resection of the articulating cartilage. **B.** Bone-to-bone apposition of the arthrodesis site of the first MPJ.

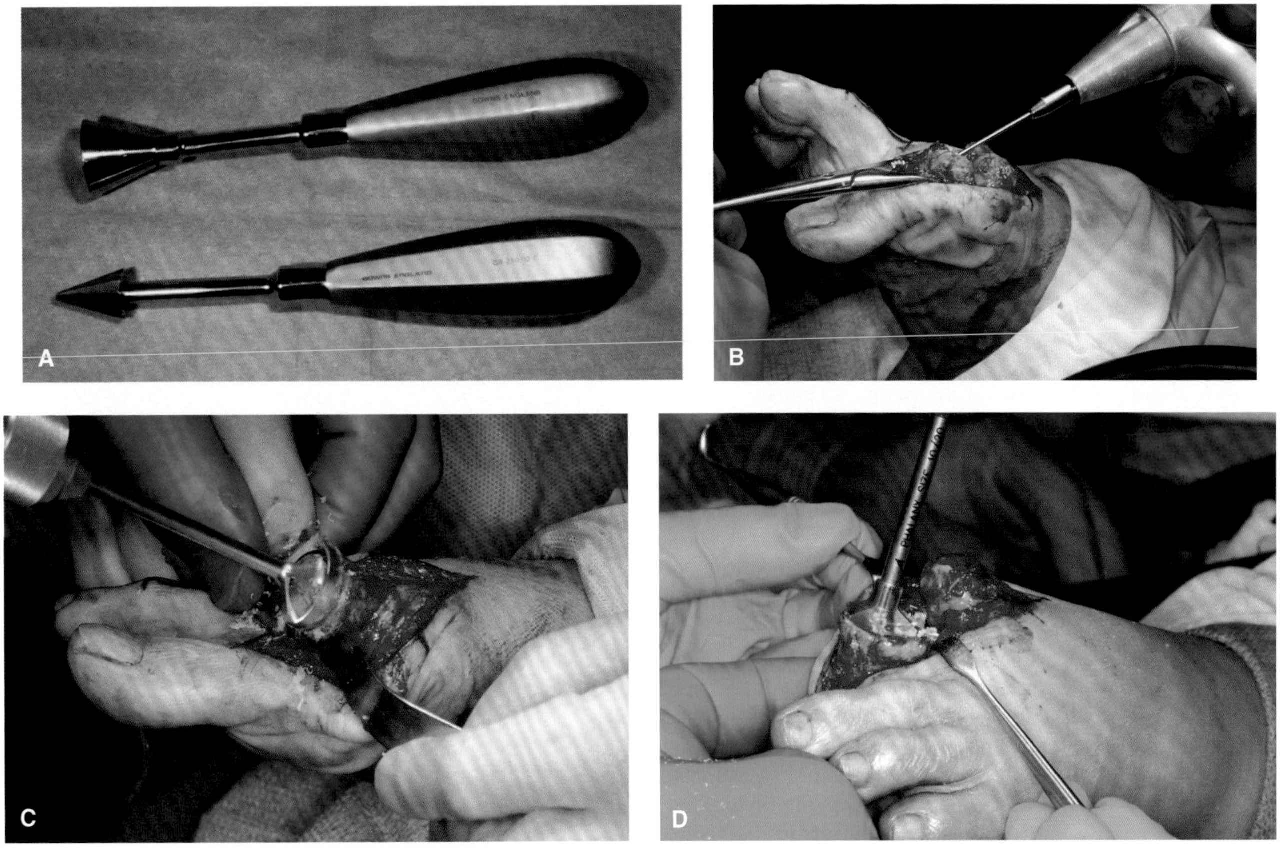

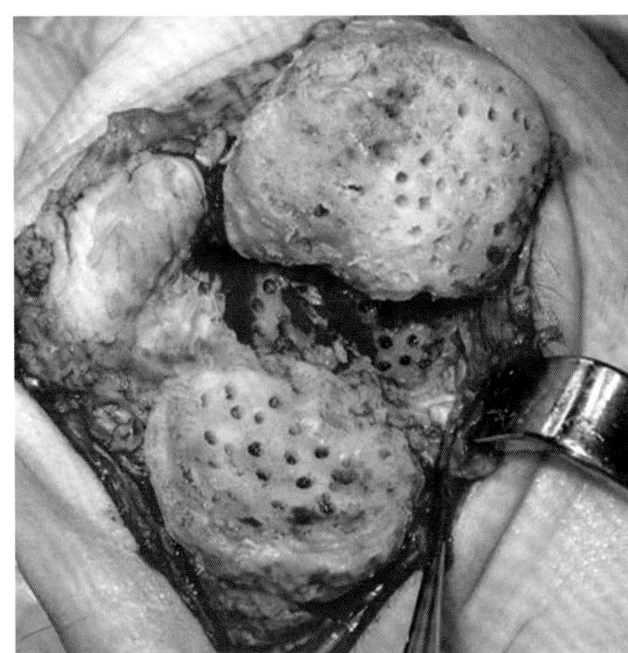

FIGURE 14.37 **A.** The cup and cone handheld reamer instruments. **B.** Placement of guide-wire down central long axis of proximal phalanx. **C.** Cup reamer under drill power to resect cartilage off of the metatarsal head. **D.** Cone power reaming of the proximal phalanx base. (Courtesy Dr. John Vanore.)

time, the cone reamer is placed over the K-wire. The cup and cone method is thought to maintain the natural alignment of the metatarsal head and proximal phalanx base to allow proper alignment with arthrodesis in all planes[62] (Fig. 14.37). The purpose of reaming is to remove all articular cartilage and get down to subchondral bone where bleeding bone or the "paprika" sign is noted. Once the joints have been prepped, subchondral drilling of the joint surfaces are often indicated. Using a 1.5- or 2.0-mm drill, multiple holes are drill ~2 mm in depth into the joint surfaces to penetrate the subchondral plate and facilitate osseous bridging during healing (Fig. 14.38). Fish scaling is another method to break the subchondral plate; although this is typically reserved for larger joint surfaces, it can be employed on the first MPJ joint surface. Using a small osteotome, the subchondral bone is penetrated at a slight angle multiple times serving to accomplish the same goal as the subchondral drilling. Some surgeons even advocate the preparation of the sesamoids for fusion to the overlying metatarsal head. Destruction of the first MPJ leaves the sesamoid apparatus of little functional benefit, but the sesamoids themselves can help fuse the joint. Preparation is typically used with curettes and subchondral drilling (see Fig. 14.38). Once the joint surfaces are prepared, the hallux (proximal phalanx) is impacted onto the metatarsal head to ensure good boney apposition of the joint surfaces. Once good apposition is achieved, osteogenic biomaterial, whether auto- or allograft, can be placed within the joint prior to fixation.

FIGURE 14.38 Completely prepped first MPJ with subchondral drilling of the metatarsal, proximal phalanx, and sesamoid bones. (Courtesy Dr. Craig Camasta.)

If performing an arthrodesis as a salvage procedure, a structural bone graft may be indicated. The authors believe that the use of osteogenic material facilitates arthrodesis and osseous bridging. One of the most common complications seen in first MPJ arthrodesis is mal- or nonunions. Roukis et al. has shown that nonunions can occur in up to 5.4% of procedures with malunion occurring at a rate of 6.1% for first MPJ arthrodesis due to any etiology.[63]

Temporary fixation with the use of K-wire can be used to ensure proper position of the hallux before permanent fixation. The hallux should be in a 10-degree dorsiflexed position, but the best way to determine proper position is to load the foot using a flat plate (Fig. 14.39). When the foot is loaded, the hallux should lightly rest on the plate, not dorsiflexed or plantar flexed, indicating proper position. An addition to this technique has been developed by the author using a single 4 × 4 in gauze. The gauze is folded in half and placed into the first interspace, which will allow the hallux to sit in proper placement in relation to the transverse plane. The gauze is then folded under the hallux and rests between the hallux and the foot plate, positioning the hallux in the proper placement in regard to the sagittal plane (Fig. 14.40).[64] Frontal plane alignment is achieved by ensuring that the hallux nail is positioned in the same plane as digits 2-5. Temporary fixation may then be achieved using a single K-wire inserted into the distal hallux and crossing the first MPJ. Fixation of the arthrodesis site can be achieved in multiple ways consisting of plates, screws, staples, or a combination of these methods. Crossing or parallel screws supply good compression across the arthrodesis site, which is of most importance (Fig. 14.41). Both techniques have reported low nonunion rate of 4.6% for crossing screws and no nonunions for parallel screws in some studies.[63] The use of a screw to provide compression along with dorsal plate is often used to supply both compression and structural support. In the setting of bone graft, structural or osteogenic, a dorsal plate is typically used to keep the graft in place. Nonunion using this technique has been reported to be as low as 5.1%.[63] Staple fixation has gained popularity over the years and is now employed for first MPJ arthrodesis. One or two staples may be used to achieve proper compression across the MPJ. If two staples are used, one is typically placed dorsally and one medially to add stability in multiple planes. The nonunion rates with staples are reported to be 5.1%, which is similar to plate fixation. Intramedullary nailing in conjunction with a dorsal staple has also been described as a solid fixation technique with no reported nonunions.[65] Rarely is a capsulotomy needed to correct in frontal or transverse planes as performed in hallux valgus surgery, but any redundant capsule can be excised prior to closure.

> ## PEARLS
> - Glissan principles of arthrodesis must be adhered to.
> - Hand instrumentation prep is preferred by authors than using a burr to properly sculp the metatarsal head and proximal phalanx base.
> - Fixation is best with an oblique threaded head screw with a dorsal locking plate designed for the MPJ.
> - Although there are specific degree guidelines for hallux placement, the hallux should be placed in most functional position for patient's foot structure and neutral in all three planes.
> - Small voids at arthrodesis site can be filled with allograft, but the authors find that filling larger grafts with autograft tends to work better.

AUTHORS' PREFERRED TREATMENT

The authors prefer to explore joint-sparing options when a patient presents with hallux limitus who has failed conservative treatments. It is important to realize that many factors come into play when discussing surgical treatment such as the grade of hallux limitus, patient's lifestyle, and patient's goals. Nonetheless, the authors' preferred treatment for these cases (stage 1-2) is a cheilectomy with a dorsiflexory phalangeal osteotomy

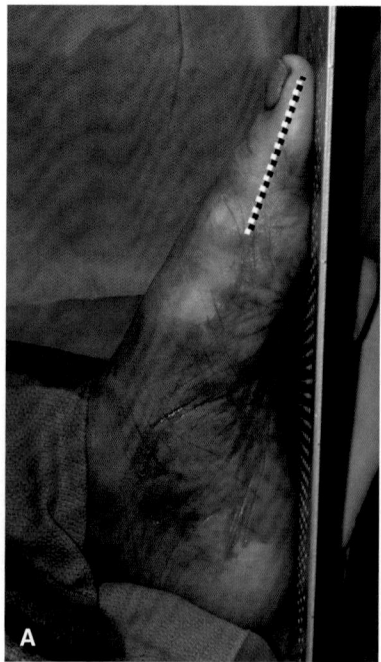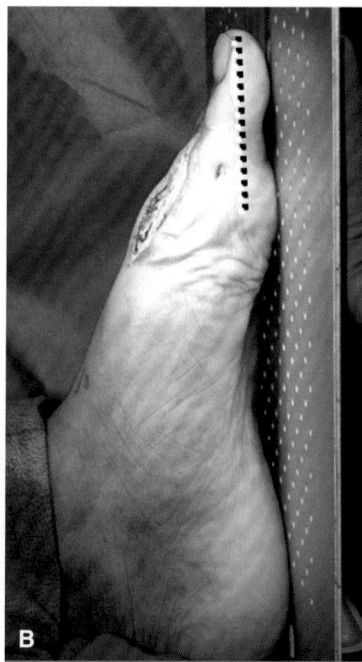

FIGURE 14.39 A. Plantar flexed hallux placing too much pressure with foot loaded by metal plate. **B.** Slightly dorsiflexed hallux position resting in neutral position upon loading of the foot.

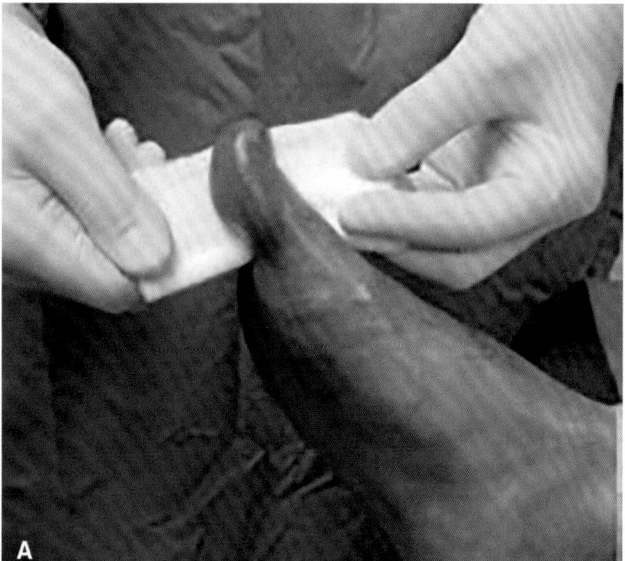

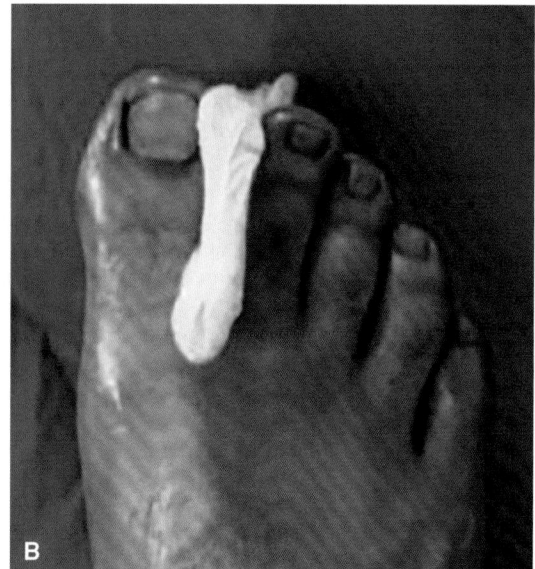

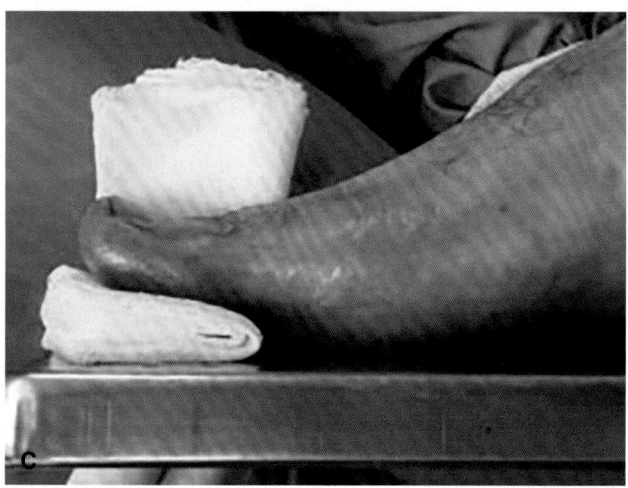

FIGURE 14.40 A. A lateral photograph of a 4 × 4 in gauze folded in half and placed in the first interspace. **B.** A dorsal to plantar photograph of the foot with the gauze in the first interspace showing proper position of the hallux in the frontal and transverse planes. **C.** Lateral photograph showing the foot resting on the flatfoot plate with the 4 × 4 gauze folded under the hallux to potion the hallux in the proper amount of dorsiflexion. (Courtesy of Thomas Roukis, DPM, PhD.)

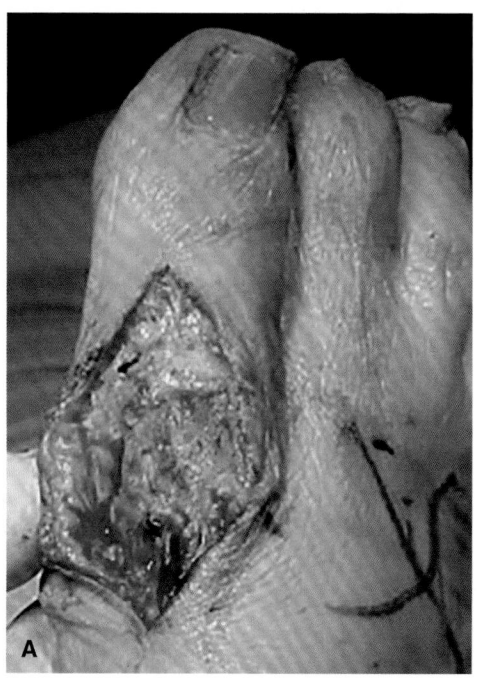

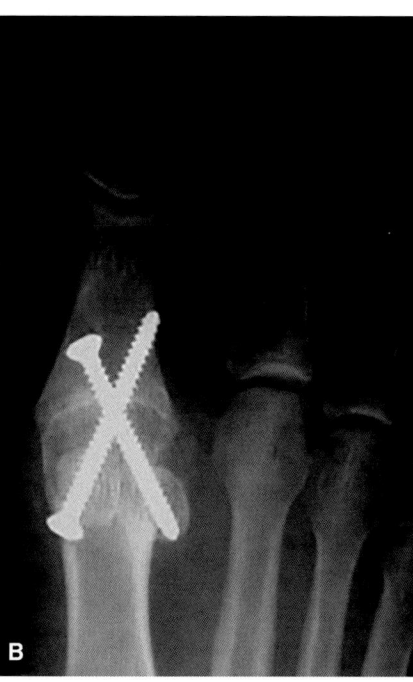

FIGURE 14.41 A. Intraoperative image of a first MPJ arthrodesis fixated with crossing screws. **B.** An AP radiograph of the first MPJ arthrodesis using the crossing screw construct. (Courtesy of Thomas Roukis, DPM, PhD.)

(ie, Moberg osteotomy). These procedures are performed per the techniques listed previously in this text. Multiple reasons exist as to why this is a preferred and often first-line surgical management for the authors. First, this procedure is a joint-sparring procedure and allows for further joint destructive procedures to be performed down the road if need be. The cheilectomy Moberg procedure overall is not technically challenging but does have good postoperative results. A systematic review performed in 2010 looked at 11 studies encompassing 374 procedures. Pain was noted to be improved in 89% of the patients at >12-month follow-up. Only 4.8% of the patient necessitated a revision surgery due to continued symptoms.[44] The removal of the dorsal metatarsal head with the cheilectomy allows greater dorsiflexion at the first MPJ. It is the author's opinion that the cheilectomy coupled with the dorsiflexory Moberg osteotomy allows the largest increase in dorsiflexion of the hallux without damaging the joint. The Moberg osteotomy is primarily to correct sagittal plane motion of the hallux; though if the hinge is broken, multiplane correction can be performed as well, especially if there is valgus deformity to the hallux.

An added benefit of this procedure is the limited restrictions during recovery. The patient is able to be weight bearing in a postoperative shoe and transition to a regular shoe around 4 weeks. It is important to note that the ability to perform weight-bearing activities greatly decreases deep venous thrombosis (DVT) risks during recovery and often negates the need for pharmacological DVT prophylaxis that may have side effects.

The cheilectomy Moberg procedure would only be indicated in grade 1-2 hallux limitus and likely an unsuccessful procedure in grades 3-4. When the first MPJ is painful and arthritic with severe joint narrowing and destruction, then the authors prefer the joint destructive procedures. Deciding on the correct joint destructive procedure involves a thorough history and physical examination along with a long discussion about patient's goals. The authors do believe that in the correct circumstances the first MPJ fusion is a predictable, good option for end-stage hallux rigidus. This procedure is performed per the technique described above. The source of patient's pain (ie, the first MPJ) is eliminated, leaving high satisfaction results.[60,61] The first MPJ arthrodesis can also be a less technically challenging procedure compared to some of the implant procedures out there. Patients who meet the criteria to undergo a first MPJ fusion can, under most circumstances, return to all normal activities they were performing prior to surgery.

PEARLS

- Adhere to original Duvries technique for the cheilectomy.
- Although unproven, cheilectomies appear to work best when the plantar first MPJ cartilage is present.
- Ensure to remove medial and lateral spurring.
- Removal of fibular sesamoid in some cases may improve range of motion and decrease pain.
- Although micro-fracturing has been described, routine use is not performed by the authors.
- Threaded head screws or dynamic compression staple is typically used for fixation.
- Patients are immediately weight bearing in a postoperative shoe until incisions heal and then transition to regular shoe gear.

positioning PEARLS

- Patient is put in supine position.
- Bump may be placed under ipsilateral hip to have first ray in rectus position.
- Pull digits into flexion upon inflation of tourniquet to neutralize any pull on the extensor or flexor tendons.
- Place ankle tourniquet just proximal to the malleoli.
- Patient's forefoot is blocked in a Mayo block type fashion.

POSTOPERATIVE CARE

All procedures discussed in this chapter can be performed as an outpatient procedure allowing the patient to return home the same day. The authors prefer to put all patients into a Sir Robert Jones soft dressing while in the operating room, which will stay clean, dry, and intact for ~2 weeks. Patients are asked to elevate their operative extremity for 45 minutes per hour to heart level or slightly above and ice behind their knee 15 minutes per hour while awake, barring any cardiovascular concerns. In absence of any wounding issues at the incision site, sutures are removed at the 2- to 3-week mark.

The weight-bearing protocol varies depending on the procedure(s) performed. Patients who undergo the joint-sparing procedures are typically placed in a postoperative shoe and permitted to perform flat foot weight bearing with or without the use of their gait aid of choice for roughly 2 weeks and then transition to regular shoe gear. Weight bearing for arthrodiastasis is typically non–weight bearing until the external fixator device is removed at ~6 weeks. Patients who undergo joint destructive procedures may have a longer period of activity restrictions, with the exception of the resection arthroplasties. Interpositional arthroplasty and implant arthroplasty patients are permitted to flatfoot weight bear in a postoperative shoe or long leg Ankilizer boot until incisions are healed at which time transition to regular shoe gear is permitted. Patients who undergo a first MPJ arthrodesis are made non–weight bearing with their gait aid of choice for 2 weeks and then weight bearing as tolerated. Radiographs are obtained at the 6-week mark to assess for osseous bridging. Depending on the radiographs and clinical course, patient may begin advancing his or her activities.

REHABILITATION

Patients who undergo surgical correction for hallux limitus or hallux rigidus typically do quite well postsurgically without rehab. Most patients, depending on the surgical procedure they underwent, are back to regular activates in 8-12 weeks. There are some instances in which rehabilitation with physical therapy (PT) is indicated. After many of the procedures discussed in the chapter, the first MPJ can become quite stiff in the postoperative period due to limited use of the joint. PT can be very helpful is working on ROM exercises or using their modalities to break up any scar formation that may have formed inhibiting motion. The therapy regimen and duration is usually left up to the physical therapist, but many times, patients can transition to a home program within a few weeks. The other instance in which PT would be sought is for gait retraining. In patients who have had medial column pain for many years and have developed a compensated gait, gait retraining may be indicated. The physical therapist will work on proper heel-to-toe walking ensuring to disperse forces in a natural manner. As noted by Elliott et al., it is important to counsel patient preoperatively that postoperative recovery could take up to 2 years to return to 100% after hallux rigidus surgeries. This is as important point as typically 6 months is the timeline stated in many podiatric offices and data as proven recovery may be longer than that.[38]

REFERENCES

1. Lau JTT, Daniels TR. Outcomes following cheilectomy and interpositional arthroplasty in hallux rigidus. *Foot Ankle Int.* 2001;22(6):462-470.
2. Berlet GC, Hyer CF, Lee TH, Philbin TM, Hartman JF, Wright ML. Interpositional arthroplasty of the first MTP joint using a regenerative tissue matrix for the treatment of advanced hallux rigidus. *Foot Ankle Int.* 2008;29(1):10-21.
3. Roukis TS. Metatarsus primus elevatus in hallux rigidus: fact or fiction? *J Am Podiatr Med Assoc.* 2005;95(3):221-228.
4. Coughlin MJ, Shurnas PS. Hallux rigidus: demographics, etiology, and radiographic assessment. *Foot Ankle Int.* 2003;21(1):731-743.
5. Lambrinudi P. Metatarsus primus elevatus. *Proc R Soc Med.* 1938;31:1273.
6. Roukis TS, Scherer PR, Anderson CF. Position of the first ray and motion of the first metatarsophalangeal joint. *J Am Podiatr Med Assoc.* 1996;86(11):538-546.
7. McMaster MJ. The pathogenesis of hallux rigidus. *J Bone Joint Surg Br.* 1978;60(1):82-87.
8. Bingold A, Collins D. Hallux rigidus. *J Bone Joint Surg.* 1950;32:214-222.
9. Shereff MJ, Baumhauer JF. Current concepts review-hallux rigidus and osteoarthritis of the first metatarsophalangeal joint. *J Bone Joint Surg.* 1998;80(6):898-908.
10. Keiserman LS, Sammarco VJ, Sammarco GJ. Surgical treatment of the hallux rigidus. *Foot Ankle Clin.* 2005;10(1):75-96.
11. Caravelli S, Mosca M, Massimi S, et al. A comprehensive and narrative review of historical aspects and management of low-grade hallux rigidus: conservative and surgical possibilities. *Musculoskelet Surg.* 2018;102(3):201-211.
12. Roukis TS, Jacobs PM, Dawson DM, Erdmann BB, Ringstrom JB. A prospective comparison of clinical, radiographic, and intraoperative features of hallux rigidus. *J Foot Ankle Surg.* 2002;41(2):76-95.
13. Coughlin MJ, Shurnas PS. Hallux rigidus: grading and long-term results of operative treatment. *J Bone Joint Surg Am.* 2003;85A:2072-2088.
14. Coughlin MJ, Shurnas PJ. Soft-tissue arthroplasty for hallux rigidus. *Foot Ankle Int.* 2003;24:661-672.
15. Giannikas AC, Papachristou G, Papavasiliou N, Nikiforidis P, Hartofilakidis-Garofalidis G. Dorsal dislocation of the first metatarso-phalangeal joint: report of four cases. *J Bone Joint Surg Br.* 1975;57(3):384-386.
16. Haines RW, McDougall A. The anatomy of hallux valgus. *J Bone Joint Surg Br.* 1954;36(2):272-293.
17. Glasoe WM, Nuckley DJ, Ludewig PM. Hallux valgus and the first metatarsal arch segment: a theoretical biomechanical perspective. *Phys Ther.* 2010;90(1):110-120.
18. Hicks JH. The mechanics of the foot: II. The plantar aponeurosis and the arch. *J Anat.* 1954;88(Pt 1):25.
19. Nawoczenski DA, Baumhauer JF, Umberger BR. Relationship between clinical measurements and motion of the first metatarsophalangeal joint during gait. *J Bone Joint Surg.* 1999;81(3):370-376.
20. Halstead J, Redmond AC. Weight-bearing passive dorsiflexion of the hallux in standing is not related to hallux dorsiflexion during walking. *J Orthop Sports Phys Ther.* 2006;36(8):550-556.
21. Payne C, Chuter V, Miller K. Sensitivity and specificity of the functional hallux limitus test to predict foot function. *J Am Podiatr Med Assoc.* 2002;92(5):269-271.
22. Zammit GV, Menz HB, Munteanu SE. Structural factors associated with hallux limitus/rigidus: a systematic review of case control studies. *J Orthop Sports Phys Ther.* 2009;39(10):733-742.
23. Vanore JV, Christensen JC, Kravitz SR, et al. Diagnosis and treatment of first metatarsophalangeal joint disorders. Section 2: hallux rigidus. *J Foot Ankle Surg.* 2003;42(3):124-136.
24. Botek G, Anderson MA. Etiology, pathophysiology, and staging of hallux rigidus. *Clin Podiatr Med Surg.* 2011;28(2):229-243.
25. Karasick D, Wapner KL. Hallux rigidus deformity: radiologic assessment. *AJR Am J Roentgenol.* 1991;157(5):1029-1033.
26. Grady JF, Axe TM, Zager EJ, Sheldon LA. A retrospective analysis of 772 patients with hallux limitus. *J Am Podiatr Med Assoc.* 2002;92(2):102-108.
27. King CK, James Loh SY, Zheng Q, Mehta KV. Comprehensive review of non-operative management of hallux rigidus. *Cureus.* 2017;9(1).
28. Pons M, Alvarez F, Solana J, Viladot R, Varela L. Sodium hyaluronate in the treatment of hallux rigidus. A single-blind, randomized study. *Foot Ankle Int.* 2007;28(1):38-42.
29. McNeil DS, Baumhauer JF, Glazebrook MA. Evidence-based analysis of the efficacy for operative treatment of hallux rigidus. *Foot Ankle Int.* 2013;34(1):15-32.
30. Gibson JA, Thomson CE. Arthrodesis or total replacement arthroplasty for hallux rigidus: a randomized controlled trial. *Foot Ankle Int.* 2005;26(9):680-690.
31. Brage ME, Ball ST. Surgical options for salvage of end-stage hallux rigidus. *Foot Ankle Clin.* 2002;7(1):49-73.
32. Maffulli N, Papalia R, Palumbo A, Del Buono A, Denaro V. Quantitative review of operative management of hallux rigidus. *Br Med Bull.* 2011;98(1):75.
33. DuVries HL. Hallux rigidus. In: DuVries HL, ed. *Surgery of the Foot.* St. Louis, MO: Mosby; 1959:341-440.
34. Roukis TS. The need for surgical revision after isolated cheilectomy for hallux rigidus: a systematic review. *J Foot Ankle Surg.* 2010;49(5):465-470.
35. Beeson P. The surgical treatment of hallux limitus/rigidus: a critical review of the literature. *Foot.* 2004;14(1):6-22.
36. Bernbach M. Hallux, McGlamry ED limitus: follow-up study. In: *Reconstructive Surgery of the Foot and Leg Update'88.* Tucker, GA: Podiatry Institute Publishing Co.; 1988:109-111.
37. Freeman BL, Hardy MA. Multiplanar phalangeal and metatarsal osteotomies for hallux rigidus. *Clin Podiatr Med Surg.* 2011;28(2):329-344.
38. Elliott AD, Borgert AJ, Roukis TS. A prospective comparison of clinical, radiographic, and intraoperative features of hallux rigidus: long-term follow-up and analysis. *J Foot Ankle Surg.* 2016;55(3):547-561.
39. Roukis TS. Clinical outcomes after isolated periarticular osteotomies of the first metatarsal for hallux rigidus: a systematic review. *J Foot Ankle Surg.* 2010;49(6):553-560.
40. Gerbert J, Moadab A, Rupley KF. Youngswick-Austin procedure: the effect of plantar arm orientation on metatarsal head displacement. *J Foot Ankle Surg.* 2001;40(1):8-14.
41. Lambrinudi C. Metatarsus primus elevatus. *Proc R Soc Med.* 1938;31:1-273.
42. Kessel L. Bonney G. Hallux rigidus in the adolescent. *J Bone Joint Surg.* 1958;40B(4):668-673.
43. Moberg E. A simple operation for hallux rigidus. *Clin Orthop Relat Res.* 1979;142:55-56.
44. Roukis TS. Outcomes after cheilectomy with phalangeal dorsiflexory osteotomy for hallux rigidus: a systematic review. *J Foot Ankle Surg.* 2010;49(5):479-487.
45. Saxena A. The Valenti procedure for hallux limitus/rigidus. *J Foot Ankle Surg.* 1995;34(5):485-488.
46. Roukis TS. The need for surgical revision after isolated Valenti arthroplasty for hallux rigidus: a systematic review. *J Foot Ankle Surg.* 2010;49(3):294-297.
47. Talarico LM, Vito GR, Goldstein L, et al. Management of hallux limitus with distraction of the first metatarsophalangeal joint. *J Am Podiatr Med Assoc.* 2005;95(2):121-129.
48. Kim YS, Park EH, Lee HJ, Koh YG, Lee JW. Clinical comparison of the osteochondral autograft transfer system and subchondral drilling in osteochondral defects of the first metatarsal head. *Am J Sports Med.* 2012;40(8):1824-1833.
49. Galli MM, Hyer CF. Hallux rigidus: what lies beyond fusion, resectional arthroplasty, and implants. *Clin Podiatr Med Surg.* 2011;28(2):385-403.
50. Title CI, Zaret D, Means KR Jr, Vogtman J, Miller SD. First metatarsal head OATS technique: an approach to cartilage damage. *Foot Ankle Int.* 2006;27(11):1000-1002.
51. Kim PJ, Hatch D, DiDomenico LA, et al. A multicenter retrospective review of outcomes for arthrodesis, hemi-metallic joint implant, and resectional arthroplasty in the surgical treatment of end-stage hallux rigidus. *J Foot Ankle Surg.* 2012;51(1):50-56.
52. Grondal L, Broström E, Wretenberg P, Stark A. Arthrodesis versus Mayo resection: the management of the first metatarsophalangeal joint in reconstruction of the rheumatoid forefoot. *J Bone Joint Surg Br.* 2006;88(7):914-919.
53. Yee G, Lau J. Current concepts review: hallux rigidus. *Foot Ankle Int.* 2008;29(6):637-646.
54. Roukis TS. Outcome following autogenous soft tissue interpositional arthroplasty for end-stage hallux rigidus: a systematic review. *J Foot Ankle Surg.* 2010;49(5):475-478.
55. Roukis TS, Landsman AS, Ringstrom JB, Kirschner F, Wuenschel M. Distally based capsule-periosteum interpositional arthroplasty for hallux rigidus: indications, operative technique, and short-term follow-up. *J Am Podiatr Med Assoc.* 2003;93(5):349-366.
56. DeHeer PA. The case against first metatarsal phalangeal joint implant arthroplasty. *Clin Podiatr Med Surg.* 2006;23(4):709-723.
57. Hasselman CT, Shields N. Resurfacing of the first metatarsal head in the treatment of hallux rigidus. *Tech Foot Ankle Surg.* 2008;7(1):31-40.
58. Carpenter B, Smith J, Motley T, Garrett A. Surgical treatment of hallux rigidus using a metatarsal head resurfacing implant: mid-term follow-up. *J Foot Ankle Surg.* 2010;49(4):321-325.
59. Mermerkaya MU, Adli H. A comparison between metatarsal head-resurfacing hemiarthroplasty and total metatarsophalangeal joint arthroplasty as surgical treatments for hallux rigidus: a retrospective study with short-to midterm follow-up. *Clin Interv Aging.* 2016;11:1805.
60. DeFrino PF, Brodsky JW, Pollo FE, Crenshaw SJ, Beischer AD. First metatarsophalangeal arthrodesis: a clinical, pedobarographic and gait analysis study. *Foot Ankle Int.* 2002;23(6):496-502.
61. Coughlin MJ, Grebing BR, Jones CP. Arthrodesis of the first metatarsophalangeal joint for idiopathic hallux valgus: intermediate results. *Foot Ankle Int.* 2005;26(10):783-792.
62. Goucher NR, Coughlin MJ. Hallux metatarsophalangeal joint arthrodesis using dome-shaped reamers and dorsal plate fixation: a prospective study. *Foot Ankle Int.* 2006;27(11):869-876.
63. Roukis TS. Nonunion after arthrodesis of the first metatarsal-phalangeal joint: a systematic review. *J Foot Ankle Surg.* 2011;50(6):710-713.
64. Roukis TS. A simple technique for positioning the first metatarsophalangeal joint during arthrodesis. *J Foot Ankle Surg.* 2006;45(1):56-57.
65. Roukis TS, Meusnier T, Augoyard M. Incidence of nonunion of first metatarsophalangeal joint arthrodesis for severe hallux valgus using crossed, flexible titanium intramedullary nails and a dorsal static staple with immediate weightbearing in female patients. *J Foot Ankle Surg.* 2012;51(4):433-436.

CHAPTER 15

Sesamoid Disorders

Sandeep B. Patel and Jason D. Pollard

DEFINITION

Hallucal sesamoid pathology can present as either an acute condition or a chronic pathological process. Disorders to the medial, or tibial sesamoid, are far more common when compared to the lateral, or fibular sesamoid. This can be attributed to the increased size of the medial sesamoid. If undiagnosed or not appropriately managed, pathology of the sesamoids can have a detrimental effect to the function of the first metatarsophalangeal joint (MTPJ) and be responsible for persistent pain, decreased push-off strength, stiffness, deformity, and degenerative arthritis.[1] The more common disorders include sesamoiditis, acute trauma, stress fracture, chondromalacia, and avascular necrosis (AVN).

CLASSIFICATION (TABLES 15.1 AND 15.2)

TABLE 15.1 Jahss Classification for First MTPJ Dislocation

Dorsal dislocation of the proximal phalanx with the metatarsal head puncturing through the plantar plate

Type I
- No sesamoid fracture and intersesamoid ligament intact
- Closed reduction blocked by plantar plate and often requires open reduction

Type IIa
- Rupture of the intersesamoid ligament
- Closed reduction often successful

Type IIb
- Intersesamoid ligament intact with transverse fracture of one of the sesamoids
- Closed reduction often successful

Type IIc
- Intersesamoid ligament intact with transverse fracture of both sesamoids
- Closed reduction often successful

Type IIIa
- Complete soft tissue disruption of the plantar complex from the proximal phalanx

Type IIIb
- Complete plantar plate disruption, including disruption of one of the sesamoids

---

ANATOMIC FEATURES

Sesamoids first appear in the 12th week of fetal development. Ossification of the hallucal sesamoids typically begins at the age of 6-8 years in girls and 7-9 years in boys and is normally completed by the age of 10 and 12, respectively.[2,3] The tibial sesamoid typically has an average size of 12-15 mm, whereas the fibular sesamoid has an average size between 10 and 12 mm. There are multiple centers of ossification, and incomplete coalescence of these growth centers can lead to either a bipartite or multipartite sesamoid (Fig. 15.1). The incidence of a bipartite or multipartite sesamoid ranges from 7% to 30%.[4] Approximately 90% of bipartite sesamoids involve the tibial sesamoid and unilateral involvement is most common.[5] Congenital absence of one or both hallucal sesamoids is extremely rare but has been previously reported.[6-8] The absence of the medial sesamoid is more commonly reported, and only limited cases have been reported with the absence of the lateral sesamoid.[7]

Both sesamoids are embedded within the flexor hallucis brevis tendon. The inner fibers of the abductor hallucis tendon in conjunction with the medial portion of the flexor hallucis brevis tendon attach to the tibial sesamoid, whereas the transverse and oblique heads of the adductor tendon and lateral portion of the flexor hallucis brevis attach to the fibular sesamoid. There is no tendinous attachment of the flexor hallucis longus tendon onto the sesamoids, but its synovial tendon sheath blends into the intersesamoid ligament as it passes between the sesamoids.[9] The sesamoids are closely connected with the fibrous layer of the joint capsule as well as the medial and lateral sesamoid ligaments, which blend with the joint capsule.[9] Sharpey fibers from the sesamoid ligaments penetrate the sesamoids on their capsular side.[1] The collateral ligaments fan out distally and plantarly from the metatarsal head and attach to the plantar aspect of the proximal phalanx. The intersesamoid ligament connects the sesamoids and consists of transverse, longitudinal, and vertical bundles.[9] The deep transverse intermetatarsal ligament extends from the neck of the second metatarsal attaching to the fibular sesamoid. The plantar plate is the most distal attachment of the sesamoid apparatus, which anchors the sesamoids to the plantar base of the proximal phalanx (Fig. 15.2).

The sesamoid arteries arise from the medial plantar artery (25%), the plantar arch (25%), or from both sources (50%) and provide the blood supply to the sesamoids.[10] These arteries penetrate the sesamoids from the plantar nonarticular surface. In addition, the arteries enter from the medial aspect of

TABLE 15.2	**Turf Toe Classification**			
Grade	Pathology	Clinical	Radiographic	MRI
I	Strain of the capsule without a loss of continuity	Localized tenderness, minimal edema, or ecchymosis	Normal	Intact soft tissue complex with surrounding edema
II	Partial tear of plantar plate or capsule	Painful motion and difficulty weight bearing	Normal	Increased signal intensity that does not extend through the full thickness of the plantar plate
III	Complete tear with loss of continuity of the plantar plate and capsule	Associated injury including sesamoid fracture, diastasis of bipartite sesamoid, or proximal migration of the sesamoids	May demonstrate avulsion fracture of the proximal phalanx, sesamoid fracture, proximal migration of the sesamoids, or MTPJ dislocation	Increased signal intensity completely traversing the plantar capsuloligamentous complex with sesamoid or chondral injury

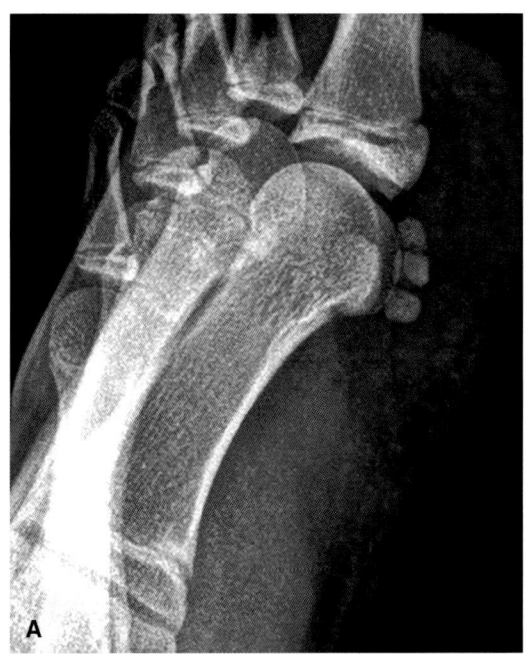

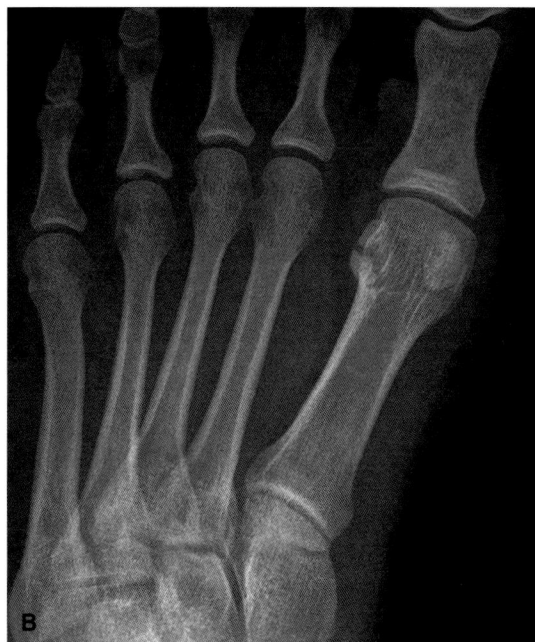

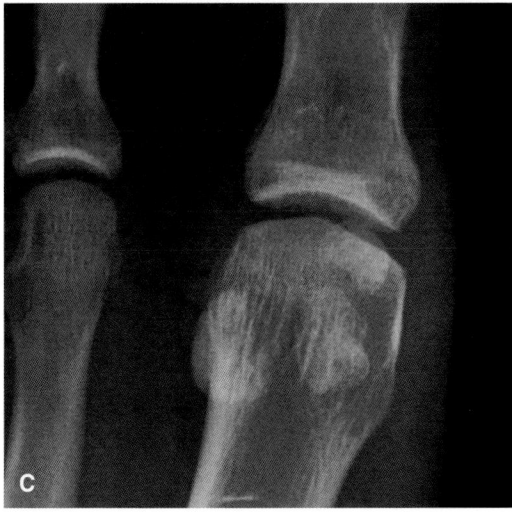

FIGURE 15.1 Example of bipartite and multipartite sesamoids. **A.** Formation of multipartite sesamoids in pediatric patient. **B.** Bipartite fibular sesamoid. **C.** Bipartite tibial sesamoid.

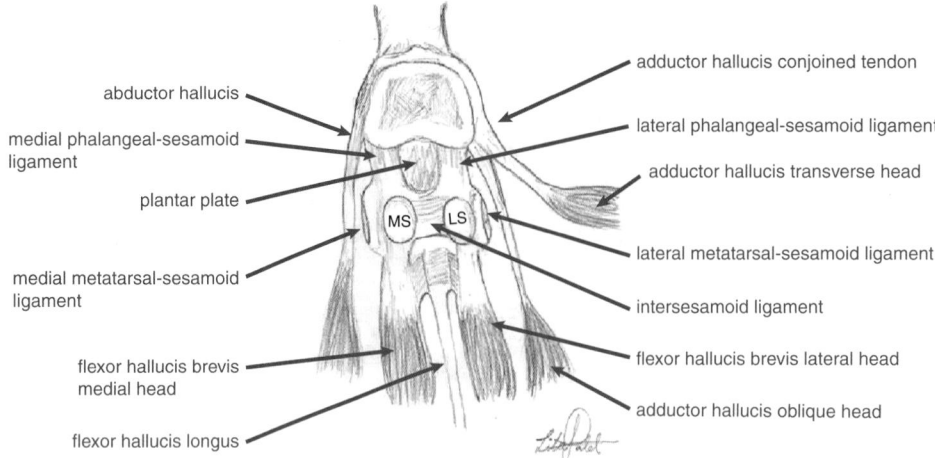

FIGURE 15.2 Anatomy of soft tissue structures surrounding the sesamoid apparatus. (Drawing courtesy of Lila S. Patel.)

the tibial sesamoid and the lateral aspect of the fibular sesamoid. This should be taken into consideration with any surgical approach to minimize the risk of vascular insult to the sesamoids. The number of sesamoidal arteries can vary from 1 (55%) to 3 (10%), with the number increasing with increasing size of the sesamoid bone.[11] Distally, the sesamoid vascular supply is tenuous and only supplied from the capsule. Innervation of the sesamoids is provided from the hallucal nerves, which run in close proximity to the sesamoids.[1] They pass underneath the crural fascia, covered by vertical fibers investing the plantar fat pad at the level of the MTPJ.[12] The plantar medial nerve runs in close proximity to the tibial sesamoid and flexor hallucis longus tendon sheath and is at risk for iatrogenic injury when surgery is performed at this location.[13]

FUNCTIONAL ANALYSIS OF THE ANATOMY

The hallucal sesamoids play a vital role in first MTPJ function and are an integral part of normal, bipedal gait. The tibial and fibular sesamoids protect the flexor hallucis longus tendon from friction as it is housed between the two bones while traversing plantar to the first metatarsal head. In addition, they serve to minimize joint forces by increasing the distance of the flexor tendons from the MTPJ.[14] Generally, sesamoid bones within a tendon act to hold the tendon further from a joint's center of rotation, thus increasing the moment arm. The sesamoid bones have been shown to increase the mechanical advantage of the flexor hallucis brevis aiding in plantarflexion of the hallux.

The sesamoidal apparatus helps to elevate the first metatarsal head, effectively decreasing plantar pressure to the metatarsal head and distribute weight bearing of the first ray. It has been estimated that 40%-60% of body weight is transmitted through the hallux MTPJ during normal gait.[14] These forces can increase to 200%-300% of body weight during athletic activities and can reach up to 800% with a running jump.[15] As mentioned before, the tibial sesamoid is larger, thus it bears the majority of the weight-bearing forces that are transmitted to the head of the first metatarsal.[16] Therefore, the tibial sesamoid is more prone to injury.[17]

There are also various anatomical variations that can result in symptoms about the sesamoid apparatus. The sesamoids can become hypertrophied resulting in painful plantar hyperkeratotic lesion. A hypertrophic fibular sesamoid can also cause pain in the first interspace due to nerve compression (Fig. 15.3).

PHYSICAL EXAMINATION

The physical examination for determining sesamoid disorders is generally straightforward. Patients will present with symptoms on the plantar aspect of the medial forefoot related to activity. The symptoms are present with weight bearing and often exacerbated by the toe off phase of gait. Pain will exist with direct palpation to the fibular or tibial sesamoid. A thorough examination of the range of motion should also be performed.

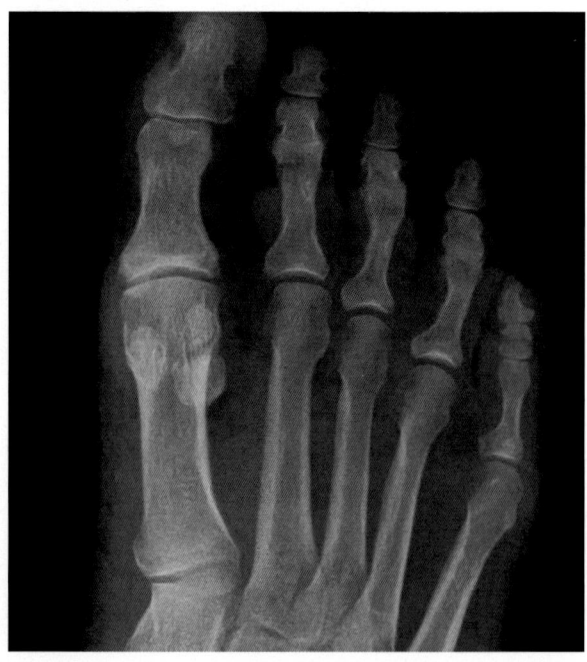

FIGURE 15.3 Example of hypertrophied fibular sesamoid.

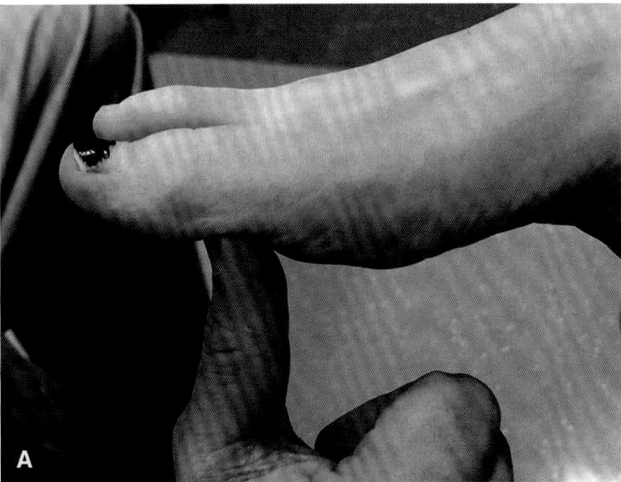

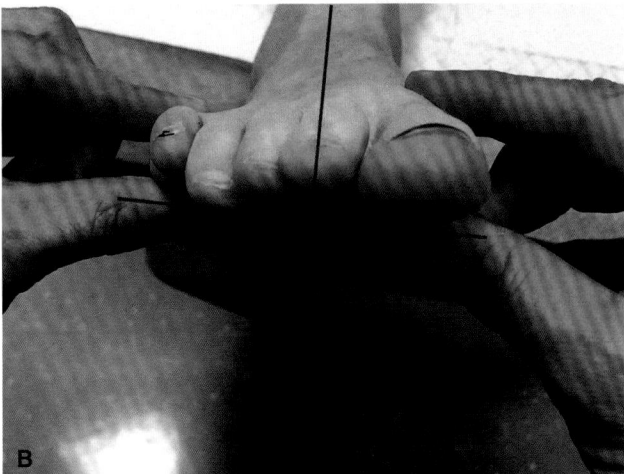
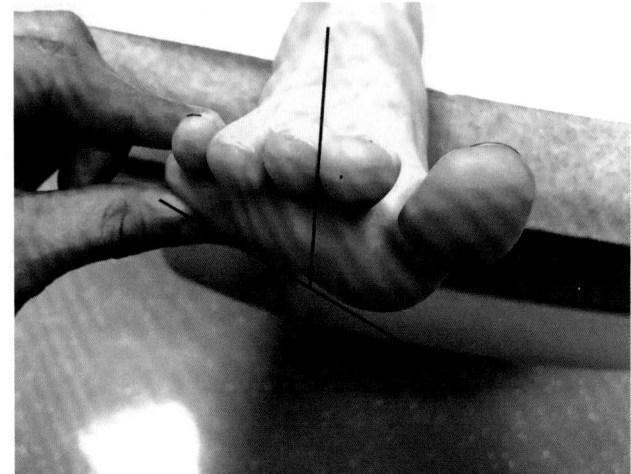

FIGURE 15.4 Muscle testing of the sesamoid complex. **A.** Isolating the flexor hallucis brevis tendon should reproduce pain in the sesamoids. Patient is asked to plantarflex the rectus hallux against resistance. **B.** Testing for peroneus longus tendon overdrive. In the resting state, all of the metatarsal heads should be aligned in the frontal plane. Once the patient is asked to fire the peroneus longus, patients with dynamic overload of the sesamoids may demonstrate a marked plantarflexion of the first ray.

Patient may have pain with range of motion of the first MTPJ, often worse with maximal dorsiflexion. This may also help assess for arthritic condition of the sesamoids or weakness of the flexor tendon. Testing the flexor hallucis brevis against resistance may also reproduce pain along the sesamoids (Fig. 15.4). Patients may also have the presence of hyperkeratotic tissue or intractable plantar keratoma on the plantar aspect of the first metatarsal head indicating increased pressure to the forefoot. In some cases, there may be the presence of a joint effusion.

A thorough biomechanical evaluation is also critical to understand the potential etiology of the symptoms and to help direct conservative and surgical management. This evaluation should differentiate between dynamic function and structural abnormalities. Specifically, the focus should be on abnormalities that would increase load to the sesamoid apparatus. Peroneal overdrive can be assessed by asking the patient to plantarflex the first ray against resistance. In the resting position, all of the metatarsal heads will be in the same frontal plane. Once the peroneus longus is fired, individuals with a hyperactivity of the tendon will demonstrate a marked plantarflexion of the first ray (Fig. 15.4). Alternatively, a structurally

plantarflexed first ray will be associated with a cavus foot type. Rigidity of the medial column can be distinguished by performing the Coleman block test.

PATHOGENESIS

Sesamoiditis is a generic term used to describe various pathologies involving the sesamoidal apparatus and first MTPJ. These conditions include osteonecrosis, chondromalacia, and mechanical overload. Sesamoiditis is more commonly seen in younger and more active individuals resulting from repetitive trauma. It has been estimated that sesamoid injuries account for 9% of all foot and ankle injuries and ~1.25% of running related injuries.[18]

There are several etiologies that can result in disorders of the sesamoids. Mechanical overload can be seen more frequently in the pes cavus foot type, a plantarflexed first ray, ankle and variations of sesamoid anatomy.[16] Scranton described several variations in sesamoid anatomy that lead to mechanical overload. The anatomical factors that can predispose patients to this include asymmetrical size, rotational malalignment, condylar malformation, and an enlarged sesamoid.[19] The tibial sesamoid is more commonly involved as it is larger and experiences more load during weight bearing.[16,17]

Osteonecrosis of the sesamoid can be a primary pathology or from repetitive trauma related to the tenuous blood supply to the sesamoid apparatus. The diagnosis of AVN of the sesamoid can be challenging and often requires a high index of suspicion. A thorough history and physical examination are essential to establish an accurate diagnosis. AVN is more

common in women in the second and third decade of life. Athletes, particularly female ballet dancers, are at an increased risk of AVN of the sesamoid due to repetitive microtrauma and increased contact pressures to the sesamoids.[20] Initial radiographs including sesamoid axial views should be obtained, but often any abnormal radiographic findings are not appreciated until the later stages of AVN. MRI can be useful in establishing the diagnosis of AVN. In cases of AVN, MRI will display low signal intensity on T1 and T2 as fibrous tissue replaces fat and hematopoietic tissue (Fig. 15.5).[21]

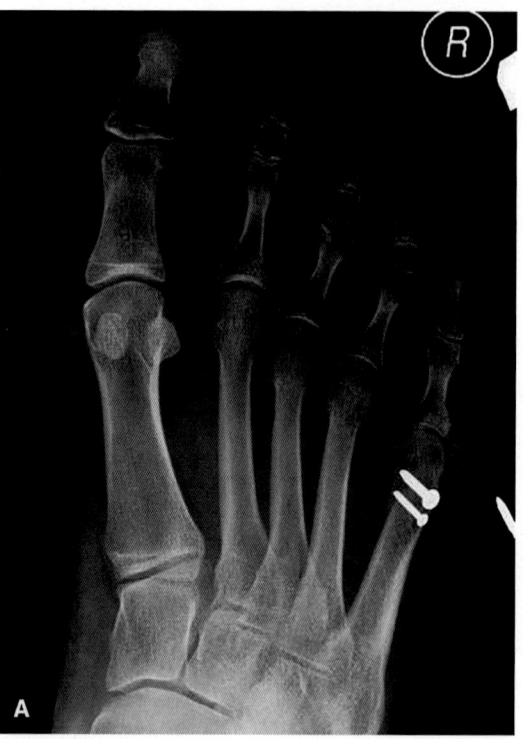

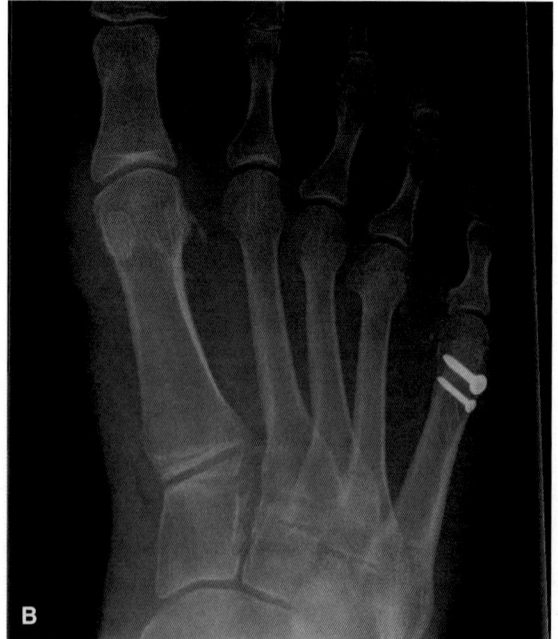

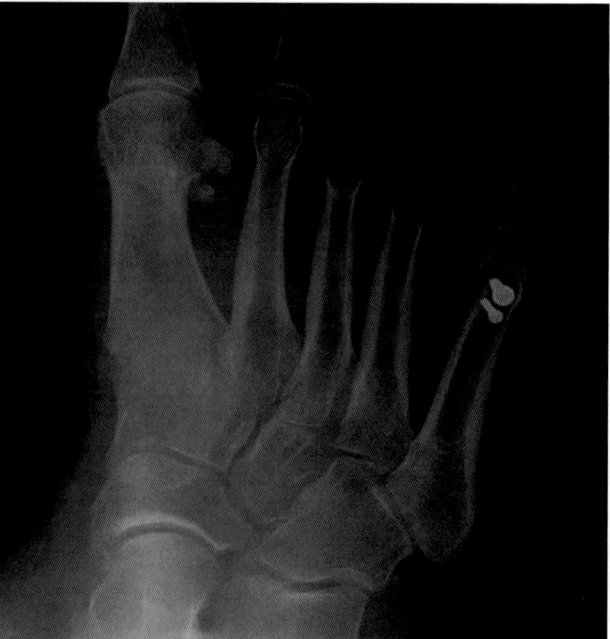

FIGURE 15.5 Example of AVN. **A.** A 30-year-old female with plantar, medial forefoot pain. Initial radiographs are normal. **B.** Continued pain at 6 months with radiographic signs of AVN of the fibular sesamoid.

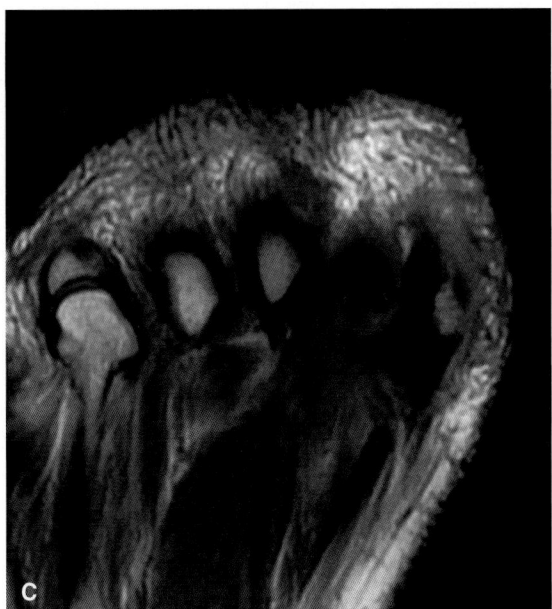
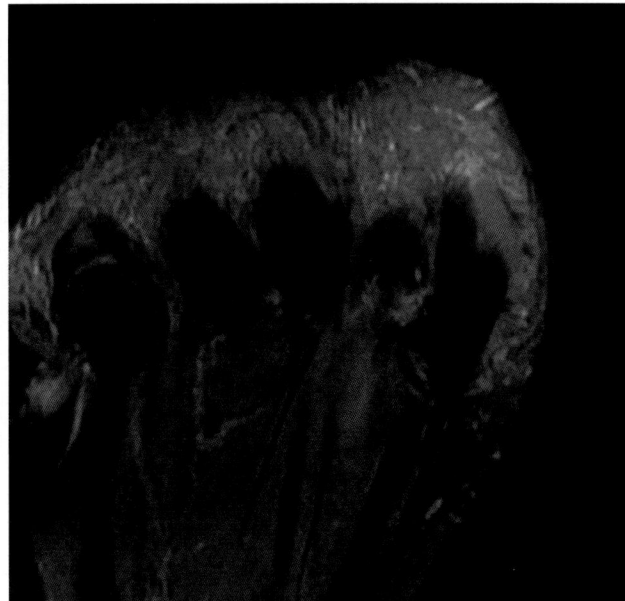

FIGURE 15.5 (*Continued*) **C.** Diagnosis is confirmed with MRI. Note the appearance of AVN on T1 and T2 images.

Traumatic injuries result in acute fractures of the sesamoid bones or separation of bipartite sesamoids. The mechanism of injury is usually secondary to forced dorsiflexion of the first MTPJ. Rarely, direct trauma or high impact load to the joint complex can result in fracture.

Acute fractures of the sesamoids are relatively uncommon injury. These injuries can present in varying manners on plain radiographs. They may appear as transverse fractures of the sesamoids, increased diastasis of the natural synchondrosis of the bipartite sesamoid, or complete fracture/dislocation of the first MTPJ (Fig. 15.6). Although it may be difficult to distinguish between an acute fracture and bipartite sesamoid, fractures of

the sesamoid will appear as a transverse fracture line with sharp, irregular edges, whereas a bipartite sesamoid will demonstrate well-defined borders. Favinger found that the dominant sesamoid interval ranged from 0 to 2 mm on a routine radiograph of the foot for bi-/multipartite sesamoids.[22] They further concluded that a sesamoid diastasis should be considered, in the appropriate clinical setting, when the sesamoid interval is >2 mm of the AP radiograph of the foot.[22] Obtaining radiographs of the contralateral foot or getting advanced imaging may assist in clarifying the diagnosis.

IMAGING AND DIAGNOSTIC STUDIES

RADIOGRAPHS

Routine weight-bearing AP and lateral radiographs are important in the initial assessment of sesamoid pathology but often are difficult to interpret or make accurate assessments due to the overlying first metatarsal on the AP projections and obstruction of the lesser metatarsals on the lateral view. A medial oblique view will provide improved visualization and evaluation of the fibular sesamoid, while a lateral oblique will improve visualization of the tibial sesamoid. Sesamoid axial views provide good visualization of both sesamoids, as well as their position and relationship to the first metatarsal. Comparison views can also be useful to evaluate for proximal migration of the sesamoids and sesamoid fracture diastasis.[1]

Favinger et al. evaluated the radiographic epidemiology and appearance of the normal bi-/multipartite hallux sesamoid bones and found an overall incidence of 14.3% in their study.[22] The medial sesamoid was involved in 82.3% of bi-/multipartite sesamoid bones, 9.2% demonstrated at least one bi-/multipartite sesamoid bone on each foot, and only 2.6% had two bi-/multipartite sesamoids on the same foot.[22] In addition, the dominant sesamoid interval ranged from 0 to 2 mm, with an average of 0.79 mm.[22] Based on their results, they concluded that when the sesamoid interval is >2 mm on the AP radiograph

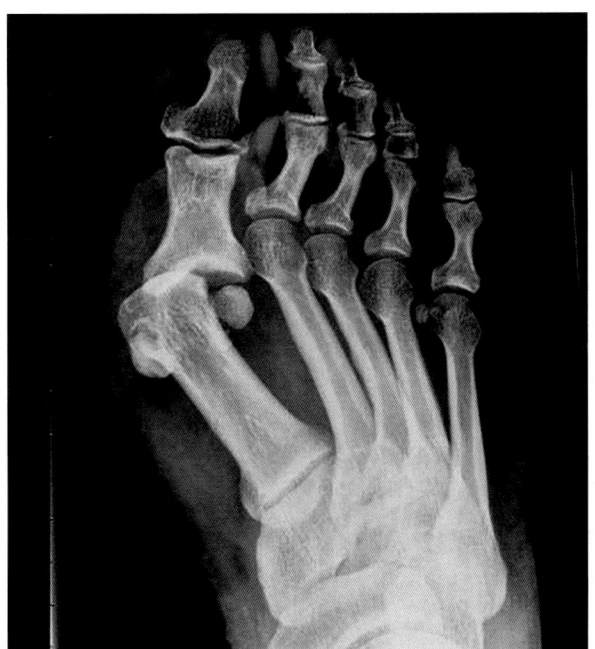

FIGURE 15.6 Complete dislocation of the MTPJ.

that a sesamoid diastasis should be considered in the appropriate clinical setting. Prieskorn et al. examined 200 normal radiographs in 100 patients to evaluate the normal distances from the distal aspect of the sesamoid to the first metatarsophalangeal joint.[23] Based on their findings, they concluded that if the distance between the distal aspect of the tibial sesamoid to the joint is >10.4 mm or the fibular sesamoid to joint distance is 13.3 mm, then there is a 99.7% chance for a plantar plate rupture.[23] In addition, they reported an incidence of a bipartite sesamoid 13.5% of the time with 37% bilateral involvement.

MRI

Magnetic resonance imaging (MRI) has been considered by some to be the investigation of choice for most sesamoid disorders given the considerable overlap in the clinical presentation and physical examination findings between various pathologic entities to the sesamoids.[24] MRI can be utilized for the evaluation of both soft tissue and bony pathology about the MTPJ. Any disruption of the plantar plate or capsular structure as well as any injury of the flexor hallucis longus tendon should be easily seen on MRI. In addition, osseous pathology such as damage of the articular surface, AVN, subchondral sclerosis, marrow edema, erosions, and subchondral cysts is readily identified with MRI. However, MRI can also overestimate the involved pathology. One such study by Dietrich et al. on 30 asymptomatic volunteers found cartilage defects, bone marrow edema-like signal changes, subchondral cysts, plantar recesses, and distal dorsal recesses as common findings on MRI of asymptomatic first MTPJs.[25] In addition, the collateral ligaments were often heterogeneous in structure and showed increased signal intensity.[25]

Although imaging parameters can vary from institution to institution, the ideal field of view should be between 10 and 14 cm, slice thickness should be 3 mm, and there should be an interslice gap of 0.3 mm (10%).[26] A thorough examination includes non–fat-suppressed T1-weighted (T1W) or proton density (PD) images in conjunction with fluid-sensitive fat-suppressed PD (PDFS) or short tau inversion recovery (STIR) images, performed in coronal, axial, and parasagittal planes.[27]

CT SCAN

A computerized tomography (CT) scan can aid in the diagnosis of acute fracture, arthritic changes, or nonunion involving the sesamoids (Fig. 15.7). There is limited research available for the use of technetium-99 (^{99m}Tc)-methylene diphosphonate (MDP) single photon emission tomography-computer tomography (SPECT-CT) for the diagnosis of sesamoid disorders, but one such case report highlighted its utility in identifying sesamoiditis as a cause of foot pain when other diagnostic imaging was otherwise unremarkable.[28]

BONE SCAN

Bone scintigraphy has previously been described to evaluate for sesamoid pathology. Bone scintigraphy is known to be highly sensitive, yet nonspecific, in detecting osseous pathology. Increased scintigraphic activity of the hallucal sesamoids is assumed to correlate with clinical pathology and can proceed radiographic findings of a stress fracture or AVN. However, previous reports conducted of both active and sedentary

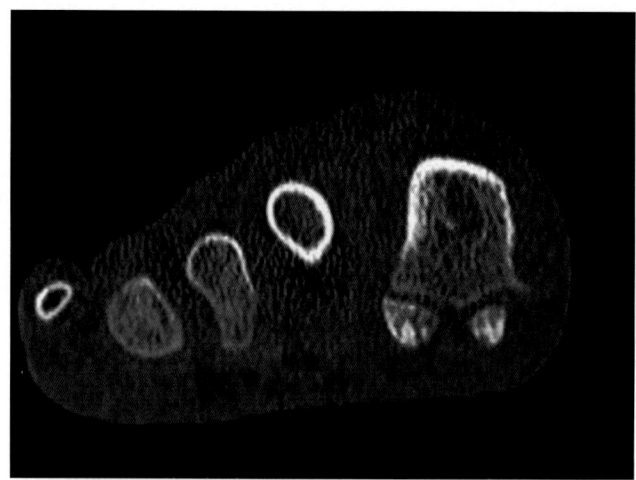

FIGURE 15.7 CT scan of sesamoid fracture. Note vertical fracture line from direct trauma. This type of injury may not be readily identified on plain radiographs.

asymptomatic individuals demonstrated 29% and 26% increased scintigraphic activity, respectively.[29] Therefore, when using scintigraphy to evaluate for sesamoid pathology, caution should be used in interpreting the meaning of increased scintigraphic activity.[29] Bone scintigraphy has also been described as a complementary examination in the diagnosis of AVN of the sesamoids.[30] Barral et al. felt that triphasic bone scintigraphy can play an important role in the early detection of AVN of the sesamoids and can, therefore, help guide the physician regarding appropriate treatment.[30] The authors feel that given more advanced imaging techniques, bone scintigraphy has a limited role in the evaluation and diagnosis of sesamoid disorders.

STRESS RADIOGRAPHS

A dorsiflexion stress radiograph can be performed under fluoroscopy as an adjunctive test to evaluate for a possible plantar plate injury when there is clinical suspicion for disruption. With complete disruption of the MTPJ complex, the sesamoids will fail to track distally with hallux MTPJ extension. A real-time view of the hallux MTPJ joint can help evaluate the sesamoids and joint complex through dynamic motion and allow comparison with the contralateral side.[21] One biomechanical study demonstrated an increase in sesamoid phalangeal distance in a simulated turf toe injury to the plantar plate. These authors noted that an increase of ≥3 mm in the distance between the sesamoids and the base of the proximal phalanx was significant and predictive of severe injury to the plantar plate.[31]

TREATMENT

NONOPERATIVE TREATMENT FOR CHRONIC SESAMOID CONDITIONS

Sesamoiditis

Initial treatment of chronic sesamoid disorders should consist of nonoperative management. Conservative treatment for acute inflammation involves an initial period of rest, ice, compression, and elevation (RICE). In addition, nonsteroidal anti-inflammatory medications should be initiated. For more severe presentations, an initial period of immobilization should be considered. Immobilization can vary from a removable walking boot to strict non–weight bearing in a short leg cast with a toe spica. Ultimately, orthotic therapy should be initiated to off-load the sesamoids and address any mechanical etiologies. Inserting a rigid forefoot insole, or a Morton extension, can reduce rocker motion of the first MTPJ to aid in both comfort and decrease the rate of recurrent injury.[1] Shoe gear modification should also include stiff sole shoes to limit hallux MTPJ extension. For lower demand patients, a metatarsal bar or rocker bottom shoe can be considered to decrease forefoot pressures. Intra-articular corticosteroid injection can be offered on a limited basis, but repeated injections should be avoided.[32]

Turf Toe

The nonoperative treatment of turf toe injuries has a high degree of success. The need for operative intervention has been previously reported as low as 2% in collegiate football players.[33] There are several different classification schemes describing turf toe based on anatomic, pathologic, and clinical symptoms (Table 15.2). The treatment strategies for turf toe are largely dependent on the grade of injury. Kadakia and Molloy found there to be sufficient evidence from several Level IV studies to support a grade B recommendation for nonoperative management in patients with grade I and II turf toe injuries.[34] However, they found insufficient evidence (grade I) to make treatment recommendations for grade III injuries.[34]

The nonoperative treatment for grade I and II injuries is similar to that of sesamoiditis. Shoe gear modification should include shoes with a rigid sole and a turf toe plate to limit first MTPJ extension. Alternatively, a custom orthotic with a Morton extension can be used. In addition, taping the hallux in slight plantarflexion can help limit pathologic motion across the joint. Gentle range of motion exercises can also be initiated as tolerated to help prevent sesamoid adhesion while protecting the soft tissue healing. Participation in explosive, push-off activities should be avoided until low impact exercises are tolerated without pain or limitations.[21] Return to near or full activity will be dictated by symptoms and the ability to reach near preinjury activity level. Grade III injuries will require a longer period of immobilization and recovery. Ideally, the hallux MTPJ should have 50-60 degrees of painless passive dorsiflexion before running or explosive activities are attempted.[21] Intra-articular corticosteroid injections will only mask or temporarily relieve symptoms and, therefore, are not recommended.[1,21]

Avascular Necrosis of the Sesamoid

Similar to other sesamoid conditions, nonoperative care should be attempted prior to any surgical intervention. The aim of nonoperative treatment for AVN is to alleviate symptoms and decrease the mechanical strain or overload to the sesamoids. This can be accomplished with RICE, orthotics with a Morton extension or off-loading accommodations to the involved sesamoid(s), stiff sole shoes, and NSAIDs. Non–weight bearing and cast immobilization can be considered for more acute or recalcitrant symptoms. However, given the low prevalence of sesamoid AVN, the success rate of nonoperative modalities is unknown. Surgical intervention can be considered after

nonoperative management has failed to alleviate symptoms or return the patient to an acceptable level of function.[21]

NONOPERATIVE TREATMENT FOR ACUTE TRAUMA

Sesamoid Fracture

Conservative management should be the initial treatment for both traumatic and chronic stress fractures of the sesamoids. Treatment of these injuries may include a period of immobilization and protected weight bearing in either a surgical shoe or a removable walking boot. However, given the recalcitrant nature of sesamoid disorders, mechanical forces transmitted through the sesamoidal apparatus during weight bearing, and the tenuous blood supply to the sesamoids, the authors recommend an initial treatment in a non–weight-bearing cast with the toe plate for 6-8 weeks, followed by weight bearing as tolerated in a removable walking boot until symptoms resolved. Ultimately, orthotics with off-loading accommodations under the MTPJ and shoe gear with a stable midsole should be initiated when there is a return to regular shoe gear. Taping can also be performed to limit the dorsiflexion of the MTPJ during strenuous activities.

However, to date there are no comparative studies that evaluate the efficacy of the various treatment modalities and the literature is limited to level V studies and case reports. The limited evidence does not allow for a recommendation with regard to a specific nonoperative treatment for sesamoid fracture (grade I recommendation).[34]

Surgical intervention for both acute and chronic sesamoid conditions should be considered if appropriate nonoperative care has failed to resolve symptoms or return the patient to desired activity level after 6 months.

First MPJ Dislocation

Dislocation of the first MTPJ occurs when the hallux in forced into dorsiflexion under an axial load. A progressive injury pattern will occur under increasing dorsiflexion and axial forces resulting in soft tissue and bony disruption across the first MTPJ. A Jahss type I injury is noted by a disruption of the weaker proximal capsular attachments, which results in a dorsal dislocation of the proximal phalanx and sesamoids with an intact intersesamoid ligament. This injury pattern is typically not amenable to closed reduction. This is due to interposition of the plantar plate and sesamoids within the joint, as well as the "noose" of the conjoined tendons encircling the metatarsal head and neck.[35] Typically, surgical intervention is required for reduction of the first MTPJ and may require transection of some of the supporting soft tissue structures proximal to the sesamoids to allow for sufficient laxity and reduction. Jahss IIa is a dorsal dislocation of the proximal phalanx and the sesamoids with a rupture of the intersesamoid ligament. On an anteroposterior radiograph, a wide separation between the sesamoids is noted and can help differentiate it from a type I injury. Jahss IIb and IIc are noted by a transverse fracture of either one or both sesamoids, respectively. Most type II injuries are amenable to closed reduction due to increased disruption of the surrounding soft tissue structures (Fig. 15.8). Jahss III injury has been described when the sesamoid complex remains intact, but there is a dorsal dislocation of the proximal phalanx with complete disruption of the plantar plate. On an

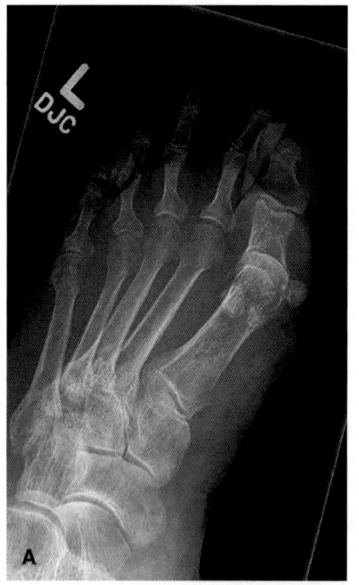

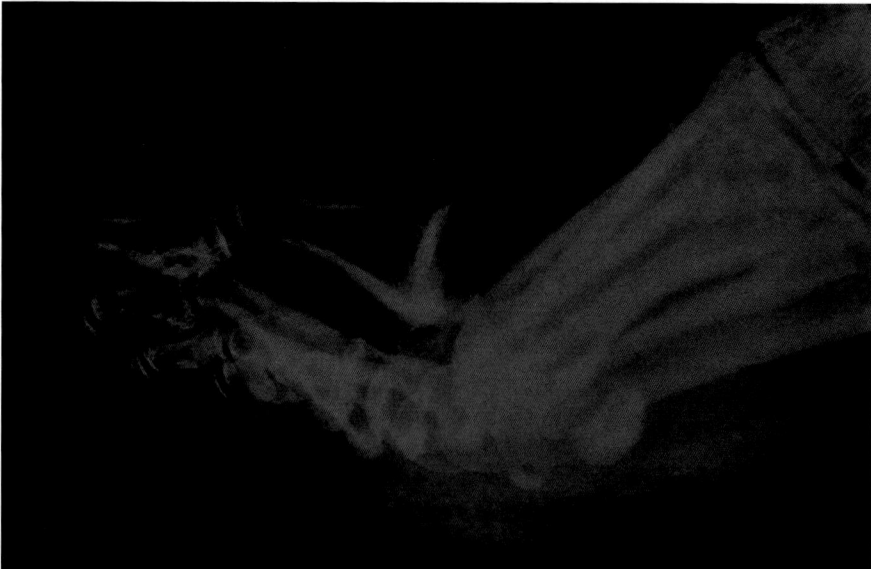

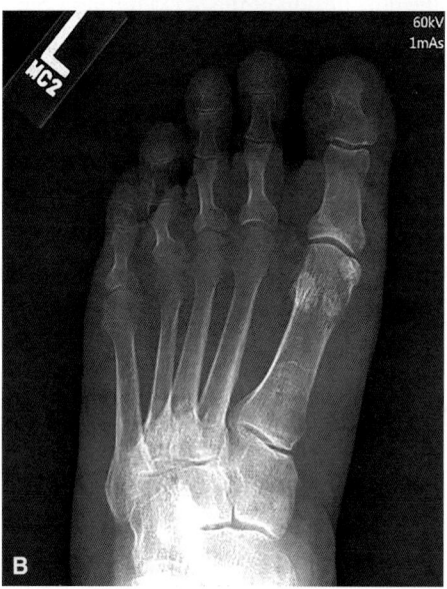

FIGURE 15.8 Sequence of type II Jahss MTPJ dislocation managed with closed reduction. **A.** Injury films demonstrating dorsal dislocation of the hallux with associated fracture of the sesamoid. **B.** Postreduction x-rays.

anteroposterior or lateral radiograph, there will be a dorsal dislocation of the proximal phalanx with a proximal retraction of the sesamoids.[35] Regardless of the classification, long-term sequelae of a first MTPJ can be expected. Adelaar noted the possibility of adhesive capsulitis resulting from excessive scar tissue formation to the plantar capsule-ligamentous structures. In addition, chondral or osteochondral defects can be seen to the first metatarsal head following the dorsal dislocation of the proximal phalanx leading to posttraumatic arthritis of the first MTPJ.

Closed reduction of first MTPJ should be attempted when indicated by the injury pattern. However, acute surgical intervention should be considered when closed reduction attempts are unsuccessful. In addition, Watson et al. recommended surgery for the following associated injuries occurred[36]:

1. Cartilaginous flaps/loose bodies noted within the joint,
2. A fracture or separated bipartite sesamoid lodged within the first MTPJ,

3. The sesamoid apparatus migrates proximally to the first metatarsal neck, and/or
4. Gross instability noted to the joint.[35,36]

> ### PEARLS
> - Patients with acute symptoms or antalgic gait secondary to pain should be immobilized for 6-8 weeks in a removable cam walker or short leg cast with toebox.
> - Goal is to
>   - Reduce mechanical load to the sesamoids
>   - Reduce traction from the attached ligaments and intrinsic muscles
> - Strenuous activities should be avoided until the patient is asymptomatic.
> - Long-term management with appropriate shoes, orthotic therapy, and taping should be anticipated to avoid recurrence.

OPERATIVE TREATMENT FOR SESAMOID CONDITIONS

The surgical management of the more common sesamoid disorders can be managed by partial or complete excision, planing, and bone grafting regardless of the etiology. The only exception is fracture of the sesamoids. This injury may be amenable to open reduction internal fixation or percutaneous pinning.[37]

Sesamoidectomy

Excision of the pathologic sesamoid may involve removal of either the entire tibial or fibular sesamoid, or partial excision in cases of symptomatic bipartite sesamoids or fracture fragments. Aper et al. demonstrated that the effective tendon moment arm of the flexor hallucis brevis did not change significantly with partial and complete removal of the tibial sesamoid.[38] When partial sesamoidectomy is performed, the distal fragment should be removed. This has resulted in good clinical outcomes.[39] In addition, the vascular supply to the sesamoid complex courses in a proximal to distal direction. Maintaining the proximal pole can theoretically result in improved healing.[40,41]

There are several incisional approaches to expose the sesamoids. A straight plantar incision can provide excellent exposure to both sesamoids. However, it is rare to excise both the fibular and tibial sesamoid. More often, the tibial sesamoid is pathologic as previously discussed. This is best approached through a medial approach (Fig. 15.9). Although this can be performed through a plantar medial or dorsomedial incision, the authors recommend a midline approach to preserve the arterial supply to this region[11] and to avoid injury to the proper digital nerve. The capsule is incised along the dorsal edge of the tibial sesamoid. The distal fragment or entire sesamoid is then sharply removed with care take to protect the capsule and flexor hallucis brevis tendon. Any redundant capsular/tendinous tissue should be imbricated in an attempt to prevent a valgus deformity and maintain function of the flexor hallucis brevis tendon.

Excision of the fibular sesamoid can either be performed through a dorsal incision in the first interspace or a plantar incision in the same interspace. The dorsal incision is only recommended when the fibular sesamoid is subluxed from the sesamoid groove, that is hallux valgus deformity. In this approach, blunt dissection is carried down to identify the lateral aspect of the of the first MTPJ complex. A lateral capsulotomy is performed. A hemostat is then inserted into the joint to isolate the fibular suspensory ligament. Once the ligament is transected, the articular surface of the fibular sesamoid comes into view. At this point, a threaded wire or specialized clamp can be used to stabilize the sesamoid, and the entire sesamoid or the distal fragment can be sharply excised (Fig. 15.10).

The plantar incision is placed between the first and second metatarsal head (Fig. 15.11). This keeps the incision from being directly on the weight-bearing surface. Dissection is carried to identify the deep intermetatarsal ligament. This landmark should allow identification of the lateral digital nerve. The nerve is retracted laterally, and the fibular sesamoid is easily identified and removed.

Bone Grafting

In the athletic population, bone grafting may be considered for a nonunion of an acute fracture, stress fracture, or symptomatic disruption of a bipartite sesamoid in order to maintain the intrinsic function of the hallux. Anderson et al. reported on their outcomes and suggested that this procedure is primarily indicated for the tibial sesamoid.[42] The procedure is approached through the medial incision as previously described with care taken to preserve the medial plantar nerve. A linear capsulotomy is performed in the interval between the tibial sesamoid and metatarsal head. At this point, the joint is assessed for any degenerative changes, significant gapping of the fragments, or instability. Any of these findings are contraindications to proceeding with the bone grafting procedure and a partial/total sesamoidectomy should be performed. In the absence of these findings, autologous cancellous bone graft is obtained from the dorsomedial aspect of the first metatarsal head. Subperiosteal dissection is then performed at the site of the nonunion, and the fibrotic tissue is curettaged to expose raw, bleeding bone.

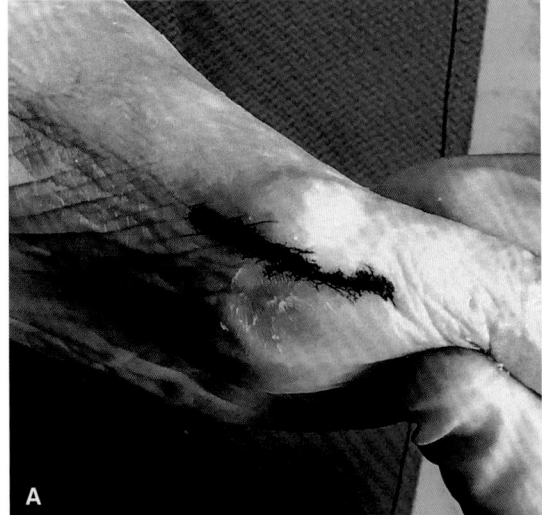

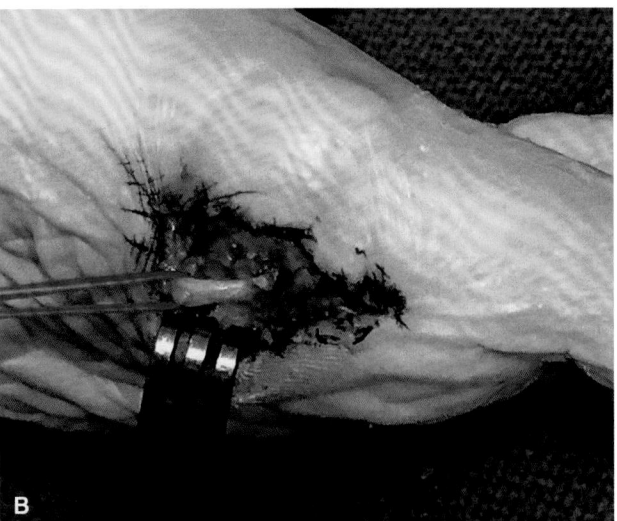

FIGURE 15.9 Medial approach to tibial sesamoid. **A.** Medial midline incision. **B.** Identification of the medial digital proper nerve. Once identified, care should be taken to maintain the nerve within the subcutaneous layer to prevent scarring of the nerve. The remainder of the procedural steps are performed dorsal to the neurovascular bundle.

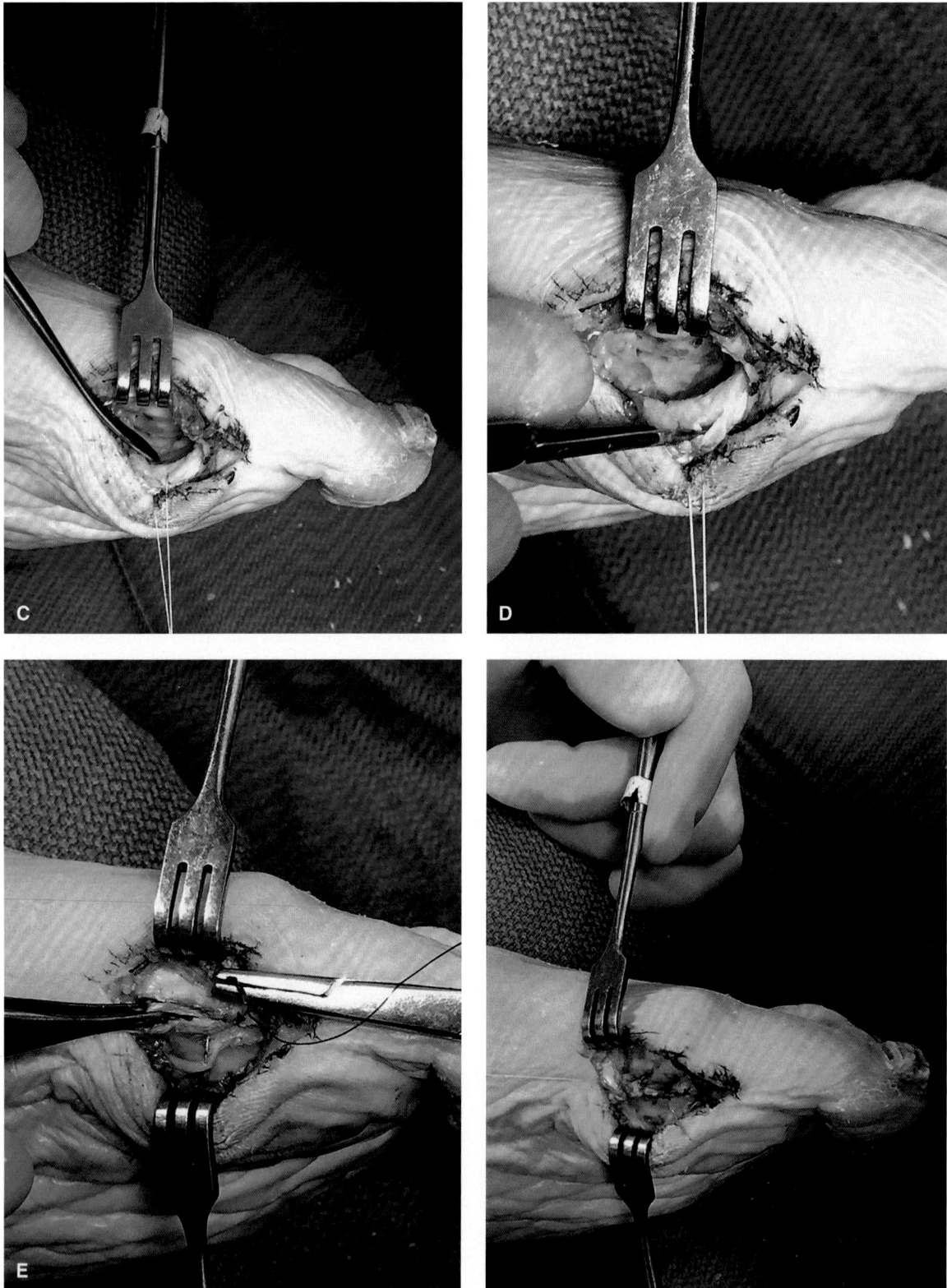

FIGURE 15.9 (*Continued*) **C.** Tibial sesamoid is visualized once the medial capsulotomy is performed. **D.** The sesamoid is excised sharply, reflecting the medial head of the flexor hallucis brevis tendon. **E.** Medial capsule and tendinous structures are imbricated and help maintain first MTPJ function and minimize risk of possible valgus deformity.

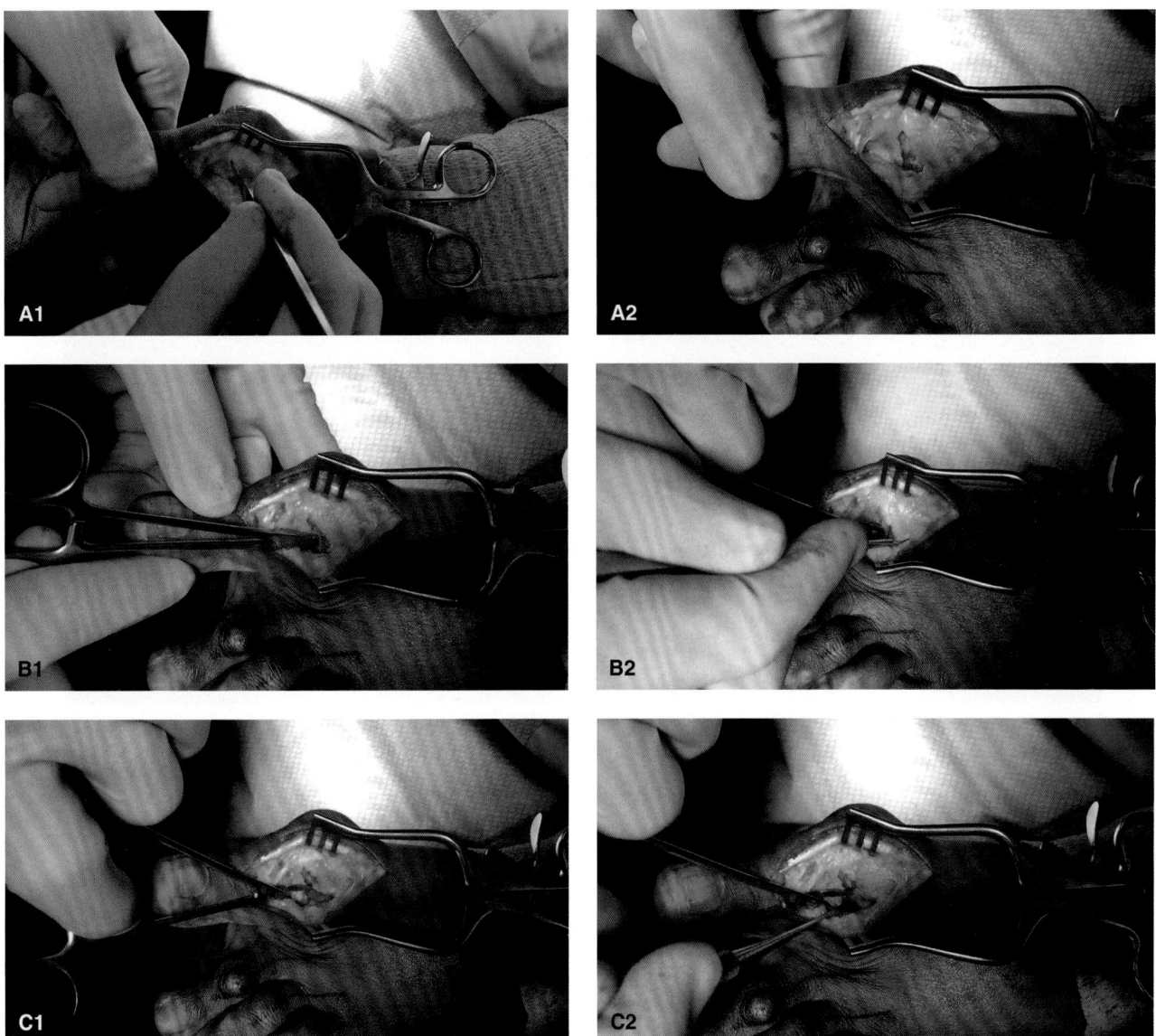

FIGURE 15.10 Dorsal approach to fibular sesamoid. This is the preferred option when there is a preexisting valgus deformity. **A.** Incision is placed through the dorsal aspect of the first interspace. Once the joint is identified, a lateral capsulotomy is performed. **B.** A hemostat is inserted deep to the fibular suspensory ligament, intra-articular. The ligament is then transected. **C.** The hemostat is opened, and the fibular sesamoid is identified. Capsular rebalancing is not generally needed once the sesamoid is removed given a preexisting valgus deformity.

The defect is then packed with the harvested bone, and the periosteal sleeve is reapproximated with suture to contain the bone graft.

First Ray Procedures

In certain cases, the increased load to the sesamoid bones may be a result of structural or dynamic plantarflexion of the first ray. It is essential to identify this during the clinical examination as it may obviate some of the morbidity and complications that may arise from sesamoid procedures. When the plantarflexed ray is structural whether idiopathic, iatrogenic, or posttraumatic, then a dorsiflexory osteotomy can be performed at the base of the first metatarsal. Alternatively, the peroneus longus may have a mechanical advantage in the

subtle cavus foot type. This can result in increased load to the sesamoids during midstance and propulsion, ultimately causing chronic sesamoiditis and stress fractures. If this is recognized during the clinical examination, a peroneus longus to brevis tendon transfer can be performed. The technique involves placing a patient supine with an ipsilateral hip bump to internally rotate the involved extremity. The incision is placed along the posterolateral ankle, just distal to the retromalleolar groove (Fig. 15.12). Dissection is carried to the peroneal tendon sheath. Once the sheath is incised, the peroneus longus and brevis tendon will be identified. Anatomic variation has been described in the literature. The most consistent way to differentiate the tendons is to take the first ray through range of motion while the ankle joint is held in a neutral position. The peroneus longus tendon will be noted to go through

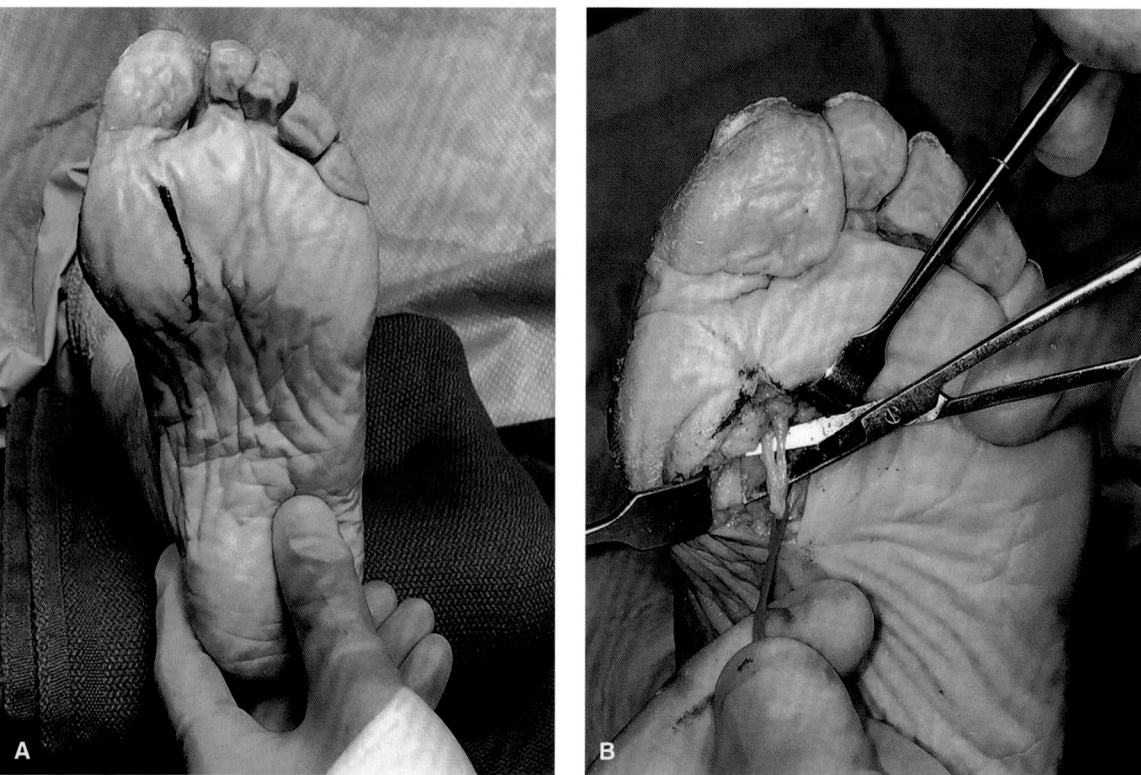

FIGURE 15.11 Plantar approach to the fibular sesamoid. **A.** Plantar incision is placed in the first interspace. **B.** Identify the lateral digital nerve. The remainder of the dissection and capsulotomy is performed medial to the nerve.

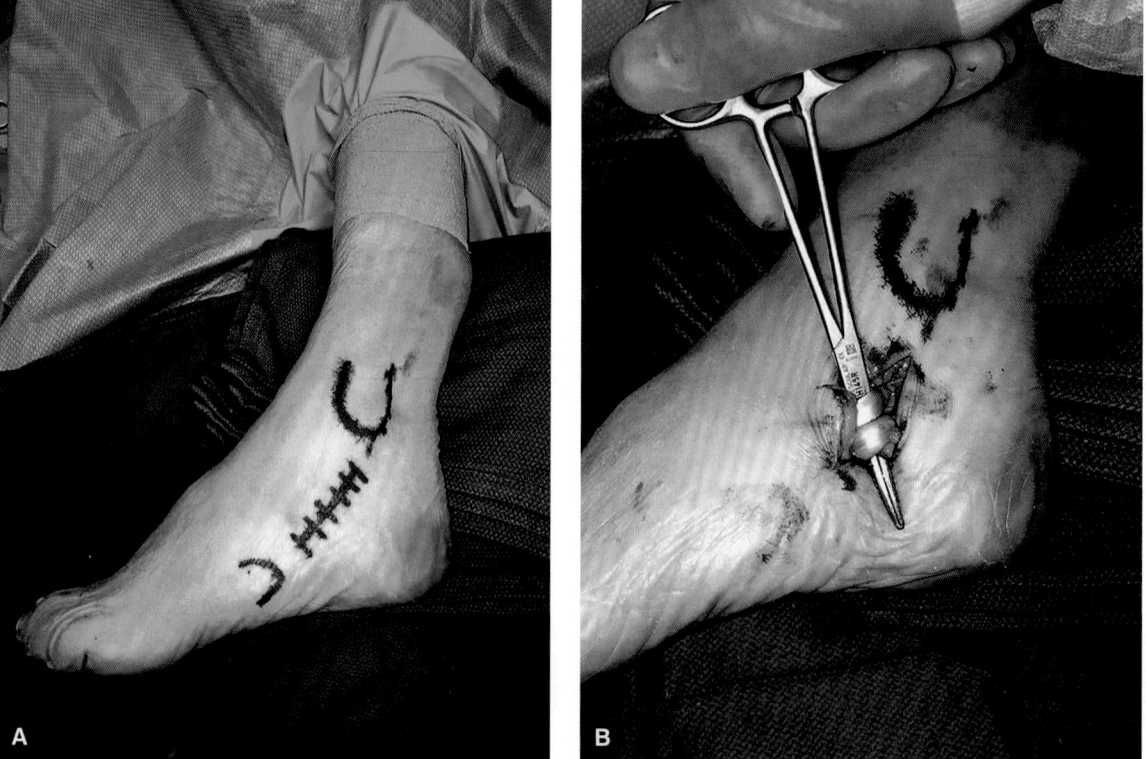

FIGURE 15.12 Peroneus longus to brevis tendon transfer. **A.** Incision is placed directly over the course of the peroneal tendons. **B.** The peroneal tendon sheath is incised, and the tendons are identified.

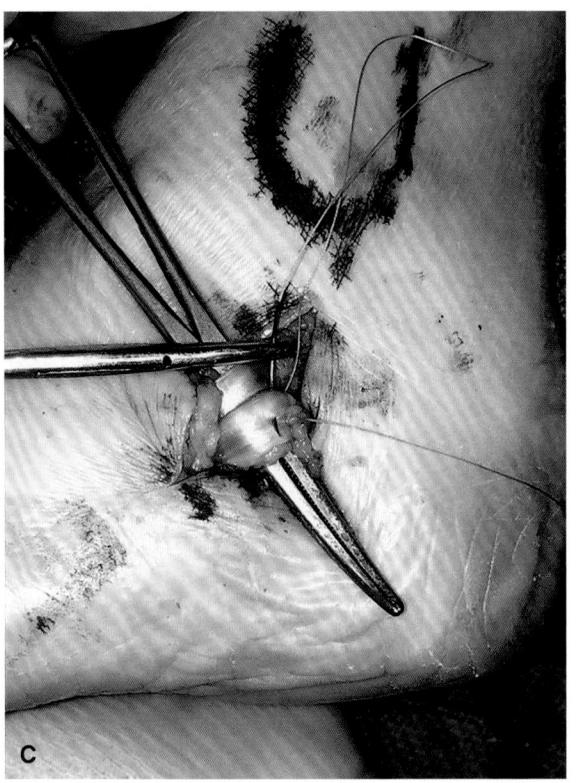

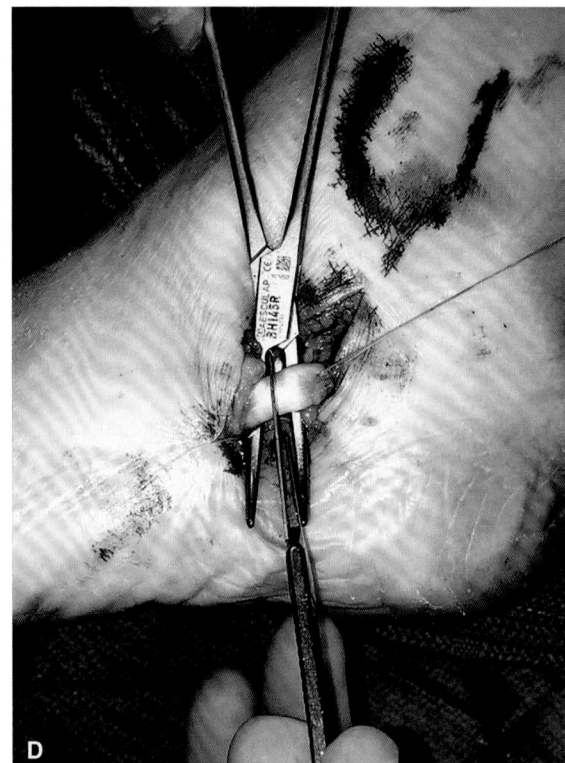

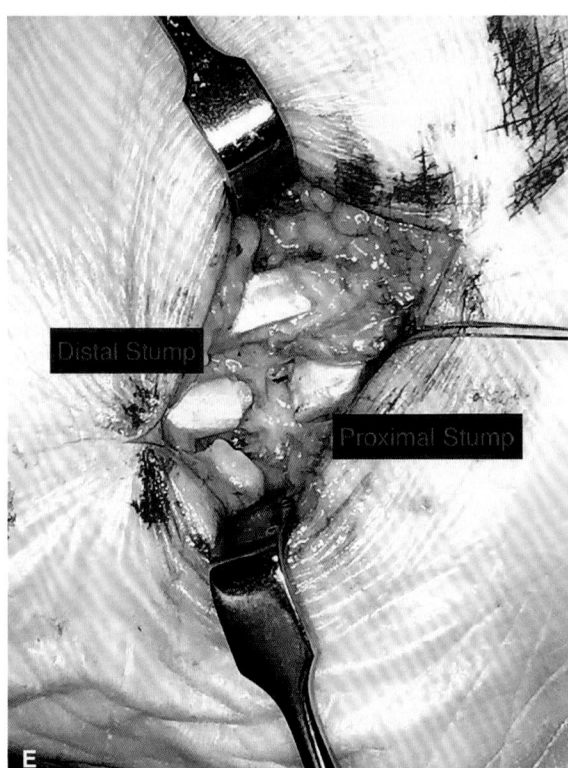

FIGURE 15.12 (*Continued*) **C.** The first ray is taken through range of motion to confirm the peroneus longus tendon. The tendon is then tagged with suture. **D.** The peroneus longus tendon is isolated and a tenotomy is performed. **E.** Once the tenotomy is performed, the first ray is positioned in the sagittal plane in line with the lesser metatarsals. Note the gap that in the peroneus longus tendon. A side to side anastomosis is performed of the proximal and distal stump to the corresponding level of the peroneus brevis tendon.

excursion. At this point, the proximal aspect of the tendon should be tagged with a suture to maintain its identity and prevent proximal migration once the tendon is transected. Next, the tenotomy is performed within the central portion of the exposure. The first ray is then slightly translated dorsally in the sagittal plane to align them evenly with the lesser metatarsals in the frontal plane while the ankle is neutral flexion.

A separation of the peroneus longus tendon stumps should be noted. At this stage, a side to side anastomosis is performed of the proximal and distal stumps of the peroneus longus to the brevis tendon at the corresponding levels. Although a simple tenotomy can also be performed, we prefer to perform the anastomosis to maintain some function of the tendon to stabilize the first ray.

COMPLICATIONS

The more common complications after sesamoidectomy occur as a result of muscular imbalance. Fibular sesamoidectomy can result in a hallux varus deformity, and tibial sesamoidectomy can result in a hallux valgus. Thus, it is critical to be meticulous with the dissection and care must be taken to reapproximate and reinforce defects upon partial or complete removal of sesamoids. Multiple studies have looked at the outcomes of sesamoidectomy procedures and reported good outcomes and return to sports in the athletic population as long as care is taken to balance the hallux upon excision of the sesamoid.[43-45] A systematic review demonstrated that 94.4% of patients returned to sports and 90.0% returned to preinjury level at an average of 12 weeks following sesamoidectomy.[46] In that same study, they also reported an overall complication rate of 22.5%, most of which involved structural deformities of varus/valgus malalignment of the hallux. However, the revision rate was only noted to be 3% at final follow-up.[46] Although not as common, when both sesamoids are removed, a cock up toe may develop.

In addition to structural deformities, these procedures are at risk for persistent neuritic pain postoperatively. The medial digital nerve is at risk during the medial approach to the tibial sesamoid. The nerve lies inferior to the abductor hallucis and is not superficial until the level of the base of the proximal phalanx. Therefore, it is important to identify this nerve and protect it throughout the case to prevent injury and scarring of the nerve. Similarly, the plantar digital nerve can be injured via the plantar lateral approach. The nerve is just lateral to the fibular sesamoid and within the subcutaneous layer. Again, identification and retraction of the nerve can prevent chronic neuritic symptoms.

POSTOPERATIVE MANAGEMENT

The usual postoperative course consists of 10-14 days of non–weight bearing in a posterior splint. The purpose of this is to manage postoperative swelling and reduce the risks of wound complications. Sutures are typically removed around this time and patients are advanced to weight bearing in a walking boot for an additional 4 weeks. During this time, patients will be encouraged to perform passive range of motion of the MTPJ in the sagittal plane to prevent capsular adhesions and scarring

of the sesamoid apparatus. Functional rehabilitation is initiated once the patient can tolerate regular shoes. High impact activities are limited for the first 3 months and are advanced per the patient's level of symptoms.

REFERENCES

1. Mason LW, Molloy AP. Turf toe and disorders of the sesamoid complex. *Clin Sports Med.* 2015;34(4):725-739.
2. Dharap AS, Al-Hashimi H, Kassab S, et al. Incidence and ossification of sesamoid bones in the hands and feet: a radiographic study in an Arab population. *Clin Anat.* 2007;20(4):416-423.
3. Leventen EO. Sesamoid disorders and treatment. An update. *Clin Orthop Relat Res.* 1991;(269):236-240.
4. Sims AL, Kurup HV. Painful sesamoid of the great toe. *World J Orthop.* 2014;5(2):146-150.
5. Munuera PV, Domínguez G, Reina M, et al. Bipartite hallucal sesamoid bones: relationship with hallux valgus and metatarsal index. *Skeletal Radiol.* 2007;36(11):1043-1050.
6. Kanatli U, Oztrk AM, Ercan NG, et al. Absence of the medial sesamoid bone associated with metatarsophalangeal pain. *Clin Anat.* 2006;19(7):634-639.
7. Le Minor JM. Congenital absence of the lateral metatarso-phalangeal sesamoid bone of the human hallux: a case report. *Surg Radiol Anat.* 1999;21(3):225-227.
8. Dennis KJ, McKinney S. Sesamoids and accessory bones of the foot. *Clin Podiatr Med Surg.* 1990;7:717-722.
9. Brenner E, Gruber H, Fritsch H. Fetal development of the first metatarsophalangeal joint complex with special reference to the intersesamoidal ridge. *Ann Anat.* 2002;184(5):481-487.
10. Boike A, Schnirring-Judge M, McMillin S. Sesamoid disorders of the first metatarsophalangeal joint. *Clin Podiatr Med Surg.* 2011;28(2):269-285.
11. Pretterklieber ML, Wanivenhaus A. The arterial supply of the sesamoid bones of the hallux: the course and source of the nutrient arteries as an anatomical basis for surgical approaches to the great toe. *Foot Ankle.* 1992;13(1):27-31.
12. Phisitkul P, Sripongsai R, Chaichankul C, et al. Anatomy of the plantarmedial hallucal nerve in relation to the medial approach of the first metatarsophalangeal joint. *Foot Ankle Int.* 2009;30(6):558-561.
13. Lui TH, Chan KB, Chan LK. Cadaveric study of zone 2 flexor hallucis longus tendon sheath. *Arthroscopy.* 2010;26(6):808-812.
14. Stokes IA, Hutton WC, Stott JR, et al. Forces under the hallux valgus foot before and after surgery. *Clin Orthop Relat Res.* 1979;142:64-72.
15. Nigg BM. Biomechanical aspects of running. In: Nigg BM, ed. *Biomechanics of Running Shoes.* Champaign, IL: Human Kinetics Publishers; 1986:1-25.
16. Dedmond BT, Cory JW, McBryde A. The hallucal sesamoid complex. *J Am Acad Orthop Surg.* 2006;14:745-753.
17. Shereff MJ, Bejjani FJ, Kummer FJ. Kinematics of the first metatarsophalangeal joint. *J Bone Joint Surg Am.* 1986;68:392-398.
18. Julsrud ME. Osteonecrosis of the tibial and fibular sesamoids in an aerobics instructor. *J Foot Ankle Surg.* 1997;36:31-35.
19. Scranton PE Jr. Pathologic anatomic variations in the sesamoids. *Foot Ankle.* 1981;1:321-326.
20. Pinto RR, Freitas D, Massada M. Hallux sesamoid osteonecrosis associated to ballet: literature review. *Rev Port Ortop Traum.* 2010;18(4):429-437.
21. Bartosiak K, McCormick JJ. Avascular necrosis of the sesamoids. *Foot Ankle Clin.* 2019;24(1):57-67.
22. Favinger JL, Porrino JA, Richardsopn ML, et al. Epidemiology and imaging appearance of the normal bi-/multipartite hallux sesamoid bone. *Foot Ankle Int.* 2015;36(2):197-202.
23. Prieskorn D, Graves SC, Smith RA. Morphometric analysis of the plantar plate apparatus of the first metatarsophalangeal joint. *Foot Ankle.* 1993;14(4):204-207.
24. Sanders TG, Rathur SK. Imaging of painful conditions of the hallucal sesamoid complex and plantar capsular structures of the first metatarsophalangeal joint. *Radiol Clin North Am.* 2008;46(6):1079-1092.
25. Dietrich TJ, da Silva FL, de Abreu MR, et al. First metatarsophalangeal joint- MRI findings in asymptomatic volunteers. *Eur Radiol.* 2015;25(4):970-979.
26. Crain JM, Phancao JP, Stidham K. MR imaging of turf toe. *Magn Reson Imaging Clin N Am.* 2008;16(1):93-103, vi. doi: 10.1016/j.mric.2008.02.002.
27. Schein AJ, Skalski MR, Patel DB, et al. Turf toe and sesamoiditis: what the radiologist needs to know. *Clin Imaging.* 2015;39(3):380-389.
28. Sharma P, Singh H, Agarwal KK, et al. Utility of (99m)Tc-MDP SPECT-CT for the diagnosis of sesamoiditis as cause of metatarsalgia. *Nucl Med.* 2012;27(1):45-47.
29. Chisin R, Peyser A, Milgrom C. Bone scintigraphy in the assessment of the hallucal sesamoids. *Foot Ankle Int.* 1995;16(5):291-294.
30. Barral CM, Félix AM, Magalhães LN, et al. The bone scintigraphy as a complementary exam in the diagnosis of the avascular necrosis of the sesamoid. *Rev Bras Ortop.* 2015;47(2):241-245.
31. Waldrop NE III, Zirker CA, Wijdicks CA, et al. Radiographic evaluation of plantar plate injury: an in vitro biomechanical study. *Foot Ankle Int.* 2013;34(3):403-408.
32. Cohen BE. Hallux sesamoid disorders. *Foot Ankle Clin.* 2009;14(1):91-104.
33. George E, Harris AH, Dragoo JL, et al. Incidence and risk factors for turf toe injuries in intercollegiate football: data from the national collegiate athletic association injury surveillance system. *Foot Ankle Int.* 2014;35(2):108-115.
34. Kadakia AR, Molloy A. Current concepts review: traumatic disorders of the first metatarsophalangeal joint and sesamoid complex. *Foot Ankle Int.* 2011;32(8):834-839.
35. Edwards CC, Malay CD. Dorsal dislocation of the first metatarsophalangeal joint: Review of the literature and case presentation of a Jahss Type III injury with rationale for surgical repair. Decatur, GA: The Podiatry Institute; 2003:320-325.

36. Watson TS, Anderson RB, Davis WH. Periarticular injuries to the hallux metatarsophalangeal joint in athletes. *Foot Ankle Clin.* 2000;5(3):687-713.

37. Blundell CM, Nicholson P, Blackney MW. Percutaneous screw fixation for fractures of the sesamoid bones of the hallux. *J Bone Joint Surg Br.* 2002;84:1138-1141.

38. Aper RL, Saltzman CL, Brown TD. The effect of hallux sesamoid resection on the effective moment of the flexor hallucis brevis. *Foot Ankle Int.* 1994;5:462-470.

39. Rodeo SA, Warren RF, O'Brien SJ, et al. Diastasis of bipartite sesamoids of the first metatarsophalangeal joint. *Foot Ankle.* 1993;14:425-434.

40. Chamberland PDC, Smith JW, Fleming LL. The blood supply to the great toe sesamoids. *Foot Ankle.* 1993;14:435-442.

41. Sobel M, Hashimoto J, Amoczky SP, et al. The microvasculature of the sesamoid complex: its clinical significance. *Foot Ankle.* 1992;13:359-363.

42. Anderson RB, McBryde AM Jr. Autogenous bone grafting of hallux sesamoid nonunions. *Foot Ankle Int.* 1997;18:293-296.

43. Saxena A, Krisdakumtorn T. Return to activity after sesamoidectomy in athletically active individuals. *Foot Ankle Int.* 2003;24(5):415-419.

44. Lee S, James WC, Cohen BE, et al. Evaluation of hallux alignment and functional outcome after isolated tibial sesamoidectomy. *Foot Ankle Int.* 2005;26(10):803-809.

45. Bichara DA, Henn RK, Theodore GH. Sesamoidectomy for hallux sesamoid fractures. *Foot Ankle Int.* 2012;33(9):704-706.

46. Shimozono Y, Hurley ET, Brown AJ, et al. Sesamoidectomy of hallux sesamoid disorders: a systematic review. *J Foot Ankle Surg.* 2018;57:1186-1190.

CHAPTER 16

Hallux Varus

Sara E. Lewis and Alan S. Banks

DEFINITION

Hallux adductus is a simple transverse plane deformity, whereby the great toe is deviated medially. Hallux varus generally refers to those patients with more advanced conditions, whereby the hallux is deviated medially and dorsiflexes at the metatarsal phalangeal joint. There is often an associated contracture at the hallux interphalangeal joint and impaired stability of the hallux.[1,2] However, most surgeons use the term hallux varus to refer to a medially deviated great toe regardless as to the severity or associated deformity.

CLASSIFICATION

The American College of Foot and Ankle Surgeons developed a clinical practice guideline for hallux varus that included a classification system based on the degree of deformity and the presence or absence of associated joint arthrosis.[2]

ACFAS CLASSIFICATION OF HALLUX VARUS

- Type 1—Adduction of the metatarsophalangeal joint
  - A, Deformity alone
  - B, Deformity plus arthritis
- Type 2—Adduction of the metatarsophalangeal joint with flexion contracture of the interphalangeal joint
  - A, Deformity alone
  - B, Deformity plus arthrosis
- Type 3—Complex multiplane deformity

To date, this appears to be the most sensible approach to classification, although most surgeons generally do not follow specific classification systems in their evaluations in a strict sense.

ANATOMIC FEATURES AND FUNCTIONAL ANALYSIS OF THE ANATOMY

In the simplest of terms, hallux abducto valgus deformity represents a loss of the normal balance of forces about the first metatarsal phalangeal joint such that those oriented laterally predominate. Surgical repair of hallux abducto valgus is designed to restore the normal balance at the joint. Over time and through experience, surgeons develop an appreciation for the techniques and approaches that are most reliable in their hands. However, like so many things, perfection is a goal that is never fully realized, and some patients will suffer from less than optimal alignment postoperatively. Complicating the process of restoring normal joint balance is the fact that the foot is a dynamic weight-bearing structure, yet surgery is performed in a static non–weight-bearing setting. Following surgery, if the balance of forces around the first metatarsal phalangeal joint is more medially oriented, then one may witness the development of a hallux varus.

PATHOGENESIS

Hallux varus most commonly is seen following repair of a hallux valgus deformity. Other causes of hallux varus are congenital, traumatic, arthritides, or neuromuscular disease.[1,2]

Pathogenesis

- Iatrogenic hallux valgus deformity
- Congenital
- Traumatic
- Arthritides
- Neuromuscular disease

IMAGING AND DIAGNOSTIC STUDIES

There are a number of factors that may be of importance when considering surgical repair of hallux varus. Joint congruity, presence or absence of arthrosis, position and status of the sesamoids, and bone quality are specific concerns when reviewing radiographs. In most patients with hallux varus, the previous surgery will usually have involved some form of first metatarsal osteotomy. Depending on overall alignment, the surgeon may need to consider some type of reverse osteotomy in order to increase the intermetatarsal angle, particularly if there is a negative intermetatarsal angle. However, the width of the first metatarsal head may limit the capacity of the surgeon to perform reverse osteotomy of the distal metatarsal if there was an aggressive resection of bone previously. In some patients, a malunion of the osteotomy may have resulted in shortening or other structural aberrations of the bone that may need to be addressed for successful repair of the hallux varus. Hallux malleus deformity is seen at times in conditions when the deformity is more severe or of greater duration. In some instances, joint salvage may not be possible without sufficient bone quality or quantity, suitable articular integrity, in the presence of hallux limitus/rigidus, or the reasonable potential to restore some semblance of normal anatomy in more advanced or rigid deformities. Medial deviation of the lesser toes is also present in some patients and generally will require concomitant surgical repair.

TREATMENT

PATIENT CONCERN

Clinicians will see an interesting spectrum of patients who present with hallux varus. For patients with a mild flexible deformity, the complaints may not be related to the hallux varus but to other unrelated conditions. However, as the hallux varus persists, and more so with advancing deformity, pain may develop secondary to shoe irritation or pain at the first metatarsal phalangeal joint due to malalignment. Patients who possess more fixed or rigid deformities are more likely to suffer from joint pain or direct irritation of the toe. Many patients will tend to develop secondary problems due to the abnormal alignment at the first metatarsal phalangeal joint; most notable is the medial deviation of the lesser toes at the metatarsal phalangeal joint level. Once a hallux malleus develops, the primary concern may be dorsal irritation at the interphalangeal joint when wearing shoes or symptoms related to increased weight-bearing pressure beneath the first metatarsal head associated with the retrograde forces from the elevated hallux. Joint symptoms, and some degree of first metatarsal phalangeal joint arthritis, may eventually develop in patients with more persistent deformity or in situations where there is associated hallux limitus.

CONSERVATIVE TREATMENT

Asymptomatic patients who present at some remote interval after their surgery and with mild or flexible deformity may require no active treatment. One study found that patients with only advanced degrees of hallux varus were dissatisfied with their outcome for repair of the original hallux valgus deformity.[3] Periodic monitoring may be a reasonable approach to identify any adverse changes that might develop in the future. This may involve serial x-rays to assess the status of the first metatarsal phalangeal joint. If symptoms develop involving the medial hallux secondary to shoe pressure, then some type of taping or light splinting may also be reasonable. Similar splinting approaches and shoe modifications may be employed for patients with greater degrees of deformity as well, but generally as the deformity advances, the success with conservative care diminishes. In patients who present with hallux varus early in the postoperative period, surgeons may employ valgus bandaging or splinting of the hallux along with monitoring of the joint alignment.[1,2,4,5]

SURGICAL TREATMENT

Surgical Options
- Osseous procedures
- Soft tissue procedures
- Arthrodesis
- Implants
- Arthroplasty

The timing of surgical intervention is based on many factors. In patients with hallux varus identified in the early postoperative interval, a more rapid revision surgery may provide a good opportunity to restore more normal joint alignment. If performed in the first 2 or 3 weeks, then there is the added benefit of limiting the ultimate recovery interval as opposed to the patient undergoing a separate intervention at a later date. However, this is not without concern, as in many instances the soft tissue and osseous segments will be more difficult to manipulate and achieving suitable correction may be more elusive than imagined at this earlier interval. Depending on the timing and situation, there are circumstances where revision surgery may be more reliable after the bone has healed, soft tissue induration has resolved, and swelling has diminished.

In patients with more chronic conditions, the presence of a painful process attributed to the hallux varus is a frequent reason for intervention. However, there are situations in which one may need to consider surgical repair of the hallux varus even with absent or more limited direct symptoms. If there is evidence of adverse change at the joint level, then surgical intervention may be considered in an attempt to prevent more rapid development of joint arthrosis. In other patients, surgical intervention of the hallux varus may be needed as part of the overall correction of other symptomatic forefoot deformities involving the lesser toes or metatarsophalangeal joints. Adverse changes in the alignment of the lesser metatarsophalangeal joints would be a reasonable indication for repair of hallux varus, with or without symptoms at the first metatarsal phalangeal joint, before progression of deformity reaches a stage whereby more advanced and aggressive intervention may be required.

INITIAL DISSECTION

Surgical dissection for repair of hallux varus deformity is more difficult due to the disruption of normal tissue planes that is anticipated with the scarring that follows any surgery. The surgeon may find that making a slightly longer incision than the existing scar, beginning the dissection in normal tissue planes, then extending into the scarred first metatarsal phalangeal joint area, facilitates dissection.

When joint salvage is contemplated, the first component of repair for hallux varus is to perform a soft tissue release about the joint.[6] This is the same philosophy employed in the repair of hallux valgus. The sequential evaluation begins at the medial aspect of the joint to identify and release those structures, which have an adverse effect on the alignment of the toe. Once the subcutaneous tissues have been separated medially from the capsule and periosteum, then the surgeon must decide how they would prefer to perform the medial capsular incision, with an awareness that as the hallux is abducted into a corrected position the medial capsule will advance. Therefore, in order to assure sufficient coverage of the joint following relocation of the hallux to the corrected position, one must plan for capsular advancement or lengthening. Techniques that have been advocated in the past include a U-shaped flap, a V-Y advancement, or a Z-plasty[6] (Figs. 16.1 and 16.2). Once the capsule has been dissected free and released, the surgeon can assess whether or not the abductor hallucis tendon needs to be lengthened or released. In some instances, the medial segment of the short flexor tendon between the distal aspect of the tibial sesamoid and the base of the proximal phalanx may require release as well. At this point, one may also assess the joint to determine the quality of the articular surface.

The next step is to evaluate the first interspace and determine if there are adhesions or scarring that limits the mobility of the first metatarsal in the transverse plane. Any tissue that is felt to be restrictive is released, and the joint position and alignment can be reassessed. At this stage, the surgeon may also elect to create an inverted L capsular incision in the lateral capsule that will facilitate tightening of the lateral tissues so as to help in the reduction or maintenance of correction.

The surgeon can evaluate the joint structures further to ensure that there are no other areas of concern as far as soft tissue restriction or maintenance of deformity. Joint alignment and mobility can be assessed and additional techniques to further enhance correction can be entertained. It is important to load the foot to simulate weight bearing and to move the great toe joint through range of motion to confirm adequate correction.

PEARLS

- Begin surgical incision proximal to previous incision so that you can develop good soft tissue planes through dissection.
- Even with bony procedures, you must balance soft tissues appropriately.

SOFT TISSUE TECHNIQUES

Perhaps the simplest soft tissue technique for help in maintaining correction in mild flexible deformities is tightening the lateral capsular structures in combination with advancement of the medial capsule. This may also be combined with any other more advanced techniques to further enhance correction. Beyond that there are a number of tendon transfer methods that have been described to provide additional support and correctional forces for hallux varus. Soft tissue techniques to repair flexible hallux varus have been reported to provide good results with few complications.[7]

The extensor hallucis longus (EHL) tendon transfer has been utilized to correct a varus deformity by aiding in plantarflexion and lateral pull of the hallux. The original description of the technique involved detachment of the EHL at its distal insertion, re-routing the tendon beneath the deep transverse intermetatarsal ligament in the first intermetatarsal space, and attachment of the extensor tendon into the plantar lateral aspect of the proximal phalanx. An interphalangeal joint fusion is an adjunct procedure used to prevent mallet toe due to the unopposed pull of the flexor hallucis longus.[8] The modified split EHL tendon transfer involves release of the lateral half of the EHL at the proximal first metatarsal, maintaining the full insertion at the interphalangeal joint. The tendon is then re-routed from distal to proximal under the deep intermetatarsal ligament and attached to the first metatarsal via a drill hole as a tenodesis.[9] The same type of transfer has also been described utilizing the extensor hallucis brevis tendon.[10] However, with all of the extensor tendon transfers, there must be an intact deep transverse intermetatarsal ligament, and this may not be the case in patients with a prior lateral release with the original bunion procedure.[1]

The abductor hallucis tendon can also been transferred to enhance lateral joint stability and correction of deformity. The tendon may be transferred dorsally across the metatarsal head and beneath the EHL and sutured into the lateral joint

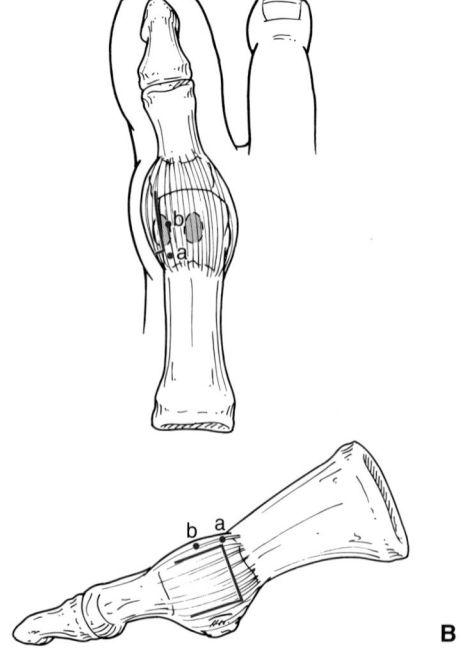
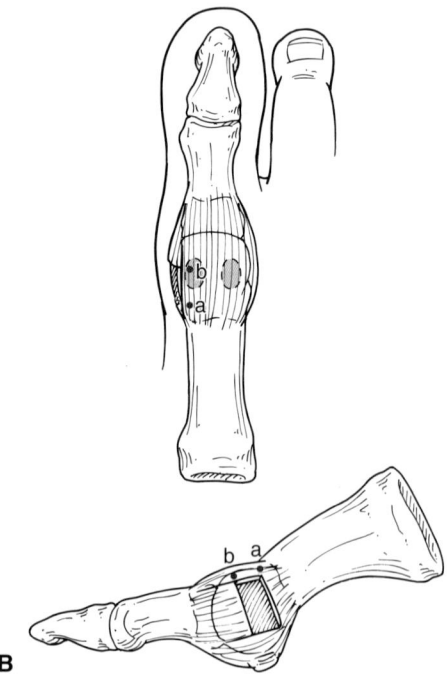

FIGURE 16.1 **A.** U-shaped medial capsular incision with the vertical arm at point *a*. **B.** Following correction of the deformity with abduction of the hallux, the capsule has advanced and will be closed in this position *b*. This leaves a small section of the first metatarsal exposed. Failure to make the vertical incision proximal to the joint will result in the residual exposure of the metatarsal joint space.

A

B

capsule.[6] Others have advocated a transfer plantarly between the metatarsal head and the short flexor tendon.[11] It may be anchored into the lateral capsule or the base of the proximal phalanx laterally.

An implantable suture-endobutton fixation technique has been used in correction of hallux varus along with other foot and ankle procedures. After a medial capsule release has been performed, bone tunnels are created through the proximal phalanx and metatarsal. Tension is applied to the tightrope

intraoperatively to ensure plantarflexion and lateral pull of the hallux leading to correct positioning of the hallux at the metatarsal phalangeal joint[12,13] (Fig. 16.3).

As a general rule, many surgeons prefer to avoid resection of the tibial sesamoid if joint salvage is preferred and possible. Usually sufficient liberation of the soft tissues will obviate the need for this approach. However, there may be patients where this could provide sufficient reduction of deformity in combination with the other components of the joint release. This may

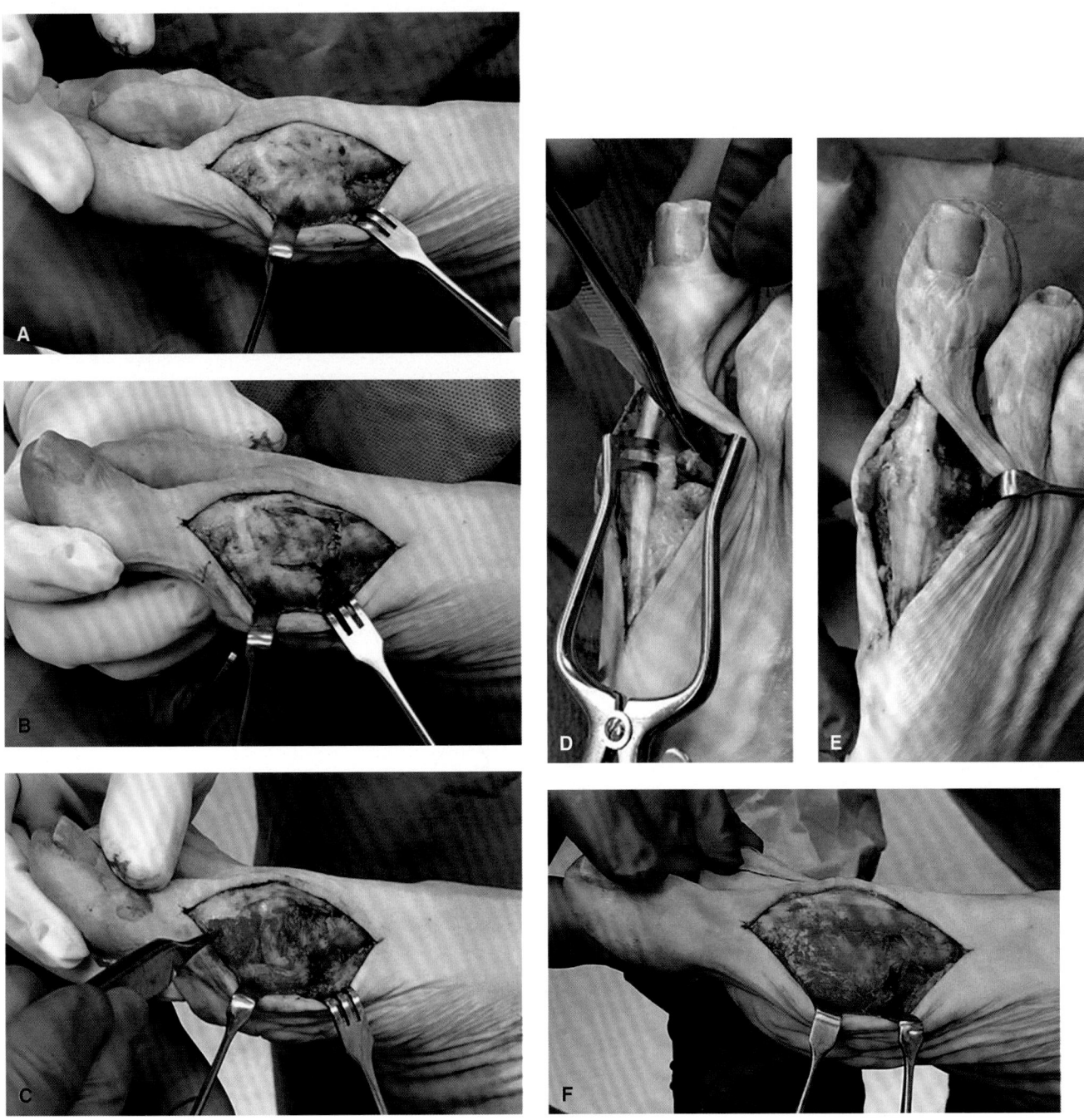

FIGURE 16.2 **A.** First MPJ dissection for hallux varus. **B.** Exposure of the medial capsule of the first MPJ. A U-shaped capsular incision is made on the medial aspect of the MPJ. **C.** Reflection of the medial capsular flap and exposure of the joint. **D.** Incision of the lateral capsule in an inverted L fashion to facilitate lateral tightening. **E.** After tightening the lateral joint capsule. **F.** Following medial capsular closure. Note the exposed area of bone proximally following capsular advancement for correction of deformity.

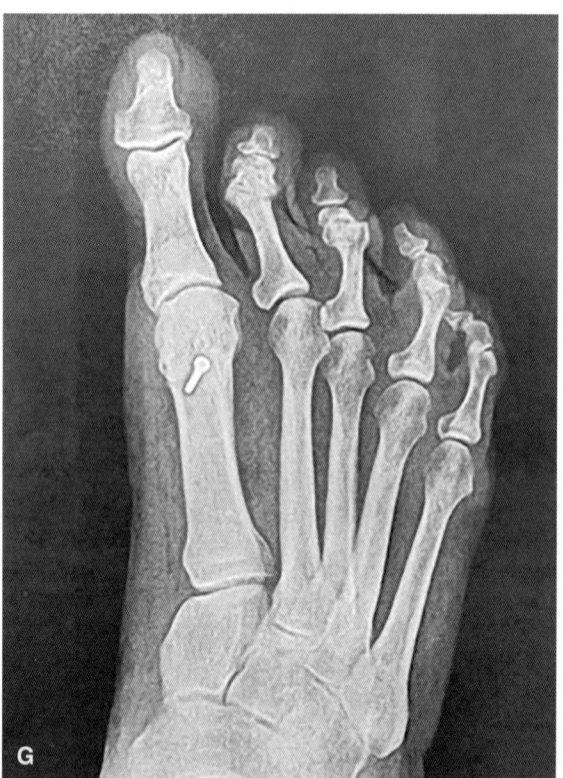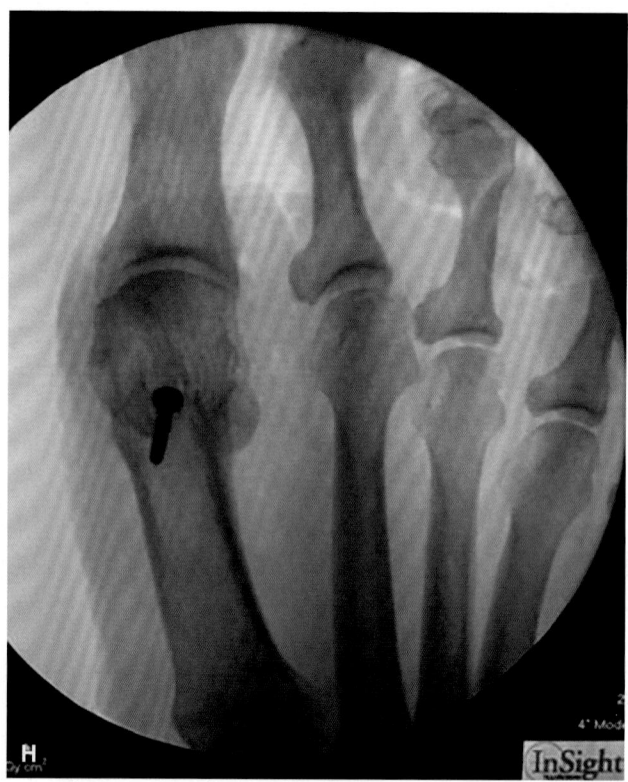

FIGURE 16.2 (*Continued*) **G.** Preoperative AP radiograph demonstrated a hallux varus.
H. Postoperative AP radiograph demonstrated correction of hallux varus with soft tissue procedure.

be a consideration in older patients where additional osteotomy might pose a greater risk due to bone quality. It may also be a consideration in an attempt to avoid more proximal osteotomy in patients with a narrow metatarsal head where non–weight bearing would be more difficult.

OSSEOUS PROCEDURES

In patients with a more resistant deformity, or cases where there is a structural problem relative to a negative intermetatarsal angle, an osteotomy may be quite helpful in restoring more normal joint balance.[1,6,12,14,15] In many instances, the options for

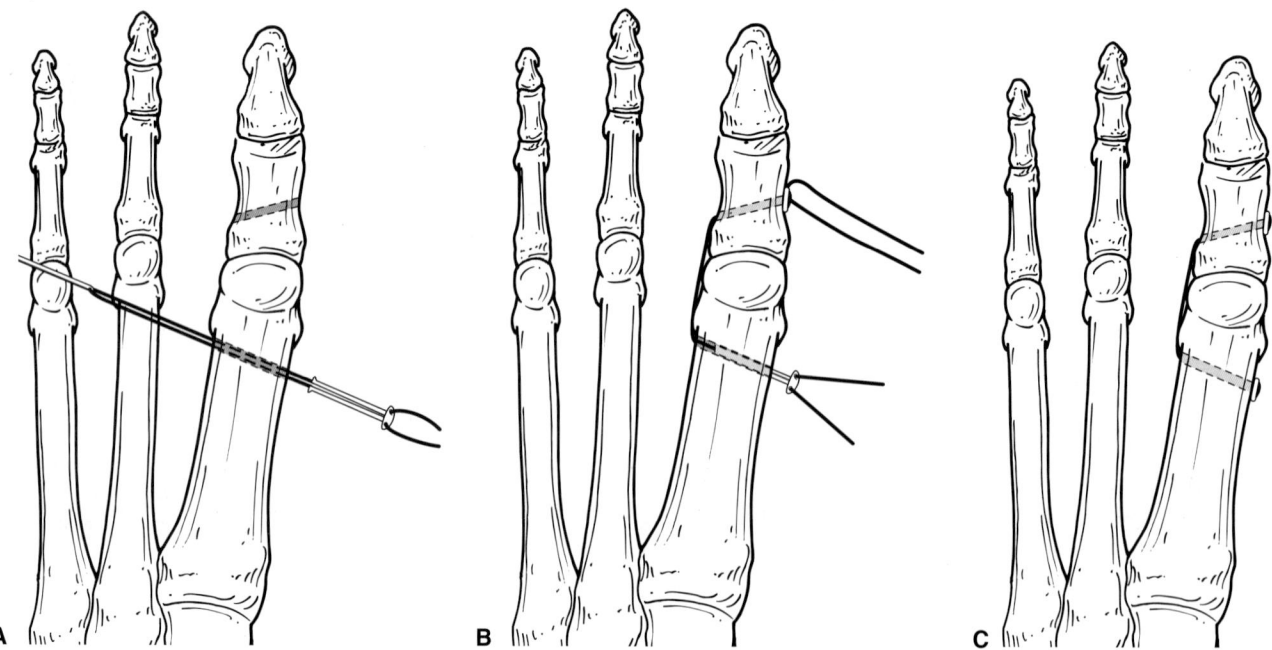

FIGURE 16.3 A-C. Use of an suture button device to repair hallux varus.

osseous procedures are the same type of osteotomy as would be performed for hallux valgus, just in reverse—with the net effect of increasing the intermetatarsal angle. However, the risk is that there may be increased prominence of the medial head of the metatarsal, or a new "bunion."

A reverse Austin osteotomy is a good stable option for many patients if the metatarsal head is of sufficient width (Fig. 16.4). If the articular surface of the metatarsal head is deviated, then a reverse Reverdin type of osteotomy may be helpful as well. In patients with significant shortening of the metatarsal, or where the metatarsal head is not of sufficient width for distal osteotomy, then a proximal or shaft osteotomy may be of benefit. Procedures may consist of variations of the Scarf, which will allow medial rotation of the distal segment with lengthening if needed. If sagittal plane orientation is a problem, then a sagittal Z osteotomy may be used to lengthen and elevate the metatarsal.

ARTHRODESIS OF THE FIRST METATARSAL PHALANGEAL JOINT

Fusion of the first metatarsal phalangeal joint offers many potential advantages for patients with hallux varus. The procedure is reliable and provides permanent correction. There is no concern for attempting to rebalance forces at the joint, and any potential issues with current or subsequent joint arthrosis are eliminated.[1,12,16,17]

IMPLANTS

The potential problem with implants in patients with hallux varus is the same in using these devices for hallux valgus. The implant itself does not provide for correction of deformity, and if placed into a joint without appropriate rebalancing of deforming forces, then the hallux varus will persist or recur. However, using these devices in combination with other techniques may be an option for patients who hope to avoid fusion.

KELLER ARTHROPLASTY

The Keller arthroplasty, or modifications thereof,[18] may be a reasonable approach in older patients with significant arthritis or in cases where there is a long hallux. This may be an alternative for patients who do not want to undergo fusion of the joint and desire some residual mobility. Maintenance of correction can be enhanced by using a K-wire to maintain (stabilize instead of maintain as you already used the word maintenance) the hallux in a corrected position for 4-6 weeks postoperatively. Anchoring the flexor hallucis longus tendon into the base of the proximal phalanx may also enhance hallux stability.

POSTOPERATIVE MANAGEMENT

The postoperative course varies depending on the procedure selection and surgical methods. Generally, this is consistent with the care provided for patients undergoing similar osteotomy types, fusion, or other procedures as would be employed for repair of hallux valgus deformity.

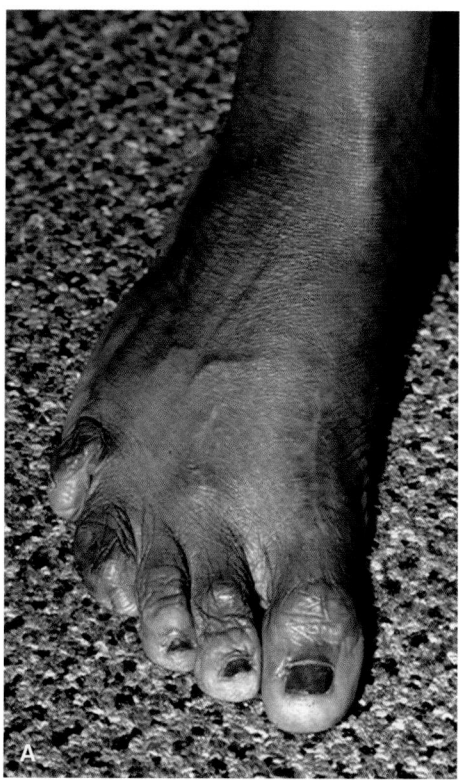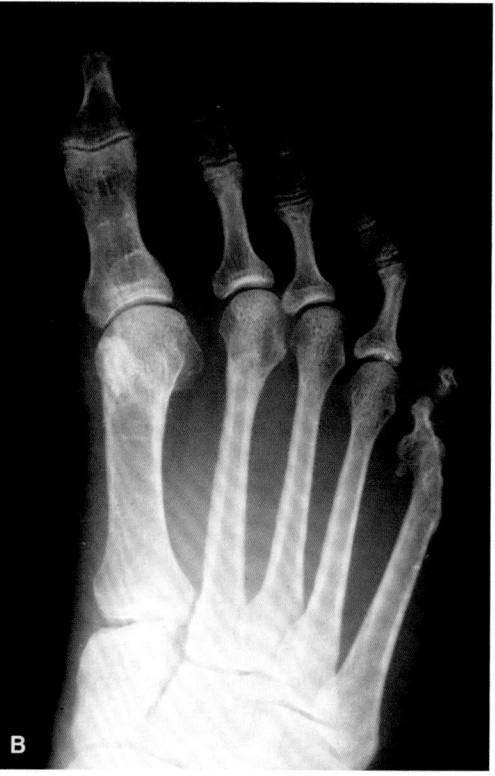

FIGURE 16.4 Preop clinical **(A)** and preop radiographic **(B)** appearance of a patient with hallux. varus.

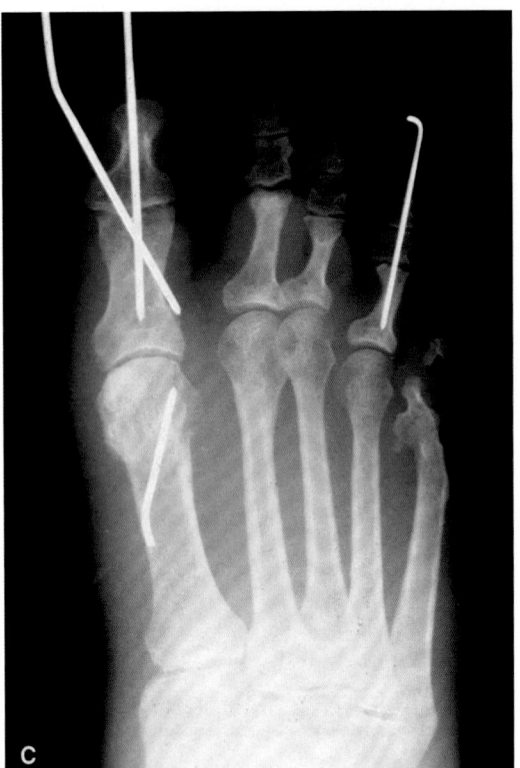

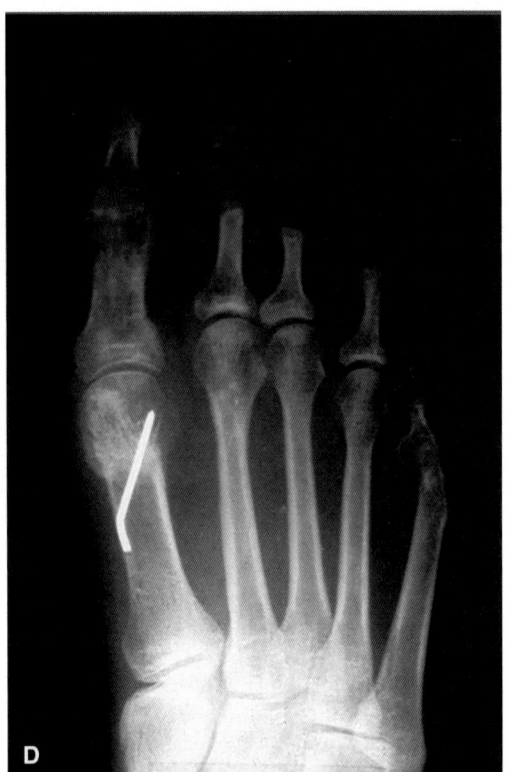

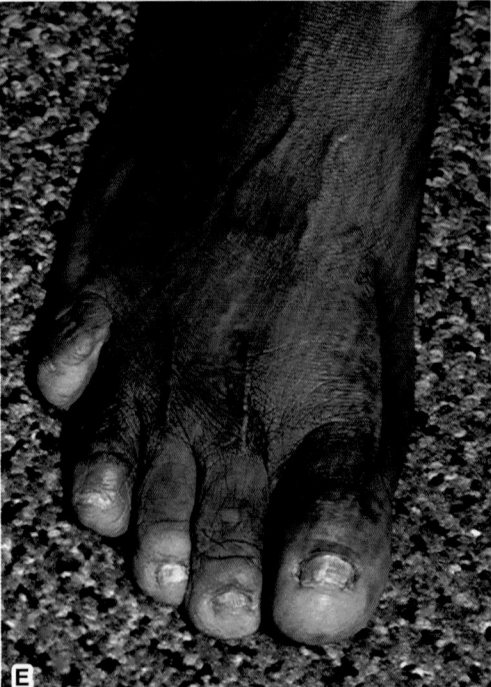

FIGURE 16.4 (*Continued*) **C.** Immediate postop view after reverse Austin procedure, hallux IPJ fusion, and soft tissue releases of the second and third MPJ. **D, E.** Following healing.

COMPLICATIONS

The common complications associated with hallux varus surgery include overcorrection with hallux valgus formation, undercorrection with failure to adequately resolve the deformity, and joint stiffness leading to arthrosis. Scar adhesions are not uncommon, especially if the surgery is a revision, and limited range of motion may be subsequently be noted.

PERILS and PITFALLS

- Recurrence after repair
- Overcorrection
- Further degeneration of the joint
- Continued pain
- Recurrence of scarring
- Limited range of motion

REFERENCES

1. Judge MA. Hallux varus. In: Southerland JT, Boberg JS, Downey MS, Nakra A, Rabjohn L, eds. *McGlamry's Comprehensive Textbook of Foot and Ankle Surgery*. 4th ed. Philadelphia, PA: Wolters Kluwer/Lippincott Williams & Wilkins; 2013:461-468.
2. Vanore JV, Christensen JC, Kravitz SR, et al.; Diagnosis and Treatment of first Metatarsophalangeal Joint Disorders. Section 3: Hallux varus. Clinical practice guideline first metatarsophalangeal joint disorders Panel of the American College of Foot and Ankle Surgeons. *J Foot Ankle Surg*. 2003;42(3):137-142.
3. Trnka HJ, Zettl R, Hungerford M, Muhlbauer M, Ritschl P. Acquired hallux varus and clinical tolerability. *Foot Ankle Int*. 1997;18(9):593-597.
4. Skalley TC, Myerson MS. The operative treatment of acquired hallux varus. *Clin Orthop Relat Res*. 1994;306:183-191.
5. Davies M, Blundell C. The treatment of iatrogenic hallux varus. *Foot Ankle Clin*. 2014;19(2):275-284.
6. Banks AS, Ruch JA, Kalish SR. Surgical Repair of hallux varus. *J Am Podiatr Med Assoc*. 1988;78(7):339-347.
7. Plovanich E, Donnenwerth M, Abicht B, Borkosky S, Jacobs P, Roukis T. Failure after soft-tissue release with tendon transfer for flexible iatrogenic hallux varus: a systematic review. *J Foot Ankle Surg*. 2012;51(2):195-197.
8. Johnson KA, Spiegl PV. Extensor hallucis longus transfer for hallux varus deformity. *J Bone Joint Surg Am*. 1984;66(5):681-686.
9. Lau JT, Myerson MS. Modified split extensor hallucis longus tendon transfer for correction of hallux varus. *Foot Ankle Int*. 2002;23(12):1138-1140.
10. Myerson MS, Komenda GA. Results of hallux varus correction using an extensor hallucis brevis tenodesis. *Foot Ankle Int*. 1996;17(1):21-27.
11. Hawkins FB. Acquired hallux varus: cause, prevention and correction. *Clin Orthop Relat Res*. 1971;76:169-176.
12. Crawford M, Patel J, Giza E. Iatrogenic hallux varus treatment algorithm. *Foot Ankle Clin*. 2014;19(3):371-384.
13. Gerbert J, Traynor C, Blue K, Kim K. Use of the Mini TightRope® for correction of hallux varus deformity. *J Foot Ankle Surg*. 2011;50(2):245-251.
14. Bilotti M, Caprioli R, Testa J, et al. Reverse Austin osteotomy for correction of hallux varus. *J Foot Surg*. 1987;26(1):51.
15. Choi KJ, et al. Distal metatarsal osteotomy for hallux varus following surgery for hallux valgus. *J Bone Joint Surg Am*. 2011;9(4):249-250.
16. Tourne Y, Saragaglia D, Picard F, et al. Iatrogenic hallux varus surgical procedure: a study of 14 cases. *Foot Ankle Int*. 1995;16(8):457-463.
17. Geaney L, Myerson M. Radiographic results after hallux metatarsophalangeal joint arthrodesis for hallux varus. *Foot Ankle Int*. 2014;36(4):391-394.
18. Castellano BD, Southerland JT. Traditional procedures for the repair of hallux abducto valgus. In: Banks AS, Downey MD, Martin DE, Miller SJ, eds. *McGlamry's Comprehensive Textbook of Foot and Ankle Surgery*. 3rd ed. Philadelphia, PA: Lippincott Williams & Wilkins; 2001:623-637.

CHAPTER 17

Digital Fractures

Mickey D. Stapp and Trevor S. Payne

DEFINITION

Digital fractures are one of the most common injuries encountered in the foot and ankle specialist clinic. Toe phalangeal fractures comprise 3.6%-8% of injuries to the lower extremity.[1] Proximal phalangeal fractures occur more often than fractures of the middle or distal phalanges. Some studies suggest that lesser digital fractures are nearly four times more common than hallux fractures,[2] while others have found that lesser digital fractures occur at rates less than double that of hallux fractures.[3]

SALTER-HARRIS FRACTURE CLASSIFICATION

Type I	Physeal injury through the same level of the growth plate
Type II	Fracture pattern from a portion of the physis exiting through metaphysis above the level of the physis
Type III	Fracture pattern from a portion of the physis exiting through the epiphysis below the level of the physis
Type VI	Fracture going through the metaphysis and traverses the physis and epiphysis
Type V	Crush injury to the physis, with high risk of permanent premature closure of the plate

INDICATIONS AND PITFALLS WHEN TREATING DIGITAL FRACTURES

- Reduction of digits should be attempted if more than 2 mm of displacement is apparent on radiographs unless there is normal clinical alignment.
- Spiral oblique fractures are the most difficult to reduce; if reduction fails after two attempts, consider a wire pinning of these to keep alignment.
- If clinical alignment of digital fractures is satisfactory, the osseous alignment will have little effect on the functional status of the digit.
- Hallux fractures also treated conservatively, most often, with immobilization and fracture boot, due to the importance of the hallux in gait and balance.
- Surgery should be reserved for displaced and clinically malaligned fractures >2 mm, open fractures, nonreducible fractures, hallux intra-articular fractures with displacement, displaced physeal fractures, painful nonunions, or arthrosis.

- Subungual hematomas encompassing more than 25% of the nail bed should be treated as an open fracture until proven otherwise.

ANATOMIC FEATURES

There are several important anatomic features to consider in the digits. All the lesser digits have a proximal, middle/intermediate, and distal phalanx. The most common synostosis is in the fifth digit between the middle and distal phalanx and is a very common finding radiographically. The hallux has a proximal and distal phalanx, but houses some of the most important tenderness structures responsible for normal gait. Perhaps the most important consideration when dealing with a digital fracture is the secondary component of possible tendinous injury and should be evaluated in the event a digital fracture is suspected or confirmed. The distal phalanx of the hallux houses the insertion for both the extensor hallucis longus (EHL) and flexor hallucis longus at its base. Simple and comminuted fractures here can have significant effects on gait if the tendinous attachments at the base of the distal phalanx of the hallux are disrupted. Furthermore, the extensor digitorum longus inserts into the middle and distal phalanx of the lateral four toes, while the flexor digitorum longus inserts exclusively into the base of the distal phalanx of the lateral four toes. Several intrinsic digital tendinous attachments are present such as the interossei and flexor/extensor brevis attachments. However, these are not readily damaged during digital fractures and are not readily fixed even in conjunction with the digital fracture. It is believed that restoration of the normal anatomic position when treating digital fractures will allow restoration of these intrinsic tendinous attachments.

FUNCTIONAL ANALYSIS OF THE DIGITS

During the gait cycle, the digits and their respective metatarsophalangeal joints (MTPJs) play a role in forward propulsion. The majority of manipulation to the digits during the gait cycle occurs from the long flexors and extensors and their attachments into the digits. In a normal heel-to-toe gait pattern, just before the forefoot hits the ground, dorsiflexion at the MTPJs causes the forefoot to become tense, firm, and pale. The long extensors acting on the digits allow this process to occur and help aid in normal gait by allowing the forefoot to share shear forces with the soft tissues and skeletal structure of the foot.

During propulsion phases of gait, the hallux acts to elongate the rigid first ray to stabilize the foot during forward motion. The lesser digits also help with propulsion phases of gait through the tendinous attachments of the long flexors and short flexors. Fractures involving the digits can compromise these tendinous attachments as well as cause pain leading to abnormal gait. Secondary evaluation of tendinous attachments in the presence of digital fractures that house these insertional tendinous attachments is vital for maintenance of normal gait.

PHYSICAL EXAMINATION

The majority of digital fractures will often present to the clinic with pain to the involved toe, and adjacent toes, that do not show fractures but may have soft tissue damage from the injury. Patients often present stating that they broke their toe. Insensate patients may present with concern of color changes and/or swelling, with no recall of injury and no complaint of pain. A thorough history and physical should be obtained with emphasis on the specific injury. How the injury occurred and mechanism of injury, if the patient is able to recall, can be beneficial. Time frame from injury to presentation for treatment will aid in the treatment plan of the digital fractures but is of critical importance in open fractures.

Upon inspection, the physician will note edema and ecchymosis of the involved digits, often extending into the forefoot (Fig. 17.1). The patient will complain of pain, painful ambulation, and difficulty with shoe gear. If any break in the skin is noted, an open fracture must be considered and treated accordingly. Neurovascular status must be evaluated in all suspected digital injuries, but especially with the less common frontal plane injuries. Palpation should be carried out to determine the exact location of pain and often to confirm the location of suspected fracture observed on radiograph. An intra-articular

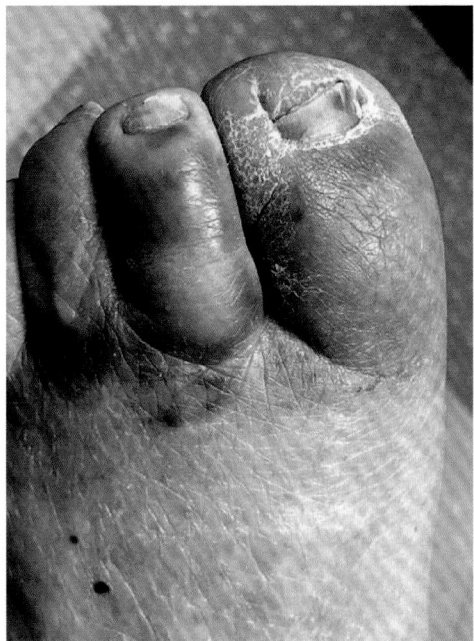

FIGURE 17.1 Clinical picture showing findings commonly seen associated with digital fractures including erythema, edema, and ecchymosis. This second digit fracture occurred in an insensate patient with concerns of "Toes turning black."

fracture will be more painful with range of motion of the involved joint, while an extra-articular fracture will be more painful with palpation of the involved phalangeal shaft.

PATHOGENESIS

The majority of digital fractures are a result of a direct injury or an indirect injury. The direct injury is typically caused by a falling object, an industrial accident, or a motor vehicle accident. The direct injury is often referred to as a crush injury. The indirect injury, causing digital fractures, is typically striking one's foot against an immobile object. An indirect injury is referred to as a stubbing injury. Van Vliet-Kappert's article on 370 phalangeal toe fractures demonstrated that three-fourths of all digital fractures in his study were from either stubbing or crush injuries, with 51.6% due to stubbing and 24% due to crush injuries.[3]

Digital fractures can manifest in a wide array of presentations and fracture patterns. They can range from simple nondisplaced injuries to open comminuted intra-articular fractures requiring emergent treatment. The old adage "it is only a broken toe" is common among lay people. Most laypersons believe that there is no "real treatment" for digital fractures. This prevalent idea often contributes to delay between initial injury and early treatment.[4] Additionally, 10%-25% of digital fractures present without pain or with only minimal symptoms, and many of these common fractures are never seen in a clinical setting.[5]

The planar force of phalangeal digital fractures will often determine the location and pattern of the fracture. Forces in the sagittal plane account for most digital fractures. A direct injury in the sagittal plane is typically associated with a crushing injury. This injury most frequently affects the hallux. This direct injury of the hallux can involve the proximal or distal phalanges, or both. When the distal phalanx is involved, a subungual hematoma is often seen concurrently. When this direct injury in the sagittal plane involves a lesser digit, it is usually the middle or distal phalanx. This injury may also be associated with a subungual hematoma of the lesser digits.[4] A hyperextension or hyperflexion force can cause an indirect injury in the sagittal plane. This injury produces a transverse fracture of the proximal phalanx of either the hallux or the lesser digits. If the transverse fracture occurs at the base, angulation may result. If not properly reduced, this abnormal angulation may lead to loss of flexion and/or extension. If the transverse fracture occurs midshaft, angulation may also exist with possible tendon adhesion. When a transverse fracture occurs at the neck of the proximal phalanx, a permanent loss of flexion is possible.[6]

The next most common plane of force causing digital fractures is an abduction or adduction force in the transverse plane. This transverse plane injury usually involves the proximal phalanx of the fifth digit and is often termed the "bedroom fracture." This force produces a short oblique or transverse fracture pattern. While the fifth toe is most commonly injured with this force, other digits can show this pattern of injury as well. Less commonly, frontal plane injury occurs with a rotational or inversion/eversion injury. This force may produce a spiral fracture, usually of the proximal phalanx. This fracture may cause shortening or rotation. Achieving closed reduction with this type of unstable fracture is more difficult and maintaining reduction can be more challenging.[4] Digital injuries occurring in the frontal plane should have careful neurovascular evaluation due to potential vessel damage.

In Van Vliet-Kappert's article of 339 consecutive patients with 370 phalangeal fractures, 33% were transverse and 41% were spiral or oblique. He found that only 13% were comminuted and 13% were an avulsion-type fracture. Intra-articular fractures, predominantly, at the base of the phalanges, accounted for 33% in his study. More interesting, 97% of the fractures were nondisplaced or minimally displaced, <2 mm. All of the 370 digital fractures were treated conservatively, with the majority of fractures being treated with splinting and/or casting. Follow-up surveys showed excellent outcomes, as measured with AOFAS (American Orthopaedic Foot and Ankle Society) and VAS (visual analog scale) scales, and high patient satisfaction.[3]

Lesser digital fractures can be divided into extra-articular or intra-articular, nondisplaced or displaced, and closed or open. Lesser digital fractures can also show isolated dislocations without fracture of the osseous structures. Nearly all extra-articular, nondisplaced or minimally displaced, closed digital fractures are amenable to conservative treatment.[7] Eves and Oddy, in their study of 74 phalangeal fractures in 65 patients over a 1-year span of their clinic, demonstrated that only 2 patients required surgery. They recommended that nondisplaced and stable toe phalangeal fractures do not need a referral to fracture clinic. Only intra-articular, displaced fractures >2 mm, physeal fractures, or open fractures require referral. At 2-year follow-up, no patients were symptomatic, demonstrated a malunion, or required future surgery.[7] Labovitz even suggests that as long as clinical alignment of the toe is satisfactory, then true osseous alignment is irrelevant and that functional outcome will be satisfactory.[8] The most common lesser digital fracture is the closed, nondisplaced or minimally displaced, transverse or short oblique fracture of the fifth proximal phalanx, usually midshaft (Fig. 17.2). This occurs with the abduction injury of stubbing one's toe. If this most common type of lesser

digital fracture is displaced >2 mm, then reduction should be attempted. This fracture pattern is more intrinsically stable, more easily reduced if required, and less likely to shorten or telescope, and hence more likely to maintain reduction. Fractures of the middle or distal phalanges of the lesser digits are seen more in the sagittal plane crush-type injury. If a subungual hematoma is present, then the nail should be avulsed to evaluate for a nail bed laceration and, if present, treated as an open fracture. Intra-articular fractures of the lesser digits occur most commonly at the proximal interphalangeal joint (PIPJ) (Fig. 17.3). Dislocations of one of the interphalangeal joints of the lesser digits, without fracture of phalanges, can usually be treated with closed reduction (Fig. 17.4).

Hallux fractures can be divided into extra-articular or intra-articular, nondisplaced or displaced, closed or open. Hallux fractures can also show only dislocation at the hallux interphalangeal joint (HIPJ) or dislocations with associated fractures. Fractures of the hallux phalanges are treated more aggressively and require open surgery more often than lesser digital fractures. The hallux plays a much more vital role in balance and propulsion in weight bearing than the lesser digits. The hallux also carries nearly 50% of the body weight in normal gait, and this force significantly increases in running and jumping.

A stubbing injury of the hallux can produce several types of fractures or no apparent fractures, yet substantial joint damage. The stubbing injury can produce a comminuted extra/intra-articular fracture of the distal phalanx, with or without a subungual hematoma. The stubbing injury can produce a dislocation of the HIPJ, with or without intra-articular fracture. Intra-articular fractures of the hallux are more important to achieve proper reduction and stable fixation due to the risk of posttraumatic

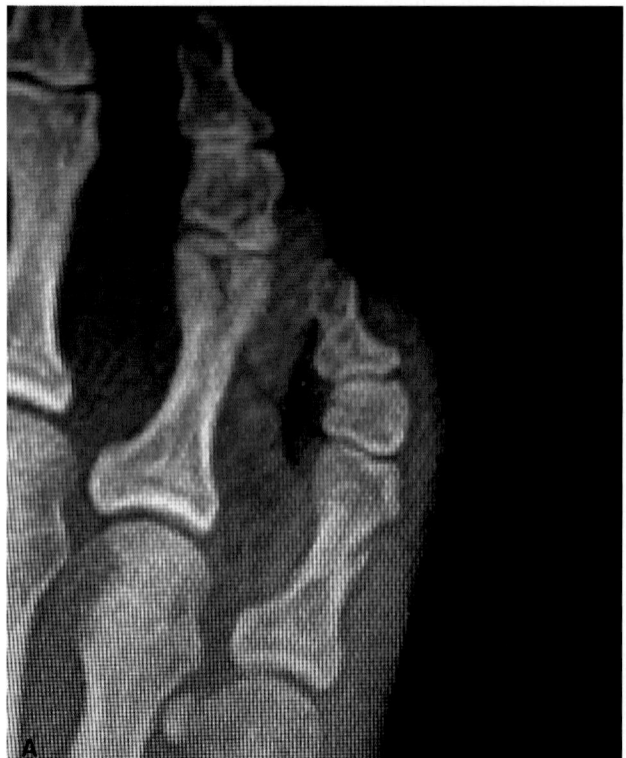
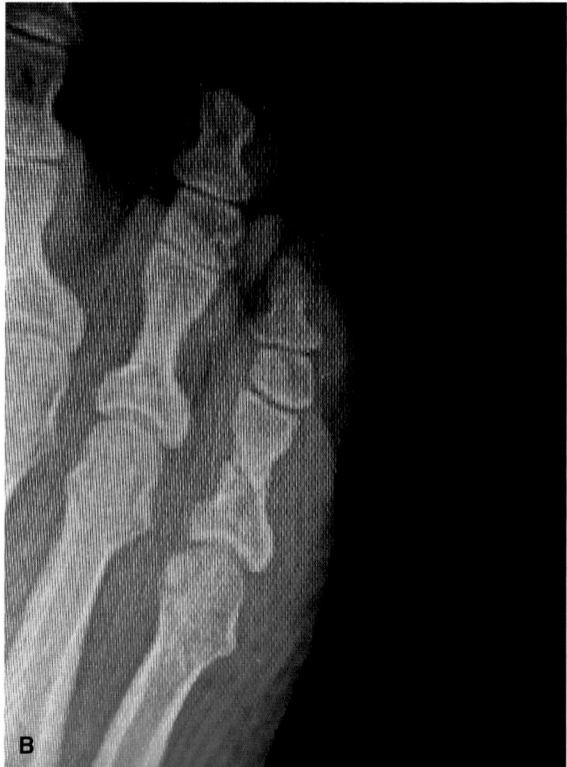

FIGURE 17.2 Extra-articular fracture of a lesser fifth digit. **A, B.** AP and MO radiographs demonstrating a fracture line in midshaft of the proximal phalanx of the fifth digit proximal phalanx. Although mildly displaced, the fracture line does not extend to the joint space in either the distal or proximal direction.

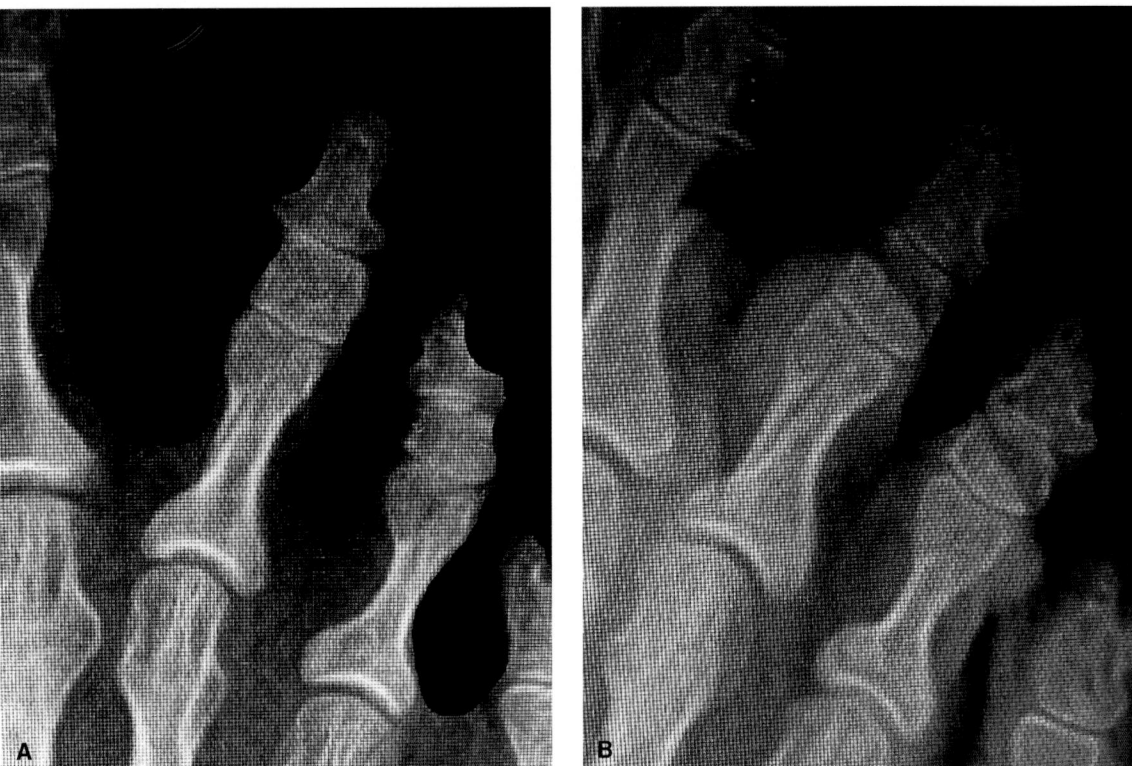

FIGURE 17.3 Intra-articular fracture of the third digit with multiple views. **A.** A fracture line can be clearly seen in this anterior-posterior radiograph in the medial aspect of the proximal phalanx of this lesser digit, but it is difficult to assess if the fracture line is intra-articular. **B.** Oblique radiograph of the same injury with clear evidence of intra-articular extension of this spiral fracture into the PIPJ.

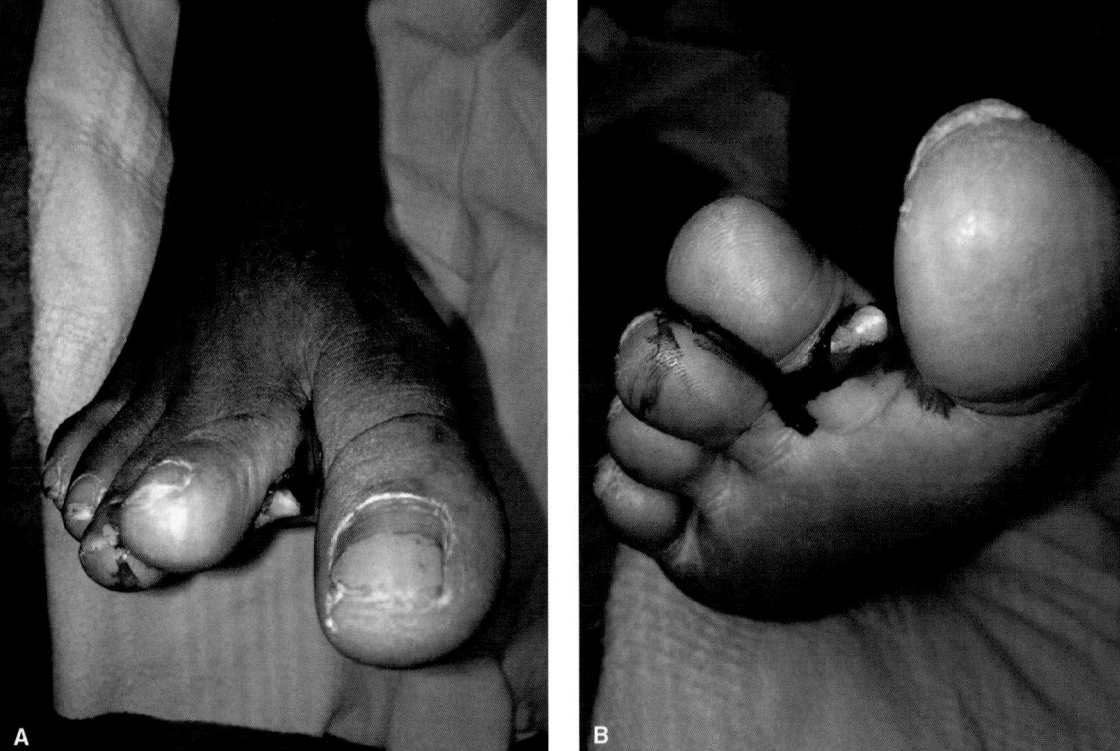

FIGURE 17.4 Open dislocation of the second digit at the level of the PIPJ. **A, B.** Clinical presentation of open displaced lesser digit at the level of the proximal interphalangeal joint.

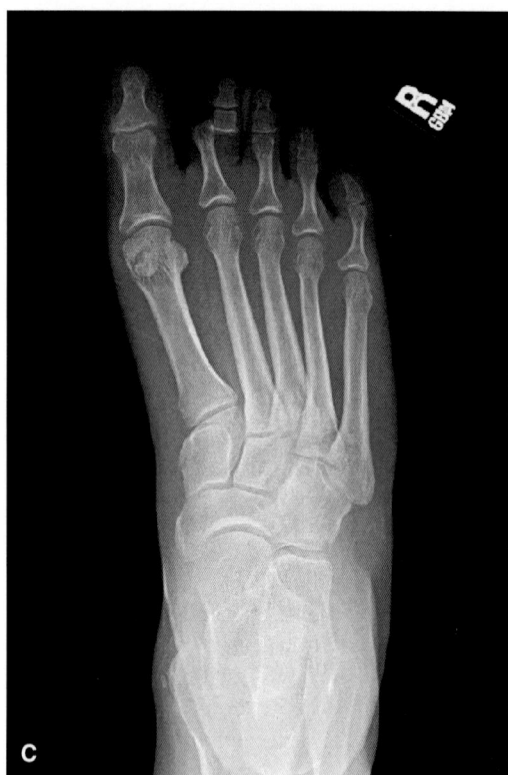

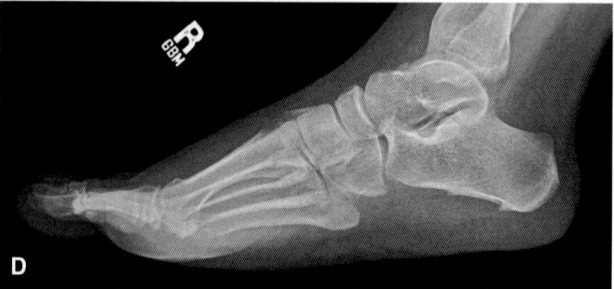

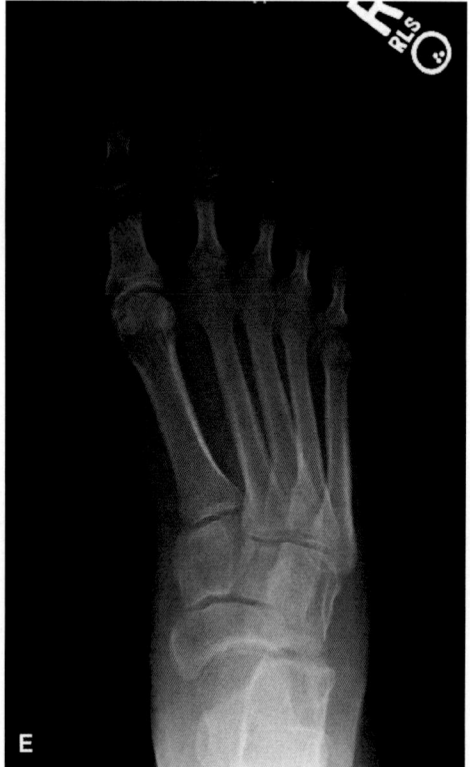

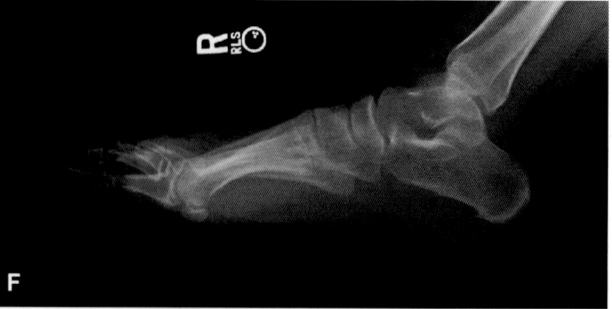

FIGURE 17.4 (*Continued*) Radiographs AP **(C)** and lateral **(D)** demonstrating lateral and dorsal displacement at the PIPJ, respectively. Post manual reduction dislocation radiographs **(E)** and **(F)** showing re-establishment of the normal joint position and alignment.

arthrosis. The crush injury, as a result of direct trauma, is the most common type of injury leading to a fracture of one of the phalanges of the hallux. This injury typically affects the distal phalanx but can affect the proximal phalanx or both. The extra-articular comminuted injury to the distal phalanx from stubbing can be treated conservatively with compression bandaging of the hallux with immobilization and protected weight bearing in a stiff-soled shoe or fracture boot for 4-6 weeks.

Indirect trauma to the hallux producing a sagittal plane fracture usually results from a hyperextension or hyperflexion injury. This fracture occurs at the base of the proximal phalanx. Anatomic reduction is critical as this type of fracture is prevalent to develop loss of dorsiflexion or plantar flexion as previously described.

A special injury to the hallux has been termed a mallet injury from its counterpart injury of the hand. The mallet injury is a hyperflexion injury where there is an avulsion fracture of the dorsal lip of the proximal aspect of the distal phalanx. The extensor hallucis tendon's (EHL) strength should be closely evaluated in this injury. Severely comminuted fracture of the distal phalanx should also have the EHL tendon closely evaluated also to prevent future loss of attachment and subsequent function (Fig. 17.5).

A particularly rare type of hallux fracture can be seen as a postoperative complication. Park reported on an avulsion fracture of the base of the proximal phalanx in 5% of 225 hallux valgus surgeries that had a distal lateral soft tissue release at the first MTPJ. Of these 12 fractures, 10 healed and 2 developed first MPJ arthrosis.[9]

Physeal fractures in children are differentiated by the Salter-Harris classification (Fig. 17.6). These fractures can have significant consequences if not identified early. If suspected,

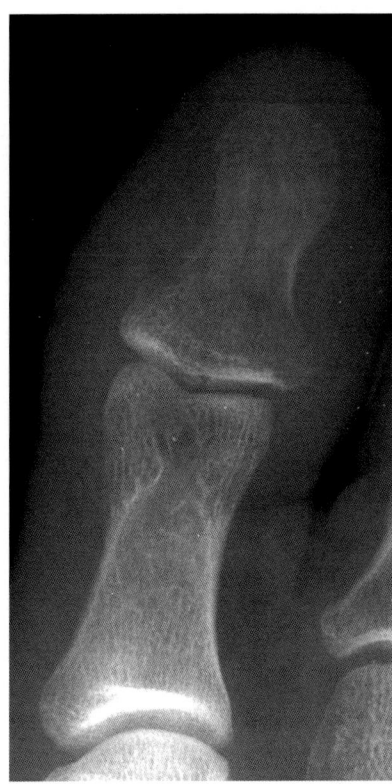

FIGURE 17.5 Comminuted open distal hallux fracture depicted with a plain AP radiograph. Evaluation for extensor hallucis longus strength should be carried out to rule out direct injury from comminuted fracture of the distal phalanx.

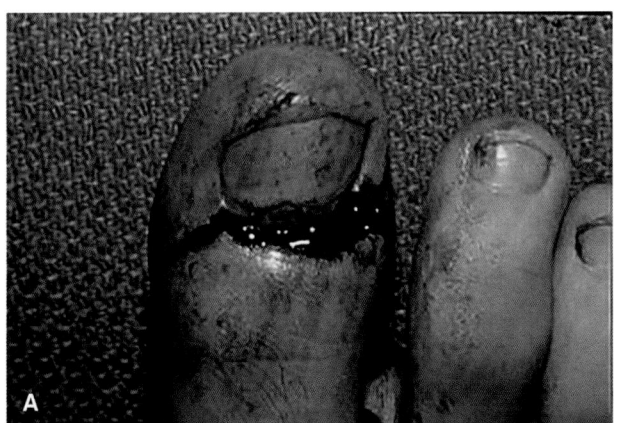

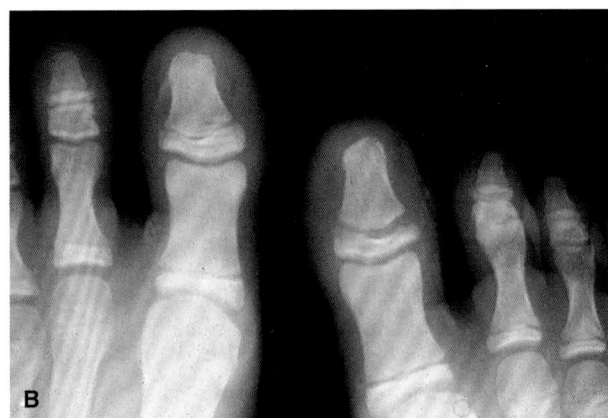

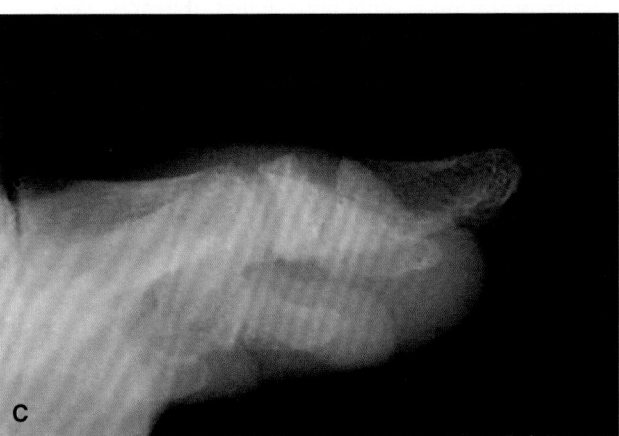

FIGURE 17.6 Assortment of pediatric physeal plate fractures in the digits. **A-C.** Clinical presentation of a hallux injury with potential open fracture involvement **(A)** and subsequent plain radiograph showing a Salter-Harris type I fracture pattern with the fracture line through the growth plate, not extending either above or below **(B,C)**. Note the incorporation of contralateral foot for in pediatric radiographs **(B)** for more accurate detection of a fracture through comparison.

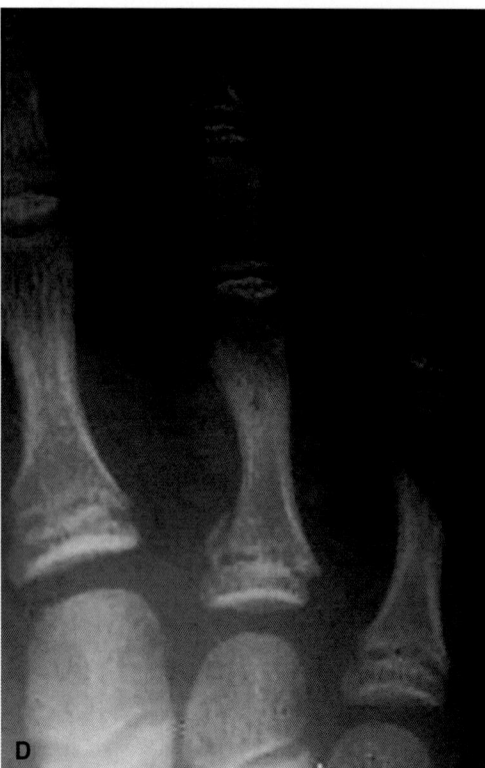
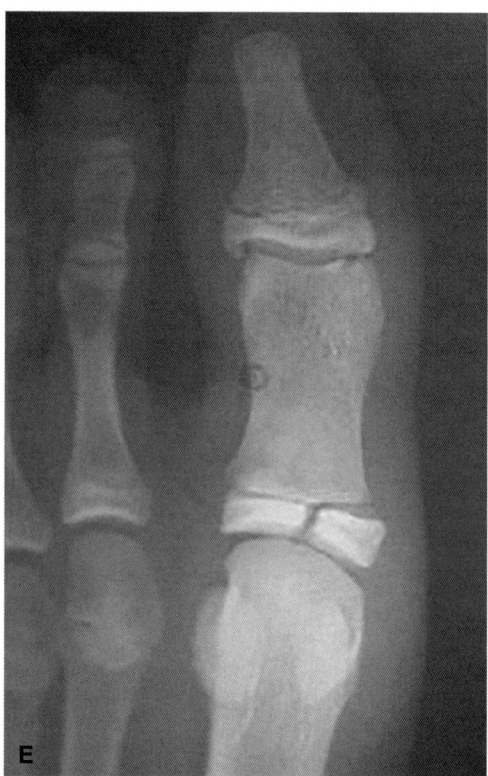

FIGURE 17.6 (*Continued*) **D.** Plain radiograph depicting a Salter-Harris type II bone injury with initial fracture line above the growth plate and exiting through the plate. **E.** Salter-Harris type III injury depicting the initial fracture line traversing in the physeal plate before exiting below and into the intra-articular space of the corresponding metatarsophalangeal joint.

clinicians should consider contralateral films to differentiate between normal variations in the growth plate architecture and true physeal plate injury. Children have a higher risk of closed or open injuries to the growth plates of the hallux. These injuries often occur while playing barefoot or participating in athletics without protective footgear. Park reported on 41 indirect injuries to the hallux in barefoot children. Hyperadduction and flexion injury produced HIPJ dislocation with skin tear representing an open fracture with the possibility of osteomyelitis. Hyperadduction and extension injury produced an avulsion fracture of the lateral condyle of the proximal phalanx. This injury had a worse prognosis with the higher possibility of nonunion and arthritis.[10]

IMAGING AND DIAGNOSTIC STUDIES

In general, plain radiographs with standard AP, oblique, and lateral images are usually sufficient in making the diagnosis and for follow-up on bone healing. Advanced imaging studies, such as CT or MRI, would rarely be indicated. While a lateral image may not be helpful in suspected lesser digital fractures due to superimposition, it should still be obtained to evaluate dorsiflexion or plantar flexion displacement. With suspected hallux fractures, an isolated view of the hallux on the lateral image, with the hallux elevated, may be especially helpful.

TREATMENT

Most digital fractures do not require surgical intervention. Lesser digital fractures are most often treated conservatively with taping the injured digit to adjacent uninjured digit/digits, often referred to as "buddy splinting." Buddy taping or splinting can be accomplished in many different ways. Care must be taken to observe the skin where any repeated use of an adhesive is used and the skin between adjacent digits. Won's study showed high percentage of use of buddy taping among surgeons, 87%, but low compliance by the patient, 65%. The above noted skin injuries were present 45% for those caused by the adhesive material and 45% interdigitally.[11] Buddy splinting and protected weight bearing in a stiff-soled shoe for 3-4 weeks is sufficient in these common digital fractures (Fig. 17.7). Follow-up radiographs may not show complete consolidation of the fracture for several months and complete remodeling of the fracture site for a year.

PEARLS
- Buddy splinting is usually all that is required to immobilize most fractured digits.
- Patients should be counseled of potential skin injury from repeated use of adhesives.

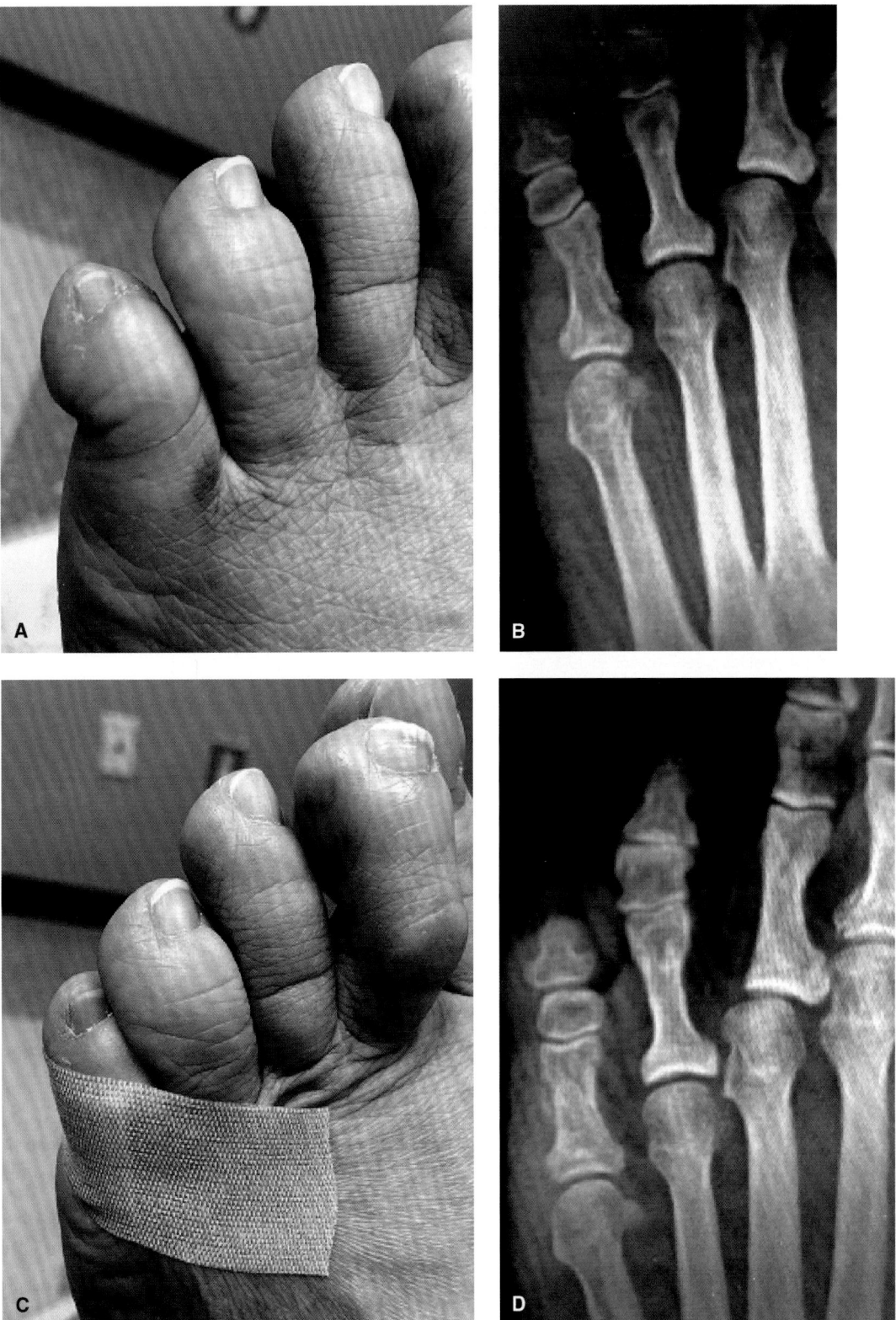

FIGURE 17.7 Example of "buddy splinting" a displaced fifth digit fracture after reduction.
A. Clinical picture showing deviation of the fifth digit after traumatic injury. Note edema and
ecchymosis present. **B.** Plain AP radiograph reiterating clinical findings with displacement of the
digit and corresponding spiral extra-articular fracture. **C.** Reduction of the deformity from resultant
fracture of the fifth digit being held in place with Band-Aid splinting to adjacent tissue structures.
D. Confirmation of postreduction position with subsequent plain AP radiograph showing restored and
maintained alignment of the fifth digit.

Reduction of intra-articular fractures of the lesser digits is not as critical as reduction of intra-articular fractures of the hallux because of the weight-bearing stress on the hallux. The majority of these fractures can also be treated conservatively with buddy splinting and protected weight bearing in a stiff-soled shoe for 3-4 weeks. If a symptomatic fracture fragment becomes present at a later date, then it can be surgically excised. If a symptomatic nonunion or arthrosis occurs at the interphalangeal joint, this can typically be treated surgically via simple arthroplasty.

Open digital fractures are more of a surgical emergency, and delay in treatment can have deleterious effects. If an open fracture is present, then tetanus prophylaxis is administered. Gram stain and aerobic and anaerobic cultures are obtained. The wound is copiously irrigated. If small fragments are encountered in the treatment of the open digital fracture, they can be excised at the time of surgery. If time to treatment was not delayed, then these wounds may be primarily closed. Nail bed lacerations, because of the granular nature of the nail bed will often close uneventfully without primary closure. Empiric antibiotics are administered and adjusted if needed based on clinical response, Gram stain, and cultures.

PEARLS
- Open fractures are surgical emergencies and should be treated accordingly in a timely fashion to reduce the risk of osteomyelitis.
- Emergent treatment should focus on early administration of antibiotics, culturing the open wound(s), irrigation, removal/debridement of nonreducible fragments of bone, and primary closure if within 6 hours of the injury.

Reduction of a displaced digital fracture or dislocated digital joint is achieved through the same principle of any displaced long bone fracture. First the injury is exaggerated, then the digit is distracted, and finally the injury is reversed. Postreduction radiographs are then again obtained to confirm reduction. The concave side of the fracture has soft tissues intact and will serve as a guide for reduction of the fracture fragment, to help prevent overcorrection by the soft tissue hinge[4] (Fig. 17.8). If the fracture site is not able to be reduced or maintain reduction, then open reduction with internal fixation (ORIF) may be required. Closed reduction with pinning would be another option in some fractures. The lesser common injury force in the frontal plane can produce the long oblique or spiral fracture. Along with the comminuted fracture, these are more intrinsically unstable.[12] It is much more difficult to achieve and maintain reduction with these injuries. Open reduction with internal or external fixation may be required. Prolonged pain may represent a nonunion, and follow-up radiographs should be obtained. Even intra-articular fractures that heal with slight angulation or develop arthrosis later can be corrected with resection arthroplasty or arthrodesis. A nonunited intra-articular fragment can be excised later if symptomatic. Occasionally after a digital fracture heals, the fracture area will develop an area of exuberant bone callus requiring surgical resection to reduce painful interdigital bony prominence that may be associated with pain and/or interdigital corns.[13]

positioning PEARLS
STEPS TO REDUCING A FRACTURED DIGIT
1. Distract and exaggerate the deformity in line with the mechanism of injury
2. Apply traction to the digit
3. Reverse the mechanism of deformity, confirm reduced position, and immobilize

Occasionally, and especially with digital dislocations, closed reduction will not be possible due to interposition of the flexor tendon.[14] In Yang's article on interphalangeal dislocations, 18 patients with dislocations of a lesser PIPJ or the HIPJ were evaluated. Approximately one-third of these dislocations involved the fifth toe and one-third involved the hallux. Most were hyperextension injuries when landing on the digit barefoot or kicking an object. Ten were closed reduced, seven required ORIF (mostly HIPJ), and one patient declined treatment.[15]

PEARLS
- Hallux hyperextension injuries have a high incidence of tendon interposition and have a lower threshold for the need of open reduction and fixation to hold a reduced position.

A pure dislocation of the HIPJ should be amenable to closed reduction, followed by splinting and protected weight bearing in a fracture boot for 4-6 weeks. If intra-articular fragments are present with the dislocation, small or minimally displaced larger fragments can be treated conservatively as a pure HIPJ dislocation. If larger fragments are present, then ORIF, closed reduction with percutaneous pinning, or external fixation methods should be carried out (Figs. 17.9 and 17.10). Jahss showed that one in six with a significant stubbing injury to the interphalangeal joint of the hallux ultimately required a HIPJ arthrodesis.[16] Sequelae of a stubbing injury of the hallux can include growth plate arrest, hallux limitus or rigidus, angulation deformities, arthrosis of the HIPJ or first MTPJ, as well as matrix damage leading to later nail abnormalities.

Treatment for a mallet injury is immobilization with splinting and a fracture boot for 6-8 weeks. York recommended ORIF if the avulsion fracture involved more than one-third of the joint surface or if the joint was unstable with plantar subluxation.[17] Complications of the mallet injury include palpable dorsal exostosis, fixed flexion deformity, and diminished range of motion at the HIPJ.[18,19]

Physeal fractures in children should be treated with more scrutiny than their adult counterparts. Timing and appropriate fixation seems to be the most important factors when treating these injuries. Perugia demonstrated four cases of proximal phalanx fractures of the hallux in young high-level gymnasts who sustained a hyperadduction mechanism of injury. All four injuries showed Salter-Harris type III or IV fractures and were treated with ORIF.[20] Banks reported on open physeal injuries to the hallux with acute hyperflexion trauma. He believed that traumatic separation of the proximal nail fold was sufficient force to fracture the open growth plate at the distal phalanx.[21] Any injury to the growth plate of the hallux can produce subsequent sequelae including premature closure of a portion or all

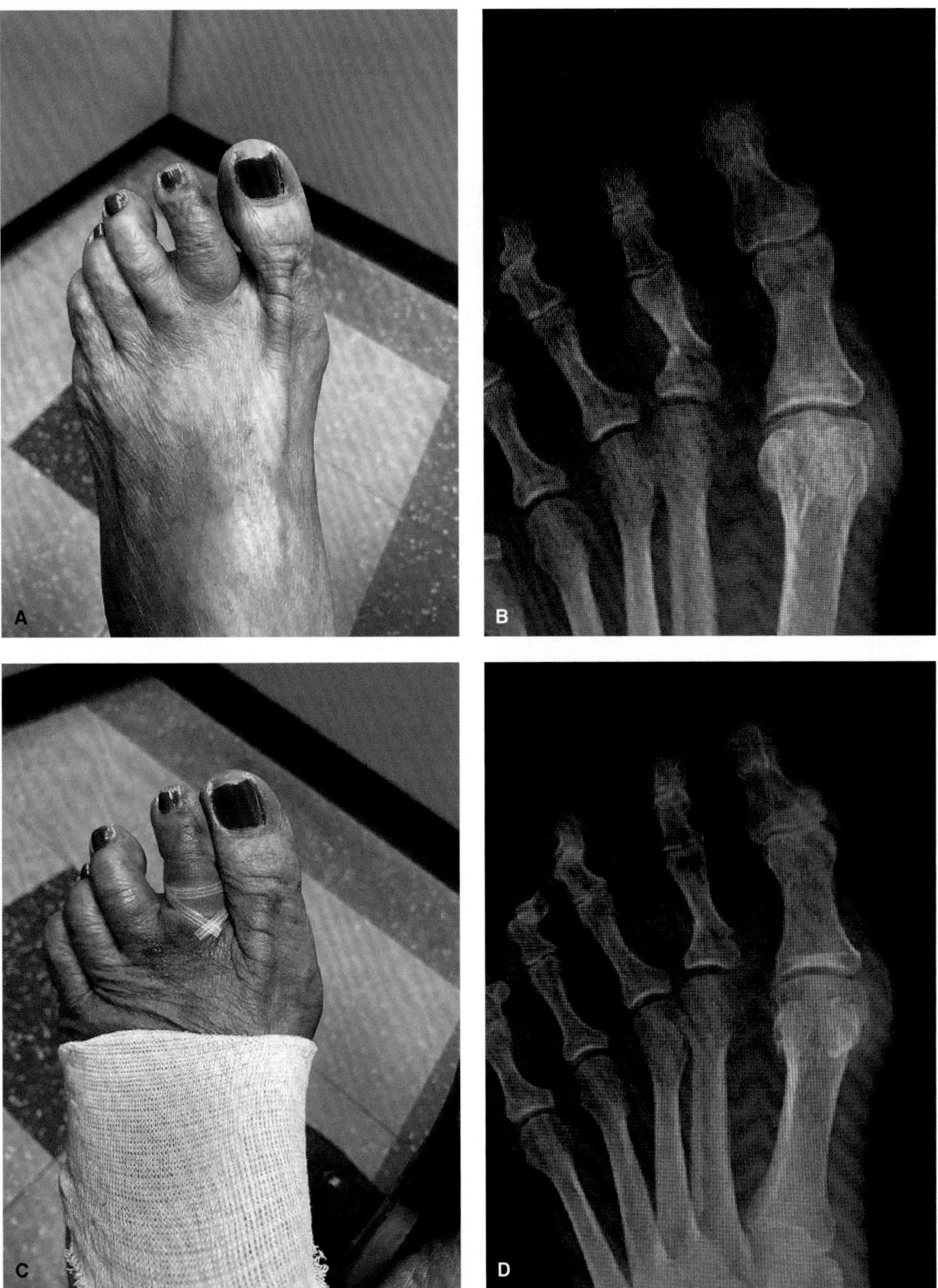

FIGURE 17.8 Displaced lesser digital fracture with subsequent manual reduction. **A.** Clinical presentation of swelling, erythema, and transverse angular deformity with lateral deviation of the second digit following traumatic injury. **B.** Prereduction radiograph confirming fracture with >2 mm displacement from normal alignment of proximal phalanx. **C.** Postreduction clinical presentation with correction of transverse angular deformity being held in place with Steri-Strip splinting and tape. **D.** Postreduction AP radiograph showing adequate reduction of displaced fracture of the proximal phalanx in the second digit.

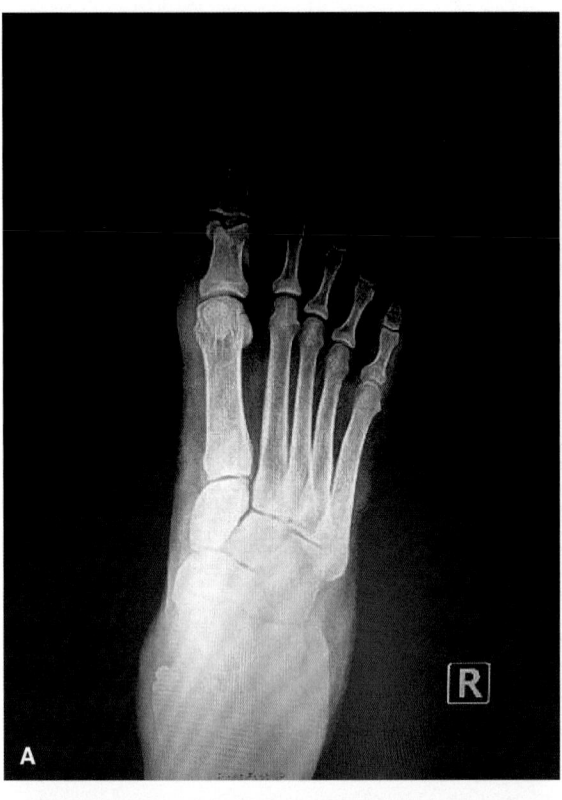

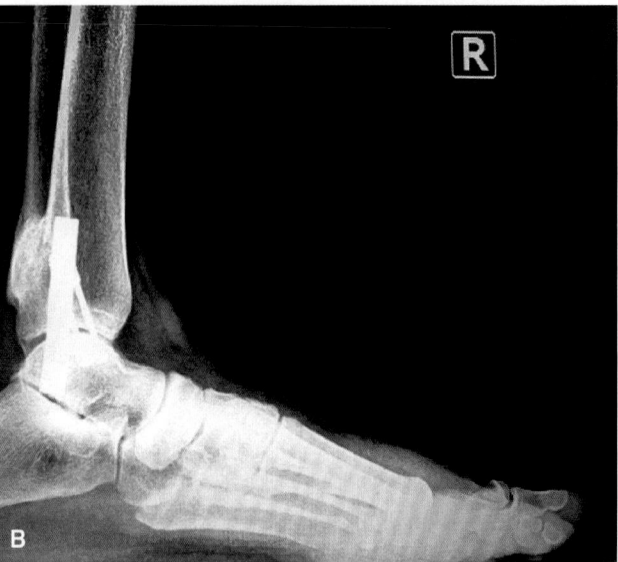

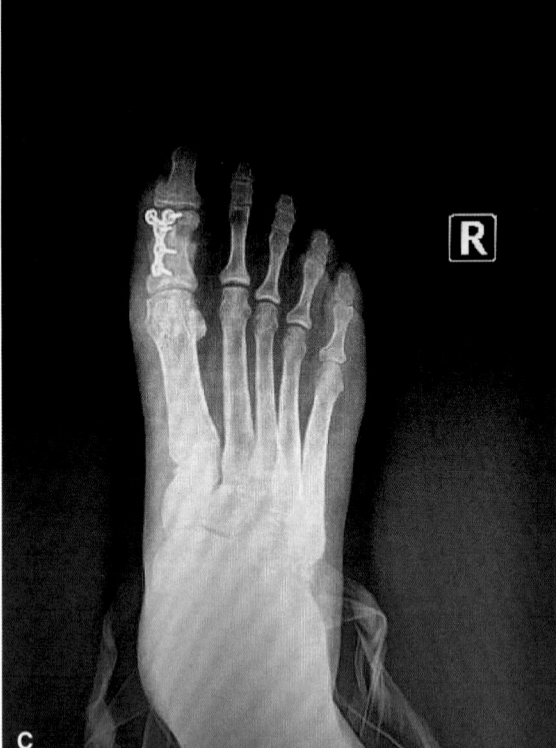

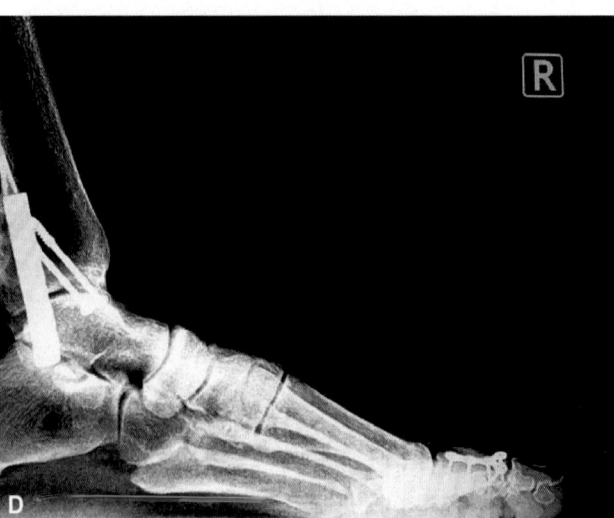

FIGURE 17.9 Intra-articular hallux fracture. **A, B.** Plain film radiographs depicting a distally oriented intra-articular hallux proximal phalanx fracture with multiple fragments and displacement in multiple planes. **C, D.** Plain film radiographs showing subsequent results of open reduction of the fracture fragments in all planes and placement held with an internal fixation plate and screws.

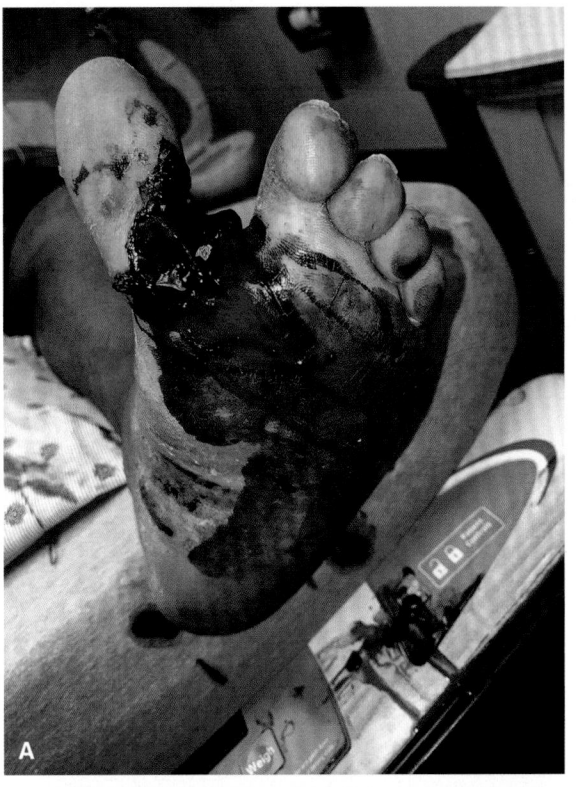

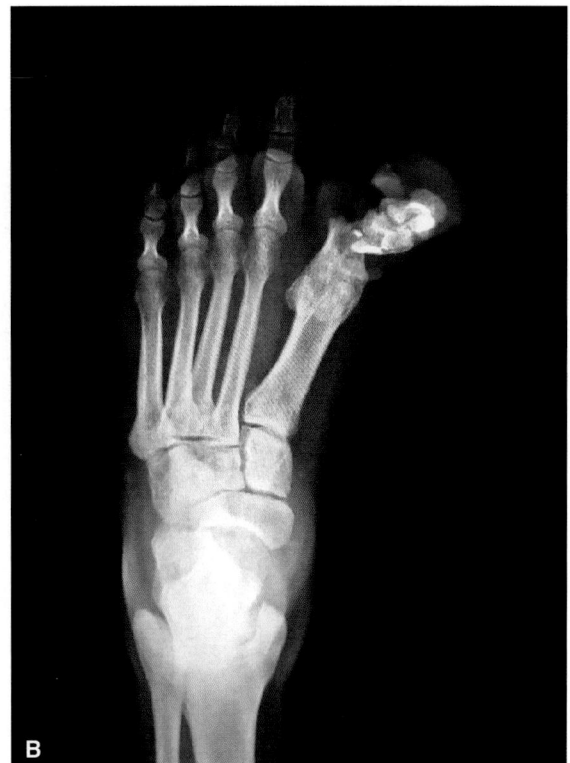

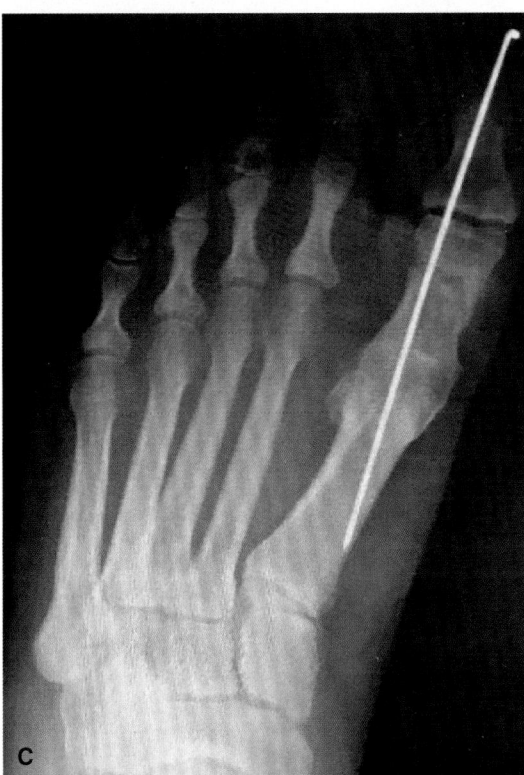

FIGURE 17.10 Open hallux fracture. **A.** Clinical presentation of full-thickness deep open wound incorporating majority of the hallux. **B.** AP plain radiograph showing obvious soft tissue defect and corresponding displacement of hallux with traumatic fracture. **C.** AP plain radiograph with reduction of the same open hallux fracture being held in place with percutaneous K-wire pinning for structural rigidity.

of the growth plate. Delay in diagnosing and treating an open growth plate injury can have more serious consequences. In Kensinger's article, three of five children with stubbing injuries with open fracture of the distal phalanx developed osteomyelitis. In follow-up, all fractures healed and no child had active infection. Four of the five children had partial or full growth plate arrest of the distal phalanx.[22] Adults can also sustain open fractures of the hallux, but less frequently, because most occur with an abduction injury while barefoot. If an open fracture of the hallux occurs in the adult, another surgical option outside the use of ORIF or percutaneous pinning is the use of external fixation to stabilize the fracture fragments (Fig. 17.11).

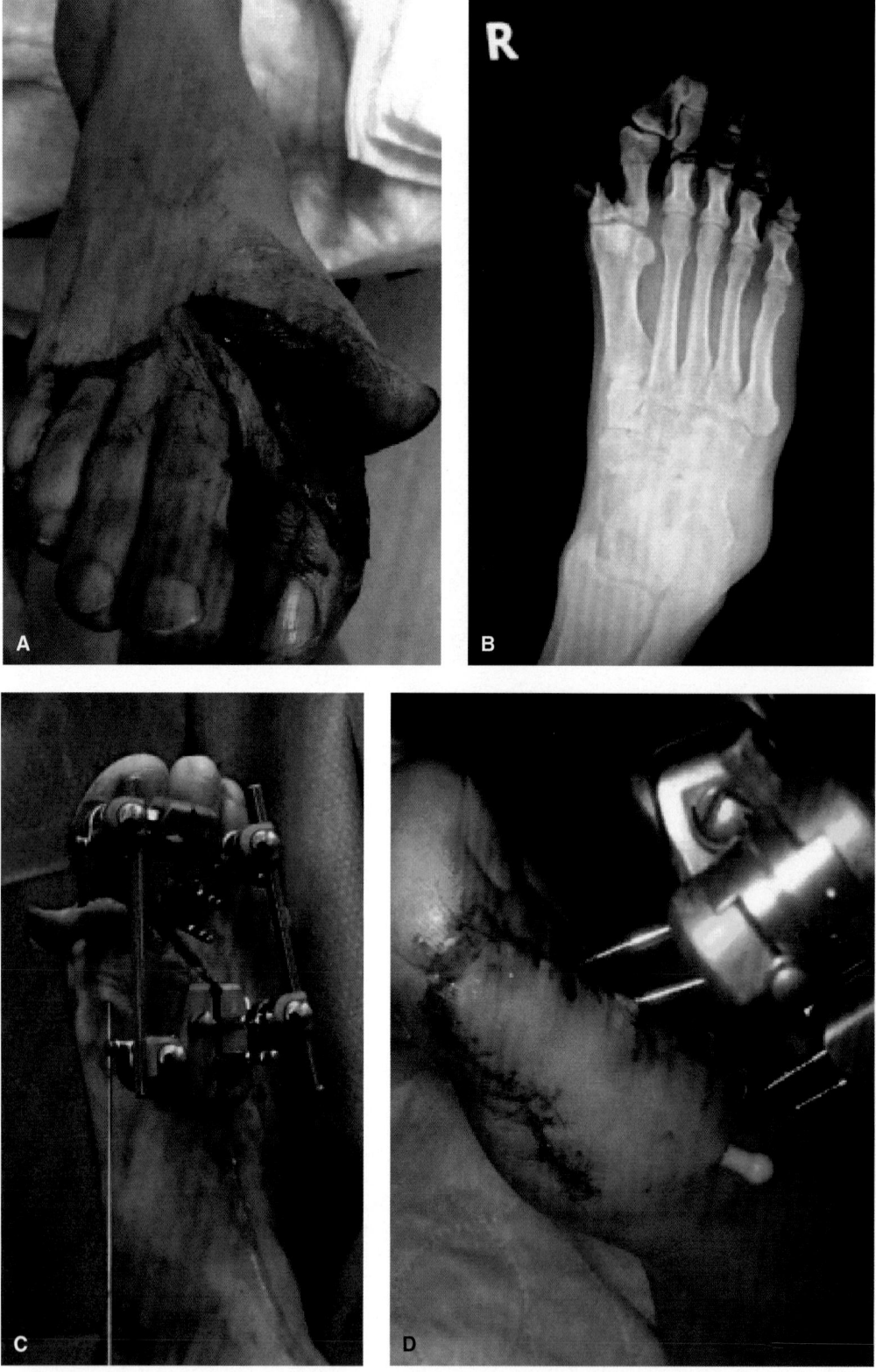

FIGURE 17.11 Another example of an open traumatic hallux fracture. **A, B.** Preoperative clinical appearance of open hallux fracture with loose skin flap. **C, D.** Reduction of subsequent open hallux fracture with MiniRail external fixation and K-wire pinning.

A rare possible fracture of the lesser digits is a stress fracture. These are seen in adolescent athletes or older athletes with osteopenia. While most of these affect the base of the hallux, they have been described as a rare cause of second MTPJ pain. These can go on to nonunion, presumably due to the difficulty in making the appropriate diagnose in a timely manner.[23,24]

AUTHOR'S PREFERRED SURGICAL PROCEDURE TECHNIQUES

Surgical intervention for reduction of fractures should follow the same general principles for open reduction and internal fixation. Surgical planning should include preoperative consideration for incision placement so that the entirety of the fracture can be observed and manipulated as needed. For instance, proximal phalanx fractures of the hallux can be exposed nicely with a lazy S-type incision dorsally. Length of the incision will depend on the digit that is affected and how many bones are affected. When accessing the underlying fractured bone from a dorsal approach, which is most commonly utilized, tendons can be temporarily transected transversely for better visualization if needed and repaired later with absorbable suture. The underlying fracture fragments should be reduced with bone reduction clamps and K-wires as needed to restore length of bones and reestablish joint congruity. For simple fractures, screw fixation is typically all that is needed. For more complex comminuted fractures, locking plates with screws can be beneficial to help hold fracture fragments in place until healing can occur. Suspected tendon injury should be examined preoperatively to measure the level of suspicion but again stressed while performing surgical intervention on those bones that house insertions for tendon attachments.

If bones involving pertinent tendinous attachments are being fixed, ruptured or displaced tendons should be treated and reapproximated with braided nonabsorbable suture or suture anchors if necessary to reattach the tendon to bone, especially if there is no insertional tendinous attachment remaining on the fractured bone. Suspected tendon injury should be examined preoperatively to measure the level of suspicion but again stressed while performing surgical intervention on those bones that house insertions for tendon attachments. All open fractures should be copiously lavaged with normal saline with the gravity lavage for pulse lavage. A more gentle lavage would be indicated when several small fragments of bone are present such as in a significantly comminuted fracture.

CONCLUSION

Digital fractures are common injuries of the foot, most often caused by crushing injuries or stubbing injuries. The large majority of these are nondisplaced or minimally displaced and will heal uneventfully with conservative care. Lesser digital fractures are treated with buddy splinting and a stiff-soled shoe. Hallux fractures are also treated conservatively, most often, with immobilization and fracture boot, due to the importance of the hallux in gait and balance. Hallux fractures will require surgical intervention more often than lesser digital fractures. Even most comminuted fractures of lesser digits and the hallux will heal satisfactorily with conservative treatment. Comminuted fractures of any distal phalanx with a subungual hematoma must be evaluated for the possibility of an open fracture. Those comminuted distal phalanges without open fracture can be treated with compression and stiff-soled shoe.

ACKNOWLEDGMENTS

We acknowledge photographic contributions from the following: Alan S. Banks, DPM; Marie-Christine Bergeron, DPM; and Sara Lewis, DPM.

REFERENCES

1. Shibuya N, Davis M, Jupiter D. Epidemiology of foot and ankle fractures in the United States: an analysis of the National Trauma Data Bank (2007 to 2011). *J Foot Ankle Surg.* 2014;53:1-3.
2. Schnaue-Constantorris E, Birres R, Grisafi P, Dellacorte M. Digital foot trauma: emergency diagnosis and treatment. *J Emerg Med.* 2002;22:163-170.
3. Van Vliet-Kappert S, et al. Demographics and functional outcome of toe fractures. *J Foot Ankle Surg.* 2011;50:307-310.
4. Downey, M, Comer-Merritt S, Sharrick-Maher C, Bernbach M. Digital and Sesamoid Fractures. In Banks A, Downey M, Matin D, Miller S, eds. *McGlamry's Comprehensive Textbook of Foot and Ankle Surgery.* Vol. 2. Philadelphia, PA: Lippincott Williams & Wilkins; 2001:1759-1773.
5. Venegas L, Rainferri J, Rzonca E. Fracture of the fifth digit. *J Am Podiatr Med Assoc.* 1995;85(3):166-168.
6. Gumann G. Lower extremity traumatology. In: Marcinko D, ed. *Medical and Surgical Therapeutics of the Foot and Ankle.* Baltimore, MD: Williams & Wilkins; 1992:821-825.
7. Eves T, Oddy M. Do broken toes need follow-up in the fracture clinic? *J Foot Ankle Surg.* 2016;55:488-491.
8. Labovitz J, et al. Classification of fractures and dislocations. In: Christman RA, ed. *Foot and Ankle Radiology.* 2nd ed. Philadelphia, PA: Lippincott Williams & Wilkins; 2015:261-310.
9. Park Y, et al. Consequences of avulsion fracture of the proximal phalanx caused by a technical failure of hallux valgus surgery. *J Foot Ankle Surg.* 2016;55:935-938.
10. Park D, Han K, Han S, Cho J. Barefoot stubbing injuries to the great toe in children: a new classification by injury mechanism. *J Orthop Trauma.* 2014;27:651-655.
11. Won SH, et al. Buddy taping: is it a safe method for treatment of finger and toe injuries? *Clin Orthop Surg.* 2014;6:26-31.
12. Anderson L. Injuries of the forefoot. *Clin Orthop Relat Res.* 1977;122:18-27.
13. Elleby DH, Marcinko DE. Digital fractures and dislocations—diagnosis and treatment. *Clin Podiatry.* 1985;2:233-245.
14. Veen M, Schipper I. Irreducible fracture of the proximal interphalangeal joint of the fifth toe. *J Emerg Med.* 2013;44:e63-e65.
15. Yang J, et al. Interphalangeal dislocation of toes: a retrospective case series and review of the literature. *J Foot Ankle Surg.* 2011;50:580-584.
16. Jahss M. Stubbing injuries to the hallux. *Foot Ankle.* 1980;1:327-332.
17. York P. Wydra F, Hunt K. Injuries to the great toe. *Curr Rev Musculoskelet Med.* 2017;10: 104-112.
18. Hennessy M, Saxby T. Traumatic "Mallet Toe" of the Hallux: a case report. *Foot Ankle Int.* 2001;22:977-978.
19. Rapoff A, Heiner J. Avulsion fracture of the great toe: a case report. *Foot Ankle Int.* 1999;20:337-339.
20. Perugia D, Fabbri M, Guidi M, Lepri M, Masi V. Salter-Harris type III and IV displaced fracture of the hallux in young gymnasts: A series of four cases at 1 year follow-up. *Injury.* 2014;45S:S39-S42.
21. Banks A, Cain T, Ruch J. Physeal fracture of the distal phalanx of the hallux. *J Am Podiatr Med Assoc.* 1988;78(6):310-313.
22. Kensinger D, Guille J, Horn D, Hermann M. The stubbed great toe: importance of early recognition and treatment of open fractures of the distal phalanx. *J Pediatr Orthop.* 2001;21:31-34.
23. Pitsis G, Perry P, Van der Wall H. Stress fracture of the proximal phalanx of the second toe. *Clin J Sport Med.* 2003;13:118-119.
24. Pitsis G, Best JP, Sullivan MR. Unusual stress fracture of the proximal phalanx of the great toe: a report of two cases. *Br J Sports Med.* 2006;38:e31.

CHAPTER 18

Metatarsal Fractures

Stephen A. Mariash

DEFINITION

Metatarsal fractures are common. They constitute 35% of all foot fractures[1] and 61% of pediatric foot fractures.[2] The fifth metatarsal is the most commonly fractured in the adult and the first metatarsal is the most commonly fractured in children under 4 years of age. Most fractures are caused by an inversion injury or fall from height.[3] Stress fractures to a metatarsal usually involve the second or third metatarsal and embody about 2.5% of all metatarsal fractures.

CLASSIFICATION

The classification of metatarsal fractures should include a description of the fracture related to several characteristics.

CLASSIFICATION OF METATARSAL FRACTURES

- Location
- Fracture Pattern
- Displacement
- Angulation
- Articular Involvement

In addition, since each of the five metatarsals functions in a different fashion, metatarsal fractures are further divided into first metatarsal fractures, central or middle metatarsal (second through fourth) fractures, and fifth metatarsal fractures. The pathophysiology and treatment will vary based on the involved metatarsal.[4]

ANATOMIC FEATURES

The first metatarsal is the largest of the five metatarsals. It articulates at its base with the anterior articular surface of the medial cuneiform and at the distal head with the base of the proximal phalanx of the hallux. The base may or may not articulate with the base of the second metatarsal by an intermetatarsal joint. The head is attached to the head of the second metatarsal by the deep transverse intermetatarsal ligament. The base of the first metatarsal is the site of the insertion of the tibialis anterior and peroneus longus tendons. The articular surface of the head of the first metatarsal extends plantarly to articulate with the superior surfaces of the medial and lateral sesamoid bones.[5]

The second through fourth metatarsals have important ligaments that interconnect each bone to its bordering lesser metatarsal. The head of each central metatarsal attaches to its neighboring metatarsal by way of an intermetatarsal ligament. The bases contain ligaments that stabilize each metatarsal with its adjoining metatarsal. The only exclusion is the lack of a ligament between the bases of the first and second metatarsals. In lieu of this ligament, the Lisfranc ligament spans from the second metatarsal to the medial cuneiform.

The fifth metatarsal has a prominent base or styloid process that serves as the attachment for the peroneus brevis tendon. The peroneus tertius attaches to the dorsum of the shaft of the fifth metatarsal. In addition, the plantar fascia has an attachment to the plantar base of the fifth metatarsal. An accessory bone at the base of the fifth metatarsal, os vesalianum, is rare, but can be confused for a fracture since it separates from the tuberosity in a transverse fashion. Likewise, an accessory ossification center may be appreciated in the pediatric patient population. This is more readily distinguished from a fracture since the epiphysis runs parallel to the shaft of the metatarsal and a fracture of the styloid process is more transversely oriented. The blood supply of the fifth metatarsal includes the nutrient artery, metaphyseal perforators, and periosteal arteries. There is a watershed area between the nutrient artery and the metaphyseal perforators. This potential area of poor vascularity may hinder fracture healing.[6]

PHYSICAL EXAMINATION

Patients will present with a history of either acute or chronic forefoot pain. Acute pain usually is the result of an injury. It is important to note the location, degree, and duration of the symptoms. A history of previous injuries, surgeries, or underlying diseases that may affect the feet is extremely helpful. It is also imperative to appreciate the patient's functional requirements related to work and recreational activities.

The neurovascular status of the foot is thoroughly evaluated. In the presence of an acute injury, if there is worsening pain, swelling, numbness or tingling, and coolness of the foot, compartment measurements may be taken to rule out compartment syndrome, which would require immediate foot compartment decompression.[7]

The patient may be able to point to a specific area of pain. Inspection of the feet and palpation will aid in determining the involved injured structures. Comparing the painful foot with the contralateral extremity, especially in regard to alignment and stability, will assist in determining any deviation from the normal state. Joints may be put through active and passive range of motion, and the associated muscles are tested for strength in order to assess the functionality of the tendons. The integument is evaluated for any open wounds that may communicate with an underlying fracture.

IMAGING AND DIAGNOSTIC STUDIES

Radiographs of the foot, anteroposterior, medial oblique, and lateral views, are usually sufficient to evaluate for metatarsal fractures. It is important to assess for intra-articular involvement and concomitant trauma such as Lisfranc injuries. Triphasic bone scans may be employed if there is a suspicion for a stress fracture that is not visualized on plain film radiographs. Furthermore, CT scans may be utilized to further evaluate intra-articular fractures or Lisfranc fracture/dislocations or to assess healing if a nonunion is suspected.

PATHOGENESIS

Metatarsal fractures may occur with either direct or indirect trauma. Crush injuries may cause these fractures as well. Stress fractures occur with a sustained increase in the intensity of activity. There may be underlying biomechanical reasons for the development of stress fractures. In addition, metabolic or endocrine deficiencies may be associated with stress fractures.

First metatarsal and central metatarsal fractures may occur at the base, shaft, or head/neck region. Displacement of the first metatarsal in any of the body planes can impair the biomechanics of the foot. The central metatarsal fractures may occur in isolation or with other metatarsals involved. Sixty-three percent of third metatarsal fractures are associated with a fracture of either the second or fourth metatarsal.[8] Often, they are the result of direct trauma, such as a crush injury. They may also be present following axial loading of a plantar flexed foot.

When the first, second, or third metatarsal bases are involved, it is important to evaluate for intra-articular involvement or a Lisfranc fracture/dislocation. Moreover, it is imperative to evaluate for compromised integument, which may signify an open fracture.

Fifth metatarsal fractures account for about 25% of all metatarsal injuries. The anatomic areas affected are exclusive to the fifth metatarsal given its shape, extrinsic tendon attachments, and unique vascular supply (Fig. 18.1).

The mechanism for zone 1 fractures involves supination and plantar flexion of the forefoot. The result is a transverse fracture of the styloid process of the fifth metatarsal. The fracture may be caused by contraction of the peroneus brevis tendon during hindfoot inversion. In addition, the lateral band of the plantar fascia may be the cause of avulsion fractures.[9] The fracture is usually nondisplaced but, in some situations, can be significantly displaced.

Zone 2 fractures occur as a result of plantar flexion and adduction of the forefoot. This is the location for the "true" Jones fracture of the fifth metatarsal.

Zone 3 injuries are often the result of chronic, repetitive overuse, usually in the presence of a cavovarus foot type.

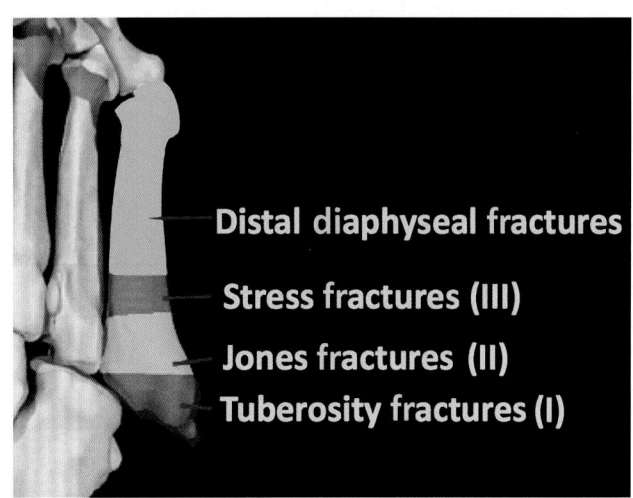

FIGURE 18.1 Location of fifth metatarsal fractures.

Distal diaphyseal fractures are present when one stands in plantar flexion (on the "tiptoes") and sustains an inversion injury. This is more common with dancers.

TREATMENT

Since each of the metatarsals functions in a different fashion, the treatment protocols require a different approach depending on the metatarsal involved. Also, the location of the fracture in the given metatarsal, amount of displacement, if there are multiple metatarsals involved, and if there is an intra-articular component, all weigh in to the decision process of whether nonsurgical or surgical treatment is indicated. Moreover, an open fracture or the presence of a compartment syndrome will require immediate surgical attention.

FIRST METATARSAL FRACTURES

Since the first metatarsal bears about one-third of the body weight through the forefoot, displacement in any direction disturbs the biomechanics of the foot. Nondisplaced first metatarsal fractures may be treated nonoperatively with immobilization. This may consist of non–weight bearing or protective weight bearing in a short-leg splint or fiberglass cast, a removable cast boot or surgical postoperative shoe for 4-6 weeks. Surgical intervention is recommended for any displacement especially in the sagittal or frontal planes. Following anatomic reduction, fixation is desired in order to stabilize the fracture fragments, which will minimize the incidence of malunion and nonunion. Depending upon the location of the fracture and the amount of displacement and comminution, various fixation techniques may be utilized. Specifically, indications for surgical intervention include angulation >10 degrees, >3-4 mm of displacement, articular involvement, and the presence of a rotational deformity or shortening (Fig. 18.2). Fixation options may include Kirschner wires, interfragmentary screws, plate, (Fig. 18.3) and cerclage wire. Postoperatively, the patient will be non–weight bearing in a short leg splint for 2 weeks. At that point, a removable boot may be employed for an additional 4 weeks while keeping the patient non–weight bearing. Weight bearing in the boot is permitted at the 6-week mark, and the

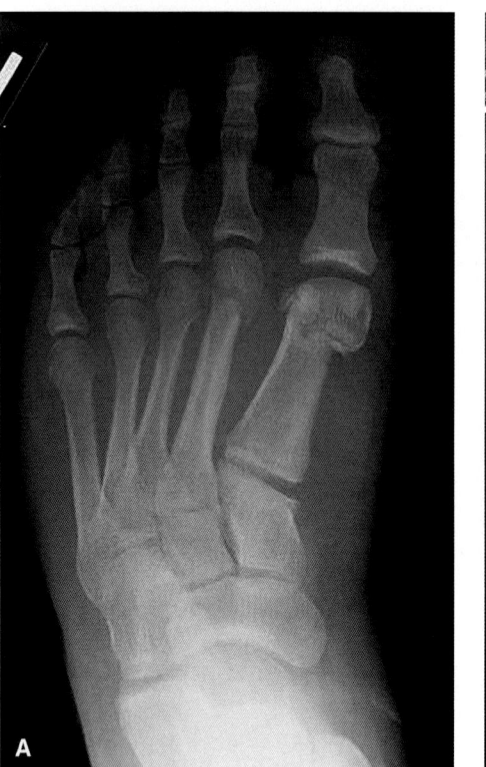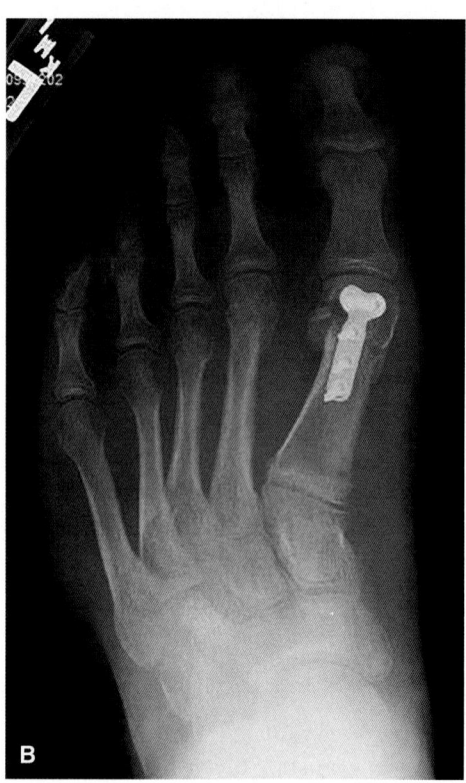

FIGURE 18.2 A. Displaced distal first metatarsal fracture. **B.** T-plate fixation of the first metatarsal fracture. Note the nondisplaced distal second metatarsal fracture treated nonoperatively.

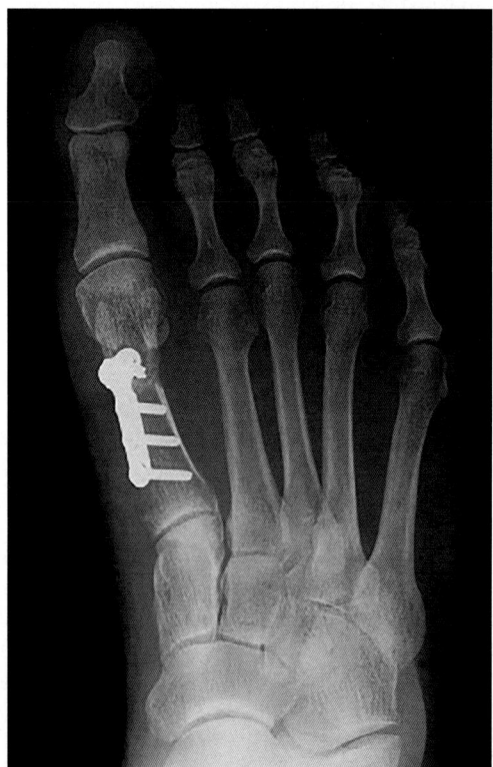

FIGURE 18.3 Screws and T-plate fixation of a diaphyseal fracture of the first metatarsal.

patient will transition into a shoe at the 8- to 9-week mark. If there is significant comminution, external fixation may be necessary in order to maintain the length of the first ray.

When to Perform Surgery—First Metatarsal

- Angulation >10 degrees
- Displacement >3-4 mm
- Intra-articular fracture
- Rotational deformity
- Shortening

CENTRAL METATARSAL FRACTURES

Central metatarsal fractures are usually the result of direct trauma. With these types of injuries, a compartment syndrome is possible; therefore it is imperative to evaluate the neurovascular status of the foot (Fig. 18.4). When appropriate, compartment pressure measurements may be obtained and a surgical release of the involved compartments may be performed. Central metatarsal fractures are located distally, centrally, or at the base. The distal and base fractures may have an intra-articular involvement. Nondisplaced fractures may be treated with conservative care consisting of non–weight bearing or protective weight bearing in a short-leg splint or fiberglass cast, a removable cast boot, or surgical postoperative shoe for 4-6 weeks. Surgical intervention is recommended if the fracture is dorsally or plantarly subluxed by 4 mm or greater.

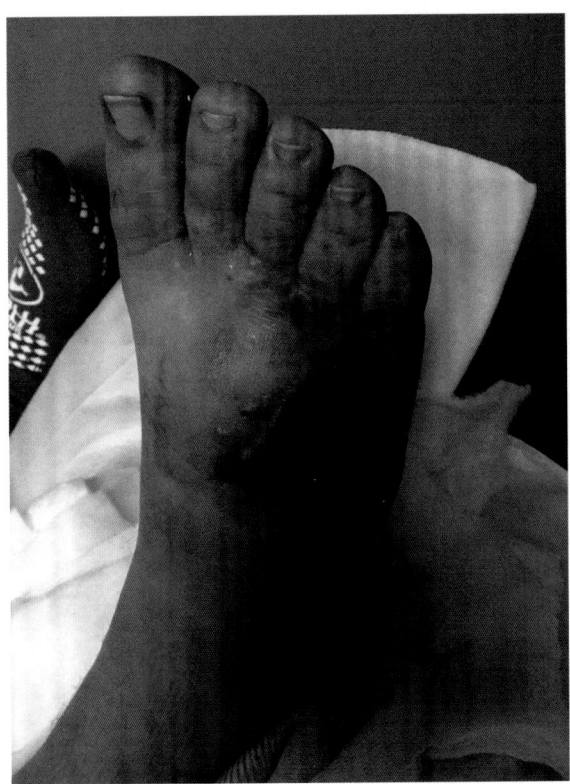

FIGURE 18.4 Compromised soft tissues with fracture blister formation following direct trauma to the foot.

When to Perform Surgery—Central Metatarsals

- Dorsal or plantar subluxation 4 mm or greater
- Intra-articular fracture with 1 mm or greater offset or separation

Then, anatomic reduction and appropriate fixation is utilized. Distracting the digit may help in reducing the fracture. Then a percutaneous Kirschner wire may be driven into the metatarsal head just plantar to the digit and advanced down the medullary canal of the metatarsal. Intraoperative fluoroscopy (anteroposterior, medial oblique, and lateral oblique views) is useful in guiding the pin correctly. If the fracture cannot be closed reduced, open reduction is performed. The fracture may be fixed with an antegrade percutaneous Kirschner wire. However, if the fracture is comminuted, internal fixation with a plate and screws is employed. Metatarsal fractures fixed with plate and screws have high rates of union and low final fracture angulation.[10] The surgeon will take into account the location of the fracture, as well as the number of metatarsals involved and if there is an intra-articular component and comminution when deciding which type of fixation is preferable (Figs. 18.5-18.9). The postoperative course is similar to first metatarsal fractures.

In some cases, there may be a combination of dislocation of one metatarsal and a displaced fracture of another metatarsal with compromised skin and soft tissue (Fig. 18.10). In these cases, the procedures may have to be staged by closed reduction of the dislocation with percutaneous pinning and then open reduction and internal fixation after the soft tissues are no longer compromised (Fig. 18.11).

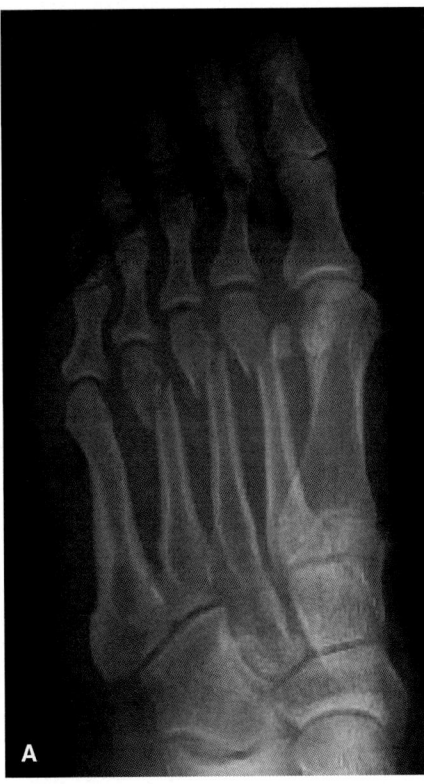 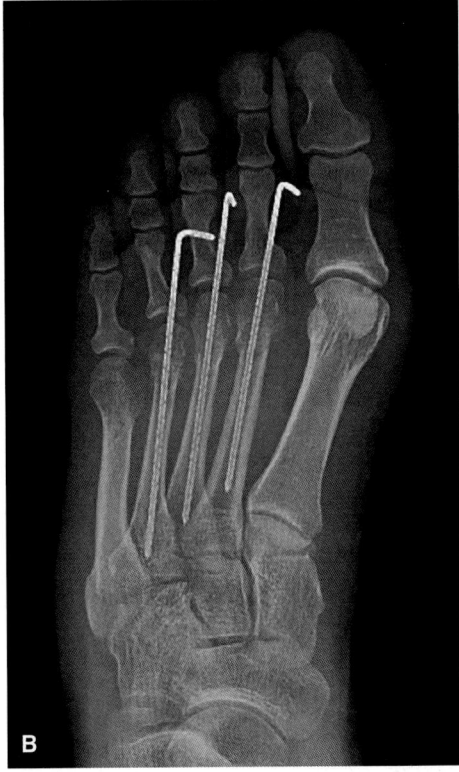

FIGURE 18.5 A. Displaced distal fractures of metatarsals 2, 3, and 4. **B.** Closed reduction and percutaneous K-wire fixation of the fractures.

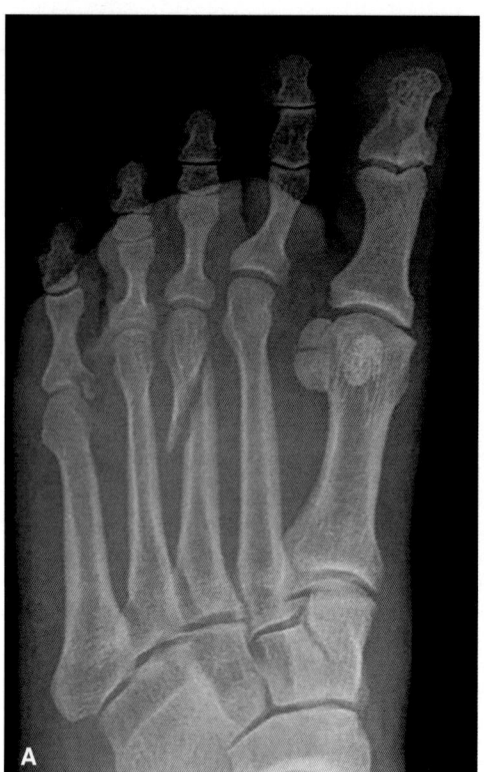
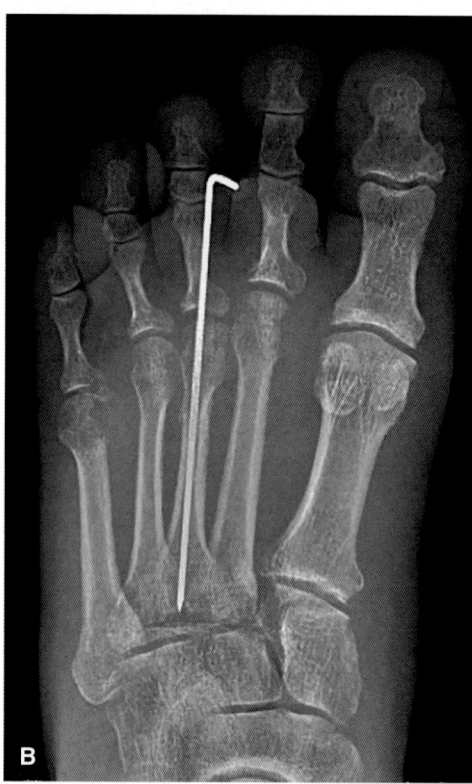

FIGURE 18.6 A. Displaced diaphyseal fracture of the third metatarsal. **B.** Percutaneous K-wire fixation.

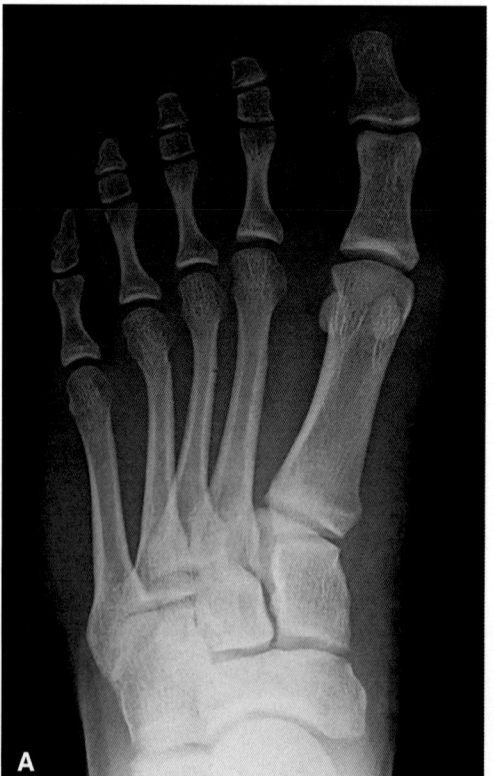
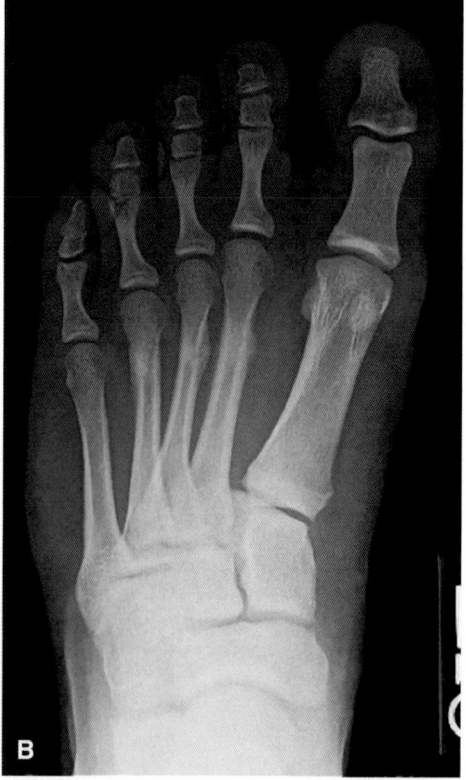

FIGURE 18.7 A. Nondisplaced diaphyseal fractures of metatarsals 2, 3, and 4. **B.** Fractures healed with nonoperative treatment.

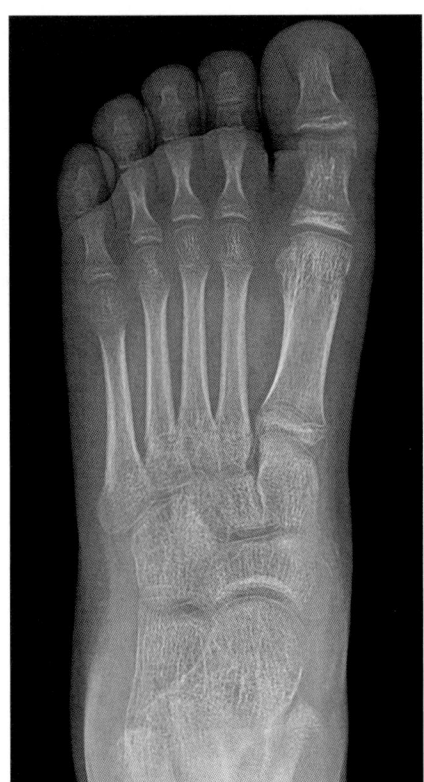
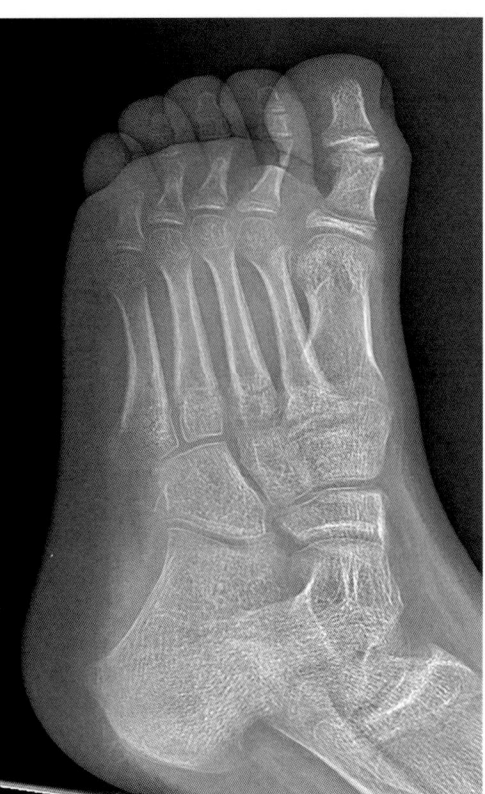

FIGURE 18.8 Nondisplaced base fractures of metatarsals 3 and 4.

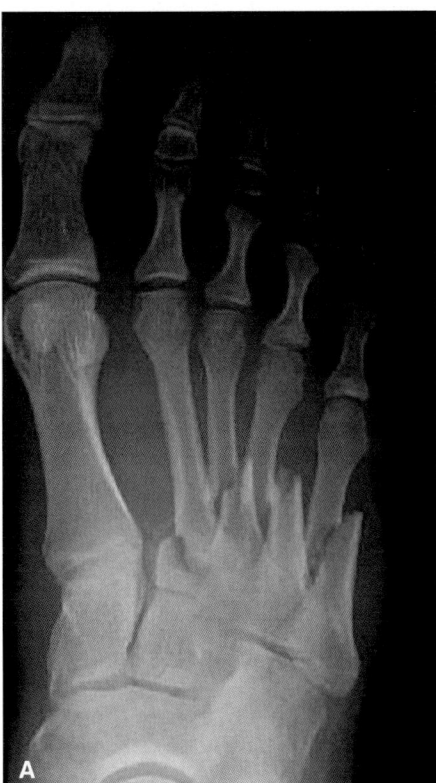
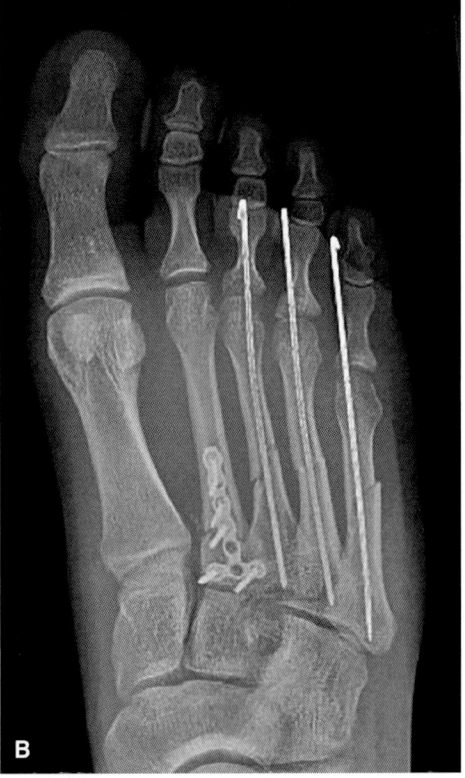

FIGURE 18.9 A. Displaced fracture of the second metatarsal base and diaphyseal fractures of metatarsals 3, 4, and 5. **B.** Open reduction and internal fixation of second metatarsal fracture with T-plate and screws. Percutaneous K-wire fixation of metatarsals 3, 4, and 5.

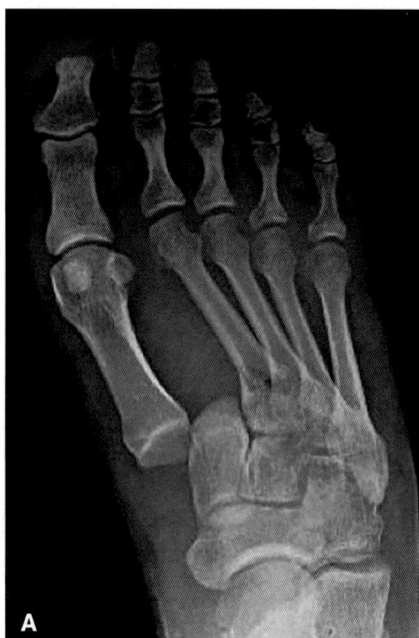
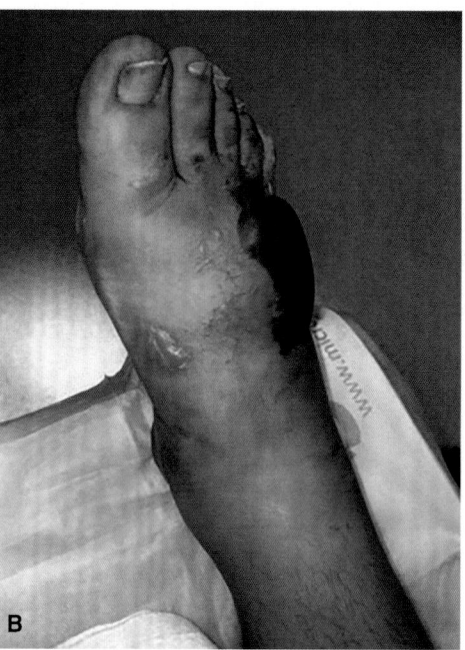

FIGURE 18.10 A. Dislocation of the first metatarsocuneiform joint and fracture of the base of the second metatarsal. **B.** Severe edema and fracture blister formation.

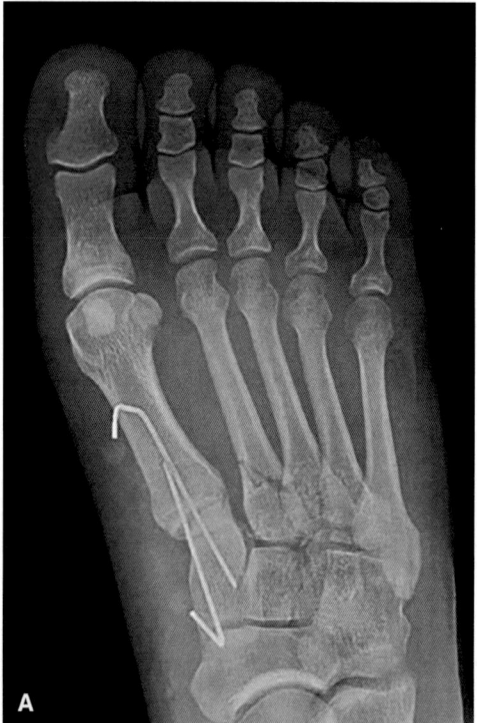
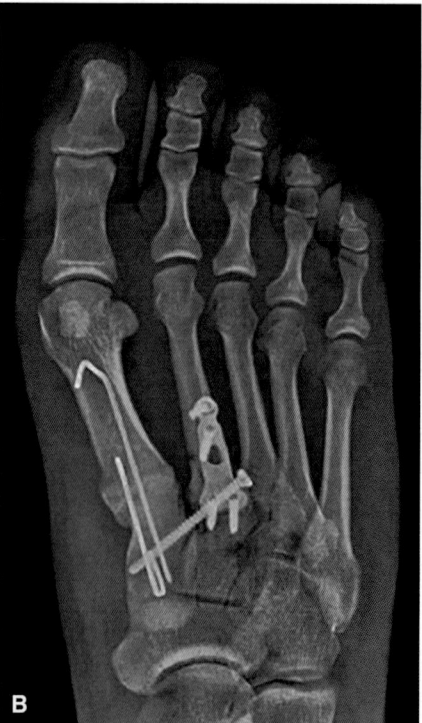

FIGURE 18.11 A. The first metatarsocuneiform joint is closed reduced and fixed with two crossed K-wires. **B.** Following satisfactory reduction of edema and healing of the fracture blisters, the second metatarsal base fracture is repaired with open reduction and internal fixation. Note the placement of a screw from the second metatarsal base to the medial cuneiform (see Chapter 24: Tarsometatarsal Fractures).

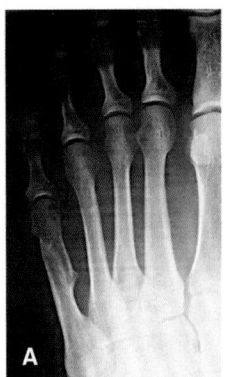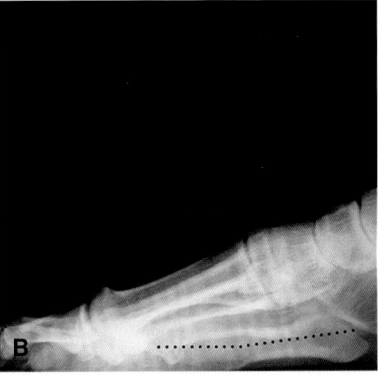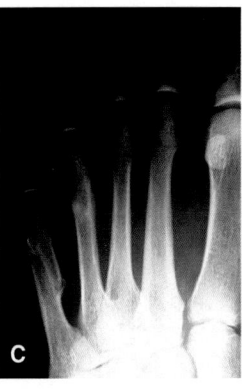

FIGURE 18.12 A. Healed diaphyseal fracture of the fifth metatarsal. **B.** Lateral radiograph demonstrating the malunion of the fifth metatarsal with dorsiflexed position of the distal fragment. **C.** Development of the fourth metatarsal stress fracture due to the biomechanical imbalance of the forefoot.

FIFTH METATARSAL FRACTURES

The management of fifth metatarsal fractures depends on the zone of injury.

When to Perform Surgery—Fifth Metatarsal
Zone 1
■ Displacement >2 mm
■ 30% or greater involvement of the joint
Zones 2 and 3
■ Displacement
■ All in athletes or highly active patients
Distal/Diaphyseal
■ Dorsal or plantar subluxation 4 mm or greater
■ Intra-articular fracture with 1 mm or greater offset or separation

Nondisplaced zone 1 or metatarsal base avulsion fractures and distal nondisplaced diaphyseal fractures have an excellent potential for healing and are usually treated nonoperatively.[11] On the other hand, zone 2 and 3 metatarsal fractures have less consistent outcomes with conservative care.

Distal diaphyseal fractures that are nondisplaced may be treated in a weight-bearing cast, removable cast boot, or surgical shoe for 4-8 weeks. The healing potential for these fractures is excellent.[12] Some authors have advocated nonoperative treatment for displaced fractures due to the capacity for healing, as well as the fact that the fifth metatarsal is very mobile and can accommodate a lot of deformity.[13] One must be cautious, however, because displacement of the distal fragment in the sagittal plane may result in a malunion with metatarsalgia.[14,15]

The metatarsalgia may be significant enough to lead to a stress fracture of an adjacent metatarsal (Fig. 18.12). Distal diaphyseal fractures that are displaced may be treated with open reduction and internal fixation utilizing screws or a small plate and screws (Fig. 18.13).

Zone 1 fractures and distal diaphyseal fractures that are nondisplaced may be treated in a weight-bearing cast, removable cast boot, or surgical shoe for 4-8 weeks (Figs. 18.14 and 18.15). Operative intervention may be considered for zone 1 fractures if displacement is >2 mm or those involving 30% or more of the joint.[2,16] In addition, if there is there is significant comminution, ORIF is indicated. Fixation options include an interfragmentary bicortical screw, a cancellous lag screw, tension band wiring, or plate fixation.

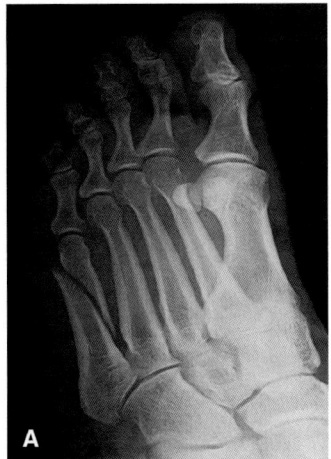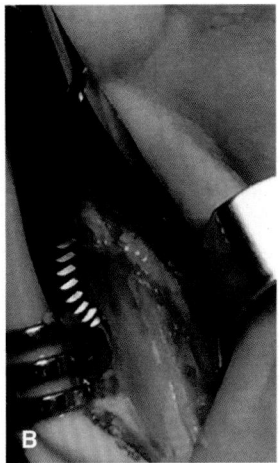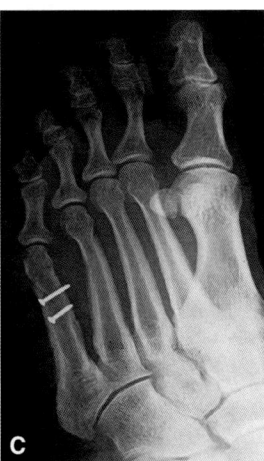

FIGURE 18.13 A. Displaced diaphyseal fracture of the fifth metatarsal. **B.** Anatomic reduction with temporary bone clamp. **C.** Screw fixation of the fracture.

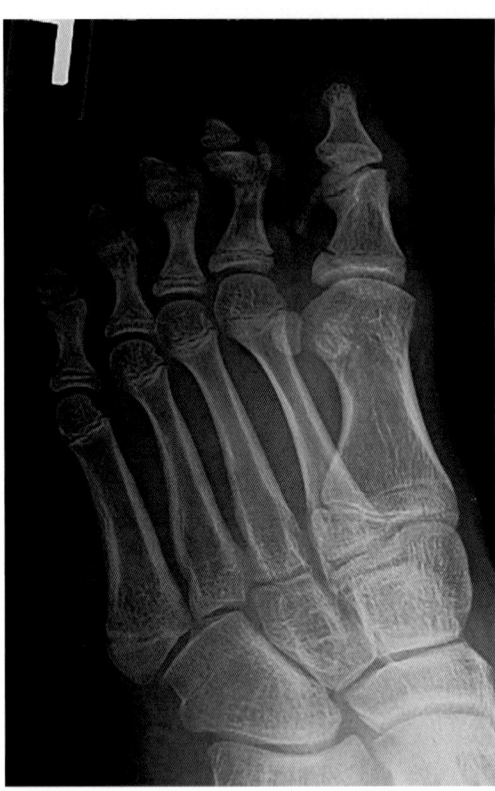

FIGURE 18.14 Nondisplaced avulsion fracture of the base of the fifth metatarsal.

PEARLS AND PITFALLS—FIFTH METATARSAL ZONE 1

Pearls	Pitfalls
▪ When temporarily stabilizing the fragment, drill a small hole in the dorsal cortex of the shaft of the metatarsal in order to accommodate the sharp tip of a bone clamp.	▪ An intramedullary screw with too small of a diameter may result in suboptimal purchase and inferior fixation.
▪ In the event of a displaced fragment with comminution, a small hook plate may yield the best fixation.	▪ With tension band technique, make sure the ends of the wire are twisting around each other, NOT one twisting around the other.

The patient may be placed in the supine position with elevation of the involved extremity or in a lateral decubitus position. An incision is placed just proximal to the base of the fifth metatarsal. For intramedullary screw fixation, a guide pin is placed from the tip of the styloid process aiming down the intramedullary canal. Two C-arm views are obtained in order to verify proper reduction and satisfactory placement of the guide pin. A cannulated 4.0- or 5.0-mm screw is then

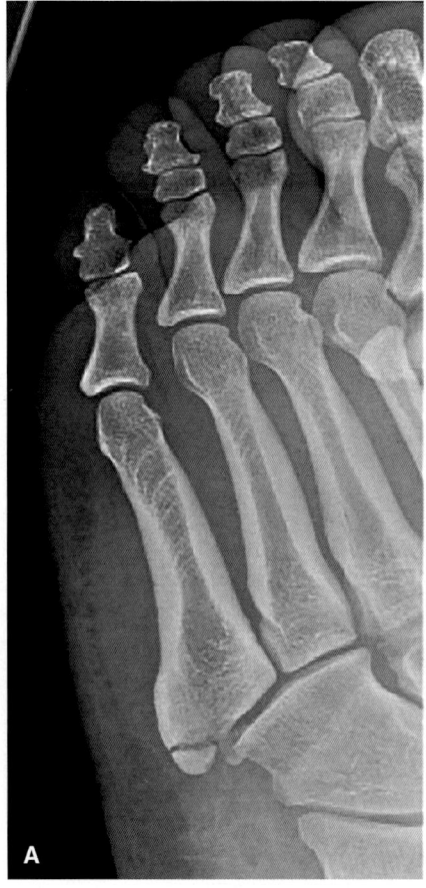
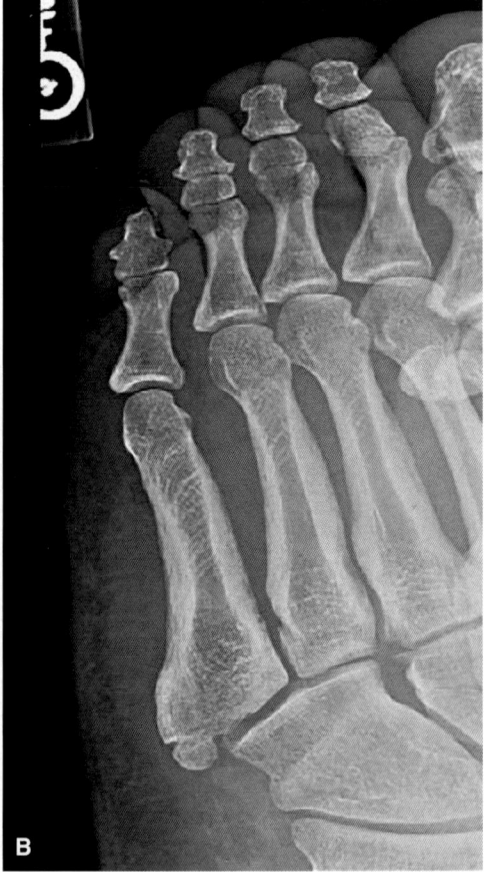

FIGURE 18.15 **A.** Small nondisplaced avulsion fracture of the fifth metatarsal base. **B.** Healed fracture treated with nonoperative measures.

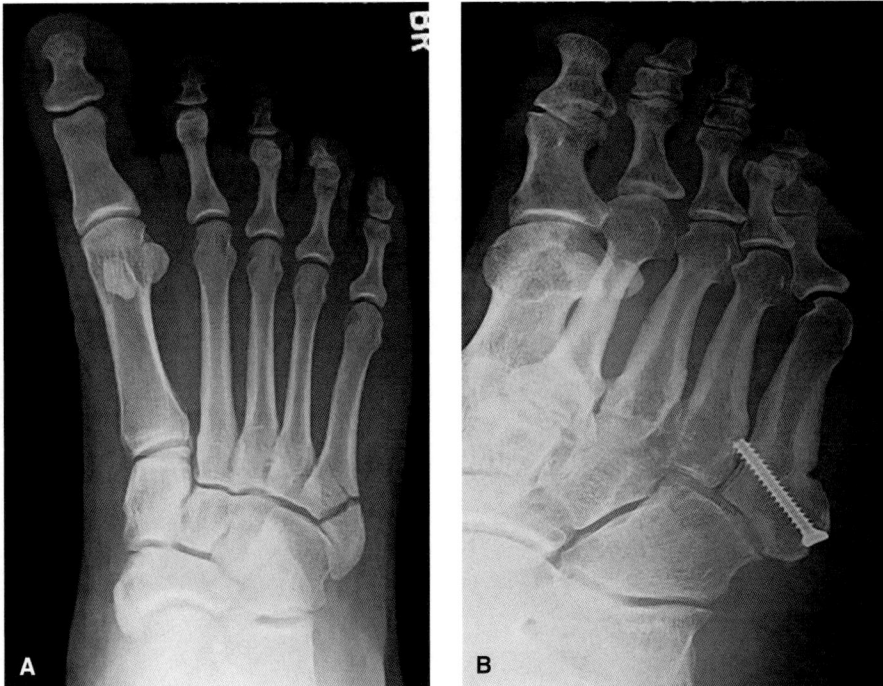

FIGURE 18.16 A. Displaced fifth metatarsal base fracture. **B.** Open reduction and internal fixation with a cortical screw crossing two cortices.

placed over the pin using standard technique (Fig. 18.16). For the bicortical technique, dissection is limited around the peroneus brevis tendon. The fracture fragment is anatomically reduced and held in place with a small bone reduction clamp. Fixation is achieved with a 3.5 cortical screw using standard AO technique. The bicortical technique has been shown to be biomechanically stronger than the intramedullary technique[17] (Fig. 18.17).

For small, displaced avulsion fractures, a standard tension band technique may be utilized[18] (Fig. 18.18). Likewise, if the fragment is comminuted, a small hook plate with screws may be used (Fig. 18.19).

The treatment of zone 2 and 3 fractures is more controversial compared to the treatment of zone 1 and distal diaphyseal fractures. Zone 2 and 3 fractures that are nondisplaced may be treated nonoperatively employing full immobilization and

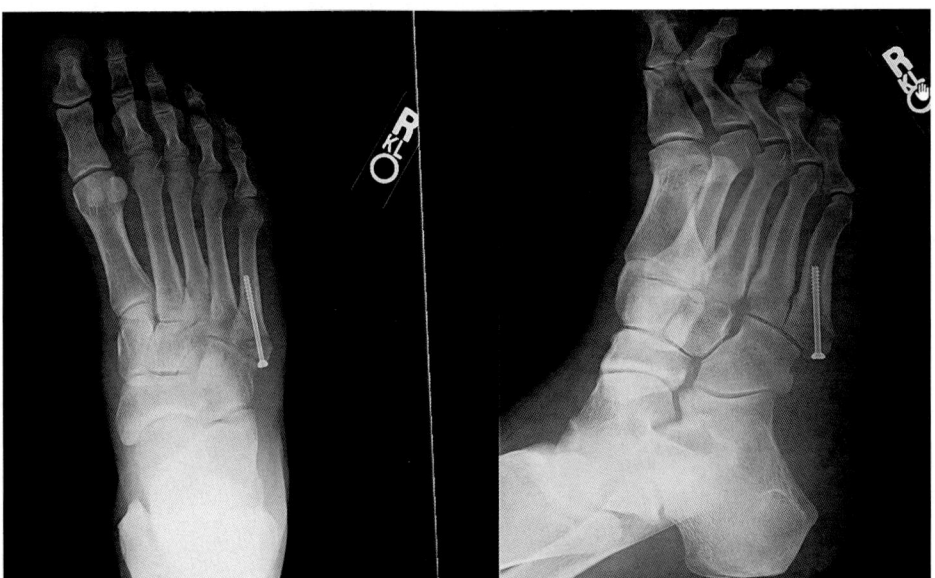

FIGURE 18.17 Open reduction and internal fixation of fifth metatarsal base fracture with a cannulated cancellous intramedullary screw.

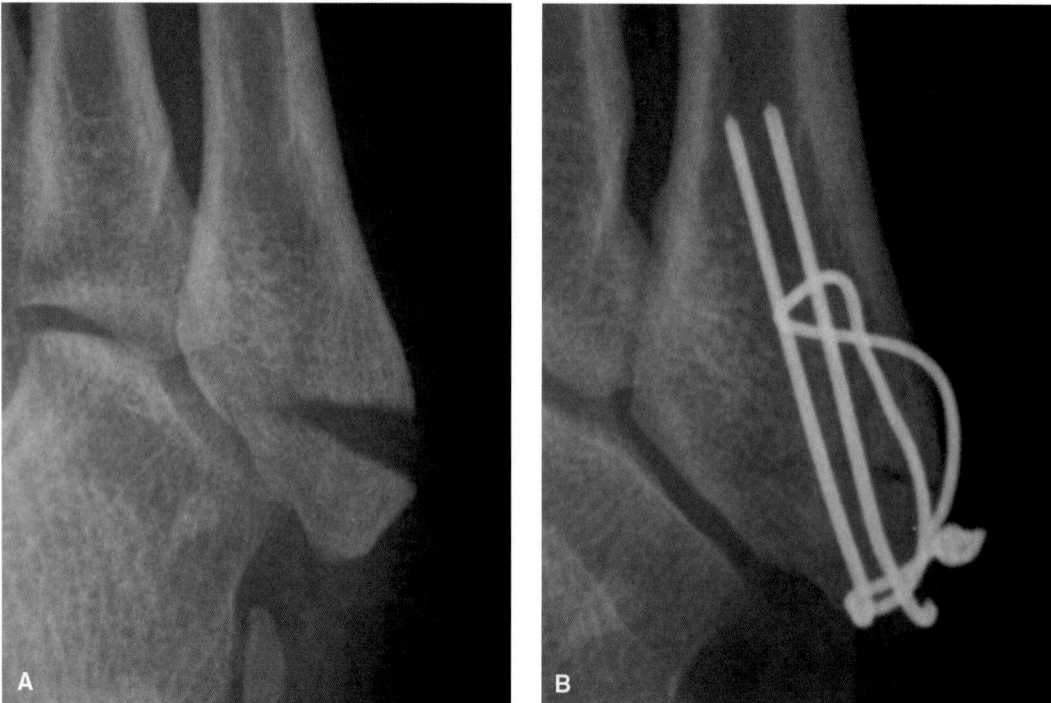

FIGURE 18.18 A. Small avulsion fracture with displacement at the fifth metatarsal-cuboid articulation. **B.** Tension band wiring of the small fracture fragment.

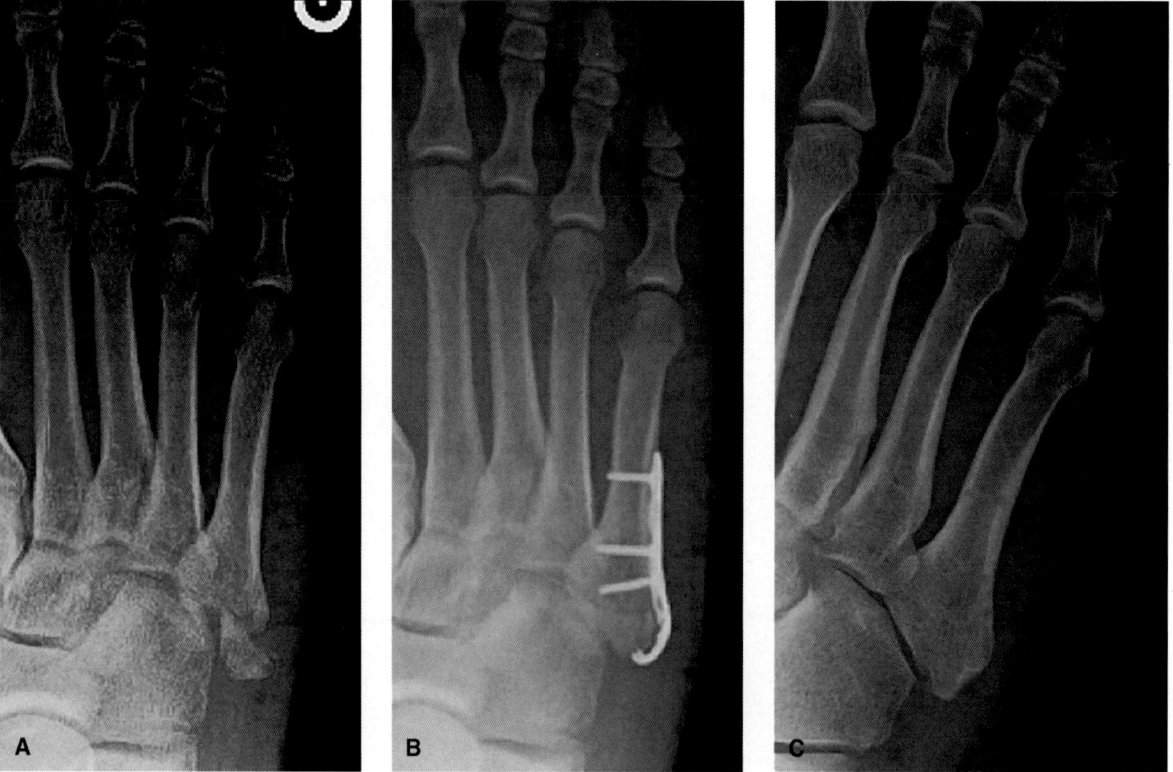

FIGURE 18.19 A. Displaced, comminuted fifth metatarsal base fracture. **B.** Open reduction and internal fixation with a small hook plate and screws. **C.** Removal of the hardware and healed fracture.

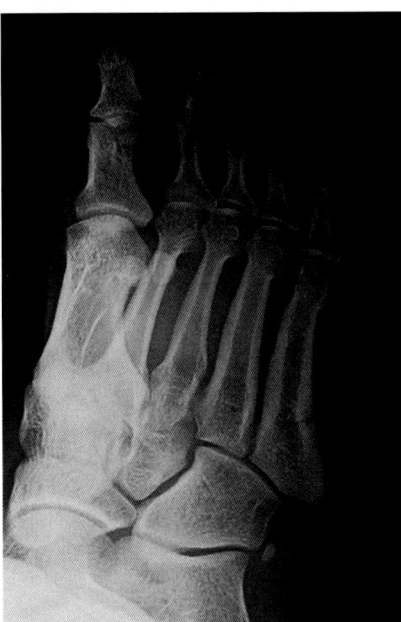

FIGURE 18.20 Nondisplaced Jones fracture (zone 2) of the fifth metatarsal.

non–weight bearing for 6-8 weeks[19] (Figs. 18.20 and 18.21). The patient is then transitioned to a boot with progressive weight bearing for an additional 3-4 weeks. In athletes and patients with a high level of activity, some surgeons prefer to proceed with operative intervention since it has been shown that in this

patient population, there is an earlier return to weight bearing with a more rapid and predictable union rate.[20]

When displacement is present with zone 2 and 3 fifth metatarsal fractures, there is less controversy in regard to treatment. Early operative intervention with intramedullary screw placement resulted in a faster clinical union by almost 50% and faster return to activity.[19,21]

Percutaneous fixation with an intramedullary screw is the preferred approach for zone 2 and 3 fractures of the fifth metatarsal. Adequate compression can be attained with little or no stripping of periosteum at the fracture site.[22] The literature has assessed what type (cannulated vs noncannulated), size, and length of screw is most appropriate[23-25] (Fig. 18.22). In general, a noncannulated screw 4.5-6.5 mm in diameter is utilized. An attempt is made to use the largest core diameter screw that fits the canal. Since the fifth metatarsal often has a lateral bend, care must be taken not to use a screw that is excessively long. The average straight-length segment of the fifth metatarsal has been shown to be 68% of the total length of the metatarsal.[24,26] The screw length is best evaluated on the lateral radiograph, while the screw diameter is best appreciated on the anteroposterior radiograph.[23]

PEARLS AND PITFALLS—FIFTH METATARSAL ZONES 2 AND 3

Pearls	Pitfalls
■ Use an intramedullary screw with the largest diameter possible in order to achieve sufficient osseous purchase and satisfactory compression. When tapping, if the threads of the tap are not engaging the bone sufficiently, change to the next larger size tap.	■ Using an excessively long screw that violates the medial cortex of the distal metatarsal.

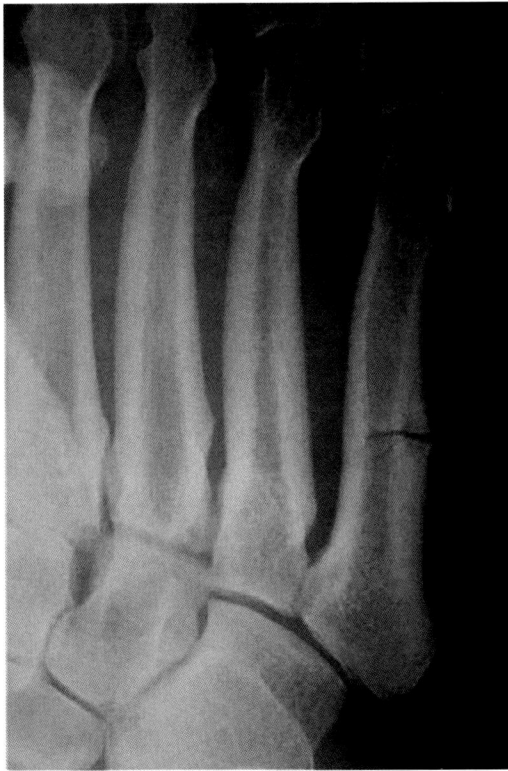

FIGURE 18.21 Nondisplaced fifth metatarsal stress fracture (zone 3).

One must also be cognizant of the foot type and morphology of the fifth metatarsal when deciding on operative vs nonoperative treatment of zone 2 and 3 fifth metatarsal fractures. The presence of a cavovarus or adducted foot type with a long, narrow, and straight fifth metatarsal, puts one at more risk for fifth metatarsal Jones fractures[27-30] (Fig. 18.23). Operative intervention in these patients may decrease the rates of nonunions and refractures. Patient obesity and fifth metatarsal protrusion may increase the incidence of refracture.[31]

For operative treatment the patient may be placed in the supine position with elevation of the affected extremity or in a lateral decubitus position. A small incision is performed just proximal to the styloid process of the fifth metatarsal, and the goal is to use cannulated instrumentation but ultimately use a noncannulated screw (Fig. 18.24). It has been accepted that the entrance point of the pin should be superior and medial at the base of the metatarsal. A recent cadaveric study[32] has shown that the ideal entrance point is at the center of the base of the fifth metatarsal at the lateral margin of the cartilage. Forefoot adduction may be

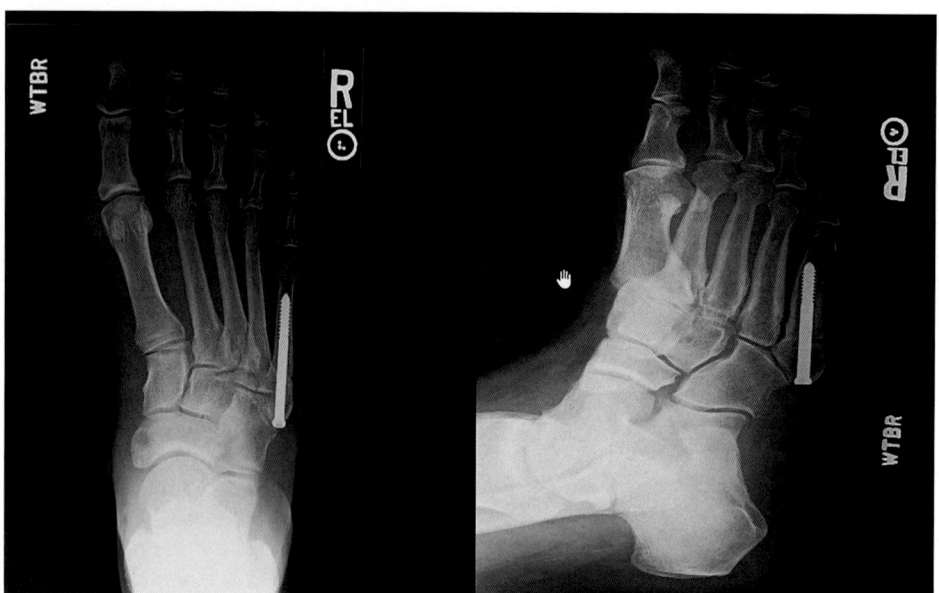

FIGURE 18.22 Percutaneous intramedullary fixation of Jones fracture.

necessary to gain access to this site. The pin is carefully advanced down the intramedullary canal. C-arm lateral, anteroposterior, and oblique views are taken to insure satisfactory pin placement. The appropriate screw length and diameter are assessed on the lateral and anteroposterior views, respectively. A cannulated drill and tap are then used. Finally, the instrumentation is removed and the screw is inserted (Fig. 18.25).

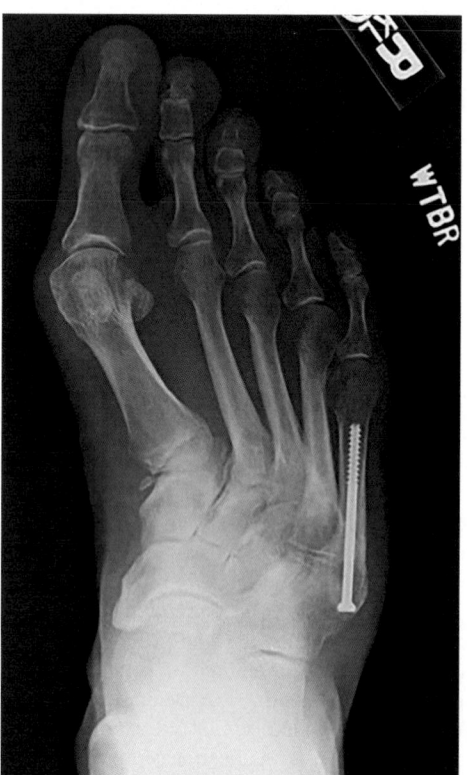

FIGURE 18.23 Healed stress fracture of the fifth metatarsal with percutaneous intramedullary screw. The patient has a cavoadductus foot type.

Postoperatively, the patient is non–weight bearing for 4 weeks and then weight bearing as tolerated in a boot for 2-4 weeks followed by return to a supportive shoe and initiation of rehabilitation. Return to activity is somewhere between 7 and 12 weeks after surgery.

STRESS FRACTURES

Stress fractures may occur in any metatarsal but more commonly occur in the second metatarsal. They are a result of increased activity, which leads to microtrauma to the affected area.[33] There are specific intrinsic factors that may contribute to the development of a stress fracture. The level of fitness of an individual can be an issue. If one is not accustomed to physical activity, the involved metatarsal may develop an insufficiency fracture. This is common in military recruits or other individuals who start a new activity, such as distance running, and do not slowly acclimate to the new activity. The anatomic alignment and morphology of the foot or specific metatarsal can result in abnormal weight-bearing forces leading to a stress fracture. The cavovarus and adducted foot have previously been discussed in regard to the development of fifth metatarsal fractures (zones 2 and 3). This has also been shown to be a factor in the development of fourth metatarsal stress fractures.[34,35] Moreover, long or short metatarsal as well as dorsiflexed or plantar flexed metatarsals may alter the biomechanics of the foot and lead to a metatarsal stress fracture. Finally, female athletes that have abnormal menstrual cycles, low bone mass (osteoporosis), and deficient energy needs, which is commonly referred to as the female athlete triad, may be predisposed to stress fractures of the metatarsals.

Several extrinsic factors can be responsible for stress fracture development. A change in the intensity of a training regimen, even in a seasoned athlete, may put abnormal stress on a metatarsal leading to a fracture. In addition, worn-out shoe gear and the playing surface itself can be contributing factors. An older shoe can result in a lack of stability and accommodation to the foot. Likewise, the playing surface, such as a banked

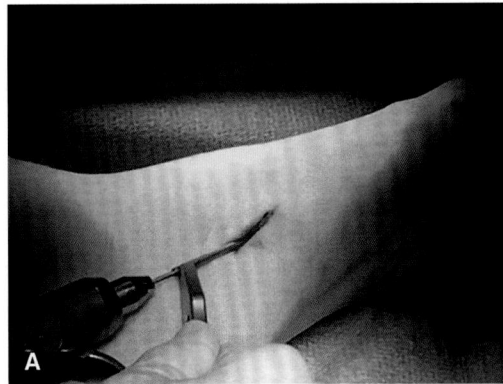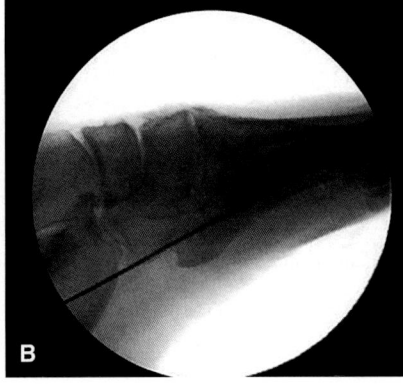

FIGURE 18.24 **A.** Placement of guide pin for Jones fracture fixation. **B.** Intraoperative C-arm view demonstrating satisfactory placement of the guide pin.

indoor track, may produce abnormal forces to the feet leading to the development of a stress fracture to a metatarsal bone.

A thorough history is important when assessing the patient. This will help to highlight any intrinsic and extrinsic factors that may be responsible for the patient's discomfort. The exam usually yields pinpoint tenderness over the involved metatarsal, and edema may be present. Plain film radiographs may show bone callus formation, which is indicative of a healing stress fracture (Fig. 18.26). However, early in the development of stress fracture, the x-rays may be negative. A triphasic bone scan or MRI may be considered, as well as treating the patient symptomatically and repeating the x-rays in about 2 weeks.

The treatment of metatarsal stress fractures usually consists of guarded weight bearing in a surgical shoe or boot. Surgical intervention is rare and possibly utilized in athletes with fifth metatarsal stress fractures (zone 3). Surgery is also considered in an established pseudarthrosis or a refracture.

NONUNIONS

The mean incidence of nonunion for the acute Jones fracture of the fifth metatarsal (Fig. 18.27) is 20.8% with nonoperative treatment.[36] One study suggested that evaluation of the plantar gap of proximal fifth metatarsal fractures on the oblique radiograph view may have prognostic value. There were significantly

longer healing times for incomplete proximal fractures of the fifth metatarsal >1 mm.[31] In the event of a refracture or nonunion of a proximal fifth metatarsal fracture, open reduction with autogenous bone grafting with screw and plate fixation (Fig. 18.28) may be considered.[37] In addition, plate fixation with autogenous calcaneal dowel graft has been used successfully in treating nonunions of proximal fourth and fifth metatarsal fractures.[38] Patients who have a history of multiple stress fractures (Fig. 18.29) may require a nutritional assessment and metabolic bone workup.[39] These patients may benefit from a referral to an endocrinologist.

Laboratory Tests for Nonunions
25-hydroxyvitamin D
Calcium
Phosphorus
Alkaline phosphatase
Magnesium
Parathyroid hormone
Growth hormone
Insulinlike growth factor 1
Thyroid function test
Cortisol (serum)
Testosterone/free testosterone
CBC

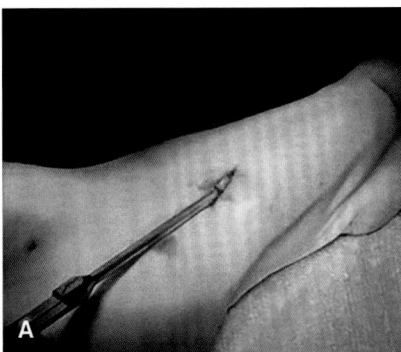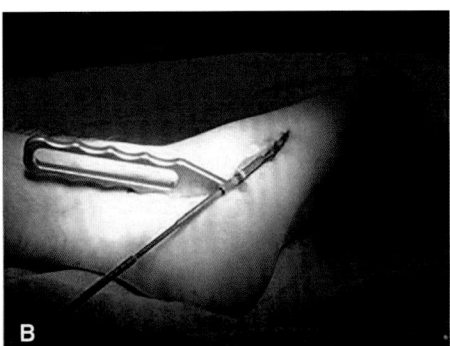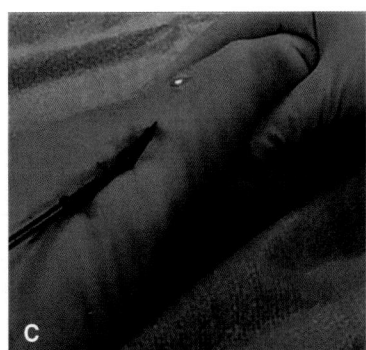

FIGURE 18.25 **A.** Depth gauge placed over the guide pin to obtain the desired screw length. **B.** Cannulated tap placed over the guide pin. **C.** Guide pin removed and placement of the solid intramedullary screw.

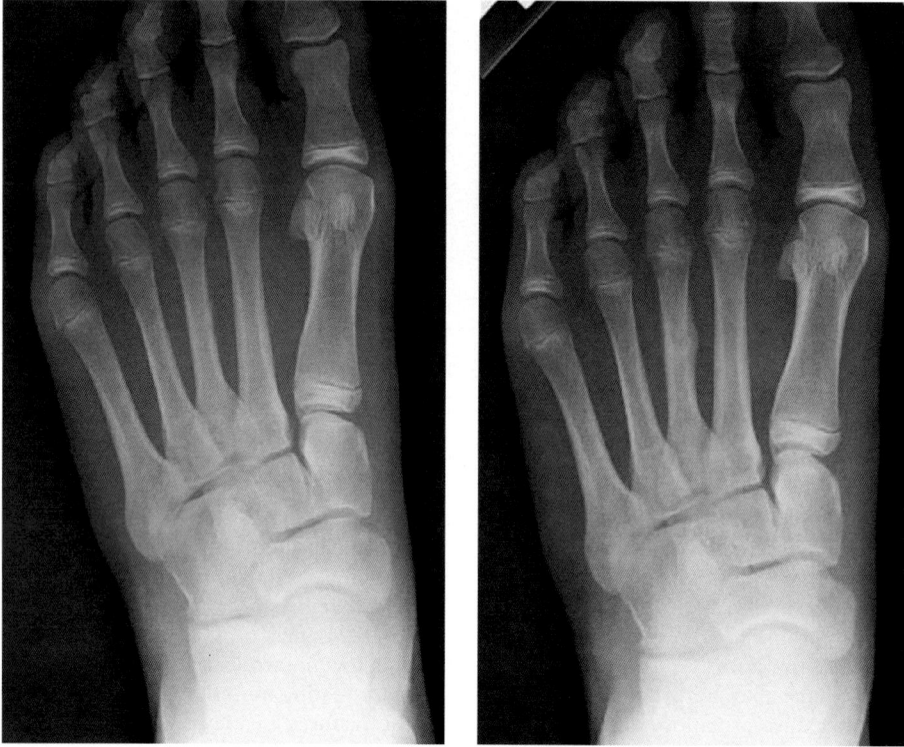

FIGURE 18.26 Healing stress fracture of the third metatarsal with bone callus.

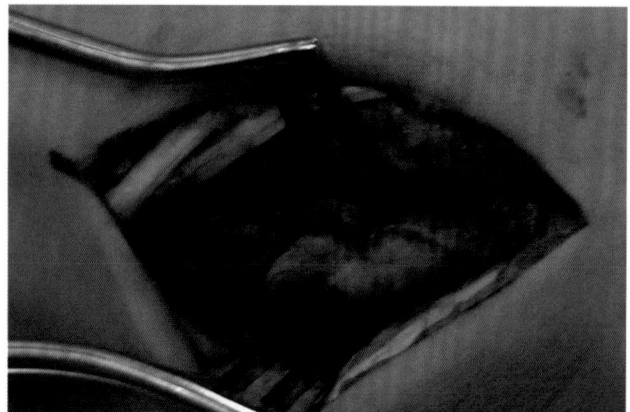

FIGURE 18.27 Nonunion of fifth metatarsal fracture.

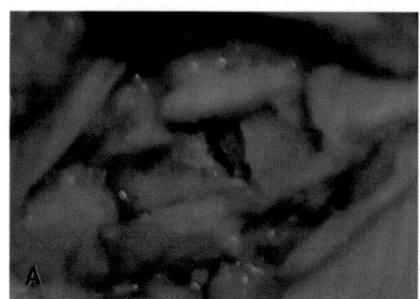
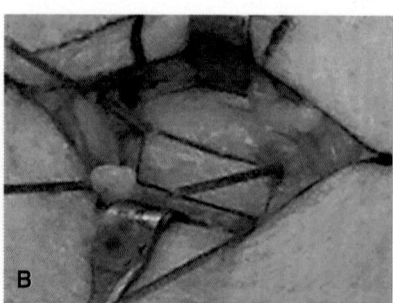
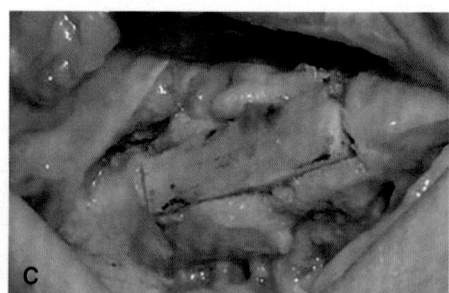

FIGURE 18.28 A. Rectangular section of bone removed at the metatarsal nonunion site. **B.** Harvest of tibial autogenous graft. **C.** Placement of autogenous graft into the metatarsal nonunion site.

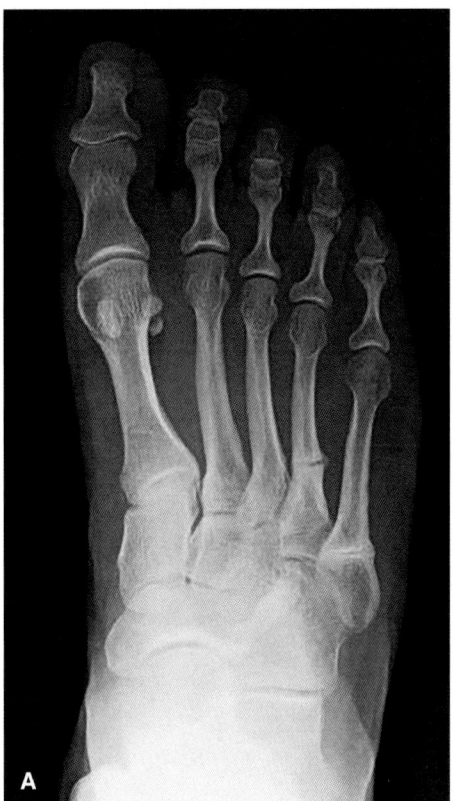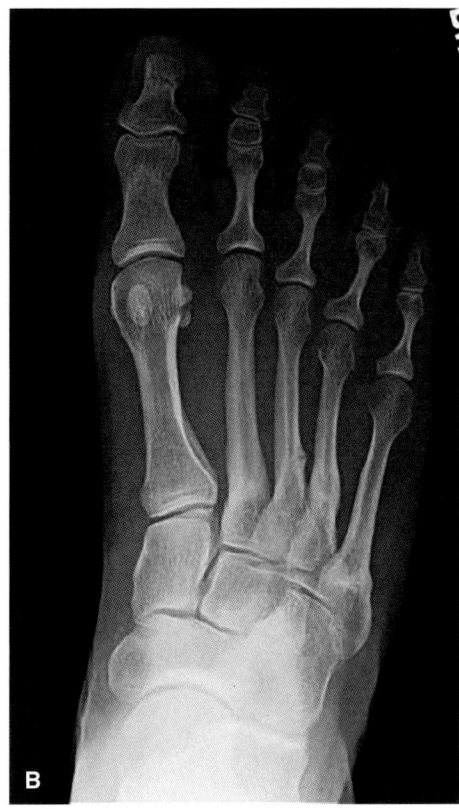

FIGURE 18.29 A. Healed fifth metatarsal stress fracture with subsequent development of a fourth metatarsal stress fracture. **B.** Same patient who now shows healing of a third metatarsal stress fracture.

CONCLUSION

Metatarsal fractures are a common injury seen by foot and ankle physicians. In most cases, nondisplaced fractures heal uneventfully with immobilization and protected weight bearing. The fifth metatarsal Jones fracture may be the exception. In patients with a high level of activity, surgical intervention may be indicated. Any metatarsal fracture that is displaced or has intra-articular involvement may require open reduction and internal fixation. Malunion and nonunion are potential complications of metatarsal fractures. Persistent metatarsal stress fractures or recurrent nonunions may require further metabolic workup.

REFERENCES

1. Pituckanotai K, Arirachakaran A, Piyapittayanun P, Tuchinda H, Peradhammanon E, Kongtharvonskul J. Comparative outcomes of cast and removable support in fracture fifth metatarsal bone: systematic review and meta-analysis. *J Foot Ankle Surg.* 2018;57: 982-986.
2. Buddecke DE, Polk MA, Barp EA. Metatarsal fractures. *Clin Podiatr Med Surg.* 2010;27: 601-624.
3. Cakir H, Van Vliet-Koppert ST, Van Lieshout EMM, De Vries MR, Van Der Elst M, Schepers T. Demographics and outcome of metatarsal fractures. *Arch Orthop Trauma Surg.* 2011;131:241-245.
4. Chou LB. *Orthopaedic Knowledge Update: Foot and Ankle 5.* Rosemont, IL: Lippincott Williams & Wilkins; 2018.
5. Draves DJ. *Anatomy of the Lower Extremity.* Baltimore, MD: Williams & Wilkins; 1986.
6. Smith JW, Arnoczky SP, Hersh A. The intraosseous blood supply of the fifth metatarsal: implications for proximal fracture healing. *Foot Ankle.* 1992;13:143-152.
7. Urteaga AJ, Lynch M. Fractures of the central metatarsals. *Clin Podiatr Med Surg.* 1995;12:759-772.
8. Petrisor BA, Ekrol I, Court-Brown C. The epidemiology of metatarsal fractures. *Foot Ankle Int.* 2006;27:172-174.
9. DeVries JG, Taefi E, Bussewitz BW, Hyer CF, Lee TH. The fifth metatarsal base: anatomic evaluation regarding fracture mechanism and treatment algorithms. *J Foot Ankle Surg.* 2015;54:94-98.
10. Bryant T, Beck DM, Daniel JN, Pedowitz DI, Raikin SM. Union rate and rate of hardware removal following plate fixation of metatarsal shaft and neck fractures. *Foot Ankle Int.* 2018;39:326-331.
11. Shahid MK, Punwar S, Boulind C, Bannister G. Aircast walking boot and below-knee walking cast for avulsion fractures of the base of the fifth metatarsal: a comparative cohort study. *Foot Ankle Int.* 2013;34:75-79.
12. Soave RL, Bleazey S, Rudowsky A, Clarke RV, Avino A Jr, Kuchar DJ. A new radiographic classification for distal shaft fifth metatarsal fractures. *J Foot Ankle Surg.* 2016;55:803-807.
13. Aynardi M, Pedowitz DI, Saffel H, Piper C, Raikin SM. Outcome of nonoperative management of displaced oblique spiral fractures of the fifth metatarsal shaft. *Foot Ankle Int.* 2013;34:1619-1623.
14. Vogler HW, Westlin N, Mlodzienski AJ, Møller FB. Fifth metatarsal fractures. Biomechanics, classification, and treatment. *Clin Podiatr Med Surg.* 1995;12:725-747.
15. Thompson P, Patel V, Fallat LM, Jarski R. Surgical management of fifth metatarsal diaphyseal fractures: a retrospective outcomes study. *J Foot Ankle Surg.* 2017;56:463-467.
16. Zwitser EW, Breederveld RS. Fractures of the fifth metatarsal; diagnosis and treatment. *Injury.* 2010;41:555-562.
17. Moshirfar A, Campbell JT, Molloy S, Jasper LE, Belkoff SM. Fifth metatarsal tuberosity fracture fixation: a biomechanical study. *Foot Ankle Int.* 2003;24:630-633.
18. The Podiatry Institute; Southerland JT, Boberg JS, Downey MS, Nakra A, Rabjohn LV. *McGlamry's Comprehensive Textbook of Foot and Ankle Surgery.* Baltimore, MD: Lippincott Williams & Wilkins; 2012.
19. Mologne TS, Lundeen JM, Clapper MF, O'Brien TJ. Early screw fixation versus casting in the treatment of acute Jones fractures. *Am J Sports Med.* 2005;33:970-975.
20. Portland G, Kelikian A, Kodros S. Acute surgical management of Jones' fractures. *Foot Ankle Int.* 2003;24:829-833.
21. Porter DA, Duncan M, Meyer SJF. Fifth metatarsal Jones fracture fixation with a 4.5-mm cannulated stainless steel screw in the competitive and recreational athlete: a clinical and radiographic evaluation. *Am J Sports Med.* 2005;33:726-733.
22. Porter DA. Fifth metatarsal Jones fractures in the athlete. *Foot Ankle Int.* 2018;39:250-258.
23. DeSandis B, Murphy C, Rosenbaum A, et al. Multiplanar CT analysis of fifth metatarsal morphology: implications for operative management of zone II fractures. *Foot Ankle Int.* 2016;37:528-536.
24. Ochenjele G, Ho B, Switaj PJ, Fuchs D, Goyal N, Kadakia AR. Radiographic study of the fifth metatarsal for optimal intramedullary screw fixation of Jones fracture. *Foot Ankle Int.* 2015;36:293-301.
25. Horst F, Gilbert BJ, Glisson RR, Nunley JA. Torque resistance after fixation of Jones fractures with intramedullary screws. *Foot Ankle Int.* 2004;25:914-919.

26. Raikin SM, Slenker N, Ratigan B. The association of a varus hindfoot and fracture of the fifth metatarsal metaphyseal-diaphyseal junction: the Jones fracture. *Am J Sports Med.* 2008;36:1367-1372.
27. Karnovsky SC, Rosenbaum AJ, DeSandis B, et al. Radiographic analysis of National Football League players' fifth metatarsal morphology relationship to proximal fifth metatarsal fracture risk. *Foot Ankle Int.* 2019;40(3):318-322.
28. O'Malley M, DeSandis B, Allen A, Levitsky M, O'Malley Q, Williams R. Operative treatment of fifth metatarsal Jones fractures (zones II and III) in the NBA. *Foot Ankle Int.* 2016;37:488-500.
29. Lee KT, Kim KC, Park YU, Kim TW, Lee YK. Radiographic evaluation of foot structure following fifth metatarsal stress fracture. *Foot Ankle Int.* 2011;32:796-801.
30. Sarpong NO, Swindell HW, Trupia EP, Vosseller JT. Metatarsal fractures. *Foot Ankle Orthopaed.* 2018;3:2473011418775094.
31. Lee KT, Park YU, Jegal H, Kim KC, Young KW, Kim JS. Factors associated with recurrent fifth metatarsal stress fracture. *Foot Ankle Int.* 2013;34:1645-1653.
32. Watson GI, Karnovsky SC, Konin G, Drakos MC. Optimal starting point for fifth metatarsal zone II fractures: a cadaveric study. *Foot Ankle Int.* 2017;38:802-807.
33. Queen RM, Crowder TT, Johnson H, Ozumba D, Toth AP. Treatment of metatarsal stress fractures: case reports. *Foot Ankle Int.* 2007;28:506-510.
34. Saxena A, Krisdakumtorn T, Erickson S. Proximal fourth metatarsal injuries in athletes: similarity to proximal fifth metatarsal injury. *Foot Ankle Int.* 2001;22:603-608.
35. Rongstad KM, Tueting J, Rongstad M, Garrels K, Meis R. Fourth metatarsal base stress fractures in athletes: a case series. *Foot Ankle Int.* 2013;34:962-968.
36. Dean BJF, Kothari A, Uppal H, Kankate R. The jones fracture classification, management, outcome, and complications: a systematic review. *Foot Ankle Spec.* 2012;5:256-259.
37. Bernstein DT, Mitchell RJ, McCulloch PC, Harris JD, Varner KE. Treatment of proximal fifth metatarsal fractures and refractures with plantar plating in elite athletes. *Foot Ankle Int.* 2018;39:1410-1415.
38. Seidenstricker CL, Blahous EG, Bouché RT, Saxena A. Plate fixation with autogenous calcaneal dowel grafting proximal fourth and fifth metatarsal fractures: technique and case series. *J Foot Ankle Surg.* 2017;56:975-981.
39. Brinker MR, O'Connor DP, Monla YT, Earthman TP. Metabolic and endocrine abnormalities in patients with nonunions. *J Orthop Trauma.* 2007;21:557-570.

Midfoot Surgery

CHAPTER 19

Surgery for Chronic Recalcitrant Plantar Fasciitis

Harry P. Schneider and Adam E. Fleischer

DEFINITION

Plantar fasciitis is characterized by thickening, hypertrophy, and degeneration of the plantar fascia, usually at the infracalcaneal origin. Patients exhibit poststatic dyskinesia with greatest pain typically during their first few steps. Plantar fasciitis is one of the most common conditions encountered by foot and ankle surgeons and accounts for over one million outpatient visits annually in the United States.[1-6] It is estimated that ~10% of the U.S. population will develop plantar fasciitis in their lifetime[7,8] and more than two million Americans experience symptoms of plantar fasciitis at any one time.[4,9-11] While nonoperative management is successful in a majority of patients, some refractory cases will go on to require surgery for relief.

It is important to recognize that some patients with refractory infracalcaneal heel pain will also have concomitant (and distinctly separate) sources of pain complicating their presentation (eg, proximal and/or distal tarsal tunnel syndrome, irregular infracalcaneal spurs, profound gastroc equinus, etc.). This chapter will discuss the workup and operative approaches to both isolated plantar fasciitis and mixed presentations as well.

ANATOMIC FEATURES

ANATOMY OF THE PLANTAR FASCIA

The plantar fascia is synonymous with the plantar aponeurosis of the foot and provides a mechanical linkage between the calcaneus and the toes. It is composed of densely compacted collagen fibers that are mainly oriented in a longitudinal direction, although some fibers run in a transverse and oblique direction.[12] The plantar fascia arises mainly from the medial calcaneal tuberosity and attaches distally, through several slips, to the plantar forefoot as well as the medial and lateral intermuscular septa. Anatomically it can be divided into the medial, lateral, and central components[13] (Fig. 19.1).

The medial band is anatomically thin and virtually nonexistent at its proximal level. Similarly, the lateral band varies in its structure from relatively thick to nonexistent in 12% of individuals.[14,15] When present, the lateral band provides a partial origin for the abductor digiti minimi muscle. The lateral band then bifurcates into the medial and lateral crura at the cuboid level.

The stronger lateral crux inserts into the base of the fifth metatarsal. The medial crux merges distally with the central band of the plantar fascia before coursing deep and inserting into the plantar plate of the third, fourth, or fifth metatarsophalangeal joint.[13]

The central band is triangular in shape and originates from the plantar medial process of the calcaneal tuberosity. The central band serves as the partial origin of the flexor digitorum brevis (FDB) as it conforms to the plantar surface of the calcaneus. Ranging from 12 to 29 mm wide at its origin, the central plantar fascial band separates at the mid-metatarsal level into five longitudinal bands.[16] Each band then divides distally to the metatarsal heads to form deep and superficial tracts. The central superficial tracts insert onto the skin and contribute to the formation of the mooring and natatory ligaments.[15] The five deep tracts separate to form medial and lateral sagittal septa, which contribute to the medial and lateral digital flexor, flexor tendon sheath, interosseous fascia, fascia of the transverse head of the adductor hallucis, the deep transverse metatarsal ligament, and the base of the proximal phalanges via the plantar plate and collateral ligaments.[13]

The plantar calcaneal spur is a bony outgrowth of the calcaneal tuberosity that occurs, with moderate regularity, even in the general population.[17] The association of the plantar calcaneal spur and plantar fascia is highly variable. The plantar calcaneal spur may be joined with all, part, or none of the plantar fascia. Tanz[18] first showed that the plantar calcaneal spur many times arises from the intrinsic muscles rather than the plantar fascia itself. This finding has later been corroborated by Forman and Green[19] and others. The plantar calcaneal spur is covered with a fibrous connective tissue layer, which is highly innervated and vascularized.[17,20,21] Rather than having an indirect periosteal attachment, the proximal attachment of the plantar fascia on the calcaneus is distinctly fibrocartilaginous.[22]

Almost all the tissue of the plantar fascia is formed of type I collagen.[23] The plantar fascia is also well innervated with both free and encapsulated nerve endings, such as Pacini and Ruffini corpuscles.[23,24] These nerve endings are particularly abundant where the plantar fascia joins with the fasciae of the abductor hallucis and abductor digiti minimi muscles and where the flexor muscles insert. These abundant innervations suggest that the plantar fascia plays a role in proprioception aiding in the stability and control of foot movements.[23,24]

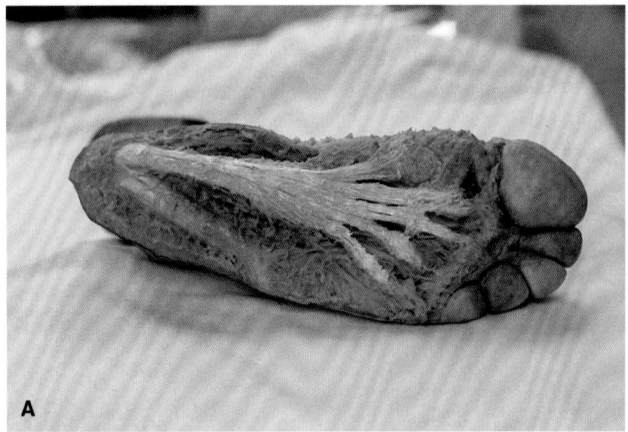

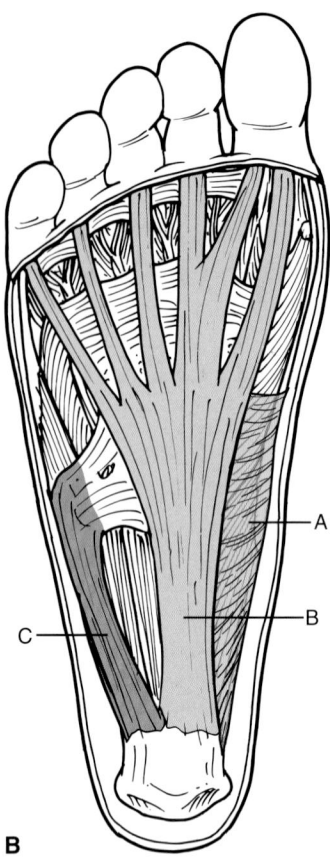

FIGURE 19.1 **A.** Anatomic specimen demonstrating the plantar fascia. Note the absence of a medial band. **B.** The plantar fascia is typically composed of an ill-defined medial band (*A*), well-defined central band (*B*), and a variable lateral band (*C*).

ANATOMY OF THE TIBIAL NERVE AND ITS BRANCHES

The tibial nerve is derived from the ventral portions of L4, L5, and S1, S2, and S3 and is the larger of the two terminal divisions of the sciatic nerve. At the heel, the medial calcaneal branches perforate the laciniate ligament and innervate the skin of the heel and medial side of the sole of the foot.[25] The tibial nerve then divides into the larger medial plantar nerve and the lateral plantar nerve. The medial plantar nerve follows the medial plantar artery and passes deep to the abductor hallucis and medial to the FDB muscle, to enter the plantar vault through the porta pedis.[25]

The lateral plantar nerve also enters the plantar vault through the porta pedis. However, before this, it gives off the "first branch," discovered in 1963 by Tanz,[18] who noticed a deep calcaneal branch at the time of a heel spur resection. He further detailed a cadaveric dissection of this nerve as it passes beneath the tuber calcanei and under the plantar fascia, where it bends laterally. In 1981, Przylucki and Jones[26] dissected the same nerve and found it to be a motor branch to the abductor digiti quinti muscle. They noted that the nerve actually passes in proximity to the calcaneal tuber. Thus, it was believed that, in patients with recalcitrant heel pain, this nerve could be the sole or concomitant cause of the painful condition, and these investigators obtained relief in three patients by nerve excision. Sections of the nerve from cadavers, as well as from surgical patients, demonstrated histologic evidence of perineural hypertrophy. This work provided the clinical confirmation for the anatomic studies performed by other investigators.[27,28] Rondhuis and Huson[28] concluded that the site of entrapment was between the deep taut fascia of the abductor hallucis muscle and the medial or caudal head of the quadratus muscle. They presented strong evidence that the nerve is a mixed type, providing sensory fibers to the calcaneal periosteum, including over the medial tuberosity, and the long plantar ligament, as well as motor fibers to the quadratus plantae, FDB, and abductor digiti quinti muscles. This evidence may help to explain the more neuralgic symptoms that are characteristic of this cause of heel pain.

PHYSICAL EXAMINATION

In patients presenting with infracalcaneal heel pain, the physical examination should include plantar palpation of the heel at the medial calcaneal tuberosity, central heel, medial palpation over the abductor hallucis muscle belly, side-to-side compression of the calcaneus, and percussion of the tibial nerve in the porta pedis. Patients should also be assessed for gastrocnemius equinus with use of the Silfverskiold test.[29] Patients with significant gastrocnemius equinus should be further evaluated for the appropriateness of a posterior muscle group lengthening.

In patients presenting with plantar fasciitis alone, the most common location of pain is at the plantar medial tubercle of the calcaneus at the plantar fascial insertion. The most common symptom is poststatic dyskinesia, with pain with the first few steps in the morning and after periods of rest. Poststatic dyskinesia differentiates plantar fasciitis from other causes of heel pain such as inferior calcaneal bursitis, calcaneal stress fracture, and neurogenic causes. Symptoms can extend along the course of the plantar fascia into the central arch, but this is a less prevalent finding. Also, lateral band and plantar lateral heel pain may be present as well but is more variable. Generally, there are minimal clinical signs of inflammation such as swelling and erythema. Pain with midfoot, hindfoot, and ankle range of motion is generally absent. Additionally, pain with side-to-side (medial-lateral) compression of the body of the calcaneus is not a component of plantar fascial–based symptoms and if present indicates the possibility of stress fracture or other primarily bone pathology.

A Tinel sign over the flexor retinaculum is indicative of proximal entrapment of the tibial nerve, while patients exhibiting maximal tenderness over the area between the abductor hallucis and quadratus plantae muscles are said to demonstrate the "hallmark of [Baxter's] compression neuropathy."[30] Patient's with proximal and/or distal nerve entrapment may also complain of "radiating" pain or describe an "afterburn" in the heel even while at rest, which is not all common in isolated proximal plantar fasciitis.

PATHOGENESIS

Plantar fasciitis is traditionally considered an overuse injury, with repetitive microtrauma and damage to the central band of the plantar fascia occurring at a rate that exceeds the body's capacity to heal.[5,31-33] While increased body mass index (BMI),[9,34-38] athletic[3,10,37,39-42] and sedentary[9] lifestyles, and a host of environmental factors are believed to contribute,[13,33-36,43] biomechanical abnormalities are what is believed to be primarily responsible for the high tensile loads and resulting injury that occurs within the fascia during static stance and gait.[13]

During the stance phase of gait, tension within the fascia gradually increases and is believed to reach peak values at the start of push off (80% of stance).[44-48] The plantar fascia is particularly susceptible to high tensile loads during stance as it works to resist arch elongation.[49] Also, as the heel begins to rise and during early push off, the fascia is again subjected to increased tension at least partially via Hicks windlass mechanism—with dorsiflexion of the toes, the plantar fascia becomes increasingly wound around the metatarsal heads, thus shortening its effective length and increasing tension in the fascia.[50-52] Elevation of the heel in late stance also produces loading of the Achilles tendon, which increases bending moments at the midfoot and increases tension in the fascia as it works to resist collapse of the arch.[49] An excessively tight or contracted Achilles tendon is also thought to produce higher tensile loads in the fascia through direct transmission of tension through the calcaneal trabecular system as proposed by Arandes and Viladot[53] and/or by increasing its passive mechanical longitudinal tension as a way of counteracting the arch flattening effect of ankle dorsiflexion stiffness.[54,55]

Entrapment of the first branch of the lateral plantar nerve can occur in one of two places: (1) as it changes direction from vertical to horizontal around the medial plantar aspect of the heel (ie, in between the deep fascia of the abductor hallucis muscle and the medial caudal head of the quadratus plantae muscle) and/or (2) as the nerve courses distal to the medial calcaneal tuberosity where spur formation in the FDB muscle can cause compression against the long plantar ligament.[28] Athletes who spend significant amounts of time on their toes appear to be more susceptible to a distal nerve entrapment by a well-developed abductor hallucis muscle belly. Similarly, those with large or irregular infracalcaneal spurs may be more susceptible to this type of nerve compression.

IMAGING AND DIAGNOSTIC STUDIES

Radiographs should be ordered prior to surgery particularly if there is a history of trauma and in patients presenting with atypical plantar fasciitis symptoms. Radiographs can also help to rule out other sources of heel pain such as calcaneal stress fractures and bony neoplasms (eg, bone cysts, intraosseous lipomas, etc.) and can help to better characterize any infracalcaneal spur if present. While spurs themselves are rarely contributing factors in infracalcaneal heel pain,[56] they sometimes need to be resected in cases of distal nerve entrapment (Baxter neuritis) and when they are irregular in morphology and believed to be contributing to the pain profile.

Point-of-care diagnostic ultrasound is particularly good at providing the surgeon with direct visualization of the plantar fascia. Normal sonographic appearance of the fascia is echogenic and fibrillar and measures no more than 4 mm in superior to inferior dimensions at the infracalcaneal origin.[57] Normal appearance of the fascia on ultrasound examination essentially rules out the presence of plantar fasciitis, and other less common sources of heel pain should be considered. Plantar fasciitis, in contrast, is demonstrated by mixed echogenicity, hypoechogenicity, biconvexity (ie, rounding), and thickening of the fascia.[58,59] Ultrasound can be used for guided injections as well. In a recent meta-analysis comparing ultrasound vs palpation-guided corticosteroid injections, Li and colleagues[60] examined five RCTs with 149 patients and concluded ultrasound-guided injection was superior with regard to VAS pain, response rate, and plantar fascia appearance on ultrasound.

Magnetic resonance imaging (MRI) can help rule out space-occupying lesions (eg, accessory soleus, ganglion cyst, and other space-occupying masses) pressing on the tibial nerve or branches, leading to a neuritic source of infracalcaneal pain. In some recalcitrant cases, calcaneal bone marrow edema seen on T2-weighted images can be filled using porous injectable calcium phosphate via Subchondroplasty technique.[61] MRI will also clearly confirm the thickened enlarged fascia, and many patients will demonstrate reactive calcaneal edema at the medial calcaneal tuberosity (Fig. 19.2).

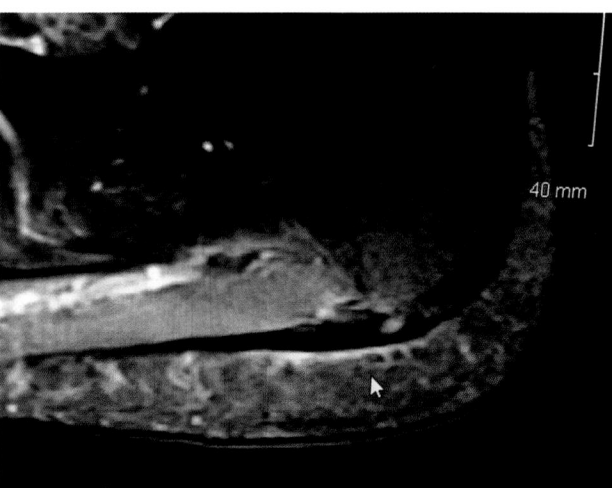

40 mm

FIGURE 19.2 Bony edema seen on T2-weighted MRI.

Nerve conduction velocity studies and electromyogram of the abductor digiti minimi can be helpful, particularly if symptoms have been long-standing. However, these are frequently not positive even in clear cases of clinical nerve entrapment.[62]

TREATMENT

NONSURGICAL

Nonsurgical treatment methods for plantar fasciitis are successful in the majority of individuals. Biomechanical support (eg, supportive shoes, taping, and over-the-counter insoles),[63-70] Achilles and plantar fascia–specific stretching,[71,72] night splints,[73,74] corticosteroid injections,[75] amniotic membrane and Botulinum toxin-A injections,[76-78] extracorporeal shockwave therapy,[79-84] physical therapy,[85-87] and custom foot orthoses[83,88,89] are all effective nonsurgical options.

SURGICAL

Surgical intervention is therefore reserved for chronic, refractory patients who have failed appropriate conservative treatment for least 6 months.[63,90-93] Surgical management of plantar fasciitis generally falls in one of three broad categories: fasciotomy, neurolysis, and posterior muscle group lengthening.

> **PEARL**
>
> Surgical intervention is reserved for chronic, refractory cases that have failed appropriate conservative therapy for at least 6 months.[63,90-93]

Fasciotomy

Release of the plantar fascia has been performed for many years whether as an isolated procedure or in combination with excision of the plantar calcaneal spur, neurolysis, and/or gastrocnemius recession. The ease of performance, generally high patient satisfaction, and faster recovery time have made this a favored approach in many patients with unremitting heel pain resulting from plantar fasciitis. The procedure can be performed as an open operation, percutaneously, or endoscopically with similar results. Comparative studies of fascial release only and spur resection reveal no major differences in outcome (although a shortened recovery period was found in some reports with the endoscopic technique).[94,95] The popularity over the last several years of performing fasciotomies to resolve heel pain resistant to conservative care has heightened awareness of the problems that may occur with loss of integrity of the plantar fascia. As weight is shifted forward and the toes dorsiflex, the fascia acts to stiffen the foot, to prepare it for propulsion. Although many ligaments and tendons contribute to this effect, the plantar fascia plays the key role.[49] Studies seem to indicate that the fascia contributes more to stability of the arch than the spring ligament, plantar ligaments, and the extrinsic flexors.[96,97] Sectioning of the plantar fascia results in decreased arch stiffness, with concomitant lowering of both the medial and lateral columns in stance.[96-100] As the distal slips of the fascia insert into the toes,

the windlass mechanism is significantly altered, as is the position of the toes, with possible claw toe formation during the propulsive phase of gait. Loss of digital stability has been attributed to a transfer in pressure from the toes to the metatarsal heads, resulting in up to an 80% increase in strain on the second metatarsal.[100,101] Work by Kitaoka et al.[102] showed that fascial release in a normal foot would not produce deformity, but in an unstable foot, markedly abnormal motion was recorded.

Although cadaveric studies are enlightening, they may not always correlate with clinical findings. Nonetheless, investigators recognize that mechanical alterations do occur as a result of plantar fasciotomy (with or without spur resection), and these changes may contribute to some of the postoperative complications reported. Calcaneocuboid pain, medial column strain, and pain in the ball of the foot have all been noted, but they are significant in only a small percentage of patients. Many surgeons have attempted to obviate this dilemma by cutting only the medial one-third to one-half of the plantar fascia. Laboratory data show that structural and mechanical aberrations will still occur,[97-101] although to a lesser extent than with complete transection of the fascia.[99,101] It is therefore recommended that no more than one-half of the fascia be transected during initial fasciotomy procedures, which is typically no more than 1.5 cm across. Complete transection can be entertained in revision cases that necessitate this. Joint-related symptoms after plantar fascia release can sometimes be improved with a well-molded orthotic device, oral anti-inflammatory medications, compression, and physical therapy.

Partial fasciotomies can be achieved using an open approach (including the medial or plantar medial incision "in-step" fasciotomy technique), endoscopically as popularized by Barrett and colleagues,[103,104] and percutaneously via radiofrequency ablation and other methods.

Open Fasciotomy Technique, Plantar Incision (Author's Preferred Method)

The patient may be placed in a supine position if other reconstructive procedures are to be performed. Alternatively, the patient may be placed in a prone position (dependent upon body habitus—authors choice) to allow natural gravity dorsiflexion. Prone position also eases positioning for a concomitant gastrocnemius recession if performed at the same operative setting. An ankle or thigh tourniquet is used based upon other procedures performed.

The central band of the plantar fascia is palpated, and a 3-cm transverse incision is planned just distal to the plantar fat pad. Incision placement can also be approximated using measurements obtained off a lateral weight-bearing x-ray. This location allows for direct dissection down to the plantar fascia insertion. The incision is also just off the weight-bearing surface to reduce scarring potential.

The incision is deepened through the skin (Fig. 19.3). There is a moderate amount of fat in this area. Blunt dissection is then continued down to the plantar fascia. The medial and lateral edges are identified. The fascia can then be resected directly with a surgical knife or with a Kelly clamp separating the fascia from the superiorly located muscle. The windlass mechanism must be engaged during the fascial incision. If the fascia does not gap wide enough, a section of the fascia may be removed at this time (ie, fasciectomy). Additionally, based upon

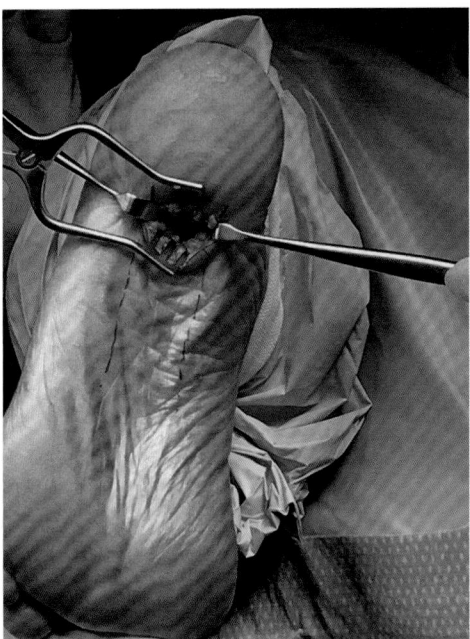

FIGURE 19.3 Exposure for open plantar fasciotomy.

the location of the incision, the inferior calcaneal spur may be removed at this time, if desired.

Closure is performed via 4-0 absorbable suture for the subcutaneous tissue and 4-0 nonabsorbable suture for the skin. The patient remains non–weight bearing for 3 weeks with the foot at 90 degrees to the leg until the sutures are removed (author's preference). Three weeks non–weight bearing avoids tension on the plantar skin to minimize hypertrophic scarring. This incision should be used with caution in smokers and keloid formers due to the potential for plantar hypertrophic scars.

Spur Removal

Although not frequently required,[56] irregular and plantarly prominent spurs can be removed through open techniques. In our experience, spur removal is perhaps most important in

patients with concomitant infracalcaneal neuralgia undergoing a Baxter decompression, but the nerve should be carefully retracted to avoid painful postoperative neuralgia. Infracalcaneal spurs are almost always located just superior to the proximal plantar fascial insertion within the FDB muscle belly.[18,19] Hemostasis can become a problem because of the cancellous nature of the spur and the disruption of the FDB muscle needed for access to the spur.

Wider exposure is typically needed for spur excision, so either a plantar approach[105-108] or longer medial incision placed lower on the heel is needed. Simply extending traditional medial incisions inevitably results in sensory loss and sometimes painful entrapments due to disruptions of the larger branches of the medial calcaneal nerve. Ruch described a modification of the DuVries[109] medial incision that offers excellent visualization with less chance of medial calcaneal nerve entrapment.[110] A medial incision is placed low on the heel to avoid cutting any large branches of the medial calcaneal nerve (Fig. 19.4). It then extends distally and laterally into the arch crossing the plantar fascia 3-4 cm distal to its origin attachment. This point is distal to the fat pad of the heel, where the plantar fascia is covered by a thin layer of subcutaneous tissue and is readily identified. The fascial plane is then followed proximally to the plantar surface of the heel, by reflecting the heel pad inferiorly. The medial edge of the fascia is then identified at its insertion into the calcaneus. The fascia is detached from the bone, and the spur is identified. The calcaneal spur is deep and difficult to get to unless part of the FDB muscle is also removed. The spur is resected with a rongeur and rasped smooth, then checked fluoroscopically. If a tourniquet is used, it is released prior to closure, and the skin is closed with interrupted nonabsorbable sutures.

Plantar Instep Open Fasciotomy

Medial (Fig. 19.5) and plantar approach instep partial fasciotomies have been employed for several decades with good success. The minimal incision technique is similar to the procedure first described by Braly in 1994.[111] Fishco et al.[112] described their findings in a retrospective study using the instep plantar fasciotomy technique on 83 patients with the main complication

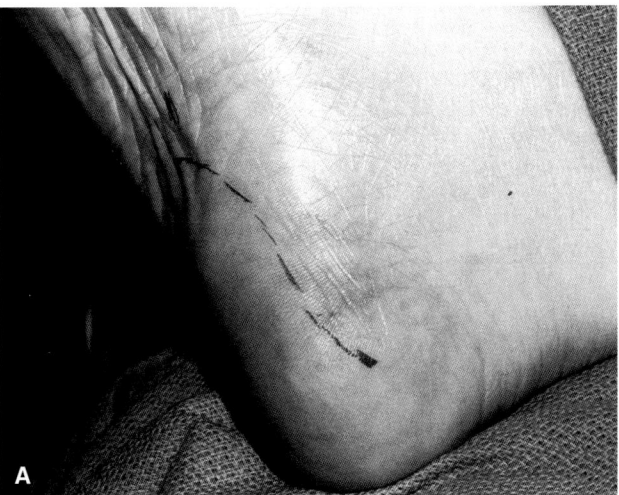

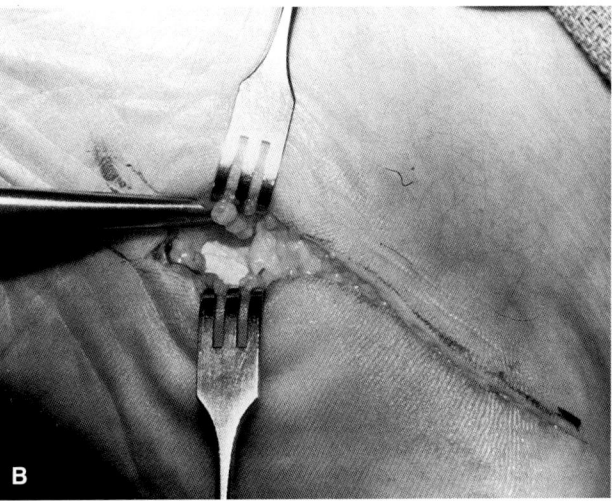

FIGURE 19.4 **A.** The low incision is designed to avoid the larger branches of the medial calcaneal nerve. **B.** It is easiest to identify the fascial plane at the distal-most aspect of the incision line.

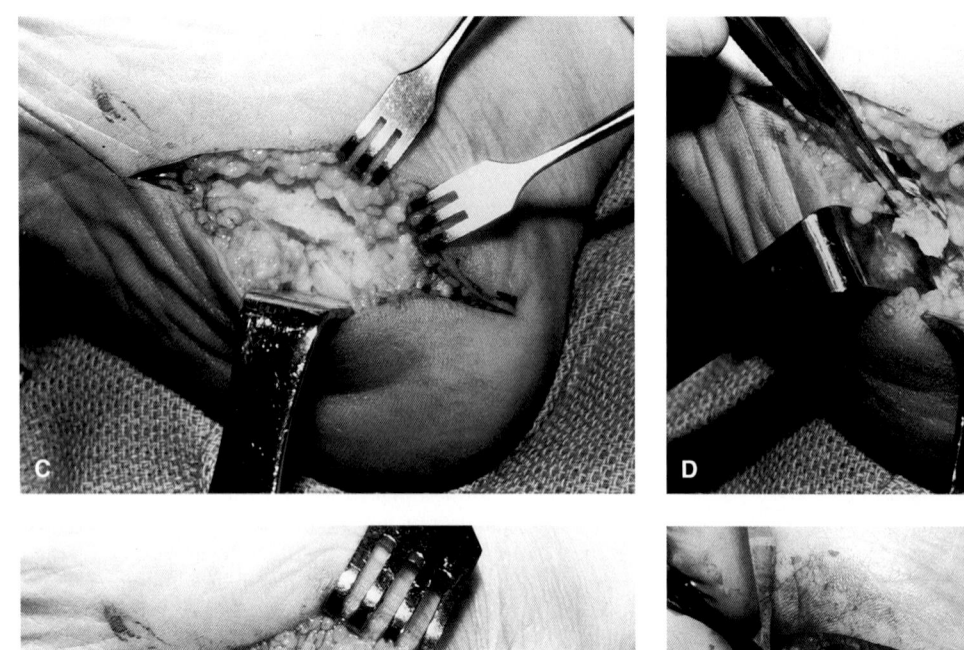

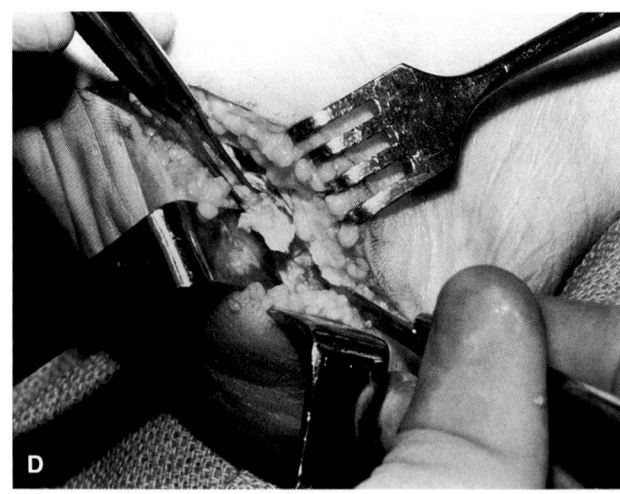

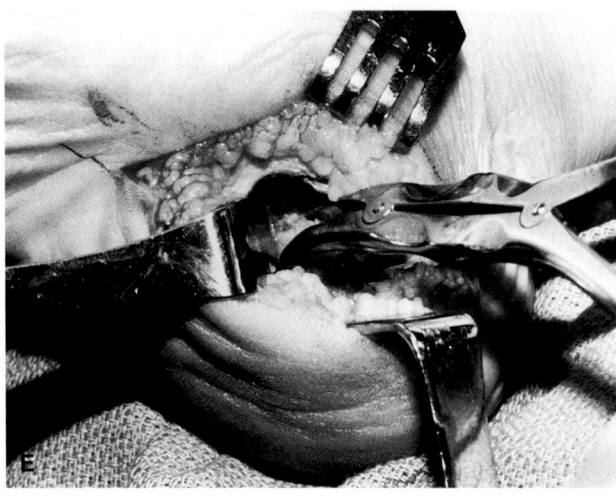

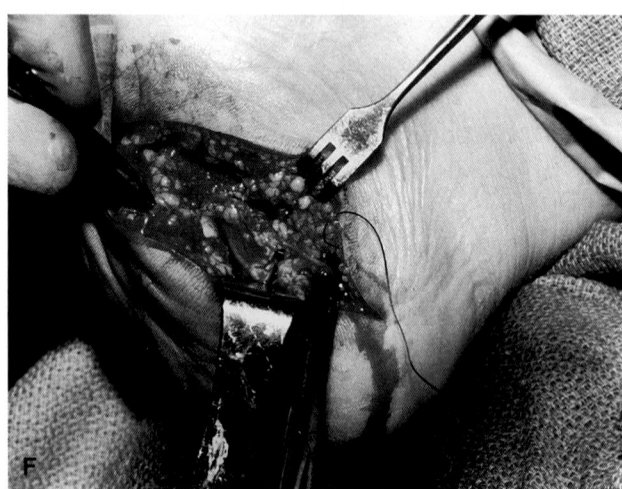

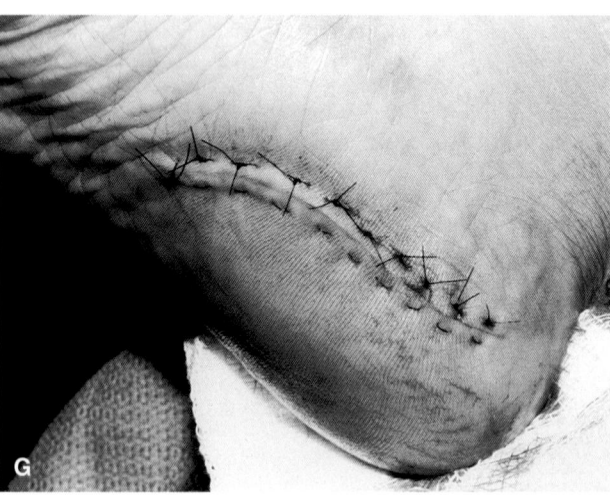

FIGURE 19.4 (*Continued*) **C.** Fascia over the abductor and plantar fascia as it inserts into the medial calcaneal tuberosity are identified. **D.** The fascial attachments to the calcaneus are incised. This can be saved for repair or a portion can be excised. **E.** The prominent spur can now be removed. **F.** The fascial defect is repaired. **G.** Wound closure. Accurate approximation of the skin edges is necessary to prevent wound dehiscence.

being scarring in 9.6% of the patients. Surgery was deemed successful 93.6% of the time, and 95.7% of the patients would recommend the procedure to someone with the same condition.[112] In 2000, Woelffer et al.[32] also published their 5-year results on patients who underwent the instep plantar fasciotomy for chronic heel pain and similarly reported a satisfaction rate of 90% or better in 30 of the 33 ft, while 3 patients did complain of pain at the surgical site at times. Similar findings were also reported by Perelman et al.[113] in 41 patients (50 ft).

The procedure is simple and can be performed in any setting, including the office, without any special instrumentation. The fascia can be well visualized without excessive dissection or disruption of vital structures. The advantages to percutaneous (and even endoscopic) methods are that they may shorten the postoperative recovery period but not significantly.

The patient is positioned supine, with surgeon's choice of anesthesia (regional, intravenous sedation, or general anesthesia). Scrub, prep, and drape the foot in the usual sterile fashion.

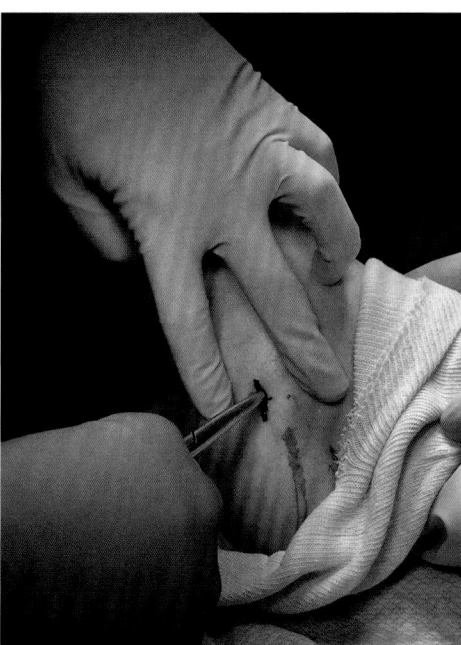

FIGURE 19.5 Incision placement for medial instep plantar fasciotomy.

Evaluate skin lines to help determine where to place the incision. Pushing the toes toward the heel exaggerates the transverse skin lines (Langer lines). Pick one of the skin creases, which is just anterior (distal) to the fat pad of the heel.

The skin incision is about 2 cm in length in a transverse to oblique orientation following the skin crease. The subcutaneous fat is usually robust in this area. A small Weitlaner retractor is used to retract the skin, and a Freer elevator is used to move the fat around. The Freer elevator can then be moved rapidly distal to proximal until the fat liquefies a little and breaks down, making visualization of the fascia easier. Additional use of Senn retractors can reposition the fat, so that an unobstructed view of the plantar fascia is achieved. Proceed to perform the plantar fasciotomy. A Metzenbaum scissors or no. 15 blade is then used to incise the fascia, taking care not to cut too deep in order to avoid violating the underlying muscle. Dorsiflexing the great toe stretches the fascia, and you can appreciate what has been cut. No more than 50% of the fascia is cut across. At this point, the wound is inspected with your index finger, feeling medially for any residual fascia fibers that may be intact.

Once the partial fasciotomy is complete, perform copious lavage and close the wound with three horizontal mattress sutures using 4-0 nylon. Do not use absorbable sutures in the fatty layer as this will increase the likelihood of developing more scarring and potential fibromas. Bandage the foot with gauze, and apply a posterior splint or fracture boot. The patient is non–weight bearing for 3 weeks with the foot at a right angle to the leg. After the first week, one can remove the sutures and allow the patient to take the fracture boot off to shower and to do some range of motion exercise. All other times, including sleeping, the foot should remain splinted in the fracture boot. After 3 weeks of non–weight bearing, full weight bearing in the fracture boot commences. After 3 weeks of walking in the fracture boot, the patient can return to regular shoes.

Endoscopic Fasciotomy

A common, minimally invasive approach to plantar fascial release is endoscopic plantar fasciotomy (EPF). The technique is associated with favorable overall outcomes and offers the possibility of earlier return to activity for some. The technique was described by Barrett and Day[103] in 1993 in 65 heels. In 1995, Tomczak and colleagues[94] performed a retrospective comparison of EPF to open plantar fasciotomy with heel spur resection. The authors concluded that both groups were asymptomatic at 9 months but that the EPF group returned to work and full activities 55 days earlier.[94] The largest group of EPF procedures reviewed to date was 652 cases by 25 surgeons by Barrett et al.[104] in 1995. In this series, all surgeons released the medial third of the band and demonstrated success and reproducibility, but the patients were only followed for 3 weeks postoperatively. O'Malley[114] in 2000 reviewed 20 ft treated by EPF found that all patients with unilateral heel pain had complete relief and that the 1 patient with bilateral heel pain reported no improvement of pain. It is important to recognize, however, that higher BMI may adversely influence EPF results. Morton et al.[91] in 2013 did a retrospective review of 105 consecutive EPF procedures on U.S. army soldiers and reviewed the outcomes based upon BMI. Those patients with a BMI at or below 25.53 kg/m^2, 96.35% had a postoperative pain level of 0, and only 44% of those with a BMI of 29.8 kg/m^2 or greater had a postoperative pain score of 0.

Endoscopic Fasciotomy, Barrett[103] Technique

The patient is placed on the operative table in a supine position. A posterior tibial and sural block or regional blocks is performed. An ankle tourniquet is generally utilized. A longitudinal incision is created medially just distal to the insertion of the plantar fascia into the calcaneus. The incision is just large enough to introduce the endoscope. The incision should be biased slightly cephalad to create increased tension on the fascia during resection. Once through the skin and subcutaneous tissue, a fascial elevator or Metzenbaum scissor (author's choice) is utilized to separate the plantar fascia from the subcutaneous fat. A small pucker in the skin will be noted laterally as the fascia is separated. The obturator and cannula are then inserted from medial to lateral. A small incision will be created laterally if a 2-incision approach is utilized. Care is taken to remain in the plane between the fascia and the subcutaneous fat. The obturator is then removed and several plastic cotton tip applicators are inserted from medial to lateral to remove any subcutaneous fat that encroached into the cannula. Plastic is preferred over wood to avoid splintering and potential foreign bodies. The endoscope is utilized to visualize the plantar fascia. A mark is made on the plantar skin approximately two-third across the foot, which is the lateral edge of the plantar fascia central band. The distance between the medial portal and the lateral mark is measured and translated onto the retrograde knife (if utilizing two portals). The translation can be noted with a marking pen (which tends to wipe off) or with use of surgical tape (Fig. 19.6). It is very important for the surgical assistant to dorsiflex the foot and engage the windlass mechanism during resection of the plantar fascia. The fascia is then released from lateral to medial (if your hand slips, you want to cut medial not lateral). Forceful pressure is applied with the thumb in a superior direction to ensure release of

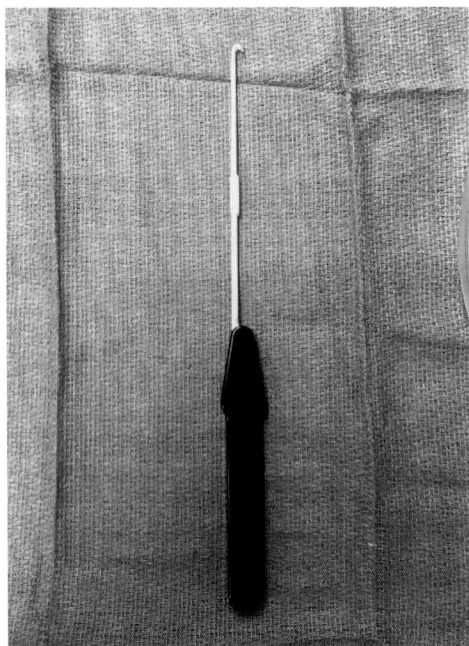

FIGURE 19.6 A wound closure strip used to mark distance between the medial portal lateral 2/3 mark.

the fascia (Fig. 19.7). One should see the muscle belly of the FDB once the fascia is fully released. It is advisable to comment on the thickness and characteristics of the plantar fascia in the operative note. Endoscopic pictures of the plantar fascia before and after resection should be taken and placed in the patient's record (Fig. 19.8). The operative field is then flushed. The author's preference is to flush with 0.5% bupivacaine with epinephrine to reduce any muscular bleeding and allow additional postoperative pain relief. The incisions are closed with 4-0 nonabsorbable suture. Usually one suture per incision.

Postoperatively, Barrett and Day[103] recommend allowing patients to ambulate in a walking boot. They suggest that immediate ambulation allows continued separation of the plantar fascial ends and prevents recurrence. Use of the walking boot allows continuous maintenance of foot 90 degrees to the leg.

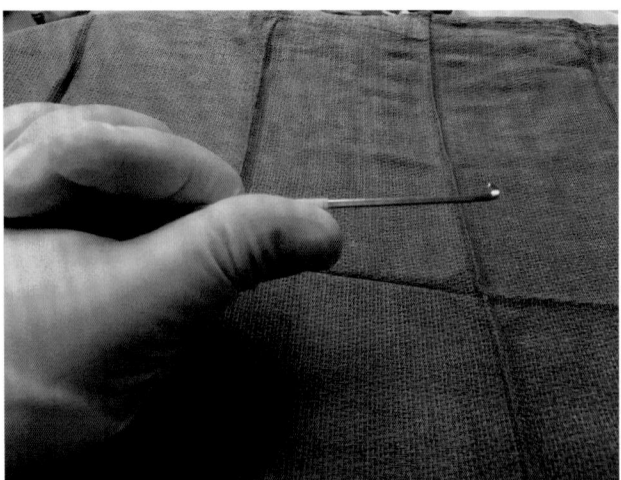

FIGURE 19.7 Thumb used to apply cephalad force to ensure resection of the deep plantar fascia fibers.

Patients may return to sneakers at 2 weeks. It is not uncommon for a patient to request a corticosteroid injection at 6 weeks postoperatively due to swelling and pain at the surgical site.

Percutaneous Bipolar Radiofrequency Fasciotomy

Radiofrequency coblation has become a popular and appealing way of addressing recalcitrant plantar fasciitis, as the procedure can be done entirely percutaneously, negating wound healing issues, and potentially offering a quicker return to activity. Radiofrequency coblation acts by exciting electrolytes in an electrolyte solution, such as normal saline, to produce energized particles in the plasma with sufficient energy to ablate soft tissues at low temperatures. Several studies suggest that this procedure yields comparable results to open and endoscopic techniques with respect to pain relief.[115-119]

Percutaneous Bipolar Radiofrequency Fasciotomy Technique[115,117]

Before the administration of any sedative or peripheral nerve block, the areas of maximal tenderness are manually probed and subsequently marked with an indelible surgical ink marker. Patients are given either general anesthesia or a posterior tibial nerve block and intravenous sedation. With the patient in the supine position, a thigh or ankle tourniquet is used to aid hemostasis. The foot is then scrubbed, prepped, and draped in a standard fashion.

Attention is directed to the area of maximal tenderness. The preoperative markings are used to further template a series of percutaneous microincisions situated at 5-mm intervals throughout the area of tenderness (Fig. 19.9). A grid pattern, ranging from 10 to 55 microincisions is used to target the underlying proximal plantar fascia. A smooth 0.062-in Kirschner wire (K-wire) is then used to puncture the skin at each specific grid mark. The microincisions created with the K-wire are made full thickness through the skin, subcutaneous fat, and down to the plantar fascia. The radiofrequency controlled ablation is achieved using the TOPAZ MicroDebrider (Smith & Nephew). The manufacturer's recommendations for settings for the delivered energy and time should be closely adhered to. The probe is then attached to a normal sterile saline drip, set to a drip rate of ~1 drop every 2-3 seconds, and then delivered sequentially through each percutaneous microincision previously made by the K-wire. The probe is advanced until resistance is felt, and the radiofrequency energy is applied. The probe is advanced further through the fascia by another radiofrequency application. In total, two radiofrequency applications are made in one percutaneous hole, one superficial and another through the thickness of the fascia; thus, varying depths of radiofrequency are applied. Adhesive skin strips are then applied with an overlying nonadherent dressing, followed by application of a modified Jones compression dressing and posterior splint.

Postoperatively, patients are kept non–weight bearing for the first 10-14 postoperative days, and at the first postoperative visit, they are placed into a CAM walker and allowed to weight bear as tolerated. In addition, the use of the night splint during non–weight-bearing activities was reinstituted. At 4 weeks postintervention, the patients are converted to supportive shoe gear with the insertion of orthoses for long-term functional support. Patients were encouraged to continue stretching and flexibility exercises to prevent potential

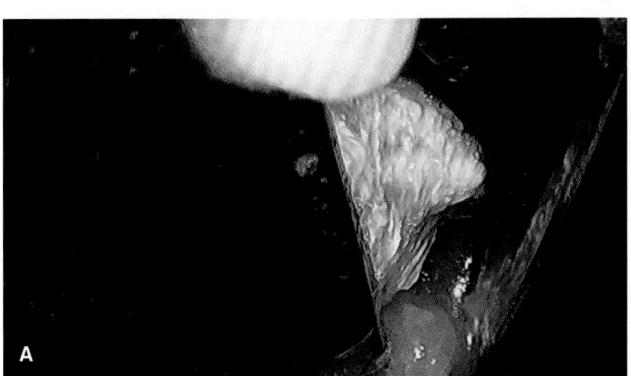

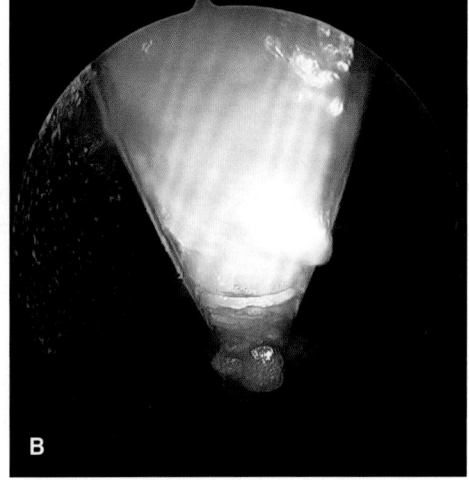

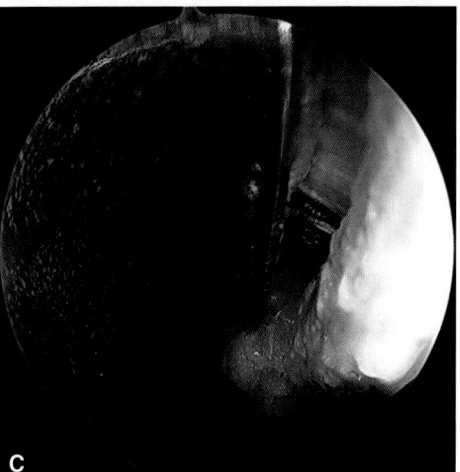

FIGURE 19.8 EPF portal visualization. **A.** Complete resection of the plantar fascia with exposed muscle belly. **B.** Visualization of the plantar fascia prior to resection. **C.** Incomplete resection of thickened plantar fascia. Deep fibers have not been transected.

scar contracture and a course of physical therapy consisting of mild resistive strengthening, range of motion exercises, and vigorous stretching. Return to regular activity is gradual and implemented as tolerated.

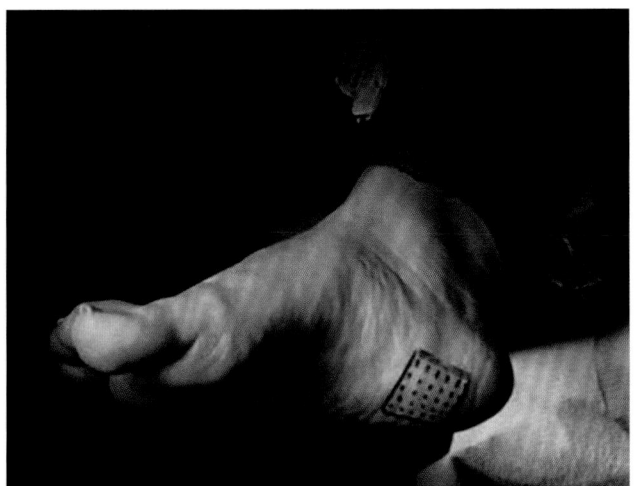

FIGURE 19.9 Grid markings to determine skin puncture sites. The grid is located in the area of maximal tenderness.

Isolated Distal Neurolysis

When there is isolated entrapment of the first branch of the lateral plantar nerve, a limited distal tarsal tunnel release and partial plantar fasciotomy can be performed. In 1981, Przylucki and Jones[26] described three patients who sustained relief of heel pain from an entrapment neuropathy of the first branch of the lateral plantar nerve by *excision* of the nerve itself. Baxter and associates[30,120] reported on the neurolysis of this nerve, and they achieved excellent to good results after an average of 49 months in 89% of the 69 heels reported in the latter study. In several cases, the fascia was severed and an occasional spur was removed if it appeared to impinge on the nerve. Other authors have reported good results with 90% success rates.[5,121] Electrodiagnostic testing was not used in any of these studies, and the decision to perform nerve release was based on clinical examinations.

Open Fasciotomy With Distal Tarsal Tunnel (aka "Baxter Nerve") Release Technique

An oblique incision is placed over the medial heel beginning at the distal medial aspect of the calcaneal fat pad and extended proximally and posteriorly (Fig. 19.10). Dissection is carried through the subcutaneous fat until the fascia overlying

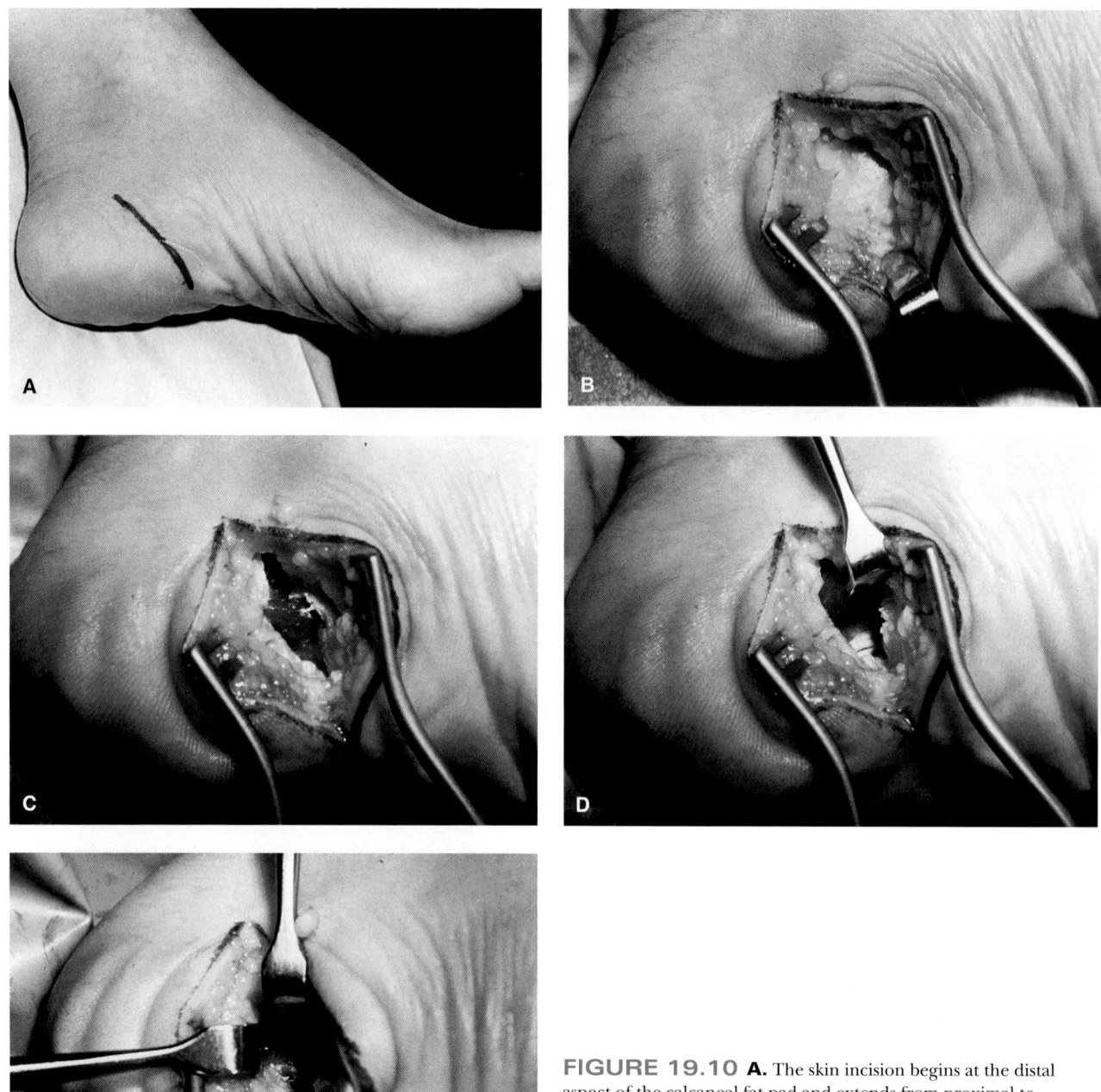

FIGURE 19.10 A. The skin incision begins at the distal aspect of the calcaneal fat pad and extends from proximal to posterior, paralleling the course of the lateral plantar nerve. **B.** The fascia over the abductor hallucis muscle is identified. Inferiorly, this blends with the plantar fascia. **C.** The fascia and medial-most part of the plantar fascia are incised. Note the bulging of the abductor through the fascia. **D.** With the abductor retracted dorsally, the fascia separating it from the quadratus plantae fibers is encountered. **E.** A small portion of this dense fascial band is excised.

the abductor hallucis muscle belly is identified. The fascia overlying the abductor muscle is then vertically incised, and the muscle is retracted plantarly or dorsally to reveal the taut, unyielding fascial band, which separates the abductor from the medial head of the quadratus plantae. This may occasionally be dense. The deeper segment of fascia is incised, and a small portion may be removed or "windowed." Generally, one attempts to incise the fascia completely from dorsal to plantar

to relieve any compression that may be present. The nerve is usually visualized at the superior margin of the fascia in a fatty bundle that typically contains an artery and one or more veins. The nerve passes plantarly on the calcaneus just anterior to the medial tuberosity and deep to the plantar fascia. The nerve then courses laterally under the FDB muscle. One may bluntly probe this channel to ensure that nothing else is binding. Similarly, the more proximal nerve channel, also known as the lower chamber of the tarsal tunnel, can be gently probed to check for any remaining fascial impingements. Next, the medial band of the plantar fascia can be partially incised, and the spur may be removed if desired. Alternatively, the plantar fascia–heel spur portion of the procedure can be accomplished before the deeper dissection for the nerve.

Proximal and Distal Neurolysis

For patients with refractory infracalcaneal heel pain who also exhibit a positive Tinel sign or positive NCVs over the flexor retinaculum, a more extensive neurolysis of the tibial nerve and its branches is recommended. In 2013, Mook et al.[122] described their outcomes in 14 patients (16 heels) using release of the tibial nerve from the proximal edge of the flexor retinaculum past the bifurcation of the medial and lateral plantar nerves deep to the abductor hallucis and including the calcaneal nerve branches along the way. Ten heels (67%) recorded an excellent or good rating at the time of the last follow-up visit. One patient reported a poor outcome. The mean VAS pain score changed from 6.3 to 1.4. Pain at rest was alleviated in all patients, while pain with activity was incompletely relieved in the cohort. There were no wound healing issues.

Open Fasciotomy With Proximal and Distal Tarsal Tunnel Release Technique

The curvilinear incision is directed on the medial ankle and foot from proximal to the laciniate ligament distally onto the plantar foot at the level of the plantar fascial incision. The incision usually starts 1-2 cm proximal and posterior to the medial malleolus and ends over the distal glabrous portion of the medial heel (Fig. 19.11). The laciniate ligament is released. To release pressure at the porta pedis, the superficial fibers of the abductor hallucis muscle belly are released, followed by the fascia deep to the muscle. Care is taken at this level to separate the deep abductor fascia from the neurovascular bundle.

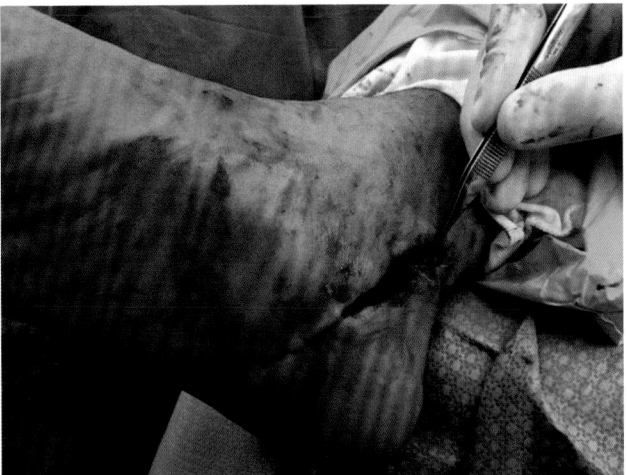

FIGURE 19.11 Incision placement and exposure for tarsal tunnel release with plantar fasciotomy.

The remaining fibers are approached from inferiorly. The abductor hallucis muscle belly is retracted dorsally, and the remaining porta pedis is released. Care is again taken to avoid damage to the neurovascular bundle. Once the tarsal tunnel component has been released, the plantar fascia is then released similar to the open plantar incision. Dissection of the nerves is avoided to prevent perineural fibrosis.

Posterior Muscle Group Lengthening

Gastrocnemius release/recession appears to be a safe and effective treatment option (in isolation and in combination) for patients with gastrocnemius contracture and chronic refractory infracalcaneal heel pain.[56] To date, there have been several studies now that have examined gastrocnemius release in patients with plantar fasciitis, some using proximal release of the medial head in the popliteal fossa and others using a distal release at the myotendinous junction. Abbassian et al.[123] looked at proximal medial gastrocnemius release (PMGR) in 21 heels (17 patients) with at least 1-year follow-up and found that 81% of the patients in the study reported total or significant pain relief at final follow-up with fast recovery and low overall morbidity. Two patients did relate subjective weakness (2/17, 12%) and 3 (17%) had some evidence of objective weakness at final follow-up, but this did not affect their outcome or satisfaction with the procedure.[123] In the case series by Maskill et al.,[124] 25 limbs underwent gastrocnemius recession for painful plantar fasciitis, and the mean VAS pain scores improved from 8.1 to 1.9 at final follow-up. Finally, in a retrospective comparative study, Monteagudo et al.[125] compared the results of open plantar fasciotomy (n = 30) with PMGR (n = 30) in the treatment of chronic recalcitrant plantar fasciitis. They found that gastrocnemius release was superior to open fasciotomy in all outcomes. Patient satisfaction in the PMGR group reached 95% (compared to only 60% in the fasciotomy group). Additionally, patients in the PMGR group were back to work and sports at 3 weeks on average, and functional and pain scores were considerably better for PMGR.[125] Huang et al.[126] studied patients who underwent percutaneous microfasciotomy (TOPAZ) and gastrocnemius recession for recalcitrant plantar fasciitis and found that the combination of radiofrequency microfasciotomy and gastrocnemius recession in patients with recalcitrant plantar fasciitis and an underlying gastrocnemius contracture shows favorable medium-term outcomes compared to performing either procedure in isolation. Techniques for posterior muscle group lengthening are described elsewhere in this text.

Additional, albeit less popular, surgical options for plantar fasciitis include **ultrasonic debridement with a microtip device and cryosurgery**. These treatment options have very little long-term data or peer-reviewed articles. Further research is needed to determine their effectiveness. Cryosurgery is a minimally invasive percutaneous procedure for plantar fasciitis that has been described by both Allen et al. and Cavazos et al.[93,127] Cryosurgery has very limited usage and clinical research to back its use. There was one retrospective study by Cavazos, which demonstrated a 77.4% success rate in a sampling of 137 ft.[93] Ultrasonic debridement with a microtip is new and does not have many peer-reviewed studies at this time (Fig. 19.12).

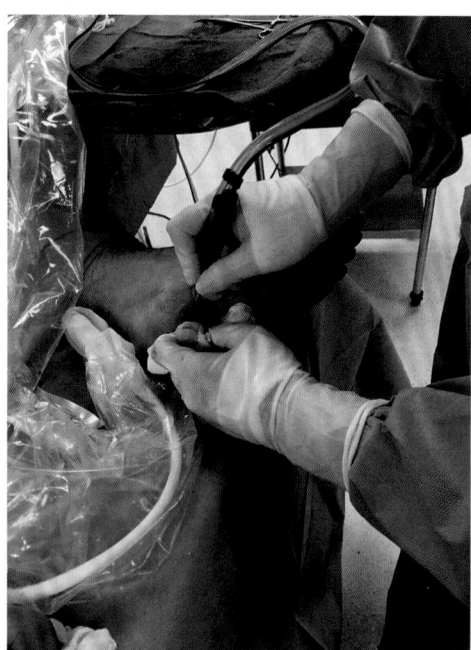

FIGURE 19.12 Ultrasonic debridement of plantar fascia.

PEARLS: PLANTAR FASCIOTOMY

- Be sure to include ancillary procedures (eg, nerve release, gastrocnemius recession) when indicated. Not addressing coexisting sources of heel pain will lead to treatment failure.
- Dorsiflex the foot and engage the windlass mechanism during resection of the plantar fascia. This makes full-thickness release easier.
- Keep patients non–weight bearing for 3 weeks postoperatively with the ankle held at 90 degrees. This allows the fascia to heal in an elongated position. This is true for open, EPF, and percutaneous techniques.

PITFALLS: PLANTAR FASCIOTOMY

- Avoid distal incisions in the arch where the subcutaneous fat is thin. Doing so decreases the chances of developing painful fibrotic nodules (fibromas) under the skin incision and minimizes the possibility for injury to the medial plantar nerve.
- Avoid sectioning more than 50% (usually no more than 1.5 cm) of the fascia across. To do otherwise results in destabilization of the foot and resulting lateral column pain, which is difficult to treat.
- Avoid blind transection ("palpation method" only) of the fascia. Even a small 2-cm instep incision still allows for direct visualization of the fascia.

PERILS: ENTRAPMENT OF BAXTER NERVE

- Diagnosis is difficult. Hallmark clinical finding is pain greatest over the abductor muscle belly and atypical plantar fasciitis symptoms (eg, pain at rest).
- The diagnosis is made on clinical grounds. NCVs and EMGs are not usually needed and frequently negative.
- Entrapment usually occurs in between the abductor fascia and quadratus plantae, but it can also be entrapped at the level of the spur as well. Important to examine and decompress all areas.

REFERENCES

1. Johal KS, Milner SA. Plantar fasciitis and the calcaneal spur: fact or fiction? *Foot Ankle Surg.* 2012;18(1):39-41. doi: 10.1016/j.fas.2011.03.003.
2. League AC. Current concepts review: plantar fasciitis. *Foot Ankle Int.* 2008;29(3):358-366. doi: 10.3113/FAI.2008.0358.
3. Pohl MB, Hamill J, Davis IS. Biomechanical and anatomic factors associated with a history of plantar fasciitis in female runners. *Clin J Sport Med.* 2009;19(5):372-376. doi: 10.1097/JSM.0b013e3181b8c270.
4. Riddle DL, Schappert SM. Volume of ambulatory care visits and patterns of care for patients diagnosed with plantar fasciitis: a national study of medical doctors. *Foot Ankle Int.* 2004;25(5):303-310. doi: 10.1177/107110070402500505.
5. Sammarco GJ, Helfrey RB. Surgical treatment of recalcitrant plantar fasciitis. *Foot Ankle Int.* 1996;17(9):520-526. doi: 10.1177/107110079601700902.
6. Thomas MJ, Roddy E, Zhang W, et al. The population prevalence of foot and ankle pain in middle and old age: a systematic review. *Pain.* 2011;152(12):2870-2880. doi: 10.1016/j.pain.2011.09.019.
7. Cole C, Seto C, Gazewood J. Plantar fasciitis: evidence-based review of diagnosis and therapy. *Am Fam Physician.* 2005;72(11):2237-2242.
8. Crawford F, Thomson C. Interventions for treating plantar heel pain. *Cochrane Database Syst Rev.* 2003;(3):CD000416. doi: 10.1002/14651858.CD000416.
9. Riddle DL, Pulisic M, Pidcoe P, Johnson RE. Risk factors for plantar fasciitis: a matched case-control study. *J Bone Joint Surg Am.* 2003;85-A(5):872-877.
10. Saxena A, Fullem B. Plantar fascia ruptures in athletes. *Am J Sports Med.* 2004;32(3):662-665. doi: 10.1177/0363546503261727.
11. Toomey EP. Plantar heel pain. *Foot Ankle Clin.* 2009;14(2):229-245. doi: 10.1016/j.fcl.2009.02.001.
12. La Porta GA, La Fata PC. Pathologic conditions of the plantar fascia. *Clin Podiatr Med Surg.* 2005;22(1):1-9, v. doi: S0891-8422(04)00074-6.
13. Wearing SC, Smeathers JE, Urry SR, Hennig EM, Hills AP. The pathomechanics of plantar fasciitis. *Sports Med.* 2006;36(7):585-611. doi: 10.2165/00007256-200636070-00004.
14. Dylevsky I. Connective tissues of the hand and foot. *Acta Univ Carol Med Monogr.* 1988;127:5-195.
15. Sarrafian SK. *Anatomy of the Foot and Ankle: Descriptive, Topographic, Functional.* New York, NY: JB Lippincott Company; 1983.
16. Hawkins BJ, Langermen RJ Jr, Gibbons T, Calhoun JH. An anatomic analysis of endoscopic plantar fascia release. *Foot Ankle Int.* 1995;16(9):552-558. doi: 10.1177/107110079501600907.
17. Nakamura A, Osonoi T, Terauchi Y. Relationship between urinary sodium excretion and pioglitazone-induced edema. *J Diabetes Investig.* 2010;1(5):208-211. doi: 10.1111/j.2040-1124.2010.00046.x.
18. Tanz SS. Heel pain. *Clin Orthop Relat Res.* 1963;28:169-178.
19. Forman WM, Green MA. The role of intrinsic musculature in the formation of inferior calcaneal exostoses. *Clin Podiatr Med Surg.* 1990;7(2):217-223.
20. Kumai T, Benjamin M. Heel spur formation and the subcalcaneal enthesis of the plantar fascia. *J Rheumatol.* 2002;29(9):1957-1964.
21. Li J, Muehleman C. Anatomic relationship of heel spur to surrounding soft tissues: greater variability than previously reported. *Clin Anat.* 2007;20(8):950-955. doi: 10.1002/ca.20548.
22. Snow SW, Bohne WH, DiCarlo E, Chang VK. Anatomy of the Achilles tendon and plantar fascia in relation to the calcaneus in various age groups. *Foot Ankle Int.* 1995;16(7):418-421. doi: 10.1177/107110079501600707.
23. Stecco C, Corradin M, Macchi V, et al. Plantar fascia anatomy and its relationship with Achilles tendon and paratenon. *J Anat.* 2013;223(6):665-676. doi: 10.1111/joa.12111.
24. Benjamin M. The fascia of the limbs and back—a review. *J Anat.* 2009;214(1):1-18. doi: 10.1111/j.1469-7580.2008.01011.x.
25. Williams P, Warnick R. *Gray's Anatomy.* 36th British ed. Philadelphia, PA: WB Saunders; 1980:612-613.
26. Przylucki H, Jones CL. Entrapment neuropathy of muscle branch of lateral plantar nerve: a cause of heel pain. *J Am Podiatry Assoc.* 1981;71(3):119-124. doi: 10.7547/87507315-71-3-119.

27. Arenson DJ, Cosentino GL, Suran SM. The inferior calcaneal nerve: an anatomical study. *J Am Podiatry Assoc.* 1980;70(11):552-560. doi: 10.7547/87507315-70-11-552.
28. Rondhuis JJ, Huson A. The first branch of the lateral plantar nerve and heel pain. *Acta Morphol Neerl Scand.* 1986;24(4):269-279.
29. Singh D. Nils Silfverskiold (1888–1957) and gastrocnemius contracture. *Foot Ankle Surg.* 2013;19(2):135-138. doi: 10.1016/j.fas.2012.12.002.
30. Baxter DE, Pfeffer GB. Treatment of chronic heel pain by surgical release of the first branch of the lateral plantar nerve. *Clin Orthop Relat Res.* 1992;(279):229-236.
31. Lemont H, Ammirati KM, Usen N. Plantar fasciitis: a degenerative process (fasciosis) without inflammation. *J Am Podiatr Med Assoc.* 2003;93(3):234-237.
32. Woelffer KE, Figura MA, Sandberg NS, Snyder NS. Five-year follow-up results of instep plantar fasciotomy for chronic heel pain. *J Foot Ankle Surg.* 2000;39(4):218-223.
33. Rompe JD, Furia J, Weil L, Maffulli N. Shock wave therapy for chronic plantar fasciopathy. *Br Med Bull.* 2007;81-82:183-208. doi: 10.1093/bmb/ldm005.
34. Irving DB, Cook JL, Young MA, Menz HB. Obesity and pronated foot type may increase the risk of chronic plantar heel pain: a matched case-control study. *BMC Musculoskelet Disord.* 2007;8:41. doi: 10.1186/1471-2474-8-41.
35. Rome K. Anthropometric and biomechanical risk factors in the development of plantar heel pain—a review of the literature. *Phys Ther Rev.* 1997;2(3):123-134. doi: 10.1179/ptr.1997.2.3.123.
36. McPoil TG, Martin RL, Cornwall MW, Wukich DK, Irrgang JJ, Godges JJ. Heel pain—plantar fasciitis: clinical practice guidelines linked to the international classification of function, disability, and health from the orthopaedic section of the American physical therapy association. *J Orthop Sports Phys Ther.* 2008;38(4):A1-A18. doi: 10.2519/jospt.2008.0302.
37. Rano JA, Fallat LM, Savoy-Moore RT. Correlation of heel pain with body mass index and other characteristics of heel pain. *J Foot Ankle Surg.* 2001;40(6):351-356.
38. van Leeuwen KD, Rogers J, Winzenberg T, van Middelkoop M. Higher body mass index is associated with plantar fasciopathy/'plantar fasciitis': systematic review and meta-analysis of various clinical and imaging risk factors. *Br J Sports Med.* 2016;50(16):972-981. doi: 10.1136/bjsports-2015-094695.
39. Taunton JE, Ryan MB, Clement DB, McKenzie DC, Lloyd-Smith DR, Zumbo BD. A retrospective case-control analysis of 2002 running injuries. *Br J Sports Med.* 2002;36(2):95-101.
40. Rome K, Howe T, Haslock I. Risk factors associated with the development of plantar heel pain in athletes. *Foot.* 2001;11(3):119-125. doi: 10.1054/foot.2001.0698.
41. Taunton JE, Ryan MB, Clement DB, McKenzie DC, Lloyd-Smith D. Plantar fasciitis: a retrospective analysis of 267 cases. *Phys Ther Sport.* 2002;3(2):57-65. doi: 10.1054/ptsp.2001.0082.
42. Messier SP, Pittala KA. Etiologic factors associated with selected running injuries. *Med Sci Sports Exerc.* 1988;20(5):501-505.
43. Buchbinder R. Clinical practice. Plantar fasciitis. *N Engl J Med.* 2004;350(21):2159-2166. doi: 10.1056/NEJMcp032745.
44. Erdemir A, Hamel AJ, Fauth AR, Piazza SJ, Sharkey NA. Dynamic loading of the plantar aponeurosis in walking. *J Bone Joint Surg Am.* 2004;86-A(3):546-552.
45. Wearing SC, Smeathers JE, Yates B, Sullivan PM, Urry SR, Dubois P. Sagittal movement of the medial longitudinal arch is unchanged in plantar fasciitis. *Med Sci Sports Exerc.* 2004;36(10):1761-1767.
46. Hunt AE, Smith RM, Torode M. Extrinsic muscle activity, foot motion and ankle joint moments during the stance phase of walking. *Foot Ankle Int.* 2001;22(1):31-41. doi: 10.1177/107110070102200105.
47. Hunt AE, Smith RM, Torode M, Keenan AM. Inter-segment foot motion and ground reaction forces over the stance phase of walking. *Clin Biomech (Bristol, Avon).* 2001;16(7):592-600. doi: 10.1016/s0268-0033(01)00040-7.
48. Cashmere T, Smith R, Hunt A. Medial longitudinal arch of the foot: stationary versus walking measures. *Foot Ankle Int.* 1999;20(2):112-118. doi: 10.1177/107110079902000208.
49. Sarrafian SK. Functional characteristics of the foot and plantar aponeurosis under tibiotalar loading. *Foot Ankle.* 1987;8(1):4-18.
50. Salathe EP Jr, Arangio GA, Salathe EP. A biomechanical model of the foot. *J Biomech.* 1986;19(12):989-1001.
51. Williams A, Vedi V, Singh D, Gedroye W, Hunt D. Hick's revisited: a weightbearing in vivo study of the biomechanics of the plantar fascia employing 'dynamic' MRI. *J Bone Jt Surg Br.* 1999;81:381.
52. Hicks JH. The mechanics of the foot. II. The plantar aponeurosis and the arch. *J Anat.* 1954;88(1):25-30.
53. Arandes R, Viladot A. Biomecanica del calcaneo. *Med Clin (Barc).* 1953;21:25-34.
54. Pascual Huerta J. The effect of the gastrocnemius on the plantar fascia. *Foot Ankle Clin.* 2014;19(4):701-718. doi: 10.1016/j.fcl.2014.08.011.
55. Amis J. The split second effect: the mechanism of how equinus can damage the human foot and ankle. *Front Surg.* 2016;3:38. doi: 10.3389/fsurg.2016.00038.
56. Schneider HP, Baca JM, Carpenter BB, Dayton PD, Fleischer AE, Sachs BD. American college of foot and ankle surgeons clinical consensus statement: diagnosis and treatment of adult acquired infracalcaneal heel pain. *J Foot Ankle Surg.* 2018;57(2):370-381. doi: S1067-2516(17)30619-1 [pii].
57. Ehrmann C, Maier M, Mengiardi B, Pfirrmann CW, Sutter R. Calcaneal attachment of the plantar fascia: MR findings in asymptomatic volunteers. *Radiology.* 2014;272(3):807-814. doi: 10.1148/radiol.14131410.
58. Fleischer AE, Albright RH, Crews RT, Kelil T, Wrobel JS. Prognostic value of diagnostic sonography in patients with plantar fasciitis. *J Ultrasound Med.* 2015;34(10):1729-1735. doi: 10.7863/ultra.15.14.10062.
59. Radwan A, Wyland M, Applequist L, Bolowsky E, Klingensmith H, Virag I. Ultrasonography, an effective tool in diagnosing plantar fasciitis: a systematic review of diagnostic trials. *Int J Sports Phys Ther.* 2016;11(5):663-671.
60. Li Z, Xia C, Yu A, Qi B. Ultrasound- versus palpation-guided injection of corticosteroid for plantar fasciitis: a meta-analysis. *PLoS One.* 2014;9(3):e92671. doi: 10.1371/journal.pone.0092671.
61. Bernhard K, Ng A, Kruse D, Stone PA. Surgical treatment of bone marrow lesion associated with recurrent plantar fasciitis: a case report describing an innovative technique using Subchondroplasty®. *J Foot Ankle Surg.* 2018;57(4):811-815. doi: S1067-2516(17)30649-X [pii].
62. Schon LC, Glennon TP, Baxter DE. Heel pain syndrome: electrodiagnostic support for nerve entrapment. *Foot Ankle.* 1993;14(3):129-135.
63. Pfeffer G, Bacchetti P, Deland J, et al. Comparison of custom and prefabricated orthoses in the initial treatment of proximal plantar fasciitis. *Foot Ankle Int.* 1999;20(4):214-221. doi: 10.1177/107110079902000402.
64. Radford JA, Landorf KB, Buchbinder R, Cook C. Effectiveness of low-dye taping for the short-term treatment of plantar heel pain: a randomised trial. *BMC Musculoskelet Disord.* 2006;7:64. doi: 10.1186/1471-2474-7-64.
65. Hyland MR, Webber-Gaffney A, Cohen L, Lichtman PT. Randomized controlled trial of calcaneal taping, sham taping, and plantar fascia stretching for the short-term management of plantar heel pain. *J Orthop Sports Phys Ther.* 2006;36(6):364-371. doi: 10.2519/jospt.2006.2078.
66. van de Water AT, Speksnijder CM. Efficacy of taping for the treatment of plantar fasciosis: a systematic review of controlled trials. *J Am Podiatr Med Assoc.* 2010;100(1):41-51. doi: 10.7547/1000041.
67. Abd El Salam MS, Abd Elhafz YN. Low-dye taping versus medial arch support in managing pain and pain-related disability in patients with plantar fasciitis. *Foot Ankle Spec.* 2011;4(2):86-91. doi: 10.1177/1938640010387416.
68. Podolsky R, Kalichman L. Taping for plantar fasciitis. *J Back Musculoskelet Rehabil.* 2015;28(1):1-6. doi: 10.3233/BMR-140485.
69. Park C, Lee S, Lim DY, Yi CW, Kim JH, Jeon C. Effects of the application of low-dye taping on the pain and stability of patients with plantar fasciitis. *J Phys Ther Sci.* 2015;27(8):2491-2493. doi: 10.1589/jpts.27.2491.
70. Wrobel JS, Fleischer AE, Matzkin-Bridger J, et al. Physical examination variables predict response to conservative treatment of nonchronic plantar fasciitis: secondary analysis of a randomized, placebo-controlled footwear study. *PM R.* 2016;8(5):436-444. doi: 10.1016/j.pmrj.2015.09.011.
71. DiGiovanni BF, Nawoczenski DA, Lintal ME, et al. Tissue-specific plantar fascia-stretching exercise enhances outcomes in patients with chronic heel pain. A prospective, randomized study. *J Bone Joint Surg Am.* 2003;85-A(7):1270-1277.
72. Kamonseki DH, Goncalves GA, Yi LC, Junior IL. Effect of stretching with and without muscle strengthening exercises for the foot and hip in patients with plantar fasciitis: a randomized controlled single-blind clinical trial. *Man Ther.* 2016;23:76-82. doi: 10.1016/j.math.2015.10.006.
73. Barry LD, Barry AN, Chen Y. A retrospective study of standing gastrocnemius-soleus stretching versus night splinting in the treatment of plantar fasciitis. *J Foot Ankle Surg.* 2002;41(4):221-227.
74. Lee WC, Wong WY, Kung E, Leung AK. Effectiveness of adjustable dorsiflexion night splint in combination with accommodative foot orthosis on plantar fasciitis. *J Rehabil Res Dev.* 2012;49(10):1557-1564.
75. David JA, Sankarapandian V, Christopher PR, Chatterjee A, Macaden AS. Injected corticosteroids for treating plantar heel pain in adults. *Cochrane Database Syst Rev.* 2017;6:CD009348. doi: 10.1002/14651858.CD009348.pub2.
76. Zelen CM, Poka A, Andrews J. Prospective, randomized, blinded, comparative study of injectable micronized dehydrated amniotic/chorionic membrane allograft for plantar fasciitis—a feasibility study. *Foot Ankle Int.* 2013;34(10):1332-1339. doi: 10.1177/1071100713502179.
77. Tsikopoulos K, Vasiliadis HS, Mavridis D. Injection therapies for plantar fasciopathy ('plantar fasciitis'): a systematic review and network meta-analysis of 22 randomised controlled trials. *Br J Sports Med.* 2016;50(22):1367-1375. doi: 10.1136/bjsports-2015-095437.
78. Cazzell S, Stewart J, Agnew PS, et al. Randomized controlled trial of micronized dehydrated human amnion/chorion membrane (dHACM) injection compared to placebo for the treatment of plantar fasciitis. *Foot Ankle Int.* 2018;39(10):1151-1161. doi: 10.1177/1071100718788549.
79. Lou J, Wang S, Liu S, Xing G. Effectiveness of extracorporeal shock wave therapy without local anesthesia in patients with recalcitrant plantar fasciitis: a meta-analysis of randomized controlled trials. *Am J Phys Med Rehabil.* 2017;96(8):529-534. doi: 10.1097/PHM.0000000000000666.
80. Thomson CE, Crawford F, Murray GD. The effectiveness of extra corporeal shock wave therapy for plantar heel pain: a systematic review and meta-analysis. *BMC Musculoskelet Disord.* 2005;6:19. doi: 10.1186/1471-2474-6-19.
81. Aqil A, Siddiqui MR, Solan M, Redfern DJ, Gulati V, Cobb JP. Extracorporeal shock wave therapy is effective in treating chronic plantar fasciitis: a meta-analysis of RCTs. *Clin Orthop Relat Res.* 2013;471(11):3645-3652. doi: 10.1007/s11999-013-3132-2.
82. Dizon JN, Gonzalez-Suarez C, Zamora MT, Gambito ED. Effectiveness of extracorporeal shock wave therapy in chronic plantar fasciitis: a meta-analysis. *Am J Phys Med Rehabil.* 2013;92(7):606-620. doi: 10.1097/PHM.0b013e31828cd42b.
83. Landorf KB. Plantar heel pain and plantar fasciitis. *BMJ Clin Evid.* 2015;2015:1111.
84. Sun J, Gao F, Wang Y, Sun W, Jiang B, Li Z. Extracorporeal shock wave therapy is effective in treating chronic plantar fasciitis: a meta-analysis of RCTs. *Medicine (Baltimore).* 2017;96(15):e6621. doi: 10.1097/MD.0000000000006621.
85. Looney B, Srokose T, Fernandez-de-las-Penas C, Cleland JA. Graston instrument soft tissue mobilization and home stretching for the management of plantar heel pain: a case series. *J Manipulative Physiol Ther.* 2011;34(2):138-142. doi: 10.1016/j.jmpt.2010.12.003.
86. Ajimsha MS, Binsu D, Chithra S. Effectiveness of myofascial release in the management of plantar heel pain: a randomized controlled trial. *Foot (Edinb).* 2014;24(2):66-71. doi: 10.1016/j.foot.2014.03.005.
87. Hansberger BL, Baker RT, May J, Nasypany A. A novel approach to treating plantar fasciitis—effects of primal reflex release technique: a case series. *Int J Sports Phys Ther.* 2015;10(5):690-699.

88. Landorf KB, Keenan AM, Herbert RD. Effectiveness of foot orthoses to treat plantar fasciitis: a randomized trial. *Arch Intern Med.* 2006;166(12):1305-1310. doi: 166/12/1305 [pii].

89. Wrobel JS, Fleischer AE, Crews RT, Jarrett B, Najafi B. A randomized controlled trial of custom foot orthoses for the treatment of plantar heel pain. *J Am Podiatr Med Assoc.* 2015;105(4):281-294. doi: 10.7547/13-122.1.

90. Davies MS, Weiss GA, Saxby TS. Plantar fasciitis: how successful is surgical intervention? *Foot Ankle Int.* 1999;20(12):803-807. doi: 10.1177/107110079902001209.

91. Morton TN, Zimmerman JP, Lee M, Schaber JD. A review of 105 consecutive uniport endoscopic plantar fascial release procedures for the treatment of chronic plantar fasciitis. *J Foot Ankle Surg.* 2013;52(1):48-52. doi: 10.1053/j.jfas.2012.10.011.

92. Wolgin M, Cook C, Graham C, Mauldin D. Conservative treatment of plantar heel pain: long-term follow-up. *Foot Ankle Int.* 1994;15(3):97-102. doi: 10.1177/107110079401500303.

93. Cavazos GJ, Khan KH, D'Antoni AV, Harkless LB, Lopez D. Cryosurgery for the treatment of heel pain. *Foot Ankle Int.* 2009;30(6):500-505. doi: 10.3113/FAI.2009.0500.

94. Tomczak RL, Haverstock BD. A retrospective comparison of endoscopic plantar fasciotomy to open plantar fasciotomy with heel spur resection for chronic plantar fasciitis/heel spur syndrome. *J Foot Ankle Surg.* 1995;34(3):305-311. doi: S1067-2516(09)80065-3 [pii].

95. Kinley S, Frascone S, Calderone D, Wertheimer SJ, Squire MA, Wiseman FA. Endoscopic plantar fasciotomy versus traditional heel spur surgery: a prospective study. *J Foot Ankle Surg.* 1993;32(6):595-603.

96. Huang CK, Kitaoka HB, An KN, Chao EY. Biomechanical evaluation of longitudinal arch stability. *Foot Ankle.* 1993;14(6):353-357.

97. Sharkey NA, Ferris L, Donahue SW. Biomechanical consequences of plantar fascial release or rupture during gait: Part I—disruptions in longitudinal arch conformation. *Foot Ankle Int.* 1998;19(12):812-820. doi: 10.1177/107110079801901204.

98. Arangio GA, Chen C, Kim W. Effect of cutting the plantar fascia on mechanical properties of the foot. *Clin Orthop Relat Res.* 1997;(339):227-231.

99. Murphy GA, Pneumaticos SG, Kamaric E, Noble PC, Trevino SG, Baxter DE. Biomechanical consequences of sequential plantar fascia release. *Foot Ankle Int.* 1998;19(3):149-152. doi: 10.1177/107110079801900306.

100. Thordarson DB, Kumar PJ, Hedman TP, Ebramzadeh E. Effect of partial versus complete plantar fasciotomy on the windlass mechanism. *Foot Ankle Int.* 1997;18(1):16-20. doi: 10.1177/107110079701800104.

101. Sharkey NA, Donahue SW, Ferris L. Biomechanical consequences of plantar fascial release or rupture during gait. Part II: alterations in forefoot loading. *Foot Ankle Int.* 1999;20(2):86-96. doi: 10.1177/107110079902000204.

102. Kitaoka HB, Luo ZP, An KN. Mechanical behavior of the foot and ankle after plantar fascia release in the unstable foot. *Foot Ankle Int.* 1997;18(1):8-15. doi: 10.1177/107110079701800103.

103. Barrett SL, Day SV. Endoscopic plantar fasciotomy: two portal endoscopic surgical techniques—clinical results of 65 procedures. *J Foot Ankle Surg.* 1993;32(3):248-256.

104. Barrett SL, Day SV, Pignetti TT, Robinson LB. Endoscopic plantar fasciotomy: a multisurgeon prospective analysis of 652 cases. *J Foot Ankle Surg.* 1995;34(4):400-406. doi: S1067-2516(09)80011-2 [pii].

105. Lewis G, Gatti A, Barry LD, Greenberg PM, Levenson M. The plantar approach to heel surgery: a retrospective study. *J Foot Surg.* 1991;30(6):542-546.

106. Boike AM, Snyder AJ, Roberto PD, Tabbert WG. Heel spur surgery. A transverse plantar approach. *J Am Podiatr Med Assoc.* 1993;83(1):39-42. doi: 10.7547/87507315-83-1-39.

107. Self TC, Kunz RE, Young G. Transverse plantar incision for heel spur surgery. Four-year follow-up survey of 35 patients. *J Am Podiatr Med Assoc.* 1993;83(5):259-262. doi: 10.7547/87507315-83-5-259.

108. Michetti ML, Jacobs SA. Calcaneal heel spurs: etiology, treatment, and a new surgical approach. *J Foot Surg.* 1983;22(3):234-239.

109. Duvries HL. Heel spur (calcaneal spur). *AMA Arch Surg.* 1957;74(4):536-542.

110. Ruch JR. Lecture presentation. In: Miller SJ, ed. *Reconstructive Surgery of the Foot and Leg: Update '98.* Tucker, GA: Podiatry Institute; 1998.

111. Braly W. Plantar fascia release. In: Johnson K, ed. *The Foot and Ankle.* New York: Raven Press; 1994:323-332.

112. Fishco WD, Goecker RM, Schwartz RI. The instep plantar fasciotomy for chronic plantar fasciitis. A retrospective review. *J Am Podiatr Med Assoc.* 2000;90(2):66-69. doi: 10.7547/87507315-90-2-66.

113. Perelman GK, Figura MA, Sandberg NS. The medial instep plantar fasciotomy. *J Foot Ankle Surg.* 1995;34(5):447-457; discussion 509-510. doi: S1067-2516(09)80020-3 [pii].

114. O'Malley MJ, Page A, Cook R. Endoscopic plantar fasciotomy for chronic heel pain. *Foot Ankle Int.* 2000;21(6):505-510. doi: 10.1177/107110070002100610.

115. Weil L Jr, Glover JP, Weil LS. A new minimally invasive technique for treating plantar fasciosis using bipolar radiofrequency: a prospective analysis. *Foot Ankle Spec.* 2008;1(1):13-18. doi: 10.1177/1938640007312318.

116. Sean NY, Singh I, Wai CK. Radiofrequency microtenotomy for the treatment of plantar fasciitis shows good early results. *Foot Ankle Surg.* 2010;16(4):174-177. doi: 10.1016/j.fas.2009.10.008.

117. Sorensen MD, Hyer CF, Philbin TM. Percutaneous bipolar radiofrequency microdebridement for recalcitrant proximal plantar fasciosis. *J Foot Ankle Surg.* 2011;50(2):165-170. doi: 10.1053/j.jfas.2010.11.002.

118. Chou AC, Ng SY, Su DH, Singh IR, Koo K. Radiofrequency microtenotomy is as effective as plantar fasciotomy in the treatment of recalcitrant plantar fasciitis. *Foot Ankle Surg.* 2016;22(4):270-273. doi: S1268-7731(15)00171-X [pii].

119. Wang W, Rikhraj IS, Chou ACC, Chong HC, Koo KOT. Endoscopic plantar fasciotomy vs open radiofrequency microtenotomy for recalcitrant plantar fasciitis. *Foot Ankle Int.* 2018;39(1):11-17. doi: 10.1177/1071100717732763.

120. Baxter DE, Thigpen CM. Heel pain—operative results. *Foot Ankle.* 1984;5(1):16-25. doi: 10.1177/107110078400500103.

121. Hendrix CL, Jolly GP, Garbalosa JC, Blume P, DosRemedios E. Entrapment neuropathy: the etiology of intractable chronic heel pain syndrome. *J Foot Ankle Surg.* 1998;37(4):273-279. doi: S1067-2516(98)80062-8 [pii].

122. Mook WR, Gay T, Parekh SG. Extensile decompression of the proximal and distal tarsal tunnel combined with partial plantar fascia release in the treatment of chronic plantar heel pain. *Foot Ankle Spec.* 2013;6(1):27-35. doi: 10.1177/1938640012470718.

123. Abbassian A, Kohls-Gatzoulis J, Solan MC. Proximal medial gastrocnemius release in the treatment of recalcitrant plantar fasciitis. *Foot Ankle Int.* 2012;33(1):14-19. doi: 10.3113/FAI.2012.0014.

124. Maskill JD, Bohay DR, Anderson JG. Gastrocnemius recession to treat isolated foot pain. *Foot Ankle Int.* 2010;31(1):19-23. doi: 10.3113/FAI.2010.0019.

125. Monteagudo M, Maceira E, Garcia-Virto V, Canosa R. Chronic plantar fasciitis: plantar fasciotomy versus gastrocnemius recession. *Int Orthop.* 2013;37(9):1845-1850. doi: 10.1007/s00264-013-2022-2.

126. Huang DM, Chou AC, Yeo NE, Singh IR. Radiofrequency microtenotomy with concurrent gastrocnemius recession improves postoperative vitality scores in the treatment of recalcitrant plantar fasciitis. *Ann Acad Med Singapore.* 2018;47(12):509-515.

127. Allen BH, Fallat LM, Schwartz SM. Cryosurgery: an innovative technique for the treatment of plantar fasciitis. *J Foot Ankle Surg.* 2007;46(2):75-79. doi: S1067-2516(07)00008-7 [pii].

CHAPTER 20

Pes Cavus Surgery

Craig A. Camasta and Michael F. Kelly

DEFINITION

Pes cavus is a sagittal plane deformity of the foot that is characterized by a high-arched foot type. Symptoms may arise in this foot type due to poor shock absorption (arch pain, intrinsic muscle fatigue, plantar fasciitis), compensation for the deformity by use of adjacent joints' range of motion (extensor substitution hammer toes, ankle joint instability/arthritis), or overuse syndromes (Achilles tendonitis/enthesiopathy, plantar fasciitis, tarsal tunnel syndrome).[1-4]

ETIOLOGY

The etiology of pes cavus is most frequently attributed to the neuromuscular disorders involving the brain, spinal cord, or peripheral nerves. Two-thirds of adults with symptomatic cavus foot have an underlying neurological condition.[5] Among them, Charcot-Marie-Tooth (CMT) disease, a hereditary sensory motor neuropathy, is most frequently reported. The probability of a patient who has bilateral cavovarus feet being diagnosed with CMT is 78%.[6]

Cavus deformity could be progressive or caused by paralytic soft tissue diseases, osteoarticular diseases, or trauma[7] (Table 20.1).

MUSCLE IMBALANCE

The progressive muscle involvement from distal to proximal most frequently affects the intrinsic muscles, the tibialis anterior, and the peroneus brevis. Extensor hallucis longus is relatively spared. Relative weakness in one of the two opposing muscles causes muscle imbalance and structural deformity. Structural deformation is more substantial when the motor imbalance begins before maturation of the skeleton.[1,8]

Muscle imbalance can occur between the extrinsic and intrinsic muscles, between the posterior tibial and the peroneus brevis muscles, and between the anterior tibial and the peroneus longus muscles. A weak anterior tibialis muscle relative to the peroneus longus muscle results in plantar flexion of the first metatarsal. The flexion power of the peroneus longus becomes much stronger as the foot is positioned in equinus.[9]

Recruitment of extensor hallucis longus produces cock-up deformity of the great toe, which further depresses the metatarsal head. With weak intrinsic muscles, the unopposed extensor digitorum longus hyperextends the unstable lesser toes at the metatarsophalangeal joint while the flexor digitorum longus and brevis flex the phalanges. The resultant claw toe deformity and plantar flexed metatarsal heads amplify forefoot equinus.[1,8]

Progressive weakness of the peroneus brevis and tibialis anterior myotendinous units causes a cavovarus foot type noted by an overpowering tibialis posterior and peroneus longus, respectively. When such overpowering occurs, the recruitment of the extensor hallucis longus and tibialis anterior myotendinous units weakens, leading to a marked increase in arch height. Footdrop and claw toe deformities will also develop as the disease worsens, and a high steppage gait is noted.[10]

The plantar flexed forefoot forces the hindfoot into varus. Hindfoot varus is initially flexible, but can gradually become

TABLE 20.1 Pes Cavus Etiology		
Cavus Foot Etiology		
Neurologic	**Osteoarticular Changes**	**Soft Tissue Contractures**
Charcot-Marie-Tooth disease	Congenital cavus foot	Ledderhose disease
Polyneuritic syndromes	Rheumatoid arthritis	Scar tissue, iatrogenic
Dejerine-Sottas disease	Trauma	Burns
Friedreich ataxia	Inadequate use of shoes	Vascular lesions
Roussy-Lévy syndrome		
Strumpell-Lorrain disease		
Pierre-Marie heredotaxy		
Cerebral palsy		
Muscular dystrophy		
Parkinson disease		
Poliomyelitis		
Myelomeningocele		
Nerve trauma		
Tumors		
Leprosy		
Hysterical cavus		

rigid over time. With the rigid hindfoot varus, the Achilles tendon becomes a secondary invertor and becomes contracted.[1,8]

Spastic conditions, such as cerebral palsy, occur as the most common form of the nonprogressive condition. Pes cavus in cavovarus foot deformities is usually accompanied by ankle equinus as well. Muscular imbalances are a critical component and involve the gastrocnemius-soleal complex, tibialis posterior, and tibialis anterior.[10]

CLINICAL MANIFESTATIONS

Cavus foot, even subtle deformity, can cause various problems throughout the foot and ankle (Table 20.2). Metatarsalgia due to forefoot overload is related to the combined effect of a cavus foot and tight heel cord. When examining a patient with metatarsalgia, cavus foot should be in the list of differential diagnoses along with Morton neuroma and long metatarsals. Overload on the first metatarsal head can lead to sesamoiditis or sesamoid fractures. Overload on the lateral border can result in a stress fracture of the fifth metatarsal. Stress fractures of the fifth metatarsal can be difficult to treat without addressing the underlying cavus deformity.[11]

Reduced shock absorption due to a rigid hindfoot and tight heel cord can lead to plantar fasciitis or Achilles tendinitis. Haglund deformity can become symptomatic more easily if the heel is in varus because the posterior superior calcaneal tuberosity will become more prominent. Rigid joints can progress to joint destruction and develop arthritis over time.[11]

Chronic lateral ankle instability and recurrent sprains are inevitable in a patient with a cavus foot. In addition, rigid joints can lead to prolonged lateral column overload and recurrent sprains can lead to peroneal tendon problems. Any attempt to repair the lateral ligamentous problems will not be successful if the osseous structures remain in varus. If left untreated, a prolonged cavus foot will eventually lead to a varus ankle deformity and osteoarthritis.[11]

Understanding the biomechanical component of each individual deformity is paramount and often difficult in a cavus foot or an ankle varus with a compensatory hindfoot. Biomechanically, a cavus foot type can be divided into several different categories. This helps the surgeon to delineate the procedure of choice.[10]

DIAGNOSTICS

Standard weight-bearing foot and ankle radiographs are utilized during the examination along with a long-leg axial view or calcaneal axial view. On an AP foot view, one can appreciate the degree of transverse plane deformity such as forefoot adduction or midfoot adduction. The calcaneal axial view is an important view to look for calcaneal varus. On a lateral foot view, one can assess for the degree of plantar flexion of the first ray or metatarsal and determine the amount of correction needed in the forefoot. Advanced imaging is used to evaluate periarticular pathology and articular damage of the midfoot and hindfoot. Computed tomography (CT) is typically ordered when determining the degree of arthritis and subchondral cysts within the involved joints. Magnetic resonance imaging (MRI) may also be utilized if there is concern for ligamentous or tendon pathology, which is common in cavus foot and ankle conditions. If the patient has any degree of footdrop or a neurologic condition, nerve conduction velocities (NCVs) and electromyographies (EMGs) are often helpful in determining the diagnosis and appropriate tendons for transfer, if indicated. The cavus foot and ankle is a complex deformity and can often present in different ways, so utilizing the appropriate diagnostic tools is key in planning surgical procedures and overall treatment.[10]

NONSURGICAL MANAGEMENT

It is crucial to correct the biomechanical anomaly present in subtle cavus foot (SCF) for nonsurgical management to succeed. In addition to other treatments prescribed, such as stretching for plantar fasciitis or proprioceptive reeducation for functional ankle instability, orthotic management of SCF may offer further benefit. LoPiccolo et al. recently reviewed 93 patients who presented with ankle instability and pain with associated SCF. They were given a custom, full-length orthosis made of ethyl vinyl acetate with a recess under the first metatarsal head, a ramp at the lateral forefoot, a lowered arch, and a heel cushion. A follow-up questionnaire conducted at 1 and 2 years after initiating orthotic management revealed a significant improvement in pain and instability events. Twenty-three of the 25 patients (92%) who had reported instability noted an improvement in their stability, with decreased episodes of "rolling the ankle" with use of the custom orthotic.[12] The principles of orthotic prescription are important because they are a deviation from the accommodative device typically offered to patients with a high arch. A shoe or orthotic with an elevated arch functions only to tip the foot into further varus. Aside from custom orthoses with a recessed first ray, a lateral wedge, and a lowered medial longitudinal arch, an over-the-counter orthosis is available, as well. This orthosis is a less expensive device that meets these same criteria; it is available by shoe size and offers an adequate amount of correction for patients with mild or true

TABLE 20.2	Clinical Manifestations of Pes Cavus
Forefoot and midfoot	
Metatarsalgia	
Callus under first, fifth metatarsal heads	
Morton neuroma	
Sesamoid problems (sesamoiditis, chondromalacia, avascular necrosis)	
Stress fracture of metatarsal bones	
Metatarsus adductus	
Midfoot arthritis ankle and hindfoot	
Plantar fasciitis	
Achilles tendinitis	
Chronic lateral ankle instability	
Subtalar instability	
Peroneal tendon problems (tear or split, rupture, tendinopathy)	
Enlarged or posteriorly placed distal fibular	
Recurrent dislocation of the peroneal tendons	
Painful os peroneum syndrome	
Painful Haglund deformity	
Varus ankle arthritis	

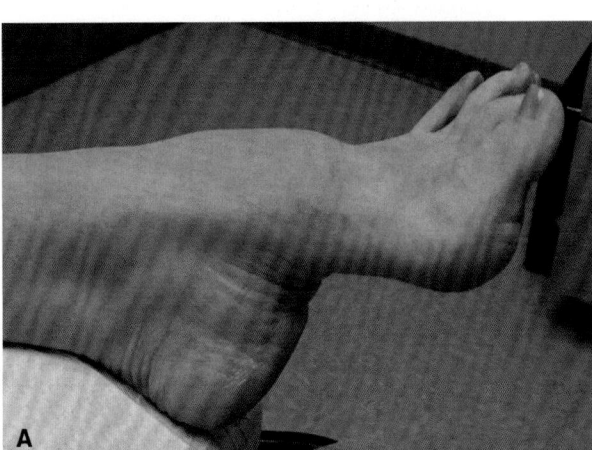
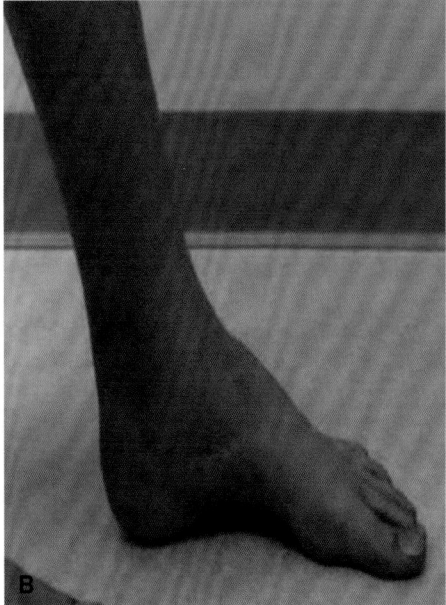

FIGURE 20.1 A. Pes cavus with plantar flexed forefoot on rearfoot. **B.** Pes equinus with plantar flexed ankle joint contracture.

SCF. Patients whose varus hindfoot is more severe would most likely benefit from custom orthoses. The benefit of a custom orthosis over a prefabricated orthosis is that the recess underlying the first metatarsal head can be made deeper and the lateral heel wedge can be of greater magnitude.[13]

EQUINUS VS CAVUS

The plantar flexed forefoot, which is a common feature of pes cavus (Fig. 20.1A), may appear similar to an equinus deformity (Fig. 20.1B) in that both exhibit limited dorsiflexion in the swing phase of gait. However, closer examination will differentiate cavus (plantar flexed foot) from equinus (plantar flexed ankle). Clinical and radiographic examinations are important to differentiate the location, dominant plane, and severity of the deformity.[1,2,14] A weight-bearing lateral foot/ankle radiograph is helpful to differentiate equinus from cavus by examination of the position of the calcaneus. In a pes cavus deformity, a lateral weight-bearing radiograph will demonstrate a higher than normal calcaneal inclination angle (>15 degrees) (Fig. 20.2A), whereas an equinus deformity will demonstrate a lower than normal to negative calcaneal inclination angle (<15 degrees) (Fig. 20.2B).[2] The importance of this differentiation relates to

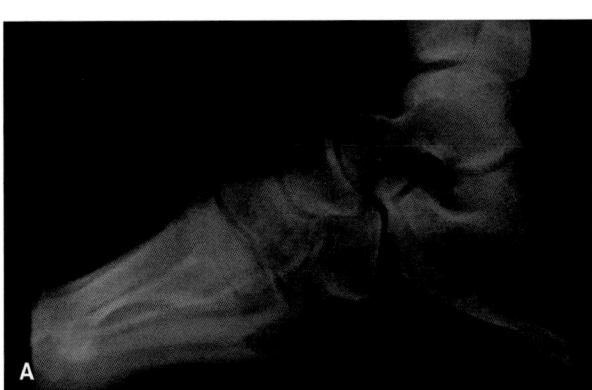
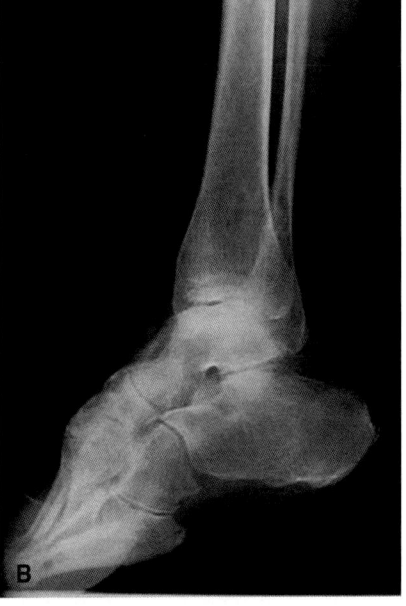

FIGURE 20.2 A. Lateral weight-bearing radiograph of a pes cavus demonstrating a greater than normal calcaneal inclination angle. **B.** Lateral weight-bearing radiograph of pes equinus demonstrating a lower than normal calcaneal inclination angle in which the heel does not contact the ground.

the method of surgical repair, with particular consideration to heel cord/Achilles tendon lengthening. An equinus deformity will frequently benefit from heel cord lengthening, enabling the heel to contact the ground. A pes cavus deformity normally does not benefit from heel cord lengthening, and in fact can be made more severe, since the heel cord is resisting further contracture within the high-arched foot.[4,14]

PEARLS

If a patient can forcefully make heel contact while in stance, then a gastrocnemius recession is typically sufficient to reduce an equinus deformity. If the patient cannot make heel contact while in a vertical stance, then a tendo-Achilles lengthening (TAL) is typically indicated (along with posterior fascia, ankle, and subtalar joint capsule release).

positioning PEARLS

A gastrocnemius recession can be performed in the supine position via a medial incision at the lower leg while externally rotating the leg. A TAL procedure may require flipping the patient intraoperatively to a prone position for appropriate exposure. It is imperative the anesthesia and operating room staff are aware of intraoperative position changes prior to case start to ensure appropriate equipment is available to prevent delays.

SURGICAL REPAIR OF PES CAVUS: COLE OSTEOTOMY

The goal of pes cavus surgery is to provide symptomatic relief while addressing the apex and plane(s) of deformity.[15,16] In a purely sagittal plane pes cavus deformity, the apex of the forefoot and hindfoot (talus and first metatarsal) intersect at the naviculocuneiform joints and cuboid bone (Fig. 20.3). The Cole

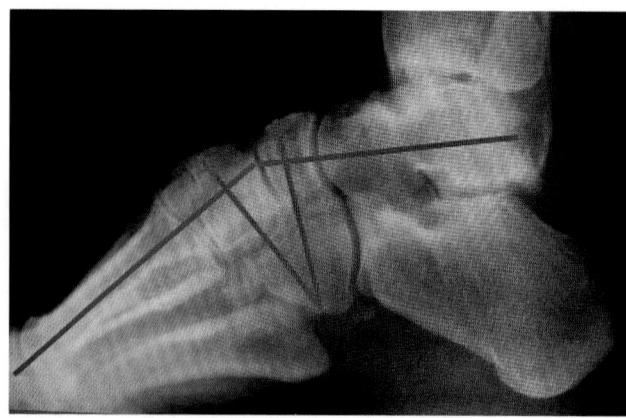

FIGURE 20.3 Pes cavus lateral radiograph demonstrating apex of forefoot and hindfoot (talus and first metatarsal) axes through the naviculocuneiform joints and cuboid bone, and location of the osteotomy/arthrodeses (*orange lines*).

osteotomy/arthrodesis is an effective procedure to reduce the sagittal plane contracture of the pes cavus foot[17-21] (Fig. 20.4).

A medial skin incision is placed longitudinal from the talonavicular joint to the metatarsal-cuneiform joints, near the dorsomedial boarder of the foot. The incision must access the top of the foot from a subcapsular/periosteal plane of dissection and thus should be high in relation to the medial bisection of the foot. Intraoperative fluoroscopy prior to surgery can assist in locating key anatomic landmarks (Fig. 20.5). A lateral skin incision is made longitudinal from the calcaneocuboid joint to the cuboid–fourth metatarsal joint, near the dorsolateral boarder of the foot, biased in a dorsal direction near the top of the cuboid bone. This incision must also access the top of the foot to allow communication between the lateral and medial dissection planes (Fig. 20.6).

Medial dissection is performed. The tibialis anterior tendon is retracted dorsally and the naviculocuneiform joint is

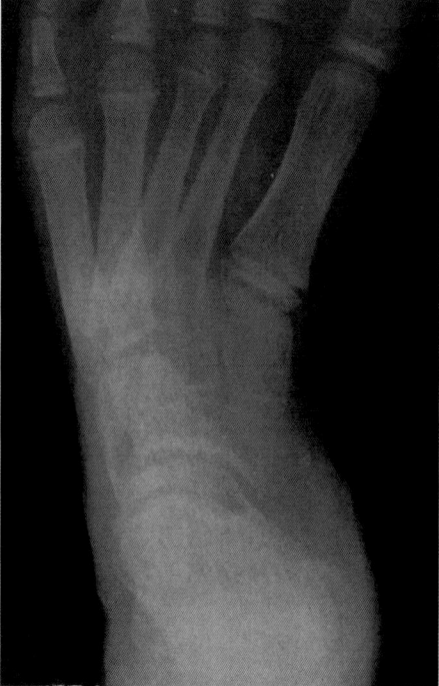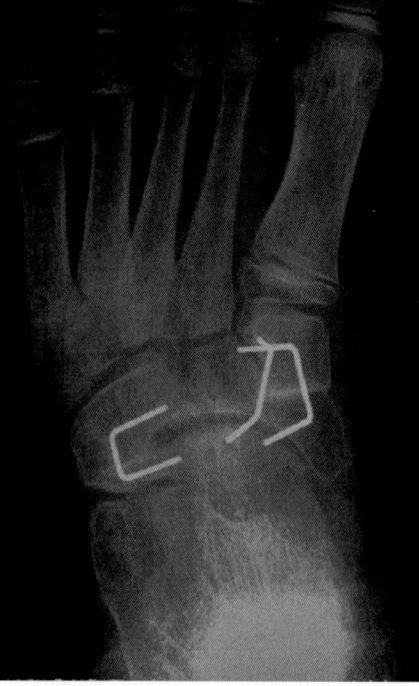

FIGURE 20.4 Dorsal-plantar view of orientation of the osteotomy location and direction of bone cuts. Note that the medial apex of the bone cuts is slightly distal to the lateral apex of the osteotomy site.

<

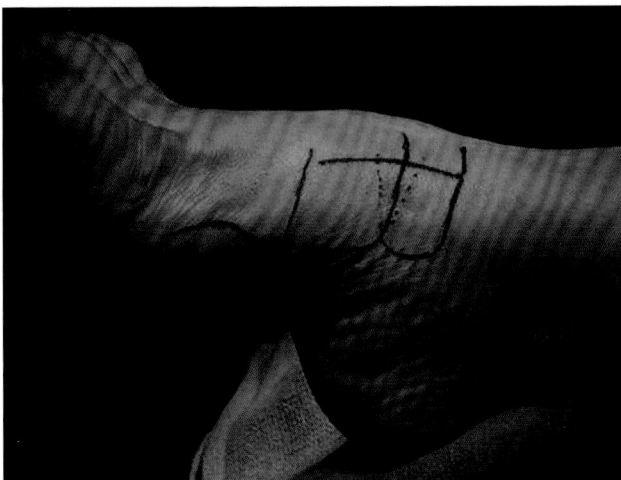

FIGURE 20.5 Medial skin incision is longitudinal from the talonavicular joint to the metatarsal-cuneiform joints, near the dorsomedial border of the foot.

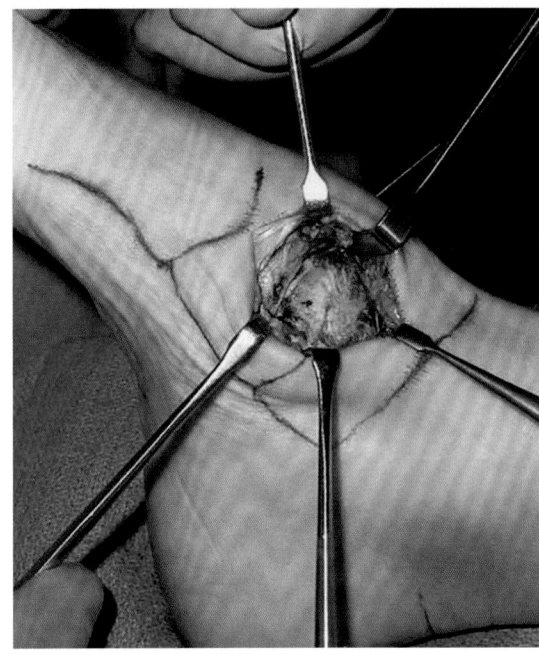

FIGURE 20.7 Medial dissection.

exposed medially and dorsally; however, the plantar ligaments are spared. Access across the dorsum of the foot must allow for adequate bone resection through a dorsal wedge of bone through the joint, one cut proximal to and one cut distal to the joint (Fig. 20.7). Next, the lateral dissection is performed. The deep fascia is divided longitudinally and the cuboid is exposed along its dorsolateral surface, retracting the extensor digitorum brevis muscle dorsally and the peroneal tendons plantarly. The cuboid is exposed from the calcaneocuboid joint to the fourth metatarsal-cuboid joint, however, care is taken to avoid violating the integrity of the periarticular ligaments. A Kirschner wire (K-wire) is then driven into the center of the cuboid to act as a reference point for making the medial bone cuts. This reference wire needs to be long enough to be viewed from the medial side of the foot (Fig. 20.8).

A sagittal saw is used to make the medial bone cuts, which consist of two cuts, one proximal and one distal to the

naviculocuneiform joint, aiming laterally proximal and distal to the cuboid reference K-wire. Use of the reference wire ensures that the medial and lateral osteotomy cuts will line up with one another, facilitating closure of the osteotomy and reduction of the deformity. Without the reference K-wire, there is a visual tendency to aim too distal with the cuts, which will not line up with the lateral cuts. Osteotomes are used to release the cut sections of bone, which will then be removed (Fig. 20.9).

For the lateral bone cuts, a similar-sized dorsal wedge is cut through the cuboid bone, with equal amounts of bone remaining on the anterior and posterior side of the osteotomy to allow

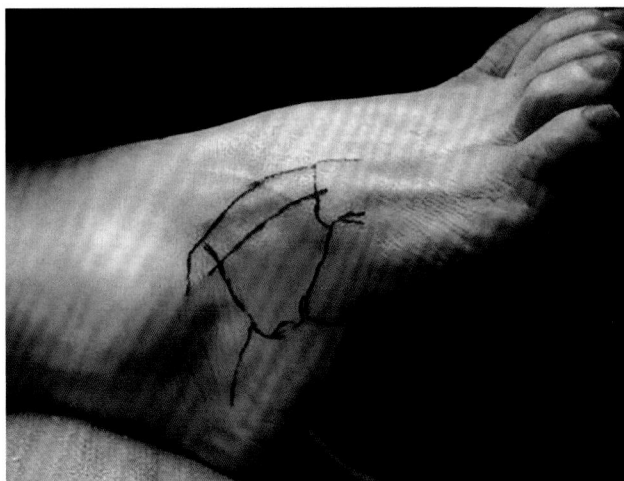

FIGURE 20.6 Lateral skin incision is made longitudinal from the calcaneocuboid joint to the cuboid–fourth metatarsal joint, near the dorsolateral boarder of the foot, biased in a dorsal direction near the top of the cuboid bone.

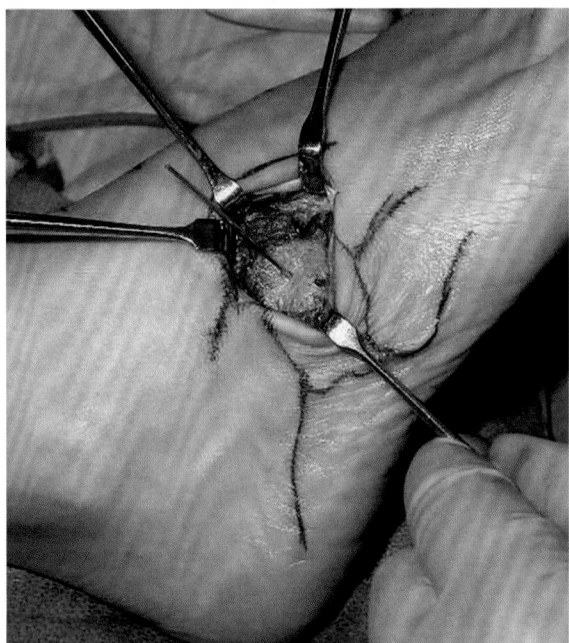

FIGURE 20.8 Lateral dissection.

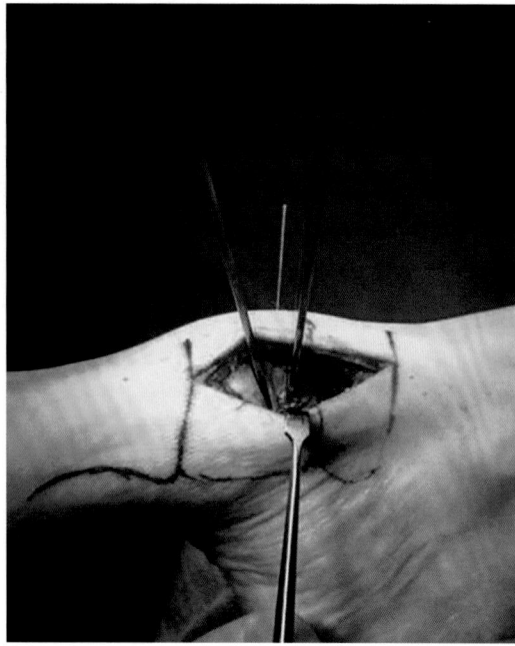

FIGURE 20.9 The medial bone cuts are performed, one proximal and one distal to the naviculocuneiform joint, aiming laterally proximal and distal to the cuboid reference Kirschner wire.

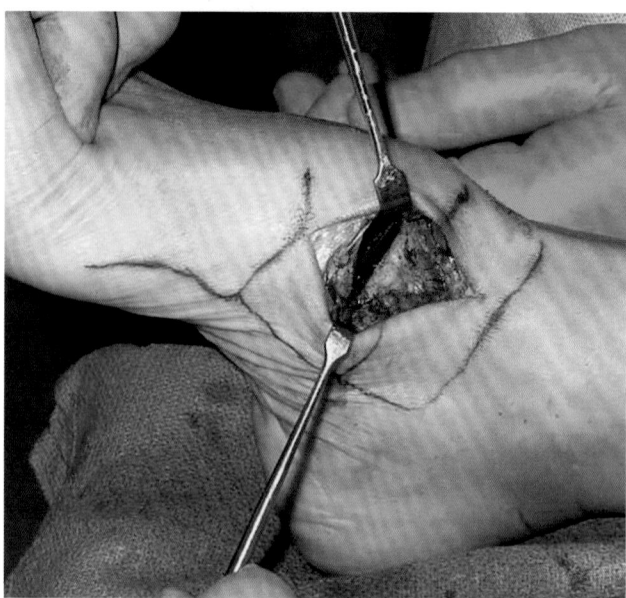

FIGURE 20.11 Additional reciprocal planing is done prior to reduction with the sagittal saw to adjust for medial and lateral correction and bone apposition.

for stable internal fixation (Fig. 20.10). Prior to reduction, additional reciprocal planing is done with the sagittal saw to adjust for medial and lateral correction and bone apposition (Fig. 20.11). Postreduction, the medial arthrodesis and lateral osteotomy sites are reduced and assessed for degree of correction (Fig. 20.12).

Staples are created using a smooth 1.1-mm K-wire, bending two right angles at the desired interaxis distance, and cutting

the arms to the desired length. The arms of the staples are abraded using the teeth of a pliers, to create a rough surface to interface with the bone, thereby securing the staple in the bone (Fig. 20.13). Staple fixation is adequate to maintain correction and allow for bone consolidation. The author fashions staples made from 1.1-mm K-wires, and uses two staples medially across the naviculocuneiform joint and one staple laterally in the cuboid bone, taking care not to enter into the adjacent joints, and confirming their location with intraoperative fluoroscopy (Figs. 20.14-20.16).

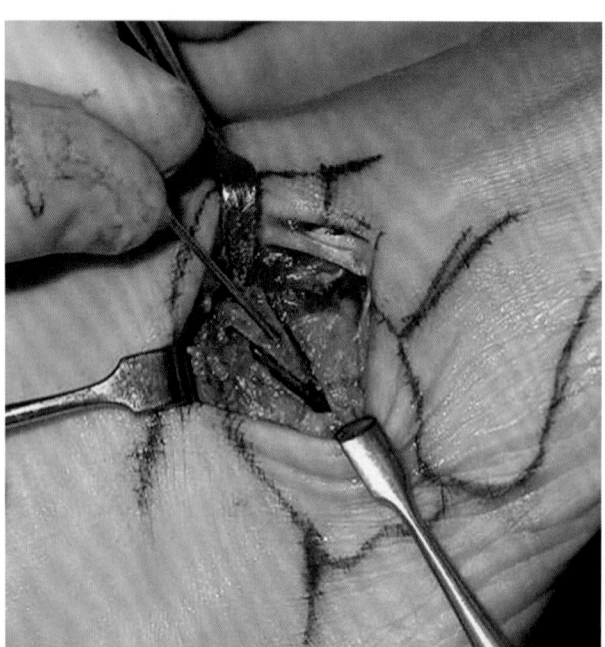

FIGURE 20.10 The lateral bone cuts are performed. A similar sized dorsal wedge is cut through the cuboid bone, with equal amounts of bone remaining on the anterior and posterior side of the osteotomy to allow for stable internal fixation.

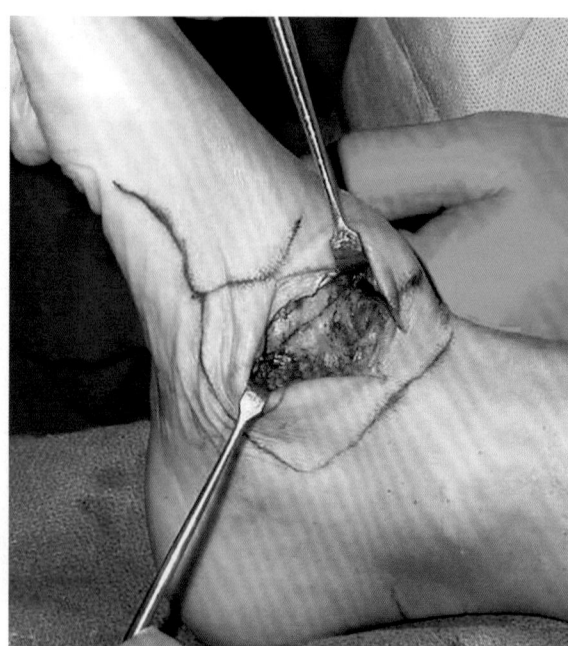

FIGURE 20.12 Postreduction, the medial arthrodesis and lateral osteotomy sites are reduced and assessed for degree of correction.

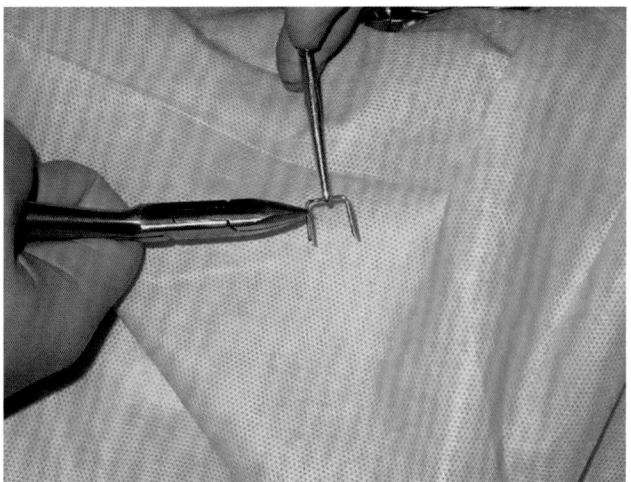

FIGURE 20.13 Staples are created using a smooth 1.1-mm K-wire, bending two right angles at the desired interaxis distance, and cutting the arms to the desired length. The arms of the staples are abraded using the teeth of a pliers, to create a rough surface to interface with the bone, thereby securing the staple in the bone. (From Kaplan JRM, Aiyer A, Cerrato RA, Jeng CL, Campbell JT. Operative Treatment of the Cavovarus Foot. *Foot Ankle Int.* 2018;39(11):1370-1382.)

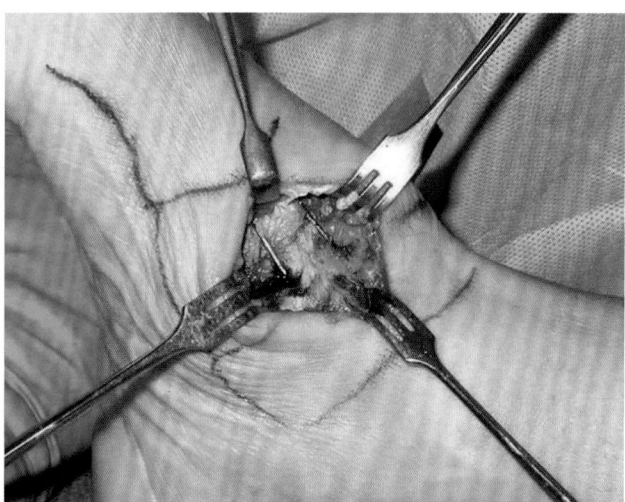

FIGURE 20.14 Staple fixation is adequate to maintain correction and allow for bone consolidation.

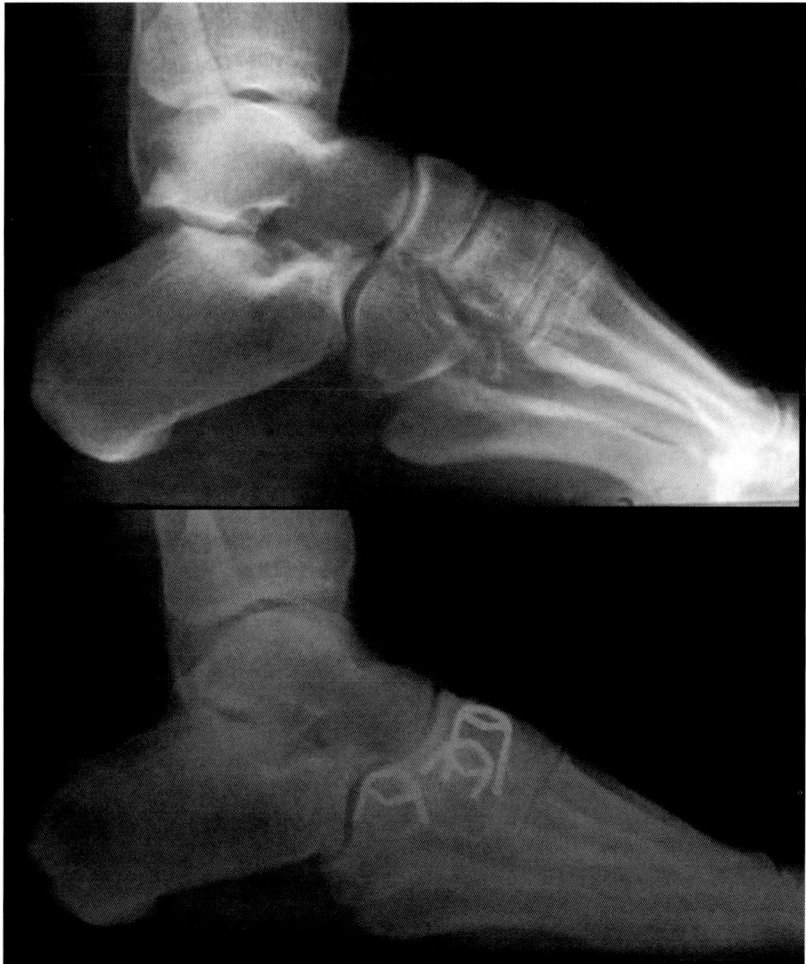

FIGURE 20.15 Lateral radiographs prior to surgery and 1 year postoperative showing correction of arch, and reduction of calcaneal inclination and talar–first metatarsal angles.

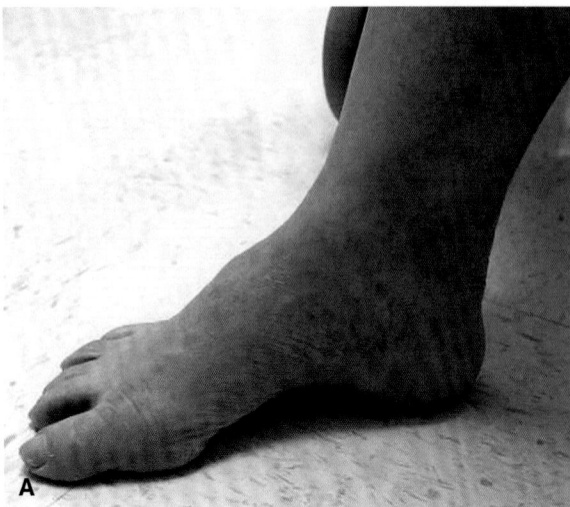
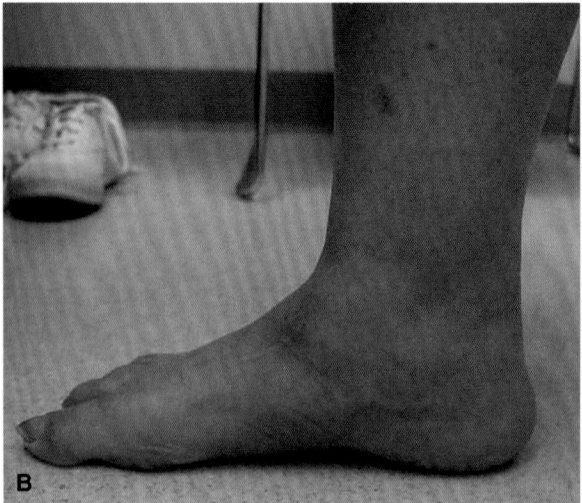

FIGURE 20.16 Preoperative **(A)** and 1-year postoperative clinical appearance **(B)** of pes cavus patient treated with a Cole osteotomy/arthrodesis. Note the resting position of the ankle before and after surgery. Prior to surgery the patient compensated for the pes cavus by stepping forward to relax tension on the tendo Achilles, and postoperative the patient stands erect with an improved alignment.

OPERATIVE AND POSTOPERATIVE MANAGEMENT

The procedure is performed under general or regional anesthesia as an outpatient. A calf tourniquet can be used for hemostasis during the procedure. If used, the tourniquet is deflated and hemostasis is achieved prior to layered closure. The patient is placed in a non–weight-bearing posterior splint or cast for 6 weeks. Radiographs are taken at the 6-week visit, and if adequate bony consolidation is achieved, the patient is then placed in a weight-bearing walker boot for an additional 3-4 weeks, followed by gradual return to regular footgear and activities. Physical therapy may be beneficial to assist with strengthening, gait training, and proprioception, particularly when tendon transfers are performed.

> ### PEARLS
>
> The incisions for a Cole osteotomy should be directed in line with the deformity and kept slightly more dorsal, so as to have access to communicate the periosteal dissection from medial to lateral. It is not necessary (and to be avoided) to dissect/ release the plantar ligaments at the osteotomy/fusion sites, as the intact plantar ligaments/periosteum act as a hinge point to allow for dorsal compression and reciprocal planning.

FRONTAL AND TRANSVERSE PLANE DEFORMITIES

Although pes cavus is defined as a sagittal plane foot deformity, frontal and transverse plane deformities are commonly associated with the high-arched foot, and require individual assessment and consideration from a surgical standpoint. Two common frontal plane deformities are encountered in patients with a pes cavus foot type; forefoot valgus, or a plantar flexed first ray (Fig. 20.17), and a varus or inverted heel. Compensation for frontal plane deformities relies on available range of motion of adjacent joints. The valgus forefoot compensates primarily in the hindfoot through the subtalar and midtarsal joints, and this leads to a varus (rigid) or inverted (flexible) heel.

Patients with frontal plane deformities are assessed with a Coleman block test prior to surgery to determine whether or not the hindfoot has the ability to pronate if the effect of the plantar flexed first ray is eliminated (Fig. 20.18). If the hindfoot is able to realign to a vertical heel position when the first ray is off-weighted, then an elevating osteotomy of the first metatarsal can be used to correct the hindfoot inversion that occurs due to the effect of the forefoot on the rearfoot. A transverse-oriented proximal dorsiflexing osteotomy of the first metatarsal (DFWO—dorsiflexing wedge osteotomy) is utilized to elevate the first metatarsal to the level of the second-fifth metatarsals[22-26] (Figs. 20.19 and 20.20).

If the heel alignment is fixed in rigid varus, then an elevating osteotomy of the first metatarsal will be insufficient to correct the varus alignment of the heel. In these instances, a valgus-realigning osteotomy of the calcaneus (Dwyer osteotomy) is used to reposition the calcaneal varus to a normal vertical alignment[27-29] (Fig. 20.21).

Various combinations of surgical procedures can be employed to address varying degrees of dominant planes of deformity in the pes cavus foot. The combination of Dwyer osteotomy and DFWO of the first metatarsal can be used to address the mild-moderate deformity that is semirigid and frontal plane dominant.[24,27] In patients with a valgus forefoot with an unstable or arthritic subtalar joint (and/or peroneal tendon pathology), a first metatarsal DFWO and subtalar joint arthrodesis can be considered[30] (Fig. 20.22). The combination of a Cole osteotomy/ arthrodesis with a first metatarsal DFWO is sufficient to treat patients with a sagittal-dominant pes cavus with mild-moderate forefoot valgus (plantar flexed first metatarsal) (Fig. 20.23).[18,20]

> ### PEARLS
>
> Complete correction of the hindfoot varus (or as we often aim to place the heel in slight valgus with the subtalar fusion) accentuates the forefoot valgus (plantar flexed first ray), requiring a more aggressive medial correction. As such, one might consider a less aggressive correction the heel valgus, and perhaps choose a subtalar joint fusion (for added stability) rather than joint-sparing osteotomies.

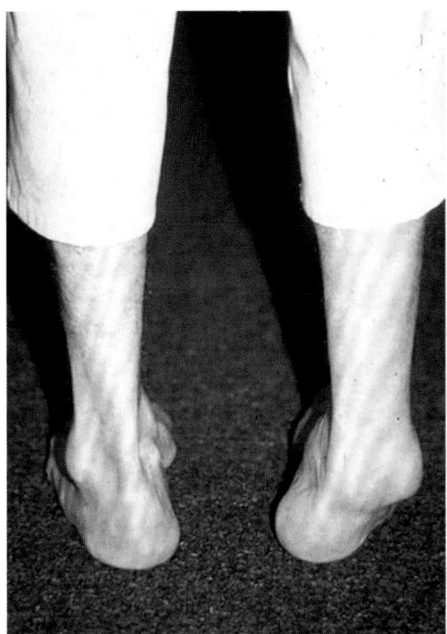 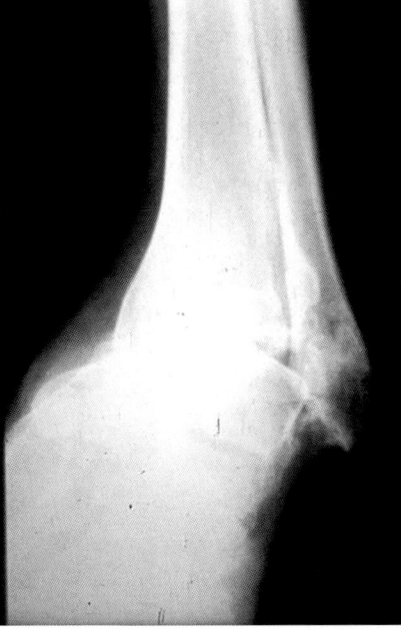 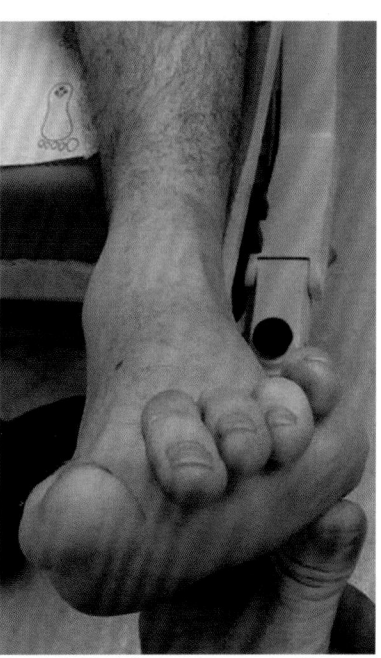

FIGURE 20.17 Rigid forefoot valgus (plantar flexed first metatarsal) increases arch height and influences hindfoot alignment by causing the heel to rotate into varus. With this foot type, compensation will occur in the hindfoot with inversion of the heel through the subtalar and midtarsal joints. If there is insufficient available range of motion in the hindfoot, compensation will occur in the ankle joint with varus subluxation of the tibiotalar articulation.

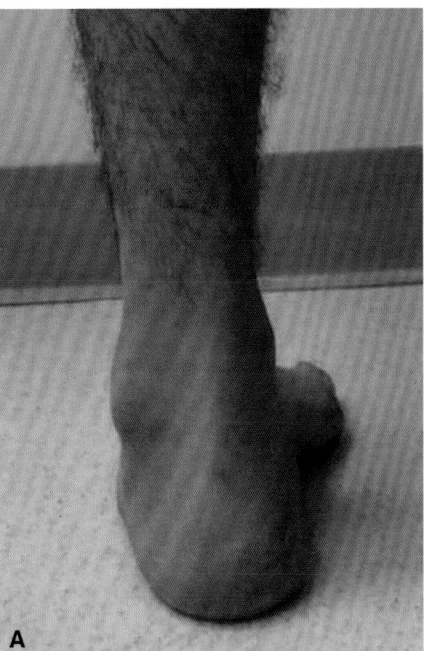 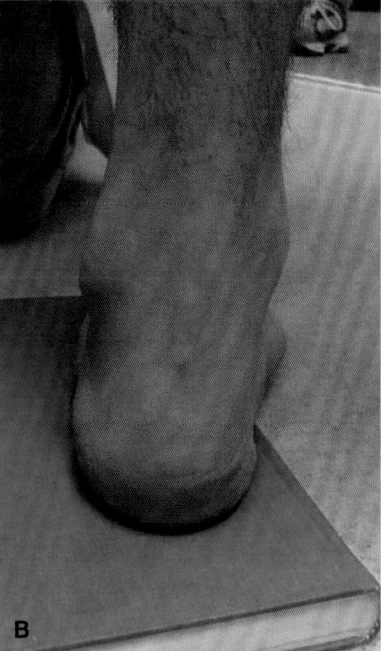

FIGURE 20.18 Coleman block test. **(A)** Posterior view of left foot with forefoot valgus (plantar flexed first metatarsal) demonstrating heel varus alignment **(B)**, and Coleman block test with the first metatarsal "floating" off the ground. This demonstrates that the rearfoot is able to realign to a vertical heel position (pronate) if the effects of the first metatarsal is reduced. This demonstrates that the varus position of the heel is secondary to the forefoot, and no heel osteotomy is necessary. This patient is a candidate for a dorsiflexing osteotomy of the first metatarsal.

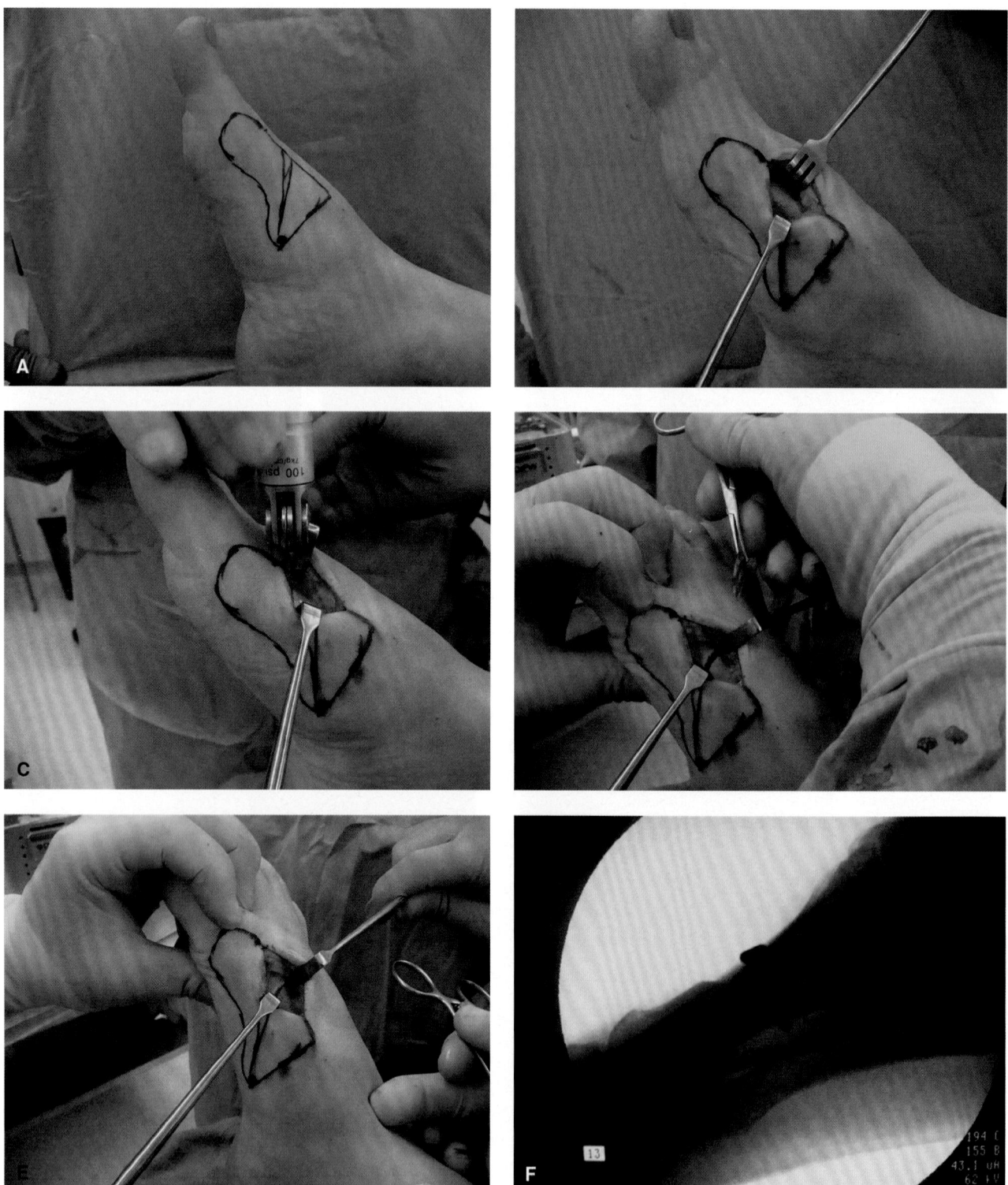

FIGURE 20.19 **A.** DFWO (dorsiflexing wedge osteotomy) of the first metatarsal. The skin incision is located dorsomedial over the proximal base of the first metatarsal, just lateral to the extensor hallucis longus tendon. Intraoperative fluoroscopy can be used to locate the base of the first metatarsal in order to avoid having the osteotomy enter into the metatarsal-cuneiform joint. A periosteal elevator is used to identify and mark the plantar metatarsal-cuneiform joint. The skin incision and osteotomy location should take into consideration avoidance of the proper dorsal digital nerve to the hallux (medial dorsal cutaneous nerve), access for osteotomy execution and wedge of bone removal, and internal fixation orientation. **B.** The dissection plane passes through the superficial fascia with care to retract the proper dorsal digital nerve to the hallux laterally. A deep fascia and periosteal incision is made longitudinally, and reflection of the periosteum is achieved to gain access to the osteotomy site as well as access for internal fixation. **C.** The osteotomy is made with a sagittal saw in an oblique orientation from dorsal-distal to plantar-proximal, converging on a point close to the base of the metatarsal-cuneiform joint.

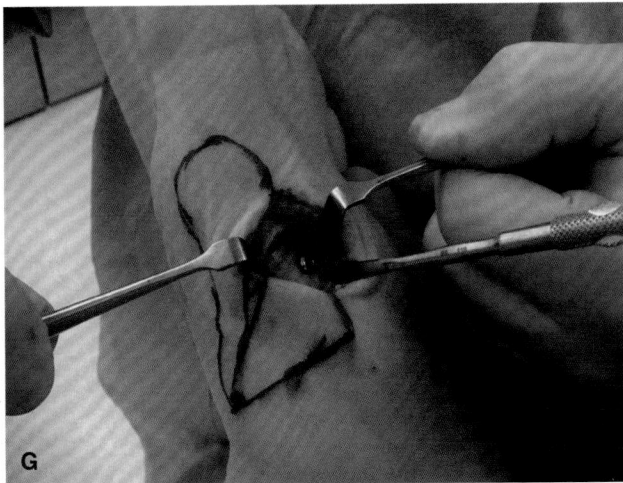

FIGURE 20.19 (*Continued*) **D.** A wedge of bone is removed, and the hinge is feathered with the saw to allow reduction of the osteotomy site. **E.** Gentle reduction is achieved manually, allowing the osteotomy to close with little tension. Additional dorsiflexion can be achieved with reciprocal planing with the saw, until the desired amount of correction is achieved. Adequate correction is obtained when the plantar aspect of the first metatarsal is realigned so that it is equal to that of the second metatarsal's weight-bearing plane. Assessment of the position of correction is done manually, and intraoperative fluoroscopy can be used to confirm the desired sagittal degree of angular correction. **F.** With the osteotomy reduced, in this case with manual compression (a bone clamp may also be employed), internal fixation is achieved with a single screw for fixation, directed dorsal-to-plantar, oblique to the osteotomy. A cortical or cancellous screw may be used for fixation, in a lag fashion, to achieve compressive stabilization of the osteotomy. Depending on the size of the bone and length of the dorsal cortical arm of the osteotomy, the chosen screw diameter can range from 2.0 to 4.0 mm. **G.** Dorsal view of screw orientation and placement. The screw should be directed from dorsal to plantar, far enough proximal to the osteotomy to avoid fracture into the osteotomy. Adequate use of the countersink will seat the screw head flush to the surface of the bone to avoid screw head prominence, and help to avoid creating a stress-riser that can fracture the dorsal cortex into the osteotomy site.

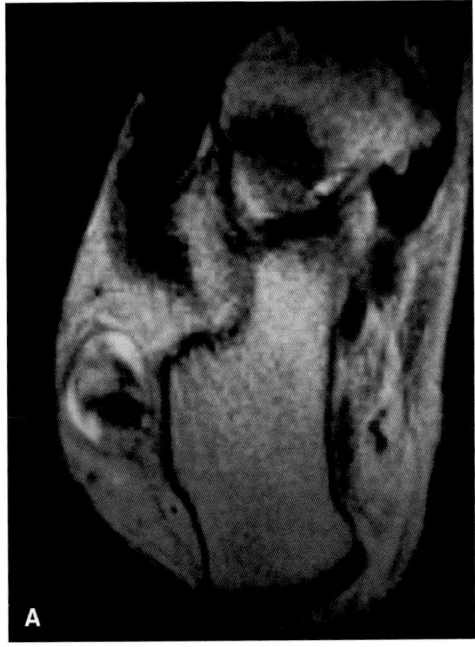

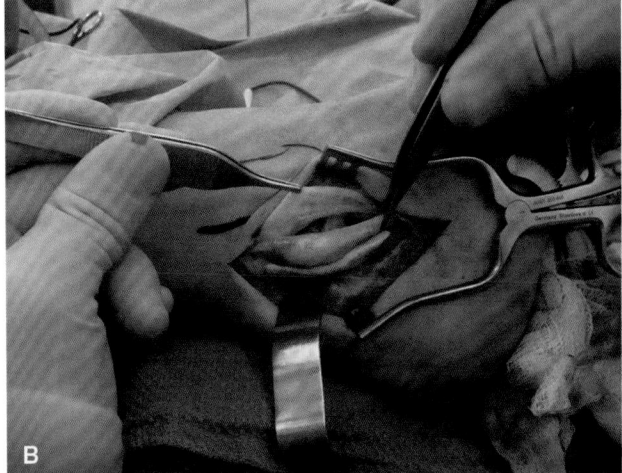

FIGURE 20.20 **A.** Dorsiflexing wedge osteotomy of the first metatarsal to correct rigid forefoot valgus (plantar flexed first metatarsal). This patient's primary complaint was peroneal tendonitis, and magnetic resonance image suggested longitudinal tears of both the peroneus longus and brevis tendons.

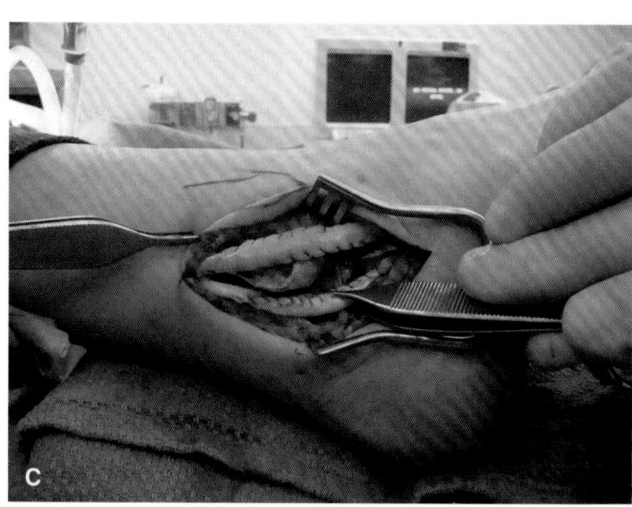

FIGURE 20.20 (*Continued*) **B, C.** The peroneal tendons were primarily repaired, and a large intratendinous calcification was débrided from within the peroneus brevis tendon (note before **B** and after **C**). A DFWO of the first metatarsal was done to realign the hindfoot in order to prevent recurrent strain on the tendons. This is the same patient shown in Figure 20.18; note the realignment of the heel to vertical postoperative, which approximates the alignment obtained with the Coleman block test of this patient prior to surgery.

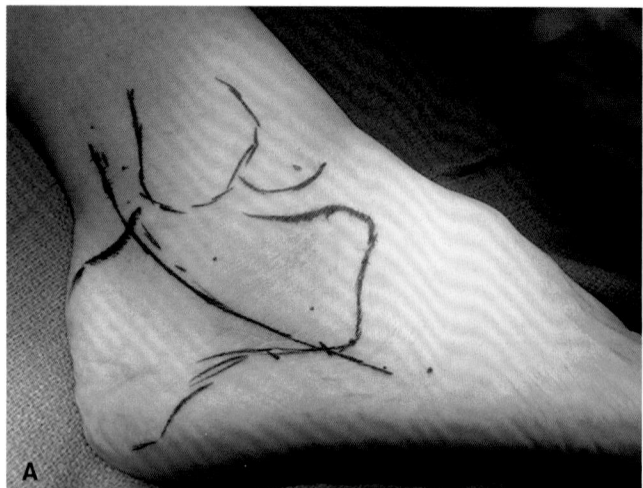

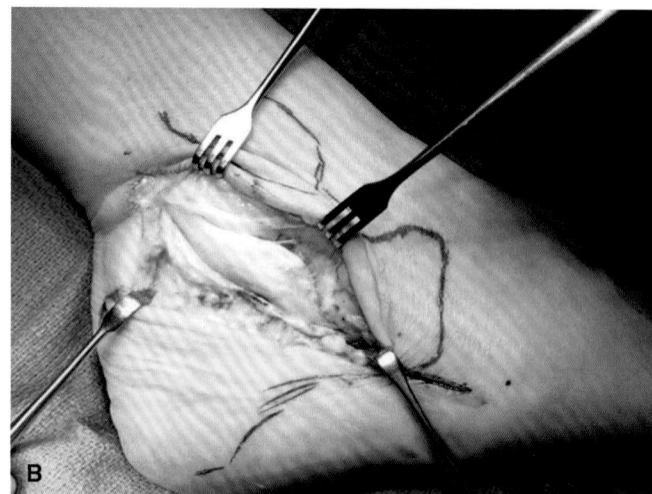

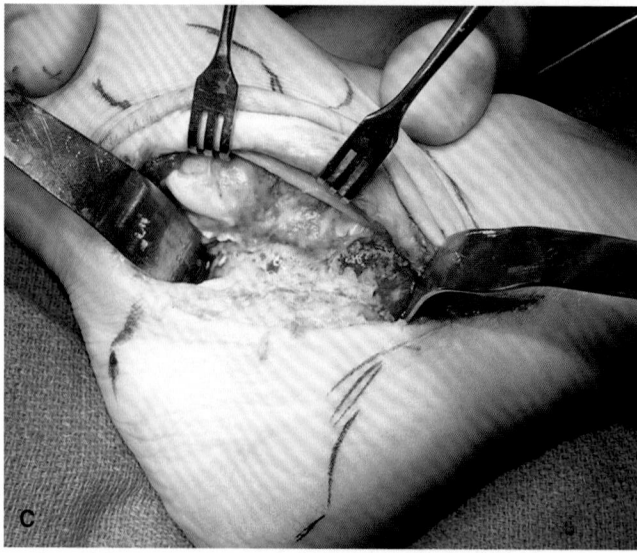

FIGURE 20.21 A. Dwyer osteotomy. A varus heel deformity is corrected by removal of a laterally based wedge of bone through the body of the calcaneus. In this case, the patient had peroneal tendon pathology as a result of the pes cavus, so the skin incision was used to both access repair of the peroneal tendons and perform a Dwyer calcaneal osteotomy. The incision should approximate the posterior course of the peroneal tendons and should be posterior to the sural nerve. **B.** Significant peroneal tendon pathology was evident. The tendons were débrided and retracted, then the osteotomy was performed, and the tendons were primarily repaired prior to closure. **C.** Periosteal reflection is performed to gain access for performing the osteotomy. The more anterior the osteotomy, the greater degree of correction can be obtained. The dorsal exit point should be 1-2 cm posterior to the subtalar joint, and the plantar exit point should be 1-2 cm proximal to the calcaneocuboid joint. Typically, a 1.0-1.5 cm lateral wedge of bone is removed, as is demonstrated below.

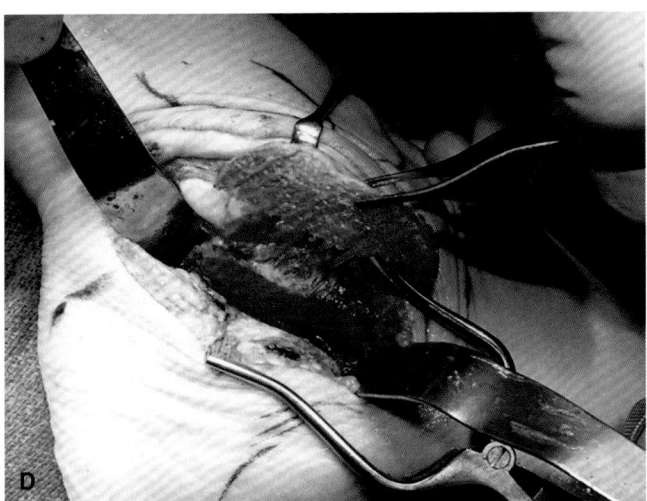
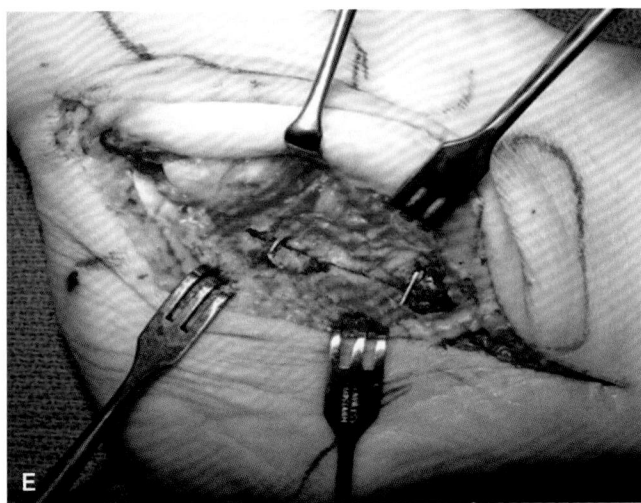

FIGURE 20.21 (*Continued*) **D.** The osteotomy is reduced and assessed for degree of correction and bony apposition, which can be adjusted by use of reciprocal planning with the saw. To aid in reducing the osteotomy, the foot is dorsiflexed on the ankle, which tensions the Achilles tendon and plantar fascia, and assists in compressing the osteotomy site. Additionally, the posterior tuber of the heel can be translated laterally to gain additional correction into the direction from varus to valgus. **E.** Staples are typically used for internal fixation of the osteotomy site. Note the improved alignment of the heel, both clinically and radiographically.

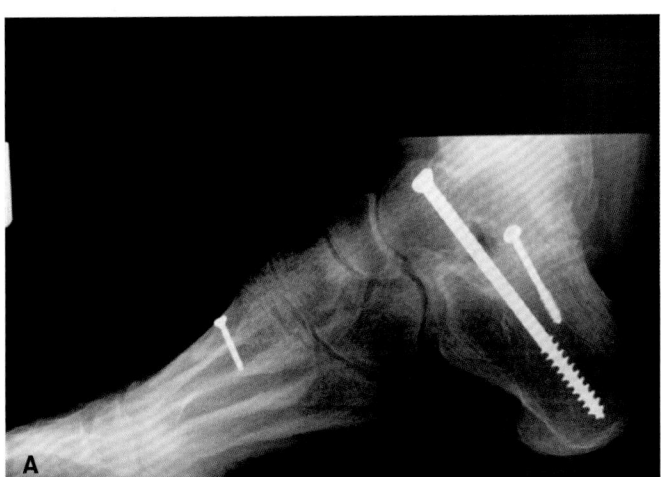
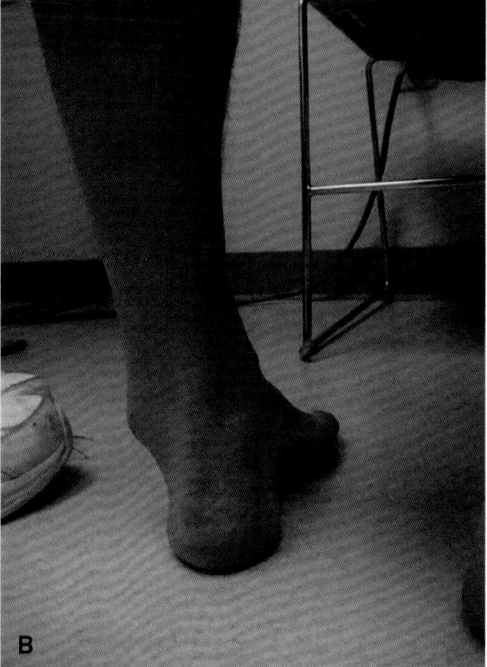

FIGURE 20.22 Subtalar joint arthrodesis and first metatarsal DFWO in a patient with an unstable subtalar joint secondary to a forefoot valgus pes cavus, and peroneal tendon pathology. The peroneal tendons were débrided and suture-repaired, and a tenosynovectomy was performed. The same incision was used to access the subtalar joint for arthrodesis. **A.** Postoperative lateral radiograph. **B.** Preoperative posterior clinical appearance of patient's left foot.

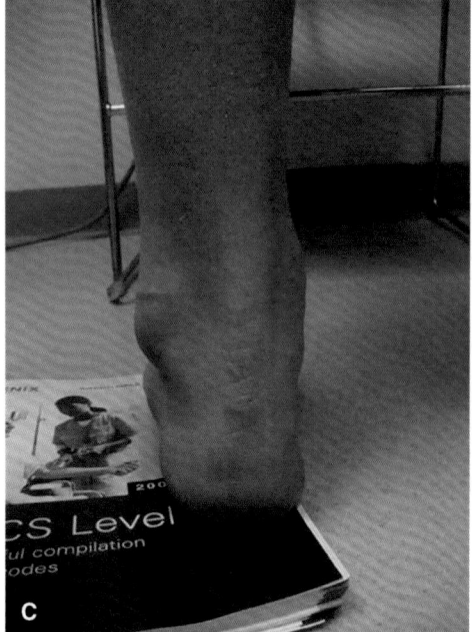

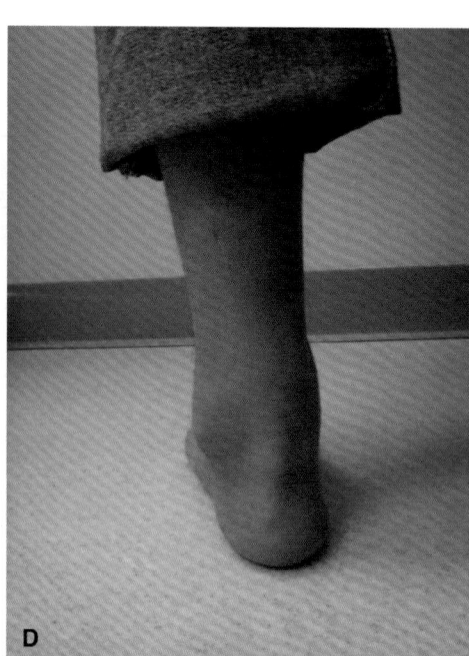

FIGURE 20.22 (*Continued*)
C. Preoperative posterior clinical appearance of patient's left foot with Coleman block test.
D. Postoperative posterior clinical appearance of patient's left foot.

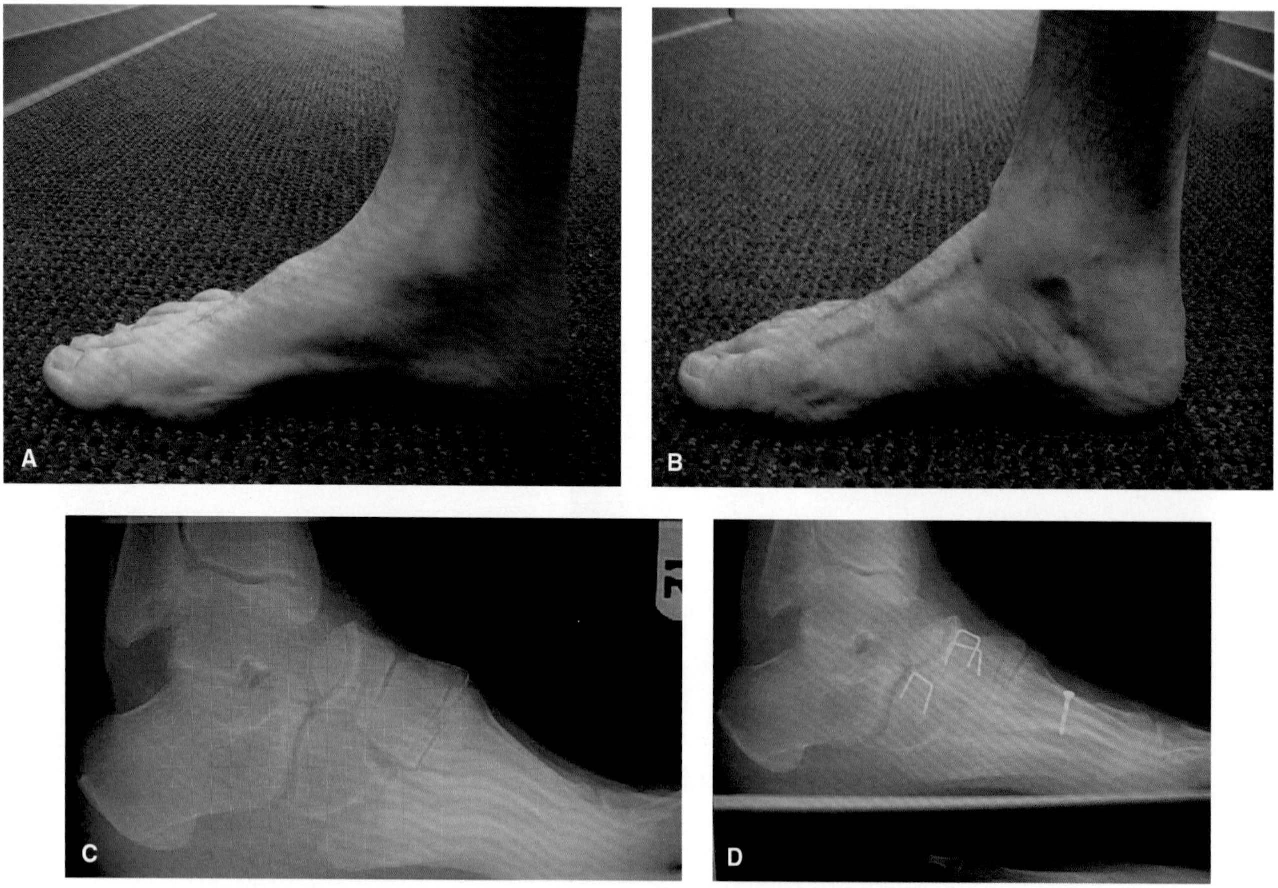

FIGURE 20.23 Cole osteotomy/arthrodesis and DFWO of the first metatarsal. Cole osteotomy/ arthrodesis to address a pes cavus deformity and a dorsiflexing wedge osteotomy of the first metatarsal to address forefoot valgus (plantar flexed first metatarsal). The Cole procedure is capable of reducing a mild-moderate degree of forefoot valgus, but in many instances, there is still a need to address the first metatarsal individually, as the peroneus longus' effect on the first ray rigidly plantar flexes the medial column. **A.** Preoperative clinical appearance. **B.** Postoperative clinical appearance. **C.** Preoperative lateral radiographs. **D.** Postoperative lateral radiographs.

SEVERE, RIGID, MULTIPLANE PES CAVUS AND ASSOCIATED DEFORMITIES

In patients with a severe deformity, rigidity, or neurologic weakness (CMT disease, post CVA, traumatic brain injury), a triple arthrodesis is required to provide deformity correction and stability to the hindfoot (Fig. 20.24). In addition to a triple arthrodesis, a first metatarsal DFWO is required in patients with residual forefoot valgus (plantar flexed first metatarsal)[23-26] (Fig. 20.25). In patients with long-standing deformity, ankle varus and degenerative arthritis occurs as a compensation for forefoot valgus malalignment. In these instances, a pan-talar arthrodesis (or ankle plus triple arthrodesis) (Fig. 20.26) may be necessary to address ankle instability and arthritis, muscular weakness, and severe multiplane deformity correction.[30]

Along with pes cavus, patients with neurologically induced muscle imbalance may demonstrate a dropfoot deformity in addition to adducto-varus foot instability, requiring a combination of bony correction (usually fusion) and muscle-tendon balancing.[28] Many of these patients benefit from a tendon transfer to assist in dorsiflexion, which also benefits the foot position if the deforming/contracted tendon is the one that is utilized to assist dorsiflexion. By this way, a deforming force can be eliminated and used to improve foot alignment and function. The most commonly utilized tendons for transfer in cavus surgery are also the most implicated in causing cavus foot deformities—tibialis posterior (Fig. 20.27) and peroneus longus tendons (Fig. 20.28). In most instances, tendon transfers are done in conjunction with bony fusion stabilization of the hindfoot, through an isolated subtalar fusion or multilevel fusion (triple arthrodesis). In lesser degree deformities where peroneus longus is at an advantage but not needing to assist with dorsiflexion, releasing peroneus longus distally and anastamosing the longus tendon to the peroneus brevis tendon eliminates its effect of plantar flexing the first metatarsal, and assists in everting the midfoot[30] (Fig. 20.29).

While pes cavus can lead to other symptoms and pathologic processes (plantar fasciitis, tarsal tunnel syndrome, metatarsalgia, ankle instability, peroneal tendon rupture, etc.), the most commonly associated condition that is addressed surgically is the extensor substitution hammer toe.[1-4] The main-

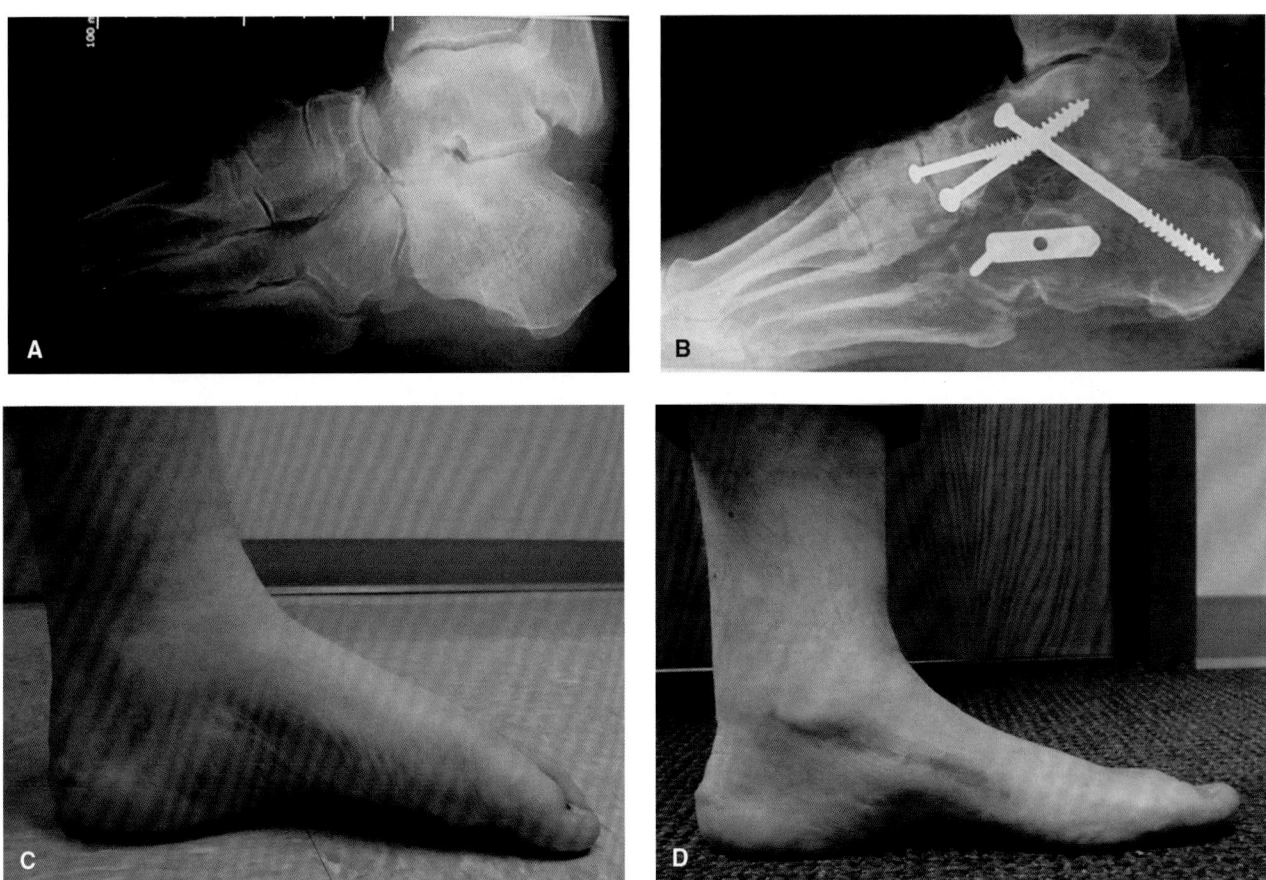

FIGURE 20.24 Triple arthrodesis is often required in treating the neurologically weak or unstable pes cavus foot. This patient also had a first metatarsophalangeal joint arthrodesis to address arthritic, spastic hallux equinus. **A.** Preoperative lateral radiograph. **B.** Postoperative lateral radiograph. **C.** Postoperative clinical appearance. **D.** Postoperative clinical appearance.

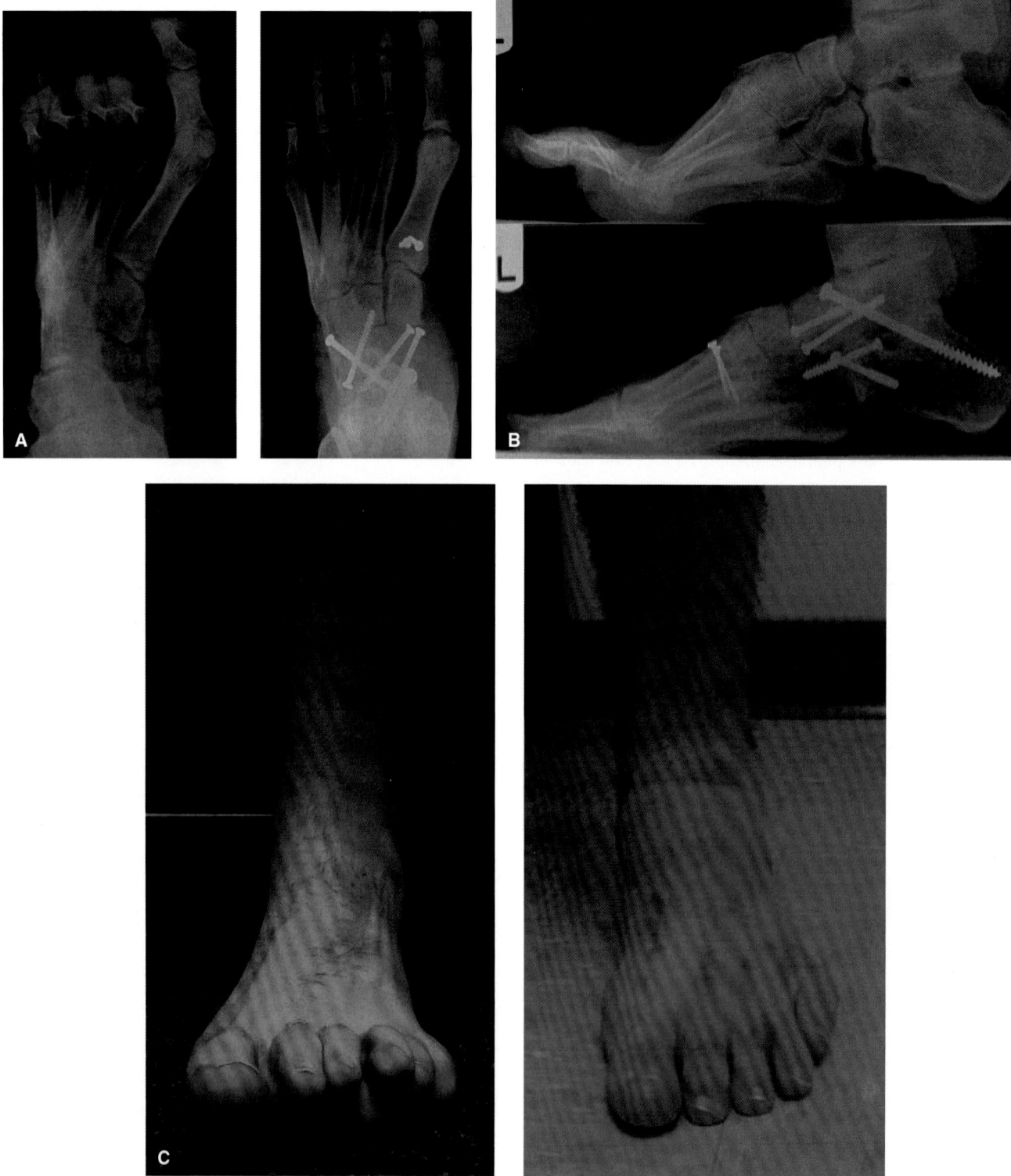

FIGURE 20.25 Triple arthrodesis plus first metatarsal DFWO. Severe pes cavus with forefoot valgus is addressed with a triple arthrodesis in addition to a first metatarsal DFWO, to address triplane structural deformities, and provide osseous stability to the foot. **A.** Pre- and postoperative AP radiograph. **B.** Pre- and postoperative lateral radiograph. **C.** Pre- and postoperative AP clinical appearance.

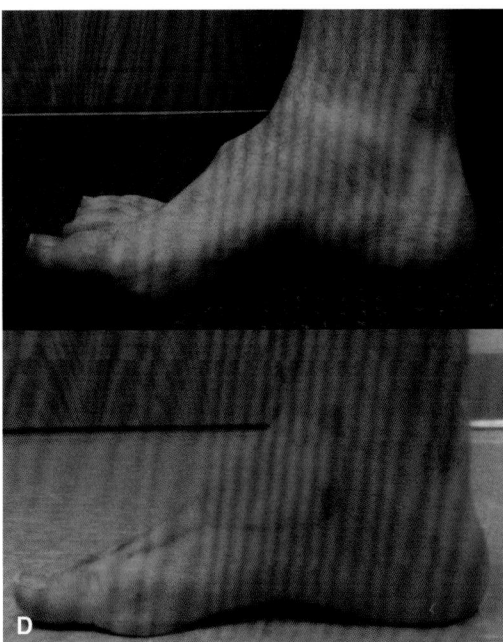

FIGURE 20.25 (*Continued*) **D.** Pre- and postoperative lateral clinical appearance.

stay procedure for addressing cavus-associated hammer toes is arthrodesis of the proximal interphalangeal joint, along with metatarsophalangeal joint capsulotomy, and extensor hood and tendon lengthening (Fig. 20.30).

PEARLS

Extensor substitution hammer toes are aggravated by cavus and equinus deformities (think of cavus as equinus within the foot).

positioning PEARLS

Most surgical procedures for the cavus foot procedures can be performed in the supine position. Operating table width extensions or applying an extra arm board to the foot end of the table can provide added space to safely externally and internally rotate the leg. Additionally, having an ipsilateral hip bump along with tilting the operating table ("lateral airplane") can assist with lateral foot exposure. Having a flat weight-bearing surface to stimulate ground contact is also important when assessing surgical fixation and foot position. Materials that can be used are instrument tray covers or sterile cutting boards.

WHAT'S NEW

A tarsal tunnel release may be necessary for cases of severe deformities requiring aggressive lateral translational calcaneal osteotomies, as these may result in subsequent tarsal tunnel syndrome and tibial nerve symptoms postoperatively. Bruce et al. performed a cadaveric study investigating medial and lateral sliding calcaneal osteotomies and found a decrease in tarsal tunnel volumes seen on MRI scan with lateral sliding osteotomies, suggesting the potential for tibial nerve compression postoperatively after lateralizing osteotomy.[31] VanValkenburg et al. in 2016 assessed patients for clinical symptoms of tarsal tunnel syndrome after a lateral calcaneal osteotomy for correction of a hindfoot varus deformity. They found an incidence of tibial nerve deficits of 33.8%, with two-thirds resolved or improved and one-third persistent at an average of 19 months of follow-up. In addition, they found a correlation between tibial nerve symptoms and location of the calcaneal osteotomy. Osteotomies through the posterior third of the calcaneal tuber had significantly lower rates of tibial nerve symptoms

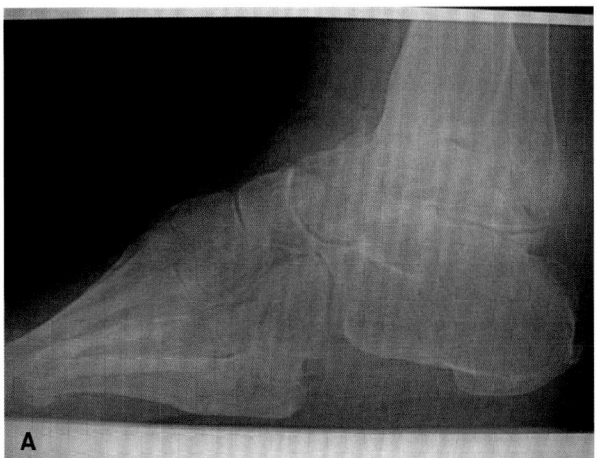
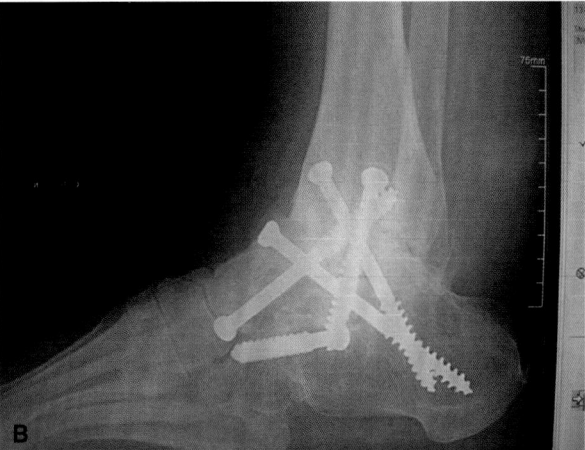

FIGURE 20.26 Ankle plus triple arthrodesis. Compensation for forefoot valgus and pes cavus can lead to degenerative arthritis of the hindfoot, and if the hindfoot has no more available range of motion to compensate for the foot deformities, the ankle joint will drift into varus and also develop degenerative arthritis and lateral ankle instability. In these cases, a pan-talar arthrodesis or ankle plus triple arthrodesis is required to correct positional concerns, muscular imbalance and weakness, as well as degenerative arthritis. **A.** Preoperative lateral radiograph. **B.** Postoperative lateral radiograph.

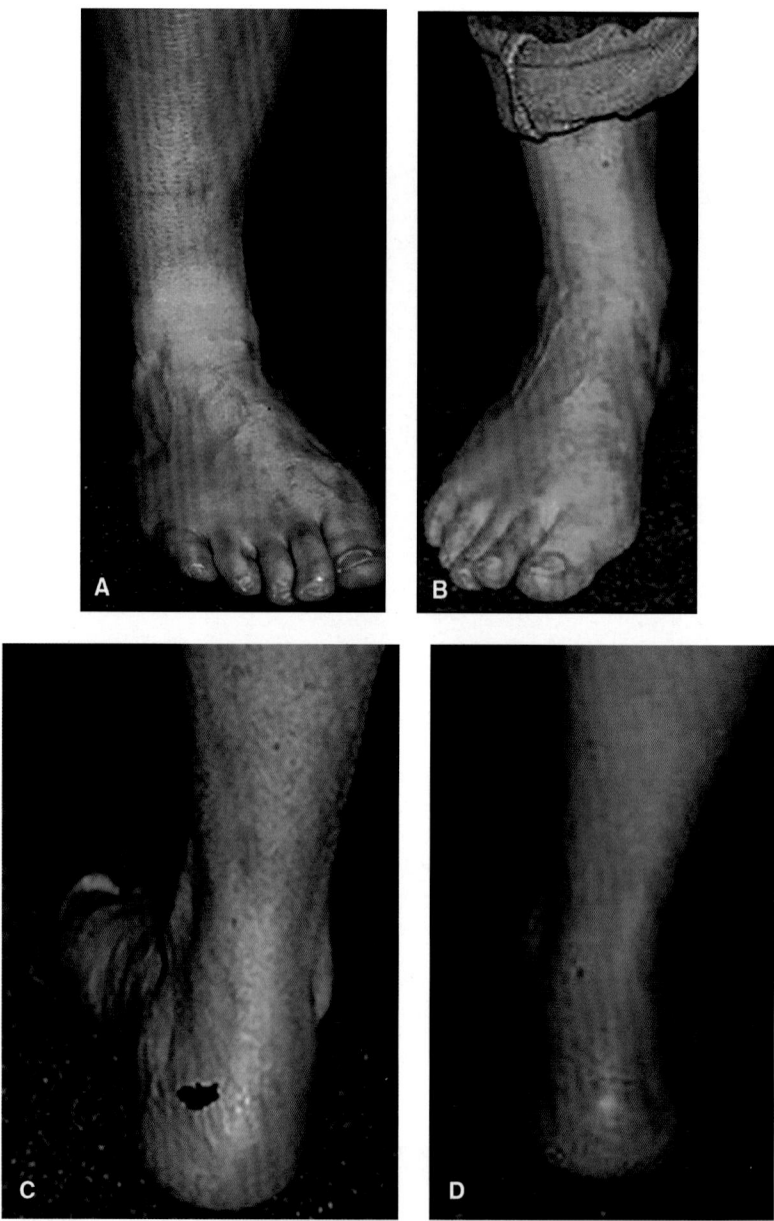

FIGURE 20.27 Patient with Charcot-Marie-Tooth disease who had a failed tibialis anterior tendon transfer, and persistent muscle imbalance and weakness and cavo-adducto-varus foot type, prior to surgery and 1 year following subtalar joint arthrodesis and tibialis posterior tendon transfer. Note the change in resting foot alignment on anterior and posterior views prior to and after surgery. **(A)** Anterior view prior to surgery. **(B)** Anterior view after surgery. **(C)** Posterior view prior to surgery. **(D)** Posterior view after surgery.

compared with osteotomies placed through the middle third of the calcaneal tuber. However, there was no significant correlation between the type of osteotomy or amount of correction and the incidence of tibial nerve symptoms. Interestingly, the authors found no significant difference in tibial nerve symptoms with or without a prophylactic tarsal tunnel release, but this could be simply due to limited patient numbers.[32] While it is believed that tarsal tunnel syndrome may occur due to a decrease in tarsal volume, alternative sources are possible, including compression of the tibial neurovascular structures on the osteotomy.[33]

It is important to recognize that the extent and severity of the cavovarus foot exists on a spectrum, and therefore the surgeon must have a comprehensive algorithm to ensure adequate correction. Pertinent concepts to consider include whether the deformity is flexible or rigid, the muscle imbalances resulting in deforming forces, and the location of the deformity.[33] Additionally, it is critical to have an understanding as to whether the deformity is forefoot driven, is hindfoot

driven, or is a combination of the two deformities.[33] Kaplan et al. have proposed the following treatment algorithm for cavus foot (Fig. 20.31).[33]

SUMMARY

Pes cavus is a sagittal plane deformity within the foot that compensates through adjacent joints' available range of motion. Symptoms can be directly related to joint strain and arthritis, but more commonly secondary to overuse conditions such as plantar fasciitis, tarsal tunnel syndrome, peroneal tendon pathology, metatarsalgia, or hammer toes.[14] Frontal plane forefoot valgus (plantar flexed first metatarsal) compensates through the hindfoot via heel inversion, which can become rigid or demonstrate adaptive bony changes within the heel bone (heel varus).[22] If the deformity exceeds the ability of the foot to compensate for frontal plane contractures, the ankle joint will become unstable and arthritic in the direction of varus.

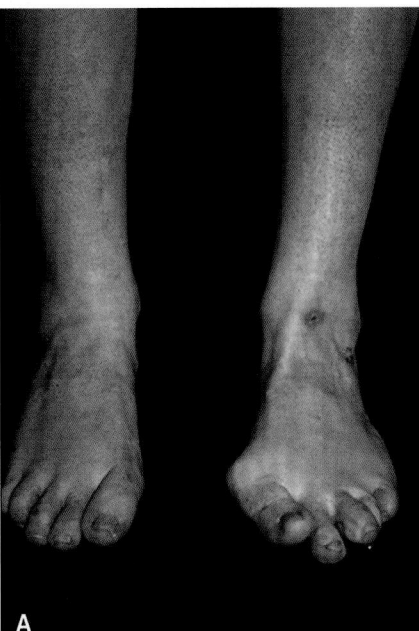
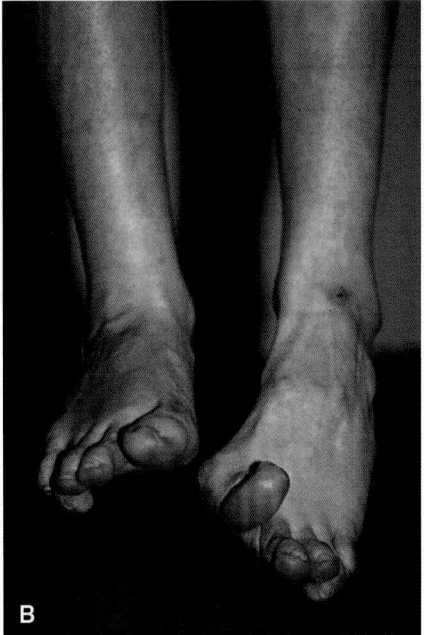

FIGURE 20.28 Peroneus longus tendon transfer. This patient underwent surgery on the right foot to address hindfoot instability and lack of dorsiflexion strength via subtalar joint arthrodesis and peroneus longus transfer to the dorsum of the foot (in addition to hallux valgus repair). **A.** Right foot standing position is improved following surgery. **B.** Right foot active dorsiflexion was achieved following tendon transfer.

Surgical correction of the pes cavus foot is individualized based on the dominant plane of deformity and degree of compensation. Hammer toes are addressed with digital PIP joint fusions and metatarsophalangeal joint/extensor tendon lengthening. A valgus forefoot is addressed by elevating the plantar flexed first metatarsal (DFWO).[26] Heel inversion or varus is assessed and characterized using the Coleman block test, and if the heel is in rigid varus, a Dwyer osteotomy can be used to realign the heel to rectus, or a subtalar joint arthrodesis can be used to treat the unstable or arthritic joint. The purely sagittal plane cavus foot deformity is treated with a Cole osteotomy/arthrodesis,[18] and a combination of procedures can be used to address individual components of the deformities that are present.[23,24] For the unstable or arthritic hindfoot with severe deformity, a triple arthrodesis is indicated. When the deformity involves the ankle, a pantalar fusion or ankle and triple arthrodesis are required to realign the foot and provide needed stability. Finally, muscle-tendon balancing for the cavus foot with a dropfoot includes isolated or combined fusions along with selective tendon transfers to weaken deforming forces and augment swing-phase dorsiflexion.[28]

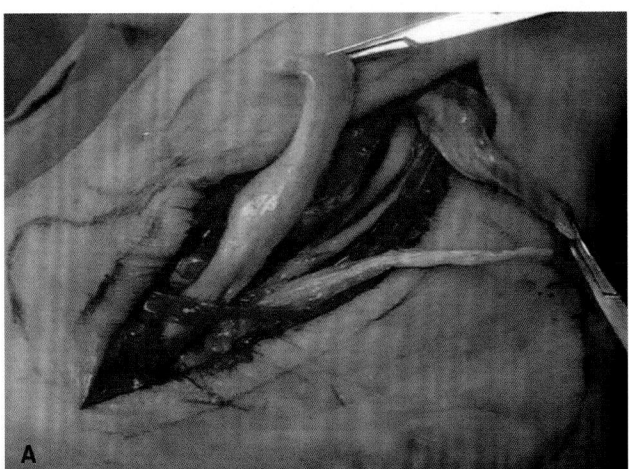
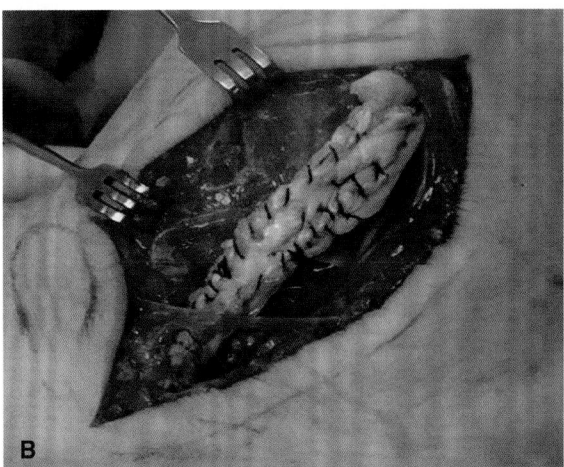

FIGURE 20.29 Peroneal tendon anastomosis. Pes cavus patients with **(A)** peroneal tendon ruptures or an overactive peroneus longus tendon (forefoot valgus) can benefit from releasing peroneus longus tendon distally and **(B)** anastomosing the longus to peroneus brevis tendon, thereby reducing its force on the first metatarsal and enhancing its pull in the direction of eversion.

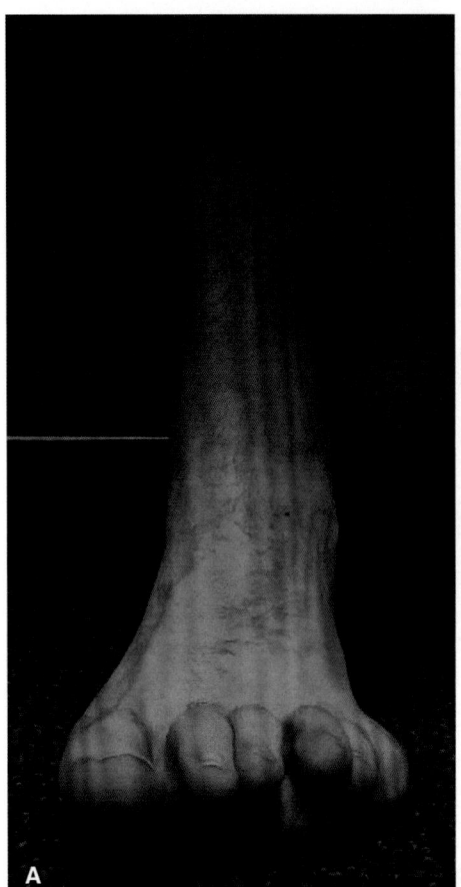
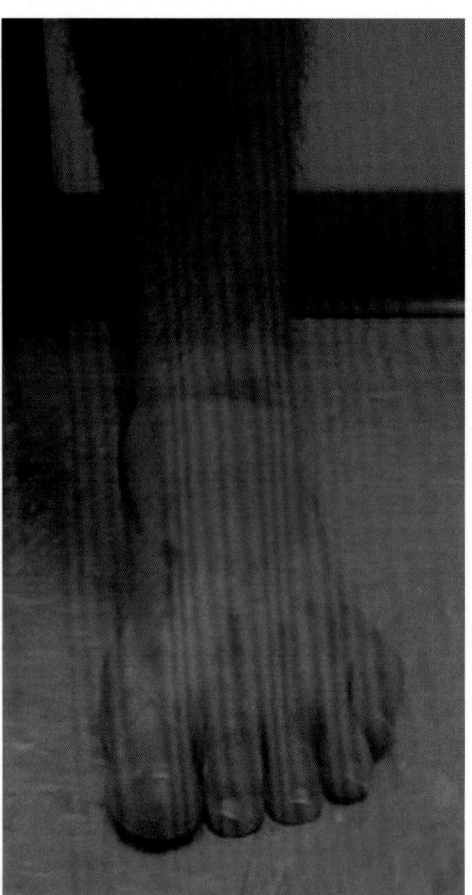
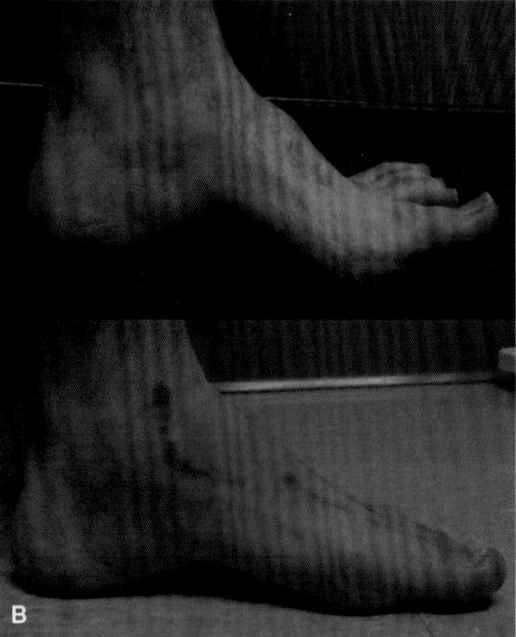

FIGURE 20.30 **A.** Extensor substitution hammer toes. The cavus foot, with a plantar flexed forefoot relative to the rearfoot, compensated for lack of swing-phase dorsiflexion by recruitment of the digital extensor tendons, which leads to swing-phase hammer toes and forefoot metatarsalgia/tylomas. Treated with a Cole osteotomy/arthrodesis and repair of the hammer toes. **B.** Proximal interphalangeal joint arthrodesis, combined with extensor tendon and metatarsophalangeal capsule lengthening, can effectively reduce the digital deformities and metatarsalgia in patients with a pes cavus deformity. Before and after photos of the same patient.

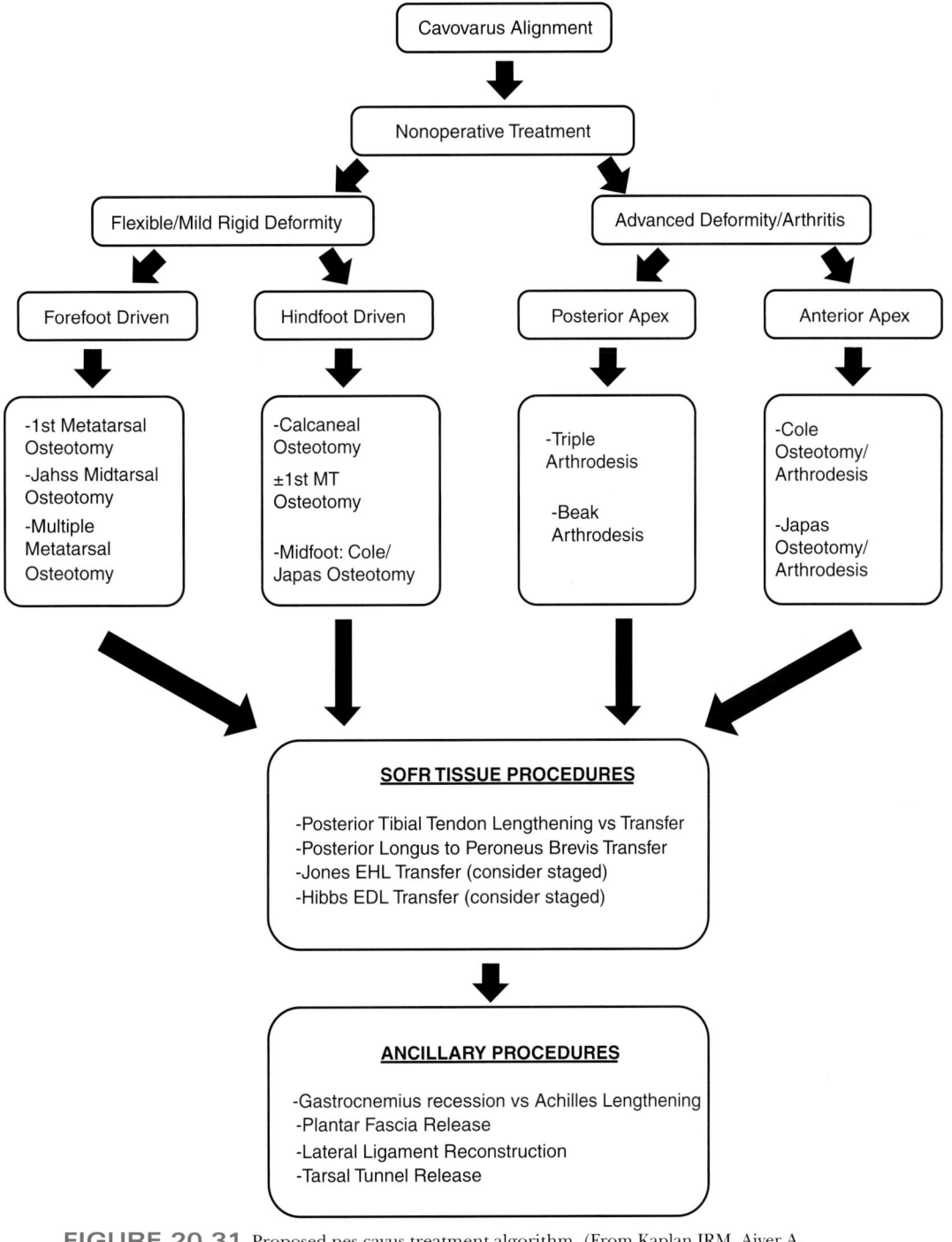

FIGURE 20.31 Proposed pes cavus treatment algorithm. (From Kaplan JRM, Aiyer A, Cerrato RA, Jeng CL, Campbell JT. Operative treatment of the cavovarus foot. *Foot Ankle Int.* 2018;39(11):1370-1382.)

The cavus foot is a challenge for the clinician, both diagnostically and surgically, but a clear and systematic approach to deformity assessment, muscle strength testing, ability to manually reduce the deformity, and balance testing will facilitate proper procedure selection and execution.

REFERENCES

1. Aminian A, Sangeorzan BJ. The anatomy of cavus foot deformity. *Foot Ankle Clin.* 2008;13:191-198.
2. Statler TK, Tullis BL. Pes cavus. *J Am Podiatr Med Assoc.* 2005;95:42-52.
3. Mosca VS. The cavus foot. *J Pediatr Orthop.* 2001;21:423-424.
4. Schuberth JM, Babu-Spencer N. The impact of the first ray in the cavovarus foot. *Clin Podiatr Med Surg.* 2009;26:385-393.
5. Alexander IJ, Johnson KA. Assessment and management of pes cavus in Charcot-Marie-tooth disease. *Clin Orthop Relat Res.* 1989;246:273-281.
6. Nagai MK, Chan G, Guille JT, Kumar SJ, Scavina M, Mackenzie WG. Prevalence of Charcot-Marie-Tooth disease in patients who have bilateral cavovarus feet. *J Pediatr Orthop.* 2006;26(4):438-443.
7. Nogueira MP, Farcetta F, Zuccon A. Cavus foot. *Foot Ankle Clin.* 2015;20(4):645-656.
8. Ortiz C, Wagner E, Keller A. Cavovarus foot reconstruction. *Foot Ankle Clin.* 2009;14(3):471-487.
9. Manoli A II, Graham B. The subtle cavus foot, "the underpronator". *Foot Ankle Int.* 2005;26(3):256-263.
10. DeVries JG, McAlister JE. Corrective osteotomies used in cavus reconstruction. *Clin Podiatr Med Surg.* 2015;32(3):375-387.

11. Kim BS. Reconstruction of cavus foot: a review. *Open Orthop J.* 2017;11:651-659.

12. LoPiccolo M, Chilvers M, Graham B, Manoli A II. Effectiveness of the cavus foot orthosis. *J Surg Orthop Adv.* 2010;19(3):166-169.

13. Deben SE, Pomeroy GC. Subtle cavus foot: diagnosis and management. *J Am Acad Orthop Surg.* 2014;22(8):512-520.

14. Gudas CJ. Mechanism and reconstruction of pes cavus. *J Foot Surg.* 1977;16:1-8.

15. McCluskey WP, Lovell WW, Cummings RJ. The cavovarus foot deformity. Etiology and management. *Clin Orthop Relat Res.* 1989;248:27-37.

16. Chilvers M, Manoli A II. The subtle cavus foot and association with ankle instability and lateral foot overload. *Foot Ankle Clin.* 2008;13:315-324.

17. Sraj SA, Saghieh S, Abdulmassih S, Abdelnoor J. Medium to long-term follow-up following correction of pes cavus deformity. *J Foot Ankle Surg.* 2008;47:527-532.

18. Ward CM, Dolan LA, Bennett DL, et al. Long-term results of reconstruction for treatment of a flexible cavovarus foot in Charcot-Marie-Tooth disease. *J Bone Joint Surg Am.* 2008;90:2631-2642.

19. Groner TW, DiDomenico LA. Midfoot osteotomies for the cavus foot. *Clin Podiatr Med Surg.* 2005;22:247-264.

20. Tullis BL, Mendicino RW, Catanzariti AR, Henne TJ. The Cole midfoot osteotomy: a retrospective review of 11 procedures in 8 patients. *J Foot Ankle Surg.* 2004;43: 160-165.

21. Wülker N, Hurschler C. Cavus foot correction in adults by dorsal closing wedge osteotomy. *Foot Ankle Int.* 2002;23:344-347.

22. Sammarco GJ, Taylor R. Combined calcaneal and metatarsal osteotomies for the treatment of cavus foot. *Foot Ankle Clin.* 2001;6:533-543.

23. Sammarco GJ, Taylor R. Cavovarus foot treated with combined calcaneus and metatarsal osteotomies. *Foot Ankle Int.* 2001;22:19-30.

24. Watanabe RS. Metatarsal osteotomy for the cavus foot. *Clin Orthop Relat Res.* 1990;252: 217-230.

25. Jolley W. Modification of midtarsal osteotomy. *J Foot Surg.* 1989;28:191-194.

26. Robinson DS, Clark B Jr, Prigoff MM. Dwyer osteotomy for treatment of calcaneal varus. *J Foot Surg.* 1988;27:541-544.

27. Samilson RL, Dillin W. Cavus, cavovarus, and calcaneocavus. An update. *Clin Orthop Relat Res.* 1983;177:125-132.

28. Suppan RJ. Repair of calcaneal varus and cavus. *J Foot Surg.* 1978;17:103-106.

29. Wang GJ, Shaffer LW. Osteotomy of the metatarsals for pes cavus. *South Med J.* 1977;70:77-79.

30. Alvik, I. Operative treatment of pes cavus. *Acta Orthop Scand.* 1953;23:137-141.

31. Bruce BG, Bariteau JT, Evangelista PE, Arcuri D, Sandusky M, DiGiovanni CW. The effect of medial and lateral calcaneal osteotomies on the tarsal tunnel. *Foot Ankle Int.* 2014;35(4):383-388.

32. VanValkenburg S, Hsu RY, Palmer DS, Blankenhorn B, Den Hartog BD, DiGiovanni CW. Neurologic deficit associated with lateralizing calcaneal osteotomy for cavovarus foot correction. *Foot Ankle Int.* 2016;37(10):1106-1112.

33. Kaplan JRM, Aiyer A, Cerrato RA, Jeng CL, Campbell JT. Operative treatment of the cavovarus foot. *Foot Ankle Int.* 2018;39(11):1370-1382.

CHAPTER 21

Flexible Valgus Surgery

Lawrence A. Ford and Francesca M. Castellucci-Garza

INTRODUCTION

The flexible pes valgus, or supple flatfoot, is a common yet challenging problem to treat. It can lead to soft tissue failure and architectural collapse (Fig. 21.1), which presents as pain and dysfunction and significant limitation in a patient's activity.

PATHOANATOMY AND BIOMECHANICS

The talus is perched on the calcaneus in such a way as to enable pronation of the triple joint complex allowing for load absorption. The large variation of potential geometric positions around the subtalar joint axis in turn is compounded by the number of positions in which the tarsal and metatarsal bones can interlock. In a foot with a medially deviated subtalar joint axis for instance, the degree of stress to the joints, ligaments, fascia, tendons, and muscles is related to the foot's ability to withstand that stress. A balanced foot is ostensibly a tripod involving the heel, first and fifth metatarsal heads. An asymmetric tripod requires strong postural muscles to overcome faulty architecture and perpetual medial column strain and lateral column impingement. In healthy patients, these postural muscles may function fine under excessive eccentric load and not necessarily lead to injury. In others, the soft tissues may fail leading to pain and dysfunction.

It is not clear what distinguishes a symptomatic pes valgus from an asymptomatic one, but several postulates have been presented. Harris and Beath in a 1948 study on young military recruits claimed that the presence of equinus was the factor that determined whether or not a flat foot was pathologic.[1] Other factors thought to influence the onset of symptoms include posterior tibial tendon insufficiency, trauma, instability, childhood and adult obesity, hypertension, collagen vascular disorders, inflammatory arthritides, neuromuscular imbalances, family history, ethnicity, genetic abnormalities, and corticosteroid injections.[2-6] Regardless of comorbidities, the underlying etiology of pes valgus deformity is the hereditary bony structure of the foot and imbalance of the supporting musculature. Similar to the reins of a horse, the foot is stabilized by the dynamic balance of muscles and tendons acting on the foot and ankle. Along with the static soft tissue structures, these impart stability in stance and gait.

In normal gait, the inverted heel contacts the ground at the beginning of the stance phase. As the lateral foot is loaded, a pronation moment is created around the triple joint complex, primarily at the level of the talonavicular joint, such that the forefoot dorsiflexes and everts around the talar head. The adaptability of the lateral column allows for shock absorption as well as flexibility while ambulating. This is facilitated by the greater mobility and independent axis of motion of the fourth and fifth tarsometatarsal joints.[7-9] The pronation is halted when the first ray makes contact with the ground, assuming the medial column is sufficiently stable. If the first ray or medial column is unstable (hypermobile, short, or elevated), then pronation can continue past the point where resupination is supposed to occur to provide a rigid lever for efficient propulsion. During this process, the posterior tibial tendon has two major roles. It lengthens as it eccentrically contracts during pronation, essentially decelerating the pronation moment arm. The posterior tibial tendon then needs to be forceful enough to shorten and contract concentrically during propulsion. In other words, it first resists overpronation and then provides a supinatory thrust during push off. Sixty percent of the physiologic cross-sectional area (PCSA) of the deep posterior group is the tibialis posterior muscle. PCSA reflects a muscle's ability to produce force.[10] In flatfeet, the tibialis posterior is less effective in raising the medial longitudinal arch because it has a decreased moment arm. More dorsal motion of the first ray is present than in a normal foot. Kinematic data of the rearfoot show flattening of the medial longitudinal arch, heel eversion, decreased stride length, and walking speed.[11] In the forefoot, there is dorsiflexion of the first ray, forefoot abduction, and limited hallux motion.[11] Chang's study of flatfeet in children found increased pressure and load on the medial foot and decreased heel contact as expected with the associated equinus.[12] EMG studies of pronated feet show decreased activity in the evertors and increased activity in the invertors, suggesting the abduction deformity is not because peroneus brevis is overpowering the posterior tibial tendon and pulling the foot into valgus. Rather, the posterior tibial tendon is even more active in order to attempt to stabilize the medial longitudinal arch.[13]

The latest research has determined that it is the talonavicular joint and not the subtalar joint that produces the majority of motion in the rearfoot. Root's theory of an oblique and longitudinal midtarsal joint axis has been questioned by researchers who have suggested that triplanar midtarsal joint motion occurs around a single triplanar helical type axis that approximates that of the talonavicular joint.[14-18] Additionally, this is supported by an earlier cadaveric simulation of selected tarsal arthrodeses that demonstrated a talonavicular arthrodesis locks up over 90% of rearfoot motion, but a subtalar joint arthrodesis only locks 50% of motion.[19]

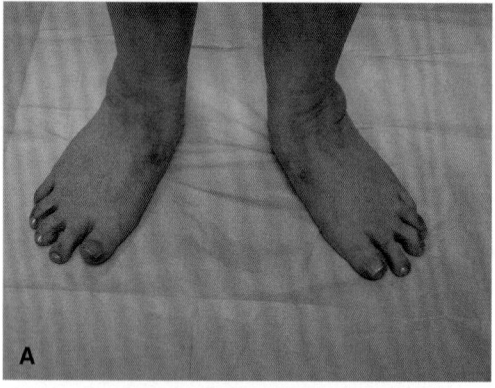

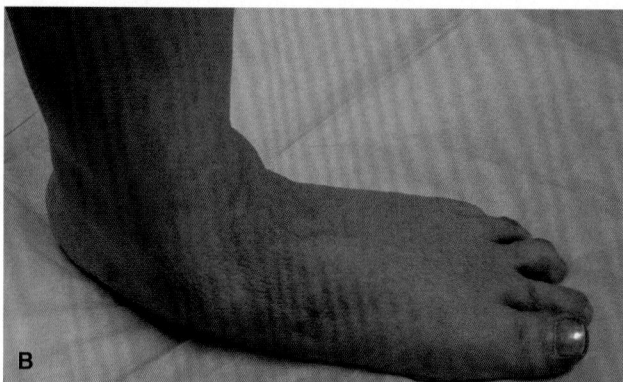

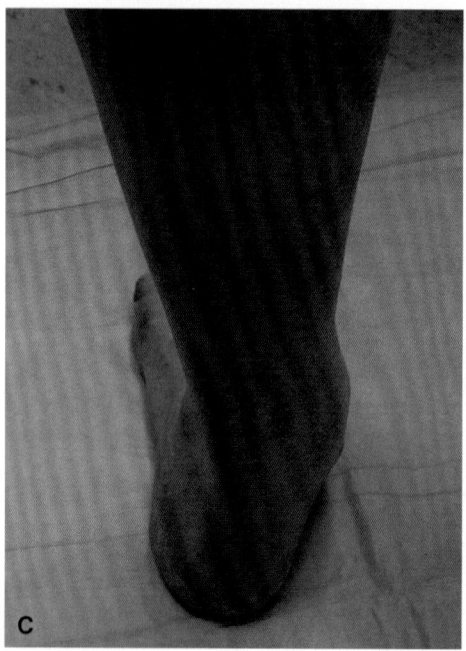

FIGURE 21.1 A-C. Symptomatic flexible pes valgus is often characterized by strain and collapse of the medial column, impingement in the sinus tarsi, medial talar head bulging, forefoot abduction, and heel eversion.

Hansen's philosophy suggests that a stable first ray is required to create a buttress to pronation and the medial deflection of body weight and to provide a propulsive lever for forward locomotion.[20] If the medial column does not provide a buttress to withstand overpronation, then the first ray will bottom out before providing any sort of leverage for push off (Fig. 21.2). In stance and gait, if the postural muscles of the foot and ankle are weak, ineffective, and cannot overcome the forces through the rearfoot and midfoot, then the retaining wall will collapse, and the medial column of the foot will strain and eventually fail.

Which structures are we talking about specifically? Adult acquired flatfoot deformity is synonymous with posterior tibial tendon dysfunction (PTTD), but it is really an incompetence of the medial soft tissue restraints. Although tibialis posterior is the main dynamic stabilizer of the rearfoot and medial longitudinal arch, it is the static structures of the arch that provide the most support.[21,22] This static support refers primarily to

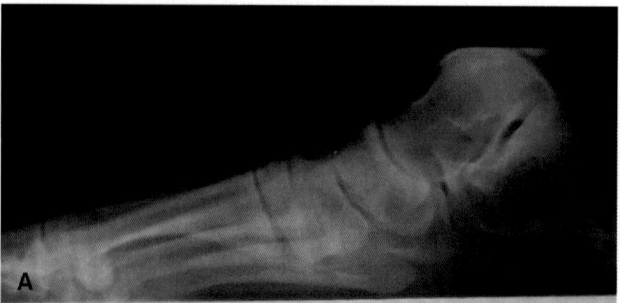

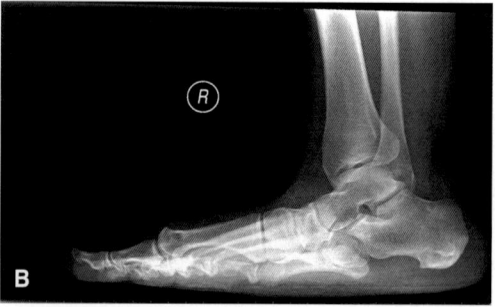

FIGURE 21.2 Instability of the first ray preventing buttressing of the medial column in midstance can be subtle **(A)** or obvious **(B)**.

the interlocking of the tarsal bones, the plantar fascia, anterior deltoid, long and short plantar ligaments, and the spring ligament. There is a threshold of strain after which tissue fails. The threshold is lower if there is an osseous architectural fault.[23] Injury is not confined to the soft tissue. The alteration of joint mechanics in the flatfoot can also have longer term deleterious consequences including arthritis and stress fractures to the fibula, navicular, and lesser metatarsals.[24]

PHYSICAL EXAMINATION

Patients with symptomatic flexible pes valgus often present with acute or chronic pain and swelling or simply arch fatigue in milder or earlier cases. Weakness is a common accompanying symptom. The pain can be located medially along the soft tissue restraints to pronation or laterally in the sinus tarsi or lateral gutter of the ankle secondary to lateral compression and impingement. As the foot is the foundation of the lower extremity, symptoms can develop proximally along the lower leg, medial compartment of the knee, hips, and lower back.

Physical examination must include the entire musculoskeletal system, not just the foot and ankle. Femoral torsion, coxa vara, genu valga, and tibial vara are important factors that can influence the position of the foot on the ground and must be considered when recommending treatment. It is important to examine both feet. Rigidity vs flexibility can distinguish arthritis and coalitions from flexible pes valgus. Manual muscle testing to assess the degree of injury to the posterior tibial tendon can help direct treatment, both conservative and surgical. The relationship of the forefoot to the rearfoot examines the integrity of the tripod and can highlight the role of the first ray in the flatfoot deformity. Every flatfoot is different due to the almost infinite number of ways the tarsal bones articulate with one another.

There are patterns of planal dominance that are apparent, particularly in the transverse and frontal planes (Fig. 21.3). Almost all flatfeet have some degree of sagittal, transverse, and frontal plane deformity. Bias toward one plane over another results in a different picture of architectural deformity, which in turn dictates a different surgical approach to restoring more normal anatomy. Heel eversion suggests more of a frontal plane component, whereas forefoot abduction suggests more transverse plane deformity. Dorsolateral peritalar subluxation is a term coined by Hansen that describes the position of the valgus foot around a plantarflexed talus.[20] Forefoot abduction is often described as the "too many toes sign" because visualization of the abducted forefoot from behind exposes more toes laterally.

Flatfoot deformity is not isolated to the triple joint complex, although deformity around the talonavicular joint is most common. Some feet collapse further distally along the medial column as demonstrated in Figure 21.4.

Johnson and Christensen simulated midstance with different degrees of equinus by increasing Achilles tension in loaded cadaveric feet.[25] Using a Polhemus 3-D radiowave tracking device, they found that increased Achilles tension resulted in bending of the medial column and flattening of the arch. The influence of equinus in pes valgus cannot be overstated. The medial column maintains a stable class II lever between the fulcrum of the forefoot and the primary input effort of the Achilles. This lever creates a bending moment through the midfoot. The ability to withstand this bending moment, or upward shear force, is critical.[26] In a subsequent study, they found that equinus dampens the effects of peroneus longus, an important stabilizer of the first ray.[27] The presence of a tight gastrocsoleal complex should be assessed upon physical examination and

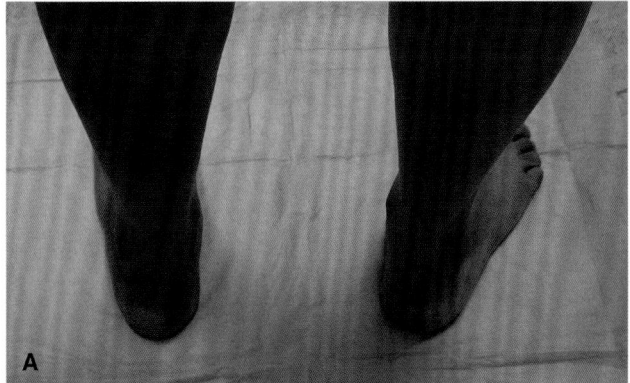
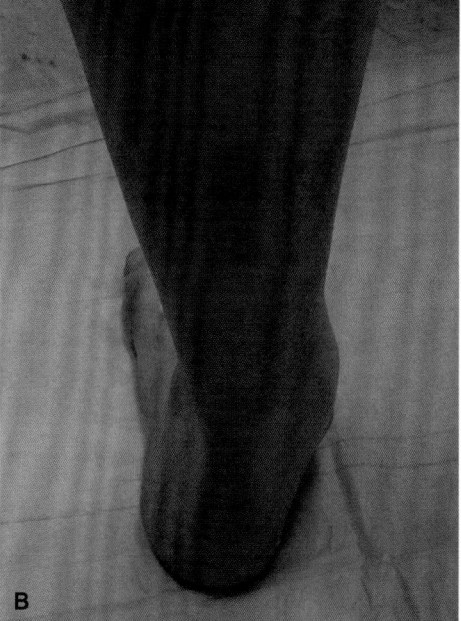

FIGURE 21.3 There are patterns of flatfeet that suggest the deformity has various influences of planal dominance. Excessive right forefoot abduction implies a predominance in the transverse plane as attested by the "too many toes sign" seen here on the right foot **(A)**, whereas heel eversion points toward more of a frontal plane contribution **(B)**.

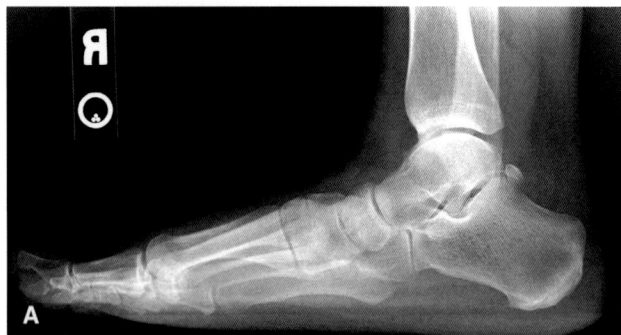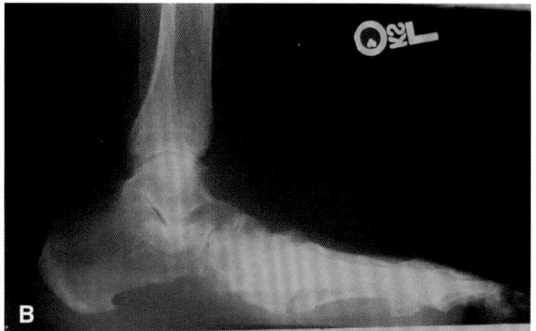

FIGURE 21.4 Collapsed pes valgus can manifest as a fault further distally in the medial column such as at the naviculocuneiform joint **(A)** and the tarsometatarsal joint **(B)**.

addressed conservatively or surgically as part of the treatment regimen. In pes valgus deformity, the majority of patients have a gastrocnemius equinus.

CLASSIFICATION

The most well-recognized staging system for PTTD is the Johnson and Strom classification with Myerson addition.[28-30] This classification system presents PTTD as a continuum of well-defined stages both clinically, pathologically, and radiographically, including proposed treatment options. Johnson and Strom defined the first three stages in 1989 with the subsequent addition of stage four by Myerson in 1997 (Table 21.1).

In stage I PTTD, the patient presents with focal pain and swelling at the medial rearfoot along the course of the posterior tibial tendon. At this stage, there is tenosynovitis; however, the length and strength of the tendon is maintained. From a clinical examination standpoint, the rearfoot alignment is normal and mobile, the patient is usually able to perform a single leg heel rise, and there is no gross biomechanical deformity. In this stage, inflammation around the tendon is present but without functional deficiencies or architectural fault.

Stage II PTTD is the stage where most controversy lies because there can exist varying levels of deformity and symptoms. The PT tendon is attenuated, torn, or ruptured, and there is a flexible, supple collapse or overpronation of the foot. Patients have difficulty performing a single heel rise. In stage II PTTD, there is disruption of the posterior tibial tendon with weakness and a clinically evident flatfoot on examination.

Stage III PTTD is a more advanced stage of tendon disruption and is highlighted by a fixed valgus position of the rearfoot as compared to stage II. Patients typically complain of lateral rearfoot pain in the setting of subfibular and sinus tarsi impingement. There are typically secondary degenerative changes in the triple joint complex. Essentially this is a semi-rigid nonreducible flatfoot with a dysfunctional PT tendon.

Distinguishing between stage II and III helps drive surgical decision-making as the former may allow for reconstruction without selected tarsal arthrodesis, whereas the latter may require it.

As described by Myerson, stage IV PTTD accounts for associated deltoid ligament disruption and medial ankle instability leading to ankle valgus. The valgus deformity at the level of the ankle joint may be either flexible or rigid in nature, with the latter being more common.

IMAGING AND DIAGNOSTIC STUDIES

RADIOGRAPHY

Weight-bearing radiographs are the first-line imaging modality for evaluation of the flatfoot. Standard radiographs are helpful to rule out concomitant structural deformities such as tarsal coalition, arthritis, previous trauma, or accessory navicular that could be contributing to the patient's pain. Standard images include weight-bearing anteroposterior (AP), lateral and oblique foot views, as well as hindfoot alignment and weight-bearing ankle AP radiographs. On the AP view of the foot, important parameters include the talocalcaneal angle, talar first metatarsal angle, talonavicular coverage, and calcaneocuboid (CC) alignment. The presence or absence of metatarsus adductus can influence treatment options. Radiographic parameters of importance on the lateral foot view include the calcaneal pitch, talar declination, Meary's angle (lateral talar first metatarsal angle), and the apex of medial column fault (Fig. 21.5). The hindfoot alignment radiograph is useful in assessing the amount of valgus deformity of the calcaneus in relation to the tibia.[31,32] It is recommended to obtain a contralateral foot radiograph for comparison purposes (Fig. 21.6). An AP view of the ankle is important for later stage PTTD if ankle valgus (stage IV) or arthritis is suspected (Fig. 21.7).

Stage	Defined by
	TABLE 21.1 PTTD Classification
I	Mild, focal medial hindfoot pain along tendon course Tenosynovitis Normal and flexible hindfoot alignment (+) single leg heel rise (−) too many toes sign
II	Increased medial hindfoot pain along tendon course Tendon elongation Valgus and flexible hindfoot alignment (+/−) single leg heel rise (+) too many toes sign
III	Medial pain +/− subfibular pain Increased tendon disruption/rupture Valgus and nonreducible hindfoot alignment (−) single leg heel rise (+) too many toes sign
IV	Stage III + ankle valgus either flexible/rigid

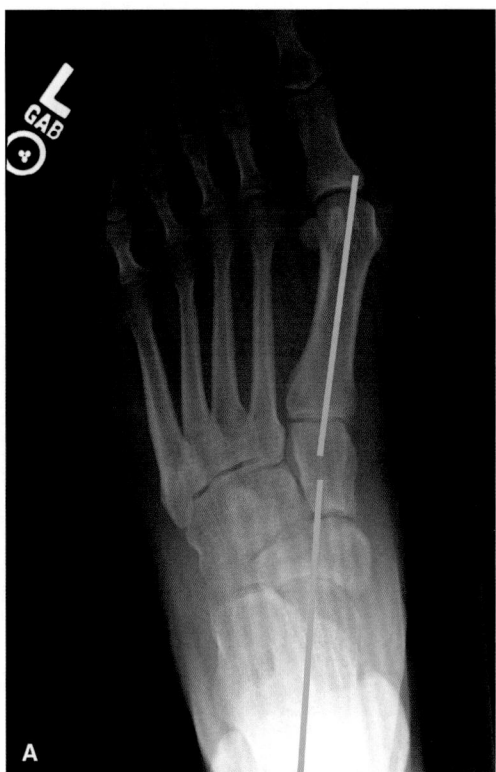

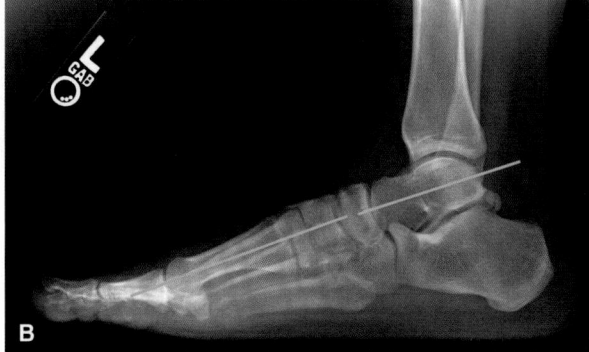

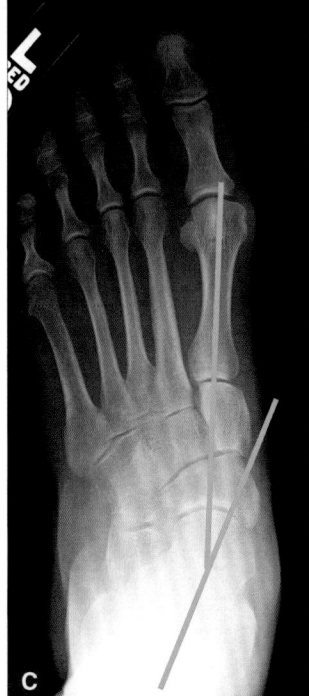

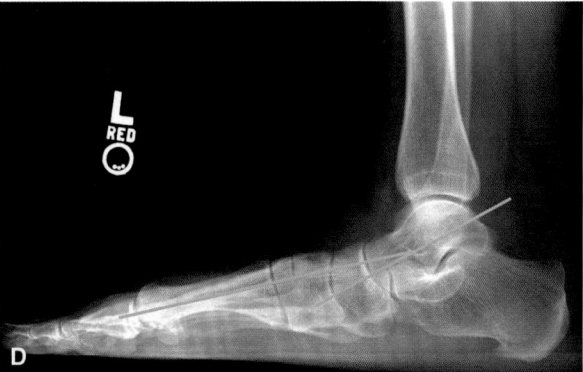

FIGURE 21.5 Important radiographic parameters to evaluate in the flatfoot deformity. Bisection of the talus is continuous with bisection of the first metatarsal on both the AP **(A)** and lateral **(B)** weight-bearing radiographs, indicating normal alignment of the rearfoot. Dorsiflexion and eversion of the foot around the talus, coined dorsolateral peritalar subluxation, are exemplified by the malalignment of the talus on both the AP **(C)** and lateral **(D)** images.

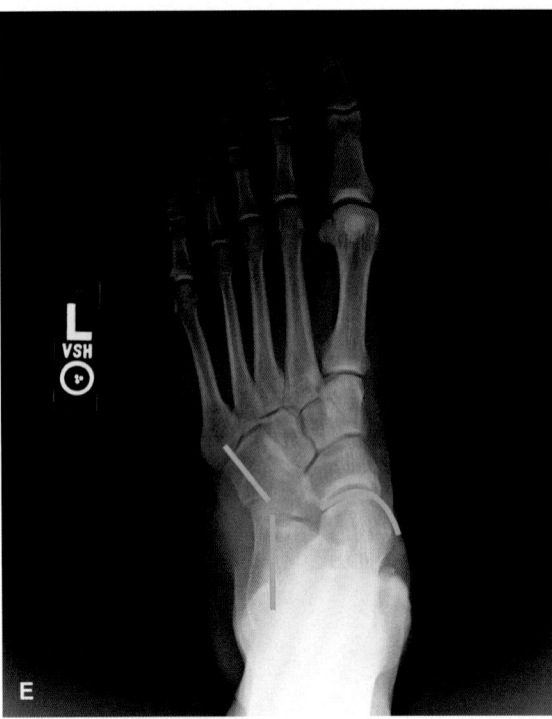

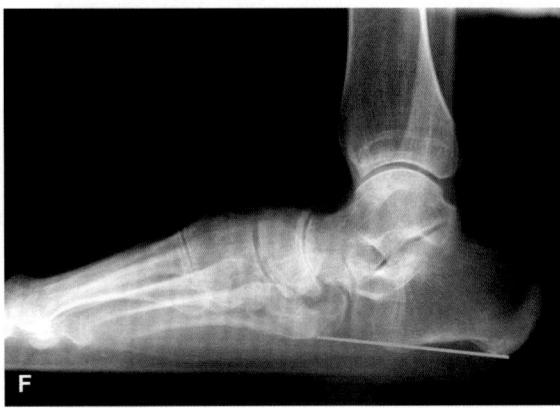

FIGURE 21.5 (*Continued*) Other radiographic parameters to evaluate the particulars of each flat foot may include increased cuboid abduction and uncovering of the talar head **(E)** and decreased calcaneal pitch **(F)**.

ADVANCED IMAGING

Advanced imaging modalities such as computed tomography (CT), magnetic resonance imaging (MRI), and ultrasound can be useful adjuncts in the diagnosis and treatment formulation for PTTD. CT scans give a more detailed evaluation of bony architecture, which can help better determine the level of arthritis in a particular joint or if there is a tarsal coalition.[33] MRI is a more powerful modality for PTTD as it allows the practitioner to evaluate the posterior tibial tendon itself, the spring ligament, deltoid ligament, and other intrinsic and extrinsic soft tissue structures in more detail.[34,35] Additionally, MRI has been used to evaluate lateral hindfoot impingement in the setting of a posterior tibial tendon tear.[36] The accuracy of MRI in the staging of PTTD has been supported by multiple studies.[35,37,38]

Ultrasound is becoming a more utilized diagnostic modality in conditions of the foot and ankle[39-41] and has been shown to have similar accuracy in comparison to MRI in the diagnosis of PTTD.[38,42] One can visualize tendon size, fluid surrounding the tendon, split tears, dynamic tendon function, and other tendon abnormalities with the use of an ultrasound in experienced hands.

However, advanced imaging is rarely indicated for flatfoot pathology unless the purpose is to rule out other causes of pain. The posterior tibial tendon is already deemed dysfunctional. The decision-making process for selecting which osseous and soft tissue procedures are indicated is based on clinical examination and standard weight-bearing radiographs rather than findings of PTTD on MRI.

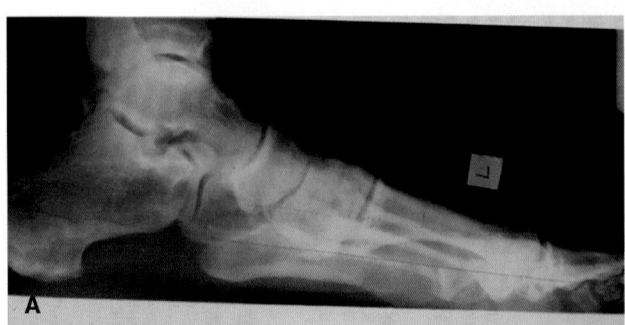

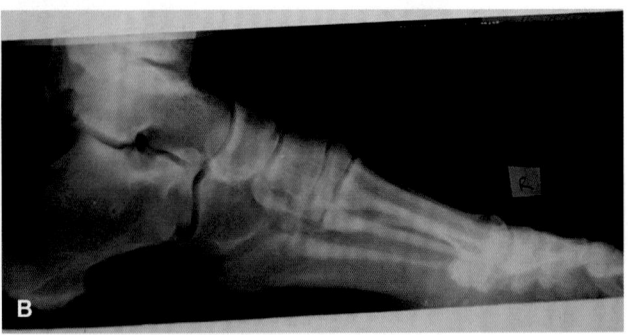

FIGURE 21.6 Contralateral weight-bearing x-rays are important to differentiate normal from pathologic anatomy. The high calcaneal inclination angle **(A, B)** is betrayed by talar equinus and NC fault seen on the symptomatic left foot **(A)**.

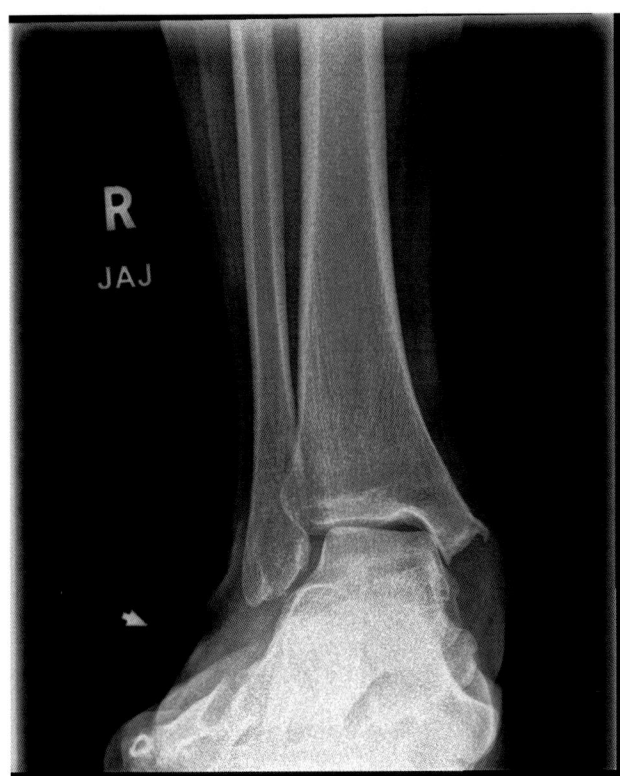

FIGURE 21.7 Ankle valgus in flatfoot deformity.

TABLE **21.2** Conservative Management	
Immobilization	Controlled ankle motion (CAM) boot Short leg cast Custom ankle foot orthoses (AFO) Over the counter ankle brace
Shoegear	1/2-1 inch heel Rigid midsole High top shoe
Orthoses	Rigid—over the counter vs custom
Medical management	NSAIDs—oral and/or topical Weight loss
Physical therapy	Stretching—gastrocsoleal complex Strengthening Proprioception

muscle group and intrinsic foot muscles should be part of a long-term ongoing treatment regimen. Conservative options are shown in Table 21.2.

OPERATIVE TREATMENT

The goal of operative treatment is essentially the same as nonoperative treatment. Realigning the foot to dampen the deleterious effects of overpronation on the osseous and soft tissue restraints is the crux of both treatments. Whether this is accomplished by externally bracing the deformity or internally fixing the faulty engineering and architecture, the concept is the same. In general, surgery is reserved for those patients who fail conservative treatment. There are many different procedures, or combination of procedures, to fix a symptomatic pes valgus. If possible, reconstructive surgery should attempt to preserve normal motion of the foot.[43]

FACTORS TO CONSIDER

In addition to shrewd analysis of the specific parameters and staging unique to the deformity, other factors are important in determining the appropriate treatment. If hallux valgus is present, then medial column work can accomplish both correction of the bunion deformity and stabilization of the first ray. If there is no hallux valgus or gross first ray malalignment, then first ray surgery may not be necessary unless it is essential for re-establishing a stable tripod. Obesity is a relative contraindication to osteotomies and reconstructive soft tissue procedures due to the higher rate of failure and recurrent collapse in this cohort. Selected tarsal arthrodeses may be preferred. Conversely, tobacco smoking increases the risk of nonunion, so osteotomies in cancellous bone are preferable to arthrodesis. Older or more sedentary patients may do better with fusions as early pain relief and stability may trump the tenet of trying to preserve normal motion. Similarly, if arthritis is present, then addressing that joint in surgery may be necessary. The ultimate goal in younger, healthier, active patients is to try to create a normal functional pain-free foot whenever possible.

SOFT TISSUE PROCEDURES

The purpose of soft tissue correction in pes valgus surgery is to address the soft tissue pathology if any, relieve a deforming force, and to assist in stability and strength. They are most

TREATMENT

The goal of treatment is to decrease pain and inflammation and increase function by providing a stable, supported foot that is able to counteract or resist the abnormal forces causing overpronation and collapse. This goal may be achieved by nonoperative and operative means.

NONOPERATIVE TREATMENT

Early conservative treatment may require a period of immobilization in a short leg cast or boot to mitigate motion of the rearfoot and stress of the injured tissue. This is in conjunction with medical management, which may include rest, ice, nonsteroidal anti-inflammatory drugs (NSAIDs), weight loss, and more. In less symptomatic patients, or in patients advancing from a cast or boot, an ankle brace or high-top shoe may be appropriate for stabilizing the ankle and rearfoot. Although the level of deformity is primarily in the rearfoot, stabilization of the ankle is important to potentiate the effects of orthotic devices and supportive shoes. Because equinus and instability of the medial longitudinal arch are important factors contributing to pes valgus deformity, shoe selection plays a critical role in nonoperative treatment. A shoe with a heel elevation requires less abnormal peritalar pronation with loading of the forefoot. A shoe with a rigid midsole helps impart stability to the medial column by providing a stable post or buttress. Rigid foot orthoses can help realign the rearfoot to forefoot relationship if used in a supportive shoe. Flat shoes without a heel, or shoes with a flexible midsole, do not provide any correction or support of the biomechanical deformity. Stretching of the gastrocsoleal complex and physical therapy to strengthen the deep posterior effective around a structurally stable platform. Soft tissue procedures alone have a high rate of failure and are inadequate in correcting pes valgus deformity. They are appropriate if there is isolated tendon pathology in an otherwise structurally stable foot such as in stage I PTTD, but this is a rare presentation. An isolated synovectomy for inflammatory tenosynovitis in a stable foot may be all that is indicated. A symptomatic accessory navicular in a well aligned foot is an example where an isolated Kidner procedure, or advancement of the posterior tibial tendon with excision of the accessory bone, could be indicated. Soft tissue procedures are also appropriate to support or balance the osseous procedures of a reconstructed foot.

Gastrocnemius recession or tendo Achilles lengthening is almost a rule rather than an exception in flatfoot reconstruction. In 1935, Morton acknowledged the deleterious effects of equinus concluding that "shortness of the calf muscles is a primary causative factor... and acts upon the medial longitudinal arch."[44] Subotnick was the first in the literature to advocate for gastrocnemius lengthening in nonspastic equinus because "equinus is the greatest symptom producer in the human foot."[45]

The spring ligament complex, made up of two to three distinct bands, is the primary restraint to talonavicular subluxation (Fig. 21.8). When the spring ligament complex was sectioned, in a cadaveric model, the posterior tibial tendon lost its ability as a dynamic stabilizer of the medial longitudinal arch.[46] An MRI study showed that the spring ligament complex is the most frequently affected ligament in PTTD.[47] Additionally, in the laboratory, an effective flatfoot model cannot be created without sectioning of the spring ligament.[47] Accordingly, its importance in the development of flatfoot deformity led to its perceived importance in flatfoot reconstruction.

Is repair of a torn spring ligament necessary for a successful surgical outcome? Perhaps not if a talonavicular arthrodesis is performed, but in the case of reconstruction without essential joint fusions, it may be necessary in order to provide support for the talar head. As the spring ligament lies inferior and lateral to the posterior tibial tendon at the level of the talonavicular joint, visualization is easy when exposing the posterior tibial tendon for repair or transfer. The spring ligament may be attenuated, torn, or ruptured. Reconstruction can take the form of direct primary repair or indirect repair by resecting redundant tissue (Fig. 21.9).

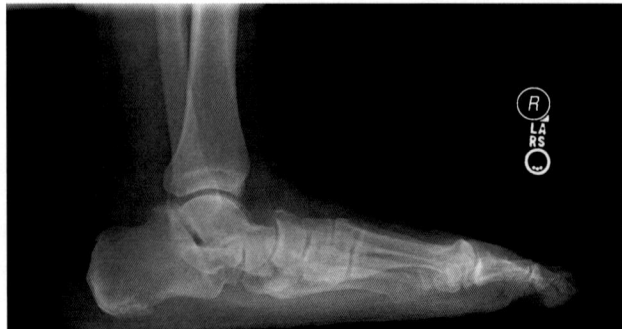

FIGURE 21.8 In contrast to a decrease in Meary's angle, true subluxation of the talonavicular joint may suggest rupture of the spring ligament or more severe deformity.

Technique for Spring Ligament Repair

- Incision is parallel and centered over the posterior tibial tendon insertion on the navicular tuberosity.
- Expose the PT tendon near its insertion by longitudinally incising the PT tendon sheath.
- Retract the PT tendon plantarly to expose the spring ligament.
- Note any tears or attenuation in the spring ligament.
- Repair torn or ruptured spring ligament with 2-0 nonabsorbable suture.
- If attenuated, perform an imbrication by sectioning the spring ligament in the frontal plane and plicating the overlapping tissue with 2-0 nonabsorbable suture with the foot and ankle in neutral position.

For many years, transfer of the flexor digitorum longus (FDL) has been advocated as an adjunctive procedure for those with stage II PTTD. An ideal tendon transfer can shift a deforming force to an advantageous one. The FDL can relieve the deforming force on the lesser toes from flexor stabilization and be used instead to assist the weakened posterior tibial tendon. It is preferable to the flexor hallucis longus (FHL) tendon as it easier to harvest immediately deep to the posterior tibial tendon and its sacrifice is less detrimental to push off in gait. FDL transfer is rarely used as an isolated procedure. Intermediate to long-term follow-up of patients with stage II PTTD who underwent FDL transfer in conjunction with medializing calcaneal osteotomy or lateral column lengthening have shown good to excellent results with high patient satisfaction rates, as well as low complication and re-operation rates.[48-53] Conversely, isolated tendon procedures on patients who do not have sufficient subtalar or transverse tarsal motion will likely fail.[54]

Because the FDL release and transfer are anatomically proximal to the master knot Henry, the lesser toes are still functional via the FHL and do not require tenodesis to the stump. As with all tendon transfers, debridement of the paratenon facilitates tenodesis. The tendon can be transferred to the PT tendon under physiologic tension in a side-to-side manner, weaved through an aperture in the PT tendon, or directly into the navicular with tendon to bone fixation.

Technique for FDL Transfer

- Similar incisional approach to spring ligament repair.
- Expose the PT tendon near its insertion by longitudinally incising the PT tendon sheath.
- Evaluate the PT tendon and sheath.
- The FDL tendon lies deep to the PT tendon sheath; it can be palpated by simultaneously moving the lesser toes.
- Incise the plantar lateral PT tendon sheath to expose the FDL tendon.
- After identifying the FDL tendon, sharply transect it as far distally as possible, proximal to the master knot of Henry.
- Debride the FDL tendon of its paratenon.
- Under physiologic tension with the foot and ankle at neutral, suture the FDL tendon to the PT tendon using 2-0 nonabsorbable suture in a side-to-side manner or weaved through an aperture in the PT tendon.
- Alternatively, the FDL can be inserted into the navicular tuberosity using a tenodesis screw or other fixation device.

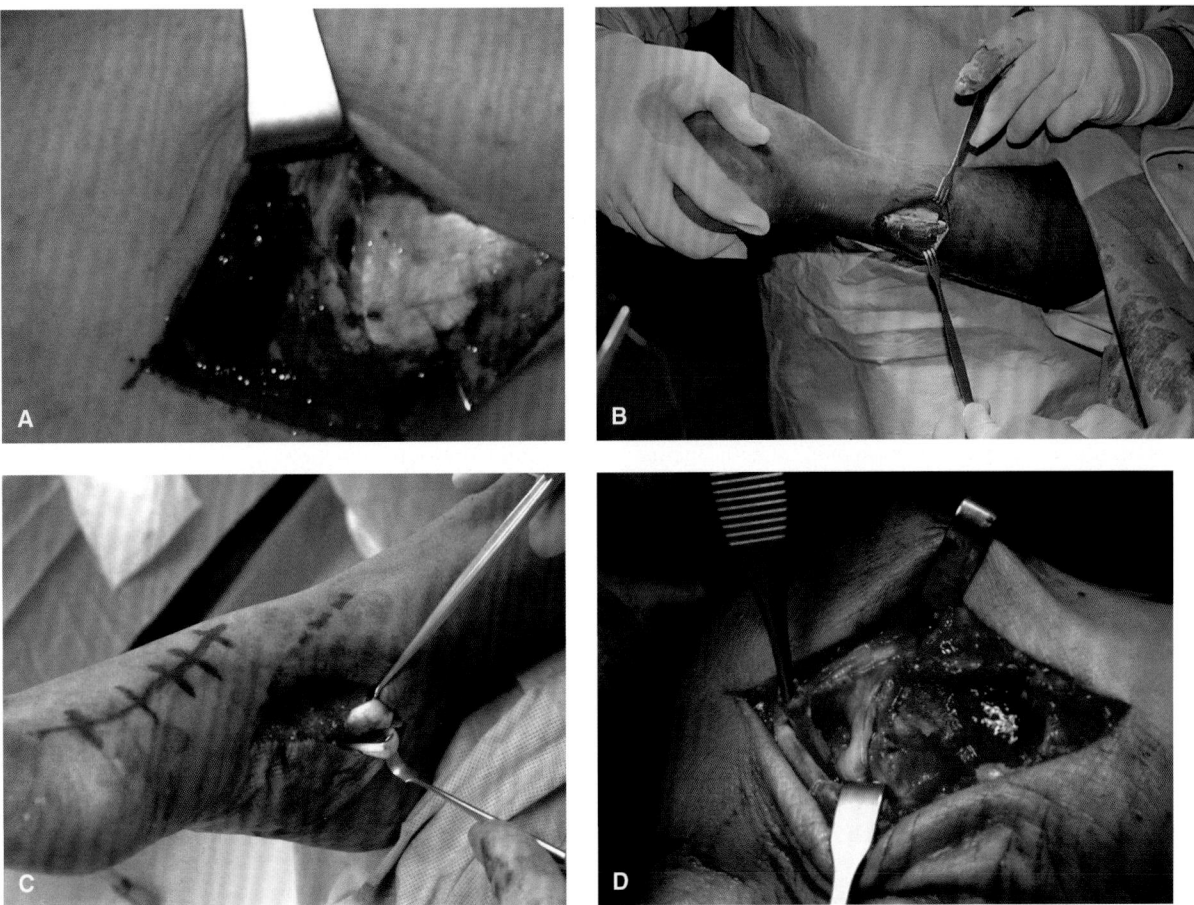

FIGURE 21.9 Tendon and soft tissue balancing are adjunctive procedures that are effective ancillary procedures around a reconstructed neutral platform. Lengthening of the triceps surae via a gastrocnemius **(A)** or gastrocsoleal **(B)** recession is usually necessary to address the underlying deforming force from the equinus. Transfer of the flexor digitorum longus to the posterior tibial tendon **(C)** and repair of the spring ligament **(D)** address the soft tissue injuries associated with pathologic flexible pes valgus.

PERILS and PITFALLS

SPRING LIGAMENT RECONSTRUCTION
- Should be used for flexible deformities
- Can be used to augment calcaneal osteotomies; rarely used alone

FLEXOR DIGITORUM LONGUS TENDON TRANSFER
- Harvest FDL as far distal as possible and just proximal to the master knot of Henry

OSSEOUS PROCEDURES

Although fusion of the rearfoot in the form of a talonavicular, subtalar, or triple arthrodesis can realign the foot and alleviate symptoms, the sacrifice of essential joint motion does not allow for a return to normal function. Triple arthrodesis and talonavicular arthrodesis can reliably correct deformity and maintain correction over time, but at a cost to normal foot mechanics. Further, adjacent joint arthrosis has been shown to develop over time following these procedures.[55-59] Because of the known complications and difficult rehabilitation, Graves and colleagues believe that rearfoot arthrodesis should be reserved for salvage operations in older adults with a fixed painful deformity.[60]

If the goal is to preserve as much normal foot function as possible, then it is preferable to realign the foot with realignment osteotomies and/or nonessential joint fusions. Hansen[20] considered the ankle, subtalar, talonavicular, lateral tarsometatarsal, and metatarsophalangeal joints as essential to mobility and function and suggested avoiding fusion of these joints if possible. Those joints with little inherent range of motion that offer stability more than functional mobility are considered nonessential joints since fusion of these joints does not adversely affect foot function. Examples are the naviculocuneiform, medial tarsometatarsal, intercuneiform, calcaneocuboid (CC), and interphalangeal joints. The flat joints in the midfoot are integral to stability of the roman arch and if collapsed may require stabilization via fusion. The subtalar and first metatarsophalangeal joints are inherent components of normal foot mechanics, but fusion does not necessarily prohibit full activities.

When considering reconstruction of the osseous architecture to realign the foot, the authors prefer to start in the rearfoot and finish in the forefoot. The object is to realign the triple joint complex such that the heel is close to perpendicular in stance and to create a stable medial column platform. Radiographically, this would equate to bisection of the talus through the first metatarsal head on both the AP and lateral projections, essentially correcting the dorsolateral peritalar subluxation associated with most flatfeet.

LATERAL COLUMN LENGTHENING

Lateral column lengthening is the most powerful procedure in flexible pes valgus surgery (Fig. 21.10). It corrects the deformity in all three planes by raising the medial longitudinal arch, adducting the forefoot, and inverting the heel.

Our understanding of how this happens is limited, but it is thought to be a result of tightening and tension of the plantar soft tissue structures acting as a tie-bar resisting dorsiflexion of the forefoot on the rearfoot. It may have more of an influence on stabilizing the medial column than other rearfoot corrective procedures as peroneus longus gains tension and an improved mechanical advantage on the first ray.

The lateral column can be lengthened as an Evans osteotomy in the distal calcaneus (Fig. 21.11) or as a CC distraction arthrodesis. Historically, the Evans osteotomy was preserved for children and the distraction arthrodesis for adults because there was concern that increased contact pressures in the CC joint after an Evans osteotomy led to painful arthrosis of that joint. Alternatively, the concern with bone block arthrodesis was a high rate of nonunion. The cause of the lateral column pain is poorly understood. One theory posed by DiNucci in 2004 suggested that it was tearing of the

long plantar ligament due to excessive graft size or aggressive dissection and destabilization of the CC joint.[61] He concluded that graft size in adults should be limited to 6 mm. Children can accommodate larger graft sizes as their soft tissues contain more elasticity to withstand increased strain of the long plantar ligament. Lateral column lengthening is no longer restricted to children as outcomes in adults have been favorable.[62,63] Distraction arthrodesis is essentially reserved for CC joint arthritis or as part of a triple arthrodesis in correcting severe deformity as results are more favorable for lateral column lengthening over CC distraction arthrodesis in stage II PTTD.[64]

Overcorrection of the flatfoot with lateral column lengthening is possible and must be avoided. Relative indications are a flexible flatfoot with medial talar head bulging, heel eversion, forefoot abduction, and a flat calcaneal pitch on radiographs. If the calcaneal pitch is not flat, then lengthening can cause subluxation of the CC joint as the forefoot plantarflexes on the rearfoot. Subluxation can be mitigated by pinning the CC joint during lengthening, but this has less chance of success if the calcaneal pitch is already relatively high. The presence of metatarsus adductus can make lateral column lengthening a contraindication or at least a more challenging proposition to avoid postoperative in-toeing. The typical parameters that are used to evaluate alignment of the rearfoot are not as reliable in a metatarsus adductus foot. Because pronation of the rearfoot is one way to compensate for metatarsus adductus, a properly corrected rearfoot may unmask metatarsus adductus. Relative overcorrection of

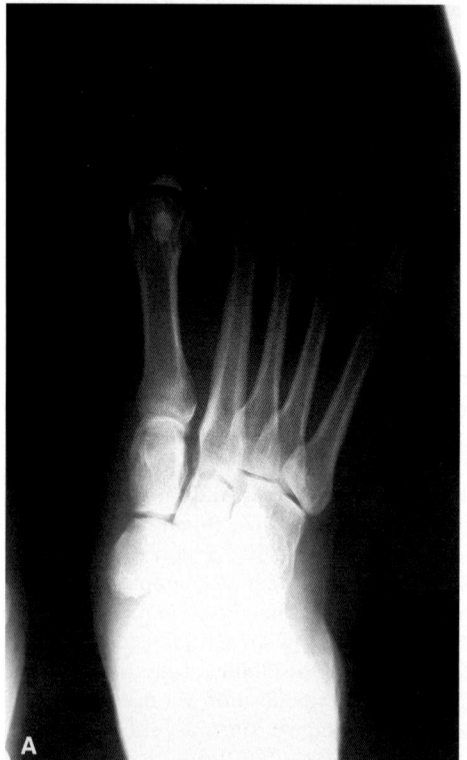
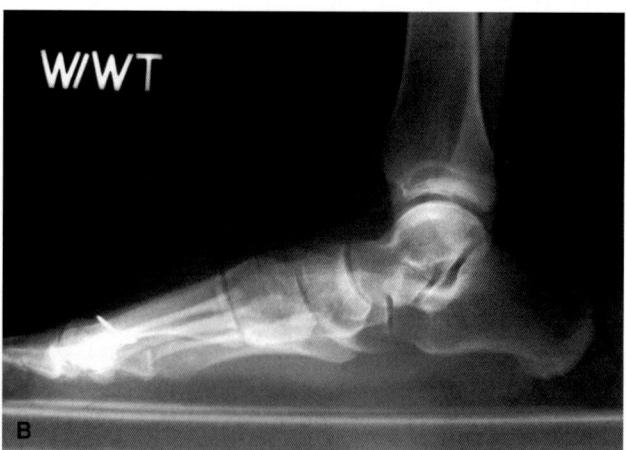

FIGURE 21.10 Lateral column lengthening is a powerful means of correcting flexible pes valgus deformity in all three cardinal planes. Preoperative AP and lateral images **(A, B)** are shown in comparison to the patients postoperative images **(C, D)**. Relative indications for the procedure are forefoot abduction or minimal met adductus, heel eversion, and a low calcaneal pitch.

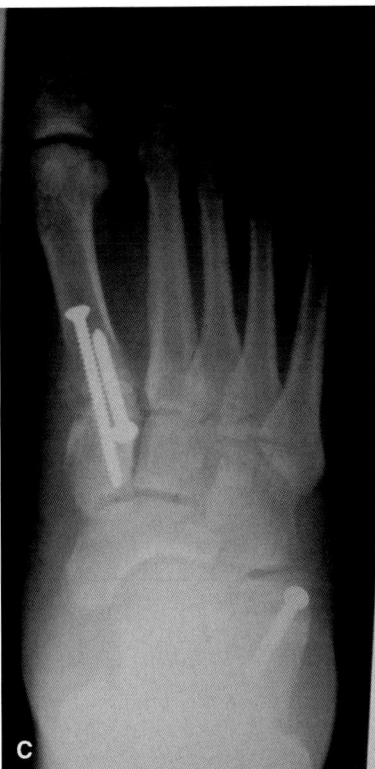
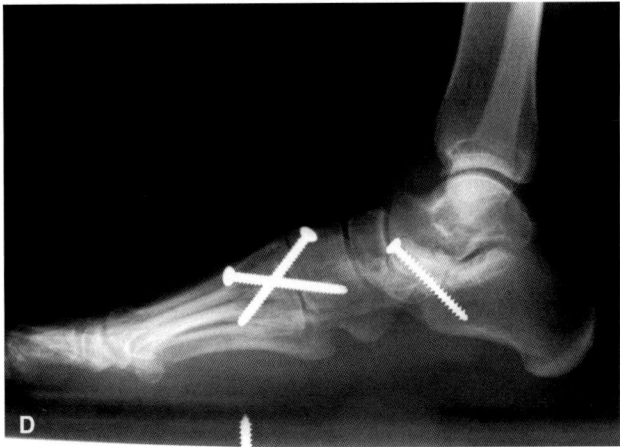

FIGURE 21.10 (*Continued*)

the rearfoot can be subtle and go unnoticed intraoperatively. The rearfoot position may be perfect, but in the presence of metatarsus adductus, it may result in overload of the lateral column and subsequent pain.

Technique for Evans Osteotomy/Lateral Column Lengthening

- Identify the sinus tarsi and location of the CC joint.
- Make a 3-4 cm longitudinal incision centered over the floor of the sinus tarsi, dorsal to the peroneal tendons.
- Retract the peroneal tendons plantarly within their sheath exposing the dorsal and plantar aspects of the calcaneus at the level of the sinus tarsi.
- Identify the CC joint without compromising its capsule.
- Temporarily pin the calcaneocuboid joint with a K-wire, if necessary, to prevent subluxation.
- Make a perpendicular through and through osteotomy ~1.5 cm proximal to the CC joint, taking care not to violate the anterior or middle facets of the subtalar joint.
- Use a laminar spreader or similar device to distract the osteotomy until the desired lengthening is achieved.
- Place a trapezoidal-shaped tricortical osseous allograft into the distracted osteotomy with the base laterally.
- If a press fit, fixation may not be necessary. Fixation can be achieved with a fully threaded positional screw placed from the anterior superior process of the calcaneus across the bone graft and into the body of the calcaneus. Alternatively, a lateral plate can be placed across the graft interfaces.

PERILS and PITFALLS

- Use a laminar spreader or pin distractor to "dial" in the desired correction.
- Use tricortical allograft or a presized allograft wedge.
- Avoid destabilization of the CC joint by temporary pinning across it.
- Authors prefer positional screw over lateral plate, as the latter is often unnecessary and can lead to hardware irritation.

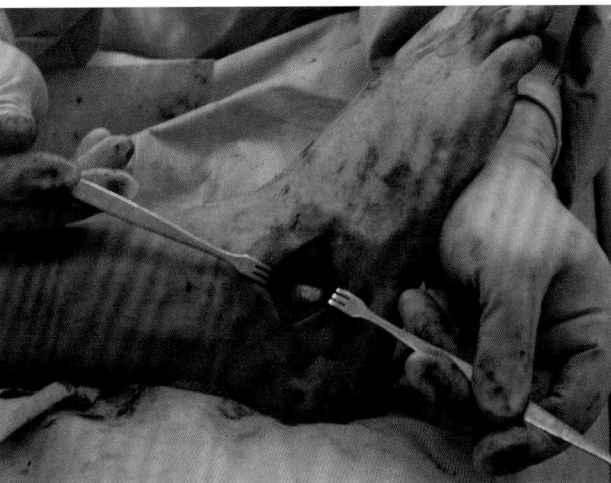

FIGURE 21.11 Intraoperative photograph showing the Evans osteotomy with bone graft placement.

CALCANEAL DISPLACEMENT OSTEOTOMY

A posterior medial calcaneal displacement osteotomy is a common procedure for addressing the heel valgus component of a flatfoot (Fig. 21.12). By translating the posterior calcaneus and its Achilles insertion medially, the center of gravity is moved more medially, and the Achilles tendon converts a pronatory moment at the rearfoot to a supinatory one.[65] At minimum it decreases the frontal plane pronatory moment arm acting on the rearfoot during heel contact and lateral foot loading. However, a medial displacement calcaneal osteotomy provides limited correction by itself. Combined with soft tissue procedures and medial column work, it can be a useful adjunct in flatfoot reconstruction.[66]

Technique for Medial Displacement Calcaneal Osteotomy

- Make an oblique incision along the lateral calcaneus immediately anterior to the Achilles tendon to just anterior to the tuber.
- Note that the course of the sural nerve averages 14 mm from the tip of the fibula.[67] Therefore, an incision that is 2 cm from the tip of the fibula should avoid the nerve and allow for adequate exposure for the planned osteotomy.
- Identify the superior and inferior margins of the calcaneus.
- Make a through and through perpendicular osteotomy of the calcaneus taking care to protect the medial soft tissue structures and the FHL tendon at the superior aspect of the calcaneus.

- Introduce a laminar spreader to the osteotomy to mobilize the tuber.
- Flex the knee as the tuber is translated medially to prevent inadvertent proximal displacement.
- The tuber can be translated medially ~1 cm.
- Make a full-thickness transverse incision at the junction of the posterior and plantar heel to deliver fixation.
- After temporarily pinning the osteotomy and confirming alignment and correction, place two 4.5-mm stacked lag screws across the osteotomy.
- Resect the overhanging ridge of bone created by the osteotomy.

PERILS and PITFALLS

- Avoid penetrating injury of the medial soft tissue structures.
- Flex the knee to eliminate the gastrocneumius' pull on the calcaneal tuber.

DOUBLE CALCANEAL OSTEOTOMY

In more severe deformity, the combination of lateral column lengthening and medial displacement calcaneal osteotomy can be more powerful than either alone, with good functional outcomes reported[68] (Fig. 21.13). It also provides a means of gaining adequate correction when lateral column lengthening is limited by concern for unmasking a metatarsus adductus.

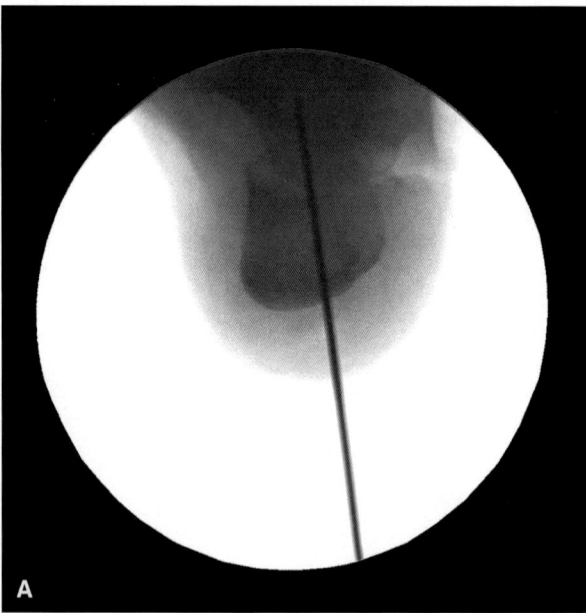

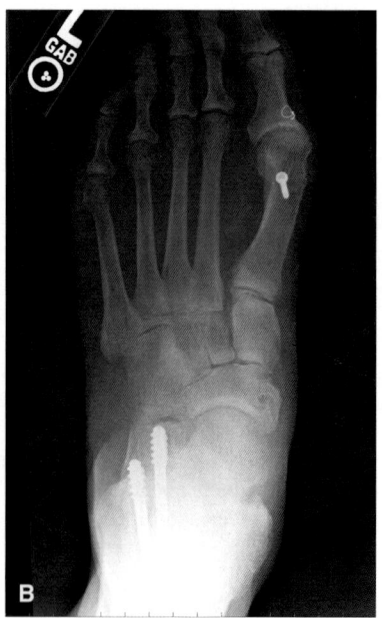

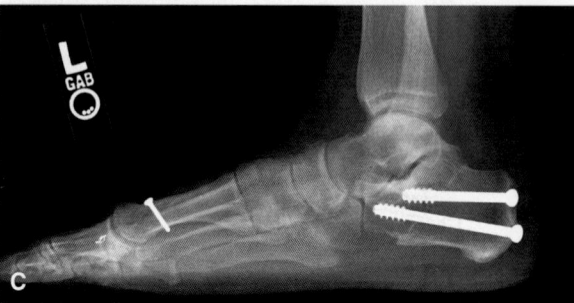

FIGURE 21.12 A medial displacement osteotomy of the posterior calcaneus can decrease the pronatory moment around the rearfoot **(A)** but does not affect the malalignment of the talus in the triple joint complex as attested by the radiographs of these postoperative images **(B, C)**.

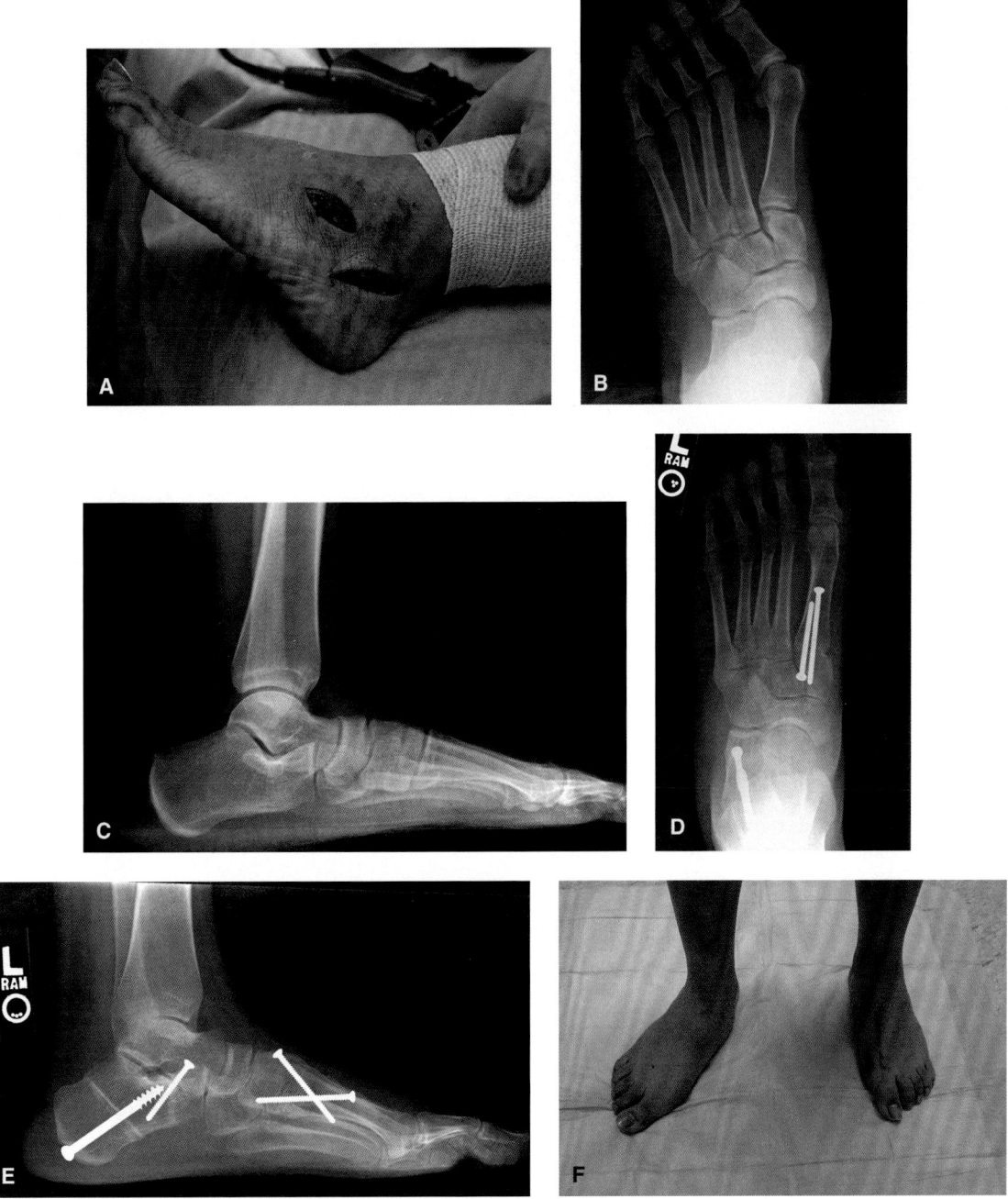

FIGURE 21.13 Double calcaneal osteotomy, combining lateral column lengthening with posterior displacement osteotomy, is utilized to either achieve more aggressive correction or avoid unmasking a met adductus with too much lateral column lengthening. **A.** The incisional approach is similar to either alone. **B-E.** Pre and postop radiographs demonstrate excellent realignment of the talus. **F.** 12 weeks postop left foot reconstruction contrasts with the contralateral pes valgus deformity.

ARTHROEREISIS

Another means of correcting frontal plane deformity of the rearfoot is with arthroereisis. An implant strategically placed in the sinus tarsi has been shown to block end-range pronatory rotation of the talus. Arthroereisis causes inversion of the calcaneus and cuboid, and dorsiflexion and internal rotation of the talus and navicular. There is some sagittal as well as frontal plane correction.[69] It does not address the medial column. The indications for arthroereisis are limited, compounded by the

potential long term effects it may have on the subtalar joint as shown in Figure 21.14.

MEDIAL COLUMN STABILIZATION

There has been increased awareness of the importance of a stable medial column in flatfoot surgery. As the medial arm of the tripod, the first ray must withstand dorsal migration and further overpronation by offering a stable platform for late midstance and early propulsion. It can be argued that once

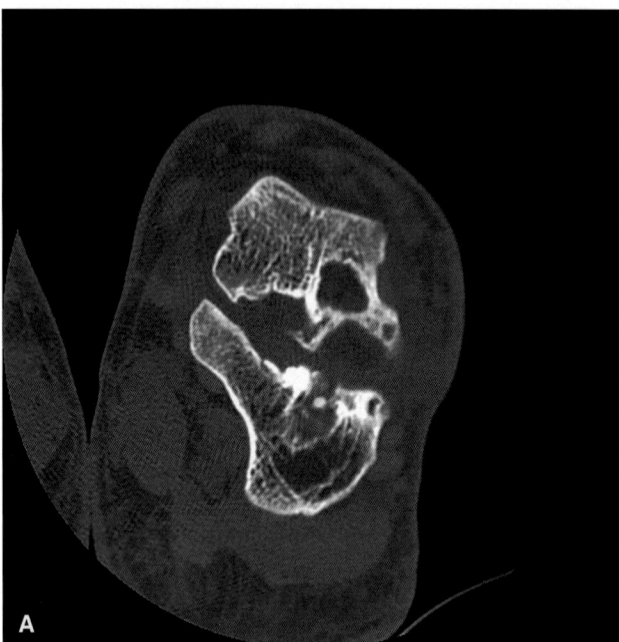 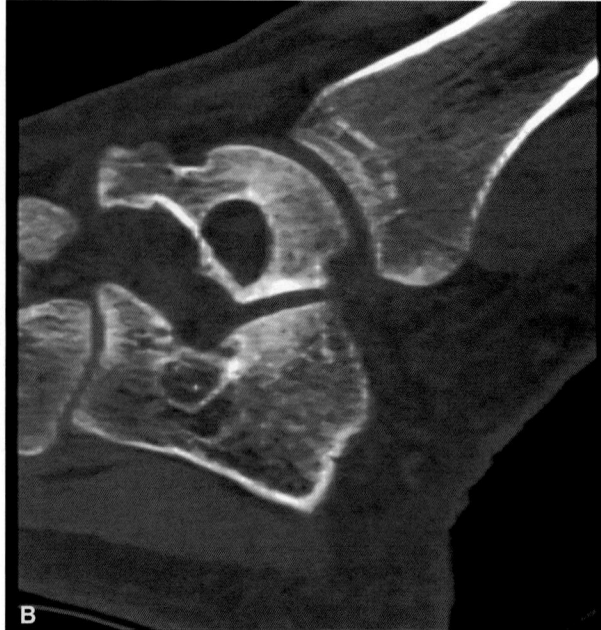

FIGURE 21.14 CT scan showing cystic changes of the subtalar joint after long-term follow-up of arthroereisis **(A, B)**.

the rearfoot is realigned around the triple joint complex, the medial column becomes stable due to the influence of peroneus longus in providing an eversion locking effect of the first ray.[27] This applies more to the juvenile flexible pes valgus before adaptation of the dorsiflexed first ray leads to a supinatus, ostensibly a reducible forefoot varus. The decision to add a medial column procedure to the flatfoot reconstruction can be made intraoperatively or preoperatively. If the first ray rests in the same sagittal plane as the fifth ray after the rearfoot is realigned, then concomitant medial column work may be unnecessary. However, if the first ray is still elevated or continues to elevate with simulated weight bearing, then addressing the medial column is necessary to provide a perpendicular forefoot. If hallux valgus or other first metatarsophalangeal joint deformity is present, stabilization of the medial column along with correction of the first MTP joint deformity can be simultaneously accomplished. Conversely, if there is minimal valgus of the heel in the presence of a collapsed medial longitudinal arch, isolated medial column work has the potential to realign the foot through the supinatory thrust provided by the stable first ray.[26]

Stabilization via arthrodesis of the nonessential joints of the medial midfoot has been shown to improve the radiographic parameters of flexible flatfoot deformity.[70-72] The first tarsometatarsal joint and naviculocuneiform joint are at the apex of the bending moment produced by ground reactive force on the first metatarsal head. Naturally, these are the joints that if fused can stabilize the medial column without adversely affecting normal foot mechanics.[20] The advantage of fusing the medial column at the first tarsometatarsal joint is if a hallux valgus or similar first ray pathology is present. Fusion of the naviculocuneiform joint, alone or in combination with the first tarsometatarsal joint, is advantageous when isolated medial column fusion is performed, if there is gross multijoint instability, or an obvious fault at the midfoot is

present (Fig. 21.15). An opening dorsal base wedge osteotomy of the medial cuneiform (Cotton procedure) provides a similar buttress to overpronation as medial column arthrodesis, and a similar supinatory moment around the triple joint complex.[72]

Technique for Medial Column Arthrodesis (Fig. 21.16)

- A frown incision is made between the PT and TA tendons for exposure of the NC joint. A second dorsal incision can be added if planning on fusing both the NC and TMT joints. The medial incision can be extended proximally along the PT tendon for any additional soft tissue work such as a flexor tendon transfer.
- The options for fusion are in situ fusion or biplanar correction. In situ is appropriate for arthritic joints without deformity.
- For deformity correction, the NC joint can be prepared by curettage of at least the medial two cuneiforms and navicular or by a biplanar osteotomy (base of the wedge is plantar and medial).
- The medial column is corrected by plantarflexing and adducting the forefoot on the rearfoot. This can correct sagittal and transverse plane deformity.
- Fixation is achieved with fully threaded screws placed in lag fashion on the tension side of the joint. Two screws are placed from the navicular tuberosity into the first and second cuneiforms.
- A third screw is placed from the medial aspect of the medial cuneiform to the second cuneiform.
- The first TMT joint can be approached and fixed similar to a Lapidus arthrodesis.

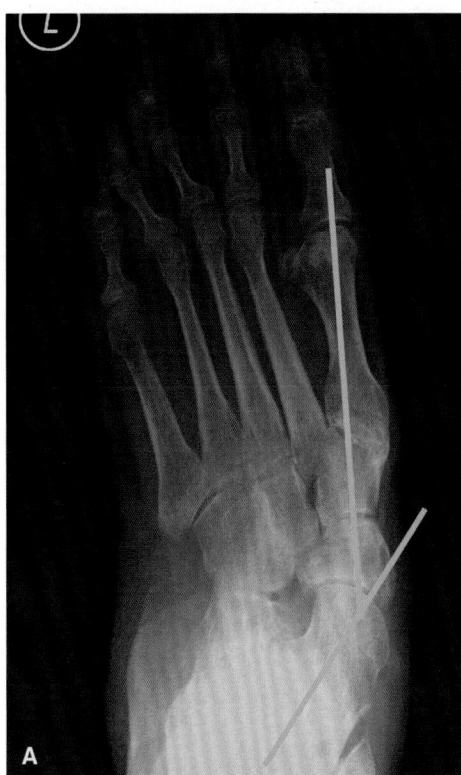

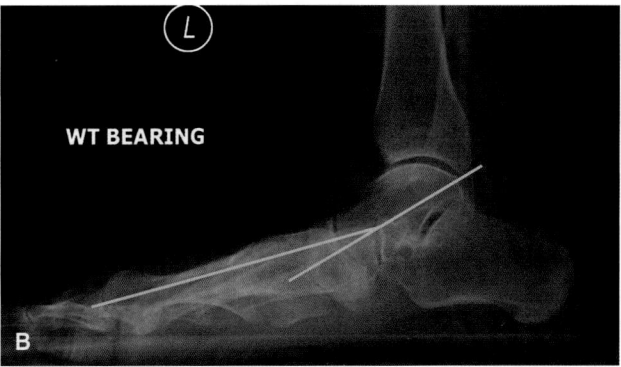

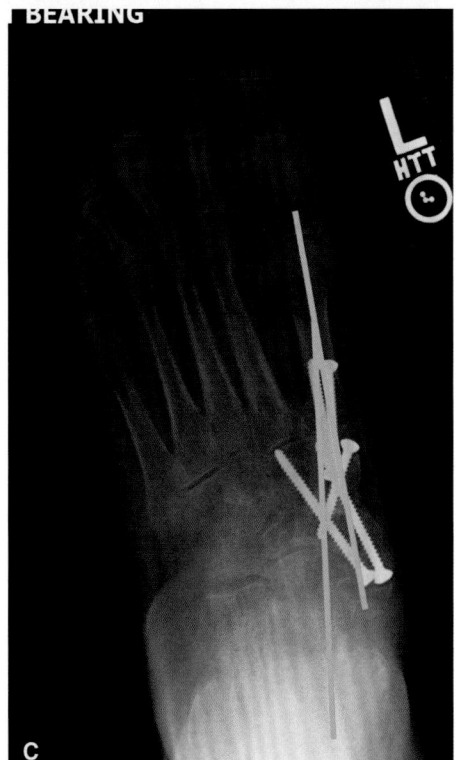

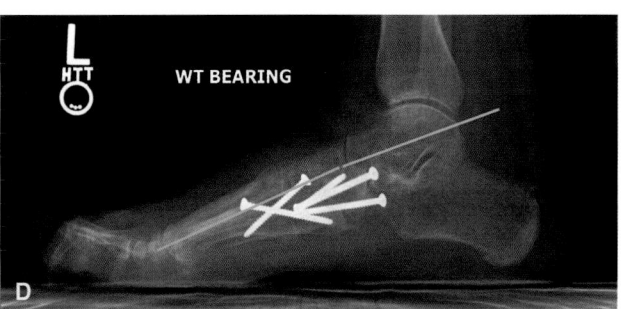

FIGURE 21.15 The ability to withstand the bending moment, or upward shear force, between the fulcrum of the forefoot and the arch flattening effect of the Achilles, requires a stable medial column. By creating a stable buttress, the medial column can provide a supinatory moment around the rearfoot, essentially realigning the talar-first metatarsal angle (**A** and **B**, preoperative; **C** and **D**, postoperative).

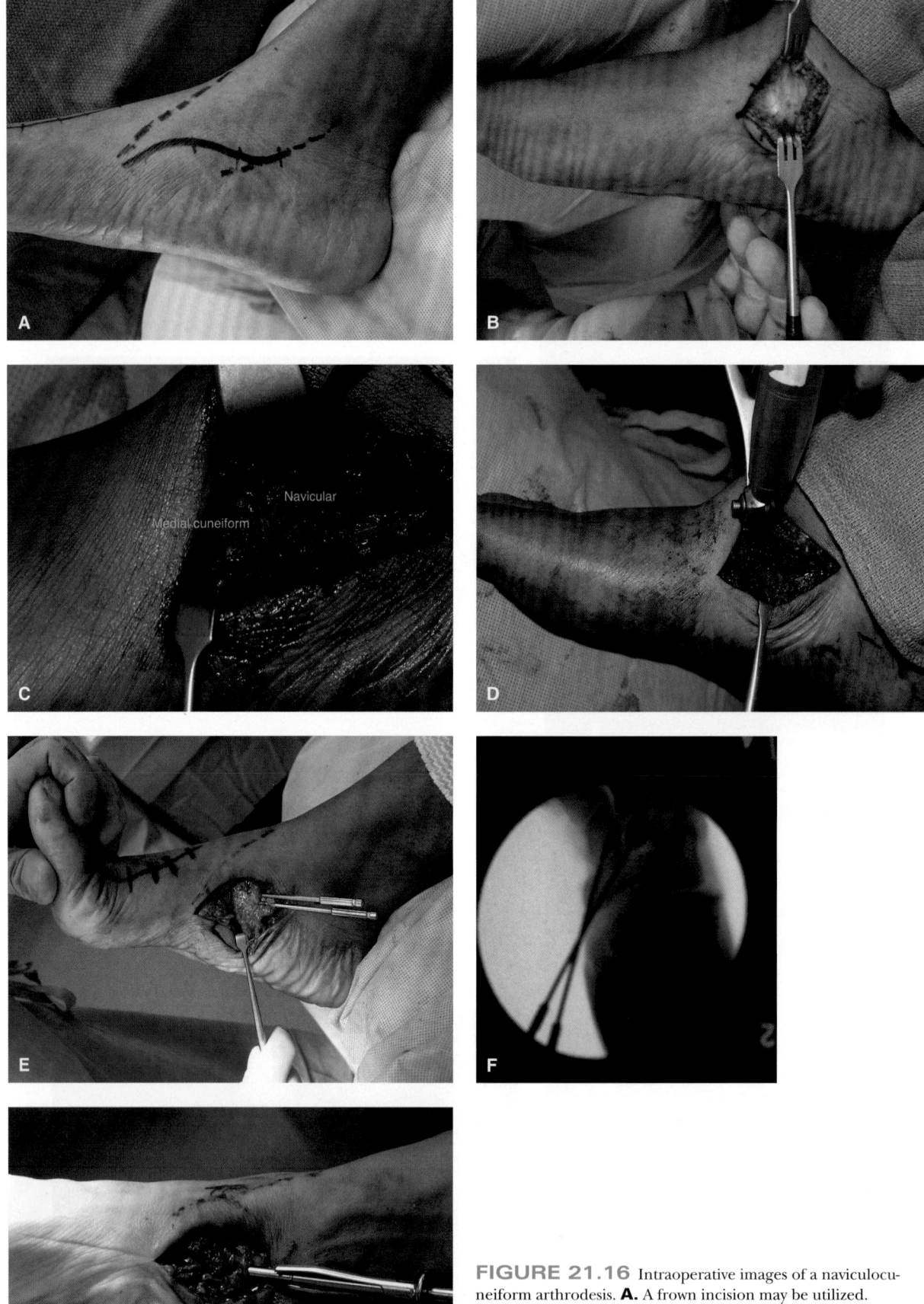

FIGURE 21.16 Intraoperative images of a naviculocuneiform arthrodesis. **A.** A frown incision may be utilized. **B, C.** Next, the NC joint can be identified just deep to the flexor retinaculum. **D.** An osteotomy vs an *in situ* fusion may be performed. **E.** After thorough joint preparation, the Hubscher maneuver facilitates apposition of the joint surfaces. Intraoperative fluoroscopy is used to ensure proper hardware placement **(F)**, and the screws should be properly buried to avoid hardware irritation **(G)**.

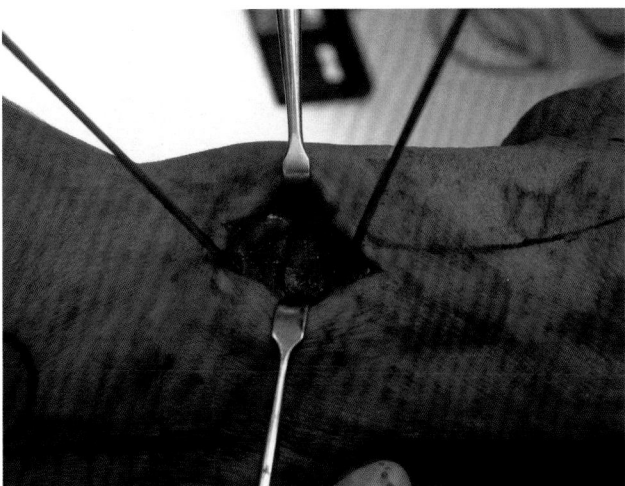

FIGURE 21.17 Intraoperative image of the Cotton osteotomy showing pin distraction and graft placement.

Technique for Cotton Osteotomy (Fig. 21.17)

- The incision is centered over the dorsal aspect of the first tarsometatarsal joint.
- Dissection is deepened lateral to the TA tendon, taking care to protect the medial dorsal cutaneous nerve and the intercuneiform joint.
- A dorsal to plantar osteotomy is performed without compromising the plantar or lateral cortex.
- A laminar spreader or similar device is used to distract the osteotomy and plantarflex the first ray to its desired position.
- Structural bicortical allograft with a dorsal base wedge is fashioned to fit in the osteotomy.
- Fixation is usually not necessary but can be achieved with K-wires if any instability is evident.

PERILS and PITFALLS

MEDIAL COLUMN ARTHRODESIS
- NC joint is easily identified just deep to the flexor retinaculum.
- To close the NC fusion, perform a Hubscher maneuver.
- Maximize compression by engaging the first cuneiform with the first screw.
- The screws should be stacked from medial and plantar to dorsal and lateral to counteract the tension forces and to provide maximum compression.

COTTON OSTEOTOMY
- Dial in correction.
- Try to not violate the plantar or lateral cortex.
- Shape of the wedge can be manipulated to affect the correction of hallux valgus deformity.

POSTOPERATIVE MANAGEMENT

In most cases, non–weight-bearing immobilization in a splint for 2 weeks followed by a short leg cast for another 4-6 weeks is appropriate. Non–weight-bearing plain film radiographs out of plaster are analyzed at 6-8 weeks postoperatively at which time the patient is advanced to weight bearing in a protective walking boot for another 2 weeks. The patient is then instructed to gradually wean off the boot into supportive shoe gear, work on physical therapy exercises, and return for weight-bearing radiographs at ~12 weeks postoperatively. Gradual increase in activities is prescribed with clinical and radiographic follow-up until healed.

COMPLICATIONS

Undercorrection and overcorrection can be mitigated by diligent preoperative evaluation and intraoperative execution. Although historically it was considered good form to position the foot with some residual valgus, the authors prefer to attempt to achieve a perpendicular heel position. This leaves less room for error with a higher chance of overcorrection. If the rearfoot is adequately corrected but the supinatus deformity in the forefoot is underappreciated, this can adversely affect the rearfoot. If the supinatus is compensated by further pronation through the rearfoot, sinus tarsi impingement can ensue, thus negating the effects of the rearfoot correction. If the supinatus is not compensated in the rearfoot, then lateral column overload develops due to the lack of weight bearing under the medial column. Similarly, overzealous plantarflexion of the medial column can lead to a forefoot-induced rearfoot varus. Varus malalignment of the heel following osteotomies or rearfoot fusions is not easily managed. Compensation is difficult. A rearfoot in varus can obviously result in too much weight bearing on the lateral column but also can cause strain and attenuation of the peroneal tendons. Other potential complications are inherent to soft tissue and osseous surgery in general, including nonunion, infection, painful scar, nerve entrapment, and continued pain and deformity.

CONCLUSION

There are many different procedures or combination of procedures to surgically fix a flexible pes valgus (Figs. 21.18 and 21.19). Choosing the right procedure or combination of procedures is the challenge. There is support in the literature for each one. If the goal of the surgeon and the patient is to attempt to preserve normal foot function, then a combination of osteotomies, nonessential joint fusions, and soft tissue balancing should be performed. This trend during the last decade has been validated by reports of long-term correction of deformity.[44]

Depending on the findings inherent to each individual case, the deformity can be addressed by lateral column lengthening, medial column stabilization, and medial displacement calcaneal osteotomies. Lengthening the lateral column essentially realigns the talonavicular joint in all three cardinal planes. A medializing calcaneal osteotomy decreases the pronatory force on the rearfoot immediately after heel strike. Stabilizing the medial column provides a rigid lever, which can act as a buttress to resist overpronation of the rearfoot and as a stable platform for effective propulsion. It dials in the third arm of the tripod. The purpose of soft tissue surgery is to augment the osseous correction and rebalance the muscles and tendons acting on the foot. Soft tissue balancing is most effective around a stable, neutrally aligned foot.

The ultimate goal when treating flexible pes valgus is to improve pain and function by either externally supporting it with shoes, orthotics, and braces or by surgically fixing the faulty engineering and architectural collapse.

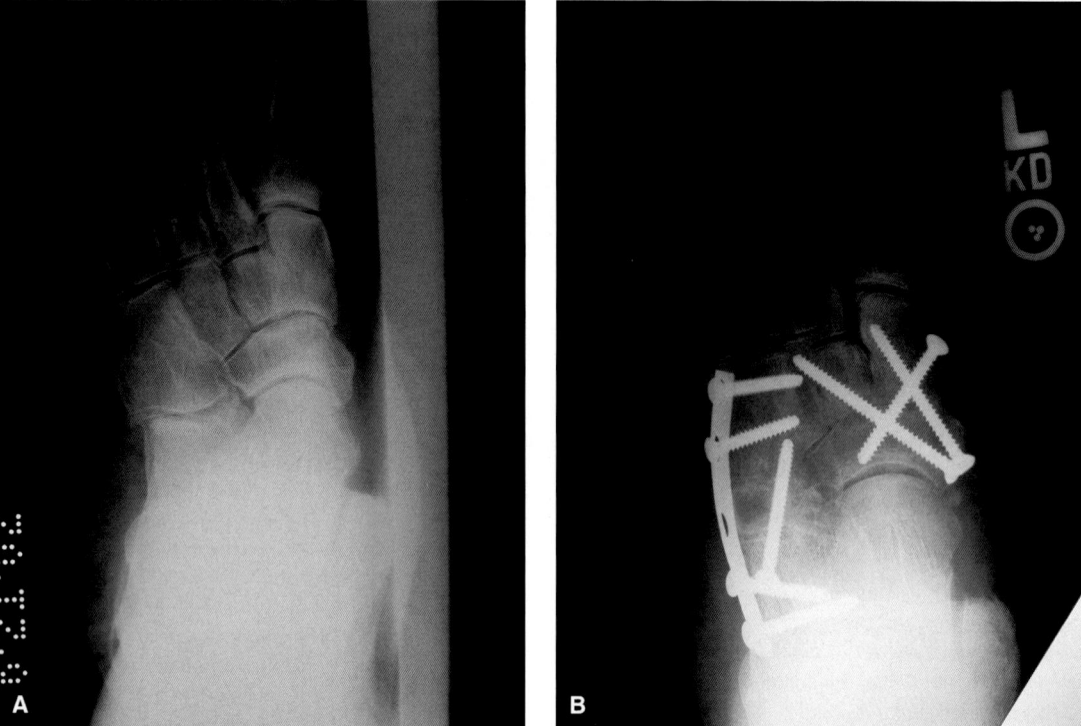

FIGURE 21.18 Patient underwent gastrocnemius recession, CC distraction arthrodesis, and NC arthrodesis. Note the correction of the talar equinus and forefoot abduction from preoperative **(A)** to postoperative **(B)**.

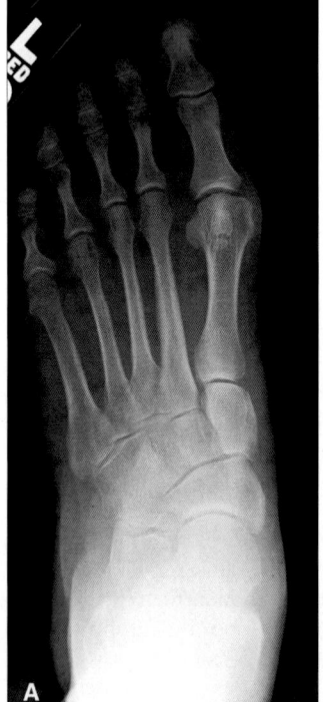
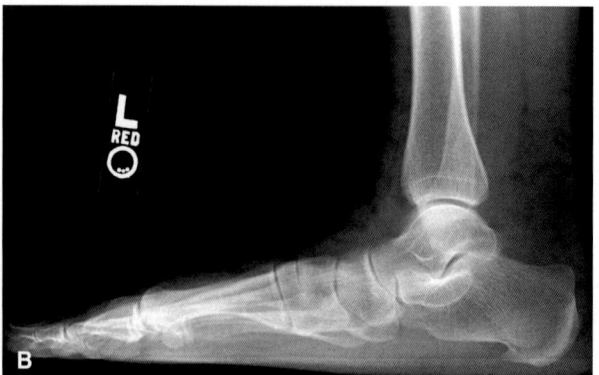

FIGURE 21.19 To preserve normal joint function, a combination of medial column arthrodesis and calcaneal slide osteotomy with gastrocnemius recession and FDL transfer to the PT tendon was performed. **A-D.** Note the improvement of radiographic parameters of flatfoot deformity, in particular the restoration of the talar-first metatarsal angle.

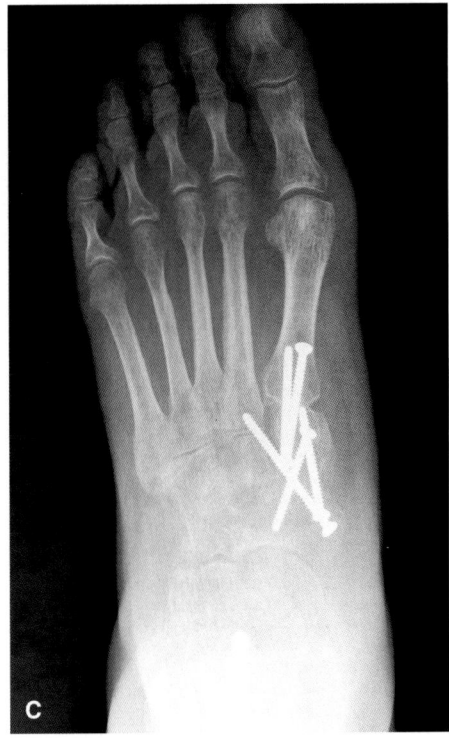
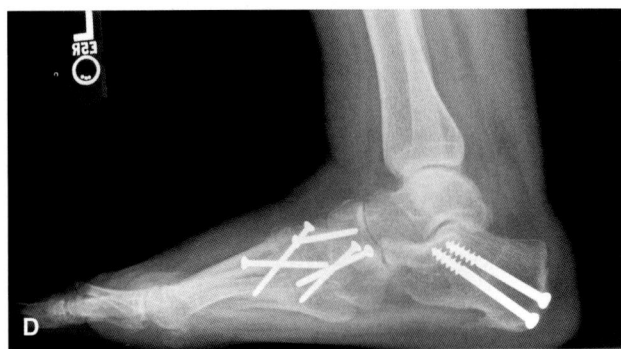

FIGURE 21.19 (*Continued*)

REFERENCES

1. Harris RI, Beath T. Hypermobile flat-foot with short tendo Achilles. *J Bone Joint Surg.* 1948;30A(1):116-150.
2. Holmes GB, Mann RA. Possible epidemiological factors associated with rupture of the posterior tibial tendon. *Foot Ankle.* 1992;13(2):70-79.
3. Myerson M, Solomon G, Shereff M. Posterior tibial tendon dysfunction: its association with seronegative inflammatory disease. *Foot Ankle.* 1989;9(5):219-225.
4. Dowling AM, Steele JR, Baur LA. Does obesity influence foot structure in prepubescent children? *Int J Obes Relat Metab Disord.* 2001;25(6):845-852.
5. Castro-Aragon O, Vallurupalli S, Warner M, Panchbhavi V, Trevino S. Ethnic radiographic foot differences. *Foot Ankle Int.* 2009;30(1):57-61.
6. Godoy-Santos A, Ortiz RT, Mattar R Jr, Fernandes TD, Santos MC. MMP-8 polymorphism is genetic marker to tendinopathy primary posterior tibial tendon. *Scand J Med Sci Sports.* 2014;24(1):220-223.
7. Ouzounian TJ, Shereff MJ. In vitro determination of midfoot motion. *Foot Ankle.* 1989;10:140-146.
8. Nester CJ, Liu AM, Ward E, et al. In vitro study of foot kinematics using a dynamic walking cadaver model. *J Biomech.* 2007;40:1927-1937.
9. Lundgren P, Nester C, Liu A, et al. Invasive in vivo measurement of rear-, mid- and forefoot motion during walking. *Gait Posture.* 2008;28(1):93-100.
10. Houck JR, Nomides C, Neville CG, Flemister AS. The effect of stage II posterior tibial tendon dysfunction on deep compartment muscle strength: a new strength test. *Foot Ankle Int.* 2008;29(9):895-902.
11. Ness ME, Long J, Marks R, Harris G. Foot and ankle kinematics in patients with posterior tibial tendon dysfunction. *Gait Posture.* 2008;27:331-339.
12. Chang HW, Chieh HF, Lin CJ, Su FC, Tsai MJ. The relationships between foot arch volumes and dynamic plantar pressure during midstance of walking in preschool children. *PLoS One.* 2014;9(4):e94535.
13. Murley GS, Menz HB, Landorf KB. Foot posture influences the electromyographic activity of selected lower limb muscles during gait. *J Foot Ankle Res.* 2009;2:35.
14. Kitaoka HB, Lundberg A, Luo ZP, An KN. Kinematics of the normal arch of the foot and ankle under physiologic loading. *Foot Ankle Int.* 1995;16(8):492-499.
15. Wulker N, Stukenborg C, Savory KM, Alfke D. Hindfoot motion after isolated and combined arthrodesis: measurements in anatomic specimens. *Foot Ankle Int.* 2000;21(11):921-927.
16. Blackwood CB, Yuen TJ, Sangeorzan BJ, Ledoux WR. The midtarsal joint locking mechanism. *Foot Ankle Int.* 2005;26(12):1074-1080.
17. Tweed JL, Campbell JA, Thompson RJ, Curran MJ. The function of the midtarsal joint: a review of the literature. *Foot (Edinb).* 2008;18(2):106-112.
18. Wang C, Geng X, Wang S, et al. In vivo kinematic study of the tarsal joints complex based on fluoroscopic 3D-2D registration technique. *Gait Posture.* 2016;49:54-60.
19. Astion DJ, Deland JT, Otis JC, Keneally S. Motion of the hindfoot after simulated arthrodesis. *J Bone Joint Surg Am.* 1997;79(2):241-246.
20. Hansen ST Jr. *Functional Reconstruction of the Foot and Ankle.* Philadelphia, PA: Lippincott Williams & Wilkins; 2000.
21. Gazdag AR, Cracchiolo A III. Rupture of the posterior tibial tendon. Evaluation of injury of the spring ligament and clinical assessment of tendon transfer and ligament repair. *J Bone Joint Surg Am.* 1997;79(5):675-681.
22. Thordarson DB, Schmatzer H, Chon J, Peters J. Dynamic support of the human longitudinal arch. A biomechanical evaluation. *Clin Orthop Relat Res.* 1995;316:165-172.
23. Kirby KA. Subtalar joint axis location and rotational equilibrium theory of foot function. *J Am Podiatr Med Assoc.* 2001;91(9):465-487.
24. Kitaoka HB, Luo ZP, An KN. Contact features of the talonavicular joint of the foot. *Clin Orthop Relat Res.* 1996;325:290-295.
25. Johnson CH, Christensen JC. Biomechanics of the first ray part V: the effect of equinus deformity. A 3-dimensional kinematic study on a cadaver model. *J Foot Ankle Surg.* 2005;44(1):114-120.
26. Rush SM, Jordan T. Naviculocuneiform arthrodesis for treatment of medial column instability associated with lateral peritalar subluxation. *Clin Podiatr Med Surg.* 2009;26(3):373-384.
27. Johnson CH, Christensen JC. Biomechanics of the first ray part I: the effects of peroneus longus function: a 3-dimensional kinematic study on a cadaver model. *J Foot Ankle Surg.* 1995;38(5):313-321.
28. Johnson KA, Strom DE. Tibialis posterior tendon dysfunction. *Clin Orthop Relat Res.* 1989;239:196-206.
29. Myseron MS. Adult acquired flatfoot deformity: treatment of dysfunction of the posterior tibial tendon. *Instr Course Lect.* 1997;46:393-405.
30. Bluman EM, Myerson MS. Stage IV posterior tibial tendon rupture. *Foot Ankle Clin.* 2007;12:341-362.
31. Saltzman CL, el-Khoury GY. The hindfoot alignment view. *Foot Ankle Int.* 1995;16(9):572-576.
32. Strash WW, Berardo P. Radiographic assessment of the hindfoot and ankle. *Clin Podiatr Med Surg.* 2004;21(3):295-304.
33. Cass AD, Camasta CA. A review of tarsal coalition and pes planovalgus: clinical examination, diagnostic imaging, and surgical planning. *J Foot Ankle Surg.* 2010;49(3):274-293.
34. Baca JM, Zdenek C, Catanzariti AR, Mendicino RW. Is advanced imaging necessary before surgical repair. *Clin Podiatr Med Surg.* 2014;31(3):357-362.
35. Mengiardi B, Pinto C, Zanetti M. Spring ligament complex and posterior tibial tendon: MR anatomy and findings in acquired adult flatfoot deformity. *Semin Musculoskelet Radiol.* 2016;20(1):104-115.
36. Donovan A, Rosenberg ZS. Extraarticular lateral hindfoot impingement with posterior tibial tendon tear: MRI correlation. *AJR Am J Roentgenol.* 2009;193:672-678.
37. Khoury NJ, el-Khoury GY, Saltzman CL, Brandser EA. MR imaging of posterior tibial tendon dysfunction. *AJR Am J Roentgenol.* 1996;167:675-682.
38. Arnoldner MA, Gruber M, Syre S, et al. Imaging of posterior tibial tendon dysfunction—comparison of high-resolution ultrasound and 3T MRI. *Eur J Radiol.* 2015;84(9):1777-1781.
39. Chen YJ, Liang SC. Diagnostic efficacy of ultrasonography in stage I posterior tibial tendon dysfunction: Sonographic-surgical correlation. *J Ultrasound Med.* 1997;16:417-423.

40. Hsu TC, Wang CL, Wang TG, Chiang IP, Hsieh FJ. Ultrasonographic examination of the posterior tibial tendon. *Foot Ankle Int.* 1997;18(1):34-38.

41. Jain NB, Omar I, Kelikian AS, van Holsbeeck L, Grant TH. Prevalence of and factors associated with posterior tibial tendon pathology on sonographic assessment. *PM R.* 2011;3(11):998-1004.

42. Nallamshetty L, Nazarian LN, Schweitzer ME, et al. Evaluation of posterior tibial pathology: comparison of sonography and MR imaging. *Skeletal Radiol.* 2005;34(7):375-380.

43. Pinney SJ, Lin SS. Current concept review: acquired adult flatfoot deformity. *Foot Ankle Int.* 2006;27:66-74.

44. Morton DJ. *The Human Foot its Evolution, Physiology and Functional Disorders.* New York, NY: Columbia University Press; 1935.

45. Subotnick SI. Equinus deformity as it affects the forefoot. *J Am Podiatry Assoc.* 1971;61(11):423-427.

46. Jennings MM, Christensen JC. The effects of sectioning the spring ligament on rearfoot stability and posterior tibial tendon efficiency. *J Foot Ankle Surg.* 2008;47(3):219-224.

47. Deland JT, de Asla RJ, Sung IH, Emberg LA, Potter HG. Posterior tibial tendon insufficiency: which ligaments are involved? *Foot Ankle Int.* 2005;26(6):427-435.

48. Fayzai AH, Nguyen HV, Juliano PJ. Intermediate term follow-up of calcaneal osteotomy and flexor digitorum longus transfer for treatment of posterior tibial tendon dysfunction. *Foot Ankle Int.* 2002;23(12):1107-1111.

49. Myerson MS, Badekas A, Schon C. Treatment of stage II posterior tibial tendon deficiency with flexor digitorum longus tendon transfer and calcaneal osteotomy. *Foot Ankle Int.* 2004;25(7):445-450.

50. Marks RM, Long JT, Ness ME, Khazzam M, Harris GF. Surgical reconstruction of posterior tibial tendon dysfunction: prospective comparison of flexor digitorum longus substitution combined with lateral column lengthening or medial displacement calcaneal osteotomy. *Gait Posture.* 2009;29(1):17-22.

51. Chadwick C, Whitehouse SL, Saxby TS. Long-term follow-up of flexor digitorum longus transfer and calcaneal osteotomy for stage II posterior tibial tendon dysfunction. *Bone Joint J.* 2015;97-B(3):346-352.

52. Silva MG, Tan SH, Chong HC, Su HC, Singh IR. Results of operative correction of grade IIB tibialis posterior tendon dysfunction. *Foot Ankle Int.* 2015;36(2):165-171.

53. Ruffilli A, Traina F, Giannini S, Buda R, Perna F, Faldini C. Surgical treatment of stage II posterior tibialis tendon dysfunction: ten-year clinical and radiographic results. *Eur J Orthop Surg Traumatol.* 2018;28(1):139-145.

54. Mann RA. Posterior tibial tendon dysfunction: treatment by flexor digitorum longus transfer. *Foot Ankle Clin.* 2001;6(1):77-87.

55. Fogel GR, Katoh Y, Rand JA, Chao EY. Talonavicular arthrodesis for isolated arthrosis: 9.5 year results and gait analysis. *Foot Ankle.* 1982;3(2):105-113.

56. Saltzman CL, Fehle MJ, Cooper RR, Spencer EC, Ponseti IV. Triple arthrodesis: twenty-five and forty-four-year average follow-up of the same patients. *J Bone Joint Surg Am.* 1999;81(10):1391-1402.

57. Thomas JL, Moeini R, Soileau R. The effects of subtalar contact and pressure following talonavicular and midtarsal joint arthrodesis. *J Foot Ankle Surg.* 2000;39(2):78-88.

58. Smith RW, Shen W, Dewitt S, Reischl SF. Triple arthrodesis in adults with non-paralytic disease. A minimum ten-year follow-up study. *J Bone Joint Surg Am.* 2004;86-A(12):2707-2713.

59. Ebalard M, Le Henaff G, Sigonney G, et al. Risk of osteoarthritis secondary to partial or total arthrodesis of the subtalar and midtarsal joints after a minimum follow-up of 10 years. *Orthop Traumatol Surg Res.* 2014;100(4 suppl):S231-S237.

60. Graves SC, Mann RA, Graves KO. Triple arthrodesis in older adults. Results after long-term follow up. *J Bone Joint Surg Am.* 1993;75(3):355-362.

61. Dinucci KR, Christensen JC, Dinucci KA. Biomechanical consequences of lateral column lengthening of the calcaneus: Part I. Long plantar ligament strain. *J Foot Ankle Surg.* 2004;43(1):10-15.

62. Hintermann B, Valderrabano V, Kundert HP. Lengthening of the lateral column and reconstruction of the medial soft tissue for treatment of acquired flatfoot deformity associated with insufficiency of the posterior tibial tendon. *Foot Ankle Int.* 1999;20(10):622-629.

63. Bolt PM, Coy S, Toolan BC. A comparison of lateral column lengthening and medial translational osteotomy of the calcaneus for the reconstruction of adult acquired flatfoot. *Foot Ankle Int.* 2007;28(11):1115-1123.

64. Haeseker GA, Mureau MA, Faber FW. Lateral column lengthening for acquired adult flatfoot deformity caused by posterior tibial tendon dysfunction stage II: a retrospective comparison of osteotomy with calcaneocuboid distraction arthrodesis. *J Foot Ankle Surg.* 2010;49(4):380-384.

65. Guha AR, Perera AM. Calcaneal osteotomy in the treatment of adult acquired flatfoot deformity. *Foot Ankle Clin.* 2012;17(2):247-258.

66. Catanzariti AR, Lee MS, Mendicino RW. Posterior calcaneal displacement osteotomy for adult acquired flatfoot. *J Foot Ankle Surg.* 2000;39(1):2-14.

67. Lawrence SJ, Botte MJ. The sural nerve in the foot and ankle: an anatomic study with clinical and surgical implications. *Foot Ankle Int.* 2004;15(9):490-494.

68. Kou JX, Balasubramaniam M, Kippe M, Fortin PT. Functional results of posterior tibial tendon reconstruction, calcaneal osteotomy, and gastrocnemius recession. *Foot Ankle Int.* 2012;33(7):602-611.

69. Christensen JC, Campbell N, DiNucci K. Closed kinetic chain tarsal mechanics of subtalar joint arthrodesis. *J Am Podiatr Med Assoc.* 1996;86(10):467-473.

70. Jordan TH, Rush SM, Hamilton GA, Ford LA. Radiographic outcomes of adult acquired flatfoot corrected by medial column arthrodesis with or without a medializing calcaneal osteotomy. *J Foot Ankle Surg.* 2011;50(2):176-181.

71. Avino A, Patel S, Hamilton GA, Ford LA. The effect of the Lapidus arthrodesis on the medial longitudinal arch: a radiographic review. *J Foot Ankle Surg.* 2008;47(6):510-514.

72. Hirose CB, Johnson JE. Plantarflexion opening wedge medial cuneiform osteotomy for correction of fixed forefoot varus associated with flatfoot deformity. *Foot Ankle Int.* 2004;25(8):568-574.

CHAPTER 22

Tarsometatarsal Joint (TMTJ) Conditions

Asim A. Z. Raja, Ronald M. Talis, and Dhaval K. Amin

INTRODUCTION

The tarsometatarsal (TMT) joint, also known as the Lisfranc joint, involves articulations between the bases of the first, second, and third metatarsals and their respective cuneiforms, and the fourth and fifth metatarsal bases with the cuboid. The TMT joint allows limited motion during the gait cycle, especially to the second metatarsal base/intermediate cuneiform articulation.[1] Primary arthritis of the TMT joint region is not common; however, trauma-related injuries can potentially elicit pain secondary to posttraumatic arthritis.[2] Operative procedures are indicated when nonoperative treatment measures have been exhausted. Goals of operative intervention include improvement of symptoms, deformity correction/plantar-grade foot realignment, and return to function as tolerated.

The views expressed herein are those of the author(s) and do not reflect the offical policy or position of the U.S. Army Medical Department, Department of the Army, Department of Defense, or the U.S. Government.

ANATOMY AND BIOMECHANICS

Traditionally, the TMT joint complex is subdivided into three separate columns: medial, middle, and lateral. The medial column involves the articulation of the first metatarsal with the medial cuneiform. The middle column involves the articulations of the second and third metatarsals with the middle (or intermediate) and lateral cuneiforms, respectively. The lateral column includes the fourth and fifth metatarsal articulation with the cuboid.

Anatomic Features		
Medial Column	**Middle Column**	**Lateral Column**
Involves the articulation of the first metatarsal with the medial cuneiform	Involves the articulations of the second and third metatarsals with the middle (or intermediate) and lateral cuneiforms, respectively	Includes the fourth and fifth metatarsal articulation with the cuboid.

These skeletal components and their respective morphologies (in concert with a vast arrangement of dorsal, interosseous, and plantar ligamentous attachments) form a polyarticular system.[3] The plantar and dorsal ligament orientations can be longitudinal, oblique, or transverse.[4] The plantar and interosseous ligamentous attachments receive supportive reinforcement by the plantar fascia, intrinsic muscles, and extrinsic tendons. Cadaveric dissection models demonstrate dorsal ligaments connecting the medial cuneiform to the first metatarsal, as being the "widest" and "longest," while the medial cuneiform to second metatarsal (ie, Lisfranc ligament), as being the thickest.[5] The Lisfranc ligament (considered the main ligamentous stabilizer of the TMT joint) originates from the lateral surface of the medial cuneiform and courses in an oblique manner to the medial aspect of the second metatarsal.[6] Thus, Lisfranc ligament integrity plays an important role in the overall preservation of articular relationships between the medial and middle TMT joint columns.[7] The second metatarsal is the most secure and limited in motion within the complex.[8] The second metatarsal sits within a "keystone" mortise configuration and is critical for TMT joint stability. As a functional unit, limited TMT joint movements are that of pronation and supination of the forefoot.[9] The second metatarsal-middle cuneiform articulation exhibits the least motion in both planes. Conversely, the fourth and fifth metatarsal-cuboid articulations (lateral column) relatively exhibit the most motion of the entire complex.

ETIOLOGY

A history of TMT joint injury can predispose a patient to painful midfoot arthrosis. Injury may be caused by both direct and/or indirect forces.[10,11] Trauma has the potential to create injury to either ligamentous and/or osseous structures in the region (Fig. 22.1). Pathologic forces can result in fractures to either the metatarsal bases or the cuneiform and cuboid regions.[12]

Pathogenesis
■ Posttraumatic injury leading to ligamentous disruption, intra-articular damage, or osseous fractures/disruption
■ Intra-articular fractures leading to posttraumatic arthrosis
■ Neuropathic joint changes leading to destruction and malreduction

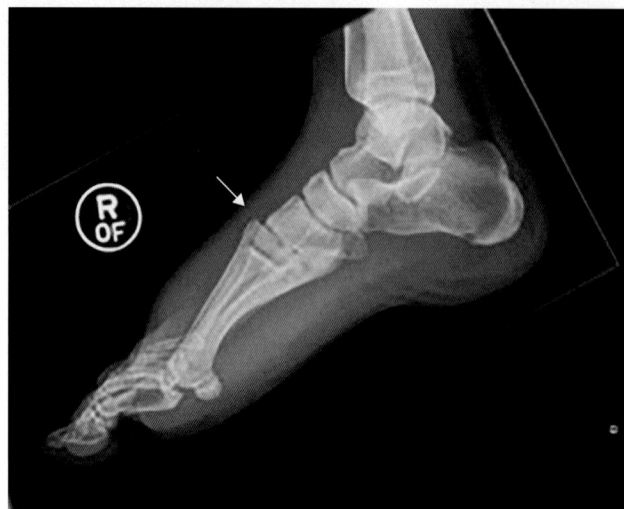

FIGURE 22.1 Lateral radiograph of the right foot with a primarily ligamentous TMT joint injury. The *white arrow* pointing to a notable dorsal migration of the second metatarsal base, relative to the adjacent metatarsal bases, and corresponding intermediate (or middle) cuneiform.

Ruling out an injury to the Lisfranc ligament complex (as part of the examination) is mandatory, especially when considering a higher reported incidence of injury than previously estimated.[13] Approximately 0.2% of all fractures reportedly involve the Lisfranc joint region, with upward of 20% of these injuries being either missed or misdiagnosed on initial radiographic assessment.[14] Lisfranc injuries generally lead to continued instability with axial loading during the gait cycle. This further potentiates the risk of arthritic change to the region. Lack of recognition is plausible, as subtle fracture-dislocation injuries may at times be misdiagnosed as sprains. The extent of articular damage may not be appreciated until the patient develops symptomatic arthritis. Conversely, more overt or higher energy injuries can lead to more significant soft tissue and vascular damage.

Lisfranc injuries on physical examination are most notable, in the form of plantar ecchymosis along the medial and central aspects of the longitudinal arch. Nonoperative treatment for these injuries has traditionally yielded less favorable results than that of open surgical management.[15] Principles for surgical management generally include an effort to achieve an anatomic reduction with stable fixation. A higher incidence of developing symptomatic degenerative changes can occur with inadequate reduction and/or inadequate stability. It is also important to keep in mind that some long-term clinical outcomes of Lisfranc injuries treated with either open reduction internal fixation (ORIF) or primary arthrodesis, demonstrate radiographic osteoarthritis, without the correlation of symptoms.[16] Furthermore, TMT joint deformity can also occur as a result of neuropathic conditions, such as Charcot neuroarthropathy[17] (Fig. 22.2A and B). Such conditions can result in both osseous and ligamentous destructive changes, to a greater extent in some cases, than of those noted in non-neuropathic patients.

PHYSICAL EXAMINATION

CLINICAL

Patient history may indicate previous injury/trauma or neuropathy. Additional history of medical comorbidities and previous attempted surgical management can further speak to potential soft tissue healing complications with additional operative intervention. Typical symptoms include chronic, deep aching pain to the TMT joint region. Neritic type symptoms or selective numbness may also be noted from direct impingement of nerves involving osseous prominences. Patients may describe problems with shoe gear, gait disturbances, or contralateral metatarsalgia secondary to compensation. Patient examination should include both non–weight-bearing and weight-bearing assessments. The patient should be asked to identify areas of maximum tenderness. Most patients present with focal pain located at one or more of the individual TMT joints, while others will also complain of pain to adjacent

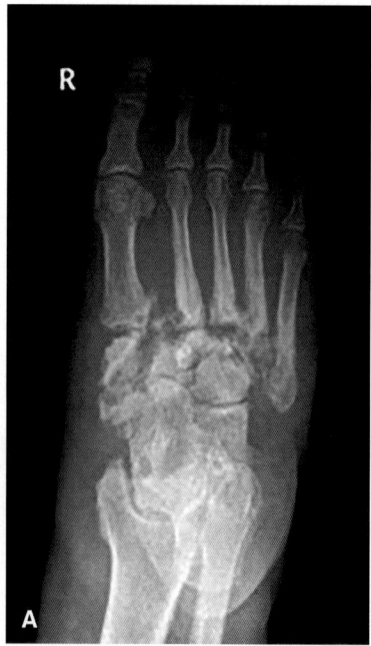

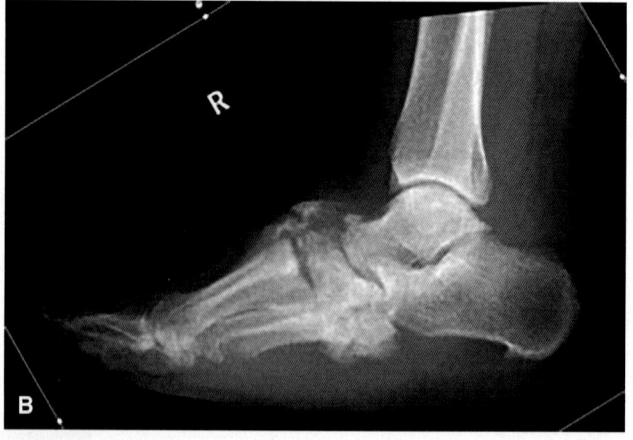

FIGURE 22.2 A. An AP view radiograph demonstrating both osseous and ligamentous destructive changes to the TMT joint, secondary to Charcot neuroarthropathy in a type II diabetic patient. **B.** A lateral view radiograph demonstrating both osseous and ligamentous destructive changes to the TMT joint secondary to Charcot neuroarthropathy in a type II diabetic patient.

regions. Passive pronation and abduction testing can be used to illicit symptoms and demonstrate instability.[18] Gentle, passive pronation and abduction of the forefoot with the hindfoot stabilized can result in increased midfoot pain. Each individual TMT joint can be palpated and manually manipulated in the sagittal plane to delineate symptomatic regions. Physical examination may reveal callosities secondary to uneven forefoot loading. Skin quality and vascular competency may be compromised if multiple prior surgical incisions have been performed or if significant crush injuries have been sustained in previous years. Noninvasive vascular studies of both lower extremities to include pulse volume recordings, ankle and digital-brachial indices, and transcutaneous oximetry should be considered when concerns of vascular sufficiency arise.

Posttraumatic or primary arthritis at the TMT joint commonly involves the medial and middle columns, with the lateral column typically being involved to a lesser extent. Patients with progressive arthritic changes can demonstrate sagittal and/or transverse plane deformity (Fig. 22.3A and B).

Physical Examination

- Both weight-bearing and non–weight-bearing evaluations
- Forefoot abduction/adduction stress examination while stabilizing the hindfoot
- Forefoot/metatarsal dorsiflexion/plantarflexion stress examination while stabilizing the hindfoot
- Patient to indicate maximum region (or) regions of tenderness
- Posterior tibial tendon strength testing for posterior muscle group weakness
- Gait analysis
- Assess for callosities, ulcerations, or multiple surgical incision sites

RADIOGRAPHIC

Weight-bearing anteroposterior (AP), oblique, and lateral radiographs of the foot should be obtained in the angle and base of gait. Angular measurements can be useful in evaluation of structural deformity, especially in unilateral conditions, when compared to the uninjured contralateral extremity. The talar-first metatarsal angle in the AP and lateral projection can be used to appreciate the degree of forefoot abduction and dorsiflexion relative to the hindfoot. Respective congruity of the dorsal and plantar aspects of each metatarsal to its corresponding cuneiform or cuboid should be assessed for malalignment within the joint complex.[19] Oblique views are useful for comparing orientation and position of the middle and lateral TMT columns (Fig. 22.4). Radiographs of the contralateral, unaffected foot should be compared to the affected foot when feasible. Manipulation under fluoroscopy, or an assessment of weight-bearing views, can both be used to determine joint gapping and joint instability patterns. For stress testing under fluoroscopy, the hindfoot is stabilized while the forefoot is manipulated, first with an abduction-adduction force, and then with plantar flexion and dorsiflexion stresses. It is important to note that there is limited standardization to both performing TMTJ stress examinations, as well as measurement parameters for assessing stress radiographs. Naguib and colleagues demonstrated an overall "fair" agreement to the reliability of interpreting stress examinations and further indicated a wide variability in eye-tracking results when assessing anatomic structures during the performance of stress testing.[20] Advanced imaging modalities such as computed tomography (CT) scans are useful in evaluating bone quality, avascular necrosis, subtle fractures, intra-articular changes, joint incongruity, and the extent of any osteoarthrosis. MRI can offer the ability to assess edematous changes to osseous structures and for assessment of the surrounding soft tissue envelope.

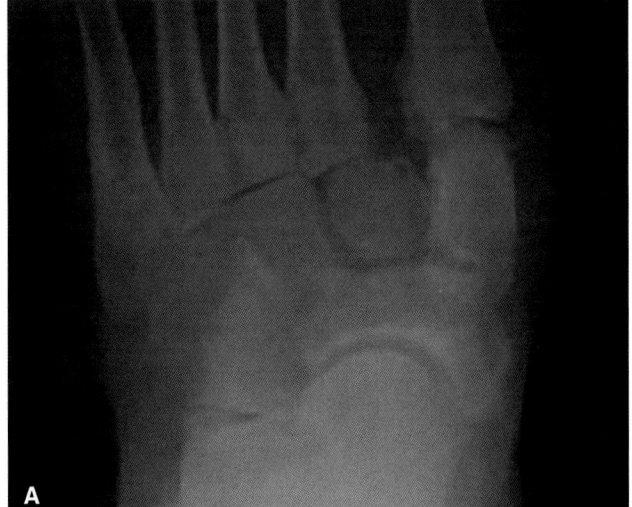
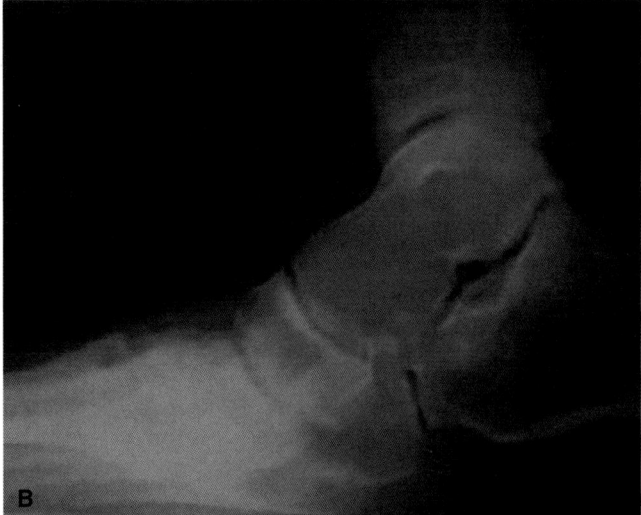

FIGURE 22.3 **A.** An AP radiograph demonstrating TMT joint instability, most notably at the second metatarsal base to intermediate cuneiform joint region. Note the lateral deviation of the medial cortex of the second metatarsal base, relative to the medial cortex of the intermediate cuneiform. **B.** Lateral radiograph demonstrating a midfoot collapse. There is combined instability of both the TMT joint and naviculocuneiform joint.

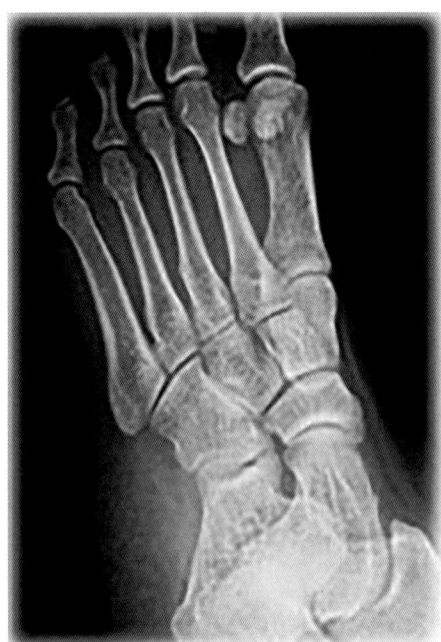

FIGURE 22.4 Note the normal alignment of the lateral cortices of second and third metatarsal bases relative to their corresponding cuneiforms. Also note the medial cortex of the fourth metatarsal base relative to the medial cortex of the cuboid.

Imaging and Diagnostic Studies

- Compare to the contralateral (uninjured) foot when feasible.
- Consider the use of advanced imaging for more detailed assessments.
- Live fluoroscopy while performing abduction/adduction forefoot stress examination.

It is always important to correlate abnormalities noted on imaging studies with patient-reported symptoms and clinical examination findings. Not all degenerative changes and/or deformity correlate with clinically appreciable symptoms and/or dysfunction.

NONOPERATIVE MANAGEMENT

TMT arthritis may be managed with conservative options, depending upon the severity of deformity. Stable Lisfranc sprains can often times mimic Lisfranc ligament rupture based on symptoms; however, stress examinations are normally negative. Nonoperative modalities can include initial immobilization, cryotherapy (for acute injuries), nonsteroidal anti-inflammatory medications (NSAIDs), injection therapy, shoe modifications, and custom-molded orthotics/braces. Orthotics ideally should act to support and accommodate the foot at the TMT joint. General recommends include a semirigid orthotics with a soft top cover. The addition of a rocker-bottom sole with an extended rigid shank (with or without a solid ankle cushion heel) can be effective during the stance phase of gait and can assist with the alleviation of pressure at the TMT joint complex. Shoes with extra depth are recommended to accommodate dorsal osteophytic prominences and avoid exacerbation of neritic symptoms. Appropriate use of orthoses and/or shoe modifications can theoretically (1) decrease compressive forces across the region of the midfoot; (2) decrease the motion through the TMT complex; (3) provide improved shock absorption; and (4) redistribute load from symptom pressure points.[21] Injections can be utilized for both diagnostic and therapeutic purposes. An important consideration when contemplating injection use is that the TMT joint region can be difficult to access in the presence of arthrosis. Local anesthetics are commonly used for diagnostic assessment. Therapeutic use of either long- or short-acting steroids are considered for temporary alleviation of symptoms. If direct injections into the joint regions prove difficult, subcapsular injections can be considered as an alternative diagnostic or therapeutic measure. Fluoroscopic guidance can be employed to assist with intra-articular (or) intracapsular needle placement. In some situations, such as the second and third tarsometatarsal/naviculocuneiform region, injecting any segment of this area will allow for the inherent articular communications to promote dispersion of the fluid throughout the region; thus, reducing the amount of injectable solution needed, and radiation exposure required for injections conducted under fluoroscopic guidance.[22,23]

SURGICAL PLANNING AND CONSIDERATIONS

Surgical management is considered when (1) conservative measures have failed; (2) the most accurate locality of TMT joint pain has been determined; and (3) concomitant malalignment has been assessed. Arthrodesis of the affected TMT joints is commonly recommended for persistent pain and/or significant deformity/instability to the TMT joint complex.

INDICATIONS FOR TMTJ-RELATED OPERATIVE INTERVENTION

- Exhausted (or) failed nonoperative treatment options
- Alleviation of symptoms with targeted diagnostic local anesthetic injections
- Concomitant malalignment
- Symptoms begin to affect quality of life or lead to compensated gait patterns
- Progressively worsening deformity leading to secondary complications
- Low to moderate risk factors for developing postoperative complications
- Preoperative counseling as to continue postoperative symptoms to a lesser extent

PERILS and PITFALLS

- Neuropathic arthropathy
- Metabolic abnormalities
- Multiple previous incisions/operative interventions
- Nerve entrapment/neuritis

Operative management of acute Lisfranc injuries can involve either primary fusion or ORIF.[24] Regardless of which surgical option is implemented, it is important to remember that anatomic reduction and stable fixation are the overall operative objective.[25,26] Coetzee and colleagues recommended Lisfranc arthrodesis when faced with either multidirectional ligamentous instability, comminuted intra-articular first or second metatarsal base fractures, or "crush"-type injuries resulting in radiographic intra-articular fractures and frank dislocation. Conversely, ORIF can be considered for more subtle (or) latent type injuries demonstrating minimal displacement, and

unidirectional (dorsally based) instability, with intact plantar ligaments[14] (Fig. 22.5A-F). "Hybrid" surgical treatment options are also possible, in which both arthrodesis and ORIF options can be implemented based on the degree of injury and instability noted on physical examination and radiographic findings.[27] In general, arthrodesis is more commonly employed for many forms of end-stage symptomatic TMTJ arthritis; Buda and colleagues noted that an overall arthrodesis nonunion

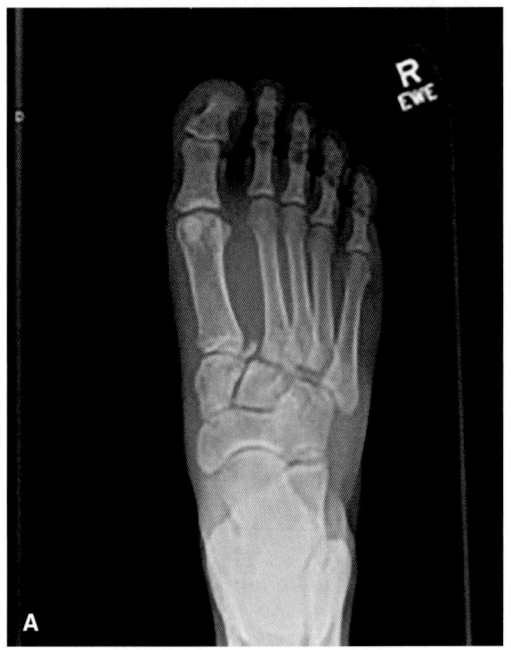

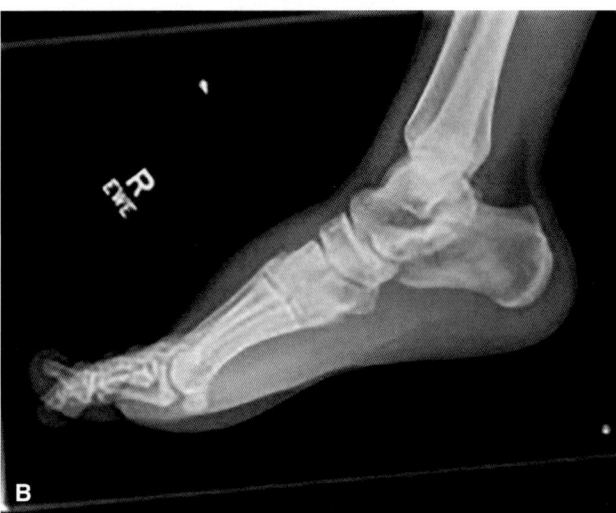

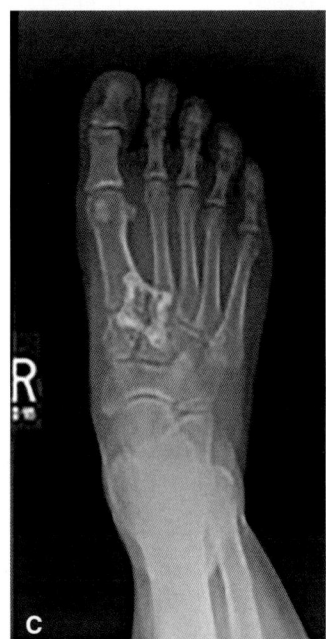

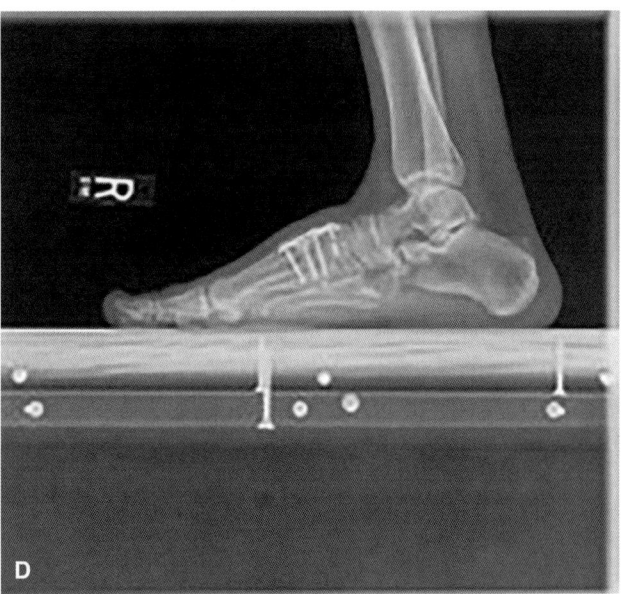

FIGURE 22.5 **A.** A 22-year-old male with an initial injury AP projection radiograph of a Lisfranc injury with a (+) fleck of the medial cuneiform and gapping between the base of the second metatarsal base and lateral aspect of the medial cuneiform. **B.** A 22-year-old male with an initial injury lateral projection radiograph of a Lisfranc injury demonstrating no frank dorsal or plantar dislocations or instability. **C.** A 22-year-old male following ORIF of a right foot Lisfranc injury. AP foot radiograph taken 4 years post-ORIF. X-rays demonstrate adequate maintenance of joint reduction. **D.** A 22-year-old male following ORIF of a right foot Lisfranc injury. Lateral foot radiograph taken 4 years post-ORIF, demonstrating maintenance of joint reduction, and broken proximal hardware.

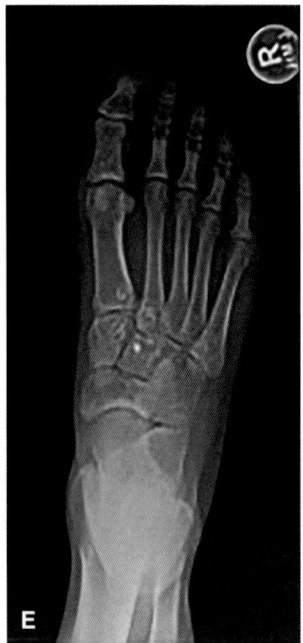
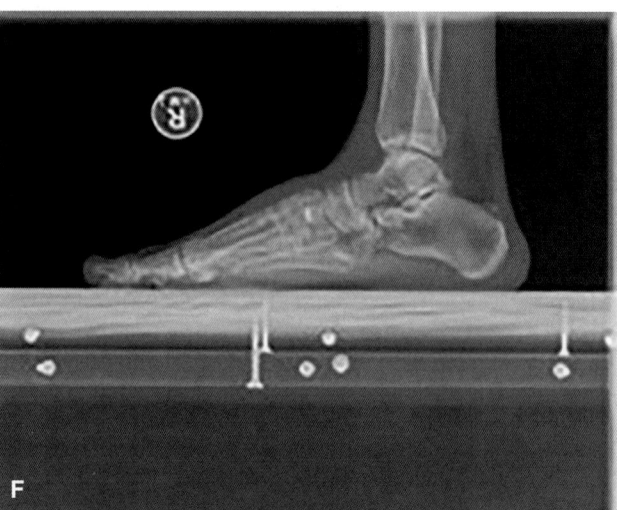

FIGURE 22.5 (*Continued*) **E.** A 22-year-old male status post 5 years from a former ORIF of a right foot Lisfranc injury and subsequent hardware removal 4 years following the initial surgery. Patient able to return to full weight-bearing activities, to include running and jumping, with 0-1/10 reported pain. **F.** Lateral foot radiograph status post 5 years from a former ORIF of a right foot Lisfranc injury and subsequent hardware removal 4 years following the initial surgery.

rate was 11.4%.[28] Global or complete arthrodesis of the TMT joint complex has limited evidence to support acceptable long-term functional outcomes.[29] Similarly, when faced with isolated lateral column pathology, arthrodesis of the lateral column alone may not consistently contribute to successful clinical outcomes.[30] Alternatives to TMTJ lateral column arthrodesis can include arthroscopic microfracture for early traumatic arthritis of the lateral TMT joints,[31] interpositional tendon arthroplasty, and metallic sphere implantation.[32,33] When TMT joint arthrodesis is accompanied with an associated deformity, then correction of the residual deformity becomes an additional consideration. Although TMT joint arthrodesis and realignment may effectively assist with improving symptoms of pain and dysfunction, complete resolution of symptoms may never truly be achieved.[34-36] Therefore, counseling patients to this fact becomes an important part of the preoperative workup.

SURGICAL TECHNIQUE CONSIDERATIONS

The procedure can be performed under intravenous sedation with a local nerve block. The use of a pneumatic tourniquet is also optional. The patient is usually placed in a supine position. The use of a preoperative Doppler may be considered to map out the dorsalis pedis artery.

positioning PEARLS
- Supine
- Ipsilateral hip bump for patients demonstrating excessive external rotation
- Operative leg on a long leg ramp (*keep the contralateral foot out of view of the lateral intraoperative fluoroscopy*)

Incisional approaches to the TMT joint region can include a medially based incision relative to the first metatarsocuneiform joint (Fig. 22.6) and a dorsal-central incision in the interval between the second and third metatarsocuneiform joint regions (Fig. 22.7). An alternative to the medially based incision, specifically when addressing Lisfranc injuries, is within the interval between the first and second metatarsocuneiform joint region. Caution should be exercised with this incision since it is in line with the deep neurovascular package, to include the deep peroneal nerve and dorsalis pedis artery (Figs. 22.8 and 22.9). The proximity of each incision when used in combination is important to keep in mind, so as to avoid multiple incisions being made too close to each other. All approaches generally provide reasonable access for joint debridement and delivery of fixation. Structures at risk can include the medial

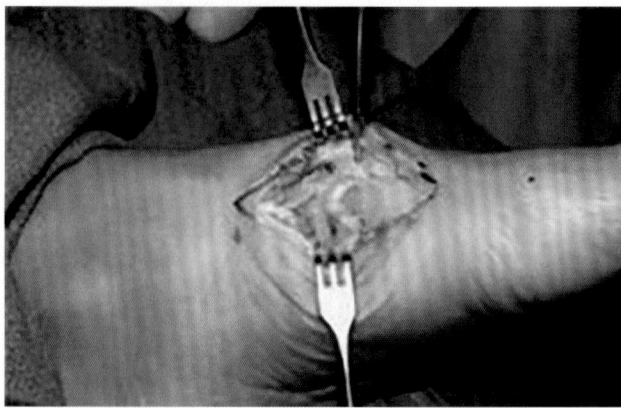

FIGURE 22.6 Medial approach to the first metatarsal base cuneiform joint. Note exposure of both the dorsal medial and plantar medial aspect of the first metatarsal base to medial cuneiform joint.

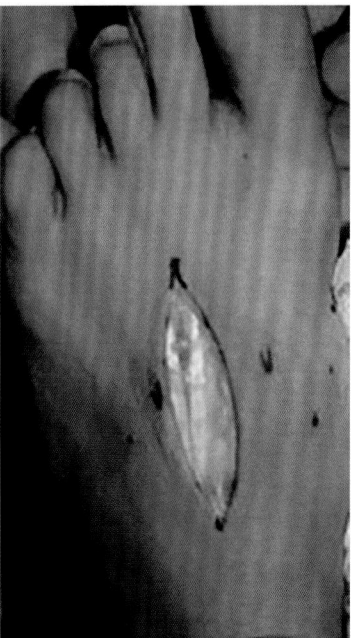

FIGURE 22.7 Dorsal approach to the TMT joint between the second and third metatarsal base region.

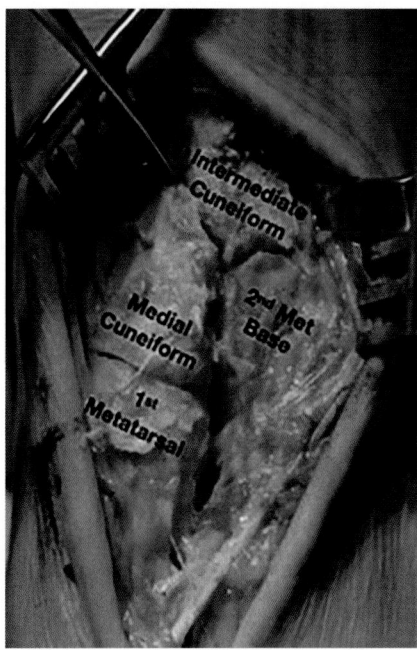

FIGURE 22.9 Alternate incision and cadaveric dissection down to the first and second metatarsal base/cuneiform joint region. Osseous and joint anatomy defining the Lisfranc complex: the base of the first metatarsal, the medial cuneiform, the base of the second metatarsal, and the intermediate cuneiform.

dorsal cutaneous nerve, the intermediate dorsal cutaneous nerve, the deep peroneal nerve, the dorsalis pedis, the extensor hallucis longus tendon, and the medial marginal vein as it joins the dorsal venous arch. A Freer elevator can be employed to identify each individual metatarsocuneiform joint (Fig. 22.10). Joint debridement may be performed with either power or hand instrumentation. Column length can be more easily

maintained, and a congruous fit more easily performed, when manual debridement with hand instrumentation is employed. Power instrumentation may be preferable with cold saline to address extensive joint arthrosis and moderate to extensive deformity correction. Close attention is afforded to the plantar surface of the joints to ensure adequate debridement of cartilage and bone. Inadequate resection of the plantar aspect of the joints can result in a dorsiflexion deformity. Manual deformity reduction becomes easier following joint resection but can be difficult with severe or long-standing fixed deformities. The use of a joint distractor may be helpful in restoring alignment in these difficult cases, especially when lateral column shortening exists secondary to previous cuboid crush injuries. Intraoperative imaging is helpful for evaluating deformity reduction in both the transverse and sagittal planes. Sagittal plane realignment is determined on the lateral projection by evaluating the

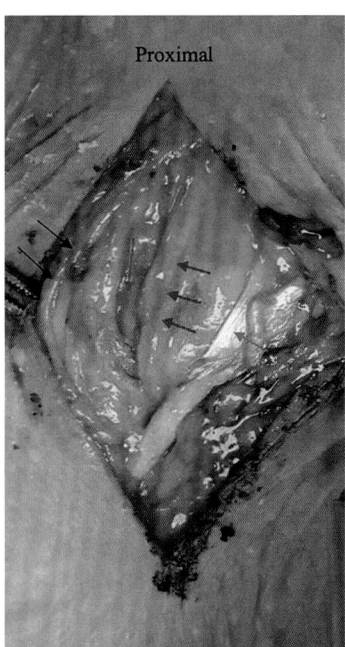

FIGURE 22.8 Alternate incision and dissection between the first and second metatarsal base/cuneiform joint region. Structures encountered from superficial to deep include the medial cutaneous nerve (*black arrows*), the extensor halluces brevis (*green arrow*), the neurovascular bundle/package (*red arrows*), and the subperiosteal layer covering the joints and osseous region (*blue arrow*).

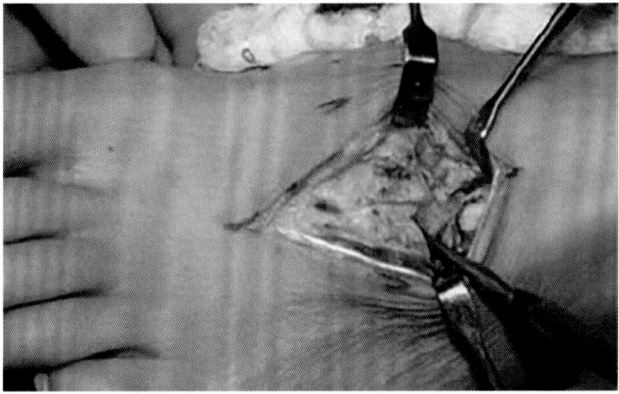

FIGURE 22.10 A Freer elevator is used here to help identify the second and third metatarsocuneiform joint.

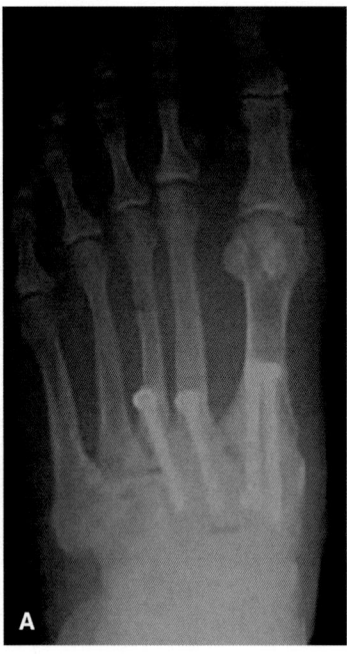

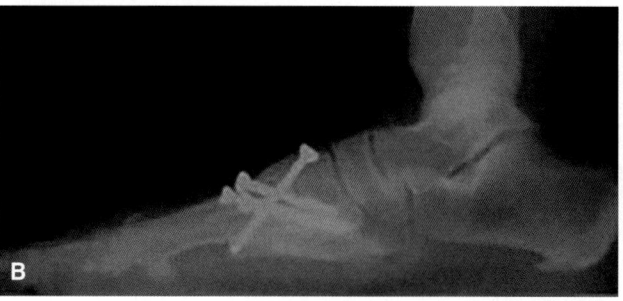

FIGURE 22.11 **A.** AP radiograph demonstrating the use of compression screw fixation of a left midfoot fusion. **B.** Lateral radiograph demonstrating the use of compression screw fixation of a left midfoot fusion.

talar-first metatarsal angle. Transverse plane re-alignment can be evaluated on an AP projection. Provisional fixation of choice is commonly utilized to maintain reduction. Fixation options for the first TMT articulation may include interfragmentary compression screws (Fig. 22.11A and B), plates (Fig. 22.12A and B), staples, or any combination thereof (Fig. 22.13A and B). External fixation may be considered when faced with lose of column length. No matter which form of fixation is selected, caution should be exercised when drilling toward the deep plantar aspects of the metatarsal base regions. Over penetration could potentially damage or interrupt blood flow in the region of the deep plantar arch.[37] Interfragmentary compression screws can be delivered in an axial fashion across the individual TMT articulations. The first TMT articulation is initially fixated, followed by the second and third, which usually moves

together as one unit. Countersinking is encouraged when screw fixation is used. Screw delivery should begin in the proximal one-third of the metatarsal shaft and extend in a proximal direction toward the plantar aspect of the corresponding cuneiform. Stress risers may develop if screw delivery is too close to the articulation. Screws can be delivered within the wound or percutaneously under image intensification. "Two screw placement" for the first TMT may be oriented from the dorsal proximal first metatarsal into the base of the medial cuneiform and the second screw from the dorsal medial cuneiform into the base of the first metatarsal. The second and third TMT joints each receive one screw oriented from the metatarsal into the corresponding cuneiform (Fig. 22.14). A supplemental screw directed from the medial cuneiform into the second metatarsal base can help maintain reduction of diastasis and also provide

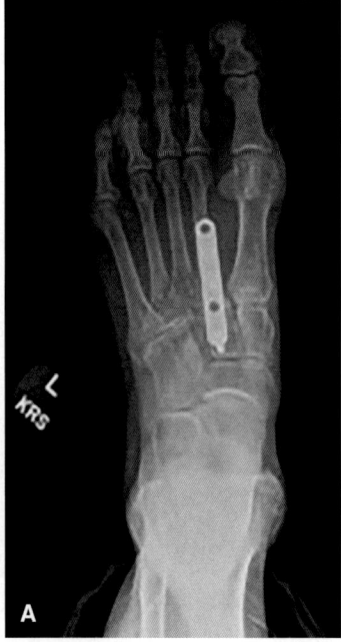

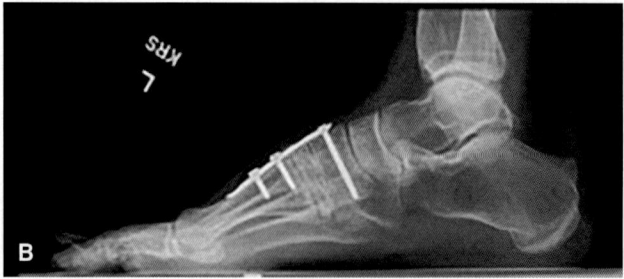

FIGURE 22.12 **A.** A 7-year follow-up AP radiograph of a 52-year-old female, demonstrating the use of dorsal plate stabilization and compression via eccentric screw placement for a left midfoot second metatarsal base to intermediate cuneiform fusion. **B.** A 7-year follow-up lateral radiograph of a 52-year-old female, demonstrating the use of dorsal plate stabilization and compression via eccentric screw placement for a left midfoot second metatarsal base to intermediate cuneiform fusion.

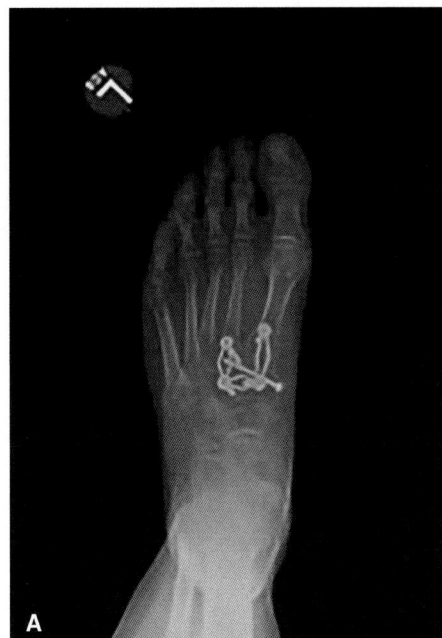

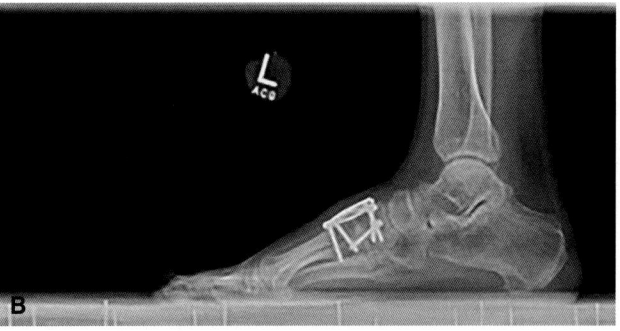

FIGURE 22.13 A. A 3-year follow-up AP radiograph demonstrating the use of a combination dorsal compression screw staple and single screw placement for a left midfoot fusion. **B.** A 3-year follow-up lateral radiograph demonstrating the use of a combination dorsal compression screw staple and single screw placement for a left midfoot fusion.

additional rigidity to the overall construct. The placement of this screw should favor the dorsal 1/3 of the region, so as to avoid injury to the deep peroneal nerve vested deep within the first interspace between the first and second metatarsals. Longer screws or plating constructs are ideal to disperse weight-bearing forces during axial loading. Any remaining defects can be packed with regional autogenous cancellous bone graft, allograft chips, or bone graft substitutes. Provisional lateral column stabilization is necessary at times to help further facilitate realignment of the medial and middle columns during arthrodesis. Pes planus deformity may require the removal of a biplanar medial-plantar–based wedge that incorporates multiple TMT joints as part of the correction.[38] The amount of wedge resection necessary for correction can be approximated preoperatively. During soft tissue closure, it is important to keep tension

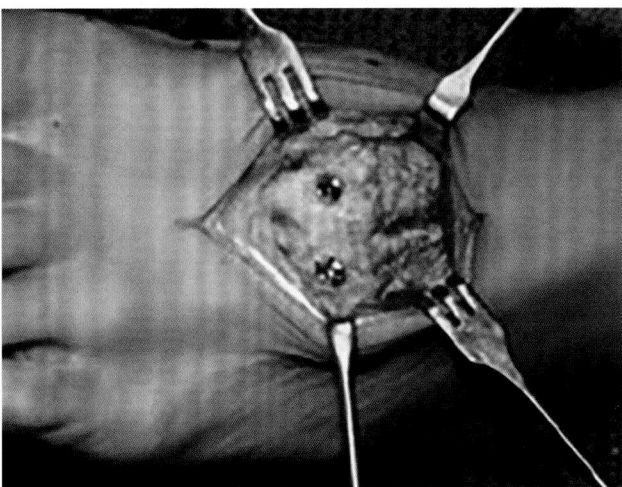

FIGURE 22.14 Demonstration of countersinking the axial screws placed for compression of the TMT joint region. Reduced prominence helps to decrease the chance of postop prominence and irritation. Also note that the distance of the final screw head placement is not close to the joint region.

off the skin edges when suturing. Ancillary procedures may include posterior muscle group lengthening, arthrodesis of the naviculocuneiform, or calcaneocuboid joints, anterior and/or posterior calcaneal displacement osteotomies, and hammer toe repair. Selection of ancillary procedures is based on the patient's individual needs and associated deformity.

POSTOPERATIVE MANAGEMENT

Patients can be placed in a standard below-knee compression dressing with a posterior splint in the immediate postop period. Postoperative neurovascular status should be monitored in sensate patients. Elevation of the leg is maintained as best as possible, until edema has resolved to a satisfactory level. Non–weight-bearing status can be maintained via the use of an assistive device (ie, crutches, four-point walker, knee scooter). Non–weight bearing is often continued for ~3-4 weeks, with eventual transition to protected weight bearing for an additional 4 weeks, or until radiographic evidence of healing is noted. Gradual return into standard shoe gear is based on continued decreases in postoperative edema and evidence of radiographic osseous consolidation. Physical therapy and rehabilitation can be incorporated for edema control, range of motion, stretching of the posterior muscle group, and gait retraining.

COMPLICATIONS

Soft tissue complications are among the most commonly experienced after TMT arthrodesis. Wound dehiscence can result with overzealous retraction, superficial skin infections, hematoma formation, or uncontrolled or prolonged postoperative edema. Skin sloughing can require debridement, local wound care, and oral antibiotics in the presence of infection. Nerve-related issues such as neuromas, neuritis, neuralgia, and entrapment can also result postoperatively. Branches of the superficial and deep peroneal nerves are within the area of correction, and injuries are at times unavoidable. Unrecognized transection of a nerve branch can result in neuroma formation. Neuralgia may develop from soft tissue dissection and overzealous retraction. Neuritis can result from entrapment within excessive fibrous scar tissue. Physical therapy modalities such as ultrasound, iontophoresis, and manual massage desensitization are useful for acute neuritis and should be initiated immediately after diagnosis of nerve complications. Surgical management of neuritis is recommended when conservative measures are unsuccessful. Malalignment or malunion can contribute to new areas of discomfort. A dorsiflexed first metatarsal can result in metatarsalgia of the lesser metatarsals. Off-loading and accommodating areas of discomfort with inserts or shoe modifications can be attempted as a nonoperative measure. Furthermore, sesamoiditis secondary to plantarflexion of the first ray has also been reported.[39] Nonunion can occur infrequently with TMT arthrodesis. Crowell and colleagues, in a systematic review, reported on a total of 443 arthrodesis, of which 16 (3.61%) were described as developing a nonunion.[40] When confronted with such a complication, patient assessments for detecting metabolic abnormalities (ie, vitamin D deficiency), tobacco use, infection, or perfusion concerns should be considered. Nonunion can be addressed with immobilization or protected weight bearing and/or the use of bone stimulators. Nonunion can be addressed surgically with revisional arthrodesis if nonoperative therapy fails or if malalignment is a continuing concern. This should include excision of scar tissue, redebridement of the bony surfaces to bleeding cancellous bone, use of autogenous bone graft, and the possible placement of both internal and external fixation constructs for better stability.

ACKNOWLEDGMENTS

Special thank you to Dr. Shine John, Dr. Alan Catanzariti, and Dr. Robert Mendicino for writing the previous Tarsometatarsal Arthrodesis chapter in the 4th Edition.

REFERENCES

1. Teng AI, Pinzur MS, Lomasney L, et al. Functional outcome following anatomic restoration of tarsal-metatarsal fracture dislocation. *Foot Ankle Int.* 2002;23(10):922-926.
2. Catanzariti AR, Mendicino RW. Technical considerations in tarsometatarsal joint arthrodesis. *J Am Podiatr Med Assoc.* 2005;95(1):85-90.
3. de Palma L, Santucci A, Sabetta SP, et al. Anatomy of the Lisfranc joint complex. *Foot Ankle Int.* 1997;18:356-364.
4. Desmond EA, Chou LB. Current concepts review: Lisfranc injuries. *Foot Ankle Int.* 2006;27(8):653-660.
5. Won HJ, Oh CS, Yoon YC. Morphologic variations of the dorsal tarsometatarsal ligaments of the foot. *Clin Anat.* 2019;32(2):212-217.
6. Peicha G, Labovitz J, Seibert FJ, et al. The anatomy of the joint as a risk factor for Lisfranc dislocation and fracture-dislocation. An anatomical and radiological case control study. *J Bone Joint Surg Br.* 2002;84(7):981-985.
7. Kura H, Luo ZP, Kitaoka HB, et al. Mechanical behavior of the Lisfranc and dorsal cuneometatarsal ligaments: in vitro biomechanical study. *J Orthop Trauma.* 2001;15:107-110.
8. Ouzounian TJ, Shereff MJ. In vitro determination of midfoot motion. *Foot Ankle Int.* 1989;10:140-146.
9. Myerson M. The diagnosis and treatment of injuries to the Lisfranc joint complex. *Orthop Clin North Am.* 1989;20:650-664.
10. Goossens M, De Stoop N. Lisfranc's fracture-dislocations: etiology, radiology, and results of treatment. A review of 20 cases. *Clin Orthop Relat Res.* 1983;176:154-162.
11. Arntz CT, Veith RG, Hansen ST. Fractures and fracture-dislocations of the tarsometatarsal joint. *J Bone Joint Surg Am.* 1988;70(2):173-181.
12. Cenatiempo M, Buzzi R, Bianco S, Iapalucci G, Campanacci DA. Tarsometatarsal joint complex injuries: a study of injury pattern in complete homolateral lesions. *Injury.* 2019; 50(suppl 2):S8-S11.
13. Ponkilainen VT, Laine HJ, Mäenpää HM, Mattila VM, Haapasalo HH. Incidence and characteristics of midfoot injuries. *Foot Ankle Int.* 2019;40(1):105-112.
14. Escudero MI, Symes M, Veljkovic A, Younger ASE. Low-energy Lisfranc injuries in an athletic population: a comprehensive review of the literature and the role of minimally invasive techniques in their management. *Foot Ankle Clin.* 2018;23(4):679-692.
15. Coetzee JC, Ly TV. Treatment of primarily ligamentous Lisfranc joint injuries: primary arthrodesis compared with open reduction and internal fixation. Surgical technique. *J Bone Joint Surg Am.* 2007;89(suppl 2 Pt.1):122-127.
16. Dubois-Ferrière V, Lübbeke A, Chowdhary A, Stern R, Dominguez D, Assal M. Clinical outcomes and development of symptomatic osteoarthritis 2 to 24 years after surgical treatment of tarsometatarsal joint complex injuries. *J Bone Joint Surg Am.* 2016;98(9): 713-720.
17. Armstrong DG, Lavery LA, Vela SA, et al. Choosing a practical screening instrument to identify patients at risk for diabetic foot ulceration. *Arch Intern Med.* 1998;148:289-292.
18. Curtis MJ, Myerson M, Szura B. Tarsometatarsal joint injuries in the athlete. *Am J Sports Med.* 1993;21(4):497-502.
19. Aronow MS. Treatment of the missed Lisfranc injury. *Foot Ankle Clin.* 2006;11(1):127-142.
20. Naguib S, Meyr AJ. Reliability, surgeon preferences, and eye-tracking assessment of the stress examination of the tarsometatarsal (Lisfranc) joint complex. *J Foot Ankle Surg.* 2019;58(1):93-96.
21. Ferris LR, Vargo R, Alexander IJ. Late reconstruction of the midfoot and tarsometatarsal region after trauma. *Orthop Clin North Am.* 1995;26(2):393-406.
22. Endo Y, Nwawka OK, Smith S, Burket JC. Tarsometatarsal joint communication during fluoroscopy-guided therapeutic joint injections and relationship with patient age and degree of osteoarthritis. *Skeletal Radiol.* 2018;47(2):271-277.
23. Hansford BG, Mills MK, Stilwill SE, McGow AK, Hanrahan CJ. Naviculocuneiform and second and third tarsometatarsal articulations: underappreciated normal anatomy and how it may affect fluoroscopy-guided injections. *AJR Am J Roentgenol.* 2019;212(4):1-9.
24. Sheibani-Rad S, Coetzee JC, Giveans MR, DiGiovanni C. Arthrodesis versus ORIF for Lisfranc fractures. *Orthopedics.* 2012;35(6):868-873.
25. Weatherford BM, Anderson JG, Bohay DR. Management of tarsometatarsal joint injuries. *J Am Acad Orthop Surg.* 2017;25(7):469-479.
26. Myerson MS. Tarsometatarsal arthrodesis: technique and results of treatment after injury. *Foot Ankle Clin.* 1996;1:73.
27. Boffeli TJ, Collier RC, Schnell KR. Combined medial column arthrodesis with open reduction internal fixation of central column for treatment of Lisfranc fracture-dislocation: a review of consecutive cases. *J Foot Ankle Surg.* 2018;57(6):1059-1066.
28. Buda M, Hagemeijer NC, Kink S, Johnson AH, Guss D, DiGiovanni CW. Effect of fixation type and bone graft on tarsometatarsal fusion. *Foot Ankle Int.* 2018;39(12):1394-1402.
29. Mulier T, Reynders P, Dereynaeker G, et al. Severe Lisfranc's injuries: primary arthrodesis or ORIF? *Foot Ankle Int.* 2002;23:902-905.
30. Raikin SM, Schon LC. Arthrodesis of the fourth and fifth tarsometatarsal joints of the midfoot. *Foot Ankle Int.* 2003;24:584.
31. Lee KB, Jeong SY. Arthroscopic microfracture for traumatic arthritis of lateral tarsometatarsal joints a case report. *J Am Podiatr Med Assoc.* 2018;108(4):344-348.
32. Russell DF, Ferdinand RD. Review of the evidence: surgical management of 4th and 5th tarsometatarsal joint osteoarthritis. *Foot Ankle Surg.* 2013;19(4):207-211.
33. Koenis MJ, Louwerens JW. Simple resection arthroplasty for treatment of 4th and 5th tarsometatarsal joint problems. A technical tip and a small case series. *Foot Ankle Surg.* 2015;21(1):70-72.
34. Sangeorzan B, Veith R, Hansen S. Salvage of Lisfranc tarsometatarsal joint by arthrodesis. *Foot Ankle Int.* 1990;10:193.
35. Mann R, Prieskorn D, Sobel M. Mid-tarsal and tarsometatarsal arthrodesis for primary degenerative osteoarthrosis or osteoarthrosis after trauma. *J Bone Joint Surg Am.* 1996;78:1376-1385.
36. Myerson MS, Fisher Burgess AR, et al. Fracture dislocations of the tarsometatarsal joints: end results correlated with pathology and treatment. *Foot Ankle.* 1986;6(5):225-242.
37. Tonogai I, Hayashi F, Tsuruo Y, Sairyo K. Distances from the deep plantar arch to the lesser metatarsals at risk during osteotomy: a fresh cadaveric study. *J Foot Ankle Res.* 2018;11:57.
38. Schon LC, Cohen I, Horton GA. Treatment of the diabetic neuropathic flatfoot. *Tech Orthop.* 2000;15:277-289.
39. Jung HG, Myerson MS, Schon LC. Spectrum of operative treatments and clinical outcomes for atraumatic osteoarthritis of the tarsometatarsal joints. *Foot Ankle Int.* 2007;28(4):482-489.
40. Crowell A, Van JC, Meyr AJ. Early weightbearing after arthrodesis of the first metatarsal-medial cuneiform joint: a systematic review of the incidence of nonunion. *J Foot Ankle Surg.* 2018;57(6):1204-1206.

CHAPTER 23

Midfoot Fractures

James Thomas and Zach Tankersley

DEFINITION

Fractures of the midfoot include fractures of the navicular, cuboid, and cuneiforms. They can occur in isolation or in various combinations. Midfoot fractures have an overall annual incidence of ~3.6/100 000 with acute traumatic navicular fractures themselves having an incidence of 1.7/10 000 yearly.[1,2] As a group, midfoot fractures account for just 10% of all foot and ankle trauma in comparison to hindfoot fractures, which account for 17%.[3] Stress fracture or acute fracture may occur, with navicular stress fracture probably being the most reported of the midfoot structures.

Acute fracture of one midfoot tarsal bone is often associated with fracture of another. In addition, they are often associated with Lisfranc injuries, as well as other lower limb, pelvic, and spine injuries.[4] Midfoot fracture and subluxations are often missed in the multitrauma patient and not identified until secondary surveys are performed. Although fractures of the midfoot may be more commonly associated with high-energy motor vehicle injuries and fall from height, fractures of the cuneiforms and tarsal-metatarsal complex are also associated with lower-energy mechanisms found in sports such as soccer, basketball, martial arts, and equestrian activities.[5]

Midfoot injuries include avulsion fractures, body fractures, and various combinations of fracture/dislocations and subluxations. Various classifications have been proposed in the past to better stratify midfoot fractures as a group as well as intra-articular fractures of the navicular.[6-8] However, many of the older classification schemes relied only on plain radiographic findings. Newer classification systems using CT findings have now been described for navicular, cuboid, and cuneiform fractures and are more helpful in defining the injury and for prognosis and treatment.[9-11]

Although stress fractures can occur in any of the bones comprising the midfoot, they seem to most commonly occur in the navicular.[12] Although the etiology of navicular stress fracture is unclear, compressive force from the talus may produce a shear type force centrally in the navicular producing a fairly consistent location of the fracture line.[13] Advanced diagnostic imaging may be needed for definitive diagnosis.

Navicular Fracture Classification[9]
- Type 1—Dorsal avulsion
- Type 2—Tuberosity
- Type 3—Fracture of the navicular with an associated Lisfranc injury
- Type 4—Fracture of the body of the navicular
- Type 5a-1—Avulsion fracture of the navicular with a lateral crush injury
- Type 5a-2—Crush fracture of the navicular with a lateral avulsion
- Type 5b—Bicolumnar fracture

Cuboid Fracture Classification[11]
- Type 1—Avulsion
- Type 2—Extra-articular
- Type 3—Intra-articular
- Type 4—Tarsometatarsal
- Type 5a—Lateral column
- Type 5b—Bicolumnar

Cuneiform Fracture Classification[10]
- Type A (1,2,3)—Injuries involving a single cuneiform
- Type B (1,2,3)—Injuries involving two cuneiforms
- Type C (1,2,3)—Injuries involving all cuneiforms

Outcome studies on navicular stress fractures have reported a return to sport in a range from 3.97 to 4.9 months in patients treated nonoperatively and 4.56-5.2 months with operative treatments.[14,15] Operative treatment was often carried out in patients with more significant fracture lines. A total of 91.9% of patients returned to their sport.[14]

Various studies have reported on the outcomes of acute navicular fractures. Evans et al. found an incidence of 43% of patients still reporting pain at follow-up of 52 weeks, and 69% of patients were able to wear normal shoes, which correlated with return to work without restriction.[16] Secondary arthritis, BMI > 35, poor fracture reduction, and pain were correlated with the inability to return to work.[17] Schmid et al. reported on 24 operatively treated navicular fractures. Outcomes were closely related to the severity of the fracture and the amount of joint involvement.[6] The quality of reduction seems to be the primary factor within surgeon control regarding the outcome of navicular fractures.[18]

Weber et al. reported good results in reconstructing the joint surfaces and lateral column length in regard to outcomes for cuboid fractures. They attributed residual symptoms usually to be related to associated midfoot injuries.[19]

Isolated fractures of the cuneiform affect the medial cuneiform most frequently. This is usually an avulsion fracture of the medial cuneiform by the anterior tibialis tendon. Isolated dislocations and fracture/dislocations involve the intermediate cuneiform 67% of the time. This is attributed to the weaker ligamentous structures.[10,19] Early osteoarthritis of the cuneonavicular joint after fracture/dislocation, but not with isolated fractures, has been reported.[20,21] Others have also observed cuneiform fractures seem to have better clinical outcomes than fracture/dislocations.[10]

INDICATIONS

- If medial midfoot injury is found, always look laterally for associated pathology. Conversely, if lateral injury is found, look medially in the midfoot for associated pathology.
- Always consider advanced imaging in the evaluation of midfoot injuries.
- Midfoot injuries are often initially overlooked or not diagnosed especially in the multitrauma patient.

ANATOMIC FEATURES

The midfoot is made up of five bones: the navicular, the medial cuneiform, the middle cuneiform, the lateral cuneiform, and the cuboid. The midfoot is bordered proximally by the transverse tarsal (Chopart's) joint and distally by the tarsal-metatarsal (Lisfranc's) joint. The midfoot bones have unique and complex morphologies. These bones are primarily cancellous with thin cortical walls. Each bone has multiple articulations and dense ligamentous attachments.

The navicular is wider dorsally and medially than it is plantarly and laterally. It is concave proximally and convex distally. Proximally it articulates with the talar head and distally with the three cuneiforms. Medially, there is a tuberosity where the tibialis posterior tendon has its primary insertion. The plantar surface is the site of the plantar calcaneonavicular (spring) ligament attachment. The dorsal surface has ligamentous attachments to each adjacent bone. These include the dorsal calcaneonavicular (medial slip of the bifurcate) ligament, the talonavicular ligament, and cuboid-navicular ligament. There are anatomic variants that involve the shape of the navicular tuberosity and the presence of an accessory navicular (os tibiale externum). These are present up to 25% of the time and 90% are bilateral.[22] Clinically, the accessory navicular is seen as a medial prominence on the foot. It can be present in one of three forms: an enlargement of the normal tuberosity, an extra bone with a flat articulation to the navicular tuberosity via a synchondrosis, and a true extra bone completely separated from the navicular. The latter two forms may be mistaken for fracture.

The cuboid articulates proximally with the anterior calcaneus via a saddle-shaped joint. It articulates distally with the fourth and fifth metatarsals. It articulates medially with the lateral cuneiform. There is a groove located on the undersurface of the cuboid, known as the peroneal groove, over which the peroneal longus tendon passes. The dorsal calcaneocuboid ligament (lateral slip of the bifurcate ligament) attaches dorsally. Plantar ligamentous attachments include the plantar calcaneocuboid (short plantar) ligament and the deep fibers of the long plantar ligament.

Each cuneiform articulates with the navicular proximally though an individual facet. Distally, the medial cuneiform articulates with the first metatarsal, the middle cuneiform articulates with the second metatarsal, and the lateral cuneiform articulates with the third metatarsal. The cuneiforms are wedge-shaped bones. The medial cuneiform has partial tendon insertions from the tibialis posterior, the peroneus longus, and the tibialis anterior. The middle and lateral cuneiforms also have partial insertions from the tibialis posterior tendon. Ligamentous attachments include the dorsal and plantar tarsometatarsal ligaments and the dorsal and plantar intercuneiform ligaments. The Lisfranc ligament also attaches the medial cuneiform to the second metatarsal.

The tibialis posterior tendon is the only tendon that has insertional attachments on all five bones of the midfoot. Its primary insertion site is the navicular tuberosity. It also extends plantarly and has insertions on the three cuneiforms, the medial metatarsals, and at times even the cuboid.

The midfoot gets its blood supply from the dorsalis pedis and the posterior tibial arteries. In particular, the navicular gets dorsal inflow from the dorsalis pedis artery and plantar inflow primarily from the medial plantar artery.[22,23] This anatomy leads to good peripheral perfusion, but relatively poor central perfusion of the navicular body. Clinically, this could explain decreased healing rates of fractures in the middle third of the navicular bone.[12,24] There are numerous small dorsal penetrating arteries, which if damaged by injury or surgery, predisposes the navicular to avascular changes.

FUNCTIONAL ANALYSIS OF THE ANATOMY

The dense ligamentous attachments of the midfoot have led many to think of the inclusion of the midfoot in terms of anatomic columns. The columns that include the midfoot have been described in two ways: a two-column version and a three-column version. The two-column version consists of a medial longitudinal column (talus, navicular, all three cuneiforms, and the first, second, and third metatarsals) and a lateral longitudinal column (calcaneus, the cuboid, and the fourth and fifth metatarsals).[25] The three-column version consists of the medial column (navicular, medial cuneiform, and first metatarsal), a middle column (middle cuneiform, lateral cuneiform, and the second and third metatarsals), and a lateral column (calcaneus, cuboid, and the fourth and fifth metatarsals).[26]

The rigidity created by the anatomy of the medial column lends itself to providing a strong lever arm that is necessary during the stance and push-off phases of the gait cycle. Conversely, the lateral column is anatomically designed to have greater mobility. This allows the forefoot to accommodate to various walking surfaces.

The bones and joints of the midfoot have limited motion and very few tendon attachments. However, they are extremely important in the overall function of the foot. The midfoot provides a biomechanical connection between the forefoot and the hindfoot. Changes in the integrity of this connection will affect the anatomic relationship of the forefoot to the hindfoot. Therefore, its structural integrity must be maintained for normal foot function to occur.[27]

PHYSICAL EXAMINATION

Examination of the patient with a suspected midfoot fracture begins with a total body survey as these fractures are often associated with other areas of injury, especially in the multi-trauma patient.[4] Once more emergent or life-threatening injuries have been ruled out or addressed, examination of the midfoot starts with evaluating for any gross deformity being present, which is indicative of dislocation or subluxation of midfoot structures. Foot deformity almost always requires shortening of either the medial and/or lateral columns. If deformity is present, one must look for any tenting of the skin or neurovascular compromise, which may necessitate emergent reduction. Doppler ultrasound may be required in assessing pulses secondary to swelling of the midfoot. In particular, the dorsalis pedis artery competency should be assured as this is the most vulnerable vascular structure in midfoot injuries. One should also test for intact superficial peroneal nerve branches in the zone of injury. Care is taken to check for proper function of the peroneal, extensor, and anterior/posterior tibial tendons. In particular, entrapment and/or compromise of the anterior tibial tendon may occur with medial column injuries. Skin must be evaluated for any compromise including abrasions or punctures and gross defects, which require open fracture protocols and possible planning for eventual soft tissue coverage. Plantar ecchymosis often indicates injury to the cuneiforms. Evaluation and monitoring for compartment syndrome should always be undertaken as injury to these areas of the foot can be associated with increased compartment pressures.

IMAGING AND DIAGNOSTIC STUDIES

Imaging of suspected midfoot fractures always starts with standard AP, oblique, and lateral views of the foot. Radiographs should be done non–weight bearing initially to prevent further displacement of possible fractures/subluxations. If minimal or no pathology is appreciated on initial non–weight-bearing views, and if the patient's symptoms allow, weight-bearing views may be considered to act as stress views to evaluate for midfoot instability. Contralateral views of the normal foot are often very beneficial for comparison. A lateral oblique view may allow for improved medial column evaluation. Care should be taken in examining for associated Lisfranc injury.

CT scan should be considered for any displaced midfoot fracture or even in nondisplaced fractures where other associated injury is suspected but not seen on plain radiographs. Indeed, CT examination often times reveals fractures in the radiographically negative midfoot injury especially along the plantar aspect of the cuneiforms. Thin cuts should be performed to not miss subtle fractures and subluxations.

MRI evaluation of midfoot injuries is beneficial in two areas. One is in the diagnosis of suspected tendon injury, especially of the anterior tibial and peroneal tendons. The other is in the definitive diagnosis of suspected stress fracture of the midfoot, in particular of the navicular. Nuclear medicine imaging may also be of benefit in this area.

TREATMENT OF NAVICULAR FRACTURES

Stress fractures of the navicular may be treated nonoperatively with a period of non–weight-bearing immobilization. Operative treatment for displaced and nonunited navicular stress fractures is indicated, possibly with bone grafting.[12,15] Operative intervention for navicular stress fracture is also considered in the treatment of the high-performance athlete.[14]

Acute fractures of the navicular include avulsion fractures, fractures of the body, and crush type injuries with or without joint dislocation/subluxation. Restoration and maintenance of medial column length is paramount. One must always look for associated lateral column injury or cuneiform injury with any fracture of the navicular. As in all fractures of the midfoot, if open treatment is required, care must be taken to allow for soft tissue recovery to occur prior to surgery.

Nondisplaced avulsion fractures of the medial aspect of the navicular may be treated nonoperatively with short leg casting/immobilization for 6-8 weeks with some of this time spent non–weight bearing. Displaced medial avulsion fractures require operative management not only to restore osseous continuity but also to avoid dysfunction of the posterior tibial tendon. Simple screw fixation is usually sufficient. Although not common, these fractures may be associated with navicular cuneiform subluxation (Fig. 23.1A-D). Small displaced medial avulsion

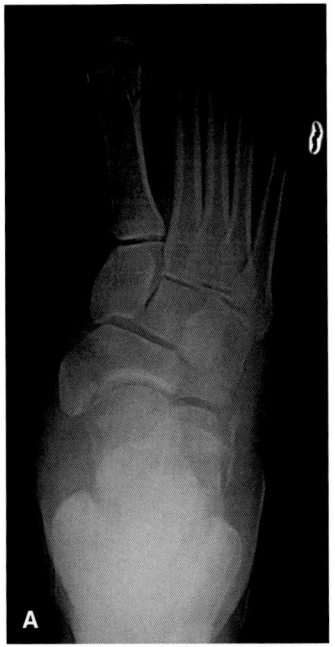

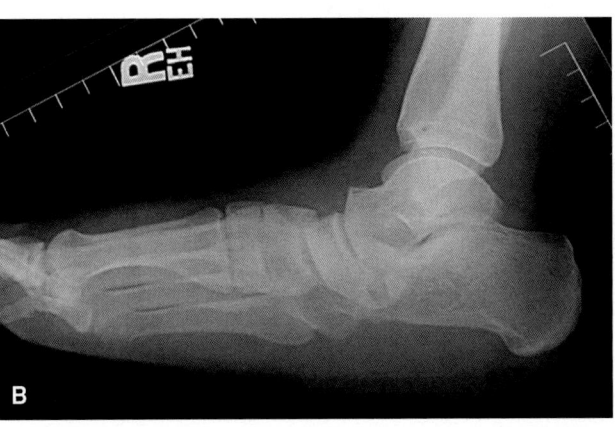

FIGURE 23.1 A, B.
AP and lateral views of medial tuberosity avulsion navicular fracture with navicular cuneiform subluxation.

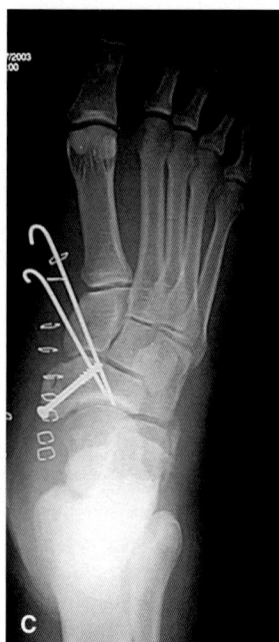

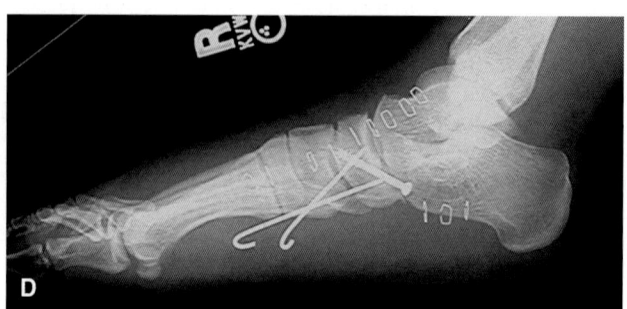

FIGURE 23.1 (*Continued*) **C, D.** AP and lateral postreduction views of single screw fixation of navicular tuberosity fracture with Kirschner wire fixation of navicular cuneiform subluxation.

fractures not large enough to accept fixation may be excised with securing of the posterior tibial tendon to the medial navicular with bone anchors if necessary. Incisional approach over the medial navicular is sufficient (Fig. 23.2).

Dorsal avulsion fractures of the navicular most often result from midfoot sprain type injuries, often with hyperflexion mechanisms. Small nondisplaced dorsal avulsion fractures can be treated nonoperatively with immobilization in a cast or walking boot. Small displaced fractures with little joint involvement may be treated with simple excision if they are symptomatic (Fig. 23.3A and B). Larger intra-articular dorsal avulsion fractures many times warrant open reduction and internal fixation. CT examination is helpful as often times fragment size is underestimated on plain radiographs. The author prefers absorbable pin fixation for these fractures as the fracture fragment shape

and articular involvement often makes small screw fixation difficult (Figs. 23.4A-C and 23.5).

Navicular body fractures are by definition intra-articular fractures of two joints (talonavicular and cuneonavicular joints) and anatomic reduction of this fracture type is required. Navicular body fractures range from simple two-part fractures to three or four-part fractures or crush type fractures. Joint dislocation or subluxation may be present.

Two-part navicular body fractures may be treated nonoperatively if 1 mm or less of displacement is confirmed on CT examination. Immobilization for 8 weeks or longer may be required until fracture healing occurs with much of this time spent non–weight bearing. If greater displacement is present, then reduction and fixation is required. Large reduction bone clamps are beneficial in aiding reduction. One or two screw fixation is usually sufficient. Either medial to lateral or lateral to medial screw direction may be used depending on the location of the larger fragment to allow proper screw thread purchase (Figs. 23.6A and B and 23.7A-E). Incisional approach is either just medial to the anterior tibial tendon or between the EHL and EDL tendons depending on need for exposure and fixation (Fig. 23.8). Occasionally, talonavicular joint subluxation may occur with two-part body fractures. In this case, Kirschner wire fixation may be used to accomplish both fracture fixation and joint stabilization (Fig. 23.9A-D). Percutaneous reduction and fixation may be considered in select cases of minimal displacement with no soft tissue interposition.

Three or more part fractures almost always require open reduction and internal fixation secondary to fracture fragment displacement and joint incongruity. Open reduction and internal fixation may need to be delayed secondary to condition of the soft tissues. Distraction via external fixation or other forms may be necessary to obtain proper medial column length. External fixation may be left in place in combination with internal fixation for added stability (Fig. 23.10). Indeed, external

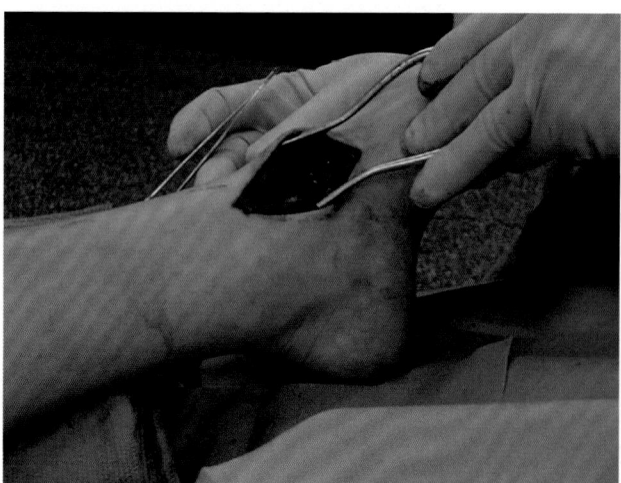

FIGURE 23.2 Medial incisional approach to navicular fracture.

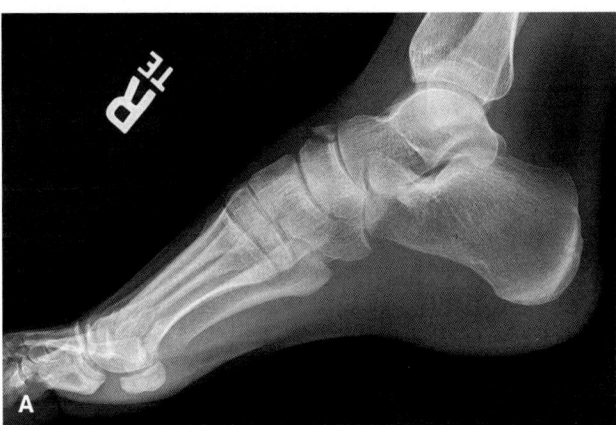
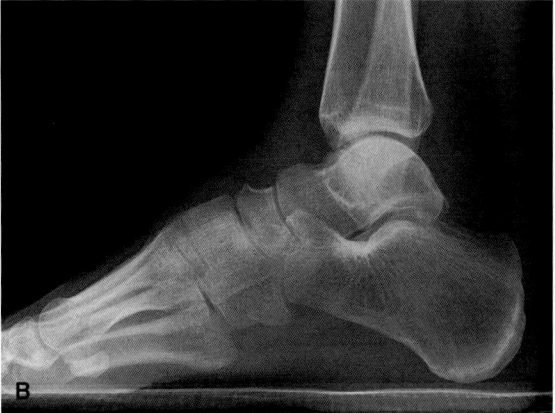

FIGURE 23.3 **A, B.** Pre- and postop views of dorsal navicular avulsion fracture treated with excision of fragment.

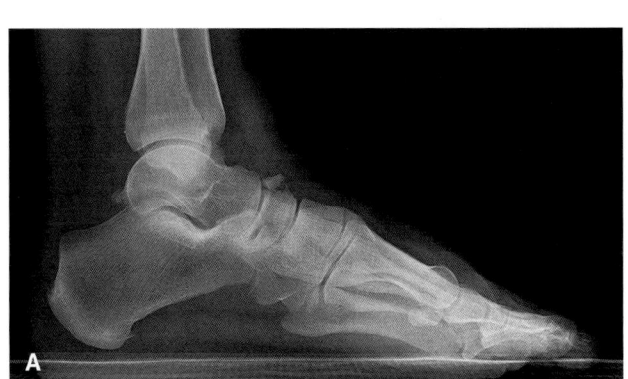
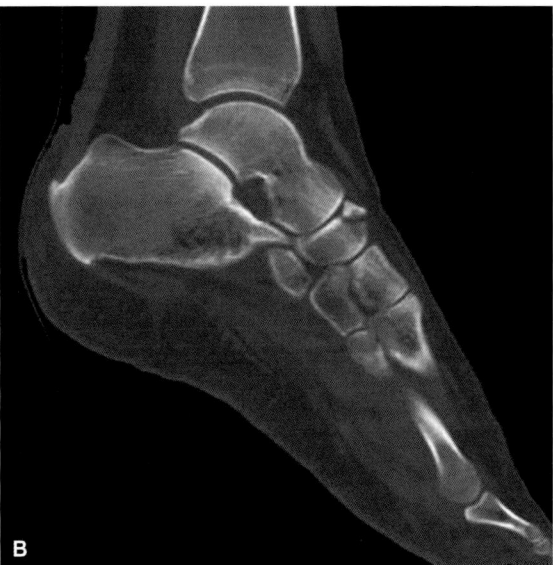

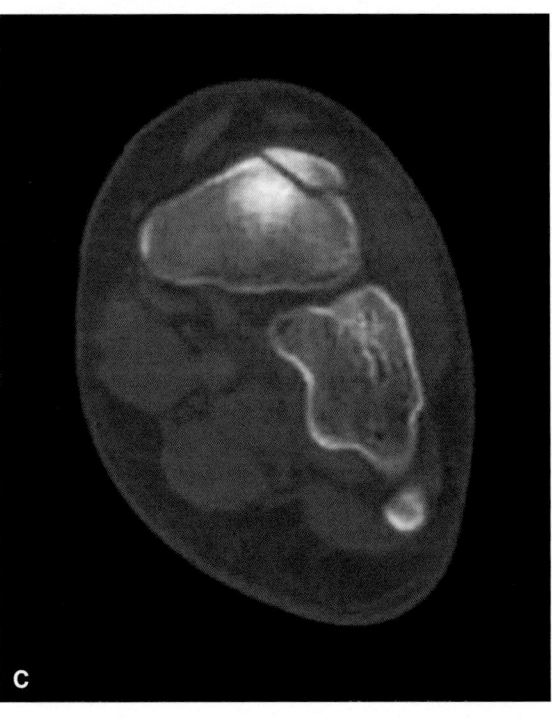

FIGURE 23.4 **A-C.** Lateral view and sagittal and coronal plane CT scans of dorsal avulsion navicular fracture. Fragment size is often underestimated on the sagittal cut.

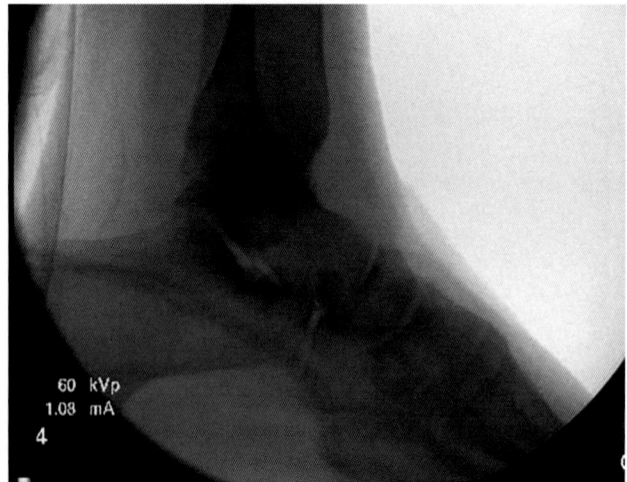

FIGURE 23.5 Intraop view of fracture fixated with absorbable fixation.

fixation may be used in isolation or with percutaneous fixation in cases of significant soft tissue compromise. Medial and lateral external fixation may be required if lateral column injury is also present (Fig. 23.11A and B). Alternatively, if open reduction and internal fixation must be delayed secondary to soft tissue condition or edema, initial reduction and fixation can be achieved by external fixation and percutaneous pin fixation, followed by postreduction CT examination. This often allows for better fracture evaluation and surgical planning. Significant plantar comminution is often seen on CT, not appreciated on plain radiographs (Fig. 23.12A-F). The author's preferred fixation method is 2 screw (3.5 or 4.0) fixation of the major fragments with smaller fixation used as supplement if necessary (Fig. 23.13A-C). Specialty plates may be considered but must be used with caution as placement of the plates may require excessive dorsal soft tissue stripping and subsequent vascular

compromise to the navicular body. Both medial and lateral incisions as previously described may be required for adequate reduction and fixation. Care must again be taken to minimize dissection over the dorsal navicular between the two incisions to prevent vascular injury to the navicular.

Crush injuries of the navicular body particularly with dislocation may only be amenable to external fixation with Kirschner wire or limited screw fixation. Restoration of medial column length must be performed. Reducing larger fragments first will aid in, or produce, reduction of smaller fragments secondary to ligamentotaxis (Fig. 23.14A-F). Primary arthrodesis may also be an alternative with crush type or highly comminuted fractures of the navicular body. Spanning plates of the medial column may be considered for highly comminuted navicular body fractures or in cases of significant bone loss from open injuries. One may span from the talus to the first metatarsal depending upon associated medial column injuries. Rotational flaps to the medial aspect of the midfoot may be accomplished for soft tissue coverage (Figs. 23.15A-C and 23.16). Dislocation of the talonavicular joint may occur often associated with small fracture fragments dorsally. Associated injuries are common. Closed reduction after musculoskeletal relaxation, along with temporary pinning to maintain reduction, is performed. Occasionally, soft tissue interposition may necessitate open reduction. These patients must also be monitored for long-term arthritic changes (Fig. 23.17A-D).

TREATMENT OF CUBOID FRACTURES

Fractures of the cuboid include simple avulsion fractures, usually of the bifurcate ligament, or compression or shear type fractures of the cuboid body with or without joint involvement and lateral column shortening. They often occur in combination with other fractures of the midfoot.

Avulsion fractures can usually be treated nonoperatively or with excision if symptomatic. Care must be taken since this

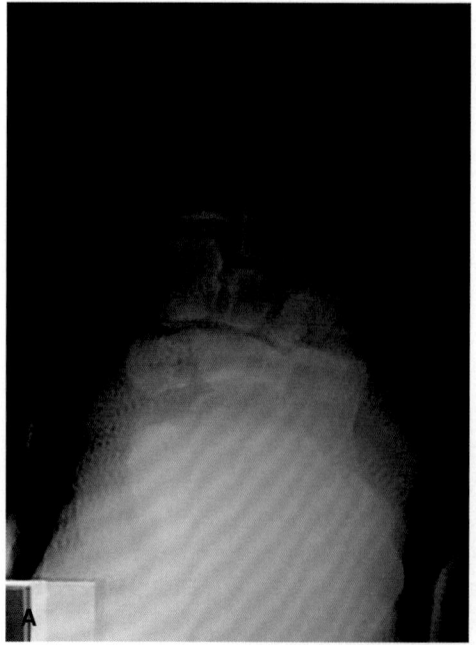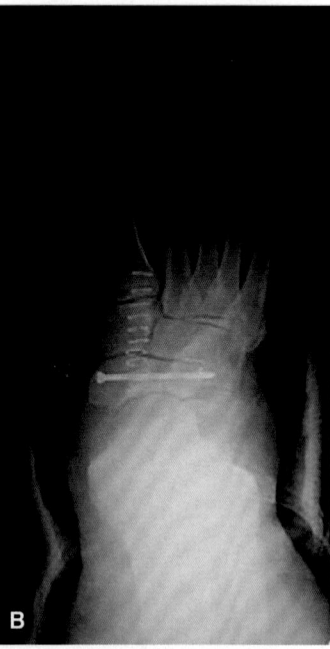

FIGURE 23.6 A. Navicular body fracture with medial-central fracture line location. **B.** Medial to lateral directed screw for fracture fixation.

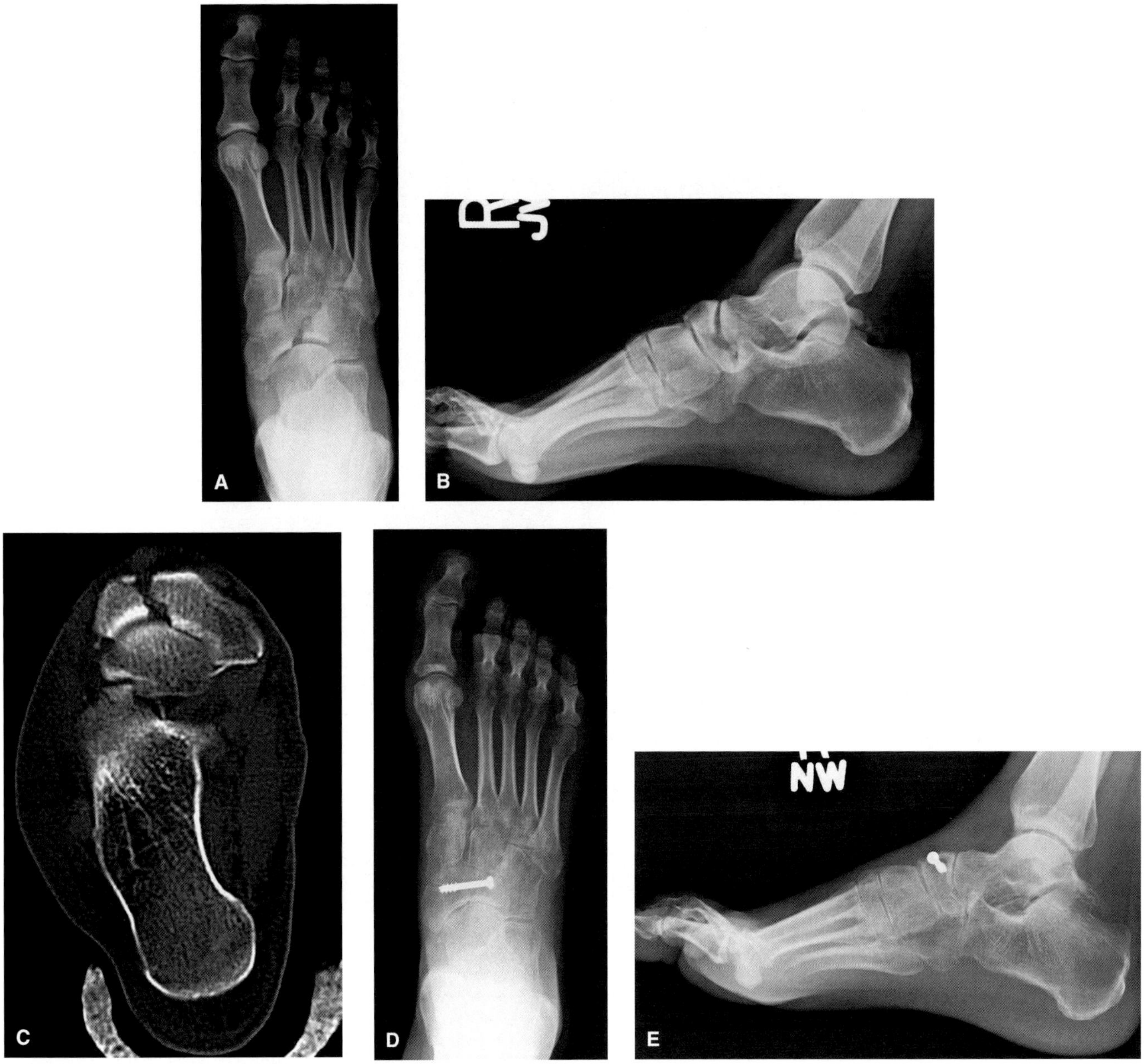

FIGURE 23.7 **A-C.** AP, lateral, and CT views of more laterally placed fracture line through navicular body. **D, E.** AP and lateral views of same fracture treated with lateral to medial screw.

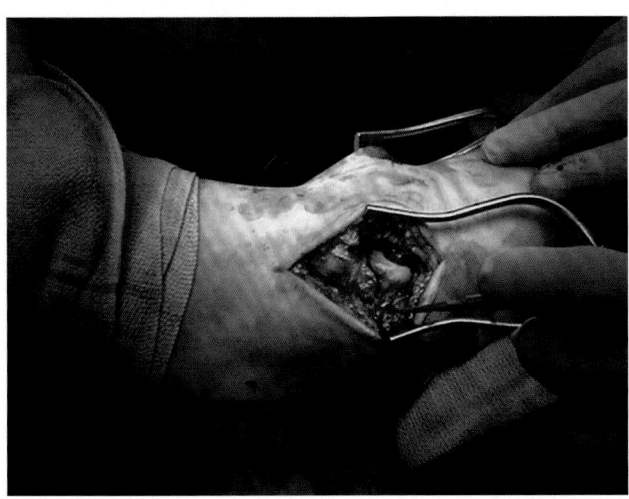

FIGURE 23.8 Lateral incisional approach for navicular body fracture. Note talar neck fracture is also present, which can be accessed through this same incision.

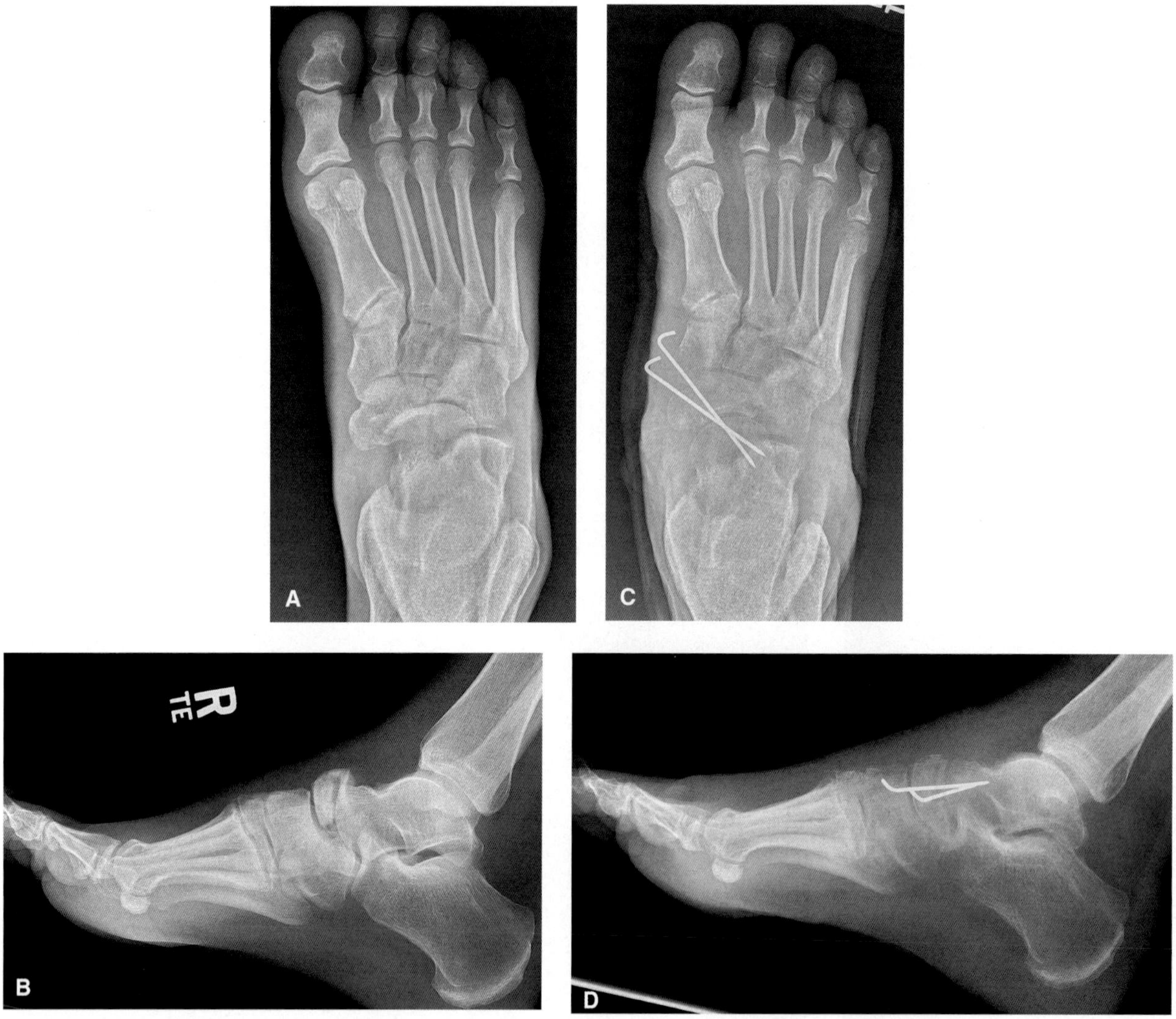

FIGURE 23.9 A, B. Preop AP and lateral views of navicular body fracture with dorsal subluxation. **C, D.** Postop AP and lateral views of Kirschner wire fixation of fracture as well as fixation of dorsal subluxation at the talonavicular joint.

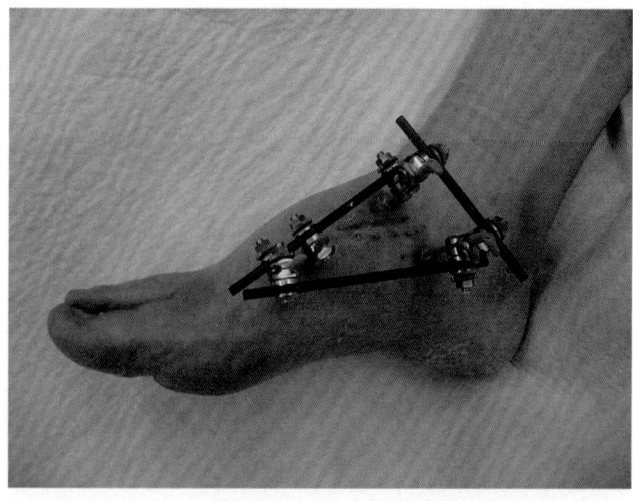

FIGURE 23.10 Example of small medial external fixator for added stability for a navicular body fracture.

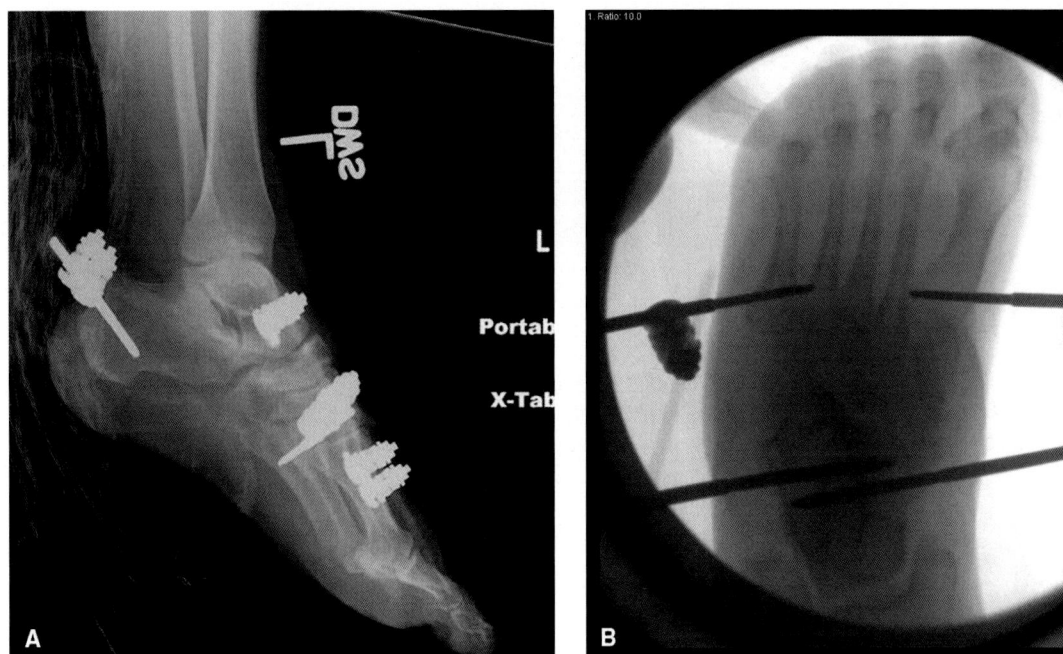

FIGURE 23.11 A, B. Examples of medial and lateral column external fixation for navicular body fracture associated with lateral column injury. External fixation may be only used to assist fracture reduction or left in place as primary or secondary fixation.

injury may be associated with ligamentous compromise to the midfoot complex in general, and proper immobilization of this injury must by undertaken.[7] This may include 6-8 weeks of immobilization/bracing and activity restriction.

Since cuboid body fractures commonly result from a compression mechanism, they may result in significant lateral column shortening. Fractures of the cuboid body may involve the calcaneal cuboid joint and/or the cuboid articulations with the

fourth and fifth metatarsals. Compromise of the peroneal longus groove may also occur. In addition to plain radiographs, CT examination is highly recommended in these fractures for better evaluation of joint congruency and degree of central body depression. Comparison contralateral radiographs are also beneficial when evaluating lateral column length. Nondisplaced cuboid body fractures without lateral column shortening may be treated with 6-8 weeks of immobilization with an

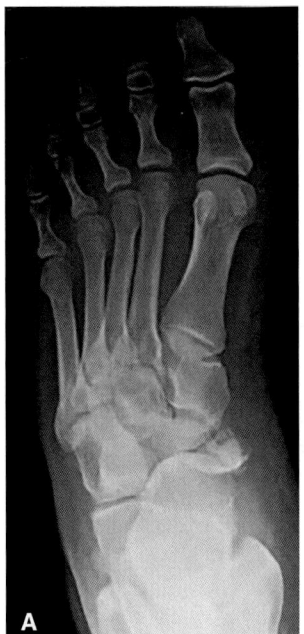

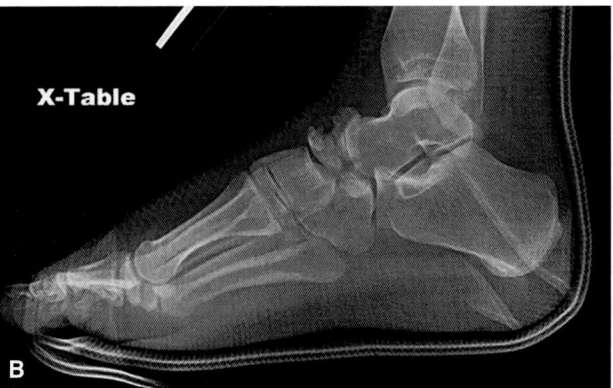

FIGURE 23.12 A-C. AP and lateral views and CT view of comminuted navicular fracture.

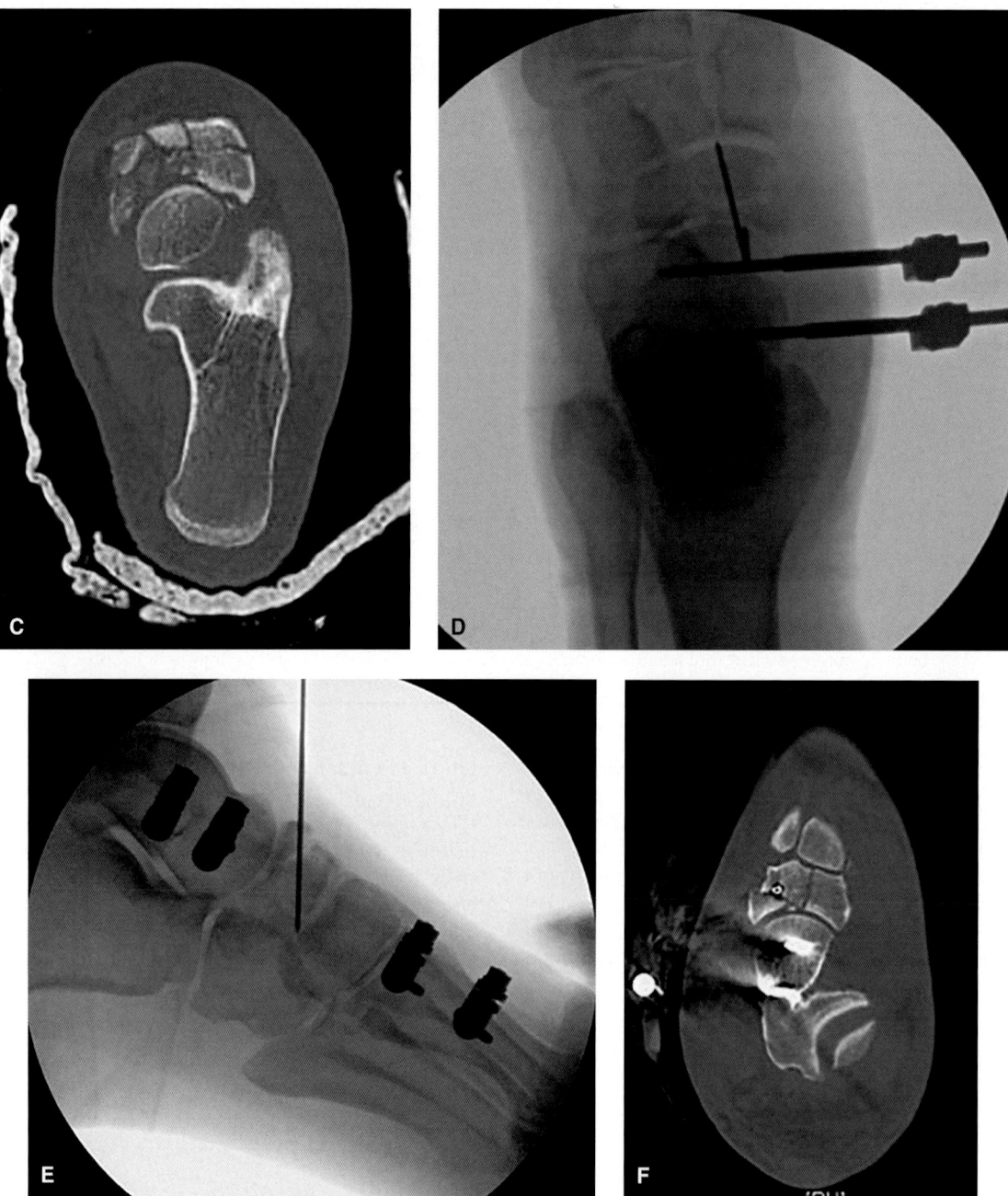

FIGURE 23.12 (*Continued*) **D-F.** AP and lateral and CT views of postreduction of same fracture with only medial external fixator and single Kirschner wire.

initial period of non–weight bearing utilized. It has been recommended that operative management is required for fractures with a more than 1 mm of joint incongruency and more than 3 mm of lateral column shortening.[28] Condition of the soft tissues may mandate delay in open treatment. Elevation of depressed articular fragments should be performed and noticeable lateral column shortening corrected. Bone grafting may be required to maintain reduction of depressed fragments and to fill voids after restoring length back to the body. Manual distraction with external fixation pins or other distraction devices are usually required to restore length to the lateral column. External

fixation may be used to not only restore length but also to serve as the primary form of fracture fixation (Fig. 23.18A and B). Bridge plating is very effective in cases of calcaneal cuboid joint involvement with comminution, as displaced intra-articular cuboid fracture fragments can be "templated" to the distal noninjured articular calcaneal surface. These can then be removed after fracture healing has occurred (Fig. 23.19A-D). Specialty plates designed to conform to the shape of the cuboid can also be utilized for fixation (Fig. 23.20A-C). At times body fractures may present with 2 primary fragments often associated with a longitudinal splint. Screw fixation with or without

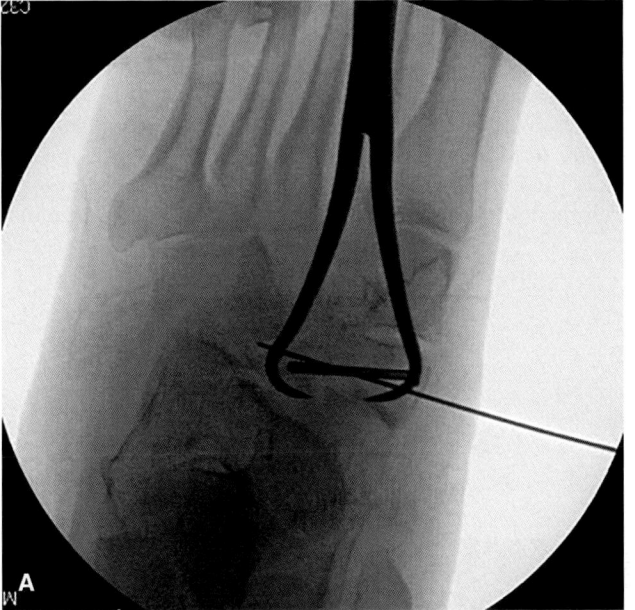

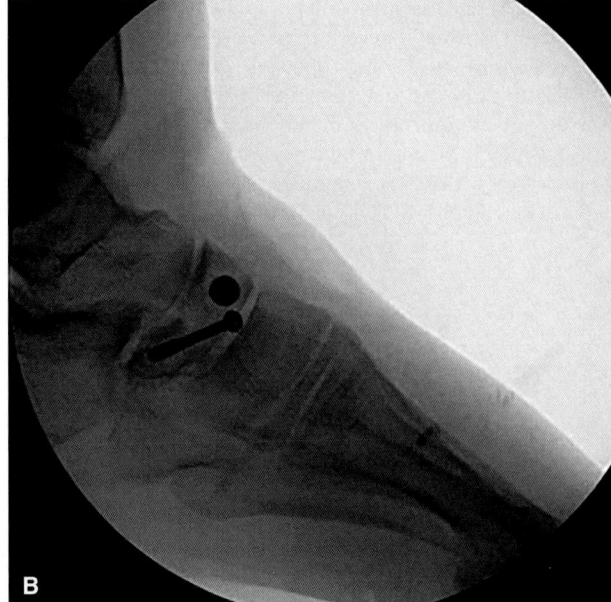

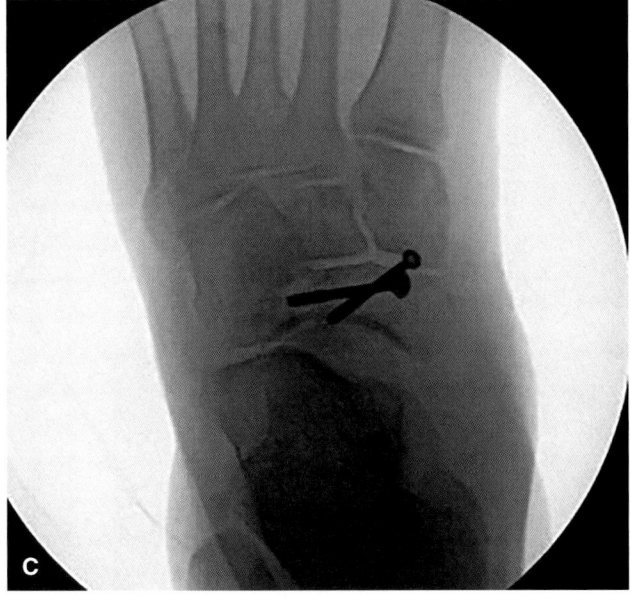

FIGURE 23.13 A-C. Reduction sequence of same fracture from Figure 23.12 with bone forceps and final 2 screw construct.

bone grafting may be sufficient in these cases (Fig. 23.21A-C). It can be quite difficult to achieve exposure for proper reduction and fixation if one of the fragments is comprised of only the most plantar, medial aspect of the cuboid. Kirschner wire fixation may be the most effective form of fixation in this instance if reduction is obtainable. In this situation, primary arthrodesis may also be an alternative especially if comminution is present. Finally, dislocation of the cuboid, although rare, can occur. Relocation of the body almost always requires distraction of the lateral column. Rail-type external fixation devices or other distraction devices are effective for distraction to aid in reduction, and external fixation devices can then be left in place for primary fixation, with or without Kirschner wire supplementation (Fig. 23.22A-D).

TREATMENT OF CUNEIFORM FRACTURES

Fracture of the cuneiforms can occur in isolation or in combination with navicular and Lisfranc injuries as well as cuboid fractures. Subluxation and/or dislocation of the tarsal metatarsal or navicular cuneiform joints may occur. Isolated fractures of the cuneiforms affect the medial cuneiform in most cases from traction of the anterior tibial tendon.[10] CT examination of cuneiform fractures is recommended in most cases to allow for proper evaluation, especially of the plantar aspect of the cuneiforms.

Nondisplaced fractures of the cuneiforms with joint congruency may be treated nonoperatively with immobilization and initial non–weight bearing for 6-8 weeks. Secondary to the anatomy and wedge-like arrangement of the cuneiforms, operative treatment is usually necessary to accomplish reduction of displaced fractures with or without join subluxation or dislocation. Restoration and maintenance of the medial column is usually the most important with cuneiform fractures. Two-part fractures, which most commonly involve the medial cuneiform, may be treated with screw fixation if fracture fragment size is sufficient (Fig. 23.23A-E). One must assure there has not been

compromise of the anterior tibial tendon insertion with fractures of the medial cuneiform. Cuneiform dislocation most commonly occurs in a dorsal direction, but plantar dislocation has been reported.[29] Oblique radiographs of the foot and ankle often give the best views of the dislocated cuneiform. Relocation of the dislocated cuneiform is usually successful with open treatment to remove any interposed soft tissue, followed by manual distraction of the forefoot. Kirschner wire fixation in multiple

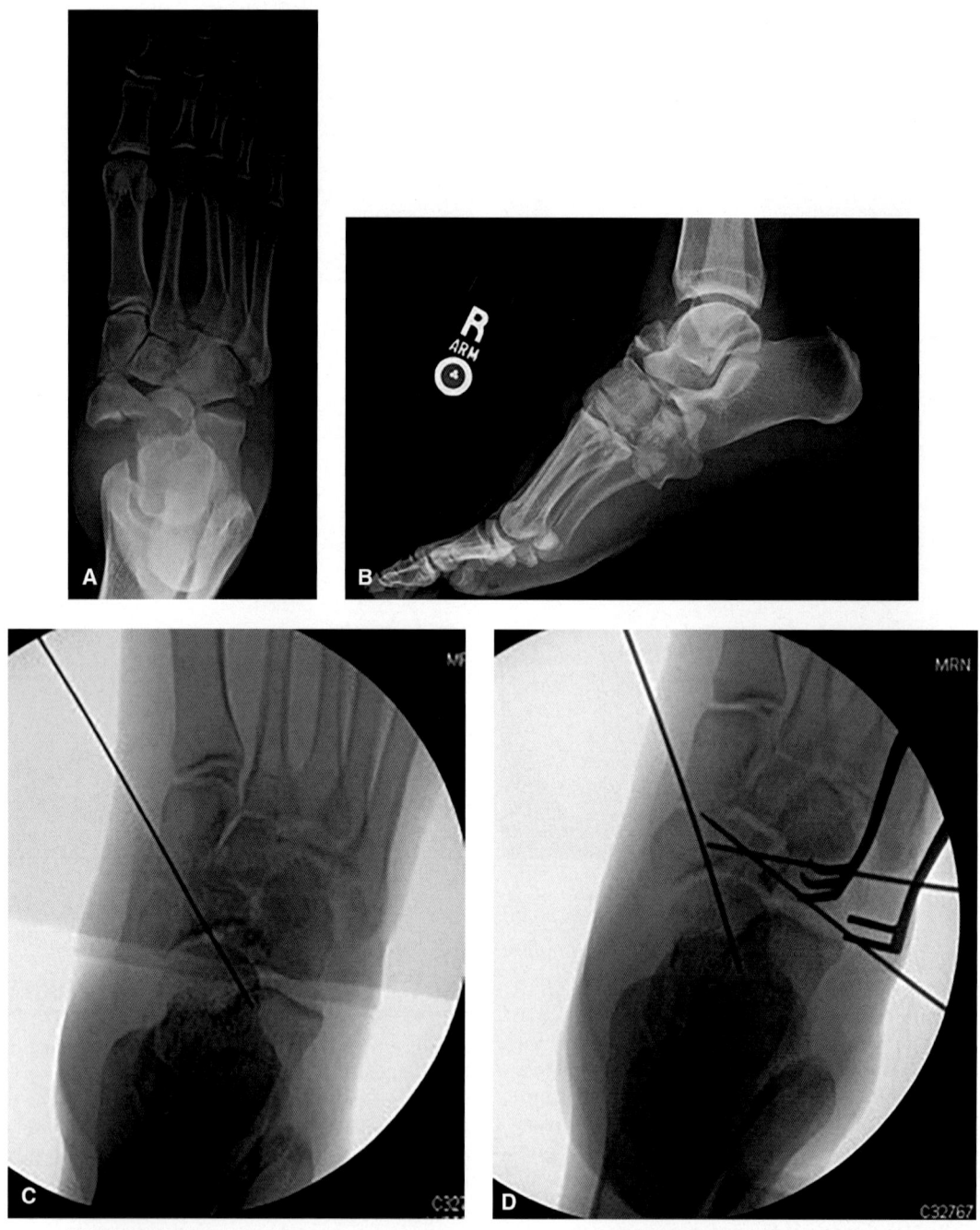

FIGURE 23.14 A-E. Reduction sequence of navicular crush injury with dislocation and associated lateral column injury. Reducing larger fragments/dislocations first aids reduction via ligamentotaxis.

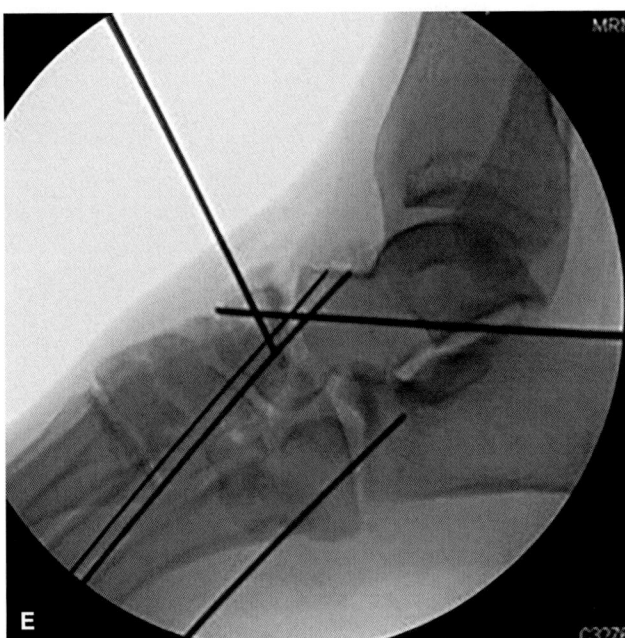
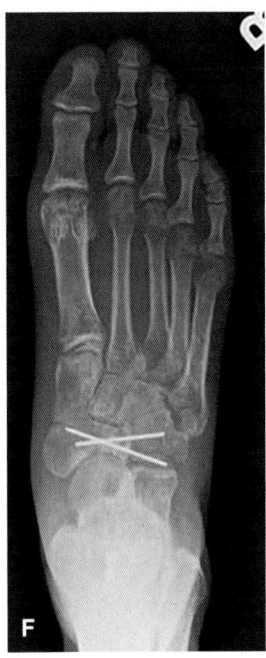

FIGURE 23.14 (*Continued*) **F.** Long-term postop AP view of same patient after partial removal of fixation. Some loss of lateral column length is present, which is a common complication of both column crush injury.

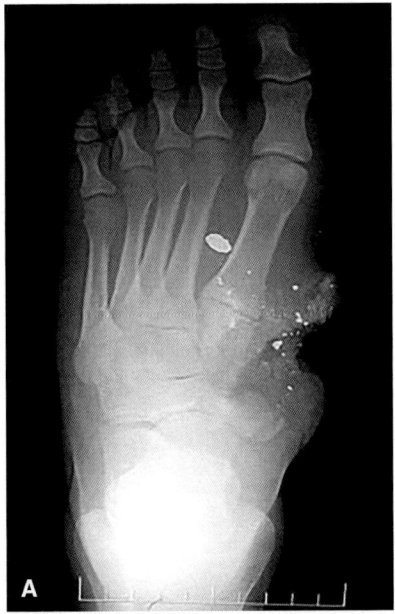
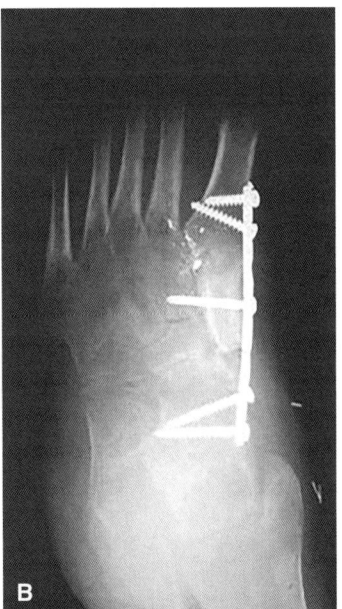
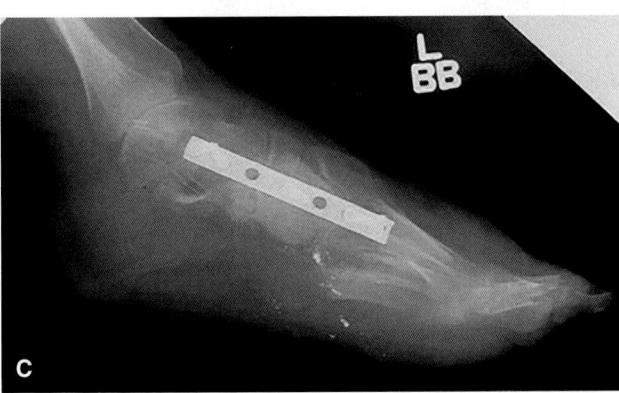

FIGURE 23.15 **A-C.** AP and lateral pre- and postop views of open comminuted navicular/medial column fracture with significant bone loss treated with iliac crest bone graft and spanning plate fixation from talus to first metatarsal.

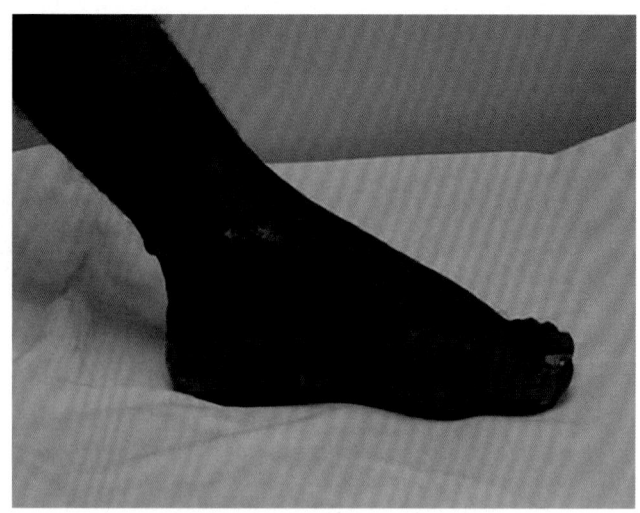

FIGURE 23.16 Sural artery rotational flap used for soft tissue coverage for open navicular fracture.

planes usually suffices along with treatment of any associated midfoot injuries to assure stabilization (Fig. 23.24A-E). Dislocation of the navicular cuneiform joint may occur in isolation from a dorsally directed force to the medial/central forefoot. Reduction requires musculoskeletal relaxation and distal traction. Open treatment may be required to remove interposed soft tissue if closed treatment is not successful. Upon relocation, the navicular cuneiform articulation is quite stable and

may be treated with cast immobilization alone or in combination with Kirschner wire fixation if deemed necessary. Avulsion fractures of the medial cuneiform may occur with this injury and one must assure competency of the anterior tibial tendon after relocation (Fig. 23.25A-D). High-energy crush type injuries of the cuneiforms almost always involve injury to adjacent structures, especially the tarsal-metatarsal complex. One must monitor closely for compartment syndrome secondary to crush

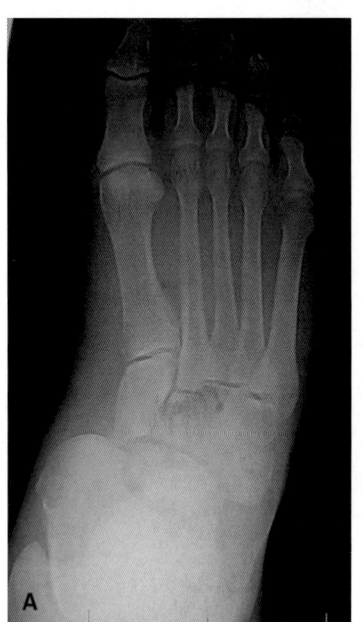

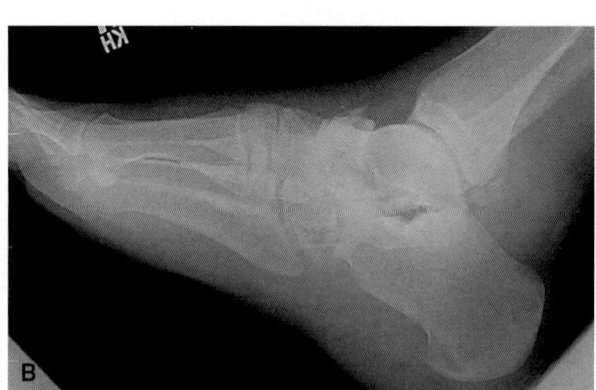

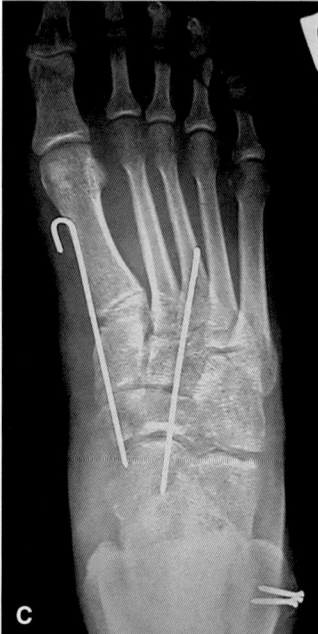

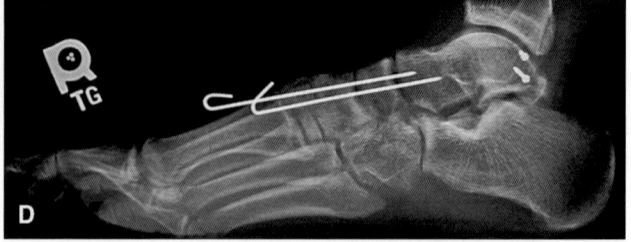

FIGURE 23.17 A-D. AP and lateral pre- and postreduction views of a talonavicular dislocation. Small dorsal avulsion fragments have been excised. Note associated fibular avulsion fracture treated with screw fixation.

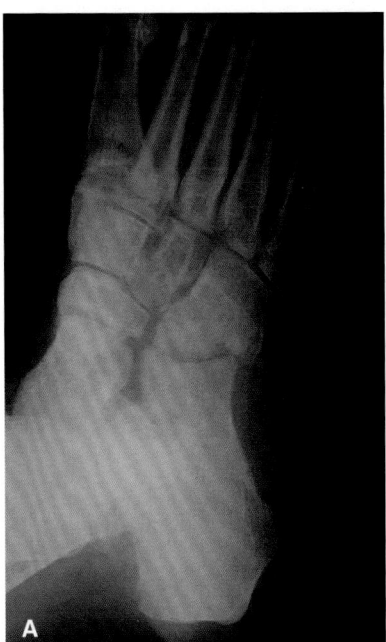 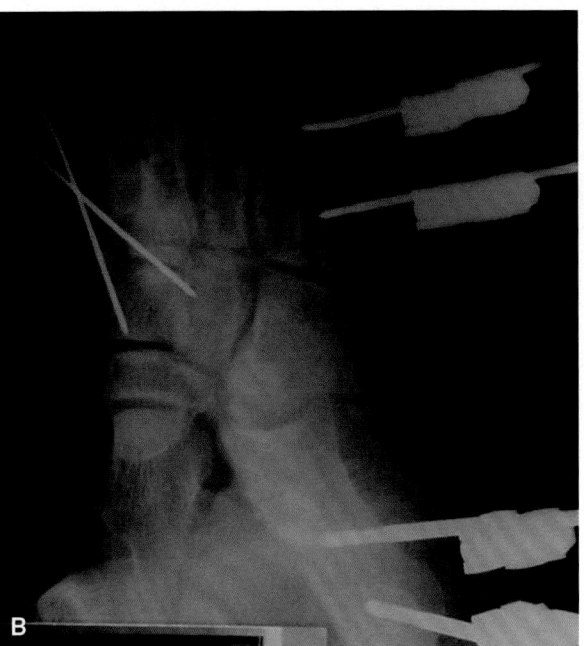

FIGURE 23.18 **A, B.** Oblique pre- and postop views of impacted cuboid body fracture treated with external fixation for both reduction aid to restore lateral column length and primary fixation. Small incision was used to elevate impacted fragments.

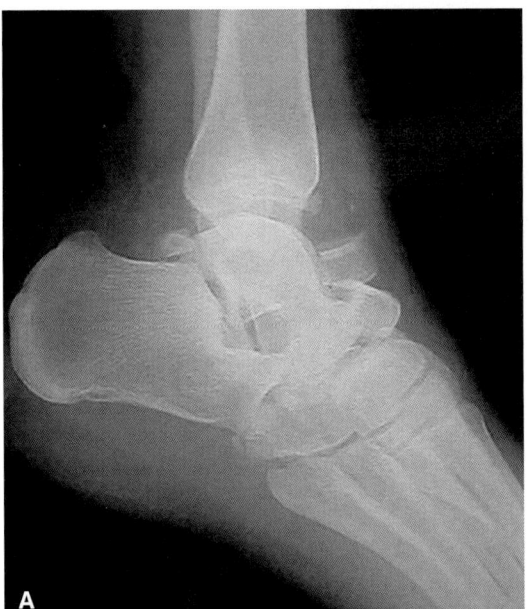 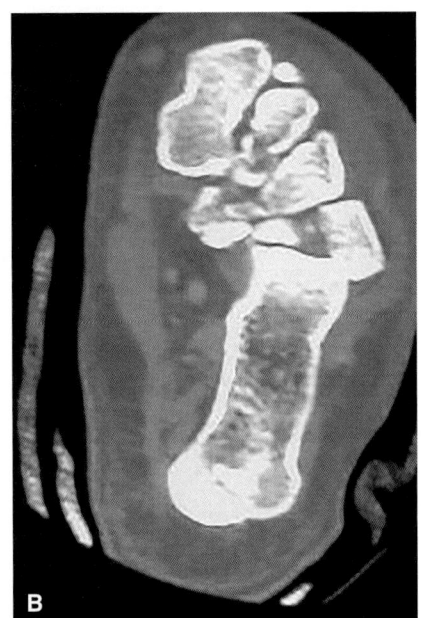 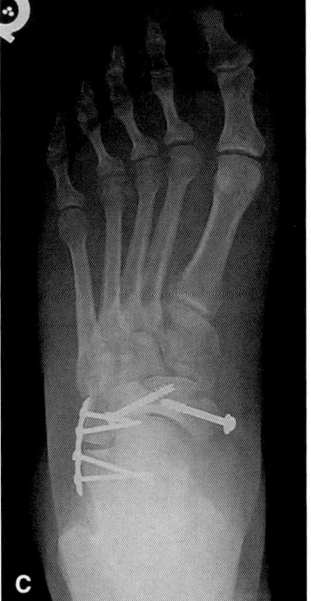

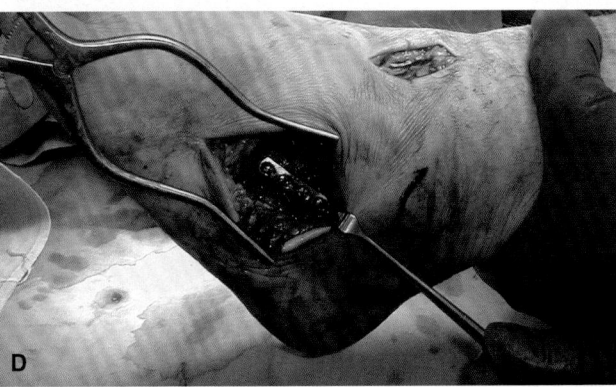

FIGURE 23.19 **A, B.** Lateral view and CT view of intra-articular cuboid body fracture with associated navicular fracture dislocation. **C, D.** AP view and intraoperative view of bridge plating of cuboid fracture and 2 screw fixation of associated navicular fracture. Associated distal tibial fracture was also fixated.

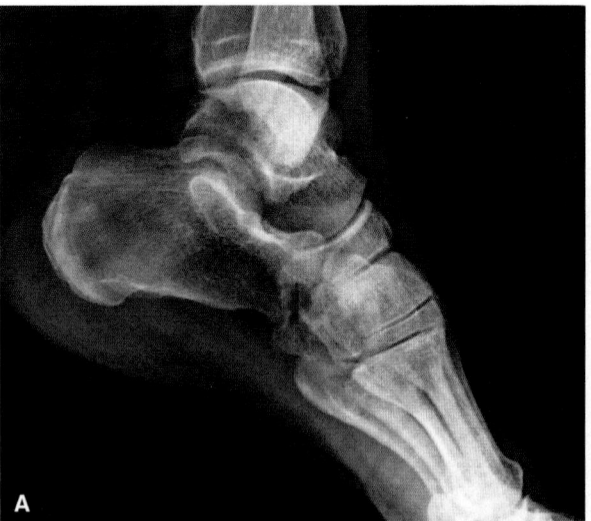

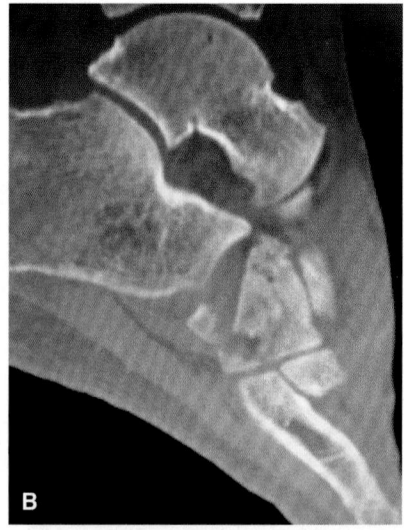

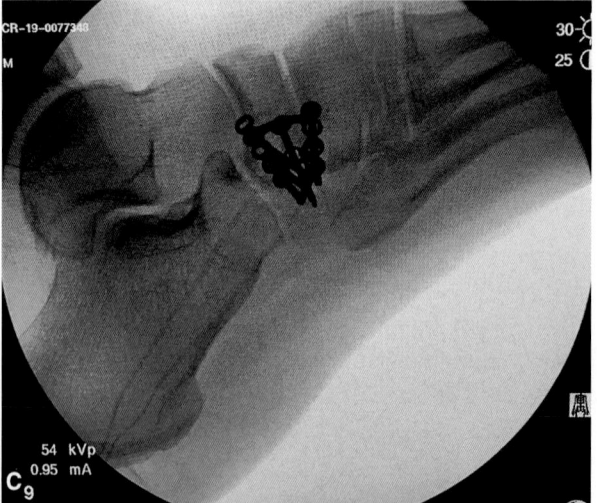

FIGURE 23.20 **A, B.** Lateral view and sagittal CT scan of displaced cuboid body fracture. **C.** Postop lateral of specialty cuboid plate fixation.

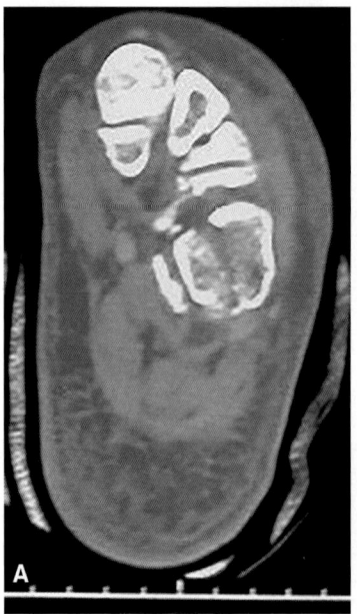

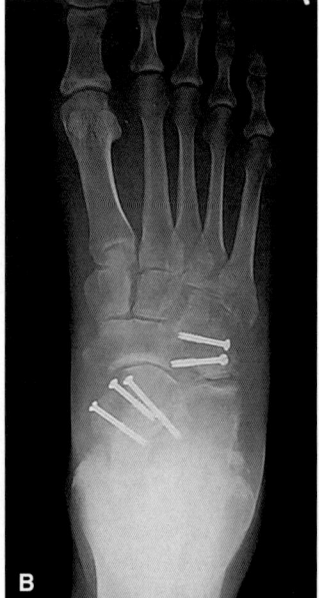

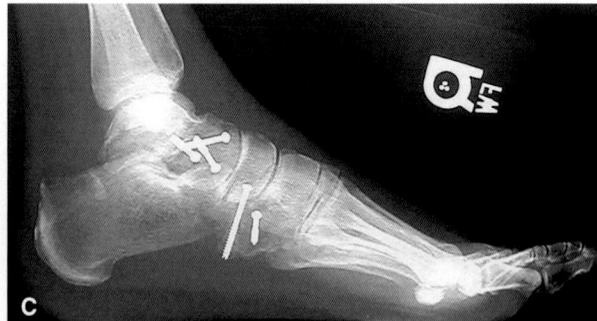

FIGURE 23.21 **A-C.** Preop CT view and postop AP and lateral views of 2-part longitudinal split fracture of the cuboid body treated with lag-screw fixation. Associated talus head fracture with minor bone loss was treated with screw fixation.

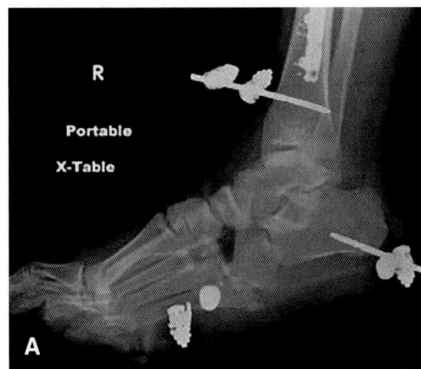
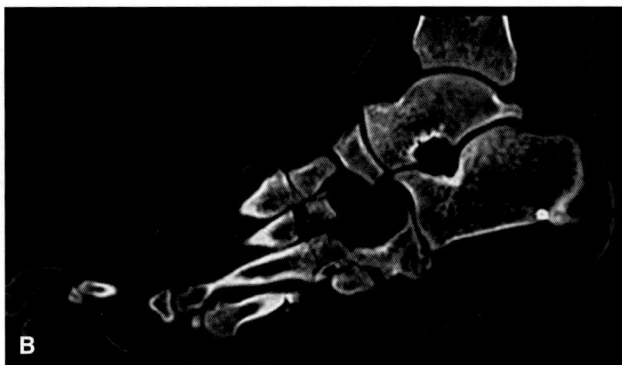
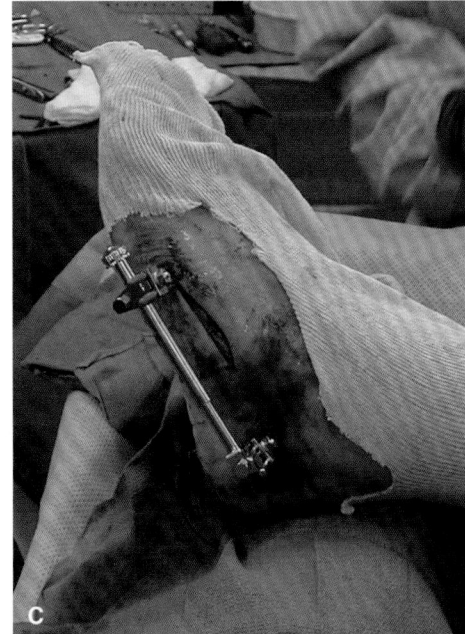
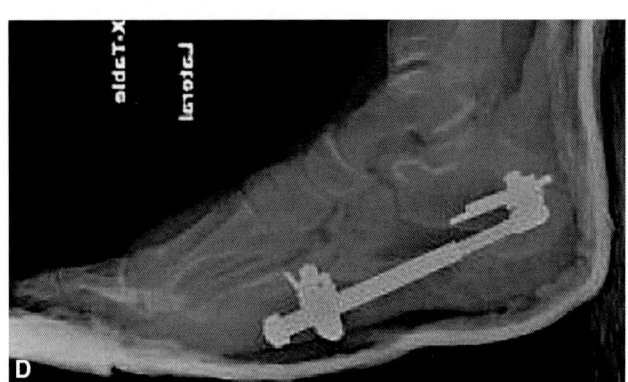

FIGURE 23.22 **A, B.** Lateral view and CT view of cuboid dislocation. **C, D.** Intraop and postop lateral view of reduction of same patient. Rail-type external fixator is used for distraction to aid in reduction and then used for primary fixation.

type injuries involving this area of the foot. Kirschner wire fixation and/or spanning bridge plate techniques may be utilized for fixation. A multiple incisional approach for reduction may be required, and these incisions can serve as access for appropriate compartment releases if indicated (Figs. 23.26A-E and 23.27A-E). Combination cuneiform/navicular fractures can produce significant medial column shortening and small external fixation distractors are often necessary to achieve reduction and restoration of medial column length and to augment internal fixation (Fig. 23.28A-D).

COMBINATION INJURIES AND LATE RECONSTRUCTION

Complex midfoot disruption can occur with injury to the medial and lateral columns as well as Lisfranc articulations. All components of the injury pattern must be addressed with reduction and fixation to assure midfoot stability (Fig. 23.29A-D). Bar to clamp or ring external fixation frames can be customized

to assure stability and alleviate need for frequent cast changes (Fig. 23.30A and B). Avascular necrosis of the navicular and significant posttraumatic arthritis are often long-term complications of these injuries. Severe combination high-energy injuries in conjunction with hindfoot and ankle dislocation are in particular limb-threatening injuries and must be treated with emergent reduction and external fixation and/or percutaneous fixation to hopefully accomplish limb salvage. These are associated with significant soft tissue damage often with open wounds; therefore, respect of the soft tissues is especially important (Figs. 23.31A-D and 23.32A-C).

Late reconstruction of midfoot fractures includes various osteotomy techniques for deformity correction. Multiplane correction can be accomplished with midfoot osteotomies. Fixation can be achieved with Steinman pins, screw, or plate fixation (Fig. 23.33A-F). Arthrodesis of the midfoot is indicated for symptomatic posttraumatic osteoarthritis having failed bracing and other nonoperative treatments (Figs. 23.34A-D and 23.35A and B). Primary arthrodesis may also be considered in crush type injuries of the midfoot with significant comminution.

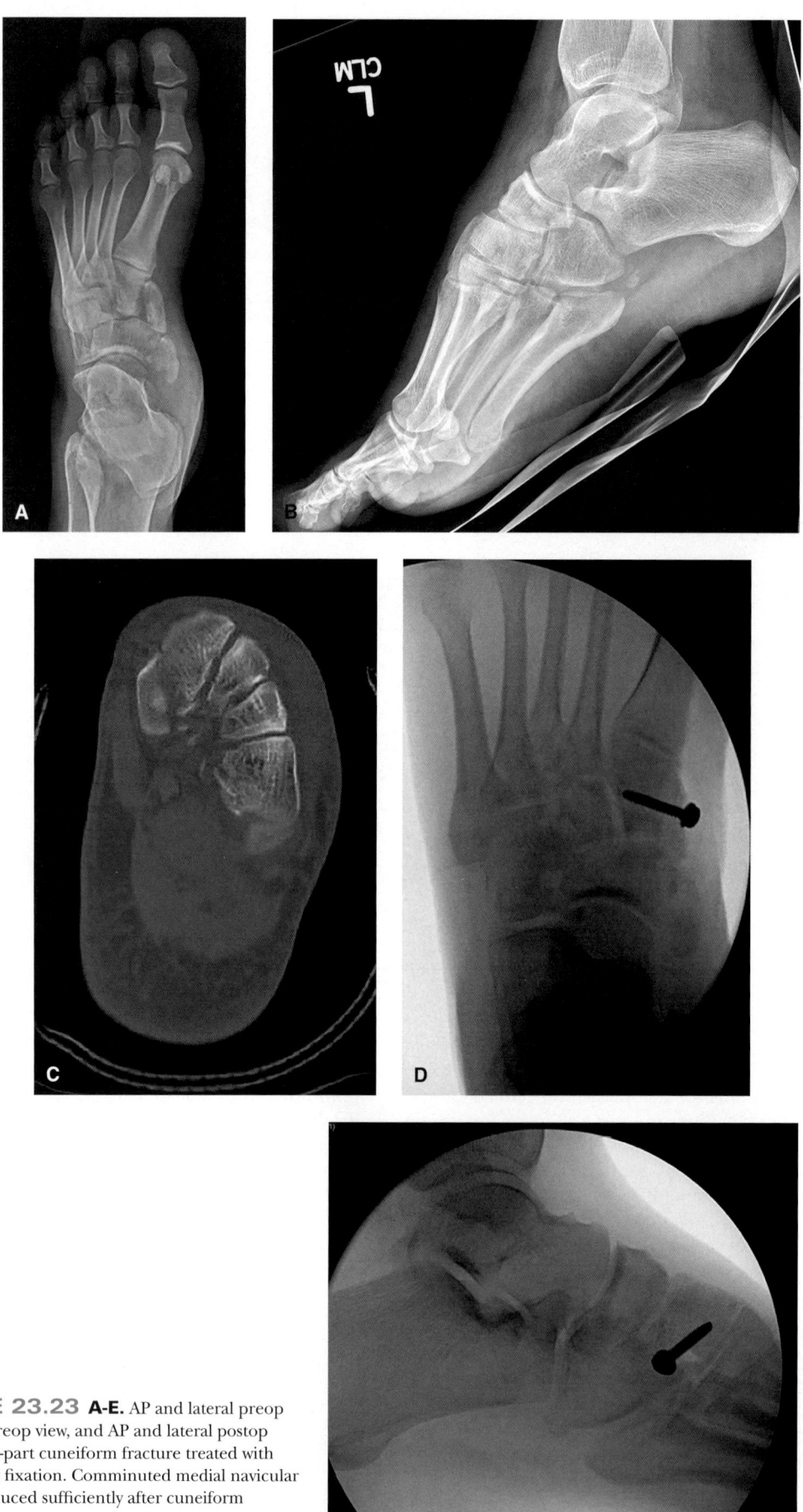

FIGURE 23.23 A-E. AP and lateral preop views, CT preop view, and AP and lateral postop views of two-part cuneiform fracture treated with single screw fixation. Comminuted medial navicular fracture reduced sufficiently after cuneiform reduction to not require internal fixation.

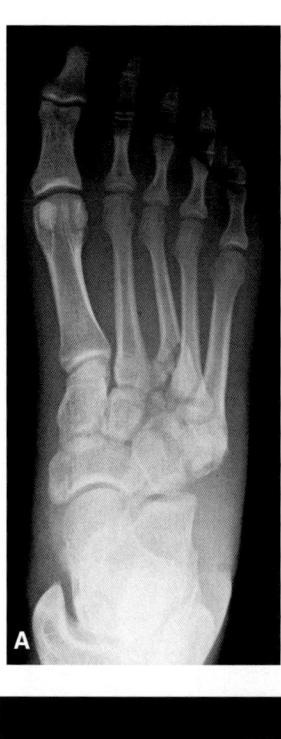
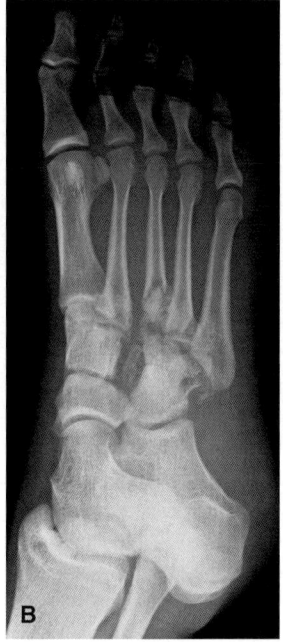
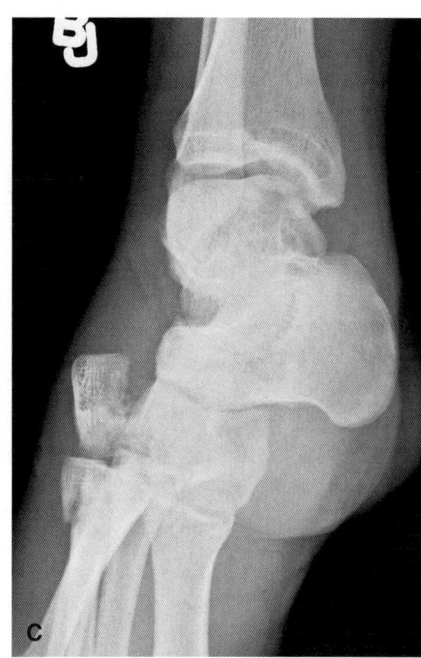
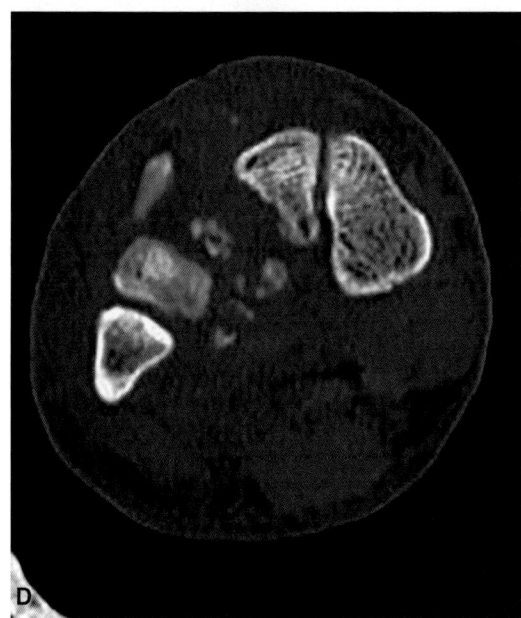
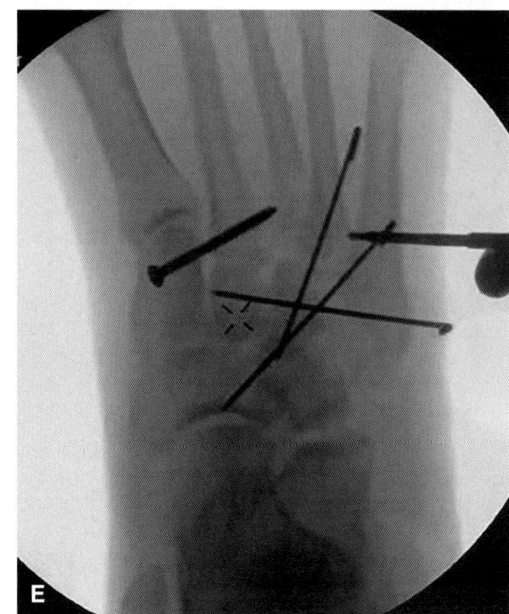

FIGURE 23.24 A-E. AP, oblique and internally rotated oblique preop views, and CT preop view of comminuted lateral cuneiform fracture/dislocation. **E.** AP postop view of Kirschner wire fixation of lateral cuneiform fracture/dislocation along with internal fixation of associated Lisfranc injury and external fixation of open cuboid fracture.

OPERATIVE TREATMENT PEARLS BOX

- Medial and lateral midfoot incisions are utilized in midfoot fractures.
- Medial incision is usually made just medial to the anterior tibial tendon and may extend across the entire medial column, if necessary, for exposure and fixation.
- Lateral incision for cuboid fractures is usually between the peroneal tendons and extensor brevis muscle belly or directly over the extensor muscle belly. It may be used to address both the lateral navicular and cuboid.

- Two incisions may be necessary in treating navicular body fractures. The lateral incision should be placed in the area between the EHL and EDL.
- Operative intervention is indicated if significant medial or lateral column shortening is present or if depressed articular fragments are present.
- Great care should be undertaken to minimize soft tissue stripping of the navicular, especially dorsally.
- Various fixation methods must be considered/employed when addressing midfoot fractures.
- Corrective midfoot osteotomy and/or arthrodesis may be performed for late reconstruction.

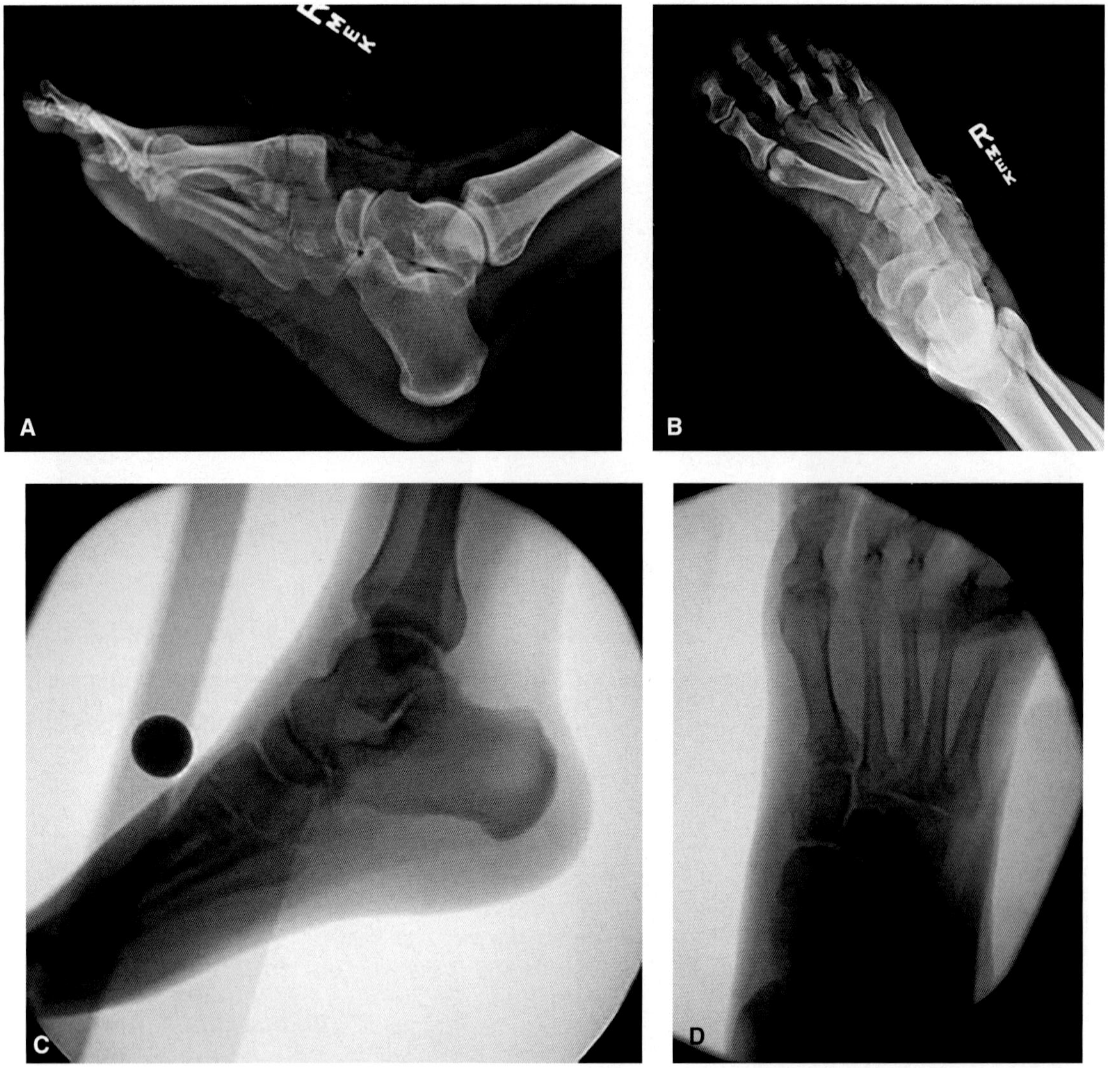

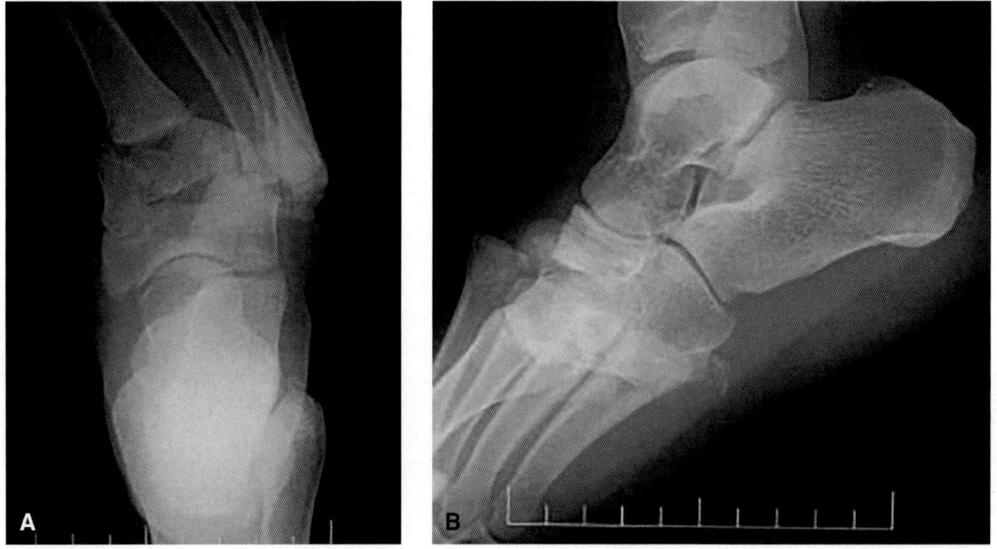

FIGURE 23.25 A-D. Lateral and AP pre- and postreduction views of navicular cuneiform dislocation. Medial avulsion fracture was present, but anterior tibial tendon insertion was not compromised.

FIGURE 23.26 A, B. Oblique and lateral views of crush type injury to cuneiforms with associated tarsal metatarsal disruption.

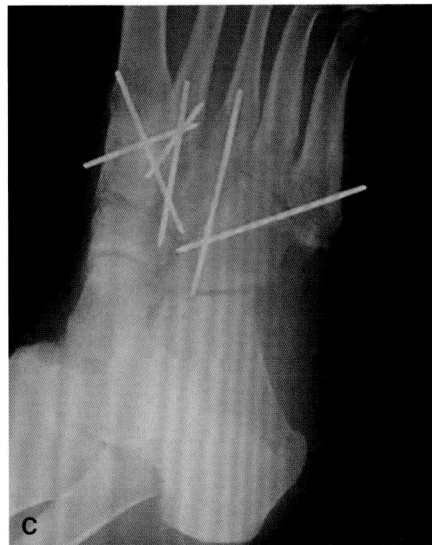
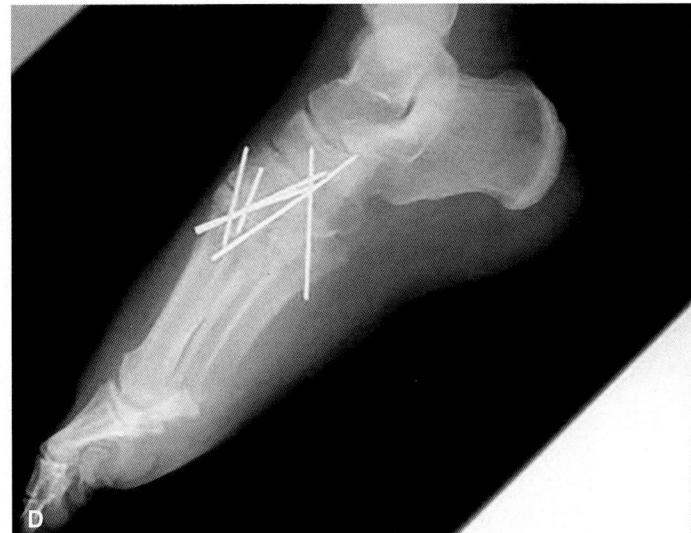
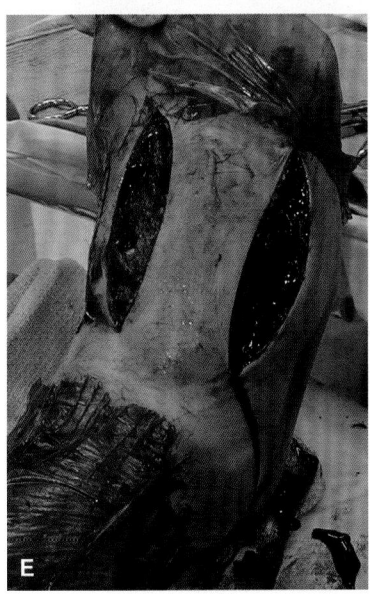

FIGURE 23.26 (*Continued*) **C-E.** Oblique and lateral postop views and intraop view of incisional approach used for reduction and compartment release of associated compartment syndrome.

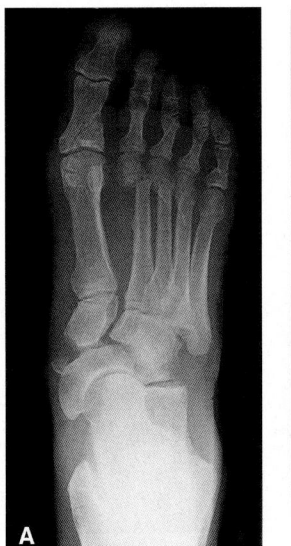
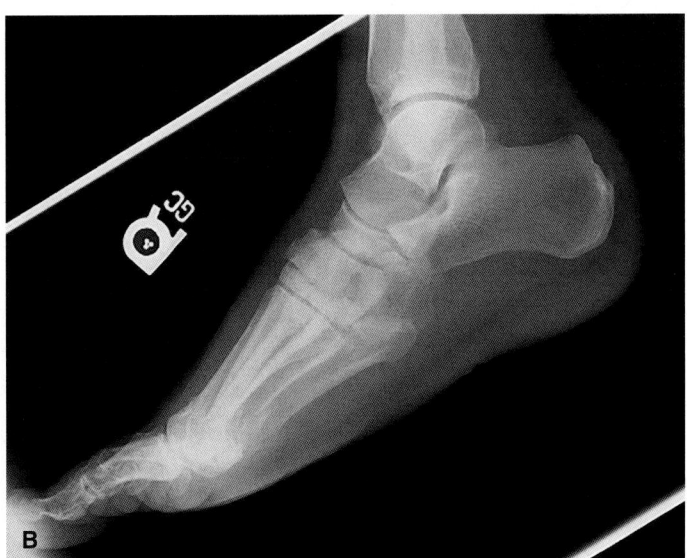

FIGURE 23.27 **A-C.** AP and lateral preop views and CT preop view of cuneiform crush type injury with other associated medial and lateral column injuries. **D, E.** Oblique and lateral postop views of same patient with bridge plating of both the medial and lateral columns.

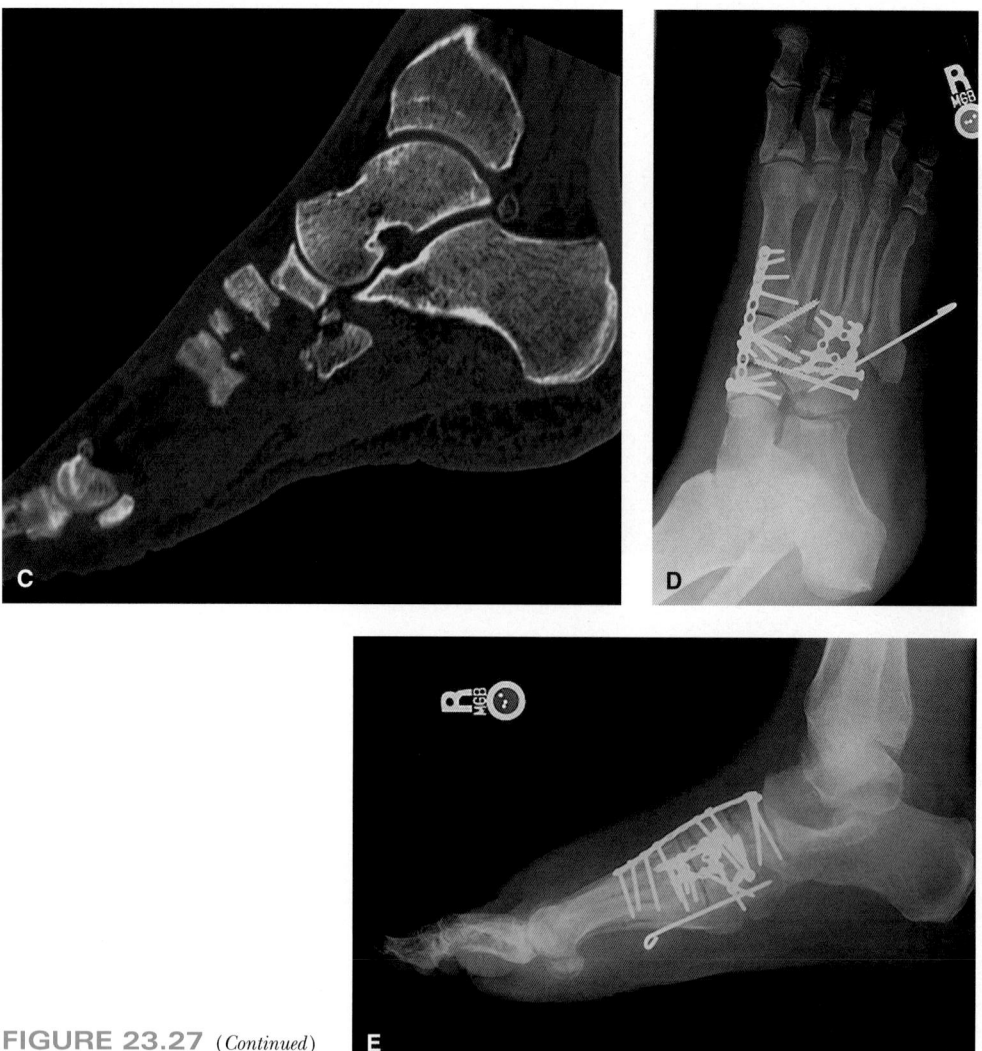

FIGURE 23.27 (*Continued*)

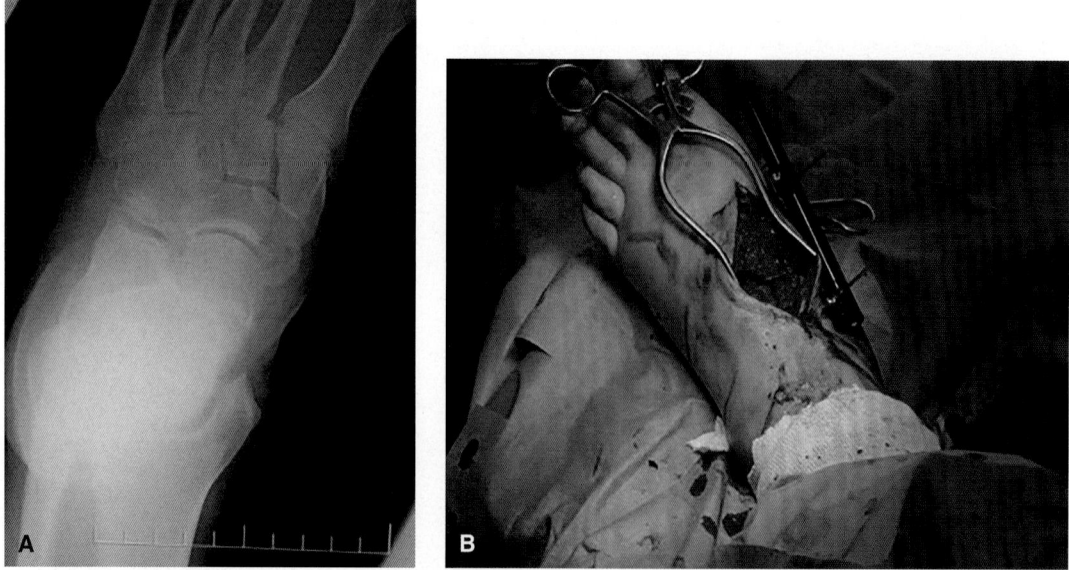

FIGURE 23.28 A, B. AP preop view and intraop view of cuneiform fracture with intercuneiform disruption, navicular fracture, and medial column shortening.

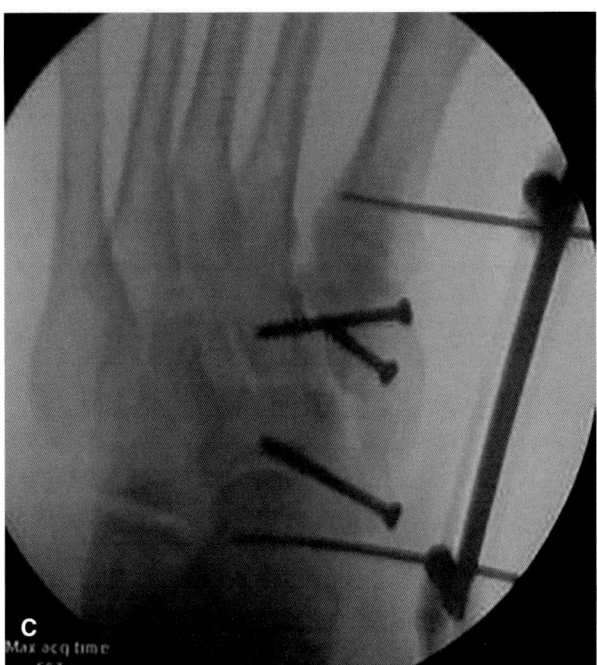

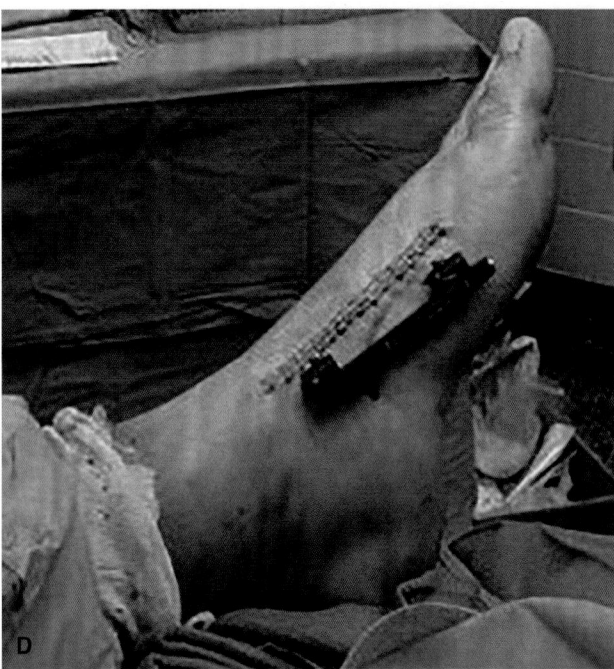

FIGURE 23.28 (*Continued*) **C, D.** AP postop view and intraop view of final fixation construct.

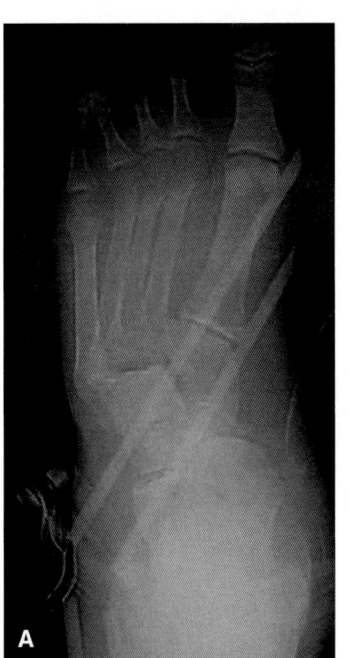

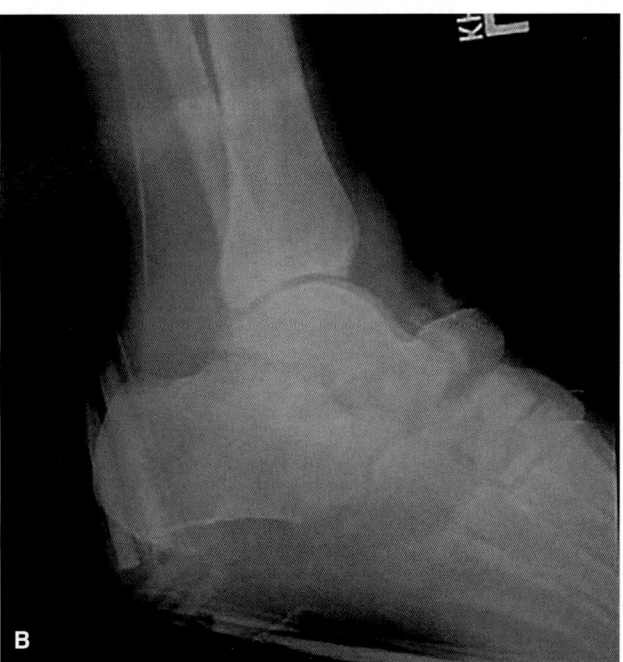

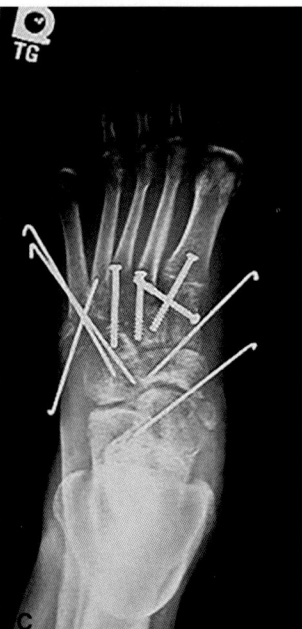

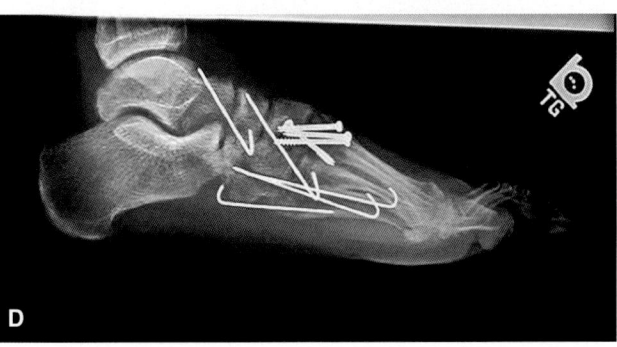

FIGURE 23.29 **A-D.** AP and lateral preop and postop views of navicular dislocation, fourth and fifth metatarsal/cuboid impaction fracture, fifth metatarsal base fracture, and Lisfranc injury.

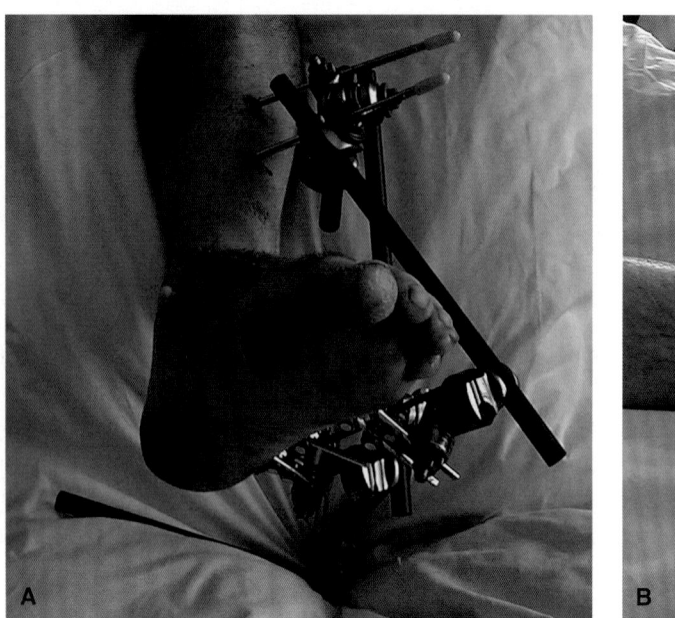
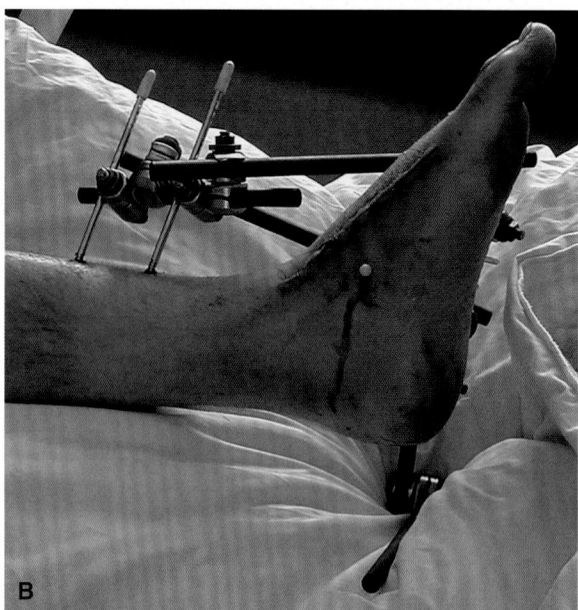

FIGURE 23.30 **A, B.** Example of bar to clamp frame for added midfoot stability and to allow for wound care if necessary.

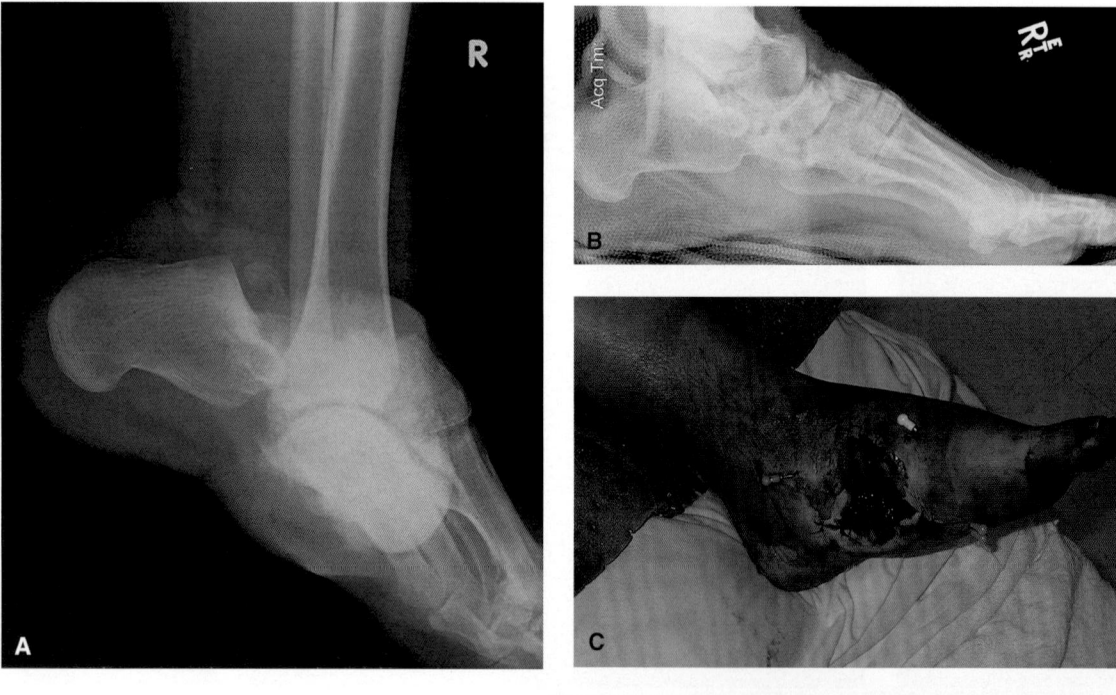

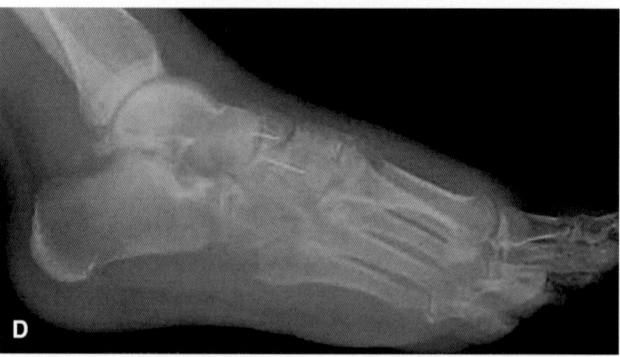

FIGURE 23.31 **A, B.** Lateral pre- and postclosed reduction views before percutaneous pinning of significant midfoot dislocation combined with subtalar dislocation. **C.** Associated open wound. **D.** Early posttraumatic arthritis at 6 months postinjury.

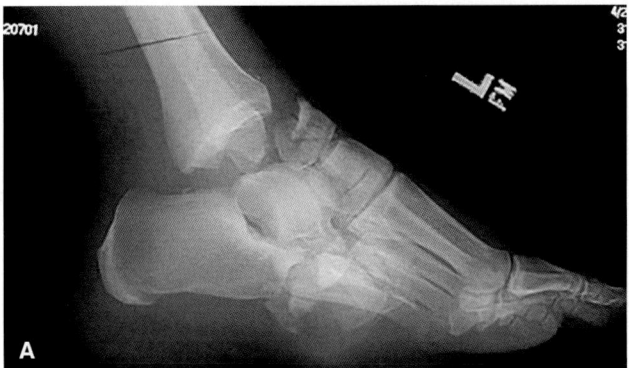

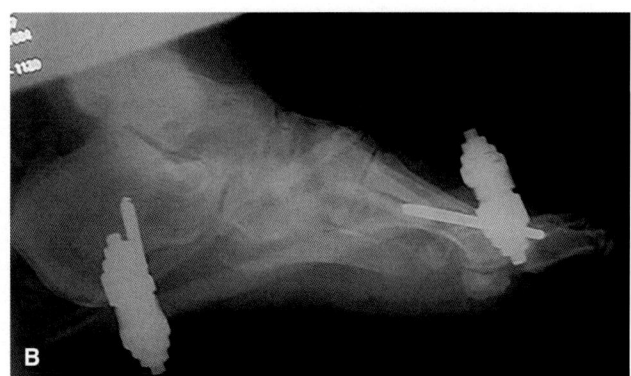

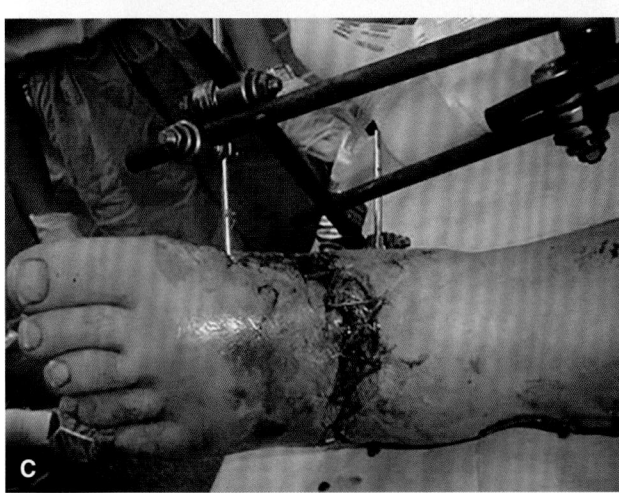

FIGURE 23.32 A-C. Lateral pre- and postclosed reduction views and associated open wound following severe midfoot dislocation combined with ankle dislocation treated with external fixation.

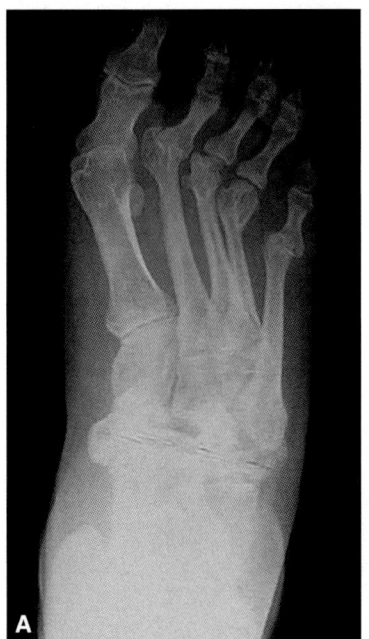

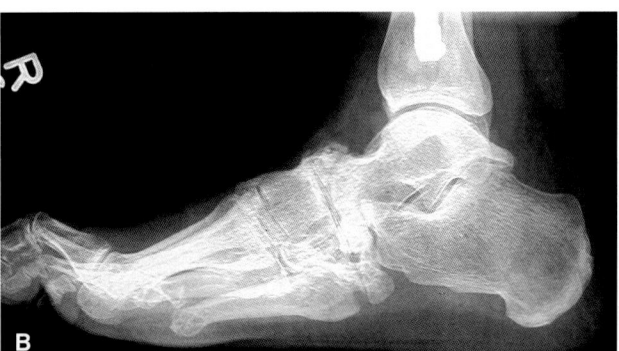

FIGURE 23.33 A, B. AP and lateral preop views of midfoot deformity after midfoot fracture. *Ink line* represents planned corrective osteotomy.

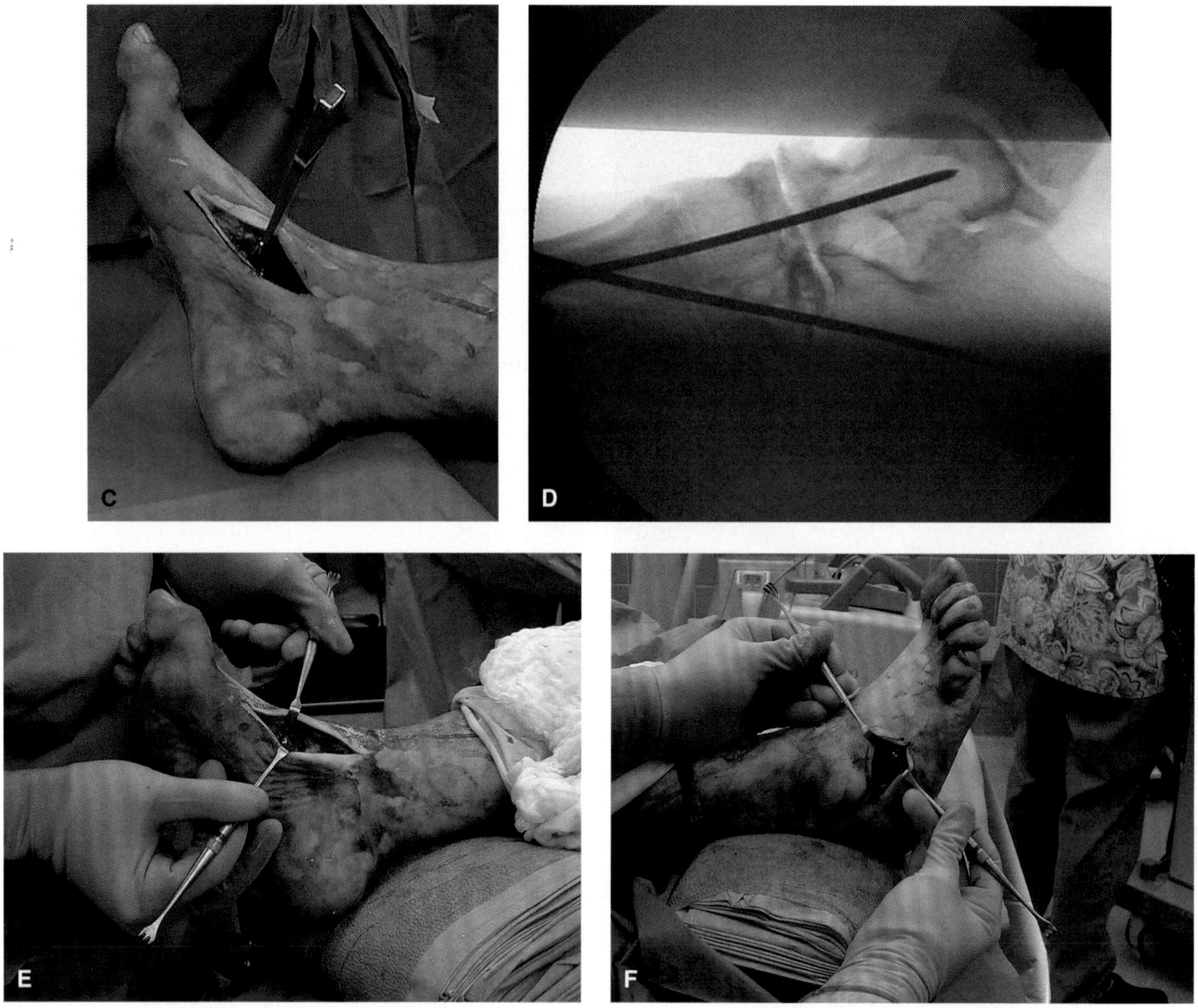

FIGURE 23.33 (*Continued*) **C.** Osteotomy is started with power saw and carefully finished with osteotomes. **D-F.** Lateral view after de-rotation of the midfoot deformity and cannulated pin fixation and medial and lateral intraop views after final cannulated screw fixation.

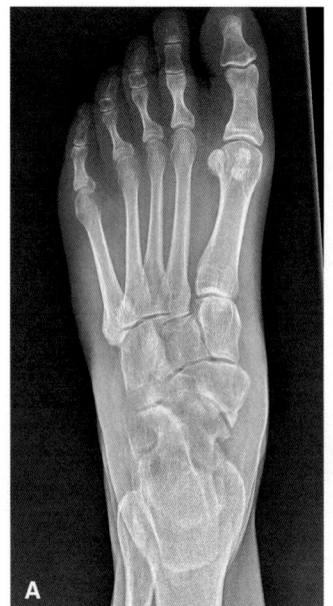
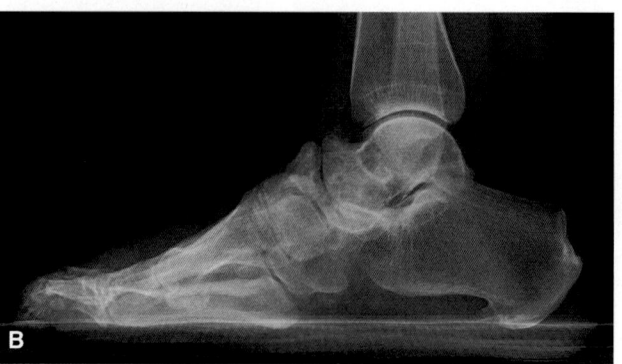

FIGURE 23.34 **A-D.** AP and lateral pre- and postop views of talonavicular joint arthrodesis for posttraumatic arthritis following intra-articular navicular body fracture.

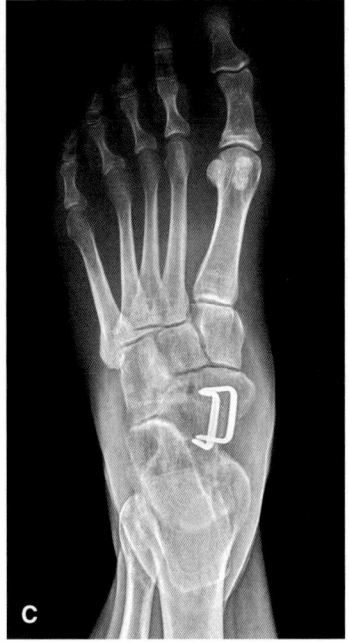

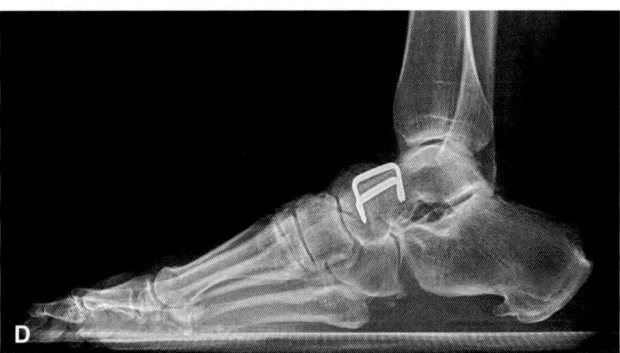

FIGURE 23.34 (*Continued*)

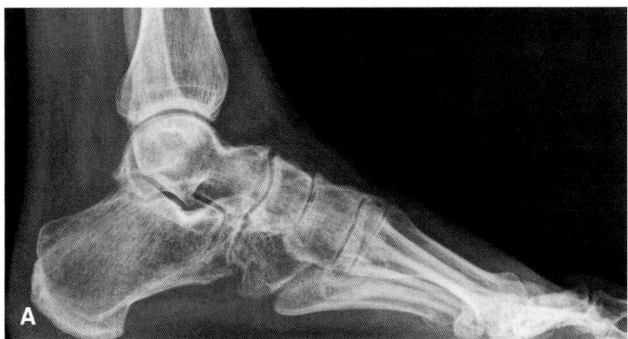

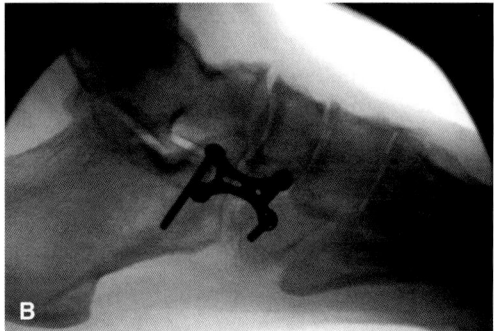

FIGURE 23.35 A, B. Lateral pre- and intraop views of calcaneocuboid joint arthrodesis for posttraumatic arthritis following intra-articular cuboid fracture.

REFERENCES

1. Court-Brown CM, Zinna S, Ekvol I. Classification and epidemiology of mid-foot fractures. *Foot.* 2006;16:138-141.
2. Pountos I, Pautel M, Giannoudis P. Cuboid injuries. *Indian J Orthop.* 2018;52(3):297-303.
3. Shibuya N, Davis ML, Jupiter DC. Epidemiology of foot and ankle fractures in the United States; an analysis of the National Trauma Data Bank (2007 to 2011). *J Foot Ankle Surg.* 2014;53(5):606-608.
4. Probst C, Richter M, Lefering R, et al. Incidence and significance of injuries to the foot and ankle in polytrauma patients—an analysis of the trauma registry of DGU. *Injury.* 2010;41(2):210-215.
5. Court-Brown CM, Ward AM, Aitken S. The epidemiology of acute sports-related fractures in adults. *Injury.* 2008;39(12):1365-1372.
6. Schmid T, Krause F, Gebel P, Weber M. Operative treatment of acute fractures of the tarsal navicular body: midterm results with a new classification. *Foot Ankle Int.* 2016;37(5):501-507.
7. Main BJ, Jowett RL. Injuries of the midtarsal joint. *J Bone Joint Surg Br.* 1975;57B:89-97.
8. Sangeorzan BJ, Benirschke SK, Mosca V, Mago KA, Hansen ST. Displaced intra-articular fractures of the tarsal navicular. *J Bone Joint Surg Am.* 1999;71(A):1504-1510.
9. Petrie MJ, Blakey CM, Chadwick C, Davies HG, Blundell CM, Davies MB. A new and reliable classification system for fractures of the navicular and associated injuries to the midfoot. *Bone Joint J.* 2018;100(B):176-182.
10. Mehlhorn AT, Schmal H, Legrand MA, Sudkamp NP, Strohm PC. Classification and outcome of fracture-dislocation of the cuneiform bones. *J Foot Ankle Surg.* 2016;55:1249-1255.
11. Fenton P, Al-Nammari S, Blundell C, Davies M. The patterns of injury and management of cuboid fractures. *Bone Joint J.* 2016;98(B):1003-1008.
12. Torg JS, Pavlov H, Cooley LH, et al. Stress fractures of the tarsal navicular. A retrospective review of twenty-one cases. *J Bone Joint Surg Am.* 1982;64(5):700-712.
13. Fitch KD, Blackwell JB, Gilmour WN. Operation for non-union of stress fracture of the tarsal navicular. *J Bone Joint Surg Br.* 1989;71(1):105-110.
14. Saxena A, Behan SA, Valerio DL, Frosch DL. Navicular stress fracture outcomes in athletes: analysis of 62 injuries. *J Foot Ankle Surg.* 2017;56(5):943-948.
15. Torg JS, Moyer J, Gaughan JP, Boden BP. Management of tarsal navicular stress fractures: conservative versus surgical treatment: a meta-analysis. *Am J Sports Med.* 2010;38(5):1048-1053.
16. Evans J, Beingessener DM, Agel J, Benirschke SK. Minifragment plate fixation of high-energy navicular body fractures. *Foot Ankle Int.* 2011;32(5):5485-5492.
17. Coulibaly MO, Jones CB, Sietsema DL, Schildhauer TA. Results and complications of operative and non-operative navicular fracture treatment. *Injury.* 2015;46(8):1669-1677.
18. Ahmed A, Westrick E. Management of midfoot fractures and dislocations. *Curr Rev Musculoskelet Med.* 2018;11:529-536.
19. Wiley JJ. The mechanism of tarso-metatarsal joint injuries. *J Bone Joint Surg Br.* 1971;53:474-482.
20. Sanders JO, McGanity PL. Intermediate cuneiform fracture—dislocation. *J Orthop Trauma.* 1990;4:102-104.
21. Saxby TS, Sharp RJ, Rosenfeld PF. Plantar fracture-dislocation of the intermediate cuneiform: a case report. *Foot Ankle Int.* 2006;27:742-745.
22. Sarrafian S. *Anatomy of the Foot and Ankle.* Philadelphia, PA: JB Lippincott; 1993.
23. Sanders R. Fractures of the midfoot and forefoot. In: Coughlin MJ, Mann RA, eds. *Surgery of the Foot and Ankle.* 7th ed. St. Louis, MO: Mosby; 1999:1574-1605.
24. Torg J, Pavlov H, Cooley L. Stress fractures of the tarsal navicular. *J Bone Joint Surg Am.* 1988;64:700.
25. Early JS, Hansen ST. Midfoot and navicular injuries. In: Helal B, Rowley DI, Cracchiolo A III, et al., eds. *Surgery of Disorders of the Foot and Ankle.* London, UK: Martin Dunitz; 1996:731-747.
26. Zwipp H, Dahlen C, Randt T, et al. Komplextrauma des Fusses. *Orthopade.* 1997;26:1046-1056.
27. Anderson RB. Injuries to the midfoot and forefoot. In: Lutter LD, Mizel MS, Pfeffer GB, eds. *Orthopaedic Knowledge Update: Foot and Ankle.* Chicago, IL: American Academy of orthopaedic Surgeons; 1994:255-268.
28. Holbein O, Bauer G, Kinzl L. Displaced fractures of the cuboid: four case reports and review of the literature. *Foot Ankle Surg.* 1997;3(2):85-93.
29. Nashi M, Bauerjee B. Isolated plantar dislocation of the middle cuneiform. *Injury.* 1997;28:704-706.

CHAPTER 24

Lisfranc Fracture/Dislocation

J. Randolph Clements and Rebekah Richards

INTRODUCTION

INDICATIONS, CONTRAINDICATIONS, SUCCESS IN LITERATURE, COMPLICATIONS IN LITERATURE

A Lisfranc injury is a fracture or ligamentous injury through the tarsometatarsal complex. They can present as a bony fracture, purely ligamentous injury, or a combination of both. The Lisfranc joint or tarsometatarsal (TMT) articulation originally received its name for Jacques Lisfranc St. Martin, who served as a French field surgeon in Napoleon's army. He described an amputation through the TMT joint (TMTJ) line performed on a soldier who suffered a midfoot injury after a fall from his horse.[1]

The Lisfranc joint is comprised of the 1st, 2nd, and 3rd metatarsal bases and corresponding cuneiforms (Fig. 24.1). The TMT serves as the junction between the forefoot and midfoot and is a critical component to both the longitudinal and the transverse arches of the foot. Injuries to the TMTJ complex are not common, but they are frequently missed and may lead to posttraumatic arthritis and long-term disability. The incidence has been published at 0.1%-0.4% of all fractures and dislocations (1 in 55 000 people each year).[2]

The mechanism of injury has a wide spectrum, ranging from low-energy falls to high-energy motor vehicle accidents. The mechanism can result from direct or indirect trauma. High-energy injuries are typically readily diagnosed, and their treatment can be more intuitive and immediate. The high-energy injuries result in multiplanar, multiarticular fracture patterns and are quickly recognized with plain radiography (Fig. 24.2). However, diagnosis of the subtle injuries is difficult and is often missed at initial presentation.[3] Low-energy injuries are often ligamentous and can be challenging to diagnose and treat. A missed diagnosis can lead to chronic pain, disability, deformity, and prolonged disability.[4]

The literature reports that the majority of TMTJ injuries occur following an axial load or twisting force applied to a plantarflexed foot.[5,6] This mechanism results in increased stress on the weaker dorsal ligaments resulting in dorsal ligaments rupturing first and resulting in dorsal subluxation and dislocation. Fracture dislocations are commonly seen between the 1st and 2nd metatarsal bases. The associated secondary medial or lateral dislocation is typically dependent upon the direction of force during the injury.

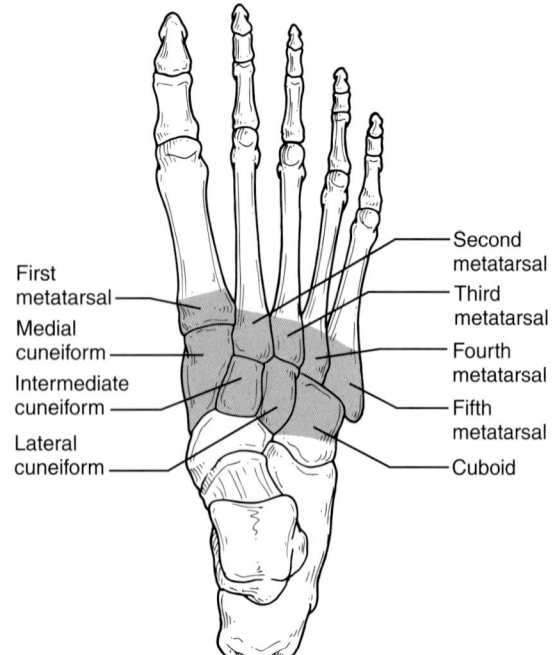

First metatarsal
Medial cuneiform
Intermediate cuneiform
Lateral cuneiform
Second metatarsal
Third metatarsal
Fourth metatarsal
Fifth metatarsal
Cuboid

FIGURE 24.1 Lisfranc complex, articulations.

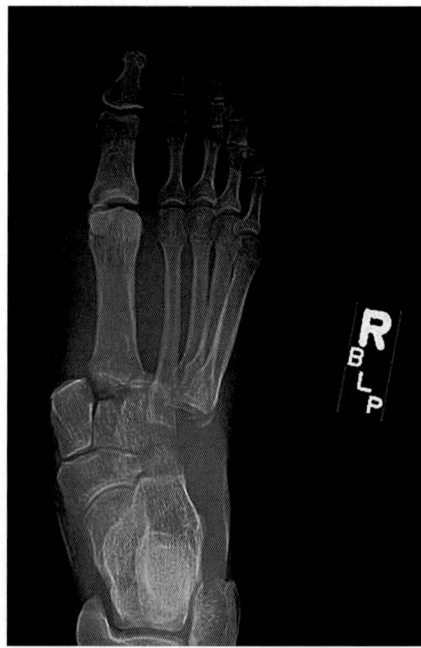

FIGURE 24.2 AP radiograph of right toot in a 22-year-old female who presented with a dorsolateral TMTJ dislocation after being thrown from a golf cart.

In high-energy events, a crush injury can produce similar injury pattern. A direct injury may also result in a fracture/dislocation across the TMTJ. These injuries that are often associated with high velocity mechanisms may result in large amounts of soft tissue damage. In these situations, the treating provider should maintain a high index of suspicion for compartment syndrome. Compartment syndrome is more commonly seen in patients with high-energy injuries; however, each injury should be treated with an astute insight for this secondary development.[7]

Subtle injuries/midfoot sprains can also occur at the TMTJ. These injuries typically occur following a low-energy twisting trauma with an indirectly applied force. Subtle injuries are more common in the athletic population especially those wearing cleats. Often these patients will report a "pop" in their midfoot followed by pain with weight bearing. The acute pain will typically subside, but the patient will often have chronic discomfort with certain movements such as pivoting or toe walking. Stable injuries may be treated nonoperatively with immobilization. Stable injuries are defined as extra-articular fractures with maintained alignment or ligamentous sprain that does not disrupt the Lisfranc ligament.

Unstable injuries should undergo operative intervention to restore alignment of the joint complex and to allow for ligamentous healing. Both primary arthrodesis and open reduction internal fixation (ORIF) have been advocated as acceptable treatment options. However, the most appropriate procedure selection remains highly debatable. The decision on surgical treatment is complicated by age, fracture pattern, mechanism of injury, severity of injury, medical comorbidities, surgeon preference, and patient goals. These are all factors in deciding ORIF and primary arthrodesis. Although no consensus has been reached on the superior treatment, we do know that the most important factor in determining good outcomes is anatomic reduction of the TMTJ. The goal for this chapter is to review patient presentation, diagnosis, and options for management of TMTJ pathology.

ANATOMY OF THE LISFRANC JOINT

The tarsometatarsal joint supports the transverse arch of the foot and serves as the junction between the forefoot and the midfoot. Although this anatomic location is frequently referred to as the "*Lisfranc Joint,*" "*Lisfranc Complex*" would be a more accurate description. The 1st, 2nd, and 3rd metatarsals articulate with the medial middle and lateral cuneiforms, respectively. The 4th and 5th metatarsals articulate with the cuboid. The Lisfranc joint can be compartmentalized based on its capsular arrangement. The medial joint capsule consists of the 1st TMT articulation, the central joint capsule consists of the 2nd and 3rd TMT articulations, and the lateral capsule consists of the 4th and 5th TMT articulations. The tarsometatarsal complex consists of a complex composite of ligamentous and osseous structures, which function synergistically to provide midfoot stability. The base of the 1st metatarsal is of reniform shape while the bases of the 2nd and 3rd metatarsal are dorsally based trapezoids. The corresponding articular surface of the cuneiforms closely resembles it corresponding metatarsal base. The 2nd metatarsal base is recessed between the 1st and 3rd metatarsal bases ~8 mm and serves as the proverbial "keystone" to central tarsometatarsal joint complex.[8] This architecture provides longitudinal support and stability to the midfoot. The 4th and 5th metatarsals articulate with individual facets located on the anterior aspect of the cuboid (Fig. 24.3).

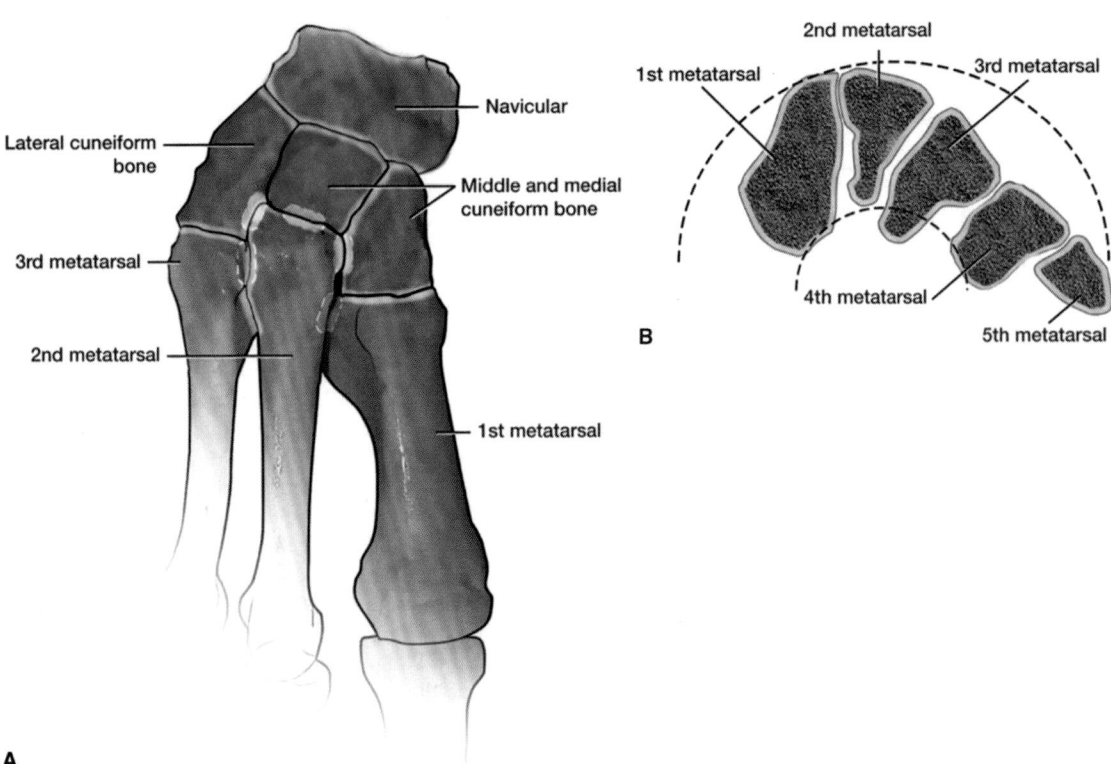

FIGURE 24.3 A. The recessed middle cuneiform allows for interposition of the second MT base between five articular surfaces. **B.** Trapezoidal MT bases form a stable arch configuration when viewed in the coronal plane. (From Schiff AP, Gross CE, Easley ME. Open reduction and internal fixation of the Lisfranc fracture-dislocation. In: *Operative Techniques in Foot and Ankle Surgery.* 2nd ed. Philadelphia, PA: Wolters Kluwer; 2017:1284-1306.)

The articular relationships are maintained by an elaborate ligamentous connection that, when intact, is inherently stable. The Lisfranc ligament (oblique interosseous ligament) extends from the plantar lateral aspect of the medial cuneiform to the plantar medial aspect of the 2nd metatarsal base and serves as the strongest of the interosseous ligaments. The ligamentous complex consists of dorsal, interosseous, and plantar ligaments. The dorsal ligaments contribute to the stability much less than the plantar ligaments. The interosseous ligaments provide the most strength and support. An osseous avulsion seen at the medial aspect of the 2nd metatarsal base is evidence of a ruptured Lisfranc ligament. Transverse ligaments connect the second through the 5th metatarsals, but there is no transverse ligament attaching the 1st to the 2nd metatarsal. This contributes to the displacement of the first metatarsal when the ligaments are injured (Fig. 24.4).

The treating provider should be considerate of the neurovascular anatomy. The surgeon should maintain awareness of the location of the dorsalis pedis artery and deep peroneal nerve between the bases of the 1st and 2nd metatarsal. These structures can be injured depending on the fracture pattern and may lead to more serious complications such as compartment syndrome.

The TMTJ complex is also strengthened by muscles coursing through the midfoot as well. The muscular attachments of the tibialis anterior and peroneus longus stabilize the 1st TMTJ. Soft tissue interposition during reduction may be an issue due to these tendons and their attachments.

The joints of the foot were divided into nonessential and essential joints by Hansen et al.[9] The tarsometatarsal joints were considered nonessential and, for this reason, a primary fusion is considered less consequential. The sagittal and frontal

TABLE 24.1	Tarsometatarsal Joint Range of Motion	
Joint	**Sagittal Plane**	**Frontal Plane**
First	3.5 mm	1.5 mm
Second	0.6 mm	1.2 mm
Third	1.6 mm	2.6 mm
Fourth	9.6 mm	11.1 mm
Fifth	10.2 mm	9.0 mm

plane motion of the TMT has been studied. The motion in the 1st, 2nd, and 3rd TMT in both sagittal and frontal planes is nominal. However, the motion demonstrated in the 4th and 5th cuboid articulation is significantly higher and supportive of joint sparring techniques. The medial and central columns consist of the more rigid keystone component while the lateral 4th and 5th TMTJ provide increased mobility, which allows for surface adaptation during gait[10] (Table 24.1).

PATIENT PRESENTATION AND RADIOGRAPHIC PARAMETERS

Patients with TMTJ complex injuries typically present with significant pain, swelling, and ecchymosis in the midfoot following acute trauma due to mechanisms that were described above. The patient will most likely be unable to bear weight and the plantar ecchymosis is often times considered pathognomonic for TMTJ injury. Midfoot pain upon exam is common and may span the majority of the midfoot. If manipulation can be performed, a pronation abduction test can be utilized to evaluate for midfoot pain or instability. In this test, pain is elicited when the forefoot is abducted and pronated while the hindfoot is kept in place.

If the patient presents with these symptoms with neuropathy and without a traumatic event, then one should consider Charcot neuroarthropathy as a differential (Fig. 24.5). Neurovascular integrity, as with all traumatic injuries, should be assessed at initial presentation. The practitioner should palpate for pedal pulses, examine sensation, and assess for compartment suppleness. If compartment syndrome is suspected, immediate intervention is required. It is important to always evaluate for concomitant injuries. It is reported that up to 40% of these injuries are associated with other tarsal bone fractures and that up to 80%-90% may also have metatarsal bone fractures.[11]

Radiographs obtained should include weight-bearing (if tolerated) anteroposterior, oblique, and lateral views of the foot. On an AP radiograph, the medial border of the medial cuneiform should align with the medial aspect of the 1st metatarsal (Fig. 24.6). The medial aspect of the intermediate cuneiform should also align with the medial aspect of the 2nd metatarsal. On the medial oblique, the medial aspect of the 4th metatarsal base should align with the medial aspect of the cuboid.[12]

Instability of the Lisfranc joint is radiographically defined as a diastasis of >2 mm noted between the medial cuneiform and 2nd metatarsal base (Fig. 24.7). The presences of a fleck fracture on plain radiographs can also indicate injury to the TMT complex.[13,14] The fleck sign represents an avulsion of the Lisfranc ligament. This is a subtle finding but represents high positive predictability of instability at that joint. In the face of a low-energy mechanism, the diastasis may be less evident unless

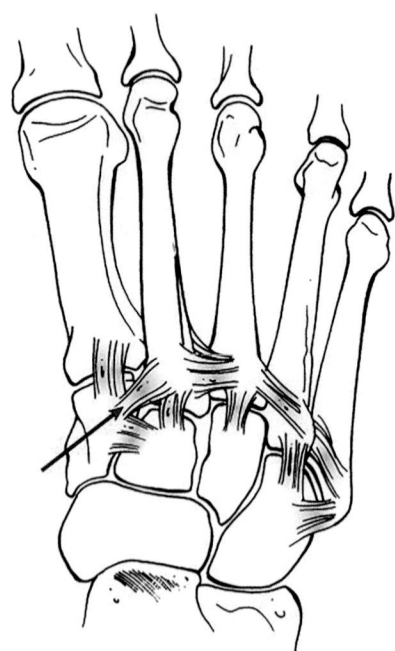

FIGURE 24.4 The plantar tarsometatarsal ligaments and plantar metatarsal ligaments are shown above. Note the absence of a plantar metatarsal ligament between the base of the 1st and 2nd metatarsals. The plantar Lisfranc ligament (*arrow*) runs obliquely from the medial cuneiform to the base of the 2nd metatarsal. (From Easley ME, Wiesel SW. *Operative Techniques in Foot and Ankle Surgery.* 2nd ed. Philadelphia, PA: Lippincott Williams & Wilkins; 2016.)

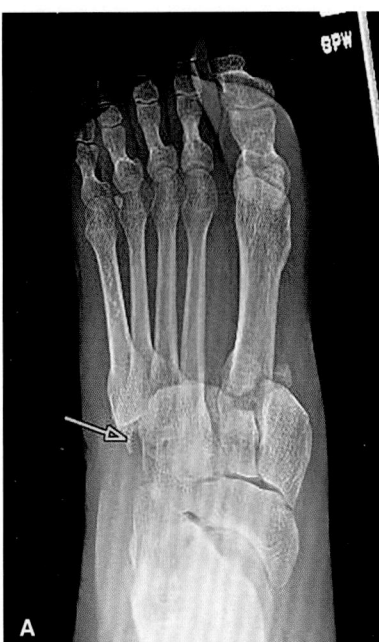

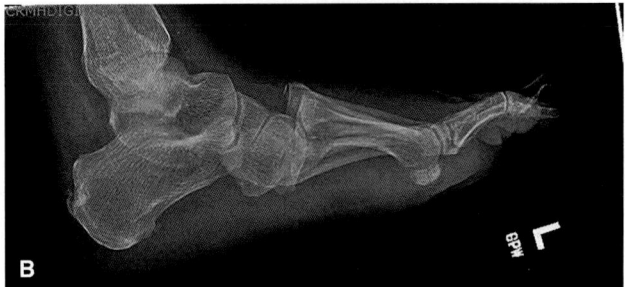

FIGURE 24.5 A. AP radiograph of left foot of a 62-year-old uncontrolled diabetic male with profound peripheral neuropathy who presented with midfoot pain, warmth, and edema. Diagnosed with Lisfranc fracture/dislocation 1 week prior by outside emergency department. **B.** Lateral radiograph of left foot of a 62-year-old uncontrolled diabetic male with profound peripheral neuropathy who presented with midfoot pain, warmth, and edema. Diagnosed with Lisfranc fracture/dislocation 1 week prior by outside emergency department. (Orthopaedic Surgery Essentials by David Thordarson ISBN 13: 9781451115963 Hardcover; LWW, 2012-10.)

stress is applied via weight-bearing radiographs.[15] Weight-bearing films are often painful, which causes the patient to guard. This may produce a false-negative result. Manual stress radiographs under anesthesia may also be considered. However, these are both inconvenient for the patient and involve some morbidity due to anesthesia risks. Stress radiographs are obtained by

dorsiflexing the ankle to neutral and applying abduction to the midfoot. A contralateral radiograph may be beneficial to detect any subtle abnormalities.

Computed tomography scans are useful in identification and evaluation of the fracture and pattern of injury. Subtle TMT injuries may require advanced imaging to confirm a

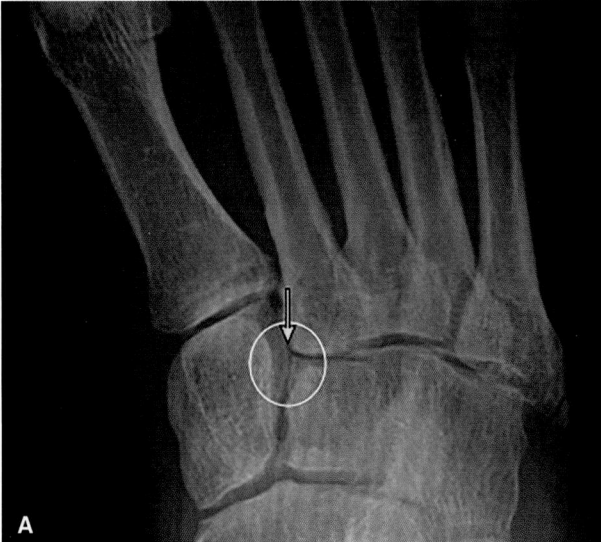

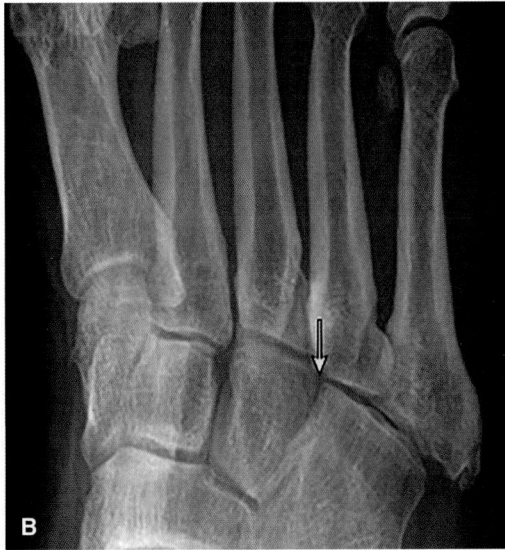

FIGURE 24.6 Normal anteroposterior and oblique non–weight-bearing radiographs of the foot. **A.** The *arrow* on the left marks the medial border of the 2nd metatarsal, which should align directly with the medial border of the middle cuneiform. **B.** The *arrow* on the right indicates the medial border of the 4th metatarsal, which should align directly with the medial border of the cuboid on the oblique radiograph of the foot.

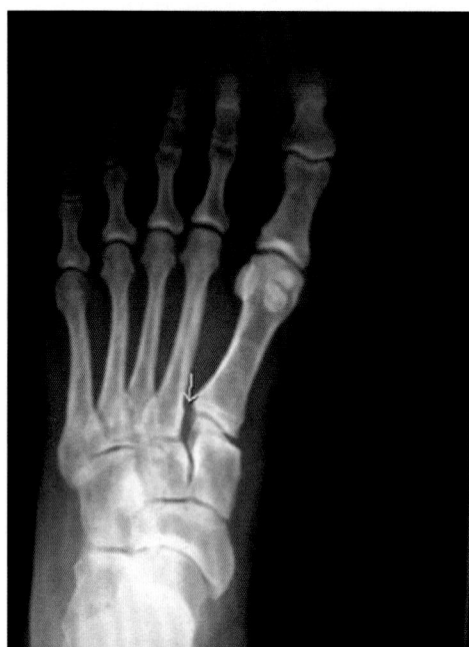

FIGURE 24.7 Greater than 2 mm of diastasis seen on an AP radiograph indicating disruption of the Lisfranc ligament and instability at the 1st TMTJ. The *arrow* indicates the diastases between the 1st cuneiform and 2nd metatarsal base.

diagnosis. Raikin et al. reported magnetic resonance imaging correctly classified 19 (90%) of 21 Lisfranc joint complexes as either stable or unstable on based on the competency of the plantar bundle of the Lisfranc ligament.[16] The appearance of a normal Lisfranc ligament was found to be highly suggestive of a stable TMT complex. An MRI can be obtained to determine integrity of the Lisfranc ligament. Patients with Lisfranc joint injuries should also be assessed for gastrocnemius tightness. An underlying equinus has been reported as a possible contributor to failure following ORIF of a Lisfranc ligament and if unaddressed, may lead to increased forces at the injured or healing TMTJ.

CLASSIFICATION

Multiple classification systems exist regarding Lisfranc injuries. In 1909, Quenu and Kuss were the first to classify specific Lisfranc injury patterns based on the direction of displacement at the TMTJ.[17] This classification was modified by Hardcastle in 1982 to describe more comprehensive energy patterns. It included three primary displacement patterns: divergent, isolated, and homolateral.[18] Hardcastle classification divided the three historical patterns: type A, total incongruity; type B, partial incongruity; and type C, divergent.

In 1986, Myerson et al.[5] further modified and subdivided Hardcastle type B and C into B1, partial incongruity w/medial displacement, B2, partial incongruity w/lateral displacement, and C1, divergent w/partial displacement, C2, total displacement (Fig. 24.8). These classification schemes describe both the fracture pattern and provide information to dictate treatment and provide prognostic outcomes.

An additional classification for more subtle Lisfranc sprain in the athletic population was described by Nunley and Vertullo.[19] These classification schemes were based on clinical findings, weight-bearing radiographs, and bone scintigraphy results. Stage I consisted of a midfoot sprain with no diastasis or arch height loss but increased uptake on bone scintigrams. Stage II sprains consisted of 1st and 2nd intermetatarsal diastasis between 1 and 5 mm with no arch height loss. Stage III displays >5 mm of diastasis on an AP weight-bearing radiograph and loss of arch height. If the midfoot injury was displaced, then one would classify the injury using the Myerson scheme as described above. This classification offers a linear connection with treatment. The stage I nondisplaced midfoot sprains were treated with a non–weight-bearing cast for 6 weeks and then transitioned to a custom-molded orthosis. Stage II and III injuries were treated with ORIF.

PATIENT WORKUP

Upon the initial presentation of a Lisfranc fracture/dislocation, one should first evaluate the neurovascular status of the lower extremity. The soft tissue envelope should also be evaluated for any skin tenting or skin necrosis. In some instances, these injuries are often related to a high-energy mechanism, which may result in soft tissue compromise. Additionally, these injuries may involve significant dislocation and displacement, which may compromise the neurovascular anatomy of the midfoot. Compartment syndrome should always be ruled out first, and if there is high suspicion, then surgical intervention should be immediate.

TMTJ fracture/dislocations should be reduced to relieve pressure on the surrounding soft tissue envelope. If compartment syndrome is ruled out and this is a closed injury, manual reduction should be attempted with subsequent application of a well-padded splint. If adequate reduction is achieved, confirmed, and maintained, then the patient may be discharged from the emergency department and definitive treatment can be planned for a later date.

AUTHOR'S PREFERRED TREATMENT: TMTJ REDUCTION

1. Reduction is easier to obtain while the patient is under conscious sedation. This mitigates patient guarding and allows the practitioner to more easily manipulate the fractures.
2. The hallux and 4th digit should be held while suspending the hindfoot and leg. An assistant should place downward pressure on the anterior aspect of the tibia. This may aid in distracting the TMTJ.
3. If the dislocation occurs in the dorsolateral direction, the provider should place his/her thumb on the medial cuneiform while holding the forefoot with the contralateral hand. Medial to lateral pressure is placed on the medial cuneiform while the forefoot and metatarsals are translated medially. A posterior sugar tong splint is then applied.

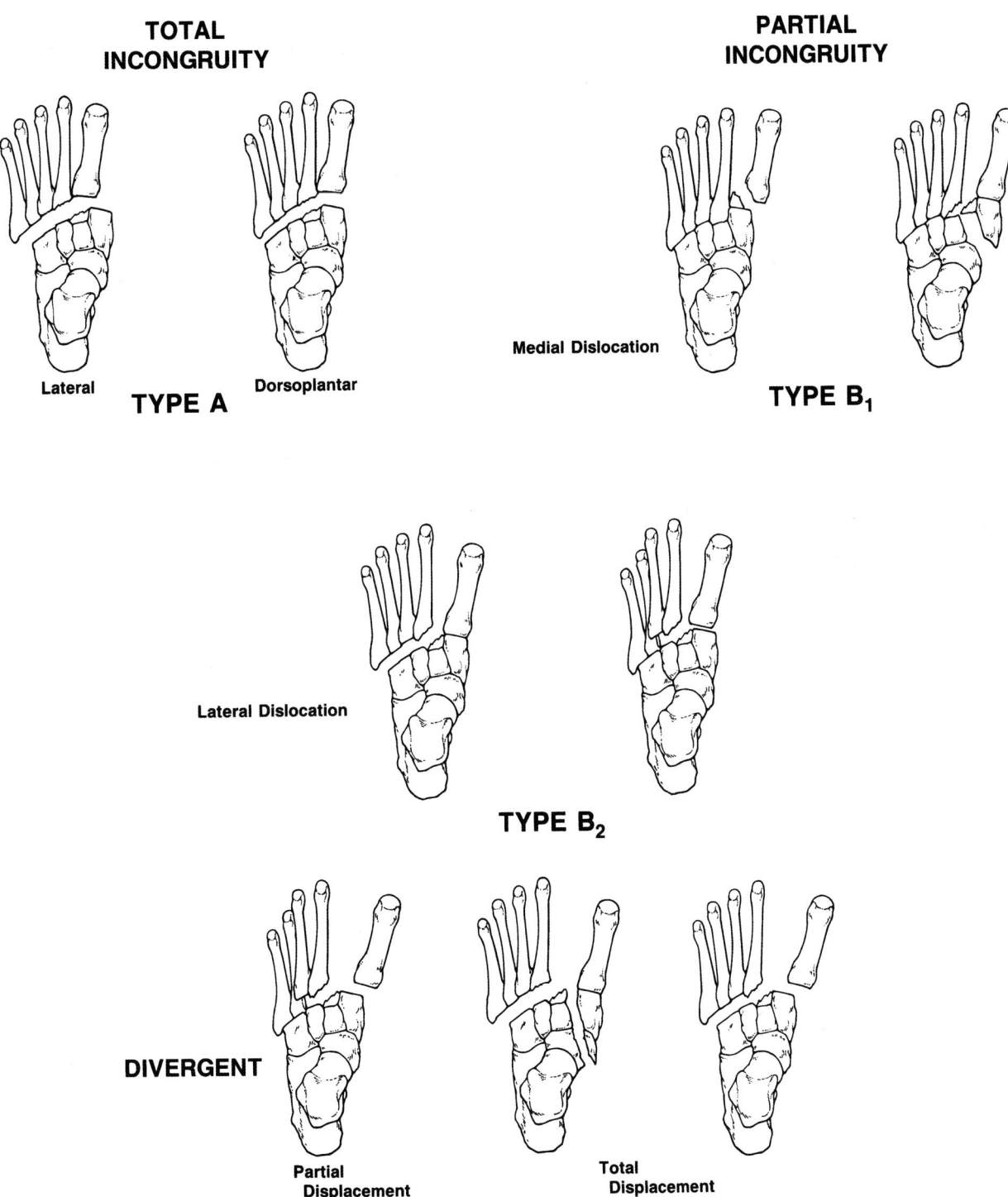

FIGURE 24.8 Myerson modification of Lisfranc dislocation classification. Reproduced with permission from DiNapoli DR, Cain TD. Lisfranc - Dislocation. In: *Update* 1988. Tucker, GA: Podiatry Institute; 1988:198-205.

Unfortunately, high-energy mechanisms are unstable and adequate closed reduction can be difficult to obtain. Lack of reduction may lead to soft tissue compromise and complicate definitive surgical care. If closed reduction attempts fail, the use of an external fixation device may be necessary to aid in reduction. If an external fixator is not available, percutaneously placed Kirschner wires are utilized to maintain reduction. External fixation is not only helpful for definitive fracture management but also soft tissue resuscitation.

One should be cautious of laterally dislocated TMT injuries. The practitioner is often attracted to the more overwhelming skeletal injury on the medial side. However, the primary focus should be restoring the lateral length first, otherwise the reduction will be futile. In order to restore anatomic congruity to the TMT, the lateral column requires length restoration. This can be achieved by distracting the lateral column with a monorail external fixator. The fixator pins are placed into the calcaneus and 5th metatarsal diaphysis. Once the fixator is secure, gentle distraction of the lateral column will create requisite length needed to reduce the medial dislocation. If this is addressed last, the reduction may prove more difficult and frustrating.

NONOPERATIVE MANAGEMENT

Nonoperative management is reserved for stable, nondisplaced injuries when the Lisfranc ligament is intact. In the case of stable injuries, the patient may be placed in a CAM boot and WB status depending on the injury and pain. Radiographs should be followed for the first 2-4 weeks to ensure there is no displacement or diastasis. The patient may transition to supportive shoe at 6 weeks if radiographs show appropriate healing.[20] Surgical management is indicated for Lisfranc ligament disruption, unstable tarsometatarsal complex, and TMT fracture dislocation.

PROCEDURE

The patient is placed in the bed in supine position with a bump positioned at the ipsilateral hip. Either a thigh or calf tourniquet is then applied for hemostasis. The author's personal preference is a thigh tourniquet set at 300 mm Hg. A popliteal block vs ankle block can be administered prior to the procedure for analgesia depending on surgeon preference. A surgical incision ~8-10 cm is then made at the 2nd TMTJ medial to the 2nd metatarsal (Fig. 24.9). This incision will typically allow access to the medial TMTJ complex (TMTJ 1-3). Care is taken to identify, mobilize, and retract the medial neurovascular bundle medially during dissection. An incision of ~8 cm is then made lateral to the base of the 4th metatarsal to access the lateral TMTJ joint complex. It is important to maintain at least a 3-cm skin bridge between both incisions in order to prevent possible skin necrosis. Incisions are deepened and carried through the tarsometatarsal joint capsule.

PATIENT POSITION AND SURGICAL SITE PREPARATION

The patient is brought to the operating room and placed on the operating room table in a supine position. An ipsilateral

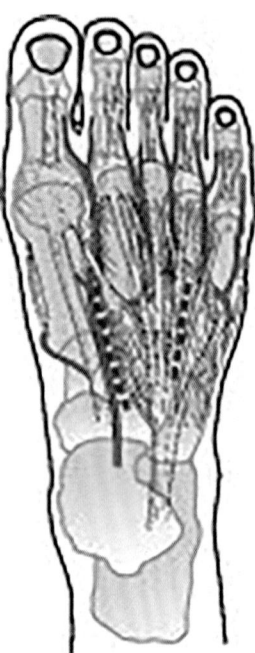

FIGURE 24.9 Incisional placement for Lisfranc ORIF or arthrodesis. (From Quenu E, Kuss G. Study on the dislocations of the metatarsal bones (tarsometatarsal dislocations) and diastasis between the 1st and 2nd metatarsals [French]. *Rev Chir.* 1909;39:281–336, 720–791, 1093–1134.)

hip bump is used. This ensures that the foot is not externally rotated. A pneumatic ankle or thigh tourniquet may be used. This author prefers a thigh tourniquet as an ankle tourniquet can interfere with insertion of some of the instrumentation. The foot is prepped and draped in sterile fashion. The foot is prescrubbed with isopropyl alcohol. A formal skin preparation is completed with chlorhexidine and alcohol. A Betadine skin preparation is also acceptable. Next, the foot, ankle, and leg are draped with standard extremity drapes. The injured extremity is elevated, exsanguinated, and the tourniquet is inflated. The tourniquet is inflated to 250 or 300 mm Hg for ankle or thigh locations, respectively. A skin marker is used to draw an 8 to 10 cm incision on the dorsal aspect of the foot. This incision is generally in line with the central 3rd of the navicular and the 2nd metatarsal. A second incision is made ~3 cm lateral to the initial incision. The skin is incised with a scalpel. Dissection scissors and Bovie electrocautery are used to dissect down to the neurovascular bundle. The neurovascular bundle including the deep peroneal nerve, distal branches of the dorsalis pedis, and deep 1st metatarsal artery are identified and protected.

Once the bone and articular surface has been exposed, the joints are reduced and provisionally pinned with a 2-mm Kirschner wire. Depending on the degree of comminution, a decision is made at this point to proceed with open reduction internal fixation, primary fusion of the tarsometatarsal joint, or bridge plating (Fig. 24.10). If the treating surgeon decides open reduction internal fixation is most appropriate, hardware can be placed once reduction is confirmed. Three-plane fluoroscopy is most helpful at confirming anatomic reduction. It is critical to ensure that all soft tissue debris is removed between the 1st and 2nd metatarsal bases.

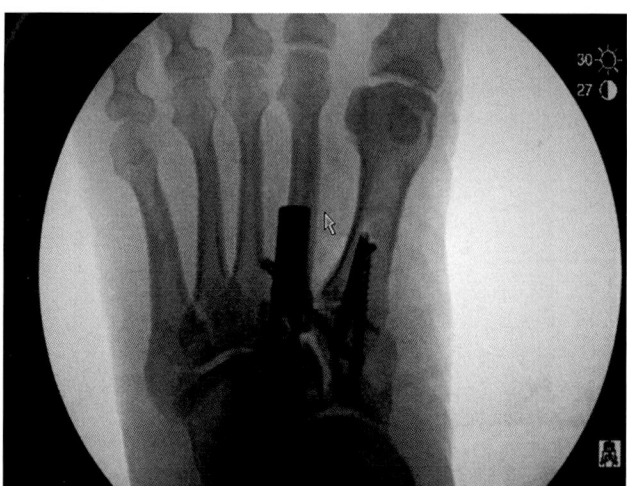

FIGURE 24.10 Combined bridge plating with screw fixation for Lisfranc arthrodesis.

If soft tissue is left interposed within this location, the surgeon will not be able to achieve anatomic reduction. Reduction of the 1st metatarsal relationship to the first cuneiform is an important initial step. Reestablishing an anatomic relationship of the first ray makes additional reduction steps simpler. Once the first ray has been reduced, it should be provisionally pinned. However, the surgeon should not proceed with placement of definitive fixation until the remaining tarsometatarsal joints are reduced.

After the 1st metatarsal and 1st cuneiform have been reduced, a pointed tenaculum is placed between the 1st cuneiform and the 2nd metatarsal base. This step is critical for restoring the 2nd metatarsal within its keystone. Once this position has been reduced, a provisional pin should be placed from the first cuneiform to the 2nd metatarsal base. Care should be taken not to advance this wire into the 3rd metatarsal as this will prevent the 3rd metatarsal from reducing. Once the 3rd metatarsal is reduced to the 3rd cuneiform, then this wire may be advanced into the 3rd metatarsal to provide additional stabilization. The author agrees with Komenda and Sangeorzan that the lateral two rays should not be fused in order to maintain mobility and adaptability of the lateral column.[21,22] Temporary stabilization may be obtained by placing a Kirschner wire across the lateral 4th and 5th TMTJs. These wires may be removed between weeks 6 and 8 postoperatively.

The use of cannulated screws allows precise hardware placement. The cannulated screws should be either 3.5 or 4.0 mm. The screws should also be fully threaded and inserted using a nonlag technique. This prevents unnecessary compression against the articular surface. The use of transarticular fixation will disrupt ~5% of the cartilage.[23] Additional compression of this cartilage is unnecessary and can lead to additional cartilage damage. If the surgeon prefers solid screw fixation, then cannulated instrumentation (guide wire, drill bit, depth gauge, countersink) may be used first, then solid screws can be placed in the prepared location. The use of partially threaded screws is discouraged, particularly between the 1st cuneiform and 2nd metatarsal base. The use of partially threaded screws conspicuously places the run out of the screw in the most unstable

anatomic landmark and predisposes the hardware to early failure (Fig. 24.11).

POSTOPERATIVE MANAGEMENT

The postoperative course is similar regardless of fixation type. The patients are placed in a well-padded posterior splint in the operating room. The patients should adhere to strict elevation and non–weight-bearing recommendations until the first postoperative visit at 2 weeks. The patients are typically seen at 10-14 days after surgery. At this time, the incision is evaluated, and depending upon the edema and skin approximation, the sutures are removed or left intact for another 7-10 days. This author will often place the patient in a short leg cast at this time to help immobilize the skin to mature the incision for an additional 7-10 days. Once the sutures are removed, the patients are placed in a short leg cast for 4-6 weeks. Any percutaneous pins are removed at 6-8 weeks again depending on radiographic findings. Radiographs are obtained at 6-8 weeks postoperatively and the patient transitions to an orthopedic boot. However, the patient should remain nonweight bearing and only remove the boot to begin gentle passive range of motion of the ankle. Subsequent radiographs are obtained at 12 weeks postoperatively. The patient's weight-bearing status can be advanced depending upon the osseous union noted. Initially, weight bearing is allowed in an orthopedic boot and the patient can begin transitioning to soft supportive shoe gear. Formal physical therapy is not required but is reserved for patients who fail to progress with weight bearing and range of motion.

COMPLICATIONS

Complications regarding Lisfranc injuries can be divided based on the type of treatment and surgical approach. The main complication on nonoperatively treated TMT injuries is the lack of recognition of injury or deformity. As stated

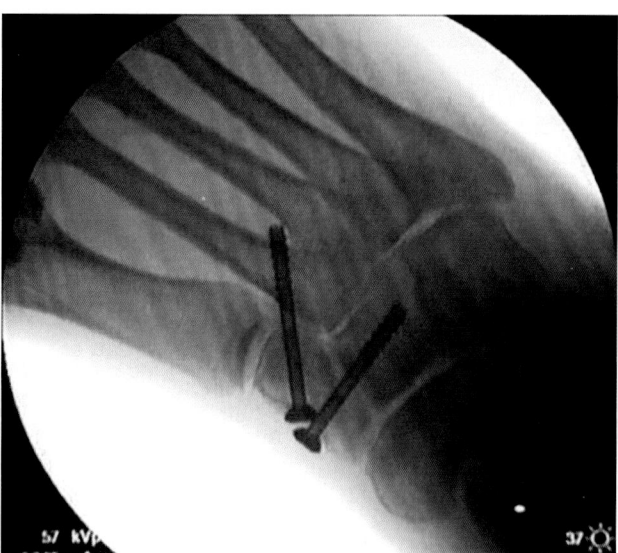

FIGURE 24.11 Partially threaded screws across Lisfranc joint place the runout of the screw at the fusion site.

earlier, up to 20% of these injuries are initially missed.[24] Many of these injuries are missed or overlooked due to the use of non–weight-bearing x-rays. In a study by Sherief et al.[25] only 61% (11/18) of Lisfranc injuries were consistently identified on plain radiographs by all nine participating clinicians. Missing the diagnosis can lead to TMT instability, pain, and premature posttraumatic arthritis.

Wound healing can become another difficult complication due to both operative technique and inappropriate surgical timing. Often the soft tissue envelope is too edematous for early ORIF and therefore may prompt the use of external fixation for fracture/dislocation reduction. This allows for soft tissue resuscitation while maintaining skeletal stability. In addition, the surgeon must take great care with incision placement. As discussed previously, an adequate skin bridge must also be utilized to avoid any possible skin necrosis. During the dissection, the surgeon should avoid injury to the neurovascular structures. Injury to the anterior tibial artery is the most common vascular injury due to its anatomic location.[26]

Compartment syndrome has been reported with high-energy TMT injury.[27] This results in poor outcomes due to pain, nerve injury, and intrinsic muscle contractures.

Following surgery, patients may complain of prominent dorsal hardware due to the thin overlying subcutaneous layer of the dorsal midfoot. Loss of reduction after hardware removal following ORIF of a purely ligamentous injury often occurs, which may lead to increased pain and the development of posttraumatic arthritis. Mulier et al. reported that, at the time of final follow-up (at 30 months), 94% of their open reduction group already had developed signs of degenerative changes of the tarsometatarsal joints radiographically.[28] In a study by Schepers et al., varying fixation constructs were studied based on their maintenance of postoperative reduction.[29] Patients treated with K-wire placement alone had a 37.5% rate of displacement, whereas 0% of displacement was found in those treated with a combination screw and plate construct. Nonunion is also a complication encountered with both arthrodesis and ORIF following Lisfranc injury. Nonunion rates for tarsometatarsal joint arthrodesis are reported anywhere from 0% to 12%.[30,31]

DISCUSSION

TREATMENT DECISION-MAKING

Over the past decade, Lisfranc injuries have been treated with immobilization, open reduction internal fixation, external fixation, percutaneous pinning, and arthrodesis. There is still debate regarding the appropriate treatment algorithm for each patient. Casting may only serve as a temporary treatment with regard to maintaining reduction of an unstable injury as well as removing any interposed soft tissues at the fracture site. As stated earlier, we do know that achieving anatomic reduction provides for the most optimal results,[32,33] which can be obtained with either ORIF or primary fusion. Operative intervention is indicated in acute fracture/dislocation injuries as well as subtle/latent Lisfranc injuries, which show widening due to weight-bearing stress. Subtle injuries may initially be treated conservatively, but unfortunately many of these patients have continued pain and ultimately require some form of open reduction (Fig. 24.12).

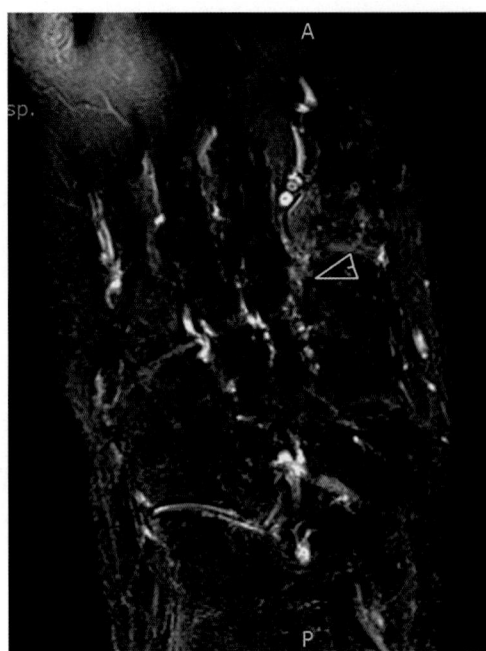

FIGURE 24.12 Patient with a subtle Lisfranc injury seen on T2-weighted image on MRI.

Crates et al. looked at operative treatment results following failure of nonoperative care in the subtle Lisfranc injury.[34] Of the 36 patients enrolled in their study, 16 (44.44%) were successfully treated nonoperatively, whereas 20 (55.56%) required operative therapy after nonoperative measures had failed. Controversy exists regarding optimal treatment of primary ligamentous Lisfranc injuries. Kuo et al. studied a group of 15 patients who underwent ORIF of a Lisfranc injury.[35] They followed these patients for 7 years and found that those with purely ligamentous injuries had suboptimal results despite anatomical reduction. Some speculate that these suboptimal results stem from incomplete and unpredictable ligamentous healing. Scar tissue forms during the healing process, which is weaker and more unstable in comparison to osseous healing. Type III collagen replaces type I collagen in the injured ligament tissue. Type III collagen is less densely packed, has small fibrils, and cross-links in an abnormal fashion, which can ultimately lead to decreased joint reduction, motion, and stability. This results in an environment that may lead to collapse and deformation at the TMTJ, which will likely end in posttraumatic arthritis. High-energy fracture dislocations with a high degree of articular disruption are often treated with fusion because of the initial cartilage damage due to severity of injury. Henning in 2009[36] randomized ORIF vs primary fusion patients and found no difference in SMFA or SF-36. One hundred percent of the ORIFs had anatomic reduction and only one of these patients needed later fusion. A higher secondary surgery rate was found, which is to be expected due to screw removal. Ly in 2006[37] compared primary arthrodesis vs open reduction and internal fixation, which showed a significant better AOFAS and return to activity score in the primary arthrodesis group. This study also showed that 25% of the ORIF group resulted in fusion and 75% of ORIF cases needed screw removal (19% in arthrodesis group). Those with late fusions were improved but unfortunately not to the level of the primary arthrodesis group. Coetzee et al. performed a qualitative, systematic review of the literature comparing ORIF vs arthrodesis results.[38] This study showed that both procedures result in satisfactory. They did find a slight advantage of primary fusion for purely ligamentous injuries. The treatment decision in choosing between ORIF and primary fusion is multifactorial. Patient history, activity level, goals for return to activity, BMI, and severity of initial injury are all considerations when choosing a treatment approach. The patient should always be informed that if planning an ORIF procedure, a surgery of screw removal and possible fusion due to arthritic changes may occur secondarily.

PEARLS and PITFALLS

- The most important factor in achieving good outcome is anatomic reduction of the TMTJ. Understanding the TMTJ anatomy is crucial.
- If compartment syndrome is suspected, immediate intervention is required. Always evaluate for concomitant injuries.
- Incision planning is very important for successful procedure.
- Reduction of the first metatarsal relationship to the first cuneiform is an important initial step. This should be provisionally pinned as an initial step.
- Use a pointed tenaculum between the first cuneiform and the second metatarsal to restore the second metatarsal within its keystone.
- The lateral two rays should not be fused in order to maintain mobility and adaptability of the lateral column. Temporary stabilization may be obtained with Kirschner wires.
- The use of cannulated screws that are fully threaded and inserted using a nonlag technique is recommended. This prevents unnecessary compression against the articular surface.
- Patient history, activity level, goals for return to activity, BMI, and severity of initial injury are all considerations when choosing a treatment approach.

REFERENCES

1. Watson TS, Shurnas PS, Denker J. Treatment of Lisfranc joint injury: current concepts. *J Am Acad Orthop Surg.* 2010;18(12):718-728.
2. Curtis MJ, Myerson M, Szura B. Tarsometatarsal joint injuries in the athlete. *Am J Sports Med.* 1993;21:497-502.
3. Buzzard BM, Briggs PJ. Surgical management of acute tarsometatarsal fracture dislocation in adults. *Clin Orthop Relat Res.* 1998;353:125-133.
4. Goosens M, De Stoop N. Lisfranc fracture dislocations: etiology, radiology, and result of treatment. A review of 20 cases. *Clin Orthop Relat Res.* 1983;176:154-162.
5. Myerson MS, Fisher RT, Burgess AR, Kenzore JE. Fracture dislocations of the tarsometatarsal joints: end results correlated with pathology and treatment. *Foot Ankle Int.* 1986;6(5):225-242.
6. Wiley JJ. The mechanism of tarso-metatarsal joint injuries. *J Bone Joint Surg Br.* 1971;53(3):474-482.
7. Manoli A. Compartment syndrome of the foot: current concepts. *FAI.* 1990;10(6):340-344.
8. Schiff AP, Gross CE, Easley ME, Easley M, Wiesel S. Open reduction and internal fixation of the Lisfranc fracture-dislocation. In: *Operative Techniques in Foot and Ankle Surgery.* 2nd ed. Philadelphia, PA: Wolters Kluwer; 2017:1284-1306.
9. Henning JA, Jones CB, Siestema DI, Bohay DI, Anderson JG. Open reduction internal fixation versus primary arthrodesis for Lisfranc injuries. *Foot Ankle Int.* 2006;27(8):653-660.
10. Ouzounian TJ, Shereff MJ. In vitro determination of midfoot motion. *Foot Ankle.* 1989;10:140-146.
11. Vuori JP. Lisfranc joint injuries: trauma mechanisms and associated injuries. *J Trauma.* 1993;35(1):40-45.
12. Tornetta, III, Paul; Wiesel, Sam W. *Operative Techniques in Orthopaedic Trauma Surgery.* 2nd ed. Philadelphia, PA: Lippincott Williams & Wilkins; 2016.
13. Foster SC, Foster RR. Lisfranc's tarsometatarsal fracture-dislocation. *Radiology.* 1976;120:79-83.
14. Norfray JF, Geline RA, Steinberg RI, Galinski AW, Gilula LA. Subtleties of Lisfranc fracture-dislocations. *AJR Am J Roentgenol.* 1981;137:1151-1156.
15. Coss HS, Manos RE, Buoncristiani A, Mills WJ. Abduction stress and AP weightbearing radiography of purely ligamentous injury in the tarsometatarsal joint. *Foot Ankle Int.* 1998;19:537-541.
16. Raikin SM, Elias I, Dheer S, Besser MP, Morrison WB, Zoga AC. Prediction of midfoot instability in the subtle Lisfranc injury. Comparison of magnetic resonance imaging with intraoperative findings. *J Bone Joint Surg.* 2009;91(4):892-899.
17. Quenu E, Kuss G. Study on the dislocations of the metatarsal bones (tarsometatarsal dislocations) and diastasis between the 1st and 2nd metatarsal. *Rev Chir.* 1909;39:281-336, 720-791, 1093-1134 (in French).
18. Hardcastle PH, Reschauer R, Kutscha-Lissberg E, Schoffmann W. Injuries to the tarsometatarsal joint. Incidence, classification and treatment. *J Bone Joint Surg Br.* 1982;64(3):349-356.
19. Nunley JA, Vertullo CJ. Classification, investigation, and management of midfoot sprains: Lisfranc injuries in the athlete. *Am J Sports Med.* 2002;30:871
20. Lattermann C, Goldstein JL, Wukich DK, et al. Practical management of Lisfranc injuries in athletes. *Clin J Sport Med.* 2007;17:311.
21. Komenda GA, Myerson MS, Biddinger KR. Results of arthrodesis of the tarsometatarsal joints after traumatic injury. *J Bone Joint Surg Am.* 1996;78:1665-1676.
22. Sangeorzan BJ, Veith RG, Hansen ST Jr. Salvage of Lisfranc's tarsometatarsal joint by arthrodesis. *Foot Ankle.* 1990;10:193-200.
23. Clements JR, Whitmer K, Nguyen H, Rich M. Cross-sectional area measurement of the central tarsometatarsal articulation: a review of computed tomography scans. *J Foot Ankle Surg.* 2018;57(4):732-736.
24. Trevino SG, Kodros S. Controversies in tarsometatarsal injuries. *Orthop Clin North Am.* 1995;26(2):229-238.
25. Sherief TI, Mucci B, Greiss M. Lisfranc injury: how frequently does it get missed? And how can we improve? *Injury.* 2007;38(7):856-860.
26. Gissane W. A dangerous type of fracture of the foot. *J Bone Joint Surg.* 1951;33(4):535-538.
27. Anton JF, Manoli A II. Acute foot compartment syndrome. *J Orthop Trauma.* 1992;6(2):223-228. doi: 10.1097/00005131-199206000-00015.
28. Mulier T, Reynders P, Dereymaeker G, Broos P. Severe Lisfranc's injuries: primary arthrodesis or ORIF? *Foot Ankle Int.* 2002;23:902-905.
29. Schepers T, Operel PP, Van Lieshout EM. Influence of approach and implant on reduction accuracy and stability in Lisfranc fracture-dislocation at the tarsometatarsal joint. *Foot Ankle Int.* 2013;34(5):705-710.
30. Mann RA, Prieskorn D, Sobel M. Mid-tarsal and tarsometatarsal arthrodesis for primary degenerative osteoarthrosis after trauma. *J Bone Joint Surg Am.* 1996;78:1376-1385.
31. Patel S, Ford LA, Etcheverry J, Rush SM, Hamilton GA. Modified lapidus arthrodesis: rate of nonunion in 227 cases. *J Foot Ankle Surg.* 2004;43(1):37-42.
32. Arntz CT, Hansen ST Jr. Dislocation and fracture dislocations of the tarsometatarsal joints. *Orthop Clin North Am.* 1987;18:105-114.
33. Adib F, Medadi F, Guidi E, et al. Osteoarthritis following open reduction and internal fixation of the Lisfranc injury. Paper presented at 12th EFORT Congress; June 1-4, 2011. Copenhagen, Denmark.
34. Crates JM, Barber FA, Sanders EJ. Subtle Lisfranc subluxations: results of operative and nonoperative treatment. *J Foot Ankle Surg.* 2015;54:350-355.
35. Kuo RS, Tejwani NC, Digiovanni CW, et al. Outcome after open reduction and internal fixation of Lisfranc joint injuries. *J Bone Joint Surg Am.* 2000;82:1609-1618.
36. Henning JA, Jones CB, Sietsema DL, Bohay DR, Anderson JG. Open reduction internal fixation versus primary arthrodesis for Lisfranc injuries: a prospective randomized study. *Foot Ankle Int.* 2009;30(10):913-922.
37. Ly TV, Coetzee JC. Treatment of primarily ligamentous Lisfranc joint injuries: primary arthrodesis compared with open reduction and internal fixation. *J Bone Joint Surg Am.* 2006;88(3):514-520.
38. Sheibani-Rad C, Giveans D. Arthrodesis versus ORIF for Lisfranc fractures. *Orthopedics.* 2012;35(6):868-873.

Hindfoot Surgery

CHAPTER 25

Triple Arthrodesis

J. Michael Miller and Andrew P. Kapsalis

DEFINITION

The triple arthrodesis is a time-tested procedure that has been performed by foot and ankle surgeons for nearly 100 years. Hoke initially described a hindfoot fusion technique to treat severe deformities in 1921. However, it was Ryerson, in 1923, who modified this technique and described the triple arthrodesis procedure as we know it today.[1,2] In its inception, the triple arthrodesis was performed to provide a pain-free and plantigrade foot in patients with severe congenital or paralytic deformities. Today, it is still regarded as a reliable procedure and is performed for a wider variety of etiologies that give rise to severe deformity, ligamentous instability, neurogenic pedal contractures, post-traumatic sequelae, or painful arthritic conditions (Table 25.1). Perhaps the biggest change in the procedure over the years has been through advancements in internal fixation. Historically, transosseous catgut suture and cast immobilization was utilized initially with the procedure. Presently, rigid metallic internal fixation is the standard. This advancement in internal fixation methods allows the procedure to be performed in a more consistent fashion with reproducible outcomes.

INDICATIONS

By definition, the triple arthrodesis procedure fuses three essential hindfoot joints: the subtalar joint, the talonavicular joint, and the calcaneocuboid joint. With our current knowledge of lower extremity biomechanics, we realize these are important, functional joints that a surgeon would prefer to maintain in their natural state. However, certain circumstances will require us to forfeit this function in order to provide a pain free foot with improved functional alignment to optimize the patient's gait. Joint sparing procedures such as periarticular osteotomies, tendon transfers, and endoprosthesis (subtalar implants) can sometimes be performed instead of rearfoot arthrodesis procedures to obtain our reconstructive goals for foot alignment and function. Sometimes, if the deformity is too severe or the joints are arthritic/painful, then a rearfoot arthrodesis may be necessary.

In general, the purpose of a triple arthrodesis is to provide a functional, plantigrade foot that is pain free. Dysfunction and deformity of the foot requiring this procedure ranges from flatfoot reconstruction, cavus reconstruction, post traumatic arthritic conditions, paralytic disorders, tarsal coalitions, and

more (Table 25.2). If the deformity or pain is located to just one of the rearfoot joints, then an isolated single joint arthrodesis procedure can be performed. Most often a triple arthrodesis is used as a salvage procedure to provide correction of rearfoot deformity by manipulation of the triple joint complex and fusing it into this corrected position in order to facilitate improved foot function.

DOUBLE VS TRIPLE ARTHRODESIS

Current treatment concepts tend to suggest that isolated or double arthrodesis may be preferable to performing a complete (triple) rearfoot fusion procedure. With this in mind, historically, a primary triple arthrodesis was often performed to achieve realignment of a severe rearfoot deformity. Fusion of the triple hindfoot complex worked well, but complete rearfoot function was sacrificed. In the early 2000s, Dr. Sigvard Hansen

TABLE **25.1** Conditions Treatable With Triple Arthrodesis
Idiopathic collapsing pes planovalgus deformity
Posterior tibialis tendon insufficiency/dysfunction
Posterior tibialis tendon rupture
Peroneal spastic flatfoot
Tarsal coalition
Idiopathic cavus and cavovarus deformities
Charcot-Marie-Tooth disease
Residual or under-corrected clubfoot
Congenital vertical talus
Joint instability
Chronic pain
Rheumatoid arthritis
Degenerative arthritis
Posttraumatic arthritis
Charcot neuroarthropathy
Hereditary familial sensorimotor neuropathies
Poliomyelitis
Spina bifida
Myelomeningocele
Muscular dystrophy
Cerebral palsy
Myelodysplasia
Friedrich ataxia
Arthrogryposis

TABLE 25.2 Indications for Triple Arthrodesis

Valgus Foot Deformities:
  Collapsing pes planovalgus deformity
  Posterior tibialis tendon insufficiency/dysfunction
  Posterior tibialis tendon rupture
  Tarsal coalition
  Progressive arthritic conditions

Varus Foot Deformities:
  Cavus deformity
  Progressive or congenital cavovarus deformity
  Talipes equinovarus deformity

Miscellaneous Conditions:
  Rearfoot arthritic conditions
  Failed previous soft tissue and other osseous surgical procedures
  Chronic pain conditions
  Joint instability
  Charcot neuroarthropathy
  Vertical talus
  Neuromuscular diseases and paralytic deformities

popularized the idea of achieving the same rearfoot correction by fusing only the subtalar and talonavicular joints. The calcaneocuboid joint was not violated unless it was painful, arthritic, or absolutely required for optimal deformity correction. This double arthrodesis is performed in the same manner as the triple arthrodesis, but deleting the calcaneocuboid arthrodesis portion of the procedure. This spares another area for potential complications to arise (ie, nonunion, hardware complications, or pain) and allows for some preservation of rearfoot motion laterally.

The double arthrodesis has been improved over time with the progress of operative technique and internal fixation and is becoming more commonly utilized by foot and ankle surgeons. Double and triple arthrodesis procedures have been well documented in their ability to sufficiently reduce deformity, both clinically and radiographically, with no differences in long-term outcomes. The double arthrodesis allows for decreased operating time, decreased cost, preservation of lateral column length, and decreased areas for potential complications as it can be done through a single medial incision in some instances.[3,4] Double arthrodesis limits rearfoot motion in all three functional planes significantly, while the triple arthrodesis completely restricts rearfoot motion in all these directions while also altering motion to adjacent joints more significantly than a double arthrodesis alone.[5] This being said, development of ankle valgus is 3.64 times higher after triple arthrodesis than when a double arthrodesis is performed.[6] Furthermore, calcaneocuboid joint osteoarthritis may be improved at least one grade after double arthrodesis, due to functional arthrodiastasis that can occur after deformity correction with fusion of the subtalar and talonavicular joints.[7]

In today's general picture, most rearfoot deformities can be corrected by the double arthrodesis (Figs. 25.1 and 25.2). Triple arthrodesis is reserved as a salvage procedure for those deformities so severe that correction is not achievable without addressing the calcaneocuboid joint, or when there is pain/significant arthrosis in this joint.

PATIENT SELECTION AND PREOPERATIVE CONSIDERATIONS

As we discussed, the triple arthrodesis is essentially a salvage procedure. Normal biomechanics of the foot rely significantly on appropriate subtalar and midtarsal joint motion. Once these joint complexes are fused, altered mechanical adaptation of the foot ensues and adjacent joints will have to compensate for this lack of motion. Therefore, if a rearfoot joint sparing procedure can be performed, one must entertain this before embarking on a rearfoot arthrodesis. The subtalar and midtarsal joints are primarily responsible for inversion and eversion of the foot as well as adaptive compensation against uneven ground reactive forces. With the triple hindfoot complex fused, this motion is transferred to the ankle joint and, to a lesser degree, the remaining midfoot joints. With this understood, premature arthritic adaptation will occur over time and adjacent joints will eventually develop arthritis. Therefore, a triple arthrodesis procedure will usually satisfy the patient in the short term but can potentially present other problems in the future. With this being understood, a triple arthrodesis may be appropriate if the deformity is significant, painful, or recalcitrant to other conservative or prior surgical efforts.

Predictable outcomes after triple arthrodesis may be attainable when specific parameters are met preoperatively, intraoperatively, and postoperatively. Preoperative considerations begin with managing patient expectations. Patient education is important when a surgeon considers a triple arthrodesis procedure. Detailed discussion regarding the recovery and postoperative course with the patient is essential (Table 25.3). The patient needs to understand that the movement and mechanics of their foot will be permanently altered after a triple arthrodesis, and it may feel "stiff" compared to the contralateral limb. However, this tradeoff is often deemed reasonable if the foot deformity is corrected, functionally improved, and pain ameliorated.

Other considerations for a triple arthrodesis include patient age, activity level, weight (body mass index), bone quality, and comorbidities that can affect healing. In general, a rearfoot fusion should be performed on skeletally mature individuals. For children and adolescents with severe rearfoot deformities, one should initially entertain soft tissue procedures combined with extra-articular osteotomies, extra-articular fusions (ie, Green-Grice procedure), or endoprosthesis via subtalar implant. This may provide corrective benefit for the short term—until age is appropriate for a definitive rearfoot fusion. Definitive arthrodesis procedures can be considered when the patient reaches a physiologic age of 14-15 years in their skeletal maturity. At this age, ~90% of the rearfoot bone growth has occurred, so a fusion of the rearfoot complex will not significantly alter overall foot size when compared to the contralateral limb.

On the other side of the age spectrum, elderly patients who are in otherwise good health are excellent candidates for a rearfoot fusion procedure if they meet the indicative criteria. These patients often have long standing deformities with arthritic changes in the rearfoot joints that make this procedure appropriate for them. Reconstruction of severe foot deformities in older patients with periarticular osteotomies and tendon transfers sometimes is not as successful due to poor soft tissue quality and osteopenic bone. Hence, an arthrodesis procedure may be a better choice for some of these individuals.

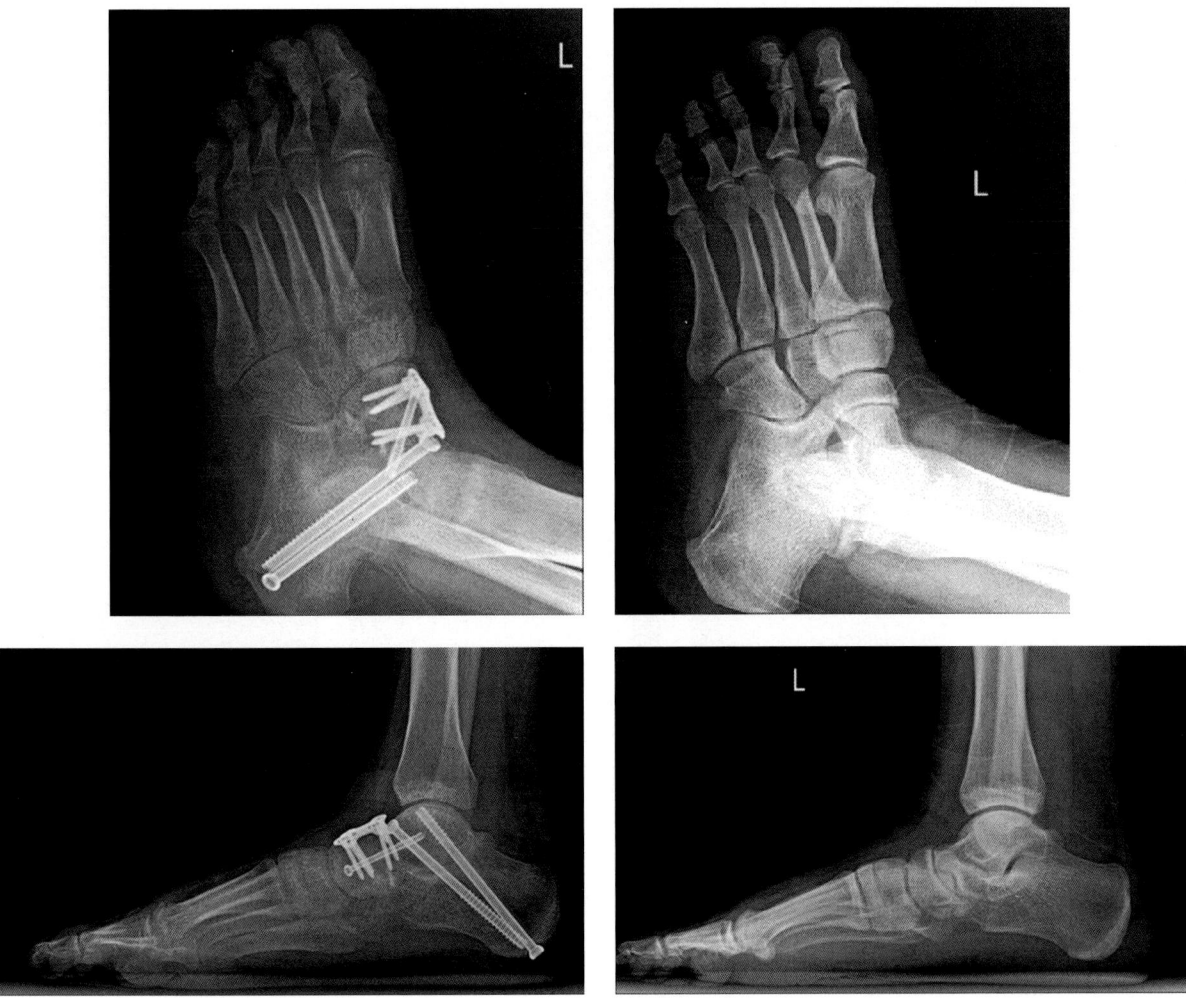

FIGURE 25.1 Calcaneonavicular coalition resection with double arthrodesis. (Pictures provided by J. Michael Miller, DPM.)

Along with older patients, obese patients are also often better candidates for rearfoot arthrodesis procedures. Increased mechanical forces about the rearfoot from excessive weight may lead to difficulty with tendon transfers holding up to significant varus or valgus stress in these patients. Because of this, an arthrodesis procedure may be a better choice for obese individuals because it "locks up" this rearfoot instability and should provide a long-lasting solution to their functional problem.

The patient's overall health, activity level, and psycho-social situation are also areas of concern that should be evaluated before recommending a reconstructive rearfoot arthrodesis. Recovery from this type of surgery can be protracted and arduous. It is often beneficial to explain to patients undergoing triple arthrodesis that it takes 6 months to a year (or more), to ultimately see the complete benefits from this surgery. Smoking, diabetes, rheumatological conditions, and osteoporosis can create prolonged healing times and may require bone grafting or prolonged non–weight-bearing to facilitate healing. So before embarking on a reconstructive procedure such as a triple arthrodesis, all these facets of patient care and recovery should be evaluated.

Preoperative assessment of the patient's ability to be non–weight-bearing with gait assistive devices is important. The patient has to be prepared to remain non–weight-bearing for 6-10 weeks, followed by protected ambulation for up to 4 months after surgery. A preoperative physical therapy consultation may be necessary for some individuals to evaluate and optimally train them for such a recovery.

Along with the physical stress of recovery from a triple arthrodesis, there are also psychological and socioeconomic stress factors to consider. Firstly, there may be an extended time away from work and social contact for these patients, which can create compliance issues and economic burden. Secondly, although most of these procedures can be performed in an outpatient setting, some patients may require inpatient management, which can drive up patient costs and inconvenience significantly.[8] Discussing these points with the patient prior to surgery is beneficial to minimize these issues during recovery. That being said, the recovery can be difficult not only on the patient but also on their family. To navigate this situation optimally, there should be a discussion of the perioperative expectations with the patient's family in the preoperative setting as well.

From a surgeon's perspective, other preoperative considerations for the patient undergoing triple arthrodesis includes a thorough evaluation of the patient's lower extremity biomechanics. Often patients with long standing rearfoot deformities will possess significant equinus deformity as well as

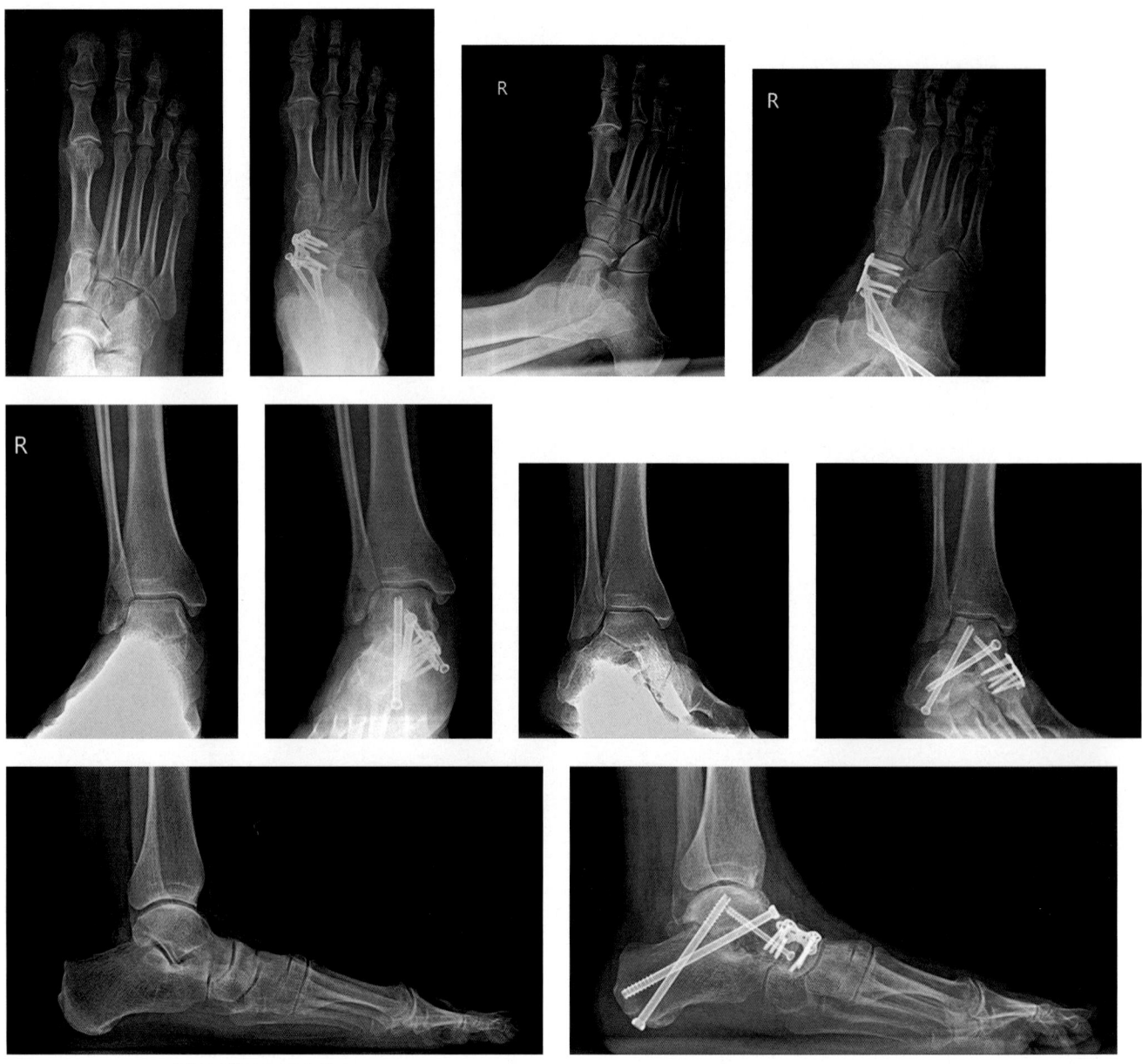

FIGURE 25.2 Double arthrodesis for severe pes valgus deformity. (Pictures provided by J. Michael Miller, DPM.)

other soft tissue contractures. Although the amount of equinus cannot fully be appreciated until the patient is on the operating room table with the foot fixated in corrected position, evaluation of gastrocnemius-soleus equinus should be performed with the foot manipulated into corrected position preoperatively. When correcting severe rearfoot valgus, gastrocnemius-soleus equinus deformity is often significant and must be addressed with either a tendo Achilles lengthening or gastrocnemius recession—pending the intraoperative evaluation. On the other end of the spectrum, when correcting a cavus deformity, the opposite can occur and correcting the deformity can sometimes correct the foot equinus position as well. This is achieved by decreasing the overall arch height and creating a more dorsiflexed position of the forefoot. If this does not occur to an appropriate extent, then a plantar soft tissue release

(ie, Steindler stripping), tendo Achilles lengthening, or gastrocnemius recession should be considered in the cavus or cavovarus foot as well.

Along with clinical examination, radiographic evaluation of the foot and ankle is necessary for appropriate procedural selection. Weight-bearing radiographs assist in evaluating bony alignment, arthritic issues, and bone quality. If the deformity is reducible, radiographs obtained with manipulation of the foot into corrected position can help guide in procedural selection as well. A flexible deformity may be corrected with soft tissue procedures combined with periarticular osteotomies. A rigid (nonreducible) deformity usually requires a rearfoot fusion procedure to allow appropriate correction. Ankle radiographs are also essential in order to make sure there is no significant valgus or varus deformity of the tibiotalar segment

TABLE 25.3 Expected Recovery and Postoperative Course

Day 0 to Week 1: Immediate Postoperative Management
- This starts with adequate layered closure and compressive dressing application
- Postoperative pain management, icing, and elevation of the operative foot
- Deformity correction and is maintained/protected using a posterior splint or below knee casting
- The patient is seen within 1 week for initial evaluation of the surgical site and to address any impending issues as early as possible (ie, infection, hematoma, venous thrombosis)
- Radiographs are obtained at this time to confirm adequate deformity correction and placement of internal fixation
- The patient remains non–weight-bearing throughout this time period

Weeks 1-4: Wound Healing
- Sutures are removed around weeks 2-3 and any as indicated wound issues are managed accordingly
- Edema control is continued using compressive support devices (ie, ACE wrap or compression sock)
- Radiographs are obtained around week 4 to confirm initial osseous healing across the fusion sites
- The patient remains non–weight-bearing throughout this time period
- The patient may perform gentle range of motion exercises across the ankle when in a resting position

Weeks 4-8: Consolidation
- At 6-8 weeks postoperatively, the patient may begin progressive transitioning to partial weight-bearing in a removable immobilization boot or short leg cast, using gait assistive devices
- More active range of motion exercises can be performed
- Radiographs are obtained around week 6-8 to confirm continued osseous healing across the fusion sites

Weeks 8-12: Return to WB
- With evidence of adequate osseous consolidation, the patient may begin slow progressive transitioning to full weight-bearing in the removable immobilization boot
- Radiographs are obtained around week 10-12 to ensure adequate fusion of the rearfoot joints

Months 3-6: Short-term Recovery
- The patient may begin progressive transitioning out of the removable immobilization boot and into regular, supportive shoe gear with use of an ankle brace and/or compressive support device
- The patient may progress to full activity without limitations during this time period
- Physical therapy may be instituted to help facilitate recovery in this time period (ie, for gait training, edema reduction, strengthening exercises)

Months 6-12+: Full Recovery
- Continued healing occurs, as discussed with the patient preoperatively
- The patient may or may not require a follow-up appointment within this time period, depending on patient and surgeon preference
- At this time, the surgeon can plan for contralateral intervention if need be

present concomitantly. If an ankle deformity is present, then it should be addressed along with the index procedure for appropriate care.

Bony equinus of the ankle from anterior exostosis or arthritic changes in the joint must also be evaluated and addressed. If the ankle is painful with arthritis or osteochondral irregularities, this may alter procedural selection due to the known problem of progressive arthrosis of the ankle joint when a triple arthrodesis is performed. Advanced imaging via MRI or CT is often necessary for proper evaluation of the rearfoot and ankle for these issues. If there is a concern of ankle pathology present in the clinical setting, a diagnostic local anesthetic injection can be given to the ankle to help discern if the pathology in the ankle is contributing to the patient's symptoms.

Moving proximally, supra-pedal deformities also need to be evaluated when considering a triple arthrodesis. If the patient has significant genu varum, genu valgum, or limb length discrepancy, rearfoot position and function can be greatly impacted. Surgical planning will have to include either addressing this proximal pathology directly, or compensating for it with our more distal procedural selection.

Ultimately, the triple arthrodesis procedure is a powerful tool to address particular foot and ankle pathology. It requires appropriate patient selection, a qualified surgeon, and appropriate patient expectations to execute the procedure. Most of the candidates for triple arthrodesis are in significant pain with deformities that have been disabling and limiting their daily activities for years. Often, they simply "want to be out of pain." With successful surgery, these patients are often the most satisfied.

OPERATIVE TECHNIQUE

The operative techniques for triple arthrodesis and double arthrodesis procedures are essentially the same. Traditionally, a double arthrodesis is performed via an incision for each joint being fused, and the same incisional approach is taken for a triple arthrodesis with the addition of a third incision for the calcaneocuboid joint. However, the subtalar and talonavicular joints can occasionally be addressed through a single medial incision (ie, the "medial double" procedure)—especially when a significant valgus deformity is present or when the calcaneocuboid joint does not have to be addressed. When considering this single medial incisional approach, one should be mindful of the deltoid ligament complex within the proximal aspect of the surgical field. Using this single incisional approach can invade the deltoid ligament complex and weaken this structure, possibly resulting in medial ankle instability. Due to this potential issue, the authors find more predictable outcomes when using two separate incisions.

SUBTALAR JOINT INCISION PLACEMENT AND DISSECTION

As stated above, the subtalar joint can be addressed via either a medial or, more commonly, a lateral incisional approach. The proximal landmark for the medial approach is the inferior pole of the medial malleolus with the incision then carried distally toward the navicular tuberosity. Often, this approach is converted into a "lazy S" configuration to help facilitate exposure for both the subtalar and talonavicular joints through this single incision (Fig. 25.3).

The lateral incisional approach to the subtalar joint is initiated from the inferior pole of the lateral malleolus and then extends distally toward the region of the fourth metatarsocuboid joint (Fig. 25.4A). This will place dissection between the sural and intermediate dorsal cutaneous neural structures. Layered dissection is carried down to the subtalar joint capsule (Fig. 25.4B and C). There is occasionally a sural nerve branch that communicates with the intermediate dorsal cutaneous nerve within the subcutaneous tissues (Fig. 25.4D). If present, this communicating nerve sometimes has to be sacrificed to gain appropriate access to the deeper landmark structures. The extensor digitorum brevis muscle is divided longitudinally and retracted dorsally, while the peroneal tendons (maintained within their tendon sheaths) and the adjacent sural nerve are carefully retracted inferiorly (Fig. 25.4E). Anteriorly within this space, the fibroadipose tissues of Hoke's tonsil in the sinus tarsi can be excised for improved visualization of the subtalar joint capsule (Fig. 25.4H). From this location, the posterior and middle facets can be accessed by tracing the superior margin of the anterior calcaneus proximally until entering these joint spaces. From the proximal aspect of the surgical site, the calcaneofibular ligament may need to be released from its fibular attachment to further facilitate exposure of the entire subtalar joint (Fig. 25.4F and G). Once the capsular and ligamentous structures are freed, now the joint complex is ready for preparation via contour resection and curettage technique as outlined below (Fig. 25.4H and I).

TALONAVICULAR JOINT INCISION PLACEMENT AND DISSECTION

The talonavicular joint is addressed by an incision coursing from the medial gutter of the ankle down to the navicular tuberosity (Fig. 25.5A). Dissection is carried down to the joint capsule in the same layered manner as described above for the subtalar joint. Important structures to identify in the dissection through subcutaneous tissues are the tibialis anterior tendon laterally, as well as the greater saphenous vein and the saphenous nerve inferiorly. These structures should be retracted and preserved. The joint capsule is entered via a longitudinal capsulotomy following the orientation of the skin incision (Fig. 25.5B). Then, joint preparation is performed via a contour resection and curettage technique as outlined below.

CALCANEOCUBOID JOINT INCISION PLACEMENT AND DISSECTION

With the evolution of our understanding of the triple rearfoot complex and utilization of joint preparation with contour resection and curettage technique, the calcaneocuboid joint is often spared from our rearfoot arthrodesis procedures. That is, unless extreme deformity is present or the calcaneocuboid joint is painful/arthritic. When arthrodesis of the calcaneocuboid joint is indicated, the incision is made central to the joint—just above the course of the peroneal tendons and the sural nerve. Often, this incision is combined with the subtalar joint approach by simply extending the subtalar incision distally on the dorsolateral foot. As mentioned above, care is taken to

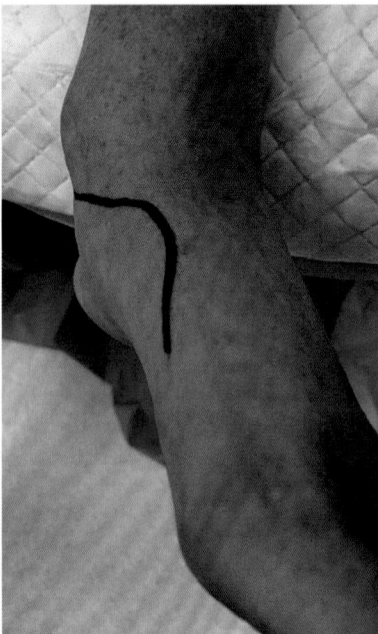
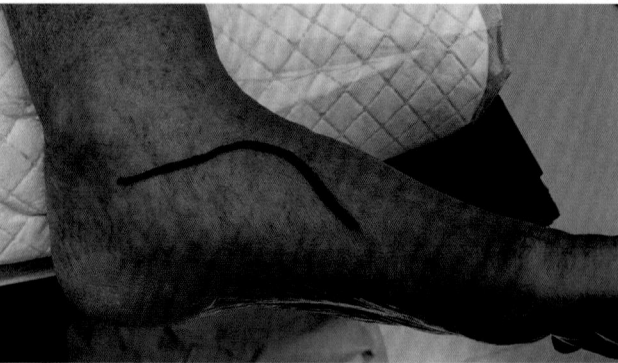

FIGURE 25.3 Modified incisional approach for medial double procedure.

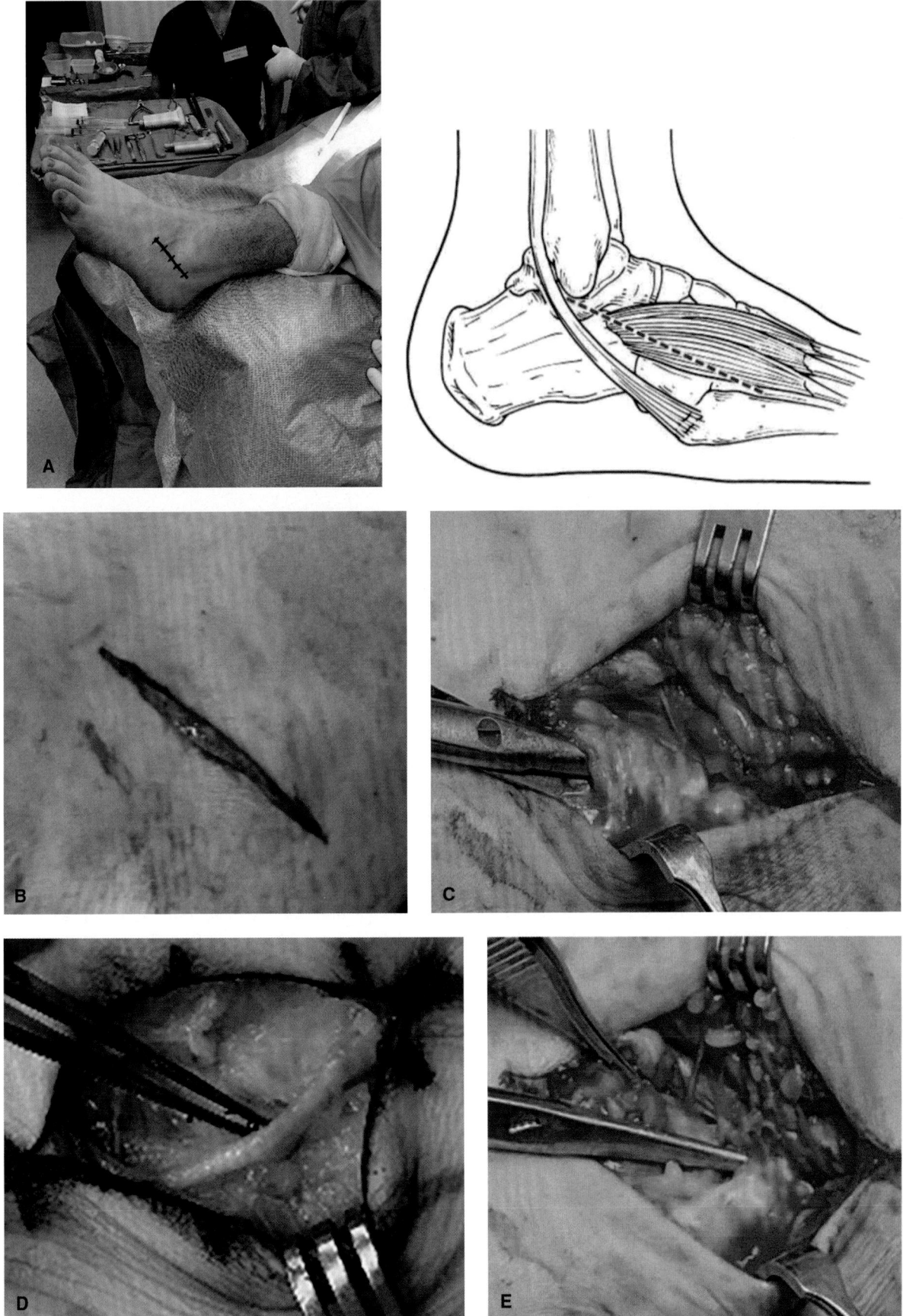

FIGURE 25.4 **A.** Lateral skin incision. **B, C.** Dissection through superficial and subcutaneous tissues. **D.** Sural nerve within surgical field (retract plantarly). **E.** Identify and retract peroneal tendons plantarly (kept in tendon sheaths).

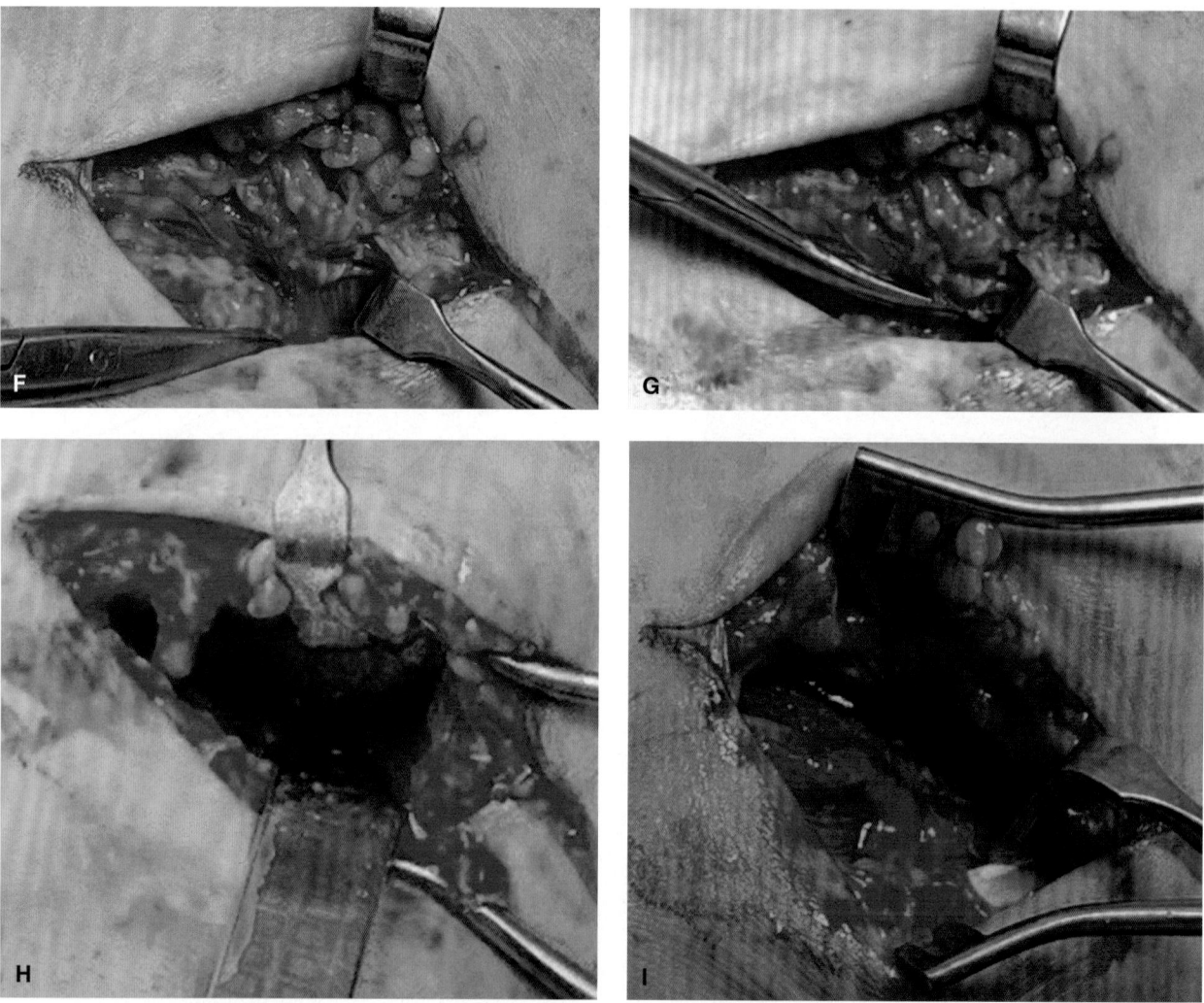

FIGURE 25.4 (*Continued*) **F, G.** Identify and transect calcaneofibular ligament. **H.** Hoke's tonsil excised for improved visualization of anterior aspect of subtalar joint. **I.** Visibility into subtalar joint.

protect the peroneal tendons and sural nerve with retraction inferiorly. The extensor digitorum brevis muscle is reflected dorsally for added exposure as well. A linear capsular incision is utilized for the calcaneocuboid joint. Subperiosteal dissection can then be performed until visualization of the cartilage is appreciated (Fig. 25.6). Preparation of the calcaneocuboid joint is performed through contour joint resection/curettage technique or sagittal saw resection depending on the requirements for correction of the deformity.

JOINT PREPARATION FOR TRIPLE ARTHRODESIS

Historically, joint resection techniques were performed on the subtalar and talonavicular joints via resection of the subchondral plate and "wedging" through angled resection utilizing a sawblade (ie, the traditional Ryerson technique). With this technique, significant shortening occurred to the triple rearfoot joint complex and to the rearfoot in general. To compensate for this shortening at the subtalar and talonavicular joints, the calcaneocuboid joint had to be violated and fused in order to gain a plantigrade foot. Now, with contour resection techniques, the joint morphology is not significantly changed

and reduction of the deformity through manipulation of only the subtalar and talonavicular joints into corrected position can often be achieved. Therefore, the calcaneocuboid joint can commonly be spared from most rearfoot reconstructive arthrodesis procedures.

For a traditional triple arthrodesis procedure, all three joints are entered and prepared in the same manner—by utilizing an osteotome for initial cartilage removal and then completing the process with a ringed curette or power burr. This technique of joint preparation is known as cartilage contour resection or, more simply, curettage technique. This technique involves removing all the nascent cartilage from the opposing joint surfaces down to, but not through, the subchondral plate. It is important not to violate the subchondral plate by creating divots or other irregularities as this technique allows for anatomical contour and apposition of the prepared joint surfaces. This curettage technique allows for better anatomic reduction of the rearfoot deformity with increased surface area contact across the joint regions when placed in its corrected position. Further, this technique minimizes bone resection, potential shortening of the limb/foot, and allows for manual deformity reduction by simple manipulation of the joint complex.

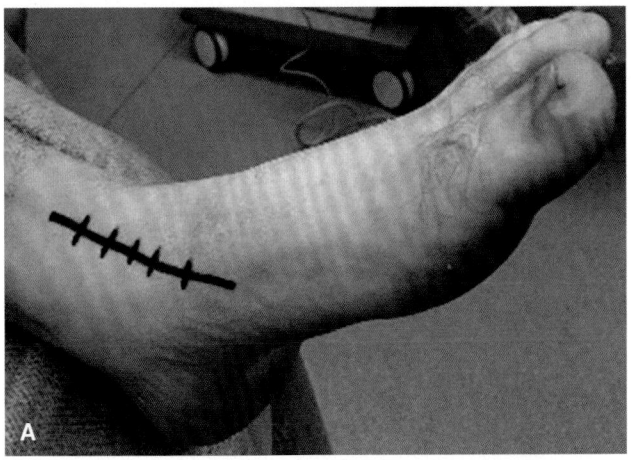

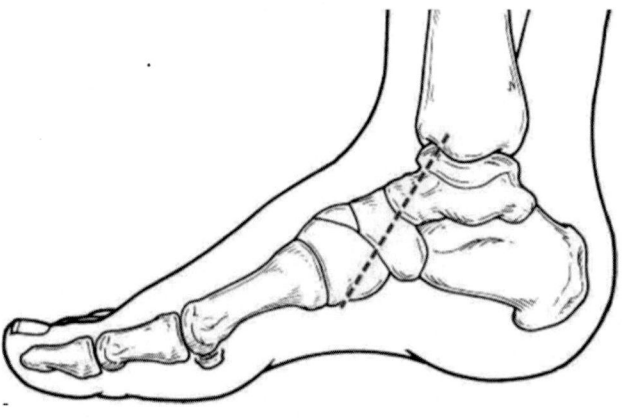

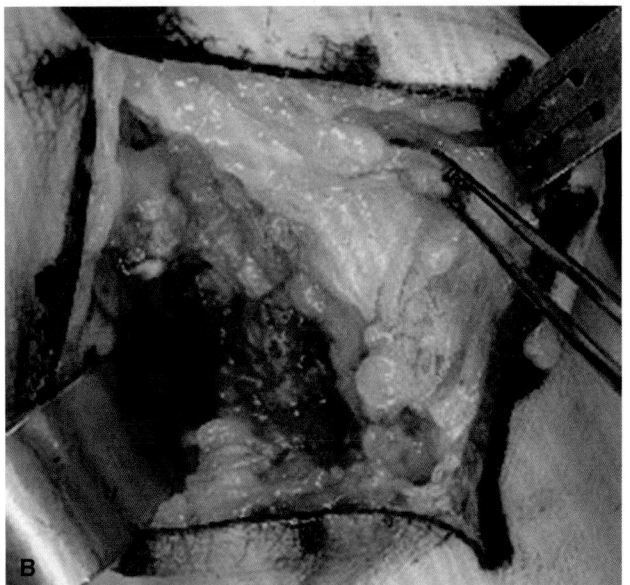

FIGURE 25.5 A. Medial skin incision. **B.** Deep dissection to talonavicular joint capsule.

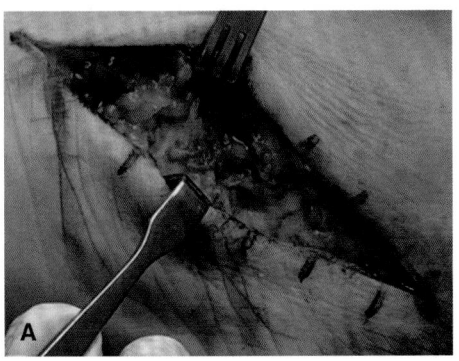

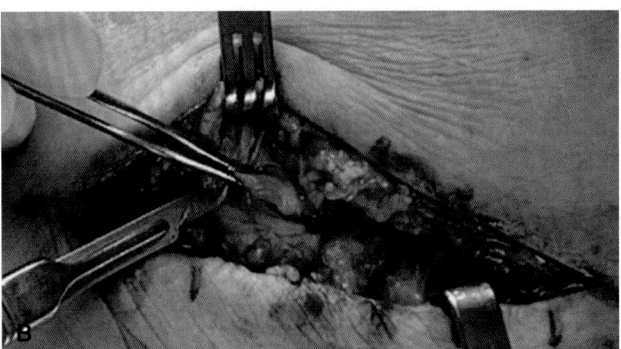

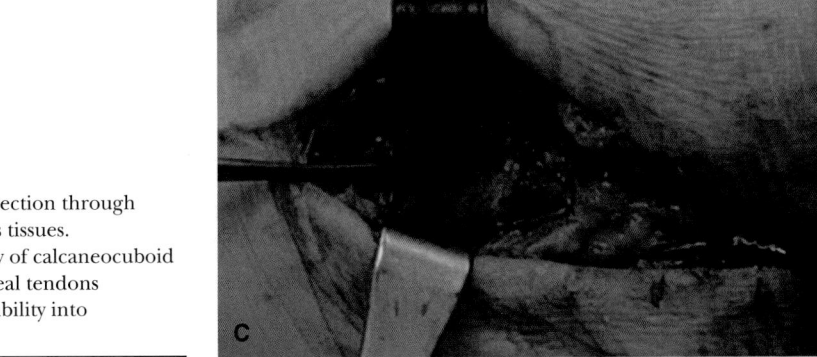

FIGURE 25.6 A. Dissection through superficial and subcutaneous tissues. **B.** Longitudinal capsulotomy of calcaneocuboid joint while protecting peroneal tendons via plantar retraction. **C.** Visibility into calcaneocuboid joint.

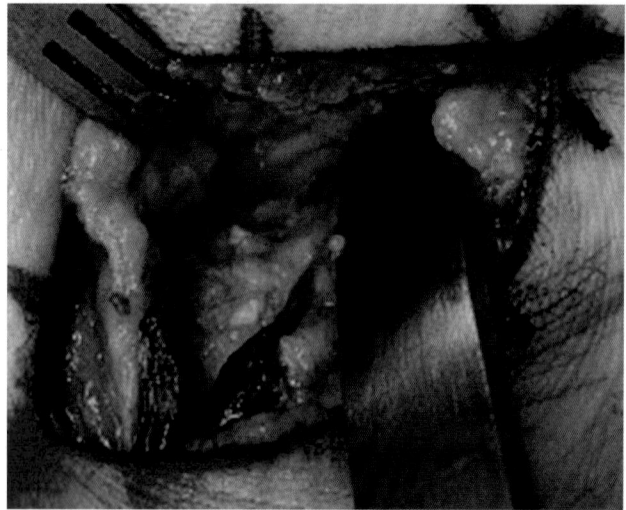

FIGURE 25.7 Osteotome dissection into subtalar joint space.

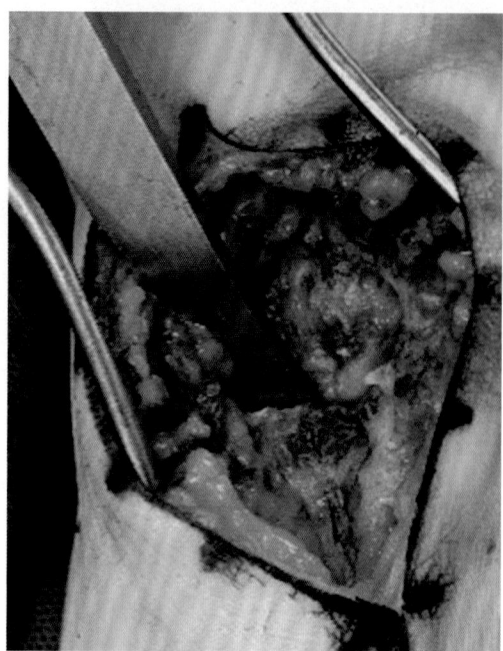

FIGURE 25.8 Osteotome dissection into talonavicular space.

Joint preparation is initiated by utilizing a ½ in. curved osteotome as a dissection tool to release capsular tissues and enter the joint surface (Figs. 25.7 and 25.8). Minimal soft tissue stripping allows for optimal preservation of periosteum to maintain vascular supply to the area for healing. It is important not to be overzealous with this maneuver, especially with the subtalar joint dissection, because medial neurovascular and posteromedial extrinsic tendon structures may be injured (especially when releasing the capsular tissues from the posterior and medial subtalar joint areas). The osteotome is also utilized to start the initial stages of cartilage removal, which is then completed with use of curettes and/or a power burr (Figs. 25.9-25.11). We have found that straight or angled ringed curettes work well within the subtalar and calcaneocuboid joints, while angled scooped curettes are best suited for the convex/concave nature of the talonavicular joint. Of note, lamina spreaders (or other distraction devices) are excellent instruments to utilize for improved visualization of the joint surfaces during this preparation stage.

Once all of the cartilage is removed from the joint surfaces, increased space and motion is obtained between the adjacent osseous structures. With this, the joint is easily manipulated and can be reduced into corrected position. Sometimes, resection of a portion of the joint is necessary to provide optimal exposure of the joint complex or to allow complete reduction of the deformity (especially with severely adapted/arthritic joints). A power saw blade can be utilized to cautiously resect a minimal amount of subchondral plate and facilitate reduction of the

rearfoot deformity with minimal segmental shortening. For example, resection of a small portion of the calcaneocuboid joint can assist in transverse plane correction with a supinated foot structure, or removal of the lateral talar process can allow for added pronation of the talus upon the calcaneus to assist in reduction of severe varus deformity as well. After achieving manual reduction of the deformity into corrected position, the final joint preparation work is now performed.

For successful joint fusion to occur, the osteochondral composite nature of the subchondral plate must be aggressively violated to the point that subchondral cancellous bone is interdigitated within the opposing joint surfaces. This is performed with the sequential combination of a 2.5-mm drill bit to aggressively fenestrate the area then utilizing a power saw or osteotome to further fish scale/microfracture the majority of the subchondral plate (Figs. 25.12 and 25.13). With this method of subchondral plate pulverization, it is important to keep the integrity of the peripheral joint margins to maintain structural rigidity of the interposing joints for hardware placement. Performing this drilling technique will pull the deep subchondral cancellous bone into the arthrodesis area to serve as autologous bone graft and assist in successful fusion across the joint surface.

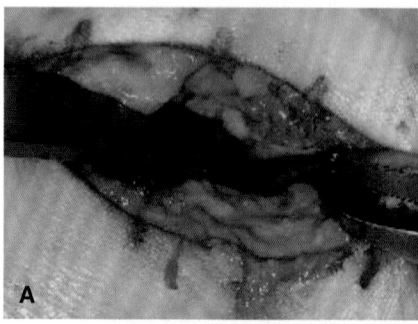

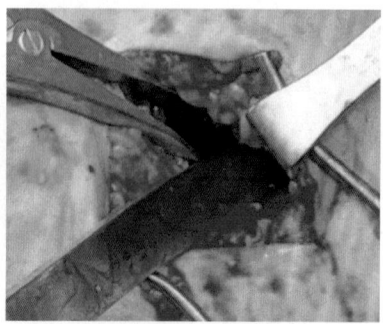

A

FIGURE 25.9 **A.** Osteotome introduced into subtalar joint for initial cartilage resection.

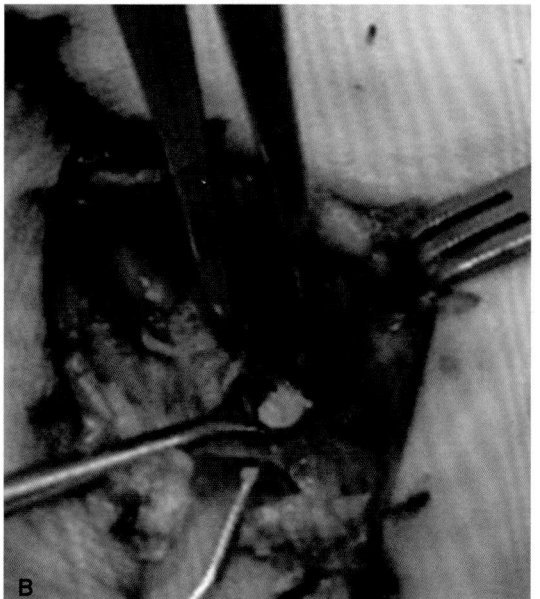

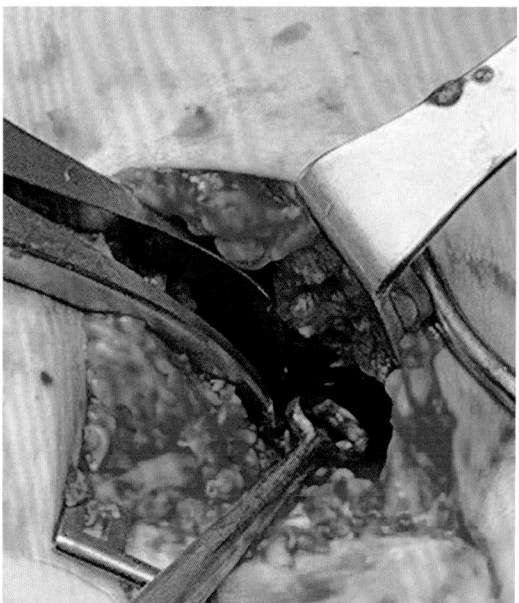

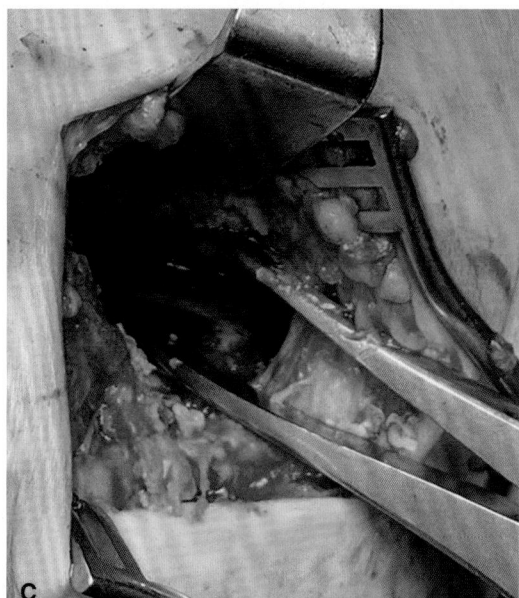

FIGURE 25.9 (*Continued*) **B.** Curette utilized to remove residual cartilage to subchondral level. **C.** Clear visualization within subtalar joint after joint preparation.

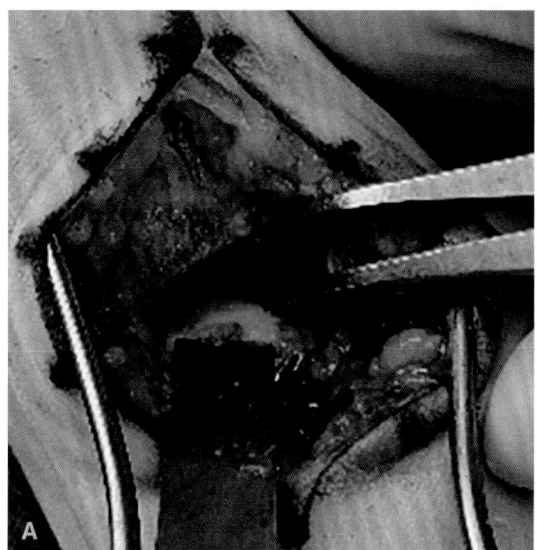

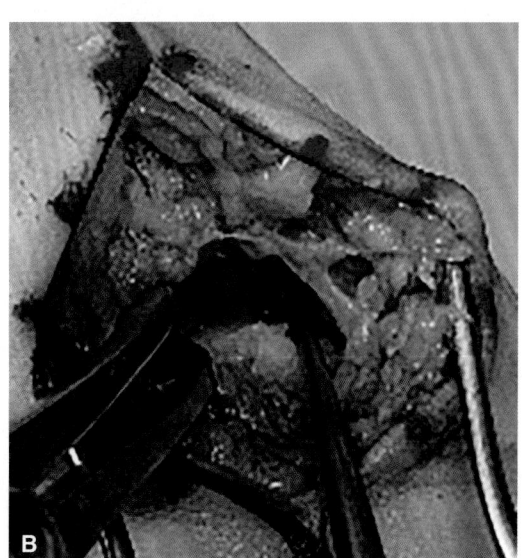

FIGURE 25.10 **A.** Osteotome introduced into talonavicular joint for initial cartilage resection. **B.** Curette utilized to remove residual cartilage to subchondral level.

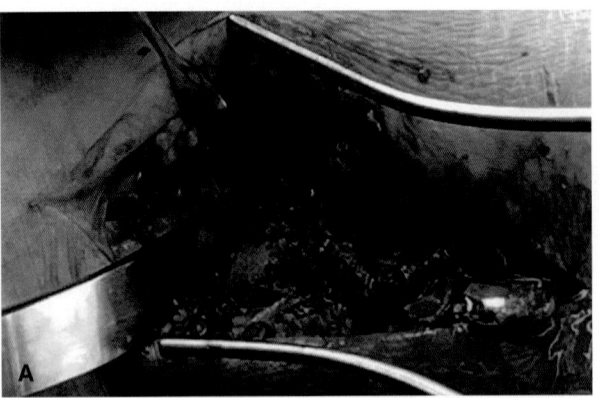
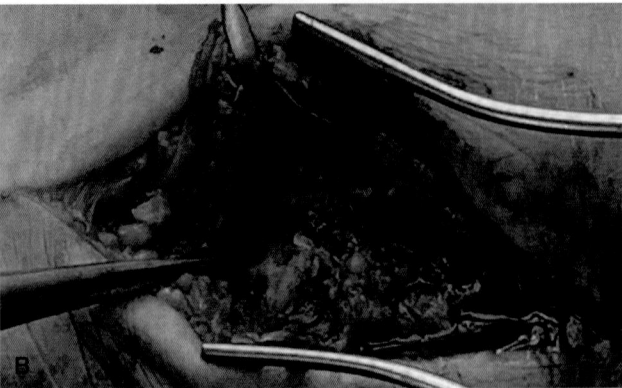

FIGURE 25.11 A. Osteotome introduced into calcaneocuboid joint for initial cartilage resection. **B.** Curette utilized to remove residual cartilage to subchondral level.

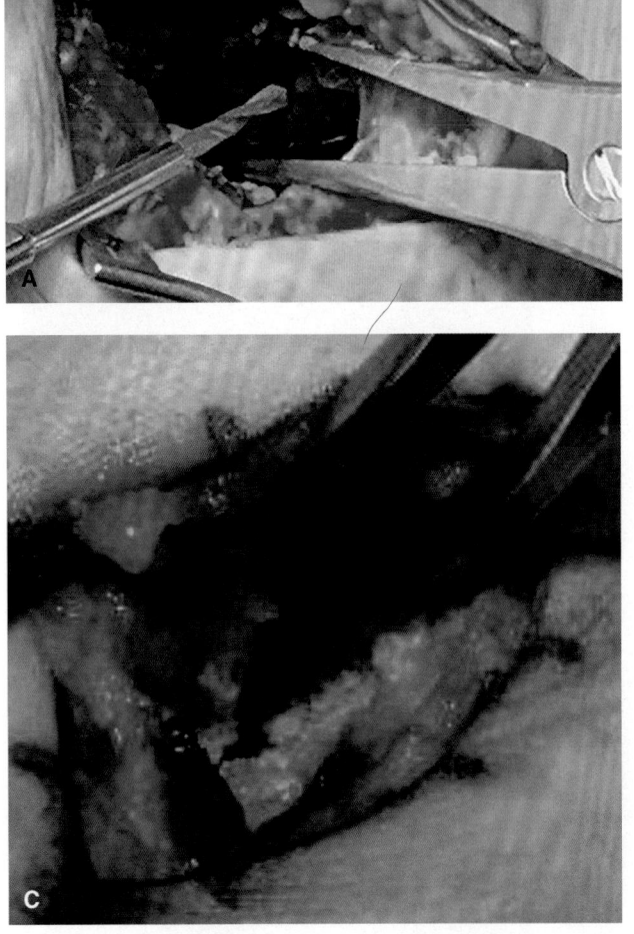
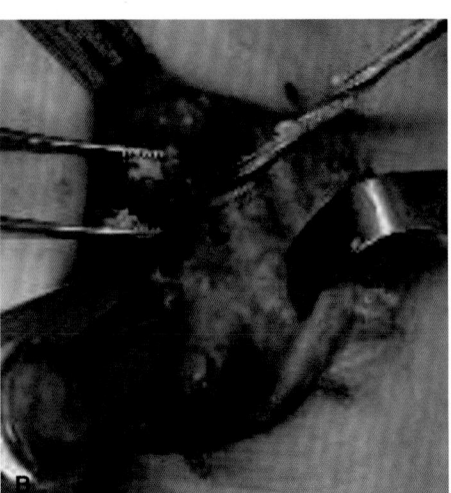

FIGURE 25.12 A. Drill bit introduced into subtalar joint for fenestration. **B.** Completion of subtalar joint microfracture. **C.** Completion of pulverizing the subtalar joint with clear subchondral autologous graft brought into joint space.

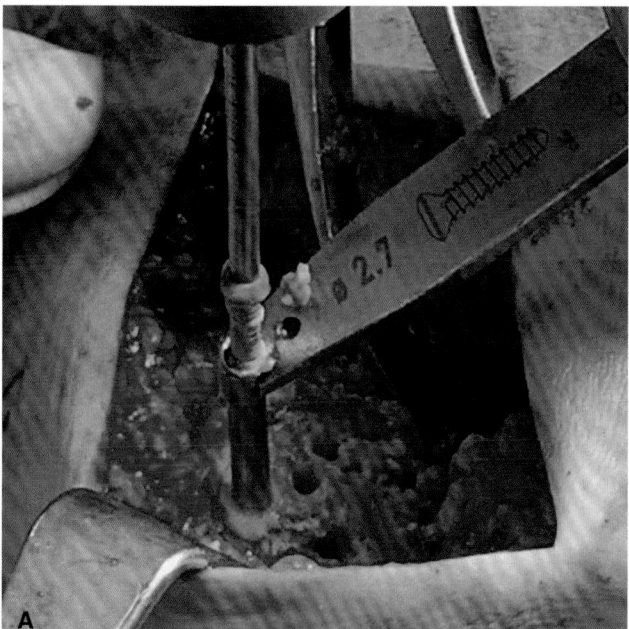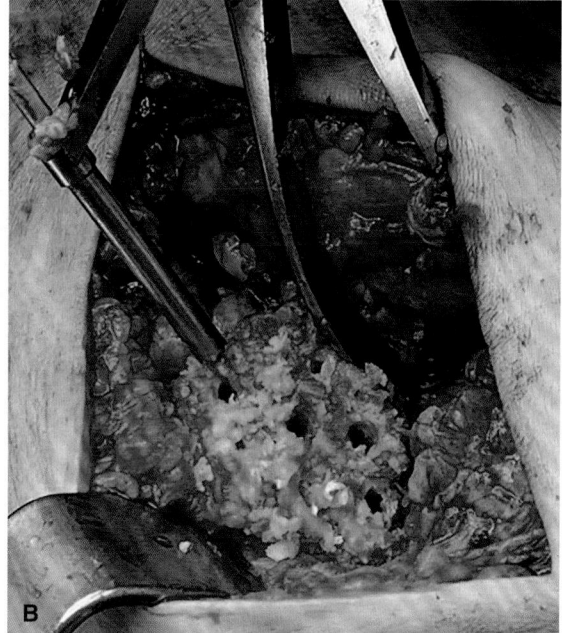

FIGURE 25.13 **A.** Drill bit introduced into talonavicular joint for fenestration. **B.** Completion of talonavicular joint microfracture with clear subchondral autologous graft brought into joint space.

Once the above joint preparation is complete, the triple rearfoot complex is once again manually manipulated into its corrected position for temporary, and then, permanent internal fixation placement.

DEFORMITY REDUCTION AND FIXATION PLACEMENT

The subtalar joint is reduced into its desired position first. Often, this corrected position is in mild valgus with the talus reduced back into a neutral position within the ankle mortise. Placing a finger or thumb into the sinus tarsi laterally while manipulating the subtalar joint can help the surgeon "feel" the reduction (Fig. 25.14). As the subtalar joint supinates, the sinus tarsi will open laterally and the surgeon will be able to feel the oval osseous tunnel to assist in placing the subtalar joint into its appropriate corrected position. K-wire/Steinmann pin fixation, or most commonly, guide pins for cannulated screws are utilized to hold position of the subtalar joint (Fig. 25.15). Most often, the subtalar joint is fixated with cannulated screws applied in a crossing manner, or two screws placed form the heel into the talar neck and body. Once the guide pins are placed and radiographic confirmation is performed for accuracy of placement, then these screws can be applied utilizing AO technique.

After the subtalar complex is temporarily fixated, reduction of deformity at the midfoot level is performed. Whether fusing the talonavicular joint alone or along with the calcaneocuboid joint, both are reduced in unison to complete the reduction of the rearfoot/midfoot complex. Manipulation and palpation of the talonavicular joint allows for the majority of overall deformity reduction due to the "ball & socket" nature of this joint complex. Ease of reduction in a triplanar manner is achieved through the talonavicular joint by, most importantly, rotating the forefoot out of its adaptive varus/valgus (Fig. 25.16). To confirm appropriate reduction of deformity, the second toe should be in line with the ipsilateral

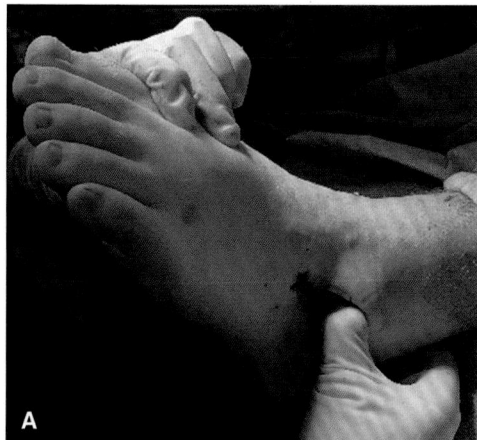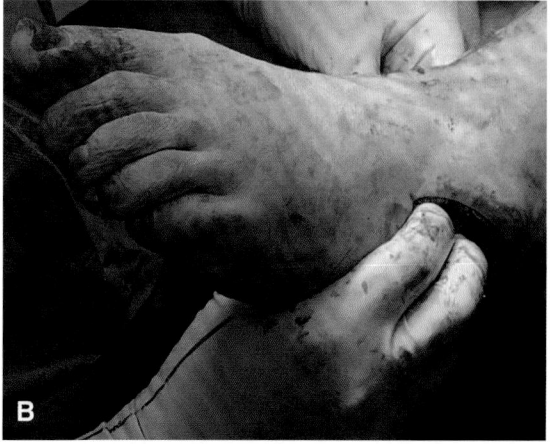

FIGURE 25.14 **A, B.** Examples of "feeling" reduction of subtalar joint utilizing thumb or index finger placed into sinus tarsi.

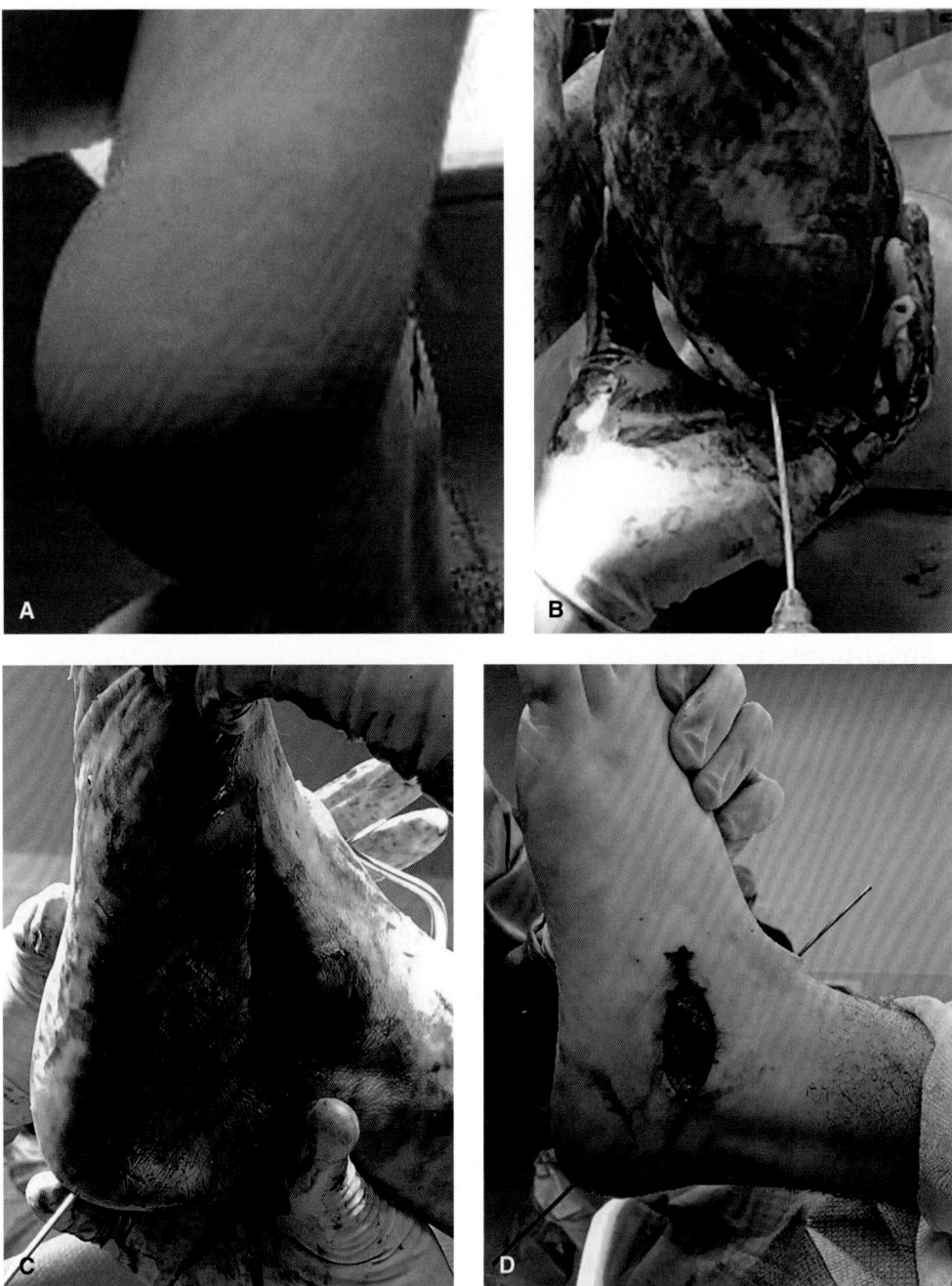

FIGURE 25.15 A. Minimally invasive incision for subtalar joint fixation through posterior calcaneal approach. **B, C.** Placement of guidewire for temporary fixation of subtalar joint. **D.** Demonstrating appropriate angulation for start and end points of subtalar joint fixation.

patella, or appropriate transverse plane position to match the contralateral limb. Temporary fixation is performed via K-wires/Steinmann pins or guide pins (Fig. 25.17), then placement of permanent fixation is performed. Since the talonavicular joint is a "ball & socket" joint that is inherently unstable, it is wise to place at least two points of fixation across this joint—especially if only performing a double arthrodesis. If performing a triple arthrodesis however, the triple rearfoot complex is inherently more stable by fusing all three joints, so less fixation can be utilized if desired. With these factors in mind, the talonavicular joint is commonly fixated with at least an interfragmentary screw along with a plate or staples to counteract rotational forces about the arthrodesis site.

The calcaneocuboid joint is the final point of fixation when performing a triple arthrodesis. This joint can be fixated with interfragmental screws, a plate/screw construct, or staples (Fig. 25.18). The flat nature of the joint complex allows for ease of placement of plates or staples laterally, so this is most commonly performed. If screws are utilized, then at least two points of fixation (ie, two screws) should be placed. However, when the calcaneocuboid joint arthrodesis is combined with a subtalar and talonavicular arthrodesis, a single screw from the calcaneus to the cuboid can be utilized because the triple rearfoot complex is "locked" together with fixation of the two adjacent joints.

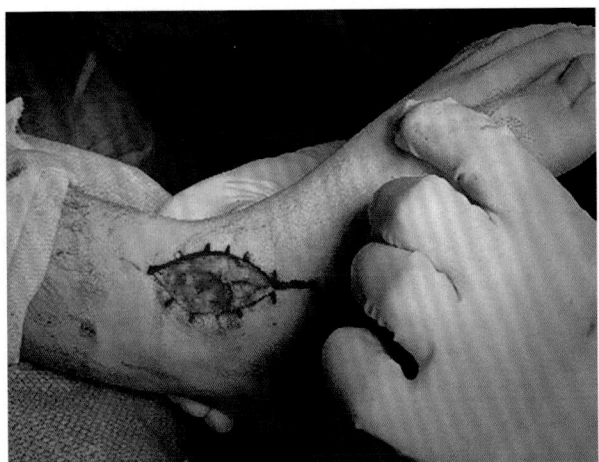

FIGURE 25.16 Reduction of forefoot through midtarsal joints (position 2nd toe in alignment with patella/or tibial crest). The forefoot is also rotated out of its adapted varus or valgus position, if need be.

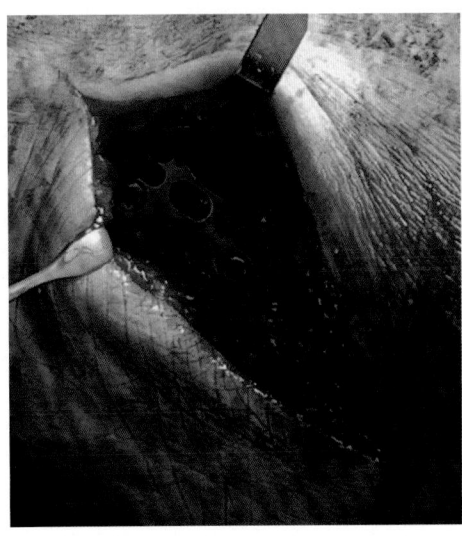

FIGURE 25.18 Permanent fixation across calcaneocuboid joint using locking plate.

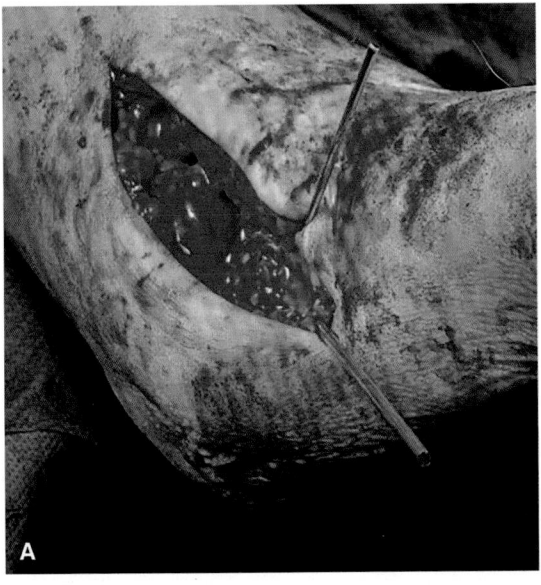

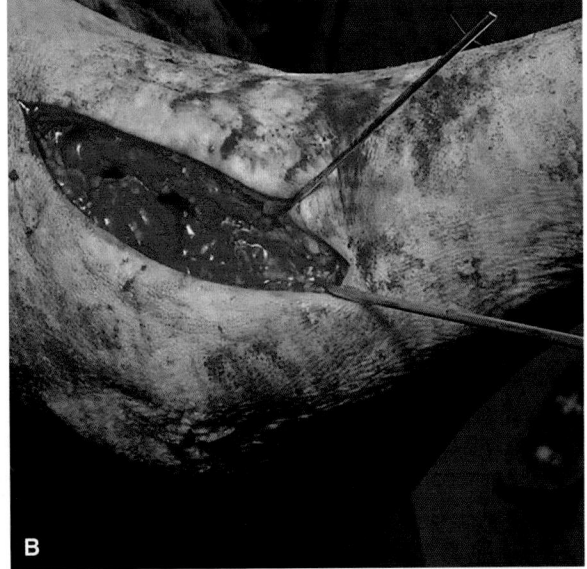

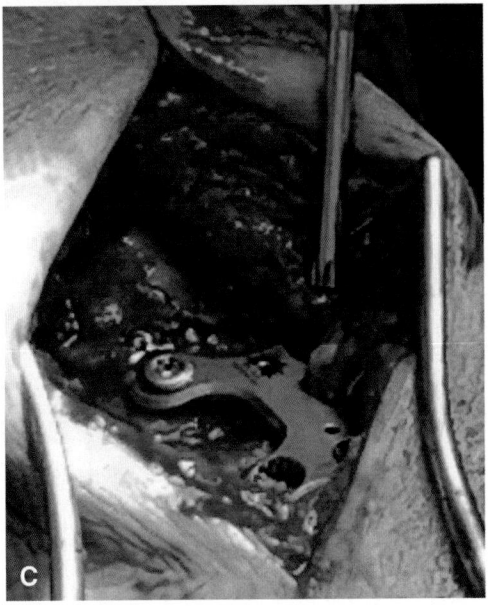

FIGURE 25.17 A, B. Temporary fixation for talonavicular joint (superior K-wire serves to hold reduction and inferior guidewire for interfragmentary screw fixation). **C.** Permanent fixation of talonavicular joint with dorsal-medial locking plate (interfragmentary screw is prior to this—not shown).

ADJUNCTIVE PROCEDURES WITH TRIPLE ARTHRODESIS

A triple arthrodesis is most commonly performed for severe, longstanding deformities that alter gait and cause adjacent adaptive deformities. Gastrocnemius-Soleus equinus deformity is commonly associated with complex rearfoot deformities, so an Achilles tendon lengthening or gastrocnemius recession is often needed in conjunction with the primary procedure to appropriately complete this type of reconstructive surgery (Fig. 25.19). Often, the amount of equinus deformity cannot be completely appreciated until the rearfoot is fixated into corrected position. With this understood, the posterior leg release should be performed after correction of the foot deformity is achieved—or at least reevaluated after the foot correction is completed if performed earlier in the procedure. Other adjunct procedures include forefoot deformity correction, tendon transfers, and other arthrodesis procedures of the midfoot and forefoot.

RADIOGRAPHIC EVALUATION

It is important to confirm placement of appropriate fixation via intraoperative radiographic evaluation prior to closure of the wounds. Positioning of the foot into a corrected plantigrade position can be identified clinically (Fig. 25.20), but confirmation of joint reduction by radiographic evaluation is also necessary. Radiographs of the foot are performed to ensure internal fixation placement is optimal (Fig. 25.21). One should also obtain ankle radiographs to make sure the subtalar screws are not entering the ankle joint, or invading the medial or lateral gutter space. If this was to happen, deterioration of the ankle joint will occur and the risk of postoperative osteoarthritis is increased dramatically.

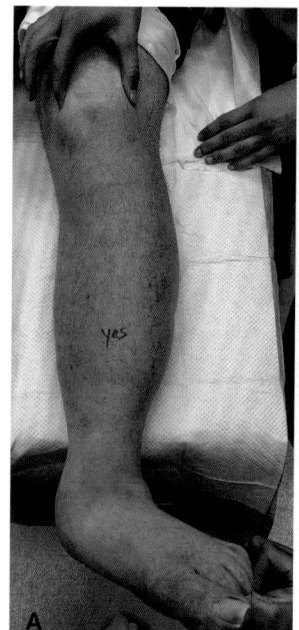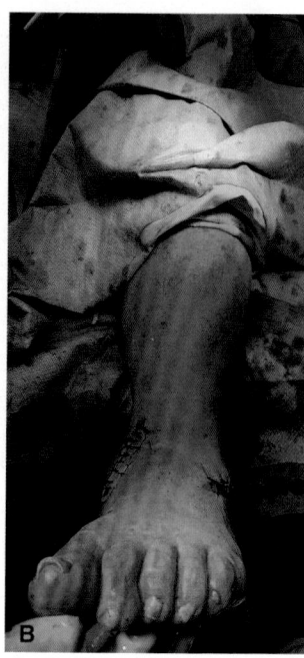

FIGURE 25.20 A. Clinical presentation of preoperative deformity. **B.** Intraoperative clinical reduction of deformity.

CLOSURE

A layered closure it performed to cover internal fixation devices and minimize potential dead space. The authors prefer to minimize deep closure by limiting the amount of absorbable suture material applied subcutaneously. This deep absorbable suture material degrades via hydrolysis and may cause increased inflammatory response within these tissue layers, so minimal deep

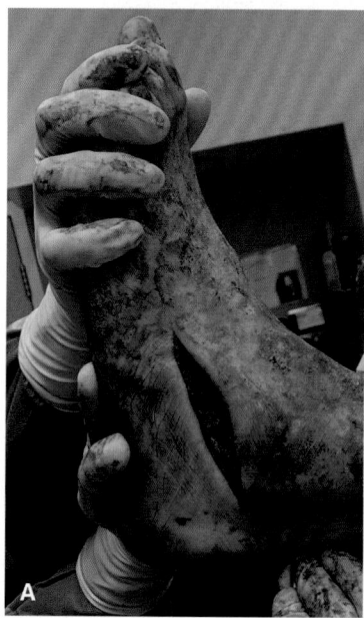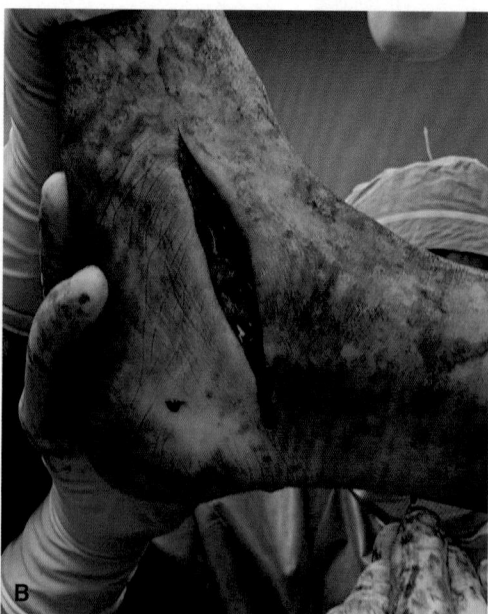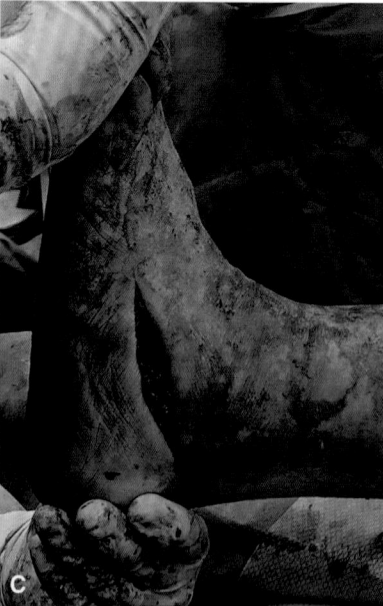

FIGURE 25.19 A. Equinus contracture appreciated (and accentuated) after correction of the rearfoot deformity. **B.** Percutaneous triple hemisection tendo Achilles lengthening with a no. 64 knife blade. **C.** Resolved equinus deformity with increased dorsiflexion after tendo Achilles lengthening.

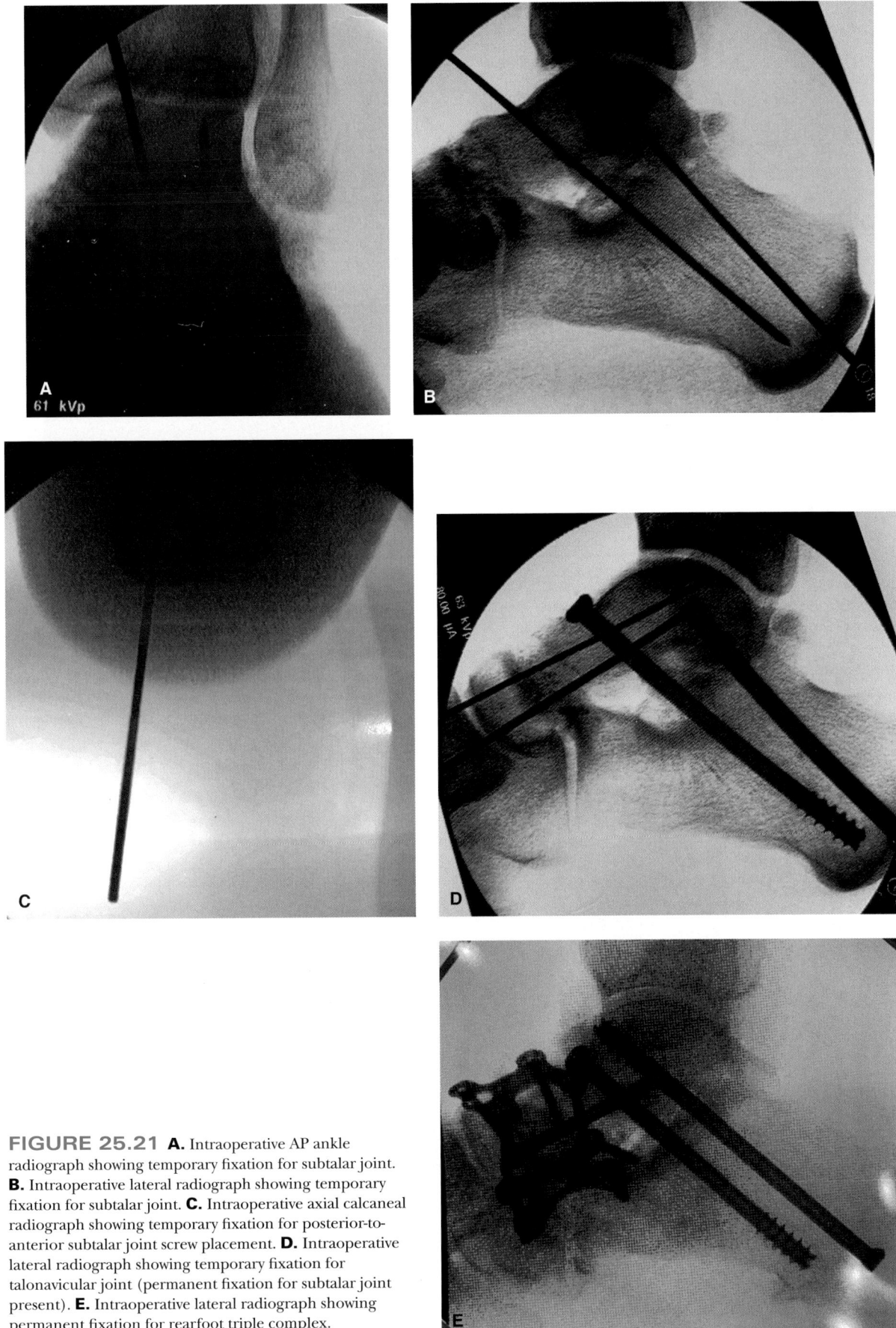

FIGURE 25.21 **A.** Intraoperative AP ankle radiograph showing temporary fixation for subtalar joint. **B.** Intraoperative lateral radiograph showing temporary fixation for subtalar joint. **C.** Intraoperative axial calcaneal radiograph showing temporary fixation for posterior-to-anterior subtalar joint screw placement. **D.** Intraoperative lateral radiograph showing temporary fixation for talonavicular joint (permanent fixation for subtalar joint present). **E.** Intraoperative lateral radiograph showing permanent fixation for rearfoot triple complex.

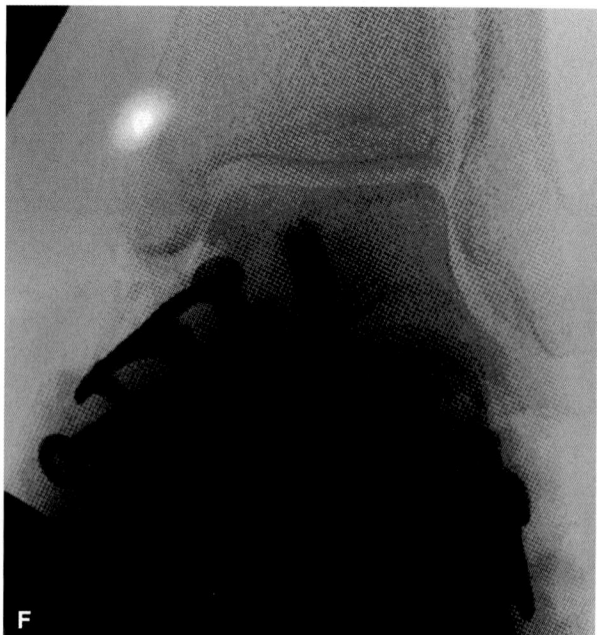
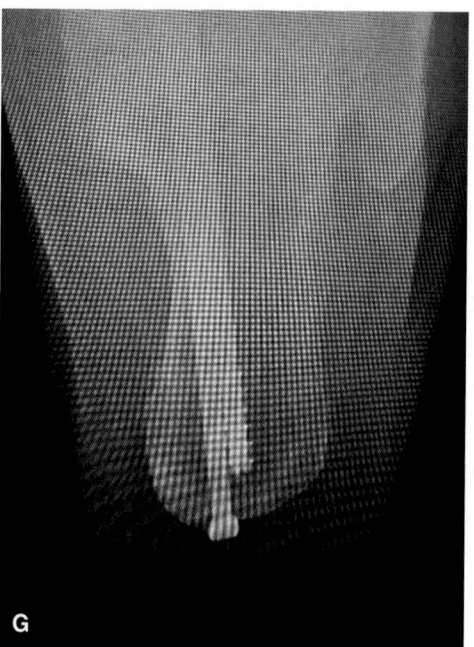

FIGURE 25.21 (*Continued*) **F.** Intraoperative AP ankle radiograph showing permanent fixation for rearfoot triple complex. **G.** Postoperative axial calcaneal radiograph showing permanent fixation for subtalar joint.

sutures are utilized. Minimal deep closure also allows for less risk of hematoma formation and less need for drain placement.

When performing skin level closure, the tourniquet is deflated for multiple reasons. Dropping the tourniquet allows the surgeon to evaluate and manage any major bleeding vessels while also providing physiologic irrigation to the surgical site via bleeding, which can decrease the risk of hematoma formation and assist in removing any bacteria/foreign micro-material that may be present in the wound. Dropping the tourniquet while closing soft tissues also allows for initial swelling to occur, hence decreasing the chances for an overly tight dressing postoperatively.

Skin closure is performed by nonabsorbable suture in a mixed simple and horizontal mattress fashion (Fig. 25.22). Once closure is complete, a regional and peri-incisional nerve block is performed for extended pain relief—if not performed prior to incision placement. Finally, a multilayer compressive dressing and well-padded below the knee posterior splint are applied as per protocol.

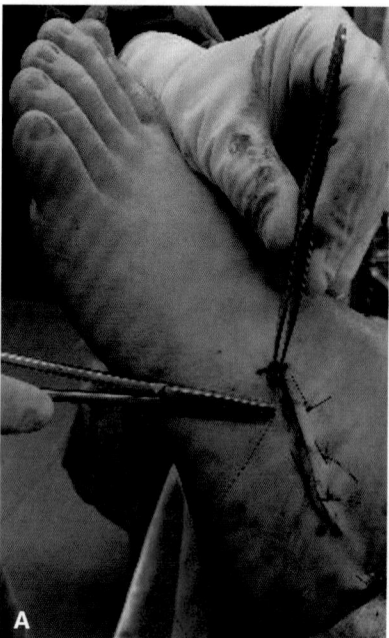
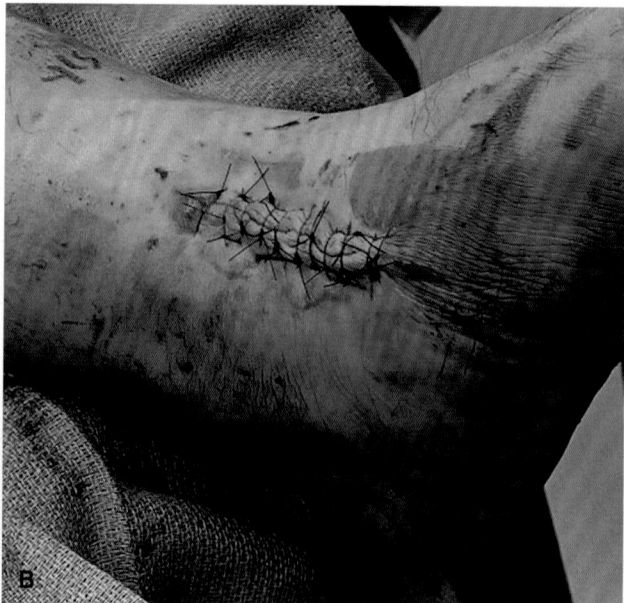

FIGURE 25.22 **A.** Lateral incision skin closure. **B.** Medial incision skin closure.

INSIGHT ON THE TRIPLE ARTHRODESIS PROCEDURE

The technical aspect of the triple or double arthrodesis is significant, and experience with performing these procedures is a prerequisite. Simple engineering principles are utilized when deciding on hardware selection and addition of adjunct procedures for our patients. The deforming forces that act about the foot in gait are significant, so placement of rigid internal fixation constructs to resist deforming/weight-bearing forces is important. Our fixation needs to hold the bone position and deformity correction in place at least to the point where the body has successfully healed the arthrodesis sites. Once the arthrodesis sites are adequately healed, most often the hardware is left in place and not removed—unless it is causing a problem for the patient. Even though we ask our patients to be non–weight-bearing for 6-10 weeks after a rearfoot arthrodesis procedure, we know appropriate compliance does not always occur. Providing secure fixation to resist weight-bearing/deforming forces may help the surgical procedure to go on to successful healing—even when the occasional patient is non-compliant to our weight-bearing restrictions.

OUTCOMES AND COMPLICATIONS

The triple arthrodesis is a time-tested procedure that can correct significant foot deformities, create stability, and improve function (Table 25.4). When performed appropriately, the procedure is very predictable and can eliminate pain and improve quality of life. In fact, long-term studies have shown

TABLE 25.4 Alternative Technical Considerations

Approach
- Most surgeons perform a triple arthrodesis procedure with pneumatic tourniquet hemostasis; however, one may perform dissection in a wet situation and inflate the tourniquet when prepping the joints
- Deflating the tourniquet when closing soft tissue is helpful to address any bleeding vessels and will reduce excessive edema in the dressing
- Incisional placement can be altered pending any previous incisions or wounds

Reduction of Deformity and Positioning
- Techniques may need to be altered when the surgeon is alone without assistant surgeon help present
- Some surgeons prefer to temporarily fixate the STJ first, while others prefer to fixate the TNJ first
- Subtalar Joint Positioning:
  - If placing a screw from dorsal to plantar, the surgeon can place their thumb in the sinus tarsi to create adequate positioning of the talus over the calcaneus and cup the back of the heel with their fingers to push the calcaneus anteriorly to assist in appropriate positioning
  - If placing screws from plantar to dorsal, the surgeon can place their index finger in sinus tarsi to create adequate positioning of the talus over the calcaneus and elevate the extremity to allow the posterior-superior heel to rest in the palm of their hand, which can assist in positioning the calcaneus anteriorly if need be
- Talonavicular Joint Positioning:
  - The surgeon can dorsiflex the hallux to engage the windlass mechanism to assist in compression across the fusion site
  - Temporary fixation with a Kirschner wire will help hold reduction while placing primary internal fixation
- Calcaneocuboid Joint Positioning:
  - The surgeon can push the cuboid superiorly when positioning the hindfoot in order to maintain lateral column length and prevent abduction of the forefoot
  - Again, temporary fixation is helpful in holding position while placing primary internal fixation

Permanent Fixation
- The surgeon may use headed or headless screws, plates, and/or staples depending on their preference
- Fixating the Subtalar Joint:
  - If placing a screw from top-down, the surgeon should start in the junction of the talar neck-body and aim for the plantar lateral calcaneus (Fig. 25.25)
  - If placing a screw from bottom-up, the surgeon should start in the plantar central calcaneus and aim for the talar body, directing fixation centrally between the malleoli or their index finger and thumb (Figs. 25.23, 25.24, and 25.26)
  - If placing a screw vertically from a lateral approach, the surgeon can start in the anterior-lateral calcaneus and aim for the junction of the talar neck-body
  - Two screw fixation of the subtalar joint is preferred, however a single screw across this joint can be utilized as fusion of the midtarsal joints may sufficiently immobilize the subtalar joint (Fig. 25.26)
- Fixating the Talonavicular Joint:
  - This may be accomplished with 1-2 screws (Figs. 25.23 and 25.26)
  - This may be accomplished with a medially based interfragmentary screw and dorsal locking plate (Figs. 25.24 and 25.25)
  - This may be accomplished with staple fixation across the fusion site
- Fixating the Calcaneocuboid Joint:
  - This may be accomplished with a screw from the posterior calcaneus into the central cuboid (Fig. 25.23)
  - This may be accomplished with a screw from the anterior-lateral calcaneus into the central cuboid (Fig. 25.24)
  - This may be accomplished with a screw from the distal-lateral cuboid into the body of the calcaneus (Fig. 25.25)
  - This may be accomplished using a lateral plate across the fusion site (Fig. 25.26)
  - This may be accomplished using staple fixation across the fusion site

Miscellaneous Considerations
- Deflate the tourniquet after deep closure to evaluate for bleeding vessels, prevent hematoma formation, allow physiologic irrigation of the surgical site, and allow some initial edema to occur prior to dressing application

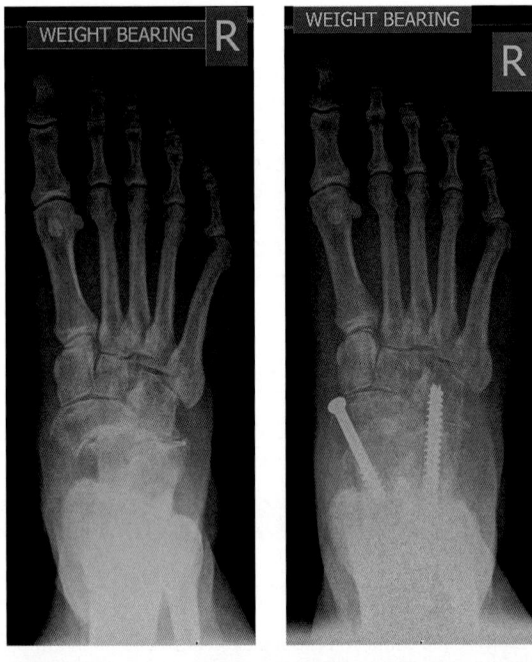

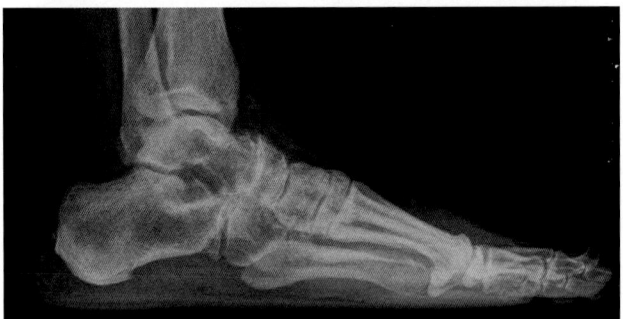

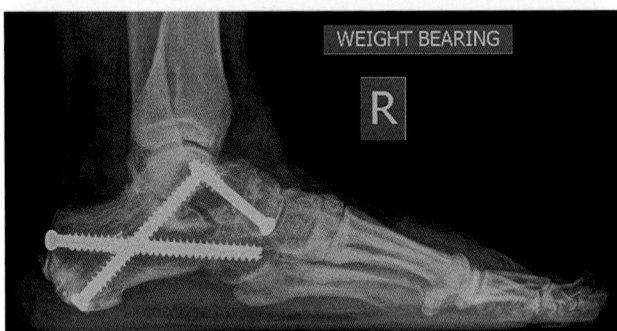

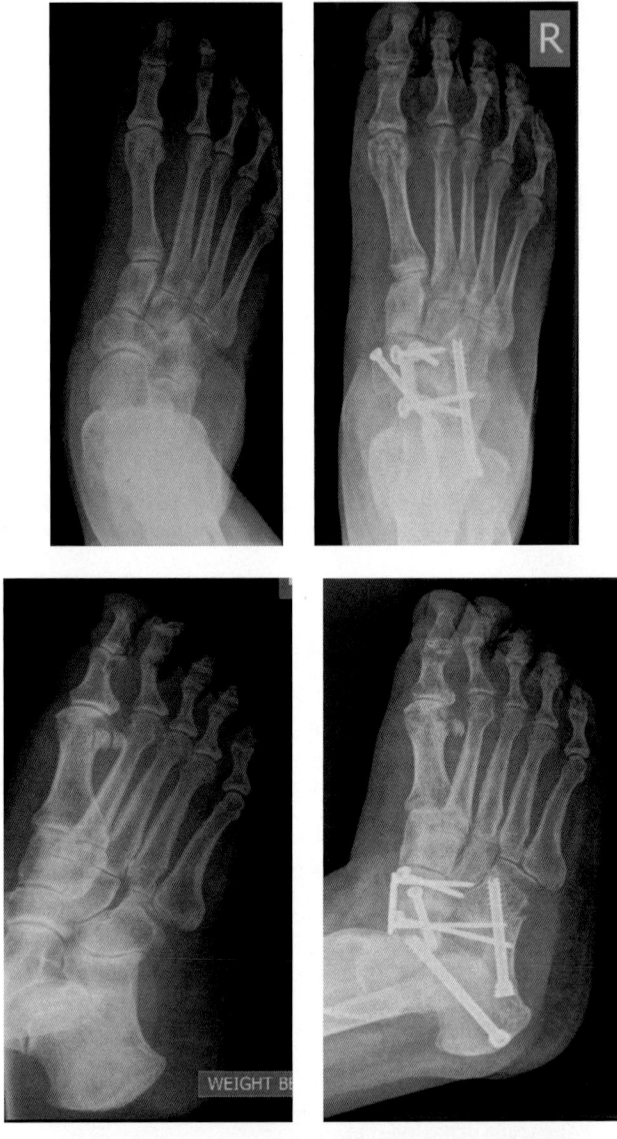

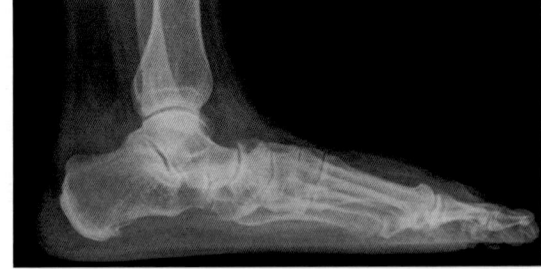

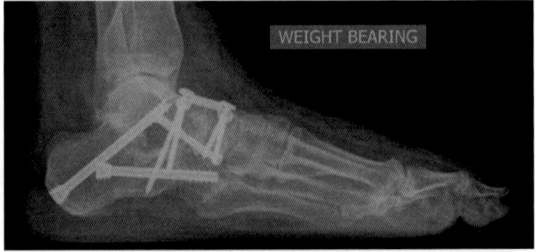

FIGURE 25.23 Correction of arthritic rearfoot with subtle cavus deformity using only three screws. (Pictures complimentary of Douglas K. Blacklidge, DPM.)

patient satisfaction and the willingness to undergo the procedure again is quite high in this patient population.[1,9,11-16,23,24] The vast majority of these patients return to full-time work and their previous level of activity.[15] The downside to the procedure is the loss of the adaptive mechanics of the rearfoot joints that, over time, can lead to premature arthritic changes in adjacent joints—especially the ankle. However, subjective satisfaction is improved with better alignment of the foot, and patient complaints of associated adjacent joint arthrosis do not always correlate with objective radiographic findings.[10-16]

FIGURE 25.24 Correction of severe valgus foot deformity using three screws and an added dorsal-medial locking plate over the talonavicular joint. (Pictures complimentary of Douglas K. Blacklidge, DPM.)

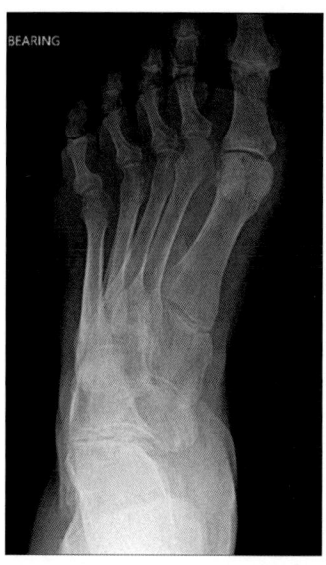
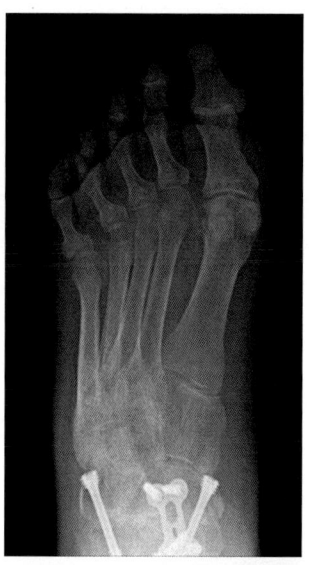
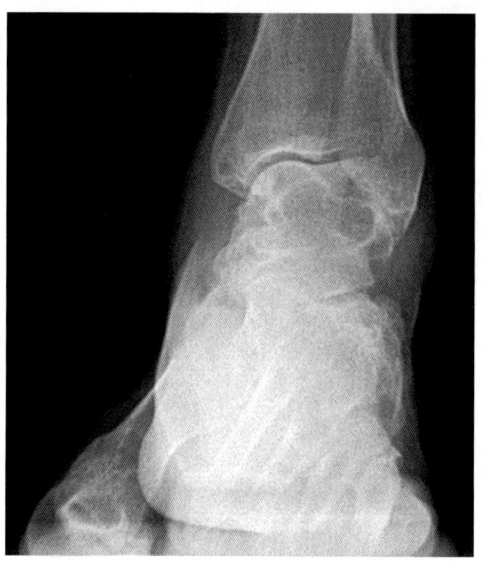
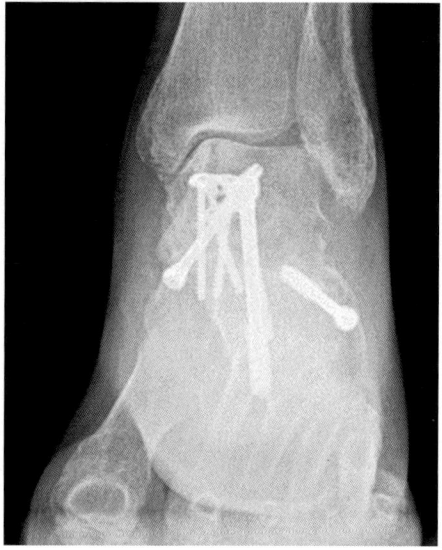
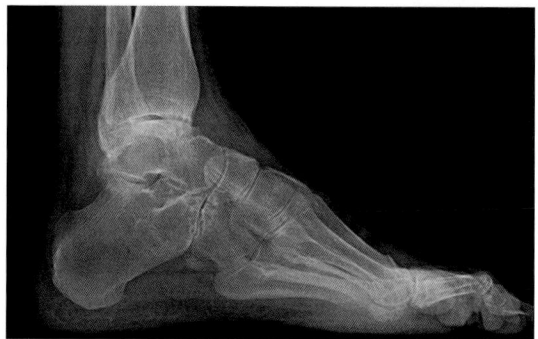
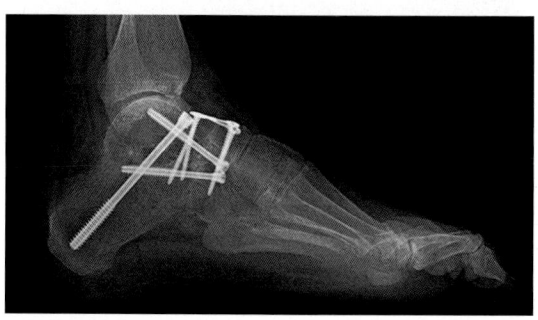

FIGURE 25.25 Correction of severe cavovarus foot deformity using three screws and an added dorsal-medial locking plate over the talonavicular joint. (Pictures complimentary of Douglas K. Blacklidge, DPM.)

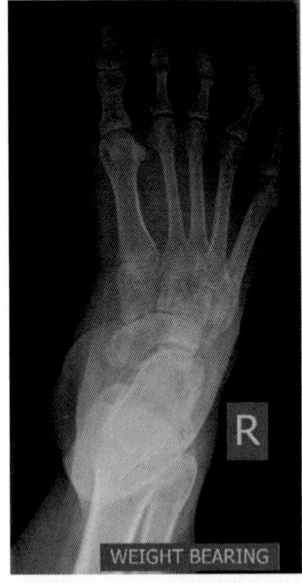
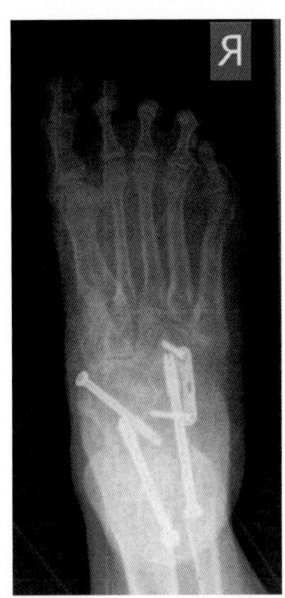
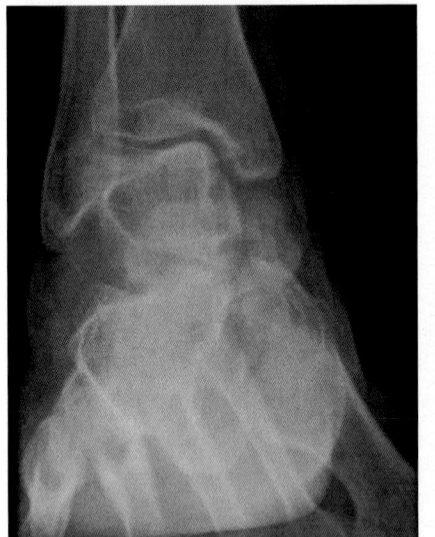
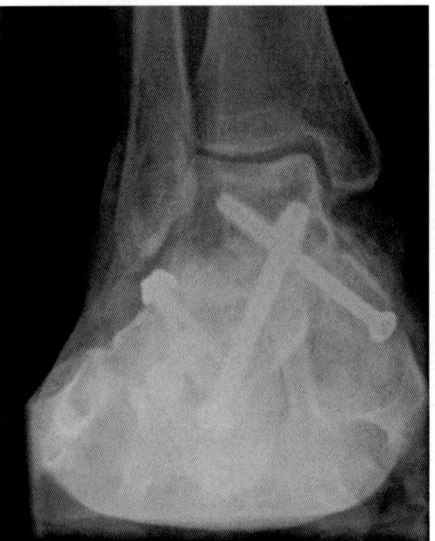
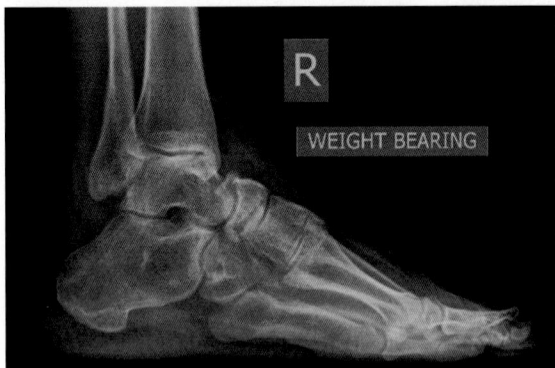
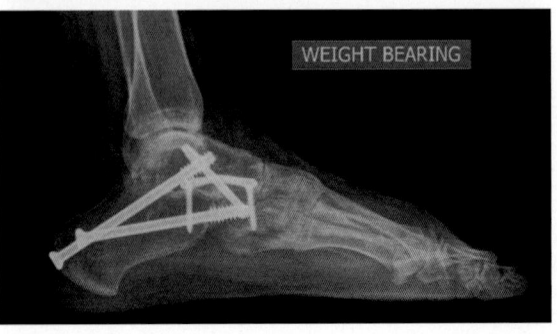

FIGURE 25.26 Correction of severe rearfoot arthritis, cavovarus foot deformity, and functional rearfoot/ankle varus using three screws and an added dorsal-lateral locking plate over the calcaneocuboid joint. (Pictures complimentary of Douglas K. Blacklidge, DPM.)

With improved instrumentation and internal fixation techniques, the triple arthrodesis procedure is very predictable with low rates of complications. Rare complications may include talar avascular necrosis, peroneal tenosynovitis, lateral ankle impingement, sural neuritis, superficial peroneal neuritis, chronic pain (RSD/CRPS), Achilles tendon rupture, acute Charcot process, and deep vein thrombosis.[1,12,13,15,16] More common complications encountered range from wound healing and hardware issues to malunion/nonunion and residual deformity. Wound dehiscence has been cited in up to 33% of these cases, and surgical site infection has been documented to occur up to 17% of the time as well.[12,15-18] Hardware removal may be required anywhere from 0% to 37.5% of the time, with subtalar screws being the most commonly removed fixation devices.[15-18] Misalignment of the arthrodesis procedure can account for up to 66% of the failures encountered postoperatively. However, interestingly enough, preoperative deformity and postoperative residual deformity are not always associated with poor long-term outcomes.[1,6,11,15,17,19]

With the above being considered, the most common significant complications are nonunion and progressive osteoarthritis of adjacent joints. The literature reports a time to bony union anywhere from 6 weeks to 6.9 months, with the majority falling between 10 and 14 weeks minimum.[9,12,13,16,20] Nonunion has been documented from 0% to 23% in children and adolescents, and 0%-46% in adults.[10-17,20-22] Pseudarthrosis accounts for 0%-22.5% of the nonunions, and debate continues as to whether the talonavicular joint or calcaneocuboid joint is most commonly affected.[10,13] Factors leading to nonunion include inadequate joint preparation, poor bony apposition, inadequate or inferior internal fixation, and early weight-bearing. These complications are not dependent on concomitant bone grafting or orthobiological use within this procedure.[9,15,17,22] Interestingly enough, a nonunion may remain asymptomatic in up to 96% of the patients when it occurs, and asymptomatic in up to 98.8% of the patients when only a single fusion site is not solidly healed.[1,9-18,20-22]

Similarly, postoperative progressive osteoarthritis may be seen in the ankle up to 60% of the time (Fig. 25.27) and in

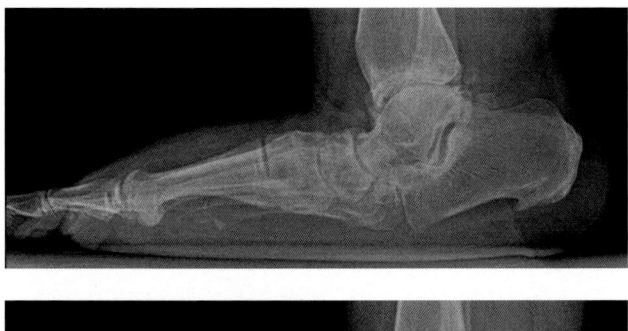

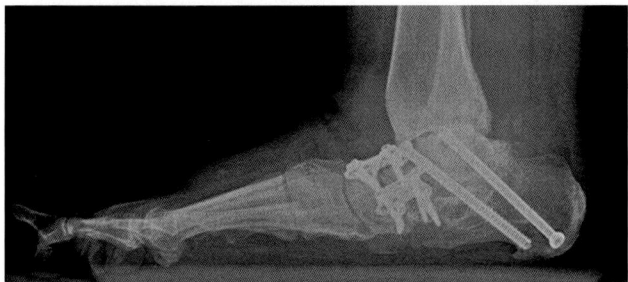

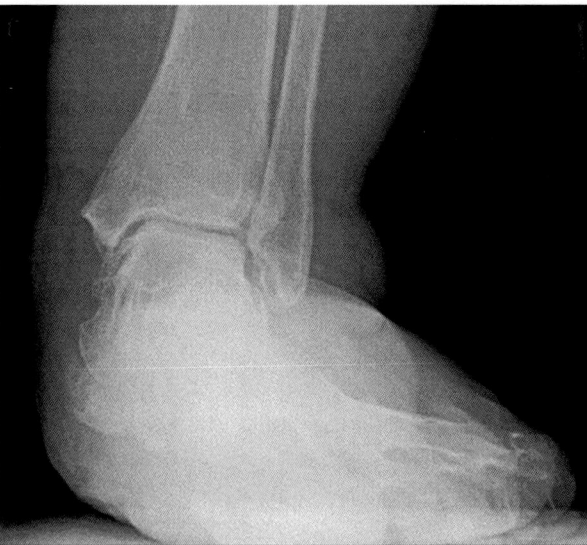

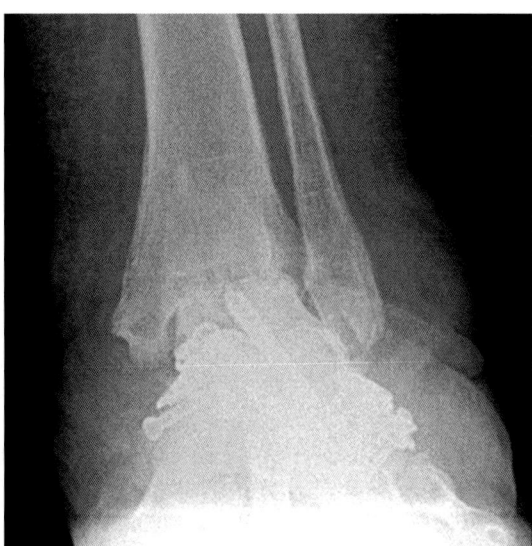

FIGURE 25.27 Radiographs depicting postoperative progressive ankle osteoarthritis after triple arthrodesis.

the midfoot up to 53.75% of the time after a triple arthrodesis procedure. Fortunately, this is often relatively asymptomatic and has little influence on the long-term function of the patient.[11,12,14,23-25] Some sources cite the ankle as becoming more arthritic postoperatively over time, while other sources cite the midfoot region as the most common area to experience postoperative arthrosis. Some surgeons feel that appropriate rearfoot alignment is critical for an optimal outcome, while other sources state it is not a major factor in good surgical results. No matter the opinion, multiple articles show that joints which develop moderate to severe progressive osteoarthritis postoperatively had preexisting degenerative changes preoperatively. Those joints that only develop mild progressive osteoarthritis postoperatively had similar radiographic findings in the same joint(s) on the contralateral limb.[1,11,12,14,15,18,21-25]

Despite the complications that may be encountered with the triple arthrodesis procedure, one thing remains constant—the importance of postoperative radiographic evaluation with this type of reconstructive surgery. Postoperative serial radiographs allow the surgeon to evaluate and ascertain the maintenance of appropriate deformity correction and document that progressive osseous consolidation/fusion across the rearfoot joints is occurring.

Historically and currently, there are many different ways to approach a triple arthrodesis procedure. The procedure can be performed utilizing multiple joint preparation techniques, as well as a variety of deformity reduction techniques and fixation methods. In the end, it all comes down to basic surgical principles that make this procedure reproducible and predictable. As long as these principles are followed, the outcome of the procedure should be satisfactory and rewarding to both the patient and surgeon.

REFERENCES

1. Angus PD, Crowell HR. Triple arthrodesis: a critical long-term review. *J Bone Joint Surg.* 1986;68(2):260-265.
2. Ryerson EW. Arthrodesing operations on the feet. *J Bone Joint Surg Am.* 1923;5:453-471.
3. DeVries JG, Scharer B. Hindfoot deformity corrected with double versus triple arthrodesis: radiographic comparison. *J Foot Ankle Surg.* 2015;54:424-427.
4. Galli MM, Scott RT, Bussewitz BW, Hyer CF. A retrospective comparison of cost and efficiency of the medial double and dual incision triple arthrodesis. *Foot Ankle Surg.* 2014;7(1):32-36.
5. Zhang K, Chen Y, Qiang M, Hao Y. Effects of five hindfoot arthrodesis on foot and ankle motion: measurements in cadaver specimens. *Sci Rep.* 2016;6:35493. doi: 10.1038/srep35493.
6. Hyer CF, Galli MM, Scott RT, Bussewitz B, Berlet GC. Ankle valgus after hindfoot arthrodesis: a radiographic and chart comparison of the medial double and triple arthrodesis. *J Foot Ankle Surg.* 2014;53:55-58.
7. Berlet GC, Hyer CF, Scott RT, Galli MM. Medial double arthrodesis with lateral column sparing and arthrodiastasis: a radiographic and medical record review. *J Foot Ankle Surg.* 2015;54:441-444.
8. Moon AS, McGee AS, Patel HA, et al. A safety and cost analysis of outpatient versus inpatient hindfoot fusion surgery. *Foot Ankle Spec.* 2019;12(10):336-344.
9. Rosenfeld PF, Budgen SA, Saxby TS. Triple arthrodesis: is bone grafting necessary? The results in 100 consecutive cases. *J Bone Joint Surg Br.* 2005;87(2):175-178.
10. Wicks ED, Morscher MA, Newton M, Steiner RP, Weiner DS. Partial of non-union after triple arthrodesis in children: does it really matter? *J Child Orthop.* 2016;10:119-125.
11. Trehan SK, Ihekweazu UN, Root L. Long-term outcomes of triple arthrodesis in cerebral palsy patients. *J Pediatr Orthop.* 2015;35:751-755.
12. Pell RF, Myerson MS, Schon LC. Clinical outcome after primary triple arthrodesis. *J Bone Joint Surg.* 2000;82-A(1):47-57.
13. Daglar B, Devect A, Delialioglu OM, et al. Results of triple arthrodesis: effect of primary etiology. *J Orthop Sci.* 2008;13:341-347.
14. Bennett GL, Graham CE, Mauldin DM. Triple arthrodesis in adults. *Foot Ankle.* 1991;12(3):138-143.
15. Bednarz PA, Monroe MT, Manli A. Triple arthrodesis in adults using rigid internal fixation: an assessment of outcome. *Foot Ankle Int.* 1999;20(6):356-363.
16. Coetzee JC, Hansen ST. Surgical management of severe deformity resulting from posterior tibial tendon dysfunction. *Foot Ankle Int.* 2001;22(12):944-949.
17. Child BJ, Hix J, Xtanzariti AR, Mendicino RW, Saltrick K. The effect of hindfoot realignment in triple arthrodesis. *J Foot Ankle Surg.* 2009;48(3):285-293.
18. Graves SC, Mann RA, Graves KO. Triple arthrodesis in older adults. Results after long-term follow-up. *J Bone Joint Surg Am.* 1993;75(3):355-362.
19. Hutchinson ID, Baxter JR, Gilbert S, et al. How do hindfoot fusions affect ankle biomechanics: a cadaver model. *Clin Orthop Relat Res.* 2016;474:1008-1016.
20. Mirmiran R, Wilde B, Nielsen M. Retrospective analysis of the rate and interval to union for joint arthrodesis of the foot and ankle. *J Foot Ankle Surg.* 2014;53:420-425.
21. Burrus MT, Werner BC, Carr JB, Perunal V, Park JS. Increased failure rate of modified double arthrodesis compared with triple arthrodesis for rigid pes planovalgus. *J Foot Ankle Surg.* 2016;55:1169-1174.
22. Klassen LJ, Weinraub GM, Shi E, Liu J. Comparative nonunion rates in triple arthrodesis. *J Foot Ankle Surg.* 2018;57(6):1-3.
23. De Heus JAC, Marti RK, Besselaar PP, Albers GHR. The influence of subtalar and triple arthrodesis on the tibiotalar joint: a long-term follow-up study. *J Bone Joint Surg Br.* 1997;79-B(4):644-647.
24. Klerken T, Kosse NM, Aarts CAM, Louwerens JWK. Long-term results after triple arthrodesis: influence of alignment on ankle osteoarthritis and clinical outcome. *Foot Ankle Surg.* 2019;25:247-250.
25. Aarts CAM, Heesterbeek PJC, Jaspers PEM, Stegeman M, Louwerens JWK. Does osteoarthritis of the ankle joint progress after triple arthrodesis? A midterm prospective outcome study. *Foot Ankle Surg.* 2016;22:265-269.

CHAPTER 26

Subtalar Joint Arthrodesis

Michael C. McGlamry and John C. Haight

DEFINITION

Subtalar joint (STJ) arthrodesis is a relatively straightforward but multifaceted procedure that can be immensely powerful in addressing arthritic and malalignment issues of the hindfoot. STJ arthrodesis is easily accomplished by closely following Glissan's principles and applying a stable fixation construct.

INDICATIONS

STJ arthrodesis is most commonly employed for correction of instability and malposition of the rearfoot including pes valgus and cavus deformities.[1-3] This procedure can also be used as for treatment of posttraumatic arthritis such as is frequently encountered following calcaneal fractures (Fig. 26.1A-D).

The author utilizes the STJ arthrodesis as the primary building block procedure for management of the flexible flatfoot deformity. Fusion of this joint often in combination with other soft tissue, osteotomy, and fusion procedures in the midfoot is capable of significant realignment and stabilization of the foot under the leg.

ANATOMIC FEATURES

The STJ is made up of three segments that must be adequately addressed for successful arthrodesis of the joint into a functional neutral position. These are the posterior, middle, and anterior facets. The posterior facet accounts for the great majority of the surface area of the joint complex. This is where the effective surgeon will focus the great majority of his or her time and attention in order to gain a successful well-positioned and functional arthrodesis of this joint complex.

Other anatomic considerations that must be managed, appreciated, and protected during the surgical approach include the sural nerve, the intermediate dorsal cutaneous nerve branches, the peroneal tendons, and the lateral ankle ligaments. All of these structures are encountered in or surround the approach for exposure of the STJ.

Anatomically, the lateral ankle gutter will be directly encountered during a standard sinus tarsi approach to the STJ, and plays a critical role in this procedure. As will later be discussed, the lateral talar process is vitally important in establishing the desired neutral position for the fusion and providing a reference for positioning after resection of the joint surfaces.

Appreciation of the ankle joint articular surface is also critical when placing definitive fixation so as to prevent violation and damage to the tibiotalar articulation.

The movement of this joint is frequently described as inversion and eversion, which suggests a pure frontal plane motion. Anatomically, however, the STJ is saddle shaped, which allows true triplanar screwing type of motion. This allows inversion and simultaneous internal rotation of the tuberosity creating movement in all three planes. In the open kinetic chain, the heel moves internally providing more support to the talus and also decreasing the available range of motion (ROM) of the mid-tarsal joint, an important and underappreciated aspect of lower extremity biomechanics.

PHYSICAL EXAMINATION

Physical examination of the STJ involves observing the patient in relaxed calcaneal stance position and noting the overall position of the heel related to the leg and weight-bearing surface. Great attention to detail must be taken at this point to insure that the patient is not guarding the position in inversion as this will potentially mask the degree of deformity.

On clinical examination, the ROM of the STJ should be evaluated for quality and extent of the motion available. Diagnostic intra-articular blocks and common peroneal nerve blocks may also be extremely helpful, even prior to any advanced imaging for evaluating the actual anatomic origin and source of pain or limitation of motion.

CONSERVATIVE TREATMENT

Conservative care alternatives for patients who may benefit from STJ arthrodesis include bracing, NSAIDs, and intra-articular injections.

Bracing can range from over the counter (OTC) lace up braces with figure 8 straps, to custom ankle foot orthosis (AFOs). Custom AFOs may be fixed ankle or articulated depending on other associated conditions being treated.

Bracing can be very successful; however, patient acceptance may be difficult often due to cosmetic reasons. Bracing can place significant burden on shoe choice as even OTC braces made out of ballistic nylon can be quite bulky while the custom leather and thermoplastic braces make shoe fit a true challenge even in the best of circumstances.

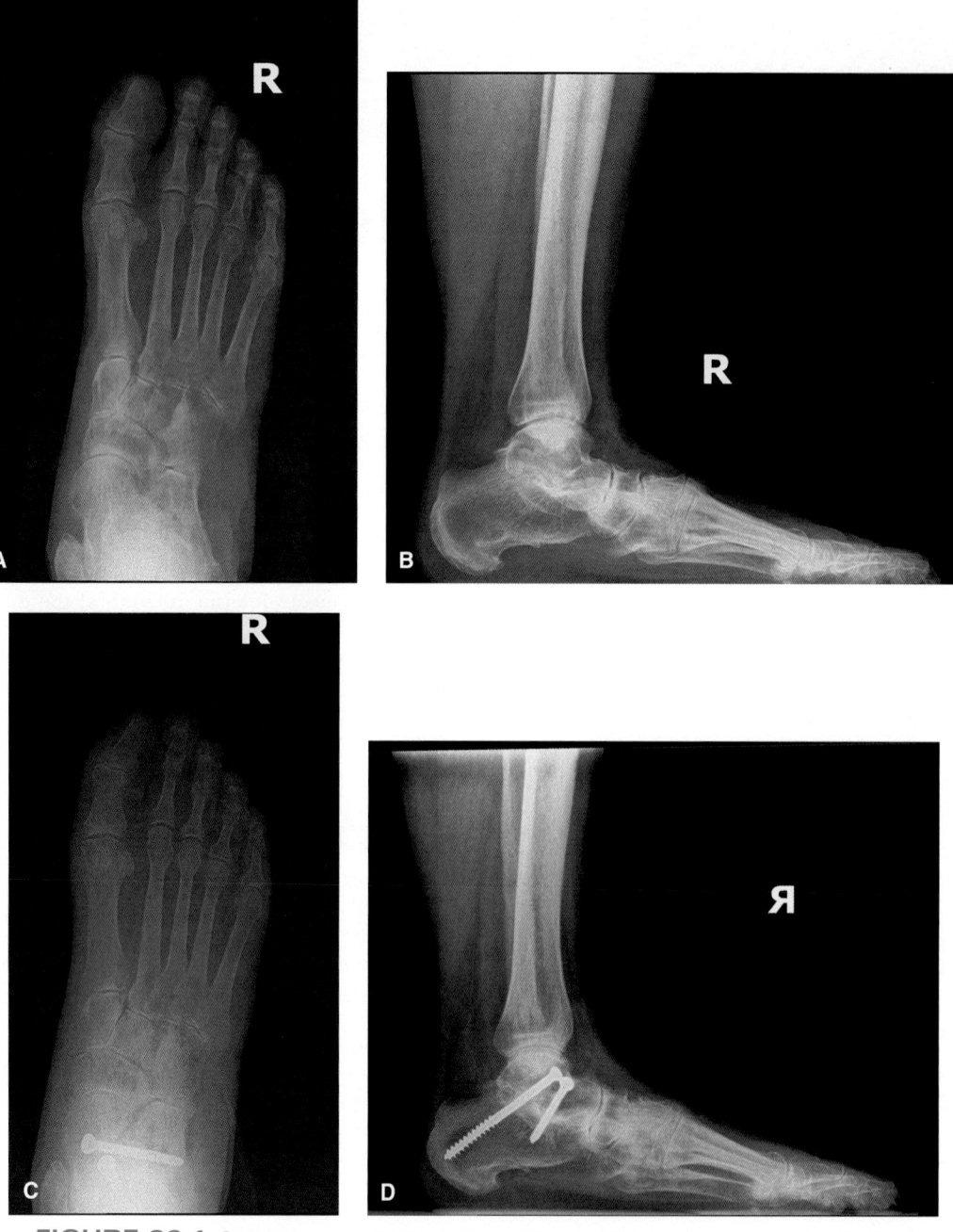

FIGURE 26.1 **A.** DP x-ray view of patient with significant peritalar subluxation associated with posterior tibial tendon dysfunction and acquired adult flatfoot deformity. **B.** Lateral x-ray view of same patient showing increased talar declination and obliteration of the subtalar joint due to the anterior displacement of the lateral talar process. **C.** DP view of the same patient following successful STJ arthrodesis. Note the increased coverage of the talar head and decreased calcaneocuboid abduction. **D.** Lateral view following successful STJ arthrodesis. Note the improved talar first metatarsal alignment and increased stacking of the metatarsals associated with realignment of the hindfoot.

PATHOGENESIS

Leading causes for the need for STJ arthrodesis include tarsal coalition, posttraumatic arthritis following calcaneal fracture, and adult pes valgus deformity associated with posterior tibial tendon dysfunction (PTTD).[4,5] The underlying pathology will guide the incisional approach for access to the joint as well as goals of the surgical intervention.

IMAGING AND DIAGNOSTIC STUDIES

Weight-bearing plain film radiographs to include AP, lateral, and medial oblique views are frequently all that is needed for evaluation of the relative alignment of the rearfoot complex. However, in order to curate a more complete understanding of the deformity, calcaneal axial and other hindfoot alignment views can be obtained as well. In the case of previous trauma or previous surgery, three-dimensional imaging such as CT scan or MRI may be necessary.

The imaging of choice is primarily based on the underlying pathology. If the STJ arthrodesis is being performed due to posttraumatic arthritis for a previous calcaneal fracture, then CT is likely more helpful. CT is also useful when performing this procedure in response to a tarsal coalition. CT allows for greater fine osseous detail due to the thinner cut thickness (as thin as 1 mm at most centers, but 2 mm is more than adequate). Alternatively if the planned procedure is for PTTD or if there is question about the viability of the bone, then MRI is the study of choice. The MRI allows a more complete examination of both osseous and soft tissue pathology in this instance. When ordering the study, use of diagrams to help guide the tech to assure that the desired field of view and orientation of the cuts is obtained to assure that the desired information can be gleaned from the study.

SURGICAL POSITIONING

Operative positioning for the STJ arthrodesis is most commonly undertaken in a traditional supine position. This allows access to the joint laterally and to the anterior medial ankle for fixation placement and causes the least amount of risk to the patient.

Alternatively those who prefer inferior approach for fixation may prefer placement of the patient in the lateral decubitus position as this also allows good direct visualization of the joint exposure and also allows easier access for placement of fixation from the inferior heel.

SURGICAL TECHNIQUE

Surgical technique for STJ arthrodesis is approached in several distinct manners. One for the virgin STJ, a separate plan of attack for the neglected calcaneal fracture, and yet another approach can be considered for rigid rearfoot deformity.

STANDARD SUBTALAR JOINT APPROACH

The virgin STJ is most commonly approached from the lateral sinus tarsi incision. This courses from the distal tip of the fibula, across the sinus tarsi and extends distally to the anterior calcaneal beak/CC joint area (Fig. 26.2). However, there has recently been a push for a more minimally invasive approach to this joint. While the minimally invasive approach does have its advantages,[6] there are concerns for an increased rate in complications due to the surgeon's inability to fully visualize this joint and thus being left with an inadequate correction or resection leading to a surgical failure. Another approach commonly utilized is the medial approach. This surgical incision placement does have its advantages, and good visualization of the joint is reported in literature.[7] However, it is not disputed by most that the lateral approach affords a better resection of the posterior facet of the STJ. Therefore, it is recommended that the medial approach be used primarily when other procedures are performed medially in conjunction with the STJ arthrodesis to eliminate the need for two incisions.

There is very limited subcutaneous tissue in most patients in this area, and caution should be taken not to prematurely

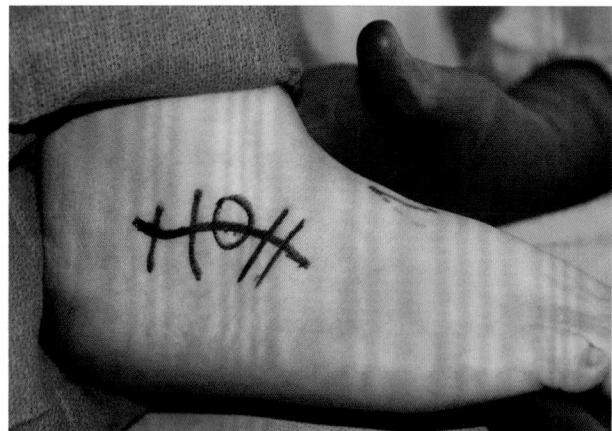

FIGURE 26.2 Intraoperative marking of standard sinus tarsi approach for STJ arthrodesis.

violate the deep fascia (Fig. 26.3). Neurovascular structures in this area should be identified and protected to the fullest extent possible as well during the anatomic dissection.

Once the subcutaneous tissue has been reflected, the deep fascia is entered along the inferior border of the extensor digitorum brevis muscle belly distally and extended proximally to the tip of the fibula. Care should be taken here not to violate the peroneal sheath inferiorly, as this may present issues with closure later in the procedure.

Full exposure for the procedure is dependent on releasing the intraosseous talocalcaneal ligament and completely excising or dorsally reflecting Hoke's tonsil. Once the ligament has been released and Hoke tonsil reflected, adequate exposure to the joint complex is gained. If all three facets are not visible, then more work needs to be done prior to beginning joint resection.

At this point, establishing the neutral position of the STJ and creating a landmark for later reference is highly advisable. Once the normal anatomy is disrupted by the joint resection, it can be more difficult to easily identify and restore the neutral position alignment of the rearfoot.

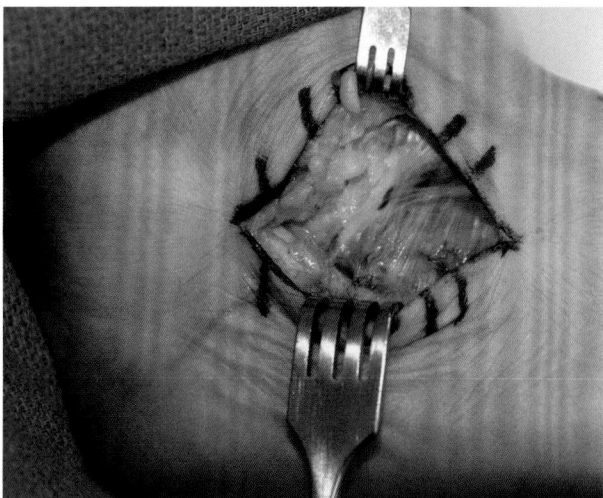

FIGURE 26.3 Intra-op appearance following reflection of the subcutaneous layer. Note that the EDB muscle belly is clearly visible below the deep fascia/extensor retinaculum.

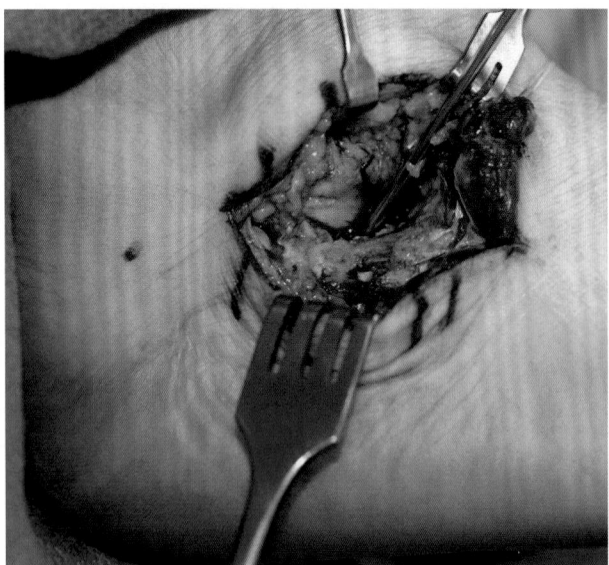

FIGURE 26.4 Intraoperative view of exposure of the sinus tarsi and lateral talar process wit neutral position 3/32 in Steinman pin in place.

The simplest way to mark the neutral position for this purpose is to place the rearfoot into neutral position based on a vertical heel position and then drill a large gauge Steinman pin into the calcaneus immediately anterior to the lateral talar process. The author utilizes a 3/32 in pin as this is larger than the smaller pins or drill bits utilized to complete preparation of the fusion site and therefore will be easier to return to once preparation is accomplished (Fig. 26.4).

With the pin inserted, the foot can be examined clinically to insure that the heel is in vertical alignment beneath the leg. One will also note significant improvement in the stability of the midtarsal joint at this time. Intra-op fluoroscopy, if performed, should show a clear view of the STJ on the lateral view with complete visualization of the anterior, middle, and posterior facets and smooth congruence of the cyma line. On the AP view, if the talar alignment has been adequately restored, one will note marked improvement in the talar-first metatarsal axis and navicular coverage of the talar head.

Distraction of the joint greatly facilitates visualization and exposure of joint surfaces. This allows for better access with instrumentation leading to a more complete resection of the articular surface. Historically a lamina spreader is utilized for STJ distraction; however, it is typically not stable and is directly in the path needed for joint resection.

A pin-based distractor, such as the AO mini distractor and Hintermann or tarsal distractor, allows larger pins to be utilized for stronger and more stable distraction and allows the pins to be placed out of the line of approach for joint distraction (Fig. 26.5). With the joint successfully distracted, débridement of the joint is a straightforward task.

There are several different techniques one could deploy for joint resection with the two main being wedge resection vs contoured resection.[8] Specifics of a certain technique are not as important as a complete resection of the cartilage. For the author, joint resection is undertaken with curved and straight osteotomes, curved and straight curettes and rongeurs in the contoured resection fashion. A pituitary rongeur and a long neck burr are also quite helpful for completing the resection into this deep joint. The goal is to resect the joint without disrupting the normal contours so that the ideal position can be dialed in without wedging or the need for graft in most cases. One aspect of this is fully understanding the shape of the facets, particularly the curvature of the posterior facet.

The author has found the sequence that best facilitates this task is:

1. Stripping of the articular cartilage typically with an 8-mm curved and straight osteotome.
2. Following initial removal of the surface, aggressive follow-up débridement is undertaken with medium to large curette. A curved curette is most helpful for accessing the posterior recess of the calcaneal portion of the posterior facet, while the straight counterpart seems to be most helpful on the inferior surface of the talus.

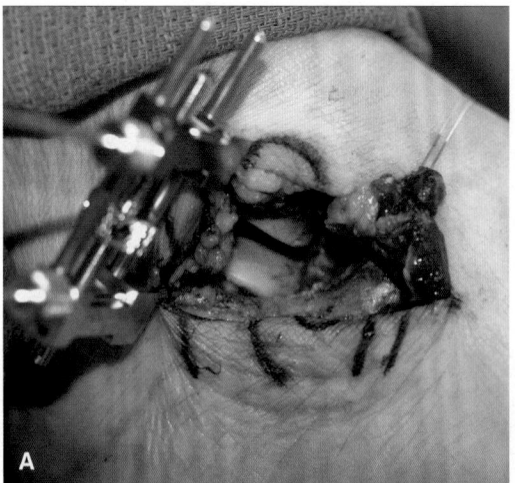
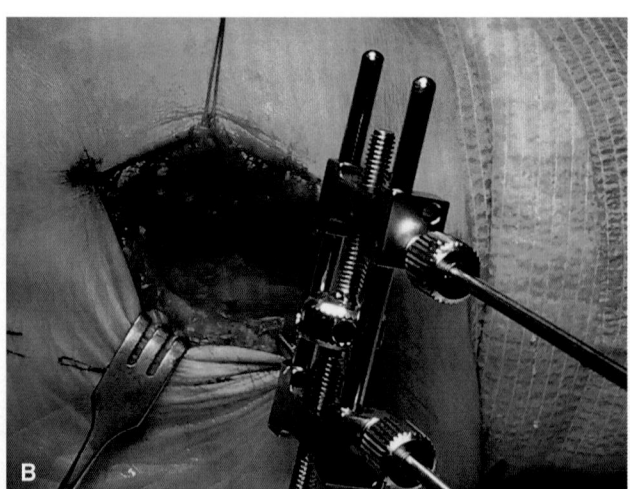

FIGURE 26.5 **A.** Intra-op view of initial distraction of the STJ in preparation for joint resection. Note the clear exposure for joint débridement with the distraction device placed more posterior and lateral to the lateral talar process. **B.** Intra-op view following initial resection of the articular surface with all three facets visible.

3. After the osteotomes and curettes, it is likely that a good portion of the subchondral bone plate may remain intact; therefore, drilling (1.6 mm wire or 2.0 drill bit) and or fish-scaling with a smaller (4-6 mm) osteotome can finish the job nicely.
4. If any remaining débridement is required at this point, a carbide burr may be used to complete the task.

With preparation of the fusion site completed, neutral to slight valgus position is restored by reinserting the neutral position pin discussed previously and loading the lateral column of the foot. This drives the lateral process of the talus forward to abut the pin. In addition to a neutral to slight valgus position being tolerated better compared to varus position of the rearfoot, it also allows for a more biomechanically advantageous ankle joint ROM in both dorsiflexion and plantar flexion.[9] The foot has now been returned to the previously established neutral to slight valgus fix-ation and temporary fixation is undertaken (Fig. 26.6).

Careful evaluation of intraoperative imaging at this time should reveal restoration of the normal cyma line, relatively neutral calcaneal cuboid angle and good coverage of the talar head on the AP view. Tight scrutiny of the lateral view will expose any errors or need for further resection (Fig. 26.7).

One example of this would be a lateral image demonstrating good apposition to the posterior facet on the magnified view and good coverage of the talar head on the AP view, but on the larger field of view, lateral incongruence of the cyma line is noted. This is typically the result of posterior displacement of the talus and can have the same effect as overcorrecting into calcaneal varus. Both result in overloading of the lateral col-umn that is poorly tolerated and almost impossible to manage conservatively.

Surgeon's choice of cannulated or solid core screw fixation is typically used for final fixation. There has been discussion of utilizing staples as the primary fixation for STJ fusion; however, better functional scores postoperatively were reported with screw fixation.[10] If cannulated screws are utilized, two divergent guide pins are placed. The author places the first pin from the talar neck, slightly lateral to midline into the posterior inferior calcaneal tuberosity. The second pin is then placed from the dorsomedial talar head/neck aiming more anterior and lateral

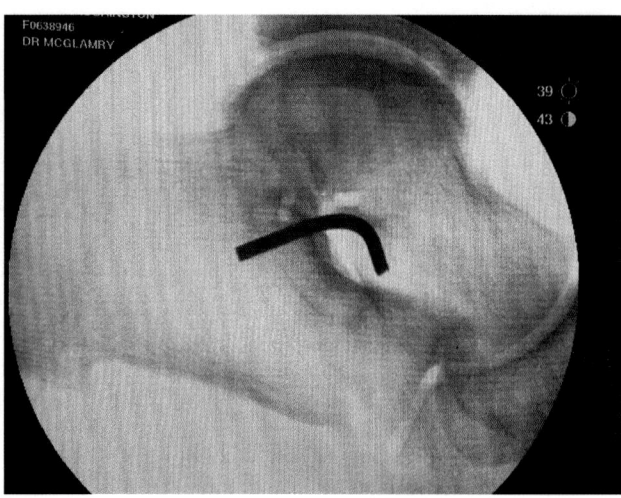
FIGURE 26.7 Intra-op lateral fluoroscopic view showing restoration of the normal cyma line and the talus sitting squarely atop the calcaneus. Particular attention should be utilized here if the neutral position pin is not employed to assure that the talus is not inadvertently displaced too far posteriorly as this will result in a functional forefoot varus by proximally displacing and effectively offloading the medial column.

from the first aiming for the plantar lateral cortex of the heel. Generally this is easily palpable and readily visualized on lat-eral oblique fluoroscopy. The first pin is generally readily pal-pable as it exits the tuberosity but again can be easily verified on lateral and calcaneal axial fluoroscopic images (Fig. 26.8A-C). Headless screws are not generally utilized for fixation cross the STJ, as it has been shown that it takes three headless screws across the STJ to approach the same compressive forces as two headed screws across the same joint.[11]

The author's preference is to use this superior to inferior fixation approach as it allows for the use of long thread profile screws for greater purchase and does not risk violation of the articular surface of the ankle. Other individuals however pre-fer a bottom up approach running fixation from the posterior inferior calcaneus up into the talar body. If this approach to fixation is chosen the surgeon should employ thorough fluoro-scopic evaluation of pins and subsequently screw placement to prevent invasion of the ankle joint as well as adequate fixation placement into the appropriate osseous structures.

The one advantage of the inferior to superior orientation of fixation is that it eliminates the second incision for place-ment of fixation used by the author. Some would argue that fixation from the top down could just as easily be delivered per-cutaneously. Percutaneous fixation of the top-down approach however is discouraged due to the number of neurovascular structures traversing this corridor in line with the direct path of the desired fixation trajectory.

After fixation is accomplished, attention should be redi-rected to the fusion site where visual inspection and palpation with a freer elevator should reveal tight apposition of the two elements contributing to the fusion mass. Any gaps noted may be packed with cancellous bone chips or filled with other ortho-biologics of choice.

Closure is then accomplished in a layered fashion. Use of closed suction drains may be helpful, especially if the patient has increased risk factors for DVT and is being anticoagulated in the immediate postoperative period. The author however

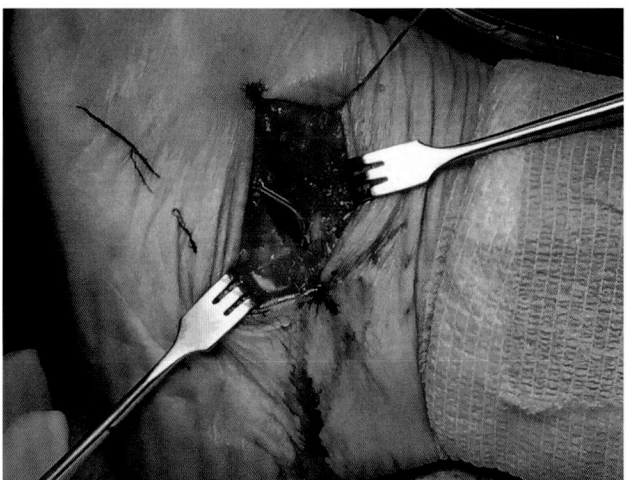
FIGURE 26.6 Intra-op appearance following complete preparation of the arthrodesis site and realignment on the neutral position pin, placed during initial exposure of the STJ complex.

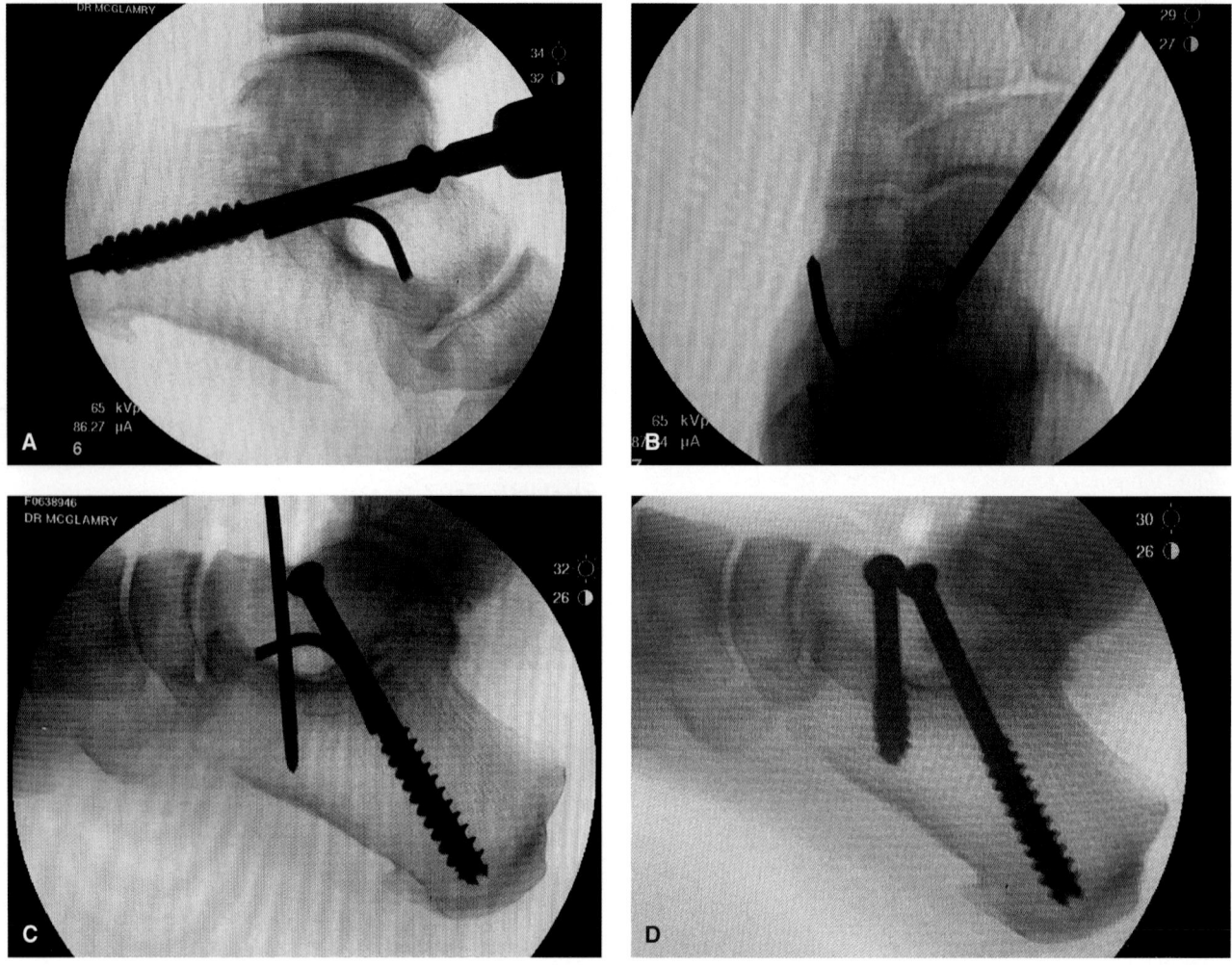

FIGURE 26.8 A. Placement of the primary fixation from the talar neck into the calcaneal tuberosity. Note that the neutral position wire remains in place while the initial screw is being delivered. **B.** DP view following placement of the primary compression screw. Coverage of the talar head is confirmed on this view prior to placement of the secondary point of fixation. **C.** Lateral intra-op fluoro image showing delivery of the guide pin for the secondary point of fixation. The neutral position pin should be removed at this point prior to placement and final tightening of the second screw. **D.** Lateral fluoro image following placement of second point of fixation and final tightening of both screws.

has gotten away from routine use of drains as even the most complicated hindfoot reconstructions are pushed into the outpatient surgical arena.

Postoperative Management of Standard STJ Approach

Postoperative management of the virgin STJ arthrodesis in a relatively healthy, uncompromised patient is fairly straightforward. The author applies compression casting in the OR and then typically replaces this with a traditional well-padded and molded below the knee synthetic cast, which is maintained up to 5-6 weeks postprocedure.

If x-rays are stable at the 5- to 6-week point, the patient is transitioned to progressive partial weight bearing in a fracture boot for the following 3-4 weeks.

Finally if post-op x-rays at the 8- to 10-week point show signs of incorporation and soft tissue healing is complete, then the patient is transitioned back to regular shoes.

As with any procedure where the patient is cast immobilized during the postoperative period for more than a week, the patient is evaluated and their risk factors stratified using the Caprini risk assessment model or some similar evaluation to reach a decision about whether full DVT prophylaxis is indicated. For all immobilized patients, the author recommends a full-strength aspirin daily (325 mg) unless contraindicated for GI risk factors or medical history reasons.

Exceptions to the Standard STJ Surgical Approach

In the authors' experience, most traditional STJ arthrodesis procedures can be managed in the above approach and technique, but as with most rules, there are almost always a few exceptions.

The primary exceptions to this rule are the neglected calcaneal fracture and the severe rigid valgus deformity that is limited to the STJ and/or its component structures.

STJ ARTHRODESIS FOR THE NEGLECTED CALCANEAL FRACTURE

Approaching the arthritic neglected calcaneal fracture for fusion and correction of the deformity requires a thorough appreciation and understanding of the original injury and also of the normal sequelae of neglected or failed treatment of the initial injury event.

A quick spin through the memory banks on the mechanism of injury and classification of severity and its corresponding prognosis is quite helpful in planning and executing a successful salvage and repair of this pathology.

If the reconstructive surgeon is not routinely managing the acute presentation of calcaneal fractures, it is helpful to remind oneself that the forces involved in the event most commonly result in a calcaneal structure that is wider, shorter, and often, but not always, rotated in the frontal plane in varus.

The goals of treatment of the arthritic STJ include the obvious primary goal of eliminating the limited amount of motion that is causing the pain. Successful treatment however will also re-establish the height and frontal plane alignment of the heel and in doing so restore the normal forces and functional position of motion to the ankle joint.

Preoperative evaluation of patients with a neglected or failed treatment of a calcaneal fracture should include relaxed calcaneal stance position clinical examination and x-rays. Special views that are also helpful include calcaneal axial and sunrise views. Views of the contralateral foot allow measurement of the loss of height of the talocalcaneal complex and will help determine the amount and type of graft required for reconstruction and restoration of more normal function (Fig. 26.9A and B).

CT or MRI scans can be very helpful for getting a detailed look at the frontal plane alignment of the heel and evaluating the viability of the bone. Additionally if there are any voids, which might not be visible on plain film, these can be volumetrically analyzed to determine the volume of allograft, autograft, or other synthetic alternatives needed to fill the defect and enhance the likelihood of a successful outcome of fusion.

If the patient is the unfortunate product of a failed or collapsed Open Reduction with Internal Fixation (ORIF), then it is highly advisable to obtain previous operative reports and clinical documentation prior to undertaking salvage. This will help avoid the ill fated discovery that the universal screw removal set is indeed not so universal after all!!

Prior treatment documentation may also reveal any hidden patient factors that may have contributed to the failure such as noncompliance with non–weight-bearing (NWB) status, smoking, or other issues that may not have been exposed on the initial H&P examination.

Finally, the author finds it strongly advised to obtain vitamin D levels on these, and all other major reconstruction patients. Even in patients with relatively normal vitamin D levels, current recommendations are for supplementation typically of 10 000 IU daily, though the disclaimer that you will need to evaluate the patient's medical status and other medications before instituting this definitely applies.

Surgical Positioning in Neglected Calcaneal Fracture

Best approach for surgical access is gained with the patient in a lateral decubitus position. This helps gain an unobstructed view of the posterolateral approach and easy access for application of fixation from the posterior inferior calcaneal tuberosity. The author utilizes a bean bag (or "Vac-Pac") for safe stabilization of the patient in this position. The surgical extremity is elevated on pillows or a foam OR positioning

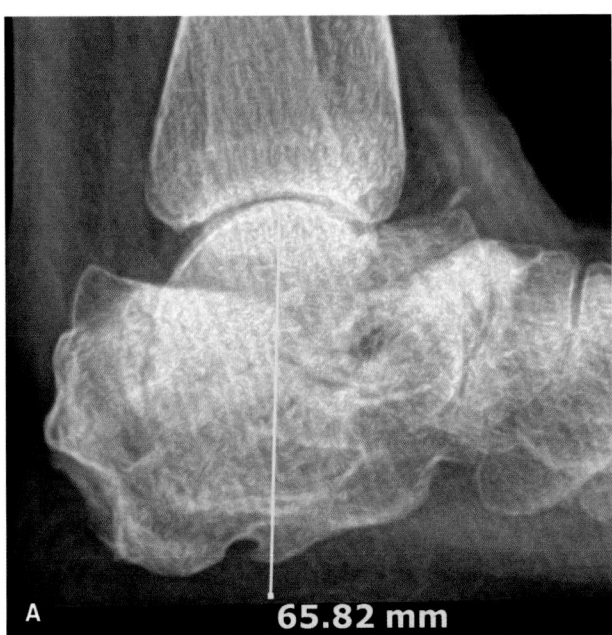
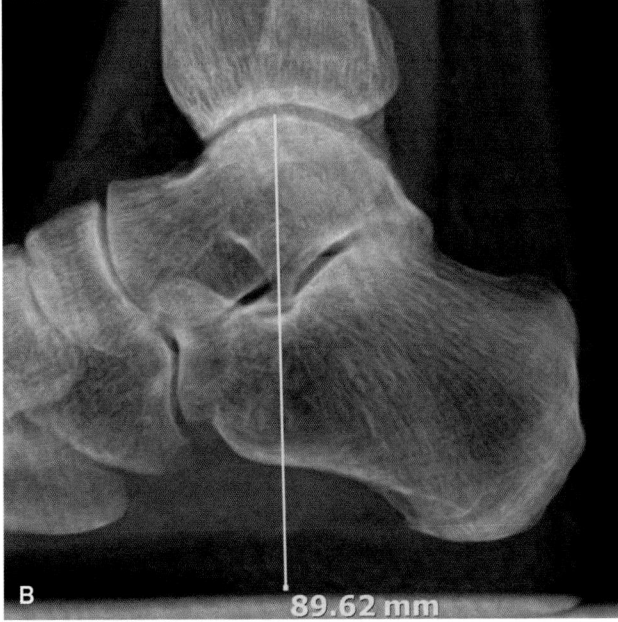

FIGURE 26.9 A. Lateral x-ray view of patient who has sustained joint depression fracture of the calcaneus. **B.** Contralateral view of the patient's heel/subtalar joint complex to establish the normal height of the talar dome and determine the amount graft necessary on the operative side. (Pre-op planning tool.)

device with the contralateral limb flexed at the hip and knee to allow unobstructed fluoroscopic evaluation during the procedure.

Anatomic Approach to the Neglected Calcaneal Fracture

Surgical approach to the neglected calcaneal fracture most often requires a posterior lateral approach instead of the typical sinus tarsi approach used for the virgin STJ arthrodesis.[12,13] The reason for this is that the associated scarring and soft tissue contracture from the injury are placed under significant tension once graft is placed and normal anatomic alignment is restored. If the standard sinus tarsi approach is used, it may result in an incision that cannot be reapproximated or potentially in a wound that is closed under tension that then results in massive wound dehiscence and its associated perils. (Fig. 26.10 showing full dehiscence of STJ arthrodesis from standard sinus tarsi approach. Image is after several weeks of negative pressure wound therapy.)

The most common approach that provides excellent exposure and successfully avoids problems of closure and dehiscence is the posterior lateral approach. The joint is accessed from an incision about 1 cm posterior to the peroneal tendons, starting at about the level of the ankle joint and curving slightly anterior at the distal aspect of the incision as it passes the distal fibula. This affords a safe pathway to access, evaluate, and reconstruct the deformity. It also naturally pulls the incision back together with placement of the graft and reestablishment of the height of the talocalcaneal complex (Fig. 26.11).

Once access to the joint is gained and location is verified under fluoroscopic guidance (keep in mind the "normal" anatomy and architecture of the joint have been destroyed by the injury), only then can the reconstruction ensue.

Once the path of the previous joint has been established and, if necessary débridement of the lateral wall of the calcaneus accomplished, it is then time to distract the joint and restore the height and rotation of the talocalcaneal complex.

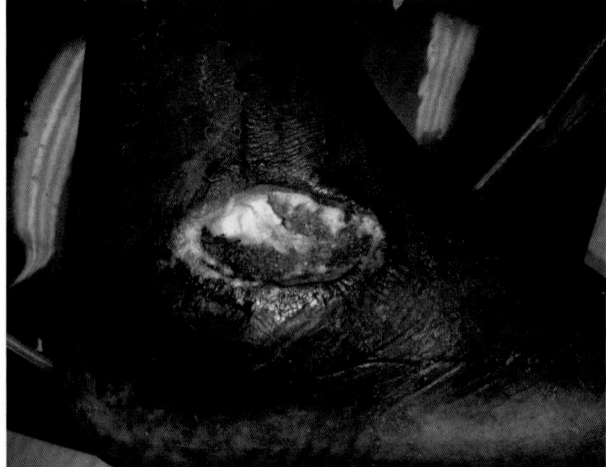

FIGURE 26.10 Lateral clinical view of wound dehiscence following sinus tarsi approach for a neglected calcaneal fracture. This image was taken after several weeks of negative pressure wound therapy and prior to rotational flap closure.

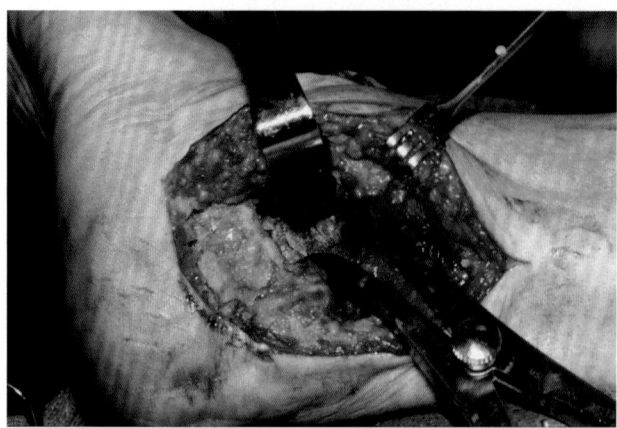

FIGURE 26.11 Posterior lateral incisional approach for the neglected calcaneal fracture. This approach affords excellent access and visualization for débridement of the site and graft placement.

Choice of distraction instrumentation remains unchanged from the virgin arthrodesis except for the restriction that the length of travel of the distractor needed is significantly greater than that needed in a traditional STJ fusion. Therefore, for these procedures, the author prefers the Hintermann or tarsal distractor as again these can be placed relatively out of the field of direct surgical access in most instances, thereby enhancing surgical access.

With the joint distracted, thorough débridement of all nonviable or questionable tissue is undertaken. The roadmap provided by the pre-op CT or MRI study is particularly helpful here.

After complete evacuation of the site and débridement back to healthy bony margins, it is time to begin to reestablish physiologic height and position of the talocalcaneal complex.

Voids in the body of the calcaneus are quite common with these mistreated or neglected injuries and if left unaddressed will greatly decrease chances of successful outcomes. In view of this, the author prefers a mixture of allograft, Demineralized Bone Matrix (DBM), and autologous Platelet Rich Plasma (PRP) and Bone Marrow Aspirate (BMA) concentrate to enhance the site.

The structural graft height should have been at least roughly determined preoperatively with comparison contralateral images and 3D imaging studies. Based on the patient's biologic activity, volume of graft required, and other logistical factors, the intercalary/interpositional bone graft source is determined.

If iliac crest autograft is being harvested for the procedure, it is highly advisable to obtain 60 cc of BMA prior to violation of the crest and concentrate this down to 5-10 cc of stem cell and growth factor rich concentrate to be utilized to augment the procedure. If iliac crest autograft is not being used, it is still desirable to obtain BMA for concentration in these cases to enhance the healing environment.

If autograft is the choice, typically we have found that we need two struts of ~2.5 cm each after the site has been prepared. Struts are placed medially and laterally so that they are interposed between the superior cortex of the calcaneal body and the inferior table of the prepared surface of the talus. Struts are typically not the same length with the discrepancy being utilized to engineer the correction of needed frontal plane malalignment.

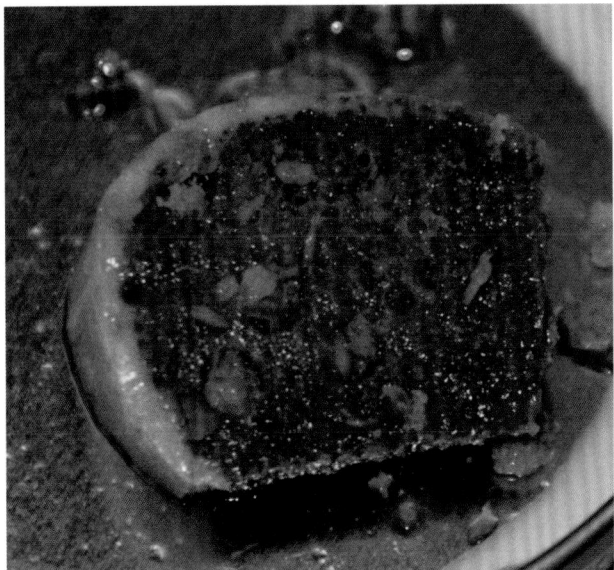

FIGURE 26.12 Intra-op photo of the fresh frozen femoral head allograft, which has been drilled and loaded with stem cell allograft material. Additionally, this graft has also been doped with BMA concentrate obtained from the proximal tibia at the start of the procedure.

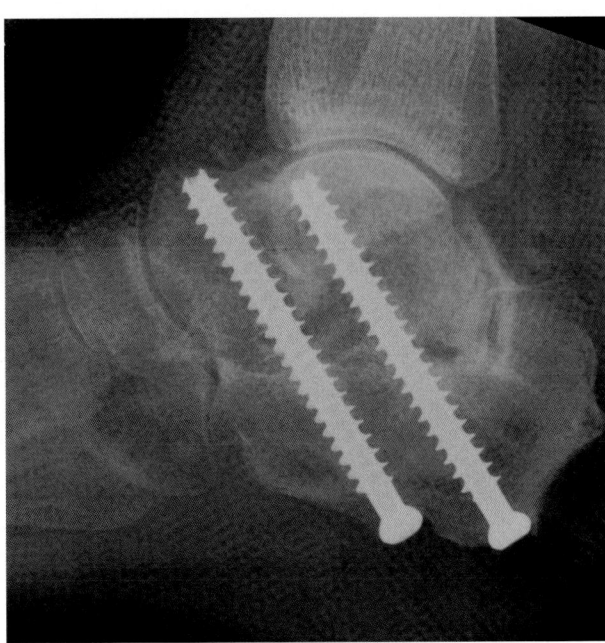

FIGURE 26.13 Lateral x-ray showing fixation of the revised neglected calcaneal fracture utilizing fully threaded large bore cannulated screws.

If allograft is the choice, the author has on numerous occasions utilized fresh frozen femoral head. This allows for a seemingly limitless supply of graft material, and after the primary graft dimensions are determined and cut, the remainder of the head can be milled or morselized and combined with the remainder of the biologics of choice to fill all remaining defects.

Another twist that the author has employed when utilizing fresh frozen femoral head is to drill the central cancellous portion of the structural graft once it has been test fitted. This is performed with a 3.5-mm drill bit. The holes that are generated are then filled with a stem cell allograft product to further enhance the healing potential of the otherwise dead structural allograft (Fig. 26.12).

Fixation of Neglected Calcaneal Fracture STJ Arthrodesis

After placement of the graft, distraction is released and the graft is naturally compressed. Further compression is not desired as this may crush the graft and compromise the correction.

Ideal fixation instead incorporates fully threaded large caliber cannulated screws. The fully threaded screw will aid in maintenance of the reestablished height and help prevent late stage collapse of the graft as forces increase throughout the postoperative period (Fig. 26.13).

If the situation arises that the fully threaded screw rack was requested but did not materialize (these are typically a special request item and are not typically available in most large cannulated screw sets), stable fixation can be accomplished by making sure that by using short- and long-thread–profile screws in combination, one can insure that threads are crossing the graft-host interface superiorly and inferiorly, thereby similarly preventing excess compression and collapse of the graft prior to incorporation. Alternatively two long thread profile screws can

be applied, but with one being introduced from superiorly and the other from the inferior approach for this procedure. Again, screw lengths are chosen so as to not compress and crush the graft (Fig. 26.14A and B).

RIGID VALGUS DEFORMITIES

The rigid valgus deformity may be due to end stage PTTD but, when isolated, is more commonly the result of a subtalar coalition.

Subtalar coalitions are most commonly described as involving the middle facet. In younger patients without other structural malalignment issues these may be successfully resected from a medial approach. CT scanning is highly encouraged to look at the frontal plane alignment of the calcaneus before assuming that the entire deformity is from peroneal spasm and ending up in an adverse surgical situation due to incomplete preoperative planning. (Fig. 26.15A-E show normal posterior facet but expected irregularity of the anterior and middle facets. Plain film lateral shows no clearly identifiable STJ space and finally Fig. 26.15E shows successful arthrodesis.)

Isolated subtalar fusion in cases of middle facet coalition can quite successfully accomplished from a medial approach; however, extreme care must be exercised so as to avoid excessive release of the deltoid ligament leading to subsequent medial ankle instability and ankle valgus.

Alternatively, the author prefers a traditional lateral approach in which the coalition is initially disrupted, typically with a 10 mm osteotome and then standard joint preparation with a more aggressive medially biased resection as needed based on the pre-op CT.

These cases rarely require grafting and are fixated in the traditional technique.

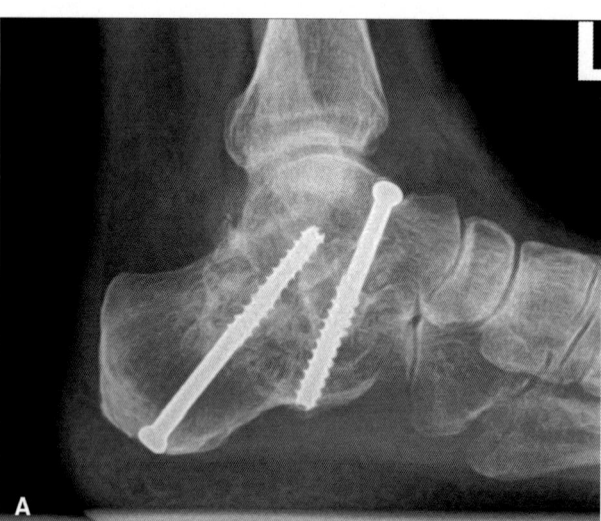

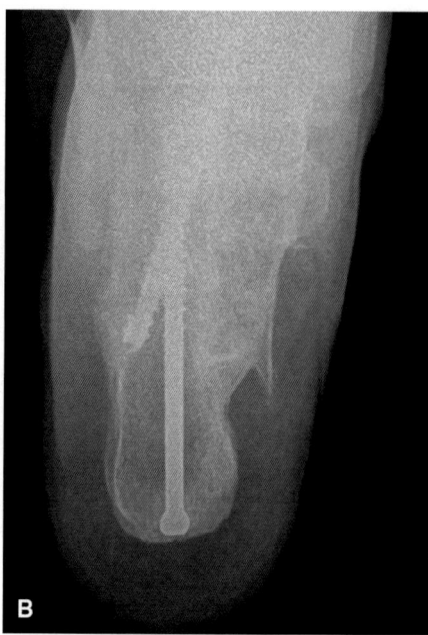

FIGURE 26.14 A. Lateral x-ray of bail out technique utilized when it was discovered that fully threaded screws were not available. Note that the threads are intentionally not completely across the fusion site, again so as to prevent over compression and collapse of the graft site. **B.** Axial calcaneal view of patient showing obliquity of the screws in addition to the intentional placement of threads across the fusion site.

PERILS and PITFALLS

- Though the overall procedure of STJ arthrodesis is relatively straightforward, there are some points that require a little extra attention to ensure success when employing this procedure.
- The most commonly seen complications of malunion and nonunion typically share a common cause, that being inadequate exposure and thus inadequate visualization of the required surfaces to resect. The revisions that the author has undertaken from St Elsewhere for nonunion and malunion/mal-position could most often be traced to inadequate surgical exposure. On reoperation, it was obvious that there were parts of the joint that had never been exposed, and if adequate exposure is not gained, then joint surface preparation cannot be achieved. For the STJ arthrodesis to be successfully executed, the surgeon must be able to have full visualization of the posterior, middle, and anterior facets. Furthermore, even if perfect preparation of the posterior facet is achieved, but the anterior and middle facets are not adequately exposed and resected, then the foot will be kicked back into valgus when the anterior and middle facets contact prematurely as they contact first when the arthrodesis sites are compressed.
- In addition to the more common frontal plane malposition issue, the surgeon should pay particular attention to the anterior/posterior translation of the talus. This issue can be entirely avoided by placing the STJ into neutral position and placing the aforementioned neutral position pin prior to starting the joint resection. The posterior displacement of the talus most commonly becomes an issue when the

surgeon is trying to neutralize the frontal plane of the heel, but disregards the cyma line and position of the lateral talar process position relative to the anterior border of the inferior surface of the posterior facet of the STJ.
- If this error occurs, though the heel is in neutral frontal plane position, it has the same effect as placing the heel in varus since the medial column is not adequately loaded and the lateral column is overloaded.
- By initially placing the foot into the STJ neutral position and drilling the neutral position pin in place just anterior to the lateral process of the talus, one can easily establish both the frontal plane position and the anterior-posterior translation neutral of the joint.
- The other most common issue that we have seen in failed STJ arthrodesis is insufficient site preparation. Though it is desirable to maintain the contour of the joint, one must make absolutely certain that the subchondral bone plate has been thoroughly disrupted to allow adequate bleeding into the site to allow for bridging between the two surfaces.

Postoperative Care and Rehabilitation

Postoperative care for the STJ arthrodesis is actually very straightforward. Patients are maintained strict NWB for about 5-6 weeks to allow for initial bridging and formation of the soft callous phase of bone healing. Fortunately, due to the axial compression on the arthrodesis site, if solid fixation is achieved and adequate bone stock is present, weight bearing can be instituted fairly early and active NWB ROM exercises instituted to restore normal ankle motion early on. The author specifically

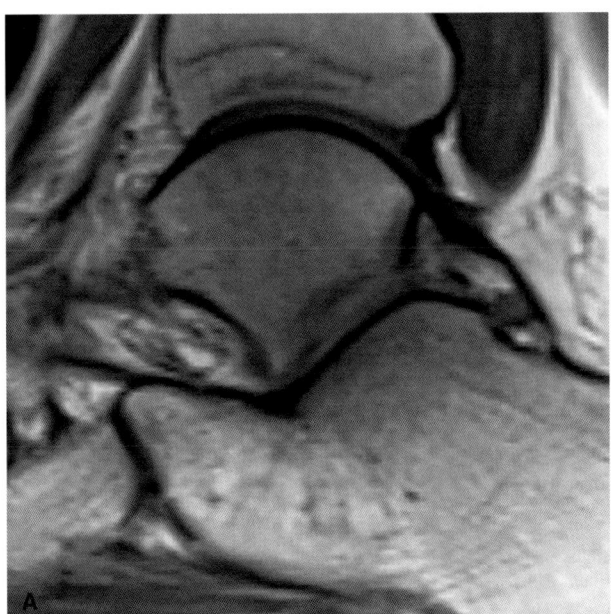

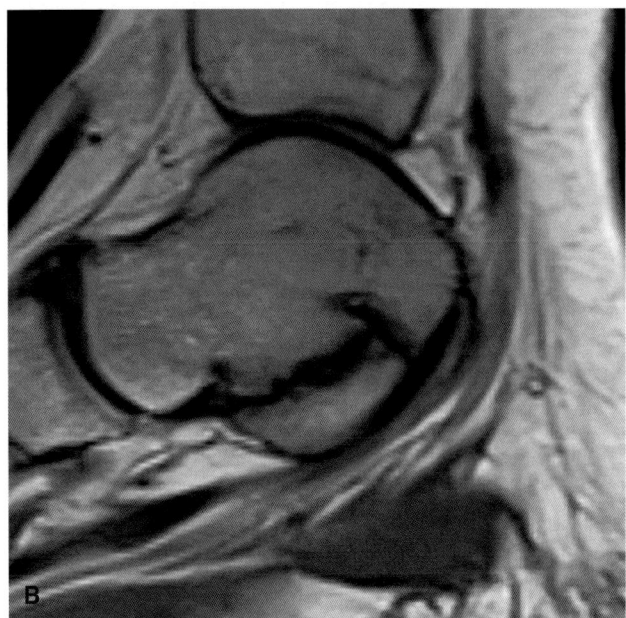

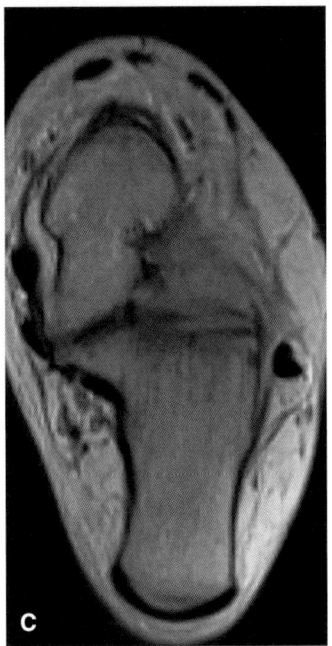

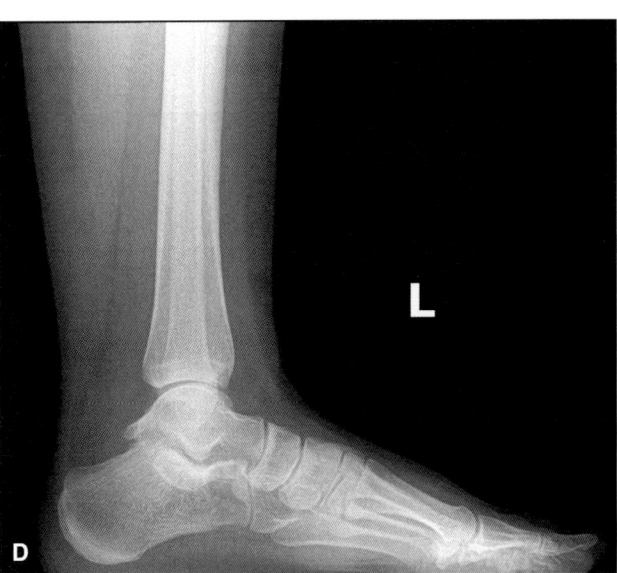

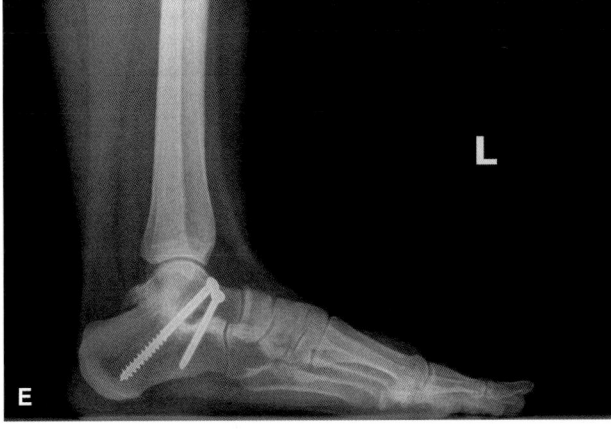

FIGURE 26.15 A. MRI showing normal posterior facet sagittal cut. **B.** Abnormal/irregular appearance of the anterior and middle facets of the STJ consistent with STJ coalition. **C.** Irregularity of the middle facet joint space and abnormal obliquity of the middle facet to the normal posterior facet. **D.** Lateral view showing relatively normal position but absence of clear joint space at the subtalar joint due to the coalition. **E.** Lateral x-ray following successful fusion of the previously painful STJ coalition.

limits early ROM to dorsiflexion/plantar flexion only so as not to prematurely stress the fusion mass.

After the initial NWB period, the patient is progressed on to progressive partial WB generally described as 50% WB the first week, 75% WB the 2nd week, and full WB as tolerated weeks 3 and 4.

Patients are also encourage to do longitudinal and cross scar massage to enhance scar mobility and aid in desensitization of any paresthesia along the incision lines

Follow-up x-rays are checked, and if good consolidation is progressing, then the patient may be returned to an athletic shoe, though activities should still be guarded until full radiographic incorporation is noted.

As a general guideline, the patient is told that full recovery will take 1 year, though many patients are more comfortable by the 3- to 4-month point than they were preoperatively.

SUMMARY

In wrapping up thoughts about the isolated subtalar fusion, the author has found it to provide a reproducible, powerful, and functional solution for posterior tibial dysfunction and other rearfoot alignment issues.

REFERENCES

1. Vulcano E, Ellington JK, Myerson MS. The spectrum of indications for subtalar joint arthrodesis. *Foot Ankle Clin.* 2015;20(2):293-310. doi: 10.1016/j.fcl.2015.02.002.
2. Didomenico LA, Butto DN. Subtalar joint arthrodesis for elective and posttraumatic foot and ankle deformities. *Clin Podiatr Med Surg.* 2017;34(3):327-338. doi: 10.1016/j.cpm.2017.02.004.
3. Roster B, Kreulen C, Giza E. Subtalar joint arthrodesis. *Foot Ankle Clin.* 2015;20(2):319-334. doi: 10.1016/j.fcl.2015.02.003.
4. Cohen BE, Johnson JE. Subtalar arthrodesis for treatment of posterior tibial tendon insufficiency. *Foot Ankle Clin.* 2001;6(1):121-128.
5. Francisco R, Chiodo CP, Wilson MG. Management of the rigid adult acquired flatfoot deformity. *Foot Ankle Clin.* 2007;12(2):317-327.
6. Carranza-Bencano A, Tejero-García S, Castillo-Blanco GD, Fernández-Torres JJ, Alegrete-Parra A. Isolated subtalar arthrodesis through minimal incision surgery. *Foot Ankle Int.* 2013;34(8):1117-1127. doi: 10.1177/1071100713483114.
7. Widnall J, Mason L, Molloy A. Medial approach to the subtalar joint. *Foot Ankle Clin.* 2018;23(3):451-460. doi: 10.1016/j.fcl.2018.04.006.
8. Hardy MA, Logan DB. Principles of arthrodesis and advances in fixation for the adult acquired flatfoot. *Clin Podiatr Med Surg.* 2007;24(4):789-813.
9. Jastifer JR, Gustafson PA, Gorman RR. The effect of subtalar arthrodesis alignment on ankle biomechanics. In: *Foot Ankle Int.* 2013;34(2):244-250. doi: 10.1177/1071100712464214.
10. Herrera-Pérez M, Andarcia-Bañuelos C, Barg A, et al. Comparison of cannulated screws versus compression staples for subtalar arthrodesis fixation. *Foot Ankle Int.* 2014;36(2):203-210. doi: 10.1177/1071100714552485.
11. Matsumoto T, Glisson RR, Reidl M, Easley ME. Compressive force with 2-screw and 3-screw subtalar joint arthrodesis with headless compression screws. *Foot Ankle Int.* 2016;37(12):1357-1363. doi: 10.1177/1071100716666275.
12. Hufner T, Geerling J, Gerich T, et al. Open reduction and internal fixation by primary subtalar arthrodesis for intraarticular calcaneal fractures. *Oper Orthop Traumatol.* 2007;19(2):155-169.
13. Poolman RW, Marti RK. Subtalar distraction bone block arthrodesis. *J Bone Joint Surg.* 2003;85(2):306.

CHAPTER 27

Talonavicular Joint Arthrodesis

Michael S. Lee, Jonathan D. Nigro, and Mary R. Brandt

DEFINITION

Fusion of the talonavicular (TN) joint can provide stability and correction for various pathologies of the foot and ankle. Typically, arthrodesis of the TN joint is considered when there is significant peritalar subluxation such as with severe pes plano valgus due to congenital deformities, the adult acquired flatfoot, neuromuscular deformities, or in cases of arthritis such as rheumatoid arthritis and posttraumatic arthritis.[1,2] In cases of isolated TN joint arthritis, such as posttraumatic arthritis, the fusion is typically an *in-situ* fusion with no deformity correction. However, in cases with significant peritalar subluxation and deformity, the "ball and socket" nature of the joint allows for triplanar correction through the fusion site.

One of the distinct advantages of the TN joint arthrodesis is it allows for significant correction of the hindfoot through one incision and one joint. This is particularly beneficial in cases of elderly patients, patients with an elevated BMI, or other compromised patients that may otherwise benefit from a double or triple arthrodesis.[3,4] Other ancillary procedures may be considered in these cases (typically to correct a forefoot varus), but ultimately an isolated TN joint fusion can provide comparable stability to a double or triple arthrodesis and delivers high patient satisfaction rates.[5]

INDICATIONS

Indications for TN joint arthrodesis may include any deformity with significant peritalar subluxation (Fig. 27.1) such as late-stage adult acquired flatfoot deformities, neuromuscular foot deformities, congenital pes valgus, or traumatic midfoot injuries. Additionally, isolated arthritis of the TN joint due to rheumatoid arthritis, posttraumatic arthritis (Fig. 27.2), navicular avascular necrosis, navicular stress fracture, and talar head or navicular fractures may serve as indications for isolated TN joint fusions.

In cases involving peritalar subluxation, particularly in cases of the adult acquired flatfoot, the TN fusion is selected in part because of the predictability and stability that it provides. The tradeoff is that it compromises significant range of motion in the hindfoot, specifically through the subtalar joint (STJ).[6] Because of this restriction in hindfoot motion, it is typically employed in later-stage deformities when a double or triple arthrodesis may also be indicated, but there are one or more relative contraindications to a more extensive procedure such

as elevated BMI or age. The TN joint arthrodesis provides an adequate alternative to these more involved procedures when needed.

ANATOMIC CONSIDERATIONS

The TN joint consists of the convex talar head fitting into the concave posterior aspect of the navicular to act as a multiaxial, functional, ball and socket joint.[7,8] The head of the talus is supported by the spring (plantar TN) ligament while the anterior deltoid ligament resides medially and the bifurcate ligament laterally. The TN joint is part of a joint complex that includes both the subtalar and calcaneocuboid joints, and it plays an important role in the motion of this triple joint complex. A TN arthrodesis will greatly reduce the motion of these associated joints, whereas significantly more motion remains after a fusion of the subtalar or calcaneocuboid joints on an isolated basis.[6] Fusion of the TN joint also limits the excursion of the posterior tibial tendon.[6]

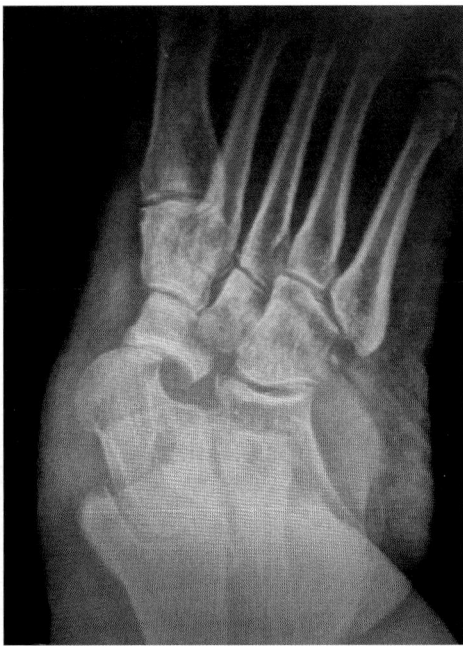

FIGURE 27.1 AP radiograph demonstrating peritalar subluxation.

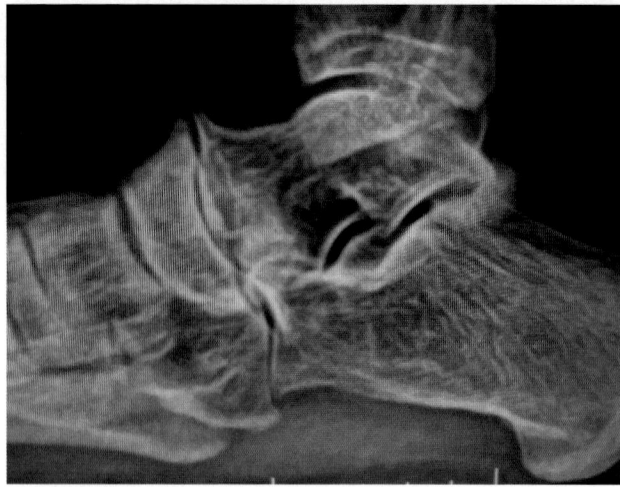

FIGURE 27.2 Post-traumatic arthritis after subtalar dislocation 10 years prior.

PHYSICAL EXAMINATION

Physical examination or evaluation of an individual requiring a TN joint arthrodesis varies based on the underlying etiology or condition causing the pain, deformity, or instability at the TN joint. For example, an individual with isolated arthritis at the TN joint may only have pain directly over the TN joint. There may be no collapse of the medial arch and no peritalar subluxation. Conversely, individuals with significant peritalar subluxation due to an adult acquired flatfoot may have little to no pain directly over their TN joint. Rather they have pain over the sinus tarsi, medially along the posterior tibial tendon, or medial arch pain.

It is always important to assess and evaluate the reducibility of the deformity. Does the STJ reduce into a neutral position?

With the STJ reduced, is there a forefoot varus or supinatus present. Assess the significance of the hindfoot valgus and forefoot abduction. One should also carefully evaluate the posterior muscle group and the significance of the equinus deformity.

IMAGING

Plain radiographs of the foot and ankle typically suffice for cases in which the surgeon is considering TN joint arthrodesis. Isolated arthritis is very easily seen and evaluated on standard radiographs. For cases involving significant deformity such as the late stage adult-acquired deformity, the degree of peritalar subluxation can easily be seen on a standard AP (DP) radiograph of the foot. The talo-first metatarsal angle on the AP and the lateral (Meary's angle) will provide details as to the severity of the deformity (Fig. 27.3). Ankle x-rays should be obtained in severe flatfoot cases to rule-out any significant ankle valgus deformity (Fig. 27.4).

Advanced imaging such as CT, MRI, or US rarely provide significant and useful information that dictate course of care when considering a TN fusion. CT may be utilized to determine the significance of the isolated arthritis or to evaluation deformity. MRI may be used early to evaluate the posterior tibial tendon and spring ligament in the adult acquired flatfoot. Additionally, in cases of navicular AVN or navicular stress fracture, MRI may be utilized to determine and evaluate navicular viability.

TREATMENT

Nonoperative treatment of a subluxated or arthritic TN joint is often dictated by the underlying etiology of the deformity. Nonetheless, consideration for various orthotics such as a UCBL or an ankle foot orthoses (AFO) may provide some relief for the patient. In cases of isolated TN arthrosis, steroid

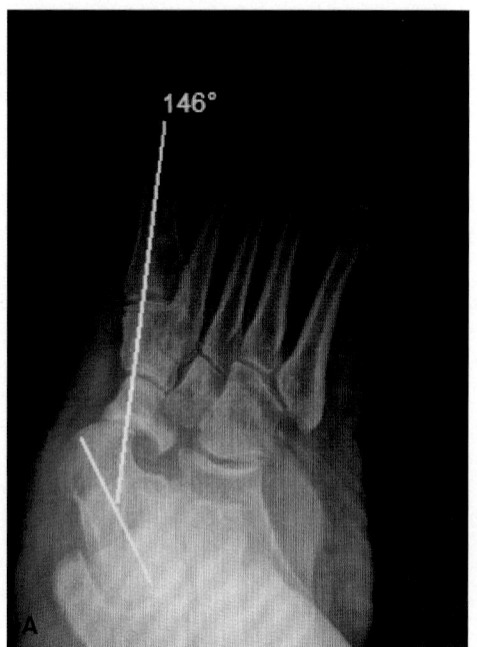

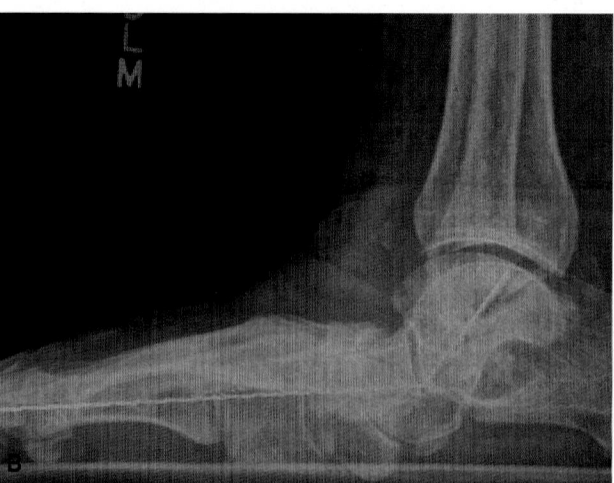

FIGURE 27.3 AP **(A)** and lateral radiographs **(B)** of a severe flatfoot demonstrating increased talo-first-metatarsal angles.

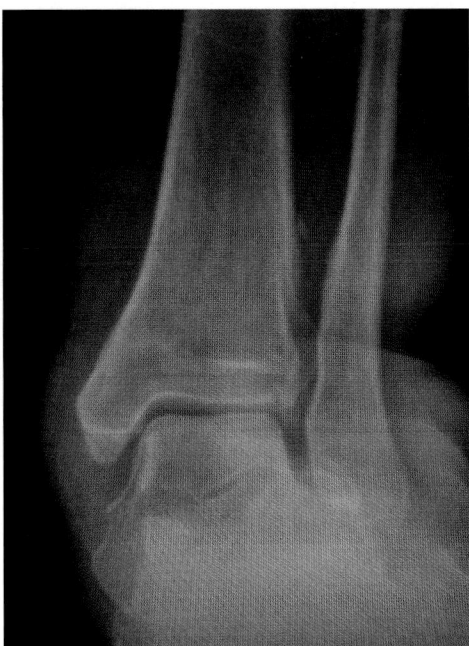

FIGURE 27.4 Ankle valgus in a sever flatfoot deformity.

injections may temporize the symptoms allowing the patient to put off surgical intervention for some time in the future.

AUTHOR'S PREFERRED SURGICAL TECHNIQUE

The procedure is typically performed under thigh tourniquet control, although this is not necessary, and it based on surgeon preference. The patient is placed in the supine position, preferably with slight external rotation of the operative extremity. In cases of adult acquired flatfoot, the posterior muscle group lengthening is completed first and is usually a medial approach gastroc recession and on rare occasions a tendo-Achilles lengthening. In isolated arthritis cases, there typically is no equinus deformity to address.

The incision is made medial to the anterior tibial tendon, extending from the ankle joint line distally to the naviculocuneiform (NC) joint. Dissection is carried deep and care should be taken to ligate any tributaries from the medial marginal vein. The dissection is carried down onto the talar neck and then exposing the TN joint. The joint and capsular tissues are exposed and elevated medially to the posterior tibial tendon and then dorsally and laterally across the TN joint. If dorsal spurring/exostosis formation is present, care should be taken while elevating the dorsal soft tissues as the deep peroneal nerve and dorsalis pedis artery are at risk.

Once the joint is properly exposed, a joint distraction device is employed to distract the TN joint to allow for proper visualization of the talar head and the navicular laterally and plantarly (Fig. 27.5). Joint preparation is carried out using the curettage method. Preparing the talar head first, including the medial and plantar aspect is critical as this is the primary fusion site once the deformity is fully corrected. By resecting the talar head, first you will gain even better visualization of the lateral extend of the navicular. Curettage of the navicular is carried out in a similar fashion. A high-speed burr is then utilized to

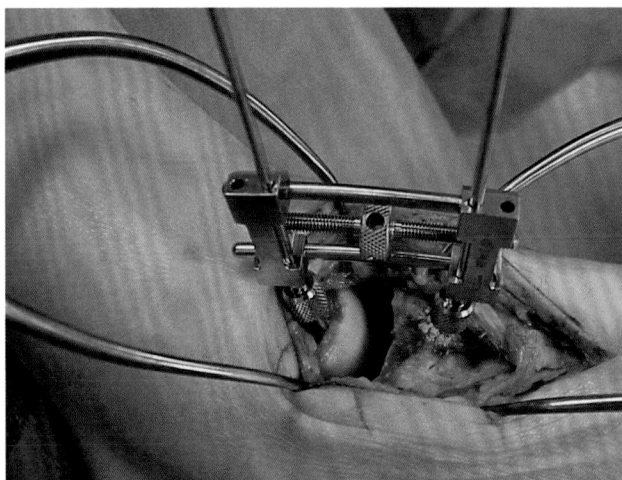

FIGURE 27.5 Joint distraction of the TN joint allowing better visualization both plantarly and laterally.

resect the subchondral plate which is always thicker and harder on the navicular. Care should be taken on the talar head as this bone is always very soft.

After joint preparation has been completed and all debris has been removed or flushed from the surgical field, the deformity is reduced (Fig. 27.6). Evoking the windlass mechanism by dorsiflexing the hallux, while adducting the forefoot against a thumb on the talar head allows the peritalar subluxation to be corrected and reduced. An anteroposterior view of the foot will help confirm that the talar head has been covered and reduced appropriately. Temporary fixation across the joint will allow visualization on the lateral view as well to confirm reduction of the deformity and proper alignment.

Fixation has traditionally been performed using 2 or 3 large caliber screw fixation (Fig. 27.7). Typically, 1 or 2 screws are placed from the medial navicular tuberosity up into the talar head, neck, and dome is utilized. Fixation of the lateral half of the TN joint is completed with either a percutaneous screw from the dorsal foot or preferably from the medial talar neck into the later navicular body (Fig. 27.8). More recently, anatomic plates with compression ramps or jigs have been

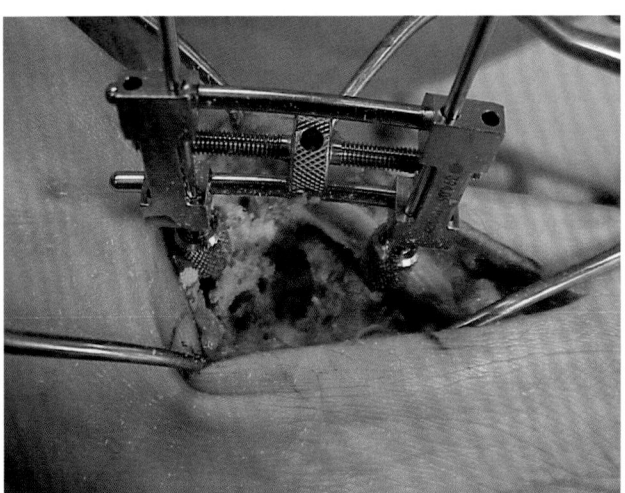

FIGURE 27.6 Joint preparation of the TN joint.

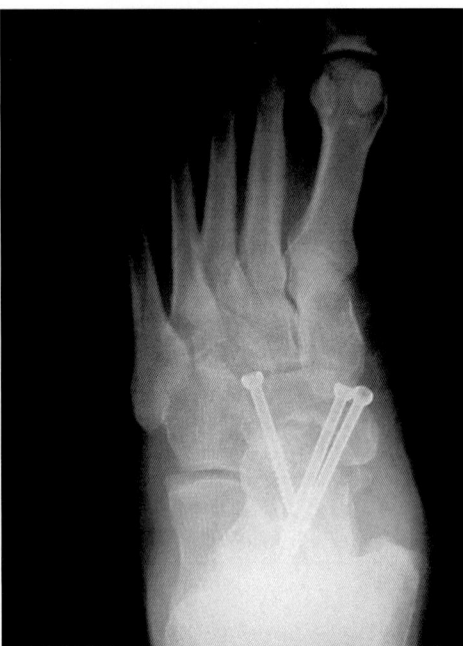

FIGURE 27.7 Three-screw fixation of the TN joint with a laterally placed percutaneous screw.

developed to provide compression and locking plate stability (Fig. 27.9). Fixation is to surgeons preference. Fluoroscopic imaging should be utilized to confirm that fixation is not violating the STJ, or the ankle joint, including the medial and lateral gutters.

A layered closure is completed according to surgeon preference. Splinting with the ankle in a neutral position is completed. Drains are not typically needed for a TN fusion.

TNJ ARTHRODESIS PEARLS

Only in *very* rare occasions should planar resection be used in arthrodesis of the TN joint. For typical fusions involving peritalar subluxation such as a severe flatfoot or in isolated arthritis of the TN joint, planar resection will typically result in significant shortening, and positioning is extremely difficult. Curettage provides a much better alternative for joint preparation. It results in significantly less shortening at the fusion site and results in a "ball and socket" that allows correction in three planes.

During joint preparation, remember that the talar head is typically very soft. Even during curettage, the subchondral plate may be violated. Care should be taken not to be too overly aggressive on the talar head, especially medially where there has been little to no articulation resulting in further softening of the subchondral bone. Using a curved rongeur in this area will often allow the surgeon to remove the cartilage and subchondral plate very efficiently.

A self-retaining distractor is critical for a TN joint arthrodesis for visualization. **A tip is to place the distractor, so the pins** are just above the posterior tibial tendon on the navicular and in line on the talar neck. This positions the distractor below your line of site and affords the surgeon plenty of working space above the distractor. A distractor is critical to visualize the lateral half of the TN joint so that this portion of the joint can be thoroughly prepped.

Finally, a tip on fixation. It is critical to achieve some compression or at least stabilization of the lateral half of the joint. This can be achieved with a percutaneous screw from the navicular into the talar neck, but this is an awkward and somewhat dangerous throw. With a little extra exposure along the medial talar neck, the same screw can be placed from proximal medial into the lateral half of the navicular. This is at a much more appropriate angle for compression and does not put the dorsal cutaneous nerves at risk. A recent alternative for fixation are the new anatomic plates, some of which provide significant compression using various compression tools while provide stability throughout the joint (including laterally).

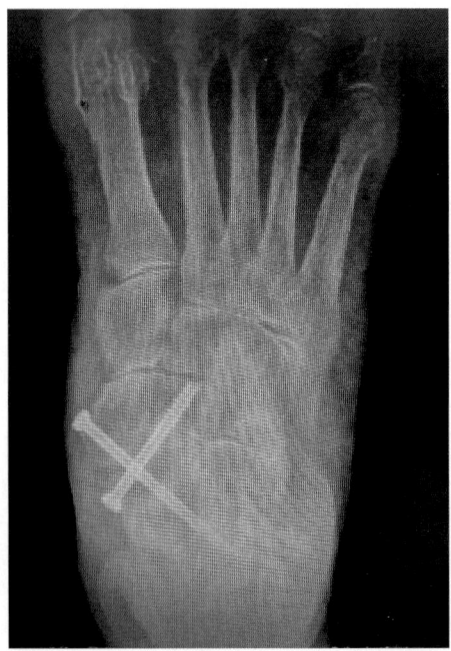

FIGURE 27.8 Fixation of the lateral half of the TN joint using a medial to lateral screw from the talar neck.

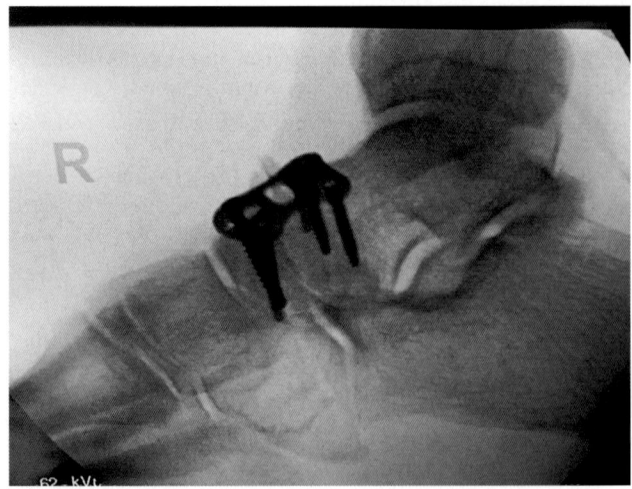

FIGURE 27.9 Anatomic compression/locking plate for TN joint arthrodesis.

POSTOPERATIVE CARE

Immediately postoperatively the patient is splinted and instructed to remain non–weight bearing on the operative extremity. The patient returns between 8 and 10 days for their first postoperative check at which time the dressing is removed, staples/stitches are removed, and the patient is placed in a below-the-knee cast at 90 degrees. They continue non–weight bearing for 5 more weeks. Typically, this is achieved with crutches and/or a knee scooter. At 6 weeks post-op, the cast is removed and x-rays are obtained which determine the progression to weight bearing from there.

Typically, the patient is placed in a CAM boot and allowed partial weight bearing which progresses to full weight in the boot over the course of the next 4 to 5 weeks. The patient is allowed to remove the boot to sleep, bathe, and begin gentle range of motion. At 10 to 11 weeks if x-rays confirm adequate bony consolidation at the fusion site, the patient is progressed from the CAM boot to a light-weight figure-of-eight ankle brace.

Physical therapy is routinely ordered to assist the patient with gait and ankle range of motion. Activities and shoe gear are progressed slowly and to tolerance. Follow-up x-rays are obtained at 4 and 6 months.

COMPLICATIONS

Nonunion and malunion are the most common complications of a TN joint arthrodesis. Nonunion is typically the result of poor joint visualization and improper joint preparation of the lateral and plantar portions of the TN joint. Distraction of the joint greatly improves visualization and therefore resection. Malalignment is more challenging and care should be taken at the time of surgery to ensure that proper alignment is achieved. The talar head should be "recovered" and on the lateral view with simulated weight bearing or loading of the foot the talo-first metatarsal ankle should be near zero (parallel). Malalignment further restricts motion and typically results in STJ arthritis and pain which often leads to triple arthrodesis. With any arthrodesis procedure, there is a risk of developing arthritis in joints proximal and distal to the surgical site due to increased stresses placed on them from the fused joint. Arthrosis of the STJ is certain with malalignment of the TN fusion.[9] When the fusion is performed, it is important to maintain neutral position in the forefoot and hindfoot (Fig. 27.10).

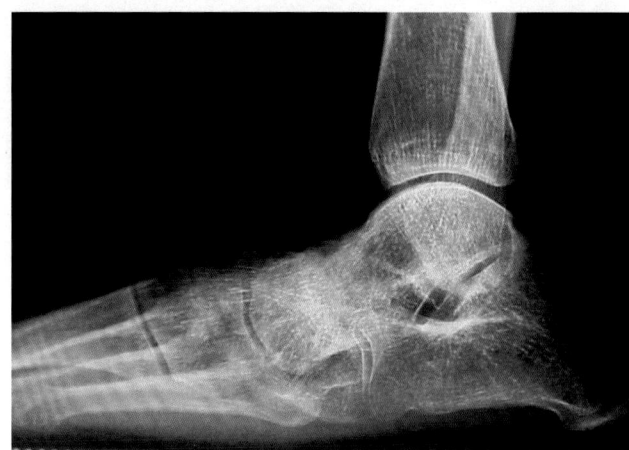

FIGURE 27.10 Malaligned TN fusion.

SUMMARY

The TN joint fusion is a proven and viable option for patients with isolated TN joint arthritis, adult acquired flat foot deformity, rheumatoid arthritis, and other deformities causing peritalar subluxation. While the procedure greatly limits STJ frontal plane motion, it has been shown to be effective in providing hindfoot stability and for deformity correction. The fusion remains a viable alternative to the triple or double arthrodesis in patients that are in some way compromised, such as the older patients and elevated BMIs. Like all fusions, appropriate joint preparation, anatomic position, and stable fixation are paramount to achieving a solid fusion and successful outcome.

REFERENCES

1. Chen CH, Huang PJ, Chen TB, et al. Isolated talonavicular arthrodesis for talonavicular arthritis. *Foot Ankle Int.* 2001;22:633-636.
2. Mothershed RA, Stapp MD, Smith TF. Talonavicular arthrodesis for correction of posterior tibial tendon dysfunction. *Clin Podiatr Med Surg.* 1999;16:501-526.
3. Weinraub GM, Schuberth JM, Lee MS, et al. Isolated medial incisional approach to subtalar and talonavicular arthrodesis. *J Foot Ankle Surg.* 2010;49:326-330.
4. Lee MS, Maker JM. Revision of the failed flatfoot surgery. *Clin Podiatr Med Surg.* 2009;26(1):47-58.
5. Ma S, Jin D. Isolated talonavicular arthrodesis. *Foot Ankle Int.* 2016;37(8):905-908.
6. Astion DJ, et al. Motion of the hindfoot after simulated arthrodesis. *J Bone Joint Surg Am.* 1997;79(2):241-246.
7. Barkatali BM, Manthravadi S. Isolated talonavicular arthrodesis for talonavicular arthritis: a follow-up study. *J Foot Ankle Surg.* 2014;53:8-11.
8. Weinraub GM, Matt HA. Isolated talonavicular arthrodesis for adult onset flatfoot deformity/posterior tibial tendon dysfunction. *Clin Podiatr Med Surg.* 2007;24:745-752.
9. Camasta CA, Menke CRD, Hall PB. A review of 51 talonavicular joint arthrodeses for flexible pes valgus deformity. *J Foot Ankle Surg.* 2010;49(2):113-118.

CHAPTER 28

Interdigital Neuroma

Thanh L. Dinh, Amish K. Dudeja, and John A. Martucci

INTRODUCTION

Dr. Thomas Morton described a condition he coined "metatarsalgia" in the late 1800s that has given rise to what the medical community now recognizes as Morton neuroma.[1] Subsequently, Dr. Morton described a generalized metatarsalgia about the fourth metatarsal phalangeal joint that was characterized by pain with shoe wear and direct palpation of the fourth metatarsal phalangeal joint. Additionally, he observed that these symptoms typically presented after an injury to the forefoot.

Yet, it would be Dr. Filippo Divining, anatomist at University of Pisa in Italy, who would first describe a "neural gangliar swelling of the foot sole" in 1835.[2] Then, in 1845, Dr. Lewis Durlacher, a surgeon-chiropodist in London, wrote a "Treatise," which more accurately describes neuromas of the foot that we know today in detail. He noted that a "neuralgic affection occasionally attacks the plantar nerve on the sole of the foot, between the third and fourth metatarsal bones…."[3]

The treatment was aggressive initially, with Dr. Morton describing surgical excision of the entire fourth metatarsal phalangeal joint and its surrounding nervous tissue to cure this metatarsalgia and neuralgia. Focusing on nonsurgical interventions, Dr. Durlacher found that simple lateral compression via a strip of plaster protected the nerve from potential pinching or compression between metatarsals during ambulation, successfully reducing the pain symptoms.[3]

ANATOMIC FEATURES

As both Drs. Morton and Durlacher described, neuromas are most commonly noted to occur on the lateral side of the foot with the third interspace traditionally the location of interdigital neuromas. While the third interspace is a regular culprit, a study by Valero et al. found that the presence of having multiple neuromas at one time was as high as 65.2%.[4] In the 182 cases of diagnosed interdigital neuromas, with isolated neuromas, the third interspace was found to be the most common. When multiple locations in a foot were identified, 100% of the cases described revealed the presence of a third interspace neuroma. Several other diagnostic studies also support the third interspace as the dominant location of interdigital neuromas.[5-8] The paper details nine other studies by groups with all but one group finding that the third

interspace is the most common site for an interdigital neuroma of the foot.

Predilection for the third interspace is thought to be due to a communicating branch between branches of the medial and lateral plantar nerves. A communication between the common digital branch of the medial plantar nerve extending into the third web space and the common digital branch of the lateral plantar nerve extending into the fourth is commonly present, leading to a larger structure to be irritated. However, the anastomosis is variable with regard to the depth, direction, and shape of the communication. Several anatomic studies have demonstrated variability in the superficial or deep location of the anastomosis to the short flexor tendons of the toes, with direction described as moving anteromedially vs laterally and observed as a single bundle or Y-shaped in configuration.[9-11]

Generally, from the dorsal aspect of the foot, the plantar nerve passes deep to the deep transverse intermetatarsal ligament and interossei muscles at the level of the metatarsal heads. Within this deep interspace, they sit in bundles of fat, atop the plantar fascia, and remain separated from neighboring interspaces by vertical fibers arising from the plantar fascia to the deep transverse metatarsal ligament on either side and the plantar plate above (Fig. 28.1). Furthermore, running alongside these neurovascular compartments are the long flexor tendons and the lumbrical muscles. Any enlargement of a neural structure is subject to compression by these many surrounding structures, with cadaveric studies supporting the development of neuromas starting at the distal portion of the bifurcation in the digital nerves and expanding proximally.[12]

Histologically, a neuroma exhibits fibrosis and thickening of the epineurium and perineurium, the outer layers of connective tissue encasing a complete nerve and its fascicles, respectively, as well as degeneration of the nerve but *not* a neoplastic process or proliferation of nerve cells. Ironically the suffix "-oma" generally denotes a tumor or abnormal growth or proliferation, which a neuroma is not. This concept is supported by a study that biopsied myomectomies from patients with pain thought to be due to neuromas with biopsies of plantar nerves from the same locations in autopsy specimens that did not have neuroma pain. The investigators found no clear differences histologically, with the only difference being that nerves excised due to pain were noticeably more swollen than those in the pain-free group.[13]

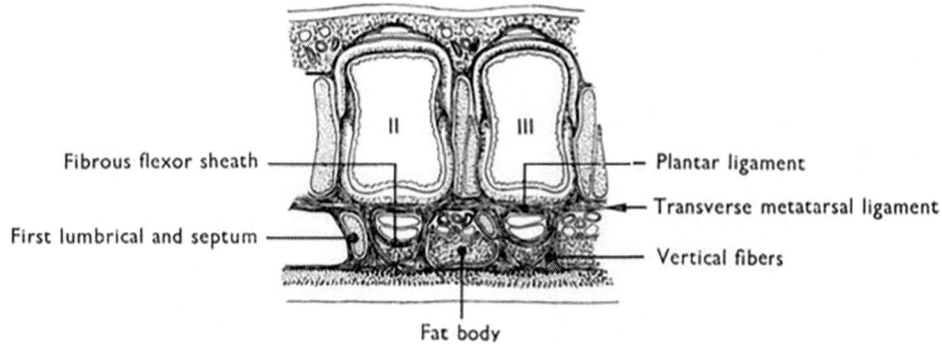

FIGURE 28.1 Neurovascular bundles within compartments (Bojsen-Moller). (From Bojsen-Moller F, Flagstad KE. Plantar aponeurosis and internal architecture of the ball of the foot. *J Anat.* 1976;121(Pt 3):599-611.)

CLINICAL PRESENTATION AND PHYSICAL EXAMINATION

The majority of patients presenting with interdigital neuromas are females between the age of 40 and 60 years.[4] It is postulated that women are predisposed to developing neuromas due to shoegear. Prolonged wearing of shoes with narrow toeboxes or high heels may aggravate the pathology by compressing, tethering, and restricting the intermetatarsal spaces.[14] Various anatomical and mechanical explanations have also been proposed to explain the development of an interdigital neuroma including ischemia, over pronation, trauma, ankle equinus, entrapment, and bursitis.[14,15] It is believed that all of these mechanisms result in increased pressure on the nerve resulting in the entrapment and subsequent pain symptoms. Additionally, as Dr. Morton observed, the fifth metatarsal phalangeal joint is observed to have increased mobility compared to the fourth metatarsal phalangeal joint, including the nerves, and perhaps predisposing to the development of mechanical pressure and pain in this area.[1]

Clinical presentation of an interdigital neuroma often includes descriptions of burning or shooting pain, numbness, and tingling that may invade the third and fourth digits or feeling as though one is walking on a pebble or rolled-up sock. These sensations can initially present following trauma and tight shoe wear or following activities with increased pressure to the forefoot. Patient will often complain of pain that is alleviated with removing the shoes or with rest from inciting activities.[16]

Common physical examination maneuvers include medial and lateral compression of the metatarsals with generation of a click upon palpation of a neuroma, or a "Mulder click." Originally described by Dr. J.D. Mulder, a Dutch surgeon and podiatrist, the technique involves simultaneous medial and lateral compression of the metatarsals about the forefoot with one hand along with a pinching pressure in the interspace from dorsal to plantar with the opposite hand. By pinching the area and restricting the neuroma's excursion dorsally or plantarly during this maneuver, a small mass may be felt to "click" or "pop" in the intermetatarsal space This maneuver may or may not produce any pain for the patient.[17]

Another technique described in the literature explicitly serves to attempt eliciting pain rather than a "click" in the interspace. This technique, known as the finger squeeze or "web space tenderness" test, involves using the sides of one's fingers to deeply compress the intermetatarsal area. To determine whether one has proper positioning and pressure, the digits neighboring the interspace should splay (Fig. 28.2). Mahadevan et al. suggest that it is a sensitive test for a neuroma at 96% compared to a Mulder click alone at 62%.[18]

In another study of various clinical maneuvers and tests for interdigital neuromas, Owens et al. note aptly that "pathognomonic diagnostic clinical tests for Morton neuroma do not exist." An accurate clinical diagnosis is best supported by an extensive patient history along with a combination of positive maneuvers such as a Mulder click and web space tenderness test.[18,19] Yet, when uncertain in clinical diagnosis or in order to explore other differentials, a clinician may utilize imaging modalities such as radiographs, ultrasound, and magnetic resonance imaging (MRI).

IMAGING AND DIAGNOSTIC STUDIES

While a history of the symptoms and physical examination of the foot is typically sufficient to diagnose interdigital neuromas, imaging modalities may be useful in elucidating a patient's etiology for pain and eliminating other possible differential diagnoses. Traditionally, plain film radiographs may be ordered first to explore for any bone pathologies such as avascular necrosis, fractures, arthropathies, to examine for foreign bodies, and to evaluate metatarsal declination and general foot structure. A significant space-occupying lesion such as a large neuroma may even produce splaying, or deviation in opposite directions in the transverse plane, of neighboring digits notable on weight-bearing films, also known clinically as "Sullivan Sign."[20] This splaying may be due to an enlargement of the intermetatarsal bursa, neuroma, or both, that put pressure on the base of the proximal phalanx.

Yet, in a study of 48 patients with neuromas, while there was no significant increase in digital divergence noticed on radiographs, there were increased intermetatarsal angles in the neuroma group compared to 100 asymptomatic controls. A more recent study by comparing 69 patients with neuromas to 32 controls found no relationship between the presence of a neuroma and metatarsal length, intermetatarsal angles, or digital divergence angles.[13]

Given that an interdigital neuroma is primarily an enlargement with swelling of a nerve in a small space, soft tissue studies are likely more helpful to rule in the diagnosis. After initial

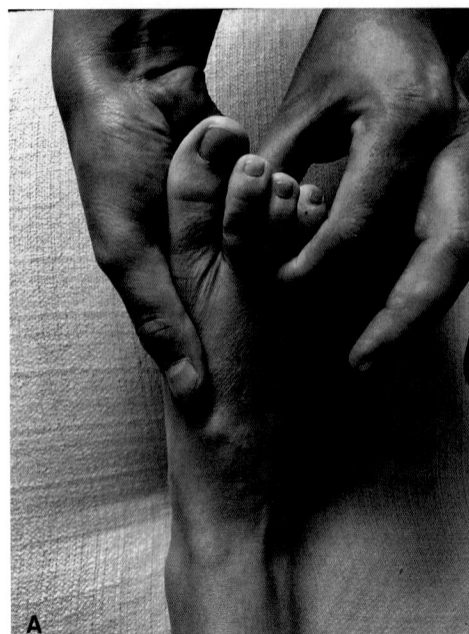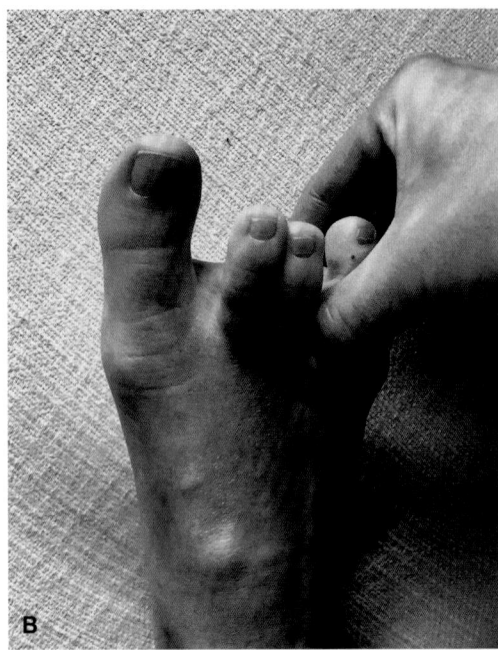

FIGURE 28.2 Clinical maneuvers for diagnosis of a neuroma. **A.** The squeeze test is performed with one hand on the medial and lateral aspects of the forefoot and another palpating the interspace with the suspected neuroma. A positive test elicits a click, or "Mulder click." **B.** The web space tenderness test is performed by using the sides of one's fingers to deeply compress the intermetatarsal area. One should see splaying of digits lining the space compressed. A positive test is when pain or the sensation of discomfort the patient experiences with ambulation is reproduced.

radiographs, ultrasound may serve as a cost-effective and readily available imaging tool for further evaluation. While allowing for visualization of the area of pain in real time and locating the enlarged nerve, this study is highly operator dependent. When performed correctly, ultrasound of a neuroma will exhibit an ovoid, hypoechoic mass consistent with thickened or enlarged nerve tissue.[21]

Alternatively, MRI also presents as highly sensitive modality for visualization of an interdigital neuroma. MRI studies often demonstrate a neuroma as an ovoid or dumbbell-shaped mass that is low signal on T1- and T2-weighted sequences due to a fibrous thickening, rather than fluid-filled content. By contrast, other differential pathologies such as schwannomas (a nerve sheath tumor) and large intermetatarsal bursae will be hyperintense on T2-weighted images.[9] While more expensive and not readily accessible in the office, MRI for interdigital neuromas is not operator dependent and with concomitant use of intravenous contrast and positioning, visualization of the lesion may be enhanced (Fig. 28.3).

While a neuroma may be visualized on all MR sequences, contrast administration for enhancement with fat suppression has been shown to provide the best visualization of a neuroma as small as 3 mm in the coronal plane.[22] It is important to remember that the normal diameter of a digital nerve is about 1-2 mm in diameter.[23] In a study of 70 asymptomatic patients, the investigators found 24 neuromas with sizes varying from 3 to 7 mm in the coronal plane using MRI. It was concluded the presence of a neuroma was established with clinical symptoms and a nerve diameter of 5 mm or more on MRI. Of note, fluid collections in the intermetatarsal bursae were frequently encountered with 67% of asymptomatic subjects demonstrating physiologic fluid collections.[24]

Additionally, patient positioning in the MRI tube can also alter neuroma visualization.[25] In a study of 20 patients, interdigital neuromas appeared to be adequately visualized in the supine and weight-bearing images. However, it was noted that when patients were positioned prone with the foot in a plantar flexed position, the diameter of the lesion was larger compared to a smaller in diameter in the other patient positions. It was also noted that the neuroma appeared to migrate distally along the metatarsal in the supine and weight-bearing positions. As a result, the authors concluded that a prone patient position may enhance the detection of an interdigital neuroma.

Diagnostic sensitivities between ultrasound and MRI have been shown to be comparable with a meta-analysis of 14 studies demonstrating that ultrasound yielded a sensitivity of 91% and MRI 90% with no significant differences between the two.[26] In a systematic review of 12 studies, the authors also noted that the diagnostic sensitivities of ultrasound compared to MRI were comparable with a sensitivity of 90% and 93%, respectively.[27] However, they also demonstrated that ultrasound yielded a specificity of 88% compared to 68% specificity with MRI. With modest differences, US had higher positive and lower negative likelihood ratios for the detection of interdigital neuromas compared to MRI only (2.77 vs 1.89; 0.16 vs 0.19, respectively). Improved specificity may be due to ultrasound's ability to distinguish between nerve and adjacent vasculature.[21,28]

Both ultrasound and MRI serve as valuable diagnostic imaging modalities. With training, practice, and access to an ultrasound machine, a practitioner can diagnose neuromas in the office with more sensitivity and specificity than MRI. However, MRI still provides reliable visualization of nerve lesions and can help evaluate other suspected pathology in the general anatomical area. Aside from the modalities discussed above, a thorough

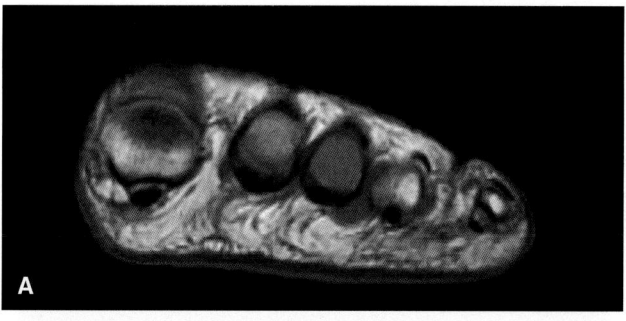
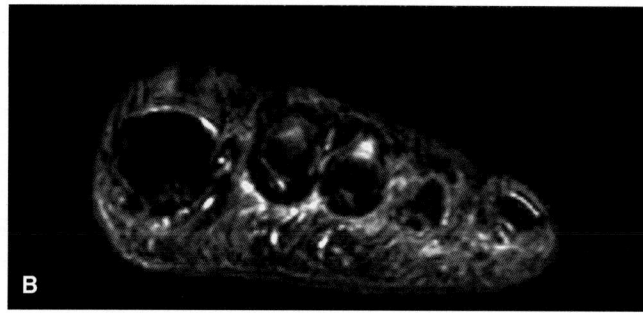
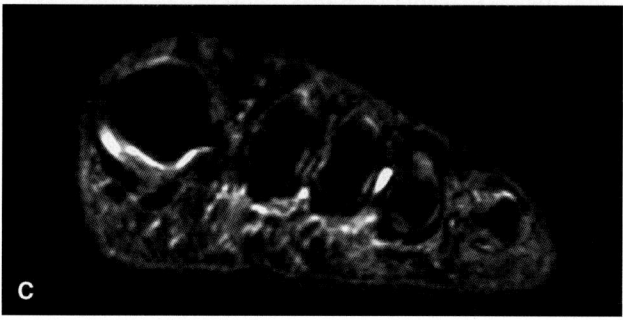

FIGURE 28.3 MRI for interdigital neuroma. **A.** Coronal T1 image showing a classic dumbbell-shaped hypointense mass between the third and fourth metatarsal heads. **B.** Coronal STIR image showing hyperintense mass between third and fourth metatarsal heads. **C.** Coronal STIR image showing a focal hyperintensity between third and fourth metatarsals representing intermetatarsal bursitis.

patient history combined with elicitation of a Mulder click with web space tenderness on physical examination remains a highly sensitive tool for diagnosis of an interdigital neuroma.[29]

TREATMENT

NONSURGICAL TREATMENT

Nonsurgical interventions for interdigital neuromas can be classified into invasive (skin penetration) and noninvasive treatments. Noninvasive measures include footwear modification, foot manipulation, orthoses, and extracorporeal shockwave therapy (ESWT).[30-34]

Manipulation and mobilization of the foot through distraction of the metatarsophalangeal joint has been shown to be effective in reducing pain symptoms in patients with interdigital neuromas. In one case series, pain reduction was demonstrated to occur by 5.5 weeks following a course of manipulation.[30] In a randomized control trial, pain reduction was reduced in the manipulation group compared to the control group at 6 weeks.[35]

Modification of footwear with a larger toe box, decreased heel height, and metatarsal head padding is thought to reduce the mechanical pressure implicated in irritating the interdigital neuroma. The use of a varus or valgus wedge insert in shoes to supinate or pronate the foot demonstrated no effect at the 12-month follow-up.[32] Footwear modification with metatarsal off-loading has also demonstrated effectiveness with a comparison study showing 63% of patients with symptom improvement. However, this intervention was inferior compared to corticosteroid injections, which was effective in 82%.[34]

ESWT is theorized to stimulate healing through the use of microsonic energy pulses. In a randomized controlled trial, patients treated with ESWT demonstrated improved pain symptoms compared to patients treated with sham ESWT.[31] However, a secondary endpoint, neuroma size, was unchanged after ESWT treatment.

Nonsurgical treatments typically consist of a combination of treatment modalities, and an algorithm for progression of each therapy has been studied to evaluate the efficacy of a staged treatment protocol.[33] In a study of 115 patients, treatment started with footwear modifications and metatarsal padding. This was followed by injection therapy and surgical intervention in the event of continued symptoms. Overall, 97 (85%) patients were pleased with the results following the staged protocol, and with 24 (21%) patients ultimately requiring surgical intervention.

INVASIVE NONSURGICAL TREATMENTS

Injection therapy provides symptomatic relief in most patients when footwear modification fails and can be performed with a number of agents. Several studies have described the risks and benefits of the particular agents as well as evaluating the efficacy of blinded vs ultrasound-guided techniques.

Corticosteroid Injections

Among the numerous invasive nonsurgical treatments for interdigital neuromas, corticosteroid injection is considered a first-line treatment, due to improved outcomes compared to shoegear modification.[34] Injection of corticosteroid is hypothesized to induce atrophy of the tissue in the interdigital space, resulting in decompression of the neuroma and inflammation reduction.[36] In one study, a single corticosteroid injection provided complete satisfaction 9 months after treatment in 38% of patients with an interdigital neuroma and 28% were satisfied with minor reservations.[37]

Despite its role as a first-line treatment, studies published to date have demonstrated unpredictable results with highly variable patient satisfaction and no clear evidence to the effectiveness of these injections.[33,34,38,39] In fact, studies examining the effectiveness of corticosteroid injections with local anesthetic compared to local anesthetic have been equivocal.

In one prospective randomized, controlled, blinded study of 131 patients with ultrasound confirmed, interdigital neuromas were treated with a single injection of corticosteroid with anesthetic or anesthetic alone.[38] At both the 1- and 3-month follow-up visits, the corticosteroid plus local anesthetic injection–treated groups were found to have better outcomes compared to the local anesthetic injection group. Furthermore, fewer patients in the corticosteroid group than the local anesthetic alone group reported that their foot was not better at all at 3 months (32% vs 52%).

Conversely, a prospective, double-blinded, randomized, placebo-controlled trial of 41 patients clinically diagnosed with an interdigital neuroma did not find that the addition of corticosteroid provided superior results compared to an injection of local anesthetic alone.[40] Instead, there were no significant differences in the pain and function scores between both injection groups at the 3- and 6-month follow-up visits. As a result, the researchers concluded that injection of a corticosteroid plus a local anesthetic was not superior to a local anesthetic alone.

Regardless of the decision to inject local anesthetic or local anesthetic with corticosteroid, studies agree that pain relief is only temporary after injection therapy and researchers have attempted to qualify what parameters influence the effectiveness of injection therapy for interdigital neuromas. Parameters such as neuroma size and patient age have been postulated as risks for predictors of poor response to treatment with corticosteroid injection.

In a study of 35 patients treated with a single corticosteroid with local anesthetic injection under ultrasound guidance, investigators found that the size of the neuroma measured on ultrasound did not correlate with pain relief.[37] In that study, 31% of the neuromas did not respond to the conservative therapy and subsequently required surgical intervention. The researchers also noted that early intervention with the corticosteroid injections proved to have increased efficacy.

Conversely, in a study of 43 patients with clinically diagnosed interdigital neuromas grouped into lesions >5 mm and lesion <5 mm, the researchers found that the corticosteroid injection appeared to be more significantly successful and longer lasting for lesions smaller than 5 mm.[41] Pain improvement following the injection was comparable between both groups at the 6-week mark; however, at the 6-month follow-up, only the group with lesions <5 mm remained symptomatically improved.

In an attempt to gain a greater understanding of the prognosis following corticosteroid injection in patients with interdigital neuromas, investigators attempted to define the cutoff values for success. In 201 patients who underwent a corticosteroid injection for an ultrasound-diagnosed interdigital neuroma, they determined the cutoff value for neuroma size in order to obtain a favorable result to be 6.3 mm or less. Additionally, the authors determined that younger age was another risk factor, but it was not associated with a specific threshold because of its low predictive value.

Pain relief after injection does not always last for a long time, and about 21%-47% of patients will require surgical treatment after injection.[37,41,42] These findings suggest that corticosteroid injection is not curative and understanding the prognosis after injection therapy is important in order to develop a protocol for treatment.

Complications following corticosteroid injections have included skin depigmentation, fat pad atrophy, local hypersensitivity and in a rare case, a resulting crossover toe.[38,43,44] These minor complications have been reported to occur in ~5% of patients. In one study, the rate of skin depigmentation reached 10%, and it was theorized that this was the result of a higher number of injections allowed within the first 3 months of follow-up.[34] The blind injection group showed a higher incidence of this complication, likely due to an inability to accurately control the placement of the corticosteroid (see Fig. 28.4 for example of hypopigmentation).

Blind Injection vs Ultrasound-Guided Injection

In nonrandomized cohort studies, blind percutaneous corticosteroid injection have shown a degree of satisfaction rates of up to 45% in blind, single infiltration[45] and 75%-80% in cases of multiple, blind injections.[33,46] The use of ultrasound-guided injections is theorized to increase the efficacy as a result of more accurate real-time placement of the injection needle into the neuroma, thus avoiding other soft tissue structures.[47]

In a study of 56 patients comparing the effectiveness of blind vs ultrasound-guided injections for interdigital neuromas, researchers demonstrated improved results and fewer complications in the ultrasound injection group.[43] Of the 56 patients included, 27 were assigned to the blind group and 29 to the ultrasound-guided group. Patient follow-up for evaluation was performed at 15 days, 1 month, 45 days, and 2, 3, and 6 months.

While both groups showed a significant reduction in pain reduction and increased function at every follow-up time point with regard to the initial vales, there was a general trend of better results in the ultrasound-guided group, reaching statistical significance at 45 days and 2 and 3 months of the follow-up.

Additionally, complications of skin discoloration were noted to be higher in the blind injection group compared to the ultrasound-guided group. As a result, the authors concluded that ultrasound-guided injections provided short-term pain relief to over 60% of the patients, led to a higher percentage of

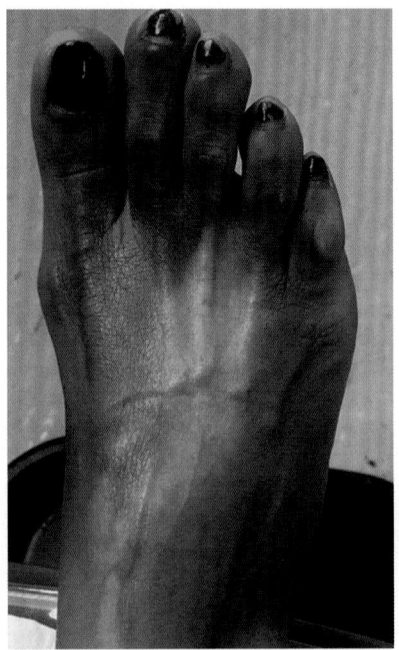

FIGURE 28.4 Hypopigmentation of skin due to corticosteroid injections.

short-term pain relief compared to blind injections and resulted in a lower percentage of skin side effects than blind injections.

Sclerosing Injections

Injection with sclerosing agents has been described for interdigital neuromas with both ethyl alcohol and phenol solutions.[48-52] The sclerosing agents act through injury to the nerve tissue cells via desiccation, necrosis, and subsequent precipitation of protoplasm. The efficacy of ethyl alcohol has been the most extensively studied and the concentration of the alcohol has been described as diluted to 4% with local anesthetic although more commonly to 20% concentration. The 20% concentration is more likely effective as this has been described as the minimum concentration to result in neural inhibition in experimental studies.[51]

Pain relief following injection with alcohol sclerosing is variable, with large case series reporting symptomatic relief in 66%-94% of patients.[49,52] In a prospective study, 101 consecutive patients with clinically diagnosed interdigital neuromas were injected with 20% ethyl alcohol under ultrasound guidance.[48] Patients received a series of 3-5 injections every 14 days with a mean follow-up of 10.5 months. The authors demonstrated a statistically significant reduction of pain symptoms with 94% of patients experiencing either total or partial symptom relief, and the authors concluded that alcohol injection treatment had a high success rate and that the results were comparable to operative treatment.

Similarly high success rates with blind alcohol sclerosing injections were found in a prospective analysis of 100 patients.[49] In this study, previously untreated interdigital neuromas were treated with 3-7 injections every 5-10 days with no additional treatment provided. Eighty-nine percent of patients demonstrated improvement of symptoms with 82 patients experiencing complete resolution of symptoms.

By contrast, a retrospective chart review of 32 patients treated with alcohol sclerosing injections found only 7 patients improved after this treatment.[53] The patients were given 20% ethyl alcohol with 0.25% bupivacaine injections without ultrasound guide. If still symptomatic at a 2 week follow-up, a patient was given another injection. These injections were given every 2 weeks until a maximum of 10 injections or if the patient declined. As a result, 25 patients considered or subsequently underwent surgical intervention, and the authors decided to eliminate alcohol injections for the treatment of interdigital neuromas in their practice.

The use of alcohol injections has reported few complications. The most common complication was complaint of increased pain symptoms after the local anesthetic effect subsided.[49] This postinjection neuritis occurred during the first 48 hours after the injection with symptoms decreasing sharply thereafter with no residual pain by the next follow-up visit. Other reported complications were rare and included an allergic reaction and poor tolerance to the pain of the injection requiring abandonment of the therapy.[52]

Most of the studies detailed weekly sclerosing injections that required up to seven injections in total. One study noted that when injections were discontinued after one or two injections, there was a high recurrence of the pain symptoms.[49] Furthermore, any injections past seven injections did not provide any additional improvement. As a result, the author advised on a minimum of three injections with a maximum of seven.

Other Injections

Injection therapy using botulinum toxin A and capsaicin has also been studied in the treatment of interdigital neuromas.[54,55] In a pilot study with 17 consecutive patients, botulinum toxin A was injected into the neuroma when 3 months of conservative care had failed.[54] After a single injection, 12 patients (70%) reported reduced pain while 5 patients (30%) reported no change in their pain symptoms. No adverse events were reported, and the authors noted that botulinum toxin A may be of use in the treatment of interdigital neuromas and further research should be considered.

Capsaicin, an agonist for the TRPV1 receptor, may act by selectively activating only nociceptor function at the level of the injection, thus relieving pain and without inducing scarring. In a randomized, double-blind, placebo study, a single 0.1 mg dose of capsaicin was injected into 58 subjects.[55] At the 4-week follow-up visit, the capsaicin injection group demonstrated significantly greater pain relief compared to the control group. This reduction was associated with the use of fewer pain medications, less functional interference in mood and walking, and trends suggesting less functional interference in sleep and life enjoyment. Postinjection adverse events (erythema, edema, and hemorrhage) occurred with similar frequencies in the capsaicin and control groups.

SURGICAL TREATMENT

In situations when nonsurgical treatment of interdigital neuromas has failed to provide adequate pain relief, operative measures may be utilized. Success of surgical intervention relies heavily on accurate diagnosis, optimal surgical technique, and appropriate assessment of complications.

As discussed previously, the diagnosis of an interdigital neuroma is largely clinical and can be complicated by the many other pathologies present in the tight anatomic space. Metatarsalgia pain associated with interdigital neuromas is common and can be present in up to 80% of patients.[56] These symptoms have been attributed to a similar biomechanical factors that can cause increased forefoot loading such as elongated lesser metatarsals, synovitis or subluxation/instability of metatarsal phalangeal joints, and tight gastrocnemius that also are implicated in the development of interdigital neuromas.[56] Thus, it is worth mentioning that unsuccessful outcomes from surgical intervention may be related to inadequately addressing all elements of the pathology present.

Conventionally, the main surgical options have included nerve decompression (with neurolysis or translocation of the affected interdigital nerve) and neurectomy (complete excision of the affected part of the interdigital nerve). Nerve decompression was first described by Gauthier in 1978,[57] in which a sharp release of the deep transverse intermetatarsal ligament was performed, rather than a complete neurectomy. Many other authors have described interdigital neuromas as a diagnosis consistent with nerve compression to address the true pathology and thus suggest that simple decompression may be sufficient treatment of pain symptoms.

There have been promising studies analyzing nerve decompression, including various minimally invasive techniques. A multicenter retrospective study of endoscopic nerve decompression for the treatment of interdigital neuromas in 193 interspaces demonstrated a high overall success with 92% of patients reporting a good or fair outcome. Complications in the study were minimal with only seven cases requiring further treatment with neurectomy.[58]

While the long-term outcomes of nerve decompression are lacking, the results of neurectomy have been more studied likely due to the popularity and consistent results of the procedure. The literature reports mostly good to excellent outcomes following neurectomy; however, the variation is broad, ranging from 45% to 86%.[59-61] In one study, only about 50% of the patients undergoing surgical neurectomy were pain-free following surgery, 30% were improved from preoperative levels but with residual pain, and 2% were worse than before surgery.[59] The authors concluded that while most symptoms improved following neurectomy, it was important to recognize that all of the procedures could not be termed successful.

In a long-term study examining the results following neurectomy in 98 ft with an average follow-up of 15.3 years, a good or excellent result was reported for 75 ft (76%).[60] Eight (8.2%) feet had a poor result. and this was attributed to the development of an amputation neuroma in all of these patients. Interestingly, only 72% of the feet following neurectomy experienced numbness along the distribution of the nerve transected and the clinical outcome did not appear to be affected by existence of sensory deficits. The authors concluded that surgical excision of an interdigital neuroma results in good clinical results with high overall patient satisfaction in the long term. Poor outcomes were attributed to amputation neuroma development, multiple neuromas in the same foot, and concomitant foot and ankle disorders unrelated to the primary diagnosis.

Similarly, a retrospective review of 82 patients with an average 5.8-year follow-up demonstrated an 85% satisfaction rate at the time of final follow-up with 65% of the patients describing themselves as "pain-free."[61] The pattern of numbness following neurectomy was variable and only bothersome in 4 ft. The patients who had had either bilateral neuroma excision or excisions of adjacent neuromas in the same foot in a staged fashion had a slightly lower level of satisfaction, but this difference was not significant. While major activity restrictions following surgery were uncommon, mild or major shoe-wear restrictions were noted in 46 patients. Although there was subjective numbness in 36 ft, the pattern of numbness was quite variable and only bothersome in only 4 ft.

Despite overall good outcomes, there remain a substantial number of patients unsatisfied with the results following neurectomy in addition to patients who reported worsening of their pain symptoms. In an attempt to improve surgical outcomes, it has been suggested that intramuscular implantation of the nerve stump may improve pain relief, particularly as a mechanism to prevent amputation neuroma.

In a comparison study, simple neurectomy was compared with neurectomy combined with intramuscular implantation.[62] Ninety-nine consecutive patients were prospectively evaluated with 66 undergoing simple neurectomy and 33 neurectomy with intramuscular implantation. All patients were followed for a minimum of 6 months postoperatively with both groups showing improvement in postoperative functional outcomes.

While both groups overall had good outcomes, the simple neurectomy group had a significantly shorter operative time compared to the implantation group. However, the implantation group demonstrated less pain at the 6-month follow-up, and the authors concluded that although the neurectomy with intramuscular implantation may require a longer operative time, it was shown to provide superior pain relief with similar complications to a simple neurectomy.

In addition to intramuscular implantation, many physicians have used other techniques to prevent stump nerve irritation including cauterization, application of chemical agents such as phenol and alcohol, suturing of the nerve fascicles to each other, and capping the nerve stump with silicone and other materials to avoid amputation neuromas.[63-66]

In a study of 69 neurectomies in 50 patients undergoing single or multiple neurectomy, the end of the resected nerve was sutured into a collagen conduit in an effort to reduce the formation of an amputation neuroma.[66] Of the 69 nerve conduits constructs, 30 (43%) were painless at final outcome, 23 (33%) had pain scores of 1-4, 6 (9%) had pain scores of 5-7, and 10 (15%) had severe symptoms with pain scores of 8-10. Satisfactory outcomes with the procedure with decreased pain symptoms and improved function occurred in 59/69 (85%). These findings demonstrated that collagen conduits were safe and generally successful adjuncts to simple excision of amputation neuromas.

Dorsal vs Plantar Approach

The dorsal approach is more common due to reports of adequate visualization, decreased potential for painful plantar scarring, and earlier postoperative weight bearing.[61,62,67,68] Disadvantages of the dorsal approach include inadequate resection of the digital nerve and damage to cutaneous nerves in the web space. The dorsal approach is implicated in having an increased incidence of amputation neuroma development.[49] Negative histological findings have also been reported in 22%-33% of cases after dorsal excision.[62] In some cases, the neuroma lies proximal to the deep transverse metatarsal ligament and may be difficult to excise by means of the dorsal approach.[69] Thus, a plantar approach has been proposed to enhance direct access to the neuroma allowing for a safe and complete neurectomy, with preservation of the vascular structures and decreased risk of amputation neuromas.[68,70]

In a randomized controlled trial evaluating incisional approach for neurectomy, 82 patients were randomly assigned to a dorsal or plantar approach. There were no significant statistically differences regarding scar tenderness, clinical outcome, and restriction in daily activities between the two approaches.[67] However, differences existed between the two groups regarding complications, with increased scar tenderness and pain with daily activities in the plantar incision group. Interestingly, histological examination of the specimens verified resection of nerves in all cases except 1, which demonstrated removal of the artery in the dorsal group, suggesting that visualization of the nerve may be improved with the plantar approach.

A long-term study evaluated patient outcomes and complications in 168 consecutive patients who underwent neurectomy through a plantar distal transverse incisional approach.[71] With an average follow-up of 7.1 years, the authors reported a good result in 89% of patients, with a fair or poor result in the remaining 11% of patients. They concluded that the plantar distal incision produced a marked reduction in pain, and high overall patient satisfaction, however, did acknowledge scar-related complications related to this approach including skin hardening, loss of sensation at the incision site, discomfort with shoes, and local paresthesias.

While the current literature does not support the superiority of a specific incisional approach, it does support good patient outcomes for neurectomy with the use of both the dorsal and plantar incisional approach. Additionally, an understanding of the risks specific to each approach may assist the surgeon in determining the appropriate approach to use for individualized patient care.

Dorsal Approach Technique

A linear dorsal incision is placed between the affected metatarsals starting just proximal to the metatarsal neck and extending distally to the web space. The intermetatarsal tissues are then dissected using a combination of sharp and blunt dissection until the deep transverse intermetatarsal ligament is adequately visualized. This ligament is then incised sharply parallel to the metatarsals.

A laminar spreader or other retractors can then be placed between the metatarsals to enlarge the operative field. Pressure is then applied plantarly to the intermetatarsal space to mobilize the thickened part of the interdigital nerve for visualization. Commonly surrounded by inflamed bursal tissue, the neuroma is first dissected distally, where the bifurcation of the two digital branches is apparent. Then, the distal nerve branches are incised distally and the plantar aspect of the nerve is traced proximally (see Figs. 28.5 and 28.6 for intraoperative images). It is at this point that any anatomic variations of the nerve branches should be handled with care. Many authors report that proximal dissection of the nerve trunk should continue proximally for at least 1-3 cm to ensure that the incised nerve ending is proximal to the weight-bearing surface of the forefoot in order to reduce the occurrence of a symptomatic amputation neuroma.[72]

Local anesthetic can be infiltrated to the nerve stump area and meticulous hemostasis should be achieved prior to incision closure. The patient is instructed to elevate the foot

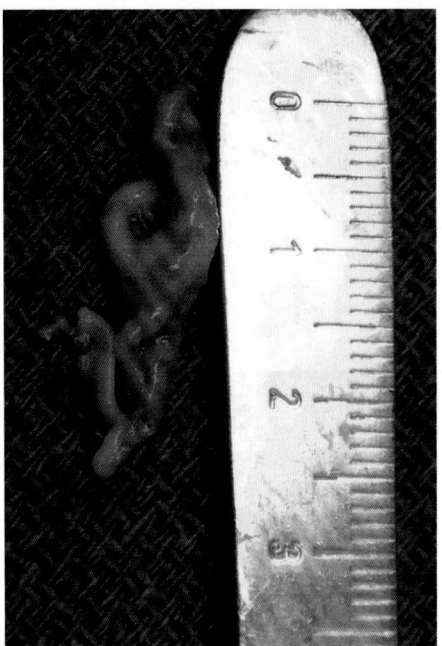

FIGURE 28.6 Neuroma specimen.

postoperatively whenever possible and to keep the surgical site dry for the first 2 weeks. It is recommended that they remain partial weight bearing for the first 48 hours in a surgical shoe and then they may transition to weight bearing as tolerated. Suture removal usually takes place 2 weeks after initial procedure if appropriate healing has taken place.

Plantar Approach Technique

A longitudinal plantar incision is performed proximal to the sulcus and just proximally between the adjacent metatarsals

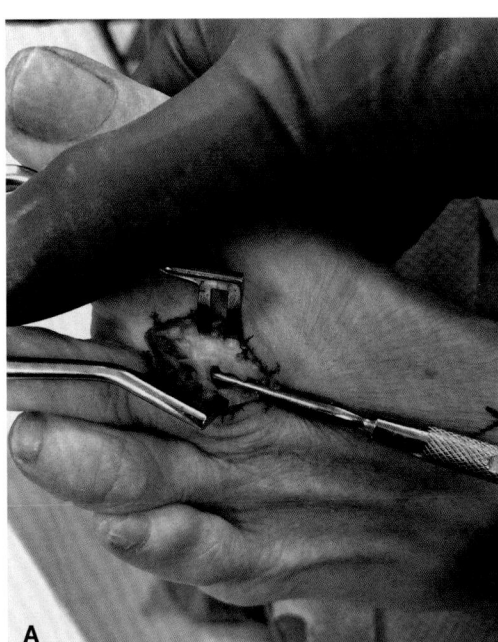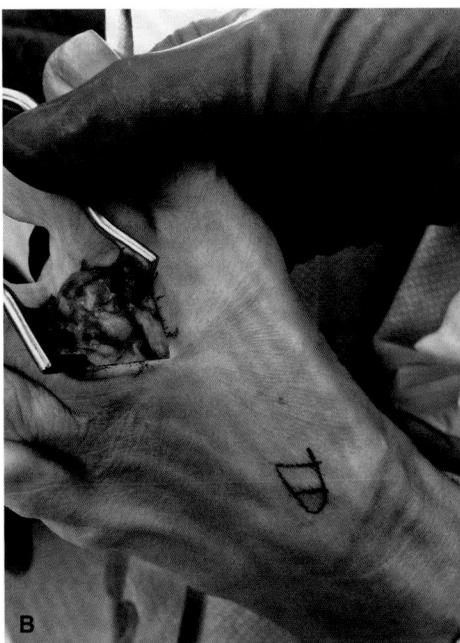

FIGURE 28.5 Intraoperative view of neuroma excision via dorsal approach. **A.** Freer elevator used to elevate deep transverse metatarsal ligament (DTML) for sectioning. **B.** Interdigital neuroma identified after DTML cut.

heads. The incision is then deepened into the subcutaneous fat layer with ease, as there are no vital structures at this depth. Using a combination of blunt and sharp dissection, the interdigital nerve is then identified.

Any accessory, communicating or plantarly directed nerve branches are protected during meticulous dissection. The interdigital nerve is then incised both 2 cm proximal to the neuroma and distally past the point of splitting into digital nerves. It is important to note that the DTIL is left intact. The proximal end of the nerve can be cauterized and allowed to retract into surrounding muscle tissue.

PEARLS and PITFALLS

- Routinely perform a comprehensive history and physical examination as this is the key basis for diagnosis and treatment. The surgical failure rate can be correlated with misdiagnosis of the condition.
- Appropriate advanced imaging modalities may be useful in elucidating a patient's etiology for pain and eliminating other possible differential diagnoses.
- Always attempt noninvasive and invasive conservative treatment prior to surgical intervention.
- Discuss with patient potential complications such as recurrence and incomplete relief.
- Resect the common digital nerve at least 3-4 cm proximal to the deep transverse metatarsal ligament. Apply gentle traction distally to allow for appropriate visualization, transect the nerve, and allow it to retract proximally.
- Hematoma formation can increase the risk of slow wound healing and infection. Release the tourniquet and obtain hemostasis prior to closure.
- For optimal outcomes, revisional surgery should be performed through a plantar approach.

The wound is then inspected for any potential bleeders and hemostasis achieved. After thorough irrigation, the wound can be closed superficially to the level of the skin using nonabsorbable single 2-0 sutures. These sutures are commonly removed at ~2-3 weeks postoperatively. Patients are encouraged to keep their operative foot elevated for the first 24 hours and can start to weight bear 1-2 days after the procedure in a forefoot off-loading shoe. A supportive sneaker with a semirigid sole is recommended after 4 weeks. The dorsal technique is the lead author's preferred approach.

Complications

As for any surgical procedure, there are a variety of potential complications. The literature has shown that formation of a hypertrophic scar, infection, dehiscence, hematoma, stump neuroma, persistent pain, missed nerves, paresthesia, etc. are a few of the potential complications with resection of an interdigital neuroma. Sensory numbness has been described by a variety of authors. It stands to reason that numbness is more common following neurectomy. Numbness can also be caused by iatrogenic damage to the dorsal sensory nerves via the incision or the aggressive use of and has a reported incidence ranging from 41% to 72% when retrospectively examining numbness in different locations of the foot.[60,73,74]

In terms of a painful scar formation, many physicians believe this to be the major disadvantage to the plantar approach. Instead, a Cochrane systematic review found little data to support the belief that dorsal incisions for resection of a plantar digital nerve resulted in fewer symptomatic postoperative scars than plantar incisions.[75] A prospective randomized control trial also demonstrated this consistent finding with 97% of patients in their plantar group experiencing no or mild tenderness to the incision compared to 100% of patients in the dorsal group, which was not statistically significant.[67] In a retrospective study by the same group, 90% of patients experience no or mild tenderness in the group with plantar incisions vs 96% in the group with dorsal incisions, again not statistically significant.[76]

Interestingly, another study evaluating plantar vs dorsal incisions demonstrated more complications in the dorsal group.[68] Four wound-related complications were reported out of 15 in the plantar incision group vs 10 complications (including 6 amputation neuromas and 1 DVT) out of 29 in the dorsal incision group. Additionally, a variety of studies have described missed nerves as potential complications, all using a dorsal incision.[67,76,77] This approach has been described as a more technically challenging procedure due to limited visibility and could potentially contribute to this complication. In fact, one study detailed a complication involving severing an artery in lieu of the intended nerve to be excised.[67]

REVISIONAL NEUROMA SURGERY

Neuromas may recur after primary neurectomy for a variety of reasons such as the failure to resect the interdigital nerve proximally enough and adherence of the neuroma to surrounding tissue. In a study investigating 37 histologic specimens following recurrent neuroma surgery, the investigators found that 21% showed characteristics of primary interdigital neuroma, while 21% showed features of a stump neuroma, illustrating a failure to resect proximally enough or continued pressure/tethering of the nerve.[69] Additionally, 46% showed features of both a stump neuroma and primary interdigital neuroma suggesting incomplete resection during the index procedure.

In order to address resected nerve adhering to surrounding tissue, one investigator described a technique in which the nerve stump is transferred through a drill hole into the metatarsal shaft.[78] Patients undergoing this procedure reported 89% good or excellent results. Further histological evaluation of the nerve buried in the bone showed that a neuroma can still form but with a more regular structure and in similar appearance to the nerve ending outside of the bone canal. As a result, the neuroma will be protected from mechanical stimulation and generation of pain with this technique.

The nerve can also be inserted into muscle, with Wolfort and Dellon describing a procedure to implant the stump neuroma into plantar intrinsic muscle belly, with a reported 80% excellent and 20% good results.[79] Historically, placing a nerve end into an innervated muscle has been shown to be successful in the upper extremity and appears to be successful in the foot as well. Histologic studies have also shown that nerve stumps buried in muscle will form little or no neuroma and will remain contained within the muscle.[80]

Colgrove and colleagues described another technique of burying the nerve stump into the intrinsic muscles of the foot. In their procedure, the nerve was transposed between the transverse head of the adductor hallucis and the interossei muscles and kept in place with a plantar suture that was removed 3-4 weeks after surgery.[81] When comparing the results of those with standard resection and transposition, they found that long-term pain scores were lower for the transposition group. Ninety-six percent of the transposition group was completely pain free, where as only 68% of the resection group was pain free. The authors believe that these positive transposition results may be due to the formation of a smaller transaction neuroma that is removed from the weight-bearing surface of the foot and cushioned by muscle.

PLANTAR VS DORSAL APPROACH FOR REVISIONAL NEUROMA SURGERY

As stated above, there are three main approaches for surgical excision of a neuroma: dorsal longitudinal, plantar longitudinal, and plantar transverse. The dorsal longitudinal approach has generally been used for primary neuroma resection due to better exposure of the distal aspect of the nerve and bursal tissue. Many have stressed its limitations in recurrent neuroma resection due to increased scar tissue and difficulty accessing the more proximal aspect of the nerve. By contrast, the plantar approach allows for better exposure along the proximal aspect of the common digital nerve where stump neuromas tend to form.

However, the literature reveals that the dorsal approach can be used successfully to resect recurrent neuromas. In a study in which 47 of 49 patients underwent a dorsal approach for recurrent neuroma resection, the investigators found that only 22% of patients were dissatisfied with their results.[82] In a study directly comparing the results of a dorsal vs plantar approach for recurrent neuromas, the plantar approach were at a higher risk for developing postoperative hematomas, wound infections, and painful scars.[6] Furthermore, patients undergoing the

dorsal approach were able to achieve weight bearing and return to work/recreational activities earlier compared to the plantar approach.

By contrast, other studies have shown that the plantar approach has been successful with little to no complications. With the use of plantar longitudinal incision, 33 of 37 patients achieved both cosmetically and functionally satisfactory incisions and scars. Only one patient experienced residual callus and scar thickening that was deemed unsatisfactory.[69]

Technique

A plantar longitudinal approach is the approach of choice for the author in revisional surgery. The patient is placed supine, intravenous anesthesia is administered, and a forefoot block is performed. Additionally, an ankle tourniquet is applied for hemostasis. A plantar longitudinal incision is made centered over the affected interspace with caution not to place the incision directly over the metatarsal head. A combination of blunt and sharp dissection is performed through the subcutaneous tissue until the plantar fascia is visualized. This is then incised longitudinally in line with the incision to reveal the common digital nerve. The nerve is then further evaluated for the presence of a stump neuroma, adherence to surrounding tissue, and accessory branches. After dissection of the nerve as proximally as possible, the nerve is resected at this proximal aspect and potentially transposed into muscle/bone as indicated (see Fig. 28.7). The skin is then irrigated with copious amounts of saline and the skin is closed using a 3-0 nonabsorbable suture with caution taken not to overly invert or evert the skin edges. The patient is maintained non–weight bearing until the sutures are removed (likely at 2 weeks) and then they may be transitioned to full weight bearing in a stiff-soled surgical shoe for the next 2 weeks.

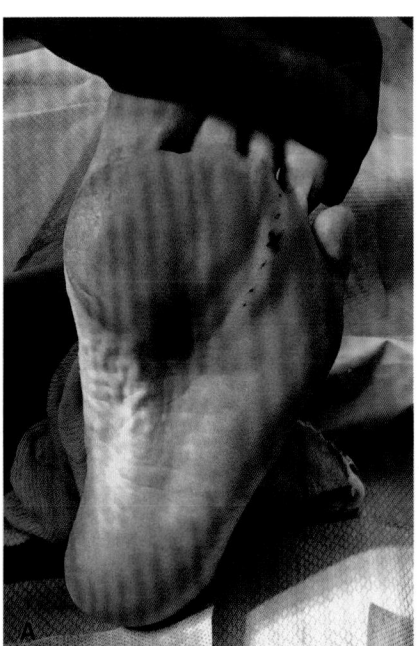 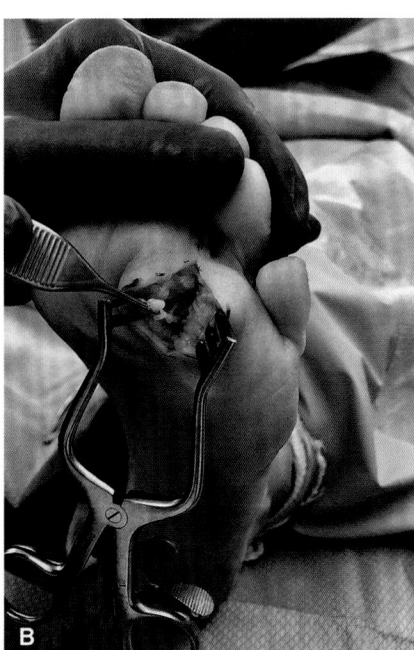 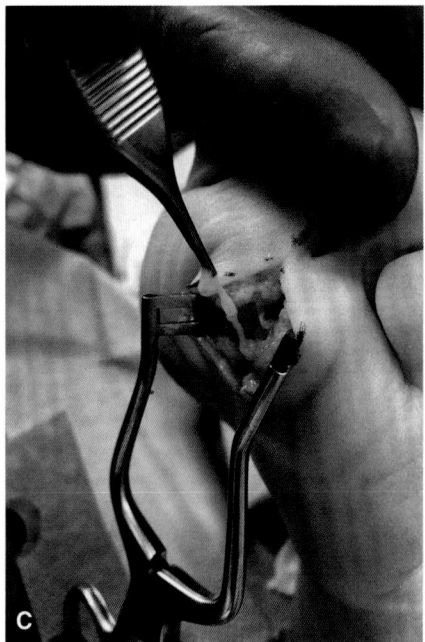

FIGURE 28.7 Plantar approach to stump neuroma excision in a revisional case. **A.** Plantar incision planned in interspace of known stump neuroma. **B.** Deep dissection through subcutaneous fat performed with blunt instruments until stump identified. **C.** Stump neuroma isolated.

REFERENCES

1. Morton TG. The classic: a peculiar and painful affection of the fourth metatarsophalangeal articulation. *Clin Orthop Relat Res.* 1979;142:4-9.
2. Pasero G, Marson P. Filippo Civinini (1805-1844) e La Scoperta del Neurinoma Plantare. *Reumatismo.* 2006;58(4):319-322.
3. Durlacher L. Soft corns. In: *A Treatise on Corns, Bunions, and the Diseases of Nails and the General Management of the Feet.* London, Simpkin, Marshall & Company, 1845.
4. Valero J, Gallart J, González D, Deus J, Lahoz M. Multiple interdigital neuromas: a retrospective study of 279 feet with 462 neuromas. *J Foot Ankle Surg.* 2015;54:320-322.
5. Addante JB, Peicott PS, Wong KY, Brooks DL. Interdigital neuromas: result of surgical excision of 152 neuromas. *J Am Podiatr Med Assoc.* 1986;76:493-495.
6. Faraj AA, Hosur A. The outcome after using two different approaches for excision of Morton's neuroma. *Chin Med J (Engl).* 2010;123:2195-2198.
7. Gudas CJ, Mattana GM. Retrospective analysis of intermetatarsal neuroma excision with preservation of the transverse metatarsal ligament. *J Foot Surg.* 1986;25:459-463.
8. Hewitt SM, Kilmartin TE, O Kane C. A Retrospective audit on the role of sonographical interpretation and localisation of intermetatarsal neuroma in the surgical management of Morton's neuroma. *Br J Podiatr.* 2007;10:99-103.
9. Adams W. Morton's neuroma. *Clin Podiatr Med Surg.* 2010;27:535-545.
10. Kelikian AS. *Sarrafian's Anatomy of the Foot and Ankle.* Philadelphia, PA: Lippincott Williams and Wilkins; 2011.
11. Jones JR, Klenerman L. A study of the communicating branch between the medial and lateral plantar nerves. *Foot Ankle.* 1984;4(6):313-315.
12. Kim JY, Choi JH, Park J, Wang J, Lee I. Anatomical study of Morton's interdigital neuroma: the relationship between the occurring site and the deep transverse metatarsal ligament (DTML). *Foot Ankle Int.* 2007;28(9):1007-1010.
13. Naraghi R, Bremner A, Slack-Smith L, Bryant A. The relationship between foot posture index, ankle equinus, body mass index and intermetatarsal neuroma. *J Foot Ankle Res.* 2016;9(46):1-8.
14. Hassouna H, Singh D. Morton's metatarsalgia: pathogenesis, aetiology and current management. *Acta Orthop Belg.* 2005;71:646-655.
15. Nissen KI. Plantar digital neuritis (Morton's metatarsalgia). *J Bone Joint Surg.* 1948;30B:84.
16. Pastides P, El Sallakh S, Charalambides C. Morton's neuroma: a clinical versus radiological diagnosis. *Foot Ankle Surg.* 2012;18:22-24.
17. Mulder JD. The causative mechanism in Morton's metatarsalgia. *J Bone Joint Surg.* 1951;33B(1):94.
18. Mahadevan D, Venkatesan M, Bhatt R, Bhatia, M. Diagnostic accuracy of clinical tests for Morton's neuroma compared with ultrasonography. *J Foot Ankle Surg.* 2015;54:549-553.
19. Owens R, Gougoulias N, Guthrie H, Sakellario A. Morton's neuroma: clinical testing and imaging in 76 feet, compared to a control group. *Foot Ankle Surg.* 2011;17(3):197-200.
20. Sullivan JD. Neuroma diagnosis by means x-ray evaluation. *J Foot Ankle Surg.* 1967;6:45-46.
21. Kankanala G, Jain AS. The operational characteristics of ultrasonography for the diagnosis of plantar interdigital neuroma. *J Foot Ankle Surg.* 2007;46(4):213-217.
22. Terk MR, Kwong P, Suthar M, Horvath BC, Colletti PM. Morton neuroma: evaluation with MR imaging performed with contrast enhancement and fat suppression. *Radiology.* 1993;189:239-241.
23. Lee M, Kim S, Huh Y, et al. Morton neuroma: evaluated with ultrasonography and MR imaging. *Korean J Radiol.* 2007;8:148-155.
24. Zanetti M, Strehle JK, Zollinger H, Hodler J. Morton neuroma and fluid in the intermetatarsal bursae on MR images of 70 asymptomatic volunteers. *Radiology.* 1997;203:516-520.
25. Weishaupt D, Treiber K, Kundert H, et al. Morton neuroma: MR imaging in prone, supine, and upright weight-bearing body positions. *Radiology.* 2003;226:849-856.
26. Bignotti B, Signori A, Sormani MP, Molfetta L, Martinoli C, Tagliafico A. Ultrasound versus magnetic resonance imaging for Morton neuroma: a systemic review and meta-analysis. *Eur Radiol.* 2015;25:2254-2262.
27. Xu Z, Duan X, Yu X, Wang H, Dong X, Xiang Z. The accuracy of ultrasonography and magnetic resonance imaging for the diagnosis of Morton's neuroma: a systematic review. *Clin Radiol.* 2015;70:351-358.
28. De Maeseneer M, Madani H, Lenchik L, et al. Normal anatomy and compression areas of nerves of the foot and ankle: US and MR imaging with anatomic correlation. *Radiographics.* 2015;35(5):1469-1482.
29. Di Caprio F, Meringolo R, Eddine MS, Ponziani L. Morton's interdigital neuroma of the foot: a literature review. *Foot Ankle Surg.* 2018;24(2):92-98.
30. Cashley DG, Cochrane L. Manipulation in the treatment of plantar digital neuralgia: a retrospective study of 38 cases. *J Chiropr Med.* 2015;14:90-98.
31. Seok H, Sang-Hyun K, Seung Yeol L, Sung WP. Extracorporeal shockwave therapy in patients with Morton's neuroma. *J Am Podiatr Med Assoc.* 2016;106:93-99.
32. Kilmartin TE, Wallace WA. Effect of pronation and supination orthosis on Morton's neuroma and lower extremity function. *Foot Ankle Int.* 1994;15:256-262.
33. Bennett GL, Graham CE, Mauldin DM. Morton's interdigital neuroma: a comprehensive treatment protocol. *Foot Ankle Int.* 1995;16:760-763.
34. Saygi B, Yildirim Y, Saygi EK, Kara H, Esemenli T. Morton neuroma: comparative results of two conservative methods. *Foot Ankle Int.* 2005;26:556-559.
35. Govender N, Kretzmann H, Price JL, Brantingham JW, Globe G. A single-blinded randomized placebo-controlled clinical trial of manipulation and mobilization in the treatment of Morton's neuroma. *J Can Chiropr Assoc.* 2007;44:8-18.
36. Read JW, Noakes JB, Kerr D, Crichton KJ, Slater HK, Bonar F. Morton's metatarsalgia: sonographic findings and correlated histopathology. *Foot Ankle Int.* 1999;20:153-161.
37. Markovic M, Crichton K, Read JW, Lam P, Slater HK. Effectiveness of ultrasound-guided corticosteroid injection in the treatment of Morton's neuroma. *Foot Ankle Int.* 2008;29(5):483-487.
38. Thomson CE, Beggs I, Martin DJ, et al. Methylprednisolone injections for the treatment of Morton neuroma: a patient-blinded randomized trial. *J Bone Joint Surg Am.* 2013;95(9):790-798, S791. for the treatment of Morton.
39. Fuhrmann RA, Roth A, Venbrocks RA. Metatarsalgia: differential diagnosis and therapeutic algorithm. *Orthopade.* 2005;34(8):767-768, 769-772, 774-775.
40. Lizano-Díez X, Ginés-Cespedosa A, Alentorn-Geli E, et al. Corticosteroid injection for the treatment of Morton's neuroma: a prospective, double-blinded, randomized, placebo-controlled trial. *Foot Ankle Int.* 2017;38(9):944-951.
41. Makki D, Haddad BZ, Mahmood Z, Shahid MS, Pathak S, Garnham I. Efficacy of corticosteroid injection versus size of plantar interdigital neuroma. *Foot Ankle Int.* 2012;33:722-726.
42. Mahadevan D, Salmasi M, Whybra N, Nanda A, Gaba S, Mangwani J. What factors predict the need for further intervention following corticosteroid injection of Morton's neuroma? *Foot Ankle Surg.* 2016;22:9-11.
43. Ruiz Santiago F, Prados Olleta N, Tomás Muñoz P, et al. Short term comparison between blind and ultrasound guided injection in morton neuroma. *Eur Radiol.* 2019;29:620-627.
44. Van Vendeloo SN, Ettema HB. Skin depigmentation along lymph vessels of the lower leg following local corticosteroid injection for interdigital neuroma. *Foot Ankle Surg.* 2016;22(2):139-141.
45. Hassouna H, Singh D, Taylor H, Johnson S. Ultrasound guided steroid injection in the treatment of interdigital neuralgia. *Acta Orthop Belg.* 2007;73:224-229.
46. Rasmussen MR, Kitaoka HB, Patzer GL. Nonoperative treatment of plantar interdigital neuroma with a single corticosteroid injection. *Clin Orthop.* 1996;326:188-193.
47. Morgan P, Monaghan W, Richards S. A systematic review of ultrasound-guided and non-ultrasound-guided therapeutic injections to treat Morton's neuroma. *J Am Podiatr Med Assoc.* 2014;104:337-348.
48. Hughes RJ, Ali K, Jones H, Kendall S, Connell DA. Treatment of Morton's neuroma with alcohol injection under sonographic guidance: follow-up of 101 cases. *AJR Am J Roentgenol.* 2007;188(6):1535-1539.
49. Dockery GL. The treatment of intermetatarsal neuromas with 4% alcohol sclerosing injections. *J Foot Ankle Surg.* 1999;38:403-408.
50. Magnan B, Marangon A, Frigo A, Bartolozzi P. Local phenol injection in the treatment of interdigital neuritis of the foot (Morton's neuroma). *Chir Organi Mov.* 2005;90:371-377.
51. Rengachary SS, Watanabe IS, Singer P, Bopp WJ. Effect of glycerol on peripheral nerve: an experimental study. *Neurosurgery.* 1983;13:681-688.
52. Musson RE, Sawhney JS, Lamb L, Wilkinson A, Obaid H. Ultrasound guided alcohol ablation of Morton's neuroma. *Foot Ankle Int.* 2012;33(3):196-201.
53. Espinosa N, Seybold JD, Jankauskas L, Erschbamer M. Alcohol sclerosing therapy is not an effective treatment for interdigital neuroma. *Foot Ankle Int.* 2011;32(6):576-580.
54. Climent JM, Mondejar-Gomez F, Rodriguez-Ruiz C, Diaz-Llopis I, Gomez-Gallego D, Martin-Medina P. Treatment of Morton neuroma with botulinum toxin A: a pilot study. *Clin Drug Investig.* 2013;33:497-503.
55. Simone DA, Nolano M, Johnson T, Wendelschafer-Crabb G, Kennedy WR. Intradermal injection of capsaicin in humans produces degeneration and subsequent reinnervation of epidermal nerve fibers: correlation with sensory function. *J Neurosci.* 1998;18:8947-8959.
56. Diez EM, Mas SM. Comparative results of two different techniques in the treatment of Morton's neuroma. *Foot.* 2004;15:14-16.
57. Gauthier G. Thoma Morton's disease, a nerve entrapment syndrome. A new surgical technique. *Clin Orthop.* 1979;142:90-92.
58. Barrett G, Rabat E, Buitrago M, Rascon V, Applegate D. Endoscopic decompression of intermetatarsal nerve (EDIN) for the treatment of Morton's entrapment—multicenter retrospective review. *Open J Orthop.* 2012;2:19-24.
59. Bucknall V, Rutherford D, Macdonald D, Shalaby H, McKinley J, Breusch SJ. Outcomes following excision of Morton's interdigital neuroma: a prospective study. *Bone Joint J.* 2016;98-B:1376-1381.
60. Coughlin MJ, Pinsonneault T. Operative treatment of interdigital neuroma: a long-term follow-up study. *J Bone Joint Surg Am.* 2001;83-A:1321-1328.
61. Kasparek M, Schneider W. Surgical treatment of Morton's neuroma: clinical results after open excision. *Int Orthop.* 2013;37:1857-1861.
62. Rungprai C, Cychosz CC, Phruetthiphat O, Femino JE, Amendola A, Phisitkul P. Simple neurectomy versus neurectomy with intramuscular implantation for interdigital neuroma: a comparative study. *Foot Ankle Int.* 2015;36:1412-1424.
63. Wagner E, Ortiz C. The painful neuroma and the use of conduits. *Foot Ankle Clin.* 2011;16:295-304.
64. Waitayawinyu T, Parisi DM, Miller B, et al. A comparison of polyglycolic acid versus type 1 collagen bioabsorbable nerve conduits in a rat model: an alternative to autografting. *J Hand Surg Am.* 2007;32:1521-1529.
65. Wangensteen KJ, Kalliainen LK. Collagen tube conduits in peripheral nerve repair: a retrospective analysis. *Hand (NY).* 2010;5:273-277.
66. Gould JS, Naranje SM, McGwin G, Florence M, Cheppalli S. Use of collagen conduits in management of painful neuromas of the foot and ankle. *Foot Ankle Int.* 2013;34(7):932-940.
67. Akermark C, Crone H, Skoog A, Weidenhielm L. A prospective randomized controlled trial of plantar versus dorsal incisions for operative treatment of primary Morton's neuroma. *Foot Ankle Int.* 2013;34:1198-1204.
68. Wilson S, Kuwada GT. Retrospective study of the use of a plantar transverse incision versus a dorsal incision for excision of neuroma. *J Foot Ankle Surg.* 1995;34:537-540.
69. Johnson JE, Johnson KA, Unni KK. Persistent pain after excision of an interdigital neuroma. Results of reoperation. *J Bone Joint Surg Am.* 1988;70:651-657.
70. Levitsky KA, Alman BA, Jevsevar DS, Morehead J. Digital nerves of the foot: anatomic variations and implications regarding the pathogenesis of interdigital neuroma. *Foot Ankle.* 1993;14:208-214.
71. Nery C, Raduan F, Del Buono A, Asaumi ID, Maffulli N. Plantar approach for excision of a Morton neuroma: a long-term follow-up study. *J Bone Joint Surg Am.* 2012;94(7):654-658.

72. Weinfeld SB, Myerson MS. Interdigital neuritis: diagnosis and treatment. *J Am Acad Orthop Surg.* 1996;4(6):328-335.

73. Giannini S, Bacchini P, Ceccarelli F, Vannini F. Interdigital neuroma: clinical examination and histopathologic results in 63 cases treated with excision. *Foot Ankle Int.* 2004;25:79-84.

74. Friscia DA, Strom DE, Parr JW, Saltzman CL, Johnson KA. Surgical treatment for primary interdigital neuroma. *Orthopedics.* 1991;14:669-672.

75. Thomson CE, Gibson JNA, Martin D. Interventions for the treatment of Morton's neuroma. *Cochrane Database Syst Rev.* 2004;(3):CD003118.

76. Åkermark C, Crone H, Saartok T, Zuber Z. Plantar versus dorsal incisions in the treatment of primary intermetatarsal Morton's neuroma. *Foot Ankle Int.* 2008;29:136-141.

77. Dereymaeker G, Schroven I, Steenwerckx A, Stuer P. Results of excision of the interdigital nerve in the treatment of Morton's metatarsalgia. *Acta Orthop Belg.* 1996;62:22-25.

78. Nelms BA, Bishop JO, Tullos HS. Surgical treatment of recurrent Morton's neuroma. *Orthopedics.* 1984;7:1708-1711.

79. Wolfort SF, Dellon AL. Treatment of recurrent neuroma of the interdigital nerve by implantation of the proximal nerve into muscle in the arch of the foot. *J Foot Ankle Surg.* 2001;40(6):404-410.

80. Mackinnon SE, Dellon AL, Hudson AR, et al. Alteration of neuroma formation by manipulation of its microenvironment. *Plast Reconstr Surg.* 1985;76:345-353.

81. Colgrove RC, Huang EY, Barth AH, et al. Interdigital neuroma: intermuscular neuroma transposition compared with resection. *Foot Ankle Int.* 2000;21(3):206-211.

82. Stamatis ED, Myerson MS. Treatment of recurrence of symptoms after excision of an interdigital neuroma. A retrospective review. *J Bone Joint Surg Br.* 2004;86(1):48-53.

83. Richardson EG, Brotzman SB, Graves SC. The plantar incision for procedures involving the forefoot: an evaluation of one hundred and fifty incisions in one hundred and fifteen patients. *J Bone Joint Surg Am.* 1993;75(5):726-731.

84. Jain S, Mannan K. The diagnosis and management of Morton's neuroma: a literature review. *Foot Ankle Spec.* 2013;6:307-317.

CHAPTER 29

Calcaneal Fractures

Jason R. Miller, Karl W. Dunn, and Christopher R. Hood Jr

DEFINITION

Calcaneal fractures, which account for 1%-2% of all fractures in the skeletal system, can be one of the most difficult fractures to manage in the lower extremity.[1,2] First described by Malgaigne in 1843, early reports of fracture management often yielded poor functional outcomes. As early as 1908, Cotton and Wilson suggested that open treatment of calcaneal fractures was contraindicated.[3] In contrast, Böhler in 1931 recommended operative management of calcaneal fractures.[4] Due to numerous inherent shortcomings of the time, including lack of antibiotics, poor surgical fixation options, and the infancy of radiographs, poor results were again noted.

Conn in 1935 described calcaneal fractures as "serious and disabling injuries in which the end results are incredibly bad."[5] The sentiment of nonoperative treatment was considered common practice up to and through the 1970s. Popularity toward open reduction internal fixation (ORIF) grew from the 1980s and 1990s as a lateral extensile incision was considered the preferred approach in the operative management of displaced calcaneal fractures.[6-8] With the advancement of imaging capabilities and implants designed specifically for the calcaneus, ORIF has gradually continued to improve outcomes over time.[9,10] Despite recent advancements, calcaneal fractures have still been considered severely incapacitating in many cases and continue to challenge both the surgeon and patient alike.

CLASSIFICATIONS

Numerous classification systems exist in literature in the description of calcaneal fractures. The authors have two preferred classifications based on their ability to accurately describe the fracture patterns and also aid the surgeon in fracture management as well as predict postoperative outcomes. Other classifications exist and display varied rates of prognostic values.[11]

Essex-Lopresti has described two distinct fracture types of the calcaneus based on the secondary fracture line (Fig. 29.1).[12,13] As described based on fracture pattern, a more inferiorly directed axial force with the foot in plantarflexion results in a tongue-type fracture while a posteriorly directed axial force with the foot in dorsiflexion results in a joint depression fracture pattern.[12] Tongue-type fracture lines run beneath the posterior facet and exit the tuber posteriorly below or through the Achilles tendon insertion. Joint depression fracture lines run

behind the posterior facet across the body of the calcaneus and exit anteriorly to the Achilles tendon insertion. In these fractures, a posterior facet fragment is created, whereas in tongue-type fractures, a variable portion of the posterior articular surface remains intact with the tuberosity fragment.

The Sanders classification is extremely useful to the foot and ankle surgeon in describing and assisting in the management of a calcaneus fracture.[6,7] A preoperative computed tomography (CT) scan is obtained and the calcaneus is viewed on a coronal section that involves the posterior facet. Four types (1-4) are used to describe the number of fractures, except type 1 where any number of fractures could exist, as long as there is <2 mm displacement of the fracture(s) (Fig. 29.2). A Sanders type 2 fracture has one displaced fracture line and then subdivided into A, B, or C. An A fracture subtype involves the lateral aspect, B central one-third of the posterior facet, and C involving a fracture through the medial one-third. The same rules apply for Sanders types 3 and 4, where the number and location of fracture fragments is easily described using this method.

INDICATIONS AND PITFALLS

Surgical intervention is not recommended for all calcaneal fractures. Nondisplaced fractures, even intra-articular (Sanders 1), are best suited for nonoperative management. Some fracture types, including beak type fractures where the Achilles tendon avulses the posterior tuberosity of the calcaneus, are considered an urgent procedure due to the possibility of skin compromise and necrosis. Open fractures are associated with higher complication rates including wound healing issues, deep soft tissue infections, and osteomyelitis. Open fractures are considered urgent cases with surgeons often electing to stage open fractures, initially employing a thorough operative debridement and irrigation, and sometimes stabilizing and spanning the fracture(s) with an external fixator device. Further management may take place 1-2 weeks thereafter as the skin begins to normalize without the presence of infection and as the skin displays a positive wrinkle sign.

At present, most displaced fractures, especially involving the posterior facet of the subtalar joint, are often recommended for surgical open reduction with internal fixation. Care is again taken to fully assess the patient, perform an accurate history and physical, and to rule out further trauma as ~10% of patients also suffer spinal injuries.[14,15] It is imperative for the surgeon

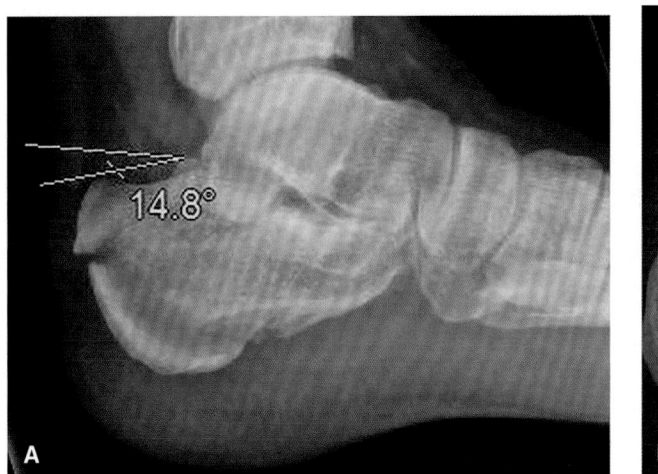 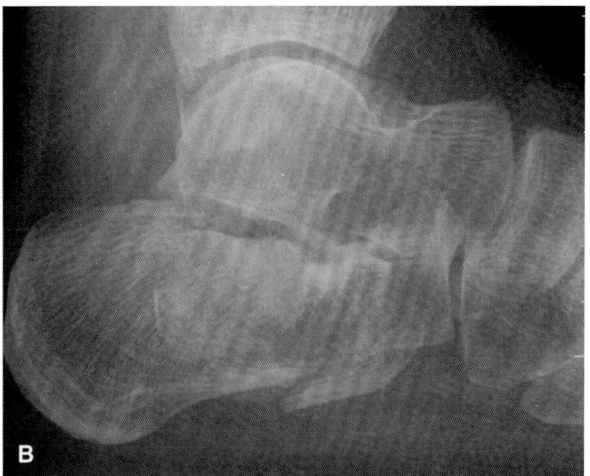

FIGURE 29.1 Essex-Lopresti classification system of tongue-type **(A)** and joint depression **(B)** fractures patterns best visualized on later plain film radiographs.

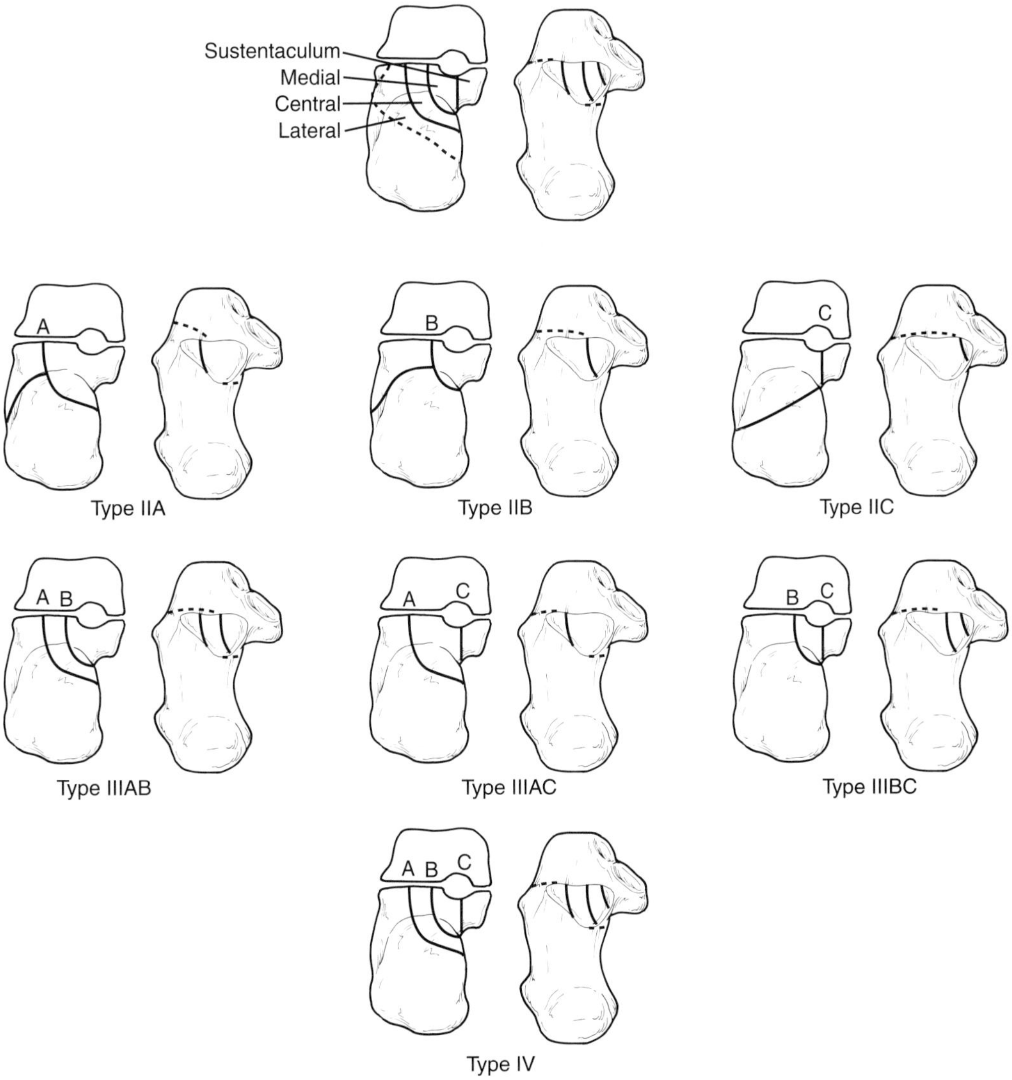

Sustentaculum
Medial
Central
Lateral

Type IIA

Type IIB

Type IIC

Type IIIAB

Type IIIAC

Type IIIBC

Type IV

FIGURE 29.2 Sanders CT calcaneal fracture classification scheme.

to obtain an accurate radiographic assessment including plain film radiographs and CT scans to visualize the extent of the fracture(s) for preoperative planning.

Another concern, especially seen more often in severe or comminuted fracture types, is that of compartment syndrome (CS). In cases with significant edema and muscular trauma in a closed compartment space, the compartment pressure could increase near that of the patient's diastolic pressure, decreasing arterial flow. Permanent sequelae secondary to CS include Volkmann contractures, deformity, chronic pain, and loss of function.[16-18] CS is commonly evaluated by using the pneumonic of the "5 Ps:" pallor, pain out of proportion, pulselessness, paralysis, and paresthesias. If there is a concern for a patient with a possible CS, there should be a low tolerance to utilize a wick catheter to assess for the condition. If the intracompartment pressure is within 30 mm Hg of the diastolic pressure, or a sustained pressure of 30 mm Hg for >30 minutes on repeated testing, an urgent fasciotomy should be employed.

Generally speaking, a sinus tarsi approach (STA) may allow the surgeon to operate sooner than with a lateral extensile approach, as there tends to be fewer wound complications associated with the former.[19-21] Approximate time to operate from a lateral extensile approach can take up to 3 weeks before the soft tissues are amendable, while it is common for a minimally invasive (MIS) or STA to be performed within the first 7-14 days.

ANATOMIC FEATURES

The calcaneus is the largest tarsal bone made up of a dense cancellous network with a thin cortical shell much like a "hard-boiled egg."[22] Within the body are both traction and compression trabecular regions whose development reflects the manner by which weight is transmitted through the bone. The tuberosity trabeculae run posteroinferior, while the anterior calcaneus trabeculae run anteroinferior. These two regions converge just below the posterior facet forming a condensation of cortical bone termed the thalamic portion, thickest under the facet.[23] Inferior to the calcaneal sulcus is the neutral triangle, a region deficient of trabeculation noted to be the weakest portion of the calcaneus and where fractures generally occur.

The superior surface contains three articular facets that correspond to matching articulations with the inferior surface of the talus. The rectangular or oval-shaped posterior facet is the largest load-bearing surface where most subtalar joint motion originates. The anterior and middle facets are much smaller and exist either distinct or one confluent facet. The anterior facet is supported by the calcaneal beak while the middle facet is supported by the sustentaculum tali. A hollow cavity termed the sinus tarsi is located between the anterior/middle and posterior facets with corresponding grooves on the calcaneal (calcaneal sulcus) and talar (sulcus tali) surfaces. Strong interosseous ligaments hold these two bones together while the cervical ligament acts as the roof of this channel at the lateral sinus tarsi opening.

The medial wall surface is cortically stronger than the lateral surface. The primary anatomic structure is the sustentaculum tali, a triangular-shaped medially projecting horizontal shelf. Its superior surface is the calcaneal middle facet, which supports the neck of the talus, while the inferior surface provides a groove for excursion of the flexor hallucis longus (FHL) tendon. Several ligaments attach here including the plantar

calcaneonavicular (spring), deltoid, and medial talocalcaneal (interosseous). In calcaneal fractures, the sustentaculum tali fragment has been termed the "constant fragment" due to these various attachments holding this anatomic structure in place despite displacement to other portions of the bone.[24-26] The neurovascular bundle also runs along the medial surface of the calcaneus, which may be injured during either fracture trauma or reduction of the sustentacular fragment.

The lateral surface is mostly flat and subcutaneous. Central to this region lay the peroneal tubercle, which serves as the insertion point for the calcaneofibular ligament (CFL). It also divides the peroneal tendons to run above (brevis) and below (longus) the tubercle on a smooth surface for gliding. The sural nerve lies posterior to the peroneal tendons and courses parallel with them until crossing superficial to them at the level of the inferior peroneal retinaculum.

FUNCTIONAL ANALYSIS OF THE ANATOMY

It is important to understand normal calcaneal anatomy, bony landmarks, and surrounding structures to better assess the extent of injuries to both the bone and surrounding soft tissue. Biomechanically, the calcaneus is the main pedal weight-bearing structure and is the foundation for bipedal gait. It functions as a lever arm transmitting the force of the gastrocnemius-soleal complex through the Achilles tendon to aid in gait and supports and maintains the lateral column of the foot. Four features of particular importance that make treating calcaneal fractures difficult include the limited area of dense bone, complex articular anatomy, the irregular medial wall with closely lying soft tissue structures, and the subcutaneous lateral wall.[8]

The critical angle or the crucial angle of Gissane is meant to describe the anatomic position of the posterior facet and of the middle and anterior facets in their relationship. Described by Gissane in 1947, this angle is formed by the angle between a line (1) parallel along the posterior facet superior surface and (2) parallel to the anterior and middle facets superior surface (Fig. 29.3). The apex of this angle is usually directly below the lateral talar process. A normal anatomic critical angle is 120 and 145 degrees. An increase in measurement represents a collapse of the posterior facet and intra-articular disruption from the lateral talar process being driven down into the critical angle apex.

Böhler angle is another well understood value, which can also aid in the diagnosis of a calcaneal fracture or in the anatomic reduction of the calcaneus. Böhler in 1931 described this angle that is formed by the angle between a line extending from (1) the most superior point on the calcaneal anterior process to the most superior point on the posterior facet and (2) the most superior point on the calcaneal tuberosity to the most superior point on the posterior facet (Fig. 29.3).[4] Böhler initially described this angle as measuring between 30 and 35 degrees while most sources will state a range from 20 to 40 degrees. The angle will decrease with displaced intra-articular calcaneal fracture and represent a collapse of the posterior facet or loss in calcaneal height. Böhler angle is often used as both a prognostic tool in predicting clinical results when measured preoperatively and is tracked postoperative to assess for loss in calcaneal height, which may lead to a variety of sequela to the patient.[27]

As mentioned earlier, the sustentaculum tali or the "constant fragment" remains relatively stable secondary to its numerous ligamentous attachments. Rarely has this fragment been noted

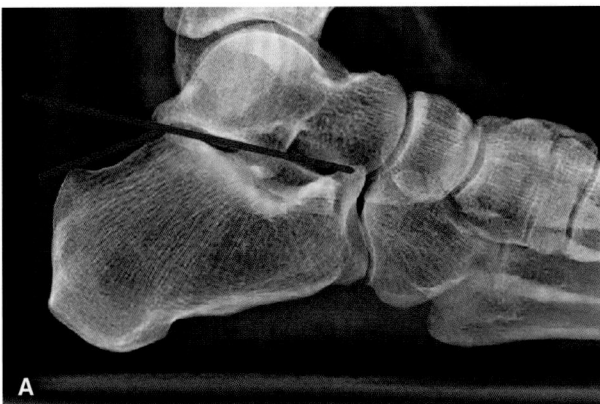

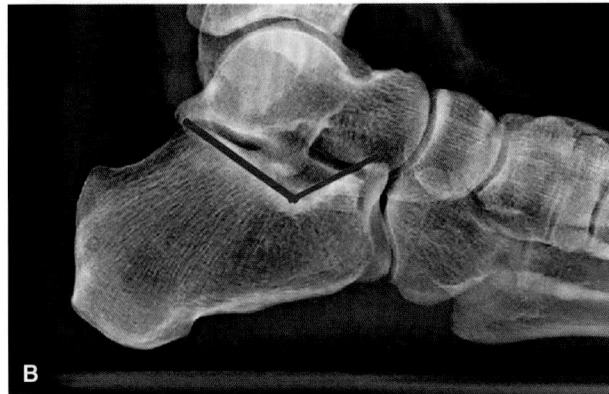

FIGURE 29.3 Böhler angle **(A)** and critical angle of Gissane **(B)**.

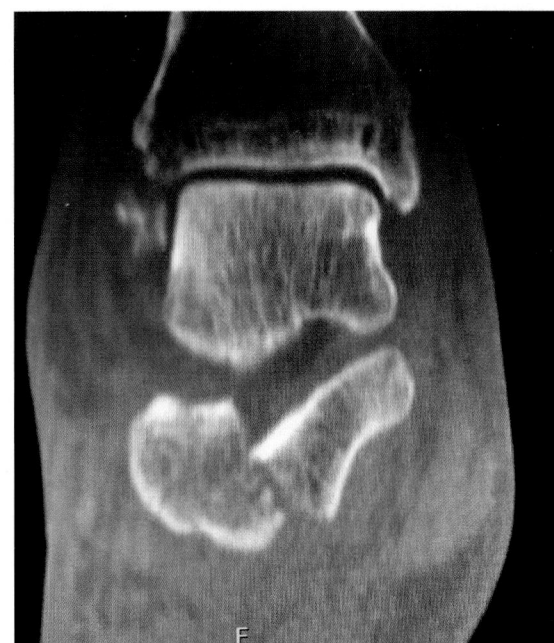

FIGURE 29.4 CT axial imaging with noted displacement and angulation of the sustentacular fragment.

to displace, which makes it a desirable area to reconstruct the fracture fragments from. The sustentaculum tali is constituted of relatively dense subchondral bone also, which can also aid the surgeon in good fixation purchase. The neurovascular bundle and FHL tendon exist just inferior to the tali, where the posterior tibial tendon and flexor digitorum longus tendon lies just superior to the osseous structure. With respect to the sustentacular "constant" fragment, the idea of its positional or anatomical consistency has been questioned in the literature. Berberian et al. and Gitajn et al. performed retrospective CT reviews of displaced intra-articular calcaneal fractures reporting rates of nonanatomic sustentaculum in 42% ($n = 100$) and 21% ($n = 212$) of cases, respectively, disproving the theory of the constant fragment.[24,25] In demonstrating high rates of calcaneal fractures with sustentacular fractures, surgeons should not assume that this important structure is anatomically aligned (Fig. 29.4).

PATHOGENESIS

The calcaneus is the most commonly fractured tarsal accounting for 60% of tarsal bone fractures.[14,15] Displaced intra-articular fractures make up 60%-75% of all calcaneal fractures in adults.[15] Associated injuries often occur in conjunction with calcaneal fractures due to the high energy nature of this trauma with rates reported as high as 70%.[28] Spinal injuries occur between 10% and 20%, most often found in the thoracolumbar region (T12-L2).[14,15] Contralateral extremity injuries occur roughly 26% of the time with bilateral calcaneal fractures occurring in

7%-10% of cases.[14,15,29] Patients are typically between 30 and 50 years of age with a 2.4—5:1 male to female rate of incidence.[14,30] However, females are more likely to sustain calcaneal fractures after the fifth decade secondary to a lower energy mechanism in osteoporotic bone.[30]

Falls from height (FFH) mechanisms represent 75% of injuries. Although the average FFH is 14 ft, distances as small as 3 ft have been reported to result in fracture.[14] Other mechanisms include motor vehicle accidents (MVAs), Achilles contracture avulsions, ligament avulsions fractures, and stress fractures.[14] One study found 21% of patients sustained injuries while intoxicated, either with alcohol or other illicit drugs, questioning the need for a toxicology lab panel upon presentation.[30] Further, the same authors found 10% of patients had a significant psychiatric history with half of the patients sustaining their injuries during a suicide attempt.[30] Both of these facts may warrant additional psychiatric consultation during the initial triage period if patient presentation warrants.

Open calcaneus fractures are relatively rare injuries representing 0.85%-10% of all calcaneal fractures most often occurring after either MVA (56%) or FFH > 6 ft (24%).[16,17,33] Worsham et al. reported 88% of open fractures were either Gustillo type II or type II with medial-based wounds, 92% of patients had ≥1 additional orthopedic fracture injury, and 58% had additional nonorthopedic injuries (eg, trauma to the head, liver, spleen, adrenal, chest).[28] Due to the high energy trauma often involved in open calcaneal fractures, a full body evaluation is warranted for these concomitant injuries, specifically to the head and chest.

INTRA-ARTICULAR FRACTURES

High-energy MVA or FFH are the two most common scenarios resulting in intra-articular fractures. The mechanism of injury involves an axial load compressing the lateral talar process into the apex of the angle of Gissane. The energy of body weight is transmitted through the talus into the calcaneal articular surface as it is forced into a hard platform such as the ground, car pedal, or floorboard. Intra-articular fracture typically produces the features of (1) loss of calcaneal height and length due to impaction; (2) rotation of the tuberosity fragment into varus; (3) increased width due to the lateral wall displacement/blowout of the tuberosity fragment; and (4) disruption of the subtalar and/or calcaneocuboid joint (CCJ).[12]

EXTRA-ARTICULAR FRACTURES

Extra-articular fractures occur between 25% and 40% of the time with reports as high as 60% in children.[15,31] They are typically the result of lower-energy trauma or a twisting mechanism.[32] These fractures have been divided into distinct regions: anterior process, plantar tubercle, tuberosity (body, avulsion "beak type," Achilles insertion, vertical shear, medial process, horizontal, apophysis), sustentaculum tali, and avulsion types.[31] Often they can be treated with cast or brace immobilization until healing has occurred radiographically.

Anterior Process of the Calcaneus

Anterior process fractures account for 15% of all calcaneal fractures and typically are one of two types: avulsion or compression.

The more common avulsion fractures are a result of foot adduction/inversion and plantarflexion with either tensioning of the Y-shaped bifurcate ligament across its origin (anterior process of the calcaneus) and insertion (calcaneocuboid and calcaneonavicular distal arms) or the calcaneocuboid interosseous ligament. Tension across the extensor digitorium brevis can also result in avulsion injuries. Both mechanisms typically result in the avulsion of bone off the calcaneal side. Compression fractures are a result of CCJ compression secondary to forefoot abduction on the hindfoot.

Due to some sort of inversion-twisting mechanism as the inciting force, one must differentiate between anterior talofibular ligament (ATFL) pain and avulsion fracture pain. This distinction is important as it is one of the reasons why these fractures are often initially missed. Typically, patients will present with point tenderness just anterior to the sinus tarsi, ~2 cm anterior and 1 cm inferior to the ATFL. Imaging consists of an x-ray with the oblique and lateral views most helpful (Fig. 29.5). MRI or CT scans may be warranted in certain situations for distinct differentiation. This fracture should be suspected in a patient who does not recover appropriately from a lateral ankle sprain due to initial misdiagnosis, and early MRI may be the best tool in differentiating between acute sprain and fracture.[33]

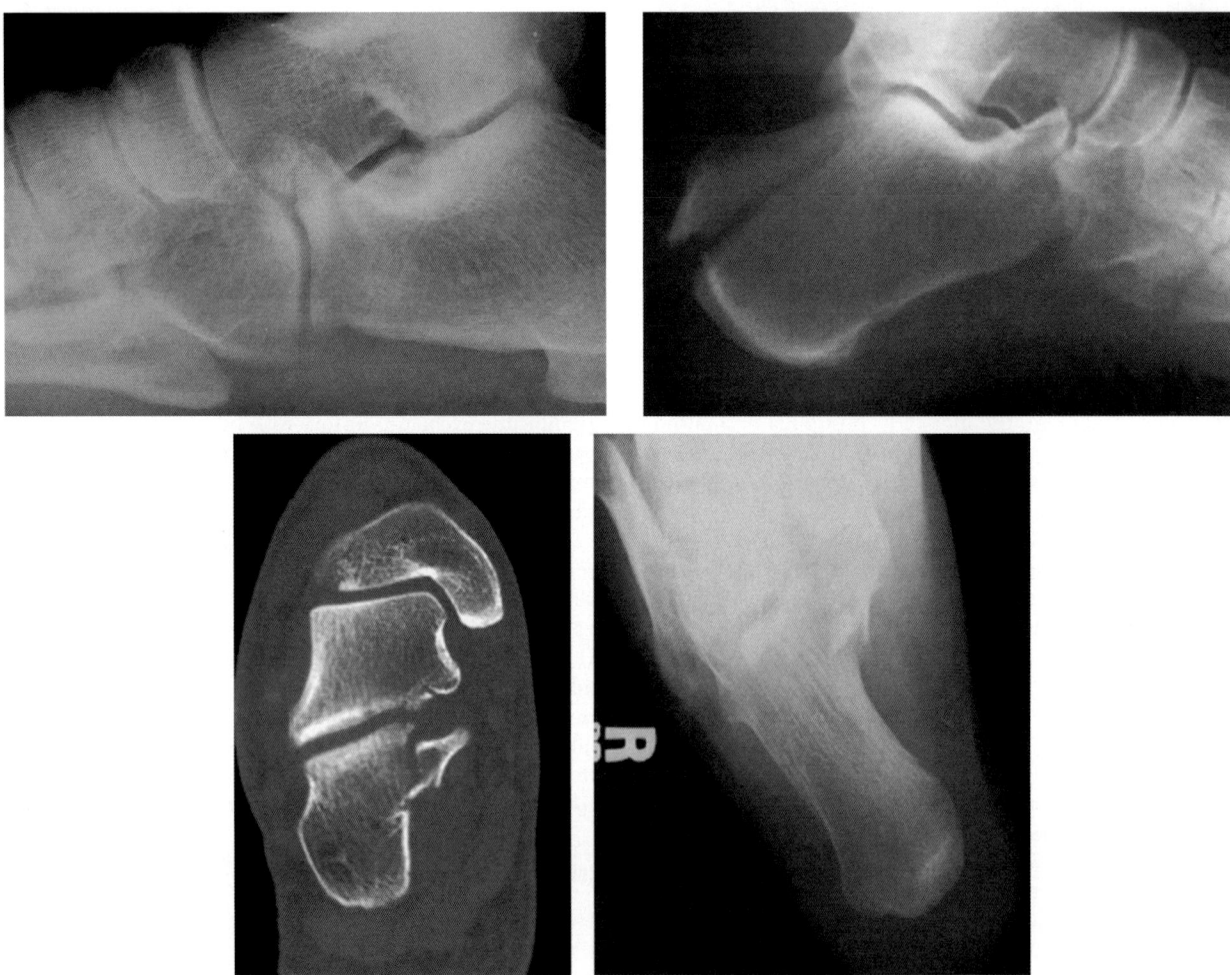

FIGURE 29.5 Extra-articular fractures of the calcaneus. Anterior process (**top-left**), calcaneal beak fracture (**top-right**), and isolated sustentaculum tali fracture on XR and CT (**bottom**).

Plantar Tubercle Fractures

The plantar weight-bearing aspect of the calcaneus contains the smaller lateral and larger medial plantar tubercles, attachment site for the plantar fascia, and multiple small intrinsic muscles of the foot. Fractures to this region typically occur through a direct ground-reactive force on the tubercles after an FFH or MVA. The position of the foot at the time of impact, pronated/valgus or supinated/varus, will result in either a medial or lateral tubercle fracture, respectively. Due to the many soft tissue attachments to this site along with the heel fat pad, fractures are often minimally to nondisplaced. Treatment includes 4-6 weeks of non–weight bearing, transitioned to full weight bearing over another 4-6 week period in a walking cast or boot. Reduction in pain and swelling typically occurs at the time walking is begun.

Tuberosity—Body

Calcaneal body fractures that do not involve an articulation are rare. They are the result of either an axial load mechanism, iatrogenic, or a missed stress fracture that progresses to a true fracture. It is important to check for possible appendicular and axial skeleton injuries when this fracture presents. Typically they are nondisplaced and undergo nonoperative treatment. Early ROM is important while consolidation occurs with patients transitioned from non–weight bearing for the first 4-6 weeks to partial then full weight bearing in a fracture boot over the following 4 weeks.

Tuberosity—Beak/Avulsion

Calcaneal beak fractures represent 1%-3% of all calcaneal fractures.[20] Of the extra-articular fractures, tuberosity avulsion fractures are considered among the most morbid and presentation is considered a surgical emergency. The cause is a violent pull from the gastrocnemius-soleus complex paired with foot dorsiflexion, often a result of a low-energy fall or sudden push-off while standing in diabetic or osteoporotic patients.[20] With a gross proximal displacement of the calcaneal tuberosity, both large amounts of hematoma can develop while the superior margin of the bone may place internal pressure on the skin. Combined, skin necrosis and wound problems may develop if not surgically reduced and drained in a timely fashion. These fractures are best seen on a lateral x-ray, and CT may be warranted to evaluate for any intra-articular extension (Fig. 29.5).

Attempted nonsurgical reduction consists of splinting with the foot in maximum plantarflexion with excess posterior ankle padding. Surgical reduction is performed either percutaneously or open through a lateral or posterior incision. When done percutaneously, a Schanz pin can be used to joystick the avulsion fragment plantar ward to reapproximate the beak fracture to the main body of the calcaneus (Fig. 29.6). The knee should be flexed, which allows the ankle to relax the Achilles tendon complex on the fragment. This Essex-Lopresti maneuver has been described for tongue-type fractures but is amenable for extra-articular tuberosity fractures.[12,13] K-wires stabilize the reduction, preloaded into the tuber just shy of the fracture with an assistant advancing them into the anterior calcaneus once reduced. A large reduction clamp may be substituted for the Schanz pin for a method of reduction and

K-wires for reduction stabilization. The technique is also accomplished open by performing just the vertical arm of the standard extensile approach. Excision of the fragment (if not of substantial size) may be performed in low-demand patients or those who may encounter significant wound healing issues.

Sustentaculum Tali Fractures

Fractures to the sustentaculum are typically a part of the joint depression fracture pattern or axial loading and inversion of the foot. They are considered extra-articular when there is no true posterior facet pathology.[32] The mechanism is an axial force applied to a supinated foot. These may be seen on lateral or calcaneal axial films, and if suspected, a CT should be ordered to evaluate an isolated fracture vs intra-articular extension (Fig. 29.5). These frequently result in a small, nondisplaced fracture that is treated nonoperatively with 3-4 weeks non–weight bearing followed by 1-2 weeks of a walking cast or boot prior to the transition to regular shoe gear. Larger, displaced fractures may require excision of the fragment or ORIF through a medial approach with either small screw or plate fixation techniques. The FHL should be evaluated intraoperatively for possible injury.

Sustentacular fractures may result in long-term sequelae such as nonunion, altered subtalar joint mechanics, or tendinopathy to the adjacent FHL tendon. While initial surgical treatment may not have been performed, it might be necessary if sequela to the fracture develops.

PHYSICAL EXAMINATION

Calcaneal fractures are primarily the result of high-level trauma. As stated, the high rates of concomitant injuries, not just orthopedic to the extremity but to the head and axial skeletal (and its organ contents) as well, warrant a full body evaluation on first examination. Once potentially more pressing injuries have been either ruled out or stabilized, a focused examination of the extremities can be performed.[34]

Pain is the most obvious symptom, either described by the patient with attempted weight bearing or with direct palpation. Deformity may be present inclusive of shortening and/or widening of the heel, the hindfoot (calcaneal tuber) in varus, and irregular bony prominences secondary to displaced fracture fragments. Deformity can result in restricted passive or active frontal plane hindfoot motion.

Skin evaluation of the extremity includes examining any abrasions, open lacerations, bruising, blisters, and swelling. Plantar arch ecchymosis coined "Mondor sign" may become present 24-48 hours after the injury and is often pathognomonic for calcaneal fractures as a result of blood extravasation from the calcaneus into the central plantar compartment (Fig. 29.7).[35] Both hemorrhagic and nonhemorrhagic blisters may develop, with the former indicating a deeper soft tissue injury. Bony prominent areas should be both evaluated by palpation and visual inspection as displaced fractures may result in pressure necrosis to the skin.

The skin should also be evaluated for the presence of tension lines and a positive "wrinkle test."[36,37] While the origin of this test is not well confounded, it is widely accepted that when

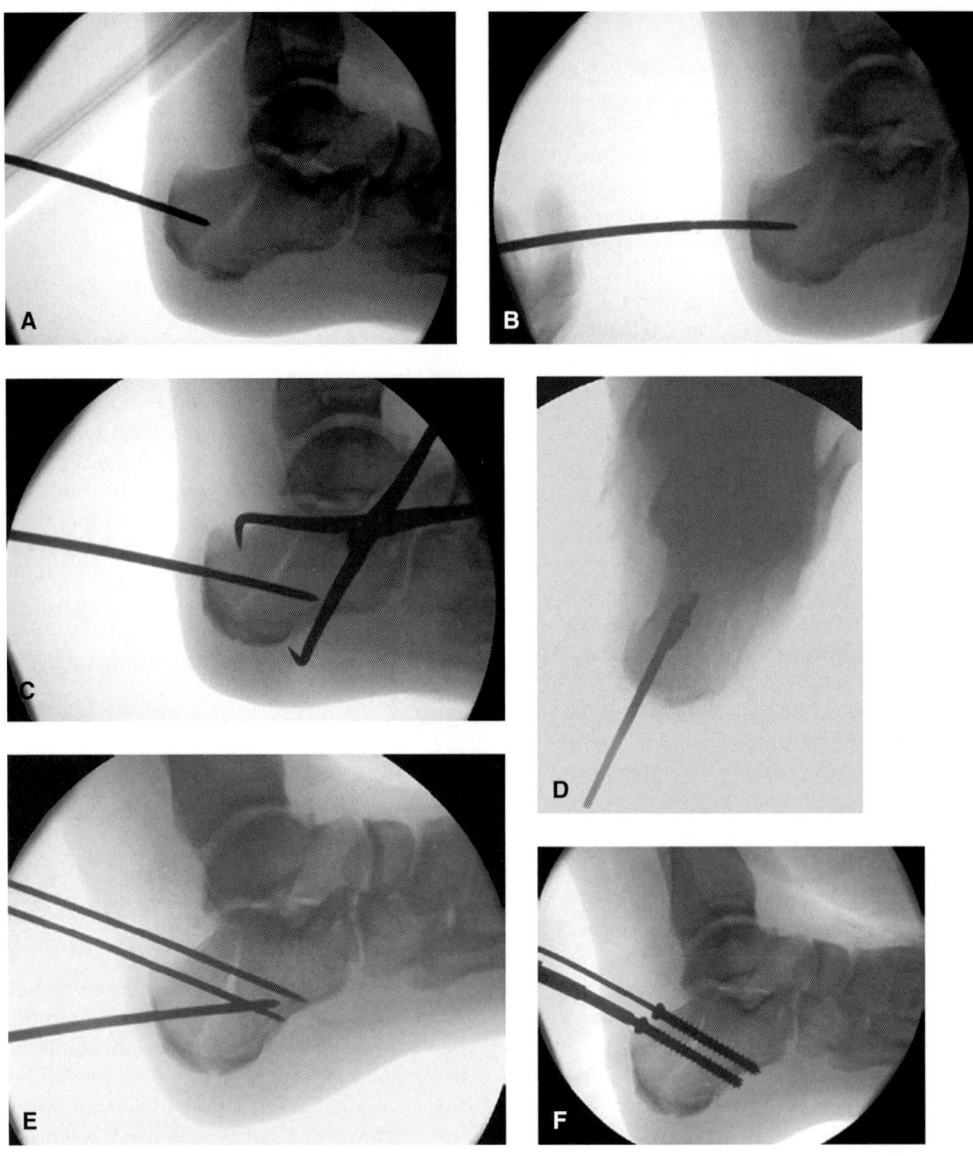

FIGURE 29.6 Reduction technique for beak fractures. A Steinman pin is inserted into the superior tuber fragment to leverage **(A)** and reduce **(B)** the fracture. A large clamp is used to hold the reduction and the Steinman pin is driven across the fracture **(C)**. Axial **(D)** and lateral **(E)** views show heel reduction and pin placement for two screws inserted percutaneously with bicortical purchase to maintain reduction **(F)**.

the surgeon attempts to squeeze or pinch the skin surface and wrinkles can be detected, the test is positive and the patients' skin is ready for surgery.[37] Loss of skin tension lines usually occurs within hours of the trauma and can take between 1 and 3 weeks to return (Fig. 29.8).

Two soft tissue–related specific instances require immediate surgical intervention: open fractures and displaced posterior tuberosity avulsion fractures. In the event of an open fracture, the standard open fracture treatment tenants hold true. Tuberosity fractures may result in pressure necrosis of the posterior skin, and prompt reduction to decrease internal pressure points is necessary to prevent wound development.

Neurovascular status should be evaluated. Patency of the lateral calcaneal artery (LCA) with Doppler is performed as injury to this structure has demonstrated increased complications in healing during open techniques.[38] Medial fracture fragments may result in either posterior tibial artery lesions or tibial nerve impingement. Furthermore, neurological deficits may pose a concern for CS, which occurs between 1% and 10% in calcaneal fractures.[16,17,39]

IMAGING AND DIAGNOSTIC STUDIES

While knowledge of anatomy, a thorough physical examination and classification systems are helpful, other imaging to consider include x-rays to the ipsilateral ankle, contralateral foot and ankle, and thoracolumbar spine due to the high rates of additional injuries in these fractures.[14,15]

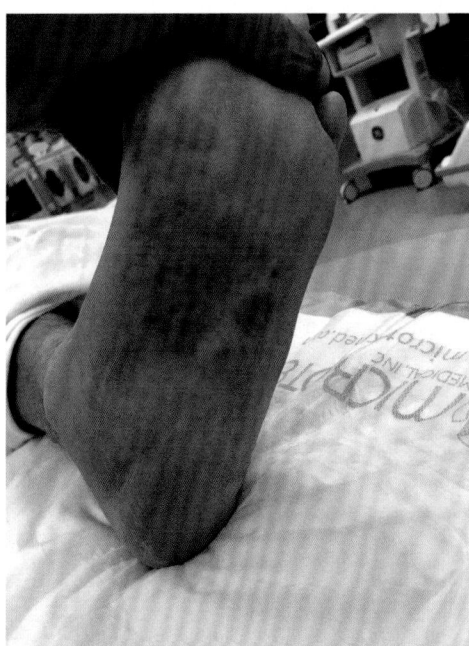

FIGURE 29.7 The Mondor sign of plantar ecchymosis seen in calcaneal fractures.

RADIOGRAPHS

A standard three-view plain x-ray series is the first imaging modality ordered in diagnosing calcaneal fractures. Anteroposterior (AP) and oblique views help evaluate lateral wall blowout, medial talar displacement or subluxation, fracture extension to the CCJ, anterior process fractures, and concomitant foot fractures. The lateral view aids in evaluating key angular relationships in the hindfoot including Böhler angle and the critical angle of Gissane (Fig. 29.3). Essex-Lopresti fractures (tongue-type and joint depression) are fairly obvious on the lateral view. A "double density" sign on the lateral view signifies a fracture through the lateral aspect of the posterior facet typically seen in joint depression fracture types (Fig. 29.9). The more superior line represents the normal anatomic position of the posterior facet, while the more inferior line represents the depressed

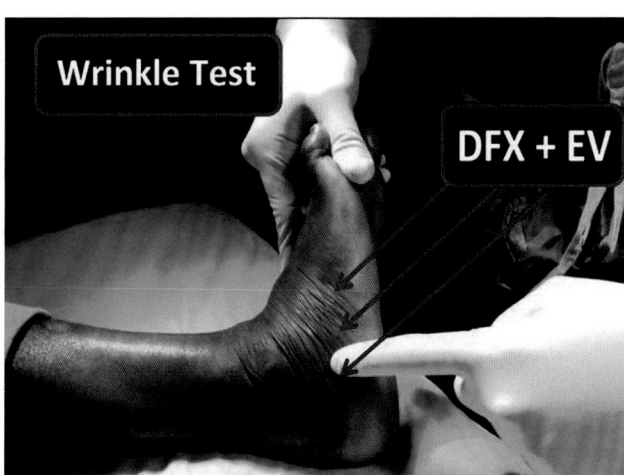

FIGURE 29.8 Positive wrinkle test ~2 weeks postinjury.

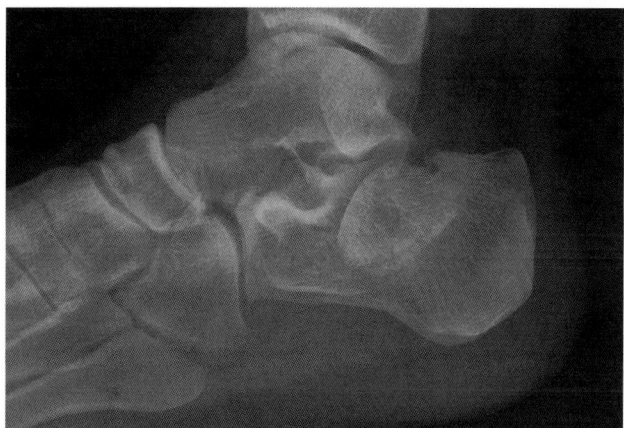

FIGURE 29.9 Double density sign on lateral radiograph.

facet fragment. Other key findings to evaluate for include calcaneal shortening and heel widening from lateral wall blowout, seen either on an AP or calcaneal axial view.

Both a Harris calcaneal axial view and Brodén views can be ordered for evaluation of the posterior facet. Understanding these studies is also helpful as they should be performed under intraoperative fluoroscopy to assess the accuracy of reduction.

A Brodén view aids in evaluating the posterior facet directly. The patient is supine and the foot is positioned resting on the film cassette x-ray plate or flat surface with the leg internally rotated 45 degrees and the foot in neutral (Fig. 29.10). The beam is directed toward the lateral malleolus, and the films are taken at 10, 20, 30, and 40 degrees of cephalic tilt to view all aspects of the posterior facet, with the 10- or 40-degree angulation demonstrating the posterior and anterior aspects, respectively.

The Harris calcaneal axial view is taken by a 45-degree heel axial view with the second toe in line with the tibia and the foot maximally dorsiflexed. These series assess any varus or valgus tuber angulation (normal is ~10-degree valgus), joint displacement, tuberosity angulation, and increased width or lateral wall blowout.

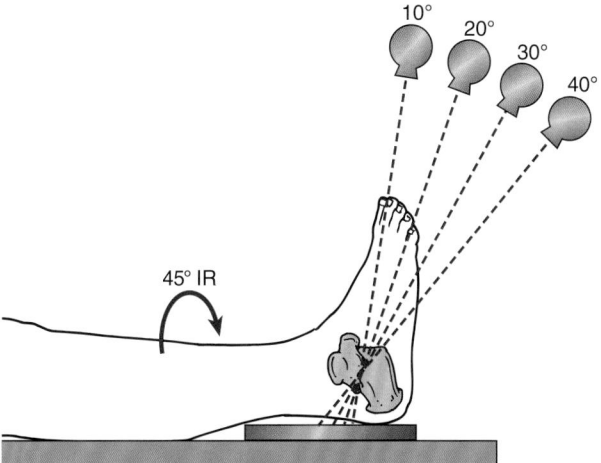

FIGURE 29.10 Brodén view radiograph with the patient's leg internally rotated 45 degrees and four projections are taken at 10-degree intervals off of the perpendicular.

COMPUTED TOMOGRAPHY

A CT scan is required if an intra-articular fracture pattern is detected on x-ray. CT imaging with three-dimensional reconstruction has advanced the understanding and thus ability to treat calcaneal fractures through better visualization and characterization of both fracture lines and fracture displacement.[40] The imaging allows assessment of the fracture pattern, specifically the personality and extent of posterior facet articular disruption, which helps the surgeon prepare in creating a surgical plan for reconstruction. Image confirmation of sustentacular position is important to recognize when using this landmark as the point of which reduction and fixation is built from.[24] Further, it may identify tendon injury or entrapment, which may be an obstacle to reduction.

The Sanders classification uses coronal CT imaging at the widest portion of the posterior facet, inclusive of the sustentaculum, to assess intra-articular calcaneal fractures (ie, involve the posterior facet).[6,7,40] This system is the most commonly used classification because it acts as a guide for treatment recommendations (ie, operative vs nonoperative), surgical recommendations (ie, ORIF vs arthrodesis, approach), and correlates with clinical outcomes (ie, risk factors, potential complications, sequela, secondary surgical requirements).[40] Implementing this system is helpful in both dictating surgical planning and giving a prognosis to the patient.[15]

In addition to assessing the articular surface of the posterior facet, the coronal series reveals sustentacular position, the shape of the heel, and position of the peroneal and FHL tendons in relation to the lateral and medial walls, respectively. Sagittal images aid in the evaluation of joint or tuberosity depression or fracture extension and fractures to the anterior process. Axial images evaluate the CCJ, anteroinferior aspect of the posterior facet, and the sustentaculum tali.

The importance of a CT scan in the treatment of calcaneal fractures cannot be understated. Referencing CT in an intraoperative manner, studies have found that use of intraoperative CT altered the surgeon's reduction or screw placement in ~40% of cases, demonstrating the power of this imaging modality in fully understanding the fracture and obtaining accurate reduction.[41,42]

OTHER IMAGING MODALITIES

Magnetic resonance imaging (MRI) and nuclear medicine imaging are used to diagnosis calcaneal stress fractures in the presence of normal x-rays, normal CT, and/or uncertain diagnosis (Fig. 29.11). In the acute fracture setting, their usefulness is limited although MRI may be helpful to assess soft tissue injuries to tendons and ligaments in calcaneal fractures.

TREATMENT

NONOPERATIVE

Nonoperative management can be employed in nondisplaced articular (Sanders type 1) and nonarticular fracture types. This is the preferred method in stress fractures and also in patients who are deemed unsuitable for surgery. Other indications for nonoperative management include patients with significant peripheral vascular disease or neuropathy, diabetes, severe immunodeficiency, significant tobacco use history, noncompliance, or other surgical contraindications.[34]

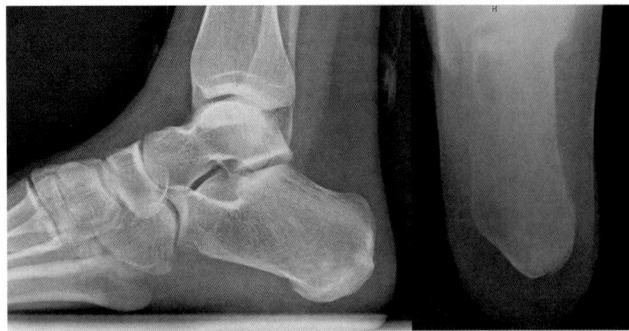

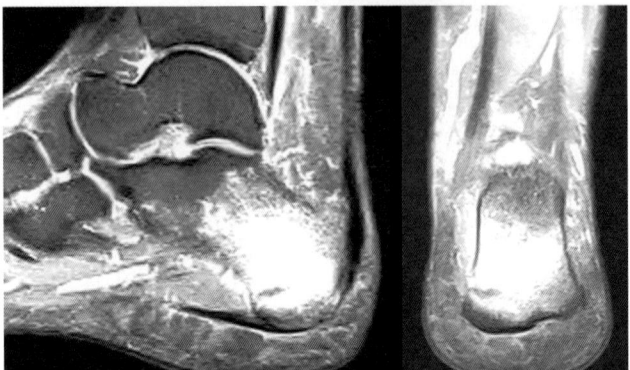

FIGURE 29.11 Radiograph without osseous findings with subsequent magnetic resonance imaging demonstrating stress fracture to the calcaneus after a fall from height.

Plain film x-rays and CT scans are still recommended to confirm the nondisplaced fracture types. Typically, cast immobilization is performed, where the patient is to remain strict non–weight bearing for 8 weeks or longer or until healing is observed across the fracture site. As the fracture continues to heal, the physician may utilize a walking boot to provide further protection and stabilization as the fracture matures.

SURGICAL PROCEDURES AND TECHNIQUES (KD/JM)

Pertinent patient past medical history and potential risk factors that may affect the healing process include the patients' age, vascular status, concurrent immunocompromised disease, bone density, and so forth. Collectively, these factors play a role in determining the best course of treatment for the patient, both conservative vs surgical, and what surgical approach.

INDICATIONS FOR ORIF

- All open fractures
- Methods include management of the open fracture site with delayed ORIF or combinations of external fixation with percutaneous fixation
- Displaced intra-articular fractures involving the posterior facet (Sanders II, III)
- Fracture-dislocation of the calcaneus
- Irreducible body fractures with >30-degree varus or > 40-degree valgus deformity
- Extra-articular fractures
- Displaced fractures of the calcaneal tuberosity
- Displaced avulsion/beak fractures placing the posterior skin at risk
- Anterior process fractures with >25% CCJ involvement

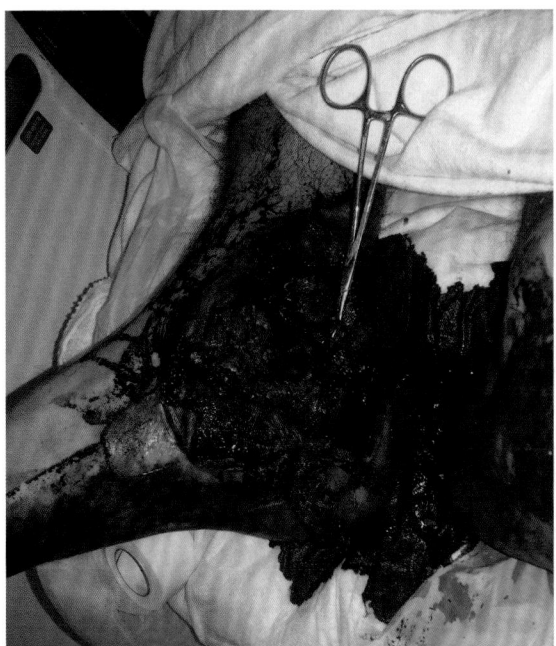

FIGURE 29.12 Open calcaneal fracture after motor vehicle rollover accident. Hemostat is ligating a lacerated tibial vein.

Open fractures of the calcaneus are high-energy injuries with a high rate of morbidity (Fig. 29.12). Open fractures are true surgical emergencies where delayed care has shown poorer patient outcomes. Treatment cornerstones include urgent copious irrigation and debridement of devitalized tissue and foreign material, antibiotic administration, and stabilization of fracture typically with external fixation and percutaneous K-wires. Reduction can be achieved through gross reduction techniques and also with the insertion of a Schanz pin in the lateral calcaneus to allow for direct leverage in aid of fracture reduction.[43,44] Commonly a staged approach is employed, where definitive fixation is reserved at a second operation on average 1-3 weeks from the initial operation as the soft tissues begin to heal without signs of infection.

By adhering to basic open fracture management principles, outcomes have improved.[43] Soft tissue management is of utmost importance in the treatment, preserving the plantar heel pad, protecting the soft tissue envelope, and closely monitoring for any possible superficial or deep infection over time.[28,45] In spite of this, limb amputation is a serious risk and is influenced based on the severity of fracture, amount of contamination in the wound, and the size of the open wound. Amputation rates following an open fracture have been reported as high as 42% in a military population.[46]

Principles of Surgical Fixation of Calcaneal Fractures[29]

- Restore calcaneal height (Böhler angle)
- Narrow calcaneal width
- Restore calcaneal length
- Correct calcaneal tuberosity varus
- Anatomically reduce the posterior facet/joint
- Anatomically reduce the lateral wall/subfibular space
- Anatomically reduce the calcaneocuboid joint (if fractured)
- Bone graft cancellous defects if deemed necessary

Lateral Extensile Approach

A formal extended lateral approach (ELA) to calcaneal fractures is still within the standard of care and may even remain the gold standard of care to achieve anatomic reduction despite newer MIS approaches and hardware systems designed for minimal approaches.[7,38,47-49] The ELA should be considered in fractures that are highly comminuted, have multiple fracture lines (Sanders grade III and IV) through the posterior facet, severe joint depression, fragment rotation or tuber migration, severe varus (>5 degrees) or valgus (>10 degrees) frontal plane deformity, significant shortening, or severe lateral or medial wall blowout.[29,38,49] Typically, these fractures require greater exposure and visualization intraoperation to achieve an appropriate reduction. Further, the ELA allows for full fracture and joint/cartilage visualization when making an intraoperative determination whether to perform ORIF vs primary fusion, or a combination of the two depending on the intra-articular destruction.

Because of the extensive incision and dissection necessary to perform the ELA, the return of skin tension lines and skin re-epithelialization postfracture blisters must be present prior to incision in order to mitigate postoperation complications (eg, incision dehiscence, flap necrosis, and infection). This typically involves a 1- to 2-week waiting period after the injury. Approach contraindications include uncontrolled diabetes, immunocompromised disease, smoking, and open fractures (relative) while more concerning conditions include vascular insufficiency, severe swelling, neuropathy, patient noncompliance, and an inexperienced surgeon.

Position and Preparation

The patient is placed on a radiolucent table in a lateral decubitus position with the operative side up (Fig. 29.13). A bean bag or padded surgical bed bars are used to position the patient with the pelvis perpendicular to the floor, the lateral aspect of the hindfoot is facing upward, and the lateral surface of the foot is parallel to the floor. The contralateral extremity should be oriented to not interfere with intraoperative imaging, typically in leg flexion at the knee to create a figure-four position. A thigh tourniquet is applied and the extremity is prepped to the tourniquet. This allows free mobility of the extremity and ability to flex and extend at the knee when necessary to manipulate the extremity for fracture reduction, hardware placement, and fluoroscopic imaging.

The prone position can be utilized in cases of bilateral calcaneal or calcaneal and concomitant contralateral extremity trauma where the surgeon elects to repair both in the same operative setting negating the need to reposition the patient after one side is complete. It also provides more convenience to obtain both lateral and calcaneal axial imaging throughout the surgery. However, the prone position does come with its own physiological risks to the patient and may not be amenable in all situations.[50] Regardless of the positioning technique used, it is important prior to draping to make sure all bony prominences, especially to the spine, pelvis, and lower extremity are well padded with gel, foam, or pillows to prevent ischemic injury to the skin or nerve palsy.

Incision (Incision/Dissection)

The standard ELA incision popularized by Benirschke and Sangeorzan resembles an "L" or "J" on a right or left foot,

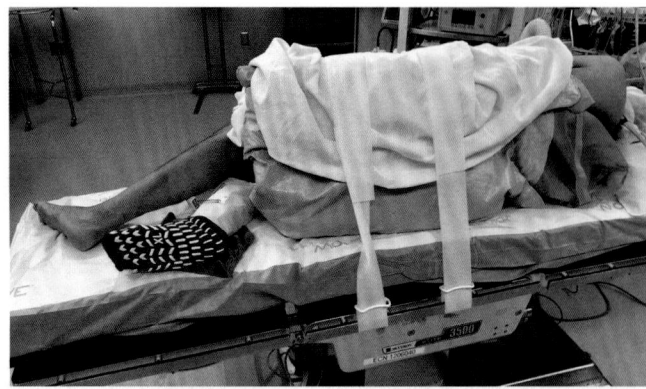

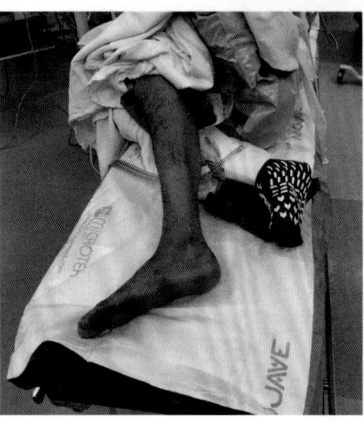

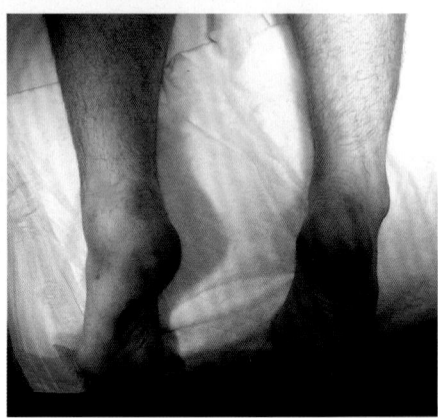

FIGURE 29.13 Positioning of the patient in a well-padded lateral decubitus position with the foot parallel to the floor (**top**, **bottom left**). A prone position is used with bilateral fracture (**bottom right**). Note the left heel in a greater varus positioning from the fracture.

respectively (Fig. 29.14).[8] In a traditional ELA, the vertical arm is centered between and parallel to the anterior edge of the Achilles tendon and posterior edge of the fibula with the horizontal arm parallel to the plantar foot at a level at or just above the glabrous border of the foot. Important structures to consider include the peroneus brevis and longus tendons, CFL, sural nerve, lesser saphenous vein, and LCA. Preoperative marking of landmarks such as an outline of the calcaneal superior, inferior, and posterior borders, the lateral malleolus, the CCJ, and the fourth-fifth metatarsal-cuboid joint under fluoroscopic guidance can assist in proper placement and course of the incision. This is especially helpful in feet that tend to be more cavus or pes planovalgus as anatomical landmarks are often distorted.

The LCA is the terminal branch of the peroneal artery and provides the main arterial supply to the flap and up to 45% of the intraosseous blood supply to the calcaneus.[38,51-53] If not injured during the initial trauma, it may be secondarily injured through edema-induced thrombosis or iatrogenically through surgical incision placement. This results in impaired microvascularization and a reduced partial pressure of oxygen to the lateral flap.[36] Bibbo et al. established a strong link between wound complications and arterial patency during the ELA for calcaneal fractures.[38] Sirisreetreerux et al. found decreased flap perfusion rates in simulated LCA injuries in cadaveric studies when comparing a standard vs modified ELA with no standard ELA demonstrating superior perfusion rates.[54] Because of the importance of this artery, others have studied modified lateral extensile approaches to avoid the LCA.[51,53,54]

The LCA pierces the deep fascia to become superficial at mean of 3.78 cm superior to a midpoint between the tip of the lateral malleolus and Achilles insertion and travels distally on average 11.6 mm anterior to the lateral border of the Achilles.[38,51,54] Recommended modifications targeted at the vertical limb suggest placement 3 cm posterior to the lateral malleolus or 0.75 cm anterior to the Achilles tendon.[51,54] Moving this incision ~1 cm posterior from the standard position of equidistance between the Achilles and fibula has been shown to decrease encountering the LCA by fourfold.[53] Sural nerve injury is also lowered as the incision is moved closer to the margin of the Achilles tendon.[18] The proximal extension and path of the vertical incision should be performed with Doppler with an incision starting point at 3-4 cm proximal to the calcaneal superior surface.[53] The linear horizontal arm terminates at the CCJ. The apex should be an obtuse angle no less than or between 100 and 110 degrees, with a distal curve superior toward the fourth or fifth metatarsal base over the calcaneal tubers posteroinferior margin at the CCJ.[36,55] Sharp angles closer to 90 degrees may increase apex necrosis.[56] Incision length is ~7-8 cm per arm depending on the technique implemented.

Use of standard superficial (layered) skin incision and dissection techniques at the regions above and below the calcaneal tuber is preferred. Over the tuber (central third of the incision about the apex), the blade can be inserted full thickness to the bone. Care must be taken for the sural nerve during dissection at the proximal and distal extent of the incision and avoidance of skiving. A full-thickness dissection is performed to lift the flap, which includes the periosteum, subcutaneous tissue, peroneal tendons, CFL, sural nerve, and LCA as one unit. The flap can be created with sharp blade dissection or use of elevator instrumentation (eg, Key, Sayre, Chandler, or Cobb). Full exposure of the

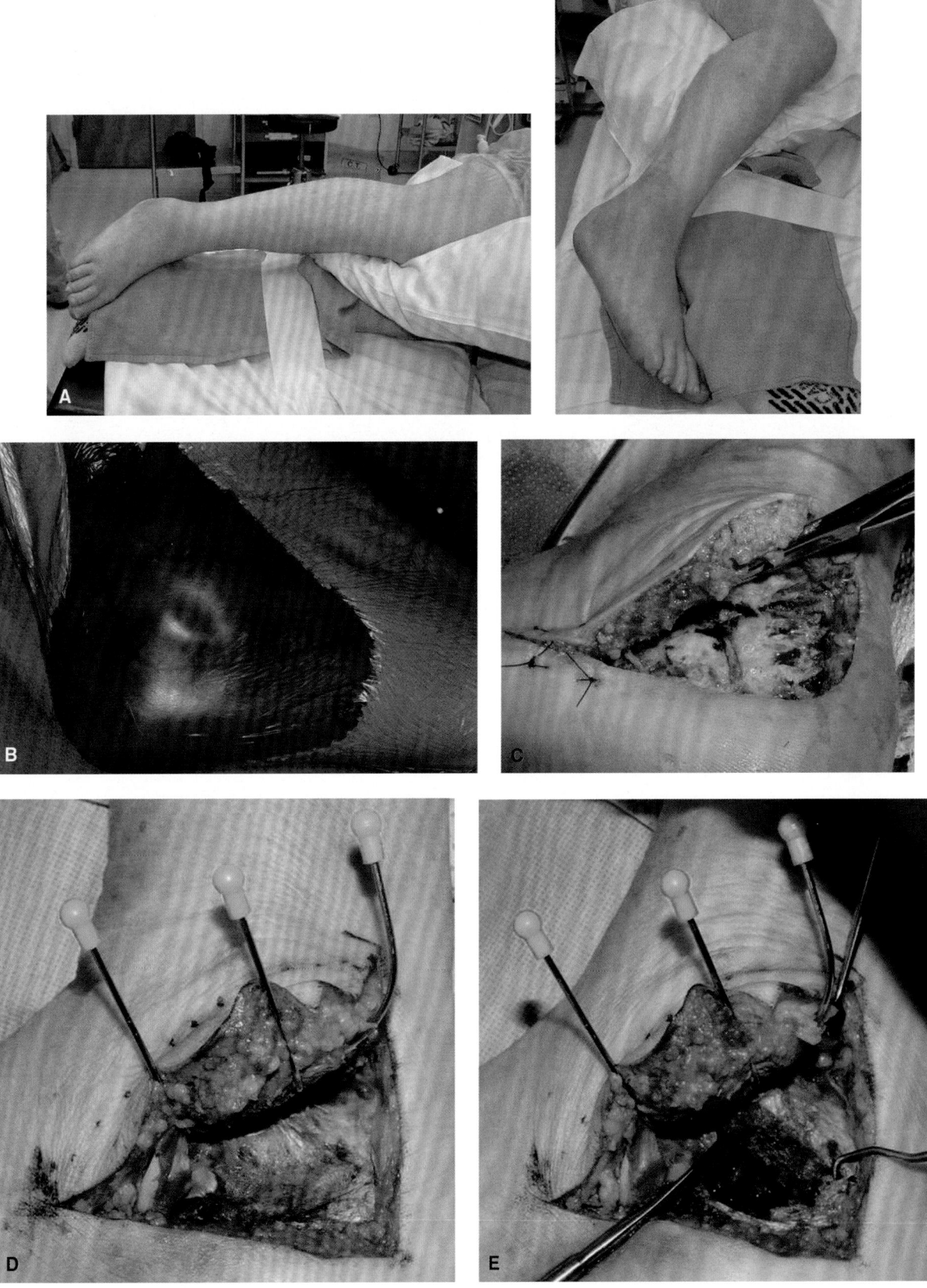

FIGURE 29.14 **A.** Positioning of the patient in a well-padded lateral decubitus position with the foot parallel to the floor allows for optimal radiographic visualization. **B.** The incision should be perpendicular to the skin, especially at the apex of the flap, to attempt to minimize wound complications. **C.** Sharp dissection is utilized to elevate the flap off of the lateral surface in a single layer. **D.** Demonstration of wires placed into the neck of body of the talus, cuboid, and distal fibula and bent superiorly to provide tension-free retraction of the flap.

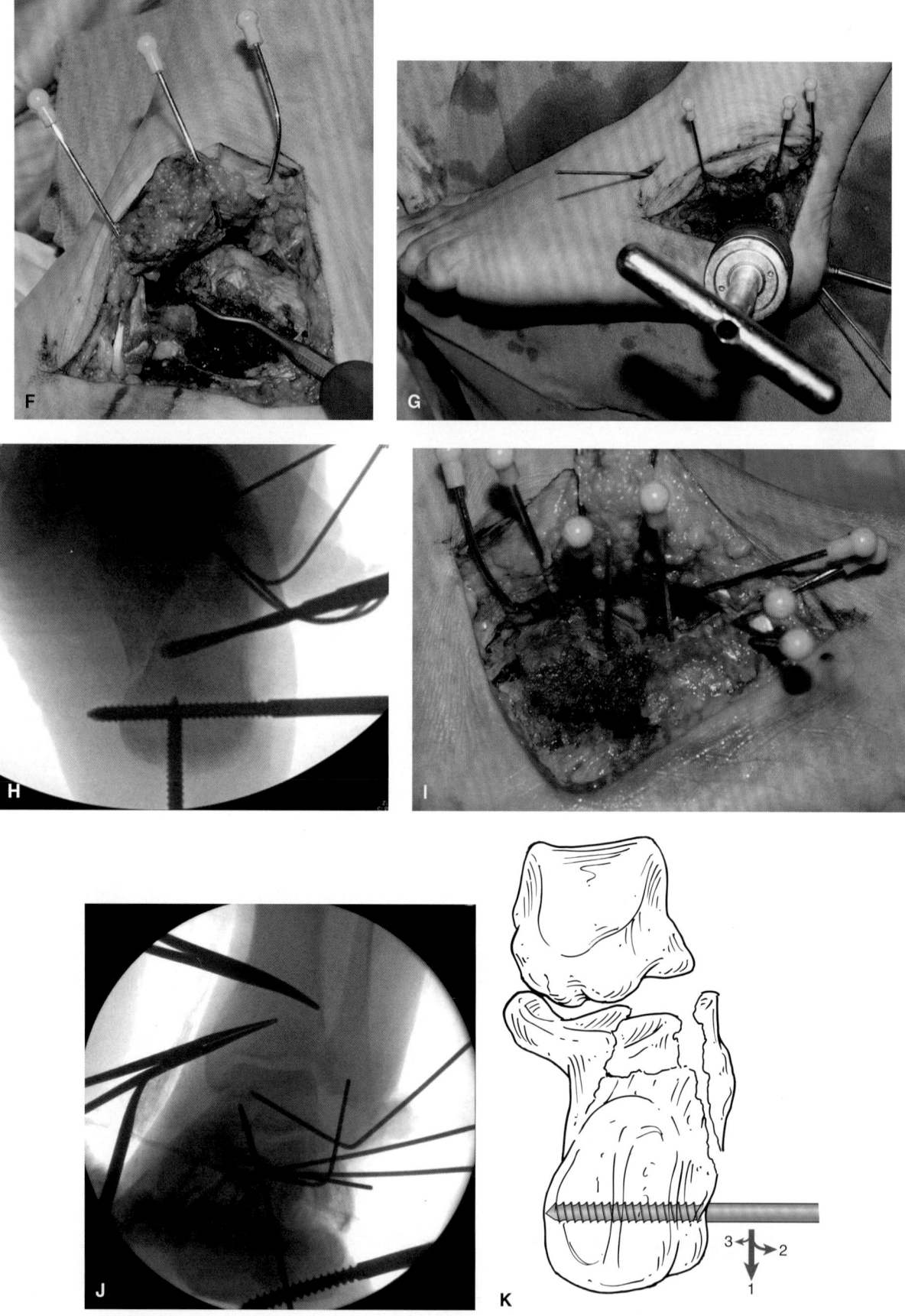

FIGURE 29.14 (*Continued*) **E, F.** Multiple articular fragments are tagged for orientation and used later in the reconstruction. **G.** A 5.0-mm Schanz pin is placed into the tuber fragment for jockeying of the tuber. This is placed from the lateral surface. **H.** The tuber is inverted to identify and evacuate the primary fracture line. **I.** The posterior facet fragments are replaced and secured under direct visualization. **J.** The intraoperative Brodén view is imperative to ensure restoration of the facet. **K.** The tuber is repositioned by mobilizing it medially and distally while derotating the varus position.

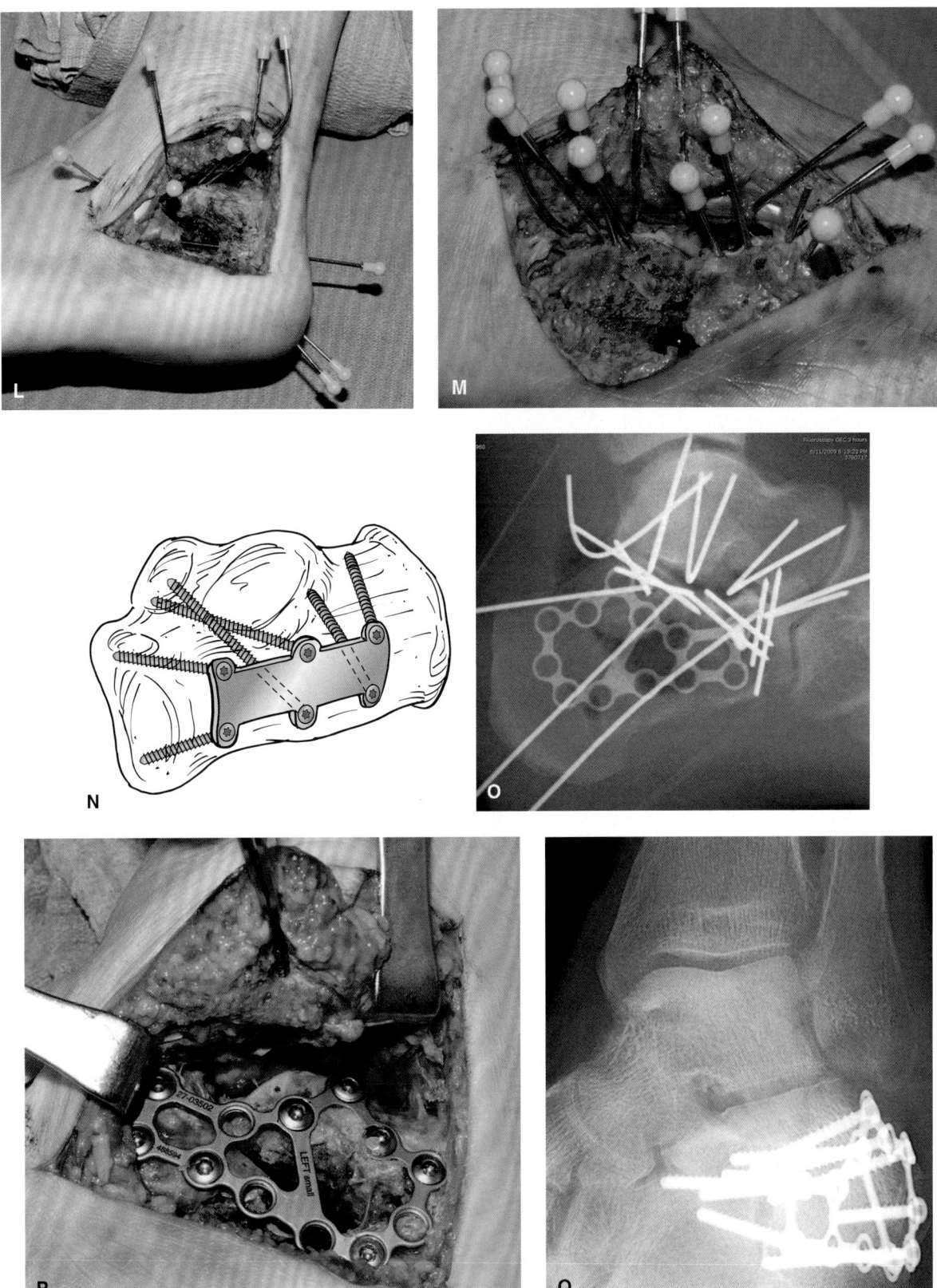

FIGURE 29.14 (*Continued*) **L.** Large K-wires are inserted from the posterior inferior aspect of the tuber into the sustentacular fragment. **M.** A K-wire should be inserted into the anterior distal edge of the anterior block, just proximal to the calcaneocuboid joint, and driven to the stable sustentacular fragment. **N.** Fixation must be targeted to areas of dense bone to attain stable fixation. **O.** Malleable plates will deform and conform to the morphology of the reduced bone, whereas the more rigid plates will have a tendency to deform the reduction.

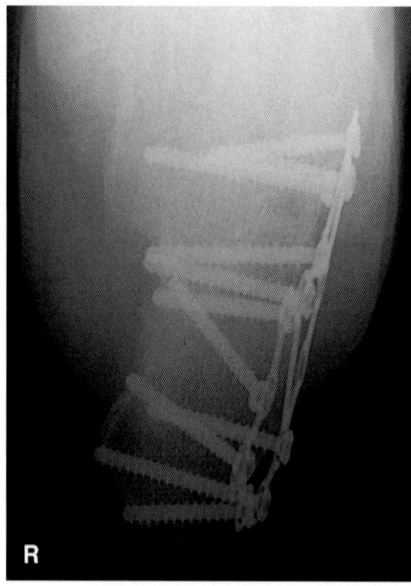

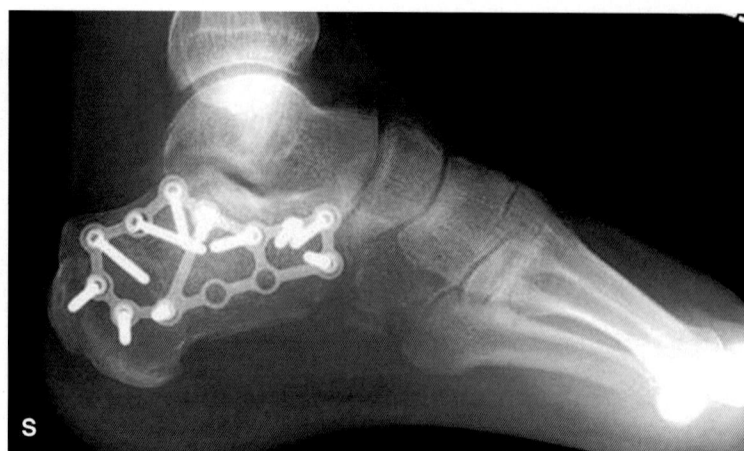

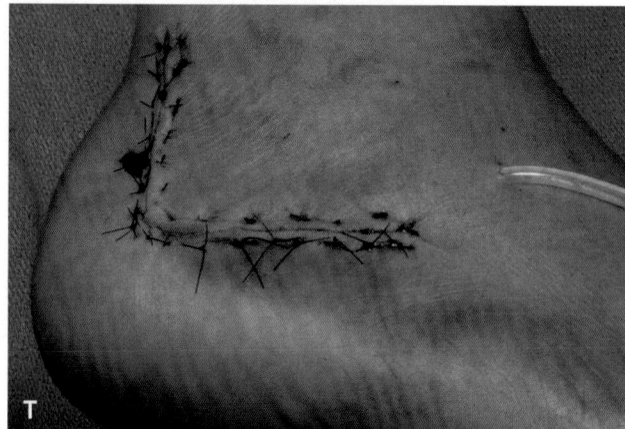

FIGURE 29.14 (*Continued*) **P–S.** Screws are placed for definitive fixation, fluoroscopy is employed to confirm placement, and K-wire temporary fixation is then removed. **T.** A hybrid apical stitch is placed as to not strangulate the apex of the incision.

lateral wall of the calcaneus should be achieved to visualize the superior calcaneus, subtalar joint, entire lateral wall, and CCJ. A "no touch technique" with respect to the flap to maintain skin edge integrity is implemented by placing 1.6- or 2.0-mm K-wires into the distal fibula, talar neck, and cuboid, bending the wires superiorly in order to retract the flap and structures contained within for the duration of the procedure without the need to handle.[29]

Other less commonly used approaches include a sustentacular incision, medial extended incision popularized by McReynolds et al. and Burdeaux et al., combined medial and lateral incisions reported on by Stephenson et al. and Romash et al., and the posterolateral (combination of the ELA and Cincinnati incisions).[29,55,57] Medial approaches allow visualization of the tuberosity to sustentacular fragment with limited visualization of the posterior facet fragment, while ELA has limited sustentacular fragment visualization.[24] The choice for additional incisions should be based upon the fracture pattern, each fraught with their own limitations. These approaches will not be described in this chapter.

PEARLS—LATERAL EXTENSILE APPROACH INCISION

- L (right foot) or J (left foot) shape incision
- Doppler map the lateral calcaneal artery to determine a safe proximal starting point
- Vertical arm is 3 cm posterior to the posterior border of the fibula
- Horizontal arm is along the lateral glabrous border of the foot
- Apex at an angle >100 degrees
- Full thickness over the calcaneus

Reduction

The principles of calcaneal fracture reduction have been well described.[8,29] Once the bone is encountered, the loose lateral wall should be reflected plantarly or removed if free and placed in a saline-soaked sponge for later replacement. Upon removal, the surgeon will be able to visualize the main fracture line(s) and fragment(s) that require reduction. Any hematoma should be evacuated to aid in visualization.

To aid in tuber manipulation, a 5.0-mm Schanz pin is placed into the tuber either from a lateral or posterior position.[8] Placement of the pin should be into what is determined to be the strongest or most intact portion of the tuber to prevent pull-out or in the correct fragment if a tuberosity fracture vs tongue-type fracture. If placed laterally (lateral to medial), a bicortical purchase should be obtained. Through utilization of a T-handle attached to the pin, the tuber can then be manipulated in varus/valgus and distraction to begin restoring the calcaneal anatomy can be performed.

The anteromedial "constant" sustentacular fragment is the foundation of which reconstruction of the posterior facet is built upon to restore joint congruity.[24,58] Once confirmed it is in the appropriate position, the pieces of the posterior facet are restored to their anatomic height and orientation using the sustentaculum tali as the foundation point. Often the posterior facet fragment needs to be disimpacted and elevated due to its depressed state. Applying a distal pull on the Schanz pin initially will aid in disimpacting the fractured posterior facet and sustentacular fragment. A periosteal or freer elevator is used to pry the fragment in a superior direction to restore articular height. As reconstruction proceeds, various K-wires are temporarily used to hold fragments in their restored anatomic locations, typically anchoring the posterior facet to the sustentaculum fragment and anterior process. The sustentacular wire should have a trajectory of starting posterior and lateral, heading anteromedial.[59] One may need to hold the tuberosity distraction until K-wire fixation between the posterior facet and sustentacular fragment is performed. Occasionally, articular pieces are removed and replaced once the reduction has been stabilized. In the presence of CCJ involvement, the reduction is performed through one or two wires placed lateral to medial, parallel with the joint surface.

If the sustentaculum tali is not in anatomic location due to fracture subluxation/displacement or it is comminuted, direct medial approach reconstruction must be performed first through either a dual medial-lateral incision approach or complete calcaneal reconstruction through a medial approach.[24]

Using the Schanz pin, the tuberosity fragment is anatomically aligned in a stepwise maneuver to reduce the joint depression, and varus/laterally translated tuber described by Benirschke et al.[8] This includes (1) pulling it distally out to length; (2) derotating it into a slight valgus (from its varus position); and (3) translating it medially to place it back underneath the long axis of the tibia.[8] The previously described Essex-Lopresti maneuver (*see Extra-articular fractures: Tuberosity—Avulsion/ Beak*) may also be implemented in tongue-type fractures with limited posterior facet involvement, whereas it is less amenable for joint depression fractures.[12,13] The surgeon should ensure to bend the knee and hold the ankle in flexion when attempting reduction to relax the Achilles/gastrocnemius muscle pull.

Provisional wires are used to hold the tuber reduction, inserted in an axial direction from the posteroinferior heel in an anterosuperior direction into the sustentacular fragment and anterior calcaneus proximal to the CCJ. This will ultimately reduce the tuberosity (body) fragment to the sustentacular fragment. Fine tuning may be required in order to achieve the main goals in reduction.

In some cases, tuberosity fragment reduction and provisional fixation are necessary to perform first to then accommodate posterior facet and anterior fragment reduction. An example of this includes a grossly comminuted posterior facet where reduction of the tuberosity first into the constant fragment provides a stable foundation for facet restoration. While there are overall many techniques and approaches for full anatomic reduction, the goals are the same and clear fluoroscopic confirmation of reduction is mandatory as direct visualization is often difficult to confirm.

With the patient in the lateral position and working on the lateral side of the foot, there is a tendency for the foot to fall into varus. The surgeon must ensure that the hindfoot remains in neutral or slight valgus on axial views throughout each step of reduction and avoid varus hindfoot at all costs. It is important to obtain not just lateral views to evaluate facet height but also Harris axial views to assess the tuber in the frontal plane and Brodén view to evaluate any articular step-off. Subtalar joint arthroscopy can be performed to evaluate for anatomic joint congruency. It is vital to have anatomic reduction and deformity correction prior to hardware placement. Once all provisional K-wire fixation has achieved these goals and fluoroscopic evaluation in multiple planes and views confirms reduction, definitive fixation can be implemented.

Bone graft (ie, autograft, cancellous allograft, polymethylmethacrylate, bone substitutes) can be packed into any deficits. Lenormant first described its use in calcaneal fracture ORIF in 1928.[60] Two common injectable synthetic bone substitutes used in periarticular fractures are calcium sulfate and phosphate due to their mechanical support and osteoconductive properties.[61] Calcium sulfate has faster integration and is recommended when there is a concern for intra-articular extravasation due to its more rapid absorption and lower risk for heterotopic ossification. The use of calcium phosphate is recommended for prolonged support secondary to its slower absorption rate and high compressive strength.

Reviewing the literature, there is no clear consensus as to which option is better: whether to graft or not to graft, with both sides offering a rationale for their choice.[8,27,60,62,63] Grafting is believed to stimulate early fracture healing, lead to earlier weight bearing, and increase mechanical strength to prevent either posttraumatic arthritis or late collapse. Others believe that the highly vascular calcaneus routinely heals radiographically in 4-8 weeks without the need of grafts. Locking plate technology offers enough mechanical strength and the use of graft actually increases infection rates, blood loss, and postoperative pain along with donor site morbidity in cases of autografting.

Various authors have noted improved variables postoperation with bone graft use inclusive of restoration and retained measurement of Böhler angle, Gissane angle, calcaneal width/height postoperation, and a quicker return to full weight bearing while seeing similar or greater functional outcomes (ie, AOFAS scores) with similar or reduced complication/infection rates (ie, wound edge necrosis, superficial or deep infection, hematoma, and sural nerve injury) between the two groups.[27,60,62,63]

A survey by Schepers et al. noted traumatologist and orthopedic surgeon responses of 20% definite graft use, 38% no graft use, and 42% grafting when deemed necessary for treatment of intra-articular calcaneal fractures.[39] As one can see, the literature is varied and the surgeon should rely on sound clinical decision-making if and/or when to use a bone graft.

Fixation

Independent screw fixation is placed in either a lag or nonlag fashion, especially in areas of high comminution where lagged compression may distort the reduction. Initially, one or two 3.5-4.0 mm cancellous screws are placed subthalamic with at least one screw into the sustentacular fragment for posterior facet reduction.[59] Screws are placed just inferior to the posterior facet with a trajectory from posterior and lateral to anterior and medial. The goal is for the threaded portion of the screw to be placed in the strong medial sustentacular cortical bone, provided it is anatomic, and without too much length to injury the medial structures. Lag fixation is preferred to compress the lateral and sustentacular fragments to obtain osseous stability and prevent gaps in the posterior facet.[29,58] This will also aid in decreasing bone substitute extravasation into the subtalar joint if utilized.

Techniques have been offered to reduce error for safe positioning of pin and screw placement in the subthalamic region. Bussewitz et al. states from a reference point 22 mm proximal to the CCJ, direct hardware (eg, temporary wire or screw fixation) starting 16 mm proximal to and at a 30-degree angle from the reference point from posterolateral to anteromedial to land in the center of the sustentaculum tali.[59] Phisitkul et al. suggest starting 15 mm inferior to the posterior facet and aiming toward the joint at a 20-degree angle less than perpendicular to the joint line with 3.5-mm diameter screws averaging 40 mm in length.[64]

The lateral wall piece is replaced last. Perimeter plate fixation can then be implemented utilizing various systems that exist offering differences in design, shape, metals, and construct with the ability to use screws, both locking and nonlocking, applied in either fixed or polyaxial orientations. Zwipp et al. found that through the use of locking plate technology, their need for bone grafting dropped to 3.8% of cases compared to 53% of cases using more traditional plating systems.[29] While all these variables exist, the plate should be long enough to cover and provide fixation into the calcaneal tuber, posterior facet, and the anterior column, while not extending above or below the bones margins especially at the subtalar joint (STJ) and CCJ. It is recommended to avoid hardware placement in the vicinity of the apex due to the areas high breakdown rate. The presence of hardware can result in either irritation from beneath or if dehiscence occurs, the visible risk of exposed hardware. Attempts should be made to place at least two screws in each major fragment or region (ie, subthalamic into the sustentaculum, tuberosity, anterior process adjacent to the CCJ).[29] If able, screws should be directed to the sustentacular fragment.[8]

Fracture extension to the CCJ can be reduced through either one or two 3.5-4.0 mm independent cancellous screws or screw through plate fixation. Smaller anterior process fractures can be fixed directly with one screw, while smaller or comminuted pieces that are not amenable to hardware can be removed or morselized into grafting material.

Closure

Prior to closure, the surgical field should be packed with wet gauze and pressure applied as the tourniquet is deflated. Bovie cauterization is used for active bleeding vessels and the wound edges, avoiding contact with the skin. This will mitigate hematoma development, which may threaten the ELA flap.

Incision closure is performed in two-layered fashion with the periosteum and subcutaneous layers closed as one using absorbable suture in a horizontal mattress pattern. Interrupted Allgöwer-Donati pattern sutures have been shown to apply the least effect on cutaneous blood flow and are recommended for flap closure to mitigate skin ischemia.[65] Starting at the proximal and distal extents, alternating closure at each arm allows for even tension as the flap is advanced to the apex. There should be no tension on the distal corner of the incision and the skin should be opposed, not strangulated. Sutures should be left in place for a minimum of 3 weeks.[66] A drain is highly recommended to prevent hematoma formation and skin embarrassment. This should be placed prior to layered closure, after tourniquet deflation and hemostasis is controlled, with the egress tube placed along the lateral wall. It is not unusual for 100-150 mL of blood to drain after calcaneal ORIF.[56] Lin et al. found that the use of non–Allgöwer-Dontai suture and lack of postoperative drain use were each a risk factor for postoperative wound infection (with an odds ratio of 2.076 and 2.994, respectively).[67]

The extremity is placed in a multilayer compression Jones splint to accommodate for tidal swelling. The ankle should be in neutral flexion to maintain mild stretch to the Achilles tendon. A below knee fiberglass cast can be used after 1-2 weeks once postoperative swelling has receded. Negative-pressure vacuum-assisted closure (VAC) utilized as an incisional VAC for preventative measures has also been recommended and can be effective at reducing wound complications and seromas.[18]

Steps: Calcaneal ORIF—Lateral Extensile Approach[68]

- Lateral extensile incision
  - Subperiosteal dissection
  - Full-thickness flap
- Lateral wall removal to visualize impacted joint
- Disimpaction and reduction through the use of Schanz pin through the tuber with an elevation of the posterior facet
- Anatomic reduction of the posterior facet with provisional, then screw fixation (lateral to medial subcortical into the sustentacular fragment)
- Tuberosity reduction through Benirschke reduction maneuver:
  - Distal traction
  - Valgus rotation
  - Medialization
- Anatomic reduction of the tuber with provisional, then screw fixation (posterior to anterior into the sustentacular fragment)
- Bone graft regions of bone loss if needed
- Replacement of the lateral wall
- Spanning plate and screw fixation
- Layered closure over a drain

PERCUTANEOUS AND MINIMALLY INVASIVE APPROACHES

Due to the high reported rates of complications with the ELA, alternative techniques have been recommended including percutaneous reduction (arthroscopic or fluoroscopic assisted), external fixation, and lateral STA with the same goals of anatomic articular reduction and restoration of Böhler angle, while minimizing risks and complications to the lateral soft tissue. The most commonly used MIS approach is the lateral STA designed

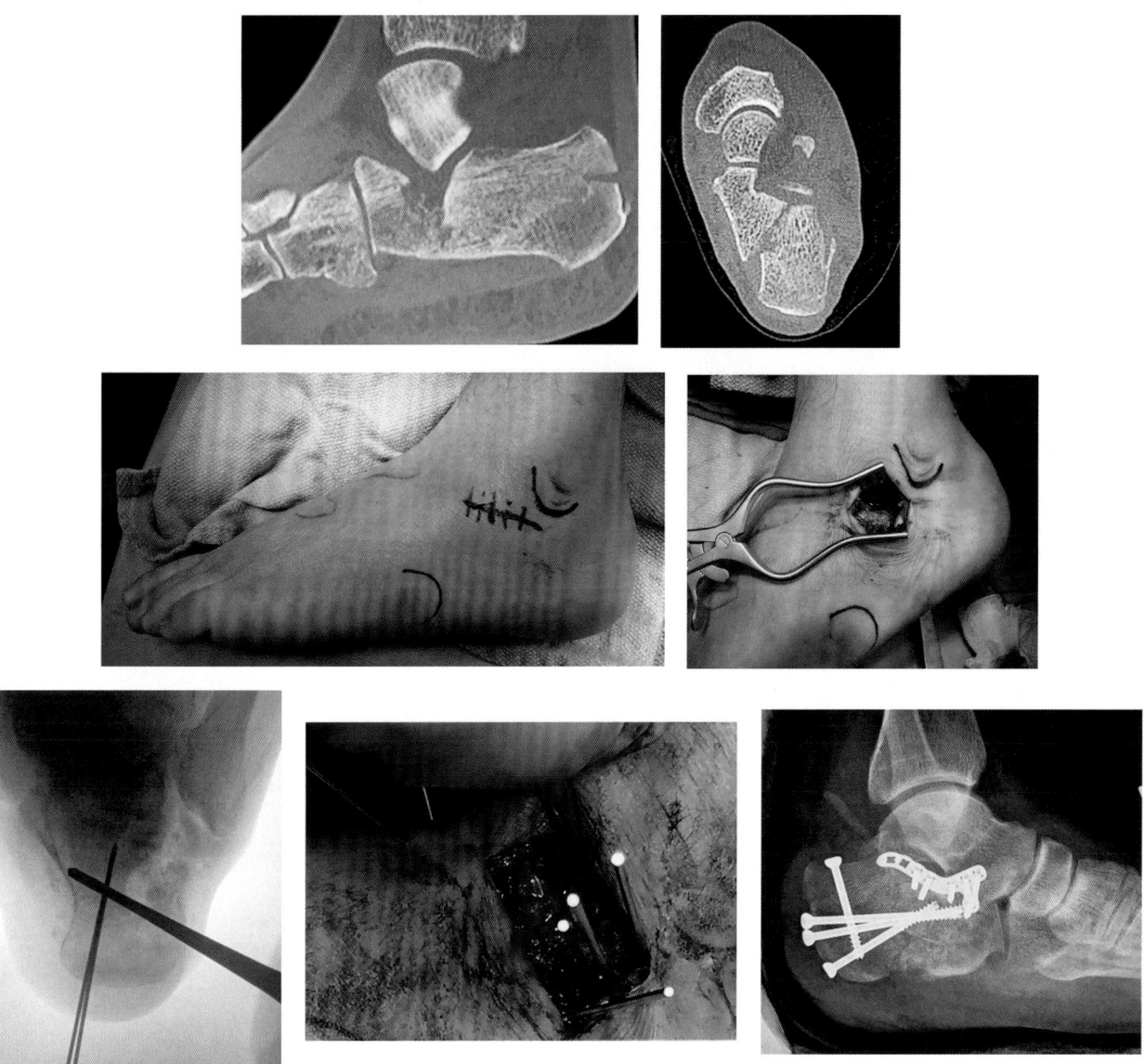

FIGURE 29.15 Minimally invasive reduction can be performed through the sinus tarsi approach. A Schanz can be introducing into the heel, or as shown here a freer through the lateral sinus tarsi incision to elevate the joint depression. Percutaneous K-wires are used to hold the reduction and a subthalamic plate placed to re-create the angle of Gissane. Additional percutaneous screws oriented toward the sustentaculum fragment to aid in reconstruction.

to evaluate the posterior facet and create a small window for achieving articular restoration while reducing neurovascular injury and subsequent wound complications (Fig. 29.15).[47]

Multiple studies have looked at comparing the ELA and less invasive approaches, bringing into question whether the ELA should still be performed.[69] Yao et al. performed a meta-analysis comparing ELA vs STA, demonstrating that latter reduces the risk of wound complications and resulted in fewer secondary surgical procedures.[47] Further, they demonstrated that despite a more limited exposure, the quality of reduction (ie, posterior facet, CCJ, Böhler angle, Gissane angle) was not jeopardized while also maintaining reduction (ie, joint congruency, calcaneal height and width, Böhler angle) postoperatively. Others have found similar or improved results in using limited approaches for Sanders type I-III fractures with respect to shorter time to surgery, postoperative wound complications

(0%-11% vs up to 33%), anatomic reduction, shorter operative times, functional outcomes, and radiographic results when comparing the STA and ELA.[19,21,47,69-72]

Depending on the technique employed, similar reduction and fixation techniques can also be instituted, especially with respect to independent screw placement and smaller, approach specific plate fixation.[73] The scenarios are variable, and it is up to the surgeon's understanding of the fracture pattern and fixation techniques to choose the most appropriate for their situation, rather than for the goal of quicker progression to ORIF or a shorter operative time. Most surgeons will agree that implementing these approaches for joint depression fractures with limited posterior facet involvement (Sanders type I-II, Sanders type IIC) and tongue-type fracture patterns is appropriate.[13,20] As surgeon experience increases, a wider range of fractures may be attempted.

Reduction

Various methods of reduction can be performed either through an STA or small percutaneous incisions depending on the technique attempted. Ultimately, the approach and reduction will dictate the fixation used. A Schanz pin is inserted into the main tuberosity fragment. Then through the incision, a freer or periosteal elevator is used to elevate the posterior facet and stabilize it to the sustentacular fragment with lateral to medial placed K-wires. This aids in restoring calcaneal height and the medial wall.[58] If this proves to be difficult secondary to impaction, a distraction force may be applied with the Schanz pin to free up the fragments. Many of the same reduction techniques described in the ELA section can be implemented during the STA or percutaneous approach for tuberosity reduction. This includes both Schanz pin manipulation of the tuberosity in either an Essex Lopresti maneuver (for tongue-type or displaced tuberosity fractures with limited posterior facet fracture) or Benirschke maneuver (for displaced calcaneal fractures).[8,12,13] The Schanz pin should be inserted into the correct portion of the tuber for reduction.

K-wires are used to fixate the tuberosity fragment to the sustentacular fragment or into the anterior calcaneus for tongue-type fractures. Small joint arthroscopy, either placed through the incision or new portals, can be implemented to either aid in or check reduction if articular congruency is questioned or difficult to ascertain by fluoroscopy.[29,58,72] After provisional K-wire or subthalamic screw fixation to the joint is performed, a varus stress can be applied through the Schanz pin in the tuberosity and a scope is introduced into the joint to evaluate for residual step-off. The CCJ reduction is performed directly with the extended incision and one or two wires placed lateral to medial are positioned parallel to the joint, prepared for cannulated screw use.

Fixation

Definitive fixation is implemented through strategically positioned free-standing screws across the various fracture lines, similar to the lateral extensile approach. There are three main methods of achieving fixation, as described below. As like other approaches to the calcaneus, these approaches require sufficient experience and multiple skills (eg, calcaneal fracture fixation, percutaneous techniques, small joint arthroscopy) to responsibly implement them in practice.[58]

Percutaneous Screws

Percutaneous reduction, wire, and screw placement have been mentioned through the discussion of calcaneal ORIF (Fig. 29.16). Strict percutaneous-only methods allow for fewer wound problems but can pose an issue making reduction more difficult and, therefore, may be more appropriate in limited fracture configurations (Sanders II and III) or tuberosity fracture patterns.[9,13,59] However, the skills of percutaneous surgery added to MIS techniques such as the STA and mixed types of hardware (eg, screws, plates, nails) can aid in the ability to perform the reconstruction.

Typical reconstruction screws are placed (1) subthalamic starting lateral in an anteromedial direction fixating the posterior fragment to the sustentacular; (2) posteroinferior to anterosuperior from the tuberosity fragment into the sustentacular fragment; and (3) lateral to medial across any anterior calcaneal fracture. Implementing techniques for the posterior facet to sustentacular fragment fixation previously described increase precision in screw placement, especially in instances of MIS techniques (eg, sinus tarsi, percutaneous) where position and fluoroscopic guidance weigh heavier than direct visualization.[59,64] Posterior to anterior tuberosity screws can be used as points of stabilization but also be used as positional screws to elevate and support the posterior facet from below at the subchondral bone plate in a "push screw" technique. The CCJ reduction is performed with one or two lateral to medial placed 3.5-4.0 mm cancellous screws, parallel with the joint, on the lower two-thirds of the anterior calcaneus.

Plating

Standard small to mid-sized footprint plates may be placed through the STA and function appropriately if well contoured. MIS hardware systems also have been created for the STA. These plates are often shaped to mirror the angle of Gissane (obtuse V-shape) with arms extending across the calcaneal tuber. Some of the screws may be placed under direct visualization through the incision, while others are inserted percutaneously with jig-assistance (Fig. 29.15).

Primary Subtalar Arthrodesis

In severely comminuted intra-articular fractures, a primary subtalar joint arthrodesis should be considered (Fig. 29.17). As the need for a secondary subtalar joint arthrodesis secondary to posttraumatic arthritis varies as high as 14%, an even higher rate is associated with Sanders type IV fractures secondary to severe, higher energy cartilage damage.[6,74,75] A subtalar joint arthrodesis should be combined with open reduction and internal fixation as restoration of normal calcaneal architecture should be a primary objective. Reduction of primary fracture fragments and reduction of a heel varus can be achieved followed by joint preparation and insertion of large diameter lag screws (6.5-8.0 mm) across the subtalar joint.

Current reports have yielded favorable outcomes over revisional surgery where osteotomies, bone grafting, and exchange of hardware are necessitated in combination with a secondary subtalar joint fusion.[74-76]

Primary Subtalar Arthrodesis

- A traditional sinus tarsi approach is utilized, starting from the tip of the lateral malleolus and continuing to the base of the fourth metatarsal.
- Evaluation of the peroneal tendons is performed and the extensor digitorum brevis is typically seen and split to gain access to the subtalar joint.
- Reduction of the large fragments is achieved in a traditional manner, special care to reduce the tuber from a varus position and restore calcaneal height.
- Once reduction is achieved, meticulous joint preparation is performed within the subtalar joint until healthy, bleeding underlying bone is encountered.
- The usage of bone grafting may be needed (autograft or allograft).
- Large diameter screws are placed in a lag technique spanning across the subtalar joint.
- Care to restore the height of the calcaneus is important and will lead to less cases of anterior ankle joint impingement.
- Secondary fixation may be required of the calcaneus fractures in addition to fusion screws.

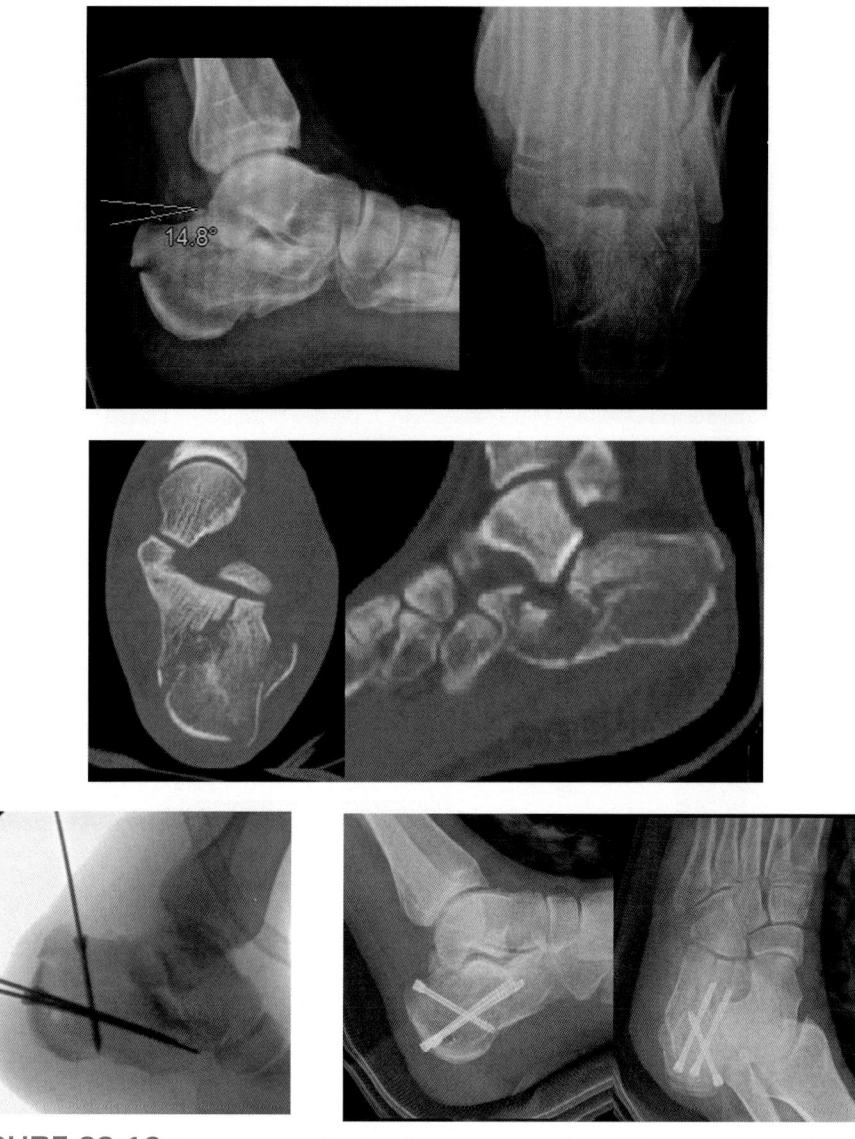

FIGURE 29.16 Percutaneous reduction of a tongue-type calcaneal fracture with extension to the CCJ. A Schanz pin was used to reduce the tuber while two screws from posterior to anterior hold the reduction with a third screw to reduce the elevated tuber.

AUTHORS PREFERRED TREATMENT— SINUS TARSI APPROACH

The STA has been gaining popularity in recent studies based on the reduction of soft tissue complications in comparison to a lateral extensile approach. Reduction has proven to be equal of the latter approach, as the STA allows for direct visualization of the articular surfaces.[19,77] Another clear advantage of the STA is the ability to operate typically at an earlier time frame than an ELA, gaining access to more mobile fracture fragments, which can aid the surgeon in anatomic reduction.[47,70]

An oblique incision is created directly over the palpable sinus tarsi, slightly extended distally as needed for any extensive anterior calcaneus fractures (Fig. 29.15). Layered dissection is performed with retraction of the peroneal tendons within their tendon sheath posteriorly or inferiorly to expose the STJ. The extensor digitorium brevis is split or can

be elevated as a full-thickness flap off the lateral calcaneus to visualize the anterior process. If encountered, the sural nerve should be protected along the inferior margin.

Bedigrew et al. found the STA exposes similar amounts of the posterior facet as the ELA with only limitations to the superomedial corner of the joint and less lateral wall exposure.[73] The STA does not provide full visualization of fractures that run more medially or for highly comminuted posterior facet fractures so arthroscopic-guided reduction with/without fluoroscopic assistance or utilization of the ELA (or conversion to the ELA) should be performed.[73,78]

A percutaneous instrument such as a key elevator is inserted or alternatively a Schanz pin drilled directly into the posterior tuber is utilized to re-establish a rectus or slightly valgus heel position. Once this has been verified with intraoperative fluoroscopy, guide pins can be advanced from the posteromedial aspect of the calcaneus, aiming at the sustentaculum tali.

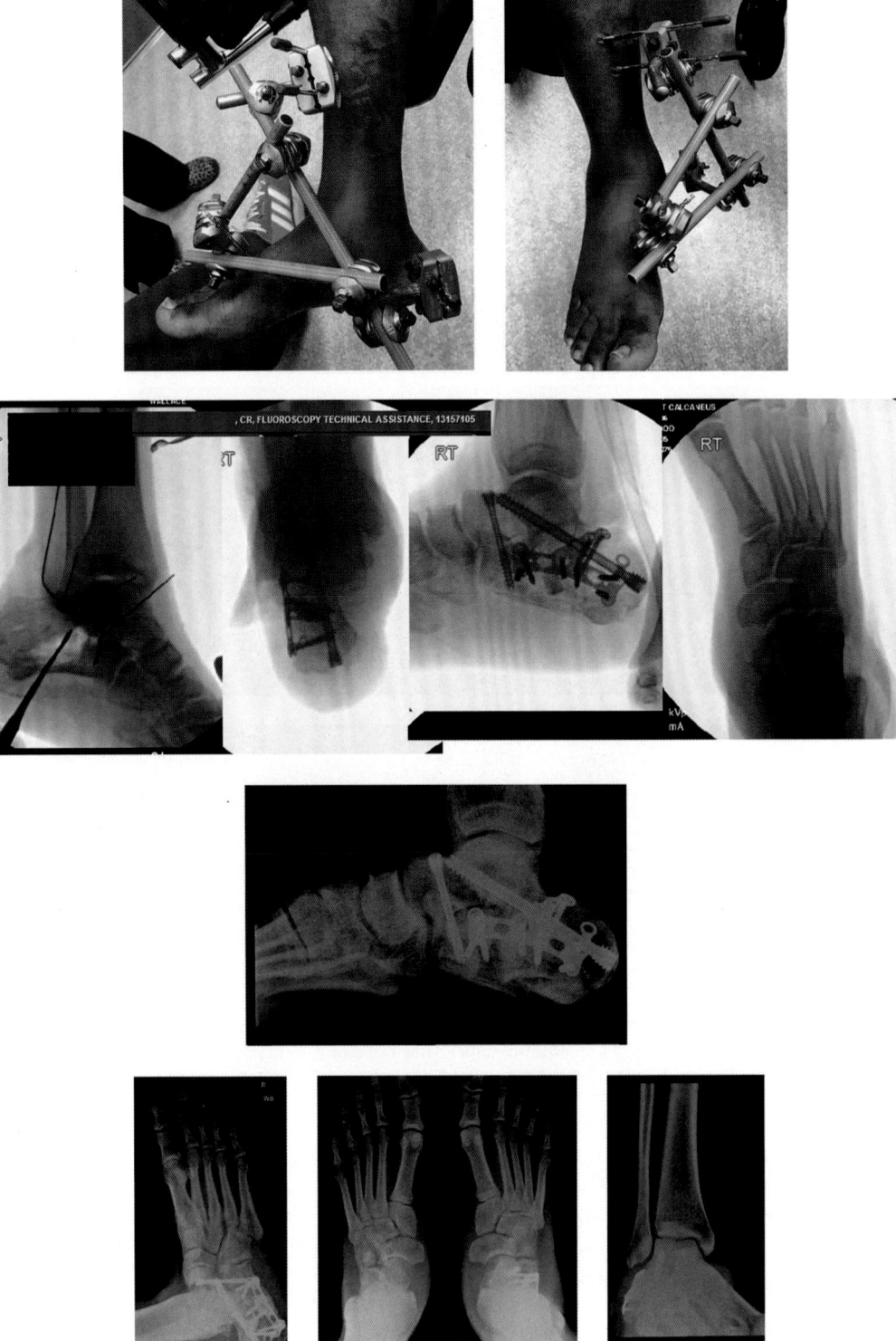

FIGURE 29.17 Primary subtalar joint fusion combined with ORIF for severely comminuted calcaneal fracture. Initial treatment for this open fracture was performed through medial frame, used to maintain and assist in reduction during the index procedure. Weight-bearing imaging at 3 months post ORIF-arthrodesis.

Next, the posterior facet is directly accessed, and the articular surface can be re-aligned and provisionally fixated at this point. Screws beneath the subchondral bone are placed from lateral to medial, with or without plate fixation. Lastly, the anterior fragment is reduced as needed and can be fixated along with final fixation from the previous two steps, with long fixation screws or an anatomic locking plate. Several anatomic locking plates have been designed to aid the surgeon when using this described approach, while other alternative forms of fixation also exist and can be utilized at the surgeon's discretion.

Sinus Tarsi Approach

- Following induction of generally anesthesia, the patient is positioned in a lateral decubitus with the aid of bean bag. Care is taken to ensure all bony prominences are well padded. A thigh tourniquet is placed.
- The sinus tarsi is palpable, and a small incision is created in an oblique manner directly to this area.
- The peroneal tendons are encountered from the posterior aspect of the incision, they are best mobilized posteriorly and plantarly.
- A Schanz pin can be placed within the tuber to aid in reduction.
- Once manipulation been performed and the tuber is reduced, K-wires are advanced from the plantar-medial aspect aiming at the sustentaculum tali. Calcaneal axial images are utilized at this time to assess the reduction.
- The posterior facet is directly accessed, reduced, and can be provisionally fixated with K-wires.
- The anterior fragment may need to be derotated or disimpacted at this time with gentle distraction. Once normal calcaneal features are re-established, intraoperative fluoroscopy is utilized prior to placing final fixation. A simulated Brodén view in additional to axial and lateral images may be useful as well.
- The authors prefer a combination of long fixation screws with a lateral anatomic locking plate.
- A layered closure is performed followed by placement of a posterior splint.

PEARLS, PITFALLS, AND COMPLICATIONS

Pearls and pitfalls to calcaneal fracture repair can be discussed in tandem and many present regardless of the type of treatment (operative or nonoperative). Often, failing to adhere to the standard techniques and guides for soft tissue protection and fracture repair lead to pitfalls and complications in treating this injury. The following sections are generalized for the aforementioned approaches and either add to or reinforce some of the stated keys in treatment. These pearls and pitfalls may be broken up into the three phases of treatment: before, during, and after surgery.

PERIOPERATIVE

Many of the perioperative pearls and pitfalls can be re-reviewed from the pathogenesis and physical examination section. This is inclusive of evaluating for concomitant injuries, monitoring neurovascular status, having a suspicion for CS, evaluating for deep vein thrombosis (DVT), and instituting measures for skin protection.

The timing of surgery is important. Surgeons will often delay the definitive surgical procedure of ORIF for anywhere between 1 and 3 weeks secondary to swelling and skin issues and the anticipated surgical approach. Attempted early fixation, in general, has been associated with skin flap necrosis, infection, and need for multiple surgical interventions. Conversely, waiting for an extended period of time may result in would closure issues and bone callus formation, making mobilization of the fragments for repair more difficult. Most MIS approaches are more difficult to perform after 1-2 weeks due to fracture consolidation and if planned should not be delayed for more than 7 days.[9] Hansen stated that primary reduction is only possible in the first 3-4 weeks, delaying any time after 4 weeks should be treated by allowing the fracture to consolidate and performing a secondary reconstruction as the symptoms and union dictates.[79] Studies have been performed looking at early fixation (<7 days) in ELA and MIS approaches demonstrating no major increase in complications or infection rates in certain patient populations.[21,80]

Acute CS should be treated as a surgical emergency with fascia compartment release performed emergently before the treatment of secondary local injuries. Highly comminuted intra-articular calcaneal fracture patterns (Sanders type IV) are a risk factor for development of CS.[16] The majority of episodes post-calcaneal fracture occur in the calcaneal compartment with the other compartments affected to a lesser degree.[17] High clinical suspicion and intracompartment pressure measurement, specifically to the calcaneal compartment, are the two most reliable methods for diagnosis.[16,17] Pain symptoms should be viewed with caution as pain from CS may be overlooked for pain from fracture with one study citing a 33% missed CS rate where all patients developed postinjury sequela.[16] Fasciotomy should be performed within 8 hours postincident to prevent permanent neurological injury. Release should focus on the calcaneal compartment through a medial incision from the origin of the abductor hallucis (3 cm above the plantar surface and 4 cm distal to the heel) that extends parallel to the plantar surface of the foot ~6 cm in length toward the first metatarsal.[17,81] The surgeon must ensure release of the fascia overlying the abductor hallucis and deeper medial intermuscular septum while taking care to identify and avoid the medial and lateral plantar nerve and vasculature. More on this topic may be found in Chapter 64.

Open fractures will undergo irrigation and debridement with reduction, but ORIF should be delayed until after fasciotomy closure.[17] Patients with calcaneal fractures who undergo prompt fasciotomy have reported similar clinical outcomes to those treated without CS and fare much better than those with a missed CS.[16]

Preoperative DVT has been reported at 12% in the ipsilateral limb after a calcaneal fracture.[82] While it may not be appropriate for chemical prophylaxis for DVT during the perioperative period, sequential compression devices and DVT education and awareness protocols should be reviewed with the patient. Park et al. did not find a significant association between antiplatelet therapy and the development of CS after calcaneal fracture despite the rationale that increased bleeding may result in increased intracompartmental or intramuscular hemorrhage and a subsequent CS episode.[16]

An inexcusable pitfall is not reviewing the imaging carefully. This includes choosing the right approach, which determines patient positioning, the type of fixation necessary, whether primary ORIF is indicated, and whether staging is required. The surgeon must ensure that the sustentacular fragment, the point at which repair is anchored to, is located in its "constant" position. A preplan with what fragment the Schanz pin will be placed into is an important point. Recognizing potential tendon entrapments that may hinder reduction should be considered. Having the appropriate hardware available for the planned ORIF is a must. Understanding the fracture pattern sets the tone for the repair and will enable the surgeon to work quickly and deliberately in the operating room.

There is a high learning curve due to the complex anatomy and the complex fracture patterns associated with injuries to the calcaneus.[6] Inexperienced surgeons and institutions may lead to iatrogenically caused complications through increased surgical time, poor soft tissue handling, and improper reduction.[66,83,84] Referral of the patient should be performed when appropriate.

Some preoperative factors may result in complications during treatment that are out of the surgeons' control but should be recognized to stratify patients' risk in determining the most appropriate treatment options. A higher Sanders classification is considered a risk factor for complications.[6,7] Folk et al. demonstrated smoking, diabetes, and open fractures as the greatest risk factors associated with operatively treated calcaneal fractures.[85] Smoking and nicotine consumption is a known risk factor to wound healing and both fracture healing and bone consolidation.[86,87] Noncompliance has also been cited as a reason for complication with Benirschke et al. attributing one-third of encountered infections related to some component of patient noncompliance.[48]

INTRAOPERATIVE

Intraoperatively, various considerations should be maintained through each step of the reconstruction. When planning the ELA incision, ensure Doppler use for avoidance of the LCA.[38,51] Appropriate incision planning, creating a full-thickness flap, and protecting it with a no-touch technique to preserve cutaneous blood supply for closure and incision healing are of paramount importance. During reduction, elevation and restoration of the posterior facet to within 1-2 mm of displacement/step-off maximum should be achieved. Obtaining multiple lateral, Harris axial, and Brodén views under fluoroscopy to assess reduction as provisional fixation is inserted will ensure successful reduction. "Thall shall not varus" should always be at the forefront of critically reviewing tuber reduction. The surgeon should always err on the side of valgus as the mobile foot adapts to this position better and shoe gear modifications can be made to adjust gait in the postoperative and rehabilitation setting. The surgeon should assure hardware placement is extra-articular, watching medial extrusion of hardware (drill, screw) to not injury the FHL about the sustentaculum tali or tibial nerve and avoid hardware beneath the apex of the ELA. The Allgöwer-Donati suturing technique is preferred with usage of a subcutaneous drain to be considered. Studies recommend reducing the operative time to 2 hours, limiting tourniquet use to 90 minutes, limiting blood loss, and reducing the number of operative room personnel (ie, surgical assists, residents, fellows, etc.) to prevent postoperation wound complications.[66,80,83]

POSTOPERATIVE

Most of the complications in the postoperative setting can be divided into early (fracture blisters, swelling, wound infection, CS, neurovascular injuries) and late (heel pain, heel deformity, tendon issues, malunion, and shoe wearing difficulties) categories.[66,88] While defining this section as postoperative complications, many of the sequela can occur with nonoperative treatment, minus points related to surgical dehiscence (Fig. 29.18).

Immediately postoperation, the main goal is skin healing and infection prevention. This can be mitigated through patient optimization perioperatively, surgical techniques, edema control to prevent skin/healing complications, and use of a drain or negative pressure incisional suction device with appropriately timed removal. Dehiscence can occur up to 4 weeks after surgery, typically beginning at the apex.[66] Therefore, sutures should be left in place to keep the edges approximated as long as possible to prevent skin retraction and

dehiscence. Early intervention is necessary to any impending skin issues with prompt local wound care. Superficial infections are managed with serial debridements (office or operative), adequately obtained culture-driven antibiosis, negative pressure wound therapy (NPWT), and tissue coverage. A postoperation hematoma should be managed with incision and debridement to avoid soft tissue loss and prevent deep infection. Attempts should be made to retain hardware for either up to 6 months or until fracture union. Whereas in the early stages, purulence is often associated with an osteitis from the adjacent wound, frank osteomyelitis can develop despite the above treatments. Unfortunately, surgical management of calcaneal fractures results in osteomyelitis in 1%-4% of closed and up to 19% of open injuries.[18] Deep infections and osteomyelitis require serial debridements, culture-driven intravenous antibiosis for 6 weeks, early hardware removal and antibiotic spacer, local or free flap coverage, and possibly amputation.[58,66,89] If the surgical site is clean, reconstruction through subtalar fusion is performed.

Late complications are often a sequela of the fracture and/or performed calcaneal ORIF and include generalized continued pain and swelling, neurological injury, peroneal impingement or dislocation, anatomic alterations, subtalar stiffness or arthritis, and malunion.[2,18,66,90]

Neurological complications occur from injury, entrapment, or syndromes directed toward the sural or tibial nerves (main nerve or its calcaneal branch), resulting from the initial injury, dissection, or reconstruction. Tibial nerve complications are more common in nonsurgical treatment compared to the sural nerve in operative treatment.[18] Common complications to the sural nerve include frank nerve injury/laceration, nerve impingement, or neuroma, occurring in up to 15% of cases.[66] The tibial nerve can be entrapped or injured secondary to medial fragment irritation, scar tissue, bony exostosis, or malunion. Errant drilling or long screws can also irritate medial structures such as the tibial nerve or FHL tendon about the sustentaculum tali. Patients may experience transient or permanent symptoms that may be distributed as a partial or complete neurological loss to the nerves region of distribution. Diagnostic nerve blocks or electrodiagnostic studies may aid in determining if a tarsal tunnel situation has developed with operative neurolysis or decompression attempted to provide relief. Conservative management includes pharmacotherapy and physical therapy. Persistent symptoms may require nerve release or neurectomy. Events of CRPS have been cited postcalcaneal fractures and so monitoring for warning signs with a prompt referral is important postoperatively.[27,66] More on this topic/CRPS may be found in Chapter 5.

Peroneal tendon issues include tendonitis, impingement/entrapment, or subluxation/dislocation.[18] Advanced imaging may be performed to evaluate the tendons, but MRI may be obscured secondary to metallic artifact and a CT, high definition MSK ultrasonography, or peroneal tenogram may be necessary. Because of this, patient symptoms and physical examination play a greater role in determining the pathology. Tenosynovitis and stenosis are more common after nonsurgical treatment due to the expanded lateral wall with tendon rubbing and impingement. It also forces the tendons more laterally, which may cause them to subluxate about the fibula. Surgical management results in soft tissue adhesions and implant irritation. Acute peroneal dislocation may be a result of the injury and should be assessed on preoperative imaging (fleck sign on x-ray) and clinical examination, with additional intraoperation evaluation and repair as

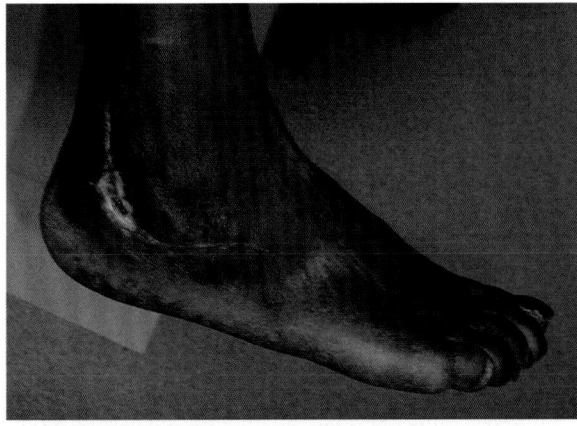
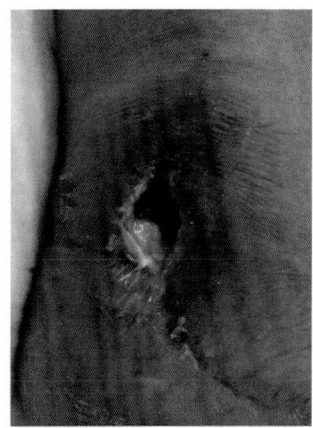
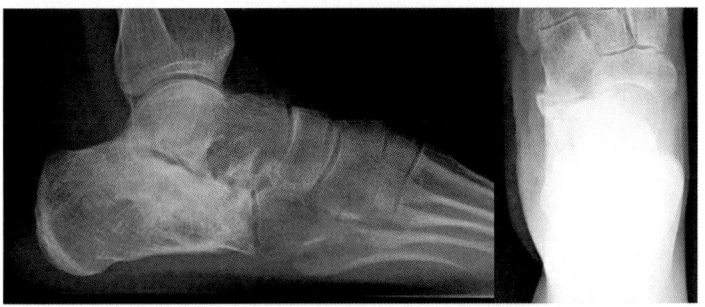
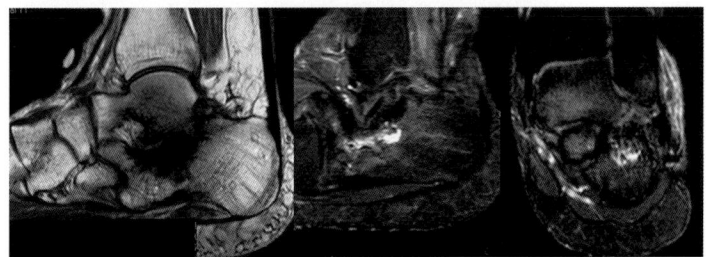

FIGURE 29.18 Various complications occur in calcaneal fracture. Common in the initial postoperative phase is superficial infection or delayed healing that may progress to a deep infection with draining sinus. Posttraumatic arthritis is a common late-stage sequela seen both on XR and MRI. Note the characteristic XR findings of sclerosis across the STJ and a flat talar declination angle.

required. Treatments include immobilization, non-steroidal anti-inflammatory drugs (NSAIDs), physical therapy (manual mobilization, stretching, frontal plane strengthening), tendon release (tenolysis and debridement), lateral wall exostectomy, or open reduction/reconstruction of the retinaculum (inferior and/or superior peroneal). After the calcaneal incision is closed to re-tension the soft tissues, and secondary incision to the distal posterolateral edge of the fibula is made to perform a superficial peroneal retinaculum repair.[18]

Alterations of the bony anatomy of the heel and the plantar fat pad may result in Achilles tendinitis (insertional or noninsertional), plantar fasciitis, and heel neuritis. Collectively this results in pain, issues finding appropriately fitting shoe gear, wearing of shoe gear, or gait alterations. Treatment recommendations include custom-molded orthotics, wider or larger shoes to accommodate the increased heel size, viscoelastic padded heel cups, and standard Achilles pathology modalities. Local heel injections should be attempted with caution due to furthering the damage to atrophied tissue, and more conservative measures like physical therapy should be implemented. Exostectomy may be performed to reshape calcaneal anatomy and reduce prominences with fascia releases or tendon lengthening

to treat the soft tissue sequela. Plantar incisions should be avoided to circumvent painful scarring. Unfortunately, there is no widely accepted effective treatment for heel pad pain.[18]

Posttraumatic joint pathology can affect the subtalar, calcaneocuboid, and/or ankle joint. Joint issues are the result of a lack of reduction in nonoperative treatment, incongruent surgical reduction, traumatic cartilage damage, errant drilling or hardware placement, and malunion. Adhesions and arthrofibrosis have been reported in 20%-25% of cases.[29] Instituting an early range of motion protocol (when appropriate) is important in preventing joint stiffness while first-line conservative treatments for arthritis include NSAIDs, joint injections, cast or fracture boot immobilization, and orthotics to limit subtalar motion (eg, deep heel cup, hindfoot posting, ankle brace, etc.). Radiographic subtalar arthritis can be seen in up to 38% of calcaneal fractures although not all patients are symptomatic, and the surgeon must correlate between x-rays and symptoms.[2] If pain persists, subtalar fusion is the procedure of choice. Calcaneocuboid arthritis can be treated by either exostectomy or arthrodesis, choosing exostectomy when only one-quarter to one-third of the joint is involved.[18]

Malunion can occur in both nonoperative and operative treatment, albeit lower with the latter. It results in loss of hindfoot height, varus or valgus heel, shortened foot and lever arm, posttraumatic subtalar and/or calcaneocuboid arthritis, ankle impingement, increased heel width, altered gait, and limb length discrepancy. Each of these issues may cause some of the aforementioned sequela (neuritis, peroneal pathology, bony prominences). Both Stephens and Sanders et al. and Zwipp and Rammelt et al. have devised classification systems with treatment algorithms for calcaneal malunion.[66,91,92] Additionally, Schepers et al. performed a systematic review of common deformities and patient complaints with treatment strategies for failed treatment of displaced, intra-articular calcaneal fractures.[93] Generally, treatments include hardware removal, lateral wall exostectomy, peroneal tenolysis, calcaneal translatory osteotomies, and *in situ* or bone block subtalar arthrodesis.

Both posttraumatic arthritis and malunion are intertwined in the development and progression of variable degrees of foot and ankle joint destruction, gait alterations, and hip/knee/back pain. Etiologies of hindfoot deformity include talar subsidence, calcaneal collapse, subchondral sclerosis, and avascular bone. The ankle can become affected due to a more relative dorsiflexed position of the talus creating anterior tibiotalar impingement. The mainstay treatment is some form of subtalar

arthrodesis with reviews noting that 5%-20% of calcaneal fractures require eventual subtalar arthrodesis on average 30 months after injury.[29,75,93] Csizy et al. noted that significant variables leading to the need for eventual subtalar fusion include workers compensation patient (odds ratio, 3×), Sanders type IV (5.5×), Böhler angle <0 degree (10.6×), and nonoperatively treated patients (5.9×).[75] Buckley et al. found similar results with nonoperatively treated patients 5.5 times more likely to need subtalar fusion.[94] Zwipp et al. reported 5.6% fusion rate at 5-year follow-up.[29]

Due to primary subtalar arthrodesis rates for postcalcaneal fracture injuries having a nonunion rate of 24%, many authors have recommended performing bone block vs *in situ* arthrodesis when undertaking fusion with the goals of restoring the talar inclination angle and reducing the rate of nonunion (Fig. 29.19).[75,93,95-97] This, in turn, should also decrease the anterior ankle joint impingement through the restoration of the talar declination angle. Due to the complexity of this reconstruction, surgeons should attempt some form of reduction to the calcaneus at initial presentation to restore anatomy, especially if nonoperative treatment is chosen, to aid in reducing multiple procedures in the late-stage salvage situation.[29,74]

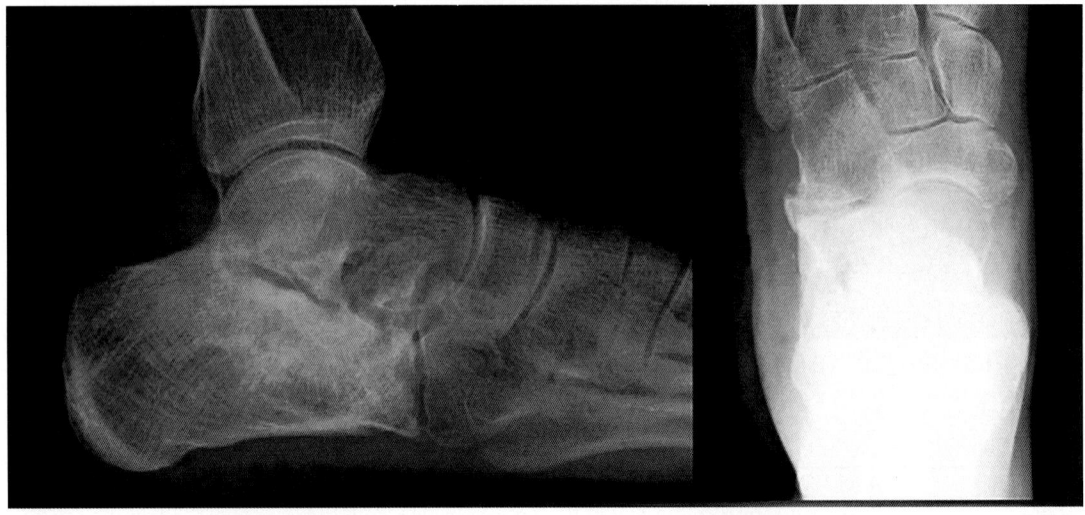

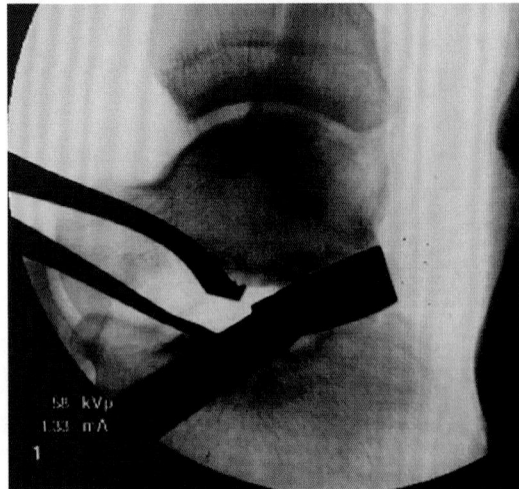
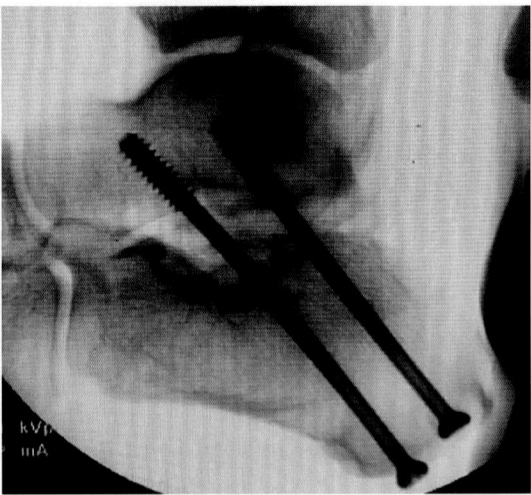

FIGURE 29.19 Patient who underwent ORIF with subsequent hardware removal after a calcaneal fracture. Noted subtalar and calcaneocuboid arthritis 2 years after the injury. Due to flattening of talar declination angle, the patient underwent bone block arthrodesis of the subtalar joint.

However, it is not uncommon to perform multiple procedures to achieve satisfactory results. A more thorough discussion of subtalar arthritis and treatment options can be reviewed in Chapter 26. Clare et al. offer a review and surgical technique description for managing calcaneal malunion.[18]

Complications of Calcaneal Fractures

Early Complications	Late Complications
▪ Fracture blisters	▪ Joint stiffness/arthritis
▪ Swelling	▪ Tendon issues
▪ Dehiscence and infection	▪ Tendinitis, impingement, dislocation
▪ Compartment syndrome	▪ Lateral ankle instability
▪ Neurovascular injuries	▪ Neurological injuries
	▪ Neuritis, CRPS

POSTOPERATIVE CARE

Most approaches to calcaneal fracture treatment will follow a similar course. Much of the progression through non–weight bearing to full weight bearing is dictated upon radiographic evidence of bone consolidation on plain films. The same can be said for union across the arthrodesis site if a subtalar fusion is performed in conjunction with ORIF. When in doubt, CT scans are more definitive to predict osseous union.

In the initial stages, soft tissue management and prevention of potential complications are the first checkpoint to pass. Perioperative cryotherapy used immediately postoperation for 72 hours has been shown to yield shorter hospital stays, lower infection rates, lower visual analog scale (VAS) pain scores at day 3, and superior foot function indices.[67] Its use along with strict elevation are a mainstay in initial edema control. If a drain has been used, removal can be performed after output has reduced to <15-25 cc/shift (8 hours) across two consecutive shifts, which typically occurs between 24 and 48 hours after surgery.[8,14,38]

Antibiotics are continued postoperation while the drain is placed and can be continued postoperation and admission based on the surgeon's preference/protocol, the nature of the fracture (ie, open vs closed), and patient's risk factors (ie, vascular compromise, immunocompromised, diabetes). Pharmacological DVT prophylaxis is typically implemented while the patient is admitted and can be continued postoperation based on the surgeon's preference, patient's comorbidities, and risk factors related to a venous thromboembolism (VTE) event.

The patient may be tracked weekly after surgery to monitor tissue healing and edema. Multilayer compression in a splint is implemented for edema control. Sutures are removed between 3 and 4 weeks. While the patient remains non–weight bearing, early range of motion to the ankle and subtalar joint can be implemented between 2 and 4 weeks postoperation to prevent stiffness. Initiation of these exercises should be delayed until full wound healing occurs, especially if any apical wound issues are present.

Historically, authors have recommended strict non–weight bearing until 12 weeks postoperation.[8] More current reviews institute partial weight bearing in a cast or fracture boot between 6 and 8 weeks at 25% of weight, increasing over the subsequent weeks to 50%, with full weight bearing by 12 weeks

provided there are clinical/radiographic signs of healing (eg, no pain or swelling, consolidation of fracture lines, maintenance of Böhler angle).

Postoperative CT has been discussed in the literature.[19] One author recommends if intraoperative arthroscopy was not performed to assess reduction, an intraoperative CT (if available) or postoperative CT should be performed to evaluate STJ congruency.[29]

Hardware removal is optional but comes with its own morbidity. It typically is not performed until at least 1 year after placement.[29] If superficial infection is present, it should be maintained until osseous union or >6 months duration, while deep infection requires prompt removal.

REHABILITATION

The recovery can be long and rates of posttraumatic arthritis resulting in subtalar fusion have been reported as high as 20%. Many reports have cited patient total incapacitation for up to 3 years and partial impairment for up to 5 years postinjury.[15] When comparing nonoperative vs operative fixation, evidence suggests that surgical restoration of anatomy is the only way for a patient to have a normal gait.[48]

Early range of motion while remaining non–weight bearing until radiographic healing can be implemented between 2 and 4 weeks after surgery, often predicated on incision healing. The goals are preventions of arthrofibrosis and adhesions both intra- and extra-articular. The use of MIS incisions such as the STA or percutaneous screw fixation can allow for an earlier range of motion exercises to the ankle with allowed motion as early as 2 days postoperation.[58]

Other non–weight-bearing modalities for extremity strengthening can be performed during home and formal physical therapy such as core and extremity muscular strengthening with continued active and passive range of motion activities while waiting to start weight bearing. Once weight bearing is allowed, gait and proprioceptive training activities can be added to the therapy regimen.

The use of variable fixation methods has changed the basic progression with respect to weight bearing. Locking plate technology has been cited to decrease the time to full weight bearing by up to 3 weeks when compared to other types of fixation.[29] Nail fixation management has cited allowing 20-kg partial weight bearing in a shoe from postoperation week 6-10 weeks, increasing weight after 10 weeks to full weight bearing as tolerated.[58]

SUMMARY

Os calcis fractures demonstrate a potential myriad of differing fracture patterns and thus require a customized treatment approach and thorough preoperative planning. Both open and closed fractures with CS or significant soft tissue impingement stemming from compressed fragment pressure are treated as surgical emergencies. Fractures that are nondisplaced, mildly displaced and extra-articular, intra-articular fractures with <2 mm displacement, and patients with contraindications to surgery are primarily treated nonoperatively. Grossly displaced extra-articular and less severe intra-articular fractures can be treated with percutaneous reduction and fixation with very successful results. In patients where more severe fracture patterns and soft tissue trauma are noted, percutaneous reduction and fixation are helpful as temporary measures to stabilize the calcaneus. ORIF is chosen for most displaced, intra-articular fractures when contraindications are not present. MIS approaches utilizing procedure-specific hardware can potentially reduce soft tissue complications while recreating anatomical reduction with secure fixation principles. These MIS surgical principles involve the surgeon utilizing either percutaneous approaches to applying hardware or utilizing small incisions to achieve fixation and hardware placement. Locking plate constructs permit the surgeon increased stability and use of unicortical fixation principles. Patients receive the best outcomes for both nonoperative and operative reduction when handled by experienced surgeons who are well versed in calcaneal fracture management. Painful malunions with impending symptomatic posttraumatic subtalar arthritis are seen in patients where fractures are not managed appropriately. It is, therefore, in the best interest of the foot and ankle surgeon to become as adept as possible in managing these difficult traumatic injuries to ensure the best possible outcomes for the patient.

REFERENCES

1. Palmersheim K, Hines B, Olsen BL. Calcaneal fractures: update on current treatments. *Clin Podiatr Med Surg.* 2012;29(2):205-220. doi: 10.1016/j.cpm.2012.01.007.
2. Lim EVA, Leung JPF. Complications of intraarticular calcaneal fractures. *Clin Orthop Relat Res.* 2001;(391):7-16.
3. Cotton FJ, Wilson LT. Fractures of the os calcis. *Boston Med Surg J.* 1908;159:559-565.
4. Böhler L. Diagnosis, pathology, and treatment of fractures of the os calcis. *JBJS.* 1931;13(1):75-89.
5. Conn HR. The treatment of fractures of the os calcis. *JBJS.* 1935;17(2):392-405.
6. Sanders RW, Fortin P, DiPasquale T, Walling A. Operative treatment in 120 displaced intraarticular calcaneal fractures. *Clin Orthop Relat Res.* 1993;(290):87-95.
7. Sanders RW. Intra-articular fractures of the calcaneus: present state of the art. *J Orthop Trauma.* 1992;6(2):252-265.
8. Benirschke SK, Sangeorzan BJ. Extensive intraarticular fractures of the foot. Surgical management of calcaneal fractures. *Clin Orthop Relat Res.* 1993;(292):128-134.
9. Rammelt S, Sangeorzan BJ, Swords MP. Calcaneal fractures—should we or should we not operate? *Indian J Orthop.* 2018;52(3):220-230.
10. Zhang F, Tian H, Li S, et al. Meta-analysis of two surgical approaches for calcaneal fractures: sinus tarsi versus extensile lateral approach. *ANZ J Surg.* 2017;87(3):126-131. doi: 10.1111/ans.13869.
11. Rubino R, Valderrabano V, Sutter PM, Regazzoni P. Prognostic value of four classifications of calcaneal fractures. *Foot Ankle Int.* 2009;30(3):229-238. doi: 10.3113/FAI.2009.0229.
12. Essex-Lopresti P. The mechanism, reduction technique, and results in fractures of the os calcis. *Br J Surg.* 1952;39(157):395-419.
13. Tornetta P III. The Essex-Lopresti reduction for calcaneal fractures revisited. *J Orthop Trauma.* 1998;12(7):469-473.
14. Jennings MM, et al. Calcaneal fractures. In: Southerland JT, ed. *McGlamry's Comprehensive Textbook of Foot and Ankle Surgery.* 4th ed. Philadelphia, PA: Lippincott Williams & Wilkins; 2012:1685-1706. http://www.dt.co.kr/contents.html?article_no=2012071302010531749001
15. Sanders RW, Rammelt S. Fractures of the calcaneus. In: Coughlin MJ, Saltzman CL, Anderson RB, eds. *Mann's Surgery of the Foot and Ankle.* 9th ed. Philadelphia, PA: Elsevier Saunders; 2014:2041.
16. Park YH, Lee JW, Hong JY, Choi GW, Kim HJ. Predictors of compartment syndrome of the foot after fracture of the calcaneus. *Bone Joint J.* 2018;100B(3):303-308. doi: 10.1302/0301-620X.100B3.BJJ-2017-0715.R2
17. Myerson MS, Manoli A. Compartment syndromes of the foot after calcaneal fractures. *Clin Orthop Relat Res.* 1993;(290):142-150.
18. Clare MP, Crawford WS. Managing complications of calcaneal fractures. *Foot Ankle Clin.* 2017;22(1):105-116. doi: 10.1016/j.fcl.2016.09.007.
19. Schepers T, Backes M, Dingemans SA. Similar anatomical reduction and lower complication rates with the sinus tarsi approach compared with the extended lateral approach in displaced intra-articular calcaneal fractures. *J Orthop Trauma.* 2017;31(6):293-298. doi: 10.1097/BOT.0000000000000819.
20. Swords MP, Penny P. Early fixation of calcaneus fractures. *Foot Ankle Clin.* 2017;22(1):93-104. doi: 10.1016/j.fcl.2016.09.006.
21. Kwon JY, Guss D, Lin DE, et al. Effect of delay to definitive surgical fixation on wound complications in the treatment of closed, intra-articular calcaneus fractures. *Foot Ankle Int.* 2015;36(5):508-517. doi: 10.1177/1071100714565178.
22. Sarrafian SK, Kelikian AS. Osteology. In: Kelikian AS, Sarrafian SK, eds. *Sarrafian's Anatomy of the Foot and Ankle: Descriptive, Topographic, Functional.* 3rd ed. Philadelphia, PA: Lippincott Williams & Wilkins; 2011:40.
23. Soeur R, Remy R. Fractures of the calcaneus with displacement of the thalamic portion. *JBJS.* 1975;57-B(4):413-421. doi: 10.1302/0301-620X.57B4.413.
24. Gitajn IL, Abousayed M, Toussiant RJ, Ting B, Jin J, Kwon JY. Anatomic alignment and integrity of the sustentaculum tali in intra-articular calcaneal fractures: is the sustentaculum tali truly constant? *JBJS.* 2014;96(12):1000-1005.
25. Berberian W, Sood A, Karanfilian R, Najarian R, Lin S, Liporace F. Displacement of the sustentacular fragments in intra-articular calcaneal fractures. *JBJS.* 2013;95(11):995-1000.
26. Harnroongroj T, Harnroongroj T, Suntharapa T, Arunakul M. The new intra-articular calcaneal fracture classification system in term of sustentacular fragment configurations and incorporation of posterior calcaneal facet fractures with fracture components of the calcaneal body. *Acta Orthop Traumatol Turc.* 2016;50(5):519-526. doi: 10.1016/j.aott.2016.08.007.
27. Duymus TM, Mutlu S, Mutlu H, Ozel O, Guler O, Mahirogullari M. Need for bone grafts in the surgical treatment of displaced intra-articular calcaneal fractures. *J Foot Ankle Surg.* 2019;56(1):54-58. doi: 10.1053/j.jfas.2016.08.004.
28. Worsham JR, Elliott MR, Harris AM. Open calcaneal fractures and associated injuries. *J Foot Ankle Surg.* 2016;55(1):68-71. doi: 10.1053/j.jfas.2015.06.015.
29. Zwipp H, Rammelt S, Barthel S. Calcaneus fractures—open reduction and internal fixation (ORIF). *Injury.* 2004;35(suppl 2):SB46-SB54. doi: 10.1016/j.injury.2004.07.011.
30. Mitchell MJ, McKinley JC, Robinson CM. The epidemiology of calcaneal fractures. *Foot (Edinb).* 2009;19(4):197-200. doi: 10.1016/j.foot.2009.05.001.
31. Schepers T, Ginai AZ, Lieshout EMM, Van Lieshout EM, Patka P. Demographics of extra-articular calcaneal fractures: including a review of the literature on treatment and outcome. *Arch Orthop Trauma Surg.* 2008;128(10):1099-1106. doi: 10.1007/s00402-007-0517-2.
32. Buddecke DE, Mandracchia VJ. Calcaneal fractures. *Clin Podiatr Med Surg.* 1999;16(4):769-791.
33. Miller JR, Dunn KW, Ciliberti LJ Jr, Eldridge SW, Reed LD. Diagnostic value of early magnetic resonance imaging after acute lateral ankle injury. *J Foot Ankle Surg.* 2017;56(6):1143-1146. doi: 10.1053/j.jfas.2017.05.011.
34. Fitzgerald J, Michael E. Protocol for lower extremity trauma. *J Foot Ankle Surg.* 1995;34(1):2-11. doi: 10.1016/S1067-2516(09)80095-1.
35. Richman JD, Barre PS. The plantar ecchymosis sign in fractures of the calcaneus. *Clin Orthop Relat Res.* 1986;207:122-125.
36. Schepers T, Den Hartog D, Vogels LM, Van Lieshout EM. Extended lateral approach for intra-articular calcaneal fractures: an inverse relationship between surgeon experience and wound complications. *J Foot Ankle Surg.* 2013;52(2):167-171. doi: 10.1053/j.jfas.2012.11.009.
37. Sanders RW. Current concepts review—displaced intra-articular fractures of the calcaneus. *JBJS.* 2000;82-A(2):225-250.
38. Bibbo C, Ehrlich DA, Nguyen HML, Levin LS, Kovach SJ. Low wound complication rates for the lateral extensile approach for calcaneal orif when the lateral calcaneal artery is patent. *Foot Ankle Int.* 2014;35(7):650-656. doi: 10.1177/1071100714534654.
39. Schepers T, van Lieshout EM, van Ginhoven TM, Heetveld MJ, Patka P. Current concepts in the treatment of intra-articular calcaneal fractures: results of a nationwide survey. *Int Orthop.* 2008;32(5):711-715. doi: 10.1007/s00264-007-0385-y.
40. Badillo K, Pacheo JA, Pauda SO, Gomez AA, Colon E, Vidal JA. Multidetector CT evaluation of calcaneal fractures. *Radiographics.* 2011;31(1):81-92.
41. Geerling J, Kendoff D, Citak M, et al. Intraoperative 3D imaging in calcaneal fracture care—clinical implications and decision making. *J Trauma.* 2009;66(3):768-773. doi: 10.1097/TA.0b013e31816275c7.
42. Franke J, Wendl K, Suda AJ, Giese T, Grutzner PA, von Recum J. Intraoperative three-dimensional imaging in the treatment of calcaneal fractures. *JBJS.* 2014;96(9):e72(1-7).
43. Mehta S, Mirza AJ, Dunbar RP, Barei DP, Benirschke SK. A staged treatment plan for the management of type ii and type iiia open calcaneal fractures. *J Orthop Trauma.* 2010;24(3):142-147.
44. Beltran MJ, Collinge CA. Outcomes of high-grade open calcaneal fractures managed with open reduction via the medial wound and percutaneous screw fixation. *J Orthop Trauma.* 2012;26(11):662-670.
45. Brenner P, Rammelt S, Gavlik JM, Zwipp H. Early soft tissue coverage after complex foot trauma. *World J Surg.* 2001;25(5):603-609. doi: 10.1007/s002680020150.
46. Dickens JF, Kilcoyne KG, Kluk MW, Gordon WT, Shawen SB, Potter BK. Risk factors for infection and amputation following open, combat-related calcaneal fractures. *JBJS.* 2013;95A(5):e24.
47. Yao H, Liang T, Xu Y, Hou G, Lv L, Zhang J. Sinus tarsi approach versus extensile lateral approach for displaced intra-articular calcaneal fracture: a meta-analysis of current evidence base. *J Orthop Surg Res.* 2017;12(43):1-9. doi: 10.1186/s13018-017-0545-8.
48. Benirschke SK, Kramer PA. Wound healing complications in closed and open calcaneal fractures. *J Orthop Trauma.* 2004;18(1):1-6.
49. Stapleton JJ, Zgonis T. Surgical treatment of intra-articular calcaneal fractures. *Clin Podiatr Med Surg.* 2014;31(4):539-546. doi: 10.1016/j.cpm.2014.06.003.
50. Malay DS. Do patients really need to be prone for foot or ankle surgery? *J Foot Ankle Surg.* 2018;57(4):643-644. doi: 10.1053/j.jfas.2018.05.002.
51. Elsaidy MA, El-Shafey K. The lateral calcaneal artery: anatomic basis for planning safe surgical approaches. *Clin Anat.* 2009;22(7):834-839. doi: 10.1002/ca.20840.
52. Andermahrl J, Helling HJ, Landwehr P, Fischbach R, Koebke J, Rehm KE. The lateral calcaneal artery. *Surg Radiol Anat.* 1998;20:419-423.
53. Kwon JY, Gonzalez T, Riedel MD, Nazarian A, Ghorbanhoseini M. Proximity of the lateral calcaneal artery with a modified extensile lateral approach compared to standard extensile approach. *Foot Ankle Int.* 2017;38(3):318-323. doi: 10.1177/1071100716674695.
54. Sirisreetreerux N, Sa-ngasoongsong P, Kulachote N, Apivatthakakul T. Location of vertical limb of extensile lateral calcaneal approach and risk of injury of the calcaneal branch of the peroneal artery. *Foot Ankle Int.* 2019;40(2):224-230. doi: 10.1177/1071100718802255.
55. Freeman BJC, Duff S, Allen PE, Nicholson HD, Atkins RM. The extended lateral approach to the hindfoot. Anatomical basis and surgical implications. *JBJS.* 1998;80(1):139-142.
56. Hollawell S. Wound closure technique for lateral extensile approach to intra-articular calcaneal fractures. *J Am Podiatr Med Assoc.* 2008;98(5):422-425.

57. Lakstein D, Bermant A, Shoihetman E, Hendel D, Feldbrin Z. The posterolateral approach for calcaneal fractures. *Indian J Orthop.* 2018;52(3):239-243. doi: 10.4103/ortho.IJOrtho.

58. Zwipp H, Pasa L, Zilka-Lubos SI, Amlang M, Rammelt S, Pompach M. Introduction of a new locking nail for treatment of intraarticular calcaneal fractures. *J Orthop Trauma.* 2016;30(3):e88-e92.

59. Bussewitz BW, Hyer CF. Screw placement relative to the calcaneal fracture constant fragment: an anatomic study. *J Foot Ankle Surg.* 2015;54(3):392-394. doi: 10.1053/j.jfas.2014.08.018.

60. Singh AK, Vinay K. Surgical treatment of displaced intra-articular calcaneal fractures: is bone grafting necessary? *J Orthop Traumatol.* 2013;14(4):299-305. doi: 10.1007/s10195-013-0246-y.

61. Gupta AK, Gluck GS, Parekh SG. Balloon reduction of displaced calcaneus fractures: surgical technique and case series. *Foot Ankle Int.* 2011;32(2):205-210. doi: 10.3113/FAI.2011.0205.

62. Zheng W, Xie L, Xie H, Chen C, Chen H, Cai L. With versus without bone grafts for operative treatment of displaced intra-articular calcaneal fractures: a meta-analysis. *Int J Surg.* 2018;59:36-47. doi: 10.1016/j.ijsu.2018.09.016.

63. Yang Y, Zhao H, Zhou J, Yu G. Treatment of displaced intraarticular calcaneal fractures with or without bone grafts: a systematic review of the literature. *Indian J Orthop.* 2012;46(2):130-137. doi: 10.4103/0019-5413.93672.

64. Phisitkul P, Sullivan JP, Goetz JE, Marsh JL. Maximizing safety in screw placement for posterior facet fixation in calcaneus fractures: a cadaveric radio-anatomical study. *Foot Ankle Int.* 2013;34(9):1279-1285. doi: 10.1177/1071100713487182.

65. Sagi HC, Papp S, Dipasquale T. The effect of suture pattern and tension on cutaneous blood flow as assessed by laser Doppler flowmetry in a pig model. *J Orthop Trauma.* 2008;22(3):171-175.

66. Koutserimpas C, Magarakis G, Kastanis G, Kontakis G, Alpantaki K. Complications of intra-articular calcaneal fractures in adults—key points for diagnosis, prevention, and treatment. *Foot Ankle Spec.* 2016;9(6):534-542. doi: 10.1177/1938640016668030.

67. Lin S, Xie J, Yao X, Dai Z, Wu W. The use of cryotherapy for the prevention of wound complications in the treatment of calcaneal fractures. *J Foot Ankle Surg.* 2018;57(3):436-439. doi: 10.1053/j.jfas.2017.08.002.

68. Herscovici D. Extensile lateral approach for the operative management of a displaced intra-articular calcaneal fracture. *JBJS Essent Surg Tech.* 2016;6(4):7-8.

69. Jansen SCP, Branse J, van Montfort G, Besselaar AT, van der Veen AH. Should the extended lateral approach remain part of standard treatment in displaced intra-articular calcaneal fractures? *J Foot Ankle Surg.* 2018;57(6):1120-1124. doi: 10.1053/j.jfas.2018.05.015.

70. Basile A, Albo F, Via AG. Comparison between sinus tarsi approach and extensile lateral approach for treatment of closed displaced intra-articular calcaneal fractures: a multicenter prospective study. *J Foot Ankle Surg.* 2016;55(3):513-521. doi: 10.1053/j.jfas.2015.11.008.

71. Yeo JH, Cho HJ, Lee KB. Comparison of two surgical approaches for displaced intra-articular calcaneal fractures: sinus tarsi versus extensile lateral approach. *BMC Musculoskelet Disord.* 2015;16(63):1-7. doi: 10.1186/s12891-015-0519-0.

72. Yeap EJ, Rao J, Pan CH, Soelar SA, Younger ASE. Is arthroscopic assisted percutaneous screw fixation as good as open reduction and internal fixation for the treatment of displaced intra-articular calcaneal fractures? *Foot Ankle Surg.* 2016;22(3):164-169. doi: 10.1016/j.fas.2015.06.008.

73. Bedigrew KM, Blair JA, Possley DR, Kirk KL, Hsu JR. Comparison of calcaneal exposure through the extensile lateral and sinus tarsi approaches. *Foot Ankle Spec.* 2018;11(2):142-147. doi: 10.1177/1938640017713616.

74. Radnay CS, Clare MP, Sanders RW. Subtalar fusion after displaced intra-articular calcaneal fractures: does initial operative treatment matter? Surgical technique. *JBJS.* 2010;92(suppl 1 Part 1):32-43. doi: 10.2106/JBJS.I.01267.

75. Csizy M, Buckley R, Tough S, et al. Displaced intra-articular calcaneal fractures: variables predicting late subtalar fusion. *J Orthop Trauma.* 2003;17(2):106-112.

76. Holm JL, Laxson SE, Schuberth JM. Primary subtalar joint arthrodesis for comminuted fractures of the calcaneus. *J Foot Ankle Surg.* 2015;54(1):61-65. doi: 10.1053/j.jfas.2014.07.013.

77. Kline AJ, Anderson RB, Davis WH, Jones CP, Cohen BE. Minimally invasive technique versus an extensile lateral approach for intra-articular calcaneal fractures. *Foot Ankle Int.* 2013;34(6):773-780. doi: 10.1177/1071100713477607.

78. Amlang M, Zwipp H, Pompach M, Rammelt S. Interlocking nail fixation for the treatment of displaced intra-articular calcaneal fractures. *JBJS Essent Surg Tech.* 2017;7(4):e33.

79. Hansen ST. Foot injuries. In: Browner BD, Jupiter JB, eds. *Skeletal Trauma.* WB Saunders; 1998:2405-2438.

80. Ho C, Huang H, Chen C, Chen J. Open reduction and internal fixation of acute intra-articular displaced calcaneal fractures: a retrospective analysis of surgical timing and infection rates. *Injury.* 2018;44(7):1007-1010. doi: 10.1016/j.injury.2013.03.014.

81. Frink M, Hildebrand F, Krettek C, Brand J. Compartment syndrome of the lower leg and foot. *Clin Orthop Relat Res.* 2010;468(8):940-950. doi: 10.1007/s11999-009-0891-x.

82. Williams JR, Little MTM, Kramer PA, Benirschke SK. Incidence of preoperative deep vein thrombosis in calcaneal fractures. *J Orthop Trauma.* 2016;30(7):e242-e245. doi: 10.1097/BOT.0000000000000568.

83. Ding L, He Z, Xiao H, Chai L, Xue F. Risk factors for postoperative wound complications of calcaneal fractures following plate fixation. *Foot Ankle Int.* 2013;34(9):1238-1244. doi: 10.1177/1071100713484718.

84. Poeze M, Verbruggen JPAM, Brink PRG. The relationship between the outcome of operatively treated calcaneal fractures and institutional fracture load. A systematic review of the literature. *JBJS.* 2008;90(5):1013-1021. doi: 10.2106/JBJS.G.00604.

85. Folk JW, Starr AJ, Early JS. Early wound complications of operative treatment of calcaneal fractures: analysis of 190 fractures. *J Orthop Trauma.* 1999;13(5):369-372.

86. Haverstock BD, Mandracchia VJ. Cigarette smoking and bone healing: implications in foot and ankle surgery. *J Foot Ankle Surg.* 1998;37(1):69-74; discussion 78.

87. Scolaro JA, Schenker ML, Yannascoli S, Baldwin K. Cigarette smoking increases complications following fracture. *JBJS.* 2014;96-A(8):674-681.

88. Ramanujam CL, Wade J, Selbst B, Belczyk R, Zgonis T. Recurrent acute compartment syndrome of the foot following a calcaneal fracture repair. *Clin Podiatr Med Surg.* 2010;27(3):469-474. doi: 10.1016/j.cpm.2010.03.005.

89. Loder BG, Dunn KW. Functional reconstruction of a calcaneal deficit due to osteomyelitis with femoral head allograft and tendon rebalance. *Foot (Edinb).* 2014;24(3):149-152. doi: 10.1016/j.foot.2014.03.010.

90. Holmes GB. Treatment of displaced calcaneal fractures using a small sinus tarsi approach. *Tech Foot Ankle Surg.* 2005;4(1):35-41.

91. Stephens HM, Sanders RW. Calcaneal malunions: results of a prognostic computed tomography classification system. *Foot Ankle Int.* 1996;17(7):395-401.

92. Zwipp H, Rammelt S. Posttraumatic deformity correction at the foot [in German]. *Zentralbl Chir.* 2003;128(3):218-226.

93. Schepers T. The subtalar distraction bone block arthrodesis following the late complications of calcaneal fractures: a systematic review. *Foot (Edinb).* 2013;23(1):39-44. doi: 10.1016/j.foot.2012.10.004.

94. Buckley R, Tough S, McCormack R, et al. Operative compared with nonoperative treatment of displaced intra-articular calcaneal fractures. A prospective, randomized, controlled multicenter trial. *JBJS.* 2002;84(10):1733-1744.

95. DeOrio JK, Leaseburg JT, Shapiro SA. Subtalar distraction arthrodesis through a posterior approach. *Foot Ankle Int.* 2008;29(12):1189-1194. doi: 10.3113/FAI.2008.1189.

96. Trnka H, Easley ME, Lam PW, Anderson CD, Schon LC, Myerson MS. Subtalar distraction bone block arthrodesis. *J Bone Joint Surg Br.* 2001;83B(6):849-854.

97. Ziegler P, Friederichs J, Hungerer S. Fusion of the subtalar joint for post-traumatic arthrosis: a study of functional outcomes and non-unions. *Int Orthop.* 2017;41(7):1387-1393. doi: 10.1007/s00264-017-3493-3.

CHAPTER 30

Talar Fractures

Amol Saxena, Louie Shou, and John Grady

INTRODUCTION

The talus is an integral part of the lower extremity that has a major role in the biomechanical function of the foot and ankle complex. Fractures involving the talus are associated with complications and functional limitations.[1] These injuries often require fixation and restoration of articular surfaces and alignment to optimize ankle and hindfoot function. Talar fractures can be challenging to the surgeon due to the difficulties in visualization and reduction. Postoperatively, patient expectations need to be managed carefully as there is a very high rate of osteonecrosis and posttraumatic degenerative joint disease. Timely diagnosis and appropriate planning are crucial to optimize outcomes. This section will give an overview of talar body and neck fractures including evaluation, treatment, and prognosis.

DEFINITION

Talar fractures are relatively uncommon and account for <1% of all fractures in the human body and about 3%-6% of all fractures in the foot.[2-4] Most talar neck and body fractures are associated with high-energy polytrauma cases such as falls or motor vehicle accidents although some can occur in lower velocity rotational ankle injuries as well. These injuries are more common in younger patients likely due to the fact that this patient population is more active and more likely to be involved in motor vehicle accidents. There is a higher incidence in males with up to 73% occurring in men. Talar neck and body fractures are traditionally considered the most common type of talar fracture.[5] Fractures of the talar head are least common and account for 5%-10% of all talar fractures. Talar body and neck fractures are high correlated with calcaneal and spine fractures, with a reported incidence of 13%-61%.[6]

ANATOMIC FEATURES

The talus is a unique bone and serves a crucial role as the osseous articulation between the leg and the foot.[7-9] The anatomy of the talus is very complex consisting of articulations with the tibia, fibula, calcaneus, and navicular. It is divided into a head, neck, and body; approximately two-thirds of the surface of the bone is articular cartilage. There are multiple ligamentous attachments but no muscular insertions. The talar head is covered with hyaline cartilage and articulates with the tarsal navicular, linking the ankle with the midfoot. The inferior surface of the talus is composed of 3 separate joints that help it articulate with the calcaneus. The superior surface of the talar body is referred to as the talar dome, which articulates with the tibia at the tibiotalar joint. The talar trochlea is broader anteriorly and inferiorly than posteriorly and superiorly. The lateral process of the talus articulates with the distal fibula. The sinus tarsi and tarsal canal lie along the inferior margin of the neck. The posterior process of the body of the talus consists of two tubercles allowing the flexor hallucis longus tendon to run in between them.

The blood supply to the talus is composed mainly of 3 distal arteries, which include the posterior tibial, anterior tibial (dorsalis pedis), and peroneal artery.[10,11] There, the posterior tibial artery gives off a branch into the deltoid ligament, and this ultimately supplies the talar dome. This arterial supply often represents the last source of blood supply in fractures or the talar neck. The posterior tibial artery also provides a significant supply via the artery of the tarsal canal, which forms an anastomosis with the artery of the sinus tarsi. The anterior tibial artery provides blood supply via the dorsalis pedis artery into the talar neck. The peroneal artery provides blood supply to the inferior talar neck and talar head via the artery of the sinus tarsi (Fig. 30.1).

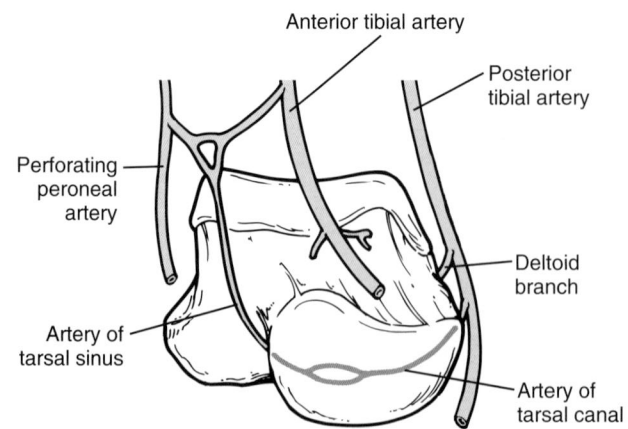

FIGURE 30.1 Blood supply to the talus.

PEARLS

Fractures of the talar neck and body are relatively rare and are usually a result of high-energy trauma. Thus, patients need to be thoroughly assessed for other injuries.

- Talar fractures can be life-changing injuries and outcomes/expectations should be tempered with patients.
- The structure of the talus and surrounding tissue is very complicated and needs to be understood well in order to restore normal anatomy.
- Advanced imaging with CT is paramount for preoperative planning.
- The soft tissue envelope of the hindfoot and ankle must be protected prior to definitive surgery. Compartment syndrome must be ruled out in high-velocity injuries.
- Early reduction is vital in long-term outcome in lowering risk of osteonecrosis. There is no relation between timing of definitive surgical fixation with relation to osteonecrosis.
- Dual incisional approaches with malleolar osteotomies help increase visualization to help facilitate accurate reduction.
- Avoid excessive dissection of the periosteal and subperiosteal structures.
- Knowledge of neurovascular structures is paramount to decrease iatrogenic injury.

CLASSIFICATION

Hawkins classification system described in 1970 is the most frequently used system to describe talar neck fractures.[5] Canale and Kelly further modified this in 1978.[2] It has proven to be useful as it provides prognostic value with respect to outcome and occurrence of avascular necrosis. The classification system is based on joint malalignment associated with vertical talar neck fractures. Talar neck fractures have a relatively high incidence due to the small cross-sectional area and vascular ingrowth, which results in a structurally weak segment of bone.[12] Type I is a nondisplaced fracture of the talar neck without any subluxation or dislocation of the peritalar joints. These injuries may be missed on initial x-rays depending on the views that are taken. Talar blood supply is usually spared in these injuries or only affecting the dorsolateral talar neck. Type II injuries involve a displaced talar neck fracture with subluxation or dislocation of the subtalar joint. In these fractures, usually 2 of the 3 sources of blood supply are interrupted. This typically will involve those talar neck branches in type I and inferiorly with the arteries in the sinus tarsi and tarsal canal. Type III injuries involve a talar neck fracture with subluxation or dislocation of the subtalar joint and tibiotalar joints. The displacement of the talus posteriorly and medially puts the medial neurovascular structures at risk.[2,12] All 3 major sources of blood supply are affected in this type of injury. Lastly, type IV injuries involve talar neck fractures with subluxation or dislocation of the ankle, subtalar, and talonavicular joints. Once again, in these injuries, all 3 major sources of blood supply are affected. There is a strong correlation between this classification and the risk of avascular necrosis. There is a 0%-15% chance of osteonecrosis in type I injuries, a 20%-50% chance of osteonecrosis in type II injuries, and a 100% chance of osteonecrosis in type II and IV injuries (Table 30.1).[13] Studies have suggested

Fracture Type	Description	Risk of Osteonecrosis (%)
I	Nondisplaced talar neck fracture	0-15
II	Talar neck fracture and talocalcaneal dislocation	20-50
III	Talar neck fracture, talocalcaneal dislocation, and tibiotalar dislocation	100
IV	Talar neck fracture and dislocation of all talar articulations	100

TABLE **30.1** **Risk of Osteonecrosis in Hawkins-Canale Type Talar Neck Fractures**

that degree of comminution, extent of soft tissue damage, and fracture displacement also influence the development of osteonecrosis[14,15] (Fig. 30.2).

The Sneppen classification is used to describe talar body fractures.[16,17] Body fractures include fractures of the talar dome, shear fractures, crush injuries, and lateral and posterior process fractures. Sneppen A fractures are defined as osteochondral dome fractures or compression fractures (Table 30.2). These are often interchangeable with the term osteochondral lesion or defect, which is further classified by Berndt and Hardy.[18] Lateral lesions are shallow and wafer shaped. They are associated with dorsiflexion and inversion injuries. Medial lesions are often asymptomatic and deep, cup shaped. These result from a plantarflexion, inversion-type mechanism. Sneppen B and C are coronal and sagittal shear fractures of the talus, respectively. These usually occur secondary to a direct axial load on a dorsiflexed foot and have a have high incidence of osteonecrosis.[19] Sneppen D fractures defined as posterior talar tubercle fractures. These can involve the medial (Cedell) and lateral (Shepherd) posterior tubercle.[20,21] These injuries usually result from a forced plantarflexion mechanism leading to compression of the posterior process between the posterior tibia and calcaneus. On examination, a "nutcracker sign" can be produced due to pain and crepitus from plantarflexion of the ankle. Often, these injuries are confused with an os trigonum (which will be discussed more later in this chapter). For reference, os trigonums are large and round with smooth surfaces. Posterior tubercle fractures generally have irregular edges. Sneppen E injuries involve the lateral talar process.[22,23] These usually occur from a forced dorsiflexion and inversion injury to the foot. Patients will complain of pain to the lateral ankle. These fractures can best be seen on AP radiograph. There is a high incidence of this in snowboarders. Lastly, Sneppen F injuries are crushed, comminuted talar body fractures and have the worst prognosis of all talar body fractures.[24]

PHYSICAL EXAMINATION

Patient history and physical examination are very important in the evaluation of talar fractures.[8,25-29] These injuries are consistently involved in trauma to the ankle. Patients will present with pain, swelling, and hematoma/ecchymosis. There is pain tenderness throughout the ankle and midfoot globally. Neurovascular

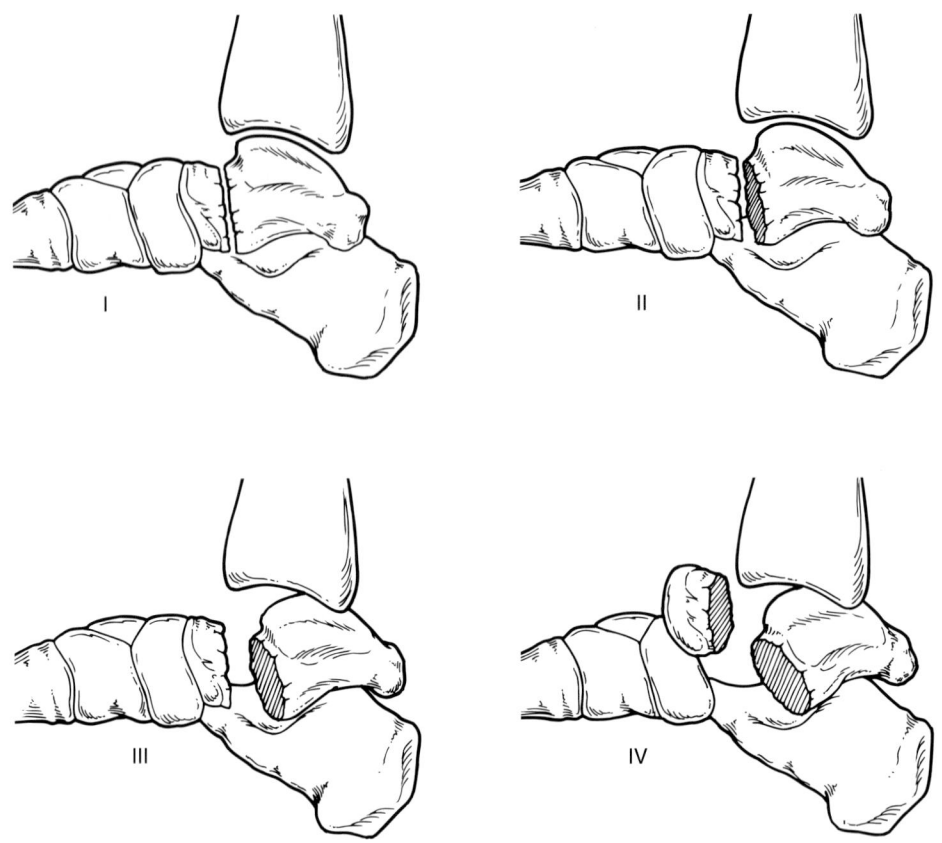

FIGURE 30.2 Types I-IV talar neck fractures.

status needs to be assessed to rule out compartment syndrome. Lateral and posterior talar fractures often present with more focal localized signs. These can sometimes be missed on initial radiograph. Lateral process fractures will present with lateral ankle pain. Posterior talar fractures are associated with pain and crepitus posteriorly with plantarflexion of the ankle joint, often described as a nutcracker sign. There will be pain associated with range of motion of the first metatarsophalangeal joint due to the flexor hallucis longus tendon. Patients will complain of either posterior ankle pain or Achilles tendon pain.

The initial radiographic evaluation of talar fractures involves anteroposterior (AP), mortise, and lateral views of the ankle as well as AP, oblique, and lateral views of the foot. A Canale view is also helpful in visualizing the talar neck. This is done with the ankle in plantarflexion with the knee bent. The foot is internally rotated ~15 degrees, and the x-ray beam is aimed at a 75-degree

angle from the floor. Furthermore, the axial Harris radiographic view is an additional image that allows for visualization for the posterior and middle portions of the subtalar joint. This is a 45-degree axial view of the heel. Harris and Canale views are less commonly used due to the availability of computed tomography (CT). CT images are vital in the treatment for talar fractures as they give the surgeon a better picture of the exact location of the fracture(s), degree of comminution, and displacement to aid in surgical planning if needed (Fig. 30.3A-C).

TREATMENT

Fractures of the talar body and neck that are nondisplaced can be treated with cast immobilization in the neutral position for 6-8 weeks. Full weight bearing is initiated in the 8-10 week period after radiographic evidence of healing. Posterior tubercle fractures are amenable to CAM boot immobilization with weight bearing to tolerance.

For displaced, intra-articular fractures of the talar head, neck, and body with or without subluxation or dislocation, surgery is recommended to restore anatomic reduction and re-align joint surfaces. Reduction of talar neck fractures, subluxations, and dislocations should be done immediately to protect the integrity of the soft tissue and prevent neurovascular compromise. Open talar fractures, talar extrusions, and irreducible dislocations warrant emergent operative treatment. Current literature states that timing of definitive fixation does not correlate with risk of avascular necrosis.[17,30-32] AVN is more likely related to the lack of initial reduction as well as the degree of

TABLE 30.2	Sneppen Classification of Talar Body Fractures
Type	**Description**
A	Compression or osteochondral dome fracture
B	Coronal shear fracture
C	Sagittal shear fracture
D	Posterior tubercle fracture
E	Lateral tubercle fracture
F	Comminuted fracture

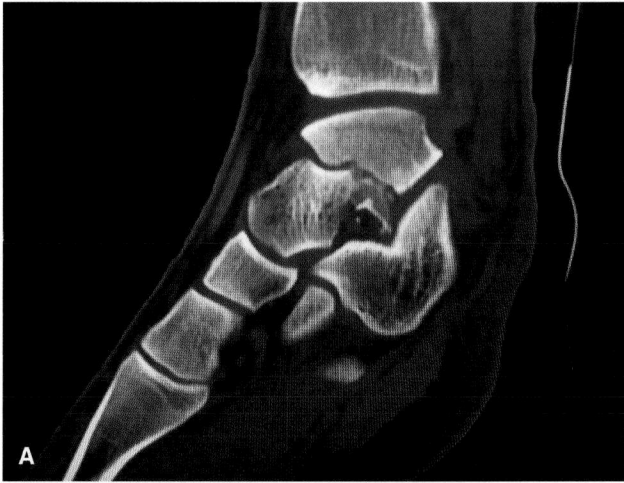

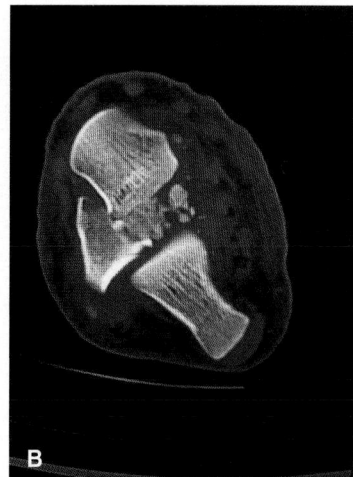

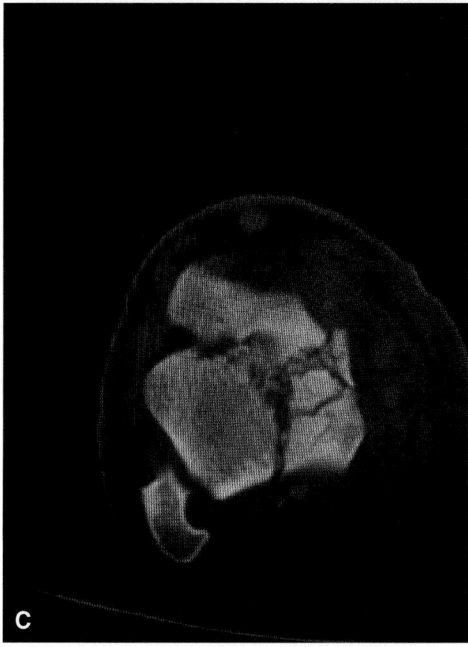

FIGURE 30.3 A-C. Preoperative CT showing intra-articular comminution of talar body fracture involving the subtalar and ankle joints.

initial injury (displacement, comminution, open fracture).[14] It is recommended to wait until soft tissue envelope is amenable for definitive fixation after the reduction of the talar fracture is completed.[17,31-33] This will help minimize postoperative complications including infection, skin necrosis, and wound dehiscence.[14,34]

There are many surgical approaches to visualization and access to the talar neck and body. To optimize visualization of the talar neck, the current standard of care is with dual incisions with an anteromedial and anterolateral approach.[14,17,25,32,33] For body fractures, these incisions are often combined with medial or lateral malleolar osteotomies for better visualization.[17,34] The patient is supine on the operative table with a bump underneath the ipsilateral hip to help position the ankle into a neutral position. The anteromedial incision is centered over the medial malleolus between the tibialis anterior tendon and the posterior tibial tendon. The incision spans from the proximal medial malleolus down to the distal talonavicular joint. This gives the surgeon access to the anteromedial talar body, the medial talar neck, and the talar head, if needed. A medial malleolar osteotomy is made if further exposure is needed of the

medial and posterior talar body.[35] The medial malleolar osteotomy is predrilled to allow for proper screw placement after talar fixation is complete. Once the medial malleolus is osteotomized, this is pulled down inferiorly to allow direct visualization of the medial talar dome for reduction and fixation. The deltoid ligament is preserved.

The anterolateral incision is anterior to the anterior border of the distal fibula just between the peroneus tertius and extensor digitorum longus tendons. The incision can be extended distally toward the talonavicular joint. Care is taken to avoid damage to the superficial peroneal nerve. The extensor digitorum brevis and longus are carefully retracted to expose the lateral talar dome, lateral talar neck, and lateral talonavicular joint.

It is important to avoid dissection of the inferior portion of the talar neck to prevent further damage to the blood supply.[36,37] Furthermore, the deltoid ligament complex should also not be violated. Provisional reductions of the talar neck and body are temporarily held with Kirschner wires. Dental picks and small point to point reduction clamps are useful in temporarily holding reduction as well. Distraction can be used as well to help with visualization and reduction. This can be achieved

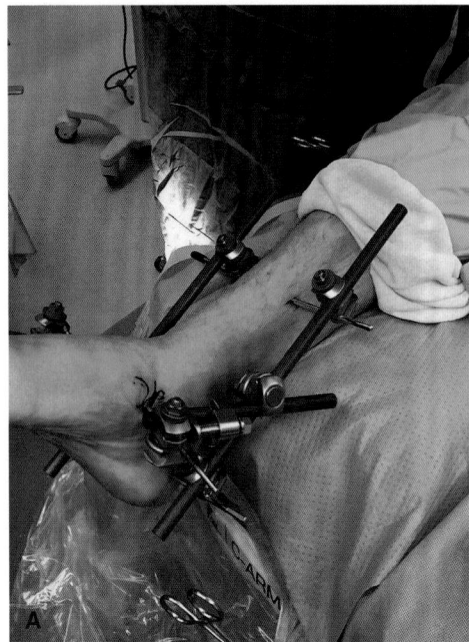

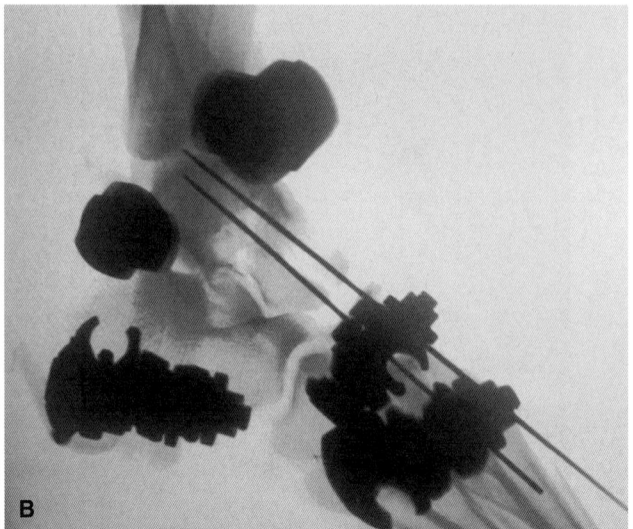

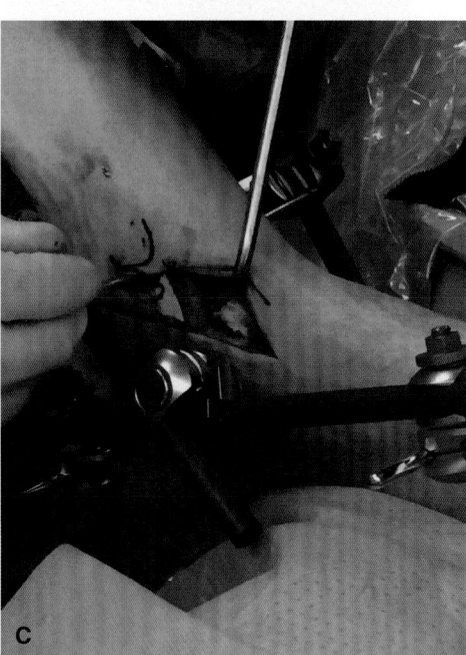

FIGURE 30.4 A-C: Initial reduction with pin fixation and placement of delta frame.

with Shanz pins, external fixators, or other distractors[14,38,39] (Fig. 30.4A-C). Radiographic assessment is used to visualize fracture alignment. AP, lateral, and oblique views of the ankle joint are imperative. Canale view must also be checked to see the reduction of the subtalar joint.[25]

Definitive fixation with small fragment or mini fragment implants is typically used to help maintain the fracture alignment and reduction. Countersunk screw heads or headless screws are preferable as they are not prominent and do not affect the gliding of the articular surfaces[14,17,33] (Fig. 30.5A and B). These are particularly useful in the setting of talar dome fractures. The talus medially and laterally are amenable to buttress plating with mini fragment locking plates to help maintain alignment and stability.[14,34,40] The lateral talus has more nonarticulating surface area and room for plating from the lateral

talar neck to the edge of the lateral process. One must be more careful medially to ensure that there is no impingement in the medial gutter. Furthermore, due to the comminution associated with many of these fractures, bone grafting of areas of the talar neck have been found to be useful to restore defects and enhance stability.[14,17] Comminution or impaction of the medial talar neck has been related to malrotation, varus deformity, and neck shortening.[36,37]

DISCUSSION

Talar fractures present with a multitude of difficulties not only for the surgeon but also for the patient's long-term prognosis. Due to tenuous blood supply and highly articular nature of the

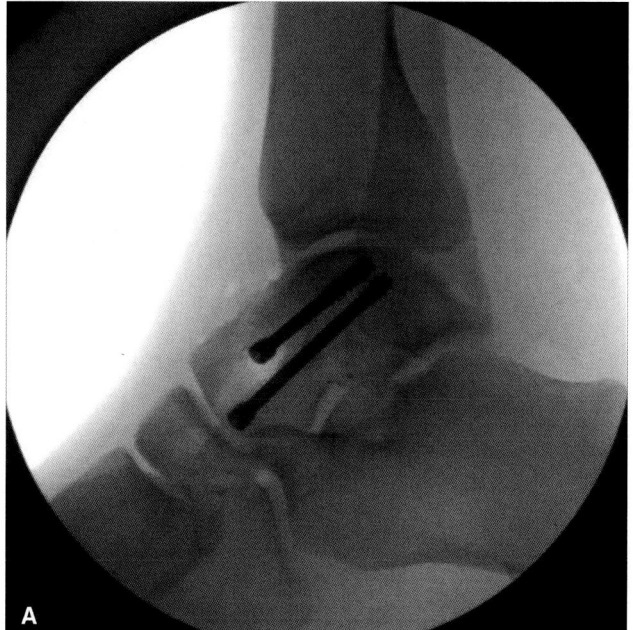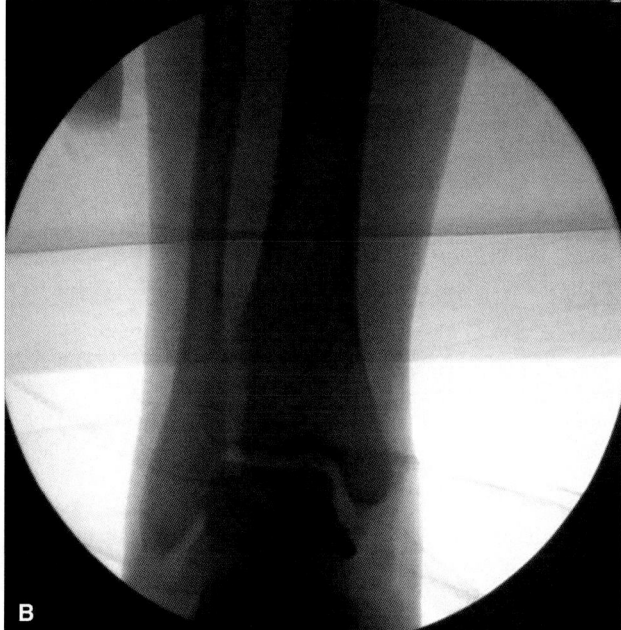

FIGURE 30.5 A, B. Postoperative x-rays showing anatomic reduction of talar fracture using crossing headless screws.

talus, patients are at a very high risk for degenerative joint disease and osteonecrosis. The high velocity nature of these injuries can cause open fractures and significant soft tissue damage as well, which will also increase risk of wound healing problems and infection. Halvorson et al. reported deep infection rates for talar neck fractures to be 21%.[30] Marsh et al. reported 38% rate of deep infection for open talar fractures.[41] The current recommendation for definitive surgical fixation to minimize risks associated with infection and wound healing problems is to wait until soft tissue swelling is improved, which can take up to 2-3 weeks.[25] Placement of external fixators can be extremely helpful in stabilizing these fractures during the acute phase. Immediate definitive surgery resulted in higher rates of wound dehiscence and infection.[5]

Osteonecrosis of the talus is notorious for these types of injuries. Overall incidence of osteonecrosis resulting from talar neck fractures varies from 26% to 33%.[30,31,42] All studies report increase in risk of osteonecrosis with increase in severity of injury. As mentioned previously, contrary to earlier belief, there is no relation between timing of surgery and definitive fixation with relation to osteonecrosis. Once again, the incidence of osteonecrosis is higher due to the severity of the injury (comminution, subtalar joint dislocation, open injuries).[17,30,31] For talar neck fractures, specifically type I, II, III, and IV fractures reported incidence of osteonecrosis of 0%-15%, 20%-50%, 100%, and 100%, respectively.[17]

Osteonecrosis is defined by increase in radiodensity between 4 weeks and 6 months postoperatively. Hawkins sign, which is a radiographic indicator for sufficient vascularity, is described as radiolucency at the subchondral bone seen at ~6-8 weeks.[5] This indicates that the progression to osteonecrosis is unlikely. It is important to keep in mind that the absence of Hawkins sign does not necessarily mean that the patient has osteonecrosis as many patients will take up to 2 years to revascularize after injury.[17,43] It is important to consider that more than half of patients who have radiographic signs of osteonecrosis are asymptomatic.[33,34]

Symptomatic osteonecrosis can be treated conservatively with restricted weight bearing, bracing, and extracorporeal shock wave therapy. Surgical repair of talar osteonecrosis depends on the amount of bone affected. Options include total ankle arthroplasty, tibiotalar arthrodesis, tibiotalocalcaneal arthrodesis, and tibiocalcaneal fusion.

Malunion is another common complication associated with talar fractures. The most common being a varus malalignment of the talar neck.[2] Dual incisional approaches to visualize both sides of the talus as well as bone grafting the defect areas reduce the risk of shortening and varus deformities.

Lastly, posttraumatic degenerative joint disease is the most common complication after talar fractures. Once again, due to the high surface area and complex nature of the talar articular cartilage, posttraumatic arthritis is almost inevitable. The overall rate of posttraumatic arthritis is reported at 51%-67%.[30,42] Of the surrounding joints to the talus, the subtalar joint is most commonly involved and reported over 80% for studies that have at least a 2-year follow-up. The current standard of care is arthrodesis of the affected joint(s). The only joint motion preserving option is a total ankle arthroplasty.

OTHER ACUTE TALAR INJURIES

SNOWBOARDER'S ANKLE

The classic "snowboarder's ankle" occurs with its namesake sport and any activity that creates the similar mechanism of injury.[44,45] This fracture typically occurs with the foot in dorsiflexion and eversion or external rotation of the calcaneus (Fig. 30.6). This mechanism of injury can occur with many sports and trauma situations.[46,47] The impact creates a compression in the region of the posterior inferior talus' lateral aspect. This can result in fracture(s) of this region from the lateral talar process to the posterior aspect of the talus. CT scan is the most

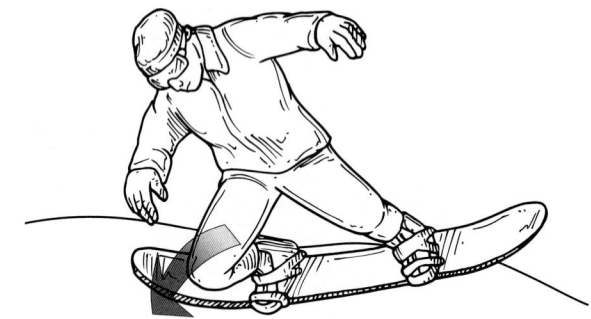

FIGURE 30.6 Snowboarder falling causing injury.

helpful examination to assess the injury. A classification system was first described by Bladin and McCrory in 1995.[47,48] These injuries are classified via CT evaluating the fracture of the lateral talar process as type A (extra-articular), B1 and B2 (incomplete or multifragment of the posterior talocalcaneal surface), and C1 and C2 (simple or multifragment involving the talofibular articular surface of the talus)[47,48] (Fig. 30.7).

Patients will have pain in the lateral foot and ankle region and often assume they have an ankle sprain. The history should include whether the patient fell with the foot fixed, such as in a snowboard binding. Pain can be produced by eversion and inversion, combined with dorsiflexion. Edema and ecchymosis are frequently noted. Weight bearing will be limited. Other concomitant injuries can occur, particularly if incurred with snowboarding, such as concussions and wrist injuries.

Initial treatment is non–weight bearing with a compression dressing, incorporated into a sugar-tong and posterior splint, ice packs proximal to the dressing (behind the knee), and pain control. Initial radiographs are taken. With an index of suspicion of a snowboarder's ankle injury, a CT is ordered as MRI may not show the true extent of the fracture and comminution. If there is significant intra-articular involvement (typically 1/3 or more) of the talar surface of the subtalar joint, along with displacement of >2 mm, surgical reduction would be recommended as well as with significantly comminuted fractures with displacement (ie, loose bodies).[44-47] Otherwise, nondisplaced fractures are treated nonoperatively with non–weight bearing in a below-knee cast or boot for 6 weeks and then weight bearing for an additional 4 weeks in a boot (Fig. 30.8A-E). Range of motion (ROM) exercises are initiated at 6 weeks, and formal physical therapy begins at 8-10 weeks.

Prior to surgical intervention, patients should have a reduction in edema and a "wrinkle sign." The patient is placed in the lateral decubitus position. A thigh tourniquet is utilized. For small nonessential fragments, arthroscopic excision may be warranted.[49] Otherwise, an open approach with a modified Ollier incision more laterally based is performed (Fig. 30.9). Smaller diameter screws (1.5-4.0 mm depending on fragment size) and plates as needed are utilized for the reduction (Fig. 30.10A-C). An endoscope can be used to verify reduction and improve visualization. Minimal deep closure is utilized. Skin is closed with interrupted nonabsorbable sutures. Postoperative care is otherwise the same as nonoperative treatment.

Despite anatomic reduction and appropriate treatment, patients with snowboarder's ankle injury can still have posttraumatic arthritis of the subtalar joint and lateral ankle impingement. The incidence of this is not as well known as with other foot and ankle injuries that are more common.[50] Nonsurgically, ankle braces, foot orthoses, and injections can be utilized. Subtalar arthrodesis is the definitive treatment.

OS TRIGONUM/POSTERIOR TALAR INJURIES

Injuries to the posterior talus can include fractures of the so-called "Stieda's process" and other portions of posterior talar tubercles. Stieda described the enlargement of the posterior lateral talar tubercle. It is implicated in posterior ankle impingement, which is common in dancers, in whom it can be found in up to 44% of that population.[51] The "os trigonum" is an accessory ossicle present up to 12% of the population, typically joined to the posterior talus by a synchondral junction.[52] Plantarflexion combined with inversion usually produce these injuries to the posterior aspect of the talus (the posterior pinching is known as a "nutcracker injury"). These posterior injuries are often initially missed with ankle injuries. There is no accepted classification system to guide treatment with os trigonum injuries. If the posterior talus is fractured more than 1/3 of the articular surface and the fragment is displaced more than 2 mm, surgical reduction is recommended. If an os trigonum injury is a first-time event, unless severely large or displaced, nonsurgical treatment is initially recommended. Below-knee cast/boot is typically recommended for at least 4 weeks.

Patients will often present in a delayed fashion. They will most often relate that they incurred a prior ankle sprain.[53,54] Pain and often edema are usually present in the posterior ankle and they may claim "Achilles pain." Symptoms will be reproduced with plantarflexion of the ankle. In addition, it can be recreated most often with range of motion of the hallux, as the flexor hallucis longus (FHL) courses on the posterior aspect of the talus. There often are significant ligamentous attachments enveloping the FHL to the posterior ankle and subtalar joint capsule.[55] Because of this, dancers especially those in ballet are among the most susceptible from an athletic and occupational aspect, due to the fact their activity produces plantarflexion at maximal ranges.[51,55]

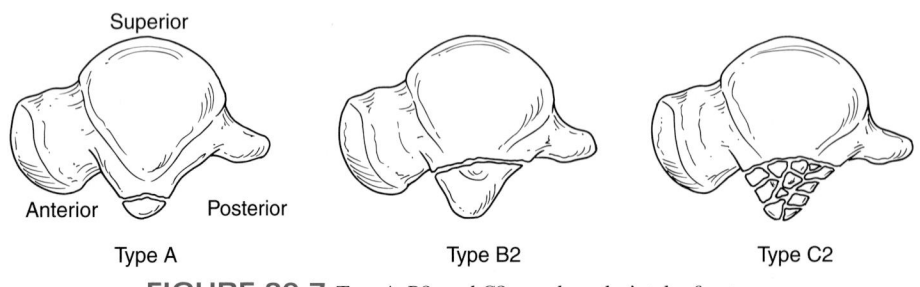

FIGURE 30.7 Type A, B2, and C2 snowboarder's talar fractures.

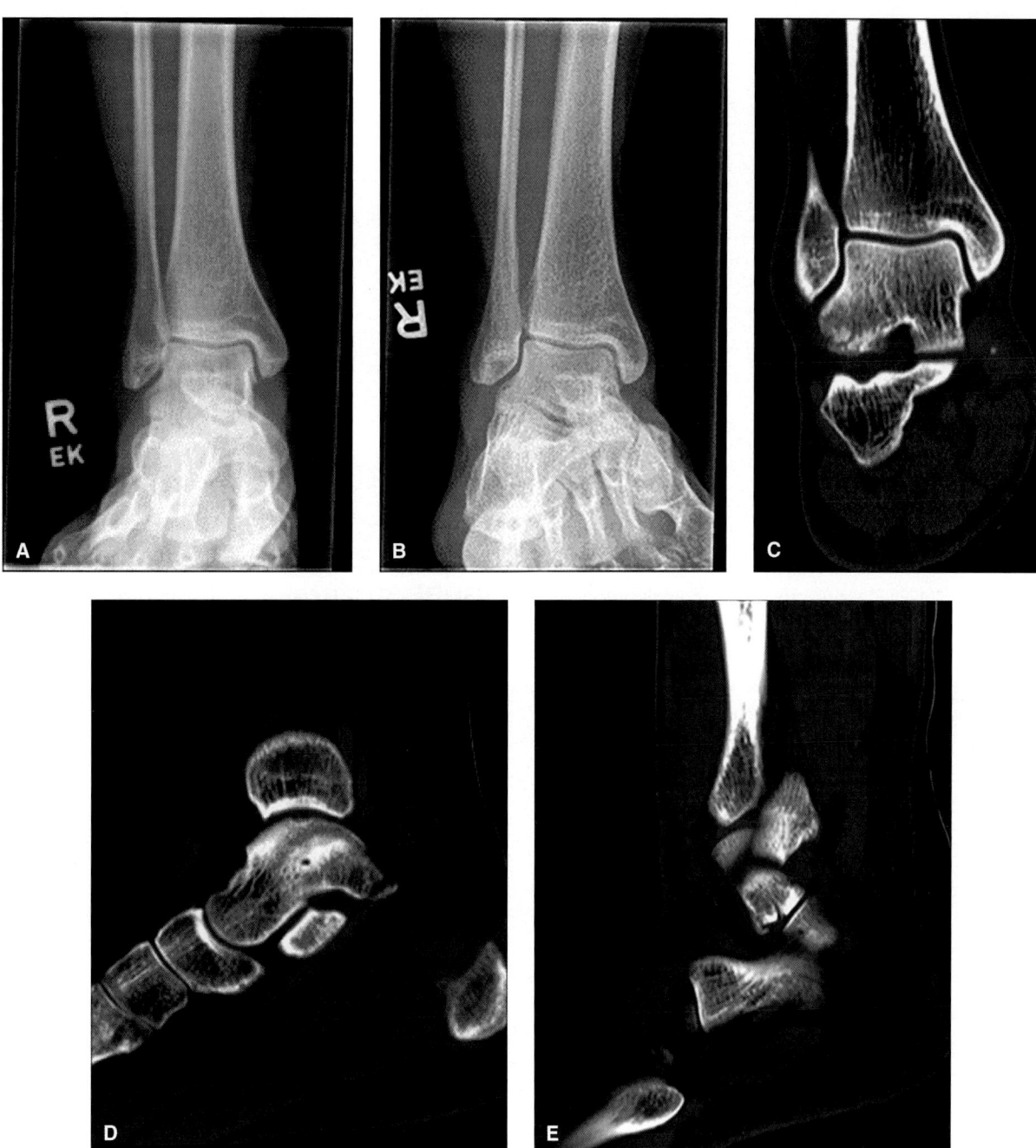

FIGURE 30.8 **A, B.** X-rays of a snowboarder's ankle injury. **C-E.** CT scan of a nondisplaced type B 2 snowboarder's ankle.

Similar to other intra-articular fractures of the foot and ankle, displacement of 2 or more mm displacement of the posterior talar/Stieda fragment can be indication for surgical intervention, particularly if it involves 1/3 of the articular surface.[56] With isolated os trigonum injuries, significant displacement is an indication for excision and can be performed arthroscopically.[55,57] Otherwise, nonsurgical treatment involves a below-knee cast/boot in neutral position for 4-6 weeks.

For surgical intervention, the patient positioning is dependent on the location of injury. Pure lateral injuries can be approached from the lateral position via an open approach. (*Arthroscopic/endoscopic approaches are described elsewhere in this text.*) An incision is placed posterior to the peroneal tendons and anterior to the sural nerve (Fig. 30.11). Care is taken to avoid excessive retraction of the neural branches posteriorly and preserve the peroneal retinaculum attachments as it must be incised. The peronei are reflected anteriorly. The posterior ankle capsule is incised to create an arthrotomy, exposing the posterior ankle and subtalar joints. A 4.0-mm endoscope or suction light source can improve visualization during excision of the posterior fragment/os trigonum. Care is taken to avoid iatrogenic laceration of the FHL. The joints are inspected for any chondral defects. The posterior talus should be rasped smooth and bone wax is applied over the exposed bony surfaces. After irrigation, intraoperative imaging should conform appropriate excision. Deep closure includes repair of the peroneal

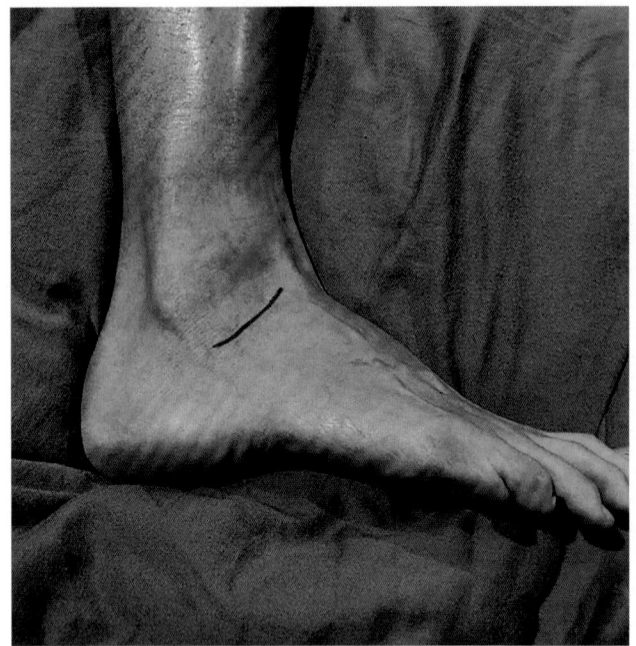

FIGURE 30.9 "Ollier" incision approach for snowboarder's ankle injury.

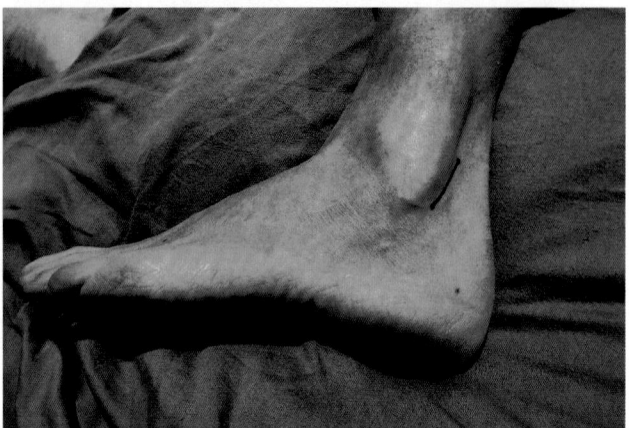

FIGURE 30.11 Posterolateral approach for open os trigonum excision.

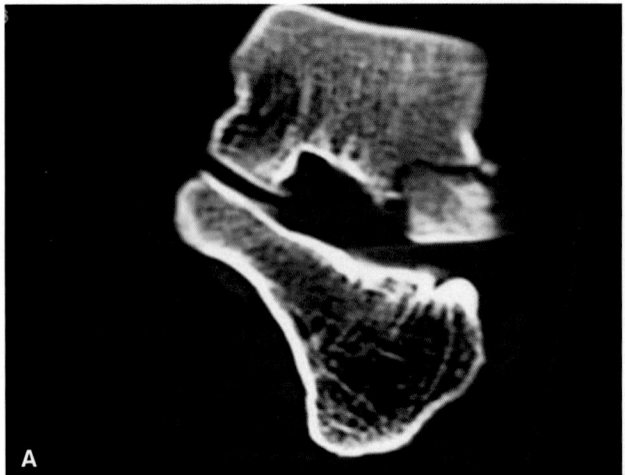

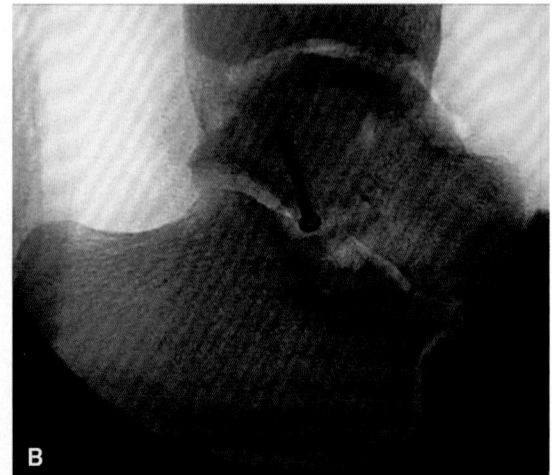

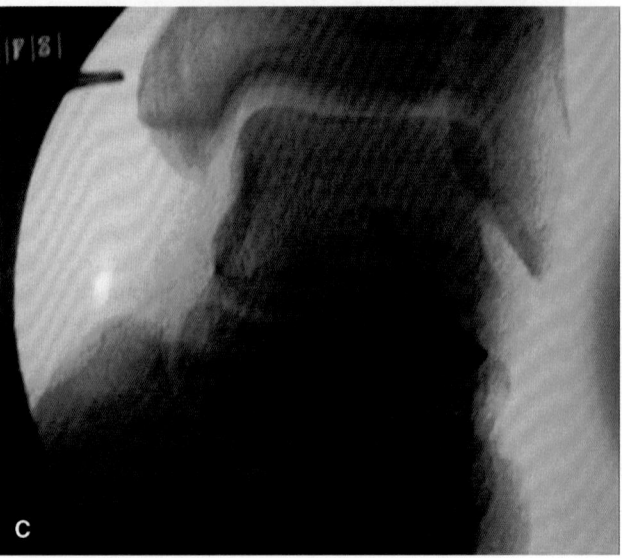

FIGURE 30.10 Preop CT of type C1 snowboarder's ankle **(A)**, and intraop post-ORIF fluoroscans **(B, C)**. (Courtesy Stephen J. Miller, DPM.)

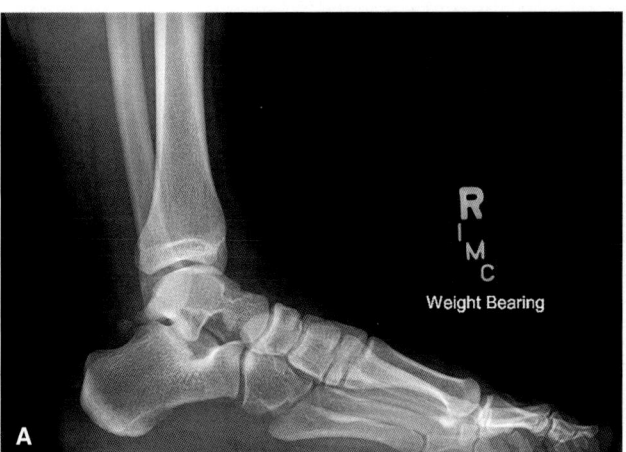

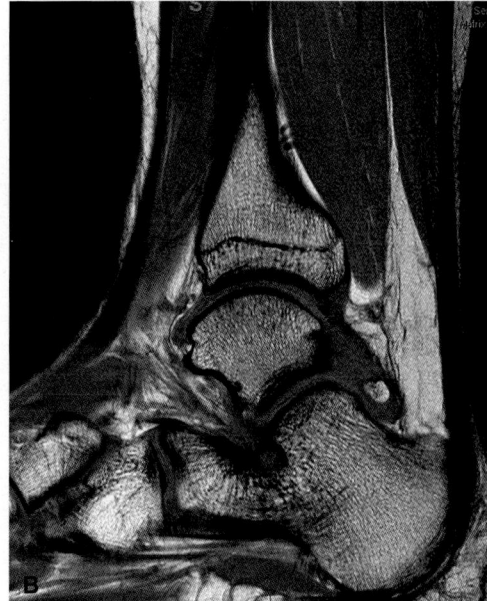

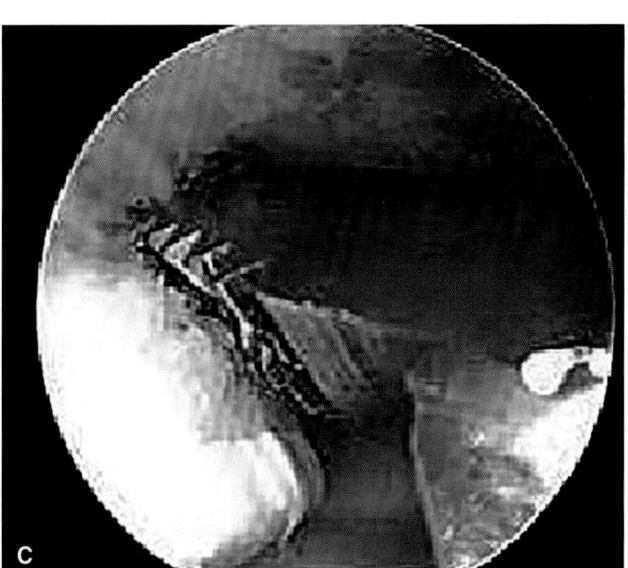

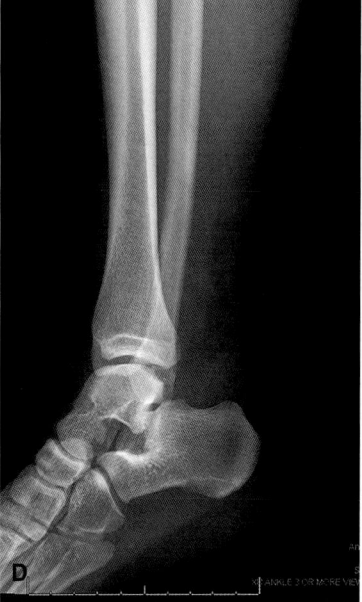

FIGURE 30.12 Preop X-ray and MRI of posterior talar impingement and displaced os trigonum injury in a dancer **(A, B)**. Arthroscopic view of rasping posterior talus postexcision of the os trigonum and posterior talus **(C)**. Postop X-ray **(D)**.

retinaculum with 2-0 braided absorbable suture. Arthroscopic approaches are generally faster healing and amenable to smaller ossicles[55,57] (Fig. 30.12A-D). Skin is closed with the foot in neutral position with 3-0 nylon.

If there is a potential the posterior fragment or os trigonum will displace medially, a prone position may be beneficial. This is particularly helpful if repair of the FHL is anticipated. For medial talar injuries and documented FHL tears, a supine position can be utilized. The medial incision is place posterior to the neurovascular bundle, which is gently retracted anteriorly[54] (Fig. 30.13). The flexor (lacinate) retinaculum attachments are maintained. Deep dissection is performed to the posterior ankle and subtalar joints. After excision of the posterior fragment/os trigonum, rasping of the posterior talus and irrigation, the FHL is repaired with nonabsorbable suture. Generally, there

is a longitudinal tear, so a buried knot cerclage technique can be utilized. Imaging is performed to confirm complete excision. The flexor retinaculum is repaired with 2-0 braided absorbable suture. The skin is repaired with the foot in neutral position.

Postoperatively, patients are placed in a below-knee cast/ boot for 4 weeks, 6 weeks if the FHL is repaired. Physical therapy is then performed and return to sports is typically at 8-12 weeks. Typically, patients wear an ankle brace or tape for the first 6-12 weeks after they remove the boot.

ACUTE TALAR DOME FRACTURES

Acute injuries to the talus can occur to the dome, involving the cartilage and underlying surface, aka "osteochondral," "transchondral" defects/lesions (OCDs, TLs). When the articular

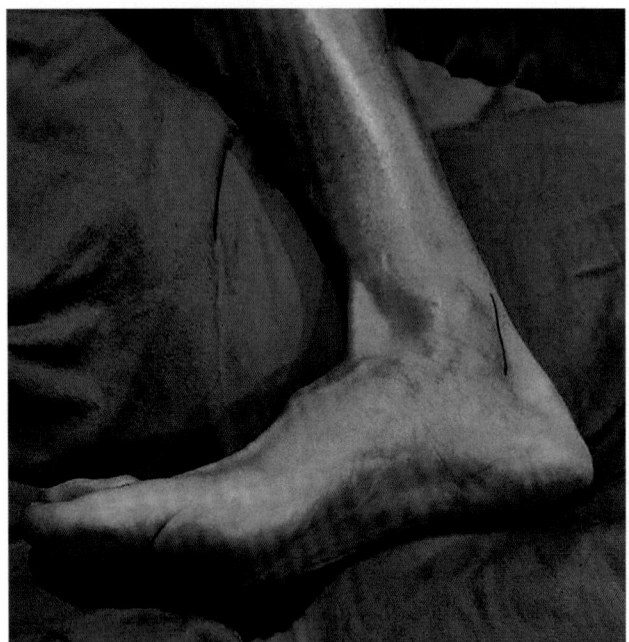

FIGURE 30.13 Posteromedial approach to repair FHL and excise posterior talus.

surface of the talus has been damaged, a determination of whether surgery should and can be performed is made. Imaging such as CT and/or MRI is often performed, in addition to plain X-rays. This chapter on talar fractures will deal with acute lesions that are displaced. Other treatment methods for talar OCDs/TLs are discussed elsewhere in this text.

Patients will present with symptoms similar to an ankle sprain or fracture. A significant percent of patients will have some degree of this injury, upward to 50% after ankle sprains and fractures.[58] It is helpful in edematous patients to perform cryotherapy and apply a compression dressing for a few days

and then re-assess the patient for tenderness on the talar dome after acute injuries. MRI or CT imaging will show a lesion in the talar dome. Sometimes, the lesion will be displaced or inverted (Fig. 30.14A-C). The size and position will be denoted via CT and/or MRI.

Large intra-articular fragments (1/3 of the dome) and significantly displaced lesions can be stabilized surgically. Small intra-articular chondral fragments can be considered potential loose bodies, which can be arthroscopically excised. Chondral defects can be treated with microfracture as well. Nondisplaced lesions < 1/3 of the articular surfaced can be treated with a period of 6 weeks non–weight bearing in a below-knee cast or boot and progressed to weight bearing based on imaging showing signs of healing. Depending on the size and location of the talar lesion, open or arthroscopic approaches can be used. Small lesions easily accessed with arthroscopic techniques can be stabilized with screws (1.5-3.5 mm, ideally low-profile head) or bioabsorbable pins (1.3-2.0 mm). Larger or significantly displaced lesions may be approached via arthrotomy (with osteotomy when needed) based on lesion location; the patient is therefore positioned appropriately. A lightened suction device or 4.0-mm endoscope can be used to improve visualization and confirm reduction with open approaches. Inverted and displaced ("LIFT") lesions are repositioned.[59] Screw or pin fixation is used to stabilize the lesion. Postoperatively, the patient is kept non–weight bearing for 6 weeks in a below-knee cast or boot and progressed to weight bearing based on imaging showing signs of healing (Fig. 30.15A and B). Physical therapy is initiated after 8 weeks though range of motion is initiated much sooner. Continuous passive range of motion (CPM) has been advocated but not critically studied for these specific talar injuries to enhance healing as in other orthopedic injuries.[59,60] Patients often use an ankle brace during the rehabilitative phase. Despite anatomic reduction, posttraumatic arthritis can occur. Treatment can include bracing, orthoses, injection therapy, and other techniques described elsewhere in this text.

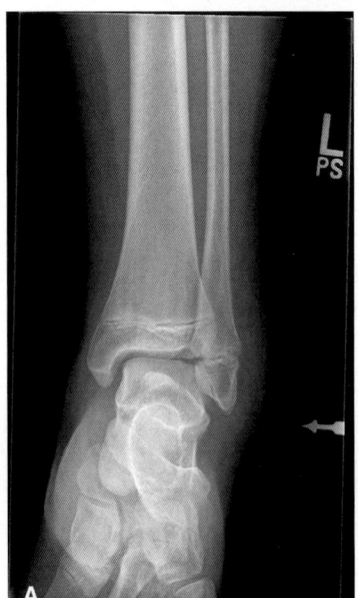
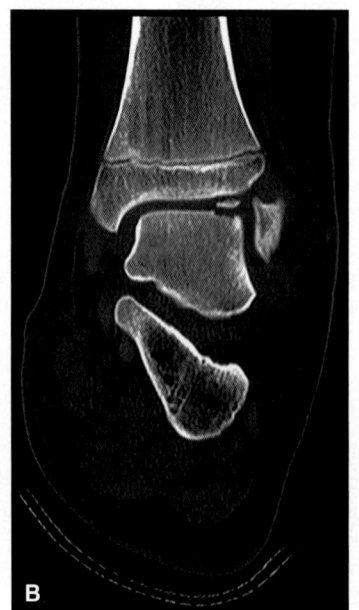
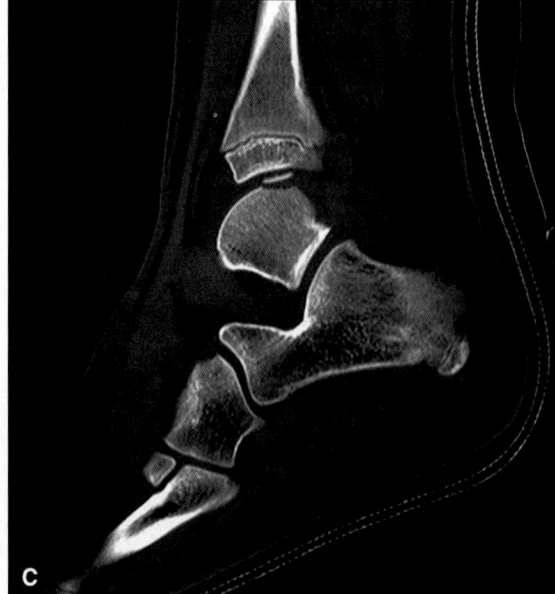

FIGURE 30.14 Preop X-ray **(A)** and CT images **(B, C)** of an inverted displaced osteochondral ("LIFT") lesion.

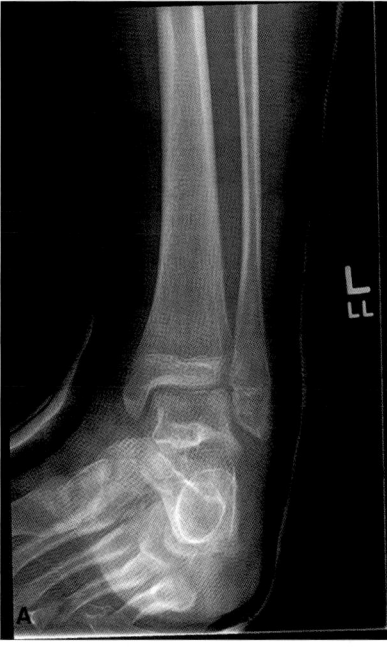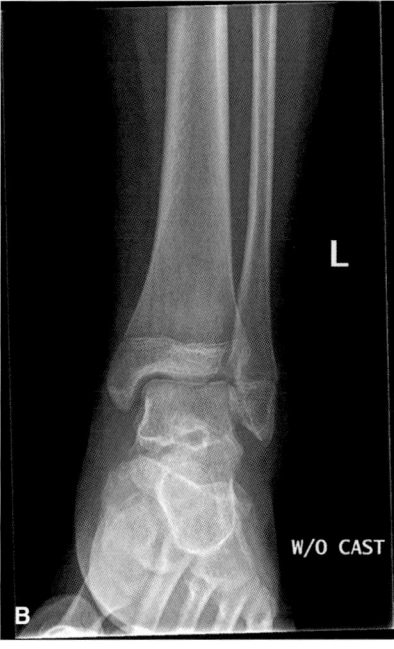

FIGURE 30.15 Immediate postreduction **(A)** and 6-week follow-up of the LIFT lesion **(B)**.

SUMMARY

Fractures of the talus are rare injuries that are usually a result of high-energy trauma. These fractures can present in a multitude of patterns due to the unique and complex shape of the talus. Patients need to be carefully assessed and major life-threatening injuries are usually occurring concomitantly. Surgical planning is paramount for improving patient outcome. Reduction of the talus and respecting the soft tissue envelope during the initial treatment are vital. Open fractures and talar extrusions need to be reduced emergently in the operative setting. Restoration of the articular surfaces and alignment of the talus are paramount in optimizing ankle and hindfoot function postoperatively. Complication rates are high due to the high surface area of articular cartilage and poor blood supply. Patients need to be aware of long-term prognosis with osteonecrosis and posttraumatic arthritis.

REFERENCES

1. Shakked RJ, Twjwani NC. Surgical treatment of talus fractures. *Orthop Clin North Am.* 2013;44:521-528.
2. Canale ST, Kelly FB. Fractures of the neck of the talus: long term evaluation of 71 cases. *J Bone Joint Surg Am.* 1978;60:143-156.
3. Lin S, Hak DJ. Management of talar neck fractures. *Orthopedics.* 2011;34:715-721.
4. Vallier HA, Nork SE, Benirsche SK, et al. Surgical treatment of talar body fractures. *J Bone Joint Surg Am.* 2003;85:1716-1724.
5. Hawkins L. Fractures of the neck of the talus. *J Bone Joint Surg Am.* 1970;52(5):991-1002.
6. Dale JD, Ha AS, Chew FS. Update on talar fracture patterns: a large level I trauma center study. *AJR Am J Roentgenol.* 2013;201:1087-1092.
7. Melenevsky Y, Mackey, RA, Abrahams, RB, Thomson NB. Talar fractures and dislocations: a radiologist's guide to timely diagnosis and classification. *Muskuloskelet Imag.* 2015;35:765-779.
8. Rammelt S, Zwipp H. Talar neck and body fractures. *Injury.* 2009;40:120-135.
9. Ebraheim NA, Sabry FF, Nadim Y. Internal architecture of the talus: implication for talar fracture. *Foot Ankle Int.* 1999;20:794-796.
10. Mulfinger GL, Trueta J. The blood supply of the talus. *J Bone Joint Surg.* 1970;52:160-167.
11. Prasarn ML, Miller AN, Dyke JP, et al. Arterial anatomy of the talus: a cadaver and gadolinium-enhanced MRI study. *Foot Ankle Int.* 2010;31(11):987-993.
12. Daniels TR, Smith JW. Talar neck fractures. *Foot Ankle.* 1993;14(4):225-234.
13. Pearce DH, Mongiardi CN, Fornasier VL, Daniels TR. Avascular necrosis of the talus: a pictorial essay. *RadioGraphics.* 2005;25(2):399-410.
14. Vallier HA, Nork SE, Barei DP, Benirschke SK, Sangeorzan BJ. Talar neck fractures: results and outcomes. *J Bone Joint Surg Am.* 2004;86-A(8):1616-1624.
15. Bellamy JL, Keeling JJ, Wenke J, Hsu JR. Does a longer delay in fixation of talus fractures cause osteonecrosis? *J Surg Orthop Adv.* 2011;20(1):34-37.
16. Sneppen O, Christensen SB, Krogsoe O, Lorentzen J. Fracture of the body of the talus. *Acta Orthop Scand.* 1977;48(3):317-324.
17. Vallier HA. Fractures of the talus: state of the art. *J Orthop Trauma.* 2015;29:385-392.
18. Berndt AL, Harty M. Transchondral fractures (osteochondritis dissecans) of the talus. *J Bone Joint Surg Am.* 1959;41-A:988-1020.
19. Abrahams TG, Gallup L, Avery FL. Nondisplaced shearing-type talar body fractures. *Ann Emerg Med.* 1994;23(4):891-893.
20. Cedell CA. Rupture of the posterior talotibial ligament with the avulsion of a bone fragment from the talus. *Acta Orthop Scand.* 1974;45(3):454-461.
21. Paulos LE, Johnson CL, Noyes FR. Posterior compartment fractures of the ankle: a commonly missed athletic injury. *Am J Sports Med.* 1983;11(6):439-443.
22. Hawkins LG. Fracture of the lateral process of the talus. *J Bone Joint Surg Am.* 1965;47:1170-1175.
23. Ebraheim NA, Skie MC, Podeszwa DA, Jackson WT. Evaluation of process fractures of the talus using computed tomography. *J Orthop Trauma.* 1994;8(4):332-337.
24. Ebraheim NA, Patil V, Owens C, Kandimalla Y. Clinical outcome of fractures of the talar body. *Int Orthop.* 2008;32(6):773-777.
25. Whitaker C, Turvey B, Illical EM. Current concepts in talar neck fracture management. *Curr Rev Musculoskelet Med.* 2018;11(3):456-474.
26. Bykov Y. Fractures of the talus. *Clin Podiatr Med Surg.* 2014;31:509-521.
27. Frawley PA, Hart JA, Young DA. Treatment outcome of major fractures of the talus. *Foot Ankle Int.* 1995;16(6):339-345.
28. Early JS. Talus fracture management. *Foot Ankle Clin.* 2008;13(4):635-657.
29. Early JS. Management of fractures of the talus: body and head regions. *Foot Ankle Clin.* 2004;9(4):709-722.
30. Halvorson JJ, Winter SB, Teasdall RD, Scott AT. Talar neck fractures: a systematic review of the literature. *J Foot Ankle Surg.* 2013;52(1):56-61.
31. Dodd A, Lefaivre KA. Outcomes of talar neck fractures: a systematic review and meta-analysis. *J Orthop Trauma.* 2015;29(5):210-215.
32. Maher MH, Chauhan A, Altman GT, Westrick ER. The acute management and associated complications of major injuries of the talus. *JBJS Rev.* 2017;5(7):1-11.
33. Buza JA, Leucht P. Fractures of the talus: current concepts and new developments. *Foot Ankle Surg.* 2017;24(4):282-290.
34. Fournier A, Barba N, Steiger V, et al. Total talar fracture—long-term results of internal fixation of talar fractures. A multicentric study of 114 cases. *Orthop Traumatol Surg Res.* 2012;98(4):48-55.
35. Ziran BH, Abidi NA, Scheel MJ. Medial malleolar osteotomy for exposure of complex talar body fractures. *J Orthop Trauma.* 2001;15(7):513-518.
36. Shakeed RJ, Tejwani NC. Surgical treatment of talus fractures. *Orthop Clin North Am.* 2013;44(4):521-528.
37. Fortin PT, Balazsy JE. Talus fractures: evaluation and treatment. *J Am Acad Orthop Surg.* 2001;9(2):114-127.
38. Patel NJ, Wansbrough G. Achieving exposure and distraction through medial malleolar osteotomy for fractures of the talus. *Tech Orthop.* 2016;31(3):207-208.
39. Liu H, Chen Z, Zeng W, et al. Surgical management of Hawkins type III talar neck fracture though the approach of medial malleolar osteotomy and mini-plate for fixation. *J Orthop Surg Res.* 2017;12(1):1-9.

40. Abdelkafy A, Imam MA, Sokkar S, Hirschmann M. Antegrade-retrograde opposing lag screws for internal fixation of simple displaced talar neck fractures. *J Foot Ankle Surg*. 2015;54(1):23-28.

41. Marsh JL, Saltzman CL, Iverson M, Shapiro DS. Major open injuries of the talus. *J Orthop Trauma*. 1995;9(5):371-376.

42. Jordan RK, Bafna KR, Liu J, Ebraheim NA. Complications of talar neck fractures by Hawkins classification: a systematic review. *J Foot Ankle Surg*. 2017;56(4):817-821.

43. Lindvall E, Haidukewych G, DiPasquale T, et al. Open reduction and stable fixation of isolated, displaced talar neck and body fractures. *J Bone Joint Surg Am*. 2004;86-A:2229-2234.

44. McCrory P, Bladin C. Fractures of the lateral process of the talus: a clinical review. Snowboarder's ankle. *Clin J Sport Med*. 1996;6:124-128.

45. Kirkpatrick DP, Hunter RF, Janes PC, et al. The snowboarder's foot and ankle. *Am J Sports Med*. 1998;26:271-277.

46. Boon AJ, Smith J, Zobitz ME, Amrami KM. Snowboarder's talus fracture. Mechanism of injury. *Am J Sports Med*. 2001;29(3):333-338.

47. Funk JR, Srinivasan SCM, Crandall JR. Snowboarder's talus fractures experimentally produced by eversion and dorsiflexion. *Am J Sports Med*. 2003;31(6):921-928.

48. Bladin C, McCrory P. Snowboarding injuries: an overview. *Sports Med*. 1995;358-364.

49. Funasaki H, Kato S, Hayashi H, Marumo K. Arthroscopic excision of bone fragments in a neglected fracture of the lateral process of the talus in a junior soccer player. *Arthrosc Tech*. 2014;3(3):e331-e334.

50. Kramer IF, Brouwers L, Brink PR, Poeze M. Snowboarders' ankle. *BMJ Case Rep*. 2014;2014.

51. Russell JA, Shave RM, Yoshioka H, Kruse DW, Koutedakis Y, Wyon MA. Magnetic resonance imaging of the ankle in female ballet dancers en pointe. *Acta Radiol*. 2010;51(6):655-661. doi: 10.3109/02841851.2010.482565.

52. Özer M, Yıldırım A. Evaluation of the prevalence of os trigonum and talus osteochondral lesions in ankle magnetic resonance imaging of patients with ankle impingement syndrome. *J Foot Ankle Surg*. 2019;58(2):273-277. doi: 10.1053/j.jfas.2018.08.043.

53. Saxena A. Os trigonum injuries. In: Saxena A, ed. *International Advances in Foot and Ankle Surgery*. Springer Berlin; 2011:273-276.

54. Heyer JH, Dai AZ, Rose DJ. Excision of os trigonum in dancers via an open posteromedial approach. *JBJS Essent Surg Tech*. 2018;8(4):e31. doi: 10.2106/JBJS.ST.18.00015.

55. Van Dijk CN, de Leeuw PAJ, Scholten PE. Hindfoot endoscopy for posterior ankle impingement: surgical technique. *J Bone Joint Surg*. 2009;91(suppl_2):287-298.

56. Majeed H, McBride DJ. Talar process fractures: an overview and update of the literature. *EFORT Open Rev*. 2018;3(3):85-92. doi: 10.1302/2058-5241.3.170040.

57. Yamakado K. Quantification of the learning curve for arthroscopic os trigonum excision. *J Foot Ankle Surg*. 2018;57(3):505-508. doi: 10.1053/j.jfas.2017.11.010.

58. Saxena A, Eakin C. Articular talar injuries in athletes: results of microfracture and autogenous bone graft. *Am J Sports Med*. 2007;35(10):1680-1687.

59. Jurina A, Delimar V, Dimnjaković D, Bojanić I. Lateral inverted osteochondral fracture of the talus: case reports and review of the literature. *Acta Clin Croat*. 2018;57(2):377-382. doi: 10.20471/acc.2018.57.02.21.

60. Rogan S, Taeymans J, Hirschmüller A, Niemeyer P, Baur H. Effect of continuous passive motion for cartilage regenerative surgery—a systematic literature review. *Z Orthop Unfall*. 2013;151(5):468-474. doi: 10.1055/s-0033-1350707 [in German].

Ankle Surgery

CHAPTER 31

Syndesmosis Injuries

George T. Liu, George S. Gumann Jr, and Robert B. Anderson

INCIDENCE

Injuries of the distal tibiofibular syndesmosis (DTFS) occur in 45% of supination–external rotation ankle fractures,[1] 58% of pronation–external rotation ankle fractures,[2] and 5.7% of all ankle injuries without fractures.[3] The overall estimated incidence of DTFS injury in the United States is 2.09 syndesmotic injuries per 100 000 person-years.[4] The most common mechanism of injury is one of contact where external rotation (ER) of the foot rotates the talus laterally forcing the fibula from tibia.

MORBIDITY OF INJURY

Both isolated and combination DTFS injuries are associated with significant morbidity with increased time to return to activity, chronic lingering pain, and disability. Compared to medial and lateral ankle sprains, DTFS injuries require significantly longer sports participation restriction times increasing the time to return to play.[5-7] At a 6-month follow-up from DTFS injury, 31.3% of patients reported lingering pain, 43.8% reported impaired function, and 56% of patients reported less than acceptable outcomes.[8]

INCIDENCE OF MALREDUCTION

Rates of DTFS malreduction after surgical repair, using standard radiographic parameters, have been reported between 15.7% and 24%.[9-11] However, other studies have shown that the rate of malreduction is largely underestimated. Computed tomographic evaluation of open reduction internal fixation (ORIF) of DTFS disruptions compared to the patient's uninjured limbs revealed that malreduction rates increase between 39% and 52% as shown in Figure 31.1.[9,12]

In general, radiographic images have been found to be insensitive in detecting DTFS ruptures. Only the absence of tibiofibular overlap (TFO) or increased medial clear space (MCS) >4 mm was associated with syndesmotic injury.[13,14]

While radiographic measures can detect DTFS widening, they have been found to be insensitive in detecting fibular translation and rotation.[15,16] The most common malalignment of the fibula in the fibula incisura was internal rotation or anterior translation.[9]

MORBIDITY OF MALREDUCTION

In addition to morbidity of DTFS injuries alone, malreduction from operative care has been shown to contribute to morbidity

and to be a risk factor for poor functional outcomes. In a 2-year follow-up, Sagi et al.[12] demonstrated significant reduction in the Short Form Musculoskeletal Assessment and Olerud/Molander functional outcomes scores in patients with malreduction of the DTFS seen in comparison ankle computed tomography (CT) between injured and uninjured limbs. Ovaska et al.[17] reported that 59% of the indication for early reoperation following ankle fracture surgery was malreduction of the DTFS. In an average 2.5-year follow-up, Naqvi et al.[18] demonstrated syndesmosis malreduction to be the only independent predictor of poor functional outcomes with the American Orthopaedics Foot and Ankle Society (AOFAS) score.

Tibiofibular malreduction has been associated with late-stage tibiotalar joint instability and has been shown to be an independent risk factor for posttraumatic arthritis as shown in Figure 31.2.[19,20] In a cadaveric study simulating an unstable syndesmosis injury sectioning both the syndesmosis and deep deltoid ligament, a widening of the DTFS by 0.73 mm was associated with a 39% decrease area of tibiotalar contact and a 42% increase in peak pressure.[21]

ANATOMY

The syndesmotic ligaments secure the fibula to the tibia stabilizing the talus in the ankle mortise for weight bearing. The DTFS complex consists of the anterior inferior tibiofibular ligament (AITFL), interosseous ligament (IOL), and the posterior tibiofibular ligament (PITFL) as shown in Figure 31.3.

The AITFL is a thick, trapezoidal ligament that originates from the anterior tubercle of the tibia (Chaput tubercle), travels inferior laterally, and inserts on the anterior border of the fibular malleolus (Wagstaff tubercle). The IOL is a collection of thick short elastic fibers that originates from the medial portion of the fibular shaft inserting along the lateral tibia. The IOL becomes a membrane of aponeurotic fibers as it ascends proximally.

The PITFL is composed of a superior and deep fascicle. The superior fascicle originates from the posterior tubercle of the tibia (Volkmann tubercle) and runs inferior laterally to insert onto the posterior aspect of the lateral malleolus. The deep fascicle, also known as the transverse tibiofibular ligament, is more fibrocartilage in content and serves as one of the principal restraints against syndesmotic widening.

Within the DTFS, the medial aspect of the fibula fits into a vertical groove along the lateral distal tibia between the anterior and posterior tibial tubercles, known as the fibular incisura

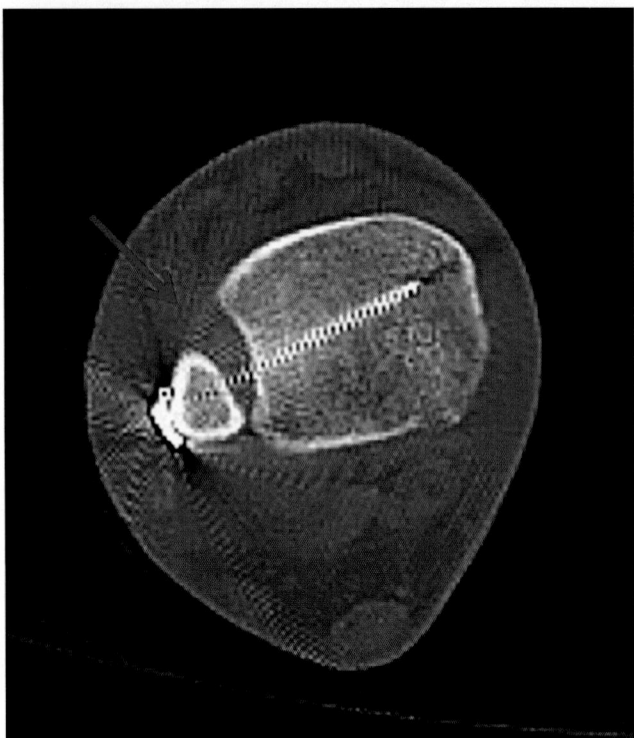
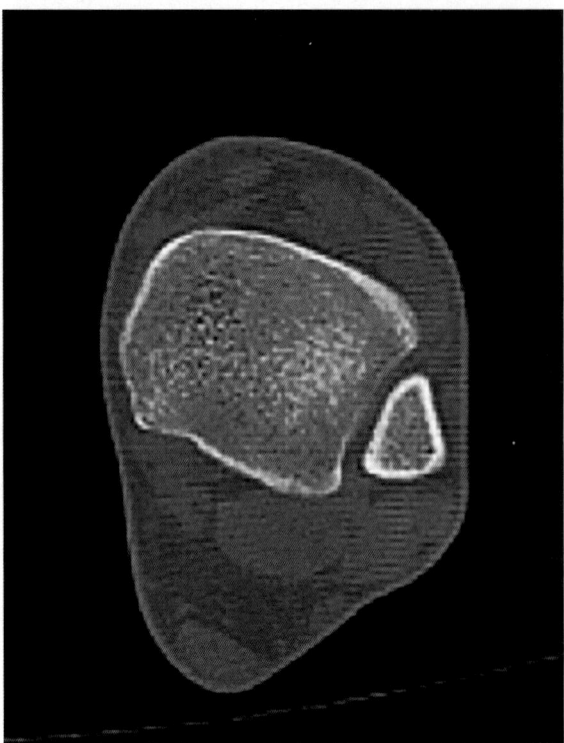

FIGURE 31.1 Bilateral computed tomographic axial cuts of syndesmosis (open reduction internal fixation on left and uninjured ankle for comparison on the right) demonstrating malreduction of the syndesmosis (widening noted by arrow) with external rotation of the fibula in the incisura of the right ankle.

of the tibia or the fibular notch. The morphology of the fibular incisura has been described as deep, shallow, crescent, rectangular, convex, or chevron.[22-31]

The morphology of the fibular incisura has been suggested as a risk factor for syndesmosis malreductions. One study reported that shallow syndesmoses were susceptible to anterior fibular sagittal plane malalignment, whereas deep syndesmoses were susceptible to posterior sagittal plane and rotational malalignment.[32]

BIOMECHANICS

The motion of the fibula within the fibular incisura of the tibia maintains the articular congruity and stability of the ankle joint.

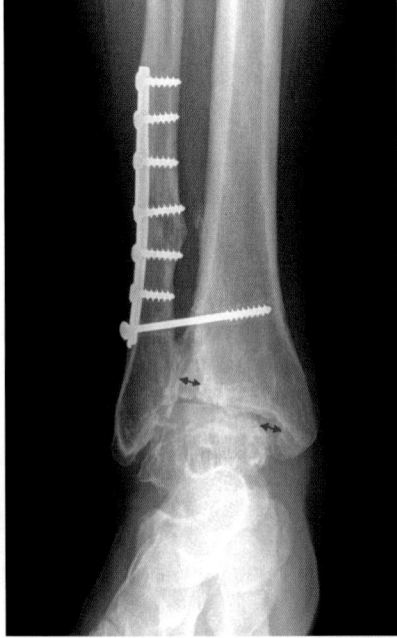

FIGURE 31.2 The ankle radiograph demonstrates posttraumatic arthritis of the ankle joint likely caused by syndesmosis malreduction. Lateral subluxation of the talus is seen evidenced by increased medial clear space and tibiofibular clear space (both shown by arrows).

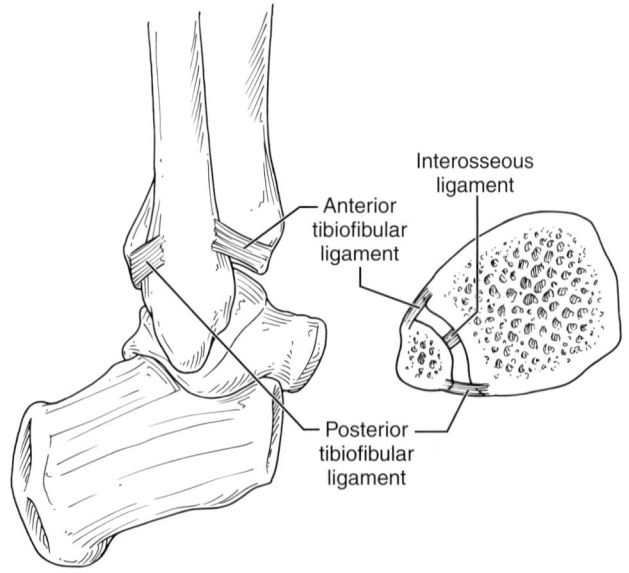

FIGURE 31.3 Anatomic illustration shows the distal tibiofibular syndesmosis.

As the ankle dorsiflexes, the intermalleolar distance increases ~1.25 mm and the fibula external rotates 2.5-3.2 degrees to accommodate the wider anterior talar dome.[32-34] In this dorsiflexed position, the DTFS ligaments tighten. Concomitant tension of the deep deltoid and lateral collateral ligaments with ankle dorsiflexion generates a secure restrained position of the talus within the ankle mortise for forward translation of body weight.

DIAGNOSTIC PARAMETERS FOR SYNDESMOSIS INJURY

RADIOGRAPHS

Plain radiographs of the ankle with anteroposterior (AP), mortise (MO), and lateral (LAT) views should be used to assess the presence and pattern of malleolar fractures and diastasis of the DTFS. Standard tibial films should assess for the presence of a high fibula fracture. On the AP and MO views of the ankle, the DTFS parameters are measured at 1 cm superior to the tibiotalar joint line. Standard radiographic parameters for the tibiotalar joint are shown in Figure 31.4.

Tibiofibular Overlap

On the AP view, the TFO represents the anterior tibial tubercle superimposed over the medial aspect of the fibular malleolus and should measure ~1 cm.[35] The consistency of the TFO measure can be affected by position of the ankle with the x-ray projection.[36] When compared to magnetic resonance imaging (MRI), TFO measures of <10 mm on the AP view had a high sensitivity but low specificity for syndesmosis injury.[14] Only the absence of TFO has high correlation with disruption of the DTFS as seen in Figure 31.5.[13]

Tibiofibular Clear Space

On both the AP and MO views, the tibiofibular clear space (TFCS) represents the space between the lateral border of the fibular incisura of the tibia and medial border of the lateral malleolus and should measure ~6 mm.[35] Though commonly used in the evaluation of DTFS injuries, the TFCS can be insensitive in identifying rotational and translational position of the fibula in the incisura fibularis of the tibia.[36] The TFCS remains unchanged on radiographs with up to 30 degrees of ER of the fibula within the incisura fibularis of the tibia shown in Figure 31.6.[16]

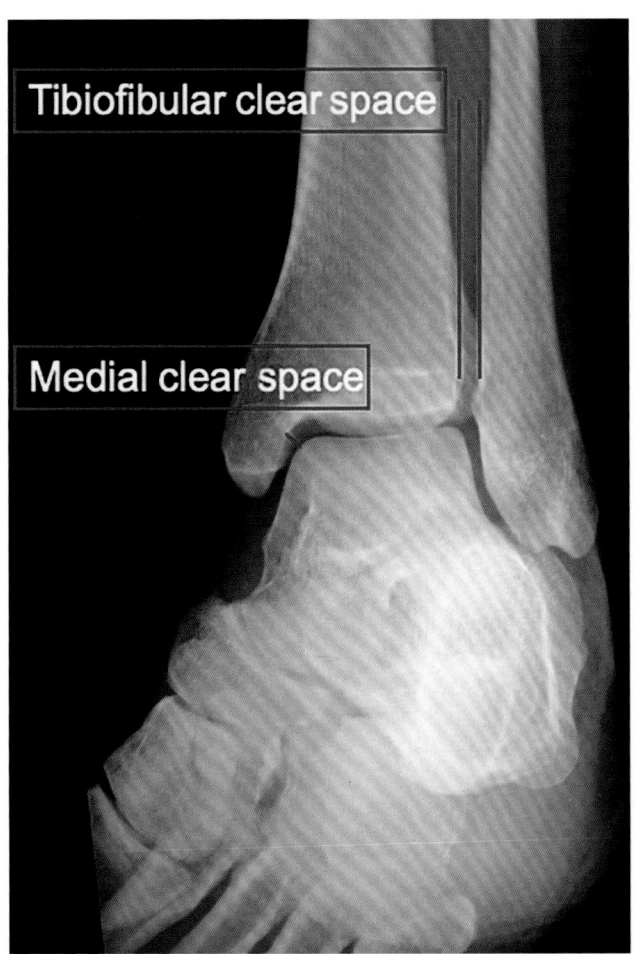
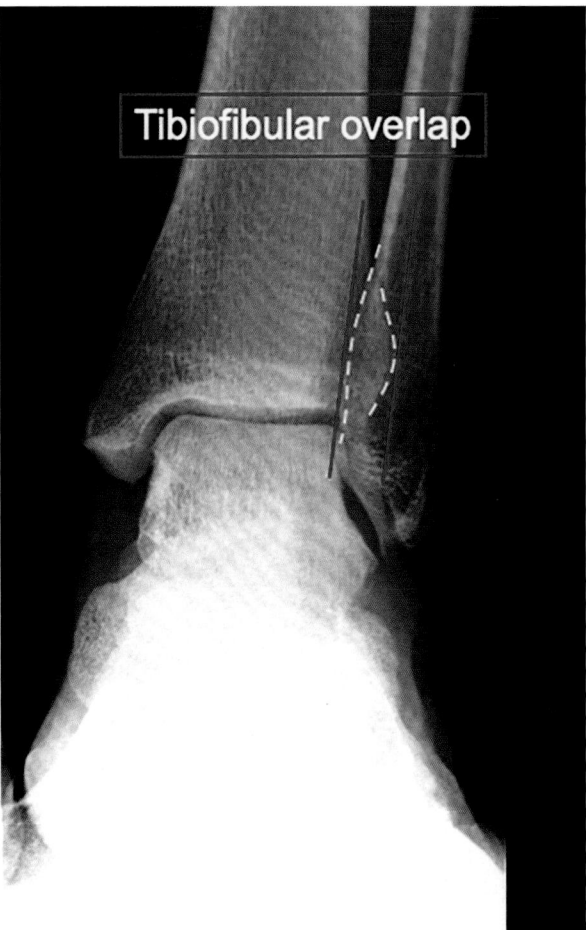

FIGURE 31.4 The ankle radiograph shows the standard radiographic measures with tibiofibular overlap, tibiofibular clear space, and the medial clear space.

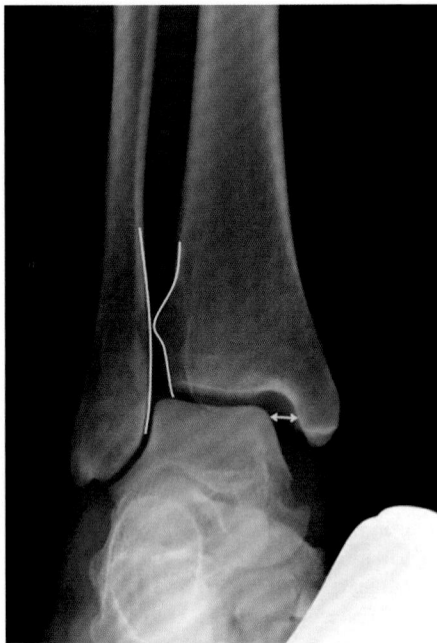

FIGURE 31.5 The ankle radiograph demonstrates absence of tibiofibular overlap, which is highly correlated with disruption of the DTFS. A medial clear space of >4 mm (arrow) correlated with disruption of both the deep deltoid ligament and DTFS.

Medial Clear Space

On the AP and MO views, the MCS is the distance between the lateral border of the medial malleolus and the medial border of the talus with the ankle joint at 90 degrees.[37] The MCS can also be affected by position of the ankle with the x-ray projection.[36] Compared to the contralateral uninjured ankle joint, an MCS > 4 mm correlated directly with deep deltoid ligament disruption and indirectly with a syndesmosis disruption as seen in Figure 31.5.[14] There is a growing clinical consensus among experts considering the threshold of 2 mm of static MCS widening as a significant deep deltoid ligament injury. Complete disruptions of the deep deltoid ligament rarely occur in isolation but in conjunction with fibular malleolar ankle fractures, proximal fibular fractures, and rupture of the syndesmotic ligaments.[38]

Other Findings

Avulsion fractures of the DTFS, such as anterior tubercle of the distal tibia (Tillaux-Chaput fragments) or anterior fibula (Wagstaffe-LaForte fragment), are attachments of the AITFL. Posterior malleolar fractures (Volkmann fragment) are the attachment site of the PITFL. These avulsion fractures of the ligamentous attachments of the DTFS are syndesmosis injury equivalents and should be assessed for ankle instability.

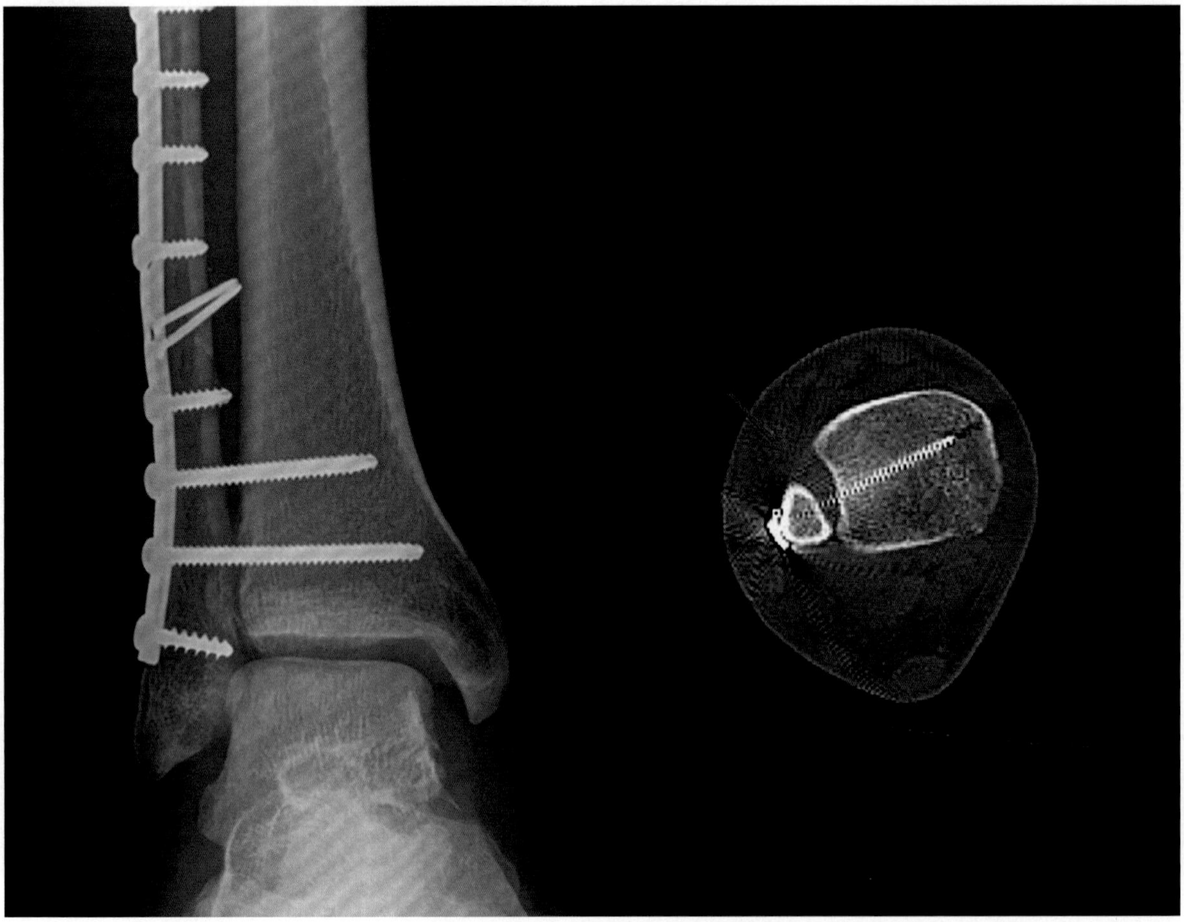

FIGURE 31.6 While the radiographs of the ankle demonstrate normal radiographic measures for the DTFS, CT scan reveals malreduction of the syndesmosis with external rotation and posterior displacement of the fibula in the incisura of the tibia resulting in widening of the syndesmosis (arrow).

ADVANCED IMAGING

The utility of diagnostic advanced imaging such as CT and MRI may be limited. One study demonstrated that CT scans were more sensitive at identifying diastasis of the DTFS that was not evident with plain film.[39] Additionally, a CT scan can also better reveal the ankle fracture patterns and the size of the posterior malleolus fragment. However, a CT scan could not identify syndesmosis instability in the absence of diastasis. MRI has been shown to have high specificity and sensitivity for DTFS ligament ruptures correlated with arthroscopic findings in two studies; however, it may not correlate with instability in the absence of diastasis.[40,41] A meta-analysis reported sensitivity and specificity for identification of syndesmosis injuries was 0.53 and 0.98 for radiographs, 0.93 and 0.87 for MRI, and 0.67 and 0.87 for non–weight-bearing CT, respectively.[42] Weight-bearing CT scans have been shown to improve diagnostic accuracy of identifying syndesmosis injuries compared to non–weight-bearing CT scans. Statistical differences in the DTFS have been shown with lateral and posterior translation and ER of the fibula within the fibular incisura of the tibia between weight-bearing and non–weight-bearing CT scans of uninjured ankles.[43]

Comparing a patient's injured to uninjured DTFS, weight-bearing CT scans were able to identify significant differences in anterior, middle, and posterior measures on axial cuts, and sagittal translation as well as dynamic increase in area within the DTFS.[44,45]

DYNAMIC STRESS IMAGING

Dynamic stress imaging with fluoroscopy or ultrasound of the DTFS can improve identification of unstable syndesmosis injuries that were previously undetected by static imaging studies. Recognizing the anatomic landmarks with imaging and interpretation of the changes in these parameters can improve detection of subtle unstable DTFS injuries.

External Rotation Stress Test

ER stress test is performed by holding the ankle in neutral flexion at a 90-degree angle and placing an external rotational force to the forefoot while stabilizing the leg as shown in Figure 31.7. Under live dynamic fluoroscopy or stress radiographic plain films, an increase in the MCS >4 mm on MO ankle view is indicative of a deep deltoid ligament rupture as demonstrated in Figure 31.8.[14] The ER stress test is commonly used to identify incompetence of the deep deltoid ligament in the presence of an isolated fibular malleolar ankle fractures classifying the ankle joint fracture as unstable (bimalleolar equivalent) requiring surgical stabilization.[46,47] The ER stress test is also employed when evaluating the stability of a high ankle sprain. Instability will be confirmed by a demonstrated widening of the MCS and the TFCS. When the ER stress test is performed in the operating room on an ankle with either an operatively stabilized fibula fracture or intact fibula, MCS widening is specifically indicative of DTFS disruption as well as deltoid ligament rupture.[48,49] The significance of identifying deep deltoid ligament insufficiency with concomitant DTFS disruption is an indication for operative stabilization of the syndesmosis as the ankle mortise is unstable. A cadaveric study demonstrated that with complete transection of the syndesmotic ligaments leaving the deltoid ligament intact, there was no significant change in

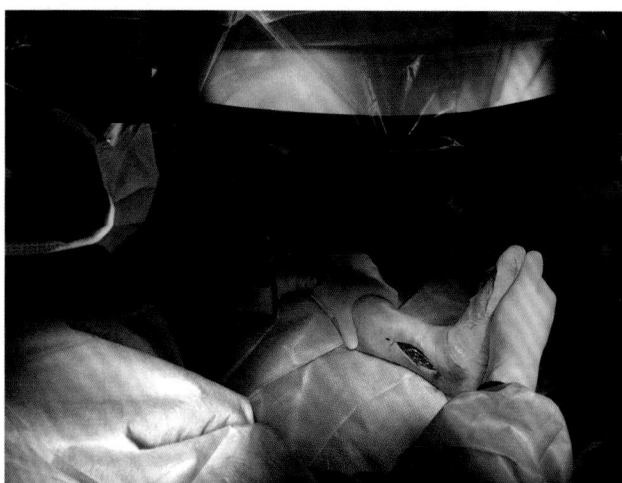

FIGURE 31.7 External rotation stress test is performed by holding the ankle in neutral flexion at a 90-degree angle and placing an external rotational force to the forefoot while stabilizing the leg.

tibiotalar contact area nor peak pressures. However, with both deep deltoid and syndesmosis ligaments transected, a syndesmotic diastasis of 0.73 mm resulted in a 42% increase in peak pressure and 39% reduction in tibiotalar contact area.[21]

The incidence of DTFS instability unpredicted by biomechanical criteria but identified through intraoperative fluoroscopic ER stress test after fibular fracture fixation was reported to be 33% of supination–external rotation ankle injuries and 57% of pronation–external rotation injuries.[50]

Several studies have demonstrated that sagittal plane movement of the fibula was a more sensitive measure of DTFS instability as seen on the lateral view with the ER stress test.[51-53] Posterior displacement of the fibula as the talus is externally rotating out of the ankle mortise was a greater indicator of

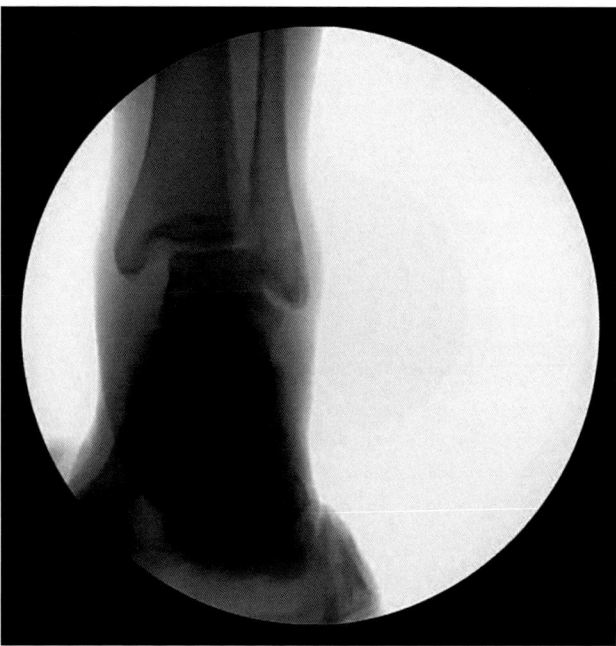

FIGURE 31.8 An increase in the MCS is seen under live fluoroscopy. An MCS >4 mm is indicative of a complete deep deltoid ligament disruption.

instability than detecting lateral displacements of the fibula on the mortise view. The primary difficulty with the ER stress test in the lateral view is stabilizing the leg adequately while externally rotating the foot not to distort the lateral view producing a false positive. Because of the difficulty obtaining a reproducible lateral view with ER stress, indicators of instability seen on both the AP and MO stress views are favored.

Lateral Stress Test

The lateral fibular stress test or "hook test" is a surgical adaptation of the Cotton test originally described as a lateral translation test of the talus to identify abnormal lateral mobility of the talus in a Pott malleolar ankle fracture.[54] This dynamic fluoroscopic stress test is used for an intact or operatively stabilized fibula fracture where a bone hook is placed on the medial cortex of the distal fibula at the superior border of the syndesmosis and lateral force is applied seen in Figure 31.9. Increased TFCS widening on the mortise view or lack of TFO on the AP view are indicative of DTFS disruption.[13,49] Though commonly used by many surgeons to assess syndesmosis instability, the lateral stress test is more sensitive for producing TFCS widening indicative of syndesmosis disruption but is not as sensitive for MCS widening, which is indicative of deep deltoid ligament disruption.[49,55]

Because the variation of the anatomic morphology of the fibular incisura of the tibia and intrarater reliability, the use of several stress tests may be necessary to identify syndesmosis instability.

Tibofibular Clear Space Widening

While insensitive with radiographs and dynamic fluoroscopy, TFCS widening can be assessed utilizing dynamic ultrasound examination with high sensitivity and specificity. The widening of the TFCS at a cutoff value of 0.4 mm measured from neutral position to ER demonstrated a sensitivity and specificity of 89%.[56] While MRI demonstrates a sensitivity of 100%, dynamic ultrasound is a quick, cost-effective, and reproducible method of diagnosing an unstable syndesmosis injury.[57]

ARTHROSCOPIC ASSESSMENT

Use of arthroscopy has been suggested as a standard for diagnosis for syndesmotic injuries; however, methods of defining instability differ greatly between studies.[41,58-64]

Lui et al.[60] reported that 66.0% rate of syndesmosis rupture in Weber type B or C ankle fractures identified by arthroscopy vs 30.2% identified by intraoperative stress fluoroscopy. The arthroscopic criterion of instability in their study was ≥2 mm of displacement of the fibula in any plane. Takao et al.[62] reported 87% rate of syndesmosis rupture in Weber B fractures through arthroscopic visualization of ligament rupture. In another study, Takao et al.[63] determined that sensitivity, specificity, and accuracy with MRI was 100%, 93.1%, and 96.2% for an AITFL tear and 100%, 100%, and 100% for a PITFL tear, using arthroscopic observation of a 2-mm gap between the tibia and fibula as a criteria for syndesmosis disruption. Only one study attempted to quantify disruption of the syndesmosis arthroscopically using a standardized measuring device.[58] In this cadaveric study with serially sectioned syndesmosis ligaments, they reported that passage of a 2.5-mm probe indicated some disruption of the syndesmosis, but had poor negative predictive value. However, passage of a 3.0-mm spherical probe had the highest likelihood of correlating with disruption of both the AITFL and IOL.

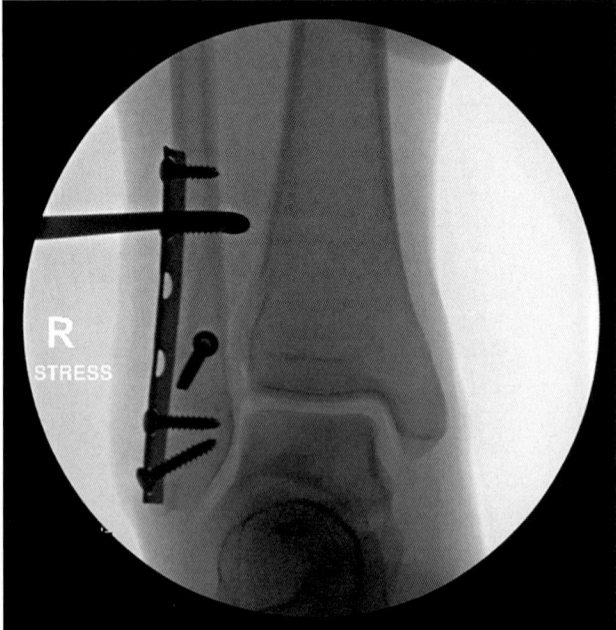

FIGURE 31.9 The bone hook test is demonstrated by applying a lateral distraction force on the distal fibula evaluating the sufficiency of the DTFS under live fluoroscopy. Increased TFCS widening on the mortise view or lack of TFO on the AP view is indicative of DTFS disruption.

> ## INDICATIONS FOR OPERATIVE INTERVENTION
> - Tibiofibular clear space widening >3 mm with Cotton test
> - Medial clear space widening >2 mm with external rotation test in the setting of an intact fibula or stabilized fibular fracture

INDICATIONS FOR SYNDESMOSIS FIXATION: WHEN FIXATION IS NEEDED AND WHEN IT IS NOT

The use of syndesmosis fixation still remains controversial based on reports that attempt to quantify instability of the syndesmosis itself vs its contribution to instability of the ankle joint. Isolated syndesmosis injuries do not constitute a direct indication for ORIF of the syndesmosis unless it contributes to instability of the talus in the ankle mortise. Syndesmosis injuries must have a concomitant deltoid ligament rupture or medial malleolar fracture to create instability of ankle joint. The principle function of the DTFS is lateral stabilization of the talus within the ankle mortise. The medial talar stabilizers are the deltoid ligament and medial malleolus. Loss of tibiotalar congruity whether from ligamentous and/or malleolar fractures are likely the cause of long-term morbidity and disability secondary to chronic ankle instability and posttraumatic arthritis. A 1-mm lateral displacement of the talus results in 42% reduction in tibiotalar contact area.[65] Therefore, syndesmosis injuries that allow the talus to shift are considered unstable and should be stabilized. Syndesmosis injuries not associated with a shift of the talus, with or without stress applied, are considered stable.

PEARLS OF REDUCING THE SYNDESMOSIS
- Place tines of the reduction forceps along the transmalleolar axis where the medial tine is along the anterior one-third of the tibia.
- Apply sufficient pressure to reduce and not "overcompress" the syndesmosis.
- Comparing radiographic parameters of the ankle joint reduction to the contralateral ankle and directly visualizing the DTFS reduction are the best methods that decrease rates of malreduction.

SYNDESMOSIS REDUCTION TECHNIQUES

Reduction of the syndesmosis continues to be a complex problem affected by insensitivity of traditional radiographic parameters,[13,14,16] inconsistency of radiographic views,[36] and variable anatomy of the fibular incisura.[24,26,28-31,66] Various techniques have been reported to address the high rate of malreduction of the DTFS.

Reduction Clamp Position

A reduction clamp is commonly used to indirectly reduce talus into the ankle mortise by reducing the fibula into the fibular incisura of the tibia. In cases of anatomically reduced malleolar ankle fractures, syndesmosis may be anatomically reduced where the use of reduction forceps are to maintain reduction while hardware is placed. Improper placement of the reduction clamp tines may cause malpositioning of the fibula in the incisura.

Placement of the tines of the reduction forceps should be through the axis between the centroid of the tibia and fibula matching the transmalleolar axis, which is ~25-30 degrees angled from posterior to anterior as the fibula is positioned on the posterior half of the tibia on the lateral view as seen in Figure 31.10A. Placement of the tines of the reduction forcep along this axis has been shown in several studies to be the most optimal orientation for anatomic reduction of the DTFS.[67-70] On the MO ankle view, the tines of the reduction clamp should be resting on the cortices of the fibula and tibia, and on the LAT ankle view, the medial tine should be about the anterior one-third of the tibia as shown in Figure 31.10B.

Position of the Ankle and Consequences of Overtightening

Though the position of the ankle joint during ORIF of DTFS disruptions does not necessarily affect ankle dorsiflexion,[71,72] positioning the ankle at 0 degree can assist reduction of the syndesmosis through the congruency of the lateral talomalleolar articulation. The reduction of the DTFS does not require significant force for reduction as manual reduction techniques have been shown to be equivocal to clamp reduction techniques.[52,70] However, overtightening has been shown to increase the rate of malreduction of the DTFS with translation or malrotation of

the fibula in the fibular incisura.[73,74] Evidence of overtightening of the syndesmosis may be demonstrated by a decrease in the MCS and TFCS compared to the contralateral uninjured limb as well as valgus tilt of the talus.

Direct Visualization

Visual confirmation of the DTFS reduction by centering the fibula within the fibular incisura of the tibia has been shown to have improved reduction rates compared to indirect reduction as shown in Figure 31.11. One CT study comparing reduction rates of DTFS disruptions demonstrated 84% anatomic reductions with direct visualization vs 48% anatomic reductions with indirect reductions.[75]

SYNDESMOSIS REDUCTION ASSESSMENT

Assessing the position of the fibula within the fibula incisura of the tibia is complicated with the use of two-dimensional imaging for a three-dimensional problem.

Contralateral Intraoperative Fluoroscopy

The use of intraoperative fluoroscopic standard three views of the contralateral ankle joint as comparison template for reduction is a simple, quick method of evaluating quality of DTFS reduction through symmetry. The fibular length and rotation are evaluated with the MO view. Fibular length is evaluated with Shenton line (confluence of the subchondral bone line of the fibula to the subchondral bone line of the lateral distal tibial plafond) and the circle sign of the distal fibula as shown in Figure 31.12. The proper rotation of the fibula is evaluated by identification of a symmetric lateral talomalleolar joint space. Increased lateral talomalleolar clear space with spoon-shaped fibula may indicate internal malrotation of the fibula, and a divergence of Shenton lines or a pointed blade-shaped appearing fibula may indicate external malrotation of the fibula.[76] The position of the fibula to the tibia is evaluated with the LAT view comparing the distance where the posterior border of the fibula overlaps the tibiotalar articular surface to the tip of the posterior malleolus.[77]

Verifying reduction with intraoperative CT scan of the operative ankle, one study reported a 94.4% anatomic reduction rate using the contralateral ankle fluoroscopy comparison method.[77]

Computed Tomography

Postoperative bilateral ankle CT scans have been recommended as the best method to assess syndesmosis reductions and to account for anatomic variations of the DTFS if there is concern for malreduction. The use of unilateral CT scans to assess syndesmosis reductions has been shown to overestimate the rate of syndesmosis malreductions by nearly 100% compared to 42% of cases with bilateral CT scans.[78] Most studies characterizing the normal morphology of the DTFS report that the fibula is internally rotated in the fibular incisura of the tibia.[22,25,29,78-83]

The use of intraoperative CT scans for the assessment of syndesmosis reductions have not been shown to effectively reduce the rate of malreductions compared to intraoperative fluoroscopy.[84]

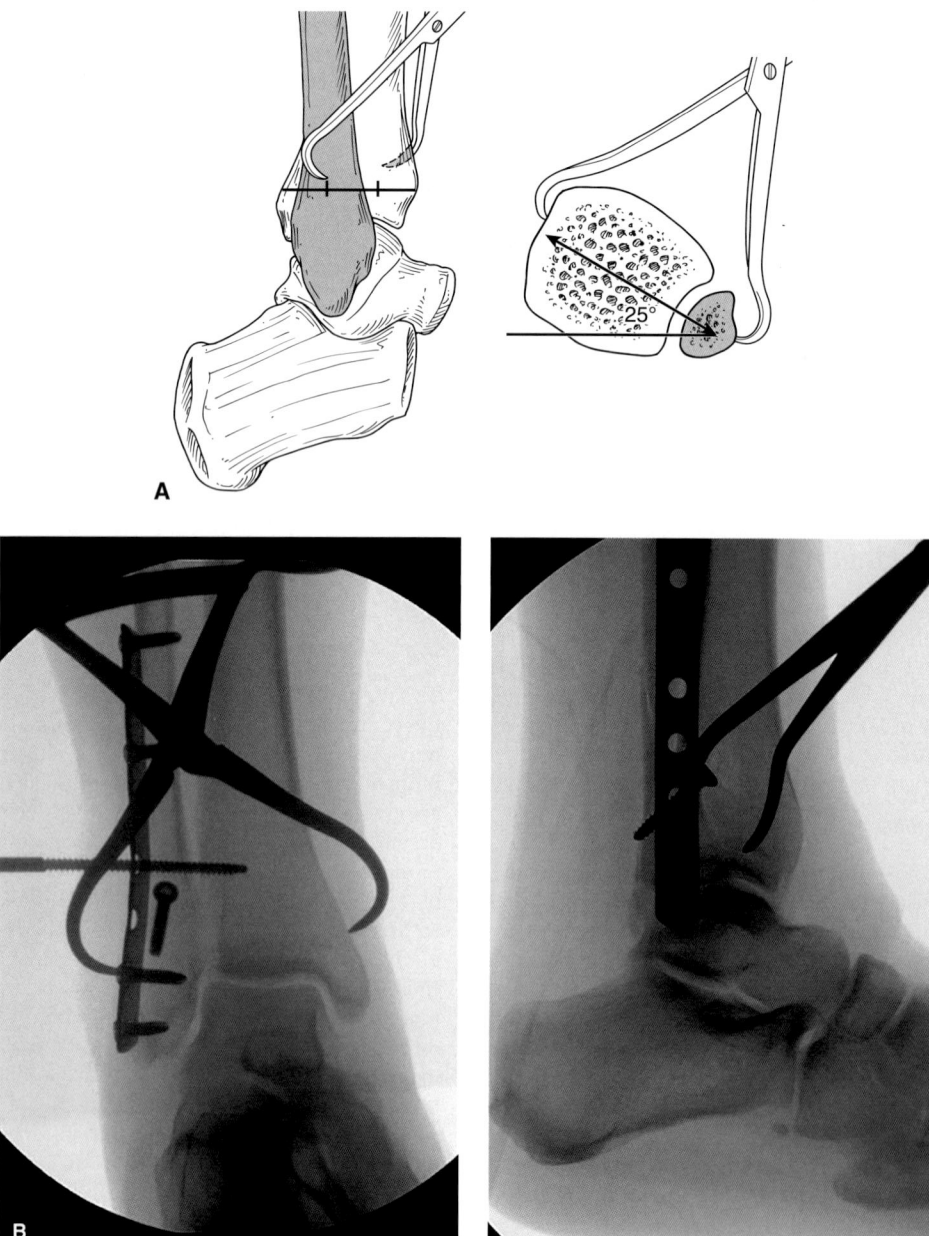

FIGURE 31.10 A. The tines of the reduction forceps are placed along the transmalleolar axis, which is ~25-30 degrees angled from posterior to anterior. The medial tine should be seen along the anterior one-third of the tibia on the lateral view. **B.** Intraoperative fluoroscopic MO ankle views show the tines of the reduction clamp placed tangentially on the cortices of the fibula and tibia (*left*). On the LAT ankle view, the medial tine should be rest along the anterior one-third of the tibia.

<table>
<tr><td>

PERILS and PITFALLS

- Malreduction of associated malleolar fractures will prevent anatomic reduction of the syndesmosis.
- Shortened or malrotation of the fibula fracture will cause lateral translation of the talus in the ankle mortise and prevent anatomic reduction of the medial aspect of fibula into the fibular incisura of the tibia.
- Malreduction of the medial malleolus often causes lateral translation of the talus in sure ankle mortise widening the syndesmosis.

</td></tr>
</table>

PITFALLS AND CONSIDERATIONS

The syndesmosis and the malleoli function as a complex to stabilize the talus in the ankle mortise; therefore, reduction of the syndesmosis should not be considered separate from the reduction the malleolar fractures. A malaligned talus within the ankle mortise secondary to a malleolar malreduction will prevent accurate reduction of the syndesmosis. Therefore, syndesmosis reductions are dependent on accurate reduction of the malleoli.

Leeds et al.[19] demonstrated that adequacy of reduction of the syndesmosis was statistically correlated with the quality of fibular malleolar reduction.

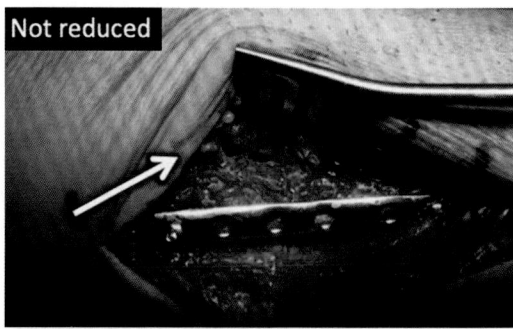

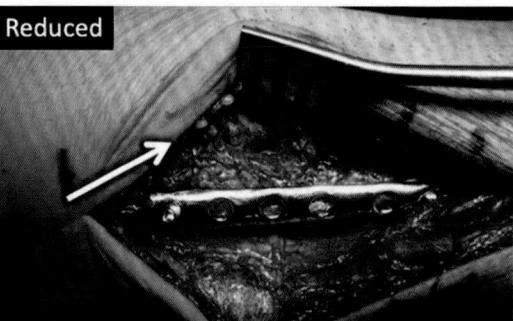

FIGURE 31.11 Visual confirmation of the DTFS reduction is seen on the bottom picture where no gap is seen at the AITFL.

In their analysis of malreduced ankle fractures that undergo reoperation, Ovaska et al.[17] found that 44.4% of the malreductions involved a combination of two malreductions, most commonly the fibula and syndesmosis.

Achieving fibular length and correct rotation may be performed through anatomic reduction of the lateral cortex and the posterior spike of the fibula. Anatomic reduction of the fibula will restore articular congruity of the lateral talomalleolar and tibiotalar articulation and secondarily allow anatomic reduction of the medial cortex of the fibula into the fibular incisura of the tibia.[85]

Malreduction of the medial malleolus can cause lateral translation of the talus in the ankle mortise widening the syndesmosis as seen in Figure 31.13. Malrotation of the medial malleolus is often evident when the MCS is not patent on both the AP and MO ankle views. Malreduction with either medial translation or valgus tilt of the medial malleolus is seen when the medial articulation is more vertically oriented. This can be seen with contralateral comparison films.

Malreduction of posterior malleolar fractures are more associated with malreduction of the syndesmosis by their connection though the PITFL and the anatomy of the incisura. In a cadaveric study, Fitzpatrick et al.[86] demonstrated that posterior malleolar malreductions did affect the reduction of the syndesmosis. Reduction of the posterior malleolus has been shown to improve syndesmosis reduction. Miller et al.[75] reported fewer

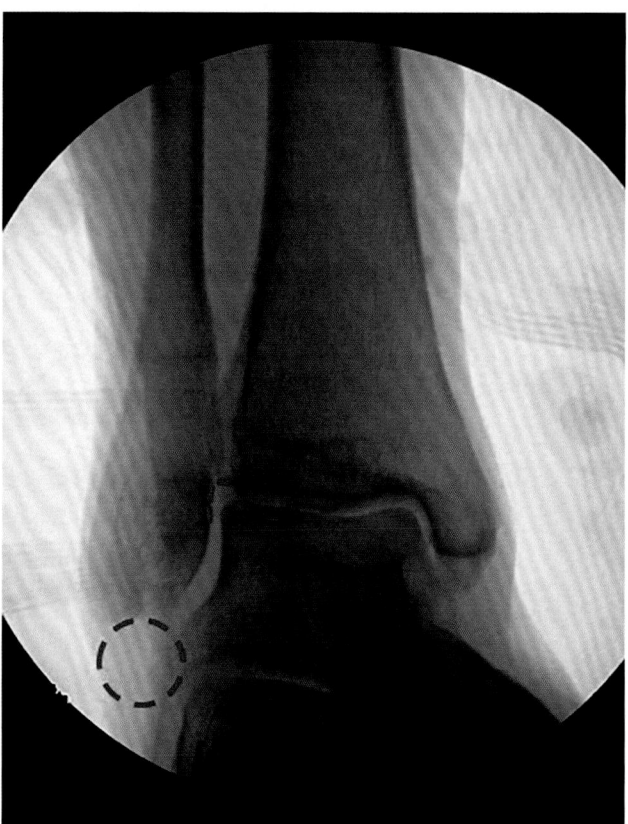

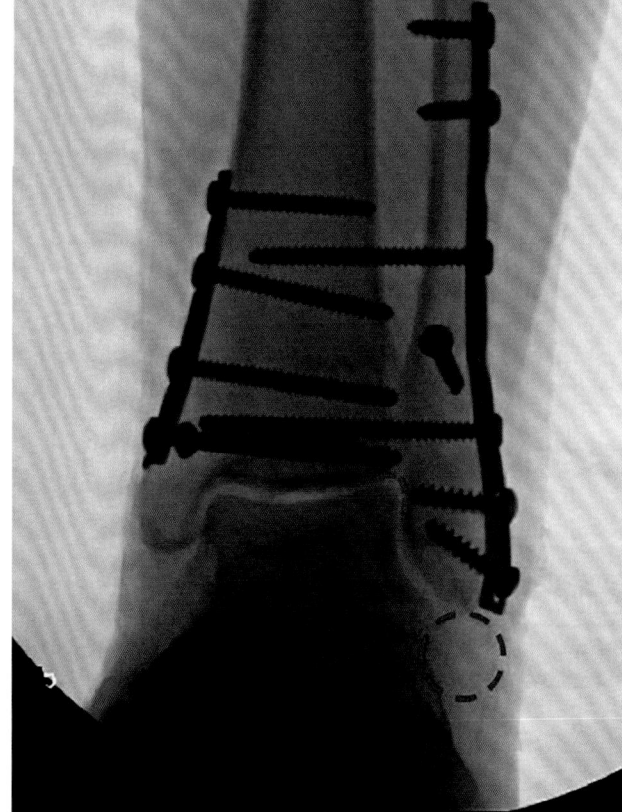

FIGURE 31.12 Contralateral fluoroscopy is used for comparison views to evaluate symmetry of the fibular length and rotation. The fibular length is evaluated with Shenton line (confluence of the subchondral bone line of the fibula to the subchondral bone line of the lateral distal tibial plafond) and the *circle* sign of the distal fibula.

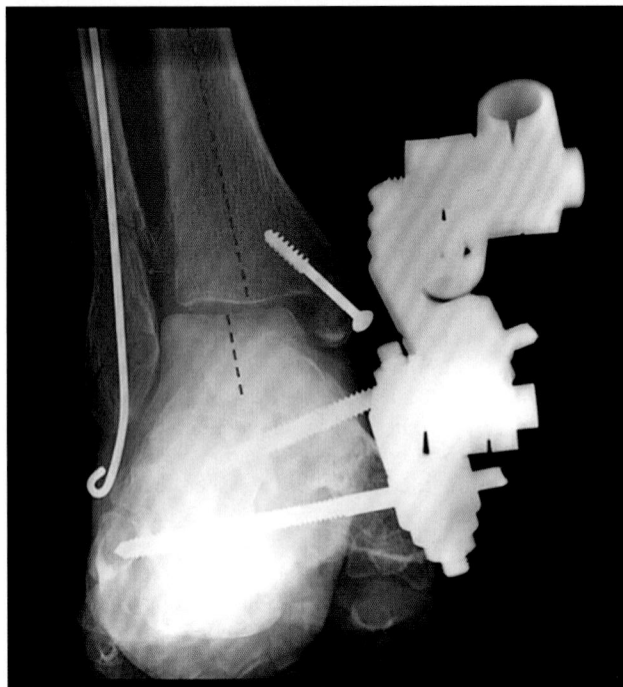

FIGURE 31.13 Postoperative ankle MO radiograph demonstrates malreduction of the lateral malleolus causing lateral translation of the talus (shown by dotted lines), malreduction of medial malleolus and widening the syndesmosis (arrow).

syndesmosis malreductions in patients with ORIF of posterior malleolar fractures compared to patients with ORIF of syndesmosis without posterior malleolar fractures (8% vs 18%).

Deep and superficial deltoid ligament injuries may be considered in patients with MCS widening and concomitant syndesmotic disruption. While functional outcomes have been comparable between syndesmotic fixation and deltoid ligament repairs in bimalleolar ankle fracture equivalents, repair of the deep deltoid ligament has been associated with lower rates of syndesmosis malreductions compared to syndesmosis fixation alone (9.09% vs 34.6%).[87,88] Repair of the superficial deltoid ligament may be indicated in similar cases when invagination of the ligament prevents reduction of MCS widening and secondary widening of the syndesmosis. Additionally, repair of the superficial deltoid ligament in professional athletes with ankle fractures has been shown to have high rate of return to play, good anatomic reduction of the ankle mortise, and no incidence of medial ankle instability or pain.[89]

Comparative studies evaluating malreduction rates after ORIF of unstable DTFS injuries have suggested that methods of fixation may be a risk factor influencing malreduction.[5,18,90-93] A meta-analysis of five randomized controlled trials comparing 143 patients with suture button fixation and 142 patients with screw fixation reported a statistically lower incidence of DTFS malreduction in suture button group vs screw fixation group (0.8% vs 11.5%).[94]

OPERATIVE TREATMENT

AUTHOR'S TECHNIQUE

Position of the patient supine with hip bump placed to position patella superiorly. The leg is elevated on foam positioner or stack of blankets to facilitate LAT fluoroscopy.

Arthroscopic evaluation of the joint is often performed via anteromedial and anterolateral portals. This is particularly valuable in those sustaining a fracture dislocation or more high-energy injury in which the articular surface may be compromised.

After anatomic reduction and internal fixation of the fibula or if the fibula is intact, the syndesmosis is stabilized with either direct manual thumb compression (with ankle internally rotated) or a reduction forceps placed ~25-30 degrees angled from posterolateral to anteromedial following the transmalleolar axis again as shown in Figure 31.10A and B. In general, this trajectory is centroid to the fibula and tibia. On the lateral view, the anterior tine should be seen positioned along the anterior one-third of the tibia. The clamp is placed while the ankle is positioned at 0 degree dorsiflexion to allow maximum contact of the lateral talomalleolar articulation reducing the probability of internal or external malrotation of the fibula in the incisura. The clamp pressure applied is just sufficient to engage the tines to the bone. Remember that the purpose of reducing the syndesmosis is to reduce the ankle joint. Application of excessive pressure and/or malposition of the clamp is the cause of malreduction of the syndesmosis and therefore the lateral talomalleolar articulation. Reduction is verified under fluoroscopy. Additionally, the anterior aspect of the syndesmosis can be directly visualized for reduction again as shown in Figure 31.11. Once syndesmosis reduction has been achieved, transyndesmotic fixation may be performed.

PEARLS FOR SCREW FIXATION

- When placing a fully threaded screw, tapping the screw holes will prevent the screw from distraction of the fibula off the tibia causing a malreduction of the syndesmosis.
- When placing a transyndesmotic screw, the screw may be left slightly protruding by 1-2 mm past the medial tibial cortex. If the screw is broken at the time of removal, both portions of the screw can be easily retrieved.
- Screw removal prior to 8 weeks resulted in higher rates of loss of syndesmosis reduction.
- Syndesmosis screw removal is only recommended in patients with intact screws at 6 months with either restricted ankle or tenderness to the syndesmosis.

SCREW FIXATION

Screw fixation has been the standard for syndesmosis stabilization. We prefer positional screw fixation without compression to maintain syndesmosis reduction. Compression screws have a higher chance of malreduction of the syndesmosis if the screw is not aligned with the centroid of the tibial and fibula.

For a 3.5- to 4.0-mm cortical fully screw fixation technique, a 2.5-mm drill bit is used to drill quadricortically along the same trajectory of the tines of the reduction forceps angled ~25-30 degrees anteriorly as seen in Figure 31.14. The drill hole is placed 1.5-2.0 cm superior and parallel to the tibiotalar joint line. Screw placement at 2.0 cm above the tibiotalar joint line was biomechanically optimal compared to 3.5 mm above the tibiotalar joint line.[95] This position also avoids iatrogenic injury to the "true" syndesmotic joint. Observe the syndesmotic joint directly, or arthroscopically, as the screw is being delivered through the fibula. Oftentimes, the screw may distract the fibula off the tibia as cutting flutes of self-tapping screws may not

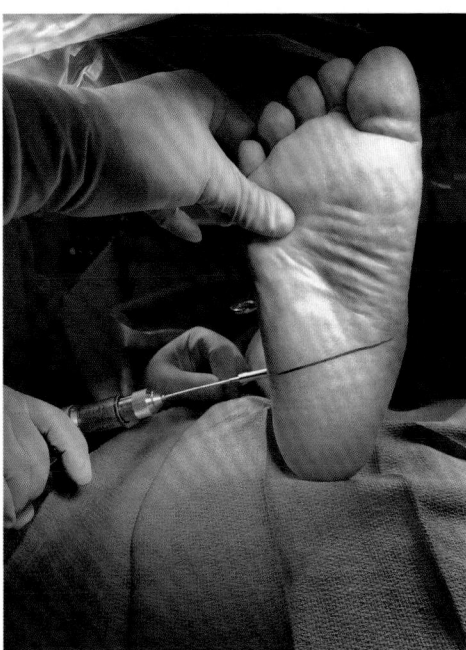

FIGURE 31.14 The direction of the drill hole is placed in the same trajectory as the tines of the reduction forceps, which is ~25-30 degrees angled from posterolateral to anteromedial following the transmalleolar axis.

engage the tibial cortex at the same rate the screw is advancing through the fibula. As a result, the screw distracts the fibula off the tibia until the screw purchases the tibia and malreduction of the syndesmosis occurs. A 3.5-mm tap is used to create the threads through the fibula and lateral tibial cortex as seen in Figure 31.15. As above, arthroscopy may be used to verify syndesmosis reduction by observing for medial gutter widening and syndesmosis widening at the synovial fringe.

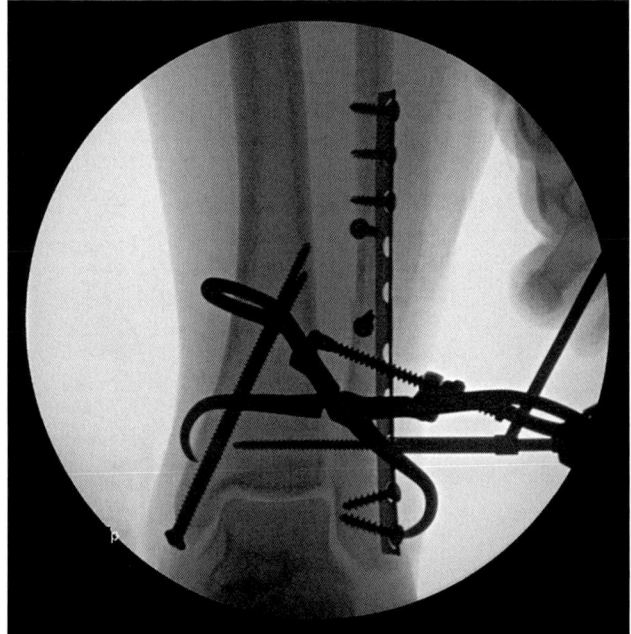

FIGURE 31.15 A tap is used to create the threads through the fibula and lateral tibial cortex for placement of the positional screw.

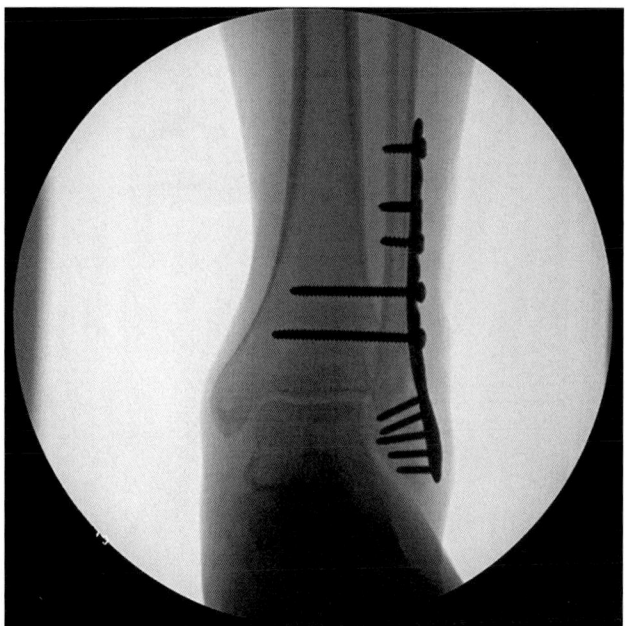

FIGURE 31.16 Two tricortical or quadricortical transyndesmotic screws may be used to stabilize the syndesmosis in severe unstable syndesmosis with deep deltoid ligament disruptions.

Transyndesmotic screws are often times delivered through a one-third tubular plate that was applied to a fibula fracture for neutralization purposes. If the distal end of the plate ends above the optimal position for the syndesmotic screw, then place the screw below the plate. In cases of significant ankle instability with syndesmosis and deep deltoid disruption, or Maisonneuve fracture, two transyndesmotic screws for stabilization may be placed as seen in Figure 31.16. In addition, a two- or four-hole fibular buttress plate can be utilized to distribute forces and protect the fibula from stress risers. For ankle fractures in patients with diabetes and sensory neuropathy, multiple transyndesmotic screws are necessary to maintain reduction of the talus as demonstrated in Figure 31.17. The multiple transyndesmotic screw configuration increases stiffness of the ankle fracture construct for anticipated delayed bone healing and unintended early weight bearing commonly encountered in patients with peripheral neuropathy.[96]

Other Considerations With Transyndesmotic Screws

1. Compression or Positional Screws?
   AO technique recommends that transyndesmotic screws be placed in as a positional screw without lag effect. Compression with lag technique or partially threaded screws is unnecessary as the purpose of fixation is to maintain and not achieve syndesmosis reduction. Use of compression screws offer little clinical or biomechanical benefit over the potential risk of malreduction if the screw trajectory is not centroid to the fibula and tibia.
2. Do Larger Screws Make a Difference?
   Cortical 3.5-mm screws are most commonly utilized screw size. Another alternative is using 4.5 mm fully threaded screw with a 3.2-mm pilot hole in patients with high body mass index. Though there is no significant difference in overall biomechanical nor clinical outcomes with fixation between 3.5 and 4.5 mm fully threaded screw fixation

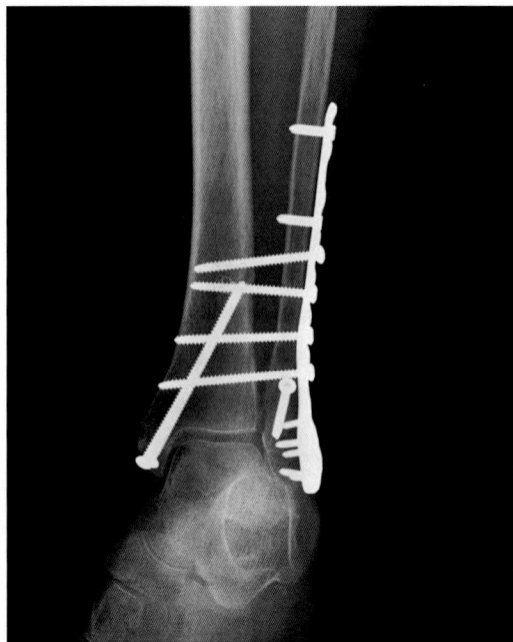

FIGURE 31.17 Multiple quadricortical transyndesmosis screw fixation improves resistance against lateral subluxation of the talus in neuropathic patients.

tricortical or quadricortical purchase, the 4.5-mm screw may be a better choice in osteoporotic bone, a patient of high body mass index, and a patient who is unable to adhere to non–weight-bearing postoperative protocol.[97-99] Cortical 4.5-mm screws resist breakage and pulling out of the bone better than do 3.5-mm screws. However, the larger screw head may cause irritation requiring removal. The larger head makes it easier to locate if removal is necessary.

3. Should Syndesmosis Screws Be Removed?

Routine syndesmosis screw removal at 8-12 weeks has been a common practice to avoid hardware failure, which some have believed to be the cause of syndesmosis pain. Several studies have disputed the common belief that retained screws and broken screws were associated with poor clinical and radiographic outcomes of syndesmosis ORIF.

One prospective randomized clinical trial compared 64 patient ankle fractures with syndesmosis instability randomized to two groups: (1) two 3.5-mm tricortical screw fixation that was not removed and (2) one 4.5-mm quadricortical screw that was removed at 2 months.[97] At 1-year follow-up, they reported that pain was significantly lower in the tricortical fixation group at 3 months, but no significant difference at 1 year. No significant difference in dorsiflexion was observed between the groups at any time, and there was no loss of fixation.

A prospective, surgeon-randomized study compared the radiographic outcomes of syndesmosis ORIF with 3.5-mm cortical screws in 59 patients with three cortical fixation vs 61 patients with four cortical fixations.[100] At a mean follow-up of 150 days, they reported there was no significant difference in loss of reduction, hardware breakage, or need for screw removal. They concluded that syndesmosis screw retention, despite screw breakage, did not result in clinical morbidity.

Manjoo et al.[101] in a mean 15-month follow-up of 76 patients who underwent ORIF of syndesmosis found a significant lower functional outcome in patients who have retained screws vs patients with broken, loosened, or removed screws. However, there was no significant difference in outcomes in patients with broken, loosened, or removed screws. Therefore, syndesmosis screw removal was only recommended for patients with intact screws at 6 months with either restricted ankle or tenderness to the syndesmosis.

Screw removal prior to 8 weeks resulted in higher rates of loss of syndesmosis reduction.[102,103]

PEARLS FOR SUTURE BUTTON FIXATION

- Avoid overtightening the suture button as malreduction with translation or rotation of the fibula in the incisura syndesmosis may occur, particularly in the presence of a posterior malleolar fracture.

SUTURE BUTTON

A 3.5-mm drill bit is used to drill quadricortically along the same trajectory of the tines of the reduction forceps centroid to the fibula and tibia. The drill hole is placed 1.5-2.0 cm superior and parallel to the tibiotalar joint line. A needle with the suture button is passed through the drill hole from lateral to medial through the skin as seen in Figure 31.18. The suture button is pulled medially passed the cortex of the tibia, while the lateral button is laid flat against the fibula as shown in Figure 31.19. Releasing the tension on the needle and pulling the suture laterally allows the suture button to lay flat on the medial cortex of the tibia as demonstrated in Figure 31.20. The suture tails are tensioned on the lateral side to create tension between the medial and lateral suture buttons maintaining reduction of the DTFS as seen in Figure 31.21. The suture is secured with 5-6 knots. Knotless suture button fixation is now available and preferred as it provides the advantage of self-retaining, self-locking braided suture system without the bulk of tied knots and potential irritation of overlying soft tissues. A single suture button

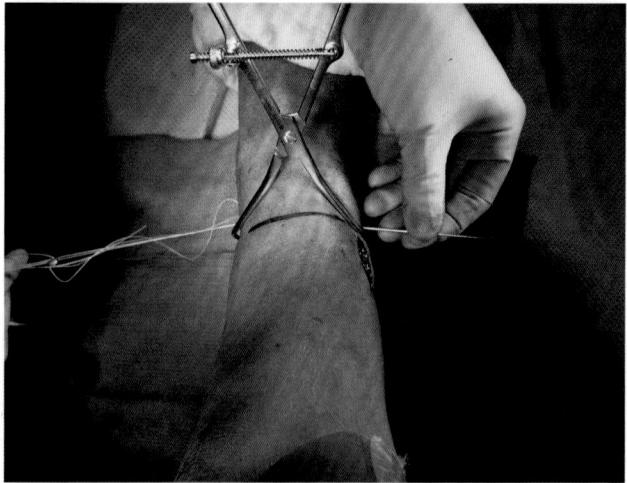

FIGURE 31.18 A needle is used to pass the suture button through a hole drilled from the fibula to the tibia.

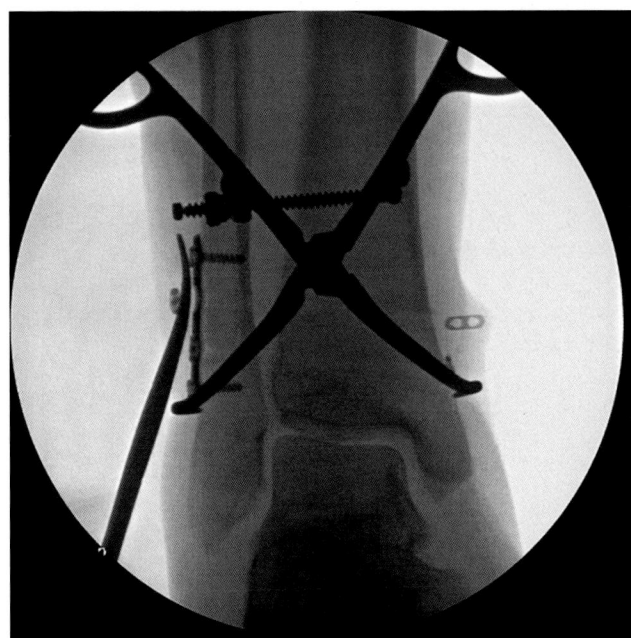

FIGURE 31.19 The suture button is pulled medially passed the tibia cortex, while the lateral button is laid flat against the fibula.

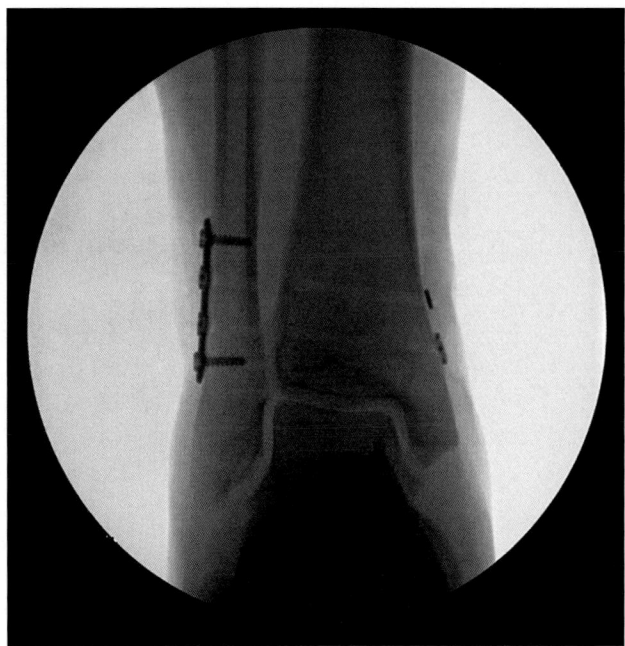

FIGURE 31.21 Suture ends are tightened on the lateral side to tension the medial and lateral buttons maintaining reduction of the DTFS.

provides sufficient stability to the syndesmosis for most patients. The addition of a second suture button may not provide added biomechanical stability but should be considered in a patient with high-activity demands such as professional or competitive athletes.[104]

One systematic review on suture button fixation and syndesmotic screw fixation reported the results of 10 studies

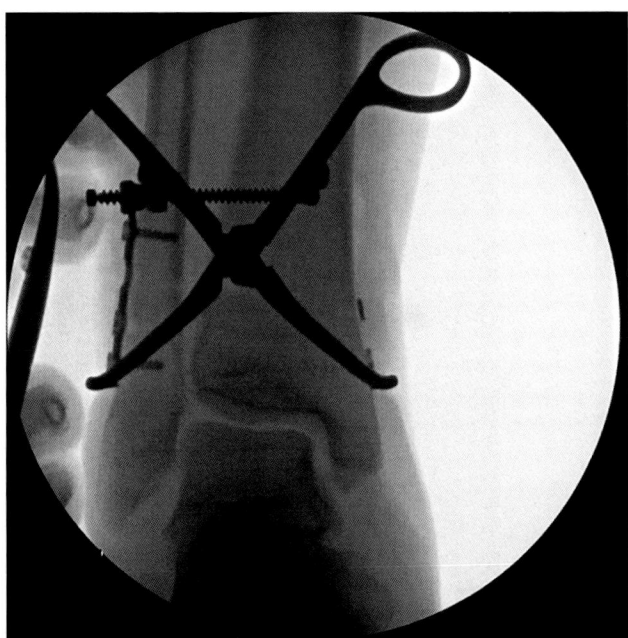

FIGURE 31.20 Releasing the tension on the needle and pulling the suture laterally allows the suture button to lay flat on the medial cortex of the tibia.

comprising 390 patients.[105] The mean AOFAS score for 150 patients with suture-button fixation was 91.06 points at an average 17.58-month follow-up. The mean AOFAS score for 150 patients with screw fixation was 87.78 points at an average 17.73-month follow-up. Malreduction was lower in patients managed with suture button (1.0%) compared to patients managed with transsyndesmotic screw (12.6%).

A systematic review and meta-analysis of five randomized controlled trials and six cohort studies suture-button fixation and syndesmotic screw fixation reported no statistical difference between MCS, TFCS, and TFO, postoperatively between the two groups.[106] However, at the 3rd, 6th, 12th, and 24th months postoperatively, the meta-analysis showed a significantly higher AOFAS score in the suture-button fixation group compared to the syndesmotic screw fixation group at each time point.

While the method of fixation has been traditionally regarded less important than method of syndesmosis reduction, some studies have suggested that method of fixation can help reduce malreduction. Flexible fixation with suture button methods has been associated with lower incidence of syndesmosis malreductions compared to rigid screw fixation methods.[90-92,107,108] A systematic review of these studies reported a malreduction rate of 12 out of 95 patients (12.6%) in the transsyndesmosis screw group and 1 out of 93 patients (1.1%) in the suture-button method.[105]

In cases of high Maisonneuve fractures or midshaft fibular fractures that are not typically directly reduced and stabilized with internal fixation, the fibula length and rotation may be restored distracting the fibula with a towel clamp applied to the distal fibula as seen in Figures 31.22 and 31.23. We recommend using static screw fixation with screws over flexible fixation with suture button as flexible fixation will not maintain the fibular length and rotation correction as seen in Figure 31.24.

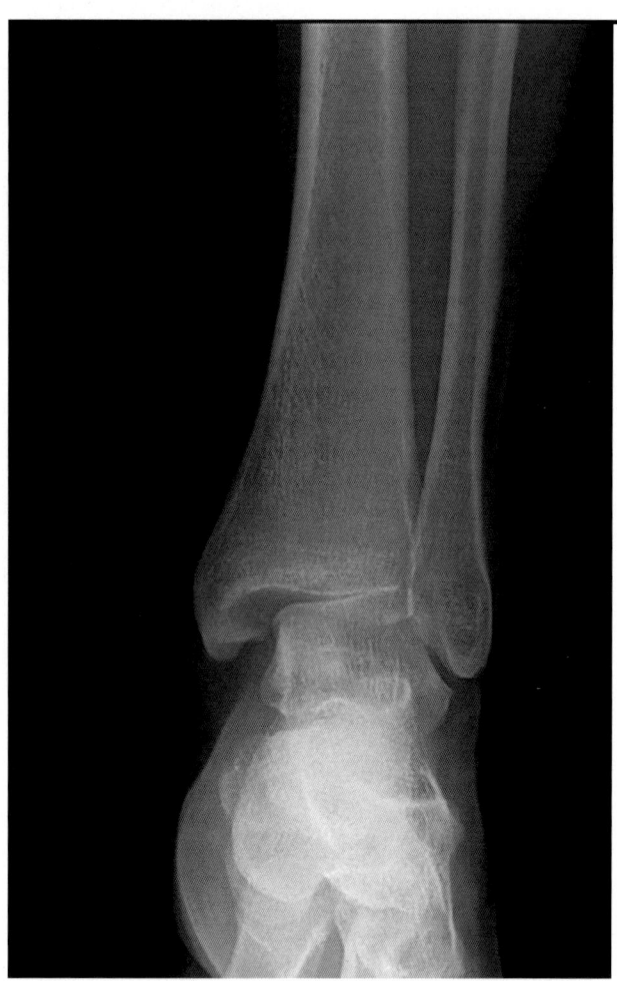
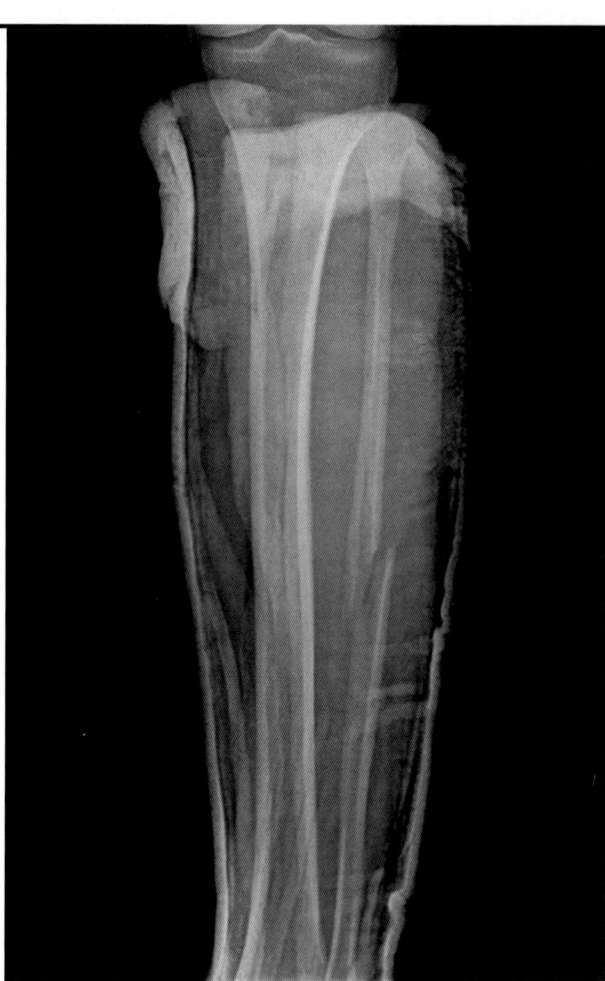

FIGURE 31.22 Radiograph demonstrates a shortened midshaft fibular fracture with syndesmosis and deep deltoid ligament rupture.

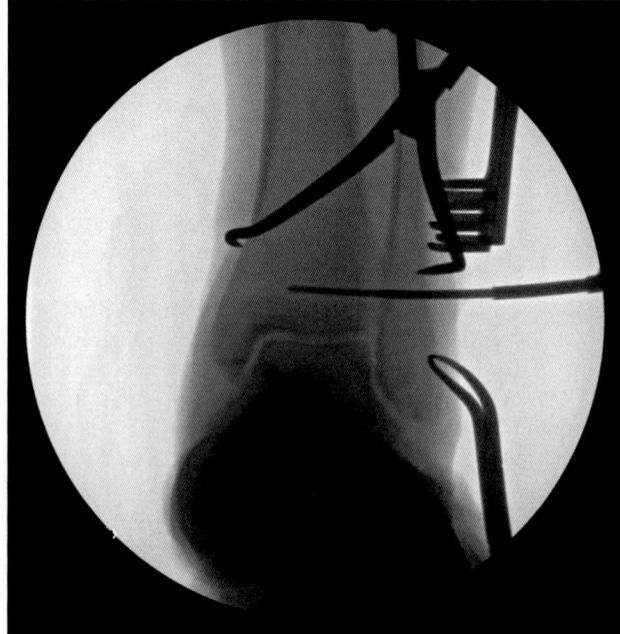

FIGURE 31.23 Intraoperative fluoroscopy shows clamp distracting the fibula to length and correcting rotation.

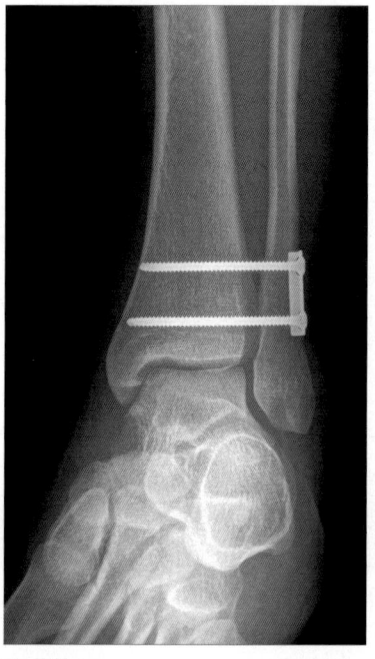

FIGURE 31.24 Intraoperative fluoroscopy shows use of static screw fixation to maintain the fibular length and rotation.

POSTERIOR MALLEOLUS

The traditional indications for posterior malleolar fixation was >25%-33% involvement of the tibial plafond.[109] However, earlier studies have demonstrated that isolated posterior malleolus fracture that involved up to 40%-50% of the tibial plafond did not cause the talus to posteriorly sublux unless the fibula and lateral ligamentous ankle restraints were compromised.[110,111]

More importantly, the reduction of the posterior malleolar fracture achieved better syndesmosis reduction compared to syndesmosis reduction alone.[75] Additionally, stabilization of the posterior malleolus provided 30% greater stiffness to the syndesmosis compared to stabilization of syndesmosis alone.[112]

The significance of the posterior malleolar fracture reduction with anatomic reduction of the syndesmosis and restoration of biomechanical stability is the PITFL, which remains intact in trimalleolar ankle fractures.[112]

If a posterior malleolus fracture is present and of sufficient size to be stabilized, it should be reduced and stabilized first to allow direct fluoroscopic visualization. Fixing the fibular fracture first will prevent visualization of the posterior malleolar reduction. Anatomic reduction of the posterior malleolus fracture will help facilitate reduction of the fibular fracture, if present, as well as reduction of the syndesmosis. Placement of the antiglide plate should be aligned over the apex of the fracture but sufficiently laterally to avoid entrapment of the flexor hallucis longus tendon or muscle belly.

Patient is placed in prone position. The leg is elevated on a stack of blankets with the knee 30 degrees flexed to facilitate LAT fluoroscopy.

Posterior lateral incisional approach is made between the peroneal tendons and flexor hallucis longus tendon. The posterior malleolus is directly visualized. In a trimalleolar ankle fracture, exposure and débridement of all fractures will facilitate reduction of the talus in the ankle mortise as well as the posterior malleolus. A reduction forceps is placed along the posterior malleolus with the anterior tine along the anteromedial distal tibia as seen in Figures 31.25 and 31.26.

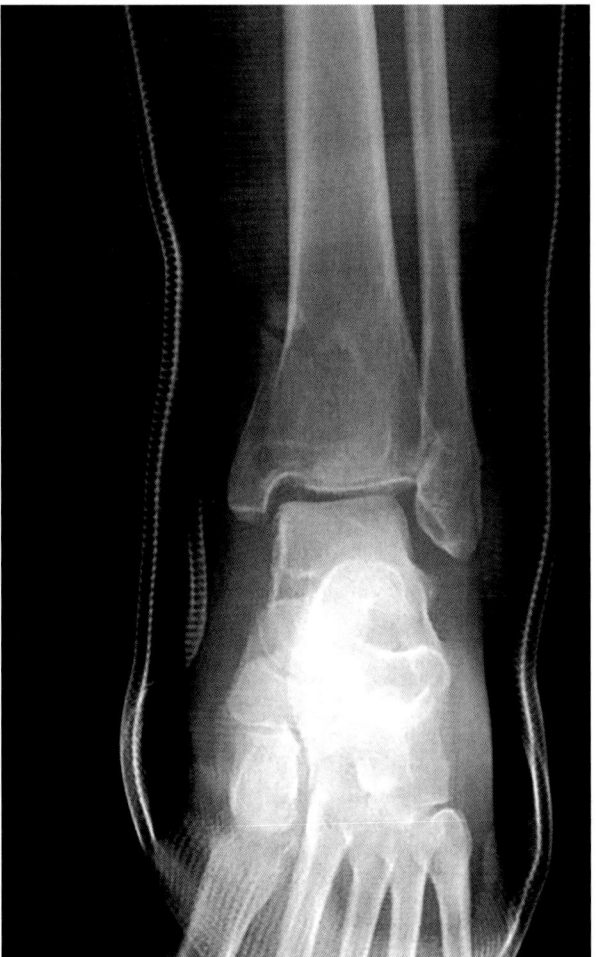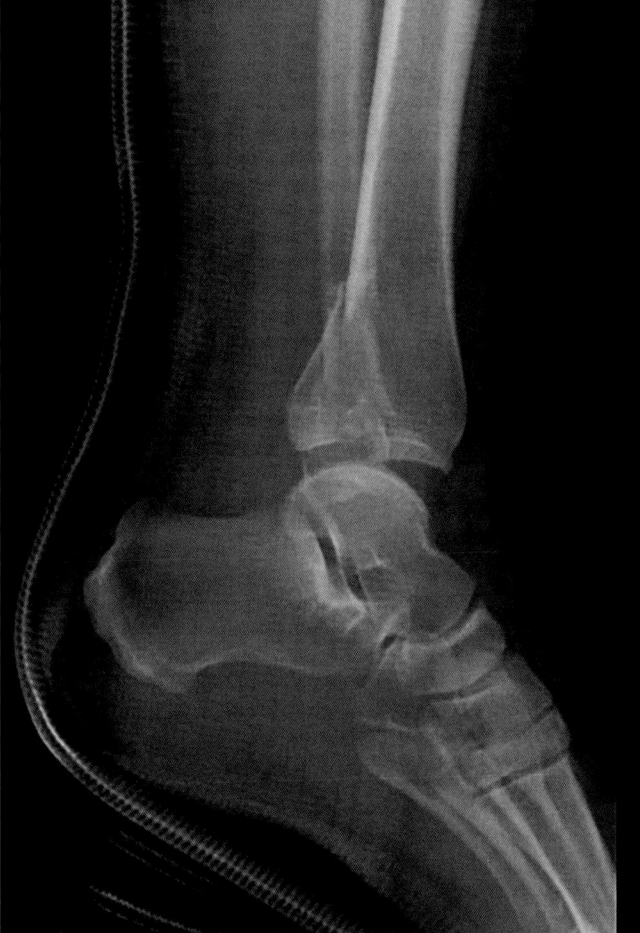

FIGURE 31.25 Radiographs show a trimalleolar ankle fracture with large posterior malleolar fragment. The posterior malleolus is attached to the fibular malleolus though the PITFL.

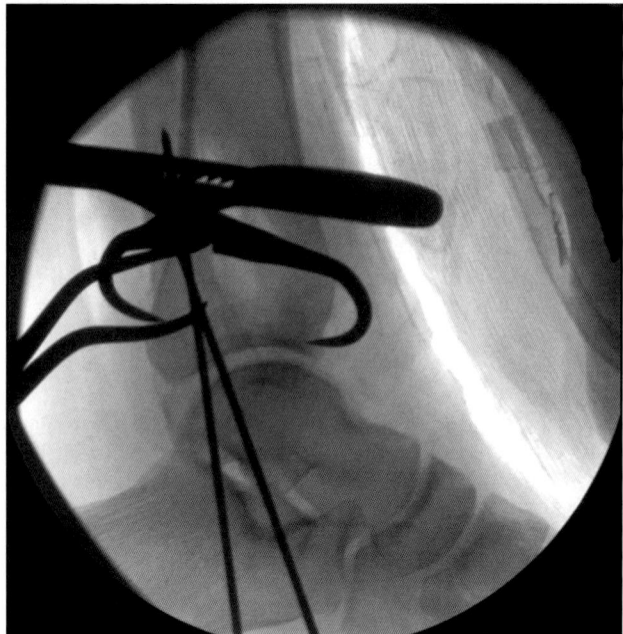

FIGURE 31.26 Intraoperative fluoroscopy shows reduction posterior malleolus fracture with the tines of the forceps placed across the posterior malleolus fracture to the anteromedial distal tibia.

Concomitant reduction of the fibular fracture will facilitate reduction of the posterior malleolus fracture through the connection of the PITFL. Once reduction of the posterior malleolus fracture is confirmed with fluoroscopy, provisional fixation is obtained with Kirschner wires placed from posterior to anterior as shown in Figure 31.27. A one-third tubular nonlocking plate is placed for antiglide function with the first screw placed at the apex of the fracture as shown in Figures 31.28-31.30.

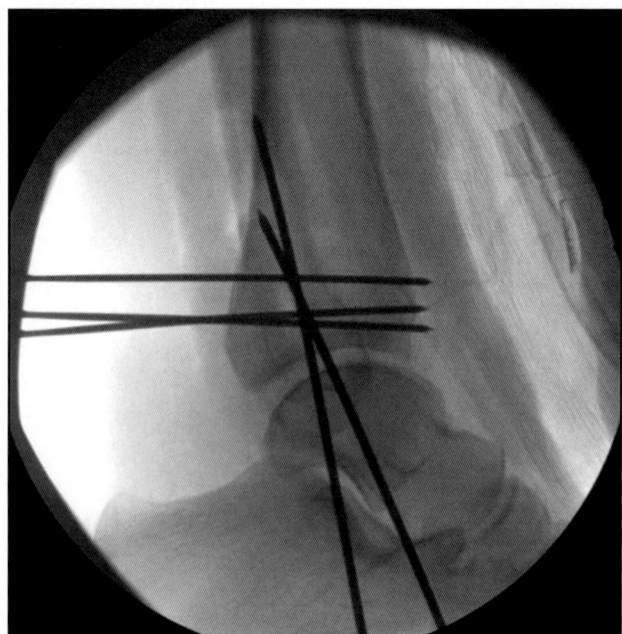

FIGURE 31.27 Reduction of the posterior malleolus fracture is confirmed with fluoroscopy and provisional fixation with Kirschner wires is placed.

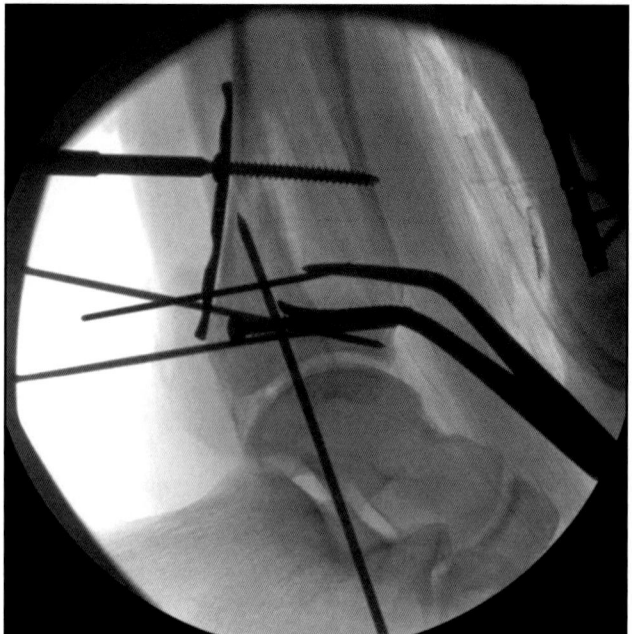

FIGURE 31.28 A one-third tubular nonlocking plate is placed for antiglide function with the first screw placed at the apex of the fracture.

An alternative choice would be to place two to three 3.5-mm fully threaded screws from posterior to anterior maintaining compression provided by the reduction forceps (AO compromise technique).

In the supine position, a standard lateral incisional approach is used for ORIF of the fibula and syndesmosis. A Weber reduction forcep is used to reduce and apply compression across the posterior malleolar fracture as shown in Figures 31.31 and 31.32. A 2.5-mm drill hole is made from the center of the anterior tibia and directed posterolaterally toward the posterior tubercle. Compression is maintained with percutaneous 3.5 mm cortical nonlag screws (AO compromise technique) placed from anterior to posterior under fluoroscopy as shown in Figures 31.33 and 31.34. Alternatively, a fully threaded cannulated screw may be used. If compression by lag technique is desired, overdrill the near cortex to the level of the fracture under fluoroscopy. Lag technique is preferred over use of partially threaded screws for smaller posterior malleolar fracture to assure passage of the screw threads across the fracture line.

POSTOPERATIVE CARE

Postoperatively, patients are placed in posterior splint with a lateral stirrup for ~2 weeks until sutures are removed. Patients are then casted for an additional 3-4 weeks non–weight-bearing. After this time period, patients are transitioned into removable fracture boot for active/passive range of motion exercises and progressive weight bearing in the boot. Patients are allowed full weight bearing in 6 weeks, assuming healing of any associated fractures and lack of significant articular surface injury. Physical therapy for range of motion, gait training, balance, and proprioceptive training is initiated at 8-10 weeks as indicated.

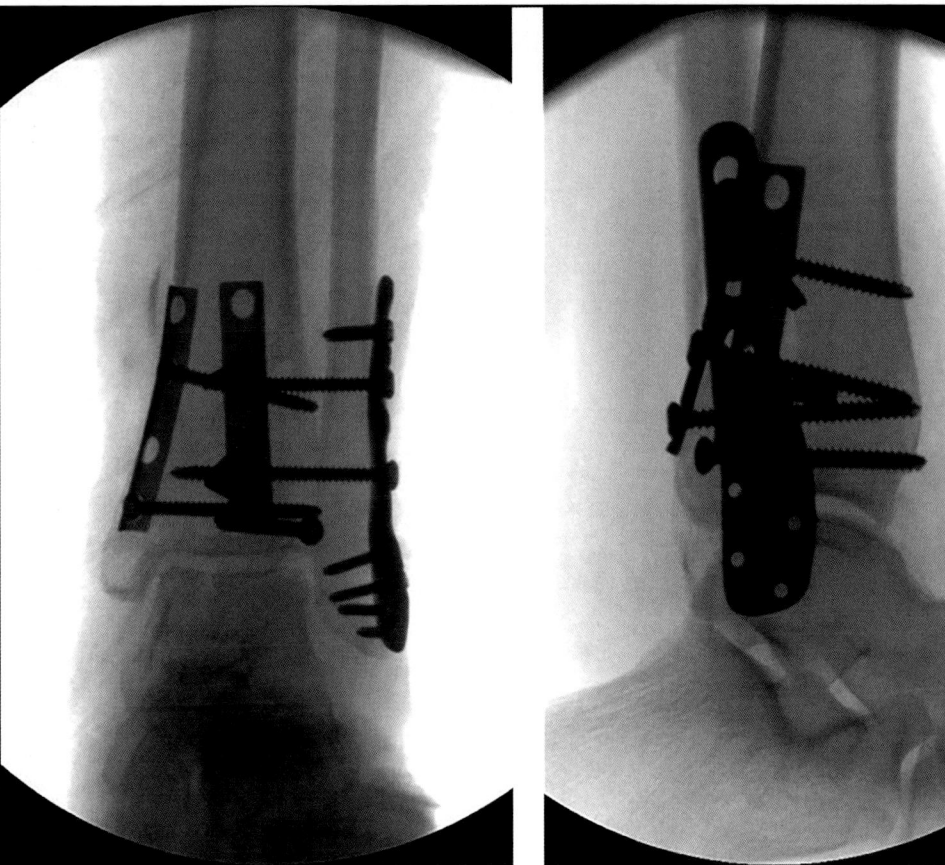

FIGURE 31.29 Final fluoroscopic views demonstrate reduction of the trimalleolar ankle fracture and syndesmosis with need for syndesmosis fixation.

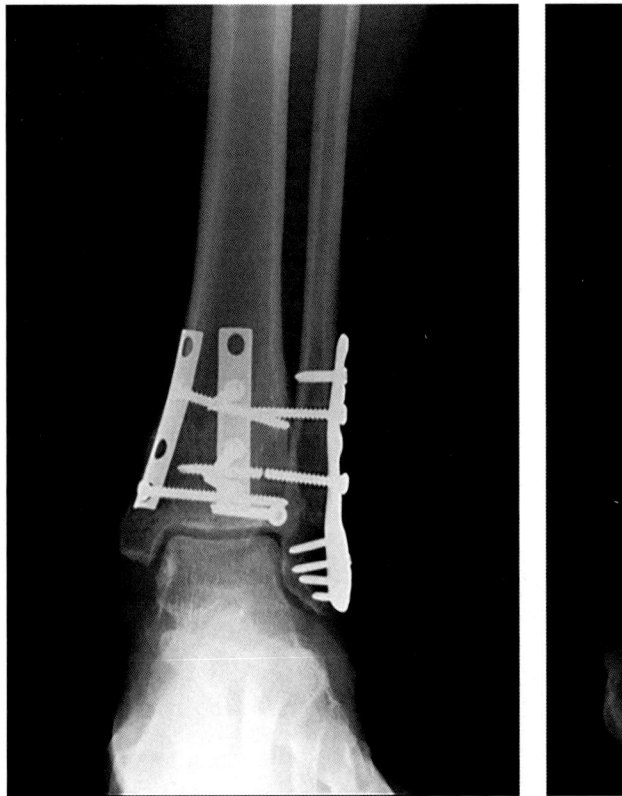 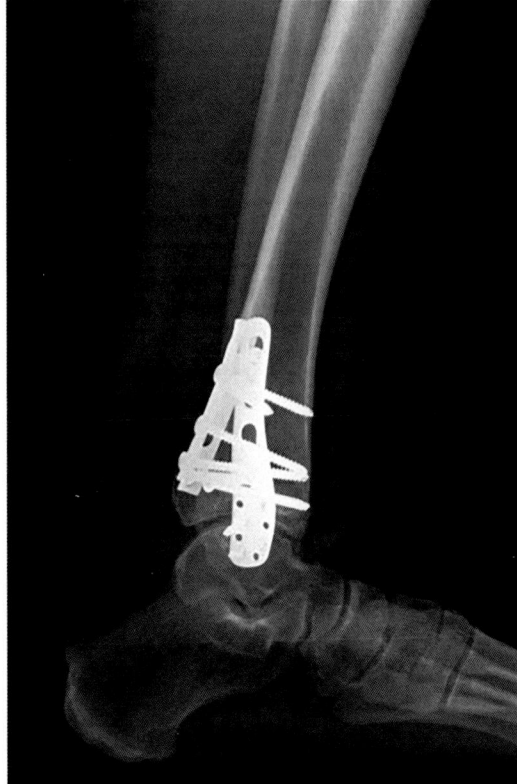

FIGURE 31.30 Weight-bearing radiographs showing 1-year follow-up status post-ORIF of trimalleolar ankle fracture and syndesmosis disruption. Transyndesmosis screw is broken but asymptomatic.

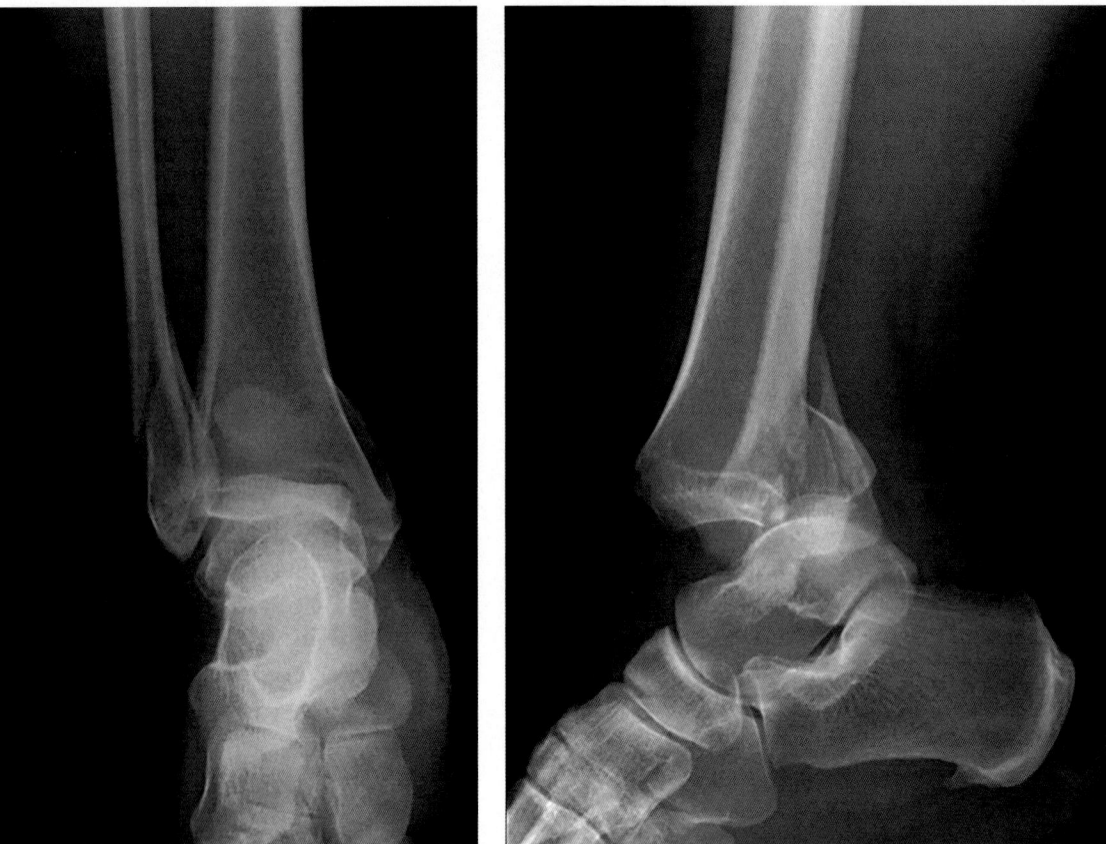

FIGURE 31.31 Radiographs show a trimalleolar ankle fracture with posterior dislocation and syndesmosis disruption.

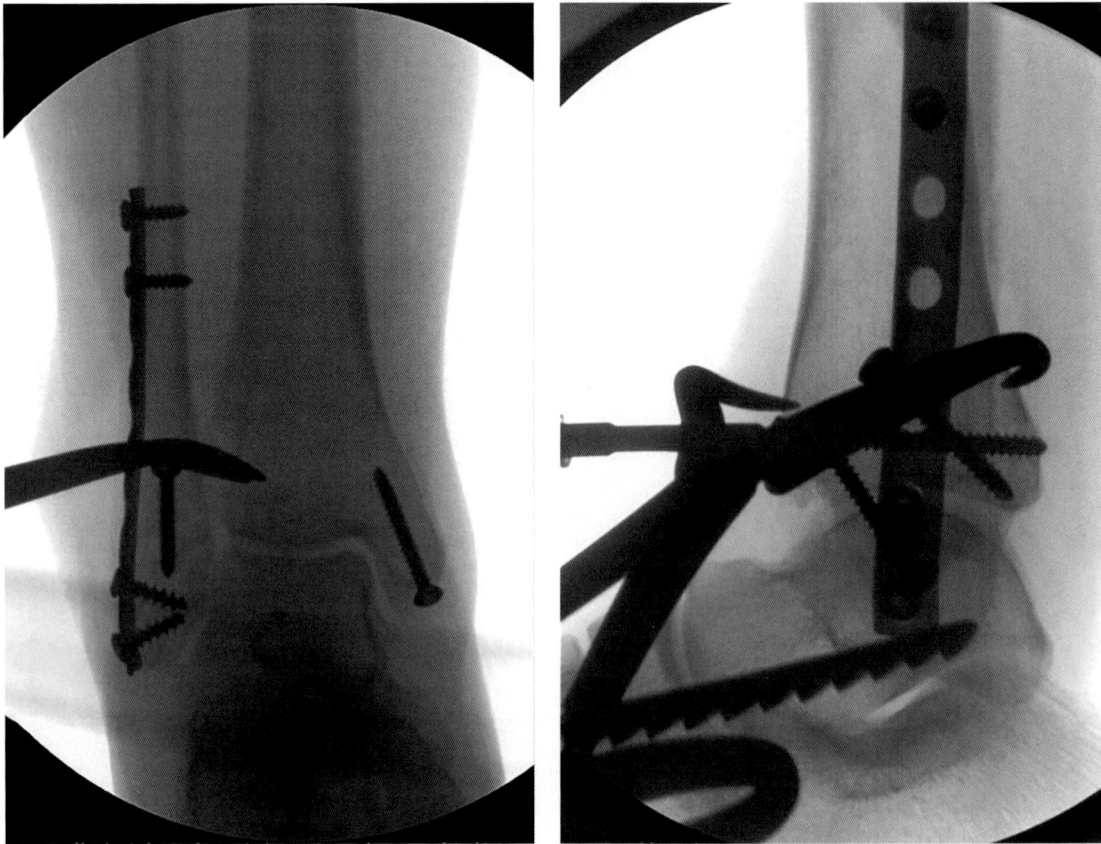

FIGURE 31.32 Intraoperative fluoroscopy demonstrates reduction posterior malleolus fracture with the tines of the forceps placed across the anterior and posterior tubercles of the distal tibia. The reduction forcep reduces and apply compression across the posterior malleolar fracture.

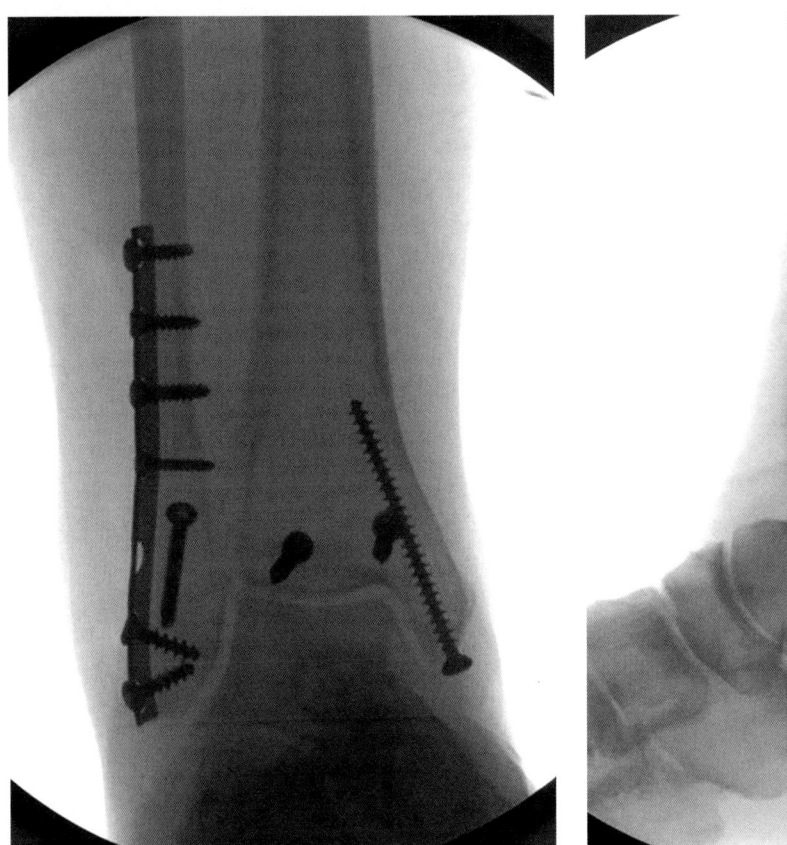
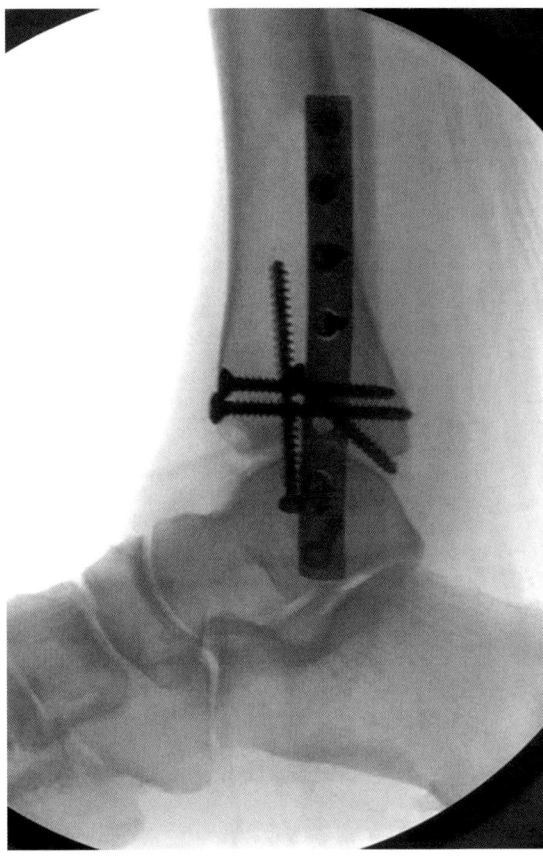

FIGURE 31.33 Intraoperative fluoroscopy shows placement of percutaneous 3.5 mm cortical nonlag screws to maintain compression achieved with reduction forceps. The syndesmosis is anatomically reduced with reduction of the posterior malleolus.

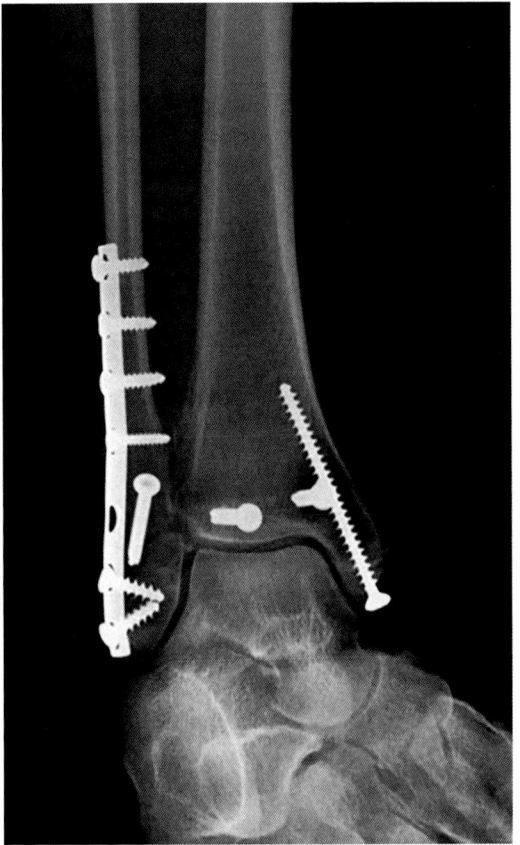
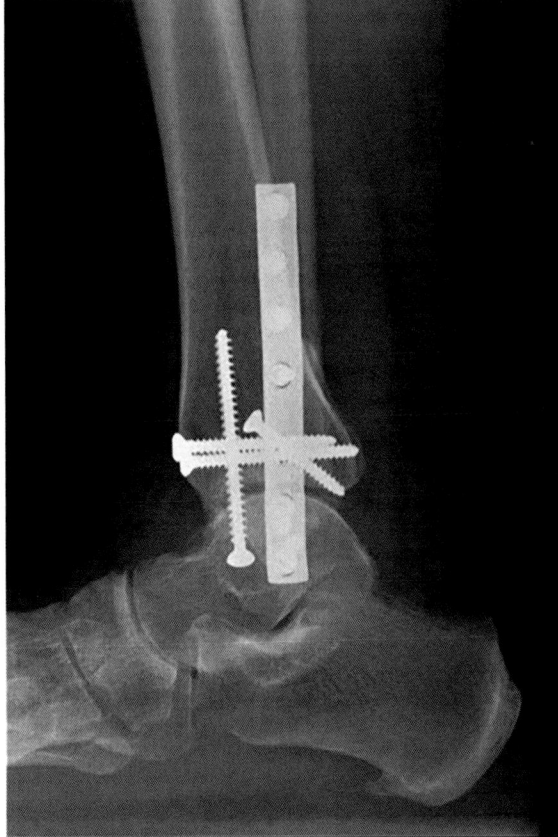

FIGURE 31.34 Radiographs showing 1-year follow-up status post-ORIF of trimalleolar ankle fracture and syndesmosis disruption.

REFERENCES

1. Tornetta P III, Axelrad TW, Sibai TA, et al. Treatment of the stress positive ligamentous SE4 ankle fracture: incidence of syndesmotic injury and clinical decision making. *J Orthop Trauma.* 2012;26(11):659-661. doi: 10.1097/BOT.0b013e31825cf39c.

2. van den Bekerom MP, Haverkamp D, Kerkhoffs GM, et al. Syndesmotic stabilization in pronation external rotation ankle fractures. *Clin Orthop Relat Res.* 2010;468(4):991-995. doi: 10.1007/s11999-009-0823-9.

3. Fallat L, Grimm DJ, Saracco JA. Sprained ankle syndrome: prevalence and analysis of 639 acute injuries. *J Foot Ankle Surg.* 1998;37(4):280-285.

4. Vosseller JT, Karl JW, Greisberg JK. Incidence of syndesmotic injury. *Orthopedics.* 2014;37(3):e226-e229. doi: 10.3928/01477447-20140225-53.

5. Kopec TJ, Hibberd EE, Roos KG, et al. The epidemiology of deltoid ligament sprains in 25 National Collegiate Athletic Association Sports, 2009-2010 through 2014-2015 academic years. *J Athl Train.* 2017;52(4):350-359. doi: 10.4085/1062.6050-52.2.01.

6. Mauntel TC, Wikstrom EA, Roos KG, et al. The epidemiology of high ankle sprains in National Collegiate Athletic Association Sports. *Am J Sports Med.* 2017;45(9):2156-2163. doi: 10.1177/0363546517701428.

7. Roos KG, Kerr ZY, Mauntel TC, et al. The epidemiology of lateral ligament complex ankle sprains in National Collegiate Athletic Association Sports. *Am J Sports Med.* 2017;45(1):201-209. doi: 10.1177/0363546516660980.

8. Gerber JP, Williams GN, Scoville CR, et al. Persistent disability associated with ankle sprains: a prospective examination of an athletic population. *Foot Ankle Int.* 1998;19(10):653-660. doi: 10.1177/107110079801901002.

9. Gardner MJ, Demetrakopoulos D, Briggs SM, et al. Malreduction of the tibiofibular syndesmosis in ankle fractures. *Foot Ankle Int.* 2006;27(10):788-792. doi: 10.1177/107110070602701005.

10. Mont MA, Sedlin ED, Weiner LS, et al. Postoperative radiographs as predictors of clinical outcome in unstable ankle fractures. *J Orthop Trauma.* 1992;6(3):352-357.

11. Weening B, Bhandari M. Predictors of functional outcome following transsyndesmotic screw fixation of ankle fractures. *J Orthop Trauma.* 2005;19(2):102-108.

12. Sagi HC, Shah AR, Sanders RW. The functional consequence of syndesmotic joint malreduction at a minimum 2-year follow-up. *J Orthop Trauma.* 2012;26(7):439-443. doi: 10.1097/BOT.0b013e31822a526a.

13. Beumer A, van Hemert WL, Niesing R, et al. Radiographic measurement of the distal tibiofibular syndesmosis has limited use. *Clin Orthop Relat Res.* 2004(423):227-234.

14. Nielson JH, Gardner MJ, Peterson MG, et al. Radiographic measurements do not predict syndesmotic injury in ankle fractures: an MRI study. *Clin Orthop Relat Res.* 2005(436):216-221.

15. Koenig SJ, Tornetta P III, Merlin G, et al. Can we tell if the syndesmosis is reduced using fluoroscopy? *J Orthop Trauma.* 2015;29(9):e326-e330. doi: 10.1097/BOT.0000000000000296.

16. Marmor M, Hansen E, Han HK, et al. Limitations of standard fluoroscopy in detecting rotational malreduction of the syndesmosis in an ankle fracture model. *Foot Ankle Int.* 2011;32(6):616-622. doi: 10.3113/FAI.2011.0616.

17. Ovaska MT, Makinen TJ, Madanat R, et al. A comprehensive analysis of patients with malreduced ankle fractures undergoing re-operation. *Int Orthop.* 2014;38(1):83-88. doi: 10.1007/s00264-013-2168-y.

18. Naqvi GA, Cunningham P, Lynch B, et al. Fixation of ankle syndesmotic injuries: comparison of tightrope fixation and syndesmotic screw fixation for accuracy of syndesmotic reduction. *Am J Sports Med.* 2012;40(12):2828-2835. doi: 10.1177/0363546512461480.

19. Leeds HC, Ehrlich MG. Instability of the distal tibiofibular syndesmosis after bimalleolar and trimalleolar ankle fractures. *J Bone Joint Surg Am.* 1984;66(4):490-503.

20. Ray R, Koohnejad N, Clement ND, et al. Ankle fractures with syndesmotic stabilisation are associated with a high rate of secondary osteoarthritis. *Foot Ankle Surg.* 2019;25(2):180-185. doi: 10.1016/j.fas.2017.10.005.

21. Burns WC II, Prakash K, Adelaar R, et al. Tibiotalar joint dynamics: indications for the syndesmotic screw—a cadaver study. *Foot Ankle.* 1993;14(3):153-158.

22. Elgafy H, Semaan HB, Blessinger B, et al. Computed tomography of normal distal tibiofibular syndesmosis. *Skeletal Radiol.* 2010;39(6):559-564. doi: 10.1007/s00256-009-0809-4.

23. Hocker K, Pachucki A. [The fibular incisure of the tibia. The cross-sectional position of the fibula in distal syndesmosis]. *Unfallchirurg.* 1989;92(8):401-406.

24. Liu GT, Ryan E, Gustafson E, et al. Three-dimensional computed tomographic characterization of normal anatomic morphology and variations of the distal tibiofibular syndesmosis. *J Foot Ankle Surg.* 2018;57(6):1130-1136. doi: 10.1053/j.jfas.2018.05.013.

25. Liu Q, Lin B, Guo Z, et al. Shapes of distal tibiofibular syndesmosis are associated with risk of recurrent lateral ankle sprains. *Sci Rep.* 2017;7(1):6244. doi: 10.1038/s41598-017-06602-4.

26. Mavi A, Yildirim H, Gunes H, et al. The fibular incisura of the tibia with recurrent sprained ankle on magnetic resonance imaging. *Saudi Med J.* 2002;23(7):845-849.

27. Sora MC, Strobl B, Staykov D, et al. Evaluation of the ankle syndesmosis: a plastination slices study. *Clin Anat.* 2004;17(6):513-517. doi: 10.1002/ca.20019.

28. Taser F, Toker S, Kilincoglu V. Evaluation of morphometric characteristics of the fibular incisura on dry bones. *Eklem Hastalik Cerrahisi.* 2009;20(1):52-58.

29. Tonogai I, Hamada D, Sairyo K. Morphology of the incisura fibularis at the distal tibiofibular syndesmosis in the Japanese population. *J Foot Ankle Surg.* 2017;56(6):1147-1150. doi: 10.1053/j.jfas.2017.05.020.

30. Yeung TW, Chan CY, Chan WC, et al. Can pre-operative axial CT imaging predict syndesmosis instability in patients sustaining ankle fractures? Seven years' experience in a tertiary trauma center. *Skeletal Radiol.* 2015;44(6):823-829. doi: 10.1007/s00256-015-2107-7.

31. Yildirim H, Mavi A, Buyukbebeci O, et al. Evaluation of the fibular incisura of the tibia with magnetic resonance imaging. *Foot Ankle Int.* 2003;24(5):387-391. doi: 10.1177/107110070302400502.

32. Close JR. Some applications of the functional anatomy of the ankle joint. *J Bone Joint Surg Am.* 1956;38(4):761-781.

33. Lepojarvi S, Niinimaki J, Pakarinen H, et al. Rotational dynamics of the normal distal tibiofibular joint with weight-bearing computed tomography. *Foot Ankle Int.* 2016;37(6):627-635. doi: 10.1177/1071100716634757.

34. Peter RE, Harrington RM, Henley MB, et al. Biomechanical effects of internal fixation of the distal tibiofibular syndesmotic joint: comparison of two fixation techniques. *J Orthop Trauma.* 1994;8(3):215-219.

35. Harper MC, Keller TS. A radiographic evaluation of the tibiofibular syndesmosis. *Foot Ankle.* 1989;10(3):156-160.

36. Pneumaticos SG, Noble PC, Chatziioannou SN, et al. The effects of rotation on radiographic evaluation of the tibiofibular syndesmosis. *Foot Ankle Int.* 2002;23(2):107-111. doi: 10.1177/107110070202300205.

37. Kristensen TB. Treatment of malleolar fractures according to Lauge Hansen's method; preliminary results. *Acta Chir Scand.* 1949;97(4):362-379.

38. Gardner MJ, Demetrakopoulos D, Briggs SM, et al. The ability of the Lauge-Hansen classification to predict ligament injury and mechanism in ankle fractures: an MRI study. *J Orthop Trauma.* 2006;20(4):267-272.

39. Ebraheim NA, Lu J, Yang H, et al. Radiographic and CT evaluation of tibiofibular syndesmotic diastasis: a cadaver study. *Foot Ankle Int.* 1997;18(11):693-698. doi: 10.1177/107110079701801103.

40. Clanton TO, Ho CP, Williams BT, et al. Magnetic resonance imaging characterization of individual ankle syndesmosis structures in asymptomatic and surgically treated cohorts. *Knee Surg Sports Traumatol Arthrosc.* 2016;24(7):2089-2102. doi: 10.1007/s00167-014-3399-1.

41. Oae K, Takao M, Naito K, et al. Injury of the tibiofibular syndesmosis: value of MR imaging for diagnosis. *Radiology.* 2003;227(1):155-161. doi: 10.1148/radiol.2271011865.

42. Chun DI, Cho JH, Min TH, et al. Diagnostic accuracy of radiologic methods for ankle syndesmosis injury: a systematic review and meta-analysis. *J Clin Med.* 2019;8(7):968. doi: 10.3390/jcm8070968.

43. Malhotra K, Welck M, Cullen N, et al. The effects of weight bearing on the distal tibiofibular syndesmosis: a study comparing weight bearing-CT with conventional CT. *Foot Ankle Surg.* 2019;25(4):511-516. doi: 10.1016/j.fas.2018.03.006.

44. Del Rio A, Bewsher SM, Roshan-Zamir S, et al. Weightbearing cone-beam computed tomography of acute ankle syndesmosis injuries. *J Foot Ankle Surg.* 2020;59(2):258-263. doi: 10.1053/j.jfas.2019.02.005.

45. Hagemeijer NC, Chang SH, Abdelaziz ME, et al. Range of normal and abnormal syndesmotic measurements using weightbearing CT. *Foot Ankle Int.* 2019;40(12):1430-1437. doi: 10.1177/1071100719866831.

46. Egol KA, Amirtharajah M, Tejwani NC, et al. Ankle stress test for predicting the need for surgical fixation of isolated fibular fractures. *J Bone Joint Surg Am.* 2004;86-A(11):2393-2398.

47. McConnell T, Creevy W, Tornetta P III. Stress examination of supination external rotation-type fibular fractures. *J Bone Joint Surg Am.* 2004;86-A(10):2171-2178.

48. Matuszewski PE, Dombroski D, Lawrence JT, et al. Prospective intraoperative syndesmotic evaluation during ankle fracture fixation: stress external rotation versus lateral fibular stress. *J Orthop Trauma.* 2015;29(4):e157-e160. doi: 10.1097/BOT.0000000000000247.

49. Stoffel K, Wysocki D, Baddour E, et al. Comparison of two intraoperative assessment methods for injuries to the ankle syndesmosis. A cadaveric study. *J Bone Joint Surg Am.* 2009;91(11):2646-2652. doi: 10.2106/JBJS.G.01537.

50. Jenkinson RJ, Sanders DW, Macleod MD, et al. Intraoperative diagnosis of syndesmosis injuries in external rotation ankle fractures. *J Orthop Trauma.* 2005;19(9):604-609.

51. Candal-Couto JJ, Burrow D, Bromage S, et al. Instability of the tibio-fibular syndesmosis: have we been pulling in the wrong direction? *Injury.* 2004;35(8):814-818. doi: 10.1016/j.injury.2003.10.013.

52. LaMothe JM, Baxter JR, Karnovsky SC, et al. Syndesmotic injury assessment with lateral imaging during stress testing in a cadaveric model. *Foot Ankle Int.* 2018;39(4):479-484. doi: 10.1177/1071100717745660.

53. Xenos JS, Hopkinson WJ, Mulligan ME, et al. The tibiofibular syndesmosis. Evaluation of the ligamentous structures, methods of fixation, and radiographic assessment. *J Bone Joint Surg Am.* 1995;77(6):847-856.

54. Cotton FJ. *Fractures and Joint Dislocations.* Philadelphia, PA: WB Saunders; 1910.

55. Monga P, Kumar A, Simons A, et al. Management of distal tibio-fibular syndesmotic injuries: a snapshot of current practice. *Acta Orthop Belg.* 2008;74(3):365-369.

56. Mei-Dan O, Kots E, Barchilon V, et al. A dynamic ultrasound examination for the diagnosis of ankle syndesmotic injury in professional athletes: a preliminary study. *Am J Sports Med.* 2009;37(5):1009-1016. doi: 10.1177/0363546508331202.

57. van Niekerk C, van Dyk B. Dynamic ultrasound evaluation of the syndesmosis ligamentous complex and clear space in acute ankle injury, compared to magnetic resonance imaging and surgical findings. *SA J Radiol.* 2017;21(1):a1191.

58. Guyton GP, DeFontes K III, Barr CR, et al. Arthroscopic correlates of subtle syndesmotic injury. *Foot Ankle Int.* 2017;38(5):502-506. doi: 10.1177/1071100716688198.

59. Han SH, Lee JW, Kim S, et al. Chronic tibiofibular syndesmosis injury: the diagnostic efficiency of magnetic resonance imaging and comparative analysis of operative treatment. *Foot Ankle Int.* 2007;28(3):336-342. doi: 10.3113/FAI.2007.0336.

60. Lui TH, Ip K, Chow HT. Comparison of radiologic and arthroscopic diagnoses of distal tibiofibular syndesmosis disruption in acute ankle fracture. *Arthroscopy.* 2005;21(11):1370. doi: 10.1016/j.arthro.2005.08.016.

61. Ogilvie-Harris DJ, Reed SC. Disruption of the ankle syndesmosis: diagnosis and treatment by arthroscopic surgery. *Arthroscopy.* 1994;10(5):561-568.

62. Takao M, Ochi M, Naito K, et al. Arthroscopic diagnosis of tibiofibular syndesmosis disruption. *Arthroscopy.* 2001;17(8):836-843.

63. Takao M, Ochi M, Oae K, et al. Diagnosis of a tear of the tibiofibular syndesmosis. The role of arthroscopy of the ankle. *J Bone Joint Surg Br.* 2003;85(3):324-329.

64. Wagener ML, Beumer A, Swierstra BA. Chronic instability of the anterior tibiofibular syndesmosis of the ankle. Arthroscopic findings and results of anatomical reconstruction. *BMC Musculoskelet Disord.* 2011;12:212. doi: 10.1186/1471-2474-12-212.

65. Ramsey PL, Hamilton W. Changes in tibiotalar area of contact caused by lateral talar shift. *J Bone Joint Surg Am.* 1976;58(3):356-357.

66. Cherney SM, Spraggs-Hughes AG, McAndrew CM, et al. Incisura morphology as a risk factor for syndesmotic malreduction. *Foot Ankle Int.* 2016;37(7):748-754. doi: 10.1177/1071100716637709.

67. Cosgrove CT, Putnam SM, Cherney SM, et al. Medial clamp tine positioning affects ankle syndesmosis malreduction. *J Orthop Trauma*. 2017;31(8):440-446. doi: 10.1097/BOT.0000000000000882.

68. Cosgrove CT, Spraggs-Hughes AG, Putnam SM, et al. A novel indirect reduction technique in ankle syndesmotic injuries: a cadaveric study. *J Orthop Trauma*. 2018;32(7):361-367. doi: 10.1097/BOT.0000000000001169.

69. Miller AN, Barei DP, Iaquinto JM, et al. Iatrogenic syndesmosis malreduction via clamp and screw placement. *J Orthop Trauma*. 2013;27(2):100-106. doi: 10.1097/BOT.0b013e31825197cb.

70. Park YH, Ahn JH, Choi GW, et al. Comparison of clamp reduction and manual reduction of syndesmosis in rotational ankle fractures: a prospective randomized trial. *J Foot Ankle Surg*. 2018;57(1):19-22. doi: 10.1053/j.jfas.2017.05.040.

71. Gonzalez T, Egan J, Ghorbanhoseini M, et al. Overtightening of the syndesmosis revisited and the effect of syndesmotic malreduction on ankle dorsiflexion. *Injury*. 2017;48(6):1253-1257. doi: 10.1016/j.injury.2017.03.029.

72. Tornetta P III, Spoo JE, Reynolds FA, et al. Overtightening of the ankle syndesmosis: is it really possible? *J Bone Joint Surg Am*. 2001;83-A(4):489-492.

73. Cherney SM, Haynes JA, Spraggs-Hughes AG, et al. In vivo syndesmotic overcompression after fixation of ankle fractures with a syndesmotic injury. *J Orthop Trauma*. 2015;29(9):414-419. doi: 10.1097/BOT.0000000000000356.

74. Haynes J, Cherney S, Spraggs-Hughes A, et al. Increased reduction clamp force associated with syndesmotic overcompression. *Foot Ankle Int*. 2016;37(7):722-729. doi: 10.1177/1071100716634791.

75. Miller AN, Carroll EA, Parker RJ, et al. Direct visualization for syndesmotic stabilization of ankle fractures. *Foot Ankle Int*. 2009;30(5):419-426. doi: 10.3113/FAI-2009-0419.

76. Marmor M, Kandemir U, Matityahu A, et al. A method for detection of lateral malleolar malrotation using conventional fluoroscopy. *J Orthop Trauma*. 2013;27(12):e281-e284. doi: 10.1097/BOT.0b013e31828f89a9.

77. Summers HD, Sinclair MK, Stover MD. A reliable method for intraoperative evaluation of syndesmotic reduction. *J Orthop Trauma*. 2013;27(4):196-200. doi: 10.1097/BOT.0b013e3182694766.

78. Mukhopadhyay S, Metcalfe A, Guha AR, et al. Malreduction of syndesmosis—are we considering the anatomical variation? *Injury*. 2011;42(10):1073-1076. doi: 10.1016/j.injury.2011.03.019.

79. Chen Y, Qiang M, Zhang K, et al. A reliable radiographic measurement for evaluation of normal distal tibiofibular syndesmosis: a multi-detector computed tomography study in adults. *J Foot Ankle Res*. 2015;8:32. doi: 10.1186/s13047-015-0093-6.

80. Lepojarvi S, Pakarinen H, Savola O, et al. Posterior translation of the fibula may indicate malreduction: CT study of normal variation in uninjured ankles. *J Orthop Trauma*. 2014;28(4):205-209. doi: 10.1097/BOT.0b013e3182a59b3c.

81. Mendelsohn ES, Hoshino CM, Harris TG, et al. CT characterizing the anatomy of uninjured ankle syndesmosis. *Orthopedics*. 2014;37(2):e157-e160. doi: 10.3928/01477447-20140124-19.

82. Nault ML, Hebert-Davies J, Laflamme GY, et al. CT scan assessment of the syndesmosis: a new reproducible method. *J Orthop Trauma*. 2013;27(11):638-641. doi: 10.1097/BOT.0b013e318284785a.

83. Warner SJ, Fabricant PD, Garner MR, et al. The measurement and clinical importance of syndesmotic reduction after operative fixation of rotational ankle fractures. *J Bone Joint Surg Am*. 2015;97(23):1935-1944. doi: 10.2106/JBJS.O.00016.

84. Davidovitch RI, Weil Y, Karia R, et al. Intraoperative syndesmotic reduction: three-dimensional versus standard fluoroscopic imaging. *J Bone Joint Surg Am*. 2013;95(20):1838-1843. doi: 10.2106/JBJS.L.00382.

85. Chu A, Weiner L. Distal fibula malunions. *J Am Acad Orthop Surg*. 2009;17(4):220-230.

86. Fitzpatrick E, Goetz JE, Sittapairoj T, et al. Effect of posterior malleolus fracture on syndesmotic reduction: a cadaveric study. *J Bone Joint Surg Am*. 2018;100(3):243-248. doi: 10.2106/JBJS.17.00217.

87. Jones CR, Nunley JA II. Deltoid ligament repair versus syndesmotic fixation in bimalleolar equivalent ankle fractures. *J Orthop Trauma*. 2015;29(5):245-249. doi: 10.1097/BOT.0000000000000220.

88. Wu K, Lin J, Huang J, et al. Evaluation of transsyndesmotic fixation and primary deltoid ligament repair in ankle fractures with suspected combined deltoid ligament injury. *J Foot Ankle Surg*. 2018;57(4):694-700. doi: 10.1053/j.jfas.2017.12.007.

89. Hsu AR, Lareau CR, Anderson RB. Repair of acute superficial deltoid complex avulsion during ankle fracture fixation in national football league players. *Foot Ankle Int*. 2015;36(11):1272-1278. doi: 10.1177/1071100715593374.

90. Andersen MR, Frihagen F, Hellund JC, et al. Randomized trial comparing suture button with single syndesmotic screw for syndesmosis injury. *J Bone Joint Surg Am*. 2018;100(1):2-12. doi: 10.2106/JBJS.16.01011.

91. Colcuc C, Blank M, Stein T, et al. Lower complication rate and faster return to sports in patients with acute syndesmotic rupture treated with a new knotless suture button device. *Knee Surg Sports Traumatol Arthrosc*. 2018;26(10):3156-3164. doi: 10.1007/s00167-017-4820-3.

92. Laflamme M, Belzile EL, Bedard L, et al. A prospective randomized multicenter trial comparing clinical outcomes of patients treated surgically with a static or dynamic implant for acute ankle syndesmosis rupture. *J Orthop Trauma*. 2015;29(5):216-223. doi: 10.1097/BOT.0000000000000245.

93. Seyhan M, Donmez F, Mahirogullari M, et al. Comparison of screw fixation with elastic fixation methods in the treatment of syndesmosis injuries in ankle fractures. *Injury*. 2015;46(suppl 2):S19-S23. doi: 10.1016/j.injury.2015.05.027.

94. Shimozono Y, Hurley ET, Myerson CL, et al. Suture button versus syndesmotic screw for syndesmosis injuries: a meta-analysis of randomized controlled trials. *Am J Sports Med*. 2019;47(11):2764-2771. doi: 10.1177/0363546518804804.

95. McBryde A, Chiasson B, Wilhelm A, et al. Syndesmotic screw placement: a biomechanical analysis. *Foot Ankle Int*. 1997;18(5):262-266. doi: 10.1177/107110079701800503.

96. Wukich DK, Joseph A, Ryan M, et al. Outcomes of ankle fractures in patients with uncomplicated versus complicated diabetes. *Foot Ankle Int*. 2011;32(2):120-130. doi: 10.3113/FAI.2011.0120.

97. Hoiness P, Stromsoe K. Tricortical versus quadricortical syndesmosis fixation in ankle fractures: a prospective, randomized study comparing two methods of syndesmosis fixation. *J Orthop Trauma*. 2004;18(6):331-337.

98. Markolf KL, Jackson SR, McAllister DR. Syndesmosis fixation using dual 3.5 mm and 4.5 mm screws with tricortical and quadricortical purchase: a biomechanical study. *Foot Ankle Int*. 2013;34(5):734-739. doi: 10.1177/1071100713478923.

99. Thompson MC, Gesink DS. Biomechanical comparison of syndesmosis fixation with 3.5- and 4.5-millimeter stainless steel screws. *Foot Ankle Int*. 2000;21(9):736-741. doi: 10.1177/107110070002100904.

100. Moore JA Jr, Shank JR, Morgan SJ, et al. Syndesmosis fixation: a comparison of three and four cortices of screw fixation without hardware removal. *Foot Ankle Int*. 2006;27(8):567-572. doi: 10.1177/107110070602700801.

101. Manjoo A, Sanders DW, Tieszer C, et al. Functional and radiographic results of patients with syndesmotic screw fixation: implications for screw removal. *J Orthop Trauma*. 2010;24(1):2-6. doi: 10.1097/BOT.0b013e3181a9f7a5.

102. Donatto KC. Ankle fractures and syndesmosis injuries. *Orthop Clin North Am*. 2001;32(1):79-90.

103. Roberts RS. Surgical treatment of displaced ankle fractures. *Clin Orthop Relat Res*. 1983;(172):164-170.

104. Tsai J, Pivec R, Jauregui JJ, et al. Strength of syndesmosis fixation: two tightrope versus one tightrope with plate-and-screw construct. *J Long Term Eff Med Implants*. 2016;26(2):161-165. doi: 10.1615/JLongTermEffMedImplants.2016016538.

105. Zhang P, Liang Y, He J, et al. A systematic review of suture-button versus syndesmotic screw in the treatment of distal tibiofibular syndesmosis injury. *BMC Musculoskelet Disord*. 2017;18(1):286. doi: 10.1186/s12891-017-1645-7.

106. Xie L, Xie H, Wang J, et al. Comparison of suture button fixation and syndesmotic screw fixation in the treatment of distal tibiofibular syndesmosis injury: a systematic review and meta-analysis. *Int J Surg*. 2018;60:120-131. doi: 10.1016/j.ijsu.2018.11.007.

107. Coetzee JC, Ebeling PB. Treatment of syndesmoses disruptions: a prospective, randomized study comparing conventional screw fixation vs TightRope fiber wire fixation—medium-term results. *SA Orthop J*. 2009;8(1):32-37.

108. Kortekangas T, Savola O, Flinkkila T, et al. A prospective randomised study comparing TightRope and syndesmotic screw fixation for accuracy and maintenance of syndesmotic reduction assessed with bilateral computed tomography. *Injury*. 2015;46(6):1119-1126. doi: 10.1016/j.injury.2015.02.004.

109. Hartford JM, Gorczyca JT, McNamara JL, et al. Tibiotalar contact area. Contribution of posterior malleolus and deltoid ligament. *Clin Orthop Relat Res*. 1995(320):182-187.

110. Harper MC. Talar shift. The stabilizing role of the medial, lateral, and posterior ankle structures. *Clin Orthop Relat Res*. 1990(257):177-183.

111. Raasch WG, Larkin JJ, Draganich LF. Assessment of the posterior malleolus as a restraint to posterior subluxation of the ankle. *J Bone Joint Surg Am*. 1992;74(8):1201-1206.

112. Gardner MJ, Brodsky A, Briggs SM, et al. Fixation of posterior malleolar fractures provides greater syndesmotic stability. *Clin Orthop Relat Res*. 2006;447:165-171. doi: 10.1097/01.blo.0000203489.21206.a9.

CHAPTER 32

Total Ankle Replacement

John M. Schuberth, Jeffrey C. Christensen, Jerome K. Steck, and Chad L. Seidenstricker

DEFINITION

Total joint arthroplasty has evolved considerably over the past 50 years, with improvement in operative technique, prosthetic materials science, and advanced engineering designs. Driven by this formative knowledge base, total ankle replacement (TAR) has emerged as a viable alternative in the surgical management of advanced ankle arthritis. Ankle replacement is more attractive to many patients than fusion, which had long been the historical standard for end-stage arthritis of the ankle.

Ankle range of motion is one of the six determinants of gait, which have been shown to be necessary to minimize energy expenditure for smooth bipedal locomotion.[1,2] Moreover, dynamic ankle plantar flexion is a critical characteristic in normal gait to optimize energy consumption.[3] Accordingly, the rationale for ankle replacement is simple: to achieve a durable and functional restoration of ankle motion that facilitates a return to the activities of daily living with reduction or elimination of pain. However, the precise manner, conditions, and limitations at which replacement arthroplasty can accomplish these aims are not fully understood. While the rationale for functional restoration is intuitive, it is important to appreciate that survivorship to date has not been similar to hip and knee arthroplasty. Many of the factors that can compromise device survivorship have been appreciated through careful observations of previous failures. Recognition of these factors has shaped refinements in selection criteria, surgical instrumentation, device design, and material selection to better combat the stressful mechanical environment of the ankle. In addition, some of the reasons for failure have not been identified or fully studied, which makes prognostication of success an imperfect science.

CLASSIFICATION

A validated ankle arthritis classification has been developed for use in ankle replacement.[4] While it is simple to use and attempts to address the spectrum of deformity, it does not address translational deformities of the ankle.[5] In the past, patients with severe and complex deformities in any plane were often relegated to ankle arthrodesis. With improvement of the prostheses and more global experience, more patients are being offered ankle replacement. To date, there is also no firm correlation of the degree of arthritis to the preferred method of treatment.

TARs have been loosely classified into generational categories based on the time frame they were brought to market. The evolutionary changes of the implants are reflected in the engineering concepts utilized with each generation of implants. Design characteristics have also been used to describe ankle replacement components, specifically, fixed and mobile bearing devices. For interested readers, previous publications have described the evolution and respective design features of historical and devices not available in the U.S. market.[6,7]

INDICATIONS

In general, the indications for TAR include posttraumatic arthritis, primary osteoarthritis, and inflammatory arthritis (ie, rheumatoid), in patients who have failed conservative treatments.[6,8,9]

INDICATIONS FOR TOTAL ANKLE REPLACEMENT

Patients with
- End-stage symptomatic ankle arthropathy
- Good bone stock
- Normal vascular status
- Good hindfoot alignment
- Sufficient collateral ligament function
- Moderate to light work or activity demands
- Coexistent midfoot and hindfoot arthrosis
- Bilateral arthritic ankles
- Inflammatory arthropathy
- Symptomatic ankle arthrodesis or nonunion of ankle fusion

Not all are good candidates for implantation based on a variety of factors. Successful implantation requires a synchronization of sound component design, astute patient selection, precise prosthetic placement and sizing, and comprehensive patient education. The concept of patient selection cannot be overemphasized insofar that each individual will have specific goals, expectations, and physical and anatomical barriers that may alter the decision-making process.

There are some clinical conditions that may increase the risk of complications in total ankle surgery. Often, these conditions cannot be quantified. The relative contraindications are listed below.

- Previous severe trauma (ie, open fracture of ankle, talar body dislocation, segmental bone loss)
- AVN talus 25%-75% of body
- Severe osteopenia/osteoporosis
- Dependence on immunosuppressive medications
- Elevated Hbg A1c levels in diabetic patients
- Demanding sport or work activities
- Obesity (especially with relatively small ankle sizes)
- Younger patients (<40 years) with intact hindfoot joint function

As such, surgeons should exercise good judgment when deciding on the optimal form of treatment for a given patient.

Although there are few absolute contraindications, the decision process should involve careful analysis of the pertinent clinical factors and a comprehensive interview with the patient.

- Charcot arthropathy
- Active or recent infection
- AVN talus (>75% of talar body)
- Severe uncorrectable deformity
- Progressive sensory or motor dysfunction of lower leg
- Open ulceration of lower extremity
- Dysvascular disease

PRIOR ARTHRODESIS

Patients with prior ankle arthrodesis can be converted to implant arthroplasty when significant symptoms develop in adjacent and/or distant joints or there is malposition or nonunion of the fusion. The primary premise is to provide some sagittal plane motion that would unload the active compensatory process. Previous reports of take down fusions and general consensus suggest that the distal fibula needs to be intact for a successful durable implantation.[10,11] Take down of ankle fusion is a challenging endeavor that has not been fully studied. However, when there is a compelling clinical situation to provide some motion and unload the compensatory joints, implant arthroplasty may be beneficial.

HISTORY OF DEEP INFECTION

A history of prior infection in the ankle is also a relative contraindication to implantation. The overwhelming majority of patients who relate a history of infection have had surgery for traumatic injuries to the lower leg. Careful probing of the nature and extent of the infection may reveal scenarios ranging from minor wound complications to frank osteomyelitis. Solicitation of details regarding treatment of the presumed infection often helps determine the likelihood of dormant infection. Advanced imaging and laboratory studies may provide assistance in determining the presence of infected foci, but through clinical history and examination with sound clinical judgment should prevail.[12] Previous joint infection does not preclude placement of a total joint prosthesis, yet the patient needs to be aware that there is still increased risk for reinfection.[13]

In patient with a history of quiescent septic arthritis, infection resolution can remain uncertain even after years of clinical resolution. Preoperative joint biopsy is recommended; however, false-negative incidence is high. Proper patient education is necessary in these cases.

PATHOANATOMIC FEATURES OF ANKLE ARTHRITIS

RANGE OF MOTION

The range of motion in patients with end-stage ankle arthritis covers a wide spectrum, from virtual ankylosis to a fluid liberal joint excursion. These latter patients typically have eburnated subchondral bone of the tibiotalar joint without significant deformity. Patients with high-energy trauma or those with prior fracture dislocations often present with a grossly limited ankle range of motion as some joints become infiltrated with pathological fibrosis and dense scar. Moreover, any unresolved deformity also negatively impacts the available range of motion. These ankles can be a challenge to restore adequate range of motion after TAR. Although not entirely linear, the attained postoperative range of motion is proportionate to the available preoperative range of motion.

SURFACE GEOMETRY AND LOAD CHARACTERISTICS

The normal ankle joint is a highly congruent joint and has a unique surface anatomy, which has been described in detail.[14,15]

In the arthritic ankle, adaptive changes to the periarticular anatomy over time with joint elongation in the AP direction with enlargement of radius of curvature in addition to typical joint destructive changes seen with any arthritis. There is often a loss of congruity due to deformity in any or all of the three cardinal body planes.[5,16]

Varus and valgus ankle deformities have been studied extensively in total ankle arthroplasty.[17-22] Most often, these frontal plane deformities are the combined result of asymmetric wear of the tibiotalar interface, ligamentous compromise, and potentiation from long-standing duration of the disease process.

Little is known about the impact of sagittal and transverse plane malalignments in the arthritic ankle.[5,23,24] During the genesis of ankle arthritis, as the ankle degenerates, the radius of the talus increases and the joint containment capacity diminishes.[25] As the ankle loses the ability to retain the talus, the talar sagittal position can drift anterior or posterior (talolisthesis). Joint adaptation can occur over time, thus making joint subluxation a poor descriptive term for this phenomenon.[5]

Foot alignment is always rotated internally (mean 21.0 ± 10.6 degrees) relative to the transmalleolar axis in arthritic ankles.[26] Adaptive changes that involve the transmalleolar axis can be subtle and go unrecognized. Most commonly rotational ankle and lower leg fractures can precipitate transverse plane malalignments, particularly if they are not accurately reduced at the time of injury. Moreover, empirical observations in patients with long-standing arthritis suggest that there is an external rotational deformity through the distal tibia-fibular joint. Patients with unilateral ankle arthritis often externally rotated their foot during gait to offload stress on the ankle. Prolonged ambulation with this compensated alignment causes maladaptive changes and distortion of the transmalleolar axis. This maladaptation can be further magnified with cavovarus feet with lateral ankle instability, which allows for external rotation of the leg relative to the foot. This type of adaptive pathology is characterized by the fibula appearing to be posteriorly displaced relative to the foot position. The accentuated and distorted transmalleolar axis may give the surgeon a spurious account of the true axis of the ankle, which could alter placement of the prosthetic components.

LIGAMENTOUS RESTRAINT

Ligamentous integrity is often compromised in patients with end-stage ankle arthritis.[27] The involved ligamentous complexes include the deltoid, syndesmosis and the lateral collateral structures. The ligaments become compromised during the original trauma or from chronic stretching due to increasing deformity. With long-standing bony adaptation of the tibial talar joint, these ligament complexes often become scarred or dormant, which can negate the necessity of reconstruction with ankle replacement. Nonetheless, the cumulative effect of planar malalignments and ligamentous insufficiency add to the complexity of reconstruction with ankle replacement. Recognition of the specific insufficient ligaments and the potential for gross instability is critical for successful reconstruction.

Arguably, the integrity of the deep deltoid is the most critical ligament for proper ankle function postimplantation; it is the primary restraint for valgus rotation of the talus and has secondary restraint function against lateral and anterior talar excursion. Yet in most TAR cases, the deltoid is compromised during preparation of the distal tibia or talus (Fig. 32.1). Most often, there is no subsequent valgus instability postimplantation, provided there is an intact lateral fibular buttress. It is also important to appreciate that asymmetric valgus wear of the tibial plafond does not necessarily correlate with deltoid compromise.[28,29]

The syndesmotic ligaments are often attenuated with end-stage arthrosis, which can lead to widening of the ankle mortise. With contemporary total ankle designs, there is no obligate invasion of the syndesmosis during implantation. But in rare cases, restoration of the fibula in the incurisa may be required particularly if there is any valgus thrust to the talar component.[30,31]

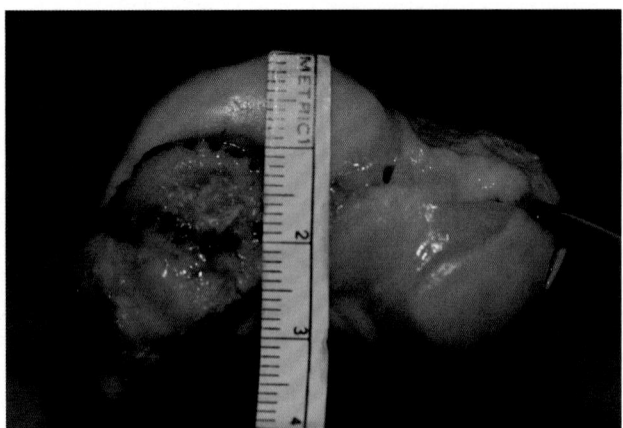

FIGURE 32.1 Photo of talus specimen; the medial side is marked in ink, which represents insertion position of deep deltoid ligament, inferior to the talomalleolar facet.

PATHOGENESIS

Patients with end-stage ankle arthritis often experience significant symptoms of progressive pain, joint immobility, deformity, and reduced activities. As a result, many are challenged to perform basic activities of daily living such as level walking, stair climbing, or stooping. The individual impairment of advanced arthritis of the ankle is severely disabling, and is comparable to that of the hip.[32] In bilateral disease, such as seen in rheumatoid arthritis, the impact can be even more devastating.[33,34]

The pathogenesis of end-stage arthritis is poorly understood and minimally covered in the TAR literature. Even though many of the patients with end-stage ankle arthritis have a common etiology, there are distinct patterns of disease and rates of degeneration (Fig. 32.2). The specific etiologies can often be explained by the patients' history but, in some instances, can only be inferred. The most prevalent etiology of ankle arthritis is trauma, unlike the hip and knee.[35-37] In most instances, the traumatic event was a rotational ankle fracture, but impaction injuries of the plafond, talus fractures, and tibiofibular fractures also can precipitate end-stage ankle arthritis.

Patients who present with incongruent varus deformities of the ankle usually have a distant history of repetitive inversion ankle injuries that have culminated in a fixed varus posture of the joint. Often, the lateral aspect of that tibiotalar articulation has not been eroded presumably because of the lack of load after the joint has adapted.

INFLAMMATORY ARTHROPATHY

In patients with inflammatory arthropathy, the clinical situation can be confusing and complex. Careful assessment is necessary to determine the overall restrictions imposed on the patient by the disease in all joints, not just the ankle. TAR may be indicated if ankle pain is restricting the ability of the patient to walk; however, other factors come into play: bone quality (presence of bone cysts, severe osteoporosis), bone loss, joint alignment, adjacent joint status, and anticipated activity level after surgery. Functional and pain relief benefits need to be weighed against surgical risks with the understanding that patients with larger levels of deformity are at higher risk for TAR failure.[38,39]

AVASCULAR NECROSIS

The presence of talar or distal tibial avascular necrosis is a relative contraindication. The designation of avascular necrosis infers that inert or dead bone would preclude biologic fixation of the components, which would lead to early loosening. However, most patients following talar neck fracture that develop end-stage arthritis do not have an avascular talar body. More commonly, the process involves the superior pole of the talus and is manifested as cystic deterioration of the dome. Whether this process is a true avascular event or represents advanced degenerative changes is unclear. If there is inconclusive evidence of talar avascular involvement, then MRI with gadolinium enhancement can be helpful to map out osseous areas where perfusion remains compromised[40] (Fig. 32.3). Some patients have similar findings on the tibial side of the ankle joint. In particular, the necrotic segment is usually on the lateral pole of the distal tibia. Although the local bone in this area may indeed be avascular, it may be preferable to consider these changes as

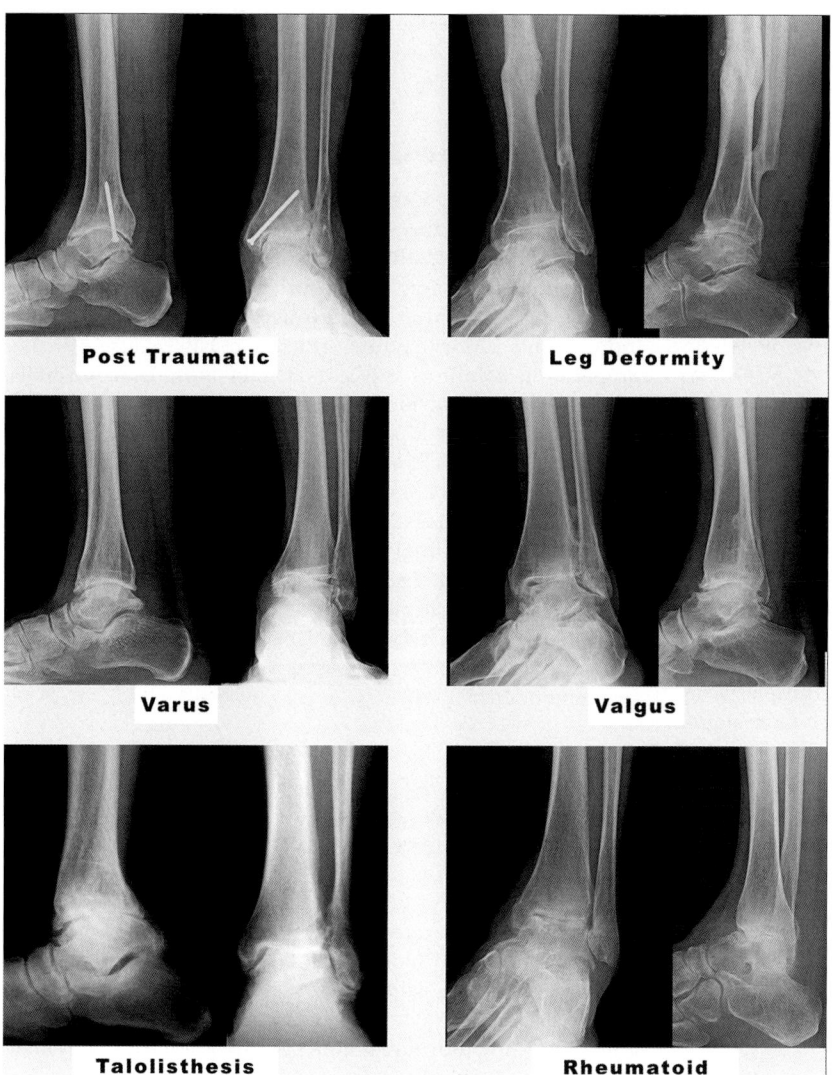

Post Traumatic

Leg Deformity

Varus

Valgus

Talolisthesis

Rheumatoid

FIGURE 32.2 Mortise and lateral radiographs of representative cases of ankle arthritis disease spectrum encountered clinically.

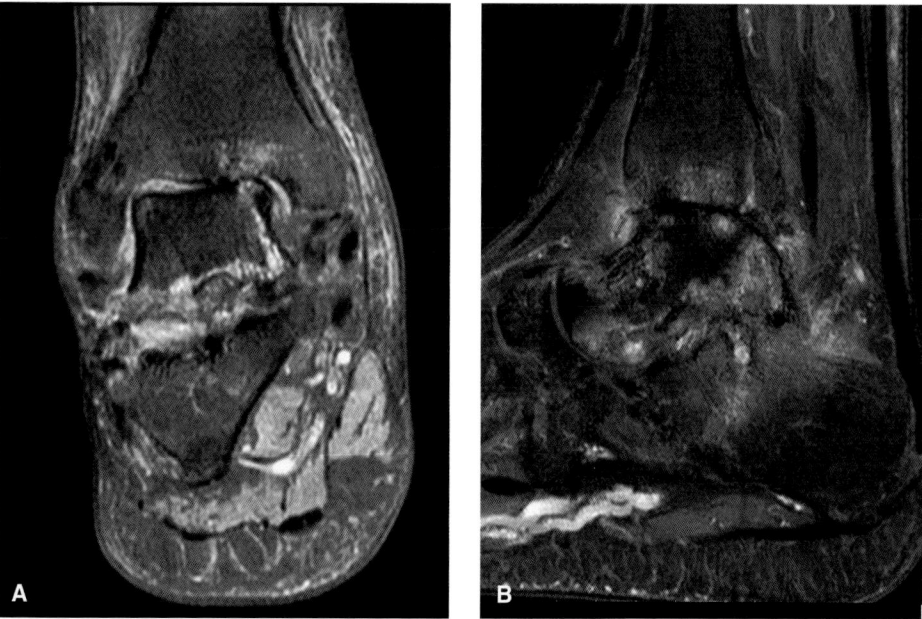

FIGURE 32.3 Magnetic resonance image after talar extrusion and relocation. Coronal **(A)** and sagittal **(B)** slices depict multifocal AVN involving the inferior talar body.

manifestations of the degenerative process.[41,42] Regardless of the location of these focal areas of necrosis or degeneration, if the diseased sections are resectable during standard implantation, then prosthetic placement can be considered. There is also early evidence that staged subtalar arthrodesis may have some protective benefit when considering TAR.[43]

PHYSICAL EXAMINATION

As with any elective reconstructive surgery, the patient should be medically stable and be appropriately evaluated to determine the overall risk for the entire surgical event. As in any total joint procedure, patients should be screened for the possibility of remote infection in the oral cavity, (poor dentition), genitourinary tract, skin ulcerations, paronychia, folliculitis, or the pulmonary system.[44,45]

In preparation for the surgery, the surgeon should perform a detailed lower extremity examination with focus on ankle ligament stability, midfoot and hindfoot alignment, soft tissue envelope (with special attention to previous ankle incisions or traumatic scars), and arterial perfusion.

Careful consideration should be given to the need for additional procedures either at the time of ankle arthroplasty or a separate surgical session. These procedures include realignment osteotomies, ligament reconstruction, equinus release, tibiotalar cyst grafting, hindfoot fusions, and tendon transfers.

IMAGING AND DIAGNOSTIC STUDIES

WEIGHT-BEARING RADIOGRAPHS

Anteroposterior, mortise, and lateral weight-bearing ankle radiographs are obligatory prior to surgery. The images should be assessed for overall alignment of the entire lower leg and for the presence of adjacent joint arthritis.

LONG LEG FILMS

When faced with malalignment issues, long leg radiographs may be helpful in deformity planning and the ultimate placement of the components. They are particularly useful in patients with ipsilateral degenerative joint disease of the knee.

ADVANCED IMAGING

CT scans may have utility for preoperative planning. In particular, the CT scan will provide more specificity into the severity of adjacent joint arthritis and the presence and location of subchondral cysts. MRI can be useful to assess the condition of the cartilage and subchondral bone when the joint space is only modestly narrowed.

SURGICAL CONSIDERATIONS

PATIENT PREPARATION

Patient Positioning

The patient should be positioned on the operating table in a supine attitude under regional or general anesthetic. A bump placed under the ipsilateral hip helps attain the malleoli on a plane parallel to the floor. The opposite limb should be secured in some fashion to prevent migration during planar deflections of the operating table.

Skin Preparation and Draping

The skin preparation and draping should extend to the knee to access and visualize the entire lower leg. Effective skin preparation with alcohol-based solutions is likely one of the most important maneuvers that will diminish the incidence of postoperative infection. While tincture of iodine, povidone-iodine, and chlorhexidine gluconate–based surgical skin preparation solutions are standard in most U.S. hospitals, there is emerging evidence that chlorhexidine scrubs show greater efficacy and longer duration in eliminating potential bacterial pathogens from the foot.[46-48] These studies also confirm at higher percentage of bacterial recolonization at the end of surgery at the digits, supporting coverage of the toes during TAR. Additional barriers to wound contamination can be obtained with the use of incise drapes, effectively isolating the skin from the surgical field. Preoperative shaving of the surgical site with a razor should be avoided. Instead, the use of a surgical clipper prior to entering the operating room is recommended.[49]

TOURNIQUET USE

The use of tourniquet during TAR has advantages and disadvantages but has not been directly studied. While placement of a thigh tourniquet for possible use is advised for all cases, the manner at which the tourniquet is used is based on surgeon preference and operative circumstances. The obvious advantages are controlled blood loss and improved visualization of the surgical field. Furthermore, if the surgeon is considering the use of bone cement, a bloodless field is needed. As in any long procedure, tourniquet time need to be appropriately managed to avoid posttourniquet syndrome.[50]

Some surgeons argue that it is important to avoid any ischemia that could compromise wound healing. While this has not been studied in the ankle, a small series on total knee arthroplasty (TKA) has detected greater wound problems in patients with tourniquets compared to patients without tourniquets.[51] Furthermore, the lack of tourniquet control allows the surgeon to monitor and control bleeding by the discovery of occult bleeders that may not have been otherwise evident. The proximity of major neurovascular structures lends support to this practice as well. However, the additional blood loss may lead to a higher incidence of blood transfusion and greater hospital expense.[52]

SURGICAL TECHNIQUE

- Long curvilinear incision following course of EHL.
- Identify and mobilize superficial peroneal nerve.
- Incise fascia just lateral to EHL.
- Take EHL and neurovascular bundle laterally and tibialis. anterior medially while preserving sheath
- Capsulotomy elevate capsule off joint to expose 180 degrees of ankle.

SURGICAL INCISION

All but one of the contemporary TAR prosthetic devices utilize an anterior midline approach between the TA and EHL tendons (Fig. 32.4). The incision should be long enough to reduce tension on incision margins and adequately expose the distal tibia and extend to the talonavicular joint. Full-thickness flaps are created. The medial branches of the superficial peroneal nerve at the distal portion of the incision are retracted laterally. The fascia is divided just lateral and parallel to the course of the EHL tendon without disturbing the synovial sheath of the tibialis anterior tendon.[53] The anterior neurovascular bundle mobilized laterally with the EHL and EDL tendons.

The anterior ankle capsule is incised longitudinally and elevated medially and laterally off the bone to gain full exposure of the ankle joint. The anterior osteophytes are removed as needed. Once accomplished, it is useful to reexamine the soft tissue restraints of the ankle and available range of motion.

BONE RESECTION

The ultimate position of the prosthesis is determined by the level and orientation of the bony resection of the respective articular surfaces. Although each manufacturer of ankle implants has a scripted technique for resection, the optimal position of the implant has not been determined. The authors recommend in most settings the device should ultimately be oriented such that when the patient is weight bearing, the components are parallel to the ground on AP and lateral views, to avoid any shearing forces.

The alignment guide (Fig. 32.5A) is typically attached to the proximal tibia either with an intraosseous pin or with an external noninvasive clamp. The slope of the distal tibia on the lateral view should be set to near 0 degrees (Fig. 32.5B).

The cutting blocks are attached to the distal alignment guide, or customized CT-generated patient-specific instrumentation (PSI) can be created and placed accordingly over the joint. While the PSI use has been recently popularized, surgeons need to be familiar with conventional alignment methods when alignment inaccuracies are discovered intraoperatively. Surgeons are encouraged to play an active role in PSI component planning with an emphasis on controlling internal/external alignment position. PSI systems may not take into account intrinsic congruent deformities of the distal tibia that are driving hindfoot malposition.

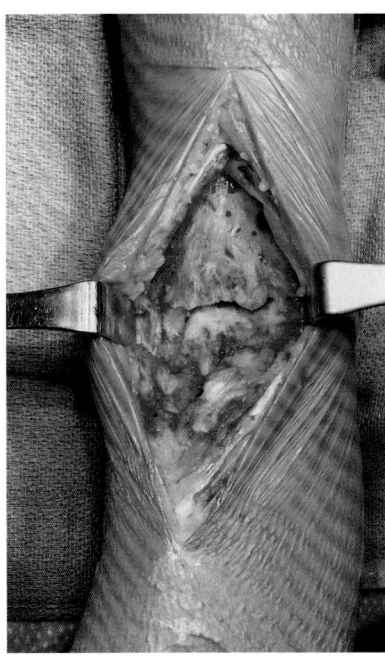

FIGURE 32.4 Surgical incision anterior ankle showing full-thickness flaps and exposed arthritic ankle.

In general, the least amount of bone should be removed, provided there is adequate range of motion after the trial components are placed. It is intuitive that more generous resection would allow for an increased range of motion but overresection of the tibia can compromise the strength of the medial malleolus due to the natural curvature of the metaphysis. Surgeon experience helps determine the optimal amount of bone resection, but there are no specific guidelines other than being conservative in the amount of initial resection. Some systems have "recut" guides if the initial bone resection does not allow for sufficient range of motion.

Lastly, the rotational orientation of the bone resection is subject to surgeon discretion. Although it is intuitive that a transmalleolar axis be replicated, the duplication of this axis may place the implant in an external attitude if the preoperative position has been altered by trauma or long-standing compensatory mechanisms. Such placement rotates the prosthesis away from the line of progression (Fig. 32.6A), which may place undue shearing forces at the talar-polyethylene interface. As such, the authors recommend erring on the side of internal rotation (Fig. 32.6B).

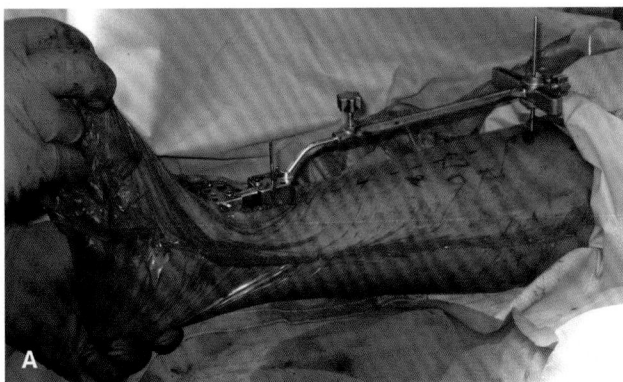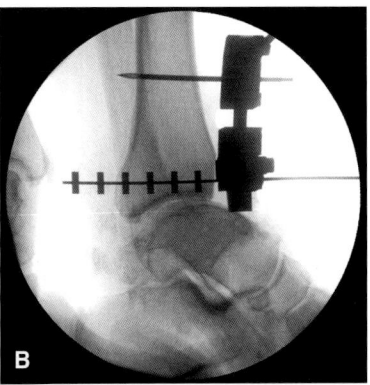

FIGURE 32.5 **A.** Alignment guide on tibia. **B.** Intraoperative radiographic image of angel wing indicating projected bone cut and relative slope.

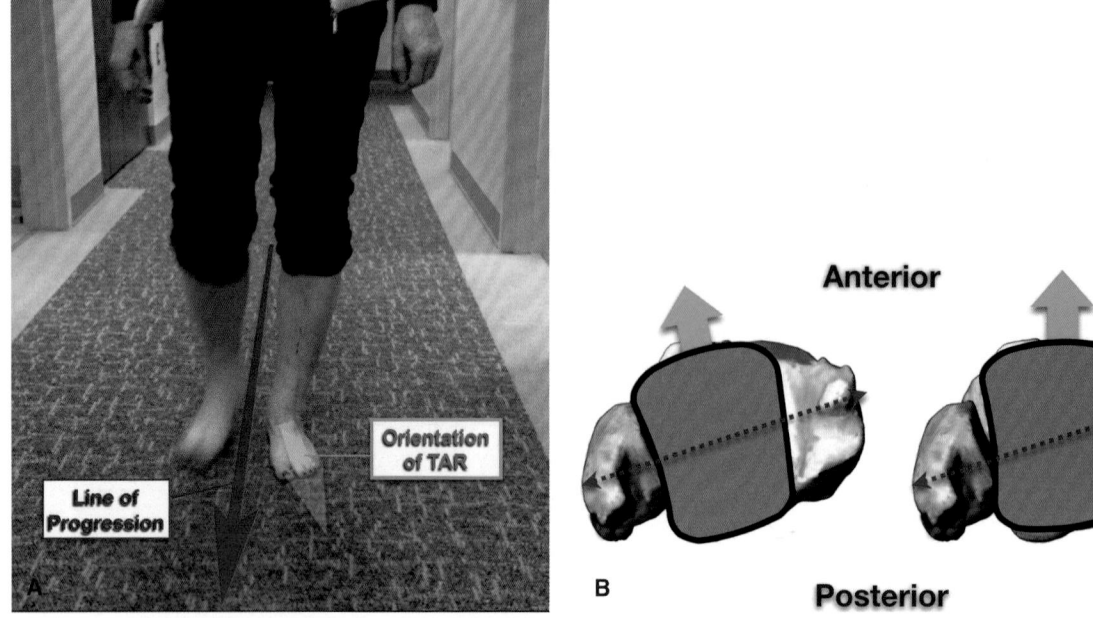

FIGURE 32.6 A. Frame grab of patient after TAR placement showing externally rotated foot position relative to line of progression. **B.** Internal-external rotation drawing illustrating variable internal-external positions when placing the TAR components.

Position alignments that differ from manufacturer guidelines should remain a judgment decision by the surgeon. Visual inspection and fluoroscopy should be used collectively to verify the ultimate position of resection. The key reference points are the intact ankle mortise and the functional axis of the collective and individual bony segments. An oscillating saw is best to make the resection. A "pecking" motion of the saw often provides adequate tactile feedback to avoid overpenetration into the posterior ankle.

Bone Excavation

The removal of bone from the distal tibia should be done in a controlled manner and with minimal levering of instruments to avoid malleolar fracture or crushing the anterior bone of the plafond. The segments can be cut into several sections to facilitate segmental removal. Residual bone in the posterior aspect of the joint can be removed after talar preparation (Fig. 32.7).

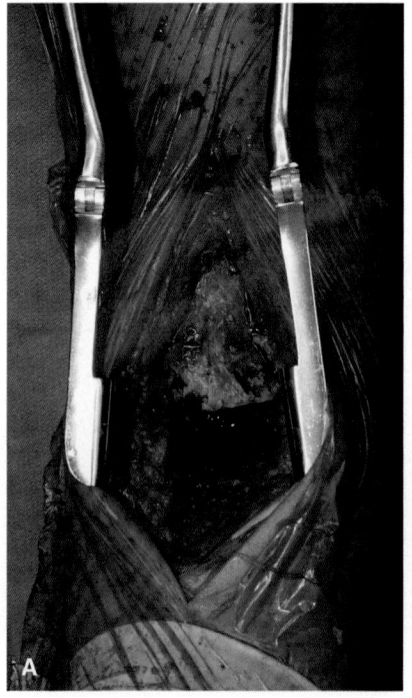
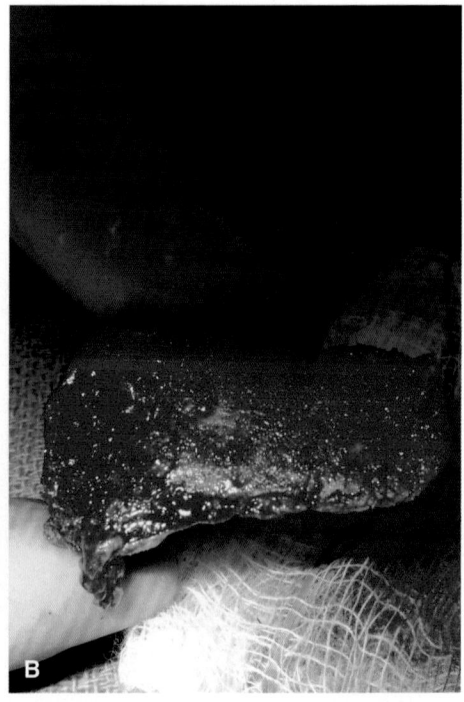

FIGURE 32.7 A. Photo of excavated bone within incision. **B.** Bone segment on sponge.

Talar Preparation

There are two basic configurations for talar preparation. The flat cut of the talar dome is an earlier design than the resurfacing components. There is generally less instrumentation needed for a flat cut component, but both designs require precision to achieve good bone-implant interfaces. Sizing of the talar component is complicated and often limited by the size of the tibial component. Nonetheless, the goal is to remove as little bone as possible and provide cortical support for the talar component if possible. Impingement of the malleoli should generally be avoided as well.

CEMENT FIXATION

Only one of the currently available implants (STAR) had been approved by the FDA without the use of cement. However, utilization of polymethyl methacrylate is not widely practiced in the other systems because contemporary implants are designed with metallic surfaces that encourage bony ingrowth or ongrowth. Cement may be indicated when there is component instability upon insertion, particularly on the tibial side, but is left to surgeon discretion. When implants are placed without cement (except [STAR]), it is an off-label application.

CLEARING THE GUTTERS

Some patients present with loss of articular cartilage on these surfaces, while others have more normal cartilage coverage. The impact of the degenerative changes of the facets on the medial and lateral aspects of the ankle has yet to be determined. As such, the specific maneuvers that remedy each specific presentation have yet to be established. Because none of the available implants completely resurface both gutters in a bimodal fashion, the potential for articular impingement on native bone remains. In any event, the talomalleolar articulations often require surgical manipulation to improve outcome.[53-55] Specifically, the medial and lateral gutters should be excavated of bony and soft tissue debris during the surgical procedure for several reasons.[56,57] The removal of bony debris allows for proper frontal plane orientation of the talus. It removes a potential source of impingement of the talomalleolar surfaces. The surgeon should be aware of the consequences of removing bone from the sides of the talus or the malleoli. These maneuvers may remove any buttressing effect of the malleoli or compromise ligamentous integrity.

POLYETHYLENE SIZING

While each system has its own scripted methodology for component stability, the concepts of balancing are basically the same for each TAR system. It is necessary for the surgeon to properly assess the quality and amount of motion upon placing the components. Balancing the periarticular ligaments can be accomplished by shaving off more bone or varying the thickness of the ultra-high molecular weight polyethylene (UHMWPE) insert. While it has been shown that wear characteristics of the UHMWPE improve with greater thickness,[58] the use of a thicker component may impart stability to the ankle as the increased cubic volume increases ligamentous tension. Paradoxically, increasing the thickness of the bearing may reduce sagittal plane motion and unmask latent frontal plane instability, particularly if the medial or lateral ligamentous complexes have been compromised. Practically, the surgeon must balance the desired effects of stability and motion based on the needs of the patient.

WOUND CLOSURE

Meticulous wound closure is necessary to assure complete soft tissue coverage over the prosthesis. A layered closure is recommended with particular attention to closure of the retinacular/fascial layer. A sound multilayer closure may be helpful to prevent prosthesis contamination when superficial wound complications are encountered.

Surgical Drains

The use of a drain in total ankle surgery has not been studied but is common in other total joint procedures. The use of a drain may reduce the incidence of hematoma.[59] Although ultimately left up to surgeon discretion, there is little evidence that the use of drains is detrimental. It has been shown that drains in knee replacements should be removed after 24 hours to reduce the risk of infection.[60,61]

ANCILLARY PROCEDURES

The incorporation of ancillary procedures in the surgical plan with TAR is often necessary, particularly when there is underlying foot deformity.

Ancillary Procedures

- Equinus release
- Tendon transfer
- Ligament reconstruction
- Calcaneal osteotomy
- Hindfoot arthrodesis
- Supramalleolar osteotomy

The timing and magnitude of the additional procedures are subject to surgeon preference, recognizing the issues of extensive reconstructions at the same surgical setting. It is sometimes more prudent to stage or modify ancillary procedures particularly those that may affect talar body blood flow in the setting of TAR.

POSTOPERATIVE CARE

At the completion of the operation, the lower extremity should be placed in some form of immobilization. Most commonly, a well-padded compressive splint is utilized that maintains the ankle joint at neutral position. Alternatively, some surgeons prefer to use a removable brace that enables the patient to mobilize the ankle in the early postoperative period.[6,62] Yet, there is no objective evidence that correlates early mobilization with an increased range of motion. Common wisdom dictates that the zeal to mobilize the ankle should be tempered with the risk of compromised wound healing or even compromised biologic fixation.

To date, the precise protocol and length of non–weight bearing after TAR has not been studied and is highly subjective. Earlier protocols suggested 6 weeks of non–weight bearing to facilitate bony ingrowth of the components. It has been shown in hip and knee arthroplasty that any shear stresses inducing micromotion of the device will prevent quality bonding of the component to bone.[63-66] Yet, empirical observation during revision total ankle surgery suggests that true bony ingrowth is remarkably uncommon even in cases where the patient was non–weight bearing for 6 weeks, in a cast, after the initial surgery. Accordingly, with improved design of the implants and more load sharing by the cortical surfaces of the talus and tibia, more aggressive strategies are being utilized. It is becoming more common practice to allow early protected weight bearing after TAR. Some surgeons will allow immediate weight bearing in a removable boot. Although additional procedures at the time of TAR may influence the weight bearing and immobilization protocols, there is a distinct trend toward earlier load bearing and functional rehabilitation. Further study is needed to determine the most optimal postoperative activity.

Some patients are not capable or motivated to perform independent ankle rehabilitation and may benefit from a more structured program with a physical therapist. However, the use of formal physical therapy has not been studied to determine its efficacy. Most surgeons generally employ some form of it, but there are few published protocols. In general, physical therapists employ modalities to improve strength, ankle range of motion, gait normalization, mobility of adjacent joints, and swelling control. They may also assist the patient in transition from a walking boot to a regular shoe.

VENOUS THROMBOEMBOLIC PROPHYLAXIS

Venous thromboembolic prophylaxis (VTE) with TAR has not been studied. However, the employment of anticoagulation in total hip and knee replacements is rather routine. Many health care facilities mandate routine prophylaxis in these patients unless there are clear contraindications. In part, the necessity is predicated on surgical manipulation of the large veins of the lower extremity during implantation. The extrapolation of similar VTE protocols to TAR is not evidenced based, but may be indicated, nevertheless. A heightened awareness of the risks and potentially grave consequences of VTE disease has been noted. Patients undergoing TAR surgery may have other established risks of VTE disease and may be best served with a VTE prophylaxis protocol. Yet, the incidence of venous thrombotic event in foot and ankle surgery is very low.[67] Therefore, risk factor analysis is recommended, and administration of VTE prophylaxis should be individualized.[68] The patient should be educated in recognizing the signs and symptoms of DVT and encouraged to practice preventative strategies. Recent evidence in total knee and hip replacements that aspirin is more effective than warfarin in preventing VTE.[69]

AUTHORS PREFERRED TREATMENT

There is a wide spectrum of deformity in patients who present for total ankle arthroplasty. Accordingly, there is an equally wide range of surgical procedures that may be needed to increase the chances of success and prolonged survivorship. Patients who have had no prior trauma or surgical procedures, and are well aligned, represent the most straightforward cases, with the lowest risk of complications. Those patients with prior trauma and/or previous surgical procedures, as well as advanced pedal or leg deformities, escalate both the complexity and risk of reconstruction.

VARUS DEFORMITY

There is considerable literature on the management of varus deformity with TAR.[18,21,70-72] It has become clear that a surgical approach tailored to the individual patient is necessary to mitigate all of the factors that potentiate the deformity and increase the risk of asymmetric poly loading, recurrence, and postoperative imbalance. The ultimate goal is to reestablish the tripod of the foot and provide tendon and ligament equilibrium.

The most critical maneuver in performing TAR with a varus deformity is to neutralize the talus in the mortise before any bone preparation. This generally requires a deltoid sleeve release coupled with resection of hypertrophic bone along the lateral gutter to unlock the varus position. In many cases, the hindfoot will be fully realigned with full talar derotation. However, with advanced intrinsic deformity of the calcaneus or a fixed varus position of the subtalar joint, a calcaneal osteotomy or subtalar fusion will be necessary to bring the heel closer to the tibial axis. If subtalar fusion is necessary, it should be done cautiously to avoid compromise of the blood supply to the talar body. Typically, we avoid dissection distal to the interosseous talocalcaneal ligament to minimize the risk of disruption of the talar blood supply from the tarsal canal.

Once the talus is neutralized in the mortise, one should anticipate some aggravation of the valgus alignment of the forefoot, particularly if there is adaptation at the midtarsal joint. If the first ray is excessively rigid, then a dorsal wedge osteotomy will be necessary to restore the tripod of the foot.[73]

In severe cavovarus foot deformities, there is likely bony adaptation of the midtarsal joint. The peroneal tendons may be dysfunctional or compromised from years of walking on the deformity. Soft tissue release or fusion of the talonavicular joint may be necessary to uncoil the foot to a plantigrade position. Transfer of the posterior tibial tendon to the peroneus brevis is a powerful technique to rebalance the ankle.[56,74]

VALGUS DEFORMITY

Valgus deformity generally is considered the most challenging and unpredictable clinical conditions, particularly if there is frank deltoid insufficiency. Accordingly, it is critical to establish whether any valgus thrust through the deltoid complex would persist after placement of the components. If so, then the chances of failure increase without correction of the pedal deformity and restoration of ligament balance. It is also important to realize that not all ankles with asymmetric tibiotalar wear have an incompetent deltoid. Yet, the deltoid complex may become compromised during preparation of the tibia and/or talus. Moreover, not all feet with a pes valgus architecture need to be reconstructed if the deformity is flexible or has adapted over time, such that there is no valgus thrust through the medial ankle. One should be aware that if a flexible or fixed valgus foot is corrected by any hindfoot or midfoot arthrodesis, it will increase the lever arm of the foot such that the valgus thrust may be potentiated.

In any event, the overall assessment of the stability of the ankle directs the surgical strategy. If the deltoid ligament is deemed incompetent in the face of a valgus foot, it is recommended that the reconstruction is staged.[20,75] The first stage typically consists of neutralization of the talus in the mortise coupled with deltoid reconstruction and hindfoot realignment. The second stage involves refinement of the alignment if necessary and placement of the prosthesis. One should also assure that there is an intact fibular buttress and stable syndesmosis. Although uncommon, syndesmotic reconstruction or fusion may be necessary to restore the lateral buttress.

TALOLISTHESIS

Talolisthesis is somewhat common in end-stage ankle arthritis and can be anterior or posterior.[5] (Fig. 32.8) The primary determinants for talar migration in the sagittal plane are the pitch of the tibial plafond and/or the primary etiology of the ankle arthritis.[5] Generally, talolisthesis will self-correct with removal of distal tibial resected bone. However, in excessive deformities, the gutters may have osteophytes and adapted bone contour that can inhibit relocation of the talus. Remodeling of the gutters is then necessary to allow relocation of the talus. In some instances, soft tissue releases along either side of the talus will allow for relocation without bone removal. One should be cautious about the use of mobile bearing implants when there is advanced talolisthesis.

HINDFOOT ARTHROSIS

Adjacent joint arthrosis is often encountered with arthritic ankles that are predictably asymptomatic after TAR. Accordingly, a conservative approach to hindfoot fusion is recommended. Joints that are unstable or have severe deformity may be fused at the time of ankle replacement with careful consideration of the impact to the blood supply of the talus. However, if there is significant concern, the involved joints can be fused either before or after TAR in a staged manner.

LEG DEFORMITY

Although beyond the scope of this chapter, suprastructural deformities of the leg may complicate the determination of the optimal position of the TAR. In some instances, patients with considerable planar deflections of the leg have adapted to the malalignment. In general, unless other circumstances are present, the ankle mortise should be in direct line with the tibial tubercle for optimal overall alignment. If surgery on the lower leg is indicated, it should be done prior to the total ankle procedure. In some cases, if the leg deformity is distal, the realignment can be done in the same setting as the total ankle. Patients with degenerative arthritis of the knee with marked varus or valgus deformity should be evaluated for TKA prior to TAR. If the TAR is done in the face of significant uncorrected frontal plane deformity of the knee, any subsequent knee replacement will alter the axis of the total ankle, which could be detrimental.

CONTEMPORARY PRIMARY TAR DESIGNS

Prosthetic device selection is another important factor that can influence the outcome for specific patients, but this is often tempered by device availability, hospital contracts, and surgeon training, industry affiliation, or personal preference. The basic design of the total ankle prosthesis has evolved considerably in the modern era, but each device has manufacturer-specific features that differentiate them. We are not recommending any specific device for use in any given clinical situation and leave implant choice to surgeon discretion.

SALTO TALARIS (INTEGRA LIFESCIENCES, PLAINSBORO, NJ, USA) (FIG. 32.9)

The Salto Talaris was introduced to the U.S. market in 2006 via 510 k FDA clearance and is approved for cemented placement. It is a two-part TAR system that was modified from the Salto mobile bearing developed in France. While it is a fixed bearing, it has considerable conformity design features that permit medial/lateral translation and internal/external rotation in addition to the sagittal ROM.[76] It has narrow bicondylar design with an exaggerated flat sulcus. The joint axis is angulated approximating Inman's axis. The talus has a resurfacing design.

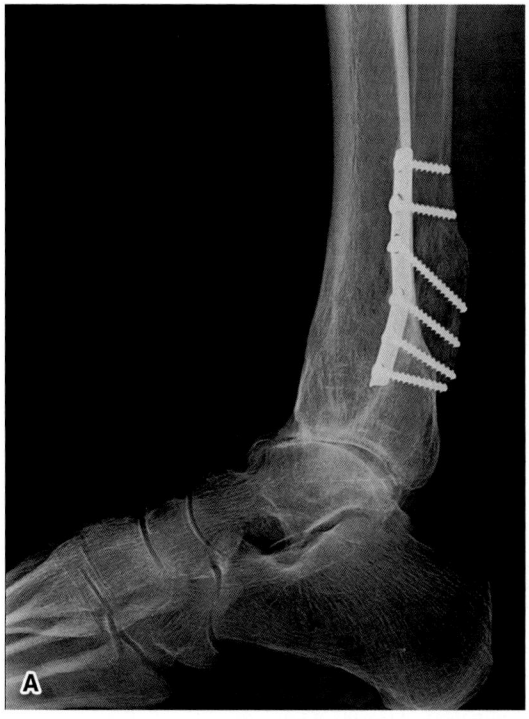
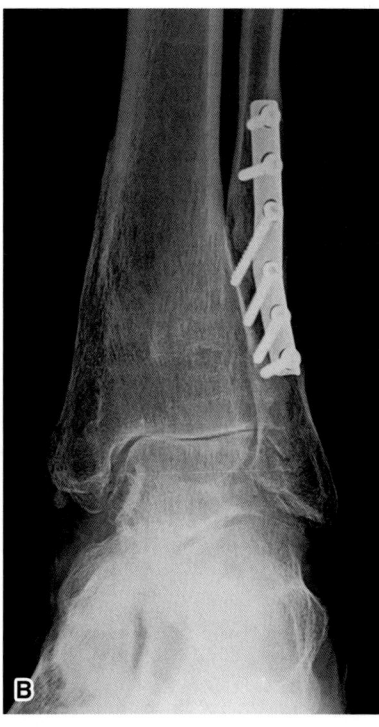

FIGURE 32.8 An example of anterior talolisthesis. The exaggerated anterior facing slope of the tibial plafond is the primary driver of this deformity. Note the lateral process of the talus that is no longer aligned with the tibial axis.

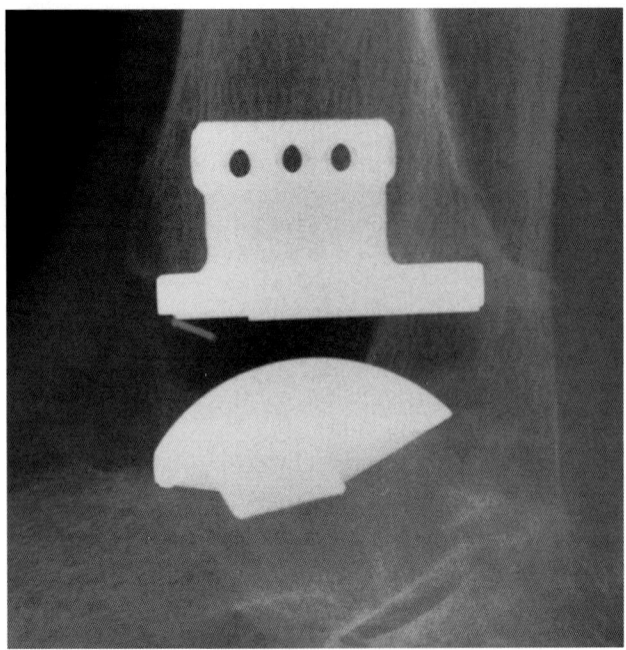

FIGURE 32.9 Salto Talaris.

Tibial component: Size range 1-3
Talar component: Size range 1-3
Flat cut option: Yes
UHMWPE Bearing
Thickness options: 8-11 (1-mm increments) also 13, 15, and 17 mm options available
Patient-specific guides: No

STAR TOTAL ANKLE REPLACEMENT (STRYKER, MAHWAH, NJ, USA) (FIG. 32.10)

The STAR is a mobile-bearing prosthesis that was introduced to the U.S. market in 2010. It went through 9 years of formal U.S.

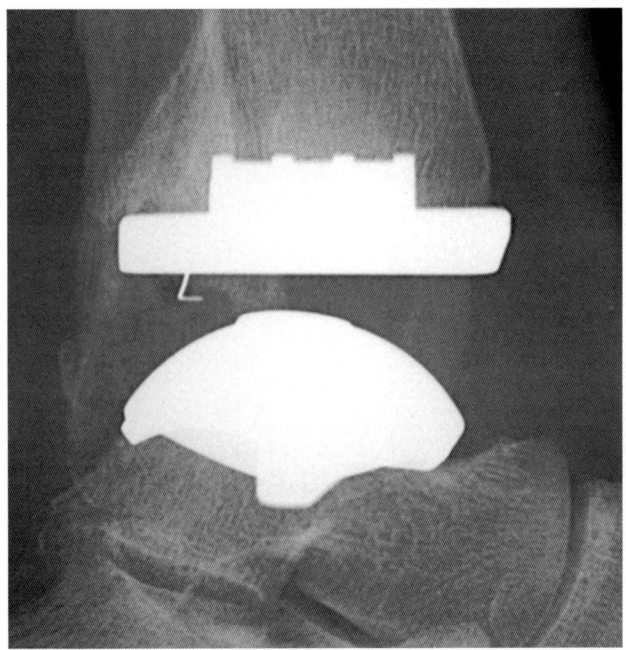

FIGURE 32.10 STAR.

clinical trials before becoming approved by FDA. It is the only ankle prosthesis that has gone through FDA type 3 trials. It can be placed on-label uncemented. It is one of the implants with a cylindrical design. It has been used for over 40 years primarily in Europe.

Tibial component: Flat glide plate that is 3 mm thick with two barrels centrally located on superior surface for osseous fixation. It comes in four sizes: small, medium, large, and extra large. It ranges from 30 to 45 mm in AP depth. There is no left or right specificity to the tibial side.
Talar component: Resurfacing design with near cylindrical shape. Enclosed cap design with recessed chamfered surfaces and a central keel. The talar components come in four sizes: large, medium, small, and extra small. There is left and right specificity to the talar side.
Flat cut option: No.
Bearing: Mobile bearing with fixed area of coverage between all components. Medium cross-linked polyethylene in 1-mm increments. It has a flat tibial surface. The talar surface has a central groove that fits over the talar crest to keep poly centralized on the talus. Superior surface can function with 3 degrees of freedom.
Patient-specific guides: No.

INFINITY TOTAL ANKLE SYSTEM (WRIGHT MEDICAL, ARLINGTON, TN, USA) TAR (FIG. 32.11) PROSTHESIS

The Infinity was introduced to the U.S. market in 2013. While it has the same bearing interface as the INBONE II, its fixed bearing design overall is more compact requiring less bone excision. It has a horizontal axis bicondylar design. Therefore, there are no left or right components. Since it has the same joint profile as the INBONE II, the system can accept the INBONE talus, which is a flat cut design.

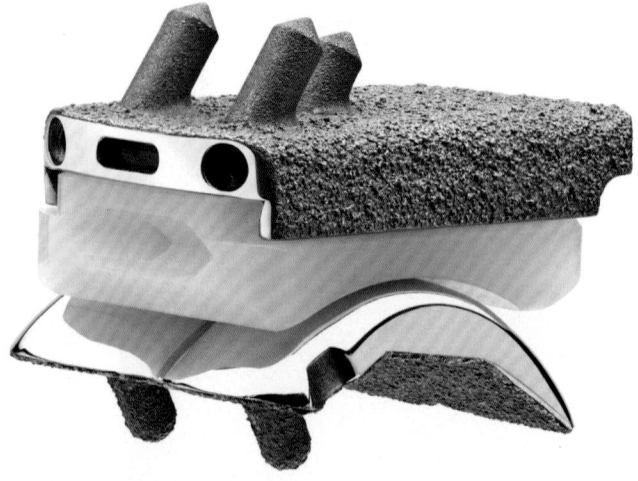

FIGURE 32.11 INFINITY™ Total Ankle System (Image courtesy of Wright Medical Group N.V.)

Tibial component: 5-mm-thick titanium with capture system for attaching polyethylene. Grit blast finish on superior surface with three angulated pegs. Size range 1-5 with size 3-5 in standard and long tray versions.
Talar component: There are 5 sizes. Cobal chrome resurfacing design with chamfer cuts open design with no sidewalls. Inferior surface features Ti plasma spray with two-angled pegs.
Flat cut option: Yes (INBONE).
Bearing: 2-mm increments. Polyethylene is non–cross-linked. It can accommodate same size components or one size down on talus.
Patient-specific guides: Yes.

CADENCE TOTAL ANKLE SYSTEM (INTEGRA LIFESCIENCES, PLAINSBORO, NJ, USA) (FIG. 32.12)

This system was FDA cleared in 2016. It is a bicondylar design with angulated joint axis. The poly layer inserts to the tibial plate via a shallow dovetail feature. Talar sizes can be downsized by one size from the tibial size used.

Tibial component: Titanium alloy with two angulated pegs anteriorly and a posterior angulated tab. Nine sizes left and right specific
Talar component: There are 5 sizes. Cobalt chrome resurfacing design with chamfer cuts open design with no sidewalls. Inferior surface features Ti plasma spray with two-angled pegs.
Bearing: Highly cross-links (UHMWPE), five sizes, seven heights left and right specific, neutral anterior and posterior biased options (6-12 mm thick poly, by 1-mm increments)
Patient-specific guides: No

HINTERMANN SERIES H2 TOTAL ANKLE REPLACEMENT SYSTEM (DT MEDTECH, LLC; BALTIMORE, MD, USA) (FIG. 32.13)

This is a semiconstrained two-part design, which is fashioned similar to the Hintegra H3. It was FDA cleared in 2018. It has the same conical configuration and talar sidewalls to control bearing tracking. The coating of the metal components is titanium plasma spray only and is indented for cemented use.

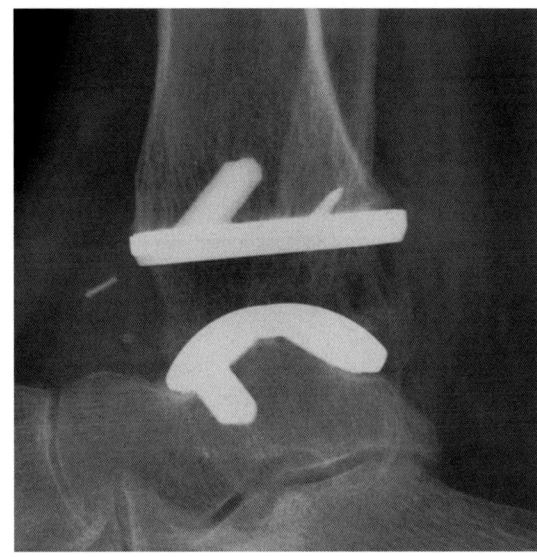

FIGURE 32.12 Cadence.

Tibial component: Sizes 2-6 right or left.
Talar component: Sizes 1-6 right or left.
Bearing: Sizes 1-6 in right or left orientation with four thicknesses (5, 6, 7, and 9 mm) and three offsets (anterior, posterior, and neutral). There are subcomponents that permit size compatibility with between tibial and talar components. The subcomponents allow for rotational error corrections before locking the poly to the tibial component.
Patient-specific guides: No.

HINTERMANN SERIES H3 TOTAL ANKLE REPLACEMENT SYSTEM (DT MEDTECH, LLC; BALTIMORE, MD, USA)

This device was FDA cleared in 2019 to use in the United States for noncemented use. This is a mobile-bearing design, which has been used in Europe for many years. This was developed by Dr. Beat Hintermann from Switzerland. It has conical design

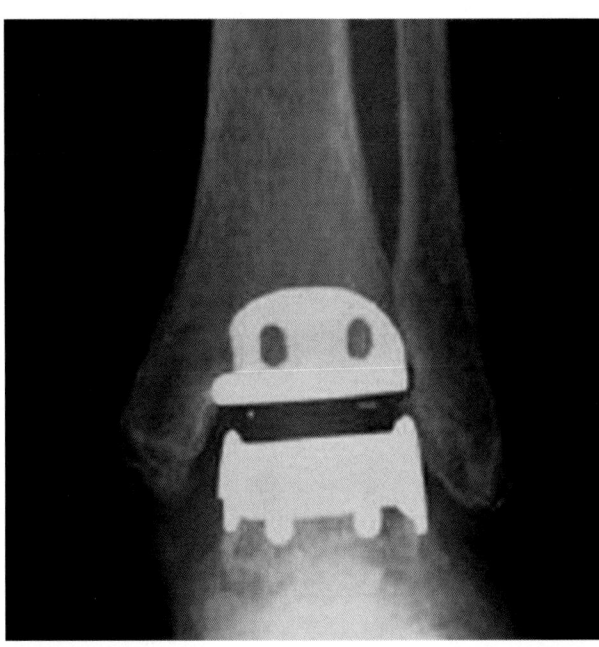

FIGURE 32.13 Hintegra H2 fixed bearing.

similar to Inman's axis. This is a dual-coated prosthesis with hydroxyapatite and titanium plasma.

> *Tibial component:* Sizes 1-6 in right or left orientation. It has an anterior shield with options for screw placement. The glide surface is flat. There are polished overhangs medially and laterally to track the bearing component.
> *Talar component:* Resurfacing design with metal sidewalls. There are six sizes 1-6.
> *Flat cut option:* Yes (sizes 1-5).
> *Bearing:* The UHMWPE bearing is available in sizes 1-6 with four thicknesses 5, 6, 7, and 9 mm. It has left and right orientations.
> *Patient-specific guides:* No.

VANTAGE TOTAL ANKLE SYSTEM (EXACTECH, GAINESVILLE, FL, USA) (FIG. 32.14)

The tibial component is anatomic design based off CT scans; however, joint axis is near horizontal and opposite to Inman's axis. The tibial tray is side specific (left and right) and provides articulation for the fibula, with central press fit bone cage and 3 plasma legs. Component sizes are interchangeable.

> *Tibial component:* Tibial sizes 1-4, right and left side specific, bicondylar articulating surface. Anterior talar shield to further prevent talar subsidence. There is no variable length to the tibial tray. Tibial component has three small pegs and one cage that is vertically oriented.
> *Talar component:* Size 1-5 right and left side specific. Available with flat cut version.
> *Bearing:* Cross-linked compression molded. Size 6-12 mm with 1-mm increments. Unique locking clip for secure fastening, designed for easy insertion and removal of the highly cross-linked net compression molded polyethylene.
> *Patient-specific guides:* No.

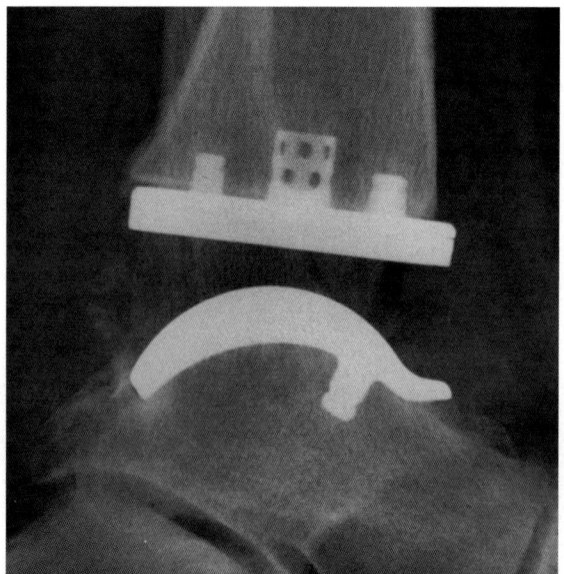

FIGURE 32.14 Vantage.

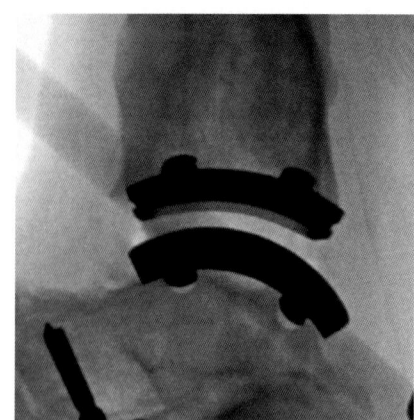

FIGURE 32.15 Zimmer.

ZIMMER BIOMET TRABECULAR METAL TOTAL ANKLE (ZIMMER-BIOMET, WARSAW, IN, USA) (FIG. 32.15)

This device was FDA cleared in 2012. It is a bicondylar, conical articulation designed to allow for more normal integration with muscular and tendon function, with two rail tibial and talar fixation oriented in the coronal plane to stabilize implant against normal joint motion. There is no size interchangeability between talar and tibial components. Metal components have a specialized metallic porous surface that is spot welded with cement. The device is placed from lateral and involves a fibular osteotomy. A specialized frame is needed to guide instrumentation.

Semi conforming articulation is designed to limit point loading from varus/valgus stress.

> *Tibial component:* Sizes 1-6 tibia.
> *Talar component:* Sizes 1-6. Curved bone-implant interface of the talar component designed to minimize subsidence.
> *Bearing:* Highly cross-linked polyethylene bearing surface to reduce volumetric wear. Three thicknesses of poly are available—highly cross-linked poly, designed to reduce surface wear and subsurface fatigue.
> *Patient-specific guides:* No.

REVISION SYSTEMS

SALTO TALARIS XT (INTEGRA LIFESCIENCES, PLAINSBORO, NJ, USA) (FIG. 32.16)

> *Tibial component:* Four symmetrical sizes, two thicknesses—4 or 10 mm (meant for either R or L).
> *Tibia:* Sizes 0-3 can upsize from 0 tibia to a 1 talus, and with each tibia 1-3, can go same size or down size 1 size on talus.
> *Talus component* (flat cut): Sizes 0-3.
> *Bearing:* Size 8-11 mm by 1-mm increments, then 13 and 15 mm (for tibial base plate 10 mm), additional poly size 17, 19, and 21 for tibial base plate 4 mm.

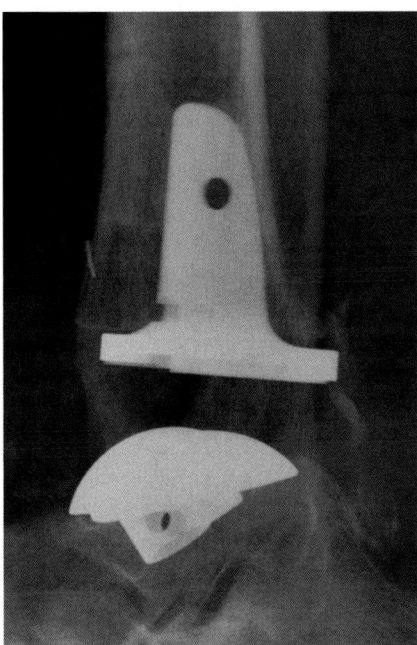

FIGURE 32.16 Salto XT.

INBONE TOTAL ANKLE SYSTEM (WRIGHT MEDICAL TECHNOLOGY, INC; ARLINGTON, TN, USA) (FIG. 32.17)

The INBONE system was brought to the U.S. market in 2005. It was initially used as a primary prosthesis but has evolved into a revision device. It originally has a saddle shaped talar component (INBONE I), which was changed later to a bicondylar shape for improved stability (INBONE II). The INBONE II talus is compatible with the Infinity system, if a flat cut talar preparation is desired. It is composed of modular segments, which can be assembled in the ankle to produce a stem of variable length.

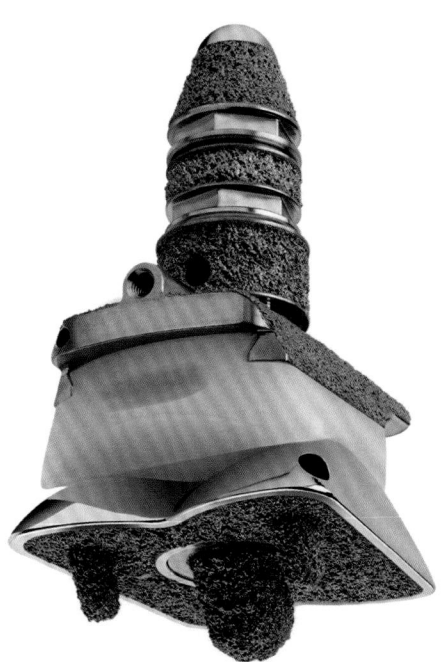

FIGURE 32.17 INBONE™ Total Ankle System (Image courtesy of Wright Medical Group N.V.)

It requires reaming and access of tools via a plantar portal. Intramedullary navigation is necessary.

Tibial component: Can use anywhere from 2 to 8 tibial stem components
Titanium stems plasma: Coated or smooth coated available
Base stem: 16-18 mm plasma coated only
Mid stem: 12, 16, and 18 mm plasma coated; 12, 14, 16, and 18 mm smooth
Top stem: 12, 14, and 16 mm smooth or plasma coated available
Talar component:
Size 1-5
1-30 wide and 32 length
2-33 wide and 34 length
3-36 wide and 36 long
4-39 wide and 39 long
5-42 wide and 42 long
Height for sizes 1-3 is 10 mm, size 4 is 11 mm, and size 5 is 12 mm
INBONE II talar stem—size 10 or 14 mm
Bearing:
Size ranges from 1+ to 5
Size 1+: 6-12 mm, 2-mm increments
Size 2: 6-12 mm, 2-mm increments
Size 2+: 8-14 mm, 2-mm increments
Size 3: 8-14 mm, 2-mm increments
Size 3+: 12-16 mm, 2-mm increments
Size 4: 9-15 mm, 2-mm increments
Size 4+: 10-16 mm, 2-mm increments
Size 5: 9-15 mm, 2-mm increments
Size 5+: 10-16 mm, 2-mm increments
Large Revision Polys
1+ and 2 sizes: 14, 16 mm
2+ and 3 sizes: 16, 18 mm
3+, 4+, and 5+: 18, 20 mm
4 and 5: 17 and 19 mm
Patient-specific guides: Yes

INVISION TAR PROSTHESIS (WRIGHT MEDICAL TECHNOLOGY, INC; ARLINGTON, TN, USA) (FIG. 32.18)

The Invision system was introduced to the U.S. market in 2017. It is a dedicated revision system that is partially compatible with the INBONE/Infinity systems. It is designed to manage bone loss of the talus or tibia. The joint interface is the same as INBONE II/and Infinity. Both the infinity and the INBONE II tibial components and polys can be utilized with the Invision talar components (in the event of talar subsidence requiring increased talar height).

Tibial components: Tibial trays (same stems as INBONE II) size 2, 3, 4, 5, and 6—tibial tray thickness can be standard INBONE II thickness, +4 mm or +8 mm in both standard and long
Talar components: Talar domes—same sulcus articulating geometry as the INBONE II—size 1-5, with standard (3 mm) and thick (6 mm) talar plate additional sizes 1-5
Male Morse taper and three anterior pegs fixate plate to the talus
Patient-specific guides: Yes (as part of the INBONE/Infinity systems)

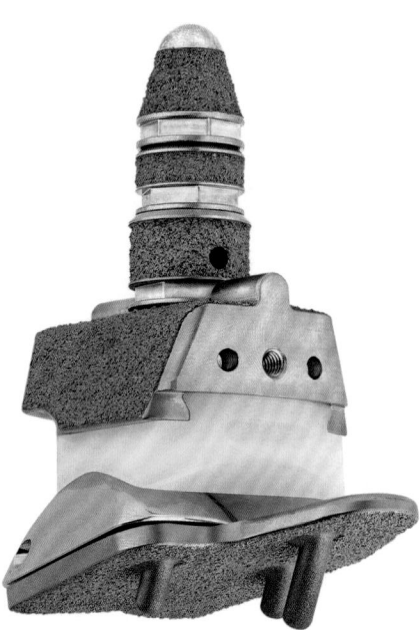

FIGURE 32.18 INVISION™ Total Ankle Revision System (Image courtesy of Wright Medical Group N.V.)

PERILS AND PITFALLS

There are known adverse events that are inherent to all total joint procedures that can prolong the postoperative course, decrease survivorship, and negatively impact the clinical outcome.

ADVERSE EVENTS THAT CAN COMPROMISE TAR OUTCOME

- Subsidence
- Aseptic loosening
- Deep infection
- Osteolysis
- Chronic pain
- Technical error
- Malalignment
- Implant failure
- Wound necrosis

It has been established that there is a higher incidence of complications early in a given surgeon's experience with TAR.[77-80] Even with perfect surgical technique and prosthetic placement combined with optimal patient selection, complications cannot be eliminated.

REPORTED COMPLICATIONS

INTRAOPERATIVE
- Artery laceration: dorsalis pedis[81]
- Component malalignment/mis-sizing[55,77-79,82-85]
- Fracture: malleolar[55,63,77,78,81,84,86-89]
- Nerve lacerations[77]
- Tendon laceration: PT[77,81]
- Tendon laceration: FDL[81]
- Tendon laceration: EHL[77,81]
- Uncorrected deformity[84]

POSTOPERATIVE
- Component dislocation: mobile bearing[63,65]
- Component fracture[82,83]
- Component subsidence/aseptic loosening[55,63,65,77,78,81-86,90,91]
- Fracture: fibular stress[81,86,92]
- Fracture: talus[90]
- Heterotopic bone formation[65,84,85,90,93]
- Infection: deep[78,81,90,94]
- Infection: superficial[63,81,82,85,90]
- Ligament insufficiency/edge loading[86,88]
- Nerve complications: CRPS[63]
- Nerve complications: incisional entrapment[82,84]
- Nerve complications: tarsal tunnel syndrome[95]
- Osteolysis/radiolucency[78,85,96]
- Pain with stiffness[55,83,84,86]
- Skin fistula[97]
- Tendon necrosis: anterior tibial[38]
- Tendonitis[84,92]
- Vascular compromise[88]
- Venous thrombotic event[84]
- Wound healing delay[55,63,77,78,81,83,84,86,90,92,98]

Further, differentiation between complications and normal attritional deterioration is often difficult and highly subjective.

JOINT STIFFNESS

The resultant range of motion after TAR is occasionally less than expected by both the patient and the surgeon. Stiffness seems to be multifactorial and often belies linear thought processes. It can be attributed to ineffective rehabilitation, poor soft tissue envelope, multiple surgeries, previous infection, overstuffing of the joint, heterotopic bone growth, and prolonged immobilization.[99] Although these factors can often be explained retrospectively, patients should be advised preoperatively that the expected ROM will probably be equal to or slightly greater than the preoperative excursion. This will help dampen patients' expectations that the motion will be normal or equal to the opposite ankle, assuming that the contralateral limb is not affected by arthrosis. In most cases, the loss of motion does not preclude smooth ambulation because the arc of motion is often in the range required for gait.

Although there are intraoperative measures can be taken by the surgeon to limit stiffness, the execution of such maneuvers may compromise stability. Surgeon experience will allow one to determine the optimal thickness of the composite implant components that maximizes both stability and range of motion. When limited motion is encountered postoperatively, there are several surgical strategies that can be employed when aggressive nonoperative care is ineffective. If the lack of motion appears to be from tight posterior structures, a posterior release of the ankle joint and triceps lengthening is often helpful. In more advanced cases, removal of heterotopic bone is often helpful provided aggressive physical therapy is utilized to preserve the regained motion. In the most severe cases, formal revision may be in order. It is often possible to revise only the talar component by removing more bone and using a flat cut prosthesis.

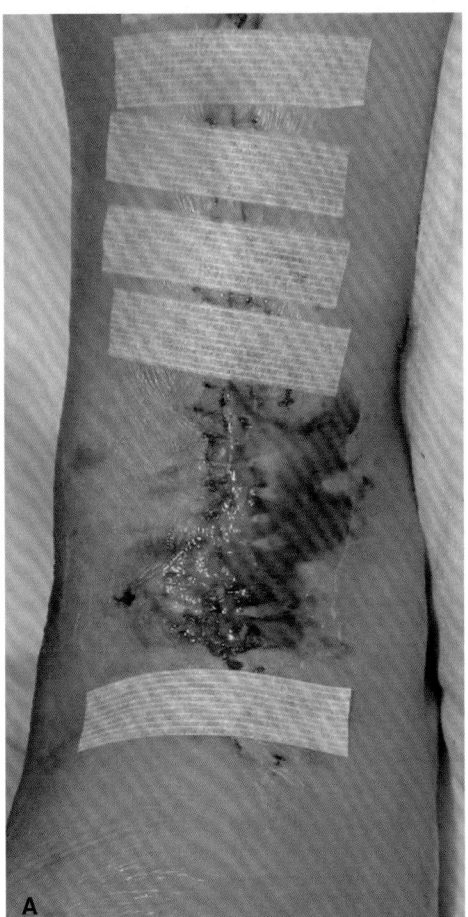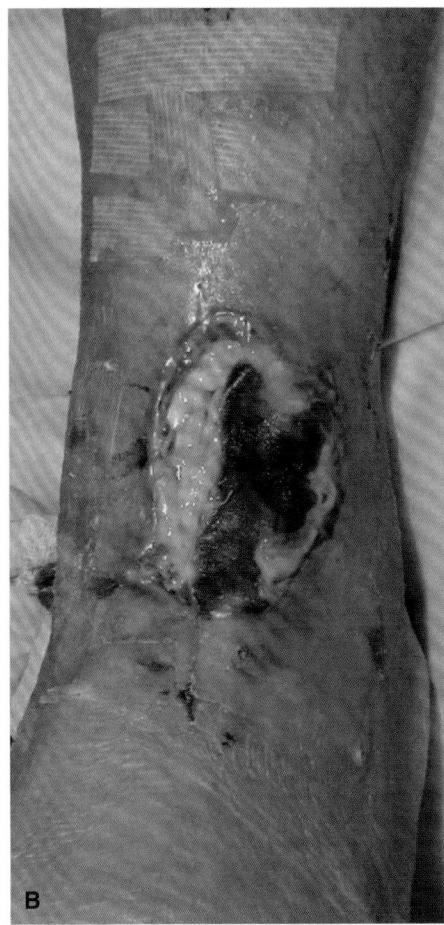

FIGURE 32.19 Wound dehiscence. **A.** Two weeks post-op early dehiscence. **B.** Four weeks post-op with full demarcation.

WOUND DEHISCENCE AND FOCAL NECROSIS

Wound dehiscence, incisional hematoma, and focal wound necrosis are predominant complications to nearly all clinical series on TAR[63,77,78,81,92,98] (Fig. 32.19). Focal necrosis typically occurs at the level of the plafond and on the medial side of the incision, most likely due to disruption of the anterior tibial angiosome.[79] However, factors of aggressive soft tissue retraction, hematoma, improper cast immobilization, shortened incisions, immune suppression, and previously traumatized soft tissue envelope can play a role in its development.

While potentially disastrous due to the risk of deep infection, these wound issues can usually be managed conservatively with parenteral or oral antibiotics, local wound care, and/or negative pressure devices. Delayed soft tissue healing can also prevent early range of motion and weight bearing, which may have a negative effect on ultimate range of motion. For larger wounds, a referral to plastic surgery may be needed for a soft tissue flap, especially if deep infection is imminent[79] (Fig. 32.20).

PROSTHETIC ALIGNMENT ERRORS

The frequency of technical error in TAR has been reported at 6%.[100] One of the more common complications is component malpositioning. Spurious alignment of the components may not be appreciated until weight-bearing x-rays of the ankle are taken. One of the most common alignment issues is misinterpretation of the tibial axis.[17,78] A constrained fluoroscopic view of only the distal tibial metaphysis can alter the surgeons' perception of the true tibial axis[78] (Fig. 32.21). Extramedullary alignment rods are inherently imprecise due to variation in tibial morphology.[101] Most often, there is unrecognized varus position of the tibial tray, although the placement of the alignment guide can lead to malposition in both the transverse and frontal plane.[102,103] Lastly, fluoroscopic images can be prone to pincushion distortion, which affects the linearity of the screen image.[104]

Minor technical component malalignments can often function very well clinically. Component malalignment tolerances remain undefined but may be subjected to increased shearing strain and are a potential cause of premature polyethylene wear. Yet, varus or valgus component positions are usually well tolerated with good osseous integration and component congruity.[105] While it has been stated that valgus malalignments are generally more tolerated than varus,[79,101] this has not been substantiated with any data.[86]

NEUROVASCULAR INJURY

Injury to the neurovascular structures during the procedure is not uncommon. Essentially, these injuries can be divided between mechanical lacerations, traction injuries or postsurgical scar entrapment. All of the major neurovascular structures crossing the ankle are at risk for injury with TAR.

The anterior and anterolateral sensory nerves are the more commonly compromised structures during performance of TAR. Evaluation of superficial nerve branches encountered

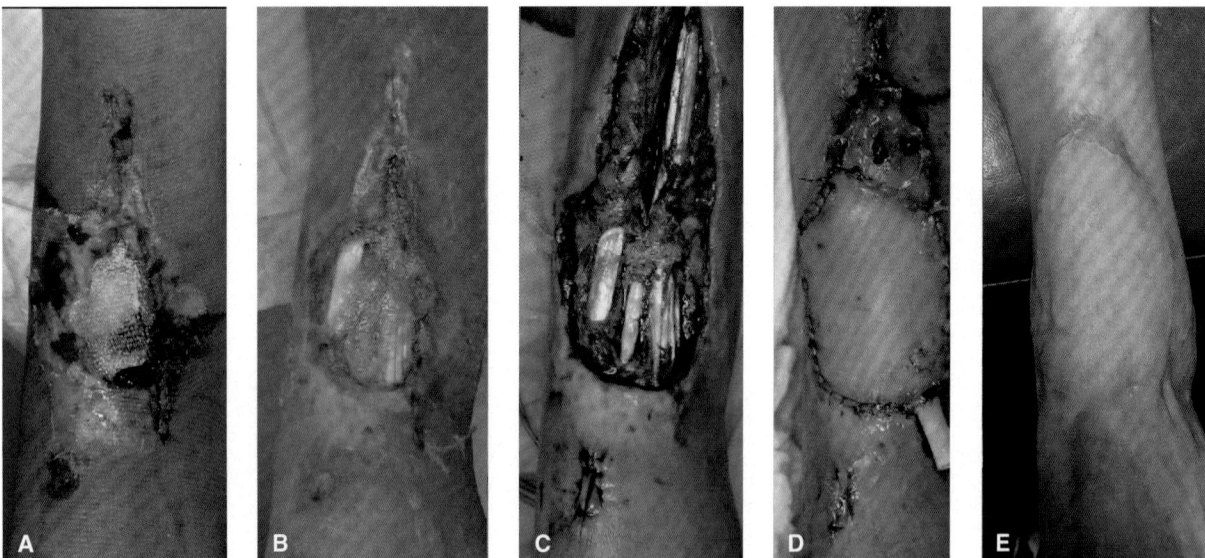

FIGURE 32.20 Free flap case. **A.** Shows initial presentation 27 days post-op, *Acinetobacter* spp. isolated. **B.** Failed aggressive wound care. **C.** Preparation for forearm free flap. **D.** Placement of flap and STSG. **E.** Five years post-op.

in the surgical field helps determine the disposition of each branch. Larger nerves should be mobilized with the skin flaps, while noncritical nerve branches at risk for traction injury should be prophylactically excised.[106] Partial nerve injury via over retraction, scarification, or suturing a nerve is a prerequisite to developing complex regional pain syndrome, while completely sectioning a nerve rarely has this response[107] (Fig. 32.22).

Many patients relate some area of sensory distortion after TAR. When the loss of normal sensation is anterior, branches of the superficial or deep peroneal nerve are usually affected. In many cases, the sensory deficit improves with time.

The posterior tibial nerve is uncommonly injured during TAR surgery, yet it resides in a vulnerable position at the posterior medial corner of the ankle. Because surgeons have a heightened appreciation of its location and impact, placement of power saw blades in the anatomic vicinity is usually a cautious venture. However, the sometimes soft bone of the distal tibia may not provide sufficient tactile feedback to determine penetration of the posterior cortex with a power saw. Although it has not been formally reported, the medial and/or lateral plantar nerves may be injured during delivery of the drill cannula or other instrumentations through the plantar heel (INBONE).

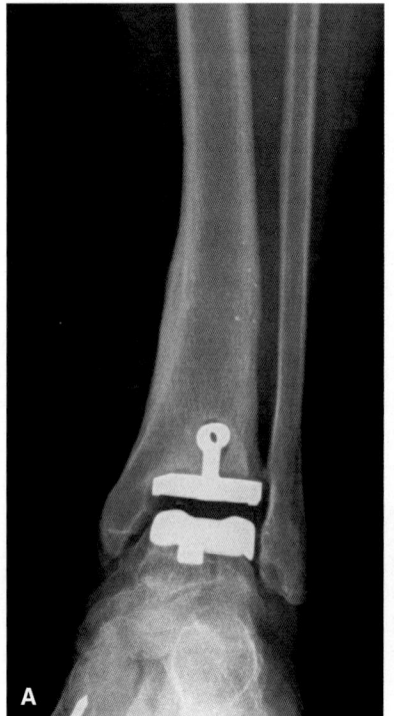
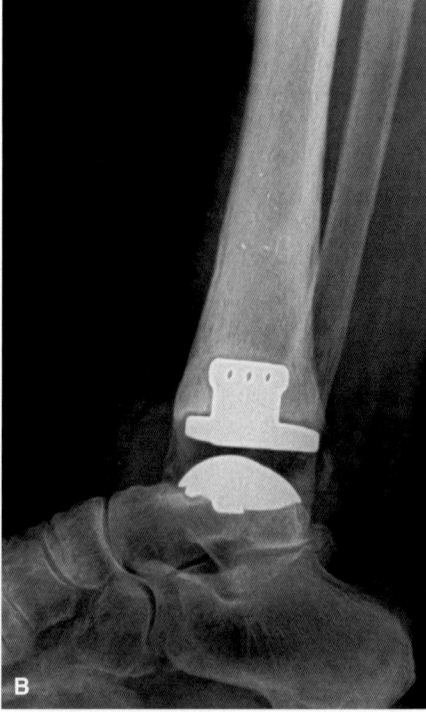

FIGURE 32.21 **A.** Mortise view showing a Salto Talaris in varus alignment. **B.** Lateral view confirms the tibial component is loose. This was confirmed with later revision.

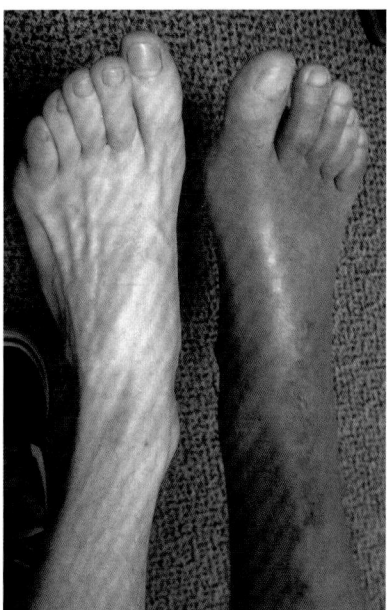

FIGURE 32.22 Complex regional pain syndrome after total ankle replacement. Pain control was an issue immediately after surgery and has been resistant to most treatments. The patient has successfully filed for disability and walks with assistive devices on a limited basis.

The potential for damage to vascular tree essentially parallels that of nerve injury because of the juxtaposition of these structures. The consequence of loss of one of the three major pedal vessels in TAR has not been determined but in all likelihood is proportionate to the degree of overall perfusion, collateral circulation, and degree of anastomotic compensation. Most commonly, the dorsalis pedis artery is compromised during the exposure. In some instances, adequate exposure to the bone cannot be attained without obligate sacrifice and mobilization of the vessel. The posterior tibial vessels are not commonly injured, but there is potentially higher risk in patients who have had extensive trauma or scar in that anatomic region as the tissue is less mobile. Lastly, the perforating peroneal artery is vulnerable during exposure of the lateral aspect of the joint.

MALLEOLAR FRACTURES

Fracture of either of the malleoli is not uncommon and can be unnerving, particularly to the low volume surgeon. The incidence of intraoperative fracture is estimated around 8%;[100] however, it seldom has appreciable impact on the surgical outcome. It has been shown that the incidence of these intraoperative mishaps diminishes with surgeon experience.[78,80] Overzealous retraction or prying type maneuvers against the malleoli can cause inadvertent fracture. Placement of the tibial cut block too medial will also potentiate the risk of fracture. If they do occur, immediate stabilization with internal fixation is recommended to prevent further displacement and distortion of the bone void that will accommodate the prosthesis. Usually simple and conventional fixatives can be utilized according to the fracture pattern. In higher-risk patients, percutaneous placement of a Kirschner wire or screw along the malleoli and away from planned saw cuts can have protective value during tibial preparation.[54,108]

Late fractures of the malleoli are distinctly uncommon. If they occur, they can be attributed to imbalance of the foot where the malleolus fractures in either a tension or avulsion mode. Alternatively, failure of the syndesmosis from valgus thrust of the foot can cause failure of the lateral malleolus (Fig. 32.23).

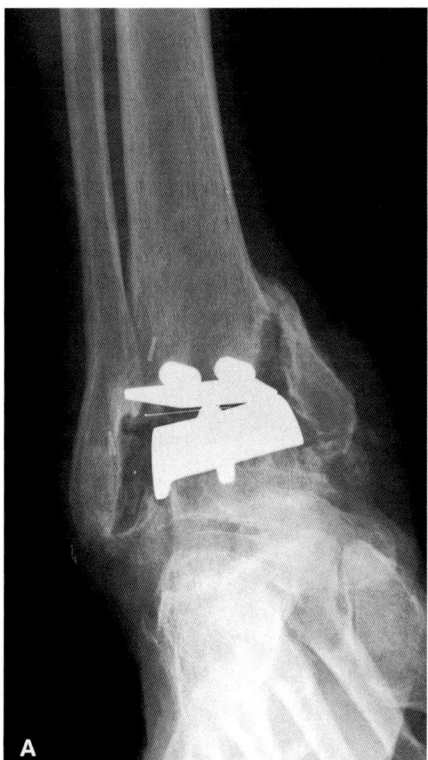
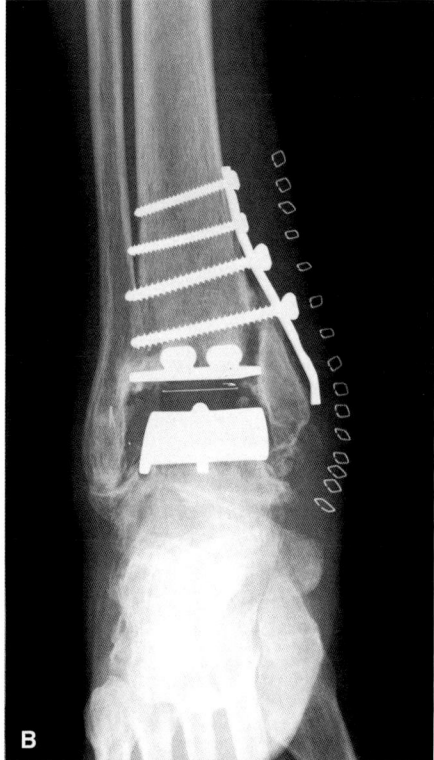

FIGURE 32.23 **A.** Radiograph of late medial malleolus fracture occurred after failure of bearing. **B.** Radiograph after ORIF and poly exchange.

SUBSIDENCE, BONY OVERGROWTH, AND COMPONENT MIGRATION

While durable fixation to bone is a desired outcome for all total ankle designs, in some instances, components can migrate within the osseous substrate. This is referred to as subsidence and can occur with the tibial or talar components (Figs. 32.24 and 32.25). Component subsidence is generally considered a late complication with a multifactorial etiology. Minor subsidence early after implantation is common as the bone remodels at the bone-prosthesis interface. It typically decreases at 3 months and stabilizes at 6 months postimplantation.[82,83,109,110] This process is associated with increased radiodensity of the adjacent bone. These local changes in bone mass have been documented with dual x-ray absorptiometry.[111]

Substantial interval component migration that persists after 6 months may be indicative of unstable bone-implant interfaces, which ultimately lead to bone loss. Although many of the newer implant designs have features to resist subsidence, the occurrence of such may not necessarily be a design-related phenomenon. Soft bone, overly aggressive bone resection, improper prosthesis placement, undersizing, and occult sepsis may all cause implant migration (Fig. 32.26).

Talar subsidence is more common than on the tibial side. Most commonly, it is due to a lack of peripheral cortical coverage.[112] In these instances, the subsidence tends to be progressive until the talar component migrates to the subtalar joint or there is impingement of the talar bone on the tibial tray (Fig. 32.24). Expectantly, motion will decrease and symptoms often evolve. These situations are difficult to remedy during revision because of the proportionate loss of bone mass as the condition progresses. The evolution of resurfacing designs, compared to flat cut talar components, has decreased the incidence of this complication.

Subsidence of the tibial component occurs infrequently and is most likely due to better design features of the implants that

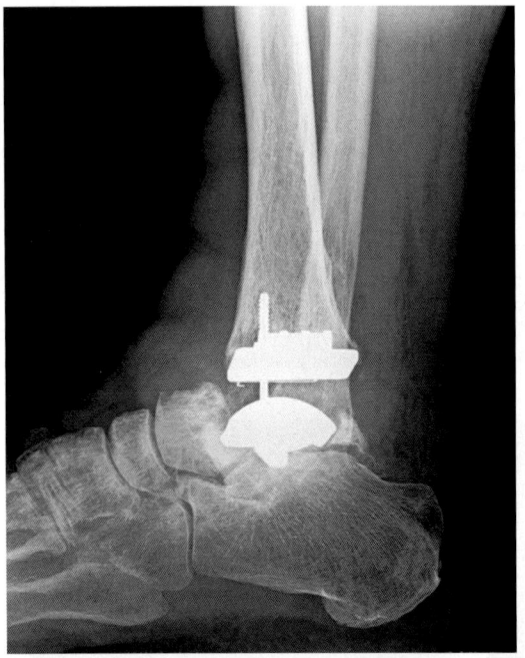
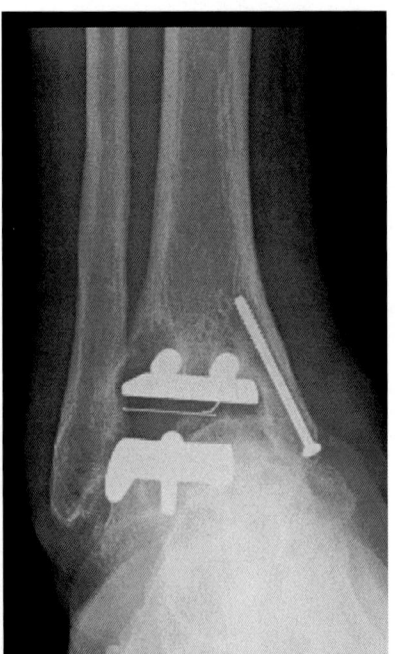
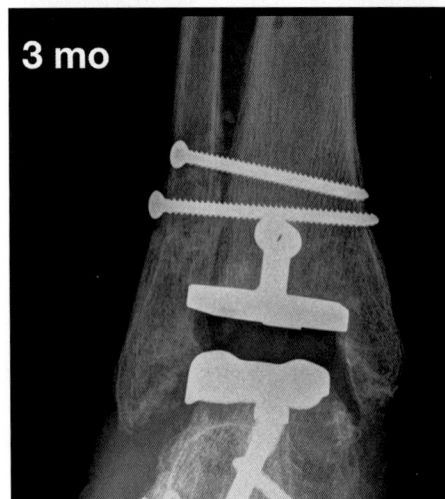
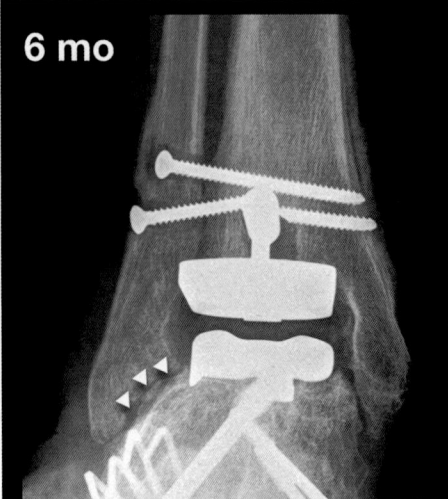

FIGURE 32.24 Talar subsidence with Salto Talaris prosthesis Note migration of talus into valgus (*arrowheads*).

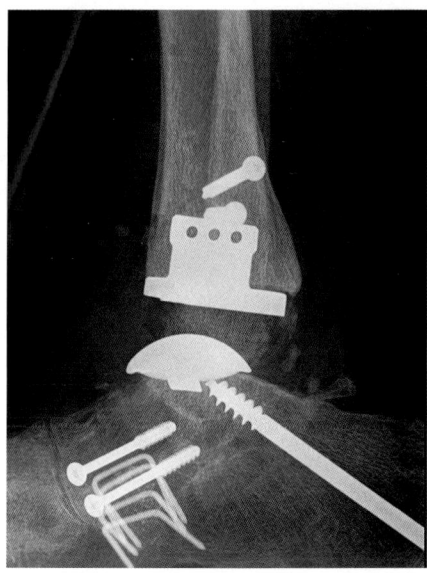
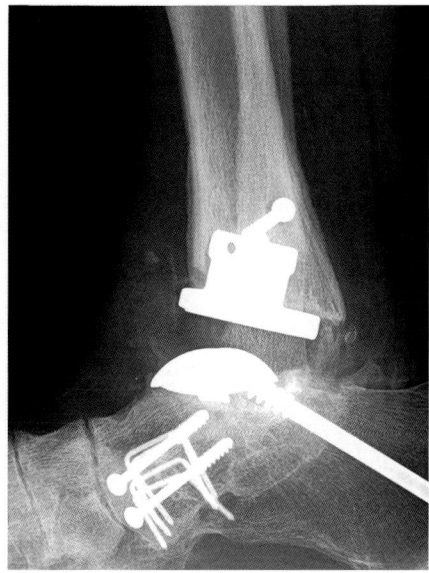

FIGURE 32.25 Tibial subsidence with 6 months of a Salto Talaris device.

encourage cortical coverage or intramedullary fixation. More commonly, bony overgrowth occurs around the margins of the tibial component. It is more common posteriorly and manifests as osseous lipping around the posterior edge of the implant.[113] Sizing issues or an enlarged posterior malleolus from long-standing deformity or trauma are often observed. Interestingly, posterior overgrowth is rarely symptomatic.[113]

Overgrowth is uncommonly observed anteriorly and can be ascribed to the fact that the anterior margin of the tibia slopes from anterior medial to posterior lateral. The obliquity virtually obligates cortical coverage of the distal tibia by the anterior portion of the tibial tray.

Any subsidence or overgrowth should be carefully monitored with postoperative radiographic surveillance. Although

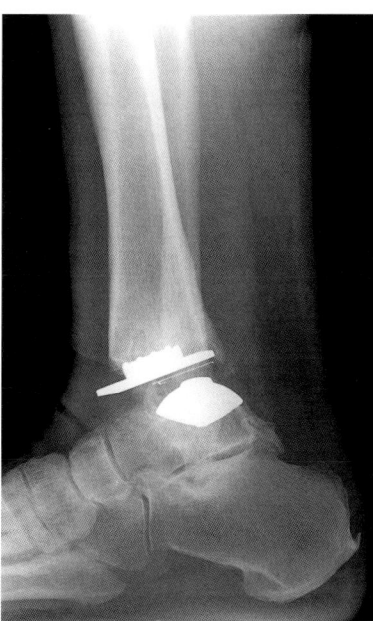

FIGURE 32.26 Posterior tibial subsidence of the STAR tibial component. Note how the mobile bearing permits posterior migration entire foot relative to the leg.

these conditions do not necessarily correlate with clinical symptoms or range of motion, the concern of progression should be reconciled.

POLYETHYLENE WEAR AND ASEPTIC LOOSENING

The fundamental limitation of UHMWPE is wear resistance. High volumetric wear leads to the generation of millions of polyethylene particles with ultimate component loosening and osteolysis.[114] In the past 20 years, tremendous knowledge of proper manufacture of the material has lead to improved practices to ensure more consistent fabrication of the material. Nonetheless, polyethylene wear is often the cause of ultimate failure of the implant (Fig. 32.27).

The wear rate of the polyethylene is influenced by many factors including patient activity, quality and design of the insert, and method of sterilization. Based on pedometer data, a sedentary to low-active individual with a TAR in a 10-year period potentially will subject their prosthesis through 9-14 million weight-bearing cycles.[115] Normal repetitive loads can be expected to cause wear of the polyethylene even under optimal conditions. Accelerated wear may cause the implant to loosen prematurely, most commonly in the second decade.[116-118]

Polyethylene wear can lead to activation of macrophages, which in turn can lead to periprosthetic osteolysis, ballooning lysis, and component loosening. There is concern in mobile-bearing designs that increased wear patterns and subsequent particulate matter are possible because of motion at the tibial component-polyethylene interface. This wear on the tibial side of the mobile bearing is sometimes referred to as backside wear.[119] It is intuitive that a larger surface area in a mobile bearing may generate more particulate matter, but it is arguable that smaller surface areas are subjected to higher pressures and less capable of dispersing the load. However, the effect of the size of any bearing in a total ankle model has not been studied.

Early prosthetic loosening is less likely caused from polyethylene wear but rather induced by failure or disruption of proper bony ingrowth (aseptic loosening).[120] This is commonly painful and radiographically can appear as a dark halo around

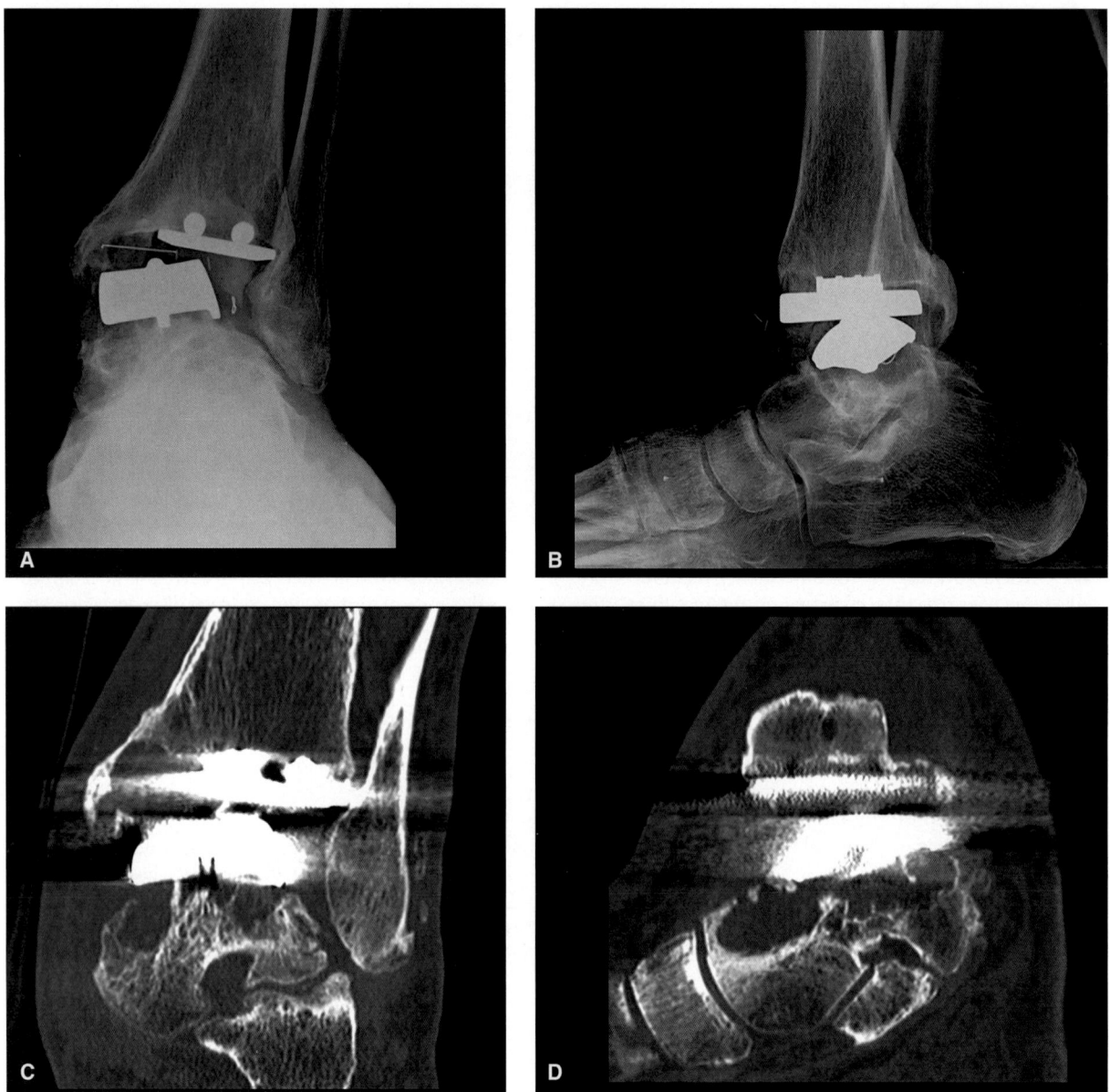

FIGURE 32.27 Diagnostic imaging illustrating a failing STAR prosthesis. **A.** Note the medial ejection of the polyethylene bearing that has eroded half of the medial malleolus and compromised the deep deltoid ligament. **B.** Hint of talar and tibial osteolysis. **C, D.** CT slices confirm significant osteolysis of the talus undermining the talar component and threatening the talonavicular joint.

the component. Patients usually complain of "start-up" pain, which may or may not subside as the ambulatory activity progresses. The cause of the lack of bony ingrowth is unknown but premature weight bearing and micromotion have been implicated. Yet, common practice is gravitating toward early postoperative weight bearing and/or range of motion.[121]

Asymptomatic aseptic loosening does not require treatment, but frequent radiographic surveillance is indicated to determine if the interface between the bone and component is increasing. If so, further investigation is warranted to rule out occult infection or frank component instability.

GUTTER IMPINGEMENT

Impingement of the medial and lateral gutter is commonly observed after TAR[56,57,90,93,122] (Fig. 32.28A and B). In many

patients, there is close apposition of either malleolus and the corresponding surface of the talus. These radiographic findings should be carefully scrutinized for signs of arthritic change of the facets. Ideally, arthritic talomalleolar facets are resected at the time of implantation, but frontal plane stability can be compromised. On the medial side, removal of the impingement at the time of the index surgery may compromise integrity of the deltoid ligament. On the lateral side, the fibula often acts as the buttress to resist talar eversion or lateral displacement and removal of either side of this articulation may permit abnormal talar migration. The correlation of radiographic findings and patient symptoms is often difficult. Patient complaints are often vague, and the clinical indications for additional surgical treatment are ill defined.[56] Patients should be advised of the possibility of an uncertain outcome until further guidelines are established.

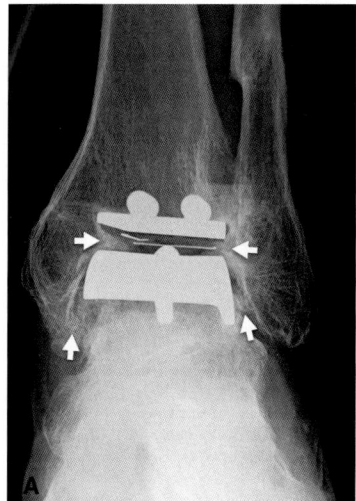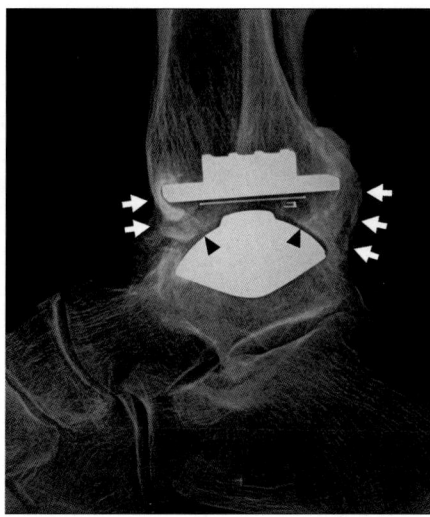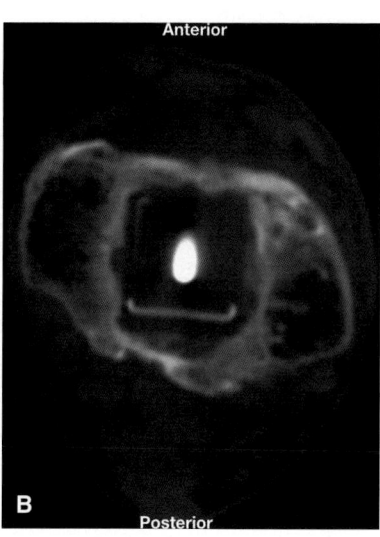

FIGURE 32.28 A. Post-op heterotopic bone growth. *White arrows* mark locations of aberrant bone growth. *Black triangles* show lucent line where heterotopic bone is contacting talar component. **B.** CT transverse cut through ankle at level of polyethylene bearing. Image confirms that a ring of heterotopic bone surrounds the polyethylene bearing.

Treatment of gutter impingement is rather straightforward provided there is reasonable evidence that the impingement is the source of the symptoms. Open and arthroscopic débridement has been reported to decompress the gutters.[56,123] Because the joint has been entered, it should be performed with the utmost precaution to prevent infection.[93] Arthroscopic treatment is more tedious, and there is risk of scuffing the metal or plastic component with the burr during débridement. Typically, the standard anteromedial and anterolateral portals are utilized. Draining portals after arthroscopic surgery can be ominous and should be carefully monitored. Open débridement can also be helpful to provide radiographic separation between the opposed surfaces. Vertical incisions directly over the involved gutter are made for exposure. Regardless of the surgical technique, sufficient space should be created such that 4.0 burr or instrument can be passed freely from the anterior capsule to the posterior capsule. Fluoroscopic imaging during the surgery is also helpful to assess the amount of bone that is removed.

DEEP INFECTION

Prosthesis-related infections are catastrophic events that are extremely difficult to treat. At best, 6 months of intensive surgical and medical care are needed to stabilize the ankle. There is significant impact to the patient in many aspects, including inability to work, financial pressure, multiple surgeries, and frequent medical visits. Unsuccessful eradication of a prosthetic joint infection can culminate in an amputation.

A pivotal factor toward the development and resistance of infection with prosthetic devices is the ability for microorganisms to adhere to biomaterials and resist antibiotic therapy. Similarly, there are many bacterial species that are capable of producing adherent biofilms as a protective mode of growth. One of the difficulties with infected total joint prosthesis is that the presentation can be latent. Although postoperative infections can manifest in the immediate postoperative period (within 6 weeks), most patients present with signs and symptoms of infection months later.[124] In part, this is due to the

sequestration of the bacterial focus at the bone-implant interface or the polyethylene liner-tibial component interface.

Prompt recognition and treatment of an infection at the time of presentation can increase the chances of complete eradication. In general, patients with symptoms suggestive of infection for <3 weeks or <30 days postimplantation can be treated with retention of the components if they are well fixed, have no draining sinuses, and the organism is sensitive to oral antibiotics. In these cases, open arthrotomy, exchange of the polyethylene liner and thorough irrigation and débridement. If the components are loose even if the presentation is relatively early, strongly suggests that the components be removed and replaced with an antibiotic impregnated cement block. Standard monitoring of the inflammatory markers, serial radiographs and overall clinical course are important to determine the success of this strategy. However, parenteral antibiotics are utilized in the initial stages.

When the presentation of infection occurs beyond the 30-day postoperative period or symptoms have persisted for more than 3 weeks, the treatment involves removal of all of the components and vigorous débridement of the entire joint. This includes any and all tissues that have communicated with the infective focus. The extent of spread of the infected material is best determined by an injection of methylene blue into the joint cavity prior to incision and drainage. All material that has been stained should be removed. Similarly, cement block insertion will provide high concentrations of antibiotics and impart some stability of the joint. Repeat irrigation and débridement may be necessary in severe cases.[94,125] The spacer should be placed at the time of the initial removal of the implant. The volume of the block of cement should approximate that of the combined components, such that the joint space is maintained for future reconstruction.[125] This is typically combined with a 6-week course of parenterally administered antibiotics and determined by the infecting organism. Once the wound has healed and there is a stable soft tissue envelope, patients can be allowed to bear full weight on the cement block while awaiting reconstruction[126] (Fig. 32.29).

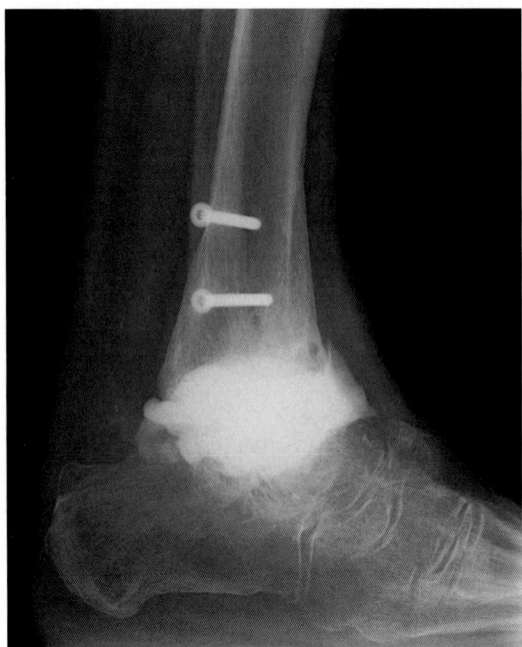

FIGURE 32.29 Bone cement spacer placed after TAR removal.

The timing of reimplantation should be governed by a reasonable assurance that the infection has been eradicated. A healed, stable soft tissue envelope should also be in place prior to any attempt at reimplantation. Laboratory values of infection markers should also be normalized. Aspirations with culture of the joint fluid are also useful in clarifying the absence of any residual infective foci. Although there is some debate regarding the safe threshold for reimplantation, in most cases, this period of time is 6 months or more. If reimplantation is not possible, a conversion to an arthrodesis is achievable.[127-129] At the time of reimplantation, a culture and biopsy of the intra-articular tissue should be obtained after the cement block has been completely removed. The bony surfaces should be prepared similar to a primary implant procedure. One should not assume that the same size prosthesis will be utilized. In some instances, a larger size implant will be necessary. Rarely longer stemmed components will be needed to bypass areas of sparse bone.[62,130]

REFERENCES

1. Perry JD, ed. *Gait Analysis: Normal and Pathological Function.* Thorofare, NJ: Slack, Inc; 1992.
2. Saunders J, Inman V, Eberhart H. The major determinants in normal and pathological gait. *J Bone Joint Surg.* 1953;35-A:543-558.
3. Kuo AD, Donelan JM, Ruina A. Energetic consequences of walking like an inverted pendulum: step-to-step transitions. *Exerc Sport Sci Rev.* 2005;33:88-97.
4. Krause FG, Di Silvestro M, Penner MJ, et al. Inter- and intraobserver reliability of the COFAS end-stage ankle arthritis classification system. *Foot Ankle Int.* 2010;31:103-108.
5. Christensen JC, Schuberth JM, Powell EG. Talolisthesis in end stage ankle arthrosis. *Foot Ankle Surg.* 2016;22:200-204.
6. Hintermann B. *Total Ankle Arthroplasty Historical Overview, Current Concepts and Future Perspectives.* Austria: Springer-Verlag/Wien; 2005:195.
7. Schuberth JM, Steck JK, Christensen JC. Ankle replacement arthroplasty. In: Southerland JT, ed. *McGlamry's Comprehensive Textbook of Foot and Ankle Surgery.* 4th ed. Philadelphia, PA: Wolters Kluwer Heath/Lippincott Williams & Wilkins; 2013:717-756.
8. Bibbo C, Deorio JK, Easley ME. Total ankle arthroplasty. *Inst Course Lect.* 2008;57:383-413.
9. Yalamanchili P, Neufeld SK, Lin S. Total ankle arthroplasty: a modern perspective. *Curr Orthop Pract.* 2009;20:106-110.
10. Greisberg J, Assal M, Flueckiger G, Hansen ST Jr. Takedown of ankle fusion and conversion to total ankle replacement. *Clin Orthop Relat Res.* 2004:80-88.
11. Schuberth JM, Christensen JC, Seidenstricker C. Takedown of ankle arthrodesis with insufficient fibula: surgical technique and intermediate-term follow-up. *J Foot Ankle Surg.* 2018;57:216-220.
12. Lee GC, Pagnano MW, Hanssen AD. Total knee arthroplasty after prior bone or joint sepsis about the knee. *Clin Orthop Relat Res.* 2002;404:226-231.
13. Jerry GL, Rand JA, Ilstrup D. Old sepsis prior to total knee arthroplasty. *Clin Orthop Relat Res.* 1988;236:135-140.
14. Inman VT. *Joints of the Ankle.* Baltimore, MD: Lippincott Williams & Wilkins; 1976.
15. Sarrafian SK, ed. *Anatomy of the Foot and Ankle.* 1st ed. Philadelphia, PA: J. B. Lippincott Company; 1983.
16. Harrington KD. Degenerative arthritis of the ankle secondary to long-standing lateral ligament instability. *J Bone Joint Surg.* 1979;61-A:354-361.
17. Greisberg J, Hansen ST Jr. Ankle replacement: management of associated deformities. *Foot Ankle Clin.* 2002;7:721-736, vi.
18. Kim BS, Choi WJ, Kim YS, Lee JW. Total ankle replacement in moderate to severe varus deformity of the ankle. *J Bone Joint Surg.* 2009;91-B:1183-1190.
19. Mayich DJ, Daniels TR. Total ankle replacement in ankle arthritis with varus talar deformity: pathophysiology, evaluation, and management principles. *Foot Ankle Clin.* 2012;17:127-139.
20. Schuberth JM, Christensen JC, Seidenstricker CL. Total ankle replacement with severe valgus deformity: technique and surgical strategy. *J Foot Ankle Surg.* 2017;56:618-627.
21. Shock RP, Christensen JC, Schuberth JM. Total ankle replacement in the varus ankle. *J Foot Ankle Surg.* 2011;50:5-10.
22. Trajkovski T, Pinsker E, Cadden A, Daniels T. Outcomes of ankle arthroplasty with preoperative coronal-plane varus deformity of 10 degrees or greater. *J Bone Joint Surg.* 2013;95-A:1382-1388.
23. Tochigi Y, Suh JS, Amendola A, Pedersen DR, Saltzman C. Ankle alignment on lateral radiographs. Part 1: sensitivity of measures to perturbations of ankle positioning. *Foot Ankle Int.* 2006;27:82-87.
24. Tochigi Y, Suh JS, Amendola A, Saltzman C. Ankle alignment on lateral radiographs. Part 2: reliability and validity of measures. *Foot Ankle Int.* 2006;27:88-92.
25. Schaefer KL, Sangeorzan BJ, Fassbind MJ, Ledoux WR. The comparative morphology of idiopathic ankle osteoarthritis. *J Bone Joint Surg.* 2012;94-A:1-6.
26. Najefi A, Ghani Y, Goldberg A. Role of rotation in total ankle replacement. *Foot Ankle Int.* 2019;40:1358-1367.
27. Hintermann B, Valderrabano V. Total ankle replacement. *Foot Ankle Clin.* 2003;8:375-405.
28. Bluman EM, Chiodo CP. Valgus ankle deformity and arthritis. *Foot Ankle Clin.* 2008;13:443-470.
29. Demetracopoulos CA, Cody EA, Adams JE, DeOrio JK, Nunley JA, Easley ME. Outcomes of total ankle arthroplasty in moderate and severe valgus deformity. *Foot Ankle Spec.* 2019;12:238-245.
30. Beumer A. Chronic instability of the anterior syndesmosis of the ankle. *Acta Orthop Suppl.* 2007;78:4-36.
31. Beumer A, Valstar ER, Garling EH. Effects of ligament sectioning on the kinematics of the distal tibiofibular syndesmosis: a radiostereometric study of 10 cadaveric specimens based on presumed trauma mechanisms with suggestions for treatment. *Acta Orthop.* 2006;77:531-540.
32. Glazebrook M, Daniels T, Younger A, et al. Comparison of health-related quality of life between patients with end-stage ankle and hip arthrosis. *J Bone Joint Surg.* 2008;90-A:499-505.
33. Alvine FGE. *Total Ankle Arthroplasty.* Philadelphia, PA: Saunders; 2000.
34. Hamblen DL. Can the ankle joint be replaced? *J Bone Joint Surg.* 1985;67-B:689-690.
35. Daniels T, Thomas R. Etiology and biomechanics of ankle arthritis. *Foot Ankle Clin.* 2008;13:341-352.
36. Saltzman CL, Salamon ML, Blanchard GM, et al. Epidemiology of ankle arthritis: report of a consecutive series of 639 patients from a Tertiary Orthopedic Center. *Iowa Orthop J.* 2005;25:44-46.
37. Valderrabano V, Horisberger M, Russell I, Dougall H, Hintermann B. Etiology of ankle osteoarthritis. *Clin Orthop Relat Res.* 2008;467:1800-1806.
38. Doets HC, Brand R, Nelissen RG. Total ankle arthroplasty in inflammatory joint disease with use of two mobile-bearing designs. *J Bone Joint Surg.* 2006;88-A:1272-1284.
39. Wood PL, Crawford LA, Suneja R, Kenyon A. Total ankle replacement for rheumatoid ankle arthritis. *Foot Ankle Clin.* 2007;12:497-508, vii.
40. Lee JH, Dyke JP, Ballon D, Ciombor DM, Tung G, Aaron RK. Assessment of bone perfusion with contrast-enhanced magnetic resonance imaging. *Orthop Clin North Am.* 2009;40:249-257.
41. Assal M, Sangeorzan BJ, Hansen ST. Post-traumatic osteonecrosis of the lateral tibial plafond. *Foot Ankle Surg.* 2007;13:24-29.
42. Rajagopalan S, Lloyd J, Upadhyay V, Sangar A, Taylor HP. Osteonecrosis of the distal tibia after a pronation external rotation ankle fracture: literature review and management. *J Foot Ankle Surg.* 2011;50:445-448.
43. Devalia KL, Ramaskandhan J, Muthumayandi K, Siddique M. Early results of a novel technique: hindfoot fusion in talus osteonecrosis prior to ankle arthroplasty: a case series. *Foot (Edinb).* 2015;25:200-205.
44. Wilson MG, Kelley K, Thornhill TS. Infection as a complication of total knee-replacement arthroplasty. Risk factors and treatment in sixty-seven cases. *J Bone Joint Surg.* 1990;72-A:878-883.
45. Maderazo ED, Judson S, Pasternak H. Late infections of total joint prostheses. A review and recommendations for prevention. *Clin Orthop Relat Res.* 1988;229:131-142.
46. Bibbo C, Patel DV, Gehrmann RM, Linn SS. Chlorhexidine provides superior skin decontamination in foot and ankle surgery: a prospective randomized study. *Clin Orthop Relat Res.* 2005;438:204-208.
47. Ostrander RV, Botte MJ, Brage ME. Efficacy of surgical preparation solutions in foot and ankle surgery. *J Bone Joint Surg.* 2005;87-A:980-985.

48. Ostrander RV, Brage M, Botte MJ. Bacterial skin contamination after surgical preparation in foot and ankle surgery. *Clin Orthop Relat Res.* 2003;406:246-252.

49. Mangram AJ, Horan TC, Pearson ML, Silver LC, Jarvis WR. Guideline for prevention of surgical site infection, 1999. Hospital Infection Control Practices Advisory Committee. *Infect Control Hosp Epidemiol.* 1999;20:250-278.

50. Sapega AA, Heppenstall RB, Chance B, Park YS, Sokolow D. Optimizing tourniquet application and release times in extremity surgery. A biochemical and ultrastructural study. *J Bone Joint Surg.* 1985;67-A:303-314.

51. Clarke MT, Longstaff L, Edwards D, Rushton N. Tourniquet-induced wound hypoxia after total knee replacement. *J Bone Joint Surg.* 2001;83-B:40-44.

52. Ewing MA, Huntley SR, Baker DK, et al. Blood transfusion during total ankle arthroplasty is associated with increased in-hospital complications and costs. *Foot Ankle Spec.* 2019;12:115-121.

53. Wood PL. Experience with the STAR ankle arthroplasty at Wrightington Hospital, UK. *Foot Ankle Clin.* 2002;7:755-764.

54. Anderson T, Montgomery F, Carlsson A. Uncemented STAR total ankle prostheses. *J Bone Joint Surg.* 2004;86-A(suppl 1):103-111.

55. Hobson SA, Karantana A, Dhar S. Total ankle replacement in patients with significant pre-operative deformity of the hindfoot. *J Bone Joint Surg.* 2009;91-B:481-486.

56. Schuberth JM, Babu NS, Richey JM, Christensen JC. Gutter impingement after total ankle arthroplasty. *Foot Ankle Int.* 2013;34:329-337.

57. Schuberth JM, Wood DA, Christensen JC. Gutter impingement in total ankle arthroplasty. *Foot Ankle Spec.* 2016;9:145-158.

58. Bartel DL, Bicknell VL, Wright TM. The effect of conformity, thickness, and material on stresses in ultra-high molecular weight components for total joint replacement. *J Bone Joint Surg.* 1986;68-A:1041-1051.

59. Saltzman CL. Perspective on total ankle replacement. *Foot Ankle Clin.* 2000;5:761-775.

60. Fletcher N, Sofianos D, Berkes MB, Obremskey WT. Prevention of perioperative infection. *J Bone Joint Surg.* 2007;89-A:1605-1618.

61. Manian FA, Meyer PL, Setzer J, Senkel D. Surgical site infections associated with methicillin-resistant Staphylococcus aureus: do postoperative factors play a role? *Clin Infect Dis.* 2003;36:863-868.

62. Myerson MS, Won HY. Primary and revision total ankle replacement using custom-designed prostheses. *Foot Ankle Clin.* 2008;13:521-538, x.

63. Buechel FF, Buechel FF, Pappas MJ. Twenty-year evaluation of cementless mobile-bearing total ankle replacements. *Clin Orthop Relat Res.* 2004;424:19-26.

64. Ducheyne P, De Meester P, Aernoudt E, Martens M, Mulier JC. Fatigue fractures of the femoral components of Charnley and Charnley-Müller type total hip prostheses. *J Biomed Mater Res.* 1977;9:199-219.

65. Hintermann B, Valderrabano V, Dereymaeker G, Dick W. The HINTEGRA ankle: rationale and short-term results of 122 consecutive ankles. *Clin Orthop Relat Res.* 2004:57-68.

66. Pilliar RM, Lee JM, Maniatopulos C. Observations on the effect of movement on bone ingrowth into porous-surfaced implants. *Clin Orthop Relat Res.* 1986;208:108-113.

67. Lim W, Wu C. Balancing the risks and benefits of thromboprophylaxis in patients undergoing podiatric surgery. *Chest.* 2009;135:888-890.

68. Richey JM, Ritterman Weinraub ML, Schuberth JM. Incidence and risk factors of symptomatic venous thromboembolism following foot and ankle surgery. *Foot Ankle Int.* 2019;40:98-104.

69. Huang RC, Parvizi J, Hozack WJ. Aspirin is as effective as and safer than warfarin for patients at higher risk of venous thromboembolism undergoing total joint arthroplasty. *J Arthroplasty.* 2016;31(9 suppl):83-86.

70. Dodd A, Daniels TR. Total ankle replacement in the presence of talar varus or valgus deformities. *Foot Ankle Clin.* 2017;22:277-300.

71. Hanselman AE, Powell BD, Santrock RD. Total ankle arthroplasty with severe preoperative varus deformity. *Orthopedics.* 2015;38:e343-e346.

72. Hennessy MS, Molloy AP, Wood EV. Management of the varus arthritic ankle. *Foot Ankle Clin.* 2008;13:417-442, viii.

73. Schuberth JM, Babu-Spencer NS. The impact of the first ray in the cavovarus foot. *Clin Podiatr Med Surg.* 2009;26:385-393.

74. Schuberth JM, Bowlby MA, Christensen JC. Combined total ankle arthroplasty with posterior tibial tendon transfer for end-stage cavovarus deformity. *J Foot Ankle Surg.* 2016;55:885-890.

75. Haddad SL. Total Ankle Arthroplasty Session: Managing Frontal Plane Deformities. American Orthopaedic Foot and Ankle Society, Summer Meeting Pre Meeting; 2009; Vancouver, BC Canada.

76. Morris CH, Christensen JC, Ching RP, Chan F, Schuberth JM. Articular congruency of the Salto Talaris total ankle prosthesis. *Foot Ankle Surg.* 2015;21:206-210.

77. Myerson MS, Mroczek K. Perioperative complications of total ankle arthroplasty. *Foot Ankle Int.* 2003;24:17-21.

78. Schuberth JM, Patel S, Zarutsky E. Perioperative complications of the Agility total ankle replacement in 50 initial, consecutive cases. *J Foot Ankle Surg.* 2006;45:139-146.

79. Conti SF, Wong YS. Complications of total ankle replacement. *Foot Ankle Clin.* 2002;7:791-807, vii.

80. Basques BA, Bitterman A, Campbell KJ, Haughom BD, Lin J, Lee S. Influence of surgeon volume on inpatient complications, cost, and length of stay following total ankle arthroplasty. *Foot Ankle Int.* 2016;37:1046-1051.

81. Saltzman CL, Amendola A, Anderson R, et al. Surgeon training and complications in total ankle arthroplasty. *Foot Ankle Int.* 2003;24:514-518.

82. Pyevich MT, Saltzman CL, Callaghan JJ, Alvine FG. Total ankle arthroplasty: a unique design. Two to twelve-year follow-up. *J Bone Joint Surg.* 1998;80-A:1410-1420.

83. Anderson T, Montgomery F, Carlsson A. Uncemented STAR total ankle prostheses. Three to eight-year follow-up of fifty-one consecutive ankles. *J Bone Joint Surg.* 2003;85-A:1321-1329.

84. Haskell A, Mann RA. Perioperative complication rate of total ankle replacement is reduced by surgeon experience. *Foot Ankle Int.* 2004;25:283-289.

85. Hurowitz EJ, Gould JS, Fleisig GS, Fowler R. Outcome analysis of Agility total ankle replacement with prior adjunctive procedures: two to six year follow up. *Foot Ankle Int.* 2007;28:308-312.

86. Wood PL, Deakin S. Total ankle replacement. The results in 200 ankles. *J Bone Joint Surg.* 2003;85-B:334-341.

87. McGarvey WC, Clanton TO, Lunz D. Malleolar fracture after total ankle arthroplasty: a comparison of two designs. *Clin Orthop Relat Res.* 2004;(424):104-110.

88. Kopp FJ, Patel MM, Deland JT, O'Malley MJ. Total ankle arthroplasty with the Agility prosthesis: clinical and radiographic evaluation. *Foot Ankle Int.* 2006;27:97-103.

89. Bonnin M, Judet T, Colombier JA, Buscayret F, Graveleau N, Piriou P. Midterm results of the Salto Total Ankle Prosthesis. *Clin Orthop Relat Res.* 2004;(424):6-18.

90. Spirt AA, Assal M, Hansen ST Jr. Complications and failure after total ankle arthroplasty. *J Bone Joint Surg.* 2004;86-A:1172-1178.

91. Knecht SI, Estin M, Callaghan JJ, et al. The Agility total ankle replacement. Seven to sixteen-year follow-up. *J Bone Joint Surg.* 2004;86-A:1161-1171.

92. Natens P, Dereymaeker G, Abbara M, Matricali G. Early results after four years experience with the S.T.A.R. uncemented total ankle prosthesis. *Acta Orthop Belg.* 2003;69:49-58.

93. Kurup HV, Taylor GR. Medial impingement after ankle replacement. *Int Orthop.* 2008;32:243-246.

94. Kotnis R, Pasapula C, Anwar F, Cooke PH, Sharp RJ. The management of failed ankle replacement. *J Bone Joint Surg.* 2006;88-B:1039-1047.

95. Bejjanki NK, Moulder E, Al-Nammari S, Budgen A. Tarsal tunnel syndrome as a complication of total ankle arthroplasty: a case report. *Foot Ankle Int.* 2008;29:347-350.

96. Harris NJ, Brooke BT, Sturdee S. A wear debris cyst following S.T.A.R. total ankle replacements—surgical management. *Foot Ankle Surg.* 2009;15:43-45.

97. Fukui A, Tanaka Y, Inada Y, et al. Turndown retinacular flap for closure of skin fistula after total ankle replacement. *Foot Ankle Int.* 2008;29:624-626.

98. Bolton-Maggs BG, Sudlow RA, Freeman MA. Total ankle arthroplasty. A long-term review of the London Hospital Experience. *J Bone Joint Surg.* 1985;67B:785-790.

99. Kitaoka HB. Complications of replacement arthroplasty of the ankle. In: Morrey BF, ed. *Joint Replacement Arthroplasty.* 3rd ed. Philadelphia, PA: Churchill Livingstone; 2003:1171.

100. Glazebrook MA, Arsenault K, Dunbar M. Evidence-based classification of complications in total ankle arthroplasty. *Foot Ankle Int.* 2009;30:945-949.

101. Conti SF, Wong YS. Complications of total ankle replacement. *Clin Orthop Relat Res.* 2001;(391):105-114.

102. Mizu-uchi H, Matsuda S, Miura H, Higaki H, Okazaki K, Iwamoto Y. The effect of ankle rotation on cutting of the tibia in total knee arthroplasty. *J Bone Joint Surg.* 2006;88-A:2632-2636.

103. Mann JA, Mann RA, Horton E. STAR ankle: long-term results. *Foot Ankle Int.* 2011;32:473-484.

104. Hendee WR, Ritenour R. *Medical Imaging Physics.* St. Louis, MO: Mosby-Year Book; 1992.

105. Hansen STJ. *Personal Communication.* Seattle, WA. 2007.

106. Christensen JC. Complex regional pain syndrome and related disorders. In: Southerland JT, ed. *McGlamry's Comprehensive Textbook of Foot and Ankle Surgery.* 4th ed. Philadelphia, PA: Lippincott Williams & Wilkins; 2013:1928.

107. Jänig W. The sympathetic nervous system in pain: physiology and pathophysiology. In: Stanton-Hicks M, ed. *Pain and the Sympathetic Nervous System.* Boston, MA: Kluwer Academic; 1990:17-89.

108. Raikin SM, Myerson MS. Avoiding and managing complications of the Agility total ankle replacement system. *Orthopedics.* 2006;29:930-938.

109. Carlsson A, Markusson P, Sundberg M. Radiostereometric analysis of the double-coated STAR total ankle prosthesis: a 3-5 year follow-up of 5 cases with rheumatoid arthritis and 5 cases with osteoarthrosis. *Acta Orthop.* 2005;76:573-579.

110. Nilsson RG, Doets HC, Valstar ER. Early migration of the tibial component of the Buechel-Pappas total ankle prosthesis. *Clin Orthop Relat Res.* 2006;448:146-151.

111. Zerahn B, Kofoed H. Bone mineral density, gait analysis, and patient satisfaction, before and after ankle arthroplasty. *Foot Ankle Int.* 2004;25:208-214.

112. Galik K. *The Effect of Design Variations on Stresses in Total Ankle Arthroplasty.* Pittsburgh, PA: University of Pittsburgh; 2002.

113. King CM, Schuberth JM, Christensen JC, Swanstrom KM. Relationship of alignment and tibial cortical coverage to hypertrophic bone formation in Salto Talaris total ankle arthroplasty. *J Foot Ankle Surg.* 2013;52:355-359.

114. Heisel C, Silva M, dela Rosa MA. Short-term in vivo wear of cross-linked polyethylene. *J Bone Joint Surg.* 2004;86-A:748-751.

115. Tudor-Locke C, Hatano Y, Pangrazi RP. Revisiting "how many steps are enough?" *Med Sci Sports Exerc.* 2008;40:S537-S543.

116. Goldring SR, Flannery MS, Petrison KK. Evaluation of connective tissue cell responses to orthopaedic implant materials. *Connect Tissue Res.* 1990;24:77-81.

117. Goldring SR, Jasty M, Roelke MS. Formation of a synovial-like membrane at the bone-cement interface. Its role in bone resorption and implant loosening after total hip replacement. *Arthritis Rheum.* 1986;29:836-842.

118. Jasty MJ, Floyd WEI, Schiller AL. Localized osteolysis in stable, non-septic total hip replacement. *J Bone Joint Surg.* 1986;68-A:912-919.

119. Schmalzried TP, Callaghan JJ. Wear in total hip and knee replacements. *J Bone Joint Surg.* 1999;81-A:115-136.

120. Sundfeldt M, Carlsson LV, Johansson CB, Thomsen P, Gretzer C. Aseptic loosening, not only a question of wear: a review of different theories. *Acta Orthop.* 2006;77:177-197.

121. Barg A, Zwicky L, Knupp M, Henninger HB, Hintermann B. HINTEGRA total ankle replacement: survivorship analysis in 684 patients. *J Bone Joint Surg.* 2013;95-A:1175-1183.

122. Stengel D, Bauwens K, Ekkernkamp A, Cramer J. Efficacy of total ankle replacement with meniscal-bearing devices: a systematic review and meta-analysis. *Arch Orthop Trauma Surg.* 2005;125:109-119.

123. Gross CE, Adams SB, Easley M, Nunley JA II, DeOrio JK. Surgical treatment of bony and soft-tissue impingement in total ankle arthroplasty. *Foot Ankle Spec.* 2017;10: 37-42.

124. Tsukayama DT, Goldberg VM, Kyle R. Diagnosis and management of infection after total knee arthroplasty. *J Bone Joint Surg.* 2003;85-A(suppl 1):S75-S80.

125. Leone JM, Hanssen AD. Management of infection at the site of a total knee arthroplasty. *J Bone Joint Surg.* 2005;87:2335-2348.

126. Ferrao P, Myerson M, Schuberth JM, McCourt MJ. Cement spacer as definitive management for postoperative ankle infection. *Foot Ankle Int.* 2012;33:173-178.

127. Carlsson AS, Montgomery F, Besjakov J. Arthrodesis of the ankle secondary to replacement. *Foot Ankle Int.* 1998;19:240-245.

128. Kitaoka HB. Fusion techniques for failed total ankle arthroplasty. *Semin Arthroplasty.* 1992;3:51-57.

129. Hintermann B, Nunley JA, Christensen JC, Steck JK, Schuberth JM. The failed total ankle. *Foot Ankle Spec.* 2013;6:434-440.

130. Hansen STJ. Total Ankle Replacement with Agility Device. Oregon Podiatric Medical Annual Meeting, Portland, OR, 2005.

CHAPTER 33

Arthroscopy of the Ankle and Foot

Chris Bourke, Meagan Jennings, and Graham Hamilton

OVERVIEW

Arthroscopy of the ankle and small joints of the foot is a useful tool in the armamentarium of the foot and ankle surgeon. As with most technological devices, a unique skill set is required to use the instrument and its accessories. The obvious advantage in arthroscopy, over traditional arthrotomy, lies in its limited dissection and disruption of the soft tissue envelope to accomplish the goals of operation. This sets the stage for reduced postoperative recovery, pain, and swelling compared with traditional open arthrotomy. Although the morbidity of arthrotomy is clearly minimized with arthroscopic technique, if similar surgical objectives are met, frequently, the long-term outcomes of arthroscopic technique parallel those of traditional open technique. In settings in which there is significant surgical pathology and surgical manipulation of the joint structures, such as osteochondral defects, this is especially true. Although it is not always as apparent as with other operations, surgical technique factors into arthroscopic surgical outcomes. It has been observed that "a technically well-performed procedure through arthrotomy is preferable to a poorly performed arthroscopic procedure."[1] The most unique requirement of the necessary skills is the ability to process a two-dimensional image to the three-dimensional anatomy at hand. An additional requirement is that this activity needs to occur without simultaneously looking at one's hands. In contrast to open surgery, in which the eyes of the surgeon usually visualize the hands of the surgeon, in arthroscopic surgery, the eyes of the surgeon are usually fixed on a monitor and the hands are removed from the operative field. The surgeon's indirect visualization of the operative field demands interpreting significant variations in magnification and alterations in visual orientation, which make objective perspective a learned skill. Additionally, the technique requires the surgeon to have indirect tactile interaction coupled with managing multiple variables (distension, manipulation, ingress-egress, control of multiple angles of attack, and orientation), all capable of causing failure of the procedure, and all in real time. Owing to the complex interrelationship of this set of variables, arthroscopy has a significant learning curve and is therefore frustrating to many surgeons.[2] Most arthroscopic surgeons regard the ankle joint and other joints of the foot as being technically difficult joints to access and perform arthroscopically guided procedures. The skill set necessary to perform arthroscopy can only be acquired in a "hands-on" setting with one experienced in the technique.[3] The authors strongly encourage serious arthroscopic training to begin with a hands-on arthroscopic course that has a dry model and a wet lab component. This chapter makes the assumption that the reader has basic knowledge regarding operative arthroscopy of the foot and ankle. The reader otherwise is referred to previously written works on the basics of the subject.[3,4]

The history of arthroscopy is quite interesting and has been well covered in previous publications.[5-7] In 1931, Burman developed an arthroscope and surveyed several joints in a cadaver study. He included the ankle as a potential joint for arthroscopy. After testing three cadaver specimens, he concluded that the joint space was too narrow for arthroscopy.[8] Clinical success and popularity came with the revolution of endoscope design.[9] The podiatric development of the arthroscope in foot and ankle surgery owes much to John Buckholz, Harold Vogler, Richard Lundeen, David Gurvis, and Leonard Janis, all visionaries in foot and ankle arthroscopy. Although Buckholz and Vogler were the first podiatric surgeons to survey the arthroscopic potential in the ankle, Lundeen and Gurvis brought surgical technique to the podiatric profession, organizing the first instructional course in arthroscopy presented to the podiatric profession in 1984.[10]

CLASSIFICATION

- Berndt and Hardy
  - Stage 1 Small area of subchondral compression
  - Stage 2 Partial fragment detachment
  - Stage 3 Complete fragment detachment but not displaced
  - Stage 4 Displaced fragment
- Modified Outerbridge grading of chondromalacia
  - **Grade I**
    - Focal areas of hyperintensity with normal contour
    - Arthroscopically: softening or swelling of cartilage
  - **Grade II**
    - Blister-like swelling/fraying of articular cartilage extending to surface
    - Arthroscopically: fragmentation and fissuring within soft areas of articular cartilage
  - **Grade III**
    - Partial-thickness cartilage loss with focal ulceration
    - Arthroscopically: partial-thickness cartilage loss with fibrillation (crab-meat appearance)
  - **Grade IV**
    - Full-thickness cartilage loss with underlying bone reactive changes
    - Arthroscopically: cartilage destruction with exposed subchondral bone

PATHOLOGY

PRIMARY SOFT TISSUE PATHOLOGY

Primary soft tissue lesions are somewhat uncommon in the ankle. Diagnosis is based on history, physical examination, and careful examination of all of the relevant structures. The consideration of intra-articular soft tissue pathology stems from the negative x-ray and or other enhanced imaging studies (CT, MRI, contrast studies, stress x-ray study). Intra-articular injections are often useful in determining whether the pathology is extra-articular (nonresponsive) or within the joint. The authors typically use 3 mL of 1% or 2% lidocaine plain for a diagnostic injection. Publications have demonstrated cartilage toxicity (chondrocyte death) with prolonged exposure to lidocaine and bupivacaine.[11-15] Even adjusting the pH of the local anesthetic has no effect of the toxic effects on cartilage.[13] Amount of 0.5% ropivacaine has been reported to have less toxicity than bupivacaine in human chondrocytes.[15] Intra-articular corticosteroids have even shown detrimental effects with higher doses and should be avoided in the joint for diagnostic purposes.[16]

A symptom complex that does not respond at least temporarily to an intra-articular injection of local anesthetic with or without steroid will not likely benefit from arthroscopy or other surgical maneuvers. Congenital bands and plicas can be found in the ankle and can cause localized symptoms usually coupled with an increase in activities (Fig. 33.1).

HEMORRHAGIC AND CHRONIC SYNOVITIS

A wide variety of abnormal soft tissue anatomy has been described in the ankle; the most common are varieties of reactive hyperplasia of the synovium commonly known as synovitis.

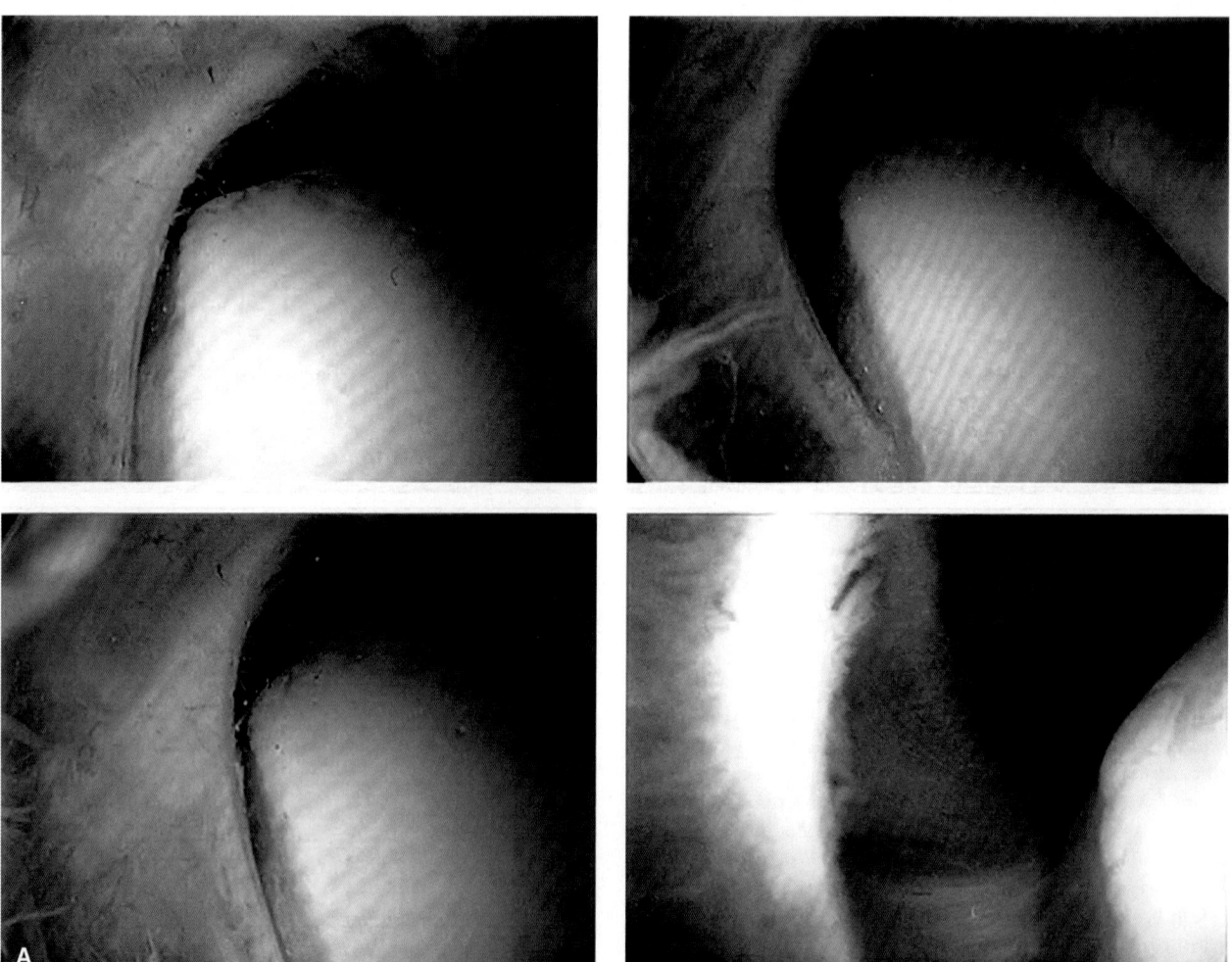

FIGURE 33.1 A. Anterior lateral ankle capsule with congenital band showing interaction with anterior talar body in different ankle positions.

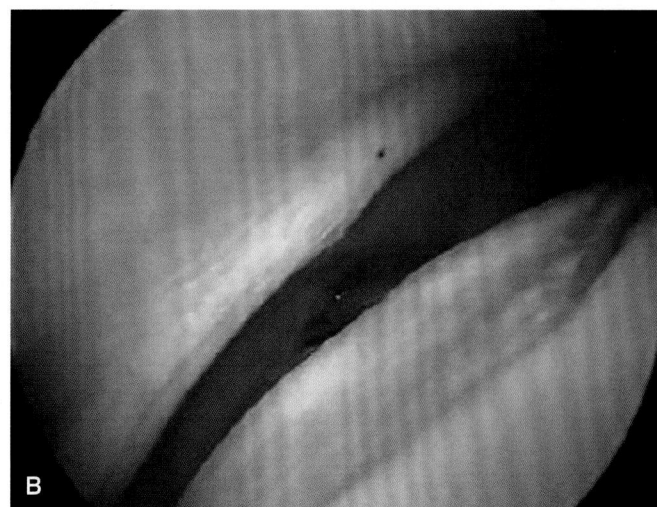

FIGURE 33.1 (*Continued*) **B.** An example of a linear-oriented congenital band causing talar dome erosion. Note these bands are localized thickenings of the joint capsule and are covered by synovium.

With several exceptions, synovitis is a reactive process and not a diagnosis. The synovium of any joint responds to intra-articular pathologic processes by inflammation characterized in the acute setting by hypertrophy, vascular injection, hyperemia, and bright erythema (Fig. 33.2A). An example of reactive synovitis is hemophilic synovitis, which is frequent in hemophilia patients who experience intra-articular bleeding secondary to trauma. Arthroscopic synovectomy of the ankle has been found to reduce the rate of episodes of hemarthrosis in these patients.[16-19] With chronic inflammatory stimulation, synovium becomes dense and fibrous, losing its bright red color and becoming white over time (Fig. 33.2B). This hypertrophic tissue can occupy a large portion of the capsular reflection. Hypertrophic synovitis, whether chronic, acute, or mixed, sometimes fills the anterior pouch completely. In some situations, the reactive tissue becomes adherent to the

juxta-articular bone and capsule. This condition is sometimes termed adhesive capsulitis because the tissue tends to contract, ultimately limiting movement and becoming impinged at the anterior joint line. Resection of adhesive capsulitis is frequently necessary to visualize the joint and define or discover the primary lesion, if it is still present. Synovial disorders that present as primary disorders include pigmented villonodular synovitis (Fig. 33.2C), rheumatoid arthritis, and related autoimmune diseases. Synovial resection for biopsy and therapy in primary synovial disorders is clearly beneficial. Synovial resection in nonspecific synovitis or in which synovitis is clearly secondary to an identifiable pathologic problem can be limited to that which is clearly impinged, obscuring or limiting the surgical procedure. Once the primary causation is resolved, one can expect spontaneous resolution of the reactive process.

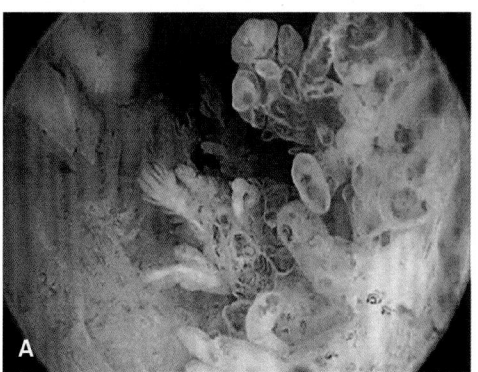
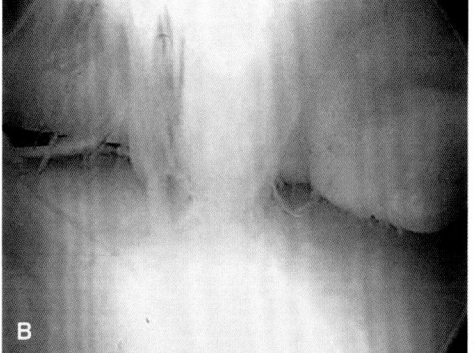
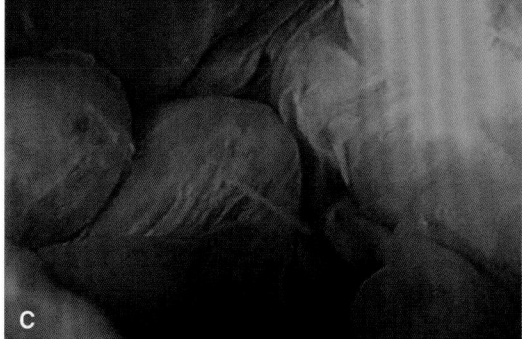

FIGURE 33.2 **A.** Hemorrhagic synovitis. **B.** Atrophic synovitis along anterior tibia in the ankle. **C.** Pigmented villonodular synovitis in the ankle.

FIBROUS BANDS AND MENISCOID LESIONS

Other soft tissue masses encountered in the ankle are not of synovial origin but are likely related to retained intra-articular blood clots secondary to trauma.[20,21] Fibrous bands, meniscoid lesions, impingement lesions, and adhesions are all similar lesions that are characterized as well-defined fibrocartilaginous bodies attached to periarticular structures, occasionally to bone and cartilage (Fig. 33.3).[22-25] Symptoms include nonspecific persistent pain and swelling, crepitus, clicking, or locking. A noninvasive diagnosis of intra-articular soft tissue lesions often demands MRI or contrast CT (Fig. 33.4). Diagnostic and therapeutic injections of local anesthetic, with or without steroids, are frequently helpful. Resection of the abnormal tissue usually leads to the resolution of symptoms. The surgeon should be wary of premature closure of the arthroscopy in situations in which a fibrous band is present because concurrent pathology may be present. Histologic evaluation of these lesions seems to point to a blood clot origin,

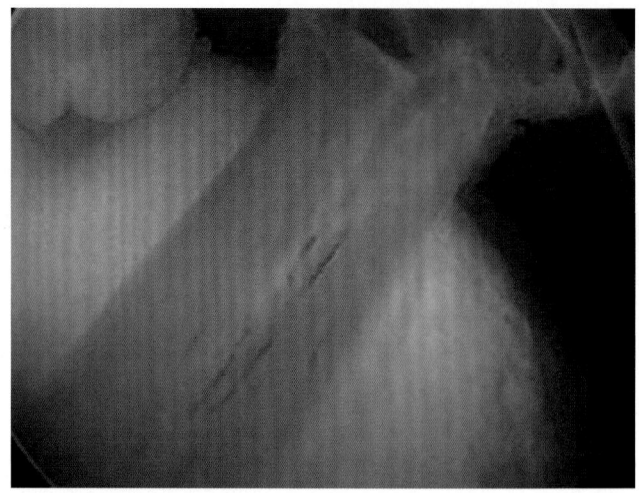

FIGURE 33.3 Fibrous band in the anterior ankle joint with transverse orientation.

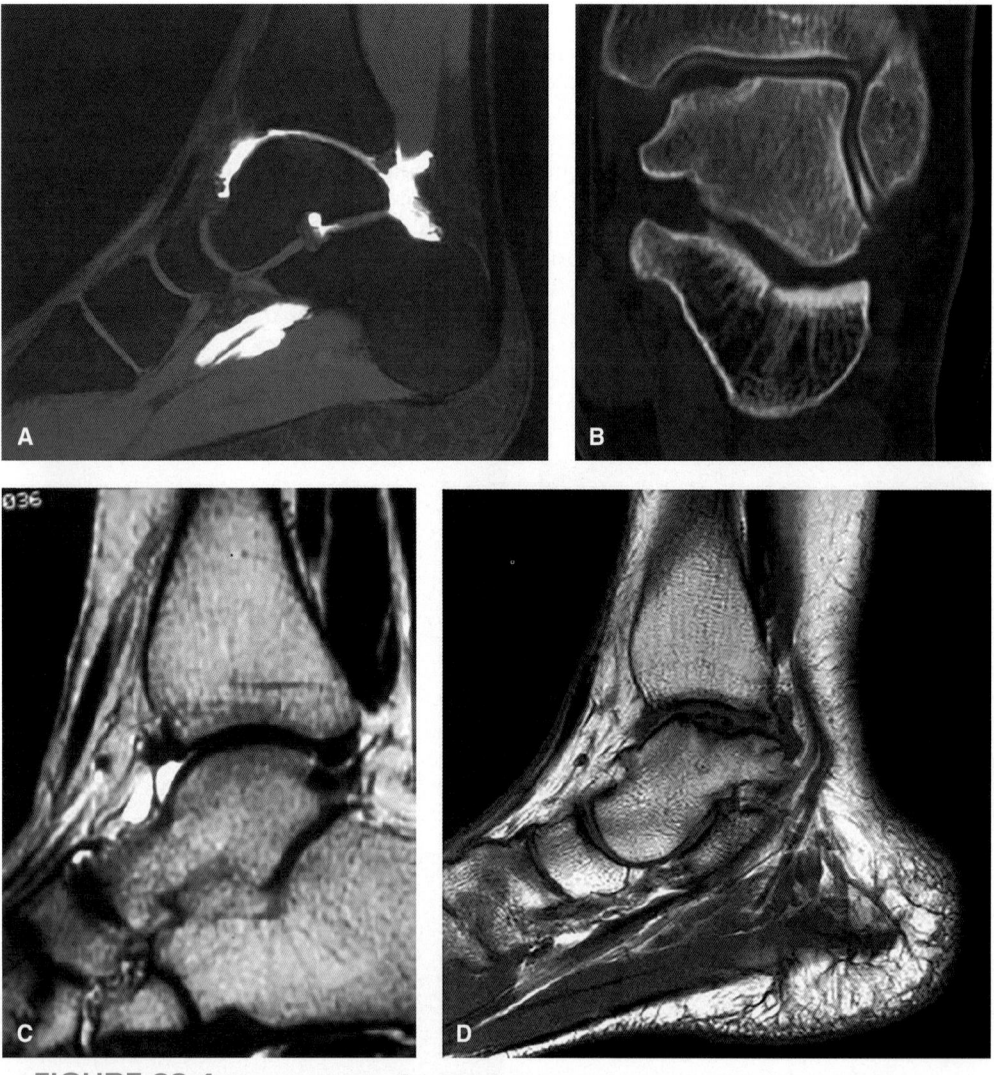

FIGURE 33.4 Diagnostic images. **A.** MRI gadolinium arthrogram sagittal STIR image that shows continuity between the ankle and subtalar joints and the flexor hallucis longus tendon sheath. Note how the study allows enhanced visualization of the cartilage surface with partial-thickness cartilage ankle joint defects on the anterior tibial and talar surfaces. **B.** CT arthrogram after arthroscopic excision of osteochondral fracture fragment. Note fibrocartilage filling of lesion site as highlighted by joint contrast agent. **C.** MRI arthrogram, sagittal slice on a T1-weighted image highlights intra-articular adhesion in the anterior joint recess. **D.** MRI demonstrating large osteochondral defect or talus.

TABLE 33.1	Organized Inventory of Ankle Anatomy
Anterior	
Medial gutter	
Anterior gutter	
Lateral gutter	
Lateral ligaments	
Anterior joint line	
Lateral interval	
Posterior	
Medial gutter	
Lateral gutter	
Posterior joint line	
Anterior ligaments	
Deltoid	
Anterior tibiofibular	
Anterior syndesmotic	
Anterior talofibular	
Posterior ligaments	
Deltoid ligament	
Posterior syndesmotic (including the transverse tibiofibular)	
Posterior talofibular	

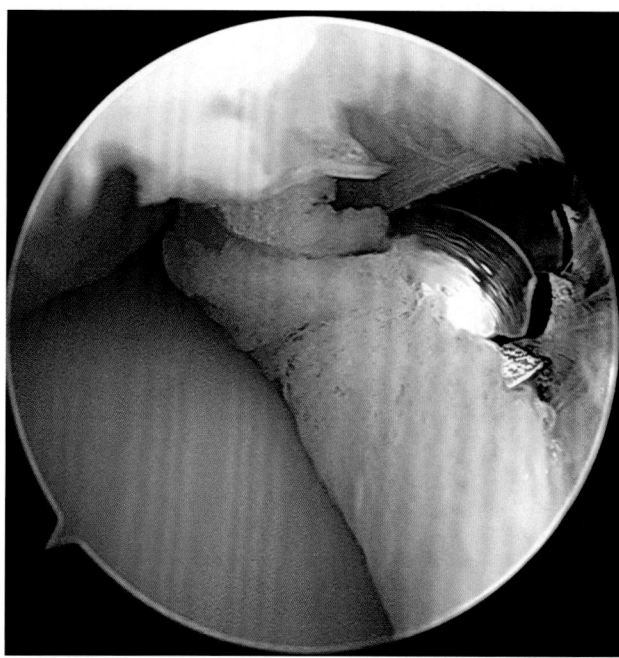

FIGURE 33.5 "Rug in front of the door"; note the hypertrophic changes to the synovial tissue that can get entrapped in the anterior ankle joint similar to a rug in the front of a door.

potentially of traumatic origin. A complete survey of the joint should be carried out to rule out other pathology of traumatic origin (Table 33.1).

SOFT TISSUE IMPINGEMENT

An impingement lesion is a posttraumatic syndrome characterized by abnormal reactive soft tissues occupying space within the capsular reflection causing chronic ankle pain that is not relieved with rest, support, and other noninvasive treatments commonly applied to posttraumatic arthralgias. Physical impingement of abnormal soft tissue between the anterior tibial lip and the dorsal talar neck is often viewable with arthroscopy. In severe cases, a "rug in front of the door" limitation of movement may occur (Fig. 33.5). The impingement lesion can take many forms, varying from a well-differentiated solitary rubbery mass attached to the joint line, to a loosely differentiated mass of soft tissue occupying space in the capsular reflection. The most common form of impingement lesion is found in the anterolateral aspect of the ankle joint about the anterior tibiofibular ligament and lateral gutter. This disorganized form of anterior impingement syndrome is perhaps end-stage synovitis or disorganized (anterior syndesmotic) ligamentous tissue that has undergone change under the influence of repetitive mechanical stimulation and reactive inflammation. This tissue is firm and fibrous and is often adherent to the anterior syndesmotic ligament and capsule of the lateral gutter. This condition is sometimes termed lateral gutter syndrome. In addition to point tenderness and inflammatory signs, frequently, there is tenderness with external rotation of the ankle in the mortise or with compression of the fibula to the tibia. MRI sometimes

demonstrates synovial thickening, although it is usually negative for well-defined pathology.[26] As with other syndromes that produce symptoms in the lateral ankle, careful differentiation from sinus tarsi syndrome and other juxtamalleolar syndromes must be made. Differential diagnostic blocks with local anesthetics are often helpful in making this determination.

Bassett Impingement Lesion

A specialized entrapment found in the anterolateral ankle is the Basset lesion. It was first described by Bassett et al.[27] and can occur after ankle trauma. This syndrome is defined by the observation of the distal fascicle of the anteroinferior tibiofibular ligament imping on the lateral shoulder of the talus, with secondary chondromalacia and mechanical erosion of the articular surface of the lateral talar shoulder (Fig. 33.6A). This observation is associated with chronic anterior ankle pain.[28] Ray and Kriz[29] determined that the distal fascicle of the anteroinferior tibiofibular ligament normally contacts the lateral shoulder of the talus. However, in the pathologic state of the Bassett lesion, there is often abnormal thickening of the fascicle and at times a change in orientation of the ligament. Change in ligament orientation can cause more severe degenerative changes of the adjacent articular cartilage (Fig. 33.6B).

Medial Impingement Lundeen has described and classified an articular irregularity that he termed a medial impingement lesion occurring on the tibial surface of the anteromedial joint line.[30,31] This lesion presents as a change in the articular profile with variable chondromalacia and a change in the articular surface of the plafond where it joins the medial malleolus (mortise angle). Although Lundeen reports this to be a pathologic lesion associated with prior trauma, Ray et al.[32] have reported a variably occurring dell in the articular surface of the plafond in this area in 77% of 77 specimens.

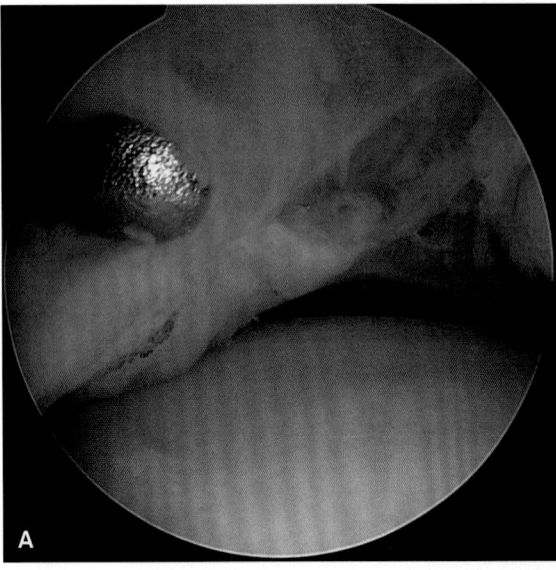
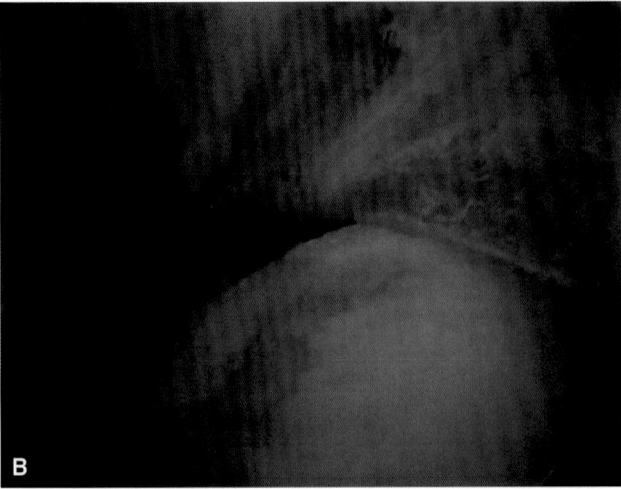

FIGURE 33.6 A. Subtle Bassett lesion with slight thickening. Orientation is normal.
B. Bassett lesion in a right ankle from an 18-year-old female with a history of severe ankle injury. Note degenerative changes of the underlying talar dome and grossly enlarged fascicle and change from a vertical to a transverse orientation.

Posterior Ankle Impingement

The ligamentous labrum of the posterior capsule may similarly be affected by trauma. This is most commonly noted at the posterolateral portion of the joint, where the posteroinferior tibiofibular ligament and the inferior transverse ligament may impinge in a "rug in front of the door"-type mechanism with ankle plantarflexion. This condition should be distinguished from other posterior ankle pathologies, including os trigonum and marsupial meniscus.[33]

Arthrofibrosis (Fig. 33.7) This is a common sequela of severe ankle trauma and multiple surgical interventions of a joint, in which hemarthrosis is involved. Prolonged immobilization in addition can further solidify the hemarthrosis. The condition cannot only clog normal synovial passage across the joint during gait, it can actually attach to the hyaline cartilage surface of the talus and the joint capsule. The scar reduces the articular capacity of the joint by eliminating synovial recesses and can occupy the entire joint cavity if severe enough.

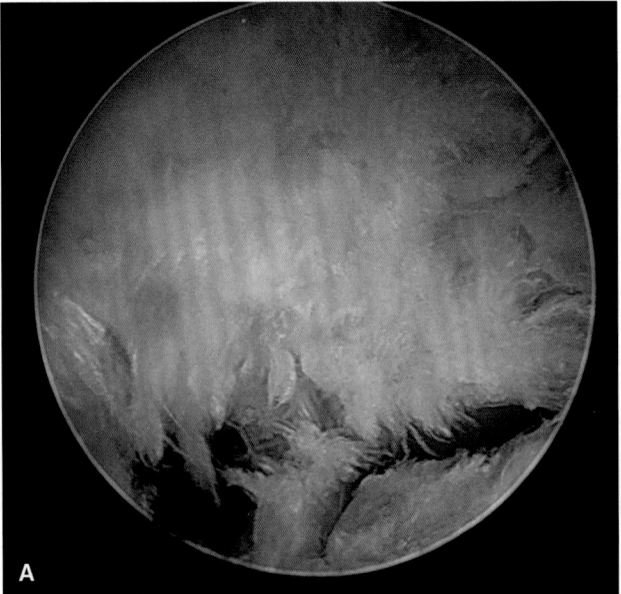
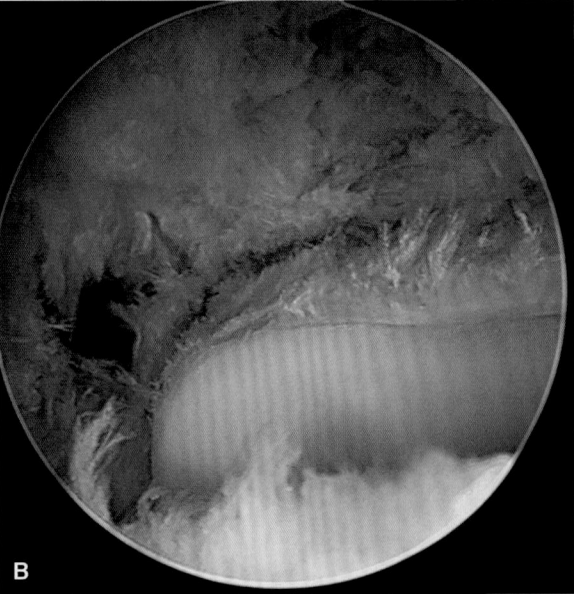

FIGURE 33.7 A, B. Arthrofibrosis; note the excessive scar tissue/synovitis from excessive collagen production and adhesion that results in restricted joint motion and pain.

OSSEOUS AND OSTEOCHONDRAL PATHOLOGY

OSTEOPHYTOSIS

The anterior osteophyte in the ankle is a frequent cause of pain and dysfunction (Fig. 33.8). This lesion is usually post-traumatic in origin and an indicator of degenerative joint disease. The osteophyte may produce bony impingement and, in severe cases, equinus deformity. The lesion may originate from the tibial surface, the talar surface, or both. Lesions extending from the talus are usually extra-articular and not amenable to arthroscopic excision. The anterior tibial lesions are almost always found within the capsular reflection and are clearly amenable to arthroscopic excision.[34-36]

AVULSIONS

Small bony masses are often identified in periarticular areas of the ankle in radiographs of patients with ankle problems. Many times, the nature of the body clearly indicates a traumatic origin. Other periarticular osseous masses may arise from ossific anlage (eg, os subfibulare or os subtibiale). Despite adequate care, these lesions can produce persistent local inflammation, occasionally becoming physically entrapped and changing normal joint mechanics and sometimes causing clicking or crepitus. Instability of the ligamentous complex with which it is associated may also be noted.

OSTEOCHONDRAL LESIONS

Transchondral fracture and similar osteochondral disorders can affect any joint surface. Arthroscopic diagnosis and treatment of these lesions are determined by skill set, technique, instrumentation, and location for each joint. Although arthroscopic treatment of osteochondral defects of the great toe joint has been reported, the clear frequency of the need to perform other reconstructive maneuvers for associated hallux limitus reduces the pool of patients who have clear indication for limited repair of the great toe.[37]

Osteochondral lesions of the talus are relatively frequent and are often associated with significant morbidity (Fig. 33.9).

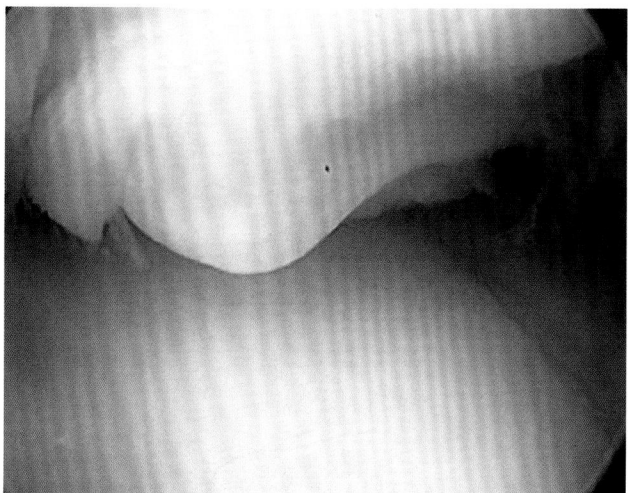

FIGURE 33.8 Anterior tibial osteophyte; note adjacent linear excoriated cartilage groove on talar surface.

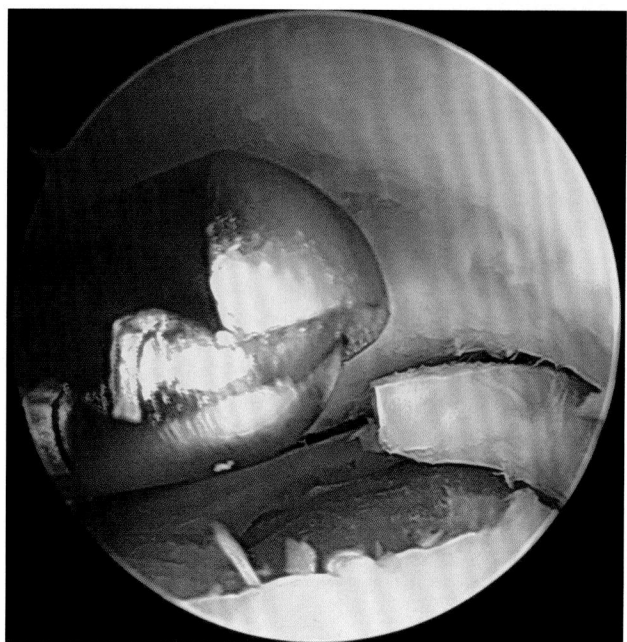

FIGURE 33.9 Anteromedial talar osteochondral lesion.

Pathologic defects involving both the articular and the associated bony portions of the talus encompass a variety of conditions. These conditions include various varieties of transchondral pathology of the talar dome. Berndt and Harty have comprehensively described transchondral fracture, and numerous other authors in the medical literature have discussed the pathophysiology of transchondral fracture at length.[38-45] The frequency of diagnosis of osteochondral fracture of the talar dome has been noted to be increasing, possibly associated with the increased sensitivity of diagnostic modalities in the treatment of foot and ankle disorders.[46] Additionally, cystic changes of the subchondral bone of the talar body and tibial plafond are frequently associated with transchondral defects, as well as other forms of degenerative joint disease.[46,47] Imaging and staging of osteochondral lesions has been greatly enhanced by CT and MRI (Fig. 33.4D).[48-50] Symptoms of osteochondral defects include pain, swelling, catching or locking, instability, and a deep ache. Often, the diagnosis is unclear until three-dimensional images are available. Even with clear delineation of a defect, the incidental finding of asymptomatic osteochondral lesions is common enough to warrant suspicion of other pathology in those cases in which the lesion is small or relatively intact. It is clear that the appearance of any given lesion, identified by any means, often does not correlate well with the symptoms exhibited by the patient.

OTHER OSTEOCARTILAGINOUS LESIONS

Synovial chondromatosis and osteochondromatosis are quite amenable to arthroscopic excision. The diagnosis is made by plain film or advanced imaging techniques. The source of the lesions should be defined and excised wherever possible. The patient should be aware of the palliative nature of this procedure and should expect recurrence over time. Arthroscopic synovectomy seems to reduce the recurrence rate in the knee.[51]

TOPOGRAPHIC ANATOMY

A solid foundation in topographical anatomy is most critical in accurately placing portals. Topographical overlay images are provided to highlight anatomic structures that pertain to common portals (Fig. 33.10). Location of these structures is necessary not only to avoid critical damage but also for proper special positioning to accomplish the surgical goals and access as much of the joint space as possible. In cases involving access of the posterior ankle from an anterior approach, the portal position if placed too high will make it impossible to access the lesion. Knowing the predicted nerve tracts relative to possible portal placement helps avoid inadvertent nerve injury, which is the most common complication. In anterior ankle arthroscopy, the anterior lateral portal can often be close to the intermediate dorsocutaneous nerve (IDCN). By plantarflexing the foot and the fourth toe, traction can be applied to the IDCN and often the nerve tract can be visualized in some patients (Fig. 33.11). Nevertheless, use of sound technique in portal development is essential in cases in which there is anatomic variation of nerves and vessels that cannot be anticipated. In subtalar joint arthroscopy, the most important topographical structure is the floor of the sinus tarsi. The entire surgery is keyed off this location. This is critical for accurate portal placement. The course of the sural nerve is important to understand in situations in which middle portal placement or large bore needles are placed to facilitate removal of air or outflow of fluid.

ARTHROSCOPIC ANATOMY

The ankle joint is divided into two distinct zones: that space between the capsule and the osteocartilaginous surfaces, termed the capsular reflection, and that space located directly between the articular structures of the talus, fibula, and tibia.

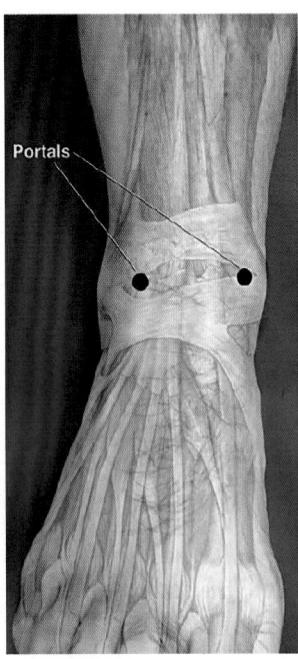

FIGURE 33.10 Topographical anatomy pertaining to portal placement for anterior ankle arthroscopy.

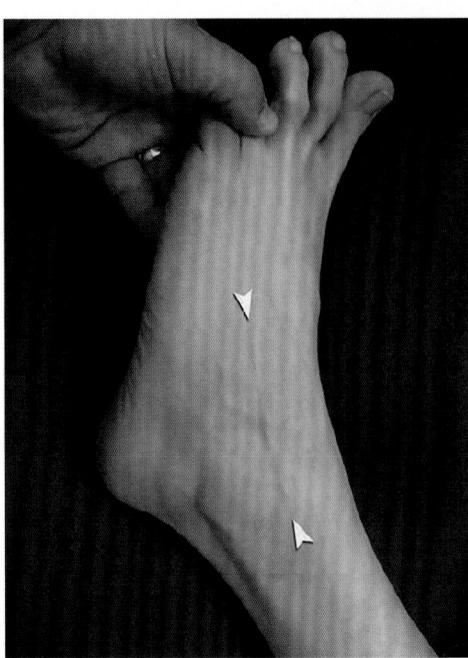

FIGURE 33.11 Passive plantarflexion of foot and fourth toe causing bow stringing (between *arrowheads*) of the IDCN.

The capsular reflection contains significant space, facilitating the arthroscope and arthroscopic instrumentation. The space between the tibial plafond and the talar dome is generally minimal. This space requires distraction or strategic manipulation to access this zone (Fig. 33.12).

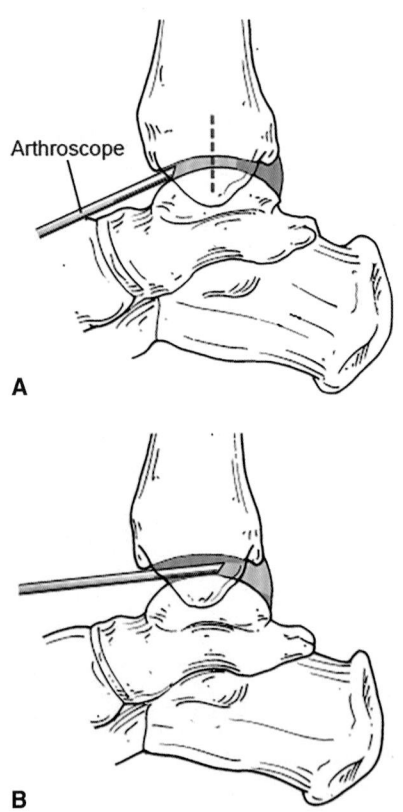

FIGURE 33.12 Diagram illustrating arthroscope access across the talar dome in undistracted joint (**A**) and distracted joint (**B**). Note how the scope orientation changes as it passes posterior.

The joint capsule and pericapsular ligaments define the capsular recesses of the ankle. This capsule is lined with synovial and subsynovial (supporting) tissue that is mainly loose connective tissue containing a network of vascular and lymphatic channels that maintain the intensely well-vascularized synovial bed. Pathologic changes of the synovial and capsular structures are often identified by hyperplasia and injection and with chronic stimulation by metaplasia to dense, space-occupying fibrous tissue. Depending on the situation, intra-articular spaces may be occupied by this pathologic tissue. The normal capsular recess of the ankle is larger anteriorly than posteriorly. The anterior capsular reflection is divided into anterior, lateral, and medial gutters. The anterior gutter is the space directly dorsal to the talar neck and anterior to the tibial surface. The anterior gutter is used to gain initial entry into the ankle joint. The cartilaginous frontier of the talus rims a plateau that rests above the talar neck just distally. The dorsal talar neck is often viewable

without synovial resection. More frequently, the anterior gutter contains proliferative synovium of varying intensity. Portions of the deep deltoid, anterior talofibular, and the distal fascicle of the anterior tibiofibular ligaments can be visualized when entering the ankle arthroscopically (Fig. 33.13). The posterior capsular reflection of the ankle has minimal volume. It is composed of thick fibrous labrum of the posterior tibiofibular ligament, the transverse ligament, and a similar capsular wall. In most patients, this feature limits mobility of the arthroscope and surgical instrumentation. In close juxtaposition to the posterior ankle pouch is the capsular reflection of the posterior facet of the subtalar joint. In the subtalar joint, the posterior capsular reflection of the posterior facet is large and easily accessed from a posterolateral approach located lateral to the Achilles tendon. The anterior portion of the posterior facet is less amply endowed with space, yet it is easily navigated by the floor of the sinus tarsi and the firm nature of the interosseous

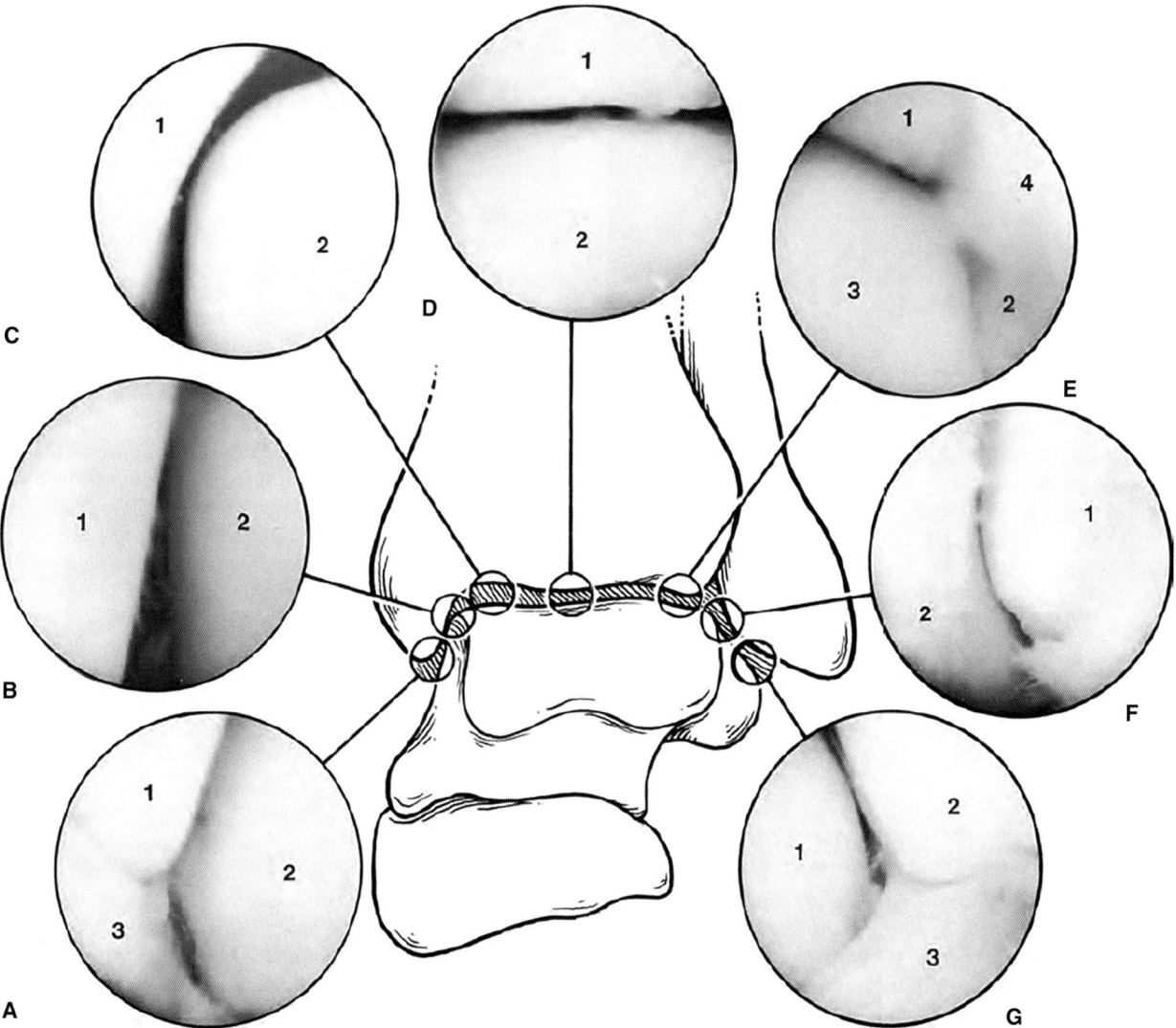

FIGURE 33.13 Normal arthroscopic intra-articular anatomy of the anterior aspect of the ankle. **A.** Deltoid ligament and inferior aspect medial malleolus, talus (*1*, tip of medial malleolus; *2*, talus; *3*, deltoid ligament). **B.** Talar medial malleolar joint (*1*, medial malleolus; *2*, talus). **C.** Medial shoulder to talotibial joint (*1*, tibia; *2*, medial shoulder of talus). **D.** Tibiotalar joint (*1*, tibia; *2*, talus). **E.** Tibiofibular-talar articulation (*1*, tibial; *2*, fibula; *3*, lateral shoulder of talus; *4*, tibiofibular synovial fringe). **F.** Talofibular joint (*1*, lateral malleolus; *2*, talus). **G.** Anterior talofibular ligament and inferior aspect of lateral malleolus, talus (*1*, talus; *2*, tip of lateral malleolus; *3*, anterior talofibular ligament).

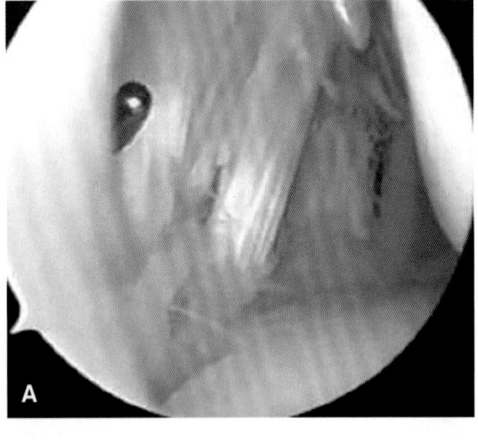
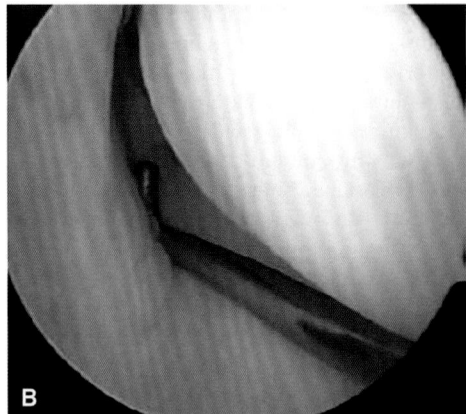
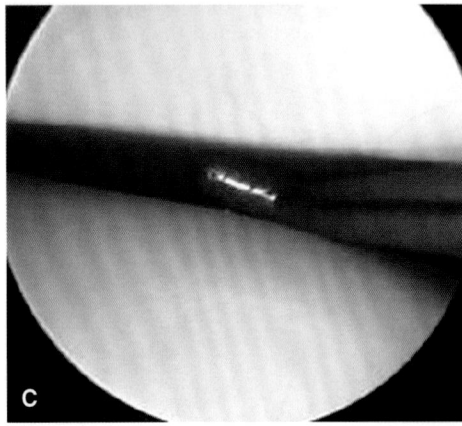

FIGURE 33.14 Arthroscopic images of the normal subtalar joint anatomy. **A.** Anterior capsule and retinacular elements of sinus tarsi. **B.** Interosseous ligament. **C.** Posterior facet.

talocalcaneal ligament, which marks the deep anterior frontier of the joint. The lateral gutter of the subtalar joint is accessible and is deep to the tip of the fibula, calcaneofibular ligament, and peroneal tendons. The instrumentation can run along the calcaneal side of the subtalar joint posterior facet. Then traversing the lateral gutter, it is possible to observe the posterior facet and the "saddle" centrally (Fig. 33.14). The posterior talofibular ligament can be visualized going parallel to the posterior half of the posterior facet and terminating at the posterior process. The posterior tibial joint is typically well visualized from lateral to medial to the flexor hallucis longus tendon sheath.

The great toe joint capsular reflection is present in significant variance of volume on the dorsal aspect of the joint. Degenerative changes associated with hallux limitus and hallux valgus frequently obscure the capsular reflection.

ARTHROSCOPIC INSTRUMENTATION

The arthroscope is essentially a telescope contained within a cannula that both protects the instrument and allows for controlled fluid flow (ingress or egress). Arthroscopes carry peripherally orientated fiberoptic bundles to illuminate the interior of the joint. These bundles are coupled with a rod lens system to carry reflected light images from the joint to the camera. The size of the arthroscope varies from smaller than 1.5 mm to as large as 7.3 mm outside diameter. The outside diameter of the cannula on a 4-mm scope varies to 5.5 mm. The space between the scope and its cannula has a purpose and allows for ingress (or less commonly egress) of fluid to the joint. The amount of fluid ingress is a function of fluid pressure and sheath size. The relative diameter of the arthroscope is important because

it affects the ease of insertion and movement in a small joint, but more importantly, it also significantly determines the functions of the scope: insufflation, illumination, and image transmission. The ability of the instrument to house light-carrying glass bundles, optical glass, and space for fluid transmission is determined by its cross-sectional area (nr). The reader should note that an exponential relationship exists between the diameter and the area available for functions of the scope. A 4-mm arthroscope has more than double the cross-sectional area and capacity of a 2.7-mm arthroscope. The significant reduction in the capacity for fluid insufflation with the smaller diameter scope can be mediated by adding additional fluid from another cannula. The available light and optical surface area are not as easily compensated for. For these reasons and the relative fragility of small arthroscopes, the most commonly used arthroscopes for the ankle and subtalar joints are the 2.9-mm and the 4-mm wide angles. In the great toe joint and other tarsal joints, the 2-2.9 mm systems are the most appropriate. An adequate light source is critical to success of an arthroscopic procedure. Typically, most systems employ controlled light generated from a halogen or metal halide light source carried to the joint cavity by fiberoptic glass bundles attached to the arthroscope. Most systems employ automatic light intensity controls and a white balance feature to optimize the video image. The tip of the scope is usually angled from the long axis of the instrument to allow for improved field of view and to allow view around corners. Common tip cut angles are 30 and 70 degrees (Figs. 33.15 to 33.17). Although there is some variability, the orientation of the tip cut is usually opposite that of the light post. The field of view of the scope is also variable between manufacturers. Improvements in optics have allowed wide angle view, facilitating small joint visualization. Some newer cameras will convert

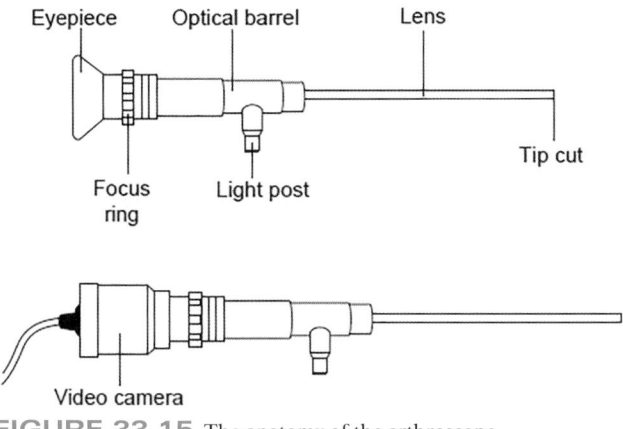

FIGURE 33.15 The anatomy of the arthroscope.

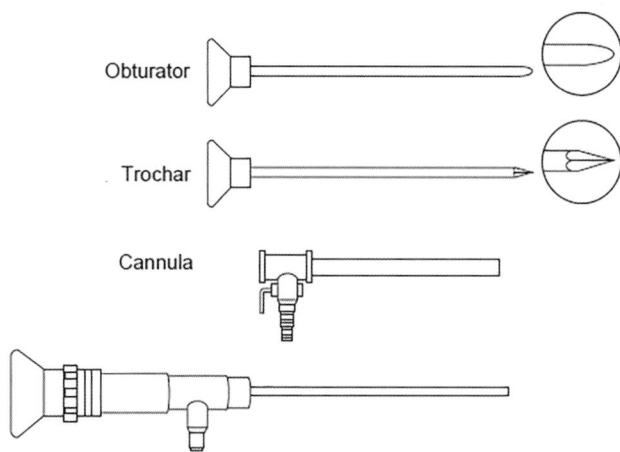

FIGURE 33.17 Instruments used to introduce the arthroscope into the joint.

the optical image received to a digitally compressed image for higher resolution. Most arthroscopy employs high-resolution video systems (camera and monitor) to allow the surgeon to visualize the optical field indirectly. This method of visualization has significantly improved the ease of viewing of the surgical field and secondarily facilitated recording.[52]

HAND INSTRUMENTS

A large variety of instruments have been developed for arthroscopy. Those instruments suited for ankle and subtalar arthroscopy generally have outside diameters smaller than 5 mm. Those that are useful in the other joints of the foot are usually smaller than 3 mm in diameter. Available nonmotorized

hand instruments include various probes, knives, graspers, and punches (Fig. 33.18). Aspirated motorized instruments (cutters, shavers, and abraders) have made a large impact on the surgeon's ability to cut, remove, and manipulate because under many circumstances, they are more efficient (Fig. 33.19).

HERMOABLATIVE TOOLS

Other tools available to the arthroscopic surgeon include arthroscopic radiofrequency wands that can vaporize, shrink, coagulate, and even weld tissue. Although arthroscopic laser technology has been available for more than 15 years, it remains as controversial as it is expensive, requires special training, and remains unproven with regard to the benefits that may be obtained.[53] The radiofrequency wand technology has advanced significantly in recent years to effectively manage soft tissue pathology, especially in a "cleanup" role after the bulk of the soft tissue has been removed. Instrument tips vary in size to adapt to small- and medium-sized joints. Proper fluid management is important to regulate intra-articular temperature with these devices; this is combined with surgeon-controlled power adjustments to match tissue density and response to thermoablation. Some radiofrequency wands are now aspirated to allow for suction application to assist with fluid flow management and to draw tissue into the wand tip (Fig. 33.20).

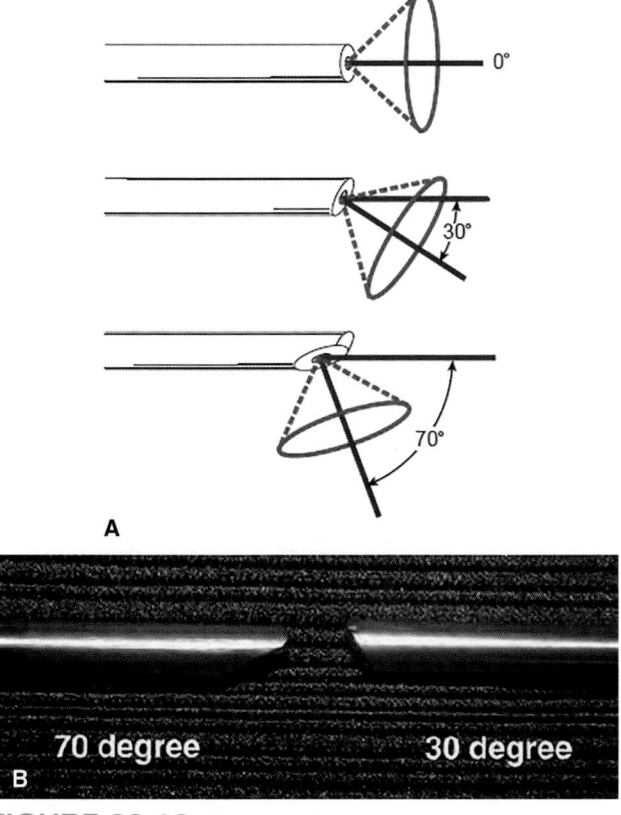

FIGURE 33.16 **A.** Effect of tip cut of various types of arthroscopes. **B.** Close-up comparison of 30- and 70-degree tip cuts.

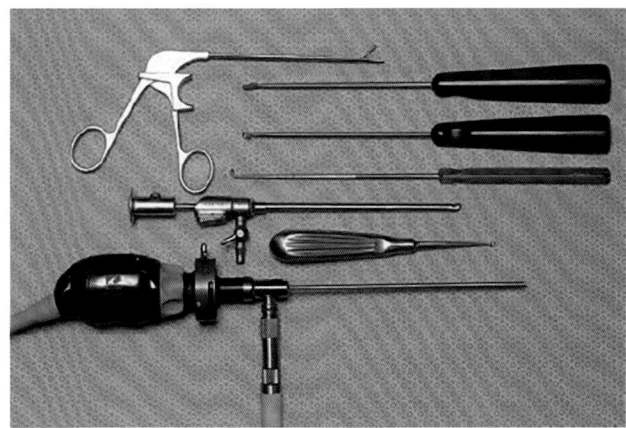

FIGURE 33.18 Appearance of a typical Mayo stand setup for foot and ankle arthroscopy.

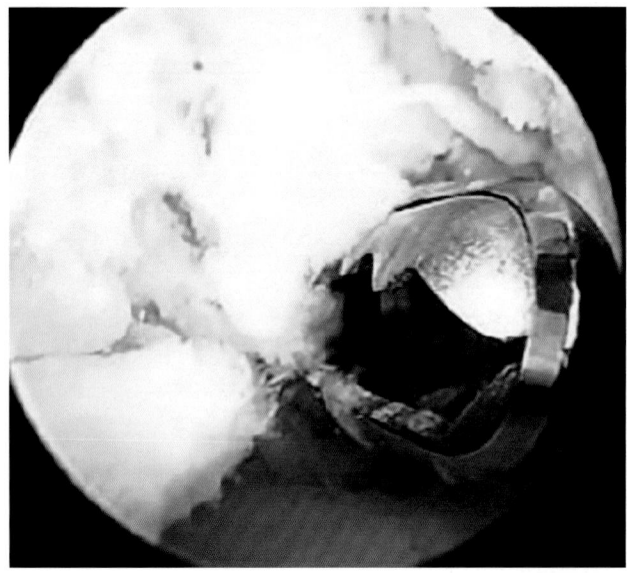

FIGURE 33.19 A 3.5-mm motorized arthroscopic shaver.

TREATMENT

ANTERIOR ANKLE ARTHROSCOPY

- General anesthesia.
- Positioned in supine position on operating room table.
- +/− placement of well-padded thigh tourniquet.
- Rolled blanket under ipsilateral hip.
- +/− placement in well-padded thigh holder.
- Preoperative local anesthetic block (adductor canal block with saphenous nerve supplementation or proximal ankle block).
- Extremity prepped and draped in usual sterile fashion with arthroscopic drape if available.
- Plantarflexion of ankle and identification/marking of intermediate dorsal cutaneous nerve.
- Confirm arthroscopy equipment is working.
  - Camera light is on and white balanced

- Cannula is connected to fluid of choice. 3L of NS or LR with or without epinephrine. Use of pump or gravity inflow
- Suction is connected to shaver
- Viewing monitor positioned for easy visualization by surgeon
- Exsanguination and tourniquet inflation (only if necessary for visualization).
- +/− application of noninvasive or invasive distractor with distraction of ankle joint.
- Insufflation of ankle joint through notch of Harty with 10-15 mL of NS or LR or local anesthetic.
  - Watch for outpouching of anterolateral capsular wall
  - Watch for slight dorsiflexion of the foot on the ankle if not in distractor
- Anteromedial portal: Use 15 blade to make vertical incision medial to anterior tibial tendon avoiding saphenous nerve and vein.
- Blunt dissection through subcutaneous tissue and capsule with curved Kelly hemostat.
- Use blunt trocar attach to cannula to enter the ankle joint with dorsiflexion of ankle joint to prevent iatrogenic scuffing of cartilage.
- Begin ingress through cannula.
- Insert 4.0- or 2.9-mm 30-degree arthroscope.
- Adjust the focus and perform brief survey of the ankle joint.
- *Anterolateral portal:* Make portal lateral to peroneus teritus and away from previously marked IDCN. A 18-gauge needle can be inserted prior incision to help adjust the appropriate height to correlate with the primary pathology in the ankle being treated. Use a 15 blade to make a vertical incision.
- Blunt dissection through subcutaneous tissue and capsule with curved Kelly hemostat with penetration into the ankle joint. Dorsiflex the ankle during this to prevent iatrogenic scuffing of cartilage.
- Insert shaver or instrumentation into anterolateral portal.
- Perform 21 point examination (Fig. 33.13). Switch portals if necessary.
- Treatment of ankle pathology visualized.
- Closure with surgeon's preference of suture.

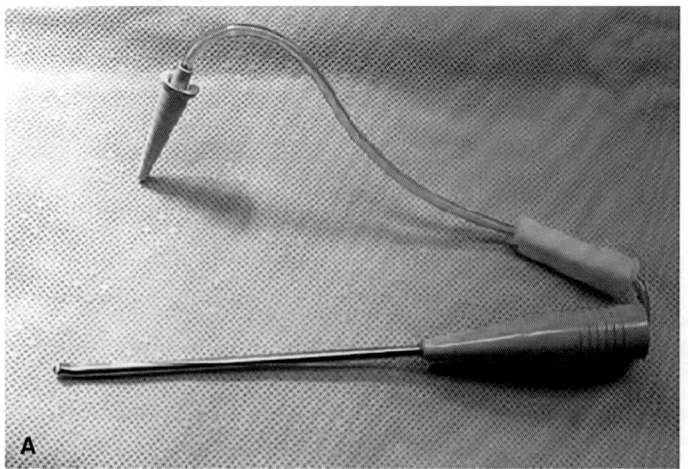
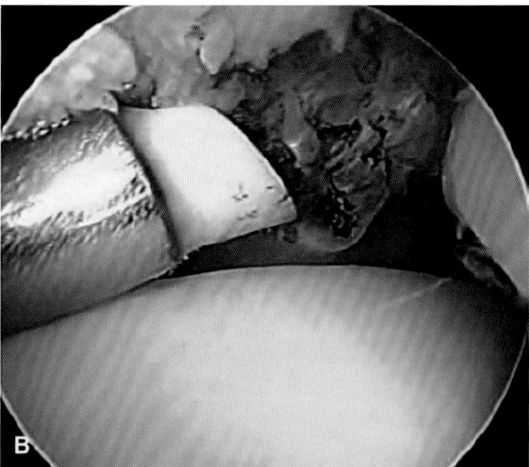

FIGURE 33.20 A. Example of a bipolar radiofrequency wand. Note 50-degree angle at tip and aspirated system. **B.** Bipolar wand being used to ablate anterolateral impingement.

SUBTALAR JOINT ARTHROSCOPY

- General anesthesia.
- Positioned in supine or lateral position on operating room table.
- +/− placement of well-padded thigh tourniquet.
- Preoperative local anesthetic block (ankle block).
- Extremity prepped and draped in usual sterile fashion with arthroscopic drape if available.
- Confirm arthroscopy equipment is working.
  - Camera light is on and white balanced
  - Cannula is connected to fluid of choice
  - Suction is connected to shaver
  - Viewing monitor positioned for easy visualization by surgeon
- Exsanguination and tourniquet inflation.
- Insufflation of subtalar joint through anterior portal with 10-15 mL of NS or LR.
- Anterior portal: ~1 cm distal to fibular tip and 2 cm anterior to the lateral malleolus. Use 15 blade to make vertical incision.
- Blunt dissection through subcutaneous tissue and capsule with curved Kelly hemostat with penetration into the anterior subtalar joint.
- Insert cannula with blunt trocar to floor of sinus tarsi.
- Begin ingress of fluid and remove trocar.
- Insert 30-degree 2.9- or 4.0-mm oblique arthroscope.
- Middle portal: Just anterior to the tip of the fibula, directly over the sinus tarsi. This can be made under direct visualization with 18 gauge needle to evaluate appropriate position prior to incision. Use 15 blade to make incision.
- Blunt dissection through subcutaneous tissue and capsule with curved Kelly hemostat.
- Insert shaver into middle portal.
- Treatment of subtalar joint pathology identified.
- Closure with surgeon's preference of suture.

POSTERIOR ANKLE ARTHROSCOPY/ARTHROSCOPIC OS TRIGONUM EXCISION

- Positioned in prone position on operating room table. Adequate padding on patients head, chest, knees, elbows, and shins. Feet are hanging off the operative table.
- +/− placement of well-padded thigh tourniquet.
- Preoperative local anesthetic block (ankle block).
- Extremity prepped and draped in usual sterile fashion with arthroscopic drape if available.
- Confirm arthroscopy equipment is working.
  - Camera light is on and white balanced
  - Cannula is connected to fluid of choice
  - Suction is connected to shaver
  - Viewing monitor positioned for easy visualization by surgeon
- Exsanguination and tourniquet inflation.
- With the ankle in neutral position, mark with a pen a line from the tip of the lateral malleolus to the Achilles tendon, parallel to the sole of the foot (para Achilles).
- Insufflation of subtalar joint through posterolateral portal with 10-15 mL of NS or LR can be performed but is not necessary.
- Posterolateral portal: Just lateral to Achilles tendon just above the line marked previously. Use 15 blade to make vertical incision.

- Blunt dissection through subcutaneous tissue and capsule with curved Kelly hemostat with penetration into the posterior ankle and subtalar joints aiming for second digit.
- Insert cannula with blunt trocar.
- Begin ingress of fluid and remove trocar.
- Insert 2.9- or 4.0-mm 30-degree oblique arthroscope.
- Posteromedial portal: Just medial to Achilles tendon at the same level of posterolateral portal. Can verify position with 18-gauge needle prior to incision. Use 15 blade to make vertical incision.
- Blunt dissection through subcutaneous tissue and capsule with curved Kelly hemostat with penetration into the posterior ankle and subtalar joints aiming for arthroscope and lateral spreading soft tissue away from the lens.
- Insert shaver with teeth of the shaver facing laterally.
- Begin initial debridement and synovectomy to create space in the posterior aspect of ankle and subtalar joint, staying lateral to FHL and medial to the peroneal tendons. Make sure to keep FHL in view during procedure to avoid damaging the medial neurovascular bundle. Passive range of motion of the hallux will help with identification of FHL.
- Debridement and removal of os trigonum can be performed with combination of shaver, burr, and graspers.
- Closure with surgeon's preference of suture.

positioning **PEARLS**

- Ankle arthroscopy
  - Supine with knee straight or bent over knee stirrup or over the end of the table
  - +/- noninvasive or invasive distractor
  - Podiatry ramp/bump (Fig. 33.21)
- Subtalar arthroscopy
  - Lateral recumbent
- Posterior joint arthroscopy
  - Prone
  - Feet hanging off the table

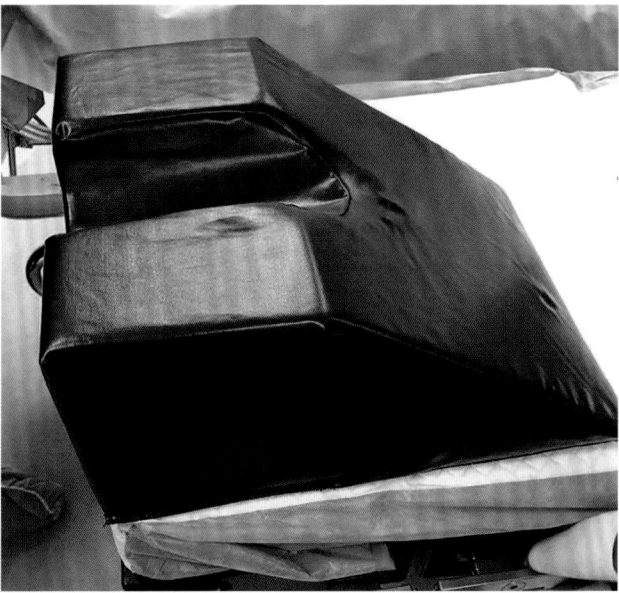

FIGURE 33.21 "Podiatry bump."

ARTHROSCOPIC FUNDAMENTALS

POSITIONING

Individual techniques in the application of arthroscopic technology may vary by surgeon, but ultimately, the basics remain the same. For ankle arthroscopy, the patient is typically placed supine, with the knee either straight or bent over a knee stirrup or over the end of the table. The author's preference is to place the knee straight, unless the noninvasive ankle distractor is used, in which case the knee and hip are flexed. Some surgeons prefer the patient supine, with the knee flexed over the end of the table, the surgeon sitting directly in front of the dependent leg and ankle. For subtalar joint arthroscopy, a lateral recumbent position facilitates access to the sinus tarsi and the posterior ankle and foot. A prone position may be desirable for situation of more involved posterior joint pathology.[54,55] These situations may require the use of both the posterior lateral and medial portals. Some authors recommend the use of an arthroscopic leg holder. This accessory device may be helpful in some cases in which additional leg stabilization or leg elevation off the operating table surface is necessary (Fig. 33.22). However, in the vast majority of cases, simple padding, straps, and sand bags offer sufficient positioning assistance and immobilization.

HEMOSTASIS

Tourniquet or pharmacologic hemostasis during arthroscopic surgery of the foot and ankle is not mandatory. Multiple studies have shown that anterior ankle arthroscopy can be adequately performed without use of a tourniquet.[56,57] The pressure of distension is usually adequate to maintain a blood-free field. To increase the pressure, raise the bag height for increased gravity inflow and better hemostasis. In those cases in which bleeding is excessive, a small quantity of 1:1000 concentration epinephrine added to the ingress fluid (3 L bag with 3 mL of epinephrine) is often sufficient to control small vessel hemorrhage. A tourniquet placed either at the thigh or proximal to the ankle is a safe method for managing bleeding when it is excessive or when epinephrine is either ineffective or contraindicated (Fig. 33.22). The use of thermoablative wands toward the end of

the procedure can facilitate a more rapid cleanup and also help manage bleeding from soft tissues. At the completion of the operative portion of the procedure, the surgical site is assessed for hemostasis. When there is any question of vascular injury associated with portal development, the tourniquet is released before application of the bandage for inspection and potential ligation of any bleeding vessels. In some situations in which significant intra-articular bleeding is noted, an active, closed suction drain is easily placed through the portal into the joint.

JOINT DISTENSION AND FLUIDS

Once the patient is anesthetized and a sterile field has been created, the ankle joint can be distended with fluid. This is usually done before portal development to permit maximal distension of the capsule. The accuracy of portal orientation is enhanced by tactile feel of the needle traversing the proposed path of the arthroscope. Because they are fundamental to joint visualization, distension and maintenance of distension are two of the most important principles of joint arthroscopy. Usually, lactated Ringer or normal saline is used because they are readily available. Questions have been raised as to which fluid is best for performing arthroscopy. Of common fluids available to the surgeon, lactated Ringer is more physiologic than normal saline in all models.[58-60] While there are solutions that may be more physiologic to cartilage cells in the laboratory setting, there is no evidence that more expensive solutions are clinically justified. Distension is maintained by balancing the ingress and egress of fluid from the joint. Gravity drainage or active pumps are used to deliver fluid, usually through the cannula of the arthroscope. When using a small-diameter arthroscopic cannula, distension is often supplemented from a separate ingress cannula. Drainage of fluid from the ankle joint is through cannulas and more commonly along the surface of the instruments inserted in the portal. Maintenance of appropriate distension pressure is sometimes a complex and changing problem, requiring the surgeon's attention as the case progresses.[61] The surgeon and the assistants should regularly take note of the periarticular soft tissues to observe for potential fluid accumulation in the fascial planes about the ankle. Although there are no reports of significant morbidity from this situation in the ankle, it is usually avoidable and should be corrected, if possible. Compartment syndrome as a result of fluid extravasation is a potential complication in knee arthroscopy but has not yet been reported in ankle arthroscopy. The distended joint is identified by a visible and palpable "bubble" of distended capsule. In ankle arthroscopy, the ankle joint is often noted to dorsiflex slightly as the end stage of capsular distension draws the foot into dorsiflexion. This phenomenon is a product of the anterior capsular structures drawing the talus up as volume within the joint is accommodated. The volume of fluid that is typically injected when meeting resistance is between 15 and 40 mL, depending on local factors including size and anatomic variation. Introduction of the arthroscopic cannula and associated instruments through the capsule is facilitated by a tautness of the capsule. This tautness can be maximized by reinflating the joint immediately before introducing the cannula, thereby simultaneously maximizing the available volume in the anterior joint pouch and the tension of the joint capsule. A distinct end point in distension will not occur when there is communication of the ankle joint with other periarticular structures. Communication

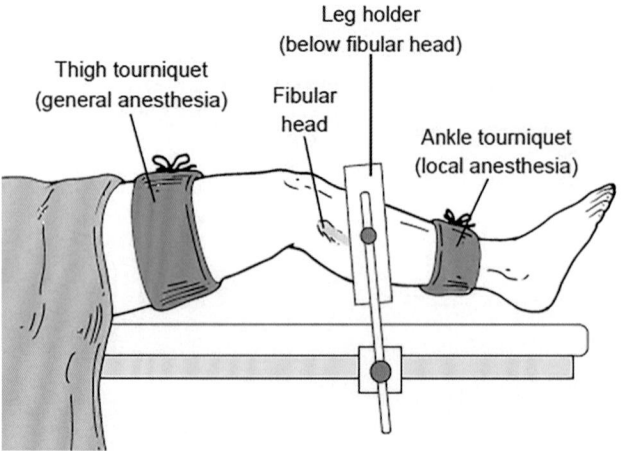

FIGURE 33.22 Illustration of one type of positioning and support of the leg with tourniquet positioning options.

Leg holder
(below fibular head)

Thigh tourniquet
(general anesthesia)

Fibular head

Ankle tourniquet
(local anesthesia)

with and extravasation into the tendon sheaths of the peroneus longus and brevis, tibialis posterior, flexor hallucis, peroneus tertius, and the subtalar joint are all possible. The lack of an end point may not necessarily be associated with a communication because a simple rent in the capsule with extravasation into the local soft tissue may also occur. Intra-articular placement of local anesthetics after completion of the arthroscopic procedure is common practice.

JOINT DISTRACTION

Separating the ankle joint surfaces to allow passage of the arthroscope is variably accomplished by a large number of arthroscopic surgeons.[62-66] Distraction permits the surgeon to manipulate the arthroscope and its associated instrumentation within the joint without inadvertently damaging or "scuffing" the joint surfaces. Keep in mind, distraction will also bring the anterior neurovascular bundle closer to the joint and risk inadvertent damage.[67] The methodology for distracting the joint is either invasive (employing a device that directly engages bone) or noninvasive (using straps or bands) to pull the articular structures apart physically. Devices vary significantly in complexity, cost, and efficacy. A simple noninvasive distraction involves using bandages or straps affixed to the foot, then applying distal traction either by attaching them to weights or to the surgeon himself, who then leans backward from the ankle (Fig. 33.23).[65,66] Commercially available noninvasive distraction systems employing mechanical distractors fastened to the operating table, then applied to a padded clove hitch strap binding the hindfoot, are available and have a proven record of safety in the adult patient (Fig. 33.24). Countertraction for most noninvasive methods is very helpful. A urologic knee stirrup placed in the popliteal fossa is often helpful in providing countertraction. As with scenarios involving positioning a patient, serious care of subcutaneous neurovascular structures are necessary to

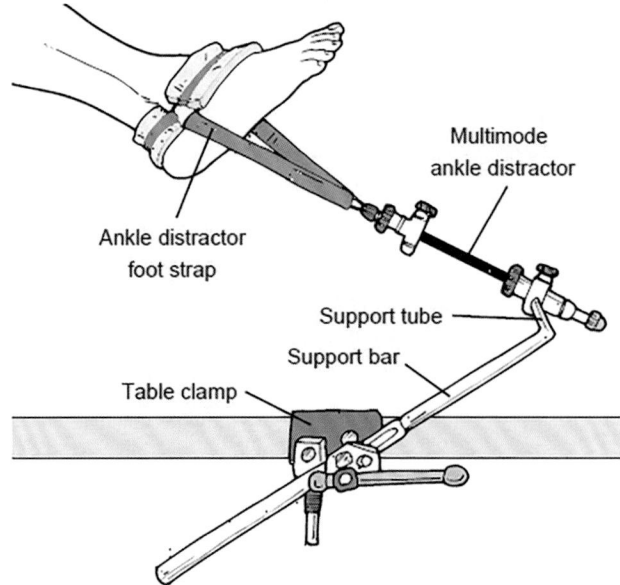

FIGURE 33.24 Illustration of joint noninvasive joint distraction setup.

prevent complications. It is quite clear that a well-distended, "loose" ankle joint will allow the experienced arthroscopic surgeon access to the majority of the pathology in the anterior two-thirds of the joint. Laxity of the collateral ligaments, allowing inversion of the talus within the mortise, facilitates entry into the lateral gutter and under the anterior syndesmotic ligament and over the talar dome. Strategic dorsiflexion and plantarflexion manipulation of the talus facilitates excellent visualization of the majority of the talar and tibial surfaces of the joint. In a minority of patients, a tight joint, especially with limited plantarflexion, requires significant physical distraction to see beyond the dorsal most portion of the talus. Degenerative joint disease with significant osteophytosis of the anterior tibial lip impairs visualization of the dome of the talus. Surgical reduction using burr, osteotome, or gouge of the impinging anterior lip is helpful in improving visualization. The combination of reduction of the anterior tibial lip and strategic manipulation allows the majority of cases to occur without the need for application of joint distraction. It is, however, recommended that an ankle joint distractor be available for use in the operative setting for all cases that may need this strategy to meet the goals of surgery. Distraction is routinely used in those situations in which the pathology is in the posterior half of the ankle compartment. Physical distraction of the subtalar joint is usually not necessary because the capsular reflection of the joint usually provides adequate room for instrumentation. Distraction of the great toe joint and intertarsal joints is usually very helpful for adequate joint visualization. A Chinese finger trap-type noninvasive distractor attached to 5-15 pounds of distraction or an invasive minirail distractor that bridges the joint is helpful in maintaining adequate working space.

PORTALS

Portals through the soft tissues to the ankle joint are required for passage of the arthroscope and instrumentation. These portals can be safely developed with careful technique and

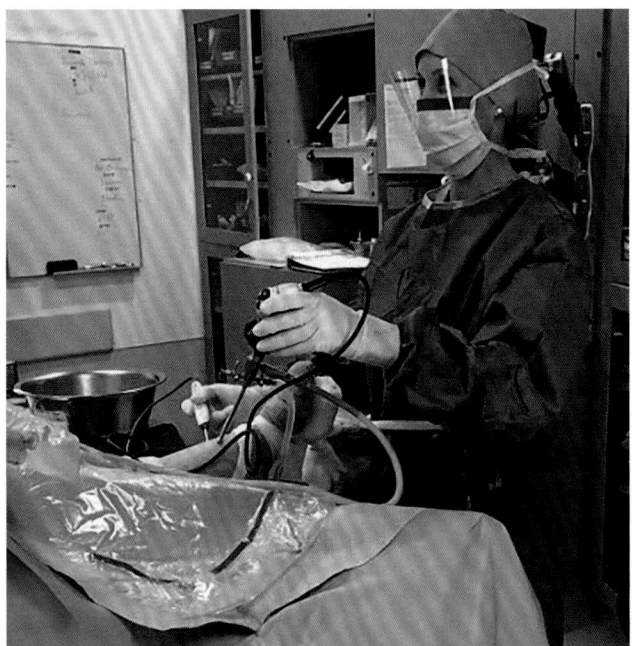

FIGURE 33.23 Demonstrating simple noninvasive distraction method with use of Kerlix roll wrapped around surgeon. The surgeon simply leans back to distract the joint.

TABLE **33.2**	**Common Foot and Ankle Arthroscopic Portals**	
Ankle	Anteromedial	Common utility portal, usually the first portal developed to inventory the anterior pathology
	Anterolateral	Common portal usually used in combination with anteromedial portal. IDCN can be in close proximity to this portal
	Central	Considered an accessory portal, higher risk portal due to proximity of dorsalis pedis and deep peroneal nerve
	Posteromedial	This portal is rarely used due to higher risk with neurovascular bundle. Safer if placed adjacent to medial border of Achilles tendon
	Posterolateral	Common portal for fluid egress or posterior ankle pathology switch stick accessible
Subtalar	Posterolateral	Common utility portal, especially for posterior subtalar joint pathology, switch stick accessible
	Anterior lateral	Main access portal located at floor of sinus tarsi. Used for anterior, lateral gutter, and posterior access
	Lateral central	This portal has higher risk due to proximity of sural nerve generally used for egress of fluids
	Accessory anterior	Common use for stacked portal technique when anterior pouch pathology encountered
	Posteromedial	Less commonly used, best placed at adjacent to medial border of Achilles. Often necessary portal when treating flexor hallucis longus pathology
First MTPJ	Dorsomedial	Utility portal used in conjunction with dorsolateral portal for dorsal pathology and plantar medial portal for plantar pathology
	Dorsolateral	Accessory portal for dorsal joint pathology
	Plantarmedial	Less commonly used but necessary for plantar or sesamoid pathology

placement. Ideally, once a portal has been developed and the cannula inserted, the cannula can be left in place for safe exchange of instrumentation. With the small instrumentation required for ankle and foot arthroscopy, this procedure is often limited by the lack of availability of instrumentation that fits. Often, instrumentation is carefully inserted into the ankle and other joints of the foot without a cannula. However, overinstrumentation of a portal can lead to creating a large breach of the joint capsule and increase the rate of fluid extravasation into the surrounding soft tissue envelope. Available portals are listed that are commonly in arthroscopic approaches of the foot and ankle (Table 33.2). It is important for the surgeon to be familiar with topographical anatomy; it is more critical to use sound technique to develop portals since superficial nerve position can be variable and prone to injury.[68] Portal position can be most critical when the scope needs to cross the articular surface deep into the joint. In this situation, the scope must be tangential to the articular surface. It is sometimes wise to use a needle to double-check portal placements, especially in extremities with large amounts of subcutaneous fat deposition and when ankles are being distracted (since this can cause shifting of topographic landmarks) (Figs. 33.25 and 33.26). Introducing a large bore needle will also allow egress for better visualization prior to making additional portals.

POSTERIOR PORTAL DEVELOPMENT (SWITCHING STICK MANEUVER)

Due to individual variation in the soft tissues surrounding the posterior ankle, it can be difficult to judge the precise location of the joint line and make accurate portal development difficult. A switching stick maneuver can be employed to develop posterior lateral ankle, as well as posterior subtalar portals. The switching stick maneuver in the ankle can be used in a loose or well-distracted joint with instrumentation and scope already present in the anterior compartment, a thin rod or probe with

a blunt tip can be directed across the joint from anteromedial to tent the posterolateral capsule. Once an appropriate opening in the skin is made, the rod can be pushed through the soft tissues.[69]

In the subtalar joint, a switching stick maneuver can be very useful in developing the posterior portal. This is accomplished by placing the obturator without the cannula in the anterior portal and advancing it along the lateral gutter through the posterior capsule and terminating adjacent to the Achilles tendon. The skin is tented up and incised to expose the obturator tip. The cannula now can be placed over the obturator and accurately placed within the joint.

GENERAL TREATMENT APPROACH

When possible, at the start of the case, it is wise to perform a survey of the entire ankle joint to inventory the pathology present. This can be performed within a couple of minutes. We recommend capturing the intra-articular pathology with photos. The pathology can then be prioritized. Since there is a finite time frame to perform the surgery (before fluid extravasation limits visibility), it is important for the surgeon to remain focused on the most important pathology.

PEARLS

- Insufflate joint
- Map out all neurovascular anatomy
- Confirm all equipment is ready for use/white balance
- Proper portal placement
- Dorsiflex ankle with obturator/curved Kelly hemostat insertion
- Direct visualization and confirmation with needle prior to portal incision

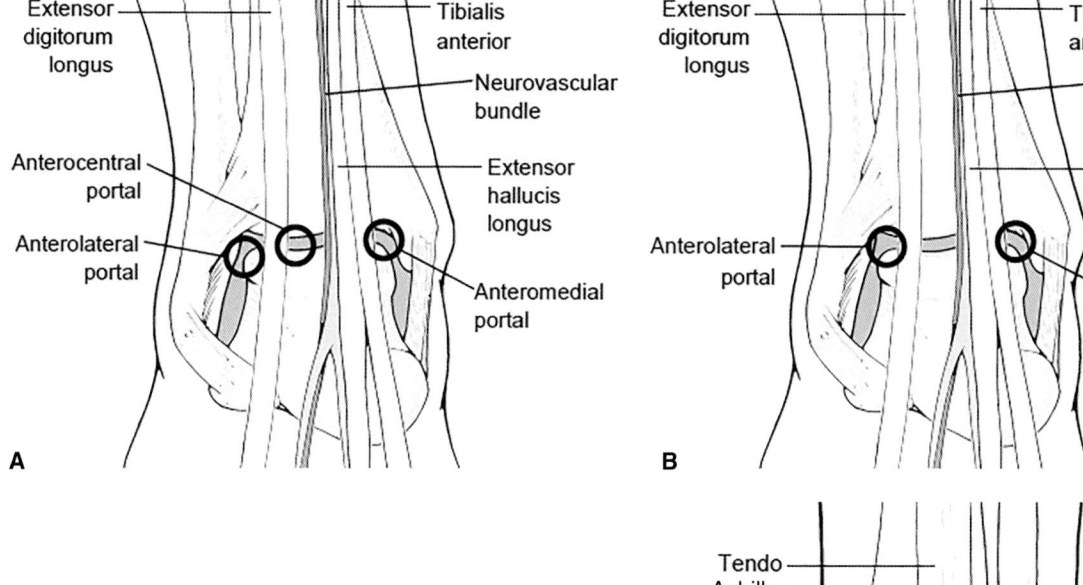

FIGURE 33.25 Classic portals of the anterior and posterior ankle. **A.** Anterior three-portal technique. **B.** Anterior two portal technique. **C.** Posterior portal placement.

ARTHROSCOPIC LAVAGE (SEPTIC ARTHRITIS)

Arthroscopic joint lavage for the acutely inflamed or "hot" joint resulting from abnormal metabolic, autoimmune, and infectious processes is often indicated. Diagnosis and debridement of tophaceous gout and pseudogout deposits of the ankle and other joints of the foot is a relatively common occurrence in foot and ankle arthroscopy. Although septic arthritis is uncommon in the foot and ankle, the arthroscope is clearly a significant tool in the surgical drainage and irrigation of the septic joint.[70,71]

DEBRIDEMENT OF IMPINGEMENT LESIONS

In most cases, debridement of the local hypertrophic synovium and other impinged pathologic soft tissues (fibrous bands, cartilaginous tissue, adhesions, poorly differentiated soft tissue) reduces symptoms (Fig. 33.2).[72-75] The more hyalinized tissue will not respond well to motorized resection. However, this tissue is very responsive to biter followed by debridement with the shaver or thermoablative energy, especially while under tension. Care should be utilized to avoid thermal injury to the adjacent cartilaginous tissue. An emphasis of local removal of impingement tissue without extensive debridement of reactive synovitis is recommended to reduce the incidence of hemarthrosis

and arthrofibrosis. Fundamental to this process is the skillful use of the motorized shaver. There are several factors that are at the control of the surgeon. First is the section of the shaver size and design. By design, there is a spectrum of aggressiveness to shaver (some designs have toothed cutting blades or larger apertures) (Fig. 33.5). Other important surgeon-controlled factors include RPMs of the shaver, shave suction and directionality, and action of the cutting blade. Counterintuitive is the concept that slower shaver speed has increased aggression. The tissue simply has more time to be drawn into the shaver aperture. However, many surgeons feel there is more shaver control at lower RPMs.

DEBRIDEMENT FOR ARTHROFIBROSIS

Treatment in these situations can be difficult. To try to salvage the situation, it becomes necessary to remove all scar tissue connections along the anterior tibial lip and both medial and lateral gutters with motorized resection often with aggressive shavers. The frayed margins of the scar should then be further reduced with thermoablative techniques. Immobilization should be avoided, and continuous passive motion can be very helpful in this situation postoperatively to guide the scar into forming a new capsule that has improved compliance and allow for unrestricted movement of articular surfaces.

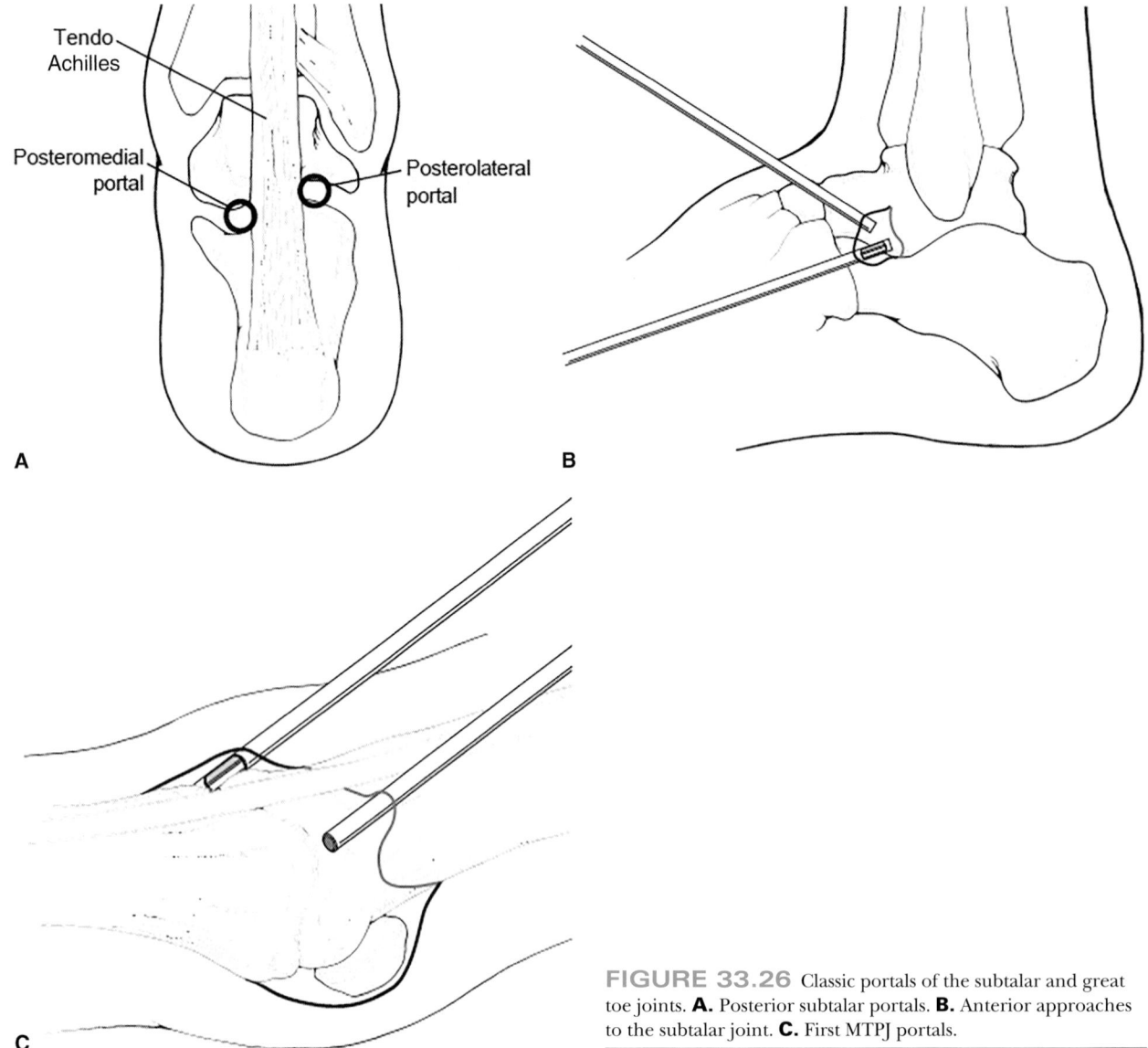

FIGURE 33.26 Classic portals of the subtalar and great toe joints. **A.** Posterior subtalar portals. **B.** Anterior approaches to the subtalar joint. **C.** First MTPJ portals.

Blind resection is the advanced technique used to treat arthrofibrosis. In this setting, the surgeon can be faced with a joint in which the capsule is scarified and there is reduced volume for normal insufflation of the joint. In the ankle, when the arthroscope is centrally placed, visualization is poor, but with experience, the surgeon can feel that the scope is properly placed. After a second portal is developed, the shaver is triangulated to the center next to the scope. Very carefully, the shaver is used to create a small pocket next to the scope and the cutting edge should face bone to protect other structures (blind resection). Once hyaline cartilage is visible and the anterior tibial lip is observed, the arthrofibrotic tissue can be successfully removed.

ANKLE STABILIZATION

The anterior talofibular ligament is a prominent anatomic feature of the anterolateral gutter. Ankle joint instability as a result of ligamentous incompetence of the talofibular ligament is both

visible and repairable by arthroscopic technique.[76-78] The surgeon considering arthroscopic repair of inversion ankle instability understands that limited repair of the anterior talofibular ligament is satisfying in that surgical morbidity is reduced with this technique as compared with formal ligament repair or reconstruction. This arthroscopic repair has shown comparable outcomes but has not shown an advantage when compared to the open technique.[78,79] The degree of soundness of the repair as to its long-term outcome and its comparison to other techniques has yet to be determined.[78] Anterior talofibular ligament repair has since been modified to an arthroscopically assisted limited suture technique.[80,81]

ANKLE OSTEOPLASTY (ARTHRITIC SPURS)

Osteoplasty is accomplished with small abraders, or for sclerotic bone, with a small osteotome or gouge guided arthroscopically while the assistant applies the mallet. Care is taken to avoid damage to the articular dome of the talus.

Aggressive resection of the tibial osteophyte is recommended (Fig. 33.7). On occasion, the osteophytic proliferation protrudes to the opposing joint surface, causing secondary linear striations or gouging of the articular surface. Findings marked by crepitus, grinding, and inflammatory symptoms that are out of proportion should lead one to consider the possibility of this lesion. Other degenerative changes within the ankle compartment, including the varying types of chondromalacia, osteophytic proliferation of the periarticular fibula, talus, and tibia, respond variably to arthroscopic arthroplasty. Although some authors have reported significant improvement in symptoms after 1 year, others have identified the procedure with poor outcomes.[81] As with open arthroplasty, debridement of osteoarthritic change is a palliative measure and continued degeneration is to be expected. Just as clearly, successful palliative arthroscopic debridement takes significant advantage of the reduced morbidity of the arthroscopic approach.

OSTEOCHONDRAL LESION TREATMENT

Arthroscopic treatment of transchondral fractures has the same surgical goals as open treatment: removal of loose bone and cartilage followed by the creation of a vascularized bed of tissue that has great potential to form fibrocartilage. The approach is with arthroscope and instruments inserted from the anterior approach in the majority of cases.[82] To clean out the defect, fragments and debris need to be carefully removed to avoid enlarging the cartilage surface defect and edges need to be resected to stable 90-degree margins. Arthroscopic graspers, angled curettes, hemostats, and motorized shavers are helpful with this process (Fig. 33.27A). Concerning lesions on the talar shoulder, it is critical to probe the gutter for cartilage debris, which can be hidden. Impacted debris can be felt with the probe and pulled out of the gutter for retrieval. Thermoablation should only be used on a limited basis when cleaning out the osteochondral defect to avoid creating a pocket of thermonecrosis and chondrocyte death, which may limit or impair the formation of high-quality fibrocartilage.[83] Posterior lesions are sometimes approached from the posterior or transosseous (transtalar or transmalleolar) approach. The use of aiming guides is extremely helpful in planning and placing portals.[84-86] Ferkel has developed a miniature C-guide for ankle and small joints, similar to larger C-guides used in knee reconstruction. Open treatment of these lesions is associated with significant morbidity including that of extensive dissection and malleolar nonunion or malunion. Arthroscopic treatment offers only a reduction of these risks. Outcomes of repair of weight-bearing articular pathology are usually less than optimal. The repair cartilage is of limited quality and often of limited quantity. Owing to increased loading in surface areas adjacent to the lesion, accelerated degeneration of the joint over time is to be expected.[87,88] Osteochondral lesions of the talus larger than 1.5 cm² and uncontained lesions were associated with a poor clinical outcome.[89] After 2 years, the outcomes of traditional open arthrotomy and arthroscopy are largely the same.[90] Techniques have been developed for treatment of partial- and full-thickness cartilage defects that involve exposing and stimulating the subchondral bone at the base of the lesion. Earlier techniques described subchondral abrasion and drilling. Another, perhaps

refinement of subchondral stimulation, is a technique of microfracture in which a sharpened contoured awl is arthroscopically placed into the defect and used to mechanically fenestrate the floor of the defect (Fig. 33.27C). Certainly, there is less risk of thermal injury. Additionally, it is thought to permit enhanced quality end tissue and cellular ingrowth and provide anchor points for fibrocartilage attachment. Cystic lesions associated with osteochondral defects can be approached arthroscopically to discharge the contents and fill the void with bone graft.[91] Alternatives to arthroscopic mechanical treatments of talar osteochondral defects are becoming more popular. There are increasing number of publications with arthroscopically assisted allograft cartilage grafting.[92-94] It is anticipated that more reports using arthroscopically placed grafts will increase as instrumentation for preparing and placing the grafts improve. In situations with cystic defects underlying intact cartilage and subchondral bone, retrograde drilling and grafting of bone has been advocated. This is usually done as an open or percutaneous technique. The technique involves evacuating the contents of the cyst and curetting the cyst lining to facilitate bleeding and incorporation of bone graft. The process can be endoscopically assisted by placing a scope in the transtalar conduit. In turning the fluid off after the field clears, one can observe pinpoint bleeding from the cyst if adequate preparation has been achieved.

AVULSION FRACTURE EXCISION

When symptoms persist despite treatment, excision of the lesion is often indicated. Arthroscopic excision can be accomplished if the lesion is identifiable from within the ankle joint. The surgeon should always be wary of the avulsion fragment that appears to be intra-articular but may in reality be extra-articular and impossible to approach without opening the area. Arthroscopic excision of avulsion fractures often requires advanced skills. Once the reactive tissue is resected and the bone fragment is identified, excision is carried out with radiofrequency wand, graspers, punches, and assorted knives. Rotating the grasping instrument along its axis is often helpful in releasing the fragment from the attached soft tissue. When the lesion is the cause of symptoms, excision is usually curative.

CHRONIC LATENT ANKLE SYNDESMOSIS DIASTASIS REPAIR

In situations of ankle trauma involving the syndesmosis, there are situations in which recognition of syndesmotic diastasis is delayed. When the condition is recognized, it is necessary to remove scar and debris within the syndesmosis to facilitate reduction of the diastasis.[95] The cleaning and removal of debris can be easily facilitated arthroscopically. A rotary shaver can be introduced and visualized at the level of the syndesmosis. The removal of debris and active bleeding of the soft tissue in proximity to the syndesmotic ligaments will allow for reduction and rebalancing of ligamentous structures postreduction. This is critical to obtain a long-lasting correction after hardware is ultimately removed.

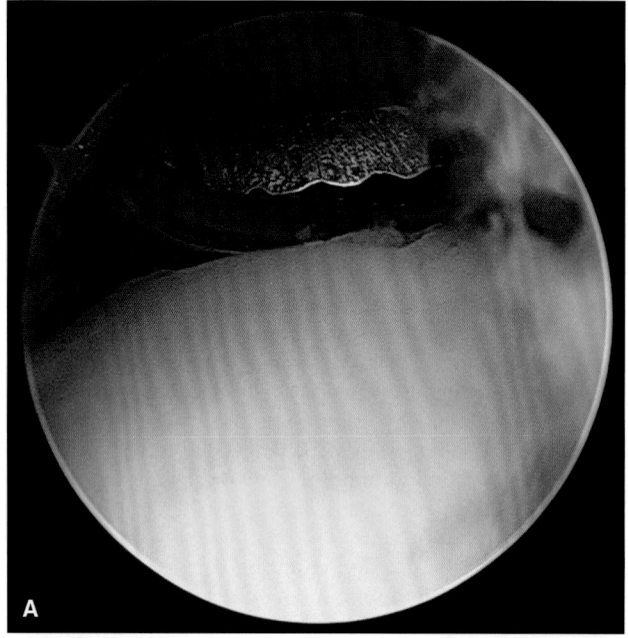

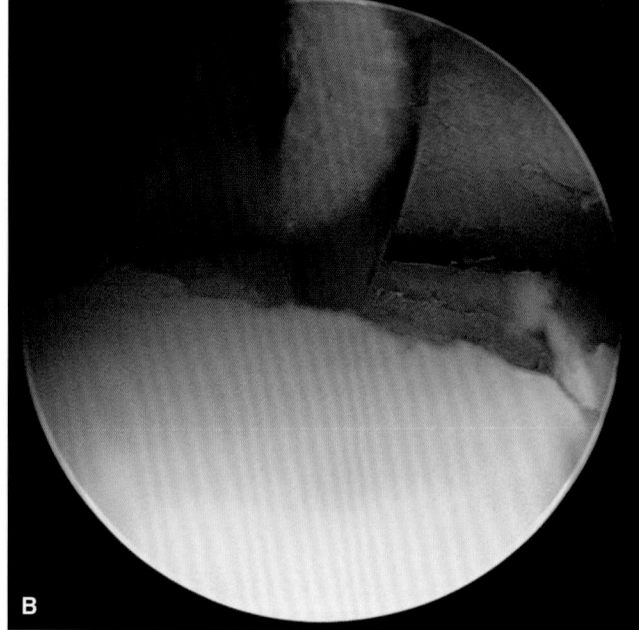

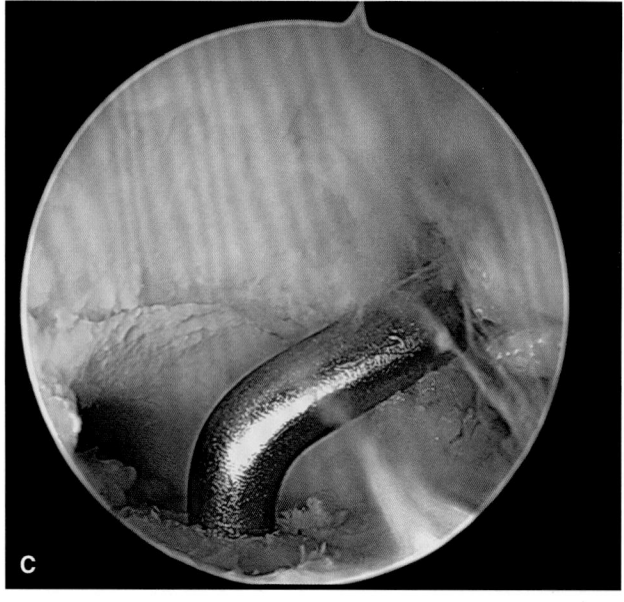

FIGURE 33.27 A. Hemostat used to grasp large osteochondral fragment. **B.** Microfracture awl placed in base of osteochondral defect use to fenestrate lesion. **C.** Penetration of osteochondral defect with awl.

ARTHROSCOPICALLY GUIDED FRACTURE REDUCTION (VIDEO 1)

Several authors have reported arthroscopically assisted fracture reduction as a means of precise fracture reduction in the ankle joint. Benefits include removal of fracture detritus, including hematoma, which may impair reduction. Usually, the reduction and repair also involves radiographic control and application of guided percutaneous pins and screws or open placement of hardware.[96-98] Arthroscopic-assisted technique in the ankle and foot can help with ligament evaluation, fragment reduction, and joint surface evaluation.[99-113] Recently, ankle arthroscopy in the setting of acute ankle fractures has gained popularity in diagnosing chondral injuries, which may negatively impact clinical outcomes.[111,112] Although, treatment of these injuries has not yet shown any improvement when compared to standard ORIF.[113] Clearly, the indications for use of the arthroscope for fractures is limited to intra-articular fractures that are amenable to reduction and fixation under the limited nature of the arthroscopic approach and the skills of the arthroscopic surgeon.

ANKLE ARTHRODESIS

Arthroscopic ankle arthrodesis has been reported by numerous authors in the last 25 years.[114-136] Interestingly, for those patients suited for arthroscopic technique, rates of fusion and time to fusion are reported as superior to traditional open methods. Preservation of local blood supply due to greatly diminished surgical dissection and periosteal stripping is thought to be the reason for the accelerated rate to fusion. This methodology also limits the shortening secondary to bony resection. Arthroscopy also limits the need for dissection in areas of marginal soft tissue in those patients with prior ankle trauma or dermal pathology and generally improves cosmesis in the otherwise normal patient. Candidates for arthroscopic fusion are those that can achieve appropriate position in situ, that is, they should have joints that do not require angular correction for optimization of their operations. Angular corrections requiring bony resection should be performed through an open approach in which accurate angular resection is simplified, measurable, and reproducible. In arthroscopic arthrodesis of the ankle, resection of the cartilage and subchondral bone plate is accomplished with larger curettes and 4-7 mm abraders. The bony portion of the joint should be taken down to bleeding or clearly viable depth, usually 1-2 mm below the cortical margin that defines the subchondral bone plate. The lateral and medial gutters should be cleared of cartilage to permit proximal advancement of the talus into the prepared ankle mortise. Many consider incorporation of the fibula into arthroscopic ankle arthrodesis optional; however, the authors preferred technique is to not place fixation through the fibula. Posterior displacement of the talus is also not possible because the posterior portion of the tibial articular surface and the nearly vertically orientated talar surface are generally geometrically resected. The contiguous surfaces of the talus

and tibia are ideally resected to maintain their convex-concave relationship in anticipation of a geometric fit. Large (6.5-8 mm) cannulated internal fixation screws in standard tripod fixation technique are then applied to the construct under fluoroscopic and arthroscopic guidance. The long-term outcomes of arthroscopic ankle fusion seem to parallel traditional open fusion techniques (Fig. 33.28).[117,136-139] There is a technique referred to as a dry ankle technique in which toward the end of the procedure, the remaining bone debris and blood form a paste that is left in place to function as a bone graft. Demineralized bone matrix paste or gel can be introduced via cannula delivery into the prepared arthrodesis site.

ARTHROSCOPIC DEBRIDEMENT AFTER TOTAL ANKLE ARTHROPLASTY

Arthrofibrosis, gutter bony and soft tissue impingement, has been increasingly diagnosed after total ankle arthroplasty.[140-142] The etiology for impingement following total ankle

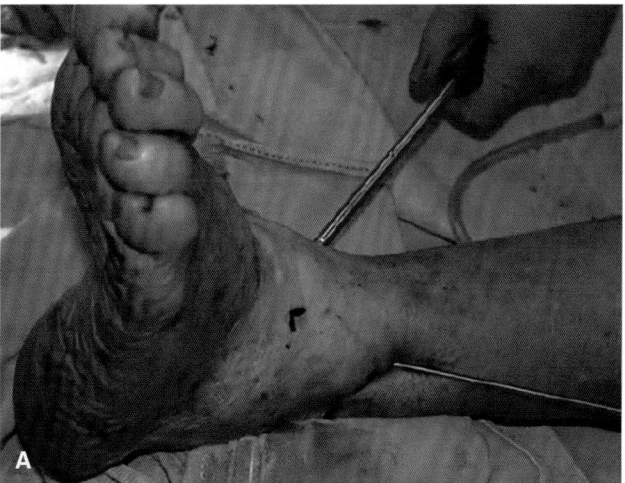
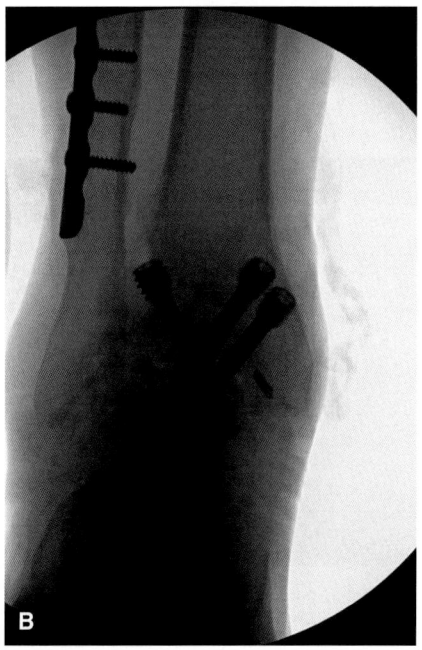
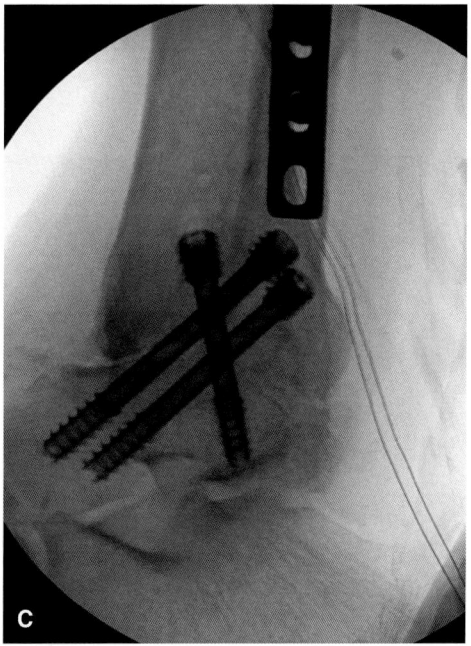

FIGURE 33.28 A. Percutaneous placement of fixation during arthroscopic ankle arthrodesis. **B, C.** Radiographs showing fixation in place.

replacement is complex due to many potential sources that exist for bony and soft tissue impingement. Both arthroscopic and open gutter debridements have been described. There is not much literature to support one treatment technique over the other, although some advocate arthroscopic approach due to earlier weight bearing and mobility.[140] In the arthroscopic procedure, standard anteromedial and anterolateral portals are created. A 3.5-mm shaver, 4.0-mm unguarded burr and curettes are utilized to perform an aggressive debridement. It may be difficult to visualize the shaver at first due to the amount of scar tissue in the ankle joint. Begin by touching the shaver to the arthroscope making sure to keep the hooded portion of the shaver in contact with the prosthesis during the anterior soft tissue debridement. Care must be taken not to be disoriented due to the shaver reflection against the prosthesis. Next, focus is turned to the medial and lateral ankle gutters once the anterior aspect of these gutters is visualized. A 4.0-mm unguarded burr creates a trough anteriorly; this trough can be followed with a 3.5-mm drill to the posterior aspect of the joint, and a curette can be used to break up the bone between the drill holes. Adequate debridement of the gutters is achieved when the posterior tibial tendon on the medial aspect and the peroneal tendons on the lateral aspect are visualized.

SUBTALAR ARTHROSCOPY SOFT TISSUE IMPINGEMENT

Soft tissue impingement of the subtalar joint can occur at any location. There can be acute and chronic types of synovitis, ligamentous tissue lesions, and scar. For lesions in the anterior compartment, usually an anterior lateral portal combined with an accessory portal is sufficient. However, a posterior lateral placement of a 70-degree scope brought anterior will allow one to visualize the anterior compartment, and use of a motorized shaver through the anterior lateral compartment will usually work; if not, the accessory portal placement can be used. There are some authors that subscribe to the diagnosis of sinus tarsi syndrome and will characterize patients with lesions in the anterior subtalar compartment into that category. However, arthrofibrosis and lesions of the interosseous ligament have been observed.[143,144] Within the confines of the subtalar joint

lateral gutter, one can encounter synovitis, which is common as well as scarification in the forms of adhesive bands and thick scarified lesions. In addition, hypertrophy of the posterior talofibular ligament can occur, and this can roll and impinge between the joint surfaces of the posterior facet. The ligament can be easily debulked with thermoablation technique. The posterior compartment of the subtalar joint similar to the lateral compartment various soft tissue lesions can be encountered. Additionally, there can be soft tissue impingement at the level of the posterior process or os trigonum as well as stenosing tenosynovitis of the flexor hallucis longus tendon.[145] All of these areas are accessible with arthroscopy with proper portal placement.

TRIGONUM/STIEDA PROCESS EXCISION

The os trigonum clinically can be a source of pain due to instability from chronic impingement or avulsion injury. Impingement from an elongated posterior process (Stieda process) has also been reported.[146] One common arthroscopic approach to the symptomatic os trigonum is from posterolateral, with arthroscopic visualization from anterolateral.[147] There have also been reports of approaching this from a prone position as well with two posterior portals, which the authors find as the easiest approach.[148-150] The flexor hallucis longus tendon borders the medial side of the os and often both guides the surgeon to the lesion and forms a medial landmark to important neurovascular structures in close proximity (Fig. 33.29). The posterior capsular reflection of the subtalar joint is much larger than the posterior capsular reflection of the ankle joint. Both open and endoscopic excision yield acceptable outcomes but endoscopic excision leads to lower complication rates and return to activity is much shorter.[151,152]

SUBTALAR ARTHRODESIS

Similar to the techniques used in arthroscopic ankle arthrodesis, the subtalar joint can be approached arthroscopically via sinus tarsi. Report of successful arthroscopic arthrodesis has been published.[150,153-155]

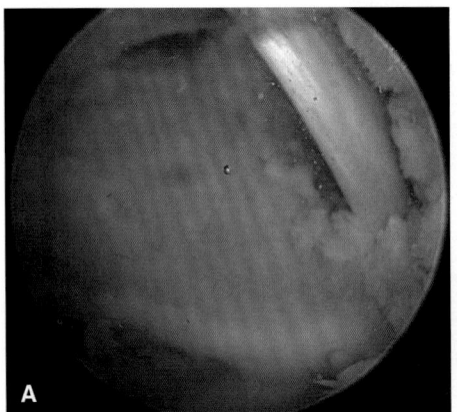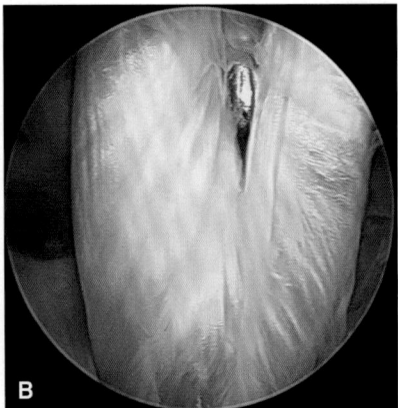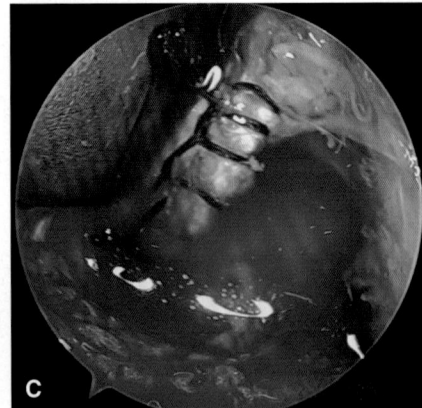

FIGURE 33.29 A. Flexor hallucis longus tendon borders the medial side of the os forms a medial landmark to important neurovascular structures. **B.** Longitudinal split tear of FHL. **C.** After retubularization repair.

OTHER ARTHROSCOPIC AND ENDOSCOPIC PROCEDURES OF THE FOOT

Arthroscopy of the calcaneocuboid joint, talonavicular joint, first metatarsophalangeal joint (MTPJ), interphalangeal joint of the hallux, and lesser MTPJs has been accomplished by various foot and ankle surgeons. Endoscopic visualization and surgical manipulation of the retrocalcaneal bursa, the Achilles tendon and aponeurosis, flexor hallucis longus tendon, tibialis posterior tendon, peroneal tendons (Fig. 33.30), plantar fascia, calcaneonavicular coalition, and the deep transverse intermetatarsal ligament, intermetatarsal nerve, or both have similarly been performed.[54,145,146,156-167] The outcomes of endoscopic release of the gastrocnemius aponeurosis,[165,166,168-172] plantar fascia,[172-176] and the deep transverse intermetatarsal ligament[164,177] would seem to indicate that it may be valuable for the patient afflicted with equinus, plantar fasciitis, and Morton neuroma, respectively. Strict indications, outcomes with direct comparisons with open procedure counterparts, and acceptance of these arthroscopic surgical procedures of the foot remain to be determined.

PERILS and PITFALLS

- Portal placement (avoid neurovascular injury)
  - Neuroma[178]
- Infection
- Inadvertant abrasion or scoring of cartilage, dorsiflex the ankle joint upon insertion of obturator
- Perforating peroneal artery injury/pseudoaneurysm
- Fluid overload
- Postoperative hemarthrosis
- Prolonged distraction
- Synovial fistula

Complications following arthroscopic surgery are infrequent but occur at a regular rate varying from 7% to 17% of cases.[179,180] As with any surgical procedure, a set of complications must be expected from the nature of the surgical procedure itself. Complications directly related to arthroscopic procedures vary from minor surface damage related to instrumentation to limb- or life-threatening arthrosepsis.[181] Articular surface injury as a result of surgical technique is common, controllable, and permanent.[182,183] Special care must be taken in "tight" joints of the foot and ankle because iatrogenic "scuffing" of the articular surfaces occurs easily. Superficial lesions of the articular surface have little potential to heal. Thankfully, these and most other complications of arthroscopy are minor and self-limiting. Experience is noted to diminish the rate of complications in arthroscopic surgery.[184,185] The most common complication following arthroscopy in any joint is local nerve injury.[186] In ankle arthroscopy, there is close proximity of a named nerve trunk with each of the standard portals. Each of these nerves and their branches are susceptible to injury including neuropraxia, axonotmesis, neurotmesis, and reflex sympathetic dystrophy. Excessive surgical manipulation of the tissue in the portal areas sets the stage for potential injury. Other complications include hemarthrosis, infection, thromboembolic disease, and local aneurysm.[187,188] The IDCN is often visible at the time of portal placement and can be avoided (Fig. 33.11). Complications unique to arthroscopy include instrument breakage and synovial fistula. Synovial fistula is recognized as a nonhealing portal wound that drains synovial fluid (Fig. 33.31). A synovial fistula usually responds well to local debridement and formal suturing. While it has not been ascertained in the literature, there are many arthroscopists that feel early weight bearing can lead to synovial fistulas. Factors increasing the frequency of complications include portal abuse and heavy manipulation of delicate (especially hinged) instrumentation. The arthroscopic surgeon must be keenly aware of the potential for complications and must recognize and treat complications appropriately.

POSTOPERATIVE CARE AND REHABILITATION

For most cases of isolated foot and ankle arthroscopy, patients are placed into a soft dressing and surgical shoe with isolated arthroscopic debridement. OCD repairs are typically placed in soft dressing with CAM boot.[189] This really depends on other procedures performed in conjunction with the arthroscopy. Early

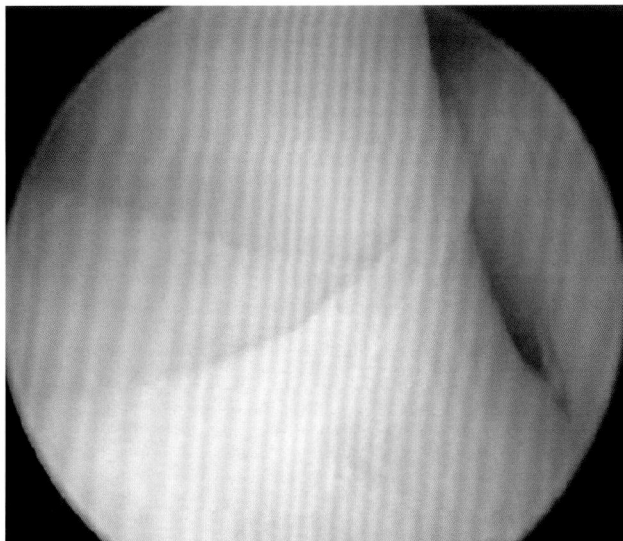

FIGURE 33.30 Oblique adhesions surrounding peroneus longus tendon that limited tendon excursion, bands changed orientation with change in ankle position.

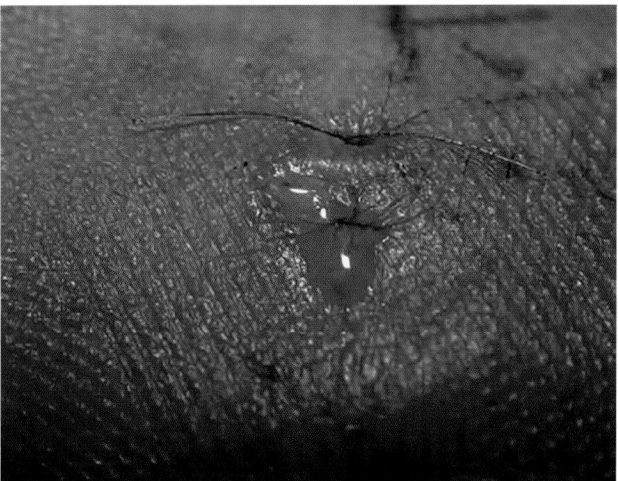

FIGURE 33.31 Synovial shunt 1 week after procedure. Compression and non–weight bearing gradually resolved condition.

passive range of motion is always encouraged unless an arthrodesis is performed. Preferably, this is started 2-5 days postoperatively. We encourage passive range of motion activities 3-4 times a day beginning at 15-20 minutes per session and increasing this over a period of 4-6 weeks postoperatively. In cases in which drilling, microfracture, or retrograde bone grafting of an osteochondral lesion is performed, a period of non–weight bearing is emphasized for 4-8 weeks although more recent studies show immediate weight bearing does not diminish patient outcomes.[189]

REFERENCES

1. Parisien JS. Arthroscopic treatment of osteochondral lesions of the talus. *Am J Sports Med.* 1986;14:211-217.
2. Voto SJ, Clark RN, Zuelzer WA. Arthroscopic training using pig knee joints. *Clin Orthop Relat Res.* 1988;226:134-137.
3. Lundeen RO. *Manual of Ankle and Foot Arthroscopy.* New York, NY: Churchill Livingstone; 1992.
4. Ferkel RD, ed. *Arthroscopic Surgery: The Foot and Ankle.* Philadelphia, PA: Lippincott-Raven; 1996.
5. Ferkel RD, ed. *Historical Developments.* Philadelphia, PA: Lippincott-Raven; 1996.
6. Guhl JF. History and development. In: Guhl JF, ed. *Foot and Ankle Arthroscopy.* Thorofare, NJ: Slack, Inc.; 1993:1-6.
7. Stienstra JJ, ed. *Arthroscopy of the Ankle and Joints of the Foot.* 3rd ed. Philadelphia, PA: Lippincott Williams & Wilkins; 2001.
8. Burman MS. Arthroscopy or the direct visualization of joints: an experimental cadaver study. *J Bone Joint Surg Am.* 1931;13A:669-695.
9. Dandy DJ. Annotation: arthroscopic surgery. *J Bone Joint Surg Br.* 1984;66-B:628-628.
10. Heller AJ, Vogler HW. Ankle joint arthroscopy. *J Foot Surg.* 1982;21:23-29.
11. Chu CR, Izzo NJ, Coyle CH, et al. The in vitro effects of bupivacaine on articular chondrocytes. *J Bone Joint Surg Br.* 2008;90:814-820.
12. Chu CR, Izzo NJ, Papas NE, et al. In vitro exposure to 0.5% bupivacaine is cytotoxic to bovine articular chondrocytes. *Arthroscopy.* 2006;22:693-699.
13. Karpie JC, Chu CR. Lidocaine exhibits dose- and time-dependent cytotoxic effects on bovine articular chondrocytes in vitro. *Am J Sports Med.* 2007;35:1621-1627.
14. Nole R, Munson NML, Fulkerson JP. Bupivacaine and saline effects on articular cartilage. *Arthroscopy.* 1985;1:123-127.
15. Piper SL, Kim HT. Comparison of ropivacaine and bupivacaine toxicity in human articular chondrocytes. *J Bone Joint Surg Am.* 2008;90:986-991.
16. Wernecke C, Braun HJ, Dragoo JL. The effect of intra articular corticosteroids on articular cartilage. *Orthop J Sports Med.* 2015;3(5).
17. Rodriguez-Merchan EC. The haemophilic ankle. *Haemophilia.* 2006;12:337-3446.
18. Dunn AL, Busch MT, Wyly JB, et al. Arthroscopic synovectomy for hemophilic joint disease in a pediatric population. *J Pediatr Orthop.* 2004;24:414-426.
19. Tamurian RM, Spencer EE, Wojtys EM. The role of arthroscopic synovectomy in the management of hemarthrosis in hemophilia patients: financial perspectives. *Arthroscopy.* 2002;18:789-79.
20. Johnson LL. Characteristics of the immediate postarthroscopic blood clot formation in the knee joint. *Arthroscopy.* 1991;7:14-23.
21. Stienstra J. Intra-articular soft-tissue masses of the ankle. Meniscoid lesions and transarticular fibrous bands. *Clin Podiatr Med Surg.* 1994;11:371-383.
22. Stone JW, Guhl JE. Meniscoid lesions of the ankle. *Clin Sports Med.* 1991;10:661-676.
23. Wolin I, Glassman F, Sideman S. Internal derangement of the talofibular component of the ankle. *Surg Gynecol Obstet.* 1950;91:193-201.
24. McCarroll JR, Schrader JW, Shelbourne KD, et al. Meniscoid lesions of the ankle in soccer players. *Am J Sports Med.* 1987;15:255-257.
25. Pritsch M, Lokiec F, Sali M, et al. Adhesions of distal tibiofibular syndesmosis. A cause of chronic ankle pain after fracture. *Clin Orthop Relat Res.* 1993;289:220-222.
26. Ferkel RD, Karzel RP, Del Pizzo W, et al. Arthroscopic treatment of anterolateral impingement of the ankle. *Am J Sports Med.* 1991;19:440-446.
27. Bassett FH III, Gates HS III, Billys JB, Morris HB, Nikolaou PK. Talar impingement by the anteroinferior tibiofibular ligament. A cause of chronic pain in the ankle after inversion sprain. *J Bone Joint Surg Am.* 1990;72:55-59.
28. Bassett FH, Gates HS, Billys JB, et al. Tatar impingement by the anteroinferior tibiofibular ligament. *J Bone Joint Surg Am.* 1990;72:55-59.
29. Ray RG, Kriz BM. Anterior inferior tibiofibular ligament. Variations and relationship to the talus. *J Am Podiatr Med Assoc.* 1991;81:479-485.
30. Lundeen RO. Medial impingement lesions of the tibial plafond. *J Foot Surg.* 1987;26:37-40.
31. Lundeen RO. Ankle arthroscopy in the adolescent patient. *J Foot Surg.* 1990;29:510-515.
32. Ray RG, Gusman DN, Christensen JC. Anatomical variation of the tibial plafond: the anteromedial tibial notch. *J Foot Ankle Surg.* 1994;33:419-426.
33. Hamilton V. Differential diagnosis. In: Guhl J, ed. *Ankle Arthroscopy: Pathology and Surgical Techniques.* Thorofare, NJ: Slack, Inc.; 1993.
34. Cutsuries AM, Saltrick KR, Wagner J, et al. Arthroscopic arthroplasty of the ankle joint. *Clin Podiatr Med Surg.* 1994;11:449-467.
35. Ogilvie-Harris DJ, Mahomed N, Demaziere A. Anterior impingement of the ankle treated by arthroscopic removal of bony spurs. *J Bone Joint Surg Br.* 1993;75:437-440.
36. Vogler HW, Stienstra JJ, Montgomery F, et al. Anterior ankle impingement arthropathy. The role of anterolateral arthrotomy and arthroscopy. *Clin Podiatr Med Surg.* 1994;11:425-447.
37. Frey C, van Dijk CN. Arthroscopy of the great toe. *Instr Course Lect.* 1999;48:343-346.
38. Berndt AL, Harty M. Transchondral fractures (osteochondritis dissecans) of the talus. *J Bone Joint Surg Am.* 1959;41:988.
39. Campbell CJ, Ranawa CS. Osteochondritis dissecans: the question of etiology. *J Trauma.* 1966;5:201.
40. Cavallaro DC, Vokasien RL, Brown JH. Osteochondritis dissecans of the talus: a review of the literature and case study. *J Am Podiatry Assoc.* 1979;69:567-570.
41. Deginder WL. Osteochondritis dissecans of the talus. *Radiology.* 1955;65:590.
42. Fairbanks HAT. Osteochondritis dissecans. *Br J Surg.* 1933;21:67.
43. Kappis M. Weiters beitrage zur traumatisch-mechanischen enstehung der "spontanen" Knorpelabiosungen. *Dtsch Z Chir.* 1922;A1:B29.
44. Konig F. Veber freie korper in den gelenken. *Dtsch Z Chir.* 1888;27:90.
45. Rendu A. Fracture intra-articulare parcellaire de Ia pulie astraglienne. *Lyon Med.* 1932;150:220.
46. Loomer R, Fisher C, Lloyd Smith R, Sisler J, Cooney T. Osteochondral lesions of the talus. *Am J Sports Med.* 1993;21:13-19.
47. Ferkel RD, Scranton PE Jr. Arthroscopy of the ankle and foot. *J Bone Joint Surg Am.* 1993;75:1233-1242.
48. Dipaola JD, Nelson DW, Colville MR. Characterizing osteochondral lesions by magnetic resonance imaging. *Arthroscopy.* 1991;7:101-104.
49. Ferkel RD, Sgaglione NA, DelPizzo W, et al. Arthroscopic treatment of osteochondral lesions of the talus: technique and results. *Orthop Trans.* 1990;14:172-173.
50. Zinman C, Wolfson N, Reis ND. Osteochondritis dissecans of the dome of the talus: computed tomography scanning in diagnosis and follow-up. *J Bone Joint Surg Am.* 1988;70A:1017-1101.
51. Ogilvie-Harris DJ, Saleh K. Generalized synovial chondromatosis of the knee: a comparison of removal of the loose bodies alone with arthroscopic synovectomy. *Arthroscopy.* 1994;10:166-170.
52. Whelan JM, Jackson DW. Videoarthroscopy: review and state of the art. *Arthroscopy.* 1992;8:311-319.
53. Brillhart AT. Lasers in arthroscopic surgery (Letter). *Arthroscopy.* 1991;7:411-412.
54. van Dijk CN. Hindfoot endoscopy for posterior ankle pain. *Instr Course Lect.* 2006;55:545-554.
55. Lui TH. Ankle arthroscopy with patient in prone position. *Arch Orthop Trauma Surg.* 2007;128:1283-1285.
56. Dimnjakovic D, Hrabac P, Bojanic I. Value of tourniquet in anterior ankle arthroscopy: a randomized controlled trial. *Foot Ankle Int.* 2017;38(7):716-722.
57. Zaidi R, Hasan K, Sharma A, et al. Ankle arthroscopy: a study of tourniquet versus no tourniquet. *Foot Ankle Int.* 2014;35(5):478-482.
58. Reagan BF, Mcinerny VK, Treadwell BV, et al. Irrigating solutions for arthroscopy. A metabolic study. *J Bone Joint Surg Am.* 1983;65:629-631.
59. Shinjo H, Nakata K, Shino K, et al. Effect of irrigation solutions for arthroscopic surgery on intraarticular tissue: comparison in human meniscus-derived primary cell culture between lactate Ringer's solution and saline solution. *J Orthop Res.* 2002;20:1305-1310.
60. Yang CY, Cheng SC, Shen CL. Effect of irrigation fluid on the articular cartilage: a scanning electron microscope study. *Arthroscopy.* 1993;9:425-430.
61. Morgan CD. Fluid delivery systems for arthroscopy. *Arthroscopy.* 1987;3:288-291.
62. Cameron SE. Noninvasive distraction for ankle arthroscopy. *Arthroscopy.* 1997;13:366-369.
63. Guhl JF. New concepts (distraction) in ankle arthroscopy. *Arthroscopy.* 1988;4:160-167.
64. Palladino SJ. Distinction systems for ankle arthroscopy. *Clin Podiatr Med Surg.* 1994;11:499-511.
65. Miyamoto W, Takao M, Komatu F, et al. Technique tip: the bandage distraction technique for arthroscopic arthrodesis of the ankle joint. *Foot Ankle Int.* 2008;29:251-253.
66. Yates CK, Gran WA. A simple distraction technique for ankle arthroscopy. *Arthroscopy.* 1988;4:103-105.
67. Tonogai I, Hayashi F, Tsuro Y, et al. Distance between the anterior tibial edge and the anterior tibial artery in distraction and nondistraction during anterior ankle arthroscopy: a cadaveric study. *Foot Ankle Int.* 2018;39(1):113-118.
68. Gumann GS Jr. Ankle arthroscopic portals and techniques. *Clin Podiatr Med Surg.* 1987;4:861-874.
69. Katchis SD, Smith RW. A simple way to establish the posterolateral portal in ankle arthroscopy. *Foot Ankle Int.* 1997;18:178-179.
70. Stienstra TI, Lamy CJ, Joseph W. Septic arthritis. In: Oloff L, ed. *Musculoskeletal Disorders of the Lower Extremity.* Philadelphia, PA: WB Saunders; 1994.
71. Thiery JA. Arthroscopic drainage in septic arthritides of the knee: a multicenter study. *Arthroscopy.* 1989;5:65-69.
72. Gusman DN, Dockery GL. Adhesive lesions of the talocrural joint. *Clin Podiatr Med Surg.* 1994;11:385-394.
73. Martin DF, Curl WW, Baker CL. Arthroscopic treatment of chronic synovitis of the ankle. *Arthroscopy.* 1989;5:110-114.
74. Palladino SJ, Chan R. Adhesive capsulitis of the ankle. *J Foot Surg.* 1987;26:484-492.
75. McCrum CL, Arner JW, Lesniak B, et al. Arthroscopic anterior ankle decompression is successful in national football league players. *Am J Orthop.* 2018;47(1).
76. Hawkins RB. Arthroscopic stapling repair for chronic lateral instability. *Clin Podiatr Med Surg.* 1987;4:875-883.
77. Lundeen RO, Hawkins RB. Arthroscopic lateral ankle stabilization. *J Am Podiatr Med Assoc.* 1985;75:372-376.
78. Brown AJ, Shimozono Y, Kennedy JG, et al. Arthroscopic repair of lateral ankle instability: a systematic review. *Arthroscopy.* 2018;34(8):2497-2503.
79. Li H, Hua Y, Li H, et al. Activity level and function 2 years after anterior talofibular ligament repair: a comparison between arthroscopic repair and open repair procedures. *Am J Sports Med.* 2017;45(9):2044-2051.

80. Kashuk KB, Landsman AS, Werd MB, et al. Arthroscopic lateral ankle stabilization. *Clin Podiatr Med Surg.* 1994;11:407-423.
81. Martin DF, Baker CL, Curl WW, et al. Operative ankle arthroscopy. Long-term follow-up. *Am J Sports Med.* 1989;17:16-23; discussion 23.
82. Lundeen RO, Stienstra JJ. Arthroscopic treatment of transchondral lesions of the talar dome. *J Am Podiatr Med Assoc.* 1987;77:456-461.
83. Lu Y, Hayashi K, Hecht P, et al. The effect of monopolar radiofrequency energy on partial thickness defects of articular cartilage. *Arthroscopy.* 2000;16:527-536.
84. Grady J, Hughes D. Arthroscopic management of talar dome lesions using a transmalleolar approach. *J Am Podiatr Med Assoc.* 2006;96:260-263.
85. Bryant DD III, Siegel MG. Osteochondritis dissecans of the talus: a new technique for arthroscopic drilling. *Arthroscopy.* 1993;9:238-241.
86. Ove PN, Bosse MJ, Reinert CM. Excision of posterolateral talar dome lesions through a medial transmalleolar approach. *Foot Ankle.* 1989;9:171-175.
87. Christensen JC, Driscoll HL, Tencer AF. Contact characteristics of the ankle joint. Part II: The effects of talar dome cartilage defects. *J Am Podiatr Med Assoc.* 1994;84:537-547.
88. Driscoll HL, Christensen JC, Tencer AF. Contact characteristics of the ankle joint, Part I: The normal joint. *J Am Podiatr Med Assoc.* 1994;84:491-498.
89. Cuttica DJ, Smith BW, Hyer CF. Osteochondral lesions of the talus: predictors of clinical outcome. *Foot Ankle Int.* 2011;32(11):1045-1051.
90. Van Buecken K, Barrack RL, Alexander H, et al. Arthroscopic treatment of transchondral talar dome fractures. *Am J Sports Med.* 1989;17:350-356.
91. Uysal M, Akpinar S, Ozalay M, et al. Arthroscopic debridement and grafting of an intraosseous talar ganglion. *Arthroscopy.* 2005;21:1269.
92. DeSandis BA, Haleem AM, Sofka CM, et al. Arthroscopic treatment of osteochondral lesions of the talus using juvenile articular cartilage allograft and autologous bone marrow aspirate concentration. *J Foot Angle Surg.* 2018;57(2):273-280.
93. Sadik B, Kolodziej L, Puskarz M, et al. Surgical repair of osteochondral lesions of the talus using biologic inlay osteochondral reconstruction: clinical outcomes after treatment using a medial malleolar osteotomy approach compared to an arthroscopically assisted approach. *Foot Ankle Surg.* 2019;25(4):449-456.
94. Ng A, Bernhard A, Bernhard K. Advances in ankle cartilage repair. *Clin Podiatr Med Surg.* 2017;34(4):471-487.
95. Schuberth JM, Jennings MM, Lau AC. Arthroscopy-assisted repair of latent Syndesmotic instability of the ankle. *Arthroscopy.* 2008;24:868-874.
96. Ferkel RD, Fasulo GJ. Arthroscopic treatment of ankle injuries. *Orthop Clin North Am.* 1994;25:17-32.
97. Guhl JF, Ferkel RD, Stone JW, eds. *Other Osteochondral Pathology Fractures and Fracture Defects.* 2nd ed. Thorofare, NJ: Slack, Inc.; 1993.
98. Whipple TL, Martin DR, Mcintyre LF, et al. Arthroscopic treatment of triplane fractures of the ankle. *Arthroscopy.* 1993;9:456-463.
99. Salvi AE, Metelli GP, Bettinsoli R, et al. Arthroscopic-assisted fibular synthesis and syndesmotic stabilization of a complex unstable ankle injury. *Arch Orthop Trauma Surg.* 2009;129:393-396.
100. Yoshimura I, Nait OM, Kanazawa K, et al. Arthroscopic findings in Maisonneuve fractures. *J Orthop Sci.* 2008;13:3-6.
101. Nehme A, Tannous Z, Wehbe J, et al. Arthroscopically assisted reconstruction and percutaneous screw fixation of a pilon tibial malunion. *J Foot Ankle Surg.* 2007;46:502-507.
102. Jennings MM, Lagaay P, Schuberth JM. Arthroscopic assisted fixation of juvenile intraarticular epiphyseal ankle fractures. *J Foot Ankle Surg.* 2007;46:376-386.
103. Panagopoulos A, van Niekerk L. Arthroscopic assisted reduction and fixation of a juvenile Tillaux fracture. *Knee Surg Sports Traumatol Arthrosc.* 2007;15:415-417.
104. Takao M, Uchio Y, Naito K, et al. Diagnosis and treatment of combined intra-articular disorders in acute distal fibular fractures. *J Trauma.* 2004;57:1303-1307.
105. Lmade S, Takao M, Nishi H, et al. Arthroscopy-assisted reduction and percutaneous fixation for triplane fracture of the distal tibia. *Arthroscopy.* 2004;20:e123-e128.
106. Schuberth JM, Collman DR, Rush SM, et al. Deltoid ligament integrity in lateral malleolar fractures: a comparative analysis of arthroscopic and radiographic assessments. *J Foot Ankle Surg.* 2004;43:20-29.
107. Loren GJ, Ferkel RD. Arthroscopic assessment of occult intra-articular injury in acute ankle fractures. *Arthroscopy.* 2002;18:412-421.
108. Hintermann B, Regazzoni P, Lampert C, et al. Arthroscopic findings in acute fractures of the ankle. *J Bone Joint Surg Br.* 2000;82:345-351.
109. Saltzman CL, Marsh JL, Tearse DS. Treatment of displaced talus fractures: an arthroscopically assisted approach. *Foot Ankle Int.* 1994;15:630-633.
110. Seo SS, Choi JS. Arthroscopic management of displaced intra-articular calcaneal fractures. In: Presented at International Society of Arthroscopy, Knee Surgery and Orthopedic Sports Medicine; May 11-16, 1997; Buenos Aires, Argentina; 1997.
111. Da Cunha RJ, Karnovsky SC, et al. Ankle arthroscopy of full thickness talar cartilage lesions in the setting of acute ankle fractures. *Arthroscopy.* 2018;34(6):1950-1957.
112. Park CH, Yoon DH. Role of subtalar arthroscopy in operative treatment of sanders type 2 calcaneal fractures using a sinus tarsi approach. *Foot Ankle Int.* 2018;39(4):443-449.
113. Gonzalez TA, Macaulay AA, DiGiovanni CW, et al. Arthroscopically assisted versus standard open reduction and internal fixation techniques for the acute ankle fracture. *Foot Ankle Int.* 2016;37(5):554-562.
114. Gougoulias NE, Agathangelidis FG, Parsons I. Arthroscopic ankle arthrodesis. *Foot Ankle Int.* 2007;28:695-706.
115. Collman DR, Raas MH, Schuberth J. Arthroscopic ankle arthrodesis: factors influencing union in 39 consecutive patients. *Foot Ankle Int.* 2006;27:1079-1085.
116. Stone JW. Arthroscopic ankle arthrodesis. *Foot Ankle Clin.* 2006;11:361-368, vi-vii.
117. Ferkel RD, Hewitt M. Long-term result of arthroscopic ankle arthrodesis. *Foot Ankle Int.* 2005;26:275-280.
118. Winson LG, Robinson DE, Allen PE. Arthroscopic ankle arthrodesis. *J Bone Joint Surg Br.* 2005;87:343-347.
119. Raikin SM. Arthrodesis of the ankle: arthroscopic, mini-open, and open techniques. *Foot Ankle Clin.* 2003;8:347-359.
120. Fleiss DJ. Arthroscopic arthrodesis of the ankle joint. *Arthroscopy.* 2000;16:788.
121. Cameron SE, Ullrich P. Arthroscopic arthrodesis of the ankle joint. *Arthroscopy.* 2000;16:21-26.
122. Wang DY. Arthroscopic ankle arthrodesis: a preliminary report. *Zhonghua Yi Xue Za Zhi.* 1998;61:694-699.
123. Fisher RL, Ryan WR, Dugdale TW, et al. Arthroscopic ankle fusion. *Conn Med.* 1997;61:643-646.
124. Glick JM, Morgan CD, Myerson MS, et al. Ankle arthrodesis using an arthroscopic method: long-term follow-up of 34 cases. *Arthroscopy.* 1996;12:428-434.
125. Jerosch J, Steinbeck J, Schroder M, et al. Arthroscopically assisted arthrodesis of the ankle joint. *Arch Orthop Trauma Surg.* 1996;115:182-189.
126. Turan I, Wredmark T, Fellander-Tsai L. Arthroscopic ankle arthrodesis in rheumatoid arthritis. *Clin Orthop Relat Res.* 1995;320:110-114.
127. Corso SJ, Zimmer TJ. Technique and clinical evaluation of arthroscopic ankle arthrodesis. *Arthroscopy.* 1995;11:585-590.
128. Yee TC, Crosby LA. Arthroscopic ankle fusions utilizing bone marrow and demineralized bone matrix: a case report. *Nebr Med J.* 1994;79:327-329.
129. Fleiss DJ. Arthroscopically assisted arthrodesis for osteoarthritic ankles. *J Bone Joint Surg Am.* 1994;76:1112.
130. Lundeen RO. Arthroscopic fusion of the ankle and subtalar joint. *Clin Podiatr Med Surg.* 1994;11:395-406.
131. De Vriese L, Dereyrnaeker G, Fabry G. Arthroscopic ankle arthrodesis. Preliminary report. *Acta Orthop Belg.* 1994;60:389-392.
132. Dent CM, Patil M, Fairclough JA. Arthroscopic ankle arthrodesis. *J Bone Joint Surg Br.* 1993;75:830-832.
133. Ogilvie-Harris DJ, Lieberman I, Fitsialos D. Arthroscopically assisted arthrodesis for osteoarthritic ankles. *J Bone Joint Surg Am.* 1993;75:1167-1174.
134. Myerson MS, Quill G. Ankle arthrodesis. A comparison of an arthroscopic and an open method of treatment. *Clin Orthop Relat Res.* 1991;268:84-95.
135. Morgan C. Arthroscopic ankle arthrodesis. In: Guhl JF, ed. *Foot and Ankle Arthroscopy.* 2nd ed. Thorofare, NJ: Slack, Inc.; 1993:161-169.
136. Jones CR, Wong E, Applegate GR, et al. Arthroscopic ankle arthrodesis: a 2-15 year follow-up study. *Arthroscopy.* 2018;34(5):1641-1649.
137. Aaron AD. Ankle fusion, a retrospective review. *Orthopedics.* 1986;13:1249-1254.
138. Baciu CC. A simple technique for arthrodesis of the ankle. *J Bone Joint Surg Br.* 1986;68B:266-267.
139. Campbell P. Arthrodesis of the ankle with modified distraction-compression and bone grafting. *J Bone Joint Surg Am.* 1990;72A:552-556.
140. Gross CE, Adams SB, Easley M, Nunley JA, et al. Surgical treatment of bony and soft tissue impingement in total ankle arthroplasty. *Foot Ankle Specialist.* 2016;10(1).
141. Gross CE, Neumann JA, Godin JA, DeOrio JK. Technique of arthroscopic treatment of impingement after total ankle arthroplasty. *Arthrosc Techn.* 2016;5(2).
142. Devos Bevernage B, Deleu PA, Birch I, et al. Arthroscopic debridement after total ankle arthroplasty. *Foot Ankle Int.* 2016;37(2):142-149.
143. Oloff LM, Schulhofer SD, Bocko AP. Subtalar joint arthroscopy for sinus tarsi syndrome: a review of 29 cases. *J Foot Ankle Surg.* 2001;40:152-157.
144. Frey C, Feder KS, DiGiovanni C. Arthroscopic evaluation of the subtalar joint: does sinus tarsi syndrome exist? *Foot Ankle Int.* 1999;20:185-191.
145. Corte-Real NM, Moreira RM, Guerra-Pinto F. Arthroscopic treatment of tenosynovitis of the flexor hallucis longus tendon. *Foot Ankle Int.* 2012;33(12):1108-1112.
146. Yumaz C, Eskanda MM. Arthroscopic excision of the talar Stieda's process. *Arthroscopy.* 2006;22:225e221-225e223.
147. Marumoto JM, Ferkel RD. Arthroscopic excision of the os trigonum: a new technique with preliminary clinical results. *Foot Ankle Int.* 1997;18:777-784.
148. Horibe S, Kita K, Natsu-ume T, et al. A novel technique of arthroscopic excision of a symptomatic os trigonum. *Arthroscopy.* 2008;24:121e121-121e124.
149. van Dijk CN, Scholten PE, Krips R. A 2-portal endoscopic approach for diagnosis and treatment of posterior ankle pathology. *Arthroscopy.* 2000;16:871-876.
150. Lombardi CM, Silhanek AD, Connolly FG. Modified arthroscopic excision of the symptomatic os trigonum and release of the flexor hallucis longus tendon: operative technique and case study. *J Foot Ankle Surg.* 1999;38:347-351.
151. Carro LP, Golano P, Vega J. Arthroscopic subtalar arthrodesis: the posterior approach in the prone position. *Arthroscopy.* 2007;23:445e441-445e444.
152. Georgiannios D, Barbinas I. Endoscopic versus open excision of os trigonum for the treatment of posterior ankle impingement syndrome in an athletic population: a randomized controlled study with 5 year follow up. *Am J Sports Med.* 2017;45(6):1388-139.
153. Glanzmann MC, Sanhueza-Hernandez R. Arthroscopic subtalar arthrodesis for symptomatic osteoarthritis of the hindfoot: a prospective study of 41 cases. *Foot Ankle Int.* 2007;28:2-7.
154. Tasto JP. Arthroscopy of the subtalar joint and arthroscopic subtalar arthrodesis. *Instr Course Lect.* 2006;55:555-564.
155. Stroud CC. Arthroscopic arthrodesis of the ankle, subtalar, and first metatarsophalangeal joint. *Foot Ankle Clin.* 2002;7:135-146.
156. Lui TH. Arthroscopic resection of the calcaneonavicular coalition or the "too long" anterior process of the calcaneus. *Arthroscopy.* 2006;22:903e901-903e904.
157. van Dijk CN, Kort N. Tendoscopy of the peroneal tendons. *Arthroscopy.* 1998;14:471-478.
158. van Dijk CN, Kort N, Scholten PE. Tendoscopy of the posterior tibial tendon. *Arthroscopy.* 1997;13:692-698.
159. Yong CK. Peroneus quartus and peroneal tendoscopy. *Med J Malaysia.* 2006;61(suppl B):45-47.
160. Poui J, Tuma J, Bajerova J. Video-assisted gastrocnemius-soleus and hamstring lengthening in cerebral palsy patients. *J Pediatr Orthop B.* 2008;17:81-84.
161. DiDomenico IA, Adams HB, Garchar D. Endoscopic gastrocnemius recession for the treatment of gastrocnemius equinus. *J Am Podiatr Med Assoc.* 2005;95:410-413.

162. Lundeen RO, Aziz S, Burks JB, et al. Endoscopic plantar fasciotomy: a retrospective analysis of results in 53 patients. *J Foot Ankle Surg.* 2000;39:208-217.

163. Barrett SL, Walsh AS. Endoscopic decompression of intermetatarsal nerve entrapment: a retrospective study. *J Am Podiatr Med Assoc.* 2006;96:19-23.

164. Saxena A, Gollwitzer H, Widtfeldt A, et al. Die endoskopische Verlangerungsoperation des Musculus gastrocnemius zur Behandlung des Gastrocnemius equinus. *Z Orthop Unfall.* 2007;145:499-504.

165. Opdam KTM, Baltes TPA, Zwiers R, et al. Endoscopic treatment of mid portion Achilles tendinopathy: a retrospective case series of patient satisfaction and functional outcome at a 2 to 8 year follow up. *Arthroscopy.* 2018;34(1):264-269.

166. Trevino S, Gibbs M, Panchbhavi V. Evaluation of results of endoscopic gastrocnemius recession. *Foot Ankle Int.* 2005;26:359-364.

167. Keeling J, Guyton GP. Endoscopic flexor hallucis longus decompression: a cadaver study. *Foot Ankle Int.* 2007;28:810-814.

168. Harris RC, Strannigan KL, Pirano J. Comparison of the complication incidence in open versus endoscopic gastrocnemius recession: a retrospective medical record review. *J Foot Ankle Surg.* 2018;57(4):747-752.

169. Saxena A, Widtfeldt A. Endoscopic gastrocnemius recession: preliminary report on 18 cases. *J Foot Ankle Surg.* 2004;43:302-306.

170. Tashjian RZ, Appel AJ, Banerjee R, et al. Endoscopic gastrocnemius recession: evaluation in a cadaver model. *Foot Ankle Int.* 2003;24:607-613.

171. Barrett SL, Day SV. Endoscopic plantar fasciotomy: two portal endoscopic surgical techniques-clinical results of 65 procedures. *J Foot Ankle Surg.* 1993;32:248-256.

172. Landsman A. Endoscopic plantar fasciotomy: a multi-surgeon prospective analysis of 652 cases. *J Foot Ankle Surg.* 1996;35:86.

173. Bazaz R, Ferkel RD. Results of endoscopic plantar fascia release. *Foot Ankle Int.* 2007;28:549-556.

174. Saxena A. Uniportal endoscopic plantar fasciotomy: a prospective study on athletic patients. *Foot Ankle Int.* 2004;25:882-889.

175. Stone PA, Davies JL. Retrospective review of endoscopic plantar fasciotomy-1992 through 1994. *J Am Podiatr Med Assoc.* 1996;86:414-420.

176. Zelent ME, Kane RM, Neese DJ, et al. Minimally invasive Morton's intermetatarsal neuroma decompression. *Foot Ankle Int.* 2007;28:263-265.

177. Barber FA, Click J, Britt BT. Complications of ankle arthroscopy. *J Foot Ankle.* 1990;10: 263-266.

178. Armstrong RW, Bolding F, Joseph R. Septic arthritis following arthroscopy: clinical syndromes and analysis of risk factors. *Arthroscopy.* 1992;8:213-223.

179. Shim JS, Lee JH, Han SH, et al. Neuroma of medial dorsal cutaneous nerve of superficial peroneal nerve after ankle arthroscopy. *PM R.* 2014;6(9):649-652.

180. Klein WW, Kurze V. Arthroscopic arthropathy: iatrogenic arthroscopic joint lesions in animals. *Arthroscopy.* 1986;2:163-168.

181. Deng DF, Hamilton GA, Lee M, et al. Complications associated with foot and ankle arthroscopy. *J Foot Ankle Surg.* 2012;51(3);281-284.

182. Lamy C, Stienstra IJ. Complications in ankle arthroscopy. *Clin Podiatric Med Surg.* 1994;11:523-539.

183. Guhl JF, Schonholtz GJ. Complications and prevention. In: Guhl JF, ed. *Foot and Ankle Arthroscopy.* 2nd ed. Thorofare, NJ: Slack, Inc.; 1993:215-230.

184. Small NC. Complications in arthroscopic surgery performed by experienced arthroscopists. *Arthroscopy.* 1988;4:215-221.

185. Rodeo SA, Forster RA, Vleiland AJ. Current concept review: neurologic complications due to arthroscopy. *J Bone Joint Surg Am.* 1993;75:917-926.

186. Gentile AT, Zizzo CJ, Dahukey A, et al. Traumatic pseudoaneurysm of the lateral plantar artery after endoscopic plantar fasciotomy. *Foot Ankle Int.* 1997;18:821-822.

187. O'Farrell D, Dudeney S, McNally S, et al. Pseudoaneurysm formation after ankle arthroscopy. *Foot Ankle Int.* 1997;18:578-579.

188. Tonogai I, Fujimoto E, Sairyo K. Pseudoaneurysm of the perforating peroneal artery following ankle arthroscopy. *Clin Rep Orthop.* 2018;2018:9821738.

189. Lundeen GA, Dunaway LJ. Immediate unrestricted postoperative weightbearing and mobilization after bone marrow stimulation of large osteochondral lesions of the talus. *Cartilage.* 2017;8(1):73-79.

CHAPTER 34

Ankle and Pantalar Arthrodesis

Steven R. Carter, Carl Kihm, and Aaron Bradley

INTRODUCTION

Ankle joint arthrodesis is a time-tested, effective, and predictable procedure for the surgical management of a variety painful conditions and pathologies of the ankle joint. It continues to enjoy popularity as a benchmark procedure.[1] A well-performed and precisely positioned arthrodesis consistently alleviates pain, corrects deformity, and improves function. Fusion of the ankle has been a useful surgical procedure for more than 100 years with more than 40 techniques and various modifications described.[2]

The Austrian surgeon, Albert, first used the term "arthrodesis" in 1878 for a fusion of the knee and ankle he performed in a 14-year-old child with lower extremity palsy. By the early 1900s, paralytic foot deformities were commonly managed surgically with ankle and subtalar joint (STJ) fusions.[3] In the 1930s, surgeons began using the procedure to manage other conditions such as posttraumatic arthritis following malunited ankle fractures.[3]

However, the procedure was not without complications and predictable fusion was not always reliable. In 1949, Glissan published four crucial principles to help ensure a successful result with greater rates of fusion.[4]

Glissan's Principles

1. Remove all interposing soft tissue.
2. Accurate and close fitting of the fusion surfaces.
3. Optimal position of (ankle) joint.
4. Maintenance of bone apposition in an undisturbed fashion until complete fusion.[5]

Additionally, we now understand the importance of not only débriding the articular cartilage but the additional step of removing the underlying subchondral bone plate to help facilitate fusion. In addition to Glissan's principles, it is important to also consider patient-specific factors that affect bone healing. Vascular status must be adequate as determined in the physical exam, with ABI studies or vascular consultation as indicated. Vascular intervention may be necessary in patients with inadequate perfusion for healing. Smoking and nicotine use inhibit vascularity and are associated with higher rates of nonunion. Therefore, patients should be educated of this and nicotine cessation encouraged. Diabetic patients with uncontrolled hemoglobin A1c levels also have higher healing risks and should be optimized to minimize infection and healing complications. Low vitamin D levels affect bone metabolism and can

be supplemented when necessary. Modification of immunosuppressive medications (steroids, chemotherapy drugs, etc.) is considered through physician collaboration. Intraoperative use of demineralized bone matrix is costly but can augment bone healing when indicated. Bone stimulation units can also be utilized in patients with high risk or delayed healing. Ultimately, regardless of patient education and instruction, the lack of patient compliance with non–weight-bearing orders can be catastrophic for bone healing and fixation construct stability.

INDICATIONS

Arthrodesis of the ankle is indicated for a variety of conditions including debilitating pain, arthritis, angular deformity, and instability that interferes with normal function and ambulation.[1] Prior to the recommendation for surgery, the surgeon is admonished to attempt substantial conservative treatment including various forms of medical as well as mechanical management. Various options include NSAIDs, corticosteroid injections, functional bracing, and physical therapy when indicated. If these treatment modalities are ineffective, the patient may become a candidate for fusion of the ankle.

ANKLE ARTHRODESIS INDICATIONS

1. Severe arthritis from a variety of conditions, as a result of trauma, an autoimmune condition such as rheumatoid arthritis, the slow progressive degeneration seen in osteoarthritis, or articular destruction from a septic arthritis
2. Neuromuscular deformity
3. Drop foot deformity
4. Deformity secondary to muscle imbalance (eg, calcaneus deformity)
5. Avascular necrosis of the talus or other disease resulting in collapse of the talar body
6. Neuropathic arthropathy often associated with diabetes or alcoholism
7. Failed implant arthroplasty of the ankle joint

ARTHRITIS

Arthrodesis of the ankle is used to treat a variety of conditions; however, posttraumatic arthritis is the most commonly reported indication, occurring most often as a result of pilon and malleolar fractures.[1] Degeneration of the joint in this scenario can be the manifestation of severe damage to the articular surface at the time of injury or inadequate reduction of the fracture fragments by either surgical or closed reduction management. Malunion that leads to posttraumatic arthritis typically occurs due to excessive shortening of the fibula and/or lateral.[1,5] Ramsey and Hamilton initially demonstrated that malreduction of the fibular fracture can allow the talus to laterally translate, and even 1mm of lateral talar shift resulted in 42% reduction of the tibiotalar surface congruency.[1] This was later confirmed in a study by Lloyd on cadaver ankles in 2006.[6] The decrease in contact area causes greater force transmitted per unit area of the ankle.[5]

Although total ankle replacement (TAR) is also a consideration in many of these situations, arthrodesis of the ankle is the gold standard. Long-term follow-up has shown favorable improvement in level of pain and degree of function. Development of adjacent joint arthritis after ankle arthrodesis with the foot positioned in neutral alignment is uncommon.[3]

Some surgeons advocate early fusion of the ankle after fracture, in the situation where there is substantial ankle pain but prior to the development of severe arthritis. This recommendation is based on the understanding that the posttraumatic arthritis is typically progressive and often resistant to conservative management.[7] However, there are also situations where radiographs demonstrate severe end-stage arthritis with complete loss of cartilage, but the patient has minimal symptoms and functions relatively well. In this scenario, arthrodesis is not indicated.[7]

NEUROLOGICAL DEFORMITIES

A number of neurological conditions can cause severe deformity and/or instability of the ankle, but are not amenable can be effectively managed with fusion of the ankle, and are often not amenable to correction with TAR. Also, many of these patients have such severe structural malalignment that successful bracing is not practically possible.

NEUROLOGICAL CONDITIONS ASSOCIATED WITH DEFORMITY OF THE ANKLE AND REARFOOT[5]

Neurological Conditions Associated With Deformity of the Ankle and Rearfoot

1. Cerebral Vascular Accident (CVA)
2. Neuropathic arthropathy
3. Charcot-Marie-Tooth Disease (CMT)
4. Spinal cord trauma
5. Myelodysplasias
6. Friedreich ataxia
7. Postpolio syndrome

In some paralytic conditions, there is frequently deformity and instability of the subtalar and midtarsal joints in addition to the ankle, necessitating a pantalar fusion as opposed to isolated arthrodesis of the ankle. An example of this is Charcot-Marie-Tooth disease, which often results in significant varus or adductus deformity of the rearfoot.[5]

FAILED AJ PROSTHESIS

TAR implant survival rate is about 69% according to the longest follow-up study known to date, which was ~10 years in length.[8] The majority of the implant failures are linked to infection, trauma, severe loss of bone stock, and inflammatory joint disease (IJD). However, one of the top factors that is an independent predictor of implant failure is ipsilateral hindfoot arthrodesis either before or after the TAR was performed, which triples the risk for revision. Another independent cause of failure is the use of an earlier generation type of implant, which leads to an eightfold higher rate of revision.[9]

Revisional ankle arthrodesis after a failed ankle implant has been found to have a union rate of 96% with noninflammatory joint disease (NIJD) subjects vs 73% of subjects with IJD.[10] A multitude of factors play a critical role in determining the appropriate procedure to perform. A failed total ankle implant can sometimes be salvaged with fusion of the ankle with autogenous bone graft and compression screw fixation.[3,5] In fact, the type of fixation is always dictated by the type of implant failure. Fixation methods include single anterior and double plating systems, internal screw fixation, and intramedullary nailing. Studies show the double plating systems offer stiffer constructs leading to higher fusion rates.[11] However, thinner screws are used with the double plating systems, which can cause them to break more easily. When substantial bone loss is present, studies show compression nail fixation is necessary. Use of the compression nails has shown a failure rate of ~17% when compared to noncompression nail fixation at 43%.[12]

AVN OF TALUS

Avascular necrosis (AVN) of the talus can occasionally be managed by fusing the ankle. The incidence of AVN ranges from 9.8% to 48%, which is dependent upon the Hawkins type of fracture.[13] Ankle trauma is linked to about 75% of the cases of AVN.[14] Conservative treatment with joint-sparing procedures has been found to help regress the process in the early stages of AVN. However, in the later stages of AVN, more extensive procedures such as arthrodesis, arthroplasty, and possible talectomy are necessary.[15]

In the case of an isolated symptomatic ankle with minimal talar collapse, the use of the open primary ankle arthrodesis with autogenous or allografts has proven successful.[16] Alternatively, when the talar body has significantly collapsed and is coupled with a symptomatic ankle, the use of the Blair fusion can be utilized. Most often, the talar body is removed and the talar neck is fused with the tibia as in the classic Blair fusion; however, some authors advocate leaving the avascular portion intact as a spacer. A sliding graft is then fashioned from the anterior tibia and inserted into the proximal neck of the talus.[7] The incidence of union rates for the Blair arthrodesis has increased to about 71%-80% as modifications have been made over the years.[17,18]

CONTRAINDICATIONS FOR ISOLATED ANKLE ARTHRODESIS

There are situations where arthrodesis of the ankle is ill-advised. Patients being scheduled for this type of surgery should be sent for preoperative medical clearance to assess medical conditions that could preclude a patient from having a major elective procedure. Examples include severe coronary artery disease, diabetes mellitus, or hypertension that is poorly controlled.

Clearly, sufficient arterial perfusion is necessary for predictable wound healing and therefore severe PAD would be a contraindication to elective surgery. However, it should be noted that there is no uniform agreement on what level of arterial insufficiency can exist and the surgery still be justified. The best advice is that if the patient has risk factors for PAD (eg, diabetes, history of tobacco use, poorly palpable pulses, or delayed capillary fill time), noninvasive vascular studies should be ordered and a vascular consult ordered to help determine the patient's risk of nonhealing. Ultimately the surgeon and the patient will have to make the final decision whether or not to proceed with surgery. The presence of PAD is not in principle, an absolute contraindication to surgery. PAD is a "risk" for nonhealing, and this risk has to be considered in the context of the degree of suffering the patient is experiencing. Some patients being considered for fusion of the ankle experience such suffering that they would consider BKA rather than to continue in daily pain. Hence, patients in this type of situation would be reasonable to accept a higher than normal risk of complication in the hope of a successful surgical outcome.

The patient's ability and willingness to comply with the postoperative protocols (eg, non–weight bearing) set forth by the surgeon must be discussed and agreed upon before surgery. It is not uncommon for a patient to be sent to physical therapy before surgery to ensure a patient's ability to remain non–weight bearing during the post-op course. Physical therapy can also be useful to help teach a patient how to ascend and descend steps when necessary.[1]

Contraindications to Isolated Arthrodesis of the Ankle

1. Severe peripheral arterial disease (PAD)
2. Unsuitable preexisting medical conditions
3. Severe osteoporosis
4. Inability to comply with post-op recommendations
5. Extensive AVN of the talus
6. Symptomatic arthritis of the subtalar joint (possibly necessitating tibiotalar calcaneal fusion) or midtarsal joint (necessitating pantalar arthrodesis)
7. Heavy tobacco use
8. Active infection

PREOPERATIVE CONSIDERATIONS

A thorough preoperative workup and consultation between the surgeon and the patient prior to major elective surgery, such as arthrodesis of the ankle, is of critical importance to help ensure optimal results. Mahan et al. have shown that patients have much higher satisfaction rates after ankle and pantalar fusions if they are sufficiently prepared prior to surgery.[2]

RADIOGRAPHY

As a part of the preoperative workup, weight-bearing views of the ankle should be taken. Those include AP, mortise, and lateral views.[3] It is also recommended to take standard DP and medial oblique to image the midfoot and tib-fib views when there is supramalleolar deformity.

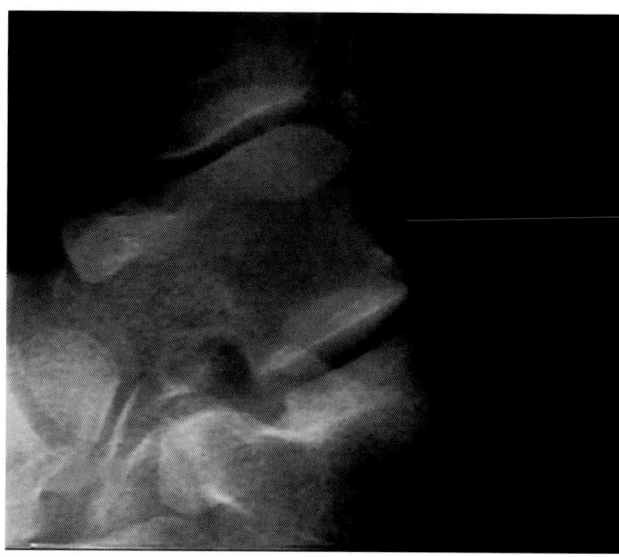

FIGURE 34.1 Broden view of the hindfoot.

Views focusing on the STJ should be considered. These include the Broden (Fig. 34.1) and Isherwood views; calcaneal-axial views can also help assess the resting calcaneal stance position.[19]

Ankle Arthrodesis Considerations

1. Incisional approach utilized
2. Optional osteotomies (medial malleolar and/or fibular)
3. Technique for articular surface removal (eg, curettage, osteotome/mallet, saw resection)
4. Fixation (internal vs external)

The described technique is the authors' preferred method, utilizing one-incision or two-incision "gutter" approach without osteotomy of the fibula to gain access to the ankle. Stabilization is achieved with internal compression screw fixation.

DOCUMENTATION CAVEATS

The medical record should clearly document substantial preoperative impairment, justifying the recommended surgery and necessary subsequent aftercare. Furthermore, a detailed list of conservative treatment that was attempted but proved unsuccessful should be documented. Although prior to surgery there is typically significant loss of motion, the long-term functional implications (both positive and negative) as they relate to the complete elimination of ankle joint motion after surgery should be discussed. It should be explained that although the motion of the ankle will be eliminated, the patient's function and activity level should be expected to improve due to the substantial decrease in pain. Although maximum benefit may not be seen for 6-9 months after surgery, the preexisting arthritic pain is usually eliminated. If other procedures, such as ankle arthroplasty or TAR are also considerations for the specific patient, these options should be discussed with the patient. With respect to the informed consent process, possible complications should be outlined including infection, wound healing problems, possible nonunion, need for bone graft, and possible need for revisional surgery.[7]

ASSESSMENT OF ADJACENT JOINT INTEGRITY

Before committing to an isolated fusion of the ankle, it is imperative to ensure that the preoperative pain is due to pathology in the ankle and not the adjacent joints. It is not infrequent that a patient has subtalar pain in addition to ankle pain and in that instance a tibiotalar-calcaneal fusion would be more suitable. The surgeon is admonished to carefully evaluate the adjacent joints through thorough examination consisting of palpation, range of motion exam, and review of plain film radiographs when there are arthritic changes in the STJ it is typically fused, even in the scenario where there is little to no preoperative pain, due to the anticipated increased stress the STJ will be expected to sustain after an isolated ankle arthrodesis. If there is uncertainty as to the amount of adjacent joint pain or pathology, further investigation can be undertaken with the use of other diagnostic imaging such as a CT scan, or selective local anesthetic blocks of the ankle and adjacent joints.[2] Ahlberg and Henricson reported that two-thirds of the patients in their study on isolated ankle arthrodesis reported pain in the region of the STJ at long-term follow-up of 12.3 years.[8,20]

PROXIMAL DEFORMITIES

A full biomechanical assessment of proximal deformities is an imperative part of any type of patient evaluation. The most common cause of ankle pathology is posttraumatic arthritis.[21,22] Fibular malleolar fractures are the leading etiological factor for ankle arthritis when compared to all lower extremity fractures.[23] Proximal deformities such as limb length discrepancies, scoliosis, spondylolisthesis, femoral anteversion, tibial torsion, genu varum, and recurvatum can have a debilitating effect on gait. It is important to treat proximal deformities prior to ankle arthrodesis because it can lead to misalignment issues and progressive arthritis postoperatively. Proximal deformity may influence which fixation option is optimal for the individual situation. Long-leg radiographs may be required to adequately assess (Figs. 34.2 and 34.3)

> ### PEARLS
>
> *Deformity or angulation proximal to the ankle joint must be assessed preoperatively. This is an example of a patient with a history of previous midtibial fracture that led to subsequent ankle osteoarthritis. In planning for tibiotalocalcaneal fusion, internal fixation was chosen over IMN fixation due to the deformity within the healed tibia.*

VITAMIN D LEVEL

Many factors contribute to Vitamin D deficiency. Disorders that alter the absorption and metabolism of vitamin D are one such cause. Certain populations, such as the elderly and others who may be unable to get proper sunlight exposure, are also at high risk.[24] Vitamin D deficiency has become a significant risk factor that has been linked to nonunion in many studies. Particular patients who have vitamin D pathology are 8 times more likely to experience a nonunion.[25] However, there have also been studies that have not demonstrated a significant relationship between vitamin D deficiency and nonunion but instead associate nonunion with multiple risk factors being present and not just vitamin D deficiency alone.[26] The majority of the associated

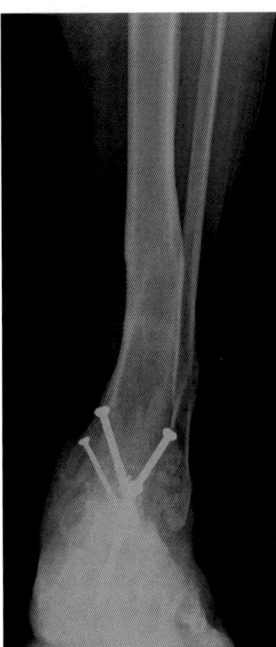

FIGURE 34.2 Anteroposterior radiograph following ankle arthrodesis with internal fixation.

risk factors include advanced age, high BMI, and the presence of osteoporosis.[27] However even with supplementation, the clinical effects of vitamin D deficiency are less well described when it comes to the relationship to nonunion and fracture healing and are inconclusive in the literature at this time.

TOBACCO USE

In addition to the adverse effects on the cardiovascular system, smoking is also known to interfere with soft tissue and bone

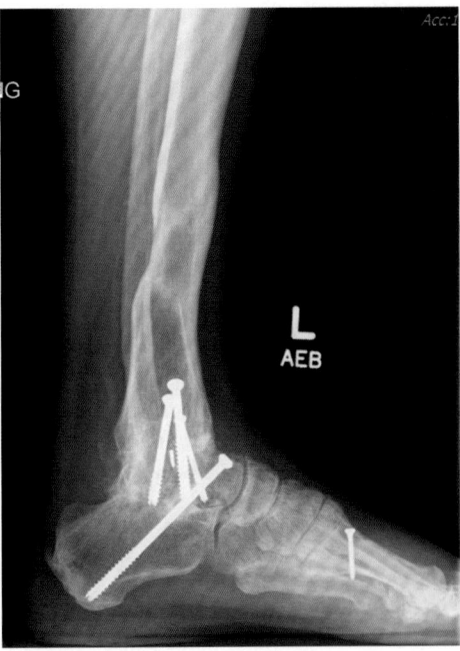

FIGURE 34.3 Lateral radiograph following ankle arthrodesis with internal fixation.

healing. Nicotine effects occur due to a combination of factors including vasoconstriction, formation of carbon monoxide, and inhibition of osteoblastic activity. Ishikawa et al., in 2002, evaluated the rate of nonunion in rearfoot fusion patients who were smokers, nonsmokers, and smokers who quit prior to surgery. The highest nonunion rate was in smokers (18.6%), and the least in nonsmokers (7.1%). Patients who discontinued smoking prior to surgery had a nonunion rate of 11.1%. These results suggest that smoking has an adverse effect on healing rates of rearfoot fusions.[28] Cobb et al. found smokers have a 3.75 times higher relative risk of nonunion compared to nonsmokers following ankle arthrodesis.[29]

Pearson performed a systematic review and meta-analysis of over 40 published studies on this subject. It was concluded that smokers have 2.2 times (1.9-2.6) the risk of delayed union and/or nonunion. In the patients in whom union did occur, it consistently took more time in the smokers, revealing an increase in time to union of 27.7 more days.[30]

There is no universal agreement on the amount of time that must pass after discontinuing smoking to offset the increased risk of nonunion that nicotine use poses. Most authors recommend tobacco abstinence for at least 30 days prior to surgery and continuing until the time bone healing is confirmed on x-rays.[31,32]

IMMUNOSUPPRESSANT THERAPY

Patients who are taking immunosuppressive medication for any disease must be fully evaluated for any potential surgical complication. A multidisciplinary approach is necessary to optimize such a patient for surgery. The only studies that have a high percentage of subjects with IJD undergoing ankle arthrodesis of 83%-89% report union rates to be at 61%-69%.[33,34] Unfortunately there are no current studies comparing the union rates of subjects with IJD and non-IJD subjects. The majority of patients with arthritis have underlying disease and are typically on disease-modifying antirheumatic drugs (DMARDs). Epidemiological studies demonstrate the prevalence of these diseases within the general population. They found the incidence of rheumatoid arthritis (RA) to be 0.5%-1%, psoriatic arthritis (PA) 0.16%, and systemic lupus (SLE) ~0.1% of the general population.[35] This demonstrates a significant population who suffer with the disease, necessitating knowledge and understanding of how to manage these patients during surgery.

It is critical to understand the pharmacodynamics and realize that patients taking these medications are at higher risk for complications. Immunosuppression therapy will increase the risk of infection, cardiovascular effects, pathological effects on clotting, and delayed wound healing.[36,37] When patients with chronic inflammatory disease reduce immunosuppression intake, it will exacerbate an inflammatory response at the wound site. This inflammatory response can present similar to an infection. When this occurs, the clinician must make a decision to treat the infection with antibiotics or instead increase the immunosuppression therapy. Both choices can have consequences; in the scenario of increasing immunosuppression medication, the underlying infection without antibiotics can lead to sepsis. Increasing immunosuppression therapy can also lead to an immunocompromised state, which can cause pneumonia and delayed wound healing. Alternatively, the scenario where the clinician starts antibiotics and reduces the immunosuppression medications can lead to a debilitating exacerbation of inflammation. This is extremely painful and

can cause patients to become sedentary, which increases risk of thrombosis.[38]

Within the current literature there is no evidence-based recommendation for the management of immunosuppressive therapy in the perioperative setting. This stems from the lack of double-blinded, randomized control trial studies available. The current recommendations suggest continuing the current dose of methotrexate, leflunomide, hydroxychloroquine, and sulfasalazine in patients with RA, ankylosing spondylothesis, and SLE.[39] However, patients taking JAk/STAT inhibitors must stop taking the medication one week prior to surgery. Communication amongst providers and a multidisciplinary approach is necessary to determine the best course of action regarding managing medications in the perioperative and postoperative settings.

TECHNIQUE

There are various technique considerations for fusion of the ankle joint. The major considerations include

1. Incisional approach utilized
2. Optional osteotomies (medial malleolar and/or fibular)
3. Technique for articular surface removal (eg, curettage, osteotome/mallet, saw resection)
4. Fixation (internal vs external)

The described technique is the authors' preferred method, utilizing one-incision or two-incision "gutter" approach without osteotomy of the fibula to gain access to the ankle. Stabilization is achieved with internal compression screw fixation.

TWO-INCISION APPROACH

The described technique employs a two-incision approach for the primary purpose of fusion of the ankle joint.[1] The patient is placed in the supine position, and a well-padded calf or thigh tourniquet is applied.

Lateral Incision

The initial incision is placed laterally over the fibula, beginning ~6 cm proximal to the tip of the lateral malleolus. Generally, the intermediate dorsal cutaneous nerve is retracted medially and is contained in the anterior flap. The incision courses distally and parallels the superior border of the peroneal tendons and ends over the sinus tarsi region. This approach provides excellent exposure of the lateral aspect of the talus (Figs. 34.4 and 34.5)

The incision courses distally and parallels the superior border of the peroneal tendons and ends over the sinus tarsi region (Fig. 34.4). This approach provides excellent exposure of the lateral aspect of the talus. Although typically not performed, osteotomy or excision of the fibula can provide further access into the tibiotalar joint surfaces (Fig. 34.5) Lateral ankle exposure offered after fibular takedown.

Although primary hemostasis is provided by use of the tourniquet, all encountered vessels that cannot be retracted should be addressed with the use of electrocoagulation and ligatures of absorbable suture. The deep fascia and lateral portion of the inferior extensor retinaculum are incised so that the extensor digitorum longus can be retracted medially (Fig. 34.6).

The periosteum is incised and subperiosteal dissection is completed along the anterior edge of the fibula and across the distal tibia and anterior ankle joint (Fig. 34.7).

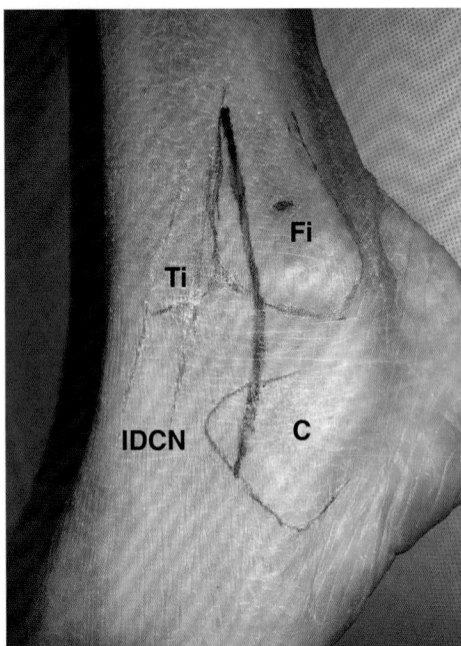

FIGURE 34.4 Lateral anatomic surgical landmarks. Ti:tibia; Fi:fibula; IDCN, intermediate dorsal cutaneous nerve; C, calcaneus.

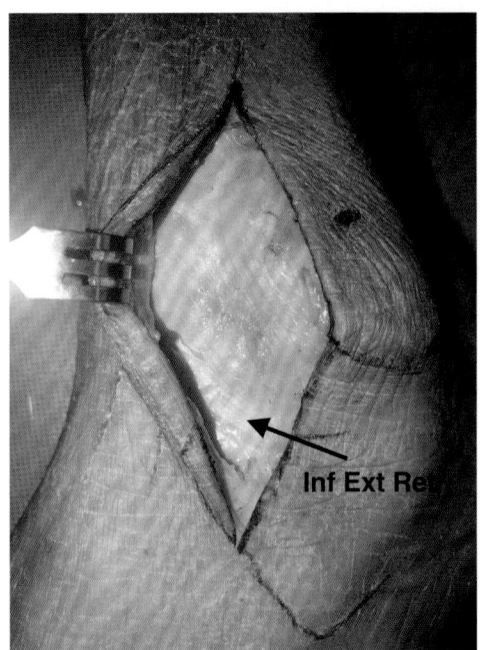

FIGURE 34.6 Lateral gutter approach showing the inferior extensor retinaculum.

It is generally not necessary to release the anterior inferior tibiofibular ligament, but if deemed helpful, it can be released to allow increased mobility of the fibula from the tibia (Fig. 34.8). The perforating peroneal artery is often encountered in the deep lateral dissection and should be ligated when encountered; otherwise, this vessel can be a source of significant bleeding after the tourniquet is deflated. The periosteum should not be completely stripped from the lateral aspect of the fibula. Maintaining periosteal attachment helps to preserve blood supply, minimizing bone healing complications.[1]

A curved osteotome can be used to release the calcaneofibular ligament (Figs. 34.9 and 34.10). This maneuver substantially improves the ability to distract the ankle joint. Excision of the ligament can aid in visualization of the posterior ankle and STJ recesses.

Medial Incision

The medial incision is placed over the medial ankle gutter and distal portion of the tibia. Most often it is oriented just anterior to the saphenous nerve and vein (Fig. 34.11).

The incision courses distally ending at the level of the navicular-cuneiform joint, to allow visualization of the anterior and medial ankle joint, the medial gutter, as well as the head and neck of the talus.[1] A curved osteotome can be used to release the deep deltoid ligament (Fig. 34.12).

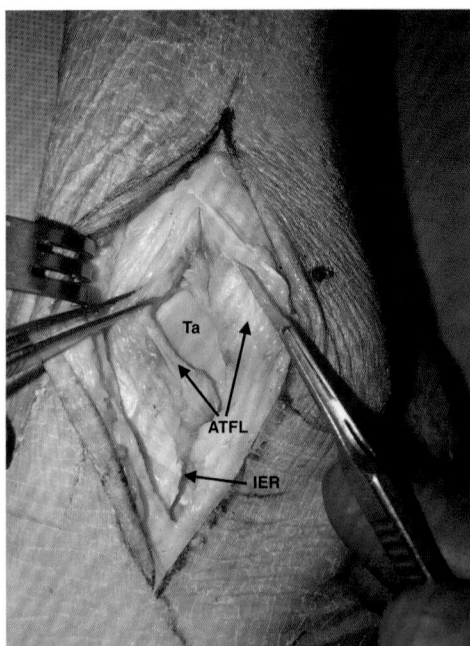

FIGURE 34.7 Lateral ankle exposure offered after fibular takedown. Ta:talus; ATFL, anterior talofibular ligament; IER, inferior extensor retinaculum.

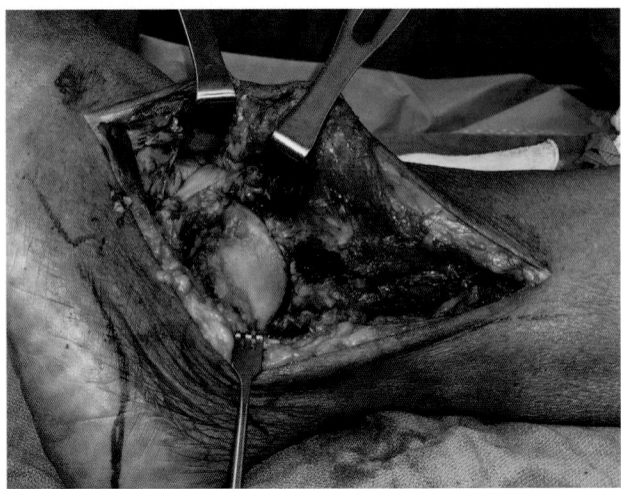

FIGURE 34.5 Lateral exposure after fibular takedown.

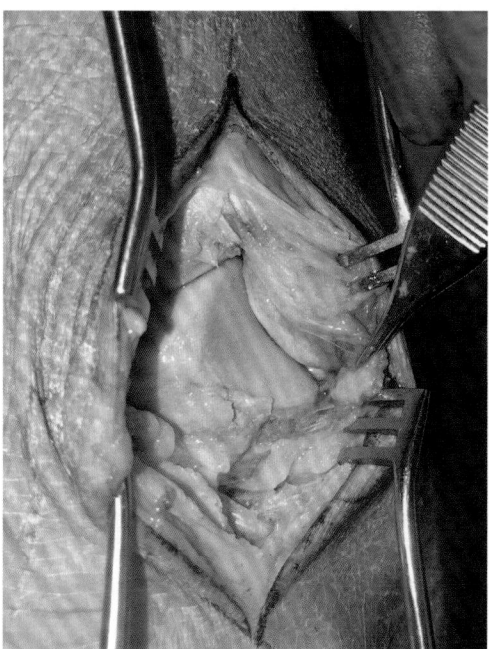

FIGURE 34.8 Visualization of the lateral shoulder of the talus. The periosteum attached to the fibular malleolus is preserved.

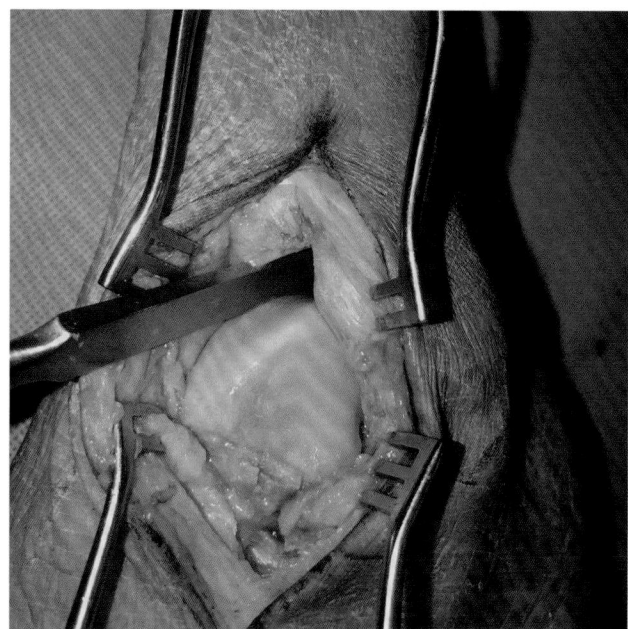

FIGURE 34.10 Dorsal and lateral exposure of the talus.

JOINT RESECTION

Once the articular surfaces are exposed, it is often necessary to remove interposed fibrous tissue and peripheral exostoses to allow sufficient visualization of the joint surfaces. Bone rongeurs typically work well to help accomplish this task. If there is preexisting varus or valgus deformity, a decision will need to be made as to whether or not the malposition can be corrected with manipulation of the joint vs a need for bony wedge resection. To help make this determination the ankle can manipulated and temporarily pinned in a desired position of fusion and evaluated under fluoroscopy prior to resection of the joint. If wedge resection is not deemed necessary, the articular

Anteriorly, the medial and lateral incisions are connected subperiosteally facilitating elevation of the tendons and neurovascular structures crossing the anterior aspects of the ankle joint. The surgeon is encouraged to preserve as much of the periosteal/capsular attachments as possible where they are attached to the distal tibia.[1] The periosteum provides ~80% of the blood supply to the bone and, therefore, should be handled carefully and maintained when possible.[40] In spite of this recommendation, it is important to remember that adequate visualization of the entire ankle joint is paramount, and sufficient dissection needs to be performed to allow precise joint resection and positioning.[1]

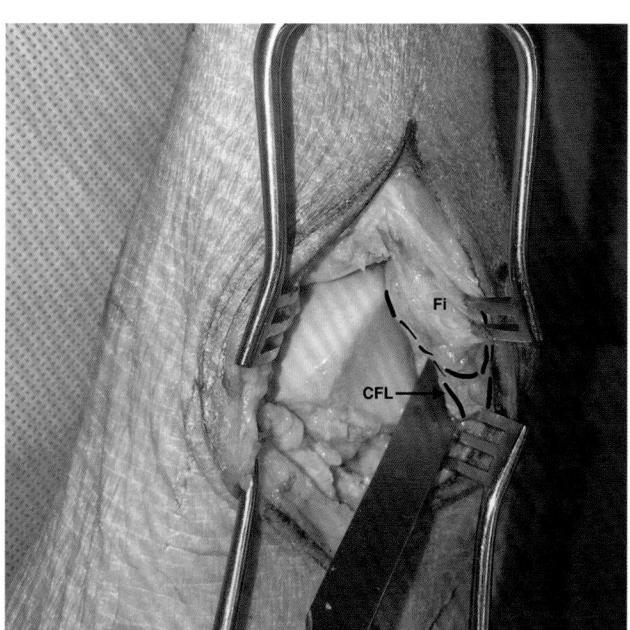

FIGURE 34.9 Calcaneofibular ligament (CFL) suspended by curved osteotome. Fi:fibula.

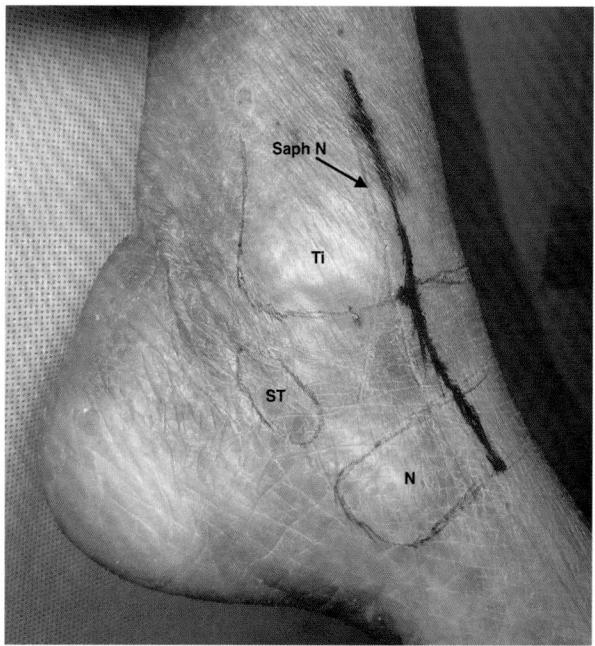

FIGURE 34.11 Medial anatomic landmarks. Saph N., saphenous nerve; Ti:tibia; ST, sustentaculum tali; N, navicular.

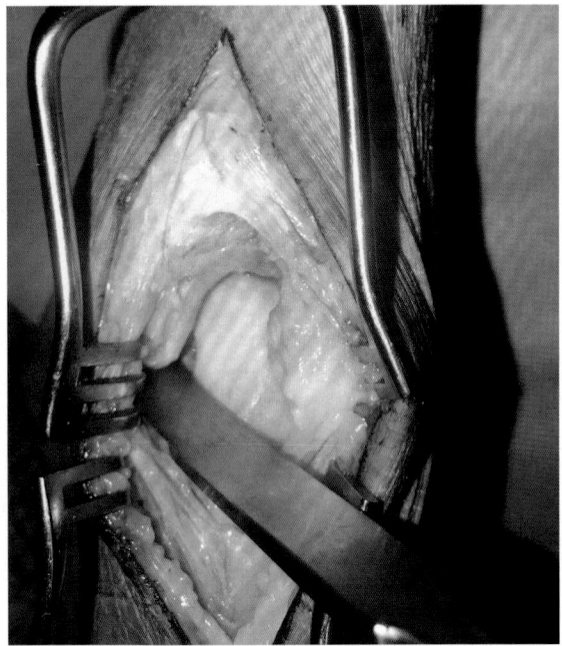

FIGURE 34.12 Curved osteotome releasing deep deltoid.

surfaces are typically removed with a combination of curettage, burring, and subchondral drilling.

If the curettage technique is chosen for joint resection, adequate distraction of the joint is imperative so that the articular surfaces can be properly visualized. There are a number of instruments to facilitate this task including lamina spreaders and small distraction devices. Generally, articular resection begins laterally, with the distraction device inserted medially (Fig. 34.13).

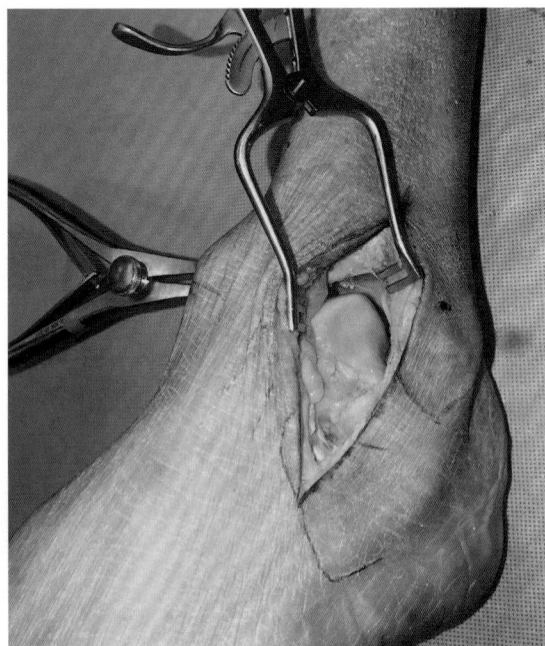

FIGURE 34.13 Weitlaner retractor maintaining lateral exposure.

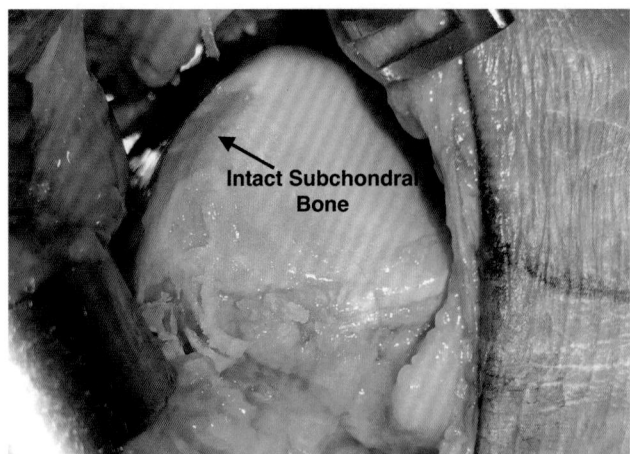

FIGURE 34.14 Initial resection of cartilage including the subchondral bone plate.

It is particularly important to not only resect the articular cartilage but also remove the dense subchondral bone plate, which if left intact can delay or prevent fusion of the joint.[1,40] (Figs. 34.14 through 34.16)

As the posterior aspect of the joint is approached, the inferior lip of the tibia should be removed so as not to interfere with proper position of the talus in the final position of fusion. If saw resection of the joint is chosen, we typically begin at the medial aspect of the joint. Before any cuts are made, it is important to ensure complete visualization of the anterior to posterior borders of the gutter so as not to create iatrogenic damage to the posterior tibial artery and tibial nerve, which are positioned just posterior to this region.[3] We begin the resection by removing the inner articular surface of the medial malleolus, followed by the adjacent comma-shaped facet on the medial body of the talus. Next, we direct our attention to the distal surface of the tibia and work from a lateral to medial direction. Unless frontal plane correction is needed, the plane of resection is perpendicular to the long axis of the distal tibia. The surgeon is cautioned to pay particular attention as the resection

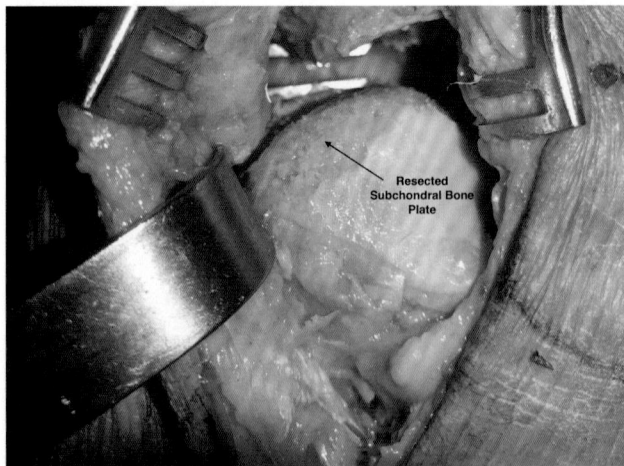

FIGURE 34.15 Further articular resection across the dorsum of the talus.

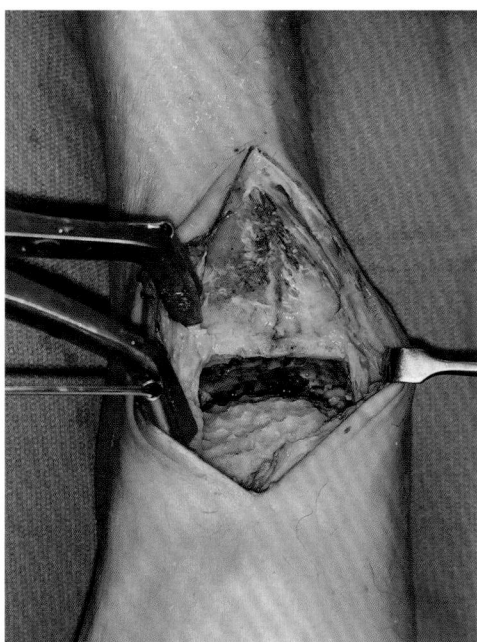

FIGURE 34.16 Completion of dorsal resection.

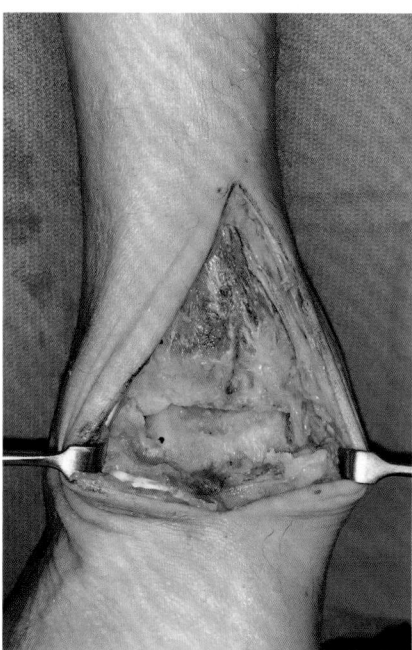

FIGURE 34.17 Medialization of the talus in the ankle mortise.

continues medially to avoid inadvertent resection of the medial malleolus.

Prior to resection of the talar dome, the ankle is held in neutral in the sagittal plane, with slight external rotation, while carefully assessing the frontal plane position of the ankle and heel. If acceptable, the dorsal surface of the talus is then removed, again working from a lateral to medial direction. If, however, slight wedging is needed, attention is redirected to the distal tibia where additional wedge resection is performed to correct frontal plane abnormalities. The focus is primarily directed to the distal tibia so as to avoid an overaggressive resection of the talar dome. When this occurs, the talus can be left excessively short making successful fixation difficult.

The fusion surfaces are resected in such a way so that when placed together, the talus can be snugly fitted against the medial malleolus (Fig. 34.17).

As the talus is translocated medially, the lateral gutter space increases. If the fibula is not being osteotomized for fibular excision or only grafting, there are three choices. Those options are to (1) pack the lateral gutter with bone graft, (2) leave the gutter open with no intention of the two surfaces fusing together, or (3) resecting the distal syndesmosis fibular onlay.[3]

After the final alignment is determined, the joint is held in the expected position of fusion and checked for stability, and a lack of rocking or gapping at the fusion site. If necessary, reciprocal planning of the joint is performed to remove high and low spots, until the adjacent surfaces are well opposed, and the construct is stable[1] (Fig. 34.18).

POSITION OF FUSION

Sagittal Plane

The ideal fused construct of the ankle is that with the foot positioned in neutral flexion in a 90-degree position to the leg. It is imperative, however, that the surgeon not pronate the STJ

while positioning the ankle in the sagittal plane. The STJ must be maintained in neutral. Some surgeons choose to temporarily pin the STJ in a neutral attitude, prior to positioning of the ankle. An ankle inadvertently fused in plantar flexion also promotes medial collateral ligament instability of the knee as well as the incidence of genu recurvatum in the stance phase of gait. Patient gait analyses and evaluation of pressure measurements within the STJ have demonstrated excessively high articular pressures when the ankle is fused in equinus instead of neutral flexion.[3,5,41]

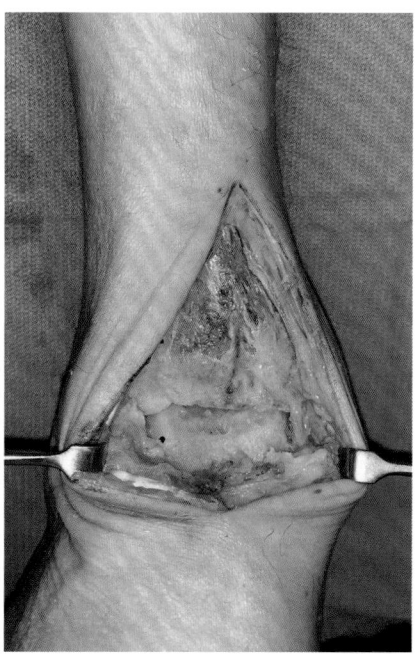

FIGURE 34.18 Final fit of the fusion construct prior to temporary fixation.

There is some disagreement in the literature as to the anteroposterior position of the talus in the ankle mortise. Buck reported fewer long-term problems with the knee and overall improved gait if the talus was translocated slightly posteriorly in the ankle mortise.[41] Other authors contend, however, that posterior shifting of the talus has a tendency to create long-term problems in the STJ due to the lengthening of the lever arm in the rearfoot.[3]

Transverse Plane

The optimal position of fusion in the transverse plane is ~15 degrees of external rotation where the foot is situated in line with the transmalleolar axis. The position of the patella should be visualized when the final transverse plane alignment is determined.[5]

Frontal Plane

The frontal plane position of the fusion should be such that the heel is oriented in slight valgus (2-5 degrees) in relation to the distal tibia when subtalar is held in a neutral position. However, this calculation has to be considered in the context of any distal tibial frontal plane deformity that may be present. As an example, if there is preexisting 10 degrees of distal tibial varum, the rearfoot may need to be fused in 12 degrees of valgus.[5,41] Visual intraoperative assessment is made easier when the entire leg, to a level just above the knee, is included in the sterile prep.

Position of Fusion

Sagittal plane: Neutral flexion in a 90-degree position to the leg
Transverse plane: ~15 degrees of external rotation
Frontal plane: Slight valgus (2-5 degrees)

INTERNAL FIXATION

Internal fixation is the most common choice made by surgeons who routinely perform ankle arthrodesis. However, external fixation is also a routine choice made by many surgeons and will also be discussed. Internal fixation offers the advantage of avoiding the common complication of pin-tract infections and also obviates the need for a mandatory second procedure to remove the external hardware.[2]

Temporary Fixation

After resection is complete and position of fusion has been set, temporary fixation is employed. One option is to percutaneously drill a smooth Steinmann pin from the plantar aspect of the heel, through the calcaneus, talus and into the distal tibia while the ankle is being held in the desired position of fusion. Another option is to temporarily fixate the joint with the guide pins, over which cannulated screws will be placed. If noncannulated screws will be used, the temporary Kirschner wires or Steinmann pins are placed adjacent to the desired position of the final screws.

Once temporary fixation is achieved, fluoroscopy is utilized to confirm proper pin placement and alignment of the fusion construct (Fig. 34.19).

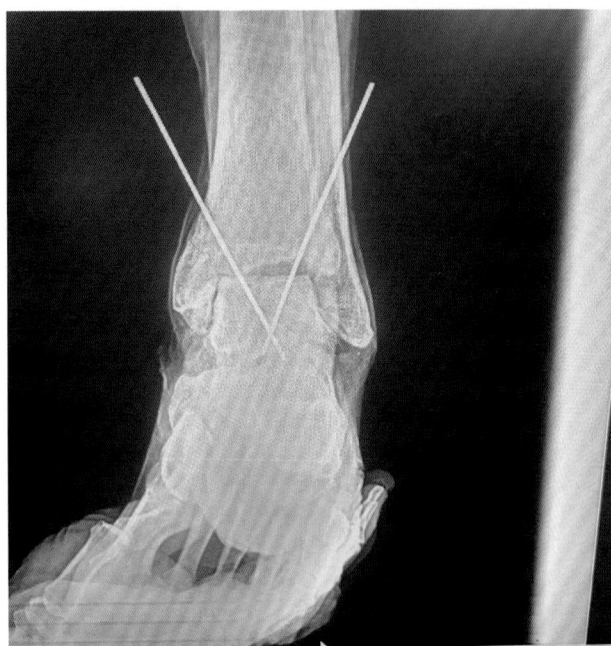

FIGURE 34.19 Anteroposterior radiograph showing temporary fixation pins.

If cannulated screws are to be used, the length of the guide pins can be adjusted and thread length selected so that the threads of a screw driven from the tibia into the talus are sufficiently within the body of the talus to maximize thread capture and joint composition. Threads of a partially threaded screw should not be within the ankle joint, and the screw must not extrude into the STJ.[5]

Final Fixation

There are a variety of screw placement options to successfully achieve stable compression fixation of an ankle arthrodesis. We will describe a 2-screw technique that is not technically difficult but is consistently reliable. We most often use two noncannulated partially threaded 6.5-mm cancellous screws. It should be pointed out, however, that specific size and number of screws should ultimately be based on individual surgeon's preference and intraoperative conditions. We begin with insertion of a screw that begins anteromedial being directed inferior and lateral. This screw is the more anteriorly positioned of the two screws and serves the purpose to compress the medial shoulder of the talus firmly against the internal surface of the resected portion of the medial malleolus. The second screw begins slightly more proximal just anterior to the fibula and is directed inferior medial (Figs. 34.20 and 34.21).

Supplemental Fixation

In some instances, it is possible or necessary to add supplementary fixation for added stability. Intraoperative assessment of local bone conditions, screw purchase, and joint compression are weighed. Partially threaded screws may not always capture enough of the talus to adequately effect compression. Patient demographics, medical comorbidities, and anticipated

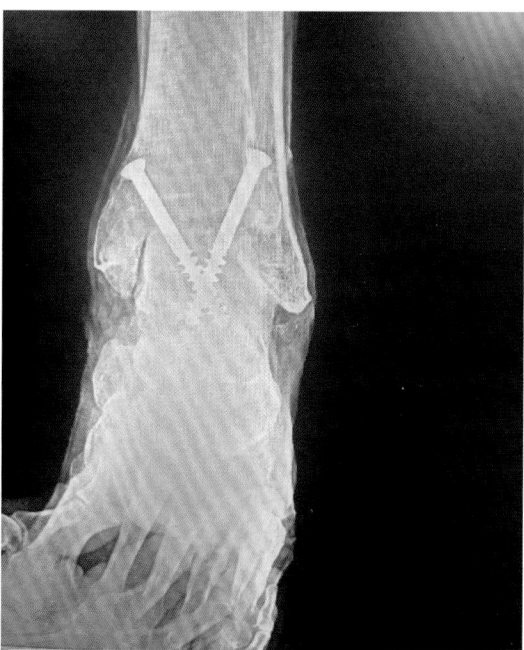

FIGURE 34.20 Anteroposterior radiograph showing internal fixation screws.

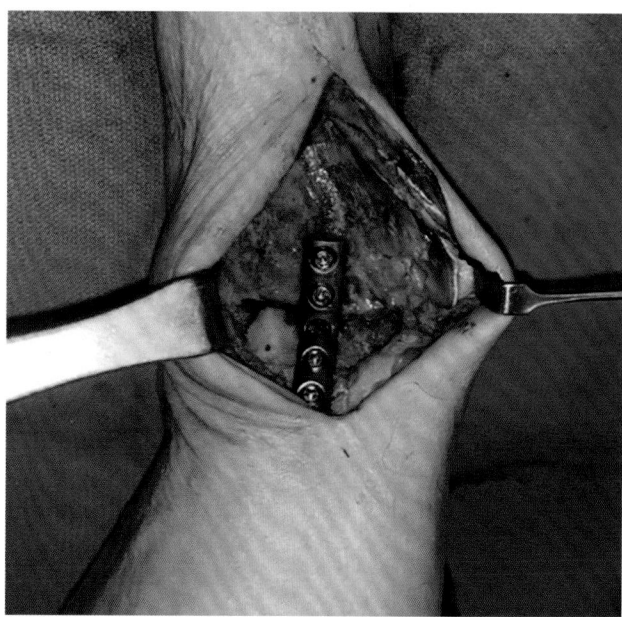

FIGURE 34.22 Through an anteromedial ankle gutter incision, the entire ankle joint surface is visualized and a plate is fixated across the anterior ankle.

non–weight-bearing compliance are considered when deciding which fixation construct is best.

When utilizing a third screw, one desirable location is to insert it from the anterior portion of the lateral talar process, directed superiorly and posteriorly into the distal tibia.[1]

Alternatively, at the anterior aspect of the joint, a small plate can be placed to fixate the distal tibia to the dorsal neck of the talus. The wide spread of fixation from front to back and side, in these constructs, increases strength (Figs. 34.22 through 34.24).

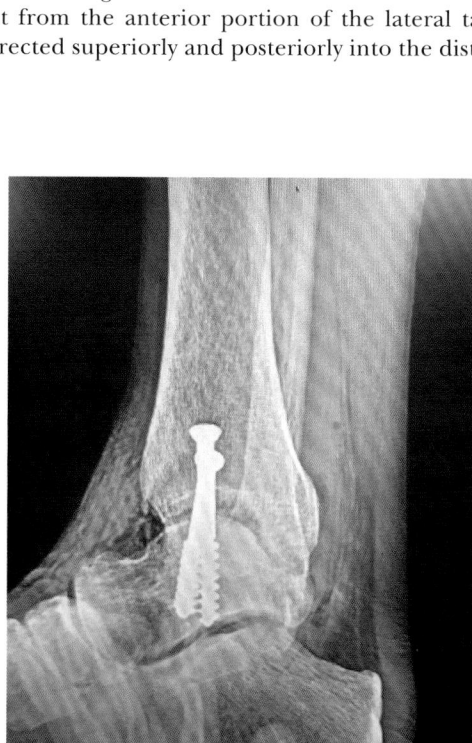

FIGURE 34.21 Lateral radiograph showing internal fixation screws.

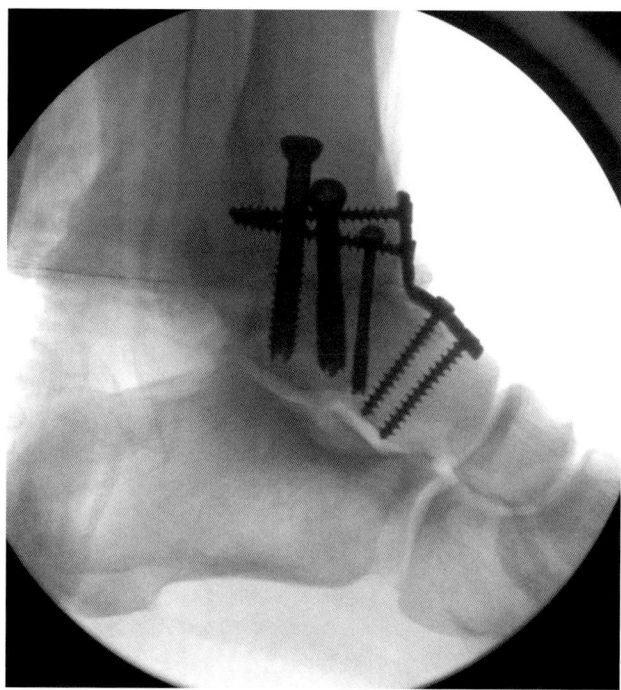

FIGURE 34.23 Lateral radiograph shows good capture across the tibiotalar joint with wide spread of fixation from front to back.

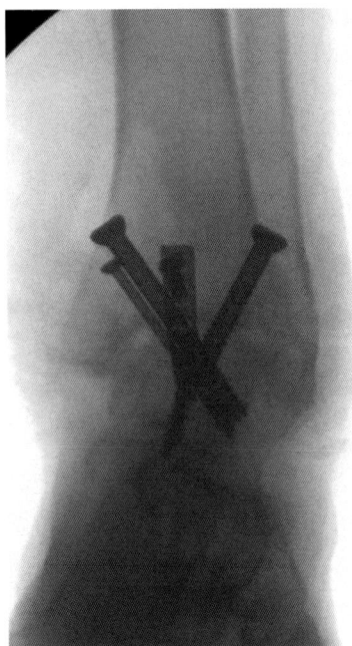

FIGURE 34.24 Anteroposterior radiograph shows good capture across the tibiotalar joint with wide spread of fixation from side to side.

Ankle/Pantalar Arthrodesis: **Pros and Cons of Fixation Options**		
	Pros	**Cons**
Internal fixation	■ Time-honored ■ Effective ■ Low expense	■ Prominent fixation ■ Requires most periosteal dissection
Intramedullary nail fixation	■ Smaller incision/minimal periosteal dissection ■ Internal compression ■ Greatest construct stiffness ■ Axial load allows early weight bearing	■ Size of bone void created ■ High rate of removal ■ Potential spread of infection ■ Risk of proximal stress risers
External fixation	■ Ability to use with ulceration ■ Ability to use if a patient has a history of infection ■ Allows early weight bearing ■ Allows postoperative dynamic manipulation	■ High expense ■ Difficult for patient ■ Pin tract infection, cellulitis

X-RAY CONFIRMATION

After final fixation is achieved and the temporary pins have been removed, intraoperative x-rays are taken, or fluoroscopy is utilized to confirm the final position of fusion and fixation placement. Multiple views should be shot while manipulating the foot to ensure that no screws are extending into the STJ.[1] Final films should include an anteroposterior, mortise, and lateral view of the ankle as well as a calcaneal axial view.[5]

FINAL TIGHTENING AND GRAFTING

Final tightening of the screws is performed once all screws have been placed and deficits packed with appropriate bone graft material as necessary.

If a fibular osteotomy was performed, the medial articular cartilage and subchondral bone plate are removed, and remodeling is performed so that the fibula is well seated against the lateral portion of the talus with the distal tibia to serve as an on-lay graft. The graft can be fixated to the talus and tibia using 4.0 mm partially threaded cancellous screws; however, attempted fixation of the fibular osteotomy is generally discouraged due to occasional painful nonunion.[5]

CLOSURE AND POST-OP CARE

After final fixation is achieved, the surgical wounds are thoroughly irrigated with sterile saline. Typically, the wounds are packed with moistened gauze sponges, the foot and ankle are wrapped with an ACE bandage, and then the tourniquet is deflated. After several minutes, the elastic bandage is removed and the amount of bleeding is determined. Hemostasis is achieved with further electrocoagulation and vessel ligation as necessary. If there is still persistent ooze and the patient is scheduled to be admitted to the hospital after surgery, a closed-suction drain can be introduced to decrease the chance of postoperative hematoma and subsequent wound healing problems.[1]

Anatomic layer closure is carried out using absorbable suture of choice. We have had excellent results with decreasing the need for postoperative narcotic analgesics by performing a popliteal block with a slow-release form of bupivacaine marketed under the name Exparel®. A sterile dressing and a well-padded Jones compression cast or splint are then applied. Most often, the Jones cast is removed 3-5 days after surgery and if there are no signs of wound healing problems, infection, or excessive edema, the permanent cast is applied. Most patients are kept non–weight bearing for 10-12 weeks or until there is radiographic evidence of consolidation followed by 2-4 weeks of protected weight bearing in a pneumatic walking boot. X-ray confirmation of fusion may not be fully apparent for 4-6 months after surgery; however there should be evidence of early consolidation at the point the patient is allowed to initiate protected, partial weight bearing.

PANTALAR ARTHRODESIS

Pantalar arthrodesis describes the surgical fusion of the ankle with the three rearfoot bones. This extensive procedure creates an osseous continuity from the leg into the foot. Through the various levels of arthrodesis, severe positional deformities can be neutralized and a more stable foot provided for better function. This extensive procedure is technically demanding and generally

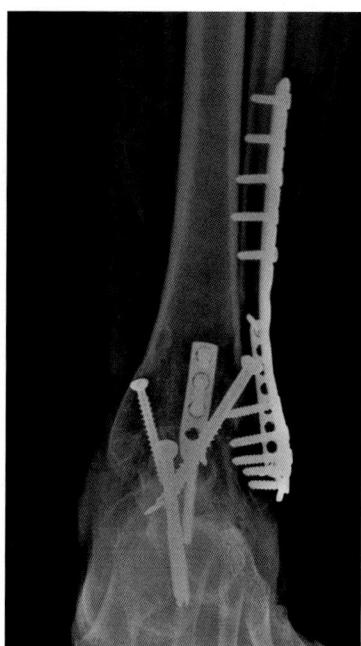

FIGURE 34.25 Posttraumatic arthritis necessitated ankle arthrodesis; however, the previous fibular fixation did not impede ankle arthrodesis. It is not always necessary to remove retained fixation.

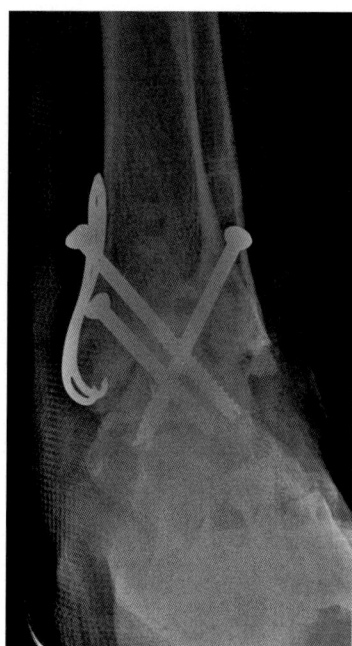

FIGURE 34.26 Another example of posttraumatic arthritis that necessitated ankle arthrodesis. Screws were removed through percutaneous incisions. The plate was not painful and did not impede ankle arthrodesis fixation, and to remove it would have required larger incisions.

reserved for complicated patients with complex deformity. The surgical goal is to reduce severe pain, deformity, and instability. This is ultimately a salvage alternative for limb amputation.[42,43]

Pantalar arthrodesis was first described in 1911 by Lorthioir as treatment for paralytic and congenital equinovarus deformities.[44] Correction of the equinovarus foot has been successful in patients affected by cerebral palsy, myelomeningocele, poliomyelitis, clubfoot and Charcot-Marie-Tooth. Ankle and rearfoot Charcot neuroarthropathies oftentimes require pantalar arthrodesis for limb salvage. Pantalar arthrodesis is preferred in cases where it is necessary to increase vascularity to an avascular bone or nonunion site. Advanced osteoarthritis, associated with systemic arthritis or extensive trauma, may also require pantalar arthrodesis to eliminate painful joints. It is not always necessary to remove all previous fixation from previous procedures (Figs. 34.25 and 34.26).

Progressive joint degeneration from the foot to the ankle can be seen long-term in triple arthrodesis patients (Figs. 34.27 through 34.30), those with advanced pes planovalgus, posterior tibial tendon dysfunction, talar AVN, osteoarthritis, rearfoot coalition, etc. (Figs. 34.31 and 34.32). Increased ankle strain in neuropathic patients may result in Charcot of the ankle instead of progressive osteoarthritic change[45,46] (Figs. 34.33 through 34.35). Alternatively, locking the ankle with an isolated ankle arthrodesis can result in increased rearfoot stress and progressive breakdown. In these situations, the patient may need to be converted to pantalar arthrodesis.

Long-term outcome studies support pantalar arthrodesis as a successful salvage procedure and alternative to limb amputation. High union rates and satisfactory results have been reported.[42,47–51] Papa reported 86% union rate at a mean of 14 weeks.[47] Patients are typically highly satisfied with significant reduction in pain and improved function.[48,49] Those with persistent pain generally benefit from shoe modifications and bracing.[47] "Takedown" of painful ankle fusions for conversion to

TAR has been reported to decrease pain and improve motion and quality of life. Although conversion patients may find some improvement, complications are frequent and improvements are not typically as dramatic as primary procedures.[52]

Arthrodesis alignment is crucial since the ankle and rearfoot joints become locked and local compensation mechanisms are eliminated. Even with proper alignment, increased strain to the midfoot, forefoot, and knee joint can lead to progressive arthritis and pain.[47,53] Provelengios found that 16 of 24 pantalar arthrodesis patients experienced ipsilateral knee pain but not until an average of 20.8 years postoperatively.[42] Although pantalar patients are generally satisfied, there are certainly

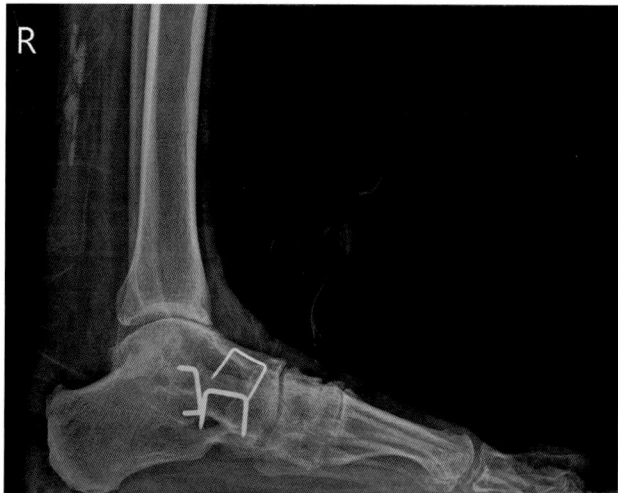

FIGURE 34.27 Lateral radiograph of a postpolio patient who underwent a triple arthrodesis 50 years ago and has since developed progressive osteoarthritis and ankle valgus deformity.

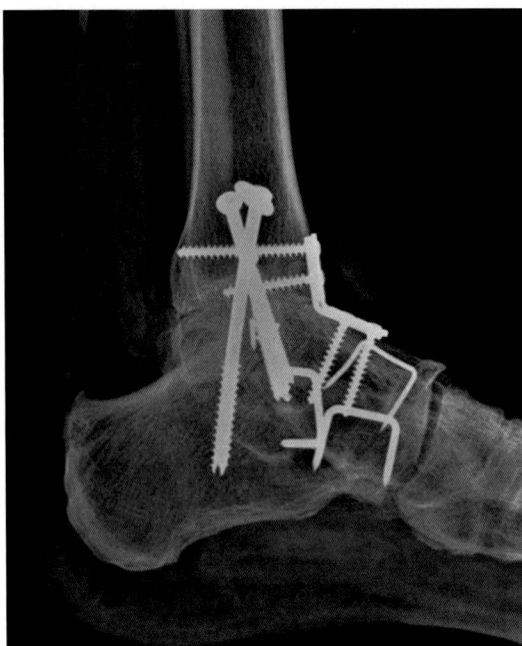

FIGURE 34.28 Patient from Figure 34.27 following ankle arthrodesis conversion to pan talar arthrodesis. Previous fixation was maintained.

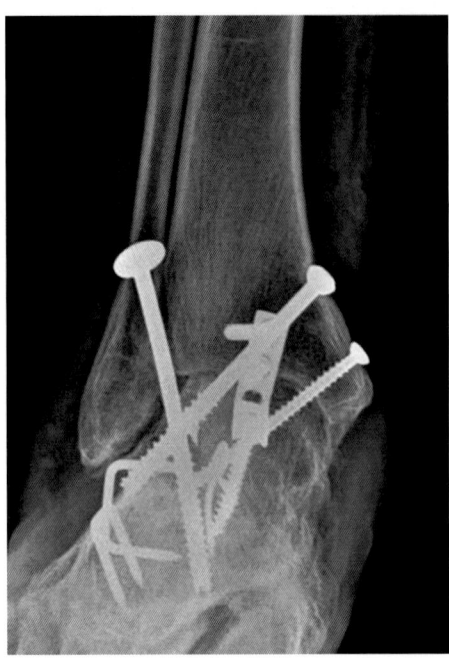

FIGURE 34.30 Anteroposterior postoperative radiograph demonstrating triple to pantalar arthrodesis conversion.

limitations in function. These include walking on uneven terrain, squatting, ascending hills, and climbing stairs. Nonetheless, these limitations are superior to the function and sequelae associated with limb amputation. It is noted that patients with tibiotalocalcaneal (TTC) arthrodesis are more mobile and have better function than do those with pantalar arthrodesis.[47] When possible, the midtarsal joints should be spared.

Operative techniques for triple arthrodesis and isolated subtalar arthrodesis are described in Chapters 25 and 26. There are

many acceptable techniques and fixation options for pantalar arthrodesis. Two incisions are generally utilized. The authors prefer a medial ankle gutter incision that is extended distally along the medial column of the foot, as necessary, and a separate lateral incision from the distal fibula to the cuboid-metatarsal junction (Figs. 34.36 and 34.37). The medial incision provides exposure to the tibiotalar joint surfaces, talonavicular joint (TNJ), and talar neck when utilizing an anterior ankle plate or superior-inferior STJ screw fixation. The lateral incision allows for STJ and calcaneocuboid joint (CCJ) resection

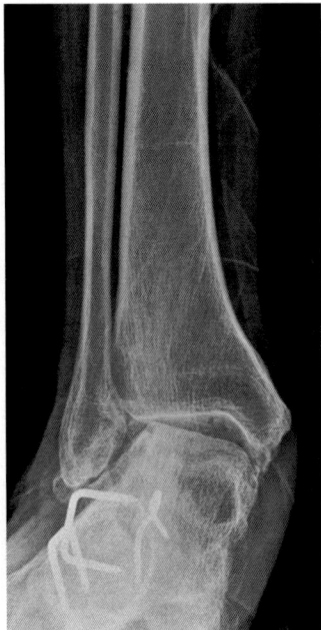

FIGURE 34.29 Anteroposterior radiograph of patient from Figure 34.27, demonstrating severity of osteoarthritis and ankle valgus deformity 50 years following triple arthrodesis.

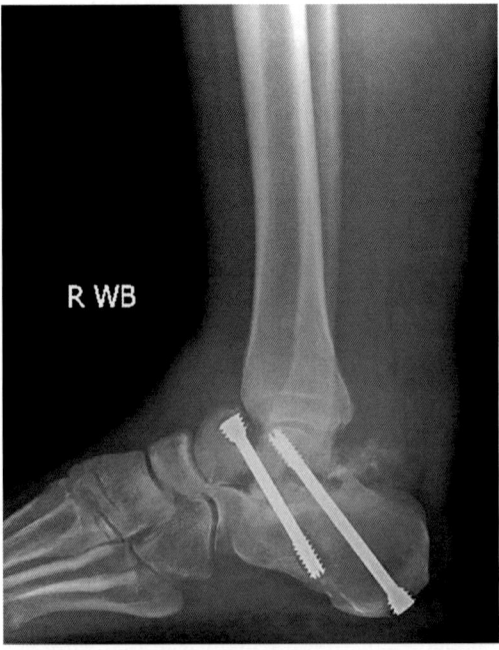

FIGURE 34.31 Arthritic STJ, due to pigmented villonodular synovitis, was managed via STJ fusion. Talar fracture, collapse, and avascular necrosis subsequently occurred.

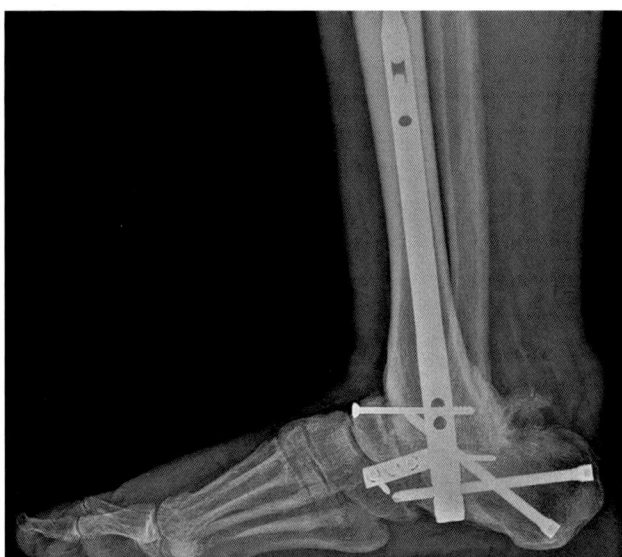

FIGURE 34.32 Patient from Figure 34.31 was managed with talectomy and tibiocalcaneal, calcaneocuboid, and tibionavicular arthrodeses.

and fixation. The distal fibula and lateral talar surfaces must not be incorporated for successful tibiotalar arthrodesis.

Historically, a longer lateral incision, which bisects the distal fibula and curves along the lateral foot, was used to expose the STJ posterior facet surfaces and CCJ. A second incision is still recommended for adequate TNJ preparation and fixation. The extensive lateral approach allows for fibular take-down and ankle joint exposure. The distal fibula can be used as a buttress onlay graft, sectioned into autogenous bone graft dowels to fill a large bony void, or morselized into cortical bone graft for smaller voids. Generally, this transfibular approach is not necessary, and the fibular malleolus can be maintained as a stable buttress even when fusion is undertaken. Other concerns with this approach include increased nonunion risk, alterations

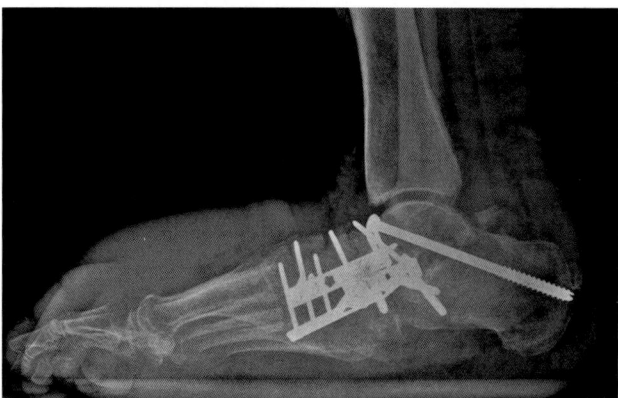

FIGURE 34.34 Patient from Figure 34.33 consolidated following reconstruction via triple arthrodesis and medial column arthrodesis.

of the ankle's overall shape and configuration, and difficulty for future conversion to TAR.

A less frequently used posterior approach for ankle arthrodesis requires the patient to be in a prone position (Figs. 34.38 through 34.40).

Although the posterior approach may be optimal at times, the prone position is not amenable for pantalar arthrodesis. Arthroscopic and minimally invasive approaches have become a more popular option for patients at high risk for healing. Smaller incisions and less invasive approaches offer less risk for infection, dehiscence, and vascular disruption. A retrospective review of TTC arthrodesis compared complications encountered in open vs arthroscopic approaches. The open group had higher rates of soft tissue infection, but the arthroscopic group had higher risk for nonunion.[54] Others who utilize minimally invasive approaches have reported successful union rates and high levels of patient satisfaction.[55,56]

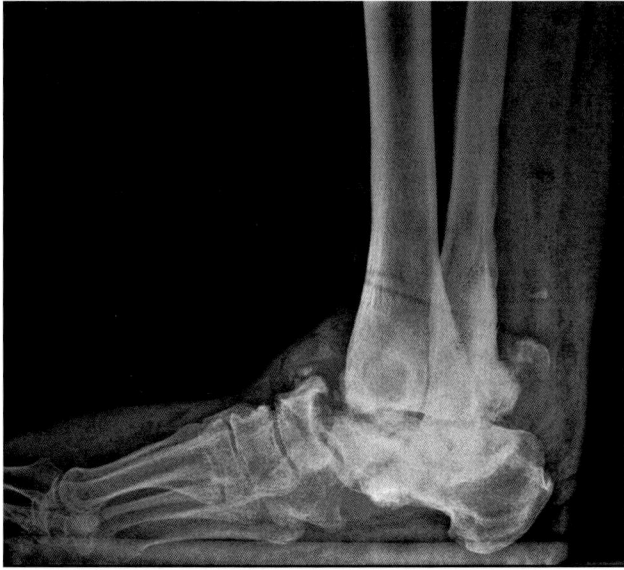

FIGURE 34.33 Peritalar subluxation and Charcot collapse in a patient with diabetic neuropathy.

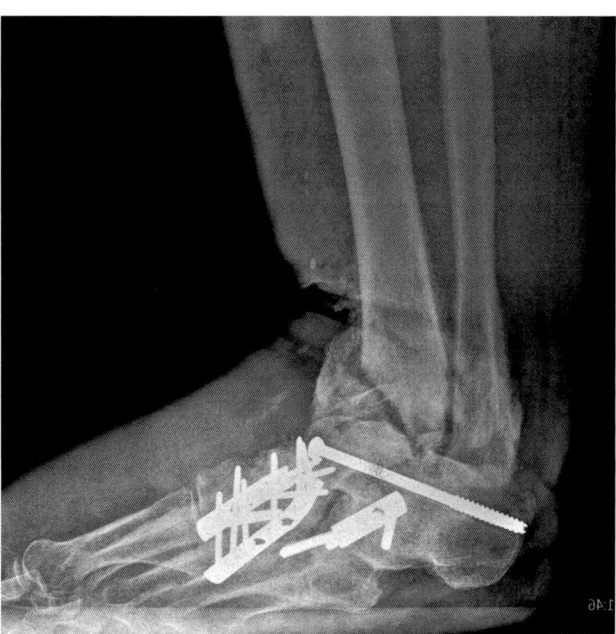

FIGURE 34.35 Patient from Figures 34.33 and 34.34 with diabetic neuropathy, following rearfoot fusion then developed a Charcot event of the ankle.

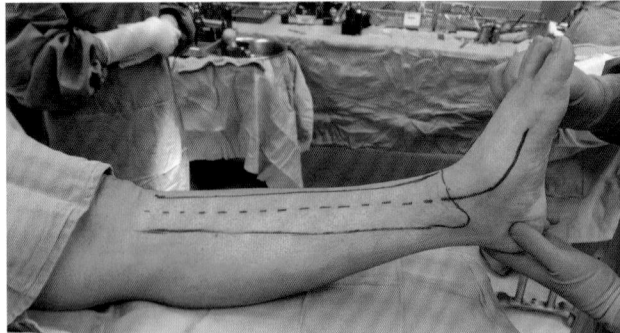

FIGURE 34.36 Ankle arthrodesis performed through a medial ankle gutter incision. This incision can be extended distally along the medial column, as necessary, for simultaneous arthrodesis procedures.

In order to achieve positional correction, shortening and wedging is sometimes necessary throughout the ankle or rearfoot. In cases of a failed TAR, talar AVN, nonunion, trauma, infection and bone lesions, voids of various sizes are generally managed with bone grafts. Fibular autograft, iliac crest autograft or allograft, femoral head allograft, and cancellous chip allograft options are considered depending on the situation.[57] Structural bone grafts have been suggested in voids larger than 2 cm to avoid limb length discrepancies.[58] Reamer-irrigator-aspirator methods have been described to obtain trabecular bone autograft from the proximal tibial metaphysis because it offers great concentrations of osteoinductive and osteoconductive cells. Blair fusion was described to preserve height after resecting the talar body, but oftentimes delayed union or nonunion occurs due to the lack of apposition between the tibia and talus neck.[17]

Once adequate joint resection and apposition is achieved, the joint segments are optimally positioned and temporarily fixated until permanent fixation is inserted. The ankle is aligned in neutral flexion with external rotation of 5-10 degrees to match the contralateral side. The heel is neutralized or positioned in slight (2-5 degrees) valgus, effecting a tibiocalcaneal position of 5-10 degrees of valgus.[59] This is most accurately assessed intraoperatively using the using the hindfoot alignment view, as described by Saltzman.[21,59] Rotation can be achieved through

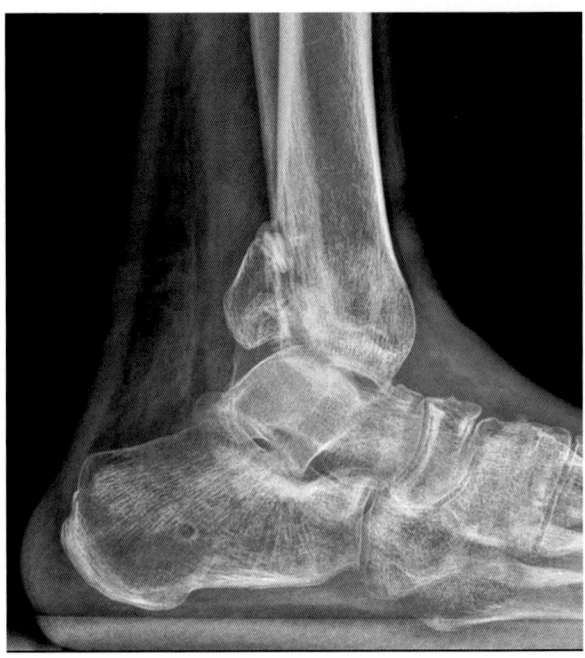

FIGURE 34.38 Neglected ankle fracture with posttraumatic arthritis and nonunion of displaced Volkmann fracture.

the midtarsal joint to align the rearfoot to the midfoot and obtain a plantargrade foot.

There are many successful fixation construct options for pantalar arthrodesis. Traditionally, screws crossing the ankle and rearfoot joints have been effective in providing compression and maintaining rigidity. This has been described separately in ankle arthrodesis and triple arthrodesis sections. Generally, pan talar arthrodesis fixation options can be categorized into: internal fixation options, retrograde intramedullary nail (IMN) options,

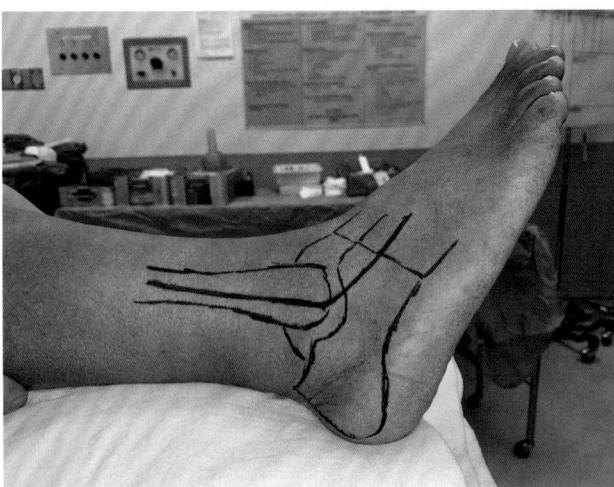

FIGURE 34.37 Lateral ankle incision technique utilized to take down a fibula or excise a fibular fracture segment. This approach allows for access into the ankle, subtalar and calcaneocuboid joints, as necessary.

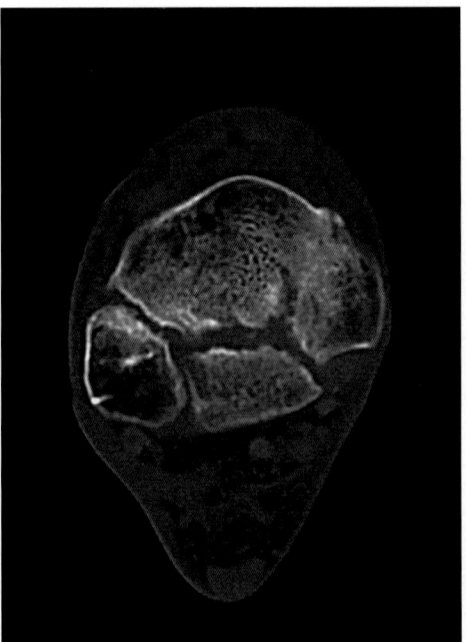

FIGURE 34.39 Patient from Figure 34.37. CT scan demonstrates a large posterior tibia nonunion. In order to incorporate this segment into the ankle arthrodesis, a posterior approach was found to be necessary.

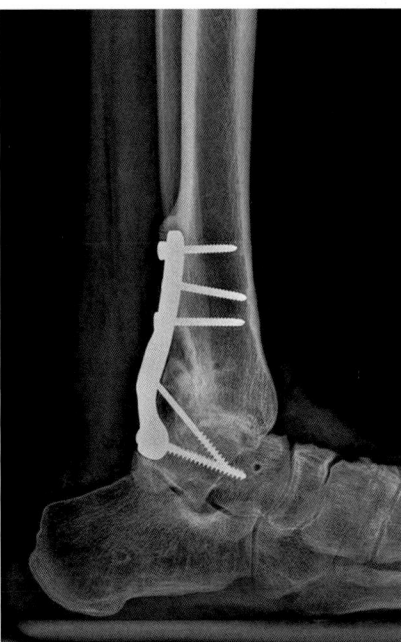

FIGURE 34.40 Patient from Figure 34.37. The Volkmann fracture nonunion segment was prepared for fusion and reduced to provide optimal tibiotalar surface apposition for arthrodesis.

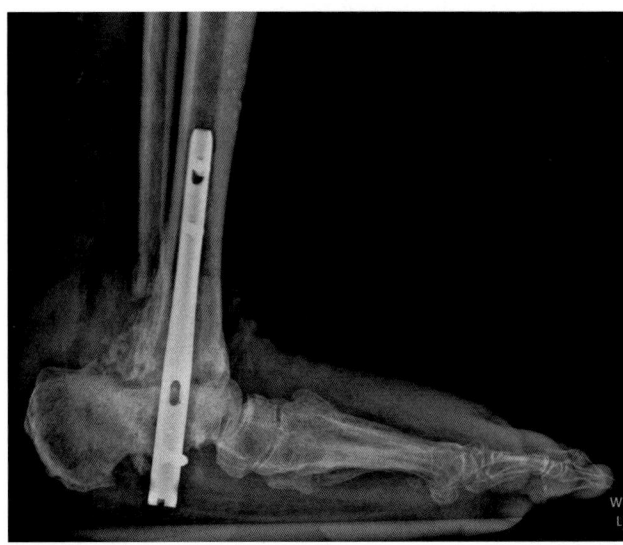

FIGURE 34.41 To maintain compression and stability, at least two screws must be incorporated into the distal nail. In this example, the nail is migrating distally out the plantar heel.

and external fixation options. Each offers advantages and disadvantages, which are considered on an individual patient basis to best meet patient demographics and arthrodesis demands.

INTRAMEDULLARY NAILS

Retrograde IMNs are commonly used in high-risk patients undergoing TTC or tibiocalcaneal arthrodesis. These procedures can be performed with or without midtarsal arthrodesis to effect pantalar arthrodesis. Since first described by Adams in 1948,[60] IMN indications have expanded and design developments allow optimization.

In high-risk patients, minimally invasive joint resection has been successfully used with the percutaneous insertion of IMN fixation.[54–56,61] Smaller incisions correlate with decreased infection rates in these patients IMN.[54] IMN insertion is more atraumatic than plate fixation methods, which require more extensive dissection and soft tissue stripping.[62] Preservation of vascularity may influence soft tissue infection and union rates. Meanwhile, IMN constructs are strong with significantly greater stiffness than crossed screws when assessed in all four bending directions and torsion.[62–64]

Axial compressive forces experienced during gait are transferred through bone via the nail, allowing for load-sharing compression across the ankle and STJ surfaces.[65,66] These constructs are stable and durable, and some investigators have even reported satisfactory fusion outcomes with early[56] and immediate postoperative weight bearing.[61]

Nail design and application ultimately determine the construct's strength and effect. Tibiotalar compression, achieved via tightening of the nail's internal compression mechanism, can provide several millimeters of internal compression. Interlocking screws are inserted into the nail to achieve static or dynamic compression, as desired. A footplate is then tightened against the heel to effect external compression of the STJ before

interlocking screws are placed within the calcaneus to maintain this compression. Biomechanical studies of cadavers have been valuable in assessing IMN compression and construct strength. A cadaver investigation has found that the IMN compression achieved across the ankle and STJ arthrodesis sites is not significantly different despite the different internal and external mechanisms to achieve compression around the joint, respectively.[67] Compressed IMN constructs have been shown to be more rigid than compressed external fixation and uncompressed IMN constructs.[68] To maintain the achieved compression, at least two screws must be interlocked at each end of the IMN (Fig. 34.41).[64]

O'neill reported that significant increase in IMN construct stiffness is achieved when augmented with a 6.5-mm TTC screw.[69,70] This may be of clinical importance when attempting to maximize construct strength for individuals with osteoporotic bone. To facilitate this, many nails are designed with a targeting arm to guide offset TTC screw fixation, as to not hit the nail or the other rearfoot interlocking screws.

Biomechanical studies also demonstrate the significance of the posteroanterior calcaneal interlocking screws on rotational stability. The perpendicular orientation of this screw, relative to the tibia and talar interlocking screws, provides angular stability and resistance to rotational forces.[71] IMN designs with two posteroanterior calcaneal screws can achieve even greater rotational stability of the nail than when only one posteroanterior calcaneal screw is used.[72] Failure to use a calcaneal posteroanterior screw increases risk for fixation failure. Therefore, when inserting the nail, it is important to assess the posterior calcaneus hole location and orientation.

Retrograde IMN for TTC have union rates reported from 74% to 93%.[45,54] Thomas' review of 59 IMN TTC arthrodeses revealed 93% union at an average of 4.17 months and 84% excellent or good functional results.[73] In the event of an ankle nonunion, the nail can be dynamized by removing the proximal static screw.

Although results are generally good for this salvage procedure, serious complications can occur. These include delayed union, nonunion, malunion, surgical site infection, osteomyelitis, fixation failure, periprosthetic fracture, ulceration, need for revision surgery, and limb amputation.[74]

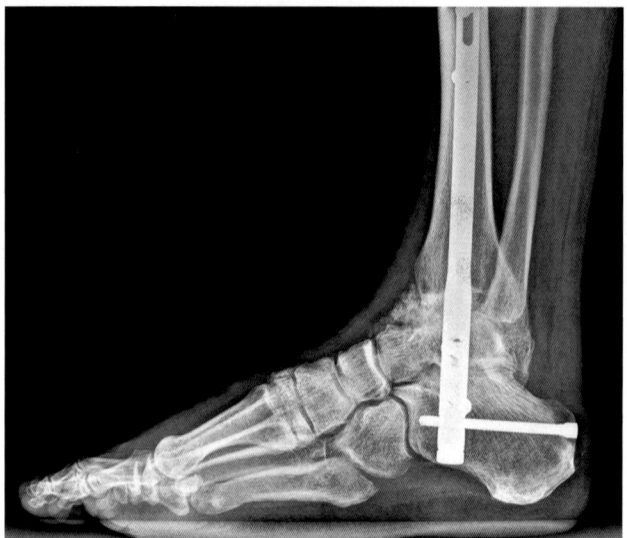

FIGURE 34.42 Example of an IM nail patient with a consolidated ankle arthrodesis and STJ nonunion that is nonsymptomatic, clinically stable, and nonproblematic.

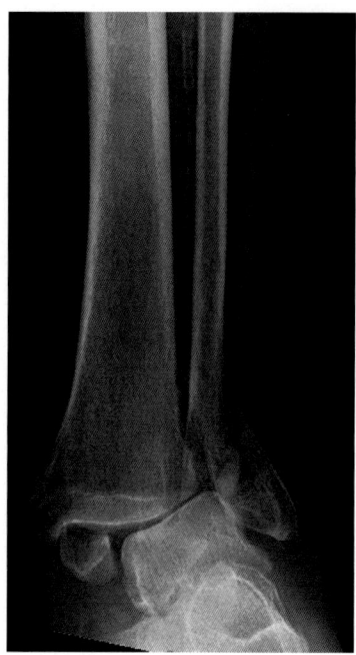

FIGURE 34.43 Traumatic ankle fracture dislocation injury in a geriatric patient.

There has been discussion as to whether STJ joint preparation is necessary. Studies have shown that STJ nonunions are usually asymptomatic and have good outcomes (Fig. 34.42).

Fenton reported on 55 IMN patients and had a 28% STJ nonunion rate; however, none of these were symptomatic or required revision surgery.[74] Griffin's assessment of 19 IMN patients found nonunion at the ankle in 12% and at the STJ in 23%; however, successful outcomes were reported in 94% and 88%, respectively.[75] A cadaver study found that only 5.89% of the talar articular surface is destructed with standard IMN reaming.[76] Long term, the joint is not destroyed, and with subsequent nail removal, STJ range of motion may be restored.[77] The use of stable IMN compression across unprepared TTC joints has now been adopted by traumatologists treating unstable ankle fractures in frail, elderly patients with mobility impairment and comorbidities.[78] In this population, a head-to-head comparison of open reduction and internal fixation (ORIF) to IMN treatment groups revealed higher complications in the ORIF group and similar functional outcomes in both groups.[79] One main advantage afforded by IMN fixation for fragility fractures is immediate postoperative partial weight bearing in this patient demographic (Figs. 34.43 through 34.45).

Due to the wide variety of surgical indications, surgical techniques, and IMN designs, direct outcome comparison is difficult.[74,80] A review of 631 IMN TTC arthrodesis patients, who underwent surgery for various indications, reported reoperation rate of 22% (137). Retrospective review of 40 patients at 1-year follow-up indicates that diabetes is associated with higher postoperative complication rates (59% vs 44%) but this difference was not statistically significant.[81] Lee's retrospective assessment of 34 IMN patients reported that uncontrolled diabetes significantly affects failure (defined as nonunion or amputation), with an odds ratio of 10 ($P = .029$).[39]

DeVries' retrospective study of 179 IMN patients produced a formula to calculate amputation risk.[82] Of the population studied, 11.7% underwent amputation. Diabetes was reported to be the most powerful predictive factor for amputation risk,

with an odds ratio of 7.01 ($P = .0019$).[82] Age between 30 and 70 years and revision surgery were also associated with increased probability for amputation. Charcot neuroarthropathy was not independently a significant risk factor for amputation; however, the authors note that diabetes is the most common cause of Charcot neuroarthropathy.

Arthrodesis of the neuroarthropathic ankle joint is difficult. Challenges include severity of deformity, poor bone stock, and propensity for wound complication and infection in patients who are oftentimes immunocompromised, with multiple medical comorbidities and low compliance. These patients are at increased risk and should expect prolonged periods of

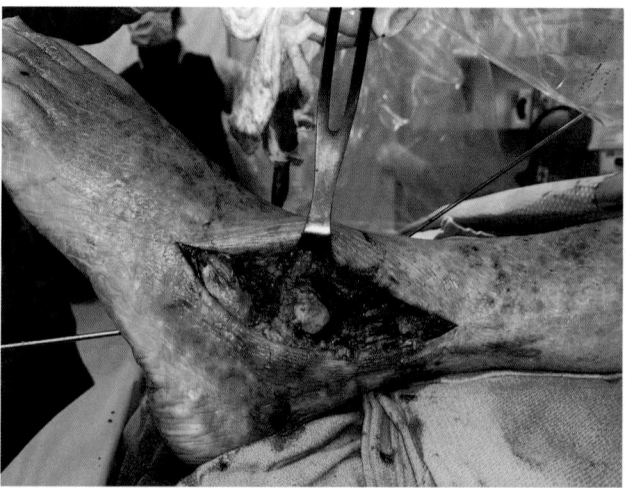

FIGURE 34.44 Patient from Figure 34.43 was treated with open management performed through a lateral incision to excise the fibular fracture, prepare the ankle and STJ joints, and insert lateral to medial IM nail screws into the talus and calcaneus (photos courtesy of Zachary Ogden DPM).

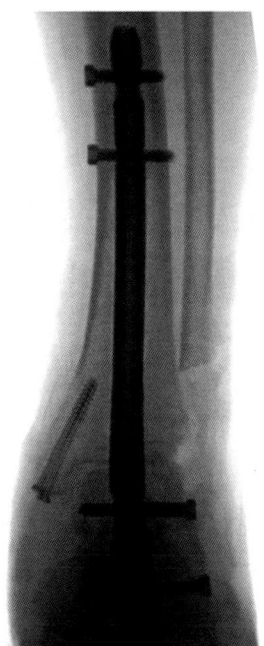

FIGURE 34.45 Anteroposterior radiograph of the geriatric ankle fracture patient from Figures 34.43 and 34.44. The IM nail construct offers stability, maintains position, and is amenable to early axial loading in the geriatric population.

postoperative immobilization and non–weight bearing.[83] Typically, these neuropathic patients are not in severe pain. Surgery is indicated as a limb salvage procedure to correct severe deformity, provide stability, minimize wound recurrence, and allow better function with a stable, plantargrade foot. Salvage of the Charcot ankle with IMN fixation has been reported in 82% or more.[65] However, only one-third of Charcot ankle IMN patients achieve uneventful and uncomplicated fusion.[61] Postoperative wound complication rates have been reported in 29%, and hardware removal necessary in 14%-21%.[65]

Ankle Charcot patients with ulceration or history of infection are at even higher risk for complication. Millet reported that once a diabetic Charcot patient ulcerates, the risk of amputation increases 12-fold.[84] Salvage surgery attempts in infected patients have traditionally utilized external fixation methods.

Amputation rate is high when IMN constructs fail, resulting in infected nonunions. If salvage is attempted, staged surgical management and long-term intravenous antibiotics are necessary. Treatment algorithms for this have been detailed.[85–87]

In the first stage of infection management, the IMN, interlocking screws and any other fixation is removed. The infected nonunion is surgically débrided. Progressive reaming of the intramedullary canal can be performed until fresh bone debris is achieved.[87] Irrigation of the nail's intramedullary canal via pulsatile lavage has been suggested.[87] Local delivery of antibiotics, via antibiotic beads or cement polymethylmethacrylate (PMMA) antibiotic nail, is recommended to augment systemic antibiotics that may have poor tissue penetration due to local ischemic conditions.[85–88] Vancomycin or tobramycin is typically chosen for their empiric coverage and elution properties. Mendicino outlined a method to create a PMMA antibiotic nail.[88] A nail maximizes bone surface contact area

within the tibial intramedullary canal for widespread antibiotic distribution. The PMMA antibiotic nail also eliminates dead space, provides stability, and can easily be removed after irradiation of infection.[88]

Bone specimens are obtained for pathology and microbiology. These indicate presence of osteomyelitis and report the infectious organisms with antibiotics sensitivities, useful to guide intravenous antibiotics selection. Typically, this is managed by an infectious disease specialist who also monitors systemic drug concentrations, drug tolerance, kidney function, etc. After completion of long-term intravenous antibiotics, the patient typically has a 2 week drug holiday prior to the next operative bone culture. If the subsequent culture and inflammatory markers are negative, definitive fixation is applied and the patient is made non–weight bearing for 3-4 months. Otherwise, the process is repeated or amputation is required.

Alternatively, Pawar presented a small case study of five Charcot ankle patients with failed, infected IMN fixation who were managed successfully in one stage.[86] Instead of using a PMMA nail in the first stage, a titanium nail coated entirely with antibiotic-impregnated PMMA was used to transfix and compress the ankle and STJ joints. This was maintained and infection was eradicated and union achieved in all five patients studied. Tomczak reported salvage in all eight patients managed with single-stage infection management using a PMMA nail and external fixation stabilization.[89]

Titanium is the most common IMN bio composite. It is infection resistant and, compared to stainless steel, has a modulus of elasticity closer to bone to better enhance stress-sharing between the implant and bone. A carbon fiber IMN has been designed with reports of good biocompatibility, and an even more optimal modulus of elasticity.[90] Carbon fiber has a stronger fatigue strength than most metal alloys, and it offers the advantage of being rather radiolucent. This allows for easier radiographic assessment of arthrodesis sites.

Even advancements in the IMN internal compression elements have optimized IMN compression. A nitinol internal compression element provides dynamic compression, which is maintained despite bone resorption in inflammatory stages of bone healing.[91,92] The nitinol compression effect has helped to achieve union rates up to 90%.[93] Alternatively, in many traditional IMN systems, dynamization to treat nonunion requires a second surgery to remove the proximal tibia's static screw. In Griffin's report on 19 IMN patients, all five nonunions encountered were treated with static screw removal to effect dynamization. This led to union in three and asymptomatic, fibrous union in the other two.[75] Head-to-head outcome studies have not directly compared IMN bio composition via cost-benefit analysis.

Nail designs also vary in size and shape. Historically, straight IMNs have been used with good outcomes.[94,95] The main advantage of the straight nail over a curved nail is that it can provide greater axial compression across the fusion sites. Most common complications of straight nails include poor rearfoot alignment, plantar neurovascular damage, poor calcaneal purchase, and tibial stress fractures.[95,96] When using a straight nail, the calcaneus is positioned under the tibia and the rearfoot alignment is set manually before temporary fixation is inserted. Due to the lateral offset of the calcaneus, optimal position can be difficult to obtain. In Brodsky's review of 30 straight IMN patients, average postoperative hindfoot position was 1.3 degrees of varus.[95]

Transient irritation of the plantar lateral nerve was reported in three (10%).[95] Shorter, straight nails around 15-16 cm in length are typically used to prevent the proximal tip of the nail from entering the tibial isthmus.[86,94] Minimizing stress here is believed to minimize stress fracture risk. Brodsky reported three (10%) proximal tibia stress fractures when a straight nail was used (lengths not reported).[95]

Curved nails have been designed to incorporate a distal valgus angulation that corresponds to the lateral position of the calcaneus under the tibia. The curve helps set valgus alignment of the rearfoot and maintains the nail's position within the tibia intramedullary canal. The nail curve is usually 5-10 degrees in valgus to allow better calcaneal purchase and a more lateral entry point.[97] Anatomic studies on cadavers suggest that the more lateral entry minimizes injury to the plantar lateral nerve and artery.[62,98,99] Neurovascular complications in curved nails still occur with 2.5% incidence.[100] Some investigations have even proposed a transverse incision of the plantar heel.[100] There is no perfect safe zone, so careful operative dissection is necessary.[100] Roukis outlined how entry position and orientation of the guidewire can most efficiently be guided by intraoperative radiographs and anatomic landmarks.[101] This study shows effective entry was achieved when the entry placement into the calcaneus was 2.0 cm proximal to the calcaneal cuboid joint (which correlates with the anterior tibia soft tissue outline). It is also our preference to map out the palpable osseous landmarks preoperatively, which will guide entry and also guidewire orientation. In most patients, the tibial crest and posterior medial tibia can be palpated and a marked bisection guides insertion angulation from anterior to posterior (Figs. 34.46 through 34.50).

There is no consensus on ideal nail length and shape (short vs long, straight vs curved). The ability to neutralize deformity and place the calcaneus under the tibia is even more important when using a straight nail. Otherwise, nail entry with incomplete calcaneus capture and proximal nail position (with increased intramedullary strain) can result in construct failure. The authors typically utilize a straight nail in tibiocalcaneal arthrodeses since the removal of the talus allows complete neutralization of the calcaneus under the tibia.

Marley's comparison study of 13 straight and 15 curved nails of different lengths reported proximal stress fracture in one

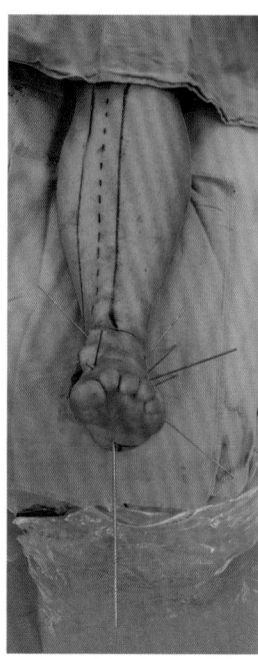

FIGURE 34.47 The surgeon inserting the guidewire can best assess the trajectory of the pin in the transverse plane. The wire is aimed along or medial to the tibia crest, to stay intramedullary in the triangle-shaped tibia canal. Aim is based on the most proximal marking so a slight error in trajectory is less devastating.

long straight IMN and one short straight IMN.[102] The authors assessed the nail's position within the canal and the cortical thickness at the level of the proximal tibial interlocking screw. Best proximal centering was found in the long straight and long curved nails. This is believed to represent overall better position, less reflection, and less strain. Proximal cortical hypertrophy, stress risers, and fractures were more likely in straight nails.[103]

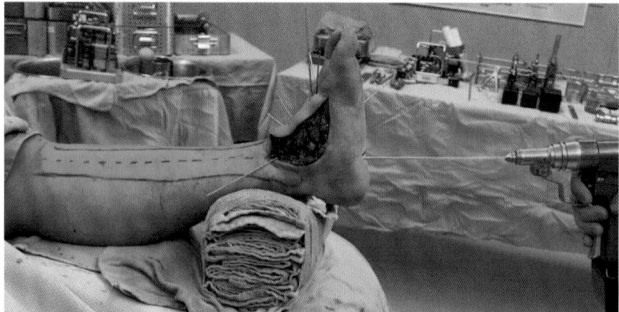

FIGURE 34.46 The palpable anterior crest and posterior border of the tibia are drawn preoperatively. Their bisection (*dotted line*) is used as a reference when inserting the IMN guide wire. An assistant looks from the side to guide the surgeon as to raise or drop their hand and trajectory of the guidewire from anterior to posterior. Notice, temporary fixation crosses the anterior ankle joint to avoid interference with this wire, reaming, and straight nail insertion.

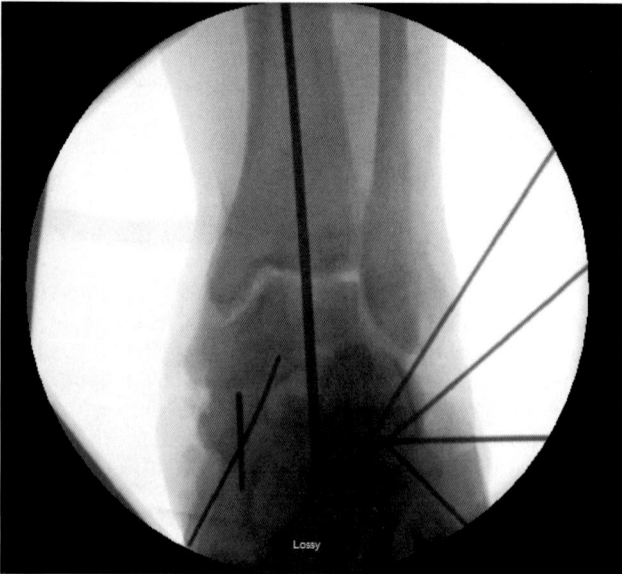

FIGURE 34.48 Anteroposterior radiograph showing central guidewire placement across the tibiotalar joint.

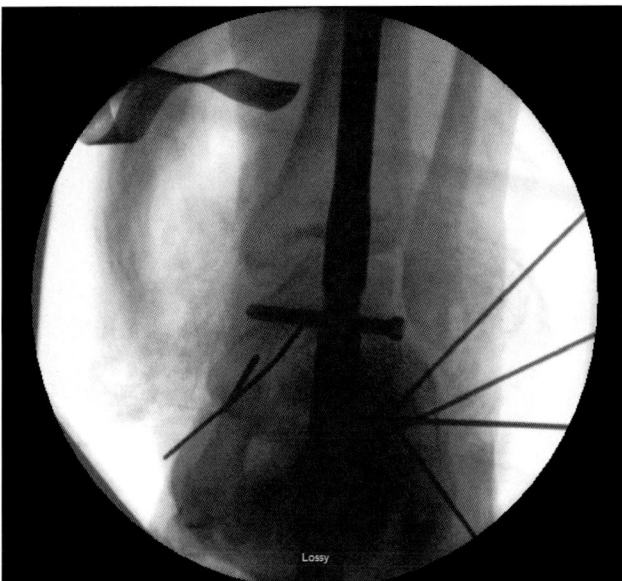

FIGURE 34.49 IM nail insertion with temporary fixation maintained across the pantalar arthrodesis. Notice the ankle joint space prior to internal compression.

Wukich's review of 117 various IMN patients revealed that 3.4% experienced a tibia stress fracture extending from the proximal nail interlocking screw. In all cases, the 15-cm-long nails were removed and the fractures were repaired with 30-cm-long nails.[104] Wukich suggested that 30-cm-long valgus nails should be used primarily to better stabilize the nail in the tibial isthmus and prevent toggle and stress.[104] We have also encountered stress fracture complications from the proximal IMN/screw. Conservative treatment is unlikely to be suitable, and nail exchange with a longer nail is generally necessary (Figs. 34.51 through 34.53).

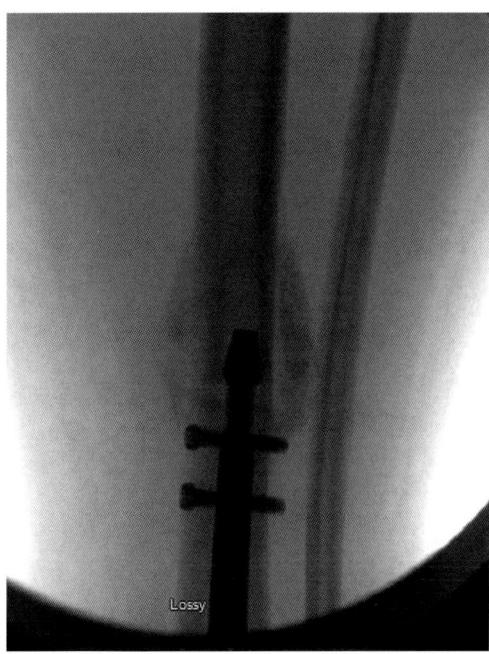

FIGURE 34.51 Anteroposterior tib-fib radiograph following Charcot rearfoot/ankle reconstruction with a straight IM nail. Once the rearfoot and ankle arthrodesis sites consolidated, the patient began protected partial weight bearing and experienced a proximal tibia stress fracture. Developing bone callus with conservative treatment is shown but not suitable to adequately stabilize the fracture site.

Proximal interlocking screw insertions in longer nails requires free-hand insertions, without assistance of a jig, which is time-consuming and challenging. Continued developments in nail design, are now incorporating up to three bends, to more optimally match the geometry of a rearfoot/tibia in attempt to better minimize stress complications.[105,106]

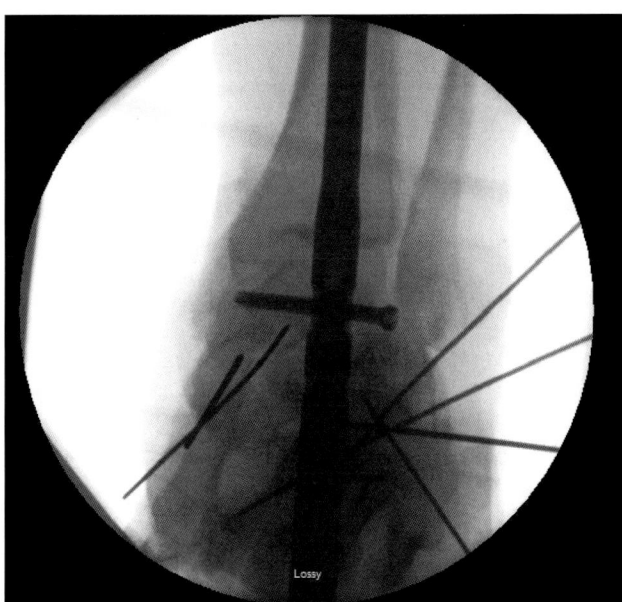

FIGURE 34.50 Following IM nail internal compression, the tibiotalar surfaces are now maximally opposed and compressed. Compare to Figure 34.49.

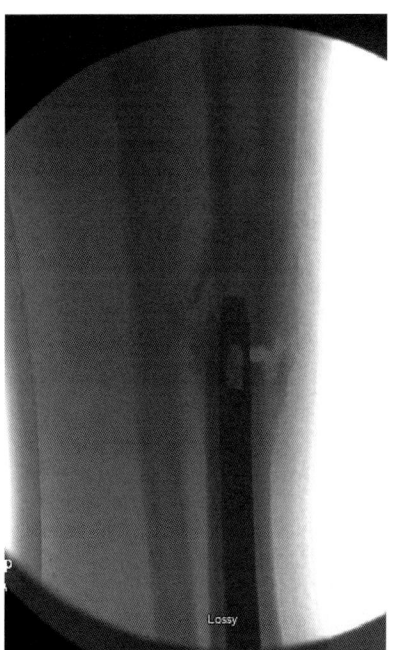

FIGURE 34.52 Lateral radiograph of patient shown in Figure 34.51.

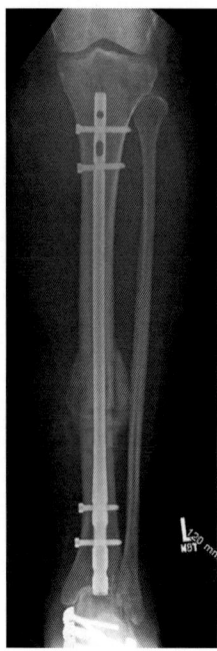

FIGURE 34.53 Patient from Figures 34.51 and 34.52 managed with IM ankle nail removal and long humeral nail insertion. This nail spanned the tibia from its proximal to distal metaphysis to allow optimal stability and bone healing (photo courtesy of Phillip Dripchak MD).

EXTERNAL FIXATION OF ANKLE FUSION

External fixation indications and techniques are detailed in Chapter 65. In regard to ankle fusion, external fixation can be used for simple primary fusion cases, but it is generally reserved for the treatment of nonunions, infection, and/or patients with preulceration.[43,107] Head-to-head outcome comparisons of external fixation, internal fixation, and IMN methods are difficult since external fixation is mainly used in clinical scenarios where limb salvage is more challenging.

External fixation is minimally invasive and does not necessitate permanent fixation in those with a history of infection. External fixation also allows for early postoperative partial weight bearing and soft tissue access if ulceration is present. Although IMN fixation provides stronger compression, a cadaver study demonstrated that 1 mm of bone resorption reduces compressive forces of IMN fixation by 90% and only 50% in external fixation constructs.[108] Some external fixation systems have incorporated computer-assisted programming to guide strut manipulations to achieve dynamic manipulation through the postoperative period.[107] Overall complication rates are significantly higher with external fixation.[109] These complications include pin loosening, pin breakage, pin tract infection, and surgical infection. The fixator is heavy and bulky and can injure the contralateral leg. The treatment duration is long, and this can lead to psychological detriment.

Fragomen's retrospective review of 101 complex ankle fusion cases with external fixation found that smokers and Charcot patients have higher nonunion rates. It was suggested that concurrent tibial lengthening should not performed while attempting to provide stability at the ankle level.[110]

Due to the poor bone stock and higher fixation failure experienced in Charcot patients, some prefer a "hybrid fixation" construct. Usually this implies IMN fixation with external

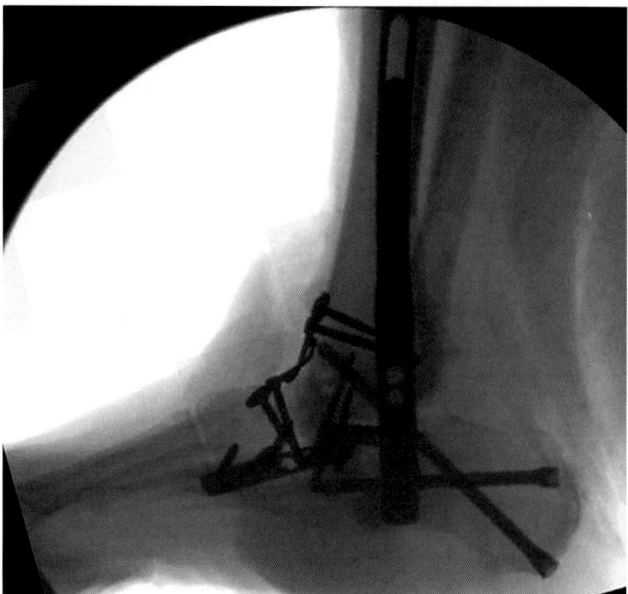

FIGURE 34.54 Example of hybrid fixation with stabilization of the ankle via an intramedullary nail construct and supplemental anterior plate internal fixation.

fixation. Utilizing an IMN with an augmented ankle plate would be another example (Fig. 34.54).

The method is analogous to wearing a "belt and suspenders" simultaneously to accomplish one job and provide backup reinforcement if one method is inadequate. El-Mowafi reviewed 24 ankle fusion hybrid patients (IMN with external fixation) and reported successful outcomes with 92% union.[102] In a head-to-head comparison study, DeVries assessed outcomes of IMN arthrodesis with and without external fixation. Amputation was required in 22% of the IMN group and 28% of the hybrid group.[111] Since the addition of external fixation did not influence salvage rate, a cost-benefit analysis must be considered.

ANKLE ARTHRODESIS IN CHILDREN

Historically, ankle arthrodesis was performed in disabled children with instability from paralytic conditions. Ankle and even pantalar arthrodesis were reported in children with poliomyelitis and other conditions as early as 6 years of age.[50,112] Children under twelve were expected to experience shortening of the limb. This was managed by fusing the ankle in plantar flexion so the foot would be able to contact the floor, making the short limb functional. When indicated, these procedures in children were reported to be successful long term; however, this is not ideal.[113–116]

In 1962, Chuinard described an ankle arthrodesis technique that does not damage the distal tibial growth plate and therefore preserves growth potential.[114] In this technique, a wedge of iliac crest autograft is impacted into the resected ankle joint via an anterior incision. The tight-fit distraction arthrodesis provided stability and internal fixation was not needed. Premature closure of the epiphysis, distortion of growth, and limb length discrepancy were not found in the 23 patients reviewed.[114]

In 1990, Campbell described a modified Chuinard technique in which a posterior approach is utilized instead. This allows for equinus correction via Achilles tendon lengthening and posterior capsular release.[115] A Steinmann pin was suggested when extra stability was needed. High union rate and good functional outcomes were reported in all 12 patients reviewed.[115]

Now, in most developed countries, advanced treatment and technologies mitigate the musculoskeletal sequelae of paralytic conditions.[117] Ankle arthrodesis in children is less frequent. The incidence of conditions like poliomyelitis and tuberculosis are decreasing worldwide as efforts for eradication continue. Ponseti casting technique and minimally invasive Achilles tenotomy now provide much better outcomes for children with clubfoot. Even when talectomy is required in the management of neglected clubfoot, ankle pseudoarthrosis is preferred over ankle arthrodesis as functional results are anecdotally good with reduced but pain-free ankle motion.

Recently, small case studies have reported ankle resection arthrodesis in children with aggressive, malignant bone tumors of the distal tibia.[118,119] These techniques offer limb salvage for children otherwise faced with below-knee amputation. After open biopsy and grading, wide "en bloc" resection was performed. An average of about 12.0 cm of bone was resected from the distal tibia and talus.[118,119] Stephane repaired the large osseous defect with vascularized fibular autograft, which was fixated via IMN or plate fixation.[119] Lou utilized Ilizarov ring fixation to perform bone transport distraction osteogenesis to reconstruct the skeletal defect over time.[118] External fixation with distraction osteogenesis, guided over an IMN, has also be described for management of bone defects larger than 8 cm.[120]

COMPLICATIONS

Common complications of ankle and pantalar arthrodesis are delayed or nonunion, malunion, superficial infection, osteomyelitis, painful fixation, and fixation failure. Although these procedures are sometimes performed in an attempt for limb salvage, postoperative complications may ultimately force limb amputation.

Nonunion is the most common complication reported in most pantalar fusion studies. Barrett assessed nonunion frequency and location in 83 children undergoing pantalar fusion for treatment of poliomyelitis or myelodysplasia. A total of 23/83 (27.7%) nonunions were reported. Frequency of nonunion per joint level was reported: ankle nonunions were most frequent with 17/83 (20.5%), TNJ nonunions in 3/83 (3.6%), CCJ (2.4%) 2/83 nonunions, and STJ (1.2%) 1/83 nonunion.[43] Partitioning the pantalar fusion into two separate, staged surgeries (ankle and rearfoot stages) does not affect union or other complication rates, as historically suggested.[42,47,48,50,51]

To prevent iatrogenic complications that lead to nonunion, the surgeon must meet demands of Glissan's principles of proper joint: preparation, apposition, position, and stability. Internal fixation, IMN fixation, and external fixation options are each considered on a cost-conscious, individual patient basis. Fixation selection should consider local bone conditions, patient systemic comorbidities and demographics, and anticipated postprocedure patient compliance.

Complications of screw fixation include stress risers, prominent screw heads, migrating screws, screw breakage, and inadequate capture of osteoporotic bone. Increased compression is available through internal and external compression offered by IMN constructs; however, IMN complications include fixation migration and periprosthetic fracture. To account for these IMN complications, advancement and optimization in nail

design (short vs long, straight vs bent, static vs dynamic internal compression components, nail bio composite options, etc.) continue to be developed.

Inherent complications of external fixation include superficial pin tract infection and deep infection; however, external fixation is usually reserved for more challenging salvage scenarios, so it is impossible to make head to head comparisons. Despite these known complications, external fixation is sometimes the best or only suitable fixation option as it allows for minimally invasive techniques, surgery in the presence of ulceration or previous infection, dynamic manipulation and deformity correction, and early non–weight bearing).

Patients must be educated about potential complications and be prepared for a postoperative journey, not a quick fix. In the postoperative healing process, patients must also be compliant with their orders. Noncompliance should be documented, and the patient should be educated and coached as necessary. Examples of patient noncompliance affecting outcome include inadequate nicotine cessation, blood sugar control, non–weight bearing, adherence of vitamin D supplementation, alteration in immunosuppressive treatment, office follow-up, etc.

Despite complications, overall limb salvage rates are high for a wide variety of indications and patients of various comorbidities. Patients groups shown to have the greatest risk for limb amputation include those with increased age, those with diabetes, those undergoing revisional surgery, and those with preoperative ulceration.[82]

REFERENCES

1. Yu G. Ankle arthrodesis master techniques. In: *McGlamry's Comprehensive Textbook of Foot and Ankle Surgery*. 3rd ed. Philadelphia, PA: Lippincott, Williams and Wilkins; 2005.
2. Mahan K. Podiatry Institute ankle fusion technique. *J Am Podiatr Med Assoc*. 1997;87(3): 101–116.
3. Grass R. Arthrodesis of the ankle joint. *Clin Podiatr Med Surg*. 2004;21:161-178.
4. Clissan DJ. The indications for inducing fusion at the ankle joint by operation; with description of two successful techniques. *Aust N Z J Surg*. 1949;19:64-71.
5. Corey S. Ankle and pantalar fusion. In: *McGlamry's Comprehensive Textbook of Foot and Ankle Surgery*. 3rd ed. Philadelphia, PA: Lippincott, Williams and Wilkins; 2002.
6. Lloyd J. Revisiting the concept of talar shift in ankle fractures. *Foot Ankle Int*. 2006;27(10):793-796.
7. Smith R. Ankle arthrodesis in the presence of large coronal plane deformity. *Orthop Proceed*. 2018;94-B.
8. Henricson A, Nilsson J-A, Carlsson A. 10-year survival of total ankle arthroplasties: a report on 780 cases from the Swedish Ankle Register. *Acta Orthop*. 2011;82:655-659.
9. Cody EA, Bejarano-Pineda L, Lachman JR, et al. Risk factors for failure of total ankle arthroplasty with a minimum five years of follow-up. *Foot Ankle Int*. 2019;40(3):249-258.
10. Kruidenier J, van der Plaat LW, Sierevelt IN, Hoornenborg D, Haverkamp D. Ankle fusion after failed ankle replacement in rheumatic and non-rheumatic patients. *Foot Ankle Surg*. 2019;25(5):589-593.
11. Kestner J, Glisson R, Nunley A. A biomechanical analysis of two anterior ankle arthrodesis systems. *Foot Ankle Int*. 2013;34:1006-1011.
12. Taylor J, Lucas DE, Riley A, Simpson GA, Philbin TM. Tibiotalocalcaneal arthrodesis nails: a comparison of nails with and without internal compression. *Foot Ankle Int*. 2016;37(3):294-299.
13. Dodd A, Lefaivre KA. Outcomes of talar neck fractures: a systematic review and meta-analysis. *J Orthop Trauma*. 2015;29:210-215.
14. Metzger J, Levin J, Clancy J. Talar neck fractures and rates of avascular necrosis. *J Foot Ankle Surg*. 1999;38:154-162.
15. Horst F, Gilbert B, Nunley J. Avascular necrosis of the talus: current treatment options. *Foot Ankle Clin*. 2004;9:757-773.
16. Backus J, Ocel D. Ankle arthrodesis for talar avascular necrosis and arthrodesis. *Foot Ankle Clin*. 2019;24(1):131-142.
17. Van Bergeyk A, Stotler W, Beals T, et al. Functional outcome after modified Blair tibiotalar arthrodesis for talar osteonecrosis. *Foot Ankle Int*. 2003;24:765-770.
18. Dennison M, Pool R, Simonis R, et al. Tibiocalcaneal fusion for avascular necrosis of the talus. *J Bone Joint Surg Br*. 2001;83:199-203.
19. Isherwood I. A radiological approach to the subtalar arthrodesis. *J Bone Joint Surg*. 1961;43B(3):566-574.
20. Ahlberg A, Henricson A. Late results of ankle fusion. *Acta Orthop Scand*. 1981;52:103-105.
21. Saltzman CL, El-Khoury GY. The hindfoot alignment view. *Foot Ankle Int*. 1995;16(9): 572-576.

22. Saltzman C, Salamon M, Blanchard G, et al. Epidemiology of ankle arthritis: report of a consecutive series of 639 patients from a tertiary orthopaedic center. *Iowa Orthop J.* 2005;25:44-46.
23. Thomas R, Daniels T. Current concepts review: ankle arthritis. *J Bone Joint Surg Am.* 2003;85:923-936.
24. Schneider D. Vitamin D and skeletal health. *Curr Opin Endocrinol Diabetes Obes.* 2006;13(6):483-490.
25. Moore KR, Howell MA, Saltrick KR, Catanzariti AR. Risk factors associated with nonunion after elective foot and ankle reconstruction: a case-control study. *J Foot Ankle Surg.* 2017;56(3):457-462.
26. Gorter E, Krijnen P, Schipper I. Vitamin D status and adult fracture healing. *J Clin Orthop Trauma.* 2017;8(1):34-37.
27. Michelson J, Charlson M. Vitamin D status in an elective orthopedic surgical population. *Foot Ankle Int.* 2016;37(2):186-191.
28. Ishikawa SN, Murphy GA, Richardson EG. The effect of cigarette smoking on hindfoot fusions. *Foot Ankle Int.* 2002;23(11):996-998.
29. Cobb TK, Gabrielsen TA, Campbell DC II, Wallrichs SL, Ilstrup DM. Cigarette smoking and nonunion after ankle arthrodesis. *Foot Ankle Int.* 1994;15(2):64-67.
30. Pearson RG, Clement RGE, Edwards KL, et al. Do smokers have greater risk of delayed and non-union after fracture, osteotomy and arthrodesis? A systematic review with meta-analysis. *BMJ Open.* 2016;6:e010303. doi: 10.1136/bmjopen-2015- 010303.
31. Campanile G, et al. Cigarette smoking, wound healing, and face-lift. *Clin Dermatol.* 1998;16:575-578.
32. Wilt M, Camasta C, Brosky T. The effect of smoking on bone healing. In: *Podiatry Institute Update on Foot and Ankle Surgery.* 2006:290-292
33. Doets H, Zürcher A. Salvage arthrodesis for failed total ankle arthroplasty. *Acta Orthop.* 2010;81:142-147.
34. Carlsson F, Montgomery J, Besjakov M. Arthrodesis of the ankle secondary to replacement. *Foot Ankle Int.* 1998;19(4):240-245.
35. Gabriel S, Michaud K. Epidemiological studies in incidence, prevalence, mortality, and comorbidity of the rheumatic diseases. *Arthritis Res Ther.* 2009;11(3):229.
36. Au K, Reed G, Curtis J, et al. High disease activity is associated with an increased risk of infection in patients with rheumatoid arthritis. *Ann Rheum Dis.* 2011;70(5):785-791.
37. Gualtierotti R. Understanding cardiovascular risk in rheumatoid arthritis: still a long way to go. *Atherosclerosis.* 2017;256:123-124.
38. Doran M, Crowson C, Pond G, O'Fallon W, Gabriel S. Predictors of infection in rheumatoid arthritis. *Arthritis Rheum.* 2002;46(9):2294-2300.
39. Lee M, Choi WJ, Han SH, Jang J, Lee JW. Uncontrolled diabetes as a potential risk factor in tibiotalocalcaneal fusion using a retrograde intramedullary nail. *Foot Ankle Surg.* 2018;24(6):542-548.
40. Dunn P, Meyer J, Ruch J. Principles of arthrodesis. In: *McGlamry's Comprehensive Textbook of Foot and Ankle Surgery.* 4th ed. Philadelphia, PA: Lippincott, Williams and Wilkins; 2013:803-809.
41. Buck P. The optimum position of arthrodesis of the ankle. *J Bone Joint Surg Am.* 1987;69(7):1052-1062.
42. Provelengios S, Papavasiliou KA, Kyrkos MJ, Sayegh FE, Kirkos JM, Kapetanos GA. The role of pantalar arthrodesis in the treatment of paralytic foot deformities. Surgical technique. *J Bone Joint Surg Am.* 2010;92(suppl 1, Pt 1):44-54.
43. Mandracchia VJ, Mandi DM, Nickles WA, Barp EA, Sanders SM. Pantalar arthrodesis. *Clin Podiatr Med Surg.* 2004;21(3):461-470.
44. Lorthioir J. Huit cas d'arthrodese du pied avec extirpation temporaire de l'astragale. *Ann Soc Belg Chir.* 1911;11:184.
45. Pinzur MS, Kelikian A. Charcot ankle fusion with a retrograde locked intramedullary nail. *Foot Ankle Int.* 1997;18:699-704.
46. Medhat MA, Krantz H. Neuropathic ankle joint in Charcot-Marie-Tooth disease after triple arthrodesis of the foot. *Orthop Rev.* 1988;17(9):873-880.
47. Papa JA, Myerson MS. Pantalar and tibiotalocalcaneal arthrodesis for post-traumatic osteoarthrosis of the ankle and hindfoot. *J Bone Joint Surg Am.* 1992;74(7):1042-1049.
48. Acosta R, Ushiba J, Cracchiolo A III. The results of a primary and staged pantalar arthrodesis and tibiotalocalcaneal arthrodesis in adult patients. *Foot Ankle Int.* 2000;21(3):182-194.
49. McKinley JC, Shortt N, Arthur C, Gunner C, MacDonald D, Breusch SJ. Outcomes following pantalar arthrodesis in rheumatoid arthritis. *Foot Ankle Int.* 2011;32(7):681-685.
50. Waugh TR, Wagner J, Stinchfield FE. An evaluation of pantalar arthrodesis. A follow-up study of one hundred and sixteen operations. *J Bone Joint Surg Am.* 1965;47(7):1315-1322.
51. Barrett GR, Meyer LC, Bray EW III, Taylor RG Jr, Kolb FJ. Pantalar arthrodesis: a long-term follow-up. *Foot Ankle.* 1981;1(5):279-283.
52. Haskell A. CORR Insights®: can a three-component prosthesis be used for conversion of painful ankle arthrodesis to total ankle replacement? *Clin Orthop Relat Res.* 2017;475(9):2295-2297.
53. Suckel A, Muller O, Herberts T, Wulker N. Changes in Chopart joint load following tibiotalar arthrodesis: in vitro analysis of 8 cadaver specimens in a dynamic model. *BMC Musculoskelet Disord.* 2007;8:80.
54. Baumbach SF, Massen FK, Hörterer S, et al. Comparison of arthroscopic to open tibiotalocalcaneal arthrodesis in high-risk patients. *J Foot Ankle Surg.* 2019;25(6):804-811.
55. Biz C, Hoxhaj B, Aldegheri R, Iacobellis C. Minimally invasive surgery for tibiotalocalcaneal arthrodesis using a retrograde intramedullary nail: preliminary results of an innovative modified technique. *J Foot Ankle Surg.* 2016;55(6):1130-1138.
56. Vilà y Rico J, Rodriguez-Martin J, Parra-Sanchez G, Marti Lopez-Amor C. Arthroscopic tibiotalocalcaneal arthrodesis with locked retrograde compression nail. *J Foot Ankle Surg.* 2013;52(4):523-528.
57. Watanabe K, Teramoto A, Kobayashi T, et al. Tibiotalocalcaneal arthrodesis using a soft tissue-preserved fibular graft for treatment of large bone defects in the ankle. *Foot Ankle Int.* 2017;38(6):671-676.
58. Gross C, Erickson BJ, Adams SB, et al. Ankle arthrodesis after failed total ankle replacement: a systemic review of the literature. *Foot Ankle Spec.* 2015;8(2):143-151.
59. Frigg A, Nigg B, Davis E, Pederson B, Valderrabano V. Does alignment in the hindfoot radiograph influence dynamic foot-floor pressures in ankle and tibiotalocalcaneal fusion? *Clin Orthop Relat Res.* 2010;468(12):3362-3370.
60. Adams JC. Arthrodesis of the ankle joint; experiences with the transfibular approach. *J Bone Joint Surg.* 1948;30B:506-511.
61. Emara KM, Ahmed Diab R, Amr Hemida M. Tibio-calcaneal fusion by retrograde intramedullary nailing in Charcot neuroarthropathy. *Foot (Edinb).* 2018;34:6-10.
62. Muckley T, Ullm S, Petrovitch A, et al. Comparison of two intramedullary nails for tibiotalocalcaneal fusion: anatomic and radiographic considerations. *Foot Ankle Int.* 2007;10(6):606-613.
63. Berend ME, Glisson RR, Nunley JA. A biomechanical comparison of intramedullary nail and crossed lag screw fixation for tibiotalocalcaneal arthrodesis. *Foot Ankle Int.* 1997;18(10):639-643.
64. Berson L, McGarvey WC, Clanton TO. Evaluation of compression in intramedullary hindfoot arthrodesis. *Foot Ankle Int.* 2002;23(11):992-995.
65. Chraim M, Krenn S, Alrabai HM, Trnka HJ, Bock P. Mid-term follow-up of patients with hindfoot arthrodesis with retrograde compression intramedullary nail in Charcot neuroarthropathy of the hindfoot. *Bone Joint J.* 2018;100-B(2):190-196.
66. Anderson RT, Pacaccio DJ, Yakacki CM, Carpenter RD. Finite element analysis of a pseudoelastic compression-generating intramedullary ankle arthrodesis nail. *J Mech Behav Biomed Mater.* 2016;62:83-92.
67. Hamid KS, Glisson RR, Morash JG, Matson AP, DeOrio JK. Simultaneous intraoperative measurement of cadaver ankle and subtalar joint compression during arthrodesis with intramedullary nail, screws, and tibiotalocalcaneal plate. *Foot Ankle Int.* 2018;39(9):1128-1132.
68. Mückley T, Hoffmeier K, Klos K, Petrovitch A, von Oldenburg G, Hofmann GO. Angle-stable and compressed angle-stable locking for tibiocalcaneal arthrodesis with retrograde intramedullary nails. Biomechanical evaluation. *J Bone Joint Surg Am.* 2008;90(3):620-627.
69. O'Neill PJ, Parks BG, Walsh R, Simmons LM, Schon LC. Biomechanical analysis of screw-augmented intramedullary fixation for tibiotalocalcaneal arthrodesis. *Foot Ankle Int.* 2007;28(7):804-809.
70. Shahulhameed A, Roberts CS, Ojike NI. Technique for precise placement of poller screws with intramedullary nailing of the metaphyseal fractures of the femur and the tibia. *Injury.* 2011;42:136-139.
71. Mann MR, Parks BG, Pak SS, Miller SD. Tibiotalocalcaneal arthrodesis: a biomechanical analysis of the rotational stability of the Biomet Ankle Arthrodesis Nail. *Foot Ankle Int.* 2001;22:731-733.
72. Richter M, Evers J, Waehnert D, et al. Biomechanical comparison of stability of tibiotalocalcaneal arthrodesis with two different intramedullary retrograde nails. *Foot Ankle Surg.* 2014;20(1):14-19.
73. Thomas AE, Guyver PM, Taylor JM, Czipri M, Talbot NJ, Sharpe IT. Tibiotalocalcaneal arthrodesis with a compressive retrograde nail: A retrospective study of 59 nails. *Foot Ankle Surg.* 2015;21(3):202-205.
74. Fenton P, Bali N, Matheshwari R, Youssef B, Meda K. Complications of tibio-talar-calcaneal fusion using intramedullary nails. *Foot Ankle Surg.* 2014;20(4):268-271.
75. Griffin MJ, Coughlin MJ. Evaluation of midterm results of the panta nail: an active compression tibiotalocalcaneal arthrodesis device. *J Foot Ankle Surg.* 2018;57(1):74-80.
76. Lowe JA, Routh LK, Leary JT, Buzhardt PC. Effect of retrograde reaming for tibiotalocalcaneal arthrodesis on subtalar joint destruction: a cadaveric study. *J Foot Ankle Surg.* 2016;55(1):72-75.
77. Lemon M, Somayaji HS, Khaleel A, Elliott DS. Fragility fractures of the ankle: stabilization with an expandable calcaneotalotibial nail. *J Bone Joint Surg.* 2005;87:809-813.
78. Persigant M, Colin F, Noailles T, Pietu G, Gouin F. Functional assessment of transplantar nailing for ankle fracture in the elderly: 48 weeks' prospective follow-up of 14 patients. *Orthop Traumatol Surg Res.* 2018;104(4):507-510.
79. Georgiannos D, Lampridis V, Bisbinas I. Fragility fractures of the ankle in the elderly: open reduction and internal fixation versus tibio-talo-calcaneal nailing: Short-term results of a prospective randomized-controlled study. *Injury.* 2017;48(2):519-524.
80. Gross JB, Belleville R, Nespola A, et al. Influencing factors of functional result and bone union in tibiotalocalcaneal arthrodesis with intramedullary locking nail: a retrospective series of 30 cases. *Eur J Orthop Surg Traumatol.* 2014;24(4):627-633.
81. Wukich DK, Shen JY, Ramirez CP, Irrgang JJ. Retrograde ankle arthrodesis using an intramedullary nail: a comparison of patients with and without diabetes mellitus. *J Foot Ankle Surg.* 2011;50(3):299-306.
82. DeVries JG, Berlet GC, Hyer CF. Predictive risk assessment for major amputation after tibiotalocalcaneal arthrodesis. *Foot Ankle Int.* 2013;34(6):846-850.
83. Herscovici D, Sammarco GJ, Sammarco VJ, Scaduto JM. Pantalar arthrodesis for post-traumatic arthritis and diabetic neuroarthropathy of the ankle and hindfoot. *Foot Ankle Int.* 2011;32(6):581-588.
84. Millett PJ, O'Malley MJ, Tolo ET, Gallina J, Fealy S, Helfet DL. Tibiotalocalcaneal fusion with a retrograde intramedullary nail: clinical and functional outcomes. *Am J Orthop (Belle Mead NJ).* 2002(31):531-536.
85. Miller J, Hoang V, Yoon RS, Liporace FA. Staged treatment of infected tibiotalar fusion using a combination antibiotic spacer and antibiotic-coated intramedullary nail. *J Foot Ankle Surg.* 2017;56(5):1099-1103.
86. Pawar A, Dikmen G, Fragomen A, Rozbruch SR. Antibiotic-coated nail for fusion of infected charcot ankles. *Foot Ankle Int.* 2013;34(1):80-84.
87. Bibbo C, Lee S, Anderson RB, Davis WH. Limb salvage: infected retrograde tibiocalcaneal intramedullary nail. *Foot Ankle Int.* 2003;24(5):420-425.
88. Mendicino RW, Bowers CA, Catanzariti AR. Antibiotic-coated intramedullary rod. *J Foot Ankle Surg.* 2009;48(2):104-110.

89. Tomczak C, Beaman D, Perkins S. Combined intramedullary nail coated with antibiotic-containing cement and ring fixation for limb salvage in the severely deformed, infected, neuroarthropathic ankle. *Foot Ankle Int.* 2019;40(1):48-55.

90. Araoye IB, Chodaba YE, Smith KS, Hadden RW, Shah AB. Use of intramedullary carbon fiber nail in hindfoot fusion: A small cohort study. *Foot Ankle Surg.* 2019;25(1):2-7.

91. Kildow BJ, Gross CE, Adams SD, Parekh SG. Measurement of nitinol recovery distance using pseudoelastic intramedullary nails for tibiotalocalcaneal arthrodesis. *Foot Ankle Spec.* 2016;9(6):494-499.

92. Hsu AR, Ellington JK, Adams SB Jr. Tibiotalocalcaneal arthrodesis using a nitinol intramedullary hindfoot nail. *Foot Ankle Spec.* 2015;8(5):389-396.

93. Ford SE, Kwon JY, Ellington JK. Tibiotalocalcaneal arthrodesis utilizing a titanium intramedullary nail with an internal pseudoelastic nitinol compression element: a retrospective case series of 33 patients. *J Foot Ankle Surg.* 2019;58(2):266-272.

94. Lucas Y Hernandez J, Abad J, et al. Tibiotalocalcaneal arthrodesis using a straight intramedullary nail. *Foot Ankle Int.* 2015;36(5):539-546.

95. Brodsky JW, Verschae G, Tenenbaum S. Surgical correction of severe deformity of the ankle and hindfoot by arthrodesis using a compressing retrograde intramedullary nail. *Foot Ankle Int.* 2014;35(4):360-367.

96. Fang Z, Claaßen L, Windhagen H, Daniilidis K, Stukenborg-Colsman C, Waizy H. Tibiotalocalcaneal arthrodesis using a retrograde intramedullary nail with a valgus curve. *Orthop Surg.* 2015;7(2):125-131.

97. Hyer CF, Cheney N. Anatomic aspects of tibiotalocalcaneal nail arthrodesis. *J Foot Ankle Surg.* 2013;52(6):724-727.

98. Moorjani N, Buckingham R, Wilson I. Optimal insertion site for intramedullary nails during combined ankle and subtalar arthrodesis. *Foot Ankle Surg.* 1998;4:21-26.

99. Knight T, Rosenfeld P, Jones IT, Clark C, Savva N. Anatomic structures at risk: curved hindfoot arthrodesis nail—a cadaveric approach. *J Foot Ankle Surg.* 2014;53(6):687-691.

100. Cesar Netto C, Johannesmeyer D, Cone B, et al. Neurovascular structures at risk with curved retrograde TTC fusion nails. *Foot Ankle Int.* 2017;38(10):1139-1145.

101. Roukis TS. Determining the insertion site for retrograde intramedullary nail fixation of tibiotalocalcaneal arthrodesis: a radiographic and intraoperative anatomical landmark analysis. *J Foot Ankle Surg.* 2006;45(4):227-234.

102. El-Mowafi H, Abulsaad M, Kandil Y, El-Hawary A, Ali S. Hybrid fixation for ankle fusion in diabetic charcot arthropathy. *Foot Ankle Int.* 2018;39(1):93-98.

103. Marley W, Tucker A, McKenna S, Wong-Chung J. Pre-requisites for optimum centering of a tibiotalocalcaneal arthrodesis nail. *Foot Ankle Surg.* 2014;20(3):215-220.

104. Wukich DK, Mallory BR, Suder NC, Rosario BL. Tibiotalocalcaneal arthrodesis using intramedullary nail: a comparison of patients with and without diabetes mellitus. *J Foot Ankle Surg.* 2015;54(5):876-882.

105. Richter M, Zech S. Tibiotalocalcaneal arthrodesis with a triple-bend intramedullary nail (A3)—2-year follow-up in 60 patients. *Foot Ankle Surg.* 2016;22(2):131-138.

106. Evers J, Lakemeier M, Wähnert D, et al. 3D optical investigation of 2 nail systems used in tibiotalocalcaneal arthrodesis: a biomechanical study. *Foot Ankle Int.* 2017;38(5):571-579.

107. Khodadadyan-Klostermann C, Raschke M, Mittlemeier T, Melcher I, Haas NP. Ankle and pan-talar arthrodesis with Ilizarov composite hybrid fixation: operative technique and review of 21 cases. *Foot Ankle Surg.* 2001;7:149-156.

108. Yakacki CM, Khalil HF, Dixon SA, Gall K, Pacaccio DJ. Compression forces of internal and external ankle fixation devices with simulated bone resorption. *Foot Ankle Int.* 2010;31(1):76-85.

109. ElAlfy B, Ali AM, Fawzy SI. Ilizarov external fixator versus retrograde intramedullary nailing for ankle joint arthrodesis in diabetic charcot neuroarthropathy. *J Foot Ankle Surg.* 2017;56(2):309-313.

110. Fragomen AT, Borst E, Schachter L, Lyman S, Rozbruch SR. Complex ankle arthrodesis using the Ilizarov method yields high rate of fusion. *Clin Orthop Relat Res.* 2012;470(10):2864-2873.

111. DeVries JG, Berlet GC, Hyer CF. A retrospective comparative analysis of Charcot ankle stabilization using an intramedullary rod with or without application of circular external fixator—utilization of the Retrograde Arthrodesis Intramedullary Nail database. *J Foot Ankle Surg.* 2012;51(4):420-425.

112. Hamsa WR. Panastragaloid arthrodesis—a study of end results in eighty-five cases. *J Bone Joint Surg.* 1936;(18);732-736.

113. Mazur JM, Cummings RJ, McCluskey WP, Lovell WW. Ankle arthrodesis in children. *Clin Orthop Relat Res* 1991;(268):65-69. Review.

114. Chuinard E, Peterson R. Distraction-compression bone-graft arthrodesis of the ankle. A method especially applicable in children. *J Bone Joint Surg.* 1963;45-A:481-490.

115. Campbell P. Arthrodesis of the ankle with modified distraction-compression and bone-grafting. *J Bone Joint Surg Am.* 1990;72(4):552-556.

116. Escalopier N, Badina A, Padovani JP, et al. Long-term results of ankle arthrodesis in children and adolescents with haemophilia. *Int Orthop.* 2017;41(8):1579-1584.

117. Chi Chuan Wu. Tibial lengthening with ankle arthrodesis in poliomyelitic patients with unilateral dysfunction of both knee extension and ankle dorsiflexion. *Acta Orthop Traumatol Turc.* 2016;50(3):284-290.

118. Lou TF, Li H, Chai YM, et al. Resection arthrodesis using distraction osteogenesis then plating as a hybrid surgical technique for the management of bone sarcomas of the distal tibia. *Int Orthop.* 2018;42(3):705-711.

119. Stéphane S, Eric M, Philippe W, Félix DJ, Raphael S. Resection arthrodesis of the ankle for aggressive tumors of the distal tibia in children. *J Pediatr Orthop.* 2009;29(7):811-816.

120. Bernstein M, Fragomen A, Rozbruch SR. Tibial bone transport over an intramedullary nail using cable and pulleys. *JBJS Essent Surg Tech.* 2018;8(1):e9.

CHAPTER 35

Ankle Fractures

Travis M. Langan, Adam L. Halverson, David A. Goss Jr, Christopher F. Hyer, and Terrence M. Philbin

DEFINITION

The ankle joint is a modified hinge joint between the talus, tibia, and fibula with complex anatomy that allows for triplane motion. Ankle fractures are a common orthopedic injury with more than 250 000 estimated occurrences per year accounting for 9% of all orthopedic injuries.[1-3] Ankle fractures are the most common intraarticular fracture of a weight-bearing joint.[4] Maintenance of congruency is essential for normal joint function and preventing posttraumatic arthritis as the joint is extremely sensitive to malalignment.[5,6] Stable, nondisplaced ankle fractures may be treated nonoperatively. Operative treatment is indicated when there is instability, displacement, or open injury.[5-10]

CLASSIFICATIONS

The two most common classifications for ankle fractures are the Danis-Weber classification and the Lauge-Hansen Classification (Tables 35.1 and 35.2).

Ankle fractures are generally high-energy injuries combined with rotation. The Lauge-Hansen classification describes the fracture pattern that will occur when the talus rotates within the mortise on a fixed tibia and fibula with the foot in either supination or pronation.[11,12] Danis-Weber classification describes the fibular fractures that result in different injury mechanisms.[13-15] There are, of course, injuries that do not follow these patterns that will be described later in the chapter.

INDICATIONS

- Stable, nondisplaced, isolated lateral malleolar injuries are generally treated nonoperatively
  - No evidence of medial injury or increased medial clear space
  - No evidence of syndesmosis injury
  - <2 mm of fibular displacement
- Unstable fracture or ligamentous injuries are treated with operative reduction and fixation
  - Medial and lateral malleolar fractures
  - Evidence of syndesmosis injury
  - Increase in medial clear space
  - >2 mm of fibular displacement
- Open fractures are treated operatively

ANATOMY FEATURES

Anatomic descriptions adapted from references.[12,16-22]

The ankle, or the talocrural joint, is the articulation between the tibia, the fibula, and the talus. It is a complex synovial hinge joint with triplanar motion. The talar dome sits within the ankle mortise created by the tibial plafond, medial malleolus, and lateral malleolus. Stability of the joint is created through the osseous medial and lateral malleoli with contributions from multiple ligament complexes.

BONY ANATOMY

Talus

The trochlea of the talus is the cartilaginous portion that includes the dorsal surface (talar dome), medial surface, and lateral surface. The dorsal surface of the talus articulates with the tibial plafond and is ~25% wider anteriorly than posteriorly. The talar dome is convex anterior to posteriorly. The medial surface articulates with the medial malleolus and the lateral surface with the lateral malleolus. The anterior neck of the talus has capsular attachments and ligamentous attachments medially and laterally. The posterior talus has a medial and lateral tubercle for ligamentous and capsular attachments with a groove in the center for the flexor hallucis longus tendon.

Tibia

The distal aspect of the tibia consists of the tibial plafond and medial malleolus. The tibial plafond is also wider anteriorly than it is posteriorly and has a concave anterior to posterior shape. The medial malleolus is the pyramidal-shaped extension of the medial tibia distal to the plafond. The inferior medial malleolus has two crests; the anterior and posterior colliculi with an intercollicular groove separating them. The medial malleolus has attachments for the deltoid ligament. There is a sulcus along the posterior border of the medial malleolus for the posterior tibial tendon and flexor digitorum longus tendon. There is a shallow grove along the posterior tibial plafond for the flexor hallucis longus tendon. The lateral surface of the distal tibia has a fibular notch where the two bones articulate. The anterior and posterior tibiofibular ligament attach along the margins of the fibular notch. The anterolateral ridge of the distal tibia is named Tillaux-Chaput tubercle for attachment of

TABLE 35.1 **Lauge-Hansen Classification**[11-13]	Supination—Adduction	Pronation—Abduction	Supination—External Rotation	Pronation—External Rotation
Stage 1 Fracture pattern	▪ Lateral ligament disruption ▪ Distal fibular avulsion fracture at or below the ankle joint	▪ Medial malleolus transverse fracture ▪ Deltoid ligament disruption	▪ Anterior inferior tibiofibular ligament or associated avulsion fracture	▪ Medial malleolus transverse fracture or disruption of the deltoid ligament
Stage 2 Fracture pattern	▪ Vertical medial malleolus fracture	▪ Anterior inferior tibiofibular ligament and posterior inferior tibiofibular ligament disruption or associated avulsion fracture	▪ Spiral oblique fibular fracture beginning at the level of the ankle joint	▪ Anterior inferior tibiofibular ligament or associated avulsion fracture
Stage 3 Fracture pattern		▪ Short oblique or transverse comminuted fracture of the fibula beginning at the level of the ankle joint	▪ Posterior inferior tibiofibular ligament disruption or associated avulsion fracture	▪ Spiral oblique fracture of the fibula above the level of the ankle joint with syndesmosis disruption
Stage 4 Fracture pattern			▪ Medial malleolus transverse fracture or disruption of the deltoid ligament	▪ Posterior inferior tibiofibular ligament disruption or associated avulsion fracture

the anterior inferior tibiofibular ligament (AITFL) and the posterolateral ridge is named Volkmann tubercle for attachment of the posterior inferior tibiofibular ligament (PITFL).

Fibula

The distal fibula is known as the lateral malleolus. This is continuous with the shaft of the fibula, and the apex of the lateral malleolus becomes bulbous before the distal tip. The lateral malleolus has two surfaces, medial that articulates with the tibia and talus, and lateral which is subcutaneous. It has two borders, anterior and posterior. The anterior border has a ridge named Wagstaffe tubercle for attachment of the AITFL. The anterior talofibular ligament (ATFL) attaches to the anterior distal border and the calcaneofibular ligament (CFL) attaches to the distal tip of the fibula. The posterior border has a groove for the peroneal tendons with medial and lateral ridges for ligamentous attachment of the posterior talofibular ligament (PTFL), PITFL, and superior peroneal retinaculum.

TABLE 35.2 **Danis-Weber Classification**[13-15]		
Type A	**Type B**	**Type C**
▪ Distal fibular avulsion fracture at or below the ankle joint	▪ Short oblique or spiral fibular fracture beginning at the level of the ankle joint	▪ Fibular fracture above the level of the ankle joint ▪ May be spiral, oblique, or complex and comminuted
▪ May have vertical medial malleolus fracture	▪ May have AITF and deltoid or medial malleolus avulsion fracture	▪ May have deltoid ligament and/or syndesmotic injuries (ie, AITFL, PITFL, IOL) associated

LIGAMENTOUS ANATOMY

Tibiofibular Joint

There are three ligaments that stabilize the distal tibiofibular joint; interosseous tibiofibular ligament, AITFL, and posterior inferior tibiofibular ligament (PITFL). The ankle syndesmosis is the strong ligament between the tibia and fibula. The interosseous tibiofibular ligament is a strong band at the distal most aspect of the syndesmosis. The syndesmotic ligaments allow for 12 degrees of fibular rotation relative to the tibia.[12] Proper alignment and reduction of the syndesmosis and tibiofibular joint is key to the success of ankle fracture surgery. The AITFL extends from the anterolateral border of the distal tibia (Tillaux-Chaput tubercle) to the anterior border of the lateral malleolus (Wagstaffe tubercle). The PITFL extends from the posterior distal tibia (Volkmann tubercle) to the posterior medial border of the lateral malleolus.

Lateral Ankle

There are three main ligaments that stabilize the lateral ankle: the ATFL, CFL, and PTFL. The ATFL and PTFL are intracapsular, while the CFL is extracapsular. The ATFL extends from the anterior margin of the lateral malleolus to the lateral neck of the talus. The PTFL extends from the posterior medial border of the lateral malleolus to the posterior lateral tubercle of the tibia (Volkmann tubercle). The CFL is a cord-like ligament that extends from the distal tip of the lateral malleolus to the lateral surface of the calcaneus.

Medial Ankle

The deltoid ligament is the medial collateral ligament of the ankle joint. It is a strong triangular-shaped ligament with superficial and deep fibers. The deltoid ligament has classically been described as four ligaments, the anterior tibiotalar ligament, posterior tibiotalar ligament, tibiocalcaneal ligament, and tibionavicular ligament. More recently, the deltoid ligament has been described as six ligaments with variability of up to eight total individual bands.[23] There are superficial and deep fibers. The deltoid ligament runs from the anterior and posterior colliculus of the medial malleolus to the dorsomedial surface of the talus, the posterior medial tubercle of the talus, sustentaculum tali, and the navicular tuberosity.

FUNCTIONAL ANALYSIS OF ANKLE JOINT ANATOMY

The described anatomic features allow for complex function of the ankle joint. The empirical axis of the ankle joint is 8 degrees from the transverse plane, 20-30 degrees from the frontal plane, and roughly perpendicular to the sagittal plane.[20,24-27] The joint axis creates mild abduction with ankle dorsiflexion and mild adduction with ankle plantarflexion. Normal gait requires ~10 degrees of dorsiflexion and 20 degrees of plantarflexion. Athletic activity may require up to 20-30 degrees of dorsiflexion.[25-27] The talar dome bears more weight per unit area than any other joint surface making it sensitive to even small tibiotalar incongruencies.[6,7,10]

The strong ligamentous anatomy provides stability of the talus within the ankle mortise. Injuries to the bony or ligamentous anatomy will result in many different fracture patterns as described in the classification systems. Close showed that with the lateral ankle ligaments sectioned, the mortise widened 2 mm.[12] When the superficial deltoid ligament was sectioned, the contact shifted laterally with an increase in peak pressure and a decrease in contact area.[7,12] When the deep deltoid was sectioned, the ankle diastasis doubled.[12] The deltoid ligament is the primary restraint against valgus talar tilting and ankle external rotation.[8-10] Yablon et al. demonstrated the importance of the lateral ankle ligaments in stabilizing the ankle. The talus will shift and follow the fibula in ankle injuries.[10] The lateral malleolus and lateral ligaments are the primary restraint of anterior and lateral talar shift as well as varus talar tilt.[10]

The syndesmosis is a complex structure that allows for normal ankle articulation by determining the precise distal tibia and fibula relationship. It can accommodate up to 120% of its length, and the intermalleolar distance fluctuates ~1.5 mm throughout dorsiflexion and plantar flexion.[12] Burns showed with disruption of the syndesmosis combined with concomitant deltoid injury, the increase in ankle diastasis resulted in a 39% reduction in contact area, and 42% increase in peak pressure.[7] Syndesmosis disruption with either medial or lateral ankle pathology results in an unstable ankle.[7]

As described in Lauge-Hansen's ankle fracture classification (see Table 35.1), the distal ankle ligaments can become disrupted or create multiple different avulsion fractures. An avulsion of the AITFL off the tibia is known as a Tillaux-Chaput fracture, while avulsion off the fibula is known as a Wagstaffe fracture.[16] An avulsion of the PITFL off the posterior tibia is known as a Volkmann fracture.[16] Somford et al. present a historical review of eponyms and classifications related to ankle fractures.[28]

PHYSICAL EXAMINATION

Focused medical history should precede any proper physical examination. Key findings include peripheral vascular disease, diabetes, peripheral neuropathy, alcohol use, tobacco use, bone density abnormalities, previous fracture history, and history of malignancy. Time from injury to presentation is also critical to note, as delayed presentation can be a sign of neuropathy or neglect.

Physical examination of the fractured ankle should include a brief skeletal survey to identify any potential concomitant injuries. Focused examination should begin with inspection of the injured extremity, first evaluating for skin changes and gross deformity. Skin color can indicate vascular compromise often associated with a dislocated joint. Any open lesions or abrasions should be noted. The contents of any fracture blisters should also be documented, including whether they are serous filled or hemorrhagic (Fig. 35.1). Abrasions or full-thickness lacerations should be probed to determine if the fracture is open.

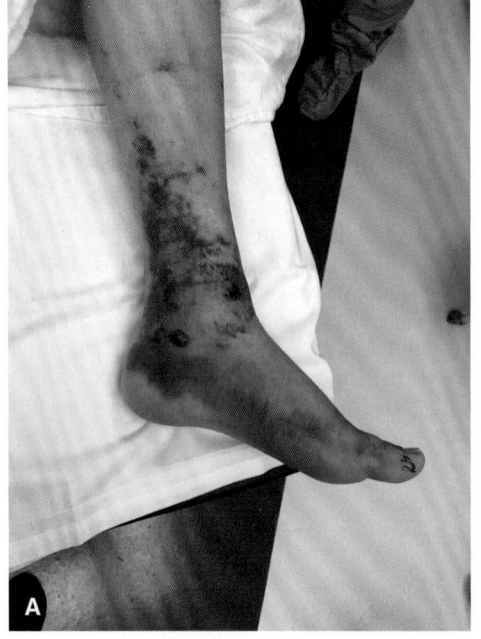
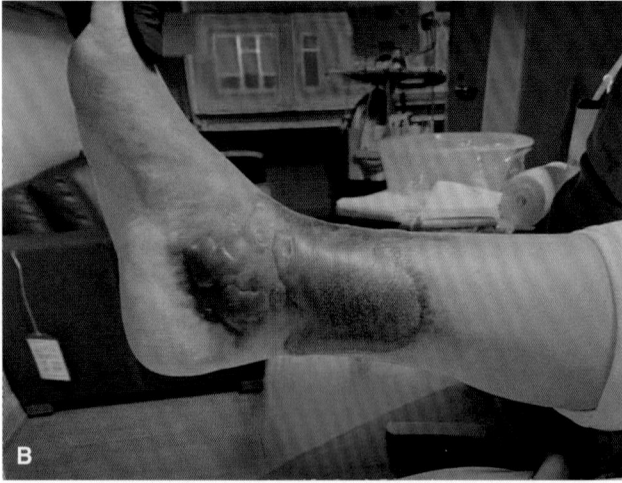

FIGURE 35.1 A, B. Fracture blisters.

Initial management should include thorough cleansing of any open skin lesion prior to splinting. Photographs of skin are helpful in communication with the treatment team as splinting can make future assessment more cumbersome, especially when they can be placed within the electronic medical record. The "wrinkle test" is a method to determine when skin and edema are ready for surgical intervention when operative stabilization is delayed from time of injury. Skin wrinkles will reappear when the swelling of the soft tissues has subsided enough to allow for wound closure following the surgery.[29,30]

Capillary refill, pulses, and temperature is assessed manually. Sensation of the foot should be tested: dorsally (superficial peroneal nerve), first web space (deep peroneal nerve), lateral foot (sural), as well as the bottom of the foot (posterior tibial nerve). Motor testing is often limited by pain, but toe range of motion can be assessed actively and passively. This examination should be repeated after reduction maneuvers.

Palpation of the medial and lateral malleoli should be performed, especially in isolated lateral malleoli fractures as medial pain can arguably give some clue toward more severe soft tissue injury patterns. Examination of the syndesmosis by palpation should be used to guide suspicions of associated syndesmotic disruption. The proximal fibula and knee should also be examined and radiographs obtained if painful to avoid missing the well-reported Maisonneuve injury which can be overlooked in the initial emergency department examination.[31-33] Achilles tendon continuity should be noted as concomitant ruptures have been reported.[34]

Compartment syndrome is rare in isolated malleolar ankle fractures but should always remain on the differential diagnosis list, especially with the Bosworth variation.[35-38] Posterior compartment syndrome is the most common to occur with ankle fractures and the most difficult to assess clinically. Painful passive dorsiflexion of the digits is the most likely clinical sign to raise suspicion in this setting.

PATHOGENESIS

Malleolar ankle fractures are most often the result of rotation of the body about a pronated or supinated foot as described by mechanistic-based classification systems. High-energy fractures about the ankle are not uncommon in motor vehicle accidents, falls from height and combat injuries, and typically do not fit as well in standard classification systems.

Ankle fractures are among the most common fractures encountered in an emergency department. Incidence is reported between 37 and 169 per 100 000 per year.[39-41] Females sustain more total fractures and have increased fracture risk with age. Multiple studies have shown increasing incidence of ankle fractures from a population level. In Finland, fractures of the ankle increased in incidence from 57 per 100 000 to 130 per 100 000 from 1970 to 1994.[42] The same authors more recently described a decrease in incidence of ankle fractures among citizens over 60 which they attribute to a healthier, older cohort, better preventative bone health, and lower smoking rates.[43]

Unimalleolar fractures comprise 70% of ankle fractures, with bimalleolar 20% and trimalleolar 10% making up the rest.[44] Over 70% of ankle fractures are caused by standing height trauma such as slip or trip and fall. Individuals at increased risk for ankle fracture are those living alone, using alcohol, sleeping <7 hours per night, and females with history of previous fracture.[41] Elsoe et al. also identified increased incidence of

ankle fractures during colder winters in Denmark, highlighting the regional and weather-related demographic differences in incidence of this common injury. Like many other fractures, there has been a bimodal distribution of incidence observed, with the young and elderly more often injured.[39]

IMAGING AND DIAGNOSTIC STUDIES

X-RAY IMAGING (A-P, MORTISE, AND LATERAL)

Standard ankle radiographs including an anteroposterior (A-P), mortise, and lateral views can provide significant information regarding the injury, especially when combined with the patient's history and physical examination. These views allow surgeons to diagnose and classify ankle fractures, formulate an advanced imaging plan when necessary, and ultimately facilitate a treatment plan. Weight-bearing images should be obtained when possible. When evaluating initial radiographs, several features can indicate additional soft tissue injuries beyond the bony disruptions that are clearly seen. Comparison contralateral ankle images are useful in evaluation of subtle soft tissue injuries, particularly of the syndesmosis or deltoid ligament.

The fibula lies just posterior to the central axial axis of the tibia. The leg is internally rotated ~15 degrees on the mortise view, aligning the beam of the x-ray perpendicular to the transmalleolar axis. When interpreting the mortise view, the medial, lateral, and superior clear spaces should be equal and congruent. Widening or incongruence of the medial clear space can be an indication of compromised deltoid integrity (Fig. 35.2). Lateral translation or external rotation of the talus can also suggest medial injury.[11,45,46] As little as 1 mm of lateral talar translation has been reported to decrease the tibiotalar contact area by ~42%.[5] When the syndesmosis is injured or laxed, talar tilt or lateral translation of the talus may occur. However, it is important to understand that the width of the medial clear space alone is not an indication of syndesmotic instability.

Fibular length is another important finding assessed on the mortise view. Several methods for assessing fibular length have been described. A concentric circle (ie, "dime sign") can be appreciated between the medial recessed contour of the distal fibula and lateral articular surface of the talus. The circle is broken when there is loss of fibular length or rotation (Fig. 35.3).[47] Another method commonly used by the authors is the level of the fibular spike. This medial spike noted on the fibula should be at the level of the tibiotalar joint line. This method may be inaccurate when fibular comminution is present at the joint level and the dime sign can be implemented. The talocrural angle can also be used to assess fibular length. This angle should be within 2 degrees of the contralateral side with an average angle of 83 ± 4 degrees.[48]

Integrity of the syndesmosis can be evaluated by interpreting the tibiofibular overlap and tibiofibular clear space. The tibiofibular clear space is not rotationally dependent and can easily be measured on both the A-P and mortise views. The measurement is taken 1 cm proximal to the tibiotalar joint, between the medial border of the distal fibula and lateral border of the tibia. This is a measurement of the joint space at the incisura (see Fig. 35.2). This distance should be <6 mm on both the A-P and mortise projections.[18] When evaluating the overlap, there should not be <6 mm of overlap between the medial border of the distal fibula and the lateral border of the anterior tibia on the A-P radiograph.

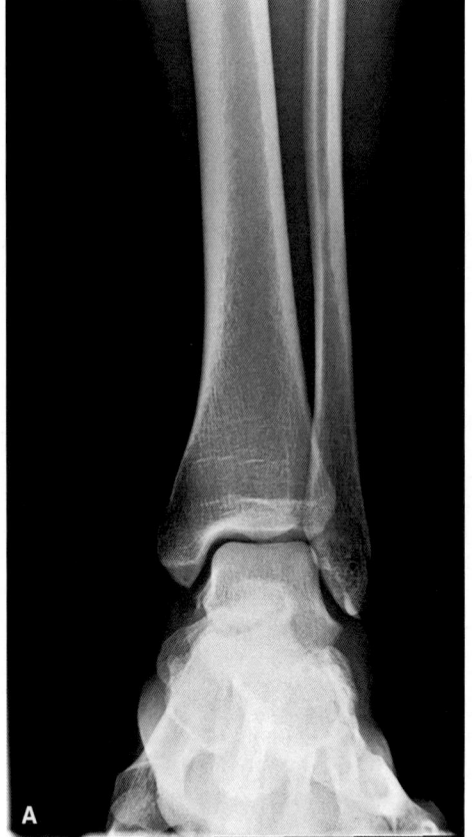
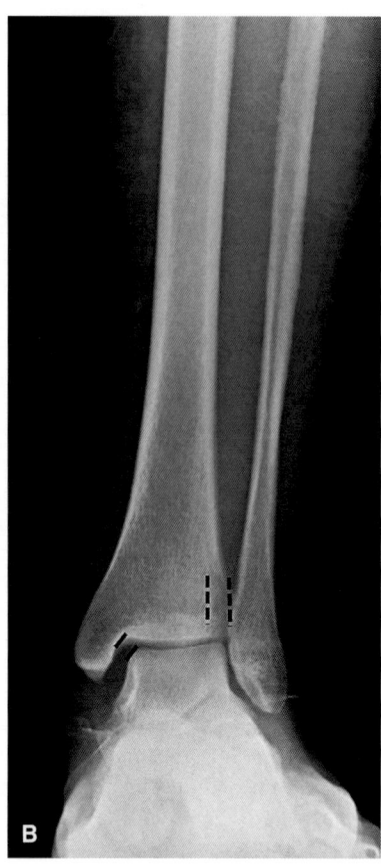

FIGURE 35.2 **A.** A normal A/P radiograph. **B.** Widening of clear space and tib/fib overlap.

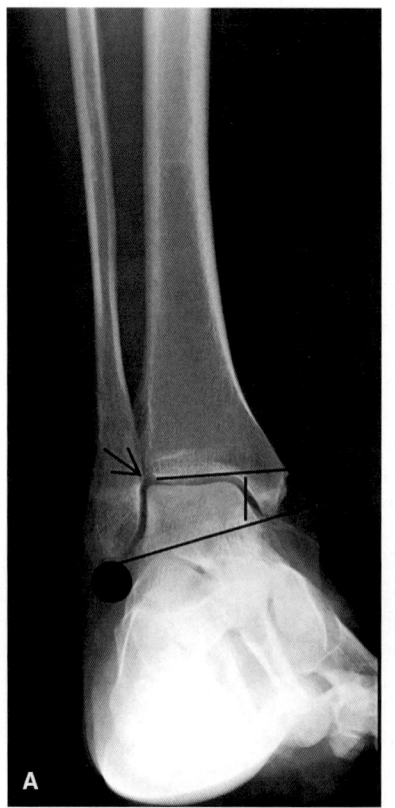
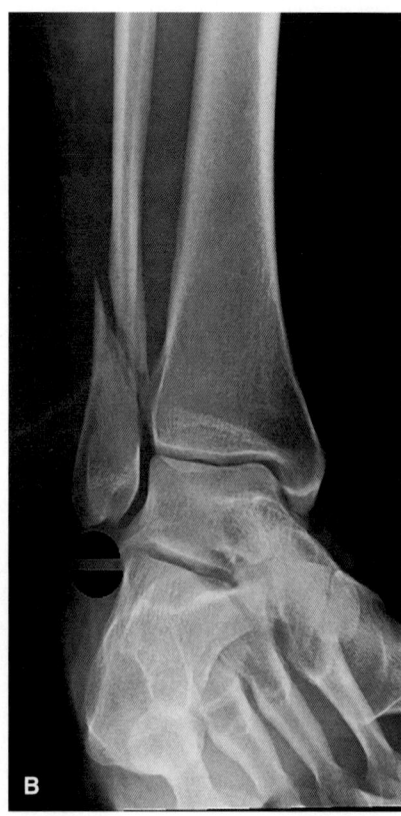

FIGURE 35.3 **A.** Dime sign intact, medial spike, talocrural angle. **B.** Dime sign broken.

The lateral view can provide valuable information regarding fracture characteristics (ie, comminution, posterior malleolar fracture) and syndesmosis integrity. Ankle subluxation or dislocation can be appreciated on a lateral view. It is important to obtain a true lateral to assess both the fracture and the position of the syndesmosis. A perfect lateral is obtained when there is concentric superior overlap of the medial and lateral borders of the talar dome (Fig. 35.4).

In patients with an isolated distal fibula fracture and an associated supination-external rotational injury, a radiographic stress examination of the medial soft tissues is indicated. Debate exists between a manually performed test and a gravity-assisted test. With both methods, an external rotation and lateral translation force is placed upon the foot and a mortise view is obtained (Fig. 35.5). It is important for the talus to be held at neutral (90 degrees) because the talus is wider anterior and a plantar flexed foot can give the appearance of medial clear space widening.

> The authors prefer a manual stress examination over gravity, despite the inconvenience of manually performing the test (see Fig. 35.5B).

CT IMAGING

Several authors have attempted to provide guidelines for when advanced bony imaging is necessary and helpful. Donohoe et al. reported a change in operative plan in 44% of CT scanned ankles and a change in fracture identification in 52% when advanced imaging was employed.[49] Kumar et al. reported that the preoperative plan was changed in 23.2% of CT scanned ankle fractures. They recommended that all ankle fracture dislocations, weber C fibula fractures, and posterior malleolar ankle fractures undergo a CT scan.[50]

> - It is the author's preference to get a CT scan when the above criteria apply.
> - See Figure 35.6.
> - Additionally, when a medial double density or "spur" sign is visualized on the distal tibia on an A-P or Mortise view, a hyper plantar flexion variant is suspected and is an indication for a CT scan (Fig. 35.7).[51]

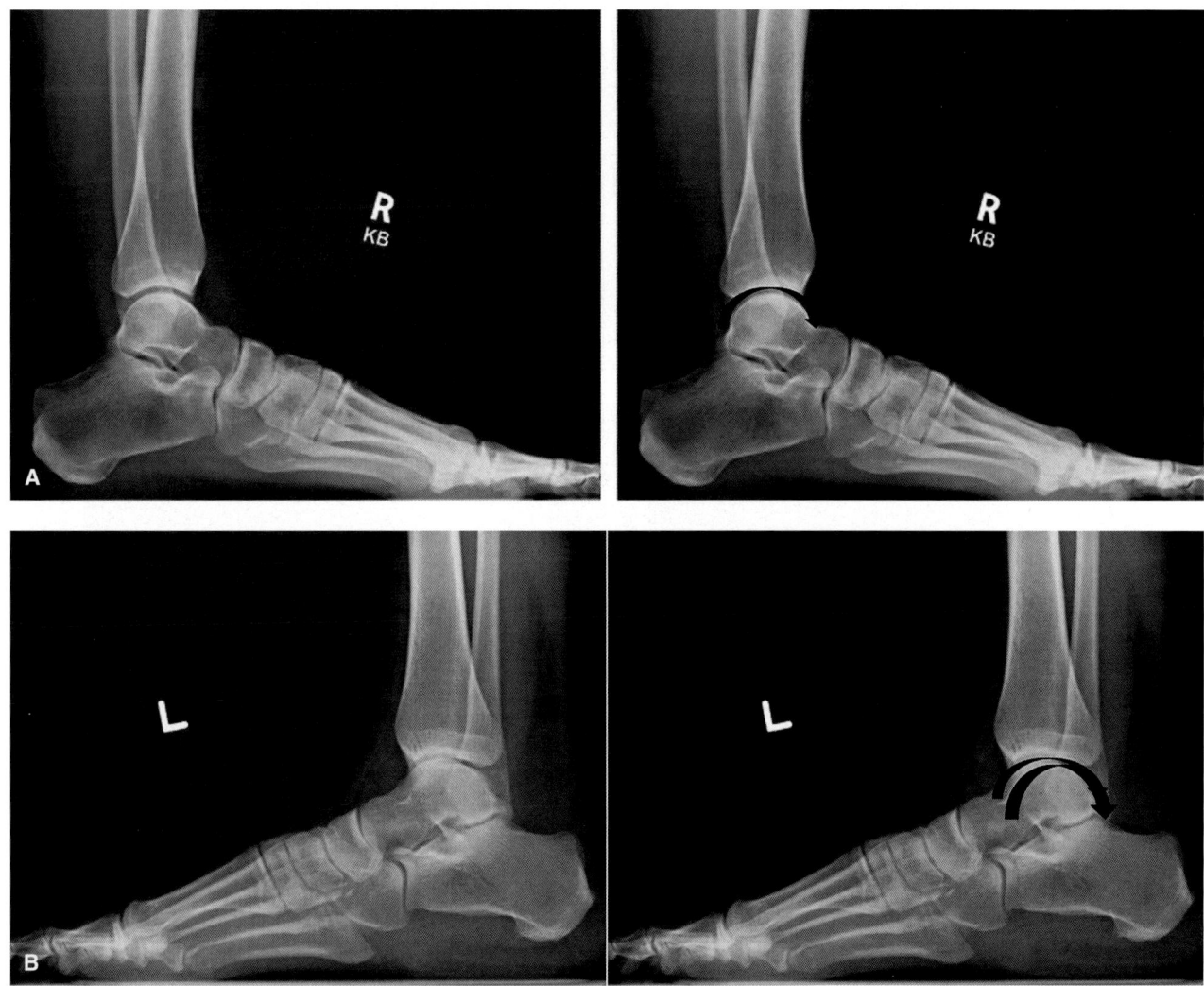

FIGURE 35.4 Lateral radiographs. **A.** True lateral projection with superimposed talar borders. **B.** Incongruent talar borders.

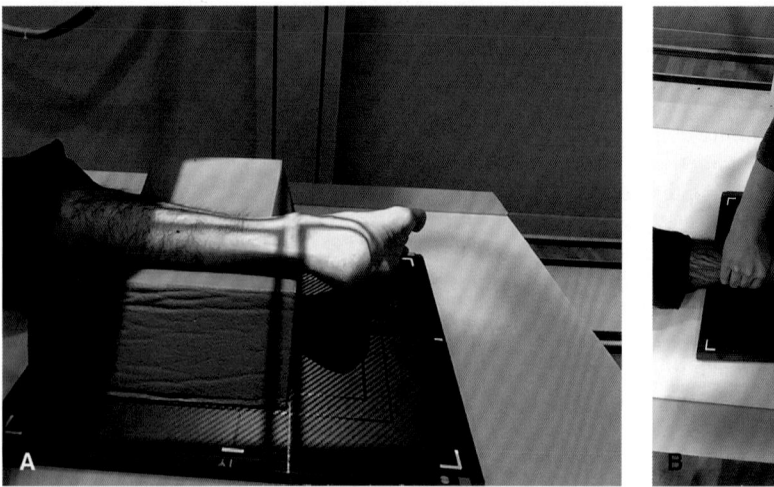
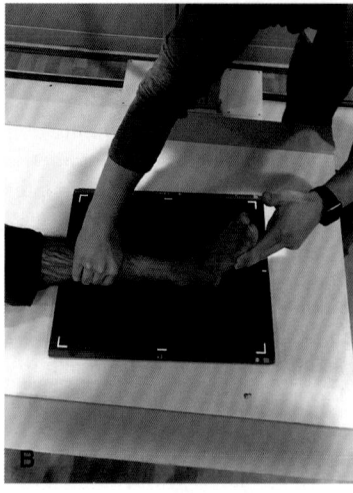

FIGURE 35.5 **A.** Gravity stress radiograph (note the plantarflexed position should be corrected to 90 degrees). **B.** Manual external rotation stress radiograph.

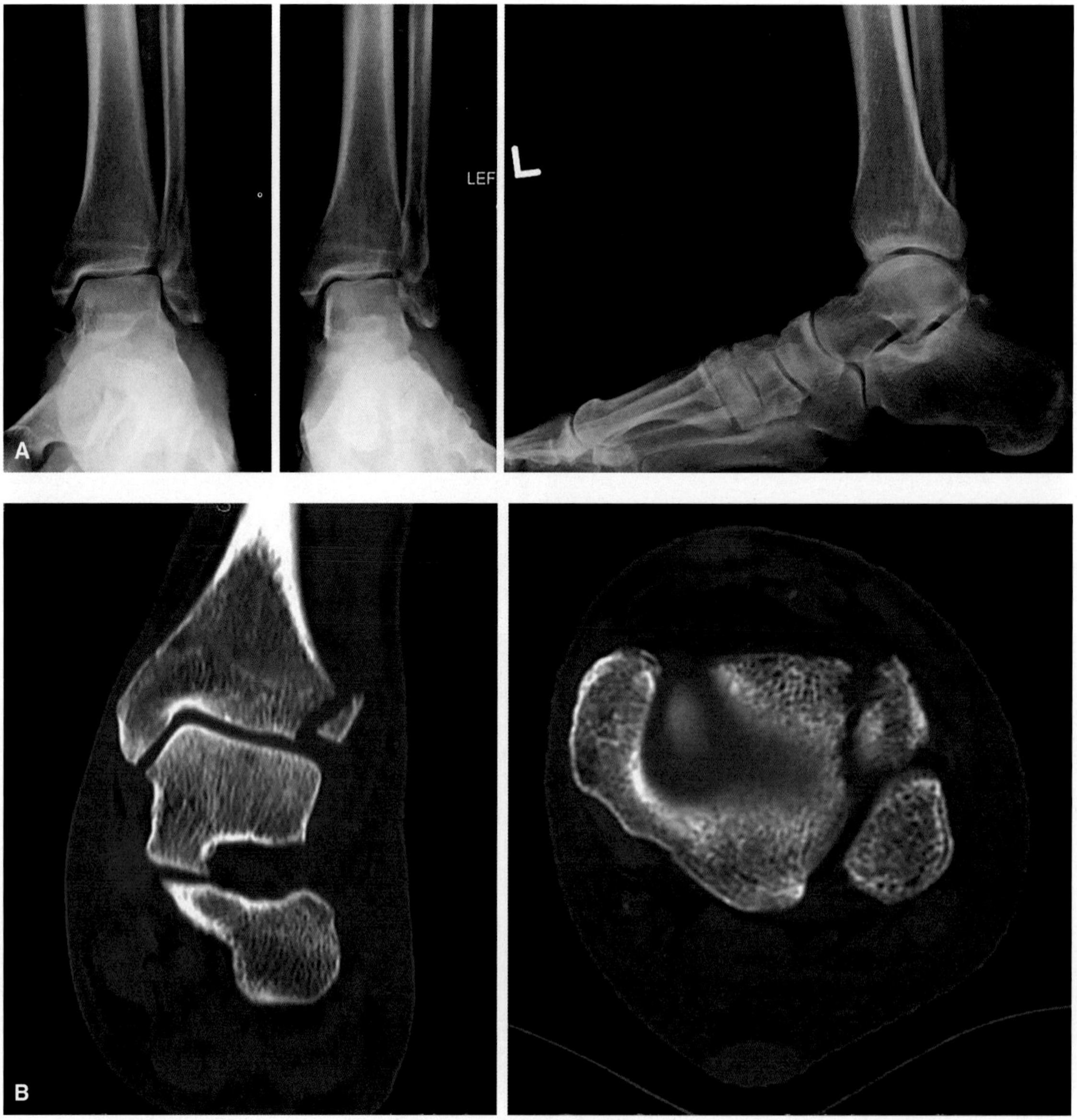

FIGURE 35.6 **A.** X-rays not clearly demonstrating Tillaux-Chaput fracture. **B.** CT scan clearly showing fracture.

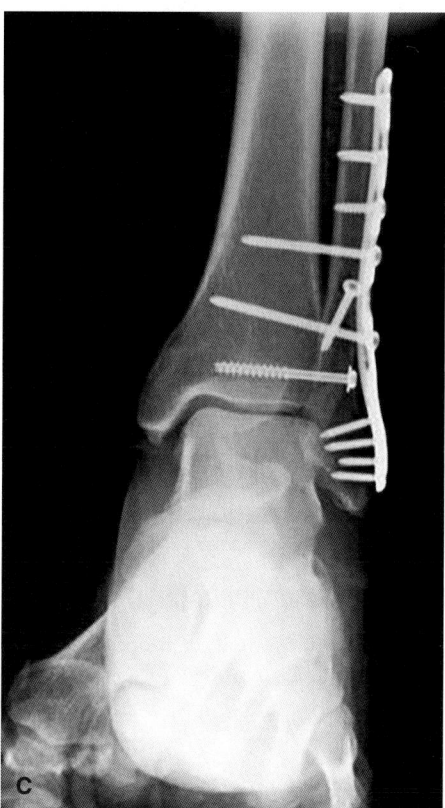

FIGURE 35.6 (*Continued*) **C.** Fixation with screw and washer.

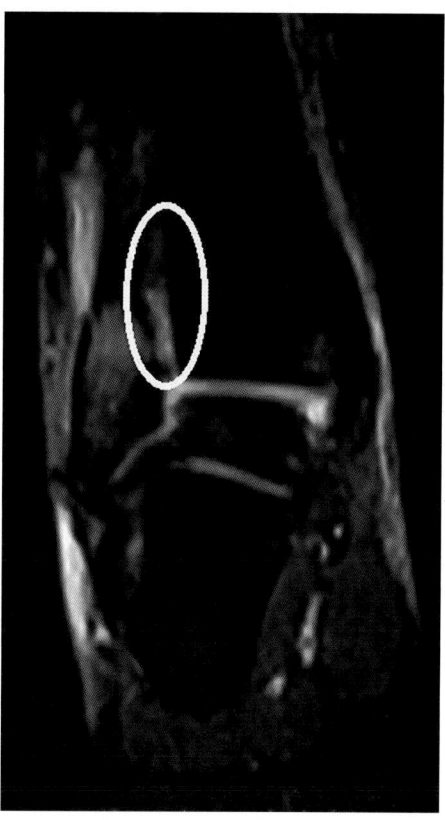

FIGURE 35.8 MRI showing fluid signal in the distal syndesmosis with a fibular fracture.

MRI

Though standard radiographs and CT images are important for determining bony fracture patterns, magnetic resonance imaging (MRI) may be useful in determining ligamentous injuries in ankle fractures. Syndesmotic injuries may not always be obvious following standard radiographs and clinical examination, particularly if the syndesmosis is incompletely disrupted.[52-55]

If there is concern for soft tissue injury following initial physical and radiographic examination, MRI can accurately diagnose acute ligamentous injuries with ankle fractures.[53,56]

The authors will utilize MRI in subtle cases where soft tissue injury or other intra-articular pathology is suspected (Fig. 35.8).

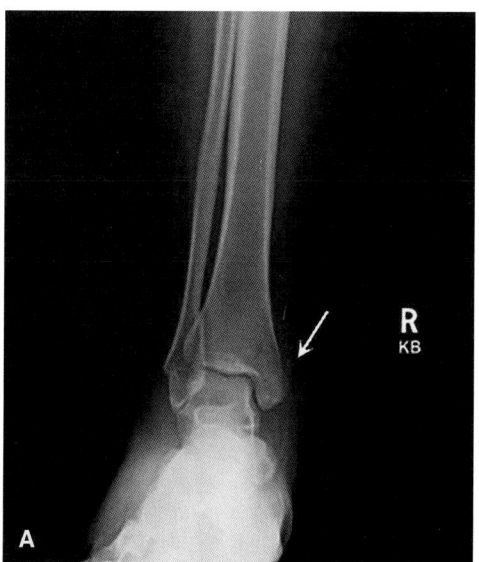

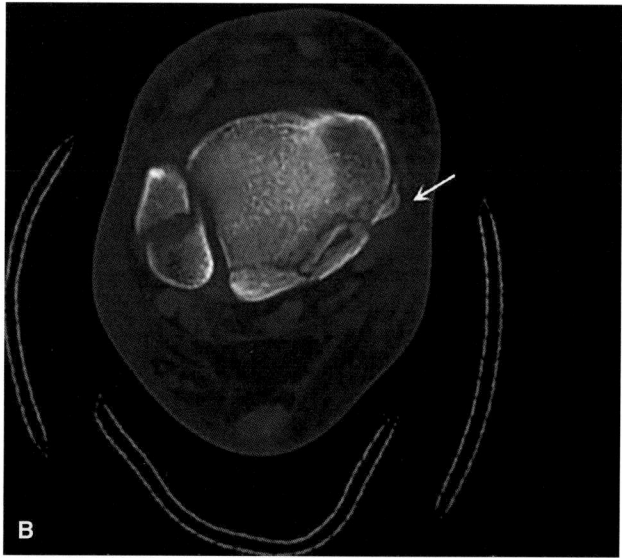

FIGURE 35.7 **A.** Posterior medial malleolar double density x-ray. **B.** Posterior medial malleolar double density CT.

ULTRASOUND

Ultrasound (US) has been shown to be useful in trauma in the lower extremity.[57] US can accurately visualize bony and soft tissue anatomy and can correlate well with MRI findings in acute foot and ankle injuries.[57-59] With an experienced musculoskeletal technician, US can offer an inexpensive alternative to diagnosing subtle soft tissue or bony pathology related to ankle fractures.[57-59]

TREATMENT

NONOPERATIVE MANAGEMENT

Unstable and displaced ankle fractures need to be treated operatively. Both bimalleolar and trimalleolar injuries are considered unstable. Unimalleolar ankle fractures that remain stable with a congruent ankle mortise can be successfully treated nonoperatively.[60-63] Isolated lateral malleolus fractures with minimal or no displacement and no evidence of medial sided injury are considered stable.

As previously mentioned, the talus will follow the fibula laterally in unstable fractures, and small amounts of displacement can lead to large differences in joint loading. The amount of fibular displacement that is tolerated for nonoperative treatment varies between 0 and 5 mm, although 2-3 mm is generally the cutoff.[60,62-64] Weber A and B fibular fractures will have stable variants, while Weber C fractures are generally unstable.

Physical examination combined with radiographic evaluation will allow for determination of fracture stability. Medial tenderness was previously used to evaluate for deltoid ligament integrity; however, it is been shown that we cannot rely on deltoid tenderness.[65,66] There is no association of the presence or absence of medial tenderness and deltoid ligament injury.[65] Grossly unstable fractures will be evident on non–weight-bearing radiographs with clear displacement. Many times, however, stability of the fracture will be less clear. Standard weight-bearing radiographs will allow for proper initial radiographic evaluation. If there is concern for medial injury or syndesmosis disruption, stress radiographs should be performed.[66-69] As previously mentioned, manual, gravity, or external rotation stress radiographs are widely used to evaluate stability of ankle fractures.[70-72] Recently, the use of standard weight-bearing radiographs rather than stress radiographs has been shown to be sufficient for evaluation of the stability of ankle fractures.[73,74] These studies show that patients with intact mortise on non-stress weight-bearing radiographs can be successfully treated nonoperatively but should have close follow-up. If the medial clear space begins to widen throughout follow-up, operative intervention should be performed.

Isolated medial malleolar ankle fractures are relatively rare. Historically, they have been treated operatively as the medial structures are important for stability.[61,75] It was also thought that medial malleolus fractures had a higher chance of nonunion.[75] There have been few reports on isolated medial malleolus fractures; however, recent literature suggests that nonoperative management of stable medial malleolus fractures is acceptable.[61] Herscovici et al. demonstrated high union rates and good functional results in 55 of 57 isolated medial malleolus fractures that were treated nonoperatively.

- The authors generally treat fractures nonoperatively if there is fibular displacement or shortening of 2 mm or less with no medial or syndesmosis widening.[63]
- Nonoperative treatment of minimally displaced fibular fractures generally consists of 3 weeks non–weight-bearing followed by protected weight-bearing in a below knee walking boot.
- Stress and serial radiographs are used to evaluate for fracture displacement (Fig. 35.9). If weight-bearing results in more than 2 mm of displacement or changes in the mortise congruency, operative treatment will be initiated.
- In higher-risk patients, nonoperative treatment consists of non–weight-bearing and serial casting for 6-8 weeks.
- The authors generally treat isolated medial malleolus fractures operatively due to the importance of medial structures for ankle stability.

OPERATIVE TREATMENT/APPROACHES

There are multiple different surgical approaches that should be used in specific fracture types. Figure 35.10 shows incisional approaches for each.

Distal Fibula Fractures

The fracture may be exposed through a standard lateral approach or through a posterolateral approach.

Standard Lateral Approach

For a standard lateral ankle incision, the patient can be in a supine position or in a lateral position. The authors prefer the lateral position for isolated distal fibular fractures and the supine position for fractures that will require additional medial exposure. The incision is centered over the lateral fibula (see Fig. 35.10). Preoperative x-rays are used to determine the distance of the fracture from distal tip of the lateral malleolus. This allows for minimal x-ray use and appropriate incision, location and length. If the fracture pattern will require a posterolateral plate, the incision can be positioned along the posterior aspect of the fibula. Dissection is carried down through the subcutaneous skin. Care should be taken to not violate the superficial peroneal nerve (SPN). The mean distance of the nerve from the tip of lateral malleolus is 10 cm; however, it has been shown to be as low as 2.5 cm from the tip of the malleolus.[76-78]

- Figure 35.11 shows a unique technique employed by the authors for dissection of the distal fibula.
- Dissection is carried down through the periosteum to bone over the distal most 1 cm of the lateral fibula. An elevator is placed subperiosteally and run proximally toward the fracture. The periosteum and fascia layer are easily elevated and split exposing the fracture site. This exposes the distal fibula efficiently and can safely expose the SPN as it courses from proximal posterior to distal anterior. If the nerve is encountered, it can be isolated and safely retracted.

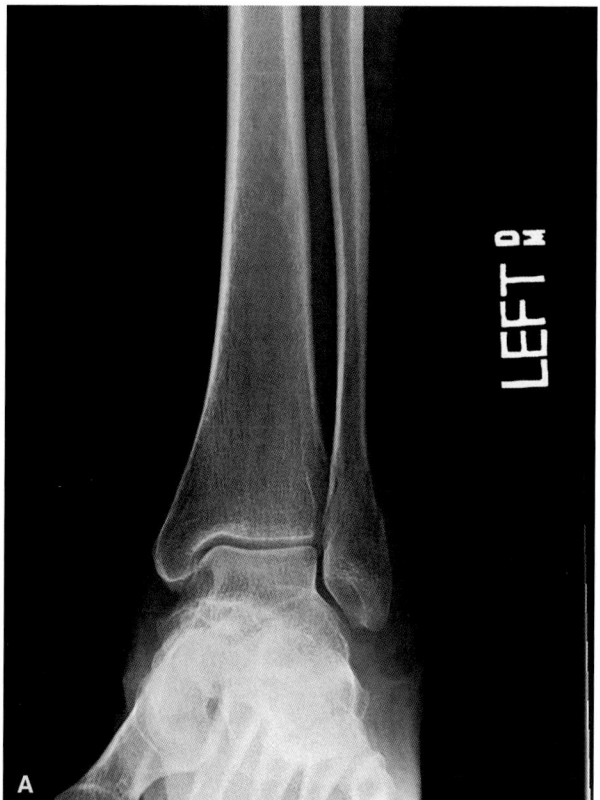

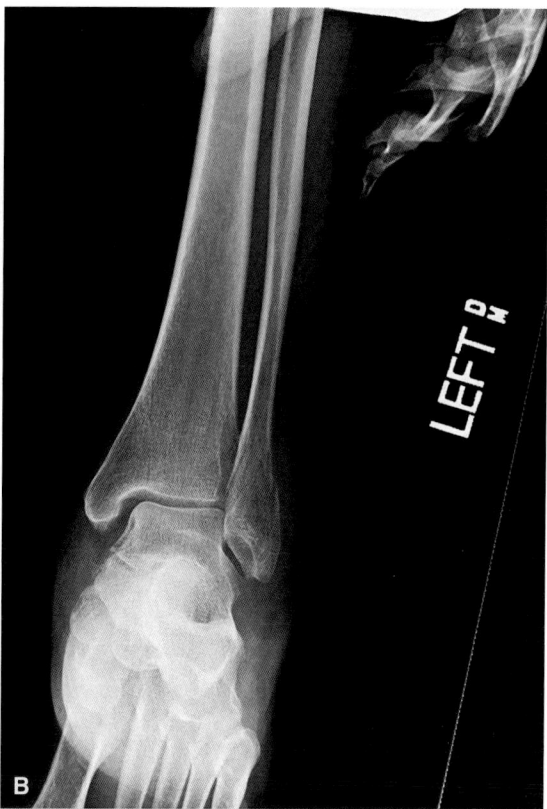

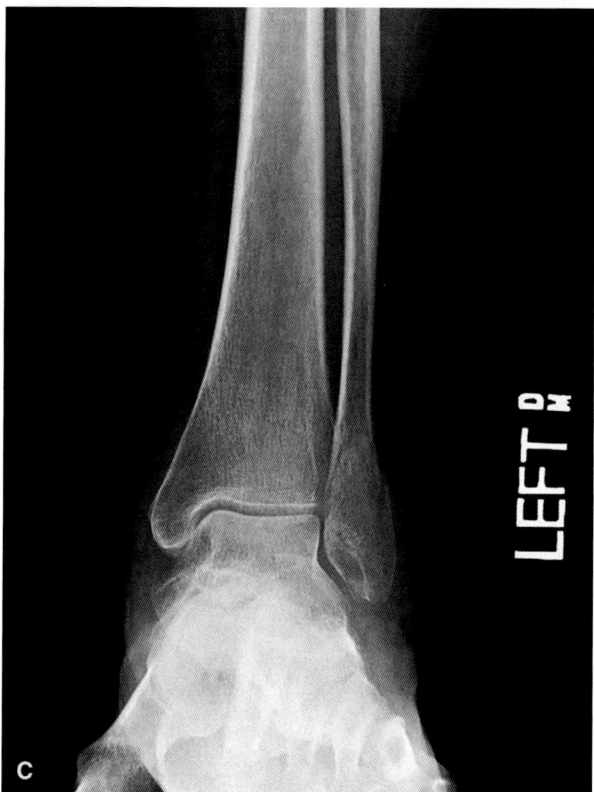

FIGURE 35.9 **A.** Standard weight-bearing examination with minimal fibular displacement. **B.** Manual stress examination showing minimal medial space opening and no fibular displacement. **C.** Nonoperative treatment was successful with no migration of the fracture or translation of the talus at 8 weeks.

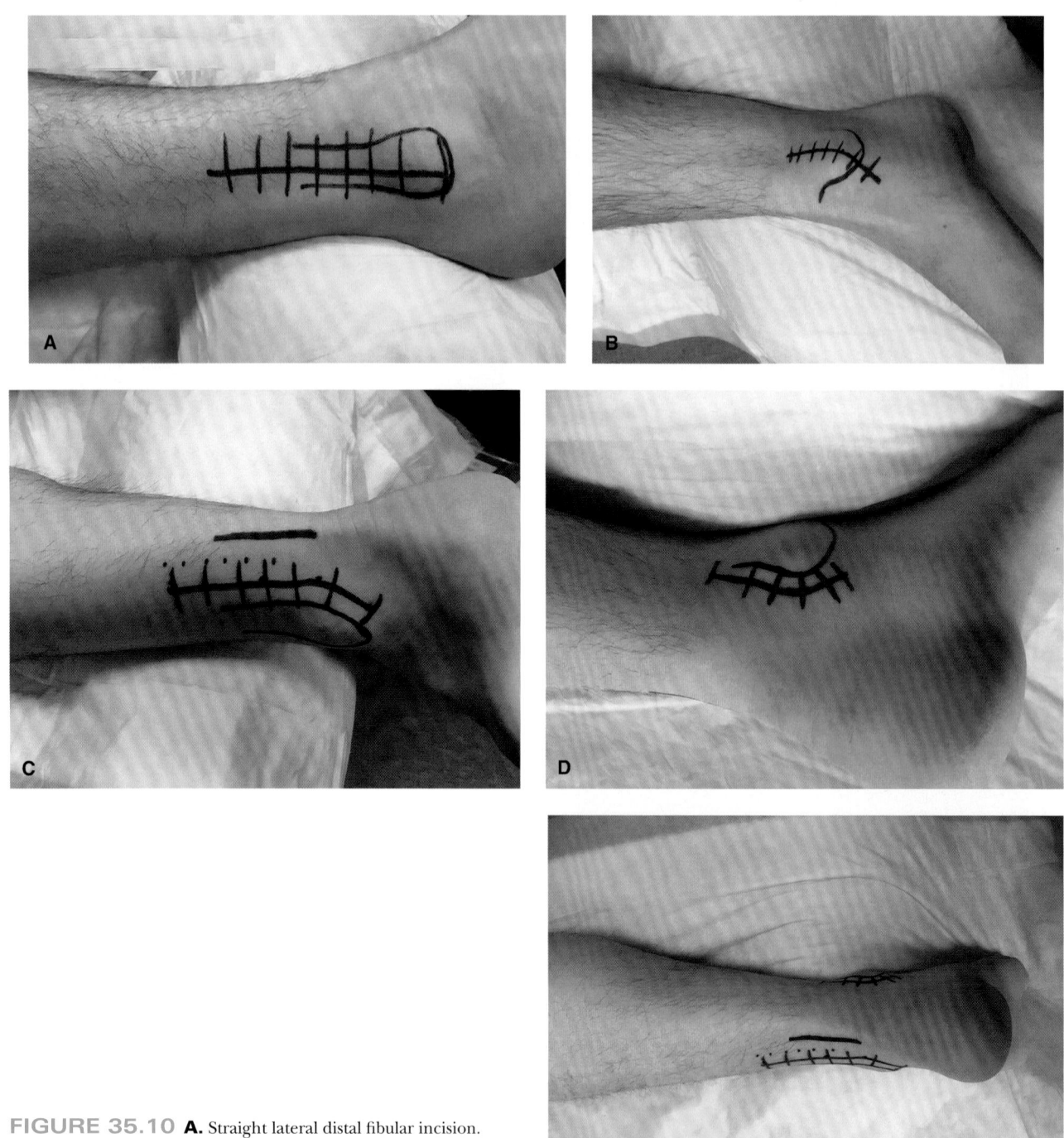

FIGURE 35.10 A. Straight lateral distal fibular incision.
B. Straight medial malleolar incision. **C.** Posterior lateral incision.
D. Posterior medial incision. **E.** Posterior view showing posterior
medial and posterior lateral incision.

Once the fracture is exposed, any hematoma and soft tissue debris are removed from the fracture site, and the fracture is mobilized (Fig. 35.12). A reduction is then performed using reduction clamps. Often the distal fragment is shortened and externally rotated. Care is taken to reduce the deformity in all planes and confirm with multiple views via fluoroscopy. Temporary fixation with K-wires can assist in holding reduction while applying fixation.

When the fracture pattern allows, one or multiple lag screws are placed across the fracture for initial fixation. The fracture is then neutralized with a plate and screw construct (see Fig. 35.12). Standard 1/3 tubular plating can be used. More recently, anatomic and locking plate designs allow for more robust fixation if needed. Anatomic locking plates are particularly useful for increased fixation for fibular fractures

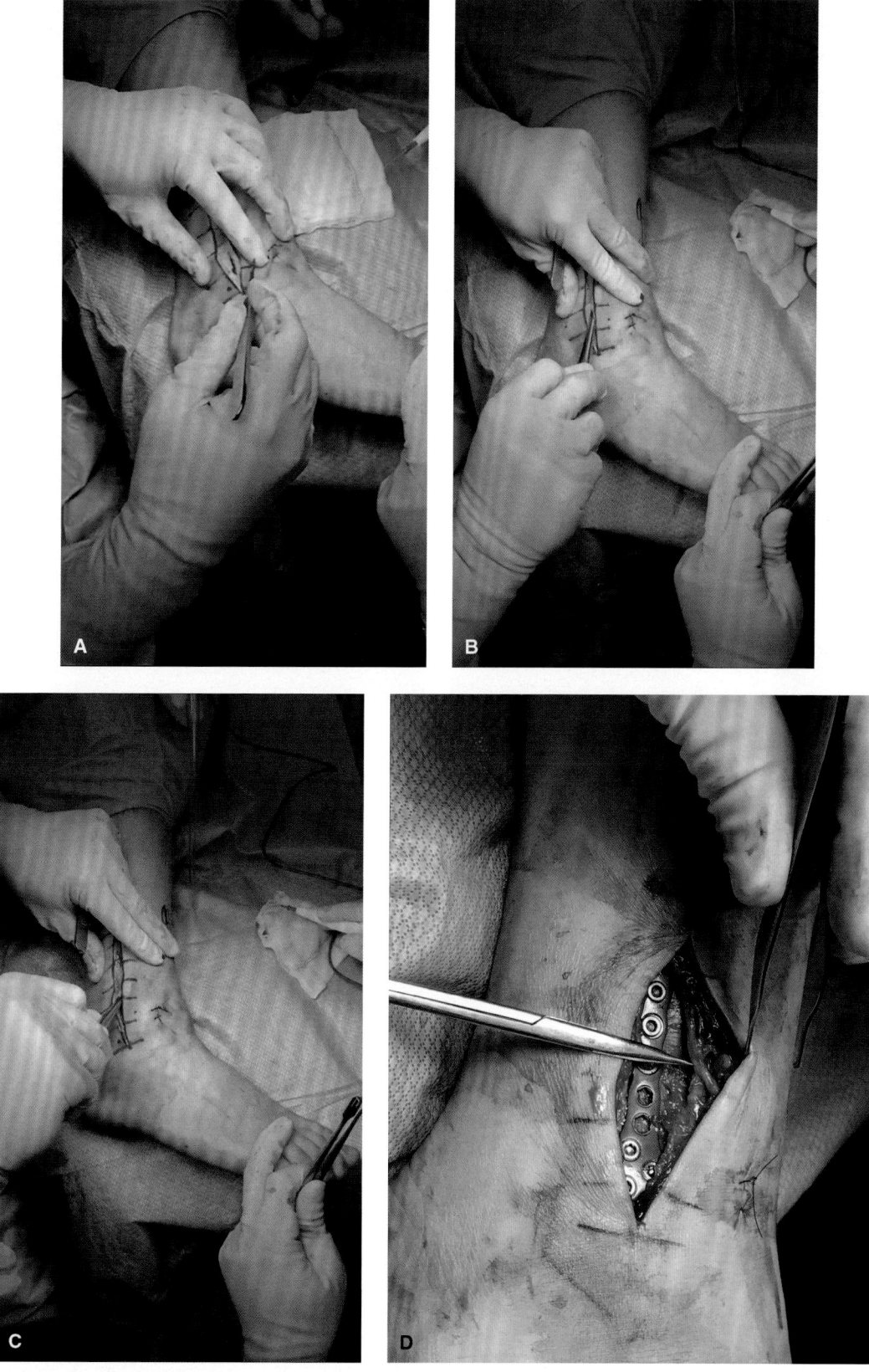

FIGURE 35.11 **A.** Incision through periosteum to bone. **B.** Introduce elevator under periosteum and run it toward the fracture. **C.** Lever the elevator to dissect through periosteum and fascia layer to expose a low-lying nerve. **D.** Low-lying SPN within the surgical field.

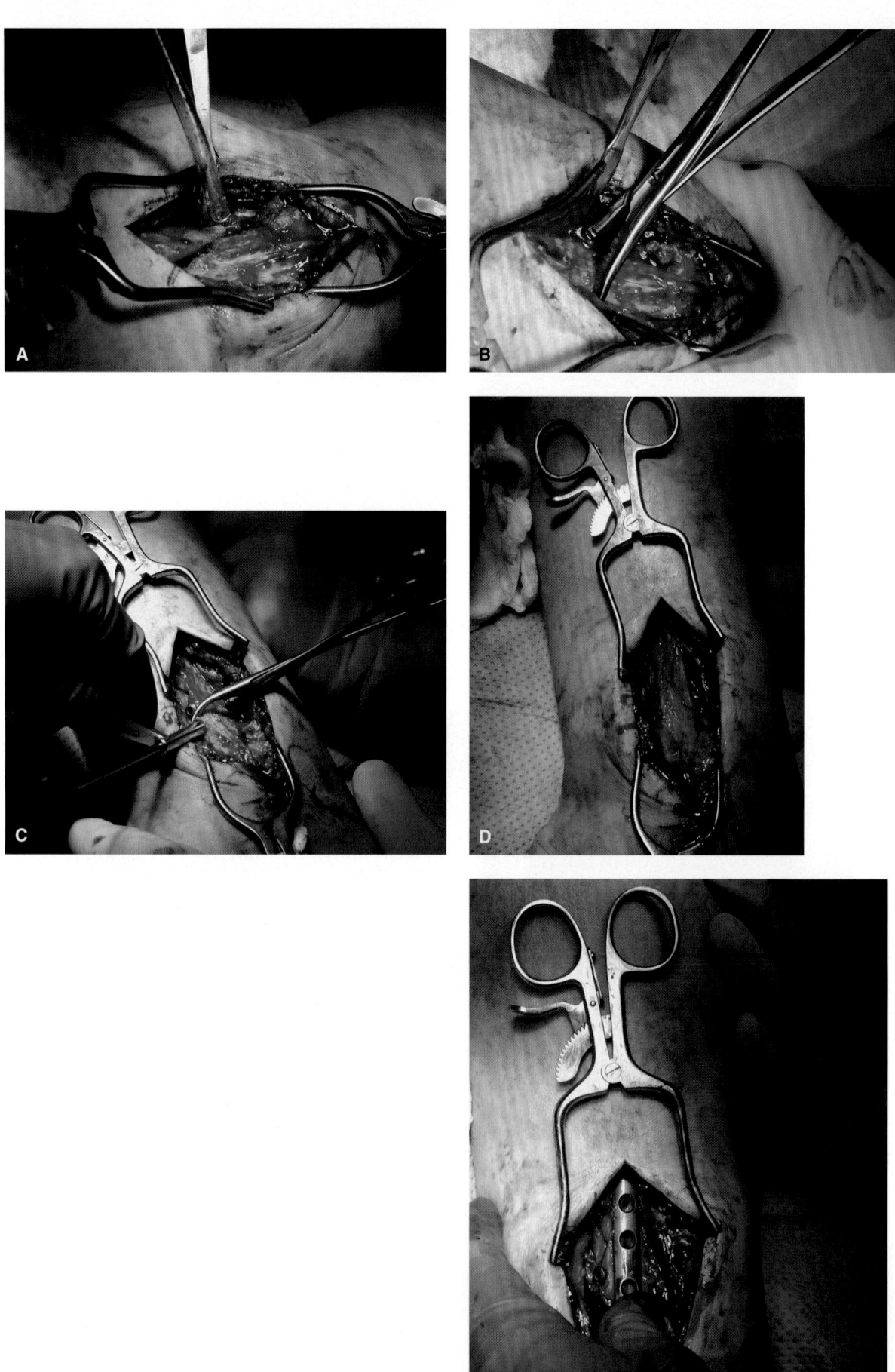

FIGURE 35.12 **A.** Identifying and cleaning fracture site. **B.** Temporary reduction with clamp. **C, D.** Fixation with lag screws. **E.** Neutralizing plate fixation.

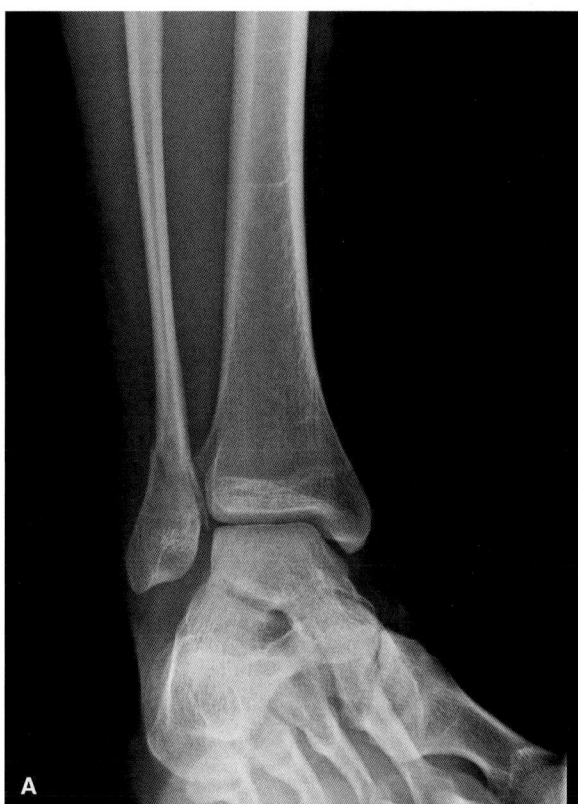
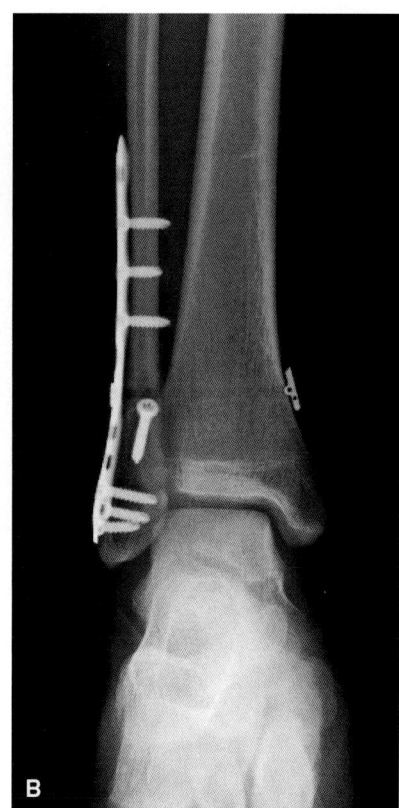

FIGURE 35.13 **A.** Distal fibular fracture with displacement. **B.** Anatomic locking plate allowing for greater fixation in distal fibula.

occurring more distal (Fig. 35.13). Intramedullary nailing has been described for distal fibula fractures, and the newer generation devices allow for syndesmotic fixation and axial stability (Fig. 35.14). These devices provide a minimally invasive option when necessary. In some instances, fragment-specific plating is needed based on the fracture characteristics (ie, Wagstaffe-Le Forte) (Fig. 35.15). Bridge plating may be needed when comminution is present as commonly seen in pronation injuries. Posterior plating can be performed for antiglide plate fixation if needed.

Posterior Lateral Approach
The posterior lateral approach can be performed when posterior fibular plating is required or when concomitant posterior malleolar fixation is required. The posterior lateral approach is performed with the patient either in a lateral or prone position. If an additional posterior medial approach is needed, then the patient is placed prone. When possible, the authors prefer to place the patient in a lateral so that ankle arthroscopy can be performed if the soft tissues allow. Lateral positioning is also more time efficient and safer from a patient positioning perspective. If a medial malleolus fracture is also present, the patient can be placed supine after fixing the posterior malleolar fracture and fibula fracture without redraping.

An incision is made half way between the fibula and the Achilles tendon (see Fig. 35.10). This incision can be extended to minimize the tension on the FHL. The sural nerve is often encountered and safely protected (Fig. 35.16). The interval between the peroneal tendons and flexor hallucis longus

tendon can be used to access the posterior fibula and the lateral aspect of the posterior tibia. Again, the fibular fracture is identified and any debris removed. This approach allows for lag screw fixation along with posterior or posterior lateral fibular

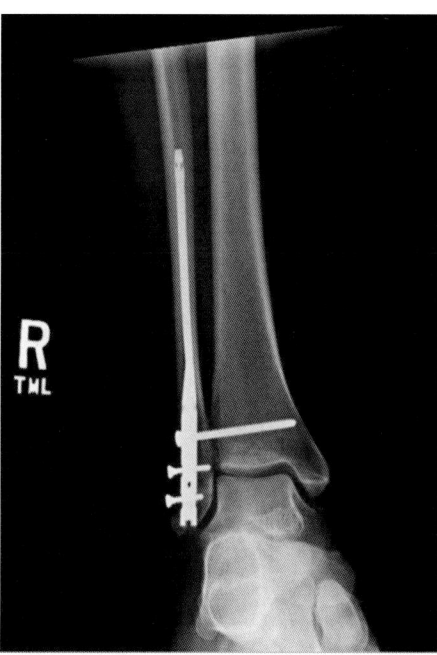

FIGURE 35.14 Intramedullary nail for fibular fracture.

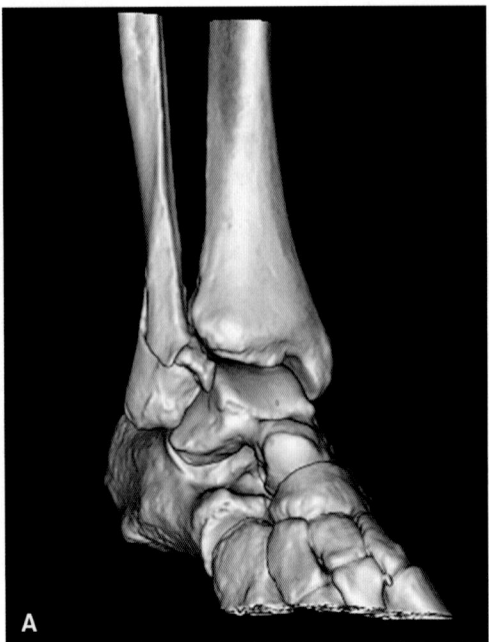

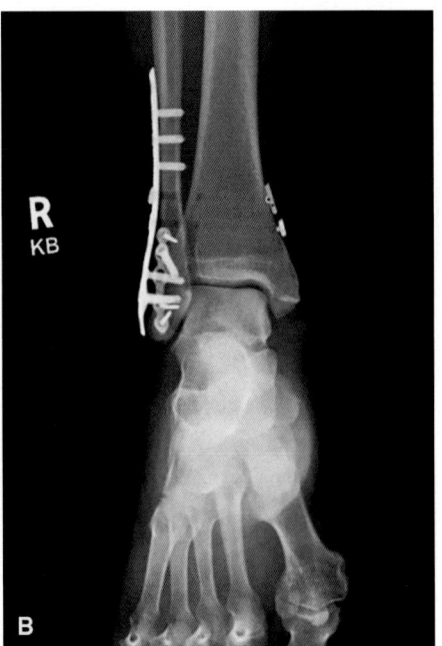

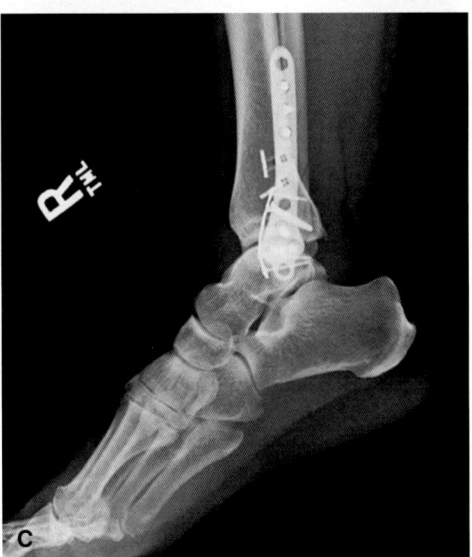

FIGURE 35.15 **A.** Wagstaffe-LeForte evident on 3-D CT. **B, C.** Wagstaffe-LeForte fixation.

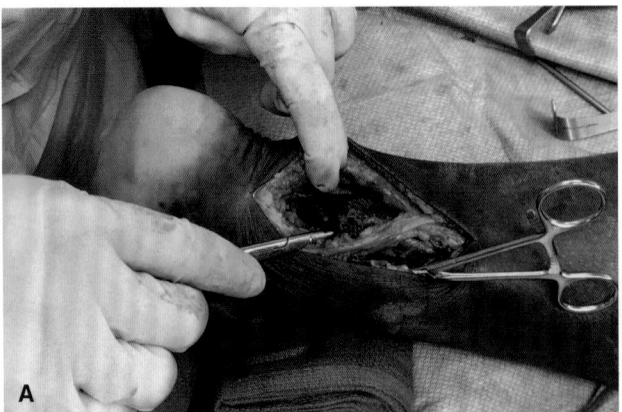

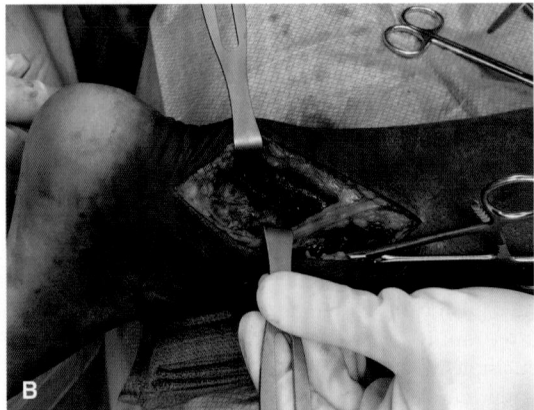

FIGURE 35.16 **A.** Posterior lateral incision with sural nerve visible. **B.** Interval between FHL and peroneal muscles exposing the posterior tibia fracture and fibula.

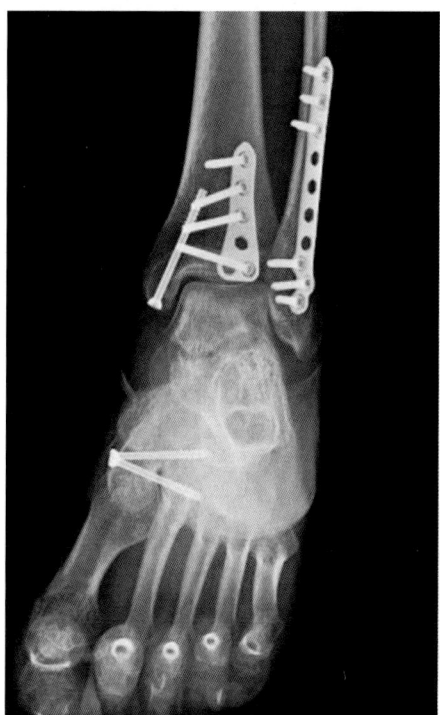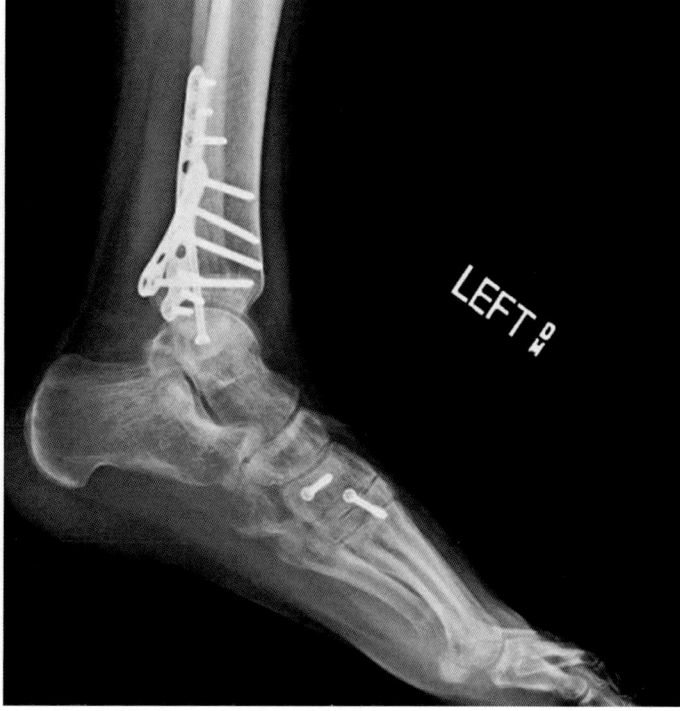

FIGURE 35.17 Posterior fibular plating from posterior lateral approach. Note the posterior lateral tibia plating as well.

plating (Fig. 35.17). Care is taken to attempt to have plate fixation terminate above the fibular groove posteriorly to reduce peroneal tendon irritation and risk of subluxation.

Maisonneuve Fracture

Fractures of the proximal 1/3 of the fibula are known as Maisonneuve fractures[79,80] (Fig. 35.18). They occur in external rotation ankle injuries and are a result of syndesmosis injury. Treatment of Maisonneuve fractures consists of indirect fixation of the fibula without addressing the fracture proximally. Fixation is performed by regaining fibular length and placing trans-syndesmotic fixation just proximal to the ankle joint. This is done with either screws alone, or screws and suture button fixation.[79,80] Riedel et al. showed that flexible fixation alone is insufficient to maintain length in unstable fibula fractures with syndesmosis disruption.[81]

Posterior Malleolus Fractures

There continues to be debate regarding the role and method of posterior malleolar fixation. If there is suspicion of a posterior malleolus fracture or it is appreciated on plain films, a CT scan is obtained to further define the fracture pattern (Fig. 35.19). Posterior lateral distal tibial fractures are typically an avulsion of the PITFL, which is part of the syndesmotic complex. By anatomically reducing and stabilizing the posterior lateral fragment, the posterior syndesmosis should be anatomically reduced and stabilized as a result.[82]

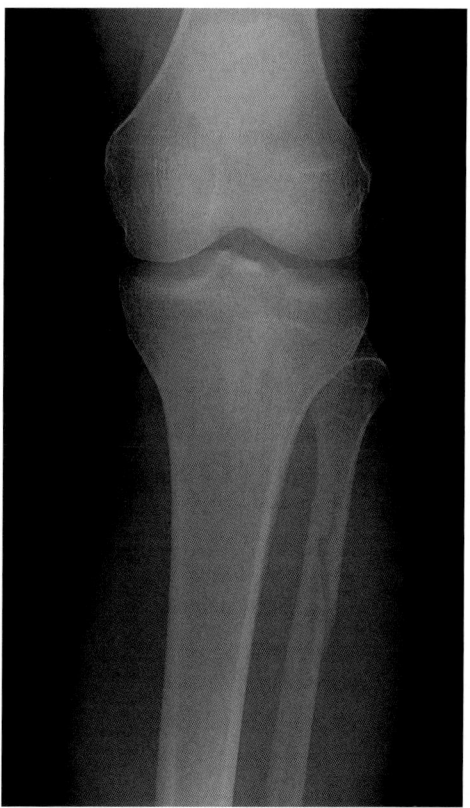

FIGURE 35.18 Maisonneuve fracture near the proximal fibula. (Photo credit Patrick Burns, DPM.)

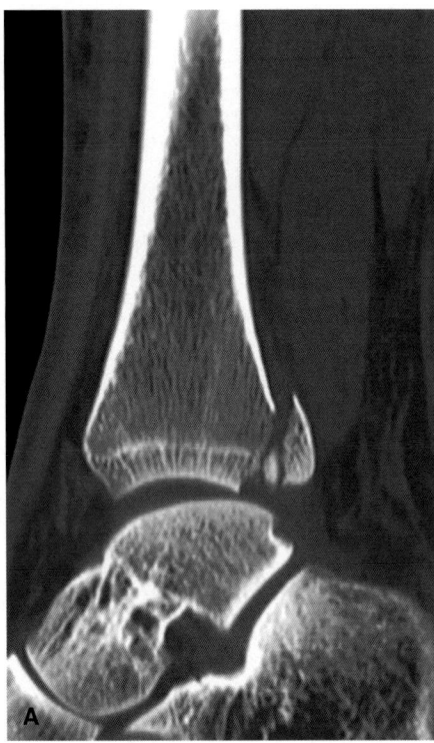 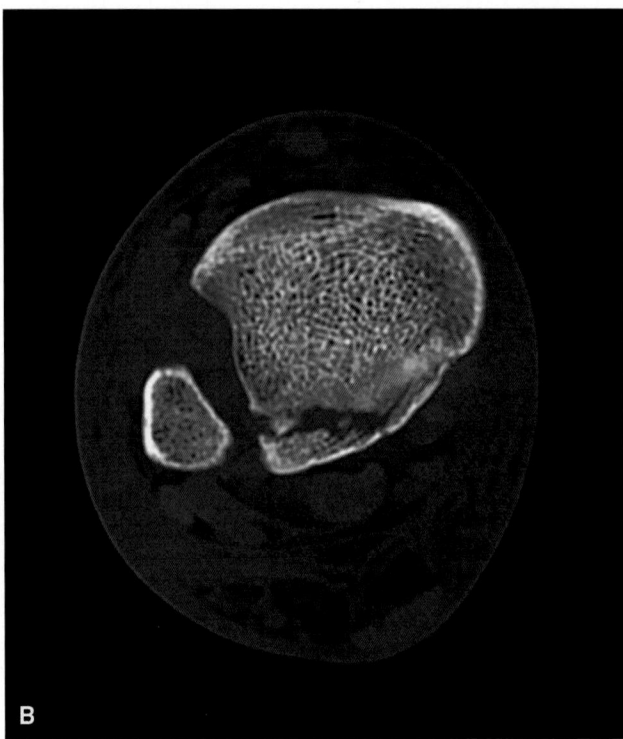

FIGURE 35.19 A. Sagittal section CT showing a posterior malleolus fracture. **B.** Coronal section CT showing posterior malleolus fracture.

Many authors suggest that fragments larger than 25%-33% of the articular surface should be treated with open reduction and internal fixation. Mcdaniel and Wilson demonstrated that restoring joint congruency was important for outcomes if >25% of the articular surface was involved.[83] In contrast, Langenhuijsen et al. retrospectively reviewed 57 patients with ankle fractures involving the posterior malleolus and found that joint congruity, with or without internal fixation, was a significant influence in patient outcome in fragments as small as 10% of the articular surface.[84] In a separate study, Van Hooff et al. found an articular step off of >1 mm, regardless of whether fixation was done, resulted in an increased risk of osteoarthritis radiographically at 7 years follow-up. They advocate the importance of obtaining an anatomic reduction of the posterior fragment.[85]

> The authors prefer fixation of the posterior malleolus of 10% or more.

Posterior Lateral Approach

Using the same interval as discussed for fibular fractures, the posterior lateral tibia can be exposed (see Fig. 35.10). The periosteum on the posterior tibia tends to be quite thick and often needs to be incised to expose the underlying fracture. Given the attachment of the PITFL to this fracture fragment, it may be difficult to reduce when the fibula is not reduced and out to length. Reduction of the fibula is performed and use reduction clamps and K-wires to provisionally hold reduction. The posterior malleolus is then reduced and fixated followed by fixation of the fibula.

> - The authors prefer to reduce and fixate the posterior tibial fragment first. The fibula fracture is then fixated with a plate and screw construct.
> - A fibular plate prior to fixation of the posterior tibia obscures visualization of the tibiotalar joint and can make it difficult for anatomic reduction of the joint.

Posterior Medial Approach

The hyperplantar flexion variant ankle fracture that consists of a posterior medial and posterior lateral fragment has been reported to occur in 6.7% of all ankle fractures.[51] There is insufficient evidence to specifically dictate which posterior malleolar fragments should be addressed. However, there is evidence to suggest the posterior hyperplantar flexion variant fractures specifically have a worse prognosis.[75,83,86-90] Despite inconclusive data regarding operative indications for the posterior medial fragment, Weber reported that failure to address and reduce this fragment may lead to talar instability, malunion, and joint incongruity.[91] In order to gain access to this fragment, a posterior medial approach is utilized.

The incision is made just posterior to the medial malleolus proximal and curved distally over the posterior tibial tendon (PTT) (see Fig. 35.10). The PTT sheath is incised and a cuff of sheath is left on the medial malleolus for repair following fracture fixation. The posterior medial fragment is often located directly under the posterior tibial tendon. Prior to incising the PTT sheath, it is important to confirm the proper tendon has been identified. This can be done by passively ranging the flexor tendons. Once located, a retractor can be placed to protect the PTT, FHL, FDL, and the neurovascular bundle. Much like the posterior lateral approach, there is often thick periosteum on the posterior tibia that needs to be incised to locate the fracture fragment. Care should be taken not strip the periosteum completely from the fragment, only what needs to be reflected to obtain an anatomic reduction. Plate and screw constructs can be used to fixate these fracture fragments (Fig. 35.20).

The authors use low profile implants in order to minimize irritation to the surrounding soft tissues, including the PTT.

Medial Malleolar Fractures

Medial Approach
Patient positioning for a medial malleolar approach is generally supine, however can be accessed with the patient prone. The location and direction of the incision is at the discretion of the surgeon and depends on the specific location and size of the medial malleolar fracture. We routinely make an incision centered over the medial malleolus and curve it slightly

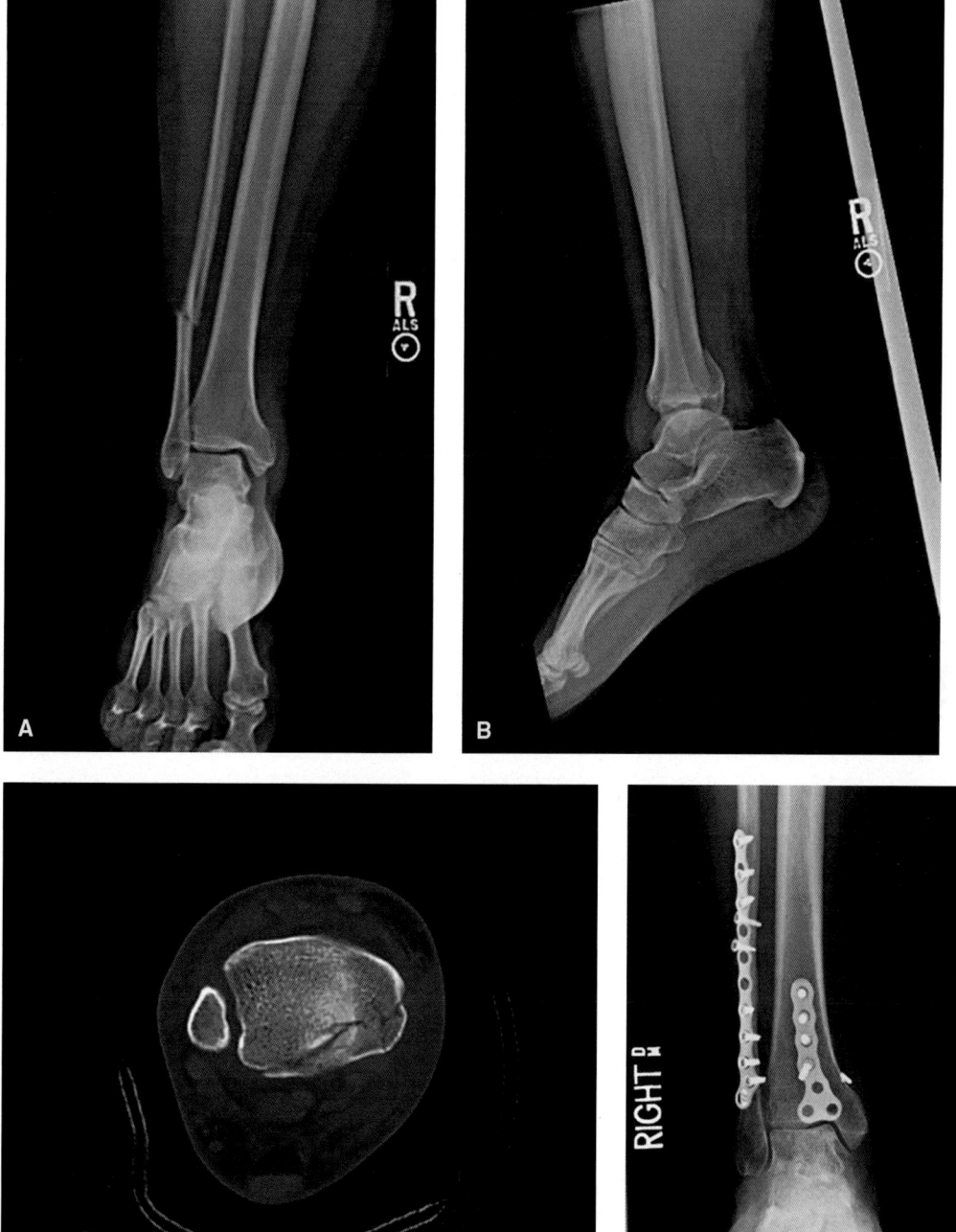

FIGURE 35.20 **A, B.** Preoperative images showing hyper-plantarflexion variant with posterior medial tibial fracture. **C.** CT image showing posterior medial tibial fracture. **D, E.** Postoperative images showing posterior medial fixation from posterior medial incision approach.

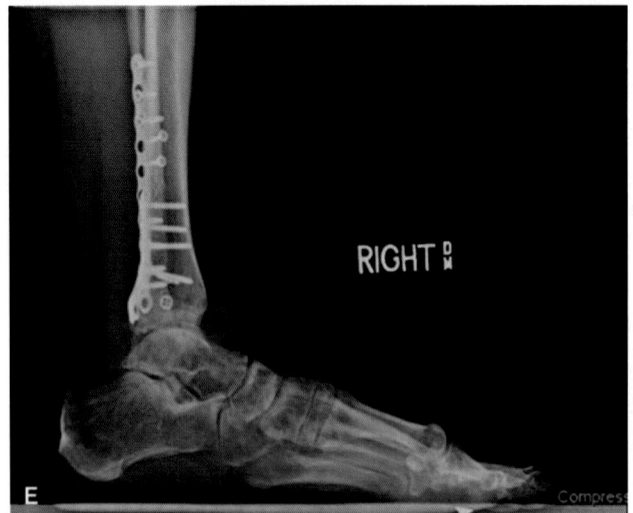

FIGURE 35.20 (*Continued*)

anterior at its distal extension (see Fig. 35.10). This allows for visualization of the tibiotalar joint, deltoid ligament, the fracture, and the PTT for tears or rupture. PTT tears are a rare but reported concomitant injury that is essential to diagnose and treat intraoperatively. In some cases of dislocation, PTT incarceration into the medial clear space is possible. If a PTT rupture is encountered, it is typically repaired in an end to end fashion or side to side for longitudinal tears.[92-94]

The medial fracture is identified, debrided/mobilized, and anatomically reduced with a clamp. Multiple fixation constructs have been described for medial malleolar fractures (ie, fully threaded bicortical screws, cannulated cancellous screws, medial malleolar plates, tension wiring, etc.) and the fracture pattern may necessitate a specific construct (Fig. 35.21). Transverse fractures may be fixated with one or two partially threaded or fully threaded screws. Small fractures can be captured with anatomic hook plates or tension wiring. Vertical fractures can be fixated with an antiglide plate.

- When a deltoid ligament tear is suspected, the authors will stress the ligament with a valgus talar tilt stress.
- If there is continued gapping, the medial approach is made and the deltoid tear identified (Fig. 35.22).
- The deltoid can then be primarily repaired or augmented with one or two suture anchors into the medial malleolus. The authors generally will use suture anchor augmentation.

Syndesmosis Fixation

When the syndesmosis is disrupted, syndesmosis fixation is indicated to create stability in the ankle joint. Two types of syndesmosis fixation can be used; syndesmosis screw fixation (static) and suture button fixation (dynamic) (Fig. 35.23). The syndesmosis is a dynamic ligament that allows for plasticity with ankle movement.[95] Screw fixation can be performed

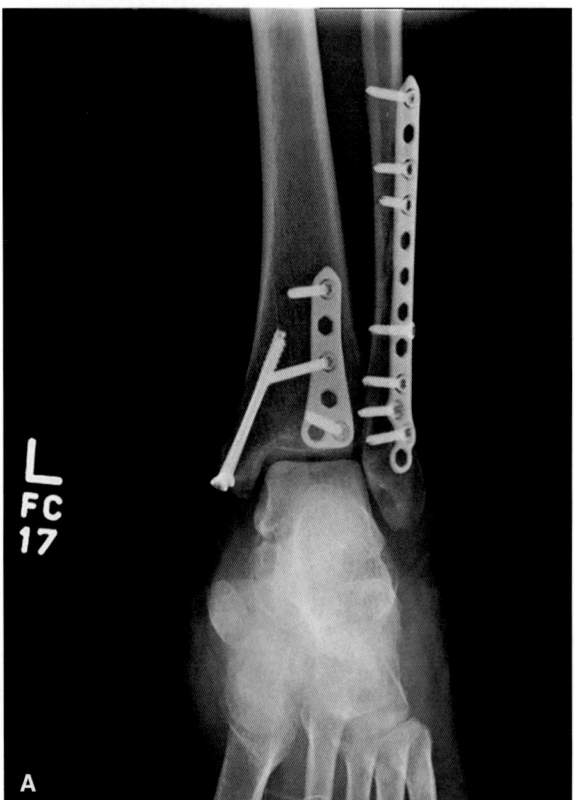

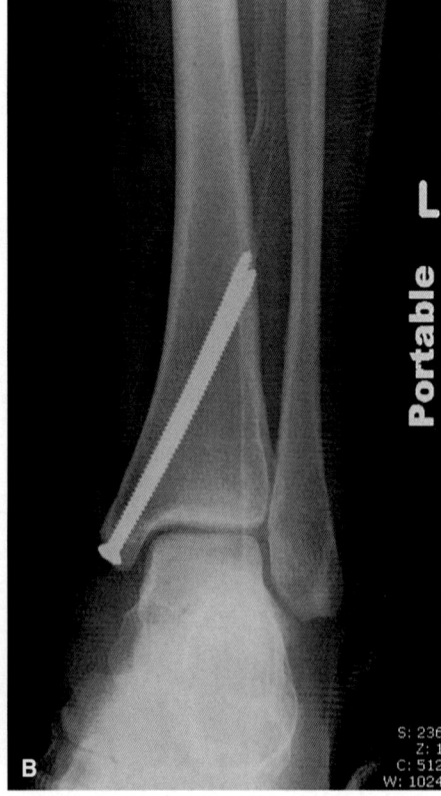

FIGURE 35.21 Medial malleolar fixation. **A.** Two partially threaded screws. **B.** Two fully threaded screws.

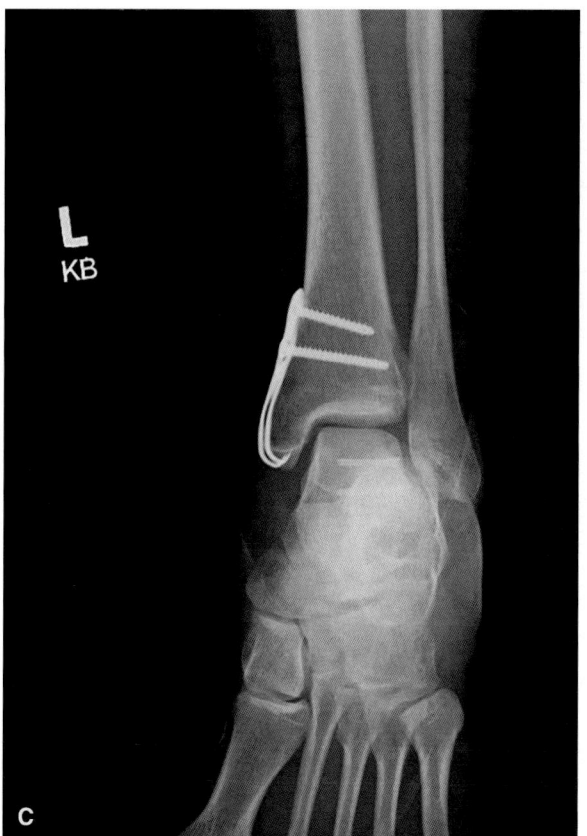

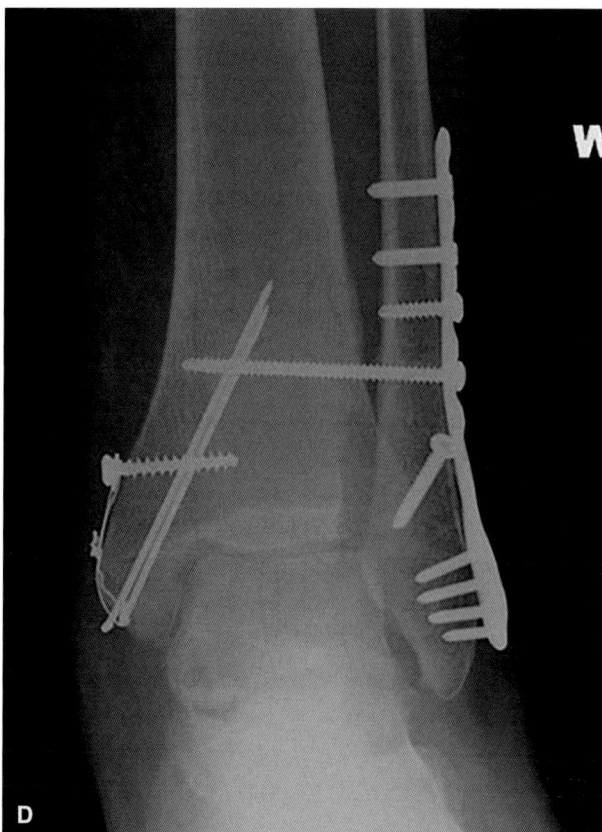

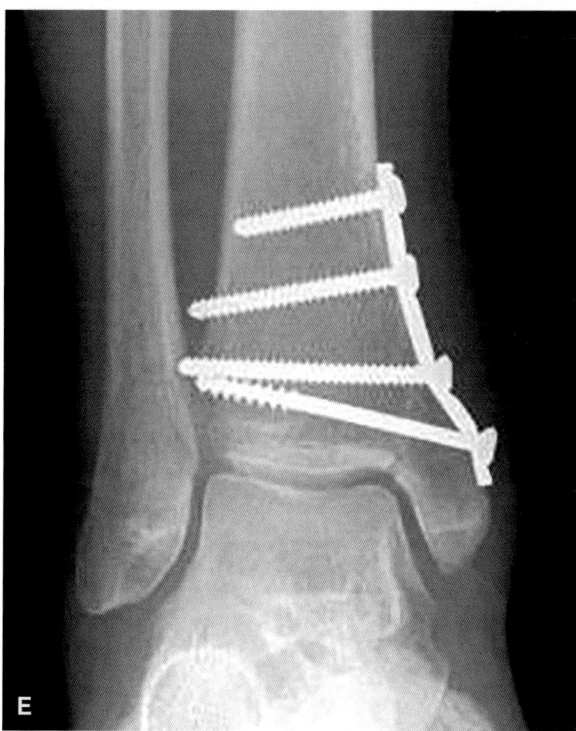

FIGURE 35.21 (*Continued*) **C.** Anatomic hook plate. **D.** Tension wiring. **E.** Anti-glide plating. (Photo B credit Ben Taylor, MD; photo D credit Patrick Burns, DPM.)

with either tricortical or quadricortical fixation with similar outcomes.[96,97] Care should be taken when utilizing screw fixation for syndesmosis reduction. Screw fixation may lead to malreduction and/or overtightening of the syndesmosis.[98,99] Some surgeons will routinely remove syndesmosis screws at

3-4 months, while others will only remove the screws if they are painful. Screw removal is recommended in painful or malreduced cases but is not necessary in patients with no syndesmotic pain.[100] Recently, suture button fixation has been utilized for syndesmosis reduction allowing for dynamic

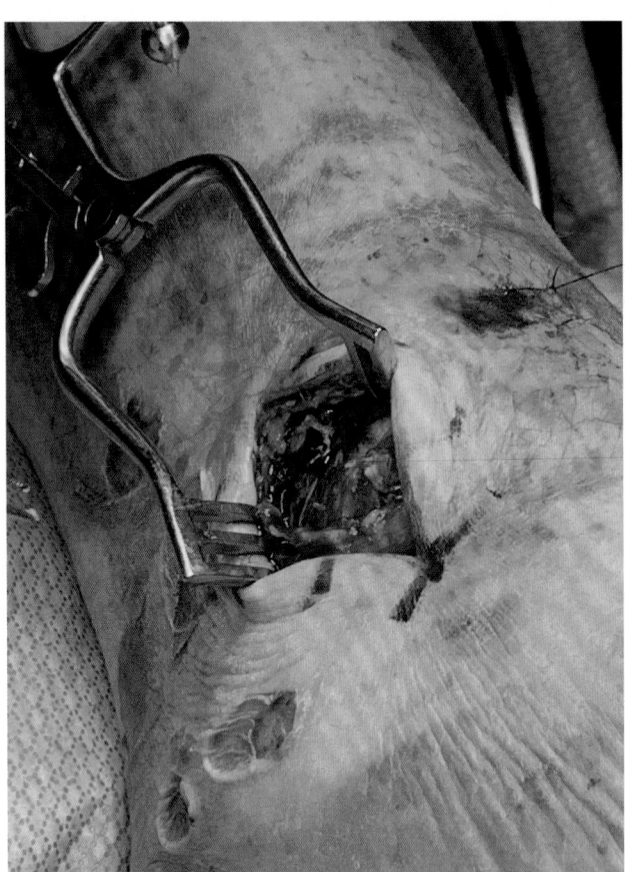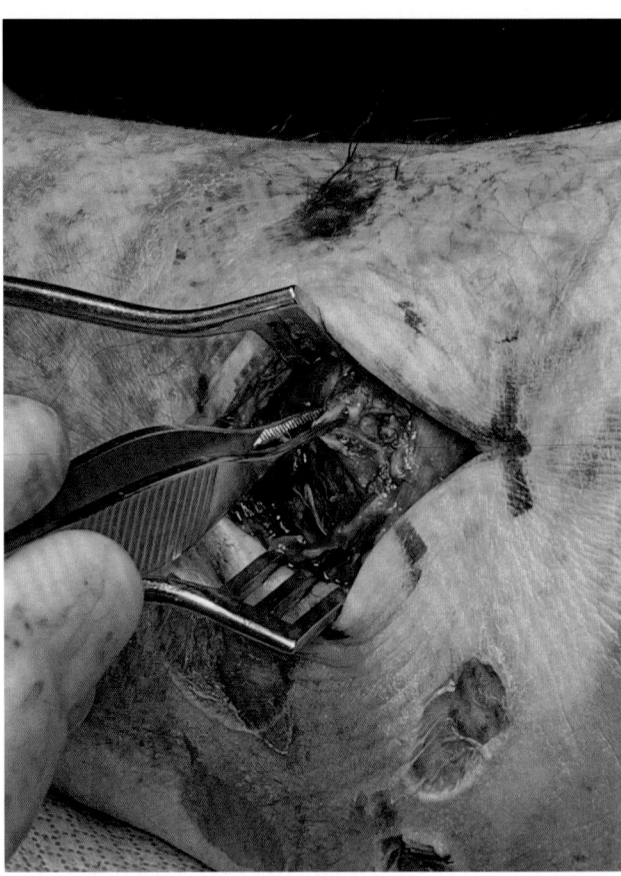

FIGURE 35.22 Deltoid ligament tear identified for repair/augmentation.

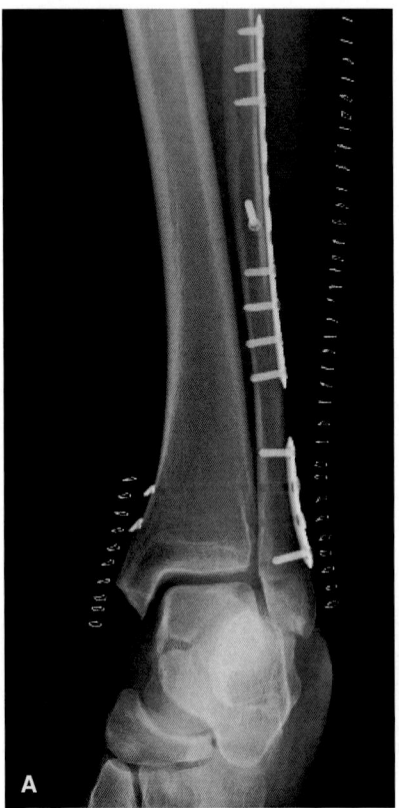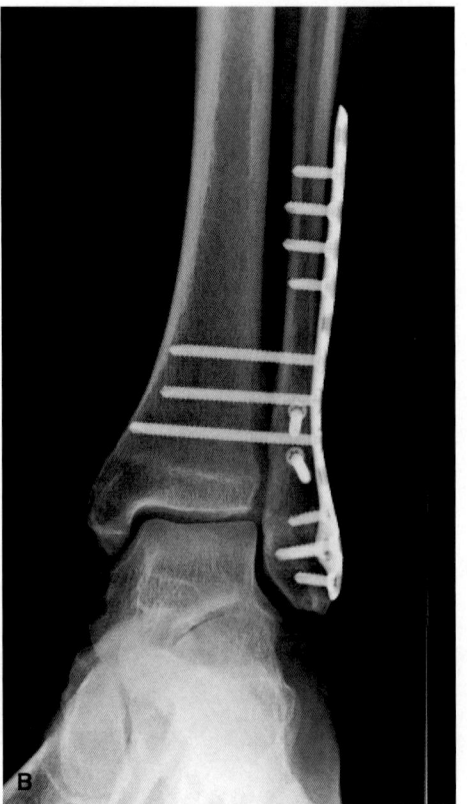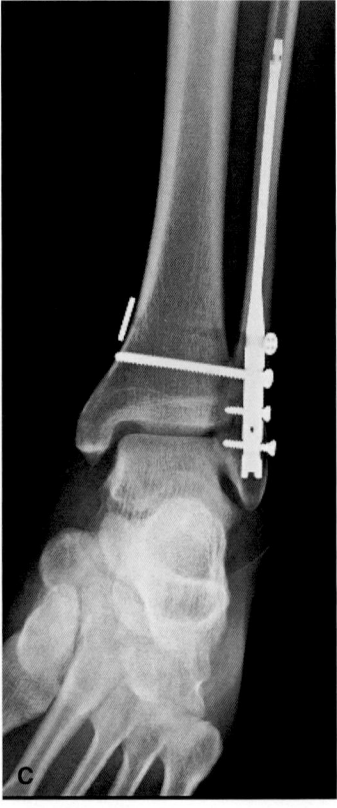

FIGURE 35.23 A. Dynamic syndesmosis fixation. **B.** Screw syndesmosis fixation. **C.** Dynamic and screw syndesmosis fixation.

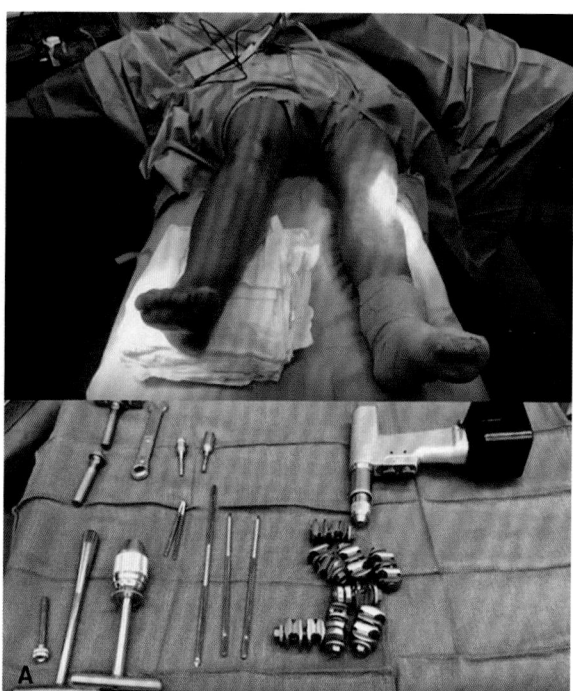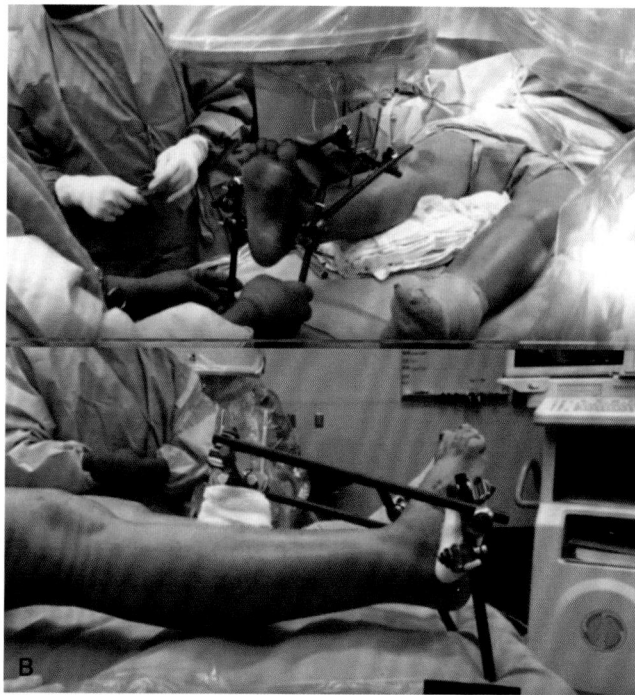

FIGURE 35.24 A. Positioning and instrument setup for external fixator application. **B.** External fixation construct with kick-stand added. (Photo credit Ben Taylor, MD.)

fixation. Suture button fixation has been shown to have good clinical and radiographic outcomes with a lower rate of hardware removal.[95,101] It should be noted that a single suture button may not provide sufficient resistance to sagittal translation of the fibula in unstable fractures.[102]

External Fixation

Temporary fixation of ankle fractures with external fixation may be necessary for some open fractures, or when significant soft tissue swelling is present. A standard Pin-To-Bar construct is generally used in the trauma setting. The patient is placed supine on a radiolucent table. A bump can be placed under the ipsilateral hip and stack of sterile towels can elevate the distal leg to better facilitate placement (Fig. 35.24). The needed instruments can be organized to allow for efficiency with frame application. A skin incision just big enough for pin placement is made for two self-drilling, self-taping pins to be placed in the tibia. The pins can be placed directly anterior or perpendicular to the medial face of the tibia and should be bicortical. The pins are placed proximal to the zone of injury, generally in the proximal ½ of the tibia. A medial to lateral trans calcaneal pin is placed next, followed by two 4.0 mm self-drilling, self-taping pins in the 1st and 5th metatarsals. A foot "steering wheel" construct is made by connecting the trans calcaneal pin and metatarsal pins. This allows the surgeon to reduce the fracture by controlling axial, coronal, and sagittal plane motion by steering the ankle under fluoroscopy. In an inpatient trauma setting, a kick-stand can be added to float the heel off the bed by extending the distal bars posteriorly (see Fig. 35.24). A transarticular, or Childress pin, can be added for additional stabilization in dislocations (Fig. 35.25). The fixator will remain in place until the soft tissues allow for incisional placement for internal fixation.

Pin Site Care: The authors prefer gentle cleaning with soap and water and chlorhexidine-soaked gauze around the pin sites for dressings.

Role of Arthroscopy

Arthroscopy can be a powerful tool when addressing ankle fractures. The patient can be positioned either supine or lateral. If the patient has an isolated distal fibula fracture, the patient can be placed laterally with arthroscopy performed in a simulated supine position facilitated by hip external rotation (Fig. 35.26). Deltoid ligament repair can be performed after a diagnostic arthroscopy with the leg remaining externally rotated and suspended in the well leg holder. If a medial malleolar fracture is present, the patient can be placed supine and standard ankle arthroscopy set up is used.

The authors routinely perform an ankle arthroscopy prior to fracture repair, especially in cases of suspected deltoid and/or syndesmotic injuries and bi- and trimalleolar fracture patterns.

Arthroscopy allows for visualization and testing of the deltoid, syndesmosis, and ATFL complex. The chondral surface can be evaluated and treated if necessary. Chondral lesions are common, reported in 78% of scoped ankle fractures. Ankle dislocation and syndesmotic injury are independent risk factors for chondral injury. Ankle fractures with chondral lesions have been correlated with decreased functional outcome, especially those of the anterolateral talus (Fig. 35.27).[103,104] It is important to note that the arthroscopic portion of the procedure should be performed quickly and with careful

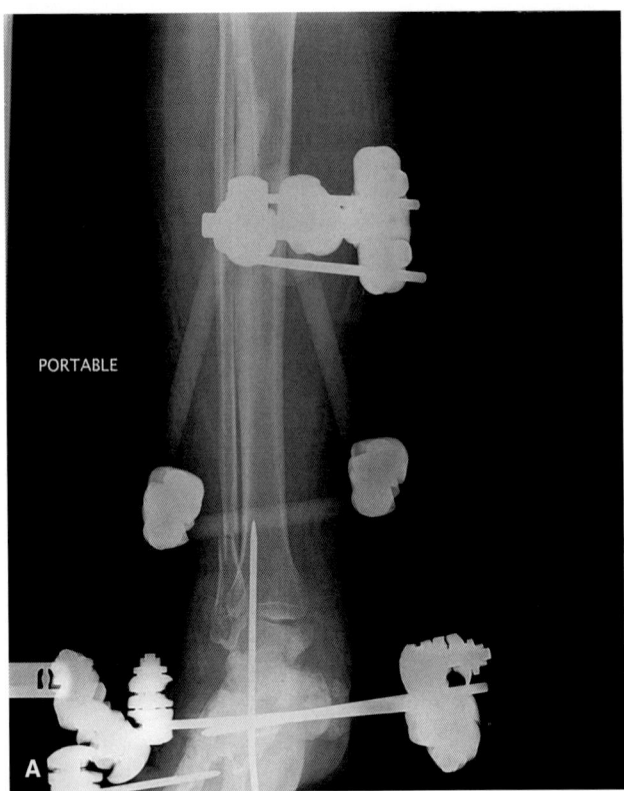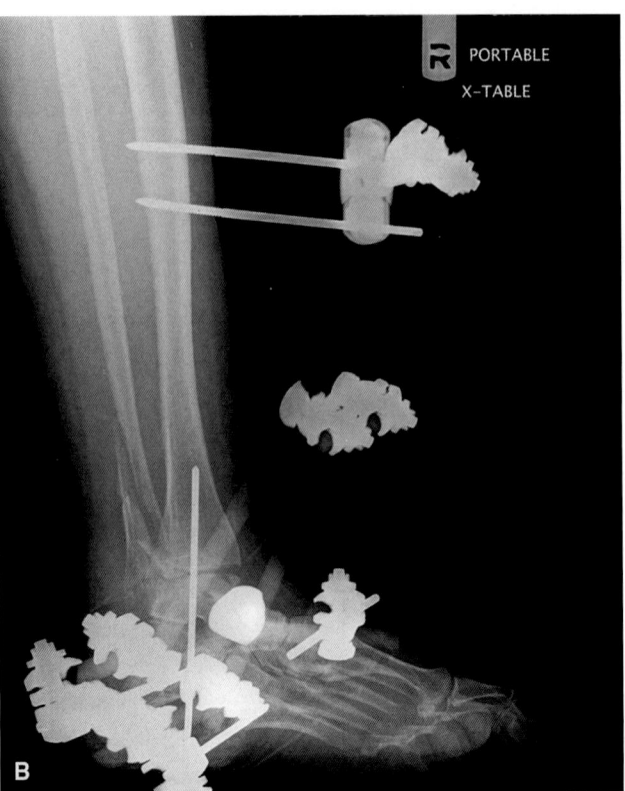

FIGURE 35.25 A, B. Radiographs showing external fixator and Childress pin. (Photo credit Patrick Burns, DPM.)

monitoring of inflow pressure and volume to avoid extravasation of fluid. When significant trauma and soft tissue destruction is present, arthroscopy should be avoided. By visualizing the deltoid and syndesmosis ligaments, the integrity of each can be assessed and the treatment algorithm adjusted accordingly. A probe is used to tension the deltoid to assess its integrity (Fig. 35.28).

When there is acute disruption of the deltoid ligament, it appears hemorrhagic and the probe often will drive around the medial malleolus. With avulsion-type injuries, a bare spot can be visualized. When evaluating the syndesmosis, a probe is placed on the anterior border of the fibula to translate the fibula posteriorly, testing its excursion. The probe is then used to translate the fibula laterally. When the syndesmosis is disrupted, the

fibula will appear unstable and freely translate in one or both planes. It is important to note the probe needs to be stressing the fibula proximal to the fracture. We also attempt to place the 3.5 mm shaver or a probe into the incisura (Fig. 35.29). If the 3.5 mm shaver can be placed in the incisura, and we can freely translate the fibula with the probe, the syndesmosis is deemed incompetent.

If traction is used during the arthroscopy, it should be decreased or released when performing dynamic diagnostic examinations. The joint is also evaluated for chondral injuries and addressed accordingly (debridement, microfracture, biologic augmentation, etc.) when indicated. Arthroscopy can also reveal subtle posterior malleolus fractures in cases where it may not be suspected (see Fig. 35.26). While arthroscopy can be used for direct visualization of syndesmotic or fracture reduction, the authors do not routinely do this due to the possibility of added fluid extravasation with extended arthroscopy and overall surgical operative time (Video 1 and 2 showing arthroscopic fracture examination).

HIGH-RISK POPULATION

Ankle fractures in elderly patients and those with multiple comorbidities can lead to a high rate of complications and morbidity.[105-108] Diabetes, specifically complicated diabetes, will lead to a higher rate of infection, delayed healing, nonunion, and charcot arthropathy following ankle fractures.[105,108] It is recommended that diabetic/neuropathic patients receive increased fixation, longer periods of non–weight-bearing, and longer

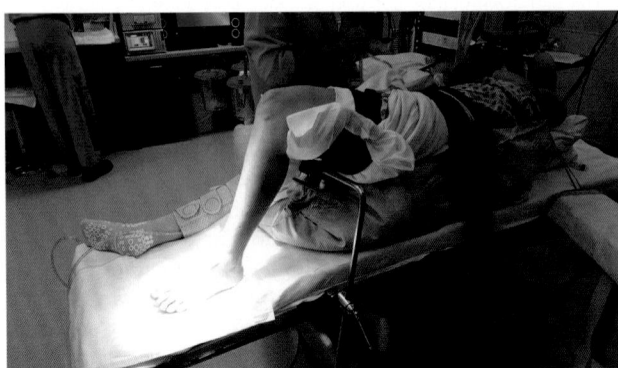

FIGURE 35.26 Arthroscopic patient positioning.

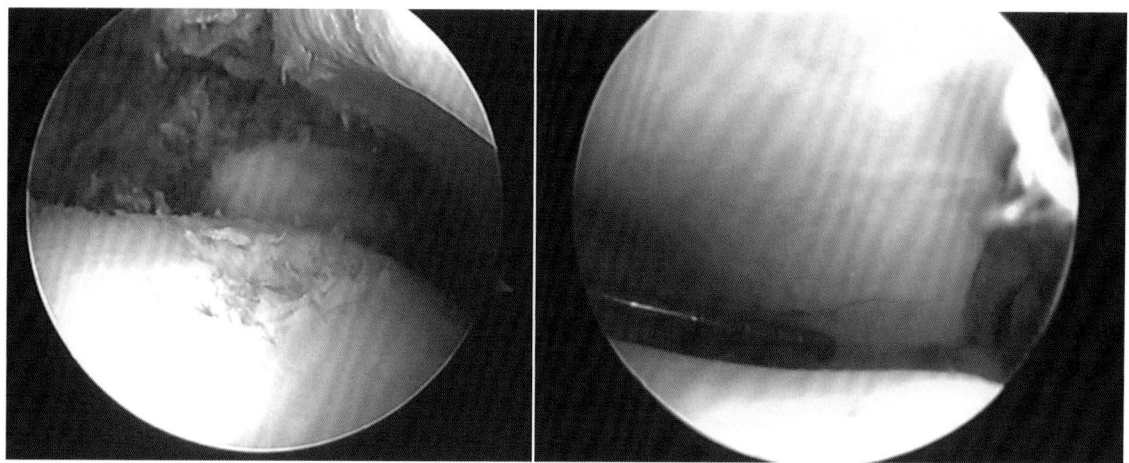

FIGURE 35.27 Arthroscopic image of anterior lateral talar lesion and posterior malleolar fracture.

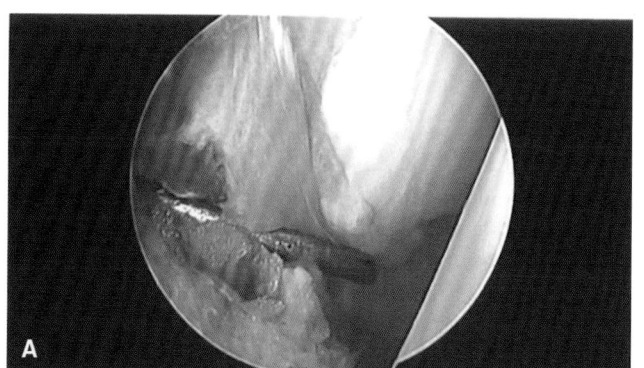

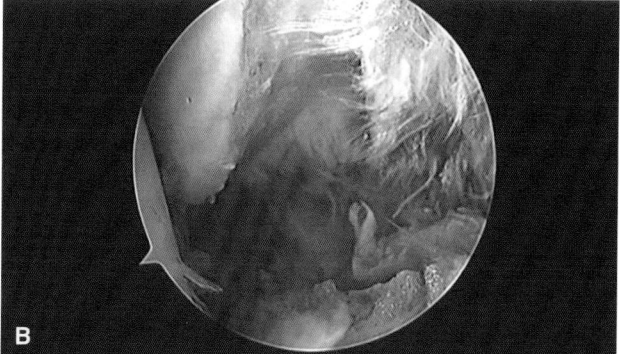

FIGURE 35.28 Arthroscopic deltoid evaluation. **A.** Tensioning an intact deltoid. **B.** Bare spot with complete deltoid disruption.

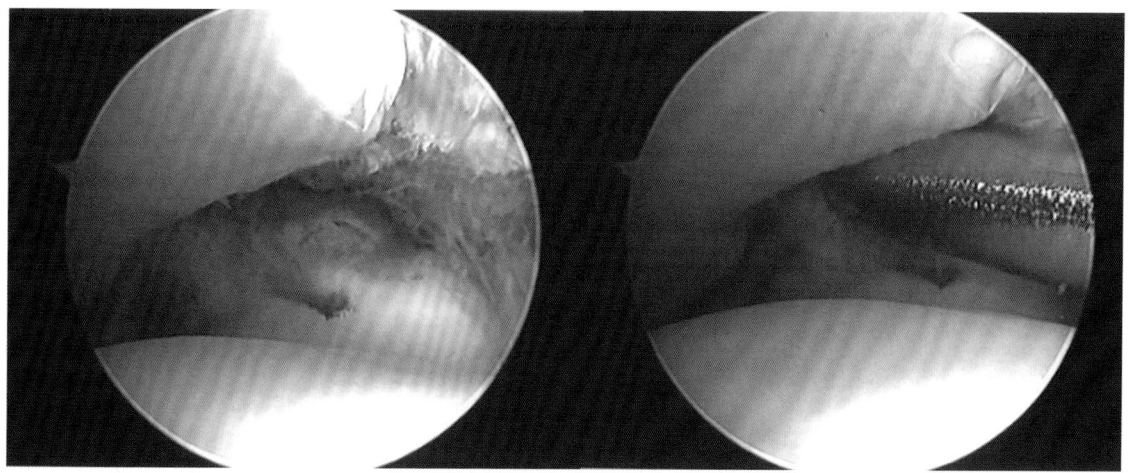

FIGURE 35.29 Arthroscopic evaluation of the syndesmosis with a 3.5-mm shaver into the incisura.

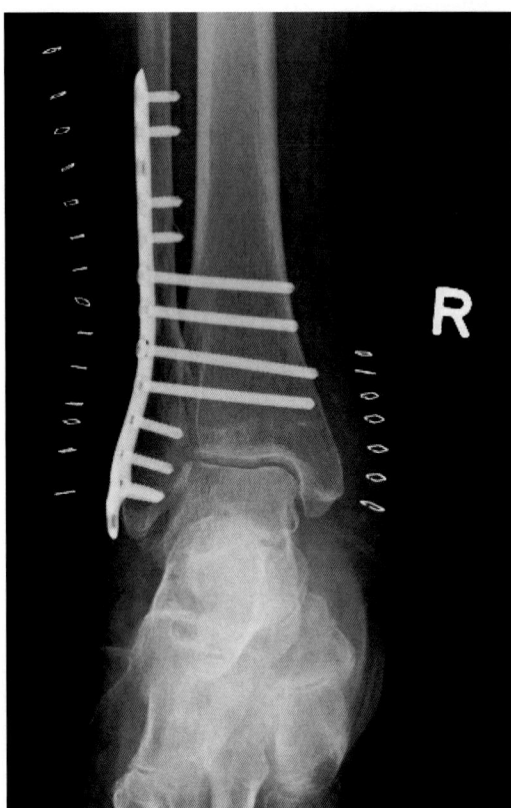

FIGURE 35.30 Increased fixation in diabetic patient.

immobilization than a healthy population (Fig. 35.30).[105,108] Fragility fractures and those in high-risk patients may be better served with closed reduction and tibiotalocalcaneal (TTC) nailing.[106] Closed TTC nailing allows for safe and effective fixation while quickly restoring function and mobility in the high-risk population.[106]

POSTOPERATIVE CARE

Ankle fractures should be splinted in a neutral position in the operating room. We typically use a modified Jones bulky soft splint with added cryotherapy device when available. Author preference is to see patients back within 1 week to remove the splint applied in operating room and place them into a non–weight-bearing cast for the next 3 weeks. At 4 weeks postoperatively, isolated lateral malleolus fractures and those with syndesmotic repair begin to weight-bear in a boot assuming satisfactory radiographs. Bimalleolar fractures are kept non–weight-bearing until week 7 when they are transitioned into a boot.

Debate surrounds prophylactic treatment for thromboembolic events after ankle fracture surgery. Foot and ankle surgery in general is associated with a much lower incidence of thromboembolic events when compared to surgery of the hip and knee. Pelet et al. reviewed 1540 ankle fractures and found a 2.9% incidence of deep venous thrombus (DVT) and 32% incidence of nonfatal pulmonary embolism (PE). This compares to a DVT incidence of 25.6% in total knee arthroplasty, 8.9% in total hip arthroplasty, and a 1.9% of nonfatal PE, even with mechanical and chemical phrophylaxis.[109]

Pelet et al. identified risk factors associated with increased thromboembolic events including neoplasia, hormone replacement therapy, pregnancy, blood dyscrasia, previous DVT, current smoking, obesity, dyslipidemia, atherosclerosis, and paralysis. Only 16% of their patients received prophylaxis, and it had no impact on incidence of thromboembolic events even when adjusting for risk factors.[110] A recent review article by Weisman et al. highlights seven studies, including 3 randomized controlled trials, none of which recommend for regular VTE (venous thromboembolism) prophylaxis in standard risk profile patients after ankle fracture fixation.[111] Jameson et al. report a PE rate of 0.22% among >10 000 nonoperatively treated ankle fractures in the UK; this incidence is similar to operatively treated ankle fractures, and they recommended against VTE prophylaxis in nonoperatively treated stable ankle fractures.[112]

> - Authors preferred VTE prevention strategy after ankle fractures includes Aspirin daily for all patients and Lovenox for patients with multiple of the previously mentioned risk factors and both are continued through the duration of non–weight-bearing.
> - In addition, we recommend use of antiembolism stockings on the opposite extremity and advice patients to get up and move about frequently, even during the nonoperative recovery period.

Postoperative antibiotic prophylaxis is another controversial topic following surgical treatment of ankle fractures. Reported rates of infection following ankle fracture surgery vary widely but average 4% in reported literature.[113-116] In a 2018 retrospective review, Lachman et al. reviewed 1442 surgically treated ankle fractures and found no difference in infection rate among patients receiving IV prophylaxis inpatient, patients discharged home with oral antibiotics, and those discharged home without antibiotics, even when controlling for risk factors.[114] A systematic review also published in 2018 reported a cumulative surgical site infection rate of 7.19% and conversely reported that use of antibiotic prophylaxis was a protective factor in prevention of infection.[117] It should be noted that SCIP protocol recommends discontinuation of prophylactic antibiotics after 24 hours following hip and knee replacement.

> Authors prefer to discharge home with 5 days of oral cephalexin after surgical treatment of ankle fractures, and inpatients receive two postoperative doses of cefazolin. Adjustments are made based on individual patient allergies as needed.

Routine postoperative radiographs are obtained by many surgeons to monitor healing and hardware position after surgical treatment of ankle fractures. McDonald et al. questioned this practice suggesting that in most cases, there is no need to obtain radiographs in the first 7-21 days postoperatively.[118] Certainly, routine imaging is warranted in later visits to assess healing as activity levels are increased. Noncompliant patients or those with questionable fixation should also be imaged early. Palmanovich et al. argue for the role of early computed tomography (CT) scans following certain fracture patterns. They scanned patients at 1 week who had syndesmotic disruptions and posterior lip fractures. Among patients scanned, 29% underwent early revision to correct issues found on the CT scan.[119]

> Authors obtain plain radiographs at the 1-week postoperative visit and again at weeks 4 and 7, weight-bearing when able.

Weight-bearing protocols after fixation of ankle fractures remains varied among surgeons. Multiple recent studies including biomechanical and randomized controlled trials suggest that early weight-bearing is beneficial in certain fracture patterns.[120-125] Some authors have gone so far as to advocate placement of soft dressing for 24 hours after surgery then allowing unprotected weight-bearing in healthy patients without syndesmotic or posterior malleoli fractures requiring fixation.[126]

Ankle fracture patterns that are fixed without fixation of posterior lip or syndesmotic instability in patients without significant comorbidities have been shown to do well with various early weight-bearing protocols. Dehghan et al. performed a randomized controlled trial comparing early and late weight-bearing and found no difference regarding wound complication, infection, or loss of reduction. Early weight-bearing patients had less hardware removal and increased early functional outcomes. In their study, the early weight-bearing patients were non–weight-bearing in splint for 2 weeks then allowed to weight bear in a boot, coming out for range of motions exercises. The late weight-bearing group was placed into a cast from weeks 2 through 6 at which point they were allowed to weight bear in a boot and begin range of motion exercises.[127]

Treating surgeons should keep in mind that accelerated postoperative protocols should not be applied to all patients. Those with impaired balance, poly trauma, medical comorbidities, unstable fixation, and other confounding variables most likely benefit from prolonged protection with cast or boot and limited or non–weight-bearing.

> - Authors prefer patients with isolated lateral malleolus or syndesmotic injuries to be splinted for 1 week then placed into a non–weight-bearing cast for 3 weeks followed by full weight-bearing in a boot at 4 weeks.
> - Bimalleolar and trimalleolar fractures are splinted for 1 week then placed into non–weight-bearing casts for a total of 6 weeks (changed at 3-week intervals), they weight bear as tolerated in a boot 7 weeks postoperatively.

REHABILITATION

Ultimate functional outcomes after fixation of ankle fractures are dependent on restoration of strength and motion, which typically requires involvement of a physical therapist. Typically, patients are placed into a well-padded compressive splint for the first 7-10 days postoperatively. During the first week after surgery, patients should focus on an aggressive protocol of Rest, Ice, Compression and Elevation (RICE). RICE therapy should be taught to all patients, and they should be encouraged to ice in 10- to 15-minute intervals throughout the day until swelling subsides. Persistent swelling is normal for several weeks.

Early range of motion (ROM) has been shown to be beneficial following ankle fracture fixation, leading to earlier return to activity, decreased pain, and improved range of motion. Physical therapy should get involved early when following these protocols. Concern exists about wound-related complications in early motion protocols and should be monitored closely by surgeon and physical therapist. A boot should always be used when not bathing or working on range of motion in order to avoid development of a problematic equinus contracture. ROM should gradually increase from gentle active to passive and eventually (after fracture union) therapist-assisted mobilizations can be employed as needed.

Functional and strengthening therapies ensue when patients have regained a more physiologic ROM. Patients are progressed from bilateral activities to split stance activities and eventually to single leg stance-based movements. A controlled single-leg squat is a good indicator for full recovery for most patients and is a time to move to more sport-specific movements when necessary.[128]

REFERENCES

1. Baron JA, Barrett JA, Karagas MR. The epidemiology of peripheral fractures. *Bone.* 1996;18:S209-S213. doi: 10.1016/8756-3282(95)00504-8.
2. Barrett JA, Baron JA, Karagas MR, Beach ML. Fracture risk in the U.S. Medicare population. *J Clin Epidemiol.* 1999;52:243-249. doi: 10.1016/S0895-4356(98)00167-X.
3. Court-Brown CM, Caesar B. Epidemiology of adult fractures: a review. *Injury.* 2006;37:691-697. doi: 10.1016/j.injury.2006.04.130.
4. Phillips WA, Schwartz HS, Keller CS, et al. A prospective, randomized study of the management of severe ankle fractures. *J Bone Joint Surg Am.* 1985;67:67-78.
5. Ramsey PL, Hamilton W. Changes in tibiotalar area of contact caused by lateral talar shift. *J Bone Joint Surg Am.* 1976;58:356-357.
6. Thordarson DB, Motamed S, Hedman T, Ebramzadeh E, Bakshian S. The effect of fibular malreduction on contact pressures in an ankle fracture malunion model. *J Bone Joint Surg Am.* 1997;79:1809-1815.
7. Burns WC, Prakash K, Adelaar R, Beaudoin A, Krause W. Tibiotalar joint dynamics: indications for the syndesmotic screw—a cadaver study. *Foot Ankle.* 1993;14:153-158.
8. Solari J, Benjamin J, Wilson J, Lee R, Pitt M. Ankle mortise stability in Weber C fractures: indications for syndesmotic fixation. *J Orthop Trauma.* 1991;5:190-195.
9. Vander Griend R, Michelson JD, Bone LB. Fractures of the ankle and the distal part of the tibia. *Instr Course Lect.* 1997;46:311-321.
10. Yablon IG, Heller FG, Shouse L. The key role of the lateral malleolus in displaced fractures of the ankle. *J Bone Joint Surg Am.* 1977;59:169-173.
11. Lauge-Hansen N. Fractures of the ankle. II. Combined experimental-surgical and experimental-roentgenologic investigations. *Arch Surg Chic Ill 1920.* 1950;60:957-985.
12. Lauge-Hansen N. Ligamentous ankle fractures; diagnosis and treatment. *Acta Chir Scand.* 1949;97:544-550.
13. Muller ME, Allgower M, Schneider R, Willenegger H. *Manual of Internal Fixation: Techniques Recommended by the AO Group.* 2nd ed. Berlin, Germany: Springer Verlag; 1979.
14. Danis R. Les fractures malleolaires. In: *Theorie et Ptactique de Osteosynthese.* Paris, France: Masson; 1949.
15. Weber BG. *Die Verletzungend des Oberen Sprungelenkes.* 2nd ed. Bern, Switzerland: Verlag Hans Huber; 1972.
16. Bixler GS, Bean M, Atassi MZ. Site recognition by protein-primed T cells shows a nonspecific peptide size requirement beyond the essential residues of the site. Demonstration by defining an immunodominant T site in myoglobin. *Biochem J.* 1986;240:139-146.
17. Golano P, Dalmau-Pastor M, Vega J, Batista J. *Anatomy of the Ankle.* Peroneal Posterior Tibial Tendon Pathol. Paris, France: Springer; 2014:1-24. doi: 10.1007/978-2-8178-0523-8_1.
18. Harper MC. Deltoid ligament: an anatomical evaluation of function. *Foot Ankle.* 1987;8:19-22.
19. Inman VT. *The Joints of the Ankle.* Baltimore, MD: Williams & Wilkins; 1976.
20. Isman RE, Inman VT, Poor PM. Anthropometric studies of the human foot and ankle. *Bull Prosthet Res.* 1969;10:97-129.
21. Khan MA, Canby C, Matz D. *Lower Limb Anatomy.* 5th ed. Des Moines: Des Mones University Osteopathic Medical Center; 2009.
22. Milner CE, Soames RW. Anatomy of the collateral ligaments of the human ankle joint. *Foot Ankle Int.* 1998;19:757-760. doi: 10.1177/107110079801901109.
23. Panchani PN, Chappell TM, Moore GD, et al. Anatomic study of the deltoid ligament of the ankle. *Foot Ankle Int.* 2014;35:916-921. doi: 10.1177/1071100714535766.
24. Barnett CH, Napier JR. The axis of rotation at the ankle joint in man; its influence upon the form of the talus and the mobility of the fibula. *J Anat.* 1952;86:1-9.
25. Lundberg A, Svensson O, Nemeth G, Selvik G. The axis of rotation of the ankle joint. *J Bone Joint Surg Br.* 1989;71-B:94-99. doi: 10.1302/0301-620X.71B1.2915016.
26. Perry J. Anatomy and biomechanics of the hindfoot. *Clin Orthop.* 1983:9-15.
27. Procter P, Paul JP. Ankle joint biomechanics. *J Biomech.* 1982;15:627-634. doi: 10.1016/0021-9290(82)90017-3.
28. Somford MP, Wiegerinck JI, Hoornenborg D, van den Bekerom MPJ. Ankle fracture eponyms. *J Bone Joint Surg Am.* 2013;95(24):e198.

29. Goost H, Wimmer MD, Barg A, Kabir K, Valderrabano V, Burger C. Fractures of the ankle joint: investigation and treatment options. *Dtsch Ärztebl Int.* 2014;111:377.
30. Hsu RY, Bariteau J. Management of ankle fractures. *R I Med J.* 2013;96:23.
31. Hirschmann MT, Mauch C, Mueller C, Mueller W, Friederich NF. Lateral ankle fracture with missed proximal tibiofibular joint instability (Maisonneuve injury). *Knee Surg Sports Traumatol Arthrosc.* 2008;16:952-956. doi: 10.1007/s00167-008-0597-8.
32. Savoie FH, Wilkinson MM, Bryan A, Barrett GR, Shelton WR, Manning JO. Maisonneuve fracture dislocation of the ankle. *J Athl Train.* 1992;27:268-269.
33. Taweel NR, Raikin SM, Karanjia HN, Ahmad J. The proximal fibula should be examined in all patients with ankle injury: a case series of missed Maisonneuve fractures. *J Emerg Med.* 2013;44:e251-e255. doi: 10.1016/j.jemermed.2012.09.016.
34. Martin JW, Thompson GH. Achilles tendon rupture. Occurrence with a closed ankle fracture. *Clin Orthop.* 1986:216-218.
35. Beekman R, Watson JT. Bosworth fracture-dislocation and resultant compartment syndrome. A case report. *J Bone Joint Surg Am.* 2003;85-A:2211-2214.
36. Ferris B. Bosworth fracture-dislocation and resultant compartment syndrome. *J Bone Joint Surg Am.* 2004;86-A:2571-2572; author reply 2572.
37. Neilly D, Baliga S, Munro C, Johnston A. Acute compartment syndrome of the foot following open reduction and internal fixation of an ankle fracture. *Injury.* 2015;46:2064-2068. doi: 10.1016/j.injury.2015.06.006.
38. Szalay MD, Roberts JB. Compartment syndrome after Bosworth fracture-dislocation of the ankle: a case report. *J Orthop Trauma.* 2001;15:301-303.
39. Elsoe R, Ostgaard SE, Larsen P. Population-based epidemiology of 9767 ankle fractures. *Foot Ankle Surg.* 2018;24:34-39. doi: 10.1016/j.fas.2016.11.002.
40. Honkanen R, Tuppurainen M, Kröger H, Alhava E, Saarikoski S. Relationships between risk factors and fractures differ by type of fracture: a population-based study of 12,192 perimenopausal women. *Osteoporos Int.* 1998;8:25-31. doi: 10.1007/s001980050044.
41. Liu S, Zhu Y, Chen W, Wang L, Zhang X, Zhang Y. Demographic and socioeconomic factors influencing the incidence of ankle fractures, a national population-based survey of 512187 individuals. *Sci Rep.* 2018;8:10443. doi: 10.1038/s41598-018-28722-1.
42. Kannus P, Parkkari J, Niemi S, Palvanen M. Epidemiology of osteoporotic ankle fractures in elderly persons in Finland. *Ann Intern Med.* 1996;125:975-978.
43. Kannus P, Niemi S, Parkkari J, Sievänen H. Declining incidence of fall-induced ankle fractures in elderly adults: Finnish statistics between 1970 and 2014. *Arch Orthop Trauma Surg.* 2016;136:1243-1246. doi: 10.1007/s00402-016-2524-7.
44. Court-Brown CM, McBirnie J, Wilson G. Adult ankle fractures—an increasing problem? *Acta Orthop Scand.* 1998;69:43-47.
45. Michelson JD. Fractures about the ankle. *J Bone Joint Surg Am.* 1995;77:142-152.
46. Morris M, Chandler RW. Fractures of the ankle. *Tech Orthop.* n.d.;2(3):10-19.
47. Weber GA, Simpson LA. Corrective lengthening osteotomy of the fibula. *Clin Orthop.* 1985;199:61.
48. Sarkisian JS, Cody GW. Closed treatment of ankle fractures: a new criterion for evaluation—a review of 250 cases. *J Trauma.* 1976;16:323-326.
49. Donohoe S, Alluri RK, Hill JR, Fleming M, Tan E, Marecek G. Impact of computed tomography on operative planning for ankle fractures involving the posterior malleolus. *Foot Ankle Int.* 2017;38:1337-1342. doi: 10.1177/1071100717731568.
50. Kumar A, Mishra P, Tandon A, Arora R, Chadha M. Effect of CT on management plan in Malleolar ankle fractures. *Foot Ankle Int.* 2018;39:59-66. doi: 10.1177/1071100717732746.
51. Hinds RM, Garner MR, Lazaro LE, et al. Ankle fracture spur sign is pathognomonic for a variant ankle fracture. *Foot Ankle Int.* 2015;36:159-164. doi: 10.1177/1071100714553470.
52. Boytim MJ, Fischer DA, Neumann L. Syndesmotic ankle sprains. *Am J Sports Med.* 1991;19:294-298. doi: 10.1177/036354659101900315.
53. Nielson JH, Gardner MJ, Peterson MGE, et al. Radiographic measurements do not predict syndesmotic injury in ankle fractures: an MRI study. *Clin Orthop.* 2005:216-221.
54. Pneumaticos SG, Noble PC, Chatziioannou SN, Trevino SG. The effects of rotation on radiographic evaluation of the tibiofibular syndesmosis. *Foot Ankle Int.* 2002;23:107-111. doi: 10.1177/107110070202300205.
55. Xenos JS, Hopkinson WJ, Mulligan ME, Olson EJ, Popovic NA. The tibiofibular syndesmosis. Evaluation of the ligamentous structures, methods of fixation, and radiographic assessment. *J Bone Joint Surg Am.* 1995;77:847-856.
56. Hermans JJ, Wentink N, Beumer A, et al. Correlation between radiological assessment of acute ankle fractures and syndesmotic injury on MRI. *Skeletal Radiol.* 2012;41:787-801. doi: 10.1007/s00256-011-1284-2.
57. Ekinci S, Polat O, Günalp M, Demirkan A, Koca A. The accuracy of ultrasound evaluation in foot and ankle trauma. *Am J Emerg Med.* 2013;31:1551-1555. doi: 10.1016/j.ajem.2013.06.008.
58. Mei-Dan O, Kots E, Barchilon V, Massarwe S, Nyska M, Mann G. A dynamic ultrasound examination for the diagnosis of ankle syndesmotic injury in professional athletes: a preliminary study. *Am J Sports Med.* 2009;37:1009-1016. doi: 10.1177/0363546508331202.
59. Morvan G, Busson J, Wybier M, Mathieu P. Ultrasound of the ankle. *Eur J Ultrasound.* 2001;14:73-82.
60. Bauer M, Bergström B, Hemborg A, Sandegård J. Malleolar fractures: nonoperative versus operative treatment. A controlled study. *Clin Orthop.* 1985:17-27.
61. Herscovici D, Scaduto JM, Infante A. Conservative treatment of isolated fractures of the medial malleolus. *J Bone Joint Surg Br.* 2007;89:89-93. doi: 10.1302/0301-620X.89B1.18349.
62. Pakarinen HJ, Flinkkil TE, Ohtonen PP, Ristiniemi JY. Stability criteria for nonoperative ankle fracture management. *Foot Ankle Int.* 2011;32:141-147. doi: 10.3113/FAI.2011.0141.
63. Van Schie-Van der Weert EM, Van Lieshout EMM, De Vries MR, Van der Elst M, Schepers T. Determinants of outcome in operatively and non-operatively treated Weber-B ankle fractures. *Arch Orthop Trauma Surg.* 2012;132:257-263. doi: 10.1007/s00402-011-1397-z.
64. Michelson JD. Current concepts review. Fractures about the ankle. *JBJS.* 1995;77:142-152.
65. DeAngelis NA, Eskander MS, French BG. Does medial tenderness predict deep deltoid ligament incompetence in supination-external rotation type ankle fractures? *J Orthop Trauma.* 2007;21:244-247. doi: 10.1097/BOT.0b013e3180413835.
66. Michelson JD, Varner KE, Checcone M. Diagnosing deltoid injury in ankle fractures: the gravity stress view. *Clin Orthop.* 2001:178-182.
67. Gill JB, Risko T, Raducan V, Grimes JS, Schutt RC. Comparison of manual and gravity stress radiographs for the evaluation of supination-external rotation fibular fractures. *J Bone Joint Surg Am.* 2007;89:994-999. doi: 10.2106/JBJS.F.01002.
68. McConnell T, Creevy W, Tornetta P. Stress examination of supination external rotation-type fibular fractures. *J Bone Joint Surg Am.* 2004;86-A:2171-2178.
69. Park SS, Kubiak EN, Egol KA, Kummer F, Koval KJ. Stress radiographs after ankle fracture: the effect of ankle position and deltoid ligament status on medial clear space measurements. *J Orthop Trauma.* 2006;20:11-18.
70. LeBa T-B, Gugala Z, Morris RP, Panchbhavi VK. Gravity versus manual external rotation stress view in evaluating ankle stability: a prospective study. *Foot Ankle Spec.* 2015;8:175-179. doi: 10.1177/1938640014565048.
71. Schock HJ, Pinzur M, Manion L, Stover M. The use of gravity or manual-stress radiographs in the assessment of supination-external rotation fractures of the ankle. *J Bone Joint Surg Br.* 2007;89:1055-1059. doi: 10.1302/0301-620X.89B8.19134.
72. Weber M, Burmeister H, Flueckiger G, Krause FG. The use of weightbearing radiographs to assess the stability of supination-external rotation fractures of the ankle. *Arch Orthop Trauma Surg.* 2010;130:693-698. doi: 10.1007/s00402-010-1051-1.
73. Hoshino CM, Nomoto EK, Norheim EP, Harris TG. Correlation of weightbearing radiographs and stability of stress positive ankle fractures. *Foot Ankle Int.* 2012;33:92-98. doi: 10.3113/FAI.2012.0092.
74. Seidel A, Krause F, Weber M. Weightbearing vs gravity stress radiographs for stability evaluation of supination-external rotation fractures of the ankle. *Foot Ankle Int.* 2017;38:736-744. doi: 10.1177/1071100717702589.
75. Broos PL, Bisschop AP. Operative treatment of ankle fractures in adults: correlation between types of fracture and final results. *Injury.* 1991;22:403-406.
76. Barrett SL, Dellon AL, Rosson GD, Walters L. Superficial peroneal nerve (superficial fibularis nerve): the clinical implications of anatomic variability. *J Foot Ankle Surg.* 2006;45:174-176. doi: 10.1053/j.jfas.2006.02.004.
77. Ducic I, Dellon AL, Graw KS. The clinical importance of variations in the surgical anatomy of the superficial peroneal nerve in the mid-third of the lateral leg. *Ann Plast Surg.* 2006;56:635-638. doi: 10.1097/01.sap.0000203258.96961.a6.
78. Huene DB, Bunnell WP. Operative anatomy of nerves encountered in the lateral approach to the distal part of the fibula. *J Bone Joint Surg Am.* 1995;77:1021-1024.
79. Sproule JA, Khalid M, O'Sullivan M, McCabe JP. Outcome after surgery for Maisonneuve fracture of the fibula. *Injury.* 2004;35:791-798. doi: 10.1016/S0020-1383(03)00155-4.
80. Stufkens SA, van den Bekerom MPJ, Doornberg JN, van Dijk CN, Kloen P. Evidence-based treatment of Maisonneuve fractures. *J Foot Ankle Surg.* 2011;50:62-67. doi: 10.1053/j.jfas.2010.08.017.
81. Riedel MD, Miller CP, Kwon JY. Augmenting suture-button fixation for maisonneuve injuries with fibular shortening: technique tip. *Foot Ankle Int.* 2017;38:1146-1151. doi: 10.1177/1071100717716487.
82. Gardner MJ, Brodsky A, Briggs SM, Nielson JH, Lorich DG. Fixation of posterior malleolar fractures provides greater syndesmotic stability. *Clin Orthop.* 2006;447:165-171. doi: 10.1097/01.blo.0000203489.21206.a9.
83. McDaniel WJ, Wilson FC. Trimalleolar fractures of the ankle. An end result study. *Clin Orthop.* 1977:37-45.
84. Langenhuijsen JF, Heetveld MJ, Ultee JM, Steller EP, Butzelaar RMJM. Results of ankle fractures with involvement of the posterior tibial margin. *J Trauma.* 2002;53:55-60.
85. Drijfhout van Hooff CC, Verhage SM, Hoogendoorn JM. Influence of fragment size and postoperative joint congruency on long-term outcome of posterior malleolar fractures. *Foot Ankle Int.* 2015;36:673-678.
86. van den Bekerom MPJ, Haverkamp D, Kloen P. Biomechanical and clinical evaluation of posterior malleolar fractures. A systematic review of the literature. *J Trauma.* 2009;66:279-284. doi: 10.1097/TA.0b013e318187eb16.
87. Berkes MB, Little MTM, Lazaro LE, et al. Articular congruity is associated with short-term clinical outcomes of operatively treated SER IV ankle fractures. *J Bone Joint Surg Am.* 2013;95:1769-1775. doi: 10.2106/JBJS.L.00949.
88. Jaskulka RA, Ittner G, Schedl R. Fractures of the posterior tibial margin: their role in the prognosis of malleolar fractures. *J Trauma.* 1989;29:1565-1570.
89. Switaj PJ, Weatherford B, Fuchs D, Rosenthal B, Pang E, Kadakia AR. Evaluation of posterior malleolar fractures and the posterior pilon variant in operatively treated ankle fractures. *Foot Ankle Int.* 2014;35:886-895. doi: 10.1177/1071100714537630.
90. Tejwani NC, Pahk B, Egol KA. Effect of posterior malleolus fracture on outcome after unstable ankle fracture. *J Trauma.* 2010;69:666-669. doi: 10.1097/TA.0b013e3181e4f81e.
91. Weber M. Trimalleolar fractures with impaction of the posteromedial tibial plafond: implications for talar stability. *Foot Ankle Int.* 2004;25:716-727. doi: 10.1177/107110070402501005.
92. Bernstein DT, Harris JD, Cosculluela PE, Varner KE. Acute tibialis posterior tendon rupture with pronation-type ankle fractures. *Orthopedics.* 2016;39:e970-e975. doi: 10.3928/01477447-20160526-04.
93. Formica M, Santolini F, Alessio-Mazzola M, Repetto I, Andretta A, Stella M. Closed medial malleolar multifragment fracture with a posterior tibialis tendon rupture: a case report and review of the literature. *J Foot Ankle Surg.* 2016;55:832-837. doi: 10.1053/j.jfas.2015.03.007.
94. Wardell RM, Hanselman AE, Daffner SD, Santrock RD. Posterior tibialis tendon rupture in a closed bimalleolar-equivalent ankle fracture: case report. *Foot Ankle Spec.* 2017;10:572-577. doi: 10.1177/1938640017704945.
95. Laflamme M, Belzile EL, Bédard L, van den Bekerom MPJ, Glazebrook M, Pelet S. A prospective randomized multicenter trial comparing clinical outcomes of patients treated surgically with a static or dynamic implant for acute ankle syndesmosis rupture. *J Orthop Trauma.* 2015;29:216-223. doi: 10.1097/BOT.0000000000000245.
96. Høiness P, Strømsøe K. Tricortical versus quadricortical syndesmosis fixation in ankle fractures: a prospective, randomized study comparing two methods of syndesmosis fixation. *J Orthop Trauma.* 2004;18:331-337.

97. Wikerøy AKB, Høiness PR, Andreassen GS, Hellund JC, Madsen JE. No difference in functional and radiographic results 8.4 years after quadricortical compared with tricortical syndesmosis fixation in ankle fractures. *J Orthop Trauma.* 2010;24:17-23. doi: 10.1097/BOT.0b013e3181bedca1.

98. Miller AN, Barei DP, Iaquinto JM, Ledoux WR, Beingessner DM. Iatrogenic syndesmosis malreduction via clamp and screw placement. *J Orthop Trauma.* 2013;27:100-106. doi: 10.1097/BOT.0b013e31825197cb.

99. Sagi HC, Shah AR, Sanders RW. The functional consequence of syndesmotic joint malreduction at a minimum 2-year follow-up. *J Orthop Trauma.* 2012;26:439-443. doi: 10.1097/BOT.0b013e31822a526a.

100. Schepers T. To retain or remove the syndesmotic screw: a review of literature. *Arch Orthop Trauma Surg.* 2011;131:879-883. doi: 10.1007/s00402-010-1225-x.

101. Anand A, Wei R, Patel A, Vedi V, Allardice G, Anand BS. Tightrope fixation of syndesmotic injuries in Weber C ankle fractures: a multicentre case series. *Eur J Orthop Surg Traumatol Orthop Traumatol.* 2017;27:461-467. doi: 10.1007/s00590-016-1882-8.

102. Clanton TO, Whitlow SR, Williams BT, et al. Biomechanical comparison of 3 current ankle syndesmosis repair techniques. *Foot Ankle Int.* 2017;38:200-207. doi: 10.1177/1071100716666278.

103. Da Cunha RJ, Karnovsky SC, Schairer W, Drakos MC. Ankle arthroscopy for diagnosis of full-thickness talar cartilage lesions in the setting of acute ankle fractures. *Arthrosc J Arthrosc Relat Surg.* 2018;34:1950-1957. doi: 10.1016/j.arthro.2017.12.003.

104. Stufkens SA, Knupp M, Horisberger M, Lampert C, Hintermann B. Cartilage lesions and the development of osteoarthritis after internal fixation of ankle fractures: a prospective study. *J Bone Joint Surg Am.* 2010;92:279-286. doi: 10.2106/JBJS.H.01635.

105. Ganesh SP, Pietrobon R, Cecílio WAC, Pan D, Lightdale N, Nunley JA. The impact of diabetes on patient outcomes after ankle fracture. *J Bone Joint Surg Am.* 2005;87:1712-1718. doi: 10.2106/JBJS.D.02625.

106. Georgiannos D, Lampridis V, Bisbinas I. Fragility fractures of the ankle in the elderly: open reduction and internal fixation versus tibio-talo-calcaneal nailing: short-term results of a prospective randomized-controlled study. *Injury.* 2017;48:519-524. doi: 10.1016/j.injury.2016.11.017.

107. Koval KJ, Zhou W, Sparks MJ, Cantu RV, Hecht P, Lurie J. Complications after ankle fracture in elderly patients. *Foot Ankle Int.* 2007;28:1249-1255. doi: 10.3113/FAI.2007.1249.

108. Wukich DK, Joseph A, Ryan M, Ramirez C, Irrgang JJ. Outcomes of ankle fractures in patients with uncomplicated versus complicated diabetes. *Foot Ankle Int.* 2011;32:120-130. doi: 10.3113/FAI.2011.0120.

109. O'Reilly RF, Burgess IA, Zicat B. The prevalence of venous thromboembolism after hip and knee replacement surgery. *Med J Aust.* 2005;182:154-159.

110. Pelet S, Roger M-E, Belzile EL, Bouchard M. The incidence of thromboembolic events in surgically treated ankle fracture. *J Bone Joint Surg Am.* 2012;94:502-506. doi: 10.2106/JBJS.J.01190.

111. Weisman MHS, Holmes JR, Irwin TA, Talusan PG. Venous thromboembolic prophylaxis in foot and ankle surgery: a review of current literature and practice. *Foot Ankle Spec.* 2017;10:343-351. doi: 10.1177/1938640017692417.

112. Jameson SS, Rankin KS, Desira NL, et al. Pulmonary embolism following ankle fractures treated without an operation—an analysis using National Health Service data. *Injury.* 2014;45:1256-1261. doi: 10.1016/j.injury.2014.05.009.

113. Hôiness P, Engebretsen L, Strömsöe K. The influence of perioperative soft tissue complications on the clinical outcome in surgically treated ankle fractures. *Foot Ankle Int.* 2001;22:642-648. doi: 10.1177/107110070102200805.

114. Lachman JR, Elkrief JI, Pipitone PS, Haydel CL. Comparison of surgical site infections in ankle fracture surgery with or without the use of postoperative antibiotics. *Foot Ankle Int.* 2018;39:1278-1282. doi: 10.1177/1071100718788069.

115. Miller WA. Postoperative wound infection in foot and ankle surgery. *Foot Ankle.* 1983;4:102-104. doi: 10.1177/107110078300400211.

116. Tantigate D, Jang E, Seetharaman M, et al. Timing of antibiotic prophylaxis for preventing surgical site infections in foot and ankle surgery. *Foot Ankle Int.* 2017;38:283-288. doi: 10.1177/1071100716674975.

117. Shao J, Zhang H, Yin B, Li J, Zhu Y, Zhang Y. Risk factors for surgical site infection following operative treatment of ankle fractures: a systematic review and meta-analysis. *Int J Surg Lond Engl.* 2018;56:124-132. doi: 10.1016/j.ijsu.2018.06.018.

118. McDonald MR, Bulka CM, Thakore RV, et al. Ankle radiographs in the early postoperative period: do they matter? *J Orthop Trauma.* 2014;28:538-541. doi: 10.1097/BOT.0000000000000052.

119. Palmanovich E, Brin YS, Kish B, Nyska M, Hetsroni I. Value of early postoperative computed tomography assessment in ankle fractures defining joint congruity and criticizing the need for early revision surgery. *J Foot Ankle Surg.* 2016;55:465-469. doi: 10.1053/j.jfas.2016.01.013.

120. Bazarov I, Peace RA, Lagaay PM, Patel SB, Lyon LL, Schuberth JM. Early protected weightbearing after ankle fractures in patients with diabetes mellitus. *J Foot Ankle Surg.* 2017;56:30-33. doi: 10.1053/j.jfas.2016.09.010.

121. Gul A, Batra S, Mehmood S, Gillham N. Immediate unprotected weight-bearing of operatively treated ankle fractures. *Acta Orthop Belg.* 2007;73:360-365.

122. Jansen H, Jordan M, Frey S, Hölscher-Doht S, Meffert R, Heintel T. Active controlled motion in early rehabilitation improves outcome after ankle fractures: a randomized controlled trial. *Clin Rehabil.* 2018;32:312-318. doi: 10.1177/0269215517724192.

123. Swart E, Bezhani H, Greisberg J, Vosseller JT. How long should patients be kept nonweight bearing after ankle fracture fixation? A survey of OTA and AOFAS members. *Injury.* 2015;46:1127-1130. doi: 10.1016/j.injury.2015.03.029.

124. Tan EW, Sirisreetreerux N, Paez AG, Parks BG, Schon LC, Hasenboehler EA. Early weightbearing after operatively treated ankle fractures: a biomechanical analysis. *Foot Ankle Int.* 2016;37:652-658. doi: 10.1177/1071100715627351.

125. Vioreanu M, Dudeney S, Hurson B, Kelly E, O'Rourke K, Quinlan W. Early mobilization in a removable cast compared with immobilization in a cast after operative treatment of ankle fractures: a prospective randomized study. *Foot Ankle Int.* 2007;28:13-19. doi: 10.3113/FAI.2007.0003.

126. Smeeing DPJ, Houwert RM, Briet JP, et al. Weight-bearing or non-weight-bearing after surgical treatment of ankle fractures: a multicenter randomized controlled trial. *Eur J Trauma Emerg Surg.* 2020;46(1):121-130. doi: 10.1007/s00068-018-1016-6.

127. Dehghan N, McKee MD, Jenkinson RJ, et al. Early weightbearing and range of motion versus non-weightbearing and immobilization after open reduction and internal fixation of unstable ankle fractures: a randomized controlled trial. *J Orthop Trauma.* 2016;30:345-352. doi: 10.1097/BOT.0000000000000572.

128. Gree A, Hayda R. *Postoperative Orthopaedic Rehabilitation.* Lippincott Williams & Wilkins; 2017.

CHAPTER 36

The Management of Pilon Fractures: Operative Principles and Approaches

Wesley Maurice Leong and J. Randolph Clements

DEFINITION

Pilon ankle fractures represent <1% of all lower extremity fractures and 1%-10% of all tibial fractures; however, 20%-25% of these injuries are open and one-third are associated with other injuries.[1,2] Originally described by Destot in 1911 as a "pilon fracture" and later as a tibial "plafond fracture" by Bonin in 1950, this injury to the distal tibial metaphysis with extension into the ankle joint is characterized by its devastating nature and considerable potential for long-term complications.[1,3] In 1959, Jergesen stated that open reduction and stabilization of severe tibial pilon fractures would be impossible, and despite improvements in surgical techniques and implants, treatment remains difficult even by today's standards.[4] Disappointing long-term results are often the result of severe damage to the articular surface as a consequence of the high energy dissipation and complications of the surgery itself. Complication rates after open reduction and internal fixation have been reported to be as high as 18% for nonunions, 42% for malunion, 23% for osteomyelitis, 20% for superficial infections, and 54% for posttraumatic arthritis.[5-10] As such, the successful management of these fractures demands attention to a number of different variables that include surgical approach, technique, timing, and postoperative care.

CLASSIFICATION

Traditionally, Ruedi and Allgower's classification (based upon displacement and comminution) and the AO/OTA alphanumeric classification (based upon anatomic location and morphological complexity) have been used to characterize pilon fractures and general prognosis and management strategies. However, these classifications have limited contribution to preoperative planning of approach or fixation. A goal of this chapter is to describe key principles of soft tissue and osseous management so as to guide the operative treatment strategy of these injuries.

Ruedi and Allgower classified pilon fractures into three groups (Fig. 36.1):

> Type 1: nondisplaced fractures
> Type 2: displaced fractures with loss of articular congruity;
> Type 3: displaced and severely comminuted fractures with impaction[8]

The AO/OTA system, which has been proven to have superior interobserver reliability, divides pilon fractures into three main groups (Fig. 36.2):

> 43-A: extra-articular; not considered to be true pilon fractures
> 43-B: partial articular fractures
> 43-C: complete articular fractures

The AO/OTA system further divides each of these three groups into subtypes 1 through 3 based upon increasing complexity of the articular and metaphyseal fragments.[11]

Lauge-Hansen described this fracture pattern with his classification of pronation-dorsiflexion injuries.[12] He divided it into four stages.

> Stage I: a fracture of the medial malleolus
> Stage II: a fracture of the anterior aspect of the distal tibia
> Stage III: a fracture of the fibula
> Stage IV: a transverse fracture of the distal tibia

The aforementioned classification systems are useful for guiding the surgeon toward making assumptions about general prognosis and deciding between conservative treatment versus open reduction internal fixation. However, they do not provide any specific recommendations to guide incision planning or placement of fixation. Traditionally, Ruedi and Allgower type 1 fractures are managed with cast immobilization. Ruedi and Allgower type 2 fractures tend to be associated with more successful outcomes when managed with ORIF. Type 3 fractures remain extremely challenging to treat due to the difficulty in achieving anatomic reduction, and for this reason, some authors have even recommended considering primary arthrodesis as a

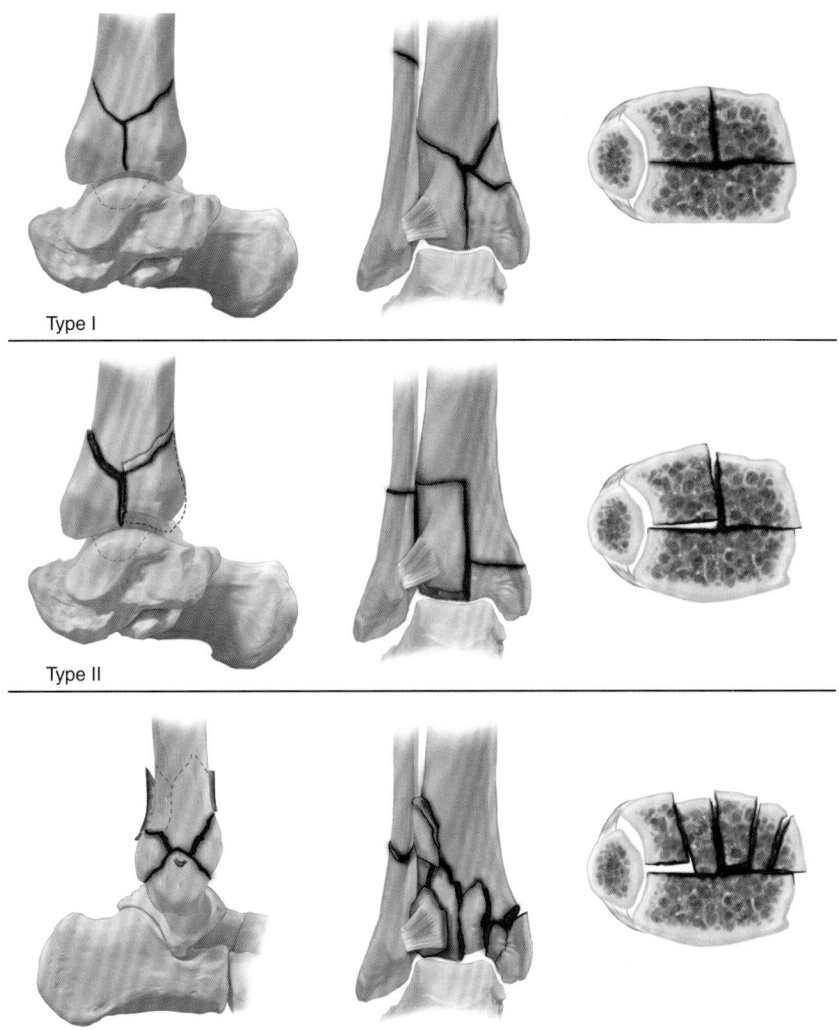

FIGURE 36.1 Ruedi and Allgower's pilon injury classification system. (Redrawn with permission from Ruedi TP, Allgower M. The operative treatment of intra-articular fractures of the lower end of the tibia. *Clin Orthop Relat Res.* 1979;138:105-110.)

treatment option in these situations.[13,14] When Ruedi and Allgower presented their study in 1969, they also provided a clear description of their treatment principles: restoration of the lateral column, anatomic joint reconstruction, autologous bone grafting, and medial buttressing of the tibia.[8]

A variety of fracture patterns can be found within a single pilon injury: usually including some combination of a distal tibial metaphyseal fracture likely with intra-articular comminution, a medial malleolar fracture, a fracture of the anterior margin of the tibia, and a transverse fracture of the posterior tibial surface.[12] Therefore, it is useful from a surgical planning point of view to determine the location of the articular injury based upon the axial CT scan findings. For this purpose, some authors have advocated for dividing the axial view of the ankle joint into columns to aid in establishing a treatment protocol driven by fracture orientation and location relative to the specific anatomic landmarks. Tang et al. proposed a four-column system (Fig. 36.3) in which anterior and posterior columns of the tibial plafond were divided by an intermalleolar line connecting the medial and lateral malleoli. The medial and lateral columns involve the medial aspect of the plafond extending to the medial malleolus and the lateral aspect of the plafond extending to the lateral fibula, respectively.[15] Assal et al. proposed a three-column system: medial, lateral, and posterior. In their system, the medial column is the continuation of the medial side of the triangular tibial diaphysis of the tibia, ending in the medial malleolus. The lateral column is a prolongation of the anterolateral side of the triangular tibial diaphysis, containing the fibular incisura and ending at the tubercle of Tillaux-Chaput, forming the anterolateral portion of the plafond. The posterior column is a continuation of the posterior triangle of the diaphysis of the tibia, ending in the posterior malleolus, which descends further than the anterior margin of the articular surface of the tibial plafond.[16]

PHYSICAL EXAMINATION

Pilon fractures can present as an isolated extremity injury or a polytraumatized patient. The examination must be complete

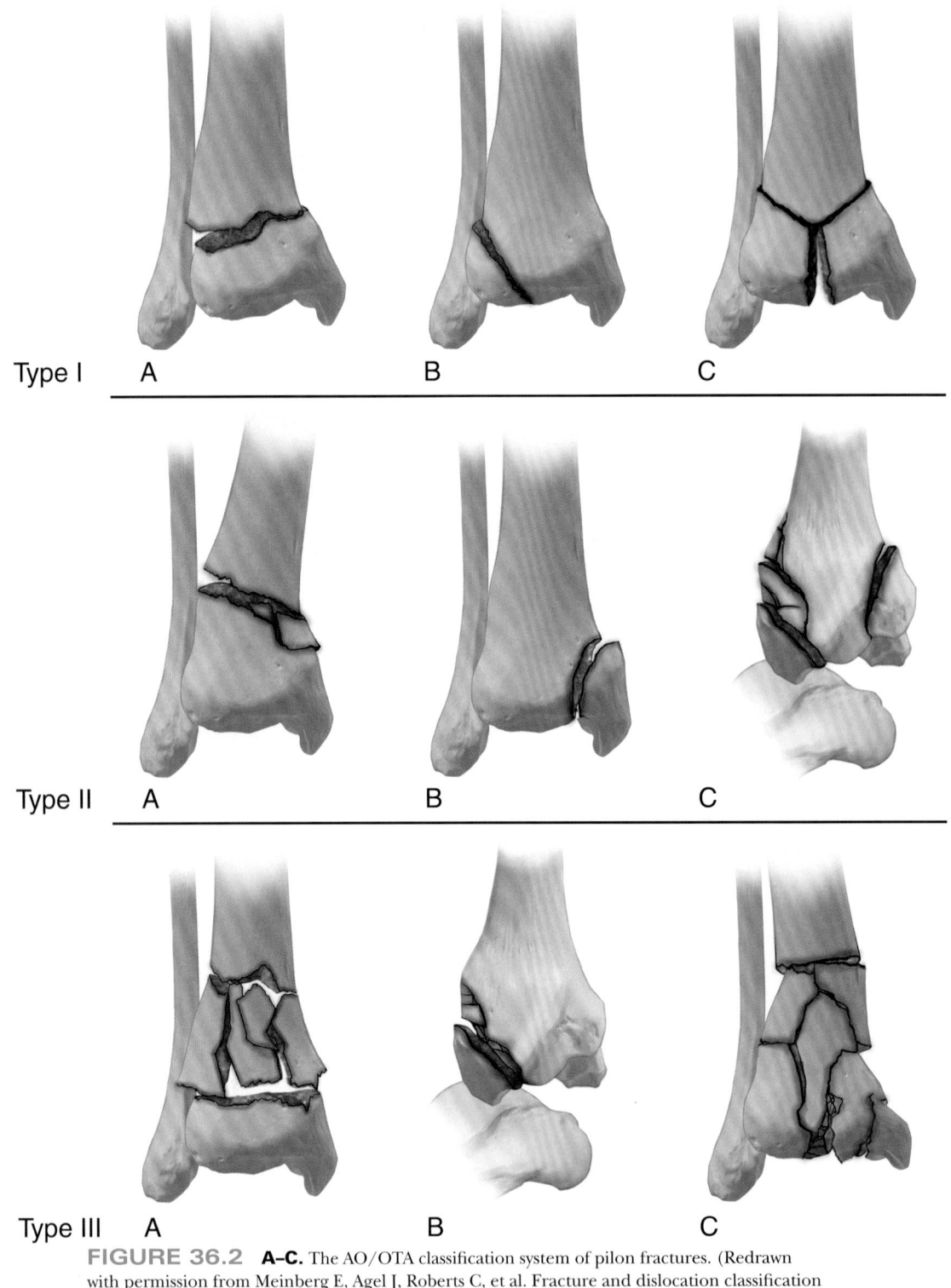

Type I   A   B   C

Type II   A   B   C

Type III   A   B   C

FIGURE 36.2 **A–C.** The AO/OTA classification system of pilon fractures. (Redrawn with permission from Meinberg E, Agel J, Roberts C, et al. Fracture and dislocation classification compendium—2018. *J Orthop Trauma.* 2018;32[1, suppl].)

and should include a primary and secondary survey. Because these injuries are impressive, they can serve as a distraction injury leaving other injuries overlooked. The practitioner should work closely with emergency department staff and other consultants to provide a comprehensive assessment of the injured.

Evaluation of the soft tissues and vascular status of the ankle is a top priority in the physical examination of pilon fractures. The location of soft tissue injuries should be noted for preoperative planning of surgical incisions. Open injuries, significant soft tissue swelling, or fracture blisters should be treated in a staged

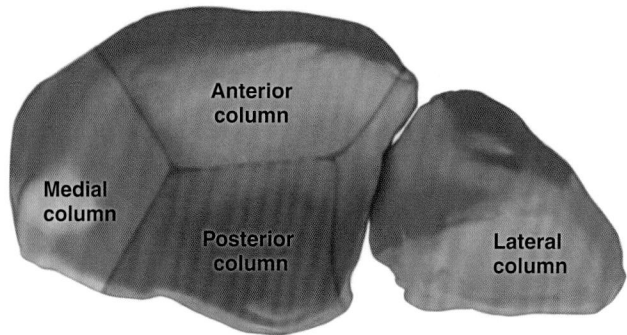

FIGURE 36.3 The four-column classification system of pilon injuries.

fashion. A systematic physical examination should be performed to identify any associated injuries involving the ipsilateral foot, knee, or other locations in cases of polytrauma. It is useful to identify patient comorbidities that predispose them toward soft tissue complications such as peripheral vascular disease, malnutrition, alcoholism, diabetes, neuropathy, tobacco use, and osteoporosis. The wound breakdown of pilon fixation can lead to the need for a free flap, and significant complications can occur that include flap failure and the ultimate need for subsequent amputation.[17,18] Any suspicion for neuropathy should be examined with 5.07-g Semmes-Weinstein monofilament testing over the plantar foot to evaluate protective sensation.

PATHOGENESIS

Two distinct mechanisms of injury are said to be responsible for these pilon fractures: low-energy rotational type forces versus high-energy trauma. Fracture of the tibial plafond caused by lower energy rotational forces are generally associated with a spiral or oblique type fracture line with minimal to moderate displacement of large articular fragments, minimal comminution, and minimal soft tissue injury. Lower energy injury patterns can be treated acutely and have shown to yield good results with open reduction internal fixation.[13,14,17] In 1979, Heim and Nasser reported that surgical treatment of a shearing, rotational-type fracture without major articular impaction yielded 84% good results.

On the other end of the spectrum, high-energy trauma can cause axial compression-type pilon fractures with extensive comminution, soft tissue injury, and articular cartilage damage.[13,14] These commonly present as one of three general types of injury as determined by the coronal plane deformity resulting from the fracture: (1) an axial failure of the tibia with an intact fibula, (2) a varus angulation of the tibia with compression medially and tension failure laterally, or (3) a valgus angulation with compression laterally. High-energy fractures with metaphyseal and diaphyseal comminution have higher reported complications rates with lower function outcome scores.[13] Heim and Nasser reported good results with surgical management of axial compression type pilon fractures with impaction and comminution in only 53% of their subjects, compared to 84% on their subjects with the rotational-type fracture pattern.[17]

IMAGING AND DIAGNOSTIC STUDIES

Radiographic evaluation should include standard ankle views and full-length images of the tibia and fibula so as to visualize the orientation of displacement of the talus, the degree of the fracture's proximal extension into the shaft, location of tibial metaphyseal comminution, and association of fibular fractures.[19,20] A retrospective study by Barei et al. determined that pilon injuries with concomitant fibular fractures were more likely to be associated with the severe type C-injuries than type B-injuries, when evaluated radiographically within the AO/OTA classification system.[21]

It is thought that the position of the foot at the time of injury can play a role in dictating the fracture pattern. If the ankle is dorsiflexed at the time of injury, the anterior part of the distal tibial articular surface is more likely to be damaged and the major fracture fragments located anteriorly. This type of injury is commonly due to landing on the ground from a great height with knee flexion and dorsiflexion of the ankle. If the ankle is plantar flexed at the time of injury, the posterior part of the distal tibial articular surface will likely be damaged and the major fracture fragments located posteriorly. This is commonly attributed to the patient slipping backward and landing upon the heel to bear the majority of the impact. If the ankle is in a neutral position at the time of injury, the full articular and metaphyseal surfaces will be compressed and impacted, commonly resulting in a Y-shaped fracture with anterior and posterior components.[22,23] Inversion of the ankle at the time of injury is likely to result in compression of the medial aspect of the joint with the major fragments medially. Eversion of the ankle at the time of injury is likely to result in compression of the lateral part of the distal tibial articular surface and major fracture fragments located laterally.[22]

A computer tomography (CT) scan is the most useful method for determining the key pattern characteristics of the injury. From this imaging modality, detailed information about the articular surface, displacement, shortening, and rotation can be obtained. Special care should be taken to examine the axial cuts, which are essential for defining the location of the main fracture lines, pattern, and number of fragments. In a study by Tornetta et al., CT was demonstrated to provide additional useful information in 82% of pilon fractures, which resulted in a change made to the surgical plan in 64% of those cases.[24] However, CT imaging prior to reduction and application of skeletal traction is of little value for surgical planning. It is advisable to wait until after the fracture has been reduced, distracted out to length, and spanned with a stabilizing external fixator before obtaining CT images in order to achieve the most useful visualization of the fracture morphology. If the CT scan is ordered prior to gross reduction, the surgeon will not be able to properly assess the intra-articular fragments and marginal impaction.

TREATMENT

If there is an associated fibular fracture, caution should be taken to avoid fixing the fibula at the same time as the application of the external fixator. This is because the incision may subsequently limit the approaches available to the surgeon before the CT scan has been obtained to allow for proper assessment of the fracture pattern and treatment approach.

A study by Topliss, Jackson, and Atkins reviewed 126 pilon fractures and classified fracture patterns as "sagittal" or "coronal" on the basis of the main fracture line as seen on the axial CT cut at the level of the tibial plafond. The sagittal patterns were more frequently associated with high-energy injuries in young patients and tended to present in varus deformity. Coronal patterns were seen more often in elderly patients and often presented with valgus deformity.[25]

HISTORICAL PERSPECTIVE ON THE TREATMENT OF PILON FRACTURES

TRADITIONAL TREATMENT VIA OPEN REDUCTION WITH INTERNAL FIXATION

Historically, pilon fractures have been considered extremely difficult to manage. Nonoperative treatment often results in malunion and operative treatment presents the treating surgeon with a large risk profile. In 1969, Ruedi and Allgower reported on a series of 84 consecutive pilon fractures treated by the principles of the Swiss Study Group/AO.[8] These principles include the following:

1. Reconstruction of the fibular fracture
2. Reconstruction of the tibial articular surface
3. Cancellous bone graft to fill the distal tibial metaphyseal defect
4. Buttress plate application to the medial aspect of the tibia

A subsequent study by Ruedi reviewed 54 of the original 84 patients 9 years after surgery.[26] Those results showed 68% of radiographs had not changed, 22% had a general improvement, and 10% of the patients showed progressively worse symptoms. These two publications provided surgeons an encouraging treatment algorithm, which led to more operative treatment of pilon fractures. Over time, the reproducibility of these favorable results was criticized, and the same authors reported another series of 75 patients.[27] In this publication, 25% were Type I fractures, 28% Type II, and 47% Type III. Interestingly, the subjective results from the patients were 80% "good." However, the author's objective criteria showed only 69.4% good results, 8% of patients had wound healing problems, and the eventual arthrodesis rate was 5.3%.

In 1979, Kellam and Waddell reported the results of 26 pilon fractures.[6] Surgical treatment of a vertically oriented shear, or rotational type fracture without major articular impaction yielded 84% good results. However, axial loading compression injuries with impaction and comminution achieved good results in only 53% of patients. These statistics suggest fracture pattern and degree of comminution had significant influence on results. Their findings also support a correlation between posttraumatic arthrosis and the degree of articular damage.

EXTERNAL FIXATION WITH LIMITED FIXATION

As the use of external fixation gained popularity, surgeons began introducing limited fragment fixation. This technique has also been advocated for other joints with severely comminuted, length unstable intra-articular fractures.[28] Originally, the fibula was treated with plating concurrent to the application of external fixation. Blauth et al. reported on 51 pilon fractures utilizing these different treatment strategies.[29] Group I with 15 fractures

had traditional ORIF using AO technique. Group II involving 28 fractures had a one-stage approach. The fibula had classic screw and plate fixation followed by distraction with an external fixator with limited ORIF of the tibia through small incisions employing screws or K-wires. Group III had eight fractures and were managed in a two-stage approach. The initial surgery involved reduction and fixation of the fibula with application of an external fixator and minimally invasive articular reduction of the tibia. Group III had the lowest infection rate. Ankle range of motion was worse in Group II and the best in Group III. No Group III patients had an arthrodesis, but the rate was 23% for Groups I and II. Wyrsch et al. published a randomized, prospective study using staged care on 38 of 58 patients.[30] Group I had 18 patients treated with ORIF. Group II had 20 patients treated with limited ORIF with external fixation. Group I had 15 complications in seven patients requiring twenty-eight additional surgeries. Group II had four complications in four patients. They concluded that limited ORIF with external fixation was less risky and as effective as traditional ORIF.

TWO-STAGE MINIMALLY INVASIVE TIBIAL PLATING

Definitive fixation with minimally invasive osteosynthesis via a staged approach is the currently recommended management technique for the treatment of compression type pilon fractures.[15,21,31] A commitment to understanding the tibial blood supply has demonstrated that the tibial blood supply has both an intrinsic (nutrient artery) and an extrinsic (tibial vessels) distribution. The extraosseous vessels supply the outer one-tenth to one-third of the tibial cortex while the intraosseous vessels contribute to the remaining cortex.[28] Borrelli's work suggested that traditional open plating of the tibia damaged the extraosseous blood supply more than minimally invasive techniques.[32] Open techniques with bicortical screw placement can compromise the periosteal biology. The evolution of locked plate designs has help mitigate these concerns. Locked plates allow for a fixed or variable ankle construct with less disruption of the periosteal biology. These plates can be placed extraperiosteal, which maintains continuity of the extraosseous blood supply. Locked plates may also be precontoured, which allows for easier minimally invasive insertion.

In 2000, Collinge and Sanders presented their experience on percutaneous plating of the lower extremity.[33] They reported on 17 fractures with an average 23-month follow-up. The tibia was fixated with a percutaneous plate, and the fibula was fixated only if it contributed to the length instability. Fourteen of the fractures consolidated. The open fracture subgroup reported three delayed unions, three nonunions, three superficial infections, one osteomyelitis, and one malunion.

Helfet et al. published a report on 20 distal tibia fractures employing a two-stage minimally invasive approach.[31] The initial operation included application of monorail external fixator with definitive fibular ORIF. The second stage of the procedure occurred in 5-6 days with percutaneous or small incision reduction and internal fixation of the tibial articular fragments followed by minimally invasive tibial plating. Average follow-up was 9 months and all fractures healed. No soft tissue complications and no implant failures were noted. There was no dehiscence, delayed wound healing, or deep infection. Two fractures healed in >5 degrees of varus and two in >10 degrees of recurvatum. This audience should keep in mind the short-term follow-up on this publication.

INITIAL SOFT TISSUE MANAGEMENT

Given the unforgiving nature of the soft tissues surrounding the ankle joint, it is widely recognized and accepted that the state of the soft tissues should dictate the timing of the surgery and degree of surgical insult. This is due to the difficulty of closing the incisions at the conclusion of the case and the postsurgical edema functioning as a secondary hit to the already severely compromised soft tissue envelope. Should the surgeon decide to perform open reduction and internal fixation on the injury, the objective of obtaining and preserving an anatomic reduction of the joint surface must be balanced with that of simultaneously preserving the integrity of the soft tissue envelope. There are many reports of wound complications after immediate open reduction and internal fixation of pilon fractures that include partial and full-thickness skin necrosis, wound dehiscence, and osteomyelitis that have even resulted in amputation.[16,34]

Evaluation of the skin should be performed at the time of initial encounter and assessed for presence or absence of skin wrinkles, degree of swelling, blistering, and open wounds.

High-energy pilon fractures are frequently associated with significant insult to the soft tissues but the lower energy variants in elderly patients with osteoporotic bone can present with soft tissue injury that is just as severe, due to age-related tissue fragility. Compression type fractures tend to lend themselves to significant edema and fracture blister formation. Due to the high-energy nature of the injury, considerable swelling can continue to increase within the first 3-5 days following the injury.[18] Fracture blister formation represents a separation of the epidermis and dermal layers (Fig. 36.4). They should not be operated through if possible. These blisters can be filled with serous or hemorrhagic fluid, the latter representing a more significant soft tissue injury. Small, unruptured, serous filled blisters away from the incisional site do not necessarily preclude surgery but hemorrhagic blisters are a contraindication to surgery. Varella et al. reported a 60% incidence of infection when surgeries were performed through open fracture blisters. Fracture blisters can be allowed to resolve on their own, or they can be decompressed

in a sterile fashion and subsequently treated with local wound care.[35] Many authors will avoid surgery until re-epithelialization of the skin blisters has been observed, and even then, any incisions will be made as far away from the damaged skin as possible. In general, the quality of the soft tissue envelope (ie, the presence of fracture blisters) will dictate the timing of the definitive procedure but not necessarily the exposure used. If it is determined that a certain approach must be used to obtain optimal fixation of the fracture, the surgeon should wait until the soft tissue has resolved and considered surgically ready based upon the previously described criteria.[36] During resolution of the soft tissue injury before surgery, the affected limb will need to be placed in a cast or splint that is windowed to allow for continued to wound care and periodic air drying.

Compartment syndrome is not common in these fracture patterns, but appropriate interval neurovascular evaluation should be prescribed when appropriate as the sequela of a missed compartment syndrome can be devastating.

External fixation has evolved into an important component in the staged care of pilon injuries. These constructs permit closed reduction and maintenance of length while the soft tissue resuscitates (Fig. 36.5). In most cases, the external fixator is a temporary device. However, these constructs may be used in an extended temporizing fashion if the soft tissue envelope remains hostile to surgical insult. The external fixator can be a monolateral pin-bar type, a hybrid, or a wire ring construct. The pin-bar external fixator is simple to apply, can distract the ankle joint via a centrally threaded pin placed through the calcaneus, and also can incorporate the foot. Some pin-bar external fixators have an articulated distal component that will allow motion. The hybrid external fixator has the advantage of being able to use transfixation wires to fixate short segment distal tibial fracture fragments. Circular external fixators employing the wire-ring construct popularized by Ilizarov are seldom used except in severe circumstances where they serve an important role in maintaining stability for a longer duration, particularly in cases of small fragment intra-articular comminution or a grievously compromised soft tissue envelope.

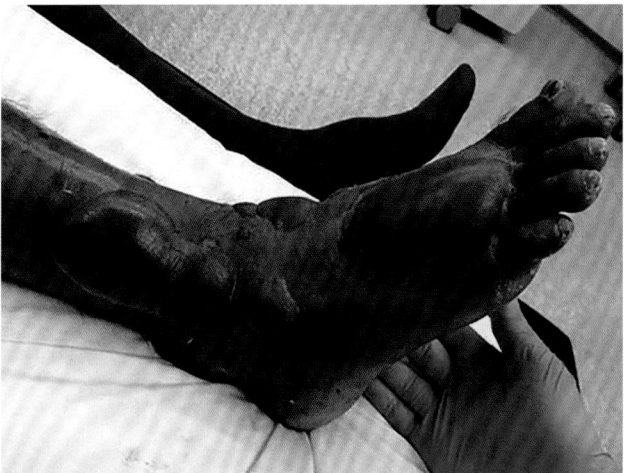

FIGURE 36.4 Photograph showing fracture blisters associated with high-energy trauma to the lower extremity.

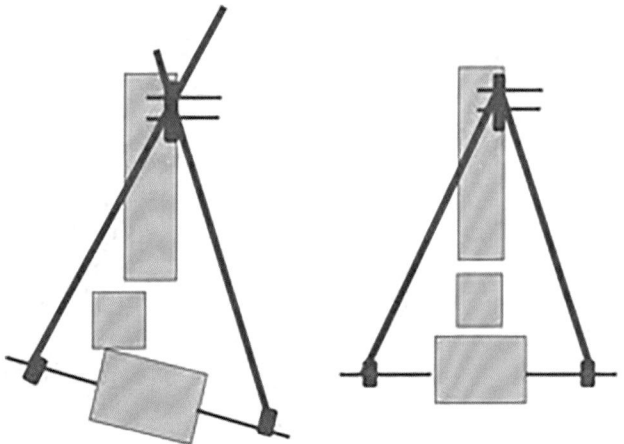

FIGURE 36.5 A style of delta frame commonly used for providing temporary spanning fixation of pilon fractures prior to definitive management.

The modern treatment of pilon fractures has popularized a staged reconstruction in order to minimize the risk of soft tissue complications.[34,37] Recent strategies have focused on staged fixation techniques that allow for initial external fixation followed by delayed, definitive ORIF of the plafond fracture. Sirkin et al. retrospectively reviewed 29 closed pilon fractures treated by definitive open reduction at an average of 12.7 days after the initial external fixation was applied. None of their patients exhibited wound dehiscence or full-thickness necrosis that required secondary soft tissue coverage postoperatively. From their data, they concluded that the historically high infection rates associated with open reduction and internal fixation of pilon fractures was likely the result of attempts at immediate fixation through swollen compromised soft tissue.[34] It is important that the pins of the initial external fixator are placed remotely from any planned surgical incisions, definitive fixation, and injured soft tissue envelope.

INITIAL MANAGEMENT: GENERAL WORKFLOW AND PRINCIPLES

The patient is initially evaluated in the emergency room; the limb is stabilized and placed into a well padded splint. If the plain radiographs reveal a tibial plafond fracture, the patient is cleared for surgical stabilization and taken into the operating room. In the case of an injury with extensive soft tissue insult, application of a spanning multiplanar external fixator is recommended for temporary stabilization prior to obtaining a CT scan. If this staged treatment plan is pursued and there is an associated fibular fracture, it has previously been accepted to fix the fibula fracture during the same procedure as the placement of the external fixator. However, one should be cautioned that fixing the fibula at this stage has the potential to be counterproductive and there is an argument to be made against it.

Taking into consideration the goals of minimizing insult to the soft tissue and maximizing opportunities for achieving articular congruity, several reasons exist for avoiding initial fibular fixation. The ideal approach for fixing the plafond fracture cannot be determined until the fracture pattern and characteristics have been reliably established using a CT scan. Therefore, an incision placed initially for the purposes of fixing the fibula could possibly prohibit the ideal placement of an incision suited to addressing the tibial plafond fracture. Additionally, it cannot be assumed that anatomic fixation of the fibula will result in successful indirect reduction of the posterior tibial plafond fragment because the fibula is often comminuted and therefore challenging to obtain anatomic reduction. Without direct inspection of the tibia and articular surface at the time of fibular fixation to confirm ideal reduction of the joint surface, it is even possible for it to be displaced superiorly in a position that makes subsequent reduction of the posterior fragment extremely difficult.[27]

DEFINITIVE MANAGEMENT: GENERAL WORKFLOW AND PRINCIPLES

The patient is positioned on a radiolucent operating room table with their feet brought to the end of the table. Whether they are positioned supine or prone will depend upon the surgeon's approach based on CT findings. Elevation of the ipsilateral or contralateral hip with a bump can be used to assist in positioning the operative limb in a neutral rotation. A tourniquet is placed on the ipsilateral thigh and intravenous antibiotics are administered before tourniquet inflation. In general, it is preferred to have the C-arm positioned on the contralateral aspect of the operative extremity (Fig. 36.6). This will minimize interference with the workspace of the surgeon and the supporting team during intraoperative imaging.

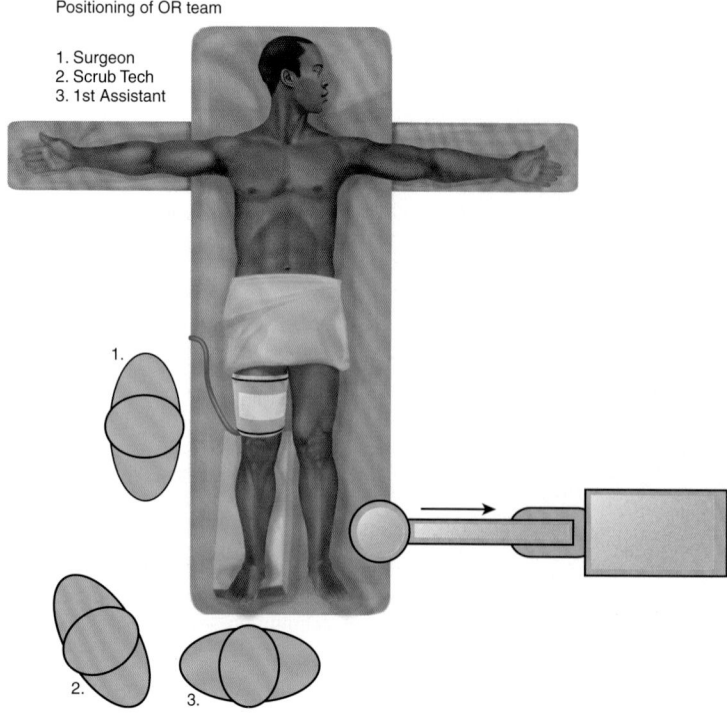

Positioning of OR team

1. Surgeon
2. Scrub Tech
3. 1st Assistant

FIGURE 36.6 Recommended intraoperative positioning of C-arm and assisting personnel.

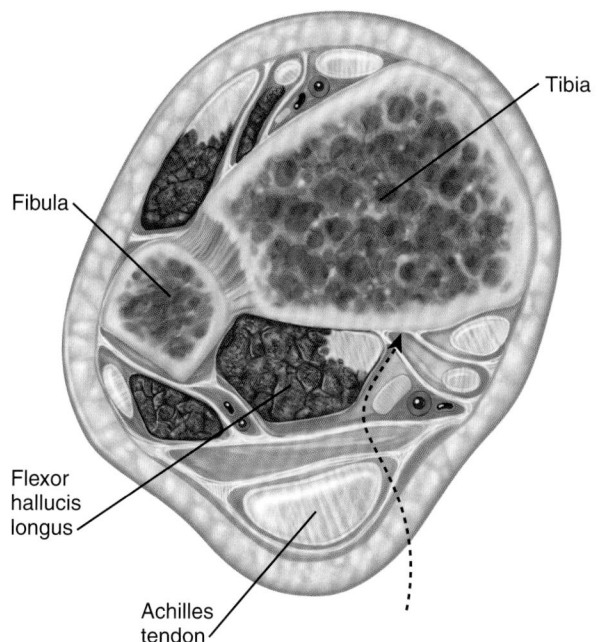

Tibia

Fibula

Flexor
hallucis
longus

Achilles
tendon

FIGURE 36.7 An appreciation of the cross-sectional anatomy surrounding the tibial plafond is necessary for proper incisional planning and ideal soft tissue preservation.

Since most pilon fractures are initially treated with an external fixator, some surgeons prefer to leave a portion of the delta frame or a medial based frame in place throughout the definitive procedure so as to help maintain length. This will allow for reduction, fixation and plating with less manipulation of the soft tissues.[18] Even if the external fixator is not maintained during the entire procedure, it is recommended that it is prepped into the sterile field so as to maintain stability of the soft tissues throughout the preparation and draping of the extremity.[36]

The skin incision should be made full thickness and undermining to create multiple subcutaneous planes is completely avoided (Fig. 36.7). Any tendon or neurovascular structures are gently retracted. Self-retaining retractors should be used sparingly. During retraction, the tension should be placed on the deeper structures whenever possible. The importance of meticulous soft tissue handling during the procedure cannot be understated and has prompted the innovation of techniques solely intended to advance this tenet. In 2008, Cannada described excellent visualization of the metaphyseal/diaphyseal region during fixation of pilon fractures utilizing a "no-touch" technique whereby the full-thickness skin flap of the incision was held in gentle retraction entirely by the deep placement of K-wires and without the use of any self-retaining retractors. These K-wires were placed proximally to the articular fracture fragments, bent at a right angle so as to protect any assistants during the procedure and removed once reduction and plate fixation was applied.[34]

The dominant fragments of the injury are approached through a major fracture line as visualized on the CT scan. This will be discussed in greater detail later in the following sections. When the fracture is visualized, there is often significant periosteal stripping as a result of the mechanism of injury. Any additional periosteal dissection should be minimal and along the edges of the fracture fragments to reduce further loss of blood supply. The major fracture fragments are reflected on

a periosteal hinge and débrided of any entrapped soft tissue and hematoma. Any hematoma can be evacuated with a bulb syringe of irrigation and a small suction tip so as to allow for better key-in of the fracture fragments. The ankle joint is visualized, and chondral injury noted. It may be difficult to fully see the articular surface and the use of an arthroscope through the incision or using standard arthroscopic portals may afford access for evaluation and aid in reduction.

PLANNING THE APPROACH AND FIXATION

As emphasized repeatedly throughout this chapter, the soft tissue envelope of the distal tibia is relatively thin and lacking in robust underlying muscle or subcutaneous tissue and is therefore especially prone to wound breakdown and blistering, especially in the setting of high-energy injuries. Postsurgical wound complications are particularly concerning because of the close proximity of internal fixation to the surface of the skin. Breakdown of the incision can necessitate soft tissue coverage with a free flap or even lead to proximal amputation secondary to infection of the exposed hardware.[18] Wyrsch et al. reported a 33% rate of wound breakdown and 28% rate of infection in pilon fractures treated by open reduction and internal fixation at 4 days; 4 of 18 patients required free flap coverage.[30] Bourne et al. reported a 13% rate of deep infection.[5]

Despite improvements in surgical techniques and implants, treatment of pilon fractures remains challenging with regard to minimizing postoperative soft tissue complications. Blauth et al. were not able to demonstrate a significant reduction in wound complications between open, staged, and minimally invasive approaches (rates: 33%, 12.5%, and 25%, respectively).[29] Pugh et al. reported a 37% rate of major wound complications in patients treated with open reduction and internal fixation and 21% rate of major complications in patients treated with external fixation.[38]

Out of respect for the potential of the soft tissue to drive the outcome of these injuries, careful consideration of the incisional approach should be taken prior to undertaking any open repair. This consideration for the soft tissue must be carefully weighed in conjunction with the surgeon's main task in treatment of a displaced articular fracture: the ability to obtain anatomic reduction of the joint. Inability to achieve perfect congruity will result in deterioration of the joint and poor long-term outcome. Direct visualization is necessary to maximize congruity of the repair, and this can only be achieved with open reduction using appropriately placed incisions. Fixation of articular fragments must precede fixation of the articular block to the metaphyseal and diaphyseal segments.[11]

After giving due consideration to the status of the soft tissue envelope, the surgical approach is dictated by the location of the articular injury (column) and the mechanically appropriate fixation. A general principle to be mindful of during incision planning is that a stable constant fragment is needed to be built upon for the reduction of complex articular fractures.[37] The surgeon will need to decide which incisional approach they are most comfortable using in order to apply this principle. For example, in calcaneal fractures, the sustentacular fragment is exploited in this fashion. In the case of a pilon fracture, a stable posterior malleolus has been described by some authors as the key to a good articular reduction. Anatomic and stable reduction of the posterior fragment could effectively convert an OTA 43C fracture to an OTA 43B fracture, which is typically associated with better outcomes.[39]

The primary fixation of a pilon fracture will generally require plate fixation on the compression (or concave) side of the deformity, thereby serving as a buttress against the deforming tendency of the fracture pattern. Despite there being multiple force vectors acting upon the joint at the time of injury, the two most common plate locations used to resist those forces are medial and anterolateral. Busel et al. characterized 103 fractures as varus or valgus based upon the orientation of the associated fibula fracture component and analyzed the outcome of medial versus anterolateral placement of the plate construct. Pilon fractures with associated fibula fractures of a transverse orientation were classified as having had a varus deforming force. Associated fibula fractures with impacted and comminuted patterns were classified as having had a valgus deforming force. The varus group presented with mechanical complications in 14.3% of patients who were plated medially and 80% of patients who were plated laterally. The valgus group saw mechanical complications in 16.7% of patients who were plated laterally and 36.4% of patients who were plated medially. They concluded that whenever the soft tissue allows, the buttress plate should be placed in such a way so as to resist the original deforming forces with medial plates for varus fractures and anterolateral plates for valgus fractures.[40]

More complex fractures with greater articular injury may require an approach that allows for visualization of the multiple columns through separate incisions. The surgeon should be comfortable with several surgical approaches as the status of the soft tissue envelope or orientation of the fracture pattern may preclude the surgeon from using the same approach every time. In the case of fracture patterns that require an approach to different sides of the articular surface via separate incisions, these can be performed in a staged fashion. Ketz et al. compared the outcomes of a staged multi-incision approach with that of a single incision anterior or anteromedial approach to treat the two groups of AO/OTA 43C tibial pilon fractures. For the multi-incisional approach group, the patients were treated with posterior plating of the tibia through a posterolateral approach, followed by a staged direct anterior approach. The single incision group was treated with an anterior or anteromedial incision. After an average follow-up of 40 months, they found that the 40% of the single incision group patients had more than 2 mm of joint incongruity on CT scans, compared to zero patients in the staged multi-incision approach group. Only 33% of patients in the staged multi-incisional approach had radiographic evidence of joint space narrowing, compared to 70% in the single incision anterior approach group. The authors concluded that this technique improved their ability to obtain an anatomic articular reduction as well as a positive correlation with improved functional outcomes scores.[37]

Described approaches in the literature include the anteromedial, anterolateral, straight anterior midline, anterior extensible, medial, direct lateral, posteromedial, and posterolateral incisions.[37,41] A systematic review, which included 733 patients, by Liu et al. sought to investigate the role of surgical approach on pilon fracture outcomes. They found that the anterior approach had one of the lowest complication rates despite having had a large proportion of OTA Type C fractures in their patient base. The medial-based approach also had a low complication rate but had a higher proportion of OTA Type B fractures. The posterolateral and anteromedial approaches were

noted to have higher complication rates; however, the authors admitted that the inability to control for differences in treatment methods (stages, timing, other procedural aspects) limited the direct establishment of a causal relationship on the role of surgical approaches on observed outcomes.[42]

Wei et al. evaluated the outcomes of a surgical strategy driven by the ankle position at the time of injury according to the patient's description of their posture at the time of injury and initial imaging finding, which were examined for direction of displacement and tilting of the articular surface. These groups were described as varus, valgus, dorsiflexion, plantar flexion, and neutral. They proposed an anteromedial approach for varus position injuries, an anterolateral approach for valgus position injuries, an anterior approach for dorsiflexion position injuries, a posterolateral approach for plantar flexion position injuries, and a combined approach for neutral position injuries.[22] Some of the most commonly used approaches will be described in this chapter as follows: anteromedial, anterolateral, straight anterior midline, and posterolateral.

ANTEROMEDIAL APPROACH

The indication for the anteromedial approach is typically for the fracture of the medial column of the distal tibia (Fig. 36.8). This approach would provide access to the medial malleolus and to the medial and middle thirds of the anterior tibiotalar joint. The anterior marginal fractures can also be addressed through this approach. It is not the approach of choice for fractures that involve the lateral column because that would require excessive traction on the fragile soft tissues to adequately visualize and reduce the Tillaux-Chaput fragment as well as perform lateral plating.

The incision begins 15 mm distal to the tip of the medial malleolus and is curved gently anterior medial crossing the tibiotalar joint and its middle third. It is extended proximally along the subcutaneous border of the tibia. If possible, the branches of the saphenous nerve and saphenous vein are spared. This developed fasciocutaneous flap is mobilized in one layer.

Once the extensor retinaculum is visualized, it should be incised vertically medial to the tibialis anterior tendon. Care should be taken to avoid opening the sheath of the tendon during this incision. Subsequently, the ankle joint is identified and opened anteriorly.

The fracture fragments are identified and reduced in standard fashion. In cases of articular impaction, the subchondral bone and articular fragments are disimpacted, anatomically reduced and temporary stabilized with K wires. The reduced articular surface can be supported by autologous bone graft harvested from the proximal tibia or iliac crest. An anatomic medial metaphyseal plate with locking screws can be applied to the medial column. If possible, independent lag screws are used to rigidly fixate the articular fragments prior to placement of this plate. The retinaculum and subcutaneous tissue will need to be closed with 2-0 resorbable sutures and the skin gently closed with interrupted nylon sutures using the Allgower Donati technique.[31]

ANTEROLATERAL

The anterolateral approach (Fig. 36.9) is indicated for pilon fractures that involve the lateral column and will give direct access to the Chaput fragment. These can present with

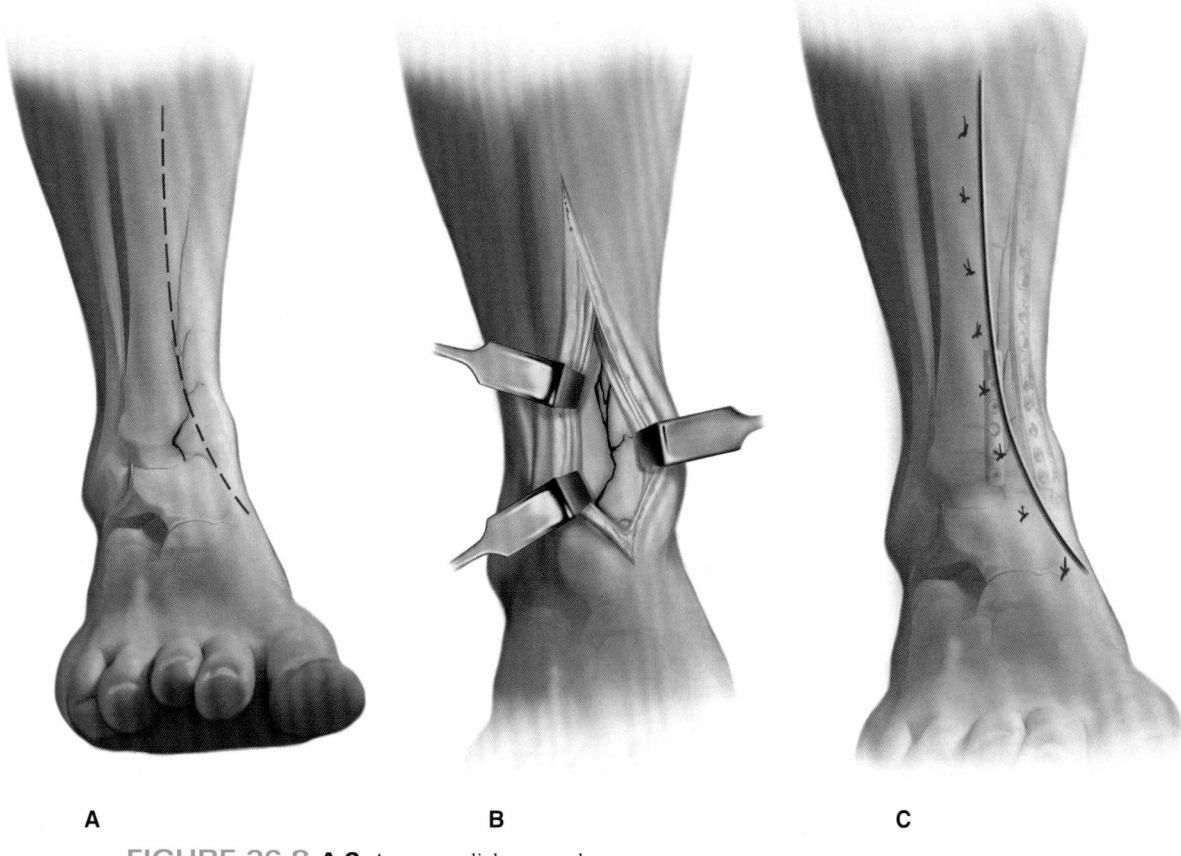

A   **B**   **C**

FIGURE 36.8 **A-C.** Anteromedial approach.

aanterior and/or lateral comminution and impaction. On plain films, this will often present as a failure into valgus. Due to lack of adequate access to the medial column, contraindications to this approach include anteromedial or medial exit of the primary fracture line and primarily medial defects and/or comminution resulting in varus deformity where a medial buttress plate would be required. If the lateral column fracture is associated with a fibular fracture, repair of both fractures can be performed through a single incision. Another advantage of the anterolateral approach is that it provides a good soft tissue envelope and allows f or the development of full-thickness flaps.[18]

Landmarks for the surgical incision include the distal fibula and the ankle joint line. The incision is made along the anterior crest of the fibula proximally and curved gently medial and toward the joint line distally. It can generally be visualized as aligned with the 4th metatarsal distally and between the tibia and fibula proximally. If there is a need to visualize the Volkmann fragment, the incision could start at the lateral subcutaneous border of the fibula and curved similarly. In cases

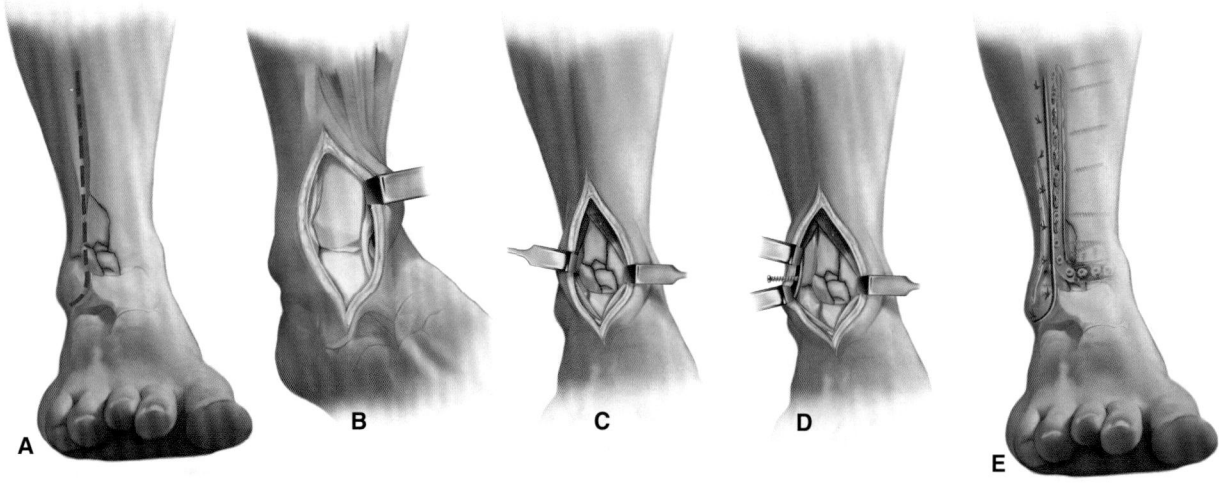

A   **B**   **C**   **D**   **E**

FIGURE 36.9 **A-E.** Anterolateral approach.

where the posterior lateral impaction and comminution is more severe, the incision may be moved more along the posterior border of the fibula with a similar curve as it moves more distal. This will allow for access to plating the posterior malleolus if the dissection is carried behind the peroneals.

After the incision is made, the subcutaneous tissues are carefully dissected and the superficial peroneal nerve branches are identified, protected, and mobilized in the anterior soft tissue flap. The fascial attachment of the anterior compartment upon the fibula is identified and sharply in size at the anterior fibular crest. A soft tissue elevator is used to bluntly dissect in this plane and follow the cortex of the fibula to the interosseous membrane over to the anterior tibial cortex.

During dissection across the interosseous membrane to the tibia, some authors have encouraged deflation of the tourniquet so as to allow the anterior tibial artery to be palpated for identification and protection of the neurovascular bundle. It is recommended to perform this blunt dissection at the level of the metaphysis so as to avoid injury of the anterior inferior tibiofibular ligament and its attachments to the Chaput fragment. Elevation of the anterior compartment can be achieved using a small Hohmann retractor to hug the tibia and also protect the neurovascular bundle in this plane of retracted tissue. The superficial peroneal nerve and anterior compartment musculature and tendons are retracted medially, exposing the distal tibial articular surface. An arthrotomy can be performed at or close to the fracture line to avoid devascularization of the distal tibia. Care should be taken not to incise the anterior tibiofibular ligament. The arthrotomy can be continued distally over the talar neck and the capsule elevated from the anterior distal tibia to properly visualize the articular segments.[36]

Once the fracture fragments are exposed, they can be reduced and temporarily fixated with Kirschner wires so as to restore the joint line. To achieve this, the usually large anterolateral Tillaux-Chaput fragment can be hinged laterally to allow visualization and reduction of the posterior articular surface and posterior column. If necessary, the articular surface is disimpacted and anatomically reduced usually progressing from posterior to anterior and lateral to medial.

A long L-shaped anatomic locking plate that connects the diaphysis to the articular block can be used to span the metaphyseal defect, placed anterolaterally just proximal to the distal tibia articular margin and passed submuscularly up the lateral surface of the tibia. Care should be taken to ensure that the proximal portion of this plate is parallel to the anterior fibular crest.[40,42] Repair of the extensor retinaculum is critical to prevent tendon bowstringing and can usually be accomplished with a running 3-0 monofilament suture. The skin can be closed with interrupted 3-0 nylon using the Allgower-Donati technique.[35]

STRAIGHT ANTERIOR MIDLINE

The anterior approach (Fig. 36.10) allows for complete visualization of the anterior medial and anterior lateral surface of the distal tibia. It allows for the placement of either an anterolateral or medial plate. This same incision is also commonly favored for an anterior approach for an ankle fusion or ankle replacement procedure.

An 8- to 10-cm incision centered over the ankle is made after identifying the interval between the anterior tibial tendon

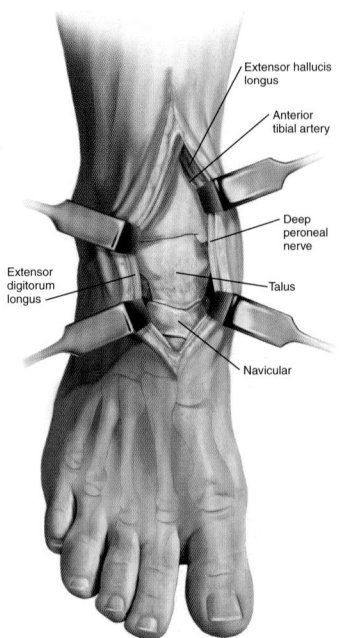

FIGURE 36.10 Straight anterior midline approach.

and extensor hallucis longus tendon. Distal to the joint, the incision is carried out 3-4 cm, stopping at the level of the talonavicular joint. After the incision, care is taken to find and protect the superficial peroneal nerve, which crosses that wound from the lateral side distal to the ankle joint. The extensor retinaculum can then be incised in line with the skin incision and tagged for closure at the end of the case. The interval between the anterior tibial and extensor hallucis longus tendons is exposed. Just medial to the extensor hallucis longus tendon at the level of the joint, the anterior tibial artery, and deep peroneal nerve should be identified and protected by retracting the neurovascular bundle laterally with the extensor hallucis longus tendon. The tibialis anterior tendon should be retracted medially to expose the ankle capsule. Subsequently, the ankle capsule can be incised in line with the skin incision. As the skin incision extends proximally, it should be placed slightly lateral to the anterior tibial crest in order to prevent formation of a painful scar.

Once the fracture fragments are identified, sequential articular reduction can be performed in a posterior to anterior manner. There is impaction or displacement of the posterior articular surface, reduction of this should be prioritized. These articular fragments can be provisionally stabilized with 1.6-mm Kirschner wires, using fluoroscopic imaging to confirm anatomic congruity. In the case of metaphyseal defects, cancellous autograft or allograft can be used. Once the anterior tibia and articular surface has been properly stabilized with Kirschner wires, independent lag screws can be used to compress the fragments together. Typically, the anterior articular fragments can be latched onto the posterior articular fragments. Subsequently, anterolateral or medial plates can be applied to attach the metaphyseal fragment to the diaphysis. Some surgeons may elect to leave the external fixator frame attached during this entire procedure to maintain length until the plate and screw construct has been applied. Once fluoroscopic imaging has confirmed attainment of stable, anatomic reduction, the external fixator pins can be removed and the surgical wounds thoroughly irrigated. The retinacular layer should be close with 0 Vicryl prior to a layered closure of the skin.[37,42]

POSTEROLATERAL

Posterior approaches to the pilon fracture are recommended when the soft tissue requires it, but this approach relies heavily upon cortical reduction and fluoroscopic assistance because it is a challenging window through which to directly visualize the articular surface. It has been hypothesized that the abundant soft tissue coverage of the posterior distal tibia would decrease the rate of wound complications. Bhattacharya et al. managed 19 consecutive pilon fractures through a posterolateral approach after initial temporary external fixation. The incidence of wound complications, nonunion, and early posttraumatic arthritis was followed for at an average of 13 months. Nine of nineteen patients (47%) developed complications and six of them (32%) sustained wound complications of which half were deep infections. It was determined that the posterolateral approach is no better than other published approaches for pilon fractures with respect to decreasing complications, and the authors did not recommend it as a routine approach for pilon fractures that did not have other indications for it.[43] Such indications would include specific fracture types in which the comminution and step-off are located in the posterior column primarily. In these cases, it is necessary to reestablish correct length and axial and rotational alignment so that the posterior column can serve as a template to reduce the anterior portion of the plafond. Soft tissue concerns may also preclude an anterior approach, although some authors have admitted that it may not be ideal to attempt reduction of the anterior pilon comminution through a posterior approach.[37]

For the posterolateral approach (Fig. 36.11), the external fixator is removed under general anesthesia and the patient placed prone on the operating table. After making a 10-cm incision between the Achilles tendon and posterolateral border of the fibula, it is extended as far proximally as required to reduce the posterior column. The sural nerve will need to be identified and protected. The approach is performed in the interval between the peroneal tendons and the flexor hallucis longus after opening the deep fascia and bluntly dissecting down to the posterior tibia. This affords excellent exposure of the posterior aspect of the distal tibia and allows for the approach to be further extended proximally if necessary. The peroneal tendons are retracted anterolaterally as the plane is developed medial to them and lateral to the FHL. The lateral fibers of the FHL can be sharply or bluntly lifted from the posterior fibula, interosseous membrane, and posterior tibia to expose the lateral portion of the tibia, posterior column, and plafond. Any large posterolateral fragments at the level of the joint can be hinged open to visualize the articular surface and reduce impacted fragments. A separate medial incision may be required for fixation of the more medial fragments, which are challenging to gain access to through this approach without extensive retraction of the soft tissue.

Articular reduction is obtained by direct manipulation of the fracture fragments under direct visualization. The large posterolateral fragments at the level of the joint can be hinged open to visualize the articular surface and reduce impacted fragments. A separate medial incision may be required for fixation of the more medial fragments, which are challenging to gain access to through this approach without extensive retraction of the soft tissue. Fluoroscopy is then used to confirm reduction with temporary Kirschner wire fixation before fixation with 3.5 mm lag screws, which is preferably done prior to the placement of a plate. The metaphyseal block can then be affixed to the diaphysis with an antiglide plate. Bone grafting in the form of acute iliac crest cancellous autograft or allograft can be used at the surgeon's discretion to provide support to the reduced articular surface. This technique is generally favored when large metaphyseal defects are found after disimpaction of the comminuted portion of the fracture. If necessary, the fibula can be plated through the same incision using a one-third tubular plate. This should generally be performed only after fixation of the tibial articular block with the posterior plate so as to allow for a confirmation of the reduction without the intraoperative imaging being obscured by the hardware in the fibula. The surgical wound is then closed primarily in layers without the routine use of suction drains.[37,41,44]

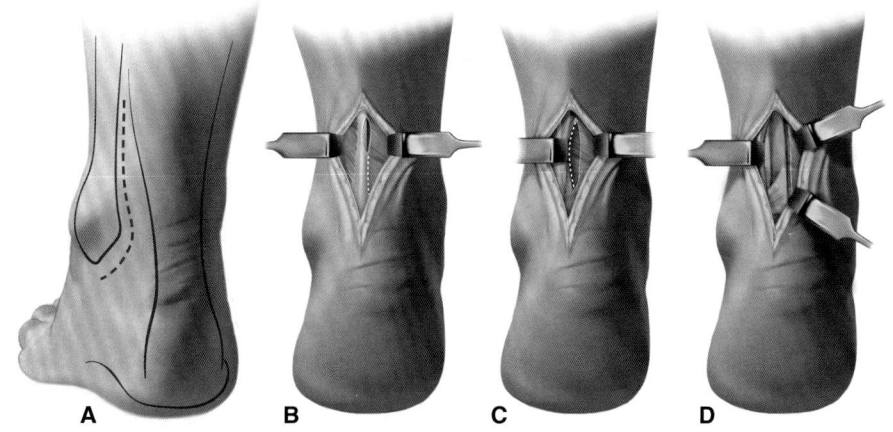

FIGURE 36.11 A-D. Posterolateral approach.

COMPLICATIONS

- The presence of persistent pain, loss of physical health, and a low return-to-work rate highlights the enormous long-term impact of tibial pilon fractures on the life of the patient. Bonato et al. followed the outcomes of 98 unilateral tibial plafond fractures prospectively for 12 months and found that only 57% had returned to work by that time and 27% continued to report moderate to severe persistent pain.[45]

- The potential risk of soft tissue complications has been emphasized repeatedly throughout this chapter. Graves et al. examined the hypothesis that the larger soft tissue envelope associated with obese patients would have a shielding effect against postoperative wound complications by providing greater area for energy distribution of the trauma and more ample coverage for subcutaneous implants. They studied a consecutive series of 176 pilon fractures with a mean follow-up of 53 weeks and found that the patients with a BMI > 30 indeed demonstrated significant increase in the ratio of soft tissue envelope to tibial bone when compared to their nonobese counterparts. However, the data did not support the hypothesis that the larger tissue envelope provided any protection against wound healing complications and in fact demonstrated the opposite trend. When compared to lean patients, the obese patients in their study had a relative risk of 1.67 for the development of a postoperative wound complication and 2.79 for the development of a complication requiring formal irrigation and débridement.[46] This finding is especially disheartening in light of several studies indicating that obesity predisposes patients to more complex ankle injury patterns.[47] A consecutive series by Strauss et al. found that there were significantly more AO/OTA type B and C fractures in their obese patients than compared to their lean patients.[48]

- Prudent incision placement plays an important role in the reduction of soft tissue complications. Howard et al. have reported that the skin bridge can be <7 cm (49). In 42 patients with 46 pilon fractures, 83% of the time the skin bridge measured from 5.0 and 6.9 cm with no increased rate of wound healing complication. Traditional ORIF has a higher incidence of infection. However, less invasive approaches have demonstrated a decreased infection rate. The worst case scenario is still an infected nonunion that can result in a protracted, complicated reconstruction or a below-knee amputation.[49]

- The most common late complication of pilon fractures is traumatic arthritis. A retrospective review by Harris et al. of 79 fractures (OTA 43B or OTA 43C) with staged tibial fixation followed for an average of 26 months found a 39% rate of posttraumatic arthritis. Early complications included two superficial complications and three deep infections. Late complications included two nonunions and four malunions.[50] A retrospective study of 47 patients with tibial plafond fractures treated operatively and followed for a mean of 5.3 years found that among the predictors of an unsuccessful outcome, the reduction quality was the only modifiable factor by the surgeon.[51] Surgical treatment for posttraumatic arthritis is ankle arthrodesis or ankle arthroplasty. These topics will be covered in other chapters of this textbook. A symptomatic malunion can be corrected along with the arthrodesis or implant arthroplasty. Other complications include loss of motion, prolonged edema, incisional scaring, skin slough, soft tissue or osseous infection, delayed union, fixation failure, nerve entrapment, and deep vein thrombosis.

- Avascular necrosis of the anterolateral corner of the distal tibia is a complication of pilon fractures that is possibly missed more often than it is diagnosed because of the expected constellation of challenges that are already being managed as a result of the injury. It can be diagnosed on plain radiographs as increased radiographic density in the anterolateral corner of the distal tibia or a segmental collapse of the overlying articular surface. Several studies have demonstrated the fragility of the vasculature supplying the anterolateral tibia, though predominantly through cadaveric study. Open plating on the medial surface of the distal tibia was found to create a significant disruption of the extra-osseous blood supply in comparison to percutaneous plating.[52] Although not able to be translated to direct clinical practice, the disruption of vascular supply from large incisions must be considered in high-impact trauma scenarios. The distal tibia contains a rich vascular supply from anastomoses of the nutrient artery and perimalleolar ring that draw their supply from the tibialis anterior and peroneal artery.[53] Disruption of all these anastomoses is required for complete loss of blood supply to the anterolateral corner of the distal tibia, and this scenario may only be produced with extremely high-energy impact. However, when combined with a large surgical exposure and plate fixation, this compounded insult to the vasculature may be sufficient to cause avascular necrosis of the tibial plafond.

POSTOPERATIVE CARE AND REHABILITATION

Patients are placed in a splint, bivalved cast, or fracture brace after surgery. Prophylactic antibiotics that were begun intravenously before surgery are usually continued for 24-48 hours in a closed fracture. If a closed suction drain is used, it is removed in 24-48 hours. The extremity is elevated, and ice is applied for edema control. Postoperative analgesics are prescribed. The operative site is examined in 3-4 days. Sutures are removed in 14-21 days. Once the edema has resolved, the extremity is placed into a short-leg nonwalking cast. It is important to maintain the ankle at 90 degrees to prevent an equinus contracture. In compression pilon fractures, the patient must refrain from weight bearing for a minimum of 3 months to allow fracture consolidation. Osseous union will be determined by clinical examination and serial radiographs. Rotation pilon fractures have been allowed to weight bear in a CAM boot in 4-8 weeks depending on stability of the internal fixation and whether the fracture entered the ankle joint or not. If radiographs do not support complete union at the abovementioned time, passive range of motion in a removable orthopedic boot can be considered. This will help promote ankle motion, while still protecting the skeleton.

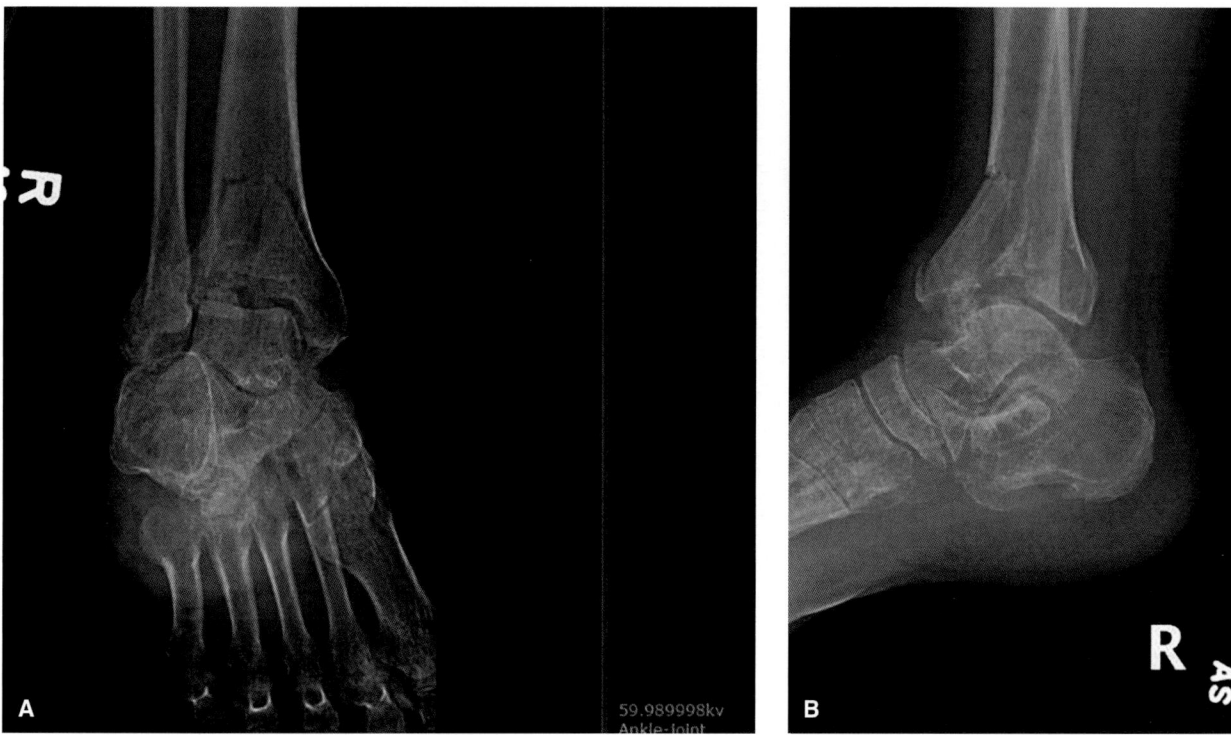

FIGURE 36.12 Case study A: preoperative AP **(A)** and lateral **(B)** radiographs.

CASE STUDY A

A 49-year-old gentleman with a prior healed calcaneal fracture sustained a right pilon fracture with significant comminution of the distal tibia after falling from a roof (Figs. 36.12 through 36.19). Plain radiographs demonstrated shortening and comminution of the lateral column of the ankle joint, associated with a valgus type deforming force. Extensive impaction of the articular surface was also appreciated. A transarticular external fixator was initially placed to re-establish length and reduce the valgus malalignment for temporary stabilization. Care was taken to place the tibial half-pins far proximal from the anticipated zone of fixation. A subsequent CT scan demonstrated a multifragmentary joint fracture of the tibia (AO/OTA 43C2) with at least one

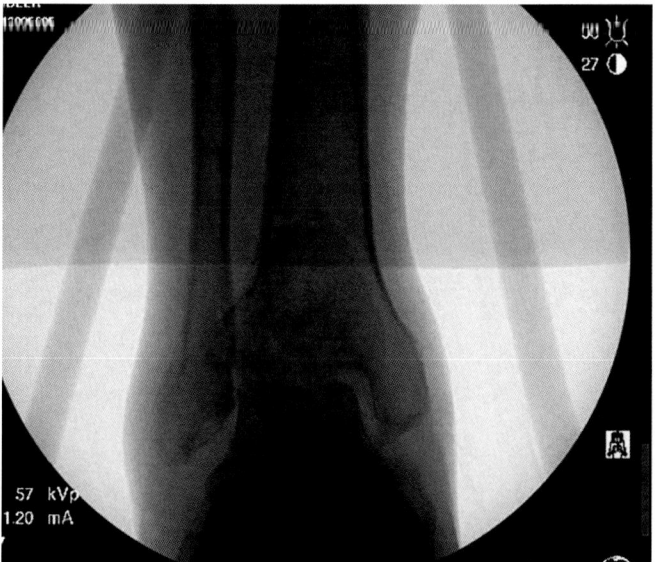
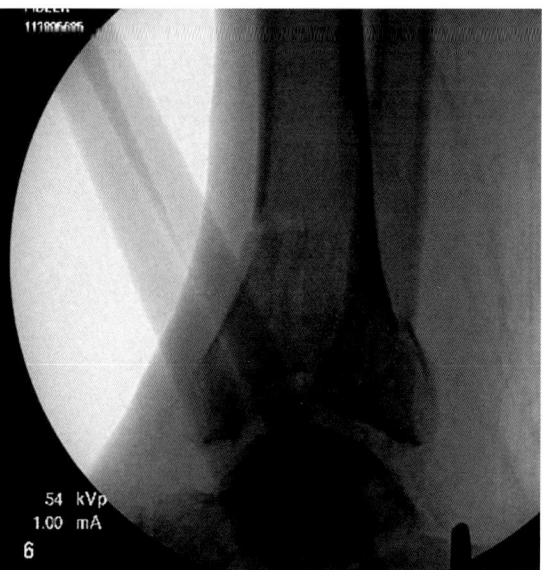

FIGURE 36.13 Case study A: the patient was brought to the operating room where the patient underwent closed reduction of injury. A spanning delta frame was applied for temporary fixation until the soft tissue had resolved adequately for open reduction internal fixation.

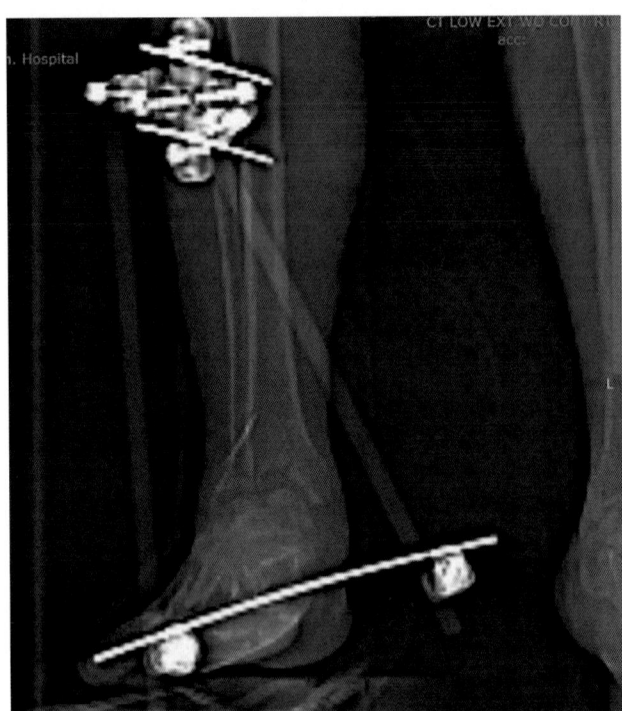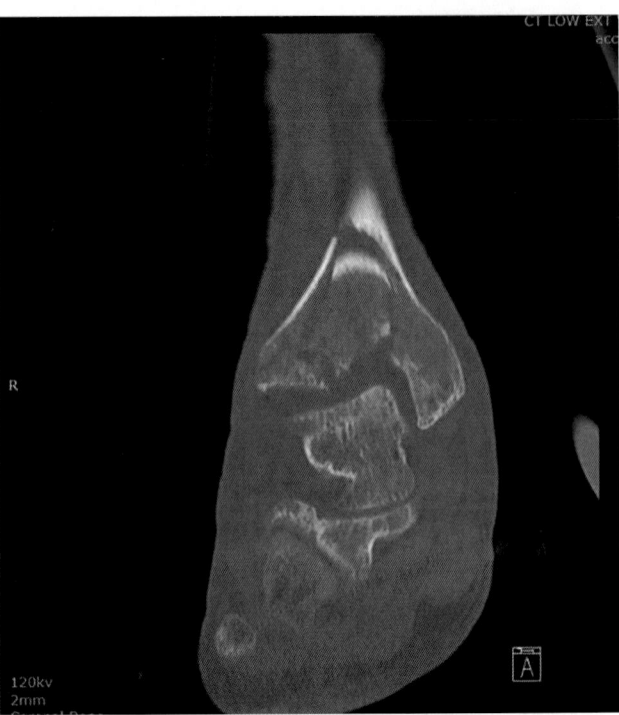

FIGURE 36.14 Case study A: significant impaction of the tibial plafond is noted on the preoperative CT scan, which was performed after application of the delta frame.

large impacted central fragment and a significant posterior malleolus fragment. The anterolateral fragment appeared to be still attached to the distal fibula by the intact anterior inferior syndesmotic ligament. A plan for staged fixation of the patient's fracture was established, with the goal of first stabilizing the posterior aspect of the tibial plafond as well as the fibula fracture through a posterolateral incision. The second portion of the staged care plan involved a return to the operating room 1 week later for fixation of the anterolateral portion of the patient's distal tibia fracture through an anterior midline incision.

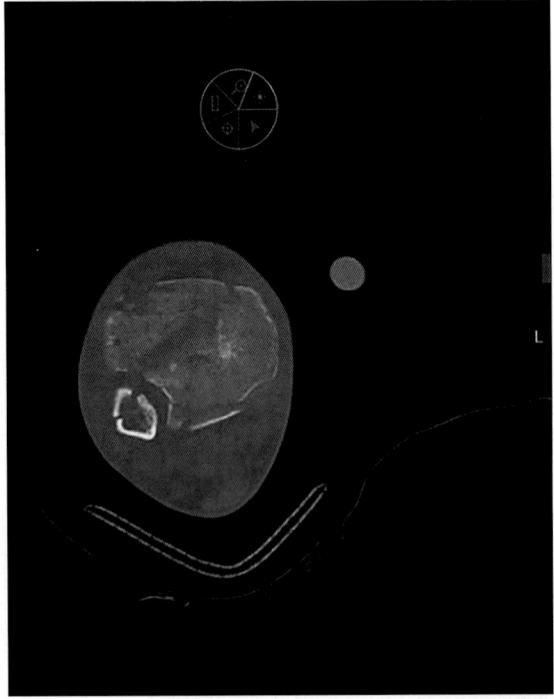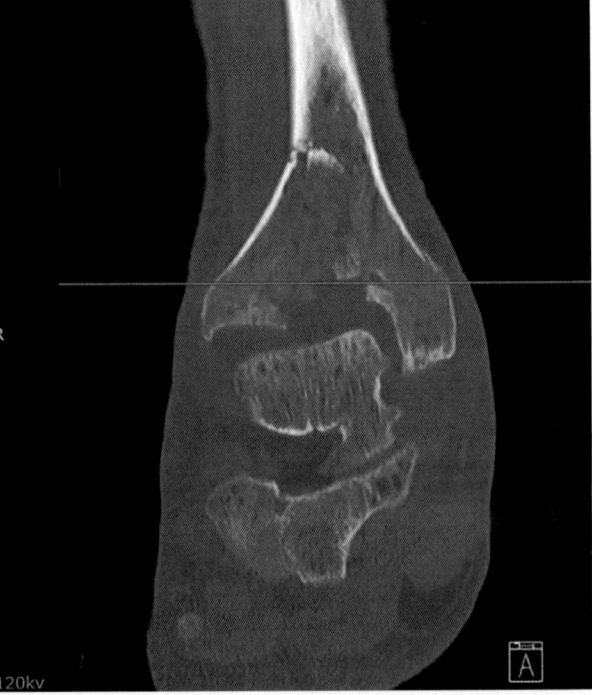

FIGURE 36.15 Case study A: significant impaction of the tibial plafond is noted on the preoperative CT scan, which was performed after application of the delta frame.

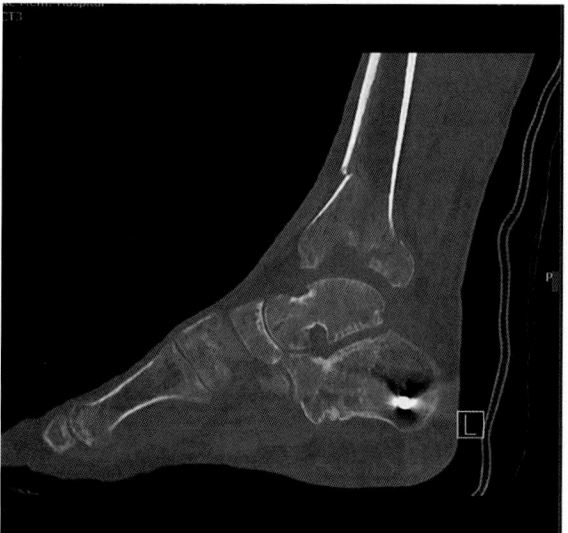
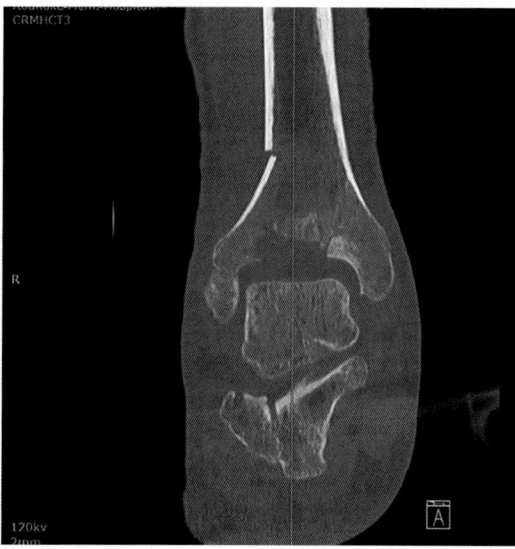

FIGURE 36.16 Case study A: significant impaction of the tibial plafond is noted on the preoperative CT scan, which was performed after application of the delta frame.

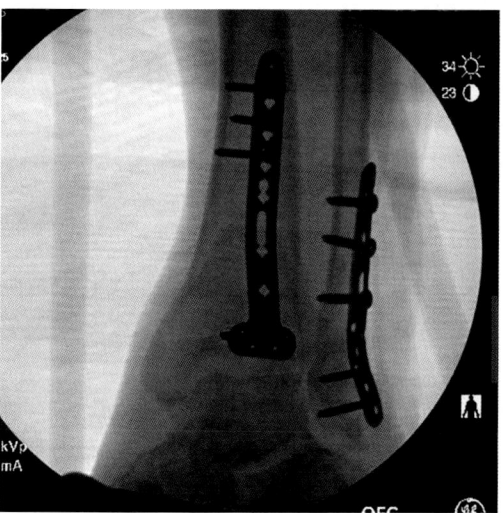
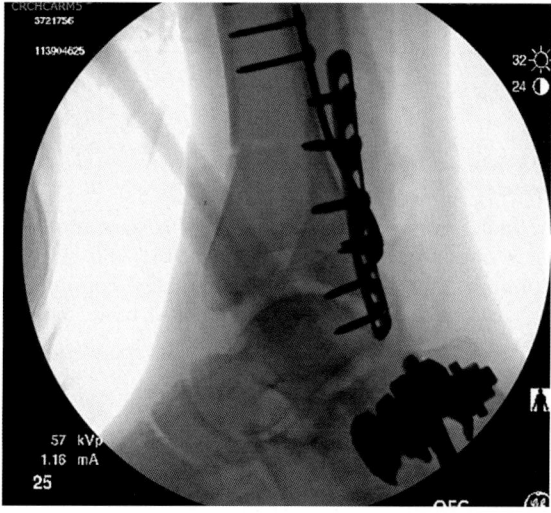

FIGURE 36.17 Case study A: a posterolateral approach was initially used for direct reduction of the posterior fragment using a buttress plate. The fibula was also addressed with a bridge plate during this stage through the same incision.

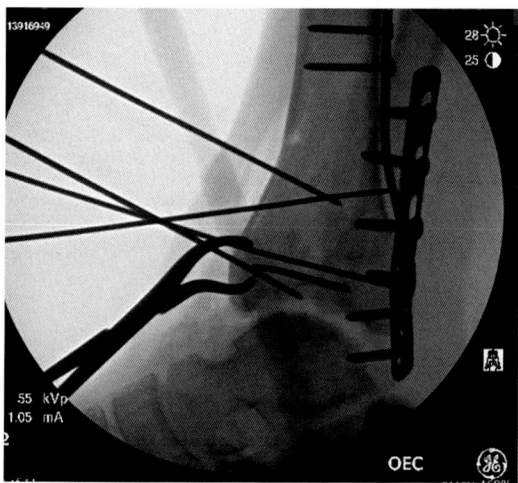
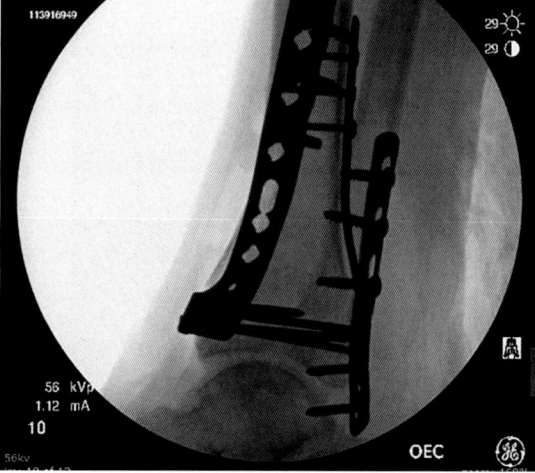

FIGURE 36.18 Case study A: the patient returned to the operating room ~1 week later for management of the anterior portion of the tibial plafond via a straight anterior approach.

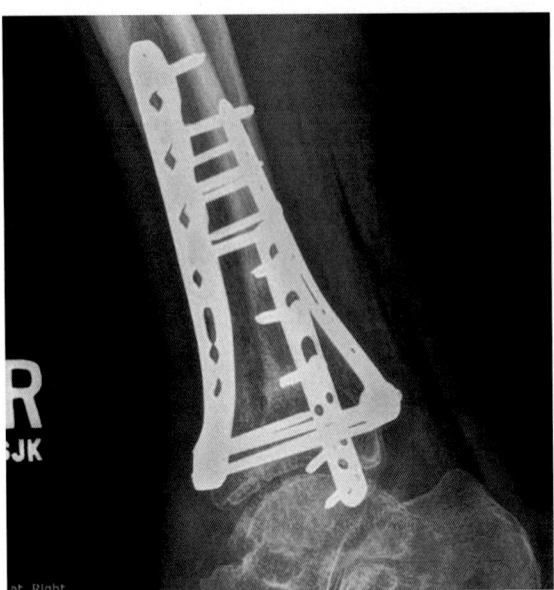
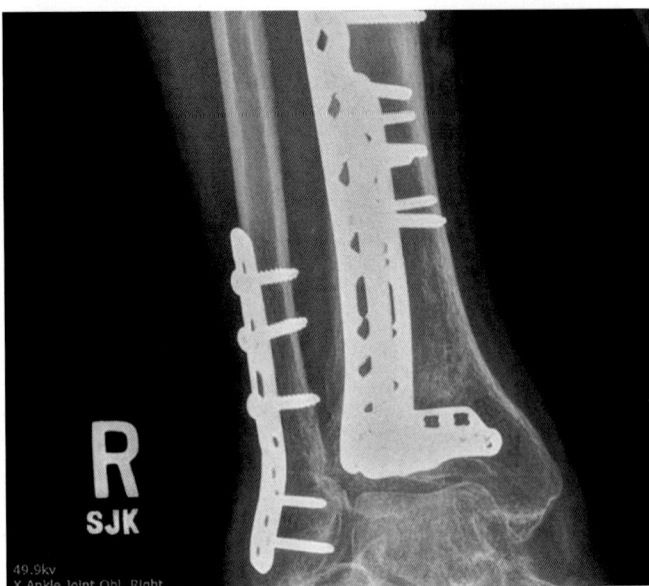

FIGURE 36.19 Case study A: final postoperative AP **(A)** and lateral **(B)** radiographs after a staged management of the open reduction.

CASE STUDY B

A 40-year-old male presented after a fall from a rooftop with significant comminution of the distal tibia and fibula. In addition to lateral column impaction and comminution, a displaced anterior fragment of cortical bone was observed clinically and radiographically to be impinging upon the skin (Figs. 36.20 through 36.31). During placement of the extra-articular external fixator, it was noted that reduction of the anterior articular fragment was being blocked by the displaced cortical fragment, so a 2-cm incision was made anteriorly to disimpact the displaced fragment.

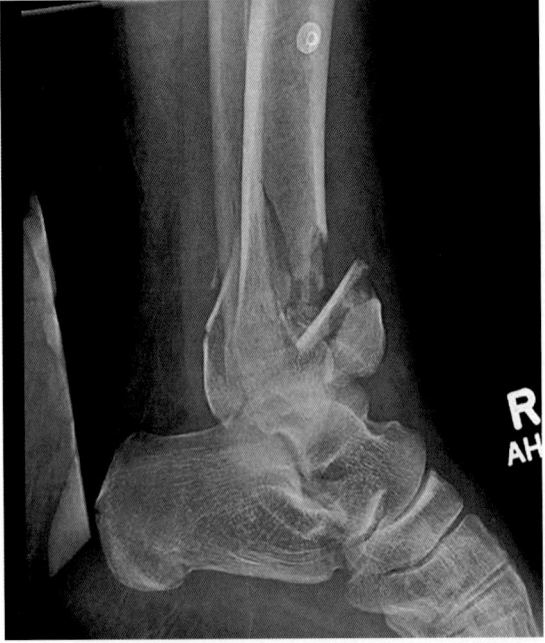

FIGURE 36.20 Case study B: preoperative lateral radiograph demonstrated a displaced cortical fragment that has been flipped out of place.

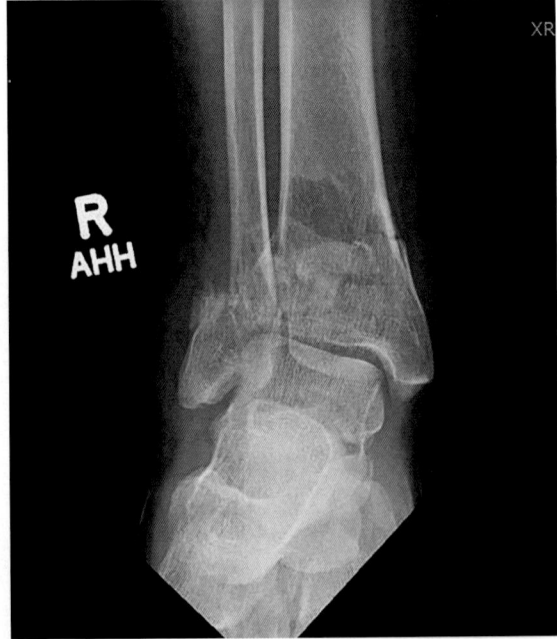

FIGURE 36.21 Case study B: preoperative AP radiograph demonstrated more lateral column comminution and shortening that is consistent with a valgus fracture pattern. This would encourage the use of anterolateral buttress plate in the final fixation construct.

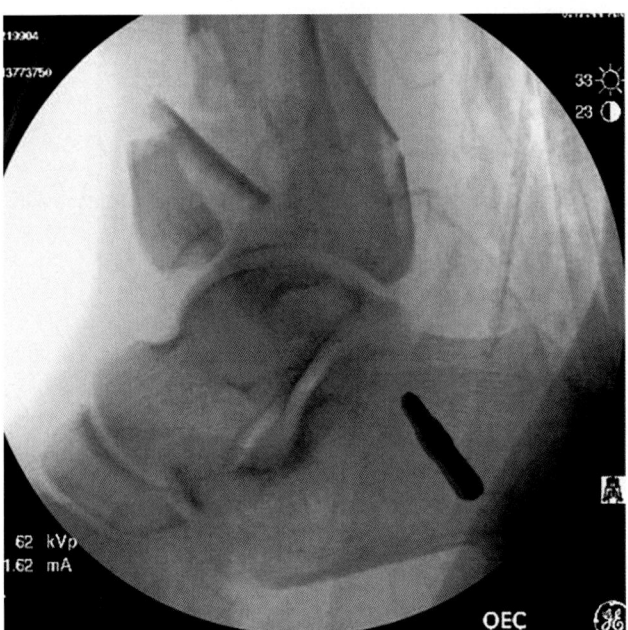

FIGURE 36.22 Case study B: during the application of the delta frame, it was noted that the proximal displaced cortical piece was blocking the reduction of the tibial plafond.

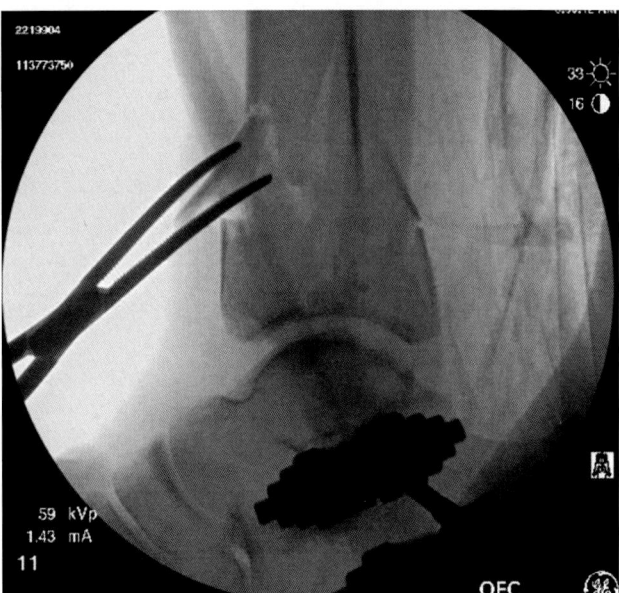

FIGURE 36.23 Case study B: a hemostat was used to manipulate the flipped fragment back into place, which allowed the reduction of the tibial plafond to proceed.

Utilizing fluoroscopic imaging and the open anterior incision, the cortical fragment was manipulated into its appropriate position that allowed reduction of the anterior articular fragment. A subsequent CT scan demonstrated a three-part comminuted fracture with an anterolateral fragment, posterolateral fragment, and a large medial fragment (AO/OTA 43C2). Extensive lateral column comminution was observed, specifically at the anterolateral metaphyseal aspect of tibia and distal fibula. An anterior midline approach was used to expose the ankle joint by extending the incision previously made to dislodge the anteriorly displaced cortical fragment. Inspection of the joint demonstrated a small impacted central articular fragment that was mobilized and reduced back down with direct pressure between the anterolateral and posterolateral fragments. The three main fragments were then reduced to one another with a combination of manual maneuvers and bone reduction forceps. Anatomic reduction was temporarily held with k-wires and interfragmentary lag screws were used to reduce from anterior to posterior in order to fully stabilize the sagittal plane reduction. An anterolateral distal tibia 3.5-mm LCP plate was applied to the bone. The plate was passed from distal to proximal, and preliminarily secured with several wires to hold position, confirmed by C-arm imaging. The plate was secured proximal to the tibia shaft fracture, before being secured distally into the articular block in order to fully stabilize the anterior and posterior components of the fracture. A medial buttress plate was then applied to capture the large medial malleolar fragment. A separate posterolateral incision was used to repair the fibular fracture using a 3.5-mm recon LCP plate during the same procedure.

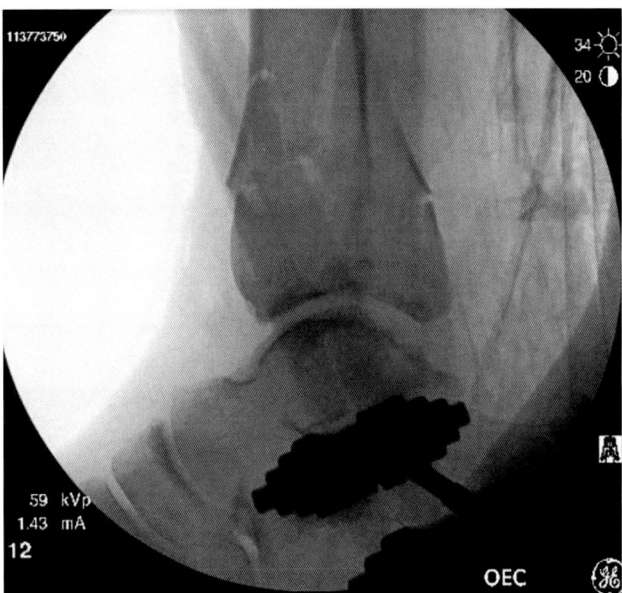

FIGURE 36.24 Case study B: This image captures the articular and cortical reduction post manipulation with hemostat.

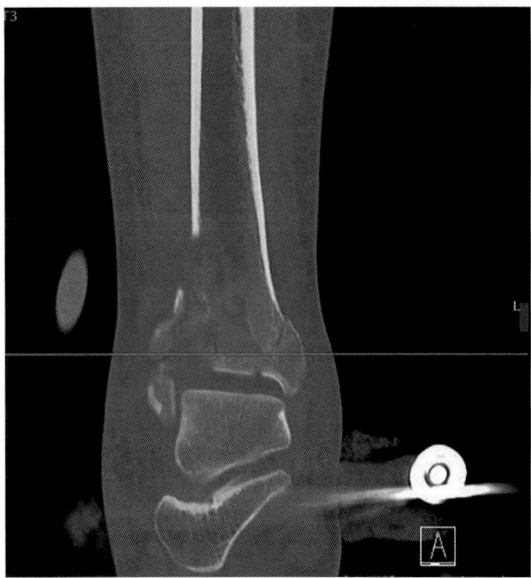
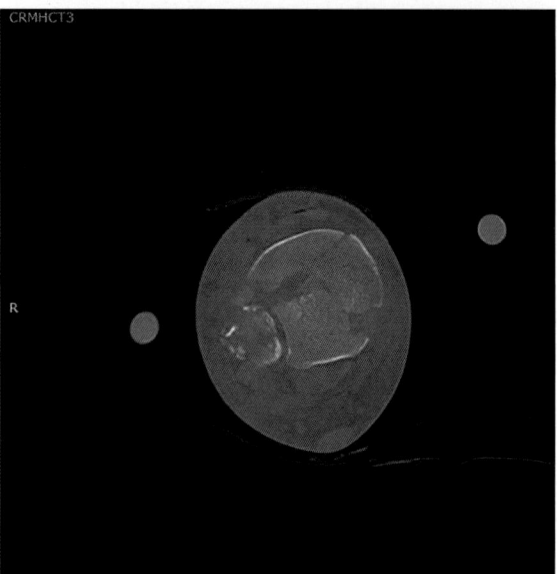

FIGURE 36.25 Case study B: a CT scan obtained after closed reduction and application of a temporizing external fixator is generally more useful for the purposes of identifying the fracture pattern.

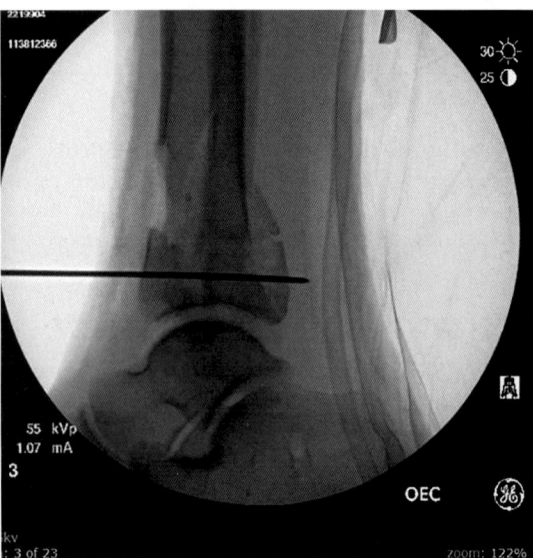
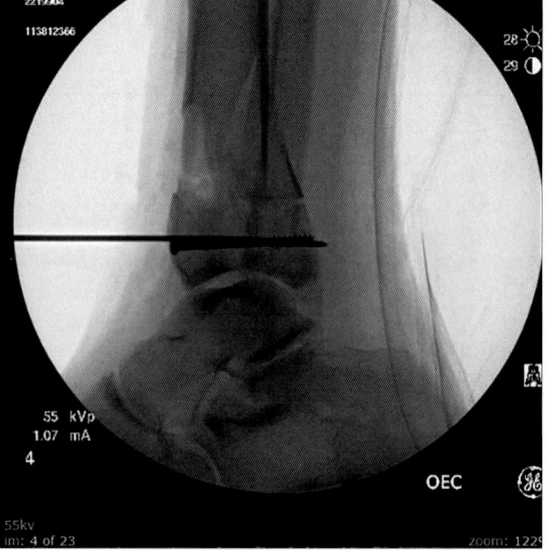

FIGURE 36.26 Case study B: Kirschner wire used to pin the anterior fragment to the posterior fragment.

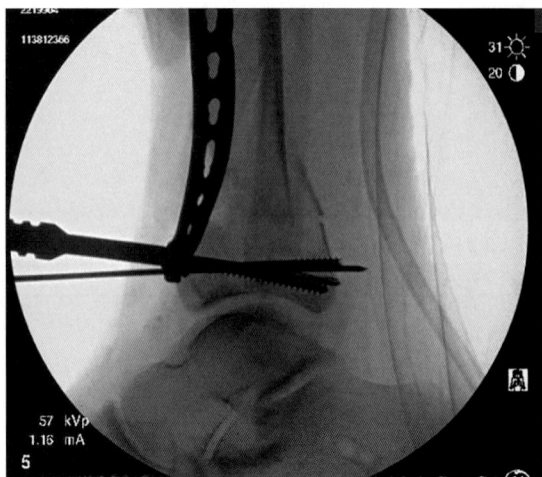
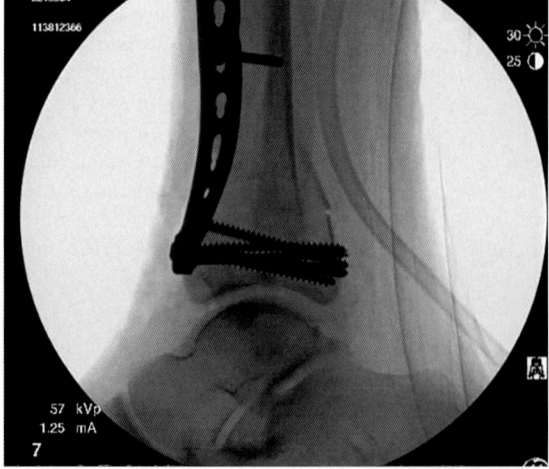

FIGURE 36.27 Case study B: an anterolateral plate was placed, along with a medial buttress plate.

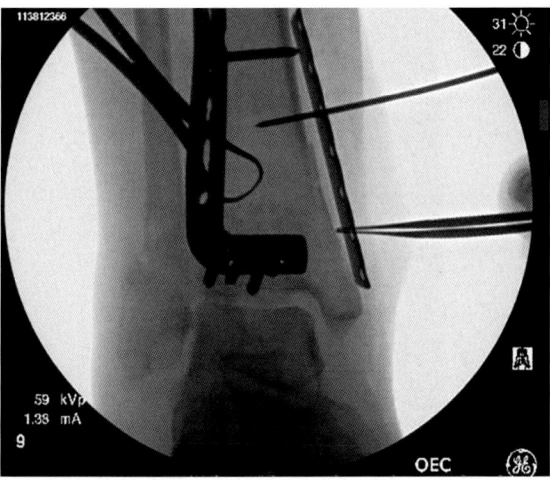 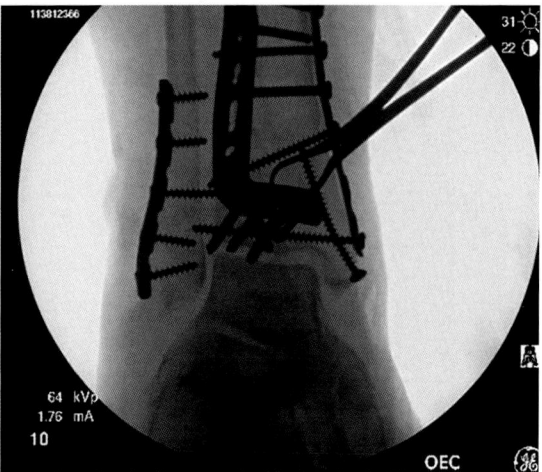

FIGURE 36.28 Case study B: a fibular bridge plate was applied subsequently.

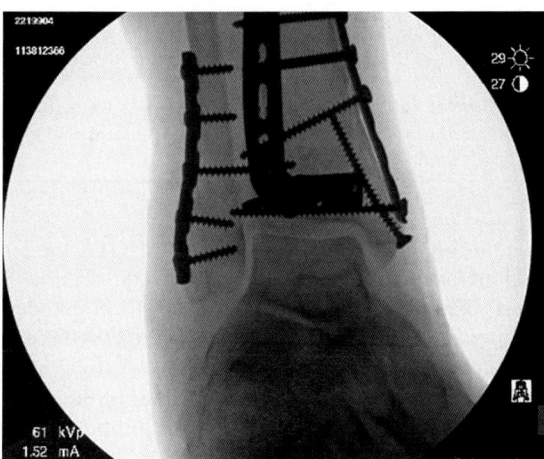 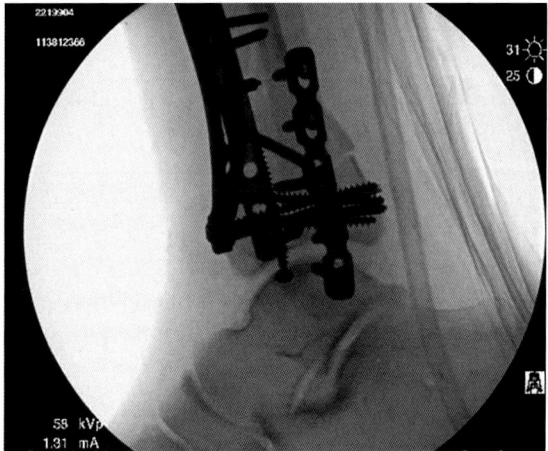

FIGURE 36.29 Case study B: several positional screws were placed from medial to lateral so as to provide additional stability.

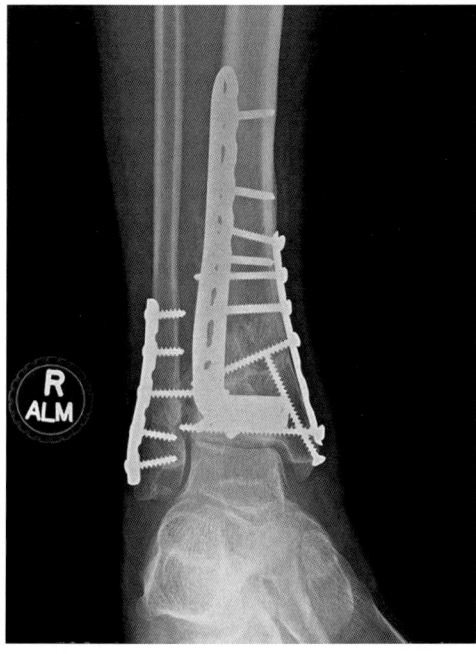 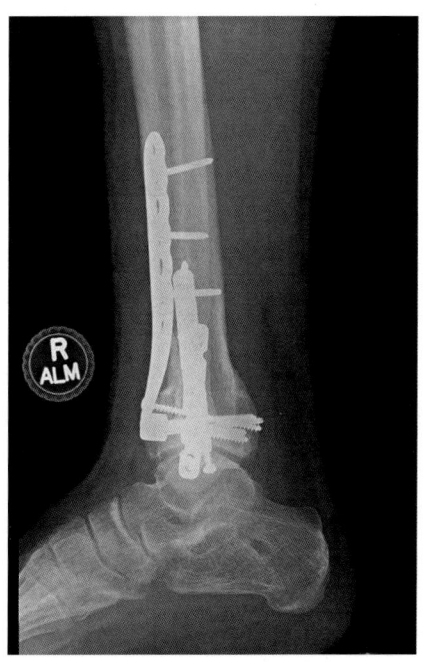

FIGURE 36.30 Case study B: postoperative AP radiograph.   FIGURE 36.31 Case study B: postoperative lateral radiograph.

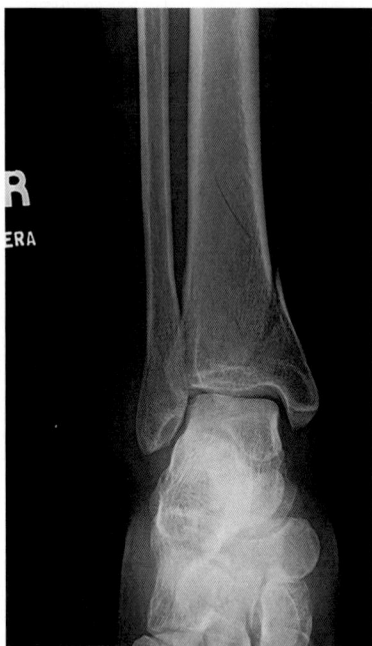

FIGURE 36.32 Case study C: preoperative AP radiograph demonstrates a large medial fragment but the true extent of the comminution and fracture pattern is unclear.

CASE STUDY C

A 32-year-old male with no significant past medical history presented to the emergency department after being struck by a motor vehicle during an altercation with a friend (Figs. 36.32 through 36.49). The plain radiographs revealed significant intra-articular destruction of the tibial plafond without a concomitant fibula injury. The subsequent CT scan demonstrated

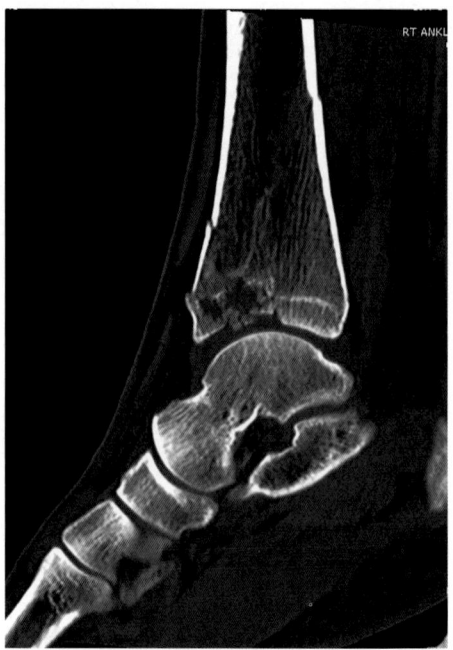

FIGURE 36.34 Case study C: preoperative sagittal CT scan clearly demonstrates impaction and comminution of the anterior tibial plafond.

a comminuted distal tibial fracture (AO/OTA 43C2) with a central impaction extending 2-3 mm into the anterior half of the tibial plafond. A large medial fragment was noted with a vertically oriented fracture pattern that exited the medial metaphysis and communicated with a fracture that extended into the posterior diaphysis. Most of the comminution was noted to be in the anterior aspect of the tibiotalar joint.

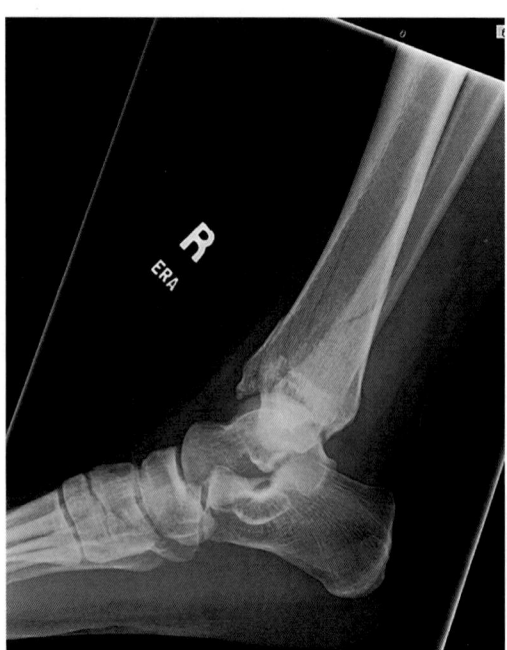

FIGURE 36.33 Case study C: preoperative lateral radiograph.

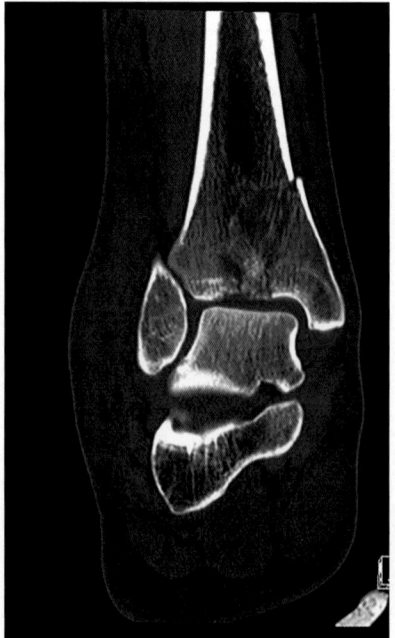

FIGURE 36.36 Case study C: preoperative coronal CT scan with significant medial fragment noted.

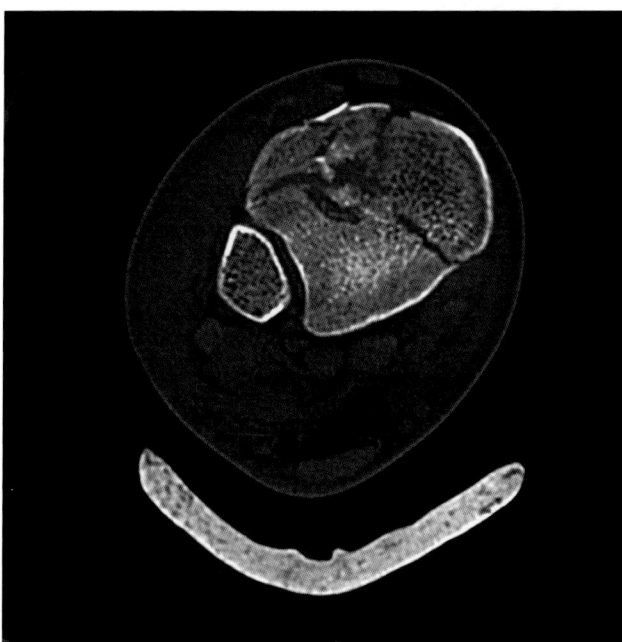

FIGURE 36.36 Case study C: preoperative axial CT scan demonstrating significant anterior comminution of the tibial plafond and confirming the presence of three major fracture lines. Also noted was a largely intact posterior fragment that was later utilized as a backstop to rebuild upon.

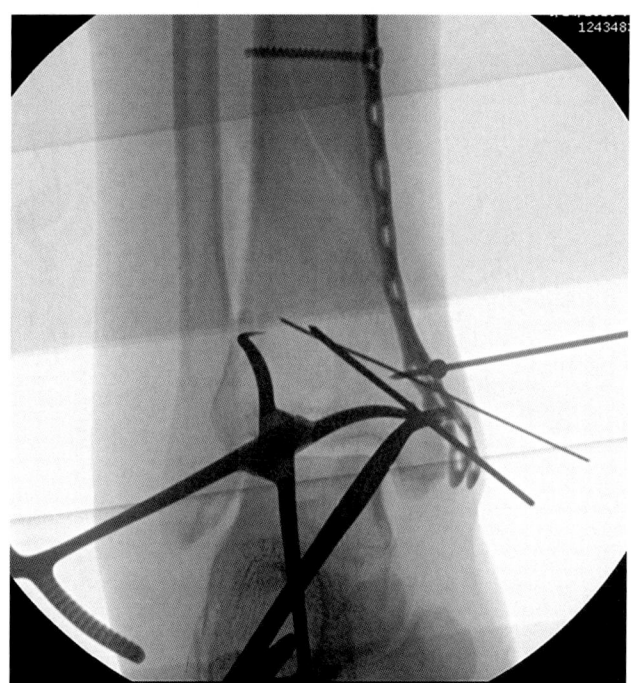

FIGURE 36.38 Case study C: the medial buttress plate was applied to the medial metaphysis via the anterior approach. Screws were placed using a minimally invasive percutaneous technique in order to minimize insult to the soft tissue adjacent to the major anterior incision.

An anterior midline approach was used to expose the ankle joint. The large anterior fragments were carefully removed and placed onto the back table to allow for inspection of the central impacted articular fragments that were subsequently disimpacted and pinned into place with K-wires. Concurrently, the

large medial fragment was reduced through the same anterior approach and pinned with K-wires. A medial buttress plate was inserted through the anterior window and pinned into place while a minimally invasive percutaneous plating technique

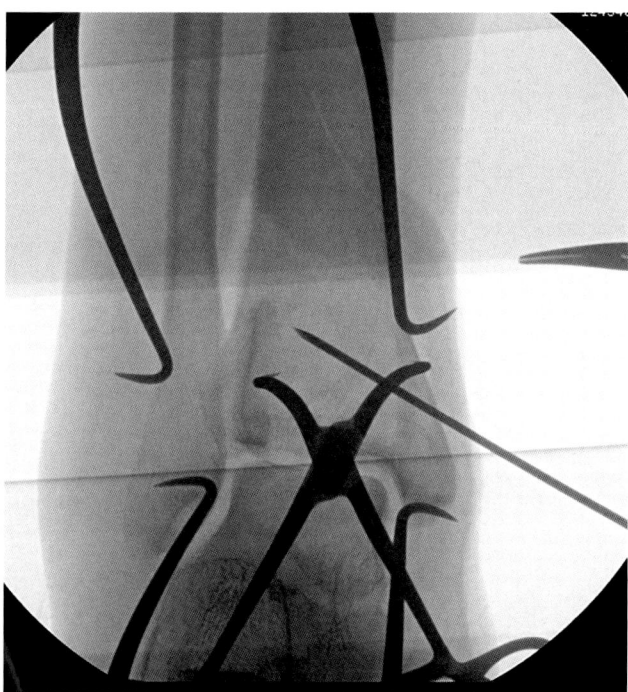

FIGURE 36.37 Case study C: reduction of the medial fragment was performed concurrently with disimpaction of the anterior tibial plafond.

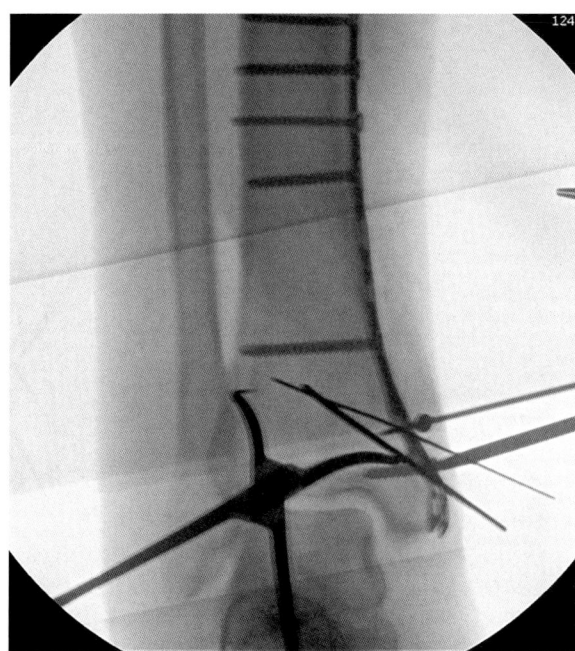

FIGURE 36.39 Case study C: the medial buttress plate was applied to the medial metaphysis via the anterior approach. Screws were placed using a minimally invasive percutaneous technique in order to minimize insult to the soft tissue adjacent to the major anterior incision.

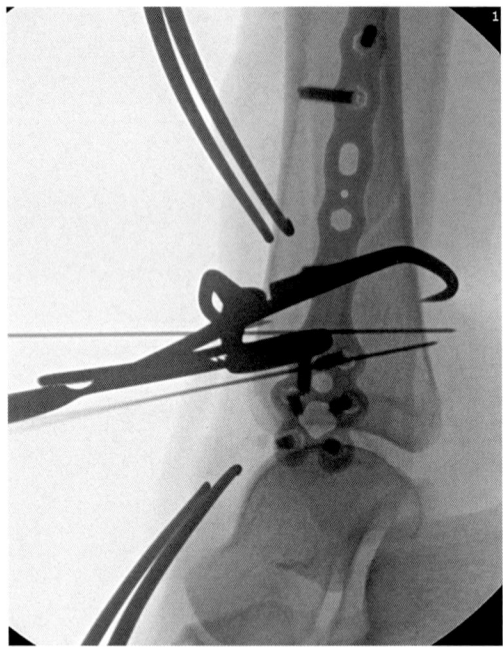

FIGURE 36.40 Case study C: large tenaculum clamp utilized to assist Kirschner wires used for temporizing fixation of the comminuted fragments prior to application of the 1.8-mm anterior bridge plate.

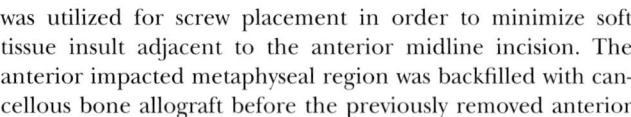

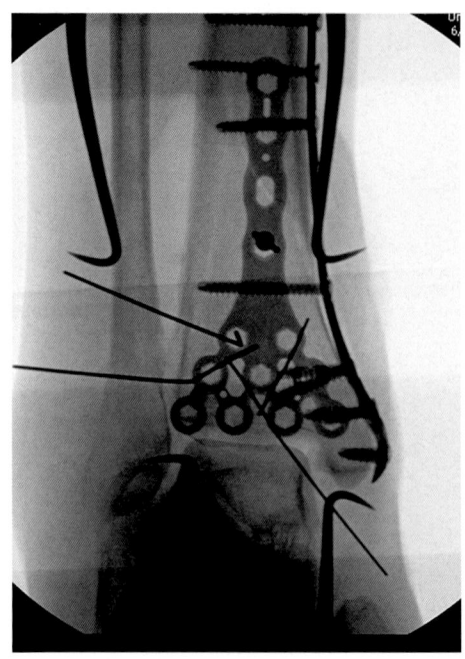

FIGURE 36.42 Case study C: Kirschner wires used for temporizing fixation of the comminuted fragments during application of the 1.8-mm anterior bridge plate.

was utilized for screw placement in order to minimize soft tissue insult adjacent to the anterior midline incision. The anterior impacted metaphyseal region was backfilled with cancellous bone allograft before the previously removed anterior

fragments were placed back into their respective positions and pinned into place. A 1.8-mm thick anterior distal tibial plate was subsequently utilized to span the entirety of the fracture in a bridge plating fashion.

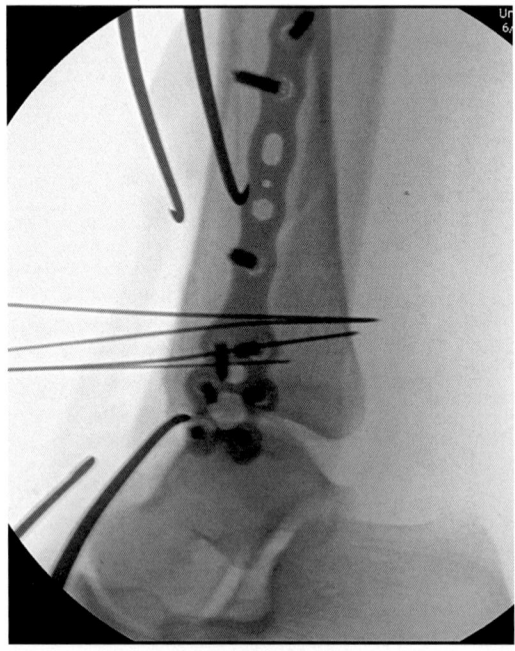

FIGURE 36.41 Case study C: Kirschner wires used for temporizing fixation of the comminuted fragments prior to application of the 1.8-mm anterior bridge plate.

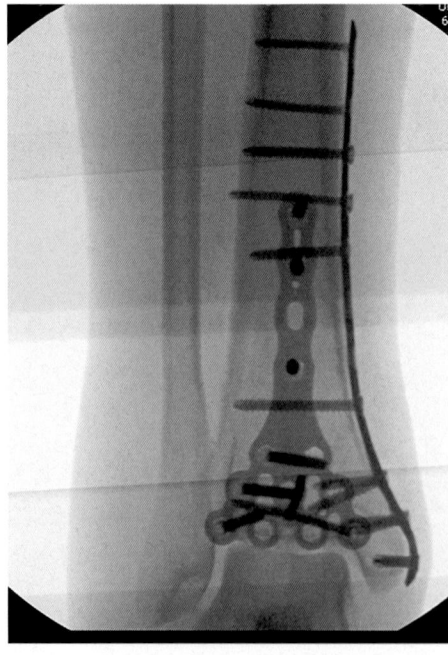

FIGURE 36.43 Case study C: final intraoperative AP view.

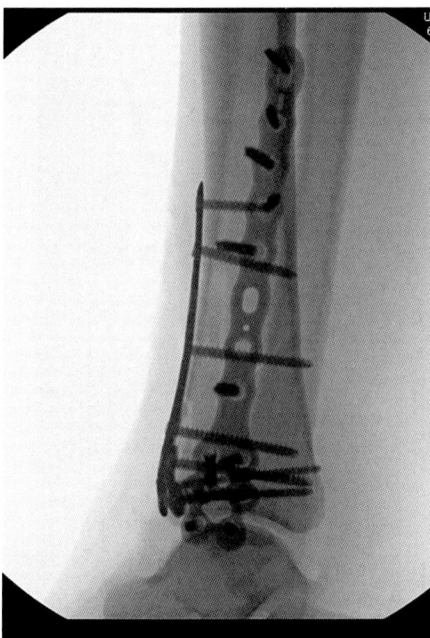

FIGURE 36.44 Case study C: final intraoperative lateral view.

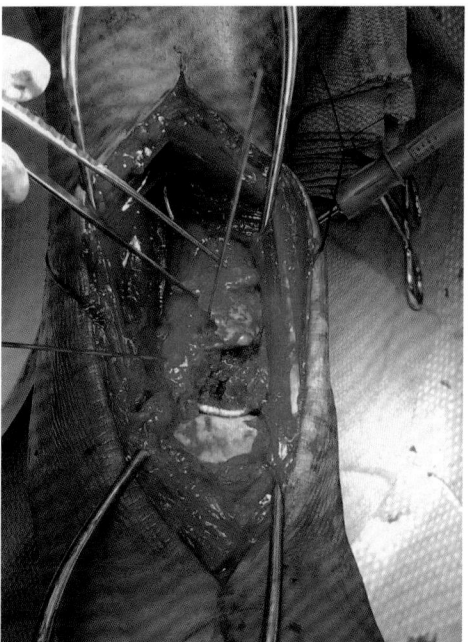

FIGURE 36.46 Case study C: anterior approach with the anterior distal tibial fragments removed in order to access the joint for direct reduction of the impacted pieces. Subsequently, the anterior distal fragments were replaced and temporarily pinned into place, utilizing the stable posterior piece as a backstop.

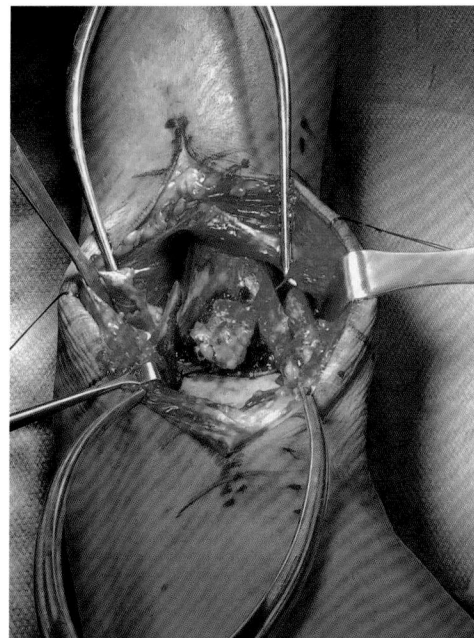

FIGURE 36.45 Case study C: anterior approach with extensive comminution of the anterior tibial plafond directly visualized.

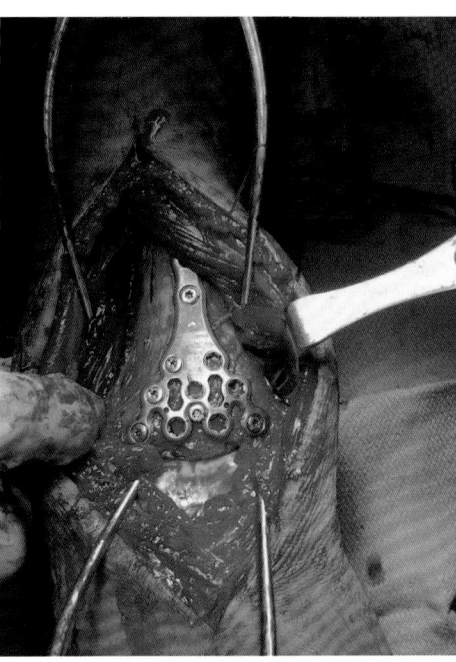

FIGURE 36.47 Case study C: spanning anterior bridge plate was placed over the distal tibial metaphysis with medial buttress plate also in view.

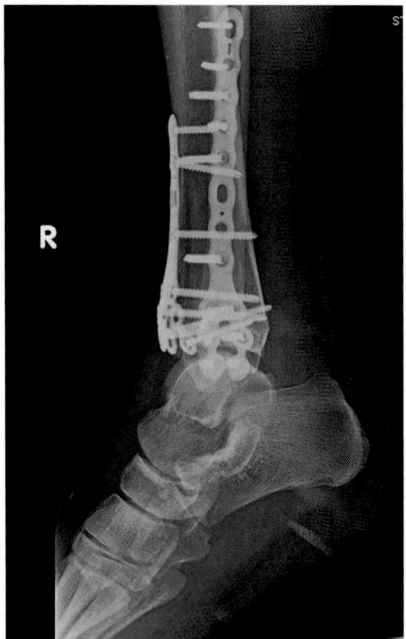

FIGURE 36.48 Case study C: final lateral view.

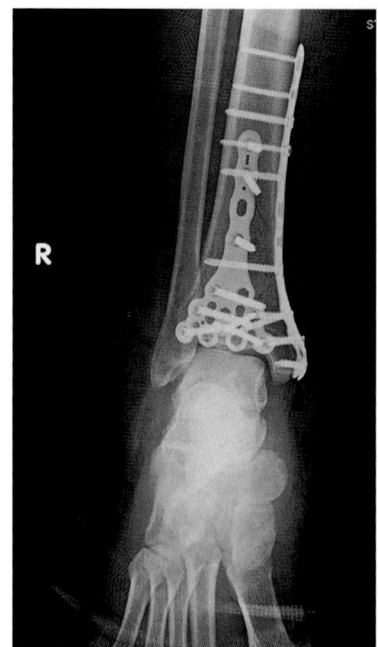

FIGURE 36.49 Case study C: final AP view.

REFERENCES

1. Destot E. *Traumatismes du pied et rayone x malleoles, astragale, calcaneum, avant-pied.* France: Massin; 1911.
2. Szyszkkowitz R, Reschauer R, Segel W. Pilon fractures of the tibia. In: Chapman MW, ed. *Operative Orthopaedics.* Philadelphia, PA: JB Lippincott; 1988:461-470.
3. Bonin JG. *Injuries to the Ankle.* London, UK: William Heinemann; 1950:248-260.
4. Jergesen F. Fractures of the ankle. *Am J Surg.* 1959;98:136.
5. Bourne RB, Rorabeck CH, Macnab J. Intra-articular fractures of the distal tibia: the pilon fracture. *J Trauma.* 1983;23(7):591-596. http://www.ncbi.nlm.nih.gov/pubmed/6876212
6. Kellam JF, Waddell JP. Fractures of the distal tibial metaphysis with intra-articular extension—the distal tibial explosion fracture. *J Trauma.* 1979;19(8):593-601. doi: 10.1097/00005373-197908000-00007
7. Sitnik A, Beletsky A, Schelkun S. Intra-articular fractures of the distal tibia. *EFORT Open Rev.* 2017;2(8):991-996. http://www.efortopenreviews.com/content/2/8/352
8. Rüedi T. Fractures of the lower end of the tibia into the ankle joint: results 9 years after open reduction and internal fixation. *Injury.* 1973;5(2):130-134. doi: 10.1016/S0020-1383(73)80089-0.
9. Teeny S, Wiss DA, Hathaway R, Sarmiento A. Tibial plafond fractures: errors, complications, and pitfalls in operative treatment. *J Orthop Trauma.* 1990;4(2):215.
10. McFerran MA, Smith SW, Boulas HJ, Schwartz HS. Complications encountered in the treatment of pilon fractures. *J Orthop Trauma.* 1992;6(2):195-200. doi: 10.1097/00005131-199206000-00011.
11. Ruedi TP, Murphy WM. *AO Principles of Fracture Management.* New York, NY: AO Publishing; 2000.
12. Lauge-Hansen N. Fractures of the ankle. *Arch Surg.* 1948;56:250.
13. Tomás-Hernández J. High-energy pilon fractures management: state of the art. *EFORT Open Rev.* 2017;1(10):354-361. www.efort.org/openreviews
14. Ho B, Ketz J. Primary arthrodesis for tibial pilon fractures. *Foot Ankle Clin North Am.* 2017;22:147-161.
15. Wheeless C. Tibial plafond fracture. http://www.wheelessonline.com/ortho/tibial_plafond_fracture. Accessed February 10, 2019.
16. Tang X, Tang P, Wang M, et al. Pilon fractures: a new classification and therapeutic strategies. *Chin Med J (Engl).* 2012;125(14):2487-2492.
17. Malige A, Yeazell S, Nwachuku C. Surgical fixation of pilon injuries: a comparison of the anterolateral and posterolateral approach. *Arch Orthop Trauma Surg.* 2019;139(9):1179-1185. doi: 10.1007/s00402-019-03145-3.
18. Cannada LK. The no-touch approach for operative treatment of pilon fractures to minimize soft tissue complications. *Orthopedics.* 2010;33(10):734-738. doi: 10.3928/01477447-20100826-16.
19. Carr JB. Surgical techniques useful in the treatment of complex periarticular fractures of the lower extremity. *Orthop Clin North Am.* 1965;25:613-624.
20. Pierce FO, Heinrich JH. Comminuted intra-articular fractures of the distal tibia. *J Trauma.* 1979;19:828-832.
21. Barei D, Nork S, Bellabarba C, Sangeorzan B. Is the absence of an ipsilateral fibular fracture predictive of increased radiographic tibial pilon fracture severity? *J Orthop Trauma.* 2006;20(1):6-10.
22. Wei S, Han F, Lan S, Cai X. Surgical treatment of pilon fracture based on ankle position at the time of injury/initial direction of fracture displacement: a prospective cohort study. *Int J Surg.* 2014;12:418-425.
23. Karas EH, Weiner LS. Displaced pilon fractures. *Orthop Clin North Am.* 1994;25:651-663
24. Tornetta PD, Weiner L, Bergman M, et al. Pilon fractures: treatment with combined internal and external fixation. *J Orthop Trauma.* 1993;7:489-496.
25. Topliss C, Jackson M, Atkins R. Anatomy of pilon fractures of the distal tibia. *J Bone Joint Surg.* 2005;87-B:692-697.
26. Assal M. Techniques d'osteosynthese des fractures du tibia distal chez l'adulte. *Rev Chir Orthop Rep L'appareil Moteur.* 2008;94S:S224-S230.
27. Ruedi TP, Allowger M. The operative treatment of intra-articular fractures of the lower end of the tibia. *Clin Orthop.* 1979;138:105-110.
28. Saleh M, Shanahan MDG, Fern ED. Intra-articular fractures of the distal tibia: surgical management by limited internal fixation and articulated distraction. *Injury.* 1993;24:37-40.
29. Blauth M, Bastian L, Krettek C, et al. Surgical options for the treatment of severe tibial pilon fractures: a study of three techniques. *J Orthop Trauma.* 2001;15:153-160.
30. Wyrsch B, McErran MA, McAndrew M, et al. Operative treatment of fractures of the tibial plafond. A randomized, prospective study. *J Bone Joint Surg Am.* 1996;78:1646-1657.
31. Helfet DL, Shonnard PY, Levine D, et al. Minimally invasive plate osteosynthesis of distal tibial fractures. *Injury.* 1997;28(suppl 1):42-48.
32. Rhinelander FW. Tibial blood supply in relation to fracture healing. *Clin Orthop.* 1974;105:34-81. doi: 10.1097/00003086-197411000-00005.
33. Collinge C, Sanders R, DiPasquale T. Percutaneous plating in the lower extremity. *J Am Acad Orthop Surg.* 2000;8:211-216.
34. Sirkin M, Sanders R, DiPasquale T, Herscovici D. A staged protocol for soft tissue management in the treatment of complex pilon fractures. *J Orthop Trauma.* 1999;13(2):S32-S38.
35. Varella CD, Vaughan KT, Carr JB, et al. Fracture blisters: clinical and pathologic aspects. *J Orthop Trauma.* 1993;7:417-427.
36. Mehta S, Gardner MJ, Barei DP, Benirschke SK, Nork SE. Reduction strategies through the anterolateral exposure for fixation of type B and C pilon fractures. *J Orthop Trauma.* 2011;25(2):116-122. doi: 10.1097/BOT.0b013e3181cf00f3.
37. Ketz J, Sanders R. Staged posterior tibial plating for the treatment of orthopaedic trauma association 43C2 and 43C3 tibial pilon fractures. *J Orthop Trauma.* 2012;26(6):341-347.
38. Pugh KJ, Wolinsky PR, McAndrew MP, et al. Tibial pilon fractures: a comparison of treatment methods. *J Trauma.* 1999;47:937-941.
39. Dunbar RP, Barei DP, Kubiak EN, et al. Early limited internal fixation of diaphyseal extensions in select pilon fractures: upgrading AO/OTA type C fracture to AO/OTA type B. *J Orthop Trauma.* 2008;22:426-429.
40. Busel G, Watson J, Israel H. Evaluation of fibular fracture type vs location of tibial fixation on pilon fractures. *Foot Ankle Int.* 2017;38(6):650-655.
41. Assal M, Ray A, Stern M. Strategies for surgical approaches in open reduction internal fixation of pilon fractures. *J Orthop Trauma.* 2015;29(2):69-79.
42. Liu J, Smith C, White E, Ebraheim N. A systematic review of the role of surgical approaches on the outcomes of the tibia pilon fracture. *Foot Ankle Spec.* 2016;9(2):163-168.
43. Bhattacharya T, Chrichlow R, Gobezie R, Kim E, Vrahas M. Complications associated with the posterolateral approach for pilon fractures. *J Orthop Trauma.* 2006;20:104-107.

44. Hickerson L, Verbeek D, Klinger C, Helfet D. Anterolateral approach to the pilon. *J Orthop Trauma.* 2016;30(8, suppl):S39-S40.

45. Bonao LJ, Edwards ER, Gosling CM, Hau R, Hofstee D, Shuen A, Gabbe B. Patient reported health related quality of life early outcomes at 12 months after surgically managed tibial plafond fracture. *Injury.* 2017;48:946-953.

46. Graves ML, Porter SE, Fagan BC, et al. Is obesity protective against wound healing complications in pilon surgery? Soft tissue envelope and pilon fractures in the obese. *Orthopedics.* 2010;33(8).

47. Bostman OM. Bodyweight related to loss of reduction of fractures of the distal tibia and ankle. *J Bone Joint Surg Br.* 1995;77(1):101-103.

48. Strauss EJ, Frank JB, Walsh M, Koval KJ, Egol KA. Does obesity influence the outcome after the operative treatment of ankle fractures? *J Bone Joint Surg Br.* 2007;89(6):794-798.

49. Howard J, Agel J, Barei D, et al. A prospective study evaluating incision placement and wound healing for tibial plafond fractures. *J Orthop Trauma.* 2008;22:299-304.

50. Harris AM, Patterson BM, Sontich JK, Vallier HA. Results and outcomes after operative treatment of high-energy tibial plafond fractures. *Foot Ankle Int.* 2006;27(4):256-265.

51. De-la-Heras-Romero J, Lledo-Alvarez A, Lizaur-Utrilla A, Lopez-Prats F. Quality of life and prognostic factors after intra-articular tibial pilon fracture. *Injury.* 2017;48:1258-1263.

52. Borrelli J Jr, Prickett W, Song E, Becker D, Ricci W. Extraosseous blood supply of the tibia and the effects of different plating techniques: a human cadaveric study. *J Orthop Trauma.* 2002;16(10):691-695. doi: 10.1097/00005131-200211000-00002.

53. Giebel GD, Meyer C, Koebke J, Giebel G. The arterial supply of the ankle joint and its importance for the operative fracture treatment. *Surg Radiol Anat.* 1997;19(4):231-235. doi: 10.1007/s00276-997-0231-3.

CHAPTER 37

Supramalleolar Osteotomies

Shannon M. Rush and Eric Shi

DEFINITION

Supramalleolar osteotomies were first described in 1936 by Speed and Boyd,[1] orthopedic surgeons who pioneered work in lower leg realignment surgeries in patients with posttraumatic deformities. Further progress was made by Russian surgeons Dzakhov and Kurochkin[2] in 1966 and Barskii and Semenov in 1979.[3] Takakura et al.[4] in 1995 were the first to report functional outcomes in patients who underwent supramalleolar osteotomies. Their work found good short-term and midterm results for pain relief, functional improvement, and return to sports and recreation activities.

Realignment osteotomy of the distal tibia is a valuable surgical procedure for the treatment of distal tibial malalignment resulting from posttraumatic malunion, physeal disturbances, congenital and metabolic diseases, and degenerative arthritis.[1-11] Juxta-articular malalignment of the distal tibia often results in hindfoot and forefoot compensation, which creates predictable patterns of joint degeneration and pain.

However, small degrees of malalignment are generally well tolerated if there is no associated stiffness or arthritis in the hindfoot.[1,2] The primary goal of the supramalleolar osteotomy (SMO) is to preserve the joints of the foot and ankle from articular degeneration and biomechanical dysfunction by realigning the hindfoot and, specifically, the spatial relationship between the talus and the tibia in order to restore normal ankle biomechanics and normalize load distribution within the ankle joint. Lastly, these procedures may serve a secondary purpose of improving postural or suprastructural symptoms of the hip, knee, and spine during gait. The absolute magnitude of necessary deformity to indicate an SMO is not clear and must be taken in the context of clinical condition.

INDICATIONS AND PITFALLS

INDICATIONS

- Tibial fracture malunion
- Ankle arthrodesis malunion
- Realignment in conjunction with total ankle replacement
- Physeal disturbances
- Congenital and metabolic diseases (rheumatoid ankle, hemophilic arthropathy, paralytic deformity)
- Asymmetric ankle osteoarthritis with angular deformity

PHYSICAL EXAMINATION

The components of the clinical evaluation include history, physical, and diagnostic testing. Although the historical features may seem irrelevant with regard to the surgical plan, some events may have importance. Events such as open fracture injuries, multiple surgical procedures, delayed healing of the soft tissue envelope, suprastructural symptoms, and others may prompt the surgeon to alter the surgical plan accordingly. These alterations may include incision placement, soft tissue coverage, fixation, osteotomy location and configuration, and whether to stage the correction or perform in a single session.

The physical examination is of the utmost importance in determining the surgical plan. In addition to the usual lower extremity examination, several additional features must be evaluated.

- *Rotational malalignment*—in particular, the *femoral foot angle* or *transmalleolar axis* should be assessed and compared with the opposite side. It is natural to strive for a normal relationship, but the contralateral limb should be considered the benchmark if there is no history of trauma or other condition that may have impacted the femoral foot relationship. There may be interval segmental rotational malalignments as well, which should be accounted for in the ultimate osteotomy.
- *Limb length inequality* should be determined. The surgeon should remember that the ultimate goals are to create a plantigrade foot and to lessen the compensatory demands of the affected extremity.
- *A complete muscle inventory* is important to ensure previous trauma or periarticular fibrosis has not diminished motor function to any significant degree.
- *Gait analysis* may often unmask subtle compensatory maneuvers as well as provide an overall assessment of the locomotion. Compensatory gait patterns such as pelvic tilt and recurvatum of the knee become evident during gait evaluation.
- The *subtalar joint* must be closely examined when planning a correctional osteotomy. Adaptive compensation for a distal tibial deformity may have resulted in degenerative arthrosis and stiffness in the hindfoot. On the contrary, frontal plane corrective osteotomies of the distal tibia may realign the ankle joint but unmask adaptive deformity in the subtalar joint, which may be poorly tolerated due to this stiffness or arthrosis.
- *Diagnostic injections* are a useful adjunct to range of motion and radiographic evaluation and can be useful to sort out the genesis of painful arthrosis.

PATHOGENESIS

Malposition of the distal tibiofibular complex can have significant functional and biomechanical consequences. These problems include accelerated focal wear of the articular surfaces of the foot and ankle and abnormal gait patterns.[12,13] There is no consensus regarding the degree of distal tibial malalignment and the potential for development of symptomatic arthritis. The degree to which the deformity influences clinical symptoms and function depends on several factors. The degree of motion in the subtalar and midtarsal joint, size of individual, severity of index injury, intra-articular fracture patterns, articular incongruity, and age all contribute to the clinical effects of the deformity. The available amount of motion in the subtalar joint is not precisely understood and can vary considerably between patients.[14,15] Paley[16] believes 30 degrees of ankle valgus and 15 degrees of ankle varus can be compensated for with a normal functioning subtalar joint. Distal tibial valgus deformity is better compensated than distal tibial varus deformity because twice as much inversion exists in the subtalar joint than eversion.

There are several etiologies that lead to a pathologic hindfoot where supramalleolar osteotomies are indicated:

- *Uncompensated subtalar joint*—when the distal tibial deformity exceeds the available frontal plane compensation in the subtalar joint, several clinical scenarios develop. When the amount of ankle varus deformity exceeds the available subtalar eversion, residual hindfoot varus deformity results. This condition creates additional forefoot pronation to maintain a plantargrade foot. The opposite occurs when a distal tibial valgus deformity is incompletely compensated with subtalar joint inversion. Complicating this condition is the progressive development of degenerative stiffness in the subtalar joint and inability to compensate for distal tibial deformity.
- *Alteration in tibiotalar contact pressures*—Tarr et al.[12] showed distal tibial deformity significantly altered the contact location, shape, and magnitude of the tibiotalar contact pressures. Sagittal plane malalignment created the most significant alterations in contact characteristics. Recurvatum (shear deformity) and procurvatum (impingement deformity) of 15 degrees resulted in changes in contact biomechanics of >40%. These cadaver studies showed how deformity near the ankle joint can focus contact pressure to small areas of the articular surface. This could explain why deformity is initially well tolerated in the distal tibia and often presents only later when painful degenerative articular wear patterns begin in the ankle and subtalar joint.
- *History of distal tibia fracture*—Kristensen and colleagues[17] looked at patients with history of distal tibia fracture with >10 degrees of malunion and found that many patients were asymptomatic and none had limitations of ankle motion. Their patients had no signs of ankle arthrosis 20 years after injury.
- *Dysfunctional flatfoot with hindfoot valgus associated with ankle valgus deformity*—This poorly compensated ankle and hindfoot valgus will predictably lead to posterior tibial tendon dysfunction and deltoid ligament failure over time. Understanding the influence of malalignment of the distal tibia and hindfoot is critical to understanding the importance of realignment osteotomy. The foot and ankle surgeon can use these techniques to restore axis alignment and joint orientation and secondarily off-load focal degenerative areas of the ankle. The clinical consequence of realignment osteotomy in preserving the tibiotalar joint in the long term is not well documented, although skeletal malalignment must be corrected prior to arthrodesis or implant arthroplasty.
- *Malpositioned ankle arthrodeses* can lead to significant degenerative changes in the subtalar and midtarsal joints with alteration in the ground reactive forces (GRFs) generated in the limb. Fusing the joint with the talus poorly aligned with the axis of the leg will lead to gait problems and forefoot overload. It is preferable in most cases to translate the talus slightly posterior to the tibial axis to alleviate these problems. In addition, sagittal plane malalignment can lead to degeneration of the midtarsal joint and generate recurvatum thrust on the knee. Corrective osteotomy for ankle malunion after arthrodesis is directed at restoring a plantargrade foot and realigning the tibiocalcaneal axis (Fig. 37.1).
- *Growth plate disturbances from fracture or infection* can result in significant secondary deformity. Often, limb length inequality is an additional consideration in these cases, and planning must take excessive shortening into account. McNicol et al.[5] and Scheffer and Peterson[6] demonstrated the use of SMO for congenital deformity in children. McNicol used SMO derotational osteotomy in children with complex equinovarus deformity and external tibial torsion. Scheffer described an opening wedge osteotomy (OWO) to correct deformity and restore length. Best[18] described a small series of four patients who had five opening wedge osteotomies using plate fixation. Autogenous bone was used in all cases, and all osteotomies had healed by 3 months.

IMAGING AND DIAGNOSTIC STUDIES

RADIOGRAPHIC ANALYSIS

Radiographic imaging must include accurate weight-bearing orthogonal projections of the ankle and foot. The importance of positioning of the extremity during the radiographic process cannot be underestimated. Malpositioned or suboptimal technique will spuriously alter the apparent deformity and surgical plan accordingly.

- The *anteroposterior* (AP) and *lateral* projections help determine the type and degree of deformity in all cardinal body planes. The center of the ankle joint relative to the long axis of the tibia is determined by subtending the mid-diaphyseal line from the distal tibia through the talus. In the normal ankle, the mid-diaphyseal line should pass through the center of the talus. On the lateral projection, the mid-diaphyseal line should pass through the superior talar dome and lateral process (Fig. 37.2).
- The *lateral distal tibial angle* (LDTA) (89 ± 3 degrees) and the *anterior distal tibial angle* (ADTA) (80 ± 2 degrees)[16] (Fig. 37.2) are joint orientation angles.

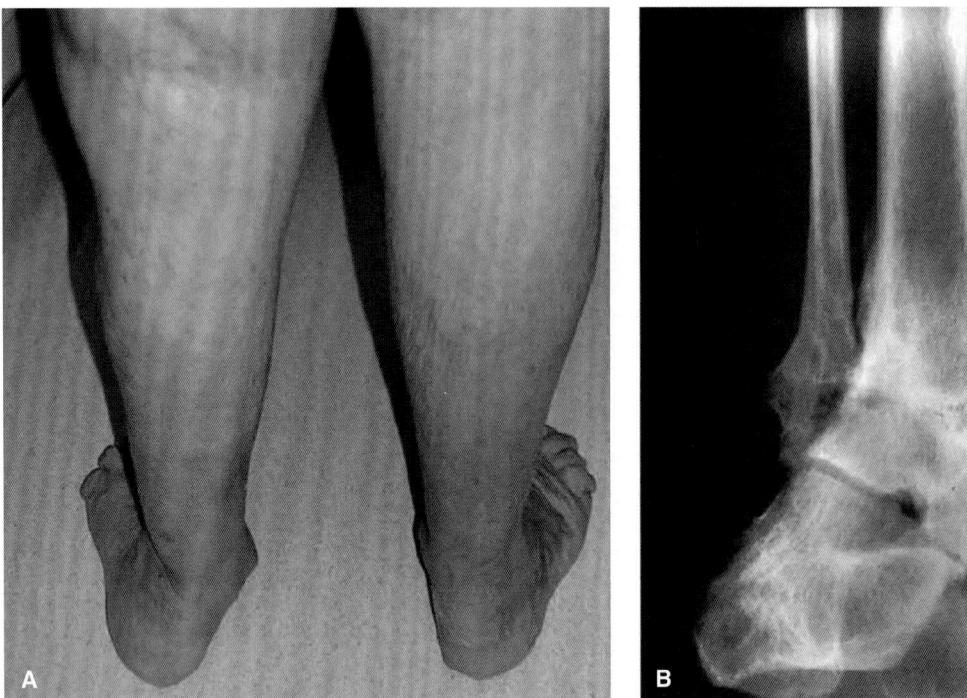

FIGURE 37.1 **A.** clinical photo shows left ankle in valgus position. **B.** left ankle radiograph shows a malunited ankle in valgus.

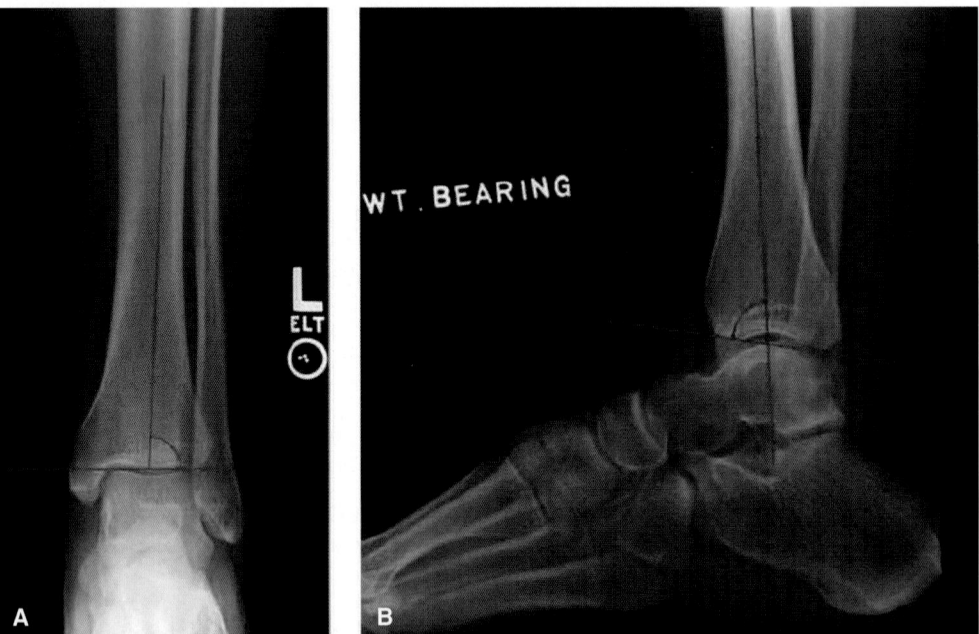

FIGURE 37.2 The center of the ankle joint relative to the long axis of the tibia is determined by subtending the mid-diaphyseal line from the distal tibia, through the talus. **A.** In the normal ankle, the mid-diaphyseal line should pass through the center of the talus. **B.** On the lateral projection, the mid-diaphyseal line should pass through the lateral process of the talus. The LDTA (89 ± 3 degrees) and the ADTA (80 ± 2 degrees) are formed with the tangent to the tibial plafond.[19]

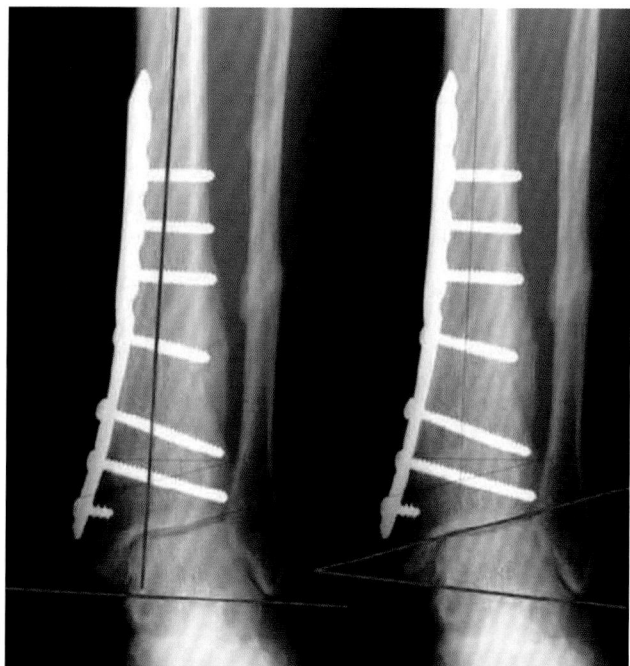

FIGURE 37.3 The talocrural angle (82 ± 3.6 degrees)[19] is the angle formed by a line connecting the tip of the medial and lateral malleolus and mid-diaphyseal line. Deformity in the distal tibia will influence this angle and is therefore not reliable. The plafond malleolar (9 ± 4 degrees)[19] angle is the angle formed by the tip of the malleoli and the tibial plafond. This angle is more reliable in the presence of distal tibial deformity.[19]

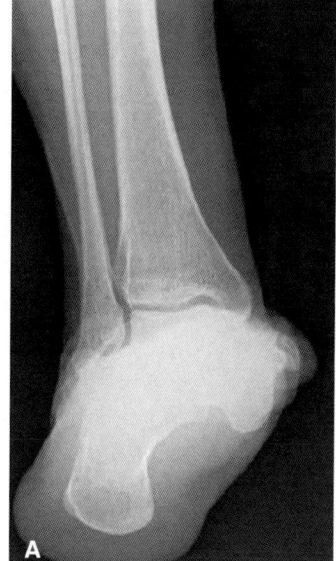 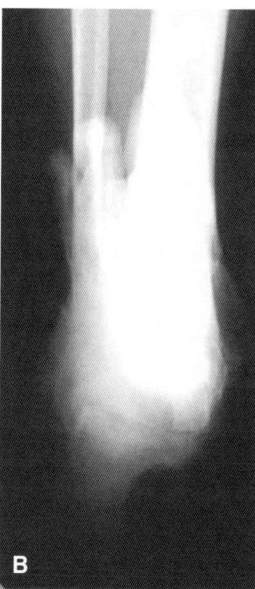

FIGURE 37.4 **A.** The hindfoot alignment view allows evaluation of the position of the calcaneus with respect to the ankle and distal tibia. The calcaneus is normally translated 1 cm lateral to the tibial mid-diaphyseal line.[12] **B.** Long leg calcaneal axial views allow assessment of the subtalar joint and the relationship of the calcaneus to the anatomic axis of the tibia.

- The *talocrural angle* (82 ± 3.6 degrees)[16] is the angle formed by a line connecting the tip of the medial and lateral malleolus and mid-diaphyseal line. Deformity in the distal tibia will influence this angle and is therefore not reliable.
- The *plafond malleolar angle* (9 ± 4 degrees)[16] is the angle formed by the tip of the malleoli and the tibial plafond. This angle is more reliable in the presence of distal tibial deformity (Fig. 37.3).
- *Hindfoot alignment views* allow evaluation of the position of the calcaneus with respect to the ankle and distal tibia. The calcaneus is normally translated 1 cm lateral to the tibial mid-diaphyseal line.[12]
- *Long leg calcaneal axial views* allow assessment of the subtalar joint and the relationship of the calcaneus to the anatomic axis of the tibia (Fig. 37.4).
- Infrequently, full-length standing films or stress views of the ankle are indicated. Advanced imaging such as MRI or CT may also be helpful to evaluate focal articular damage and periarticular pathology.

TREATMENT

PREOPERATIVE DEFORMITY EVALUATION AND OSTEOTOMY PLANNING

The clinical and radiographic evaluation of deformity and execution of corrective osteotomy has been described in a comprehensive way by Paley et al.[16,20] Using concepts of vector trigonometry, SMO can be planned and executed with predictable results. Various osteotomy techniques can be employed to restore alignment. The best osteotomy for any particular deformity is determined by several factors. Supramalleolar osteotomies can be utilized to correct any deviations from any of the three cardinal body planes. Frontal and sagittal plane deviations are more common presenting complaints than rotational ones, but there is frequently a transverse plane component to each deformity. When compound deformities are present, there is more difficulty in attaining the ultimate and optimal alignment, and more sophisticated techniques are often indicated to attain coaxial alignment of the foot and leg.

- *Manipulation of GRF*—often, only a portion of the articular surface of the joint is involved, and corrective osteotomy can unload the degenerative articular surface by redistribution of pathologic wear patterns on the joint. Steffensmeier[21] demonstrated the focal areas of the talar dome could be off-loaded with shift in center of pressure of 1 and 1.58 mm with lateral and medial displacement osteotomy of 1 cm, respectively. Normally, GRF passes through the heel and lateral aspect of the ankle joint, creating a valgus torque in the hindfoot.[18] The lateral position of the calcaneal axis with respect to the tibial axis explains this mechanical principle. Additionally, abnormal lateral translation (>1 cm) of the calcaneus can cause detrimental hindfoot valgus forces.
- The restoration of articular alignment and joint orientation is critical for dampening abnormal degenerative wear patterns on the articular surface and diminishing secondary subtalar and midtarsal compensation.[12,13]

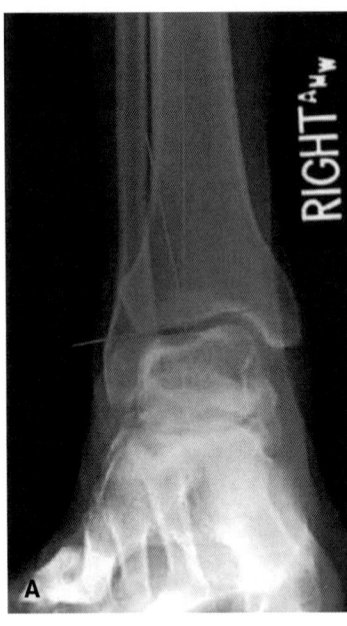
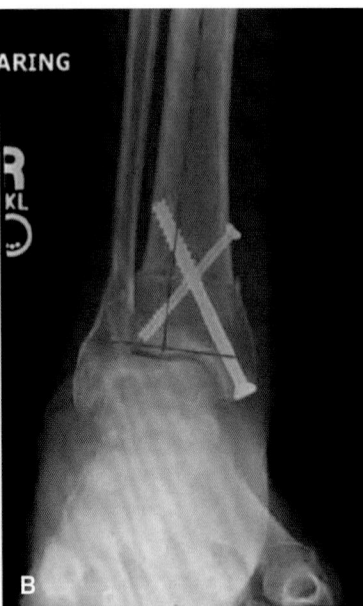

FIGURE 37.5 **A.** CORA analysis for articular varus deformity. The mid-diaphyseal line cannot be accurately drawn in the distal tibia. In these cases, a reference joint orientation angle is utilized. The LDTA (89 degrees) and the ADTA (80 degrees) are determined and extended proximally to intersect with the mid-diaphyseal line proximal to the deformity. The intersection of these lines is the CORA. This articular ankle varus deformity was secondary to a hereditary motor-sensory neuropathy. **B.** Treated with lateral closing wedge osteotomy of tibia and calcaneus. An oblique osteotomy of the fibula made in the frontal plane was not stabilized with internal fixation. Note the mid-diaphyseal bisection is coaxial with the center of the talus.

CENTER OF ROTATION OF ANGULATION ANALYSIS

Every deformity has a geometric center that defines the apex of the deformity. This apex is referred to as the center of rotation of angulation (CORA) and serves as an important reference point in osteotomy planning. Generally, the diaphyseal bisection on each side of the deformity will define the location of the CORA. For juxta-articular deformity, the mid-diaphyseal line cannot be accurately drawn in the distal tibia (Fig. 37.5). In these cases, a reference joint orientation angle is utilized. The LDTA (89 degrees) and the ADTA (80 degrees) are determined and extended proximally to intersect with the mid-diaphyseal line proximal, which is extended toward the ankle, forming an angle that represents the magnitude of the deformity and defining the level of the CORA. Often, the level of the CORA will be different on the anteroposterior and lateral films. This is the result of translation in a different plane from the plane of the angulation deformity. Translation is common in fracture malunion deformity of the distal tibia after spiral oblique fractures (Fig. 37.6).

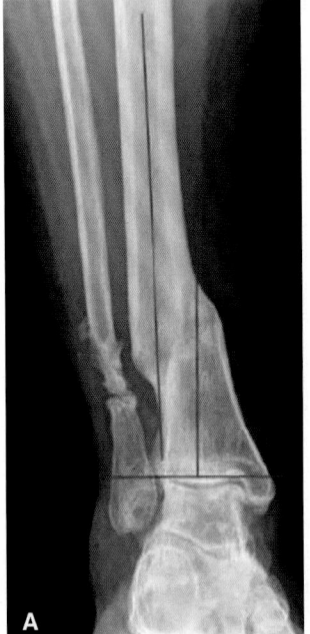
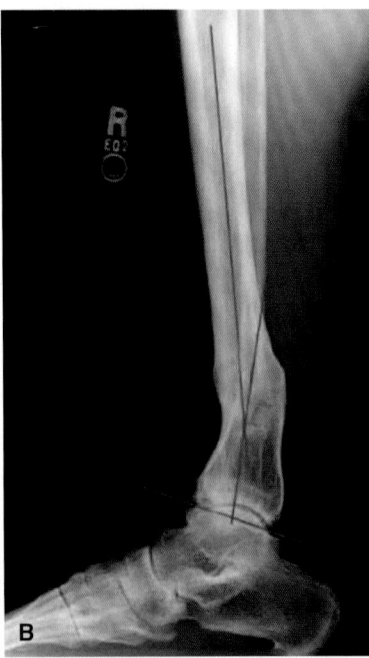
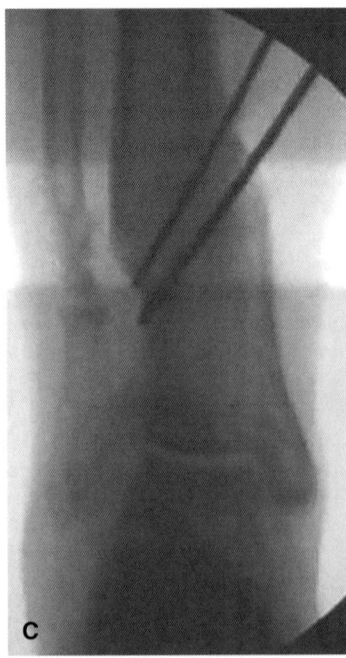

FIGURE 37.6 **A.** A medially translated ankle joint relative to the long axis of the tibia.
B. Recurvatum deformity formed by the axis of the ankle joint relative to the long axis of the tibia
C. two guide pins are used to make the medially based truncated wedge osteotomy

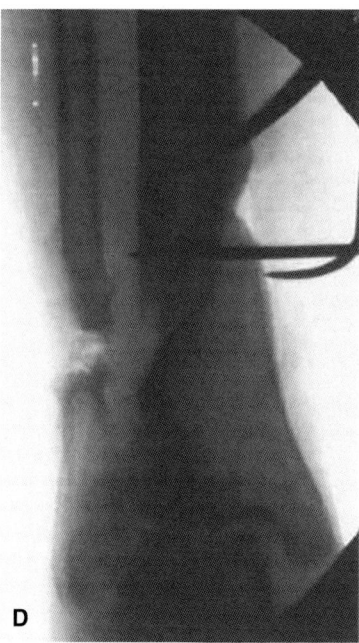
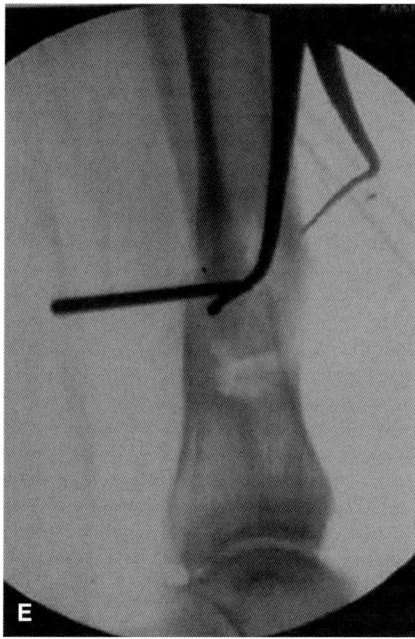

FIGURE 37.6 (*Continued*) **D & E.** Correction of the deformity in all three planes.

Once the surgeon has defined the deformity, level of the CORA, and hindfoot position, clinical examination should determine rotation, soft tissue contracture, and ligament instability. With this complete information, proper deformity correction with the appropriate procedures can be performed.

SURGICAL PROCEDURES AND TECHNIQUES: STEP-BY-STEP NARRATIVE

Although there are several techniques available for correction of supramalleolar deformity, the simplest and most common are the opening and closing wedge techniques. Irrespective of the technique, in general, SMO is preferably performed at or in close proximity to the CORA.

- In general, supramalleolar osteotomies are performed through a medial, anterior, or lateral approach. It is important to evaluate the local soft tissue conditions and the presence of previous incisions or wounds.
- It is important to avoid stripping excessive amounts of the periosteal layer to prevent devascularization of the osteotomy site.
- The transverse design and metaphyseal location of the osteotomy is helpful, because it is inherently stable in an area of good blood supply for rapid healing.
- Kirschner wires (K-wires) or other pins can be used to transcribe the expected amount of resected bone. The distal pin is placed parallel to the tibial plafond and the proximal pin is perpendicular to the tibial axis.
- When the resultant wedge is removed, the tibial articular surface should be near perpendicular to the long axis of the tibia. Slight deflections of the saw blade can provide correction in the sagittal plane in the case of varus or valgus deformity.

CLOSING WEDGE OSTEOTOMY

- A medial linear approach is developed, and subperiosteal dissection about the medial, anterior, and posterior horizon of the distal tibia is performed.

- A half pin percutaneously placed as near to the CORA as possible in the distal vascular metaphyseal region of the tibia serves as the center of rotation for the osteotomy. This allows for pure angular correction without translation of the distal fragment, which would compromise coaxial alignment. When the CORA falls at the ankle joint, the pin cannot be placed in the joint but can be placed just proximal, which will cause some translation.
- The amount of bone to be removed is transcribed with two K-wires placed from medial to lateral under fluoroscopic guidance. The apex of the resultant wedge should be at the lateral border of the distal tibia. The distal wire should be parallel to the articular surface, and the proximal wire should be perpendicular to the long axis of the bone.
- Prior to cutting and resecting the tibial bone, the fibula is exposed with a lateral midline approach, and a transverse osteotomy is performed directly through the periosteum. The level of the osteotomy should also be close to the CORA, but if possible, the dissection and exposure should not communicate with the expected tibial osteotomy to diminish the chance of a synostosis.
- If there is an insufficient syndesmosis that needs to be corrected, it should be done at this time. Excavation of the bony, osteocartilaginous, or fibrous debris is necessary to oppose the distal fibula to the incurisa. In this instance, confluence of the exposures may be beneficial to impart some stability to the restored syndesmotic relationship (Fig. 37.7).
- Once the osteotomy is completed and the distal fibula can be mobilized to its desired position, the closing wedge is completed from the medial exposure of the distal tibia. Mobilization and apposition of the distal tibial segment is accomplished with manual manipulation. Some translational and rotational correction is possible and done if necessary, followed by temporary K-wire or Steinmann pin fixation in the ultimate position.
- With apposition of the osteotomy fragments, the distal fibula will migrate with the distal tibial fragment. However,

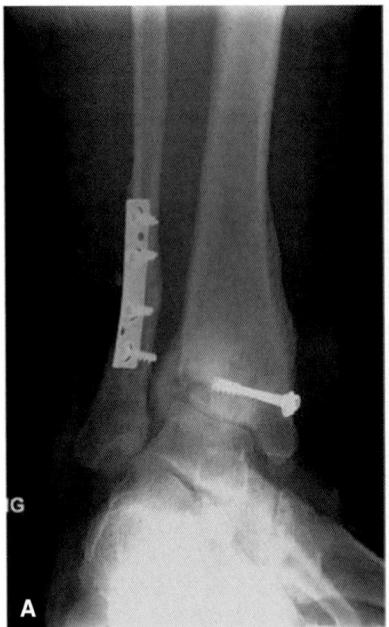 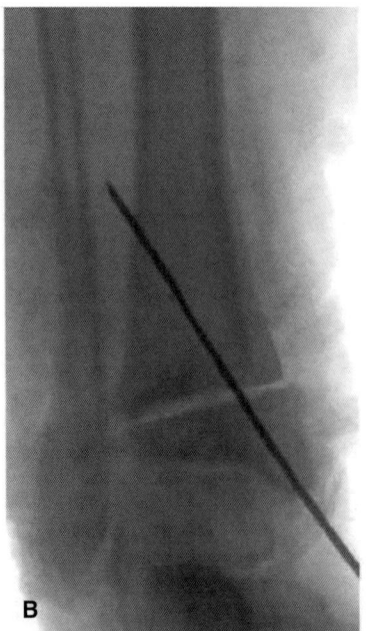 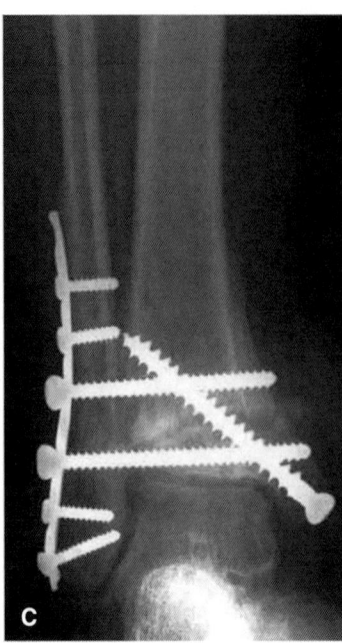

FIGURE 37.7 A. Valgus ankle malunion with syndesmotic instability. Collapse of the lateral tibial plafond with valgus angulation. The deformity in this case is articular and makes the CORA the ankle joint. **B.** A medial closing wedge is performed above the plafond to correct the articular and axial alignment. **C.** The syndesmosis is then débrided, reduced, and stabilized after fibular osteotomy.

the resultant defect in the fibula may be irregular, and mobilization of the osteotomy may cause the two fibular segments to be out of coaxial alignment. Nevertheless, the tibiofibular relationship is now restored and temporarily stabilized as well.

- The entire fibula is stabilized with a tubular plate if possible, and the resultant defect is backfilled with bone graft. If the syndesmosis requires internal fixation, it is done at this time with transsyndesmotic screws.
- Lastly, the distal tibial osteotomy is fixated with either a small tubular plate or an obliquely directed screw from the medial malleolus into the lateral distal tibial cortex. Additional points of fixation are delivered based on the degree of instability in any of the cardinal body planes and the configuration of the medial surface of the tibia.

PEARLS

- To further capitalize on the healing features of the local anatomy, any of the available methods can be performed with limited surgical exposure.
- When varus or valgus deformity is being corrected, it is technically easier to select a surgical approach that is directly over the base of the proposed wedge resection. However, when varus deformity is the issue, a laterally based closing wedge must violate the relationship of the tibia and fibula.
- In rare instances in the varus ankle, there is need to address tibiofibular malposition, and a lateral approach may be more prudent. However, more commonly, the varus deformity can be corrected with an opening wedge technique from the readily accessible medial cortex of the distal tibia.

OPENING WEDGE OSTEOTOMY

OWO is executed in a similar fashion as the closing wedge osteotomy. Indications include osteotomy of the distal tibia requiring angulation and modest amounts of length. This type of osteotomy is usually used to treat physeal disturbances and malunion resulting in varus deformity or modest valgus postures of the ankle. There is little additional translation correction after the opening wedge is completed, unless the lateral cortex is divided, but this is at the expense of stability and apposition. A potential problem with OWO is the tensioning of the soft tissues with correction.

- Make a linear midline incision over the base of the opening wedge along the distal medial metaphysis (Fig. 37.8).
- Subperiosteal dissection around the visible circumference of the distal tibia exposes the target area for insertion of the bone graft wedge.
- Based on preoperative planning, the location of the osteotomy is selected and should be as close to the CORA as possible, but should remain within the confines of the cancellous bone substrate of the tibial metaphysis.
- Fluoroscopy is utilized to synchronize the osteotomy site with the preoperative plan, and a guide wire is placed to transcribe the desired amount of correction (Fig. 37.9).
- Once the guide wire is in the proper location, an osteotome or power saw is utilized to divide the distal tibia. The cutting instrument should not be rotated from the pure transverse plane, unless a triplanar configuration is desired.
- When the osteotomy is close to or at completion across the distal tibia, a wide osteotome is used to pry the osteotomy open. Additional feathering or finesse may be required for distal mobilization of the distal fragment. A lamina spreader or other distraction instrument can be used to dial in the amount of desired correction (Fig. 37.10).

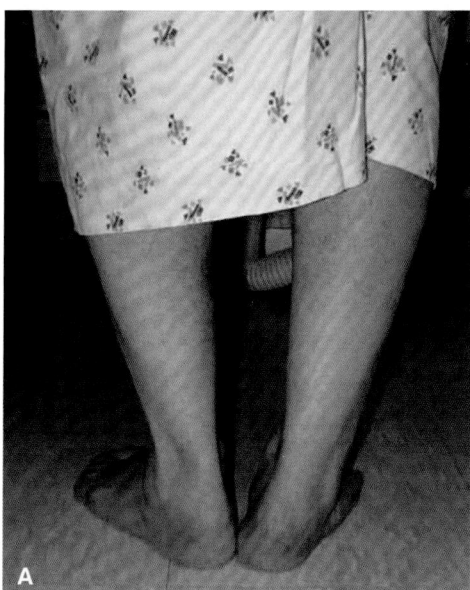
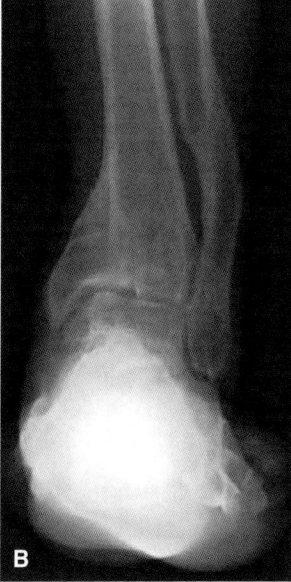
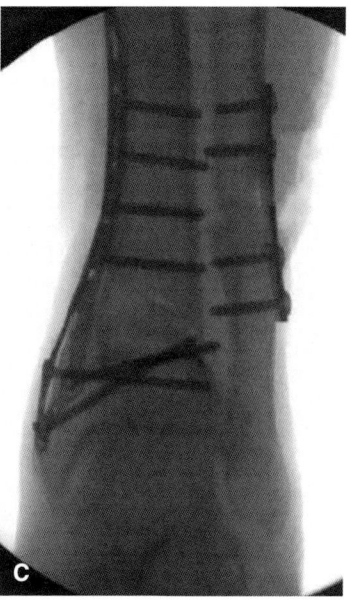

FIGURE 37.8 **A, B.** Varus malunion of distal tibia and fibular fracture resulting in chronic lateral ankle instability and lateral column overload. **C.** Treated with metaphyseal OWO and closing wedge fibular osteotomy. An autogenous iliac crest graft is placed into the open wedge and stabilized with a medial plate.

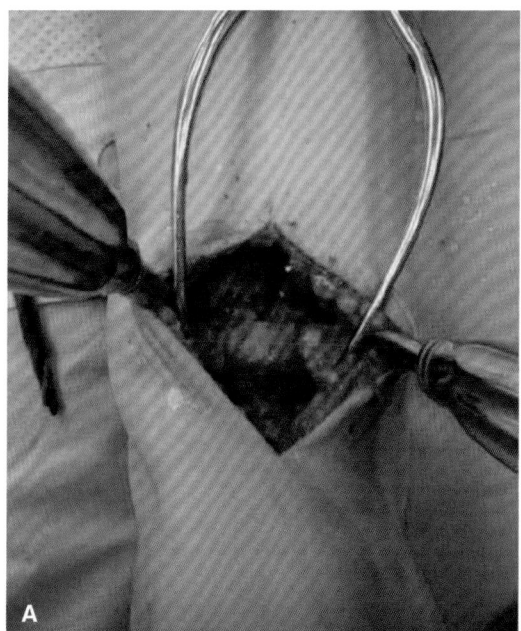
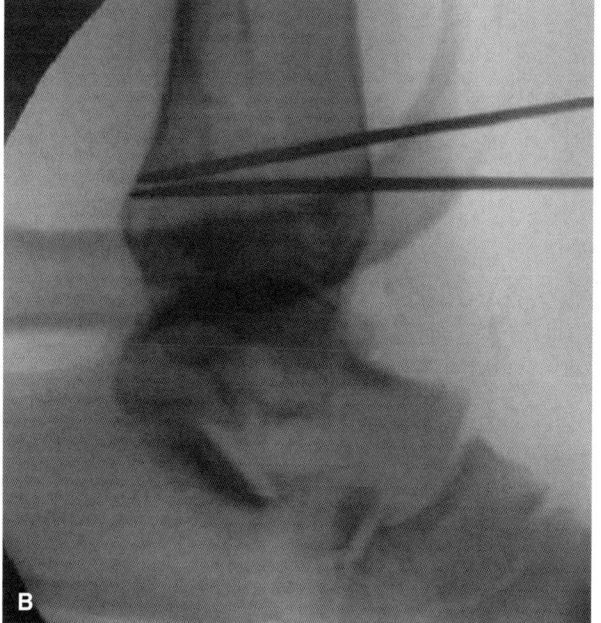

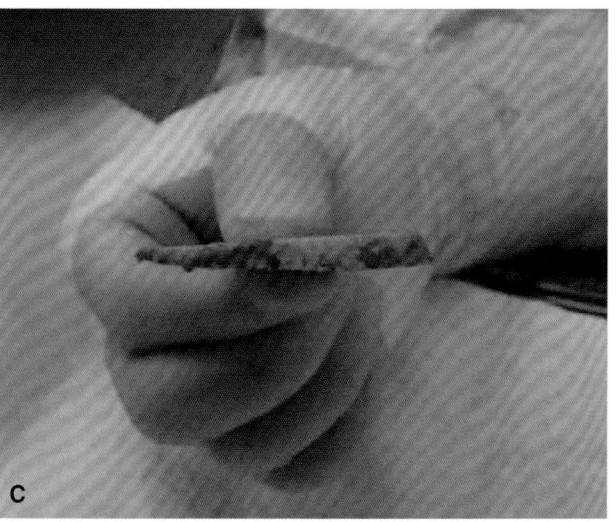

FIGURE 37.9 **A.** K-wires or other pins can be used to transcribe the expected amount of resected bone. **B.** The distal pin is placed parallel to the tibial plafond and the proximal pin is perpendicular to the tibial axis. When the resultant wedge is removed, articular angles of the tibial plafond should be restored. **C.** This example shows an anterolateral wedge to correct a posttraumatic varus and procurvatum deformity.

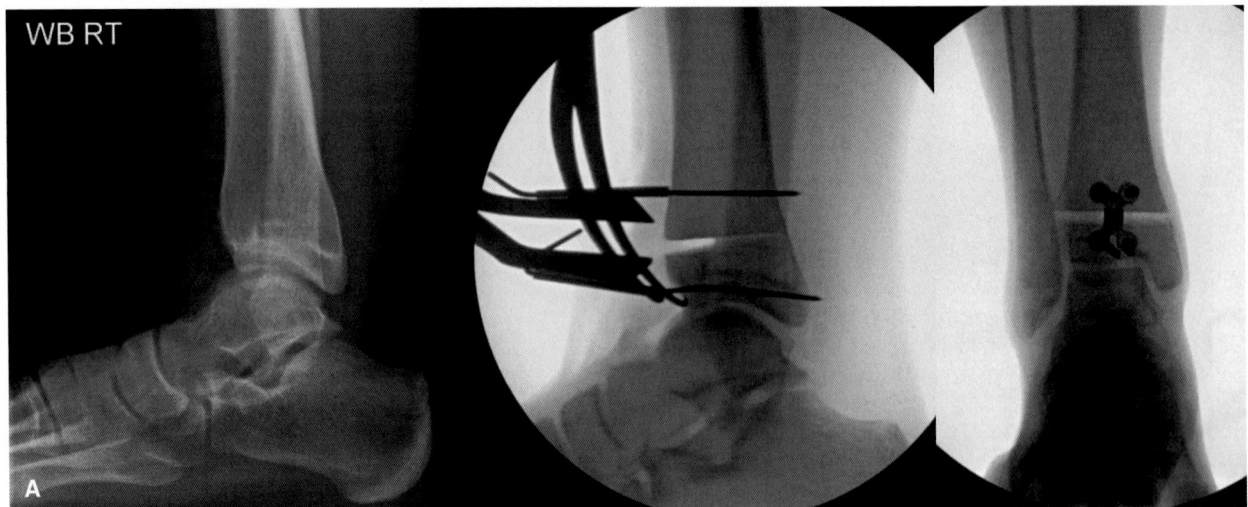

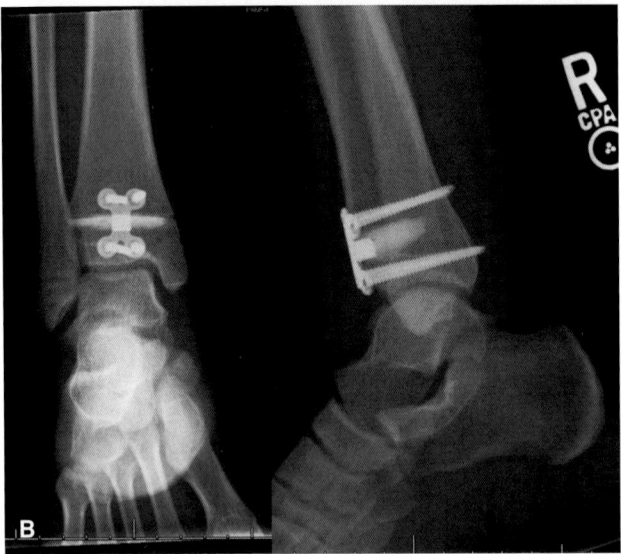

FIGURE 37.10 A. A prior growth plate injury resulted in early closure of the anterior distal tibial physis and an increased anterior distal tibia angle. Intraoperative fluoroscopic images show the Weinraub distractor used to obtain the desired correction prior to holding the correction open with an opening wedge plate and back-filling the osteotomy with bone cement. **B.** Postoperative images show correction of the deformity.

- Using fluoroscopic monitoring, the distal fragment is manipulated into a position such that the articular surface is perpendicular to the long axis of the tibia. Once the optimal and most functional position is attained, reassessment of the need for horizontal or other translational manipulations is done.

- Because the procedure is optimally performed in the distal tibial metaphysis from a bone graft incorporation standpoint, it may not be proximate enough to the CORA for optimal coaxial alignment. If necessary, the osteotomy is completed through the lateral cortex, and these planar deviations are executed so that the final position is realized.

- The final posture is maintained with some form of temporary fixation, but it should be placed such that it will not interfere with the permanent fixatives. Most commonly, a large-caliber K-wire or small Steinmann pin is delivered obliquely across the osteotomy from the medial malleolus through the lateral tibial cortex.

- Bone graft is utilized to backfill the resultant defect, most commonly a hybrid of tricortical iliac crest allograft and crushed cancellous bone fragments. The tricortical graft is sculpted to fit the defect, and the superior cortex of the iliac crest graft is positioned most medially to absorb the

natural compression from the distraction process. The graft should have a press fit rather than sit loosely in the void. The remaining defect is filled with crushed cancellous chips that are packed tightly within (Fig. 37.11).

- Once the defect is filled with biologic substrate, the permanent fixation is applied. Given the natural tendency for bone resorption with incorporation, the selected fixation should be designed to resist compressive or settling forces. If there is any rotatory instability or shear across the interfaces, the fixation should also be capable of dampening these forces. However, with an intact fibula, a simple construct is usually sufficient.

- Most commonly, a tubular-type plate is applied to the medial surface the tibia. The number of points of purchase should be maximized, particular distal to the osteotomy. If necessary to increase the number of holes, a T-type or Y-type plate can be applied, if a simple straight tubular plate does not suffice. A number of various plates can be used for this purpose. Locked plates are also valuable to maintain the osteotomy and minimize compression across the bone graft (Fig. 37.12).

- The periosteal sleeve helps secure the bone graft but is not sufficient to maintain the ultimate position, as it is usually not possible for complete reapproximation.

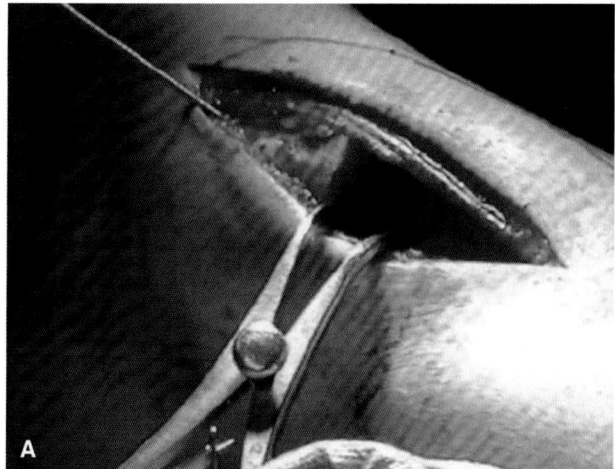

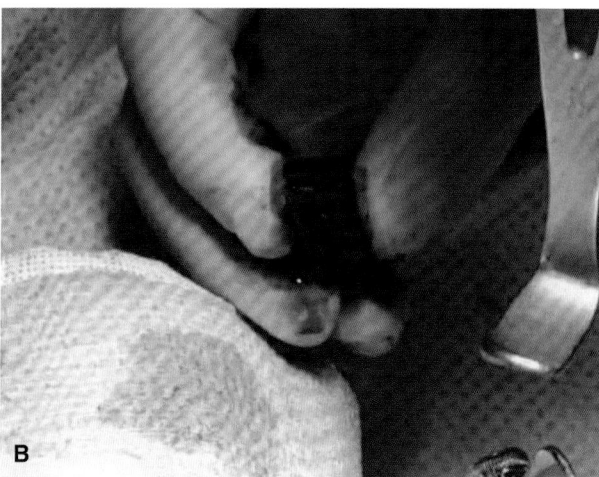

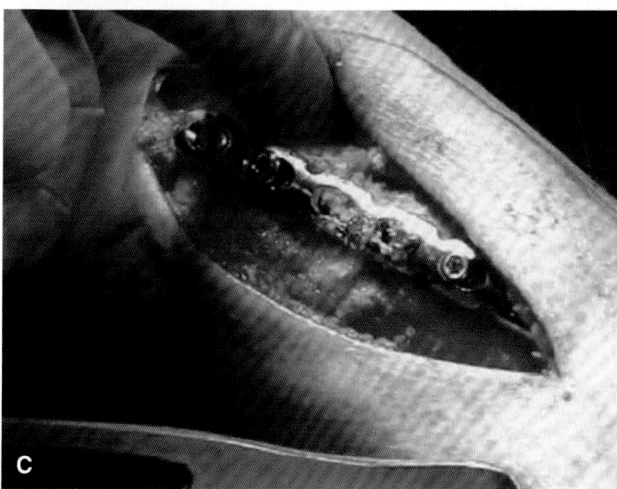

FIGURE 37.11 A. OWO of distal tibia. The osteotomy is executed in cancellous bone of the distal tibia to facilitate healing. This should be done as closely as possible to the CORA. Intraoperative photo, showing opening wedge of distal tibia using a lamina spreader to dial in the amount of desired correction and held with a temporary wire to maintain position. **B.** Autogenous corticocancellous bone graft is harvested and hand milled to fill the wedge. Additional allograft chips and demineralized bone matrix are used to fill any additional voids. **C.** A medial 3.5-mm locking reconstruction plate is used for stabilization. This locked plate and cortical bone strut resists the settling of bone graft during incorporation.

PEARLS

- Intraoperative assessment of axial alignment, to assess the center of the talus, with respect to the axis of the tibia, in both the frontal and sagittal planes is important prior to definitive fixation.
- The authors prefer intraoperative imaging to better assess alignment. If there is residual translational deformity, the distal tibia can be translated to realign the talus beneath the tibial axis.
- Fixation can be delivered in a percutaneous method. In some circumstances, a medial plate can be used, but often there is a cortical step-off at the level of the osteotomy, which makes plating impractical.
- Use of an opening wedge technique helps restore the loss of length, but soft tissue tension may preclude complete correction in a one-stage operation.
- Those patients with severe deformities may be better served by alternate techniques such as callus distraction or a focal dome technique. Although the former can restore limb length, the latter technique cannot. Furthermore, because of the large planar deflections, the fibula almost always needs to be shortened.

COMBINATION OF MEDIAL OPENING AND LATERAL CLOSING WEDGE OSTEOTOMY

A combination medial opening and lateral closing wedge osteotomy can be accomplished, which affords several advantages (Fig. 37.13). Larger degrees of deformity can be addressed with less tension on the medial soft tissue structures. The transverse nature of half of the osteotomy affords enhanced stability. Less bone graft is required to backfill the opening wedge.

- The surgical approach is done through a medial and lateral approach in the same manner as the OWO. Under fluoroscopic guidance, wires are placed to plan the opening and closing wedges.
- The technique is done with provisional wires as osteotomy guides. The intersection of the wires should ideally converge at the CORA in distal metaphyseal bone. Once correction has been achieved and temporarily stabilized with wires, permanent fixation is achieved both medially and laterally.
- Fibular plating is ideal, and a spanning medial plate is placed. Bone graft is then used to backfill the void as previously mentioned.

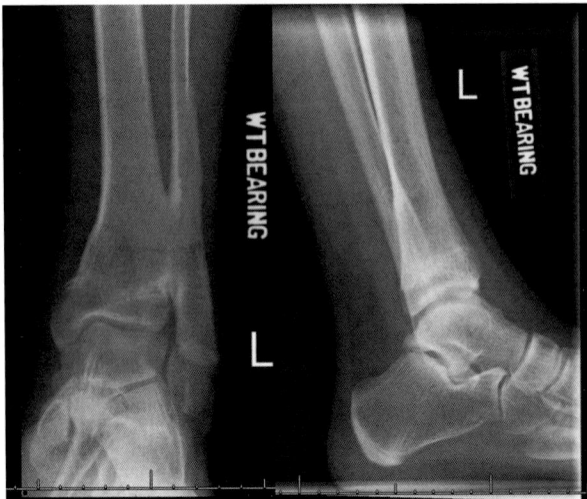
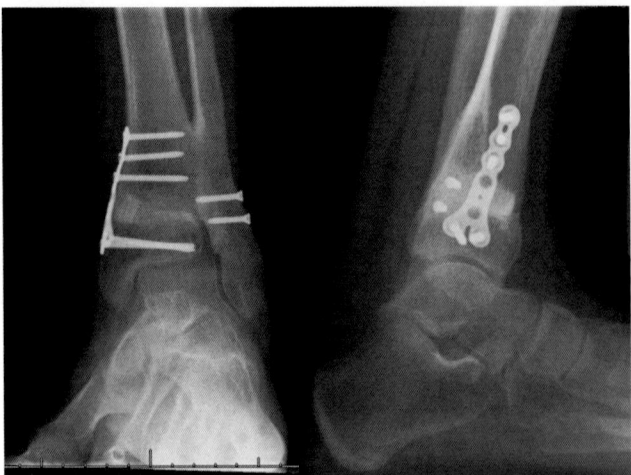

FIGURE 37.12 Preoperative and postoperative images of an opening wedge osteotomy of the distal tibia to correct a varus ankle deformity after prior growth plate injury. In this case, an oblique fibular osteotomy was made to shorten the fibula as well as rotate the talus into a more valgus position.

FOCAL DOME OSTEOTOMY

The focal dome osteotomy (FDO) is performed for angular deformity at or near the ankle joint. It is generally not suited for proximal, midshaft, or even distal third deformities because correction of rotational or translational deformities is not possible with the configuration of the osteotomy, which subtends a portion of a circumference of a circle. As such, the FDO is most appropriate for frontal or sagittal plane correction. The FDO capitalizes on the enhanced healing potential of cancellous, metaphyseal bone but requires a more treacherous anterior exposure to correct frontal plane varus deformities. Furthermore, because of the large planar deflections, the fibula almost always needs to be shortened (Fig. 37.14).

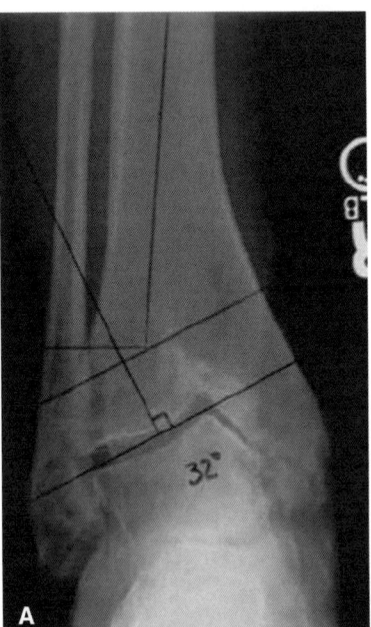
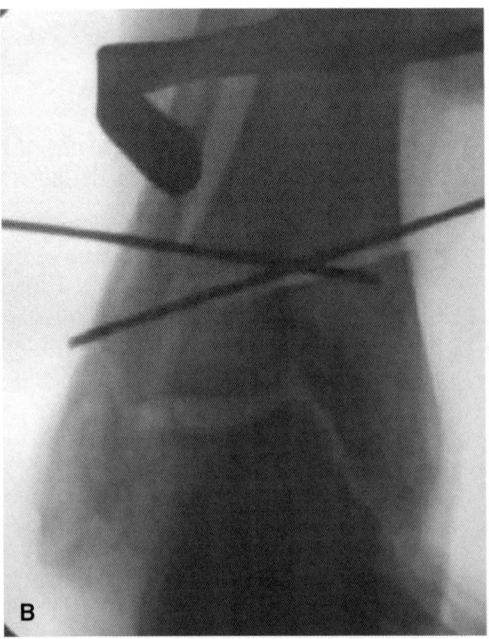
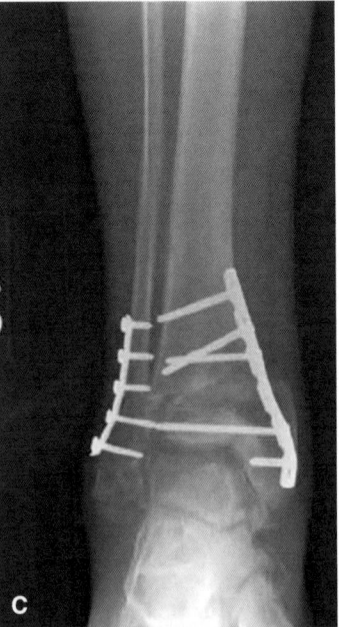

FIGURE 37.13 A. Distal tibial varus resulting from physeal injury. **B.** A combined medial opening wedge and lateral closing wedge allows for correction near the CORA and maintains length. A lateral closing wedge is performed through the fibula and lateral tibia. The apex is completed from the medial side. The amount of lateral wedge is proportional to the amount of desired correction. **C.** The lateral bone is removed, correcting the varus malunion. The lateral plate is placed, maintaining the correction. The medial side is then bone grafted and plated.

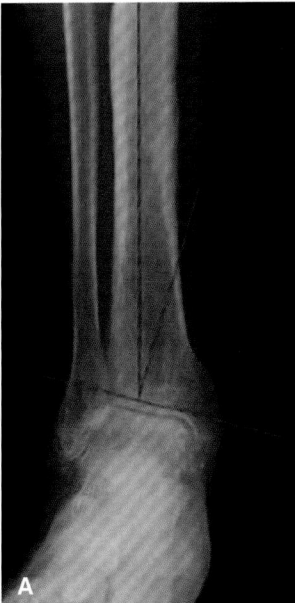
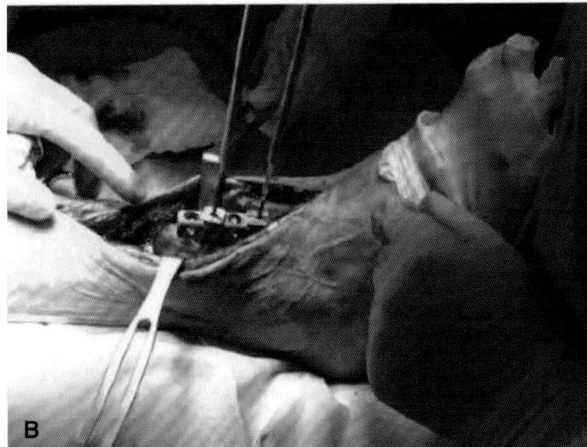
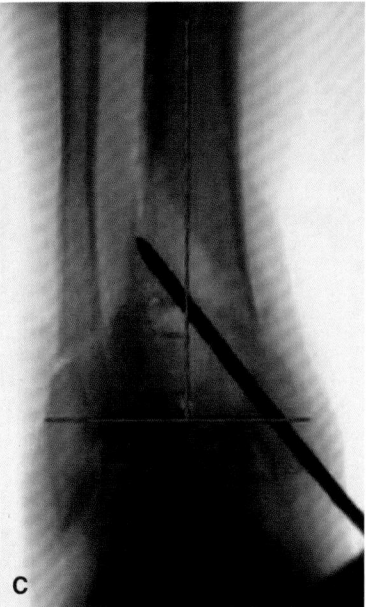

FIGURE 37.14 A. Distal tibial valgus deformity with CORA very near the ankle joint. No translational or sagittal plane correction needed. **B.** This patient underwent a frontal plane FDO to realign the articular angle with the tibial axis. **C.** The axis pin is placed just above the articular surface. The fibular osteotomy is performed in an oblique orientation.

- To correct frontal plane deformity with an FDO, a straight anterior incision is used. The surgical exposure should be between the extensor hallucis longus (EHL) and extensor digitorum longus (EDL) tendons.
- The anterior compartment is divided and the neurovascular bundle is mobilized laterally with the EDL. The tibialis anterior and EHL are mobilized medially to provide access to the distal tibial metaphysis.
- The axis of rotation is selected based on the requirements of the osteotomy, and an axis pin is placed at the center of the arc. This is ideally placed at the CORA, thereby not introducing any secondary deformity.
- A Rancho cube with drill sleeve is placed over the pin. This provides for circular rotation and transcribes the arc of the osteotomy. The holes in the cube are used as a drill guide, and intraoperative fluoroscopy is employed to ensure that the arc of the osteotomy penetrates the medial and lateral cortices of the distal tibia.
- Sequential drill holes are placed completely through the tibia along the transcribed arc and are then connected with an osteotome, completing the osteotomy. Some manual manipulation may be necessary to disengage the proximal and distal portions of the tibia.
- A large pin placed in the distal fragment is helpful to disengage the osteotomy and facilitate correction. Before mobilization of the distal fragment can occur, the fibula also requires an osteotomy, same as for the closing medial wedge of the distal tibia. It can be performed in an oblique fashion in the same plane as the planned correction but should be located at the same level as the tibial osteotomy.
- Alternatively, a cylindrical shortening may be done but requires sequential resections to attain optimal apposition of the fragments.

PEARLS

- The FDO is performed for angular deformity at or near the ankle joint. It is generally not suited for proximal, midshaft, or even distal third deformities because correction of rotational or translational deformities is not possible with the configuration of the osteotomy, which subtends a portion of a circumference of a circle.
- The FDO capitalizes on the enhanced healing potential of cancellous, metaphyseal bone but requires a more treacherous anterior exposure to correct frontal plane varus deformities. Furthermore, because of the large planar deflections, the fibula almost always needs to be shortened.

TRIPLANE OSTEOTOMY

The triplane osteotomy is a technique that allows for deformity correction in all three planes with a single bone cut[22,23] (Fig. 37.15). The osteotomy is based on the principle that any deformity has one axis of rotation around which the deformity can be corrected. Sangeorzan et al.[23] described a mathematical model for deformity planning and correction based on vector trigonometry. A carefully planned and executed osteotomy can realign the deformity in all three planes. The osteotomy is ideally centered at the level of the CORA. The principle of the technique is that the degree of correction in any plane is proportional to the amount of deviation from that plane. For example, a long oblique osteotomy made in the frontal plane affords frontal plane correction

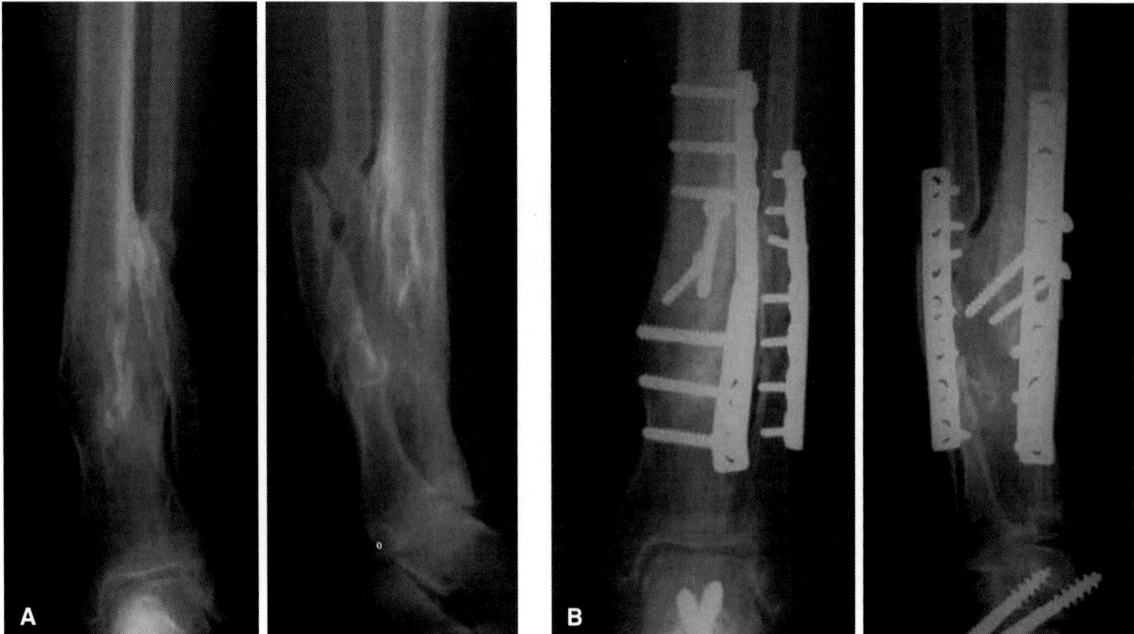

FIGURE 37.15 **A.** Distal tibial malunion with valgus and recurvatum. **B.** Treated with oblique triplane osteotomy and fixated with a lateral tension plate to correct valgus and recurvatum.

with little transverse or sagittal plane correction. In contrast, a 45-degree osteotomy with respect to all three planes will afford equal correction in all three planes. This osteotomy is only useful for tibial malunion above the metaphysis. This approach affords excellent exposure of the tibia at the level of the deformity and CORA.

- The incision is just lateral to the anterior tibial crest. This exposure affords exposure to the anterior compartment of the leg.
- The osteotomy is made based on the type and degree of deformity.
- One lag screw is placed across the osteotomy to act as a rotational hinge, and the correction is dialed in.
- Radiographs are taken to ensure proper correction.
- A second screw is placed across the osteotomy, and the tibia is then plated using standard fixation techniques.
- The fixation for this type of osteotomy is done with a lateral tension plate on the tibia, which is nicely hidden in the anterior compartment.

CALLUS DISTRACTION

The use of callus distraction for correction of distal tibial malposition should be considered whenever the deformity is such that a single-stage correction would be difficult. Single-stage corrections may be difficult due to scarring from previous trauma, poor soft tissue coverage such as skin grafting, or severe degrees of deformity. In addition, if there is multiplanar deformity or loss of axial length, then this technique is most versatile and capable of optimal correction in all planes. Although any adjustable ring external fixator may be utilized, the Taylor Spatial Frame (TSF) is exceptionally useful in these situations because the proprietary software allows for computer-governed surveillance of the correction. It also affords for triplanar deformity correction while allowing weight bearing to proceed for the duration of the deformity correction and healing process.

The general technique using the TSF involves the application of a circular frame that matches the distal tibial deformity (crooked frame on crooked leg) with tensioned wires. In essence, the configuration of the frame mimics the configuration of the deformity in all plans. The software is then used to create a plan of incremental correction that takes into account optimal rates of distraction and soft tissue structures at risk during correction. Essentially, the distal fragment is mobilized to the proximal or reference fragment in three dimensions until the optimal alignment is realized (Fig. 37.16). Periodic radiographs will assess the spatial relationships of the respective fragments. The software program can be adjusted periodically to optimize the ultimate position of the distal fragment. There are several advantages to using callus distraction. In addition to the ability to correct multiple plane deformity and restore length, the frame can be readjusted to achieve the optimal degree of correction. The ability to weight bear on the operated limb is also possible using circular frames.

- The osteotomy or corticotomy is performed in a minimally invasive method with a Gigli saw or osteotome. Preservation of the periosteal sleeve is critical to achieve healthy regenerate bone during the bone mobilization process. Ideally, the corticotomy is done at the level of the CORA to minimize translatory effects. However, any tendency for translation can be neutralized by incorporation into the prescription.
- The tibia can be exposed either before or after frame application to the leg. If done after frame application, exposure is facilitated by removing two or three adjacent struts to complete the tibial cut. In either event, the tibial cut is not executed until the frame is completely intact, to prevent loss of existing alignment.
- Several issues must be reconciled during distal tibial correction. First, the surgeon must ensure that equinus contracture does not evolve with progression of the correction. Active weight bearing helps obviate this

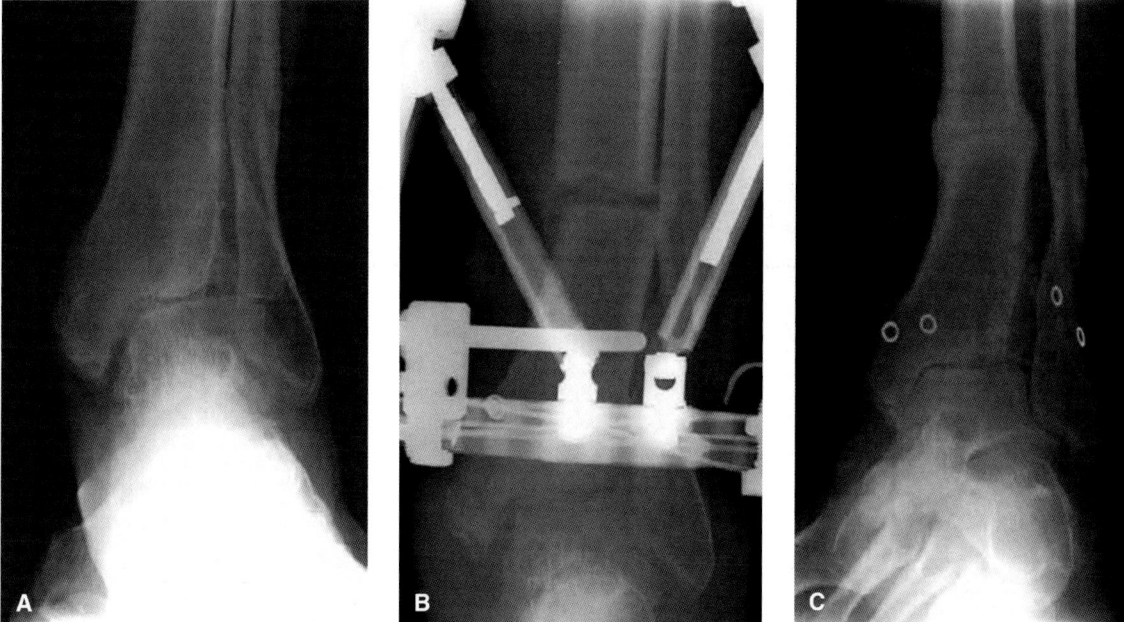

FIGURE 37.16 **A.** Multiplane deformity with rotation. Single-stage osteotomy correction is not attainable. **B.** Gradual correction is achieved with corticotomy and application of TSF. The distal fragment is mobilized to the proximal or reference fragment in three dimensions until the optimal alignment is realized. **C:** Postop radiograph.

concern, but preoperative planning will help anticipate the necessity to address at the time of the index operation.

- If equinus becomes significant, it may be necessary to address before final correction or frame removal is attained. Generally, four points of fixation (wires) are utilized in the distal metaphyseal fragment to allow for full and immediate weight bearing. Strategic positioning of these wires is necessary to avoid transfixion of the extrinsic tendons that otherwise would impede ankle motion. One of the olive wires should be placed across the syndesmosis from lateral to medial to capture and maintain the anatomic relationship of the tibiofibular articulation. Strict adherence to technique in the application of the frame must be followed. Whether using half pins with or without tensioned wires, the proximal and distal must be adequate to achieve adequate fixation, facilitate correction of the deformity, and maintain the correction until complete consolidation of the regenerate bone.

ADDRESSING THE DISTAL TIBIOFIBULAR COMPLEX

When an SMO is indicated, most commonly the distal tibiofibular complex should be mobilized as a unit, even though there may be malposition of the fibula within the fibular incurisa of the tibia. In those cases, apposition and stabilization of the fibula to the tibia are done in conjunction with the osteotomy of the tibia and fibula. If possible, the fibular osteotomy is made in an oblique fashion in the same plane as the correction. This is performed in the frontal plane for varus and valgus tibial osteotomy and the sagittal plane for procurvatum and

recurvatum osteotomy. For these simple osteotomy designs, the fibula is cut above the syndesmosis to maintain the tibiofibular relationship. However, in those instances in which the fibula must be lengthened or there is any translation of the tibiofibular segment, the most optimal maneuver is a transverse osteotomy with or without filling the resultant defect with bone graft. If direct apposition of the cut ends of the fibula is possible, it should not be at the expense of disrupting the tibiofibular relationship at the level of the syndesmosis.

CORRECTION OF VARUS DEFORMITY

The presenting symptoms of a patient with intrinsic ankle varus typically revolve around lateral overload (Fig. 37.17). Most often, the chronicity of the varus posture correlates with the severity of the symptoms, particularly if asymmetric wear of the tibiotalar joint occurs. Rarely is a significant varus ankle malunion fully compensated in the subtalar joint with eversion, and residual hindfoot varus results. Furthermore, the concomitant hindfoot varus and a sense of lateral instability often dictate additional procedures such as calcaneal osteotomy and lateral ankle ligament reconstruction to achieve complete coaxial alignment and a stable ankle.

- There are essentially three strategies to correct the varus ankle, opening or closing wedge osteotomy and FDO.
- The most direct technique is an OWO of the distal tibia, with or without fibular osteotomy. In most cases, the fibula can be left undisturbed, unless there is significant bony debris or stiffness at the tibiofibular joint or syndesmotic area that would preclude mobilization of the distal tibial metaphyseal segment around the syndesmotic ligament hinge.

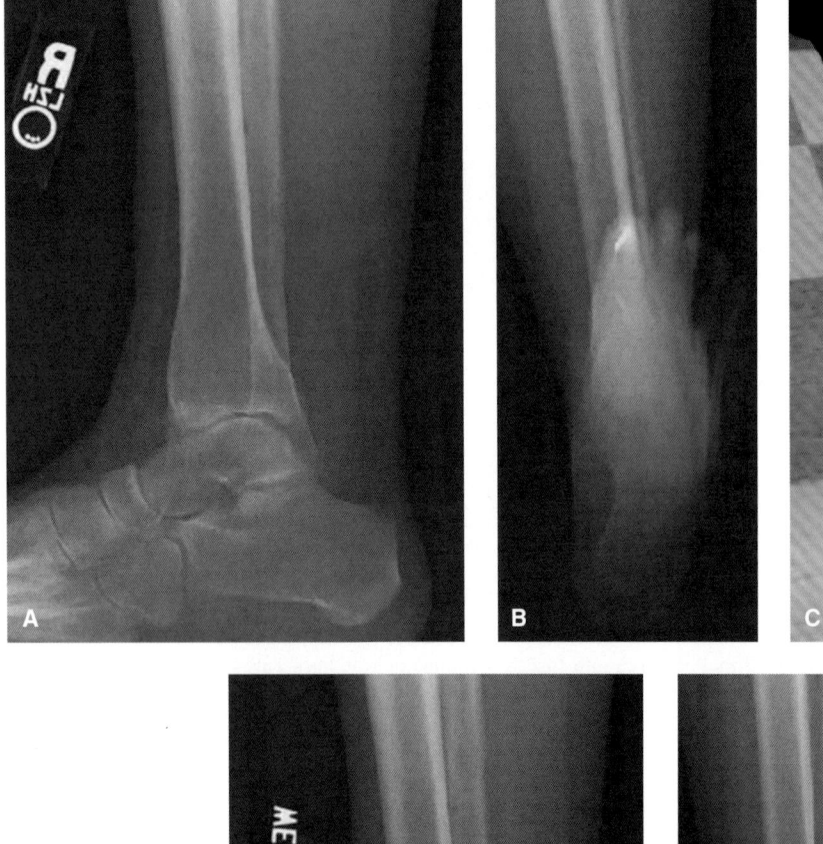
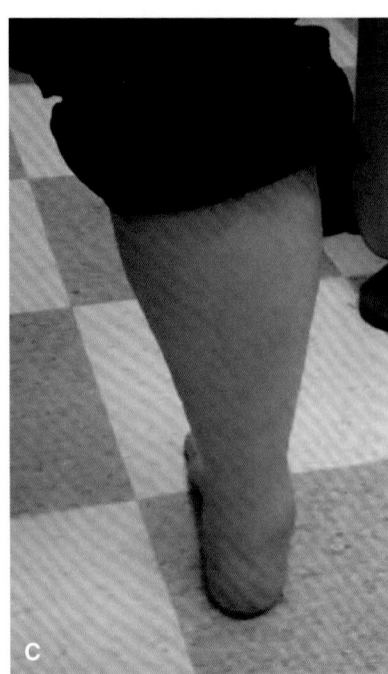
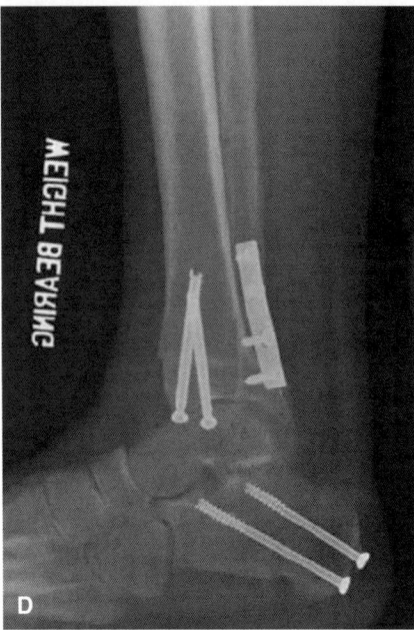
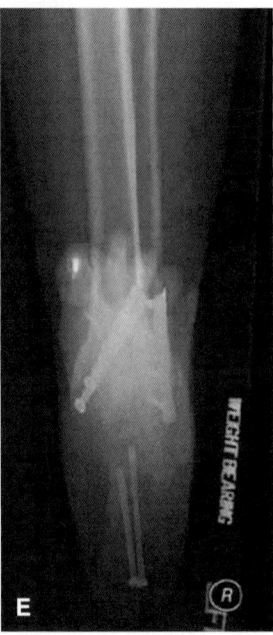

FIGURE 37.17 A, B. Malunion of posterior malleolar fracture resulting in osseous anterior ankle impingement and compensatory hindfoot varus in a 22-year-old female. **C.** Clinical photo showing hindfoot varus position. Deformity treated with an anterior closing wedge osteotomy of the tibia and lateral closing wedge calcaneal osteotomy. Postoperative lateral **(D)** and long leg calcaneal **(E)** axial views. Note the posterior translation of the tibial osteotomy to maintain coaxial alignment of the talus and tibia.

PEARLS

- There are essentially three strategies to correct the varus ankle, medial opening wedge or lateral closing wedge osteotomy and focal dome osteotomy (FDO). The most direct technique is an OWO of the distal tibia; however, in a patient with preoperative varus deformity of more than 10, an appropriate correction often cannot be achieved with a tibial osteotomy alone because the fibula may restrict the degree of supramalleolar correction.

- In most cases, the fibula can be left undisturbed, unless there is significant bony debris or stiffness at the tibiofibular joint or syndesmotic area that would preclude mobilization of the distal tibial metaphyseal segment around the syndesmotic ligament hinge.
- The location of the osteotomy is selected and should be as close to the CORA as possible, but should remain within the confines of the cancellous bone substrate of the tibial metaphysis.

ADJUNCTIVE PROCEDURES FOR VARUS DEFORMITY

When correcting varus deformity with any of the available techniques, there are several conditions that require attention.

- *Posterior tibial nerve damage*—the posterior tibial nerve is at risk for traction neuropathy, proportional to the degree of preoperative deformity. As the deformity is reduced, the nerve remains tethered to the distal tibial segment. Although there is risk of mechanical nerve irritation with correction of any planar deviation such as procurvatum, equinus, or internal rotation, the tibial nerve is most vulnerable during correction of varus deformity. Prophylactic tarsal tunnel release is generally recommended for any significant degree of correction.[1,16] Care should be taken with release of the tarsal tunnel and porta pedis to adequately decompress the medial and lateral plantar nerves as they pass beneath the abductor hallucis muscle. Sanders et al.[22] used neuromonitoring for any lengthening procedures to avoid iatrogenic nerve injury with deformity correction.
- *Hindfoot varus*—with long-standing varus deformity, there may be cavovarus adaptation to the foot that may require additional procedures to attain a plantigrade foot. In particular, the heel is often in a varus posture and requires calcaneal osteotomy for resolution. Most commonly, this is performed from a lateral incision inferior to the peroneal tendons using a closing wedge technique. However, it can be performed from a medial approach, especially if a tarsal tunnel release is performed during the surgical session. Generally, more correction can be obtained from a medial exposure because an opening wedge technique is utilized. Additional corrective osteotomies or fusions of the hind and midfoot complex may be indicated to achieve the ultimate goal of a stable plantigrade foot.
- *Lateral ankle stabilization*—it is also common to encounter lateral collateral ligament instability in long-standing varus deformity of the lower extremity. Often, secondary soft tissue reconstruction such as peroneal tendon repair or lateral ankle stabilization is warranted. Clinical examination and diagnostic testing will guide one to the appropriate procedures.

CORRECTION OF VALGUS DEFORMITY

Correction of valgus deformity is typically more complicated than correction of the varus ankle because the syndesmosis is more frequently involved in the pathologic relationship. This is due to the frequent posttraumatic etiology of the valgus ankle. As such, the tibiofibular relationship should be either maintained or corrected during the normalization of the distal tibial plafond. In addition, there is frequently asymmetric wear on the lateral aspect of the distal tibia as a consequence of focal avascular necrosis. The easiest surgical technique for the valgus ankle is a medial closing wedge of the distal tibial metaphysis (Fig. 37.18).

CORRECTION OF SAGITTAL PLANE DEFORMITY

There are three prevailing strategies for correction of sagittal plane deformities. These techniques are similar to those utilized for varus or valgus deformities. In many cases of the varus or valgus ankle, there is some component of sagittal plane malalignment. Uniplanar deformities of procurvatum or recurvatum are uncommon in the distal aspect of the tibia as

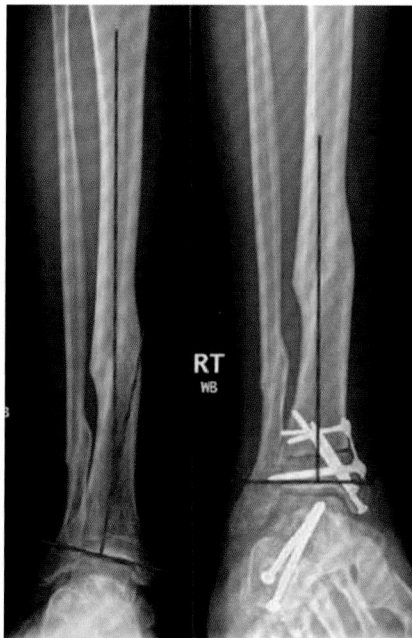

FIGURE 37.18 Posttraumatic ankle valgus malunion with subtalar arthritis. The osteotomy was performed slightly distal to the CORA in the metaphyseal region of the tibia. The fibula was left intact, and a medial H-plate was used for fixation. Subtalar arthrodesis was also performed for painful arthritis.

most of the patients that present with sagittal plane deformities have had a history of a tibia fracture that was treated without surgical intervention.

- *Recurvatum deformity* is seemingly more prevalent after a tibia fracture. When this deformity is long-standing, degenerative joint disease develops rapidly due the shear forces that are in effect across the ankle with attempts at dorsiflexion during gait. The resultant loss of motion causes the recognized compensatory mechanisms. These compensatory mechanisms may actually be the presenting complaint, as the symptoms in the ankle joint may be modest or minimal because of the lack of excursion.
- *Procurvatum deformity* is less common than recurvatum deformity, but is more likely to manifest as impingement pain in the anterior ankle joint and lack of ankle dorsiflexion. Malunited posterior malleolar fractures often present with anterior impingement with lack of dorsiflexion and anterior impingement symptoms.
- *Anterior impingement following pediatric clubfoot surgery*—often, the talus is small and hypoplastic, and in some instances flattened. This dysmorphic shape of the talus results in loss of height in the ankle and can lead to anterior osseous equinus. Often, unsuccessful attempts at correction of the equinus have been undertaken with Achilles lengthening (Fig. 37.19).

The end result of sagittal plane osteotomy for recurvatum and procurvatum (restoring the ADTA) should be adequate dorsiflexion and a plantargrade foot and restoration of the axial alignment of the center of the talus beneath the axis of the leg. Recurvatum deformities usually have more anterior translation associated with them, and planned osteotomy must account for this.

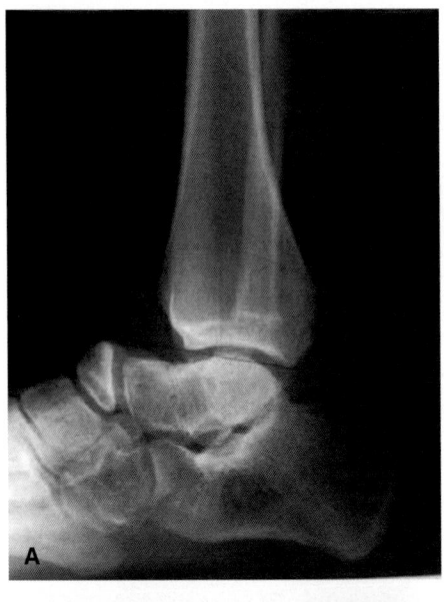
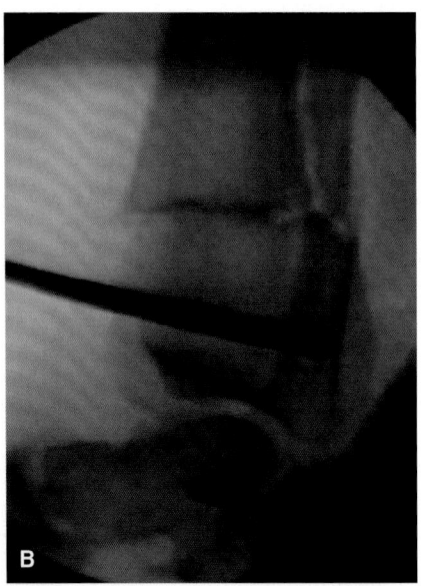
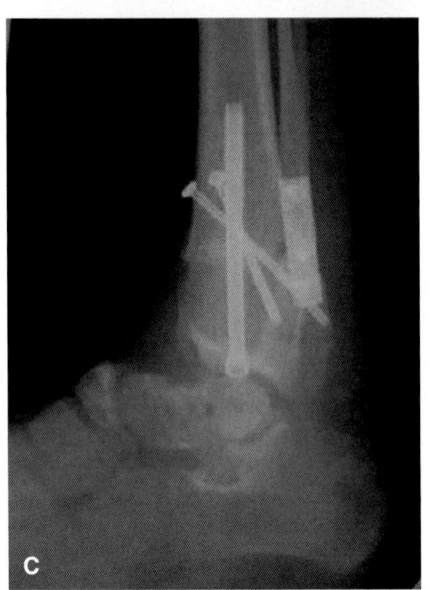
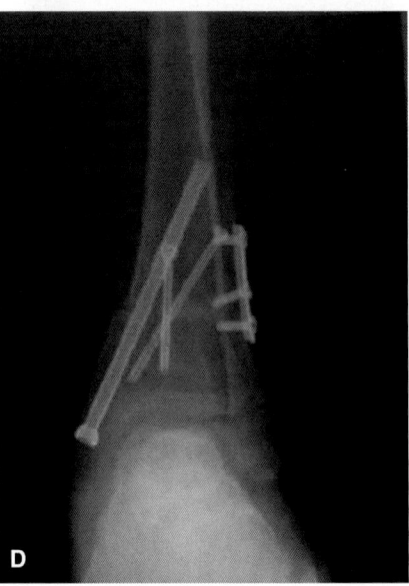

FIGURE 37.19 A. Anterior ankle impingement resulting from clubfoot talus and loss of height in the ankle mortise leading to anterior plafond impingement. Treated with FDO in the sagittal plane. **B.** A large pin in the distal segment facilitates disengaging the osteotomy and achieving correction. **C&D.** Fixation is delivered in a percutaneous method.

- The fibular osteotomy is done in an oblique fashion in the same plane of the desired correction. The osteotomy should generally be above the syndesmosis and at approximately the same level as the tibial osteotomy.
- After removal of the wedge, the distal tibia can be translated to restore the axial alignment of the joint.
- Fixation can be accomplished in a percutaneous method with screw fixation.
- Fixation of the fibula is not always necessary and if needed is accomplished with screws as plating is difficult due to cortical step-off.

SUMMARY

SMO for posttraumatic malunion, developmental or physeal deformities, congenital malalignment, as well as focal articular degenerative problems in the ankle is a useful surgical technique. Accurate clinical evaluation of the distal tibial deformity,

soft tissue for contractures and instability, and weight-bearing radiographs will guide the surgeon to the proper surgical plan. Osteotomy planning must involve all components of the deformity including the foot and respect osteotomy principles. Most often, juxta-articular deformities can be corrected with a single-stage corrective osteotomy. Multiple plane deformity often requires gradual correction with external fixation.

REFERENCES

1. Speed JS, Boyd HB. Operative reconstruction of malunited fractures about the ankle joint. *J Bone Joint Surg Am.* 1936;18(2):270-286.
2. Dzakhov SD, Kurochkin I. Supramalleolar osteotomies in children and adolescents. *Ortop Travmatol Protez.* 1966;27(12):41-48.
3. Barskii AV, Semenov NP. Methods of the supramalleolar osteotomy in ununited fractures of the malleoli. *Ortop Travmatol Protez.* 1979;7:54-55.
4. Takakura Y, Tanaka Y, Kumai T, et al. Low tibial osteotomy for osteoarthritis of the ankle. Results of a new operation in 18 patients. *J Bone Joint Surg Br.* 1995;77(1):50-54.
5. Mendicino RW, Catanzariti AR, Reeves CL. Percutaneous supramalleolar osteotomy for distal tibial (near articular) ankle deformities. *J Am Podiatr Med Assoc.* 2005;95(1):72-84.
6. Napiontek M, Nazar J. Tibial osteotomy as a salvage procedure in the treatment of congenital talipes equinovarus. *J Pediatr Orthop.* 1994;14:763-767.

7. Abraham E, Lubicky JP, Songer MN. Supramalleolar osteotomy for ankle valgus in myelo-meningocele. *J Pediatr Orthop.* 1996;16:774-781.

8. Graehl PM, Hersh MR, Heckman JD. Supramalleolar osteotomy for the treatment of symptomatic tibial nonunion. *J Orthop Trauma.* 1987;1:281-292.

9. McNicol D, Leong JC, Hsu LC. Supramalleolar derotation osteotomy for lateral tibial tor-sion and associated equinovarus deformity of the foot. *J Bone Joint Surg Br.* 1983;65:166-170

10. Scheffer MM, Peterson HA. Opening-wedge osteotomy for angular deformities of long bones in children. *J Bone Joint Surg Am.* 1994;76:325-334.

11. Harstall R, Lehmann O, Krause F, et al. Supramalleolar lateral closing wedge osteotomy for the treatment of varus ankle arthrosis. *Foot Ankle Int.* 2007;28(5);542-548.

12. Heywood AW. Supramalleolar osteotomy in the management of the rheumatoid hind-foot. *Clin Orthop.* 1983;177:76-81.

13. Pearce MS, Smith MA, Savidge GF. Supramalleolar tibial osteotomy for hemophilic arthropathy of the ankle. *J Bone Joint Surg Br.* 1994;76B:947-950.

14. Merchant TC, Dietz FR. Long term follow up after fractures of the tibial and fibular shafts. *J Bone Joint Surg Am.* 1989;71A:599-606.

15. Kristensen KD, Kiaer T, Blicher J. No arthrosis of the ankle 20 years after malaligned tibial-shaft fracture. *Acta Orthop Scand.* 1989;60:208-209.

16. Paley D. Ankle and foot considerations. In: Paley D, ed. *Principles of Deformity Correction.* New York, NY: Springer; 2002.

17. Tarr RR, Resnick CT, Wagner KS. Changes in tibiotalar joint contact areas follow-ing experimentally induced tibial angular deformities. *Clin Orthop.* 1985;199:72-80.

18. Takakura Y, Tanaka Y, Kumai T. Low tibial osteotomy for osteoarthritis of the ankle. Results of a new operation in 18 patients. *J Bone Joint Surg Br.* 1995;77:50-54.

19. Sammarco GJ. Biomechanics of the foot. In: Nordin M, Frankel VH, eds. *Basic Biomechan-ics of the Musculoskeletal System.* 2nd ed. Philadelphia, PA: Lea & Febuger; 1989

20. Inman VT. *The Joint of the Ankle.* Baltimore, MD: Williams and Wilkins; 1976.

21. Ting AJ, Tarr RR, Sarmiento A. The role of subtalar motion and ankle contact pressure changes from angular deformities of the tibia. *Foot Ankle.* 1987;7:290-299.

22. Steffensmeier SJ, Saltzman CL, Berbaum KS. Effects of medial and lateral displace-ment calcaneal osteotomies on tibiotalar joint contact stresses. *J Orthop Res.* 1996;14:980-985.

23. Best A, Daniels TR. Supramalleolar tibial osteotomy secured with the Puddu plate. *Ortho-pedics.* 2006;29(6):537-540.

24. Takakura Y, Takaoka T, Tanaka Y. Results of opening wedge osteotomy for the treatment of a post traumatic varus deformity of the ankle. *J Bone Joint Surg Am.* 1998;80;213-218.

Note: Page numbers followed by "*f*" refer to figures; page numbers followed by "*t*" refer to tables.

VOLUME TWO

McGLAMRY'S
Foot and Ankle Surgery

FIFTH EDITION

VOLUME TWO

McGLAMRY'S

Foot and Ankle Surgery

FIFTH EDITION

BRIAN CARPENTER, DPM, FACFAS

Professor
Department of Orthopaedics
The University of North Texas Health Science Center
Fort Worth, Texas

MICHELLE L. BUTTERWORTH, DPM, FACFAS

Williamsburg Foot Center
Williamsburg Regional Hospital
Kingstree, South Carolina

WILLIAM D. FISHCO, DPM, MS, FACFAS

Faculty
The Podiatry Institute
Decatur, Georgia
Adjunct Site Director and Clinical Instructor
Creighton University PMSR/RRA
Private Practice
Anthem, Arizona

JOHN T. MARCOUX, DPM, FACFAS

Program Director, Podiatric Medicine and Surgery Residency
Department of Surgery
Steward–St. Elizabeth's Medical Center
Brighton, Massachusetts

DANIEL F. VICKERS, CAE

Executive Director
The Podiatry Institute
Decatur, Georgia

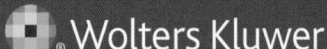 Wolters Kluwer

Philadelphia · Baltimore · New York · London
Buenos Aires · Hong Kong · Sydney · Tokyo

Executive Editor: Brian Brown
Development Editor: Stacey Sebring
Editorial Coordinator: Julie Kostelnik/Emily Buccieri
Marketing Manager: Phyllis Hitner
Production Project Manager: David Saltzberg
Design Coordinator: Stephen Druding
Manufacturing Coordinator: Beth Welsh
Prepress Vendor: SPi Global

Fifth Edition

Cataloging-in-Publication Data available on request from the Publisher

ISBN: 978-1-9751-3606-2

CCS0621

CONTENTS

CONTRIBUTORS

Sharif Abdelfattah, DPM, AACFAS
Foot and Ankle Surgeon
Sullivan Community Hospital
Sullivan, Indiana

Rachel H. Albright, DPM, MPH, AACFAS
Physician
Stamford Health Medical Group
Stamford, Connecticut

Dhaval K. Amin, DPM, DABPM
Staff Podiatric Foot and Ankle Surgeon
Department of Orthopaedics and
    Rehabilitation
Womack Army Medical Center
Fort Bragg, North Carolina

Robert B. Anderson, MD
Director, Foot and Ankle Service
Titletown Sports Medicine and Orthopaedics
Co-Chairman, Musculoskeletal Committee for
    the National Football League
Associate Team Physician, Green Bay Packers
Green Bay, Wisconsin

Peter J. Apel, MD, PhD
Assistant Professor
Department of Orthopaedic Surgery
Institute for Orthopaedics and Neurosciences,
    Carilion Clinic
Roanoke, Virginia

Albert V. Armstrong Jr, DPM, MS, BSRS
Professor of Radiology
Director of Advanced Medical Imaging
Former Dean
Barry University of School of Podiatric
    Medicine
Miami Shores, Florida

Christopher E. Attinger, MD
Professor, Georgetown University School of
    Medicine
Codirector, Center for Wound Healing
Department of Plastic and Reconstructive
    Surgery
MedStar Georgetown University Hospital
Washington, District of Columbia

Jayson N. Atves, DPM, AACFAS
Assistant Professor, Georgetown University
    School of Medicine
Program Director, MedStar Georgetown
    University Hospital Foot and Ankle Research
    Fellowship
Attending Physician, MedStar Health Podiatric
    Surgery Residency
Department of Plastic and Reconstructive Surgery
MedStar Georgetown University Hospital
Washington, District of Columbia

Alan S. Banks, DPM, FACFAS
Faculty
The Podiatry Institute
Decatur, Georgia
Private Practice
Tucker, Georgia

Luke C. Bates, DPM
Resident
Carilion Clinic Department of Orthopaedics
Roanoke, Virginia

Tzvi Bar-David, DPM, FACFAS
Director of Podiatric Surgery Service
Department of Orthopedic Surgery
Columbia University Medical Center
New York Presbyterian Hospital
New York, New York

Eric A. Barp, DPM, FACFAS
The Iowa Clinic-Foot and Ankle Surgery
Director of Foot and Ankle Surgery-Unity Point
    Hospital
Des Moines, Iowa

Peter A. Blume, DPM, FACFAS
Medical Director/HVC/Ambulatory Surgery
Yale New Haven Health Systems
Assistant Clinical Professor of Surgery
Anesthesia and Cardiology
Yale School of Medicine
New Haven, Connecticut

Troy J. Boffeli, DPM, FACFAS
Residency Program Director
HealthPartners Institute/Regions Hospital
Department Chair
HealthPartners Foot and Ankle Surgery
St. Paul, Minnesota

Allan M. Boike, DPM, FACFAS
Dean—CEO
Professor, Division of Foot and Ankle Surgery
Kent State University College of Podiatric
    Medicine
Independence, Ohio

Chris Bourke, DPM, AACFAS
Foot and Ankle Surgeon
Department of Orthopedics and Podiatry
Mid-Atlantic Permanente Medical Group
Kaiser Permanente
Springfield, Virginia

Aaron Bradley, MD
Private Practice
Glen Allen, Virginia

Mary R. Brandt, BA
Fourth Year Podiatric Medical Student
College of Podiatric Medicine and Surgery
Des Moines University
Des Moines, Iowa

Stephen A. Brigido, DPM, FACFAS
Section Chief, Foot and Ankle Reconstruction
Director, Foot and Ankle Fellowship
Coordinated Health at Lehigh Valley Health
    Network
Bethlehem, Pennsylvania
Clinical Professor of Surgery
The Geisinger Commonwealth
    Medical College
Scranton, Pennsylvania

Thomas A. Brosky II, DPM, FACFAS
Adjunct Faculty
Podiatric Medicine and Surgery Residency
Emory School of Medicine
Decatur, Georgia

William Brownell, DPM, MA, AACFAS
Fellow, Lower Extremity Plastic &
    Reconstructive Surgery
Division of Plastics & Reconstructive
    Surgery
Hospital of the University of
    Pennsylvania
Philadelphia, Pennsylvania

Amy E. Bruce, DPM
Chief Resident
Division of Podiatric Medicine & Surgery
University of Pennsylvania Health System–
  Penn Medicine
Philadelphia, Pennsylvania

Jennifer Buchanan, DPM, MS, FACFAS
Department of Surgery
Cambridge Health Alliance
Cambridge, Massachusetts

Michelle L. Butterworth, DPM, FACFAS
Hospital Employee
Williamsburg Foot Center
Williamsburg Regional Hospital
Kingstree, South Carolina

Jarrett D. Cain, DPM, MSc, FACFAS
Associate Professor
Department of Orthopaedics
University of Pittsburgh School of
  Medicine
University of Pittsburgh Physicians
Pittsburgh, Pennsylvania

David J. Caldarella, DPM, FACFAS
Foot and Ankle Surgery
ORTHO Rhode Island
Assistant Clinical Professor
Department of Orthopaedic Surgery
Warren Alpert School of Medicine
Brown University
Providence, Rhode Island
AO Scholar
Harborview Medical Center
Department of Orthopedic Surgery
Foot, Ankle and Amputee Service
University of Washington School of Medicine
Seattle, Washington
Alumnus, Faculty Member
The Podiatry Institute
Atlanta, Georgia

**Craig A. Camasta, DPM, FACFAS,
FABPS, FACSP**
Private Practice
Section Chief
Department of Surgery
Emory Saint Joseph's Hospital
Atlanta, Georgia
Faculty, The Podiatry Institute
Decatur, Georgia

Steven R. Carter, DPM, FACFAS
Department of Surgery
Piedmont Hospital
Private Practice
Covington, Georgia

Andrea D. Cass, DPM, FACFAS
Faculty, The Podiatry Institute
Decatur, Georgia
Assistant Director
Atlanta Reconstructive Surgery and Limb
  Preservation Fellowship
Smyrna, Georgia

**Francesca M. Castellucci-Garza, DPM,
AACFAS, MS**
Podiatric Surgery
Department of Orthopedics
Kaiser Permanente
Attending Surgeon
Kaiser San Francisco Bay Area Foot and Ankle
  Residency Program
Walnut Creek, California

Gage M. Caudell, DPM, FACFAS
Faculty, The Podiatry Institute
Decatur, Georgia
Fort Wayne Orthopedics
Fort Wayne, Indiana

David Chan, DPM
Private Practice
Leesburg, Virginia

Thomas J. Chang, DPM, FACFAS
Faculty, The Podiatry Institute
Decatur, Georgia
Clinical Professor and Past Chairman
Department of Podiatric Surgery
Samuel Merritt College of Podiatric Medicine,
  Formerly CCPM
Oakland, California
Redwood Orthopedic Surgery Associates
Santa Rosa, California

Jeffrey C. Christensen, DPM, FACFAS
Founder, Ankle & Foot Clinic of Everett
Past Foot & Ankle Section Chair/Attending
  Surgeon
Department of Orthopedics
Swedish Medical Center
Seattle, Washington

Robert A. Christman, DPM, EdM
Professor
College of Podiatric Medicine
Western University of Health Sciences
Pomona, California

J. Randolph Clements, DPM
Associate Professor of Orthopaedic
  Surgery
Virginia Tech Carilion School of Medicine
Roanoke, Virginia

David R. Collman, DPM, FACFAS
Site Director, Kaiser San Francisco Bay Area
  Foot and Ankle Residency Program
Assistant Chief, Podiatry/Foot and Ankle
  Surgery
Department of Orthopedics, Podiatry, Injury,
  Sports Medicine
The Permanente Medical Group, Inc.
Kaiser Foundation Hospital San Francisco
San Francisco, California

James C. Connors, DPM, FACFAS
Assistant Professor
Division of Foot and Ankle Surgery
Kent State University College of Podiatric
  Medicine
Independence, Ohio

Dustin Constant, DPM
Foot and Ankle Surgeon
Palm Beach Sports Medicine and Orthopedics
Palm Beach, Florida

**Emily A. Cook, DPM, MPH, CPH,
FACFAS**
Assistant Professor of Surgery
Harvard Medical School
Director of Resident Education
Department of Surgery
Mount Auburn Hospital
Cambridge, Massachusetts

**Jeremy J. Cook, DPM, MPH, CPH,
FACFAS**
Assistant Professor of Surgery
Harvard Medical School
Director of Research and Quality Assurance
Department of Surgery
Mount Auburn Hospital
Cambridge, Massachusetts

Guillaume Cordier, MD
Past President
Group of Research and Study in Minimally
  Invasive Surgery of the Foot/Minimal Invasive
  Foot Surgery
Foot and Ankle Surgeon
Clinique du Sport Bordeaux-Mérignac,
  Chirurgie du Sport–Foot and Ankle
Merignac, France

Judd Cummings, MD
Clinical Assistant Professor
Department of Orthopaedic Surgery
University of Arizona
Orthopaedic Surgical Oncology of Arizona
Scottsdale, Arizona

Miki Dalmau-Pastor, PhD, PT, DPM
Human Anatomy and Embryology Unit
Department of Pathology and Experimental
  Therapeutics
University of Barcelona
Foot and Ankle Unit
Hospital Quirón Barcelona
Barcelona, Spain

Paul Dayton, DPM, MS, FACFAS
Surgeon
Foot & Ankle Center of Iowa/Midwest Bunion
  Center
Ankeny, Iowa

Lawrence A. DiDomenico, DPM, FACFAS
Director of Residency Training
East Liverpool City Hospital
Director of Fellowship Training
NOMS (Northern Ohio Medical Specialist)
  Ankle and Foot Care Centers
Section Chief
Mercy Health St. Elizabeth Medical Center
Boardman, Ohio
Adjunct Professor
Kent State University College of Podiatric
  Medicine
Independence, Ohio

Thanh L. Dinh, DPM, FACFAS
Assistant Professor of Surgery
Harvard Medical School
Program Director
Podiatric Surgical Residency Program
Beth Israel Deaconess Medical Center
Boston, Massachusetts

Matthew B. Dobbs, MD, FACS
Director, Dobbs Clubfoot Center
Paley Orthopedic & Spine Institute
West Palm Beach, Florida
Senior Editor, Clinical Orthopaedics and
  Related Research
President, United States Bone and Joint Initiative
Secretary, Association of Bone and Joint Surgeons
Park Ridge, Illinois

Michael S. Downey, DPM, FACFAS
Chief, Division of Podiatric Surgery
Department of Surgery
Penn Presbyterian Medical Center
University of Pennsylvania Health System
Clinical Professor, Department of Surgery
Temple University School of Podiatric Medicine
Philadelphia, Pennsylvania
Private Practice
Penn Podiatry
Philadelphia, Pennsylvania and Mt. Laurel,
  New Jersey

Matthew D. Doyle, DPM, MS
Fellow
Silicon Valley Reconstructive Foot and Ankle
  Fellowship
Palo Alto Medical Foundation
Mountain View, California

Amish K. Dudeja, DPM, AACFAS
Foot and Ankle Surgical Fellow
Atlanta Reconstructive Surgery and Limb
  Preservation Fellowship
Village Podiatry Centers
Atlanta, Georgia

Karl W. Dunn, DPM, FACFAS
Compass Orthopedics
An Affiliate of Compass Rehabilitation
East Lansing, Michigan

Jordan J. Ernst, DPM, MS, AACFAS
Fellow, Foot and Ankle Deformity Correction
Fellow, Limb Lengthening and Reconstruction
Paley Orthopedic and Spine Institute
West Palm Beach, Florida

William D. Fishco, DPM, MS, FACFAS
Adjunct Site Director and Clinical Instructor
Creighton University PMSR/RRA
Private Practice
Anthem, Arizona

Adam E. Fleischer, DPM, MPH, FACFAS
Associate Professor
Dr. William M. Scholl College of Podiatric Medicine
Rosalind Franklin University of Medicine and
  Science
North Chicago, Illinois
Director of Research
Weil Foot & Ankle Institute
Mount Prospect, Illinois

Lawrence A. Ford, DPM, FACFAS
Chief of Podiatric Surgery
Department of Orthopedics
Kaiser Permanente
Attending Surgeon
Kaiser San Francisco Bay Area Foot and Ankle
  Residency Program
Oakland, California

Robert Fridman, DPM, FACFAS, CWSP
Faculty Podiatric Surgery Service
Department of Orthopedic Surgery
Columbia University Medical Center
New York Presbyterian Hospital
New York, New York

Ajay K. Ghai, DPM, AACFAS
Fellow, NOMS Ankle and Foot Care Center
Visalia Medical Clinic
Visalia, California

David A. Goss Jr, DO
Orthopedic Foot and Ankle Surgeon
Associates of Orthopedics and Sports Medicine
Dalton, Georgia

John Grady, DPM, FFPM RCPS (G), FASPS, FAAPSM
Residency Director
Advocate Christ Medical Center
Great Lakes Foot & Ankle Institute
Oak Lawn, Illinois

David W. Gray, MD, FAAOS
Professor
Department of Surgery
Texas Christian University Medical School
Cook Children's Department of Orthopedics and
  Spine Surgery
Fort Worth, Texas

George S. Gumann Jr, DPM, FACFAS
Retired Chief, Foot and Ankle Service
Orthopedic Clinic
Martin Army Hospital
Fort Benning, Georgia

Adam L. Halverson, DO
Consultant Surgeon
Orthopedic Surgeon: Foot and Ankle
  Specialist
Bone and Joint
Wausau, Wisconsin

John C. Haight, DPM
Chief Resident
Podiatric Medicine and Surgery Residency
Emory University School of Medicine
Decatur, Georgia

Patrick B. Hall, DPM, FACFAS
Faculty, The Podiatry institute
Decatur, Georgia
Private Practice
The Bone and Joint Clinic of Baton Rouge
Baton Rouge, Louisiana

Graham Hamilton, DPM, FACFAS
Foot and Ankle Surgeon
Department of Orthopedic and Podiatric
  Surgery
Sutter Health–Palo Alto Foundation Medical
  Group
Dublin, California

Mark A. Hardy, DPM, FACFAS
Division Head, Foot and Ankle Surgery
Kent State University College of Podiatric
  Medicine
Independence, Ohio

Carl T. Hasselman, MD, FAAOS, FAOFAS
Vice Chairman of Orthopedics, UPMC St. Margaret
Clinical Associate Professor, University of
  Pittsburgh
Professor, Saint Vincent College
Pittsburgh, Pennsylvania

Daniel J. Hatch, DPM, FACFAS
Director of Surgery
North Colorado Podiatric Surgical Residency
Greeley, Colorado
Private Practice
Foot and Ankle Center of the Rockies
Denver, Colorado

Christopher R. Hood Jr, DPM
Foot and Ankle Surgery
Hunterdon Podiatric Medicine
Hunterdon Healthcare System
Flemington, New Jersey

Byron Hutchinson, DPM, FACFAS
Medical Director
CHI/Franciscan Advanced Foot & Ankle
  Fellowship
Franciscan Foot & Ankle Associates: Highline
  Clinic
Burien, Washington

Christopher F. Hyer, DPM, MS, FACFAS
Codirector
Foot and Ankle Reconstructive Fellowship
Orthopedic Foot and Ankle Center
Worthington, Ohio

Trusha Jariwala, DPM, AACFAS
Associate Podiatrist
Moore Foot and Ankle Specialists, PA
Asheville, North Carolina

Meagan Jennings, DPM, FACFAS
Foot and Ankle Surgeon
Department of Orthopedics and Podiatry
Sutter Health–Palo Alto Foundation Medical Group
Mountain View, California

Molly S. Judge, DPM, FACFAS
Mercy Foot & Ankle Residency Program
  Cleveland, Ohio
Adjunct Faculty; Colleges of Podiatric
  Medicine, USA
Faculty; Graduate Medical Education
Mercy Health Partners
Toledo, Ohio

Daniel C. Jupiter, PhD
Associate Professor
Department of Preventive Medicine and
  Population Health
Department of Orthopaedic Surgery and
  Rehabilitation
Assistant Dean for Recruitment
Graduate School of Biomedical Sciences
The University of Texas Medical Branch
Galveston, Texas

Andreas C. Kaikis, DPM, AACFAS
Staff Surgeon
University Hospital Health System
Augusta, Georgia

Andrew P. Kapsalis, DPM, AACFAS
Research Coordinator for Fellowship Training
Foot and Ankle Reconstructive Surgical
  Services
American Health Network
Indianapolis, Indiana

Navita Khatri, DPM
Resident
Podiatric Medicine and Surgery Residency
Emory University School of Medicine
Decatur, Georgia

Michael F. Kelly, DPM, AACFAS
Foot and Ankle Surgeon
Department of Podiatry
St. Joseph Hospital–Covenant Health
Nashua, New Hampshire

Jason M. Kennedy, MD, FAAOS
Clinical Faculty, John Peter Smith Residency
  Program
Clinical Faculty, Baylor University Residency
  Program
Cook Children's Department of Orthopaedics
  and Sports Medicine
Fort Worth, Texas

Ansab Khwaja, MD
Resident Physician
University of Arizona Orthopaedic Surgery
  Residency
Tucson, Arizona

Carl Kihm, DPM, FACFAS
Attending Surgeon
Norton Audubon Hospital Residency
  Program
Private Practice
Louisville, Kentucky

Christy M. King, DPM, FACFAS
Program Direction
Kaiser San Francisco Bay Area Foot and Ankle
  Residency Program
Attending Physician, Kaiser Foundation
  Hospital–Oakland
Department of Orthopedics and Podiatry
Oakland, California

Alex J. Kline, MD, FAAOS, FAOFAS
Clinical Associate Professor
University of Pittsburgh
Chairman
Department of Orthopedics
UPMC St. Margaret
Professor
Saint Vincent College
Pittsburgh, Pennsylvania

Bradley M. Lamm, DPM, FACFAS
Chief, Foot and Ankle Surgery
St. Mary's Medical Center & Palm Beach
  Children's Hospital
Director, Foot and Ankle Deformity Center and
  Fellowship
Paley Orthopedic and Spine Institute
West Palm Beach, Florida

Travis M. Langan, DPM
Fellowship Trained Foot and Ankle Surgeon
Carle Orthopedics and Sports Medicine
Champaign, Illinois

Michael S. Lee, DPM, MS-HCA, FACFAS
Foot and Ankle Surgery
Capital Orthopaedics & Sports Medicine, PC
Des Moines, Iowa

Wesley Maurice Leong, DPM
Podiatric Surgeon
Department of Foot and Ankle Surgery
Monument Health Orthopedics and Specialty
  Hospital
Rapid City, South Dakota

Sara E. Lewis, DPM, AACFAS
Faculty
The Podiatry Institute
Decatur, Georgia
Health First Medical Group
Melbourne, Florida

Chandler J. Ligas, DPM
Resident
Podiatric Medicine and Surgery Residency
Emory University School of Medicine
Decatur, Georgia

George T. Liu, DPM, FACFAS
Associate Professor
Department of Orthopaedic Surgery
University of Texas Southwestern Medical Center
Dallas, Texas

Samantha A. Luer, DPM
Staff Surgeon
Department of Foot and Ankle Surgery/
  Orthopedics
Avera Medical Group, St. Anthony's Hospital
O'Neill, Nebraska

**Caitlin Mahan Madden, DPM,
AACFAS**
Associate Foot and Ankle Surgeon
Podiatry Care Specialists, PC
West Chester, Pennsylvania

**Kieran T. Mahan, DPM, FACFAS,
FABFAS, FCPP**
Professor
Department of Surgery
Temple University School of Podiatric Medicine
Chair, Department of Foot and Ankle Surgery
Temple University Hospital
Philadelphia, Pennsylvania

D. Scot Malay, DPM, MSCE, FACFAS
Faculty, The Podiatry Institute
Decatur, Georgia
Staff Surgeon and Director of Podiatric
  Research
Penn Presbyterian Medical Center
Philadelphia, Pennsylvania

Joshua J. Mann, DPM, FACFAS
Director
Podiatric Medicine and Surgery Residency
Emory University School of Medicine
Adjunct Assistant Professor
Department of Family and Preventive
  Medicine
Emory University School of Medicine
Private Practice
Ankle and Foot Centers of Georgia
Snellville, Georgia

John T. Marcoux, DPM, FACFAS
Program Director, Podiatric Medicine and
  Surgery Residency
Department of Surgery
Steward–St. Elizabeth's Medical Center
Brighton, Massachusetts

Stephen A. Mariash, DPM
Podiatric Surgeon
St. Cloud Orthopedics
Sartell, Minnesota

John A. Martucci, DPM
Resident Physician, Podiatric Medicine and
 Surgery
Division of Podiatric Surgery
Department of Surgery
Beth Israel Deaconess Medical Center
Clinical Fellow in Surgery
Harvard Medical School
Boston, Massachusetts

Stephen A. McCaughan, DO
Associate Professor
Department of Anesthesiology
Lewis Katz School of Medicine
Philadelphia, Pennsylvania

Michael C. McGlamry, DPM, FACFAS
Faculty, The Podiatry Institute
Private Practice
Cumming, Georgia

Andrew J. Meyr, DPM, FACFAS
Clinical Professor
Department of Surgery
Temple University School of Podiatric Medicine
Philadelphia, Pennsylvania

J. Michael Miller, DPM, FACFAS
Director of Fellowship Training
Foot and Ankle Reconstructive Surgical Services
American Health Network
Indianapolis, Indiana

Jason R. Miller, DPM, FACFAS
Director, Pennsylvania Intensive Lower
 Extremity Fellowship Program
Residency Director, Tower Health/Phoenixville
 Hospital PMSR/RRA
Adjunct Associate Professor
Department of Surgery
Temple University School of Podiatric Medicine
Philadelphia, Pennsylvania
Premier Orthopaedics
Malvern, Pennsylvania

Kelsey Millonig, DPM, MPH, AACFAS
Foot and Ankle Deformity Correction and
 Orthoplastics Fellow
Rubin Institute Advanced Orthopedics
International Center for Limb Lengthening
Baltimore, Maryland

Jeanne Mirbey, DPM
Physician
Emory Decatur Hospital
Decatur, Georgia

Roya Mirmiran, DPM, FACFAS
Foot and Ankle Surgeon
Sutter Medical Group
Sacramento, California

Travis A. Motley, DPM, MS, FACFAS
Professor, Department of Orthopaedic Surgery
Program Director, Podiatry Surgical Residency
Acclaim Physician Group
John Peter Smith Hospital
Fort Worth, Texas

Benjamin Meyer, DO
Resident Physician
MountainView Regional Medical Center
 Orthopaedic Surgery Residency
Las Cruces, New Mexico

Gina H. Nalbandian, DPM, AACFAS
Clinical Fellow of Surgery
Tufts University School of Medicine
Clinical Fellow of Surgery
University of California, Los Angeles
Los Angeles, California

Alan Ng, DPM, FACFAS
Foot & Ankle Surgeon, Advanced Orthopedic
 and Sports Medicine Specialists
Fellowship Director
The Rocky Mountain Reconstructive Foot &
 Ankle Fellowship at Advanced Orthopedic
Sports Medicine Specialists
Division of Orthopedic Centers of Colorado and
 Presbyterian/St. Luke's Medical Center/HCA
Residency Committee Member
Highlands-Presbyterian/St. Luke's Medical
 Center Podiatric Surgical Residency Program
Denver, Colorado

Jonathan D. Nigro, BS
Fourth Year Podiatric Medical Student
College of Podiatric Medicine and Surgery
Des Moines University
Des Moines, Iowa

Selene G. Parekh, MD, MBA, FAOA
Director of Digital Strategy & Innovation
Professor, Department of Orthopaedic Surgery
Partner, North Carolina Orthopaedic Clinic
Adjunct Faculty, Fuqua Business School
Duke University
Durham, North Carolina

Sandeep B. Patel, DPM, FACFAS
Chief of Podiatric Surgery
Department of Podiatric Surgery and Orthopedics
The Permanente Medical Group, Diablo
 Service Area
Kaiser San Francisco Bay Area Foot and Ankle
 Residency Program
Walnut Creek, California

Trevor S. Payne, DPM
Private Practice
Augusta, Georgia

Terrence M. Philbin, DO, FAOAO
Orthopedic Foot and Ankle Center
Worthington, Ohio

Alfred J. Phillips, DPM
Chief of Podiatry
St. Elizabeth Medical Center
Action, Massachusetts

Jason D. Pollard, DPM, FACFAS
Director of Research and Assistant Program
 Director
Department of Podiatric Surgery
Kaiser San Francisco Bay Area Foot and Ankle
 Residency Program
Oakland, California

Adam D. Port, DPM
Adjunct Faculty
Podiatric Medicine and Surgery Residency
Emory School of Medicine
Decatur, Georgia

Asim A. Z. Raja, DPM, FACFAS, DABPM
Director, Podiatric Medical Education (PMSR/RRA)
Department of Orthopaedics and Rehabilitation
Womack Army Medical Center
Fort Bragg, North Carolina

Nilin M. Rao, DPM, PhD, AACFAS
Fellow
Silicon Valley Reconstructive Foot and Ankle
 Fellowship
Department of Podiatric Surgery
Sutter Health–Palo Alto Medical Foundation
Mountain View, California

Rahn Ravenell, DPM, FACFAS
Assistant Professor
Medical University of South Carolina
Faculty, Podiatry Institute
Mount Pleasant, South Carolina

Christopher L. Reeves, DPM, FACFAS
Research Coordinator, Department of Podiatric
 Surgery, Advent Health System
Faculty, Advent Health East Podiatric Surgical
 Residency
Orlando Foot and Ankle Clinic/Upperline
 Health
Orlando, Florida

Rebekah Richards, DPM
Richards Orthopedic and Sports Medicine
Chambersburg, Pennsylvania

**Douglas H. Richie Jr, DPM, FACFAS,
FAAPSM**
Associate Clinical Professor
California School of Podiatric Medicine at
 Samuel Merritt University
Oakland, California

Ryan B. Rigby, DPM, FACFAS
Fellowship Trained Foot and Ankle Surgeon
Department of Orthopedics
Logan Regional Hospital
Logan Regional Orthopedics & Sports Medicine
Logan, Utah

Shayla A. Robinson, DPM
Resident
Podiatric Medicine and Surgery Residency
Emory University School of Medicine
Decatur, Georgia

Thomas S. Roukis, DPM, PhD, FACFAS
Past President (2014–2015), American College
of Foot and Ankle Surgeons
Editor-in-Chief, Foot & Ankle Surgery:
Techniques, Reports & Cases
Clinical Professor
Division of Foot & Ankle Surgery
Department of Orthopaedic Surgery and
Rehabilitation
College of Medicine–Jacksonville
University of Florida
Jacksonville, Florida

Laura P. Rowe, DPM
Private Practice,
Valley Foot & Ankle Specialty Providers
Fresno, California

Shannon M. Rush, DPM, FACFAS
Tri-Valley Orthopedics Specialists, Inc
Pleasanton, California
Adjunct Professor
California College of Podiatric Medicine at
Samuel Merritt University
Fellowship Director
Tri-Valley Foot and Ankle Reconstruction
Fellowship
Pleasanton, California
Surgical Staff
Stanford Valley Care
Pleasanton, California

Hannah J. Sahli, DPM
Chief Resident
Advent Health East Orlando Podiatric Surgical
Residency
Orlando, Florida

Laura E. Sansosti, DPM, AACFAS
Clinical Assistant Professor
Departments of Surgery and Biomechanics
Temple University School of Podiatric Medicine
Philadelphia, Pennsylvania

**Amol Saxena, DPM, FFPM, RCPS (G),
FACFAS, FAAPSM**
Fellowship Director Foot and Ankle Surgery
Department of Sports Medicine
Sutter Health–Palo Alto Division
Palo Alto, California

Harry P. Schneider, DPM, FACFAS
Assistant Professor of Surgery
Harvard Medical School
Residency Program Director
Cambridge Health Alliance
Cambridge, Massachusetts

John M. Schuberth, DPM
Staff Surgeon
Dept Orthopedic Surgery, Sports Medicine &
Podiatry
Kaiser Foundation Hospital
San Francisco, California

Josh Sebag, DPM
Chief Resident
Department of Podiatric Surgery
Advent Health East Orlando Podiatric Surgical
Residency
Orlando, Florida

Matthew J. Seidel, MD
Surgeon Department of Orthopedic Surgery
Honor Health Hospital System
Clinical Assistant Professor of Orthopedic
Surgery University of Arizona
Scottsdale, Arizona

Chad L. Seidenstricker, BS, DPM
Foot & Ankle Surgeon
New Mexico Orthopaedics
Albuquerque, New Mexico

Michael L. Sganga, DPM, FACFAS
Chief of Podiatry Milford Regional Medical
Center
Foot and Ankle Surgeon
Orthopedics New England
Natick, Newton, and Hopkinton,
Massachusetts

Amber M. Shane, DPM, FACFAS
Chair, Department of Podiatric Surgery, Advent
Health System
Faculty, Advent Health East Podiatric Surgical
Residency
Orlando Foot and Ankle Clinic/Upperline Health
Orlando, Florida

Eric Shi, DPM
Foot and Ankle Surgeon
Department of Podiatry
Sutter East Bay Medical Foundation
Castro Valley, California

Naohiro Shibuya, DPM, MS, FACFAS
Professor
College of Medicine
Texas A&M University
Temple, Texas

Sara Shirazi, DPM
Podiatric Surgeon
Pasadena Orthopedics, Inc.
Los Angeles, California

Louie Shou, DPM, AACFAS, FAAPSM
Reconstructive Orthopedics
Medford, New Jersey

Clay Shumway, DPM AACFAS
Fellow, Pennsylvania Intensive Lower Extremity
Fellowship
Premier Orthopaedics & Sports Medicine
Malvern, Pennsylvania

Mickey D. Stapp, DPM, FACFAS
Private Practice
Augusta, Georgia

Jerome K. Steck, DPM
Chief of Podiatric Surgery
Carondelet Medical Group: Orthopedics
Carondelet St. Joseph's Hospital
Tucson, Arizona

John S. Steinberg, DPM, FACFAS
Professor, Georgetown University School of
Medicine
Program Director, MedStar Health Podiatric
Surgery Residency
Codirector, Center for Wound Healing
Department of Plastic and Reconstructive
Surgery
MedStar Georgetown University Hospital
Washington, District of Columbia

N. Jake Summers, DPM, FACFAS
Chief of Podiatry Dartmouth-Hitchcock
Manchester
Faculty - New England Musculoskeletal
Institute
Dartmouth-Hitchcock
Manchester, New Hampshire

Ronald M. Talis, DPM, FACFAS
Staff Podiatric Foot and Ankle Surgeon
Department of Orthopedics and Rehabilitation
Womack Army Medical Center
Fort Bragg, North Carolina

Zach Tankersley, DPM, FACFAS
Associate Professor of Orthopaedic Surgery
Joan C. Edwards School of Medicine
Marshall University
Huntington, West Virginia

Robert P. Taylor, DPM, FACFAS
Stonebriar Foot & Ankle
Firsco, Texas

Michael H. Theodoulou, DPM, FACFAS
Chief
Division of Podiatric Surgery, Cambridge Health
Alliance
Department of Surgery
Instructor of Surgery
Harvard Medical School
Cambridge, Massachusetts

James Thomas, DPM, FACFAS
Chief, Foot and Ankle Surgery
Professor of Orthopaedic Surgery
Joan C. Edwards School of Medicine
Marshall University
Huntington, West Virginia

Mitchell J. Thompson, DPM
Podiatric Medicine & Surgery Resident
Podiatric Medicine and Surgery
Gundersen Medical Foundation
LaCrosse, Wisconsin

Michael Van Pelt, DPM, FACFAS
Associate Professor
Department of Orthopaedic Surgery
UT Southwestern Medical Center Dallas
Dallas, Texas

Tracey C. Vlahovic, DPM, FFPM, RCPS (Glasg)
Clinical Professor
Department of Podiatric Medicine
Temple University School of Podiatric
 Medicine
Philadelphia, Pennsylvania

Mitzi L. Williams, DPM, FACFAS
Pediatric Foot and Ankle Surgery
Department of Podiatric Surgery and
 Orthopedics
Attending Surgeon
Kaiser Permanente
Oakland, California

The presentation of the fifth edition of *McGlamry's Foot and Ankle Surgery* is a time to look back as well as forward. I look back to the genesis of this textbook and realize that it is one of the most satisfying chapters in my career in Podiatric Medicine and Surgery.

From 1972 to 1982, I was privileged to serve as editor of *The Journal of the American Podiatry Medical Association*. In that capacity, I made frequent visits to meet with our publisher, Williams and Wilkins Medical Publishers, in Baltimore, Maryland. This resulted in a close relationship with Norville Miller, the executive responsible for the final production and printing and distribution of the journal. Norville frequently reminded me that Podiatric Surgery was yet to produce its own textbook.

When I retired as editor of *JAPMA*, Norville called asking to meet with me in Atlanta. He was very forthright in saying that he wanted to talk about a textbook on Foot and Ankle Surgery. He also said that Williams and Wilkins (W and W) was willing to make an attractive arrangement.

Norville flew to Atlanta and met with me and two of my residents, Drs. Kieran Mahan and John Ruch. He presented the idea of doing the first medical textbook ever, with the entire book being written in computer instead of typed. The idea was to complete the book and turn over the floppy discs to W and W instead of submitting a typed manuscript. He said that W and W would purchase for us an IBM Computer, a printer, a computer desk, and most important, would purchase a support contract whereby we could call for computer instruction and technical assistance at any time of day or night. Remember, the personal computer was then new. There were no ribbons with commands at the top of the page. There was no mouse.

Dr. Mahan, Dr. Ruch, and I accepted the challenge on behalf of the relatively young Podiatry Institute. We also got a commitment from Becky McGlamry that she would serve as Author's Editor. And for the next 5 years that embryo book drove our lives and that of many of our colleagues and former residents of our program in Podiatric Surgery.

Each addition of the textbook has shown progressive maturity. This edition is no exception to that trend, and it is so written and organized as to facilitate immediate access to virtually any challenge confronting the Podiatric or Orthopedic Surgeon as they deal with foot and ankle surgery. This should provide the most accessible and in-depth information of any of the five editions, an appropriate accomplishment for the fifth edition. My personal congratulations to the editors and to the publisher, now Lippincott, Williams & Wilkins.

E. Dalton McGlamry, retired

PREFACE

We are delighted and honored to write the preface for the fifth edition of *McGlamry's Foot and Ankle Surgery*. E. Dalton McGlamry recognized the need for a complete and well-referenced textbook in foot and ankle surgery and published the first edition in 1987. Through the centuries, physicians and surgeons have been engaged in preservation of normal foot and ankle function. In ancient times, the normal functioning foot was vital to survival. Aristotle (384-322 BC) studied movement and analyzed the degeneration of muscles and the defective development of human beings, and it was believed that individuals possessing these attributes could not survive. In ancient Rome, those with disabilities were treated as objects of scorn. As early as 400 BC, Hippocrates described clubfoot and recommended nonoperative treatments using manipulation and bandaging techniques not dissimilar to the techniques utilized today.

In recent times, an abundance of medical knowledge and innovations have been unveiled and the dynamic nature of medical science continues to evolve. Professionals among the medical disciplines work collectively as interdisciplinary teams and are the cornerstone of medical organizations and health care systems representing the future of medicine. Well-trained, successful, foot and ankle surgeons exert a large influence within medicine and represent departmental chairs, current and past presidents of major medical associations, journal authors and editors, researchers, and reviewers.

This textbook is intended for use by residents in training with a focus on foot and ankle pathology as well as surgeons with interest in the foot and ankle; both nonoperative and operative techniques are described with quick reference text boxes highlighted as an educational tool for the reader.

The esteemed authors represented in this textbook were carefully selected for their educational, clinical, and surgical acumen, contributions to research and achievements in their selected subject matter. The editorial board endeavored to ensure that the information provided is accurate and current.

It is our hope and expectation that this book will provide an effective learning experience and referenced resource for all foot and ankle specialists and ultimately lead to improved patient care and outcomes.

Brian Carpenter, DPM, FACFAS
Michelle L. Butterworth, DPM, FACFAS
William D. Fishco, DPM, MS, FACFAS
John T. Marcoux, DPM, FACFAS

ACKNOWLEDGMENTS

I would like to acknowledge the authors and reviewers, Dr. Butterworth, Dr. Fishco, and Dr. Marcoux, for their dedication to this project. You have provided countless hours in bringing this to fruition and have remained steadfast friends and supportive colleagues. The world of medicine is enhanced by your contributions to academic medicine, your zeal in sharing your talent, and your ability to incentivize others by your mentorship. Your gift of time and sacrifice is immeasurable.

To the individuals with whom I have been blessed to work and serve with and those who I have had the opportunity to train and educate, I thank you for inspiring me to undertake this project. Being part of the Podiatry Institute is one of the highlights of my career being allowed to enhance the quality of life for patients with foot, ankle, and leg disorders through innovative education, research, and service is humbling. Without the experiences and support I have garnered from students, residents, and peers throughout the years, this publication would not exist.

I would be remiss if I didn't highlight those who have been instrumental in my own personal development and professional career. Physicians, nurses, and fellow residents were an integral part of my education and I am reminded of you whenever I reduce and fixate a fracture by nail or plate or when powering up a saw. I want to give special recognition and thanks to my mentors: Jeff Coen, DPM; A. Edward Mostone, DPM; Raymond Igou, MD; Michael Corbett, MD; Stephen Tubridy, DPM; Francis Wolfort, MD; and Ted Hansen, MD, who provided innumerable educational opportunities. During my training, they challenged me to never be content with my knowledge and skills. I am grateful for their stewardship and now call them friends.

Seek knowledge, serve as an ambassador for your patients, do the right thing and ultimately, your life will be blessed. I pay homage to God; without him none of this would be possible.

Brian Carpenter, DPM, FACFAS

INTRODUCTION

I am honored to have been chosen to write this introduction to the fifth edition of *McGlamry's Foot and Ankle Surgery*.

I vividly remember 30 years ago, as Dennis Martin and I began our residency at Doctors Hospital in Tucker, Georgia, the publishing of the first edition of the *McGlamry's Foot and Ankle Surgery*. No other comprehensive textbook on foot surgery had been written. The textbook included three separate volumes. The first was a text entitled the "Fundamentals of Foot Surgery" that reviewed anatomy, surgical materials, sutures, etc., and essentially provided the reader with a framework to learn the cornerstones of foot surgery. Another two volumes entitled "Comprehensive Textbook of Foot Surgery" reviewed specific pathologics of the foot and ankle and the surgical procedures associated with them. As a new resident, I looked up to the authors with reverence: E. Dalton McGlamry, John Ruch, Kieran Mahan, Gerard Yu, among others. To me, they were larger than life characters and I was humbled to be associated with them.

I remember how useful the text was as I began to learn and develop my surgical skills. In my first year, the fundamental text was invaluable to me as I learned the various biomechanical and surgical principles as well as memorizing suture materials and surgical instrumentation. The comprehensive texts were more valuable to me in my second and third years as I developed my surgical skills in the operating room and understanding complex surgical dilemmas. I am sure that my experience as an aspiring foot and ankle surgeon during this time period was not different to others in our field of expertise. The text quickly became a required text in all podiatric medical schools and remains so.

The second, third, and fourth editions built on the edition it followed. Although the editors and the authors have changed with each edition, the message and goal has been the same: to create a premier up-to-date text to teach students, residents, and attending podiatric and orthopedic surgeons foot and ankle surgery.

The fifth edition of the *McGlamry's Foot and Ankle Surgery* is a result of a collaboration of well-renowned faculty of the Podiatry Institute as well as accomplished podiatric and orthopedic foot and ankle surgeons throughout our surgical specialty. The fifth edition documents the most up-to-date information on foot and ankle surgery and does so in a unique way. As you will see, the textbook includes technique-driven color photography of surgical procedures in order to share the operative experience as well as author-specific techniques and pearls. The fifth edition also includes links in the eBook to videos illustrating surgical procedures discussed in the text, a feature not available in previous editions.

There are numerous chapters covering material that was not present in the previous texts. These include 3D imprinting, caging, cartilage replacement technology, and others.

I congratulate the editors in providing a truly new addition to the foot and ankle literature. I specifically thank Brian Carpenter, the lead editor, and the contributing editors Michelle Butterworth, William Fishco, and John Marcoux who provided endless hours reviewing and editing each chapter. I also thank Dan Vickers for his tireless work as the authors' editor. The work that they have accomplished together has provided a manuscript of supreme quality. I am certain that it will be enjoyed and treasured by all those who seek to perform foot and ankle surgery at a higher standard.

Alfred J. Phillips, DPM, FACFAS
Chairman of the Podiatry Institute 2019-2020

Special Surgery Conditions

Charcot Neuroarthropathy

Lawrence A. DiDomenico, Ajay K. Ghai, Sharif Abdelfattah, Clay Shumway, and David Chan

DEFINITION

Neuropathic osteoarthropathy has been an intensely misunderstood condition since its discovery and initial description by Musgrave in 1703. At that time, this process was thought to be an arthralgia resultant of venereal disease.[1] Jean-Martin Charcot made the connection of neuropathies in observance of spinal cord damage resulting from tabes dorsalis. The French neurologist in his publication *Demonstration of arthropathic affections of locomotor ataxy* in 1881 established the disease as a pathological one.[2] He described this disease process as a progressive neurodegeneration of the joints of the foot and ankle.[3] It was not until the mid-1930s that the connection to diabetes mellitus was made as a possible etiology of Charcot neuroarthropathy (CN).[4] CN of the foot and ankle is rare; however, it remains a devastating complication of diabetes that the health care community often fails to diagnose despite its pathognomonic clinical appearances.[5] Despite the wealth of research and literature published regarding Charcot, the disease process to this day remains enigmatic and often confusing given the diverse range of professional opinions available with no clearly defined standard of care. This syndrome has the potential to be a limb-threatening complication of diabetes. Jean-Martin Charcot once stated that "to learn how to treat a disease, one must learn how to recognize it. The diagnosis is the best trump in the scheme of treatment."[6]

The most commonly cited etiologies leading to Charcot arthropathy are diabetes mellitus, alcoholic neuropathy, syringomyelia, injuries to the spinal cord, and syphilis.[7] The common thread being that neuropathy is a preceding complication of Charcot joints.[8] In the past, hyperglycemia—known to cause axonal and microvascular injury—was thought to be a primary pathologic mechanism that set the stage for diabetic peripheral neuropathy; however, the pathology appears now to be multifactorial. This list of factors has grown to include oxidative stress, mitochondrial dysfunction, adipose toxicity, activation of the polyol pathway, elevation of inflammatory markers, and accumulation of advanced glycation end products (AGEs).[9,10] That being said, despite good glucose control, some patients manage to develop neuropathy. Tesfaye et al. found that patients with HbA1c of <5.4% are at risk of developing peripheral neuropathy.[11] Tesfaye et al. later found that there are probable connections to hypercholesterolemia, hypertension, hypertriglyceridemia, cardiovascular disease, obesity, and smoking.[12] No matter the etiology of peripheral neuropath, the resultant effect is nerve injury and subsequent loss of sensation.[13]

It is important to understand the epidemic of diabetes when discussing Charcot. An estimated 30.3 million people (9.4% of the population) in the United States had diabetes in 2015 according to the National Diabetes Statistic Report of 2017. Overall, the prevalence was higher among American Indians/Alaska Natives (15.1%), non-Hispanic blacks (12.7%), and people of Hispanic ethnicity (12.1%) than among non-Hispanic whites (7.4%) and Asians (8.0%). In 2015, an estimated 1.5 million new cases of diabetes were diagnosed in US adults over the age of 18 of which more than half of these new cases were among adults ages 45-64 years. An estimated 33.9% of all US adults over the age of 18 had prediabetes in 2015. Nearly half of adults ages 65 years or older had at least prediabetes.[14] In the diabetic population, the prevalence of Charcot has been contested in previous literature. Larson et al. suggested the prevalence of diagnosed Charcot arthropathy in diabetic patients is reported to be 0.08%-7.5%.[15] Chisholm et al. found a higher prevalence with as many as 13% of diabetic patients and 29% of neuropathic patients affected.[16] Armstrong and Schon have proposed that prevalence of this condition increases dramatically among patients with diabetes and peripheral neuropathy, ranging from 29% to 35% in this specific population.[17,18] It is the senior authors opinion and personal experience that the amount of patients suffering from CN at all stages is much higher than reported and often misdiagnosed.

The pathophysiology of the Charcot foot in diabetes is complicated with numerous contributing factors. Two of the prevailing theories in the past have been the neurotraumatic and the neurovascular theory.

The neurotraumatic theory is attributed to the German researcher, Volkmann who hypothesized that in the setting of peripheral neuropathy, there are significant sensory deficits resulting in impaired pain perception allowing for repetitive acute minor injury or chronic injury to the foot and ankle.[19] Since the patient has the inability to sense pain and prevent this from happening, a response is initiated to the trauma in the form of microfracture or microdislocations.[20] This repetitive microtrauma may be enough to change the distribution of forces on adjacent structures.[21] In this instance, obesity and weight bearing has been implicated in direct correlation with detrimental progression of the neuroarthropathy.[22]

Alternatively, the neurovascular theory implicates autonomic neuropathy in the stead of peripheral neuropathy as the culprit responsible for Charcot. In this theory, autonomic neuropathy results in impaired vascular reflexes with arteriovenous (AV) shunting and results in increased arterial perfusion.[23-25]

Increase in blood flow to the foot has been implicated in an increased bone resorption with reduction of bone mineral density predisposing these patients for fractures and collapse.[26] It has been suggested that neuropathic patients have a higher prevalence of calcification within the smooth muscle of the arterial walls.[27] Intravascular trauma was thought to be a nonspecific consequence of sympathetic denervation due to a decrease in peripheral vascular resistance and progressive widening of the pulse pressure.[27-30] The pathophysiology of Charcot is a continuously growing pool of research and literature. More recently, there has been evidence to suggest that traumatic and vascular theories may play a part in the development of CN. The theory that results is one that is based on an inappropriate inflammatory response. Trauma to the neuropathic foot results in unrecognized minor injury that can lead to a local inflammation and infection. Variations in gene expression can help to explain the tendency of a neuropathic patients' proinflammatory status and ultimately may provide an answer as to why not all neuropathic patients develop Charcot arthropathy.[31]

From a molecular standpoint, there may be some pathways that offer explanations for the link between diabetes and Charcot osteoarthropathy. Receptor activator of nuclear factor kappaB ligand or RANKL is produced by osteoblasts and interacts with the RANK receptors on precursor and mature osteoclast cells. In healthy patients, this ligand is expressed by osteoblasts and vital to osteoclast function in bone resorptions. Osteoprotegerin or OPG is also secreted by osteoblasts and also plays an important role in inhibition of bone resorption by actively inhibiting RANKL. In diabetics with CN, there is increased expression of nuclear transcription factor NF-kappaB. Cell injury initiates the process leading to expression of RANKL production on the surface of osteoblasts and T cells. In its activated form, the RANK receptor is expressed on the surface of the osteoclasts. As the transduction cascade continues, IK kinase is inducted resulting in the phosphorylization of nuclear factor kappaB, which once activated acts as a transcription factor promoting increasing osteoclast activity and generation. Additionally, RANKL has been found to increase expression of bone matrix proteins in vascular smooth muscle cells. Overexpression of the RANKL pathway may be responsible for calcifications of the vascular endothelial smooth muscle cells as well as predispose these patients to osteopenia through the activation of osteoclast activity.[22,31-40] Bruhn-Olszewska et al. showed in a 2017 study that the OPG-RANKL-RANK axis regulating bone metabolism can be associated with development of Charcot. Their results showed that the genotypes of specific single nucleotide polymorphisms have a direct correlation and provide for a marker of Charcot and these genotypes expressions.[39]

It is the senior authors' opinion and experience that CN of the foot and ankle is a combination of the neurovascular and neurotraumatic theories resulting in a significant mechanical breakdown secondary to a tight posterior muscle group. A tight posterior muscle causes significant increase in pressure to the osseous, ligamentous, and tendinous structures to a focused area of the foot and/or ankle resulting in a localized trauma. In a nonpathologic foot and ankle, the osseous, ligamentous, and tendinous structures are neatly cohesively aligned. When one experiences a "Charcot event," it is a direct result of this increase in pressure and fault in this very well organized, well-aligned structure resulting in loosening and a beginning of a "domino effect" leading to significant local and regional destruction to the osseous structures and soft tissues of the foot and/or ankle. Unfortunately, this is often easily unidentifiable

until significant destruction is grossly obvious. The senior author highly recommends advanced imaging early in the process if this condition is suspected to assist with the more complete observation of this condition.

Based on 26 years of experience with Charcot arthropathy, the senior authors' opinion is bullish for those patients who suffer from Charcot neuropathy. Not every case will be successful; however, the majority can be successfully treated if appropriately managed. In order to successfully treat these complicated patients, the surgeon should have in depth knowledge on the disease process, vascular disease, and infectious disease. They should also have excellent surgical skills with both internal and external fixation and be well versed and able to apply various plastic surgery and bone grafting techniques.

CLASSIFICATION

EICHENHOLTZ

The Charcot foot has multiple classification systems based on staging, radiographic, anatomical, and clinical presentations. Radiographically, the widely recognized classification is the Eichenholtz classification with stages I through III described initially.[41] Stage 0 or the prodromal phase was added by Shibata et al., in which the radiographic imaging is negative.

In the later stages, radiographically, there is often a breakdown of bony architecture in the affected joints and surrounding skeleton. The Eichenholtz classification is widely used to describe the pathophysiologic presentation of diabetic neuroarthropathy into three radiographic stages[42]:

EICHENHOLTZ CLASSIFICATION

Stage I (bone dissolution): subchondral osteopenia, fragmentation of bone with accompanying intra-articular loose bodies, and joint malalignment due to ligamentous laxity.

Stage II (coalescence): debris absorption, subchondral sclerosis, periosteal bone formation, and fusion of larger fragments of bone.

Stage III (reconstruction): remodeling of deformity with rounding and smoothing of bone fragments and fibrous ankyloses.

Shibata et al. added a stage 0 consisting of inflammatory foot edema without radiographic changes as with stage I.[43]

There may be clinical symptoms such as swelling, erythema, and warmth along with joint effusion. Bone scans may be positive in all stages. In order to effectively monitor the progression, serial imaging as well as protected weight bearing should be initiated. In stage I or the development/fragmentation stage, radiographically, there are signs of fragmentation, dislocations, or joint subluxations as well as osteopenia. The clinical presentation will be similar to that of stage 0; however, there may be some perceived ligamentous laxity. At this stage, protected weight bearing in a total contact cast (TCC) or pneumatic brace should be initiated. Bracing should be utilized until there appears to be resolution on radiographs of fragmentation and presence of normal skin temperature. This process can take upward of 4 months. In stage II, the coalescence phase, it is radiographically characterized by adsorption of debris, sclerosis, and fusion of larger fragments. Clinically, there is decreased

warmth, swelling, and erythema. The preferred conservative treatment at this stage is total contact casting, pneumatic bracing, Charcot restraint orthotic walker (CROW), or clamshell ankle foot orthosis (AFO). Stage III is referred to as the reconstruction phase. Radiographically, there is consolidation of deformity, joint arthrosis, fibrous ankyloses, and rounding and smoothing of bone fragments. The clinical presentation at this stage should be consistent with absence of warmth, swelling, and erythema, as well as a stable joint with or without a fixed deformity. In a plantigrade foot, recommendations for custom inlay shoes with a rigid shank and rocker bottom sole may be made. However, in a nonplantigrade foot or with ulceration, surgical intervention is indicated in the form of debridement, exostectomy, deformity correction, or arthrodesis with internal and/or external fixation.[41]

SANDERS AND FRYKBERG

The anatomical classification that was proposed by Sanders and Frykberg categorizes Charcot based on the involved areas of the foot and ankle. In pattern I, the metatarsophalangeal and interphalangeal joints are affected. This pattern has an occurrence of about 15% of Charcot foot. In pattern II, the tarsometatarsal (TMT) joint or Lisfranc joint is affected. This pattern has an occurrence of 40% and is the most common pattern. In pattern III, naviculocuneiform, talonavicular, and the calcaneocuboid joint or Chopart joint is affected. This pattern has an occurrence of 30%. Pattern IV has involvement at the ankle and subtalar joints and has an occurrence of 10%. Pattern V involves the calcaneus and is the least common with a 5% occurrence rate.[44]

BRODSKY

Brodsky classification is another anatomical classification that has been used.

The Brodsky classification describes the incidence of diabetic CN among different anatomical regions of the foot and ankle.[45]

BRODSKY CLASSIFICATION	
Type I	■ Involves the tarsometatarsal and lesser tarsus joints. ■ This is the most common type to cause plantar ulceration. ■ It accounts for ~70% of the cases.
Type II	■ Involves the midtarsal and subtalar joints. ■ This accounts for ~20% of the cases.
Type IIIA	■ Involves the ankle and accounts for ~10% of the cases
Type IIIB	■ Avulsion at the insertion of the tendo-Achilles. ■ This accounts for <10% of the cases.
Type IV	■ A combination of type I, II, and III. Type V is characterized by involvement of the forefoot.[46,47]

SCHON

Schon developed a classification system, which further categorized midfoot deformities. They concluded that midfoot deformities can be classified as one of four types based on the anatomic location. These patterns include Lisfranc,

naviculocuneiform, perinavicular, and transverse tarsal patterns of deformity. The Lisfranc pattern will have significant involvement at the metatarsocuneiform joints. One may see the naviculocuneiform pattern when the deformity occurs more proximally at the naviculocuneiform joint. The perinavicular pattern includes the navicular and its adjacent bones, and the transverse tarsal pattern involves significant deformity at the talonavicular joint.

Schon also included three stages of severity (A-C) based on the degree of collapse in the sagittal plane as shown on lateral weight-bearing radiographs. Stage A is the least severe as the deformity does not collapse to the level of the plantar surface of the foot. Stage B deformities collapse to the level of the plantar surface of the foot.

Stage C represents the most severe deformity in which the midfoot is collapsed beneath the level of the plantar foot. This deformity represents a rocker bottom foot and is often associated with plantar ulcerations.

PHYSICAL EXAMINATION

The diagnosis is typically made from the appearance of the foot and ankle dislocation or fracture dislocation on radiographs in combination with a lack of normal sensation on physical examination. An equinus contracture is highly associated with this presentation. In the general medical community, there tends to be a high association of diabetics with vascular disease and possible infection leading to a misdiagnosis. Many neuropathic fractures and dislocations associated with swelling and inflammation are often misdiagnosed as infection or as osteomyelitis. Additionally, this is associated with hyperemia, which is often misinterpreted as osteomyelitis. A good physical examination and an experienced foot and ankle surgeon should be able to recognize the problem based on clinical examination, radiographs, blood work, and advanced imaging.

DIFFERENTIATING ACUTE VS CHRONIC CHARCOT

The classic presentation of the initial stages of Charcot arthropathy (stage I in the Eichenholtz classification) is a grossly swollen, warm, painless foot (with occasional complaints of mild to moderate discomfort) in a long-standing diabetic. In the setting of peripheral neuropathy, concern for trauma is unreliable.[48] Most patients who present with Charcot are in their fifth or sixth decade of life and are overweight. There is often a significant temperature difference between the contralateral extremity with the affected limb. On average, the area is about 2°C warmer.[49] As for vascularity, pulses are characteristically 4/4 or bounding in nature.

The lower extremity is unique in its ability to adapt to weight-bearing changes. In a nonosteoarthropathic individual, there is a durable soft tissue envelope surrounding a network of small bones that allow for a plantigrade foot to accept the weight-bearing load. However, in the process of Charcot arthropathy, the ability of this mechanism is diminished. As the disease progresses, there may have been subluxations or dislocations and microfractures that occur along the midfoot, typically resulting in a classic rocker bottom foot. In the setting of continued weight bearing, this may further result in plantar ulceration.[50-53]

The acute Charcot joint typically features erythema, edema, and increased warmth. It is sometimes misdiagnosed as acute

gout, cellulitis, or a deep venous thrombosis (DVT). A Doppler ultrasound can help rule out a DVT. To rule out cellulitis, one can perform a rubor of dependency test by elevating the affected limb above the level of the heart for a few minutes, and if the erythema recedes, it is likely Charcot arthropathy, whereas, if the erythema remains, it is probably cellulitis.[54] Additionally, antibiotics can be started, and if the erythema resolves, Charcot is ruled out.

The acute Charcot foot is usually several degrees warmer than the contralateral foot.[55,56] Similar to Petrova et al., Ruotolo et al. found that the average initial temperature difference between the affected foot and a similar site on the contralateral foot was ~3°C.[57] With the chronic Charcot joint, the patient will often display musculoskeletal deformities. The characteristic deformity for this condition is the rocker bottom foot in which the talus is plantarflexed and medially deviated with a collapse of the midfoot.

However, it can present in other joints and lead to a medial arch collapse, bony prominence, and/or ligamentous laxity. The deformity may be slightly or grossly evident depending on the chronicity of the disease.

Clinical suspicion should be raised in patients over the age of 40, with a diabetes diagnosis >10 years,[58] with obesity, and/or with peripheral neuropathy. Patients may describe a "crunching" sensation with ambulation.[59] The patient will usually have palpable, often bounding pedal pulses, provided the foot is not too edematous. The key clinical risk factor for Charcot arthropathy is diabetic peripheral neuropathy as tested by Semmes-Weinstein 5.07 monofilament.[60]

IMAGING AND DIAGNOSTIC STUDIES

RADIOGRAPH AND CT

Plain weight-bearing radiographs and computed tomography images of the foot and ankle may be negative in the early stages of the disease, but they can be useful in identifying chronic pathologic changes. Plain radiography has low sensitivity and specificity rates (<50%) in detection of early findings of Charcot arthropathy.[61-63] In the early stages of Charcot arthropathy, focal demineralization[42] and degenerative changes can mimic osteoarthritis or septic arthritis.[63]

Some critics believe that the Eichenholtz classification is outdated due to the emergence of newer imaging modalities like magnetic resonance imaging (MRI), which can detect Charcot changes earlier than plain radiographs, allowing for earlier diagnosis, staging, and intervention.[64,65] Additionally, interobserver variability is present when using the classification's stages, as it can be difficult to distinguish when one stage ends, and another begins.[66]

MAGNETIC RESONANCE IMAGING

MRI is a very useful imaging modality in detecting early changes of acute Charcot arthropathy in the form of soft tissue edema,[67] cortical fractures, joint effusion, and subchondral bone marrow edema.[43,54,68,69] Many of these manifestations can precede Eichenholtz stage I by weeks. Therefore, its utility is advantageous because early diagnosis can lead to early immobilization and offloading, which can prevent a full-blown Charcot attack.

MRI is also beneficial in differentiating between abscesses and soft tissue swelling, but it lacks utility in distinguishing between osteomyelitis and Charcot arthropathy. Anatomically, Charcot arthropathy primarily affects joints, whereas osteomyelitis is typically an extension from a skin ulcer.[70] If the diagnosis is in question, a bone biopsy is considered the gold standard for diagnosis of osteomyelitis,[71] and its sensitivity and specificity are 95% and 99%, respectively.[72]

NUCLEAR IMAGING

Three phase bone scans are ineffective in distinguishing between osteomyelitis and neuroarthropathy due to bone remodeling present in both conditions. The uninfected Charcot joint may have increased activity on bone scan due to hematopoietically active marrow, rather than inflammation itself.[73] However, with combined technetium-99m sulfur colloid imaging, osteomyelitis can be determined when there is accumulation of leukocytes in bone, but without the accumulation of sulfur colloid. These images are said to be spatially incongruent or positive for infection.[73-75]

Positron emission tomography (PET) can distinguish between inflammatory and infectious soft tissue and between osteomyelitis and neuroarthropathy. A comparison of MRI, ring PET, and hybrid PET in evaluation of CN found ring PET to be preferable to MRI in that it can differentiate between inflammatory and infectious soft tissue lesions, as well as between Charcot lesions and osteomyelitis.[76] Basu et al. compared the sensitivity and specificity of FDG PET scan vs MRI in distinguishing Charcot foot from osteomyelitis in diabetic patients. They found the FDG PET scan to be 100% sensitive and 93.8% specific and the MRI to be 76.9% sensitive and 75% specific.[77]

Single photon emission computerized tomography-computed tomography (SPECT-CT) combines anatomical imaging with scintigraphic studies. It is a highly sensitive and specific tool in diagnosing and localizing CN.[77] Positive SPECT-CT scans identify where cortical fractures have occurred with significant subchondral bone turnover consistent with CN.[78]

DIAGNOSTIC STUDIES

When a patient presents with a red, hot, swollen foot with no skin breakdown, the white blood cell count is within normal limits, and the erythrocyte sedimentation rate (ESR) and C-reactive protein (CRP) are normal or slightly raised, clinical suspicion for Charcot should be present.[79] However, an ESR that is significantly elevated (>70 mm/h), without other probable cause, is likely a diabetic foot infection.[80-82] Acute Charcot and osteomyelitis can be present concomitantly, and if any doubt is present, a bone biopsy should be taken for definitive diagnosis.

DIFFERENTIATION OF OSTEOMYELITIS AND CHARCOT ARTHROPATHY

Osteomyelitis and Charcot are difficult to differentiate from one another and in fact can occur concurrently, which makes diagnosis even more challenging. Chantelau et al. reported that 80% of patients who have sought out care for concern over their Charcot were misdiagnosed with CRPS, osteomyelitis, rheumatoid arthritis, and sprains. If in fact osteomyelitis is present, the infection needs to be addressed and more importantly eliminated prior to addressing the Charcot if reconstruction is to be considered and successful. In this respect, a staged approach to addressing these issues should be employed. In the setting

of a patient presenting with an ulceration on presentation, a full infection work up should be performed prior to determining whether to perform surgical reconstruction or brace. The work up should consist of ESR, CRP, bone biopsy, and advanced imaging as needed.[83]

INDICATIONS, TREATMENT, AND PITFALLS

NONOPERATIVE MODALITIES

TCC is the nonoperative treatment of choice when dealing with stage 0 or stage I CN.[84,85] If the patient has a plantigrade foot, then a non–weight-bearing below the knee (BK) cast or TCC is acceptable for 8-12 weeks during the acute phase.[86] If the TCC is employed, then it should be changed every 1-2 weeks while in the acute stage, until the edema and warmth stabilize (around 2-4 months). If the patient also has ulcerations, the cast changes should be weekly for evaluation and debridement. Radiographs should be taken monthly to monitor progression. Katz et al. found that using a removable cast walker rendered irremovable (by wrapping a single layer of fiberglass casting material around the walker) was equally efficacious to TCC but was easier to use, faster to apply, and less expensive.[87]

After the fragmentation and coalescence phases, the patient will need accommodative long-term bracing. Examples include accommodative shoes, foot orthoses, and AFOs. The CROW is a custom ankle-foot orthosis meant to reduce all motion, while supporting the foot and ankle architecture during the remodeling phase of the disease.

Another device is the patellar tendon-bearing brace, which is a custom-molded plastic brace meant to unweight the foot and ankle. However, Saltzman et al. found that while load transmission was reduced to the hindfoot, it was not reduced to the midfoot or forefoot.[88]

For patients with minimal deformity, extra-depth shoes and custom foot orthotics are recommended. A rocker bottom outsole can be beneficial for redistributing plantar pressures during gait. A double rocker bottom shoe will help to offload plantar midfoot prominence. For patients with moderate to severe Charcot collapse, custom-made footwear with custom-made orthosis is recommended.

- TCC has been considered as the gold standard in the treatment of neuropathic diabetic plantar foot ulcers.[89-92]
- According to Coughlin and Mann, a Brodsky type II deformity averages 18 months of non–weight bearing. They also stated that most type I deformities can be treated conservatively.[93]
- If ulceration occurs after failed conservative treatment, exostectomy of an ulcer-inciting bony prominence can be considered.[94] Brodsky and Rouse's studies indicated that limb-salvage rates reached 90% with exostectomy.[95] Exostectomy techniques have been performed successfully in many studies on surgical treatment in Charcot midfoot deformities and ulcers.[96,97] Even when exostectomy is performed for a TMT deformity (Brodsky type 1), Achilles tendon lengthening should also be considered for the patient with concomitant recurrent plantar ulceration and severe equinus contracture. Lengthening of the Achilles tendon or gastrocnemius recession can decrease the forefoot pressures and improve the alignment of the ankle and hindfoot to the midfoot and forefoot.[94] Catanzariti et al. reported that an Achilles tendon lengthening,

in addition to an osteotomy in Charcot patients with lateral midfoot ulcers, healed primarily with a rate of 38%. However, in the same study, the rate of primary healing in medial midfoot ulcers was 92%.[96] A randomized study by Mueller et al. showed that in patients with Charcot arthropathy and midfoot deformity, TCC with Achilles tendon lengthening were 75% less likely to have ulcer recurrence at 7 months. They recommended an Achilles tendon lengthening in patients for equinus contracture and with recurrent plantar ulceration.[98,99]

SURGICAL INDICATION

The vascular supply of the patient must be assessed prior to making any surgical plans for elective reconstructive surgery. A noninvasive vascular examination can provide sufficient information to establish whether the patient is well vascularized in order to undergo the reconstructive surgery successfully. A full and thorough noninvasive vascular examination coupled with digital pressures or transcutaneous oxygen should be performed to evaluate the diabetic patient. The diabetic patient can have falsely elevated ABIs because of Monckeberg medial calcific sclerosis. The digital vessels are spared from these calcifications; therefore, the digital pressures may provide a more accurate reflection of the perfusion to the patient's given extremity. If there is uncertainty, or less than optimal results from the testing, a referral to a vascular specialist should be provided for the patient.

The senior author suggests that the surgeons who surgically treat this very complicated patient possess himself/herself with a multiple skill set to address all aspects of this complex deformity. The surgeon should be well versed with external fixation and should understand and be experienced with pin-bar external fixation as well as ring circular external fixation. The surgeon should also be very experienced and proficient with internal fixation. The surgeon should also have a good knowledge base on vascular conditions of the lower extremity. The surgeon needs to be well skilled in orthoplastic procedures and plastic surgery techniques in order to manage many of the soft tissue complications experienced with this patient population. These skill sets are necessary in order to predictably have continuous success with this patient population. If the surgeon does not possess all of these skills, he/she must surround himself/herself with other skilled surgeons who possesses these skills who are willing to treat this patient population.

Indications for reconstructive surgery are to lower the incidence of wounds, ulcers, infection, and amputation for this patient population and condition. This is accomplished most often with surgical intervention addressing the underlying deforming forces and deformities. The earlier treatment is initiated, the less likely it is that ulcers and infection will occur since the deforming cause and focal pressure have been eliminated. These problems should be managed as early as possible to balance the weight distribution in the foot and ankle to try to prevent ulcerations. These deformities within this patient population, in combination with diabetic peripheral neuropathy, are considerably more prone to ulceration and potential amputation. Diabetic peripheral neuropathy is the typical common component of this pathological process and because of this, surgical intervention is even more strongly recommended and needed to correct underlying pathology. These problems are amenable to both prophylactic and therapeutic surgery.

In the experience of the senior author, the best results with Charcot foot and ankle are achieved when the deformity is

managed early. When these deformities are managed earlier, there is less secondary destruction to the bone and soft tissues. These consist of smaller wounds/infections, less soft tissue changes such as contractures, diseased skin malalignment, fractures, fragmentation, bony destruction, and smaller deformities. The bone integrity in a patient who recently developed Charcot deformity compared to a long-standing chronic Charcot foot and/or ankle is grossly different. When the condition is chronic, the deformity is typically more severe and there is more severe malalignment and often times the deformities are fixed in a malposition. When there is a larger deformity, there is usually more diseased soft tissues associated with the large bony deformity. The bone integrity appears to be more sclerotic, diseased, and avascular in nature throughout a larger geographic area in comparison to an acute scenario. In the acute scenario, there is much less secondary destruction involving both the soft tissue and bone. Because of these reasons, it has been the authors' experience to address the Charcot foot and ankle earlier in the disease process. We have found that earlier intervention, with surgical treatment including and a posterior muscle lengthening, prior to significant malalignment may halt the process resulting in much less secondary destruction to both the bone and soft tissues. With earlier surgical intervention, there is less need for bone resection, resulting in less shortening, thus less need for bone grafting and there is more solid bone to manage with fixation.

Patients who are clinically plantigrade without any ulcerations or indication of infection at time of presentation are initially treated nonoperatively until the foot and ankle is stable. This includes offloading casting, a TCC followed by a CROW, an AFO with weight bearing. These devices reduce plantar surface pressure as well as reducing the motion at the foot and ankle to prevent further degradation of the joints. In the case of a CROW boot, there is additional reduction of motion at the ankle with a rocker bottom sole.[100] These patients are often progressed once the acute phase has resolved and consolidated into a pneumatic walking boot and then progressively into custom diabetic shoes. Patients who remain unstable or present with a nonplantigrade foot/ankle progress on to surgery. Gross instability with dislocations and subluxations of the bones and joints tend to apply stress to the soft tissues and in turn can develop a wound and infection of the foot and ankle and this becomes a surgical indication. Surgical correction is pursued to prevent break down and ulceration and infection.

Surgical treatment and procedure selection is reliant on the surgeon's opinion and experience and the patient's presentation. Recurrent ulcerations, a potential for soft tissue compromise, joint instability from dislocation or collapse, prominent exostosis, and a nonbraceable/shoeable ankle and foot are all indications for surgical intervention. The surgeon must take into account the patient's deformity location and severity, medical comorbidities, malalignment, biomechanical instability, and the ability to comply with the intended treatment protocol. Infection must be ruled out before proceeding using blood work, imaging and bone cultures, and biopsy if needed. It is the senior authors' opinion and experience that a patient with CN with an open wound is viewed as more likely than not of having a bone infection until proven otherwise.

SURGICAL TREATMENT

Regardless of the location of the deformity, as a principle in surgical treatment, the authors recommend working from proximal to distal as the proximal structures are typically aligned and stable. This provides the surgeon a stable, firm anatomic reference to realign the unstable deformed anatomy.

In most typical scenarios, the patient is placed in the supine position. After administration of anesthesia, cotton padding is placed over the upper thigh of the foot undergoing surgery, and a pneumatic thigh tourniquet is applied. The foot is then prepared and draped in the usual sterile manner above the knee. The tourniquet is applied and elevated. The appropriate draping is performed, and the knee should be exposed. Exposing of the knee and partial thigh provides the surgeon exposure to the lower extremity and assists the surgeon in reference of the more stable proximal anatomy.

EQUINUS/POSTERIOR MUSCLE ANKLE AND FOOT CONTRACTURE

In almost every case, the posterior muscle lengthening is mandatory in order to appropriate, correct, and reduce the deformity. When evaluating the contracted or the functional short posterior muscle group, the surgeon should routinely check to see if the contracture is from the gastrocnemius muscle alone or if the contracture is a gastrocnemius and soleus combined deformity when considering reconstructive surgery. Performing the Silfverskiold test appropriately should be done to identify whether the patient is experiencing a bony block equinus, a gastrocnemius muscle, or a gastrocnemius and soleus contracture. When contracture is limited to an isolated gastrocnemius muscle, the gastrocnemius aponeurosis should be lengthened to preserve the full power of the soleus muscle. The senior author prefers an endoscopic technique when possible as this limits the exposure of the soft tissues in an already compromised patient.[101]

Alternatively, the Baumann procedure consists of intramuscular lengthening (recession) of the gastrocnemius muscle in the deep interval between the soleus and gastrocnemius muscles. The Baumann procedure treats equinus contracture of the gastrocnemius muscle by improving ankle joint dorsiflexion.

When a gastrocnemius-soleus equinus is noted, a tendon Achilles lengthening should be performed. The senior author again prefers a percutaneous technique in an attempt to reduce the soft tissue stresses on complicated and compromised patients.[102] In the experience of the senior author, most equinus contracture deformities are isolated to the gastrocnemius muscle as compared to the gastrocnemius-soles contracture, thus yielding more gastrocnemius recessions needing to be performed than tendo-Achilles lengthening procedures.

In the early stages of CN, before collapse (Eichenholtz stage 0) and deformity, the posterior muscle group should be lengthened, and the patient should be immobilized. The goal of this technique is to lengthen the posterior muscle group, decrease intraosseous pressure and necrosis, and manage the patient through this acute phase of this induced hyperemia with the foot and ankle being free of any significant deformity. This treatment should be maintained for several months until the foot and ankle is stabilized. When the foot and ankle is stabilized and maintains anatomic shape and alignment, an accommodated shoe/brace (AFO) can be provided. On the other hand, if the deformity is large and causes excessive pressure and ulceration and cannot be prevented, reconstructive surgery should be performed.

For more advanced deformities, surgical treatment options include posterior muscle group lengthening, bone debridement, realignment osteotomies/arthrodesis, external fixation, and or internal fixation consisting of possible screws/plates,

beaming, nailing, etc. based on the stage and location of the deformity. Arthrodesis can be accomplished with internal and/or external fixation.[103] The timing of the surgeries as well as the possible staging of the surgeries also should be taken into consideration based on each individual case. It has been the senior authors' experience to perform the reconstructive surgery as early as possible in the "Charcot Joint Process." The senior author has found that the amount of bone needing resected is less in these earlier stages. Also, the quality of the remaining bone following aggressive resection appears to exhibit better integrity following the resection of the diseased bone. This healthier remaining bone is capable of maintaining the fixation much better. With the need of reduced bone resection, there is less need for bone grafting, which results in more naturally remaining bone to bone contact, which improves the rate of arthrodesis. When an arthrodesis is performed in later stages with a more advanced Charcot arthropathy, there is a need for more aggressive bone resection, thus there is more instability because of the secondary effects of the amount of diseased bone needing resection. When Charcot arthropathy is more advanced, typically, there is more notable bone loss resulting in more instability, which usually requires more bone grafting.

Surgical correction of this disease process is difficult; however, contrary to some beliefs, Charcot arthropathy typically demonstrates good blood supply and can heal fairly well. Good surgical technique, restoring anatomical alignment, associated with good fixation is critically important.

STAGING OF SURGERIES

It has been the experience of the senior author to stage the reconstructive surgery when there is an open wound or a history of a previous open wound, a large deformity with secondary soft tissue adaptations, or a compromise to the soft tissue envelope. If there is an open wound caused by a bony deformity and malalignment, the recommendation is to perform osseous debridement while obtaining cultures and a biopsy of the bone to rule out osteomyelitis. One should consider an infectious disease consult as well. Additionally, bony resection, osteotomy, or chiseling of the bone allows the surgeon to reduce/manipulate the deformity along with aggressive soft tissue debridement in order to create healthy clean margins of both bone and soft tissue. The soft tissues should be cultured and biopsied too. Moreover, the tight heel cord should be lengthened typically performing a gastrocnemius recession or an Achilles tendon lengthening based on the results of a Silfverskiold test. An aggressive resection, debridement of the diseased bone, and chiseling of the malaligned fused or fibrous bony deformity allows for reduction of the deformity into anatomic alignment. The extremity should then be placed in an external fixator with an adequate reduction and into anatomic alignment. The calcaneal inclination angle should be restored or improved in the sagittal plane as well as the frontal and transverse planes if needed. The hindfoot and ankle should be maintained in a neutral alignment in all three planes and the forefoot and midfoot should be dialed into a neutral position in the frontal, sagittal, and transverse planes as well. A "three legged bar stool" should be created placing the first and fifth metatarsals on the same plane as the calcaneus creating a tripod effect of the foot. This should limit and offload any midfoot, hindfoot, and/or ankle deformities.

If the deformity has no open wounds and the deformity is reducible (this typically only occurs in an acute or early stage) and is unstable, then there is typically no need for a staged approach and/or external fixation. In this scenario, an open reduction and primary arthrodesis can be performed. Every case is very unique and must be evaluated on a case by case basis. In this scenario, an acute primary arthrodesis is performed in the early stages of the "Charcot Process."

When a patient presents with an open wound/ulcer and the wound has not healed as expected, advanced alternative care must be considered. Rarely does a wound heal in the presence of a large deformity before correction of the deformity. In cases such as this, we recommend immediate and staged surgical correction. The goal of the staged surgical reconstruction is to restore anatomic alignment by stabilizing the fractures and dislocations of the deformity, thus offloading the pressure necrosis/wound. This should be done as soon as possible in order to prevent severe infections and the potential for limb loss. Good surgical principles should be carried out with debridement of bone, cartilage, and fibrous tissue in order to achieve a reduction of the deformity, anatomic alignment, followed by application of an external fixation device. The external fixation device is utilized to maintain the anatomic alignment. This is followed by wound care for those patients who possess an ulcer.

Wound care is accomplished with weekly wound debridement, possible negative pressure therapy, and other possible procedures such as hyperbaric oxygen and other advanced therapies. Additionally, compressive wraps of the lower extremity to control the edema is often needed. Once the wound has healed, the serum markers are reduced and treatment with intravenous or oral antibiotics is completed, then definitive surgical reconstructive is performed. The wounds typically heal without complication as the deforming forces will be alleviated.

Following wound healing, evidence of reduced serum markers and consultation with infectious disease, the reconstructive surgical phase can be initiated. In the reconstructive phase, the diseased bone must be resected. Whether the bone is "Charcot bone" or previously infected bone or a combination, it must be resected and eradicated. The "diseased Charcot/infected bone and soft tissues" need to be thought of as a cancer and wide aggressive resection of the soft tissues and bone are mandatory. There needs to be clean/healthy margins of soft tissues and bone remaining in order to be successful with the surgical reconstruction. This aggressive soft tissue and bone resection should limit the chance of remaining infection or diseased "Charcot" bone. The "Charcot bone" is essentially diseased and avascular, therefore, elimination of the diseased bone is essential for adequate healing. Relative to the bony infection, aggressive bony resection along with intravenous antibiotic treatment, now becomes a "surgical cure" in hopes of complete irradiation of the infection/diseased bone and only allows for the healthy bone to remain.

EXTERNAL FIXATION

- External fixation should be utilized in patients with open wounds or possible infection to span the area of compromise. It is useful in staging complex reconstruction efforts to decrease operating room time and the stress on the patient. It is also useful for patients with poor bone quality, inadequate vascular supply, and/or a compromised soft tissue envelope. External fixation may be combined with internal fixation for added stability. Additionally, it has been the senior authors' experience that stability is greatly helpful with wound healing and infection.

- Patients with Charcot arthropathy of the midfoot and open ulcers have an extremely high risk for infection when using internal fixation for arthrodesis. In a study by Thompson and Clohissy, the deep infection rate was 40% and the amputation rate was 15% in patients with open ulcerations where internal fixation was used to stabilize the arthrodesis.[104,105] Therefore, a staged approach is recommended so the infection is eradicated both surgically and medically.

- Daniel et al. found in a cadaveric study that there was 186% more compression capability for transverse tarsal arthrodesis using external ring fixator vs three lag screws.[106] Compression across the fusion sites may be from a Taylor spatial frame with adjustable struts or by employing a bent wire technique, also termed "Russianing."[107] Other techniques include gradual correction with adjustable struts and CT-guided correction, with the allowance of weight bearing. The weight bearing is designed for the deconditioned patient and may also be used in a staged approach. An in-depth discussion of external fixation techniques is outside the scope of this chapter but certainly has important applications that may be used in the surgical correction of Charcot deformity. This technique may be utilized in cases in which the surgeon cannot utilize internal fixation.

- External fixation can be used in combination when a patient presents who cannot be non–weight bearing. In cases such as this, the senior author will use internal fixation coupled by circular ring fixation to allow patients to weight bear postoperatively.

- The surgeon should be skilled in using pin-bar external fixation as well as circular multilevel external fixation (Fig. 38.1).

AUTHORS PREFERRED TREATMENT

MIDFOOT OSTEOTOMY

The midfoot osteotomy is not a common procedure with Charcot reconstruction. Typically, there is a lot destruction throughout the midfoot in the presence of Charcot. In a few cases, there may be a midfoot that is fused in a malaligned position

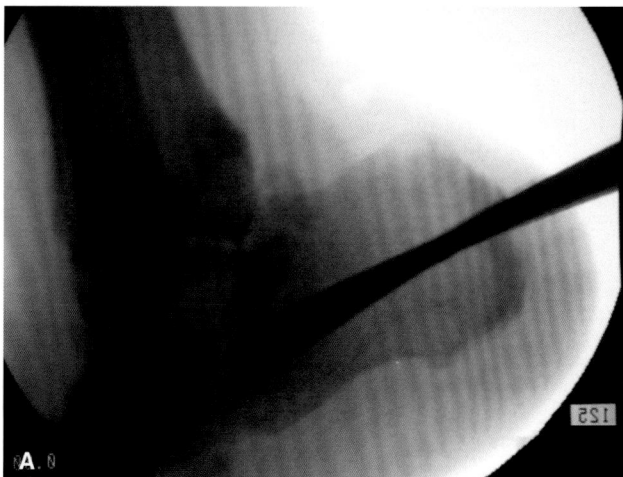
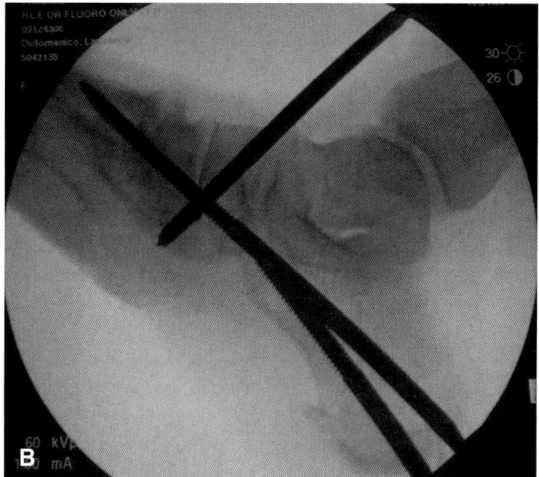
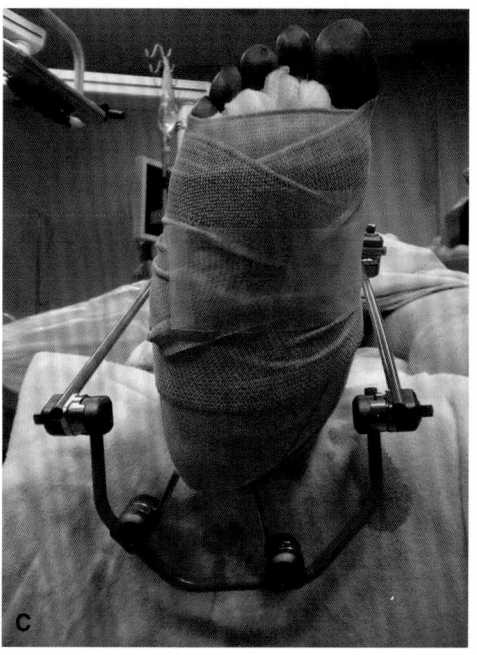

FIGURE 38.1 **A.** Placement of calcaneal external fixator pins in a posterior-to-anterior direction instead of a medial to lateral direction provides advantages. Inserting the pins from posterior to anterior will provide two to three times as much pin length in comparison to medial to lateral. With the classic medial-lateral pins, the calcaneus tends to develop loosening and in turn pin track infection can occur. Additionally, this orientation lessens the risk of damage to the neuromuscular structures, increases stability within the calcaneus, and it allows for more leverage in all three cardinal planes when reducing a deformity. Additionally, it prevents calcaneal wounds and may provide for decreased pin tract infections. Care should be taken to ensure that they are placed in a slightly convergent vector and at two distinct levels of insertion, with one pin superior to the other. **B.** The pins can be advanced more distally to provide additional stability to the midfoot if needed. **C.** A variety of partial rings can be applied, including 5/8 ring and a U-shaped bar. This U-shaped bar becomes like a "steering wheel" and allows one to have better control and leverage during a reduction. (From DiDomenico LA, Giganacova A, Cross D, Ziran B. Alternative techniques for transosseous calcaneal pinning in external fixation. *J Foot Ankle Surg.* 2012;51:528-530. Ref.[108].)

in the frontal, transverse, and sagittal planes but possess good medial and lateral column length. The goal of a midfoot osteotomy in a Charcot patient is to re-establish a plantigrade foot and prevent ulceration. The goal is to get the heel, the first metatarsal, and the fifth metatarsal into anatomic alignment and all on the same plane creating the "three legged stool/tripod effect." A single medial incision may be used depending on the deformity. If needed, a second lateral incision may be utilized. A triplane wedge is removed from the central midfoot at the apex of the deformity. The deformities typically present in three planes so the apex of the resected bones needs to be thought out well. The goal is to reverse the deformity in the sagittal plane as well as correct any transverse and frontal plane deformity. In order to reverse a deformity with a "classic" rocker bottom deformity, more bone must be removed plantarly than dorsally resulting in bone resected at the base of the deformity. One may use Kirschner-wires (K-wires) as guide rails for appropriate bone resection. The wedge of bone is removed and the osteotomy is closed down, placed in anatomic alignment and temporarily fixated with 2.0 K-wires. The diseased bone is resected, leaving good, healthy bleeding bone. The surgeon may then use various internal methods of fixation and/or external fixation to stabilize the osteotomy for fusion.[109] The senior author typically uses screw and plate fixation and places the patient in a BK cast.

Multiple internal and external fixation constructs have been described, with variable levels of success.[110] "Beaming" is a relatively new technique used to achieve medial column stability and arthrodesis.[111] If required based on the extent of the deformity, the senior author utilizes a long solid bolt typically placed antegrade through the posterior talus through the midfoot and into the first metatarsal. Advantages include restoration of Meary angle in all planes with focus on the sagittal plane. Additional application of intraosseous hardware and medial or plantar plating may be used in combination. A medial based or plantar plate may also be used independently with intraosseous fixation.[112] The nonplantigrade foot with progressive deformity that is at high risk for ulceration is an excellent indication for midfoot arthrodesis and internal fixation with the "beaming" technique[113] and/or plantar- or medial-based plating.

RECONSTRUCTING THE MIDFOOT

Following the lengthening of the posterior muscle group, typically a medial-based incision is made in order to stabilize the medial column. In most cases, the authors have found that the lateral column does not need to be arthrodesed. Because of this, the focus is on the medial aspect of the foot and most of the reduction and fixation has been able to be achieved through one medial-based utility incision. If more exposure is needed, however, a lateral incision can be employed or a Z type of incision can be utilized.

LISFRANC CHARCOT (ISOLATED)

Indications

The indications for surgical treatment include chronic ulcers associated with bony deformities or contractures, unstable joints of the foot and ankle that cannot be treated with a shoe or brace, recurrent infected ulcers with bony prominences, and

acute displaced fractures in neuropathic patients with adequate circulation. Traditionally, surgical treatment has been limited to the inactive phase of the disease; however, it has been the experience of the senior author to perform this procedure in the acute phase as well. When performed in the acute phase, there is less secondary soft tissue and bony deformity and less need for bone resection and bone grafting.

Gross instability at the TMT articulation will lead to the characteristic symptomatic medial and plantar bony prominences, which can cause ulceration and infection, often resulting in amputation of the limb. Ostectomy alone does not address the biomechanical instability and thus does not provide long-term benefit.

Procedure

Attention is then directed medially where an incision is made beginning at the talonavicular joint and extending to the distal one-third of the first metatarsal shaft. The incision is deepened by sharp and blunt dissection down to the first metatarsal, medial cuneiform, and navicular. A full-thickness tissue flap is then retracted off of the TMT joints. Attention is directed toward the base of the Lisfranc articulation. An osteotome is used to remove approximately a 1-cm block of necrotic bone or the amount needed to identify healthy bone. This is performed across the Lisfranc joint, down to good, healthy, bleeding bone. If all of the diseased Charcot bone cannot be resected through the medial incision, a second incision is made on the lateral aspect of the foot between the fourth and fifth metatarsals. This incision is deepened down to the base of the metatarsals and cuboid. All necrotic bone is removed, completing the resection of the Charcot bone across the Lisfranc joint. The Lisfranc joint is adducted, rotated, and plantarflexed into anatomic position using 2.0-in K-wires for temporary fixation. Next, a 3.5-mm reconstruction plate is eccentrically loaded and applied to the plantar aspect of the first metatarsal, medial cuneiform, and navicular. One 3.5/4.0-cm cortical screw is placed outside the plate in an oblique fashion, seating on the medial wall of the first metatarsal and aiming at the lateral edge of the navicular. Its length depends on the extension of the bone debrided. A second cortical screw is inserted outside the plate from the medial cuneiform or navicular into the second and/or third metatarsal base. No fixation is used on the fourth and fifth rays. Alternatively, in case there is difficulty with obtaining plantar plating, a medial-based plate can be utilized. The plantar plate is preferred as applying the plate to the plantar aspect is biomechanically more stable.[112] Shear strain relief graft is used to "gap fill" and place bone in any visible defects.

A drain is inserted and the deep tissues and skin are closed. Autogenous or allogenic cancellous bone can be used to fill any void or space at the arthrodesis site. The incisions are then dressed with a multilayered compression bandage and an univalved cast is applied.[114]

An aggressive resection of the diseased bone needs to be performed. If there was a bone infection from and/or open wound, this will also serve as a surgical correction/cure. If there is no bone infection and there is only Charcot bone, this must be removed. Charcot bone is diseased bone, and it cannot predictably maintain the hardware; therefore, it needs to be resected. The resection needs to be performed to where the remaining bone is very firm, clinically stable/strong, and there

is good bleeding to the bone demonstrating good vascularity to the bone. This is often times referred to as "An Internal Amputation."

The reduction needs to be completed in all three planes. In most cases, the forefoot is adducted, plantarflexed, and rotated in the frontal plane getting the first ray down on the same plane as the fifth metatarsal head and calcaneus creating a plantigrade foot. This is called the "Tripod Effect" of a "Three Legged Stool."

The goal of this surgery is to fuse the medial aspect of Lisfranc joint. Once the medial TMT joints are reduced, TMT-4 and TMT-5 will follow and find their natural anatomic locations relative to the new reduction and alignment of the TMT-1–TMT-3. This reduction is similar to the "Vassal Principle" with ankle fractures. Once the dominant fracture (TMT-1) is reduced, the lesser TMT joints will reduce the remaining fractures/dislocations because of the soft tissues (Figs. 38.2 and 38.3).

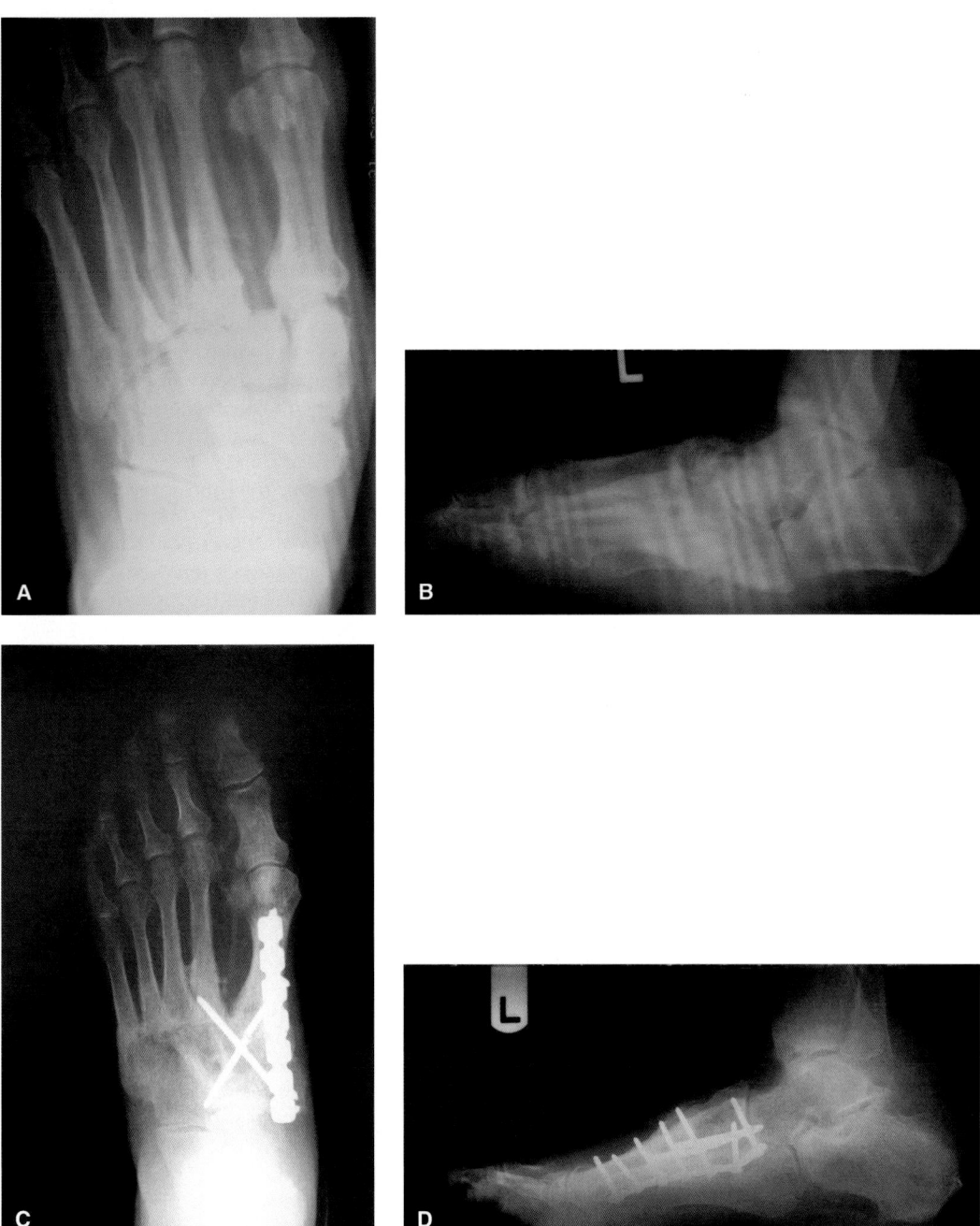

FIGURE 38.2 A. An AP preop radiograph demonstrating displacement at Lisfranc joint with malalignment. **B.** A lateral radiograph demonstrating preop malalignment and rotation of the forefoot. **C.** An AP postop radiograph demonstrating good anatomic alignment and good fixation with a solid bony fusion 12 years postop (plantar plating with intraosseous fixation). **D.** A lateral postop radiograph demonstrating good anatomic alignment and good fixation with a solid bony fusion 12 years postop.

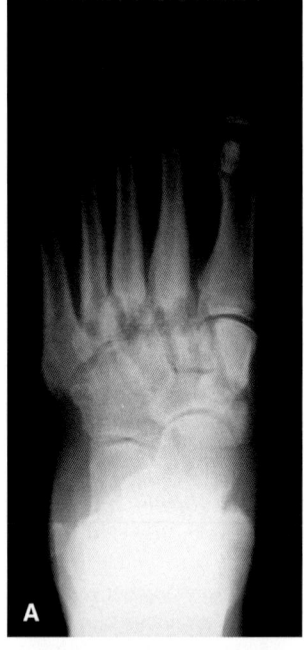
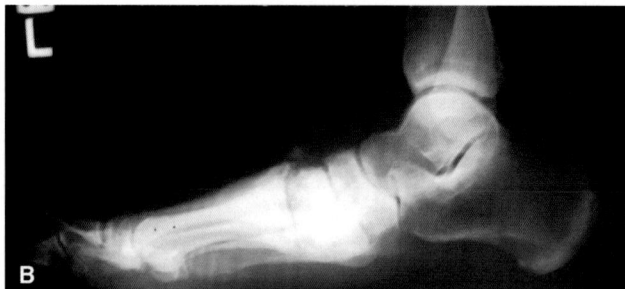
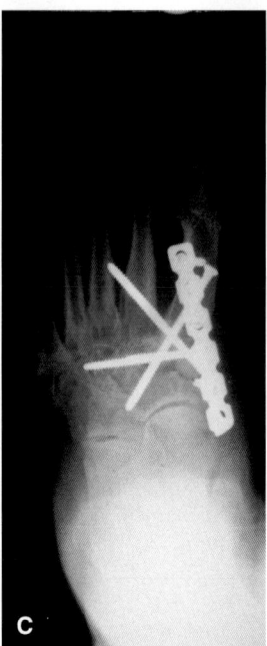
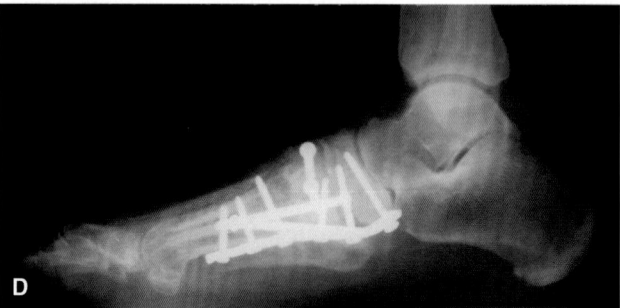

FIGURE 38.3 A. An AP preop radiograph demonstrating bony breakdown at Lisfranc joint with malalignment. **B.** A lateral radiograph demonstrating preop malaligment and bony fragmentation at Lisfranc joint. **C.** An AP postop radiograph demonstrating good anatomic alignment and good fixation with a solid bony fusion at Lisfranc joint. **D.** A lateral postop radiograph demonstrating good anatomic alignment and good fixation with a solid bony fusion at Lisfranc joint. Note that Meary angle is maintained.

An alternative to the plantar plate is to use a medial-based plate. The plantar plate is stronger and is applied to the tension side; therefore, biomechanically, it should provide a better construct. In the cases where it is difficult to place a plate plantarly, a medial-based plate can be applied.

The postoperative course included serial radiographs every 3 weeks, and the patients are kept non–weight bearing, depending on the radiographic and clinical appearance. The patients are placed in a walking cast or controlled ankle motion (CAM) walker for an additional 2-3 months, after the initiation

of weight bearing with physical therapy. This is followed by a CROW boot and subsequently and AFO. If all is very stable and the bone is well consolidated, our goal is to allow the patient to ambulate in a more regular shoe such as a diabetic shoe with custom inserts.

MIDFOOT CHARCOT (ISOLATED)

Midfoot Charcot arthropathy may or may not involve Lisfranc joint. If the scenario of a given Charcot case does not involve

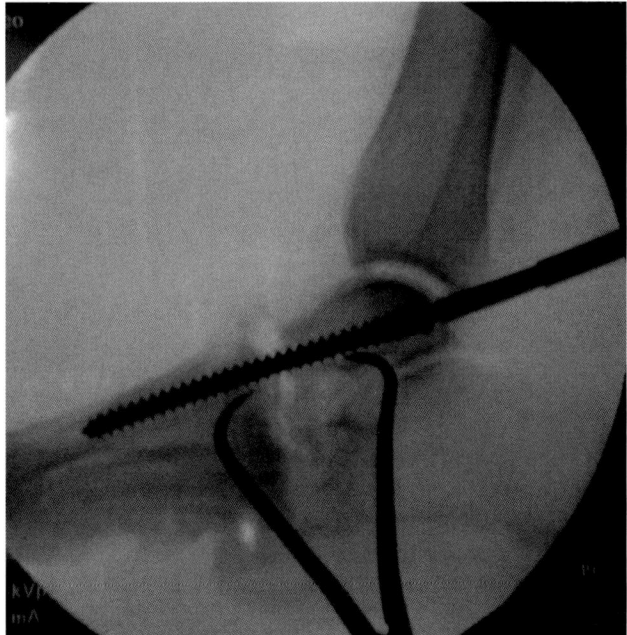

FIGURE 38.4 Following the posterior muscle lengthening (this allows for the calcaneal pitch angle to improve) and the internal amputation, the reduction is made and insertion of a solid 6.5-mm bolt is inserted from the posterior talus into the medullary canal of the first metatarsal re-creating Meary angle.

Lisfranc joint, then essentially a double or triple arthrodesis is required with a posterior muscle lengthening. In the senior authors' experience, it is more common that Lisfranc joint is involved with most midfoot Charcot arthropathy cases. In these cases, the procedure is very similar to the Lisfranc approach with the addition of arthrodesis being performed more proximally. We typically attempt to use intramedullary beaming with 6.5-mm solid bolt from the posterior talus to the mid shaft of the first metatarsal coupled with a plantar plate or a medial-based plate. Inserting the intramedullary fixation from the posterior talus is a very difficult insertion (Fig. 38.4).

One needs to work around the Achilles tendon. The amount of space between the posterior skin and posterior talus is substantial. Additionally, to re-create Meary angle, the fixation has to be placed anatomically. When the hardware is placed from posterior to anterior, the length of the fixation is shorter and stronger. With midfoot Charcot, the load is more proximal (closer to the posterior midfoot). When hardware is placed from distal to proximal, that is, the first metatarsophalangeal joint (MTPJ), the hardware is longer and not as strong. Additionally, in order to get into the first MTPJ, one has to expose an already "diseased foot" and disrupt normal anatomy. Because it is easier to do, does not mean it is better.

The authors' recommendation is to use intramedullary fixation with a combination of plantar plate or medial-based plating. We recommend inserting the hardware through the posterior talus down into the medial column. This provides a stronger construct, and there is less collateral damage to the other soft tissues. Also, this allows the surgeon to place the alignment of the osseous structures into anatomic alignment and re-align Meary angle. Typically, this is done with is a solid 6.5-mm noncannulated bolt. This is a difficult insertion; however, this is much more effective than inserting the bolt from distal to proximal. Additionally, it is recommended that multiple intraosseous screws be inserted for fixation from medial to lateral. The concept is to make this a rigid construct similar to rebar. The anatomic structures need to have tremendous fixation while the bone and bone graft slowly consolidate (Figs. 38.5-38.8).

The midfoot fusion can be made with one medial-based incision or with an additional lateral-based incision. We recommend attempting one medial utility incision to lessen the secondary soft tissue effects of a second lateral-based incision.

TIBIOTALAR FUSION

Indications

The indications for surgical treatment include chronic ulcers associated with bony deformities or contracture, unstable joints of the ankle that cannot be treated with a shoe or brace, recurrent infected ulcers with bony prominences, and acute displaced fractures in neuropathic patients with adequate circulation. The procedure is performed when there is enough talar body remaining and the subtalar joint remains healthy and well aligned. Ostectomy and/or simple bony resection alone does not address the biomechanical instability and thus does not provide long-term benefit.

Procedure

Prior to embarking on an isolated tibial-talar, tibial-fibular fusion, the surgeon should have performed a thorough

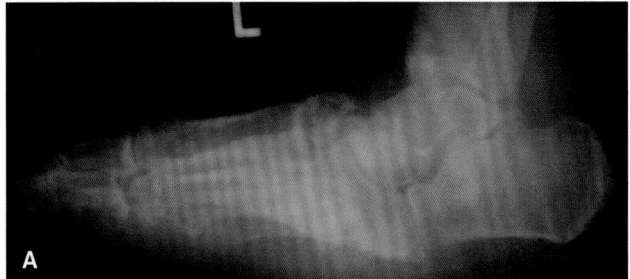

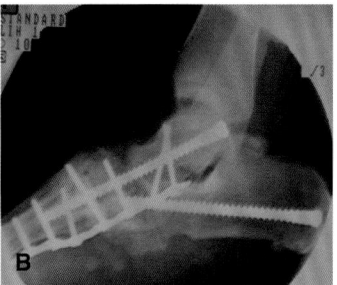

FIGURE 38.5 A. A lateral preoperative radiograph demonstrating significant malalignment throughout the midfoot. **B.** A lateral intraoperative fluoroscopy demonstrating re-alignment following an internal amputation, insertion of a bolt posteriorly and plantar plating.

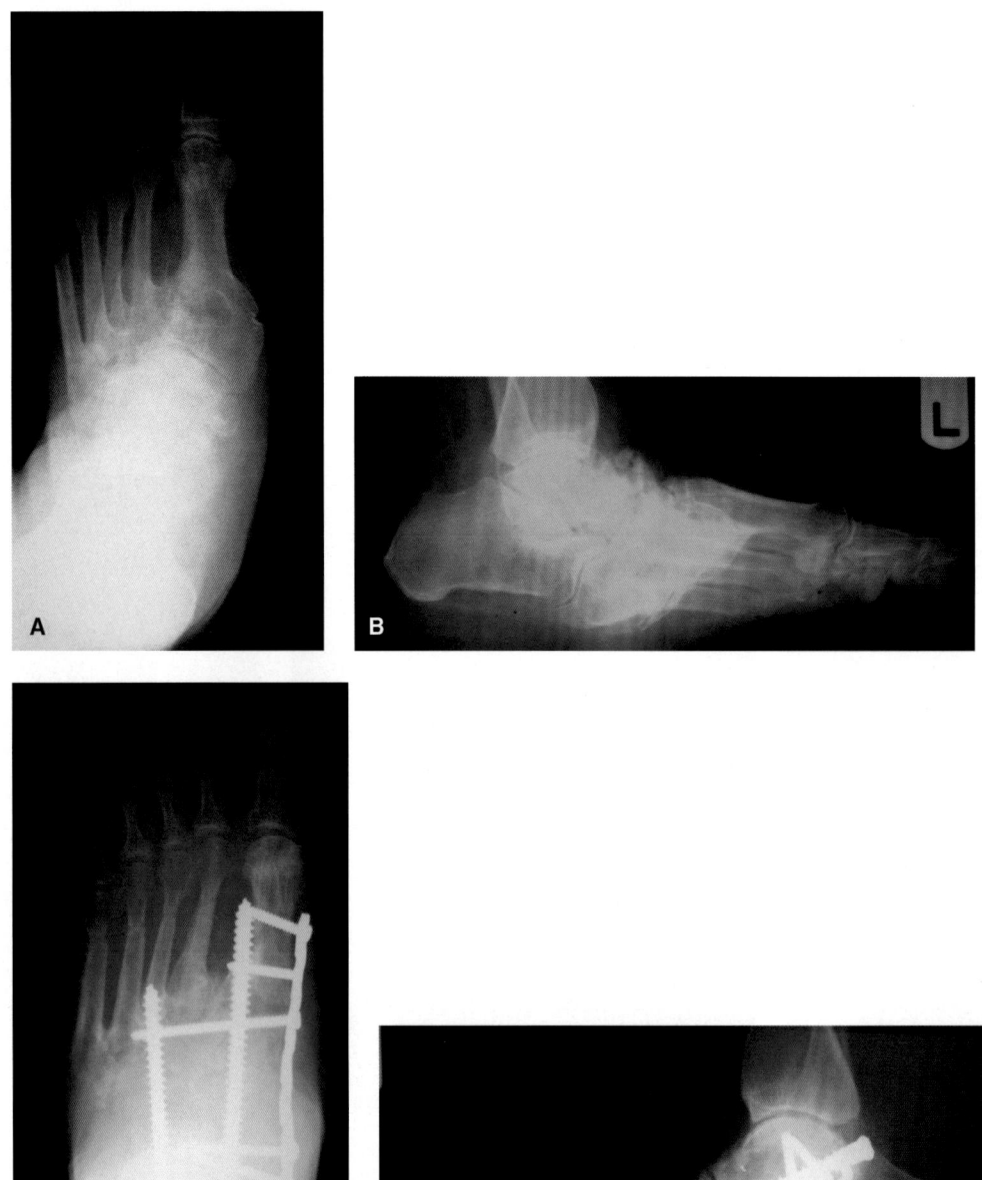

FIGURE 38.6 A. An AP radiograph demonstrating significant midfoot destruction and malalignment. Note the malaligned and fused Lisfranc joint. **B.** A lateral radiograph demonstrating significant midfoot destruction, malalignment, and midfoot displacement. Note the forefoot varus and significant malalignment. **C.** An AP radiograph demonstrating anatomic alignment with 6.5-mm solid bolt fixation and a medial-based plate. **D.** A postoperative lateral radiograph demonstrating long-term bony fusion and alignment. Note the changes in comparison of the preop radiographs while comparing Meary angle, the calcaneal inclination angle and the forefoot varus are corrected.

clinical and radiographic evaluation with or without advanced imaging. The surgeon needs to identify if there is enough talar body in order to successfully hold the fixation required to accomplish a tibial-talar arthrodesis. If there is not enough talar body to house the necessary hardware, instability will result. If there is insufficient bone, then a tibial-talar-calcaneal or a tibial-calcaneal arthrodesis may need to be performed.

APPROACHES

Anterior Approach

An incision is made over the anterior ankle joint and carried down to the talonavicular joint. The incision is carried deep to the level of the joint, avoiding all neurovascular structures. At this time, all soft tissues are retracted to allow for complete visualization of the bony anatomy of the tibial-talar joint as well

as the tibial-fibular joint. The fibula is left intact and the syndesmosis is taken down. This provides excellent exposure to the ankle joint, and the lateral aspect of the distal tibia and medial aspect of the fibula are prepared for fusion. The cortices of the tibia and fibula are debrided in preparation for arthrodesis. An osteotome is used to takedown the syndesmosis and to remove the diseased bone and any remaining cartilage as needed until healthy bleeding bone is identified. This is performed across the tibial-talar and tibial-fibular joints. All diseased Charcot bone needs to be resected to ensure adequate healing. This anterior approach allows for great exposure to the ankle joint and good reduction in the coronal plane.

The ankle joint is placed in a neutral position with the lateral process of the talus under the midpoint of the tibia on a lateral fluoroscopy. In the coronal plane, the talus needs to be placed directly under the tibia. The foot must also be in a plantigrade position. Often, when there is significant Charcot deformity of the tibial-talar joint, osseous deficits result. They must be back filled with bone graft to fill the voids. Next, guidewires for large cannulated cancellous screws are inserted from the tibia into the talus. One can also be inserted from the posterior malleolus into the talar head and neck if enough bone is present, to create a tripod of fixation. Again, there needs to be enough talus remaining in order for this procedure to be successful. If there is not enough talus remaining, then a tibial-talar-calcaneal or a tibial-calcaneal procedure will need to be performed. When there is enough talus remaining, the large cannulated cancellous screws are inserted from proximal to

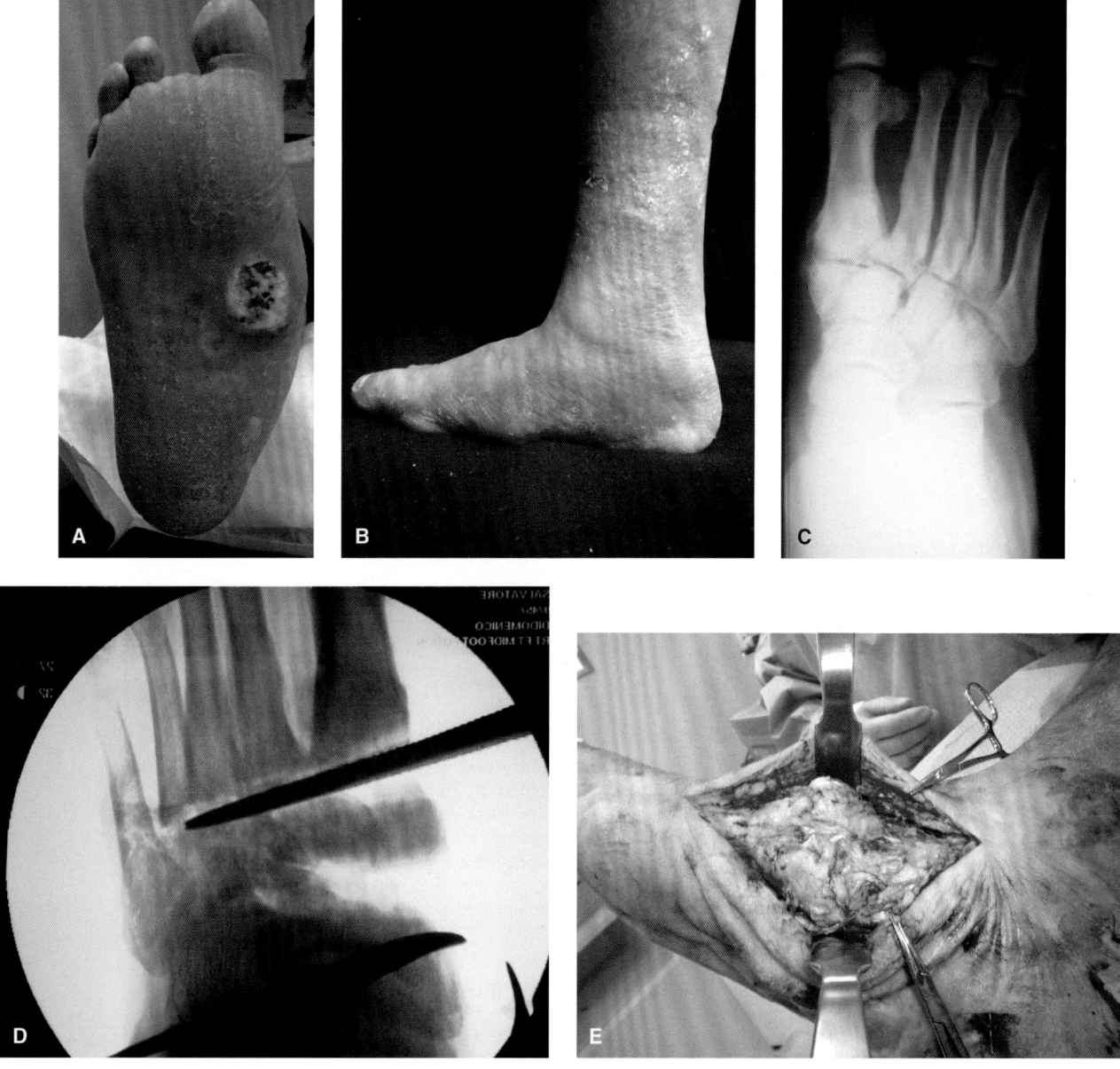

FIGURE 38.7 A, B. A clinical photo demonstrating an ulcer from a Charcot midfoot secondary to malalignment. **C.** An AP preoperative radiograph demonstrating a Charcot midfoot with malalignment and displacement of the midfoot. **D, E.** An intraoperative clinical photo demonstrating diseased, avascular Charcot bone and a AP fluoroscopy demonstrating an "internal amputation" resecting all of the diseased Charcot bone.

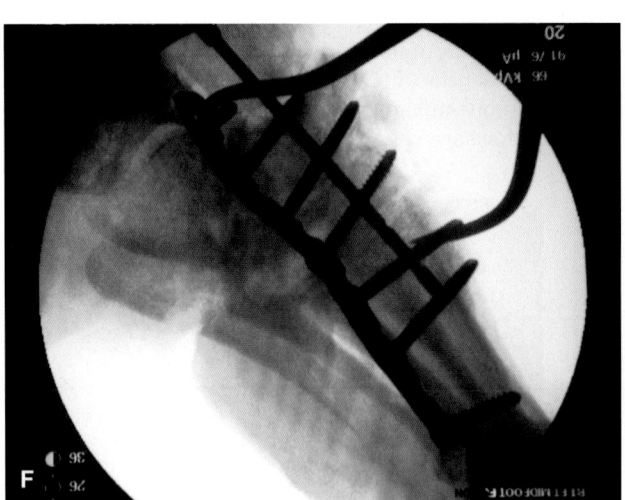

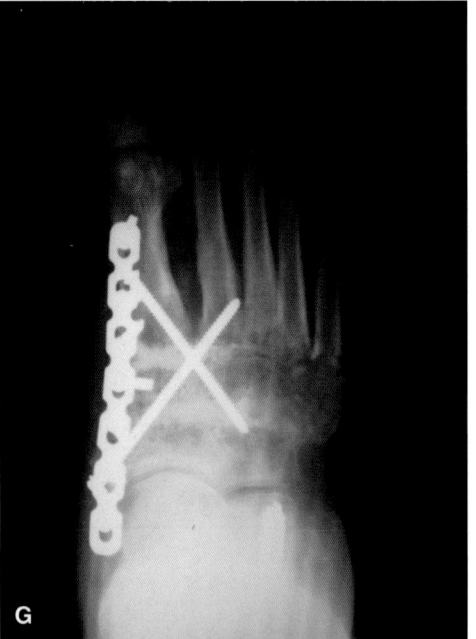

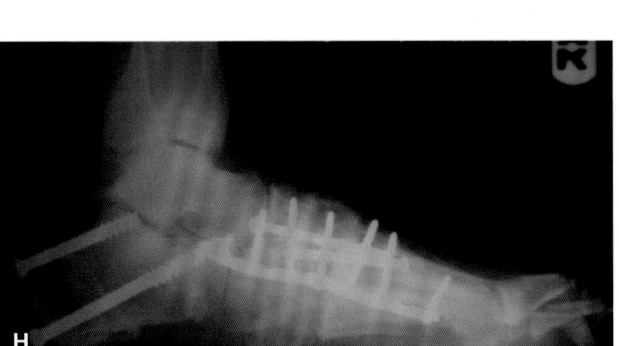

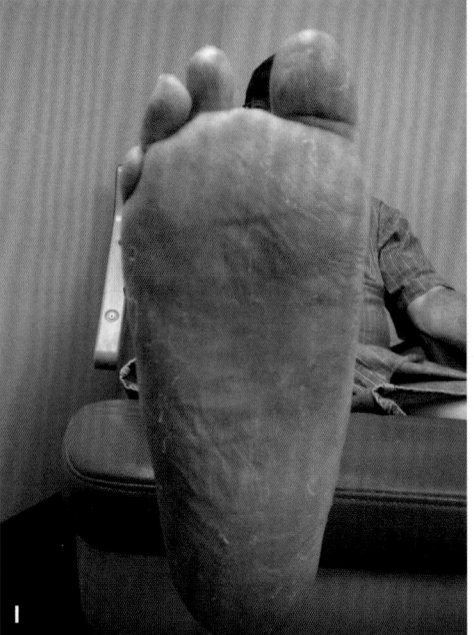

FIGURE 38.7 (*Continued*) **F.** An intraoperative fluoroscopy demonstrating a reduction and a plantar plate and intraosseous screw fixation following the "internal amputation" of the midfoot. **G, H.** An AP and lateral radiographic view following successful re-alignment and fixation. **I.** A clinical view demonstrating anatomic alignment, and good bony fusion post midfoot Charcot reconstruction. Note the shape of the foot and the ulcer is healed. An AP preop x-ray demonstrating fracture and dislocation of the midfoot.

distal (tibia-talus) to the inferior aspect of the talus (far cortex) preserving the healthy remaining subtalar joint. The screws are then inserted creating compression. In a case where there is little or any bone loss, then compression is required and partially threaded screws are used. In cases where there is substantial bone loss, the goal is to obtain some bone-bone (tibial-talus) contact and insert fully threaded large cancellous screws across as a positional screw and then back fill the voids with bone graft. An anterior based locking plate is then applied (Fig. 38.9).

Lateral Approach

An incision is made over the distal portion of the fibula and carried down to the ankle joint. The lateral incision is carried deep to the level of the fibula, avoiding all neurovascular structures. At this time, all soft tissues are retracted to allow for complete visualization of the fibula anatomy. A fibular osteotomy is performed and retraction of the fibula from the distal tibia is performed taking down the syndesmosis providing excellent

exposure to the ankle. A benefit of the lateral approach is relatively easy access to the tibial-talar joint. One of the challenges of the lateral approach is even resection of the ankle joint in the frontal plane. Errors are made with less bone resection medially and more laterally as there may be more difficulty reaching the medial aspect of the ankle joint, thus resulting in a valgus position.

Bone debridement is performed at the medial aspect of the fibula and the lateral aspect of the tibia for fusion until good, healthy, bleeding bone is identified. This is also performed across the tibial-talar joint and all diseased Charcot bone is resected. The ankle joint is placed in a neutral position with the lateral process of the talus under the midpoint of the tibia on a lateral fluoroscopy image. In the coronal plane, the talus needs to be placed directly under the tibia. The foot must also be in a plantigrade position. Often when there is significant Charcot deformity of the tibial-talar joint, the surgeon needs to back fill the deficits with bone graft to fill the voids or irregular deficits of bony topography. Two guidewires for large cannulated cancellous screws can be percutaneously inserted from the anterior

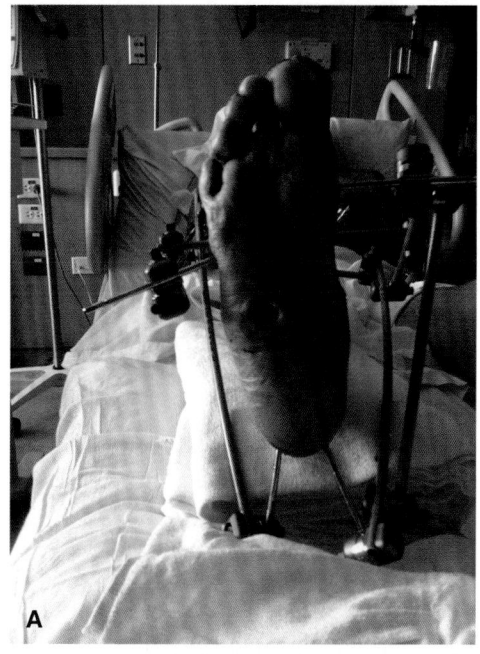
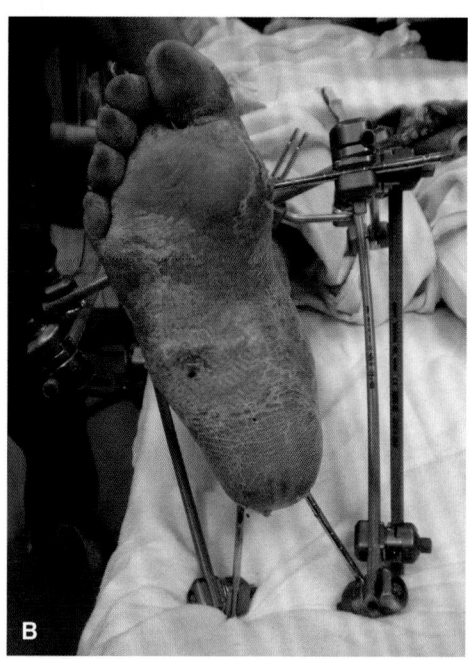
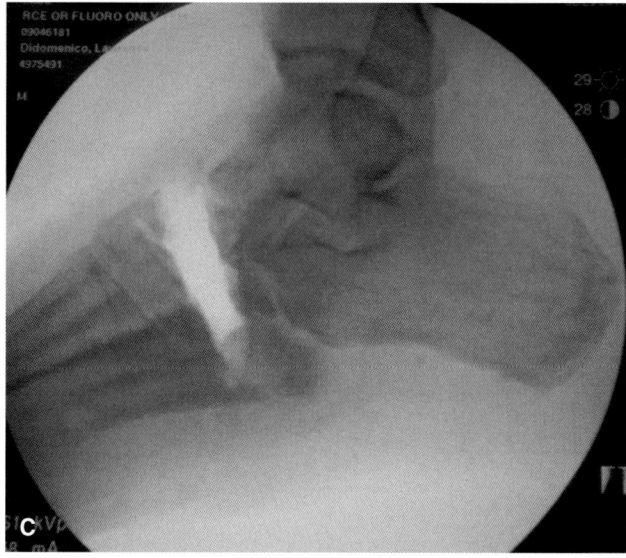
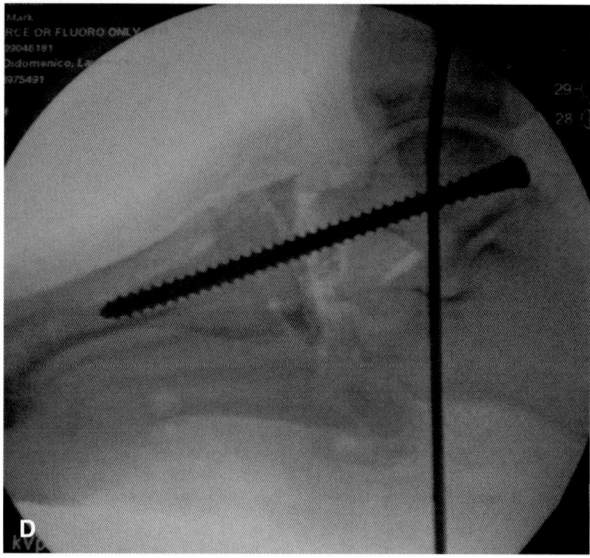

FIGURE 38.8 A. Preoperatively this patient suffered from a rocker bottom Charcot midfoot with an infected ulcer. A posterior muscle lengthening was performed, and soft tissue and bone debridement along with cultures and biopsies were performed. Fracturing and chiseling of the midfoot deformity was performed through the wound allowing for reduction of the deformity. A pin to bar external fixator was used to stabilize the deformity in the corrected position and infectious disease prescribed the antibiotics. **B.** Approximately 8 weeks later, the wound had healed, the serum markers improved, and the patient was prepared for the staged reconstruction. **C.** A lateral intraoperative view demonstrating an "internal amputation" resecting all of the diseased bone and preparing for arthrodesis of the midfoot. **D.** A lateral intraoperative view demonstrating insertion of a solid fully threaded bolt inserted from the talus into the first metatarsal.

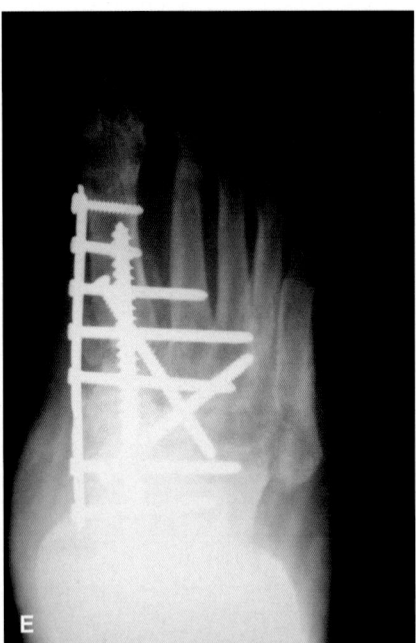
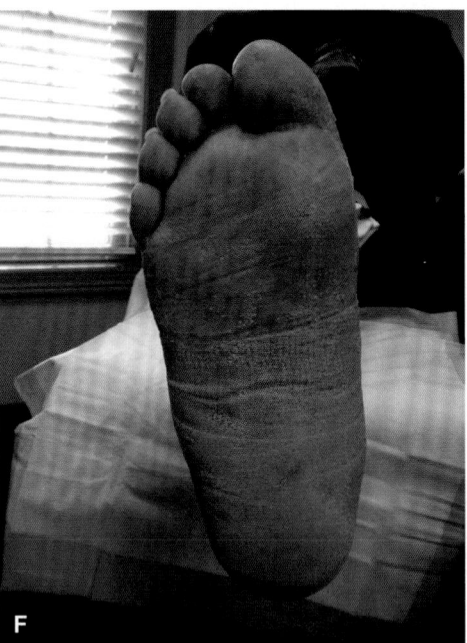

FIGURE 38.8 (*Continued*) **E.** A postoperative view demonstrating good anatomic alignment and good fixation with a solid arthrodesis across the midfoot. **F.** A postoperative clinic view demonstrating a long-term follow-up of a healed wound.

medial and lateral tibia into the talus, and one can be inserted from the posterior malleolus into and the talar head and neck if a talar head and neck are present to create a tripod of fixation. Again, there needs to be enough talus remaining in order for this procedure to be successful. If there is not enough talus remaining, then a tibial-talar-calcaneal or a tibial-calcaneal procedure will need to be performed. When there is enough talus remaining, the large cannulated cancellous screws are inserted from proximal to distal (tibia-talus) to the inferior aspect of the talus preserving the healthy remaining subtalar joint. The screws are then inserted creating compression. In a case where there is little bone loss, then compression is required and partially threaded crews are used. In cases where there is significant bone loss, the goal is to obtain some bone-bone contact and insert fully threaded large cancellous screws across as a positional screw and then back fill the voids with bone graft.

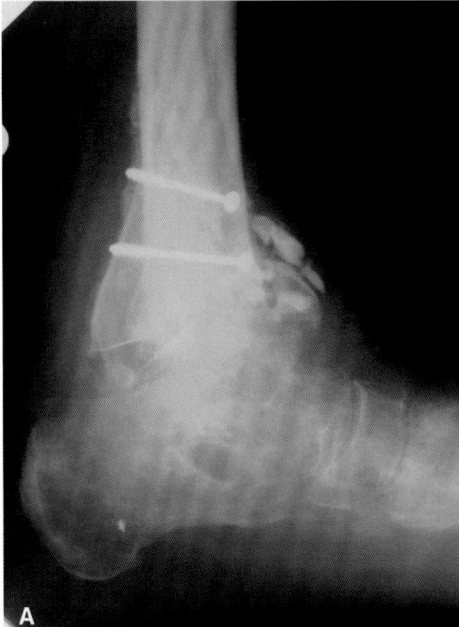
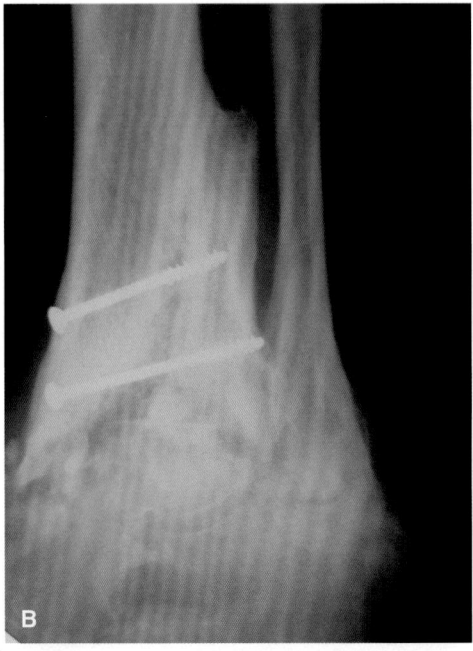

FIGURE 38.9 **A.** A lateral radiograph demonstrating an isolated Charcot joint of the tibial-talar joint. This patient was in a motor vehicle accident, had a prior open reduction and internal fixation at a trauma center, and developed an isolated tibial-talar Charcot joint. **B.** An oblique radiograph of the isolated tibial-talar Charcot joint.

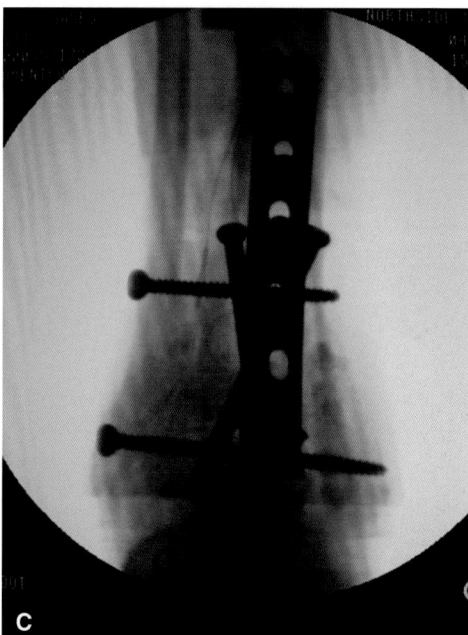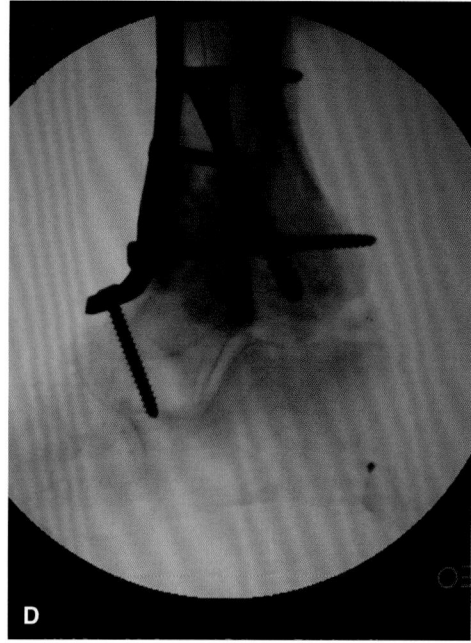

FIGURE 38.9 (*Continued*) **C.** An intraoperative AP radiograph following bone grafting of the tibial-talar joint and screw and plate fixation. **D.** An intraoperative lateral radiograph following bone grafting of the tibial-talar joint with screw and plate fixation.

Next, the fibula can be used as an onlay graft or an inlay graft depending on the goals of the surgery. If an inlay graft is desired, then time is spent creating a groove on the lateral aspect of the tibia and talus so insertion of the prepared medial cortex of the fibula is press fitted into the groove inlaying the fibula as a biological plate. Using a large Weber clamp, compression is created along the tibial-fibular joint and two solid 4.0-mm cortical or a solid 4.5-mm malleolar screws are inserted at the distal fibula into the distal tibia above the ankle joint obtaining four cortices and a 4.0-mm or a 4.5-mm screw is inserted from the distal fibula across the talus and into the medial malleolus exiting out the far cortex of the medial malleolus in attempt for fusion. If an onlay graft is utilized, the fibula is laid onto the tibia and talus and the same screw fixation technique is completed. Following this fixation, all bone voids are packed tightly with bone graft into the distal tibia-fibula joint. A drain is inserted and the deep tissues and skin are closed. Autogenous or allogenic cancellous bone can be used to fill any void or space at the arthrodesis site. The incisions are then dressed with a multilayered compression bandage and an univalved cast is applied[114] (Fig. 38.10).

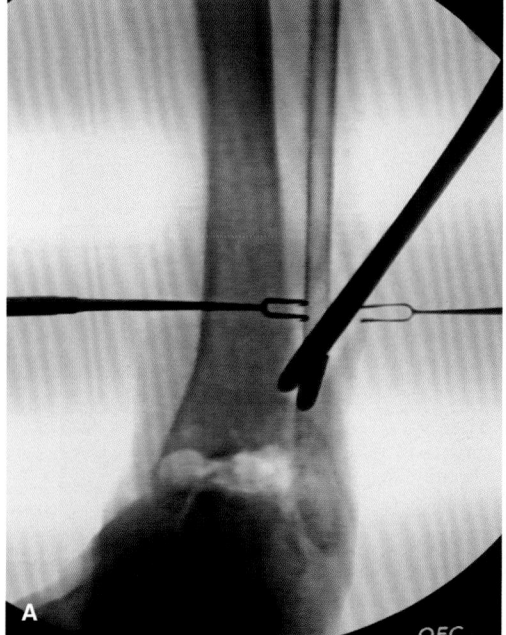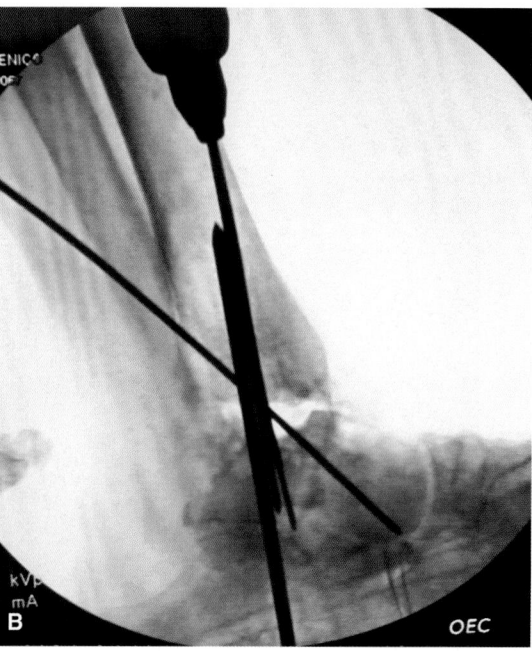

FIGURE 38.10 **A, B.** This patient's Charcot arthropathy was diagnosed early and limited to the tibial-talar and tibial-fibular joints. Radiographically the subtalar joint is preserved, and clinically it is not affected.

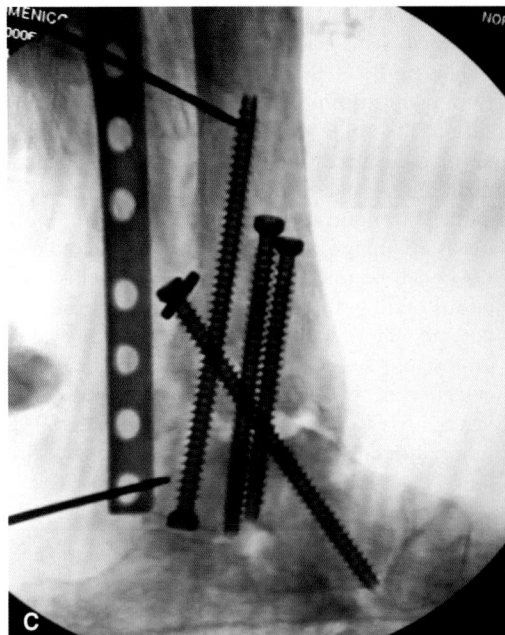

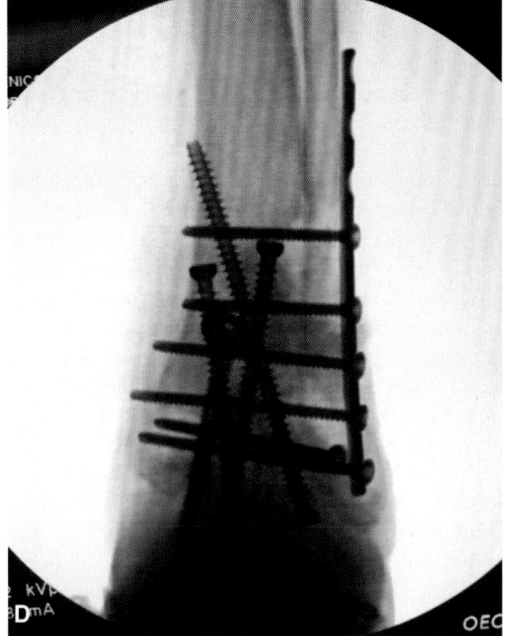

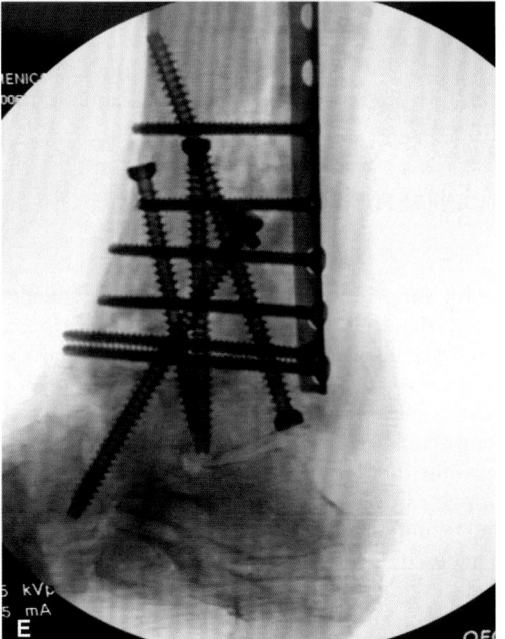

FIGURE 38.10 (*Continued*) **C.** Due to the severe osteopenia, multiple screws are inserted within the tibial-talar joint while preserving the subtalar joint. A lateral plate is temporized to buttress the fibula to the tibia for a tibial-fibular fusion. The hardware is in place and stabilizing the ankle prior to inserting the bone graft. **D, E.** Multiple screws are inserted from the tibia to the talus and from the talus to the tibia with additional screw and plate fixation for the severely osteopenic Charcot artropathy ankle joint. The bone graft was inserted to fill the bone voids following the rigid fixation insertion of the hardware.

Posterior Approach

When there is a diseased soft tissue envelope anteriorly or laterally from previous wounds, infection, or surgeries, the posterior approach provides an excellent corridor as an alternative approach as it provides good access to the posterior ankle joint.[115] A posterior incision is made directly over the Achilles tendon. Next the subcutaneous tissue is incised to the level of the Achilles tendon. A "Z" pasty of the Achilles tendon is performed in order to expose the deep fascia. A full-thickness tissue flap is then retracted off the ankle joint.

The surgeon can easily reach the fibula from the posterior approach if needed and perform a fibular osteotomy or perform a takedown of the tibia and fibula syndesmosis to prepare for fusion if needed. The posterior approach provides better soft tissue coverage and vascularity to the osseous and soft tissues because of the well-vascularized low lying flexor hallucis longus muscle. This provides a good vascular supply to the soft tissues resulting in less soft tissue and bony complications with this patient population.

Attention is directed toward the tibial-talar joint and the lateral aspect of the tibia and the medial aspect of the fibula. An osteotome is used to takedown the syndesmosis and to remove the diseased bone and any remaining cartilage as needed. As described earlier, it is important to perform an aggressive debridement of the tibial-fibular joint as well as the tribal-talar joint for successful arthrodesis. Next the alignment needs to be evaluated under fluoroscopy for anatomic alignment ensuring the foot and ankle are in a plantigrade position.

Next, guidewires for large cannulated cancellous screws are inserted from the tibia into the talus and one can be inserted from the posterior malleolus into and the talar head and neck if a talar head and neck are present. If a talar head and neck are not present, then this can be placed into the remaining body of the talus.

If there is not enough talus remaining, then a tibial-talar-calcaneal or a tibial-calcaneal procedure will need to be performed. Based on the given anatomy, the surgeon will apply either compression screws or positional screws with bone graft.

Next, a large Weber clamp is utilized to create compression along the tibial-fibular joint and percutaneously a solid 4.0-mm solid cortical or a solid 4.5-mm malleolar screws are inserted at the distal fibula into the distal tibia above the ankle joint in attempt for fusion. We typically place two of these syndesmotic fusion screws above the ankle joint from the fibula into the tibia while obtaining four cortices. Next, at the inferior fibula, a 4.0-mm or a 4.5-mm screw is inserted from the distal fibula across the talus and into the medial malleolus exiting out the far cortex of the medial malleolus. Following this fixation, all bone voids are packed tightly with bone graft into the distal tibia-fibula joint. This can be followed by a locking plate. The locking plates assist in creating a stable construct from multiple directions.

A drain is inserted and the deep tissues and skin are closed. Autogenous or allogenic cancellous bone can be used to fill any void or space at the arthrodesis site. The incisions are then dressed with a multilayered compression bandage and an uni-valved cast is applied.[114]

TIBIOTALOCALCANEAL FUSION

Indications

The indications for surgical treatment include chronic ulcers associated with bony deformities or contractures, unstable joints of the foot and ankle involving both the subtalar and ankle joints that cannot be treated with a shoe or brace, recurrent infected ulcers with bony prominences, and acute displaced fractures in neuropathic patients with adequate circulation. Gross instability at the hindfoot and/or ankle will lead to bony prominences, which can cause ulceration and infection, often perhaps resulting in amputation of the limb. Ostectomy and/or simple bony resection alone does not address the biomechanical instability and thus does not provide long-term benefit.

All corrective procedures should begin by starting more proximal and lengthening the needed posterior muscle group. Optimal placement of the ankle and foot consist of 10-15 degrees externally rotated and/or maintain alignment that is consistent with the contralateral limb in the transverse plane. Align the tibial tuberosity and the second toe. Relative to a lateral radiograph, a neutral position of the ankle joint should align the lateral process of the talus with the midline of the tibia. In the frontal plane, the patient should be in a neutral position (most desirable) to 0-5 degrees of valgus.

Approaches

Lateral Approach
Following the appropriate posterior muscle lengthening, the lateral incision is made over the distal portion of the fibula and carried out to the calcaneus. The lateral incision is carried deep to the level of the bony structures, avoiding all neurovascular

structures. At this time, all soft tissues are retracted to allow for complete visualization of the bony anatomy. A fibular osteotomy is performed and retraction of the fibula from the distal tibia taking down the syndesmosis providing excellent exposure to the ankle and subtalar joints.[116] A benefit of the lateral approach is relatively easy access to the tibial-talar, tibial-calcaneal, and subtalar joints. Additionally, there is less chance of damage to neurovascular structures. Also, one can use the fibula as an onlay graft, or an inlay graft (biological plate), or the fibula can be put into a bone mill and this can provide autogenous bone graft. The distal portion of the fibula can also be cut and split in half. This provides a bicortical cancellous bone graft strut. One of the downsides of the lateral approach is even resection of the joints in the frontal plane. Errors are made in less bone resection medially and more laterally as there may be more difficulty reaching the medial aspect of the STJ and ankle joint (Fig. 38.11).

Posterior Approach
Following the appropriate posterior muscle lengthening, the posterior incision is made over the Achilles tendon and carried out to the calcaneus. The posterior approach provides excellent access to both the posterior facet of the STJ and ankle joint.[115] The surgeon can easily reach the fibula from the posterior approach if needed and perform a fibular osteotomy or perform a takedown of the tibia and fibula syndesmosis to prepare for fusion if needed. The posterior approach provides a better soft tissue envelope. With the low lying flexor hallucis longus muscle belly, this allows for much less soft tissue injuries resulting in less bony complications with this patient population.

An Achilles tendonectomy is performed in order to expose the deep fascia. With a tibial-talar-calcaneal arthrodesis, the Achilles tendon has essentially very little blood supply; therefore, it is completely removed. Similar to the posterior approach for a tibia-talar arthrodesis, the incision approach provides good visualization of the anatomy of the tibial-fibular joint, the tibial-talar, and the talar-calcaneal joints. As previously described, it is required by the surgeon to execute an aggressive debridement of the tibial-fibular joint, the tibial-talar, and the talar-calcaneal joints.

The anatomy needs to be appropriately aligned and the foot and ankle in a plantigrade position as previously stated.

Fixation consists of two fully threaded screws. In cases where there is good bone loss, the goal is to obtain some bone-bone contact and insert fully threaded large cancellous screws across as a positional screw and then back fill the voids with bone graft. If the fibula is present, a large Weber clamp is utilized to create compression along the tibial-fibular joint and percutaneously a solid 4.0-mm or a solid 4.5-mm screw is placed as previously described.

An alternative fixation is an intramedullary nail. Screws and plates is the senior authors' primary form of fixation. The two long, large fully threaded screws are typically wider in diameter than the largest intramedullary nail on the market. These two long, large fully threaded screws purchase two cortices and provide more stability than an intramedullary nail with only one cortical purchase. The addition of a posterior placed locking plate provides tremendous stability to the fully threaded screw construct. Additionally, if the fibula is still present, then additional points of fixation and fusion involving the tibial-fibula joint allows for a very stable, solid construct. The senior author reserves the use of most intramedullary nails for revision

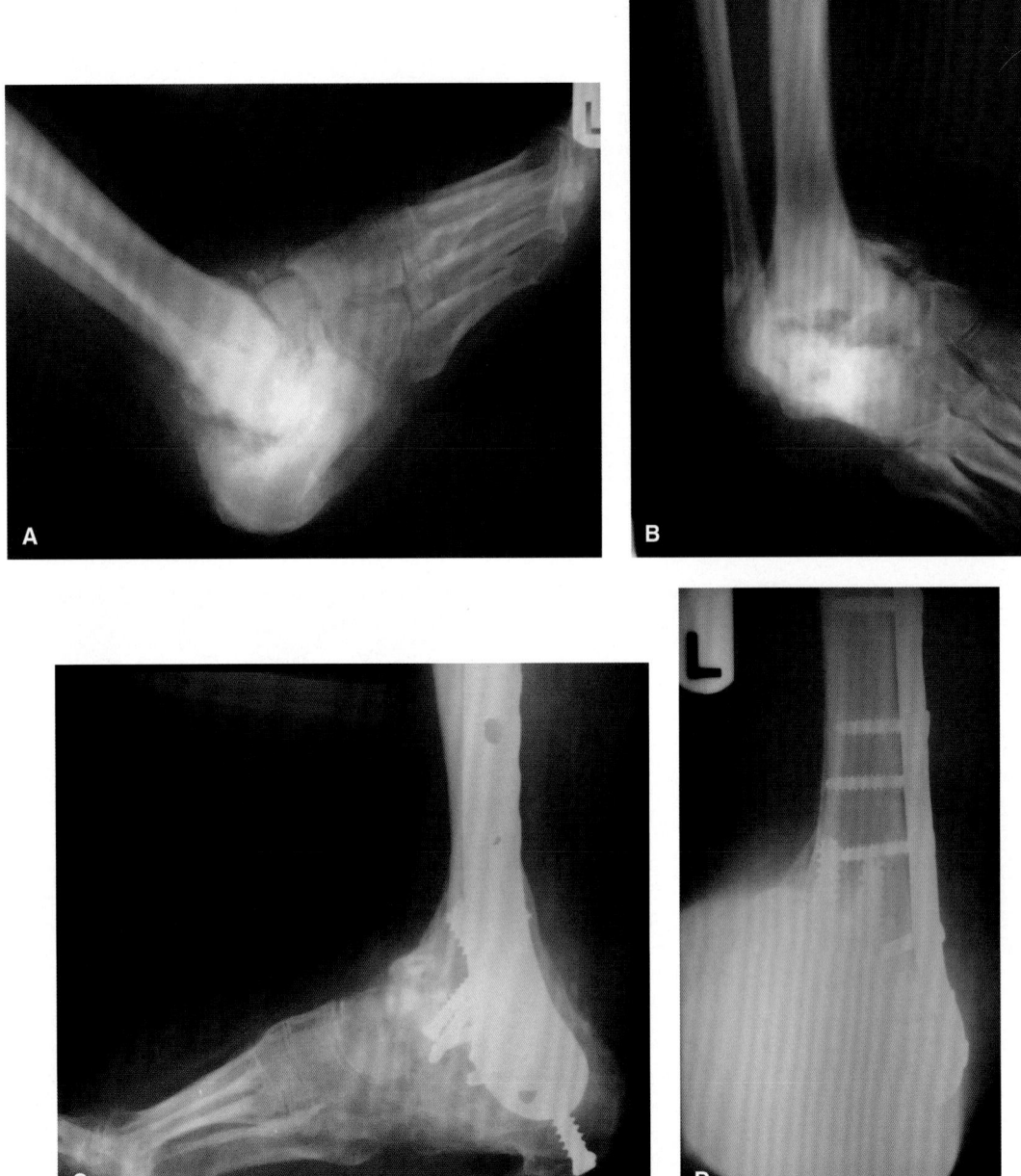

FIGURE 38.11 **A.** This patient suffers from Charcot arthropathy of the tibial-talar, talar-calcaneal, and talar-navicular malalignment. **B.** An oblique radiograph demonstrating the comminution and fractures of the tibial-talar, talar-calcaneal, and talar-navicular malalignment. **C, D.** Eleven months postsurgery, a solid plantigrade tibial-talar, talar-calcaneal arthrodesis utilizing two fully threaded cannulated cancellous screws with a femoral locking plate with anatomic alignment maintained.

surgery and for those patients who have a poor soft tissue envelope in cases where most of the surgery can be performed percutaneously or through small incisions (Fig. 38.12).

A drain is inserted and the deep tissue and skin are closed. Autogenous or allogenic cancellous bone can be used to fill any void or space at the arthrodesis site. The incisions are then dressed with a multilayered compression bandage and an uni-valve cast is applied.[114]

LATERAL APPROACH UTILIZING THE FIBULA AS A BIOLOGIC PLATE

In cases when a patient presents with a previous history soft tissue and bone infection and the surgeon is concerned the hardware need to secure fixation may increase the chance of infection, the use of the fibula as a biologic plate may decrease the likelihood of infection.

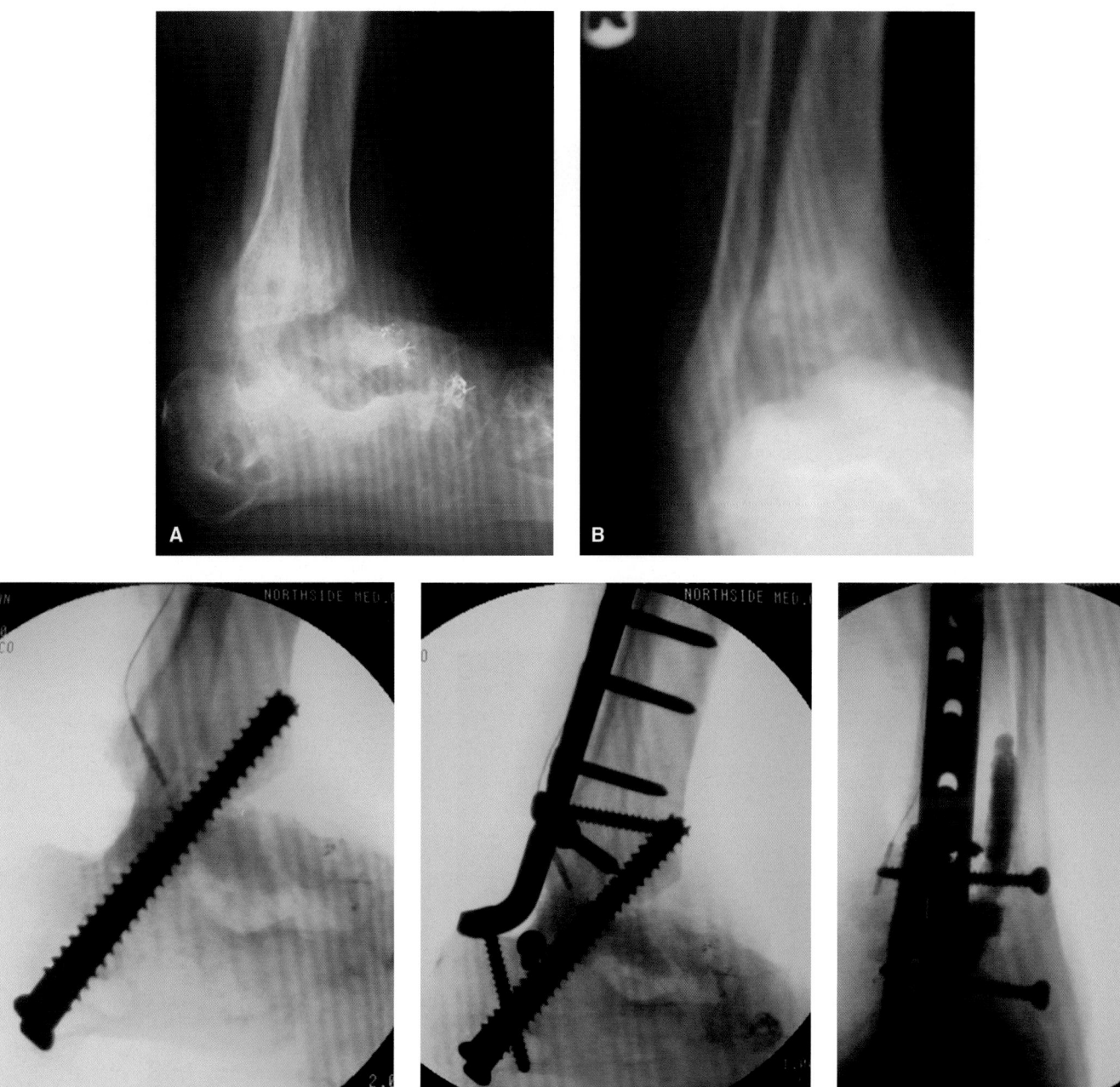

FIGURE 38.12 A. A preoperative lateral radiograph of a Charcot joint in a patient with a healthy soft tissue envelope posteriorly and collapse of the talar body. **B.** A preoperative oblique radiograph demonstrating collapse of the talar body. **C.** An intraoperative lateral radiograph demonstrating the use of bone graft to fill the void. Two fully threaded screws inserted from the calcaneus into the distal tibia obtaining two cortices for stability of good purchase of the fixation. **D.** An intraoperative lateral radiograph demonstrating the use of bone graft, two fully threaded screws inserted from the calcaneus into the distal tibia and an anterior ankle locking plate utilized on the posterior ankle and subtalar joint. **E.** An intraoperative posterior to anterior radiograph demonstrating the use of bone graft and bone graft substitute (*darken area*) to fill the void. Two fully threaded screws inserted from the fibula into the distal tibia for a syndesmotic fusion.

A fibular osteotomy ~12-13 cm proximal to the distal tip of fibula is made. The distal fibula is then completely removed and placed on the back table in sterile saline. The fibula is to be used as an autograft, as well as a fibular plate. The ankle and subtalar joints are debrided sand prepped for fusion. Once the joints are adequately debrided, the angular deformity of the ankle and subtalar joints are re-aligned and corrected into anatomic position. Guidewires are utilized as temporary fixation from the posterior inferior calcaneus to the anterior distal tibia. The position is checked under fluoroscopy with AP, lateral, and calcaneal axial views. Attention is then directed to the lateral distal tibia, lateral talus, and lateral calcaneus, where bone is debrided and

prepped for fusion. This is accomplished with a V-cut depression/bone debridement that is created with osteotomes and a mallet to the lateral aspect of tibia, talus, and calcaneus.

Next the fibular graft is prepared where the medial portion of fibula graft is decorticated to expose the medial portion of the fibular graft to allow for fusion with the lateral tibia, talus, and calcaneus. The debrided medial fibular graft is morsalized and the fibular graft is to be used as the biological plate for the fusion. The fibula is then placed on the lateral aspect of the fusion site (tibia, talus, and calcaneus). The entire fibula is inserted into the inlay "V cut depression" of the tibia, talus,

and calcaneus. The fibula is translated inferiorly from its natural position ~3-4 cm. The fibula functions as a biological plate and an inlay autogenous bone graft. Next, two large cannulated, fully threaded, cancellous screws are placed from posterior inferior to superior anterior obliquely across the ankle and subtalar joints for adjunct fixation. The fibular plate (bone graft) is fixated with bicortical lag screw fixation using 4.0-mm solid critical screws. At this time, any remaining bone graft is then packed into the fusion sites. The surgical site is then closed in standard fashion and placed in a plaster univalve cast (Fig. 38.13).

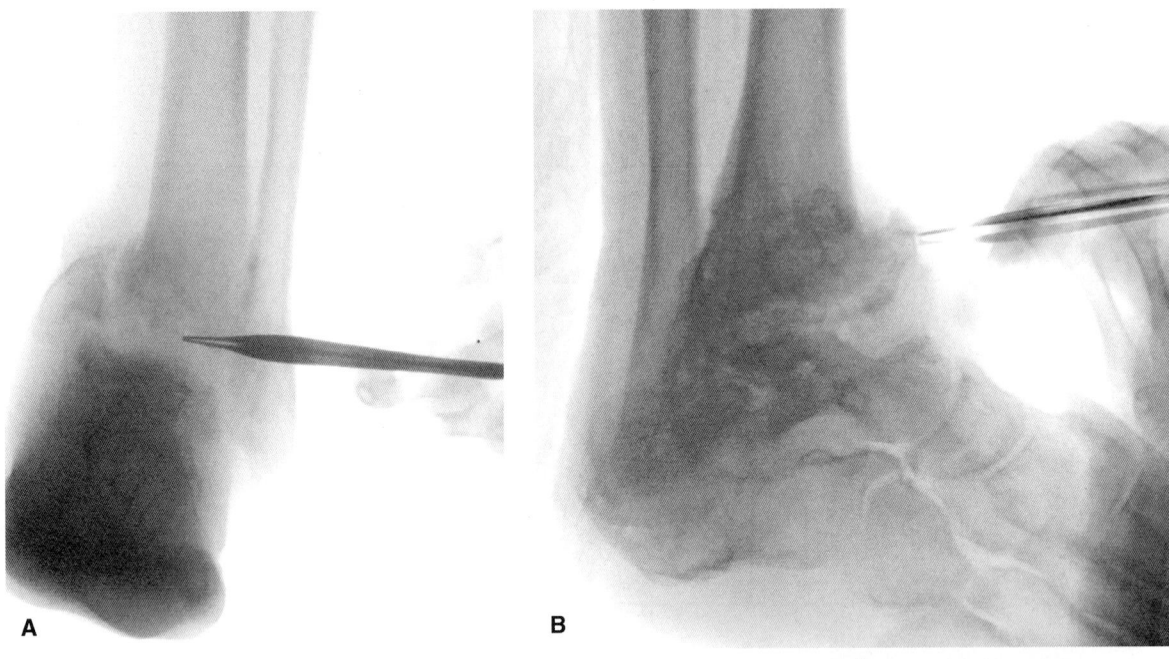

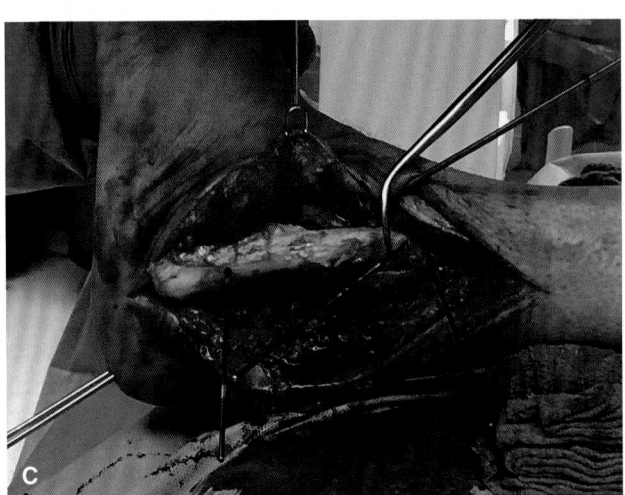

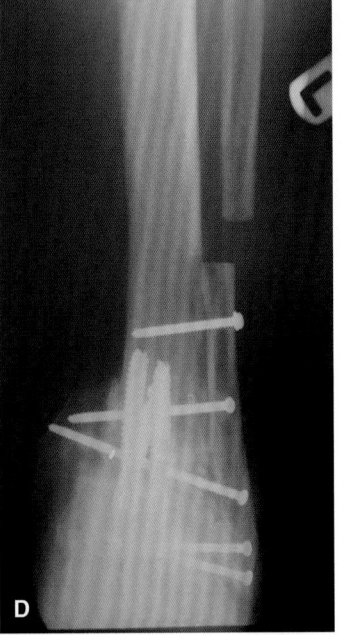

FIGURE 38.13 A. An AP intraoperative fluoroscopy demonstrating Charcot arthropathy of the ankle and subtalar joint. **B.** A lateral intraoperative fluoroscopy demonstrating Charcot arthropathy of the ankle and subtalar joint. **C.** An intraoperative view demonstrating the "fibular biologic plate" inserted into the lateral tibia, talus, and calcaneus in preparation for screw fixation. **D.** A postoperative AP ankle radiograph demonstrating good bony fusion and alignment.

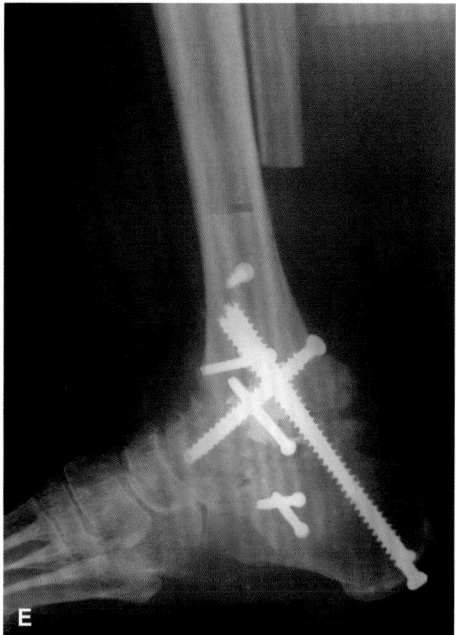
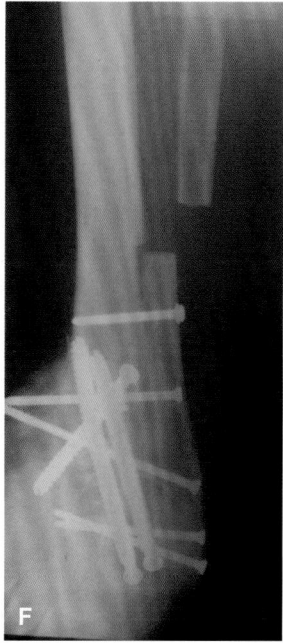
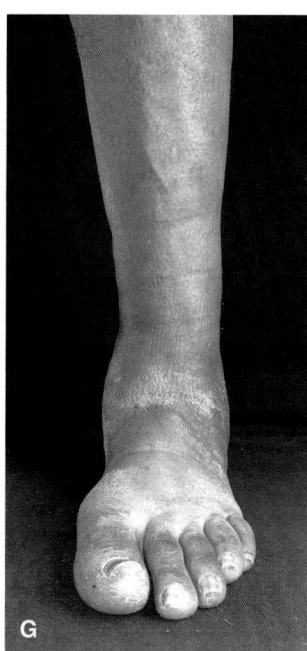
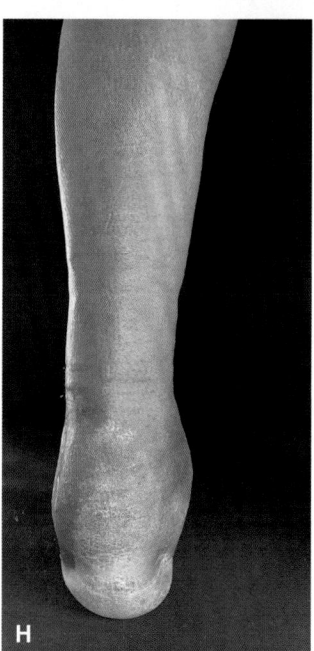

FIGURE 38.13 (*Continued*) **E.** A postoperative lateral ankle radiograph demonstrating good bony fusion and alignment. **F.** A postoperative oblique ankle radiograph demonstrating good bony fusion and alignment. **G.** A postoperative anterior clinical photo demonstrating good bony fusion and alignment. **H.** A postoperative posterior clinical photo demonstrating good bony fusion and alignment.

LIMITED JOINT RESECTION TECHNIQUE

This technique is used in patients with little to no deformity and/or a poor soft tissue envelope.

Boer et al. in their series of 50 patients performed tibial-talocalcaneal (TTC) arthrodesis without STJ preparation and only percutaneous ankle joint preparation reported an average time of fusion was 20 weeks for both joints with patient satisfaction rate was 92%. They concluded that STJ preparation was unnecessary and the ankle joint could be performed percutaneously with excellent results.[117]

In a multicenter study, Mulhern et al. similarly found a decline in pain and high rate of union comparable to TTC arthrodesis with and without STJ joint preparation with a decrease in operative time when the STJ preparation was not performed in 40 patients.[118]

TIBIAL-CALCANEAL FUSION

Indications

The indications for surgical treatment include chronic ulcers associated with bony deformities or contractures, unstable joints of the foot and ankle involving both the subtalar and ankle joints that cannot be treated with a shoe or brace, recurrent infected ulcers with bony prominences, and acute displaced fractures in neuropathic patients with adequate circulation. This procedure is performed when the talus is not salvageable or is significantly comminuted. In cases when the talar body is not salvageable, the surgeon should attempt to preserve the talar head and neck as this will provide some stability given the cubic volume of bone loss with the talar body.

Following joint resection, the calcaneus is often medialized as its natural anatomy sits lateral to the midline or weight-bearing axis of the tibia.[119-127]

The ankle and foot should be 10-15 degrees externally rotated and/or maintain alignment that is consistent with the contralateral limb. Align the tibial tuberosity and the second toe. Relative to a lateral fluoroscopy view, a neutral position in terms of the ankle should align the lateral process of the talus with the midline of the tibia, and the hindfoot frontal plane should be in a neutral position (most desirable) to 0-5 degrees of valgus.

TIBIAL-TALAR, TIBIAL-TALAR-CALCANEAL AND TIBIAL-CALCANEAL ARTHRODESIS

- On a lateral radiograph, it is important to have the talus under the tibia; this effectively decreases the lever arm applied during the terminal stance phase of gait.[116]
- Posterior approach—The patient is placed in a prone position. The Achilles tendon may be split or resected. The syndesmosis can be debrided through the posterior approach. The medial aspect of the fibula is debrided and the lateral aspect of the tibia is debrided to allow for bony fusion of the tibia and fibula. Alternatively, the fibula can be taken down and may be used as inlay or onlay autogenous bone graft. The distal aspect of the fibula makes for an excellent cortical cancellous bone graft. The senior author will often cut off the distal two-three centimeters of the fibula. It is then cut it in half within the sagittal plane leaving excellent cortical cancellous bone graft, which can be utilized for inlay or onlay autogenous bone graft. The proximal fibula can be taken down and placed in a bone mill as morselized graft. This can be mixed with the patient's blood soaking with allogenic cancellous bone chips creating a nice bony slurry for back filling any bone defect/loss. Additionally, the proximal fibula may also be used at struts from the calcaneus to the tibia to maintain length of the extremity[128] or used as an onlay graft buttressing the lateral aspect of the tibia and talus providing additional structural support.
- Ultimately the surgical approach should be based on the soft tissue envelope and the deformity that needs to be corrected.
- Many deformities require a staged approach. For example, a patient with a long-standing rigid contracted ankle in significant varus deformity, and a wound, would typically need a prophylactic tarsal tunnel release, a bone debridement and bone biopsy, posterior muscle lengthening, and reduction of the rigid deformity and stabilized with external fixation. This is necessary to allow the soft tissues to adapt and normalize, especially the neurovascular bundle, to function appropriately at its lengthened position. Additionally, this will allow time to treat any underlying infection in preparation and before the final reconstruction consisting of internal fixation.
- Soft tissue preparation is often underemphasized but is key to obtaining would closure. Using a staged approach and weekly compressive dressing changes can greatly improve the chances of adequate soft tissue closure by optimizing the patient for surgery and decreasing subcutaneous fluid retention. If the soft tissue has difficulty healing, then a muscle transfer and split-thickness skin grafting can be performed.

RETROGRADE INTRAMEDUALLARY NAIL

- There are a variety of intramedullary (IM) nails to choose from and there is no one size that fits all; however, when deciding which nail to use, there are some important factors to consider (Fig. 38.14).
- Marley et al. demonstrated that a long nail had less stress risers than a short nail and a valgus nail had less stress risers than a straight nail.[129,130]
- Pinzur and Noonan found 19 of 21 Charcot ankles went on to a successful fusion with a retrograde locked IM nail.[129]
- During the reaming process, the surgeon should experience "chatter." Chatter occurs when maximal diameter has been obtained and the reamer fits "tight" within the cortical walls. It is very important to reach this point in order to avoid the "wiper blade affect." The wiper blade affect occurs when too small of a diameter nail is inserted into the distal tibia allowing for toggle to occur with eventual loosening; therefore, it is desirable to obtain the largest diameter nail that will fit within the medullary canal for most favorable results.[119,131]
- The author prefers not to fixate the proximal portion of the nail and to stabilize only the distal aspect of the nail to the foot to allow for dynamic compression during ambulation. One may place a screw in the proximal aspect of the dynamic hole and remove before weight bearing to dynamize the nail.
- In their cadaveric study, Means et al. demonstrated that anterior to posterior screws used in an IM nail had a significantly higher stiffness and load to failure providing a more stable construct than using medial to lateral screws.[130]
- Mendicino et al. reported 95% fusion rate with IM nail for TTC fusions in both diabetic and nondiabetic patients. As expected, major complications, average time to fusion, average time to full weight bearing, and overall compilations were higher in the diabetic group.[131]
- Percutaneous IM nailing provides stable fixation for tibiotalocalcaneal arthrodesis without extensive soft tissue damage.[119]
- Pellegrini et al. showed a 17% periprosthetic stress fracture in patients undergoing TTC arthrodesis with IM nailing.[132] The authors have observed this complication though with screw and plate fixation too and prefer to reserve a long IM nail for revision of periprosthetic fractures. Chapman stated that reaming and nailing embolizes marrow contents into the systemic circulation and reduces blood flow to the total bone and cortex by 30%-80%.[133] Additionally, the authors have reserved the usage of an IM nail for revision and minimally invasive approaches.

PLATE AND SCREW FIXATION

- Femoral locking plate—lateral approach—DiDomenico et al. described the use of a femoral locking plate with a fully threaded screw fixation hybrid construct. This construct provides a good option for patients with poor bone quality.[134] The senior author favors this form of fixation as the femoral locking plate is large and stiff. This technique utilizes two or three long fully threaded screws from the

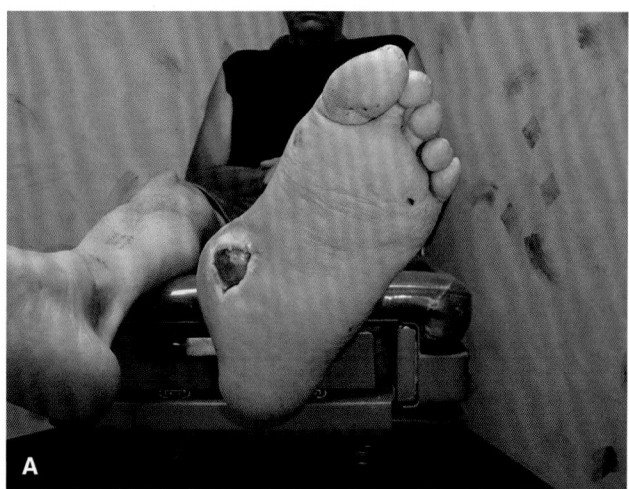

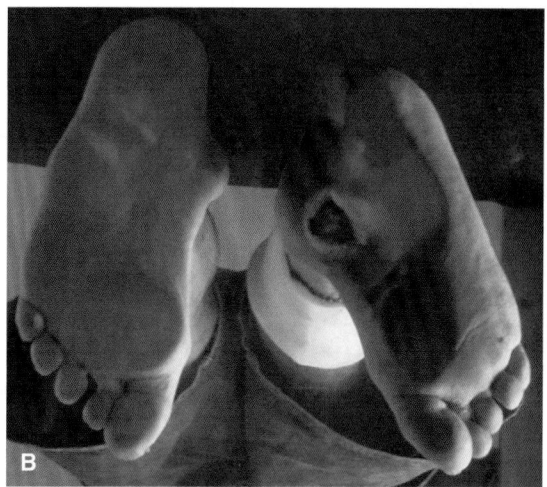

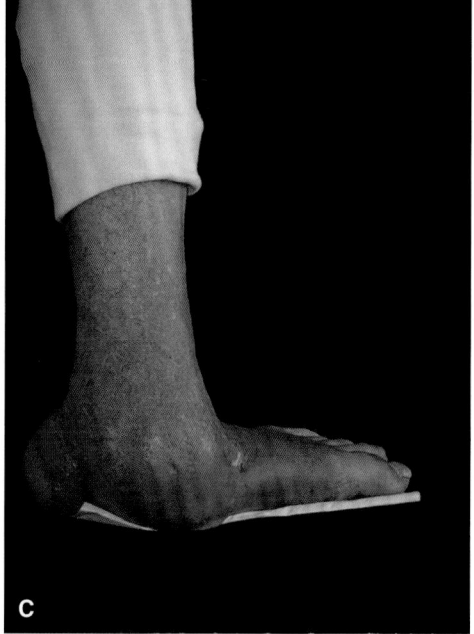

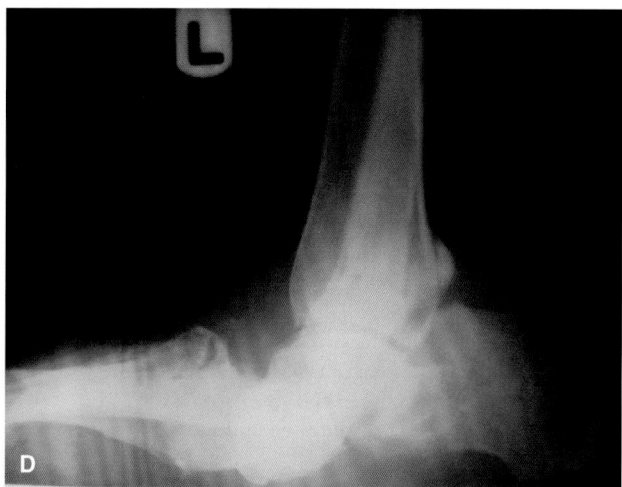

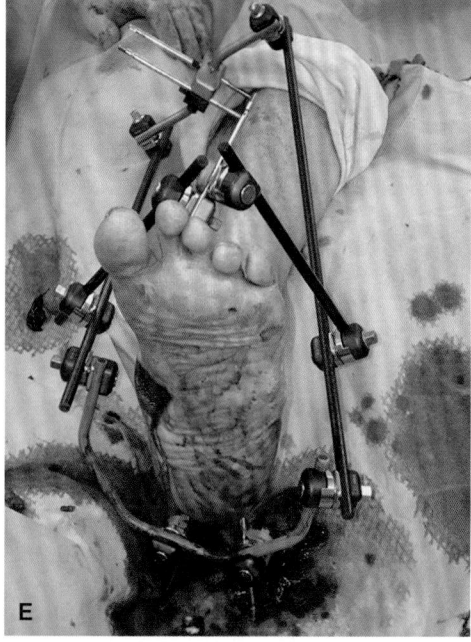

FIGURE 38.14 A-C. Patient who suffers from a tight posterior muscle group and Charcot arthropathy of the ankle, subtalar, and midtarsal joint. Pressure necrosis is present from significant malalignment causing pressure necrosis resulting in ulceration and osteomyelitis. **D.** A lateral radiograph demonstrating a progressed Charcot arthropathy. **E.** A posterior muscle lengthening was performed with wound and bone debridement and cultures. A reduction of the deformity was performed and fixated and stabilized with the external fixator.

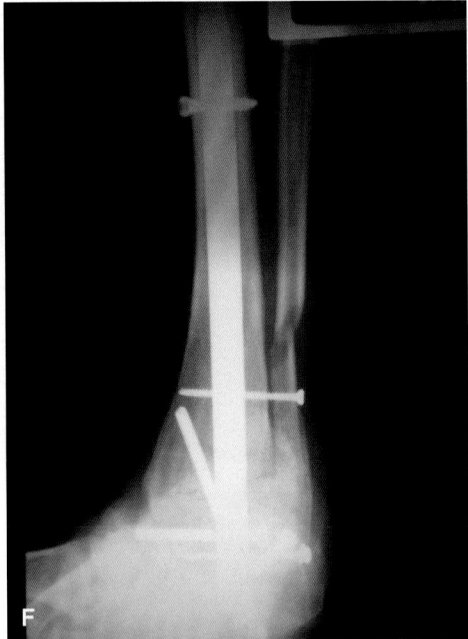
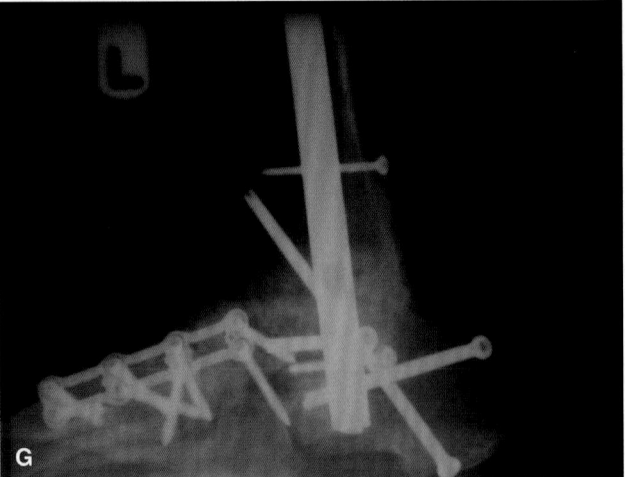

FIGURE 38.14 (*Continued*) **F, G.** A complete talectomy was performed because of osteomyelitis. A tibial-calcaneal arthrodesis with an IM nail was performed. The senior author recommends using adjunctive fixation with an IM nail. In this case, a fully threaded independent screw was placed outside of the nail construct. Additionally, the fibula was used as a biological plate.

inferior posterior and anterior calcaneus cortices to the distal tibia cortex providing bicortical purchase. In most of these cases, there is significant malalignment preoperatively leaving minimal bone to bone contact and the need for back filling with bone graft. Because of this, the senior author does not want compression across the bone graft but would rather obtain stability with bicortical purchase of the long, large fully threaded cancellous screws maintaining position. The thought is two or three large cancellous bicortical purchased screws result in excellent stability coupled by a laterally based locking plate. Advantages of the femoral locking plate in addition to stability are the multiple holes of bicortical fixation afforded with this construct. The weakest bone in this deformity is the calcaneus with a highly populated area of cancellous bone coupled by a very thin cortex. The multiple points of bicortical fixation in the calcareous enhance the stability of the construct in an already compromised patient population. Performing TTC arthrodesis with a femoral locking plate takes advantage of the added stability and alignment. Once the plate is fixated to the tibia, the plate maintains the alignment of the calcareous relative to the tibia ensuring there is no varus or valgus (Fig. 38.15).

■ Posterior plating has the benefit of a thick and more robust soft tissue envelope. The flexor hallucis longus has a low lying muscle belly, and this covers the majority of the hardware with a posterior approach.
■ Blade plates
  ■ Chiodo et al. found that blade-plate-and-screw fixation resulted in significantly higher mean initial and final stiffness and decreased plastic deformation than did IM rod fixation.[135]

■ IM nailing and the use of blade plates were comparable in terms of stability, and the IM nailing method was also considered inferior to the locking plate construct.[135,136] Conversely, Lee et al. found that the IM nail provided a stiffer and more stable construct.[137]
■ Blade plates were a precursor to locking plates and are no longer widely used.
■ Humeral locking plate—Ahmad et al. reported a rate of nonunion of ~6% in 18 patients who underwent TTC arthrodesis using a humeral locking plate.[138]
■ Anterior plate
  ■ In their systemic review, Kusnezov et al. reported 97.6% of 164 patients with isolated tibiotalar arthrodesis went on to uneventful union.[139]
  ■ Anterior plating may be used as primary fixation or for revision procedures. Matson et al. described the use of an anterior plate in isolated ankle nonunions after IM nailing. Their study included six patients using the anterior plate with retention of the IM nail. All six patients achieved tibiotalar fusion at an average of 9.3 weeks (range, 5.4-16.1 weeks) postoperatively and average pain scores significantly improved (7.8-5.3, $P = .019$) postoperatively.[140]
■ Locking plate technology enables a rigid, stable construct, while preserving the biologic principles of bone such as the blood supply that are typically lost with conventional plating due to locking plate design with less direct plate to bone contact. The screwhead threads into and rigidly purchases the plate, which acts as an "internal" external fixator, maintaining an established distance between the plate and bone. With plate holes that can accommodate both locked and unlocked screws, "hybrid" constructs can

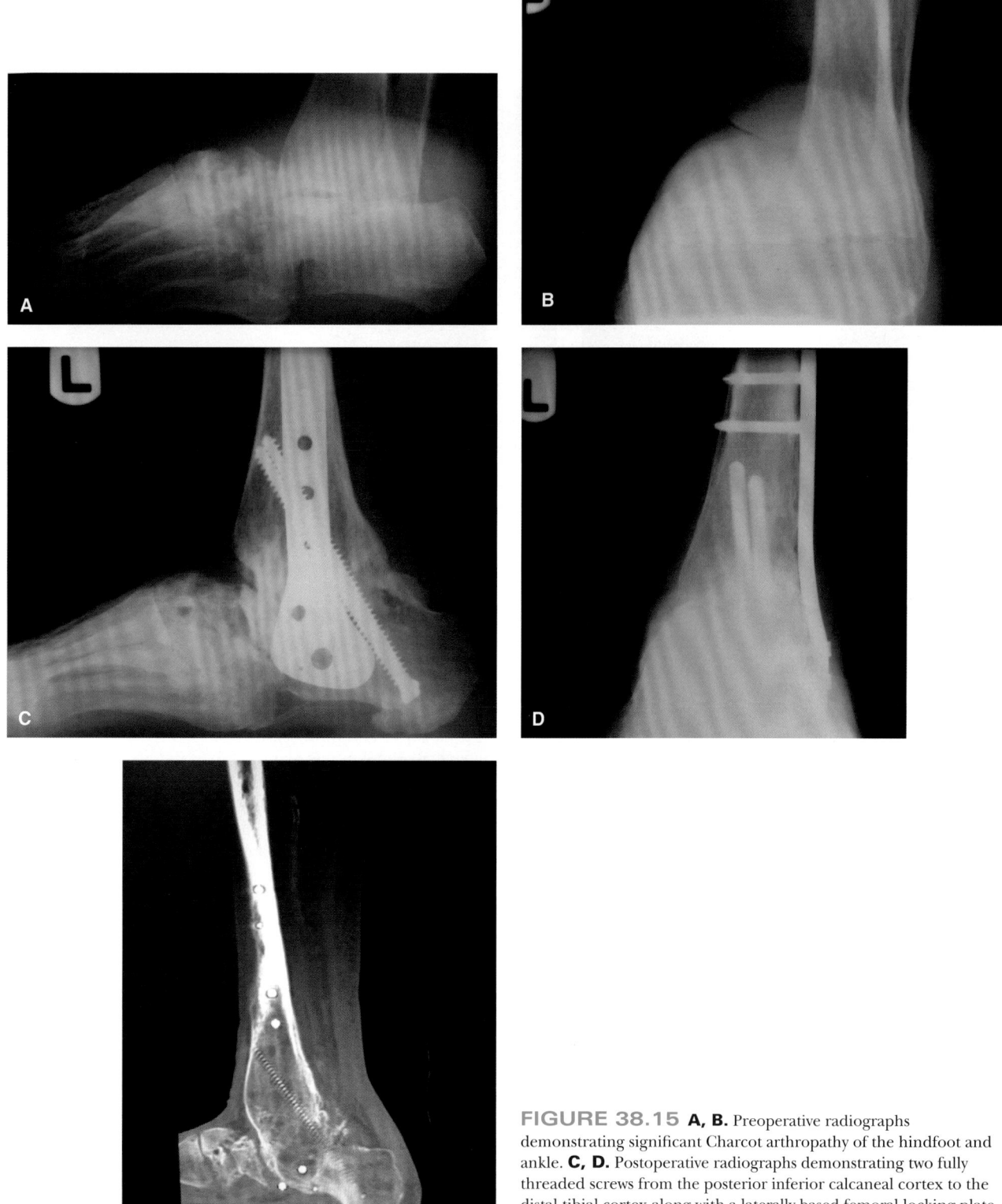

FIGURE 38.15 **A, B.** Preoperative radiographs demonstrating significant Charcot arthropathy of the hindfoot and ankle. **C, D.** Postoperative radiographs demonstrating two fully threaded screws from the posterior inferior calcaneal cortex to the distal tibial cortex along with a laterally based femoral locking plate. **E.** A CT scan demonstrating good bony union and alignment of a complex hindfoot and ankle Charcot joint.

be achieved, thereby using lag screws to assist with achieving the reduction and locked screws to aid in maintaining the reduction.[141]

- Smith et al. had a high failure rate with a lateral plate and screw construct postulating that a construct that is too stiff

may lead to higher failure rates in part due to excessive bone resorption from stress shielding.[142]

- For a lateral approach, the authors prefer the use of a femoral locking plate. When applying the plate, it is not uncommon to use nonlocking screws for the initial

reduction and then add locking screws for stabilization. One can obtain many points of bicortical fixation in the calcaneus to spread the forces. Because of the very thin cortex and vastly cancellous bone within the calcaneus, IM nails tend to fail within the calcaneus.

The senior author prefers a femoral locking plate with independent long fully threaded screws construct over an IM nail for the following reasons. An IM nail is IM and in order to insert it, the surgeon has to ream the bone of the most healthy portion of the bone leaving a cortical shell. The fixation is not cortical and is IM. IM does not provide as much stability as cortical purchased fixation. Based on what nail is used, there is very limited availability for fixation to the calcaneus. The calcaneus is where most nails fail as the calcaneus has a very thin cortex and mostly cancellous bone. A femoral locking plate construct is built with two independent fully threaded screws that purchase two cortices (the calcaneus and tibia). Two large screws are larger than any IM nail on the market with the addition of cortical purchase. Based on the femoral locking plate utilized, most plates offer multiple fixation positions within the calcaneus and the screws can be bicortical increasing the strength of the construct. Lastly, using a screws and plate construct does not disturb the medullary bone.

PERILS AND PITFALLS

- Typically, most Charcot patients present with edema from many causes before and after surgery. Compression bandages are essential for skin preparation and optimizing the soft tissue envelope prior to surgery. By reducing the edema preoperatively, the surgeon optimizes the soft tissues and there is less stress on the soft tissues, which leads to less postoperative wound complications. Wound complications are relatively common in this patient population and controlling the edema pre- and postoperatively is essential. Additionally, if the surgeon is able to control the edema postoperatively, this risk of DVT and wound issues are reduced.
- Autogenous bone graft is utilized when available.
- Allograft bone chips have been proven to be an effective means of bone replacement in the acetabulum for total hip revision surgery,[143-145] and these authors have found similar usefulness in the foot and ankle.
- Fixation should be solid. The construct needs to be very stable and sturdy for the given fixation.
- A drain should be considered in most cases. There is a lot bony work done with these cases and often times there will be significant blood loss.
- The patient must understand that this is a salvage procedure to avoid a more proximal amputation, such as BK or an above the knee amputation. They must understand the length of non–weight bearing required and that solid bony fusion is not guaranteed. The long-term goal is to have a plantigrade foot. Some of the extremities may require some form of bracing.
- Goals for patients with regard to target HgA1c before surgery and smoking status are physician dependent but may be a strong motivator for patients to improve their overall health and surgical outcomes. Wukich et al. in a prospective study demonstrated that neuropathy and poorly controlled DM (hemoglobin A1c >8%) were associated with increased rates of surgical site infection.[146]

- The surgeon must also realize that not all patients are candidates for surgery because of medical comorbidities. The ability to remain non–weight bearing and patient willingness to go through multiple surgeries is mandatory.
- Wukich et al. reported that the overall likelihood of deep surgical sight infection were 80% less likely in patients who received vancomycin powder. The authors recommended foot and ankle surgeons consider applying 500-1000 mg of vancomycin powder prior to skin closure in diabetic patients undergoing reconstructive surgery.[147]
- It is the senior authors' experience and opinion that all retraction should be done with fine skin hook retractors and/or Hohmann retractors. The assistant needs to be very cognizant of where the surgeon is working and retract with Hohmann or fine skin tooth retractors applying the minimal amount of tension on the skin as possible. Paying attention to this detail should assist with adequate soft tissue healing.
- The senior authors' experience and recommendation is to use as much autogenous bone graft as possible. With many of the Charcot arthropathy cases, there will be large voids. The senior author recommends using as much autogenous bone graft as possible and then using cancellous bone chips mixed with the patient's blood. The senior author typically will ask the anesthesia team for ~20 cc of blood from the patient's arm once the patient is asleep. This allows the patient's blood to sit and soak into the cancellous chips, allowing all the natural growth factors, to saturate the porous cancellous chips with the patient's own blood and begin clotting into a slurry of bone and blood to fill any voids or large bone defects. Sites for harvesting are the calcareous, the distal tibia, the fibula, and the proximal tibia (Gerdy tubercle).

POSTOPERATIVE CARE

- The postoperative dressings are left intact for ~14-17 days. When the surgical wound is dressed in the operating room, it is considered to be a sterile environment thus it makes most sense to leave the wound dressing intact. Additionally, a postoperative compressive dressing is applied, and this minimizes the postoperative edema if left intact. Also, if the wound is not disturbed and maintains its stability, this allows for good wound healing. This is consistent with the wound healing cycle in terms of days of wound healing. If one removes the dressing earlier, that is, 7 days, this disturbs the wound healing cycle; therefore, we recommend leaving the dressing intact for 14-17 days. The patient is seen at 1 week postsurgery, however, to evaluate for any gross signs of infection or other pathology. The univalve cast is left intact during this evaluation. The patient is assessed for shortness of breath, leg pain, and calf pain to ensure that there are no signs for DVT and/or pulmonary embolism (PE). They are also evaluated for fever, chills, drainage, or foul odor to assess for any signs of infection.

In the operating room, a univalve BK plaster cast is applied. The univalve BK cast is made of plaster in place of fiberglass because it molds better to the leg. A 1-2 in strip is removed from the anterior aspect of the cast and the cast is slightly spread apart and an ace badge is applied. This allows for some swelling to occur and to decrease the

chance of a compartment syndrome. Also, if the compression bandage is too tight, there is access to the bandage without having to take down the entire cast and the treating doctor can cut the bandage if needed. Even though a small anterior strip is removed, the cast is still as protective as complete cast should the patient fall or experience some sort of trauma. The univalve cast is very stable in comparison to a sugar tong or posterior splint. Another benefit of the large plaster cast is that it is heavy and it hopefully will assist in keeping the patient more compliant since it is heavier than fiberglass.[114]

- Postoperatively, a hematocrit and hemoglobin should be done to evaluate for blood loss.
- DVT and PE prevention should also be employed. Each individual patient needs to be evaluated independently. Mechanical prophylaxis should be utilized all the times. This includes antiembolism support hose on the contralateral side as well as pneumatic sequential compression pumps. These should be prescribed during surgery and postoperatively. Incentive spirometry should also be ordered postoperatively. Pharmacologic prophylaxis should be considered and individualized according to risk factors.
- Radiograph evaluation should be performed at ~3 week intervals until bony consolidation can be observed.
- The patient is then transitioned to partial protected weight bearing in a CAM boot followed by full weight bearing in a CROW boot for 6 months. This is followed by 6 months in an AFO and then into a rocker bottom shoe as tolerated. Some patients may need a CROW boot or AFO permanently.
- A patient may stay in the CROW boot indefinitely with the understanding that a braceable, plantigrade foot is considered a success.
- Mendicino et al. reported the major complications, average time to fusion, average time to full weight bearing, and overall complications to be higher in diabetics undergoing TTC arthrodesis through IM nail.[113]
- A complete medical team is needed to optimize nutrition, blood glucose, vascular status, infection control, and to manage the patients' other comorbidities. Patients will need physical therapy at all levels of care as the patient transitions from weight bearing to non–weight bearing to partial weight bearing and back to weight bearing. They may need to use some or all of the following: wheel chairs, non–weight bearing roll about to walkers, crutches, CROW boots, fracture boots, AFO, CFO, and other various braces and supports.

REHABILITATION

- The authors' preferred protocol is to consult PT/OT prior to surgery if possible. When this is not possible, PT/OT is consulted for gait training and non–weight bearing postoperatively.
- Social service is consulted following surgical intervention. Placement to a rehabilitation facility is highly recommended. This is typically opposed by most patients and sometimes the patients' family members. The rehabilitation is recommended for the postoperative period. Many

of these patients are deconditioned and are not able to take care of themselves nor are their family members able to appropriately manage the patient. Placement into a facility is also recommended for the safety of the patient, as they may be unstable postoperatively and subject to falls and subsequent injuries.

- The patient may also benefit from placement into an appropriate facility if intravenous antibiotics are needed postoperatively.
- Following successful surgical reconstruction, the goal is to have the patient progress from advanced bracing to accommodative shoes. Although this is not accomplished in all cases, limb salvage with minimal assistance with a device is achieved in many patients. Patients do not typically like to wear braces and prosthetics but there is a progression they must go through postoperatively. They are in a non–weight bearing cast immediately postoperatively and then transitioned to a Cam boot. After a course of time, they are then placed into a CROW boot, followed by an AFO, and then hopefully into a shoe with a rocker bottom sole. The decision-making is made on each patient's progress and outcome. This may be a 12- to 24-month process, as it takes a long time for the bone to remodel and consolidate permanently in anatomic alignment.

REFERENCES

1. Gupta R. A short history of neuropathic arthropathy. *Clin Orthop Relat Res.* 1993;296: 43-49.
2. Charcot JM. Sur quelques arthropathies qui paraissent dependre d'une lesion du cerveau ou de la moelle epimere. *Arch physiol norm et pathol.* 1868;1. Article 161.
3. Jeffcoate W. The causes of the Charcot syndrome. *Clin Podiatr Med Surg.* 2008;25(1): 29-42, vi.
4. Jordan WR. Neuritic manifestations in diabetes mellitus. *Arch Intern Med.* 1936;57(2): 307-366.
5. Nather A, Bee CS, Huak CY, et al. Epidemiology of diabetic foot problems and predictive factors for limb loss. *J Diabetes Complications.* 2008;22(2):77-82.
6. Kundu AK. Charcot in medical eponyms. *J Assoc Physicians India.* 2004;52:716-718.
7. McInnes AD. Diabetic foot disease in the United Kingdom: about time to put feet first. *J Foot Ankle Res.* 2012;5:26.
8. Gouveri E, Papanas N. Charcot osteoarthropathy in diabetes: a brief review with an emphasis on clinical practice. *World J Diabetes.* 2011;2:59-65.
9. Singh R, Kishore L, Kaur N. Diabetic peripheral neuropathy: current perspective and future directions. *Pharmacol Res.* 2014;80:21-35.
10. Callaghan B, Feldman E. The metabolic syndrome and neuropathy: therapeutic challenges and opportunities. *Ann Neurol.* 2013;74(3):397-403.
11. Tesfaye S, Stevens LK, Stephenson JM, et al. Prevalence of diabetic peripheral neuropathy and its relation to glycaemic control and potential risk factors: the EURODIAB IDDM Complications Study. *Diabetologia.* 1996;39(11):1377-1384.
12. Tesfaye S, Chaturvedi N, Eaton SE, et al.; EURODIAB Prospective Complications Study Group. Vascular risk factors and diabetic neuropathy. *N Engl J Med.* 2005;352(4):341-350.
13. Chantelau E, Onvlee GJ. Charcot foot in diabetes: farewell to the neurotrophic theory. *Horm Metab Res.* 2006;38:361-367.
14. Centers for Disease Control and Prevention. *National Diabetes Statistics Report, 2017.* Atlanta, GA: Centers for Disease Control and Prevention, U.S. Dept of Health and Human Services; 2017.
15. Larson SA, Burns PR. The pathogenesis of Charcot neuroarthropathy: current concepts. *Diabet Foot Ankle.* 2012;3.
16. Chisholm KA, Gilchrist JM. The Charcot joint: a modern neurologic perspective. *J Clin Neuromuscul Dis.* 2011;13(1):1-13.
17. Schon LC, Easley ME, Weinfeld SB. Charcot neuroarthropathy of the foot and ankle. *Clin Orthop.* 1998;(349):116-131.
18. Armstrong DC, Todd WF, Lavery LA, Harkless LB, Bushman TR. The natural history of acute Charcot arthropathy in the diabetic foot specialty clinic. *Diabet Med.* 1997;24:357.
19. Tesfaye S, Boulton AJ, Dyck PJ, et al. Diabetic neuropathies: update on definitions, diagnostic criteria, estimation of severity, and treatments. *Diabetes Care.* 2010;33:2285-2293.
20. Jeffcoate WJ. Charcot neuro-osteoarthropathy. *Diabetes Metab Res Rev.* 2008;24(suppl 1): S62-S65.
21. Jeffcoate WJ. Abnormalities of vasomotor regulation in the pathogenesis of the acute Charcot foot of diabetes mellitus. *Int J Low Extrem Wounds.* 2005;4(3):133-137.
22. Kimmerle R, Chantelau E. Weight-bearing intensity produces Charcot deformity in injured neuropathic feet in diabetes. *Exp Clin Endocrinol Diabetes.* 2007;115:360-364.
23. Vinik AI, Ziegler D. Diabetic cardiovascular autonomic neuropathy. *Circulation.* 2007;115:387-397.

24. Gilbey SG, Walters H, Edmonds ME, et al. Vascular calcification, autonomic neuropathy, and peripheral blood flow in patients with diabetic nephropathy. *Diabet Med.* 1989;6:37-42.
25. Papanas N, Maltezos E. Etiology, pathophysiology and classifications of the diabetic Charcot foot. *Diabet Foot Ankle.* 2013;4:20872. doi: 10.3402/dfa.v4i0.20872.
26. Edmonds ME, Clarke MB, Newton S, Barrett J, Watkins PJ. Increased uptake of bone radiopharmaceutical in diabetic neuropathy. *Q J Med.* 1985;57:843-855.
27. Sinha S, Munichoodappa C, Kozak GP. Neuro-arthropathy (Charcot joints) in diabetes mellitus. *Medicine (Baltimore).* 1972;51:191-210.
28. Hofbauer LC, Schoppet M. Osteoprotegerin: a link between osteoporosis and arterial calcification? *Lancet.* 2001;358:257-259.
29. Collin-Osdoby P. Regulation of vascular calcification by osteoclast regulatory factors RANKL and osteoprotegerin. *Circ Res.* 2004;95:1046-1057.
30. Jeffcoate W. Vascular calcification and osteolysis in diabetic neuropathy: is RANK-L the missing link? *Diabetologia.* 2004;47:1488-1492.
31. Korzon-Burakowska A, Jakóbkiewicz-Banecka J, Fiedosiuk A, et al. Osteoprotegerin gene polymorphism in diabetic Charcot neuroarthropathy. *Diabet Med.* 2012;29(6):771-775.
32. Lam J, Nelson CA, Ross FP, Teitelbaum SL, Fremont DH. Crystal structure of the TRANCE/RANKL cytokine reveals determinants of receptor-ligand specificity. *J Clin Invest.* 2001;108(7):971-979.
33. Whyte MP. The long and the short of bone therapy. *N Engl J Med.* 2006;354(8):860-863.
34. Buckley KA, Fraser WD. Receptor activator for nuclear factor kappaB ligand and osteoprotegerin: regulators of bone physiology and immune responses/potential therapeutic agents and biochemical markers. *Ann Clin Biochem.* 2002;39(Pt 6):551-556.
35. Collin-Osdoby P. Regulation of vascular calcification by osteoclast regulatory factors RANKL and osteoprotegerin. *Circ Res.* 2004;95(11):1046-1057.
36. Anandarajah AP, Schwarz EM. Anti-RANKL therapy for inflammatory bone disorders: mechanisms and potential clinical applications. *J Cell Biochem.* 2006;97(2):226-232.
37. Baud'huin M, Duplomb L, Ruiz Velasco C, Fortun Y, Heymann D, Padrines M. Key roles of the OPG-RANK-RANKL system in bone oncology. *Expert Rev Anticancer Ther.* 2007;7(2):221-232.
38. Boyce BF, Xing L. Biology of RANK, RANKL, and osteoprotegerin. *Arthritis Res Ther.* 2007;9(suppl 1):S1.
39. Bruhn-Olszewska B, Korzon-Burakowska A, Węgrzyn G, Jakóbkiewicz-Banecka J. Prevalence of polymorphisms in OPG, RANKL and RANK as potential markers for Charcot arthropathy development. *Sci Rep.* 2017;7:501.
40. Yogo K, Ishida-Kitagawa N, Takeya T. Negative autoregulation of RANKL and c-Src signaling in osteoclasts. *J Bone Miner Metab.* 2007;25(4):205-210.
41. Rosenbaum AJ, DiPreta JA. Classifications in brief: Eichenholtz classification of Charcot arthropathy. author information. *Clin Orthop Relat Res.* 2015;473(3):1168-1171. doi: 10.1007/s11999-014-4059-y.
42. Eichenholtz SN. *Charcot Joints.* Springfield, IL: Charles C. Thomas; 1966.
43. Shibata T, Tada K, Hashizume C. The results of arthrodesis of the ankle for leprotic neuroarthropathy. *J Bone Joint Surg Am.* 1990;72-A:749-756.
44. Ergen FB, Sanverdi SE, Oznur A. Charcot foot in diabetes and an update on imaging. *Diabet Foot Ankle.* 2013;4. doi: 10.3402/dfa.v4i0.21884.eCollection 2013.
45. Brodsky JW. The diabetic foot. In: Coughlin MJ, Mann RA, Saltzman CL, eds. *Surgery of the Foot and Ankle.* 8th ed. St Louis, MO: Mosby; 2006:1281-1368.
46. Sella EJ, Barrette C. Staging of Charcot neuroarthropathy along the medial column of the foot in the diabetic patient. *J Foot Ankle Surg.* 1999;38:34-40.
47. Petrova NL, Edmonds ME. Charcot neuro-osteoarthropathy-current standards. *Diabetes Metab Res Rev.* 2008;24(suppl 1):S58-S61. doi: 10.1002/dmrr.846.
48. Rogers LC, Frykberg RG, Armstrong DG, et al. The Charcot foot in diabetes. *Diabetes Care.* 2011;34(9):2123-2129.
49. Petrova NL, Edmonds ME. Charcot neuro-osteoarthropathy-current standards. *Diabetes Metab Res Rev.* 2008;24(suppl 1):S58-S61. doi: 10.1002/dmrr.846.
50. Rosenbaum AJ, DiPreta JA. Classifications in brief: Eichenholtz classification of Charcot arthropathy. *Clin Orthop Relat Res.* 2015;473(3):1168-1171. doi: 10.1007/s11999-014-4059-y.
51. Kelikian AS. *Operative Treatment of the Foot and Ankle.* Stamford, CT: Appleton & Lange; 1999:153.
52. Brodsky JW. Outpatient diagnosis and care of the diabetic foot. *Instr Course Lect.* 1993;42:121-139.
53. Faglia E, Caravaggi C, Clerici G, et al. Effectiveness of removable Walker Cast versus nonremovable fiberglass off-bearing cast in the healing of diabetic plantar foot ulcer. *Diabetes Care.* 2010;33(7):1419-1423.
54. van der Ven A, Chapman CB, Bowker JH. Charcot neuroarthropathy of the foot and ankle. *J Am Acad Orthop Surg.* 2009;17(9):562-571.
55. Armstrong DG, Lavery LA. Monitoring healing of acute Charcot's arthropathy with infrared dermal thermometry. *J Rehabil Res Dev.* 1997;34:317-321.
56. McGill M, Molyneaux L, Bolton T, Ioannou K, Uren R, Yue DK. Response of Charcot's arthropathy to contact casting: assessment by quantitative techniques. *Diabetologia.* 2000;43:481-484.
57. Ruotolo V, Di Pietro B, Giurato L, et al. A new natural history of Charcot foot: clinical evolution and final outcome of stage 0 Charcot neuroarthropathy in a tertiary referral diabetic foot clinic. *Clin Nucl Med.* 2013;38(7):506-509.
58. Ergen FB, Sanverdi SE, Oznur A. Charcot foot in diabetes and an update on imaging. *Diabet Foot Ankle.* 2013;4. doi: 10.3402/dfa.v4i0.21884.
59. Burson LK, Schank CH. Charcot neuroarthropathy of the foot and ankle. *Home Healthc Now.* 2016;34(3):135-139.
60. Lee S, Kim H, Choi S, Park Y, Kim Y, Cho B. Clinical usefulness of the two-site Semmes-Weinstein monofilament test for detecting diabetic peripheral neuropathy. *J Korean Med Sci.* 2003;18(1):103-107.
61. Chantelau E, Poll LW. Evaluation of the diabetic Charcot foot by MR imaging or plain radiography—an observational study. *Exp Clin Endocrinol Diabetes.* 2006;114(8):428-431.
62. Rajbhandari SM, Jenkins RC, Davies C, Tesfaye S. Charcot neuroarthropathy in diabetes mellitus. *Diabetologia.* 2002;45(8):1085-1096.
63. Jones EA, Manaster BJ, May DA, Disler DG. Neuropathic osteoarthropathy: diagnostic dilemmas and differential diagnosis. *RadioGraphics.* 2000;20(suppl_1):S279-S293.
64. Chantelau EA, Richter A. The acute diabetic Charcot foot managed on the basis of magnetic resonance imaging: a review of 71 cases. *Swiss Med Wkly.* 2013;143:w13831.
65. Rosenbaum AJ, DiPreta JA. Classifications in brief: Eichenholtz classification of Charcot arthropathy. *Clin Orthop Relat Res.* 2014;473(3):1168-1171.
66. de Souza LJ. Charcot arthropathy and immobilization in a weight-bearing total contact cast. *J Bone Joint Surg Am.* 2008;90:754-759. doi: 10.2106/JBJS.F.01523.
67. Ergen FB, Sanverdi SE, Oznur A. Charcot foot in diabetes and an update on imaging. *Diabet Foot Ankle.* 2013;4. doi: 10.3402/dfa.v4i0.21884.
68. Greenstein AS, Marzo-Ortega H, Emery P, O'Connor P, McGonagle D. Magnetic resonance imaging as a predictor of progressive joint destruction in neuropathic joint disease. *Arthritis Rheum.* 2002;46:2814-2816.
69. Edmonds ME, Petrova NL, Edmonds A, Elias A. Early identification of bone marrow oedema in the Charcot foot on MRI allows rapid intervention to prevent deformity (Abstract). *Diabet Med.* 2006;23(suppl 2):70.
70. Low KT, Peh WC. Magnetic resonance imaging of diabetic foot complications. *Singapore Med J.* 2015;56(1):23-33; quiz 34.
71. Butalia S, Palda VA, Sargeant RJ, Detsky AS, Mourad O. Does this patient with diabetes have osteomyelitis of the lower extremity? *JAMA.* 2008;299(7):806-813.
72. Lavery LA, Sariaya M, Ashry H, Harkless LB. Microbiology of osteomyelitis in diabetic foot infections. *J Foot Ankle Surg.* 1995;34(1):61-64.
73. Palestro CJ, Mehta HH, Patel M, et al. Marrow versus infection in the Charcot joint: indium-111 leukocyte and technetium-99m sulfur colloid scintigraphy. *J Nucl Med.* 1998;39:346-350.
74. Palestro CJ, Kim CK, Swyer AJ, Capozzi JD, Solomon RW, Goldsmith SJ. Total-hip arthroplasty: periprosthetic indium-111-labeled leukocyte activity and complementary technetium-99m-sulfur colloid imaging in suspected infection. *J Nucl Med.* 1990;31:1950-1955.
75. Palestro CJ, et al. Combined labeled leukocyte and technetium 99m sulfur colloid bone marrow imaging for diagnosing musculoskeletal infection. *Radiographics.* 2006;26(3):859-870.
76. Höpfner S, et al. Preoperative imaging of Charcot neuroarthropathy in diabetic patients: comparison of ring PET, hybrid PET, and magnetic resonance imaging. *Foot Ankle Int.* 2004;25(12):890-895.
77. Basu S, Chryssikos T, Houseni M, et al. Potential role of FDG PET in the setting of diabetic neuro-osteoarthropathy: can it differentiate uncomplicated Charcot's neuroarthropathy from osteomyelitis and soft-tissue infection? *Nucl Med Commun.* 2007;28:465-472.
78. Bilal A, Boddu K, Hussain S, et al. Evaluation of acute Charcot foot using SPECT/CT imaging. *Orthop Proceed.* 2018;96B(17).
79. Ahluwalia R, Ahmed B, Mullhollad N, Vivian J, Kavarthapu V, Edmonds M. The evaluation of SPECT-CT in the early management of acute Charcot osteoarthropathy (CN). *Foot Ankle Orthop.* 2016;1. doi: 10.1177/2473011416S00300.
80. Fleischer AE, Didyk AA, Woods JB, Burns SE, Wrobel JS, Armstrong DG. Combined clinical and laboratory testing improves diagnostic accuracy for osteomyelitis in the diabetic foot. *J Foot Ankle Surg.* 2009;48(1):39-46.
81. Butalia S, Palda VA, Sargeant RJ, Detsky AS, Mourad O. Does this patient with diabetes have osteomyelitis of the lower extremity? *JAMA.* 2008;299(7):806-813.
82. Kaleta JL, Fleischli JW, Reilly CH. The diagnosis of osteomyelitis in diabetes using erythrocyte sedimentation rate: a pilot study. *J Am Podiatr Med Assoc.* 2001;91:445-450.
83. Donegan R, Sumpio B, Blume PA. Charcot foot and ankle with osteomyelitis. *Diabet Foot Ankle.* 2013;4.
84. Frykberg RG, Zgonis T, Armstrong DG, et al.; American College of Foot and Ankle Surgeons. Diabetic foot disorders. A clinical practice guideline (2006 revision). *J Foot Ankle Surg.* 2006;45(5 suppl):S1-S66.
85. Pinzur MS. Current concepts review: Charcot arthropathy of the foot and ankle. *Foot Ankle Int.* 2007;28:952-959.
86. Sanders LJ, Frykberg RG. The Charcot foot (Pied de Charcot). In: Bowker JH, Pfeifer MA, eds. *Levin and O'Neal's the Diabetic Foot.* 7th ed. Philadelphia, PA: Mosby Elsevier; 2007:257-283.
87. Katz IA, Harlan A, Miranda-Palma B, et al. Randomized trial of two irremovable off-loading devices in the management of plantar neuropathic diabetic foot ulcers. *Diabetes Care.* 2005;28(3):555-559.
88. Saltzman CL, Johnson KA, Goldstein RH, Donnelly RE. The patellar tendon-bearing brace as treatment for neurotrophic arthropathy: a dynamic force monitoring study. *Foot Ankle.* 1992;13(1):14-21.
89. Güven MF, Karabiber A, Kaynak G, Öğüt T. Conservative and surgical treatment of the chronic Charcot foot and ankle. *Diabet Foot Ankle.* 2013;4:1.
90. Van der Ven A, Chapman CB, Bowker JH. Charcot neuroarthropathy of the foot and ankle. *J Am Acad Orthop Surg.* 2009;17:562-571.
91. Armstrong DG, Peters EJ. Charcot's arthropathy of the foot. *J Am Podiatr Med Assoc.* 2002;92:390-394.
92. Shibata T, Tada K, Hashizume C. The results of arthrodesis of the ankle for leprotic neuroarthropathy. *J Bone Joint Surg Am.* 1990;72:749-756.
93. Coughlin MJ, Saltzman CL, Mann RA. *Mann's Surgery of the Foot and Ankle E-Book: Expert Consult-Online.* Elsevier Health Sciences; 2013.
94. Güven MF, Karabiber A, Kaynak G, Öğüt T. Conservative and surgical treatment of the chronic Charcot foot and ankle. *Diabet Foot Ankle.* 2013;4:1.
95. Brodsky JW, Rouse AM. Exostectomy for symptomatic bony prominences in diabetic Charcot feet. *Clin Orthop Relat Res.* 1993;296:21-26.
96. Catanzariti AR, Mendicino R, Haverstock B. Ostectomy for diabetic neuroarthropathy involving the midfoot. *J Foot Ankle Surg.* 2000;39:291-300.
97. Laurinaviciene R, Kirketerp-Moeller K, Holstein PE. Exostectomy for chronic midfoot plantar ulcer in Charcot deformity. *J Wound Care.* 2008;17:53-59.

98. Mueller MJ, Sinacore DR, Hastings MK, Strube MJ, Johnson JE. Effect of Achilles tendon lengthening on neuropathic plantar ulcers. A randomized clinical trial. *J Bone Joint Surg Am*. 2003;85:1436-1445.

99. Mueller MJ, Sinacore DR, Hastings MK, Strube MJ, Johnson JE. Impact of Achilles tendon lengthening on functional limitations and perceived disability in people with a neuropathic plantar ulcer. *Diabetes Care*. 2004;27:1559-1564.

100. Sella EJ, Barrette C. Staging of Charcot neuroarthropathy along the medial column of the foot in the diabetic patient. *J Foot Ankle Surg*. 1999;38:34-40.

101. DiDomenico LA, Adams HB, Garchar D. Endoscopic gastrocnemius recession for the treatment of Gastrocnemius Equinus. *J Am Podiatr Med Assoc*. 2005;95(4):410-413.

102. Haro A, DiDomenico LA. Frontal plane-guided percutaneous tendo Achilles lengthening. *J Foot Ankle Surg*. 2007;46(1):55-61.

103. DiDomenico L, Flynn Z, Reed M. Treating Charcot arthropathy is a challenge: explaining why my treatment algorithm has changed. *Clin Podiatr Med Surg*. 2018;35(1):105-121.

104. Thompson RC, Clohissy DR. Deformity following fracture in diabetic neuropathic osteoarthropathy. Operative management of adults who have Type I diabetes. *J Bone Joint Surg*. 1993;75-A:1765-1773.

105. Misson JR, et al. External fixation techniques for foot and ankle fusions. *Foot Ankle Clin*. 2004;9(3):529-539.

106. Latt LD, et al. Biomechanical comparison of external fixation and compression screws for transverse tarsal joint arthrodesis. *Foot Ankle Int*. 2015;36(10):1235-1242.

107. Panagakos P, Ullom N, Boc SF. Salvage arthrodesis for Charcot arthropathy. *Clin Podiatr Med Surg*. 2012;29(1):115-135.

108. DiDomenico LA, Giganacova A, Cross D, Ziran B. Alternative techniques for transosseous calcaneal pinning in external fixation. *J Foot Ankle Surg*. 2012;51:528-530.

109. Stapleton JJ, DiDomenico LA, Zgonis T. Corrective midfoot osteotomies. *Clin Podiatr Med Surg*. 2008;25:681-690.

110. Pinzur MS. Current concepts review: Charcot arthropathy of the foot and ankle. *Foot Ankle Int*. 2007;28(8):952-959.

111. Rooney J, Hutabarat SR, Grujic L, Hansen ST. Surgical reconstruction of the neuropathic foot. *Foot Ankle*. 2002;12(4):213-223.

112. Garchar D, DiDomenico LA, Klaue K. Reconstruction of Lisfranc joint dislocations secondary to Charcot neuroarthropathy using a plantar plate. *J Foot Ankle Surg*. 2013;52:295-297.

113. Jones CP. Beaming for Charcot foot reconstruction. *Foot Ankle Int*. 2015;36(7):853-859.

114. DiDomenico LA, Sann P. Univalve split plaster cast for postoperative immobilization in foot & ankle surgery. *J Foot Ankle Surg*. 2013;52:260-262.

115. Rausch S, Loracher C, Fröber R, et al. Anatomical evaluation of different approaches for tibiotalocalcaneal arthrodesis. *Foot Ankle Int*. 2014;35(2):163-167.

116. Paul J, et al. Tibiotalocalcaneal arthrodesis with an intramedullary hindfoot nail and pillar fibula augmentation: technical tip. *Foot Ankle Int*. 2015;36(8):984-987.

117. Boer R, et al. Tibiotalocalcaneal arthrodesis using a reamed retrograde locking nail. *Clin Orthop Relat Res*. 2007;463:151-156.

118. Mulhern JL, et al. Is subtalar joint cartilage resection necessary for tibiotalocalcaneal arthrodesis via intramedullary nail? A multicenter evaluation. *J Foot Ankle Surg*. 2016;55(3):572-577.

119. DiDomenico LA, Thomas GW, Saxsena A. Intramedullary nail fixation for tibiotalocalcaneal arthrodesis. In: *International Advances in Foot and Ankle Surgery*. London, England: Springer; 2012:453-465.

120. Chou LB. Tibiotalocalcaneal arthrodesis. *Foot Ankle Int*. 2000;21:804-808.

121. Cooper PS. Complications of ankle and tibiotalocalcaneal arthrodesis. *Clin Orthop Relat Res*. 2001;391:33-44.

122. Buck P, Morrey B, Chao E. The optimum position of arthrodesis of the ankle: a gait study of the knee and ankle. *J Bone Joint Surg Am*. 1987;69-A:1052-1062.

123. Bennett GL, Cameron B, Njus G, Saunders M, Kay DB. Tibiotalocalcaneal arthrodesis: a biomechanical assessment of stability. *Foot Ankle Int*. 2005;26:530-536.

124. Berend ME, Glisson RR, Nunley JA. A biomechanical comparison of intramedullary nail and crossed lag screw fixation for tibiotalocalcaneal arthrodesis. *Foot Ankle Int*. 1997;18:639-643.

125. Maurer RC, Cimino WR, Cox CV, Satow GK. Transarticular cross screw fixation: a technique of ankle arthrodesis. *Clin Orthop Relat Res*. 1991;268:56-64.

126. Scranton PE Jr. An overview of ankle arthrodesis. *Clin Orthop Relat Res*. 1991;268:96-101.

127. Roukis TS. Determining the insertion site for retrograde intramedullary nail fixation of tibiotalocalcaneal arthrodesis: a radiographic and intraoperative anatomical landmark analysis. *J Foot Ankle Surg*. 2006;45(4):227-234.

128. Marley D, Tucker A, Mckenna S, Wong-Chung J. Pre-requisites for optimum centering of a tibiotalocalcaneal arthrodesis nail. *Foot Ankle Surg*. 2014;20(3):215-220.

129. Pinzur MS, Noonan T. Ankle arthrodesis with a retrograde femoral nail for Charcot ankle arthropathy. *Foot Ankle Int*. 2005;26(7):545-549.

130. Means KR, Parks BG, Nguyen A, Schon LC. Intramedullary nail fixation with posterior-to-anterior compared to transverse distal screw placement for tibiotalocalcaneal arthrodesis: a biomechanical investigation. *Foot Ankle Int*. 2006;27(12):1137-1142.

131. Mendicino RW, Catanzariti AR, Saltrick KR, et al. Tibiotalocalcaneal arthrodesis with retrograde intramedullary nailing. *J Foot Ankle Surg*. 2004;(2):82-86.

132. Pellegrini MJ, Schiff AP, Adams SB Jr, DeOrio JK, Easley ME, Nunley JA II. Outcomes of tibiotalocalcaneal arthrodesis through a posterior Achilles tendon-splitting approach. *Foot Ankle Int*. 2010;37:312-319.

133. Chapman MW. The effect of reamed and nonreamed intramedullary nailing on fracture healing. *Clin Orthop Relat Res*. 1998;355:S230-S238.

134. DiDomenico LA, Wargo-Dorsey M. Tibiotalocalcaneal arthrodesis using a femoral locking plate. *J Foot Ankle Surg*. 2012;51(1):128-132.

135. Chiodo CP, Acevedo JI, Sammarco VJ, et al. Intramedullary rod fixation compared with blade-plate-and-screw fixation for tibiotalocalcaneal arthrodesis: a biomechanical investigation. *J Bone Joint Surg Am*. 2003;85:2425-2428.

136. Alfahd U, Roth SE, Stephen D, Whyne CM. Biomechanical comparison of intramedullary nail and blade plate fixation for tibiotalocalcaneal arthrodesis. *J Orthop Trauma*. 2005;19:703-708.

137. Lee AT, Sundberg EB, Lindsey DP, Harris AH, Chou LB. Biomechanical comparison of blade plate and intramedullary nail fixation for tibiocalcaneal arthrodesis. *Foot Ankle Int*. 2010;31(2):164-171.

138. Ahmad J, Pour AE, Raikin SM. The modified use of a proximal humeral locking plate for tibiotalocalcaneal arthrodesis. *Foot Ankle Int*. 2007;28:977-983.

139. Kusnezov N, et al. Anatomically contoured anterior plating for isolated tibiotalar arthrodesis: a systematic review. *Foot Ankle Spec*. 2017;10(4):352-358.

140. Matson AP, et al. Anterior plating with retention of nail for ankle nonunion after tibiotalocalcaneal arthrodesis. *Tech Foot Ankle Surg*. 2017;16(1):41-45.

141. Gardner MJ, Griffith MH, Demetrakopoulos D, et al. Hybrid locked plating of osteoporotic fractures of the humerus. *J Bone Joint Surg Am*. 2006;88:1962-1967.

142. Smith K, Araoye I, Jones C, Shah A. Outcomes of locking-plate fixation for hindfoot fusion procedures in 15 patients. *J Foot Ankle Surg*. 2017;56(6):1188-1193.

143. Comba F, Buttaro M, Pusso R, Piccaluga F. Acetabular reconstruction with impacted bone allografts and cemented acetabular components: a 2- to 13-year follow-up study of 142 aseptic revisions. *J Bone Joint Surg Br*. 2006;88-B:865-869.

144. Garcia-Cimbrelo E, Cordero J. Impacted morsellised allograft and cemented cup in acetabular revision surgery: a five to nine year follow-up study. *Hip Int*. 2002;12:281-288.

145. Buckley SC, Stockley I, Hamer AJ, Kerry RM. Irradiated allograft bone for acetabular revision surgery: results at a mean of five years. *J Bone Joint Surg Br*. 2005;87-B:310-313.

146. Wukich DK, Crim BE, Frykberg RG, Rosario BL. Neuropathy and poorly controlled diabetes increase the rate of surgical site infection after foot and ankle surgery. *J Bone Joint Surg Am*. 2014;96(10):832-839.

147. Wukich DK, et al. Topically applied vancomycin powder reduces the rate of surgical site infection in diabetic patients undergoing foot and ankle surgery. *Foot Ankle Int*. 2015;36(9):1017-1024.

CHAPTER 39

Surgical Considerations in the Rheumatoid Foot and Ankle

Thomas A. Brosky II, Adam D. Port, and Jeanne Mirbey

INTRODUCTION

Rheumatoid arthritis (RA) is an inflammatory, symmetric, peripheral polyarthritis that commonly manifests with forefoot and rearfoot deformities.[1] The etiology of RA is unknown, but it commonly leads to deformity through a mechanism of laxity of soft tissue structures including tendons and ligaments, along with the destruction of joints through bone and cartilage erosion. Untreated or unresponsive RA can lead to loss of joint function, difficulty with maintaining employment, and inability to carry out activities of daily living. Patients who are rheumatoid factor positive have disease progression two times faster than rheumatoid factor negative patients.[2] C-reactive protein is also a predictor of disease progression[3,4] as patients with higher levels of inflammation have worse clinical outcomes.[5] Patients with RA also suffer with "chronic wasting disease" with high energy expenditure due to abnormal anatomy.[5]

The prevalence of RA is 0.5% of the population in Europe and the United States.[6,7] This progressive disease affects women three to four times more often than men, at any age, but especially between 50 and 70 years old. Symptoms related to the foot and ankle are the first manifestations of RA in 20% of cases,[7,8] and during the course of the disease, the foot is affected in 50%-90% of cases.[6,9,10] There is controversy as to whether the rearfoot is more often affected than the forefoot.[10] However, when it comes to the chronology of manifestations of RA in the foot, forefoot symptoms usually appear first.[6,7,9,11] Typical deformities of the forefoot are hallux abducto valgus and dorsolateral dislocations of the lesser metatarsophalangeal joints (MPJs), while polyarthritis of the hindfoot often leads to a pes planovalgus deformity. Foot and ankle surgery represents 20% of all surgeries performed on the musculoskeletal system in patients with RA.[12] Early surgery, often in the form of arthrodesis, is effective in treating pain and deformity and can sometimes prevent disease progression. The postoperative satisfaction rate of patients is high despite a slightly higher complication rate than that of foot surgery in general. While specific surgical techniques are discussed elsewhere in this book, this chapter will review alterations of foot and ankle surgery in RA and discuss the necessity, varying results, and unique complications associated with surgery in the rheumatoid foot.

PATHOPHYSIOLOGY AND DISEASE PROGRESSION

Inflammatory synovitis is the deformative cause of the rheumatoid foot by resulting in a weakening of stabilizing capsuloligamentous structures, which leads to musculotendinous imbalances.[6,11] These deformities generate pain and biomechanical abnormalities, which in turn worsen the deformity, thus constituting a degenerative cycle (Fig. 39.1).

Difficulties in walking in the rheumatoid rearfoot are based on painful instability, which is particularly felt on uneven surfaces. The disease progression of RA typically begins in the forefoot and moves proximally as disease severity increases. Forefoot symptoms usually develop with pain and generalized edema. The most frequently involved joint in the foot occurs in the first MPJ, whereas the Lisfranc joint is less frequently involved. The ankle joint is the least affected joint of the hindfoot, whereas the subtalar joint is frequently involved.[7] In the midfoot, pes planovalgus has a reported prevalence of between 46% and 64% in the RA population.[13] Unlike congenital flatfoot deformities, RA pes planovalgus does not result from isolated degeneration of the posterior tibial tendon but additionally from the loss of intrinsic stability of the joints of

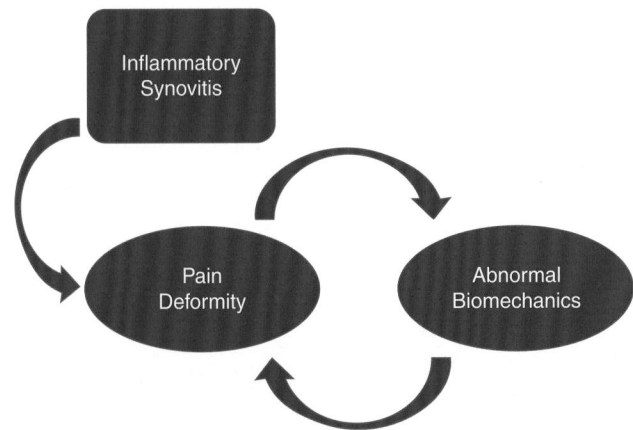

FIGURE 39.1 Pathophysiology and disease progression of rheumatoid arthritis.

the hindfoot (subtalar, talonavicular, and calcaneocuboid) by inflammatory destruction.[6,9,14] Inflammatory synovitis and dysfunction of the peritalar joints and the tibialis posterior muscle-tendon unit are postulated mechanisms leading to instability of the subtalar and midtarsal joints.[15] Studies conclude that the ankle joint is involved late in the disease as severity increases.[16] Often, changes to the ankle joint are secondary to stress from abnormal positional changes after breakdown of the midtarsal and subtalar joint complexes.[17]

Ankle equinus is frequently seen in the RA population and is related to increased forefoot pressures.[18] This coupled with periarticular changes of the midfoot and hindfoot leads to collapse of the medial longitudinal arch. This gastroc-soleus contracture should be evaluated and addressed when considering reconstruction.

Early stages of collapsing pes planovalgus deformity can be treated in RA patients with conservative bracing techniques. In later stages where deformity impedes ambulation, soft tissue and osseous procedures are employed to address any arthritic joints. The goals of the RA rearfoot or forefoot surgery are to improve function and decrease pain, while biomechanically protecting surrounding joint structures.

Typically, severe deformity is less likely in juvenile rheumatoid arthritis (early-onset RA) patients. In these patients, there is increased involvement in certain joints including proximal interphalangeal, metacarpal phalangeal, metatarsophalangeal, elbow, and ankle joint.[19] Patients diagnosed after the age of 60 are considered adult onset and tend to have more serious deformity and instability.[20] The RA case rate of geriatric patients is ~2%.[21]

CONSERVATIVE MANAGEMENT

Medical therapy is vital to the long-term management of RA. Traditional therapies include nonsteroidal anti-inflammatory drugs (NSAIDs) and corticosteroids. More recently, disease modifying antirheumatic drugs (DMARDS) and biologic agents are playing an important role in medical management and, as their name suggests, modification of progression of disease. These medications are discussed later in this chapter.

Customized orthotics and ankle-foot orthoses (AFOs) are also useful to accommodate the later stages of the deformity including pes planovalgus deformity. These are especially useful in the management of the geriatric population and/or other nonsurgical candidates.

Symptomatic relief of chronically painful rheumatoid joints can be managed with intra-articular cortisone injections to relieve symptomatic synovitis and the pain associated with joint destruction. The authors recommend fluoroscopic-guided injections (Fig. 39.2), which are far superior to blind injections, particularly in the midfoot joints.[22]

PREOPERATIVE CONSIDERATIONS

Surgery is indicated in the rheumatoid patient in the presence of pain that alters activities of daily living after aggressive, unsuccessful medical and conservative therapy. Additionally, extensive deformity or instability leading to loss of function indicates surgery in rheumatoid patients. In the absence of preoperative pain or deformity, rheumatoid patients have a poor postoperative prognosis. Patients should be counseled on the specific

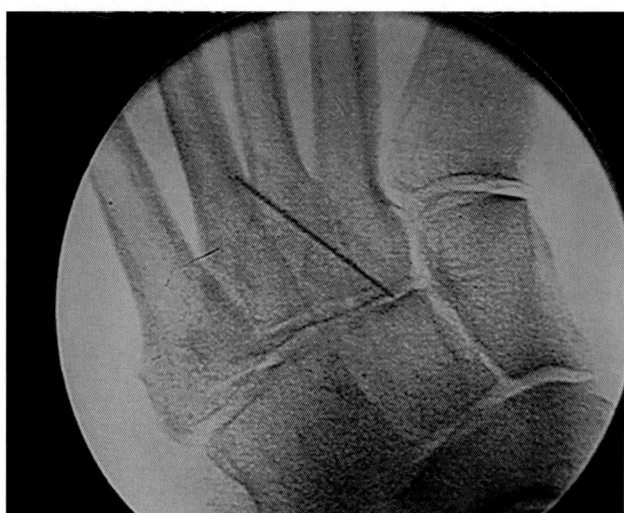

FIGURE 39.2 Fluoroscopic-guided injection.

risks associated with surgery in the rheumatoid foot, including increased infection rates, longer recovery, failure of hardware, continued pain, possible need for revision or further surgery, and continued progression of deformities.

A "whole patient" multidisciplinary approach should be taken with the surgical management of RA patients. The rheumatologist and/or primary care physician should be consulted to give input into surgical planning and appropriate perioperative management.

Preoperative history and physical examination is very important in the rheumatoid patient. A thorough history should include the patient's ability or inability to perform activities of daily living along with pain level. This is paramount in determining whether surgery is indicated, and vital to appropriate procedure selection. On physical examination, forefoot MPJ function and position should be evaluated. In the rearfoot examination, the extent of the pes planovalgus deformity, which is common in RA, should be determined along with determining the extent of ankle joint involvement. On gait examination, patients often have a slower gait with longer double support phase.[13,23] A rigorous examination to determine the level of pain with range of motion, and extent of function loss is necessary for adequate surgical planning.

These patients should be evaluated for undiagnosed arterial and venous disease, especially in the presence of a sedentary lifestyle. Claudication symptoms can be mistaken for articular or muscular pain, and therefore, vascular referral is crucial in the preoperative planning process.[24,25] It is also helpful to evaluate the venous system since many patients have considerable edema. It is important to control edema in the postoperative period to avoid wound healing complications. RA has also been associated with a higher risk for thromboembolic events following foot and ankle surgery.[26] Therefore, it is important to collaborate with the patient's primary care physician for medical management and a potential need for anticoagulation therapy postoperatively.

From a preoperative standpoint, it is important for the surgeon to evaluate the RA patient's medication profile. With the advent of the newer biologic medications, the inflammatory process of RA can be well controlled, but there can be negative side effects of poor wound healing and an increased risk of

infection. There are four categories of biologics: tumor necrosis factor (TNF); interleukin (IL) inhibitors; B-cell inhibitors; and T-cell inhibitors. It is beneficial to coordinate each patient's medication regime with the rheumatologist preoperatively.

Peripheral sensory neuropathy must also be considered in the RA population.[27] Certain medications have been implicated in the cause of peripheral neuropathy that include infliximab, leflunomide, gold salts, and methotrexate.[28] Peripheral neuropathy in RA is also associated with increasing age, duration of disease, and increased disease severity.[29] Overt neuropathy symptoms can be detected with clinical examination, whereas subacute symptoms typically need electrophysiologic testing with nerve conduction studies. Referral to neurology for a comprehensive workup should be considered prior to surgery. This is an important diagnostic step to take preoperatively in order to prevent and safeguard the development of Charcot neuroarthropathy in this patient population.

Traditionally, plain film radiographs have been used in diagnosis and monitoring of progression of RA in the foot. Soft tissue swelling, periarticular osteopenia, marginal joint erosion, subluxation, and osteoarthritic changes should be evaluated. Over the last two decades, significant attention has been focused on ways to harness advanced imaging such as CT, PET, and MRI for the evaluation of RA. Prior to the advent of effective structure-modifying therapies, little attention was paid to advanced methods of monitoring the progression of RA. Plain film radiographs have been the standard for evaluating RA, but this method alone is fundamentally limited in its ability to visualize nonosseous features of the disease.[30] Plain film radiographs can be used to effectively evaluate bone erosion, joint space narrowing, and osseous position, but these findings are only evident late in the disease process. The Larsen score is used to determine the extent of radiographic changes due to RA. This method scores the amount of spacing between joints, bony outlines, and level of joint erosion.[31] Radiographically, patients often have a lower calcaneal inclination angle, lower medial arch height, greater peak eversion in stance, and lower peak plantar flexion. Osteopenia should be taken into consideration when determining fixation method. MRI and ultrasound can be useful in evaluation of synovitis, bursal changes, and damage to soft tissue structures such as tendons and ligaments, including enthesopathies. If surgery is deemed necessary, DEXA scanning can be utilized to determine bone quality. However, the authors tend to assume poor bone quality prior to any rheumatoid boney procedure. Therefore, while DEXA scanning is useful in the chronic management of patients with RA, it may not be necessary in all preoperative patients.[32]

PEARLS

When considering surgical necessity, pain is not always the only factor to consider, it is also crucial to evaluate the present deformity and understand that it could lead to further breakdown of adjacent joints. Therefore, early intervention may help limit the necessity for further surgery by preventing disease progression.

Since this disease process can cause muscular insufficiency, it is important to stage forefoot and hindfoot procedures when possible because ambulation and off-loading can be challenging in this patient population. It is important to evaluate each patient for specific off-loading techniques prior to surgical intervention. Prior to procedures that will require non–weight

bearing, physical therapy should be considered for assessment of the patient's ability to use safe ambulatory assistive devices, especially with patients involving severe hand deformities that are common in this population. Atlantoaxial damage is common in rheumatoid patients and should be taken into consideration with surgical positioning and postoperative mobility.[33]

In surgical planning, forefoot surgery is often indicated first and early, with the goal of pain free ambulation.[20] Knowledge of essential and nonessential joints is also important in surgical planning. The ankle, subtalar, talonavicular, and lesser MPJs are essential in regular gait.[18] Because of this, arthroplasty should be a consideration in the ankle and lesser MPJs. In addition to osseous considerations, soft tissue abnormalities should be accounted for, including tendon, ligamentous, and capsular imbalance, and addressing bursae that are prevalent in the rheumatoid foot.

PEARLS

It is important to strongly consider obtaining preoperative consults to physical therapy, neurology, vascular surgery, pain management, and rheumatology. In addition, due to the increased complexity of rheumatoid patients, the authors recommend not to neglect early surgical intervention. While complication rates are increased in this population, surgery is often necessary and patient satisfaction rates are similar to the general patient population.

OPERATIVE CONSIDERATIONS

Traditionally, the decision to proceed with surgical intervention is only made after conservative means have been exhausted. This does not always apply to the rheumatoid foot. In cases of rapid progression of pathology, or moderate to severe development of deformities, early intervention is necessary to arrest progression of the disease. Severe deformity, even with minimal pain, generates abnormal biomechanical stresses on adjacent joints that lead to increased inflammation and the possibility of rapid joint destruction. Surrounding joints are threatened by both inflammatory and mechanical mechanisms. It is therefore paramount to consider these processes, and not merely current pain and function levels, when determining whether to operate.

The authors note that specific surgical procedures generally do not vary when dealing with progressive joint destructive diseases. Surgical reconstruction of the rheumatoid foot involves much more than improved cosmesis. The aim of reconstruction of the rheumatoid foot is to restore as much function as possible to allow the patient to return to his or her normal daily activities by reducing pain and leaving the patient with a plantigrade foot. Anatomic reconstruction, while a worthy goal, if often not achievable in the rheumatoid foot due to extensive destruction and deterioration of osseous and soft tissue structures as a result of the disease. Patient and surgeon expectations should be managed with the goals of improvement of function and reduction of pain, while providing foot and ankle stability. Often, smaller procedures can yield more satisfactory results for rheumatoid patients.[20] At the same time, an early and more aggressive approach to performing surgery, prior to extensive progression of deformities, can yield better outcomes.

Over the past few decades, there has been a trend away from joint destructive surgery and toward joint preservation in essential joints. Twenty years ago, the Keller procedure with pan met

head resections was the standard for forefoot reconstruction in the rheumatoid patient.[34] Currently, the use of a first MPJ arthrodesis along with lesser MPJ joint sparing periarticular releases or pan met head resections in patients with extensive articular damage are recommended by the authors due to more consistent long-term results with first MPJ arthrodesis.

There are several surgical options for the correction of the rheumatoid foot, many of which are not specific to RA itself including synovectomy, arthrodesis, arthroplasty, and joint replacement. In the forefoot, first MPJ arthrodesis with lesser MPJ arthroplasty via metatarsal head resection is a common and reliable surgical option for treatment in the presence of severe deformity. Other options, including first MPJ replacement, along with lesser MPJ soft tissue rebalancing with or without metatarsal osteotomies are beneficial in the presence of less severe deformity. In the rearfoot, total ankle arthroplasty (TAA), ankle arthrodesis, and tibiotalocalcaneal (TTC) arthrodesis via intramedullary (IM) nail are all reliable options.

Surgical technique should be altered to account for abnormal anatomy. Precise anatomical dissection is utilized particularly in this patient population due to the fact that most of these patients are immunocompromised from long-term steroid or other medication use. Wound complications are not uncommon in this patient population and should be considered carefully in the preoperative and intraoperative phase. Skin incision should be deepened into the dermal and subcutaneous junction. The subcutaneous tissue should be opened with blunt dissection and appropriate hemostasis applied with care to avoid unnecessary destruction of vasculature. Severe digital contractures should be approached with caution. These digits have a high rate of ischemia and careful dissection should be utilized throughout the procedure.

Due to osteopenia, screws must engage the cortex, and appropriate countersink should be accomplished if possible to avoid stress risers that can more easily occur in osteopenic bone. Kirschner wires and Steinmann Pins[20] are an excellent option for fixation in rheumatoid patients and can be used as a primary or augmentary fixation option. Locking plate fixation is strongly encouraged when plate fixation is used due to poor bone quality and the superior stability of locking plates.[35] The use of external fixation during staged procedures can aid with soft tissue rebalancing.

PEARLS

Poor bone quality and the presence of neuropathy in some patients will increase the likelihood of hardware failure. Therefore, a more solid fixation construct may be necessary in the rheumatoid patient. The authors recommend locking plates that could also be reinforced with K-wire or Steinmann pins for increased fixation solidity.

FOREFOOT RECONSTRUCTION

There are many issues that need to be addressed when contemplating forefoot reconstruction. These include the length of the metatarsals, the degree of subluxation and/or dislocation of the lesser metatarsal phalangeal joints, and the extent of pathology to the first metatarsal phalangeal joint. It has been well documented that arthrodesis is more reliable in providing long-term patient satisfaction when compared to generalized

arthroplasties.[11] Arthrodesis offers increased stability to the first MPJ segment and the entire forefoot. This stability translates into improved long-term maintenance of the structural integrity of the forefoot and digits as well as overall functional results.[36]

FIRST METATARSOPHALANGEAL JOINT ARTHRODESIS WITH PAN-METATARSAL HEAD RESECTION

INCISIONAL APPROACHES

There are many different incisional approaches described for this procedure. The dorsal approach using five longitudinal incisions overlying each metatarsal and respective digit is effective in minimizing surrounding dissection. A three–longitudinal-incision approach can be utilized and is described in the literature, but significant dissection is needed and thereby increases the risk of hematoma and wound complications. The dorsal approach may be difficult when there are existing metatarsal phalangeal joint dislocations. When significant metatarsal phalangeal joint dislocations are present, a single longitudinal approach over the first metatarsal is utilized with a single transverse plantar approach over the lesser metatarsal heads (Fig. 39.3).

If any existing rheumatoid nodules are present, an elliptical incision can be utilized plantarly over the metatarsal heads, thereby debulking the area and providing stability to the lesser digits. When the plantar approach is utilized, small longitudinal incisions may be placed over the proximal interphalangeal joints of each digit for arthrodesis or arthroplasty. The most challenging aspect of the plantar incision is Kirschner wire placement. Fluoroscopy is utilized when retrograding a Kirschner wire out the respective digit and crossing the metatarsal phalangeal joint down each respective metatarsal.

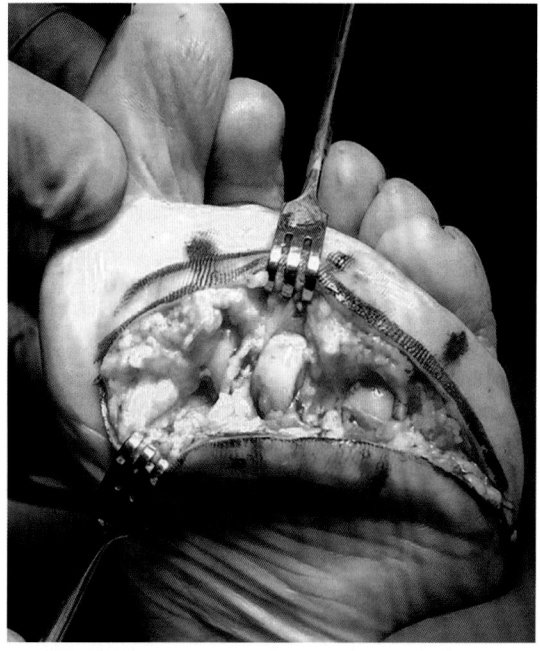

FIGURE 39.3 Single transverse plantar incision.

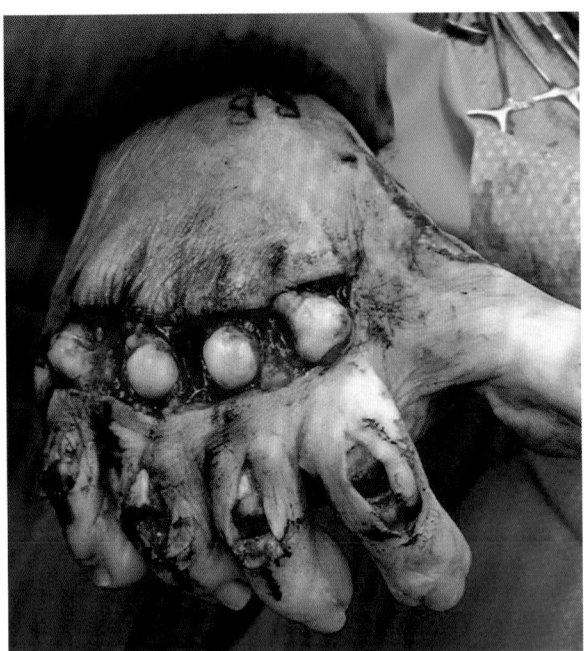

FIGURE 39.4 Dorsal transverse incision.

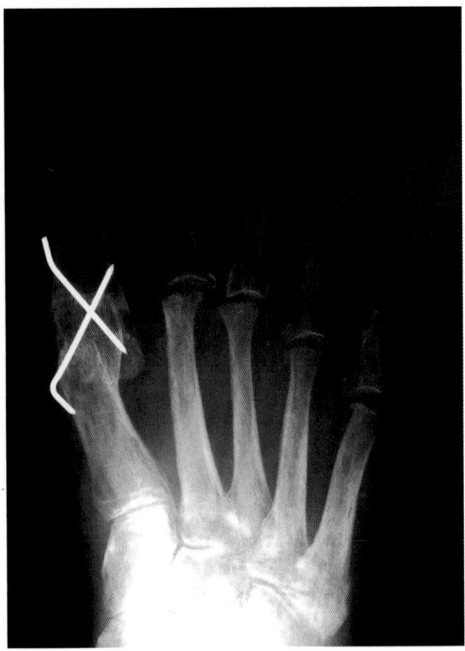

FIGURE 39.5 Radiographic metatarsal parabola.

An alternative incisional placement that seems to minimize hematoma and wound dehiscence complications consists of a longitudinal incision over the first metatarsal phalangeal joint followed by a dorsal transverse incision over the lesser metatarsal phalangeal joints (Fig. 39.4). This allows for anatomical access to the metatarsal heads with direct visualization of the parabola for resection. Secondary small incisions are placed over the dorsal proximal interphalangeal joints of each digit to carry out arthrodesis or arthroplasty.

> ## PEARLS
>
> The authors recommended a dorsal transverse incision for the metatarsal phalangeal joints 2-5 (pan metatarsal head resection), which can minimize postoperative complications including wound dehiscence and edema. This also gives the ideal visualization for the parabola correction.

The authors utilize arthrodesis for all digital procedures for the benefit of long-term results as previously mentioned.

The dissection surrounding each metatarsal phalangeal joint is eased by the use of a McGlamry elevator. This assists in freeing the metatarsal head and allowing easier access for resection. The process for maintaining the parabola is calculated beginning with the second metatarsal, which should remain the longest. The first and third metatarsals are usually the next longest in creating the new metatarsal parabola. This is followed by the fourth metatarsal and then the fifth, which should be the shortest (Fig. 39.5).

A power saw should be utilized when transecting the metatarsal heads (Fig. 39.6). The cut should be made from dorsal distal to plantar proximal, thereby limiting any sharp protrusion of bone plantarly, which may cause plantar lesions or discomfort. Once the parabola is evaluated under fluoroscopy and found to be adequate, positioning of the first MPJ arthrodesis site is then utilized with a flat plate (Figs. 39.7 and 39.8).

Once the first MPJ arthrodesis site is stabilized with the surgeon's preference for fixation, keeping in mind the generally poor bone quality in rheumatoid patients, attention is directed to stabilizing the lesser digits with Kirschner wire fixation. Stabilization occurs from the second digit in sequence to the fifth digit. Once the proximal interphalangeal joints are inspected for appropriate apposition, attention is then directed to deep closure. Each metatarsal phalangeal joint is approximated with nonabsorbable suture, along with the capsule around each Kirschner wire. This stabilizes the metatarsal phalangeal joint and allows for fibrosis to occur, thereby keeping the digit in a more rectus position. Layered closure of soft tissue with subcuticular closure of the skin is then carried out.

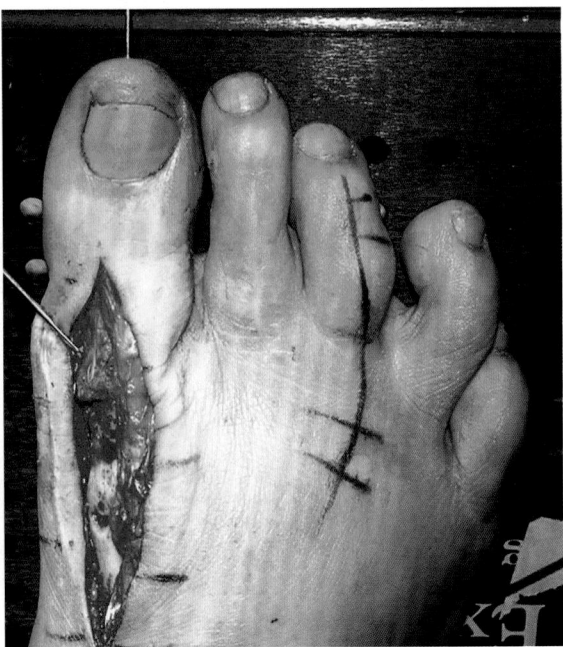

FIGURE 39.6 Saw resection of metatarsal head.

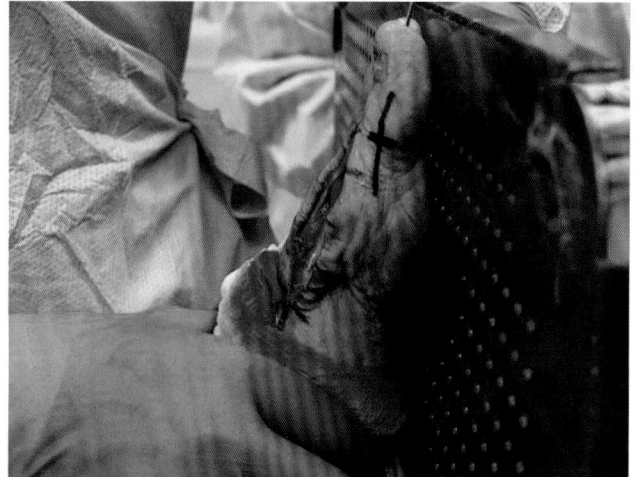

FIGURE 39.7 Utilization of a flat plate for adequate joint positioning.

FOREFOOT ARTHROPLASTY OPTIONS

Resection arthroplasty has been shown as a viable alternative to arthrodesis in rheumatoid patients. Traditionally, the Keller arthroplasty has been used as a go-to option for arthritic first MPJs as a joint destructive procedure. However, shortening of the digit and loss of joint stability can occur due to disruption of the plantar plate and intrinsic musculature attachments at the base of the proximal phalanx.[30] As an alternative, the Hueter-Mayo resection arthroplasty (resection of the metatarsal head of the first MTP joint) has been shown to relieve joint pain while maintaining joint stability about the first MPJ and without disruption of the plantar plate.[30]

Implant arthroplasty of the first MPJ using silicone implant has been performed since the late 1960s for treatment of hallux rigidus and hallux valgus. These procedures allow for maintenance of mobility and minimal joint resection. Material concerns and high complication rates including wear, particulate

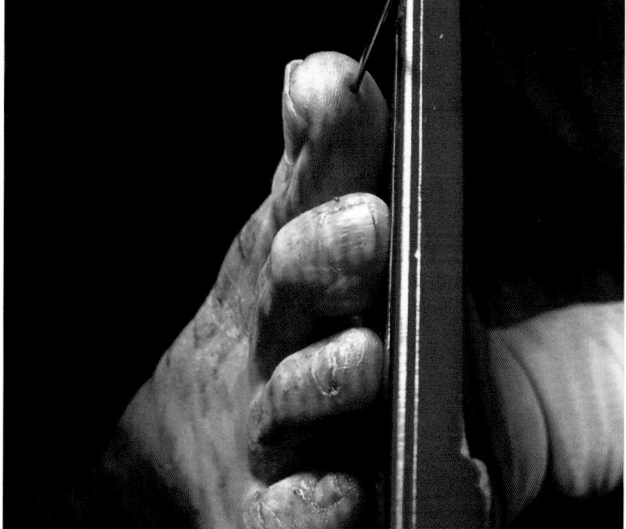

FIGURE 39.8 Utilization of a flat plate for adequate hallux positioning.

release, implant fracture, and patient reactions including synovitis and cyst formation have led to much debate in literature as to the efficacy of these procedures.[1,37] Salvage of failed implant arthroplasty often requires interpositional bone block arthrodesis due to cystic osteolysis and peri-implant bone loss.

SYNOVECTOMY

Relief of pain and reduction of periarticular edema are the goals of synovectomy as they may limit disease progression.[38] Persistent synovitis in the rheumatoid population leads to chronic inflammation and chronic painful deformity. This can involve forefoot and/or hindfoot joints. Ligamentous and capsular damage can occur, which is caused by release of catabolic cytokines, such as TNF, interleukin, and protease.[39] This long-term synovial damage causes ligamentous instability and joint position compromise, which leads to further deformity. In the end stage of disease, synovectomy is less likely to succeed as articular destruction has already occurred. Physical therapy postoperatively may be helpful in enhancing postoperative range of motion and maintaining joint motion.

MIDFOOT RECONSTRUCTIVE SURGERY

Midfoot deformities are less dramatic and often less symptomatic than those in the forefoot or rearfoot. This is because they are sometimes obscured by the symptoms of the hindfoot. Arthritis of the midfoot, although rarely seen in isolation, is nevertheless common in RA. It leads to collapse of the medial longitudinal arch.[6,40] Rheumatoid midfoot surgery essentially consists of isolated or multi-joint arthrodeses (Lisfranc, intercuneiform, naviculo-cuneiform), which are effective at reducing pain and providing stability. These procedures, often when utilized in conjunction with forefoot or rearfoot procedures, allow for improved correction of deformity, which is often the collapse of the longitudinal arch. The nature and rate of complications associated with this surgery are similar to those of the forefoot and so is patient satisfaction.[41]

RHEUMATOID REARFOOT CONSIDERATIONS

It is important to evaluate each hindfoot joint: talonavicular, calcaneocuboid, subtalar, and tibiotalar joints. Each joint must be evaluated for erosive and positional changes that may warrant bracing or surgery in the future. The frequency of talonavicular involvement is predominant and involves 30%-40% of cases, followed by subtalar, which involve 20%-30% of cases.[7,9] Rheumatoid involvement of the ankle is rarer and often a later finding. It results either from direct inflammatory joint destruction or from abnormal stresses caused by the deformation of the hindfoot. Early in the progression of disease, inflammatory processes are predominant and lead to disability.[13]

In the event of isolated involvement of the talonavicular joint, and in the case of a rectus rearfoot, arthrodesis of this joint alone may be considered. Talonavicular arthrodesis alone decreases the mobility of the hindfoot complex by 75%. In the event of even moderate damage to the subtalar or calcaneocuboid joints, a double (talonavicular and subtalar) or

triple (talonavicular, subtalar, and calcaneocuboid) arthrodesis should be considered to give further stability to the hindfoot.[6,7]

Isolated ankle involvement is rare. The most commonly performed rheumatoid ankle procedure is arthrodesis, which is associated with a union rate >90% and a complication rate equivalent to that of hindfoot arthrodesis in other patient populations.[4,20,25] With the goal of maintaining mobility at the ankle and reducing the compensatory stresses on neighboring joints in patients with a low functional demand, TAA has shown encouraging results on the moderate to long-term basis. An additional advantage of ankle replacement over arthrodesis is the ability of immediate weight bearing while arthrodesis requires immobilization with non–weight bearing and partial weight bearing for 10-12 weeks. This is a particularly important consideration in rheumatoid patients with upper extremity loss of function. The TAA also has its place when deformity is present in both the rearfoot and ankle joints as an alternative to pantalar arthrodesis.

ARTHROSCOPY

Arthroscopic surgery of the ankle is a valuable treatment option for rheumatoid patients with ankle synovitis early in the disease process when osseous deformity is absent. Arthroscopic treatments have shown significant benefits and improvements in pain and edema, as well as in return to daily activities and sports.[42] Advantages of ankle arthroscopy are the direct visualization of the pathology, minimal dissection required for the placement of the ankle portals, and minimal disruption of the soft tissue envelope. These advantages aid in the reduction of healing time, which is particularly important in rheumatoid patients.[43]

POSTOPERATIVE CONSIDERATIONS

Coordination with PCP and/or rheumatologist in postoperative management is essential in providing the patient with the best chance for osseous and soft tissue wound healing. Serial radiographs can be used to monitor progression both preoperatively and postoperatively. Often, extended non–weight bearing is needed, especially when external fixation is utilized. Careful management of ambulatory status and the use of assistive devices such as rolling knee scooters or four point walkers are helpful in assisting patients to maintain non–weight-bearing status. Pain management should be carefully coordinated with the patient's rheumatologist. It is not uncommon for patients to be on an extended pain management plan due to pain at the operative or other nonoperative joints prior to surgery. This may necessitate the need for pain management consultation due to build up of tolerance after long-term pain medication use. The long-term postoperative course will likely require augmentation in the form of shock-absorbing plantar supports, spacious orthopedic shoes, orthotic or AFO support, physical therapy, and possibly staged procedures or other further surgical intervention.[44–46]

In forefoot reconstruction, Kirschner wire fixation is generally left in place for 6-8 weeks. In these patients, early weight bearing is encouraged with support from a postoperative shoe or pneumatic walking boot. Patients should be educated to avoid the propulsive phase of gait on the operative limb.

The postoperative course for rearfoot surgical intervention in the rheumatoid foot includes 6-8 weeks of non–weight bearing followed by transition to partial weight bearing and physical therapy. Rearfoot arthrodesis has a high rate of union (90%-98%) and patient satisfaction. Ultimately, however, ankle changes are seen in 30%-60% of cases.[7,9,11] Complications include 2%-10% nonunion, 0%-5% infections, and 0%-17% delayed wound healing.[41]

CONCLUSION

The key goals of rheumatoid foot and ankle reconstructive surgery are correction of deformity, stabilization, and reduction of pain. In the majority of cases, this surgical mission is fulfilled by performing arthrodesis. When essential joints of the foot are involved, alternatives to arthrodesis must be considered. Surgical results are associated with a high rate of patient satisfaction despite a higher complication rate than foot surgery in the general population. Early surgical management is encouraged to limit the mechanical consequences on neighboring joints. The "whole patient" needs to be considered to ensure appropriate expectations, comprehensive perioperative management, and successful surgical outcomes.

REFERENCES

1. Granberry WM, Noble PC, Bishop JO, Tullos HS. Use of a hinged silicone prosthesis for replacement of the first metatarsophalangeal joint. *J Bone Joint Surg.* 1991;73-A:1453-1459.
2. Bukhari M, Lunt M, Harrison BJ, et al. Rheumatoid factor is the major predictor of increasing severity of radiographic erosions in rheumatoid arthritis: results from the Norfolk Arthritis Register Study, a large inception cohort. *Arthritis Rheum.* 2002;46:906-912.
3. Amos RS, Constable TJ, Crockson RA, et al. Rheumatoid arthritis: relation of serum C-reactive protein and erythrocyte sedimentation rates to radiographic changes. *Br Med J.* 1977;22:195-197.
4. Stenger AA, Van Leeuwen MA, Houtman PM, et al. Early effective suppression of inflammation in rheumatoid arthritis reduces radiographic progression. *Br J Rheumatol.* 1998;37:1157-1163.
5. Chehata JC, Hassell AB, Clarke SA, et al. Mortality in rheumatoid arthritis: relationship to single and composite measures of disease activity. *Rheumatology (Oxford).* 2001;40:447-452.
6. Bouysset M, Tourné Y, Tillmann K. *Le pied et la cheville rhumatoïdes.* Paris, France: Springer; 2004.
7. Jaakkola JI, Mann RA. A review of rheumatoid arthritis affecting the foot and ankle. *Foot Ankle Int.* 2004;25:866-874.
8. Fleming A, Crown JM, Corbett M. Early rheumatoid disease. I. Onset. *Ann Rheum Dis.* 1976;35:357-360.
9. Mann RA, Horton GA. Management of the foot and ankle in rheumatoid arthritis. *Rheum Dis Clin North Am.* 1996;22:457-476.
10. Michelson J, Easley M, Wigley FM, Hellmann D. Foot and ankle problems in rheumatoid arthritis. *Foot Ankle Int.* 1994;15:608-613.
11. Trieb K. Management of the foot in rheumatoid arthritis. *J Bone Joint Surg Br.* 2005;87:1171-1177.
12. Hamalainen M, Raunio P. Long-term follow-up of rheumatoid forefoot surgery. *Clin Orthop Relat Res.* 1997;(340):34-38.
13. Turner DE, Helliwell PS, Emery P, et al. The impact of rheumatoid arthritis on foot function in the early stages of disease: a clinical case series. *BMC Musculoskelet Disord.* 2006;7:102.
14. Masterson E, Mulcahy D, McElwain J, McInerney D. The planovalgus rheumatoid foot—is tibialis posterior tendon rupture a factor? *Br J Rheumatol.* 1995;34:645-646.
15. Jernberg ET, Simkin P, Kravette M, Lowe P, Gardner G. The posterior tibial tendon and tarsal sinus in rheumatoid flat foot: magnetic resonance imaging of 40 feet. *J Rheumatol.* 1999;26:289-293.
16. Belt EA, Kaarela K, Maenpaa H, et al. Relationship of ankle joint involvement with subtalar destruction in patients with rheumatoid arthritis. A 20 year follow up study. *Joint Bone Spine.* 2001;68:154-157.
17. Mann R, Coughlin M, eds. *Surgery of the Foot and Ankle.* Vol. I. St. Louis, MO: Mosby; 1992.
18. Hansen S. *Functional Reconstruction of the Foot and Ankle.* Philadelphia, PA: Lippincott Williams & Wilkins; 2000.
19. Healey LA. Rheumatoid arthritis in elderly patients. *Clin Rheum Dis.* 1986;12:173-179.
20. Shuberth JM. Pedal fusions in the rheumatoid patient. *Clin Podiatr Med Surg.* 1988;5:227-247.
21. Rasch EK, Hirsch R, Paulose-Ram R, et al. Prevalence of rheumatoid arthritis in persons 60 years of age and older in the United States: effect of different methods of case classification. *Arthritis Rheum.* 2003;48:917-926.

22. Amin A, Cullen N, Singh D. Rheumatoid forefoot reconstruction. *Acta Orthop Belg.* 2010;76(3):289-297.
23. Khazzam M, Long JT, Marks RM, et al. Kinematic changes of the foot and ankle in patients with systemic rheumatoid arthritis and forefoot deformity. *J Orthop Res.* 2007;25:319-329.
24. Henke PK, Sukheepod P, Proctor MC, et al. Clinical relevance of peripheral vascular occlusive disease in patients with rheumatoid arthritis and systemic lupus erythematosus. *J Vasc Surg.* 2003;38:111-115.
25. Hafner J, Schneider E, Burg G, et al. Management of leg ulcers in patients with rheumatoid arthritis or systemic sclerosis: the importance of concomitant arterial and venous disease. *J Vasc Surg.* 2000;32:322-329.
26. Hanslow SS, Grujic L, Slater HK, et al. Thromboembolic disease after foot and ankle surgery. *Foot Ankle Int.* 2006;27:693-695.
27. Mold JW, Vesely SK, Keyl BA, et al. The prevalence, predictors, and consequences of peripheral sensory neuropathy in older patients. *J Am Board Fam Pract.* 2004;17:309-318.
28. Metzler C, Arlt AC, Gross WL, et al. Peripheral neuropathy in patients with systemic rheumatic diseases treated with leflunomide. *Ann Rheum Dis.* 2005;64:1798-1800.
29. Kaeley N, et al. Prevalence and patterns of peripheral neuropathy in patients of rheumatoid arthritis. *J Family Med Prim Care.* 2019;8(1):22.
30. Grondal L, Brostrom E, Wretenberg P, Stark A. Arthrodesis versus Mayo resection: the management of the first metatarsophalangeal joint in reconstruction of the rheumatoid forefoot. *J Bone Joint Surg.* 2006;88-B:914-919.
31. Larsen A. How to apply Larsen score in evaluating radiographs of rheumatoid arthritis in long-term studies. *J Rheumatol.* 1995;22(10):1974-1975.
32. Hafez EA, et al. Bone mineral density changes in patients with recent-onset rheumatoid arthritis. *Clin Med Insights Arthritis Musculoskelet Disord.* 2011;4:87-94.
33. Wineld J, Young A, Williams P, et al. Prospective study of the radiological changes in hands, feet, and cervical spine in adult rheumatoid disease. *Ann Rheum Dis.* 1983;42:613-618.
34. Belt EA, Kaarela K, Lehto MU. Destruction and arthroplasties of the metatarsophalangeal joints in seropositive rheumatoid arthritis: a 20-year follow-up study. *Scand J Rheumatol.* 1998;27(3):194-196.
35. Bastias C, Henríquez H, Pellegrini M, et al. Are locking plates better than non-locking plates for treating distal tibial fractures? *Foot Ankle Surg.* 2014;20(2):115-119. doi:10.1016/j.fas.2013.12.004.
36. Vandeputte G, Steenweckx A, Mulier T, Peeraer L, Dereymaeker G. Forefoot reconstruction in rheumatoid arthritis patients: Keller-Leliévre-Hoffmann versus arthrodesis MTP-1 Hoffmann. *Foot Ankle Int.* 1999;20:438-443.
37. Rahmann H, Fagg PS. Silicone granulomatous reactions after first metatarsophalangeal joint hemiarthroplasty. *J Bone Joint Surg.* 1993;75-B:637-639.
38. Caputi RA. Synovectomy. *Clin Podiatr Med Surg.* 1988;5:249-257.
39. Nakamura H, Tanaka H, Yoshino S. Long-term results of multiple synovectomy for patients with refractory rheumatoid arthritis. Effects on disease activity and radiological progression. *Clin Exp Rheumatol.* 2004;22:151-157.
40. Vidigal E, Jacoby RK, Dixon AS, Ratliff AH, Kirkup J. The foot in chronic rheumatoid arthritis. *Ann Rheum Dis.* 1975;34:292-297.
41. Nassar J, Cracchiolo A. Complications in surgery of the foot and ankle in patients with rheumatoid arthritis. *Clin Orthop Relat Res.* 2001;(391):140-152.
42. Epstein DM, Black BS, Sherman SL. Anterior ankle arthroscopy: indications, pitfalls, and complications. *Foot Ankle Clin.* 2015;20(1):41-57.
43. Han G, Xu B, Geng C, Cheng X. Effectiveness of arthroscopy for ankle impingement syndrome. *Zhongguo Xiu Fu Chong Jian Wai Ke Za Zhi.* 2014;28(6):673-676.
44. Lelièvre J. *Podologie.* Paris, France: Expansion scientifique française; 1968.
45. Woodburn J, Barker S, Helliwell PS. A randomized controlled trial of foot orthoses in rheumatoid arthritis. *J Rheumatol.* 2002;29:1377-1383.
46. Kavlak Y, Uygur F, Korkmaz C, Bek N. Outcome of orthoses intervention in the rheumatoid foot. *Foot Ankle Int.* 2003;24:494-499.

Amputations

Robert P. Taylor and Michael Van Pelt

INTRODUCTION

Lower extremity amputation (LEA) is one of the oldest known surgical procedures. 130,000 lower extremity amputations on diabetic patients alone accounting for 5.6 per 1,000 persons with diabetes in the United States.[1] Medical advancements have significantly improved the outcome and prognosis of distal LEAs. Advancements that help the surgeon more accurately predict wound healing of distal amputations at various levels include the ability to assess various wound healing parameters, such as the patient's vascular, nutritional, and medical status. In the nonemergent setting, appropriate consultations can positively influence many of these parameters and increase the patient's healing potential following the amputation. Other advancements involve the improvements in wound care and the availability and refinements of wound healing products such as wound dressings, bioengineered tissues, and appliances such as wound vacuum systems. These products allow more distal amputations to be considered that otherwise would have required more proximal amputations in order to provide tissue coverage for closure. Advancements in the materials, methods and techniques used to manufacture prosthetic devices, have also improved functional outcomes for the lower extremity amputee.[2]

While amputation surgery is performed to remove nonviable or diseased tissue, it requires no less preoperative planning than any complex reconstructive surgical procedure. A comprehensive preoperative patient assessment is essential as well as adhering to fundamental surgical principles such as proper tissue handling, hemostasis, and appropriate closure techniques.

The initial step in the patient assessment is an overall examination to determine if infection or sepsis is present. Septic patients require emergent incision and drainage and obtaining cultures of the infected foot. The patient should be medically stabilized, and if available, an infectious disease consultation obtained. In the septic patient, the definitive level of amputation may not be performed as the initial procedure. Septic patients often require multiple debridements, and the definitive level of amputation is not considered until all nonviable tissue has been removed.[3] Prior to amputation, appropriate consultations should also be obtained to optimize the patient's medical status, maximize nutrition, control diabetes if present, and control the specific infecting organism as well.[4]

Imaging studies should include foot and ankle radiographs, CT scans or MR imaging to assess the extent of diseased, infected, and nonviable tissue involved. This information will form the foundation for surgical planning to help ensure that the surgical margins are clear of devitalized and infected tissue.

Imaging Studies

- Radiographs 3 views of foot and ankle
- MRI of foot and ankle
- CT scan

The ability of the patient to heal must also be assessed. The patient's healing capacity can be assessed by indices that were described by Dickaut and Pinzur et al., which were modifications of the original work by Wagner.[2,5] From a nutritional and immunological competence standpoint, commonly used indices are total lymphocyte count and albumin level. Generally, a patient is felt to be deficient, with regard to the needed immune and/or nutritional levels to adequately promote healing, with a total lymphocyte count of <1500/μL and an albumin level of <3.0 mg/24 hours.[2,3] A total lymphocyte count of <1500/μL indicates immune deficiency and increases the possibility of infection. A serum albumin level of 39.2 g/L or less, or a serum pre albumin level of 186 mg/L or less.[6] A total protein level of 6.0 g/dL or higher is required to assure a minimum level of tissue nutrition. None of the indices should be used singly as indicators of nutritional status. Serum prealbumin levels should be considered in all patients with a borderline or questionable nutritional competence. Normal prealbumin levels range from 6 to 35 mg/dL. Levels under 10 mg/dL are indicative of moderate to severe nutritional deficiency. The prealbumin level is not generally influenced by external factors; therefore, it can provide an accurate representation of nutritional status. The prealbumin level can also be used to monitor the effect of dietary supplementation. All patients not meeting these minimum guidelines should receive a consultation with a dietician and undergo nutritional supplementation.

Other useful laboratory studies include C-reactive protein, erythrocyte sedimentation rate (ESR), and hemoglobin levels. A hemoglobin level >10 g/dL is generally considered necessary for wound healing. Increased C-reactive protein levels can be an indicator of infection. A normal range for ESR is typically 0-22 mm/hour for men and 0-29 mm/hour for women. In a study by Lavery et al., an ESR of 60 mm/hour and a CRP level

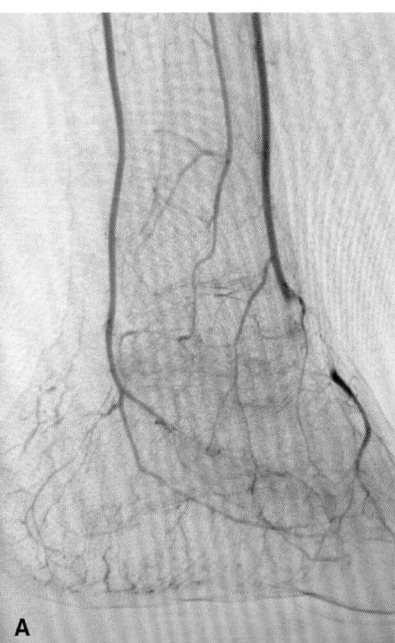 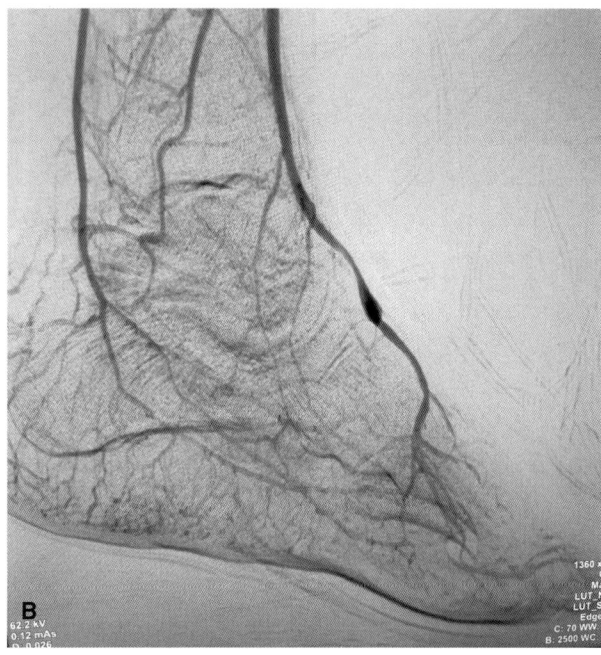

FIGURE 40.1 **A.** Arteriogram of a patient with vascular disease of the distal anterior tibial artery preprocedure. **B.** Arteriogram of the same patient showing significant increased arterial flow after vascular procedure.

of 7.9 mg/dL have been shown to be the optimal cutoff points for predicting osteomyelitis based on results of the receiver operative characteristic (ROC) analysis. The ESR threshold of 60 mm/hour demonstrated a sensitivity of 74% (95% confidence interval [CI], 67-80) and specificity of 56% (95% CI, 48-63) for osteomyelitis, whereas the CRP threshold of 7.9 mg/dL had a sensitivity of 49% (95% CI, 41-57) and specificity of 80% (95% CI, 74-86). If the ESR is < 30 mm/hour, the likelihood of osteomyelitis is low. However, if ESR is >60 mm/hour and CRP level is >7.9 mg/dL, the likelihood of osteomyelitis is high, and treatment of suspected osteomyelitis should be strongly considered.[7]

Lab Tests for Wound Healing Potential

- Total lymphocyte count >1500/μL
- Serum albumin >3.5 g/dL
- Total protein level of >6.0 g/dL
- Prealbumin level range from >10 mg/dL

The presence of peripheral vascular disease (PVD) requires evaluation and revascularization considered when possible. The leading indication for limb amputation in the United States is PVD.[6] In the patient with vascular disease, considerations include preservation of limb length, wound healing ability, and the potential for ambulation. When clinical signs and symptoms of PVD are present, a vascular evaluation and consultation is beneficial to determine the feasibility of vascular reconstruction in the hope of the patient healing with the best possible functional outcome.

Poor vascular status distally has been a primary reason for many transtibial or transfemoral amputations. However, recent advancements in cardiovascular surgery and intervention now offer the ability to improve the vascularity of the limb distally often with minimally invasive procedures, which can be done

on patients who are not viable medical candidates for invasive vascular reconstruction (Fig. 40.1).

Advancements in technology and increased affordability of those technologies now allow many community providers to obtain vascular indices that aid in the operative planning. Some of these indices include transcutaneous oxygen pressure, Doppler ultrasonography, toe pressures, ischemic index, and ankle-brachial index (ABI).

Vascular Testing for Amputation Level

- ABI, TBI, toe pressures
- Transcutaneous oxygen pressures
- Indocyanine green fluorescence imaging agent intraoperative

Intraoperative techniques are available to help determine level of adequate tissue healing. Intraoperative injection with a nonionizing radiation solution that utilizes a fluorescence imaging agent (indocyanine green) with a very short half-life can allow surgeons to repeat intraoperative perfusion assessment numerous times throughout the procedure. The imaging system can allow you to visualize the microvascular blood flow and level of soft tissue perfusion for adequate healing. This can help reduce postoperative complications such as wound dehiscence and wound necrosis.

AMPUTATION SURGICAL PRINCIPLES AND PREOPERATIVE SURGICAL PLANNING

Extent of diseased tissue, assessment of the patient's healing potential, changes in functional anatomy as a result of the amputation, and the patient's socioeconomic responsibilities should be addressed in preoperative surgical planning to

determine which level of amputation offers patient the best overall prognosis. If these parameters are not addressed, the patient can be left with a limb that is continuously prone to ulceration and infection or is not shaped well to accommodate an orthotic or prosthetic device. The complications of ulceration, infection, and deformity have caused many surgeons to move to more proximal transtibial or transfemoral amputations and abandon partial foot or foot amputations.

The primary objective of LEA surgery should be to remove all diseased tissue while maintaining a functional stump.[8] The benefits of preserving a portion of the foot include the ability to stand and walk for short distances without an orthotic or prosthetic device, and for those who have a preexisting contralateral limb amputation, the ability to transfer with less effort and requiring less oxygen consumption with activities.[9]

Amputation Goals
- Remove abscess.
- Remove nonviable tissue and bone.
- Maintain a functional stump.
- Balance the foot.

Amputation Principle Hints
- Preserve length.
- Correct equinus.
- Biomechanically balance the foot.
- Remove bony prominences.

FUNCTIONAL ANALYSIS OF THE ANATOMY

When performing a partial foot amputation, you must adhere to certain biomechanical tenets. The surgeon should attempt to preserve the greatest length possible in the foot. The ability to preserve limb length, functional segments, and joints helps reduce energy expenditure. Preserving a functional segment can help with shoe fit after amputation. If the foot is shortened through amputation, the musculature responsible for dorsiflexion and plantar flexion must be rebalanced to compensate for the shorter lever arm acting on the triceps surae. If a resultant equinus is present, the surgeon should consider performing a tendo-Achilles lengthening or tenotomy.[10,11] If the amputation is performed at the level of the Lisfranc joint or at a more proximal level, there will be disruption of the primary inverters and everters of the foot and balance between these should be reestablished.[4]

INCISION PLACEMENT AND TISSUE HANDLING

Several factors are considered when determining the appropriate incision placement for the definitive amputation. First and foremost, all diseased tissue must be removed until the remaining surface appears to be clear and viable.[3] When able, the weight-bearing areas should be covered with healthy skin that is specifically adapted for weight bearing.[4] The surgeon should plan incisions parallel to the relaxed skin tension lines if possible. Anatomic dissection and proper tissue handling is essential in preventing wound complications.[11]

HEMOSTASIS

A tourniquet can be placed on the limb prophylactically and used on a discretionary basis.[6] The use of a tourniquet until wound closer has not been shown to have a detrimental effect on healing following surgery.[3] The authors recommend a tourniquet not be used in patients who have recently undergone vascular surgery restorative procedures to the affected limb. A tourniquet can occlude the vessels that have recently undergone recannulization. Blood vessels should be cauterized or ligated; however, efforts should be made to limit the amount of absorbable suture utilized in the operative wound. Frequent lavage with cool saline and positioning the patient in a slight Trendelenburg may assist with hemostasis.[11]

CARTILAGE REMOVAL

Amputation surgeons differ on their opinions regarding removing cartilage at the level of amputation vs leaving it intact. Those that choose to remove the cartilage claim getting down to bleeding surface of bone leads to a significant improvement in tissue healing.[10] Definitive reasons for removal of cartilage include the presence of gout, dysvascular cartilage, or infection. Those that prefer leaving the cartilage intact claim the cartilage and subchondral bone serve as a barrier to infection. Another cited advantage to leaving the cartilage intact is that it allows shear mobility of the soft tissues over the bone, and breakdown of the tissue is less apt to occur.[3]

WOUND CLOSURE

When a wound is closed after debridement, a nonreactive material such as monofilament suture can be used, with no tension placed on the wound edges.[11] The surgeon should avoid inversion of the skin margins to help prevent delayed healing or would dehiscence. The optimal skin closure should be end to end with direct approximation of the skin margins of the wound and slight eversion of the skin margins. Sutures, which are too tight and too few in number, are also potential causes of delayed healing, which may lead to wound dehiscence.[11]

In partial foot amputations, the foot may need to be debrided multiple times prior to wound closure until the wound is clean. Once the surgeon is convinced the wound is clean, a delayed primary closure can be performed. When in doubt, the surgeon should leave the wound open.[11] Delayed primary closure significantly shortens healing time that otherwise without closure may take many months of granulation and wound contracture. Delayed primary closures can be performed under local anesthetic. The cost and potential morbidity of an additional procedure can be significantly offset by the reduction in healing time. Even if the wound cannot be closed entirely, converting a large open wound to a small open wound offers the same benefit.[3]

Split-thickness skin grafts may be used to complete wound coverage or decrease tension on the wound closure, while maintaining limb length. When placed over soft tissue, these grafts can function quite well; however, often these skin-grafted areas do not tolerate the axial and shear stresses within the prosthesis and may require removal at a later date.[6]

POSTOPERATIVE MANAGEMENT

With any foot amputation, it is very important that meticulous attention is given to the initial and subsequent postoperative bandages that are applied after the amputation. It is the authors' experience that many complications involving the operative wound as well as new wounds are caused when the initial dressing or subsequent dressing changes are not applied carefully. Improper bandaging may significantly increase healing time as well as produce severely delayed or nonhealing wounds over poorly vascularized areas.

Compression dressings, when applied appropriately, can help control excessive postoperative edema. The compressive bandage should be applied in concentric layers utilizing increased compression distally at the level of the digits, and decreased compression proximally. It is important to have adequate gauze coverage to minimize any direct contact of inelastic materials on the skin. The Jones compression dressing is an excellent adjunct in the postoperative care. Concentric layers of 4-6 in cast padding and 4-6 in elastic wraps are utilized to immobilize the foot and lower leg in a supportive, yet very comfortable surgical dressing that controls postoperative edema.[11]

Resting an injured area or surgical site postoperatively for the first several days not only prevents excessive bleeding but also promotes healing of damaged tissue. Simple elevation of the operative limb can be the single most important factor in controlling excessive edema and preventing other complications.[11]

Mobility enhancement devices such as canes, walkers, and crutches offer amputees assistance and stability during ambulation; however, they increase oxygen consumption, heart rate, and energy expenditure due to the strength required to use these devices. Careful consideration must be taken when planning the postoperative course of weight bearing and prosthetic management in high-risk individuals.[2]

Advances in prosthetic materials and technology have enabled the creation of highly functional prosthetic devices. It is important to remember that creating a quality device requires an experienced prosthetist in the management of amputation particularly those with Chopart or Syme level amputations. The surgeon must ensure that a qualified prosthetist is available to ensure a well-fitting, functional device.[2]

A physical therapy consultation for transfers and assisted ambulation should be considered as well as a consultation for psychosocial and emotional support. Support groups for people who have undergone amputations and discussion with someone who has undergone amputation can be invaluable.

Care does not end after the amputation. Amputees need to be under the care of a surgeon for the remainder of their life to periodically evaluate the remaining limb and the prosthetic device to determine appropriate timing for palliative care and prosthetic replacement.

DIGITAL AMPUTATIONS

HALLUX

Traditionally, a racquet type incision is made with the arm of the racquet oriented medially with the two diverging semi-elliptical incisions progressing around the base of the hallux connecting laterally (Figs. 40.2 and 40.3A-C). The arm of the racquet allows for extension to evaluate the first metatarsophalangeal joint and head of the first metatarsal. When adequate skin coverage is available, and the diseased or infected tissue does not extend proximally, the proximal metaphysis of the proximal phalanx should be preserved. This phalangeal base is the attachment site of the abductor hallucis, the extensor hallucis brevis, the adductor hallucis, the flexor hallucis brevis, the sesamoids, and the plantar fascia. Because the sesamoids bear approximately one-third of the weight in the forefoot, they should be preserved whenever possible. When the base of the hallux must be sacrificed, it is surgeon's preference as to whether or not to denude the cartilage from the head of the first metatarsal or leave it intact. Some advocate denuding the distal inferior cartilage and attaching the tendons to the capsule by means of tenodesis as well as arthrodesis of the sesamoids in their correct position.[4] All nerves and tendons should be incised sharply proximally and allowed to retract proximally. Layered closure of the tissue and skin should be done as previously discussed.

LESSER DIGIT

The most common indications for amputation of the middle three digits are injury, deformity, sepsis, and gangrene. Amputation of just one digit, particularly the second, can have an adverse effect on the adjacent digits, which drift into the empty space.[4] If you perform an isolated digit amputation, it is imperative that the patient wear a spacer postoperatively, and with

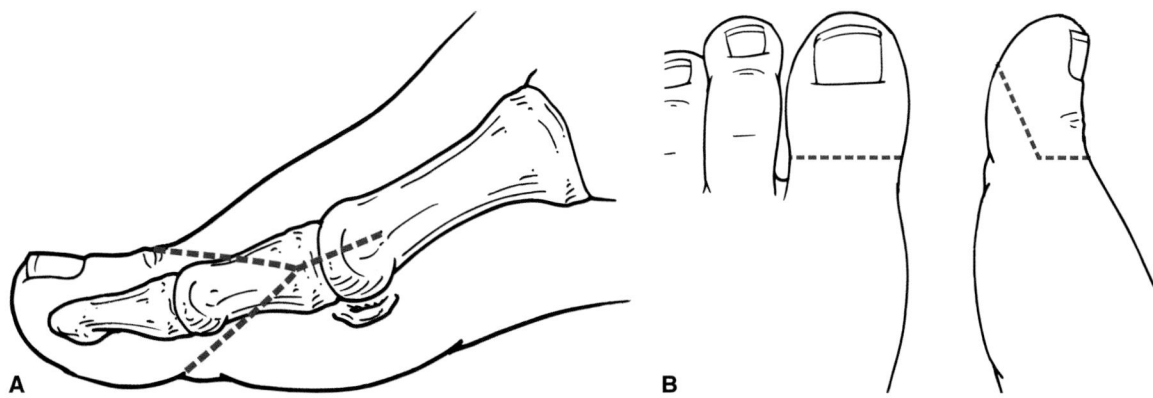

FIGURE 40.2 **A.** Racquet type incision can be used for total or partial amputation of the hallux. **B.** Example of incision for partial hallux amputation creating plantar flap to aid in closure.

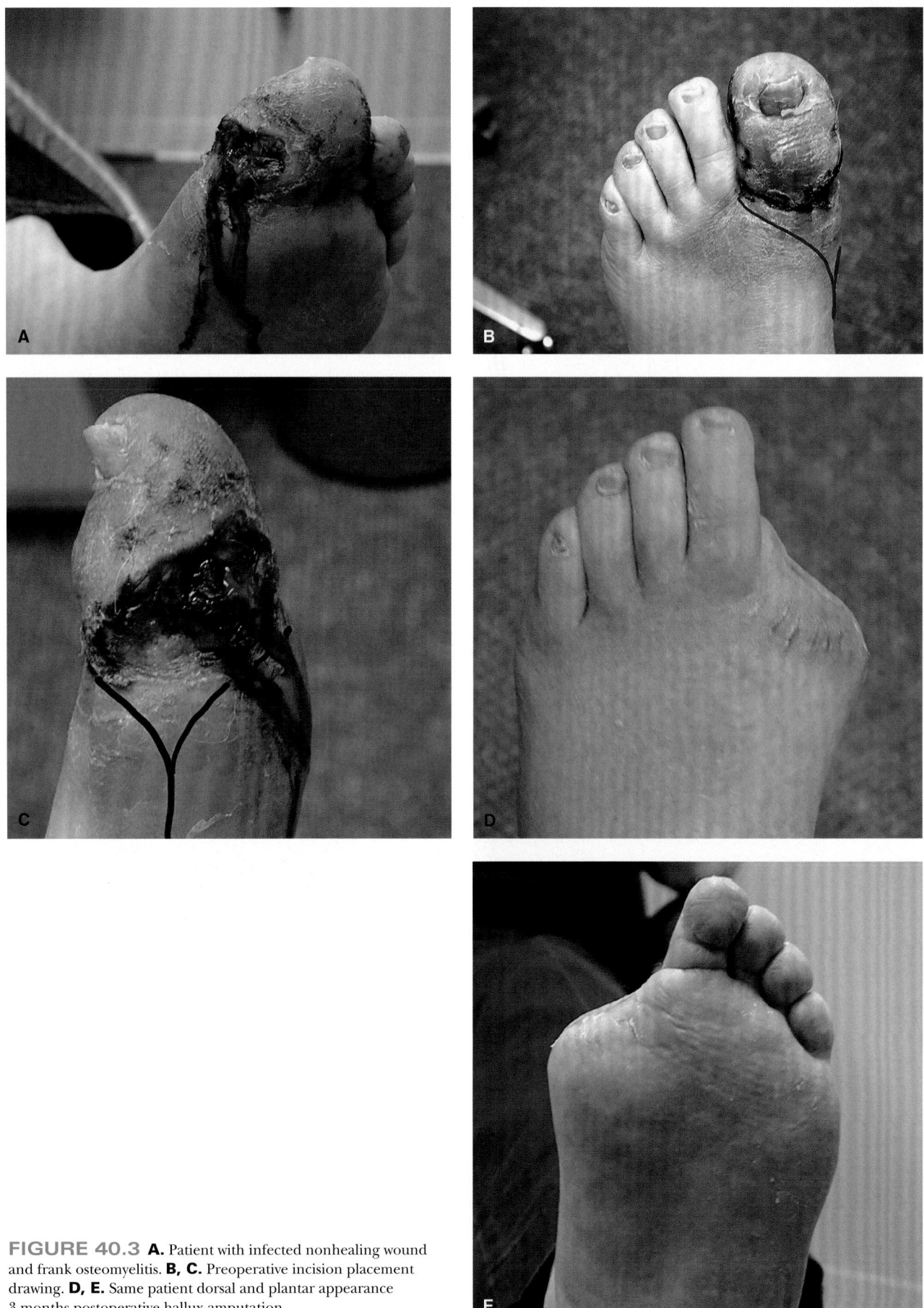

FIGURE 40.3 A. Patient with infected nonhealing wound and frank osteomyelitis. **B, C.** Preoperative incision placement drawing. **D, E.** Same patient dorsal and plantar appearance 3 months postoperative hallux amputation.

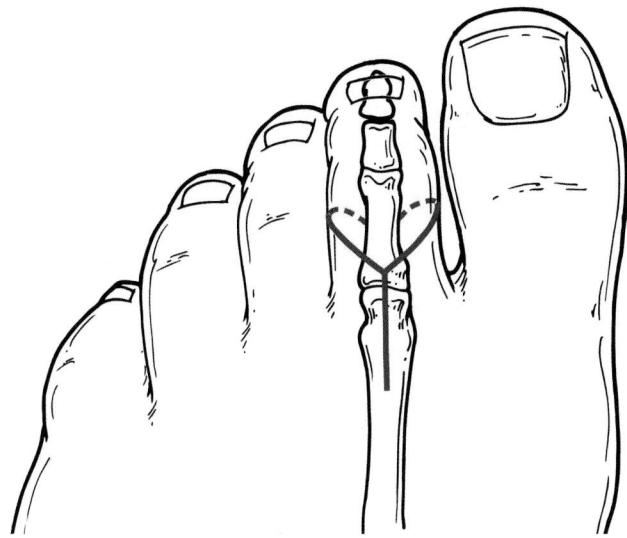

FIGURE 40.4 Incision placement for isolated partial or total lesser digital amputation. Incision can also be carried proximally for isolated partial or total ray amputation.

second digit amputations, this is very important as a rapidly progressing bunion deformity may ensue.

A distal Syme type of incision or racquet type incision works well for digital amputations. Two semi-elliptical incisions are made starting midline on the dorsal aspect of the digit joining

plantarly and distally in a transverse fashion (Fig. 40.4A). The start of the incisions is determined by the level of the amputation. If the digit is being disarticulated and inspection of the metatarsal phalangeal joint is indicated, a midline arm can be made to convert the incision to a racquet type incision. If the amputation is being performed because of an interphalangeal joint lesion, the contralateral incision to the lesion side can be made more distal to create a flap for tissue coverage (Fig. 40.5A-C). Incision placement may vary and the surgeon must always take into account creating a flap to allow closure if possible (Fig. 40.5D-G). Nerves and tendons should be incised sharply proximally and allowed to retract proximally.[8]

RAY AMPUTATIONS

The primary indication for a ray resection is to remove infection or nonviable soft tissue or bone that involves the phalanges and the metatarsal. In general, the entire ray is not removed to allow for salvage of the base of the metatarsal. If the infection extends into the base of the metatarsal, and the base must be sacrificed, this can cause instability to the Lisfranc joint. This instability in the neuropathic patient can result in the development of Charcot osteoarthropathy.[3]

In general, fourth and fifth ray amputations tend to be more predictable and have a better prognosis than medial ray amputations. Experience has shown that partial fourth and fifth ray amputations may be performed without significant

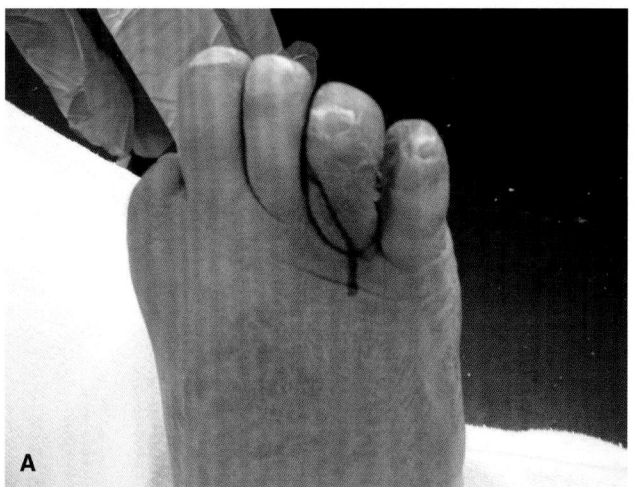

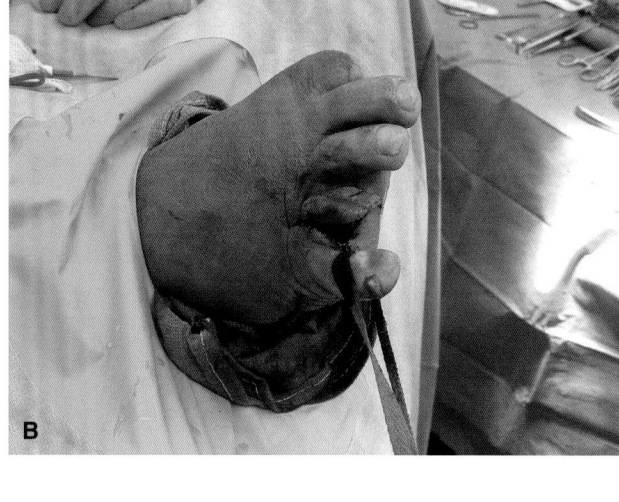

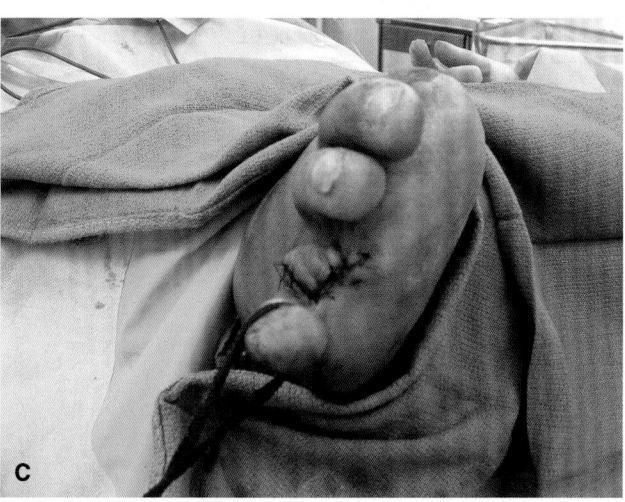

FIGURE 40.5 **A.** Offset racquet incision to create a flap medial for coverage of an ulcer on lateral fourth toe. **B.** Postamputation with adequate tissue for closure. **C.** Closed operative area.

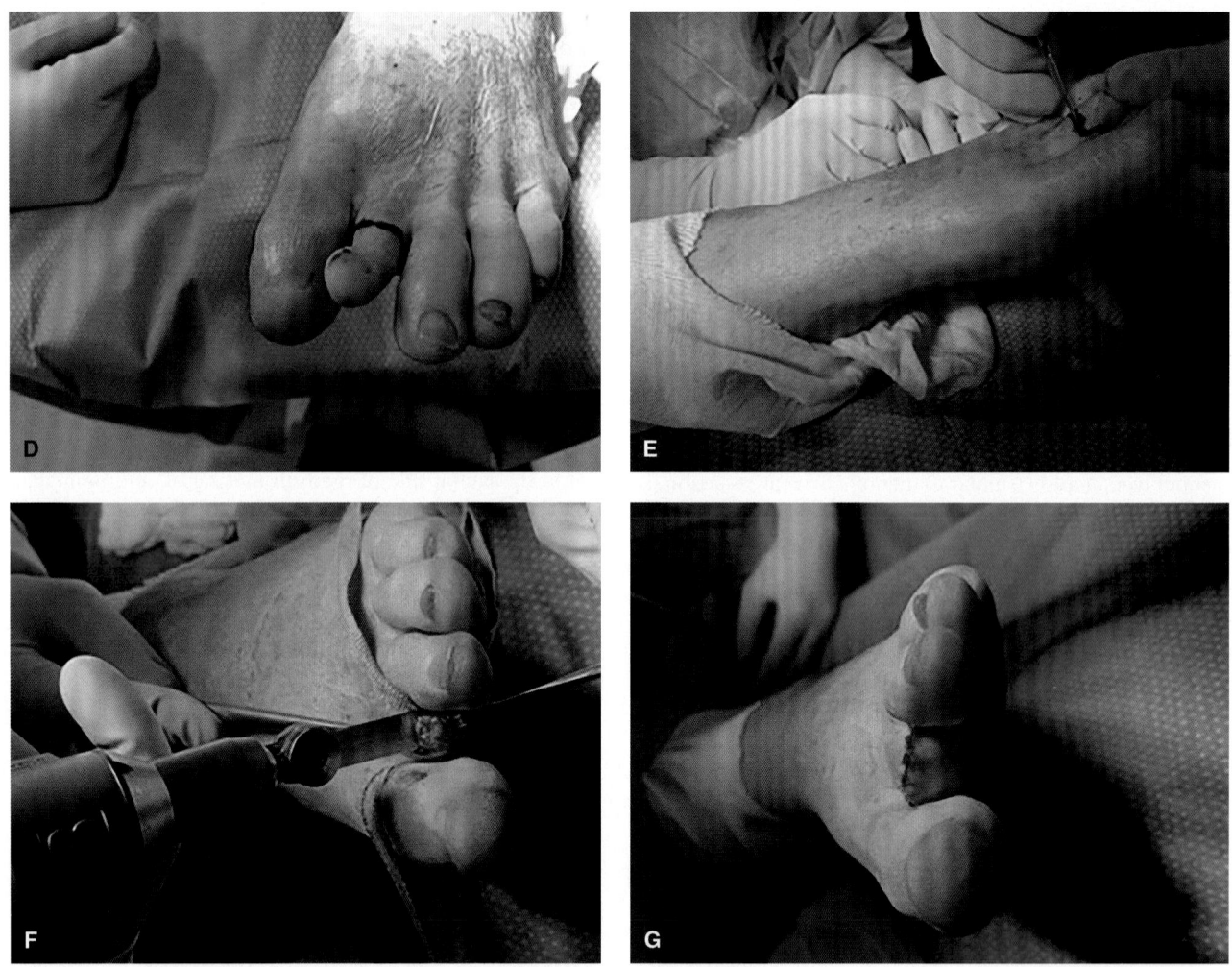

FIGURE 40.5 (*Continued*) **D,E:** Surgical incision plan to create plantar flap for closure.
F: removing portion of proximal phalanx with power instrumentation. **G:** closure of the surgical wound.

compromise of foot function. When choosing between length and width of the foot, length is preferred.[3] Foot function may be significantly altered with a first ray resection and orthotic devices can be more difficult to fit. Transfer lesions are the most common sequelae of ray amputations. If removal of three or more metatarsals is anticipated, the surgeon should consider a transmetatarsal amputation (TMA).[3]

Regardless of which ray is resected, the surgeon should adhere to basic surgical tenants. As discussed earlier, these include delicate management of soft tissues, debridement of all necrotic or infected tissue, prevention of dead space, and suturing without undue tension.

Authors' Preferred Amputation Level

- Transmetatarsal amputation
- Digital amputation

FIRST RAY

Traditionally, a racquet type incision similar to that of a hallux amputation is made with the arm of the racquet oriented medially with the two diverging semi-elliptical incisions progressing around the base of the hallux connecting laterally. The arm of the racquet allows for extension proximally to evaluate the first metatarsal to determine appropriate level of resection. Reasonable measures should be considered to salvage as much of the first ray as possible. These measures include sesamoidectomy, extensor tenotomy, and Achilles tendon lengthening (TAL) procedures.

If a partial first ray amputation is indicated, and the diseased tissue seems to be localized to the metatarsal head and base of the proximal phalanx of the hallux, one of the authors has applied an external mini-fixator to maintain the length of the ray while resecting the head of the metatarsal and base of the proximal phalanx. While there will still be significant shortening of the ray, this can help lessen some of that shortening as more granulation tissue is allowed to form in the site acting as a spacer.

Unless it is significantly infected, leaving the hallux on a partial first ray amputation serves as a vestigial digit and can help to function as a spacer in a shoe. The toe looses normal function, but cosmetically, the foot may appear close to normal. When the hallux is amputated, the surgeon can anticipate hammering of the second digit. The use of a buttress pad or toe sling can help minimize the effects of the hammering, as well as appropriate extra depth shoes.

SINGLE RAY RESECTION OF THE SECOND, THIRD, OR FOURTH METATARSAL

With internal ray resection, an incision is made dorsal and plantar that splits the foot and often circumscribes the involved digit. This incision allows inspection of all of the tissue planes to ensure removal of all infected tissue. If the surgeon is confident that all necrotic and infected tissue has been removed, the plantar incision can be closed leaving the dorsal incision to granulate in or delayed primary closure. When amputation surgical principles are adhered to, particularly closing down the dead space and all diseased tissue is removed, healing often occurs quickly and the patient can maintain close to normal foot function.

FIFTH RAY RESECTION

A racquet type incision, similar to that of a first ray resection, is made with the arm of the racquet oriented laterally with the two diverging semi-elliptical incisions progressing around the base of the fifth digit connecting medially. The arm of the racquet allows for extension proximally to evaluate the fifth metatarsal to determine appropriate level of resection. In a fifth ray amputation, it is desirable to leave the base of the fifth metatarsal to keep the attachment of the peroneus brevis intact, as well as

providing structural integrity to the Lisfranc joint. Obviously, if the diseased or infected bone extends into the base of the fifth metatarsal, the entire metatarsal should be removed; however, this can destabilize the Lisfranc joint triggering a Charcot osteoarthropathy breakdown. Stabilizing the fourth metatarsal-cuboid joint with pins or screws may reduce this instability.

TRANSMETATARSAL AMPUTATIONS

TMAs are often performed when more distal amputations of digits have failed, or plantar head metatarsal ulcerations have progressed to osteomyelitis and the patient is not a good candidate for a single ray resection.

The incision is initiated on the dorsum of the foot across the metatarsal bases, from the medial side of the first metatarsal to the lateral side of the fifth metatarsal, and immediately deepened to bone. Any vascular structures should be cauterized or tied as deemed necessary. Tendons are distracted, incised to bone, and allowed to retract proximally. A plantar flap is created by extending the dorsal transverse incision at ~90-degree angles along the medial and lateral aspects of the foot, then distally across the sulcus at the level of the distal metatarsals (Fig. 40.6A-F). If a plantar ulcer is present, the surgeon may

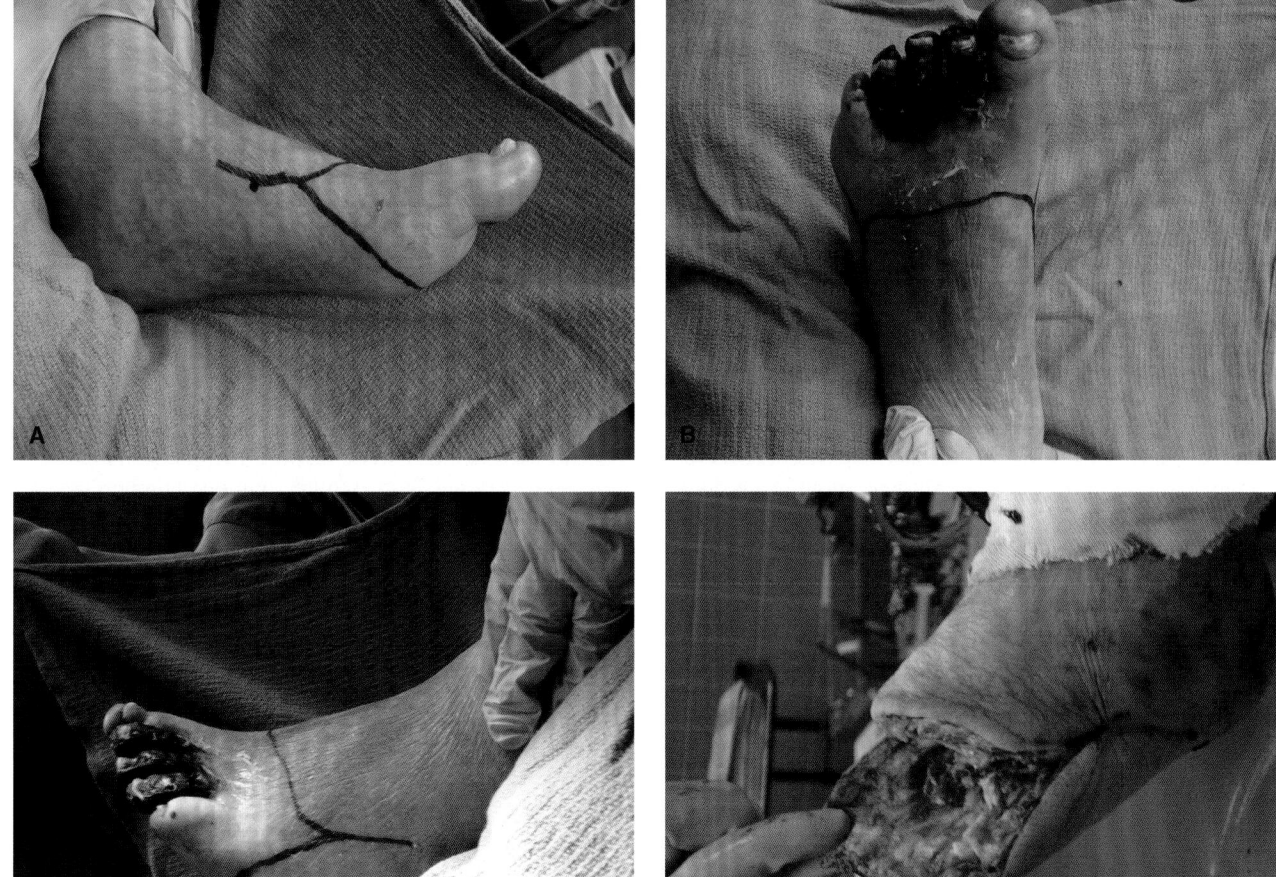

FIGURE 40.6 A. Incision placement for TMA medial view. **B.** Incision placement for TMA dorsal view. **C.** Incision placement for TMA lateral view. **D.** Clinical view of TMA after diseased tissue has been débrided.

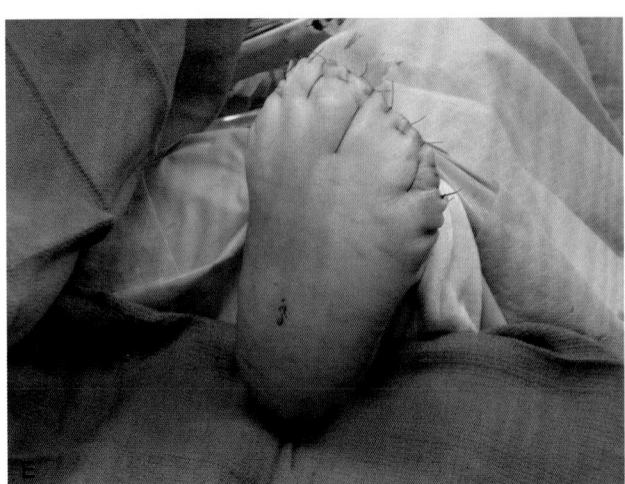
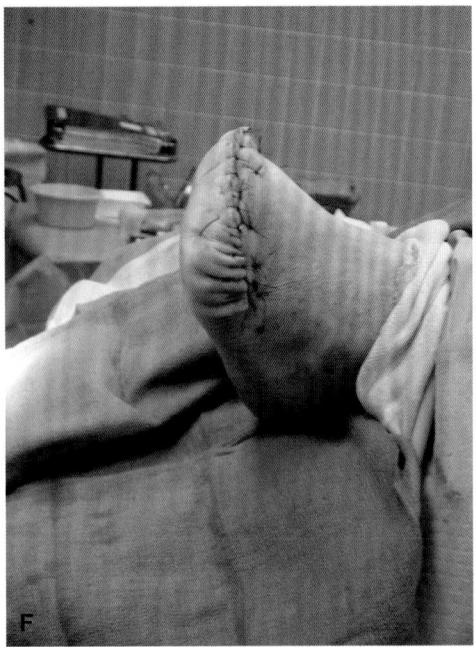

FIGURE 40.6 (*Continued*) **E.** Closed TMA plantar view. **F.** Closed TMA dorsolateral view.

compromise the plantar flap by excising the ulceration using a wedge incision as described by Sanders, with the base at the sulcus and the apex proximal to the ulcer[12] (Fig. 40.7). When this is closed, it takes on a T-incision appearance.

The periosteum can be stripped from the metatarsal bases, and the metatarsal osteotomized at the proximal metaphyseal-diaphyseal area. Meticulous care and attention must be taken to create a smooth metatarsal parabola. The second metatarsal should maintain the longest length with the third, first, fourth, and fifth following in that order. The metatarsals should be beveled from dorsal-distal to plantar-proximal to avoid leaving a sharp edge of resected bone plantarly where the patient will bear weight. The metatarsals should be cut in a metatarsal protrusion similar to normal metatarsal protrusion. Each metatarsal should be cut slightly shorter in a staircase fashion. The most common metatarsal to cause problems is the fifth; therefore, it should be cut shorter and beveled laterally. The first metatarsal is beveled medially, and the fifth metatarsal is beveled laterally. A handheld rasp or reamer may be used to smooth off the edges of the remaining metatarsal bases. The insertions of the tibialis anterior, tibialis posterior, and the peroneal tendons should be left intact when possible, as varus and/or equinus deformity of the stump may occur if their insertions are released. The extensor digitorum longus tendons may be sutured into the peroneus tertius or the lateral dorsal fascia. This can help negate potential varus deformity, especially in the absence of peroneus tertius on examination of the opposite side.[4] The metatarsals are dissected and removed from the plantar flap, taking care to preserve vascular structures. Any loose remaining tendinous or capsular structures are dissected away. The flap is then brought over the metatarsal ends and closed in layers. If there is concern of any dead space or bleeding, a Penrose or suction drain may be used, to prevent hematoma or seroma formation, but this is usually not necessary with this amputation.

Postoperatively, a compression dressing is applied with a posterior splint or below knee cast to protect the wound from

tension associated with range of motion of the ankle joint. The patient should be kept nonweight bearing until the skin is healed. The authors' experience is this usually occurs ~4 weeks postoperatively. Physical therapy is helpful for instruction on transfers, aerobic conditioning, and upper body strengthening.

Wound failures can occur, and if muscle imbalance occurs, the foot remains at risk for new ulcer formation over any residual bony prominences, particularly plantar-laterally. If reulceration occurs, it should be treated similar to any nonhealing wound or ulceration, and consideration should be made to possibly readdress tendon balancing issues. These include a revisional TAL or tenotomy of the Achilles tendon and transfer or split transfer of the tibialis anterior tendon.

LISFRANC AMPUTATION

Lisfranc amputation involves disarticulating the foot at the tarsometatarsal joint. The incision design is similar to that of the TMA, just oriented more proximal on the foot (Fig. 40.8A-E). It is a viable choice if the amount required for adequate resection eliminates a TMA as a surgical option. As with most amputations, normal biomechanics of the foot are altered, and subsequent equinovarus deformities of the foot have been seen postoperatively with the Lisfranc amputation.[13] This resulting deformity is due to the shortened lever arm and unantagonized function of the tibialis anterior and Achilles tendon function. An attempt to prevent these complications can be done by lengthening or tenotomy of the Achilles, and transferring the tibialis posterior to the third cuneiform.[5,10] An alternative surgical option is to leave the base of the fifth metatarsal intact with the peroneus brevis attachment. Another adjunctive procedure is leaving a portion of the insertion of the tibialis anterior and peroneus longus tendons intact as they insert on either side of the first metatarsocuneiform joint, as well as leaving a small portion of the second metatarsal base to serve as a keystone.

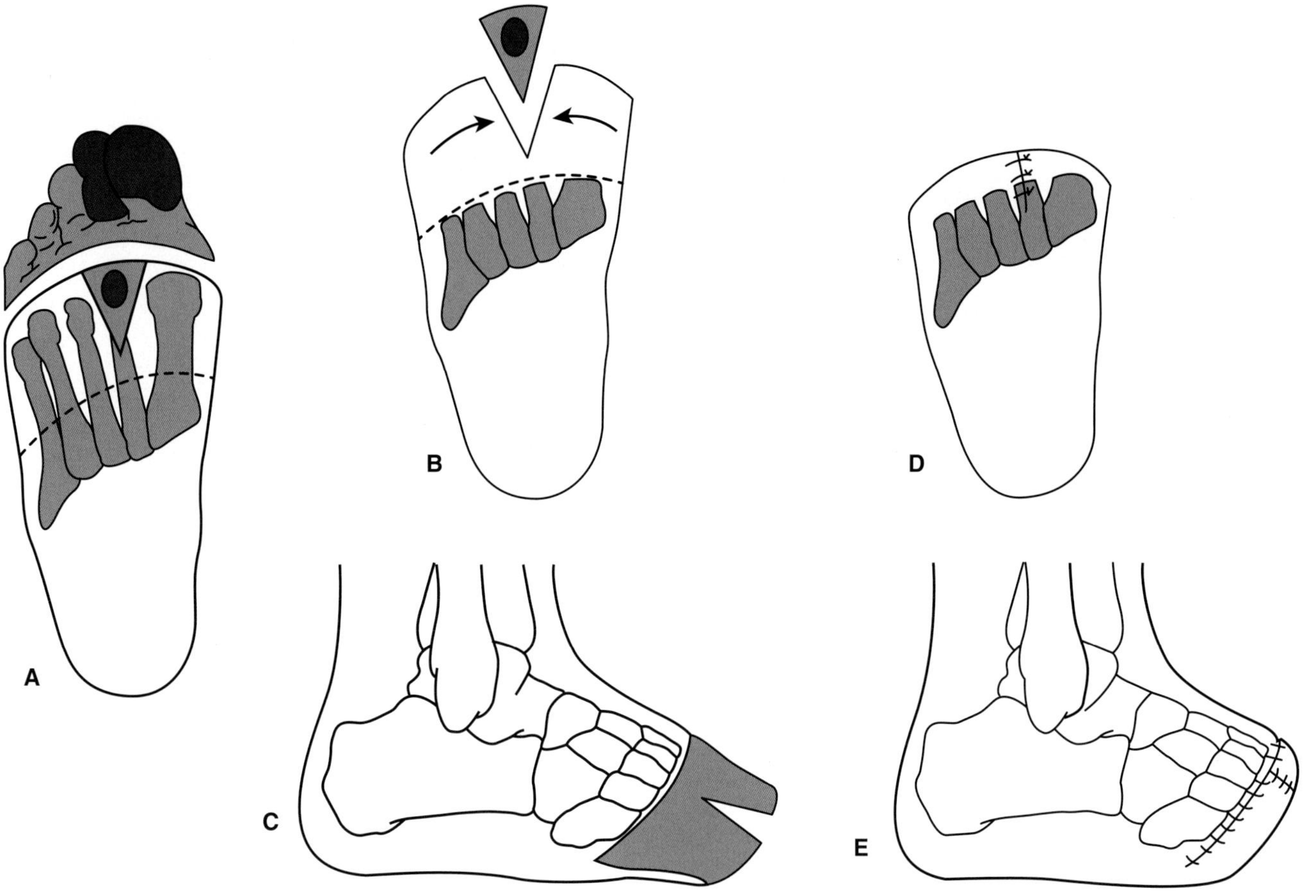

FIGURE 40.7 **A-E.** Sanders method for preservation of the transmetatarsal flap in the presence of plantar ulceration. (Redrawn from Sanders LJ. Transmetatarsal amputation and midfoot amputations. *Clin Podiatr Med Surg.* 1997;14:741-762.)

Despite keeping the peroneus brevis intact, the pull of the tibialis anterior can still produce a varus deformity; therefore, some surgeons transfer the tibialis anterior into the lateral cuneiform or cuboid to provide for a more balanced foot.[3] While these transfers may improve the balance and alignment of the foot, they do require increased tissue dissection that could potentially complicate healing.

CHOPART AMPUTATION

Chopart amputation is the disarticulation of the foot at the midtarsal joint between the talonavicular and the calcaneocuboid joints. Many abandoned the Chopart amputation as a definitive procedure citing complications such as inevitable equinovarus deformity and subsequent ulceration, or

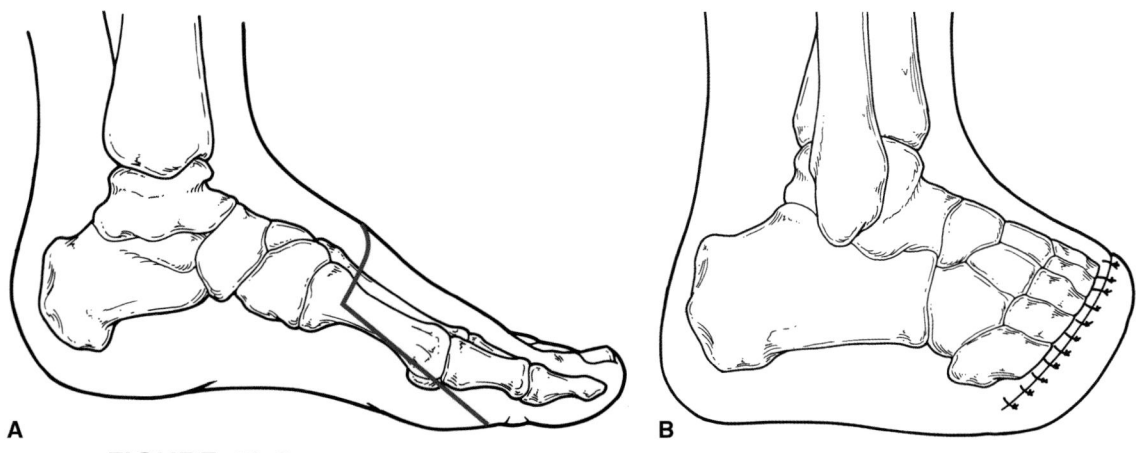

FIGURE 40.8 A, B. Typical incision placement for Lisfranc amputation and closure.

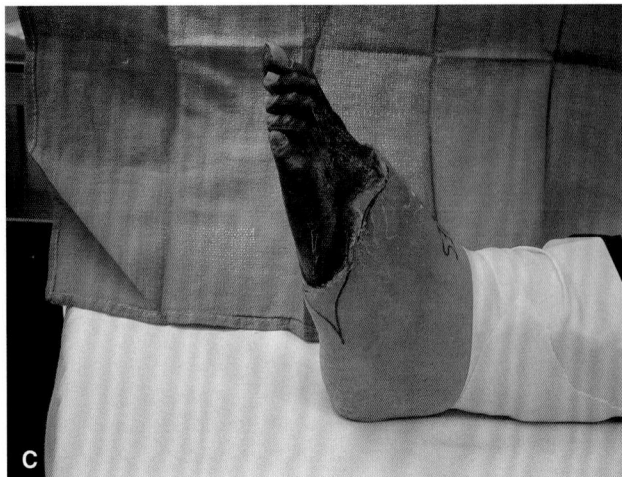

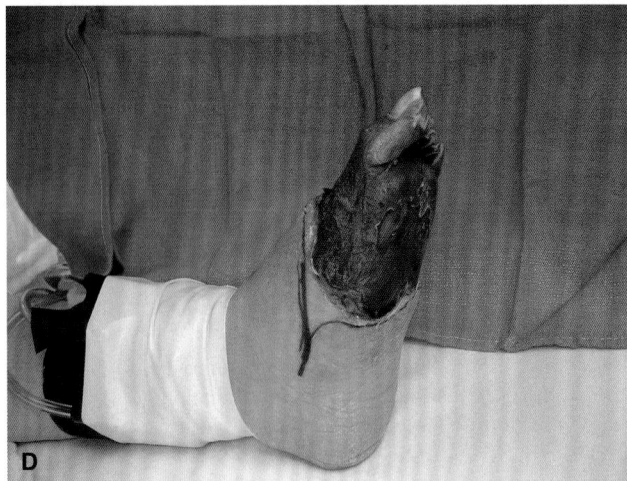

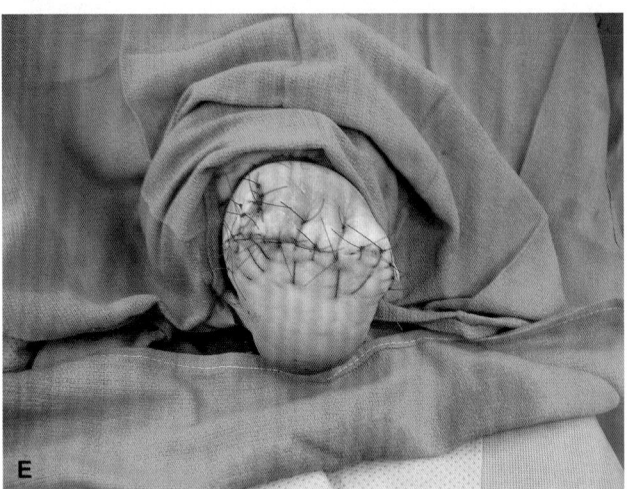

FIGURE 40.8 (*Continued*) **C, D.** Clinical images and incision placement of gangrenous foot requiring Lisfranc amputation. **E.** Closure following Lisfranc amputation.

difficulty with prosthetic fitting.[13] The equinovarus deformity complication is the result of a shortened distal lever arm and an unopposed gastroc-soleus complex posteriorly and the anterior tibial tendon medially. Despite its bad reputation in previous literature, more recent studies, as well as validation of contemporary amputation surgeons, have shown the Chopart amputation to be a viable option to more proximal procedures.[14,15] The recent increase in utilization and the improved outcomes are primarily due to adjunctive

procedures such as tendon transfers, TAL or tenotomy, and improved prosthetic devices.

The surgical approach is similar to that of the TMA just more proximal on the foot (Fig. 40.9A-B). The tibialis anterior, tibialis posterior, and the peroneal tendons should be tenotomized distally and tagged for possible transfer. If a TAL procedure is going to be performed, it should be done prior to disarticulating the foot at the midtarsal joint as this provides a lever arm to obtain lengthening of the Achilles tendon. If the TAL is performed after

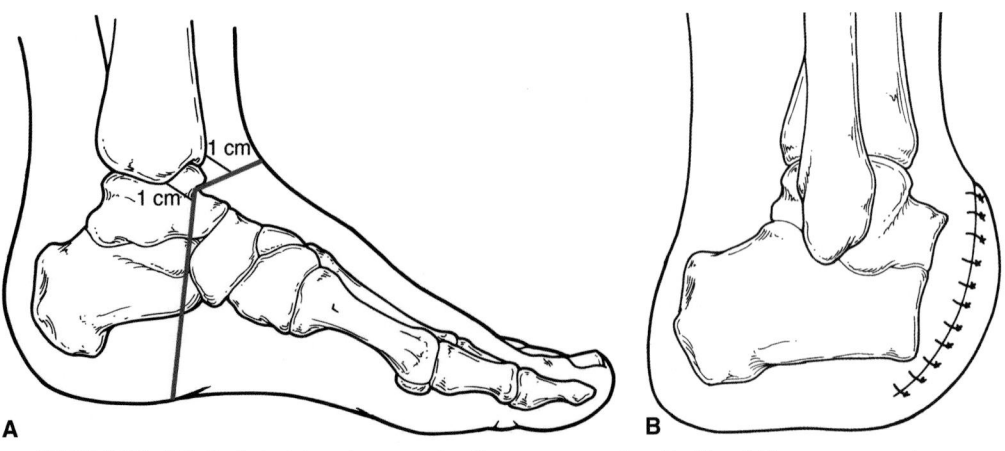

FIGURE 40.9 **A.** Incision placement for Chopart amputation. **B.** Closed Chopart amputation.

the forefoot is disarticulated, it can be very difficult to dorsiflex the hindfoot to gain length of the Achilles tendon. Despite doing a TAL, equinus has been still shown to develop; therefore, a tenotomy of the Achilles tendon or even excising a 2-3 cm portion of the Achilles tendon have been utilized and recommended. Experience has shown that loss of Achilles tendon function has not caused significant problems since these patients are going to be ambulating in an ankle-foot orthosis (AFO).[16] After the Achilles tendon has been addressed, the foot can now be disarticulated at the talonavicular and calcaneocuboid joints. Distal tension is applied to tendon and nerve structures, which are cut proximally and allowed to retract.

Once the distal tissues and bone are removed, the Achilles tendon addressed, adjunctive tendon balancing procedures can be considered. The tibialis anterior tendon can be transferred into or through the lateral neck of the talus. In an effort to further balance the foot, Cohen et al. have recommended also transferring the peroneal tendons to the lateral wall of the calcaneus instead of simple transaction and allowing them to retract.[10,17] Other described adjunctive procedures include contouring the anterior calcaneus and talus, and arthrodesis of the ankle and subtalar using an intramedullary nail. Advocates claim this method provides rigid control to the rearfoot while prohibiting posterior calcaneal extension.[18]

Besides the previously stated benefits of foot amputations over leg amputations, the Chopart amputation can also provide the amputee multiaxial movement when the patient is fitted with a multiaxial prosthesis. Long-term success of this amputation is dependent on patient compliance and follow-up, as well as the skill of the prosthetic and the quality of the prosthetic the patient is fitted with.[9]

SYME AMPUTATION

The Syme amputation is a disarticulation of the foot at the ankle joint. This amputation may be employed in any patient suffering from a wide range of foot and ankle conditions including congenital deformities, trauma/crush injury, soft tissue and osseous malignancies of the foot, ischemia, frostbite, and osteomyelitis. Today, the procedure is primarily performed in patients suffering from gangrene, severe Charcot osteoarthropathy, nonhealing dysvascular ulcers, and nonsalvageable diabetic foot infections.[11,19]

The main advantages of the Syme procedure are a potentially fully weight-bearing stump of near normal length, a swift return to functional activity, and decreased mortality when compared to transtibial amputation.[2] This can be explained by the functional advantage Syme amputees have as ambulation will not require the same level of energy as in patients with higher levels of amputation.[20,21] Another advantage of Syme amputation is the durability of the stump. Below knee amputates frequently suffer stump irritation from prosthesis use; however, the biomechanical and tissue features of the plantar heel pad make this complication uncommon with Syme amputees. Also, the almost full-length extremity can be used for emergency ambulation and transfers for daily life activities.[2,22]

The reasons for underutilization of the Syme procedure are similar to that of the Chopart amputation, which are the perceptions that wound healing is routinely difficult and prolonged, varus, cavovarus, or equinus deformities are inevitable, or that the residual stump is prone to ulceration or difficult to fit with a prosthesis.[2] Many of these concerns, however, have

been greatly diminished with the use of adjunctive surgical procedures, advances in wound healing modalities, prognostic tests and evaluations, and the improvement in prosthetic devices and materials. These advances have caused a recent resurgence by amputation surgeons to utilize the Syme amputation.

Contraindications to performing a Syme procedure are similar to all amputations including inadequate blood flow to the area, infection, ascending cellulitis, lymphangitis, severely immunocompromised patients, or malnutrition. An intact, ulcer-free heel pad is paramount to the success of this procedure as lesions of the heel pad should be considered a significant contraindication. Modifications to the standard incisional approach have been described using an anterior ankle flap; however, the anterior ankle flap does not contain the same shock-absorbing qualities of the plantar fat pad and may result in an uncomfortable stump that may be more prone to irritation or possible ulceration.[11] With any of these contraindications, a transtibial amputation should be considered.[2,3,11]

Wagner recommended the procedure be performed in two stages, first disarticulating the foot, then a subsequent procedure for removal of the malleoli and fashioning the stump for prosthesis use.[10] Pinzur et al. performed the amputation utilizing the single-stage technique.[23,24,25,26,27] Most contemporary amputation surgeons advocate performing the procedure in a single stage. In either instance, it is crucial that the procedure be performed in an area free of infection.[22] The single-stage approach includes an anterior ankle incision to essentially connect the tips of the malleoli and a conjoined transverse incision across the more anterior portion of the plantar heel pad (Fig. 40.10A-B). The exact location of these incisions is determined in part by the amount of viable tissue remaining at the heel pad, which must be intact. Because most of these patients have diseased or infected anterior portions of their foot, contamination might be prevented by disarticulating the foot at the midtarsal joint, and starting with a "clean hind foot" section. After resection of the talus, the calcaneus is then dissected free from the Achilles tendon and surrounding soft tissues. Meticulous care must be taken not to pierce or buttonhole the skin on the posterior heel. Care should also be given to preserve the medial arterial vessels. Placing a Steinman pin in the talus and calcaneus and using a joystick technique can significantly improve stability and control during this crucial portion of the dissection (Fig. 40.10C). The malleoli are then remodeled to surgeon's preference ranging from leaving them intact or obliquely removing portions to create a tapering stump, or a more aggressive resection as originally described (Fig. 40.10D). Resection of the cartilage from the tibial plafond is to surgeon's discretion as well. Tendon ends and redundant or nonviable soft tissue is resected and the plantar flap is fashioned for closure. Soft tissue anchors or drill holes are placed in the distal anterior tibia to secure the heel pad in proper position with nonabsorbable sutures (Fig. 40.10F). Tension-free closure is required; however, too long of a plantar flap will result in an unstable or "floppy stump." Final closure is achieved over a drain (Fig. 40.10H).

Postoperatively, the first several weeks are critical as it is during this time that the wound is most at risk for dehiscence, slough, or other related complications. During this time, hematoma and seroma formation are common occurrences and must be managed appropriately.[2] A Jones compression type dressing with a fiberglass splint works well for these patients. Patients should remain nonweight bearing until the sutures are removed at ~3 weeks postoperatively. At this time, some surgeons will place patients in a total contact walking cast for partial weight

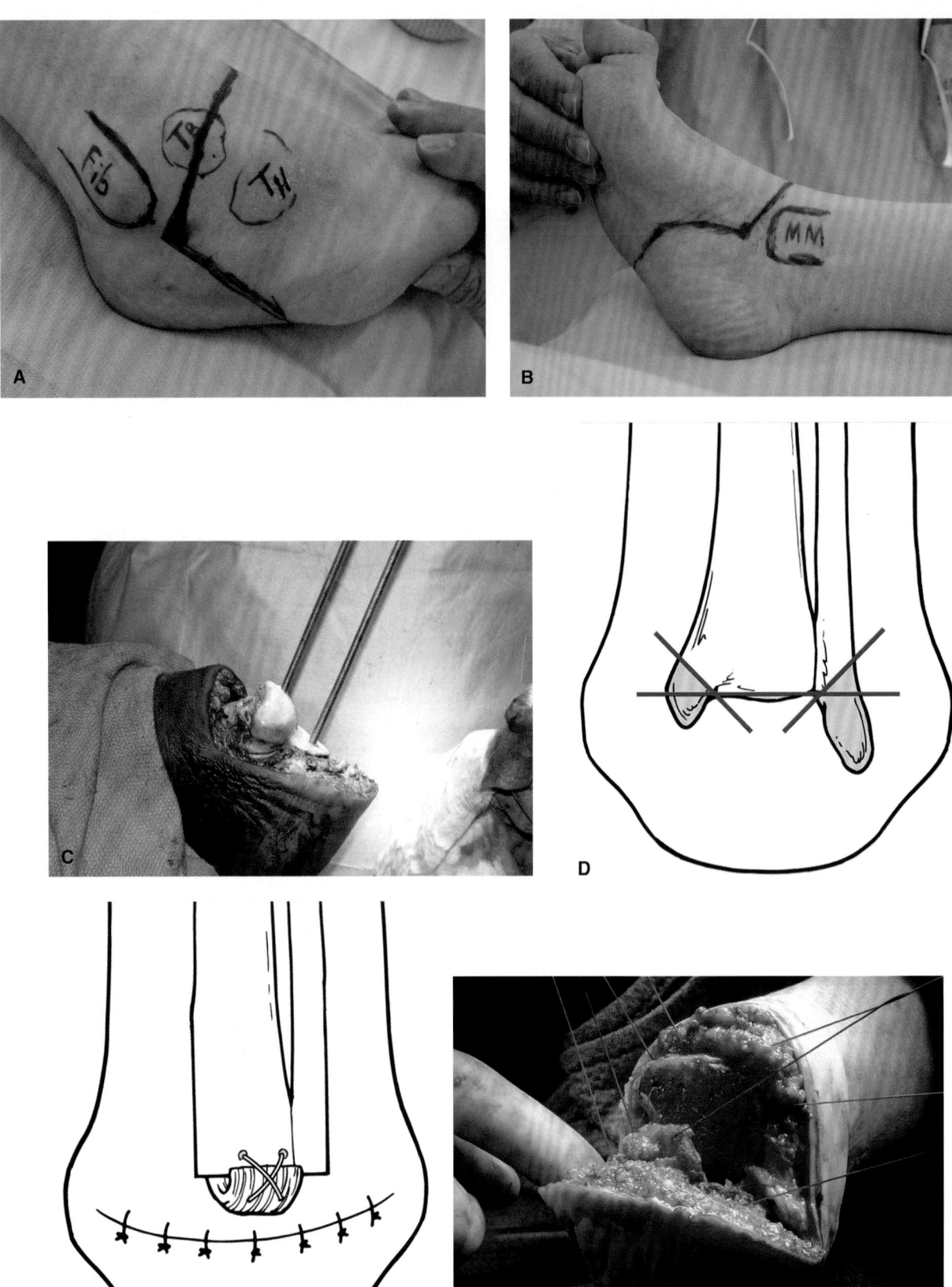

FIGURE 40.10 **A.** Incision placement for a Syme amputation, lateral view showing relationship to the fibula, talar dome, and head. **B.** Incision placement for Syme amputation, medial view showing relationship with the medial malleolus. **C.** Intraoperative view showing the use of large pins placed in the remaining talus and calcaneus. This technique can increase the surgeon's ability to extricate the bones while protecting the remaining soft tissue. **D.** Appearance of tibia and fibula after modified osteotomies. **E.** Modified osteotomy placement for Syme amputation. Anchor and drill hole placement in the anterior tibia to secure heel pad. **F.** Intraoperative view after all adequate bone has been débrided. Suture placement is shown prior to advancement of the plantar and posterior tissues.

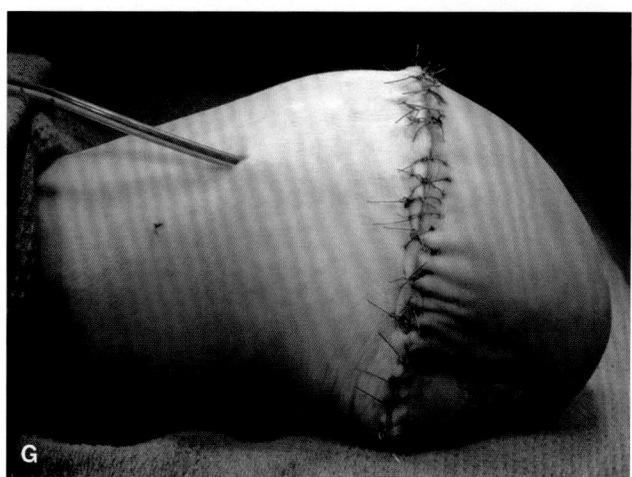

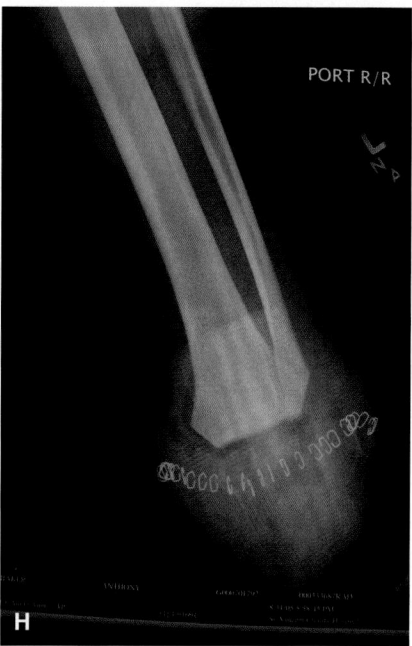

FIGURE 40.10 (*Continued*) **G.** Closure of Syme amputation with drain placement. **H.** Postoperative radiograph following Syme amputation.

bearing, while others will keep the patient completely off of the limb until all wounds are completely healed. When incisions have healed and edema has sufficiently resolved, prosthetic fitting can be performed.[19]

A wobbly or floppy stump or pad is a possible complication of the Syme amputation. It may be necessary to go back and trim either medially or laterally by removing a wedge of pad tissue and to drill more holes in the tibia to attach the fascia and tighten it up. Tissue resection medially and laterally reduces the mobility of the pad from side to side. The drill holes in the anterior tibia reduce mobility from anterior to posterior. The floppy stump is one reason surgeons minimize malleolar resection so as to give a wider base to support the stump. A floppy pad is no reason to abandon the Syme amputation in lieu of a Below Knee Amputation (BKA) or Above Knee Amputation (AKA). Revisional procedures are often successful to correct the problem.

A consultation with a prosthetician experienced with this level of amputation and prosthesis is crucial. The prosthetic should address several objectives. It should compensate for the loss of foot and ankle motion while providing the propulsive energy required for ambulation. It is also necessary to compensate for the limb length discrepancy created by this level of amputation and to suspend the prosthesis adequately during swing phase of gait.[2]

REFERENCES

1. *National Diabetes Statistics Fact Sheet.* U.S. Department of Health and Human Services and the CDC; 2020.
2. Yu GV, Schinke TL, Mezaros A. Syme's amputation: a retrospective review of 10 cases. *Clin Podiatr Med Surg.* 2005;22:395-427.
3. Myerson MS, Bowker JH, Brodsky JW, et al. Symposium: partial foot amputations. *Contemp Orthop.* 1994;29:139-157.
4. Hansen S. Amputation techniques. In: *Functional Reconstruction of the Foot and Ankle.* 1st ed. Philadelphia, PA: Lippincott Williams & Wilkins; 2000:273-279.
5. Pinzur M, Kaminsky M, Sage R, et al. Amputations at the middle level of the foot. *J Bone Joint Surg Am.* 1986;68:1061-1064.
6. Loftus TJ, Brown MP, Slish JH, Rosenthal MD. Serum Levels of Prealbumin and Albumin for Preoperative Risk Stratification. *Nutr Clin Pract.* 2019;34(3):340-348. doi: 10.1002/ncp.10271. Epub 2019 Mar 25. PMID: 30908744.
7. Lavery LA, Ahn J, Ryan EC, et al. What are the optimal cutoff values for ESR and CRP to diagnose osteomyelitis in patients with diabetes-related foot infections? *Clin Orthop Relat Res.* 2019;477(7):1594-1602.
8. Bouchard JL. Forefoot amputations: alternative to AK/BK. In: Vickers NS, Miller SJ, Mahan KT, Yu GV, Camasta CA, Ruch JA, eds. *Reconstructive Surgery of the Foot and Leg, Update 2005.* Tucker, GA: Podiatry Institute Publishing; 2004.
9. Zernich G, Dowell T, Rothenberg GM, Cohen M. Surgical pearls: how to achieve improved results with the Chopart's amputation. *Podiatr Today.* 2007;20(7):36-42.
10. Wagner FW. Amputations of the foot and ankle. *Clin Orthop.* 1977;122:62-69.
11. Bouchard JL. Delayed primary closure techniques for complex foot and ankle wounds. In: Vickers NS, Miller SJ, Mahan KT, Yu GV, Camasta CA, Ruch JA, eds. *Reconstructive Surgery of the Foot and Leg, Update 2005.* Tucker, GA: Podiatry Institute Publishing; 2005.
12. Sanders LJ. Transmetatarsal amputation and midfoot amputations. *Clin Podiatr Med Surg.* 1997;14:741-762.
13. Zgonis T. *Surgical Reconstruction of Diabetic Foot and Ankle.* 1st ed. Philadelphia, PA: Lippincott Williams & Wilkins; 2009.
14. Reyzelman A, Hadi S, Armstrong D. Limb salvage with Chopart's amputation and tendon rebalancing. *J Am Podiatr Med Assoc.* 1999;89:100-103.
15. Schade V, Roukis T, Yan J. Factors associated with successful Chopart's amputation in patients with diabetes: a systemic review. *Foot Ankle Spec.* 2010;3:278-284.
16. Dillingham TR, et al. Limb amputation and limb deficiency: epidemiology and recent trends in the United States. *South Med J.* 2002;95:875-883.
17. Cohen-Sobel E, Caselli AM, Rizzuta J. Prosthetic management of a Chopart amputation variant. *J Am Podiatr Med Assoc.* 1994;84:505-510.
18. DeGere MW, Grady JF. A modification of Chopart's amputation with ankle and subtalar arthrodesis by using a intramedullary nail. *J Foot Ankle Surg.* 1999;44(4):281-286.
19. Frykberg R, Abraham S, Tierney E, et al. Syme amputation for limb salvage: early experience with 26 cases. *J Foot Ankle Surg.* 2007;46(2):93-100.
20. Waters RL, Perry J, Antonelli D, et al. Energy cost of walking of amputees: the influence of level of amputation. *J Bone Joint Surg Am.* 1976;58(1):42-46.
21. Pinzur M, Gold J, Schwartz D, et al. Energy demands for walking in dysvascular amputees as related to the level of amputation. *Orthopedics.* 1992;15:1033-1037.
22. Aulivola B, Hile CN, Hamdan AD, et al. Major lower extremity amputation; outcome of a modern series. *Arch Surg.* 2004;139:395-399.
23. Sage R. Limb salvage and amputations. In: Banks AS, Downey MS, Martin DE, Miller SJ, eds. *McGlamry's Comprehensive Textbook of Foot & Ankle Surgery.* 3rd ed. Philadelphia, PA: Lippincott Williams & Wilkins; 2001.
24. Pinzur MS, Sage R, Abraham M, et al. Limb salvage in infected lower extremity gangrene. *Foot Ankle.* 1988;8:212-215.
25. Choudhury SN, Kitaoka HB. Amputations of the foot and ankle: analysis of techniques and results. *Orthopedics.* 1997;20:446-457.
26. Syme J. Surgical cases and observations. Amputation at the ankle joint. 1843. *Clin Orthop Relat Res.* 1990;(256):3-6.
27. Pinzur MS, Stuck RM, Sage R, Hunt N, Rabinovich Z. Syme ankle disarticulation in patients with diabetes. *J Bone Joint Surg Am.* 2003;85-A:1667-1672.

Bone Lengthening

Byron Hutchinson and Kelsey Millonig

HISTORY AND INTRODUCTION

The past 100 years have seen incredible advances in the surgical lengthening of bone. Some of the early pioneers left their mark on the development of various techniques for bone lengthening that helped revolutionize treatments available today.[1-3] In the past 30-40 years, there have been three noteworthy technical advances in bone lengthening:

1. "Distraction osteogenesis" using fine wire circular fixation popularized by Ilizarov[4]
2. Computerized program-assisted hexapod multiplanar fixator deformity correction
3. Recent development of motorized intramedullary lengthening nails[5,6]

In modern bone lengthening, Heinz Wagner became internationally renowned in 1978 for use of monolateral external fixator along with an aggressive osteotomy, acute intraoperative distraction of up to 2 cm, and then a fairly rapid distraction until desired length was achieved.[3] Ultimately this led to a distraction gap with minor bone formation, and subsequent reports on "The Wagner method of lengthening" showing high complication rates.[7]

In 1989, De Bastiani and colleagues understood the high rate of complications and revision surgeries associated with the Wagner method. They were also aware of the work being done by Ilizarov and subsequently developed an external fixator along with improved osteotomy and distraction techniques that became very popular.[8]

Gavriil Ilizarov, arguably the father of the revolution of limb lengthening and deformity correction, began his influence in Italy. Professors Roberto Cattaneo, Alessandro Villa, and Maurizio Catagni embraced many of his concepts and taught his unique method to many eager young orthopedic surgeons in the Western hemisphere.[9] Ilizarov's own publications eventually became published in English, and his detailed animal work confirming the osseous and soft tissue neogenesis effect of tension-stress was revolutionary.[4,10]

Another major advancement in the evolution of circular fixation has been the introduction of the computer-assisted hexapod multiplanar circular fixator.[11] These devices and associated computer software allow for simultaneous correction of complex multiplanar deformities. The indications for these devices have been expanding and now include a wide range of foot- and ankle-related conditions (Fig. 41.1).

Historically, one of the largest challenges with circular fixation for bone lengthening has been the extent of possible complications. For example, such complications have included soft tissue scarring, muscle tethering, associated joint deformity, and pin tract inflammation or infection.[12,13]

Lengthening via intramedullary nails was developed to help eliminate some of the challenges with external fixation. Early intramedullary nail designs had many additional problems including mechanical failure.[14] The introduction of motorized nails has revolutionized long bone lengthening especially in the femur.[15] These nails are activated transcutaneously and do not require external manipulations that can be challenging with patient education and compliance.

The art and science of bone lengthening is a dynamic process and continues to evolve as more technological advances and indications are realized.

INDICATIONS

In addition to limb length discrepancies (LLD), one of the most common indications for lengthening bone is the presence of a segmental bone defect. One of the leading causes

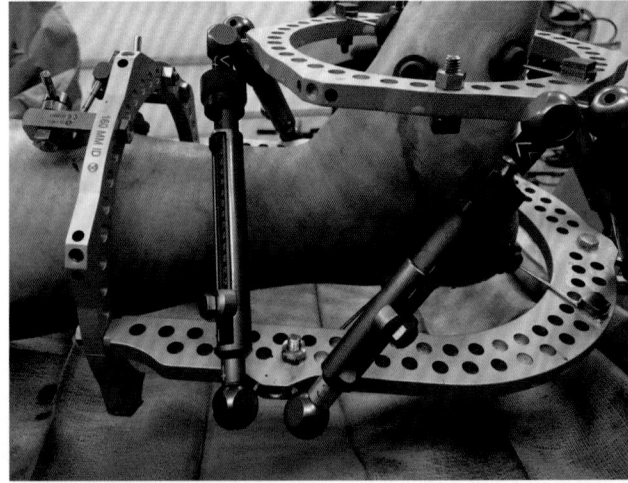

FIGURE 41.1 Diabetic patient undergoing gradual correction of a midfoot Charcot reconstruction utilizing computer-assisted multiplanar hexapod external fixation.

TABLE 41.1	Indications for Bone Lengthening
Segmental bone defects	Neoplasm
Osteomyelitis	Hardware explantation
Trauma	Avascular necrosis
Endoprosthesis	Limb length discrepancy

of these segmental bone defects in the foot and ankle occurs with explantation of a total ankle replacement (TAR) or avascular necrosis (AVN). Currently, several solutions for these large defects are being explored, and no standard of care exists (Table 41.1).

One of these solutions for segmental bone defects is to consider a primary tibiocalcaneal fusion with a proximal or distal tibial lengthening (Figs. 41.2 and 41.3). There are several advantages to this technique. Including need for incorporation of a large bone graft, which has shown marginal results in the literature.[16] The lengthening procedure with a frame allows for dynamization, which is a process for promoting bone healing by allowing axial micromotion with compressive load of the extremity. Components of the external fixator can be removed or loosened to allow more loading of the bone segment to help consolidate the regenerate bone. The authors have found that the consolidation of the regenerated bone is more predictable than incorporation of a large bone graft.

AVN can produce fairly large segmental bone defects that can be difficult to manage. Talar AVN poses the same problems seen with TAR explant with vascular compromise and a sizable defect. Navicular AVN poses a different set of challenges.

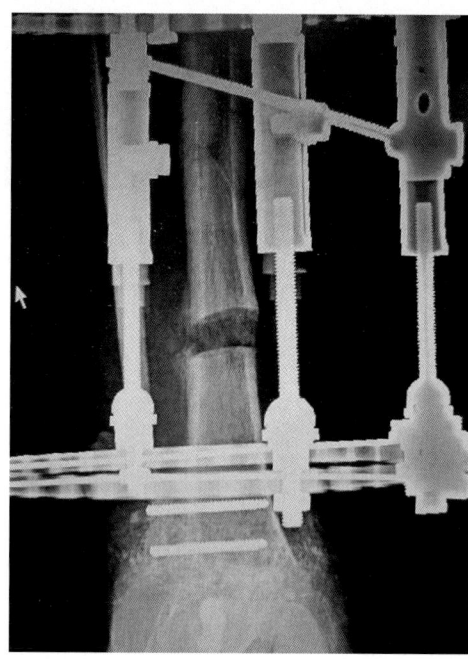

FIGURE 41.3 Postoperative radiographs of total ankle arthroplasty explantation in a 43-year-old female with primary tibiocalcaneal fusion. The foot plate was removed for patient to begin dynamization of the distal tibial lengthening.

The size of the segmental bone defect is usually smaller than with talar AVN, and bone lengthening is not possible, so utilization of a bone graft is necessary. An additional challenge is the loading of a navicular segmental bone defect is not axial loading, but rather tension compression type of loading. This tension compression dynamic requires the utilization of different fixation techniques that neutralize the tension forces on the bone graft (Figs. 41.4 and 41.5).

LLD can be problematic in the lower extremity. Discrepancies of >10 mm can contribute to functional deficits including low back pain and hip pain.[17-19] These discrepancies can

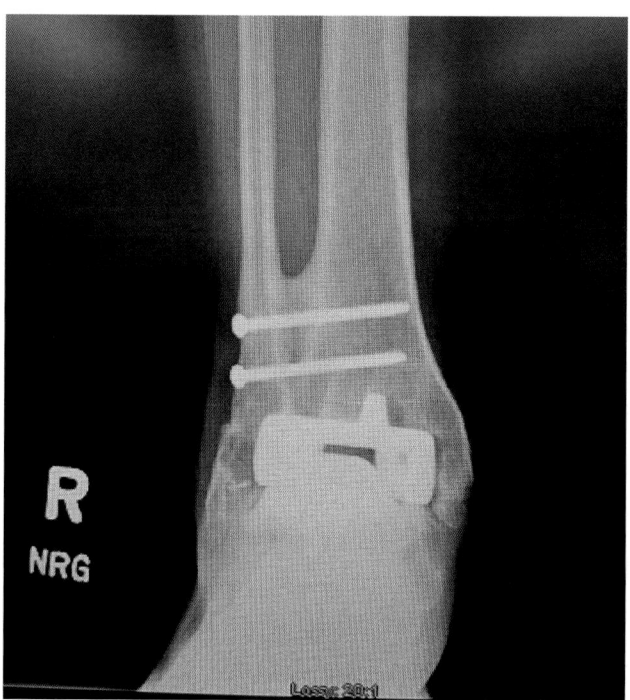

FIGURE 41.2 Postoperative radiographs of failed total ankle arthroplasty implant in a 43-year-old female with a 4-year survival with one polyexchange.

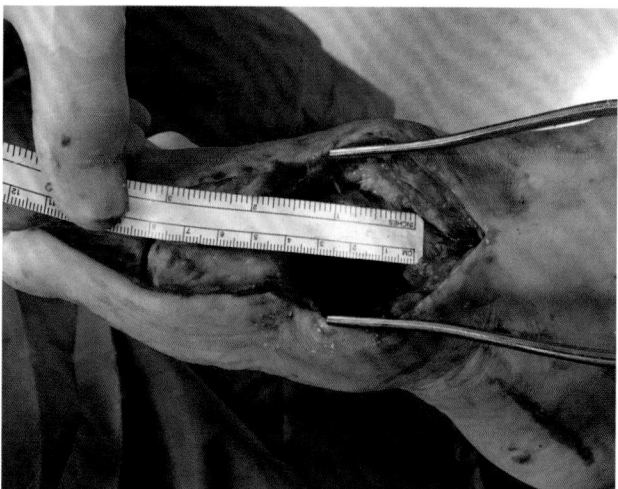

FIGURE 41.4 Resection of infected navicular and subsequent spacer explant with segmental bone defect of ~5 cm.

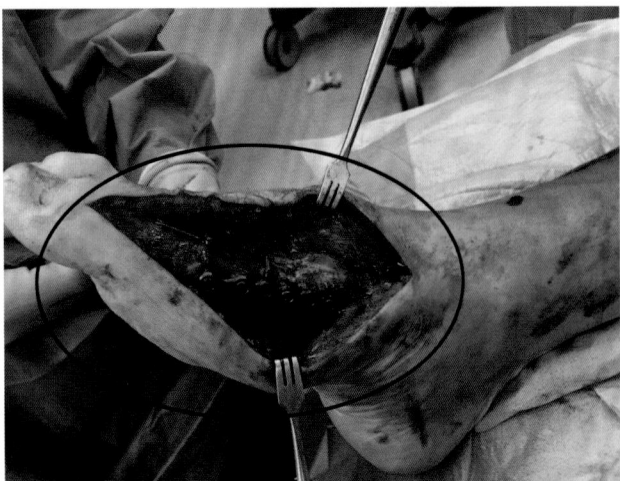

FIGURE 41.5 Utilization of fresh femoral head, BMAC, PRP, and intramedullary screw fixation with a straddle plate.

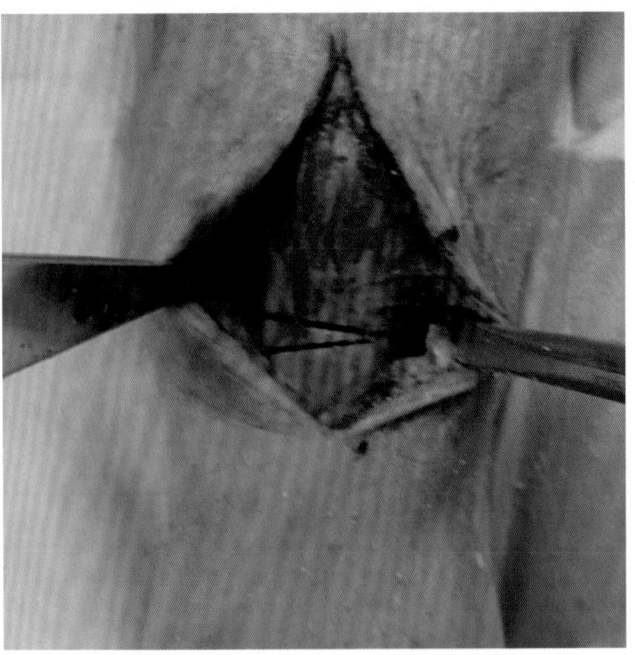

FIGURE 41.7 Acute correction of frontal plane deformity.

be the result of congenital deformities, growth plate arrest, or trauma. LLD are particularly challenging when there is associated trauma that has created deformity through malunion or nonunion. The authors see this quite commonly following pilon and midshaft tibial fractures. The deformity can be treated with acute correction followed by gradual lengthening or gradual deformity correction and lengthening from a percutaneous approach (Figs. 41.6, 41.7, 41.8, and 41.9).

PEARLS

The authors finds it easier for both the surgeon and patient if a two-plane deformity can be acutely corrected. This leaves only one deformity for gradual correction.

It is the author's opinion that management of short metatarsals with congenital brachymetatarsia or iatrogenic shortening has been treated inadequately in the past with intercalary bone grafting. This technique results in inadequate length and potential vascular compromise or impaction of the distal joint due to the acute lengthening process.[20] Gradual bone lengthening with a mini external fixator has become favored to avoid these specific complications and has improved outcomes.

Foot and ankle reconstruction or revision is another example where bone lengthening techniques can be utilized to improve outcomes. The only limit is one's creativity when applying good external fixation principles to a set of

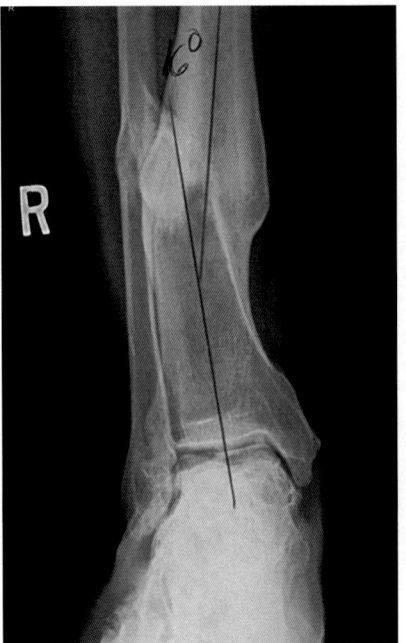
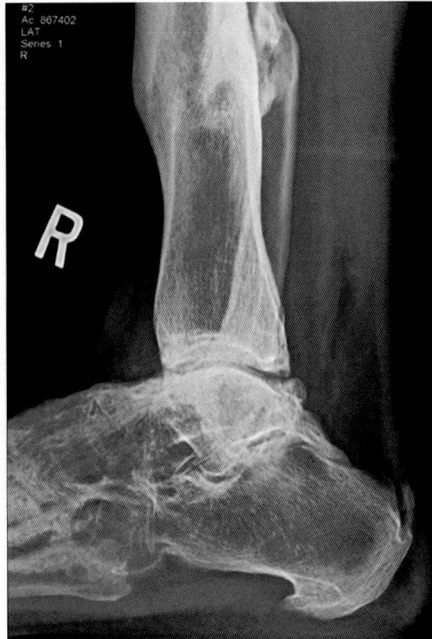

FIGURE 41.6 Status post triple arthrodesis with malunion tibia in varus and tibial shortening in a 65-year-old male.

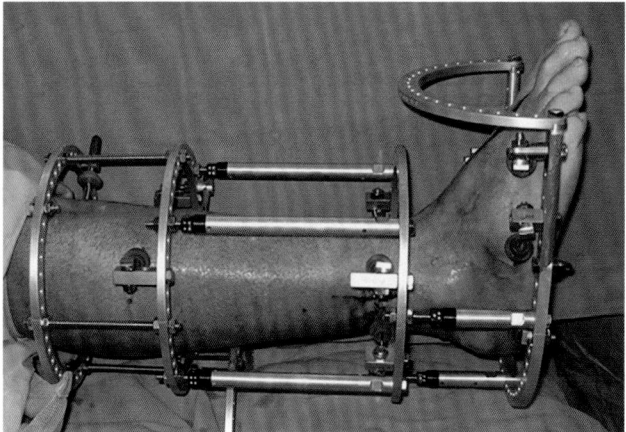

FIGURE 41.8 Gradual distal tibial lengthening.

clinical challenges often seen in revisional surgery. A good example of this is a failed first metatarsal phalangeal implant that requires a revisional procedure whereby the surgeon is converting this to a bone graft fusion either in one or multiple staged procedures. The problem is the predictability of incorporation of a large intercalary bone graft. The authors' experience with large bone grafting in the first metatarsal phalangeal joint (MPJ) fusion is not as predictable as one may originally think. A primary first MPJ fusion with proximal corticotomy and distraction osteogenesis in the authors' experience provides a more reproducible and improved outcome (Figs. 41.10, 41.11, and 41.12). Malposition in hindfoot and ankle surgery can also require repositioning along with bone lengthening (Figs. 41.13, 41.14, 41.15, 41.16, and 41.17).

PEARLS

One-stage revision such as a first MPJ fusion with proximal lengthening is desirable, but sometimes, a two-stage approach is necessary because of vascular compromise to the digit acutely.

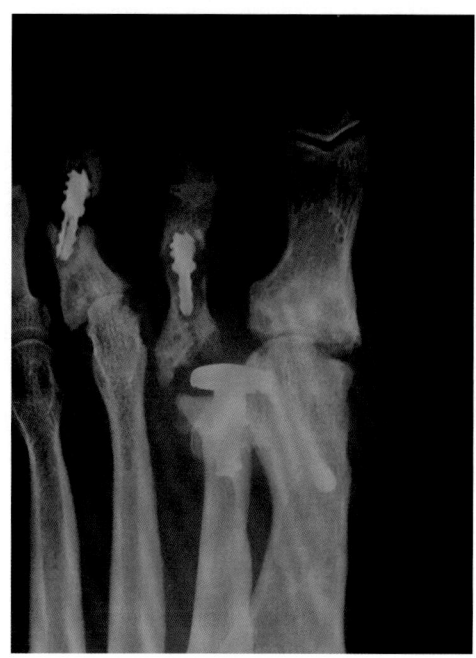

FIGURE 41.10 Initial presentation after multiple forefoot surgeries.

TECHNIQUE

Corticotomy

The foundation for success of new bone formation is an appropriate osteotomy technique. To accomplish this, one must prevent thermal damage and respect the periosteum, thereby creating good vascular bone surfaces to allow for new bone formation. Most surgeons today perform corticotomies with varying technical details depending on personal preference, but all adhere to the principles outlined.

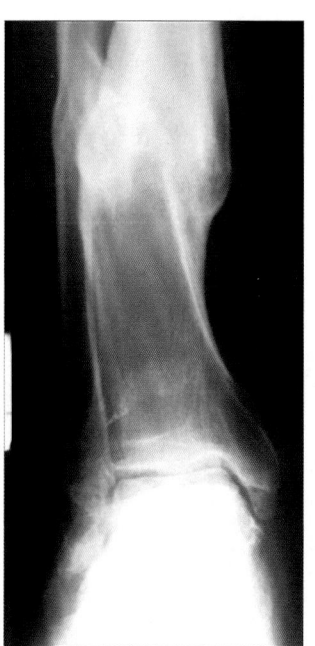

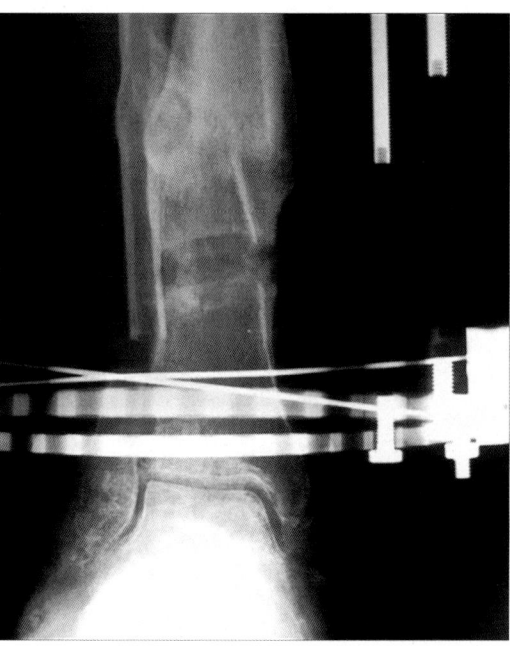

FIGURE 41.9 Preoperative and postoperative radiographs demonstrating realignment of ankle joint with establishment of length. Patient is considering future TAR following deformity correction.

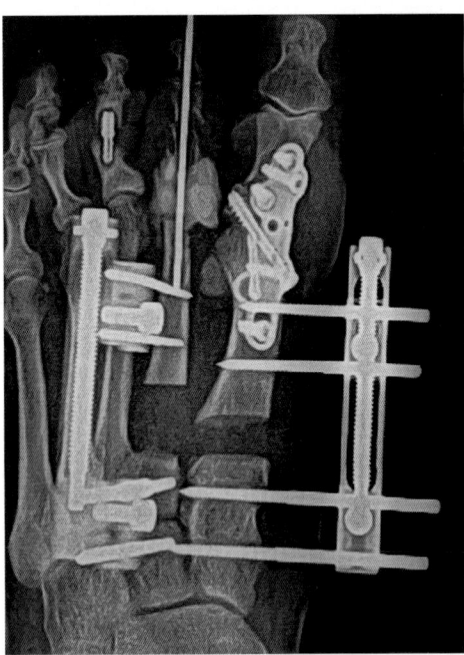

FIGURE 41.11 Lengthening of first and second metatarsal with primary fusion of first MPJ and Masquelet technique of the second MPJ.

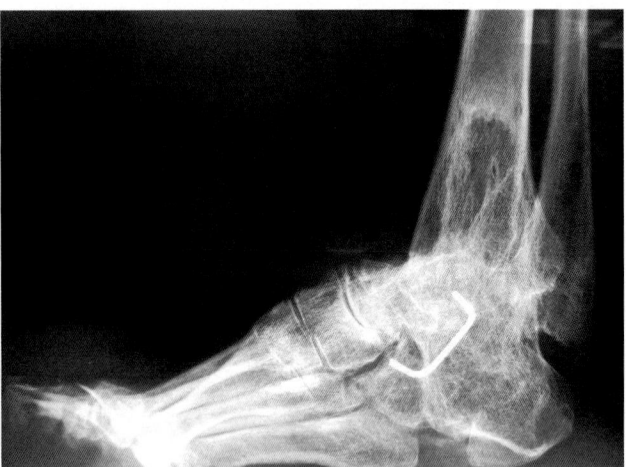

FIGURE 41.13 Post polio 62-year-old female with subsequent malpositioned pantalar arthrodesis and significant limb length discrepancy preoperative imaging.

Ilizarov described corticotomy as a means of surgical division of the bone with a low-energy osteotomy of the cortex. This technique was based on interrupting the cortex of the long bone without violating the medullary vascularity or the periosteum. He believed that preservation of the medullary circulation enhanced bone formation and was necessary for successful osteogenesis.[4,10,21]

Since that time, other techniques briefly outlined below have been described to accomplish the same goal providing

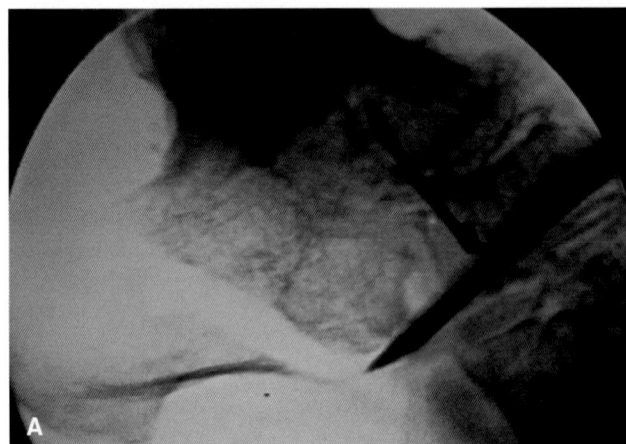

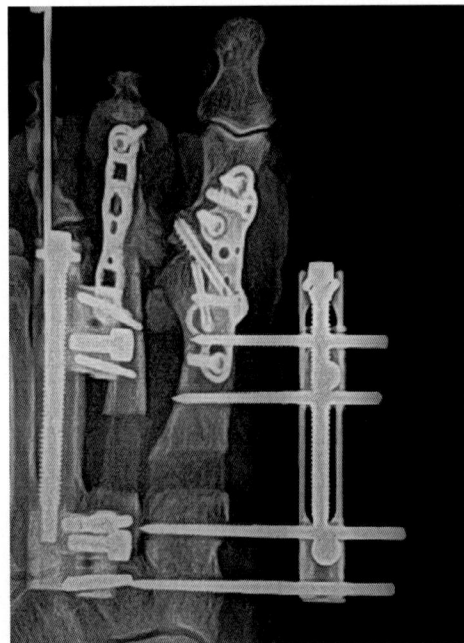

FIGURE 41.12 Stable regenerate of the first and second metatarsal with good alignment and length maintained.

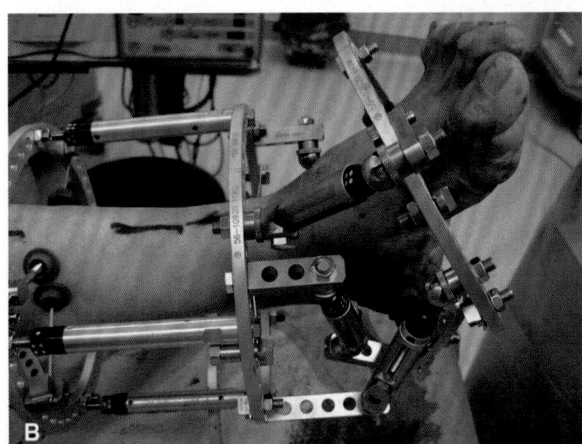

FIGURE 41.14 A. Percutaneous "V" osteotomy performed to dorsiflex forefoot, lengthen calcaneus, correct varus of malunion pantalar arthrodesis. **B.** External fixation construct to allow movement of forefoot and hindfoot independently. Distal corticotomy of the tibia for lengthening.

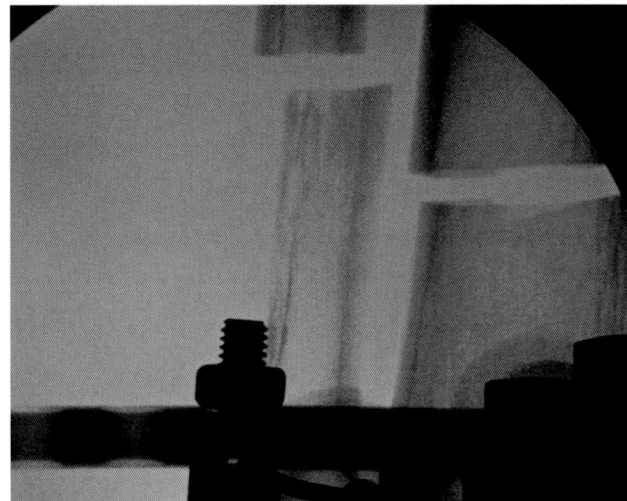

FIGURE 41.15 Distal tibial distraction for lengthening.

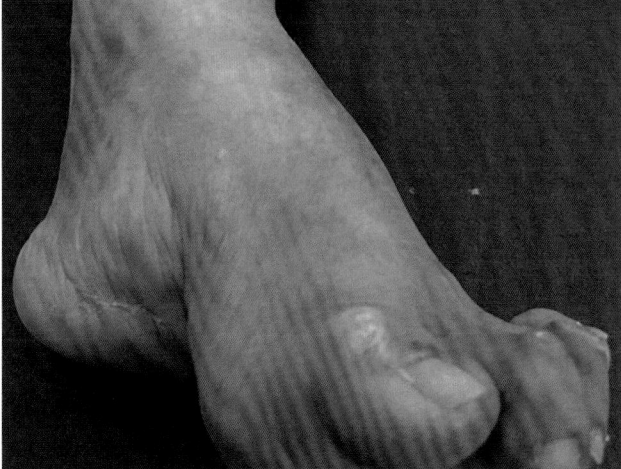

FIGURE 41.16 Malposition of foot and ankle prior to revisional surgery.

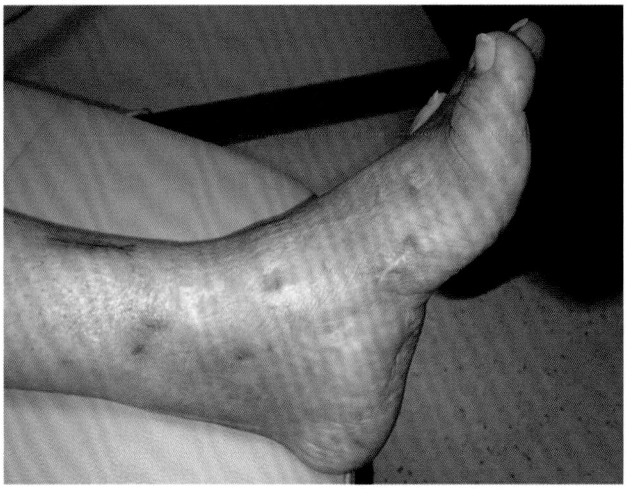

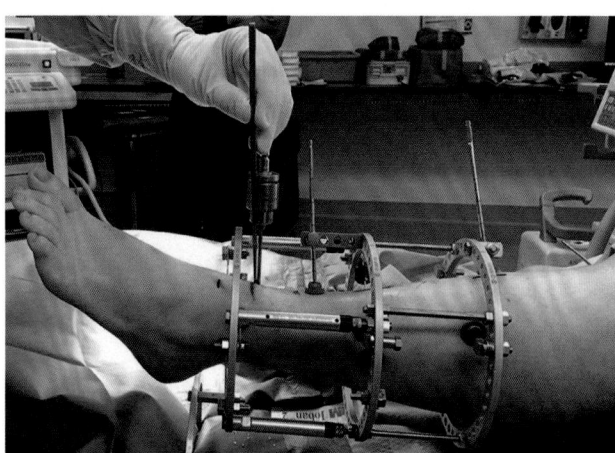

FIGURE 41.17 Final foot and ankle position following correction.

new bone formation over a segment with quality regenerate as the end point.[22,23]

The classic corticotomy technique in the tibia has historically been described in the proximal tibia. It begins with a 5-10 mm longitudinal incision over the lateral border of the tibia and elevation of the periosteum. The anterior half of the lateral tibial cortex is then osteotomized, the medial cortex of the tibia is osteotomized in a similar manner, and the remaining lateral cortex is divided. All of these osteotomies are done with protection of the soft tissue with an elevator. The final portion of the corticotomy is completed with rotational osteoclasis utilizing the circular rings with no connecting rods. This is performed by stabilizing the proximal tibial ring, while rotating the distal ring. This rotation completes the osteotomy across the posterior tibial cortex.

The multiple drill hole osteotomy technique was popularized in the 1980s by De Bastiani et al.[8] This technique has been found to be more precise than the historical "corticotomy technique" and is generally less technically demanding with an easier learning curve. A small anterior incision is made over the proximal tibia, and a 4- to 5-mm diameter drill is used to create a series of drill holes around the anterior two-thirds of the bone circumference (Figs. 41.17, 41.18, 41.19, and 41.20). Numerous methods can be utilized to achieve the desired orientation of the drill holes including setting the alignment with a Steinmann pin or using a drill guide or rancho cube. An osteotome is then utilized to complete the osteotomy by connecting the drill holes. The posterior cortex is then broken.

PEARLS

The authors utilizes drill holes and connects them with a sharp osteotome. The author keeps a set of osteotomes for use only for corticotomy and sharpens the blade prior to every case. The author has also used a surgical saw with similar results in general over osteotome method especially for a straight bone cut. The author prefers the drill and osteotome for focal domes while often utilizing the Gigli saw for midfoot or derotation of the tibia.

FIGURE 41.18 Distal tibial corticotomy using multiple drill holes and a small osteotome to complete the corticotomy.

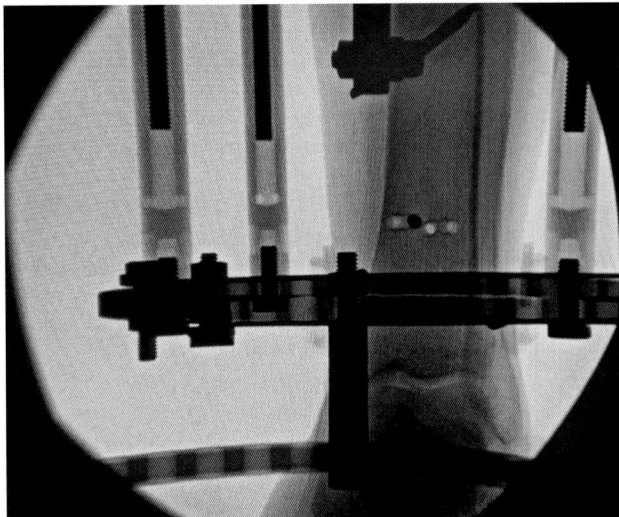

FIGURE 41.19 Note the drill in place for reference to perform additional drill holes that can now be connected with the osteotome.

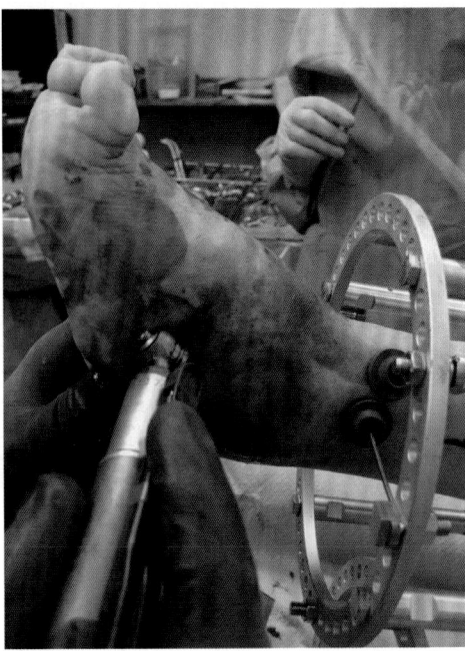

FIGURE 41.21 Midfoot osteotomy for deformity correction utilizing a power saw. The forefoot portion of the frame will then be applied and the osteotomy will then be manipulated through the frame.

The percutaneous Gigli saw technique is a popular method of creating a corticotomy in any long bone and is particularly popular in the foot.[24,25] It is especially useful in metaphyseal bone. Two transverse incisions are made, and subperiosteal tunnels are created. Protection of the soft tissues is paramount since the osteotomy is completed in a "blind" fashion. The Gigli saw is then tied to a suture and passed from one transverse incision to the other close to the bone. There are several advantages to this osteotomy. It is a low-energy osteotomy that leaves a very smooth cut, and this can be extremely beneficial for rotational correction.

The focal dome osteotomy is a semicircular-shaped cut in the bone again utilizing drill holes and osteotomes to complete. The center of rotation of angulation (CORA) corresponds to the center of the circular cut and the point of rotation for the dome. This osteotomy is best done in metaphyseal bone, which provides the widest diameter of bone. The dome osteotomy is used primarily for angular deformities but can be used to acutely correct a deformity and then lengthen through the dome gradually.

The power saw osteotomy is a popular approach, especially in the foot. Typically, there is more open exposure for this method for direct visualization and is often relatively simple. The disadvantages include greater disruption of blood supply from soft tissue exposure and potential thermal necrosis of the bone. Irrigation and pecking techniques during the creation of the osteotomy can mitigate these potential complications. This technique can also be used for acute wedge correction followed by gradual lengthening (Fig. 41.21).

Latency Period

These low-energy, minimally invasive osteotomies can be compared to a closed low-energy fracture whereby secure fixation such as a circular fixator or an intramedullary lengthening device provides an optimal local environment for the initial healing response. This is critical in the latency phase prior to distraction. The length of the latency is often dictated by age, anatomical site, and surrounding soft tissues. Generally the length of the latency period is 3-10 days.[26-29] Factors such as previous infection, radiation, immunosuppressive therapy, smoking, certain comorbidities, previous surgery locally, and anti-inflammatory medications or steroid use may necessitate a longer latency period.

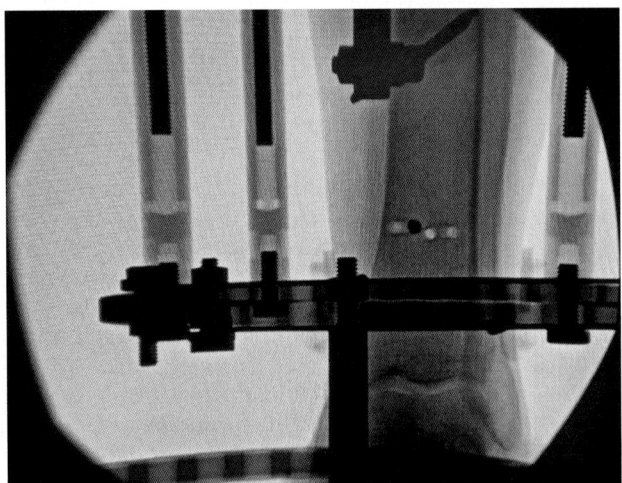

FIGURE 41.20 Osteotome being used to complete the corticotomy.

PEARLS

The authors will typically increase the latency period around the distal tibia especially with previous surgery locally and with the presence of comorbidities. Generally, metatarsals can be the typical 3-7 days.

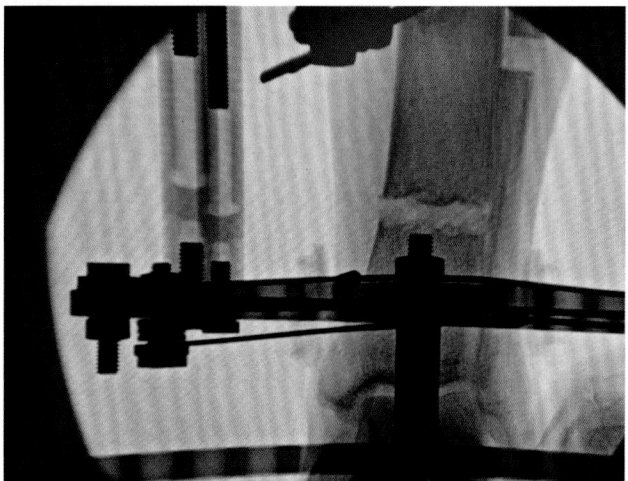

FIGURE 41.22 Distraction osteogenesis is occurring during lengthening.

Distraction

The distraction phase begins at the conclusion of the latency period. Generally, the amount of lengthening per day is set at 1 mm. This is achieved in increments of 0.25 mm four times per day (Figure 41.22). Increasing the rhythm (decreasing increments) leads to better bone formation.[10] Many factors can change this general distraction rate, and at times, it is dependent on the location of distraction and the health of the soft tissue envelope (Table 41.2). The stability of the two bony segments is extremely important as well as the location of the corticotomy.

For example, a typical brachymetatarsia responds to a 1-mm/day distraction rate, and the resultant regenerate bone formation is consistent with very few complications. If you compare this to a distal distraction of the tibia in an individual with multiple ankle surgeries and a compromised soft tissue envelope, a 1-mm/day distraction rate may be too fast to lay down proper regenerate, and bone healing may be compromised. Metabolic aspects of bone formation and metabolic bone diseases can certainly have a profound effect on distraction and regenerate formation. Common conditions such as vitamin D deficiency and thyroid disorders should be optimized prior to lengthening. In the author's experience, patients with osteogenesis imperfecta may be poor candidates for bone lengthening.

> **PEARLS**
>
> The authors generally slows the rate and rhythm for any procedure that is being done with previous violation of the soft tissue envelope specifically about the distal ankle.

TABLE 41.2	Influences on Bone Lengthening and Regenerate	
Bone Disease	**Medication**	**Substance Abuse**
Diabetes mellitus	Corticosteroids	Alcoholism
Anorexia	Heparin	Smoking
Celiac disease	NSAIDs	
Gastric bypass		

Regenerate

Outlining the entire process of regenerate formation in detail is beyond the scope of this chapter. Understanding the numeric parameters, variables and milestones in the development of a stable and consolidated regenerate is vitally important.

At the end of the distraction phase, the regenerate begins to consolidate, and bone remodeling occurs until the normal corticomedullary architecture is reached and full, unprotected weight-bearing is possible. The events building up to consolidation of regenerate are very complex, and many factors can influence the success of the final consolidation.

For example, the location of the corticotomy can directly affect regenerate formation. The metaphyseal area is better vascularized, has a larger bony surface, and heals faster than diaphyseal bone. A circular fixator that is not orthogonal can also negatively impact the consolidation of the regenerate.

During distraction osteogenesis, the renewal of bone is enhanced by gradual stretching of the soft tissues in the gap area between the bone segments. The process of bone regeneration involves a complex system of biological changes whereby mechanical stress is converted into a cascade of signals that activate cellular behavior resulting in enhanced formation of bone.

Intramembranous bone formation is the underlying biological process of callotasis.[4,10,21,30] The bone formation evolves in defined radiographic and histological zones. Controlled axial load and dynamization help to consolidate the regenerate. The most common definition of consolidation and stability to allow for the removal of the frame is tricortical radiographic consolidation on two orthogonal radiographs.[31] Quantitative CT can also be useful as well as a "clinical test" defined by detaching the ring blocks and stressing the regenerate bone segment with intraoperative fluoroscopy under anesthesia to visualize any possible movement.

> **PEARLS**
>
> The authors have found that CT can be useful especially when frame removal is being considered. Stimulation of the regenerate early on with orthobiologics can also avoid problems. If the regenerate is slow to form, then compress the segment and start distraction again. Dynamization is always a beneficial strategy.

Numeric parameters can be employed to quantify the quality and speed of bone formation. The two most popular parameters are the distraction-consolidation time (DCT) and the healing index (HI). Generally, the consolidation time is about twice as long as the distraction time in children and may be three to four times longer in adults. The healing index (DCT/cm) is the most widely used parameter and is typically 1 month/cm in children and 2-3 months/cm in adults.[31] The authors have found that much of the bony consolidation assessment is a clinical judgment and due to the particular situation rather than reliance on objective data and formulas. There are many variables to consider such as location of the corticotomy, complexity of correction, previous trauma, and age of the patient.

EFFECT OF BONE LENGTHENING ON SURROUNDING SOFT TISSUE

Gradual bone lengthening impacts the surrounding tissues. Muscles may be stretched which can cause pain and affect the lengthening process. Skinny wires and half pins might impale certain soft tissues causing pain and inflammation. There are significant effects due to muscle distraction and subsequent decreased joint range of motion directly proportional to the amount of lengthening.[32-34] Nerves and vessels seem to adapt during the lengthening process and generally recover 2-3 months after distraction is halted.[35]

> ### PEARLS
> Providers must recognize that external bone transport is always going to be hard on the soft tissues. Internal bone transport should be considered with large defects such as 6-8 cm (Figure 41.23: Example of bone transport for a 12-year-old male road trauma with infected tibial nonunion. Courtesy of Mikhail Samchukov, MD, Texas Scottish Rite Hospital).

Providers must be cognizant that excessive gradual (>20%-30%) or acute distraction (>15%) can lead to nerve damage.[36,37] The typical distraction speed previously outlined is about four to eight times faster than during adolescent growth spurts.[26] This is why some unique complications occur in various locations during lengthening. For example, proximal tibial lengthenings can develop procurvatum because of the powerful muscles working around the knee joint particularly the posterior muscle group. In contrast, a distal tibial lengthening may show poor regenerate formation anteriorly because of the less favorable soft tissue envelope in this region of the

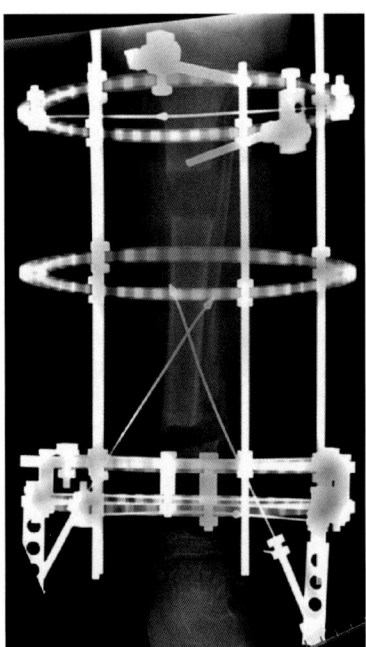

FIGURE 41.23 Example of bone transport for a 12-year-old male road trauma with infected tibial nonunion. Courtesy of Mikhail Samchukov, MD, Texas Scottish Rite Hospital

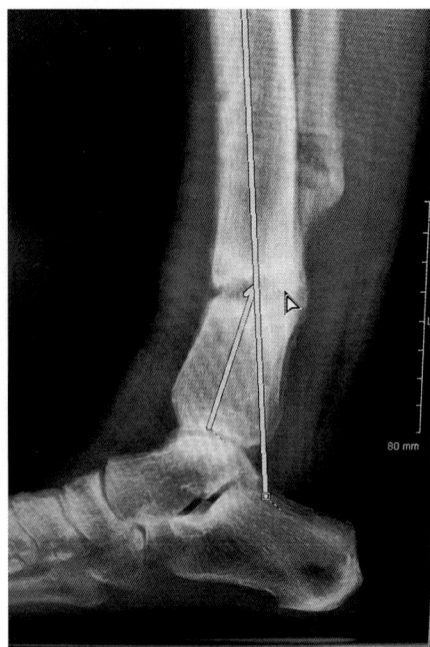

FIGURE 41.24 Note the sagittal plane displacement that occurred in this distal lengthening procedure. Three quarters of the cortex consolidated while the anterior aspect of the tibia failed. This was remedied with an anterior bone graft during a second surgery. Patient outcome was successful despite the complication.

tibia (Fig. 41.24). During lengthening in brachymetatarsia, unless the digit is appropriately stabilized with an external fixator or a K-wire, a nonfunctional flail toe can result.

TECHNICAL OPTIONS AND FRAME BIOMECHANICS

A stable construct is extremely important to the distraction process. The device should be orthogonal and adherence to proper frame biomechanics is paramount. Wires and pins need to be placed properly to avoid failure of the frame. Even the most experienced surgeons with many years of frame experience can apply a suboptimal frame. Stability needs to be maintained for consolidation of the regenerate to occur with axial loading and eventual dynamization.

> ### PEARLS
> The author encourages everyone to be familiar with frame biomechanics. It has been the author's experience that most frame failures are due to a poorly applied frame.

UNILATERAL FIXATORS

A monolateral fixator is indicated for simple lengthening of a short to medium distance. Ease of application has made these devices popular, especially in femoral lengthening (Fig. 41.25). Unilateral fixators are more likely to cause angular deviation of the regenerate.[38] Another extremely popular use of unilateral fixators is seen in forefoot surgery including primary lengthening such as brachymetatarsia or in revisional situations in the forefoot as previously outlined.

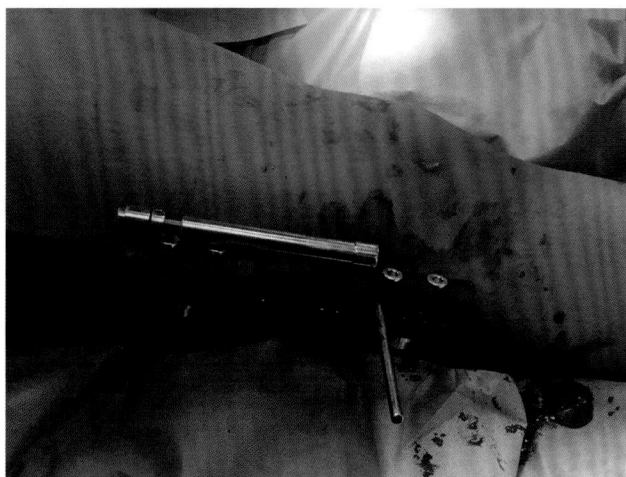

FIGURE 41.25 Example of monolateral fixator for distal femoral lengthening.

CIRCULAR FIXATORS

Circular fixation is especially useful in tibial lengthening of any distance and in tibial deformity correction. Straight lengthening can be controlled very effectively with circular fixation. Deformity correction is more complex and is beyond the scope of this chapter. Understanding hinge placement and other deformity correction principles is paramount in obtaining successful outcomes. Computer assisted hexapod multiplanar circular fixators have become popular in treating these extremely complex deformities from the tibia to the foot. The author has not found these devices to be necessary in the vast majority of tibial lengthening procedures, however, computer-assisted planning may make it easier to address any angular deformity that may be created during the lengthening process.

> **PEARLS**
>
> If you know that you are eventually going to treat the traumatic or nontraumatic segmental bone loss with a circular fixator start with the circular fixator.

INTRAMEDULLARY FIXATION

Over the past 20 years, several new techniques have been developed to decrease the time in an external fixator. The fixator is removed at the end of the distraction phase and replaced with internal fixation to provide stability during the consolidation of the regenerate bone. Lengthening over a nail (LON) was first introduced by Paley and his colleagues in 1997.[39] An intramedullary nail is inserted at the time of frame application. At the end of distraction, the fixator is removed and the nail is locked statically. Lengthening and then nailing (LATN) was introduced by Rozbruch et al. in 2008.[40] In this technique, a circular external fixator is used for gradual distraction. Once the length has been obtained, an intramedullary nail is inserted and the fixator is removed. Dynamization of the nail or using the nail statically is generally a decision made by the surgeon. The author has used both of these techniques in tibial lengthenings with or without segmental bone defects with predictable

results. Lengthening over plates and lengthening then plating techniques have also been described.[41,42]

LENGTHENING BY INTRAMEDULLARY DEVICES

Historically, motorized intramedullary lengthening devices relied on mechanical means to obtain distraction. Distraction was initiated by rotating the leg. The problem with these devices was that the rate and rhythm of distraction were inconsistent and these initial devices have since been abandoned. There are several newer devices in use today. These devices allow for greater lengthening when compared to external devices.[43] Lengthenings of up to 80 mm in the femur and 60 mm in the tibia may be achieved. A high implant reliability and success rate has been reported in clinical series.[15,44,45] Patient satisfaction is high because the device is internal and lengthening occurs with a transmitter. In the author's opinion, these devices will revolutionize lengthening procedures, especially in the femur within the next decade.

COMPLICATIONS AND OUTCOMES

All surgeries and techniques present their own unique complications, but for the most part many complications with bone lengthening can be remedied because the frame allows for dynamic adjustments to be made during the process. Certainly the more severe deformities have higher complication rates than straight forward lengthening procedures.[28]

Pain is a common complaint during the distraction phase and can persist even in the consolidation phase. The pain is initially caused by stretching of the periosteum, muscle spasms, contractions due to wire or pin transfixion, and later also due to pin and wire related soft tissue and bone inflammation. Sometimes the pain is significant enough to require cessation of the lengthening for a time. Patients can also develop mental challenges coined "cage rage," especially if the fixator is on for a prolonged period of time. Discussing this phenomenon before surgery is important so patients know what to expect during the lengthening process. Central mediated pain is rare but needs to be recognized early on and treated appropriately. The author has had success treating this pain problem with gabapentin (eg, Neurontin) or pregabalin (eg, Lyrica).

Nerve palsies are reported to occur in up to 2%-5% of patients and mostly affect the deep peroneal nerve. Identification of a direct nerve palsy from wire or pin placement needs to be recognized immediately so that adjustments may be made to avoid permanent damage to the nerve. During the lengthening process, traction on any nerve can occur. This is of particular concern in revision cases where there is previous scar formation. The surgeon should also be aware of the risk of compartment syndrome during lengthening, especially when lengthening the tibia.

Poor regenerate formation is rare in the pediatric population but can occur in adults undergoing deformity correction along with lengthening. There are many factors that can delay regenerate formation. Smoking, corticotomy at the site of previous trauma, and fast distraction are examples of some factors that may contribute to poor regenerate formation. There are several strategies to deal with poor regenerate formation. The surgeon can cease distraction and start over. Another option is to stimulate the regenerate bone by injecting

BMAC and PRP into the regenerate.[46] Further dynamization or attempting the accordion maneuver can also help to stimulate bone healing.[47]

With external fixation (circular and monolateral) there is always concern for infection. Pins and wires can show initial irritation that can rapidly progress to infection if not addressed. Typically, if there is irritation to the skin from a wire, the wire is loose and/or the skin is sliding on the wire. Tightening wires (re-tensioning) in the office often can prevent infections. Bolstering around the pin can mitigate the movement of the skin on the wire, which helps decrease skin irritation and prevent infection. If erythema and edema surrounding the pin are observed, antibiotics are appropriate as well. One must be prepared to remove wires if necessary and at times adjustments to the frame must be made in the operating room.

The versatility of bone lengthening has allowed surgeons to manage LLD as well as very complicated segmental bone defects. Understanding the variables that can affect regenerate bone formation and strategies to aid in consolidation, allows for better outcomes.

CASE PRESENTATIONS

TIBIAL LENGTHENING WITH FOCAL DOME

- A 39-year-old male with distal tibial deformity secondary to a gunshot wound at 25 years of age.
- Difficulty walking and pain in his ankle. Wears a 3-cm heel lift that helps his hip pain while he is wearing the lift.
- 3 cm LLD, lateral translation of tibia, and severe recurvatum.

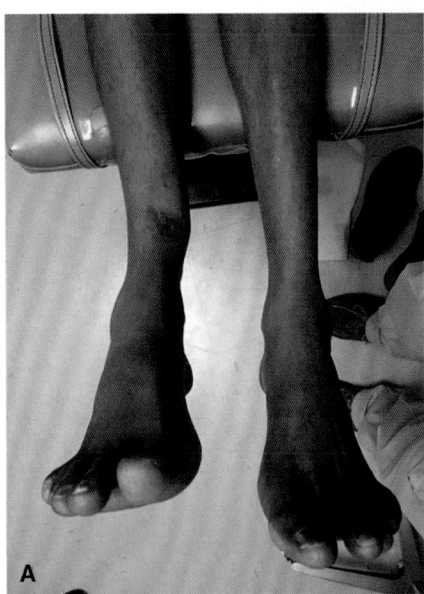
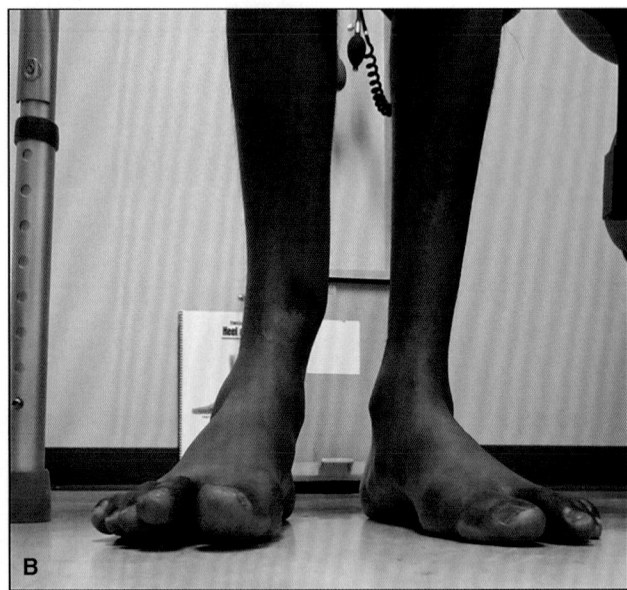
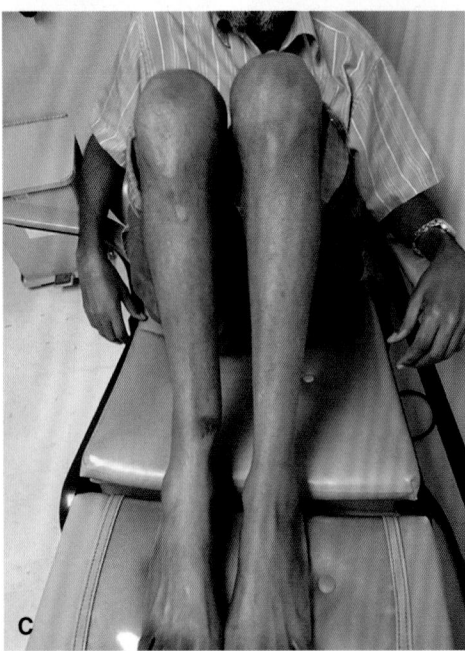

FIGURE 1 **A.** Preoperative LLD. **B.** Preoperative weightbearing stance. **C.** Preoperative clinical presentation.

Pertinent medical history:

- Expatriate from Somalia
- Gunshot wound treated with debridement
- Tibial fracture closed reduced and casted

- Entry wound: skin adhesion to bone
- LLD accommodated with external shoe lift
- PMH: healthy patient nonsmoker and taking no medications
- Previously offered a BKA

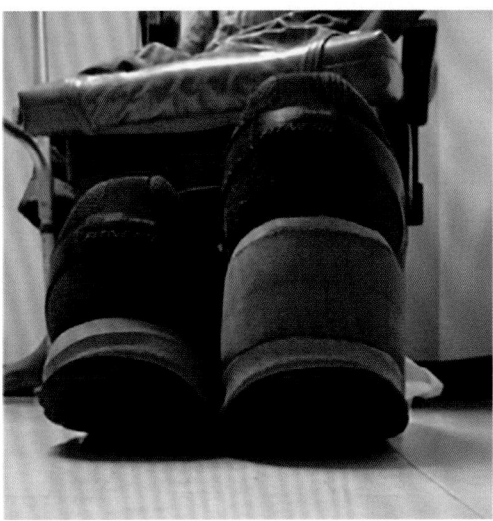

FIGURE 2 Patients preoperative shoegear wear for LLD.

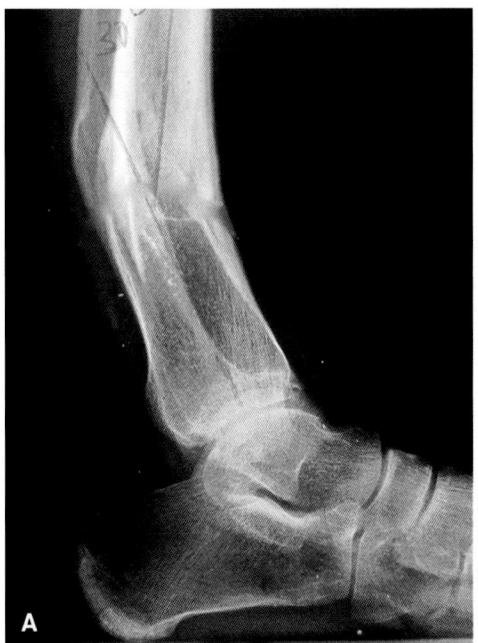
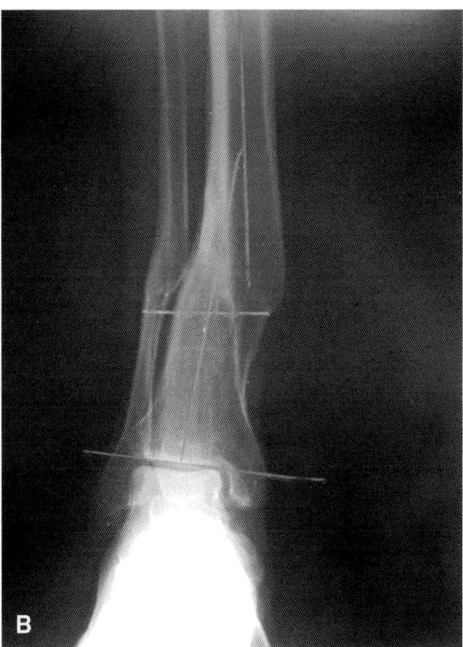

FIGURE 3 **A.** Preoperative lateral ankle radiograph. **B.** Preoperative AP ankle radiograph.

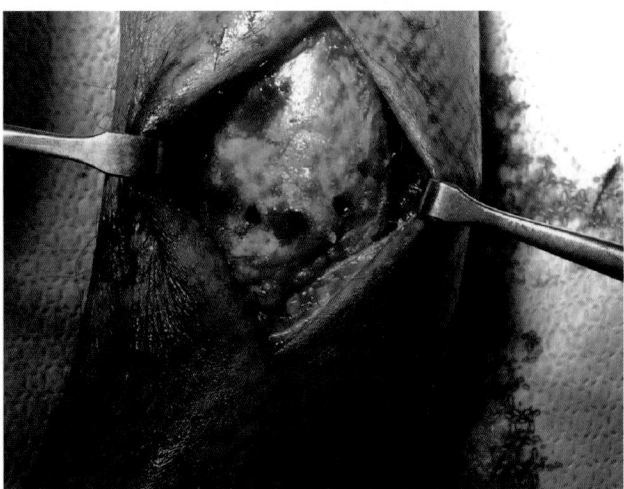

FIGURE 4 Intraoperative focal dome corticotomy.

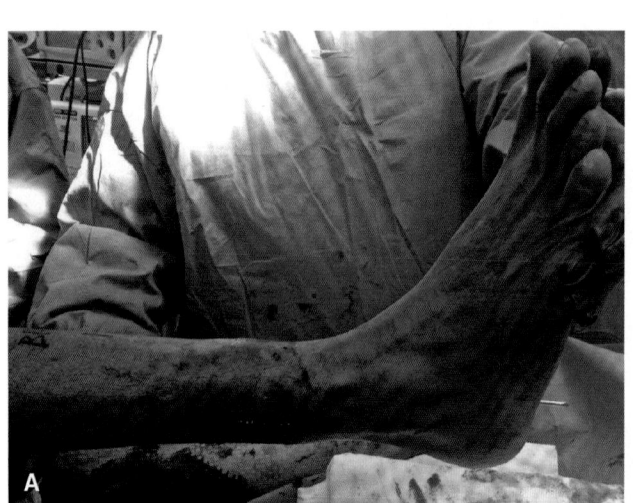

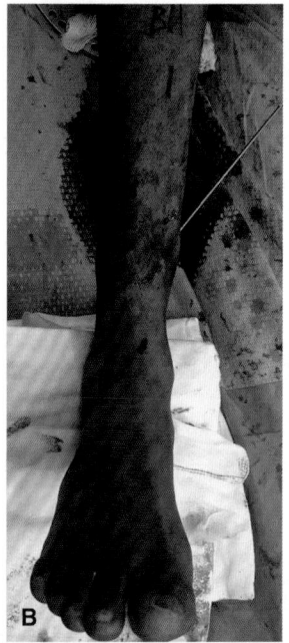

FIGURE 5 A, B. Intraoperative deformity correction.

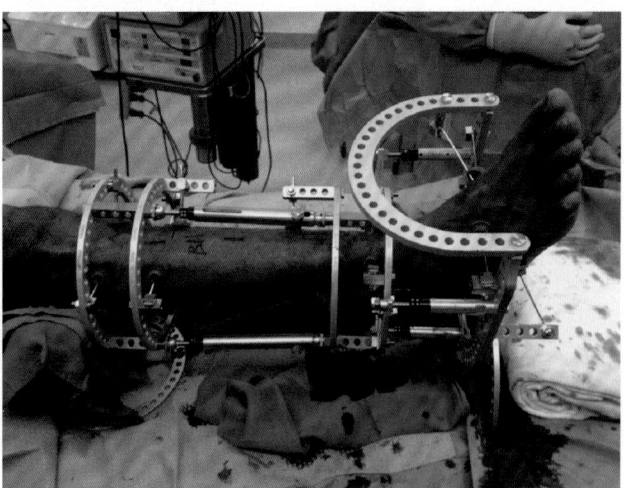

FIGURE 6 External fixation construct.

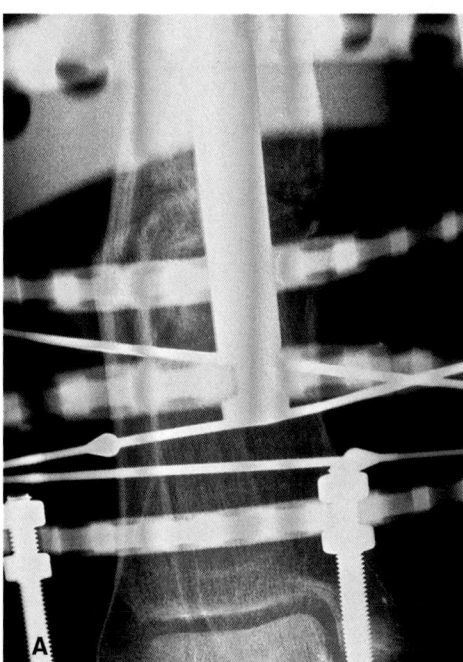
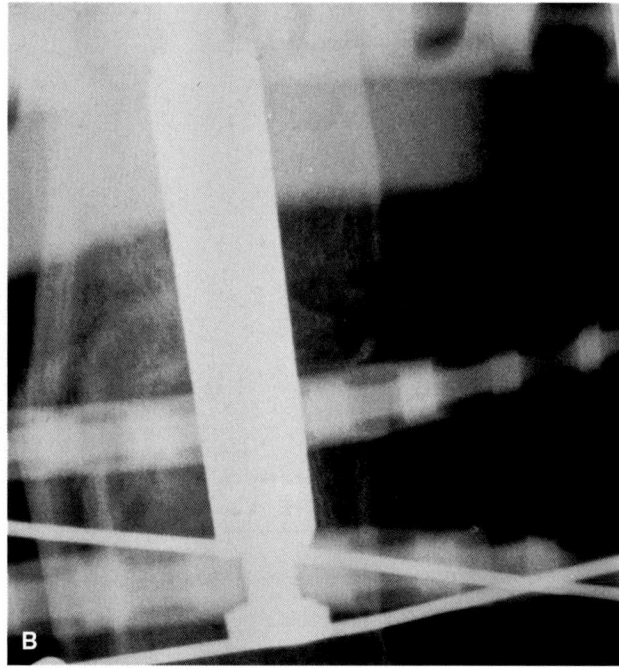

FIGURE 7 **A.** Postoperative radiographs. **B.** Postoperative radiograph of corticotomy site.

TIBIOCALCANEAL FUSION WITH DISTAL TIBIAL LENGTHENING

A 74-year-old female 5 months s/p closed talar fracture
(Case courtesy of Kevin McKann, DPM, St. Cloud Orthopedics)

- Primary spanning delta frame
- Delayed ORIF
- 8 weeks non–weight-bearing cast

9 months s/p injury

- Ankle crepitus, pain, and <20 degrees total range of motion of the ankle joint
- Rearfoot and ankle deformities

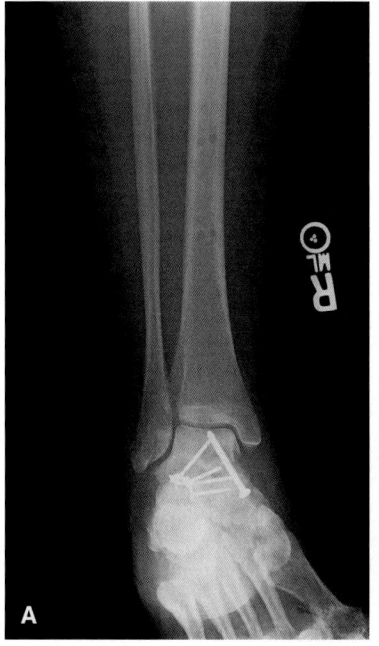
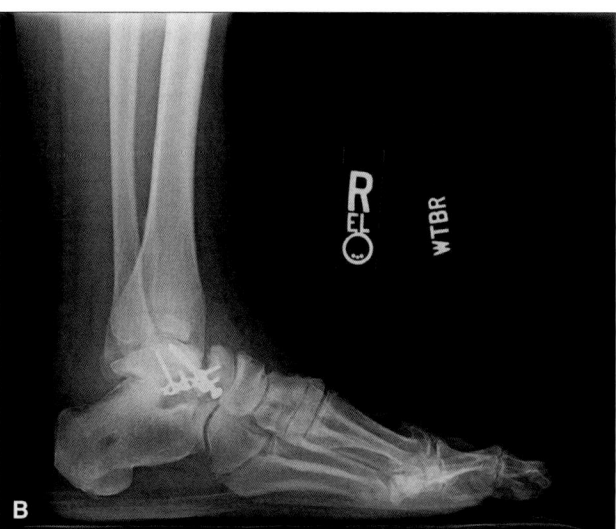

FIGURE 1 **A.** Preoperative AP ankle radiograph. **B.** Preoperative lateral ankle radiograph.

11 months s/p initial injury

- Talectomy and tibial calcaneal arthrodesis
- Distal tibial corticotomy to address 23 mm LLD

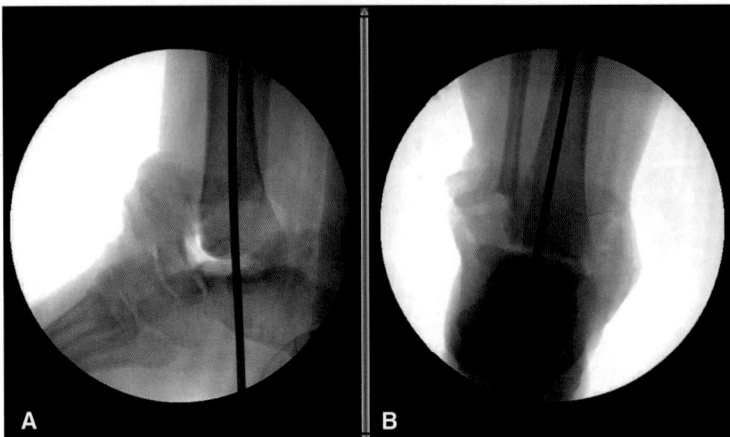

FIGURE 2 **A.** Intraoperative lateral view of talectomy with positioning. **B.** Intraoperative AP view of talectomy with positioning.

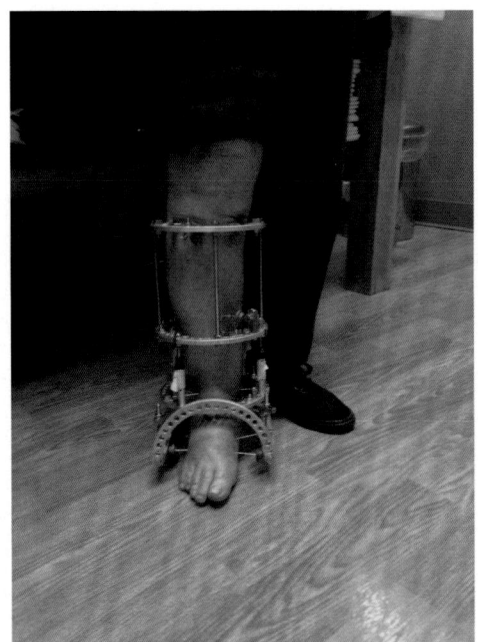

FIGURE 3 Clinical external fixation positioning 12 weeks postoperatively.

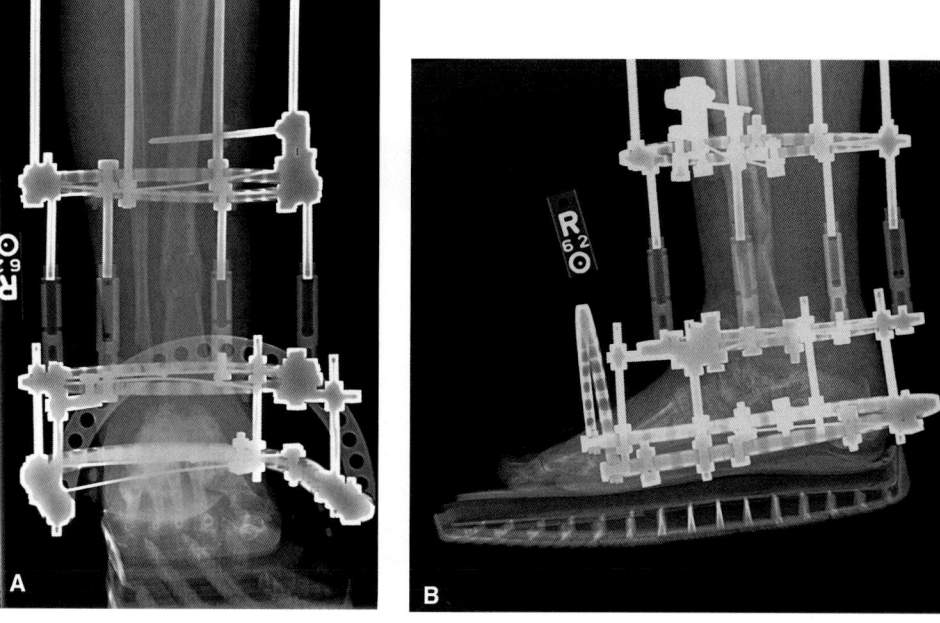

FIGURE 4 A. AP radiographs 12 weeks postoperatively. **B.** Lateral radiographs 12 weeks postoperatively.

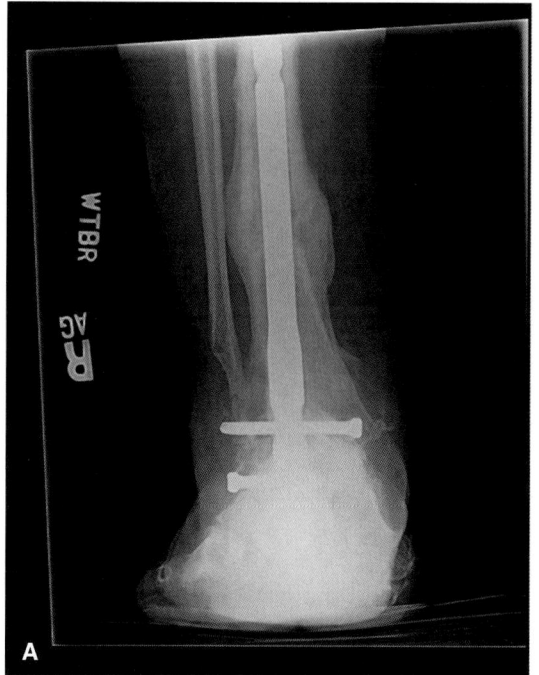
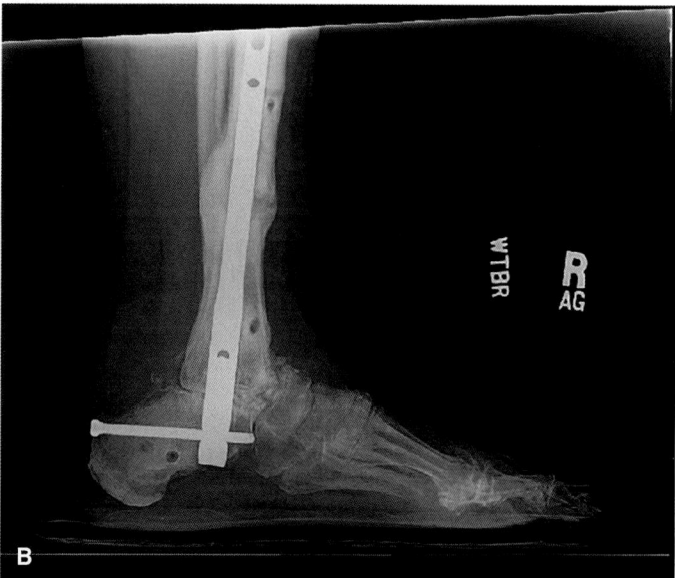

FIGURE 5 A. AP radiograph six month follow-up after intramedullary fixation. **B.** Lateral radiograph six month follow-up after intramedullary fixation.

REFERENCES

1. Cordivilla A. On the means of lengthening, in lower limbs, the muscles and tissues which are shortened through deformity. *J Bone Joint Surg Am.* 1905;s2-2:353-369.
2. Putti V. The operative lengthening of the femur. 1921. *Clin Orthop Relat Res.* 1990;250:4-7.
3. Wagner H. Operative lengthening of the femur. *Clin Orthop Relat Res.* 1978;136:125-142.
4. Ilizarov GA. The tension-stress effect on the genesis and growth of tissues: Part II. The influence of the rate and frequency of distraction. *Clin Orthop Relat Res.* 1989;239:263-285.
5. Stewart D. A platform with six degrees of freedom. *Proc Inst Mech Eng.* 1965;180:371-378.
6. Guichet JM, Deomedis B, Donnan LT, et al. Gradual femoral lengthening with the Albizzia intramedullary nail. *J Bone Joint Surg Am.* 2003;85-A:838-848.
7. Aaron AD, Eilert RE. Results of the Wagner and Ilizarov methods of limb-lengthening. *J Bone Joint Surg Am.* 1996;1:20-29.
8. De Bastiani G, Aldegheri R, Renz-Brivio L, et al. Limb lengthening by callus distraction (callotasis). *J Pediatr Orthop.* 1987;7:129-134.
9. Ilizarov GA, Green SA. *Transosseous Osteosynthesis.* Berlin/Heidelberg: Springer-Verlag; 1992.
10. Ilizarov GA. Clinical application of the tension-stress effect for limb lengthening. *Clin Orthop Relat Res.* 1990;250:8-26.
11. Paley D. History and science behind the six-axis correction external fixation devices in orthopedic surgery. *Oper Tech Orthop.* 2011;21:125-128.
12. Velazquez RJ, Bell DF, Armstrong PF, Babyn P, Tibshirani R. Complications of use of the Ilizarov technique in the correction of limb deformities in children. *J Bone Joint Surg Am.* 1993;75(8):1148-1156.
13. Paley D. Problems, obstacles, and complications of limb lengthening by the Ilizarov technique. *Clin Orthop.* 1990;250:81-104.
14. Cole JD, Justin D, Kasparis T, et al. The intramedullary skeletal kinetic distractor (ISKD): first clinical results of a new intramedullary nail for lengthening of the femur and tibia. *Injury.* 2001;32(suppl 4):SD 129-SD 136.
15. Baumgart R, Betz A, Schweiberer L. A fully implantable motorized intramedullary nail for limb lengthening and bone transport. *Clin Orthop Relat Res.* 1997;343:135-143.
16. Jeng CL, Campbell JT, Tang EY, Cerrato RA, Myerson MS. Tibiocalcaneal arthrodesis with bulk femoral head allograft for salvage of large defects in the ankle. *Foot Ankle Int.* 2013;34(9):1256-1266.
17. Gurney B. Leg length discrepancy. *Gait Posture.* 2002;15(2):195-206.
18. Defrin R, Ben Benyamin S, Aldubi RD, Pick CG. Conservative correction of leg-length discrepancies of 10 mm or less for the relief of chronic low back pain. *Arch Phys Med Rehabil.* 2005;86(11):2075-2080.
19. Kujala UM, Kvist M, Osterman K, Friberg O, Aalto T. Factors predisposing army conscripts to knee exertion injuries incurred in a physical training program. *Clin Orthop Relat Res.* 1986;210:203-212.
20. Choi IH, Chung MS, Baek GH, et al. Metatarsal lengthening in congenital brachymetatarsia: one stage lengthening versus lengthening by callotasis. *J Pediatr Orthop.* 1999;19(5):660-664.
21. Delloye C, Delefortrie G, Coulter L, et al. Bone regenerate formation in cortical bone during distraction lengthening. An experimental study. *Clin Orthop Relat Res.* 1990;250:34-42.
22. Cattaneo R, Villa A, Catagni MA, et al. Lengthening of the humerus using Ilizarov technique. Description of the method and report of 43 cases. *Clin Orthop Relat Res.* 1990;250:117-124.
23. Green SA. Complications of external skeletal fixation. *Clin Orthop Relat Res.* 1983;180:109-116.
24. Paley D, Tetsworth K. Percutaneous osteotomies. Osteotome and Gigli saw techniques. *Orthop Clin North Am.* 1991;22:613-624.
25. Lamm BM, Gourdine-Shaw MC, Thabet AM, Jindal G, Herzenberg JE, Burghardt RD. Distraction osteogenesis for complex foot deformities: Gigli saw midfoot osteotomy with external fixation. *J Foot Ankle Surg.* 2014;53(5):567-576.
26. Aronson J. Experimental and clinical experience with distraction osteogenesis. *Cleft Palate Craniofac J.* 1994;31:473-481.
27. Bonnard C, Favard L, Sollogoub I, et al. Limb lengthening in children using the Ilizarov method. *Clin Orthop Relat Res.* 1993;293:83-88.
28. Dahl MT, Gulli B, Berg T. Complications of limb lengthening. A learning curve. *Clin Orthop Relat Res.* 1994;301:10-18.
29. Paley D. Current techniques of limb lengthening. *J Pediatr Orthop.* 1988;8:73-92.
30. Aronson J, Good B, Stewart C, et al. Preliminary studies of mineralization during distraction osteogenesis. *Clin Orthop Relat Res.* 1990;250:43-49.
31. Fischgrund J, Paley D, Suter C. Variables affecting time to bone healing during limb lengthening. *Clin Orthop Relat Res.* 1994;301:31-37.
32. Kawamura B, Hosono S, Takahashi T, et al. Limb lengthening by means of subcutaneous osteotomy. Experimental and clinical studies. *J Bone Joint Surg Am.* 1968;50:851-878.
33. Lee DY, Choi IH, Chung CY, et al. Effect of tibial lengthening on the gastrocnemius muscle. A histopathologic and morphometric study in rabbits. *Acta Orthop Scand.* 1993;54:688-692.
34. Matano T, Tamai K, Kurokaea T. Adaptation of skeletal muscle in limb lengthening: a light diffraction study on the sarcomere length in situ. *J Orthop Res.* 1994;12:193-196.
35. Ippolito E, Peretti G, Bellocci M, et al. Histology and ultrastructure of arteries, veins, and peripheral nerves during limb lengthening. *Clin Orthop Relat Res.* 1994;308:54-62.
36. Lee DY, Han TR, Choi IH, et al. Changes in somatosensory-evoked potentials in limb lengthening. An experimental study on rabbits' tibiae. *Clin Orthop Relat Res.* 1992;285:273-279.
37. Strong M, Hruska J, Czyrny J, et al. Nerve palsy during femoral lengthening: MRI, electrical and histologic findings in the central and peripheral nervous systems. A canine model. *J Pediatr Orthop.* 1994;14:347-351.
38. Hamdy RC. Evolution in long bone deformity correction in the post-Ilizarov era: external to internal devices. *J Limb Length Reconstr.* 2016;2(2):61-67.
39. Paley D, Herzenberg JE, Paremain G, Bhave A. Femoral lengthening over an intramedullary nail. A matched-case comparison with Ilizarov femoral lengthening. *J Bone Joint Surg Am.* 1997;79:1464-1480.
40. Rozbruch SR, Kleinman D, Fragomen A, Ilizarov S. Limb lengthening and then insertion of an intramedullary nail: a case matched comparison. *Clin Orthop Relat Res.* 2008;466:2923-2932.
41. Oh CW, Kim JW, Baek SG, et al. Limb lengthening with a submuscular locking plate based on an original article. *J Bone Joint Surg Br.* 2009;91:1394-1399.
42. Harbacheuski R, Fragomen AT, Rozbruch SR. Does lengthening and then plating (LAP) shorten duration of external fixation? *Clin Orthop Relat Res.* 2012;470:1771-1781.
43. Garcia-Cimbrelo E, Curto de la Mano A, et al. The intramedullary elongation nail for femoral lengthening. *J Bone Joint Surg Br.* 2002;84:971-977.
44. Krieg AH, Speth BM, Foster BK. Leg lengthening with a motorized nail in adolescents: an alternative to external fixators? *Clin Orthop Relat Res.* 2008;466:189-197.
45. Krieg AH, Lenze U, Speth BM, et al. Intramedullary leg lengthening with a motorized nail. *Acta Orthop.* 2011;82:344-350.
46. Lee DH, Ryu KJ, Kim JW, et al. Bone marrow aspirate concentrate and platelet-rich plasma enhanced bone healing in distraction osteogenesis of the tibia. *Clin Orthop Relat Res.* 2014;472(12):3789-3797.
47. Baruah RK. Accordion maneuver: a bloodless tool in Ilizarov. *J Limb Length Reconstr.* 2018;4(1):11-19.

CHAPTER 42

Dislocations

Travis A. Motley and Eric A. Barp

METATARSAL PHALANGEAL JOINT DISLOCATIONS (FIRST VS LESSER)

DEFINITION

- Injury to the metatarsophalangeal complex is a common injury in athletics and the third leading cause of missed participation in university athletes as noted by Clanton and Ford. George et al. examined the National Collegiate Athletic Association database and identified several risk factors associated with injury in football players including playing surface, time of the season, position, and activities on the field.[1,2]
- Injury occurs when there is hyperdorsiflexion of the metatarsophalangeal joint when the foot is in a plantar flexed position resulting in a stretch or tearing of the plantar capsular structures.
- Strains or stretching injuries with dorsal dislocation of the hallux are frequently reported in ballet dancer and football players, who refer to these injuries as "turf toe."[3] Plantar dislocations of the hallux have been coined "sand toe" after the injury was reported in 12 sand volley ball players.[4]

CLASSIFICATION

- Jahss[5]:
  - ▶ Type 1: dorsal dislocation of the hallux/sesamoid apparatus without disruption of the sesamoid apparatus. Cannot be closed reduced
  - ▶ Type 2a: dorsal dislocation with disruption of the intersesamoidal ligament. Able to closed reduced
  - ▶ Type 2b: transverse fracture of the sesamoids. Able to closed reduce
  - ▶ Type 2c: combination of types 2a and 2b. Will not be able to closed reduce

INDICATIONS

- Turf toe injuries
- Traumatic dislocations of the MPJs

ANATOMIC FEATURES

- The metatarsophalangeal joint involves the articulation between the rounded head of the metatarsal bone and the concave base of the proximal phalanx. The first metatarsophalangeal joint is unique in that there are sesamoids situated in the plantar groves of the first metatarsal head on each side of the median crista within the flexor apparatus. The presence of accessory sesamoid osicicle can be seen in the lesser metatarsophalangeal joints, but this is variable and occurs infrequently. The metatarsal is joined to the proximal phalanx by a thick fibrous capsule circumferentially with strong medial and lateral collateral ligaments. The tibial and fibular sesamoids of the first metatarsal bone are held together by the intersesamoidal ligament. These ossicles are firmly attached distally to the proximal phalanx by the medial and lateral heads of the flexor hallucis brevis tendon and have bands of the abductor hallucis and adductor hallucis tendons both medially and laterally, respectively.[6] The joint is a ginglymoarthrodial joint that acts as both a hinge and sliding joint. During dorsiflexion and plantar flexion of the first metatarsal phalangeal joint, the central axis of rotation changes to provide full range of motion. The natural range of motion of the first metatarsophalangeal joint with dorsiflexion is 65-75 degrees and >15 degrees plantar flexion.[7]
- The lesser metatarsophalangeal joints are composed of the metatarsal and their respective proximal phalanx. The capsule maintains the integrity of the joint which is supported medially and laterally by collateral ligaments, dorsally by the extensor expansion formed by the tendons of intrinsic and extrinsic muscles of the foot, as well as the thick fibrocartilaginous band known as the plantar plate. Trauma that can result in capsular disruption can result in lesser metatarsophalangeal joint dislocation, which can be magnified by the change in the normal anatomic axis of the supporting tendinous structures.

FUNCTIONAL ANALYSIS OF THE ANATOMY

- In dorsal dislocations, the thick plantar fibrocartilaginous plate becomes locked in position and the proximal phalanx remains subluxed over the metatarsal head. If the intersesamoidal ligament remains intact, closed

reduction attempts often fail. If the intersesamoidal ligament becomes disrupted or detached, often times closed reduction is successful.[6]

- There have been reports of hyperplantarflexion injuries, coined "sand toe," which occurs as a result of fixed plantar flexed position of the hallux in respect to the metatarsal with forward movement of the foot causing the proximal phalanx to slide over the metatarsal head.[4]

PHYSICAL EXAMINATION

- Instability with dorsiflexion and plantar flexion of the metatarsophalangeal joint with slight dorsiflexion of the digit.[6]
- The metatarsal head is prominent plantarly with a commonly noted dorsomedial dimple in the skin.[3]
- Severe pain with inability to bear weight and a prominent metatarsal head.
- Dorsoplantar drawer test, Lachman test, should be performed to assess the plantar plate with a varus and valgus stress if tolerated to look for instability.
- Patients often have ecchymosis and swelling to the digit.

PATHOGENESIS

- Metatarsophalangeal joint dislocations can occur when there is a high-energy or low-energy force from distal to proximal that causes hyperextension of the proximal phalanx on the first metatarsal bone, which disrupt the metatarsophalangeal joint and potentially the sesamoidal apparatus as well. Prompt relocation is essential for these types of injuries to prevent vascular compromise and skin tenting.[3]

IMAGING AND DIAGNOSTIC STUDIES

X-RAYS[3]

- Anteroposterior, lateral, medial oblique, axial sesamoid weight-bearing radiographs.
- Stress radiographs with 3 mm of movement of the sesamoids relative to the contralateral side have been shown to be highly predictable for injuries involving the plantar ligaments.[8]
- In type 1 dislocations, the sesamoids are situated dorsal to the first metatarsal head without evidence of widening or fractures of the sesamoids.
- Type 2
  - Type 2a dislocations have the same appearance as the type 1 dislocation but do demonstrate widening of the sesamoids, which represents a tear of the intersesamoidal ligament.
  - Type 2b radiographs have evidence of a sesamoid fracture without widening.
  - Type 2c dislocations have both widening of the intersesamoidal complex with fracturing of the sesamoid.

MRI

- MRI can be used to identify plantar ligament and capsule tears as well as to assess the integrity of the flexor tendons, which are best seen on coronal and transverse views.[9] This modality can also detect possible cartilaginous damage or avascular changes of the osseous structures.

TREATMENT

NONOPERATIVE

- Closed reduction is often successful in Jahss type 2 and 3 injuries as the intersesamoidal ligament or fracture of a sesamoid has occurred, which allows for relocation. Relocation can often be accomplished under local anesthetic blockade.
- An initial period of non–weight-bearing immobilization is recommended. Taping or bracing the digit in rectus alignment can help stabilize the joint and allow these patients to ambulate in a stiff-soled shoe or CAM boot to prevent excessive motion at the joint.[3] Gradual progression to normal shoes can take some time, but patients tend to return to activity in 2-6 weeks with mild to moderate injuries.[10]

SURGICAL PROCEDURES AND TECHNIQUES: STEP-BY-STEP NARRATIVE

- Surgical procedures are dependent on the pathology and location of the dislocation.
- It is important to get postreduction radiographs to confirm adequate reduction and restoration of the normal joint.

First Metatarsal Phalangeal Joint

- A medial approach has been recommended by many surgeons to provide direct visualization of the impeding structures and avoids a painful weight-bearing scar, which can be seen with the plantar approach.
- A 4- to 5-cm longitudinal incision is made on the medial aspect of the foot slightly inferior to midline to prevent injury to the neurovascular bundle. The incision extends from the first metatarsal neck to the flexor sulcus of the hallux with a 90-degree lateral curve proximally to form a flap. The flap is retracted inferior to have full visualization of the capsule and sesamoid complex.
- Longitudinal capsulotomy is then made to provide visualization of the metatarsal-sesamoid complex.
- If there is no disruption of the intersesamoidal ligament, the ligament can be transected to allow for reduction. Exaggeration of the dorsiflexion deformity is performed with distal traction to reduce the metatarsophalangeal joint into the correct position. The intersesamoidal ligament is primarily repaired with suture to reapproximate the plantar plate.
- If there is a concomitant tear of the plantar plate with deviation, a separate incision is made dorsally over the metatarsal phalangeal joint (MPJ) and the proximal phalanx just lateral to the EHL tendon. Dissection is carried down to the EHL. The EHL is retracted medially to provide exposure of the dorsal capsule. Once the collaterals are released distally from the proximal phalanx for exposure, a 0.062-in K-wire can be used to create two medial and two lateral holes in the base of the proximal phalanx. Using a suture passing device, two strands can be placed

in the capsule medially and laterally then passed through the drill holes from a plantar to dorsal fashion.

- If the joint is unstable, a 0.062-in K-wire can be placed percutaneously to maintain position during the healing process.[11]
- The capsule is closed with an absorbable suture with a slight plantar flexion of the joint and the skin closed in layers.

Lesser Metatarsophalangeal Joint

- Rarely do these need to be reduced surgically in the OR unless there is a plantar plate tear.
  - A linear incision is made from a dorsal approach, which spans from the distal one-third of the metatarsal to the head of the proximal phalanx just medial to the extensor digitorum tendon.
  - Once the tendon is visualized and freed, it is retracted laterally and the incision is carried down to the joint capsule.
  - The collateral ligaments are released distally from the proximal phalanx to provide exposure.
  - Distal traction is applied to the digit to assess for possible tear of the plantar plate.
  - If torn, multiple techniques or devices have been described in the literature to repair this structure.

Plantar Approach

- An incision is made in a linear fashion in the intermetatarsal space to prevent possible plantar scar complication with a slight curve in the plantar digital sulcus.
- Mechanical dissection is performed until the flexor tendons are noted. Once visualized, they are retracted, and the plantar plate is easily visualized.
- The plantar plate can be repaired in various ways including primary repair with suture or even a small suture anchor placed in the proximal phalanx.

> **positioning PEARLS**
> - Postrepair, the digit should be placed in a slight plantar flexed position while the skin is closed in layers.
> - The digit should also be placed in slight plantar flexion postoperatively to allow for healing to occur and strengthen your repair.

AUTHORS' PREFERRED TREATMENT

- Obtain Kerlix gauze roll from the storage cabinet once the patient is locally anesthetized or under conscious sedation. Wrap the Kerlix gauze around the affected digits. Used the Kerlix gauze roll to apply dorsodistal traction to exaggerate the deformity and then immediate distal traction to relocate the affected digits simultaneously.[10]
- Splint the digits where the proximal phalanx is slightly plantar flexed on the corresponding metatarsal head. A stiff-soled postoperative shoe or CAM boot is recommended to prevent excessive motion at the metatarsophalangeal joints.

> **PERILS, TIPS, AND PITFALLS**
> - Intra-articular steroid injections are not advised as they can cause weakening to the capsule and only provide temporary relief in disguising symptoms.
> - Jahss type 1 injuries usually require open reduction as the soft tissue structures remain intact making closed reduction extremely difficult.
> - Type 2 dislocations can usually be reduced under local anesthetic or conscious sedation if needed to restore the normal joint structure.
> - If a lesser metatarsophalangeal joint dislocation occurs, closed reduction is usually successful and the digit can be buddy taped to the adjacent digit and then placed in a stiff-soled shoe for ~4 weeks.

POSTOPERATIVE CARE

Surgically repaired patients can be splinted or placed in a soft dressing postoperatively. Surgeons may choose to allow for partial weight bearing or a period of non–weight bearing before transferring the patient to a hard-soled surgical shoe or CAM boot for ~4-6 weeks.

REHABILITATION

- Passive plantar flexion exercises are to be performed once incision has healed and passive dorsiflexion to commence 6 weeks postoperatively once patient has been transferred to a hard-soled shoe.
- Return to activity can begin 3 months postoperatively with a slow gradual progression to full activity with a graphite insole for at least 6 months.

LISFRANC DISLOCATIONS

DEFINITION

Tarsometatarsal joint injuries are commonly referred to as Lisfranc injuries, after the Napoleonic era field surgeon who described disarticulation amputations at these joints without ever defining injuries at the corresponding levels.[12]

CLASSIFICATION

> **QUENU AND KUSS[13]/HARDCASTLE[14]/MYERSON[15]**
> - Type A—total incongruity homolateral or homomedial
> - Type B1—partial incongruity medial
> - Type B2—partial incongruity lateral
> - Type C1—partial displacement divergent
> - Type C2—total incongruity divergent

ANATOMIC FEATURES

Lisfranc joint complex includes the tarsometatarsal joints and the proximal intermetatarsal and anterior intertarsal articulations. It is stabilized by its unique bone structure and by strong capsular and ligamentous attachments as well as the surrounding plantar soft tissues. Movement across these articulations is characterized by 10-20 degrees of sagittal plane motion at the fifth tarsometatarsal joint, with progressively less mobility in the medial joints.[16] The exception is the first tarsometatarsal articulation, which also allows significant sagittal and coronal plane motion.

FUNCTIONAL ANALYSIS OF THE ANATOMY (PEICHA[17] AND RAIKIN[18])

The tarsometatarsal joints are formed by the proximal articular surfaces of the five metatarsals and the distal articular surface of the corresponding three cuneiforms and cuboid. The tarsometatarsal joints are weight-bearing structures with numerous ligamentous and tendon insertions. The forefoot is relatively mobile compared to the stable midfoot. The midfoot bones function as a single unit with minimal motion between the bones. These stable joints help form the longitudinal medial arch. The first tarsometatarsal joint is stabilized by its shape, size, and strong ligamentous attachments. The peroneus longus and anterior tibial tendons also provide stability through its dynamic tension on the joint. There is varying degrees of dorsal and plantar motion through this joint. In nonpathologic feet, the second and third tarsometatarsal joints are essentially immobile. Their osseous configuration and strong plantar intermetatarsal ligaments stabilize these joints. The fourth and fifth tarsometatarsal joints are mobile adapters; they have immense gliding motions to allow for adjustments with uneven surfaces and align the rear foot with the forefoot.

- **Bony anatomy:** The tarsometatarsal complex is made up of the three cuneiforms, metatarsals, and cuboid. Two arches are formed in the frontal and transverse planes. The second and third cuneiforms are situated more dorsally than plantarly. They are wedge shaped with the base of the wedges situated dorsally and the apex plantarly. The second metatarsal is recessed between the adjacent metatarsocuneiform joints, forming the "key stone" effect.
- **Ligamentous anatomy:** A strong transverse, oblique, and interosseous ligament, except between the base of the first and second metatarsals, connects each metatarsal base. The designated Lisfranc ligament is an extremely strong and thick ligament extending from the medial base of the second metatarsal obliquely into the medial cuneiform. It is roughly 1.5 cm in length, 0.5 cm thick. In 22% of cases, it has been found to consist of two portions; one obliquely and the other longitudinally. The ligaments are stronger plantarly than dorsally. The plantar fascia, tendons, and muscles also support the joints on the plantar aspect.

PHYSICAL EXAMINATION

A high index of suspicion for injury to Lisfranc joint complex must be maintained with all foot injuries, no matter how trivial, because of the many causes and injury types. Severe injuries with wide displacement are usually obvious and are usually accompanied by significant midfoot swelling, ecchymosis, deformity, and obvious radiographic abnormalities. Many patients go misdiagnosed with a foot sprain or unrecognized due to spontaneous reduction of the injury, however; close examination will still show some displacement. An individual may present with swelling, tenderness, and instability along the tarsometatarsal joints. Weight-bearing radiographs can be difficult to obtain as pain may prevent patients from fully weight bearing. A stress test may be performed by grasping both the first and second metatarsals and performing dorsiflexion and plantar flexion motions. A positive test is one that elicits pain with minimal stress. Harwood and Raikin[19] suggested maintaining the hindfoot in an inverted position during stress testing to eliminate subtalar joint motion.

PATHOGENESIS

The majority of Lisfranc injuries occur in males around 30-40 years old.[20] Injuries can be either high or low impact. High-energy injuries result in severely displaced fracture-dislocations, whereas less severe twisting injuries can cause more subtle sprains and subluxations. High-impact injuries can occur from a direct load to the dorsal midfoot as seen in crush injuries or more commonly an indirect injury from a longitudinal force on the foot in plantar flexion as seen in motor vehicle accidents. MVA are the leading cause of Lisfranc fracture-dislocation and are responsible for nearly two-thirds of all cases.[15] Others include crush injuries, falls from ground level with or without twisting injuries to the foot, and falls from a height. The mechanism of injury has been classified as either direct or indirect. Direct injuries are those with forces applied directly to Lisfranc articulations, as with direct blows or industrial crush injuries. The direction of displacement is predicated on the applied force rather than on the inherent bony architecture and soft tissue restraints. Plantar displacement of the metatarsal bases as well as significant soft tissue disruption is common with this mechanism. Indirect injuries occur more often and result from a combination of twisting and axial loading of the extremely plantar flexed foot. Dislocation typically occurs at the site of least resistance, with dorsal dislocation of the metatarsals and secondary medial or lateral displacement.[21-23]

IMAGING AND DIAGNOSTIC STUDIES

Diagnostic imaging: Normal plain radiographs will show alignment of the medial aspect of the base of the second metatarsal with the medial border of the intermediate cuneiform on AP. A space may be present between the base of the first and second metatarsals that can be normal; however, if there is a step off at the base of the second metatarsal and intermediate cuneiform, this may be evidence of injury. A distance between the first and second metatarsals of >2 mm is suggestive of injury. Myerson identified a "fleck" sign that can be seen at the medial base of the second metatarsal or lateral base of the first metatarsal. This is indicative of an avulsion fracture. In cases of subtle injuries, it is recommended obtaining bilateral weight-bearing radiographs for comparison as well as advanced imaging such as CT, which can be useful in surgical planning, and MRI, which can be useful in subtle injuries as studies have found a sensitivity and predictive value of up to 94% of determining instability of the Lisfranc joint.[15,24]

TREATMENT

The goal of treatment is a stable, painless, plantigrade foot. Nondisplaced injuries with negative weight-bearing radiographs and stress test are managed well with a CAM boot. Anatomic reduction is required with displacement of 2 mm or greater of any portion of the Lisfranc complex. Closed reduction should be attempted. Postreduction radiographs are needed to ensure adequate reduction. If closed reduction is maintained, a below knee cast can be applied and non–weight bearing maintained for 6-8 weeks.[25] If closed reduction cannot be maintained due to instability, screw/pin fixation should be performed. Percutaneous fixation with K-wire fixation can provide a stable construct. If closed reduction cannot be obtained, soft tissue impingement such as the tibialis anterior, Lisfranc ligament, or bony fragments could be implicated in hindering reduction. Open reduction internal fixation should be considered within 6 weeks of injury. Surgical correction after 6 weeks of injury generally results in poor functional outcomes.[26] Fractures with bony displacement should be treated with ORIF to achieve anatomical reduction.

Fixation technique consists of ORIF with lag screw fixation of the second tarsometatarsal joint from the proximal superior medial corner of the medial cuneiform to the base of the second metatarsal. This is followed by lag screws placed from the bases of the involved metatarsals into their respective cuneiforms. If there is comminution of the metatarsal bases, plates spanning the fractures should be utilized. The standard incisional approach is a curvilinear incision slightly lateral and parallel with the second metatarsal starting at the distal one-third metatarsal and extending to the navicular. This provides excellent exposure to the first, second, and third tarsometatarsal joints while avoiding deep neurovascular structures. To access the lateral side of the Lisfranc complex, a linear incision should be made over the fourth metatarsal shaft. If instability is identified between the intercuneiform joints, an intercuneiform lag screw should be utilized from medial to lateral.

Malalignment of the Lisfranc joint complex can lead to posttraumatic arthritis, deformity, and degenerative changes. Primary arthrodesis is an alternative to ORIF in some cases where the risk of instability, deformity, and degenerative changes are high or likely to occur. Typically, the first through third tarsometatarsal joints are fused. Incision approach is the same as for ORIF.

AUTHORS' PREFERRED TREATMENT

PERILS, TIPS, AND PITFALLS

- Spontaneous reduction can occur, and make identification of an injury difficult.
- Perform stress radiographs and bilateral weight-bearing radiographs when there is suspicion of injury.
- Evaluate the neurovascular status. Prolonged vascular compromise could lead to severe necrosis and amputation.
- Evaluate for compartment syndrome, which can develop after trauma.

POSTOPERATIVE CARE

A posterior splint should be applied for the first 2 weeks to allow for soft tissue swelling and surgical incisions to heal. A below knee fiberglass cast can then be applied for an additional 4-6 weeks followed by full weight bearing in a CAM boot with physical therapy for 4 weeks. If screws have been placed, they should be removed at ~12 weeks. Full-unprotected weight bearing should not be permitted until hardware is removed.

CHOPART DISLOCATIONS

DEFINITION

Francois Chopart described the articulation of the talonavicular and calcaneal cuboid joint as an area of amputation. The components of Chopart joint include the more rigid calcaneal cuboid joint and the more flexible talonavicular joint (also referred to as the coxa pedis). These joints are also collectively referred to as the midtarsal joint and separate the hindfoot from the midfoot. Like other joints with a robust ligamentous network, isolated pure dislocations without associated avulsion fractures or associated complex fractures are rare. If there is a suspicion of isolated injury to a single bone of the midtarsal joint, advanced imaging is necessary.

Simple Chopart joint injuries can occur with low-energy mechanisms, but more complex injuries commonly occur with high-energy mechanisms. Midtarsal joint injuries are mostly combined injuries across the talonavicular and calcaneocuboid joints due to their coupled motion.[27] Understanding the anatomy, mechanism of injury, likelihood of associated injuries, and treatment options will help the practitioner provide a plan for treatment of these complex injuries.

ANATOMY

The midtarsal joint allows rearfoot motion when the forefoot is stationary on the ground. The midtarsal joint works with the subtalar joint to invert and evert the foot. As the heel everts, the axes of the calcaneocuboid and the talonavicular joints become more parallel allowing motion across the midtarsal joint.[28] Likewise, as the heel inverts, those axes diverge and the calcaneocuboid and talonavicular joints become more immobile.

The talonavicular joint is an enarthrodial joint with thin ligaments. Dorsally, the joint is covered by extensor tendons. The talonavicular joint lacks ligamentous attachment plantarly but is reinforced by the spring ligament.[29,30] Due to the paucity of ligamentous support, the talonavicular joint may be the weakest link in the Chopart complex.[30]

The calcaneocuboid joint is an arthrodial joint and is supported by more robust ligaments and the peroneus longus tendon plantarly.[31] Plantar ligaments are the strongest around the midtarsal joint, which is stabilized by the long and short plantar ligaments, bifurcate ligament (calcaneocuboid and calcaneonavicular), medial calcaneocuboid ligament, plantar cubonavicular ligament), and the spring ligament.[32]

DIAGNOSIS

Clinical examination will demonstrate pain at the midtarsal joint with direct palpation and with inversion/eversion of the midfoot. Clinical examination can be difficult due to associated pain and swelling. It is important to also examine the subtalar joint as well as the tarsometatarsal joint complex to evaluate for associated pain and injuries. Mondor sign (plantar ecchymosis) can be pathognomonic for midfoot injuries due to the hematoma that forms after avulsion/rupture of the strong plantar ligaments. Due to the often high-energy forces that can produce midtarsal joint injuries, initial and subsequent examinations must rule out compartment syndrome. In a series by Rammelt et al., half of the patients with acute injuries had fractures at more than one bone in the Chopart joint.[33] The rate of additional fractures (local and remote) in patients with a talonavicular joint dislocation has been reported to range between 75% and 90%.[34] It is important for the physician to remember that any isolated dislocation of Chopart joint likely includes at least avulsion fractures of the navicular, cuboid, talus, and calcaneus in addition to significant ligamentous injury.

Chopart sprains with associated avulsion fractures may not show any significant deformity. Significant injuries to the midfoot may not demonstrate any significant gross deformity of the foot due to spontaneous reduction. Unreduced dislocation of the midtarsal joint usually presents with demonstrable foot deformity of forefoot adduction or abduction. Standard three view x-ray images may range from small avulsion fractures at the joint margins to small impaction fractures to severely comminuted fractures with profound dislocation. Traditionally, the Cyma line on lateral projection is referenced for evaluation of joint incongruity or adjacent avulsion fractures in Chopart joint. However, the value of disruption in the Cyma line for subtle injuries is predominantly on weight-bearing images, which can rarely be obtained after Chopart injuries due to pain. Some injury mechanisms result in only small avulsions or spontaneous reductions and likely help to explain why prior studies have estimated that Chopart injuries are initially missed 20%-41% of the time.[34,35] Detection of midfoot fractures or subtle dislocations with conventional radiographs has been shown to be poor.[36] Schmitt et al.[27] emphasized the importance of even a small dorsal navicular fracture as a sign of significant Chopart injury. Even with the presence of small avulsion fractures surrounding the midtarsal joint, advanced imaging (CT/MRI) is necessary as these x-ray findings may be indicative of spontaneous reduction of a significant injury.

Diagnosis can be challenging in patients who present with a history of remote Chopart injury with persistent pain. In these cases, diagnostic injections can be used to isolate a specific joint as a source of pain. Stress x-rays (abduction and adduction of the forefoot with rearfoot stabilized) can be beneficial to rule out instability in those with delayed presentation as well as in those with subtle acute injuries. Stress x-rays can provide additional information regarding midtarsal joint stability even if advance imaging (CT/MRI) are normal, especially in delayed presentation with chronic pain at or near Chopart joint.[37]

MECHANISM

There are multiple mechanisms of injury to the midtarsal joint that result in different clinical and radiographic findings. Main and Jowett[38] described five different types of Chopart fracture dislocations based on mechanism in 71 patients (Table 42.1). Forced adduction of forefoot leads to medial stress and fractures of the navicular and/or talar head with the navicular dislocating medially and plantarly. Some authors have speculated that a cavus foot type may be a predisposing factor with this type of injury. Because of the anatomic proximity and the related function, sprains can be associated with injuries to the calcaneal cuboid and subtalar joints. Isolated dislocation of the talonavicular joint has been termed a "swivel" dislocation (of the talonavicular or subtalar joints). Medial talonavicular dislocation is a more common finding with a reported prevalence of 30% of Chopart joint injuries.[39] Axial loads along the medial column result in protrusion of the talonavicular joint with the navicular dislocating dorsolaterally and rupture of the plantar spring (plantar calcaneonavicular) ligament. Medial and axial forces have been reported to be the most common followed by lateral dislocations in prior studies.[38,39]

Forced abduction of the forefoot leads to lateral stress and fractures of the anterior process of the calcaneus and the cuboid (Fig. 42.1). Compression forces at one side (lateral) result in distraction forces at the other (medial).[40,41] Forced abduction of the midfoot leads to lateral dislocation and compression of the lateral column and can result in a compression fracture of

TABLE **42.1**	**Main and Jowett Classification Based on Mechanism**
Force	**Result**
Medial directed force to forefoot resulting in adduction (sprain)	Dorsal avulsion talar head, dorsal navicular, "swivel" subtype with rotation/dislocation, medial dislocation with fracture of the lateral navicular body, cuneiforms, or talus
Axial along the first ray	Central navicular fracture/s
Lateral directed force with dislocation (forefoot abduction)	Cuboid or anterior process calcaneal fracture
Dorsiflexion force with plantar displacement of forefoot	Talonavicular and calcaneocuboid dislocation or talonavicular and talocalcaneal dislocation
Crush injury (high velocity/energy)	Random

From Main BJ, Jowett RL. Injuries of the midtarsal joint. *J Bone Joint Surg Br.* 1975;57-B:89-97.

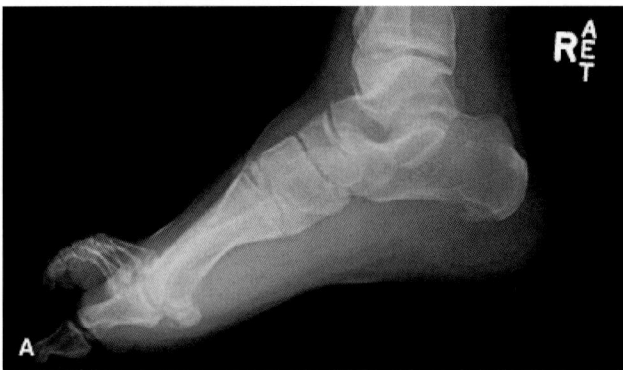

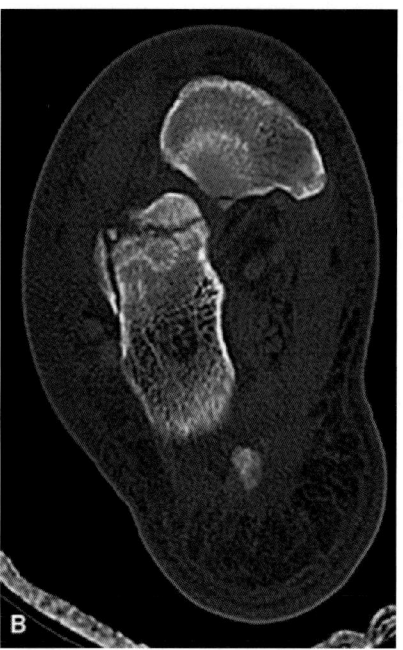

FIGURE 42.1 **A.** Lateral projection demonstrating subtle lucency in the anterior process of the calcaneus occurring after a twisting injury. **B.** Frontal plane CT imaging demonstrating compression fracture of the anterior process of the calcaneus as well as a small plantar avulsion of the navicular.

the cuboid (the "nutcracker fracture" coined by Hermel and Gershon-Cohen[42]) or a compression fracture of the anterior calcaneal process.

Dorsally directed forces result in plantar dislocation of the talonavicular and calcaneocuboid joints or the talonavicular and talocalcaneal joints. High-energy crush injuries result in complex injuries and are usually accompanied by significant soft tissue injuries.

Other mechanisms in addition to those described by Main and Jowett[38] have been described for Chopart joint injuries as a result of higher-impact/extreme sports and their related injuries. Isolated dorsal midtarsal dislocation is a result of plantar flexion of the forefoot on the dorsiflexed hindfoot first.[43,44] Zwipp[45] also described a classification system based on the fractured components (Table 42.2) with subsequent studies reporting transnavicular and transcuboid patterns being the most common.[33]

TABLE 42.2	Zwipp Classification According to Fractured Components

- Transligamentous
- Transcalcaneal
- Transcuboidal
- Transnavicular
- Transtalar
- Combination pattern of other groups

Data from Zwipp H. *Chirurgie de Fuβes.* New York, NY: Springer Wien; 1994.

TREATMENT

positioning PEARLS

- Supine
- Thigh tourniquet
- Patient secured to the bed as reduction may require significant force

EXPOSURE PEARLS

- Open injuries may determine or limit surgical approach.
- Open injuries may require extension of skin tears for irrigation and debridement and subsequent fixation.
- Closed injuries are amenable to approaches that allow reduction and fixation of deformities.
- When making an incision for any temporary fixation, always consider what incisions will be required for definitive fixation to prevent small skin bridges.
- Attention to skin bridges of 3 cm will help prevent ischemic skin islands.

PEARLS

- Attention to soft tissues with gentle retraction is paramount to preventing further skin injury or ischemia.
- Reducing the deformities and stabilizing osseous structures will allow relaxation of the soft tissues.
- Stabilize the deformity from medial to lateral. Once the medial column is stabilized, it can be used as a reference to reduce and stabilize the central and lateral columns.
- Bridge plating or external fixation techniques can be used to span the zone of comminuted injuries.
- Compartment syndrome can still occur in open injuries.
- Open treatment is preferable to closed treatment.

After appropriate evaluation of the injury and completion of the secondary survey for evaluation of local and remote injuries, the goal of Chopart injuries is immediate joint reduction to restore alignment to the medial, central, and lateral columns of the foot and to release tension of the soft tissues. Initially, closed reduction technique should be attempted by increasing the deformity, axial distraction, then reducing the deformity. Closed reduction of a midtarsal dislocation can be challenging. If initially unsuccessful, the practitioner should have a low threshold for operative reduction as intervening soft tissue structures and tension from surrounding soft tissues can prevent reduction.[46-48] If operative reduction is not an immediate option, continuous evaluation for compartment syndrome is necessary. Attempted closed reduction may be bypassed in those patients with severe open and/or contaminated wounds that will proceed promptly to the operating room.

Older reports advocated for conservative treatment with isolated dislocation or only small avulsion fractures with non–weight-bearing below knee cast 6-8 weeks followed by a transition to protected weight bearing and physical therapy.[49] Richter et al.[50] evaluated a large series of Chopart joint injuries with pure joint dislocation without related fracture (17% of 110 patients) that were treated with closed reduction without internal fixation produced good results. Likewise, Garafalo et al.[51] reviewed 18 patients with 13 medial and 5 lateral talonavicular joint dislocations. They suggested that medial talonavicular dislocations were lower-energy injuries than lateral talonavicular dislocation. Medial talonavicular dislocations were more amenable to closed treatment and had a better prognosis. Others have reported that low-energy midtarsal joint sprains that were treated conservatively had difficulty returning to their previous activity level.[49]

However, more recent studies suggest that internal or external fixation of even isolated dislocations or small avulsion fractures may provide better results.[41,52] They indicate that early anatomic reduction and stable internal fixation is the single most important prognostic factor in the treatment of Chopart joint injuries. Closed reduction, delayed or inadequate fixation, and the presence of concomitant fractures of the lower leg or foot especially with severe soft tissue damage, such as crush injuries, have been shown to be negative prognostic factors. Closed reduction and cast immobilization often yields unacceptable results with frequent redislocations and painful malunions.

Richter et al.[50] evaluated 110 Chopart joint dislocations by four treatment categories: closed reduction no internal fixation, closed reduction with internal fixation, open reduction internal fixation and optional external fixation, and amputation. Pure joint dislocation without related fracture were treated with closed reduction without internal fixation. No statistically significant difference were found in the follow-up Hannover scores considering different methods of treatment (operative vs nonoperative, internal fixation with Kirschner wires vs Kirschner wires and screws). They did find that open reduction led to a better score than closed reduction with percutaneous fixation and that patients who required surgical intervention had better AOFAS midfoot scores if they were addressed within 24 hours. Other studies have also noted better results with open treatment compared to percutaneous treatment.[52] Generally, there is agreement that more profound injuries require surgical intervention. Kutaish has described an algorithm of evaluation, diagnosis, and treatment based on increasing severity of injury[52] (Table 42.3).

Closed injuries may require a period of immobilization and compression to allow the soft tissues to be receptive to surgical incisions. Open injuries will require operative debridement. In open injuries, definitive fixation may not be necessary, but temporary fixation with pins, wires, or external fixation can be placed to assist with relaxing the soft tissues including neurovascular structures (Fig. 42.2). Surgical treatment should focus on the goals of any fracture or dislocation surgery with restoration of articular surfaces and restoring alignment to the medial, central, and lateral columns of the foot. If the columns are not restored, a cavus or planus foot type may result and will be poorly tolerated.

Surgical approaches are tailored to address not only the Chopart dislocation but also the skin and associated injuries. Standard longitudinal incisions with appropriate width of skin bridges are typically used. Generally, both medial and lateral incisions are needed. Alternative anterior medial (medial cuneiform to sustentaculum tali) and anterolateral (oblique sinus tarsi) incisions have been described by Klaue.[53]

TABLE 42.3	Treatment Algorithm			
	Value of Radiography			
CCI Injury Type	**Rx**	**CT**	**MRI**	**Diagnosis and Treatment**
Ligaments	No value	No value	Valuable	Conservative
Bony contusion	No value	No value	Valuable	Conservative
Extra-articular avulsion	Little value	Valuable	Valuable	Conservative
				Casting
Intra-articular fracture	Little value	Valuable	Valuable	Nondislocated => conservative
				Dislocated => ORIF
Dislocation	Valuable	Valuable	Valuable	ORIF
Intra-articular impaction	Little value	Valuable	Valuable	ORIF
Combined[a]	Valuable	Valuable	Valuable	ORIF

[a]Combined injury is any combination of the above-listed injuries.

From Kutaish H, Stern R, Drittenbass L, Assal M. Injuries to the Chopart joint complex: a current review. *Eur J Orthop Surg Traumatol.* 2017;27:425-431.

Definitive operative reduction of dislocations can require significant force even when utilizing the appropriate technique of accentuating the deformity and distraction. If difficulty in achieving or maintaining reduction, the surgeon must evaluate for any intervening soft tissues that prevent reduction. Operative reduction of Chopart dislocations usually begins with the talonavicular joint then progresses to the calcaneocuboid joint.[53] Maintaining joint alignment may require temporary fixation with Kirschner wires/Steinman pins prior to final fixation. Threaded pins, wires, or those from an external fixation set can also be utilized to "joy stick" fragments to their correct alignment. If external fixator pins are used, they can be incorporated into unilateral or multiplanar external fixation constructs (Fig. 42.3). Additionally, the external fixation construct can be used to hold distraction across joints to allow direct visualization for better reduction of articular surfaces and fracture fragments for placement of screws and/or plates.[34]

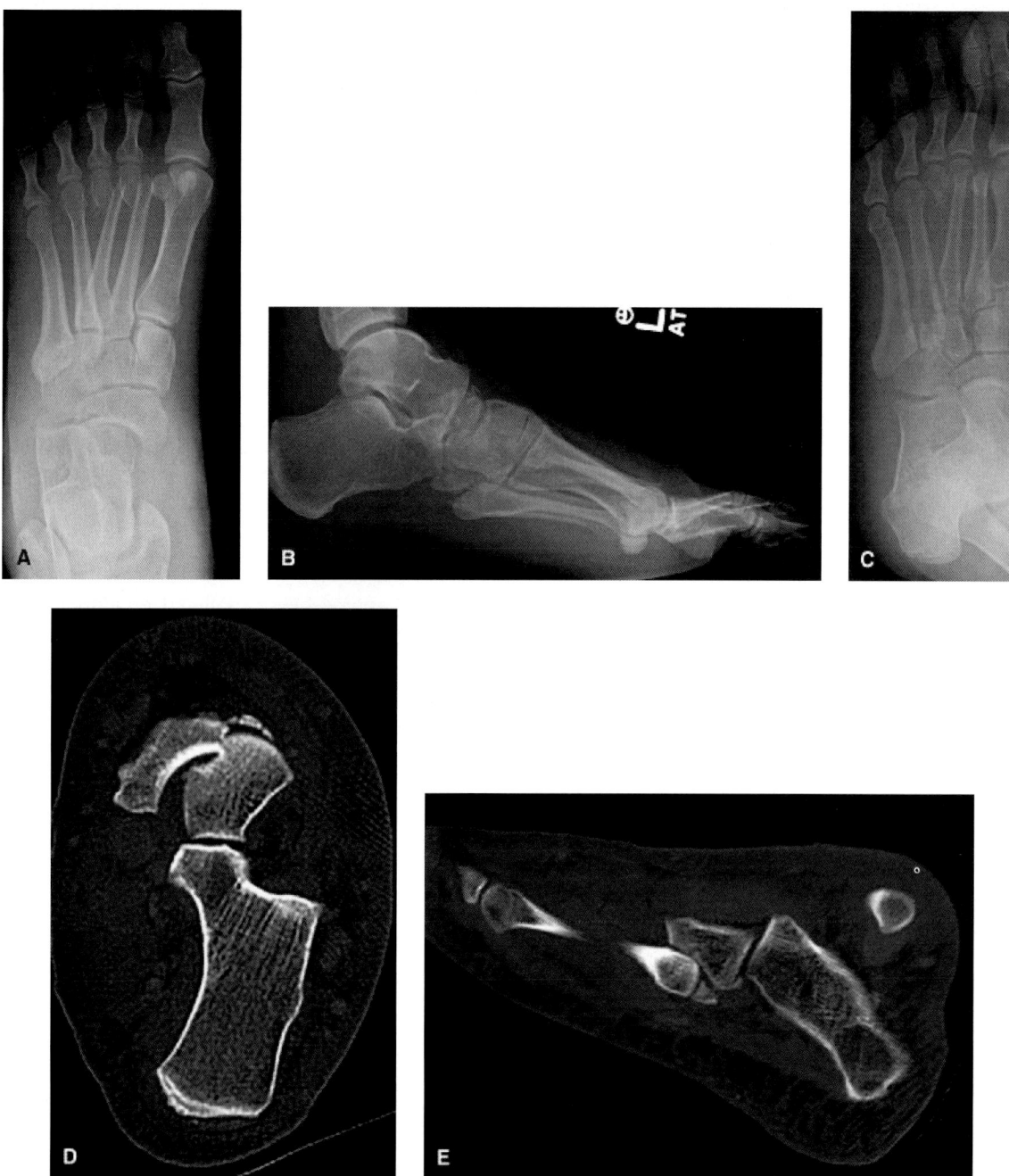

FIGURE 42.2 A–C. Injury films of the left foot after a motor vehicle accident demonstrating Chopart joint incongruity and multiple associated fractures. Coronal and sagittal CT images demonstrating medial navicular dislocation with impaction of the medial talar head **(D)** and plantar dislocation of the cuboid **(E)** with small avulsion fragment and associated injury of plantar dislocation of the fifth metatarsal.

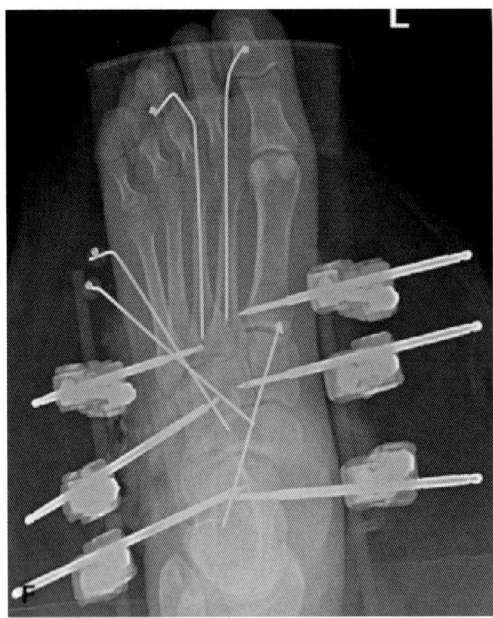

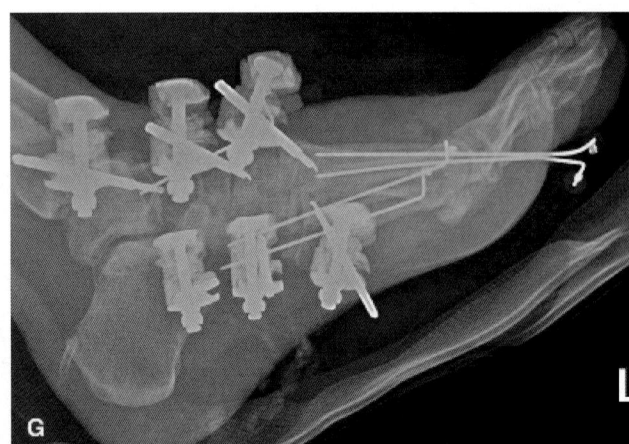

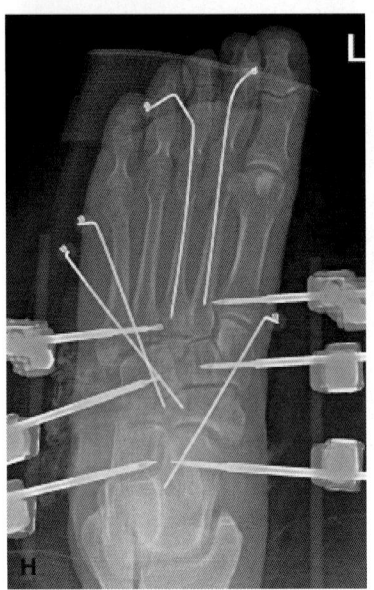

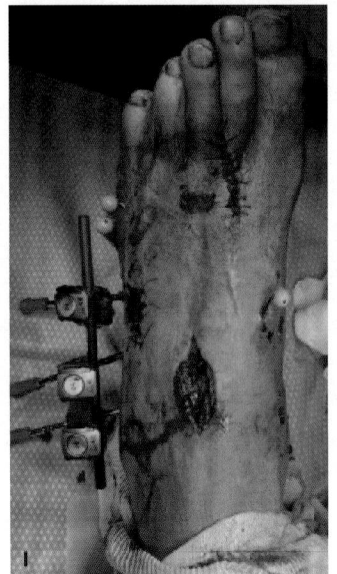

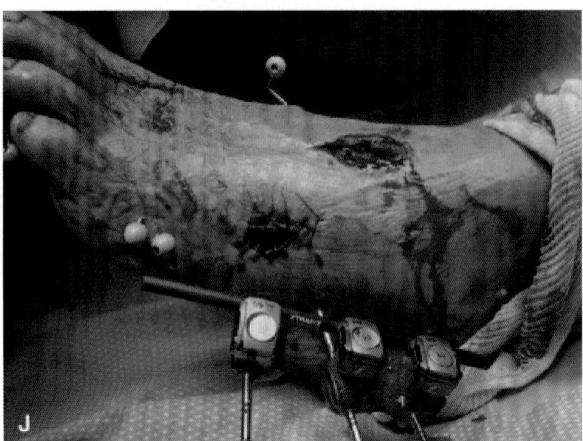

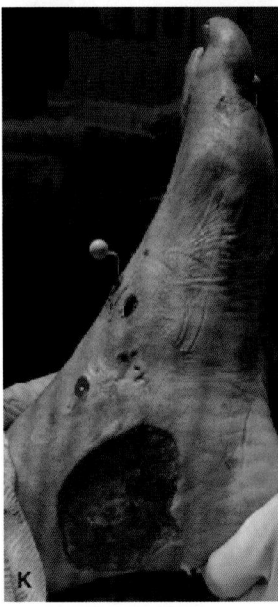

FIGURE 42.2 (*Continued*) **F–H.** Postreduction films demonstrating multiple transarticular pin placement and medial and lateral unilateral external fixation placement with restoration of the medial, central, and lateral column. **I–K.** Two weeks after initial fixation, the patient returned to the operating room for repeat debridement of ulcerated fracture blisters and removal of the medial external fixator due to infection.

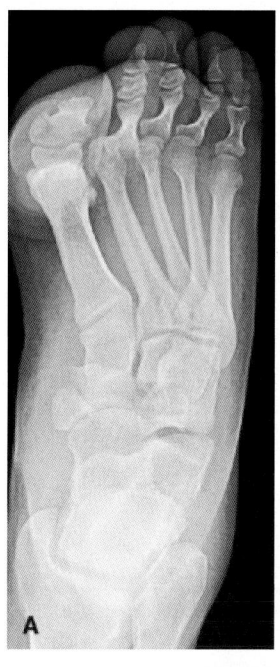
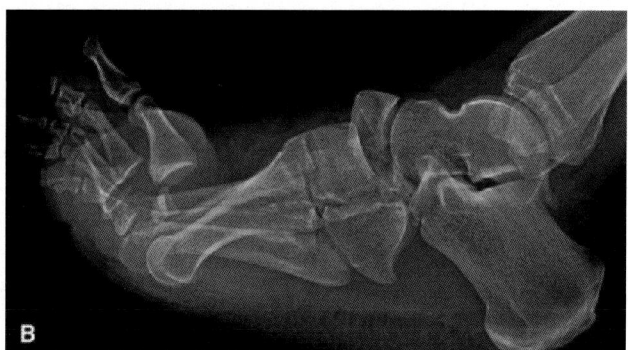
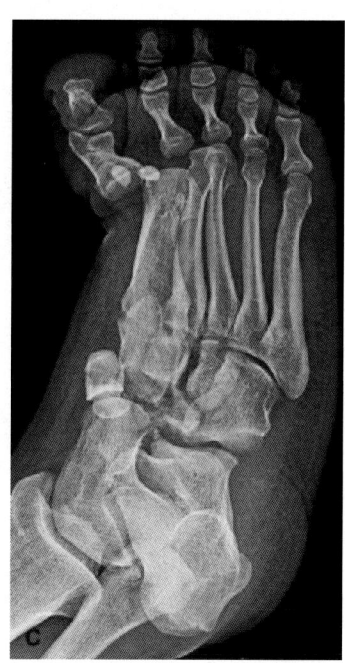
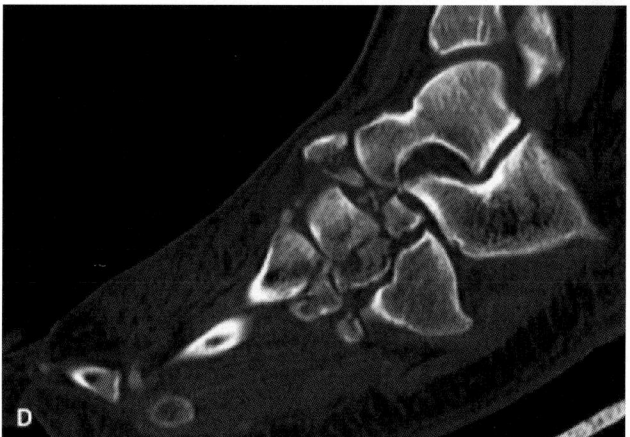
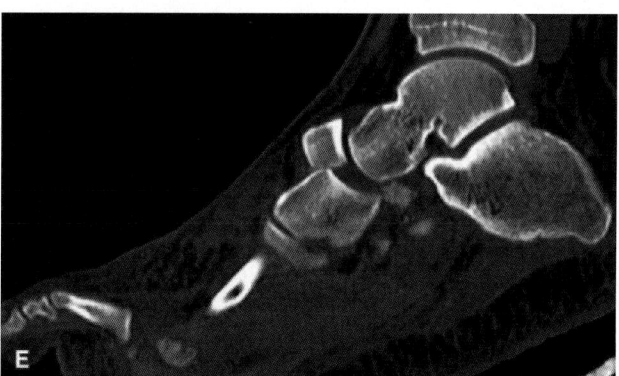
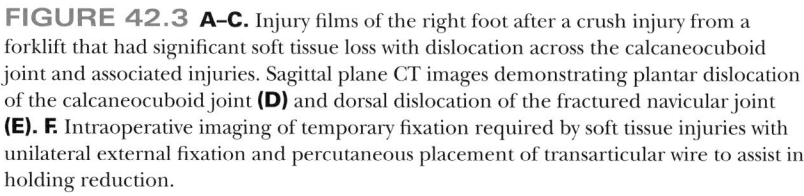
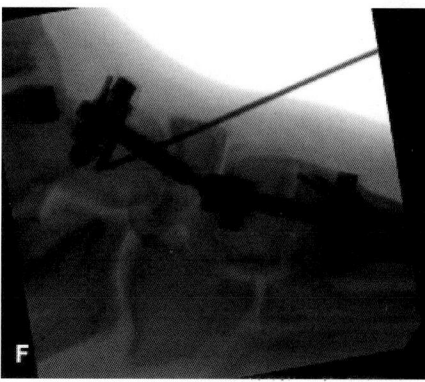

FIGURE 42.3 A–C. Injury films of the right foot after a crush injury from a forklift that had significant soft tissue loss with dislocation across the calcaneocuboid joint and associated injuries. Sagittal plane CT images demonstrating plantar dislocation of the calcaneocuboid joint **(D)** and dorsal dislocation of the fractured navicular joint **(E). F.** Intraoperative imaging of temporary fixation required by soft tissue injuries with unilateral external fixation and percutaneous placement of transarticular wire to assist in holding reduction.

Operative fixation of fracture fragments can be achieved with direct fixation from mini or small fragment sets. Comminuted fracture fixation can be achieved with small standard or specialized plates from many manufacturers that are specific to the area or bone involved, which are available in both standard and locking constructs. Some fracture fragments may be too small for direct fixation with wires and screws and should be removed. Ligamentous injuries associated with these small avulsion fractures can be repaired directly with suture to bone or with small anchors. Alternatively, these ligaments can heal based on stability to the surrounding bones/joints provided by direct fixation and immobilization.

In cases with severe comminution, ligamentous instability, and severe soft tissue injuries, final fixation restoring the column lengths of the foot may be with Kirschner wires in multiple planes and crossing multiple joints. While this fixation may not

TABLE **42.4**	**Rammelt Classification of Posttraumatic Deformities at the Midtarsal Joint**

I: joint incongruity
II: nonunion
III: I/II with arthritis at the CCJ
IV: I/II with arthritis at the TN joint
V: bilateral arthritis and complex deformity

From Rammelt S, Zwipp H, Schneiders W, et al. Anatomical reconstruction after malunited Chopart joint injuries. *Eur J Trauma Emerg Surg.* 2010;36(3):199. Ref.[56]

be rigid, it will allow for ligamentous healing without further compromise of the skin. Likewise, bridge plating techniques can also be employed to span the unstable joints and fractures (talar neck to metatarsals).[54,55] Creative combinations of wires, pins, plates, and external fixation may be necessary.

Arthrodesis should be reserved for severely comminuted fractures with significant articular incongruity that will likely progress toward some degree of avascular necrosis of fracture fragments, profound cartilage injury, or persistent midtarsal joint laxity after fixation. The goal of primary (or delayed) arthrodesis is appropriate alignment and stability of the columns of the foot to prevent subsequent deformity. Disruption in column length leads to deformity: short medial column can lead to cavus, and short lateral column can lead to pes planus.

Patients with Chopart joint injuries appropriately treated conservatively or surgically will likely report stiffness. More severe injuries will likely develop arthritic changes or have persistent ligamentous instability with recurrent subluxations or dislocations. Ip and Lui[44] pointed out the importance of significant damage to ligamentous structures after a dorsal midfoot dislocation that allowed persistent instability of Chopart joint even after open reduction and subsequent hardware removal. Rammelt[40] described a classification of posttraumatic deformities at the midtarsal joint. Types 1 or 2 posttraumatic deformities in a compliant patient with appropriate bone quality and articular cartilage may benefit from corrective osteotomies or resection of fibrous nonunion with secondary anatomic reconstruction with the goal to preserve the talonavicular and calcaneocuboid joints (Table 42.4).[40,57] Posttraumatic OA develops more rapidly in the talonavicular joint[40] and requires fusion with realignment of incongruity joints. Isolated talonavicular joint fusions required by instability or pain will result in loss of motion in adjacent calcaneocuboid joint by 81%-92% and the subtalar joint by 62%-86%.[58,59]

CONCLUSIONS

Correct diagnosis of Chopart joint injuries requires basic foot views as well as an index of suspicion by the physician. Often, advanced imaging is required to establish the extent of the injury, particularly in those injuries that appear to only demonstrate subtle signs such as small avulsion fractures. More recent studies suggest that even the small avulsion fractures indicate significant joint instability and may require stabilization with fixation. Older and newer studies agree that prompt alignment of joint surfaces and stabilization produces better results in more complex injuries. Regardless of treatment, patients often develop stiffness and can progress to posttraumatic arthritis

that will require arthrodesis. Even isolated joint arthrodesis will result in more stiffness of the midtarsal and the subtalar joint but should be geared toward the goal of pain reduction and maintaining appropriate lengths of the medial, central, and lateral columns of the foot to prevent deformity.

SUBTALAR JOINT DISLOCATIONS

DEFINITION

Subtalar joint dislocations are rarely encountered injuries accounting for <2% of all dislocations.[60] These injuries were originally described by DuFaurest and Judcy in 1811. This injury pattern is defined as simultaneous dislocation of the subtalar and talonavicular joints without dislocation of the calcaneocuboid or tibiotalar joints and without fracture. These injuries most commonly occur in men in their fourth decade of life.[61]

CLASSIFICATION

BROCA 1853,[62] MODIFIED BY MALGAIGNE

- Medial (80%), lateral (17%), posterior (2.5%) in descending order of frequency[63]
- Modified by Malgaigne in 1856: added rare anterior dislocations (1%)
- Some argue that posterior and anterior dislocations do not exist and only result from secondary displacement after medial or lateral dislocation
- Prognostic

ANATOMIC FEATURES

STJ has three articular facets with the calcaneus (anterior, posterior, medial), which provide bony structural support. The STJ is also stabilized by a number of strong soft tissue structures: interosseous talocalcaneal ligament within the sinus tarsi, individual facet capsules, the deltoid ligament medially, and calcaneal fibular ligament laterally. The posterior talar tubercles as well as the FHL provide posterior stabilization.

FUNCTIONAL ANALYSIS OF THE ANATOMY

Cadaveric studies have shown that the CF, superficial deltoid, TC ligaments all must tear for dislocation to occur. Generally, the bifurcate ligament and spring ligament are not disrupted during subtalar joint dislocation injuries.[64] The tubercles are subject to avulsion fractures due to the insertions of the deep deltoid ligament medially and posterior talofibular ligament laterally.

PHYSICAL EXAMINATION

Neurovascular examination is very important. Vascular compromise is uncommon; however, tented skin can break down quickly.

PATHOGENESIS

Fifty to eighty percent occur from high-energy injuries such as motor vehicle accident or falls from a height.[65] Generally speaking, higher-energy injuries result in poorer outcomes.[66]

- The majority of STJ dislocations are classified as medial dislocations, which have also been described in the text as acquired flatfoot deformity or basketball foot due to the clinical appearance. This injury results from forceful inversion of a plantar flexed foot. The initial trauma results in dislocation of the talar head from the navicular, followed by subluxation of the subtalar joint as the talus rotates on the calcaneus. Forty percent result in open injuries.[67]
- Lateral dislocations are the result of forceful eversion of a plantar flexed foot. These require a much greater energy force and often result in more substantial injuries including open injuries (>50%) or fracture.[61,66,68]
- Posterior dislocation: severe plantar flexion forces. Prolonged or continued force can result in tibiotalar dislocation.

IMAGING AND DIAGNOSTIC STUDIES

Radiographic evaluation: three views of the foot or ankle will obviously demonstrate dislocation of the STJ. These should be obtained prior to attempted reduction. Following reduction, additional radiographs should be taken. Postreduction radiographs may make associated fractures more visible. CT scans may be useful following reduction to rule out any additional fractures.

TREATMENT

- Prompt reduction of the dislocation to prevent skin breakdown and neurovascular injuries. Sedation will assist in relaxation. Flexion of the knee will relax the pull of the gastrocsoleus complex and ease reduction. Reduction of the STJ is focused on relation of the TN joint. As with any reduction, the steps include exaggerating the deformity, applying traction, and placing gentle pressure on the talar head to reduce it.
- Open reduction should be performed if you have failed two attempts at closed reduction or one attempt with an open physis. Open reduction is more common in lateral dislocations (15%-20%) compared to medial dislocations (5%-10%) and is often required if closed reduction was delayed. Medial dislocation reduction can be impaired by buttonholing the talar head through the extensor retinaculum, TN capsule, interposition of the neurovascular bundle or peroneal tendon, and bony impaction. Incisions can be made from the medial aspect of the talar head extending proximally to allow visualization of all the potentially intruding structures. A separate incision can be made laterally from the distal aspect of the fibula to the sinus tarsi may aid in reduction.
- Open injuries are treated as surgical urgencies and require formal irrigation and debridement. Immediate irrigation can be performed in the emergency room if

tolerated. Due to the potential risk of spreading contaminants or foreign debris, we prefer to delay reduction until a formal irrigation and debridement can be completed, unless neurovascular compromise is present. We do not recommend delaying reduction if other life-threatening injuries will delay formal irrigation and debridement.

- Fractures can cause instability and may require stabilization through the fragments or through the previously dislocated joints.
- Fixation can be performed with K-wires or Steinman pins. Use of external fixation has also been described in the literature.
- If vascular injury is identified, vascular surgery may be advised. Generally, soft tissue is amenable to closure. If severe deficits are noted, negative pressure dressings or plastic surgeon involvement may be necessary.

POSTOPERATIVE CARE

- Following closed reduction, the joint is usually stable and does not require further fixation. Open injuries result in more severe soft tissue damage and are more likely to result in instability. Range of motion can evaluate stability of the STJ.
- If fixation is required, it should be left in place for 4-6 weeks while the patient is non–weight bearing. Serial x-rays should be used to evaluate healing of any fractures identified.
- Stable immobilization for up to 1-4 months is recommended. Easily reduced injuries without fracture can usually begin protected partial weight bearing in 4-6 weeks. Prolonged immobilization can result in increased stiffness, where early range of motion is associated with recurrent dislocation and chronic instability.
- Confirm adequate reduction with repeat radiographs. Reduction films will provide better evaluation for other injuries including avulsion fractures or OCDs. Postreduction CT scan can also be useful in identifying OCDs.

REHABILITATION

Physical therapy can be a helpful adjuvant therapy to regain motion of the subtalar joint, as well as the adjacent ankle and midtarsal joints. If chronic instability is noted, orthotic therapy or bracing may be used for first-line therapy; however, arthrodesis may eventually be required.

COMPLICATIONS

- Acute complications include neurovascular compromise, wound healing issues, or infection with open injuries. Neurovascular injury is seen most commonly in open injuries. If vascular compromise is noted, ligation of the vessels can be performed. Consider urgent vascular surgery involvement if indicated. Prompt reduction to reduce skin tenting can aid in reducing wound complications. Infection has been shown to be a potentially serious complication in approximately one-third of open dislocations. IV antibiotics should be given for a minimum of

24-48 hours after formal debridement. Repeat debridement may be required depending on the amount of contamination and patient response. Intraoperative cultures can help guide antibiotic therapy. Infection rate and subsequent amputation have been shown to be rare in subtalar dislocations.[69]

- Other long-term complications include instability, posttraumatic arthritis, and avascular necrosis. Chronic instability is more common in younger patients who were immobilized <4 weeks following injury.[70] This can often be initially treated with orthotics, bracing, and aggressive PT. If continued instability is noted, arthrodesis may be required. AVN of the talus is relatively uncommon following STJ dislocation. This is attributed to the lack of disruption of blood supply through the deltoid ligament. Incidence of AVN has been shown to increase with infection, premature weight bearing, open injuries, and talar fractures. OCDs are common precursors to posttraumatic osteoarthritis. Medial: 50%-71% will have an accompanying OCD. Lateral: up to 100% will have OCDs.[61,63,68,71] Posttraumatic arthritis is found in nearly all cases of STJ dislocation.[68] This is treated symptomatically as needed and may require arthrodesis of the primary joint, as well as adjacent joints as needed. Total ankle replacement can also be considered in these patients; however, correct patient selection is encouraged.

ANKLE DISLOCATIONS

INTRODUCTION

Ankle dislocations without associated fractures are rare. The ankle is stabilized by the osseous structures, joint capsule, and four main ligaments: anterior talofibular, posterior talofibular, calcaneofibular, and deltoid ligament complex.[72] These rare injuries are predominantly caused by motor vehicle accidents (usually motorcycle) followed by sports trauma. In sports, ankle dislocation is associated with jumping sports such as volleyball and basketball.[73] Ankle dislocations can present as a closed injury, although more than 50% of ankle dislocations are open.[74-79]

DIAGNOSIS

Ankle Dislocation According to Direction of Dislocation[80]
- Anterior
- Posterior
- Medial
- Lateral
- Combined (posteromedial is most common)

Ankle dislocations present with a gross deformity. Standard views of the ankle are sufficient for diagnosis but may be inadequate to determine any associated injuries such as avulsion fractures. Small avulsion fractures may occur with associated ligament tears most commonly involving the anterior talofibular and calcaneofibular ligaments.[81,82] Associated soft tissue damage can include avulsion of the extensor digitorum brevis, rupture of the ankle capsule, and torn anterior inferior tibiofibular ligament.[83] CT scanning after ankle reduction has been recommended to evaluate for other osseous injuries that have been reported such as avulsion at the posterolateral talar process and nondisplaced calcaneal anterior process fractures.[83] Repeat physical examination after reduction may help to diagnose other reported injuries such as avulsion fractures, syndesmotic injury, neurovascular damage, skin necrosis, and chondrolysis of the talus and/or tibia.[75,83-85]

Classification of ankle dislocations have been described[80] that recognize five types according to the direction of dislocation: anterior, posterior, medial, lateral, and combined. The most common dislocations are posteriomedial.[86]

MECHANISM

Mechanism is usually a high-energy forced inversion or eversion of the foot with the ankle in plantar flexion.[81] This mechanism was reproduced by Fernandes[81] by stressing the foot into inversion or eversion in maximal ankle plantar flexion resulting in ankle dislocation without associated fracture. These studies demonstrated rupture of the anterior talofibular and calcaneofibular ligaments. Fernandes suspected the talus and foot were pulled posteriorly by the Achilles tendon.

Patients with ankle dislocation may have an entirely normal-appearing ankle joint without a history of injury. Some predisposing factors are considered to be medial malleolus dysplasia, lack of talar coverage, ligamentous laxity, previous sprains, and weakness of the peroneal muscles.[79,85,87-92] Some reports describe these predisposing factors in detail. Elise et al.[78] reported on relative shortness of the medial malleolus in two cases, and described a ratio between the length of the medial and lateral malleoli. Different reports focus on particular factors. The findings of a short medial malleolus have been reported by others as well.[85,93] In patients with ankle dislocations, talar coverage was found to be normal.[78,85] Other reports describe ankle dislocations in patients with ligamentous laxity on a secondary physical examination.[82,83]

TREATMENT

PERILS, TIPS, AND PITFALLS
- Spontaneous or partial reduction of deformity can occur and may falsely make the injury appear less severe.
- Prompt reduction of deformity will allow relaxation of soft tissues. This remains important in the polytraumatized patient when extremity injury is not the initial priority. If closed reduction is possible in these patients, a bulky Jones type dressing will help prepare the soft tissues for surgical intervention.
- Intervening soft tissues can prevent appropriate reduction.

Reduction of an ankle dislocation requires an understanding of the mechanism of injury. Reduction is achieved by longitudinal traction with the knee flexed and reduction of the deformity. In the more common posteromedial ankle dislocations, the rearfoot is held and the knee is flexed to allow relaxation of the triceps surae. Dorsiflexion of the foot is followed by longitudinal traction for reduction. Lazarettos[73] has shown reduction with hematoma block, while others use general anesthesia with complete muscle relaxation.

Most authors recommend closed treatment of closed ankle dislocations. The goal is to promptly restore articular congruity and remove tension from the soft tissues. Open dislocations will require operative debridement followed by reduction of the ankle joint. There is no agreement on the necessity to repair the surrounding ligamentous injuries. Syndesmotic fixation has been recommended in those with torn anterior inferior tibiofibular ligament and an unstable syndesmosis.[83] Some authors[76,78,90] recommend repair of lateral but not medial ligaments in open injuries at the time of initial debridement. Some advocate surgical repair of damaged ligaments in the younger active athlete but can be performed later with good results.[87] Moehring[75] reported that most (10/12) patients who had surgical ligament repair had good and excellent results, no patient had signs or symptoms of instability at follow-up.

Kannus and Renstrom[94] found no differences between patients with or without ligament repair when comparing return to work or physical activity, functional instability, pain, swelling, stiffness with activity, ankle mobility, muscle atrophy, return to preinjury activities, repeat injury, objective mechanical stability of the ankle, and complication. Similar findings have been found in patients with closed ankle dislocations treated non-operatively.[76,95] Other studies[80,96] reported syndesmotic disruption with ankle dislocation but neither recommended surgical treatment, favoring cast immobilization, although both of these studies are from a time when syndesmosis fixation was not considered as necessary as today. Wroble[77] reported long-term follow-up conservative care in eight patients with all results good to excellent, no patient reported instability, all returned to sports, and some had decreased range of motion. Reproducible favorable results have been seen following prompt closed reduction of ankle dislocation injuries and application of a non–weight-bearing short leg cast for 6-8 weeks followed by progressive protected weight bearing.[73,75,84,85,95]

COMPLICATIONS

Joint instability, stiffness, degenerative changes, and capsular calcification can present as late complications of ankle dislocation.[80] Several authors reported stiffness in dorsiflexion after ankle dislocation, with a loss of 10-15 degrees of motion.[82,85] Persistent instability may require stress views to determine if there is any ligamentous instability that may need to be addressed surgically. Elise[78] reported degenerative arthritis in 25% of ankle dislocations and that arthritis was more common in open dislocation or if transarticular pins were placed.

Avascular necrosis of the talus has been reported with both open and closed injuries. Open injuries have a propensity for neurovascular deficits and underscore the need for prompt lavage, debridement, and reduction to minimize the sequelae to the soft tissue and osseous structures.[75,95] Reports of injury to the tibial, superficial peroneal, or sural nerves range from 10% to 25%.[78,83,85,97] Hatori[82] described paresthesias of the superficial peroneal nerve that resolved with time. The incidence of parenthesis in the tibial, deep peroneal, and intermediate dorsal cutaneous nerve has been reported to be 25%.[78]

DISCUSSION

The literature on isolated ankle dislocations without associated fractures are mainly isolated case reports in the literature with the largest reported series by Toohey and Worsing.[95] The consensus is for prompt reduction of the deformity to restore articular alignment and relieve tension of the soft tissues (Fig. 42.4). Postreduction x-rays and advanced imaging are utilized to evaluate for associated injuries. Open injuries require debridement. Most authors report good results with reduction of ankle dislocation without repair of associated ligament disruptions, favoring cast immobilization and non–weight bearing. Repair of ligament ruptures is controversial but has been reported.

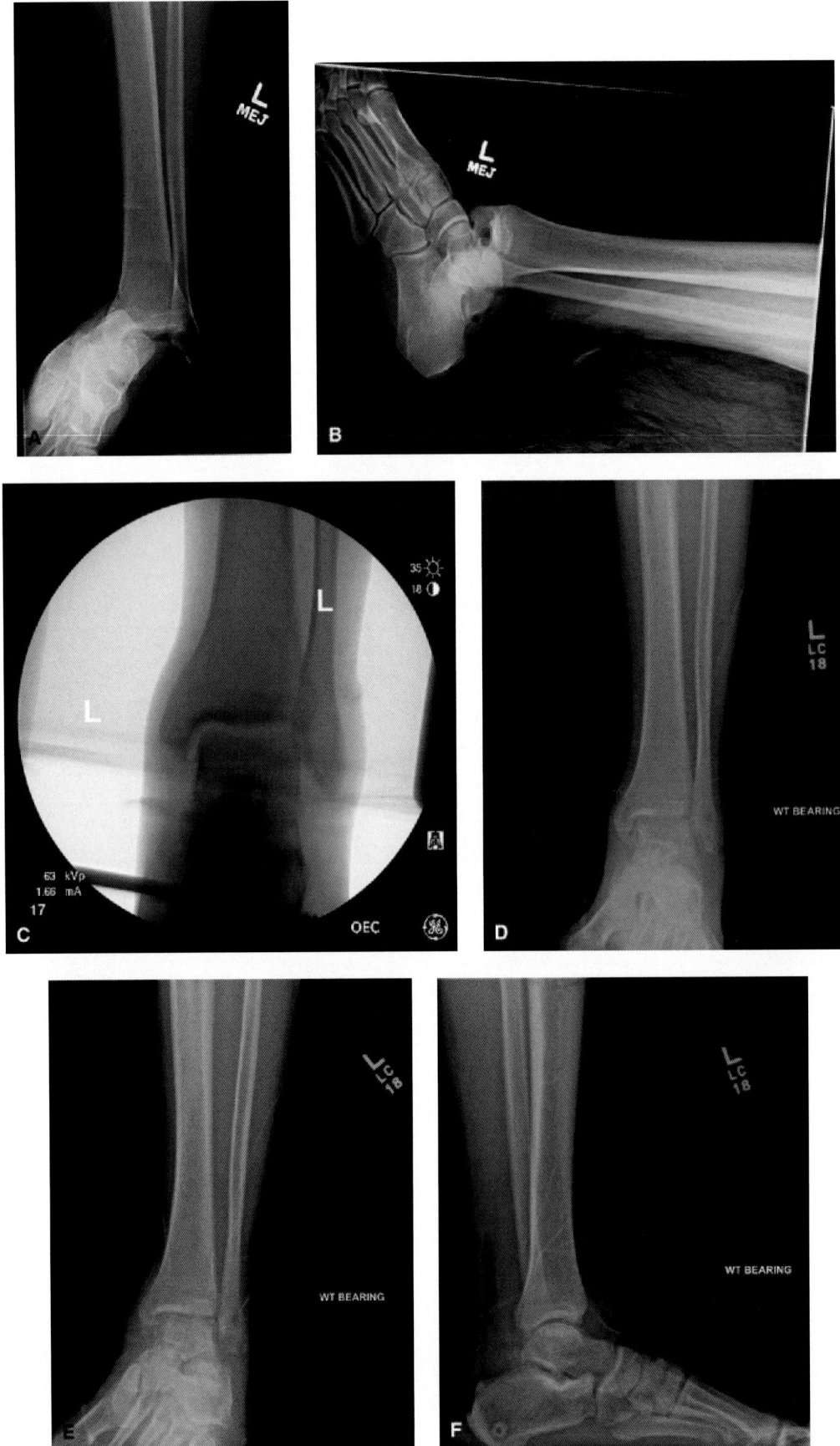

FIGURE 42.4 A, B. AP and lateral injury films of posterior medial ankle dislocation sustained after motor vehicle collision. This ankle dislocation was open laterally. **C.** Intraoperative fluoroscopy after irrigation and debridement demonstrating reduction of dislocation and placement of delta external fixator. **D–F.** Four months after injury demonstrating normal ankle alignment.

REFERENCES

1. Clanton TO, Ford JJ. Turf toe injury. *Clin Sports Med.* 1994;13(4):731-741.
2. George E, Harris AH, Dragoo JL, et al. Incidence and risk factors for turf toe injuries in intercollegiate foot: data from the National Collegiate Athletic Association injury surveillance system. *Foot Ankle Int.* 2014;35(2):108-115.
3. Hamilton GA, Ford LA, Richey JM. "Chapter 102: Dislocations of the Foot and Ankle" in *McGlamry's Comprehensive Textbook of the Foot and Ankle.*, 4th ed. Wolters Kluwer Health / Lippincott Williams & Wilkins, Philadelphia PA: 2013.
4. Frey C, Anderson D, Feder K. Plantarflexion injury of the metatarsophalangeal joint ("Sand Toe"). *Foot Ankle Int.* 1996;17(9):576-581.
5. Jahss MH. Traumatic dislocations of the first metatarsophalangeal joint. *Foot Ankle.* 1980;1:15-21.
6. Mason LW, Molloy AP. Turf toe and disorders of the Sesamoid complex. *Clin Sports Med.* 2015;34:725-739.
7. Finney FT, Cata E, Holmes JR, Taulsen PG. Anatomy and physiology of the lesser metatarsophalangeal joint. *Foot Ankle Clin North Am.* 2018;23:1-7.
8. Waldrop NE, Zirker CA, Wijdicks CA, et al. Radiographic evidence of plantar plate injury: an in vitro biomechanical study. *Foot Ankle Int.* 2013;34(3):403-408.
9. Nery C, Baumfeld D, Umans H, Yamada A. MR imaging of the plantar plate. *Magn Reson Imaging Clin N Am.* 2017;25(1):127-144.
10. Johnson J, Mansuripur PK, Anavian J, Born CT. Closed reduction of the metatarsophalangeal joint dislocations in acute and subacute presentations: a novel technique. *Am J Emerg Med.* 2015;33(9):1333.e3-1333.e7.
11. Doty JF, Coughlin MF. Turf toe repair: a technical note. *Foot Ankle Int.* 2013;6(6):452-456.
12. Cassebaum WH. Lisfranc fracture-dislocations. *Clin Orthop Relat Res.* 1963;30(30):116-129.
13. Quénu EG. KüssEtude sur les luxations du métatarse (luxations métatarso-tarsiennes). *Rev Chir.* 1909;39:281-336
14. Hardcastle PH, Reschauer R, Kutscha-Lissberg E, Schoffmann W. Injuries to the tarsometatarsal joint: incidence, classification and treatment. *J Bone Joint Surg Br.* 1982;64:349-356.
15. Myerson MS, Fisher RT, Burgess AR, Kenzora JE. Fracture dislocations of the tarsometatarsal joints: end results correlated with pathology and treatment. *Foot Ankle.* 1986;6(5):225-242.
16. Coetzee JC. Making sense of Lisfranc injuries. *Foot Ankle Clin.* 2008;13:695-704.
17. Peicha G, Labovitz J, Seibert FJ, et al. The anatomy of the joint as a risk factor for Lisfranc dislocation and fracture-dislocation. An anatomical and radiological case control study. *J Bone Joint Surg Br.* 2002;84(7):981-985.
18. Raikin SM, Elias I, Dheer S, et al. Prediction of midfoot instability in the subtle Lisfranc injury. Comparison of magnetic resonance imaging with intraoperative findings. *J Bone Joint Surg Am.* 2009;91(4):892-899.
19. Harwood MI, Raikin SM. A Lisfranc fracture-dislocation in a football player. *J Am Board Fam Med.* 2003;16:69-72.
20. Desmond EA, Chou LB. Current concepts review: Lisfranc injuries. *Foot Ankle Int.* 2006;27(8):653-660.
21. Trevino S, Kodros S. Controversies in tarsometatarsal injuries. *Orthop Clin North Am.* 1995;26(2):229-237.
22. Vuori J, Aro H. Lisfranc joint injuries: trauma mechanisms and associated injuries. *J Trauma.* 1993;35(1):40-45.
23. Wilson DW. Injuries of the tarsometatarsal joints. *J Bone Joint Surg Br.* 1972;54(4):677-686.
24. Nunley JA, Vertullo CJ. Classification, investigation, and management of midfoot sprains: Lisfranc injuries in the athlete. *Am J Sports Med.* 2002;30(6):871-878.
25. Hatem S, Davis A, Sundaram M. Diagnosis: midfoot sprain: Lisfranc ligament disruption. *Orthopedics.* 2005;28:75-77.
26. Aronow MS. Treatment of the missed Lisfranc injury. *Foot Ankle Clin.* 2006;11(1):127-142.
27. Schmitt JW, Warner CML, Ossendorf C, Wanner GA, Simmen HP. Avulsion fracture of the dorsal talonavicular ligament: a subtle radiographic sign of possible Chopart joint dislocation. *Foot Ankle Int.* 2011;32(7):722-726.
28. De Asla RJ, Deland JT. Anatomy and biomechanics of the foot and ankle. In: Thodarson DB, ed. *Orthopaedic Surgery Essentials: Foot and Ankle.* Philadelphia, PA: Lippincott Williams & Wilkins; 2004:1-23.
29. Milch H. Astragalo-Scaphoid dislocation. *Ann Surg.* 1929;89(3):427-434.
30. O'Donoghue AF. Astragalo-Scaphoid dislocations of the foot: report of five cases from the Orthopedic Service, Iowa State University College of Medicine. *J Bone Joint Surg.* 1920;2:327-328.
31. Kollmannsberger A, De Boer P. Isolated calcaneo-cuboid dislocation: brief report. *J Bone Joint Surg Br.* 1989;71(2):323.
32. McMinn RMH. *Last's Anatomy: Regional and Applied.* 8th ed. London, UK: Churchill Livingstone; 1990:204-207.
33. Rammelt S, Grass R, Schikore H, Zwipp H. Injuries of the Chopart joint. *Unfallchirurg.* 2002;105:371-385 (in German).
34. Swords MP, Schramski M, Sitzer K, Nemec S. Chopart fractures and dislocations. *Foot Ankle Clin North Am.* 2008;13:679-693.
35. Bernirschke SK, Meinberg E, Anderson SA et al. Fractures and dislocations of the midfoot: Lisfranc and Chopart injuries. *J Bone Joint Surg.* 2012;94:1325-1337.
36. Haapamaki VV, Kiuru MJ, Koskinen SK. Ankle and foot injuries: analysis of MDCT findings. *Am J Roentgenol.* 2004;183:615-622.
37. Milgram JW. Chronic subluxation of the midtarsal joint of the foot: a case report. *Foot Ankle Int.* 2002;23(3):255-259.
38. Main BJ, Jowett RL. Injuries of the midtarsal joint. *J Bone Joint Surg Br.* 1975;57-B:89-97.
39. Miller CM, Winter WG, Bucknell AL, Jonassen EA. Injuries to the midtarsal joint and lesser tarsal bones. *J Am Acad Orthop Surg.* 1998;6:249-258.
40. Rammelt S, Zwipp H, Schneiders W, et al. Anatomic reconstruction of malunited Chopart joint injuries. *Eur J Trauma Emerg Surg.* 2010;36:196-205.
41. Rammelt S, Schepers T. Chopart injuries: when to fix and when to fuse? *Foot Ankle Clin North Am.* 2017;22(1):163-180.
42. Hermel MB, Gershon-Cohen J. The nutcracker fracture of the cuboid by indirect violence. *Radiology.* 1953;60:850-854.
43. Puthezhath K, Veluthedath R, Kumaran CM, Patinharayil G. Acute isolated dorsal midtarsal (Chopart's) dislocation: a case report. *J Foot Ankle Surg.* 2009;48(4):462-465.
44. Ip KY, Lui TH. Isolated dorsal midtarsal (Chopart) dislocation: a case report. *J Orthop Surg.* 2006;14(3):357-359.
45. Zwipp H. *Chirurgie de Fußes.* New York, NY: Springer Wien; 1994.
46. Richter M, Wippermann B, Krettek C, Schratt HE, Hufner T, Thermann H. Fractures and fracture dislocations of the midfoot: occurrence, causes and long term results. *Foot Ankle Int.* 2001;22:392-398.
47. Pehlivan O, Akmaz I, Solakoglu C, Rodop O. Medial peritalar dislocation. *Arch Orthop Trauma Surg.* 2002;122:541-543.
48. Salvi AE, Metelli GP, Domeneghini E, Florschutz AV, Bettinsoli R. Diagnostic imaging and unforeseen associated lesions in astragalo-scaphoid dislocation: a case report. *Arch Orthop Trauma Surg.* 2010;130:1129-1132.
49. Van Dorp KB, de Vries MR, van der Elst M, Schepers T. Chopart joint injury: a study of outcome and morbidity. *J Foot Ankle Surg.* 2010;49:541-545.
50. Richter M, Thermann H, Huefner T, Schmidt U, Goesling T, Krettek C. Chopart joint fracture-dislocation: initial open reduction provides better outcome than closed reduction. *Foot Ankle Int.* 2004;25:340-348.
51. Garafalo R, Moretti B, Ortoano V, et al. Peritalar dislocations: a retrospective study of 18 cases. *J Foot Ankle Surg.* 2004;43:166-172.
52. Kutaish H, Stern R, Drittenbass L, Assal M. Injuries to the Chopart joint complex: a current review. *Eur J Orthop Surg Traumatol.* 2017;27:425-431.
53. Klaue, K. Treatment of Chopart fracture-dislocations. *Eur J Trauma Emerg Surg.* 2010;3:191-195.
54. Schildhauer TA, Nork SE, Sangeorzan BJ. Temporary bridge plating of the medial column in severe midfoot injuries. *J Orthop Trauma.* 2003;17:513-520.
55. Apostle KL, Younger AS. Technique tip: open reduction internal fixation of comminuted fractures of the navicular with bridge plating of the medial and middle cuneiforms. *Foot Ankle Int.* 2008;29(7):739-741.
56. Rammelt S, Winkler J, Heineck J, Zwipp H. Anatomical reconstruction of malunited talus fractures: a prospective study of 10 patients followed for 4 years. *Acta Orthopaedica.* 2005;76(4):588-596. doi: 10.1080/17453670510041600.
57. Schneiders W, Rammelt S. Joint-sparing corrections of malunited Chopart joint injuries. *Foot Ankle Clin.* 2016;21:147-160.
58. Astion DJ, Deland JT, Otis JC, et al. Motion of the hindfoot after simulated arthrodesis. *J Bone Joint Surg.* 1997;79:241-246.
59. Wülker N, Stukenborg C, Savory KM, et al. Hindfoot motion after isolated and combined arthrodesis: measurements in anatomic specimens. *Foot Ankle Int.* 2000;21:921-927.
60. Leitner B. Obstacles to reduction in subtalar dislocations. *J Bone Joint Surg Am.* 1954;36(A-2):299-306.
61. Heppenstall RB, Farahvar H, Balderston R, Lotke P. Evaluation and management of subtalar dislocations. *J Trauma.* 1980;20:494-497.
62. Broca P. Mémoire sur les luxations sous-astragaliennes. *Mem Soc Chir.* 1853;3:566-656.
63. Zimmer TJ, Johnson KA. Subtalar dislocations. *Clin Orthop Relat Res.* 1989;238:190-194.
64. Buckingham WW Jr, LeFlore I. Subtalar dislocation of the foot. *J Trauma.* 1973;13:753-765.
65. Bibbo C, Anderson RB, Davis WH. Injury characteristics and the clinical outcome of subtalar dislocations: a clinical and radiographic analysis of 25 cases. *Foot Ankle Int.* 2003;24:158-163.
66. Goldner JL, Poletti SC, Gates HS III, Richardson WJ. Severe open subtalar dislocations. Long-term results. *J Bone Joint Surg Am.* 1995;77(7):1075-1079.
67. Dunn AW. Peritalar dislocation. *Orthop Clin North Am.* 1974;5(1):7-18.
68. Christensen SB, Lorentzen JE, Krogsoe O, Sneppen O. Subtalar dislocation. *Acta Orthop Scand.* 1977;48:707-711.
69. Smith CS, Norke SE, Sangorzan BJ. The extruded talus: results of reimplantation. *J Bone Joint Surg Am.* 2006;88A(11):2418-2424.
70. Larsen HW. Subastragalar dislocation (luxatio pedis sub talo). *Acta Chir Scand.* 1957;113:380.
71. DeLee JC, Curtis R. Subtalar dislocation of the foot. *J Bone Joint Surg Am.* 1982;64(3):433-437.
72. Schuenke M, Schulte E, Schumacher U. *General Anatomy and the Musculoskeletal System: THIEME Atlas of Anatomy.* 1st ed. Germany: Thieme; 2006.
73. Lazarettos I, Brilakis E, Efstathopoulos N. Open ankle dislocation without associated malleolar fracture. *J Foot Ankle Surg.* 2013;52:508-512.
74. Larsen J, Burzotta J, Brunetti V. Ankle dislocation without fracture in a young athlete. *J Foot Ankle Surg.* 1998;37:334-348.
75. Moehring H, Tan R, Marder R, Lian G. Ankle dislocation. *J Orthop Trauma.* 1994;8:167-172.
76. Colville MR, Colville JM, Manoli A. Posteromedial dislocation of the ankle without fracture. *J Bone Joint Surg Am.* 1987;69:706-711.
77. Wroble RR, Nepola JV, Malvitz TA. Ankle dislocation without fracture. *Foot Ankle.* 1988;9:64-74.
78. Elise S, Maynou C, Mestdagh H, Forgeois P, Labourdette P. Simple tibiotalar luxation, apropos of 16 cases. *Acta Orthop Belg.* 1998;64:25-34.
79. Soyer AD, Nestor BJ, Friedman SJ. Closed posteromedial dislocation of the tibiotalar joint without fracture or diastasis: a case report. *Foot Ankle Int.* 1994;15:622-624.
80. Fahey JJ, Murphy JL. Talotibial dislocation of the ankle without fracture. *Surg Clin North Am.* 1965;45:80-101.
81. Fernandes TJ. The mechanism of talotibial dislocation without fracture. *J Bone Joint Surg Br.* 1976;58:364-365.

82. Hatori M, Kotajima S, Smith RA, Kokubun S. Ankle dislocation without accompanying malleolar fracture. A case report. *Uppsala J Med Sci.* 2006;111(2):263-268.

83. Thangarajah T, Giotakis N, Matovu E. Bilateral ankle dislocation without malleolar fracture. *J Foot Ankle Surg.* 2008;47:441-446.

84. Shaik MM, Tandon T, Agrawal Y, Jadhav A, Taylor LJ. Medial and lateral rotatory dislocations of the ankle after trivial trauma—pathomechanics and management of two cases. *J Foot Ankle Surg.* 2006;45:346-350.

85. Rivera F, Bertone C, Dem Martino M, Pietrobono D, Ghisellini F. Pure dislocation of the ankle: three case reports and literature review. *Clin Orthop Relat Res.* 2001;382:179-184.

86. Grotz MR, Alpantaki K, Kagda FH, Papcostidis C, Barron D, Biannoudis PV. Open tibiotalar dislocation without associated fracture in a 7-year old girl. *Am J Orthop.* 2008;37:E116-E118.

87. Finkemeier C, Engebresten L, Gannon J. Tibial-talar dislocation without fracture: treatment principles and outcome. *Knee Surg Sports Traumatol Arthrosc.* 1995;3:47-49.

88. Garrick JG. The frequency of injury, mechanism of injury, and epidemiology of ankle sprains. *Am J Sports Med.* 1977;5:241-242.

89. Georgilas I, Mouzopoulos G. Anterior ankle dislocation without associated fracture: a case with an 11 year follow-up. *Acta Orthop Belg.* 2008;74:266-269.

90. Kaneko K, Muta T, Mogami A, et al. Vertical dislocation of the talus without malleolar fracture. *Eur J Orthop Surg Traumatol.* 2000;10:207-209.

91. Krasin E, Goldwirth M, Otremski I. Complete open dislocation of the talus. *J Accid Emerg Med.* 2000;17:53-54.

92. Palomo-Traver JM, Cruz-Renovell E, Granell-Beltran V, Monzonis-Garcia J. Open total talus dislocation: case report and review of the literature. *J Orthop Trauma.* 1997;11:45-49.

93. Tarantino U, Cannata G, Gasbarra E, Bondi L, Celi M, Iundusi R. Open medial dislocation of the ankle without fracture. *J Bone Joint Surg Br.* 2008;90:1382-1384.

94. Kannus P, Renstrom P. Treatment for acute tears of the lateral ligaments of the ankle: operation, cast, or early controlled mobilization. *J Bone Joint Surg Am.* 1991;73:305-312.

95. Toohey JS, Worsing RA Jr. A long-term follow-up study of tibiotalar dislocations without associated fractures. *Clin Orthop Relat Res.* 1989;239:207-210.

96. Kelly PJ, Peterson LFA. Compound dislocation of the ankle without fracture. *Am J Surg.* 1962;103:170-172.

97. Rios-Luna A, Villanueva-Martinez M, Fahandezh-Saddi H, Pereiro J, Martin-Garcia A. Isolated dislocation of the ankle: two cases and review of the literature. *Eur J Orthop Surg Traumatol.* 2007;17:403-407.

Open Fracture Management

Mark A. Hardy and James C. Connors

DEFINITION

Open fractures are defined as a trauma where the injury force fractures the bone and extends to the soft tissue to the outside environment.[1] This distinct injury, formerly known as a compound fracture, is an emergent condition necessitating urgent medical damage control. Fracture communication beyond the soft tissue increases the risk of osteomyelitis. This serious injury carries a potential limb and life-threatening prognosis. The pillars of treatment include immediate therapeutic antibiotic treatment, tetanus prophylaxis, and early irrigation with extensive wound debridement combined with fracture stabilization and soft tissue coverage. The ultimate goals of open fracture management are prevention of wound sepsis and restoration of anatomic function by providing staged fracture stability for eventual reduction and fixation. Without strict adherence to these critical principles, ensuing return to preinjury activity is unlikely.

CLASSIFICATION

Gustilo and Anderson instituted a standardized format to stratify tibial open fracture severity based on size of soft tissue deficit and time of injury.[1,2] Based on their study, type I injuries are clean wounds that are <1 cm in diameter, and type II injuries are clean wounds >1 cm in diameter. Type III wounds are >5 cm in diameter or a small injury that is >8 hours old. These type III wounds underwent further subcategorization by soft tissue coverage, contamination, and the presence of arterial injuries.[2] While useful for a baseline assessment and antibiotic initiation, the Gustilo and Anderson classification system is rather flawed when tested for observational bias.[3,4] The true assessment of smaller wounds is limited and requires intraoperative consideration to appreciate the true accuracy of the injury extent following debridement of nonviable tissue. High-velocity injuries such as gunshot wounds cause soft tissue cavitation, bone fragmentation, and lead to misjudgment of the injury severity at first glance.[5,6]

GUSTILO-ANDERSON CLASSIFICATION OF OPEN FRACTURES

- Type I
  - ▶ Clean wound; wound diameter <1 cm
- Type II
  - ▶ Wound diameter >1 cm but <5 cm
- Type III
  - ▶ Segmental fracture with a wound diameter >5 cm or a type I or II injury that is >8 hours old; may have extensive soft tissue damage

GUSTILO'S CLASSIFICATION OF TYPE III OPEN WOUNDS

- Type IIIa
  - ▶ 4% infection rate; adequate soft tissue coverage despite soft tissue laceration or flaps
- Type IIIb
  - ▶ 52% infection rate; periosteal stripping; usually has massive contamination
- Type IIIc
  - ▶ 42% infection rate; arterial injury requiring repair; high rate of primary amputation

INDICATIONS AND PITFALLS

INDICATIONS

- All open fractures regardless of anatomic site require immediate damage control starting with antibiotic therapy with urgent irrigation and evaluation to assess soft tissue viability.

ANATOMIC FEATURES

Due to the thin soft tissue envelope and shallow subcutaneous layer overlying the osseous anatomy, the lower leg and

foot are susceptible to open fractures. Environmental factors including proximity to lawn care equipment place the foot and ankle in the vicinity to unprotected exposure to mechanical force.

FUNCTIONAL ANALYSIS OF THE ANATOMY OF THE CHAPTER

The lack of musculature origin or other soft tissue attachment leads to an increased propensity for fracture communication through the thin soft tissue envelop overlying osseous anatomy such as the medial aspect of the distal tibia or the lateral aspect of the fibula. The relative stability of the ankle mortise creates a higher propensity for rotation force to be transferred to the osseous structures opposed to solely ligamentous disruption.

PHYSICAL EXAMINATION

Due to the innate force present with open fractures, the overall patient stability and vital assessment is required prior to lower extremity treatment initiation. The presence of polytrauma in patients with a concomitant extremity fracture is relatively common and dictates treatment stratification based on severity.[7] The entire soft tissue envelope including skin, neurovascular structures, tendons, and ligaments necessitates inspection. The presence of an insensate limb in the setting of an open fracture accelerates the need for reduction and stabilization due to nerve traction.[8] Evaluation and removal of gross debris by irrigation allows better visual assessment and prevents embedment into deeper tissue. One must also rule out adjacent compartment syndrome utilizing compartmental pressures or near-infrared spectroscopy, which shows an acute drop in tissue oxygenation.[9] The presence of fracture blisters requires documentation and drainage by dependent technique. The blister roof is preserved while the gravity-dependent quadrant is incised, and the liquid is evacuated. The maintained roof functions as an autogenous barrier and aids in underlying skin healing. The addition of a nonadherent intermediate dressing and a well-padded compressive multilayer dressing quickens soft tissue recovery.

PATHOGENESIS

The development of open fractures arises in the traumatic setting. The injury force exceeds the patient's osseous integrity and is transmitted through the soft tissue. These injuries are most likely to occur at anatomic locations that lack muscular attachments such as the medial leg as well as overlying osseous prominences in the foot. Rotational foot injuries in the setting of a fixed leg position place significant stress on the soft tissue structures. An axial force through the foot in a fixed knee position drives the talus into the tibial plafond, which may fracture through medial malleolus and exit the skin.[7] Lower extremity crush injuries result in the traumatic force finding the path of least resistance to exit the body through the soft tissue envelope. Puncture wounds that are initiated by a projectile, such as

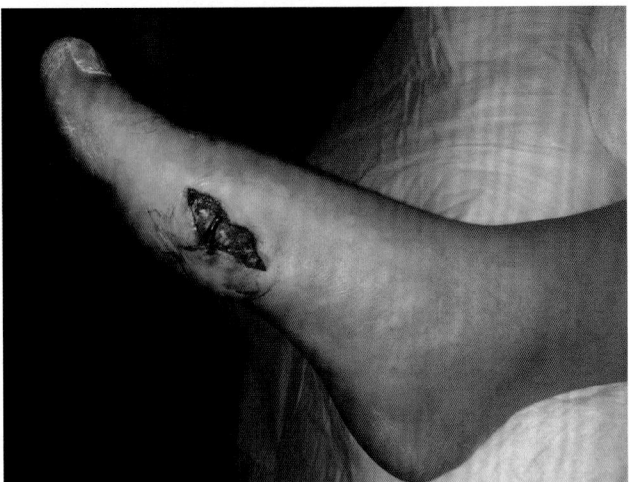

FIGURE 43.1 A 55-year-old male with rheumatoid arthritis fell down his basement stairs suffering an open dislocation of the right foot.

a gunshot, that lead to a fractured bone are considered an open fracture.[5] High- and lower-energy environmental injuries that expose the surrounding soft tissue and osseous structures must be treated as an open fracture.[10]

Rotational foot injuries are shown in Figures 43.1-43.3. Rotational lower extremity injuries in the setting of pilon fracture or ankle fractures are shown in Figures 43.4 and 43.5. Impact crush injuries in the leg, foot, and digits are shown in Figures 43.6-43.14.

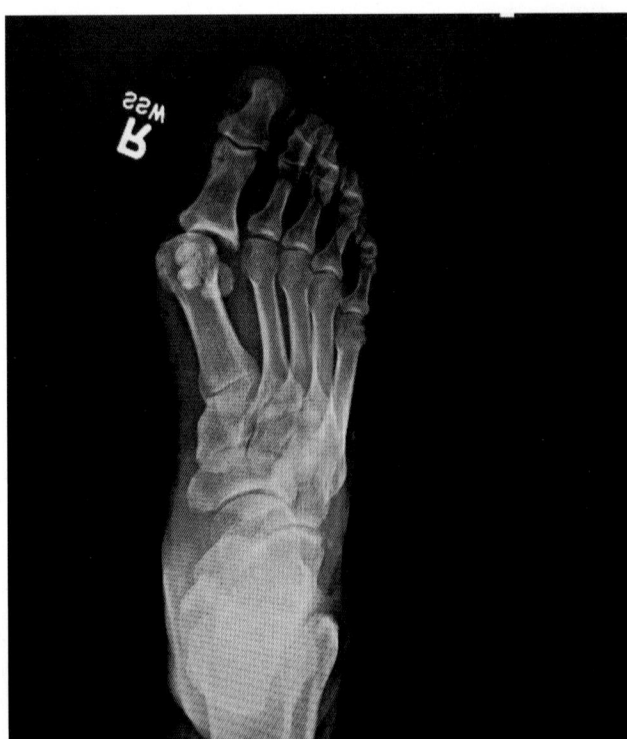

FIGURE 43.2 He suffered a first metatarsal dislocation with entrapment of the extensor hallucis longus tendon in the MTP joint and tibial sesamoid fracture.

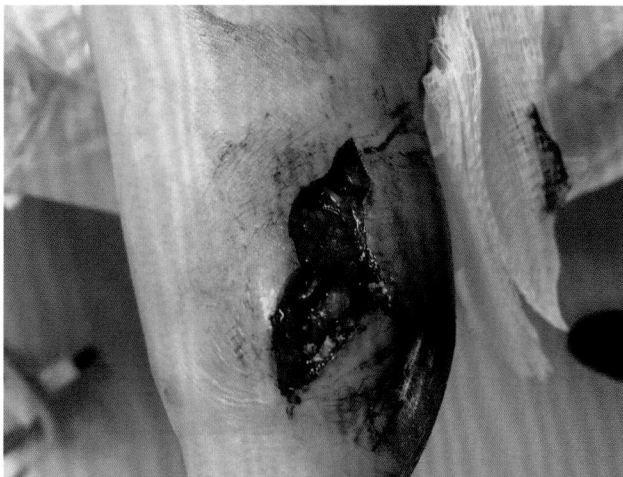

FIGURE 43.3 The soft tissue defect after dislocation reduction.

IMAGING AND DIAGNOSTIC STUDIES

Initial multiple view plain film radiographs are required to evaluate the amount of fragmentation, degree of angulation, and the severity of displacement of the fracture(s). Computed tomography (CT) is an essential component of surgical planning and eventual reconstruction. Both postreduction CT imaging and subsequent CT imaging following temporary fracture stabilization are necessary to plan for fracture realignment and judge the true extent of the osseous defect.

TREATMENT

During the preliminary assessment, preferably in the emergency department setting, neurovascular compromise is evaluated,

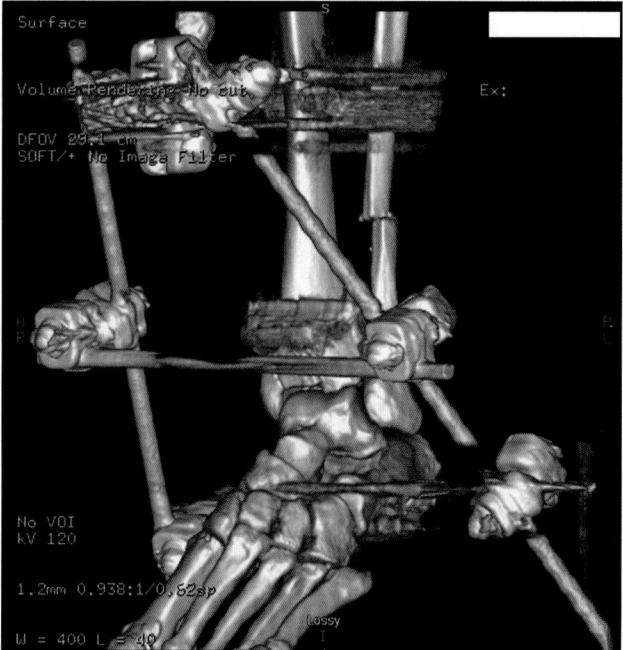

FIGURE 43.4 A 40-year-old male suffered a rotational leg injury when the foot became lodged in hole.

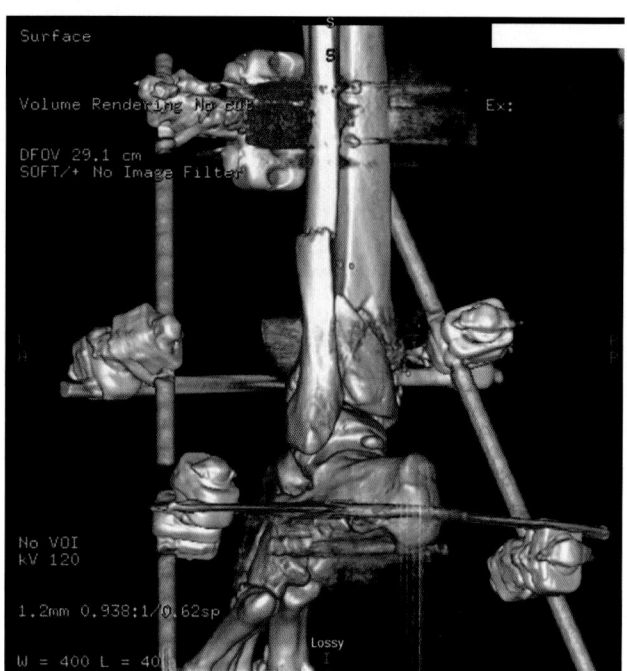

FIGURE 43.5 Posterior view of 3D reconstruction CT.

pictures of the injury are obtained, and copious amounts of irrigation is cycled through the defect to remove large debris before the temporary dressing is applied. The overall severity needs to be accessed with the possibility of amputation are discussed with the patient.[11,12] The classic guideline of emergent need for surgical debridement within a 6-hour window has been revised to an urgent operative debridement and irrigation inside of a 24-hour period from the initial injury.[13,14] The immediate initiation of broad-spectrum antibiotics is required and considered paramount for reducing the risk of sepsis.[15,16] The open defect is colonized at the time of injury by bacteria either from the opportunistic natural skin flora or by the outside contact. The updated recommendation to limit wound exposure to the outside and nosocomial contamination includes a "one-look technique" for initial evaluation.[17] The timing of antibiotic

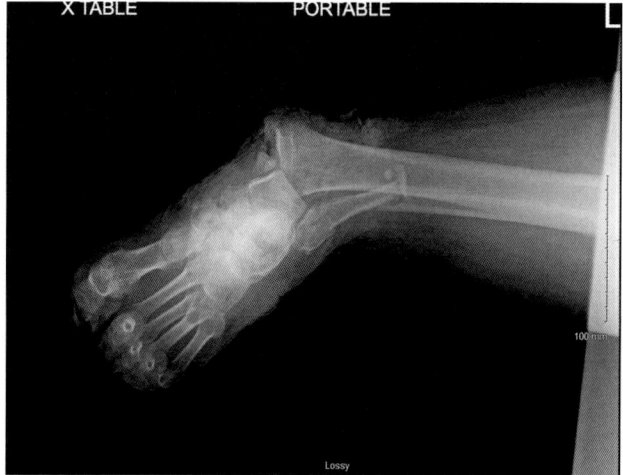

FIGURE 43.6 A 61-year-old male involved in a motor vehicle accident where he was side swiped sustaining a lateral force fracture dislocation.

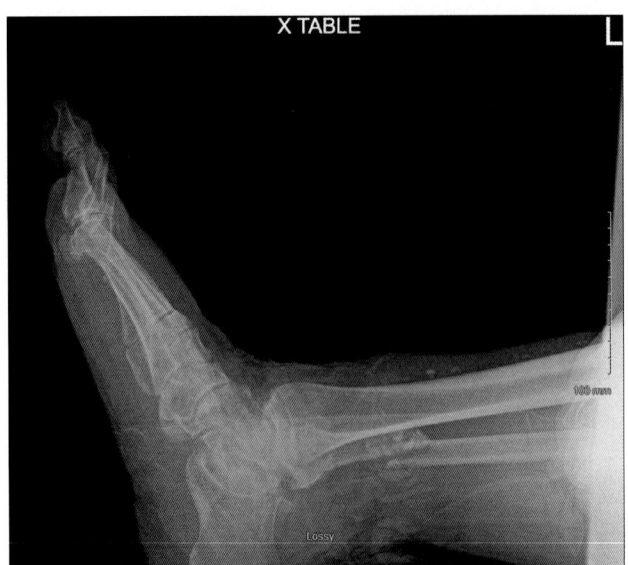

FIGURE 43.7 Lateral radiographic view.

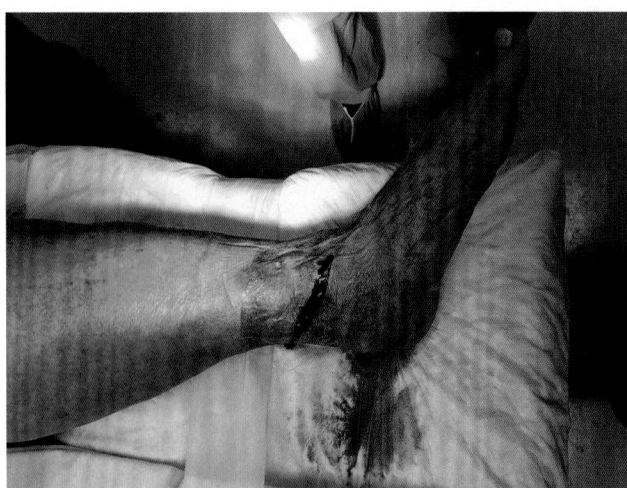

FIGURE 43.9 Poor soft tissue envelope but relatively free of debris following irrigation.

therapy is vital to reduce the risk of inherent complications.[18] Delayed antibiotic coverage increases infection rates independent of surgical debridement timing.[19] Antibiotics delayed >3 hours has been shown to increase the overall infection risk.[20] The lower extremity must be placed in elevation and a well-padded compressive dressing applied to prevent fracture blister formation. The presences of hemorrhagic fracture blisters warrant caution and dictates alternate incisional placement. Untimely, incision placement without full soft tissue injury appreciation can potentiate the "Pandora's Box" effect and greatly increase the risk of wound infection.

ANTIBIOTIC THERAPY

The modern intention to direct antibiotic therapy has been modified from the previously advised cefazolin in type I and type II injuries with the addition of gentamicin in type III wounds, as well as penicillin G for fecal and clostridium exposure. The paradigm shift is rooted in new evidence-based studies that advocate the use of modern broad-spectrum antibiotic therapy.[21] Recent studies confirm the higher likelihood of gram-positive infections.[22] Grade I/II: cefazolin (clindamycin if allergic); grade III: ceftriaxone (clindamycin and aztreonam if allergic) for 48 hours. The past recommendations of aminoglycosides, vancomycin, and penicillin have been removed.[23] The authors advocate the use of facility-targeted antibiotic treatment utilizing hospital-specific antibiogram aimed to include the potential nosocomial infectious pathogen. Cefazolin with the addition of piperacillin/tazobactam is recommended opposed to adding the classically recommended gentamicin.[24] Current studies have demonstrated that concerns for resistant organism infection are valid in specific patient settings, but the overall general implementation of resistance-targeted antibiotics is unwarranted.[25] The presence of antibiotic-resistant bacteria remains low but must be considered in relation to injury setting and patient factors.[26,27] Prophylactic antibiotics should be discontinued at 24 hours post wound closure without evident clinical symptoms.[21] Tetanus prophylaxis is required regardless of exposure dependent on previous immunization status.[16]

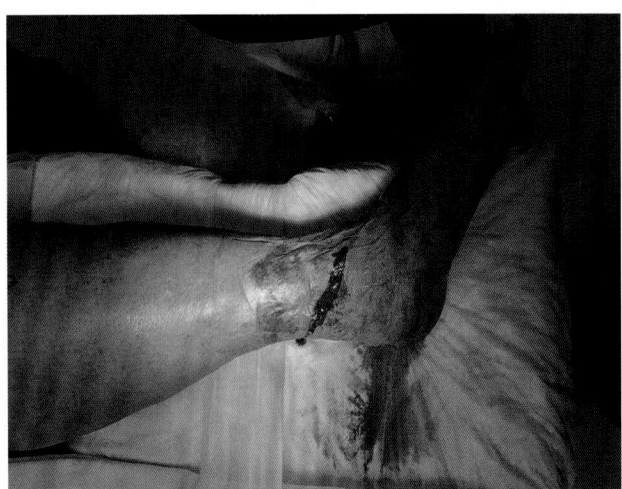

FIGURE 43.8 Soft tissue defect, medial aspect.

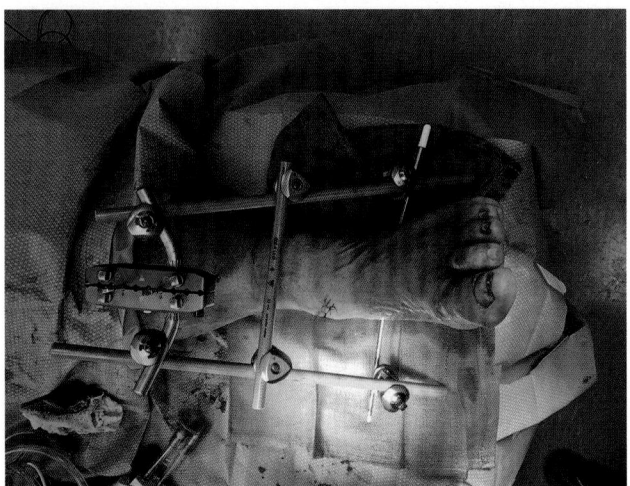

FIGURE 43.10 Temporary fracture stabilization and primary closure.

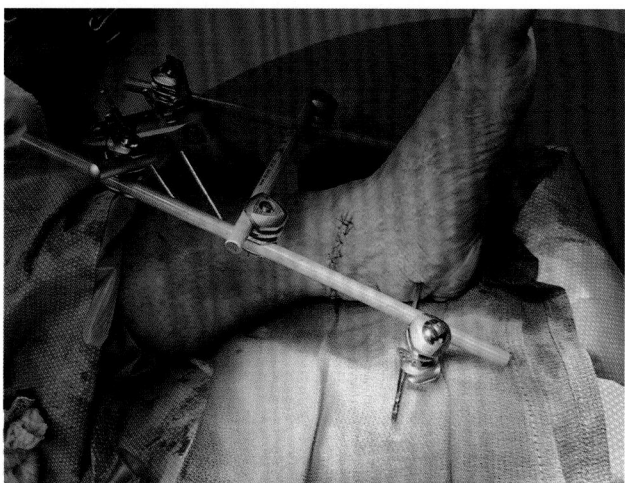

FIGURE 43.11 Lateral intraoperative view.

Antibiotics

Type I: cefazolin (clindamycin if allergic)
- Can add piperacillin/tazobactam

Type II: cefazolin (clindamycin if allergic)
- Can add piperacillin/tazobactam

Type III: ceftriaxone (clindamycin and aztreonam if penicillin allergy)

*Patient history of antibiotic resistance modify therapy as necessary[23,24,25]

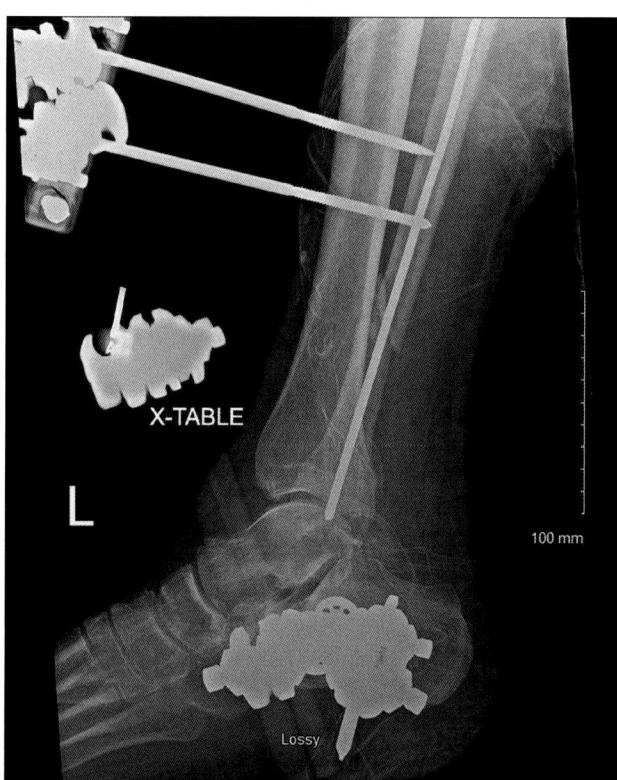

FIGURE 43.12 Postoperative radiographs showing intramedullary fibular fixation and delta frame external fixator application.

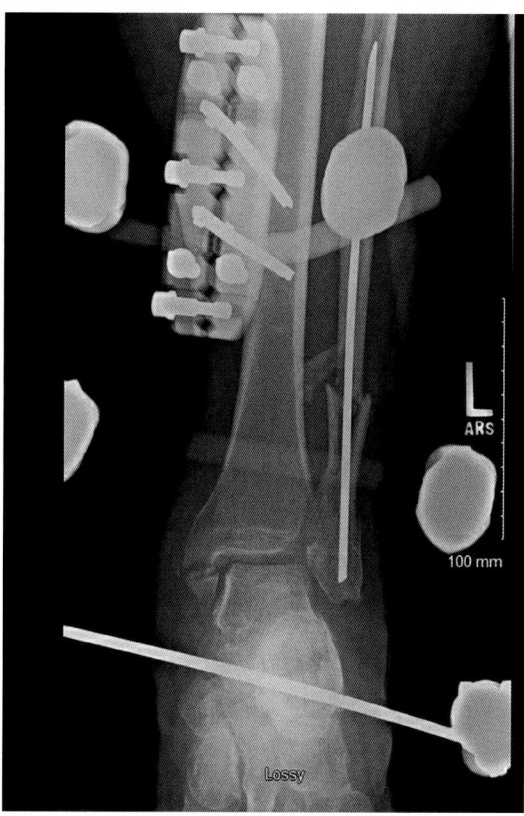

FIGURE 43.13 Anterior posterior view after fixation.

SURGICAL DEBRIDEMENT

Following antibiotic therapy, tetanus update, and full body evaluation, the patient is optimized for lavage irrigation, debridement, and provisional fracture stabilization. Timing of the "golden period" surgical debridement is currently open for debate. Recent evidence suggests that the 6-hour rule for increased bacterial growth is unreliable with the enactment of decisive antibiotic therapy.[28,29] Initial washout employs mechanical debridement that functions to reduce environmental contaminates encountered during the initial trauma.[30] Initial surface wound swabs are unlikely to be accurate and must be

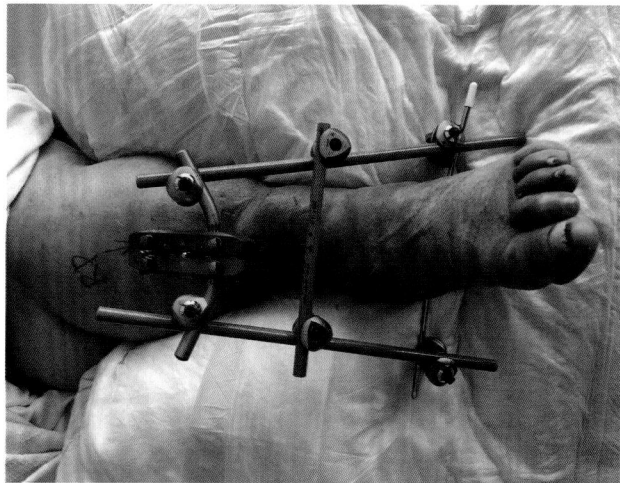

FIGURE 43.14 Postoperative clinical view.

held in lieu of deep tissue cultures.[31] The use of pulse lavage at 30 lbs per square inch (PSI) is classically recommended without a true basis of support. Current studies have shown no significant reduction in infection rates utilizing highly pressurized irrigation.[32,33] The use of Cysto tubing, commonly employed by urology, allows gravity flow irrigation to lavage the site of the injury without the potential of driving the debris and bacteria deeper into the unaffected tissue.[33] The true volume of irrigation is subjective and injury dependent. The authors recommend copious amounts of isotonic saline solution or sterile distilled water. The use of antiseptic additives lacks supportive evidence to recommend the use and has the potential of being caustic to viable surrounding tissue.[34] The amount of irrigate and the functional debridement properties of the fluid are more important than chemical additives.[34]

Wound Irrigation

- The greater the size of soft tissue defect or the longer duration the wound is untreated necessitates a higher volume of irrigation. The liquid irrigate delivers mechanical lavage flow to the injury site that reduces the bacterial contamination as well as the gross environment debris.

FRACTURE STABILIZATION

The use of spanning external fixation creates a damage control setting for the soft tissue wound to subside and minimize further osseous injury.[35] The ability to span deficits and reduce anatomic osseous malalignment and skin tension with pin-to-bar external fixation without the use of permanent internal fixation greatly reduces the risk of seeding a deep infection in the setting of contamination. The proper use of pin-to-bar external fixation in delta frame configuration permits wound access for easy negative pressure wound vacuum-assisted closure (VAC) therapy and periodic dressing changes. Spanning external fixation permits nonanatomic reduction by ligamentotaxis.[36] When large osseous defects are encountered, the use of antibiotic spacers provides a temporary void filler to maintain anatomic length. The placement of antibiotic spacers also affords local delivery of antibiotics while occupying dead space, which eliminates potential abscess formation.[21] The authors prefer a combination of polymethylmethacrylate (PMMA) cement and heat stable antibiotic powder such as vancomycin for temporary prevention of length deficits.[37,38]

Studies have shown that there is no clinical advantage to performing fracture internal fixation within 6 hours of the injury vs 6-24 hours on preventing nonunions.[39,40] Immediate placement of permanent fixation produces a potential nidus for bacterial colonization and eventual infection.[39,40] The authors advocate staging the treatment procedures dependent on severity. Concerning injuries with a high index of suspicion for infection, permanent fracture fixation is delayed until adequate soft tissue coverage is achievable as well as elimination of clinical signs of infection regardless of time. The fundamental goal is to accomplish definitive reduction and fixation as well as skin closure within 24-72 hours if possible. The overall soft tissue envelope is the limiting factor for definitive fixation timing. Incision planning necessitates proper anatomic access while minimizing the complications associated with skin bridges <6-7 cm. Plate and screw fixation to aim to restore congruency to the articular surfaces as well as reestablish anatomic length to the fracture site.

The use of locking plate fixation adds stability in the setting of poor bone quality.[40] In cases where osseous deficits are present, small defects are filled acutely while larger voids are addressed by structural cortical grafts to reduce subsidence and restore osseous integrity. The caveat being the need for large deficit bone grafting before 8 weeks to reduce the increased risk of delayed union or nonunions.[41,42] The use of autogenous bone graft provides osteogenic, osteoinductive, as well as osteoconductive factors. Masquelet demonstrated the use of biologic membrane formation by first utilizing an antibiotic cement spacer to induce biomembrane casing while providing temporary structural support to the osseous deficit site.[43] Following adequate membrane development, the spacer is removed while the casing is preserved to aid in vascularization of the autogenous graft foundation.[44,45]

WOUND COVERAGE

Early wound coverage is advised. Gustilo originally recommended delaying primary closure but subsequent studies showed a significant decreased infection rate with wound closure or flap application in <3 days.[46,47] Recent studies have demonstrated that delayed wound closure has the opposite effect and increases the occurrence of deep space infections.[48,49]

A recent study investigated incision closure in the primary time frame opposed to delaying closure.[50] A level of subjectivity remains regarding immediate wound closure following permanent fixation. In smaller wounds that lack clinic signs of infection, primary closure should be considered but with the caveat of close postoperative period monitoring. In larger wounds, the decision for primary incision closure is less obvious and requires consideration of patient comorbidities.[51] The addition of negative pressure VAC is recommended to augment expeditious closure in the setting of larger soft tissue deficits or at the very least to prepare the site for eventual skin graft placement or flap transfer.[52,53] The evidence supporting wound VACs in clean surgery is unfortunately limited and does not defend the overall cost of the adjunctive therapy.[54] Negative pressure VAC applied for 5 days provides wound moisture balance control, stimulates blood flow to the skin edges, and reduces the potential for bacterial contamination while also keeping a physical barrier against nosocomial contamination.[55]

positioning PEARLS

- The patient should be positioned appropriately on the operating room table based on the injury site. The use of posterior elevation under the tibia allows the talus to fall into the ankle mortise while eliminating contralateral limb interference with intraoperative fluoroscopic imaging.

Infected Hardware

- In the setting of infected internal fixation, hardware removal is indicated while maintaining fracture stability. If incomplete fracture healing is noted, antibiotics are required to suppress the infection until stability is achieved. The use of external fixation offers the ability to span the fracture site while providing stability but has the potential to lead to secondary osseous healing.

AUTHORS PREFERRED TREATMENT

The patient's neurovascular status is evaluated with the initial "one-look," including pictures completed in the ED. Large debris is removed by irrigation, and a compressive posterior splint is applied. Antibiotic therapy consisting of broad-spectrum antibiotics is started immediately. The first stage of treatment consists of urgent OR debridement as well as extensive irrigation followed by temporary fracture stabilization utilizing delta frame external fixator configuration. Once adequate soft tissue coverage is possible and clinical signs of infection are absent, definitive fracture fixation and osseous defect grafting are accomplished. Consider adjunctive wound VAC closure in cases of tenuous closures.

PERILS and PITFALLS

- "One-look" ED evaluation
- Immediate initiation of broad-spectrum antibiotics
- Intraoperative assessment to determine severity
- Irrigation and debridement
- Temporary spanning external fixation as indicated
- Infection risk minimized, discontinue antibiotics
- Soft tissue reconstruction and permanent fixation
- Regular postoperative imaging monitoring
- Maintain hardware until fracture stability achieved

POSTOPERATIVE CARE

Following incisional wound VAC placement, skin edge viability needs to be reassessed after 5 days.[52,53] In cases of primary closure, the wound must be inspected weekly until suture removal. Caution must be taken to control postoperative edema with regular applications of compressive dressings. The requirement for nonweight bearing to the lower extremity is dictated by fracture location and on average should be based upon radiographic indications of fracture healing.

Regular plain film radiographic evaluation for hardware lucency, fracture reduction, and periosteal reactions is needed to monitor for latent infections. In the setting of infection seeded at the time of permanent fixation, initiate antibiotic therapy until fracture stabilization is achieved.[56] Upon anatomic healing, the hardware removal is mandatory with mechanical debridement and further treatment as directed by tissue viability.

REHABILITATION

The length and intensity of physical therapy and rehabilitation is determined by the severity of the injury. The degree of hardship and privation exponentially increases with the extent of surgical debridement and required postoperative course. A comprehensive rehabilitation program with the goal of returning to everyday function shows benefits with early commencement. Following soft tissue healing, passive range of motion to pain tolerance potential reduces postinjury stiffness. Introduction of timely protected weight bearing may reduce muscle atrophy as well as adjacent joint and muscle decompensation.

REFERENCES

1. Gustilo RB, Anderson JT. Prevention of infection in the treatment of one thousand and twenty-five open fractures of long bones: retrospective and prospective analyses. *J Bone Joint Surg Am.* 1976;58:453-458.
2. Gustilo RB, Mendoza RM, Williams DN. Problems in the management of type III (severe) open fractures: a new classification of type III open fractures. *J Trauma.* 1984;24(8):742-746.
3. Brumback RJ, Jones AL. Interobserver agreement in the classification of open fractures of the tibia. The results of a survey of two hundred and forty-five orthopaedic surgeons. *J Bone Joint Surg Am.* 1994;76:1162-1166.
4. Horn BD, Rettig ME. Interobserver reliability in the Gustilo and Anderson classification of open fractures. *J Trauma.* 1993;7:357-360.
5. Fackler ML, Surinchak JS, Malinowski JA, Bowen RE. Bullet fragmentation: a major cause of tissue disruption. *J Trauma.* 1984;24(1):35-39.
6. Hospenthal DR, Murray CK, Anderson RC, et al. Guidelines for the prevention of infections associated with combat-related injuries: 2011 update: endorsed by the Infectious Diseases Society of America and the Surgical Infection Society. *J Trauma.* 2011;71(2):S210-S234.
7. Pape HC, Giannoudis P, Krettek C. The timing of fracture treatment in polytrauma patients: relevance of damage control orthopedic surgery. *Am J Surg.* 2002;183:622-629.
8. Bosse MJ, McCarthy ML, Jones AL; the Lower Extremity Assessment Project (LEAP) Study Group. Severe lower extremity trauma: an indication for amputation? *J Bone Joint Surg Am.* 2005;87:2601-2608.
9. Schmidt AH. Acute compartment syndrome. *Injury.* 2017;48(suppl 1):S22-S25.
10. Court-Brown CM, Honeyman C, Bugler K, McQueen M. The spectrum of open fractures of the foot in adults. *Foot Ankle Int.* 2013;34(3):323-328.
11. Working ZM, Elliott I, Marchand LS, et al. Predictors of amputation in high-energy forefoot and midfoot injuries. *Injury.* 2017;48(2):536-541.
12. Agel J, Rockwood T, Barber R, Marsh JL. Potential predictive ability of the orthopaedic trauma association open fracture classification. *J Orthop Trauma.* 2014;28(5):300-306.
13. Enninghorst N, McDougall D, Hunt JJ, Balogh ZJ. Open tibia fractures: timely debridement leaves injury severity as the only determinant of poor outcome. *J Trauma.* 2011;70(2):352-356, discussion 356-357.
14. Prodromidis AD, Charalambous CP. The 6-hour rule for surgical debridement of open tibial fractures: a systematic review and meta-analysis of infection and nonunion rates. *J Orthop Trauma.* 2016;30(7):397-402.
15. Hull PD, Johnson SC, Stephen DJ, Kreder HJ, Jenkinson RJ. Delayed debridement of severe open fractures is associated with a higher rate of deep infection. *Bone Joint J.* 2014;96-B(3):379-384.
16. Melvin JS, Dombroski DG, Torbert JT, Kovach SJ, Esterhai JL, Mehta S. Open tibial shaft fractures: I. Evaluation and initial wound management. *J Am Acad Orthop Surg.* 2010;18(1):10-19.
17. Manway J, Highlander P. Open fractures of the foot and ankle: an evidence-based review. *Foot Ankle Spec.* 2015;8(1):59-64.
18. Penn-Barwell JG, Murray CK, Wenke JC. Early antibiotics and debridement independently reduce infection in an open fracture model. *J Bone Joint Surg Br.* 2012;94:107-112.
19. Patzakis MJ, Wilkins J. Factors influencing infection rate in open fracture wounds. *Clin Orthop Relat Res.* 1989;(243):36-40.
20. Patzakis MJ, Harvey JP Jr, Ivler D. The role of antibiotics in the management of open fractures. *J Bone Joint Surg Am.* 1974;56(3):532-541.
21. Carver DC, Kuehn SB, Weinlein JC. Role of systemic and local antibiotics in the treatment of open fractures. *Orthop Clin North Am.* 2017;48(2):137-153.
22. Carsenti-Etesse H, Doyon F, Desplaces N, et al. Epidemiology of bacterial infection during management of open leg fractures. *Eur J Clin Microbiol Infect Dis.* 1999;18:315-323.
23. Rodriguez L, Jung HS, Goulet JA, Cicalo A, Machado-Aranda DA, Napolitano LM. Evidence-based protocol for prophylactic antibiotics in open fractures: improved antibiotic stewardship with no increase in infection rates. *J Trauma Acute Care Surg.* 2014;77(3):400-407.
24. Redfern J, Wasilko S, Groth ME, McMillian WD, Bartlett CS. Surgical site infections in patients with type 3 open fractures: comparing antibiotic prophylaxis with Cefazolin Plus Gentamicin Versus Piperacillin/Tazobactam. *J Orthop Trauma.* 2016;30(8):415-419.
25. Torbert JT, Joshi M, Moraff A, et al. Current bacterial speciation and antibiotic resistance in deep infections after operative fixation of fractures. *J Orthop Trauma.* 2015;29:7-17.
26. Saveli CC, Belknap RW, Morgan SJ, Price CS. The role of prophylactic antibiotics in open fractures in an era of community-acquired methicillin-resistant *Staphylococcus aureus.* *Orthopedics.* 2011;34:611-616.
27. Chen AF, Schreiber VM, Washington W, Rao N, Evans AR. What is the rate of methicillin-resistant Staphylococcus aureus and gram-negative infections in open fractures? *Clin Orthop Relat Res.* 2013;471:3135-3140.
28. Skaggs DL, Friend L, Alman B, et al. The effect of surgical delay on acute infection following 554 open fractures in children. *J Bone Joint Surg Am.* 2005;87:8-12.
29. Schenker ML, Yannascoli S, Baldwin KD, Ahn J, Mehta S. Does timing to operative debridement 23 affect infectious complications in open long-bone fractures? A systematic review. *J Bone Joint Surg Am.* 2012;94:1057-1064.
30. Crowley DJ, Kanakaris NK, Giannoudis PV. Irrigation of the wounds in open fractures. *J Bone Joint Surg Br.* 2007;89(5):580-585.
31. Bhandari M, Guyatt GH, Swiontkowski MF, Schemitsch EH. Treatment of open fractures of the shaft of the tibia. *J Bone Joint Surg Br.* 2001;83:62-68.
32. Draeger RW, Dahners LE. Traumatic wound debridement: a comparison of irrigation methods. *J Orthop Trauma.* 2006;20:83-88.
33. Hassinger SM, Harding G, Wongworawat MD. High-pressure pulsatile lavage propagates bacteria into soft tissue. *Clin Orthop.* 2005;439:27-31.
34. Anglen JO. Comparison of soap and antibiotic solutions for irrigation of lower-limb open fracture wounds: a prospective, randomized study. *J Bone Joint Surg Am.* 2005;87-A:1415-1422.

35. D'Alleyrand JC, O'Toole RV. The evolution of damage control orthopedics: current evidence and practical applications of early appropriate care. *Orthop Clin North Am.* 2013;44(4): 499-507.

36. Kapoor SK, Kataria H, Patra SR, Boruah T. Capsuloligamentotaxis and definitive fixation by an ankle-spanning Ilivaroz fixator in high energy pilon fractures. *J Bone Joint Surg Br.* 2010;92(8):1100-1106.

37. Wukich DK, Dikis JW, Monaco SJ, Strannigan K, Suder NC, Rosario BL. Topically applied vancomycin powder reduces the rate of surgical site infection in diabetic patients undergoing foot and ankle surgery. *Foot Ankle Int.* 2015;36:1017-1024.

38. Singh K, Bauer JM, LaChaud GY, Bible JE, Mir HR. Surgical site infection in high energy peri-articular tibia fractures with intra-wound vancomycin powder: a retrospective pilot study. *J Orthop Traumatol.* 2015;16:287-291.

39. Charalambous CP, Siddique I, Zenios M, et al. Early versus delayed surgical treatment of open tibial fractures: effect on the rates of infection and need of secondary surgical procedures to promote bone union. *Injury.* 2005;36:656-661.

40. Harley BJ, Beaupre LA, Jones CA, et al. The effect of time to definitive treatment on the rate of nonunion and infection in open fractures. *J Orthop Trauma.* 2002;16:484-490.

41. Blick SS, Brumback RJ, Lakatos R, Poka A, Burgess AR. Early prophylactic bone grafting of high-energy tibial fractures. *Clin Orthop Relat Res.* 1989;(240):21-41.

42. Trabulsy PP, Kerley SM, Hoffman WY. A prospective study of early soft tissue coverage of grade IIIB tibial fractures. *J Trauma.* 1994;36:661-668.

43. Masquelet AC, Fitoussi F, Begue T, et al. Reconstruction of the long bones by the induced membrane and spongy autograft. *Ann Chir Plast Esthet.* 2000;45(3):346-353.

44. Azi ML, Teixeira AA, Cotias RB, Joeris A, Kfuri M Jr. Membrane induced osteogenesis in the management of posttraumatic bone defects. *J Orthop Trauma.* 2016;30(10):545-550.

45. Demitri S, Vicenti G, Carrozzo M, Bizzoca D, De Franceschi D, Moretti B. The Masquelet technique in the treatment of a non-infected open complex fracture of the distal tibia with severe bone and soft tissue loss: a case report. *Injury.* 2018;49:S58-S62.

46. Godina M. Early microsurgical reconstruction of complex trauma of the extremities. *Plast Reconstr Surg.* 1986;78:285-292.

47. Gopal S, Majumder S, Batchelor AG, Knight SL, De Boer P, Smith RM. Fix and flap: the radical orthopaedic and plastic treatment of severe open fractures of the tibia. *J Bone Joint Surg Br.* 2000;82:959-966.

48. Blum ML, Esser M, Richardson M, Paul E, Rosenfeldt FL. Negative pressure wound therapy reduces deep infection rate in open tibial fractures. *J Orthop Trauma.* 2012;26: 499-505.

49. Liu DS, Sofiadellis F, Ashton M, MacGill K, Webb A. Early soft tissue coverage and negative pressure wound therapy optimizes patient outcomes in lower limb trauma. *Injury.* 2012;43:772-778.

50. Hohmann E, Tetsworth K, Radziejowski MJ, Wiesniewski TF. Comparison of delayed and primary wound closure in the treatment of open tibial fractures. *Arch Orthop Trauma Surg.* 2007;127(2):131-136.

51. Rajasekaran S, Dheenadhayalan J, Babu JN, Sundararajan SR, Venkatramani H, Sabapathy SR. Immediate primary skin closure in type-III A and B open fractures: results after a minimum of five years. *J Bone Joint Surg Br.* 2009;91(2):217-224.

52. Hou Z, Irgit K, Strohecker KA, et al. Delayed flap reconstruction with vacuum-assisted closure management of the open IIIB tibial fracture. *J Trauma.* 2011;71(6):1705-1708.

53. Schlatterer DR, Hirschfeld AG, Webb LX. Negative pressure wound therapy in grade IIIB tibial fractures: fewer infections and fewer flap procedures? *Clin Orthop Relat Res.* 2015;473(5):1802-1811.

54. Bhattacharyya T, Mehta P, Smith M, Pomahac B. Routine use of wound vacuum-assisted closure does not allow coverage delay for open tibia fractures. *Plast Reconstr Surg.* 2008;121:1263-1266.

55. Stannard JP, Volgas DA, Stewart R, McGwin G Jr, Alonso JE. Negative pressure wound therapy after severe open fractures: a prospective randomized study. *J Orthop Trauma.* 2009;23(8):552-557.

56. Berkes M, Obremskey WT, Scannell B, Ellington JK, Hymes RA, Bosse M; Southeast Fracture Consortium. Maintenance of hardware after early postoperative infection following fracture internal fixation. *J Bone Joint Surg Am.* 2010;92(4):823-828.

Tarsal Coalition

Michael S. Downey

DEFINITION

Tarsal coalition is an abnormal condition that exists when there is partial or complete union between two or more tarsal bones causing restricted motion or absence of motion between the tarsal bones. Coalitions can produce a dramatic, and often pathognomonic, symptom complex that may ultimately be identified as rigid peroneal spastic flatfoot. A basic understanding of tarsal coalitions and their associated symptom complexes will enable the clinician to diagnose tarsal coalitions more readily and accurately and to initiate appropriate treatment.

HISTORICAL REVIEW

Tarsal coalitions have been identified and recorded for several hundred years or more. Heiple and Lovejoy[1] reported a tarsal coalition in the foot of a pre-Columbian Indian skeleton *circa* 1000 AD. Coe and Broman[2] found an even older specimen in the ruins of a Mayan temple in Guatemala. More recently, in 2005, Silva[3] reported two cases of nonosseous calcaneonavicular coalition in older specimens from Portuguese burial sites dating back to between the late Neolithic period and the early Bronze age (ie, between 3600 and 2000 BC).

Historically, the first written description of tarsal coalition is attributed to Buffon[4] in 1769. Sir Robert Jones[5] provided the first detailed clinical recounting of peroneal spastic flatfoot in 1897, but he did not associate it with tarsal coalition. The first radiographic demonstration of tarsal coalition was by Kirmisson[6] in 1898, only 3 years after Roentgen's discovery of x-rays.

Many years passed between the earliest anatomic descriptions and the discovery of x-rays, and many more years elapsed before the identification of the relationship between tarsal coalition and peroneal spastic flatfoot. In this sense, the two most common tarsal coalitions—calcaneonavicular and talocalcaneal—were identified in similar fashion. First they were identified anatomically, then radiographically, and, more recently, they were related to peroneal spastic flatfoot.

Calcaneonavicular coalition was first described anatomically by Cruveilhier[7] in 1829. Slomann,[8] in 1921, reported five cases of calcaneonavicular bar and demonstrated the coalition on an oblique radiographic view of the foot. Not until 1927, however, when Badgley[9] resected a calcaneonavicular coalition, was the deformity associated with peroneal spastic flatfoot.

Similarly, Zuckerkandl[10] first anatomically identified *talocalcaneal coalition* in 1877. Korvin,[11] in 1934, used an axial radiographic view of the calcaneus to demonstrate a talocalcaneal coalition. In 1948, Harris and Beath[12] popularized Korvin's axial or ski-jump view of the calcaneus and recognized talocalcaneal coalition as a cause of peroneal spastic flatfoot.

Other tarsal coalitions are less frequent but have been reported. *Talonavicular coalition* was first reported by Anderson[13] in 1879. *Calcaneocuboid coalition* was first recognized by Holland[14] in 1918. *Cubonavicular coalition* was first reported by Waugh[15] in 1957, and Lusby[16] first identified *naviculocuneiform coalition* in 1959. Multiple and massive coalitions involving several tarsal bones also have been reported.[17,18] Farid and Faber[19] recently described a case of bilateral talocalcaneal, calcaneonavicular, talonavicular coalitions, further confirming that varying combinations of tarsal coalition occur in rare instances.

Before the advent of radiography, earlier clinicians had to rely on clinical examination alone to diagnose a tarsal coalition. Today, with advanced radiographic and diagnostic imaging techniques, the demonstration and diagnosis of tarsal coalition are simplified. However, although much has been written about tarsal coalition and much is understood, numerous diagnostic and therapeutic questions remain unanswered.

ETIOLOGY

Tarsal coalition is clearly the most common cause of peroneal spastic flatfoot. However, the cause of tarsal coalition is not always so clear. Many authors have attempted to attribute all tarsal coalitions to one etiologic factor. It is now certain that the condition has many causes, and tarsal coalitions may be either congenital or acquired.

Congenital coalition is more frequently identified and reported, although the mechanism of congenital coalition is not conclusively known. Pfitzner[20] suggested that a congenital tarsal coalition is formed from the incorporation of accessory ossicles into the normal tarsal bones on either side of a joint or in close approximation with one another. Many authors have supported this theory, and the primary evidence has been that the os sustentaculum proprium accessory bone occurs at the side of the middle facet of the subtalar joint, where many coalitions occur. In addition, other investigators have described a tarsal coalition occurring in the area of the os trigonum accessory bone.[21-23] This evidence strongly suggests that any accessory bone may fuse to one or more tarsal bones and may result in a tarsal coalition (Fig. 44.1). Although this has been shown to be one possible cause of coalition, Harris[24] disproved it as the sole

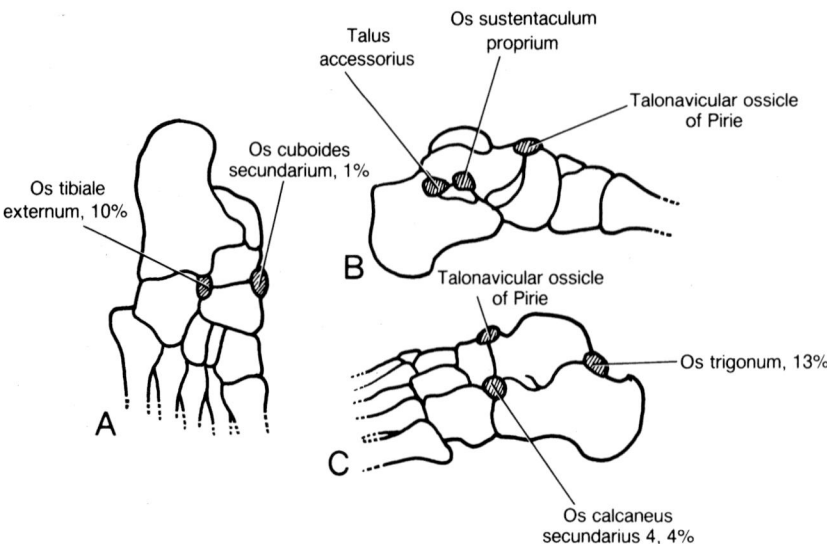

FIGURE 44.1 A-C. Ossicles responsible for formation of tarsal coalitions according to Pfitzner. (Reprinted with permission from Farid A, Faber FWM. Bilateral triple talocalcaneal, calcaneonavicular, and talonavicular tarsal coalition: a case report. *J Foot and Ankle Surg.* 2019;58:374-376.)

cause by demonstrating a tarsal coalition in a fetus. The appearance of a tarsal coalition in a fetus, in which development and incorporation of accessory ossicles would not have had time to occur, certainly works against Pfitzner's theory.

Harris's finding supports the theory proposed by Leboucq,[25] who suggested that congenital coalition results from the failure of differentiation and segmentation of primitive mesenchyme. This concept, which is now widely accepted as the most common etiology of tarsal coalition, attributes congenital coalitions to a heritable defect or to an insult in the first trimester of pregnancy. Subsequently, numerous authors have reported hereditary patterns of coalitions.[17,26-34] A large field study by Leonard[35] concluded that tarsal coalition was a unifactorial disorder with autosomal dominant inheritance. Kawashima and Uhthoff[36] examined 20 cartilaginous talocalcaneal bridges in 16 embryos and fetuses ranging from 7 to 20 weeks and concluded that coalition was caused by a failure or delay in differentiation of mesenchymal tissue between the posterior portion of the sustentaculum tali and the corresponding area of the talus during the 7.5-8.5 postovulatory weeks. More recently, histopathologic evidence has been found to support Leboucq's theory further.[37] Most evidence supports a gene mutation for coalition formation, which is then passed on to future generations as an autosomal dominant gene. Recently, Takano and associates[38] have demonstrated that mutations of the human Noggin (NOG) gene, a gene associated with bone and joint development, is associated with tarsal-carpal coalition syndrome. The exact genetic expression of tarsal coalition has not yet been elucidated. Today, the generally accepted theory is that congenital tarsal coalitions are caused by a genetic mutation to an autosomal gene that results in the failure of differentiation and segmentation of primitive mesenchyme.

Tarsal coalition may also be acquired. *Acquired tarsal coalition* may result from arthritis, infection, trauma, neoplasms, or other conditions.[39] Acquired coalition is less common in pediatric and adolescent patients.[40] The acquired coalition typically starts as a diminished range of motion within the involved joints, with varying progression to complete fusion.[41] A talonavicular coalition in a 24-year-old patient has been described secondary to osteoarthritis, which resulted from a previous tuberculosis septic arthritis of the tarsus when the patient was 11 years of age.[42] A case of restricted subtalar joint motion and

peroneal spastic flatfoot that occurred secondary to a fibrosarcoma has also been noted.[43] Healey and Willkens[44] reported 2 patients with juvenile rheumatoid arthritis with resultant tarsal arthritis and eventual tarsal coalition. In a retrospective review of 88 patients with juvenile rheumatoid arthritis and 97 patients with classic or adult rheumatoid arthritis, 16% of the patients with juvenile rheumatoid arthritis and 10% of the patients with adult rheumatoid arthritis had intertarsal ankylosis.[45] Roth[46] reported a case of massive tarsal ankylosis in a patient with juvenile ankylosing spondylitis. Talonavicular coalition has also been reported after Köhler disease (ie, avascular necrosis of the navicular).[47] In addition, subtalar joint limitus and eventual coalition are known to result from a joint depression calcaneal fracture.[48,49] Thus, when all age groups are considered, it is clear from these examples that acquired coalition is common and is a frequent cause of peroneal spastic flatfoot.

INCIDENCE

The incidence of tarsal coalition in the general population is not known. Rankin and Baker[50] reported a 0.04% incidence (24 cases in 60 000 young adults) in a large population of military personnel. Shands and Wentz[51] reported an incidence of 0.9% (11 cases in 1232 children) in a population of children in a clinic. Vaughan and Segal,[52] studying army personnel, found the incidence to be ~1.4% (28 cases in 2000 patients). This is the highest reported incidence to date. However, one may argue that these studies were not conducted on representative populations in regard to age or sex and may suffer from selection bias. Thus, the actual incidence in the general population may be higher or lower.

Nonetheless, the incidence of tarsal coalition is not the same as the incidence of peroneal spastic flatfoot. Peroneal spastic flatfoot is usually a sequela of the tarsal coalition. A tarsal coalition may be present without symptoms or without peroneal spastic flatfoot. In addition, peroneal spastic flatfoot may be present without tarsal coalition. Harris and Beath[12] examined 3619 Canadian army enlistees and found ~2% incidence of peroneal spastic flatfoot, with a correspondingly lower incidence of tarsal coalition of 0.03%.

Tarsal coalition has been reported to have no racial preference.[50] Further, roughly 50% of the cases have been reported as bilateral,[50] although Leonard[35] reported that the incidence of bilateral involvement was as high as 80%.

Several authors have suggested a greater incidence of tarsal coalition in male patients, with male-to-female ratios reported in two different studies as 12:5[53] and 4:1.[54] Investigators have theorized that this unequal sex predilection may reflect selection bias as the studies were performed on army personnel.[55] Indeed, if these studies are correct in their suggested predilection, the theory of mutation of an autosomal dominant gene must be reconsidered. Leonard[35] reported a more equal sex incidence in his large study. Thus, the actual sex predilection remains uncertain.

Talocalcaneal coalition and calcaneonavicular coalition are by far the most common anatomic types of this condition. These two forms account for ~90% of all tarsal coalitions.[56] However, controversy exists about which of these two coalitions is most prevalent. Leonard[35] reported an extremely skewed study in which 27 of 31 patients (87%) with coalitions had calcaneonavicular involvement. Conversely, Harris[57] reported 66 talocalcaneal coalitions (65%) and 29 calcaneonavicular coalitions (28%) among the total of 102 coalitions found. Other studies have demonstrated a more even distribution.[49,58-62] Stormont and Peterson,[62] after reviewing the literature, tabulated the relative incidence of talocalcaneal and calcaneonavicular coalitions reported in all articles they found that included cases of more than one type of coalition. The calculated relative incidence was 48.1% for talocalcaneal coalitions, 43.6% for calcaneonavicular coalitions, and 8.3% for other coalitions. Thus, the current consensus is that talocalcaneal and calcaneonavicular coalitions account for about 90% of all coalitions, and talocalcaneal coalition is slightly more common.

Talonavicular coalition appears to be the third most common type of tarsal coalition. This type is rare, with fewer than 50 cases reported in the literature.[13,26,32,49,54,57,58,61,63-80] Calcaneocuboid,[14,57,61,81-85] cubonavicular,[15,49,86-93] naviculocuneiform,[16,94-104] metatarsocuneiform,[105-107] combination tarsal coalitions,[19] and massive coalitions occur with even less frequency.[55,103]

ASSOCIATED ABNORMALITIES

The association of tarsal coalition with other skeletal abnormalities and syndromes is well documented. Once a tarsal coalition has been identified, one should query and examine the patient to rule out the presence of these coincidental deformities.

Symphalangism, or ankylosis of the interphalangeal joints, has been shown to be associated with tarsal coalition (Fig. 44.2). In 1917, Drinkwater[108] described proximal interphalangeal joint anarthrosis transmitted through 14 generations but did not associate tarsal coalition with the digital deformity. Later, Austin[109] reported a case of bilateral symphalangism of the distal interphalangeal joints of the third, fourth, and fifth toes associated with bilateral talocalcaneal and calcaneocuboid coalitions. Symphalangism associated with fusion of the second through fifth metatarsals with the cuneiforms and cuboid has been noted in one family.[34] Two families with symphalangism of the hands and concomitant talonavicular coalitions have also been described.[67] Investigators suggested that the two deformities were determined by a single gene, because in both kindreds, the inheritance followed an autosomal dominant pattern. Harle

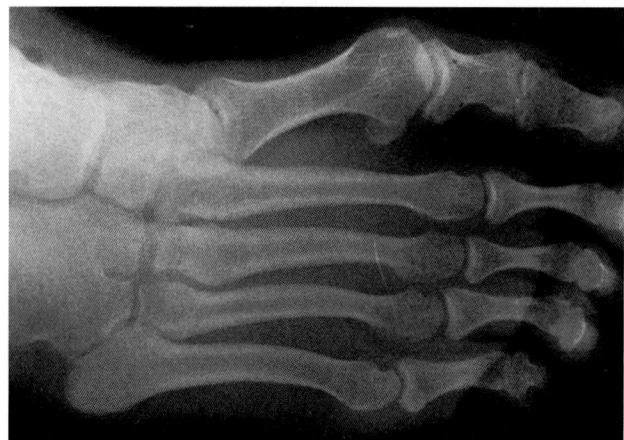

FIGURE 44.2 Synostosis of proximal and middle phalanges of fourth and fifth digits. This patient also had talonavicular and cuboid-third cuneiform coalitions.

and Stevenson[110] also believed that a coupling effect of genes was responsible for the two conditions, along with metatarsal and midtarsal fusions. Gaal and others[111] described three distinct ethnic pedigrees that they believed confirmed that symphalangism was an autosomal dominant genetic trait. Castle et al.[112] reviewed 4 generations of a family with 15 family members exhibiting symphalangism with associated tarsal synostosis and hypophalangism. Typically, symphalangism is not identifiable at birth, because the involved phalanges have not ossified. With growth, however, the affected bones show a faster rate of epiphyseal closure than the nonaffected bones. After epiphyseal closure, the joint space narrows until complete bony fusion occurs.

Tarsal coalitions have also been associated with *metatarsal abnormalities* and massive coalitions. Bersani and Samilson[17] reported a mother and two children who had bilateral massive coalitions involving the talus, navicular, cuboid, second and third cuneiforms, and second, third, and fourth metatarsals. A case of lesser tarsal ankylosis involving the cuneiforms and cuboid and a synostosis between the bases of the fourth and fifth metatarsal bones has also been reported[113] (Fig. 44.3). Illievitz[69] reported a unilateral case in a boy with four toes, four metatarsals, and coalition of the talonavicular joint.

In addition, *tarsal and carpal coalitions* may coexist. O'Rahilly[114] claimed that fusions of almost every possible combination in the carpal and metacarpal region and in the corresponding portion of the foot have been found. However, despite the developmental similarity of the carpus and tarsus, and despite a recent report suggesting a genetic mutation may be associated with tarsal-carpal coalitions syndrome,[38] the coalitions in the two areas may be unrelated.[42,70]

Less commonly, tarsal coalitions have been reported with other *major limb anomalies.* Tarsal and carpal coalitions have been noted in cases of phocomelia[114] (ie, defective development of the arms or legs so the hands or feet are attached close to the body), and tarsal coalitions have been noted in patients with and fibular and tibial hemimelia (ie, absence of a portion of a limb).[114-118] Lamb[119] reported the association of a ball-and-socket ankle joint with tarsal coalition, but whether the ankle change is an isolated congenital anomaly or is secondary to compensation for the tarsal coalition itself is debatable.[120]

Further, multiple or massive tarsal coalitions may be part of a more complex syndrome. In 1944, Nievergelt[121] described a

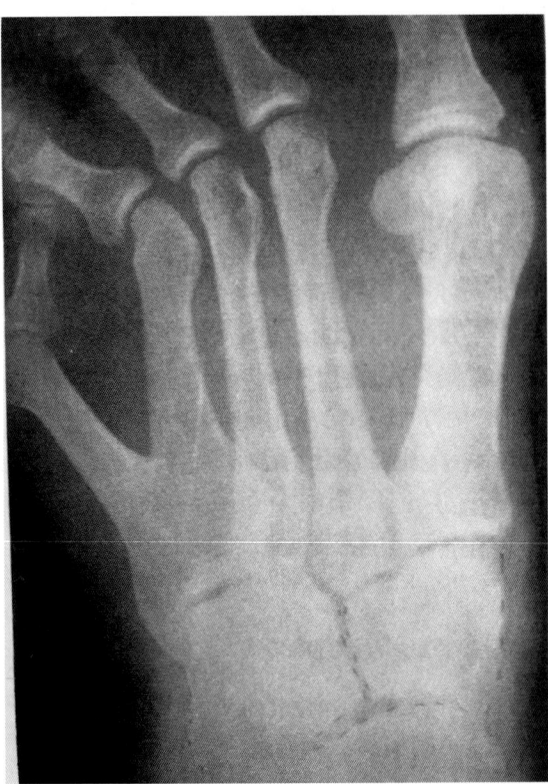

FIGURE 44.3 Congenital synostoses of fourth and fifth metatarsals and first and second cuneiforms, as well as the lateral cuneiform and cuboid. (From Boccio JR, Dockery GL, LeBaron S. Congenital metatarsal synostosis. *J Foot Surg*. 1984;23:42, with permission.)

syndrome occurring in both sexes in three successive generations of a family. The syndrome consisted of elbow dysplasia with radioulnar synostosis and subluxation of the radial head, dysplasia of the tibia and fibula with the fibula remaining longer because of lesser involvement, and tarsal synostosis associated with atypical clubfoot. Twenty years later, Pearlman and associates[122] reported a similar combination of deformities in a mother and daughter. Their patients did not have dysplasia of the tibia, but they did have concomitant carpal synostosis, symphalangism, and associated brachydactylia (ie, short fingers), camptodactyly (ie, flexion deformity of the fingers), and clinodactyly (ie, angular deformity of the fingers). These investigators termed the combined deformity *Nievergelt syndrome*. Later, Dubois[123] reported an additional case and suggested that *Nievergelt-Pearlman syndrome* would be a more appropriate name. In 1975, Murakami[124] reported three additional cases in a family with impairment of hearing resulting from bony fusion of the ossicles in the middle ear. In 1978, Nixon[125] reviewed Nievergelt-Pearlman syndrome and believed it would be better termed *multiple synostoses syndrome*. He concluded that this syndrome appeared to be inherited in an autosomal dominant fashion and was probably caused by a single gene abnormality.

Similarly, in *Apert syndrome*, patients may have massive synostosis of the tarsal bones. Tachdjian[126] described an example of the resulting condition with craniosynostosis, midfacial hypoplasia, osseous or cutaneous syndactyly of all digits (or commonly of the second, third, and fourth fingers and toes), and a broad distal thumb and hallux. Collins et al.[127] used computed tomography (CT) to define the dysmorphology of the foot in three patients with Apert syndrome. These investigators found

five consistent findings among the three pairs of feet: (1) anomalous great toes with phalangeal and metatarsal pathologic features, (2) syndactyly of toes 2-5, (3) fusions between metatarsals, (4) tarsal coalitions, and (5) limitations in shoes.

Osebold-Remondini syndrome is yet another skeletal dysplasia, first described in 1985.[128] Mesomelic shortness of limbs and associated shortness of stature, absence of hypoplasia of the middle phalanges with synostosis of the remaining phalanges, and carpal and tarsal coalitions are the typical anomalies associated with this syndrome. Although rare, these syndromes are seen because affected persons have normal health and life spans.[129]

A relationship between tarsal coalition and *clubfoot deformity* has also been reported.[130-134] Turco[134] reported 8 feet in a series of 240 resistant clubfeet to have tarsal coalitions in the region of the sustentaculum tali. Callahan[130] reported a single clubfoot discovered intraoperatively to have an absent tibialis posterior tendon and a middle facet talocalcaneal coalition. Five cases of arthrogryposis multiplex congenita have been described in association with tarsal coalition.[131] Spero et al.[132] reported 18 cases (14 patients) of rigid equinovarus deformity with a tarsal coalition. In their series, preoperative radiographs demonstrated the coalition in only a single case, and the coalitions in the other cases were identified at surgery or at morbid dissection. These authors suggested the possible preoperative use of magnetic resonance imaging (MRI) studies to identify the presence of any coalition before surgical treatment.

Takakura et al.[135] in 1991 reported a possible association between tarsal coalition and *tarsal tunnel syndrome*. In 23 of 67 feet with symptomatic talocalcaneal coalitions, these investigators found tarsal tunnel syndrome to be present. They believed that the bony eminence in the area of the middle facet most likely accounted for the external compression on the posterior tibial nerve. In a later paper, Takakura and associates[136] discussed seven cases of tarsal tunnel syndrome that were believed to be caused by a medial talocalcaneal coalition and a concurrent ganglion. They excised the coalition and ganglion in six of the seven cases with mixed results. In 2002, Lee and others[137] described the ultrasonic findings of tarsal tunnel syndrome caused by a talocalcaneal coalition. In 2009, Yoo and associate[138] described a failed tarsal tunnel decompression that they attributed to a tarsal coalition. In 2016, Alaia et al.[139] reviewed 67 ankle MRIs with talocalcaneal coalition and performed a retrospective review of the tarsal tunnel tendons and nerves for any abnormalities. Entrapment of the flexor hallucis longus (FHL) tendon by bony prominences was seen in 14 of 67 cases (21%). Attenuation, split tearing, tenosynovitis, or tendinosis of the FHL was present in 26 cases (39%). Attenuation or tenosynovitis was seen in the flexor digitorum longus (FDL) tendon in 18 cases (27%), and tenosynovitis or split tearing of the posterior tibial (PT) tendon was present in 9 cases (13%). Markedly increased signal and caliber of the medial plantar nerve (MPN), indicative of neuritis, was seen in 6 of the 67 cases (9%). The researchers concluded that talocalcaneal coalitions may be associated with soft tissue abnormalities in the tarsal tunnel, implicating in decreasing order, the FHL, FDL, and PT tendons, as well as the MPN. In 2017, Bhat and colleagues[140] reported a case of bilateral tarsal tunnel syndrome that they attributed to bilateral talocalcaneal coalitions and associated symmetrical hypertrophy of the sustentaculum tali.

Further, one study noted that patients with tarsal coalition had significantly *lower bone densities* than normal patients. The trabecular bone density was ~17% lower, on average, in patients with a tarsal coalition. These investigators concluded

that the pain and gait changes associated with a tarsal coalition may lead to inactivity, resulting in a decrease in bone density.[141] More recently, in 2018, Kilicoglu et al.[142] reported a high rate of psychiatric disorders and below normal mental capacity associated with peroneal spastic flatfoot. Their series described 16 patients, but only 6 had a documented tarsal coalition. The most common reported psychiatric disorders were social phobia and attention deficit–hyperactivity disorder (ADHD).

CLASSIFICATION

Tarsal coalitions may be classified in several ways: (1) etiologic type, (2) anatomic type, (3) tissue type, and (4) according to articular involvement. Downey[143,144] proposed the last classification (ie, according to articular involvement) as a surgically based classification system that relates criteria associated with a particular tarsal coalition to the likelihood of surgical success with a proposed procedure.

Tarsal coalitions may be classified according to their origin, either congenital or acquired.[56] This classification is not generally helpful in ascertaining the best possible treatment plan. Tarsal coalitions may be classified according to their anatomic constituents. Tachdjian[126] provided a classification that subdivides coalitions into the bones that are abnormally united or, infrequently, part of a complex malformation (Table 44.1). Although only descriptive, Tachdjian's classification suggests the importance of assessing other areas of the foot and the remainder of the body when an apparently local or isolated coalition is identified.

Another common way of grouping tarsal coalitions is to classify them according to the tissue type of their union. In this way, a coalition may be a *synostosis* (osseous union), a *synchondrosis* (cartilaginous union), a *syndesmosis* (fibrous union), or a combination of these. A synostosis may evolve from a synchondrosis or a syndesmosis. Investigators have theorized that this occurs with age or possibly after trauma to the coalition.[37,40] A synostosis is also referred to as a *complete coalition*, because all motion is necessarily absent. An *incomplete coalition* is fibrocartilaginous and has varying amounts of interposed cartilaginous or fibrous tissue that may allow motion between the bones involved. The tissue type of the coalition may be important when one is attempting to diagnose this condition.

By combining the aforementioned classifications, one may make a useful description of a tarsal coalition. For example, a tarsal coalition may be described as a congenital synchondrosis of the middle facet of the talocalcaneal joint. Given this information (ie, the cause, tissue type, and anatomic constituency), one may more accurately understand the tarsal coalition present. However, these classification systems, even when combined, are only descriptive and provide only a small amount of information helpful to the development of a surgical treatment plan.

Identifying this deficiency, Downey[143,144] proposed the *Articular Classification System* based on the articular relationship of the bones involved in the coalition and the indirect effect of the coalition on surrounding joints (Table 44.2). This articular classification system, when combined with the descriptive parameters already discussed, may serve as a basis for communication about possible surgical treatment. The classification assumes that the most important criteria for determining treatment are the age of the patient, the type of coalition, and the degree of secondary arthritic changes. The classification begins by distinguishing between juvenile (osseous immaturity) and adult (osseous maturity) tarsal coalitions. These conditions are then further subdivided into the types of coalition, whether extra-articular or intra-articular (Table 44.3). *Extra-articular coalitions* are those that occur outside a normal joint. These coalitions are commonly called *bars*, and the calcaneonavicular coalition is the most frequently occurring example. *Intra-articular coalitions* occur at normal joint sites and have been referred to as *bridges*. A talocalcaneal coalition of the middle facet of the subtalar joint is the most common example of an intra-articular coalition. Finally, the classification is subdivided

TABLE 44.1	Tachdjian's Classification of Tarsal Coalitions

Isolated anomaly
 Dual between two tarsal bones
  Talocalcaneal
   Middle
    Complete
    Incomplete
    Rudimentary
   Posterior
   Anterior
  Calcaneonavicular
  Talonavicular
  Calcaneocuboid
  Naviculocuneiform
 Multiple: combinations of the above
 Massive: all tarsal bones fused together
Part of a complex malformation
 In association with other synostoses
  Carpal coalition
  Symphalangism
 As one of manifestations of a syndrome
  Nievergelt-Pearlman
  Apert's
 In association with major limb anomalies
  Absence of toes or rays
  "Ball-and-socket" ankle joint
  Fibular hemimelia
  Phocomelia
  Proximal focal femoral deficiency

Modified from Tachdjian MO. *The Child's Foot.* Philadelphia, PA: WB Saunders; 1985:262, with permission.

TABLE 44.2	Articular Classification System[a]

Juvenile (Osseous Immaturity)
 Type I: Extra-articular coalition
  A: No secondary arthritis
  B: Secondary arthritis
 Type II: Intra-articular coalition
  A: No secondary arthritis
  B: Secondary arthritis
Adult (Osseous Maturity)
 Type I: Extra-articular coalition
  A: No secondary arthritis
  B: Secondary arthritis
 Type II: Intra-articular coalition
  A: No secondary arthritis
  B: Secondary arthritis

[a]Classification of tarsal coalitions based on age, articular involvement, and secondary arthritic changes. The classification may be used as a foundation for the discussion of surgical management.

TABLE 44.3	Division of Tarsal Coalitions into Extra-articular and Intra-articular Coalitions[a]

Extra-articular Coalitions
  Calcaneonavicular
  Cubonavicular
Intra-articular Coalitions
  Talocalcaneal
    Middle
    Posterior
    Anterior
    Combination
  Talonavicular
  Calcaneocuboid
  Naviculocuneiform

[a]Multiple and massive coalitions are usually intra-articular coalitions and most frequently are associated with adaptive or degenerative changes.

into the presence or absence of significant secondary arthritic or adaptive changes within surrounding joints. As an example, a middle facet talocalcaneal coalition occurring in an adult with secondary arthritic changes at the talonavicular or calcaneocuboid joints would be an "adult IIB" coalition or an "adult intra-articular coalition with secondary arthritic changes" (Fig. 44.4). A calcaneonavicular coalition occurring in a child with no secondary arthritic changes would be a "juvenile IA" coalition or a "juvenile extra-articular coalition without secondary arthritic changes" (Fig. 44.5). In this manner, treatment plans may be related to the classification system.

While the Articular Classification System is not meant to be all inclusive, it does describe important considerations used in the development of any treatment regimen. As noted, the original description included several parameters: patient age, articular involvement, and the extent of secondary adaptive or arthritic changes.[143,144] In addition to these factors, Downey[145] has more recently recommended that the size of the coalition, and possibly the degree of heel valgus, also be considered when developing a surgical treatment plan, especially with talocalcaneal coalitions.

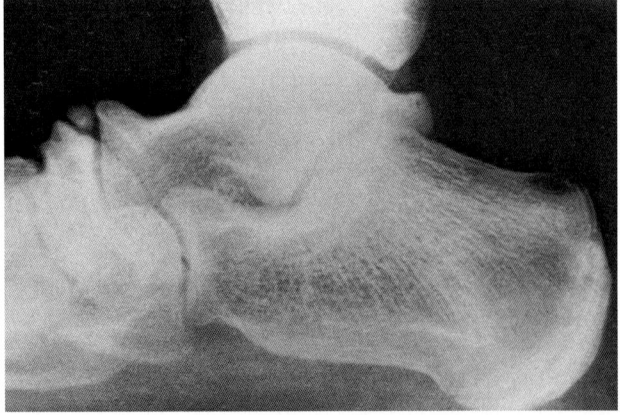

FIGURE 44.4 Middle facet talocalcaneal coalition in a 34-year-old patient. Note the secondary degenerative changes at the subtalar and talonavicular joints. This would be "adult IIB" or "adult, intra-articular coalition with secondary arthritis" in the articular classification system.

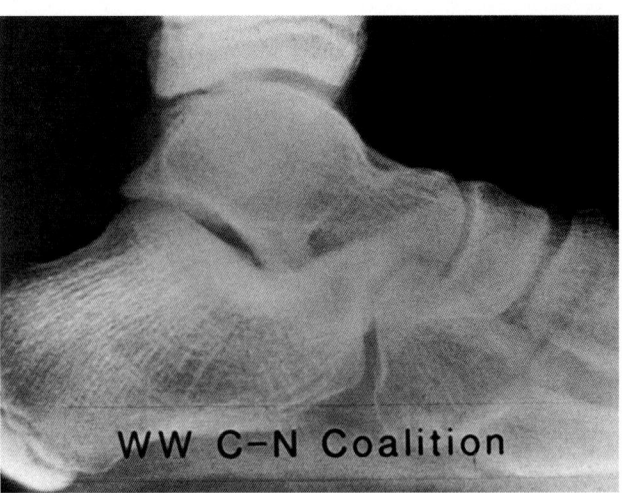

FIGURE 44.5 Calcaneonavicular bar in an 11-year-old patient. No secondary arthritic changes are noted. This would be "juvenile IA" or "juvenile, extra-articular coalition without secondary arthritis" in the articular classification system.

CLINICAL FINDINGS

Tarsal coalition may be completely without symptoms and an incidental finding on routine radiographs. In a study of 23 patients with tarsal coalition, Jack[60] found that 5 (22%) had no symptoms. Three clinical findings—pain, limitation of motion, and muscle spasm—should make the clinician suspect a tarsal coalition. Unfortunately, these patients are often erroneously treated for recurrent ankle sprains, sinus tarsi syndrome, tarsal tunnel syndrome, or other problems that may cause pain in the hindfoot and ankle. A thorough understanding of the common clinical findings associated with tarsal coalitions, at the very least, permits a high index of suspicion for possible coalition after a routine history and physical examination.

Pain is a common finding in patients with tarsal coalition. The pain is usually deep and aching and is frequently in the area of the tarsal coalition. Rarely, it is neuritic. Kumai et al.[37] examined 55 coalitions histologically and found that no nerve endings existed in the coalition itself, but numerous nerve endings were present in the periosteum around the coalition site and in the articular capsule surrounding affected tarsal bones. Further, their study found histologic evidence of vascular proliferation, bleeding caused by vascular damage, osteoblastic and osteoclastic activity, interposition of fibrous connective tissue containing large amounts of cellular components, and irregularity of the cartilaginous bony interface at the boundary between the coalition site and the bone tissue involved. Thus, the pain in a tarsal coalition does not appear to be mediated by nerve endings in the coalition site and is more likely secondary to repeated mechanical stress, with cycles of microfracture and remodeling, with the associated pain mediated by free nerve endings in the surrounding periosteum and strained articular capsules. Katayama and colleagues[146] also discussed a case that showed an association of symptoms and progressive ossification seen on diagnostic imaging. Their patient developed his symptoms simultaneously with ossification of the coalition, which suggested that his pain was caused by mechanical stress.

The patient often can localize the pain to the sinus tarsi, the medial or lateral hindfoot, the anterolateral part of the ankle, or the dorsum of the midfoot. With a middle facet talocalcaneal

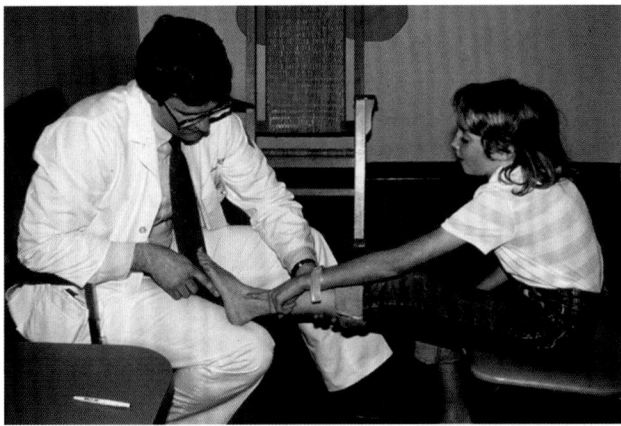

FIGURE 44.6 Young patient with middle facet talocalcaneal coalition localizes pain to sinus tarsi.

coalition, the patient may indicate that the pain encompasses the entire hindfoot and localized the pain to the sustentaculum tali medially and the sinus tarsi laterally (Fig. 44.6). If significant secondary arthritic changes are present, the pain may be greatest in those areas. If the patient is unable to pinpoint the pain, the clinician can usually localize it accurately with firm palpation.

The onset of the pain is usually insidious, developing after some unusual activity (eg, excessive walking, hiking, or running) or innocuous trauma (eg, minor ankle sprain). Rarely, trauma to the foot or ankle injures the area of the coalition.[147-149] This symptom-producing injury has been termed "awakening" trauma.[150] Further, investigators have stated that all coalitions are initially fibrocartilaginous and eventually ossify and have suggested that the different coalitions ossify at different ages and the pain begins as this ossification process occurs. Colwell stated that a talonavicular coalition ossifies from the ages of 3-5 years, a calcaneonavicular coalition ossifies from the ages of 8-12 years, and a talocalcaneal coalition ossifies from the ages of 12-16 years[151] (Table 44.4).

The pain associated with a tarsal coalition is usually aggravated by activity and is relieved with rest. On questioning, the patient frequently relates pain associated with walking over rough, uneven terrain, with prolonged standing especially on hard surfaces, or with athletic activity. Investigators have hypothesized that the decreased hindfoot motion associated with a tarsal coalition may cause an increase in laxity of the ankle ligaments and may result in more frequent sprains in the patient with a coalition.[152] Evidence to support this hypothesis came from Snyder and associates,[153] who, in 1981, retrospectively examined the radiographs of patients with sprained ankles (no other clinical criteria were used) and reported a 63% incidence of calcaneonavicular abnormalities. However, the radiographic criteria used for their assessment were marginal. In a study of 48 patients with tarsal coalition, Gonzalez

TABLE 44.4	Age When Ossification Begins in Most Common Tarsal Coalitions[a]
Talonavicular coalition: 3-5 y	
Calcaneonavicular coalition: 8-12 y	
Talocalcaneal coalition: 12-16 y	

[a]Beginning of ossification may correlate with the onset of symptoms.

and Kumar[154] reported that 9 (19%) were initially seen because of repeated ankle sprains. Appropriately, investigators have suggested that any active adolescent with recurrent ankle sprains or strains should be considered as potentially having a tarsal coalition until proven otherwise.[155,156]

Limitation of subtalar and midtarsal joint motion is common with tarsal coalition and is typically the most obvious clinical finding. Usually, the subtalar joint is limited in the direction of inversion. This limitation becomes even more apparent when peroneal muscle spasm is present. In the case of an incomplete coalition, as ossification progresses, range of motion at the subtalar and midtarsal joints decreases. Clinical examination for subtalar and midtarsal joint motion may be performed with the patient both seated and standing. While the patient is seated, the examiner may assess the subtalar and midtarsal joints passively for the amount of motion available. A decrease in motion may be found in either or both joints. In unilateral cases, the motion may be compared with that of the contralateral limb. Similarly, it is easy to evaluate the patient while he or she is standing. If a pes valgo planus deformity is present, as is seen with the typical peroneal spastic flatfoot, the *Hubscher maneuver* or the *toe test of Jack* may be used to assess the flexibility of the deformity. These maneuvers involve passive dorsiflexion of the hallux while the patient stands in a normal, relaxed position. When the hallux is dorsiflexed, the medial strand of the plantar fascia and the FHL are tightened via the windlass mechanism. If the deformity is flexible, the medial longitudinal arch will increase in height and the hindfoot will supinate (Fig. 44.7A and B). If the deformity is rigid, as typically seen with a tarsal coalition, no change in the longitudinal arch will be seen (Fig. 44.7C and D). Cass and Camasta[157] described how performing the Hubscher maneuver in a patient with a flexible pes planovalgus deformity and concomitant ankle equinus might result in the inability to recreate the arch. They surmised that the posterior equinus contracture could preclude the ability to reproduce the arch height in an otherwise flexible deformity. Therefore, they recommended that a "step-forward" Hubscher maneuver be performed. In this way, the patient stands and steps forward with the extremity to be examined. This "step forward" plantarflexes the foot on the leg and negates the effect of the ankle equinus. With the gastrocsoleus complex relaxed, a more accurate Hubscher maneuver can be performed.

Another method of assessing subtalar joint motion is to ask the patient to roll to the outside of the feet (ie, invert the feet) and then to roll to the inside of the feet (ie, evert the feet). In patients with a tarsal coalition, inversion is diminished (Fig. 44.8). Koeweiden et al.[158] advocated a similar test, which they termed the *heel-tip test*, and in nine patients with known talocalcaneal coalitions, they found 8.4 degrees of motion as compared with 27 degrees of motion in 60 anatomically normal control feet. Other investigators have proposed that measurement of hindfoot movement helped to quantify the extent of restriction and aided in the earlier detection of coalition.[159]

With tarsal coalition, *tonic muscle spasm* may occur. It should be clearly understood that this is a tonic muscle spasm and *not* clonic muscle spasticity. Electrodiagnostic studies have confirmed the absence of true neurologic clonic spasm.[160] The peroneus brevis is usually the muscle that is most significantly involved. However, spasm of the peroneus longus, tibialis anterior, tibialis posterior, gastrocnemius, and soleus may occur.[161-163] Investigators have theorized that as subtalar joint motion becomes painful, the peroneus brevis attempts to guard

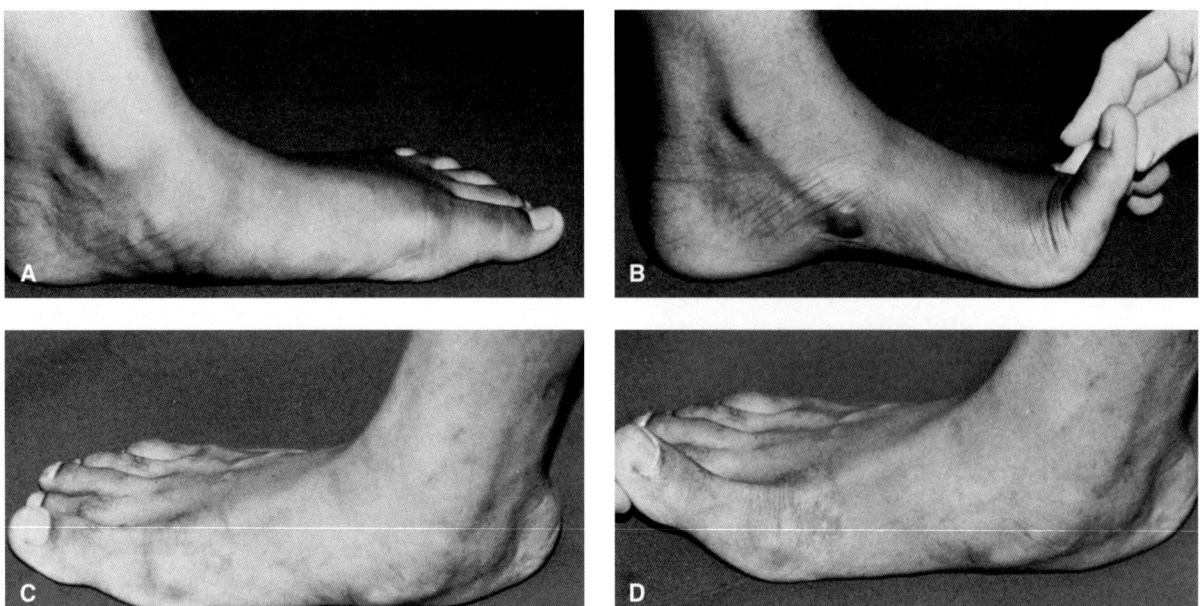

FIGURE 44.7 Clinical demonstration of the Hubscher maneuver in flexible pes valgo planus **(A, B)** and rigid pes valgo planus **(C, D)**. **A.** Patient standing relaxed with severe pes valgo planus deformity. **B.** The Hubscher maneuver is performed. Note the increase in the longitudinal arch. The patient has a flexible pes valgo planus deformity and no tarsal coalition. **C.** Patient standing relaxed with a severe pes valgo planus deformity. **D.** The Hubscher maneuver is performed. Note no change in the longitudinal arch. The patient has a rigid pes valgo planus deformity secondary to a tarsal coalition.

or restrict this motion. This tonic spasm resembles abdominal muscle guarding in a patient with appendicitis. In the simplest sense, it is a subconscious attempt by the peroneus brevis to limit painful motion. This spasm is not neurologic, as in clonic spasticity, but represents simply an increase in tension of the peroneus brevis muscle-tendon unit (ie, tonic spasm). The muscle spasm, like pain associated with the coalition, is precipitated by activity and is relieved by rest.

The peroneus brevis muscle spasm may be intermittent or continuous. As the symptoms progress, the muscle guarding or tonic spasm generally becomes more intense. As the peroneus brevis contracts, subtalar joint motion is further restricted, and the taut tendon may be palpated or observed laterally (Fig. 44.9). The hindfoot is maintained in a valgus position with depression of the medial longitudinal arch and abduction of the forefoot. The hindfoot valgus occurs because this is the position of comfort of the foot. Kyne and Mankin[164] tested the intra-articular pressure of the subtalar joint during range of motion. They found that pressure within the subtalar joint is increased with inversion. When joint effusion was present, a

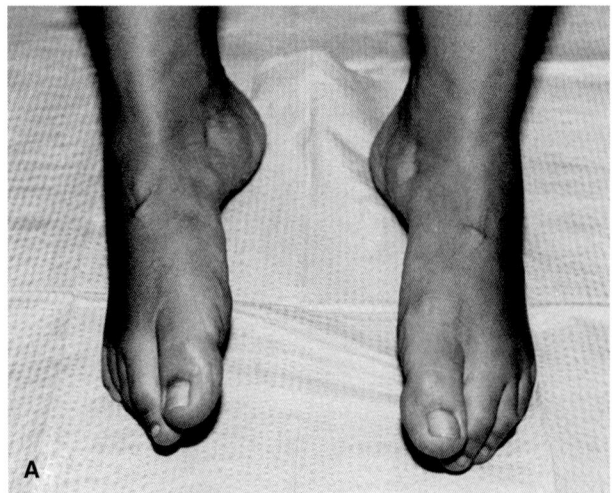
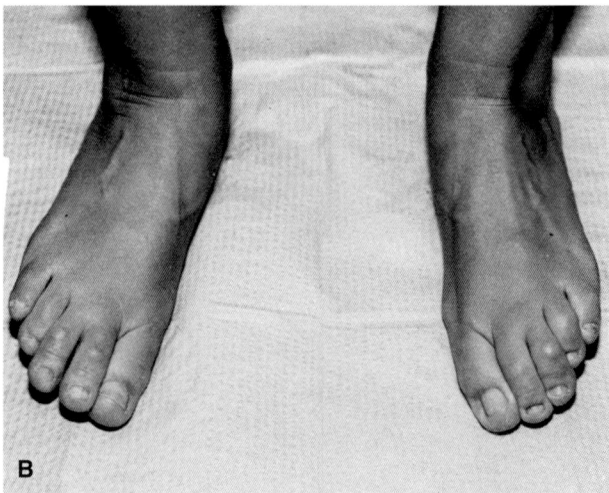

FIGURE 44.8 **A.** Active inversion motion of the subtalar joint is evaluated by having the patient stand and attempt to invert the foot (ie, roll to outside of foot). **B.** Active eversion movement of the foot is evaluated by having the patient stand and attempt to evert the foot (ie, roll to inside of feet as far as possible). The flexibility demonstrated strongly suggests a flexible deformity and no tarsal coalition.

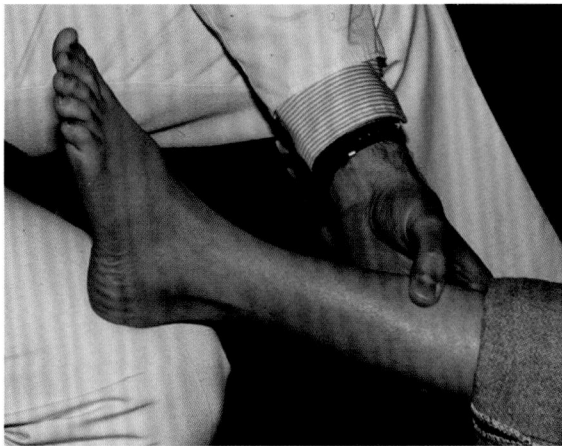

FIGURE 44.9 Tonic spasm of the peroneus brevis observed in the inferolateral leg in a patient with peroneal spastic flatfoot secondary to a tarsal coalition.

reflex mechanism to limit painful inversion ensued. Thus, the peroneus brevis spasm is nothing more than reactive immobilization of a swollen, painful joint to maintain that joint in the position of maximum capsular capacity (ie, eversion). With time, and if left untreated, the valgus deformity will become more rigid. In this manner, tarsal coalition may become associated with rigid peroneal spastic flatfoot. Further, significant forefoot supinatus, forefoot abductus, and changes secondary to associated ankle equinus may become apparent. Clinical identification of these secondary adaptive changes is imperative to the development of an appropriate treatment plan (Fig. 44.10). Cass and Camasta[157] described a "Gray Zone" group of patients who have an incomplete tarsal coalition that has not yet ossified and therefore have varying degrees of motion available in the hindfoot. These patients do not have a rigid pes valgo planus deformity and do not have a flexible pes valgo planus deformity either. These "Gray Zone" patients have signs and symptoms lying somewhere in between the extremes and a semirigid pes valgo planus deformity.[157]

Peroneal spastic flatfoot does not always occur with tarsal coalition, and peroneal spastic flatfoot may result from other conditions.[165] Occasionally, other muscles may be spastic in patients with a tarsal coalition. If other muscles are involved, the foot may not develop a pes valgo planus attitude. Several authors have reported a varus position of the heel in patients

with a tarsal coalition[54,143,154,163,166-170] (Fig. 44.11). Further, peroneal spastic flatfoot may occur secondary to other causes, including arthropathies, inflammation, infection, and osteochondral fractures.[171] These may also be considered acquired causes of tarsal coalition in certain instances. Lowy[165] outlined a suggested protocol for evaluating and treating patients with peroneal spastic flatfoot deformities with or without associated tarsal coalitions and advocated the use of a common peroneal nerve block to reduce the spastic muscular contracture and to allow better evaluation of joint motion.

Similarly, during evaluation of a patient who has a tarsal coalition associated with restricted motion or muscle spasm, a local anesthetic injection in the area of the coalition or to a proximal nerve segment (eg, a common peroneal block) may provide valuable diagnostic information. The anesthetic block may relieve the pain and muscle spasm sufficiently to allow more accurate assessment of joint motion. This technique not only allows direct confirmation of the extent of the coalition (ie, complete vs incomplete) but also may afford information on the quality and quantity of joint motion. This information may be helpful if surgery is considered and resection of the coalition is contemplated.

Finally, if a patient presents with a middle facet talocalcaneal coalition, he or she may demonstrate prominence in the area of the sustentaculum tali. Rocchi and associates[172] coined the term "double medial malleolus" to describe the appearance of the normal medial malleolus and the submalleolar boney protuberance of the medial talocalcaneal coalition. When present, this can be another clinical finding associated with this coalition type.

RADIOGRAPHIC AND ADVANCED IMAGING FINDINGS

Roentgenographic evaluation of a suspected tarsal coalition should be performed in a systematic, cost-effective manner. In most instances, routine radiographs lead to an accurate diagnosis of tarsal coalition.[173] Crim and Kjeldsberg[174] found that standard radiographs had 88% specificity for talocalcaneal coalitions and 97% specificity for calcaneonavicular coalitions. More sophisticated studies such as CT or MRI are usually reserved for when standard radiographs are inconclusive or when one wishes to assess the identified tarsal coalition in more detail.

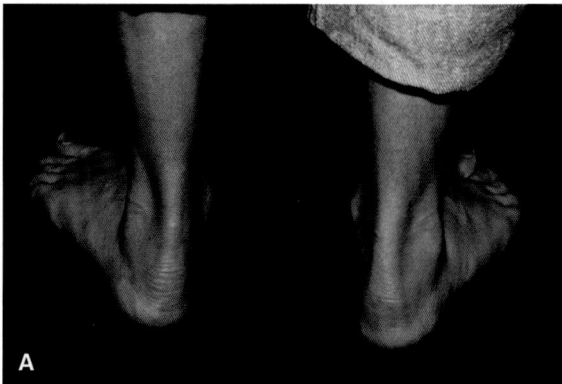
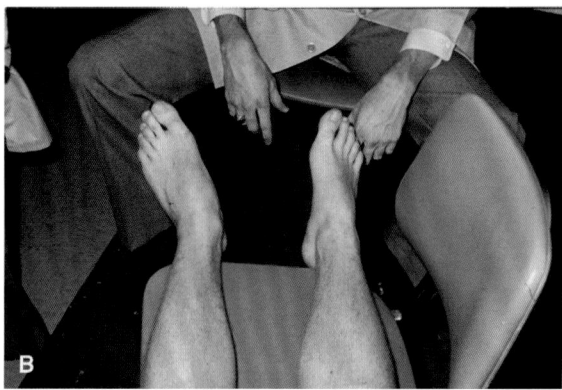

FIGURE 44.10 A, B. Peroneal spastic left flatfoot. Note the increased hindfoot and forefoot abductus associated with the deformity.

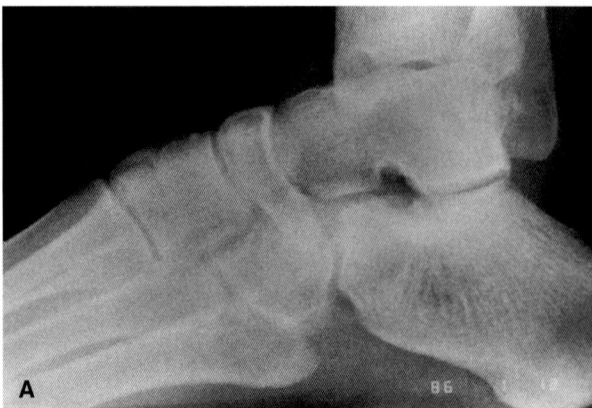
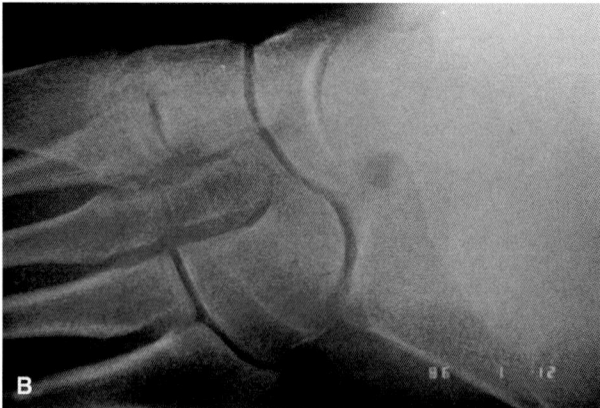

FIGURE 44.11 Cavovarus foot deformity in a patient with a calcaneonavicular bar. **A.** Cavus deformity on the lateral view. **B.** Calcaneonavicular synostosis (ie, complete coalition) noted more readily on the medial oblique view (lateral oblique projection).

RADIOGRAPHIC EVALUATION

When the clinical findings suggest a possible tarsal coalition, initial routine radiographs should be obtained. These may include the anteroposterior, lateral, and medial oblique views. In the majority of cases, these routine films clearly portray a tarsal coalition and confirm the diagnosis. However, a thorough appreciation of the normal radiographic anatomy and the radiographic pathologic features expected with tarsal coalition is necessary if one is to use routine radiographs to maximum benefit. In this sense, different views are more helpful for different coalitions.

As stated earlier, the calcaneonavicular coalition was first demonstrated radiographically on an oblique view.[8] This coalition is still most readily appreciated on the medial oblique view (ie, lateral oblique projection), although it may be identified on an anteroposterior or lateral view. The protrusion of the calcaneus toward the navicular has been termed the "comma sign" on the medial oblique view or the "anteater nose sign," due to its similarity to an anteater's nose, on the lateral view.[175] Nalaboff and Schweitzer[176] described the "anteater nose sign," also known as the "anteater sign," as a hyperplastic anterior calcaneal process with anterior elongation and the "reverse anteater sign" as a hyperplastic navicular with posterior elongation. The connecting bar between the calcaneus and navicular may be osseous, cartilaginous, fibrous, or mixed. Complete osseous union is easiest to diagnose (Fig. 44.11B), but diagnosis of an incomplete union can be more difficult. In these cases, the calcaneus and the navicular are frequently in close proximity to one another, and their contiguous cortical surfaces appear flattened and irregular, like a pseudarthrosis (Fig. 44.12). Moreover, the head of the talus may be underdeveloped or hypoplastic in a foot with a calcaneonavicular coalition.[58] Thus, secondary signs of an incomplete calcaneonavicular coalition include (1) close proximity of the calcaneus and navicular, (2) irregularity of the lateral cortical surface of the navicular, (3) flattening of the navicular as it approaches the calcaneus, and (4) hypoplasia of the head of the talus. Lysack and Fenton[177] described four different calcaneonavicular morphologies according to their appearance on a medial oblique radiographic view. Type 1 in their morphologic grouping is characterized by a wide calcaneonavicular gap and smooth, rounded, and well-defined calcaneal and navicular cortices. Type 2 is defined by a narrow gap, flattening and widening of the calcaneus where it approaches the navicular, and smooth, regular, and well-defined cortical surfaces. Type 3 is visualized as a narrow calcaneonavicular gap, flattening and widening of the calcaneus where it approaches the navicular, and rough, irregular, and poorly defined calcaneal and navicular cortices. Finally, in type 4, the morphology is characterized by a completely continuous osseous structure spanning the calcaneus and navicular. The authors described these morphologic types as a histopathologic continuum with type 1 being normal, types 2 and 3 being intermediate incomplete types, and type 4 representing a complete calcaneonavicular bar. In their series of 460 patients presenting with acute foot pain to an emergency department, Lysack and Fenton[177] found 94.3% were type 1 (normal), 5.6% were types 2 and 3 (incomplete calcaneonavicular coalition), and 0% were type 4 (complete calcaneonavicular coalition).

A talocalcaneal coalition may usually be identified and diagnosed from a lateral radiograph if the normal radiographic anatomy of the subtalar joint is well understood (Fig. 44.13A).

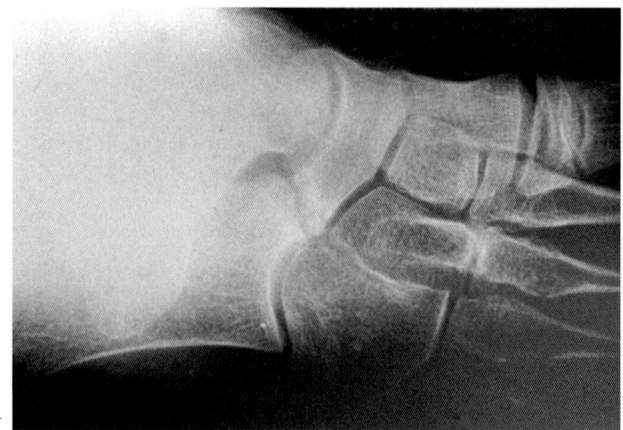

FIGURE 44.12 Incomplete calcaneonavicular coalition noted on the medial oblique view (lateral oblique projection). The adjacent surfaces of the navicular and calcaneus resemble a pseudarthrosis.

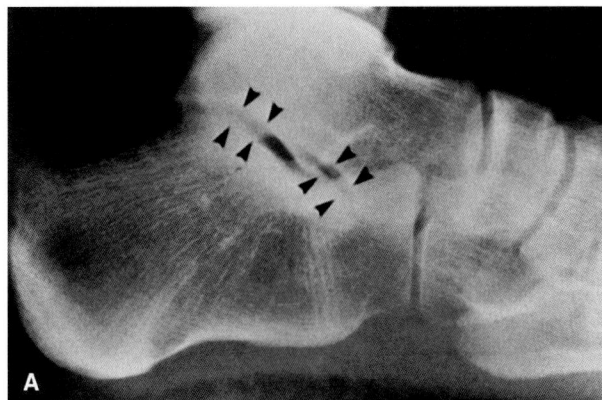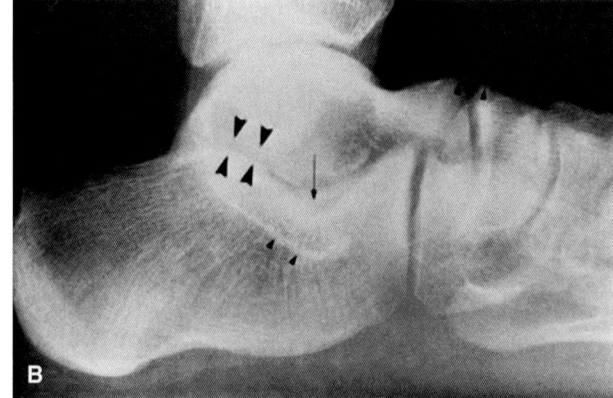

FIGURE 44.13 Lateral radiographic views. **A.** Normal right foot. The *arrowheads* delineate the middle and posterior facets of the subtalar joint. **B.** Right foot with middle facet talocalcaneal coalition. Note the four classic features of such a coalition: (1) halo sign (*small arrowheads*, most inferior), (2) loss of subtalar joint clarity (*large arrowheads*), (3) talonavicular joint beaking, and (4) flattening of lateral talar process (*arrow*).

The middle and posterior facets of the subtalar joint may be visualized on a properly taken lateral view. The anterior facet cannot be visualized because its obliquity causes it to be obliterated by other osseous structures.[31,178] A talocalcaneal coalition involving the middle or posterior facets may be directly visualized on a lateral radiograph as a joint space that is absent or diminished. It may only be suggested if it involves the anterior facet.

When coalition of the subtalar joint occurs, it is predominantly of the middle facet. The common radiographic hallmarks of a middle facet talocalcaneal coalition seen on a lateral radiograph are (1) a halo sign or "C" sign representing a circular sclerotic enhancement of the talar dome and inferior margin of the sustentaculum tali, (2) narrowing of the middle and/or posterior facets of the subtalar joint with loss of subtalar joint clarity, (3) talonavicular joint beaking, and (4) flattening of the lateral talar process (Fig. 44.13B).[40,53,179] These findings may also be seen in varying degrees with coalitions that involve the anterior and posterior subtalar joint facets or with other tarsal coalitions. Additionally, a short talar neck or the "drunken waiter" sign (ie, an incomplete talocalcaneal coalition with an enlarged, dysmorphic sustentaculum tali with a convex joint space such as the hand of drunken waiter holding a tray awkwardly) have been described as radiographic findings.[180] The lateral radiograph must be taken properly to allow for the diagnosis of a talocalcaneal coalition. Shaffer and Harrison[181] described a "pseudocoalition" seen on a lateral radiograph that is caused by positional artifact created by either slight abduction or inversion of the foot when the radiograph is taken. The "pseudo" or false appearance of the coalition is created by overlap of normal osseous structures in such a foot position.

Harris and Beath views (ie, axial or ski-jump views) may be taken to obtain additional information concerning the status of the middle and posterior facets of the subtalar joint. If a complete osseous coalition is present, the involved facets will not be visualized. If an incomplete coalition is present, the facets involved will usually demonstrate osseous irregularity, joint space narrowing, and facet obliquity. In the normal foot, the posterior and middle facets are parallel to the ground and to one another (Fig. 44.14A). If a facet

is angulated more than 25 degrees from the ground or its neighboring facet, a talocalcaneal coalition may be strongly suspected[151] (Fig. 44.14B).

Isherwood views may also provide information on a talocalcaneal coalition. Unfortunately, the views require exact positioning of the patient and are difficult to obtain properly.[182-184] These views are no longer routinely used to evaluate tarsal coalitions.

Further, neutral position radiographs, radiographs taken during the performance of the Hubscher maneuver, and lateral stress dorsiflexion ankle radiographs may provide evidence of the flexibility of the deformity. In complete talocalcaneal coalitions, the deformity frequently results in a rigid pes valgo planus deformity, whether or not it is associated with peroneal muscle spasm.

In the valgus foot, neutral position radiographs and radiographs taken during the Hubscher maneuver may be used to evaluate the supinatory flexibility of the subtalar joint. In this manner, the subtalar joint may be placed in its neutral position and radiographs may be taken. When compared with the weight-bearing radiographs with the subtalar joint everted, an assessment of flexibility may be made. No change in the talocalcaneal relationship will be noted on the neutral position radiographs if the deformity is rigid, whereas radiographic signs of subtalar joint supination (eg, decreased talocalcaneal or Kite's angle, decreased talar declination angle, improved cyma line) will be noted if the deformity is flexible. Similarly, the Hubscher maneuver may be used to assess the flexibility of the pes valgo planus foot deformity. While the examiner holds the hallux in a dorsiflexed position, a lateral radiograph may be taken in an attempt to demonstrate an increase in the medial longitudinal arch and a change in the lateral talocalcaneal relationship representing hindfoot supination (ie, a decrease in the lateral talocalcaneal angle) (Fig. 44.15). If this does not occur, the deformity is rigid. However, in most instances, radiographs are not required to determine the reducibility or irreducibility of the deformity.

Conversely, a lateral stress dorsiflexion view of the ankle may be taken. This should place a dorsiflexory force on the subtalar and midtarsal joints. In a flexible pes valgo planus deformity, this causes pronation of the subtalar joint, and

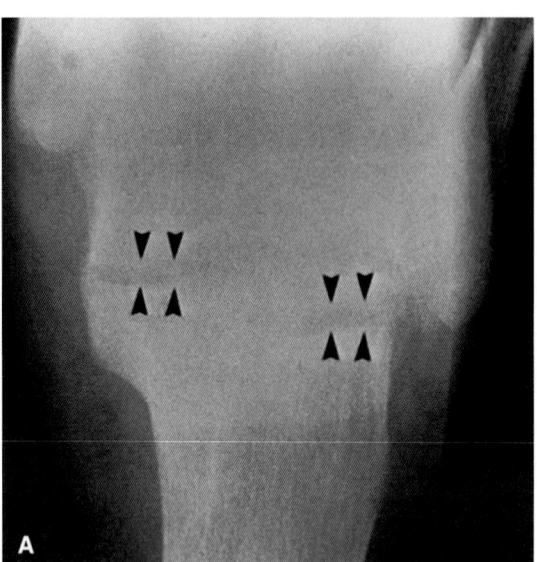
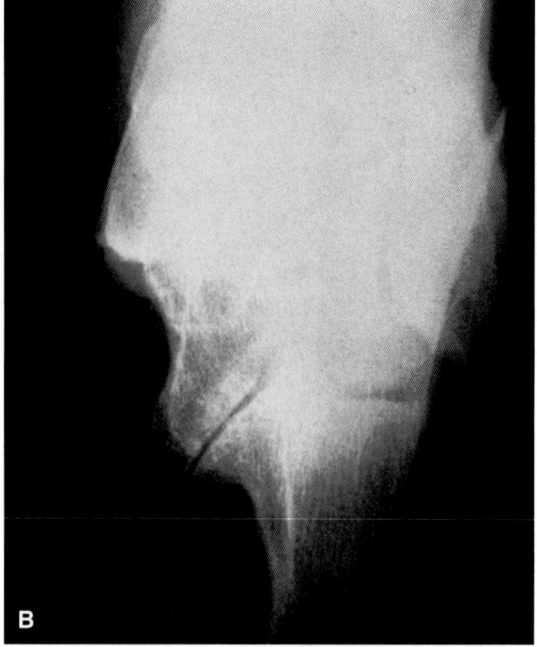

FIGURE 44.14 **A.** Harris and Beath normal view of the right foot. The middle and posterior facets (*arrowheads*) are parallel to the ground and to one another. The middle facet is slightly superior to the posterior facet in the normal foot. **B.** Abnormal Harris and Beath view in a patient with incomplete middle facet talocalcaneal coalition of the right foot. Note the angulation of the middle facet with the weight-bearing surface and the posterior facet.

the lateral radiograph should demonstrate a decrease in the medial longitudinal arch and a change in the talocalcaneal relationship representing hindfoot pronation (ie, an increase in the lateral talocalcaneal angle) (Fig. 44.16). Further, any osseous impingement of the talus and tibia may be documented with this view. Any talotibial exostoses should be differentiated from the talonavicular beaking associated with a tarsal coalition.

Talonavicular and other more rare coalitions are usually readily seen on standard radiographs. In most cases, the anteroposterior and lateral views clearly demonstrate these coalitions (Fig. 44.17). Both feet may need to be evaluated for other coalitions when any tarsal coalition is found. This information may

suggest a complex malformation and is helpful in the construction of a treatment plan.

Routine radiographs may also be used to evaluate the foot for secondary adaptive, compensatory, or arthritic changes related to the tarsal coalition. These secondary changes include joint beaking, osteoarthritis with diminished joint space, and secondary adaptive changes. Debate continues on whether *joint beaking*, which may also be referred to as lipping, spurring, molding, or cresting, is an arthritic change. Outland and Murphy[185] believed that talar beaking arose from the force of the navicular, by crushing the soft talar head and causing it to remodel. Conway and Cowell[54] suggested that the talar beak is secondary to repeated minute elevations of the periosteum of

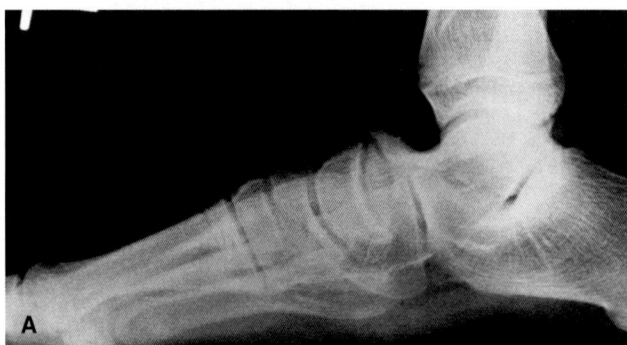
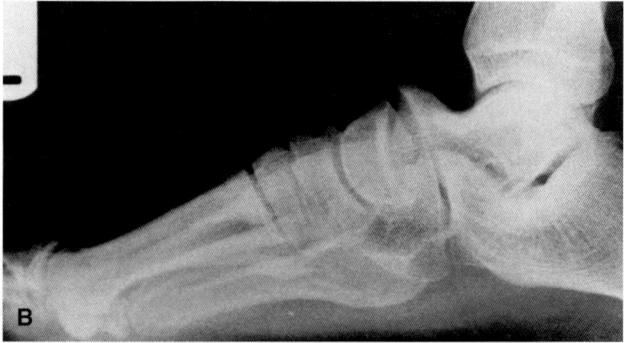

FIGURE 44.15 **A.** Lateral weight-bearing view of the left foot in a patient with pes valgo planus deformity. **B.** Lateral view of the same foot while the Hubscher maneuver is performed. While the Hubscher maneuver is performed, no change occurs in the talocalcaneal relationship. The lateral talocalcaneal angle has remained the same. This is a rigid pes valgo planus deformity secondary to a middle facet talocalcaneal syndesmosis. If the deformity were flexible, a decrease in the lateral talocalcaneal angle would be noted.

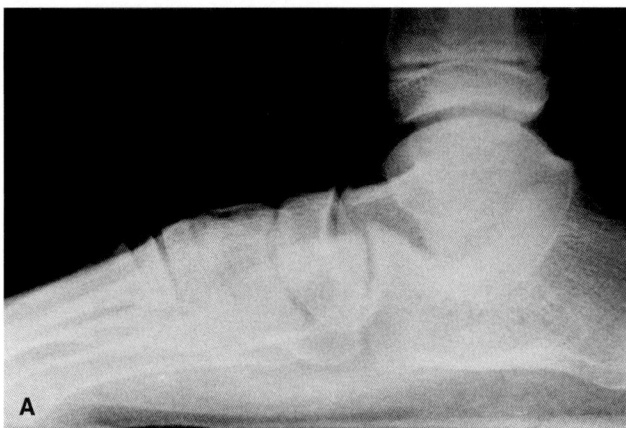
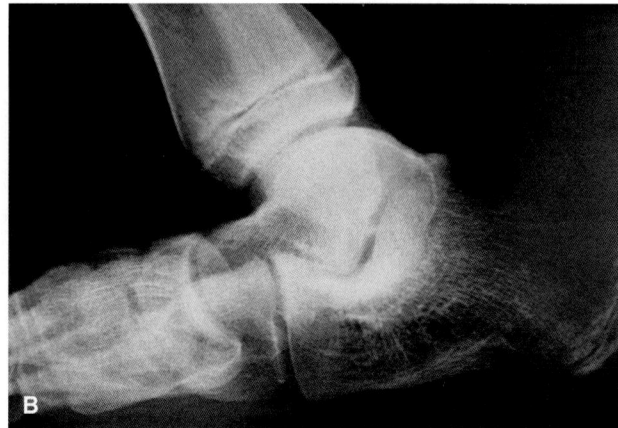

FIGURE 44.16 A. Lateral weight-bearing view of the left ankle and hindfoot demonstrating a pes valgo planus deformity. **B.** Lateral stress dorsiflexion view of the same ankle and hindfoot. No change in the talocalcaneal relationship is noted. If the deformity were flexible, an increase in the lateral talocalcaneal angle would be noted. Thus, this is a rigid deformity that was subsequently diagnosed to be secondary to a middle facet talocalcaneal coalition.

the talus resulting from stress on the talonavicular ligament. Other investigators have described it as an osteoarthritic spur secondary to degeneration of the talonavicular joint.[58,186,187] However, one typically sees no narrowing of the talonavicular joint. Usually, no subchondral sclerosis or cystic bone changes are noted within the talus or the navicular. Thus, the beaking appears to develop as a remodeling process secondary to altered motion of the talonavicular joint. In support of this assumption, similar joint beaking is seen with pathologic talonavicular joint motion in patients with diffuse idiopathic skeletal hyperostosis, acromegaly, rheumatoid arthritis, hypermobile flatfoot, and overzealous cast correction of clubfoot, as well as in long-term follow-up after a Grice extra-articular arthrodesis of the subtalar joint.[54,188]

Joints directly involved in an incomplete coalition typically demonstrate osteoarthritic changes. Close apposition, eburnation, or subchondral sclerosis of adjacent articular surfaces implies fibrous or cartilaginous union. The *halo sign* or *C-sign* are examples of bony sclerosis that occurs around the middle facet with a middle facet subtalar coalition. Close apposition or narrowing of the posterior talocalcaneal joint space is another common example of osteoarthritic change associated with a middle facet subtalar joint coalition.

Secondary adaptive changes also may occur with a tarsal coalition. Valgus angulation of the calcaneus, as seen with many tarsal coalitions, causes abnormal pressure on the lateral talar process. With prolonged pressure, broadening or rounding of the lateral talar process is seen as it adapts to the

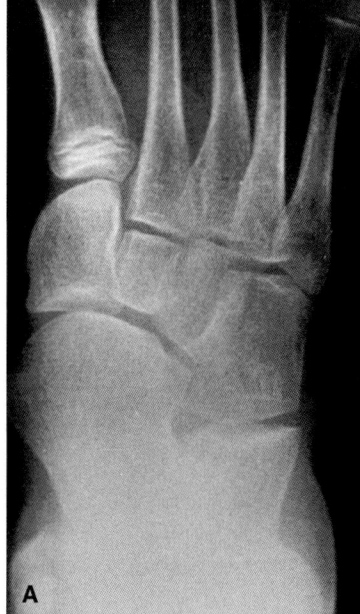
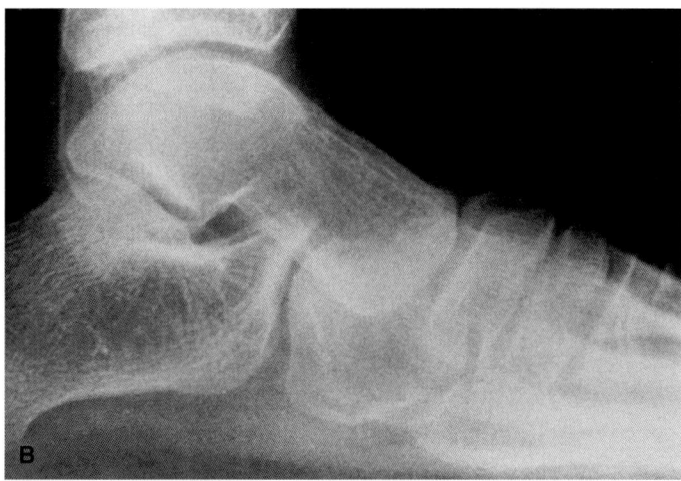

FIGURE 44.17 Anteroposterior **(A)** and lateral **(B)** views of talonavicular coalition. Note the adaptive rounding and increased joint space of the naviculocuneiform joints.

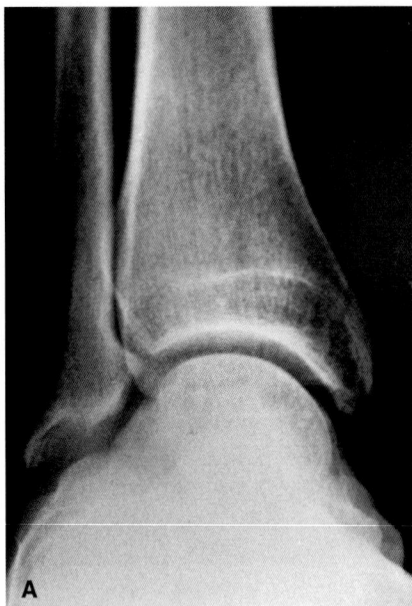
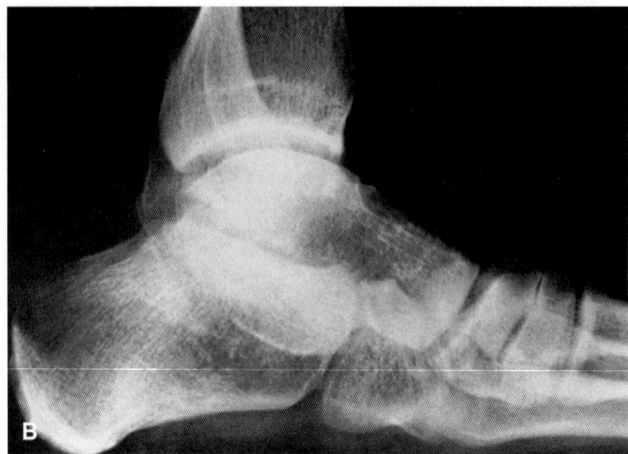

FIGURE 44.18 Anteroposterior (**A**) and lateral (**B**) views of the ankle demonstrating the ball-and-socket ankle joint. The talus appears dome-shaped in the anteroposterior view and in the lateral view. The patient has talocalcaneal and a talonavicular synostosis.

abnormal subtalar joint mechanics. Furthermore, in the presence of a tarsal coalition, particularly of the talocalcaneal joint, the functions of supination and pronation may be assumed by other joints. Common examples include a ball-and-socket ankle joint in a talocalcaneal coalition (Fig. 44.18)[120,189-194] and increased joint motion at the naviculocuneiform joint in a talonavicular coalition. The extent of these secondary arthritic or adaptive changes frequently determines the prognosis and treatment plan.

CROSS-SECTIONAL IMAGING

Standard tomography, CT, and MRI offer the ability to obtain multiplanar cross-sectional images of the foot with minimal bony overlap. These modalities are optimally indicated for cases in which radiographs are inconclusive, or for evaluation of the size, type of union and secondary arthritic changes associated with a tarsal coalition. Information gathered from these modalities can aid in surgical decision-making.

Conventional lateral plane tomography is rarely used today but does afford improved visualization of the subtalar joint by minimizing the problem of osseous superimposition that occurs with conventional radiography.[29,195] In 1969, Conway and Cowell[54] first described the use of tomography to evaluate the anterior facet of the subtalar joint. However, Beckly and associates[53] more recently indicated that the plantar medial obliquity of the anterior facet makes the joint space cross the sagittal tomographic plane at a different angle than the optimal 90 degrees. These investigators stated that this obliquity would be further accentuated by the valgus foot and could lead to the false appearance of an anterior facet subtalar joint coalition with standard lateral plane tomography. These authors suggested lateral oblique tomography to demonstrate the anterior facet. In view of this positioning difficulty and with the advent of CT, standard tomography is rarely used to evaluate tarsal coalitions today.

Smith and Staple[196,197] were the first to describe the use of CT for the evaluation of a tarsal coalition. Today, CT scans, along with MRI studies are the consensus-preferred imaging modalities for the cross-sectional evaluation of a tarsal coalition, and many descriptions of their use have been published.[198-217] Advantages of CT scanning include noninvasiveness, precise evaluation of adjacent osseous structures and soft tissues with superior cortical definition, potential for demonstration of associated abnormalities, and the ability to simultaneously image the opposite foot.[201] In addition, the anterior facet of the subtalar joint is imaged in a predictable fashion,[210] and some investigators have found that CT scans occasionally identified talocalcaneal coalitions not seen with Harris and Beath views.[204] Coronal or frontal plane CT scans are used for the evaluation of a suspected talocalcaneal coalition with contiguous sections 2- to 4-mm thick obtained from the posterior aspect of the subtalar joint to just distal to the midtarsal joint (Fig. 44.19A and B). Three-dimensional (3D) CT scans are also becoming more widely available and can offer superior morphology of the joints and any coalition present (Fig. 44.19C-E). Some authors have advocated that a CT scan of the hindfoot be ordered in 1-mm sections with no gap between the slices to provide even greater detail.[157] This can be helpful if a coalition is incomplete and it is difficult to ascertain whether or not a coalition is present. Frontal plane or 3D CT scans may also be used to image other coalitions (Fig. 44.20). However, transverse plane or 3D CT scans are generally preferred for imaging other tarsal coalitions, including calcaneonavicular and talonavicular coalitions. Stoskopf et al.[214] reported that the normal transverse plane CT scan of the foot shows a triangle of soft tissue density anterior to the calcaneus. These investigators found this to be uniformly absent in calcaneonavicular coalitions.

Because of its superior ability to image cartilage and soft tissue, MRI has also proven to be a useful, and increasingly preferred, cross-sectional imaging modality for coalitions. In 1989, Bonk and Tozzi[63] demonstrated a talonavicular synostosis

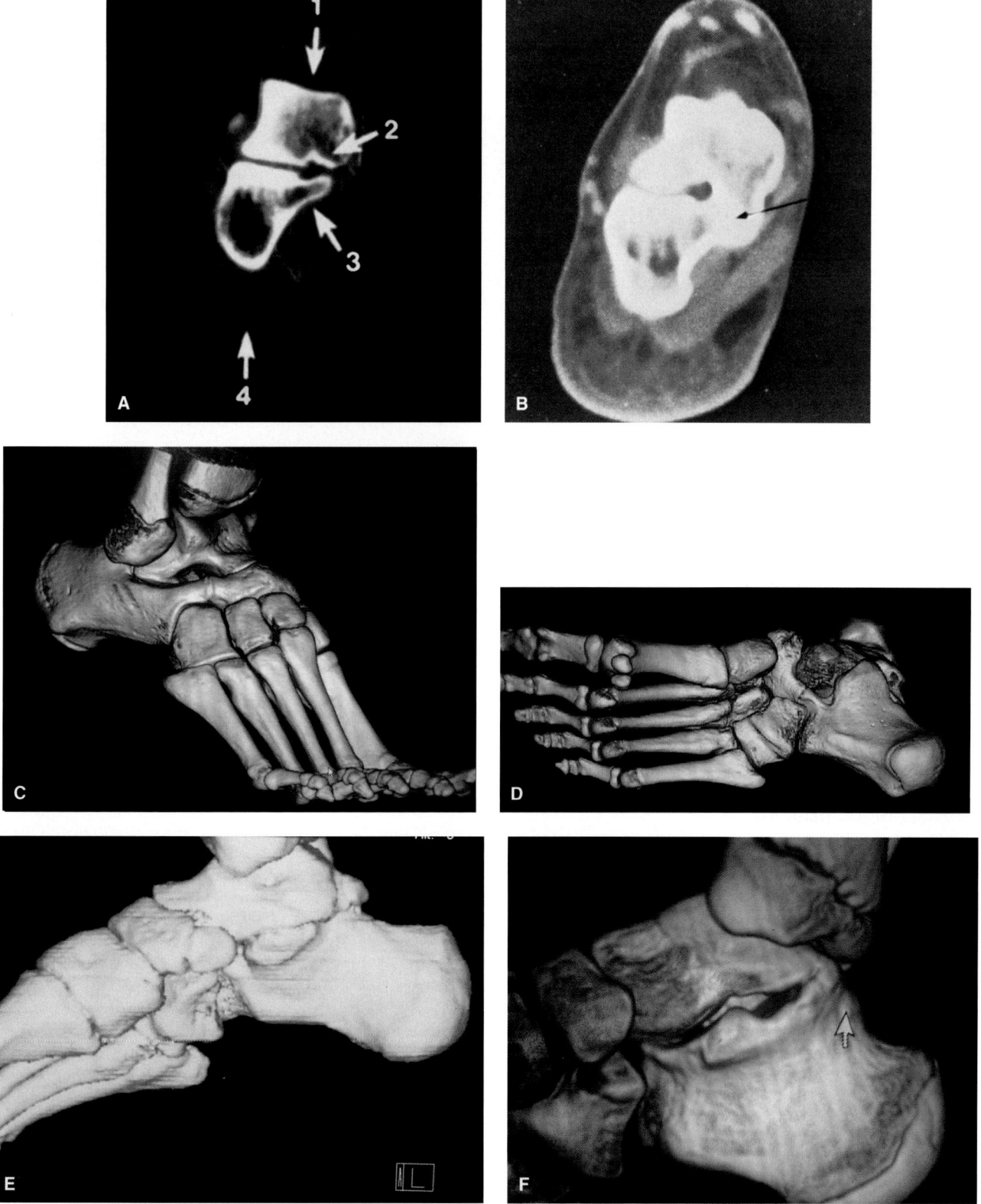

FIGURE 44.19 A. Coronal or frontal plane computed tomography image through the subtalar joint area in a normal foot: *1*, dorsal talus; *2*, sinus tarsi; *3*, inferior aspect of the sustentaculum tali; *4*, plantar calcaneus. **B.** Coronal or frontal plane computed tomography image of a middle facet talocalcaneal synostosis (*arrow*). The sinus tarsi and posterior facet are clearly visible. **C, D.** Three-dimensional (3D) CT scan of complete calcaneonavicular coalition. **E.** Three-dimensional (3D) CT scan of incomplete middle facet talocalcaneal coalition. Note accessory navicular bone is also present. **F:** Three-dimensional (3D) CT scan of incomplete posterior facet talocalcaneal coalition (*arrow*).

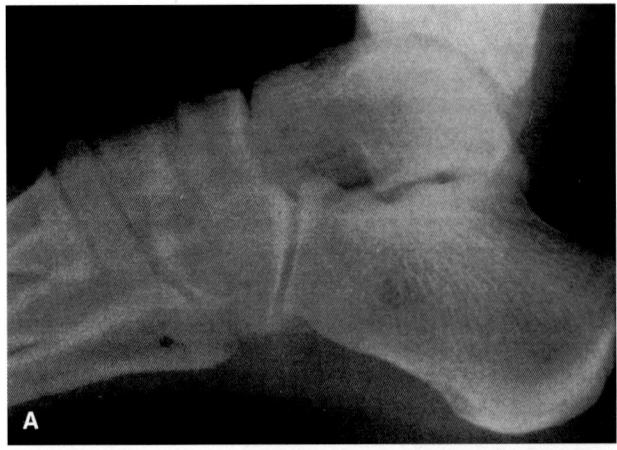

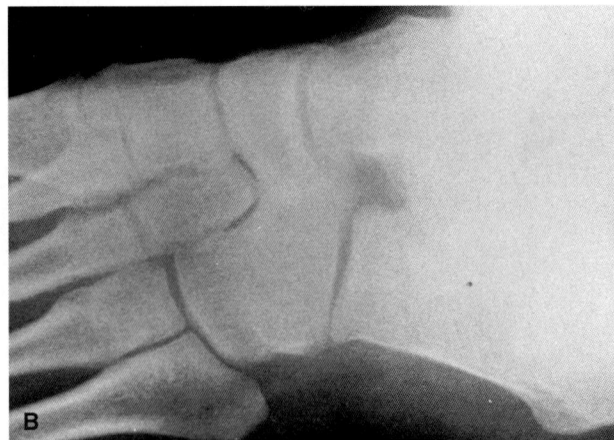

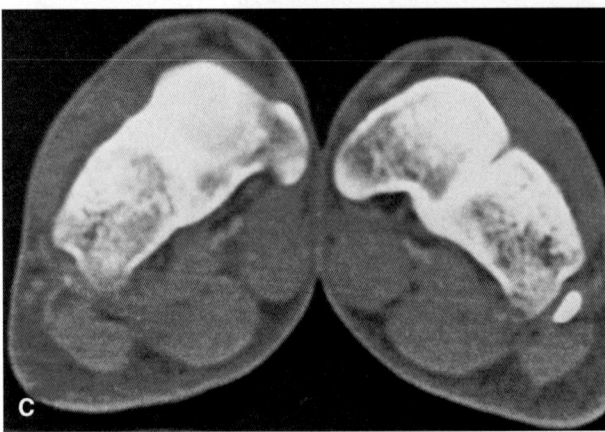

FIGURE 44.20 A, B. Lateral and oblique radiographs of the left foot in a patient with bilateral cubonavicular synostosis. **C.** Coronal or frontal plane computed tomography image through the midfoot area of both feet demonstrating bilateral cubonavicular coalitions.

with MRI. CT scanning still seems to be the preferred modality for complete coalitions. MRI, meanwhile, appears to be a useful alternative for evaluating an incomplete coalition (ie, synchondrosis or syndesmosis), especially when the CT scan is equivocal[217-219] (Figs. 44.21 and 44.22). MRI is clearly becoming more popular. Pachuda and associates[220] demonstrated a fibrous talocalcaneal coalition in a 10-year-old patient with an apparently normal Harris and Beath view and suggested that MRI may be the study of choice for all coalitions. Similarly, Bresnahan and Fung[221] demonstrated an incomplete coalition in a 9-year-old patient on MRI scans and thought that MRI helped to identify nonosseous coalitions earlier. MRI has also been used to identify fibrous coalitions in patients with heel pain.[222] Masciocchi and associates[223] believed that MRI was preferred because it allowed the evaluation of changes in the ankle and subtalar joint cartilage associated with a tarsal coalition.

In 2008, Nabaloff and Schweitzer[176] described the primary and secondary signs typically seen on an MRI of a tarsal coalition (Table 44.5). Secondary MRI changes seen with an incomplete calcaneonavicular coalition were similar to those seen with standard radiographs and included a blunted or flattened anterior calcaneal process, "anteater sign," "reverse anteater sign," and talar beaking proximal to the talonavicular joint. Secondary MRI signs of an incomplete talocalcaneal coalition include the "drunken waiter sign," which Nabaloff and Schweitzer[176] described as a dysplastic sustentaculum tali occurring with an incomplete talocalcaneal coalition. The authors felt that the abnormal morphology of the sustentaculum tali associated with

the talocalcaneal coalition appeared like a waiter having trouble carrying his tray (either an upturned or downturned hand and plate) while intoxicated, where the body of the calcaneus is considered the waiter and the sustentaculum tali is the tray. Other secondary MRI signs included talar beaking, bone marrow edema and cystic changes around the suspected coalition, and fractures.[176]

ULTRASOUND EVALUATION

Although traditionally used for evaluation of soft tissue structures in the foot and ankle, ultrasound has been described for the evaluation of tarsal coalitions in young children or for incomplete coalitions. Ultrasonography allows 3D movement of the tarsal joint complex during the imaging process, and this can be particularly helpful in evaluating for the presence or absence of normal motion between the tarsal bones.[137,224]

INVASIVE STUDIES AND EVALUATION

Radionuclide scanning and arthrography have also been used in the diagnosis of tarsal coalitions. A bone scan obtained with technetium-99m-methylene diphosphonate (^{99m}Tc) may be sensitive to the presence of a tarsal coalition. Magnification or pinhole images with their higher resolution are best.[225] Positive findings include augmented radionuclide accumulation in the region of the subtalar joint as well as in the talonavicular joint

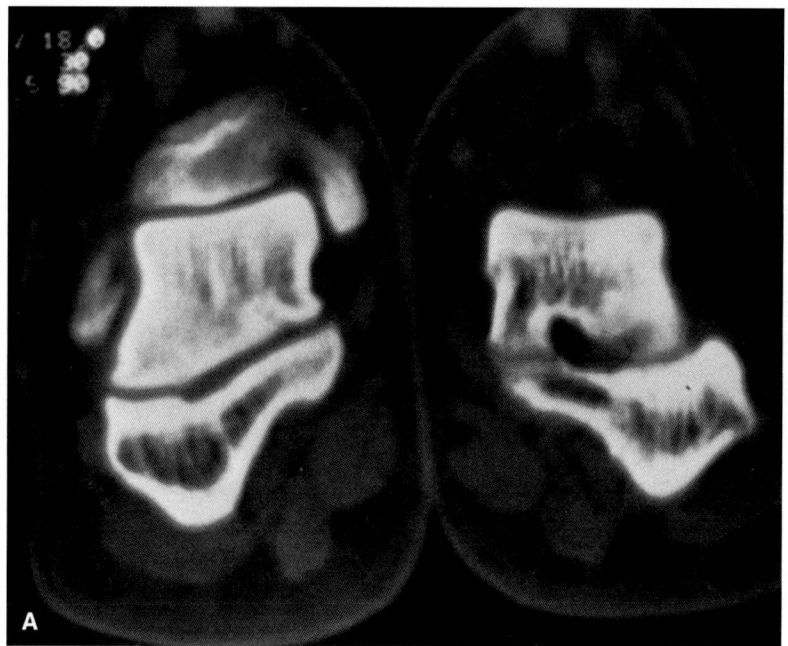

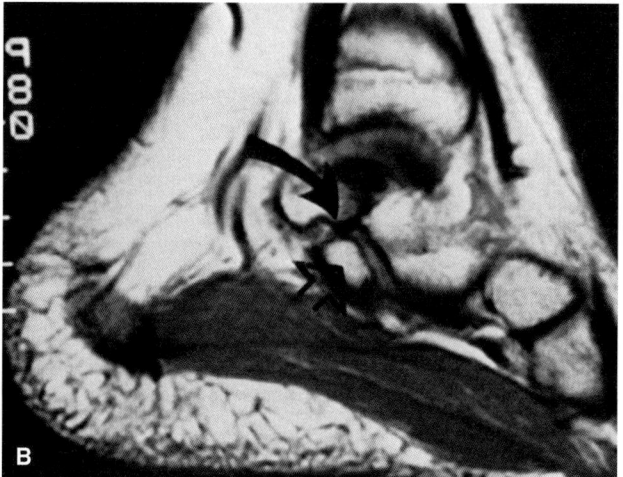

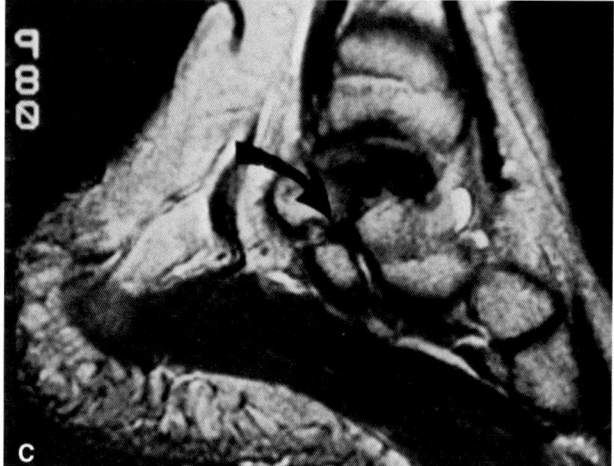

FIGURE 44.21 **A.** Frontal plane computed tomography image through both feet of a patient with peroneal spastic flatfoot and suspected incomplete coalition. Note the hazy definition of subchondral bone at the middle facet of the subtalar joint. **B.** Sagittal plane T1-weighted magnetic resonance imaging (MRI) scan. The *open arrow* points to the sustentaculum tali. **C.** Sagittal plane T2-weighted MRI scan. Both MRI scans are oriented along the medial border of the foot through the middle facet of the subtalar joint. Note the consistent low signal intensity at the posterior aspect of the middle facet on both images (*curved arrows*). This finding is consistent with fibrous tissue and suggests a middle facet talocalcaneal syndesmosis. This diagnosis was confirmed at surgery.

(Fig. 44.23). The subtalar joint collection probably represents bone activity generated by the abnormal biomechanical stress placed on the joint, whereas the talonavicular accumulation is probably secondary to the same mechanism that produces dorsal talar and navicular excrescences. Because many conditions may cause similar activity, a ⁹⁹ᵐTc bone scan is nonspecific for tarsal coalition and should be used only as a screening study.[201,226,227] El Rassi et al.[228] described the use of technetium-99m bone scintigraphy and single photon emission computed tomography (SPECT) for imaging of arthrofibrosis of the talocalcaneal joint when traditional radiographs and CT or MRI are inconclusive.

Arthrography of the talocalcaneonavicular joint may be used to detect a talocalcaneal coalition when routine radiographs are inconclusive.[229] When contrast medium is injected dorsally into the talonavicular joint, the dye usually spreads throughout the thin joint space of the entire talocalcaneonavicular articulation, including the anterior and middle facets of the subtalar joint but not the posterior facet (Fig. 44.24). When dye can be seen filling the area above the sustentaculum tali, the diagnosis of coalition of the middle facet is excluded. When a middle facet talocalcaneal coalition is present, a filling defect is noted between the sustentaculum tali and the talus. Normally, no communication exists between the talocalcaneonavicular

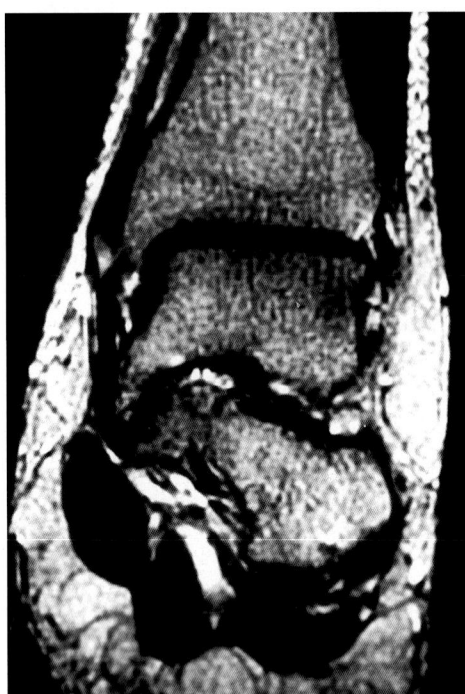

FIGURE 44.22 Frontal (coronal) plane magnetic resonance imaging of an incomplete middle facet talocalcaneal coalition. Note the marked obliquity of the middle facet and the intermediate to low signal intensity of the coalition, which is consistent with fibrocartilage.

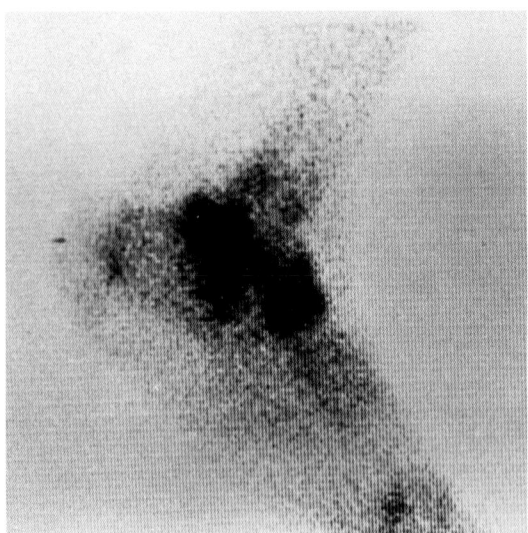

FIGURE 44.23 Technetium-99m bone scan (third phase) of a foot with a middle facet talocalcaneal coalition. Note activity in area of the subtalar and talonavicular joints secondary to abnormal biomechanical stress.

joint and the calcaneocuboid, posterior subtalar, and naviculocuneiform joint cavities.[230,231] When dye is injected into the posterior subtalar joint, a thin line of contrast material is normally noticed between the talus and the calcaneus (Fig. 44.25). In ~10% of the cases, communication and exchange of contrast occur between the subtalar and ankle joints. If a posterior facet coalition is present, a filling defect will be noted.[29] The main disadvantage of arthrography is that the technique is invasive and is often difficult to interpret. Conversely, the use of cross-sectional imaging techniques is more accurate and noninvasive. MRI arthrography can be used if the clinician wishes to combine the advantages of both MRI and arthrography to evaluate small joints for the presence of a potential coalition or other related disorder.

TREATMENT

Not all tarsal coalitions cause symptoms. Moreover, not all coalitions that are symptomatic necessarily remain so. Therefore, in most cases, conservative treatment should be attempted initially. If this proves unsuccessful, then surgical intervention may be considered.

CONSERVATIVE TREATMENT

Conservative therapy is directed toward immobilization, off-loading, and anti-inflammatory medications. The goal of immobilization and off-loading is the restriction of subtalar and midtarsal joint motion, thereby reducing pain and muscle spasm. This approach may be combined with physical therapy and anti-inflammatory medication as needed.

Subtalar and midtarsal joint motion may be limited with shoe modifications, padding, orthotic devices, bracing, immobilization boots, or casting. Shoe modifications may include a Thomas heel, a medial heel wedge, or a longer medial heel

TABLE 44.5 MRI Signs of Tarsal Coalition					
	Osseous	**Cartilaginous**	**Fibrous**	**Calcaneonavicular**	**Talocalcaneal**
Primary MR criteria	Continuity of marrow space between the suspect bones	Loss of joint space, with signal intensity of cartilage or joint fluid between the suspect bones	Areas of intermediate or low signal intensity bridging the adjacent bones	Loss of marrow fat between calcaneus and navicular	Loss of marrow fat between talus and calcaneus Irregularity of the talocalcaneal articulation
Secondary MR criteria				Blunted anterior calcaneal process, "Anteater" sign, "reverse anteater" sign, talar "beak," marrow edema, fracture	"Drunken waiter" sign, talar "beak," marrow edema, fracture

With permission from Nalaboff KM, Schweitzer ME. MRI of tarsal coalition: frequency, distribution, and innovative signs. *Bull NYU Hosp Jt Dis*. 2008;66:14-21.

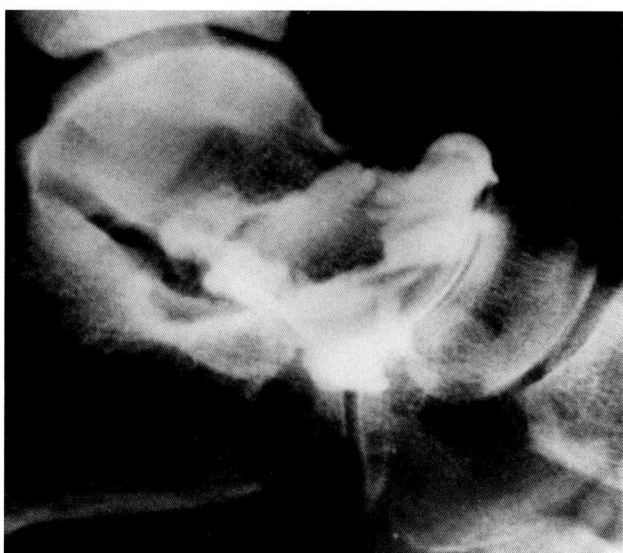

FIGURE 44.24 Normal arthrogram of the talocalcaneonavicular joint space.

counter. Padding in the shoe may include a heel wedge, a medial longitudinal support, or a Plastazote insole. Orthoses should be specifically constructed to limit subtalar joint motion. A neutral position device with a long rearfoot post, or in some cases an orthotic device posted in valgus, may prove to be beneficial. Many authors have suggested even more restrictive orthoses, such as UCBL (University of California Biomechanical Laboratories) type orthoses or ankle foot orthoses (eg, Arizona anklefoot orthotic or Richie brace).[232,233] If these fail or if the patient has significant symptoms, a soft cast, strapping, immobilization boot (eg, CAM-walker boot), or below-knee walking cast may be considered.[234] If desired, these devices may be applied after a local corticosteroid injection to the area of the coalition. The below-knee cast is applied with the ankle and subtalar joints in their neutral positions and is kept intact for 3-6 weeks. In more severe cases, or if initial casting fails, a non–weight-bearing cast may be attempted. In this sense, more than one trial of cast

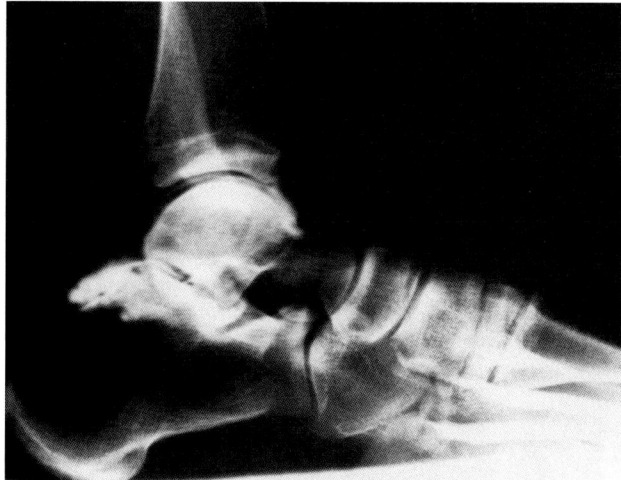

FIGURE 44.25 Normal arthrogram of the posterior subtalar joint space. Communication is noted between the ankle and the subtalar joints.

therapy may be necessary to attempt to render the patient free of symptoms if this approach is going to be effective.[235,236] Casting has been reported to produce symptomatic improvement in ~25%-33% of patients.[55,187] However, although symptoms may resolve with a course of casting, the symptoms may recur at any time in the future and may necessitate repeated casting or surgical intervention.

In addition, symptomatic relief of a coalition may be afforded by physical therapy or anti-inflammatory medication. Therapeutic modalities such as heat, warm soaks, paraffin baths, or whirlpool baths may be beneficial. Kendrick[237] suggested manipulation under anesthesia as a possible treatment, but this concept has not been supported.[173] Local injections of a corticosteroid or local anesthetic may provide relief. Further, injection of a local anesthetic agent into the area of an incomplete coalition may allow increased motion. This may be helpful when one is evaluating a patient for a coalition and determining a possible surgical treatment plan. Oral anti-inflammatory medication may also provide symptomatic relief.

Unfortunately, conservative treatment often fails to alleviate the symptom complex associated with a tarsal coalition. Morgan and Crawford[155] reported a series of 12 adolescent athletes with tarsal coalitions treated conservatively with restricted weight bearing, 3-week immobilization, physical therapy, and occasionally shoe inserts and injection of the subtalar joint. None of their patients had lasting relief, and 8 of the 12 elected to proceed with surgical intervention. Shirley and others[238] studied the results of nonoperative treatment for symptomatic tarsal coalitions. Pain relief was achieved with conservative measures in 53% of the 81 patients they followed, with the greatest success achieved with supportive measures (ie, shoe inserts and physical therapy) as opposed to immobilization. These authors did conclude that although conservative treatment has the potential to achieve pain relief, some patients (and their families) may elect to forgo conservative treatment measures knowing that surgery may eventually be required. In yet another study, Birisik et al.[239] performed a retrospective study of the natural course of pain in patients with symptomatic tarsal coalitions. These researchers found that in the 30 patients they followed, 16 patients (53%) failed conservative modalities and underwent surgery. They also found that patients who started with lesser pain (visual analog scale [VAS] score: <6) were more likely to respond to nonoperative measures. These authors concluded that in patients who presented with an initial VAS score of 6 or greater early surgery might be preferred since conservative treatment was more likely to fail in alleviating their pain. Conclusively then, when conservative treatment fails or is not likely to be successful, surgery is often the next option.

SURGICAL TREATMENT

Direct surgical treatment of a tarsal coalition is essentially confined to either resection of the coalition or fusion of the involved joint complex. In a large cohort study published in 2015, Khoshbin and colleagues[240] reviewed 304 patients who underwent tarsal coalition resection at an average age of 24.2 years. At a mean follow-up of 9 years, 85% of the patients had not required any additional operative intervention. However, there are many variables when considering resection of a tarsal coalition, and many adjunctive procedures that are often

performed, including correction of associated heel valgus, collapsed arch, ankle equinus, or out-toeing deformity. Significant controversy remains concerning the indications for the procedures and the results to be expected with these varied surgical approaches. For this reason, Downey[48,49,143-145] has attempted to create a classification system, which may be used as a framework for the construction of an appropriate surgical treatment plan. The classification system is not meant to be all inclusive but considers several important parameters used in the development of any treatment regimen: patient age, articular involvement, and the extent of secondary adaptive or arthritic changes. Certainly, other factors not included in the original description of the classification system need to be considered. Recently, Downey[145] described the inclusion of coalition size and degree of heel valgus as additional factors to consider, particularly with talocalcaneal coalitions.

The age of a patient is invariably a factor when the surgical treatment of a tarsal coalition is contemplated. Ideally, in all patients, one would like to be able to resect the tarsal coalition and to restore normal or near-normal function to the involved tarsal joints, although from a practical standpoint this often is not possible. Thus, the surgeon must balance the likelihood of success of resection of the coalition against the possible need for additional surgery (ie, arthrodesing procedures), should the resection procedure fail. In the juvenile patient who has not yet achieved osseous maturity (ie, physeal growth plates are still open), resection would initially seem to be preferred for most tarsal coalitions. The remodeling potential of the growing juvenile patient should not be underestimated. For example, the immature patient is much more likely than an adult to achieve an acceptable subjective and objective return of function after a severe, joint depression calcaneal fracture. Similarly, in the juvenile patient with a tarsal coalition, it is hoped that the increased joint motion achieved with resection of the coalition, combined with continued osseous growth and remodeling, will result in a more normal, less painful, joint complex in the area of the coalition. If, after resection, symptoms and limited function remain or recur in this immature patient, major arthrodesis procedures can be performed at a later date (ie, after osseous maturity has been achieved). In mature or adult patients, resection of a tarsal coalition may also be considered but is more prone to failure. The reality of limited remodeling potential in the adult patient diminishes the probability of recovery to a functional, symptom-free state. Therefore, mature patients who undergo coalition resection are at greater risk of recurrent or increased joint limitation and symptoms in the area of the excised tarsal coalition. Arthrodesis may eventually be necessary to treat the condition and diminish the symptom complex. With this understood, resection of the coalition may be attempted in the adult patient, but arthrodesis procedures may also be considered as primary treatment options in some cases.

The articular involvement, or the joint affected by the tarsal coalition, reasonably may be considered the most important factor when one is assessing the surgical management of a tarsal coalition. Tarsal coalitions may be divided into those that are extra-articular (ie, occurring outside normal joints) and those that are intra-articular (ie, occurring within normal joints). Extra-articular coalitions would practically be expected to be more responsive to resection, because their excision does not destroy or alter the existing tarsal joints. Conversely, resection of an intra-articular tarsal coalition does remove a portion or all

of an existing joint, and logically would be expected to be more prone to failure. For this reason, the intra-articular tarsal coalition is generally considered less amenable to resection, because its excision destroys or alters an already abnormal tarsal joint. Despite this rationale, recent studies have suggested that the outcome differences between resection of extra-articular and intra-articular coalitions may not be as dramatic as previously thought. In a series of 19 calcaneonavicular coalition (extra-articular) resections and 13 talocalcaneal coalition (intra-articular) resections, Khoshbin et al.[240] reported similar long-term functional and patient satisfaction outcomes at a mean of 14.4 years postoperative. Mahan and others[241] also reported no differences in activity and outcome scores between their 43 calcaneonavicular coalition (extra-articular) resections and 20 talocalcaneal coalition (intra-articular) resections at an average of 4.62 years after surgery.

The presence or absence of arthritic changes in the joints surrounding a tarsal coalition has a significant impact on the selection of a surgical remedy. These changes often are considered to be secondary to the restricted motion and altered biomechanics created by the tarsal coalition and are therefore termed secondary arthritic or adaptive changes. Many of these changes are classically seen in patients with tarsal coalitions. For example, talonavicular joint arthritis is a secondary change that is occasionally seen with a middle facet talocalcaneal joint coalition. Narrowing of joint spaces, joint lipping, or osteophyte formation and adaptive changes in osseous structures (eg, wedging of the navicular) and joints (eg, ball-and-socket ankle joint) are all frequent secondary arthritic or adaptive changes that may be associated with a tarsal coalition. Obviously, the greater the quantity and severity of the secondary arthritic changes present in conjunction with a tarsal coalition, the more difficult will be the surgical procedure for correction of that coalition. Further, with more secondary arthritic changes, the tarsal area will likely be less responsive to simple resection of the tarsal coalition. Secondary adaptive changes, which are deemed nonarthritic, are less problematic and have less of an effect on the foot after surgical resection of the coalition. Resection of a tarsal coalition in the presence of significant secondary arthritic changes could necessitate further biomechanical adjustment in an already mechanically compensated foot. This generally results in further aggravation of any existing symptom complex. Thus, when significant secondary arthritic changes are associated with a tarsal coalition, an arthrodesis type of procedure is usually considered the operation of choice. Kernbach et al.[242] utilized CT scans to grade and stage the severity of talocalcaneal degenerative joint disease associated with a series of middle facet talocalcaneal coalitions. They then made treatment recommendations based upon their staging system.

The size of a tarsal coalition has also been assumed to impact the success rates of resection, particularly with intra-articular coalitions such as the middle facet talocalcaneal coalition. Researchers have made attempts using preoperative CT scans to determine whether the size of a talocalcaneal coalition affects the result obtained with resection. Wilde and colleagues[243] examined 20 feet in 17 patients, all <16 years of age and each undergoing resection of a talocalcaneal coalition. These investigators reported excellent or good results in 10 feet (50%) in patients in whom the preoperative coronal views on the CT scan showed <50% involvement of the posterior facet of the subtalar joint. These patients also had <16 degrees of heel valgus and no radiographic signs of arthritis of the

posterior facet of the talocalcaneal joint. In the 10 feet (50%) with fair or poor results, coronal CT sections showed >50% involvement of the posterior facet. The patients also had >16 degrees of heel valgus and radiographic changes of the posterior facet consistent with arthritis. These investigators concluded that one could obtain excellent or good results if the coalition involved <50% of the joint, but fair or poor results occurred with attempts at resection of larger coalitions.[243] Similarly, Comfort and Johnson[244] found that the clinical results obtained with resection correlated well with the size of the coalition. These authors reviewed a series of 20 feet undergoing resection of talocalcaneal coalitions (16 patients). There were preoperative CT scans for 17 feet. The average patient age was 14.2 years and the mean follow-up was 2.4 years postoperatively. Unlike Wilde and associates, these authors evaluated all three facets of the subtalar joint and not just the posterior facet. They found 77% excellent or good results when the coalition involved less than one-third of the entire subtalar joint as measured on a coronal CT view.[244] Based upon these results, the size of a talocalcaneal coalition was deemed to have relevance in the choice of a surgical plan for patients with intra-articular tarsal coalitions. Arbitrarily, many surgeons then concluded that >50% involvement of the talocalcaneal joint by the coalition precluded an attempt at surgical resection of the coalition. More recently, many investigators have called this conclusion into question and concluded that there is no definitive coalition size that renders an attempt at coalition resection unacceptable.[240,241,245]

More recently, the shape or morphology of the talocalcaneal coalition may be a factor in the success of its resection. In 2010, Rozansky and associates[246] first described a variety of talocalcaneal coalition configurations based on 3D CT scan reconstructions. Bixby and others[247] studies 138 talocalcaneal coalitions and found 97 of them (70%) affected the middle facet, 39 (28%) affected the posteromedial aspect of the joint, and 2 (1.4%) involved the posterior facet. The posteromedial talocalcaneal coalition is associated with an intact but shorter middle facet with a long sustentaculum tali. In 2017, Mahan and colleagues[248] then reported the resection in 51 feet (36 patients) with talocalcaneal coalitions—15 feet with posteromedial talocalcaneal coalition and 36 feet with middle facet talocalcaneal coalition. At a mean follow-up of 2.6 years, the authors reported that the patients with the posteromedial variant had better clinical outcomes, with less pain and higher AOFAS scores (95.7 vs 86.5), than the middle facet coalition type. The researchers concluded that the differences in outcome were likely not only due to the typical smaller size of the posteromedial variant but also due to its simpler and more superficial anatomic location. Whether preoperative identification of the joint morphology can improve patient outcomes and expectations following coalition resection requires further study.

Finally, many investigators have suggested that failure of tarsal coalition resection may be due to the degree of hindfoot valgus present. Wilde and colleagues[243] found that more than 16 degrees of heel valgus correlated with a poor outcome after resection of talocalcaneal coalitions. Luhmann and Schoenecker[249] found no problems with 16 degrees of heel valgus but did find poorer outcomes with resection of talocalcaneal coalitions in patients with more than 21 degrees of heel valgus. These authors suggested either a medializing calcaneal osteotomy or a lateral column lengthening along with resection of a talocalcaneal coalition associated with severe hindfoot val-

gus. More recent research has called the negative relationship between heel valgus and the success of coalition resection into question. Numerous authors did not find increased hindfoot valgus predictive of outcome in their series of tarsal coalition resections.[240,241,250]

Calcaneonavicular Coalition

Traditionally, extra-articular coalitions, such as a calcaneonavicular coalition, have been considered more amenable to surgical resection. This is particularly true when no secondary degenerative changes have occurred and no other coalitions are noted in the same foot. Resection of a calcaneonavicular bar should be performed as early as possible. Thus, in the younger patient with an extra-articular coalition and minimal secondary arthritic changes (ie, juvenile IA coalition), resection arthroplasty is generally preferred (Fig. 44.26). In the older patient with a calcaneonavicular coalition and minimal secondary changes (adult IA coalition), resection arthroplasty may be strongly considered, but one should recognize that failure is more likely.

The classic procedure, as first described by Slomann[8] in 1921 and performed by Badgley[9] in 1927, involves excision of the coalition with interposition of the extensor digitorum brevis muscle belly in the void created between the calcaneus and the navicular (Fig. 44.27). The procedure has been referred to as an *extensor digitorum brevis arthroplasty*.

Surgical Technique

The approach for this procedure is through a lateral curvilinear or Ollier type of incision, beginning over the lateral calcaneus or sinus tarsi area and extending medially to the lateral aspect of the talonavicular joint (Figs. 44.27A and 44.28A). Blunt dissection is carried deep through the subcutaneous layer, with hemostasis obtained as necessary. Care is taken to avoid the intermediate dorsal cutaneous nerve, which courses across the medial extent of the incision and the sural nerve (lateral dorsal cutaneous nerve), which may be visualized in the lateral margin of the incision. These nerves are uniformly preserved and, if identified, are gently retracted. Occasionally, a small neural communicating branch between the sural (lateral dorsal cutaneous) and intermediate dorsal cutaneous nerves is noted. In some cases, this small branch may have to be sacrificed to afford optimal exposure.

The subcutaneous tissue is then bluntly reflected from the deep fascia revealing the extensor digitorum brevis muscle belly. The peroneus tertius and extensor digitorum longus tendons are often noted in the medial portion of the incision (Figs. 44.27B and 44.28B). The origin of the extensor digitorum brevis is then reflected off the calcaneus and is retracted distally. All soft tissue is freed from the calcaneonavicular bar. Care is taken to preserve the talonavicular and calcaneocuboid joint ligaments, to minimize future instability and degenerative changes of these articulations (Figs. 44.27C and 44.28C).

The calcaneonavicular bar is generously resected, with removal of as much bone as possible. The coalition is not a thin bar but a deep, substantial block. The coalition should not be removed as a triangular or trapezoidal-shaped wedge. Preferably, a 1- to 1.5-cm uniform, rectangular thickness of bone should be removed (Figs. 44.27D and 44.28D). Any remaining prominences of bone may be rasped smooth. If desired, bone wax may be applied after the area is rasped or cauterized. Frequently, an immediate improvement in midtarsal and subtalar joint motion is apparent (Fig. 44.28E).

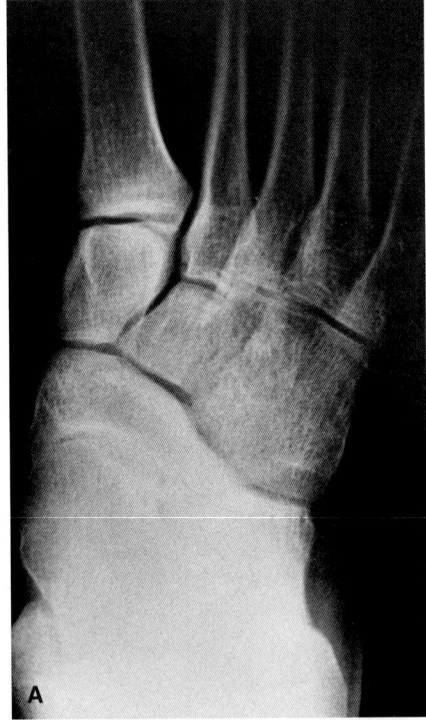

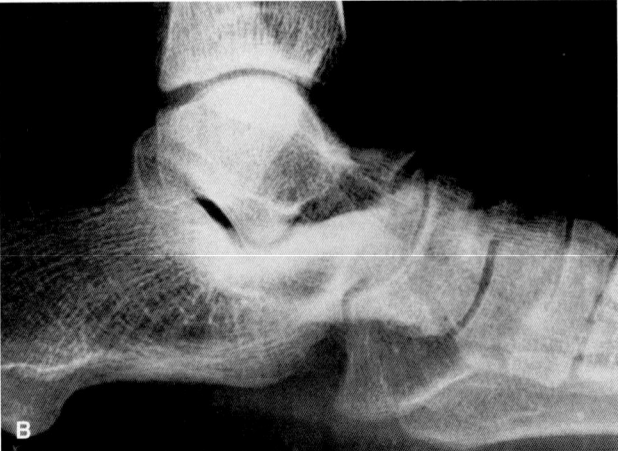

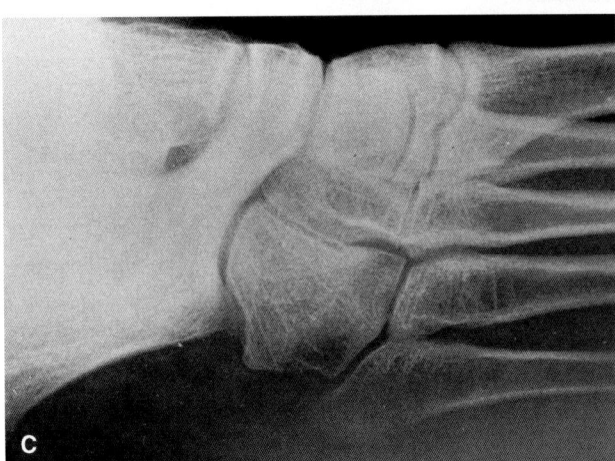

FIGURE 44.26 Anteroposterior **(A)**, lateral **(B)**, and medial oblique **(C)** views of a patient with a complete calcaneonavicular bar. The "anteater nose sign" is readily apparent on the lateral view, and the "comma sign" is readily apparent on the oblique view.

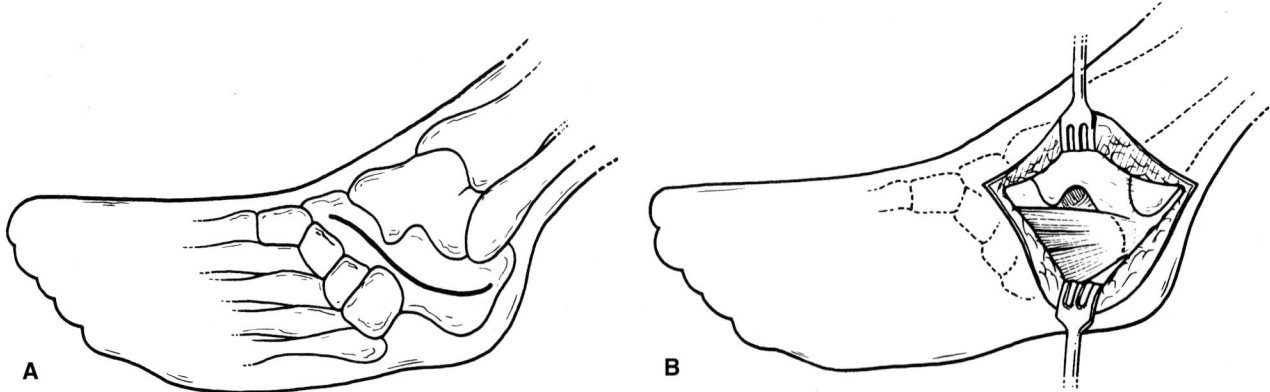

FIGURE 44.27 Diagrammatic representation of resection of a calcaneonavicular bar. **A.** Skin incision. **B.** The extensor digitorum brevis muscle belly is identified.

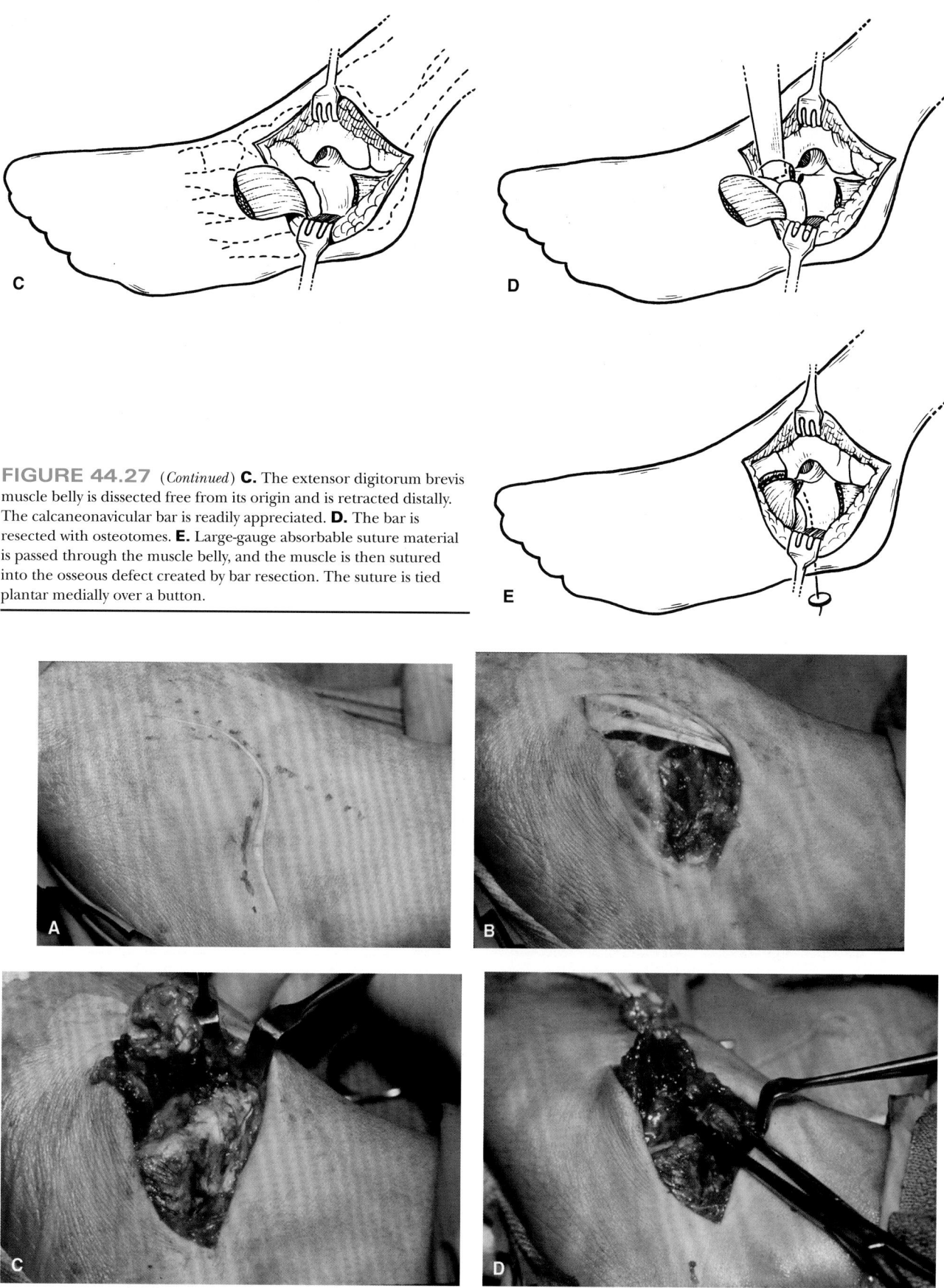

FIGURE 44.27 (*Continued*) **C.** The extensor digitorum brevis muscle belly is dissected free from its origin and is retracted distally. The calcaneonavicular bar is readily appreciated. **D.** The bar is resected with osteotomes. **E.** Large-gauge absorbable suture material is passed through the muscle belly, and the muscle is then sutured into the osseous defect created by bar resection. The suture is tied plantar medially over a button.

FIGURE 44.28 Surgical demonstration of resection of a calcaneonavicular bar. **A.** Skin incision. The intermediate dorsal cutaneous nerve was identified and was marked with a skin marker before the surgical incision (*dotted line*). **B.** Dissection is carried to the level of the deep fascia. The belly of the extensor digitorum brevis muscle is apparent in the plantar portion of the wound, and the peroneus tertius and extensor digitorum longus tendons are visible in the medial portion of the wound. **C.** The belly of the extensor digitorum brevis muscle is freed from its origin and is reflected distally. The calcaneonavicular bar is readily appreciated. **D.** The bar is resected in the form of a rectangular piece of bone.

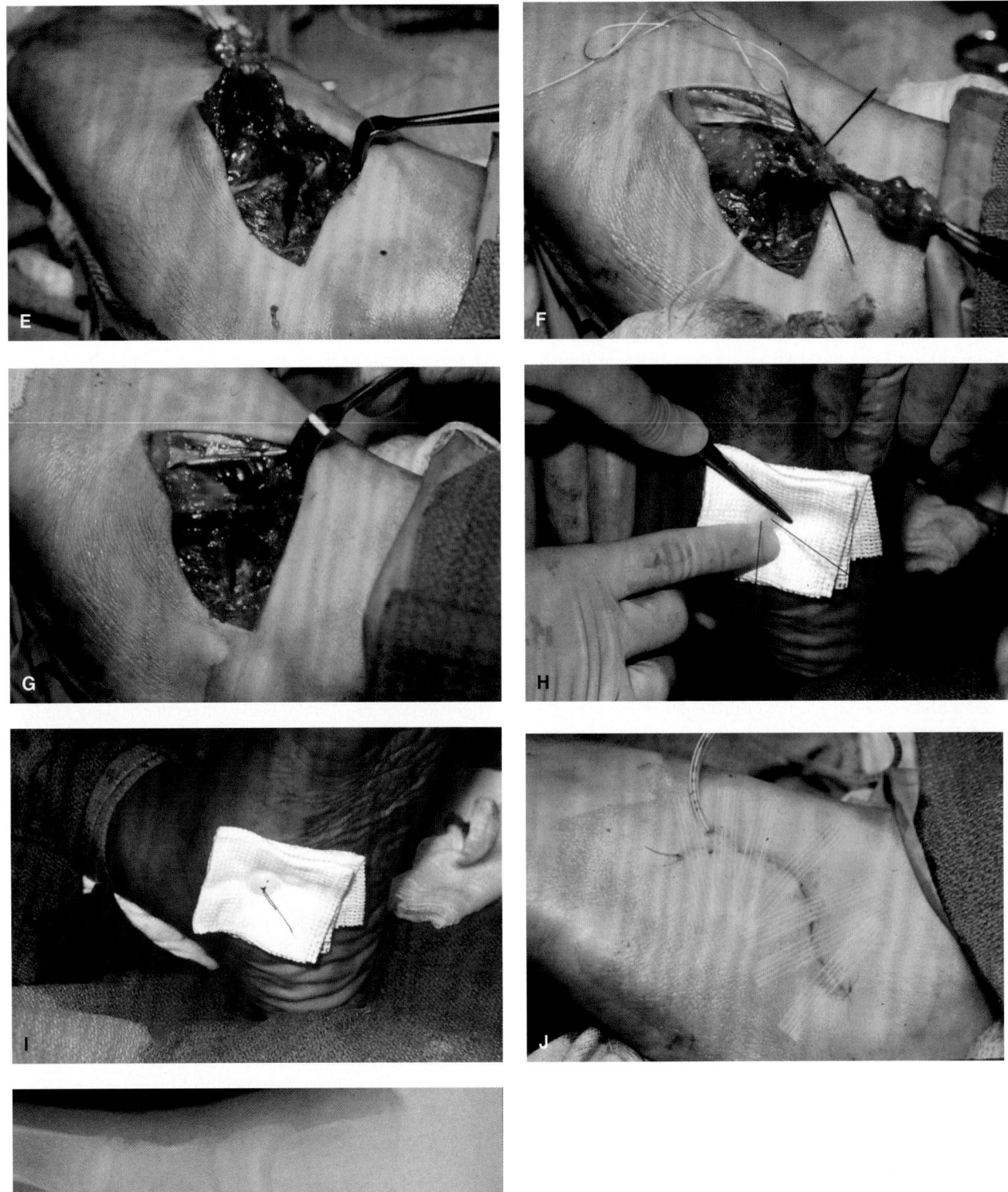

FIGURE 44.28 (*Continued*) **E.** Any remaining prominences of bone are removed, and motion is assessed. Note the resection void. **F.** Large-gauge absorbable suture is placed through the muscle belly. **G.** The muscle is sutured into the osseous void created by bar resection. **H, I.** Keith needles are used to pass the suture through the bottom of the foot, and the suture is tied to a button and a gauze square. **J.** Layer wound closure is achieved with insertion of a closed suction drain. **K.** Postoperative radiograph demonstrating the resected coalition.

A large absorbable suture is then placed through the proximal portion of the muscle belly (Fig. 44.28F). With the use of straight Keith needles, the extensor digitorum brevis muscle belly is then passed into the defect (Fig. 44.28G). The suture may be directed plantar medially and sutured over a button on the plantar medial aspect of the foot (Figs. 44.27E and 44.28H and I). Alternatively, an internal suture technique or bone anchor in which the muscle is anchored to soft tissue or bone may be employed. With any reinsertion method, the origin of the extensor digitorum brevis muscle is used to fill the dead space created by the bony resection. The goal of this reinsertion is to use the muscle belly as both a filler and a spacer between the navicular and calcaneus to prevent hematoma formation and recurrent growth of the bar. Alternatively, the muscle may simply be reapproximated to its normal anatomic position without being inserted as a spacer between the calcaneus and the navicular. Advocates of this alternative prefer the earlier range of motion achieved without a muscle transfer to the benefits of the muscle as a filler and a spacer.[55,251] Still another equivalent is to use another material or method to limit hematoma formation or recurrent bar formation. Coagulation of the bone ends,[152,252] the use of bone wax on the bone ends,[29,253] the insertion of adipose tissue instead of the muscle belly between the bone ends,[152,171,250] and the insertion of a silicone implant or other synthetic or nonsynthetic materials instead of the muscle belly between the bone ends[254-257] have all been espoused.

Once the muscle is sutured in the defect, a closed-suction drain may be inserted, and anatomic layer closure is performed (Fig. 44.28J). If concomitant talar beaking is present, it may be resected if desired, before closure or through a separate medial incision. Postoperatively, a below-knee non–weight-bearing cast is applied for 3-4 weeks. The cast may be split or bivalved at any point desired, and subtalar and midtarsal joint range-of-motion exercises may be begun. Continuous passive motion may be used, if desired. Weight bearing is initiated after ~43-6 weeks (Fig. 44.28K).

Since the operation was first described in the 1920s, many authors have reported success with this procedure.[154,155,187,250,252,253,258-276] In 1967, Mitchell and Gibson[252] reported on 48 patients followed for 4-13 years (mean, 6.6 years) after calcaneonavicular bar resection. Seventy-five percent of their patients had satisfactory results, with the best results unquestionably occurring in children <14 years of age who had no secondary adaptive or arthritic changes at the time of operation.

In 1968, Andreasen[260] reported on 30 calcaneonavicular bar resections in 25 patients. Subjectively, 13 of the 30 feet were free of symptoms, and 9 other feet had only slight pain, which did not interfere with work. Thus, 73% had subjectively satisfactory results. Objectively, 22 feet initially had mild or no pronation, and 8 had severe pronation. At long-term follow-up 10-22 years after surgery, 6 feet had undergone eventual triple arthrodesis. Of the remaining 24 feet, 19 had mild or no pronation and 5 had severe pronation. Preoperatively, subtalar joint motion was markedly reduced in 8 feet and was absent in 22 feet. At follow-up, 4 feet continued to have no motion, 9 had reduced motion, and 11 had normal motion. Recurrence of bar formation was noted in 16 of 24 cases. In addition, at follow-up, osteoarthritic changes were noted in the subtalar joint of 11 feet, in the talonavicular joint of 19 feet, and in the calcaneocuboid joint of 19 feet. Because of these arthritic changes, and despite

a reasonable success rate, Andreasen recommended triple arthrodesis as the primary procedure for all patients with calcaneonavicular coalition.

In another study, 23 of 26 patients were free of symptoms after resection arthroplasty.[187] Thirteen patients had partial recurrent formation of the bar, but 10 of these retained satisfactory motion without symptoms. The length of follow-up in this group of patients was not clear. However, it appeared that the ideal criteria for resection included a young patient, a painful foot, limited subtalar joint motion, and an incomplete coalition. A complete coalition was believed to be a relative contraindication to resection arthroplasty because degenerative changes were likely to be present in surrounding joints.

In 1983, Swiontkowski and associates[275] reported 39 cases of calcaneonavicular bar resection. After an average of 4.6 years, 35 feet (90%) were improved. They found no correlation between talar beaking and long-term results.

Contrary to this finding, Inglis et al.[268] reported on 16 feet in 11 patients who underwent calcaneonavicular bar resection between the ages of 10 and 14 years. They observed their patients for an average of 23 years after surgery and found that 11 feet (69%) were free of symptoms. These authors concluded that talar beaking was a prognosticator of probable failure, because 2 of 3 feet with preexistent talar beaks eventually required triple arthrodesis.

In 1990, Gonzalez and Kumar[154] reported their long-term findings in 48 patients (75 feet). When results were evaluated from 2 to 23 years after resection, these investigators found satisfactory results in 58 feet (77%), with the best outcome in patients <16 years of age who had an incomplete coalition. These authors also did not believe that talar beaking was a contraindication to surgery.

In 1991, Alter and others[258,259] reported their results in 14 patients (16 feet) who were evaluated on average 4.5 years after resection arthroplasty. The mean patient age was 19.5 years (range, 11-68 years), and 12 of the 16 feet (75%) were judged to have a satisfactory result. In the 4 feet in patients assessed as having unsatisfactory results, each had continued moderate to severe pain with no reduction in the preoperative symptoms. Two of the 4 unsatisfactory results were determined to have had inadequate initial resection of the calcaneonavicular bar, and 2 of the feet had significant associated degenerative joint disease in the subtalar and midtarsal joints.

In 1993, Cohen et al.[262] reported their success with resection arthroplasty with interposition of the extensor digitorum brevis in 10 patients (13 feet) with an average age of 12.3 years (range, 10-14 years). The mean postoperative follow-up was 5.5 years (range, 8 months to 11.75 years); 12 feet (9 patients) (92.3%) had good or excellent results, and 1 patient (1 foot) (7.7%) reported a fair result. The patient with the fair result described swelling and stiffness with strenuous activity and only a mild reduction in symptoms compared with the preoperative level.

In 1998, Fuson and Barrett[253] reported good results in resection arthroplasty with the use of bone wax on the ends of the resected bones. These authors used no interpositional material in 23 of their 24 cases (20 of 21 patients). They reported good results in 20 of the 24 procedures (83.3%) and concluded that the interposition of the extensor digitorum brevis muscle was unnecessary and may actually alter the muscle's function in assisting subtalar joint motion.

In a unique study, Cohen and associates[263] reviewed the success of resection arthroplasty for calcaneonavicular coalition

in a group of 12 adults (13 feet). Unlike previous studies, their average patient age was 33 years (range, 19-48 years). The authors initially applied bone wax to the resected surfaces and interposed the extensor digitorum brevis muscle into the defect. However, after experiencing 3 cases of lateral wound dehiscence using this technique, the authors switched to using bone wax and an absorbable gelatin sponge (Gelfoam) and returning the extensor digitorum brevis muscle to its anatomic position. At a mean follow-up of 3 years (range, 17-54 months), subjective relief of preoperative symptoms was achieved in 10 of the 12 patients (83.3%). The authors identified degenerative arthritic changes in 75% of the feet preoperatively. The naviculocuneiform joint was involved in 3 patients, the subtalar joint in 3 patients, and the talonavicular joint in 6 patients. The arthritic changes could actually have been adaptive changes, because they consisted of only minimal peripheral joint osteophytes in all but a single patient. No changes in activity level or occupation were found in their patients. The authors concluded that the resection of a calcaneonavicular coalition in an adult, with minimal arthritic changes, can be successful.

Scott and Tuten[273] reported excellent results in their study with seven adult patients (8 feet) with a mean age of 41 years old. The authors performed surgical resection with extensor digitorum brevis interposition with no evidence of degenerative changes. The mean postoperative follow-up was 56.5 months, and the average AOFAS (American Orthopedic Foot and Ankle Society) Ankle-Hindfoot scale score was 87. The authors admitted that a limitation of their study was that no preoperative scaled score was obtained. Despite this low number of patients, this is a promising study for adult patients.

In 2009, Mubarak and associates[250] reported their results on 69 patients (96 feet) with a mean age of 12 years old at the time of surgery. They resected the calcaneonavicular bar and then inserted a 1-cm × 3-cm fat graft obtained from a gluteal cleft or the abdomen. The extensor digitorum brevis was sutured back into its normal anatomic position. The mean postoperative follow-up was 29 months. The majority of the patients (74%) had improved subtalar joint motion postoperatively, and the degree of hindfoot valgus present before surgery did not affect the outcome. The significant majority of patients (89%) related markedly reduced pain and 13% of the feet had some recurrent growth of the coalition.

In a retrospective study performed via questionnaire, Van Renterghem and De Ridder[276] evaluated 22 patients who underwent calcaneonavicular resection with interposition of the extensor digitorum brevis muscle belly. These authors found that 95% of their patients were subjectively satisfied with the procedure.

In 2017, Masquijo and associates[277] concluded that after resection of a calcaneonavicular coalition, the interposition of a fat graft or bone wax in the resection defect provided better functional outcomes and lower reossification rates than extensor digitorum brevis muscle interposition. In their series of 48 patients (56 feet), 23 feet had fat graft interposition (the fat grafts were obtained from the posterior or posteromedial crease of the buttocks), 18 feet had bone wax placed on the resected bone surfaces, and 15 feet had extensor digitorum brevis muscle interposition. The authors reported 6 of 15 feet (40%) undergoing the extensor digitorum brevis muscle interposition had radiographic evidence of reossification with 5 of the 15 feet (33%) being symptomatic. The fat graft

interposition cases resulted in only 1 of 23 (4%) demonstrating radiographic evidence of reossification, and the bone wax technique resulted in only 1 of 18 (6%) cases demonstrating radiographic evidence of reossification. None of the fat graft interposition cases or bone wax cases had a recurrence of symptomatology.

In 2006, Lui[278] described using an arthroscope to resect a calcaneonavicular coalition. He advocated using two small arthroscopy portals to resect the calcaneonavicular coalition. One portal, created at the angle of Gissane, was the "primary visualization portal" through which a 2.7-mm 30-degree arthroscope was inserted. This "primary visualization portal" was the subtalar anterolateral portal as described by Parisien and Vangness.[279] A second portal, the "working portal," was located at the space between the talonavicular and calcaneocuboid joints or directly over the coalition. No fluid was used for distention, and the procedure would be better described as an endoscopic approach. A shaver was introduced through the "working portal," and the soft tissues overlying the coalition were debrided. An arthroscopic burr was then used through the "working portal" to resect the coalition. The foot was manipulated during this process to allow full exposure and resection. A "secondary visualization portal" was sometimes created medially (at the medial side of the extensor hallucis longus tendon at the level of the talonavicular joint) to allow full visualization. In his report, Lui[278] did not describe using any interposition material, and he did not report any results.

Subsequent to this report, Bernardino and associates[280] performed several cadaver dissections and determined that portals to resect a calcaneonavicular coalition could be safely made and the coalition safely resected. They then described performing the procedure on a 12-year-old patient through two arthroscopic portals, initially using a 4.0-mm arthroscope, arthroscopic shaver, and a 3.5-mm arthroscopic burr. During the procedure, they noted difficulty resecting the fibrous component of the coalition and had to remove the fibrous tissue with a combination of soft tissue resector and radiofrequency device. No material was interposed into the defect created. The authors felt the procedure was technically demanding but advocated future investigation into the approach.[280]

In 2010, Bauer et al.[281] reported their success with the two-portal endoscopic resection of a calcaneonavicular synostosis using a 4.0-mm arthroscope, 4.0-mm arthroscopic shaver, and a 4.0-mm arthroscopic burr. These authors stressed that portal placement was the "key" to successful coalition resection with avoidance of damage to the terminal branches of the superficial peroneal nerve. In 2011, Knorr and associates[282] reported performing an arthroscopic resection of three calcaneonavicular coalitions. At a mean follow-up of 1 year, these authors noted that the mean AOFAS score rose from 58 preoperatively to 91 at follow-up. These authors felt that their arthroscopic approach reduced the risk of recurrence due to its less traumatic nature and ability to explore deeper into the foot. More recently, Bonasia and colleagues[283] provided a detailed description of the surgical technique for endoscopic tarsal coalition resection. In 2018, Bourlez et al.[284] described arthroscopic resection of a "too-long anterior process" of the calcaneus in children and adolescents. They reported a series of 10 patients (11 feet) undergoing the procedure with a minimum of 6-month follow-up. The mean AOFAS score increased from a preoperative mean of 61.9 to a postoperative mean of 89.1. The arthroscopic/endoscopic approaches for tarsal coalition resection clearly are

more technically demanding than open approaches, but the minimally invasive nature of the approaches along with the potential lesser need for immobilization and earlier restoration of full weight bearing may prove to be advantages.

Currently, the consensus seems to be that calcaneonavicular bar resection or extensor digitorum brevis arthroplasty is most successful in the immature patient with an incomplete coalition, but it can be considered in an adult without significant subtalar or midtarsal joint arthritis or in a complete coalition. The most frequent postoperative problem reported has been a varying amount of recurrent bone growth of the bar. This generally has not been a problem when a generous resection was initially performed. Talar beaking may or may not increase the failure rate, and the presence of a complete synostosis or significant arthritic change in surrounding joints certainly increases the probability of failure. The procedure may be attempted when factors that suggest failure are present, but one should recognize the possible need for eventual triple arthrodesis. Arthroscopic and endoscopic approaches and their reported results for resection of a calcaneonavicular coalition are in their infancy. Larger and more long-term studies are still needed, but the initial reports suggest that these approaches have a steep learning curve but are likely to be safe and reproducible.

When resection of the calcaneonavicular bar has failed, or when significant arthritic changes are present (ie, juvenile IB, adult IB), triple arthrodesis may be considered the procedure of choice. An extra-articular coalition with secondary arthritic changes is less amenable to simple surgical resection. In the younger patient, however, the resection procedure should be strongly considered, with arthrodesis presented as a possible future option. When triple arthrodesis is to be performed, the coalition may be left intact if it is complete. However, if the coalition is incomplete or if significant positional abnormalities exist, the coalition should be resected to obtain optimal postoperative position and fusion. Triple arthrodesis is usually performed after the patient reaches osseous maturity.

Several authors have discussed the possibility of performing a varus-producing osteotomy of the calcaneus for treatment of a tarsal coalition.[285,286] Dwyer[286] believed that the valgus position of the hindfoot, commonly seen with a tarsal coalition, produced an "oblique strain of the ligaments" in the hindfoot and ankle with resultant pain. He suggested an opening wedge calcaneal osteotomy with a bone graft inserted through a lateral approach. Cain and Hyman[285] reported success in treating coalitions with a similar procedure. Instead of an opening osteotomy, Cain and Hyman performed a closing osteotomy through a medial approach. None of these authors suggested resection of the coalition along with the calcaneal osteotomy. Certainly, the osteotomy alone would seem to be of limited benefit, as demonstrated by orthotic devices that maintain the heel in a varus position and yet afford only minimal relief of symptoms. However, if significant heel valgus is present, a varus-producing calcaneal osteotomy combined with resection of the coalition may be of some benefit.

More recently, Quinn and associates[287] compared a group of isolated calcaneonavicular coalition resections (20 feet) with a group of calcaneonavicular coalition resections with concomitant pes planovalgus reconstruction (7 feet). The pes planovalgus reconstruction procedures varied but included combinations of gastrocnemius recessions, anterior calcaneal osteotomies, posterior calcaneal osteotomies, and midfoot

osteotomies. The mean age at the time of surgery was 18.1 years, and the mean follow-up was 10.2 months. Preoperative and postoperative radiographic angular assessment was done, and the groups were compared. Both groups demonstrated a statistically significant reduction in talar head uncoverage (mean 22.9 degrees preoperatively to mean 18.9 degrees postoperatively). The group undergoing the simultaneous calcaneonavicular coalition resection and pes planovalgus reconstruction also demonstrated a statistically significant increase in the calcaneal inclination angle (mean increase of 2.7 degrees). No other statistically significant differences were noted between the two groups, including no differences in talo-first metatarsal angle on lateral or anterior-posterior radiographs. The authors concluded that the combined approach improved some radiographic parameters but that longer follow-up and patient satisfaction scores would be desirable goals in a future study.

Talocalcaneal Coalition

Although extra-articular coalitions are generally believed to be more amenable to resection, intra-articular coalitions are traditionally considered an indication for arthrodesis. However, recently, the literature has shown that many talocalcaneal coalitions may also be amenable to resection. Arguably, the best example of an intra-articular coalition that would be responsive to resection is the "juvenile IIA" coalition, an intra-articular coalition that occurs in a younger patient with minimal or no secondary degenerative changes. If small enough and/or if incomplete, this coalition is very amenable to resection arthroplasty. However, future arthrodesis may still be necessary.

A common example is a middle facet coalition of the subtalar joint (Fig. 44.29). Typically, resection of this coalition leaves a defect and an irregular area in an articular facet of a major weight-bearing joint. However, several authors have described resection of the coalition with or without the interposition of fat grafts or tendon and have reported satisfactory results.[48,49,126,135,143,155,187,200,235,242-244,249,275,288-315] Simply stated, when a middle facet talocalcaneal coalition is resected, the area of the dysmorphic middle facet (and likely the anterior facet as well) is obliterated and the weight-bearing function of

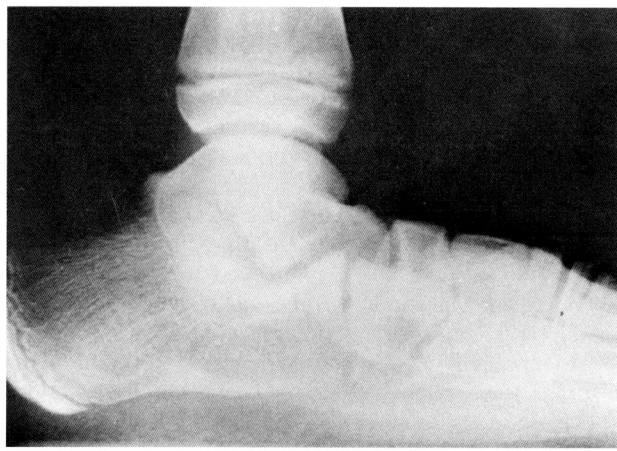

FIGURE 44.29 Lateral radiograph of an immature patient with a middle facet talocalcaneal coalition. No secondary arthritis is noted. This is a "juvenile IIA" coalition or a "juvenile, intra-articular coalition without secondary arthritis."

the subtalar joint postoperatively is reliant entirely upon the remaining posterior facet of the joint.

Surgical Technique

Resection of the coalition is most easily accomplished through a medial approach. A linear or slightly curvilinear incision is made, extending from just posterior and inferior to the medial malleolus to the plantar medial aspect of the medial cuneiform (Fig. 44.30A). The incision is carried bluntly deep to the level of the deep fascia. The tendons and neurovascular bundle that comprise the tarsal tunnel are palpated, and the incision is carried deep between the FDL tendon and the neurovascular bundle. The tibialis posterior and FDL tendons are retracted dorsally, and the neurovascular bundle and the FHL tendon are retracted plantarly. A Keith needle, small osteotome, or other flat instrument is then used to identify the area of the middle facet (Fig. 44.30B). If necessary, intraoperative radiographs or fluoroscopic studies are used to localize the coalition.

Recently, Field and Ng[296] described the concomitant use of subtalar joint arthroscopy to help localize the coalition. They inserted a 2.7-mm arthroscope through an anterior subtalar joint portal and directed it posteromedially to inspect the anterior edge of the posterior facet, as well as the quality and extent of the middle facet coalition and synovitic proliferation. They then evaluated the amount of subtalar motion present by putting the joint through a full range of motion with the arthro-scope in place. The synovitis within the joint was then resected using a 2.0-mm or a 2.7-mm arthroscopic shaver. Once the synovitis was adequately debrided, more precise visualization of the middle facet could be appreciated and the type of coalition determined. Once the location of the middle facet was adequately visualized, the shaver was removed and a 0.062-in Kirschner wire (K-wire) was driven through the facet from lateral to medial, in a perpendicular fashion, under arthroscopic guidance. The K-wire was advanced until it caused a tenting of the skin along the medial side of the foot. The medial tenting of the K-wire was then used to assist in medial incisional placement. The actual coalition was then resected in open fashion with continued use of the arthroscope to support the resection and joint evaluation.[296]

Another method of demarcating the talocalcaneal coalition is with the K-wire technique described by Edmonds and associates.[316] These surgeons first made the traditional medial incision over the sustentaculum tali and exposed the general area of the coalition. Then, a second, ancillary, lateral incision was made extending from just distal to the fibula, over the sinus tarsi, toward the fourth metatarsal base. The extensor digitorum brevis muscle was then dissected and the sinus tarsi exposed. Next, 0.045-in K-wires were inserted from lateral to medial outlining and localizing the coalition. The medial incisional approach was then used to identify the K-wires and directly expose and resect the talocalcaneal coalition.

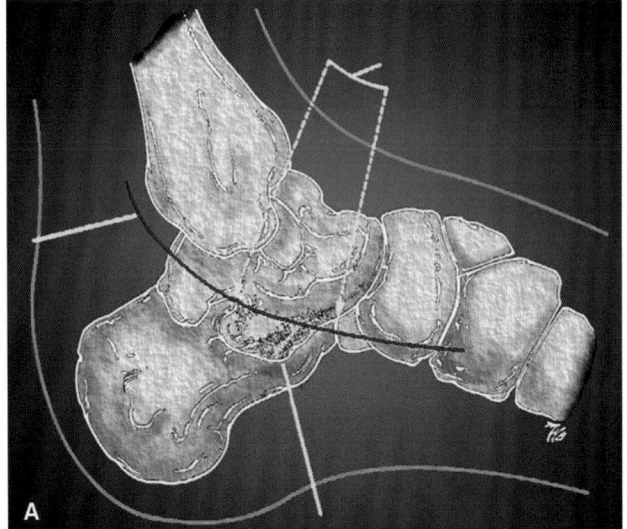

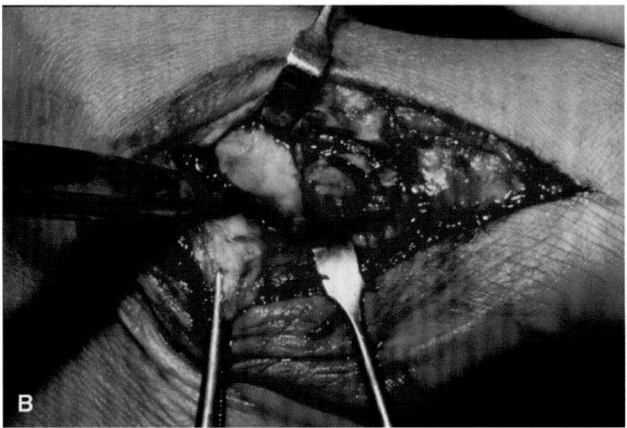

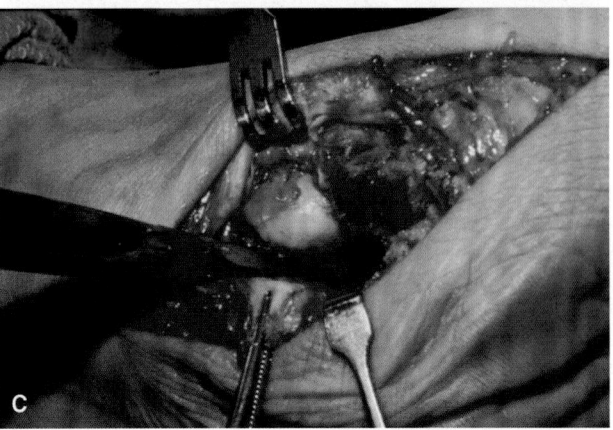

FIGURE 44.30 A. Diagrammatic representation of the incisional approach for resection of a middle facet talocalcaneal coalition. The incision is similar to the medial arm of a Cincinnati incision. **B.** Surgical demonstration of an anterior and middle facet talocalcaneal coalition in a left foot approached through a medial incision. Note the flat instrument placed into the slightly visible portion of the subtalar joint. **C.** The same foot after resection of the coalition.

Once identified, the coalition is resected with hand instrumentation. Typically, an osteotome and mallet and/or sagittal saw are used for the bulk of the resection. Any remaining prominence is removed with a rongeur, sharp curette, or is rasped or burred smooth. Care is taken to preserve the substance, or at the very least the inferior margin, of the sustentaculum tali. The coalition must be generously resected with the width of the resection slightly larger than the coalition itself. This width can vary from as little as 4 mm to as great as 1 or 2 cm. An immediate increase in subtalar joint motion is typically observed after resection of the coalition (Fig. 44.30C).

Recently, Aibinder et al.[317] described a technique of intraoperative CT-guided navigation for the resection of the talocalcaneal coalition. The technique described requires the placement of a reference frame and performing two intraoperative CT scans. The first CT scan is used to mark the coalition, and the second CT scan is done after a navigated burr has been used to resect the coalition. The authors hypothesize that the technique both decreases the risk of over-resection of the medial bone and decreases the risk of incomplete resection. The noted disadvantages of the technique are the radiation exposure and increased cost of using the intraoperative CT scans. Although this technique is not in common use, it clearly merits further

investigation with studies assessing the clinical outcomes and comparing them to traditional surgical approaches.

If the surgeon desires, after resection, bone wax may be used on the resected bone margins, and fat may be interposed into the defect created. This autogenous fat may be harvested from the area between the tendo Achilles and the deep flexor compartment (ie, Kagar triangle), from incisional subcutaneous fat, from a gluteal fold, or from any other area where subcutaneous fat can be readily harvested with minimal potential sequelae. Alternatively, the FHL may be split longitudinally and the superior one-half interposed into the resection site (Fig. 44.31). Once interposition has been accomplished, layer closure is performed.

In younger patients, one may consider performing medial resection of the middle facet talocalcaneal coalition, with or without fat or tendon interposition, in conjunction with the lateral insertion of a subtalar joint arthroereisis to maintain distraction of the resected joint space indirectly. In such cases, the aforementioned medial incision is used to resect the coalition. A second incision is placed laterally over the sinus tarsi. This incision is used to insert the arthroereisis, but it may also be used to aid in anatomic localization of the coalition. A small osteotome, K-wire, or other instrument can be introduced

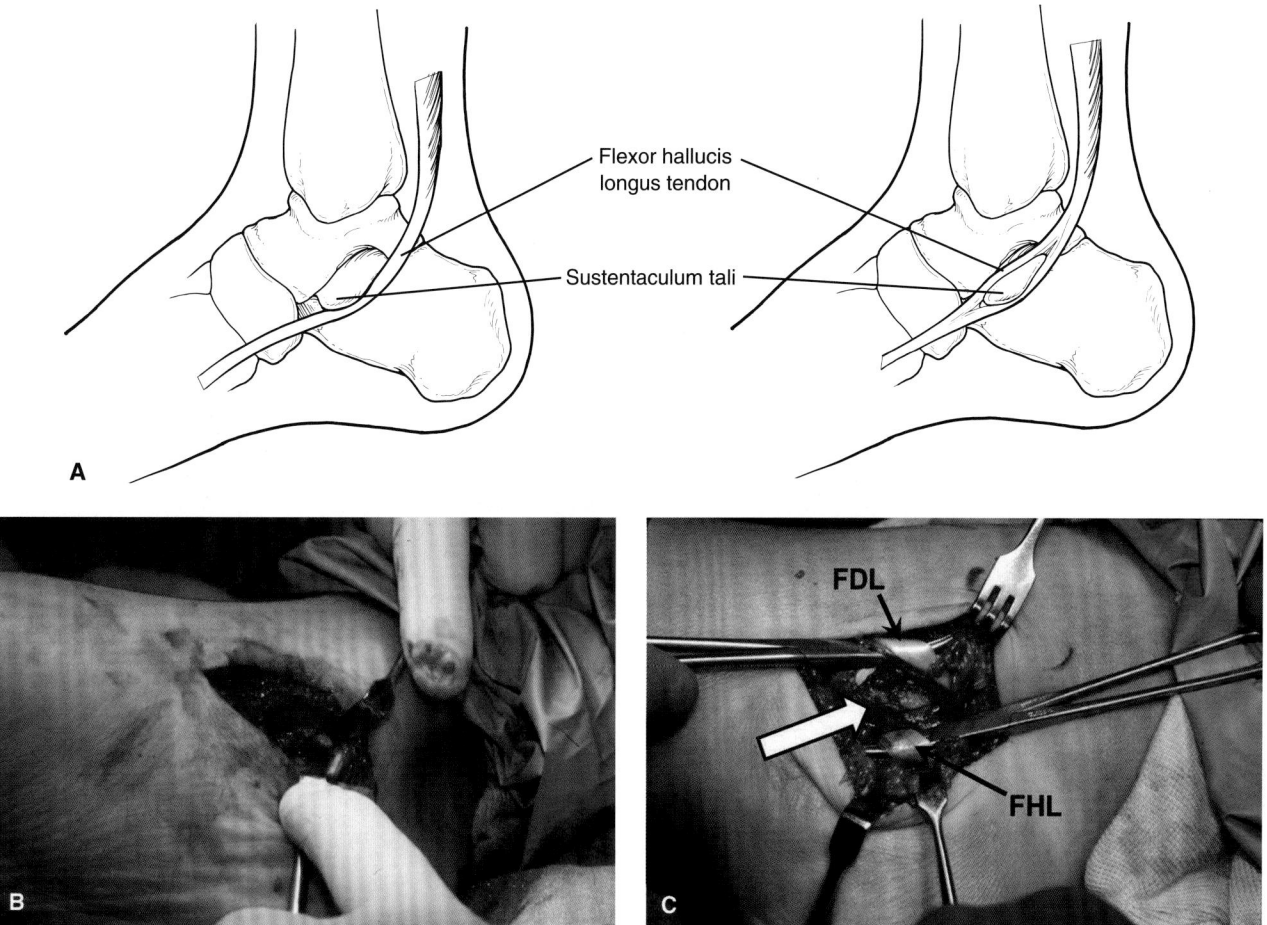

Flexor hallucis longus tendon

Sustentaculum tali

A

FDL

FHL

B

C

FIGURE 44.31 A. Diagrammatic representation of the technique for flexor hallucis longus (*FHL*) tendon splitting and interposition. The FHL tendon is split longitudinally, and the superior half is interposed through the resection site above the sustentaculum tali, and the inferior half is left in its normal channel below the sustentaculum tali. The periosteum in the area is closed to maintain the split FHL tendon in its new position. **B.** Surgical approach to middle facet talocalcaneal coalition. **C.** Middle facet talocalcaneal coalition exposed (*large white arrow*) between flexor digitorum longus (*FDL*) tendon and FHL tendon.

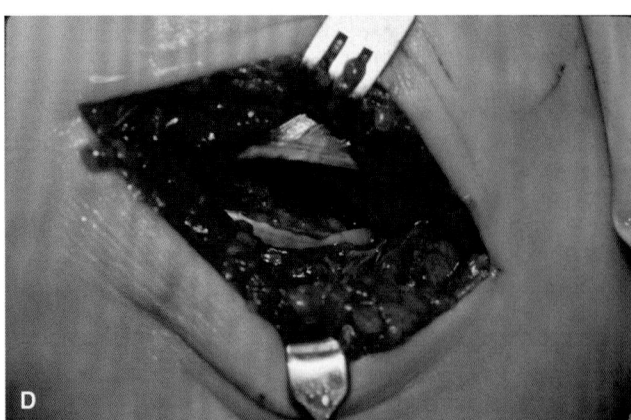 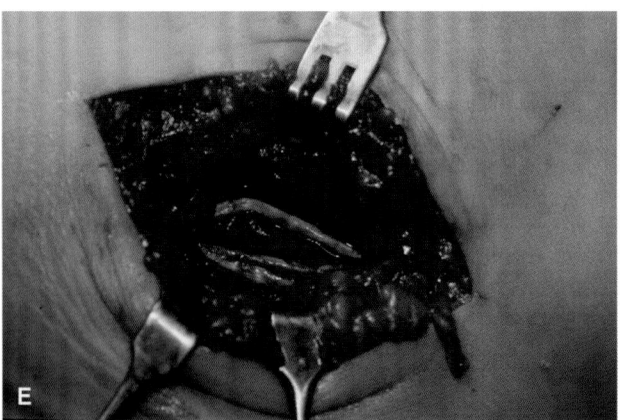

FIGURE 44.31 (*Continued*) **D.** Appearance immediately after coalition resection. Note space where coalition previously existed. **E.** FHL tendon is split longitudinally with one-half of the tendon now passing through the resection site and one-half of the tendon left below the remaining sustentaculum tali. (NB: The FDL tendon is being retracted dorsally and is not visible in **E**).

through the lateral incision and gently passed medially. The instrument can then be manually felt medially, and the surgeon will have a better idea of the location of the coalition. In cases involving larger coalitions, the small osteotome can be introduced through the lateral incision and then struck medially through the coalition until the tip of the osteotome is palpated medially. The medial incision can then be centered over the palpated osteotome. Once the middle facet talocalcaneal coalition has been resected, an arthroereisis is inserted into the sinus tarsi laterally. Used in this fashion, the arthroereisis helps to maintain a space where the coalition has been resected and aids in the prevention of ossification or recurrent formation of the coalition.[48,49,294,297]

Postoperatively, a below-knee non–weight-bearing cast is applied for 2-4 weeks. If pes valgus was present preoperatively, the subtalar joint is maintained in a neutral or supinated position within the cast. The cast may be split or bivalved at any point desired, and subtalar and midtarsal joint range-of-motion exercises may be started. Weight bearing is initiated after ~3-6 weeks. Aggressive physical therapy, including aggressive range-of-motion exercises, is typically recommended. A continuous passive motion device may be used, if desired.[317] In the long term, the patient is fitted with functional orthoses to attempt to maintain the motion achieved intraoperatively.

Many different approaches and success rates have been described for the resection of middle facet talocalcaneal coalitions. The most popular surgical approach in the literature is a medial resection of the coalition with subsequent interposition of autogenous fat into the defect. Other approaches involve similar resection, but they vary in how the space created between the talus and calcaneus is managed. Whether the insertion of organic or nonorganic material is necessary in an attempt to maintain the resection space remains unknown.[303] The diversity of the surgical approaches, the small case series, and the criteria for grading the results at follow-up make concise conclusions difficult.

In 1987, Olney and Asher[309] reported their results on middle talocalcaneal coalition resections in 10 feet (9 patients). They used a medial approach and, after resection, pressed bone wax onto the resected surfaces and packed the defect with a free autogenous-fat graft obtained from the buttocks. Their patients ranged in age from 10.5 years to 22 years, with a mean age of

13 years, 7 months. Their mean length of follow-up was 3.5 years, and in 8 of the 10 feet (80%), the results were excellent (ie, no pain) or good (ie, occasional pain but no limitation of activity). In addition, these authors quantitated the subtalar joint motion postoperatively and found that the motion in the surgically treated foot was roughly 81% of the normal range of motion in the contralateral foot without any apparent coalition. Subjectively, they noted that all their patients believed that their motion had increased. These investigators noted no correlation between the age, sex, or tissue type of the coalition and the results obtained by coalition resection.

In another retrospective study, Scranton[313] reported on 14 feet (9 patients) that underwent middle or posterior talocalcaneal coalition resection. Of these 14 feet, 10 feet (7 patients) were resections of middle facet coalitions. Scranton approached the coalition through a medial incision and, like Olney and Asher, used bone wax on the bleeding osseous surfaces and an autogenous-free fat graft to fill the defect. Fat grafts were harvested from behind the calcaneus through the superior portion of his incision. The patients undergoing middle facet talocalcaneal resection varied in age from 12 to 24 years, with a mean age of roughly 15 years, 8 months. Scranton did not determine the average postoperative follow-up for just his middle facet coalition resections, but the results on the patients in his study were evaluated from 2 to 9 years (mean, 3.9 years), regardless of whether the treatment was conservative or surgical. Of the patients undergoing resection of the middle facet, 9 feet (90%) in 6 patients were considered to have good results (ie, no limitation of function, some motion of the talocalcaneal joint, and no pain during everyday activity), 1 foot (10%) had a satisfactory result (ie, some limitation of function, motion of the talocalcaneal joint could be absent, and pain could be present after prolonged standing and walking), and none had a poor result (ie, definite functional limitation, no motion of the talocalcaneal joint, and pain with standing, walking, or at rest). Although these results appeared promising, the criteria for the procedure were selective. Scranton believed that degenerative arthritis in the talonavicular joint, but not talar beaking, was a contraindication to resection. Further, he arbitrarily reasoned that a coalition involving more than one-half of the surface area of the subtalar joint, as determined preoperatively with a CT scan, precluded a good result with resection. Thus, middle facet

talocalcaneal resections were all done in patients with less than one-half of their middle facet involved and with no degenerative narrowing at the talonavicular joint.

In a study published in 1992, Salomao et al.[312] reviewed their series of 32 feet (22 patients) undergoing resection of a middle facet talocalcaneal coalition. These authors resected the coalition through a medial approach, used electric cautery and bone wax on the bleeding bone surfaces, and interposed a free autogenous fat graft (obtained from the subcutaneous tissues through the same incision) between the talus and the calcaneus. Their mean patient age was 14 years, with a range of 10-23 years. Their average follow-up was 2 years, 1 month. They noted that 25 feet (78.1%) had no pain, and the remaining 7 feet (21.8%) had residual pain that was less intensive than before surgery. The mobility of the subtalar joint increased in 24 (75%) of the 32 feet. They concluded that surgical resection of the coalition produced "gratifying results."

Also in 1992, Kumar et al.[304] reported their results of resection on 18 feet (16 patients) with middle facet talocalcaneal coalition. In their series, the coalition was resected through a medial approach, bone wax was applied to the bleeding ends of bone, but then the method of managing the space created varied. In 3 feet, nothing was interposed into the space; in 6 feet, fat obtained from the gluteal area or heel pad was interposed; and in 9 feet, the FHL was split, and one-half of the tendon was interposed into the defect. When the FHL tendon was used, the tendon was split in half longitudinally, and the superior half was placed into the resected area. Continuity of the FHL tendon was maintained superior and inferior to the split, so when the muscle contracted, the split tendon moved in its normal groove inferior to the sustentaculum tali and through the resection site. In this study, the average patient age at the time of surgery was 14 years (range, 7-19 years). The average length of follow-up was 4 years (range, 2-8 years). The results of resection arthroplasty were excellent (75% or more of subtalar joint motion, no symptoms, and no recurrence of the coalition) in 8 cases, good (50%-74% of subtalar joint motion, no symptoms, and little cortical irregularity in the area of resection) in 8 cases, fair (25%-49% of subtalar joint motion, pain at the end of the day) in 1 case, and poor (limited subtalar joint motion, constant pain, or reformation of the coalition) in 1 case. Thus, 88.9% of their patients achieved excellent or good results. In their patient with a poor result, a second attempt at resection was undertaken because the coalition was believed to have recurred, and the authors reported an excellent result after the revisional surgical procedure. The authors in this study did not believe that the patient's age, the type of coalition (ie, osseous, cartilaginous, or fibrous), or the type of material interposed influenced the result of the procedure.

Similarly, other authors have studied the use of the split FHL interposition after resection of a middle facet talocalcaneal coalition.[289,311] In 1998, the preliminary report of one study was described by Blakemore et al.[289] with the final report published by Raikin et al.[311] in 1999. These papers reviewed the results of a series of 10 patients (14 feet). At a mean follow-up of 4.3 years, excellent results were noted in 11 feet (78.6%), there was 1 good result (7.1%), 1 fair result (7.1%), and 1 poor result (7.1%). The fair and poor results occurred in feet with mild degenerative changes in the posterior talocalcaneal facet noted preoperatively. These authors noted that none of their patients had any loss of motion of the great toe, and no weakness in toe-off was detected manually or during observation of the patient's gait.[311]

Computerized gait analysis has been used to study a series of patients undergoing resection of middle facet talocalcaneal coalitions.[303] In 11 patients (14 feet), the average age was 17 years, and the average length of follow-up was 6 years. Five feet had resection of the coalition with interposition of fat or tendon, and 9 feet had nothing interposed. Nine feet had excellent or good results (64.3%), and 5 had fair or poor results (35.7%). Gait analysis demonstrated decreased motion of the subtalar joint and ankle in comparison with motion in the contralateral, uninvolved foot (when available) and in comparison with anatomically normal subjects. The authors of this study found no consistent relationship between the result obtained and the age of the patient at the time of operation, no correlation between the clinical result and the duration of symptoms, and no correlation between the tissue interposed (or lack of interposed tissue) and the result obtained. From their data, these researchers concluded that most of the patients improved symptomatically and functionally after resection of the talocalcaneal coalition but that most had a residual functional deficit with abnormal subtalar and ankle joint motion.

Lyon et al.[161] evaluated dynamic plantar pressures and electromyography in patients who underwent resection compared with normal subjects. They found that there was abnormal activity in the peroneal, gastrocnemius, and soleus muscles and increased plantar pressures to the fifth metatarsal head as compared with the normal subjects. They suggest that coalition resection success does not correlate with restoration of normal foot alignment.

Conversely, several other authors have found that activity levels and plantar pressures improved in patients who underwent surgical resection as compared with nonsurgical patients.[211,318-320] Saxena and Erickson[211] performed a retrospective study of 31 patients with 39 coalitions and had a mean follow-up of 3 years. Fifteen patients (17 feet) underwent surgical resection of their tarsal coalition, but the authors did not distinguish between talocalcaneal and calcaneonavicular coalitions. The authors reported no statistically significant difference in the return-to-activity time between talocalcaneal and calcaneonavicular coalitions and found that tarsal coalition resection did not correlate with failure of patients to reach desired activity levels. They concluded that surgical resection of tarsal coalitions has a positive outcome.[211] Giacomozzi and associates[318] performed a prospective study evaluating eight patients (11 feet) with talocalcaneal coalitions. Five patients underwent surgical resection and three did not. The authors also studied five patients without coalitions as a control group. The authors used a Mazur scoring system for clinical and functional assessment. Their results showed improved Mazur scores in surgical patients as well as more normal subtalar and forefoot motion and loading patterns.

Hetsroni and colleagues[319,320] performed a kinematic analysis of subtalar joint motion in three groups. The first group had nine patients with painful tarsal coalitions, three calcaneonavicular and six talocalcaneal. The second group was identical but had undergone surgical resection 2-4 years earlier. The third group was nine patients (18 feet) with no tarsal coalition used as a control group. Passive motion of the subtalar joint was measured, and kinematic analysis of subtalar motion in the coronal plane and in the sagittal plane was performed using a computerized gait analysis system. A statistically significant increase in passive subtalar joint range of motion was noted in the postresection group (group 2) compared to the preoperative group

(group 1). However, the kinematic results performed during walking revealed similar, severe restriction of the subtalar coronal plane motion (ie, inversion and eversion) in both the postoperative group (group 2) and preoperative group (group 1). Angular velocity of the subtalar motion was also similar in both groups 1 and 2 and was significantly increased compared with the control (group 3). The kinematic results of subtalar joint sagittal plane motion revealed that there was partial improvement in subtalar joint position in group 2 as compared to group 1. The authors concluded that despite the favorable clinical outcomes they observed in tarsal coalition patients undergoing resection (AOFAS scale: group 1—54, group 2—81, group 3—100), normal foot kinematics were not recreated. The abnormal kinematics were expressed as severe subtalar motion restriction during walking. The long-term significance of this motion restriction was not studied, but the authors felt one possible implication might be further deterioration of the subtalar joint and adjacent joints.

Attempts have been made using CT scans preoperatively to try to determine whether the size of the coalition affects the result obtained with resection.[243,244] Wilde et al.[243] examined 20 feet in 17 patients, all <16 years of age and each undergoing resection of the coalition. These investigators reported excellent or good results in 10 feet (50%) in patients in whom the preoperative coronal views on the CT scan showed <50% involvement of the posterior facet of the subtalar joint. These patients also had <16 degrees of heel valgus and no radiographic signs of arthritis of the posterior facet of the talocalcaneal joint. In the 10 feet (50%) with fair or poor results, coronal CT sections showed >50% involvement of the posterior facet, and the patients also had >16 degrees of heel valgus and radiographic changes of the posterior facet consistent with arthritis. Like previous authors, these investigators concluded that excellent or good results can be obtained if the coalition involves <50% of the joint, but fair or poor results occur with attempts at resection of larger coalitions.[313]

Similarly, Comfort and Johnson[244] found that the clinical results obtained with resection correlated well with the size of the coalition. These authors reviewed a series of 20 feet undergoing resection of talocalcaneal coalitions (16 patients) in which 17 feet had preoperative CT scans performed. The average patient age was 14.2 years, and their mean follow-up was 2.4 years postoperatively. Unlike Wilde et al.,[243] these authors evaluated all three facets of the subtalar joint and not just the posterior facet. They found 77% excellent or good results when the coalition involved less than one-third of the entire subtalar joint as measured on a coronal CT view. These authors also found that other clinical factors such as the patient's age and weight and plain radiographic findings (talar beaking, talonavicular spur, and narrowing of the posterior facet) did not correlate with the results obtained with resection.

Other authors have also studied the relationship between the size of the talocalcaneal coalition and the outcome following resection and found no direct correlation.[240,241,245] Khoshbin and associates[321] presented a series of 13 talocalcaneal coalition resections with a mean patient age of 11.9 years at the time of operation. These investigators reported reviewing preoperative CT scans on 9 of the feet and noted the mean involvement of the talocalcaneal joint as 57.6% with an average of 16.8 degrees of hindfoot valgus. They reported consistently good functional outcomes at a mean follow-up of 13.1 years, with no noted degradation of outcome in patients with more involvement of the

talocalcaneal joint or larger degrees of heel valgus. Mahan and colleagues[241] reported the results of resection of talocalcaneal coalition in 16 patients (21 feet). CT scans of the feet were reviewed where available and the mean involvement of the talocalcaneal joint was 47%. At a mean follow-up of 4.62 years after surgery, the average AOFAS score was 88.3 with 73% of the patients reporting no restrictions to their activities caused by foot pain. These authors also found no correlation between the size of the coalition or the amount of hindfoot valgus relative to the long-term functional outcome.

Several other reports on smaller series described good results in patients undergoing resection of the coalition through a medial approach with or without autogenous fat graft interposition.[155,200,235,275,288,292,300,305,308,315] In the largest series reported to date, Takakura et al.[135] reported excellent or good results in 31 of 33 (93.9%) talocalcaneal resections at an average of 5.3 years postoperatively.

In 1997, McCormack, Olney, and Asher[307] reevaluated the same series of patients previously reported on by Asher and Mosier[288] in 1983. The eight patients (nine feet) reevaluated had a mean follow-up of 11.5 years, with a minimum follow-up of 10 years. The authors found no deterioration of the results initially reported. At long-term follow-up, the patients had maintained their subtalar joint motion, had no further degenerative changes on plain radiographs, and seven feet in six patients (77.8%) continued to have excellent results.

Several small case reports have advocated the insertion of varying autogenous tissue into the talocalcaneal coalition resection defect. Miyamoto and colleagues[322] described their experience of interposition of a pedicle fatty flap harvested just distal to the resection site from local subcutaneous tissue. Hubert and associates[323] described a series of 12 feet (10 patients) where a pediculated flap of the tibialis posterior tendon sheath was interposed into the resection site. Their mean age at the time of surgery was 12.2 years, and their mean follow-up was 57.2 months. They noted statistically significant reductions in pain at follow-up as measured by preoperative and postoperative VAS scores (mean preoperative score, 7.3; mean postoperative score, 0.3) and AOFAS hindfoot scores (mean preoperative score, 62.9; mean postoperative score, 95.8).

Other authors have reported resection of the coalition with varying additional procedures performed to attempt to decrease the likelihood of recurrent coalition formation and to attempt to maintain improved subtalar joint motion and pedal alignment. Lepow and Richman[305] reported a case treated successfully with resection and arthroereisis. Collins[292] described resection of the coalition through a medial approach with insertion of a condylar implant into the plantar aspect of the talar surface of the resection site. He reported success in five cases that were followed up from 1 to 4 years. Downey[48,49,294,295] also reported the successful resection of tarsal coalitions with the use of an arthroereisis (Fig. 44.32).

In the largest reported series to date incorporating an arthroereisis with resection of the talocalcaneal coalition, Giannini et al.[297] assessed 12 patients (14 feet) after the resection of a talocalcaneal coalition with the insertion of a bioreabsorbable subtalar arthroereisis. Preoperative and postoperative AOFAS scores were obtained with a median improvement from 29 to 90, respectively. They did separate patients under 14 years of age from patients over 14 years and found that age was inversely proportional to the AOFAS score. They also reported improvement in the subtalar joint range of motion, and postoperative

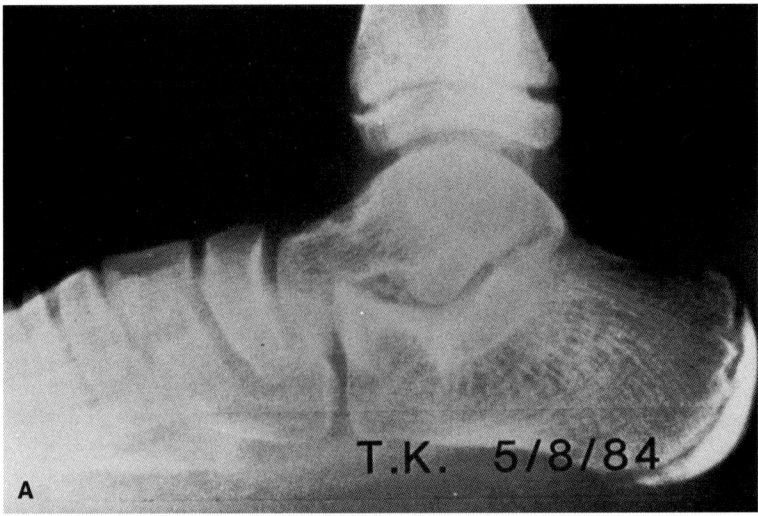

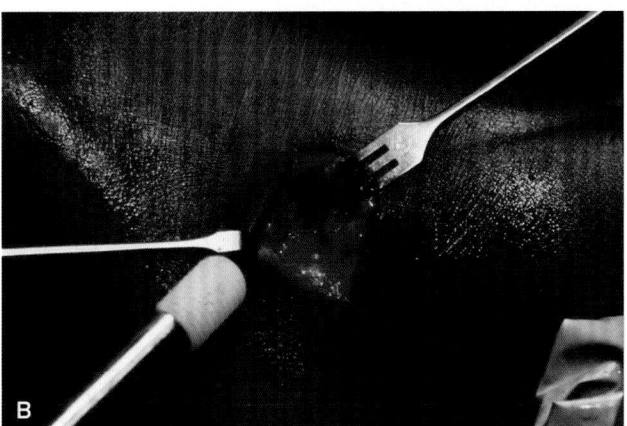
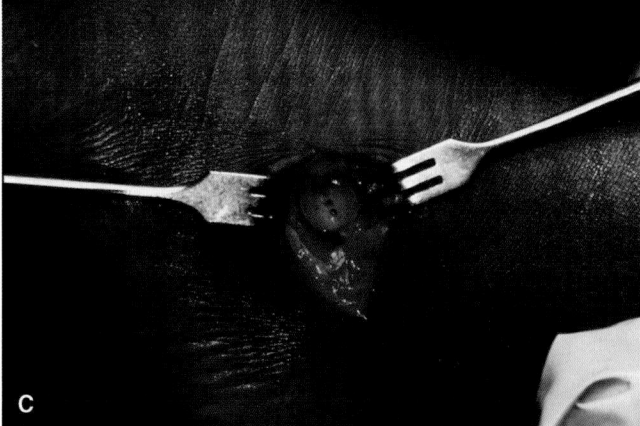

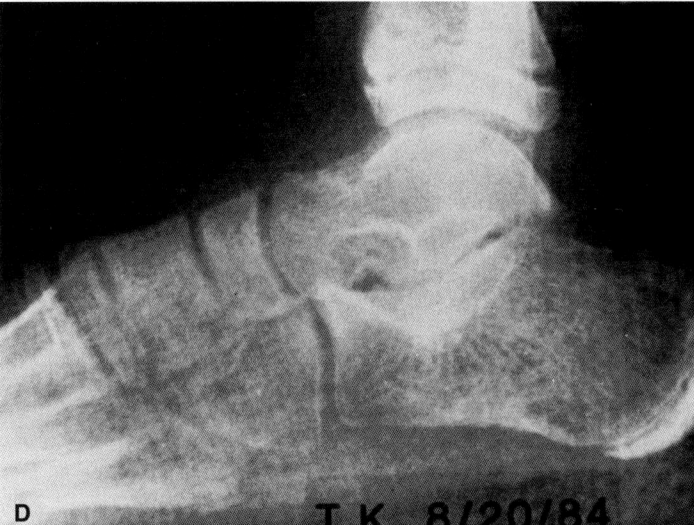

FIGURE 44.32 A. Preoperative lateral view of the left foot in a 12-year-old patient with middle facet talocalcaneal coalition. **B, C.** Insertion of a subtalar joint arthroereisis through a lateral incision over the sinus tarsi. A separate medial incision was used to resect the coalition. **D.** Postoperative lateral view of the foot. Note the improved talocalcaneal relationship and the decrease in the lateral talocalcaneal angle.

CT scans and radiographs performed at a mean of 7 years postoperative demonstrated no recurrence.[297] More recently, in 2016, Krief et al.[324] described the interposition of a silicone sheet into the talocalcaneal resection defect in three cases. They inserted a 0.5-mm reinforced, nondegradable, silicone sheet into the resected space and covered the areas of bone resection. The material was sutured in place with absorbable suture. At a mean follow-up of 48 months, the authors reported an AOFAS score of 100 in their patients.

As with other types of tarsal coalitions, several reports have indicated that varus-producing osteotomies of the calcaneus may afford relief of symptoms in tarsal coalitions without significant secondary arthrosis.[243,249,285,286,298] Many of these authors have suggested that failure of talocalcaneal coalition resection

is due to the degree of hindfoot valgus present. Wilde and associates[243] found that more than 16 degrees of heel valgus correlated with a poor outcome after resection. Luhmann and Schoenecker[249] found no problems with 16 degrees of heel valgus but did find poorer outcomes with resection of talocalcaneal coalitions in patients with more than 21 degrees of heel valgus. These authors suggested either a medializing calcaneal osteotomy or a lateral column lengthening along with resection of a talocalcaneal coalition associated with severe hindfoot valgus. These procedures may be useful adjuncts if concomitant resection of the coalition is attempted, but they should not be performed alone.

With the resection of any tarsal coalition, a preexisting pes valgo planus deformity may potentially become more problematic and/or symptomatic. Kernbach, Blitz, and colleagues[242,290,301,302] have advocated and provided rationale for a single-stage approach with resection of the talocalcaneal coalition and flatfoot reconstruction. They reported good results in six cases in three patients.[302] Lisella et al.[306] reported on a retrospective series of seven consecutive patients (eight feet) who underwent talocalcaneal coalition resection with simultaneous pes valgo planus reconstruction. The authors stated that the clinical and radiographic hindfoot malalignment was reliably corrected. Their reported average increase in medial longitudinal arch height was 8.7 mm. After 2 years, their average AOFAS hindfoot score was 88. The authors concluded that coalition resection and concomitant hindfoot reconstruction is a better option than resection alone or hindfoot fusion in patients with talocalcaneal coalition and painful pes valgo planus deformity. When a tarsal coalition is associated with severe hindfoot valgus, one must address the valgus either conservatively or surgically if the coalition is going to undergoing resection. Whether this should occur in one stage or in two stages is still open to debate.

To summarize, the consensus of current results and opinion supports the conclusion that surgical resection of a symptomatic middle facet talocalcaneal coalition is a reasonable and viable procedure. Some other consensus findings from the literature regarding middle facet talocalcaneal coalition resection include the following:

1. Most studies have been on younger patient populations, and although age does not appear to be a contraindication to resection, younger patients are generally deemed more amenable to resection.
2. The presence of talonavicular joint beaking does not seem to be a contraindication to resection. Narrowing of the talonavicular joint and degenerative changes of the talonavicular joint do appear to be contraindications to resection.
3. The tissue type of the coalition does not seem to be a limiting factor regarding whether resection may or may not be considered. However, incomplete coalitions are generally thought to be more amenable to resection than complete coalitions.
4. Debate continues on whether the size of the coalition may or may not be a contraindication to resection. Patients with coalitions involving <50% of the talocalcaneal joint are considered good candidates for resection. Coalitions involving more than 50% of the talocalcaneal joint may or may not be amenable to resection. The argument over the amount of the joint that may be involved has been arbitrarily set at 50%. Further studies involving resections in coalitions involving more than 50% of the talocalcaneal joint, and specifically looking at the architectural shape of the coalition and composition of the coalition are needed to determine what composition, shape, and percentage of joint involvement preclude a reasonable chance of a good long-term functional outcome with resection.
5. The material interposed in the defect after coalition resection does not appear to influence the results obtained.
6. The degree of pes valgo planus deformity present may affect the postoperative result. The concomitant correction of a pes valgo planus deformity may be appropriate for tarsal coalitions associated with significant and/or painful pes valgo planus deformity.

In the older patient with a talocalcaneal coalition and minimal secondary arthritic changes (adult IIA), arthrodesis is usually the preferred approach. However, if both the patient and the surgeon wish to try resection and realize the potential for failure, then it may be attempted.

In patients with significant arthritic or adaptive involvement or failed resection, arthrodesis is the procedure of choice. Certainly, in the older patient with an intra-articular coalition and arthritic changes (adult IIB), arthrodesis is the procedure of choice. In most instances, triple arthrodesis is preferred. With talocalcaneal coalitions involving the middle facet and without secondary arthritic changes, debate continues on the preferred arthrodesis: isolated subtalar joint arthrodesis or triple arthrodesis. Evidence suggests that isolated subtalar joint arthrodesis generally provides a superior functional result[143,325-329] (Fig. 44.33). Schwartz et al.[329] reported on nine feet (eight patients) who underwent subtalar joint distraction arthrodesis to concomitantly address the talocalcaneal coalition and associated heel valgus. Their patients had a mean age of 11.9 years at the time of surgery. A subtalar joint arthrodesis was performed with the insertion of a wedge-shaped, allogeneic, tricortical, iliac crest bone graft. The graft was inserted into the resected posterior facet of the joint, decreasing the preoperative heel valgus. At a mean follow-up time of 25.5 months, the authors noted a mean AOFAS score of 90.1.

Double or triple arthrodesis may be reserved for cases in which the coalition, although not associated with secondary degenerative changes, demonstrates significant structural abnormalities (eg, profound forefoot varus, hindfoot valgus, or equinus). In such cases, a double or triple arthrodesis is necessary to obtain a structurally acceptable relationship between the forefoot and hindfoot. Most patients with an intra-articular coalition with moderate to severe secondary arthritic changes are optimally treated with a triple arthrodesis after osseous maturity[330] (Fig. 44.34).

Talonavicular Coalition

Talonavicular coalition is another example of intra-articular coalition. The talonavicular coalition is the third most common type of congenital tarsal coalition. Patients are frequently asymptomatic, and the coalition is often discovered only as an incidental finding on radiographs. The absence of the dorsal portion of the normal cyma line is noted on the lateral radiograph. Severe pes valgo planus is frequently associated with a talonavicular coalition.[70-72,75,77,79,80,331]

Surgical resection of the coalition is not a practical alternative in the foot with a symptomatic talonavicular coalition.

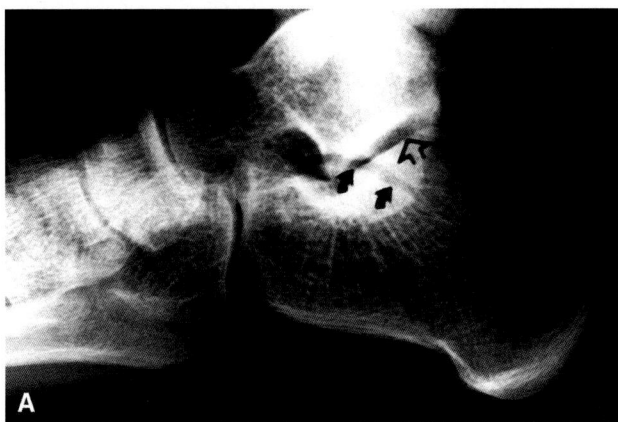

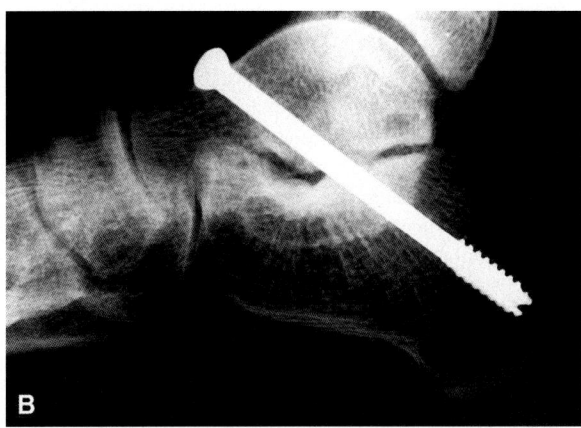

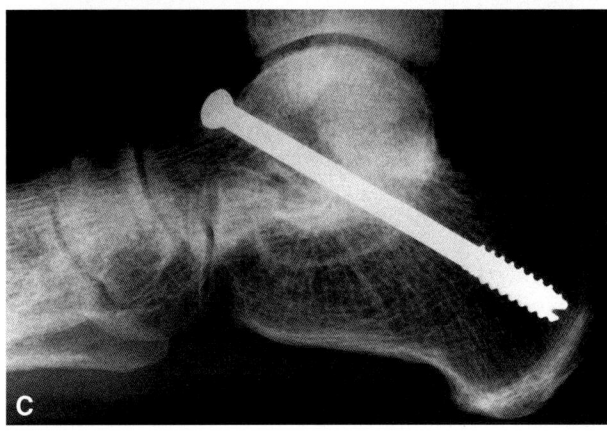

FIGURE 44.33 A. Preoperative lateral radiograph of a 25-year-old patient with an incomplete middle facet talocalcaneal coalition. Note the large and tortuous middle facet (*closed arrows*) and the minimal secondary adaptive and arthritic changes. This is an "adult IIA" coalition or an adult, intra-articular coalition without secondary arthritis. *Open arrow*, posterior subtalar joint facet. **B.** Postoperative lateral view immediately after isolated subtalar joint arthrodesis. **C.** A 1-year postoperative lateral view.

David et al.[331] reported excellent results with the use of orthotic management. If the talonavicular coalition is complete and the subtalar and calcaneocuboid joints are arthritic or demonstrate severe adaptive change, then double arthrodesis of the two joints may be considered. If the talonavicular coalition is incomplete, it may be resected, and a triple arthrodesis may be performed. Occasionally, a talonavicular coalition is associated with severe structural forefoot varus and arthritis of the subtalar and calcaneocuboid joints. If the coalition is a synchondrosis or syndesmosis, the coalition may be resected, and a correctional

triple arthrodesis, including arthrodesis of the resected coalition site, can be achieved. If the coalition is a synostosis or complete coalition, an osteotomy may be made through the coalition and a similar correctional triple arthrodesis may be performed (Fig. 44.35).

In many cases of talonavicular coalition, secondary adaptive or arthritic changes occur at the naviculocuneiform joints. If symptoms occur at the level of the naviculocuneiform joint, isolated naviculocuneiform arthrodesis may be considered.[332]

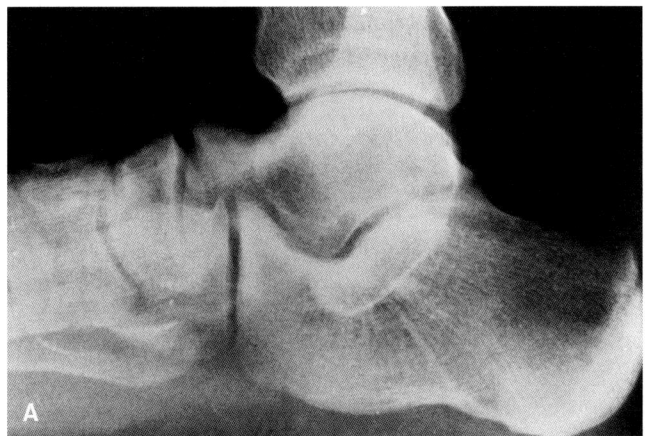

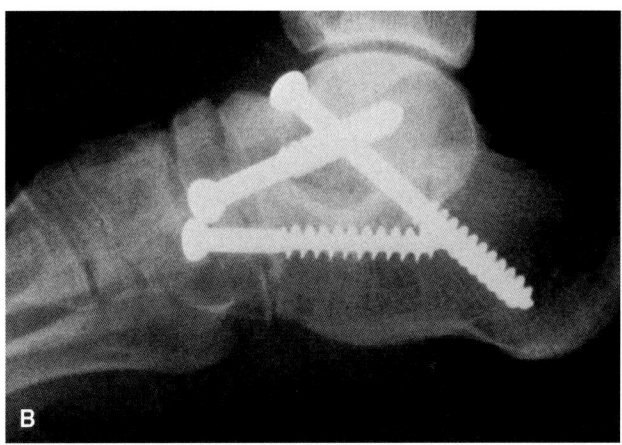

FIGURE 44.34 A. Preoperative lateral radiographic view of middle facet talocalcaneal coalition in a 17-year-old patient. Note the arthritic and adaptive changes including talonavicular and calcaneocuboid joint beaking. This is an "adult IIB" coalition or an "adult, intra-articular coalition with secondary arthritis." **B.** Postoperative lateral view after triple arthrodesis with internal screw fixation.

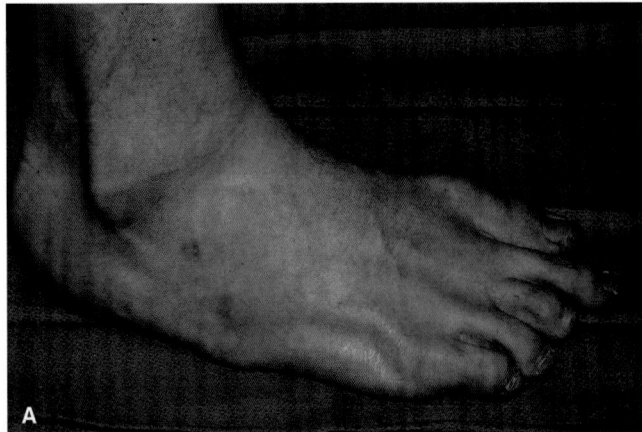

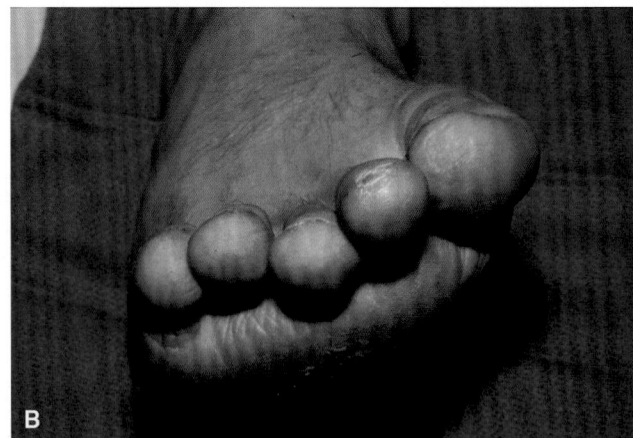

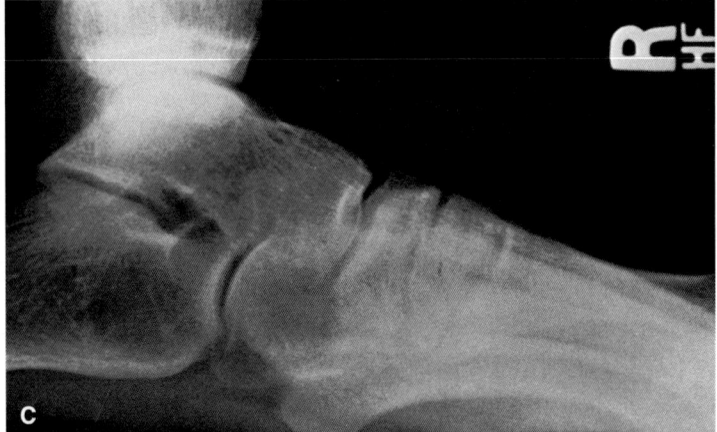

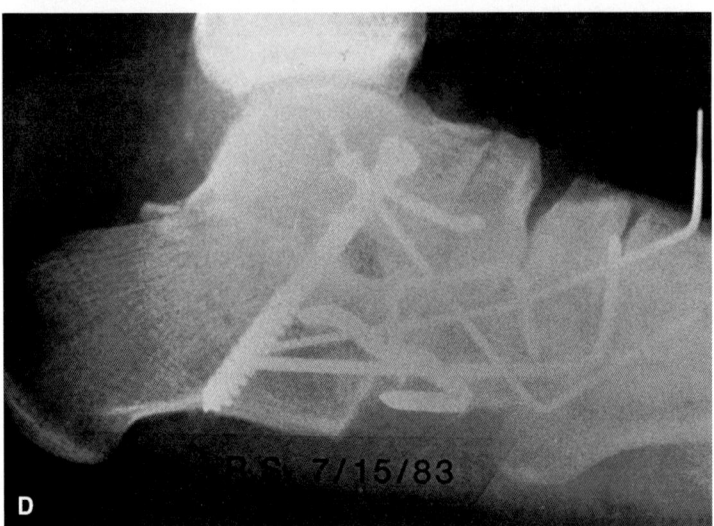

FIGURE 44.35 A, B. Preoperative clinical views of a patient with severe structural forefoot varus secondary to a talonavicular synostosis. The patient complained of pain along the lateral border of the foot. **C.** Preoperative lateral radiograph. Note the elevatus of the medial column. **D.** Postoperative lateral radiograph. Rotational osteotomy was performed through talonavicular coalition with plantar flexion of the medial column. A triple arthrodesis was performed concomitantly.

In other cases of talonavicular coalition, pain may be caused by the presence of a medial navicular prominence or even an accessory navicular. In such cases, the prominence may be resected or the accessory navicular may be excised.[333] Adjunctive surgery for pes valgo planus deformity, if present, may be performed simultaneously.[334]

Calcaneocuboid Coalition

Calcaneocuboid coalitions represent a rare type of intra-articular coalition (Fig. 44.36). When present, they are associated

with a decreased range of motion at the subtalar and midtarsal joints. In addition, other forms of intertarsal strain (eg, forefoot abductus with transverse naviculocuneiform breech) may be noted. Absence of the plantar portion of the normal cyma line is noted on a lateral radiograph.

If conservative therapy does not successfully resolve symptoms, then single arthrodesis of the talonavicular joint or double arthrodesis of the talonavicular and subtalar joints may be considered.[83-85] If significant planus deformity exists, or if the coalition is incomplete, the coalition may be corrected by osteotomy or resection, and angulational correction may be

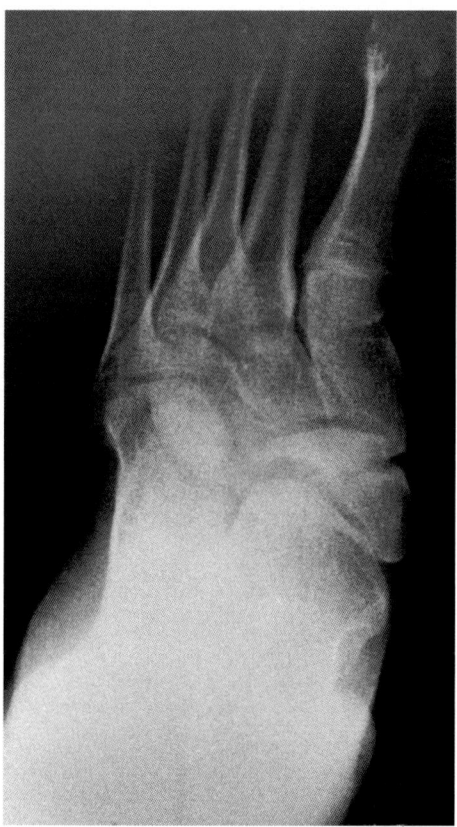

FIGURE 44.36 Example of calcaneocuboid coalition.

achieved with a triple arthrodesis. Isolated resection of a calcaneocuboid coalition has not been reported to be successful.

Cubonavicular Coalition

Cubonavicular coalition is another type of extra-articular coalition, and it usually involves symptoms similar to those of a calcaneonavicular coalition. The coalition is readily visible on a lateral or oblique radiograph and, if desired, can be confirmed with a CT scan or MRI.

Treatment of a cubonavicular coalition is similar to that of a calcaneonavicular coalition. Surgically, Cavallaro and Hadden[86] presented the first detailed description of cubonavicular bar resection. They described a two-incision approach. The first incision was slightly curvilinear and extended from the inferior margin of the talonavicular joint to the first metatarsocuneiform joint. Through this incision, the belly of the abductor hallucis muscle was identified and was retracted plantarly. Dissection was carried laterally along the inferior surface of the navicular. All soft tissue was reflected plantarly until the medial margin of the coalition was encountered. An osteotomy was then performed through the coalition flush with the plantar surface of the navicular. A second curvilinear incision was then made over the dorsolateral aspect of the calcaneocuboid joint. The belly of the extensor digitorum brevis muscle was exposed and was reflected distally from its origin on the calcaneus. Dissection was carried medially over the cuboid until the lateral margin of the coalition was noted. A second osteotomy was then performed in the sagittal plane along the medial surface of the cuboid. The bar was freed and was removed through the plantar medial incision. Any remaining bony prominences were

rasped smooth. If desired, bone wax was used on the bleeding bone ends, and the belly of the extensor digitorum brevis muscle or an autogenous-free fat graft was interposed in the osseous defect. Closure was then afforded over a closed-suction drain. Postoperatively, a below-knee non–weight-bearing cast was applied for 3-4 weeks. The cast could be split or bivalved at any point desired, and subtalar and midtarsal joint range-of-motion exercises begun. Weight bearing was initiated after ~3-6 weeks.

Piqueres et al.[92] reported surgical resection as treatment of a cubonavicular coalition but did not describe their surgical procedure. Johnson et al.[90] presented a case of surgical resection of a cubonavicular coalition through a single lateral incision. The incision placement was similar to the lateral approach for a triple arthrodesis, with the incision extending from just below the lateral malleolus to the fourth metatarsal base. The extensor digitorum brevis was retracted identifying the calcaneocuboid joint and cubonavicular coalition. The coalition was resected, and the remaining bone ends were covered with bone wax. These authors reported that their patient returned to normal activity without pain despite some limitation in subtalar joint and transverse tarsal joint motion.

More recently, several surgeons have recommended resection with the interposition of fat and/or allogenous graft material into the defect. Sarage and colleagues[93] described a small series of cubonavicular coalitions in which they exposed the coalition through a dorsolateral, longitudinal incision centered over the cuboid, and then reflected the extensor digitorum muscle belly distally. The cubonavicular coalition was then resected followed by the insertion of an autogenous adipose tissue graft, they harvested from the anterior lower leg, into the defect. Postoperatively, these authors reported uniformly excellent results in their four cases. Ehredt and associates[88] described a case of an incomplete cubonavicular coalition that they resected with the interposition of cryopreserved amniotic membrane and autogenous fat tissue. These authors advocated a dorsolateral, curvilinear incision that extended from the sinus tarsi to the cubonavicular region distally. The extensor digitorum muscle belly was then freed from its origin on the calcaneus and reflected distally. The cubonavicular coalition was then identified and resected with sharp osteotomes. Next, fibrofatty tissue (Hoke's tonsil) was harvested from the sinus tarsi and wrapped with a 3- × 3-cm piece of cryopreserved amniotic membrane allograft. The combined graft was then interposed in the resection site between the cuboid and navicular. At 2-year follow-up, the authors noted their patient demonstrated the maintenance of increased midfoot motion, no pain upon ambulation, and radiographic preservation of the resection space between the cuboid and navicular.

Surgical Technique

The author's preferred approach for resection of a cubonavicular coalition is similar to the author's preferred approach for a calcaneonavicular coalition resection, as the two coalitions share anatomic proximity. The procedure is done through a lateral curvilinear or Ollier type of incision, beginning over the lateral calcaneus or sinus tarsi area and extending medially to the lateral aspect of the cubonavicular area (Fig. 44.37A). Blunt dissection is carried deep through the subcutaneous layer, with hemostasis obtained as necessary. Care is taken to avoid the intermediate dorsal cutaneous nerve, which courses across the medial extent of the incision, and the sural nerve (lateral dorsal cutaneous nerve), which may be visualized in the lateral margin of the incision. These nerves are uniformly preserved and,

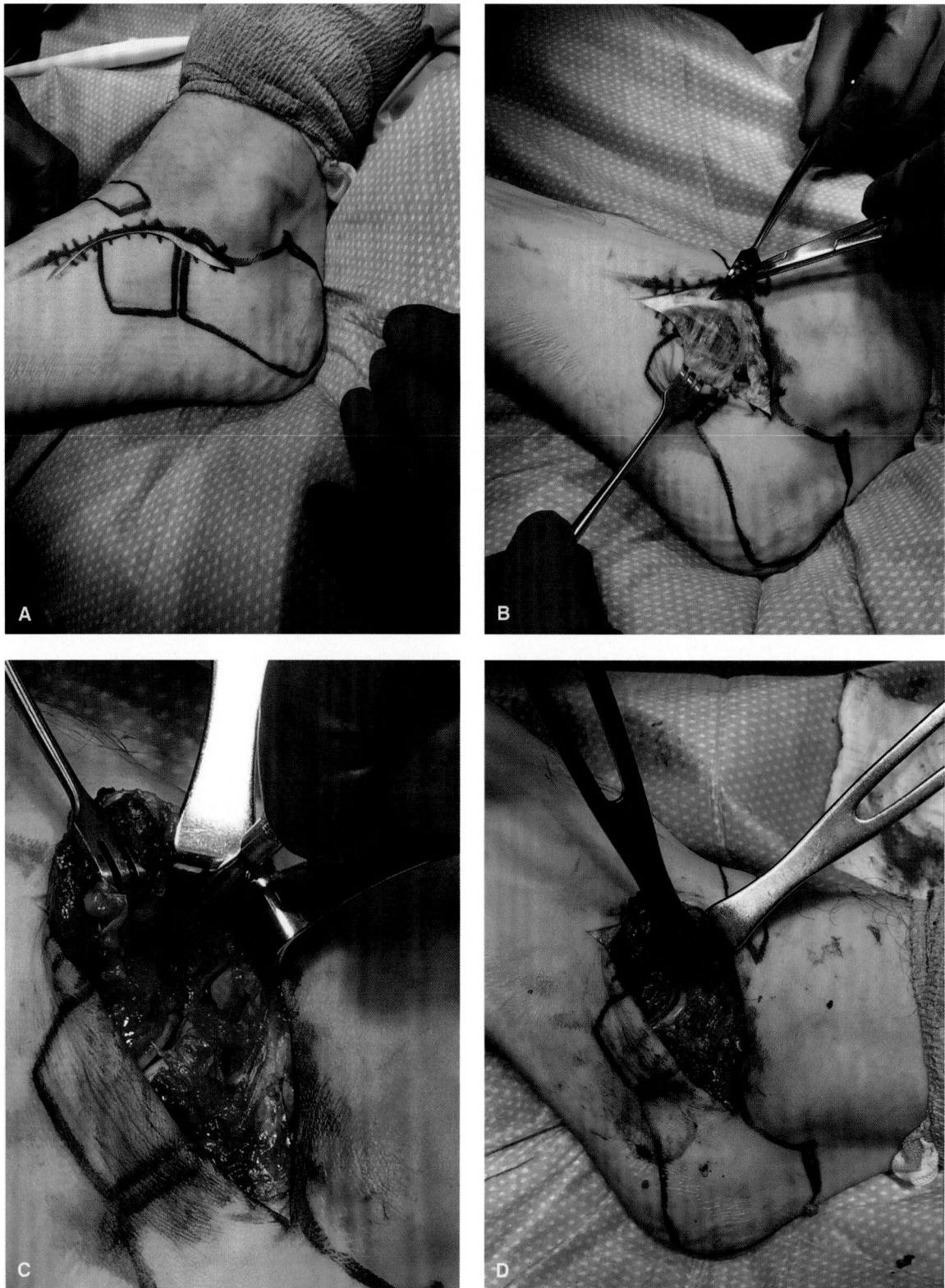

FIGURE 44.37 Surgical demonstration of resection of a cubonavicular bar. **A.** Skin incision placement. Dorsolateral, curvilinear approach starting at the sinus tarsi and extending medially to the lateral aspect of the cubonavicular area. **B.** Dissection is carried to the level of the deep fascia. The belly of the extensor digitorum brevis muscle is apparent as is the peroneus tertius in the dorsomedial portion of the wound. **C.** The belly of the extensor digitorum brevis muscle is freed from its origin and is reflected distally. The cubonavicular bar is readily appreciated between the cuboid and navicular. **D.** The bar is resected in the form of a rectangular piece of bone and the resultant defect between the cuboid and navicular is appreciated.

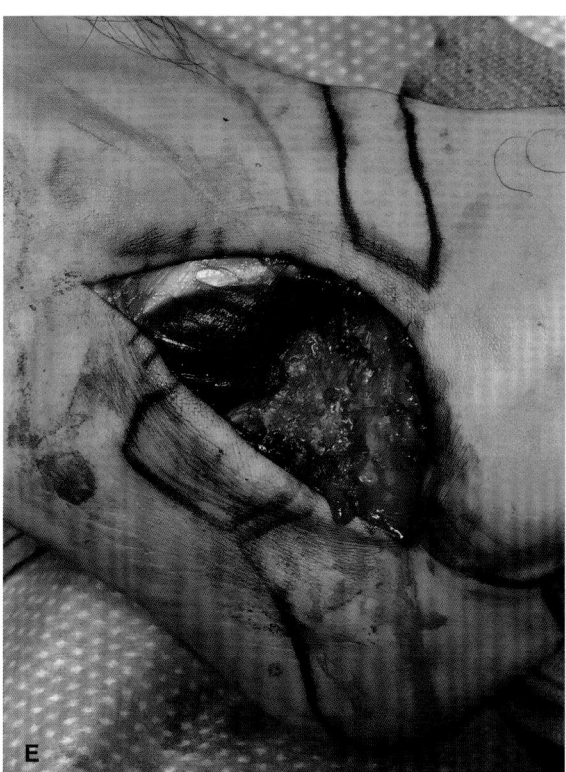
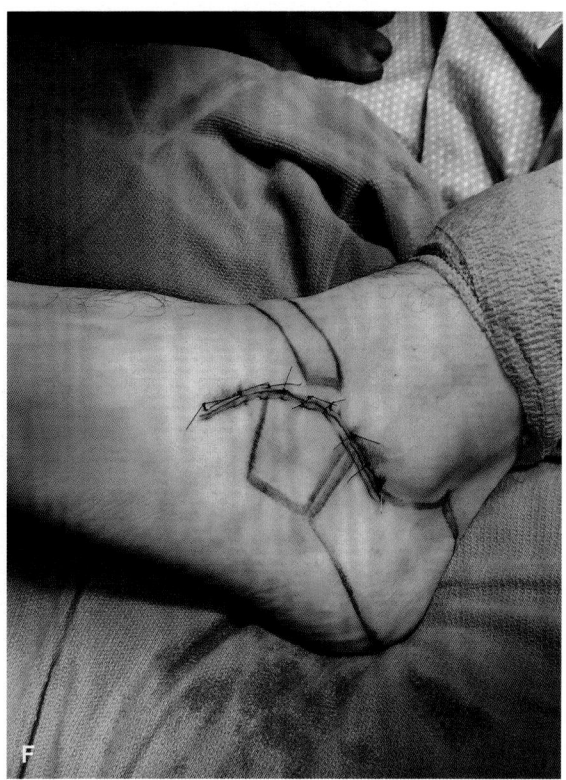

FIGURE 44.37 (*Continued*) **E.** The muscle is sutured into the osseous void created by the bar resection. **F.** Layer wound closure is achieved.

if identified, are gently retracted. Occasionally, a small neural communicating branch between the sural (lateral dorsal cutaneous) and intermediate dorsal cutaneous nerves is noted. In some cases, this small branch may have to be sacrificed to afford optimal exposure. The subcutaneous tissue is then bluntly reflected from the deep fascia revealing the extensor digitorum brevis muscle belly (Fig. 44.37B). The origin of the extensor digitorum brevis is then reflected off the calcaneus and is retracted distally. All soft tissue is freed from the cubonavicular coalition (Fig. 44.37C). The cubonavicular bar is generously resected, with removal of as much bone as possible without damaging the supportive structure of either bone (Fig. 44.37D). Any remaining prominences of bone may be rasped smooth. If desired, bone wax may be applied after the area is rasped or cauterized. A large absorbable suture is then placed through the proximal portion of the muscle belly. With the use of straight Keith needles, the extensor digitorum brevis muscle belly is then passed into the defect (Fig. 44.37E). The suture may be directed plantar medially and sutured over a button on the plantar medial aspect of the foot. Alternatively, an internal suture technique or bone anchor in which the muscle is anchored to soft tissue or bone may be employed. The author does not typically insert any other tissue in the resected area. Once the muscle is sutured in the defect, a closed suction drain may be inserted if desired, and anatomic layer closure is performed (Fig. 44.37F). Postoperatively, a below-knee, non–weight-bearing cast is applied for 3-4 weeks. The cast may be split or bivalved at any point desired, and subtalar and midtarsal joint range-of-motion exercises may be initiated. Weight bearing is initiated after ~3-6 weeks.

Other Coalitions

Naviculocuneiform, first cuneometatarsal, multiple, and massive coalitions are rare. When they are present and cause symptoms, a treatment plan is devised to limit abnormal motion. If conservative treatment fails, then appropriate arthrodesis procedures are performed. Using the articular classification system, one may formulate an acceptable approach for almost any type of coalition (Table 44.6).

TABLE 44.6 Possible Surgical Procedures Based on Articular Classification System[a]
Juvenile: IA
Resection alone
Resection with interposition of EDB muscle
Resection with interposition of adipose tissue
Resection with varus-producing calcaneal osteotomy
Resection with insertion of implant
Varus-producing calcaneal osteotomy alone
Juvenile: IB
Resection alone
Resection with interposition of EDB muscle
Resection with interposition of adipose tissue
Resection with varus-producing calcaneal osteotomy
Resection with insertion of implant
Varus-producing calcaneal osteotomy alone
Double arthrodesis/triple arthrodesis

TABLE 44.6	Possible Surgical Procedures Based on Articular Classification System[a] (*Continued*)

Juvenile: IIA
  Resection alone
  Resection with interposition of adipose tissue
  Resection with interposition of arthroereisis
  Resection with varus-producing calcaneal osteotomy
  Varus-producing calcaneal osteotomy alone
  Isolated/single arthrodesis
  Double arthrodesis/triple arthrodesis

Juvenile: IIB
  Resection alone
  Resection with interposition of adipose tissue
  Resection with interposition of arthroereisis
  Resection with varus-producing calcaneal osteotomy
  Varus-producing calcaneal osteotomy alone
  Isolated/single arthrodesis
  Double arthrodesis/triple arthrodesis

Adult: IA
  Resection alone
  Resection with interposition of EDB muscle
  Resection with interposition of adipose tissue
  Resection with varus-producing calcaneal osteotomy
  Resection with insertion of implant
  Varus-producing calcaneal osteotomy alone
  Double arthrodesis/triple arthrodesis

Adult: IB
  Resection with isolated/single arthrodesis
  Double arthrodesis/triple arthrodesis

Adult: IIA
  Isolated or single arthrodesis
  Double arthrodesis/triple arthrodesis

Adult: IIB
  Double arthrodesis/triple arthrodesis

[a]Procedures listed in **bold type** are currently recommended.

EDB, extensor digitorum brevis.

SUMMARY

An in-depth review of tarsal coalitions, including a surgical articular classification system with specific references to treatment, has been presented. A working knowledge of the clinical findings, roentgenographic findings, and advanced diagnostic imaging findings is imperative to the construction of a logical treatment plan. When based on the articular classification system, recommended surgical procedures and the report of long-term results may be more accurately related and reported. The management of tarsal coalitions continues to evolve and as larger and more long-term results are elucidated, treatment protocols will continue to be modified and improved.

REFERENCES

1. Heiple KG, Lovejoy CO. The antiquity of tarsal coalition: bilateral deformity in a pre-Columbian Indian skeleton. *J Bone Joint Surg Am.* 1969;51:979-983.
2. Coe WR, Broman VL. *Excavations in Stella 23 Group.* University of Pennsylvania Museum Monographs. Tikal reports, no. 2. Philadelphia, PA: University Museum, University of Pennsylvania; 1958.
3. Silva AM. Non-osseous calcaneonavicular coalition in the Portuguese prehistoric population: report of two cases. *Int J Osteoarchaeol.* 2005;15:449-453.
4. Buffon GLL de C. *Histoire naturelle, générale et particulière: avec la description du cabinet du roy.* Vol. 3. Paris: Imprimerie-royale; 1769:47.
5. Jones R. Peroneal spasm, and its treatment. *Liverpool Med Chir J.* 1897;17:442.
6. Kirmisson E. Double pied bot varus par malformation osseuse primitive associé à des ankyloses congenitales des doigts et des orteils chez quarte membres d'une meme famille. *Rev Orthop.* 1898;9:392-398.
7. Cruveilhier A. *Anatomie pathologique du corps humain.* Vol. 1. Paris: JB Baillière; 1829.
8. Slomann HC. On coalitio calcaneo-navicularis. *J Orthop Surg.* 1921;3:586-602.
9. Badgley CE. Coalition of the calcaneus and the navicular. *Arch Surg.* 1927;15:75-88.
10. Zuckerkandl E. Uber einen fall von Synostose zwischen Talus und Calcaneus. *Allgemeine Weine Med Zeitung.* 1877;22:293-294.
11. Korvin H. Coalitio talocalcanea. *Z Orthop Chir.* 1934;60:105-110.
12. Harris RI, Beath T. Etiology of peroneal spastic flat foot. *J Bone Joint Surg Br.* 1948;30:624-634.
13. Anderson RJ. The presence of an astragalo-scaphoid bone in man. *J Anat Physiol.* 1879–1880;14:452-455.
14. Holland CT. Two cases of rare deformity of feet and hands. *Arch Radiol Electrother.* 1918;22:234-239.
15. Waugh W. Partial cubonavicular coalition as a cause of peroneal spastic flat foot. *J Bone Joint Surg Br.* 1957;39:520-523.
16. Lusby HLJ. Naviculo-cuneiform synostosis. *J Bone Joint Surg Br.* 1959;41:150.
17. Bersani FA, Samilson RL. Massive familial tarsal synostosis. *J Bone Joint Surg Am.* 1957;39:1187-1190.
18. Clarke DM. Multiple tarsal coalitions in the same foot. *J Pediatr Orthop.* 1997;17:777-780.
19. Farid A, Faber FWM. Bilateral triple talocalcaneal, calcaneonavicular, and talonavicular tarsal coalition: a case report. *J Foot Ankle Surg.* 2019;58:374-376.
20. Schwalbe G, ed. Morphologisches Arbeiten. In: Schwalbe G, ed. *Beitrage zur Kenntnis des mensch-lichen Extremitatenskelets. VII. Die Variationem im aufbau des Fuskelets.* Vol. 6. Jena, Germany: Gustav Fischer; 1896:245-257.
21. Bentzon PGK. Bilateral congenital deformity of the astragalocalcanean joint: bony coalescence between os trigonum and the calcaneus? *Acta Orthop Scand.* 1930;1:359-364.
22. Outland T, Murphy ID. The pathomechanics of peroneal spastic flat foot. *Clin Orthop.* 1960;16:64-73.
23. Galinski AW, Crovo RT, Ditmars JJ Jr. Os trigonum as a cause of tarsal coalition. *J Am Podiatry Assoc.* 1979;69:191-196.
24. Harris BJ. Anomalous structures in the developing human foot (abstract). *Anat Rec.* 1955;121:399.
25. Leboucq H. De la soudure congenitale de certains os du tarse. *Bull Acad R Med Belg.* 1890;4:103-112.
26. Boyd HB. Congenital talonavicular synostosis. *J Bone Joint Surg.* 1944;26:682-686.
27. Glessner JR Jr, Davis GL. Bilateral calcaneonavicular coalition occurring in twin boys: a case report. *Clin Orthop.* 1966;47:173-176.
28. Hodgson FG. Talonavicular synostosis. *South Med J.* 1946;39:940-941.
29. Schlefman BS. Tarsal coalition. In: McGlamry ED, Banks AS, Downey MS, eds. *Comprehensive Textbook of Foot Surgery.* Baltimore, MD: Lippincott Williams & Wilkins; 1987:483-507.
30. Pensieri SL, Jay RM, Schoenhaus HD, et al. Bilateral congenital calcaneocuboid synostosis and subtalar joint coalition. *J Am Podiatr Med Assoc.* 1985;75:406-410.
31. Plotkin S. Case presentation of calcaneonavicular coalition in monozygotic twins. *J Am Podiatr Med Assoc.* 1996;86:433-438.
32. Rothberg AS, Feldman JW, Schuster OF. Congenital fusion of astragalus and scaphoid: bilateral; inherited. *N Y State J Med.* 1935;35:29-31.
33. Webster FS, Roberts WM. Tarsal anomalies and peroneal spastic flatfoot. *JAMA.* 1951;146:1099-1104.
34. Wray JB, Herndon CN. Hereditary transmission of congenital coalition of the calcaneus to the navicular. *J Bone Joint Surg Am.* 1963;45:365-372.
35. Leonard MA. The inheritance of tarsal coalition and its relationship to spastic flat foot. *J Bone Joint Surg Br.* 1974;56:520-526.
36. Kawashima T, Uhthoff HK. Prenatal development around the sustentaculum tali and its relation to talocalcaneal coalitions. *J Pediatr Orthop.* 1990;10:238-243.
37. Kumai T, Takakura Y, Akiyama K, et al. Histopathological study of nonosseous tarsal coalition. *Foot Ankle Int.* 1998;19:525-531.
38. Takano K, Ogasawara N, Matsunaga T, et al. A novel nonsense mutation in the NOG gene causes familial NOG-related symphalangism spectrum disorder. *Hum Genome Var.* 2016;3:16023.
39. Page JC. Peroneal spastic flatfoot and tarsal coalitions. *J Am Podiatr Med Assoc.* 1987;77:29-34.
40. Downey MS, Ruch JA. Juvenile spastic flatfoot: tarsal coalition. In: McGlamry ED, ed. *Categoric Foot Rehabilitation.* Tucker, GA: Doctors Hospital Podiatric Education and Research Institute; 1985:56-60.
41. Gold GS Jr. Tarsal coalitions: clinical significance, diagnosis and treatment. *J Am Podiatry Assoc.* 1971;61:409-422.
42. Lapidus PW. Congenital fusion of the bones of the foot: with a report of a case of congenital astragaloscaphoid fusion. *J Bone Joint Surg.* 1932;14:888-894.
43. Johnson JC. Peroneal spastic flatfoot syndrome. *South Med J.* 1976;69:807-809.
44. Healey LA, Willkens RF. Tarsal arthritis with ankylosis in late onset Still's disease. *Arthritis Rheum.* 1982;25:1254-1256.
45. Garcia-Morteo O, Gusis SE, Somma LF, et al. Tarsal ankylosis in juvenile and adult onset rheumatoid arthritis. *J Rheumatol.* 1988;15:298-300.
46. Roth RD. Tarsal ankylosis in juvenile ankylosing spondylitis. *J Am Podiatr Med Assoc.* 1986;76:514-518.
47. Ertel AN, O'Connell FD. Case report: talonavicular coalition following avascular necrosis of the tarsal navicular. *J Pediatr Orthop.* 1984;4:482-484.
48. Downey MS. Tarsal coalition. In: Banks AS, Downey MS, Martin DE, Miller SJ, eds. *McGlamry's Comprehensive Textbook of Foot and Ankle Surgery.* 3rd ed. Philadelphia, PA: Lippincott Williams & Wilkins; 2001:993-1031.

49. Downey M, DeWaters AM. Tarsal coalition. In: Southerland JT, Boberg JS, Downey MS, Nakra A, Rabjohn LV, eds. *McGlamry's Comprehensive Textbook of Foot and Ankle Surgery.* 4th ed. Philadelphia, PA: Wolters Kluwer/Lippincott Williams & Wilkins; 2013:598-635.
50. Rankin EA, Baker GI. Rigid flatfoot in the young adult. *Clin Orthop.* 1974;104:244-248.
51. Shands AR Jr, Wentz IJ. Congenital anomalies, accessory bones, and osteochondritis in the feet of 850 children. *Surg Clin North Am.* 1953;33:1643-1666.
52. Vaughan WH, Segal G. Tarsal coalition, with special reference to roentgenographic interpretation. *Radiology.* 1953;60:855-863.
53. Beckly DE, Anderson PW, Pedegana LR. The radiology of the subtalar joint with special reference to talo-calcaneal coalition. *Clin Radiol.* 1975;26:333-341.
54. Conway JJ, Cowell HR. Tarsal coalition: clinical significance and roentgenographic demonstration. *Radiology.* 1969;92:799-811.
55. Ehrlich MG, Elmer EB. Tarsal coalition. In: Jahss MH, ed. *Disorders of the Foot and Ankle: Medical and Surgical Management.* Philadelphia, PA: WB Saunders; 1991:921-940.
56. Perlman MD, Wertheimer SJ. Tarsal coalitions. *J Foot Surg.* 1986;25:58-67.
57. Harris RI. Follow-up notes on articles previously published in the journal: retrospect—peroneal spastic flat foot (rigid valgus foot). *J Bone Joint Surg Am.* 1965;47:1657-1667.
58. Braddock GTF. A prolonged follow-up of peroneal spastic flat foot. *J Bone Joint Surg Br.* 1961;43:734-737.
59. Coventry MB. Flatfoot, with special consideration of tarsal coalition. *Minn Med.* 1950;33:1091-1103.
60. Jack EA. Bone anomalies of the tarsus in relation to "peroneal spastic flat foot." *J Bone Joint Surg Br.* 1954;36:530-542.
61. Kneifati A, Frankovitch KF. Operative intervention for symptomatic tarsal coalition. *Orthop Rev.* 1981;10:87-88.
62. Stormont DM, Peterson HA. The relative incidence of tarsal coalition. *Clin Orthop.* 1983;181:28-36.
63. Bonk JH, Tozzi MA. Congenital talonavicular synostosis: a review of the literature and a case report. *J Am Podiatr Med Assoc.* 1989;79:186-189.
64. Bullitt JB. Variations of the bones of the foot: fusion of the talus and navicular, bilateral and congenital. *Am J Surg.* 1928;20:548-550.
65. Challis J. Hereditary transmission of talonavicular coalition in association with anomaly of the little finger. *J Bone Joint Surg Am.* 1974;56:1273-1276.
66. Frost RA, Fagan JP. Bilateral talonavicular and calcaneocuboid joint coalition [Letter]. *J Am Podiatr Med Assoc.* 1995;85:339-341.
67. Geelhoed GW, Neel JV, Davidson RT. Symphalangism and tarsal coalitions: a hereditary syndrome. A report on two families. *J Bone Joint Surg Br.* 1969;51:278-289.
68. Gill PW, Sullivan RW. Talonavicular coalitions: a review and case report. *J Am Podiatr Med Assoc.* 1985;75:443-445.
69. Illievitz AB. Congenital malformations of the feet: report of a case of congenital fusion of the scaphoid with the astragalus and complete absence of one toe. *Am J Surg.* 1928;4:550-552.
70. Lapidus PW. Bilateral congenital talonavicular fusion: report of a case. *J Bone Joint Surg.* 1938;20:775-777.
71. Lewis SD, Chew FS. Incidental discovery of isolated talonavicular coalition: report of two cases. *Radiol Case Rep.* 2019;14:1156-1158.
72. Macera A, Teodonno F, Carulli C, Frances Borrego A, Innocenti M. Talonavicular coalition as a cause of foot pain. *Joints.* 2017;5(4):246-248.
73. Migues A, Slullitel GA, Suarez E, Galan HL. Case reports: symptomatic bilateral talonavicular coalition. *Clin Orthop Relat Res.* 2009;467:288-292.
74. Person V, Lembach L. Six cases of tarsal coalition in children aged 4 to 12 years. *J Am Podiatr Med Assoc.* 1985;75:320-323.
75. Pontious J, Hillstrom HJ, Monahan T, et al. Talonavicular coalition: objective gait analysis. *J Am Podiatr Med Assoc.* 1993;83:379-385.
76. Rosen JS. Tarsal coalitions: rare or not. *J Am Podiatry Assoc.* 1984;74:572-574.
77. Sanghi JK, Roby HR. Bilateral peroneal spastic flat feet associated with congenital fusion of the navicular and talus: a case report. *J Bone Joint Surg Am.* 1961;43:1237-1240.
78. Schreiber RR. Talonavicular synostosis. *J Bone Joint Surg Am.* 1963;45:170-172.
79. Shtofmakher G, Rozenstrauch A, Cohen R. An incidental talonavicular coalition in a diabetic patient: a podiatric perspective. *BMJ Case Rep.* 2014;10:1136.
80. Spector AJ, Schoenhaus HD. Gait analysis of a unilateral talonavicular synostosis: a case study. *J Am Podiatr Med Assoc.* 1991;81:267-275.
81. Brobeck O. Congenital bilateral synostosis of the calcaneus and cuboid and of the triquetral and hamate bones: report of a case. *Acta Orthop Scand.* 1957;26:217-221.
82. Craig CL, Goldberg MJ. Calcaneocuboid coalition in Crouzon's syndrome (craniofacial dysostosis): report of a case and review of the literature. *J Bone Joint Surg Am.* 1977;59:826-827.
83. Mahaffey HW. Bilateral congenital calcaneocuboid synostosis: a case report. *J Bone Joint Surg.* 1945;27:164-165.
84. Veneruso LC. Unilateral congenital calcaneocuboid synostosis with complete absence of a metatarsal and toe. *J Bone Joint Surg.* 1945;27:718-719.
85. Wagoner GW. A case of bilateral congenital fusion of the calcanei and cuboids. *J Bone Joint Surg.* 1928;26:220-223.
86. Cavallaro DC, Hadden HR. An unusual case of tarsal coalition: a cuboid navicular synostosis. *J Am Podiatry Assoc.* 1978;68:71-75.
87. Del Sel JM, Grand NE. Cubo-navicular synostosis. *J Bone Joint Surg Br.* 1959;41:149.
88. Ehredt DJ, Zulauf EE, Kim HM, Connors J. Cryopreserved amniotic membrane and autogenous adipose tissue as an interpositional spacer after resection of a cubonavicular coalition: a case report and review of the literature. *J Foot Ankle Surg.* 2020;59:173-177.
89. Garcia-Mata S, Hidalgo-Ovejero A. Cuboid-navicular tarsal coalition in an athlete. *An Sist Sanit Navar.* 2011;34:289-292.
90. Johnson TR, Mizel MS, Temple T. Cuboid-navicular tarsal coalition—presentation and treatment: a case report and review of the literature. *Foot Ankle Int.* 2005;26:264-266.
91. Palladino SJ, Schiller L, Johnson JD. Cubonavicular coalition. *J Am Podiatr Med Assoc.* 1991;81:262-266.
92. Piqueres X, de Zabala S, Torrens C, Marin M. Cubonavicular coalition: a case report and literature review. *Clin Orthop Relat Res.* 2002;296:112-114.
93. Sarage AL, Gambardella GV, Fullem B, Saxena A, Caminear DS. Cuboid-navicular tarsal coalition: report of a small case series with description of a surgical approach for resection. *J Foot Ankle Surg.* 2012;51:783-786.
94. Green MR, Yanklowitz B. Asymptomatic naviculocuneiform synostosis with a ganglion cyst. *J Foot Surg.* 1992;31:272-275.
95. Gregersen HN. Naviculocuneiform coalition. *J Bone Joint Surg Am.* 1977;59:128-129.
96. Hynes RA, Romash MM. Bilateral symmetrical synchondrosis of navicular first cuneiform joint presenting as a lytic lesion. *Foot Ankle.* 1987;8:164-168.
97. Kumai T, Tanaka Y, Takakura Y, et al. Isolated first naviculocuneiform joint coalition. *Foot Ankle Int.* 1996;17:635-640.
98. Miki T, Oka M, Shima M, et al. Naviculo-cuneiform coalition: a case report. *J Foot Surg.* 1979;18:81-82.
99. Miki T, Yamamuro T, Iida H, et al. Naviculo-cuneiform coalition: a report of two cases. *Clin Orthop.* 1985;196:256-259.
100. Nakajima Y, Hasegawa A, Kimura M, et al. Naviculo-first cuneiform coalition occurring in a family. *J Jpn Soc Surg Foot.* 1994;15:107-110.
101. Ross JR, Dobbs MB. Isolated navicular-medial cuneiform tarsal coalition revisited: a case report. *J Pediatr Orthop.* 2011;31:e85-e88.
102. Sato K, Sugiura S. Naviculo-cuneiform coalition: report of three cases. *J Jpn Orthop Assoc.* 1990;64:1-6.
103. Wiles S, Palladino SJ, Stavosky JW. Naviculocuneiform coalition. *J Am Podiatr Med Assoc.* 1988;78:355-360.
104. Zwierzchowski H, Bartkowich E, Zalech H. Congenital cuneiform-navicular synostosis. *Chir Narzadow Ruchu Ortop Pol.* 1980;45:49-52.
105. Day FN III, Naples JJ, White J. Metatarsocuneiform coalition [Letter]. *J Am Podiatr Med Assoc.* 1994;84:197-199.
106. Fujishiro T, Nabeshima Y, Yasui S, Fujita I, Yoshiya S, Fujii H. Coalition of bilateral first cuneometatarsal joints: a case report. *Foot Ankle Int.* 2003;24:793-795.
107. Stevens BW, Kolodziej P. Non-osseous tarsal coalition of the lateral cuneiform-third metatarsal joint. *Foot Ankle Int.* 2008;29:867-870.
108. Drinkwater H. Phalangeal anarthrosis (synostosis, ankylosis) transmitted through fourteen generations. *Proc R Soc Med.* 1917;10:60-68.
109. Austin FH. Symphalangism and related fusions of tarsal bones. *Radiology.* 1951;56:882-885.
110. Harle TS, Stevenson JR. Hereditary symphalangism associated with carpal and tarsal fusions. *Radiology.* 1967;89:91-94.
111. Gaal SA, Doyle JR, Larsen IJ. Symphalangism in Hawaii: a study of three distinct ethnic pedigrees. *J Hand Surg [Am].* 1988;13:783-787.
112. Castle JE, Bass S, Kanat IO. Hereditary symphalangism with associated tarsal synostosis and hypophalangism. *J Am Podiatr Med Assoc.* 1993;83:1-9.
113. Boccio JR, Dockery GL, LeBaron S. Congenital metatarsal synostosis. *J Foot Surg.* 1984;23:41-45.
114. O'Rahilly R. A survey of carpal and tarsal anomalies. *J Bone Joint Surg Am.* 1953;35:626-642.
115. Baek GH, Kim JK, Chung MS, Lee SK. Terminal hemimelia of the lower extremity: absent lateral ray and a normal fibula. *Int Orthop.* 2008;32:263-267.
116. Grogan DP, Holt GR, Ogden JA. Talocalcaneal coalition in patients who have fibular hemimelia or proximal femoral focal deficiency: a comparison of the radiographic and pathological findings. *J Bone Joint Surg Am.* 1994;76:1363-1370.
117. Searle CP, Hildebrand RK, Lester EL, Caskey PM. Findings of fibular hemimelia syndrome with radiographically normal fibulae. *J Pediatr Orthop B.* 2004;13:184-188.
118. Turker R, Mendelson S, Ackman J, et al. Anatomic considerations of the foot and leg in tibial hemimelia. *J Pediatr Orthop.* 1996;16:445-449.
119. Lamb D. The ball and socket ankle joint: a congenital abnormality. *J Bone Joint Surg Br.* 1958;40:240-243.
120. Cetinus E, Uzel M, Bilgic E, Karaoguz A. [A case of ball-and-socket deformity of the ankle joint]. *Acta Orthop Traumatol Turc.* 2003;37:406-409.
121. Nievergelt K. Positiver Vaterschaftsnachweis auf grund erblicher Missbildungen der Extremitaten. *Arch Kalus Stift Verebungforsch.* 1944;19:157-195.
122. Pearlman HS, Edkin RE, Warren RF. Familial tarsal and carpal synostosis with radial-head subluxation (Nievergelt's syndrome). *J Bone Joint Surg Am.* 1964;46:585-592.
123. Dubois HJ. Nievergelt-Pearlman syndrome: synostosis in feet and hands with dysplasia of elbows. Report of a case. *J Bone Joint Surg Br.* 1970;52:325-329.
124. Murakami Y. Nievergelt-Pearlman syndrome with impairment of hearing: report of three cases in a family. *J Bone Joint Surg Br.* 1975;57:367-372.
125. Nixon JR. The multiple synostoses syndrome: a plea for simplicity. *Clin Orthop.* 1978;135:48-51.
126. Tachdjian MO. *The Child's Foot.* Philadelphia, PA: WB Saunders; 1985:261-294.
127. Collins ED, Marsh JL, Vannier MW, et al. Spatial dysmorphology of the foot in Apert syndrome: three-dimensional computed tomography. *Cleft Palate Craniofac J.* 1995;32:255-261.
128. Osebold WR, Opitz JM, Remondini DJ, et al. An autosomal dominant syndrome of short stature with mesomelic shortness of limbs, abnormal carpal and tarsal bones, hypoplastic middle phalanges, and bipartite calcanei. *Am J Med Genet.* 1985;22:791-809.
129. Opitz JM, Gilbert EF. Autopsy findings in a stillborn female infant with the Osebold-Remondini syndrome. *Am J Med Genet.* 1985;22:811-819.
130. Callahan RA. Talipes equinovarus associated with an absent posterior tibial tendon and a tarsal coalition: a case report. *Clin Orthop.* 1980;146:231-233.
131. Grant AD, Rose D, Lehman W. Talocalcaneal coalition in arthrogryposis multiplex congenita. *Bull Hosp Jt Dis Orthop Inst.* 1982;42:236-241.
132. Spero CR, Simon GS, Tornetta P III. Clubfeet and tarsal coalition. *J Pediatr Orthop.* 1994;14:372-376.

133. Stocker B, Reichel H, Nelitz M. [Tarsal coalitions: a rare differential diagnosis of congenital clubfoot]. *Z Orthop Unfall.* 2009;147:424-426.

134. Turco VJ. Resistant congenital club foot-one-stage posteromedial release with internal fixation: a follow-up report of a fifteen-year experience. *J Bone Joint Surg Am.* 1979;61:805-814.

135. Takakura Y, Sugimoto K, Tanaka Y, et al. Symptomatic talocalcaneal coalition: its clinical significance and treatment. *Clin Orthop.* 1991;269:249-256.

136. Takakura Y, Kumai T, Takaoka T, Tamai S. Tarsal tunnel syndrome caused by coalition associated with a ganglion. *J Bone Joint Surg Br.* 1998;80:130-133.

137. Lee MF, Chan PT, Chau LF, Yu KS. Tarsal tunnel syndrome caused by talocalcaneal coalition. *Clin Imaging.* 2002;26:140-143.

138. Yoo JH, Kim EH, Kim BS, Cha JG. Tarsal coalition as a cause of failed tarsal tunnel release for tarsal tunnel syndrome. *Orthopedics.* 2009;32.

139. Alaia EF, Rosenberg ZS, Bencardino JT, Ciavarra GA, Rossi I, Petchprapa CN. Tarsal tunnel disease and talocalcaneal coalition: MRI features. *Skeletal Radiol.* 2016;45:1507-1514.

140. Bhat AK, Madi S, Mane PP, Acharya A. Bilateral tarsal tunnel syndrome attributed to bilateral fibrous tarsal coalition and symmetrical hypertrophy of the sustentaculum tali. *BMJ Case Rep.* 2017;10:1136.

141. Gilsanz V, Gibbens DT, Carlson M, et al. The effect of limping on vertebral bone density: a study of children with tarsal coalition. *J Pediatr Orthop.* 1989;9:33-36.

142. Kilicoglu OI, Salduz A, Birisik F, et al. High rates of psychiatric disorders and below normal mental capacity associated with spastic peroneal flatfoot: a new relationship. *J Foot Surg.* 2018;57:501-504.

143. Downey MS. Tarsal coalition: current clinical aspects with introduction of a surgical classification. In: McGlamry ED, ed. *Reconstructive Surgery of the Foot and Leg: Update '89.* Tucker, GA: Podiatry Institute; 1989:60-77.

144. Downey MS. Tarsal coalitions: a surgical classification. *J Am Podiatr Med Assoc.* 1991;81:187-197.

145. Downey MS. Keys to treating tarsal coalitions. *Podiatry Today.* 2011;24:48-56.

146. Katayama T, Tanaka Y, Kadono K, Taniguchi A, Takakura Y. Talocalcaneal coalition: a case showing the ossification process. *Foot Ankle Int.* 2005;26:490-493.

147. Miller AR, Lehman WB. Subtalar dislocation associated with calcaneonavicular coalition: a case report. *Bull Hosp Jt Dis Orthop Inst.* 1989;50:84-87.

148. Richards RR, Evans JG, McGoey PF. Fracture of a calcaneonavicular bar: a complication of tarsal coalition. A case report. *Clin Orthop.* 1984;185:220-221.

149. Tanaka Y, Takakura Y, Akiyama K, et al. Fracture of the tarsal navicular associated with calcaneonavicular coalition: a case report. *Foot Ankle Int.* 1995;16:800-802.

150. Scranton PE Jr, McDermott JE. Pathologic anatomic variations in subtalar anatomy. *Foot Ankle Int.* 1997;18:471-476.

151. Cowell HR. Talocalcaneal coalition and new causes of peroneal spastic flatfoot. *Clin Orthop.* 1972;85:16-22.

152. Cowell HR. Diagnosis and management of peroneal spastic flatfoot. *Instr Course Lect.* 1975;24:94-103.

153. Snyder RB, Lipscomb AB, Johnston RK. The relationship of tarsal coalitions to ankle sprains in athletes. *Am J Sports Med.* 1981;9:313-317.

154. Gonzalez P, Kumar SJ. Calcaneonavicular coalition treated by resection and interposition of the extensor digitorum brevis muscle. *J Bone Joint Surg Am.* 1990;72:71-77.

155. Morgan RC Jr, Crawford AH. Surgical management of tarsal coalition in adolescent athletes. *Foot Ankle.* 1986;7:183-193.

156. Kean JR. Foot problems in the adolescent. *Adolesc Med State Art Rev.* 2007;18:182-191.

157. Cass AD, Camasta CA. A review of tarsal coalition and pes planovalgus: clinical examination, diagnostic imaging, and surgical planning. *J Foot Ankle Surg.* 2010;49:24-293.

158. Koeweiden EM, Van Empel FM, Van Horn JR, et al. The heel-tip test for restricted tarsal motion. *Acta Orthop Scand.* 1989;60:481-482.

159. Percy EC, Mann DL. Tarsal coalition: a review of the literature and presentation of 13 cases. *Foot Ankle.* 1988;9:40-44.

160. Kaplan EG, Kaplan GS, Vaccari OA. Tarsal coalition: review and preliminary conclusions. *J Foot Surg.* 1977;16:136-143.

161. Lyon R, Liu XC, Cho SJ. Effects of tarsal coalition resection on dynamic plantar pressures and electromyography of lower extremity muscles. *J Foot Ankle Surg.* 2005;44:252-258.

162. Maudsley RH. Spastic pes varus. *Proc R Soc Med.* 1956;49:181.

163. Simmons EH. Tibialis spastic varus foot with tarsal coalition. *J Bone Joint Surg Br.* 1965;47:533-536.

164. Kyne PJ, Mankin HJ. Changes in intra-articular pressure with subtalar joint motion with special reference to the etiology of peroneal spastic flat foot. *Bull Hosp Joint Dis.* 1965;26:181-186.

165. Lowy LJ. Pediatric peroneal spastic flatfoot in the absence of coalition: a suggested protocol. *J Am Podiatr Med Assoc.* 1998;88:181-191.

166. Barrett SE, Johnson JE. Progressive bilateral cavovarus deformity: an unusual presentation of calcaneonavicular tarsal coalition. *Am J Orthop (Belle Mead NJ).* 2004;33:239-242.

167. Charles YP, Louahem D, Dimeglio A. Cavovarus foot deformity with multiple tarsal coalitions: functional and three-dimensional preoperative assessment. *J Foot Ankle Surg.* 2006;45:118-126.

168. Keh RA, Krych SM, Harkless LB. Middle facet talocalcaneal coalition presenting with a subtalar varus deformity. *J Am Podiatr Med Assoc.* 1991;81:506-508.

169. Knapp HP, Tavakoli M, Levitz SJ, Sobel E. Tarsal coalition in an adult with cavovarus feet. *J Am Podiatr Med Assoc.* 1998;88:295-300.

170. Nabeshima Y, Fujii H, Ozaki A, Nishiyama T, Takakura Y. Tibialis spastic varus foot with tarsal coalition: a report of five cases. *Foot Ankle Int.* 2007;28:731-734.

171. Mosier KM, Asher M. Tarsal coalitions and peroneal spastic flat foot: a review. *J Bone Joint Surg Am.* 1984;66:976-984.

172. Rocchi V, Huang MT, Bomar JD, Mubarak S. The "double medial malleolus": a new physical finding in talocalcaneal coalition. *J Pediatr Orthop.* 2018;38:239-243.

173. James AE Jr. Tarsal coalitions and peroneal spastic flat foot. *Australas Radiol.* 1970;14:80-83.

174. Crim JR, Kjeldsberg KM. Radiographic diagnosis of tarsal coalition. *Am J Roentgenol.* 2004;182:323-328.

175. Oestreich AE, Mize WA, Crawford AH, et al. The "anteater nose": a direct sign of calcaneonavicular coalition on the lateral radiograph. *J Pediatr Orthop.* 1987;7:709-711.

176. Nalaboff KM, Schweitzer ME. MRI of tarsal coalition: frequency, distribution, and innovative signs. *Bull NYU Hosp Jt Dis.* 2008;66:14-21.

177. Lysack JT, Fenton PV. Variations in calcaneonavicular morphology demonstrated with radiography. *Radiology.* 2004;230:493-497.

178. Schlefman BS, Ruch JA. Diagnosis of subtalar joint coalition. *J Am Podiatry Assoc.* 1982;72:166-170.

179. Lateur LM, Van Hoe LR, Van Ghillewe KV, Gryspeerdt SS, Baert AL, Dereymaeker GE. Subtalar coalition: diagnosis with the C sign on lateral radiographs of the ankle. *Radiology.* 1994;193:847-851.

180. Klammer G, Espinosa N, Iselin LD. Coalitions of the tarsal bones. *Foot Ankle Clin.* 2018;23:435-449.

181. Shaffer HA Jr, Harrison RB. Tarsal pseudo-coalition: a positional artifact. *J Can Assoc Radiol.* 1980;31:236-237.

182. Isherwood I. A radiological approach to the subtalar joint. *J Bone Joint Surg Br.* 1961;43:566-574.

183. Pinsky MJ. The Isherwood views: a roentgenologic approach to the subtalar joint. *J Am Podiatry Assoc.* 1979;69:200-206.

184. Schlefman BS. Radiology. In: McGlamry ED, ed. *Fundamentals of Foot Surgery.* Baltimore, MD: Lippincott Williams & Wilkins; 1987:136-173.

185. Outland T, Murphy ID. Relation of tarsal anomalies to spastic and rigid flatfeet. *Clin Orthop.* 1953;1:217-224.

186. Harris RI. Rigid valgus foot due to talocalcaneal bridge. *J Bone Joint Surg Am.* 1955;37:169-183.

187. Jayakumar S, Cowell HR. Rigid flatfoot. *Clin Orthop.* 1977;122:77-84.

188. Resnick D. Additional congenital or heritable anomalies and syndromes. In: Resnick D, Niwayam G, eds. *Diagnosis of Bone and Joint Disorders with Emphasis on Articular Abnormalities.* Philadelphia, PA: WB Saunders; 1981:2559-2565.

189. Bettin D, Karbowski A, Schwering L. Congenital ball-and-socket anomaly of the ankle. *J Pediatr Orthop.* 1996;16:492-496.

190. Channon GM, Brotherton BJ. The ball and socket ankle joint. *J Bone Joint Surg Br.* 1979;61:85-89.

191. Erlemann R, Wuisman P, Just A, et al. [Deformities and trauma sequelae of the ankle joint in children and adolescents.] *Radiologe.* 1991;31:601-608.

192. Pistoia F, Ozonoff MB, Wintz P. Ball-and-socket ankle joint. *Skeletal Radiol.* 1987;16:447-451.

193. Takakura Y, Tanaka Y, Kumai T, Sugimoto K. Development of the ball-and-socket ankle as assessed by radiography and arthrography. A long-term follow-up report. *J Bone Joint Surg Br.* 1999;81:1001-1004.

194. Takakura Y, Tamai S, Masuhara K. Genesis of the ball-and-socket ankle. *J Bone Joint Surg Br.* 1986;68:834-837.

195. Schlefman BS, Katz FN. Tomographic interpretation of the subtalar joint. *J Am Podiatry Assoc.* 1983;73:65-69.

196. Smith R, Staple T. CAT scan evaluation of the hindfoot: an anatomical and clinical study. *Foot Ankle.* 1982;2:346(abst).

197. Smith RW, Staple TW. Computerized tomography (CT) scanning technique for the hindfoot. *Clin Orthop.* 1983;177:34-38.

198. Cataldi A, Caputo M. [Chronic pain in the hindfoot: computed tomography as a complement in clinico-radiographic evaluation. A study of 38 cases.] *Radiol Med (Torino).* 1996;91:22-27.

199. Crim J. Imaging of tarsal coalition. *Radiol Clin North Am.* 2008;46:1017-1026, vi.

200. Danielsson LG. Talo-calcaneal coalition treated with resection. *J Pediatr Orthop.* 1987;7:513-517.

201. Deutsch AL, Resnick D, Campbell G. Computed tomography and bone scintigraphy in the evaluation of tarsal coalition. *Radiology.* 1982;144:137-140.

202. Emery KH, Bisset GS III, Johnson ND, Nunan PJ. Tarsal coalition: a blinded comparison of MRI and CT. *Pediatr Radiol.* 1998;28:612-616.

203. Floyd EJ, Ransom RA, Daily JM. Computed tomography scanning of the subtalar joint. *J Am Podiatry Assoc.* 1984;74:533-537.

204. Herzenberg JE, Goldner JL, Martinez S, et al. Computerized tomography of talocalcaneal tarsal coalition: a clinical and anatomic study. *Foot Ankle.* 1986;6:273-288.

205. Kulik SA Jr, Clanton TO. Tarsal coalition. *Foot Ankle Int.* 1996;17:286-296.

206. Marchisello PJ. The use of computerized axial tomography for the evaluation of talocalcaneal coalition: a case report. *J Bone Joint Surg Am.* 1987;69:609-611.

207. Martinez S, Herzenberg JE, Apple JS. Computed tomography of the hindfoot. *Orthop Clin North Am.* 1985;16:481-496.

208. Migliori V, Papp J, Kanat IO. Computerized tomography as a diagnostic aid in middle facet talocalcaneal coalition. *J Am Podiatr Med Assoc.* 1985;75:490-492.

209. Newman JS, Newberg AH. Congenital tarsal coalition: multimodality evaluation with emphasis on CT and MR imaging. *Radiographics.* 2000;20:321-332.

210. Pineda C, Resnick D, Greenway G. Diagnosis of tarsal coalition with computed tomography. *Clin Orthop.* 1986;208:282-288.

211. Saxena A, Erickson S. Tarsal coalitions. Activity levels with and without surgery. *J Am Podiatr Med Assoc.* 2003;93:259-263.

212. Sarno RC, Carter BL, Bankoff MS, et al. Computed tomography in tarsal coalition. *J Comput Assist Tomogr.* 1984;8:1155-1160.

213. Solomon MA, Gilula LA, Oloff LM, et al. CT scanning of the foot and ankle. II. Clinical applications and review of the literature. *Am J Roentgenol.* 1986;146:1204-1214.

214. Stoskopf CA, Hernandez RJ, Kelikian A, et al. Evaluation of tarsal coalition by computed tomography. *J Pediatr Orthop.* 1984;4:365-369.

215. Warren MJ, Jeffree MA, Wilson DJ, et al. Computed tomography in suspected tarsal coalition: examination of 26 cases. *Acta Orthop Scand.* 1990;61:554-557.

216. Wechsler RJ, Karasick D, Schweitzer ME. Computed tomography of talocalcaneal coalition: imaging techniques. *Skeletal Radiol.* 1992;21:353-358.
217. Wechsler RJ, Schweitzer ME, Deely DM, et al. Tarsal coalition: depiction and characterization with CT and MR imaging. *Radiology.* 1994;193:447-452.
218. Munk PL, Vellet AD, Levin MF, et al. Current status of magnetic resonance imaging of the ankle and hindfoot. *Can Assoc Radiol J.* 1992;43:19-30.
219. Lawrence DA, Rolen MF, Haims AH, Zayour Z, Moukaddam HA. Tarsal coalitions: radiographic, CT, and MR imaging findings. *HSS J.* 2014;10:153-166.
220. Pachuda NM, Lasday SD, Jay RM. Tarsal coalition: etiology, diagnosis, and treatment. *J Foot Surg.* 1990;29:474-488.
221. Bresnahan PJ, Fung J. Magnetic resonance imaging of the foot and ankle in the pediatric patient. *J Am Podiatr Med Assoc.* 1991;81:112-118.
222. Hall RL, Erickson SJ, Shereff MJ, et al. Magnetic resonance imaging in the evaluation of heel pain. *Orthopedics.* 1996;19:225-229.
223. Masciocchi C, D'Archivio C, Barile A, et al. Talocalcaneal coalition: computed tomography and magnetic resonance imaging diagnosis. *Eur J Radiol.* 1992;15:22-25.
224. Hamel J, Grossmann P, Schramm J, et al. [Sonographic diagnosis of the juvenile tarsus: clinical application possibilities demonstrated by examples.] *Z Orthop Ihre Grenzgeb.* 1995;133:43-49.
225. Mandell GA, Harcke HT, Hugh J, et al. Detection of talocalcaneal coalitions by magnification bone scintigraphy. *J Nucl Med.* 1990;31:1797-1801.
226. Goldman AB, Pavlov H, Schneider R. Radionuclide bone scanning in subtalar coalitions: differential considerations. *AJR Am J Roentgenol.* 1982;138:427-432.
227. Sartoris DJ, Resnick DL. Tarsal coalition. *Arthritis Rheum.* 1985;28:331-338.
228. El Rassi G, Riddle EC, Kumar SJ. Arthrofibrosis involving the middle facet of the talocalcaneal joint in children and adolescents. *J Bone Joint Surg Am.* 2005;87:2227-2231.
229. Kaye JJ, Ghelman B, Schneider R. Talocalcaneonavicular joint arthrography for sustentacular-talar tarsal coalitions. *Radiology.* 1975;115:730-731.
230. Resnick D. Radiology of the talocalcaneal articulations: anatomic considerations and arthrography. *Radiology.* 1974;111:581-586.
231. Pavlov H. Talocalcaneonavicular arthrography. In: Freiberger RH, ed. *Arthrography.* New York, NY: Appleton-Century-Crofts; 1979:257-260.
232. Blakemore LC, Cooperman DR, Thompson GH. The rigid flatfoot. Tarsal coalitions. *Clin Podiatr Med Surg.* 2000;17:531-555.
233. Lemley F, Berlet G, Hill K, Philbin T, Isaac B, Lee T. Current concepts review: tarsal coalition. *Foot Ankle Int.* 2006;27:1163-1169.
234. Tisa LM, Brandreth DL, Reinherz RP. Talocalcaneal coalitions: a review and discussion of past and current therapy. *J Foot Surg.* 1987;26:425-428.
235. Elkus RA. Tarsal coalition in the young athlete. *Am J Sports Med.* 1986;14:477-480.
236. Musgrave RE, Goldner JL. Results of triple arthrodesis for rigid (spastic) flat feet. *South Med J.* 1956;49:39.
237. Kendrick JI. Tarsal coalitions. *Clin Orthop.* 1972;85:62-63.
238. Shirley E, Gheorghe R, Neal KM. Results of nonoperative treatment for symptomatic tarsal coalitions. *Cureus.* 2018;10:7.
239. Birisik F, Demirel M, Bilgili F, Salduz A, Yeldan I, Ismet Kilicoglu O. The natural course of pain in patients with symptomatic tarsal coalitions: a retrospective clinical study. *Foot Ankle Surg.* 2020;26:228-232.
240. Khoshbin A, Bouchard M, Wasserstein D, et al. Reoperations after tarsal coalition resection: a population-based study. *J Foot Ankle Surg.* 2015;54:306-310.
241. Mahan ST, Spencer SA, Vezeridis PS, Kasser JR. Patient-reported outcomes of tarsal coalitions treated with surgical excision. *J Pediatr Orthop.* 2015;5:583-588.
242. Kernbach KJ, Barkan H, Blitz NM. A critical evaluation of subtalar joint arthrosis associated with middle facet talocalcaneal coalition in 21 surgically managed patients: a retrospective computed tomography review. Investigations involving middle facet coalitions-part III. *Clin Podiatr Med Surg.* 2010;27:135-143.
243. Wilde PH, Torode IP, Dickens DR, et al. Resection for symptomatic talocalcaneal coalition. *J Bone Joint Surg Br.* 1994;76:797-801.
244. Comfort TK, Johnson LO. Resection for symptomatic talocalcaneal coalition. *J Pediatr Orthop.* 1998;18:283-288.
245. Gantsoudes GD, Roocroft JH, Mubarak SJ. Treatment of talocalcaneal coalitions. *J Pediatr Orthop.* 2012;32:301-307.
246. Rozansky A, Varley E, Moor M, Wenger DR, Mubarak SJ. A radiologic classification of talocalcaneal coalitions based on 3D reconstruction. *J Child Orthop.* 2010;4:129-135.
247. Bixby SD, Jarrett DY, Johnston P, Mahan ST, Kleinman PK. Posteromedial subtalar coalitions: prevalence and associated morphological alterations of the sustentaculum tali. *Pediatr Radiol.* 2016;46:1142-1149.
248. Mahan ST, Prete VI, Spencer SA, Kasser JR, Bixby SD. Subtalar coalitions: does the morphology of the subtalar joint involvement influence outcomes after coalition excision? *J Foot Ankle Surg.* 2017;56:797-801.
249. Luhmann SJ, Schoenecker PL. Symptomatic talocalcaneal coalition resection: indications and results. *J Pediatr Orthop.* 1998;18:748-754.
250. Mubarak SJ, Patel PN, Upasani VV, Moor MA, Wenger DR. Calcaneonavicular coalition: treatment by excision and fat graft. *J Pediatr Orthop.* 2009;29:418-426.
251. Mercado OA. Rearfoot surgery. In: *An Atlas of Foot Surgery.* Oak Park, IL: Carolando Press; 1987:162-168.
252. Mitchell GP, Gibson MC. Excision of calcaneo-navicular bar for painful spasmodic flat foot. *J Bone Joint Surg Br.* 1967;49:281-287.
253. Fuson S, Barrett M. Resectional arthroplasty: treatment for calcaneonavicular coalition. *J Foot Ankle Surg.* 1998;37:11-15.
254. Bright RW. Resection of calcaneo-navicular coalition with insertion of a Silastic spacer. *Orthop Trans.* 1983;7:150.
255. Hounshell CR. Regenerative tissue matrix as an interpositional spacer following excision of a cuboid-navicular tarsal coalition: a case study. *J Foot Ankle Surg.* 2011;50:241-244.
256. Schechter RS, Sollitto RJ, Kittay JM. The use of a silicone implant following resection of a calcaneonavicular coalition: a case report. *J Foot Surg.* 1979;18:124-127.
257. Sperl M, Saraph V, Zwick EB, Kraus T, Spendel S, Linhart WE. Preliminary report: resection and interposition of a deepithelialized skin flap graft in tarsal coalition in children. *J Pediatr Orthop B.* 2010;19:171-176.
258. Alter SA. Calcaneonavicular bar resection. *Clin Podiatr Med Surg.* 1991;8:469-483.
259. Alter SA, McCarthy BE, Mendicino S, et al. Calcaneonavicular bar resection: a retrospective study. *J Foot Surg.* 1991;30:383-389.
260. Andreasen E. Calcaneo-navicular coalition: late results of resection. *Acta Orthop Scand.* 1968;39:424-432.
261. Chambers RB, Cook TM, Cowell HR. Surgical reconstruction for calcaneonavicular coalition: evaluation of function and gait. *J Bone Joint Surg Am.* 1982;64:829-836.
262. Cohen AH, Laughner TE, Pupp GR. Calcaneonavicular bar resection: a retrospective review. *J Am Podiatr Med Assoc.* 1993;83:10-17.
263. Cohen BE, Davis WH, Anderson RB. Success of calcaneonavicular coalition resection in the adult population. *Foot Ankle Int.* 1996;17:569-572.
264. Cowell HR. Extensor brevis arthroplasty. *J Bone Joint Surg Am.* 1970;52:820.
265. Daumas L, Morin C, Leonard JC. [Congenital tarsal synostosis.] *Arch Pediatr.* 1996;3:900-905.
266. Dungl P. [Calcaneonavicular coalition and its treatment.] *Acta Chir Orthop Traumatol Cech.* 1989;56:408-418.
267. Dutoit M, Rigault P, Padovani JP, et al. [Primary synostosis of the tarsus in children: apropos of 32 cases in 20 patients.] *Rev Chir Orthop Reparatrice Appar Mot.* 1984;70:231-243.
268. Inglis G, Buxton RA, Macnicol MF. Symptomatic calcaneonavicular bars: the results 20 years after surgical excision. *J Bone Joint Surg Br.* 1986;68:128-131.
269. Kendrick JI. Treatment of calcaneonavicular bar. *JAMA.* 1959;172:1242-1244.
270. Montsko P, Kranicz J, Than P. [Management of calcaneonavicular coalition and results.] *Magy Traumatol Ortop Kezseb Plasztikai Seb.* 1994;37:229-233.
271. Moyes ST, Crawfurd EJP, Aichroth PM. The interposition of extensor digitorum brevis in the resection of calcaneonavicular bars. *J Pediatr Orthop.* 1994;14:387-388.
272. Rouvreau P, Pouliquen JC, Langlais J, et al. [Synostosis and tarsal coalitions in children: a study of 68 cases in 47 patients.] *Rev Chir Orthop Reparatrice Appar Mot.* 1994;80:252-260.
273. Scott AT, Tuten HR. Calcaneonavicular coalition resection with extensor digitorum brevis interposition in adults. *Foot Ankle Int.* 2007;28:890-895.
274. Stoller MI. Tarsal coalitions: a study of surgical results. *J Am Podiatry Assoc.* 1974;64:1004-1015.
275. Swiontkowski MF, Scranton PE, Hansen S. Tarsal coalitions: long-term results of surgical treatment. *J Pediatr Orthop.* 1983;3:287-292.
276. Van Renterghem D, De Ridder K. Resection of calcaneonavicular bar with interposition of extensor digitorum brevis. A questionnaire review. *Acta Orthop Belg.* 2011;77:83-87.
277. Masquijo J, Allende V, Torres-Gomez A, Dobbs MB. Fat graft and bone wax interposition provides better functional outcomes and lower reossification rates than extensor digitorum brevis after calcaneonavicular coalition resection. *J Pediatr Orthop.* 2017;37:e427-e431.
278. Lui TH. Arthroscopic resection of the calcaneonavicular coalition or the "too long" anterior process of the calcaneus. *Arthroscopy.* 2006;22:903.e1-903.e4.
279. Parisien JS, Vangsness T. Arthroscopy of the subtalar joint: an experimental approach. *Arthroscopy.* 1985;1:53-57.
280. Bernardino CM, Golano P, Garcia MA, Lopez-Vidriero E. Experimental model in cadavera of arthroscopic resection of calcaneonavicular coalition and its first in-vivo application: preliminary communication. *J Pediatr Orthop B.* 2009;18:347-353.
281. Bauer T, Golano P, Hardy P. Endoscopic resection of a calcaneonavicular coalition. *Knee Surg Sports Traumatol Arthrosc.* 2010;18:669-672.
282. Knorr J, Accadbled F, Abid A, et al. Arthroscopic treatment of calcaneonavicular coalition in children. *Orthop Traumatol Surg Res.* 2011;7:565-568.
283. Bonasia DE, Phisitkul P, Amendola A. Endoscopic coalition resection. *Foot Ankle Clin.* 2015;20:81-91.
284. Bourlez J, Joly-Monrigal P, Alkar F, et al. Does Arthroscopic resection of a too-long anterior process improve static disorders of the foot in children and adolescents? *Int Orthop.* 2018;42:1307-1312.
285. Cain TJ, Hyman S. Peroneal spastic flat foot: its treatment by osteotomy of the os calcis. *J Bone Joint Surg Br.* 1978;60:527-529.
286. Dwyer FC. Causes, significance and treatment of stiffness of the subtaloid joint. *Proc R Soc Med.* 1976;69:97-102.
287. Quinn EA, Peterson KS, Hyer CF. Calcaneonavicular coalition resection with pes planovalgus reconstruction. *J Foot Ankle Surg.* 2016;55:578-582.
288. Asher M, Mosier K. Coalition of the talocalcaneal middle facet: treatment by surgical excision and fat graft interposition. *Orthop Trans.* 1983;7:149-150.
289. Blakemore LC, Cooperman DR, Thompson GH. The rigid flatfoot: tarsal coalitions. *Foot Ankle Clin.* 1998;3:609-631.
290. Blitz NM. Pediatric & adolescent flatfoot reconstruction in combination with middle facet talocalcaneal coalition resection. *Clin Podiatr Med Surg.* 2010;27:119-133.
291. Bonasia DE, Phisitkul P, Saltzman CL, Barg A, Amendola A. Arthroscopic resection of talocalcaneal coalitions. *Arthroscopy.* 2011;27:430-435.
292. Collins B. Tarsal coalitions: a new surgical procedure. *Clin Podiatr Med Surg.* 1987;4:75-98.
293. De Vriese L, Dereymaeker G, Molenaers G, Fabry G. Surgical treatment of tarsal coalitions. *J Pediatr Orthop B.* 1994;3:96-101.
294. Downey MS. Tarsal coalition. In: McGlamry ED, Banks AS, Downey, MS, eds. *Comprehensive Textbook of Foot Surgery.* 2nd ed. Baltimore, MD: Lippincott Williams & Wilkins; 1992:898-930.
295. Downey MS. Resection of middle facet talocalcaneal coalitions. In: Miller SJ, Mahan KT, Yu GV, et al., eds. *Reconstructive Surgery of the Foot and Leg: Update '98.* Tucker, GA: Podiatry Institute; 1998:1-5.
296. Field C, Ng A. Resection of middle facet coalition with arthroscopic guidance. *J Foot Ankle Surg.* 2009;48:273-276.
297. Giannini S, Ceccarelli F, Vannini F, Baldi E. Operative treatment of flatfoot with talocalcaneal coalition. *Clin Orthop.* 2003;411:178-187.

298. Hamel J. [Resection of talocalcaneal coalition in children and adolescents without and with osteotomy of the calcaneus]. *Oper Orthop Traumatol.* 2009;21:180-192.

299. Hark FW. Congenital anomalies of the tarsal bones. *Clin Orthop.* 1960;16:21-25.

300. Jimenez AL, Taylor RP. Surgical excision of tarsal coalitions in juvenile athletes: three case reports. In: Camasta CA, Vickers NS, Carter SR, eds. *Reconstructive Surgery of the Foot and Leg: Update '95.* Tucker, GA: Podiatry Institute; 1995:37-40.

301. Kernbach KJ, Blitz NM. The presence of calcaneal fibular remodeling associated with middle facet talocalcaneal coalition: a retrospective CT review of 35 feet. Investigations involving middle facet coalitions—Part II. *J Foot Ankle Surg.* 2008;47:288-294.

302. Kernbach KJ, Blitz NM, Rush SM. Bilateral single-stage middle facet talocalcaneal coalition resection combined with flatfoot reconstruction: a report of 3 cases and review of the literature. Investigations involving middle facet coalitions—part 1. *J Foot Ankle Surg.* 2008;47:180-190.

303. Kitaoka HB, Wikenheiser MA, Shaughnessy WJ, et al. Gait abnormalities following resection of talocalcaneal coalition. *J Bone Joint Surg Am.* 1997;79:369-374.

304. Kumar SJ, Guille JT, Lee MS, et al. Osseous and non-osseous coalition of the middle facet of the talocalcaneal joint. *J Bone Joint Surg Am.* 1992;74:529-535.

305. Lepow GM, Richman HM. Talocalcaneal coalition: a unique treatment approach in case report. *Podiatr Tracts.* 1988;1:38-43.

306. Lisella JM, Bellapianta JM, Manoli A II. Tarsal coalition resection with pes planovalgus hindfoot reconstruction. *J Surg Orthop Adv.* 2011;20:102-105.

307. McCormack TJ, Olney B, Asher M. Talocalcaneal coalition resection: a 10-year follow-up. *J Pediatr Orthop.* 1997;17:13-15.

308. O'Neill DB, Micheli LJ. Tarsal coalition: a followup of adolescent athletes. *Am J Sports Med.* 1989;17:544-549.

309. Olney BW, Asher MA. Excision of symptomatic coalition of the middle facet of the talocalcaneal joint [published erratum appears in *J Bone Joint Surg Am* 1987;69:1111]. *J Bone Joint Surg Am.* 1987;69:539-544.

310. Philbin TM, Homan B, Hill K, Berlet G. Results of resection for middle facet tarsal coalitions in adults. *Foot Ankle Spec.* 2008;1:344-349.

311. Raikin S, Cooperman DR, Thompson GH. Interposition of the split flexor hallucis longus tendon after resection of a coalition of the middle facet of the talocalcaneal joint. *J Bone Joint Surg.* 1999;81-A:11-19.

312. Salomao O, Napoli MMM, de Carvalho AE Jr, et al. Talocalcaneal coalition: diagnosis and surgical management. *Foot Ankle.* 1992;13:251-256.

313. Scranton PE Jr. Treatment of symptomatic talocalcaneal coalition. *J Bone Joint Surg Am.* 1987;69:533-539.

314. Westberry DE, Davids JR, Oros W. Surgical management of symptomatic talocalcaneal coalition by resection of the sustentaculum tali. *J Pediatr Orthop.* 2003;23:493-497.

315. Wright EM, Lieberman R, Brekke M, et al. Tarsal coalition. In: Vickers NS, ed. *Reconstructive Surgery of the Foot and Leg: Update '97.* Tucker, GA: Podiatry Institute; 1997:151-163.

316. Edmonds WB, Wiley K, Panas K. Technique article: tarsal coalition resection using Kirschner wires across the subtalar Joint in a two-incision approach. *J Foot Ankle Surg.* 2019;58:337-340.

317. Aibinder WR, Young EY, Milbrandt TA. Intraoperative Three-Dimensional Navigation for Talocalcaneal Coalition Resection. *J Foot Ankle Surg.* 2017;56:1091-1094.

318. Giacomozzi C, Benedetti MG, Leardini A, Macellari V, Giannini S. Gait analysis with an integrated system for functional assessment of talocalcaneal coalition. *J Am Podiatr Med Assoc.* 2006;96:107-115.

319. Hetsroni I, Ayalon M, Mann G, Meyer G, Nyska M. Walking and running plantar pressure analysis before and after resection of tarsal coalition. *Foot Ankle Int.* 2007;28:575-580.

320. Hetsroni I, Nyska M, Mann G, Rozenfeld G, Ayalon M. Subtalar kinematics following resection of tarsal coalition. *Foot Ankle Int.* 2008;29:1088-1094.

321. Khoshbin A, Law PW, Caspi L, Wright JG. Long-term functional outcomes of resected tarsal coalitions. *Foot Ankle Int.* 2013;34:1370-1375.

322. Miyamoto W, Takao M, Uchio Y, Ochi M. Technique tip: interposition of the pedicle fatty flap after resection of the talocalcaneal coalition. *Foot Ankle Int.* 2007;28:1298-1300.

323. Hubert J, Hawellek T, Beil FT, et al. Resection of medial talocalcaneal coalition with interposition of a pediculated flap of tibialis posterior tendon sheath. *Foot Ankle Int.* 2018;39:935-941.

324. Krief E, Ferraz L, Appy-Fedida B, et al. Tarsal coalitions: preliminary results after operative excision and silicone sheet interposition in children. *J Foot Ankle Surg.* 2016;55:1264-1270.

325. Catanzariti AR, Mendicino RW, Saltrick KR, Orsini RC, Dombek MF, Lamm BM. Subtalar joint arthrodesis. *J Am Podiatr Med Assoc.* 2005;95:34-41.

326. Mann RA, Baumgarten M. Subtalar fusion for isolated subtalar disorders: preliminary report. *Clin Orthop.* 1988;226:260-265.

327. Mann RA, Beaman DN, Horton GA. Isolated subtalar arthrodesis. *Foot Ankle Int.* 1998;19:511-519.

328. Peterson HA. Dowel bone graft technique for triple arthrodesis in talocalcaneal coalition: report of a case with 12-year follow-up. *Foot Ankle.* 1989;9:201-203.

329. Schwartz JM, Kihm CA, Camasta CA. Subtalar joint distraction arthrodesis to correct calcaneal valgus in pediatric patients with tarsal coalition: a case series. *J Foot Ankle Surg.* 2015;54:1151-1157.

330. Weinraub GM, Schuberth JM, Lee M, et al. Isolated medial incisional approach to subtalar and talonavicular arthrodesis. *J Foot Ankle Surg.* 2010;49:326-330.

331. David DR, Clark NE, Bier JA. Congenital talonavicular coalition. Review of the literature, case report, and orthotic management. *J Am Podiatr Med Assoc.* 1998;88:223-227.

332. Berkey SF, Clark B Jr. Tarsal coalition: case report and review of the literature. *J Am Podiatry Assoc.* 1984;74:31-37.

333. Lahey MD, Zindrick MR, Harris EJ. A comparative study of the clinical presentation of tarsal coalitions. *Clin Podiatr Med Surg.* 1988;5:341-357.

334. Jacobs AM, Sollecito V, Oloff L, et al. Tarsal coalitions: an instructional review. *J Foot Surg.* 1981;20:214-221.

Benign and Malignant Tumors of Soft Tissue and Bone

Matthew J. Seidel, Judd Cummings, Ansab Khwaja, and Benjamin Meyer

BENIGN

FIBROUS TUMORS

FIBROMA

Fibromas are firm-fixed lesions on the medial border of the plantar fascia and produce discomfort with weight bearing. It can occur at any age, males are affected more than females, and people of northern European ancestry more than other races.[1] Lesions grow slowly up to 2 cm and have a similar histology of myofibroblasts similar to Dupuytren lesions.[2] Fibromas can be small and isolated but can range to extensive fibromatosis. Treatment starts with nonsurgical management including footwear modification with accommodative arch and nonsteroidal anti-inflammatory medications. Eradication is difficult with surgical management and recurrence is common.[3] In 1996, Aluisio et al. reviewed a variety of surgical options from local excision, wide excision, and subtotal fasciectomy both with and without skin grafting and each group had recurrence, with evidence of disease within 14 months (6.9 months average). In a more recent review of patients who underwent surgical excision, an operative staging system was developed, which incorporated plantar fascia involvement, presence of skin adherence, and depth of tumor extension. Recommendations included incisions in non–weight-bearing portion of plantar arch, use of loupe magnification, and avoiding full-thickness resection even with dermal infiltration and local wound care with avoidance of early skin grafting. Eighteen of 21 patients reported that they would have surgery done again and there were 2 recurrences in this series.[4]

DESMOID FIBROMATOSIS

This is a benign but locally aggressive tumor characterized by proliferation of fibroblasts. This disease is more common in women than man, and the largest numbers arise from the abdominal viscera, but are also seen in the extremities.[5] It presents as an enlarging painless mass with symptoms related to compression of anatomical structures. It does not metastasize, but has a tendency to recur, and surgical excision has been recommended for treatment, but recurrence rates vary from 13% to 77%.[6] There is no clear role for endocrine treatment, radiation therapy, or chemotherapy,[7] though radiation has been espoused as an adjunct to surgery, which may reduce likelihood of recurrence.[5] It is now realized that desmoid fibromatosis can have periods of stable size and even regression,[8] and it is also noted that positive margins on microscopic evaluation do not have an adverse effect on recurrence rates.[9] Thus, treatment is trending toward more nonoperative management initially, and acceptance of microscopic positive margins to maintain important anatomical structures.

DERMAL TUMORS

DERMATOFIBROMA

A common cutaneous lesion, defined as a "fibrosing dermatitis characterized by increased number of fibrocytes in dermis…with a mixture of inflammatory cells…with coarse collagen bundles and hyperplasia of adjacent structures."[10] It can develop at any age with multiple variants and thought to be a local response to some type of inflammation or trauma (ie, bite, ruptured hair follicle). Early lesions are red or red-brown, and chronic lesions brown to skin colored with darker peripheral rim, well circumscribed, and firm. Histology shows dense infiltrate of fibrocytes and/or macrophages in the reticular dermis. Fitzpatrick sign is present on exam, which is dimpling of the skin with lateral compression next to the lesion caused by smooth pressure forcing the dermatofibroma into the subcutis.[11] Patients should be provided reassurance about the benign nature of this condition, though resection has been reported with low recurrence rate.[10]

GRANULOMA ANNULARE

In the subcutaneous form, nodules appear alone or with other intradermal lesions. They are more frequent in children and young adults, females greater than males with no inflammatory appearance at the skin surface.[12] The dermal form presents with papules. On histology, there is basophilic degeneration of collagen bundles with palisading granulomas, with subcutaneous granuloma having a larger area of necrobiosis.[13] Eosinophils are more common in the subcutaneous form. Biopsy can help provide diagnosis, but lesions usually resolve spontaneously and there is generally no role for resection.

VASCULAR TUMORS

HEMANGIOMA AND LYMPHANGIOMA

A developmental abnormality of the vascular system, which presents as a soft mass with blue discoloration when superficial. Anatomic location and overall size predict symptoms. Subcutaneous hemangiomas irritate sensory nerves, intramuscular lesions can increase compartment pressure, intra-articular lesions cause recurrent hemarthrosis, and peri-articular or large lesions can cause hypertrophy or limb length discrepancy.[14] Radiographs may show calcified phleboliths. Magnetic resonance imaging demonstrates "cluster of grapes" appearance.[15] Lymphangiomas are similar to hemangiomas in histology and presentation, with malformation of the lymphatic system.[16] The port wine type of hemangioma is the most common vascular anomaly of the foot. Initial treatment is observation and compression stockings for symptomatic lesions. Oral propranolol was effective in children up to 5 years of age in a randomized control trial treating children for facial or otherwise cosmetically disfiguring lesions.[17] Sclerotherapy with polidocanol has been effective in a series that included 87 children and adolescents being treated for rapidly growing facial hemangiomas, requiring up to three injections.[17] While excision under tourniquet control is possible, it has a high rate of recurrence, reported at up to 48%.[14] Recurrence is improved with wide marginal excision. A 2007 review of intramuscular hemangiomas noting 5-year recurrence of 67% with gross residual tumor, 35% when intralesional without any gross remaining tumor, and 7% with wide margins.[18]

GLOMUS TUMOR

Thought to arise from cutaneous arteriovenous anastomoses, these structures are composed of vessels and glomus cells embedded in a stroma. They usually present as painful, firm, purplish solitary nodule, especially in the nail bed, and occur sporadically presenting as multiple or solitary forms.[19] Multiple glomus tumors are rare and are described as softer, more compressible, bluish nodules, and are often inherited in an autosomal-dominant pattern.[20] Radiographs may show bony erosion over the dorsal surface of the distal phalanx. Symptoms include intense burning pain at the tumor site, which may be spontaneous or be precipitated by touch and temperature changes.[21] Treatment is surgical resection, with a described technique of creating a full-thickness flap down to bone with subperiosteal dissection. The glomus is noted to be obvious as an egg-shaped semi-elastic structure, which is then excised. Pain relief and low recurrence rates can be expected after surgical treatment.

NEURAL TUMORS

SCHWANNOMA

Benign tumor of the nerve sheath Schwann cell, with peak age 40-60.[22] Exam generally shows a mobile soft mass with a markedly positive Tinel sign. The distribution of the Tinel sign may indicate the nerve involved. Although the mass is noted to have a plane between the tumor and nerve fascicles themselves, some level of nerve damage is usually seen after resection. Recurrence is rare after surgical excision. Malignant schwannoma in the foot has occurred in the setting of neurofibromatosis.[23]

NEUROFIBROMA

A spindle cell tumor of peripheral nerves, with the majority being solitary and 10% associated with neurofibromatosis.[24] In patients who present with this entity, the foot and ankle surgeon should evaluate for cutaneous manifestations of neurofibromatosis type 1 (NF1), which include café-au-lait spots, as well as pseudoarthrosis of the tibia and scoliosis.[25] Plexiform neurofibromas can occur in setting of NF1. These are large neurofibromas, which permeate between nerve fibers, with no clear plane of dissection compared to schwannomas.[26] Surgical excision, therefore, requires patient-centered decision-making on the impact of the tumor vs impact of extensive resection and resulting motor and/or sensory deficits. Ten percent of patients with NF1 develop malignant peripheral nerve sheath tumors from malignant transformation of a neurofibroma, necessitating close observation and routine monitoring of these patients.

FATTY TUMORS

LIPOMA

While benign lipomatous lesions of the soft tissue are common throughout the musculoskeletal system (50% of all soft tissue tumors), they are rare in the foot. Nine subtypes are identified in the literature (lipoma, lipomatosis, lipomatosis of nerve, lipoblastoma or lipoblastomatosis, angiolipoma, myolipoma of soft tissue, chondroid lipoma, spindle cell lipoma and pleomorphic lipoma, and hibernoma).[27] These can be infiltrative vs noninfiltrative, are soft, nontender, mobile, and asymptomatic until local compression of anatomic structures. Diagnosis on MRI is generally straightforward in that the lesion should appear as the normal subcutaneous tissue on every sequence. A few septations may be seen in benign masses. More septations or signal other than lipomatous tissue may indicate a more aggressive lesion such as atypical lipomatous tumor or liposarcoma. Treatment for symptomatic lipomas is local excision, with low recurrence.

SYNOVIAL TUMORS AND TUMORLIKE CONDITIONS

GANGLION

A cystic lesion with thin wall and gelatinous fluid inside, the ganglion is the most common soft tissue mass in the foot, where it is usually found on the dorsum of the foot and ankle. The majority originate from the tendon sheath, and secondarily from a joint capsule. While it is most common in the dorsum of the hand and wrist, 11% of all ganglia occur in foot and ankle.[28] The etiology is thought to be a result of myxoid degeneration in connective tissues, and cysts develop at sites of ligamentous or capsular stress.[29] Diagnosis is clinical, but ultrasound or magnetic resonance imaging can be helpful for those located deep in the tarsal tunnel or plantar aspect of the foot. Treatment is generally nonoperative, unless there is symptomology from compression of local structures or making shoe wear difficult and painful. Additionally, ganglia in the foot tend to be larger than the wrist. Pain is the most common reason for surgery, which is marginal excision of entire cyst and surrounding degenerative joint capsule or tendon sheath. Recurrence is reported from 5% to 30%, especially when the cyst originates from the tendon sheath.[28] In one subset, recurrence occurred

when cases originated from the tendon sheath and had satellite masses, which may have led to recurrence. Nerve injury during cyst removal is the greatest risk, and it is recommended to use loupe magnification and bipolar cautery.[30] Surgery for ganglia in the tarsal tunnel has been associated with tibial nerve injury, and cutaneous nerve branches have been attached to the mass requiring meticulous dissection or sacrificing nerve branches.

GIANT CELL TUMOR OF TENDON SHEATH

A well-defined solitary benign soft tissue tumor that arises from synovial lining of tendon sheaths. It presents clinically as a small painless mass that slowly enlarges but may become painful due to mass effect as the tumor enlarges.[31] Grossly the mass has a brown/orange appearance and is often attached to the synovium or tenosynovium. The microscopic appearance is characterized by pleomorphic cells, including lipid laden foam cells, multinucleated giant cells often with deposits of hemosiderin in a collagenous stroma. It is more common in the upper extremities; however, the foot and ankle are frequent sites of involvement. Surgical excision provides good results with low recurrence, though admittedly it has not been extensively studied.[32]

PIGMENTED VILLONODULAR SYNOVITIS

A benign entity of unknown etiology, characterized by synovial metaplasia producing villi with hemosiderin accumulation.[33] There is both a localized and diffuse type with intra-articular or extra-articular locations. Patients present with intermittent swelling without a history of trauma. On histology, PVNS is identical to tenosynovial giant cell tumor, histologically characterized by both small histiocyte like cells and larger cells with dense cytoplasm as well as multinucleated giant cells and macrophages overloaded with hemosiderin.[33] MRI is the imaging modality of choice, with low T1 and low T2 signal due to the paramagnetic activity of hemosiderin.[34] X-ray and CT are nonspecific, but they can be used to evaluate disease progression and treatment response. When there is joint destruction or a lesion is symptomatic, then arthroscopic or open synovectomy can be performed. Localized disease has lower recurrence than diffuse variants.[35] Radiation has been used as an adjuvant after synovectomy with one case series of recurrent cases treated with radiation had no further recurrence at medium-term follow-up average of 3.5 years.[36] Caution must be used when using radiation in that there is a small chance of postradiation malignancy and the tissue changes make any further surgeries more complicated. More recently, treatment with antitumor necrosis factor antibodies has been suggested, after finding TNF-alpha expression in arthroscopic synovial tissue samples. Treatment with the monoclonal antibody (infliximab) at dose of 5 mg/kg has demonstrated reduction in macrophage numbers and TNF-alpha expression in the synovium.[37] As such, moving forward rheumatological management of PVNS may play a central role in the treatment, especially of the diffuse subtype or with recurrent disease.

SYNOVIAL CHONDROMATOSIS

A condition where the synovial lining of joints, bursae, or tendon sheaths undergoes metaplasia and ultimately forms cartilaginous loose bodies.[38] It can occur in the foot and ankle but is much more common in the hip and knee. Patients may present with pain, swelling, sprains, paresthesias, and/or a palpable mass. Radiographs are nonspecific but can show calcified juxta-articular bodies. MRI shows low signal on T1, high signal on T2, and the disease can even be extra-articular.[38] Treatment with synovectomy and loose body removal has reported to be successful and has shown these masses have the potential for malignant transformation.[38] Arthroscopic and open treatment have both been reported as successful in treatments for this disease.[26,39] Synovial chondromatosis that is longstanding and untreated may lead to degenerative arthritis characterized by peri-articular erosions and joint inflammatory changes.

METABOLIC DEPOSITION LESIONS

XANTHOMA OF TENDON

Low-density lipoproteins (LDLs) may accumulate from the circulation into the tendons. Transformation of the LDL into its oxidized form with the subsequent invasion of macrophages within the tendon forms the xanthoma. The Achilles tendon being the most common site[40] and usually presents as painless nodules. These may be associated with familial hypercholesterolemia or sporadic hypercholesterolemia. Treatment is geared toward managing the basic metabolic disorder of lipid metabolism. Surgical debulking, if necessary due to pain, is challenging due to the infiltration of the disease and risk for postoperative tendon rupture.

TOPHACEOUS GOUT

A common rheumatological disorder, gout is caused by a biochemical derangement leading to hyperuricemia, with deposition of uric acid crystals into the joints and soft tissues. Tophaceous gout is the chronic phase of this disease but is occasionally the initial presentation for a patient. A tophus is a mass of either crystalline or amorphous urates, surrounded by tissue showing increased vascularity and intense inflammatory reaction. The acute phase of gout can mimic infection due to erythema and swelling while a solitary chronic tophus can be confused for a neoplastic process, especially when bone erosion or pain is present.[41] Treatment of the underlying metabolic condition and rheumatological management is the cornerstone of management. In the acute flare setting, colchicine can be used as an oral agent while intra-articular steroid injection may also be helpful.

MALIGNANT

SOFT TISSUE SARCOMAS

Soft tissue sarcomas (STS) are a heterogeneous group of malignant tumors of mesenchymal origin. They are classically classified based on their differentiation according to the adult tissue they resemble (Figs. 45.1 and 45.2). Benign neoplasms of soft tissues out number malignant cases by a factor of 50. The annual incidence is about 300 new cases per 100 000 persons, whereas STS have an annual incidence of about 6 per 100 000 persons, accounting for 1.5% of all malignant tumors in adults and 7.4% in children.[42] While they often arise in the lower extremities, they rarely do so below the ankle.[43]

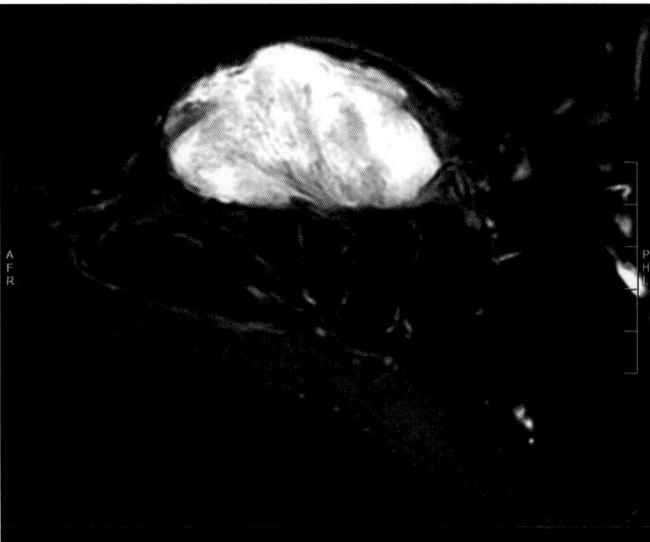
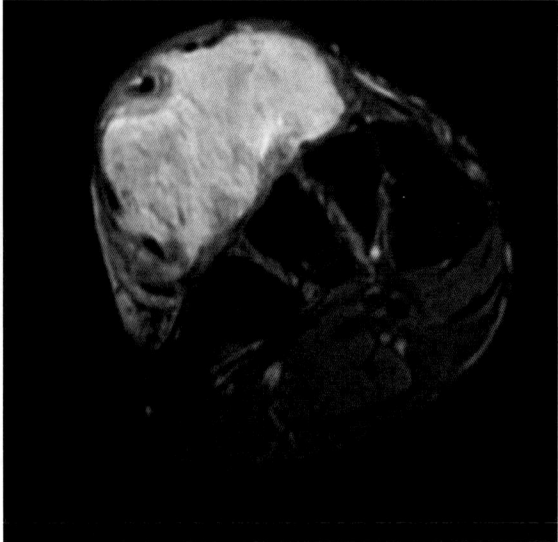

FIGURE 45.1 Sagittal and coronal T2 MRI images showing a synovial sarcoma of the dorsum of the midfoot. Note the classic high T2 signal appearance.

Soft tissue sarcoma is best managed with wide marginal surgical resection. Radiation therapy is often added to enhance local control of the disease. With this management, the local recurrence rate is reported to be below 10%.[44] Unsurprisingly, incompletely resected tumors (positive histologic margins) have been linked with increased local recurrence.[45] Subcutaneous or superficial tumors more amenable to wide resection tend to have favorable local control rates. Tumors penetrating the deep fascia and for those located extracompartmentally, complete surgical resection can often be challenging without sacrificing normal limb function (Fig. 45.3). These patients tend to have higher recurrence rates and should be considered for adjuvant therapy. Unplanned surgery for STS of the foot and ankle often results in the need for more aggressive surgery and/or adjuvant radiotherapy, which may impact oncologic outcome. Limb salvage may still be possible in these cases and does not necessarily result in worse functional outcomes.[46]

KAPOSI SARCOMA

Kaposi sarcoma is caused by human herpes virus 8 (HHPV8) and is predominant in patients with acquired immunodeficiencies, including acquired immunodeficiency syndrome and iatrogenic immunosuppression including organ transplantation, but can also develop in elderly.[47] It is endothelial in origin from blood and lymph vessels.[48] It often presents on the skin of the feet as bluish skin papules. Treatment for Kaposi sarcoma is palliation and rarely involves surgery. Patients are often limited because of discomfort ambulating and difficulty with shoe wear. Radiation therapy has been reported with response rate up to 90% in the literature. Patients sometimes have discomfort relating to the radiation itself and increased pedal edema, but this usually resolves within 2 weeks.[49]

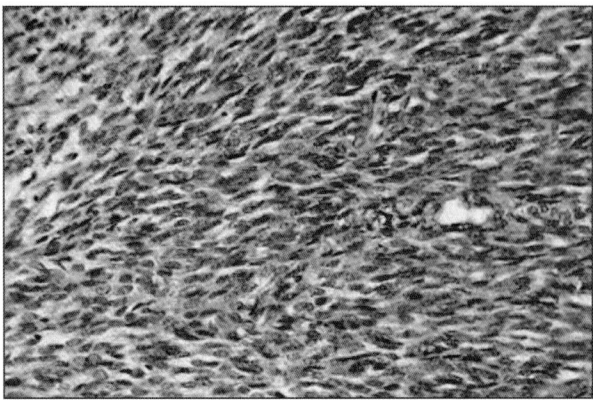
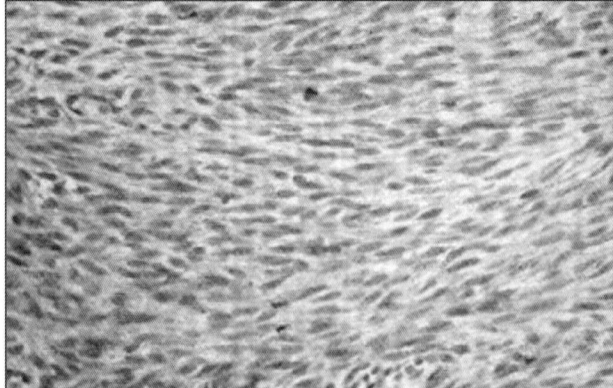

FIGURE 45.2 Photomicrograph showing a monophasic synovial sarcoma. Note the hypercellular tissue with large hyperchromatic nuclei.

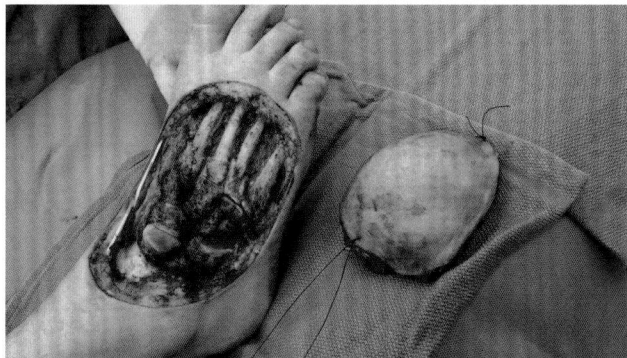

FIGURE 45.3 Intraoperative photograph after resection of the sarcoma to the level of the bone. The patient required free flap soft tissue reconstruction.

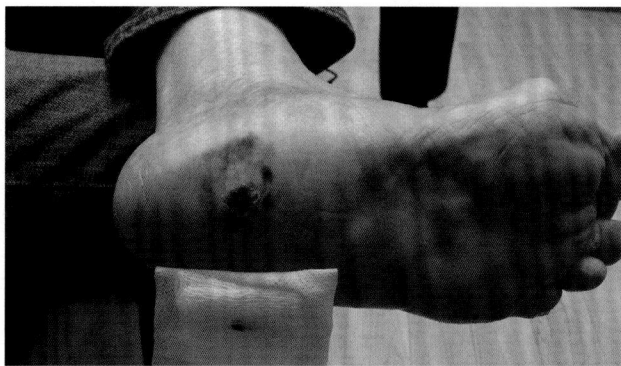

FIGURE 45.4 Clinical photograph of plantar malignant melanoma of the skin with ulceration.

MALIGNANT MELANOMA

Melanoma is a malignant tumor arising from the pigment producing cell of the skin, the melanocyte. There are four main types: acral lentiginous, nodular, superficial spreading, and lentigo maligna. The acral lentiginous is characterized by an extensive component running as a layer of malignant melanocytes within the basal layer of the epidermis. It represents about half of the melanoma occurring on the hands and feet. In the early stages, the clinical symptoms for this type of melanoma can be very subtle such as an ill-defined macule or patch of light brown or gray discoloration of the skin. Nodular melanoma has vertical invasion when viewed microscopically and macroscopically appears as a pigmented lesion, which may appear nodular to the naked eye. The superficial spreading variant is the most common of the four subtypes and most frequently reported on the dorsum of the foot. It has lateral spread before becoming invasive. Lentigo maligna is usually a result of sun damage in geriatrics. A small proportion of melanoma lack pigmentation and are hence labeled amelanotic melanoma. These are more likely to arise on acral areas and can be fleshy in color. Such lesions are more likely to arise on acral areas such as the feet and be misdiagnosed as other skin disorders as they may be fleshy in color.[50]

There is an increasing burden of melanoma in the United states, with incidence increasing by an average of 3.1% per year between 1992 and 2004.[51] Melanoma on the hand and foot tends to have a poorer prognosis than melanoma elsewhere, likely due to later diagnosis.[52] While non-whites have an overall lower rate of melanoma, they have a higher rate in acral regions such as palm, plantar foot, and nailbed.[53] In a review of 66 patients, the mean age of presentation was 57 years, overall 5-year survival rate of 63% and 10-year survival rate of 51%. The mean duration of survival for the patients who had a plantar or subungual lesion was significantly shorter than that for the patients who had a lesion at another site on the dorsal aspect of the foot or on the ankle (47 compared with 72 months). Lesions at plantar and subungual sites were also associated with a higher prevalence of clinical misdiagnosis compared with lesions on the dorsal aspect of the foot or on the ankle[54] (Fig. 45.4). Early recognition is difficult given the inconspicuous location of the plantar foot. A standard teaching for assessing pigmented lesions is the evaluation of ABCDE: Asymmetry, Border irregularity, Color heterogeneity, Diameter, and Evolution over time.[50]

Subungual lesions are in particular difficult to identify and are often confused for hematoma. Because melanocytes are limited to the matrix and nail folds, if pigment change occurs within a structurally normal nail or nail bed, with no continuity with the nail folds or matrix, then it is not likely to be melanocytic and cannot be a melanoma. Additionally, blood may present as small irregular pools in nail bed, whereas longitudinal melanoma arises as well-organized bands of similar width throughout the longitudinal axis.[50] Surgical treatment is determined by site, depth, and stage of the lesions and ranges from wide local excision with skin grafting to amputation.[54] Chemotherapy, radiation, and immunotherapy are all potential treatment options for advanced cases.

BASAL CELL CARCINOMA

Basal cell carcinoma (BCC) is the most common cancer in the United States, with annual incidence of 0.5%,[55] and defined as malignant tumor of follicular germinative cells.[56] Basal cancer can grow aggressively causing local tissue damage,[57] with low rate of generalized dissemination, but cases of metastasis to lung, bone, liver, and lymph nodes have been reported. Ultraviolet exposure is thought to cause the majority of damage leading to development of BCC. Surgical excision is the primary mode of treatment, though scarring, tissue loss, and pigmentation changes are associated. Photodynamic therapy, imiquimod cream, and cryotherapy are now also being investigated as options for treatment with lower comorbidity and improved cosmetic results.[58] Data from Europe with 5-year follow-up show histological clearance rates of 90 in patients who used imiquimod cream five times a week for 6 weeks[59] and clearance of 80% with both cryotherapy and photodynamic therapy.[60]

SQUAMOUS CELL CARCINOMA

Squamous cell carcinoma (SCC) is the second most common cancer and again related to ultraviolet light and more frequent in fair skinned individuals. It appears as a red scaly papule or patch, which can bleed spontaneously. Chronic leg ulcers are associated with SCC, as are burns, traumatic wounds, diabetic wounds, and osteomyelitis.[61] One study noted 10.4% skin cancer frequency in patients with chronic leg ulcers, with the recommendation to biopsy ulcers that do not respond to 3 months of treatment.[62] Patients who have had solid organ transplants

have up to a 250 times increased risk of SCC vs general population, though this is reported in the scalp.[63] Treatment is generally surgical, either by excision or Mohs micrographic surgery, though curettage and electrodessication or cryosurgery is described.[64] Tumor thickness divides SCC into three main risk categories for metastasis: 2 mm or less with no detectable risk, 2.1-6.0 mm with low risk, and >6.0 mm with high risk for metastasis.[65]

SOFT TISSUE METASTASES

Metastatic tumors presenting as soft tissue masses in the foot and ankle are uncommon. In one review of a 30-year period at a large academic medical center, there was one case of metastatic disease to the foot and one to the ankle, from 118 identified cases.[66] Treatment consists of radiation therapy vs surgical resection or prophylactic stabilization depending on the location of the lesions.

BENIGN

BONE FORMING

OSTEOCHONDROMA

Osteochondromas are the most common benign bone lesion, and their true incidence is likely underreported as many are asymptomatic. The cartilage cap of an osteochondroma resembles physeal cartilage, and they are thought to be developmental anomalies stemming from the growth plate itself. Osteochondromas migrate away from the growth plate as patients' age and rarely continue to grow after skeletal maturity. Approximately 1:50 000 patients have a condition known as multiple hereditary exostosis (MHE) also known as multiple osteochondromatosis, an autosomal-dominant condition affecting males more than females. MHE is caused by mutations of EXT genes on chromosomes 8 and 11.[67] Changes in an osteochondroma after adulthood are concerning for malignant transformation termed secondary chondrosarcoma. Malignant transformation occurs in <1% of solitary osteochondromas, and in the case of MHE has been reported as high as 25% in older series. A 2015 wide multicenter survey reported only a 2.7% risk, and most of these involved the pelvis and scapula.[68]

Less than 1% of osteochondromas appear in the foot and ankle, while the most common location is around the knee.[69] Patients usually present with a hard painless mass. When pain is noted, it is usually due to mechanical symptoms or inflammation of an overlying bursa. Radiographs will reveal a bony outgrowth usually growing away from the adjacent physis. The base may be sessile or pedunculated. Characteristically, there is continuity between the marrow cavities of the normal bone and the lesion. CT can help to better define the bony anatomy, and MRI can help to determine the size of the cartilage cap and evaluate the extent of local soft tissue irritation.

Treatment is observation in most cases. Symptomatic treatment may be warranted if there is local irritation. Surgical resection is required if more conservative measures fail, and surgeons should ensure removal of the entire cartilage cap. If reasonable, surgery should be delayed until after skeletal maturity to decrease the risk of recurrence or growth disturbance.[70] Patients with MHE can develop multiple skeletal deformities, including hindfoot valgus deformities from intertibiofibular osteochondromas, which may require surgical correction before skeletal maturity.[71]

OSTEOID OSTEOMA

Osteoid osteomas are small, usually <1.5 cm benign bone tumors that have a peak incidence during the second decade of life. They account for 10%-12% of all benign bone tumors and have a male to female ratio of 2-3:1. They most commonly occur in the metadiaphysis of long bones.[72] A recent systematic review that included 94 studies and 223 cases of foot and ankle osteoid osteomas reports that the talus is overall the fourth most commonly affected bone in the body with an incidence of 2%-10%. They also report that the calcaneus is involved in 2.7% of cases, the phalanges 2%, and the metatarsals 1.7%.[73]

The classic clinical vignette is one of achy pain that is worse at night, nonmechanical, and rapidly but temporarily relieved by NSAIDs or aspirin. The typical radiographic appearance is that of a small sclerotic nidus surrounded by an area of lucency with a sclerotic rim. In some cases, the lesion might not be visible but rather a significant amount of reactive cortical bone may be present visualized on radiographs as diffuse thickening of the cortex. Because of their small size, high-resolution CT is helpful in visualizing and characterizing the nidus. MRI reveals bone marrow inflammation and may lead to misdiagnosis if radiographic and CT findings are not taken into account. Bone scan is highly sensitive in identifying the nidus.[72]

Osteoid osteomas have been known to "burn out" or resolve over time, but in the case of unmanageable discomfort, intervention is warranted. The nidus is thought to produce highly inflammatory cytokines that cause the pain so complete eradication of the nidus is of paramount importance. This can be accomplished by radiofrequency ablation (RFA) of the nidus or surgical excision. RFA is generally done in an interventional radiology setting, is minimally invasive, and generally results in rapid pain relief and high success rates. Local curettage can also result in high success rates but is more invasive.[72] En block excision is rarely used now but has been in the past. Arthroscopy has been reported to be successful for removal of osteoid osteomas near the articular surface in the ankle.[74] The author's preferred method of treatment is RFA, which we also believe to be the gold standard of osteoid osteoma treatment in the modern era.

OSTEOBLASTOMA

Osteoblastomas are benign bone tumors related to osteoid osteoma but differentiated by their greater growth potential. They account for approximately 3% of all benign bone tumors and arise in similar age and sex distributions as osteoid osteoma.[72] A total of 12.5% of osteoblastomas occur in the foot and ankle, with the talus being the most frequently involved.[75] Most patients present with pain, but the nonmechanical night pain relieved by NSAIDs that is typical with osteoid osteoma is less consistent. Local tenderness or swelling may also exist. Radiographs reveal a central lytic lesion with a rim of reactive sclerotic bone similar to osteoid osteoma but exceeds 1.5 cm in size, with some documented lesions reaching up to 10 cm. CT is the imaging modality of choice. Bone scan is sensitive but not specific. MRI plays a role in osteoblastomas of the spine but

may be less useful in lesions of the foot.[72] Osteoblastoma does not typically resolve without intervention. Treatment of symptomatic lesions consists of extended intralesional curettage and bone grafting. Internal fixation to augment stability or mitigate fracture risk should be used when deemed necessary for all of the lesions in this chapter. Recurrence may require repeat local excision or en bloc resection.[72]

BPOP

Bizarre parosteal osteochondromatous proliferation (BPOP or Nora lesion) was first described as "peripheral skeletal osteochondromatous tumefaction" by Nora et al. in 1983.[76] It is a benign primary bone tumor that has a propensity to affect the tubular bones of the hands and feet. BPOP has been diagnosed throughout a wide age range and affects males and females equally.[76] Patients with BPOP present with a palpable mass or pain. Foot deformities due to mass effect have also been reported.[77] Radiographs reveal an osteocartilaginous outgrowth from the cortex that, unlike osteochondroma, lacks medullary continuity with normal bone.[78] The typical histologic features of BPOP include cartilaginous, osseous, and fibrous tissue and the presence of "blue bone," which has been described as "unusual mineralized cartilaginous matrix," and enlarged, binucleated chondrocytes.[79,80] BPOP has been mistaken for low-grade chondrosarcoma, and some authors have argued for reclassifying BPOP as a neoplastic process.[81-83] Berber et al. reported a 27.3% recurrence rate after excision and also suggest that more aggressive surgical excision does not necessarily decrease the rate of recurrence.[83] Long-term follow-up is recommended.[83]

SUBUNGUAL EXOSTOSIS

Subungual exostosis is a relatively uncommon osteochondral tumor, which arises from the dorsal aspect of the distal phalanx. It can occur on any toe, but 80% of cases involve the hallux.[84] It is thought to be a reactive lesion that is secondary to trauma or infection.[84,85] The cartilage cap is composed of fibrocartilage in contrast to the hyaline cartilage of osteochondromas.[86] Patients present with pain, erythema, or deformity of the nail bed, and radiographs will reveal a pedunculated calcified mass on the dorsal aspect of the distal phalanx.[86] A systematic review of surgical treatment found that complete marginal excision using a fish-mouth incision and protecting the nail led to satisfactory clinical results and a recurrence rate of only 4%.[86] Onychodystrophy, a common complication of treatment, can be prevented with careful wound management aimed at minimizing disruption to the nail bed.[86]

CARTILAGE FORMING

ENCHONDROMA

Enchondromas are benign growths of hyaline cartilage in medullary bone. Half of all enchondromas appear in the hands and feet, and overall it is the most common bone tumor of the foot. The majority are found in the phalanges and metatarsals.[87] They are found most frequently in the second through fourth decades of life. A majority are asymptomatic and discovered incidentally on radiographs, but they can also rarely present with pathologic fracture or stress fractures. Radiographs reveal

a central lesion with uniformly prominent mineralization commonly described as arcs and rings. Generally there is a lack of endosteal scalloping but some minimal scalloping can occur. Cortical breakthrough is generally not seen and if present raises the possibility of neoplastic process. CT and MRI are useful in evaluating symptomatic enchondromas and can help to distinguish between a simple benign enchondroma and a more aggressive lesion. Asymptomatic enchondromas can be monitored radiographically, typically yearly.[88] Those that are symptomatic respond well to curettage and bone grafting. Stress fractures should be allowed to heal prior to curettage and bone grafting. Enchondromas may have a potential for malignant transformation to secondary chondrosarcoma and would be heralded by pain and or growth. Biopsy of cartilage tumors has been shown to be inaccurate due to the heterogenicity of the tumor. Cartilage tumors of the foot that exceed 5 cm^2 display any aggressive features, or those arising in the midfoot or hindfoot should be considered for surgical removal.[89]

Several forms of multiple enchondromatosis have been classified such as Ollier disease (Spranger type I) and Maffucci syndrome. Cheirospondyloenchondromatosis (Spranger type VI) in particular has marked hand and foot involvement.[90] Patients with these conditions have a 40% lifetime risk of malignant degeneration.[91]

Periosteal (juxtacortical) chondromas are histologically similar to enchondromas but appear on the surface of the bone.[92] Radiographs reveal a radiolucent lesion that abuts and erodes the cortical bone in the shape of a saucer, a so-called "saucerization." In the foot, they occur most frequently in the tubular bones, a case in the cuboid with a secondary aneurysmal bone cyst (ABC) has also been described.[93,94] If symptomatic, excision is usually curative.

CHONDROBLASTOMA

Chondroblastomas are benign tumors of cartilage consisting of chondroid matrix and fibroblasts. They occur almost exclusively in the epiphysis of long bones in patients with an average age of 17.3 years. A 2018 review of 40 cases involving the foot reported a slightly older age, 20-25 years, location in the hindfoot, and a slight male predominance.[95] Patients typically present with pain and swelling. Radiographs reveal a radiolucent lesion and are sharply demarcated with a thin sclerotic border (Fig. 45.5). MRI can help to differentiate the chondroid matrix and assess for soft tissue involvement (Fig. 45.6). CT may be useful to further assess bony anatomy. Biopsy or intraoperative frozen section is recommended prior to or during treatment (Fig. 45.7). Extended intralesional curettage and bone grafting has been shown to be curative in most cases[95] (Fig. 45.8). RFA has been reported to be an effective alternative to surgery. A retrospective analysis of 25 consecutive patients treated with RFA reported a 12% local recurrence rate during a mean follow-up period of 49 months.[96] Because of local recurrence and small chance of pulmonary metastasis, annual follow-up with radiographs of the original lesion and chest are recommended.

CHONDROMYXOID FIBROMA

Chondromyxoid fibromas (CMFs) are rare, benign neoplasms that are thought to arise from or mimic fetal cartilage canals.[97] Most arise in the second to third decade of life

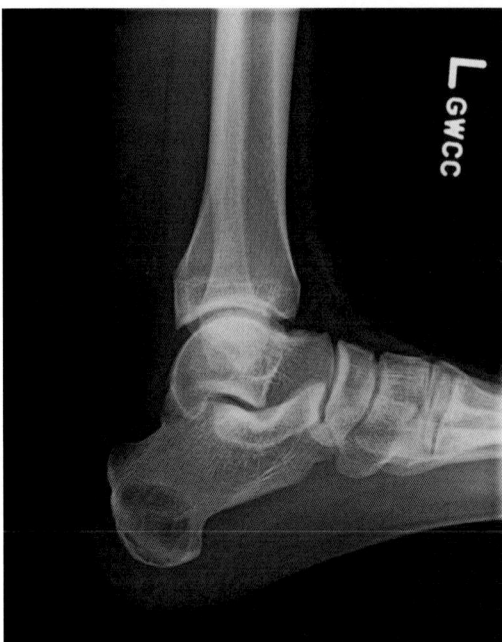

FIGURE 45.5 A 17-year-old male with heel pain. Lucent lesion seen in the posterior calcaneus.

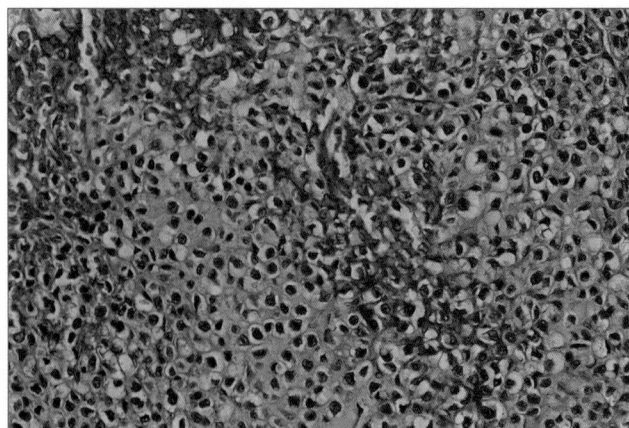

FIGURE 45.7 Photomicrograph of chondroblastoma. Note scattered (not regular as in giant cell tumor of bone) multinucleated giant cells through a "sea" of mononuclear chondroblasts. The thin calcification between groups of cell is known as "chicken wire" calcifications.

with a second peak in the fifth to seventh decade and have a slight male predominance. CMFs are most common in the metaphysis of long bones. The knee is the most common location followed by the foot, which is involved in 17%-20% of cases.[98] As the name suggests, CMFs have variable histologic features composed of chondroid, myxoid, and fibrous elements. CMFs can be confused with chondrosarcoma, which is the most common misdiagnosis.[98] Secondary lesions such as ABCs have been reported and may complicate the diagnosis and treatment.[99]

Patients typically present with pain and may have soft tissue swelling but rarely a mass. Radiographs reveal a lytic, eccentric lesion with sharp sclerotic borders. Lesions involving the feet may show cortical erosion or expansion into surrounding tissues.[98] MRI is useful to delineate the fibrous and myxoid components. Biopsy is required to confirm the diagnosis.

Curettage and bone grafting is the mainstay of treatment. Grossly, CMF is a rubbery, gray/blue or white/tan multilobulated tissue. Recurrence rates up to 25% have been reported, and those treated with curettage and bone grafting have lower rates than those treated with curettage alone.[100] En bloc resection may be required for smaller bones of the foot. A minimum of 3-year follow-up has been suggested.[98]

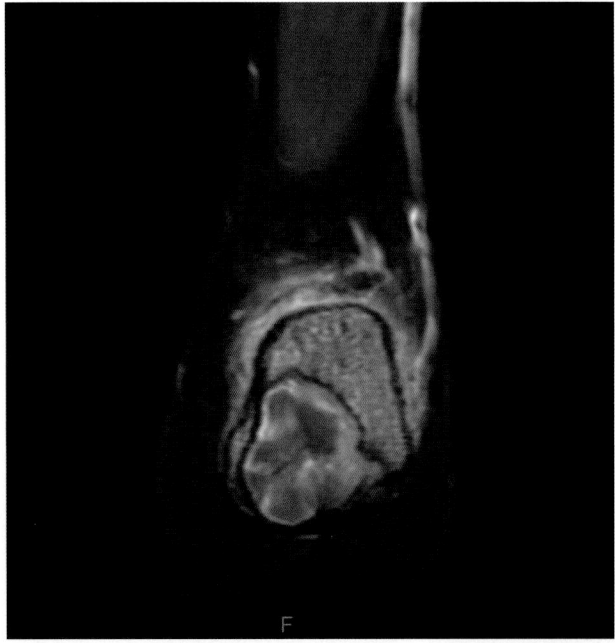
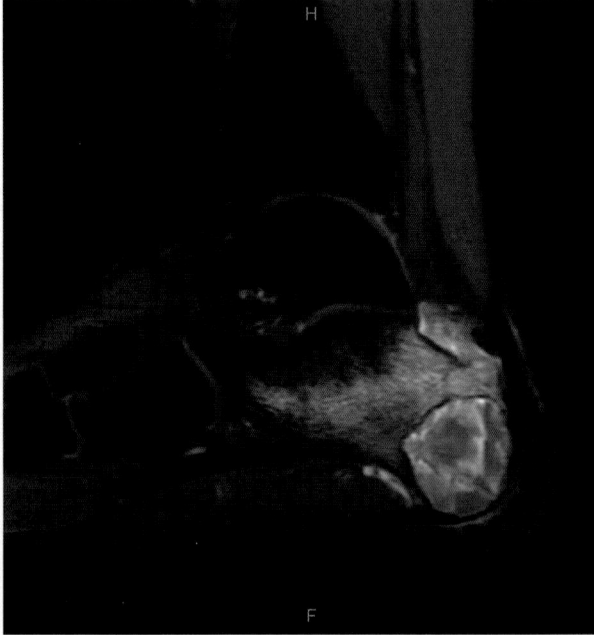

FIGURE 45.6 Sagittal and coronal T1 fat-suppressed MR images revealing a geographic lesion with mixed contrast enhancement.

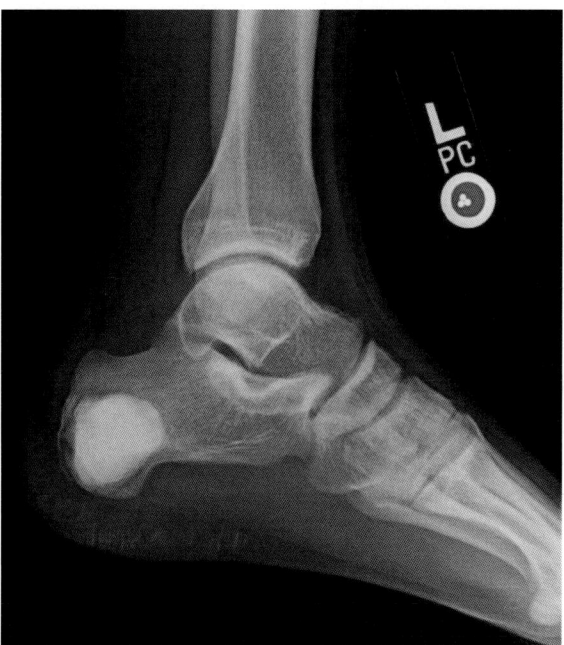

FIGURE 45.8 Postop images after extended curettage and bone grafting. Patient went on to full graft incorporation and relief of pain while back to full activity.

BENIGN AGGRESSIVE

ANEURYSMAL BONE CYSTS

ABCs are cystic neoplasms that typically affect the proximal metaphysis of long bones in patients younger than 20 with a slight female predominance. They can be either a primary lesion or as a component of another bone lesion. ABCs were historically thought to be a reactive process, but translocation of ubiquitin-specific protease fusion protein USP6 on chromosome 17

has also been implicated.[101] In the foot and ankle, the distal fibula is the most common location with reported incidence between 1.5% and 7.1% of all ABCs.[102] Patients may present with pain due to fracture or impending fracture and may have a prominent lateral malleoli in more expansile lesions. Radiographs will show an eccentric, lucent, multiloculated, expansile lesion with a thin cortical rim (Fig. 45.9). MRI or CT may reveal the classic "fluid-fluid levels" within the multiloculated chambers (Fig. 45.10). Biopsy prior to treatment may be useful and will reveal chronic inflammatory cells, hemosiderin-laden macrophages, and scattered giant cells. This is in contrast to telangiectatic osteosarcoma, an important inclusion on the differential diagnosis as on MRI they also present with fluid-fluid levels, and would demonstrate malignant pleomorphic cells and atypical mitotic figures.[103]

Curettage and bone grafting is the standard of treatment (Figs. 45.11 and 45.12). Recurrence rates up to 31% have been reported and are associated with factors such as periarticular location and open growth plates.[104] Adjuvant therapy such as phenol, liquid nitrogen, high-speed burring, and argon beam have been suggested but none show conclusive reduction of recurrence rates.[105] Radiation therapy was historically used but is no longer recommended. Alternative therapies such as sclerotherapy and embolization have shown some promise.[106,107]

GIANT CELL TUMORS OF BONE

Giant cell tumors of bones (GCTBs) are benign, locally aggressive epiphyseal lesions that most commonly occur in the distal femur, proximal tibia, and distal radius. The incidence peaks between the third and fourth decades of life and has a slight female predominance. The foot and ankle are involved in 4% of cases, most commonly the distal tibia and hindfoot.[108,109] It has been suggested that GCTB of the foot is more aggressive than other forms, but a recent series showed that this is likely not due to more aggressive biologic behavior but due to

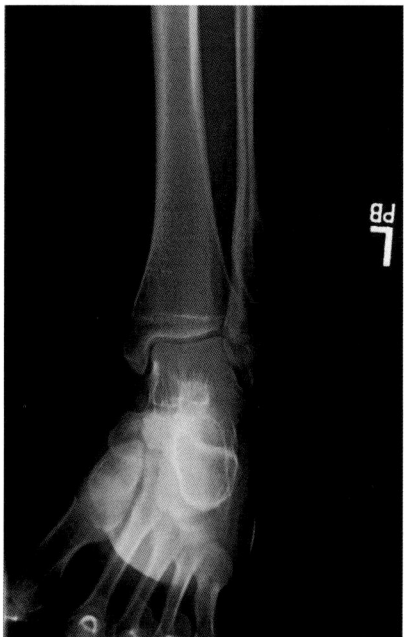
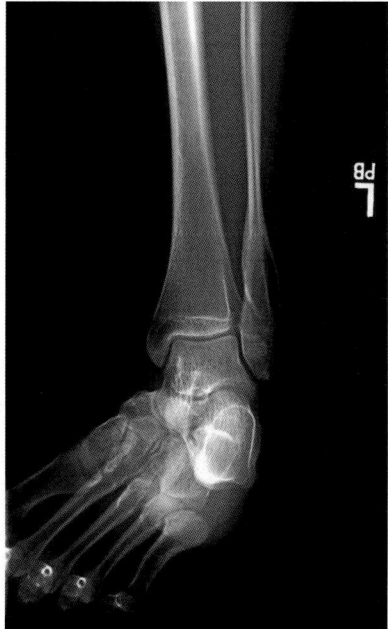
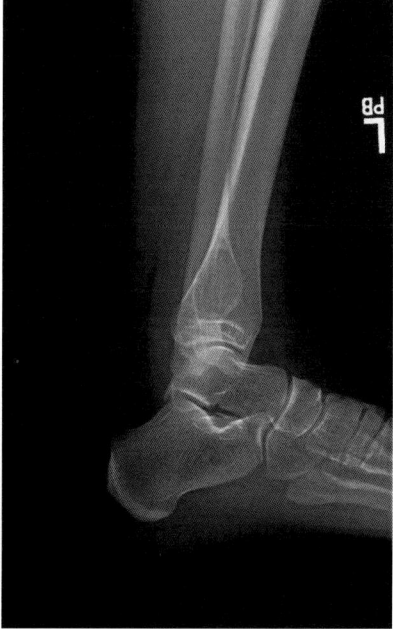

FIGURE 45.9 Preoperative radiographs of fibular ABC in a 17-year-old male.

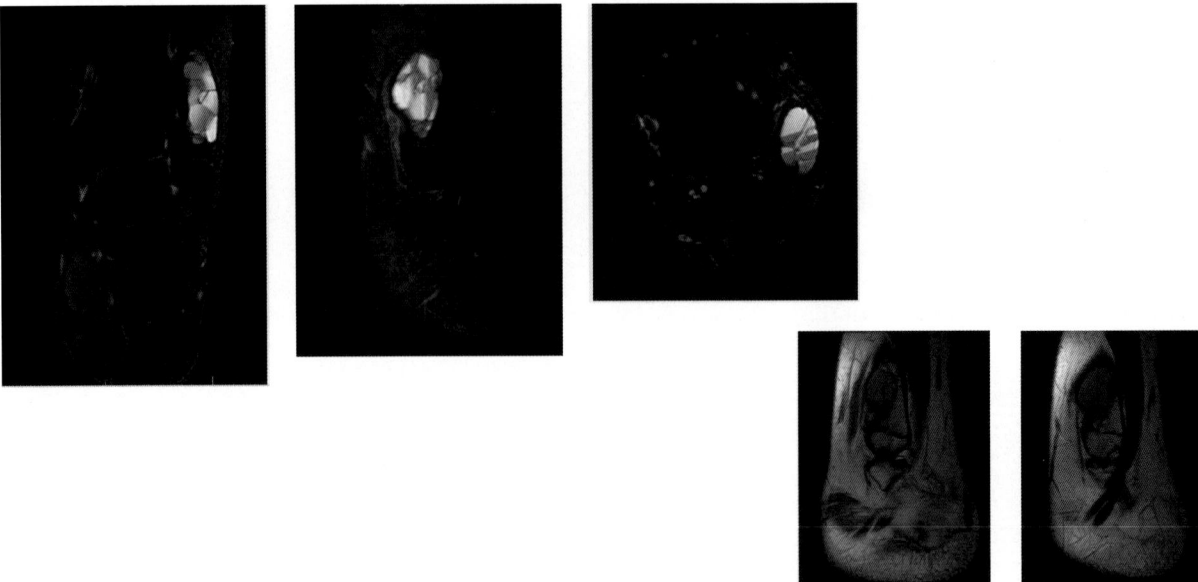

FIGURE 45.10 MRI of fibular ABC demonstrating classic fluid-fluid levels.

delayed presentation and diagnosis as well as difficult surgical resections.[110]

Patients typically present with localized dull ache, swelling, or pathologic fracture. Radiographs demonstrate an eccentric, geographic, radiolucent lesion plus or minus a thin sclerotic rim opposite from the fading border. MRI helps to characterize the extent of soft tissue and marrow involvement (Fig. 45.13). CT scan can be helpful to distinguish between malignancy as GCTB typically has a thin sclerotic border on CT scan. Chest radiograph or CT is recommended as there is a 2%-4% chance of pulmonary metastasis, which occurs more frequently in recurrent disease.[111]

Biopsy will reveal the classic multinucleated giant cells scattered amid a background of mononuclear cells (Fig. 45.14). Surgery is the treatment of choice for GCTB. Initially, local curettage and bone grafting was used, but with high recurrence rates, the pendulum has shifted to large en bloc resections, which many argued were too aggressive for a benign disease. Now, surgical treatment consists of extended intralesional curettage with local adjuvant therapies such as high-speed burring, argon beam, and phenol with local recurrence rates reported between 6% and 25%[112-114] (Figs. 45.15 and 45.16). En bloc resection is reserved for recalcitrant cases. Systemic therapy such as bisphosphonates and denosumab are currently being investigated and show promise in decreasing recurrence rates. The National Comprehensive Cancer Network has published guidelines for the treatment and surveillance of GCTB.[115]

CYSTIC

SIMPLE BONE CYST

Unicameral (one chamber) bone cysts (UBCs) (simple bone cyst, solitary bone cyst) are thought to be caused by abnormal pressure during growth, which leads to necrosis and cavity formation followed by subsequent accumulation of fluid.[103] The most common sites of involvement are the metaphysis of the proximal humerus and proximal femur. Within the foot, the calcaneus is most commonly involved and accounts for 2%-11% if simple cysts. UBCs of the medial cuneiform and talus have also been described.[116-118] Radiographs show a lucent cystic lesion with only one chamber that is centrally located within the bone. The cortices may be thinned, and if it does expand the contour of the bone, only does so minimally in comparison to ABCs. Radiographs of a pathologic fracture may reveal the classic "fallen leaf" sign, which is a portion of the cortex that has broken off has settled to a dependent position within the lesion. In the absence of pathologic fracture, the cyst contains "straw colored" proteinaceous fluid, which is nonbloody in contrast to the grossly bloody fluid of ABCs.[119]

UBCs of the long bones are typically discovered in the first two decades of life and may heal spontaneously with skeletal maturity. Lesions within the calcaneus are discovered more often in middle age and are less likely to spontaneously resolve.[116,120] Intralesional steroid injections have been suggested but have not proven to be as effective for calcaneal lesions as it is in other locations.[121] Levy et al. in their systematic review of UBCs of the calcaneus recommend open curettage with autograft augmentation as the most effective surgical treatment for symptomatic lesions.[116] Internal fixation may be indicated in the case of pathologic fractures.

DEGENERATIVE BONE CYST

Historically thought to be separate entities, the terms "degenerative bone cyst," "intraosseous ganglion," "intra-osseous lesion," "subchondral cyst," "pseudo-cyst," and "goede" are now used interchangibelly.[122] Two conflicting hypotheses of the pathophysiology are the "synovial intrusion" theory caused by articular cartilage defects and the "bone contusion" theory caused by microdamage and necrosis of subchondral bone.[123,124] Either way, these lesions are caused by abnormal stress on the subchondral bone due to trauma or arthritis. The most common locations in the foot and ankle are the talar dome and the medial malleolus.[125] Typical presentations may be an incidental

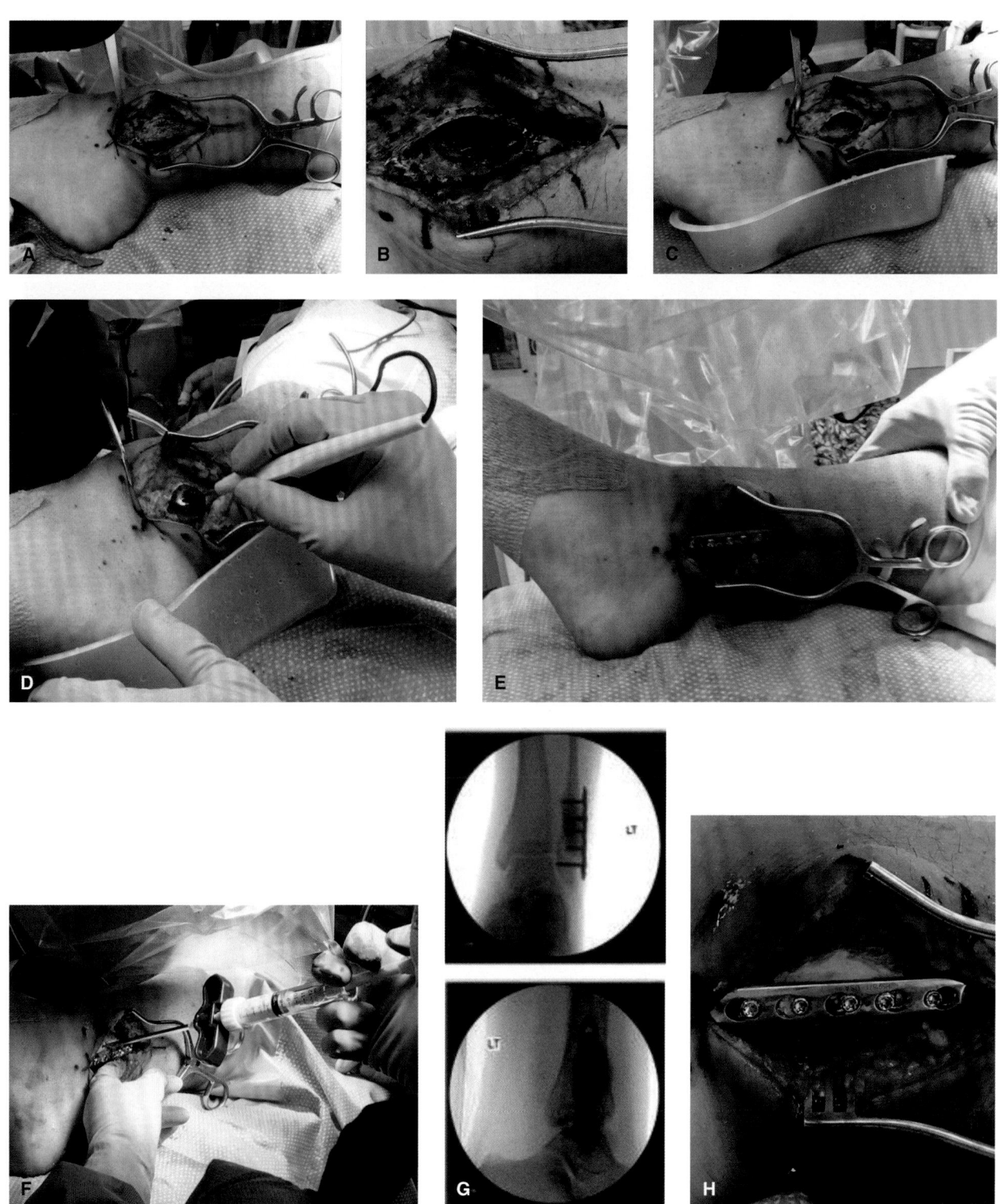

FIGURE 45.11 Intraoperative photographs of surgery to treat aneurysmal bone cyst of the fibula. **A.** Exposed distal lateral fibula. **B.** Decorticated lesion. **C.** s/p use of high-speed burr. **D.** Electrocautery within lesion. **E.** Application of plate and screws. **F.** Synthetic bone grafting. **G.** Intraoperative fluoroscopic images. **H.** Prior to wound closure.

finding on imaging, activity-related pain, or found in the presence of a chronically painful, arthritic joint. Radiographs show a well-defined subchondral bone defect with a sclerotic border, often in association with an arthritic joint. MRI shows a fluid-filled cavity with a dense border. Treatment is observation and management of underlying joint condition. Larger lesions are treated with curettage and bone grafting. Internal fixation is

rarely required. Arthroscopic debridement and bone grafting has been successful in the ankle.[126]

EPIDERMOID INCLUSION CYST

Epidermoid inclusion cysts are benign lesions, which can develop after a portion of epidermis becomes "included" in the

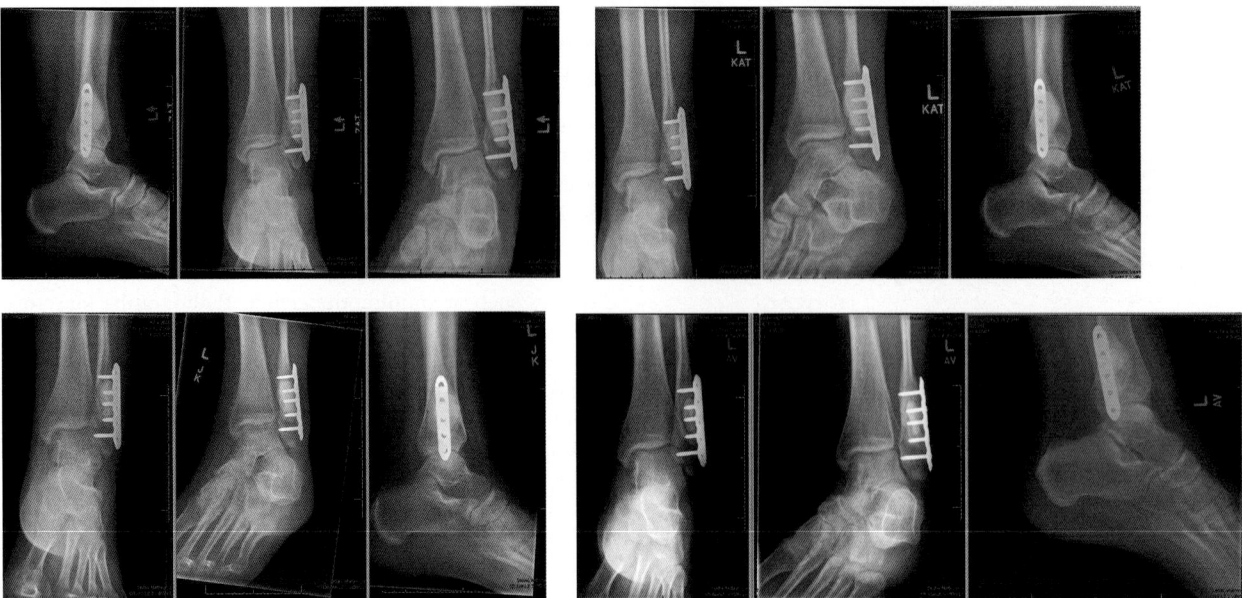

FIGURE 45.12 Postoperative radiographs (from left to right) at 2, 6, 12, and 20 weeks.

dermis or deeper tissues.[127] This can be a result of trauma or surgery.[128,129] When they occur in the feet, they are typically a result of trauma to the nail bed.[130] Ectopic cells can proliferate and form a keratin-lined cyst.[127] Patients present with pain, and radiographs reveal a radiolucency in the subungual distal phalanx.[129] Treatment is curettage with or without bone grafting.[131] Giant epidermal inclusion cysts are a rare variant, which can mimic malignancy, and several cases have been reported in the foot, including the medial aspect of the hallux with underlying osseous changes.[132]

INTRAOSSEOUS LIPOMA

Intraosseous lipomas are rare and constitute <0.1% of bone tumors.[133] Campbell et al. reported on 35 new cases and their meta-analysis revealed only 110 previously reported cases in the English literature.[134] The calcaneus is most commonly affected.[134] The etiology of these lesions is controversial, but the consistent location in the calcaneus at the critical angle of Gissane suggests that biomechanical stresses may be involved.[134] Most are asymptomatic and discovered inciden-

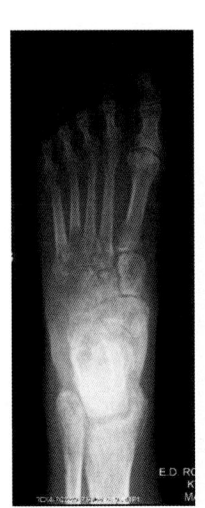
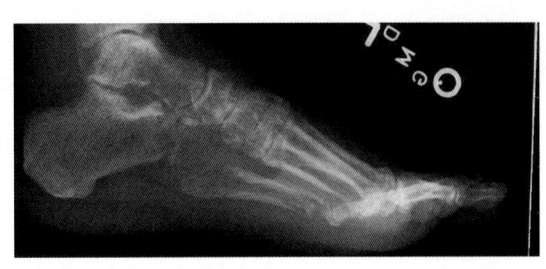
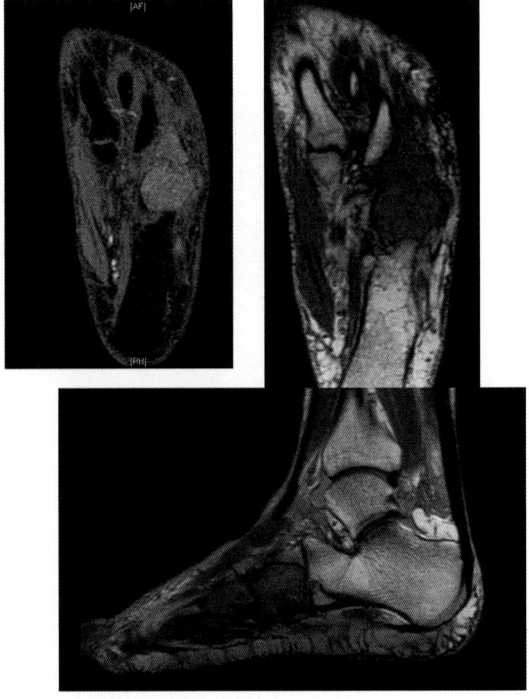

FIGURE 45.13 AP and lateral radiographs and MRI images of a giant cell tumor of bone. Note the destructive nature of the tumor extending across multiple bones in the midfoot.

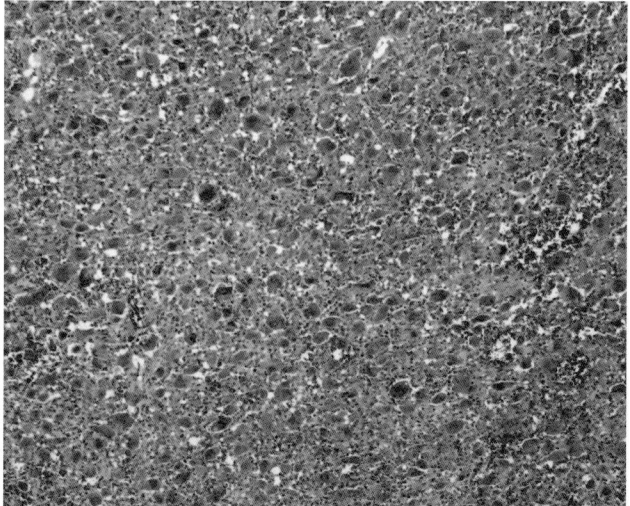

FIGURE 45.14 Photomicrograph of the biopsy of the foot lesion showing giant cell tumor of bone. Note the many giant cells in a background of smaller cells.

tally on radiographs as a well-defined lesion with marginal sclerosis (61%) and central calcifications (62%) and are often confused with a simple bone cyst[134,135] (Fig. 45.18). Observation is recommended for asymptomatic lesions. Advanced imaging modalities can confirm the presence of fat but are rarely necessary (Fig. 45.17). As is the case with other fatty tumors, biopsy results can be variable.[136] In patients with pain suspected to be related to the intraosseous lipoma, curettage and bone grafting has shown reliable decrease in pain and improved functional scores[79,136] (Fig. 45.18). Neither recurrence nor malignant change during follow-up were reported in a single institution analysis of 21 patients over 17 years.[133]

TUMORLIKE CONDITIONS

INFECTION

It is important to consider infection in the differential diagnosis of suspected bone tumors. Classic signs of infection such as warmth, redness, and drainage may not be present, especially in the scenario of chronic or subacute osteomyelitis. Children are more likely to develop hematogenous osteomyelitis than adults. A thorough history is important to assess risk factors such as immunodeficiency. Radiographs may reveal a geographic lesion, periosteal elevation, or a permeative appearance. Gadolinium-enhanced MRI can aid in the diagnosis and help to differentiate infection from tumor. Complete blood count, erythrocyte sedimentation rate, and C-reactive protein are important laboratory tests in cases of suspected infection, and cultures should be obtained at the time of biopsy. Once the diagnosis of osteomyelitis is confirmed, treatment should consist of appropriate antibiotic therapy with aggressive surgical debridement indicated for recalcitrant cases or with subperiosteal abscess.

EOSINOPHILIC GRANULOMA

Langerhans cell histiocytosis (LCH) (histiocytosis X) is a group of disorders characterized by the proliferation of macrophages (histiocytes). This has been previously referred to as eosinophilic granuloma (EG) with disease process limited to bones, but this presentation is now recognized as a variation of LCH. In the majority of cases, the skull, spine, pelvis, and ribs are involved. Foot and ankle involvement is rare, and isolated involvement of the foot and ankle has not been reported. EG has classically been referred to as the "great mimicker" as radiographs can demonstrate various degrees of lucency, sclerosis, and even periosteal reaction. Most cases are seen in individuals under 21 years of age, and the mean age at presentation is 8.9 years.[137] While LCH is a non-neoplastic

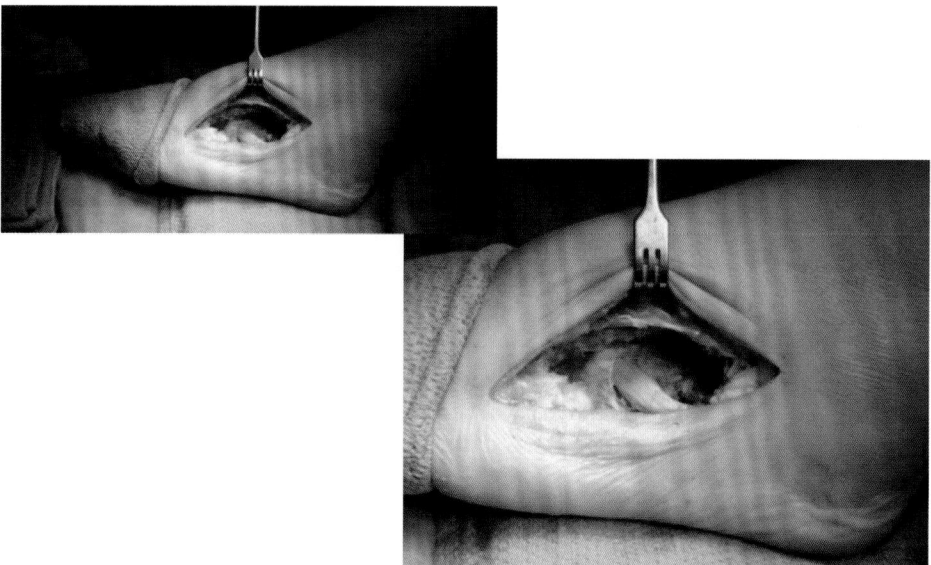

FIGURE 45.15 Intraoperative photograph after complete removal of the giant cell tumor of bone and after adjuvant treatment with argon beam cautery.

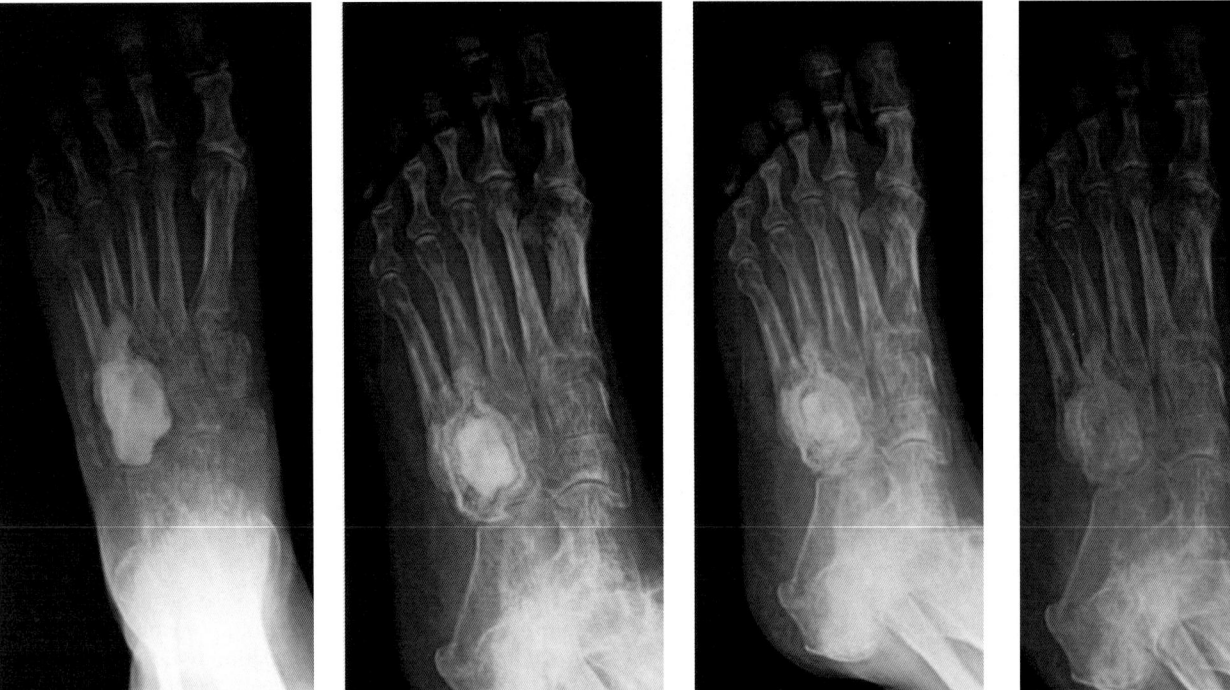

FIGURE 45.16 Radiographs at 2 weeks, 6 weeks, 3 months, and 1 year after curettage and bone grafting of a giant cell tumor of bone of the midfoot.

entity, studies suggest a higher rate of additional malignancies in adults with LCH.[138,139] Aggressive lesions in the absence of an established diagnosis require biopsy. Treatment of disseminated disease requires referral for medical management. Chemotherapy, immunosuppression, and external beam radiation have all been utilized.[140] Intralesional corticosteroid injection has been shown to be successful for symptomatic lesions.[141]

FIBROUS DYSPLASIA

Fibrous dysplasia is a developmental anomaly characterized by fibrous and fibro-osseous tissue replacing bone marrow and normal cancellous bone. Manifestations are variable, ranging from isolated lesions to diffuse involvement leading to significant deformities. There are four recognized categories of fibrous dysplasia: monostotic, polyostotic, McCune-Albright syndrome, and Mazabraud syndrome.[142] The majority of skeletal lesions manifest in the first decade of life and can persist through adulthood. Fracture rates peak between 6 and 10 years of age.[142] Radiographs reveal a characteristic "ground glass" appearance with a sharp border in the metaphysis or diaphysis of long bones.[143] Bones in the foot are involved in 73% of cases.[144] Lesions in the foot are most commonly treated conservatively. However, curettage, bone grafting, and internal fixation may be necessary in the face of pathologic fracture or impending fracture but are associated with a high recurrence rate (Fig. 45.19).

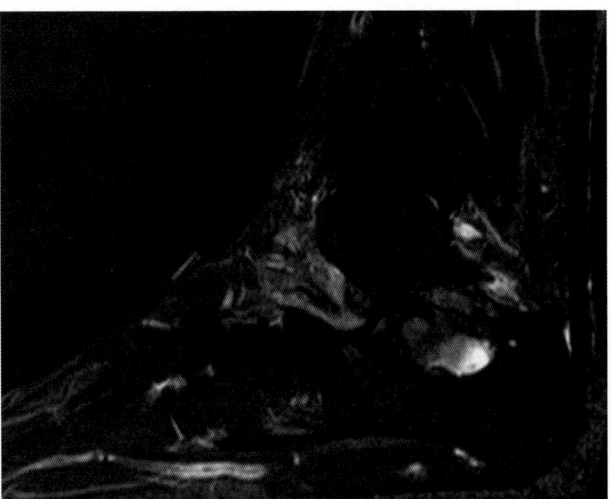
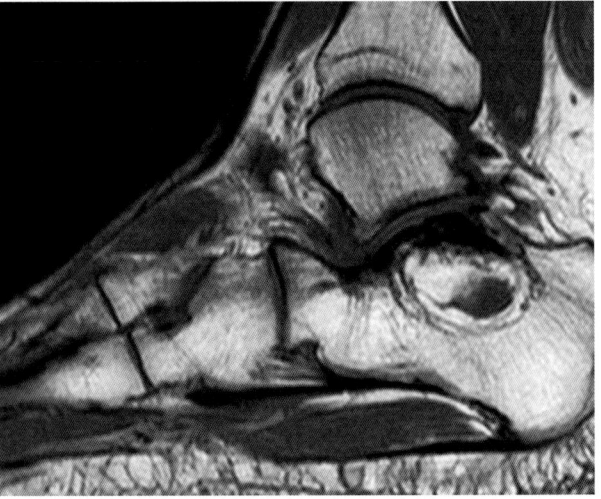

FIGURE 45.17 T2 and T1 images of an intraosseus lipoma of the calcaneus.

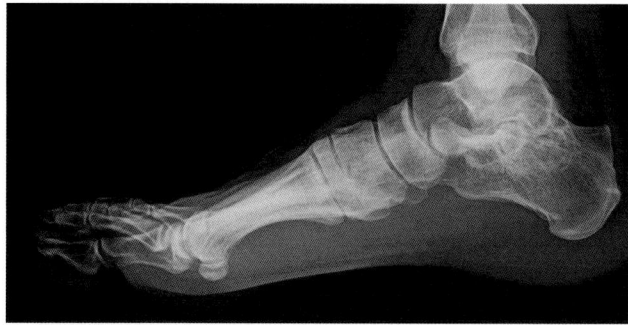

FIGURE 45.18 Lateral radiograph showing intraosseus lipoma of the calcaneus.

HYPERPARATHYROIDISM (BROWN TUMOR)

Elevated levels of parathyroid hormone, no matter the cause, lead to disordered bone metabolism. This can manifest as generalized osteoporosis, subperiosteal bone resorption, and occasionally reactive bone lesions known as Brown tumors. Named for the color of hemosiderin deposits, the so-called Brown tumor develops during the bone remodeling process. These tumors are seen in 4.5% of patients with primary and 1.5% to 1.7% of patients with secondary hyperparathyroidism.[145] The most common location is the pelvis, ribs, or clavicle, and they are exceedingly rare in the foot and ankle.[145,146] Multiple giant cells are seen histologically and therefore are occasionally confused with giant cell tumor of bone.[147] Treatment should focus on medical management of hyperparathyroidism. Surgical treatment is rarely indicated.[147]

CHONDROSARCOMA

Among primary malignant bone tumors of the foot and ankle, chondrosarcoma is the most common.[148] However, <5% of all chondrosarcomas appear in this location.[149,150] The calcaneus and hallux are the most common sites in the foot.[149,150] It is important to understand that chondrosarcoma is highly variable, and disease can range from indolent to fulminant. Establishing an appropriate radiographic/histologic grade is of utmost importance in determining an appropriate treatment plan. Axial lesions are much more likely to metastasize, regardless of grade, and are treated more aggressively. Low-grade chondrosarcomas, particularly those in the extremities, have low incidence of metastasis.[151]

Chondrosarcomas can either arise de novo (primary) or from malignant transformation of an enchondroma (secondary). The typical clinical presentation is either pain and a new mass or change in an existing mass. Radiographs are variable depending on the grade of the lesion and range from the appearance of an enchondroma with atypical features such as bone erosion to change in bone morphology to a highly destructive lesion (Fig. 45.20). MRI is useful in determining the amount of marrow and soft tissue involvement (Fig. 45.21). CT

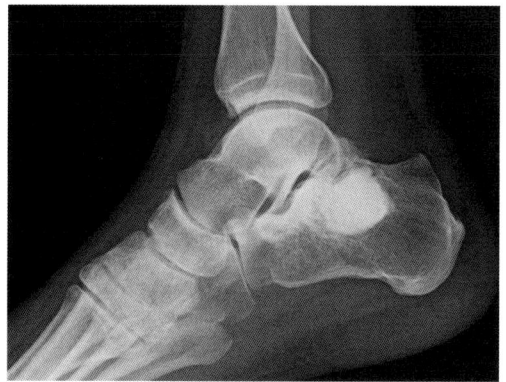
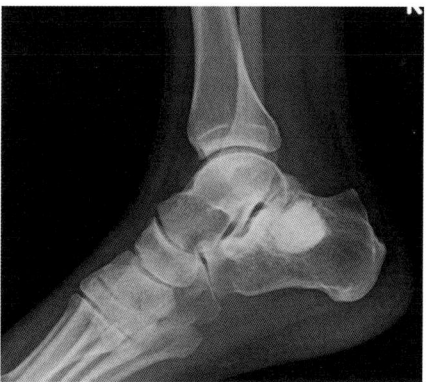
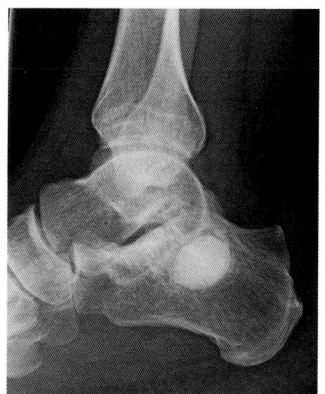
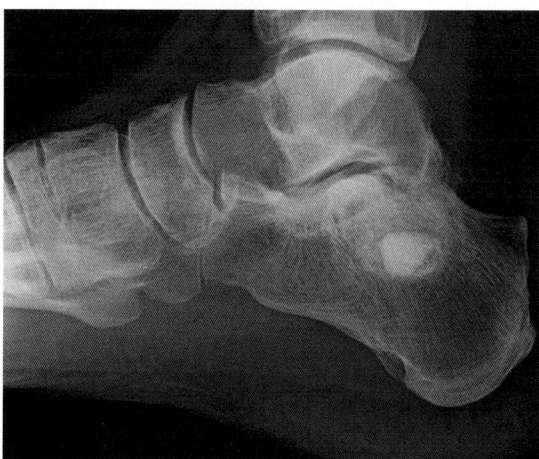
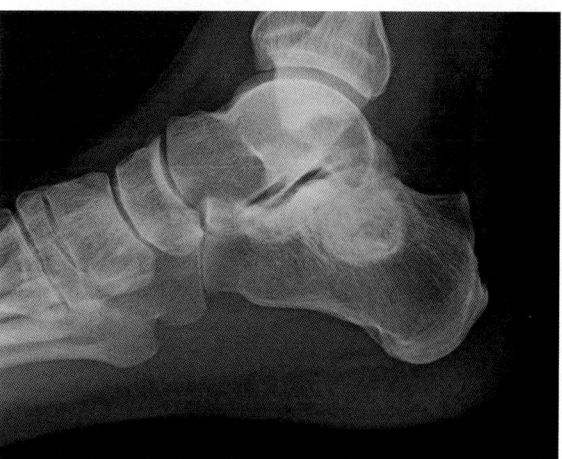

FIGURE 45.19 Treatment of calcaneus intraosseous lipoma with curettage and bone grafting at 2 weeks, 6 weeks, 10 weeks, 14 weeks, and at 1 year.

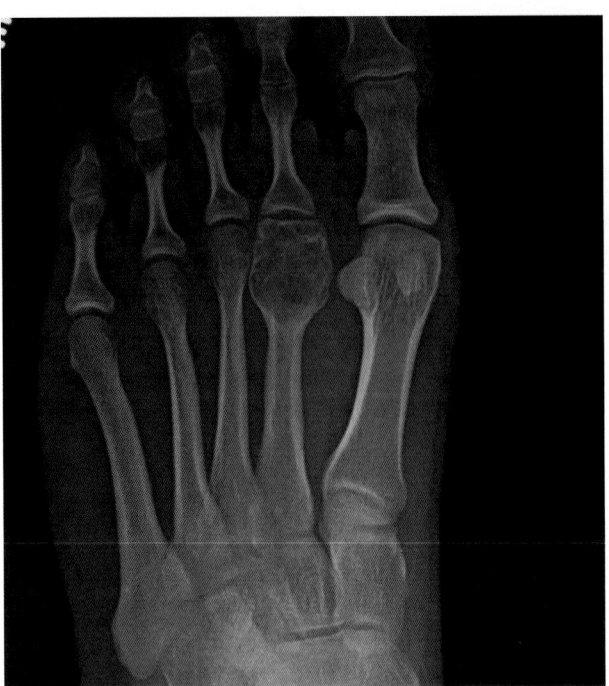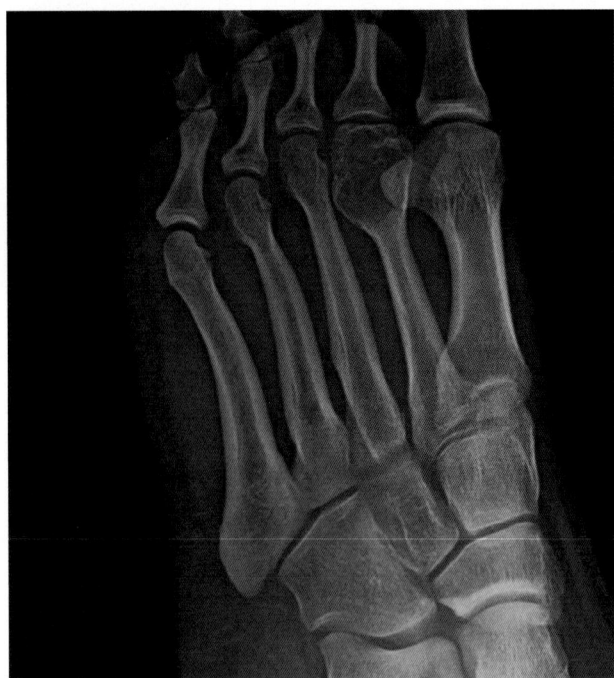

FIGURE 45.20 Radiographs of a 21-year-old male with a painful second metatarsal bone lesion. Note the expansion of the bone.

is the modality of choice for assessing cortical integrity.[152] Standard bone scan or PET scan is helpful for staging.

Because of the high level of heterogeneity within the tumor, biopsy if done should consist of multiple cores from multiple locations as some areas of a high-grade lesion may appear less aggressive or benign[153] (Fig. 45.22). Both radiologic appearance and histologic grade should be taken into consideration when developing a treatment plan.

Chondrosarcoma is generally resistant to chemotherapy and radiation, and treatment is primarily surgical. The appropriate surgical intervention is based on histologic grade and

anatomical factors and can range from intralesional curettage to limb salvage or amputation[154] (Fig. 45.23).

EWING SARCOMA

Ewing sarcoma (ES) is a primary malignant bone tumor. Overall, it is less common than osteosarcoma but is more common than osteosarcoma in the foot.[155,156] It is primarily a pediatric condition with most cases presenting before 20 years of age. ES is a small round blue cell tumor, which expresses CD99. The

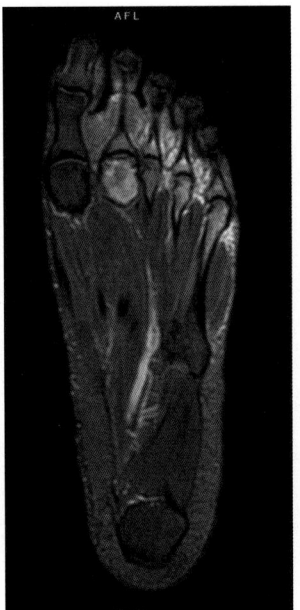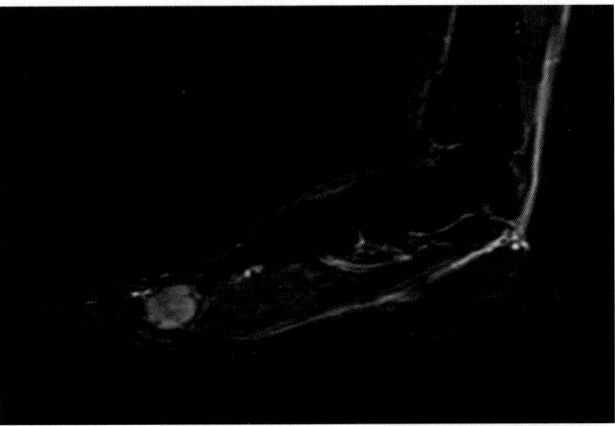

FIGURE 45.21 MRI images showing a high T2 signal lesion in the second metatarsal with bone expansion.

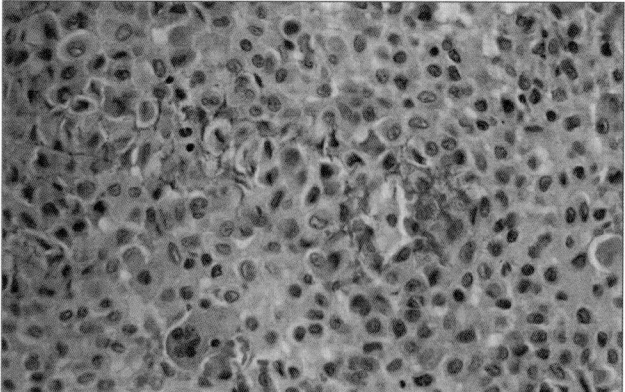

FIGURE 45.22 Photomicrograph of the biopsy specimen from Figure 45.20 showing clear cell chondrosarcoma.

pathognomonic 11:22 translocation is present in a vast majority of cases.[157] Yang's series found 20 patients with Ewing sarcoma of the foot. Six involved the hindfoot, 2 the midfoot, 8 the rays, and 3 the hallux.[150] Twenty-nine cases involving the calcaneus were reported between 1921 and 2006.[158] Patients typically present with regional pain. Ewing sarcoma is often misdiagnosed, and even more so when it occurs in an atypical location such as the foot. Unfortunately, treatment is often delayed >9 months from initial presentation.[159] ES can present similarly to infection including systemic symptoms and elevated inflammatory markers. Radiographs often underestimate the extent of the lesion, which often has a large soft tissue component (Fig. 45.24A). Advanced imaging should be considered early in the presence of pain without a history of trauma[158] (Fig. 45.24B). Appropriate biopsy, staging, and multidisciplinary approach to treatment is required (Fig. 45.25). Local control involves surgery, radiation, or a combination, with systemic neoadjuvant and adjuvant chemotherapy.[157] Surgical resection with a wide margin is necessary and often requires some level of amputation in the foot and ankle.[155,156]

OSTEOSARCOMA

Osteosarcoma is the most common primary bone tumor in both adults and children, but it is the least common in the foot and ankle.[150] The majority of cases of osteosarcoma are seen about the knee and proximal humerus with a peak incidence in the second decade of life. A recent review of the Cooperative Osteosarcoma Study Group (COSS) between January 1980 and April 2016 found 23 patients with primary osteosarcoma of the foot. The median age in this group was 32 years, and the tarsus was most commonly affected.[160] Of these 23 patients, 10 were female and 13 were male. The clinical presentation of osteosarcoma of the foot is similar to that in other areas of the body and involves pain or pathologic fracture. Plain radiography will reveal a destructive lesion (Fig. 45.26A). MRI with contrast is the advanced imaging modality of choice and is useful in surgical planning to determine the extent of bone and soft tissue involvement (Fig. 45.26B). Histology will show malignant osteoid forming tumor and is further differentiated into osteoblastic, chondroblastic, and fibroblastic subtypes (Fig. 45.27). Once the diagnosis is confirmed, treatment involves a multidisciplinary approach. Neoadjuvant chemotherapy followed by wide surgical resection and adjuvant chemotherapy is standard treatment for high-grade osteosarcomas.

METASTATIC CARCINOMA

Metastatic carcinoma involving the bones of the foot and ankle is rarely seen. Lung and genitourinary origin has been described most often.[161,162] Renal cell and colon cancer have also been described as common sources.[163] A recent review of a 40 000 patient tumor database over a 30-year period revealed only 15 patients with osseous metastatic lesions within the foot. The sites of their primary tumors were as follows: 4 lung, 2 breast, and 9 infradiaphragmatic including 2 bladder, 2 melanoma, 1 uterine, 1 anal, 1 vaginal, and 1 rhabdomyosarcoma.[150]

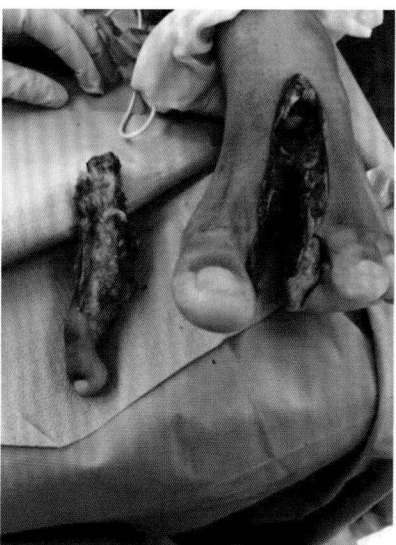 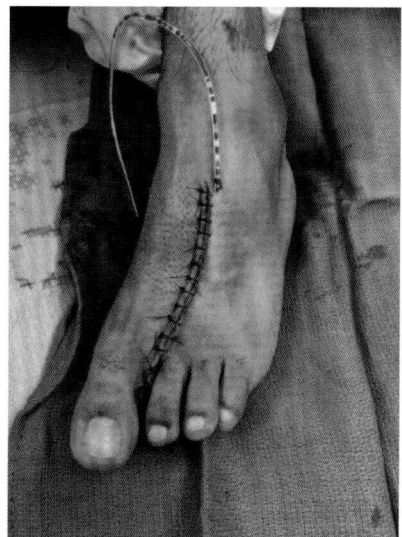 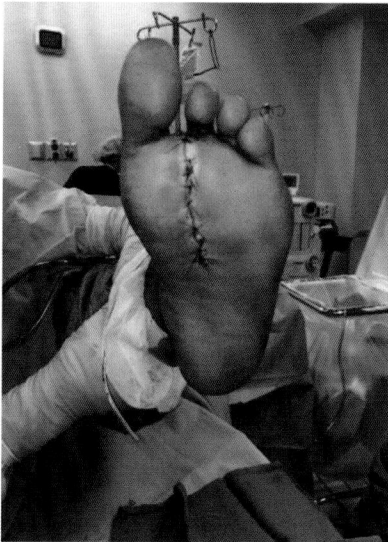

FIGURE 45.23 Intraoperative photographs of a second ray resection for chondrosarcoma of the second metatarsal.

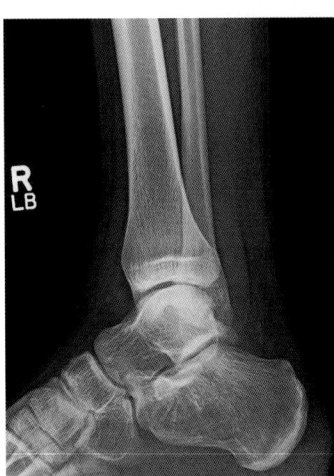
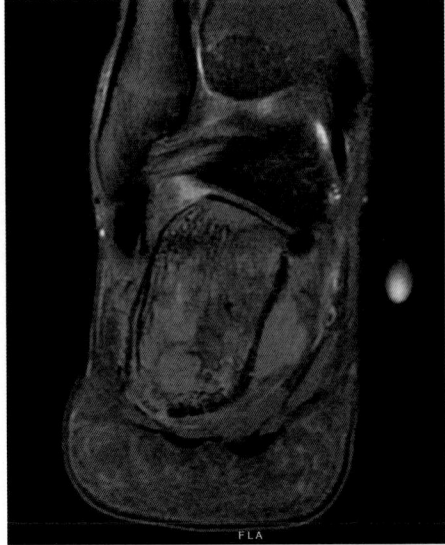
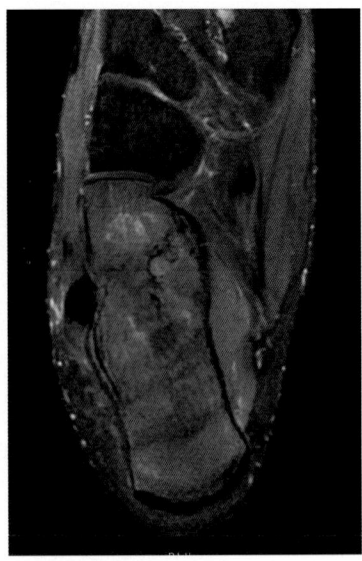

FIGURE 45.24 Lateral x-ray and coronal and axial images of a 17-year-old male with ankle pain. Note the subtle changes in the calcaneus on x-ray. On MRI, there is a marrow replacing bone lesion with extra-osseous extension indicating an aggressive process.

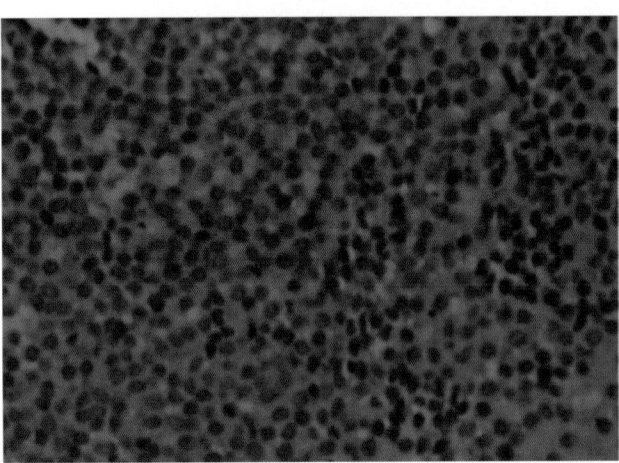

FIGURE 45.25 Biopsy specimen showing sheets of small round blue cells consistent with Ewing sarcoma. Treatment consisted of chemotherapy and below knee amputation.

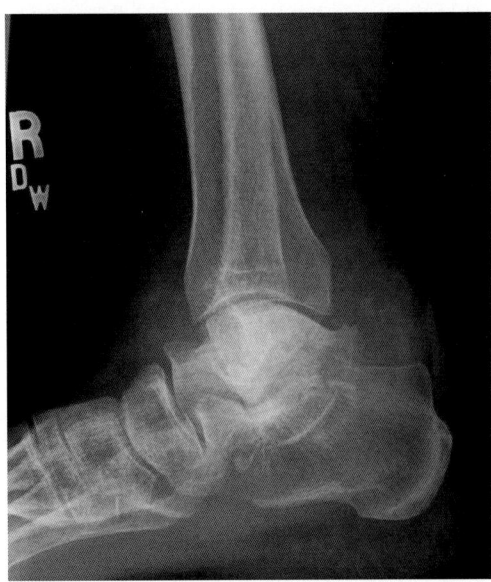
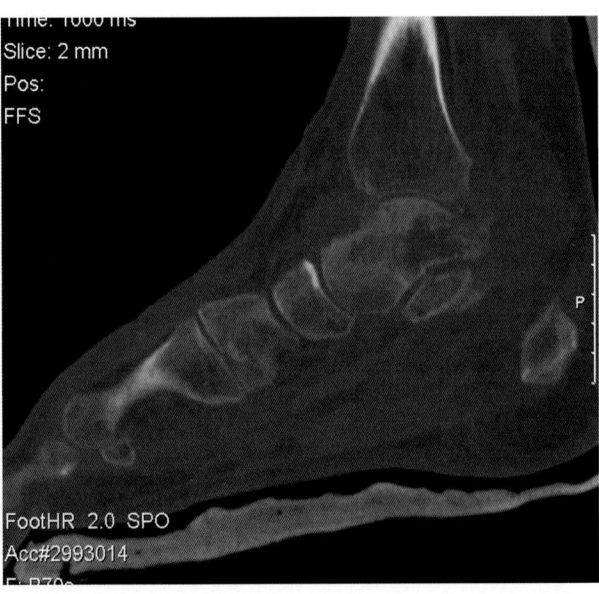

FIGURE 45.26 A 25-year-old male. Lateral ankle x-ray and sagittal CT image show a lytic destructive lesion in the right talus. Note periosteal reaction on posterior talus. Biopsy consistent with osteosarcoma.

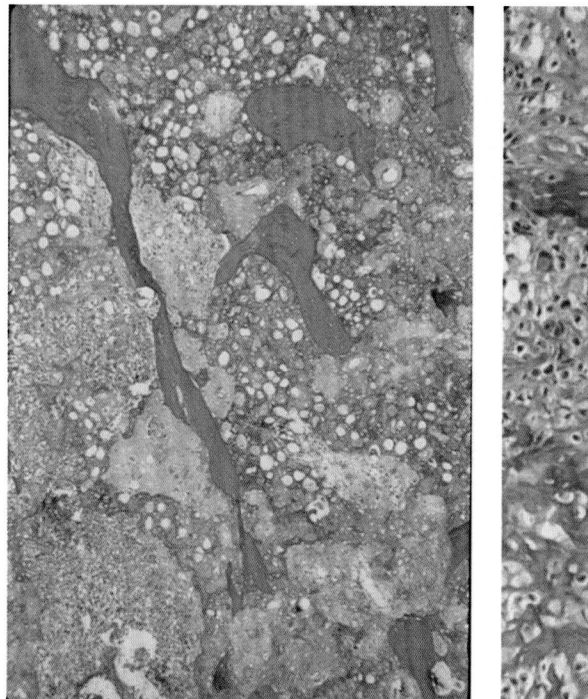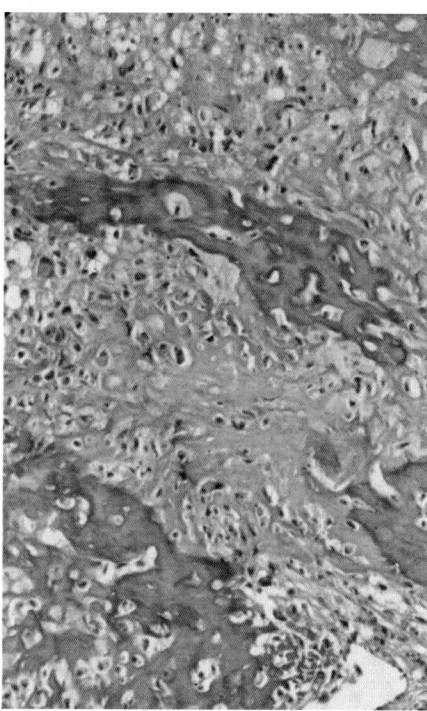

FIGURE 45.27 Photomicrographs of osteogenic osteosarcoma. Note large cells with irregular hyperchromatic nuclei. The background of light pink material indicates production of osteoid, one of the hallmarks of osteosarcoma. Treatment consisted of chemotherapy followed by below knee amputation.

The calcaneus is the most commonly affected bone. Lesions in the hindfoot and midfoot are more common than those of the forefoot.[150] Treatment is based on the severity of symptoms and likelihood of pathologic fracture. Nonoperative treatment options include radiation, bisphosphonates, and denosumab. Embolization can be effective in renal cell carcinoma and other hypervascular tumors. Curettage, bone grafting, and internal fixation are indicated for larger lesions and pathologic fractures or impending fractures. Amputation may be appropriate for refractory lesions of metatarsals and phalanges.

REFERENCES

1. Fetsch JF, Laskin WB, Miettinen M. Palmar-plantar fibromatosis in children and preadolescents: a clinicopathologic study of 56 cases with newly recognized demographics and extended follow-up information. *Am J Surg Pathol.* 2005;29(8):1095-1105.
2. Cummings JE, Smith RA, Heck RK. Argon beam coagulation as adjuvant treatment after curettage of aneurysmal bone cysts: a preliminary study. *Clin Orthop Relat Res.* 2010;468(1):231-237.
3. Aluisio FV, Mair SD, Hall RL. Plantar fibromatosis: treatment of primary and recurrent lesions and factors associated with recurrence. *Foot Ankle Int.* 1996;17(11):672-678.
4. Sammarco GJ, Mangone PG. Classification and treatment of plantar fibromatosis. *Foot Ankle Int.* 2000;21(7):563-569.
5. Mankin HJ, Hornicek FJ, Springfield DS. Extra-abdominal desmoid tumors: a report of 234 cases. *J Surg Oncol.* 2010;102(5):380-384.
6. De Bree E, Zoras O, Hunt JL, et al. Desmoid tumors of the head and neck: a therapeutic challenge. *Head Neck.* 2014;36(10):1517-1526.
7. Okuno SH, Edmonson JH. Combination chemotherapy for desmoid tumors. *Cancer.* 2003;97(4):1134-1135.
8. Fiore M, Rimareix F, Mariani L, et al. Desmoid-type fibromatosis: a front-line conservative approach to select patients for surgical treatment. *Ann Surg Oncol.* 2009;16(9):2587-2593.
9. Gronchi A, Casali PG, Mariani L, et al. Quality of surgery and outcome in extra-abdominal aggressive fibromatosis: a series of patients surgically treated at a single institution. *J Clin Oncol.* 2003;21(7):1390-1397.
10. Zelger B, Zelger BG, Burgdorf WH. Dermatofibroma—a critical evaluation. *Int J Surg Pathol.* 2004;12(4):333-344.
11. Fitzpatrick TB, Gilchrest BA. Dimple sign to differentiate benign from malignant pigmented cutaneous lesions. *N Engl J Med.* 1977;296(26):1518.
12. Requena L, Fernández-figueras MT. Subcutaneous granuloma annulare. *Semin Cutan Med Surg.* 2007;26(2):96-99.
13. Ramappa AJ, Lee FY, Tang P, Carlson JR, Gebhardt MC, Mankin HJ. Chondroblastoma of bone. *J Bone Joint Surg Am.* 2000;82-A(8):1140-1145.
14. Rogalski R, Hensinger R, Loder R. Vascular abnormalities of the extremities: clinical findings and management. *J Pediatr Orthop.* 1993;13(1):9-14.
15. Papp DF, Khanna AJ, McCarthy EF, Carrino JA, Farber AJ, Frassica FJ. Magnetic resonance imaging of soft-tissue tumors: determinate and indeterminate lesions. *J Bone Joint Surg Am.* 2007;89(suppl 3):103-115.
16. Wu KK. Lymphangioma of the ankle region. *J Foot Ankle Surg.* 1996;35(3):263-265.
17. Hogeling M, Adams S, Wargon O. A randomized controlled trial of propranolol for infantile hemangiomas. *Pediatrics.* 2011;128(2):e259-e266.
18. Bella GP, Manivel JC, Thompson RC, Clohisy DR, Cheng EY. Intramuscular hemangioma: recurrence risk related to surgical margins. *Clin Orthop Relat Res.* 2007;459:186-191.
19. Kuru I, Oktar SO, Maralcan G, Yaycioğlu S, Bozan ME. [Familial glomus tumor encountered in the same finger and localization in four family members]. *Acta Orthop Traumatol Turc.* 2005;39(4):365-368.
20. Moor EV, Goldberg I, Westreich M. Multiple glomus tumor: a case report and review of the literature. *Ann Plast Surg.* 1999;43(4):436-438.
21. Heje M, Bang C, Jensen SS. Glomus tumours causing limb hypoplasia?. *J Bone Joint Surg Br.* 1992;74(5):779-780.
22. Kehoe NJ, Reid RP, Semple JC. Solitary benign peripheral-nerve tumours. Review of 32 years' experience. *J Bone Joint Surg Br.* 1995;77(3):497-500.
23. Zivot ML, Pitzer S, Pantig-felix L, Nathan LE. Malignant schwannoma of the medial plantar branch of the posterior tibial nerve. *J Foot Surg.* 1990;29(2):130-134.
24. Reed TS, Marty JA. Peripheral nerve tumors. Large neurofibroma of the foot. *J Am Podiatr Med Assoc.* 1995;85(10):552-554.
25. Vitale MG, Guha A, Skaggs DL. Orthopaedic manifestations of neurofibromatosis in children: an update. *Clin Orthop Relat Res.* 2002;(401):107-118.
26. Bojanic I, Bergovec M, Smoljanovic T. Combined anterior and posterior arthroscopic portals for loose body removal and synovectomy for synovial chondromatosis. *Foot Ankle Int.* 2009;30(11):1120-1123.
27. Grivas TB, Savvidou OD, Psarakis SA, et al. Forefoot plantar multilobular noninfiltrating angiolipoma: a case report and review of the literature. *World J Surg Oncol.* 2008;6:11.
28. Ahn JH, Choy WS, Kim HY. Operative treatment for ganglion cysts of the foot and ankle. *J Foot Ankle Surg.* 2010;49(5):442-445.
29. Angelides AC, Wallace PF. The dorsal ganglion of the wrist: its pathogenesis, gross and microscopic anatomy, and surgical treatment. *J Hand Surg Am.* 1976;1(3):228-235.
30. Rosson GD, Spinner RJ, Dellon AL. Tarsal tunnel surgery for treatment of tarsal ganglion: a rewarding operation with devastating potential complications. *J Am Podiatr Med Assoc.* 2005;95(5):459-463.
31. Jones FE, Soule EH, Coventry MB. Fibrous xanthoma of synovium (giant-cell tumor of tendon sheath, pigmented nodular synovitis). A study of one hundred and eighteen cases. *J Bone Joint Surg Am.* 1969;51(1):76-86.

32. Vargaonkar G, Singh V, Arora S, et al. Giant cell tumor of the tendon sheath around the foot and ankle. A report of three cases and a literature review. *J Am Podiatr Med Assoc.* 2015;105(3):249-254.
33. Fałek A, Niemunis-sawicka J, Wrona K, et al. Pigmented villonodular synovitis. *Folia Med Cracov.* 2018;58(4):93-104.
34. Iovane A, Midiri M, Bartolotta TV, et al. Pigmented villonodular synovitis of the foot: MR findings. *Radiol Med.* 2003;106(1-2):66-73.
35. Bisbinas I, De Silva U, Grimer RJ. Pigmented villonodular synovitis of the foot and ankle: a 12-year experience from a tertiary orthopedic Oncology Unit. *J Foot Ankle Surg.* 2004;43(6):407-411.
36. Brien EW, Sacoman DM, Mirra JM. Pigmented villonodular synovitis of the foot and ankle. *Foot Ankle Int.* 2004;25(12):908-913.
37. Ioannidis JP. Large scale evidence and replication: insights from rheumatology and beyond. *Ann Rheum Dis.* 2005;64(3):345-346.
38. Galat DD, Ackerman DB, Spoon D, Turner NS, Shives TC. Synovial chondromatosis of the foot and ankle. *Foot Ankle Int.* 2008;29(3):312-317.
39. Young-In Lee F, Hornicek FJ, Dick HM, Mankin HJ. Synovial chondromatosis of the foot. *Clin Orthop Relat Res.* 2004;(423):186-190.
40. Tsouli SG, Kiortsis DN, Argyropoulou MI, Mikhailidis DP, Elisaf MS. Pathogenesis, detection and treatment of Achilles tendon xanthomas. *Eur J Clin Invest.* 2005;35(4):236-244.
41. Yu JS, Chung C, Recht M, Dailiana T, Jurdi R. MR imaging of tophaceous gout. *AJR Am J Roentgenol.* 1997;168(2):523-527.
42. Ferrari A, Sultan I, Huang TT, et al. Soft tissue sarcoma across the age spectrum: a population-based study from the Surveillance Epidemiology and End Results database. *Pediatr Blood Cancer.* 2011;57(6):943-949.
43. Popov P, Tukiainen E, Asko-Seljaavaara S, et al. Soft tissue sarcomas of the lower extremity: surgical treatment and outcome. *Eur J Surg Oncol.* 2000;26(7):679-685.
44. Davis AM, O'Sullivan B, Turcotte R, et al. Late radiation morbidity following randomization to preoperative versus postoperative radiotherapy in extremity soft tissue sarcoma. *Radiother Oncol.* 2005;75(1):48-53.
45. Latt LD, Turcotte RE, Isler MH, Wong C. Case series. Soft-tissue sarcoma of the foot. *Can J Surg.* 2010;53(6):424-431.
46. Thacker MM, Potter BK, Pitcher JD, Temple HT. Soft tissue sarcomas of the foot and ankle: impact of unplanned excision, limb salvage, and multimodality therapy. *Foot Ankle Int.* 2008;29(7):690-698.
47. Bhutani M, Polizzotto MN, Uldrick TS, Yarchoan R. Kaposi sarcoma-associated herpesvirus-associated malignancies: epidemiology, pathogenesis, and advances in treatment. *Semin Oncol.* 2015;42(2):223-246.
48. Uldrick TS, Whitby D. Update on KSHV epidemiology, Kaposi Sarcoma pathogenesis, and treatment of Kaposi Sarcoma. *Cancer Lett.* 2011;305(2):150-162.
49. Gressen EL, Rosenstock JG, Xie Y, Corn BW. Palliative treatment of epidemic Kaposi sarcoma of the feet. *Am J Clin Oncol.* 1999;22(3):286-290.
50. Bristow IR, De Berker DA, Acland KM, Turner RJ, Bowling J. Clinical guidelines for the recognition of melanoma of the foot and nail unit. *J Foot Ankle Res.* 2010;3:25.
51. Linos E, Swetter SM, Cockburn MG, Colditz GA, Clarke CA. Increasing burden of melanoma in the United States. *J Invest Dermatol.* 2009;129(7):1666-1674.
52. Durbec F, Martin L, Derancourt C, Grange F. Melanoma of the hand and foot: epidemiological, prognostic and genetic features. A systematic review. *Br J Dermatol.* 2012;166(4):727-739.
53. Bellows CF, Belafsky P, Fortgang IS, Beech DJ. Melanoma in African-Americans: trends in biological behavior and clinical characteristics over two decades. *J Surg Oncol.* 2001;78(1):10-16.
54. Fortin PT, Freiberg AA, Rees R, Sondak VK, Johnson TM. Malignant melanoma of the foot and ankle. *J Bone Joint Surg Am.* 1995;77(9):1396-1403.
55. Rubin AI, Chen EH, Ratner D. Basal-cell carcinoma. *N Engl J Med.* 2005;353(21):2262-2269.
56. Krüger K, Blume-peytavi U, Orfanos CE. Basal cell carcinoma possibly originates from the outer root sheath and/or the bulge region of the vellus hair follicle. *Arch Dermatol Res.* 1999;291(5):253-259.
57. Patel RV, Frankel A, Goldenberg G. An update on nonmelanoma skin cancer. *J Clin Aesthet Dermatol.* 2011;4(2):20-27.
58. Dessinioti C, Antoniou C, Katsambas A, Stratigos AJ. Basal cell carcinoma: what's new under the sun. *Photochem Photobiol.* 2010;86(3):481-491.
59. Gollnick H, Barona CG, Frank RG, et al. Recurrence rate of superficial basal cell carcinoma following treatment with imiquimod 5% cream: conclusion of a 5-year long-term follow-up study in Europe. *Eur J Dermatol.* 2008;18(6):677-682.
60. Basset-seguin N, Ibbotson SH, Emtestam L, et al. Topical methyl aminolaevulinate photodynamic therapy versus cryotherapy for superficial basal cell carcinoma: a 5 year randomized trial. *Eur J Dermatol.* 2008;18(5):547-553.
61. Kerr-valentic MA, Samimi K, Rohlen BH, Agarwal JP, Rockwell WB. Marjolin's ulcer: modern analysis of an ancient problem. *Plast Reconstr Surg.* 2009;123(1):184-191.
62. Senet P, Combemale P, Debure C, et al. Malignancy and chronic leg ulcers: the value of systematic wound biopsies: a prospective, multicenter, cross-sectional study. *Arch Dermatol.* 2012;148(6):704-708.
63. Cooper JZ, Brown MD. Special concern about squamous cell carcinoma of the scalp in organ transplant recipients. *Arch Dermatol.* 2006;142(6):755-758.
64. Lansbury L, Leonardi-bee J, Perkins W, Goodacre T, Tweed JA, Bath-hextall FJ. Interventions for non-metastatic squamous cell carcinoma of the skin. *Cochrane Database Syst Rev.* 2010;(4):CD007869.
65. Brantsch KD, Meisner C, Schönfisch B, et al. Analysis of risk factors determining prognosis of cutaneous squamous-cell carcinoma: a prospective study. *Lancet Oncol.* 2008;9(8):713-720.
66. Plaza JA, Perez-montiel D, Mayerson J, Morrison C, Suster S. Metastases to soft tissue: a review of 118 cases over a 30-year period. *Cancer.* 2008;112(1):193-203.
67. Beltrami G, Ristori G, Scoccianti G, Tamburini A, Capanna R. Hereditary multiple exostoses: a review of clinical appearance and metabolic pattern. *Clin Cases Miner Bone Metab.* 2016;13(2):110-118.
68. Czajka CM, DiCaprio MR. What is the proportion of patients with multiple hereditary exostoses who undergo malignant degeneration? *Clin Orthop Relat Res.* 2015;473(7):2355-2361.
69. Whitaker JM, Craig GC, Winship S. Osteochondroma of the cuboid: a case report. *J Foot Ankle Surg.* 2017;56(6):1269-1275.
70. Chin KR, Kharrazi FD, Miller BS, Mankin HJ, Gebhardt MC. Osteochondromas of the distal aspect of the tibia or fibula. Natural history and treatment. *J Bone Joint Surg Am.* 2000;82(9):1269-1278.
71. Appy-Fedida B, Krief E, Deroussen F, et al. Mitigating risk of ankle valgus from ankle osteochondroma resection using a transfibular approach: a retrospective study with six years of follow-up. *J Foot Ankle Surg.* 2017;56(3):564-567.
72. Atesok KI, Alman BA, Schemitsch EH, Peyser A, Mankin H. Osteoid osteoma and osteoblastoma. *J Am Acad Orthop Surg.* 2011;19(11). https://journals.lww.com/jaaos/Fulltext/2011/11000/Osteoid_Osteoma_and_Osteoblastoma.4.aspx
73. Jordan RW, Koc T, Chapman AWP, Taylor HP. Osteoid osteoma of the foot and ankle—a systematic review. *Foot Ankle Surg.* 2015;21(4):228-234.
74. Jurina A, Dimnjakovic D, Smoljanovic T, Bojanic I. Removal of osteoid osteoma of the calcaneus using subtalar arthroscopy. *Foot Ankle Spec.* 2017;10(4):359-363.
75. Temple HT, Mizel MS, Murphey MD, Sweet DE. Osteoblastoma of the foot and ankle. *Foot Ankle Int.* 1998;19(10):698-704.
76. Nora FE, Dahlin DC, Beabout JW. Bizarre parosteal osteochondromatous proliferations of the hands and feet. *Am J Surg Pathol.* 1983;7(3):245-250.
77. Noguchi M, Ikoma K, Matsumoto N, Nagasawa K. Bizarre parosteal osteochondromatous proliferation of the sesamoid: an unusual hallux valgus deformity. *Foot Ankle Int.* 2004;25(7):503-506. doi: 10.1177/107110070402500710.
78. Gruber G, Giessauf C, Leithner A, et al. Bizarre parosteal osteochondromatous proliferation (Nora lesion): a report of 3 cases and a review of the literature. *Can J Surg.* 2008;51(6):486-489.
79. Cocks M, Helmke E, Meyers CA, Fayad L, McCarthy E, James AW. Bizarre parosteal osteochondromatous proliferation: 16 cases with a focus on histologic variability. *J Orthop.* 2018;15(1):138-142.
80. Doganavsargil B, Argin M, Sezak M, Kececi B, Pehlivanoglu B, Oztop F. A bizarre parosteal osteochondromatous proliferation (Nora's lesion) of metatarsus, a histopathological and etiological puzzlement. *Joint Bone Spine.* 2014;81(6):537-540. http://www.sciencedirect.com/science/article/pii/S1297319X14001894
81. Zambrano E, Nose V, Perez-Atayde AR, et al. Distinct chromosomal rearrangements in subungual (Dupuytren) exostosis and bizarre parosteal osteochondromatous proliferation (Nora lesion). *Am J Surg Pathol.* 2004;28(8):1033-1039.
82. Endo M, Hasegawa T, Tashiro T, et al. Bizarre parosteal osteochondromatous proliferation with a t(1;17) translocation. *Virchows Arch.* 2005;447(1):99-102.
83. Berber O, Dawson-Bowling S, Jalgaonkar A, et al. Bizarre parosteal osteochondromatous proliferation of bone. *J Bone Joint Surg Br.* 2011;93-B(8):1118-1121. doi: 10.1302/0301-620X.93B8.26349.
84. Russell JD, Nance K, Nunley JR, Maher IA. Subungual exostosis. *Cutis.* 2016;98(2):128-129.
85. Lee SK, Jung MS, Lee YH, Gong HS, Kim JK, Baek GH. Two distinctive subungual pathologies: subungual exostosis and subungual osteochondroma. *Foot Ankle Int.* 2007;28(5):595-601. doi: 10.3113/FAI.2007.0595.
86. DaCambra MP, Gupta SK, Ferri-de-Barros F. Subungual exostosis of the toes: a systematic review. *Clin Orthop Relat Res.* 2014;472(4):1251-1259.
87. Chun KA, Stephanie S, Choi JY, Nam JH, Suh JS. Enchondroma of the foot. *J Foot Ankle Surg.* 2015;54(5):836-839.
88. Deckers C, Schreuder BHW, Hannink G, de Rooy JWJ, van der Geest ICM. Radiologic follow-up of untreated enchondroma and atypical cartilaginous tumors in the long bones. *J Surg Oncol.* 2016;114(8):987-991.
89. Gajewski DA, Burnette JB, Murphey MD, Temple HT. Differentiating clinical and radiographic features of enchondroma and secondary chondrosarcoma in the foot. *Foot Ankle Int.* 2006;27(4):240-244. doi: 10.1177/107110070602700403.
90. Pansuriya TC, Kroon HM, Bovee JVMG. Enchondromatosis: insights on the different subtypes. *Int J Clin Exp Pathol.* 2010;3(6):557-569.
91. Verdegaal SHM, Bovee JVMG, Pansuriya TC, et al. Incidence, predictive factors, and prognosis of chondrosarcoma in patients with Ollier disease and Maffucci syndrome: an international multicenter study of 161 patients. *Oncologist.* 2011;16(12):1771-1779.
92. Zheng K, Yu X, Xu S, Xu M. Periosteal chondroma of the femur: a case report and review of the literature. *Oncol Lett.* 2015;9(4):1637-1640.
93. Parodi KK, Farrett W, Paden MH, Stone PA. A report of a rare phalangeal periosteal chondroma of the foot. *J Foot Ankle Surg.* 2011;50(1):122-125. doi: 10.1053/j.jfas.2010.10.003.
94. Rolvien T, Zustin J, Amling M, Yastrebov O. Periosteal chondroma of the cuboid with secondary aneurysmal bone cyst in a setting of secondary hyperparathyroidism. *Foot Ankle Surg.* 2018;24(1):71-75.
95. Angelini A, Arguedas F, Varela A, Ruggieri P. Chondroblastoma of the foot: 40 cases from a single institution. *J Foot Ankle Surg.* 2018;57(6):1105-1109.
96. Xie C, Jeys L, James SLJ. Radiofrequency ablation of chondroblastoma: long-term clinical and imaging outcomes. *Eur Radiol.* 2015;25(4):1127-1134.
97. Zustin J, Akpalo H, Gambarotti M, et al. Phenotypic diversity in chondromyxoid fibroma reveals differentiation pattern of tumor mimicking fetal cartilage canals development: an immunohistochemical study. *Am J Pathol.* 2010;177(3):1072-1078.
98. Roberts EJ, Meier MJ, Hild G, Masadeh S, Hardy M, Bakotic BW. Chondromyxoid fibroma of the calcaneus: two case reports and literature review. *J Foot Ankle Surg.* 2013;52(5):643-649.
99. Toda Y, Sonohata M, Ikebe S, Uchihashi K, Mawatari M. Chondromyxoid fibroma with a secondary aneurysmal bone cyst of the distal radius: a case report. *J Orthop Sci.* 2018.

100. Lersundi A, Mankin HJ, Mourikis A, Hornicek FJ. Chondromyxoid fibroma: a rarely encountered and puzzling tumor. *Clin Orthop Relat Res.* 2005;439:171-175.

101. Ye Y, Pringle LM, Lau AW, et al. TRE17/USP6 oncogene translocated in aneurysmal bone cyst induces matrix metalloproteinase production via activation of NF-kappaB. *Oncogene.* 2010;29(25):3619-3629.

102. Lampasi M, Magnani M, Donzelli O. Aneurysmal bone cysts of the distal fibula in children. *J Bone Joint Surg Br.* 2007;89-B(10):1356-1362. doi: 10.1302/0301-620X.89B10.19375.

103. Mascard E, Gomez-Brouchet A, Lambot K. Bone cysts: unicameral and aneurysmal bone cyst. *Orthop Traumatol Surg Res.* 2015;101(1 suppl):S119-S127.

104. Cottalorda J, Bourelle S. Modern concepts of primary aneurysmal bone cyst. *Arch Orthop Trauma Surg.* 2007;127(2):105-114.

105. Steffner RJ, Liao C, Stacy G, et al. Factors associated with recurrence of primary aneurysmal bone cysts: is argon beam coagulation an effective adjuvant treatment? *J Bone Joint Surg Am.* 2011;93(21):e1221-e1229.

106. Batisse F, Schmitt A, Vendeuvre T, Herbreteau D, Bonnard C. Aneurysmal bone cyst: a 19-case series managed by percutaneous sclerotherapy. *Orthop Traumatol Surg Res.* 2016;102(2):213-216.

107. Rossi G, Mavrogenis AF, Facchini G, et al. How effective is embolization with N-2-butyl-cyanoacrylate for aneurysmal bone cysts? *Int Orthop.* 2017;41(8):1685-1692.

108. O'Keefe RJ, O'Donnell RJ, Temple HT, Scully SP, Mankin HJ. Giant cell tumor of bone in the foot and ankle. *Foot Ankle Int.* 1995;16(10):617-623. doi: 10.1177/107110079501601007.

109. Errani C, Ruggieri P, Asenzio MAN, et al. Giant cell tumor of the extremity: a review of 349 cases from a single institution. *Cancer Treat Rev.* 2010;36(1):1-7.

110. Co HL, Wang EH. Giant cell tumor of the small bones of the foot. *J Orthop Surg (Hong Kong).* 2018;26(3):2309499018801168.

111. Rosario M, Kim H-S, Yun JY, Han I. Surveillance for lung metastasis from giant cell tumor of bone. *J Surg Oncol.* 2017;116(7):907-913.

112. Algawahmed H, Turcotte R, Farrokhyar F, Ghert M. High-speed burring with and without the use of surgical adjuvants in the intralesional management of giant cell tumor of bone: a systematic review and meta-analysis. *Sarcoma.* 2010;2010.

113. Lin W-H, Lan T-Y, Chen C-Y, Wu K, Yang R-S. Similar local control between phenol- and ethanol-treated giant cell tumors of bone. *Clin Orthop Relat Res.* 2011;469(11):3200-3208.

114. Becker WT, Dohle J, Bernd L, et al. Local recurrence of giant cell tumor of bone after intralesional treatment with and without adjuvant therapy. *J Bone Joint Surg Am.* 2008;90(5):1060-1067.

115. Bierman J, Adkins D, Agulnik M, Al E. Bone cancer—giant cell tumor. *J Natl Compr Canc Netw.* 2013;11(6):688-723.

116. Levy DM, Gross CE, Garras DN. Treatment of unicameral bone cysts of the calcaneus: a systematic review. *J Foot Ankle Surg.* 2015;54(4):652-656.

117. Schick FA, Daniel JN, Miller JS. Unicameral bone cyst of the medial cuneiform. *J Am Podiatr Med Assoc.* 2016;106(5):357-360.

118. Wu KK. A surgically treated unicameral (solitary) bone cyst of the talus with a 15-year follow-up. *J Foot Ankle Surg.* 1993;32(2):242-244.

119. Komiya S, Kawabata R, Zenmyo M, Hashimoto S, Inoue A. Increased concentrations of nitrate and nitrite in the cyst fluid suggesting increased nitric oxide synthesis in solitary bone cysts. *J Orthop Res.* 2000;18(2):281-288.

120. Polat O, Saglik Y, Adiguzel HE, Arikan M, Yildiz HY. Our clinical experience on calcaneal bone cysts: 36 cysts in 33 patients. *Arch Orthop Trauma Surg.* 2009;129(11):1489-1494.

121. Glaser DL, Dormans JP, Stanton RP, Davidson RS. Surgical management of calcaneal unicameral bone cysts. *Clin Orthop Relat Res.* 1999;(360):231-237.

122. Li G, Yin J, Gao J, et al. Subchondral bone in osteoarthritis: insight into risk factors and microstructural changes. *Arthritis Res Ther.* 2013;15(6):223.

123. Durr HD, Martin H, Pellenghar C, Schlemmer M, Maier M, Jansson V. The cause of subchondral bone cysts in osteoarthrosis: a finite element analysis. *Acta Orthop Scand.* 2004;75(5):554-558.

124. Ondrouch AS. Cyst formation in osteoarthritis. *J Bone Joint Surg Br.* 1963;45(4):755-760.

125. Murff R, Ashry HR. Intraosseous ganglia of the foot. *J Foot Ankle Surg.* 1994;33(4):396-401.

126. Lui TH. Arthroscopic bone grafting of talar bone cyst using posterior ankle arthroscopy. *J Foot Ankle Surg.* 2013;52(4):529-532.

127. Weir CB, St.Hilaire NJ. *Epidermal Inclusion Cyst.* 2020 Aug 11. In: StatPearls. Treasure Island (FL): StatPearls Publishing; 2020. PMID: 30335343.

128. Tsai T-C, Lo S-P, Lien F-C. Epidermal inclusion cyst following percutaneous trigger finger release. *J Hand Microsurg.* 2018;10:143-145.

129. Wadhams PS, McDonald JF, Jenkin WM. Epidermal inclusion cysts as a complication of nail surgery. *J Am Podiatr Med Assoc.* 1990;80(11):610-612.

130. Van Tongel A, De Paepe P, Berghs B. Epidermoid cyst of the phalanx of the finger caused by nail biting. *J Plast Surg Hand Surg.* 2012;46(6):450-451.

131. Kumar U, Lamba S. Intraosseous epidermal inclusion cyst of the great toe: masquerading as bone tumour. *J Clin Diagn Res.* 2017;11(6):EJ01-EJ02.

132. Paparella T, Fallat L. A rare presentation of a giant epidermoid inclusion cyst mimicking malignancy. *J Foot Ankle Surg.* 2018;57(2):421-426.

133. Kang HS, Kim T, Oh S, Park S, Chung SH. Intraosseous lipoma: 18 years of experience at a single institution. *Clin Orthop Surg.* 2018;10(2):234-239.

134. Campbell RSD, Grainger AJ, Mangham DC, Beggs I, Teh J, Davies AM. Intraosseous lipoma: report of 35 new cases and a review of the literature. *Skeletal Radiol.* 2003;32(4):209-222. doi: 10.1007/s00256-002-0616-7.

135. Narang S, Gangopadhyay M. Calcaneal intraosseous lipoma: a case report and review of the literature. *J Foot Ankle Surg.* 2011;50(2):216-220. doi: 10.1053/j.jfas.2010.12.004.

136. Aycan OE, Keskin A, Sokucu S, Ozer D, Kabukcuoglu F, Kabukcuoglu YS. Surgical treatment of confirmed intraosseous lipoma of the calcaneus: a case series. *J Foot Ankle Surg.* 2017;56(6):1205-1208.

137. Arkader A, Glotzbecker M, Hosalkar HS, Dormans JP. Primary musculoskeletal Langerhans cell histiocytosis in children: an analysis for a 3-decade period. *J Pediatr Orthop.* 2009;29(2):201-207.

138. Ma J, Laird JH, Chau KW, Chelius MR, Lok BH, Yahalom J. Langerhans cell histiocytosis in adults is associated with a high prevalence of hematologic and solid malignancies. *Cancer Med.* 2019;8(1):58-66.

139. Egeler RM, Neglia JP, Arico M, et al. The relation of Langerhans cell histiocytosis to acute leukemia, lymphomas, and other solid tumors. The LCH-Malignancy Study Group of the Histiocyte Society. *Hematol Oncol Clin North Am.* 1998;12(2):369-378.

140. Thacker NH, Abla O. Pediatric Langerhans cell histiocytosis: state of the science and future directions. *Clin Adv Hematol Oncol.* 2019;17(2):122-131.

141. Yasko AW, Fanning CV, Ayala AG, Carrasco CH, Murray JA. Percutaneous techniques for the diagnosis and treatment of localized Langerhans-cell histiocytosis (eosinophilic granuloma of bone). *J Bone Joint Surg Am.* 1998;80(2):219-228.

142. Robinson C, Collins MT, Boyce AM. Fibrous dysplasia/McCune-Albright syndrome: clinical and translational perspectives. *Curr Osteoporos Rep.* 2016;14(5):178-186.

143. Caro-Dominguez P, Navarro OM. Bone tumors of the pediatric foot: imaging appearances. *Pediatr Radiol.* 2017;47(6):739-749.

144. Hillock RZC. Fibrous dysplasia. *Orthop Knowl Online.* 2007;5(4).

145. Brabyn P, Capote A, Belloti M, Zylberberg I. Hyperparathyroidism diagnosed due to brown tumors of the jaw: a case report and literature review. *J Oral Maxillofac Surg.* 2017;75(10):2162-2169.

146. Yazgan P, Ozturk A, Orhan I, Sirmatel O, Baba F. Third metatarsal brown tumor with secondary hyperparathyroidism. *J Am Podiatr Med Assoc.* 2008;98(4):314-317. doi: 10.7547/0980314.

147. Triantafillidou K, Zouloumis L, Karakinaris G, Kalimeras E, Iordanidis F. Brown tumors of the jaws associated with primary or secondary hyperparathyroidism. A clinical study and review of the literature. *Am J Otolaryngol.* 2006;27(4):281-286. http://www.sciencedirect.com/science/article/pii/S0196070905002218

148. Chou LB, Ho YY, Malawer MM. Tumors of the foot and ankle: experience with 153 cases. *Foot Ankle Int.* 2009;30(9):836-841. doi: 10.3113/FAI.2009.0836.

149. Mascard E, Gaspar N, Brugières L, Glorion C, Pannier S, Gomez-Brouchet A. Malignant tumours of the foot and ankle. *EFORT Open Rev.* 2017;2(5):261-271. doi: 10.1302/2058-5241.2.160078.

150. Yang P, Evans S, Bali N, et al. Malignant bone tumours of the foot. *Ann R Coll Surg Engl.* 2017;99(7):568-572.

151. Leddy LR, Holmes RE. Chondrosarcoma of bone. *Cancer Treat Res.* 2014;162:117-130.

152. Gholamrezanezhad A, Basques K, Kosmas C. Peering beneath the surface: juxtacortical tumors of bone (part I). *Clin Imaging.* 2018;51:1-11.

153. Qian X. Updates in primary bone tumors: current challenges and new opportunities in cytopathology. *Surg Pathol Clin.* 2018;11(3):657-668.

154. Chen X, Yu LJ, Peng HM, et al. Is intralesional resection suitable for central grade 1 chondrosarcoma: a systematic review and updated meta-analysis. *Eur J Surg Oncol.* 2017;43(9):1718-1726.

155. Leeson MC, Smith MJ. Ewing's sarcoma of the foot. *Foot Ankle.* 1989;10(3):147-151. doi: 10.1177/107110078901000306.

156. Mikel S-J, Julio D, Pablo Diaz de R, Luis S. Limb salvage in Ewing's sarcoma of the distal lower extremity. *Foot Ankle Int.* 2008;29(1):22-28. doi: 10.3113/FAI.2008.0022.

157. Bernstein M, Kovar H, Paulussen M, et al. Ewing's sarcoma family of tumors: current management. *Oncologist.* 2006;11(5):503-519.

158. Şahin K, Bayram S, Salduz A. Calcaneal Ewing's sarcoma with skip metastases to tarsals and lymph node involvement: a case report. *J Foot Ankle Surg.* 2018;57(1):162-166. doi: 10.1053/j.jfas.2017.07.002.

159. Sneppen O, Hansen LM. Presenting symptoms and treatment delay in osteosarcoma and Ewing's sarcoma. *Acta Radiol Oncol.* 1984;23(2-3):159-162. doi: 10.3109/02841868409136005.

160. Tocpfcr A, Harrasscr N, Rcckcr M, Lcnzc U, Pohlig F. Distribution patterns of foot and ankle tumors: a university tumor institute experience. *BMC Cancer.* 2018:1-10.

161. Kemnitz MJ, Erdmann BB, Julsrud ME, Jacobs PM, Ringstrom JB. Adenocarcinoma of the lung with metatarsal metastasis. *J Foot Ankle Surg.* 1996;35(3):210-212. doi: 10.1016/S1067-2516(96)80098-6.

162. Maheshwari A V, Chiappetta G, Kugler CD, Pitcher JD, Temple HT. Metastatic skeletal disease of the foot: case reports and literature review. *Foot Ankle Int.* 2008;29(7):699-710. doi: 10.3113/FAI.2008.0699.

163. Hattrup SJ, Amadio PC, Sim FH, Lombardi RM. Metastatic tumors of the foot and ankle. *Foot Ankle.* 1988;8(5):243-247. doi: 10.1177/107110078800800503.

Skin Tumor Management

Tracey C. Vlahovic

As many skin conditions and possible skin cancers are clinically difficult to distinguish, a biopsy provides a histopathologic diagnosis, which ultimately helps to support the treatment plan. It can also clarify the skin disorder when a treatment plan is not yielding the appropriate results. Lastly, a biopsy can be curative or even lifesaving if one excises the lesion *in toto* or when the biopsy helps identify a treatable malignant diagnosis. Ultimately, a biopsy can both complement and confirm the diagnosis.

The techniques of performing a shave, punch, and incisional/excisional biopsies to diagnose and manage skin tumors are straightforward; however, choosing the correct procedure is important to aid in the diagnosis. The aim of this chapter is to present a basic guideline that one can use in daily practice when confronted with challenging wounds, rashes, and pigmented lesions.

WOUNDS

Understanding the etiology of a wound is imperative in its management. Besides establishing a diagnosis, one of the most important reasons for performing a wound biopsy is to rule out the presence of malignancy. Chronic wounds that are the site of long-standing inflammation such as from a burn or a sinus tract may transform into a malignant lesion. A squamous cell carcinoma arising in an area of an old scar, burn, or wound is termed a Marjolin ulcer and is more often seen in the lower extremity.[1] This transformational process may take anywhere from 1 year to 25 years to develop.[2] In addition, lesions that are malignant (both *de novo* and metastasis) may present as wounds and can easily be misdiagnosed as a chronic wound.

Reasons to biopsy a wound include the following: the treated area has been present for over 3 months and has not responded to standard treatment, the wound bed has become exophytic and hypergranular, and in the absence of infection, the wound has become painful, malodorous, and changed in the amount of drainage.[3]

For the clinician who works in a wound care center, a scenario of a patient who presents with a painful medial leg ulcer that has been present for 25 years, been treated as a venous stasis ulcer, and has not changed is suggestive of performing a biopsy during the first visit. After performing a thorough history and physical examination, the clinician may perform a wound biopsy not only to rule out malignancy but also to determine if the wound has an inflammatory basis. Painful leg wounds, such as pyoderma gangrenosum, arising in the presence of rheumatoid arthritis, inflammatory bowel disease, or hematological disorders may not have specific histopathologic identifiers in their chronic state. In the case of pyoderma gangrenosum, this diagnosis of exclusion can be just as helpful to place the patient along the course of appropriate treatment. Other inflammatory-based ulcers include those seen in vasculitis, anticoagulant syndromes, and drug reactions. In those cases, it might be helpful to do a second biopsy that will be sent for direct immunofluorescence, which will help in elucidating the underlying cause.

When performing a biopsy for a suspected basal cell carcinoma or squamous cell carcinoma, a deep punch or incisional biopsy of the base and the wound edge may be performed.[3] For pyoderma gangrenosum, two biopsies (punch or incisional) that include the wound edge (with partial ulcer bed) and the central base will be useful. With an ulcer associated with vasculitis, the center of the lesion is best to biopsy, but a punch of newly formed palpable purpura would also be diagnostic. A specimen for direct immunofluorescence staining should be sent in a special media (Michel fixative), which the pathology lab of choice can assist the clinician in obtaining a kit for easy transport. Otherwise, all other specimens for histopathology should be sent in 10% formalin solution.

Overall, a wound that has not decreased in size after several months of standard care, has changed in a negative manner, has a suspected etiology beyond the original diagnosis, and has a potential for being malignant should be sampled and sent for a histopathologic review.

DERMATITIS NONRESPONDING TO STANDARD OF CARE

All of us have experienced a patient whose red, scaly rash has not responded to our prescription topical therapy. Not only is this challenging to us as practitioners but also to the patient. Failure to respond to conventional therapy warrants a skin biopsy. In these cases, a punch biopsy is an appropriate choice. This procedure can be utilized in patients who have seen numerous practitioners prior to a visit with me, have a long list of failed medications, and have not had a skin biopsy to define the skin condition. In these cases, performing the skin biopsy prior to initiating any further treatment will refine the management plan and reduce patient frustration of purchasing yet another possible failed therapy.

TABLE 46.1	Inflammatory Skin Conditions and Biopsy	
Disease	**Stage of Lesion**	**Location**
Atopic eczema (dermatitis)	Acute	Intact vesicle
Atopic eczema (dermatitis)	Chronic	Lichenified skin
Contact dermatitis	Acute	Intact vesicle
Contact dermatitis	Chronic	Lichenified skin
Erythema multiforme	Target lesion	One from center, one from edge
Lichen planus	Any time	Papule
Necrobiosis lipoidica	Any time	Atrophic center
Psoriasis, plaque	Scaly plaque	Any part of plaque
Psoriasis, pustular	Early pustule	Entire pustule
Tinea pedis	Untreated	Scale or vesicle

Routine biopsy of all skin rashes is not recommended, but if a new-onset rash does not correspond to the conventional presentations of psoriasis, eczema, and lichen planus, a punch biopsy can be a useful diagnostic tool (Table 46.1). In the case of a psoriatic like plaque, differential diagnoses can range from plaque psoriasis to cutaneous T-cell lymphoma. Treatment plans for these two diagnoses are varied in approach and prognosis.

SUSPICIOUS PIGMENTED LESIONS

Over the course of a career, the podiatric practitioner will be faced with diagnosing benign lesions (nevi, dermatofibroma), precancerous lesions (actinic keratosis), non-melanoma skin cancer (basal cell and squamous cell), and melanoma (Table 46.2).

When faced with a pigmented lesion, it is important first to establish if the lesion is melanocytic. Examples of melanocytic lesions are nevi, lentigines, atypical nevi, and melanoma. Early detection of a melanoma is ideal, but choosing which melanocytic lesion to biopsy can be difficult. A biopsy of every pigmented lesion on a patient would be "disfiguring and unnecessary."[4] The combination of clinical examination

TABLE 46.2	Pigmented Lesions and Biopsy	
Disease	**Stage of Lesion**	**Location**
Malignant melanoma	Anytime	Most infiltrated area
Basal cell carcinoma	Anytime	Most infiltrated area
Squamous cell carcinoma	Anytime	Most infiltrated area
Nevi (junctional, compound intradermal)	Anytime	Entire lesion or thickest part

Adapted from Sina B, Kao G, Deng A, Gaspari A. Skin biopsy for inflammatory and common neoplastic skin diseases: optimum time, best location, and preferred techniques. A critical review. *J Cutan Pathol.* 2009;36(5):505-510.

and choosing the appropriate biopsy type for the lesion can aid in diagnosis and management.

After performing a thorough history and physical examination and prior to the biopsy, a dermatologist can add dermoscopy and confocal microscopy to the examination when trying to determine if and where to biopsy. Dermoscopy requires special instrumentation and education, but it is a valuable technique in refining the decision whether to biopsy. As with any technique, there are limitations, and the dermoscopy examination can yield questionable and vague results; therefore, the *in vivo* reflectance confocal microscope has been utilized as a tool increasingly to evaluate pigmented lesions. The microscope works in a similar principle to ultrasound, but instead of sound waves, it uses laser optics to visualize melanocytic lesions. The confocal microscope is mainly found in large academic medical centers and is a valuable resource for dermatologists specializing in identifying and managing pigmented lesions.

Beyond these advanced instruments available to specialists, it is still important to ask the patient pertinent questions regarding the lesion, look at the lesion carefully, and then biopsy when appropriate to have the best overall outcome.

Questions that the clinician should ask the patient include the following: how and if the lesion has changed; if it has developed over the age of 40; if it is pruritic; if it is a previous (or current) site of a nevi, ulcer, or scar; and importantly, if it is an area that does not heal. A lesion that has not healed despite conventional therapies should be biopsied to rule out a malignant process.

Following the patient interview, the clinician next needs to perform the examination utilizing the ABC's of melanoma and the "ugly duckling" sign.

The ABC's of melanoma are a guide when investigating a suspicious melanocytic lesion and are as follows:

A—Asymmetry: one side of the lesion is different from the other side.
B—Border: notching and irregularity are uncommon in benign lesions.
C—Color: shades of red, whites, and blue, along with black, may indicate a superficial spreading melanoma type.
D—Diameter: lesions under 6 mm in diameter are more likely to be benign.
E—Evolving: any changing mole warrants careful observation and probable biopsy.
F—Family or personal history of skin cancer.

The ABC's of subungual melanoma are as follows:

A = age (fifth to seventh decade is peak)
B = brown to black discoloration with a breadth of 3 mm or greater
C = change in the nail plate or lack of change with treatment
D = digit most commonly affected (hallux)
E = extension of pigment into proximal nail fold or lateral nail fold (Hutchinson sign)
F = family or personal history of skin cancer

Also relevant is the "ugly duckling" sign. Most nevi in an individual tend to resemble each other. A melanocytic lesion that appears grossly different from the others should be viewed with suspicion. Both of these visual techniques are guides, are not perfect, but are solid places to begin the decision-making process of whether or not to biopsy a lesion.

TABLE 46.3	Suggested areas on where to obtain a biopsy specimen	
Disease	**Stage**	**Location**
Malignant melanoma	Anytime	Complete lesion or thickest part
Basal cell carcinoma	Anytime	Complete lesion or thickest part
Squamous cell carcinoma	Anytime	Complete lesion or thickest part
Nevi	Anytime	Complete lesion or thickest part

Adapted from Sina B, Kao G, Deng A, Gaspari A. Skin biopsy for inflammatory and common neoplastic skin diseases: optimum time, best location, and preferred techniques. A critical review. *J Cutan Pathol.* 2009;36(5):505-510. Ref.[5]

If the question of whether or not to biopsy after using both the ABC's of melanoma and the "ugly duckling" sign as guidelines continues, a referral to a dermatologist is recommended.

Once the determination to sample a suspicious pigmented lesion has been made, the clinician should determine the type of biopsy to be performed. The AAD (American Academy of Dermatology) and NCCN (National Comprehensive Cancer Network) have suggested, when possible, to perform a total excisional biopsy (Table 46.3). Fully realizing that larger lesions and various anatomical areas (soles, digits, subungual) are not always amenable to a total excision with a 1- to 3-mm border, their recommendations then include incisional and punch. They reserve a deep shave technique for when the index of suspicion of melanoma is low to none.

Throughout the years, clinicians have shared the concern of creating metastasis during the initial biopsy procedure of a melanocytic lesion. Various studies have been unable to show differences in survival and sentinel lymph node metastasis between those who had an excisional procedure vs those who had an incisional, punch, or deep shave procedure.[4] The major concern that the NCCN and AAD have regarding the nonexcisional procedures is the possible lack of procuring the deep margin of the tumor. The deep margin helps to determine the Breslow depth, which allows for staging of the lesion and ultimately the prognosis. Ultimately, the guidelines recommend excision when possible and nonexcisional biopsy of an area that best represents the lesion in difficult anatomic areas and large lesions.[4]

REVIEW OF THE SKIN BIOPSY TECHNIQUES FOR SKIN TUMORS

In order to have the best biopsy result, physicians must ensure that all three layers of skin (epidermis, dermis, and subcutaneous tissue) are present. A "scraping" of the skin, in which one sends the scales of the lesion to pathology, is not appropriate to diagnose any inflammatory skin disorder or neoplasm. Physicians should only use this "scraping" technique when doing a KOH test to determine the presence of a dermatophyte.

Podiatrists should also avoid superficial shave biopsies as they do not involve the deep dermis or subcutaneous tissue, which is needed for many histopathologic diagnoses and staging of the neoplastic disease.

Both the "scrape" and superficial shave ultimately delay a true diagnosis and create a lot of frustration for the patient. Additionally, physicians should never perform the scrape and superficial shave if they suspect a malignant lesion.

In addition to choosing and performing the appropriate procedure, giving the pathologist sufficient clinical information is important in order to receive an accurate diagnosis.[6] When filling out the pathology form, one should provide sufficient detail on the evolution of the lesion or dermatitis, the clinical description, the specific anatomic location of the biopsy site, and the differential diagnosis.

Podiatrists should always obtain consent and forewarn the patient about the possible need for further surgery. For example, a second excision may be necessary for an atypical or malignant lesion. One should also counsel the patient about the possibility of a painful scar, especially when the lesion in question involves the plantar foot.

To reiterate, the location of biopsy and use of the proper fixative medium are also imperative for optimum results.

PUNCH BIOPSY

The punch biopsy can offer a useful and simple way of supporting a clinical diagnosis. One can perform this biopsy in minutes with little discomfort to the patient. Podiatrists should reserve the punch biopsy for neoplasms, vesicles, and inflammatory skin disorders.

After consent is obtained and the site prepared, one can perform a local infiltrative intradermal injection of local anesthetic. Using a 30-gauge, ½-in needle (with the bevel facing up), an injection 1 mL of lidocaine with epinephrine can be given for an appropriately sized lesion. There is a blanching effect of the area due to the epinephrine and minimal pain with an intradermal technique. Ultimately, the intradermal technique offers immediate anesthesia by raising a small wheal, which enables one to perform the biopsy without delay.

Prior to infiltration, the skin should be gently pinched in order to find the relaxed skin tension lines.[7] One can subsequently use these lines as a guide to direct the biopsy in order to minimize the impact of scarring.

Once one has obtained anesthesia for the patient, apply a 4- or 6-mm disposable punch tool to the skin. Use the dominant hand to hold the punch instrument while using your other hand to place a gentle perpendicular force to the relaxed skin tension lines away from the lesion. This enables you to avoid "dog ears" when closing the defect.

When it comes to the dorsum of the foot, be careful about controlling the depth of the biopsy to avoid important structures deep to the lesion. On the plantar foot, use the entire cutting edge of the punch. Once you have performed the punch, gently lift the circular button of skin and subcutaneous tissue. Using an iris scissor, cut the fatty attachment as deeply as possible in order to give all three levels of skin to pathology.

Proceed to suture the defect. Have the patient return in 10-14 days for both suture removal and diagnosis review. Steri-Strips may be utilized in place of sutures per the surgeon's preference. For most skin lesions, one can send the specimen in formalin.

INCISIONAL AND EXCISIONAL BIOPSIES

When one can completely excise a lesion with a margin of unaffected skin, an excisional biopsy is warranted. In circumstances in which just a part of the lesion is required, an incisional elliptical biopsy is warranted.

With both of these biopsies, one often draws an ellipse with the 3:1 parameters (with the length being three times the width) and a 2-mm border around the lesion.

As with the punch biopsy, it is important to consider relaxed skin tension lines in order to facilitate the best scar outcome and complete the biopsy down to subcutaneous tissue. Once you have obtained consent and prepared the surgical site, use the intradermal anesthesia technique. If the lesion is larger than 4 mm, one can also use a diamond block to create anesthesia around the area of the ellipse.

The elliptical incision should be parallel to the relaxed skin tension lines for the best scar. After the first pass of the no. 15 blade, deepen the incision to include the subcutaneous tissue. Proceed to dissect the ellipse of skin carefully in one plane and send the specimen in formalin (or another media if a vesicle). One may employ simple interrupted or running sutures to close the defect.

The technique for incisional biopsy is the same as the excisional biopsy. The only exception is the incisional biopsy does not remove the lesion completely.

If a lesion is too large to remove completely in the office, the thickest portion of the lesion with a margin of normal skin is the ideal place for biopsy. The incisional biopsy is also best for ulcers. For example, if a podiatric physician suspects a venous stasis ulcer has elements of squamous cell carcinoma, an incisional biopsy of the fungating granulation tissue with a margin of the periwound skin is an ideal place to start when it comes to confirming the diagnosis.[8,9]

CURETTAGE AND ELECTRODESICCATION

When it comes to verruca or previously biopsied basal cell carcinomas that are superficial in nature, physicians may use curettage and electrodesiccation.

One can prep the area without an alcohol wipe and use the anesthesia infiltration technique. With firm strokes, the physician should apply the curette over the lesion. Only send the first pass with the curette in formalin to pathology. Following curettage, apply topical hemostasis with a handheld electrocautery device. Perform curettage and electrodessication twice more to complete the procedure. Bear in mind that sending the curetted material after electrodesiccation will not aid in the diagnosis at all.

Curettage provides a fragmented specimen to the pathologist and does not aid in diagnosing inflammatory skin disorders, neoplasms, and other diseases.[7] One should only use curettage for the two indications above. Also be aware that the affected area will heal by secondary intention and leave a minimal scar.

NAIL BIOPSY

The nail biopsy is underutilized in podiatric medicine. When it comes to biopsy of the nail, physicians generally use the punch biopsy or incisional/excisional biopsies.

When a patient presents with a dark brown to black longitudinal line (longitudinal melanonychia) in the nail, the physician must use his or her best judgment on whether to do a punch biopsy. These lines are present in every toenail and fingernail in 100% of African American patients by the age of 50.[10]

However, if the longitudinal melanonychia changes in these patients or if the patient is Caucasian, one should obtain a punch biopsy. The podiatric physician should not wait for the pigmentation to spill out onto either the distal or proximal digit. This pigmentation, or Hutchinson sign, signals extensive disease and usually yields a poor prognosis.

Generally, longitudinal melanonychia presents for the entire length of the nail. When it comes to planning of a punch biopsy of that lesion, the physician should always involve the most proximal part of pigmented area due to the pigmentation originating from melanocytes in the matrix portion of the nail unit. Therefore, one should dissect the proximal nail fold back carefully to expose the nail matrix.

Direct a 4-mm punch (or smaller/larger depending on the size of the lesion) to the most proximal part of the pigmented area. Using a gentle motion, excise a small circular area.[11] Remember that there is no subcutaneous tissue deep to the nail unit. The punch instrument will most likely touch the distal phalanx. One can fill the circular defect with Gelfoam or another hemostatic agent, and close the proximal nail fold with appropriate suture technique or Steri-Strips.

Regarding the small button of nail plate and nail bed, do not tease them apart and be sure to send the specimen in formalin for processing. Due to the disturbance of the matrix during this procedure, it is imperative to discuss with the patient during the informed consent process that permanent dystrophy may occur as the nail grows distal. However, if a neoplasm is uncovered, it is unlikely that the patient will be disturbed by this fact.

If a patient presents with a nail bed neoplasm, one may obtain an incisional or excisional biopsy depending on the size of the lesion. Surgical planning involves first removing the nail plate in order to gain access to the nail bed.[11,12]

Regarding excising a neoplasm from the nail bed, this is unlikely to cause permanent nail dystrophy due to the distance from the matrix. Once one has excised the lesion, place it in formalin and send it for histopathologic processing. The physician may also send the nail plate if he or she feels it would aid in the diagnosis.

PATHOLOGY RESULTS

If podiatric physicians have any questions regarding the histopathologic diagnosis, they should not hesitate to speak with the pathologist for clarification. Proper and prompt communication will only benefit the patient.

If the lesion is malignant with Clark level, Breslow depth, and affected margins noted, the podiatric physician may choose to send the patient to an oncological surgeon, a Mohs surgeon, or a plastic surgeon for further care.

If the lesion returns as *in situ* (superficial epidermis), the physician may choose to re-excise the lesion using the excisional biopsy method in order to have a pathology report return with "margins clear" of neoplasm. One should also refer the patient to a dermatologist for a full body skin check to determine if there are any similar lesions to those on the lower extremity.

OVERVIEW

Skin biopsies are simple procedures to do, but they can yield a great result. Often, a biopsy will prevent a delayed or incorrect diagnosis. Overall, the punch, incisional, and excisional biopsies should become part of the podiatric armamentarium and not be underutilized any longer.

In general, choosing when to biopsy can prove to be a challenge to the practitioner. After a thorough history and clinical examination, the clinician needs not only to choose which lesion to biopsy but also what type of biopsy to perform. Overall, a wound, rash, or lesion that does not meet general criteria should be biopsied. Also, a lesion that has not responded to standard therapy should also be met with suspicion and sampled. In conclusion, biopsy of these conditions is a valuable technique that allows the practitioner to refine a diagnosis and direct further course of treatment.

Optimal Conditions/Lesions for a Punch Biopsy

- Skin dermatoses/rashes
- Small nevi
- Wounds
- Pigmented streak (longitudinal melanonychia) in a nail

Optimal Conditions/Lesions for an Excisional Biopsy

- A lesion that anatomically and closure-wise can be excised *in toto* on the lower extremity.
- Otherwise, an incisional or punch may be appropriate until a more optimal surgical situation can be done, or the lesion can be closed in a staged manner.

Optimal Conditions for a Shave Biopsy

- Exophytic lesions like a skin tag or nodular lesion that is benign.
- It is best for suspected malignant lesions to perform a punch, incisional, or excisional biopsy.

A Quick Overview of Biopsy Techniques

- For all types: Inject with appropriate anesthetic: whether that is 1 mL in an intradermal manner or 3 mL or more in a local block (depending on size and area targeted).
- For a shave biopsy: Use a BioBlade or a no. 15 or 10 blade parallel to the lesion and shave; place lesion in formalin, apply topical hemostasis, apply dressing.
- For a punch biopsy: Find relaxed skin tension lines by pinching, then apply the appropriately sized punch tool to the lesion with the dominant hand while the nondominant hand spreads the relaxed skin tension lines perpendicular to their course. Remove specimen and send in formalin. Close defect in skin as physician deems appropriate. Apply dressing.
- For an incisional or excisional biopsy: A 3:1 elliptical incision is standard, followed by careful dissection. Submit lesion in formalin-filled container for processing. Close with surgeon's choice of suture. Apply dressing.

REFERENCES

1. Cocchetto V, Magrin P, de Paula RA, et al. Squamous cell carcinoma in chronic wound: Marjolin ulcer. *Dermatol Online J.* 2013;19(2):7.
2. Pavlovic S, Wiley E, Guzman G, et al. Marjolin ulcer: an overlooked entity. *Int Wound J.* 2011;8(4):419-424.
3. Alavi A, Niakosari F, Sibbald RG. When and how to perform a biopsy on a chronic wound. *Adv Skin Wound Care.* 2010;23(3):132.
4. Tran KT, Wright NA, Cockerell CJ. Biopsy of the pigmented lesion—when and how. *J Am Acad Dermatol.* 2008;59:852-871.
5. Sina B, Kao G, Deng A, Gaspari A. Skin biopsy for inflammatory and common neoplastic skin diseases: optimum time, best location, and preferred techniques. A critical review. *J Cutan Pathol.* 2009;36(5):505-510.
6. Mehregan D, Dooley V. How to get the most out of your skin biopsies. *Int J Dermatol.* 2007;46(7):727-733.
7. Olbricht S. Biopsy techniques and basic excisions. In: Bolognia JL, Rapini RP, et al., eds. *Dermatology.* 1st ed. London, UK: Mosby; 2003:2269-2286.
8. Jankovic A, Binic I, Ljubenovic M. Basal cell carcinoma is not granulation tissue in the venous leg ulcer. *Int J Low Extrem Wounds.* 2008;7(3):182-184.
9. Spear M. Pyoderma gangrenosum: an overview. *Plast Surg Nurs.* 2008;28(3):154-157.
10. Dawber R, De Berker D, Baran R. Science of the nail apparatus. In: Baran R, Dawber R, eds. *Diseases of the Nails and Their Management.* 2nd ed. Oxford, UK: Blackwell Scientific Publications; 1994:1-34.
11. Rich P. Nail surgery. In: Bolognia JL, Rapini RP, et al., eds. *Dermatology.* 1st ed. London, UK: Mosby; 2003:2321-2330.

CHAPTER 47

Excision of Accessory Bones

Adam E. Fleischer and Rachel H. Albright

DEFINITION

Accessory bones, or ossicles, are normal anatomical variants. Typically arising from failure of secondary ossification centers to achieve union, these bones are usually asymptomatic and discovered only incidentally. However, since these ossicles exist adjacent to a main osseous body, they are susceptible to fracture, dislocation, irritation, impingement, degenerative changes, soft tissue tumors, and osteonecrosis. This chapter will cover the two most clinically important accessory bones encountered in the foot and ankle—the accessory navicular and os trigonum.

ACCESSORY NAVICULAR

CLASSIFICATION

ACCESSORY NAVICULAR (OS TIBIALE EXTERNUM, PREHALLUX)

Geist Classification:

Type I—Sesamoid bone within the tibialis posterior tendon, separated from the navicular bone, but within 3 mm from the body

Type II—Accessory bone up to 1.2 cm in diameter with a synchondrosis between the bone and the navicular

Type III—Accessory bone fused to the main body of the navicular, resulting in a large cornuate-shaped navicular

---

ANATOMIC FEATURES

The incidence of an accessory navicular ossicle in radiographic and cadaveric studies varies from 2% [1] to more than 20%.[2] The incidence is evenly divided between men and woman, and the condition is typically bilateral in presentation. The accessory navicular is the second most frequently occurring accessory bone of the foot behind the os peroneum and ahead of the os trigonum.[3] The accessory bone is known by a multitude of synonyms including accessory navicular, os tibiale externum, navicular secundum, prehallux, bifurcate navicular, accessory tarsal scaphoid, extrascaphoid, and divided navicular.

There are three types of accessory ossicle, described similarly by Geist.[4] The type I navicular deformity presents as small 4- to

6-mm round ossicle proximal to and distinctly separate from the navicular tuberosity (Fig. 47.1A). It is a true sesamoid within the deep substance of the tibialis posterior tendon. This discrete round ossicle is generally referred to as os tibiale externum. It is typically separated from the navicular by 5-7 mm.

The type II navicular deformity is a separate ossicle appearing radiographically as an extension of the navicular tuberosity, but connected to it by a radiolucent nonossified zone (Fig. 47.1B). This condition is sometimes referred to as a bifurcate navicular. A type II navicular deformity presents as a clinical enlargement of the navicular resulting in a medial arch prominence over the tuberosity of the navicular or slightly more proximally overlying the talonavicular joint. The ossicle may be triangular or heart shaped. The radiolucent or nonossified zone can measure 1-3 mm and may be fibrous, cartilaginous, fibrocartilaginous, or partially osseous.[5] Lemont et al.[6] found this area to represent a true joint within the navicular. Histologic specimens from symptomatic patients simulated microfracture and cellular proliferation suggestive of attempted repair. Weight-bearing forces across this area of compromised bone, which is similar to a nonunion, can result in a deep achy type of medial arch pain. The size and extent of the type II navicular can vary. The nonosseous zone of the ossicle is typically nonarticular with the talus, but it can involve the talonavicular joint.

The type III navicular deformity is united by a bony ridge producing a cornuate navicular (Fig. 47.1C). The type III navicular deformity may actually represent a type II where the various ossification centers within the navicular bone have actually bridged with bone. The bone is enlarged both medially forming the clinical bump and extending proximally to overlie the head of the talus. Type II and type III accessory naviculars represent 70% of navicular deformities.[7]

PHYSICAL EXAMINATION

TYPE I

There are really no clinical findings specific to a type I accessory ossicle, as this bone is rarely symptomatic and does not typically cause irritation with shoegear. It can however become symptomatic particularly if associated with an intrasubstance posterior tibial tendon tear, in which case the attenuation or thickening of the posterior tibial tendon with resultant compromise in strength and function is more of a clinical issue than the ossicle itself.

940

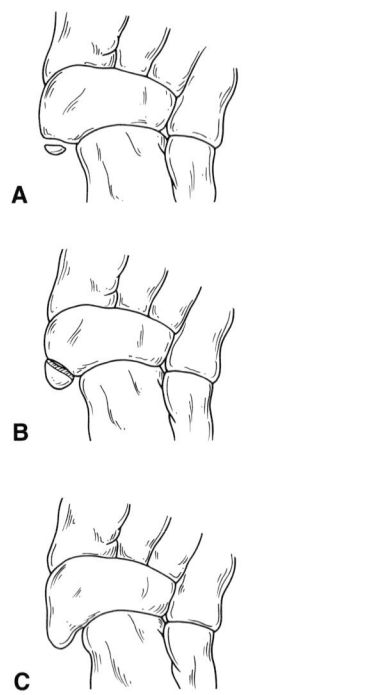

FIGURE 47.1 Geist classification system for accessory navicular taxonomy. (Adapted from Geist ES. Supernumerary bone of the foot: A roentgen study of the feet of 100 normal individuals. *Am J Orthop Surg.* 1914;12:403.)

TYPE II

Patient complaints may include not only medial midfoot prominence shoe irritation but also a deep achy soreness within the navicular itself. Single heel raise performance is sometimes affected in those patients in whom a large portion of the posterior tibial tendon is inserting into the accessory ossicle and

not to the main navicular body. If not present preoperatively, resection of a type II navicular can result in posterior tibial tendonitis and progressive pes valgo planus postoperatively.[8]

TYPE III

The primary complaint in patients suffering with type III navicular deformities is medial "bump" pain and shoegear irritation. Patients sometimes report, "I seem to have two ankle bones on the inside of my foot." The deep aching pain seen in a type II presentation is usually not reported, unless associated with significant pes valgoplanus with a degree of arthrosis or soft tissue strain. They change little in size clinically with subtalar joint pronation and supination. Type III naviculars are typically noted with pes valgoplanus but can present in rectus feet as well.

PATHOGENESIS

Symptomatic type II accessory naviculars are frequently caused by an injury. This may be due to tension shearing and/or compression forces transmitted through the posterior tibial tendon to the fibrous and/or cartilaginous interface. Symptoms related to a type III navicular are shoegear mediated, predominantly.

IMAGING AND DIAGNOSTIC STUDIES

Diagnostic testing can assist in isolating the exact pathology associated with a navicular prominence. The accessory navicular becomes apparent radiographically at about the age of 9-11 years. Plain film evaluation, particularly the lateral oblique view, helps to confirm that the clinically observed medial foot prominence is, in fact, an accessory navicular, and not a prominent medial talar head or neoplasm (Fig. 47.2).

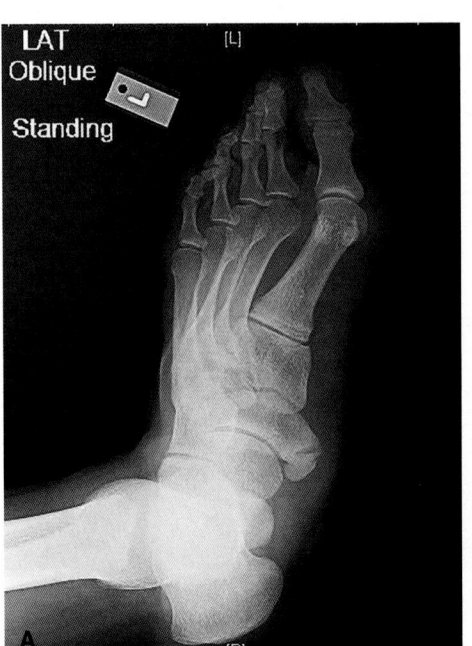
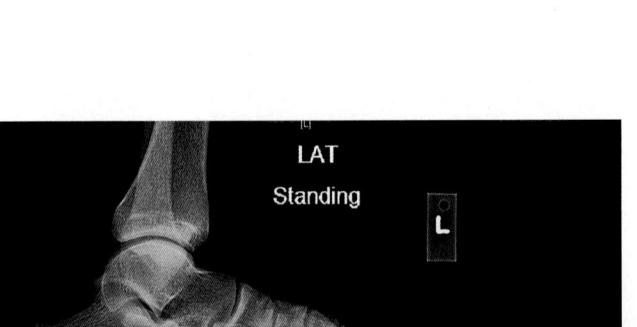

FIGURE 47.2 A. The lateral oblique view is perhaps the most informative view when visualizing the accessory navicular. Seen here is moderate-sized type II variant with clear radiolucent zone separating the ossicle from the main body of the navicular. **B.** The standing lateral view shows what appears to be an exaggerated navicular tuberosity superimposed on the anterior calcaneus.

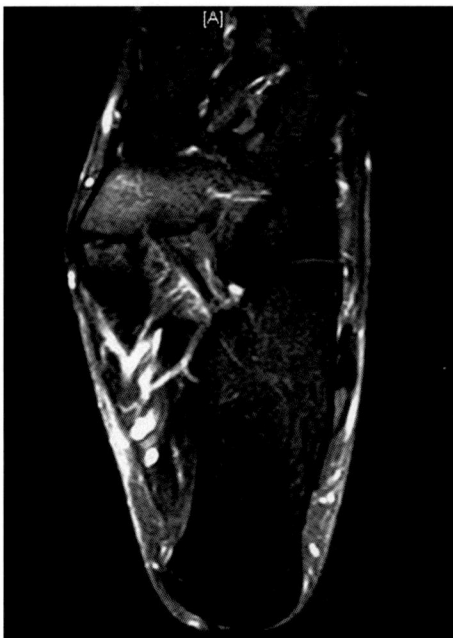

FIGURE 47.3 Symptomatic patients will typically exhibit bone marrow edema (BME) on fat-suppressed MR images. Seen here is a type II variant demonstrating extensive BME within both the ossicle and within the body of the navicular itself. Asymptomatic patients will typically not exhibit this BME pattern.

The type II navicular prominence on the lateral radiograph extends rather proximally overlapping the distal calcaneus far more than a normal navicular contour (Fig. 47.2B). The size and location of the radiolucent zone within the navicular can be assessed to determine whether the zone is articular or nonarticular with the talus. Although infrequently needed, CT scanning can also help identify the size and shape of the accessory bone as well as the degree of possible talonavicular joint involvement.

Magnetic resonance imaging (MRI) can be helpful to evaluate for the presence of possible associated posterior tibial tendonitis and/or tendon ears.[9] Bone marrow edema on MRI, as an indication of stress within the navicular, is a consistent finding in symptomatic type II ossicles (Fig. 47.3).[10] MRI can also be used to assess the location of the posterior tibial tendon with respect to the ossicle and may help surgeons anticipate how much tendon disruption will be needed upon complete excision (Fig. 47.4A and B). This also helps in managing preoperative patient expectations regarding their recovery. In virtually all cases, bone scans show increased uptake in painful accessory naviculars; however, this modality has largely been supplanted by MRI. When used, increased uptake will only be observed on the symptomatic side in bilateral presentations.[11-14]

TREATMENT

CONSERVATIVE (NONSURGICAL) CARE

Type I ossicles are rarely, if ever, by themselves symptomatic. Nonoperative care of the painful type II ossicle centers around immobilization (particularly if there is a traumatic onset) for 4-6 weeks, then addressing any tendon dysfunction that may be present with custom-molded foot orthoses. For type III ossicles, nonoperative care generally involves shielding and padding as little change in the size of the medial prominence is noted with custom foot orthoses and splinting.[15]

SURGERY FOR TYPE I NAVICULAR

The os tibiale externum may be a factor in the development or exaggeration of a posterior tendonitis, but its excision alone as a surgical option is rarely indicated. The os tibiale externum is considered more of a coincidental finding and not necessarily the reason for pain when posterior tibial tendonitis and tears are present. With that said, removal of the ossicle itself can

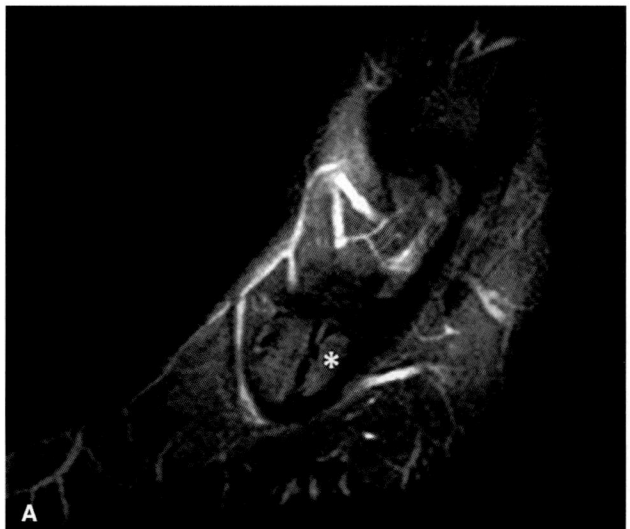

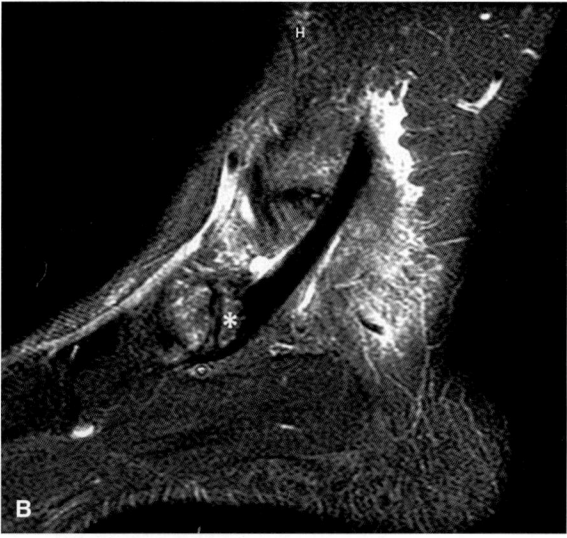

FIGURE 47.4 MR imaging can be useful for preoperative planning and incision placement. **A.** Seen here is a type II accessory navicular (white asterisk [*]) that lies superior to the posterior tibial tendon. When this is encountered, excision can be performed many times with only limited disruption to the posterior tibial tendon insertion. **B.** In this example, the accessory navicular (white asterisk [*]) can be seen serving as the primary insertion point for the posterior tibial tendon. When this is encountered, greater disruption to the posterior tibial tendon insertion is typically needed and greater efforts for re-attachment and advancement of the tendon will be required intraoperatively.

be performed as part of the tendon repair process when large intrasubstance tears are present and the ossicle is felt to be compromising tendon integrity.

Excision of a type I accessory navicular may be accomplished by exposing the superior margin of the posterior tibial tendon in the medial arch from the surface of the navicular, distally to the talar neck area proximally. This sesamoid bone is then carefully shelled out from the deep surface of the posterior tibial tendon proximal to the insertion into the navicular. Identification can be difficult if the sesamoid is buried deep within the tendon. If visual inspection or palpation of the os tibiale externum is inconclusive, assistance with C-arm fluoroscopy can be helpful to verify the location and avoid further damage of the posterior tibial tendon. The insertion of the posterior tibial tendon need not be compromised to effect excision. Surgical exposure of the talonavicular joint is not necessary since the sesamoid does not articulate with the joint.

SURGERY FOR TYPE II NAVICULAR

Surgical exposure for resection of a type II navicular generally extends from just distal to the naviculocuneiform joint distally to the talar neck proximally on the medial surface of the midfoot (Fig. 47.5A–J). The skin, deep fascia, and capsular-periosteal layers are incised superior to the tibialis posterior tendon. The tibialis posterior tendon is then reflected plantarly with the

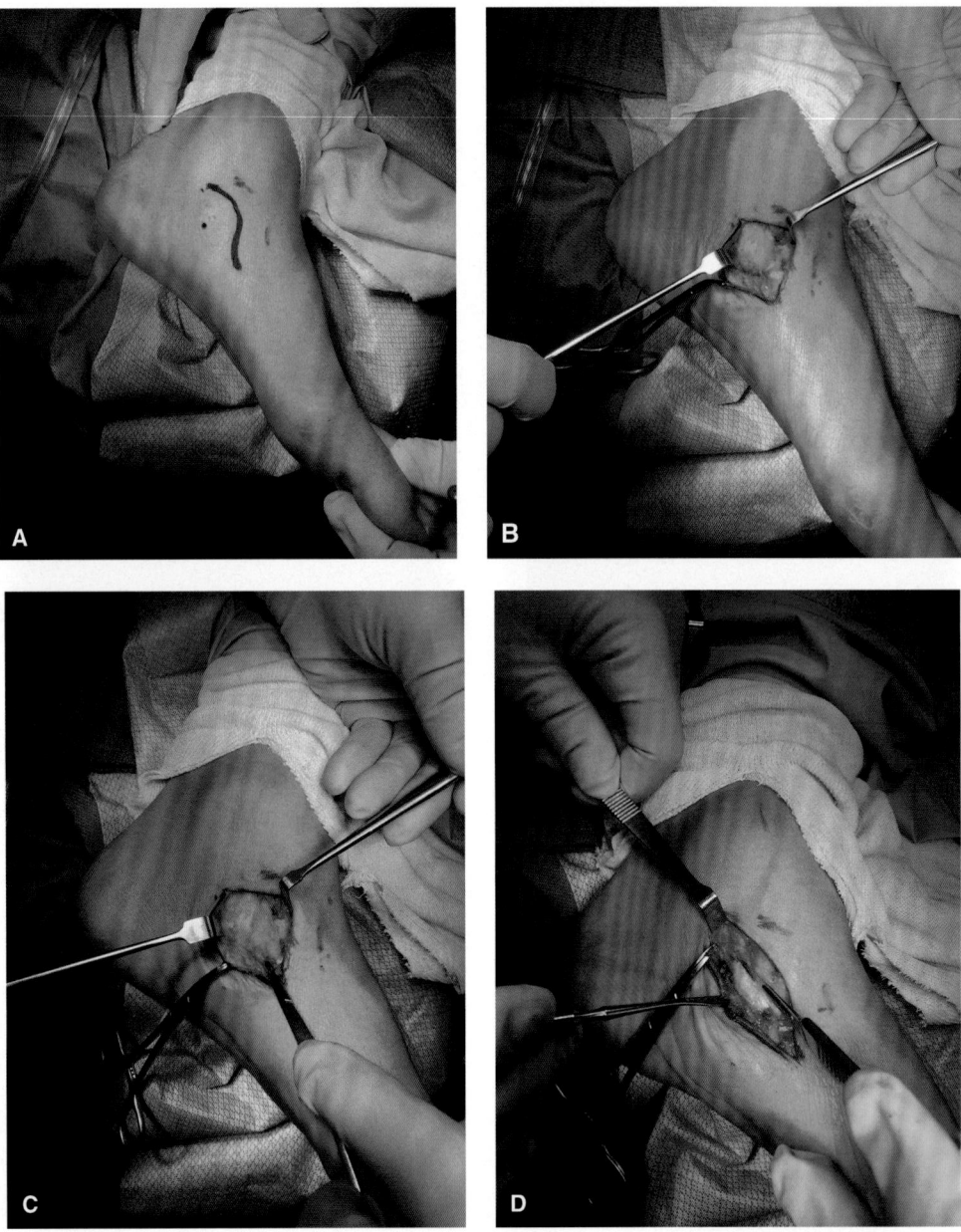

FIGURE 47.5 Surgical excision of a type II accessory navicular. **A)** A curvilinear incision on the medial foot is utilized, extending from the talar head to just past the naviculocuneiform joint. The incision courses just superior to the posterior tibial tendon and accessory navicular. **B)** Dissection is carried through the skin and subcutaneous tissue until the sheath of the posterior tibial tendon, and the periosteum and capsule of the accessory ossicle and navicular body can be visualized. **C)** The tendon insertion point on the navicular is now identified. **D)** The capsular-periosteal layers are incised superior to the tibialis posterior tendon.

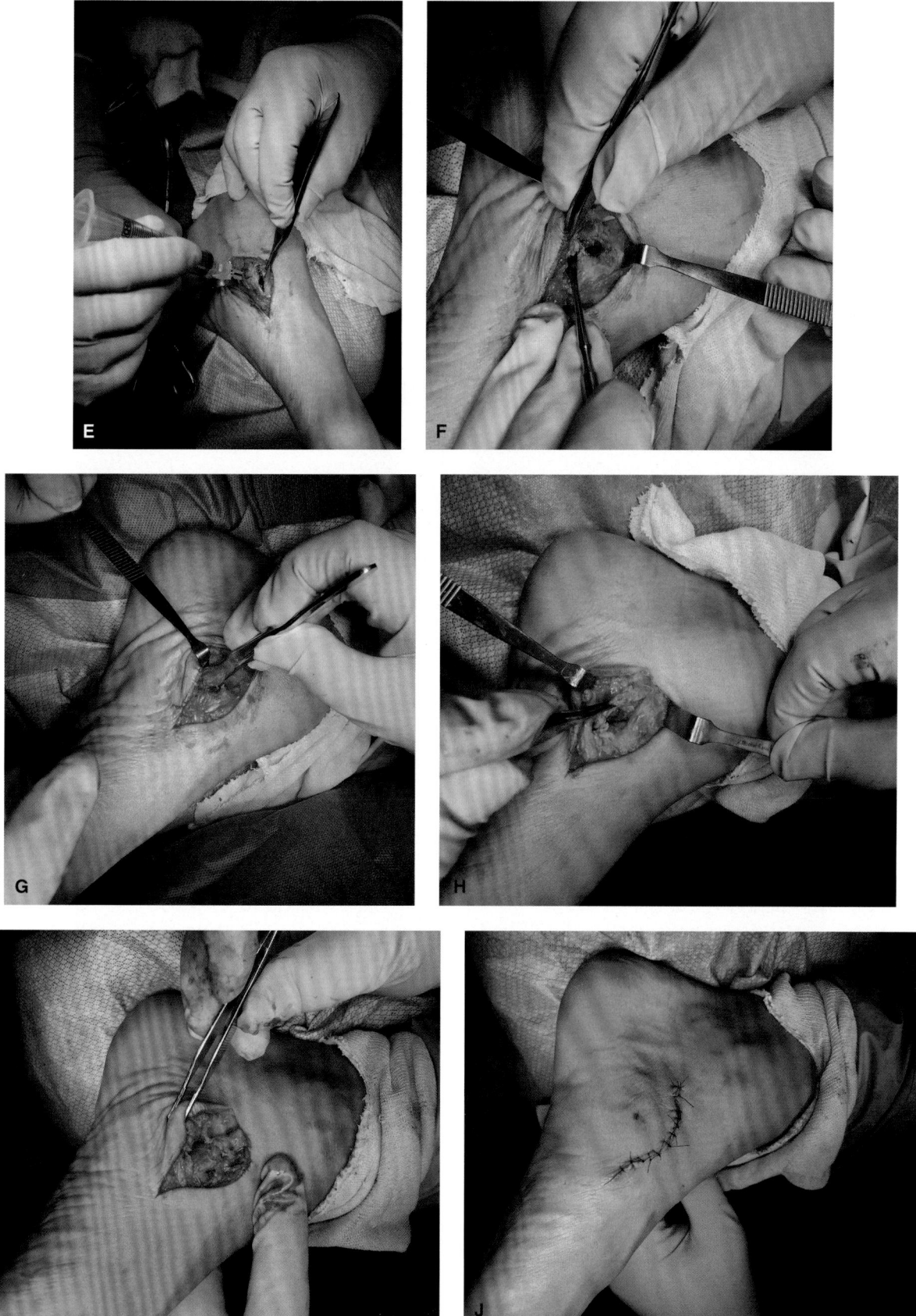

FIGURE 47.5 (*Continued*) **E)** The synchondrosis is identified with a large bore needle. **F)** The accessory ossicle is sharply dissected while reflecting the tibialis posterior and the periosteum/joint capsule inferiorly. **G)** The accessory bone is now shelled out and delivered from the wound. **H)** Inevitably some portion of the posterior tibial tendon medial navicular insertion is compromised with excision, but it is important to preserve as much of the plantar insertion and the lateral slip as possible. **I)** The compromised portion of the tibialis posterior tendon insertion is then secured back to the navicular either through drill holes and suture or with the use of bone anchors. Imbrication and repair of the spring ligament may be also be required. **J)** A layered closure completes the procedure.

periosteum and joint capsule compromising only the medial navicular insertion, while maintaining the plantar insertion and the lateral slip. The entire navicular medially needs to be visualized to assess the degree of medial bone resection necessary. The medial navicular redundancy is resected relative to the medial surface of the first cuneiform and the medial margin of the head of the talus. The talar head must be protected from injury during resection. The enlarged navicular tuberosity typically extends both medially as well as proximally onto the talar head. The nonossified zone can be difficult to appreciate and gentle probing with a freer elevator can help with identification. A large-bore needle can also be used to identify the nonossified zone and confirmed with fluoroscopy. Once identified, the ossicle may be shelled out and the integrity of the remaining soft tissues assessed. If a larger ossicle is present, the nonossified zone is resected without ossicle excision and is internally fixated back to the main body of the navicular. If a large plantar fragment of the navicular is removed, repair or reinforcement of the spring ligament may be required.[16] The degree of navicular resection is assessed with the foot held in a neutral to pronated position to be assured an even contour to the medial arch has been created with enough navicular remaining to protect and articulate with the talar head. Resection typically does not include any proximal articular surface of the navicular. The actual resection can be performed with the midtarsal joint supinated to protect the talar head. The compromised portion of the tibialis posterior tendon insertion is then secured back to the navicular either through drill holes and suture or with the use of bone anchors.[17,18] Generally, the anchors can be placed more distally in the navicular closer and parallel to the naviculocuneiform joint to avoid violating the hidden convex proximal contour of the navicular.

Resection of the nonunion zone with internal fixation without ossicle excision is not unreasonable.[19,20] This approach is probably best reserved for patients who report an injury, and when the primary posterior tibial tendon attachment to the navicular is via the accessory ossicle. This approach avoids exposing a portion of the talar head that would then be nonarticular with navicular thus protecting and maintaining talonavicular joint congruity. Navicular repair over resection helps to maintain ligamentous insertions that can be compromised with removal of especially larger type II navicular fragments. Resection of type II naviculars first involves resecting any enlarged medial navicular prominence, then excision of the accessory bone through the nonossified zone or repair by resection of the nonossified zone with internal fixation. Most of the nonossified zone can be expected to lie from within the medial redundancy of the navicular tuberosity extending laterally proximal to the talonavicular joint, but not necessarily the entire width of the navicular. A portion of the nonossified zone may lie within the normal confines of the navicular itself or extend into the talonavicular joint. The degree of exposed talar head that can be safely left nonarticular following resection of an intra-articular type II navicular is unknown, but fortunately in most cases if present, it is rather small. If the accessory bone is deemed too large for excision including a substantial portion of the normal navicular or involving a significant portion of the talonavicular joint, it can be preserved and fixated back to the body of the navicular to preserve ligamentous integrity, maintain articulation with the head of the talus, and close dead space.[19,20] If the fragment is large and significant preoperative talonavicular arthrosis exists, talonavicular arthrodesis is a reasonable

surgical approach. Talonavicular arthrodesis is a consideration in situations where an enlarged type II navicular presents with preoperative posterior tibial tendonitis and weakness with progressive pes valgoplanus deformity.[21-23]

Debate exists concerning whether ossicle resection can result in weakness to the tibialis posterior tendon, potentially worsening preexisting pes valgoplanus deformity. Kidner, supported by other early authors, felt this was possible and advocated advancing the posterior tibial tendon following ossicle resection.[24-26] Giannestras noted type II naviculars in nonpronated feet that did well without tendon advancement.[27] Other authors have agreed with this finding noting no advantage to tendon advancement.[28,29] There has been no evidence of pes valgoplanus correction with tibialis posterior advancement alone.[30,31] If significant pes valgoplanus deformity is present preoperatively with a type II navicular, it is not unreasonable to include additional procedures to correct or at a minimum prevent progression of the pes valgoplanus deformity following excision. If the foot is relatively rectus preoperatively with a type II navicular, then advancement of the tibialis posterior tendon to the navicular to maintain functional tension would be a reasonable approach.[17,18,32,33] However, advancement is much better tolerated in children, than in adults.

SURGERY FOR TYPE III NAVICULAR

Symptomatic type III navicular prominences generally require surgical remodeling. Surgical resection of both type II and type III naviculars requires exposure and visualization of the entire medial navicular from just distal to the naviculocuneiform joint distally to the talar neck proximally. The skin incision is placed superior to the tibialis posterior tendon and inferior to the saphenous vein over the medial midline of the arch. Dissection is carried through the superficial fascia to the deep fascia. An incision is then made through the deep fascia including the periosteal and capsular structures superior to the tibialis posterior tendon from the talonavicular joint area to the naviculocuneiform joint. A tag of tissue is maintained superior to the posterior tibial tendon for later closure. The posterior tibial tendon is not necessarily isolated but reflected sandwiched within the deep fascial and periosteal layer. This deep incision is executed with the subtalar joint supinated to prevent damage to the articular cartilage of the medial head of the talus. The dissection is begun proximally at the talonavicular joint within the pocket of the medial articular head of the talus. Dissection is carried distally and subperiosteally, exposing the medial surface of the navicular to the naviculocuneiform joint. Like the talonavicular joint, the naviculocuneiform joint is just visualized without overly dissecting or weakening the medial ligamentous and joint capsular tissues. Special care is taken in the pediatric patient to avoid reflecting the appositional bone growth layer of cartilage over the navicular with the soft tissues. The tibialis posterior tendon insertion into the medial navicular is incised, but maintained distally into the first cuneiform, inferiorly into the navicular, and laterally as the lateral slip. Medial navicular resection is performed to reduce the clinical prominence, but not expose the medial head of the talus creating a new medial talar prominence. Excessive navicular resection can occur if the talonavicular joint is overly supinated during resection assessment. Inadequate resection can occur if the talonavicular joint is positioned overly pronated during resection assessment. Intraoperative assessment prior to resection should be with the foot held in

a neutral stance position or the expected neutral stance position if other pes valgoplanus procedures are planned. Postoperative radiographs should demonstrate an even, flattened contour from cuneiform distally to the talus proximally, not involving or exposing joint margins. Actual navicular resection should occur with the rear foot held in exaggerated supination to avoid damage to the talar head. The posterior tibial tendon may then be advanced and reattached to the navicular to recreate physiologic tension. If excessive tendon laxity is noted, an advancement or Z-plasty shortening may be performed. Reattachment of the posterior tendon under physiologic tension can be aided with drill holes and suturing or with bone anchors. The bone anchors should be inserted to avoid the talonavicular joint. The surgical wound is then closed in layers. Patients are kept non–weight bearing in a removable CAM boot for 3-4 weeks followed by progressive increase in weight bearing until rehabilitation is complete. Resection of type III naviculars or excision and resection of type II naviculars can impact performing tibialis anterior tendon transfers, or Young's procedure, as part of a combined pes valgoplanus reconstruction. The outer medial cortical shell of the navicular is weakened following resection of a type III navicular making these types of tendon transfers impractical.

INDICATIONS AND PEARLS

ACCESSORY NAVICULAR EXCISION

- Type I ossicles rarely, if ever, warrant excision as the primary procedure. They may however need to be excised as an adjunct to repairing tears/ruptures in the posterior tibial tendon.
- Progressive pain, usually after a history of trauma/injury and a period of nonsurgical management, is usually a good time to remove a symptomatic type II accessory navicular ossicle.
- Avoid, if possible, advancing the posterior tibial tendon in adult patients. In children advancement of the tendon is better tolerated and can help to prevent ensuing symptomatic flatfoot.
- Many times the posterior tibial tendon will sit well inferior to the ossicle, in which case minimal tendon disruption is needed during ossicle excision, and postoperative rehabilitation can be accelerated.
- When structural, symptomatic, flatfoot is occurring concomitantly, then osseous procedures (eg, calcaneal and medial cuneiform osteotomies) should be included.

OS TRIGONUM

ANATOMIC FEATURES

An os trigonum is an ossicle present adjacent to the posterolateral tubercle of the talus. When an os trigonum exists, it can be difficult to differentiate from the posterolateral tubercle itself (Fig. 47.6). The posterolateral tubercle is typically larger than the medial tubercle and can vary in size. The os trigonum articulates anteriorly with the posterolateral tubercle and may be attached via a fibrous, fibrocartilaginous, or cartilaginous tissue. A fused os trigonum is called a trigonal process. Separation

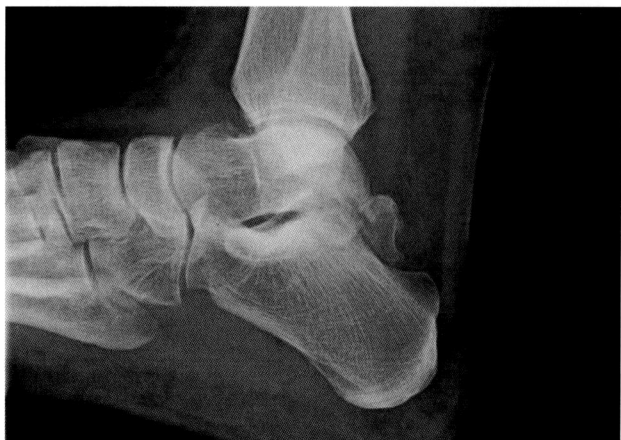

FIGURE 47.6 Irregular os trigonum visualized on the lateral radiograph.

of the os trigonum from the posterolateral tubercle may present as a normal variant and can often be mistaken for a fracture of the ossicle, known as a Shepherd fracture. The frequency of occurrence of os trigonum in adults is between 2.7% and 7.7%.[34-38] Prevalence of this accessory ossicle has been reported from 3% to 13% when taking into account clinical case reports found within the literature.[39,40] In one sports medicine clinic, 100 consecutive ankle radiographs revealed a 14% occurrence of the os trigonum, suggesting this ossicle may be even more prevalent than previously reported in an athletic population.[41] Children and adolescents are generally spared of injury to the ossicle as the os trigonum does not ossify until the second decade of life and usually fuses within 1 year of its radiographic appearance (between the ages of 8 and 10 years in females and 11 and 13 years in males). In this age group, the ossicle is rarely symptomatic as its attachment to the talus is cartilaginous until the time of ossification. Its incidence of appearance is found unilaterally twice as often as bilaterally.[42]

PATHOGENESIS

A symptomatic os trigonum is commonly caused by an overuse injury/insult when the ankle is plantar flexed forcefully. Chronic repetitive injury to the ossicle and posterior ankle capsule and supporting ligaments is frequently termed posterior ankle impingement syndrome. This mechanism is common in certain sports (eg, ballet, soccer, and gymnastics) where ankle plantar flexion and toe pointing is required.[40,41,43-49] A less common presentation is previous lateral ankle sprain that has failed to fully respond to conservative care, or subjective symptoms of ankle instability (ie, feeling like the ankle is giving way) that manifest as os trigonum syndrome. One study reported an incidence of os trigonum syndrome in a cohort of patients diagnosed with ankle sprains of 0.2%.[50]

The posterior talar process itself becomes more susceptible to injury when an os trigonum is present. This ossicle is positioned in close proximity to the subtalar joint, with some describing articulation with the joint itself; however, traditionally, the ossicle articulates with the posterior lateral tubercle of the talus. Varying histories of trauma can ultimately present with pain to the os trigonum. The most common mechanism of

injury is forced plantar flexion of the ankle where the posterior process is compressed between the posterior malleolus of the tibia and the tuber of the calcaneus. This force can result in fracture of the tubercle, especially, if the present os trigonum, is fused to the talar body. If the os trigonum is not fused, this force could then cause further separation of the ossicle from the talar body, with disruption of the fibrous tissue in the area. The talofibular ligament, inferior transverse ligament, posterior talocalcaneal ligament, and the flexor hallucis longus tendon are in close proximity to this area, and can thus influence the degree of symptoms. Despite damage that may occur to the adjacent soft tissues in an acute trauma, a fracture only of the os trigonum should not result in subtalar joint instability. However, if the fracture involves a large portion of the talus, then instability may occur and should be evaluated in the clinical examination. While planning surgical intervention, the surgeon should keep this concept in mind when considering how much of the os trigonum or posterior talus to resect. Iatrogenic disruption of the ligamentous structures in this area can further contribute to instability. Impingement of the posterior soft tissues could cause synovitis, provoked further by repetitive plantar flexion of the ankle joint. Activities and sports that encourage a plantar flexed ankle are most commonly implicated (eg, ballet, soccer).[41,43] It can often be difficult to differentiate between an acute fracture and impingements of the posterior region, when an os trigonum is present. Although it can be difficult to differentiate between an acute fracture and impingement by the os trigonum, the true etiology is not essential to establish.

PHYSICAL EXAMINATION

The differential diagnosis for posterior ankle pain is extensive (eg, ankle capsulitis, flexor tendonitis and/or tenosynovitis, lateral ankle instability, syndesmotic injury, osteochondral lesions of the talus, ankle impingement, posttraumatic arthritis, Achilles tendonitis, gout, peroneal tendinopathy). Concomitant conditions are common, especially flexor hallucis longus tenosynovitis. The goal of the clinical examination is to determine the principal diagnosis and determine associated pathology contributing to the chief complaint, including structural and dynamic pathologies.

Common complaints relating to os trigonum syndrome include pain with prolonged weight-bearing activities, vague aching within the posterior ankle, lateral ankle stiffness, discomfort to the peroneal group, pain stemming from the back of the heel, and poststatic dyskinesia to the posterior ankle. Activities involving increase subtalar joint motion, such as walking on uneven surfaces, walking up or down ramps/hills, and descending stairs may aggravate pain. Athletes may complain of pain when pushing off on the ball of their foot, but not necessarily with standing or walking. Pain can also be present at rest, given the plantar flexed position of the ankle which naturally occurs while resting.

The physical examination associated with a suspected symptomatic accessory ossicle involves ankle range of motion assessment, ligamentous integrity at the foot and ankle, and isolating the point of maximal tenderness. These assessments are encouraged to be completed in a stepwise fashion. For a suspected os trigonum, tenderness with deep palpation in the most distal extent of Kager triangle is typical. Encouraging the patient to point to the target area of tenderness with one finger will typically lead

to this area and should be confirmed with the physician's objective examination. Having the patient use one finger is important, because it minimizes confusion that may revolve around lack of patient's ability to differentiate pain stemming from the ankle versus the rearfoot. Evidence of joint crepitation, restriction in motion, or tenderness should be isolated to a specific location. Rearfoot range of motion may be limited if an associated peroneal spasm is present, indicating a possible malunion of the os trigonum to the posterior subtalar joint facet.[51] Manual muscle testing may additionally reveal crepitation, or impingement.[43,46,52] The examination does not typically demonstrate edema, erythema, or calor, unless an acute trauma is present. Even with localization of pain to the posterior process of the talus, it is uncommon to witness an actual acute fracture of the process.

Examination findings for os trigonum syndrome are best evaluated with the hyper-plantar flexion test, described by Van Dijk.[53] The patient is placed in a sitting position, or may lie supine on an examination table. The foot is placed in the neutral position, slightly internally rotated or slightly externally rotated in relation to the tibia. The distal tibia is stabilized with the examiner's left hand, and the foot forcefully plantar flexed with the right hand. The quick, passive force should mimic the impingement syndrome caused by the ossicle between the posterior inferior aspect of the tibia, and the superior aspect of the calcaneus. A negative test is when no pain is elicited with the maneuver, and this helps to exclude os trigonum syndrome. A positive test will reproduce pain at the posterior ankle and should reproduce the pain described in the patient history. This test can be performed again after a diagnostic block to confirm the diagnosis[54]; however, these injections can be difficult given the close proximity to the subtalar and ankle joints. These adjacent joints make it difficult to be sure the injection has targeted the pain caused by the os trigonum, or of these adjacent joints. Ultrasound guidance may help alleviate this problem. Diagnostic blocks are performed at the area of maximal tenderness in small amounts, posterior to the peroneal tendons.[55] The "nutcracker" sign (ie, similar to the hyper-plantar flexion test) is one of the more reliable clinical examination features indicating an acute fracture may be present (Fig. 47.7). It can be elicited with forced plantar

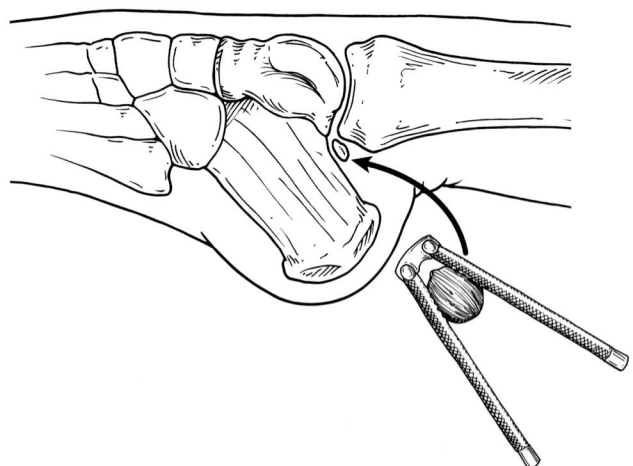

FIGURE 47.7 "Nutcracker" test. Forced plantarflexion of the ankle joint results in pain in the posterior ankle and talus. (From Easley ME. *Operative Techniques in Foot and Ankle Surgery*. Philadelphia, PA: Wolters Kluwer; 2010, Chap. 89, Figure 2, p. 750, with permission.)

flexion of the ankle joint, resulting in pain to the posterior talus. Less reliable clinical features of a fracture include direct pain on palpation to the posterior talus and pain with dorsiflexion, or active range of motion, of the hallux. Despite dorsiflexion of the hallux being a popular clinical sign, the literature suggests that this examination finding has high rates of false negatives.

IMAGING AND DIAGNOSTIC STUDIES

The os trigonum can be visualized on several views on plain radiographs. The ossicle typically has a smooth, rounded appearance with distinct cortical borders, and radiolucent line between it and the posterolateral tubercle of the talus. The os can typically be seen easily on the lateral view. It can be helpful to establish the proximity the os has to the subtalar joint. Fractures of the posterior talus are difficult to identify radiographically. Irregular borders between the fragment and talar body may indicate a fracture, whereas smooth cortical borders are more indicative of an ossicle. A Shepherd fracture refers to an acute fracture of the os trigonum, viewed radiographically as separation of the ossicle from the talus. If the ossicle is fused to the talus, there may be a larger portion of the talus involved in the fracture, making it easier to differentiate from a simple os trigonum. Several custom views can be obtained to better visualize the relationship between the ossicle and talus. A stress lateral view, where the ankle is maximally plantar flexed, may display further separation of the ossicle from the talus than a typical lateral view.[56] A modified lateral projection taken at 30 degrees to the subtalar joint may help differentiate an acute fracture from an os trigonum.[41] Serial x-rays may aid the diagnosis if increased separation of the fragment and the body is noted, or signs of osseous healing (ie, bone proliferation) is present.

Advanced imaging studies can be helpful in making a diagnosis but should be interpreted within the context of the clinical picture. CT scans offer detailed three-dimensional configurations of the osseous structures and may be helpful when clinical examination and plain radiographs are elusive. MRI is more helpful to evaluate the soft tissue structures and should therefore be reserved for when the os trigonum syndrome is complicated by tendonitis of the flexor hallucis longus, or posterior capsulitis.[57,58] Low signal intensity on T1 within the ossicle and increased signal intensity on T2 and/or STIR images is suggestive of marrow edema and can therefore be associated with os trigonum syndrome with a posterior ankle impingement (Fig. 47.8). Increased signal intensity within the sheath of the flexor tendon, increased intensity to the posterior ankle, and synovitis to the subtalar joint may also be present on MRI.[59] Findings on the MRI should not sway the provider to treat a condition that was not identified on the physical examination. These MRI findings will serve little purpose and may complicate the picture for an examiner who has not adequately identified the chief complaint on physical examination and is unaware of associated pathologies. The MRI should therefore be used to supplement the clinical examination and not be performed in lieu of thorough examination. Finally, technetium bone scans, although rarely indicated, can be helpful in equivocal cases to rule out a fracture if the scan is negative. A positive

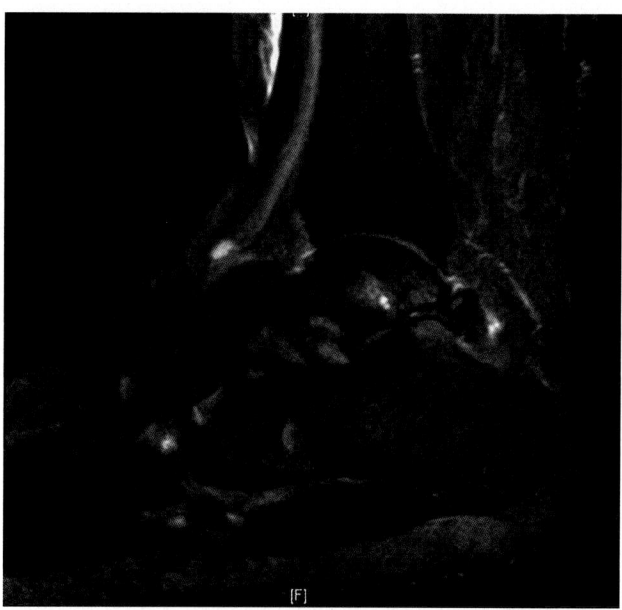

FIGURE 47.8 The marrow edema seen on this STIR sagittal image within the posterior talus, os trigonum, and the adjacent posterior superior calcaneus suggests a symptomatic os trigonum syndrome.

bone scan, however, provides little additional information, as they lack any real specificity.

TREATMENT

Treatments, regardless of the cause if the symptomatic os trigonum (eg, fracture or impingement), are targeted at alleviation of symptoms. Typical nonsurgical care involves a period of protected weight bearing with a cast walker, or removable ankle brace. Chronic conditions may present with an arthritic component, in which case anti-inflammatories, deep heat therapy, cold compression, and physical therapy can be helpful. Therapy should be aimed at decreasing stiffness in adjacent joints and preventing adhesions in the posterior ankle, further exacerbating impingement symptoms. For conditions recalcitrant to conservative treatment, surgical intervention may be warranted, consisting of ossicle excision.

Treatment for the acute fracture will involve a period of immobilization in a cast walker, or fiberglass cast depending on degree of symptoms. It may take several weeks to see full pain resolution (ie, 4-6 weeks). Early range of motion of the hallux is encouraged to prevent tendon adhesions. Oftentimes, the fragment and talar body will not achieve complete osseous union, secondary to separation of the fragment with ankle dorsiflexion. Severe separation is prevented via surrounding ligamentous structures. This nonunion is typically asymptomatic. Fractures of the os trigonum will rarely need surgical intervention, unless a large portion of the talus is involved. Smaller fragments will typically require less immobilization than larger fragments. For persistent symptoms, a corticosteroid injection may be beneficial. In a small percentage of patients, when conservative treatment is unsuccessful, surgical excision of the fragment may be required.

Surgical results for symptomatic os trigonum and posterior ankle impingement syndrome are quite good and highly consistent. Removal of a symptomatic os trigonum can be achieved using open techniques or endoscopic retrieval. Open surgery, in our experience, allows for a more complete release and/or débridement when there is significant concomitant FHL pathology. While endoscopic excision has a steep learning curve, when performed well the advantages include improved visualization during the procedure, less overall morbidity,[60-64] and faster return to activity.[64,65] Most studies comparing open verses endoscopic removal demonstrate a complication rate (including postoperative neuropraxia) that is 50% less with endoscopic techniques. Endoscopic excision is also clearly preferable in athletes and military personnel, when possible. The reported mean time to return to training following endoscopic excision ranges from 3 to 7.5 weeks[54,61,64,66-70], while open techniques may require 10+ weeks.[64,65]

It is important to counsel patients that the deep arthritic pain sensation related to the preoperative condition may take months to fully resolve even after the most successful of resections.[51] The potential complications of excision of the os trigonum are most commonly associated with the incision or portal placement, that is, the development of infection, capsulitis, rear foot stiffness, peroneal stiffness, sural neuritis, lesser saphenous vein disruption, or the development of a painful or unsightly scar. Sural neuritis is perhaps the most commonly reported complication.[71] On the whole, the literature is largely devoid of significant permanent complications from excision of the os trigonum regardless of the technique performed, that is, open or endoscopic.

OPEN EXCISION OF OS TRIGONUM

There are reasons to gravitate to an open procedure when addressing this pathology, and those conditions generally involve compound deformity: symptomatic os trigonum in the presence of chronic lateral ankle instability, flexor hallucis longus (FHL) tenosynovitis, peroneal tendon dysfunction or osteoarthritis of the rear foot, and/or midfoot complexes. Both posteromedial and posterolateral open approaches are described in the literature. When using the calcaneal bisection as a reference, the ossicle lies more medially, pushing some surgeons to choose a medial approach despite the close proximity to the neurovascular bundle. It is not required to obtain advanced imaging before pursuing surgery. If, however, a MRI or CT scan is obtained preoperatively, these images can be used to determine where fracture fragments lie, or if an associated tendon tear should be repaired, and therefore, help direct incision placement. Preoperative considerations are similar to all osseous surgeries and should include weight-bearing status, risk factors for deep vein thrombosis, time needed off work, and social determinants that may affect the postoperative course (eg, financial constraints to obtaining prescription drugs, transportation barriers to postoperative appointments). These considerations will vary depending on the surgical plan.

When considering your approach and execution for excision of a symptomatic os trigonum, it is critical to maintain ankle and subtalar joint stability. Iatrogenic disruption of one or a combination of ligaments about the posterior subtalar joint can destabilize a previously solid joint. Paulos[41] described a bifurcate ligament traversing the posterior subtalar joint consistently present in his dissections. This ligament tethers the posterior process of the talus both medially and laterally. Once the posterior process was osteotomized, it became evident that the ligament would distract the posterior fragment as the ankle was put through sagittal plane range of motion. This ligament attaches to the lateral process along with the posterior talofibular ligament, while the medial attachment is the posterior talocalcaneal ligament.[41] The FHL runs through this bifurcate ligament, and it is within this tethered arrangement that that the FHL comes into contact with the os trigonum. In viewing this arrangement from the posterior subtalar and ankle joints, it is easy to appreciate how FHL tenosynovitis and/or tendinopathy may develop in conjunction with a hypertrophic tubercle or an irritated and inflamed os trigonum. It is suspected that the distraction effect of the bifurcate ligament is the culprit for the nonunion of a fractured os trigonum or posterior process of the talus. In Shepherd's dissections, he noted that the deeper the groove for the FHL tendon, the larger the process of the talus.[72] That observation is consistent with the current philosophy that the hypertrophic posterior process and/or irritated ossicle are often associated with the repetitive mechanical stress from the FHL tendon seen in dancers with os trigonum syndrome.

OPEN POSTEROLATERAL APPROACH TECHNIQUE

Under general anesthesia or epidural, the patient is positioned in the lateral decubitus position to allow exposure of the posterior lateral rear foot and ankle.[71,73] A mid-calf tourniquet is placed atop multiple layers of cast padding material. Ample padding is applied to the contralateral knee, proximal fibula, and ankle region to eliminate pressure about these bone prominences, reducing the risk of postoperative neuritis of the contralateral peroneal or sural nerve. To gain access to the os trigonum, a posterior lateral incision is made beginning ~2 cm posterior and 6 cm superior to the distal tip of the fibula. The incision is made parallel to the posterior border of the peroneal tendons and anterior to the sural nerve. This incision should run along the posterior border of the peroneal tendons extending distally along the inferior aspect of the subtalar joint. This curvilinear incision will provide a relaxed skin flap allowing excellent exposure and direct access to the posterior lateral aspect of the talus, the region of the os trigonum, and the proximal aspect of the posterior subtalar joint facet. Blunt dissection is performed to identify and isolate the predictable structures of this area, the sural nerve, and lesser saphenous vein, which should be identified and retracted. The superior surface of the calcaneus and posterior subtalar joint capsule are then identified. With manipulation of the great toe joint, the FHL tendon can be identified, isolated, and protected as it rests deep and slightly medial to the ossicle. Prior to the capsular incision, it is frequently helpful to use fluoroscopy to first identify the location of the ossicle. This will also allow prompt confirmation of complete excision once the offending ossicle or fragment has been removed. The posterior ankle and subtalar joint capsule can now be visualized and a capsular incision can be made over the osseous prominence adjacent to the posterior subtalar joint. Often the ossicle is palpable and the capsular incision is then made in line with the posterior facet extending superiorly at the most proximal lip of the posterior subtalar joint facet.

With the capsule reflected, the ossicle may be found as an extension of the posterior lateral tubercle of the talus. I typically

use a small key elevator to free the fragment from the posterior talus, and rongeur to deliver the fragment. If it is united, an osteotome can be used as well-being sure to protect the medially positioned FHL and neurovascular bundle. This osseous body should be resected in toto, and the surrounding surfaces should be rasped smooth to ensure that there are no residual osteophytes to cause impingement or adhesion. Manipulation of the rear foot at this time will reveal unrestricted motion of the subtalar joint. Once satisfied with the excision, copious irrigation and final exploration of the region is completed. The posterior ankle joint can be inspected by putting the foot through a full range of motion from extreme plantar flexion and then extreme dorsiflexion. In the plantar flexed position, ensure adequate decompression has been performed by deeply palpating for any remaining bony impingement.

The wound should be closed in layers, ensuring that the foot is placed at 90 degrees to the leg for best approximation of the tissues. Closure of the posterior capsule can be completed after copious irrigation using 2-0 undyed absorbable suture material. While the FHL tendon can be approached from the lateral incision, it is considerably difficult and not advised by some.[74] The subcutaneous layer is closed with the benefit of 4-0 undyed absorbable suture and consideration for using a drain should be entertained at this time. Dermal closure using 5-0 undyed absorbable suture material is perhaps best tolerated when applied in a running subcuticular manner. While overconstriction will impede range of motion regardless of the technique used, external sutures, such as skin staples or an interrupted mattress technique, may prove more restrictive due to superficial skin sensitivity.

OPEN POSTEROMEDIAL APPROACH TECHNIQUE

Under general anesthesia or epidural, the patient is positioned in the decubitus position to allow exposure of the posterior medial rear foot and ankle.[75] A mid-calf tourniquet is placed atop multiple layers of elasticized cast padding material also applying ample padding to the lateral knee and ankle region to eliminate pressure about those bone prominences, reducing the risk of postoperative neuritis of the ipsilateral common peroneal or sural nerve. The medial approach incision plan is often required in athletes, ballet dancers in particular, as they often present with a concomitant FHL tenosynovitis or other FHL tendinopathy. This approach is more challenging than the lateral incision due to the proximity of the medial neurovascular bundle and the flexor tendons. The incision begins proximally and is placed ~2 cm posterior and 4 cm proximal to the sustentaculum tali. This incisional approach will allow optimal visualization of the os trigonum while allowing full access to the FHL tendon. Caution is exercised while bluntly dissecting to identify, isolate, and transect the thin flexor retinaculum that overlies the posterior tibial neurovascular bundle. The ligament should be tagged with 3-0 silk suture and retracted in preparation for later repair. Manipulation of the great toe joint confirms the location of the FHL tendon, and it is retracted posteriorly along with the neurovascular bundle to expose the posterior aspect of the subtalar joint and ankle capsule. The capsular incision begins with identification of the natural synovial recess along the posterior medial border of the joint capsule where the FHL tendon courses posteriorly and distal to the sustentaculum tali. The fibro-osseous tunnel of the FHL tendon should then be identified and released down to

the sustentaculum tali.[75] The FHL tendon is then inspected, and débridement of diseased tendon may be performed at that time. Once completed, the repaired FHL tendon and the neurovascular bundle are retracted posteriorly. The posterior ankle and subtalar joint capsules are now visualized, and the capsular incision can be made over the ossicle. Often the ossicle is palpable and the capsular incision is made in line with the posterior facet beginning superiorly at the most proximal lip of the posterior subtalar joint facet. With the capsule reflected, the ossicle may be found as an extension of the posterior lateral tubercle of the talus united, malunited, or fractured. The ossicle is then identified and should be sharply resected in toto. The surrounding bone and joint surfaces should inspected and rasped smooth when warranted to prevent residual adhesion and osteophytic degeneration. Manipulation of the rear foot at this time will reveal unrestricted motion of the subtalar joint in the absence of a coalition. Crepitation from within the subtalar joint, discolored joint fluid, or middle facet fusion are suggestive of chronic degenerative joint disease and are indications of progressive joint dysfunction. These intraoperative findings should be disclosed in the operative report accordingly. Ancillary procedures such as resection of middle facet coalition and interpositional tendon transfer should be considered when warranted. Once satisfied with the excision of the ossicle and peripheral joint débridement, a copious irrigation and final exploration of the region are completed. The posterior ankle joint can be inspected at this time, and osteochondral defects can be débrided or drilled as desired. The wound should be closed in layers ensuring that the foot is placed at 90 degrees to the leg for best approximation of the tissues. Closure of the posterior capsule can be completed using a small amount of 2-0 undyed absorbable suture material. The subcutaneous layer is closed with the benefit of 4-0 undyed absorbable suture, and consideration for using a drain should be entertained at this time. When resection of a posterior coalition is necessary, exposed bleeding bone surfaces may warrant a drain for 24 hours to prevent hematoma formation. The dermal edges can be reapproximated in a running subcuticular fashion using 5-0 undyed absorbable suture. While over constriction by any skin suture technique will impede range of motion, external sutures, such as skin staples, or an interrupted mattress technique may be more restrictive due to superficial skin sensitivity. The dressing preparation and postoperative course are the same as that for the lateral approach technique. If an extensive FHL tendon débridement and tendon repair are performed, then a prolonged course of non–weight bearing will be required to allow for sufficient tendon healing.

ENDOSCOPIC EXCISION OF OS TRIGONUM, VAN DIJK[76] TWO-PORTAL TECHNIQUE

General anesthesia is typically used. The patient is positioned prone on the operating table with both feet suspended off the end of the table so the surgeon can fully dorsiflex the ankle (Fig. 47.9). A thigh tourniquet is applied. The cutaneous landmarks for posterior ankle arthroscopy and hindfoot endoscopy are drawn out. With a marking pen, a reference line is drawn from the tip of the lateral malleolus to the Achilles tendon, parallel to the sole of the foot. Posteromedial and posterolateral portals are made just above this line, at the same level in the horizontal plane, and just medial and lateral to the Achilles tendon (Fig. 47.10A). Additionally, it is helpful to also draw out the path of the posterolateral portal by tracing a line that starts at

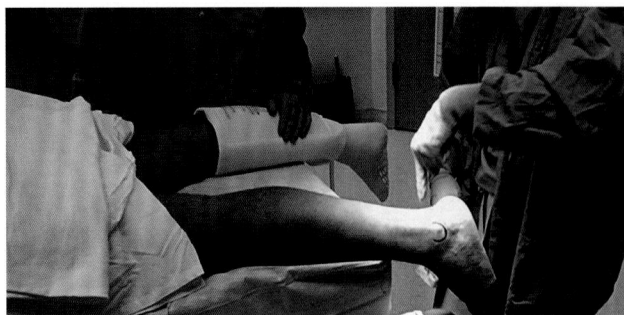

FIGURE 47.9 Positioning for endoscopic excision of os trigonum. The patient is placed prone on the operating table with both feet suspended off the end of the table so the surgeon can fully dorsiflex the ankle.

the plantar heel, lateral to the Achilles, and extending it distally along the sole of the foot into the first web space (Fig. 47.10B). The foot and leg is scrubbed, prepared, and draped.

The posterolateral portal is made first at the level or slightly above the tip of the lateral malleolus, just lateral to the Achilles tendon. A vertical stab incision is made, and a mosquito hemostat is directed anteriorly, pointing in the direction of the first interdigital space. When the tip of the hemostat touches bone, it is exchanged for a 4.5-mm arthroscope shaft with blunt trocar pointing in the same direction. The blunt trocar is situated extra-articularly at the level of the ankle joint, but it is not necessary to enter the joint capsule. The trocar is exchanged for the 4-mm arthroscope; the direction of view is 30 degrees to the lateral side.

The posteromedial portal is made just medial to the Achilles tendon at the same level as the posterolateral portal in the horizontal plane. A vertical stab incision is made, and a mosquito hemostat is directed toward the arthroscope shaft at a 90-degree angle. When the hemostat touches the shaft of the arthroscope, the shaft is used as a guide for the hemostat to move anteriorly in the direction of the ankle joint, touching

the arthroscope shaft until it reaches bone. The scope is pulled back until the tip of the hemostat comes into view. The mosquito hemostat is exchanged for a 5-mm full radius shaver.

The tip of the shaver is directed in a lateral and slightly plantar direction toward the posterior subtalar joint. When the tip of the shaver has reached this position, shaving can begin. The fatty tissue and adhesions overlying the joint capsule are partially removed, and the posterior compartment of the subtalar joint can be visualized, including the posterior talar process and the FHL tendon. With manual distraction of the calcaneus, the posterior aspect of the ankle joint is opened, and synovectomy and capsulectomy are performed as needed. The talar dome is inspected and any osteochondral defects are débrided, and drilled as necessary.

The posterior syndesmotic ligaments are inspected and partially resected if hypertrophic. Removal of a symptomatic os trigonum or nonunited fracture requires partial detachment of the posterior talofibular ligament and release of the flexor retinaculum Figure 47.11, both of which attach to the posterior talar prominence. Release of the FHL tendon involves detachment of the flexor retinaculum from the posterior talar prominence by means of a punch. A tight, thick crural fascia, if present, can hinder the free movement of instruments. It is helpful to enlarge the hole of the fascia using a punch or shaver.

Bleeding is controlled by electrocautery at the end of the procedure. After removal of the instruments, the stab incisions are closed with 4-0 nylon. A sterile compression dressing is applied. Ankle immobilization is not needed nor recommended after surgery. As soon as possible after surgery, the patient is advised to start range of motion exercises. The patient is weight bearing with crutches (as tolerated) for the first 3 days or so, then encouraged to weight bear without crutches. At 2 weeks postoperatively, formal physical therapy for muscle strengthening, ROM, and proprioceptive exercises is started. Return to activity/training is advisable when full ROM and muscle strength has been achieved.

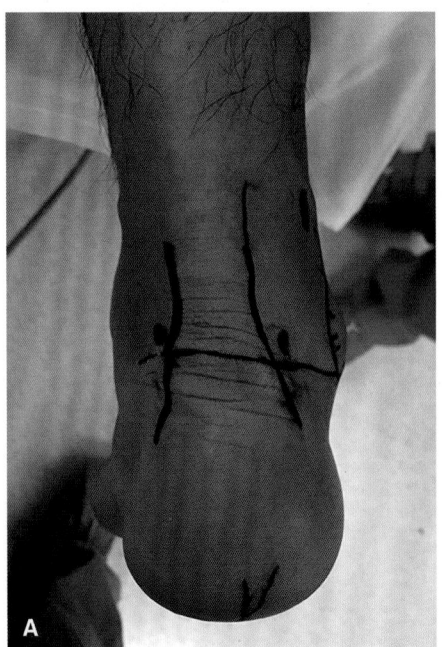
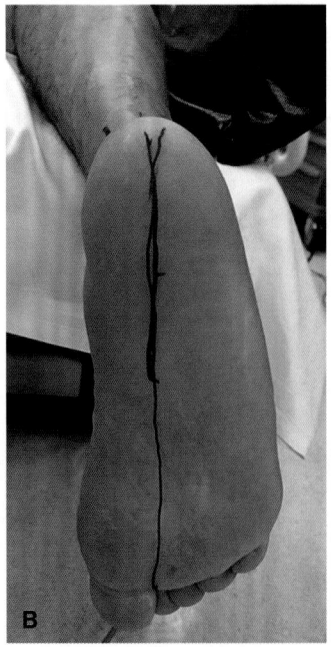

FIGURE 47.10 Cutaneous landmarks for 2 portal posterior ankle endoscopy. **A)** Posteromedial and posterolateral portals are planned just medial and lateral to the Achilles, just superior to a reference line that is drawn parallel to the sole of the foot extending from the tip of the fibula to the Achilles tendon. **B)** It is helpful also to draw out the path of the posterolateral portal by tracing a line that starts at the plantar heel, lateral to the Achilles, and extending it distally along the sole of the foot into the 1st web space.

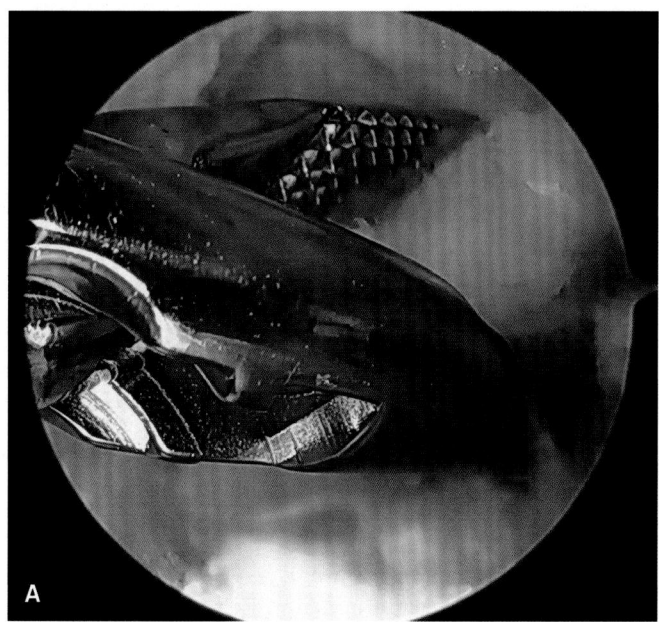 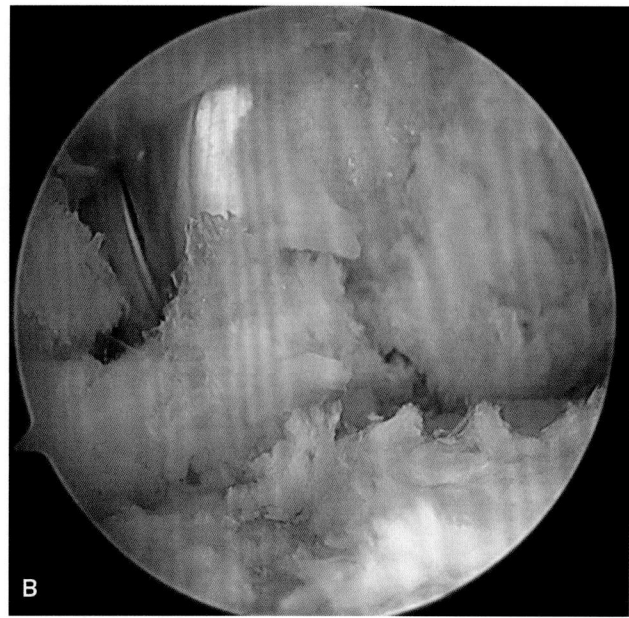

FIGURE 47.11 **A.** Endoscopic excision of the os trigonum requires freeing of the ossicle fully from its soft tissue attachments, prior to extraction, seen here. **B.** The flexor hallucis longus tendon can be completely visualized from the posterolateral portal once the osscile is removed.

PEARLS: OS TRIGONUM EXCISION

- Patients who have failed nonsurgical management but responded favorably initially to a diagnostic/therapeutic injection are perhaps the best candidates for isolated os trigonum excision.
- Be sure to determine whether FHL tenosynovitis is contributing. If so, open release is typically required (via posteromedial approach).
- The FHL is an important landmark. Motion of the great toe can help to identify the FHL tendon in the posterior ankle.
- Check FHL tendon excursion prior to closure to ensure there is unobstructed movement of the tendon. Place the ankle through a range of motion also to ensure there is no evidence of bony impingement remaining upon maximal plantar flexion.
- Fibrous adhesions due to a hypertrophic crural fascia can restrict instrumentation and exposure of the posterior rear foot and ankle when using the arthroscopic technique. This thickening, known as the ligament of Rouviere, is often encountered during this procedure as it has natural attachments to the trigonal process of the talus. A shaver, punch, or, as Van Dijk suggests, arthroscopic scissors can be used to enlarge the opening of the fascia and enhances visualization.[53]
- Keeping the instrumentation lateral to the FHL tendon will facilitate work within this trouble-free zone as there are no major neurovascular elements within this posterior margin of the rear foot and ankle.

REFERENCES

1. Bizarro AH. On sesamoid and supernumerary bones of the limbs. *J Anat.* 1921;55(Pt 4): 256-268.
2. Tsuruta T, Shiokawa Y, Kato A, et al. [Radiological study of the accessory skeletal elements in the foot and ankle (author's transl)]. *Nihon Seikeigeka Gakkai Zasshi.* 1981;55(4): 357-370.
3. Kruse RW, Chen J. Accessory bones of the foot: clinical significance. *Mil Med.* 1995;160(9):464-467.
4. Geist E. Supernumerary bones of the foot—a roentgen study of the feet of one hundred normal individuals. *Am J Orthop Surg.* 1914;12:403-414.
5. Zadek I, Gold AM. The accessory tarsal scaphoid. *J Bone Joint Surg Am.* 1948;30(4): 957-968.
6. Lemont H, Travisano VL, Lyman J. Accessory navicular: appearance of a synovial joint. *J Am Podiatr Assoc.* 1981;71(8):423-425.
7. Sella EJ, Lawson JP. Biomechanics of the accessory navicular synchondrosis. *Foot Ankle.* 1987;8(3):156-163.
8. Mahan K. In: Vickers N, ed. *Reconstructive Surgery of the Foot and Leg: Update'96.* Tucker, GA: The Podiatry Institute; 1996.
9. Wong MW, Griffith JF. Magnetic resonance imaging in adolescent painful flexible flatfoot. *Foot Ankle Int.* 2009;30(4):303-308.
10. Miller TT, Staron RB, Feldman F, Parisien M, Glucksman WJ, Gandolfo LH. The symptomatic accessory tarsal navicular bone: assessment with MR imaging. *Radiology.* 1995;195(3):849-853.
11. Grogan DP, Gasser SI, Ogden JA. The painful accessory navicular: a clinical and histopathological study. *Foot Ankle.* 1989;10(3):164-169.
12. Sella EJ, Lawson JP, Ogden JA. The accessory navicular synchondrosis. *Clin Orthop Relat Res.* 1986(209):280-285.
13. Romanowski CA, Barrington NA. The accessory navicular—an important cause of medial foot pain. *Clin Radiol.* 1992;46(4):261-264.
14. Lawson JP, Ogden JA, Sella E, Barwick KW. The painful accessory navicular. *Skeletal Radiol.* 1984;12(4):250-262.
15. Smith TM, Jones J. Flatfoot: kidner procedure. In: Jay R, ed. *Current Therapy in Podiatric Surgery.* Toronto, ON: BC Decker; 1989:242.
16. Jennings MM, Christensen JC. The effects of sectioning the spring ligament on rearfoot stability and posterior tibial tendon efficiency. *J Foot Ankle Surg.* 2008;47(3):219-224.
17. Dawson DM, Julsrud ME, Erdmann BB, Jacobs PM, Ringstrom JB. Modified Kidner procedure utilizing a Mitek bone anchor. *J Foot Ankle Surg.* 1998;37(2):115-121; discussion 174.
18. Yu GV. The Kidner Procedure revisited. In: Camasta C, ed. *Reconstructive Surgery of the Foot and Leg: Update'93.* Tucker, GA: The Podiatry Institute; 1993:209.

19. Scott AT, Sabesan VJ, Saluta JR, Wilson MA, Easley ME. Fusion versus excision of the symptomatic Type II accessory navicular: a prospective study. *Foot Ankle Int.* 2009;30(1):10-15.

20. Chung JW, Chu IT. Outcome of fusion of a painful accessory navicular to the primary navicular. *Foot Ankle Int.* 2009;30(2):106-109.

21. Mothershed RA, Stapp MD, Smith TF. Talonavicular arthrodesis for correction of posterior tibial tendon dysfunction. *Clin Podiatr Med Surg.* 1999;16(3):501-526.

22. Cohen BE, Ogden F. Medial column procedures in the acquired flatfoot deformity. *Foot Ankle Clin.* 2007;12(2):287-299, vi.

23. Tellisi N, Lobo M, O'Malley M, Kennedy JG, Elliott AJ, Deland JT. Functional outcome after surgical reconstruction of posterior tibial tendon insufficiency in patients under 50 years. *Foot Ankle Int.* 2008;29(12):1179-1183.

24. Chater EH. Foot pain and the accessory navicular bone. *Irish J Med Sci.* 1962;442:471-475.

25. Leonard MH, Gonzalez S, Breck LW, Basom C, Palafox M, Kosicki ZW. Lateral transfer of the posterior tibial tendon in certain selected cases of pes plano valgus (kidner operation). *Clin Orthop Relat Res.* 1965;40:139-144.

26. Kidner FC. The prehallux (accessory scaphoid) in its relation to flat-foot. *J Bone Joint Surg.* 1929;11(4):831-837.

27. Giannestras N. *Foot Disorders: Medical and Surgical Management.* 2nd ed. Philadelphia, PA: Lea & Febiger; 1973.

28. Ray S, Goldberg VM. Surgical treatment of the accessory navicular. *Clin Orthop Relat Res.* 1983(177):61-66.

29. Macnicol MF, Voutsinas S. Surgical treatment of the symptomatic accessory navicular. *J Bone Joint Surg Br.* 1984;66(2):218-226.

30. Prichasuk S, Sinphurmsukskul O. Kidner procedure for symptomatic accessory navicular and its relation to pes planus. *Foot Ankle Int.* 1995;16(8):500-503.

31. Veitch JM. Evaluation of the Kidner procedure in treatment of symptomatic accessory tarsal scaphoid. *Clin Orthop Relat Res* 1978(131):210-213.

32. Kopp FJ, Marcus RE. Clinical outcome of surgical treatment of the symptomatic accessory navicular. *Foot Ankle Int.* 2004;25(1):27-30.

33. Jasiewicz B, Potaczek T, Kacki W, Tesiorowski M, Lipik E. Results of simple excision technique in the surgical treatment of symptomatic accessory navicular bones. *Foot Ankle Surg.* 2008;14(2):57-61.

34. Sarrafian SK, Kelikian AS. Osteology. In: Kelikian A, ed. *Sarrafian's Anatomy of the Foot and Ankle.* 3rd ed. Philadelphia, PA: Lippincott Williams & Wilkins; 2011.

35. Thompson A. Report of Committee of Collection Investigation of the Anatomical Society of Great Britain and Ireland for the year 1899-1890. *J Anat Physiol.* 1891;25:89-101.

36. Stieda L. Der Talus und das Os Trigonum Bardelebens beim Menschen. *Anat Anz.* 1899;4:336.

37. Pfitzner W. Beitrage zur Kenntniss des Menschlichen Externitatenskelets: VI. Die Variationen in Aufbau des Fusskelets. In: Schwalbe G, ed. *Morphologische Arbeiten.* Jena, Germany: Gustav Fischer; 1896:245.

38. Grant J. *Grant's Atlas of Anatomy.* Baltimore, MD: Williams & Wilkins; 1962.

39. Ecker ML, Ritter MA, Jacobs BS. The symptomatic os trigonum. *JAMA.* 1967;201(11):882-884.

40. Marotta JJ, Micheli LJ. Os trigonum impingement in dancers. *Am J Sports Med.* 1992;20(5):533-536.

41. Paulos LE, Johnson CL, Noyes FR. Posterior compartment fractures of the ankle. A commonly missed athletic injury. *Am J Sports Med.* 1983;11(6):439-443.

42. Grant J. *Method of Anatomy.* Baltimore, MD: Williams & Wilkins; 1958.

43. Brodsky AE, Khalil MA. Talar compression syndrome. *Am J Sports Med.* 1986;14(6):472-476.

44. Hamilton WG. Stenosing tenosynovitis of the flexor hallucis longus tendon and posterior impingement upon the os trigonum in ballet dancers. *Foot Ankle.* 1982;3(2):74-80.

45. Oloff LM, Schulhofer SD. Flexor hallucis longus dysfunction. *J Foot Ankle Surg.* 1998;37(2):101-109.

46. Quirk R. Talar compression syndrome in dancers. *Foot Ankle.* 1982;3(2):65-68.

47. Wredmark T, Carlstedt CA, Bauer H, Saartok T. Os trigonum syndrome: a clinical entity in ballet dancers. *Foot Ankle.* 1991;11(6):404-406.

48. Clanton TO, Porter DA. Primary care of foot and ankle injuries in the athlete. *Clin Sports Med.* 1997;16(3):435-466.

49. Kolettis GJ, Micheli LJ, Klein JD. Release of the flexor hallucis longus tendon in ballet dancers. *J Bone Joint Surg Am.* 1996;78(9):1386-1390.

50. Fallat L, Grimm DJ, Saracco JA. Sprained ankle syndrome: prevalence and analysis of 639 acute injuries. *J Foot Ankle Surg.* 1998;37(4):280-285.

51. Galinski AW, Crovo RT, Ditmars JJ Jr. Os trigonum as a cause of tarsal coalition. *J Am Podiatr Assoc.* 1979;69(3):191-196.

52. Marumoto JM, Ferkel RD. Arthroscopic excision of the os trigonum: a new technique with preliminary clinical results. *Foot Ankle Int.* 1997;18(12):777-784.

53. van Dijk CN, de Leeuw PA, Scholten PE. Hindfoot endoscopy for posterior ankle impingement. Surgical technique. *J Bone Joint Surg Am.* 2009;91(suppl 2):287-298.

54. van Dijk CN. Hindfoot endoscopy. *Foot Ankle Clin.* 2006;11(2):391-414, vii.

55. Karasick D, Schweitzer ME. The os trigonum syndrome: imaging features. *AJR Am J Roentgenol.* 1996;166(1):125-129.

56. Hamilton WG. Foot and ankle injuries in dancers. In: Mann RC, Coughlin MJ, eds. *Surgery of the Foot and Ankle.* 7th ed. St. Louis, MO: Mosby; 1999.

57. Wakeley CJ, Johnson DP, Watt I. The value of MR imaging in the diagnosis of the os trigonum syndrome. *Skeletal Radiol.* 1996;25(2):133-136.

58. Sanders TG, Ptaszek AJ, Morrison WB. Fracture of the lateral process of the talus: appearance at MR imaging and clinical significance. *Skeletal Radiol.* 1999;28(4):236-239.

59. Bureau NJ, Cardinal E, Hobden R, Aubin B. Posterior ankle impingement syndrome: MR imaging findings in seven patients. *Radiology.* 2000;215(2):497-503.

60. Donnenwerth MP, Roukis TS. The incidence of complications after posterior hindfoot endoscopy. *Arthroscopy.* 2013;29(12):2049-2054.

61. Jerosch J, Fadel M. Endoscopic resection of a symptomatic os trigonum. *Knee Surg Sports Traumatol Arthrosc.* 2006;14(11):1188-1193.

62. Ribbans WJ, Ribbans HA, Cruickshank JA, Wood EV. The management of posterior ankle impingement syndrome in sport: a review. *Foot Ankle Surg.* 2015;21(1):1-10.

63. Smyth NA, Murawski CD, Levine DS, Kennedy JG. Hindfoot arthroscopic surgery for posterior ankle impingement: a systematic surgical approach and case series. *Am J Sports Med.* 2013;41(8):1869-1876.

64. Georgiannos D, Bisbinas I. Endoscopic versus open excision of os trigonum for the treatment of posterior ankle impingement syndrome in an athletic population: a randomized controlled study with 5-year follow-up. *Am J Sports Med.* 2017;45(6):1388-1394.

65. Guo QW, Hu YL, Jiao C, Ao YF, Tian DX. Open versus endoscopic excision of a symptomatic os trigonum: a comparative study of 41 cases. *Arthroscopy.* 2010;26(3):384-390.

66. Ahn JH, Kim YC, Kim HY. Arthroscopic versus posterior endoscopic excision of a symptomatic os trigonum: a retrospective cohort study. *Am J Sports Med.* 2013;41(5):1082-1089.

67. Calder JD, Sexton SA, Pearce CJ. Return to training and playing after posterior ankle arthroscopy for posterior impingement in elite professional soccer. *Am J Sports Med.* 2010;38(1):120-124.

68. Noguchi H, Ishii Y, Takeda M, Hasegawa A, Monden S, Takagishi K. Arthroscopic excision of posterior ankle bony impingement for early return to the field: short-term results. *Foot Ankle Int.* 2010;31(5):398-403.

69. Weiss WM, Sanders EJ, Crates JM, Barber FA. Arthroscopic Excision of a Symptomatic Os Trigonum. *Arthroscopy.* 2015;31(11):2082-2088.

70. Willits K, Sonneveld H, Amendola A, Giffin JR, Griffin S, Fowler PJ. Outcome of posterior ankle arthroscopy for hindfoot impingement. *Arthroscopy.* 2008;24(2):196-202.

71. Abramowitz Y, Wollstein R, Barzilay Y, et al. Outcome of resection of a symptomatic os trigonum. *J Bone Joint Surg Am.* 2003;85-a(6):1051-1057.

72. Shepherd FJ. A hitherto undescribed fracture of the astragalus. *J Anat Physiol.* 1882;17(Pt 1):79-81.

73. Yu GVM, Mezzaro A, Schinke A, et al. Os trigonum syndrome in update. Proceedings of the Annual Meeting of the Podiatry Institute; 2005.

74. Hamilton WG, Geppert MJ, Thompson FM. Pain in the posterior aspect of the ankle in dancers. Differential diagnosis and operative treatment. *J Bone Joint Surg Am.* 1996;78(10):1491-1500.

75. Chao W. Os trigonum. *Foot Ankle Clin.* 2004;9(4):787-796, vii.

76. van Dijk CN, Scholten PE, Krips R. A 2-portal endoscopic approach for diagnosis and treatment of posterior ankle pathology. *Arthroscopy.* 2000;16(8):871-876.

Nonunions and Malunions

Michelle L. Butterworth and Laura E. Sansosti

Foot and ankle surgical procedures, whether it be a straightforward first metatarsal osteotomy or a complex rearfoot arthrodesis, are not without potential complications. Nonunion and malunion of an osteotomy or fusion site are not uncommon and are potential postoperative complications that every surgeon should be well versed in, not only in how to manage them postoperatively when they occur but also in how to try to prevent them from happening through patient selection, preoperative planning, and proper intraoperative technique. In this chapter, concepts surrounding the diagnosis and management of both nonunion and malunion will be discussed. The basic science of bone healing, risk factors for developing a nonunion, and a comprehensive patient evaluation are all important concepts when dealing with these complications and will be reviewed in detail. Finally, conservative and surgical treatment of nonunions and malunions will be discussed including bone stimulation devices, recommended surgical protocols and pearls, bone grafting options, and the proper use of orthobiologics. This is an all-encompassing chapter, and it is the hope of the authors that providing this useful information will supply surgeons with a complete armamentarium to deliver superior care to their patients when these devastating complications occur.

NONUNION

Nonunion is a complex complication, where the biologic mechanisms of bone healing cease to function appropriately, and there is absence of healing across two opposing bony surfaces.[1] Nonunion is a chronic condition that can result from a fracture, osteotomy, or arthrodesis procedure and typically produces pain, deformity, and instability in the lower extremity. Previous reports have described a nonunion as a fracture that is unable to heal within 6-8 months of observation.[2-4] Campbell's Operative Orthopedics uses a timetable of 6 months to differentiate between a delayed and nonunion, stating that if the osteotomy site does not show any radiographic signs of healing by 6 months, it can be called a nonunion[5] (Figs. 48.1 and 48.2). Currently, the Food and Drug Administration (FDA) characterizes nonunion as "established when a minimum of 9 months has elapsed since injury, and the fracture site shows no visibly progressive signs of healing for a minimum of 3 months."[1,6] Although a time frame of 9 months might be helpful in certain situations, treatment should not be delayed until this time frame has passed simply for purposes of complying with a recommended definition. A good understanding of bone

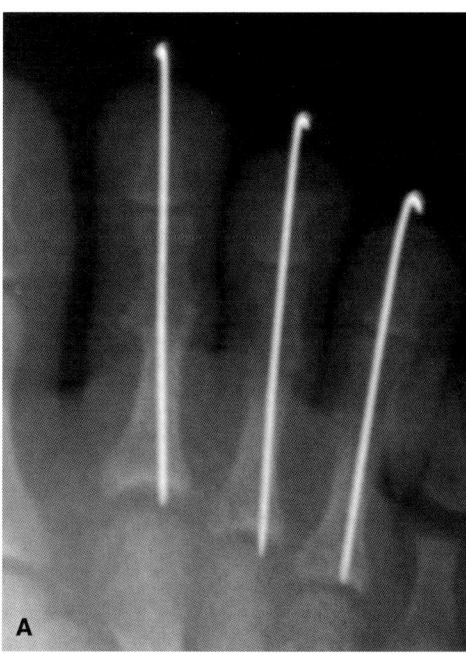
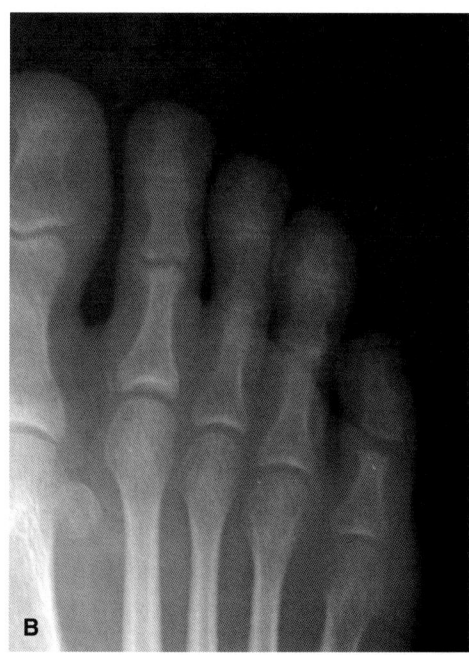

FIGURE 48.1 A. A 16-year-old female status post (S/P) arthrodesis of toes 2, 3, and 4 with external Kirschner wires (K-wires) placed. She bumped her second toe, and the wire loosened and came out at 4 weeks post-op. The toe was splinted. **B.** At 8 weeks post-op, there is gapping at the arthrodesis site on the second toe denoting a delayed union. Notice the third and fourth toes are healed.

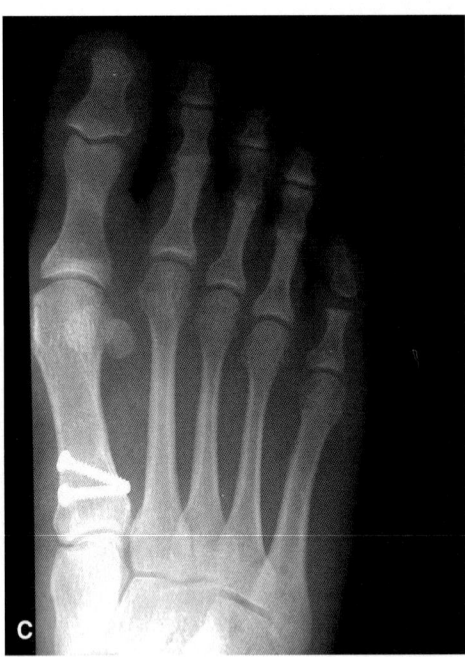

FIGURE 48.1 (*Continued*) **C.** Fortunately, at 4 months post-op, the second toe is healed and a nonunion was avoided.

healing, patient physical examination, and serial radiographs should enable the surgeon to determine if a nonunion is present and when adjunctive treatment is necessary.

Despite increased knowledge and advancing surgical techniques, the rates of nonunion remain relatively consistent. The rate of developing a nonunion following a long bone fracture is ~5%, resulting in about 100 000 nonunions in the United States annually.[7] Nonunion rates of arthrodesis procedures vary based on age and the specific joints involved and range from 2% to 3% in young triple arthrodesis patients to 17%-30% in adult triple arthrodesis patients, upward of 30% in isolated calcaneocuboid joint fusions, 20% in talonavicular fusions, and as high as 41% in ankle fusions.[7–10] Klassen et al. performed a retrospective, radiographic review and assessed the rate of osseous union following triple arthrodesis. One hundred and fifty-seven procedures were included in the study, and they found an overall nonunion rate of 29.9%. When broken down by joint, the talonavicular joint had the highest nonunion rate at 20.4%, followed by the calcaneocuboid joint at 17.2%, and the subtalar joint with a nonunion rate of 8.9%[10] (Figs. 48.3 and 48.4). The smaller joints of the foot typically have lower nonunion rates with the first metatarsophalangeal joint (MTPJ) and the first tarsometatarsal joint (TMTJ) arthrodesis being reported below 10%[11–16] (Fig. 48.5). Surprisingly, however, a recent systematic review of hallux interphalangeal joint arthrodesis revealed a nonunion rate of 28.3% and an overall complication rate of 33%.[17]

CLASSIFICATION

Weber and Cech classified nonunions by their vitality and osteogenic potential.[18] Their work was performed on long bones, and they subdivided nonunion types into hypervascular (hypertrophic) and avascular (atrophic). This classification scheme is important because it will guide the physician's treatment plan. While many of the hypervascular nonunions have the potential to heal with conservative measures, the symptomatic, avascular nonunions typically require surgical intervention to restore the vascular supply and viability to the osseous surfaces.

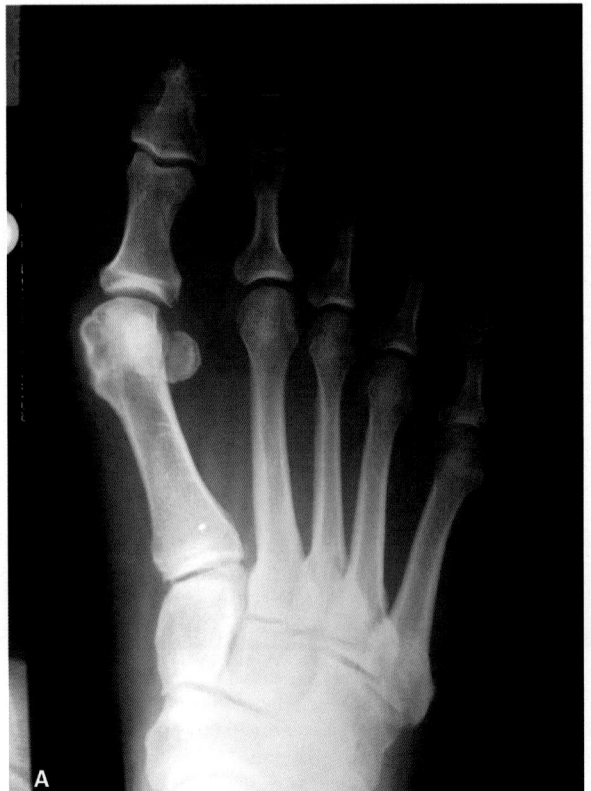
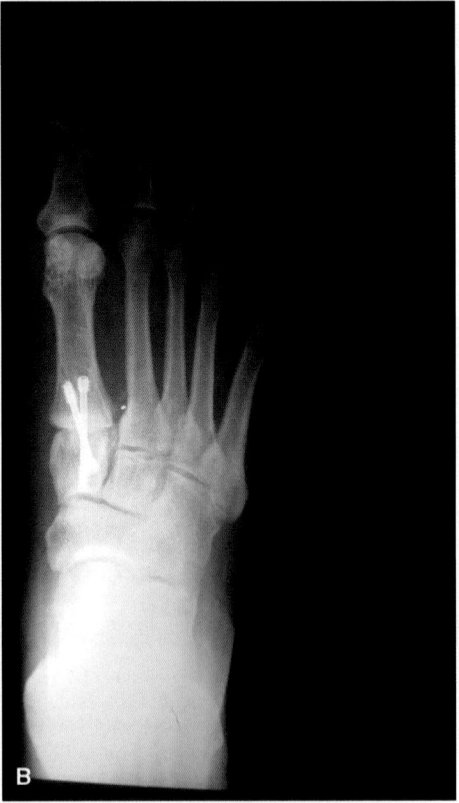

FIGURE 48.2 **A.** Preoperative radiograph of a large bunion deformity. Surgical procedure selection was a first metatarsal cuneiform arthrodesis. **B.** Immediate post-op radiograph reveals good alignment.

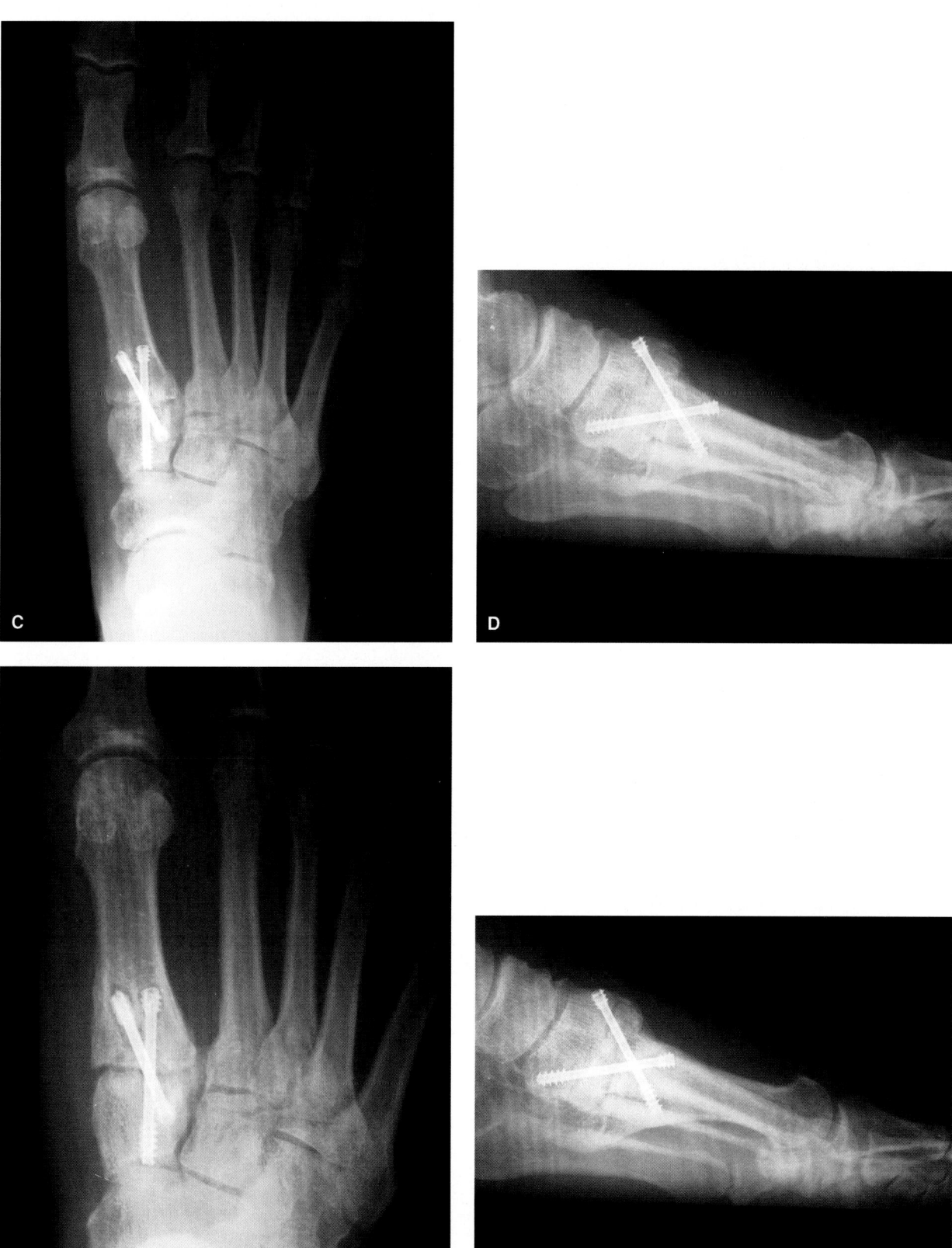

FIGURE 48.2 (*Continued*) **C, D.** At 10 weeks post-op, there are signs of healing with crossing trabeculation and increased consolidation. **E, F.** At 4 months post-op, however, there is lucency and resorption at the arthrodesis site. This is classified as a delayed union because of the timing but the nonhealing ensues, and the end result is a nonunion at 6 months post-op. Also, notice the position change with increased dorsiflexion of the first metatarsal signifying instability at the arthrodesis site.

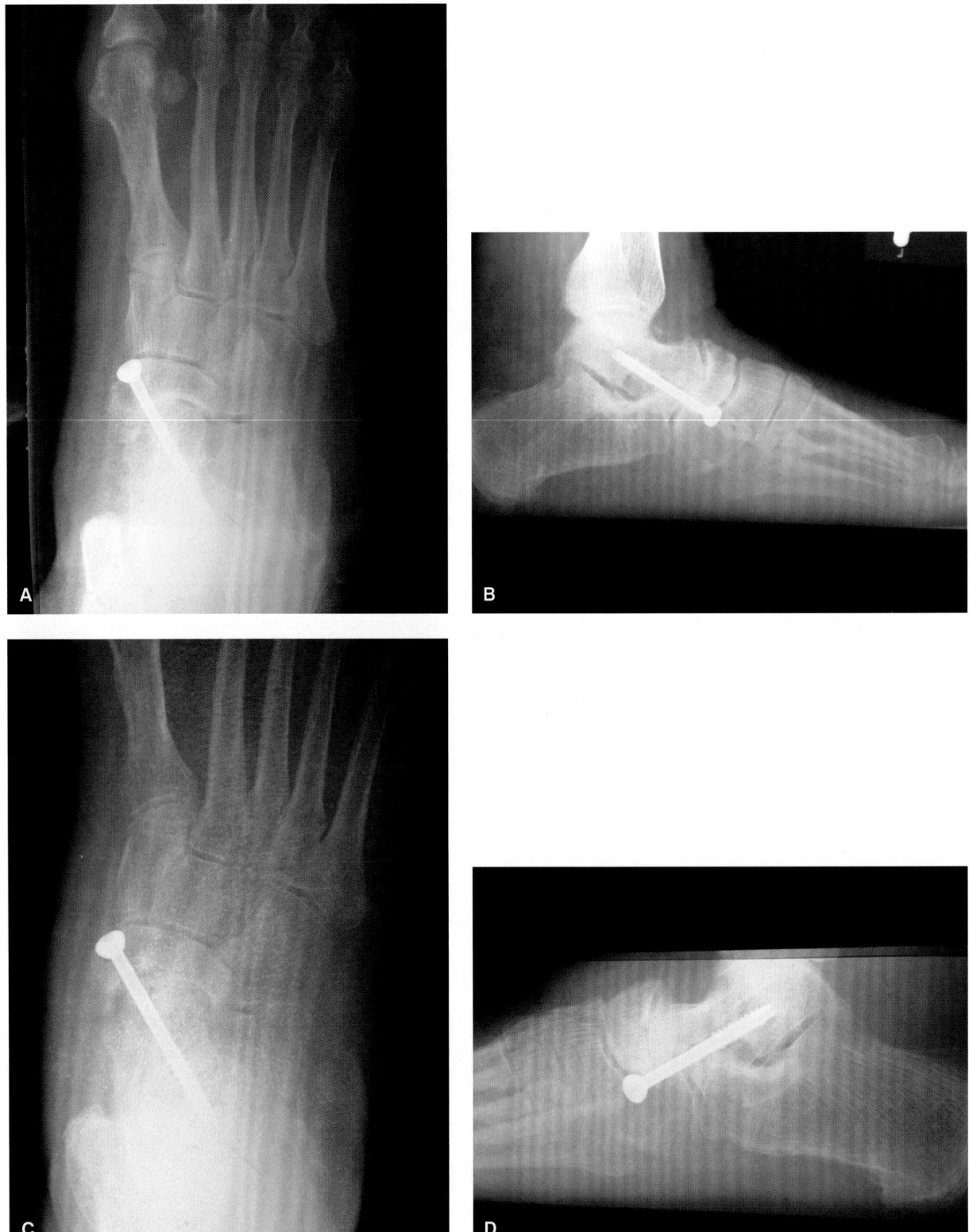

FIGURE 48.3 A, B. DP and lateral radiograph 3 months post-op of a talonavicular arthrodesis. Notice there is only one point of fixation, and there is gapping and lucency laterally and dorsally where there is no compression along the arthrodesis site. **C, D.** At 6 months post-op, there is incomplete healing and a nonunion is diagnosed.

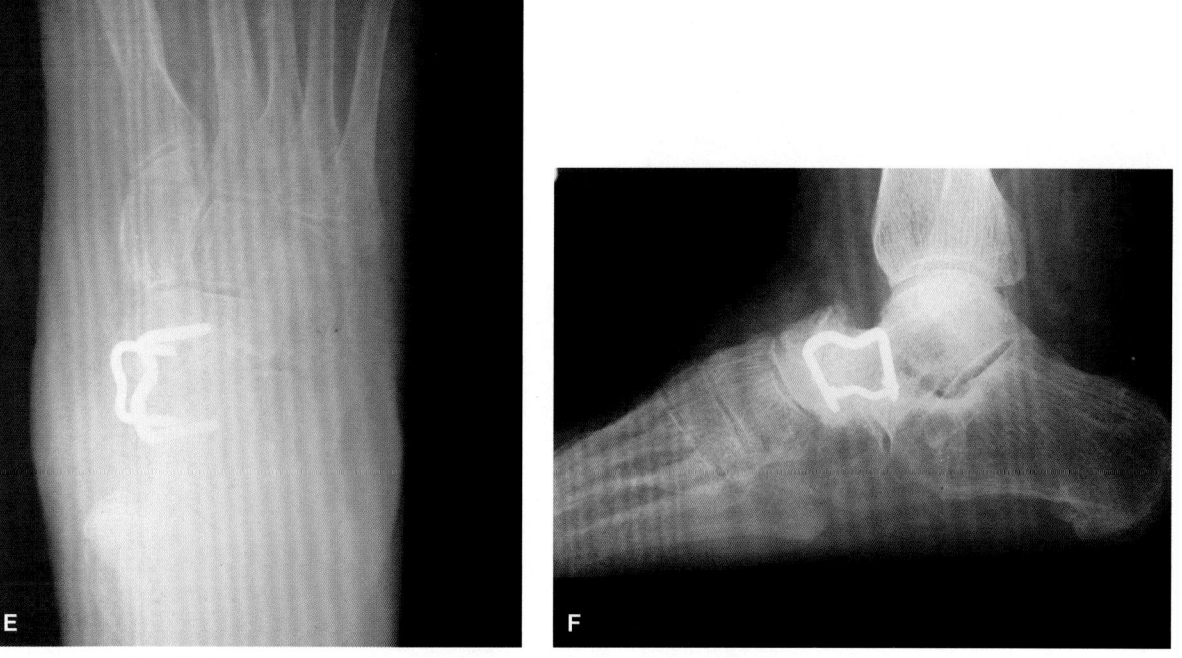

FIGURE 48.3 (*Continued*) **E, F.** Revisional surgery was performed with two points of staple fixation. Complete consolidation was achieved.

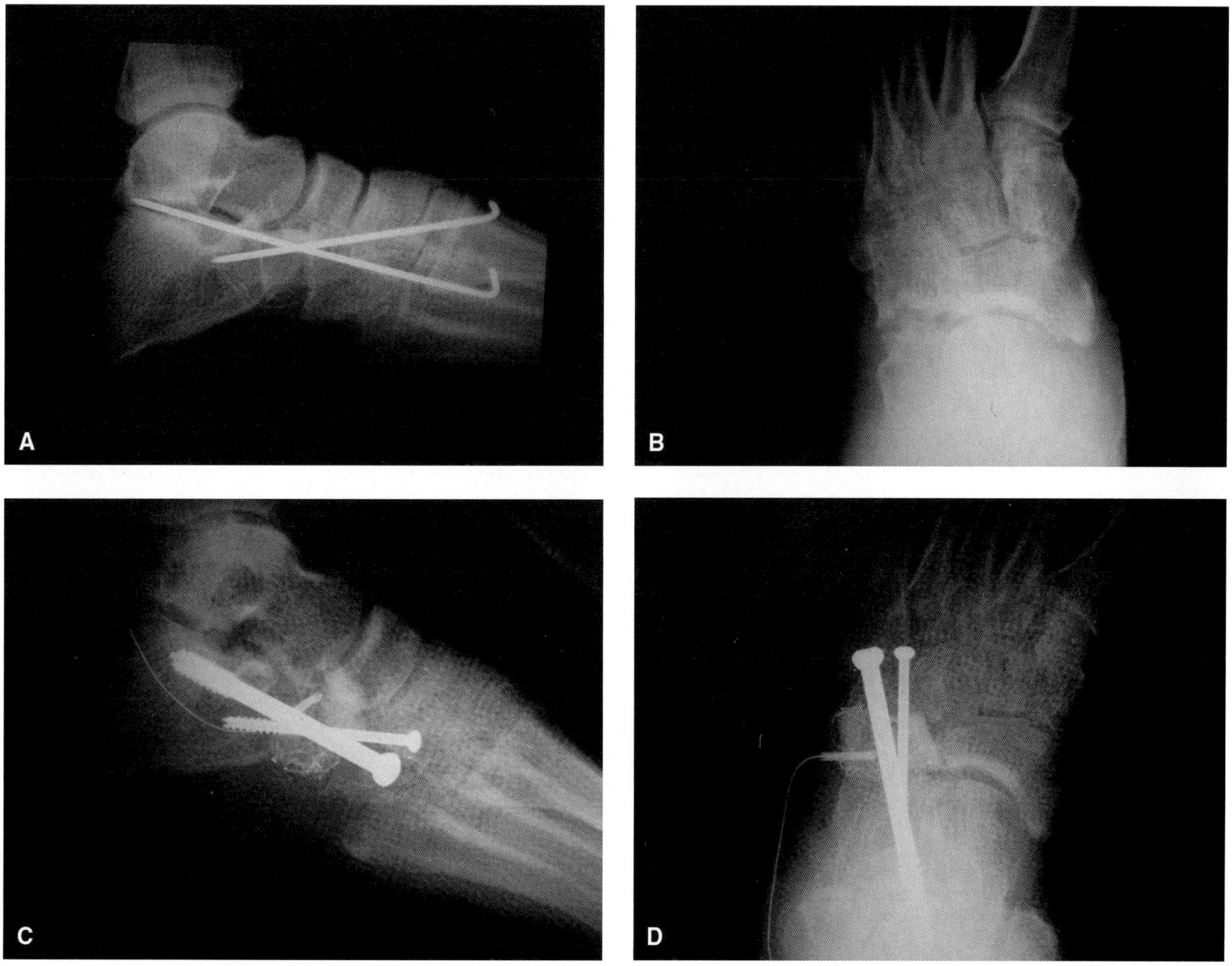

FIGURE 48.4 **A.** Lateral radiograph of a calcaneocuboid distraction arthrodesis. **B.** DP radiograph showing resorption and nonunion at the distal graft site. **C, D.** Revisional surgery was performed with autogenous bone graft, implantable bone stimulation, and screw fixation.

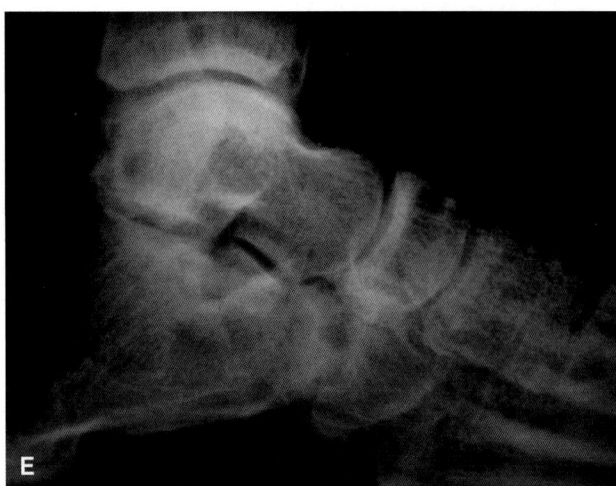

FIGURE 48.4 (*Continued*) **E.** Healed at 9 months post-op from the revisional surgery. Notice the fixation has been removed, and there is diffuse osteopenia from extended non–weight bearing.

CLASSIFICATION OF NONUNIONS

- Hypervascular nonunions
  ▸ Elephant's foot
  ▸ Horse's hoof
  ▸ Oligotrophic
- Avascular nonunions
  ▸ Torsion wedge
  ▸ Comminuted
  ▸ Defect
  ▸ Atrophic

Hypervascular nonunions are associated with continuing proliferation of blood vessels at the fracture ends and have capable biologic activity to promote callus formation and osseous healing. These nonunions have the potential to heal if treated appropriately. There are three subsets of hypervascular nonunions: elephant's foot, horse's hoof, and

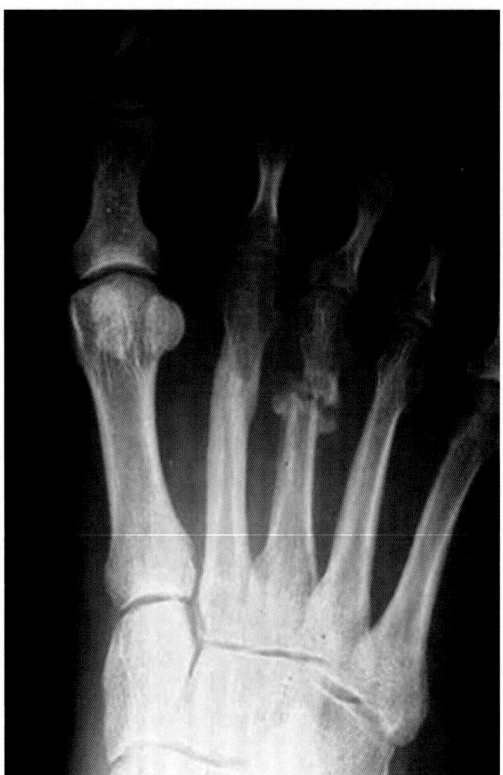

FIGURE 48.6 Elephant's foot nonunion of the third metatarsal with viable osseous fragments and abundant bone callus formation. This resulted secondary to weight bearing and lack of fixation.

oligotrophic. The elephant's foot nonunion is rich in vascular supply and has viable osseous fragments with an abundance of callus formation (Fig. 48.6). These nonunions usually result from premature weight bearing or insufficient fixation and typically only require improved stability to facilitate osseous union. The horse's hoof nonunion also displays viable bone ends but has a marked decrease in callus formation, which may display sclerotic densities at the ends of the bony surfaces (Fig. 48.7). These nonunions usually result

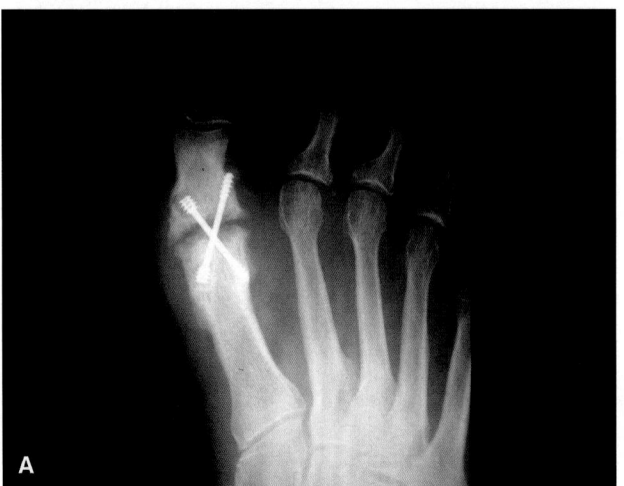

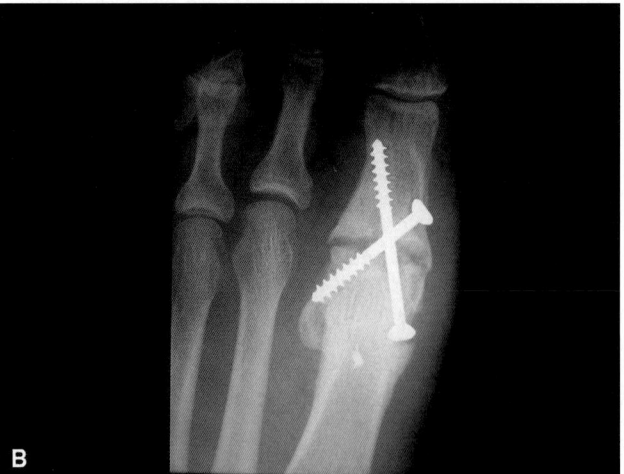

FIGURE 48.5 **A.** Nonunion of a first metatarsophalangeal joint (first MTPJ) arthrodesis with headless screw fixation. Notice lucency around the fixation confirming instability and resorption and nonhealing at the fusion site. **B.** First MTPJ nonunion at 6 months with 2-screw fixation. Good alignment was maintained, and fixation appeared stable. A bone stimulator was applied.

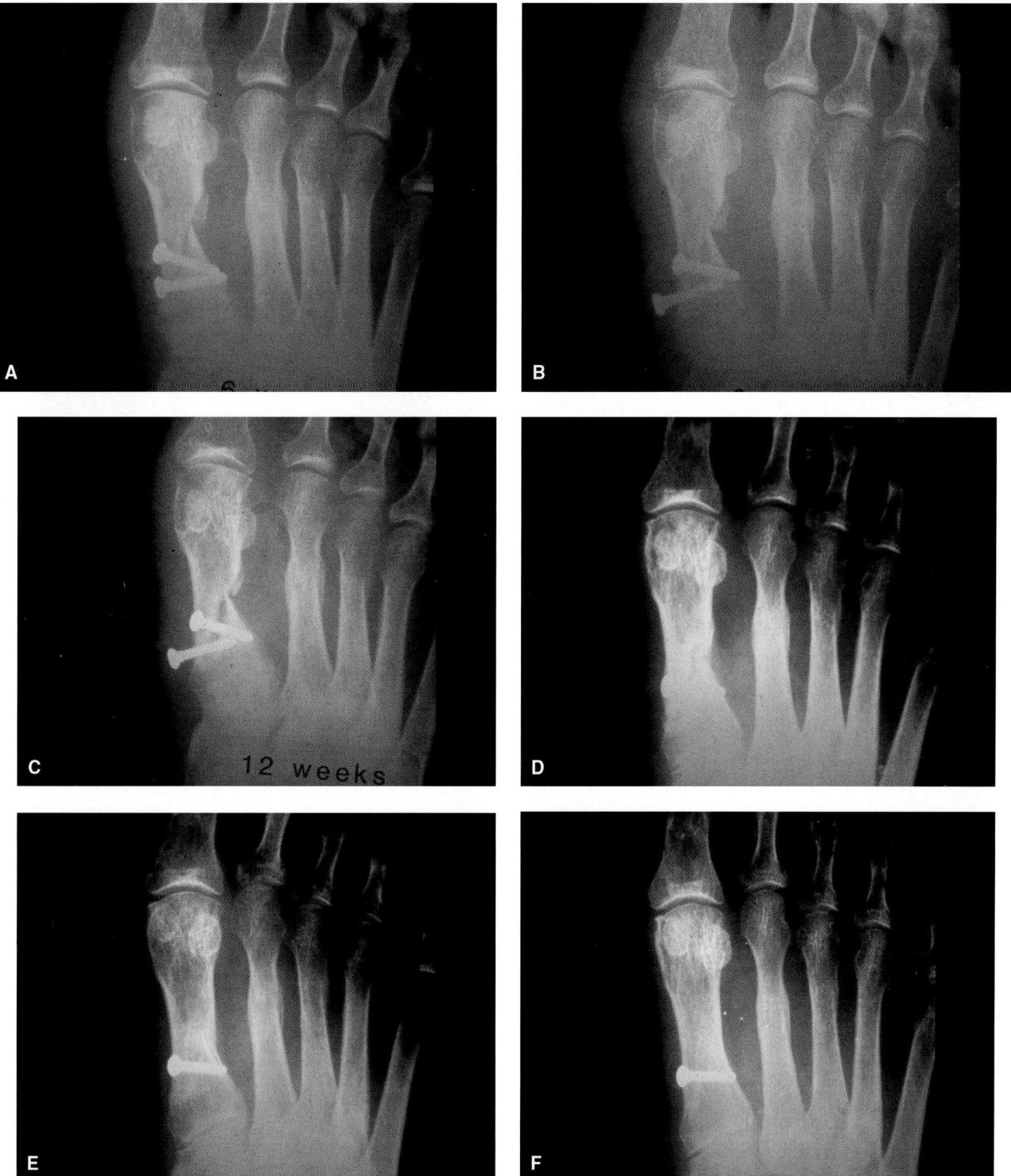

FIGURE 48.7 **A.** Six weeks post-op closing base wedge osteotomy (CBWO). Note the fragment along the distal aspect of the osteotomy. **B.** Eight weeks post-op. There is some consolidation of the osteotomy, but the proximal screw is unstable and backing out. **C.** At 12 weeks post-op, some consolidation is noted but there is persistent lucency along the osteotomy and the proximal screw is still unstable. The bone ends appear viable, however, and there is minimal bone callus formation. These are the signs of a horse's hoof nonunion. The patient was kept non–weight bearing. **D.** At 6 months post-op, the osteotomy is almost completely healed, and the proximal screw was removed. **E.** At 8 months post-op, consolidation is complete. Notice that even the distal fragment has healed. **F.** At 2.5 years post-op, excellent healing and alignment is shown. Fortunately, although the proximal screw failed, the distal screw and intact osteotomy hinge helped maintain enough stability to achieve consolidation.

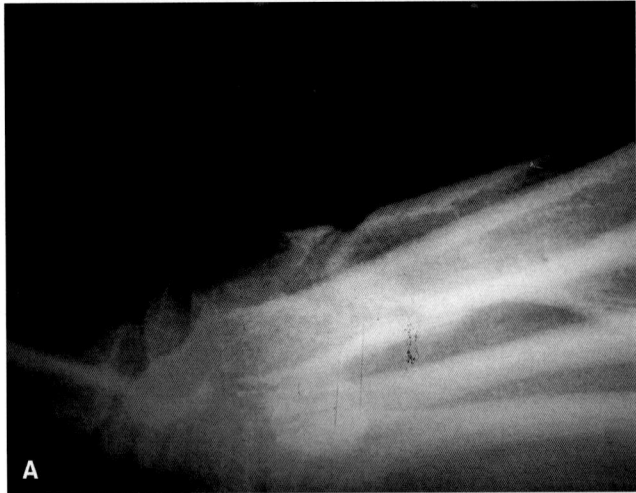

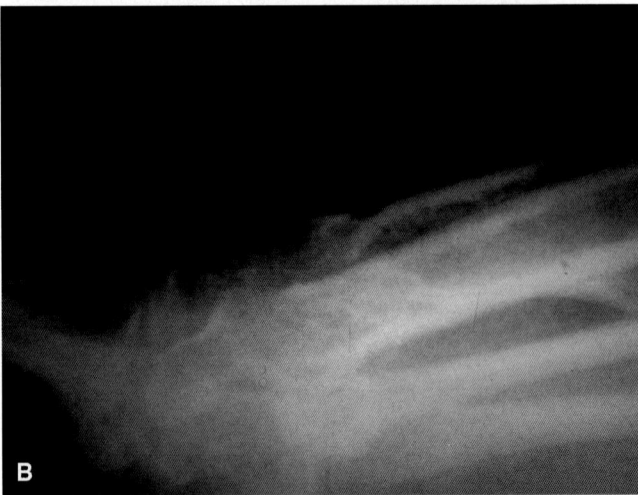

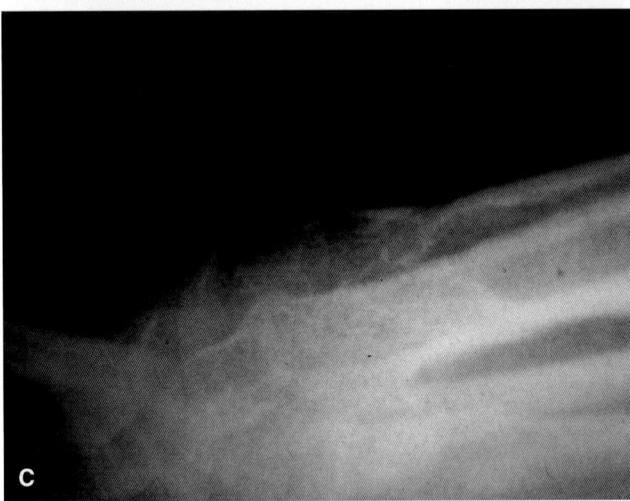

FIGURE 48.8 A. Eight weeks post-op Austin osteotomy. Notice the poor approximation of the osteotomy site with gapping. **B.** Six months post-op shows continued healing but consolidation is still not complete. This is an oligotrophic nonunion resulting from poor apposition of the osseous surfaces during the initial surgery. This is still a hypertrophic nonunion, however, with viable bone ends. **C.** Complete consolidation and healing at 9 months post-op. Notice, there was no bone callus formation.

from fatigue of internal fixation. Finally, the oligotrophic nonunion also displays viable bone ends; however, callus formation is minimal or absent in this subtype; therefore, biologic activity is much less than the other two hypertrophic nonunions described (Fig. 48.8). These nonunions usually result from poor initial apposition of osseous surfaces or distraction of the bony fragments.

Avascular nonunions have little or no vascular supply and exhibit poor osteogenic potential and are considered nonviable. There are four different types reported: torsion wedge, comminuted, defect, and atrophic. Torsion wedge nonunions occur in the presence of a butterfly fragment at the fracture site. There is diminished blood supply to this fragment, and it will typically only unite with one side of the fracture. Comminuted nonunions have multiple intervening fragments that may exhibit necrosis and persistent gapping at the fracture site. Defect nonunions occur when there is complete loss of bone substance and significant gapping remains at the fracture site (Fig. 48.9). As the distance between bone fragments is too great for healing this type of nonunion, union is only possible with replacement of bone (Fig. 48.10). These nonunions commonly result from excessive bone resection secondary to infection or open fracture. Finally, atrophic nonunions result from necrosis of an intervening fragment with fibrous tissue

filling the void. Partial absorption of the osseous surfaces, osteoporosis, and atrophy are commonly seen. The term pseudoarthrosis is oftentimes used for this type of nonunion (Figs. 48.11 and 48.12). Gudas and Cann have defined a pseudoarthrosis as a false fluid- and tissue-filled space between two fracture fragments.[19]

SCIENCE OF BONE HEALING

Bone healing is an orchestrated set of events mediated by systemic and local factors at a cellular level.[20] There are two types of bone healing: primary (direct) and secondary (indirect). Most osseous injuries that are treated conservatively heal by secondary intention. This indirect healing uses an initial intermediate connective or fibrocartilage tissue bridge that is secondarily replaced by bone. This secondary healing is a result of some degree of motion at the fracture site and is typically characterized by abundant callus formation, temporary widening of the fracture site resulting from osteoclastic resorption, and a slow disappearance of the fracture line as fibrocartilage mineralizes into bone.[20–23]

Heppenstall described six different stages of secondary bone healing.[24] The initial impaction phase is characterized

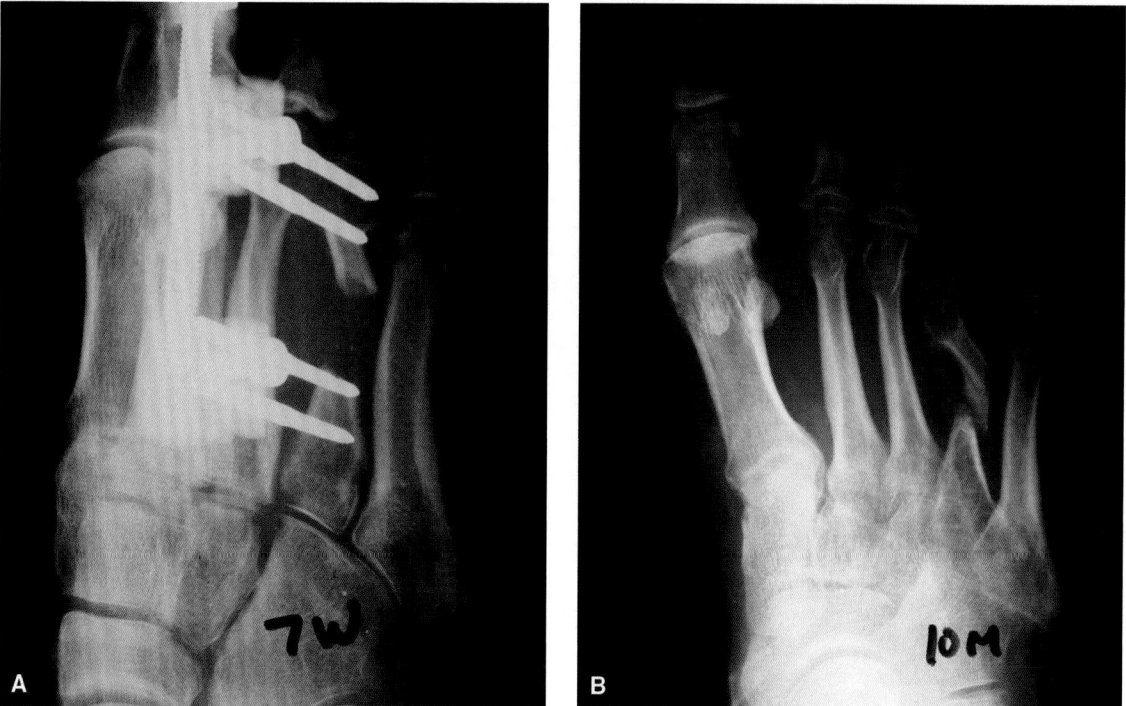

FIGURE 48.9 A. Brachymetatarsia repair was performed with callus distraction. At 7 weeks post-op, there is minimal callus formation and a large osseous defect and malalignment. **B.** At 10 months post-op, some bone formation is noted but nonunion and malunion result.

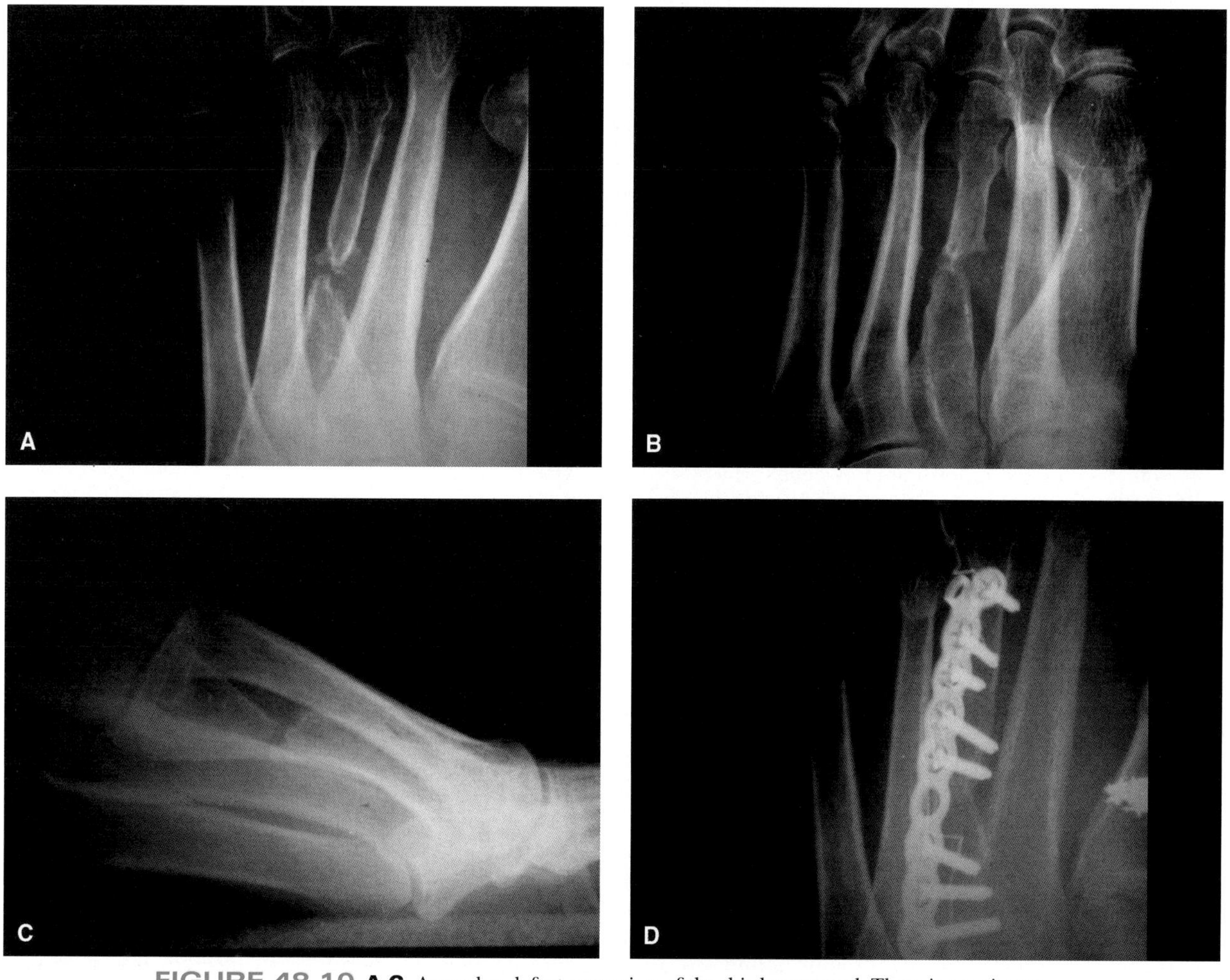

FIGURE 48.10 A-C. Avascular, defect nonunion of the third metatarsal. There is gapping at the fracture site with sclerotic bone ends. **D-F.** Surgical reconstruction with plate and screw fixation, autogenous calcaneal bone graft, and implantable bone stimulation.

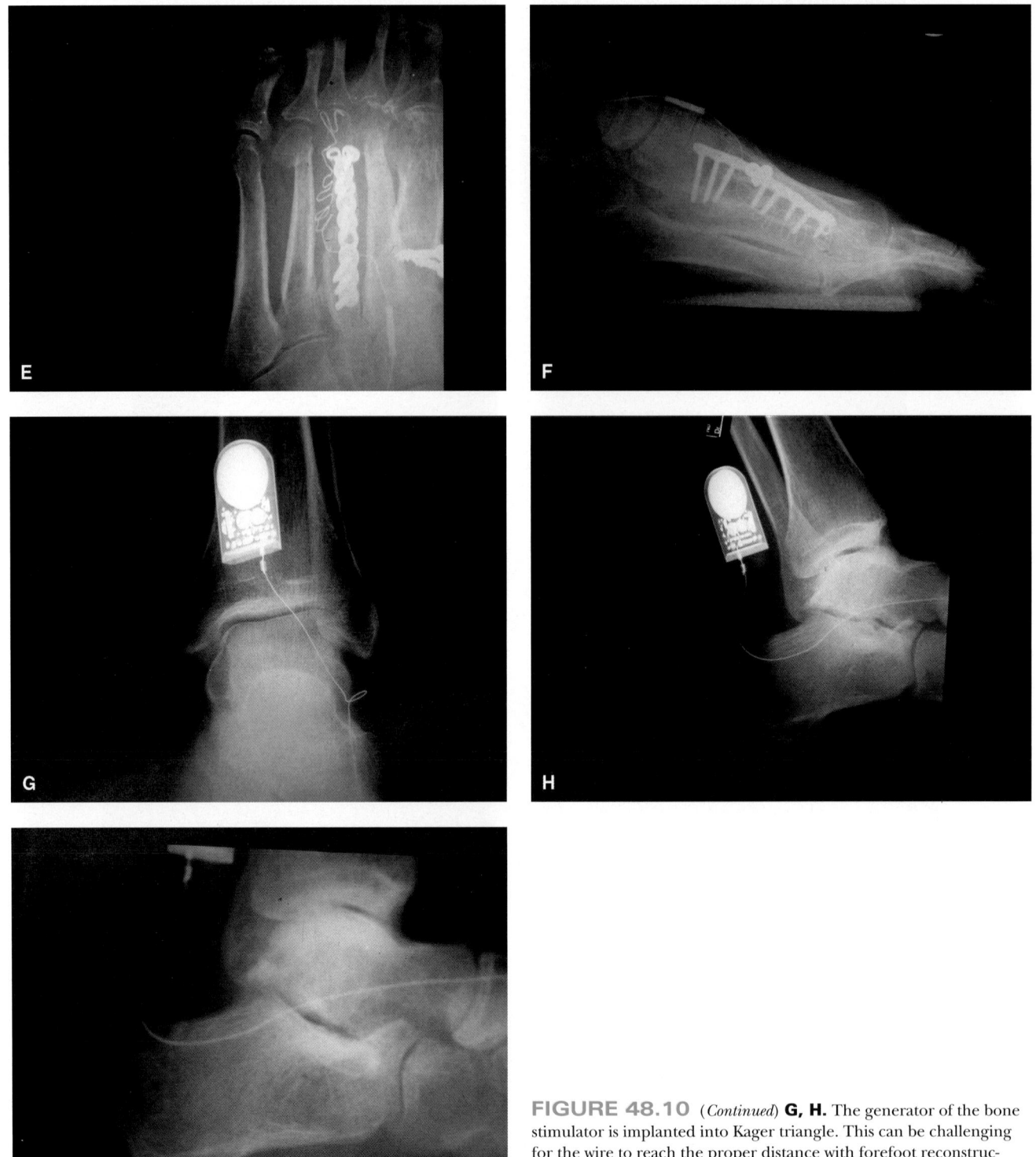

FIGURE 48.10 (*Continued*) **G, H.** The generator of the bone stimulator is implanted into Kager triangle. This can be challenging for the wire to reach the proper distance with forefoot reconstructions. **I.** Consolidation of the calcaneal bone graft donor site is noted at 3 months.

by disruption of the bone and starts the cascade of events hopefully resulting in successful bone healing. The induction phase follows and is characterized by osteogenic precursor cells being recruited to the site of injury. Urist discovered bone morphogenetic protein, and subsequently a myriad of growth factors, responsible for the recruitment of these osteoprogenitor cells and mesenchymal cells in the periosteum and surrounding soft tissues.[25] The value of these growth factors is significant in bone healing; therefore, the surgeon must utilize meticulous atraumatic technique to preserve the blood supply and ensure an environment rich in these osteoprogenitor cells. The inflammatory phase is marked by increased pain and edema when inflammatory cells invade the area and usually lasts 3-5 days from the inciting event. The soft callus

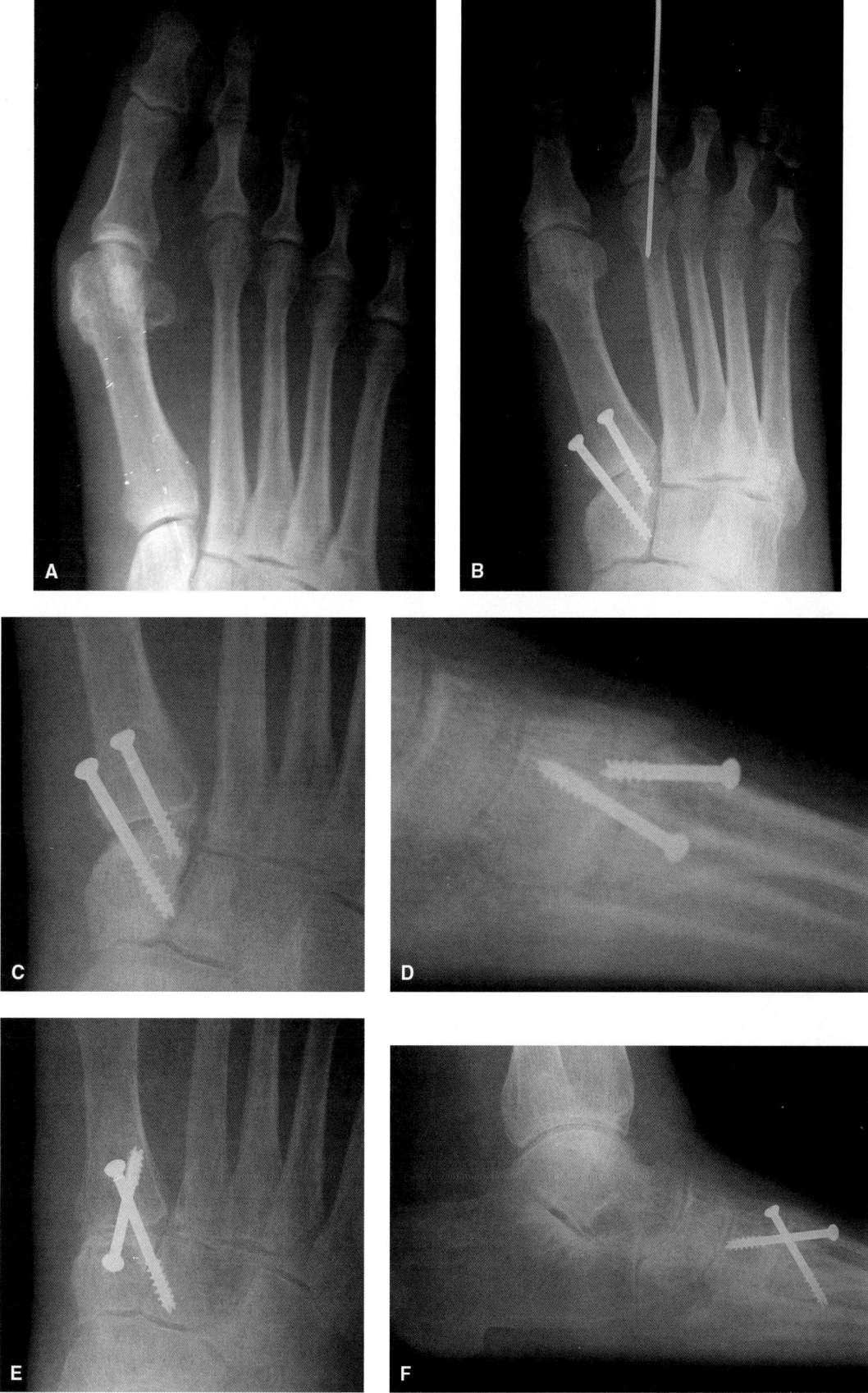

FIGURE 48.11 A. Preoperative radiograph. Surgical plan is a first metatarsal cuneiform arthrodesis. **B.** Full reduction of the intermetatarsal angle is not obtained, and the screw placement is not ideal. The most lateral screw is short, and the threads are not completely crossing the arthrodesis site. **C, D.** Atrophic nonunion has developed 6 months post-op. The bone ends are sclerotic with bone resorption. An external bone stimulator was applied but the arthrodesis still failed to heal. **E, F.** Six-month post-op revisional surgery with autogenous calcaneal bone graft, 2-screw fixation, and continuation of the external bone stimulator, still does not show complete consolidation.

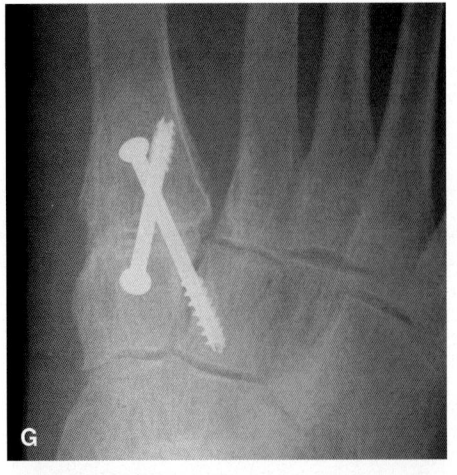

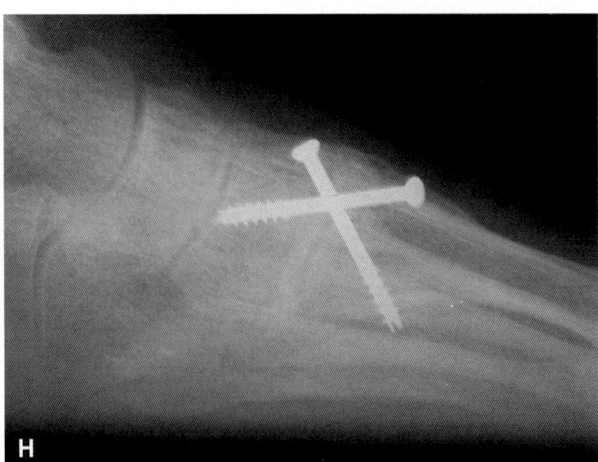

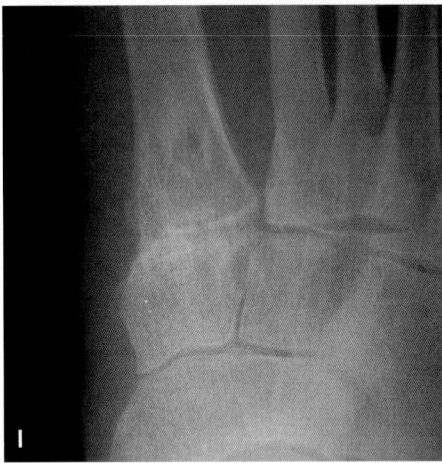

FIGURE 48.11 (*Continued*) **G, H.** Increased consolidation at 12 months post-op but still lucency seen at the arthrodesis site. **I.** Fifteen-month post-op revisional surgery with complete consolidation and screw removal. Patient was finally asymptomatic.

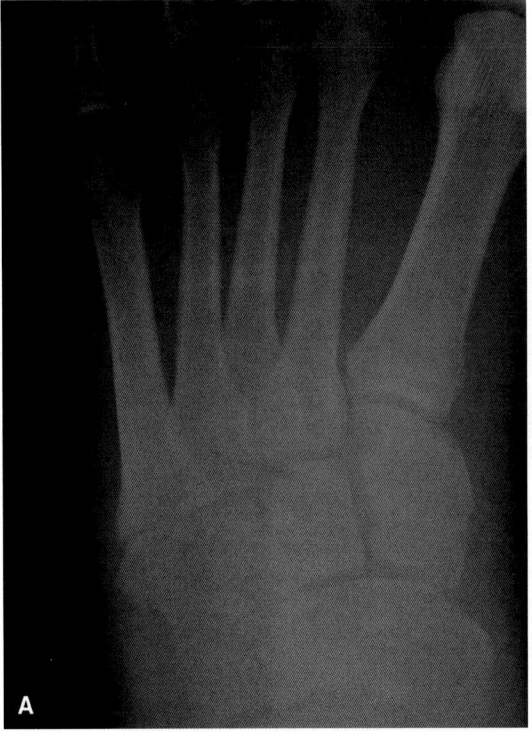

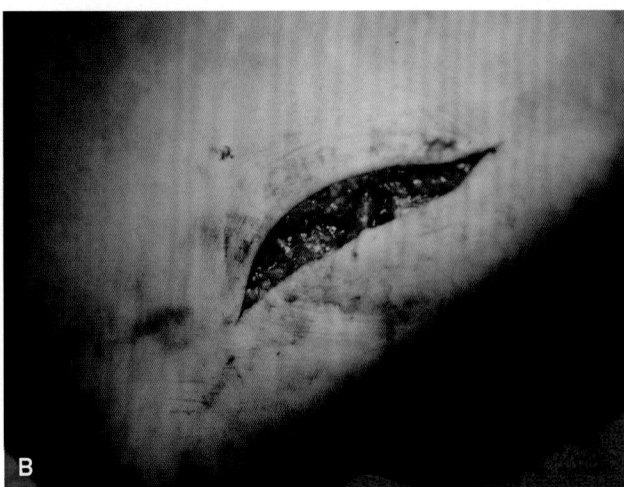

FIGURE 48.12 **A.** Nonunion of a fifth metatarsal avulsion fracture. Required surgical repair. **B.** Incision over the fifth metatarsal base.

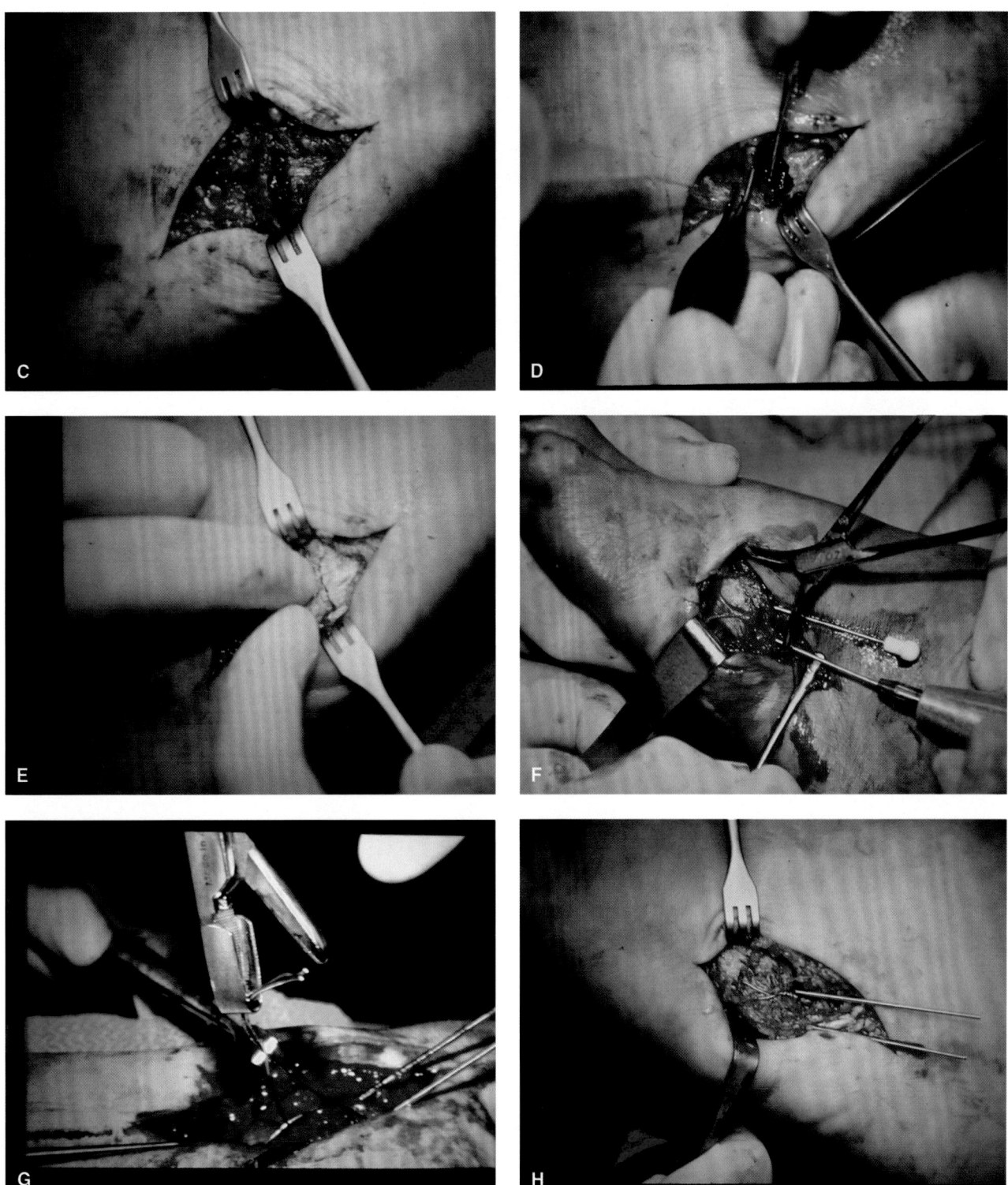

FIGURE 48.12 (*Continued*) **C.** Intra-op view of the nonunion site. **D.** Débridement of the sclerotic bone in the nonunion. **E.** Realignment of the fracture fragments. **F-I.** Tension band technique was utilized for fixation.

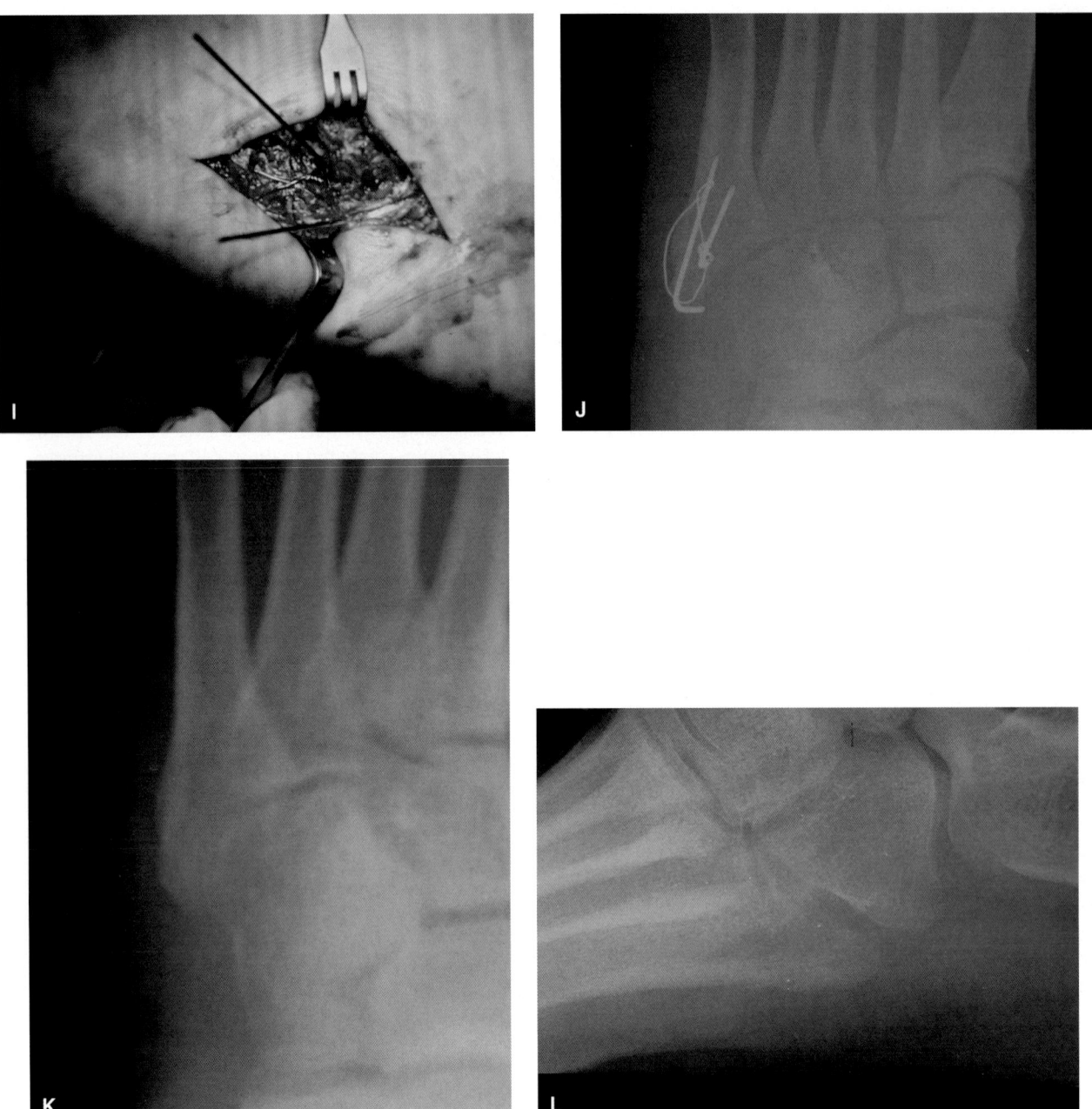

FIGURE 48.12 (*Continued*) **J.** Eight weeks post-op with complete healing. **K, L.** Six months post-op after fixation removal shows complete consolidation.

then begins to form through the organization of hematoma and the bone is "splinted" in an attempt to decrease motion across the fracture or surgical site. This process can take up to 16 weeks to develop. The hard callus phase is then witnessed as this cartilaginous callus is woven into bone. This phase begins in the first 7-10 days and can last up to 1-4 years. Finally, during the remodeling phase, immature woven bone is resorbed by the osteoclasts and replaced with lamellar bone by osteoblasts.

In contrast to secondary bone healing, primary bone healing is the desired method of healing for our elective surgical reconstructions, including osteotomies and arthrodesis procedures. This repair is characterized by the absence of bone callus formation and the lack of widening at the osteotomy or arthrodesis site. The surgeon must adhere to a myriad of criteria in order for this direct healing to ensue. First, close anatomic reduction of the adjacent bone segments is critical; therefore, the osseous surfaces need to be in direct contact.[1] Second, stable fixation is required in order to resist deforming forces and facilitate adequate compression across the surgical site. When these criteria are met, the opposing osseous surfaces undergo internal remodeling and new lamellar bone is laid down along the path of osteoclasts. This cutting cone phenomenon facilitates the ingrowth of new vasculature and the delivery of bone forming cells producing a "bridged" bony segment.[26] One millimeter of new

bone can be seen across the fracture, osteotomy, or arthrodesis site at ~2-3 weeks as the cutting cones advance at a rate of 50-80 μm/day.[26] Following the union of the osseous surfaces, this newly formed bone then begins the remodeling process according to Wolff law.[27]

ETIOLOGY OF A NONUNION

Factors leading to a nonunion can include infection, poor vascularity, patient comorbidities, medications, inadequate joint preparation and/or poor osseous alignment, soft tissue interposition, unstable or inadequate fixation, and improper postoperative management including patient noncompliance.[7,28] In order for a surgeon to successfully manage a nonunion, they must determine the etiology of this complication so that they are able to provide proper intervention to address the deficiency.

RISK FACTORS

Risk Factors for Nonunions

- Diabetes
- Rheumatoid arthritis
- Vitamin D deficiency
- Immunocompromised state
- Smoking
- Obesity
- Medications
  - NSAIDs
  - Bisphosphonates
- Inadequate joint prep
- Inadequate fixation
- Malposition
- Revisional surgery
- Infection
- Noncompliance

Comorbidities

Patient comorbidities are an ever-prevalent consideration in the preoperative planning phase with conditions such as diabetes, rheumatoid arthritis, vitamin D deficiency, and immunocompromised states on the rise.[9,29] The American Diabetes Association's 2015 data indicate 30.3 million Americans, or 9.4% of the population, have diabetes. Although a direct link between diabetes and bone healing has not been established, it does have the potential to slow the healing process. This comes in the form of altering normal osteoblastic and proliferative activity, as well as collagen synthesis, which negatively impacts callus formation and overall biomechanical strength.[9,29] Several studies have demonstrated that peripheral neuropathy and hemoglobin A1c of >7 are risk factors for the development of complications, including nonunion, postoperatively.[30] In a retrospective study by Perlman and Thordarson on 67 ankle fusions, a higher rate of nonunion was demonstrated in diabetic patients (38%) compared to those without (27%).[31] Loder and colleagues demonstrated a substantial delay in healing in diabetic patients with closed lower extremity fractures, at 163% of the expected

healing time.[32] A recent systematic review noted that diabetes was cited as a risk factor for nonunion in 71% of studies included, with 97% of surgeons identifying it as a risk factor.[33] One study on Type I and II diabetic patients with long or short bone fractures had roughly double the risk of nonunion.[34]

Aside from being a known risk factor for fracture, osteoporosis has the potential to impact bone healing as well. Osteoporosis tends to affect an elderly population; however, it may also be present in patients with arthritis and autoimmune disorders. Much of the research on this topic has been via animal studies. In rat models, studies have shown that fracture healing may be delayed in regards to biomechanical strength and callus formation.[35,36] Parker et al. demonstrated age was predictive of nonunion following open reduction internal fixation (ORIF) of femoral neck fractures.[37] A study by Nikolaou and colleagues looking at femoral fracture patients demonstrated increased time to union in those over 65 with osteoporosis (19.4 weeks) as compared to those <40 years old without osteoporosis (16.2 weeks).[38] A systematic review performed by Zura et al. also noted patient age and osteoporosis to be confirmed risk factors for nonunion after fracture in 61% and 40% of studies reviewed, respectively, with 82% of surveyed surgeons recognizing age as such.[33] One could potentially make the link with age and osteoporosis that an increased rate of nonunion in an elderly population is related to difficult fixation in osteoporotic bone, thus making it difficult to isolate age specifically as an independent risk factor.

Rheumatoid arthritis may have implications in bone healing as well, both from the disease state itself and the effects of medications used to treat the condition. Resultant osteoporosis, as discussed previously, may predispose to nonunion and other healing complications. Rheumatoid patients are often managed on medications such as steroids and immunomodulators such as methotrexate. Several studies have looked at fusion rates of the rearfoot in the setting of rheumatoid arthritis, noting nonunion rates between 0% and 26%.[39-43]

Other genetic, metabolic and endocrine disorders such as osteogenesis imperfecta, Vitamin D deficiency, thyroid disorder, and hyperparathyroidism may predispose a patient to higher rates of nonunion. Moore and colleagues noted that 76% of patients with endocrine disease, including diabetes, developed a nonunion following foot and ankle arthrodesis procedures as opposed to 26% of those in the nonendocrine disease group.[28] They also noted that patients with Vitamin D deficiency or insufficiency were 8.1 times more likely to develop a nonunion postoperatively.[28] Osteogenesis imperfecta is characterized by malformation of type I collagen, which can result in increased rates of nonunion.[44]

Patient-Derived Risk Factors

Smoking is a well-established perioperative risk factor for the development of complications. It has been demonstrated that smoking affects tissue oxygenation and impedes wound healing.[9,29] According to a study by Ishikawa and colleagues, the rate of developing a nonunion was 2.7 times higher in smokers compared to nonsmokers.[45] Schmitz et al. performed a level II prospective study of 146 patients with tibial fractures that demonstrated a 69% delay in radiographic union in smokers.[46] Numerous other studies support these findings. In 2006, Chahal et al. showed that smokers were 3.8 times more likely to develop a nonunion following subtalar arthrodesis than

nonsmokers.[47] Castillo and colleagues led a prospective multicenter study on 268 open tibial fractures revealing smokers were 37% more likely to develop a nonunion.[48] The relative risk of developing a nonunion in smokers following ankle arthrodesis was 3.75 times higher than nonsmokers according to a study by Cobb et al.[49] In 2000, Easley et al. demonstrated in a study of 184 subtalar arthrodeses a fusion rate of 92% vs 73% in nonsmokers compared to smokers.[50] Zura and colleagues noted smoking as a confirmed risk factor in 64% of studies included in their systematic review, although its prevalence varied based on anatomic location and several studies on the same anatomic region were in disagreement. Ninety-eight percent of surgeons surveyed identified smoking as a risk factor for nonunion.[33]

Alcohol may be considered an indirect risk factor for development of nonunion given its association with osteoporosis in the setting of chronic consumption. Those partaking in excessive consumption may also have a higher fall risk and predisposition for fracture. This form of osteopenia is thought to be caused by suppression of new bone formation and inhibition of osteoblastic activity.[51] Animal studies have demonstrated negative effects of alcohol on bone healing. Ethanol-fed rats had deficient bone repair in comparison to those with a standard diet.[52] Nyquist and colleagues found statistically significant decreases in bone mineral density and mechanical strength at fracture sites in rats given ethanol as opposed to the control group.[53] Zura et al. reported alcoholism as a confirmed risk factor in 80% of studies reviewed; however, they noted that there was much disagreement between studies and specific anatomic regions.[33]

Obesity is a rising epidemic throughout the country and certainly a factor in procedural selection and perioperative management. Although there is a paucity of evidence to support obesity as a risk factor for nonunion, there are several challenges that this may create, especially in the postoperative period. For patients with a significantly elevated body mass index (BMI), it may be difficult to achieve proper bracing/casting and to remain non–weight bearing. This could certainly compromise internal fixation constructs leading to hardware loosening, disruption, or breakage and subsequent unwanted motion at the procedure site.[29] In a follow-up study, Thevendran and colleagues developed a nonunion risk assessment model and subsequent application. They found that a BMI of >30 was associated with nonunion, with data suggesting nonunion is four times more likely in this cohort of patients.[54]

A final patient-derived risk factor is overall noncompliance with the prescribed course of treatment. Following fracture repair or arthrodesis, patients are routinely immobilized and maintained in a state of non–weight bearing for a duration related to the surgery that was performed. Early weight bearing may result in unwanted micromotion at the repair or fusion site, which can lead to disruption of primary bone healing and failure of the hardware construct (Fig. 48.13). More recent literature has demonstrated that early weight bearing does not have a negative impact on healing rates[55,56]; however, in an at-risk foot/ankle and those with other risk factors, noncompliance and early weight bearing may have an additive effect to a poorer outcome.

Medications

Nonsteroidal anti-inflammatory drugs (NSAIDs) are frequently prescribed medications for many lower extremity pathologies, including postoperative pain management. Patients may also be taking these (and other steroid-based

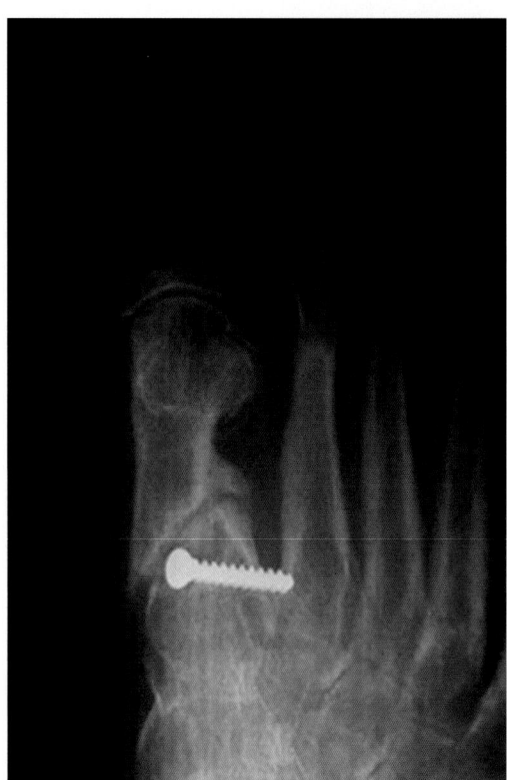

FIGURE 48.13 CBWO with fixation failure and delayed union secondary to early weight bearing.

medications) on a chronic basis for other comorbidities or musculoskeletal complaints. NSAIDs can have an inhibitory effect on prostaglandins, especially during the early inflammatory phase of healing. This, in turn, has the potential to compromise bone formation.[57] Animal studies have been conducted, which have shown a deleterious effect of NSAIDs on healing[58]; however, evidence in human studies is lacking and controversial.[59–62] Giannoudis demonstrated an increased risk of nonunion at the femoral diaphysis with the use of ibuprofen and diclofenac,[61] whereas Reuben and colleagues found no effect on the rate of spinal fusion with the use of celecoxib, rofecoxib, or low-dose ketorolac.[62] NSAIDs and steroids were identified as a risk factor for nonunion by 86% and 96% of surgeons, respectively, according to a systematic review by Zura et al.[33] Hernandez noted the use of NSAIDs, 12 months prior to fracture, was linked to a 2.6-fold higher odds ratio of nonunion or delayed union.[34]

In relation to patients with osteoporosis, some may be treated with bisphosphonates. The use of this class of medications has been associated with decreased fracture union. With a mechanism of action of inhibition of formation and breakdown of bone, in the setting of injury or surgery, there may be decreased callus formation leading to an increased rate of nonunion.[29] Solomon and colleagues showed a nearly two-fold increase of humeral fracture nonunion in an elderly population treated with bisphosphonates.[63] A 2007 study involving hip fractures demonstrated those who received bisphosphonate therapy within 90 days of fracture had a 3.2% nonunion rate as compared to 2.7% in the placebo group.[64] As there is relatively limited evidence, a definitive conclusion cannot be drawn in regard to the risk of nonunion with concurrent use of bisphosphonates.

Methotrexate may be a part of the medication regimen for those with certain types of cancers and rheumatoid arthritis. This and other classes of immunosuppressive drugs, such as cyclosporine, may have negative effects on bone healing, especially in the setting of long-term use. These medications may slow bone healing and result in weaker bone formation. Patients taking these medications typically have many other risk factors for surgery and should receive additional evaluation and clearance from their prescribing physician to determine if they are a candidate to undergo the planned surgical intervention and if these medications can be suspended in the perioperative setting.

Local and Iatrogenic Risk Factors

There are a host of local and iatrogenic risk factors to consider. From an intraoperative standpoint, there are many things that the surgeon can control to optimize patient outcomes and decrease the likelihood of nonunion. Surgeons learn early on the principles of AO fixation including preservation of vascular supply, restoring alignment, and rigid internal fixation, all of which are critical to a successful outcome (Fig. 48.14). Maintenance of vascularity to the affected site is crucial for proper bone healing. Vascular endothelial growth factor (VEGF) is responsible for angiogenesis and has been demonstrated to play a role in bone healing. Inhibition of this prevents intramembranous and endochondral osteogenesis[65,66] and nonunion can result. Meticulous intraoperative technique is paramount in order to maintain vascularity to the surgical site. The surgeon must avoid excessive periosteal stripping, be cautious of thermal necrosis with an overzealous saw, and protect the local soft tissue envelope.

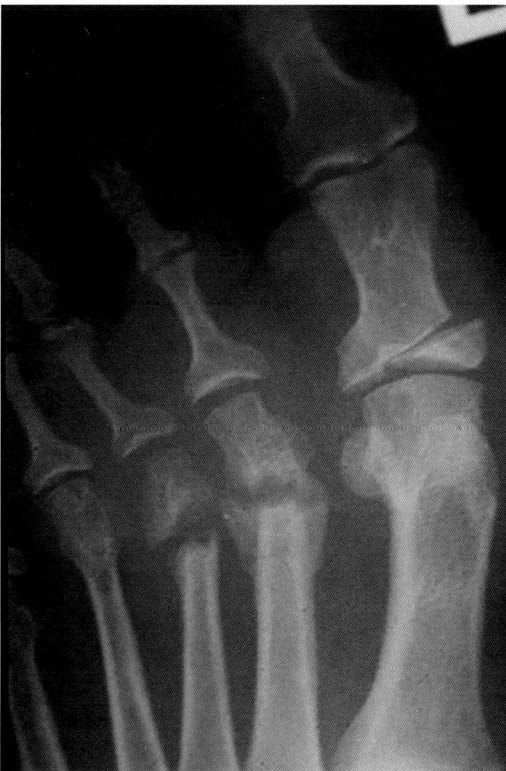

FIGURE 48.14 Second and third metatarsal osteotomies performed without rigid internal fixation. The second metatarsal is a hypertrophic nonunion with bone callus formation, and the third metatarsal is shortened with an atrophic nonunion.

Appropriate joint preparation is also essential to achieve osseous union. Adequate resection of all cartilage and subsequent fenestration of the subchondral bone plate down to cancellous bleeding bone is critical and is a significant determining factor for successful bone healing (Figs. 48.15 and 48.16). Good osseous apposition of the bony surfaces and proper alignment of the fracture, osteotomy, or arthrodesis site is also crucial for bone healing as malalignment can generate abnormal stress across the surgical site and interrupt the phases of bone healing. Finally, stable fixation is necessary for adequate bone healing in order to avoid excessive motion at the surgical site (Fig. 48.17). Although micromotion at the bone-to-bone interface has been shown to positively affect healing, gross instability due to insufficient fixation can be detrimental to achieving osseous union.[21,67–69] Choosing an appropriate hardware construct should be based on individual patient characteristics as well as surgical site demands. Patients with certain comorbidities such as diabetes, obesity, or osteoporosis may require more fixation and a sturdier construct than a healthy individual. It is up to the surgeon to decide the best form of fixation to utilize based on that particular patient, their risk factors, and the surgical procedure itself.

Once the patient enters the postoperative period, consideration must be made as to when the patient may begin to bear weight on the operative site. Wolff law must be taken into account, as an immobilized site that has not been placed under physiologic stress may be at higher risk for failure if not gradually stressed.[27] The anatomic location of the surgical site and the procedure performed plays a role in this decision-making process. For example, a fibular ORIF is not subject to the same stresses as a first metatarsal osteotomy or a first TMTJ fusion when weight bearing is initiated. Although radiographic healing may be observed, the site may not be able to withstand physiologic loading at that point. Therefore, gradual transition to weight bearing in a protective device such as a CAM walker should be considered to allow the bone to adapt to the applied force.

Previous surgery, or revisional surgery, in a given area may increase the risk of nonunion as well. This likely stems from the previous disruption in vascularity and decreased bone stock. In a study of failed first MTPJ arthrodeses, the nonunion rate was significantly higher in those who had undergone previous surgery in the area.[70] Similarly, Easley and colleagues demonstrated that an initial failure of a subtalar arthrodesis was a significant predictor for nonunion in the revisional case.[50] Vascularity of the region may also be compromised in patients with peripheral arterial disease, smokers, and those who have sustained significant tissue loss in the setting of injury.[29] If a patient has a questionable vascular examination, further studies such as arterial brachial indices and pulse volume recordings should be obtained, with a referral to vascular surgery if needed to ensure the patient is optimized.

Infection either in the pre- or postoperative setting can be detrimental to bone healing. Baldwin et al. noted up to a 3.5-fold risk of infection in open fractures with an increased time to union as the fracture severity increased.[71] A 2016 study however, examining posttraumatic subtalar arthrodesis, failed to correlate risk factors associated with nonunion, including postoperative wound infection.[72] Although a direct link has not been established between infection and nonunion, it is well known that infection can lead to necrosis and a dysvascular environment. It is also known that infection of the bone weakens its structural integrity and can cause failure of the fixation construct, resulting in instability of the surgical site. Diseased fibrous tissue and necrotic bone surfaces can be barriers to the ingrowth of healthy vascular channels and can inhibit the delivery of growth factors.[73]

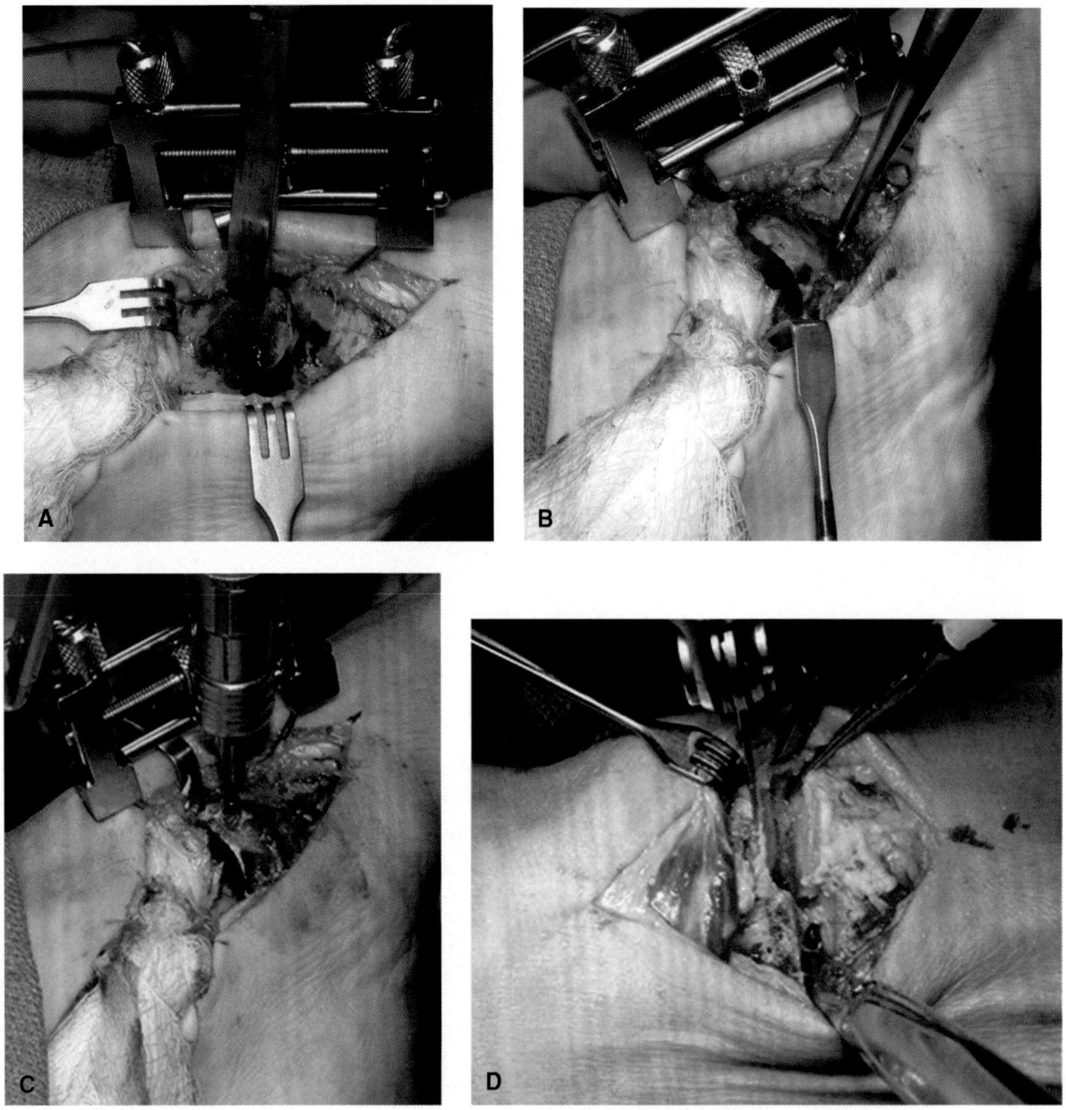

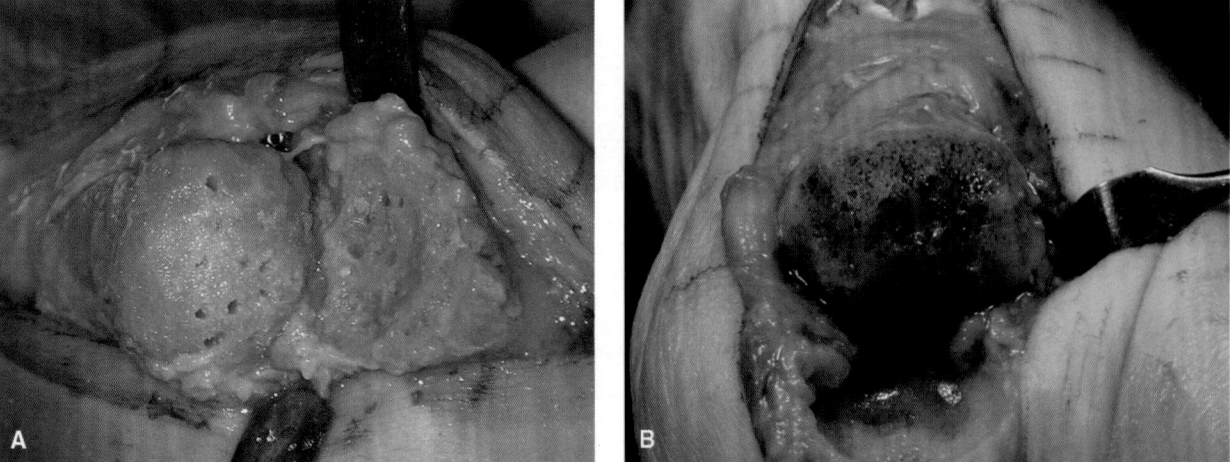

FIGURE 48.15 **A-C.** Débridement of cartilage, in preparation for joint arthrodesis, can be performed with many different instruments. Utilizing an osteotome and mallet, curette, and/or power burr is preferable as minimal bone resection can be performed more easily with these instruments, which helps maintain length and the normal contour of the joint. **D.** Planal resection can also be performed with a power saw, but care should be taken to minimize bone resection to prevent shortening, gapping, and malalignment at the arthrodesis site.

FIGURE 48.16 **A.** All cartilage has been débrided, and fenestration of the subchondral bone plate has been achieved with a 0.062-in. K-wire. **B.** Notice the bleeding, cancellous bone. This is known as the paprika sign and signifies adequate cartilage resection and successful penetration of the subchondral bone plate. This will help ensure adequate vascularity to the arthrodesis site.

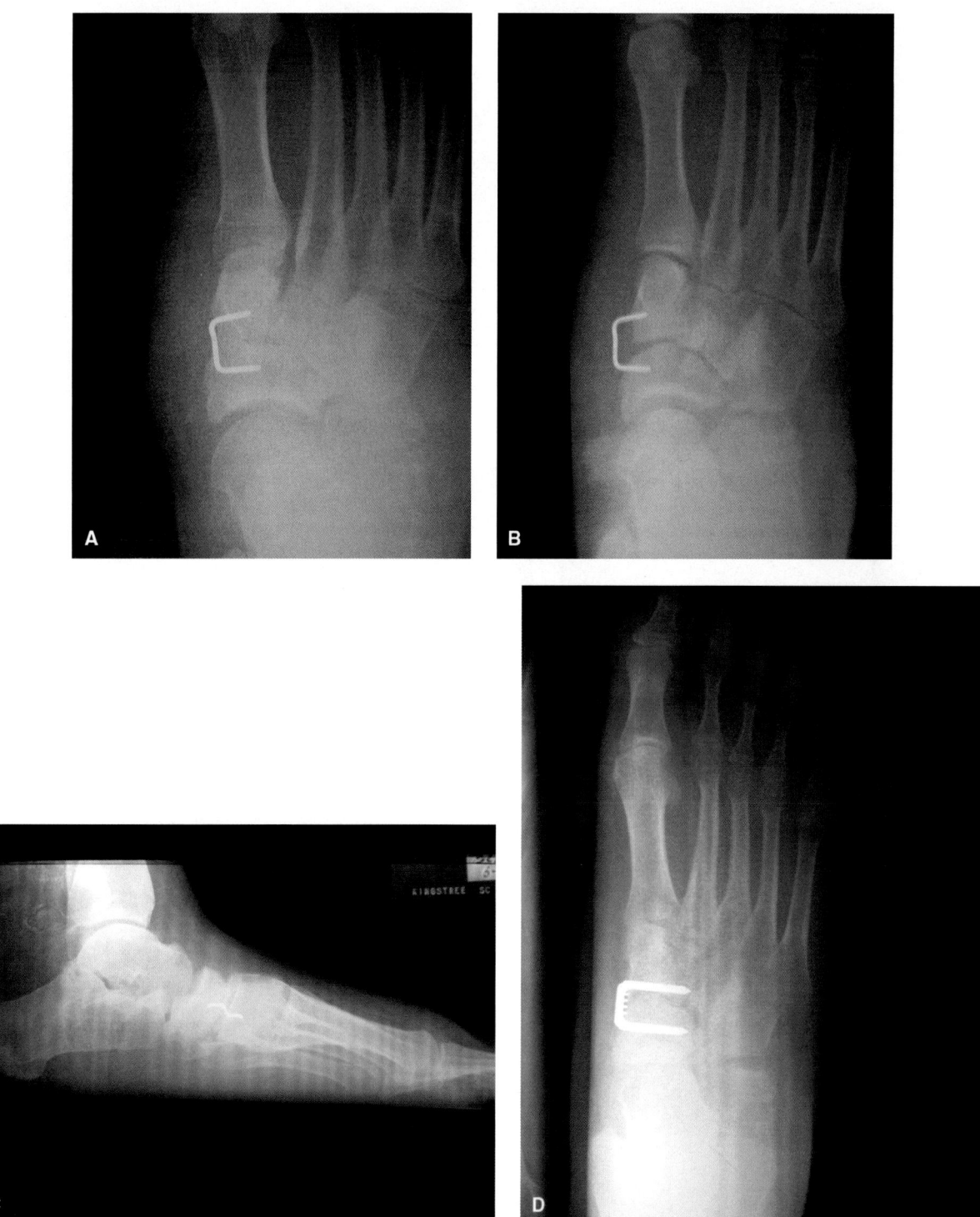

FIGURE 48.17 A. A naviculocuneiform arthrodesis in a 16-year-old female was performed with one staple fixation, as part of a flatfoot reconstruction. Good osseous apposition is seen on this immediate post-op radiograph. **B, C.** Two-week post-op radiographs show failure of the staple fixation, gapping at the arthrodesis site, and collapse of the naviculocuneiform joint with a recurrent fault. This staple was not strong enough nor were the arms long enough to maintain adequate compression for this arthrodesis. **D.** Revisional surgery with a larger and stronger staple fixation was performed and osseous union was achieved.

Surgeon experience and knowledge may also have an impact on perioperative planning and surgical outcomes. Each surgeon has criteria for which they use to determine candidacy and risks for various procedures, largely based on experience and evidence-based medicine. Thevendran and colleagues

sought to assess perceived risk factors for nonunions among an international group of foot and ankle surgeons from journal editorial boards and organizational executive committees. The greatest perceived risk factors were smoking more than 2 packs per day, lack of hardware construct stability, and poor local

vascular supply. The least important were increased age, rheumatoid arthritis, and osteoporosis. When asked in regard to absolute contraindications for arthrodesis, the most common responses were infection, poor vascular supply, and smoking.[9]

Overall, the literature has many disparities and is inconclusive at times in determining the above as definite risk factors for nonunion. It can be hard to draw conclusions secondary to inherent limitations in the scientific literature. Regardless, the topics discussed should certainly be given great consideration in the perioperative setting. Each patient should be individually assessed and educated based on their comorbidities and modifiable factors. It is imperative to counsel patients appropriately, and disclose their risk for complications, taking the above factors into account. Patients are often unaware of the implications of surgery and may see it as a quick fix to their complaint; however, realistic expectations of the risks vs benefits, as well as potential complications, to the proposed surgical interventions should be thoroughly reviewed to optimize patient outcomes.

EVALUATION

PATIENT EVALUATION

When a nonunion is suspected, the physician must be very thorough in their evaluation including a complete history of events leading up to the present clinical scenario. Details of the initial surgery or injury, including the initial date of the operation or traumatic episode should be documented. If surgery was performed, the operative report needs to be obtained so the surgeon will have the knowledge of the surgical procedures performed and any fixation utilized. Details regarding the postoperative course must also be discussed including the immobilization and weight-bearing status throughout this treatment phase, medications utilized for pain and inflammation, and any

physical therapy modalities instilled. Any postoperative complications, such as infection, must also be ascertained.

A thorough review of the patient's past medical history, including current and previous medial issues, all previous surgeries, current medications, and social aspects, such as smoking and disability and work status also need to be reviewed. Particular emphasis should be placed on the patient's comorbidities and risk factors for developing a nonunion as discussed above. The etiology of the nonunion needs to be identified, and the surgeon needs to determine if this can be corrected in order to try to obtain a successful osseous union. If the risks of further surgical intervention are too high, or the etiology cannot be properly addressed, the surgeon must seriously consider delaying any further surgery until the patient factors are optimized.

PHYSICAL EXAMINATION

A complete physical examination should be performed, including a thorough neurovascular examination. Pain is usually the most common complaint when dealing with a nonunion but other physical signs such as edema, erythema, and temperature variations may also be present, especially when compared to the nonaffected limb. The patient will typically have pain to palpation at the nonunion site and pain also with attempts at range of motion. The area should be manually stressed to assess for any motion present and gross instability. The surrounding joints should also be palpated and put through a range of motion to assess for the presence of pain and crepitus and any degenerative changes that may be present. If surrounding joints have been affected, the surgeon must consider this in their overall treatment plan. Assessing alignment of the joint or osteotomy is also critical. If malalignment is present, this may need to be addressed regardless of whether osseous union is achieved (Fig. 48.18). Of course, malalignment may also affect surrounding joints as they try to compensate for a poor position. Manual

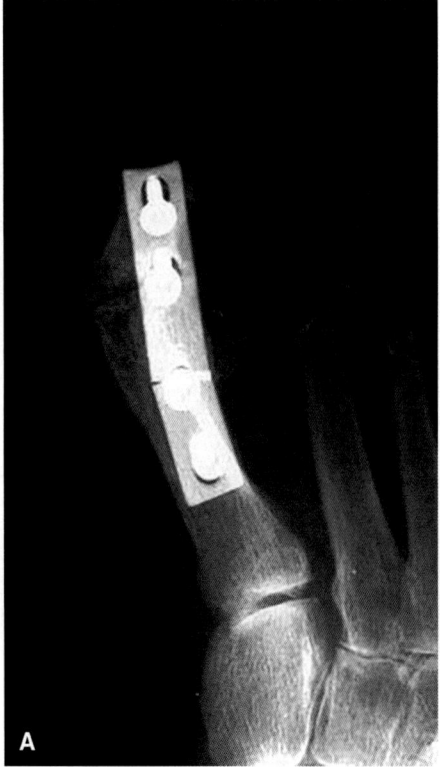

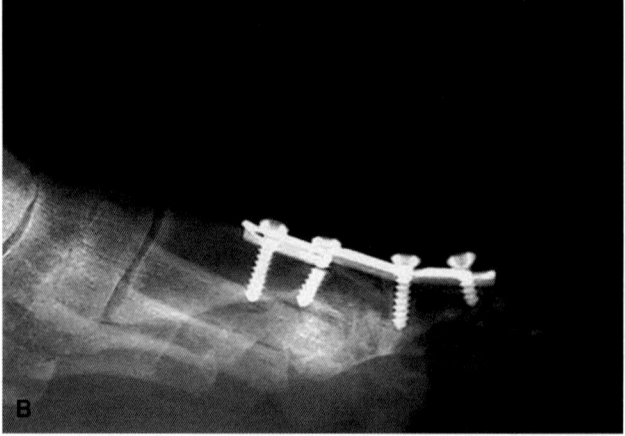

FIGURE 48.18 **A, B.** First MTPJ arthrodesis in malalignment with broken plate and screws. The arthrodesis site appears to be hypertrophic with the potential for complete consolidation if the patient is kept non–weight bearing; however, revisional surgery will be necessary secondary to the malunion.

muscle testing should also be performed to assess any effects the nonunion has had on strength of the extremity. In addition, the skin should also be evaluated for any areas of irritation or wounds that have resulted from infection or possibly loosened and unstable or broken hardware. If the patient has been allowed to weight bear, a gait analysis should be performed. The patient will typically have an antalgic gait and limp on the affected side. They often have weak propulsion and are very guarded on the affected extremity.

LABORATORY EVALUATION

Laboratory evaluation is typically aimed at trying to identify the etiology of the nonunion and then trying to make sure the patient is medically optimized prior to any further surgical intervention. Updated chemistry and hematology panels should be obtained including Hemoglobin A1c for diabetic patients. Nicotine levels can be evaluated for smokers to assess their compliance with cessation and nutritional levels can be assessed on patients focusing on albumin, prealbumin, transferrin, and vitamin D levels.

In scenarios where infection is suspected, or if infection was diagnosed and treated previously and monitoring or assessment for resolution is needed, acute phase reactant testing with erythrocyte sedimentation rate (ESR) and C-reactive protein (CRP) tests can be helpful. Both of these tests have a high sensitivity and specificity for the diagnosis of osteomyelitis.[74,75] Stucken et al. compared ESR and CRP in the diagnosis of infection in nonunion patients and found that the combination of both tests was a significantly accurate predictor of infection in these cases.[76] Of course, bone biopsy still remains the gold standard for diagnosis of osteomyelitis and should be performed if there is any suspicion of infection prior to any further surgical reconstruction.

IMAGING MODALITIES

Plain film radiographs are the mainstay for assessing bone healing in fractures, osteotomies, and arthrodesis procedures.

Osseous union is noted to have occurred when there is trabecular bridging across the fracture or surgical site. This is usually concurrent with the patient's reduction of symptoms including pain and edema. Serial radiographs should be assessed in a chronological manner to evaluate for continued increased bone healing, maintenance of proper alignment, and stability of fixation as the postoperative or postinjury course progresses. If there is progression of radiolucent lines, absence of crossing trabeculation at the union site, sclerosis of the osseous fragments, and/or bone callus formation identified on serial postoperative radiographs, the physician should be highly suspicious of the development of a possible nonunion (Fig. 48.19). The presence of hardware loosening, migration, or breakage is indicative of motion at the surgical site and again the physician should be highly suspicious of an impending nonunion and possible presence of an infectious process.

Computed tomography (CT) scanning can also be useful and employed as an adjunct to radiographs when trying to assess and diagnose a nonunion. Visualizing crossing trabeculation of an osteotomy or arthrodesis can be difficult when internal fixation is utilized. The hardware can obscure the area of interest making it difficult to adequately evaluate bone healing. Hindfoot joints can also be difficult to assess on standard radiographs since they are nonplanar. The joints in the midfoot have significant superimposition making them difficult to assess as well. CT scanning can be useful in these areas and be an adjunct for evaluation if the physician is suspicious of healing problems. In 2006, Coughlin and colleagues prospectively compared standard radiographs to CT scans in the evaluation of union in hindfoot arthrodesis. They found a significant difference in the reliabilities of true bone union between CT scans and radiographs.[77] A more recent study by Krause et al. evaluated nonunions of hindfoot and ankle fusions with a blinded CT assessment. They identified 67 nonunions out of 370, or 18%, compared to 21 out of 389 patients, or 5%, found by surgeon assessment alone.[78] CT scanning can be very helpful if a patient has persistent pain and swelling but the radiographic assessment displays probable osseous union. CT scans can help identify partially united fusions that may give the appearance

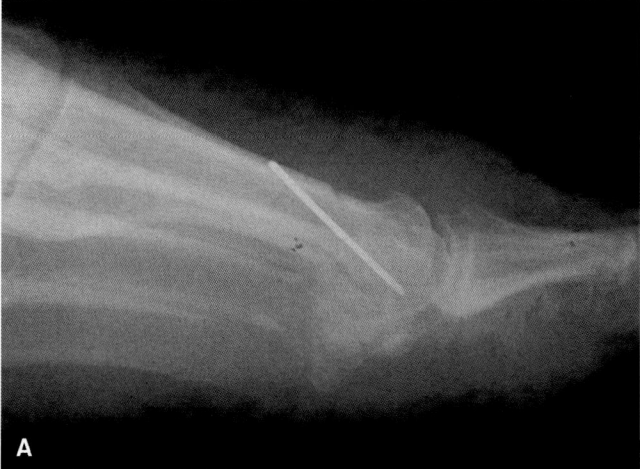 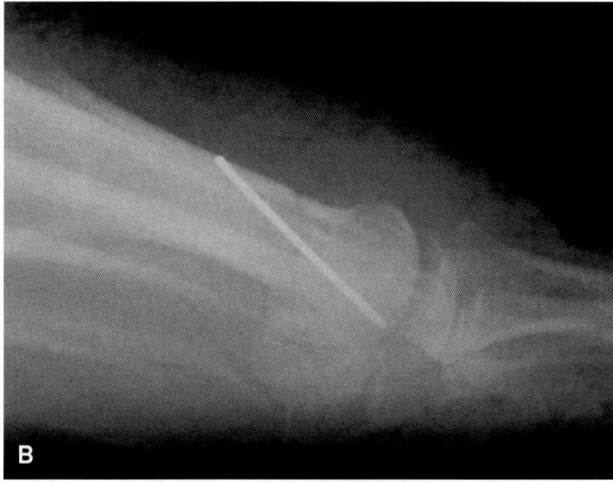

FIGURE 48.19 A. Immediate postop radiograph of an Austin osteotomy with 0.045 in. K-wire fixation. **B.** Six week post-op radiograph shows almost complete consolidation of the osteotomy except the most dorsal cortex.

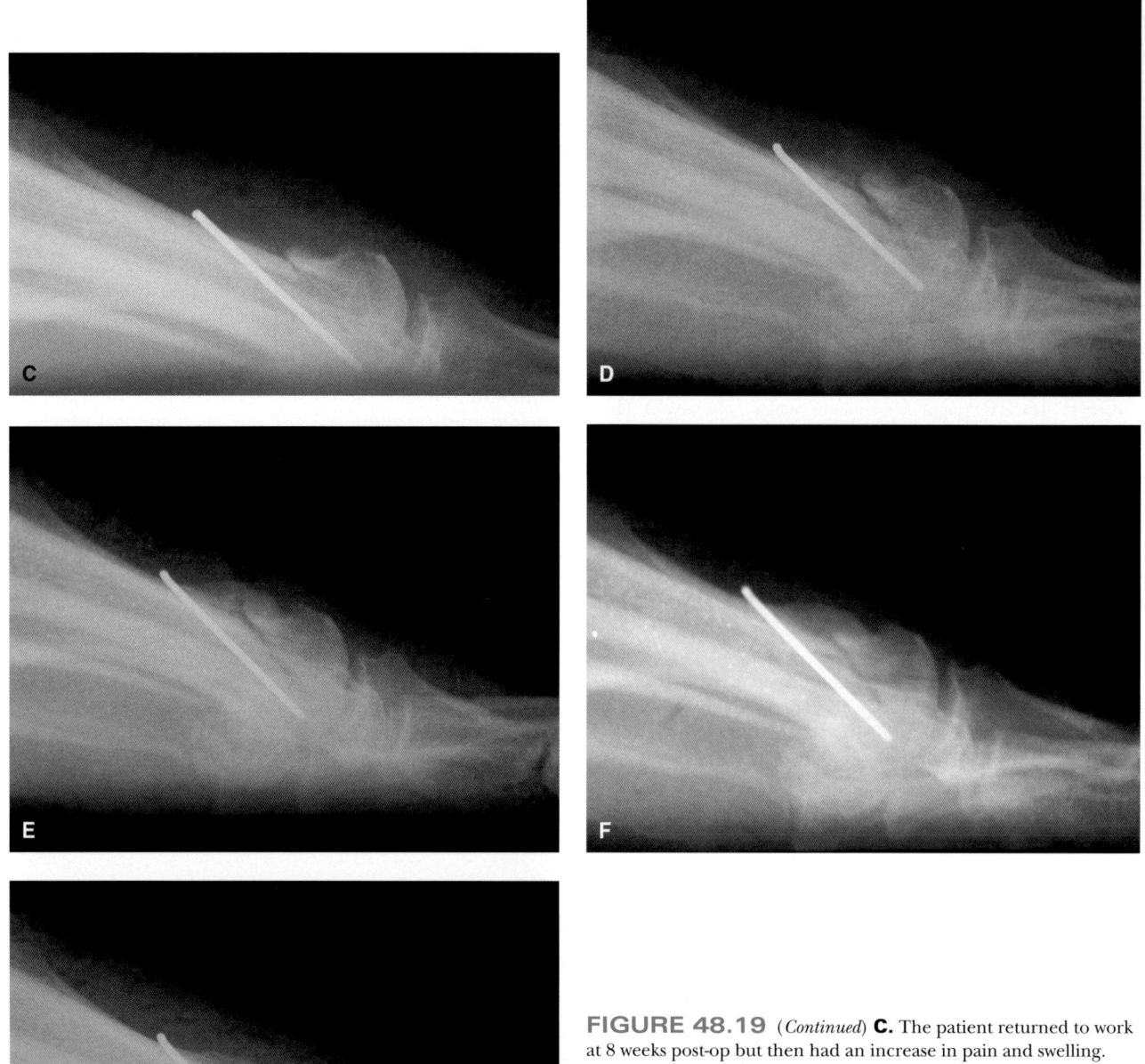

FIGURE 48.19 (*Continued*) **C.** The patient returned to work at 8 weeks post-op but then had an increase in pain and swelling. This radiograph is 3 months post-op. Notice the lucency seen along the dorsal wing of the osteotomy and bone callus formation. Mild dorsal displacement of the first metatarsal head is also seen. The 0.045 in. K-wire failed to maintain alignment and osseous apposition. **D.** Six-month post-op radiograph shows a hypertrophic nonunion with bone callus formation. An external bone stimulator was applied. **E, F.** Eight and ten-month post-op radiographs show good consolidation of the bone callus, but the dorsal wing of the osteotomy is still apparent. **G.** Complete consolidation of the osteotomy at 12 months post-op.

of adequate fusion on standard radiographs. They can quantify the percentage of fusion mass, whereas this can be very difficult with standard radiographs. It is recommended that 50% or more bridging at an arthrodesis site be achieved before it is considered a successful union on CT scan.[79]

It is of the utmost importance that vascularity be maintained to achieve osseous union. When viability and vascularity of the fracture, osteotomy, or arthrodesis site is in question, magnetic resonance imaging (MRI) and bone scintigraphy have

been demonstrated to be useful.[80–82] MRI has been shown to be nearly 100% sensitive in the detection of avascular necrosis (AVN) in the foot and ankle.[83] One drawback of the use of MRI, in assessment of nonunions, is the potential artifact and scatter produced on the images secondary to retained hardware (Fig. 48.20). When there is significant internal fixation impeding visualization of the nonunion site, bone scintigraphy can be utilized to evaluate vascularity of the site. The delayed phase of a Technetium-99 bone scan should demonstrate increased

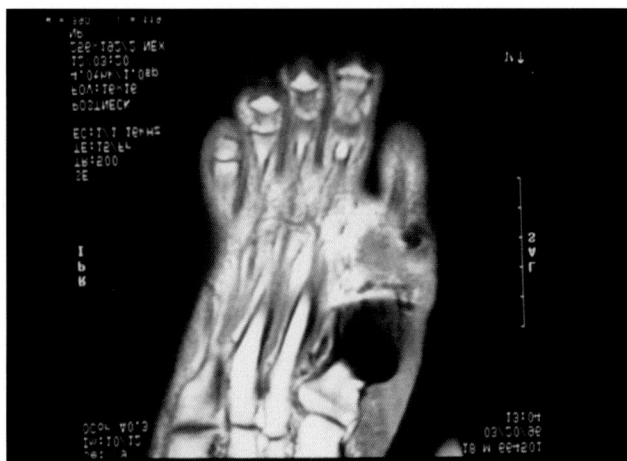

FIGURE 48.20 Magnetic resonance imaging of a CBWO. The black void at the surgical site is artifact from the screw fixation. This makes it difficult to evaluate for a nonunion at the site.

activity with a hypertrophic nonunion (Fig. 48.21). This type of nonunion is characterized by hypervascularity; therefore, there would be a high potential for osseous union. By contrast, an atrophic nonunion would lack isotope uptake since the bone fragments are avascular; therefore, there would be a very low healing potential in these cases.[84]

Advanced imaging modalities, described above, can also be used to help evaluate and potentially rule out or aid in the diagnosis of other complications such as infection. When infection is suspected, however, bone biopsy still remains the gold standard for diagnosis of osteomyelitis. In patients for whom there is underlying osteopenia, and osteoporosis is suspected, bone densiometry can be helpful and deliver useful

information to the surgeon regarding bone healing potential. When there is a bone mass deficiency present in a patient with a nonunion, the surgeon should consider utilization of additional orthobiologics and alternative fixation devices, such as locking plate constructs and/or external fixation, both of which are helpful when dealing with osteoporotic bone.

TREATMENT

Before treatment of a nonunion can be initiated, the etiology of the complication must be identified and addressed. As described above, there are many risk factors for nonunions. Without knowing the cause of the nonunion, treatment cannot be specifically directed to correct the problem and further complications and continued nonunion may result. Patient risk factors must be addressed and any prior surgical procedures should be evaluated for iatrogenic causes. Viability of the osseous fragments must be assessed and internal fixation must be thoroughly evaluated to determine its continued effectiveness. Finally, bone and joint alignment must also be examined. If malunion is present, correction of the deformity must be implemented in the treatment plan.

The ultimate goal of treating a nonunion is a painless, well-aligned, and functional foot and ankle. This goal may be challenging, and a realistic prognosis and treatment plan must be thoroughly communicated with the patient. While some nonunions heal rather quickly, others may require a longer period of time and even multiple surgical interventions. If patient risk factors have been successfully corrected, the bones are viable, there is good stable fixation, and overall alignment is good, conservative therapy may be all that is warranted to achieve osseous union. Unfortunately, however, even in the most favorable of

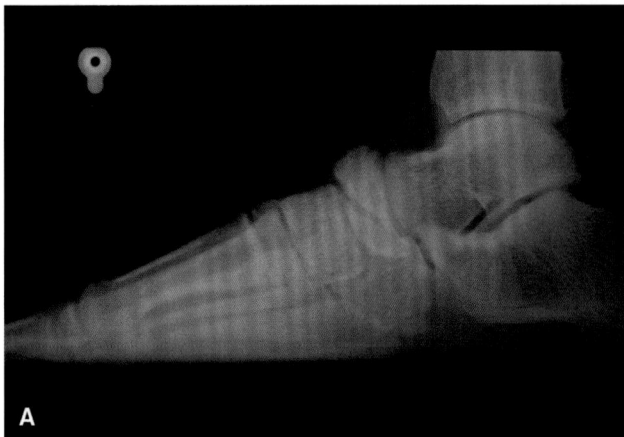

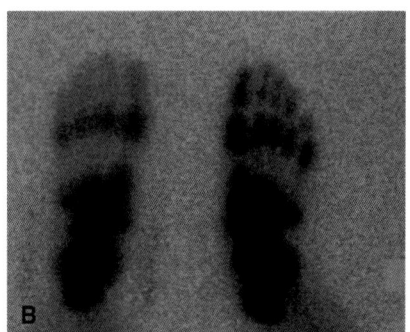

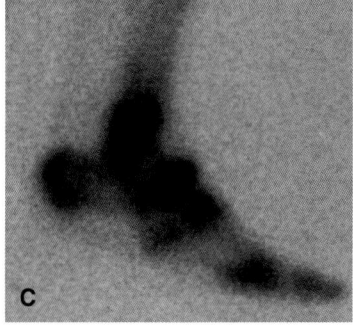

FIGURE 48.21 A. Nonunion of a navicular fracture. **B, C.** Technetium-99 bone scan shows increased isotope uptake in the navicular signifying a hypervascular nonunion that indicates the potential for osseous union.

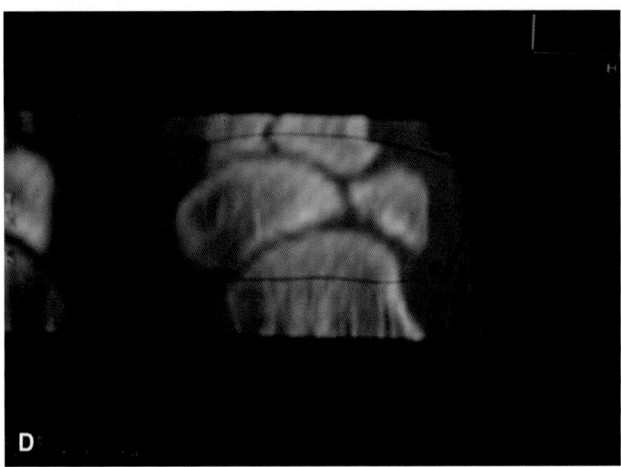
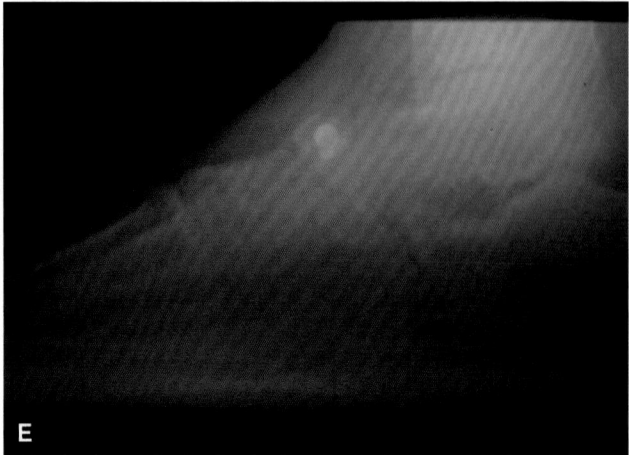

FIGURE 48.21 (*Continued*) **D.** CT scan confirming the navicular nonunion. **E.** Four-week post-op radiograph of the open reduction internal fixation (ORIF) of the navicular fracture nonunion. Crossing trabeculation and signs of some osseous consolidation is noted.

conditions, a nonunion still persists. If the patient is asymptomatic however, even if a nonunion persists on imaging studies, the authors recommend clinical treatment of the patient. This means if there are no clinical symptoms of a nonunion, primarily pain, then no further treatment is necessary. This is called an asymptomatic nonunion and is an acceptable result if the patient is satisfied. If the patient is symptomatic however, further intervention is typically required and a treatment plan should be developed on an individual basis depending on the etiology of the nonunion and the other risk factors described above.

CONSERVATIVE THERAPY

Ideally, treatment should begin when a delayed union is suspected to try to avoid the progression to a nonunion. Non–weight bearing and immobilization is the mainstay of initial, conservative therapy. This of course is assuming there is rigid, stable internal fixation, viability to the bone ends, and good alignment. If internal fixation has failed, and/or there is lack of viability to the bone surfaces, osseous healing is highly unlikely, regardless of weight-bearing status and immobilization. In these patients, surgical intervention may be warranted for successful healing. Also, as mentioned earlier, if the risk factors that lead to the nonunion are not addressed, the bone healing potential remains low until these issues are corrected. Finally, if malalignment is present, even if bone healing is achieved, there may be an unsuccessful outcome secondary to poor position and surgical intervention may be necessary to achieve a good result and satisfied patient.

Bone Stimulation

Biophysics of Bone Healing
When there are limited or no signs of progressive bone healing with immobilization and non–weight bearing, application of a bone growth stimulator is typically the next conservative treatment option. Bone growth stimulation is a well-known treatment modality to aid in bone healing for nonunions.[85–87] The utilization of electrical energy to achieve bone healing dates back to 1812, when Birch used electrical fluid to heal a tibial

nonunion.[88] Periodic reports utilizing electricity for successful treatment for bony nonunions continued[89] but it was not until 1957 when Fukada and Yasuda demonstrated that mechanical deformation of bone produced electrical potentials that bone growth stimulation really became a topic of interest.[90]

It is well known that bone adapts in response to environmental factors explained by Wolff law, which states, "The law of bone remodeling is that mathematical law according to which observed alterations in the internal architecture and external form of bone occur as a consequence of the change in shape and/or stressing of the bone."[91] Fukada and Yasuda demonstrated that electrical potentials occur within a bone when an external force is applied and they referred to this as a piezoelectric property.[90] The electrical signals generated within bone in response to stress are biphasic, producing current flow in one direction when stress is applied and in the opposite direction when stress is removed. These potentials are of a negative polarity in areas of compression and a positive polarity in areas of tension (Fig. 48.22). Further research on the understanding of these potentials has found that bone production is increased in regions of negative polarity, the compression side, and bone resorption is increased in regions of positive polarity, the tension side.[92]

In addition to stress-related potentials, areas of increased cellular activity, including growing and remodeling bone seen in the physis or freshly fractured bones, have a greater association with electronegativity.[93–95] It has also been shown that the use of electrical fields results in an increase in bone morphogenetic proteins (BMP), transforming growth factor (TGF) beta, and insulinlike growth factor II and a subsequent increase in the extracellular matrix of bone and cartilage.[96–99]

Devices and Method of Application
Electrical and mechanical bone growth stimulators all consist of a power source, and/or signal generator, and a delivery source that is a coil, cathode wire, or transducer. Both invasive, or implantable devices, and noninvasive, or externally applied devices, exist. The subcategories of these devices include direct current (DC), capacitive coupling (CC), pulsed electromagnetic fields (PEMFs) also known as inductive coupling, and low-intensity pulsed ultrasound (LIPUS).

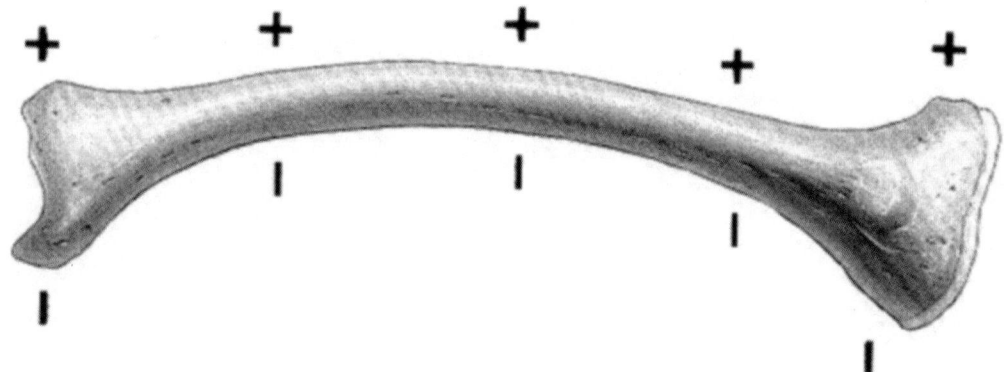

FIGURE 48.22 Electrical potentials are created when an external force is applied to bone. A negative polarity is produced on the compression side and a positive polarity on the tension side.

> **Bone Stimulation Devices**
> - Internal
>   - Direct current
> - External
>   - Capacitive coupling
>   - Pulsed electromagnetic fields (PEMF)
>   - Low-intensity pulsed ultrasound (LIPUS)

Direct Current

DC electrical stimulation requires invasive/internal application. It is included here, under conservative therapy, for completeness as a bone growth stimulator device; however, this bone stimulator should only be considered if the patient is undergoing revisional surgery.

With this device, a metallic cathode is surgically implanted at the nonunion site and an anode is placed in nearby subcutaneous tissues producing a direct electrical current between them. In 1971, Friedenberg was the first to report successful healing of a medial malleolar nonunion with an implantable cathode,[100] but it was not until a few years later, in 1974, that Dwyer and Wickham first described a totally implantable DC bone stimulator.[101] Brighton et al. later performed a multicenter study on the use of constant DC for nonunions. They found an 84% union rate with DC and immobilization in a series of 178 nonunions.[102] In 2005, Saxena et al. also carried out a multicenter study using DC stimulation in 26 high-risk patients (28 hindfoot fusions). Twenty-four of twenty-eight procedures showed radiographic union at an average of 10.3 weeks.[103]

Surgical Technique

The electrode wires (cathode) can be configured into a variety of shapes and can be single, double, or meshed. Common configurations for insertion of the cathode into the bone include zigzag, helix, and straight or fishscale into a drill hole to maximize surface area. It is important to ensure that the cathode does not come into contact with any metallic fixation devices during its implantation. The generator is then implanted in subcutaneous tissue about 8-10 cm from the nonunion site. This is typically in the distal calf or Kager triangle (Fig. 48.23). It is also imperative to discontinue the use of a Bovie, and any

other electrical device within the surgical field, prior to insertion of the bone stimulator, as this may damage the stimulator's settings and circuitry.

The advantage to these DC devices is that they are implantable; therefore, patient compliance and operator error are not risk factors. They do require surgical implantation however, and subsequent explantation of the generator so there are basic surgical risks involved. Also, the placement of the cathode is surgeon dependent and there is risk of displacement or breakage of the wire.

Capacitive Coupling

CC is similar to DC since both theorize that a DC adjacent to the nonunion is more effective than a current applied further from the site. CC is believed to enhance bone union by creating a low voltage, alternating or oscillating current. CC is applied with an external device and is noninvasive. The device consists of a power source and two electrode cables connecting to electrode pads that are applied directly to the skin on either side of the nonunion. The devices success is dose dependent and, therefore, should be worn 24 hours per day (Fig. 48.24). As a result of this recommended continuous application of the device, patient compliance can be an issue with this method of bone stimulation. Also, skin irritation can be of concern and the power source (battery) may need to be changed frequently.

There are several controlled studies supporting the effectiveness of CC devices. Brighton and Pollack treated 22 nonunions with CC and obtained a union rate of 77%.[104] Sarmiento et al. claim a 73% union rate when treating nonunions with CC[105] The only randomized controlled trial (RCT) assessing bone healing with CC was by Scott and King. Of the 23 patients randomly selected, 55% of the nonunions healed in the CC group, compared to only 8% healed in the placebo group.[106]

Pulsed Electromagnetic Fields: Inductive Coupling

PEMF devices rely on the delivery of pulsed electrical charges through soft tissue and bone utilizing a broad electromagnetic field rather than a direct, focused current. These devices utilize a low-level, time varying, programmed current, supplied to a treatment transducer, which is a wire coil. The coils come in different sizes and shapes. They are placed externally and

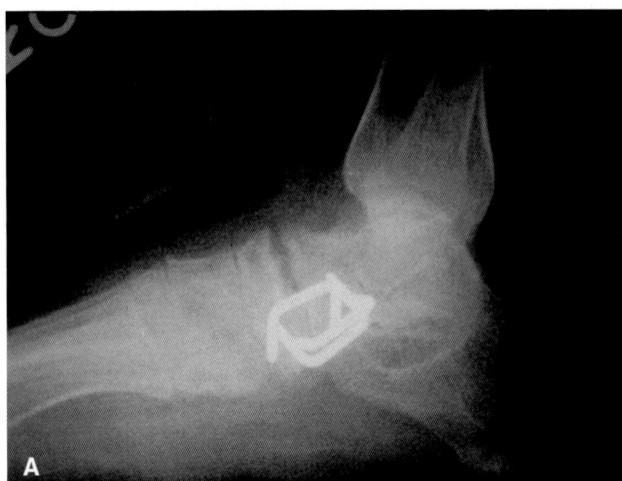

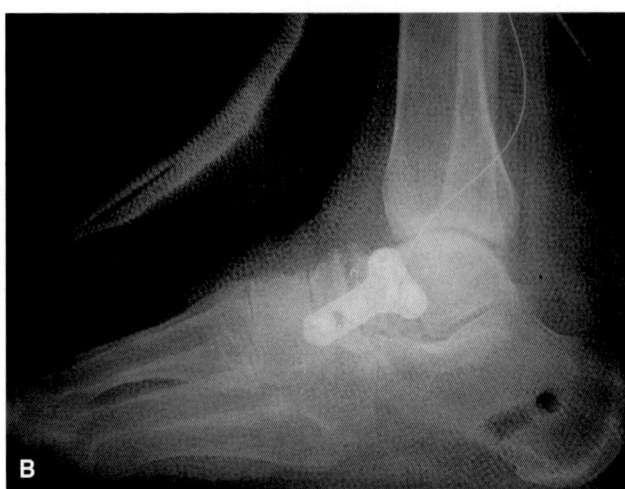

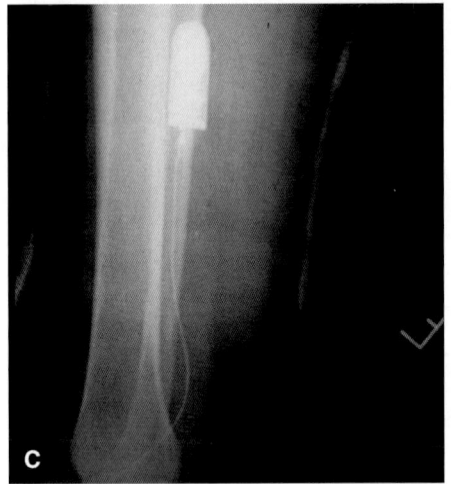

FIGURE 48.23 **A.** Lateral radiograph of a nonunion of a talonavicular joint arthrodesis. **B.** Revisional surgery performed with débridement of the nonunion site, autogenous calcaneal bone graft, plate and screw fixation, and an implantable bone stimulator. Notice the cathode wire is around the nonunion site. **C.** The anode (generator) is placed in the subcutaneous tissues in the lower leg away from the cathode.

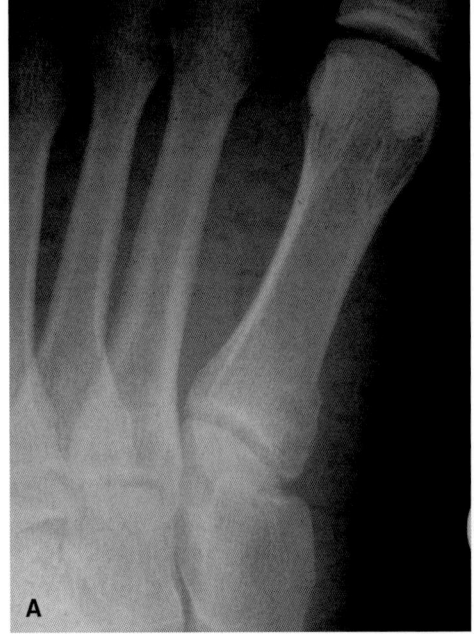

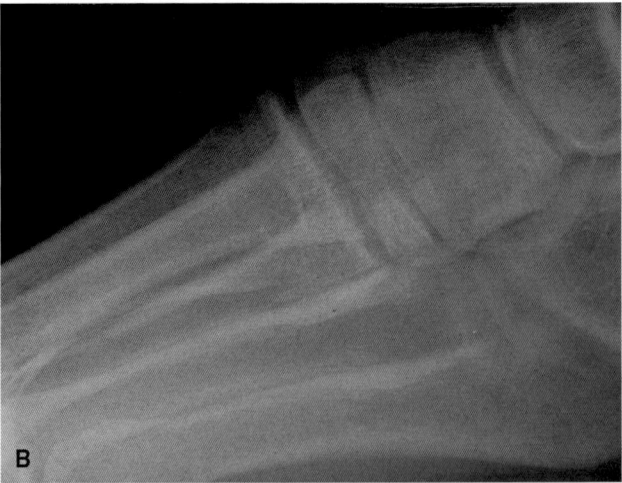

FIGURE 48.24 **A, B.** First metatarsal base fracture in a 17-year-old cheerleader. She fell from a lifted position.

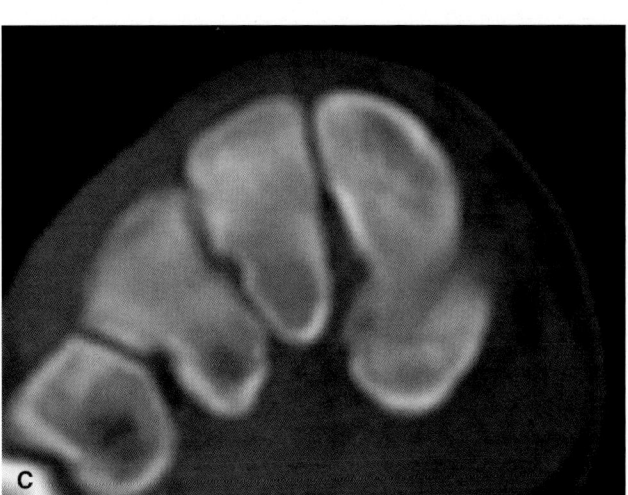

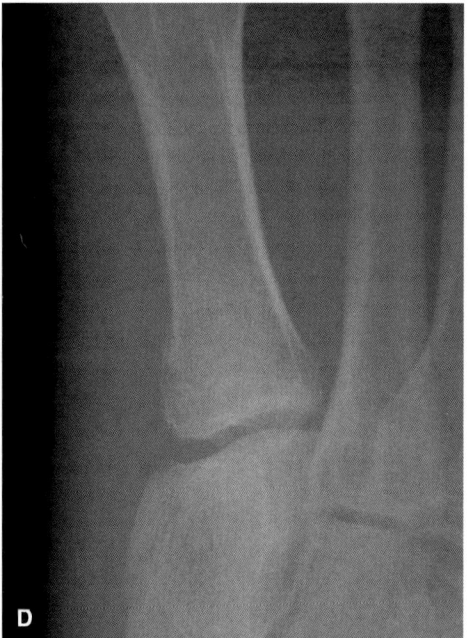

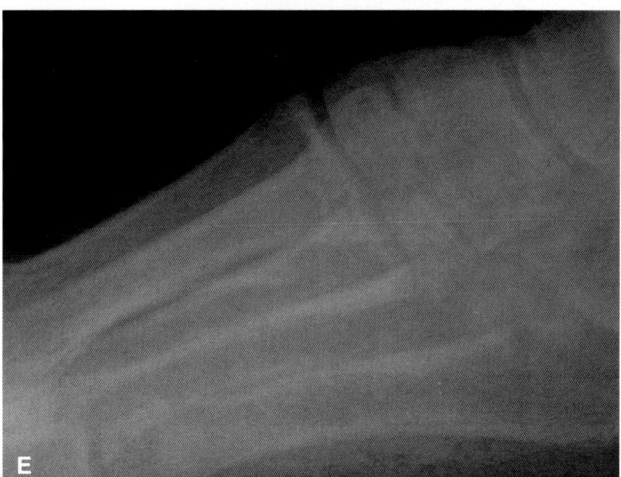

FIGURE 48.24 (*Continued*) **C.** CT scan confirming the first metatarsal base fracture. **D, E.** A capacitive coupling bone stimulator was applied, the patient was immobilized, and osseous consolidation was achieved in just 4 weeks.

can be applied over casts and splints. The device is powered by a rechargeable battery pack. PEMF devices are advantageous since they are noninvasive but patient compliance can be an issue as with the other external devices. This device is typically worn between 3 and 10 hours daily depending on product type, so it does require less time application than with CC (Fig. 48.25).

In 1981, Basset et al. was the first to apply a noninvasive bone growth stimulator utilizing PEMFs to treat tibial nonunions.[107] They achieved an 87% union rate of 127 patients utilizing PEMF. Sharrard reported on a multicenter, double-blind trial in 45 tibial shaft nonunions. A total of 9 out of 20 patients in the PEMF group achieved union, compared to only 3 out of 25 patients in the placebo group.[108] Heckman et al. reported that out of 149 nonunions, 96 (64%) progressed to complete union utilizing PEMF.[109] They stated patient noncompliance as contributory to the lower union rate. Fox and Smith applied PEMF to metatarsal nonunions and reported positive results.[110] Holmes demonstrated time to healing of 3 months utilizing PEMF and a non–weight-bearing cast for proximal fifth metatarsal fractures, compared to a mean healing time of 4.5 months for those patients treated with PEMF and a weight-bearing cast.[111]

Although most of these studies found increased healing utilizing PEMF, there are still some questions regarding its effectiveness. A systematic review in 2013 found that although PEMF had the greatest volume of published literature, it consisted primarily of level IV studies and could only provide grade C recommendations for delayed unions and nonunions.[112] Griffin and colleagues concluded that there may be benefit to bone healing utilizing PEMF, but most of the quality studies are focused on the tibia and there was not enough evidence to definitively determine its clinical usefulness.[113]

Low-Intensity Pulsed Ultrasound

LIPUS produces a mechanical signal that is sent through soft tissues and bone creating micromotion at the nonunion site.[114] The theory is that this micromotion stimulates a cascade of events leading to bone healing. These low-intensity ultrasound devices are placed directly over the nonunion, typically for about 20 minutes per day. The most common target frequency is 1.5 MHz but some utilize up to 3 MHz.[115,116] Although the time of application per day is significantly lower than the

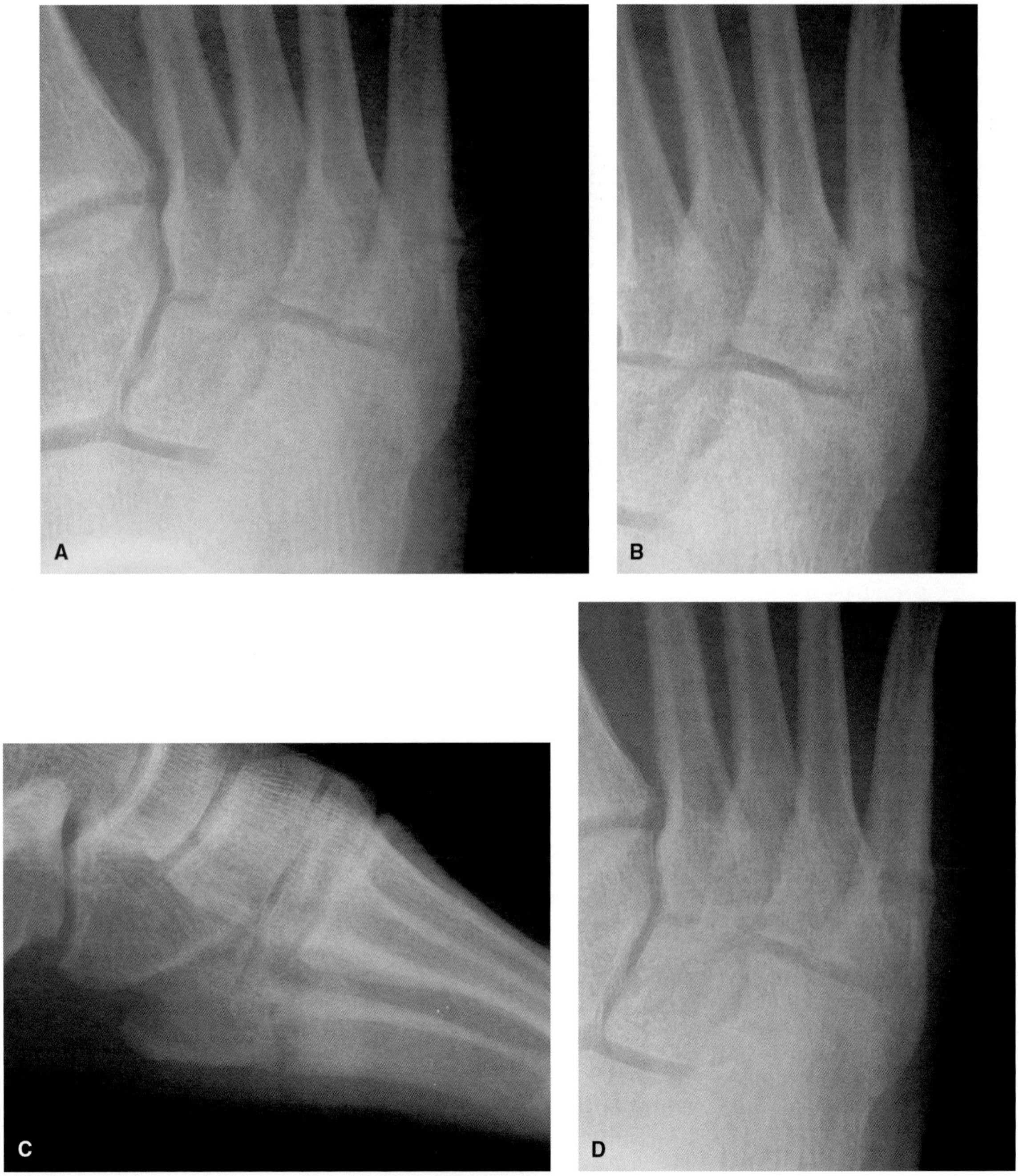

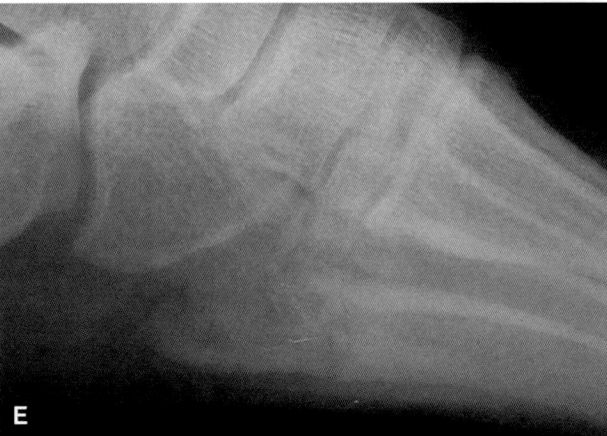

FIGURE 48.25 A. Jones fracture in a high school football player. He had persistent pain for over 1-month duration. A pulsed electromagnetic field (PEMF) bone stimulator was applied, and the patient was immobilized. **B, C.** Four weeks of utilization of the PEMF device shows increased consolidation and healing. **D, E.** Six weeks of PEMF bone stimulation produced significant osseous healing and consolidation is almost complete.

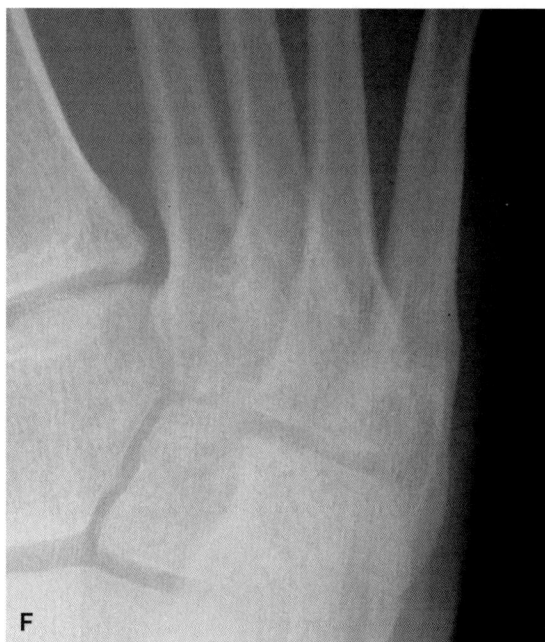
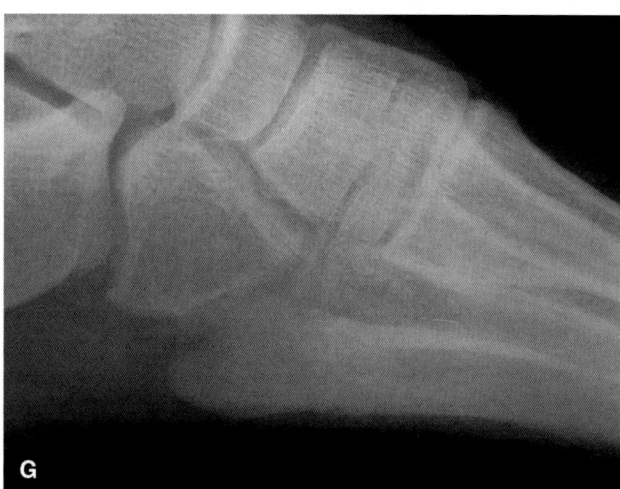

FIGURE 48.25 (*Continued*) **F, G.** Eight weeks of PEMF bone stimulation and immobilization resulted in complete osseous union.

other external devices, patient compliance is still a factor. Also, the device must come in contact with the skin and cannot be applied over casts. Roussignol and colleagues[117] and Watanabe and Arai[118] both stressed that the success of LIPUS was also dependent upon stable fixation, decreased time to treatment, and small interfragment gapping.

LIPUS has been extensively studied in the animal model as early as 1950 by both Buchtala and Maintz[119,120] and in later studies most notably by Dyson and Brookes.[115] Human trials soon followed these early reports. While most data favor the use of LIPUS in improving bone healing and consolidation,[121–123] some show no difference when using this ultrasound technique.[124] Katano et al. believed that LIPUS improved bone healing by promoting endochondral ossification, therefore decreasing the time required for complete ossification.[125]

There is wide ranging support for the use of LIPUS for delayed and nonunions but also for acute fractures. Heckman et al.[121] reported a 24% reduction in time to clinical healing for acute fractures treated with LIPUS, which supported similar findings reported by Kristiansen and colleagues[122] and Leung and colleagues.[126] A systematic literature review and meta-analysis by Hannemann et al. also reported evidence that LIPUS can significantly shorten the time to radiographic healing in acute fractures.[127] Hemery et al.[123] and Jingushi and colleagues[128] report data to support increased success rates when using LIPUS for the treatment of delayed unions and nonunions within 6 months of the most recent surgery vs a more delayed time to initial treatment. A recent study by Mirza et al. reviewed the use of LIPUS in 18 patients who had arthrodesis procedures in the foot and ankle diagnosed with delayed union or nonunion. Twelve patients (67%) were treated successfully with radiographic union, four patients required surgical revision, and two patients were treated conservatively. They concluded that LIPUS may have a role as a treatment modality for delayed union of isolated small joints of the foot since they demonstrated a higher incidence of fusion (9/10; 90%), but

they would not recommend its use in large or multiple joints of the foot and ankle since they demonstrated only a 38% (3/8) union rate utilizing LIPUS in these joints.[129]

Device Selection
Although there is basic science and clinical evidence to support the use of bone growth stimulators, as has been shown here for each device, there are no high-level comparative studies to guide the foot and ankle surgeon on the most effective bone stimulator. A retrospective study of 271 tibial nonunions over 24 years compared outcomes using bone grafting, DC, or CC and found that as the patient risk factors increased, the likelihood of osseous healing decreased, regardless of the bone stimulator utilized.[130] A study on rat fibular osteotomies comparing percutaneous DC and LIPUS did not show any significant difference in healing times between the two devices.[131] Finally, a systematic literature review and meta-analysis showed evidence from RCTs, suggesting that both PEMF and LIPUS can significantly shorten the time to radiographic healing in acute fractures; however, there was little evidence found to support any risk reduction in the development of nonunions.[127]

All of these bone growth stimulators have their own advantages and disadvantages. DC requires surgical implantation and therefore acquires surgical risk; however, patient compliance is not an issue. CC is an external device but requires 24-hour application directly on the skin. PEMF is an external application that can be applied over casts and splints and only has to be applied between 3 and 10 hours per day. LIPUS is advantageous because it is only a 20 minutes per day external application, but again it has to be applied directly to the nonunion site and cannot go over a cast. It can, however, be incorporated into a cast if desired.

Bone stimulation should be viewed as an adjunctive modality available to the surgeon to try to maximize the healing potential of a nonunion. The surgeon must realize, however, that there are other factors dependent on the success of these bone growth stimulators including gap size of the nonunion site,

stable fixation, time to initial treatment, and weight-bearing status of the patient. The surgeon must then decide which device is most favorable for the specific clinical and radiographic presentation and patient risk factors.

SURGICAL INTERVENTION

For persistent nonunions, despite conservative therapy, the surgeon needs to reevaluate the etiology of the nonunion. If there is unstable fixation, questionable viability to the bone fragments, and/or malalignment, surgical intervention is typically required to obtain osseous union. However, the surgeon must determine the pros and cons of further surgical intervention. Identifying and correcting patient risk factors is imperative to achieving adequate bone healing. If patient risk factors, such as increased glucose or continued nicotine usage are not corrected, a poor outcome and continued nonunion is usually inevitable, and the surgeon should take this into consideration prior to any further surgery. Sometimes, no further surgical intervention is the best treatment we can offer our patients, even if it means not reaching our treatment goals. Minimizing pain and optimizing function through bracing techniques may be the best treatment option when the risk for surgical intervention is too high.

Revisional surgery for nonunions requires a lot of planning, patient education, and many times referrals and consultations. Depending on patient risk factors and examination findings, these consultations may include infectious disease, endocrinology, vascular surgery, plastic surgery, and pain management. The patient needs to be medically optimized, correcting all risk factors, before any further surgery is performed. Physical therapy should also be considered for gait training to maximize the patient's compliance with non–weight bearing postoperatively. Long-term rehabilitation and placement may also be an option for some elderly and less mobile patients, especially if there is not a good support system at home.

Nonunion surgery should include a comprehensive roadmap to address all of the aspects that played a role in the resulting nonunion. Revisional surgery can be technically difficult and the surgeon should not only be prepared to carry out the proposed surgical plan, but also be prepared to address any potential complications that may be encountered intraoperatively. The surgeon should have a solid surgical plan to correct any deformity present and increase vascularity to the site. Good, stable fixation is the cornerstone for maintenance of correction, and bone grafting and orthobiologics can assist with increasing viability of the nonunion site. The surgeon must be familiar with the advantages and disadvantages to different fixation constructs and to the many and various bone grafts and bone graft substitutes available to aid in the healing process. The use of these fixation devices and implantable materials are surgeon preference, but selection of these materials should be individualized according to patient needs and assessment. The surgeon should also have a back-up plan if additional or different fixation or grafting materials are needed.

The surgical plan for a nonunion may involve surgery to additional anatomic locations, or the need to involve multiple or staged surgeries. For example, if there is failure of a single joint fusion, such as a subtalar joint, the surgeon may want to consider arthrodesis of additional joints, such as a triple arthrodesis, for overall increased stability. If infection is a concern, biopsy, débridement, removal of hardware, placement of antibiotic materials, and possible application of an external fixator may be the first phase of surgery. Intravenous antibiotics are typically employed and then once the infection has resolved, surgical reconstruction can be undertaken. Likewise, if there are significant osseous defects and challenging hardware removal, the first surgery may involve explantation of fixation and filling of bone defects with grafting materials in an effort to optimize bone quality. Once osseous consolidation is maximized, and bone voids are minimized, the second, surgical reconstruction can be pursued.

Surgical Techniques and Principles

Regardless of the anatomical location of where the nonunion has occurred, whether it be a fracture, osteotomy, or failed arthrodesis, surgical techniques and principles remain the same. The goal of revisional surgery, as previously stated, is to produce a painless, functional foot and ankle. To achieve this, vascularity to the site must be restored, stable fixation must be provided, and proper alignment must be maintained.

SURGICAL PEARLS FOR REPAIR OF NONUNIONS

- Identify and manage/correct risk factors.
  - Consults and referrals as appropriate.
- Perform meticulous dissection.
  - Avoid disruption of the blood supply.
- All interposing soft tissue, any remaining cartilage, and all devitalized bone, must be débrided and excised.
  - Débridement down to good bleeding bone is paramount.
- Use of distractors can aid in joint access and visualization.
- Fenestration of the subchondral bone plate is crucial.
  - Look for the "Paprika Sign."
- Proper alignment is critical to success.
  - Any malunion needs to be corrected.
  - Wedge resection may be needed.
  - Bone grafting can help maintain length.
- Apply good rigid fixation, internal and/or external, specific for the patient's deformity, bone stock, and risk factors.
- Adjunctive bone grafts and/or orthobiologics can be utilized as needed.

Full-thickness skin incisions down to bone are typically utilized. Undermining of the skin, and excessive retraction on the tissues, should be avoided. The goal is to avoid disruption of the blood supply and necrosis or dysvascularity to the tissues. Meticulous dissection is then utilized, taking care to identify and avoid all vital structures including nerves, vessels, and tendons. Significant scar tissue may be encountered, and it is essential to débride and evacuate all nonviable tissue. Once scar tissue has been successfully removed, tension around the surgical site is often reduced, making it easier for the surgeon to identify the nonunion site.

Once the nonunion site is identified, all devitalized and necrotic bone, and any remaining cartilage in the joint, should be removed. This includes any soft tissue that was interposed within the surgical site initially impeding bone healing. It is imperative that the bone ends be débrided down to bleeding surfaces. This may create significant gaps and shortening

requiring grafts; dysvascular bone, however, cannot be left in the surgical site. This will doom the procedure to failure once again. Joint access is very important so the surgeon can visualize that all devitalized material has been successfully removed. There are many types of distractors available that can be utilized to aid in this maneuver. A lamina spreader without teeth can also be very useful in gaining visualization of the surgical site while not compromising the osseous integrity or creating multiple drill holes where fixation may need to be placed (Fig. 48.26).

Following bone débridement, fenestration through the subchondral tissues is performed. This is typically done with drill bits or Kirschner wires (K-wires) depending on the size of the area to be fenestrated. The authors usually prefer a 2.0-mm drill bit at medium speed. This technique should also be performed with constant saline irrigation to minimize burning and necrosis of the bone. Fenestration through this subchondral bone plate cannot be overemphasized, as it creates the vascular channels for the delivery of the osteoprogenitor and bone healing cells, bone marrow, and various growth factors, all of which provide good vascularity and the mechanism for successful osseous union.

Once the osseous surfaces have been adequately prepared, alignment and fixation are the final steps in the surgical revision. Appropriate alignment of the nonunion site is of paramount importance. The bone ends need to have good apposition and contact and be free of any angular deformities. This will maximize the healing potential and neutralize stress along the union site. Fixation should provide a stable construct, eliminating motion across the union site, as well as maintaining proper alignment. Motion during healing impedes osseous consolidation and can also prevent incorporation of bone grafts utilized.

The choice of fixation is usually surgeon preference but there are many factors that may influence one's choices. The location of the nonunion, proximity of surrounding joints, previous fixation, degree of bone loss, bone grafts and grafting materials utilized, osteopenia, patient compliance and risk factors, and postoperative non–weight-bearing capabilities should all be taken into consideration. Recent advances in technology have provided many excellent options for fixation. Locking plates are a good option for osteopenic or poor-quality bone, as they create a more stable construct in this patient population. Similarly, beaming techniques are commonly employed for Charcot arthropathy reconstructions, as they also provide increased stability for these patients. Alternatively, external fixation can be utilized in place of, or in addition to, internal fixation in many patient populations, as it provides rigid fixation without interrupting the immediate surrounding soft tissues and blood supply. External fixators are commonly utilized in cases where infection has been present or is being treated, poor quality bone, Charcot arthropathy, and for patients that may not be able to maintain a completely non–weight-bearing attitude postoperatively.

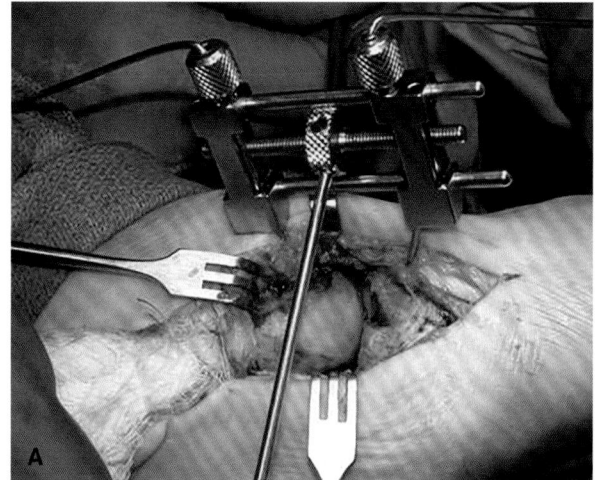

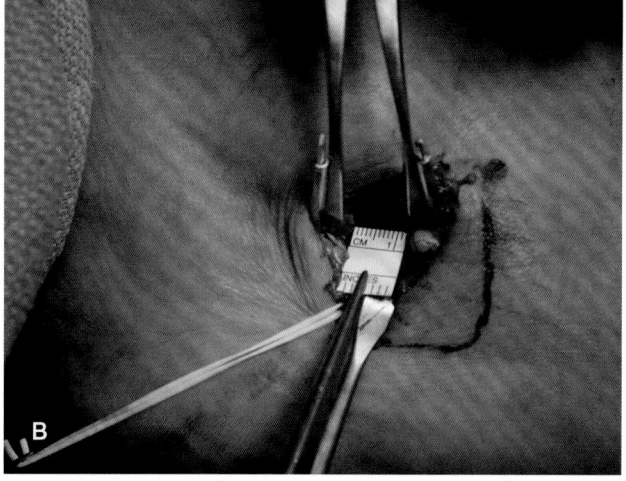

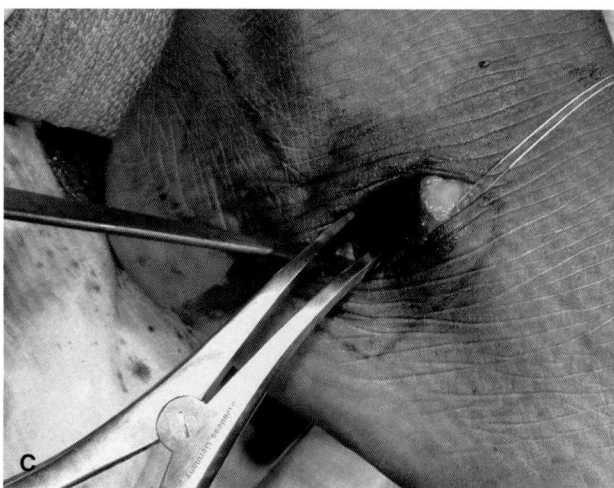

FIGURE 48.26 A, B. Mini distractors used to gain better visualization of the surgical area. This helps to ensure all cartilage and dysvascular bone has been successfully removed, which is necessary to achieve osseous union. **C.** A lamina spreader without teeth can also be utilized to gain better access and visualization to the surgical site.

They are also commonly utilized in staged procedures to correct for significant angular deformities.

Finally, osseous defects and bone voids need to be filled in with bone grafts and/or bone graft substitutes. This will help maintain length and structural integrity and maximize viability to the nonunion site. There are advantages and disadvantages to each type and the selection should be individualized for each patient scenario. The surgeon should also consider the best fixation options when bone grafts are utilized, as a stable construct is very important to maximize graft incorporation.

BONE GRAFTS

Bone grafts and bone grafting materials play a very important role in the treatment of nonunions. Oftentimes, after the débridement of nonviable bone, there is significant shortening and large voids at the nonunion site. Bone grafts and orthobiologics can be utilized to fill the osseous defects, maintain structural integrity, and increase vascularity and viability to the union site. There are many different types of bone grafts and bone grafting materials available. The surgeon should be familiar with the advantages and disadvantages of each, and know their indications, so these materials can be used appropriately and most effectively.

Again, an understanding of the biology of bone healing will allow selection of the proper substance/material to augment the surgical procedure at hand. Autogenous grafts, allografts, and even xenografts have all been utilized in the treatment of nonunions. Autogenous grafts, however, are still widely considered the gold standard, as they have osteogenic, osteoconductive, and osteoinductive properties.[132–137] They can provide either cortical or cancellous bone, and the majority of the time a combination of both is utilized. Cortical bone provides greater mechanical strength and therefore, is preferred when structural maintenance is necessary. Cancellous grafts, however, have a greater abundance of bone morphogenetic protein, which mediates induction of osteoprogenitor and mesenchymal cells, allowing for quicker incorporation of the graft. Common sites of autogenous bone graft harvest in the foot and ankle are the calcaneus, the distal and proximal tibia, and the fibula. When the fibula is utilized, it is commonly employed as a long cortical strut. Autogenous iliac crest is also an excellent source of corticocancellous bone that can be utilized in many different locations in the foot and ankle.

Autogenous grafts are commonly utilized to fill voids, provide structural integrity, and provide viable cells for healing. One common example of this is revisional first MTPJ arthrodesis, secondary to nonunion and failed implants or arthroplasty (Fig. 48.27). Oftentimes there is significant shortening with this procedure requiring a bone graft. An autogenous, corticocancellous calcaneal bone graft is ideal for this surgical revision as it provides both structural integrity and viable cells to the surgical site. Small amounts of autogenous bone can also be obtained utilizing a percutaneous trephine technique. This is usually a combination of corticocancellous bone and can be used to fill small defects or mixed in with other biologic materials to create a bone slurry/paste. Although autogenous grafts have many advantages, they are not without risks and potential complications associated with their use both at the donor and application sites.

Regarding technique, the most common use of an autograft is as a free, interposed section of bone. Typically, an autogenous bone graft can fill a maximum gap of up to about 2.5 cm and provide adequate healing and graft incorporation.[138] However, for gaps larger than this, other techniques including onlay/inlay grafting, bone transport, and vascularized grafts may need to be employed.[139–143]

Allograft bone and orthobiologic materials only harness one or two of the desired properties of bone healing, osteogenic, osteoinductive, and/or osteoconductive, unless combined or in conjunction with a native substance. Allografts provide equivalent osteoconductive properties, but their osteoinductive properties are diminished compared to autografts. They are a good alternative to autogenous grafting when the risk of an

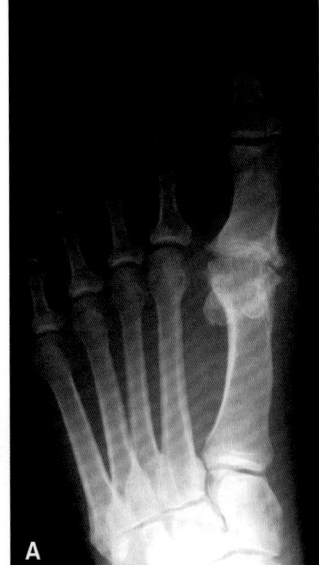
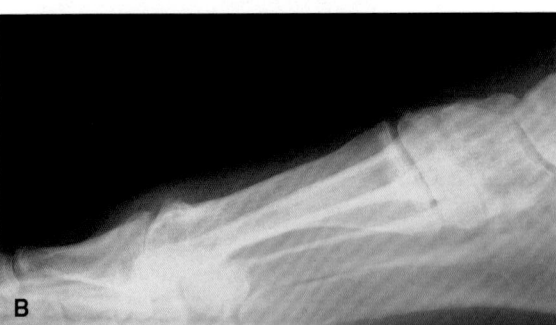

FIGURE 48.27 A, B. This 62-year-old female had previous first MTPJ surgery, which resulted in limited and painful joint motion.

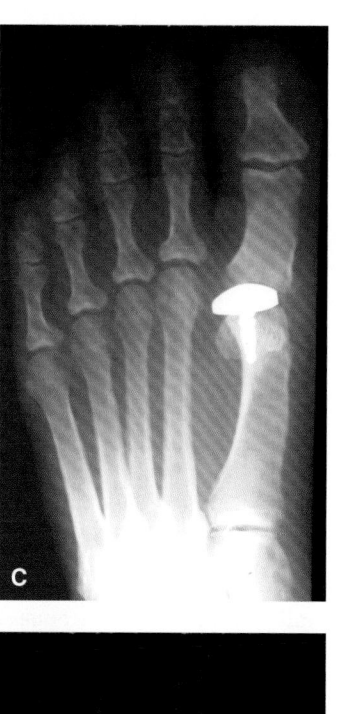

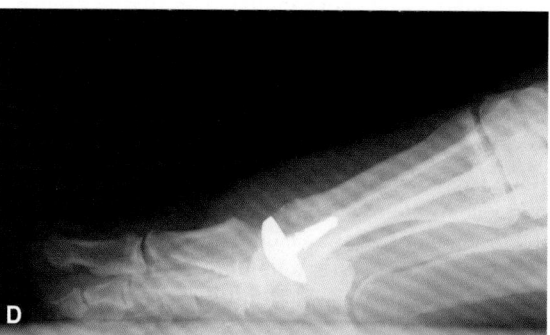

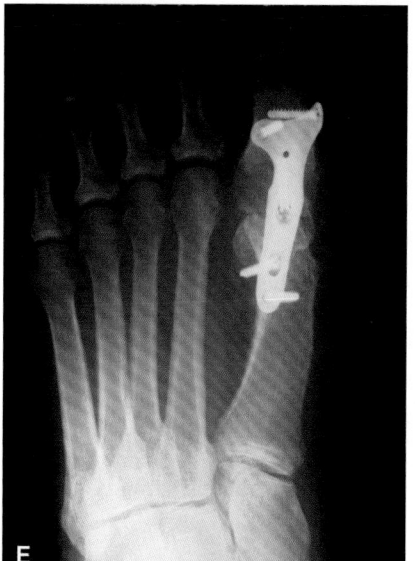

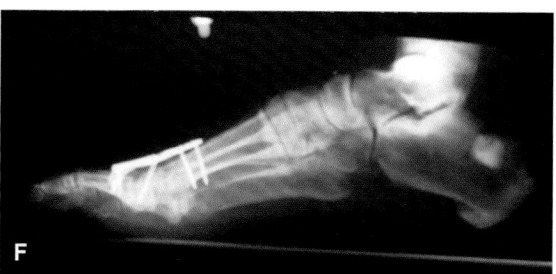

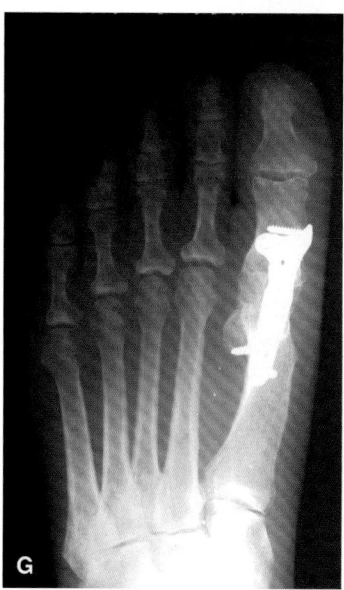

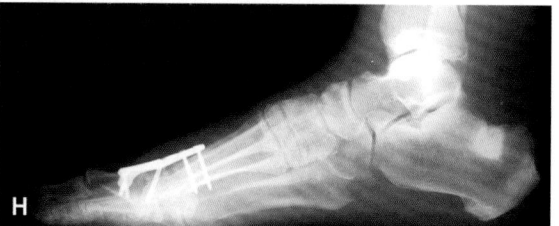

FIGURE 48.27 (*Continued*)
C, D. A first MTPJ implant was performed, but the patient's pain and limited motion persisted. Note the lateral angulation of the implant in the first metatarsal head and the absence of joint space. **E, F.** The implant was removed producing a large gap in the first MTPJ. A first MTPJ arthrodesis with autogenous calcaneal bone graft was performed, and length of the first ray was maintained. **G, H.** Three-month postop radiographs show osseous consolidation of the first MTPJ and the donor site of the calcaneus, which was backfilled with calcium hydroxyapatite.

autograft is too high, or when the advantageous properties of an autograft are not necessary for the specific clinical scenario. Allografts and orthobiologics can also be used concomitantly with autografts. Allografts are available in many different sizes and shapes and in different combinations/percentages of cortical and cancellous bone. Although allografts do not have any osteogenic properties, the advantage they have over autografts is no donor site morbidity and decreased surgical and anesthesia time.[144]

ORTHOBIOLOGICS

In recent years, there has been growing interest in the use of orthobiologic materials to augment musculoskeletal healing. Orthobiologics are founded on the biology of bone healing, working to supplement and engage the body's healing pathways. Use of orthobiologics implies surgical intervention with adequate preparation, restoration of anatomic alignment of a fracture or fusion site with application of stable fixation under which primary bone healing can occur. The aforementioned are the keys to successful healing; however, in patients with risk factors for poor healing or nonunion, use of orthobiologics may optimize outcomes. While many have incorporated orthobiologic application routinely in practice, others may reserve their use for specific cases, especially those that are revisional. Various classes of orthobiologics exist such as platelet-rich plasma, bone morphogenetic protein, demineralized bone matrix (DBM), bioglass, calcium-based bioceramics, and mesenchymal stem cells (MSC). This sector of medicine and surgery will only continue to grow with much research being devoted to development and investigation of these products. Knowledge of orthobiologics and their properties and application will provide the foot and ankle surgeons with additional resources in their arsenal to promote optimal outcomes for their patients.

The different orthobiologic materials tap into the properties of osteogenesis, osteoconduction, and osteoinduction with a goal of supplementing healing whether it be a primary or revisional procedure.[145,146] The local factors contributing to healing, such as vascularity and stability, are critical to the success of the orthobiologics as well. Bony healing progresses through several phases including inflammatory, proliferative/fibroblastic, and remodeling with each phase varying in duration based on the host and local factors. Orthobiologics, when chosen strategically, have the potential to augment the host's natural mechanisms throughout the various phases of healing.

Orthobiologics

- Osteoinductive
  - PRP
  - BMP
  - Growth factors
- Osteoconductive
- DBM
  - Bioceramics
  - Bioglass
- Osteogenic
  - Mesenchymal stem cells

OSTEOINDUCTIVE MATERIALS

As the name implies, these substances induce bone healing. MSC are stimulated to multiply and differentiate into progenitor cells. When combined with other growth factors and proteins, formation of cartilage and/or bone occurs. The most widely used materials in this category are platelet-based products, BMP, and various growth factors. DBM may double as both osteoinductive and conductive.

Platelet-Rich Plasma

Platelet-rich plasma (PRP) has gained popularity in use for bone, ligament, and tendon healing. PRP is generated by centrifuging the patient's blood to separate out and obtain a gel-like concentration of growth factors. The PRP is then injected in and around the surgical site.[147,148] Numerous studies advocate its use, noting improved outcomes compared to controls.[149,150] While PRP provides a concentrated application of autologous growth factors, the actual product may be variable, depending on the method of preparation, and even if standardized, may yield insufficient quantities of desired growth factors and include white blood cells and other substances that might impede bony healing.[151,152] Gandhi et al. published a study on ankle fracture nonunions in which PRP and autograft were utilized in the revisional surgery. Union was achieved in all patients with a mean time to union of 60 days.[153] The release of platelet associated growth factors following application may provide the essential growth factors that may otherwise be reduced, especially at nonunion sites. Bibbo et al. performed a study evaluating the use of PRP in elective foot and ankle surgery on high-risk patients. Sixty-two patients were followed for 6 months following intervention. Some patients also received autogenous graft if indicated as part of the procedure. Ninety-four percent union was achieved with a mean time to union of 41 days.[149] A 2014 systematic review of various applications for PRP in the foot and ankle did not note any clear or specific indications for use of PRP.[154] A more recent 2018 review echoed the same sentiment, but acknowledging its possible benefit and future potential.[155]

Bone Morphogenetic Proteins

BMPs were first described by Marshall Urist[25] when he discovered de novo bone formation in rabbits after application of decalcified bone. Now, more than 20 BMPs have been recognized, 7 of which have shown a significant role in bone formation.[156-159] These proteins are within the TGF-beta superfamily, which participate in and contribute to tissue formation and regeneration.[158] Numerous studies support the use of BMPs in the management of fractures and nonunions throughout the body.[160-164] In a 2009 study, Schuberth et al. examined the use of BMP in 38 cases involving patients at a high risk for healing complications. The rate of successful healing was observed at 84.21%.[165] Bibbo and colleagues reported hindfoot fusion rates of 96% in rhBMP-2-treated fusion sites as compared to 48% in fusion alone.[166] Subtalar, talonavicular, and calcaneocuboid fusions were individually examined with fusion rates of 95% across the procedures when rhBMP-2 was applied either in isolation or in combination with allo- or autograft.[166] A retrospective study of 82 ankle fusions treated with rhBMP-2 noted

a fusion rate of 93% compared to 53% in the control group. In addition, greater bony bridging was noted on CT scans.[167] Similarly, Bibbo et al. reported a 100% fusion rate in a group of 24 high-risk ankle fusions with a mean time to union in 9.1 weeks.[166] A 2014 investigation on 51 cases of fusion or fracture nonunion demonstrated a revisional procedure union rate of 92.2% with use of rhBMP-2 with a mean time to union of 111 days.[168] DeVries and colleagues published a 2018 study that examined 68 patients undergoing hindfoot and ankle arthrodesis. They noted a 10.3% and 17.9% nonunion rate in patients managed with a BMP allograft vs those without. This was not statistically significant; however, 13.8% and 35.9% of patients in the respective groups developed a complication.[169] While no significant adverse effects have been directly attributed to BMPs, nonunions and other postoperative complications may arise. Some literature has reported development of heterotopic and ectopic bone formation in sites of application.[170] Despite the high initial cost of some of these products, the potential exists for this to be a cost saving option if the literature continues to demonstrate that their use decreases nonunions and expedites healing.[170]

Growth Factors

Numerous growth factors contribute to bone and soft tissue healing. Platelet-derived growth factor (PDGF) contributes to angiogenesis, macrophage activation, chemotaxis, proliferation of fibroblasts, and collagen synthesis. TGF is responsible for proliferation of fibroblasts, collagen synthesis, bone matrix formation, and inhibition of bone resorption. Insulinlike growth factor (IGF) promotes chemotaxis of fibroblasts, proliferation and differentiation of osteoblasts, bone matrix formation, as well as growth and repair of skeletal muscle. VEGF stimulates angiogenesis, migration and mitosis of endothelial cells, chemotaxis of macrophages and granulocytes, and vasodilation. Lastly, epidermal growth factor (EGF) promotes proliferation and differentiation of epithelial cells.[148] These are all naturally occurring and are prominent at various phases of the healing process. Some of these growth factors, particularly PDGF, are being incorporated into orthobiologic compounds. PDGF is a protein released from platelets and macrophages in response to tissue injury. The PDGF-BB dimer is the most potent form and is chemotactic and mitogenic for osteoblast progenitor cells and osteoblasts. It has also been demonstrated to promote angiogenesis even in regions of compromise, which allows for an influx of pro-inflammatory and osteogenic agents to the surgical site/area of injury.[171] When combined with tricalcium phosphate, an osteoinductive and conductive substrate is produced. Several studies comparing this orthobiologic compound to autogenous bone graft noted a larger percentage of patients achieving radiographic union at designated intervals in the orthobiologic group.[172,173] A follow-up study of 573 hindfoot arthrodesis cases by DiGiovanni et al. noted a comparable rate of nonunion of 31% in the rhPDGF BB/tricalcium phosphate group and 27% in the autograft group.[174]

OSTEOCONDUCTIVE MATERIALS

Osteoconductive materials serve as a scaffolding or framework in which bone can proliferate. These are porous substances that can be used as a filler for structural deficits. These products can allow fusion/incorporation to take place without resorption of

the fusion site. However, they are not as strong initially as trabecular bone and lack a collagen matrix.[175] When autograft is limited, these may be incorporated as an adjunct. These materials alone may have limited efficacy in addressing nonunions, but when used in combination with autograft or osteoinductive materials, these orthobiologics can be effective.[145,146]

Demineralized Bone Matrix

As a processed allograft, DBM lacks mineralization but retains growth factors and collagen. The continued presence of growth factors will stimulate osteoblast formation. These grafts are prepared with combinations of acids or detergents and solvents. Antibiotics and freeze drying have not been found to have adverse effects on the processing of the grafts.[175–177] Given the properties of these grafts, they can be both osteoinductive and osteoconductive (Fig. 48.28). However, it is important to be aware of the sterilization methods, as gamma irradiation, formaldehyde, or ethylene oxide prep will strip the osteoinductive properties.[175] DBM may come in many forms such as gel, putty, sheets, and chips, with different strengths and pliability, and may be selected based on the desired application (Fig. 48.29). A study by Michelson et al. examined use of DBM in subtalar and triple arthrodeses with a comparison to iliac crest bone graft. They noted that union, and time to union, were similar in both groups, concluding that DBM performed at least as well as the iliac graft but without the donor site morbidity and complications.[178] Thordarson and Kuehn compared patients receiving DBM putty and DBM with allograft in 63 ankle/hindfoot fusions. They noted nonunion rates at 14% and 8%, respectively, which did not constitute a statistically significant difference, and was comparable to the historic nonunion rate of 10% for iliac crest bone graft.[179] Collman and colleagues reviewed 39 arthroscopic ankle arthrodeses that received PRP or DBM. A union rate of 87.2% was achieved by

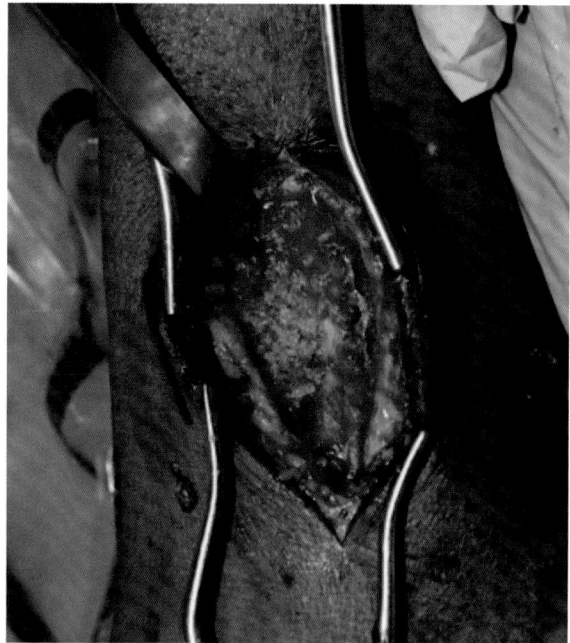

FIGURE 48.28 Repair of a fibular nonunion utilizing demineralized bone matrix (DBM) putty along the nonunion site and syndesmosis.

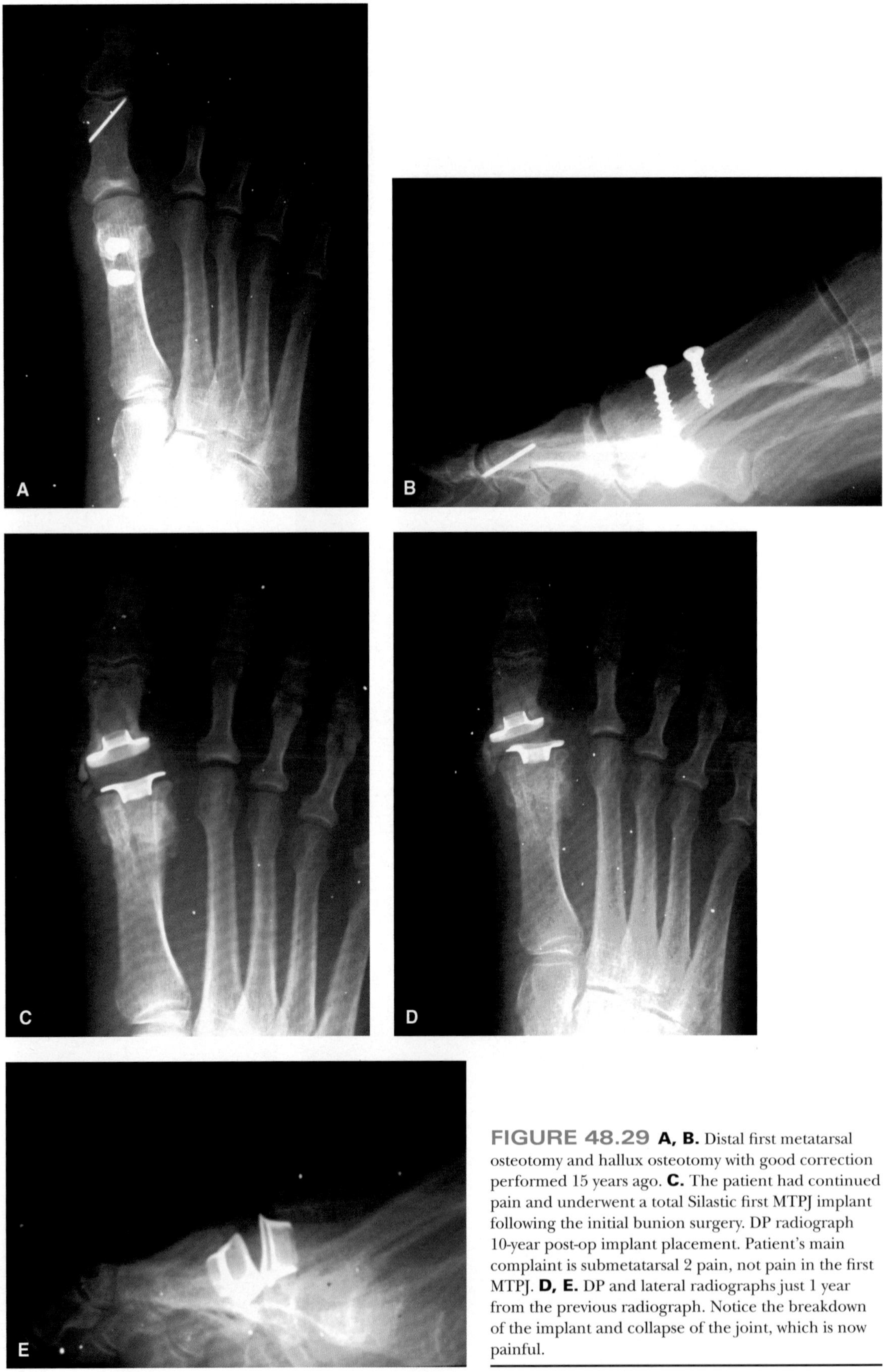

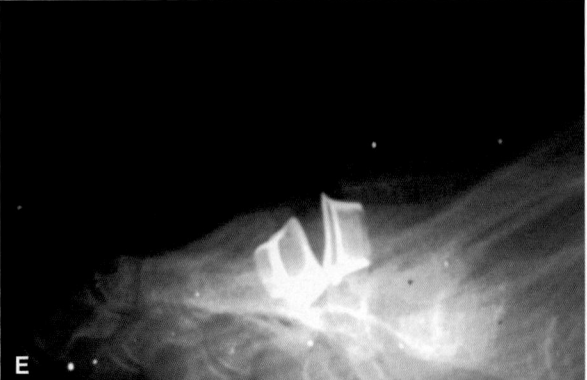

FIGURE 48.29 A, B. Distal first metatarsal osteotomy and hallux osteotomy with good correction performed 15 years ago. **C.** The patient had continued pain and underwent a total Silastic first MTPJ implant following the initial bunion surgery. DP radiograph 10-year post-op implant placement. Patient's main complaint is submetatarsal 2 pain, not pain in the first MTPJ. **D, E.** DP and lateral radiographs just 1 year from the previous radiograph. Notice the breakdown of the implant and collapse of the joint, which is now painful.

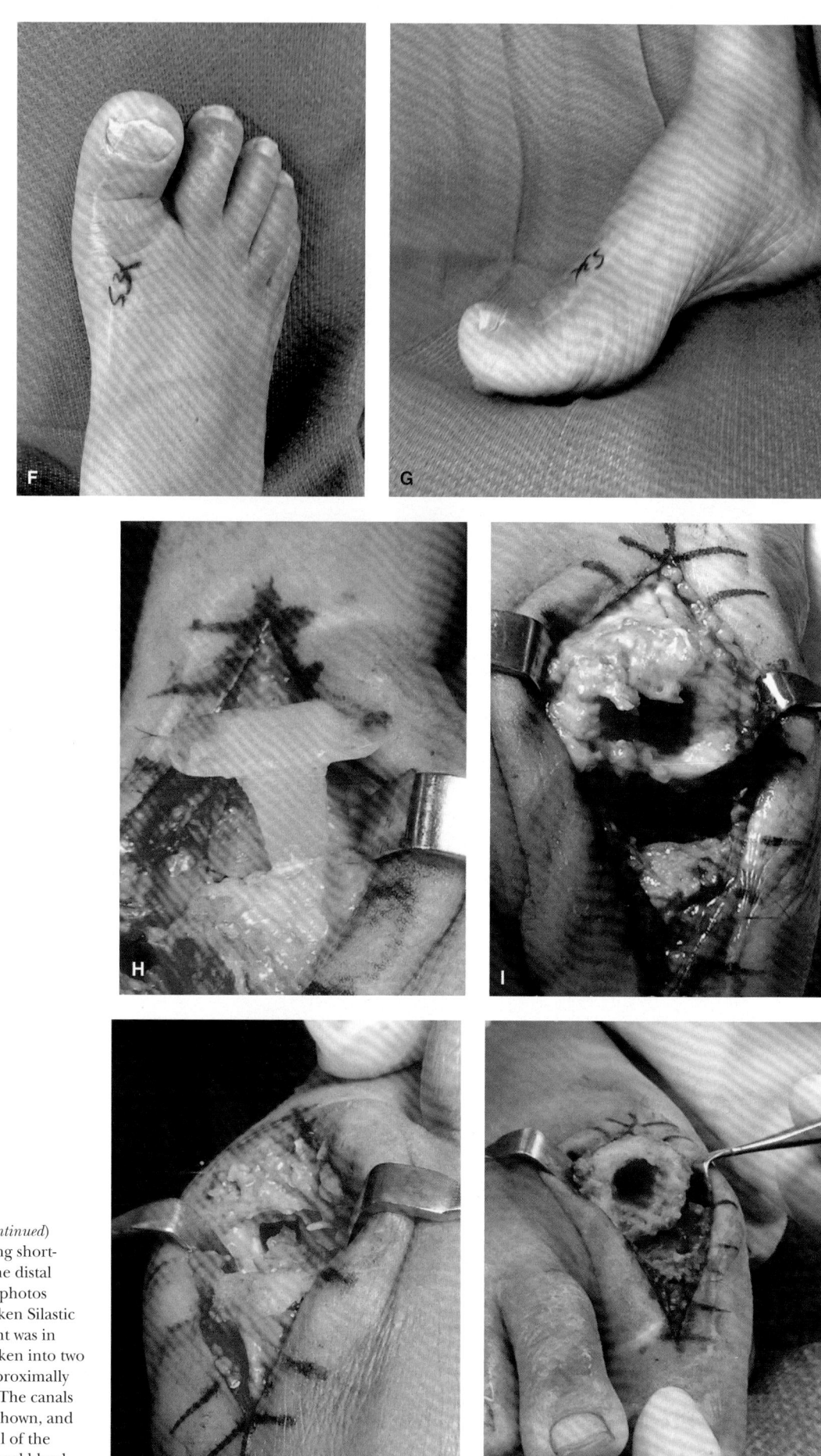

FIGURE 48.29 (*Continued*)
F, G. Clinical photos showing shortening and dorsiflexion of the distal hallux. **H-L.** Intraoperative photos showing removal of the broken Silastic implant. Overall, the implant was in good condition but was broken into two main pieces with one stem proximally and the other stem distally. The canals proximally and distally are shown, and these were débrided until all of the fibrotic tissue was removed and bleeding was encountered.

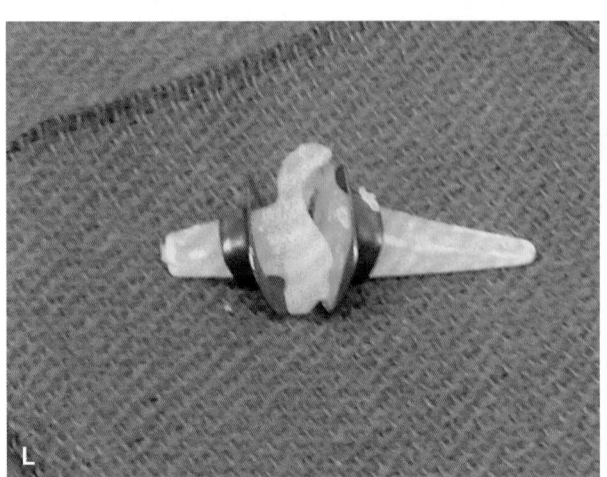

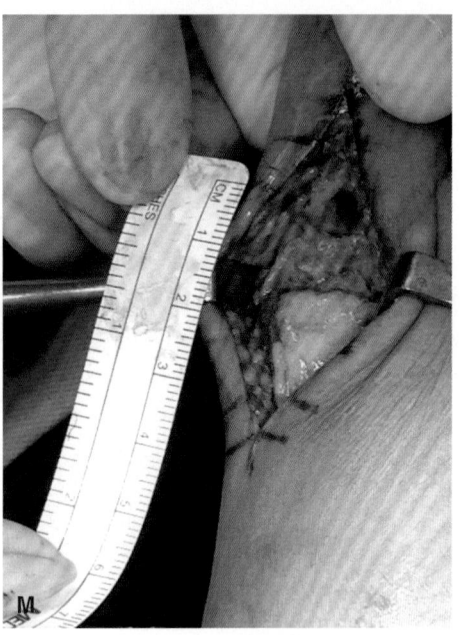

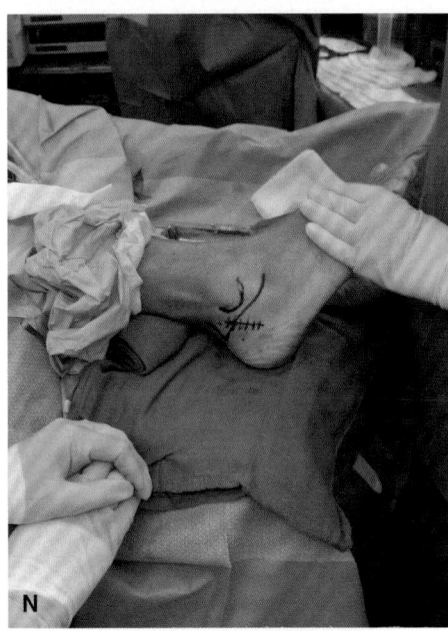

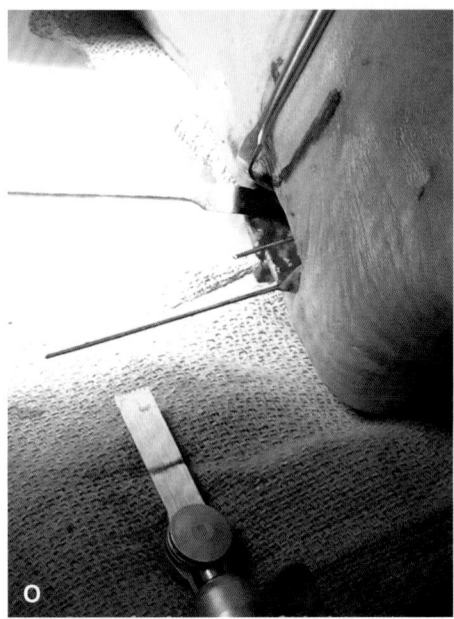

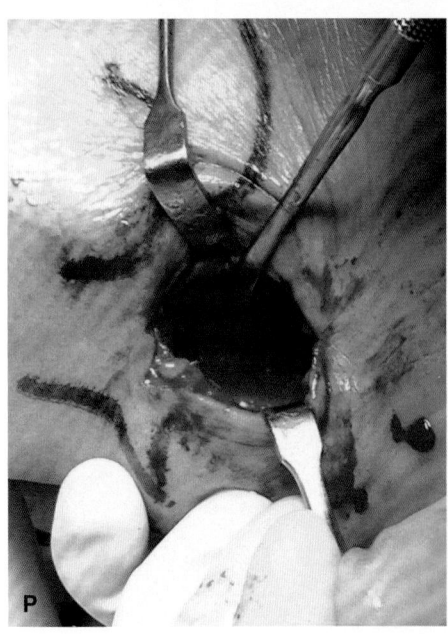

FIGURE 48.29 (*Continued*) **M.** Intra-op view measuring a 1.5-cm gap created in the first MTPJ after removal of the implant and débridement of devitalized bone. **N.** In order to maintain appropriate length of the first ray, an autogenous calcaneal bone graft was procured for the first MTPJ arthrodesis. The incision for harvesting of the bone graft is over the proximal lateral superior calcaneus, posterior to the peroneal tendons and sural nerve and anterior to the Achilles tendon.

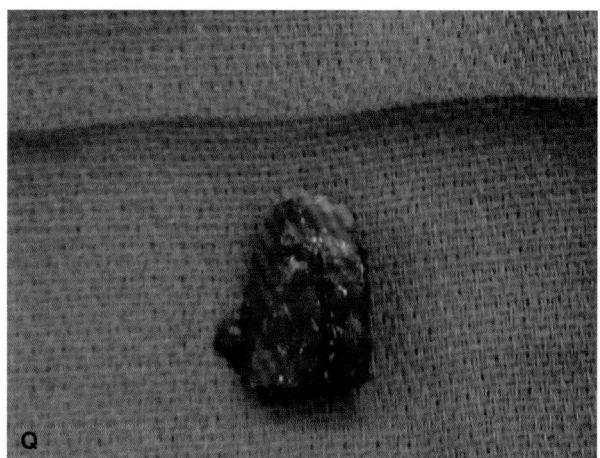

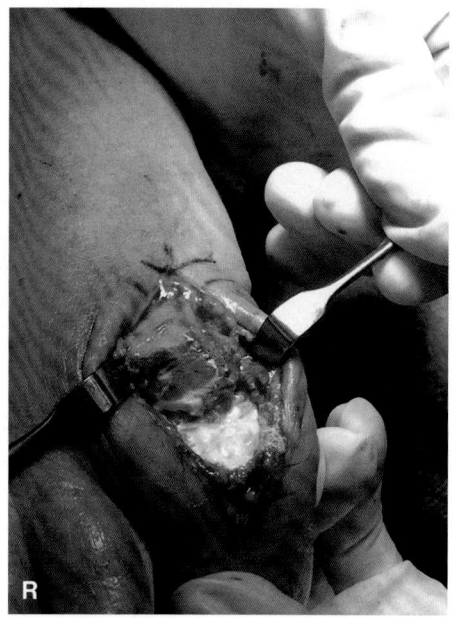

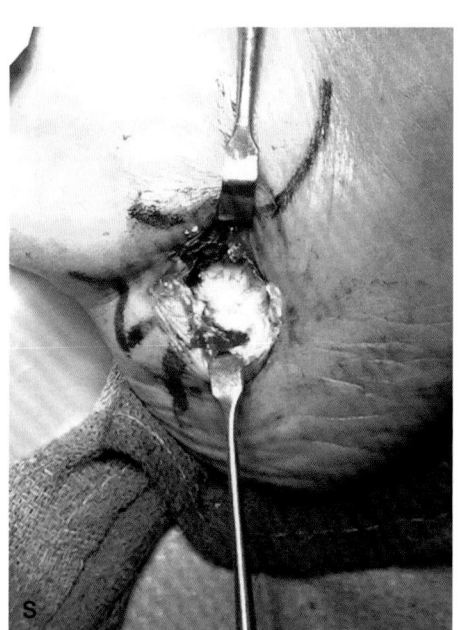

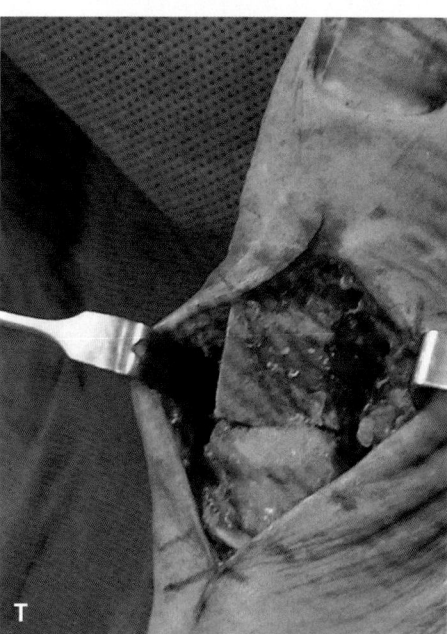

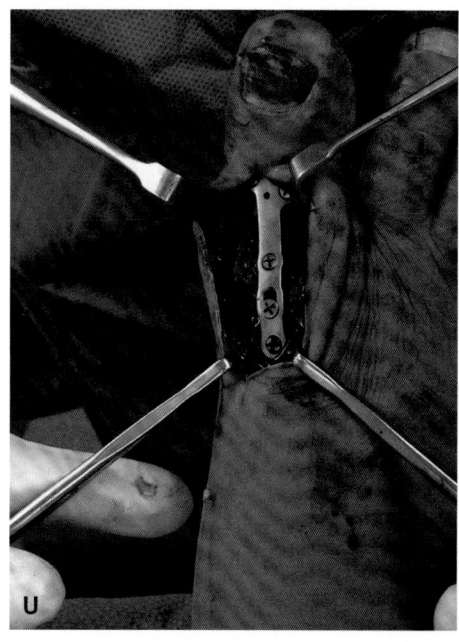

FIGURE 48.29 (*Continued*) **O-Q.** A total of three bone cuts are made in the calcaneus after measuring the proper graft size needed. Two vertical cuts; one proximal and one distal and one horizontal cut connecting the two vertical ones together. Two guide pins are placed along the inferior corners of the osteotomies to ensure proper angulation of the saw. The saw blade is also marked so that the depth of each cut will be the same. A curved osteotome is then utilized to greenstick the superior cortex and the graft should be removed as one whole piece. **R, S.** Bone voids are created at the calcaneal graft donor site and the first metatarsal and hallux where the implant was removed. These voids are backfilled with a tricalcium sulfate bioceramic combined with DBM to aid in healing and help maintain stability. **T, U.** Placement of the calcaneal bone graft in the arthrodesis site, which is secured with plate and screw fixation.

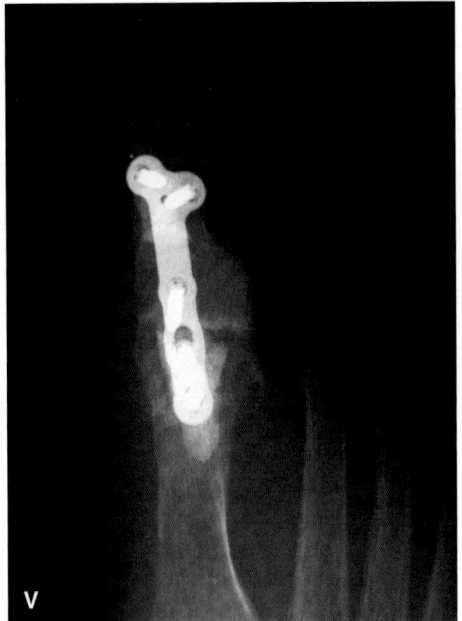

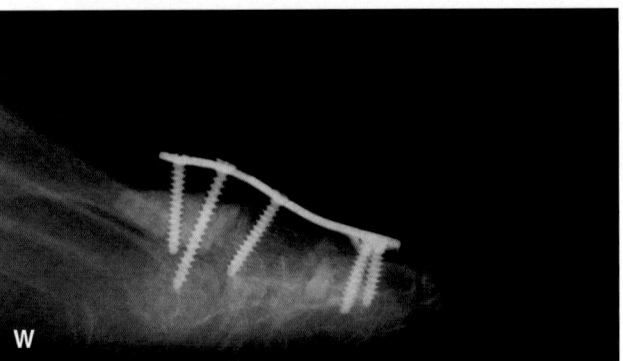

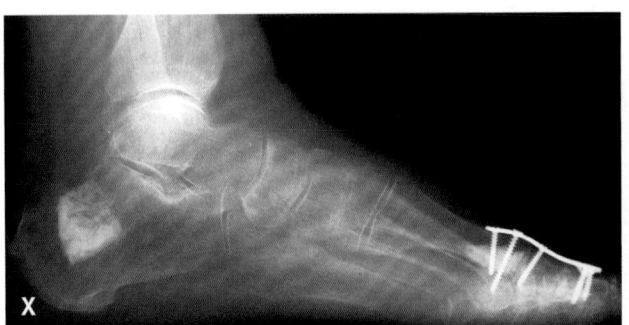

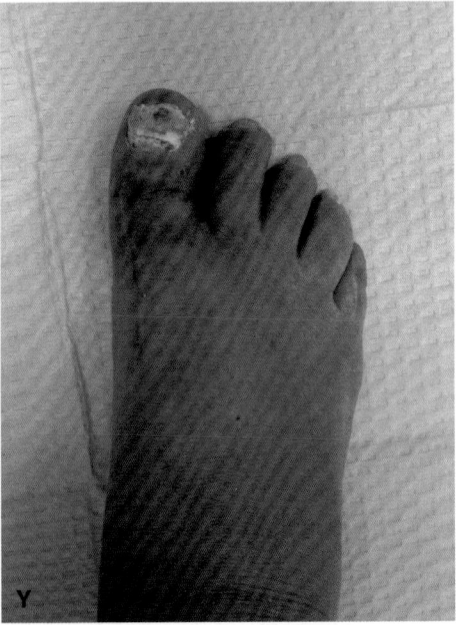

FIGURE 48.29 (*Continued*) **V-X.** Three-month post-op radiographs showing good consolidation of the first MTPJ arthrodesis site with graft incorporation. Increased density and incorporation of the bioceramic and DBM used to fill the voids of the calcaneal graft site and the canals of the first metatarsal and hallux is also seen. **Y.** Post-op clinical photo with good positioning and length of the hallux.

an average of 47 days. They did not conclude, however, that these substances improved the rate of fusion.[180]

Calcium-Based Bioceramics

Calcium-based bioceramics come in many formulations. The most common materials are combinations of hydroxyapatite, tricalcium phosphate, ceramics, fibrillar collagen, and/or coralline hydroxyapatite.[175,181] When selecting a graft, consideration should be given to the calcium-phosphate ratio as this dictates its rate of absorption. When used for filling a bone void,

rate of resorption cannot exceed the rate of bone deposition. Products with a ratio of 1.5-1.67 are most widely accepted. Pore size of the graft is also critical to allow influx of appropriate cells and growth factors and subsequent osteogenesis.[182] Pores of 300 μm or greater have yielded better angiogenesis and healing.[183] In a study of 267 long bone fractures, no difference in results or radiographic parameters were noted when comparing these grafts with iliac crest bone graft. They also noted decreased operative time as there was no harvest involved with use of the bone graft substitute.[177] Numerous studies support these compounds as safe, viable alternatives to fill bone voids

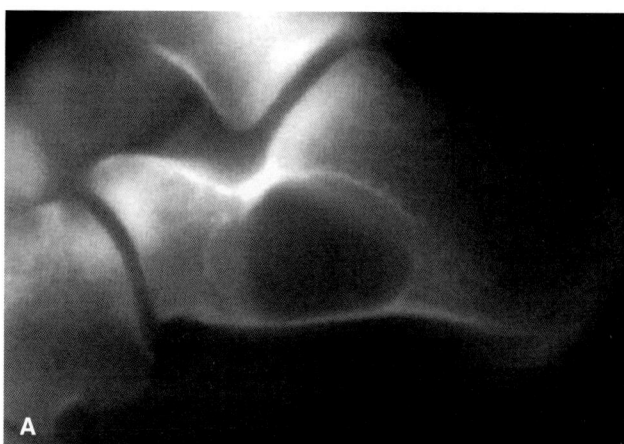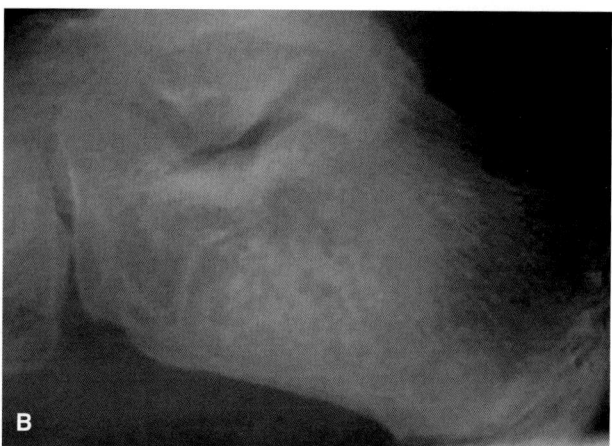

FIGURE 48.30 A, B. A calcaneal bone cyst filled with tricalcium phosphate bioceramic. This is an excellent orthobiologic to fill large voids as it acts as a scaffold for osseous incorporation.

at surgical sites and to act as a scaffold for healing and incorporation[176,177,184] (Figs. 48.30 and 48.31). Calcium sulfate and calcium phosphate in combination may yield greater compressive strength as shown in an animal study by Urban, with noted properties similar to bone.[185] Hydroxyapatite is one of the most commonly used synthetic calcium-based compounds. Its porous surface allows ingrowth and development of new bone, which, once incorporated, can tolerate loading.[181] Bioceramics may serve a dual purpose as they can be combined with antibiotics to treat infection while serving as a filler. Several studies have reported on the efficacy of antibiotic impregnated bioceramics and/or DBM in promoting healing, treating infection, and decreasing the need for autogenous graft.[186–189] Additionally,

these materials may offer an advantage over polymethylmethacrylate beads, as they are absorbable and do not necessitate removal.

Bioglass

Bioactive glass is a solid, nonporous, inorganic material comprised of calcium, phosphorous, and silicon dioxide. It demonstrates both osteoconductive and osteointegrative properties by binding with hydroxyapatite forming a scaffold for healing, which is subsequently resorbed during the bone deposition process. The calcium phosphate deposition attracts osteoblasts. This in turn results in electrical

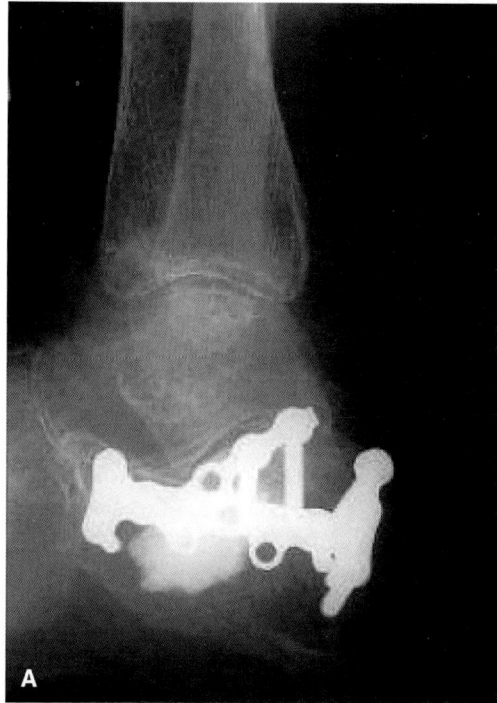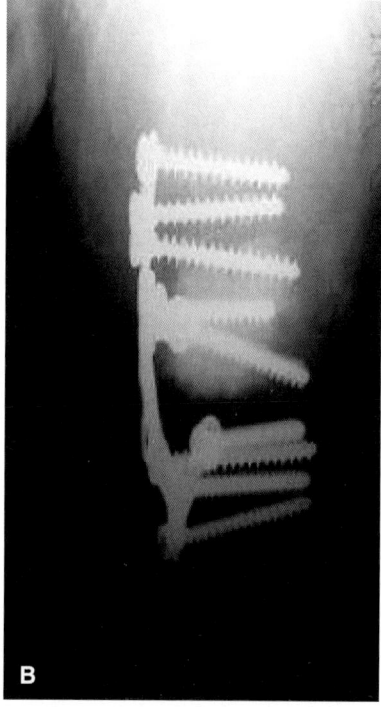

FIGURE 48.31 A, B. ORIF of a calcaneal fracture. Unfortunately, there was significant bone loss, so the void was backfilled with tricalcium sulfate bioceramic combined with DBM.

bone growth stimulation.[190] There are several studies examining its use in other anatomic locations, particularly the lumbar spine; however, research pertaining to the lower extremities is more limited. Shi and colleagues noted a 25% nonunion rate in 48 joints supplemented with bioactive glass with a mean interval to union of 13.2 ± 2 weeks. A total of 66.7% of the nonunions involved the ankle joint, with the majority of these cases being revisional. Risk factors for nonunion were identified as previous history of revision and age >65 years.[190] Over the last several years, research has looked into introduction of additional properties, such as antimicrobial activity, to bioactive glass. Some traditional compositions had noted antimicrobial properties; however, addition of ions such as silver, copper, and strontium impart additional bactericidal activity and possibly enhance bone tissue regeneration. However, the compositional change may affect the degradation rate.[191] Godoy-Santos et al. presented a case study of a staged reconstruction of a Charcot foot with use of bioactive glass, noting complete bone healing and incorporation of the bioactive glass. They advocate its use in the setting of limb salvage to aid with bone void filling and fighting infection.[192]

OSTEOGENIC MATERIALS

Mesenchymal Stem Cells

Osteogenesis is the formation of new bone through proliferation and development of osteoblasts and other precursor cells. Only tissue and bone from the host have this specific property. Autograft harvest may not be an option for some patients; however, combining an osteoinductive or osteoconductive orthobiologic with the patient's own stem cells may be a viable option. MSC can differentiate into osteoblasts and chondroblasts. A common source of MSCs is bone marrow aspirate (BMA). BMA can be harvested from various locations, with numerous options in the lower extremity. While the option exists for the BMA to be harvested and undergo additional processes including expansion, more often, this is something that is typically harvested and applied in the same surgery. The proximal or distal tibia metaphyses are popular sites for harvest, which can be accomplished with the use of a Jamshidi needle and syringe. The BMA is often then combined with DBM or a calcium-based bioceramic. Allogeneic MSCs are available for use, and in large quantities, however, there is always a chance for cross-reactivity. Studies have shown low potential for rejection, as well as noting a high content of viable cells at time of implantation with resultant osteogenesis.[193–195] Melick and colleagues reviewed use of MSC in the foot and ankle, noting potential for use in patients with osteoarthritis, rheumatoid arthritis, and other degenerative processes to mitigate inflammation and promote new cartilage growth.[196] Some advocate for intra-articular injection of MSCs as this would allow for a more direct effect on a pathologic area. In a 2016 study, Lamo-Espinosa et al. report on intra-articular knee injection with MSC-based compounds in different concentrations. Patients were noted to have increased range of motion, decreased pain, and improved function with no adverse events noted.[197] Another study was performed by Vega and colleagues, noting similar findings and improved cartilage on MRI.[198] Studies focal to the foot and ankle have demonstrated improved pain and functional outcomes in ankle arthritis patients treated with MSC injections as an ancillary procedure coupled with surgical interventions as opposed to surgery alone.[199,200] Hernigou et al. investigated use in relation to talar AVN noting improved pain and less frequent talar collapse. Those who went on to talar collapse and arthrodesis demonstrated faster healing.[201]

Orthobiologics are an important addition to the foot and ankle surgeon's arsenal. These products should always be considered as a complement to proper surgical principles and construct, not a substitute. Autogenous bone still remains the gold standard due to its osteogenic, inductive, and conductive properties. If autograft is not an option and allograft is intended for use, consideration should be given to combining it with an orthobiologic. Osseous healing relies on intrinsic and extrinsic factors, including a stable hardware construct, adequate nutritional and vascular status, and proper surgical technique. When all necessary factors are not present, nonunion may result. Understanding the mechanisms of bony healing contributes to the selection of available orthobiologics, which give the foot and ankle surgeon additional tools to enhance the healing process.

MALUNION

Deformity is invariably associated with nonunion in the foot and ankle. In addition to addressing nonunion, surgeries must also address any deformity and malunion present. Malunion can result either from initial surgical positioning or it can be an eventual development over time secondary to a failed union or potentially noncompliance of the patient in the postoperative period (Fig. 48.32). If malalignment is not corrected, there will be an unevenly distributed amount of stress across the nonunion site and there will be an increased risk of nonhealing once again.

While each physician may have a slightly different set of criteria, a malunion is any osteotomy or fusion that has healed in

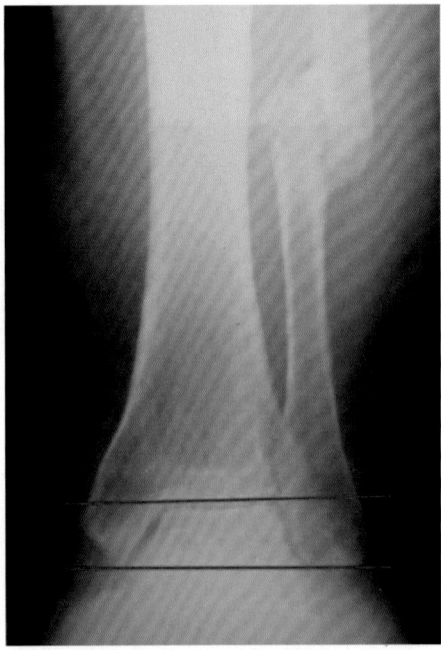

FIGURE 48.32 Fibular malunion. There is lateral displacement and significant shortening.

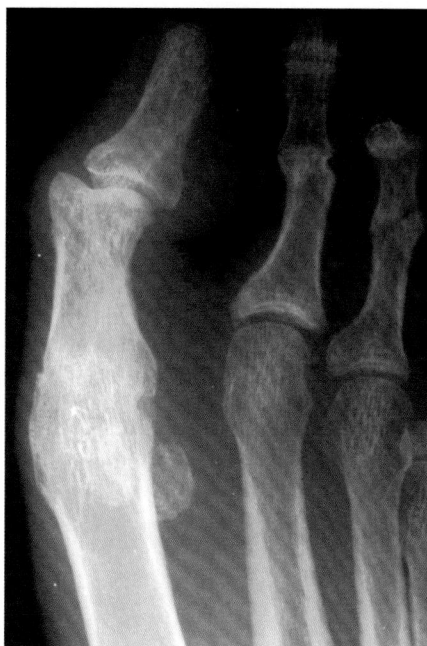

FIGURE 48.33 Although the first MTPJ arthrodesis has complete consolidation and the joint is in rectus alignment, there is significant abduction at the hallux interphalangeal joint (IPJ). The hallux could have been fused in a more abducted position to try to avoid the adaptation of the surrounding joint.

a poor position, potentially undercorrecting deformity or creating new deformity that may be symptomatic or impeding function.[202] Depending on the anatomic location, some malunions may be more symptomatic than others and may require immediate management, while others may be subtler or not have an effect on the patient's overall functional capacity. General principles and definitions exist for optimal positions for some procedures; however, it would be difficult to find a set of fixed guidelines for positioning of fusions or osteotomies that could

be adhered to universally. As surgeons, we often have to adapt to the individual patient's anatomy.[202]

Looking at common procedural sites, several points can be made. Involving the first MTPJ, the classic triad for positioning is between 5 and 15 degrees of dorsiflexion, 5-10 degrees of abduction, and no frontal plane rotation. Sagittal plane positioning is critical and malunion in the sagittal plane will be apparent when assessing function postoperatively. Failure to correct the deformity and position in any of the planes could be considered a malunion[202] (Figs. 48.33 and 48.34). First metatarsal osteotomies may be considered a malunion if there is failure to correct or overcorrect in the transverse plane, as well as if there is alteration to the sagittal plane alignment (Fig. 48.35). Recurrence of deformity does not automatically constitute a malunion.

First TMTJ arthrodeses have a higher risk of malposition in the sagittal plane (Figs. 48.36 and 48.37). If attention is not paid to the first MTPJ and TMTJ when positioning the fusion site, resultant deformity may occur. For example, malposition resulting in dorsiflexion of the distal metatarsal can result in first MTPJ jamming as well as compensatory pronation to get the medial column down to the ground. By contrast, excessive plantar flexion will create a metatarsus primus equinus with subsequent supinatory compensation, assuming that motion is available at the subtalar joint.[202]

Subtalar malposition is often frontal plane dominant. Patients who have significant deformity preoperatively may be at higher risk for this. Traditionally, 0-5 degrees of valgus is recommended to allow for some adaptability. To fuse the joint in >5 degrees of valgus, or potentially worse in varus, has a higher likelihood to cause greater functional problems for the patient. Any deviation from neutral sagittal, slight valgus frontal, and slight external rotation positioning will have lasting consequences for the patient secondary to proximal and distal compensation.[202,203]

Ankle malunion may be seen in instances such as ankle fractures or fusions (Fig. 48.38). For patients with ankle fractures requiring surgical intervention, restoration of anatomic

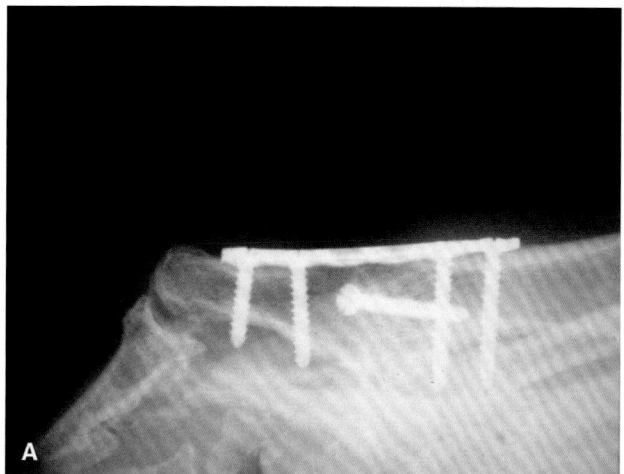

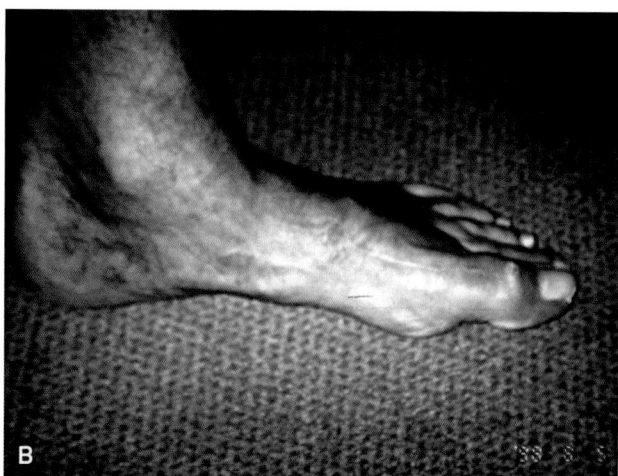

FIGURE 48.34 **A, B.** Radiograph and clinical photo showing complete consolidation of the first MTPJ arthrodesis; however, the hallux was fused in too much dorsiflexion so there is subluxation and plantar flexion at the hallux IPJ to accommodate for this position. Notice the skin irritation at the dorsal hallux IPJ.

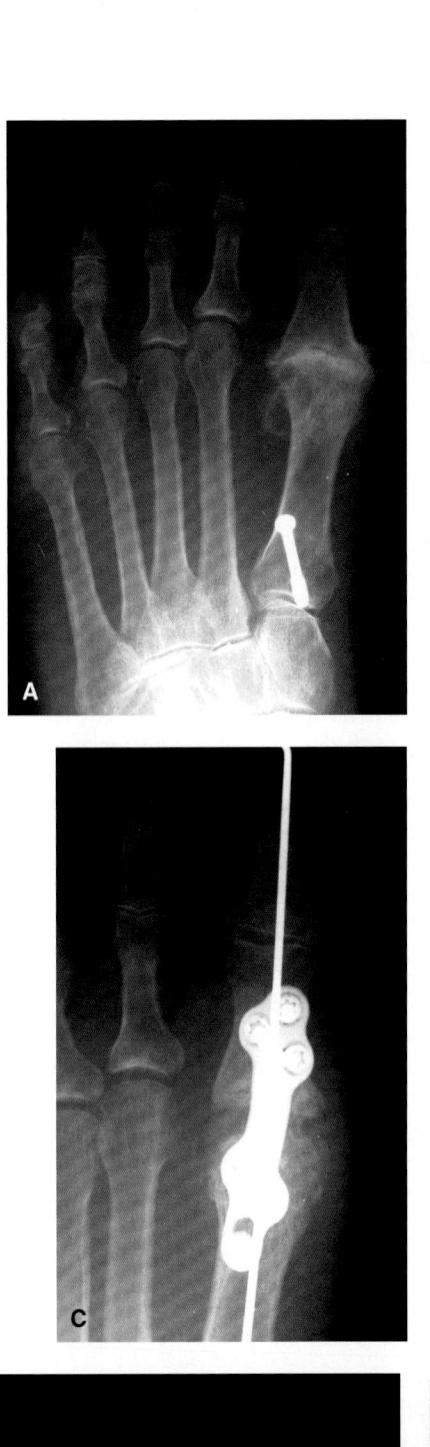

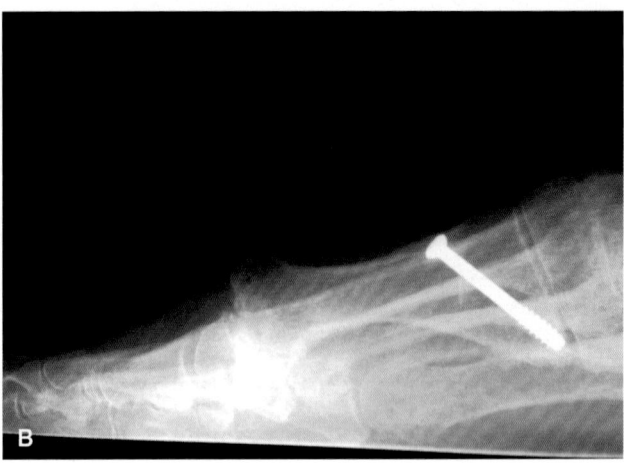

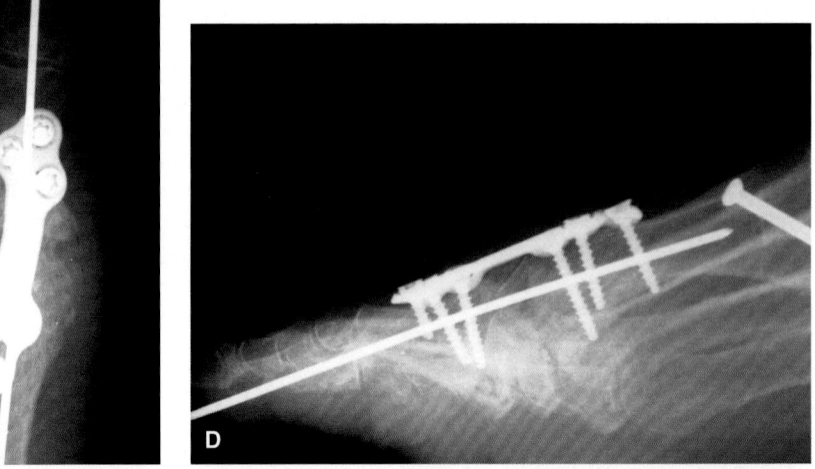

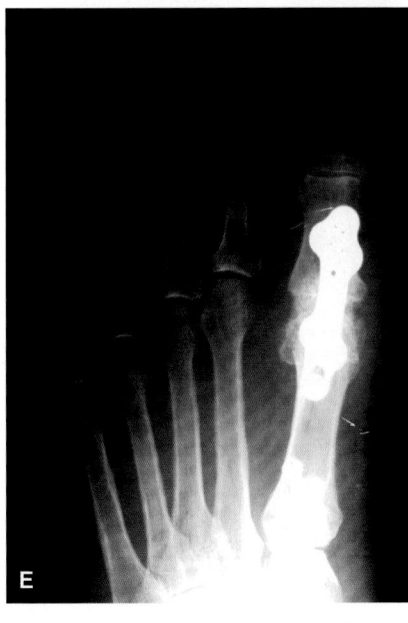

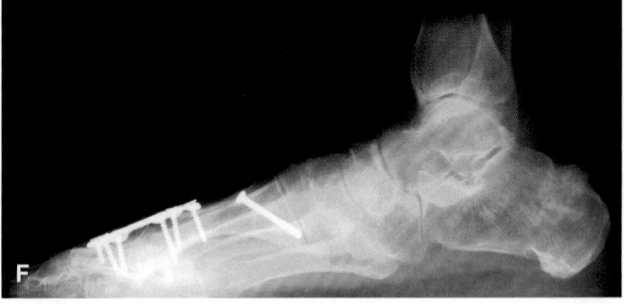

FIGURE 48.35 A, B. A crescentic osteotomy was performed on the first metatarsal base over 15 years ago producing significant dorsiflexion of the first metatarsal. This resulted in hallux limitus and significant degeneration of the first MTPJ. **C, D.** Post-op radiographs of revisional surgery with a first MTPJ arthrodesis with autogenous calcaneal bone graft. Realignment of the first MTPJ was restored. **E, F.** Three months post-op with consolidation of the first MTPJ arthrodesis and calcaneal graft site. The first MTPJ alignment remains good.

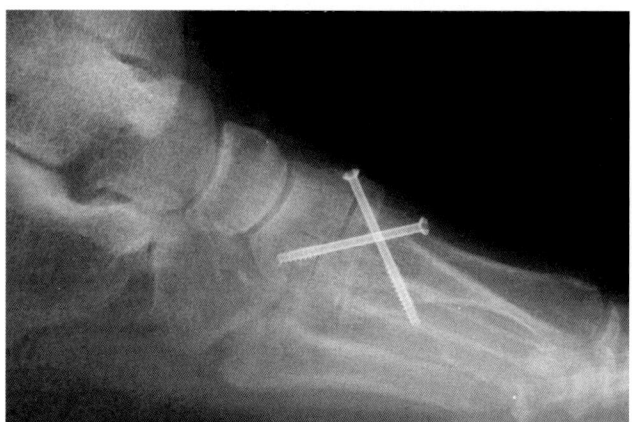

FIGURE 48.36 Elevation of the first metatarsal after a first metatarsal cuneiform arthrodesis. This can produce lesser metatarsalgia and hallux limitus.

alignment is paramount. Fixation in a malaligned position, whether it be the medial or lateral malleolus, can lead to significant planal deformities. Failure to reduce a lateral malleolar fracture may lead to healing in a shortened position and resultant tipping of the ankle into a valgus orientation. This compensation can lead to additional pathologies and symptoms.[204] A similar malunion may occur in nonoperatively managed ankle fractures. When it comes to ankle fusions, triplanar positioning standards include neutral sagittal plane alignment with slight external rotation and valgus of no more than 5 degrees. Again, deviation from these parameters will result in proximal and distal compensation.[202]

Malunion is typically a result of iatrogenic factors and, as illustrated above, patient outcomes are largely dependent on surgeon technique and experience. Prevention from the surgeon's standpoint includes careful preparation of the surgical site, ensuring proper alignment with use of visual inspection and fluoroscopy, and rigid internal fixation. Knowing the patient's preoperative anatomy and anticipating ahead of time what difficulties may be encountered is critical. This may include the need to recommend adjunctive procedures or grafting in the preoperative planning phase. However, malunions may also be the result of an insult to the area in the postoperative period. Patient noncompliance may contribute to failure at a surgical site. Maintaining a prescribed weight-bearing status may be extremely difficult for patients to adhere to, especially non–weight bearing. Despite proper fixation and casting, excessive loading, tension, or shear forces at a surgical site may result in disruption and malalignment.

Once a malunion has occurred, the first step in addressing the issue is to have an open and honest conversation with the patient to review the current problem, why it might have occurred, and how to best treat it. Depending on the severity and symptoms associated with the malunion, some patients may be able to be managed conservatively. This would come in the form of orthotic options, mostly for forefoot and midfoot malunions, to accommodate/alleviate resultant biomechanical imbalances. Heel lifts may be added for an ankle in plantar flexion and bracing may be used for rearfoot and ankle malposition.[202]

While conservative options are usually trialed first, surgery may be required either in the more immediate or delayed setting. In the instance of noncompliance in the early postoperative period with gross displacement or failure, corrective surgery would often be pursued right away. Those patients who have a healed, malunited site, and failed conservative management, may be counseled on a revisional procedure at that time. In preparation for revisional surgery, great care must be taken to

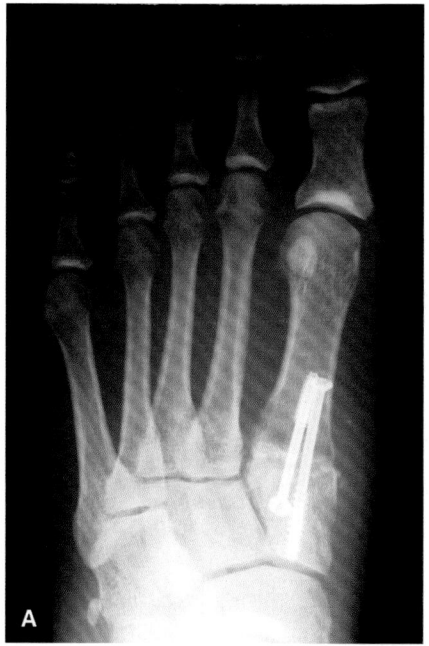
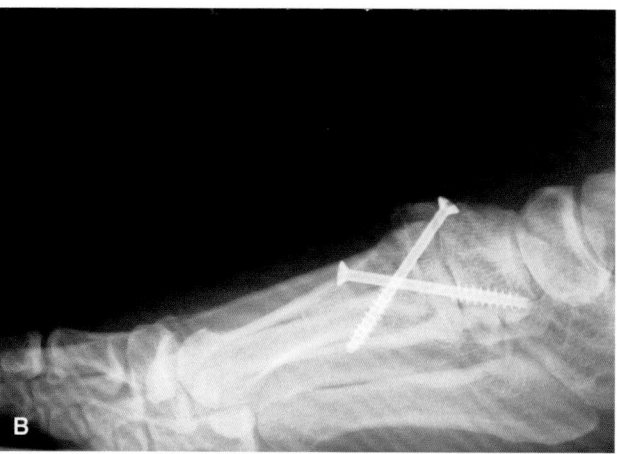

FIGURE 48.37 A, B. Although dorsiflexion of the first metatarsal is more common with a first metatarsal cuneiform arthrodesis, plantar flexion following this procedure can occur as well, and can produce significant sesamoiditis. Also, notice the genetic absence of the tibial sesamoid.

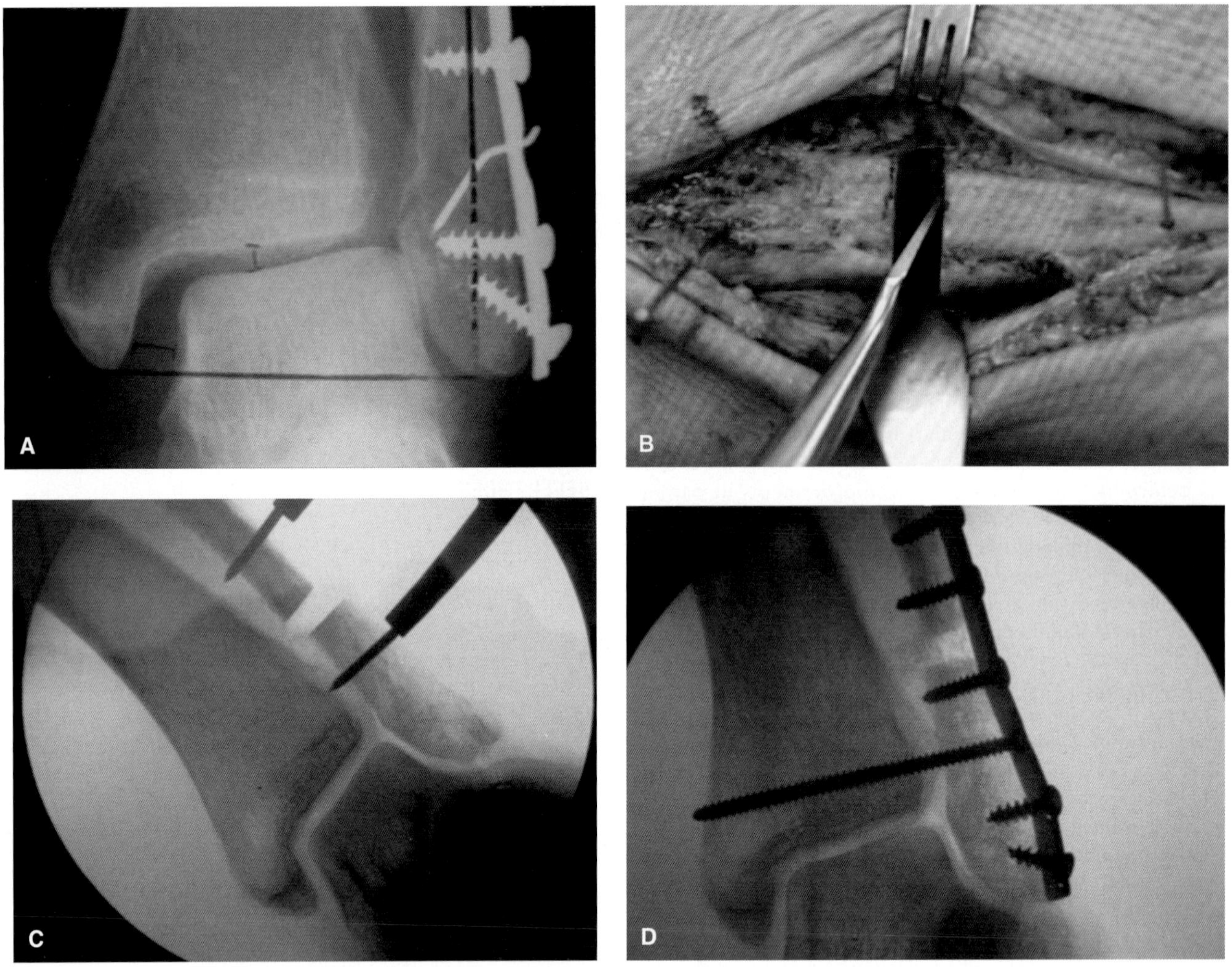

FIGURE 48.38 **A.** Ankle valgus has resulted after ORIF of the fibula. **B, C.** An osteotomy is made in the fibula, and it is lengthened and held in proper position to correct for the ankle valgus. **D.** The post-op radiograph shows good alignment of the ankle joint. A corticocancellous allogeneic bone graft was placed in the fibular gap. Fixation of the syndesmosis was also warranted to maintain full correction of the malunion.

thoroughly evaluate the clinical and radiographic deformity. Identifying the center of rotation and angulation (CORA) of the deformity is also essential, as the corrective osteotomy should be planned so that the point of rotation of the osteotomy is as close to the CORA as possible to maximize correction. This may be in the form of a closing or opening wedge osteotomy, with the latter requiring additional planning for graft placement[202] (Fig. 48.39). Additionally, in the preoperative planning phase, adjunctive procedures beyond a correctional osteotomy may need to be performed. For example, patients who have been in a deformed position for some time have likely acquired soft tissue adaptation where a capsule release, tendon lengthening, or potentially a tarsal tunnel release might be required to allow for reduction of the deformity and prevent excessive traction on a neurovascular bundle once the new position is acquired.

As with nonunion surgery, débridement of the site to healthy bone, confirming restored alignment and applying an appropriate fixation construct are paramount to success. Patients should be counseled thoroughly on postoperative expectations, and

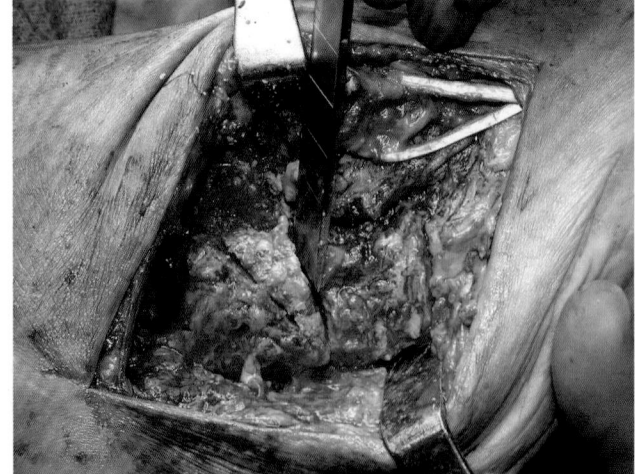

FIGURE 48.39 Wedge resection performed in order to restore proper joint alignment.

they should be made aware that that they are prone to a higher rate of complication. Perfect alignment may not be achieved, a length discrepancy may exist, and they may still require bracing or orthoses.[202,203]

In order to maximize surgical success, it is imperative to correct all angular deformities and neutralize any deforming forces. Nonunion, continued pain, and subsequent deformities are highly likely when malalignment is present. Guo and colleagues published a study in 2017 examining realignment surgery in malunited ankle fractures. They noted statistically significant improvements in tibiotalar tilt angle, tibial anterior surface angle, and AOFAS and VAS scores, concluding that realignment surgery can decrease pain, improve function, and delay onset of arthrosis, which might necessitate fusion or implant.[204] In a 2018 study, Guo et al. advocated for a combined supramalleolar and intra-articular osteotomy for treatment of malunited medial impacted ankle fractures associated with varus deformity. They noted similar improvements in parameters of the 2017 study.[205] A surgeon should be able to recognize the presence of malalignment, determine the etiology, understand the consequences of not addressing these deformities, and be able to treat them appropriately, so that the best patient outcome can be obtained.

POSTOPERATIVE MANAGEMENT

Revisional nonunion and malunion surgeries typically require extended periods of non–weight bearing. Since many of these surgeries utilize bone grafts and bone grafting materials, healing time is often lengthened for full graft incorporation. It is helpful to obtain a physical therapy consultation preoperatively for gait training so the patient will have the necessary assistive device, to help reduce/eliminate pressure and weight on the affected extremity after the surgery. Oftentimes, this is a combination of knee walkers and wheelchairs for full compliance. Deep venous thrombosis prophylaxis may be recommended and is dictated by the patient's risk factors. When employed, the authors recommend continued prophylaxis during the entire period of immobilization. Also, any risk factors addressed preoperatively, such as elevated blood glucose, calcium deficiencies, and smoking should continue to be addressed postoperatively. Bone growth stimulators, in addition to being utilized as an adjunct to conservative therapy preoperatively, can also be utilized to aid in healing postoperatively. Progression of union should be monitored closely with serial radiographs and advanced imaging if necessary.

CONCLUSION

Nonunion and malunion of a fracture, osteotomy, or arthrodesis site are not uncommon and are potential complications that every surgeon should be able to diagnose and treat appropriately. Successful management of these entities requires an understanding of basic bone healing and appropriate evaluation of the risk factors involved with the nonunion and/or malunion, including both patient-dependent and iatrogenic causes. The etiology of the nonunion/malunion needs to be identified so that it can be corrected, and a comprehensive treatment plan implemented. For hypervascular nonunions, with stable fixation, and good alignment, immobilization and possible bone stimulation may be all that is warranted to achieve adequate union. In more complex cases, however, or in avascular nonunions, revisional surgery is often necessary. Treating a nonunion and malunion is often a multidisciplinary approach, and the patient must be medically optimized prior to any additional surgery. Surgical revisions can be very complex and the surgeon should have a good plan with the availability of various fixation options, and access to bone grafts and bone grafting materials, and should be prepared to address any intraoperative complications that may arise. It is imperative that the patient be well educated as to their prognosis, goals of treatment, and the need for compliance of the chosen treatment plan for the best possible outcome. A comprehensive evaluation and a patient-specific treatment plan will maximize the potential for a successful osseous union and hopefully produce a satisfied patient.

REFERENCES

1. Brinker MR. Nonunions: evaluation and treatment. In: Browner BD, Levine AM, Jupiter JB, Trafton PG, eds. *Skeletal Trauma: Basic Science, Management, and Reconstruction.* 3rd ed. Philadelphia, PA: W.B. Saunders; 2002:507-604.
2. Muller ME, Allgower M, Schneider R, et al. *Manual of Internal Fixation: Techniques Recommended by the AO Group.* 2nd ed. Berlin, Germany: Springer Verlag; 1979.
3. Lack WD, Starman JS, Seymour R, et al. Any cortical bridging predicts healing of tibial shaft fractures. *J Bone Joint Surg Am.* 2014;96(13):1066-1072.
4. Nicoll EA. Fractures of the tibial shaft: a survey of 705 cases. *J Bone Joint Surg Br.* 1964;46:373-387.
5. Crenshaw AH. *Cambells Operative Orthopedics.* Vol. 1. St. Louis, MO: C.V. Mosby; 1974:761.
6. Bishop JA, Palanca AA, Bellino MJ, et al. Assessment of compromised fracture healing. *J Am Acad Orthop Surg.* 2012;20(5):273-282.
7. Mandracchia VJ, Nickles WA, Mandi DM, et al. Treatment of nonunited hindfoot fusions. *Clin Podiatr Med Surg.* 2004;21:417-439.
8. Toolan BC, Sangeorzan BJ, Hansen ST Jr. Complex reconstruction for the treatment of dorso-lateral peritalar subluxation of the foot: early results after distraction arthrodesis of the calca-neocuboid joint in conjunction with stabilization of and transfer of the flexor digitorum longus tendon to the midfoot to treat acquired pes planovalgus in adults. *J Bone Joint Surg Am.* 1999;81:1545-1560.
9. Thevendran G, Shah K, Pinney SJ, et al. Perceived risk factors for nonunion following foot and ankle arthrodesis. *J Orthop Surg.* 2017;25(1):1-6.
10. Klassen LJ, Shi E, Weinraub GM, et al. Comparative nonunion rates in triple arthrodesis. *J Foot Ankle Surg.* 2018;57:1154-1156.
11. Goucher NR, Coughlin MJ. Hallux metatarsophalangeal joint arthrodesis using dome-shaped reamers and dorsal plate fixation: a prospective study. *Foot Ankle Int.* 2006;27(11):869-876.
12. Doty J, Coughlin M, Hirose C, et al. Hallux metatarsophalangeal joint arthrodesis with a hybrid locking plate and a plantar neutralization screw: a prospective study. *Foot Ankle Int.* 2013;34(11):1535-1540.
13. Roukis TS. Nonunion after arthrodesis of the first metatarsalphalangeal joint: a systematic review. *J Foot Ankle Surg.* 2011;50(6):710-713.
14. Catanzariti AR, Mendicino RW, Lee MS, et al. The modified Lapidus arthrodesis: a retrospective analysis. *J Foot Ankle Surg.* 1999;38(5):322-332.
15. Donnenwerth MP, Borkosky SL, Abicht BP, et al. Rate of nonunion after first metatarsal-cuneiform arthrodesis using joint curettage and two crossed compression screw fixation: a systematic review. *J Foot Ankle Surg.* 2011;50(6):707-709.
16. Thompson IM, Bohay DR, Anderson JG. Fusion rate of first tarsometatarsal arthrodesis in the modified Lapidus procedure and flatfoot reconstruction. *Foot Ankle Int.* 2005;26(9):698-703.
17. So E, Wilson MD, Chu AK, et al. Incidence of nonunion of the hallux interphalangeal joint arthrodesis: a systematic review. *J Foot Ankle Surg.* 2018;57:776-780.
18. Weber BG, Cech O. *Pseudarthrosis: Pathophysiology, Biomechanics, Therapy, Results.* New York, NY: Grune and Stratton; 1976.
19. Gudas CJ, Cann JE. Nonunions and related disorders. *Clin Podiatr Med Surg.* 1991;8:321-339.
20. Mandracchia VJ, Nelson SC, Barp EA. Current concepts of bone healing. *Clin Podiatr Med Surg.* 2001;18:55-77.
21. McKibbin B. The biology of fracture healing in long bones. *J Bone Joint Surg Br.* 1978;60(2):150-162.
22. Ham AW. A histological study of the early phases of bone repair. *J Bone Joint Surg Am.* 1990;12(4):827-844.
23. Charnley J. *The Closed Treatment of Closed Fractures.* 3rd ed. Edinburgh and London, UK: E & S Livingston Ltd; 1975.
24. Heppenstall RB. *Fracture Treatment and Healing.* Philadelphia, PA: W.B. Saunders; 1980.
25. Urist MR. Bone formation by autoinduction. *Science.* 1965;150:893.
26. Schenk RK, Willenegger H. Morphological findings in primary fracture healing. *Symp Biol Hung.* 1967;7:75.
27. Wolff J. *The Law of Bone Remodeling (translated from the 1892 original, Das Gesetz der Transformation der Knochen, by P. Maquet and R. Furlong).* Berlin, Germany: Springer Verlag; 1986.

28. Moore KR, Howell MA, Saltrick KR, et al. Risk factors associated with nonunion after elective foot and ankle reconstruction: a case-control study. *J Foot Ankle Surg.* 2017;56:457-462.

29. Thevendran G, Younger A, Pinney S. Current concepts review: risk factors for nonunions in foot and ankle arthrodeses. *Foot Ankle Int.* 2012;33(11):1031-1040.

30. Shibuya N, Humphers JM, Fluhman BL, et al. Factors associated with nonunion, delayed union, and malunion in foot and ankle surgery in diabetic patients. *J Foot Ankle Surg.* 2013;52(2):207-211.

31. Perlman MH, Thordarson DB. Ankle fusion in a high risk population: an assessment of nonunion risk factors. *Foot Ankle Int.* 1999;20:491-496.

32. Loder RT: The influence of diabetes mellitus on the healing of closed fractures. *Clin Orthop Relat Res.* 1988;232:210-216.

33. Zura R, Mehta S, Della Rocca GJ, et al. Biological risk factors for nonunion of bone fracture. *J Bone Joint Surg Rev.* 2016;4(1):e2.

34. Hernandez RK, Do TP, Critchlow CW, et al. Patient-related risk factors for fracture-healing complications in the United Kingdom General Practice Research Database. *Acta Orthop.* 2012;83(6):653-660.

35. Namkung-Matthai H, Appleyard R, Jansen J, et al. Osteoporosis influences the early period of fracture healing in a rat osteoporotic model. *Bone.* 2001;28:80-86.

36. Walsh WR, Sherman P, Howlett CR, et al. Fracture healing in a rat osteopenia model. *Clin Orthop Relat Res.* 1997;342:218-227.

37. Parker MJ. Prediction of fracture union after internal fixation of intracapsular femoral neck fractures. *Injury.* 1994;25(suppl 2):3-6.

38. Nikolaou VS, Efstathopoulos N, Kontakis G, et al. The influence of osteoporosis in femoral fracture healing time. *Injury.* 2009;40(6):663-668.

39. Anderson T, Linder L, Rydholm U, et al. Tibio-calcaneal arthrodesis as a primary procedure using a retrograde intramedullary nail: a prospective study of 26 patients with rheumatoid arthritis. *Acta Orthop.* 2005;76(4):580-587.

40. Anderson T, Maxander P, Rydholm U, et al. Ankle arthrodesis by compression screws in rheumatoid arthritis: primary nonunion in 9/35 patients. *Acta Orthop.* 2005;76(6):884-890.

41. Cracchiolo A III, Cimino WR, Lian G. Arthrodesis of the ankle in patients who have rheumatoid arthritis. *J Bone Joint Surg Am.* 1992;74(6):903-909.

42. Fujimori J, Yoshino S, Koiwa M, et al. Ankle arthrodesis in rheumatoid arthritis using an intramedullary nail with fins. *Foot Ankle Int.* 1999;20(8):485-490.

43. Knupp M, Skoog A, Tornkvist H, et al. Triple arthrodesis in rheumatoid arthritis. *Foot Ankle Int.* 2008;29(3):293-297.

44. Agarwal V, Joseph B. Non-union in osteogenesis imperfecta. *J Pediatr Orthop B.* 2005;14(6):451-455.

45. Ishikawa SN, Murphy FA, Richardson EG. The effect of cigarette smoking on hindfoot fusions. *Foot Ankle Int.* 2002;23:996-998.

46. Schmitz MA, Finnegan M, Natarajan R, et al. Effect of smoking on tibial shaft fracture healing. *Clin Orthop Relat Res.* 1999;365:184-200.

47. Chahal J, Stephen DJG, Bulmer B, et al. Factors associated with outcome after subtalar arthrodesis. *J Orthop Trauma.* 2006;20(8):555-561.

48. Castillo RC, Bosse MJ, MacKenzie EJ. Fracture healing and risk of complications in limb-threatening open tibia fractures. *J Orthop Trauma.* 2005;19:151-157.

49. Cobb TK, Gabrielsen TA, Campbell DC, et al. Cigarette smoking and non-union after ankle arthrodesis. *Foot Ankle Int.* 1994;15(2):64-67.

50. Easley M, Trnka HJ, Schon LC, et al. Isolated subtalar arthrodesis. *J Bone Joint Surg Am.* 2000;82:613.

51. Friday KE, Howard GA. Ethanol inhibits human bone cell proliferation and function in vitro. *Metabolism.* 1991;40:562-565.

52. Chakkalakal DA, Novak JR, Fritz ED, et al. Inhibition of bone repair in a rat model for chronic and excessive alcohol consumption. *Alcohol.* 2005;36(3):201-214.

53. Nyquist F, Halvorsen V, Madsen JE, et al. Ethanol and its effects on fracture healing and bone mass in male rats. *Acta Orthop Scand.* 1999;70:212-216.

54. Thevendran G, Wang C, Pinney SJ, et al. Nonunion risk assessment in foot and ankle surgery: proposing a predictive risk assessment model. *Foot Ankle Int.* 2015;36(8):901-907.

55. Blitz NM, Lee T, Williams K, et al. Early weight bearing after modified Lapidus arthrodesis: a multicenter review of 80 cases. *J Foot Ankle Surg.* 2010;49(4):357-362.

56. Lampe HI, Fontijne P, van Linge B. Weight bearing after arthrodesis of the first metatarsophalangeal joint. A randomized study of 61 cases. *Acta Orthop Scand.* 1991;62(6):544-545.

57. Kawaguchi H, Pilbeam CC, Harrison JR, et al. The role of prostaglandins in the regulation of bone metabolism. *Clin Orthop Relat Res.* 1995;313:36-46.

58. Simon AM, Manigrasso MB, O'Connor JP. Cyclooxygenase 2 function is essential for bone fracture healing. *J Bone Miner Res.* 2002;17:963-976.

59. Adolphson P, Abbaszadegan H, Jonsson U, et al. No effects of piroxicam on osteopaenia and recovery after Colles' fracture. A randomized, double-blind, placebo controlled prospective trial. *Arch Orthop Trauma Surg.* 1993;112:127-130.

60. Bhattacharyya T, Levin R, Vrahas M, et al. Nonsteroidal anti-inflammatory drugs and non-union of humeral shaft fractures. *Arthritis Care Res.* 2005;53(3):364-367.

61. Giannoudis PV, MacDonald DA, Matthews SJ, et al. Nonunion of the femoral diaphysis. The influence of reaming and non-steroidal anti-inflammatory drugs. *J Bone Joint Surg Br.* 2000;82(5):655-658.

62. Reuben SS. Considerations in the use of COX-2 inhibitors in spinal fusion surgery. *Anesth Analg.* 2001;93:798-804.

63. Solomon DH, Hochberg MC, Mogun H, et al. The relation between bisphosphonate use and non-union of fractures of the humerus in older adults. *Osteoporosis Int.* 2009;20:895-901.

64. Lyles KW, Colon-Emeric CS, Magaziner JS, et al. Zoledronic acid and clinical fractures and mortality after hip fracture. *N Engl J Med.* 2007;357(18):1799-1809.

65. Jacobsen KA, Al Aqi ZS, Wan C, et al. Bone formation during distraction osteogenesis is dependent on both VEGFR1 and VEGFR2 signalling. *J Bone Miner Res.* 2008;23(5):596-609.

66. Keramaris NC, Calori GM, Nikolaou VS, et al. Fracture vascularity and bone healing: a systematic review of the role of VEGF. *Injury.* 2008;39:S2, S45-S57.

67. Perren SM. Physical and biological aspects of fractures healing with special reference to internal fixation. *Clin Orthop Relat Res.* 1979;138:175-196.

68. Perren SM. Evolution of internal fixation of long bone fractures. The scientific basis of biological internal fixation: choosing a new balance between stability and biology. *J Bone Joint Surg Br.* 2002;84(8):1093-1110.

69. Hak DJ, Toker S, Yi C, et al. The influence of fracture fixation biomechanics on fracture healing. *Orthopedics.* 2010;33(10):752-755.

70. Hope M, Savva N, Whitehouse S. Is it necessary to re-fuse a non-union of a hallux metatarsophalangeal joint arthrodesis? *Foot Ankle Int.* 2010;31(8):662-669.

71. Baldwin KD, Babatunde OM, Russell Huffman G, et al. Open fractures of the tibia in the pediatric population: a systematic review. *J Child Orthop.* 2009;3(3):199-208.

72. Dingemans SA, Backes M, Goslings JC, et al. Predictors of nonunion and infectious complications in patients with posttraumatic subtalar arthrodesis. *J Orthop Trauma.* 2016;30:e331-e335.

73. Catanzariti A, Moore K. Complication management: nonunions. In: Lee MS, Grossman JP, eds. *Complications in Foot and Ankle Surgery.* Cham, Switzerland: Springer; 2017:29-53.

74. Rabjohn L, Roberts K, Troiano M, et al. Diagnostic and prognostic value of erythrocyte sedimentation rate in contiguous osteomyelitis of the foot and ankle. *J Foot Ankle Surg.* 2007;46(4):230-237.

75. Fleischer AE, Didyk AA, Woods JB, et al. Combined clinical and laboratory testing improves diagnostic accuracy for osteomyelitis in the diabetic foot. *J Foot Ankle Surg.* 2009;48(1):39-46.

76. Stucken C, Olszewski DC, Creevy WR, et al. Preoperative diagnosis of infection in patients with nonunions. *J Bone Joint Surg Am.* 2013;95(15):1409-1412.

77. Coughlin MJ, Grimes JS, Traughber PD, et al. Comparison of radiographs and CT scans in the prospective evaluation of the fusion of hindfoot arthrodesis. *Foot Ankle Int.* 2006;27(10):780-787.

78. Krause F, Younger ASE, Baumhauer JF, et al. Clinical outcomes of nonunions of hindfoot and ankle fusions. *J Bone Joint Surg Am.* 2016;98:2006-2016.

79. Jones C, Coughlin M, Shurnas P. Prospective CT scan evaluation of hindfoot non-unions treated with revision surgery and low-intensity ultrasound stimulation. *Foot Ankle Int.* 2006;27(4):229-235.

80. Buchan CA, Pearce DH, Lau J, et al. Imaging of postoperative avascular necrosis of the ankle and foot. *Semin Musculoskelet Radiol.* 2012;16(3):192-204.

81. Solicito V, Jacobs AM, Oloff L, et al. The use of radionucleotide bone and joint imaging in arthritic and related diseases. *J Foot Ankle Surg.* 1984;23(2):173-182.

82. Visser HJ, Jacons AM, Oloff LM, et al. The use of differential scintigraphy in the clinical diagnosis of osseous and soft tissue changes affecting the diabetic foot. *J Foot Surg.* 1984;23(1):74-85.

83. Mont MA, Ulrich SD, Seyler TM, et al. Bone scanning of limited value for diagnosis of symptomatic oligofocal and multifocal osteonecrosis. *J Rheumatol.* 2008;35(8):1629-1634.

84. Weber BG, Brunner C. The treatment of nonunions without electrical stimulation. *Clin Orthop.* 1981;161:24-32.

85. Cook JJ, Summers NJ, Cook EA. Healing in the new millennium: bone stimulators. An overview of where we've been and where we may be heading. *Clin Podiatr Med Surg.* 2015;32:45-59.

86. Latham W, Lau JTC. Bone stimulation: a review of its use as an adjunct. *Tech Orthop.* 2011;26:14-21.

87. Ramanujam CL, Belczyk R, Zgonis T. Bone growth stimulation for foot and ankle nonunions. *Clin Podiatr Med Surg.* 2009;26:607-618.

88. Peltier LF. A brief historical note on the use electricity in the treatment of fractures. *Clin Orthop.* 1981;161:4-7.

89. Lente RW. Cases of un-united fracture treated by electricity. *NY State J Med.* 1850;5:317-319.

90. Fukada E, Yasuda I. On the piezoelectric effect of bone. *J Phys Soc Japan.* 1957;12:1158-1162.

91. Brand RA. Biographical sketch: Julius Wolff, 1036-1902. *Clin Orthop.* 2010;468:1047-1049.

92. Pollack SR. Bioelectric properties of bone. Endogenous electrical signals. *Orthop Clin North Am.* 1984;15:3-14.

93. Bodamyali T, Kanczler SM, Simon B, et al. Pulsed electromagnetic fields simultaneously induce osteogenesis and upregulate transcription of bone morphogenic proteins 2 and 4 in rat osteoblasts in vitro. *Biochem Biophys Res Commun.* 1998;250:458-461.

94. Brighton CT, McCluskey WP. Cellular response and mechanisms of action of electrically induced osteogenesis. *J Bone Miner Res.* 1986;4:213-254.

95. Simon J, Simon B. Electrical bone stimulation. In: Pietrzak WS, ed. *Musculoskeletal Tissue Regeneration, Biological Materials and Methods.* 1st ed. Totowa, NJ: Humana Press; 2008:259-287.

96. Haddad JB, Obolensky AG, Shinnick P. The biologic effects and the therapeutic mechanism of action of electric and electromagnetic field stimulation on bone and cartilage: new findings and a review of earlier work. *J Altern Complement Med.* 2007;13(5):485-490.

97. Aaron RK, Boyan BD, Ciombor DM, et al. Stimulation of growth factor synthesis by electric and electromagnetic fields. *Clin Orthop Relat Res.* 2004;419:30-37.

98. Brighton CT, Wang W, Seldes R, et al. Signal transduction in electrically stimulated bone cells. *J Bone Joint Surg Am.* 2001;83A:1514-1523.

99. Guerkov HH, Lohmann CH, Lui Y. Pulsed electromagnetic fields increase growth factor release by nonunion cells. *Clin Orthop.* 2001;384:265-279.

100. Friedenberg ZB, Harlow MC, Brighton CT. Healing of a non-union of the medial malleolus by means of direct current: a case report. *J Trauma.* 1971;11:883-885.

101. Dwyer AF, Wickham GG. Direct current stimulation in spinal fusion. *Med J Aust.* 1974;1:73-75.

102. Brighton CT, Black J, Friedenberg ZB, et al. A multi-center study of the treatment of non-union with constant direct current. *J Bone Joint Surg Am.* 1981;63:2-13.

103. Saxena A, DiDomenico LA, Widtfeldt A, et al. Implantable electrical bone stimulation for arthrodesis of the foot and ankle in high risk patients: a multicenter study. *J Foot Ankle Surg.* 2005;44:450-454.

104. Brighton CT, Pollack SR. Treatment of recalcitrant non-union with a capacitively coupled electrical field. A preliminary report. *J Bone Joint Surg Am.* 1985;67:577-585.
105. Sarmiento A, Gersten LM, Sobol PA, et al. Tibial shaft fractures treated with functional braces. Experience with 780 fractures. *J Bone Joint Surg Br.* 1989;71:602-609.
106. Scott G, King JB. A prospective, double-blind trial of electrical capacitive coupling in the treatment of non-union of long bones. *J Bone Joint Surg Am.* 1994;76:820-826.
107. Bassett CA, Mitchell SN, Gaston SR. Treatment of ununoted tibial diaphyseal fractures with pulsing electromagnetic fields. *J Bone Joint Surg Am.* 1981;63:511-523.
108. Sharrard WJ. A double-blind trial of pulsed electromagnetic fields for delayed union of tibial fractures. *J Bone Joint Surg Br.* 1990;72:347-355.
109. Heckman JD, Ingram AJ, Loyd RD, et al. Non-union treatment with pulsed electromagnetic fields. *Clin Orthop.* 1981;161:58-66.
110. Fox IM, Smith SD. Bioelectric repair of metatarsal nonunions. *J Foot Surg.* 1983;22(2):108-115.
111. Holmes GB Jr. Treatment of delayed unions and nonunions of the proximal fifth metatarsal with pulsed electromagnetic fields. *Foot Ankle Int.* 1994;15:552-556.
112. Behrens SB, Deren MA, Monchik KO. A review of bone growth stimulation for fracture treatment. *Curr Orthop Pract.* 2013;24(1):84-91.
113. Griffin XL, Parson N, Smith N. Electromagnetic field stimulation for treatment delayed union or non-union of long bone fractures in adults. *Cochrane Database Syst Rev.* 2011;(4):CD008471.
114. Rubin C, Bolander M, Ryaby JP, et al. The use of low-intensity ultrasound to accelerate the healing of fractures. *J Bone Joint Surg Am.* 2001;83A:259-270.
115. Dyson M, Brookes M. Stimulation of bone repair by ultrasound. *Ultrasound Med Biol.* 1983;2:61-66.
116. Wang S, Lewallen D, Bolander M, et al. Low-intensity pulsed ultrasound treatment increases strength in a rat femoral fracture model. *J Orthop Res.* 1994;12:40-47.
117. Roussignol X, Currey C, Duparc E, et al. Indications and results for the Exogen ultrasound system in the management of nonunion: a 59-case pilot study. *Orthop Traumatol Surg Res.* 2012;98:206-213.
118. Watanabe Y, Arai Y. Three key factors affecting treatment results of low-intensity pulsed ultrasound for delayed unions and nonunions: instability, gap size, and atrophic nonunion. *J Orthop Sci.* 2013;18:803-810.
119. Buchtala V. Present state of ultrasound therapy. *Diabet Med.* 1950;22:2944-2950.
120. Maintz G. Animal experiments in the study of the effect of ultrasonic waves on bone regeneration. *Strahlentherapie.* 1950;82:631-638.
121. Heckman JD, Ryaby JP, McCabe J, et al. Acceleration of tibial fracture-healing by noninvasive, low-intensity pulsed ultrasound. *J Bone Joint Surg Am.* 1994;76A:26-34.
122. Kristiansen TK, Ryaby JP, McCabe J, et al. Accelerated healing of distal radial fractures with the use of specific, low-intensity ultrasound: a multicenter, prospective double-blind, placebo-controlled study. *J Bone Joint Surg Am.* 1997;79:961-973.
123. Hemery X, Ohl X, Saddiki R, et al. Low-intensity pulsed ultrasound for nonunion treatment: a 14-case series evaluation. *Orthop Traumatol Surg Res.* 2011;97:51-57.
124. Emami A, Petren-Mallmin M, Larsson S. No effect of low-intensity ultrasound on healing time of intramedullary fixed tibial fractures. *J Orthop Trauma.* 1999;13:252-257.
125. Katano M, Natuse K, Uxhida K, et al. Low-intensity pulsed ultrasound accelerates delayed healing process by reducing the time required for the completion of endochondral ossification in the aged mouse femur fracture model. *Exp Anim.* 2011;60(4):385-395.
126. Leung KS, Lee WS, Tsui HF, et al. Complex tibial fracture outcomes following treatment with low-intensity pulsed ultrasound. *Ultrasound Med Biol.* 2004;30:389-395.
127. Hannemann PF, Mommers EH, Schots JP, et al. The effects of low-intensity pulsed ultrasound and pulsed electromagnetic fields bone growth stimulation in acute fractures: a systematic review and meta-analysis of randomized controlled trials. *Arch Orthop Trauma Surg.* 2014;134(8):1093-1106.
128. Jingushi S, Mizuno K, Masushita T, et al. Low-intensity pulsed ultrasound treatment for postoperative delayed union or nonunion of long bone fractures. *J Orthop Sci.* 2007;12:35-41.
129. Mirza YH, Teoh KH, Golding D, et al. Is there a role for low intensity pulsed ultrasound (LIPUS) in delayed or nonunion following arthrodesis in foot and ankle surgery? *Foot Ankle Surg.* 2019;25(6):842-848.
130. Brighton CT, Shaman P, Heppenstal RB. Tibial nonunion treated with direct current, capacitive coupling, or bone graft. *Clin Orthop Relat Res.* 1995;321:323-334.
131. Zorlu U, Tercan M, Ozyazgan I, et al. Comparative study of the effect of ultrasound and electrostimulation on bone healing in rats. *Am J Phys Med Rehabil.* 1998;77:427-432.
132. Janis L, Krawetz L, Wagner S. Ankle and subtalar fusion utilizing a tricortical bone graft, bone stimulator, and external fixator after avascular necrosis of the talus. *J Foot Ankle Surg.* 1996;35(2):120-126.
133. Zwipp H, Grass R, Rammelt S, et al. Arthrodesis non-union of the ankle. Arthrodesis failed. *Chirurg.* 1999;70(11):1216-1224.
134. Deyerle WM. Etiology and treatment of non-union of the femoral neck by grafting and rigid fixation. II. *Am J Orthop.* 1965;7:50-53.
135. Deyerle WM. Etiology and treatment of non-union of the femoral neck by grafting and fixation. A review of 14 cases. I. *Am J Orthop.* 1965;7:18-23.
136. Henry RT. Fractures of the shaft on the tibia: types and treatment, bone grafts, and nonunion. *R I Med J.* 1948;31(5):299-301.
137. Fitch KD, Blackwell JB, Gilmour WN. Operation for non-union of stress fracture of the tarsal navicular. *J Bone Joint Surg Br.* 1989;71(1):105-110.
138. Nicholl EA. The treatment of gaps in long bones by cancellous insert grafts. *J Bone Joint Surg Br.* 1956;38:70.
139. Dawson WJ, Mead NC, Sweeney HJ, et al. Onlay fibular bone grafting in treatment of tibial fracture non-union. *Clin Orthop Relat Res.* 1978;130:247-253.
140. Hansson G, Jerre R, Markhede G, et al. Treatment of non-union after tibial shaft fracture with a full cortical thickness inlay bone graft. *Ups J Med Sci.* 1992;97(2):169-176.
141. Takeuchi N, Oka Y, Arima T. Clinical significance of the free vascularized bone grafts in fractures with large bone defects and non-unions. *Tokai J Exp Clin Med.* 1989;14(1):35-43.
142. Fernandez DL, Eggli S. Non-union of the scaphoid. Revascularization of the proximal pole with implantation of a vascular bundle and bone grafting. *J Bone Joint Surg Am.* 1995;77(6):883-893.
143. Kirkeby L, Baek Hansen T. Vascularized bone graft for the treatment of non-union of the scaphoid. *Scan J Plast Reconstr Surg Hand Surg.* 2006;40(4):240-243.
144. Sammarco VJ, Chang I. Modern issues in bone graft substitutes and advances in bone tissue technology. *Foot Ankle Clin.* 2002;7:19-41.
145. DiDomenico LA, Thomas ZM. Osteobiologics in foot and ankle surgery. *Clin Podiatr Med Surg.* 2015;32:1-19.
146. Wallace GF. Current orthobiologics for elective arthrodesis and nonunions of the foot and ankle. *Clin Podiatr Med Surg.* 2017;34:399-408.
147. Pinzur MS. Orthobiologics in foot and ankle surgery. *Curr Orthop Pract.* 2013;24(5):457-460.
148. Mehta SK, Sood A, Lin SS. Role of platelet-rich plasma in foot and ankle surgery: current concepts. *Tech Foot Ankle Surg.* 2012;11(1):3-8.
149. Bibbo C, Bono CM, Lin SS. Union rates using autologous platelet concentrate alone and with bone graft in high-risk foot and ankle surgery patients. *J Surg Orthop Adv.* 2005;14:17-22.
150. Coetzee JC, Pomeroy GC, Watts JD, et al. The use of autologous concentrated growth factors to promote syndesmosis fusion in the Agility Total Ankle replacement. A preliminary study. *Foot Ankle Int.* 2005;26:840-846.
151. Hsu WK, Mishra A, Rodeo SR, et al. Platelet-rich plasma in orthopedic applications: Evidence-based recommendations for treatment. *J Am Acad Orthop Surg.* 2013;21:739-748.
152. Proucznik MA. PRP an Unproven Option, Agree Forum Experts. AAOS Now. http://www.aaos.org/news/aaosnow/mar11/cover1.asp. Accessed April 26, 2019.
153. Gandhi AVGJ, Berberian WS, et al. Platelet releasate enhances healing in patients with a non-union. Orthopaedic Research Society 49th Annual Meeting. New Orleans, LA, 2003.
154. Vannini F, Di Matteo B, Filardo G, et al. Platelet-rich plasma for foot and ankle pathologies: a systematic review. *Foot Ankle Surg.* 2014;20(1):2-9.
155. Henning PR, Grear BJ. Platelet-rich plasma in the foot and ankle. *Curr Rev Musculoskelet Med.* 2018;11(4):616-623.
156. Lieberman JR, Daluiski A, Einhorn TA. The role of growth factors in the repair of bone. Biology and clinical applications. *J Bone Joint Surg Am.* 2002;84A:1032-1044.
157. Termaat MF, Den Boer FC, Bakker FC, Patka P, Haarman HJ. Bone morphogenetic proteins. development and clinical efficacy in the treatment of fractures and bone defects. *J Bone Joint Surg Am.* 2005;87A:1367-1378.
158. Sampath TK, Coughlin JE, Whetstone RM, et al. Bovine osteogenic protein is composed of dimers of OP-1 and BMP-2A, two members of the transforming growth factor-beta superfamily. *J Biol Chem.* 1990;265:13198-13205.
159. Food and Drug Administration. Document H010002-OP-1 Implant. October 17, 2001. www.fda.gov/OHRMS/DOCKETS/98fr/03-7817.pdf. Accessed April 26, 2019.
160. Yasko AW, Lane JM, Fellinger EJ, et al. The healing of segmental bone defects, induced by recombinant human bone morphogenetic protein (rhBMP-2). *J Bone Joint Surg Am.* 1992;74A: 659-671.
161. Friedlaender GE, Perry CR, Cole JD, et al. Osteogenic protein-1 (bone morphogenetic protein-7) in the treatment of tibial nonunions. *J Bone Joint Surg Am.* 2001;83A(suppl 1, Part 2):151-158.
162. Kain M, Einhorn T. Recombinant human bone morphogenetic proteins in the treatment of fracture. *Foot Ankle Clin.* 2005;10:639-650.
163. Mont MA, Ragland PS, Biggins B, et al. Use of bone morphogenetic proteins for musculoskeletal applications. *J Bone Joint Surg Am.* 2004;86A(suppl 2):41-55.
164. Bibbo C, Haskell MD. Recombinant bone morphogenetic protein-2 (rhBMP-2) in high-risk foot & ankle surgery: techniques and preliminary results of a prospective, intention to treat study. *Tech Foot Ankle Surg.* 2007;6:71-79.
165. Schuberth JM, DiDomenico LA, Mendicino RW. The utility and effectiveness of bone morphogenetic protein in foot and ankle surgery. *J Foot Ankle Surg.* 2009;48(3):309-314.
166. Bibbo C, Patel DV, Haskell MD. Recombinant bone morphogenetic protein-2 (rhBMP-2) in high-risk ankle and hindfoot fusions. *Foot Ankle Int.* 2009;30(7):597-603.
167. Fourman MS, Borst EW, Bogner E, et al. Recombinant human BMP-2 increases the incidence and rate of healing in complex ankle arthrodesis. *Clin Orthop Relat Res.* 2014;472(2):732-739.
168. Rearick T, Charlton TP, Thordarson D. Effectiveness and complications associated with recombinant human bone morphogenetic protein-2 augmentation of foot and ankle fusions and fracture nonunions. *Foot Ankle Int.* 2014;35(8):783-788.
169. DeVries JG, Scharer B. Comparison and use of allograft bone morphogenetic protein versus other materials in ankle and hindfoot fusions. *J Foot Ankle Surg.* 2018;57:707-711.
170. Hreha J, Krell ES, Bibbo C. Role of recombinant human bone morphogenetic protein-2 on hindfoot arthrodesis. *Foot Ankle Clin.* 2016;21:793-802.
171. Krell ES, DiGiovanni CW. The efficacy of platelet-derived growth factor as a bone-stimulating agent. *Foot Ankle Clin.* 2016;21:763-770.
172. Digiovanni CW, Baumhauer J, Lin SS, et al. Prospective, randomized, multi-center feasibility trial of rhPDGF-BB versus autologous bone graft in a foot and ankle fusion model. *Foot Ankle Int.* 2011;32(4):344-354.
173. DiGiovanni CW, Lin SS, Baumhauer JF, et al. Recombinant human platelet-derived growth factor-BB and beta-tricalcium phosphate (rhPDGF-BB/beta-TCP): an alternative to autogenous bone graft. *J Bone Joint Surg Am.* 2013;95(13):1184-1192.
174. DiGiovanni CW, Lin SS, Daniels TR, et al. The importance of sufficient graft material in achieving foot or ankle fusion. *J Bone Joint Surg Am.* 2016;98:1260-1267.
175. Arner JW, Santrock RD. A historical review of common bone graft materials in foot and ankle surgery. *Foot Ankle Spec.* 2014;7(2):143-151.
176. Elsinger EC, Leal L. Coralline hydroxyapatite bone graft substitutes. *J Foot Ankle Surg.* 1996;35:396-399.
177. Cornell CN, Lane JM, Chapman M, et al. Multicenter trial of Collagraft as bone graft substitute. *J Orthop Trauma.* 1991;5:1-8.
178. Michelson JD, Curl LA. Use of demineralized bone matrix in hindfoot arthrodesis. *Clin Orthop Relat Res.* 1996;325:203-208.
179. Thordarson DB, Kuehn S. Use of demineralized bone matrix in ankle/hindfoot fusion. *Foot Ankle Int.* 2003;24:557-560.

180. Collman DR, Kaas MH, Schuberth JM. Arthroscopic ankle arthrodesis: factors influencing union in 39 consecutive patients. *Foot Ankle Int.* 2006;27:1079-1085.

181. Dux KE. Implantable materials update. *Clin Podiatr Med Surg.* 2019;36(4):535-542.

182. Lemons JE. Ceramics: past, present, and future. *Bone.* 1996;19(1 suppl):121S-128S.

183. Karageorgiou V, Kaplan D. Porosity of 3D biomaterial scaffolds and osteogenesis. *Biomaterials.* 2005;26:5474-5491.

184. Bucholz RW, Carlton A, Holmes R. Interporous hydroxyapatite as a bone graft substitute in tibial plateau fractures. *Clin Orthop Relat Res.* 1989;240:53-62.

185. Urban RM, Turner TM, Hall DJ, et al. Increased bone formation using calcium sulfate-calcium phosphate composite graft. *Clin Orthop Relat Res.* 2007;459:110-117.

186. Beardmore AA, Brooks DE, Wenke JC, et al. Effectiveness of local antibiotic delivery with an osteoinductive and osteoconductive bone-graft substitute. *J Bone Joint Surg Am.* 2005;87:107-112.

187. Niikura T, Tsujimoto K, Yoshiya S, et al. Vancomycin-impregnated calcium phosphate cement for methicillin-resistant *Staphylococcus aureus* femoral osteomyelitis. *Orthopedics.* 2007;30(4):320-321.

188. Joosten U, Joist A, Frebel T, et al. Evaluation of an in situ setting injectable calcium phosphate as a new carrier material for gentamicin in the treatment of chronic osteomyelitis: studies in vitro and in vivo. *Biomaterials.* 2004;25(18):4287-4429.

189. Scharer BM, Sanicola SM. The in vitro elution characteristics of vancomycin from calcium phosphate-calcium sulfate beads. *J Foot Ankle Surg.* 2009;48(5):540-542.

190. Shi E, Carter R, Weinraub GM. Outcomes of hindfoot arthrodesis supplemented with bioactive glass and bone marrow aspirate: a retrospective radiographic study. *J Foot Ankle Surg.* 2019;58:2-5.

191. Fernandes JS, Gentile P, Pires RA, et al. Multifunctional bioactive glass and glass-ceramic biomaterials with antibacterial properties for repair and regeneration of bone tissue. *Acta Biomater.* 2017;59:2-11.

192. Godoy-Santos AL, Rosemberg LA, de Cesar-Netto C, et al. The use of bioactive glass S53P4 in the treatment of an infected Charcot foot: a case report. *J Wound Care.* 2019;28(suppl 1):S14-S17.

193. Arinzeh TL, Peter SJ, Archambault MP, et al. Allogenic mesenchymal stem cells regenerate bone in a critical-sized canine segmental defect. *J Bone Joint Surg Am.* 2003;85-A(10):1927-1935.

194. Kraus KH, Kirker-Head C. Mesenchymal stem cells and bone regeneration. *Vet Surg.* 2006;35(3):23-242.

195. Caplan AI. Adult mesenchymal stem cells for tissue engineering versus regenerative medicine. *J Cell Physiol.* 2007;213(2):341-347.

196. Melick G, Hayman N, Landsman AS. Mesenchymal stem cell applications for joints in the foot and ankle. *Clin Podiatr Med Surg.* 2018;35(3):323-330.

197. Lamo-Espinosa JM, Mora G, Blanco JF, et al. Intra-articular injection of two different doses of autologous bone marrow mesenchymal stem cells versus hyaluronic acid in the treatment of knee osteoarthritis: multicenter randomized controlled clinical trial (phase I/II). *J Transl Med.* 2016;14(246):1-9.

198. Vega A, Martín-Ferrero MA, Del Canto F, et al. Treatment of knee osteoarthritis with allogeneic bone marrow mesenchymal stem cells: a randomized controlled trial. *Transplantation.* 2015;99:1681-1690.

199. Kim YS, Lee M, Koh YG. Additional mesenchymal stem cell injection improves the outcomes of marrow stimulation combined with supramalleolar osteotomy in varus ankle osteoarthritis: short-term clinical results with second-look arthroscopic evaluation. *J Exp Orthop.* 2016;3(12):1-10.

200. Kim YS, Koh YG. Injection of mesenchymal stem cells as a supplementary strategy of marrow stimulation improves cartilage regeneration after lateral sliding calcaneal osteotomy for varus ankle osteoarthritis: clinical and second-look arthroscopic results. *Arthroscopy.* 2016;32(5):878-889.

201. Hernigou P, Dubory A, Flouzat Lachaniette CH, et al. Stem cell therapy in early post-traumatic talus osteonecrosis. *Int Orthop.* 2018;42(12):2949-2956.

202. Chiodo CP, Cicchinelli L, Kadakia AR, et al. Malunion and nonunion in foot and ankle surgery. *Foot Ankle Spec.* 2010;3(4):194-200.

203. Casillas MM, Allen M. Repair of malunions after ankle arthrodesis. *Clin Podiatr Med Surg.* 2004;21:371-383.

204. Guo C, Li X, Hu M, et al. Realignment surgery for malunited ankle fracture. *Orthop Surg.* 2017;9:49-53.

205. Guo C, Liu Z, Xu Y, et al. Supramalleolar osteotomy combined with an intra-articular osteotomy for the reconstruction of malunited medial impacted ankle fractures. *Foot Ankle Int.* 2018;39(12):1457-1463.

Infections

David R. Collman and Christy M. King

DEFINITION

The effective treatment of musculoskeletal infection is a significant challenge for the medical professional and the multidisciplinary care team. Humans are increasingly vulnerable to infection. There are a number of complex primary drivers for this public health problem: a rise in immune system compromise, socioeconomic factors that alter disease transmission, significant technologic advances producing nosocomial infections and biofilm formation in orthopedic surgery, disease reservoirs in long-term care facilities, and the proliferation of microorganism resistance and adaptation to the mainstays of antimicrobial therapy.

The human immune system is designed to destroy microorganism invasion by the collaborative response of humoral and cellular responses. The immune response of a healthy host is both innate and adaptive. However, the impaired host more easily succumbs to evolved microorganisms with unique virulence factors capable of thwarting human immune response. Even the healthy host is challenged by the serious modern-day problems of implant-associated infection and multidrug-resistant microorganisms.

This chapter first explores general principles in the recognition, diagnosis, and treatment of orthopedic infections. Pathogen virulence, the influence of patient host factors, and guidelines for the selection of antimicrobial therapy are addressed. Then the scope and complexity of soft tissue infections, native joint infections, adult and pediatric osteomyelitis, and diabetic foot infections (DFIs) are evaluated with close attention to the principles and techniques of surgical treatment when indicated.

GENERAL PRINCIPLES

The prompt and accurate assessment of musculoskeletal infections is critical to timely successful treatment and the prevention of complications. Diagnosis is based on evaluation of the patient's clinical presentation, laboratory assessment, imaging modalities, cultures, and intraoperative findings/histopathology when surgery is indicated. Close attention must be paid to the patient's health and capacity to combat infection. There is wide clinical variation in the mode of presentation for orthopedic infections.

HISTORY AND PHYSICAL EXAMINATION

A careful patient history will often provide important information about possible pathogens and potential clinical course of lower extremity infections. A history of events should be noted, including recent or remote trauma and surgery, travel, and potential exposure to disease. A thorough patient examination is critical for successful diagnosis and treatment. Changes to the soft tissues suggest different types of infection: fluctuance indicates an abscess; anaerobic bacteria cause crepitus; tissue necrosis results from advanced arterial disease or a necrotizing process. The extent of erythema may be outlined on the foot or leg to help monitor the course of the infection and patient response to treatment. Wounds should be measured, probed, and assessed for undermining or tunneling. Sinus tracts typically represent a deep infection. The volume, consistency, and odor of any fluid drainage should be noted: serous fluid may be aseptic, while purulent fluid is highly cellular and typically indicates infection. Toe web spaces should be carefully inspected for fissures or wounds. The pedal arch and leg compartments should be compressed to evaluate for possible deep space extension. Adjacent joints should be palpated and assessed for the presence of effusion, pain, range of motion, and stability. The course of adjacent tendons should be evaluated for potential extension of the local process. The proximal limb should be evaluated for lymphadenopathy. Finally, pedal pulses, potential venous insufficiency, sensation, and motor function must be assessed.

Physical examination must also include patient vital signs and assessment of mental status. Fever or temperature below 36°C, malaise, chills, night sweats, tachycardia, hypotension, and tachypnea may suggest a deeper soft tissue infection and early sepsis, particularly if the patient's mental status is altered. Systemic examination is also necessary to rule out other sources of infection that may skew accurate interpretation of laboratory data. Other pertinent systems that may harbor infection and complicate the diagnosis of musculoskeletal infection are the pulmonary, cardiovascular, and gastrointestinal systems and the urinary tract.

PATHOGENESIS

Orthopedic infections typically result from a breach of the soft tissue and less commonly a hematogenous source. Microorganisms release antigens that trigger a host immune response, culminating in the recruitment of inflammatory cells and eradication of the invading microbe. Infection occurs when microorganism invasion overwhelms host mechanisms of protection. Soft tissue defenses are able to combat 10^5 microorganisms per gram of tissue before infection arises.[1] This pathogenic process

TABLE 49.1 **Cardinal Signs of Infection**
Erythema
Warmth
Edema
Pain
Impaired function

is dependent on microorganism virulence, which determines the capacity of some microbes to produce infection, while others fall to host defenses. *Staphylococcus aureus*, one of the most common opportunistic pathogens that resides on human skin, is particularly virulent and capable of producing a wide range of infections, including a simple cellulitis, osteomyelitis, or life-threatening sepsis. By contrast, coagulase-negative staphylococci are low-virulence microorganisms but they abundantly form biofilms. Increased vascular permeability and local blood flow produces the clinical manifestation of the host defense process: erythema, temperature increase, edema, and pain. These cardinal signs of inflammation typically indicate infection (Table 49.1). Some infections are mild, superficial, and slowly progressive, while others can be severe with rapid advancement and deep tissue extension, and may cause life-threatening systemic complications without immediate treatment. Still others are chronic and may lie dormant for years, persisting in a subclinical state until they become pathogenic much later.

The etiology, local skin compromise and blood supply, and systemic disease are risk factors that impair wound healing and influence the course of lower extremity infections (Table 49.2). Systemic disease often impairs the host response to the microorganism. Multiple patient risk factors are associated with more resistant pathogens and portend worse outcomes.[2] Peripheral neuropathy and peripheral arterial disease (PAD) compound soft tissue infection risk. The distal lower extremity is susceptible to rapid progression of infections in such patients. The management of DFIs, a distinct challenge for the foot and ankle specialist, is reviewed in the last section of this chapter.

LABORATORY ASSESSMENT

Routine blood analysis is an integral part of patient assessment in infections. Yet reliable interpretation of serum markers

TABLE 49.2 **Risk Factors for Infections in the Foot and Ankle**		
Etiology	**Local Factors**	**Systemic Compromise**
Trauma mechanism	Peripheral arterial disease	Immunocompromise (disease or suppression)
Surgery	Peripheral neuropathy	Diabetes mellitus
Environmental exposure	Venous stasis	Renal/liver disease
	Wounds	Malnutrition
	Significant scar	Malignancy
	Colonization with *S aureus*	Obesity
	Fungal disease	Hypoxia
		Organ failure
		Age (>65 years)
		Substance abuse
		Tobacco/nicotine use

TABLE 49.3 **Standard Laboratory Assessment of Infection and Patient Health**	
Blood Markers	**Host Status Markers**
White blood cell (WBC) count	Complete blood count
Leukocyte manual differential	Chemistry panel
C-reactive protein (CRP)	Coagulation studies
Erythrocyte sedimentation rate (ESR)	HgA1c
Blood cultures	Albumin/Prealbumin
	Transferrin
	Total lymphocyte count
	Total protein

depends on host response to the pathogen. Bacterial infections are a common cause of elevated white blood cell (WBC) count, which may be normal in the immunocompromised host. Standard laboratory assessment for infection and patient health is depicted in Table 49.3.

CRP and ESR are also useful in the assessment of deep infection. Both are widely available, easy to perform, and inexpensive. CRP levels rise and normalize quickly in response to inflammation, including surgery. Serial CRP measurements are necessary to track the clinical course of infection and evaluate the patient's response to treatment. Additional markers of evaluation for deep infection are found in Table 49.4. If necrotizing soft tissue infection suspected, serum creatinine kinase helps monitor tissue and muscle destruction. Procalcitonin may helpful to rule in the diagnosis of septic arthritis and acute osteomyelitis at a cutoff level of 0.4 ng/mL.[3] Interleukin-6 (IL-6), like CRP, normalizes quickly once infection resolves. Yet IL-6 is not widely available and is more expensive than other inflammatory markers. Forthcoming research is exploring immunology to identify assays for host immunity to *Staphylococcus aureus*, the leading microorganism in implant-associated infections.[4]

IMAGING

Musculoskeletal imaging is essential in the evaluation of infections. Plain radiography is always advisable as the first imaging study. Radiography is a relatively quick, inexpensive, and often effective means to rule out gas and many foreign bodies (metal and most glass objects) retained in the soft tissue, evaluate for the presence of implants, and assess for potential bone involvement. Ultrasonography is a useful modality to evaluate the size and location of an abscess. It may have the most utility for necrotizing fasciitis because it can demonstrate fluid about the fascia, where other imaging studies fall short. Ultrasound may help visualize soft tissue changes suggestive of infection in the presence of orthopedic implants. It is also highly sensitive for revealing various retained foreign bodies in soft tissue that radiographs seldom detect, such as plastic and wood.[5] Computed tomography (CT) scans and magnetic resonance imaging (MRI) help define the precise location and extent of an abscess or deep infections. CT with

TABLE 49.4 **Biomarkers for Deep Infection**
Creatinine kinase
Procalcitonin
Interleukin-6

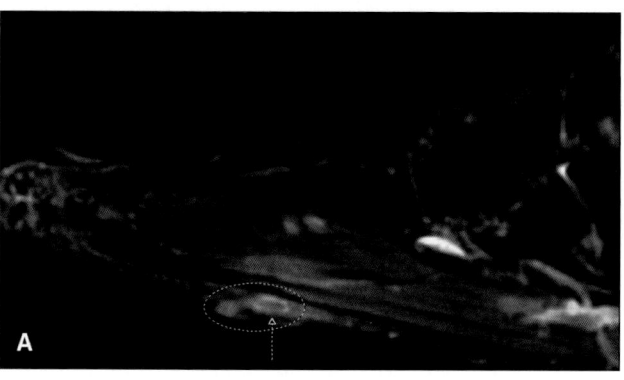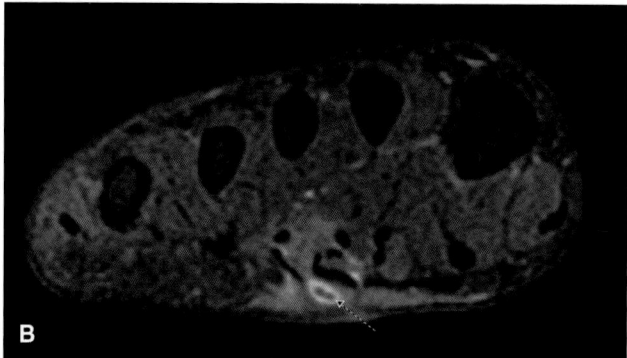

FIGURE 49.1 A, B. MRI fat saturation images depicting small abscess and retained wood fragment in sole of the foot (*arrows*).

intravenous contrast helps determine soft tissue changes in response to infection, including the presence of gas. Gadolinium-enhanced MRI is useful for identifying sinus tracts and ruling out abscess in the presence of cellulitis.[6] These imaging modalities are also useful for the detection of retained wood fragments in soft tissues[7] (Fig. 49.1). Table 49.5 depicts advantages of common imaging for assessment of soft tissue infections. Imaging for osteomyelitis, including nuclear medicine, is presented in a later section.

CULTURES

Microorganism identification is essential for targeted therapy in musculoskeletal infection. Cultures are the standard because they produce rapid results at generally little expense. Culture and antimicrobial sensitivities must be accurate for effective treatment. Yet culture yield may be diminished by insufficient specimen, confounded by contaminants that mask true pathogens, influenced by existing antimicrobial therapy, or adversely impacted by transport time and laboratory media or plating methods.

Normal human flora is abundant with potentially pathogenic microorganisms. *Staphylococcus aureus*, a particularly

virulent pathogen that is increasingly resistant to common antibiotic therapy, may be shed in high quantities from operating room personnel.[8] The operating field is often culture positive, and the surgical wound may be contaminated with microorganisms.[9] Meticulous tissue sampling technique is critical to ensure that specimens accurately reflect potential microorganisms at the site of biopsy. Cross-contamination is avoided by careful tissue dissection and biopsy with separate clean curettes and rongeurs that remain covered until they are needed. Sampling several tissue specimens from different sites of high probability for infection optimizes culture yield (Table 49.6). Adequate tissue sample volume from high-probability sites is imperative for reliable culture results (Fig. 49.2). The samples should be at least several millimeters in diameter or several milliliters in volume.[10-12] If antibiotics are added to irrigation, wound lavage must wait until tissue specimens have been harvested. The tissue should be immediately transferred to a screw-cap specimen container without transport medium, which is closed and sent to the laboratory within 2 hours. Bacteria lose viability within 1-2 hours if they are not contained within ample tissue or fluid, which underscores the importance of procuring adequate tissue volume.[10-12] In cases where tissue débridement is not necessary to treat infection, an image-guided percutaneous bone biopsy under sterile conditions is the sampling method of choice. Specimens should be tested for Gram stain, for the presence of aerobic and anaerobic bacteria, and for atypical microorganisms such as acid-fast bacilli and fungus. Information about the tissue source, history of infection, and antibiotic treatment should be provided with the tissue samples, which must be correctly

TABLE 49.5	The Merits of Common Imaging Studies in Evaluation of Soft Tissue Infection	
Radiographs	**Ultrasound**	**CT/MRI**
Quick	Quick	Precision abscess
Inexpensive	Relatively	assessment:
Evaluate for gas	inexpensive	location and
Rule out foreign	Superior for foreign	depth
body	body	Assess for wood
Determine implants	Determine abscess	fragments
Assess for bone	size	Gas (CT w/contrast)
involvement	Assess infection	Sinus tracts (MRI w/
	with implant	contrast)
	Evaluate for	
	epifascial	
	fluid: rule out	
	necrotizing	
	fasciitis	

TABLE 49.6	Tissue Sites for Optimal Culture Yield
Biopsy Source	
Purulent soft tissue or bone	
Necrotic soft tissue or bone	
Sequestrum	
Intramedullary canal ends	
Thick synovium	
Implants	
Foreign material	
Periprosthetic membrane	
Component interface exudate	

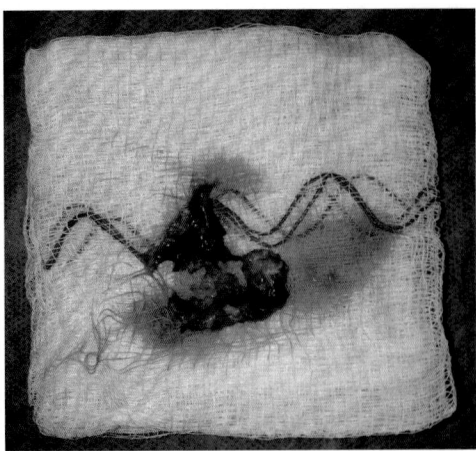

FIGURE 49.2 Tissue samples are preferred to swabs for culture.

labeled. Culture analysis is based on the suspected pathogen. Cultures should be kept for a minimum of 5-7 days unless low-virulence microorganisms are suspected or joint aspirate is negative, in which case they are held for 14-21 days because longer periods of incubation provide higher yield.[10,12]

Swab cultures are not reliable for accurate microorganism analysis. Swab fibers retain most of the microorganisms, and the handle is often contaminated. Swab cultures of sinus tract or wound drainage typically detect colonizing microorganisms rather than true pathogens.

Antimicrobial treatment should ideally be withheld until tissues are cultured, yet in many cases of infection this not possible. However, in chronic orthopedic infections, antimicrobial therapy should be stopped at least 2-3 weeks prior to tissue culture in order to minimize false-negative results.

Despite holding antibiotics before the operation and close attention to careful culture methods, the yield may still be low or the results unreliable. Unfortunately, alternative sophisticated testing measures are expensive and not yet widely available. Sonication may improve culture yield by low-intensity ultrasound disruption of biofilm on implant surfaces.[13] Microorganisms may also be directly identified in some cases by a number of different culture-independent DNA-based techniques and methods of genetic amplification such as polymerase chain reaction (PCR), though false-positive results occur.[14]

Interpretation of culture results and decision-making about antimicrobial therapy is based on an understanding of microorganism virulence, and the patient's clinical presentation. Consultation with an infectious disease specialist is recommended in order to fully understand microorganism significance and virulence, appropriate antimicrobial therapy, and the host response to treatment.

HISTOPATHOLOGY

Histopathology is important for diagnosis in orthopedic infections because it complements microbiologic findings. Although the pathogen(s) cannot be identified by histology alone, the

negative predictive value is 90%-100%. Identification of acute inflammatory cells in tissue specimens is particularly valuable where culture yield is low, prompting other methods of microorganism identification. In such cases paired samples should be harvested from the same site.

The value of intraoperative frozen section for detecting infection is dependent on the skill of the pathologist and clear communication from the surgeon. The frozen section is diagnostic if 10 or more neutrophils are present per high-powered field based on the five most cellular fields evaluated. If there are <5 neutrophils per high-powered field, absence of infection is likely in 91% of cases.[15] It is important to correlate the results of frozen section with microbiologic and histopathologic findings.

TREATMENT

The effective treatment of musculoskeletal infection is based on optimizing the patient's immune response, addressing the manifestations of inflammation, and targeted antimicrobial therapy. The basic principles of treating infection are depicted in Table 49.7. Guidelines for the selection of an antimicrobial agent and administration pathways are based on infection severity (Table 49.8, Fig. 49.3). Antimicrobial susceptibility testing allows selection of first- and second-line therapeutic agents based on their bioavailability and target tissue penetration, along with drug toxicity, patient allergies, and expense. Short antibiotic courses – often a week or less – are typically effective for common bacterial infections. This approach helps reduce antibiotic resistance and minimizes untoward effects of treatment. While most minor soft tissue infections respond to nonsurgical management, antimicrobial therapy is not effective for the treatment of many orthopedic infections. The cornerstone of surgical management of infection is the evacuation of pus, which dates back to Hippocrates. The quality of surgical débridement is the most important tenant of successful treatment.[16] Close attention to detail guides the drainage of purulence, removal of all foreign and devitalized tissue, and careful soft tissue handling. The goal is to establish a clean, viable wound (Fig. 49.4). Serial wound débridement is often necessary to this end. If any contaminated tissue remains, microorganisms can persist. Devitalized tissue creates cellular hypoxia, which impairs the healing process. In some instances, staging débridement is necessary to permit demarcation of viable

TABLE 49.7	Principles of Infection Diagnosis and Treatment		
Source Control	**Examination and Diagnostics**	**Optimize Host Response**
Surgery as necessary ■ Incision and drainage ■ Débridement and lavage Wound dressings	Vital signs Examination Laboratory data Imaging Cultures/pathology	Medical/fluid management Antimicrobial therapy Nutritional status Stable environment Monitor treatment: CRP/ESR

TABLE 49.8 Antibiotic Selections for Nonpurulent Mild and Moderate Soft Tissue Infections	
Mild: Oral Antibiotics	**Moderate: IV Antibiotics**
Penicillin	Penicillin
Clindamycin	Clindamycin
Cephalosporin (first/second generation)	Cefazolin
	Ceftriaxone
Trimethoprim-Sulfamethoxazole	Vancomycin

Adapted from IDSA Guidelines 2014.

tissues. The wound and surrounding soft tissues must be closely evaluated for healing potential, and vascular tests may be necessary. Planning for soft tissue coverage of any existing or anticipated defect(s) begins early in the course of treatment, including consultation with a vascular surgeon and a plastic surgeon as necessary.

In addition to addressing the infection at it source, close attention must be paid to the patient's health to optimize host immune response to microorganisms and mitigate the impact of treatment. Nutritional status should be assessed with protein and vitamin supplementation as necessary. The influence of venous insufficiency and PAD should be addressed. Diabetes mellitus should be optimized (blood glucose between 110 and 180 mg/dL or hemoglobin A1c 7.5% or below). Patients with autoimmune disorders, and those on immunosuppressive therapy—corticosteroids or chemotherapeutic agents—are at higher risk of infection. Obese patients also carry a greater risk of infection. Consultation with internal medicine, rheumatology, endocrinology, vascular surgery, and oncology should be considered based on underlying disease and risk factors in the patient.

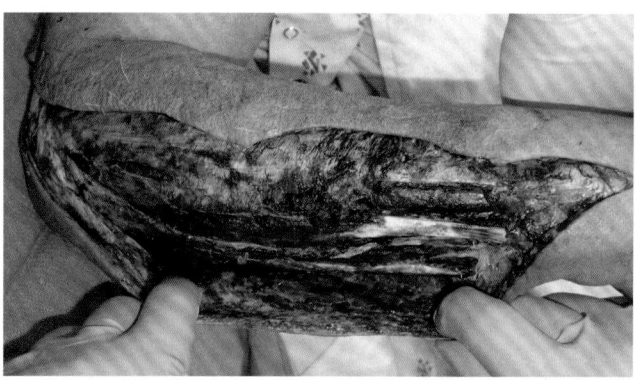

FIGURE 49.4 Clean, viable wound bed after incision, drainage, lavage, and débridement of necrotizing fasciitis subsequent to multiple cat bites in the forearm.

PEARLS FOR DIAGNOSIS AND TREATMENT OF SOFT TISSUE INFECTIONS

- Complete patient host assessment: vital signs, medical history, physical examination.
- Low threshold for diagnosis of necrotizing soft tissue infection.
- Obtain CBC, ESR, CRP, and blood cultures; consider advanced laboratory markers as necessary.
- Imaging appropriate to nature of infection.
- Empiric/targeted antibiotic selection based on IDSA guidelines.
- Optimize host health for immune response.
- Closely monitor patient during treatment.

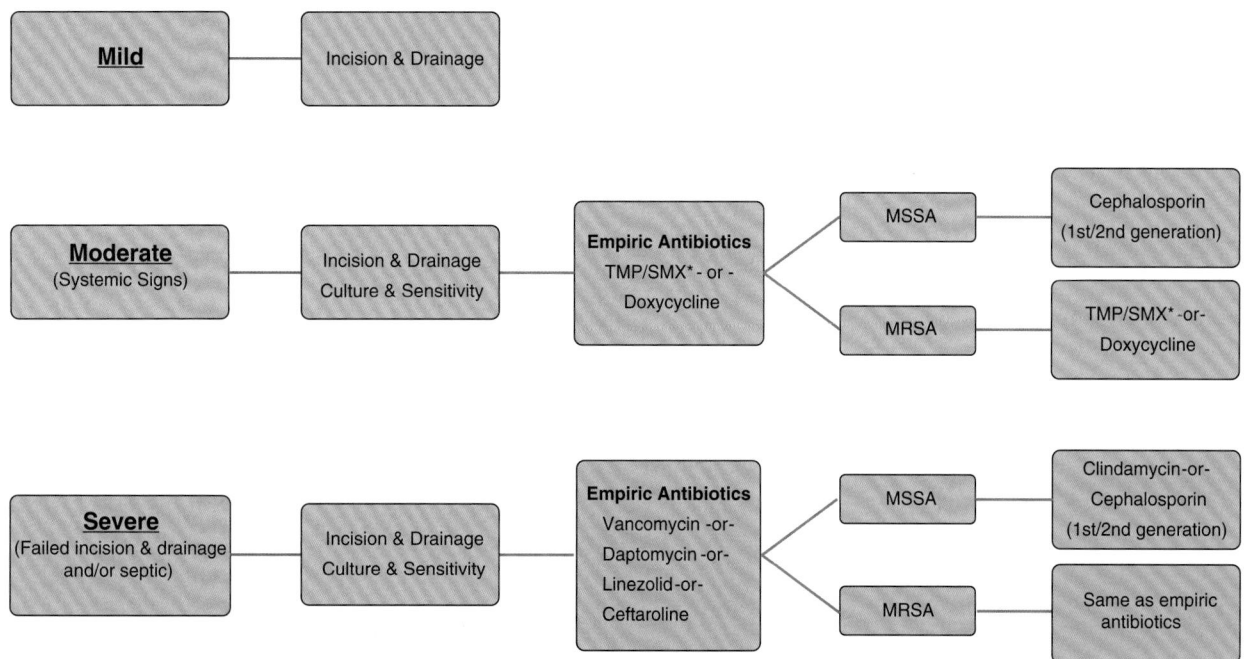

FIGURE 49.3 Algorithm for treatment of purulent soft tissue infections. (Adapted from IDSA Guidelines 2014.) *TMP/SMX, trimethoprim-sulfamethoxazole.

- As more diffuse tissue involvement abates, a more focal infection nidus may become evident.
- Appropriate wound care as indicated.
- Adequate course of antibiotic therapy/monitor response: examination, CBC, CRP.
- If surgical treatment necessary:
  - Obtain clean tissue specimens from high-probability sites.
  - Plan for soft tissue coverage: collaboration with vascular and plastic surgeon as necessary.
  - Thorough débridement (repeat as necessary) and careful soft tissue handling.
- Postoperative care: appropriate limb protection/elevation.
- Physical therapy to minimize deconditioning and avoid joint contractures.

SOFT TISSUE INFECTIONS

The scope of soft tissue infections is broad, encompassing the skin and all underlying structures over the bone. The Infectious Disease Society of America (IDSA) established guidelines for the diagnosis and treatment of soft tissue infections.[17] Such infections are increasingly common due to the proliferation of microorganisms resistant to antibiotics. In the early part of this century alone, soft tissue infections were cause for a 27% increase in U.S. hospital admissions.[17]

CLASSIFICATION

Most classification schemes for soft tissue infection have limited clinical utility. IDSA guidelines differentiate such infections into those with purulence and those without, which dictates surgical treatment.[17] A pertinent classification that prioritizes the timeline for surgery based on the clinical progress of foot and ankle infections is depicted in Table 49.9.

TABLE 49.9 Classification of Soft Tissue Infections Pertinent to Foot and Ankle Based on Clinical Progress and Timeline for Surgical Intervention		
Soft Tissue Infections	**Clinical Progress**	**Surgical Timeline**
Limited cellulitis Erysipelas Folliculitis/furuncle	Slow	Nonsurgical
Diffuse cellulitis Paronychia Abscess Septic bursitis	Moderate	Urgent
Necrotizing soft tissue infections: Necrotizing fasciitis Gas gangrene Toxic shock syndrome Rabies	Rapid	Emergent

Modified from Kingston D, Seal DV. Current hypothesis on synergistic microbial gangrene. *Br J Surg.* 1990;77:260-264.

PATHOGENESIS

Soft tissue infection severity is based on depth. Differentiating more localized soft tissue infections from those with the potential for deeper levels of tissue destruction is essential to minimize patient morbidity. The foot and ankle are uniquely at risk for soft tissue infection.

The foot is predisposed to microorganism contamination because of exposure to moisture from sock and shoe wear, limited web space aeration, and higher distribution of eccrine glands.[18] Load-bearing stress and prominent bone may lead to mechanical soft tissue irritation such as skin fissures. Penetrating trauma and the condition of the skin may impact infection severity. The concentration of pedal microorganisms is increased in older and immunocompromised patients, those with peripheral vascular disease, and those with existing wounds.[19,20]

SPECIFIC CONDITIONS

Cellulitis and Erysipelas

Cellulitis is an acute pyogenic inflammation of the dermis and subcutaneous tissues.[21] In the foot and ankle, the genesis is most often contiguous—violation of the skin from an obvious or obscure wound—and less commonly hematogenous. Cellulitis presents as a progressive area of warmth, erythema, and edema without well-defined borders. Lymphangitis may be present (Fig. 49.5). Cellulitis may manifest with cutaneous hemorrhage and bullae, which can be a warning sign for deeper infection.[17] Left untreated, cellulitis may lead to the formation of an abscess. Older patients are more susceptible to cellulitis.[22] Source identification is useful for determining the organism: wounds from human or animal bite, fresh or salt water exposure, penetrating farm injury, and those in the diabetic foot are each contaminated with unusual bacteria.[21] The

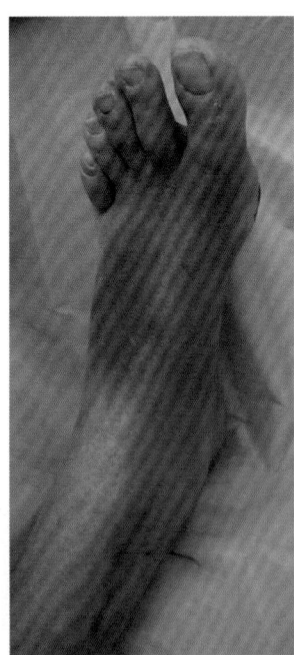

FIGURE 49.5 Foot/ankle cellulitis and lymphangitis caused by a plantar wound.

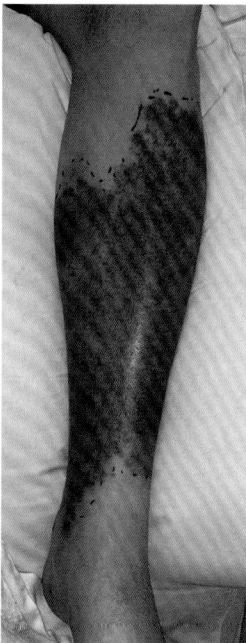

FIGURE 49.6 Erysipelas of the ankle and leg. Note the intense erythema and well-demarcated border.

most common bacteria causing cellulitis are β-hemolytic Streptococci (often group A or B), and methicillin-sensitive *Staphylococcus aureus* (MSSA), less commonly group C or G *Streptococcus* and methicillin-resistant *S aureus*.[21] MSSA and streptococci commonly colonize toe web spaces.[23]

Erysipelas is a more superficial infection than cellulitis, typically limited to the upper layer of the dermis and superficial lymphatic system, though it may extend into subcutaneous fat. Its characteristic presentation is indurated, fiery erythema with elevation of the affected tissue and a well-demarcated raised border, similar to an intense rash[17,24] (Fig. 49.6). It most commonly afflicts the lower extremity[25] in patients with poor skin condition such as venous insufficiency.[26] Erysipelas is caused by β-hemolytic streptococci, most commonly *S pyogenes,* less frequently group B, C or G *Streptococcus* and *S aureus*.[25]

The diagnosis of cellulitis and erysipelas is made by a thorough patient history and clinical examination. Standard infection labs may be necessary. Imaging is seldom indicated, except in cases concerning for more significant infection. These common soft tissue infections are treated with rest, ice, elevation, limb immobilization, oral or parenteral antibiotics, compression as appropriate, and local dressings for skin lesions. Close monitoring for patients at risk of necrotizing soft tissue infection is critical.

Common Pedal Skin Infections

Some common skin infections in the foot may lead to deeper infection and require surgical management if overlooked or left untreated. These include tinea pedis (athlete's foot) and toe paronychia. Folliculitis and furuncles are less common cutaneous infections that may afflict the foot and have similar consequences. Patients with diabetes and those undergoing surgery are particularly at risk of more significant infection from these conditions.

Tinea Pedis

Tinea pedis (athlete's foot) is a cutaneous dermatophyte infection most commonly caused by *Trichophyton rubrum.* The genesis is direct contact to fomites, which can persist for years in areas of moisture accumulation. Tinea pedis commonly presents in an asymptomatic moccasin distribution with hyperkeratotic scales overlying erythematous plaques along the heel and sole. The most common complication of tinea pedis is onychomycosis and cellulitis.[27] Vesiculobullous tinea pedis presents with tiny pruritic vesicles along the arch, is often caused by *Trichophyton mentagrophytes*, and may become infected with *S aureus* or *S pyogenes*.[27] Young, active patients are prone to infection with *T mentagrophytes*.[27] Toe web spaces are of particular concern for bacterial infection because they are prone to contamination by *T mentagrophytes*, which can produce maceration, fissures, and subsequent wounds (Fig. 49.7). β-Hemolytic streptococci are common in interdigital tinea pedis.[28] However, in some cases of web space involvement, superimposed bacterial infection is caused by gram-negative microorganisms. Dermatophytes may produce changes in normal bacterial flora and give rise to microorganisms that can result in a significant deep space infection.[29] Careful patient examination, early treatment, and follow-up are critical to minimize the risk of a bacterial superinfection. Tinea pedis is typically diagnosed by clinical examination. Potassium hydroxide analysis of skin scrapings from the border of an active lesion will present as multiple, branched, septate hyphae.[30]

Educating patients about appropriate foot hygiene through moisture reduction is important for both treatment of tinea pedis and reducing transmission of the infection.[31] Simple approaches include ventilated shoe gear, moisture-wicking socks, use of antifungal powders, and avoiding barefoot activity in public areas. About one-third of cases can be cured with proper foot hygiene alone, but high-quality studies show superior outcomes with topical antifungal agents compared with no treatment.[32] Terbinafine is typically the most effective topical medication. It should be used for 4 weeks or until symptom

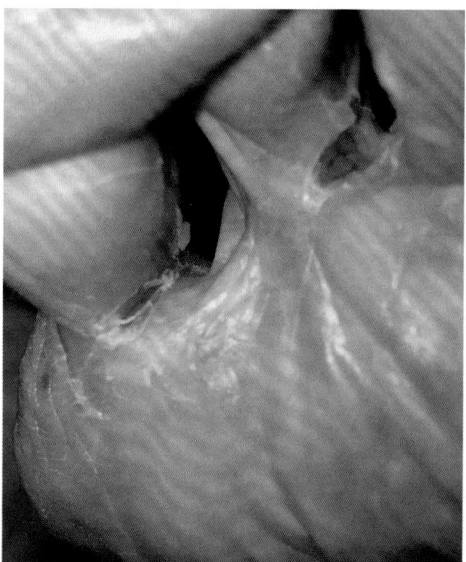

FIGURE 49.7 Web space tinea pedis infection: fissure wounds and macerated scales amidst erythematous patches.

resolution. If a bacterial infection is present, a broad-spectrum topical antibiotic and antibacterial wash may be necessary. Topical corticosteroids may help address pruritus and inflammation.[27] In severe dermatophyte infections, systemic antifungal therapy may be necessary. In rare cases of deep space infection, incision and drainage is necessary for successful treatment.

Paronychia

Paronychia is infection of the periungual skin resulting from ingrowth of the nail into the adjacent skin fold. The firm nail plate penetrates the soft tissue and essentially causes a foreign body reaction.[33] The toes are frequently affected because of increased bacterial flora and poor hygiene, which produces a nidus for infection. Characteristic findings include pain, erythema, edema, and serous or purulent drainage. Sometimes pyogenic granuloma is present. In severe cases an abscess or felon may arise. Common bacteria include *S aureus*, *Streptococcus* species, and *Pseudomonas* species.[34] The etiology includes variation in toenail morphology, shoe gear, trauma, and improper nail trimming. Diagnosis is made by history and physical examination. In severe presentations (Fig. 49.8), radiographs should be obtained to rule out osteomyelitis.

The most effective treatment for paronychia is avulsion of the offending toenail margin and drainage of an abscess if present. Oral antibiotics do not improve patient outcomes.[34,35] In chronic cases there may also be a role for topical corticosteroids and antifungal medication.[36] Matrixectomy may not be indicated in severe paronychia but may be helpful for recurrent cases. Failure to treat this condition can result in cellulitis, osteomyelitis, and even gangrene. Patients with poorly controlled diabetes mellitus and PAD are particularly at risk for such complications. Toenail avulsion in patients with advanced PAD may lead to tissue necrosis. Recommended treatment in such cases includes warm water soaks, topical antifungal and corticosteroid therapy, oral antibiotics, and draining the abscess.

Folliculitis and Furuncles

Folliculitis is a superficial infection of hair follicles. A furuncle is a form of folliculitis that may develop into a painful abscess. Since the foot is prone to moisture and friction, it is particularly at risk.[37] Initially the lesions present as dense, erythematous, painful papules. In some cases necrotic tissue may be present.[17] Furuncles are caused by *S aureus*. Recurrent cases are associated with patients in whom immune response is compromised and the skin is colonized with *S aureus*, including the methicillin-resistant strain.

Diagnosis is made by patient history and examination. Mild folliculitis and smaller furuncles can be treated with warm water compresses to promote drainage and topical antibiotics.[17] Larger lesions may require incision and drainage with culture and oral antibiotics, particularly if cellulitis is present.[17,30] In recurrent cases the patient may require application of mupirocin to colonized areas.[38]

Septic Bursitis

Septic bursitis is inflammation typically caused by bacteria inoculation—usually *S aureus*—via skin lesion(s), through it is rarely hematogenous or due to adjacent cellulitis.[39] It most commonly presents in the olecranon and prepatellar bursa. It is extremely rare in the foot and ankle.[40] Although it can be difficult to differentiate the condition from nonseptic bursitis, clinical criteria include bursal warmth, increasing pain, skin lesions, and fever.[41] The diagnosis of septic bursitis is made by clinical examination, common infection labs, radiographs, and ultrasound or MRI/CT as necessary for deep infection.[42] Careful bursal aspiration under adequate skin preparation will show purulence, which should be sent for Gram stain, bacterial culture, WBC, and glucose.[43]

Treatment for septic bursitis is early empiric oral antibiotic therapy, rest, ice, compression, elevation, and nonsteroidal anti-inflammatory medication for about 2 weeks, along with bursal aspiration as a method of pain reduction and antibiotics targeted to the responsible microorganism.[44] Two weeks of oral antibiotic therapy is recommended for mild to moderate cases. In severe cases, parenteral antibiotic therapy for 10 days may be necessary. Bursectomy is indicated only in those patients recalcitrant to antibiotics with surrounding cellulitis, abscess, or systemic infection.[44]

Trauma

Trauma may contaminate the soft tissue injury and produce a wound infection, which is most common after penetrating insults (Fig. 49.9), including burns and bites.

Infection After Open Fractures

A breach in the soft tissue envelope significantly increases the risk of infection. Infection risk is based on fracture severity—the energy of the injury/degree of soft tissue crush and the

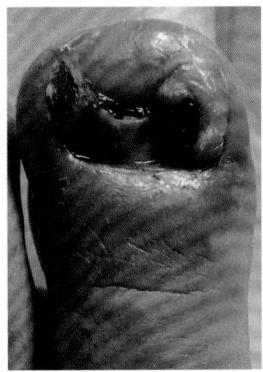

FIGURE 49.8 Advanced paronychia of the hallux with marked pyogenic granuloma at the toenail margins.

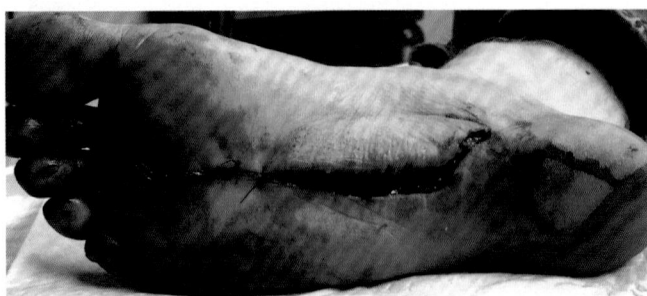

FIGURE 49.9 Deep plantar foot laceration from broken dirty glass. Such penetrating trauma poses greater infection risk.

extent of contamination—along with patient comorbidities and response to injury. Infection is the primary driver of fracture nonunion and loss of limb function.[45] Deep tissue specimens from the fracture wound should be cultured only after débridement to increase identification of potential pathogens.[46] Four treatment tenets reduce infection rates in open fractures: early administration of empiric systemic antimicrobial therapy (with local antibiotic depots as necessary), timely thorough wound débridement and lavage, skeletal stabilization, and soft tissue coverage. The principles of diagnosis and treatment of open fractures are covered in Chapter 43.

Puncture Wound Infections

Pedal puncture wounds are relatively common injuries. Infections develop in up to 15% of cases.[47,48] Those sustained in the region of the metatarsal head to toes are more prone to complications.[49] Retained foreign bodies are relatively uncommon but may produce a granuloma and in some cases latent infection (Fig. 49.10). Patient history provides worthy clues to potential microorganisms that may produce infection. *S aureus* or Group A β-hemolytic streptococci commonly cause infections that arise from puncture wounds in the unshod patient. In patients wearing shoes, *P aeruginosa* and other gram-negative bacteria are commonly isolated from puncture wounds on the sole of the foot. *Aeromonas*, *Vibrio*, and *Mycobacterium* species often produce infections in puncture wounds sustained in water. Infected puncture wounds from plant material are caused by a number of rare microorganisms, while animal bowel flora typically causes those inflicted on a farm. Following a thorough patient history, the next steps are assessing the patient's tetanus status, ruling out potential neurovascular injury, and careful evaluation of the puncture site.

Many patients who sustain a plantar puncture wound have a benign outcome. The rate of infection is relatively low, perhaps even lower than reported because not all patients seek medical care after the injury.[49] There is disagreement about the best treatment for pedal puncture wounds. Some suggest simply cleaning the puncture site, minimizing activity on the injured foot, and an oral antibiotic if a cellulitis arises.[49,50] Others advocate surgery for thorough débridement and wound exploration, removal of foreign material, and irrigation to minimize infection and other complications.[51-53] A prudent treatment protocol is wound cleaning and irrigation, attempted foreign body removal if it is easily accessible, protecting the foot, and close observation with follow-up for additional care as necessary. If the wound is prone to tetanus, a toxoid booster injection is recommended in patients whose last injection was a >1 year prior to the injury.[54]

Bite Wound Infections

Bite wounds afflict about half of people in the United States during their lifetime and are responsible for ~1% of emergency department visits annually.[55] Most bite wounds are minor, but some are severe and may cause significant morbidity, influenced by organisms from the biter and/or the victim. About 2% of patients require hospitalization.[56] Bite injuries to the foot are relatively uncommon.[57] However, patients with peripheral vascular disease and diabetes mellitus are at high risk for complications from bite wounds. Children are also at significant risk.[58] Domestic cat bites produce focal puncture wounds that are directly inoculated and harbor bacterial growth. Infection results in approximately half of all cases.[58] Dogs account for the majority of bite injuries in the United States, causing both puncture wounds and tearing of the soft tissue (Fig. 49.11). Infection occurs in only 15%-20% of dog bites because the wound is typically open and is easily irrigated and débrided.[59] *Pasteurella multocida* is the cause of infection in ~50% of dog bites and 90% of cat bites, along with a number of other small domestic animals.[60,61] *P multocida* is particularly virulent, causing a local cellulitis within 24 hours of injury, often followed by purulence, lymphadenopathy, and fever.[62] Other causative microorganisms are depicted in Table 49.10.

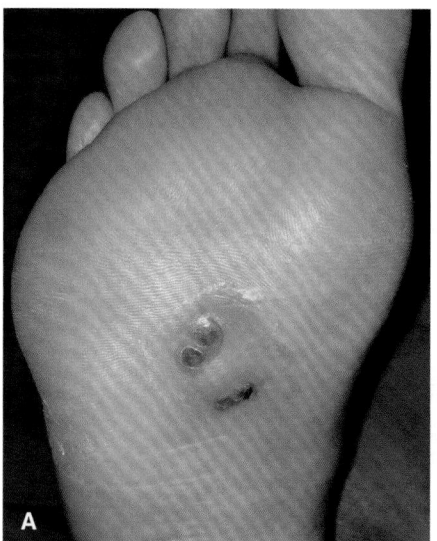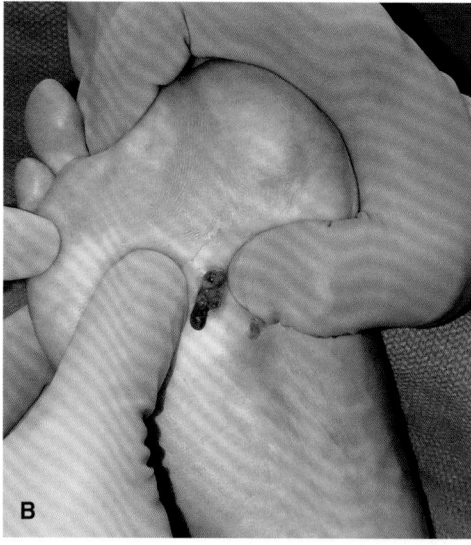

FIGURE 49.10 **A.** Foreign body granulomas with surrounding erythema on the plantar aspect of the foot 2 months after puncture wound through shoe. **B.** Small abscess appreciated prior to granuloma excision and soft tissue exploration, which demonstrated retained wood material.

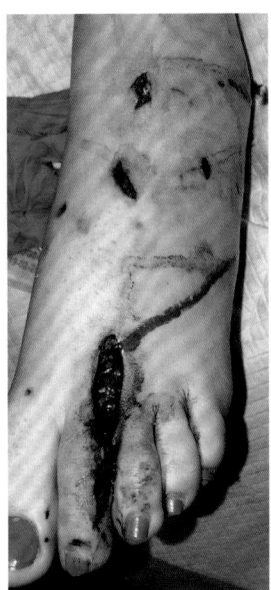

FIGURE 49.11 Dog bite wounds: characteristic torn tissue and open wounds, prior to treatment.

Local rabies prevalence must also be considered in animal bite wounds. Bat bite wounds are high risk for rabies transmission. Human bite wounds may produce significant morbidity if infected. They introduce many aerobic and anaerobic bacteria, also listed in Table 49.10. *Eikenella corrodens*, a gram-negative facultative anerobic organism similar to *P multocida*, is commonly found in human bite wounds. They also pose a low risk for hepatitis B/C and HIV transmission.[63,64]

Snake bites are most often inflicted by a rattlesnake, copperhead, or cottonmouth. *Clostridium perfringens* and *Bacteroides fragilis* are the most common organisms in snake bite wounds, but *Shigella* or *Salmonella* may also be present. Envenomation occurs in ~80% of poisonous snake bites.[65] Minimal envenomation produces pain, edema, and discoloration absent systemic signs. Extensive limb edema, rapidly progressive symptoms, and coagulopathy are signs of moderate envenomation, while severe cases produce these symptoms along with abnormal vital signs and systemic symptoms.[65] Rodent bites can also cause significant morbidity. *Streptobacillus moniliformis* is the bacteria in rat bite fever, causing fever, rigors, polyarthralgia, and if untreated, mortality in 10% of cases.

TABLE 49.10	Microorganisms in Infected Dog/Cat and Human Bite Wounds
Cat and Dog Bite Wounds	**Human Bite Wounds**
Pasteurella multocida	*Streptococcus anginosus*
Streptococci	*S aureus*
Staphylococci	*Eikenella corrodens*
Moxarella	*Fusobacterium nucleatum*
Neisseria	*Prevotella melaninogenica*
Fusobacterium species	*Candida* species
Bacteroides species	
Peptostreptococcus species	
Actinomyces species	
Porphyromonas species	
Veillonella parvula	

There is often in a delay in diagnosis because specific clinical findings are not initially present and the bacterium is difficult to culture.[66]

Infections following marine life injuries to the foot and ankle typically result from seawater organisms, typically gram-negative bacteria. Stings and puncture wounds may produce tissue necrosis. Their toxins may cause significant systemic symptoms and shock. Sea urchins, stingrays, catfish, jellyfish, and even coral are common causes of injury. *Vibrio vulnificus*, an organism found in warm coastal waters, may cause a rapidly progressing necrotizing limb infection after inoculating a wound sustained from a shark bite or while harvesting or cleaning shellfish, typically in the immunocompromised patient.[67] Such infections are associated with a high rate of limb amputation and mortality.

Most spider bites produce a local reaction. The exception is a brown recluse spider bite, which causes substantial tissue necrosis and in some cases a systemic response. Black widow spider bites produce little injury to the local tissue but significant systemic symptoms because of the neurotoxin in the venom.

The early administration of antibiotic prophylaxis is recommended for 3-5 days in most extremity bite wounds, particularly in the following situations: the immunocompromised patient, for deep bites at risk for penetrating joint capsule or bone, all cat bites, patients with developing edema, and for all moderate or severe injuries.[17] Recognition of the microorganism is the cornerstone of treatment. If infection develops after an animal bite, amoxicillin-clavulanate is the first line of treatment.[17] Antibiotics active against both aerobic and anaerobic bacteria should be considered since many dog or cat bite wounds contain anaerobic microogranisms.[68] Human bite victims should receive treatment for possible HIV or hepatitis B/C transmission in addition to antibiotic prophylaxis for aerobic and anaerobic organisms. Amoxicillin-clavulanate is the initial antibiotic of choice for human bite wounds. Rabies vaccination should be considered as appropriate. It is important to maintain a low threshold for surgical débridement and irrigation of all bite wounds. Irrigation and open wound care may be sufficient for dog bite wounds larger than a puncture, whereas infected cat bite wounds are more likely to require incision and drainage. Infected human bite wounds often require incision and lavage with thorough débridement. Bite wounds on the extremity are never closed primarily.[17] Care of marine bite, puncture, or sting wound requires antibiotic and tetanus prophylaxis, prompt removal of retained spines with débridement and irrigation, and pain control when necessary. In the treatment of snake bites, the most important factor is to determine whether the bite was envenomated.[65] Snake size, species, and age should be considered. Patient symptoms, the rate of progression, and the severity of envenomation should be established by closely monitoring the wound site and extremity. A complete blood count (CBC), coagulation markers, and metabolic studies should be obtained. Ice and tourniquet application should be avoided. Antivenin should be administered in cases of moderate or severe envenomation. Tetanus prophylaxis should be considered. Broad-spectrum antibiotics are administered if the wound appears infected. Incision and irrigation of the site is seldom indicated. Spider bite wounds should be treated with local wound care; antibiotics are administered only if infection is present.

Abscesses

Incision and drainage with ample lavage is typically adequate for the treatment of a simple abscess. So long as the extremity or host is not compromised, evacuation of pus provides for adequate reduction in bacterial load such that host defense and antibiotics will eliminate the infection. Abscess puncture aspiration or stab incision and drainage is a simple initial approach that can be executed in the clinic or at the bedside. This method not only confirms the presence of an abscess but also facilitates early decompression and can provide some initial symptom relief. In the insensate foot, this may allow for significant evacuation of purulence prior to formal exploration, débridement, and lavage in the operating room.

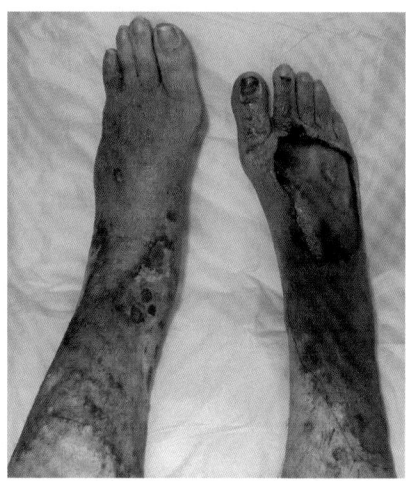

FIGURE 49.12 Necrotizing soft tissue infection in the foot and ankle. Cutaneous hemorrhage and bullae are also common in some presentations of cellulitis, but the skin necrosis seen in the right foot is a clear indication of a serious infection.

PERILS AND PITFALLS IN TREATMENT SOFT TISSUE INFECTION

- Failure to recognize a more subtle presentation of infection
- Incomplete patient assessment
- Delay in recognition of necrotizing soft tissue infection
- Inappropriate choice of antimicrobial therapy
- Failure to optimize host status and monitor response to treatment
- Failure to follow patient during symptom resolution/ observe for focal infection nidus
- If surgery is necessary:
  - Insufficient specimens for culture
  - Hesitancy in time to or quality of débridement/repeat débridement
  - Absence of or ill-conceived planning for coverage or soft tissue defect
- Lack of attention to postoperative wound care, limb protection, physical therapy

Necrotizing Soft Tissue Infections

Necrotizing soft tissue infections produce necrosis of multiple tissue layers including skin/subcutaneous tissue, fascia, and muscle, either limited to each layer or manifesting in combination.[69] These infections are rare with an incidence of 0.4-0.5 cases per 100 000 people.[70] They are often associated with traumatic wounds or bites, yet in many cases the skin lesion is minor or cannot be identified.[17,71] Necrotizing soft tissue infections initially resemble a cellulitis, but the patient may present with severe pain and the rapid spread of erythema in spite of antibiotic therapy, followed by subcutaneous hemorrhage, draining bulla, and skin necrosis[72,73] (Fig. 49.12). Necrotizing fasciitis causes necrosis of fascia and subcutaneous fat as it rapidly spreads along fascial planes and may be life threatening. Type I necrotizing fasciitis is caused by aerobic and anaerobic bacteria in synergy and most commonly occurs following surgery or in patients with diabetes mellitus or peripheral vascular disease. It commonly presents in the lower extremity, and the foot is at high risk. Type II is typically caused by group A streptococci and commonly presents with toxic shock syndrome. Gas gangrene is equally deadly as necrotizing fasciitis and may have a similar clinical presentation—soft tissue crepitus and pain out of proportion—but more often produces muscle necrosis and is caused by *C perfringens* or *Bacillus* species.

The hallmarks of a swift diagnosis for necrotizing fasciitis are careful patient examination, a high index of suspicion, and clinical judgment, all of which is critical for timely and successful treatment of this potentially devastating soft tissue infection. Patient history and risk factors such as intravenous or subcutaneous drug use and chronic disease should be considered. Physical examination helps differentiate the early presentation of necrotizing fasciitis from cellulitis or erysipelas because the subcutaneous tissues are palpable and yield, often with crepitus.[17,74] Yet diagnosis in the early stages is often complicated by cutaneous hemorrhage and minor skin bullae (which may resemble cellulitis) along with the absence of systemic manifestations. Severe pain out of proportion is the most sensitive diagnostic sign, present in almost all cases.[75] As the infection progresses the skin bullae drain serosanguineous (and later hemorrhagic) fluid, tissue inflammation rapidly advances, and necrosis of the skin and fat develops. Signs of systemic toxicity are present, and the other key components of a through patient evaluation are vital signs, assessment of mental status, and laboratory markers for sepsis.[17] Ultrasound will demonstrate epifascial fluid. Plain radiography, MRI, and CT are typically low-yield for early diagnosis. Vascular occlusion in the proximal limb should be ruled out.

Prompt surgical intervention is critical for treatment of necrotizing soft tissue infections. Radical débridement of necrotic skin and subcutaneous tissue immediately reduces inflammatory and bacterial tissue load (Fig. 49.13).

In cases of necrotizing fasciitis, the resection of nonviable fascia is also necessary to mitigate the risk of the limb infection progressing to the trunk, where prognosis significantly worsens. In such instances, limb amputation may be necessary. Repeat tissue exploration is typically necessary within 12-36 hours, followed by serial tissue débridement based on the patient's response to surgery and medical care, including early empiric antibiotic therapy that covers both aerobic and anaerobic bacteria.[17] Consultation with an infectious

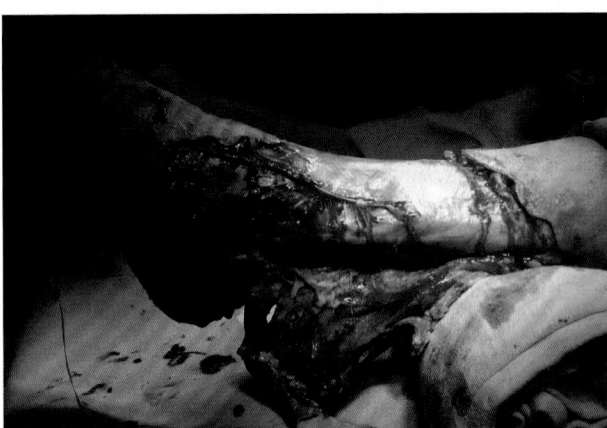

FIGURE 49.13 Radical débridement is essential for severe necrotizing soft tissue infection.

disease specialist will guide targeted antibiotic treatment once microorganisms are identified. Critical care management is essential for addressing fluid management and treatment of multisystem organ failure as necessary. Table 49.11 summarizes the approach to these infections in the patient with sepsis. Table 49.12A and B depicts empiric and targeted antibiotic selection for necrotizing soft tissue infections. Negative pressure wound therapy provides an aseptic dressing that is useful for wounds of varying size (Fig. 49.14). Hyperbaric oxygen therapy may be considered, though there is little evidence to support this modality.[76,77]

Authors' Preferred Treatment of Soft Tissue Infections

- Thorough patient history, examination, laboratory, and imaging assessment
- Low threshold of suspicion for necrotizing soft tissue infections
- Optimize patient host
- Antibiotic selection based on IDSA guidelines
- Carefully monitor patient response to treatment
- Timely thorough débridement as indicated/ample tissue culture from high yield sites
- Plan for soft tissue coverage
- Appropriate postoperative wound care, limb protection, and physical therapy plan

POSTOPERATIVE CARE AND REHABILITATION

The care of the patient with a lower extremity soft tissue infection is focused on measures to reduce the risk of recurrent

TABLE 49.11 Treatment of Necrotizing Soft Tissue Infections With Sepsis

Radical surgical débridement
Prompt high-dose empiric antibiotic therapy
Critical care management

TABLE 49.12A Empiric Antibiotic Therapy for Necrotizing Soft Tissue Infections: Treat With One Antibiotic From Each Group

Empiric Antibiotics 1	Empiric Antibiotics 2
MSSA - Clindamycin	**MSSA** - Piperacillin-tazobactam - Carbapenem - Third-generation cephalosporin[a] - Moxifloxacin[b]
MRSA - Vancomycin - Linezolid - Daptomycin	**MRSA** - Piperacillin-tazobactam - Carbapenem - Third-gen. cephalosporin and metronidazole - Fluoroquinolone and metronidazole

[a]May combine with metronidazole instead of clindamycin.

[b]May combine with linezolid instead of clindamycin.

Adapted from IDSA Guidelines 2014.

infection, rehabilitate the limb, and minimize deconditioning of the patient. Open wounds should be covered with regular dressing changes based on wound care principles. If bed rest is required, pressure wounds must be avoided. The extremity should be regularly elevated to the level of the heart to help minimize edema. The limb is immobilized in a splint, boot, or rigid shoe with a period of non– or protected weight bearing as necessary. A physical therapist should assist with joint motion so long as the wound does not cross the joint, strengthening maneuvers, and gait training. An adequate course of antimicrobial therapy should be completed with regular assessment of the patient's clinical response along with laboratory markers.

TABLE 49.12B Targeted Antibiotic Therapy for Necrotizing Soft Tissue Infections: Treat With One Antibiotic From Each Group

Microorganism	Targeted Antibiotics 1	Targeted Antibiotics 2
S aureus	Nafcillin Oxacillin Cephalosporin (first-generation) Clindamycin Vancomycin (for MRSA)	
Streptococcus spp. *Clostridium* spp.	Penicillin	Clindamycin
Polymicrobial	Piperacillin-tazobactam Cefotaxime	Vancomycin Carbapenem Clindamycin Metronidazole

Adapted from IDSA Guidelines 2014.

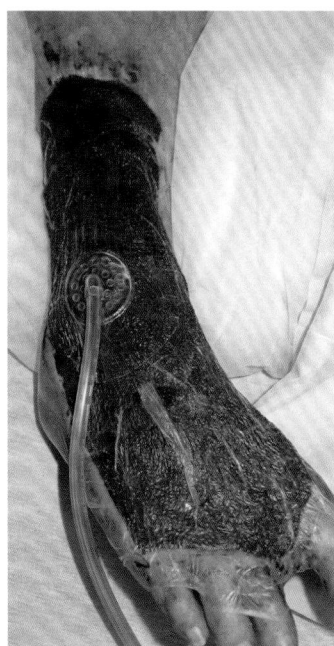

FIGURE 49.14 Negative pressure wound therapy is appropriate for temporary wound dressing, even for large soft tissue defects. In some cases of smaller lesions, an additional soft tissue coverage plan may not be necessary.

NATIVE JOINT SEPTIC ARTHRITIS

Native septic arthritis results from microorganism invasion into the synovial joint. One or more joints may be affected, but the disease is monoarticular in 90% of patients: the knee is affected in nearly half of all cases. The annual incidence is 2-10 per 100 000 people and 5-10 per 10 000 hospitalized patients. Patients with rheumatoid arthritis are affected at 28-38 per 100 000 each year.[78] The adult ankle is affected in 10%-15% of cases and the child's ankle in 4%-13% of cases.[79,80] Septic arthritis is a medical emergency. Left untreated, irreversible cartilage destruction and sepsis can result.[81] Even with timely and appropriate treatment, loss of joint function occurs in 25%-50% of patients.[82] The adult mortality rate is upwards of 10%.[83,84]

Risk factors are important determinants of septic arthritis. Existing inflammatory or degenerative joint disease is the most significant.[85,86] The rheumatoid joint is at higher risk for infection because the synovial leukocytes have diminished phagocytic activity.[87] Other risk factors include advanced age, immunosuppression, trauma, indwelling vascular catheters, intravenous drug use, endocarditis, rheumatoid arthritis, and infections that increase the risk of bacteremia.[88,89] The risk of septic arthritis after joint aspiration is <0.01%[85] and similarly low after arthroscopy (0.01%-0.6%).[90,91] However, the administration of intra-articular steroids after arthroscopy puts the patient at 27 times the risk of infection than without such injection.[92]

PHYSICAL EXAMINATION

Over 80% of patients with septic arthritis present with pain at rest, made worse with load, and limited joint motion, while less than half of patients have fever.[83,93] The ankle is effused, warm, often erythematous, and markedly tender with significant pain on even slight motion.[83,94] About half of patients with the condition have another focus of infection on presentation. In addition to ruling out more distant primary infection, the surrounding skin should be carefully examined. The aforementioned risk factors should be considered, including acute ankle trauma. In cases of soft tissue injury that is suspected to violate the ankle joint capsule, patients should undergo a saline-load test, which is 99% sensitive.[95] The presentation in children can be confounded by transient synovitis, where symptoms surge and regress and load bearing is still tolerated. By contrast, septic arthritis in children is marked by severe pain, unrelenting symptoms, and refusal to move the joint or bear load.[96] Vital signs should also be attained.

PATHOGENESIS

Three pathways drive the pathogenesis of septic arthritis: hematogenous seeding, contiguous spread, or direct inoculation. The most common cause is hematogenous dissemination from a distant focus of microorganisms owing to the highly vascularized synovial tissue without a basement membrane, which allows for rapid organism transfer from blood into the joint. Synovial fluid is poorly immunogenic. Contiguous focus septic arthritis is most common in infants under 1 year of age where there are vascular anastomoses between the epiphysis and metaphysis. Direct inoculation may occur with open joint injury, trauma, intra-articular injections, or surgery. A sinus located near a joint should be assumed to communicate with the joint. Introduction of microorganisms into a joint produces an acute synovial inflammatory response. As inflammatory cells fill the joint, they release enzymes and cytokines that gradually destroy articular cartilage, exacerbated by microorganism toxins. In addition to chemical injury, increased joint pressure from the inflammatory effusion produces physical damage to the cartilage.[78,97] After 5 days of infection, cartilage damage is irreversible.

Staphylococcus and streptococcus species are the primary pathogens in septic arthritis. Mycobacterium or fungal organisms may also cause infection, though such cases usually develop slowly. Viral arthritis may be intra-articular or present as an immune response with arthralgia.[98] In infants under 2 months of age, *Streptococcus agalactiae* and other gram-negative organisms may cause septic arthritis; *S pyogenes* and *S pneumonia* are more likely pathogens in children ages 2-5 years.[99] *Haemophilus influenza* is now a rare cause of infection in young children because of widespread immunization. Causative microorganisms in septic arthritis based on patient risk factors are depicted in Table 49.13.

DIAGNOSTIC STUDIES

Laboratory blood tests include a CBC, ESR, and CRP, although these makers have poor specificity. As noted earlier in this chapter, CRP is helpful for evaluating the patient's response to treatment. Procalcitonin may have value to rule in the diagnosis of septic arthritis at a cutoff level of 0.4 ng/mL.[3] Blood cultures should be drawn because of the high incidence of hematogenous dissemination, but they are positive in only about half of patients. The definitive diagnosis is typically made by synovial fluid aspiration under sterile skin preparation before initiating

TABLE 49.13	Microorganisms Responsible for Septic Arthritis Based on Patient Risk

Microorganism/Incidence	Risk Factors
Staphylococcus aureus (50%) (including coag-negative staphylococci)	Healthy older adult, risk factors: diabetes mellitus, skin compromise/infection, arthritis, endocarditis
Streptococcus spp. (20%-30%)	Joint aspiration, cortisone injection, arthroscopy
Neisseria gonorrhoeae	Youth, sexually active, associated tenosynovitis
Pseudomonas aeruginosa/ Serratia spp.	Intravenous drug users, immunocompromised patient
Enterobacteriaceae	Elderly, immunocompromised patient, gastrointestinal or urogenital infection
Mycoplasma hominis Candida spp.	Immunocompromised patient IV drug users, immunocompromised patient
Polymicrobial (5%-15%)	Extra-articular polymicrobial infection, trauma in immunocompromised patient

antimicrobial treatment, with caution to avoid an area of cellulitis. The synovial aspirate is sent for leukocyte count (via EDTA tubes to prevent clotting), Gram stain, aerobic and anaerobic bacterial culture, as well as protein and crystals.

Table 49.14 presents synovial fluid markers for the differential diagnosis of septic arthritis. Although a synovial WBC count of >50 000 cells/mm^3 is the accepted cutoff for septic arthritis, this criterion is only 64% sensitive for infection.[100] Furthermore, a much lower synovial WBC count threshold (>20 000 cells/mm^3) should be considered for immunocompromised patients. In cases where crystals are present, septic arthritis may not be excluded.[101] Synovial protein levels of 40 mg/dL or lower than the level of serum protein is indicative of septic arthritis.

The sensitivity of synovial fluid Gram stain for diagnosing septic arthritis is 50%-75%, while synovial fluid culture is positive in 75%-90% of patients.[102] If the synovial fluid is inoculated into pediatric blood culture tubes (BACTEC Peds Plus/F vial)

the diagnostic yield increases.[103] Yet cultures may be negative in cases of insufficient fluid sample, early antibiotic treatment prior to fluid aspiration, or due to fastidious or atypical microorganisms.[78] Arthrocentesis detects planktonic bacteria but not bacteria in biofilm. In a study of 132 native septic joints, synovial cultures were negative in 36% of cases.[104] Septic ankle arthritis was shown to be culture negative in up to 20% of patients in one series.[105] In such instances, arthroscopic synovial tissue biopsy from multiple high-probability sites may improve culture yield compared to joint fluid aspirate alone.

In culture-negative cases, molecular testing methods such as PCR to identify bacterial DNA may be considered.[106] However, some recent periprosthetic joint infection literature suggests that PCR may be no more sensitive than traditional cultures for bacterial detection.[107,108] Next-generation sequencing (NGS) is a recent and relatively inexpensive high-volume rapid genomic sequencing method that has demonstrated high sensitivity for detecting microorganisms in synovial fluid.[109] However, these advanced diagnostic methods are not widely available.

IMAGING

Imaging is seldom necessary for the diagnosis and treatment of acute septic arthritis in the native joint. Radiographs are often normal but they can establish existing joint disease - including evidence joint destruction in late presentation cases of septic arthritis - and they may demonstrate an effusion as well as retained implants.[110] Ultrasound may be useful in the child because it is quick and diagnostic for effusion in all cases. CT will show surrounding soft tissue infection and joint effusion and is more sensitive than radiographs for ruling out abscess and bone erosion. MRI is the most sensitive study for depicting joint effusion and surrounding osteomyelitis (Fig. 49.15). A radionucleotide scan may be the best imaging modality for septic arthritis. A technetium 99m methylene diphosphonate (MDP) bone scan may demonstrate diminished tracer uptake early in the infection process and increased tracer uptake later owing to the hyperemic response.[111] Yet image production is often delayed in scintigraphy, and timing of the diagnosis in septic arthritis is critical. Positron emission tomography (PET) scan with intravenous fluorine-18 fluorodeoxyglucose (FDG) injection is an excellent alternative because the scan can be completed in 2 hours since FDG is rapidly absorbed by leukocytes.[112] It is less expensive than leukocyte scintigraphy and has a relatively high diagnostic accuracy. A systematic and meta-analysis study

TABLE 49.14	Synovial Fluid Analysis for Diagnosis of Arthritis				
Fluid Marker	Normal Joint	Degenerative Arthritis	Inflammatory Arthritis	Crystal-Based Arthritis	Septic Arthritis
Clarity	Transparent	Transparent	Opaque–turbid	Turbid	Turbid
WBC[a]	<1000	<2000	5000-75 000	>20 000	>50 000[b]
PMNs[c]	<25%	25%-75%	>50%	>50%	>75%
Culture	Negative	Negative	Negative	Negative	Positive

[a]White blood cell count.

[b]Immunocompromised patients may not have an elevated synovial WBC so a lower cutoff should be considered at >20 000.

[c]Polymorphonuclear cells.

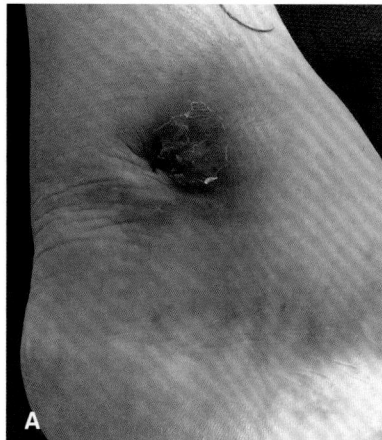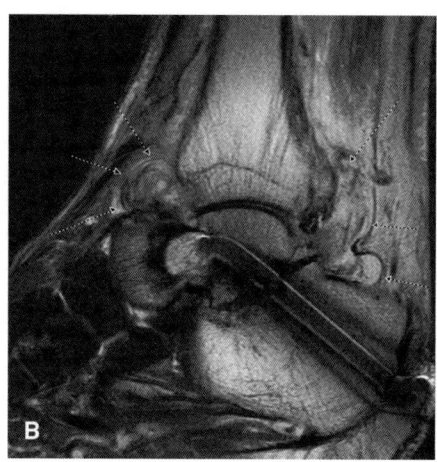

FIGURE 49.15 A. Chronic ankle sinus tract. **B.** MRI fat saturation sequence depicting matter about the ankle (*arrows*), erosions along the anterior tibiotalar joint, and retained talocalcaneal screw. Cultures grew coccidioidomycosis.

demonstrated the combined sensitivity and specificity of FDG PET scan to be 96% and 91%, respectively.[113] Furthermore, antibiotic administration is unlikely to skew the sensitivity of infection sites visible by the tracer.

PERILS AND PITFALLS IN DIAGNOSIS AND TREATMENT OF NATIVE ANKLE SEPTIC ARTHRITIS

- Delayed recognition or joint aspiration
- Failure to differentiate ankle pyarthrosis from gouty arthritis or rheumatoid flare
- Delay in administration of intravenous antimicrobial therapy
- Synovectomy in mild stages (limits tissue levels of antibiotic)
- Inadequate joint débridement in advanced stages
- Insufficient volume of synovial tissue samples for culture
- Inattention to patient's postoperative clinical course and lab monitoring
- Prolonged joint immobilization

TREATMENT

Successful treatment of native joint septic arthritis is based on early identification of the patient's clinical presentation, immediate joint aspiration, swift administration of antimicrobial therapy, and surgical débridement and lavage. Initial arthrocentesis is not only necessary for the diagnosis; it is the first step in therapy by evacuation of inflamed synovial fluid rich with enzymes and toxins that cause cartilage demise.[78] Early intravenous administration of antimicrobial therapy following a clean arthrocentesis is essential for successful treatment. Early antibiotic therapy reduces the risk of cartilage damage.[114] The highly vascularized synovium that allows for rapid microorganism invasion into the joint also facilitates high levels of antibiotic tissue perfusion. The intra-articular administration of antibiotics may produce a chemical synovitis and is contraindicated.[81]

Empiric intravenous antibiotic therapy should target staphylococci and streptococci based on their prevalence (see Table 49.13). Vancomycin should be considered because MRSA is increasingly common in native joint septic arthritis.[104] Bactericidal antibiotics are recommended. The choice of antibiotic agent and duration of microorganism-targeted treatment is determined based on synovial culture results and consultation with an infectious disease specialist (Table 49.15). Oral antibiotics are not recommended for empiric therapy in adult cases of native joint septic arthritis. However, conversion from targeted intravenous therapy to an oral regimen with superior bone penetration and high bioavailability (such as rifampin) may be considered within 1-2 weeks if the patient demonstrates clinical improvement and normalized WBC and inflammatory markers.

TABLE 49.15 Empiric and Targeted Antibiotic Therapy for Native Ankle Septic Arthritis

Microorganism	Empiric Antibiotic	Targeted Antibiotic and Suggested Duration
S aureus	Nafcillin or cefazolin[a,b] - or - vancomycin (MRSA prevalence)	**MSSA**[c] Nafcillin or cephalosporin (first-gen) 4-6 weeks **MRSA**[c] Vancomycin 4-6 weeks
Streptococci	Nafcillin or cefazolin[a]	Penicillin or ampicillin 2-4 weeks
N gonorrhoeae	Ceftriaxone	Ceftriaxone 7-10 days
P aeruginosa Enterobacteriaceae	Piperacillin[b] + Gentamicin[a]	Piperacillin + aminoglycoside 4-6 weeks

[a]The addition of an aminoglycoside is indicated for empiric therapy in patients under 3 months of age, in cases of nosocomial infection, or if the patient is treated with immunosuppressive therapy.

[b]In intravenous drug abusers empiric therapy should cover both *S aureus* and *P aeruginosa*.

[c]Patients who are immunocompromised or who demonstrate a slow response to treatment require 6 weeks of antibiotic therapy.

PEARLS FOR DIAGNOSIS AND TREATMENT OF NATIVE JOINT SEPTIC ARTHRITIS

- Clinical suspicion based on risk factors
- Rapid joint aspiration for synovial decompression and pathogen identification (use pediatric blood culture tubes to increase culture yield)
- Prompt empiric intravenous antimicrobial therapy
- If aspirate culture negative consider [99m]TC MDP bone scan + ^{111}In-labeled WBC scan
- Serial arthrocentesis if poor surgical candidate or unsalvageable joint
- Surgical débridement and lavage: arthroscopy or arthrotomy
  - Avoid synovectomy in mild stages to maximize antibiotic tissue perfusion.
  - Avoid arthroscopy in advanced stages for adequate débridement.

Following empiric intravenous antibiotic therapy, one of three definitive treatment approaches is necessary: serial joint aspiration, arthroscopic joint débridement and lavage, or joint arthrotomy, débridement, and lavage. Retrospective studies comparing needle aspiration with surgical drainage of the joint show good results with serial arthrocentesis.[115] Joint aspiration should be performed once or twice daily with a large-bore needle under aseptic conditions until there is resolution of clinical symptoms, joint cultures are negative, and synovial leukocyte counts, serum WBC, and inflammatory markers normalize. Although serial arthrocentesis is a good option for patients who are poor surgical candidates or whose joint may not be salvageable based on imaging assessment, there is increasing evidence that initial arthrocentesis should be followed by aggressive arthroscopic joint lavage.[116-118] The joint should be irrigated with at least 9 L of lactated Ringer solution or NaCl 0.9% solution. Antiseptic irrigation should be avoided because it may cause chondrolysis.[119]

There is no high-level evidence to show arthroscopic débridement is superior to arthrotomy for the treatment of native joint septic arthritis, yet there are intuitive advantages. Arthroscopy facilitates joint visualization, facilitates staging of the infection (Table 49.16), allows for a thorough débridement, and permits early joint range of motion. Synovectomy is not recommended for Gächter stage 1 and 2 infections because it limits the synovial perfusion of antimicrobial therapy. Arthrotomy is necessary for adequate débridement if the infection

cannot be controlled by serial arthroscopic débridement and lavage, in Gächter stage 3 infections where the synovium is thick, or if there is evidence of osteomyelitis (Gächter stage 4).[116,120] Arthrotomy is also indicated in the presence of periarticular implants or retained suture within the joint capsule, which must be removed in order to eliminate biofilm.

There are limited data comparing arthroscopy and arthrotomy in the treatment of native septic arthritis. In the knee, both approaches demonstrated successful treatment in 80%-100% of cases but the risk for infection relapse and poorer functional outcome was more common in the arthrotomy group.[121,122] A review of limited reports in the literature a small case series on treatment of septic arthritis in the native ankle shows a high cure rate with arthroscopic débridement and lavage.[117] Single surgical débridement has a higher success rate in smaller joints, including the ankle.[104,123] Finally, immediate surgical drainage and lavage may not be necessary for successful treatment. A recent survey of 204 culture-positive cases of native septic arthritis at a median 2-year outcome showed that surgery delayed up to 48 hours after diagnosis produced the same functional outcome as surgery within 6 hours of diagnosis.[124]

In children who present with acute uncomplicated septic arthritis, arthrocentesis and antimicrobial therapy may be sufficient treatment providing MRSA is not the cause.[125,126] Two to three weeks of oral antibiotic therapy may follow only 3-5 days of targeted intravenous antibiotic therapy based on clinical improvement and a significant reduction of CRP.[127] In cases complicated by host compromise or more virulent microorganisms, a longer period of intravenous antimicrobial therapy is often necessary. In MRSA infections, 4-6 weeks of antibiotic therapy is recommended.[128] So long as the child's clinical course is improving, a CRP below 2 mg/dL is an indication to stop antibiotic therapy.[129] Consultation with a pediatric infectious disease specialist is advisable.

Surgical drainage and lavage of the septic joint is necessary in neonates, in immunocompromised children, for isolation of virulent pathogens (MRSA or *Salmonella* spp.), and in cases not responsive to antimicrobial therapy. Arthroscopic débridement and lavage is safe and effective for large and small joints in very young children.[130]

Authors' Preferred Treatment Protocol for Native Ankle Septic Arthritis

- Immediate joint aspiration under aseptic skin preparation and fluid analysis
  - If low fluid yield: arthroscopic synovial biopsy
  - If purulence: arthroscopic débridement/lavage
- Other diagnostics: blood cultures, CBC, CRP, radiographs
- Saline-load test if traumatic arthrotomy suspected
- Early empiric intravenous antibiotics
- If fluid aspirate diagnosticbut subchondral erosions on x-ray: arthrotomy, débridement/lavage, bone biopsy
- Culture-directed antimicrobial therapy: consult infectious disease specialist
- Close patient monitoring: examination, WBC, serial CRP until normal
- Mobilize joint

Low threshold for repeat joint irrigation/débridement

TABLE 49.16	Gächter Staging Criteria for Native Joint Septic Arthritis
Stage	**Intraoperative Findings**
1	Synovitis, cloudy fluid
2	Purulence, hemorrhagic synovium, fibrin collections
3	Synovial membrane thickening with adhesions and pouch formation
4	Aggressive synovitis, pannus, subchondral erosion

From Stutz G, Kuster MS, Kleinstück F, et al. Arthroscopic management of septic arthritis: stages of infection and results. *Knee Surg Sports Traumatol Arthrosc.* 2000;8:270-274.

Periprosthetic joint infection is covered in Chapter 32.

POSTOPERATIVE CARE AND REHABILITATION

As with soft tissue infections, an adequate course of antimicrobial therapy should be completed with regular assessment of the patient's clinical response along with laboratory markers. In the acute phase of recovery the patient should be kept non–weight bearing. Early ankle range of motion is important to maintain joint health. In some cases the joint may be temporarily immobilized to mitigate any complications relative to healing the surgical wound. However, passive range of motion and isometric exercise should commence for joint reconditioning as soon as the surgical wound has closed and symptoms permit. Incremental return to ankle load is permitted as tolerated.

ADULT OSTEOMYELITIS

Osteomyelitis is an infection of bone and the medullary canal.[131] The incidence of osteomyelitis in the United States is not well understood. A Minnesota population-based study over 40 years found the annual prevalence to be 21.8 cases per 100 000 person-years; in patients without diabetes the incidence of pedal osteomyelitis was 15%.[132] The most common causes of adult osteomyelitis are trauma and surgery, which are the genesis of contiguous focus infection that is most prevalent in the lower extremity. Prior surgery, wounds following trauma, and diabetic foot ulcers are the primary causes of osteomyelitis in the foot and ankle. Up to half of all cases of osteomyelitis are posttraumatic and the infection is polymicrobial: S aureus, coagulase-negative staphylococci, gram-negative bacilli, and anaerobic organisms have been shown to account for over 75% of microorganisms.[133] MRSA is increasingly prevalent, isolated in upwards of 50% of adults hospitalized for osteomyelitis. Postsurgical osteomyelitis is typically caused by coagulase-negative staphylococci and S aureus. The pathogenic organisms may also be based on the epidemiologic factors or the environment in which the injury occurred (Fig. 49.16). Table 49.17 presents common microorganisms in adult osteomyelitis based on patient risk factor. Hematogenous osteomyelitis primarily afflicts children but may also occur in older adults over 65 years, where gram-negative rod organisms are often isolated.[134]

CLASSIFICATION AND ANATOMIC FEATURES

Established in 1983, the Cierny-Mader classification for chronic osteomyelitis defines the natural history of the disease by describing the extent of infection, the physiologic status of the host, and effective protocol-based treatment.[135] This clinical staging system describes three host classes and four anatomic types of infection, defining 12 different categories of adult osteomyelitis to stratify risk factors for treatment (Table 49.18).

The condition of the host determines appropriate patient selection for treatment. A single physiologic class is established based on host health, the impact of the disease, and response to treatment. A patient with a strong immune system who has a normal physiologic response to stress and infection is categorized as an A-host. Any patient with comorbidities that may

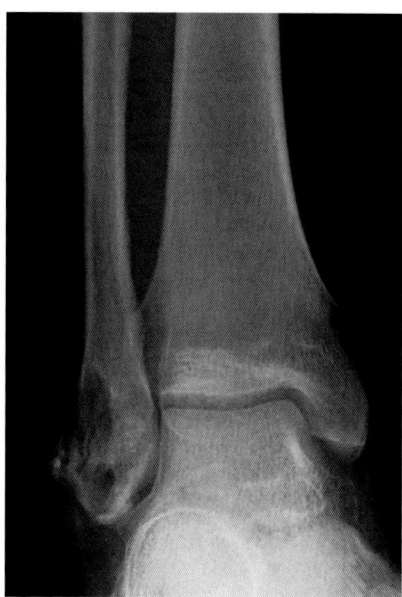

FIGURE 49.16 Ankle radiograph demonstrates fibular malleolus rarefaction and a cloaca in a patient with valley fever.

compromise wound healing and response to treatment is considered a B-host. In the C-host class the treatment plan may be more detrimental to the patient than the disease. These cases warrant observation or antibiotic suppression. However, if the disease worsens or there is an opportunity to improve the patient's quality of life by a new treatment, the C-host may be

TABLE 49.17	Common Microorganisms in Adult Osteomyelitis
Risk Factor	**Microorganisms**
Trauma/open fracture	Staphylococcus aureus Gram-negative bacilli Clostridium spp. Bacillus spp.
Implant-associated	Coagulase-negative staphylococci Staphylococcus aureus Corynebacterium spp. Propionibacterium spp.
Nosocomial infection	Enterobacteriaceae Pseudomonas spp.
Immunocompromise	Aspergillus spp. Candida spp. Mycobacterium avium complex
Intravenous drug use	Staphylococcus aureus Pseudomonas aeruginosa Enterobacteriaceae Candida spp.
HIV infection	Bartonella henselae Bartonella quintana
Sickle cell disease	Salmonella spp. Streptococcus pneumoniae
Pedal puncture wound	Pseudomonas aeruginosa
Bite wound	Pasteurella multocida Eikenella corrodens

From Lew DP, Waldvogel FA. Osteomyelitis. *Lancet.* 2004;364:369-379.

TABLE 49.18	Cierny-Mader Classification for Chronic Osteomyelitis
Host Class	**Anatomic Type**
A—Normal physiologic response	I—Medullary
B—Compromised healing capacity	II—Superficial
C—Treatment worse than disease	III—Localized
	IV—Diffuse

From Cierny G III, Mader JT, Pennick JJ. A clinical staging system for adult osteomyelitis. *Clin Orthop Relat Res.* 2003;414:7-24.

reclassified. The impact of treatment on the host must also be closely monitored so B-hosts do not fall to C-host class.

The impact of the disease is also based on the extent of bone involvement. Anatomic types I-IV characterize the natural history of osteomyelitis in increasing order of severity based on the scope of infection (Fig. 49.17). Type I (medullary osteomyelitis) is defined by an infection nidus confined to endosteal bone, often with involvement of the surrounding soft tissue envelope. A common instance in the adult is the infected intramedullary implant. Hematogenous osteomyelitis in the adult is uncommon and occurs primarily in the immunocompromised host. Type II (superficial osteomyelitis) is a contiguous focus lesion that is most common in the foot and ankle. The infection nidus affects only the superficial aspect of exposed bone at the base of a wound and does not extend to the medullary canal. Type III (localized osteomyelitis) is a full-thickness but often discrete cortical sequestrum within a stable osseous segment. The infection nidus extends into the medullary canal. A soft tissue defect may be present. It is most common in cases of retained hardware with infection following osteosynthesis. In type IV

(diffuse osteomyelitis) the infection nidus is permeative, compromising the soft tissue, multiple cortices, and the medullary canal. It represents the culmination of types I through III with the morbid addition of skeletal instability, established either by the disease or following surgical treatment.

PHYSICAL EXAMINATION

The clinical presentation of a patient with osteomyelitis is highly variable. The spectrum encompasses acute infection with pain and bone tenderness, swelling, warm, fluctuance from the production of pus, and fever. Yet in some chronic infections none of these clinical features are present. Such variability is a result of both pathogen virulence and host immune response. Physical examination must consider all factors that will influence treatment: a close evaluation of the local process, the quality of the overlying soft tissue envelope, careful assessment of the wound when present, limb deformity, and joint contractures. Signs of vascular compromise in the limb or local tissues will determine the indications for angiography and transcutaneous oxygen assessment for soft tissue coverage when necessary. Finally, a complete history and physical examination is essential to assess the health of the patient and determine factors that may complicate the host response to the disease and the treatment.

PATHOGENESIS

Normal bone is resistant to infection, which is caused by either a sudden tissue breach or the introduction of microorganisms through hematogenous dissemination that overwhelms the host immune response. The infection begins with a suppurative inflammatory process with neutrophil recruit-

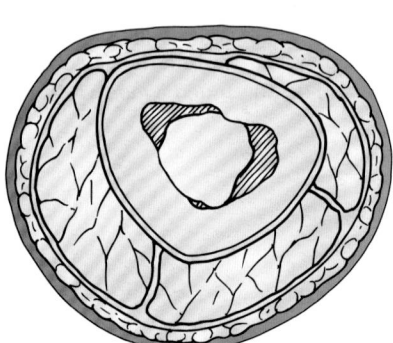
I Medullary osteomyelitis

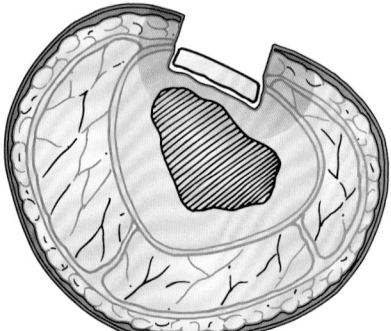
II Superficial osteomyelitis

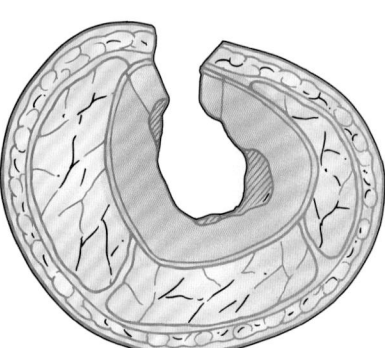
III Localized osteomyelitis

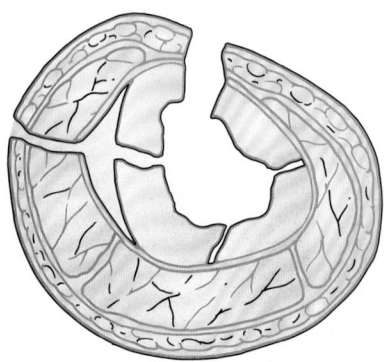
IV Diffuse osteomyelitis

FIGURE 49.17 Graphic depiction of the four anatomic types of osteomyelitis based on the Cierny-Mader classification scheme. (From Cierny G III, Mader JT, Pennick JJ. A clinical staging system for adult osteomyelitis. *Clin Orthop Relat Res.* 2003;414:7-24.)

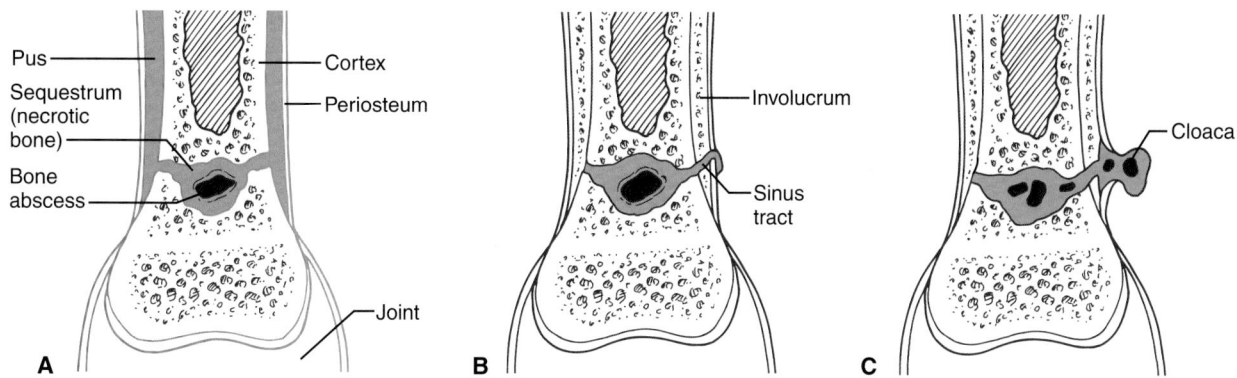

FIGURE 49.18 Graphic depiction of the pathogenesis of bone destruction in osteomyelitis. **A.** Development of sequestrum (necrotic bone) and extrusion of necrotic debris into subperiosteal space. **B.** Reactive new periosteal bone (involucrum) forms to contain infection and a tract often develops from sequestrum. **C.** A cloaca forms through involucrum for sequestrum egress.

ment and phagocytosis. Local blood supply is compromised by vascular congestion and small vessel thrombosis. A complex cascade of innate immune response and bacterial toxins leads to osteoclast-mediated bone resorption.[136-138] Over time, healthy bone is gradually lost to infection and the process becomes chronic, characterized by the persistence of necrotic bone and biofilm. Figure 49.18 depicts the pathogenesis of bone destruction in osteomyelitis. The sequestrum of necrotic bone becomes isolated from the surrounding live bone through segmentation and resorption. At the same time reactive new bone formation—the involucrum—develops around the infection nidus or sequestra to isolate the pathogen(s). As the infection progresses it may advance into the subperiosteal space, which is more common in children. If the process is close to the joint capsule, a septic arthritis may arise. Tracts often develop from the sequestrum into the involucrum, allowing a cloaca to form for the extrusion of necrotic debris. This process is often visible on imaging but may also manifest on clinical examination (Fig. 49.19). A chronic draining sinus may persist (Fig. 49.20).

Pathogen Virulence

Disease severity and course are influenced by pathogen virulence. *Staphylococcus aureus* and *Staphylococcus epidermidis* are two common bacteria ubiquitous on human skin with significant virulence factors. Both pathogens have numerous modes of survival afforded by their capacity to evade human immune response, live within host cells, and adapt to the host environment. *S aureus* is responsible for most cases of osteomyelitis and is capable of causing acute infection due to coagulase, which enables the bacteria to avoid phagocytosis. *S aureus* produces a multitude of protein secretions that alter or inhibit both innate and adaptive mechanisms of host immune response.[139] Some of these proteins facilitate attachment to both implants and bone.[140,141] In the animal model *S aureus* is capable of initiating biofilm formation soon after infection that matures within 1-2 weeks.[142] Other secretions are bone-resorbing toxins that allow *S aureus* to invade, multiply within, and destroy osteoblasts.[143,144] *S aureus* may also utilize sequestra as a reservoir for survival.[145] Transmission electronic microscopy of sequestra has also demonstrated *S aureus* in cana-

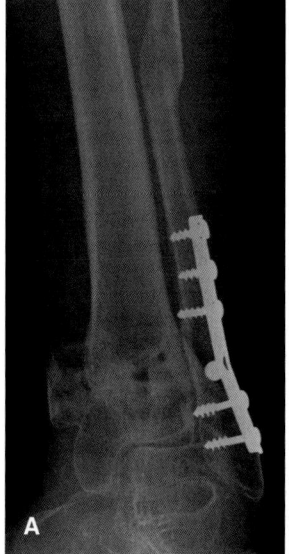

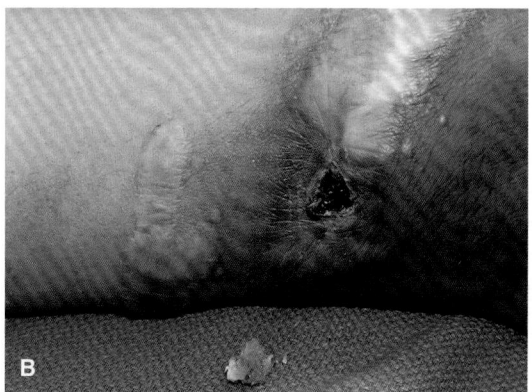

FIGURE 49.19 A. Ankle radiograph demonstrating distal tibial chronic osteomyelitis 2 years following surgery: sequestrum, involucrum, and cloaca as depicted in Figure 49.18. **B.** Clinical photograph of same patient demonstrating the cloaca along the medial ankle.

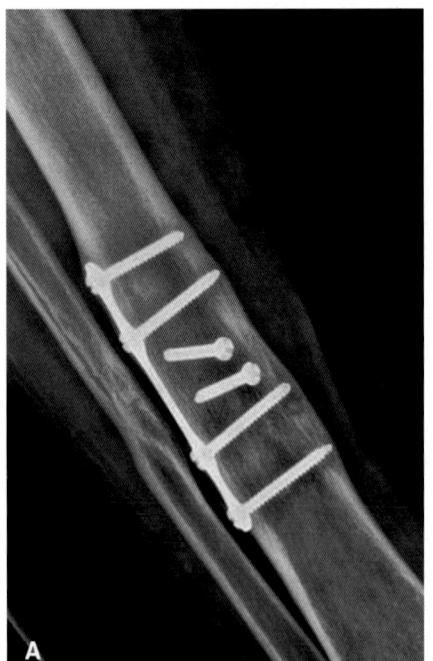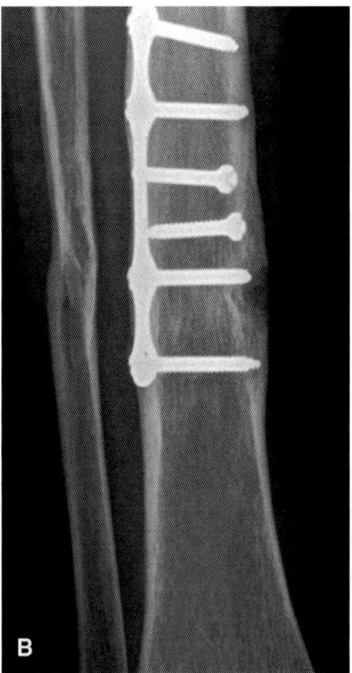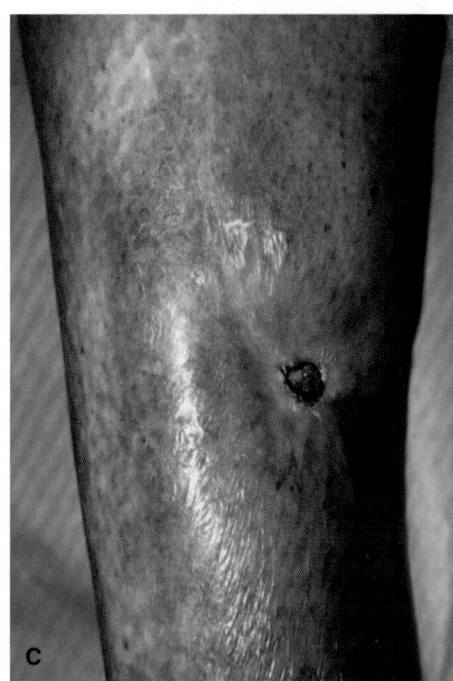

FIGURE 49.20 Healed tibia fracture with chronic osteomyelitis 45 years after surgery. **A.** Leg radiograph demonstrates tibial sequestra and involucrum along medial cortex adjacent to the retained implant. **B.** Follow-up radiograph depicts the cloaca. **C.** Clinical photograph of draining sinus, which has closed and reopened for decades.

liculi.[146] These mechanisms demonstrate the tenacity of *S aureus* for chronic and relapsing infection. In comparison, *S epidermidis* is low virulence in terms of its toxin activity, but it is capable of rapidly forming a dense biofilm and is a significant pathogen for implant-related infection. It has also been shown to invade osteoblasts.[147] *S epidermidis* infection may not clinically manifest for many months to years.[148]

Biofilm

William Costerton, an early pioneer of important biofilm research, described the entity as bacterial cells that establish a structured immobile community enclosed in a self-produced polymeric extracellular matrix adherent to an inert or living surface.[149] Biofilm is essentially an alternative lifestyle for microorganisms that enables enhanced growth and protection from host defenses and antimicrobial therapy.[149] All biofilms are dynamic with a life cycle of microorganism attachment, maturation, and dispersal within weeks (Fig. 49.21). Some biofilms are complex communities composed of multiple bacterial species. Many microorganisms have virulence factors that enable biofilm formation (Table 49.19). Persistent infection is the result of two mechanisms of microorganism survival: biofilm maturation facilitates mutations of some bacteria that allow them become dormant and resist antibiotics,[150] while other bacterial cells respond to virulence factors that promote dissemination for biofilm growth or disassembly to establish new communities.[151,152]

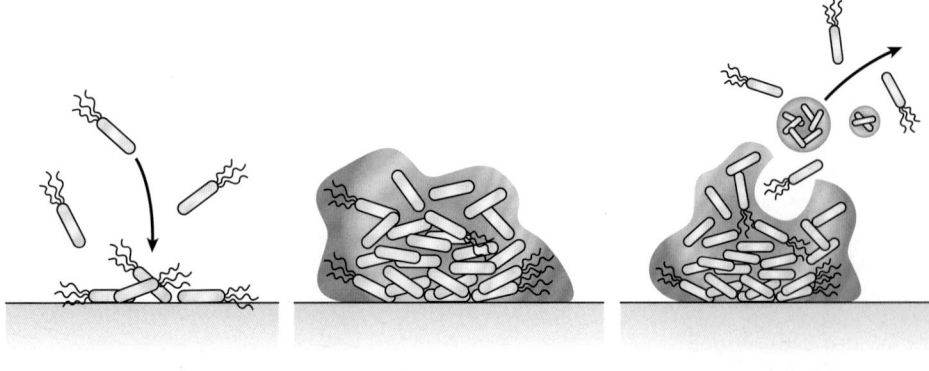

1 Attachment   2 Maturation   3 Dispersal

FIGURE 49.21 Graphic depiction of the life cycle of a biofilm.

TABLE 49.19	Microorganisms Capable of Forming Strong Biofilms

Staphylococcus aureus
Coagulase-negative staphylococci: *S epidermidis, S lugdunensis*

Streptococci: *S agalactiae, S pyogenes, S pneumonia, S viridans*

Enterococci: *E faecalis, E faecium*

Enterobacteria: *Enterobacter* spp., *E coli, Klebsiella* spp., *Proteus* spp., *Citrobacter* spp., *Serratia* spp., *Morganella* spp., *Salmonella* spp.

Pseudomonas aeruginosa
Fungi: *Candida species* or *Aspergillus*

Bacterial biofilms constitute at least 65% of human bacterial infections.[153] The vast majority of orthopedic infections are biofilm infections because of the presence of implants and dead bone sequestrate. Implants provide microorganisms with surfaces for secure attachment and access to host factors, both of which facilitate biofilm growth. In some cases, implant colonization is asymptomatic and host defenses may suppress microorganisms in the biofilm indefinitely. Yet pathogens may produce infection after existing in a sessile state for years (Fig. 49.22). In other cases, microorganisms seed a retained implant because of a vascular response to the device or the mechanical influence of the implant on the bone.

DIAGNOSTIC STUDIES

Similar to evaluation of the native septic joint, WBC count, ESR, and CRP are standard serum inflammatory markers for the evaluation of osteomyelitis. A meta-analysis study of these markers for the diagnosis of late fracture-related infection demonstrated each to lack sufficient accuracy: CRP showed a sensitivity and specificity of 67.8% and 77% respectively; ESR was 45.1% and 79.3%, respectively; WBC was 51.7% and 67.1%, respectively.[154] In that study, combined scores improved diagnostic accuracy for fracture-related infection but the sensitivity was not sufficiently compelling. However, another study evaluated diagnostic value of WBC, CRP, and ESR for infection in fracture nonunion and showed the value of each marker to be additive: the probability of infection with one, two, and three positive

tests was 18.8%, 56%, and 100%, respectively.[155] Yet CRP and ESR have demonstrated poor combined sensitivity (33%) and specificity (84%) in the diagnosis of osteomyelitis in the nondiabetic foot.[156] As noted earlier in this chapter, procalcitonin may also serve to rule in the diagnosis of acute osteomyelitis at a cutoff level of 0.4 ng/mL.[3] While there are conflicting data regarding the utility of serum inflammatory markers for the diagnosis of osteomyelitis in the ankle and foot, the diagnosis is not made by laboratory analysis alone. There is value in combining all three markers in the context of clinical evaluation of the patient and the judgment of the treating physician. Furthermore, serial CRP measurements are important for monitoring the clinical course of the infection and evaluating the patient's response to treatment.

Traditional culture methods remain the gold standard for diagnosis of osteomyelitis. Yet the accuracy of intraoperative tissue samples for microorganism detection is highly variable, from 65% to 95%.[157] To increase culture yield, a minimum of 3-5 tissue samples for different sites should be sampled.[158] Adequate tissue sample volume is also important[10-12] (Fig. 49.23). More tissue samples may be necessary in cases of low-grade infection. It is critical to follow meticulous tissue procurement methods described earlier in this chapter and to have the microbiology laboratory hold specimens for at least 2 weeks. Yet even with a sufficient number of tissue samples from high-probability sites it may be impossible to identify any pathogens. Suppurative infections typically contain ample planktonic (free-living) bacteria, which can be readily grown in the laboratory. However, bacteria in biofilm are sessile and very difficult to grow in the laboratory.[159] These bacteria are often resistant to identification by conventional cultures, hence the prevalence of culture-negative infection.[160]

Modern methods of molecular diagnosis such as PCR and fluorescent in situ hybridization (FISH) may be considered for microorganism identification in culture-negative infections.[161] However, as noted earlier in this chapter, there are conflicting data about the efficacy of PCR compared with traditional cultures for bacterial detection in periprosthetic infections.[107,108] NGS has shown promise in detecting microorganisms in

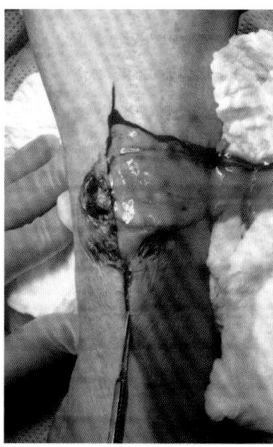

FIGURE 49.22 A Brodie abscess 20 years following open tibia fracture.

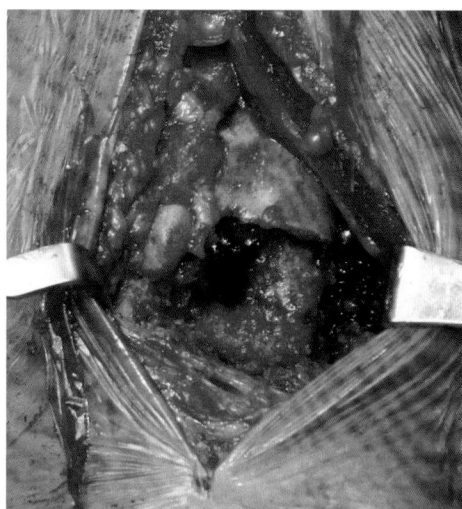

FIGURE 49.23 Intraoperative photograph depicting the harvest site of multiple tissue blocks from the distal tibia and ankle for diagnosis of chronic osteomyelitis.

culture-negative periprosthetic joint infections.[162] Yet it remains to be determined if this culture-independent testing method is effective for diagnosing other prosthetic infections. Sonication is a low-intensity ultrasound process that disrupts bacterial biofilm and improves culture sensitivity compared to conventional methods.[13,163] It is not yet known whether this method is effective for the identification of fungal organisms or mycobacteria. Although sonication is expensive and not yet prevalent, it is increasingly utilized in the diagnosis of periprosthetic joint infection. There is a role for sonication in the diagnosis of osteomyelitis where implants are present. Unfortunately these advanced diagnostic tests are not widely available.

The histopathologic findings in osteomyelitis vary based on a number of factors including the microorganism, blood supply, involved bone, host immunity, and patient age. Neutrophils are most common in acute suppurative osteomyelitis, but they are also often identified from tissue samples in chronic osteomyelitis, along with chronic inflammatory cells such as macrophages, lymptocytes, and plasma cells.[164] The neutrophilic response is seen in infections that have been dormant for years and may be related to biofilm shedding from necrotic bone, suggesting recurrence of infection.[165] As noted earlier in this chapter, histological analysis and fresh frozen sections are a useful adjunct for the diagnosis of infection and may rule out other granulomatous or neoplastic processes.

IMAGING

Conventional radiographs are the first step in imaging for the diagnosis of osteomyelitis because they are inexpensive, are readily available, and are useful for excluding other diagnoses such as trauma or neoplasm.[166] Yet radiographs are insensitive for detection of the early stages of osteomyelitis because 30%-50% of bone destruction is necessary before abnormalities are visible on x-ray.[167] Initial findings include localized soft tissue swelling, osteolysis, and periosteal reaction. Serial x-rays are useful for assessing skeletal changes over time, which may be high yield in cases of acute osteomyelitis. As the infection progresses, bone rarefaction, erosion, sequestra, and reactive bone formation are visible as depicted in Figures 49.18-49.20. However, radiographs do not demonstrate these findings until 2-3 weeks after the onset of infection. The sensitivity and specificity of radiography for the diagnosis of osteomyelitis is limited (Table 49.20). Radiographs cannot distinguish between an infectious and aseptic process, such as avascular necrosis, arthrosis, osteolysis, or new bone formation evident in fracture healing (Fig. 49.24). Osteomyelitis in the presence of implants is typically evident by device loosening with or without the aforementioned bone changes (Fig. 49.25).

CT imaging is far superior to radiography in defining bone pathology.[172] In acute osteomyelitis, the features of periosteal reaction and increasing density of the medullary canal from edema can be identified by CT.[168] Common features of chronic osteomyelitis—sequestrum, involucrum, and cloaca—are well demonstrated by CT.[173] CT is also useful for surgical planning because it defines available bone volume, integrity, and the status of a nonunion if present.

MRI is highly sensitive for osteomyelitis and is often considered the imaging modality of choice for diagnosis, particularly in the early stages of the disease. MRI delineates margins of inflammation within soft tissue, cortical bone, and the medullary canal.[174] This makes the imaging modality valuable for localizing bone compromise and determining the necessary extent of bone débridement and resection. In the acute phase, medullary inflammation and edema produces decreased signal intensity on T1-weighted images and increased signal intensity on T2-weighted and fat suppression sequences (short T1 inversion recovery or fat saturation); in chronic osteomyelitis cortical thickening and defects may be visible (Fig. 49.26). However, fibrovascular scar, Charcot neuroarthropathy, and neoplasm may show similar signal changes and

TABLE 49.20 Imaging Diagnostic Accuracy for Osteomyelitis		
Study	**Sensitivity**	**Specificity**
Radiography[113]	67%	60%
CT[168]	66%	97%
MRI[113]	84% (69%-92%)	60% (38%-78%)
Bone scintigraphy[113]	82% (70%-89%)	25% (16%-36%)
Leukocyte scintigraphy[113]	61% (43%-76%)	77% (63%-87%)
Combined bone and leukocyte scintigraphy[113]	78% (72%-83%)	84% (75%-90%)
FDG PET-CT[169]	86%-94%	76%-100%
SPECT CT[170]	100%	89%
SPECT CT + combined bone and leukocyte scintigraphy[171]	50%-87%	43%-71%

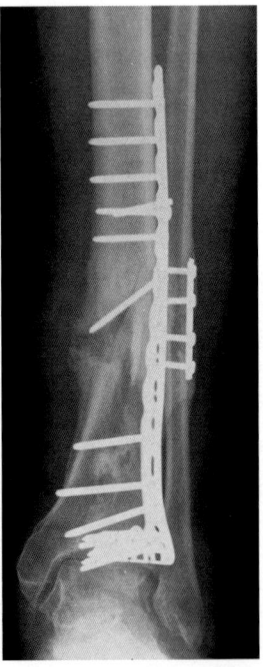

FIGURE 49.24 Radiograph demonstrating medullary and cortical changes suggestive of either callus formation or chronic osteomyelitis following plate osteosynthesis of a grade IIIA tibia fracture. The patient was asymptomatic, had no concerning clinical examination findings, and was found to have normal serum inflammatory markers, bone cultures, and histopathologic results.

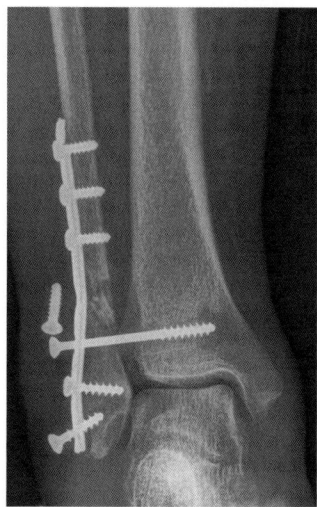

FIGURE 49.25 Radiograph depicting chronic osteomyelitis following osteosynthesis of a distal fibula fracture: implant loosening, bone rarefaction in the distal medial tibia, and sequestrum in the fibula.

produce false-positive readings for osteomyelitis. Gadolinium is indicated when an abscess or sinus tract is suspected.[175] Artifact from the presence of metal implants also obscures signs of infection on MRI. There are a number of proposed metal artifact reduction sequence techniques to improve bone depiction.[176,177] Although some of these metal artifact suppression modalities may improve image quality, no studies demonstrate the diagnostic accuracy of MRI for osteomyelitis in the presence of metal implants. A systematic review and meta-analysis demonstrated that the diagnostic accuracy of MRI was similar to leukocyte scintigraphy and combined bone and leukocyte scintigraphy[113] (Table 49.20). In cases where MRI produces false positive results, artifact precludes reliable interpretation, or the study is contraindicated, nuclear medicine may be necessary.

Nuclear medicine provides a number of effective imaging modalities to aid in the diagnosis of osteomyelitis. It is based on the evaluation of an injected radioactive tracer that localizes in tissue through its binding to certain cell types. Nuclear medicine scans depict cellular activity and therefore help define the extent of nonviable bone. One of the most common bone scintigraphy studies is a technetium-99m methylene diphosphate (Tc-99m MDP) scan, where the altered metabolic activity of the involved bone demonstrates increased tracer uptake.[178] MDP collects in areas of bone metabolism by absorbing onto the hydroxyapatite crystals. This scan helps discriminate between cellulitis vs osteomyelitis and helps define the extent of bone infection.[179] Increased activity on all three phases measured over time—blood flow (60 seconds), blood pool (5-10 minutes), and delayed (2-4 hours)—is consistent with osteomyelitis. The delayed phase demonstrates tracer uptake only in bone (Fig. 49.27). Absence of tracer uptake in well-vascularized tissue essentially rules out osteomyelitis. Yet false-negative scans may result in tissue with impaired blood supply, commonly seen in acute hematogenous osteomyelitis (AHO). False positive scans may occur due to normal uptake in vascularized tissue at areas of bone remodeling, trauma, Charcot neuroarthropathy, and neoplasm.

Leukocyte-labeled radionucleotide scans were developed to improve the specificity of scintigraphy for diagnosis in musculoskeletal infection. A technetium-99m hexamethyl-propyleneamine oxime (HMPAO)-labeled leukocyte scan (Ceretec) is superior to bone scintigraphy alone and has replaced most indium-111-labeled leukocyte scans because of diminished radiation, increased speed, and high-quality images. This scan is more specific for neutrophil production and bone marrow reaction that are present in infection. Tc-99m HMPAO scans are useful for complex cases where there is a history of trauma, surgery, or Charcot neuroarthropathy. Tc-99m sulfur colloid scanning may also improve leukocyte scan specificity for infection in complex cases by an inverse correlation of diminished medullary bone activity on the sulfur colloid scan compared to increased uptake on the leukocyte scan.

Introduced earlier in this chapter, an effective alternative scintigraphy technique is fluorine-18 fluorodeoxyglucose positron emission tomography (FDG PET). A radiolabeled glucose analog is utilized to identify intracellular glucose metabolism as well as leukocyte activity. It is most often combined with

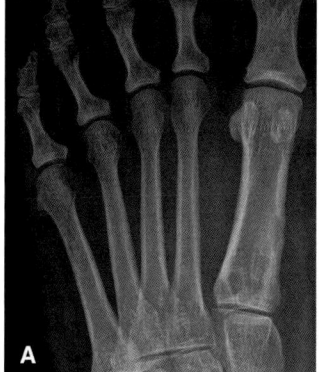 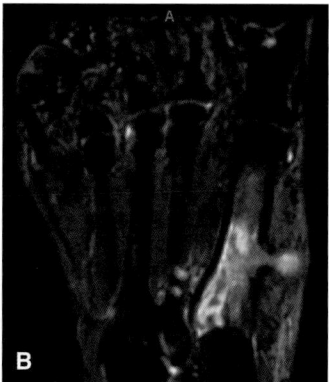 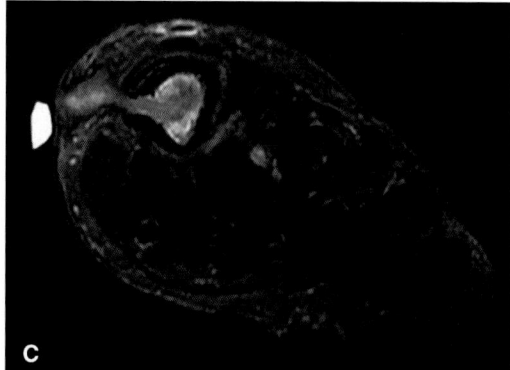

FIGURE 49.26 Chronic osteomyelitis of the first metatarsal. **A.** AP foot radiograph demonstrates cystic changes in the proximal metaphysis and disruption of the medial cortex at the diaphysis. MRI axial short T1 inversion recovery (STIR) sequence **(B)** and coronal fat saturation sequence **(C)** depict hyperintensity of the reactive medullary canal, cortical thickening, and an obvious breach in the cortex consistent with a cloaca.

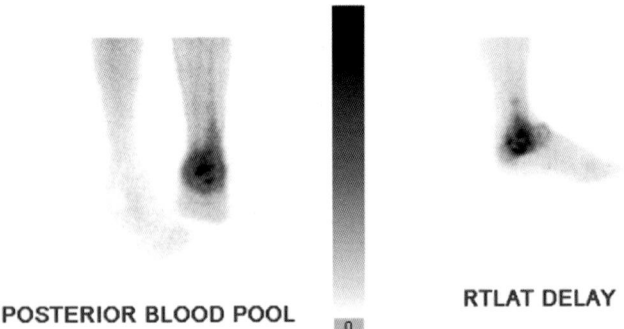

POSTERIOR BLOOD POOL   **RTLAT DELAY**

FIGURE 49.27 Tc-99 MDP scan consistent with ankle/hindfoot osteomyelitis. The blood pool flow phase is not shown. In the blood pool phase, the tracer uptake is more diffuse. In the delayed phase the tracer uptake is localized to bone.

computed tomography (FDG PET-CT) to provide good spatial resolution and better localize infection. The study is much faster and less expensive than leukocyte scintigraphy, and it has a relatively high diagnostic accuracy. As noted previously, FDG PET-CT scanning is also advantageous for the diagnosis of osteomyelitis because the sensitivity of infection sites visible by the tracer is not likely to be influenced by antibiotic therapy.

Single photon emission computed tomography (SPECT) CT combines imaging of altered bone physiology in scintigraphy with volume-rendered structural detail of bone afforded by CT. SPECT CT enables differentiation of infection at the level of the medullary canal, cortex, and subperiosteal space.[170] This study may also be combined with leukocyte scintigraphy to provide a more accurate picture of the location and extent of osteomyelitis.[180]

TREATMENT

Successful treatment of osteomyelitis is based on careful manipulation of the patient host, the pathogen, the soft tissue envelope, and the bone. The extent of disease, the anatomic site, patient impairment, the experience of the care team, and available resources will dictate whether the treatment plan is reconstructive, palliative, or ablative (Table 49.21). Physician experience and clinical judgment determines whether the path to limb salvage is justified, which is largely determined by patient comorbidities (Table 49.2). The impact of multiple comorbidities compounds the risk of limb reconstruction.[181,182] Once patient risk factors are defined, the host response must be optimized. In a 15-year outcome study of nearly 2000 patients treated for chronic osteomyelitis, Cierny and DiPasquale demonstrated that host deficiencies could be improved to the point where B-host outcomes approached those of A-hosts.[180] If the B-host response cannot be improved, surgical methods that minimize patient morbidity are often successful, such as protocols for staged treatment that include local antibiotic therapy and atraumatic exposure.[184]

Robust modern treatment protocols for chronic osteomyelitis have demonstrated the capacity to achieve infection-free functional outcome in over 90% of patients, minimize the incidence of C-hosts, and diminish amputation rates to well below 10% despite the steady increase in B-hosts over time.[183] This is in stark contrast to the persistent infections and chronic wounds that defined poor outcomes with 36%-50% treatment failure before the mid-1970s.[185,186] Yet suppressive therapy is necessary when reconstruction poses too great a risk to patient health and function. However, if palliation is neither safe nor practical for the patient, amputation is indicated. Some cases of pedal osteomyelitis provide for a unique intersection of reconstruction and ablation for a curative outcome. Isolated ray or transmetatarsal amputations are a prime example, as many patients function quite well after these operations. In such cases a curative outcome is also functional, yet in many instances of treatment a functional outcome alone is an acceptable result. Indeed, the tenacity of some pathogens in the setting of inept host response may make a cure for osteomyelitis simply impossible in many cases of limb preservation. Yet, with modern regimented treatment protocols, most patients will see a significant improvement in the quality of their life.

TABLE 49.21	Key Factors in the Treatment of Adult Osteomyelitis
Host status	
Functional impairment	
Anatomic site	
Extent of bone necrosis	

From Cierny M, Mader JT, Pennick JJ. A clinical staging system for adult osteomyelitis. *Clin Orthop Relat Res.* 2003;414:7-24.

PEARLS FOR DIAGNOSIS AND TREATMENT OF ADULT OSTEOMYELITIS IN THE DISTAL LOWER EXTREMITY

- Recognize patient host factors that may complicate or preclude treatment
- Host/disease assessment based on Cierny-Mader scheme (Table 49.19)
- Collaborate with internist to optimize host
- Obtain serum inflammatory markers + WBC count
- Imaging assessment: radiographs, MRI, +/− Tc-99m HMPAO scan
- Stop antibiotics at least 3 weeks prior to culture
- Obtain sufficient number of tissue samples from high-probability sites
- Special attention to pathogen virulence
- Recognize pathogens with unique antibiotic resistance mechanisms
- Application of antibiotic depots with vancomycin + gentamicin or tobramycin
- Careful surgical planning and execution: Cierny-Mader treatment protocols
- Special attention to challenges of thin soft tissue envelope about the ankle and foot
- Specialist collaboration: infectious disease, vascular surgery, plastic surgery
- Frequent patient monitoring/close follow-up: examination and serum inflammatory markers
- Long-term follow-up

Systemic Antimicrobial Therapy

Many planktonic bacteria can be destroyed by competent host defenses and targeted antimicrobial therapy. Yet some pathogens have unique survival strategies. Antimicrobial resistance remains a significant challenge in the treatment of osteomyelitis. Certain bacteria demonstrate intrinsic antibiotic resistance. The resistance of *S aureus* to methicillin is ubiquitous. Enterococci modify proteins to which penicillin binds, hence the resistance to β-lactam antibiotics.[187] *E cloaca* is a good example. Vancomycin-resistant enterococci (VRE) have probably arisen from the transfer of genetic information necessary for antibiotic resistance from other bacterial strains or mutation.[188] *S epidermidis* and Pseudomonas species also demonstrate antibiotic resistance. Intracellular bacterial survival is another method of antimicrobial resistance. Many antibiotics are not active inside human cells and are effectively resisted by the intracellular accumulation of *S aureus* within osteoblasts.[189] Other bacteria demonstrate altered phenotype of small colonies with slow growth described as small-colony variants, which are also capable of intracellular survival.[190] Staphylococci, *E coli*, *P aeruginosa*, and salmonella species may all exist as small colony variants.

Biofilm is one of the most significant barriers to the medical treatment of osteomyelitis. Necrotic bone may form as early as 10 days postinfection, and some bacteria rapidly form biofilm within this period of time. Bacteria in a biofilm are resistant to most antibacterial agents owing to diminished antibiotic penetration of the extracellular matrix, reduced metabolic activity of bacteria, and phenotypic bacterial transformation that evades antibiotic agents.[144] Microcolonies may be another reservoir for chronic infection. They are described as patches of biofilm associated with soft tissue observed in recurrent soft tissue infections.[191] Although they have not yet been observed in human osteomyelitis, microcolonies have been demonstrated in animal models.[192]

Two antibiotic agents are particularly effective for treatment of bone infection. Rifampin has superb activity against *S aureus* and enterococci, making it a mainstay of antibiotic therapy in osteomyelitis.[193,194] Rifampin is also uniquely suited to treat osteomyelitis because it is the only antibiotic capable of targeting gram-positive biofilm.[195,196] It has also been shown to destroy intracellular *S aureus* replication within osteoblasts.[197] The quinolones have demonstrated activity against gram-negative biofilms.

Targeted antimicrobial therapy is selected based on the identified pathogens. At least 6 weeks of parenteral antibiotic therapy is often recommended for most cases of osteomyelitis. Increasingly patients may be converted from intravenous to oral antibiotics earlier in the course of treatment. The patient's response to treatment must be closely assessed based on examination, serial serum inflammatory markers, and in some cases imaging. In some cases of osteomyelitis chronic antimicrobial suppression may be necessary.

Rarely can adult osteomyelitis be treated effectively without an operation because of the aforementioned pathogen virulence and survival mechanisms. Furthermore, there are wide variations in bacterial strain, inoculum volume, and the host response to infection. In some instances of acute contiguous osteomyelitis (Cierny-Mader stage II lesion), targeted antibiotic therapy and wound care may be effective so long as early treatment is initiated.[135] However, the infection site should be observed for bone sequestra and the patient should be closely monitored for treatment failure with a low threshold for

débridement if either scenario is discovered. It is very difficult to differentiate between acute and chronic infection, where treatment is far more challenging. Cierny, Mader, and Pennick described an entity called minimal necrosis osteomyelitis where the chronic infection nidus is necrotic scar tissue rather than bone sequestra.[135] This situation arises because of the incapacity of the host to eliminate the nonviable tissue, which typically persists until the host response is improved.

SURGICAL TREATMENT

Surgery is essential for the treatment of chronic osteomyelitis. The fundamental tenant of the operation is the replacement of dead bone and soft tissue scar with durable, vascular tissue.[135] This approach establishes a clean wound, revascularizes the bone, and facilitates antimicrobial therapy. The sessile pathogens protected by a resilient biofilm at the substrate must be physically eradicated. Only a thorough débridement will achieve healthy, bleeding bone. Targeted local and systemic antimicrobial therapy follows. Over the past four decades the surgical treatment of osteomyelitis has seen significant advancements owing to innovations in bone stabilization and fixation, wound coverage through negative pressure therapy and various flaps, discovery of biofilm and methods to isolate sessile pathogens, improved understanding of tissue transfer methods, the local delivery of antibiotics, and antimicrobial therapy for resistant microorganisms.[198-207] These innovations established a new foundation for the effective management of bone and soft tissue defects.

Maintaining or restoring the soft tissue envelope is critical for the successful treatment of osteomyelitis. Secondary intention healing is avoided whenever possible because the resulting scar becomes devascular.[135] Reliable coverage of the soft tissue defect was historically realized by muscle flaps, which date back to the 1940s. Flap coverage of the defect prevents microorganism recolonization, eliminates dead space, revascularizes bone and adjacent soft tissue structures, assists host defense mechanisms, enhances antibiotic delivery, and facilitates reexposure of the site (Fig. 49.28). In cases where flap coverage is delayed, fails, or is otherwise not an option, negative pressure wound therapy is a good alternative.[208,209] However, larger defects will often require a more definitive treatment plan.

Antibiotic Depots

The development of antibiotic depots has been one of the most important advances in the treatment of osteomyelitis. An antibiotic depot is the implantation of bone cement in the local tissue site loaded with antibiotic selected for the known or suspected pathogen(s). Antibiotic depots facilitate the local delivery of extremely high levels of antibiotics—50-100 times the concentration of parenteral therapy—often necessary to eliminate most microorganisms.[210] The depot helps destroy residual pathogens surrounding the infection site following a thorough surgical débridement, thereby diminishing some of the burden on host defenses.[211] Antibiotic depot protocols allow for staged treatment of chronic osteomyelitis similar to protocol treatments in orthopedic oncology.[212-214]

Polymethylmethacrylate (PMMA) is the most commonly used nonbiodegradable carrier. PMMA was first introduced in the 1970s to help minimize the risk of infection in total joint surgery and as a method of salvage for periprosthetic infection.[215] Commercially available bone cements are designed only

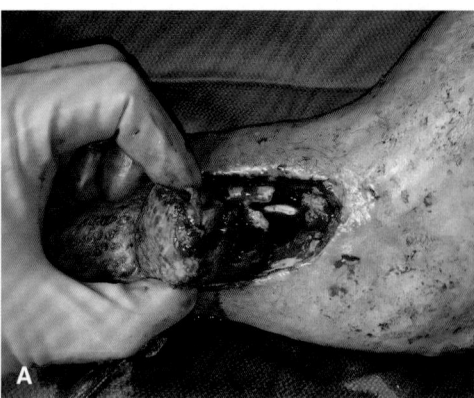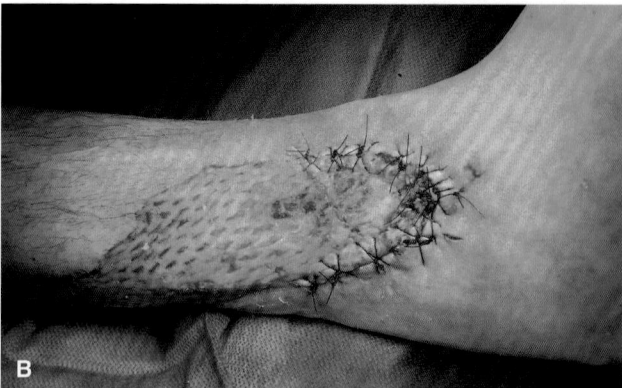

FIGURE 49.28 A. Mature gracilis free flap raised over the site of distal tibial osteomyelitis for decortication and débridement after removal of a hindfoot intramedullary nail, canal reaming, and placement of an antibiotic-loaded intramedullary nail (visible deep in wound). **B.** Flap reattachment.

for infection prophylaxis in total joint arthroplasty and should not be used in antibiotic depots because they contain a much lower antibiotic concentration. Palacos bone cement (Zimmer, Warsaw, IN) is preferred because of its elution kinetics.

The antibiotic mixed with PMMA must be available in pharmaceutical grade powder, heat stable, low toxicity, and demonstrate bioactivity against both gram-positive and gram-negative bacteria. Liquid antibiotics substantially weaken PMMA strength.[216] Bactericidal antibiotics are preferred: gentamicin, tobramycin, and vancomycin are most commonly utilized to load PMMA cement because of their elution characteristics and the synergy between vancomycin and the aminoglycosides. Clindamycin is less commonly utilized but is equally advantageous because it too demonstrates high tissue levels upon release.[217] Rifampin can be used only with carriers that are bioabsorbable, not PMMA.

Antibiotic elution from PMMA occurs rapidly in the initial phase—largely concentrated in the first 24 hours after implantation—followed by diminishing release over the subsequent weeks.[218] Increasing the monomer in the mixture will decrease the elution concentration, so less monomer is recommended to improve antibiotic release kinetics.[219] If cement exchange is planned it should transpire by 4 weeks after implantation because the much lower concentration of antibiotics by that time could harbor microorganism resistance and become an infection reservoir.[220] Ultimately the antibiotic depot is typically replaced with a bone graft, flap, or hardware.[211]

PMMA beads are an effective strategy for treatment of smaller defects or implantation about the soft tissue-bone interface. The high surface area to volume ratio increases antibiotic elution.[221] Suitable antibiotic dosage for treatment of osteomyelitis with handmade PMMA cement beads is found in Table 49.22.

If the ratio of antibiotic powder exceeds 24 to 120 mL per 40 g of cement the cement will not reliably harden.[135] Gentamicin-loaded PMMA beads are commercially available, but the advantage of handmade beads is the addition of other antibiotics to achieve synergy, reduced cost, and the ability to control bead size. The beads may be strung onto a stainless steel wire or a heavy nonabsorbable suture, which often simplifies their extraction. In some cases the soft tissue may be closed around a bead chain so it may be removed without a second operation, but it is important to keep the area sealed so the antibiotic elution remains in the tissues. In other instances, the nature of the soft tissue defect lends itself to delayed wound closure, and a bead pouch may be established (Fig. 49.29).

Resorbable antibiotic depots are also very useful for the treatment of osteomyelitis. Calcium sulfate beads are commercially available. They do not require removal, release antibiotic more uniformly over time, and, unlike PMMA, may be loaded with rifampin. However, they are limited in the type and amount of antibiotic they can deliver, they lack the integrity to function as a structural spacer, and they have a tendency to produce draining wound fistulas.[222] Calcium sulfate has been combined with nanoparticulate hydroxyapatite in solid pellet form and has demonstrated superior biocompatibility compared to calcium sulfate alone.[223] Bioactive glass is a relatively new resorbable carrier option that has osteoinductive, angiogenic, and antibacterial properties by virtue of

TABLE 49.22	Antibiotic Dosage for Handmade PMMA Beads
Antibiotic	**Dosage**
Gentamicin	1 g/40 mg PMMA powder
Tobramycin	1 g/40 mg PMMA powder
Vancomycin	2 g
+ Gentamicin	0.5 g/40 mg PMMA powder

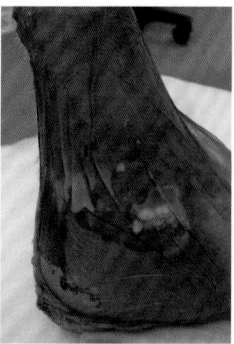

FIGURE 49.29 Antibiotic bead pouch within an ankle/hindfoot defect sealed by adhesive dressing.

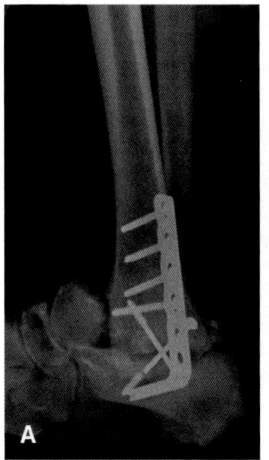 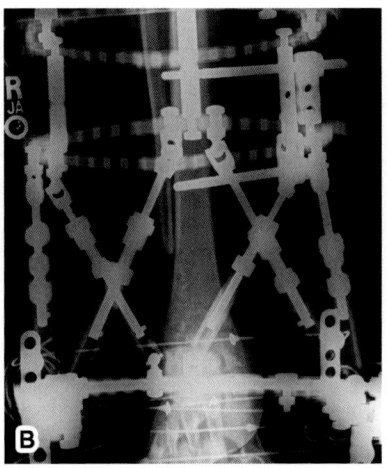 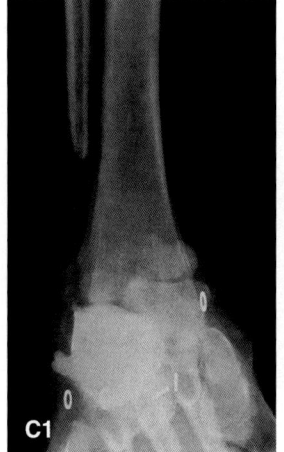 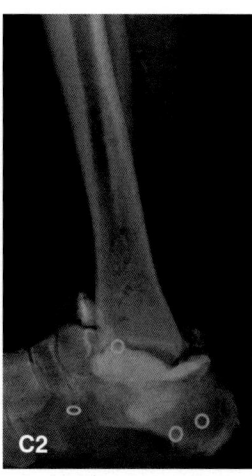

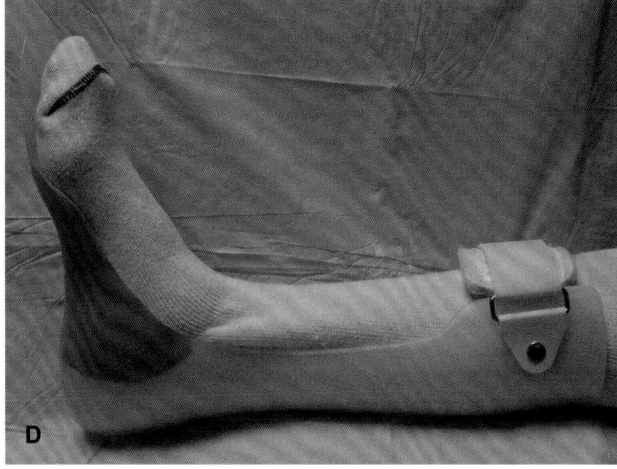

FIGURE 49.30 A. Ankle radiograph depicts attempted tibiocalcaneal arthrodesis in a diabetic patient with talar body fracture and collapse. **B.** An osteomyelitis developed, all nonviable bone was removed, and the patient was treated with a PMMA spacer. Temporary stability was achieved with a ring external fixator. Reconstruction options were limited in this B-host, so the PMMA block was retained **(C1-C2)**. Follow-up ankle radiographs years later depicting a stable cement block. Note that some of the restoration of length has been maintained and the block seated within the calcaneus has not migrated. The tibia articulates with the block, affording some motion. **D.** Ankle-foot orthosis for stability in same patient.

creating an uninhabitable environment.[224-226] Early outcomes are promising in a small series of patients treated for chronic osteomyelitis.[227]

A structural PMMA cement spacer helps maintain bone length and prepares defect for late reconstruction. In some cases the cement spacer may be permanently retained. This approach has been shown to be effective in cases of ankle/hindfoot osteomyelitis with a substantial void.[228] The success of the cement block is based on both surgical technique and patient monitoring (Fig. 49.30). The entire void must be filled, ensuring the cement reaches all interstices while distracting the segment until the cement hardens. It is important to keep the cement at the level of the bone so it is not proud against the overlying soft tissue envelope, which can make it difficult to establish a seal for healing. Segment stability is typically maintained by bracing, and the patient must be monitored over time with serial x-rays to ensure the cement does not migrate, since it may gradually erode surrounding bone. The cement block is strong enough to withstand normal loading forces in gait.

Masquelet developed an induced membrane technique that harnesses the antibiotic depot to generate a host response for bone healing (Fig. 49.31). First introduced in 1986 for the management of large bone defects, this technique has been increasingly utilized over the past two decades. The method achieves a vascularized membrane that contains growth factors—vascular endothelial growth factor (VEGF), transforming growth factor β-1 (TGF β-1), and bone morphogenic protein-2 (BMP-2)—that are conducive for bone growth.[229] The first stage of the protocol involves implantation of an antibiotic-loaded PMMA spacer in a bone defect following resection and débridement. The spacer should be formed to overlap the bone ends. Various fixation methods may be used to maintain bone stability as a vascularized synovium-like membrane grows on the spacer surface over 4-8 weeks. During the second stage the spacer is explanted with care to preserve the surrounding membrane, the medullary cavity is débrided, the bone ends are roughened, the defect is grafted with small pieces of cancellous bone graft, and the membrane is closed. The membrane secretes the aforementioned growth factors, which serve as a biologic chamber, and also prevents graft resorption. The highest growth factor expression has been reported at 4 weeks following cement spacer implantation, which suggests this interval is optimal for the bone grafting stage.[230] The technique is technically challenging and may require several cycles of bone grafting and multiple operations. A systematic review and meta-analysis of the Masquelet technique demonstrated an 89.7% union rate, a 91.1% cure rate, and an 18% persistence of nonunions or infections.[231]

Some caution should be exercised with implantation of PMMA. It may compromise the local immune response by decreasing leukocyte migration to the site as well as reducing

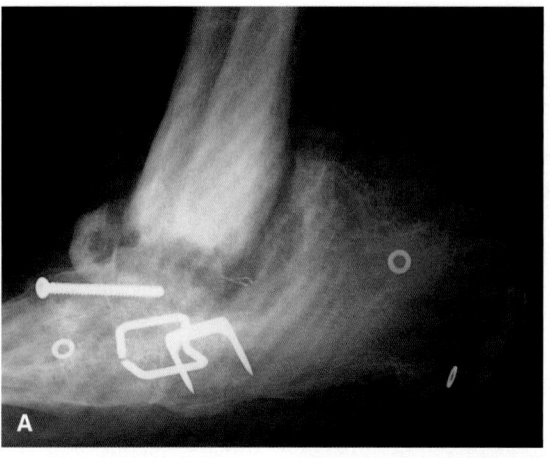
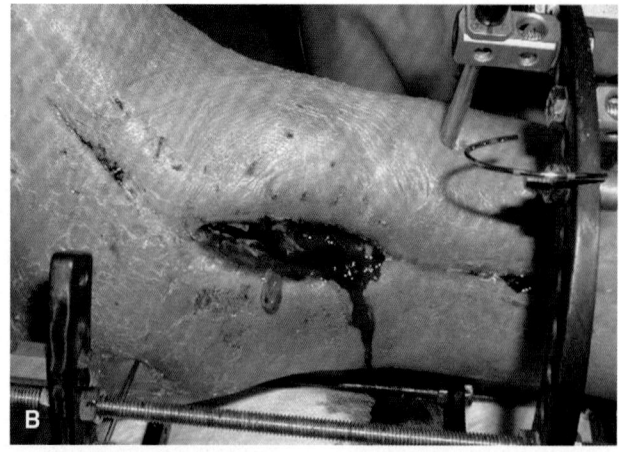
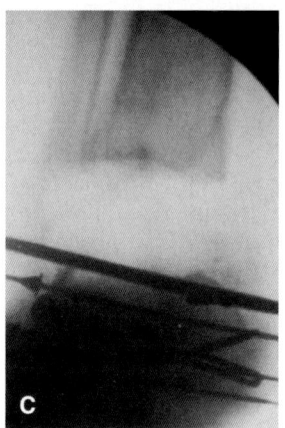
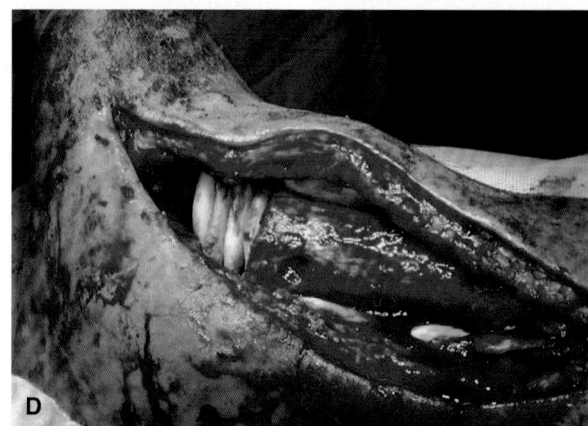
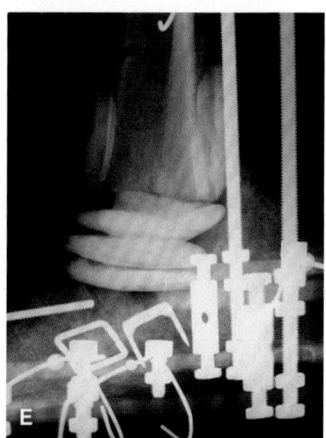
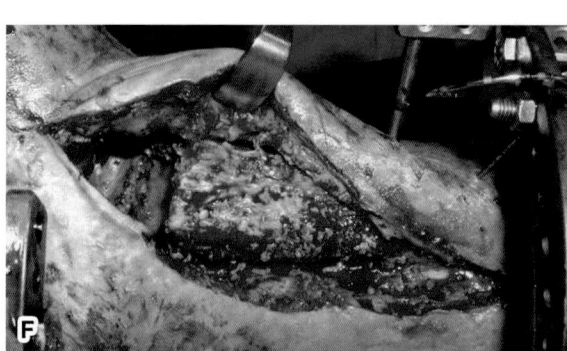
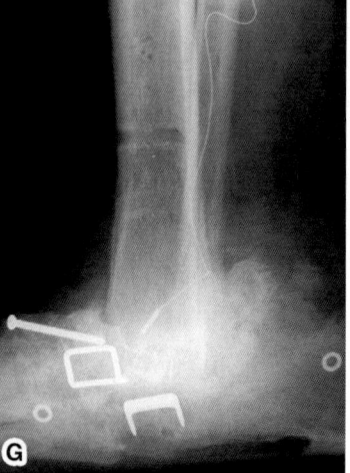

FIGURE 49.31 Modification of the Masquelet technique to treat an infected ankle nonunion in a B-host. **A.** Ankle radiograph depicting nonunion. **B.** Initial arthrodesis attempt failed and became infected. Clinical photograph of large draining soft tissue lesion. **C.** Intra-operative fluoroscopy demonstrating significant bone defect following débridement. **D.** Intra-operative photograph of clean tissue bed and antibiotic-loaded PMMA spacer in the form of wafers to improve surface area for elution. A good soft tissue seal was established by primary closure alone. **E.** Ankle radiograph demonstrating spacer maintained for 6 weeks, the time required for the serum inflammatory markers to normalize. **F.** Intra-operative photograph of the tissue bed following spacer removal during the second stage. Note the thin membrane near the retractor and in the depths of the defect. **G.** Radiograph of union following late bone graft.

the phagocytic capacity of neutrophils.[232] As noted previously, the intracellular residence of *S aureus* cannot be targeted with the standard concentration of gentamycin available in most preloaded PMMA because it does not penetrate the osteoblasts. Much higher antibiotic concentrations are necessary, yet there are also concerns about antibiotic potency on bone healing. There is animal model evidence to show that tobramycin may impair fracture healing.[233] Moreover, although retained antibiotic-loaded cement elutes very little antibiotic within 4-6 weeks following implantation, it may release more antibiotic when disturbed even years later.[234] Cultures should be obtained prior to evacuating the cement so as to minimize the risk of compromising the culture yield. It is also important to monitor patient renal function when treating with high concentrations of antibiotic because there is a risk of nephrotoxicity.[235] Lastly, it is important to thoroughly débride the tissue immediately surrounding retained PMMA beads because biofilm can form on their surface.

PERILS AND PITFALLS IN THE TREATMENT OF ADULT OSTEOMYELITIS

- Insufficient patient host assessment
- Decision to treat host with insufficient reserve to combat infection
- Failure to optimize host response and revisit host during course of treatment
- Avoiding patient discussion about the merits of primary amputation
- Incorrect disease staging or treatment protocol
- Inadequate débridement of all necrotic tissue
- Failure to procure adequate volume and number of tissue specimens from high-yield sites
- Inadequate incubation period for cultures
- Reluctance to repeat cultures for pathogens with known intrinsic antibiotic resistance
- Failure to consult with other specialists: infectious disease, vascular surgery, plastic surgery
- Improper management of dead space and soft tissue defects
- Inattention to need for stabilizing bone and methods to achieve it
- Implantation of foreign bone graft materials, which risk biofilm formation
- Avoiding necessary surgery dictated by protocol-directed care
- Lack of patient monitoring during treatment and over the long term
- Entrenchment with limb salvage: cannot admit defeat

Treatment Protocol Based on Disease Staging

The cornerstone of the surgical approach to osteomyelitis is the methodical and meticulous débridement of nonviable bone to a healthy bleeding tissue bed. The Cierny-Mader treatment protocol for chronic osteomyelitis defines this approach based on the staging of the disease (Tables 49.23 and 49.24). The protocol complexity increases based on anatomic type but the fundamental principles remain constant.

TABLE 49.23 Cierny-Mader Treatment Protocol for Chronic Osteomyelitis based on Anatomic Type

Type	Treatment	Reconstruction Method (Additive)
I	Deroofing	Dead space management
II	Decortication	+ Soft tissue coverage
III	Sequestrectomy	+ Bone grafting
IV	Stabilization	+ Fixation

From Cierny G III. Chronic osteomyelitis: results of treatment. *Instr Course Lect.* 1990;39:495-508.

The infection nidus in medullary osteomyelitis (type I) is accessed either by reaming the canal or by direct excision of the overlying cortex. A combination of these techniques is usually necessary. Débridement and soft tissue closure over the dead space is often accomplished in a single stage.[135] If the soft tissue is not as supple a short delay before closure may be necessary. An antibiotic depot is ideal, and a PMMA-coated plate or nail is commonly utilized to maintain segment stability. Handmade fabrications of antibiotic cement nails and coated plates have been described previously.[236,237] Removal of a hindfoot nail requires reaming to a diameter that meets the cortex (usually 0.5-1.5 mm larger than the nail) and copious canal lavage prior to insertion of an antibiotic cement nail (Figs. 49.28 and 49.32). If the segment is unstable following nail removal it typically requires support with an external fixator. If the soft tissue is compromised, the cortical entry point to the canal should be offset from the site of soft tissue coverage to prevent wound margin inversion and persistent drainage.[135] If a medullary infection is present in type III or IV osteomyelitis, the type I treatment protocol is followed.

In superficial osteomyelitis (type II) the soft tissue defect is the initial point of focus. Consultation with a plastic surgeon experienced in free flap transfers is usually necessary unless the defect is small and the surrounding soft tissues are sufficiently supple for wound excision and primary closure or local tissue advancement. Vascular studies assist in planning

TABLE 49.24 Treatment Protocol for Limb Salvage in Adult Osteomyelitis

1. Patient evaluation: history, examination, laboratory studies
2. Disease staging: determine host class and anatomic type
3. Optimize patient host
4. Thorough débridement to eradicate biofilm and establish viable tissue bed
5. Identify microorganism(s)/select targeted antibiotic therapy
6. Antibiotic depot placement (beads/spacer) as necessary
7. Manage dead space: cement spacer +/− flap as necessary
8. Stabilize bone segment as necessary: cement spacer +/− fixation
9. Reconstruct soft tissue defect as necessary
10. Monitor patient: examination/laboratory markers/imaging
11. Repeat débridement for viable tissue bed +/− cement exchange as necessary
12. Late reconstruction dictated by laboratory markers
13. Annual follow-up

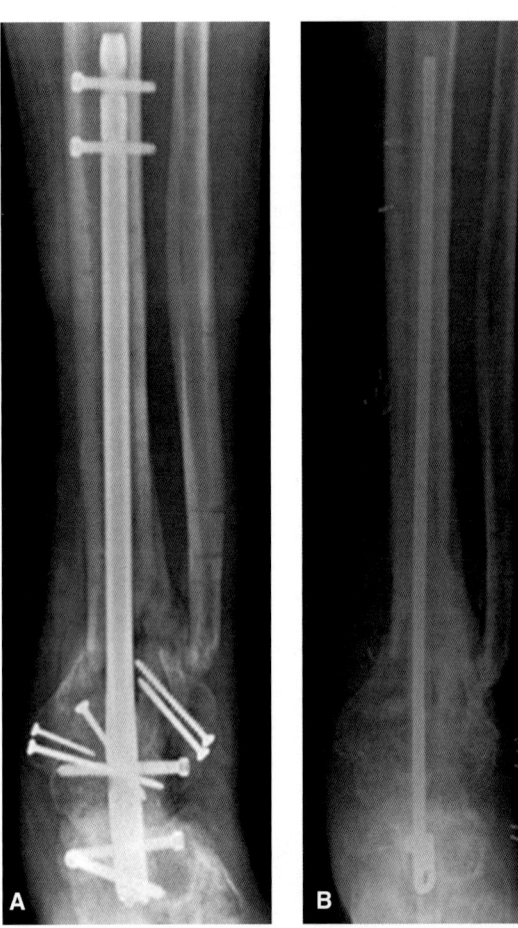

the approach to soft tissue coverage. Following excision of the nonviable soft tissues, the exposed bone is decorticated until a bleeding base (paprika sign) is established.[238] The wound bed must be clean and healthy if the soft tissue coverage plan is to succeed.[135]

Type III (localized osteomyelitis) is treated by sequestrectomy. The infection nidus typically involves soft tissue and bone. The devitalized soft tissue is removed, the necrotic cortical and medullary bone is excavated, and the reconstruction is planned based on resulting dead space, remaining skeletal integrity, and location of the infection.[135] In some cases the bone segment must be stabilized with an antibiotic-loaded cement spacer or fixation device. Strategies for filling the soft tissue defect may follow the protocol for type II osteomyelitis as part of a larger multistage reconstruction. Late bone grafting is often necessary. Yet the treatment of some type III lesions results in only a limited healthy bone defect with minimal dead space. Here primary closure without an antibiotic depot may be successful. Most cases of localized osteomyelitis result from previous surgery and are often posttraumatic. Fracture stability is afforded by the implant and helps to reduce microbial growth at the site, yet microorganism colonization ensues and biofilm is typically established. However, the fracture may heal despite infection. Serial radiographs should be followed for implant stability and fracture healing. If there are progressive signs of fracture healing without implant loosening, the implant should be retained until the fracture heals, at which point sequestrectomy can be performed (Fig. 49.33). In some cases, the period of implant retention may extend over a number of months. Parenteral antibiotics should be administered during this time. If the fracture is not healing or there are signs of implant loosening, treatment is as described above.

FIGURE 49.32 A. Distal tibial osteomyelitis treated by hindfoot nail removal, medullary reaming, and decortication at the infection nidus. **B.** Placement of antibiotic-impregnated PMMA coated nail.

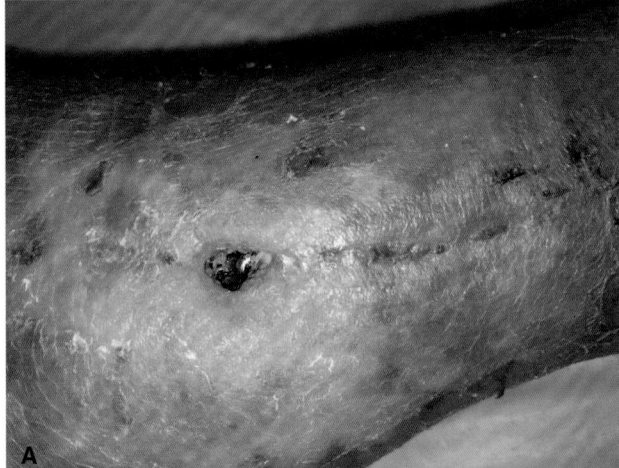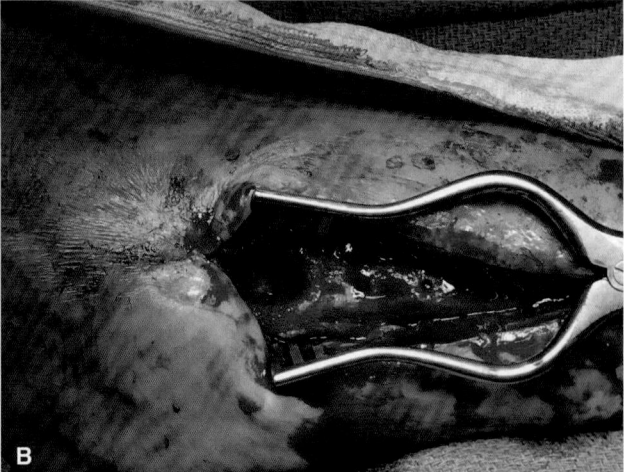

FIGURE 49.33 Immunocompromised and malnourished patient (B-host) developed a deep lateral ankle wound 4 weeks after surgical care for an unstable trimalleolar fracture. **A.** Close-up clinical photograph of exposed screw, plate, and bone. Radiographs showed well fixed fibular implants without loosening. Implants were retained until the fracture healed while the patient's wound was treated with local care and suppressive oral antibiotics (stopped 3 weeks prior to surgery). **B.** Intra-operative photograph depicting fibula implant removal and sequestrectomy in the metaphysis. The defect was small and the remaining bone was healthy and strong with sufficient volume, obviating the need for additional stability to prevent insufficiency fracture. Primary closure was achieved, the patient was treated with targeted antibiotic therapy for confirmed osteomyelitis, and the soft tissue envelope healed.

In diffuse osteomyelitis (type IV), either the infection or the operation produces instability of the affected segment. Surgical strategies are based around bone stabilization. The hallmarks of this stage are significant soft tissue lesions and bone loss that limit fixation options and require staged reconstruction with external fixation (see Fig. 49.31).[135] Soft tissue restoration and dead space management is often necessary before bone reconstruction (Fig. 49.34). Antibiotic depots are common in type IV osteomyelitis. Methods of Ilizarov for distraction osteogenesis or the Masquelet technique may be necessary to fill larger bone defects. In some cases host status or the size/location of the bone defect precludes late reconstruction. In such instances permanent cement spacers may be appropriate (see Fig. 49.30).

POSTOPERATIVE CARE AND REHABILITATION

Postoperative care is based on the mode of treatment. The common feature is regular follow-up intervals for patient monitoring through examination, serum inflammatory markers and other laboratory assessment as indicated, and imaging. Collaboration with an infectious disease specialist is recommended. An internist should help optimize host response when treatment is associated with greater morbidity. Limb protection is

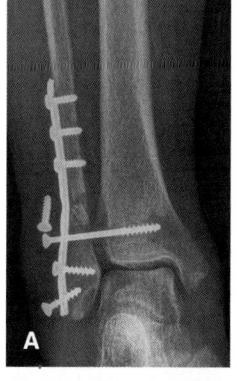
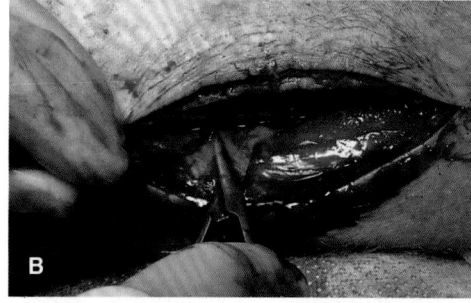
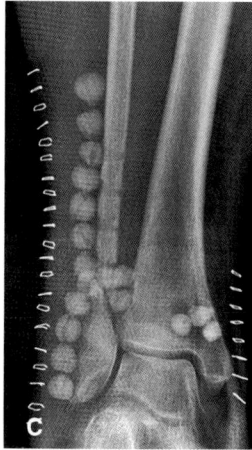
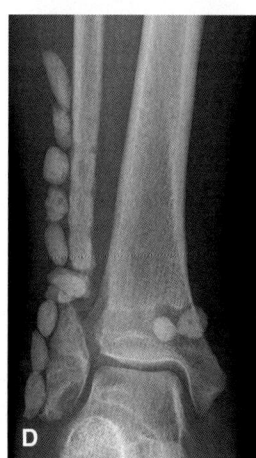
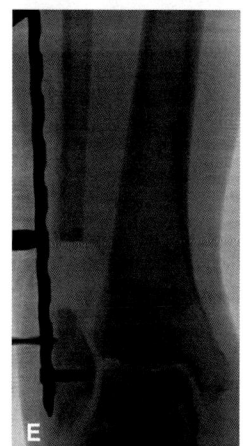
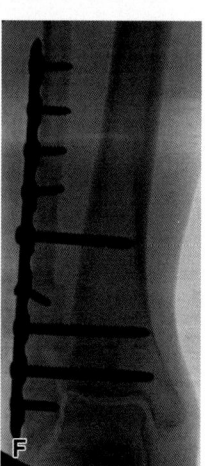
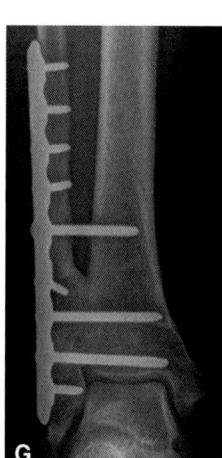

FIGURE 49.34 Type IV osteomyelitis in poorly controlled diabetic patient (B-host) 10 weeks after fracture repair. The patient presented with a draining sinus. **A.** Ankle radiograph depicts implant loosening, bone rarefaction in the distal medial tibia, and sequestrum in the fibula. **B.** Intraoperative photograph of purulent material during incision and drainage. **C.** Ankle radiograph demonstrates implant removal, elimination of sequestra, and placement of antibiotic depot. The soft tissues were closed primarily. A short leg splint was sufficient for stability because the distal tibia infection compromised very little bone. **D.** Repeat débridement and antibiotic bead exchange 3-4 weeks later. **E.** Reconstruction via plate osteosynthesis after serum inflammatory markers normalized 4 weeks later. **F.** Intercalary autogenous iliac crest bone graft for fibular defect. **G.** Final radiograph demonstrates incorporation of bone graft and functional ankle.

dictated by fixation. The remaining care elements are similar to the patient recovering from soft tissue infection. The principles of rehabilitation after treatment for osteomyelitis are also similar to those established for soft tissue and joint infection with a focus on reconditioning. The primary difference is the importance of stabilizing the affected limb. Physical therapy is guided by bone integrity and segment stability afforded by the necessary fixation, along with the nature of soft tissue defect coverage and the limb protection required for successful healing.

PEDIATRIC OSTEOMYELITIS

Children are most often afflicted with AHO. The rate of disease is between 1:5000 and 1:10 000; boys are affected twice the rate of girls.[239,240] Half of children are under the age of 5 years.[240] Multifocal infection is less common than single bone involvement.[239,240] The infection is usually focused in the metaphysis of the tibia or femur.[241] AHO involves the distal tibia in at least half of cases.[242] Pediatric calcaneal osteomyelitis occurs in 3%-10% of cases.[243] Adjacent septic arthritis presents in one-third of cases.[244] The ankle is one of the most commonly affected joints.[245] Prompt recognition of the problem is crucial for timely and effective treatment, particularly because the virulence of *S aureus* and other pathogens has increased.[246] Yet the diagnosis of pediatric AHO is difficult and the clinician must have a high index of suspicion for this problem.

PHYSICAL EXAMINATION

Physical examination of the child is essential to make the diagnosis of AHO. The typical signs of inflammation do not present until the infection progresses through the porous metaphyseal cortex into the subperiosteal space (Fig. 49.35).[247] Pain, guarding of the limb, and tenderness over the bone are common. The most significant area of pain is usually the site of infection.[248] Significant swelling of the soft tissue is an important early sign of AHO. Impaired mobility is a sensitive clinical indicator for tibial osteomyelitis, with weight-bearing status altered in 81% of patients and refusal to load the limb in 67% of patients.[242] Fever

is a less reliable symptom, absent in one-third of presenting patients.[249]

PATHOGENESIS

The rich metaphyseal blood supply of the tibia predisposes to hematogenous osteomyelitis because bacteria are thought to collect here due to rather tortuous blood flow that results from an avascular growth plate.[250,251] Metaphyseal exudate is produces and forms a bone abscess. The purulence transudes through the porous metaphysis and elevates the thick periosteum, which is not as well adhered to bone as it is in the adult. Reactive bone formation occurs along the periosteum and an involucrum may form, while the underlying cortex may form sequestra (Figs. 49.18 and 49.36). The exception to this process is in infants (age 12-18 months) where the epiphysis may receive arterial supply from blood vessels that cross the growth plate.[248] In these cases infection bone deformity may result because the infection destroys the physeal plate.[252]

Some children are more prone to develop AHO than others, though the process is poorly understood. Transient bacteremia is thought to be implicated, the result of otitis media, pharyngitis, and even teeth brushing.[251] However, transient bacteremia must occur in the setting of the genetic up-regulation of microorganism virulence and iron metabolism genes, which helps sustain bacteria in the bloodstream.[253] Trauma is a precursor to pediatric tibial osteomyelitis in over one-third of cases.[242] Most children with AHO typically present within a few days of symptom onset.[254,255] Neonatal osteomyelitis is often multifocal and is typically seen in children of low birth weight who require invasive procedures.[248] Pathogens differ based on the age of the child, although *S aureus* and streptococci are seen in all age groups (Table 49.25).

DIAGNOSTIC STUDIES

Blood cultures, WBC, CRP, and ESR should be obtained. CRP is a highly sensitive acute phase reactant, helps differentiate septic arthritis from osteomyelitis alone, and has prognostic value for determining length of parenteral antimicrobial therapy.[240]

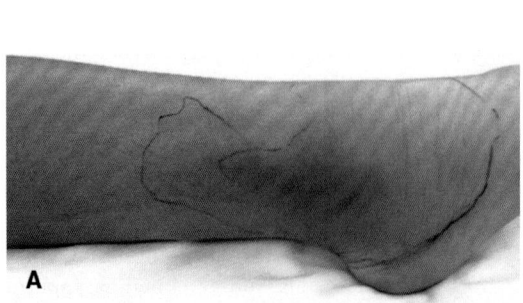
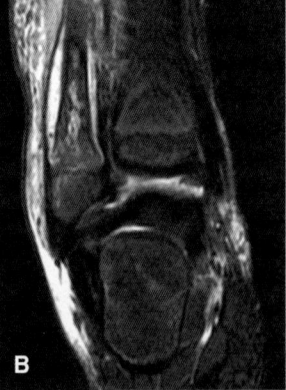

FIGURE 49.35 A. Clinical signs of inflammation in a 6-year-old with AHO of the distal fibula. **B.** MRI image demonstrating subperiosteal abscess and meta-diaphyseal osteomyelitis. The lifted periosteum is clearly depicted on this scan by hypointense signal with enhancing underlying purulence.

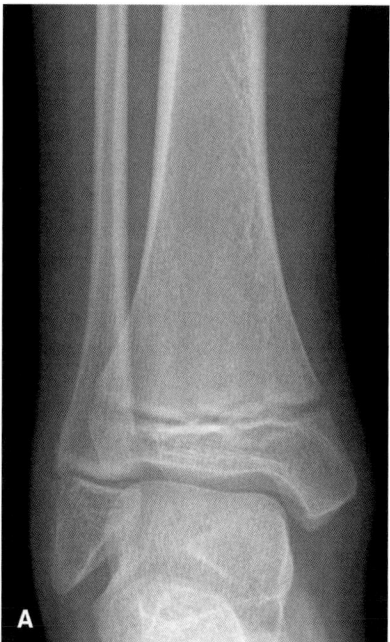
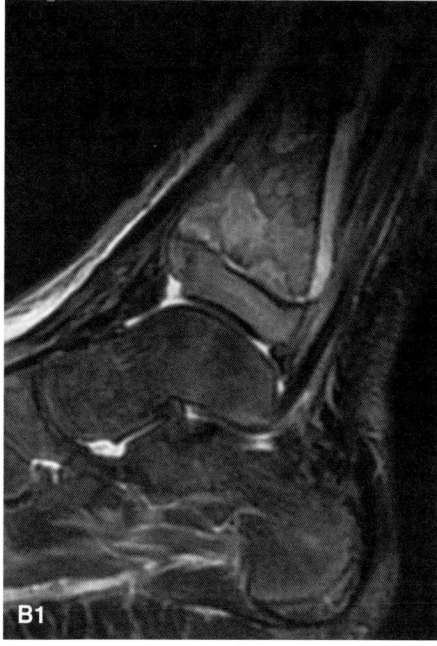
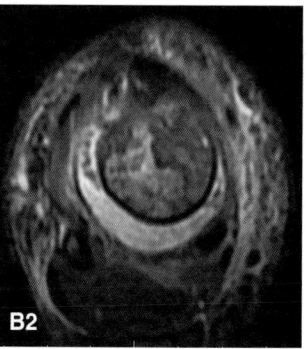

FIGURE 49.36 A 13-year-old boy who presented with fever, refusal to walk, focal distal tibial/ankle tenderness, edema, and erythema. He sustained an ankle sprain 10 days prior. **A.** Ankle radiograph demonstrate subtle shadow around the distal tibia and fibula consistent with periosteal lifting. **B.** MRI fat saturation sequences demonstrate superiosteal abscess and osteomyelitis of the distal tibial metaphysis.

Blood cultures are positive in only up to half of cases of AHO. WBC is also a poor diagnostic indicator, elevated in only 30%-40% of cases.[240,256] Leukocytosis and elevated inflammatory markers are not reliable indications of AHO in the neonate.

TABLE 49.25	Microorganisms Commonly Identified in Pediatric Osteomyelitis based on Patient Age
Child's Age	**Microorganisms**
2-18 mo	*Staphylococcus aureus* Coagulase-negative staphylococci Streptococci: *S agalactiae, S pneumoniae* *Klebsiella kingae* *Haemophilus influenzae* type b (nonimmunized)
18 mo to 3 y	*Escherichia coli* *Staphylococcus aureus* *Streptococcus pneumonia* *Klebsiella kingae* *Neisseria meningitides* *Haemophilus influenzae* type b (nonimmunized)
3-12 y	*Staphylococcus aureus* *Streptococcus pyogenes* *Mycobacterium tuberculosis*
12-18 y	*Staphylococcus aureus* *Streptococcus pyogenes* *Neisseria gonorrhoeae*

Modified from Funk SS, Copley LA. Acute hematogenous osteomyelitis in children: pathogenesis, diagnosis, and treatment. *Orthop Clin North Am.* 2017;48:199-208.

IMAGING

Radiographs are of little value in the diagnosis of AHO. They will demonstrate deep soft tissue swelling in the early stages.[172,257] Ultrasound can identify subperiosteal fluid and may be useful for diagnosis of early osteomyelitis in children,[258] particularly in instances where MRI may be more difficult. Ultrasound may also be used to guide needle aspiration of a suspected subperiosteal abscess for purposes of earlier microorganism determination. MRI is the imaging study of choice. MRI without contrast should be considered within 24 hours for any child with symptoms suspicious for AHO (Fig. 49.36). It is an excellent screening study and is also recommended in cases of septic arthritis to rule out adjacent osteomyelitis prior to arthrotomy.[259] Gadolinium is indicated when the epiphyseal plate may be affected, such as in infants.[175] MRI is superior for determining abnormal bone marrow involvement compared to radiographs, CT scan, and bone scans.[260] CT has limited application in the diagnosis of pediatric osteomyelitis. Bone scintigraphy may be useful for diagnosis provided it does not delay treatment, a concern given the time required for some of these scans. Radiation exposure must also be considered. A Tc-99m MDP scan is helpful in some cases of AHO, but the frequency of false negative results is 4%-20%.[178] This study may be difficult to interpret in the foot owing to multiple growth plates in a relatively small area.[261] The Tc-99m HMPAO scan may have advantages in this age group because of diminished radiation, shorter imaging time, faster results, and a smaller blood sample required. The most compelling application of bone scintigraphy may be for the evaluation of multifocal AHO in the neonate. There are insufficient data on FDG PET-CT on its use in the diagnosis of pediatric AHO.

PEARLS FOR DIAGNOSIS AND TREATMENT OF PEDIATRIC AHO IN THE DISTAL LOWER EXTREMITY

- AHO is suspected in any child with bone pain, fever, and refusal to walk
- If signs of inflammation are present, an abscess may have already developed
- CRP and MRI are diagnostic tests of choice
- Prompt empiric intravenous antimicrobial therapy must cover *S aureus*
- If MRI depicts abscess: surgery
- If fever persists and CRP does not diminish: surgery
- Anticipate conversion to oral antibiotics by downtrending CRP
- Always consider repeat débridement/lavage

TREATMENT

Systemic Antimicrobial Therapy

Antimicrobial therapy is essential for the treatment of AHO. Empiric antibiotics are typically nafcillin, oxacillin, or cefazolin. In patients who are not immunized for *H influenzae*, cefotaxime or cefuroxime should be added. Patients with a disseminated gonococcal infection are treated with doxycycline. If the infection is nosocomial or community acquired, gentamicin should be added.[246] Culture-negative AHO in communities with a high prevalence of MRSA has been successfully treated with clindamycin.[262,263]

The optimal duration of antimicrobial therapy is not known.[264] Twelve prospective studies that evaluated IV antimicrobial treatment demonstrated a cure rate of 95% (<7 days) vs 98.8% (>7 days) at 6 months' follow-up.[265] A prospective study of 70 patients demonstrated that the vast majority of children could be converted from IV to oral antimicrobial therapy within 3-5 days, guided by CRP monitoring, with a 100% cure rate.[127] Since treatment of pediatric osteomyelitis with parenteral antibiotics is not always benign, it is reasonable to convert the child to oral therapy within 2-3 weeks based on serial CRP values. This marker is the lab of choice in treatment of pediatric AHO and returns to baseline within a week if treatment is effective. Consultation with a pediatric infectious disease specialist should be considered, particularly in children with persistent bacteremia, fever, disseminated infection, and atypical

or antimicrobial-resistant organisms and infants or the immunocompromised.[246] Nonoperative treatment involves bone marrow biopsy needle aspiration of the affected site (bone and subperiosteal abscess) based on imaging along with the adjacent joint effusion, if present.[246] AHO in the calcaneus typically responds to antibiotics with occasional need for curettage.[266]

Authors' Preferred Treatment Protocol for Pediatric AHO

- Suspect AHO: hospital admission, blood cultures, CBC, CRP
- Empiric IV antibiotics
- Imaging: radiographs and MRI
- If moderate to severe abscess: surgery
- If mild abscess: attempt needle drainage/assess response to antibiotic
- If fever persists and CRP is static or escalating despite IV antibiotics: surgery
- Culture-directed antimicrobial therapy: consult pediatric infectious disease specialist
- Close patient monitoring: examination/temperature, blood cultures as necessary, WBC, serial CRP
- Downtrending CRP determines conversion to oral antibiotics. Monitor CRP for 1 year

Low threshold for repeat joint irrigation/débridement

Surgery

Surgical intervention is often indicated in the treatment of AHO, with operation rates ranging between 43% and 92%.[242,255,267] Surgery is necessary when a subperiosteal abscess, sinus, or sequestrum is identified on imaging.[267] Children who present with moderate to large abscesses or do not respond to 48-72 hours of intravenous antibiotic therapy should go to surgery.[268] The mainstay of surgical management for pediatric AHO is decompression of the abscess and a thorough tissue débridement down to a healthy wound bed (Fig. 49.37). If the subperiosteal abscess is not resolved, the periosteum may not survive. Metaphyseal cortical windows for drainage of all purulent material within the bone are typically necessary, though this can often be accomplished with a large curette because the

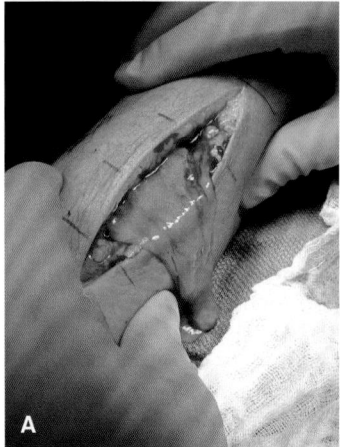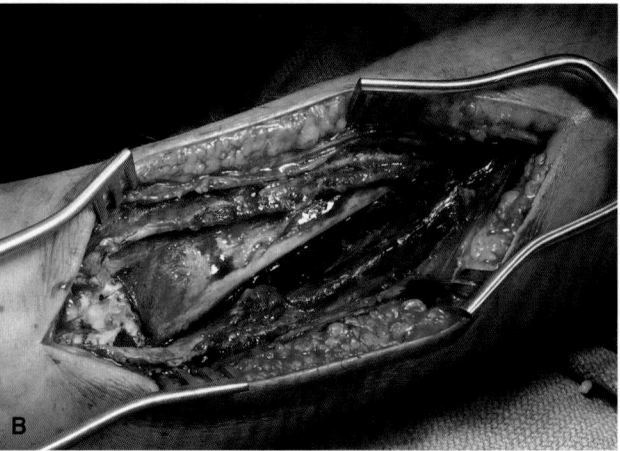

FIGURE 49.37 A. Distal tibial AHO abscess decompression. **B.** Clean wound after thorough débridement and lavage. The deep muscle compartment of the leg is opened. Note the thick periosteum, which was lifted off the bone by extravasated purulence from the metaphysis.

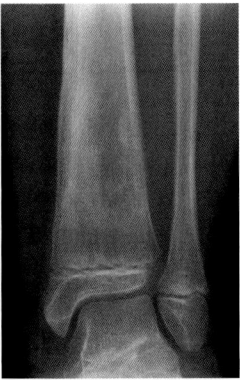

FIGURE 49.38 Bony remodeling in 11-year-old boy treated for distal tibial osteomyelitis 18 months prior. Asymptomatic, no leg or ankle tenderness, and normal inflammatory markers.

bone is typically soft or porous. The addition of fenestration of the cortical bone with antibiotic irrigation of the medullary canal has been shown to be effective alternative for the treatment of pediatric tibial osteomyelitis.[269] Care must be taken to avoid injury of the growth plate. For larger abscesses, the wound is often packed and the margins loosely approximated for repeat irrigation and delayed primary closure. If the abscess is smaller, primary closure over a drain is possible. However, repeat débridement and irrigation is indicated if the child demonstrates persistent fever and static or rising CRP.[246] Treatment of AHO in the neonate follows the same principles as in the older child. Hospital discharge is appropriate if two blood cultures are negative 48 hours prior and the child is afebrile, in addition to the typical signs of clinical improvement.

The treatment of AHO is successful with a high cure rate in the vast majority of cases.[127,270] Hospital readmission occurs in ~25% of pediatric patients with acute osteomyelitis, though a recent study demonstrated 17% of cases were due to infection relapse, many of which were culture negative.[242] Approximately 6% of children experience treatment complications, including chronic infection, avascular necrosis, growth disturbance, pathologic fractures, deep vein thrombosis, and sepsis.[251,268,271,272] Chronic osteomyelitis typically develops in <5% of children following with recurrent infection in 6.8% of cases.[268,273,274] The rate of pathologic fracture is below 2% and typically occurs in children with more severe infections and who underwent surgical débridement.[268,275] Children should be followed closely within the first year of treatment with examination, radiographs (Fig. 49.38), and serial CRP values. The incidence of premature arrest of the epiphyseal plate is below 2%.[268,276] Following the child for several years after the infection is recommended, but not necessarily through skeletal maturity.

PERILS AND PITFALLS IN TREATMENT OF PEDIATRIC AHO

- Low suspicion/delayed recognition
- Delay in administration of intravenous antimicrobial therapy
- Delay in early MRI
- Inattention to patient clinical course and lab monitoring
- Inadequate surgical decompression of periosteum and bone débridement
- Prolonged intravenous antimicrobial therapy despite downtrending CRP
- Failure to monitor patient over several years

POSTOPERATIVE CARE AND REHABILITATION

The principles of postoperative care and rehabilitation for the child after treatment for AHO in distal lower extremity are similar to those established for adult osteomyelitis. The major difference is a shorter period of limb protection, which is typically accomplished with a short leg splint, cast, or boot. Return to protected load is usually possible within a few weeks because bone integrity is sufficient to withstand weight bearing. However, it is important to control limb edema and avoid high impact activity for at least several months.

DIABETIC FOOT INFECTIONS

DFI is responsible for significant morbidity and mortality, causing a serious burden on the patient, their family, the workforce, and the health care system. Among the 30.3 million people with diabetes mellitus in the United States, it is reported that 19%-34% of those will develop an ulcer in their lifetime.[277-279] Fifty percent of patients with a diabetic foot ulcer have the possibility of subsequent infection.[278] DFIs are a common cause of hospital admission, reported to be about 20% of all primary admissions and 40% of readmissions.[280,281] One in six patients admitted for a diabetic infection will die in 1 year.[281] The direct and indirect cost of treating patients with diabetes in the United States is estimated to cost $245 billion dollars per year.[282] A DFI plagues a compromised host and is often polymicrobial, both of which make treatment a significant challenge.

DEFINITION

DFI is an invasion and multiplication of microorganisms in host soft tissue or bone of a person with diabetes that induces a host inflammatory response, usually followed by tissue destruction.[283]

CLASSIFICATION

There are multiple classification systems that have been developed in an attempt to capture the complexity of a diabetic host and foot infection. The Wagner Classification was one of the earliest adopted systems. It is based on wound depth along with the presence of osteomyelitis, gangrene, and extent of tissue necrosis.[284] Unfortunately, due to its simplicity, it does not fully represent the severity of the peripheral vascular disease and it does not distinguish gangrene caused by infection vs vascular compromise.[284]

The University of Texas (UT) Classification has gained popularity over the years because it is more comprehensive, capturing the effects of both infection and ischemia (Table 49.26). The UT classification pairs the depth of the ulceration with separate consideration for infection and vascular compromise. While this makes it a better predictor of outcome compared to the Wagner classification, the system lacks proper differentiation of tissue perfusion and infection.[284]

The IDSA-IWGDF classification combines systems from the Infection Disease Society of America (IDSA) and the International Working Group on Diabetic Foot Infection (IWGDF) for the evaluation of pedal ulcerations and infection. Its portrayal of each infection category is complex and utilized more frequently in research rather than clinical practice. It has been shown to predict need for hospitalization and lower extremity amputation.[285]

TABLE 49.26 University of Texas Diabetic Foot Ulcer Classification System				
	Grade			
	0	**I**	**II**	**III**
Stage	**Pre- or Postulcerative Lesion Completely Epithelized**	**Superficial Wound not Involving Tendon, Capsule, or Bone**	**Wound Penetrating to Tendon or Capsule**	**Wound Penetrating to Bone or Joint**
A	No infection or ischemia	No infection or ischemia	No infection or ischemia	No infection or ischemia
B	Infection	Infection	Infection	Infection
C	Ischemia	Ischemia	Ischemia	Ischemia
D	Infection and ischemia	Infection and ischemia	Infection and ischemia	Infection and ischemia

From Oyibo SO, Jude EB, Tarawneh I, et al. A comparison of two diabetic foot ulcer classification systems: the Wagner and the University of Texas wound classifications systems. *Diabetes Care*. 2001;24:84-88.

The Wound Ischemia foot infection (WIfI) classification is the most comprehensive diabetic foot classification system to date (Table 49.27A and B). It captures a complete evaluation of the wound, the level of ischemia, and the degree of infection. These factors are combined to determine the risk of amputation: very low, low, moderate, and high (Table 49.28).[286,287] The WIfI system can predict hospital duration and cost, wound healing rates, and need for revascularization.[286-288]

INDICATIONS

- Swift identification and management of a diabetic foot infection are crucial to minimize morbidity and mortality.
- All manifestations of diabetes mellitus should be considered and addressed by a multidisciplinary team to optimize host response and maximize treatment success.
- The primary goal of incision and drainage or amputation is to eliminate the infection. A secondary goal is to heal the wound and establish a plantigrade foot to help minimize the risk of recurrent ulceration or infection.

PHYSICAL EXAMINATION

The distal lower extremity physical examination of a diabetic patient is important not only for evaluation of potential tissue compromise and infection but also for assessment of the patient's overall health and the patient's capacity to heal. It is thought that 60% of diabetic foot ulcerations are infected on presentation. Early clinical suspicion and prompt identification of the problem with swift treatment may mitigate the impact of the infection, save tissue, and ultimately extend the patient's life.[289]

Patients with diabetes mellitus typically have some degree of PAD. Signs of more advanced ischemia include nonpalpable pulses, sluggish capillary refill, cool and shiny atrophic skin, and lack of pedal hair. An arterial Doppler examination is essential in patients with nonpalpable pulses; more advanced vascular assessment may also be necessary. Peripheral neuropathy is the most common of all the neuropathies in patients with diabetes. Evaluation of gross sensation with a 5.07-g Semmes Weinstein monofilament and vibratory sensation should be utilized to determine the level of neuropathy. Vibratory sensation deteriorates first while loss of sensation with 5.07 Semmes Weinstein monofilament occurs in the later stages of neuropathy. Skin integument should be carefully evaluated for defects, wounds, or calluses that could predispose to ulcers. Skin ulceration is the most common precursor to infection in the diabetic foot.[280] If an ulcer is identified it must débrided to more accurately assess the size, depth, and other characteristics that may risk deep infection. Musculoskeletal deformity must also be evaluated. Muscle imbalances associated with motor neuropathy

TABLE 49.27A WIfI Classification				
	0	**1**	**2**	**3**
Wound (W)	No ulcer No gangrene	Small ulcer No gangrene	Deep ulcer; forefoot gangrene (limited)	Extensive ulcer or gangrene
Ischemia (I)				
TcPO$_2$ (mm Hg)	>60	40-59	30-39	<30
Ankle pressure (mm Hg)	>100	70-100	50-70	<50
ABI	>0.80	0.60-0.79	0.40-0.59	<0.40
Foot Infection (fI)	Not infected	Mild (<2 cm cellulitis)	Moderate (>2 cm cellulitis and purulence)	Severe (systemic response/sepsis)

Adapted from Aboyans V, Ricco JB, Bartelink MEL, et al. 2017 ESC Guidelines on the Diagnosis and Treatment of Peripheral Arterial Diseases, in collaboration with the European Society for Vascular Surgery (ESVS): document covering atherosclerotic disease of extracranial carotid and vertebral, mesenteric, renal, upper and lower extremity arteries. *Eur Heart J*. 2018,39:763-816.

TABLE 49.27B WIfI Classification

Estimated Risk of Pedal Amputation at 1 Year															
	Ischemia 0				Ischemia 1				Ischemia 2				Ischemia 3			
W-0	VL	VL	L	M	VL	L	M	H	L	L	M	M	L	M	M	H
W-1	VL	VL	L	M	VL	L	M	H	L	M	H	H	M	M	H	H
W-2	L	L	M	H	M	M	H	H	M	H	H	H	H	H	H	H
W-3	M	M	H	H	H	H	H	H	H	H	H	H	H	H	H	H
	fI-0	fI-1	fI-2	fI-3	fI-0	fI-1	fI-2	fI-3	fI-0	fI-1	fI-2	fI-3	fI-0	fI-1	fI-2	fI-3

W, wound; fI, foot infection; H, high risk; L, low risk; M, moderate risk; VL, very low risk.

Adapted from Aboyans V, Ricco JB, Bartelink MEL, et al. 2017 ESC Guidelines on the Diagnosis and Treatment of Peripheral Arterial Diseases, in collaboration with the European Society for Vascular Surgery (ESVS): document covering atherosclerotic disease of extracranial carotid and vertebral, mesenteric, renal, upper and lower extremity arteries. *Eur Heart J.* 2018,39:763-816.

often result in toe contractures and abnormal load along the plantar forefoot, which can increase ulceration risk. In some cases more significant imbalance along the midfoot, hindfoot, or ankle may occur.

Local Infection

The International Disease Society of America (IDSA) guidelines define infection as the presence of obvious purulent drainage (Fig. 49.39) or the presence of two or more signs of inflammation (erythema, pain, tenderness, warmth, or induration). Other symptoms of local infection include edema, odor, presence of necrosis, friable or discolored granulation tissue, or failure of wound to heal.[285,290] Dependent rubor is a common finding in advanced PAD (Fig. 49.40). It may be confused with erythema, but it will resolve on elevation of the limb.[291] Risk factors for DFI include ulcers that probe to bone, have been present over 30 days, recurrent ulcerations, traumatically induced ulcerations, and systemic disease such as neutrophil dysfunction, chronic renal failure, and the presence of PAD.[292,293]

Systemic Infection

Diabetes mellitus depresses the host's inflammatory response. A DFI may progress unrecognized until it has overwhelmed the host and becomes a more serious systemic infection. In addition to the common systemic signs of infection established earlier in the section on general principles, the diabetic patient may exhibit vomiting, anorexia, and changes in glycemic control.[291]

Osteomyelitis in the Diabetic Foot

Pedal osteomyelitis is typically the result of contiguous spread from an ulcer to bone. A number of physical examination findings are suggestive of osteomyelitis in the diabetic foot. The ability to penetrate to bone with a probe from an ulcer has a strong correlation with osteomyelitis (Fig. 49.41). The sensitivity and specificity of this test have been shown to be 66% and 85%, respectively.[294] The inability to probe to bone has a 98% negative predictive value compared to a 57% positive predictive value.[292] Clinical suspicion with the probe to bone test, underlying bony prominence, failure to heal an ulcer, erythema with

TABLE 49.28	Differentiating Osteomyelitis From Charcot Neuroarthropathy			
	Osteomyelitis	**Acute Charcot**	**Chronic Charcot**	**Osteomyelitis + Charcot**
Physical examination	Erythema, edema, warmth, ulceration	Erythema, edema, warmth	Edema	Erythema, edema, warmth, ulceration or sinus tract
Location	Forefoot, MTP joint, hindfoot, calcaneus	Midfoot, subarticular	Midfoot	Midfoot or forefoot
ESR	>70 mm/h	Normal or possibly elevated	Normal	>70 mm/h
CRP	>3.2 mg/dL	Normal or possibly elevated	Normal	>3.2 mg/dL
X-ray	*Early* (day 1-41): normal *Late*: cortical erosions, demineralization, and periosteal reaction (typically near site of ulceration, sequestrum, involucrum, cloacae)	*Early*: Normal or focal demineralization, subchondral or periarticular changes	Joint fragmentation, deformity, and destruction	Joint deformity and destruction
MRI	Marrow edema, bone destruction T1 weighted: Local focal intensity T2: High focal signal STIR: High bone barrow signal	Marrow edema, periarticular and subchondral T1 and T2: Low signal intensity in subchondral bone Cortical fragmentation Joint deformity	No marrow edema	Marrow edema near site of ulceration
Bone scintigraphy	Focal hyperperfusion, hyperemia, bony uptake	Focal hyperperfusion, hyperemia, bony uptake	No focal uptake	Focal hyperperfusion, hyperemia, bony uptake
Combined bone and leukocyte scintigraphy	Leukocyte activity corresponds to abnormal activity on 3-phase bone scan	No focal uptake	No focal uptake	Leukocyte activity corresponds to abnormal activity on 3-phase bone scan

dactylitis (Fig. 49.42), and other local signs of infection have shown a positive and negative likelihood ratio of 5.5 and 0.54, respectively.[295,296]

PATHOGENESIS

The genesis of a DFI is often based on a number of influencing factors, including peripheral neuropathy, motor neuropathy, autonomic neuropathy, vasculopathy, and immunopathy. It is imperative to identify and treat a diabetic infection quickly before it overwhelms the host.

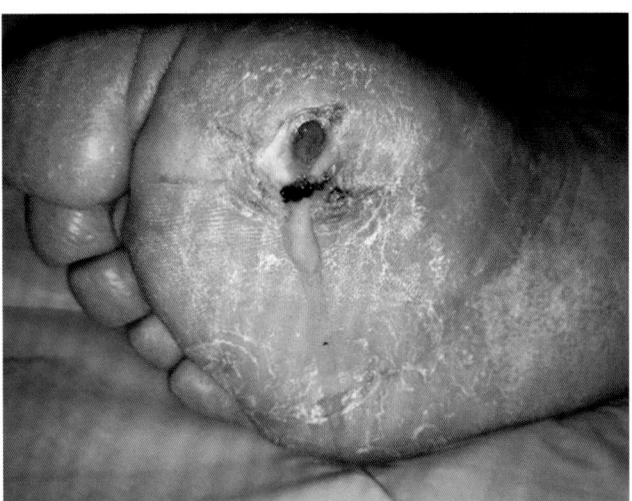

FIGURE 49.39 Diabetic foot wound with draining purulence.

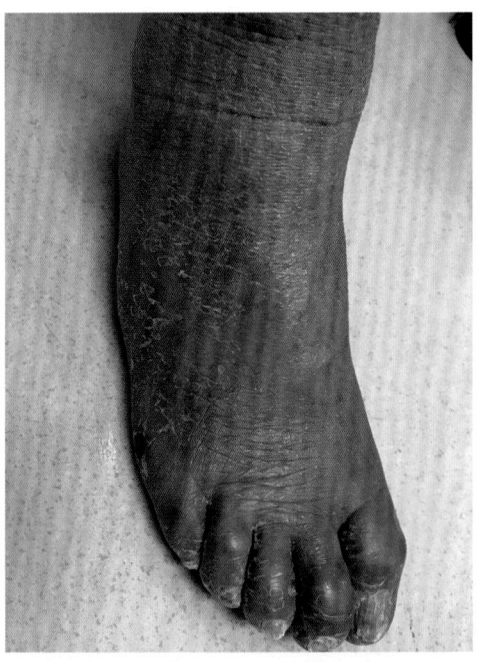

FIGURE 49.40 Dependent rubor is common in advanced peripheral arterial disease. Unlike cellulitis, it resolves with elevation of the limb.

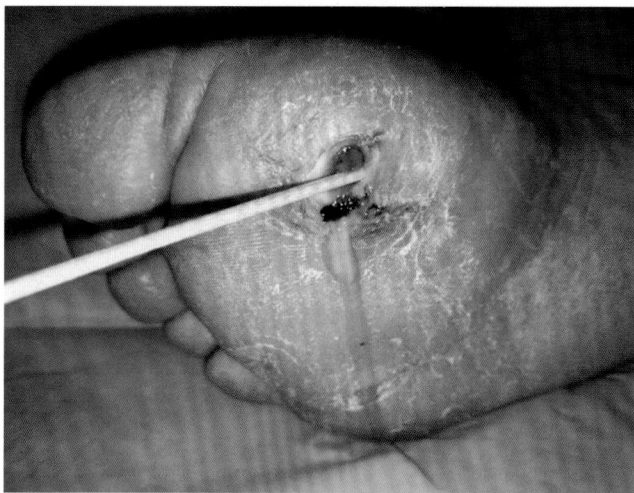

FIGURE 49.41 The probe to bone test shows strong correlation for osteomyelitis.

Neuropathy

Peripheral neuropathy is considered the most significant risk factor for a diabetic foot ulcer.[297] An impaired or absent feedback mechanism for the sensation of pain makes patients with diabetes highly susceptible to trauma or repetitive pressure from common forces like ill fitting shoe gear or foreign bodies.[291] Neuropathy is also a complicating factor after elective foot and ankle surgery, increasing the infection risk by 1.78 times.[297] Motor neuropathy may produce muscle weakness or imbalance that can lead to foot deformities that subsequently increase pressure, causing a callus, blister, or ulceration.[291] The intrinsic muscles weaken and the larger muscles overpower, creating common deformities like hammer toes and metatarsal head prominences. This allows for abnormal pressure distribution in the foot, leading to local site overload that may progress to a wound. Autonomic neuropathy leads to changes in microvasculature blood flow and arteriolar-venous shunting, decreasing skin perfusion, and elevating skin temperature.[291] This also leads to decreased sweat and oil gland function, resulting in dry, keratinized skin, which can contribute to formation of an ulcer.

Vasculopathy

Vascular compromise, both macroangiopathy and microangiopathy, have been reported as the most common cause

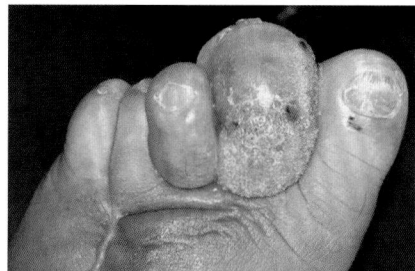

FIGURE 49.42 Dactylitis is suggestive of osteomyelitis.

of morbidity and mortality in diabetic patients.[298] Impaired lower extremity arterial inflow is a significant risk factor for tissue necrosis and delayed wound healing. Macroangiopathy is typically present as diffuse multisegmental disease, more typical to the infrapopliteal vessels, leading to compromised collateral circulation to the lower extremity. Microangiopathy involves thickening of the basement membrane, altered nutrient exchange, tissue hypoxia, and ultimately microcirculation ischemia.[291]

PAD can prolong the presence of a wound and increases the risk of wound infection.[293,299] There is a 5.5-increased risk of DFI in patients with PAD.[300] Ischemia can also complicate treatment by inhibiting antibiotic delivery to infected tissue.[301]

Immunopathy

Hyperglycemia impairs host defenses by diminishing the normal host inflammatory response to impending pathogens. Chronic hyperglycemia increases advanced glycation end products, allowing for chronic inflammation and increasing apoptosis.[302] Bacteria are attracted to glucose. Once established, the infection further escalates serum glucose and glycemic control becomes more difficult. Elevated blood glucose antagonizes neutrophils, leading to increased reactive oxygen species, free fatty acids, and inflammatory mediators, which cause cell damage, further potentiating vascular and immune malfunction.[303]

DIAGNOSTIC STUDIES

Diagnostic studies for evaluation of the DFI follow the same principles established for soft tissue, native joint, and bone infection as described in the previous sections of this chapter. Beyond the standard laboratory and imaging studies for infection in the diabetic patient, special attention must be also directed to serum glucose levels, nutrition status, limb perfusion, renal function, and cardiac reserve.

Glycemic Assessment

Glycemic control provides a measure of infection risk. Patients with glucose levels >200 mg/mL have demonstrated more wound complications in elective surgery, while patients with glucose levels >220 mg/mL were seven times more likely to develop infection after trauma than those without diabetes.[304,305] Hemoglobin A1c (HgbA1c) measures glycemic control over a 3-month period. HgA1c levels over 7%—corresponding average glucose level 154 mg/dL—suggest poor glycemic control. Preoperative HgbA1c > 6.7 correlates with an increased risk of wound complications or infection, while levels >7%-8% were associated with increased mortality and postoperative complications.[304,306-308] A comprehensive study of risk factors associated with complications after surgery in diabetic patients found there was a 5% increased risk of complication for every 1% increase in HgbA1c.[297] For every 1% reduction of HgbA1c, there is a 25% reduction in complication rate.[309] One limitation of HgA1c is that it cannot provide an accurate assessment of glycemic control in a shorter time interval. Serum fructosamine allows for such assessment. This test was demonstrated to be good indicator of infection risk in patients with diabetes at a level of ≥ 292 μmol/L and is a useful alternative to HgA1c for preoperative glycemic evaluation.[310]

Nutrition

Prealbumin and albumin not only are useful for evaluating the nutritional status of the hostbut also may decrease in the presence of infection. Patients with DFIs who ultimately required an amputation compared to those who did not had significantly lower serum albumin levels.[311] Patients with a serum albumin level of 3.5 g/dL had a higher likelihood of failure to heal their wound as compared to those with a serum albumin level of 3.8 g/dL.[291]

Neurologic Assessment

The Semmes Weinstein 10-g monofilament and vibratory sensation with the 128 Hz tuning fork are the most commonly utilized tools to evaluate for peripheral neuropathy.

Vascular Assessment

Ankle- and Toe-Brachial Indices

The IWGDF recommends the consideration of further vascular testing in wounds that do not improve over a 6-week period regardless of palpable pulses.[312] Ankle-brachial index (ABI) is a common noninvasive, rapid, and cost effective test to evaluate for PAD. An ABI < 0.9 or >1.3 is considered impaired and diagnostic for PAD. However, patients with diabetes may demonstrate falsely elevated ABI values due to arterial calcification. Toe-brachial index (TBI) is a more specific measurement for healing capacity. A normal TBI is >0.7. A TBI < 0.4 is predictive or poor healing while a TBI of 0.11 is associated with ischemic rest pain.[313] Absolute toe pressures may be useful as well. A toe pressure below 30 mm Hg is predictive of nonhealing while >60 mm Hg is predictive of healing.[314]

Transcutaneous Oxygen Tension Measurements

Transcutaneous oxygen ($TcPO_2$) tension measurements are far more advanced for estimating the microvascular perfusion of the toes. They are predictive of wound failure when levels are below 25 mm Hg.[314] The $TcPO_2$ is an important factor in the WIFI wound classification system and can help predict the risk of amputation.[286,287] Urgent imaging and revascularization are recommended with $TcPO_2 < 25$ mm Hg or toe pressure <30 mm Hg.[314] A low $TcPO_2$ had been linked to increased mortality rates and an increased risk of major cardiovascular events.[315,316]

Endovascular Procedures

Inadequate arterial perfusion to the foot impairs wound healing and is associated with increased mortality. In a recent study of patients who underwent a TMA, those with a nonpalpable pedal pulse had a 46.2% chance of mortality as compared to 21.3% in those with palpable pulses.[317] Angiography is an excellent diagnostic tool to determine both the level of occlusion and viable targets for limb revascularization, which are based on the patient's anatomic pattern of disease, patient risk, and wound complexity. Vascular occlusions in diabetic patients are most common below the knee.[318] Collaboration with a vascular surgeon is essential in the care of these patients to assist with healing and antibiotic delivery.[319]

Bone Biopsy and Culture

Bone biopsy and culture are the traditional gold standard for pathogen identification in diabetic pedal osteomyelitis, with a sensitivity and specificity of 95% and 99%, respectively.[320] Selection of appropriate antibiotic treatment has been based on this approach. A study that correlated the microbiologic results of deep wound culture with bone biopsy demonstrated that the identical bacterial strain was identified in 73.5% of cases.[321] Yet cultures may demonstrate false-positive detection of osteomyelitis because of bacterial contaminates. A recent study correlated bone swab culture and bone biopsy histopathology results: 65% of the cultures grew bacteria while only 27% of the samples were histologically positive.[322] Superficial wound cultures may contain bacterial contaminates and do not correlate well with the pathogens identified on bone biopsy and cultures.[323,324] As established in the section on general principles, multiple tissue samples from high-yield sites should be obtained and swab cultures should be avoided. Despite best practices, pathogen identification is not always reliable. Clinical judgment will help determine whether antimicrobial therapy is necessary based on both local factors and the patient host status. Clinically uninfected wounds should not be cultured or treated with antibiotics. This practice leads to antibiotic resistance.

IMAGING

Osteomyelitis vs Charcot Neuroarthropathy

Differentiating osteomyelitis from Charcot neuroarthropathy is often very difficult (Table 49.28). Both processes may occur simultaneously. Bone biopsy is the definitive method to rule out osteomyelitis, but this approach may not be necessary in all cases. While there are various laboratory tests and imaging modalities to help distinguish the two entities, they may be equivocal. Clinical suspicion may be the best tool. Both entities may present as a red, hot, swollen foot. Yet osteomyelitis typically results from a contiguous ulceration that probes to bone, which is less common in isolated acute Charcot neuroarthropathy. The midfoot is most commonly affected in Charcot neuroarthropathy, while the forefoot and metatarsophalangeal joints are the most common site for osteomyelitis in the diabetic foot.[325] Serum inflammatory markers may provide some clarity: an ESR > 70 mm/h and CRP >3.2 mg/dL are more suggestive markers for osteomyelitis compared to Charcot neuroarthropathy.[291]

A number of imaging studies may also help differentiate between these conditions (Table 49.29). Radiographic changes in osteomyelitis have been established in that section of this chapter (Fig. 49.43). Charcot neuroarthropathy may demonstrate similar radiographic signs in the early phase (Fig. 49.44), but the later stages demonstrate gross bone destruction, fragmentation, and dislocation.[325]

MRI is the most sensitive imaging study for distinguishing osteomyelitis from Charcot neuroarthropathy and helps define the extent of bone affected.[326,327] MRI demonstrates a sensitivity and specificity of 90% and 79%, respectively, for diagnosis of osteomyelitis in the diabetic foot.[296] Osteomyelitis appears as low focal signal intensity on T1-weighted images and high focal intensity on T2-weighted images, while Charcot

TABLE 49.29	Common Microorganisms Associated With Diabetic Wound Infections
Type of Infection	**Microorganism**
Mild Infection	*S aureus* Group B Streptococcus
Deep, limb-threatening infection	Aerobic gram-positive cocci Gram-negative bacilli: *E coli,* *Klebsiella* spp., *Proteus* spp. Anaerobes: *Bacteroides* spp. and *Peptostreptococcus* spp.
Pathogenic colonizers and contaminants	Coagulase-negative staphylococcus Enterococcus *Corynebacterium* spp.
Previously treated with antimicrobials OR Chronic ulcers	Typically polymicrobial *Enterococcus* spp. *Pseudomonas aeruginosa* *Enterobacteriaceae* *Anaerobic bacteria*
Fungal infections	*Candida parapsilosis* *Zygomycetes* *M tuberculosis*

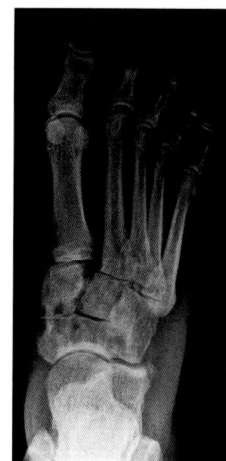

FIGURE 49.44 Radiograph depicting early signs of midfoot Charcot neuroarthropathy, which are similar to some late findings in osteomyelitis.

neuroarthropathy demonstrates low signal intensity in both T1 and T2 phases. A significant MRI finding suggestive of osteomyelitis is a sinus tract communicating directly from the ulcer to bone.

Bone scintigraphy has a high sensitivity (80%-100%) but low specificity (25%-60%) for differentiating osteomyelitis from Charcot neuroarthropathy.[328] A Tc-99m MDP scan is not commonly performed due to high false positives. A leukocyte-labeled Tc-99m HMPAO bone scan may help confirm osteomyelitis: the positive predictive value for osteomyelitis is 75%-90%, the negative predictive value is 80%, and sensitivity and specificity are 86% and 85%, respectively.[329,330]

COMMON MICROORGANISMS IN DIABETIC FOOT INFECTIONS

The DFI is often polymicrobial (Table 49.29). Gram-positive bacteria are the most common pathogens.[320,323,324,331-334] *Staphylococcus aureus* is the most frequent pathogen, responsible for 26.4%-81.9% of infections, while methicillin-resistant *Staphylococcus aureus* (MRSA) is found in 9.6%-28.9% of infections.[320,323,324,332-334] The incidence of MRSA osteomyelitis appears to be decreasing with time, with a peak incidence in 2005.[334,335] *Streptococcus* species are another common pathogen.[323,324,334] Gram-negative bacteria are found in 18.4%-50% of osteomyelitis cases; *Pseudomonas* is the most common gram-negative bacteria.[323,324,334] Anaerobic bacteria, including *Peptostreptococcus magnus* and *Bacteroides fragilis*, increase based on wound duration, with an incidence ranging from 4.8% to 14%.[324,332,334,336] Patients with peripheral vascular disease have been found to

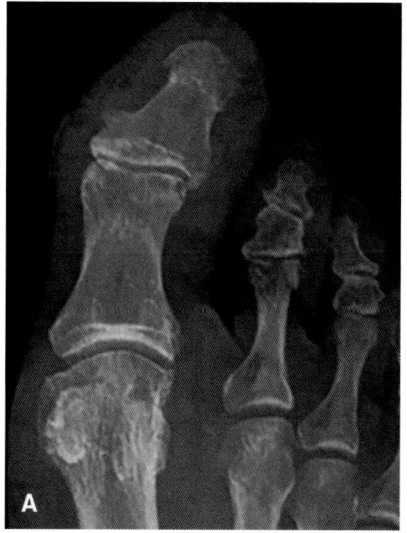 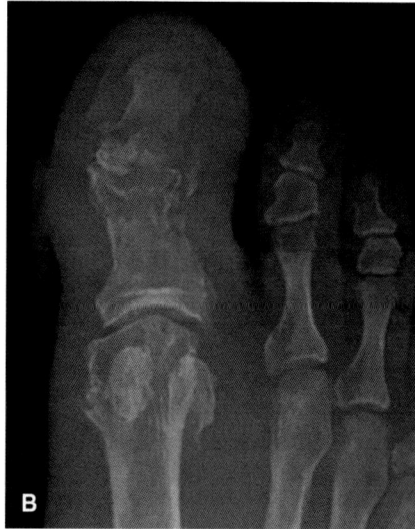

FIGURE 49.43 Radiograph depicting osteomyelitis of the hallux. **A.** Early stages show subtle rarefaction, cystic changes, and periosteal reaction about the interphalangeal joint. **B.** Late stages show obvious bone erosion and collapse.

have a higher incidence of gram-negative bacteria, which may be a result of the longevity of the wound.[334] Polymicrobial infection occurs in 15%-31.8% of the cases of osteomyelitis,[320,324,332,334] which often makes antibiotic selection more challenging. Fungal infections are less common but may occur with a bacterial infection, typically called a superinfection. Candida, Zygomycetes, and *M tuberculosis* are the most common fungal pathogens in the diabetic foot.[331] Consultation with an infectious disease specialist is recommended in the treatment of most DFIs.

TREATMENT

A multidisciplinary team approach is essential to maximize success in the treatment of a DFI. The team should include a foot and ankle specialist and surgeon, vascular surgeon, infectious disease specialist, internal medicine physician, endocrinologist, plastic surgeon, prosthetist, and pharmacist. Some infections may be successfully treated with oral antibiotics, wound care and off-loading as necessary, and frequent clinical follow-up. However, a low threshold for hospital admission is advisable. Many DFIs are often more sinister than their initial appearance.

Systemic Antibiotic Therapy

Antibiotic therapy should be initiated as soon as a DFI is suspected. Some mild infections may be treated with appropriate oral antibiotics, but if a more significant infection is suspected, parenteral antibiotics are necessary to achieve rapid therapeutic serum levels[285] (Table 49.30). Since gram-positive bacteria are the most common pathogen, antibiotic therapy should be directed accordingly, with special consideration of host risk factors for MRSA, anaerobic, and gram-negative infection. Prior to initiation of antibiotic therapy, deep tissue cultures should be obtained as indicated and according to clean methods as previously described, though this is not always possible. Ultimately, antibiotic therapy should selectively target the pathogen, which is best identified by deep cultures or the gold standard, bone biopsy and culture.[285,291] Typically 1-2 weeks of antibiotic therapy is adequate to treat a soft tissue infection in the diabetic foot.[285]

Foot and ankle surgeons have a unique opportunity to surgically eradicate infection through amputation. If the infected bone is removed, no more than a week of oral antibiotics may be necessary.[285] If there is a residual infection but the bone appears to be healthy, 6 weeks of parenteral antibiotics may be adequate for treatment.[337] If osteomyelitis is confirmed yet clean margins cannot be attained, at least 12 weeks of antibiotic therapy is recommended. Serum inflammatory markers should be followed to determine the duration of antibiotic therapy. Antibiotic stewardship helps weigh the risks of infection treatment against potential side effects of the antibiotic, such as *C difficile* colitis. Extended or suppressive antibiotic therapy should be considered if it is impractical to excise the infected bone, such as in more extensive cases of midfoot/hindfoot osteomyelitis, or if surgical treatment is precluded as in cases of advanced PAD or the C-host patient.

Surgery

Surgical treatment of the diabetic foot or ankle infection may vary from simple incision and débridement to amputation. Swift

TABLE 49.30	**Antibiotic Selection for Diabetic Foot Infections**	
Infection Severity	**Common/Suspected Organisms**	**Antibiotic Recommendation**
Mild	Staphylococcus and Streptococcus species	Cephalexin Dicloxacillin Amoxicillin/clavulanate Clindamycin
	MRSA	Clindamycin Septra Minocycline Linezolid
	Gram negative	Septra + amoxicillin/ clavulanate Clindamycin + fluoroquinolone
Moderate to Severe	Streptococcus	Ceftriaxone
	MRSA	Vancomycin Linezolid Daptomycin
	Aerobic gram negative bacilli	Ampicillin-sulbactam Zosyn Meropenem Ertapenem
	Anaerobes	Ceftriaxone Cefepime Levofloxacin Moxifloxacin Aztreonam Metronidazole

and aggressive débridement of necrotic soft tissue and bone is vital for infection control, limb salvage, and in severe DFIs, to prevent mortality (Fig. 49.45). A patient with severe infection will often require serial débridement, especially as the extent of necrosis declares itself over time. Upon initial evaluation of the patient, it may be useful to decompress an obvious abscess prior to the operation. In the presence of significant PAD vascular intervention may be necessary. However, initial decompression of the infection takes priority.

Amputations in the diabetic foot are an effective means of infection control and allow for preservation of some pedal function (Figs. 49.46 and 49.47). It is important to consider how the residual foot will function over the long term. To this end, it is necessary to balance the foot in an effort to minimize pressure points and the development of new wound. A well-balanced transmetatarsal amputation is quite functional, particularly if the plantar flap is robust (Fig. 49.47).

Surgical emergencies include gas gangrene (Fig. 49.48), necrotizing fasciitis, infection causing sepsis, and on rare occasions, compartment syndrome.[285] In some cases, the infection severity precludes limb salvage. In other cases, the infection may advance into the leg and may require a below the knee (BKA) or above the knee (AKA) amputation. Early surgical treatment may help to decrease the chance of a major amputation.[338]

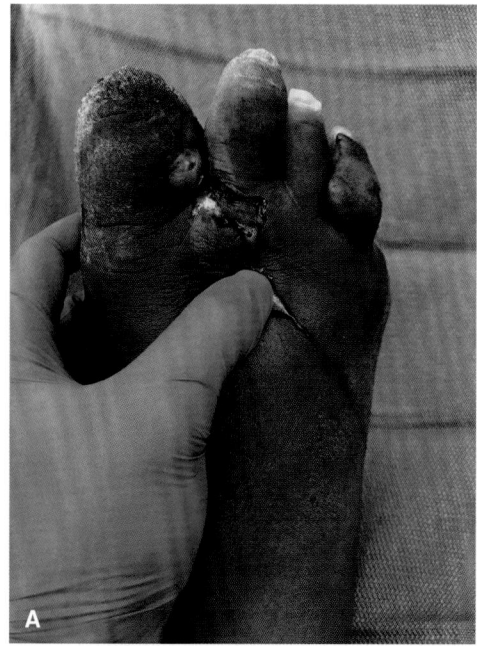
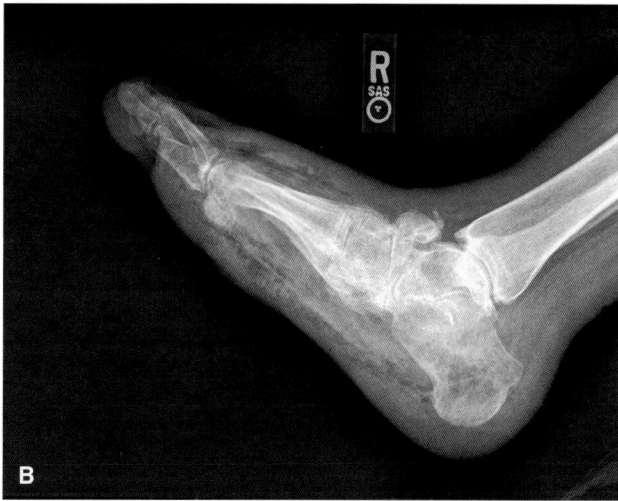
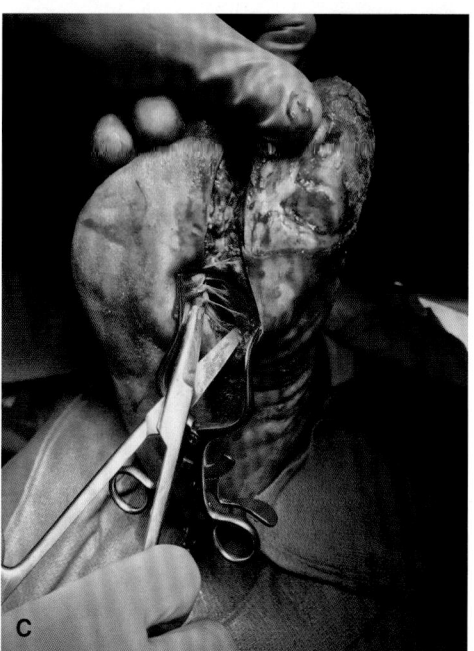
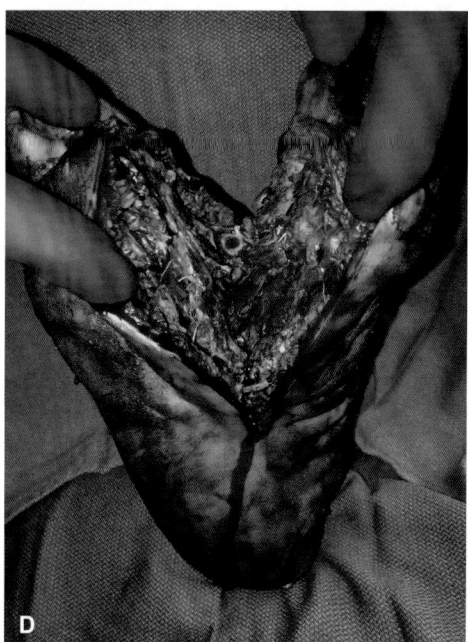

FIGURE 49.45 Extensive diabetic foot infection originating at the second interspace. **A.** Gas bubbles consistent with *Clostridium* spp. **B.** Radiograph demonstrating gas throughout the soft tissue planes. **C.** Urgent intermetatarsal space and pedal arch decompression. **D.** Radical débridement to establish a clean tissue bed. The foot was ultimately salvaged after serial débridement with a transmeta tarsal amputation.

Antibiotic Depots

The surgical resection of necrotic bone in some diabetic foot and ankle infections may result in large defects that may compromise skeletal integrity. Antibiotic-loaded cement spacers may be used to fill the deficit and treat the infection until a definitive procedure can be attempted[339] (Fig. 49.49). In some cases, the cement spacer is retained permanently for structural support (Fig. 49.30). Antibiotic-impregnated beads or pellets are an effective means to deliver high concentration of antibiotic directly to the infection site in the diabetic foot.[340]

Soft Tissue Management

The elimination of nonviable bone and soft tissue in the diabetic foot or ankle may also produce substantial dead space and soft tissue defects. Soft tissue voids on the load-bearing surface of the insensate foot are particularly difficult to manage. Planning for soft tissue coverage begins during the initial débridement. Careful attention to preservation of all viable tissue and avoiding the disruption of local arterial supply is vital. Local tissue is typically robust and often preferred to the scar that forms as a result of secondary intention healing, particularly on the plantar aspect of the foot. Once a clean wound has been

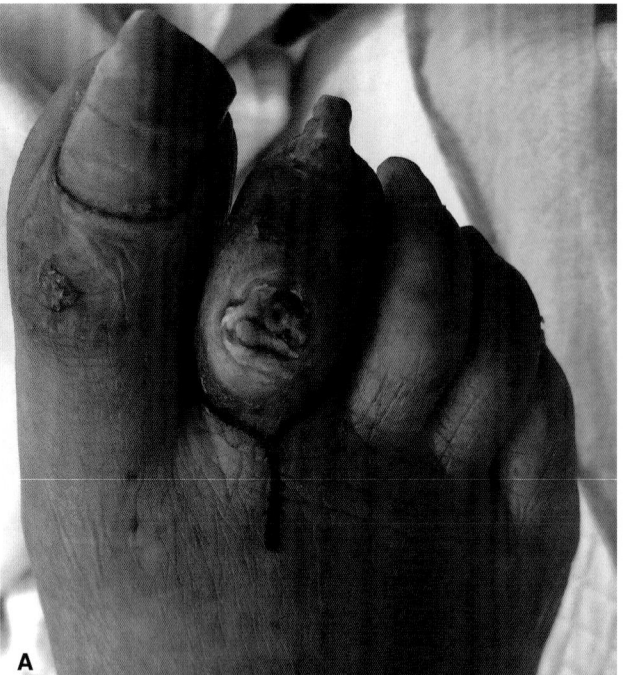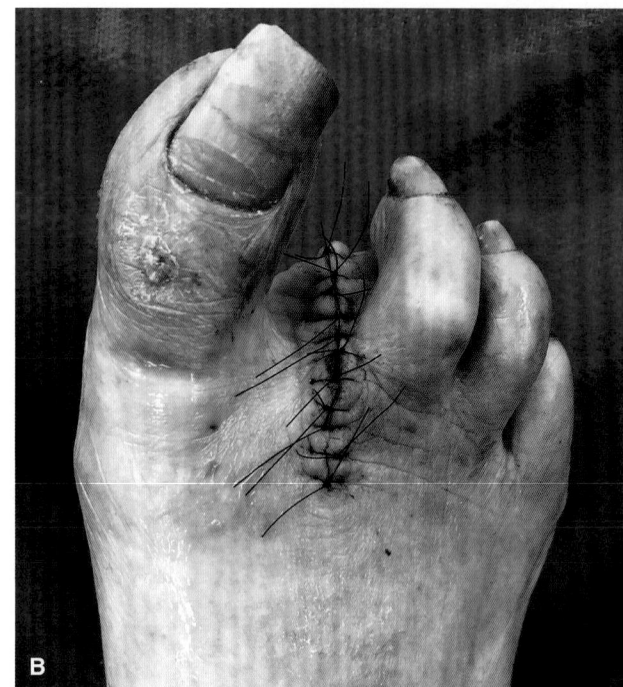

FIGURE 49.46 Toe amputation to eradicate infection. **A.** Photograph of second toe with exposed bone at the head of the proximal phalanx with osteomyelitis. **B.** Photograph following second toe amputation and primary closure.

established, various local flaps may be utilized for coverage (Figs. 49.50 and 49.51). Consultation with the plastic surgery team may be necessary for large or complex wounds that preclude local tissue coverage, though in many cases the B-host patient is a poor candidate for more significant flap reconstruction, including free tissue transfer.

Negative pressure wound therapy is an important adjunct method for delayed wound closure techniques in the diabetic foot. A systematic review of negative pressure wound therapy vs standard of care for diabetic foot wounds reported a higher rate of complete healing, shorter time to healing, greater reduction in ulcer area and depth, fewer amputations, and few adverse effects.[341]

POSTOPERATIVE CARE AND REHABILITATION

The ongoing multidisciplinary care of diabetic patient following a foot or ankle infection is paramount to prevent further complications. The patient should see the primary care physician, diabetes nurse educator, and endocrinologist as necessary. Follow-up with the infectious disease specialist and vascular surgeon is also important. Wound care is dictated by the nature of the surgical site. In patients undergoing toe amputations, weight bearing in a postoperative shoe is typically sufficient for protection. For ray resection, transmetatarsal amputation, or plantar wounds, a non–weight bearing splint or cast is initially recommended unless it places undue pressure on the flap.

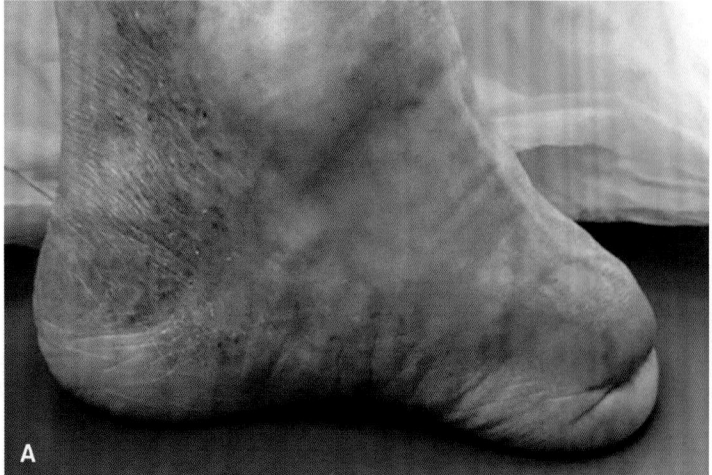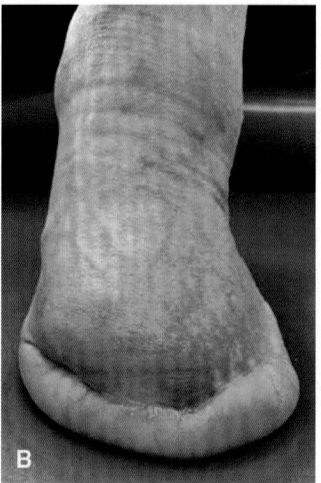

FIGURE 49.47 A, B. Plantigrade, well-balanced transmetatarsal amputation.

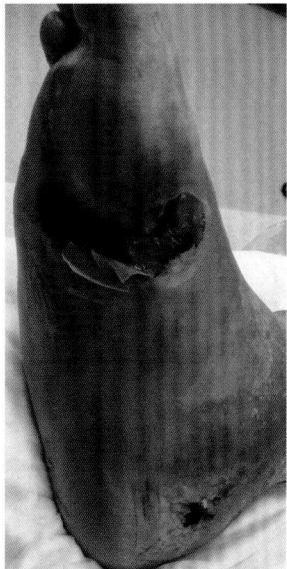

FIGURE 49.48 Gas gangrene is a surgical emergency.

A boot is an alternative, but wear adherence may be problematic. If the patient is a fall risk or unstable, protected heel load may be necessary. Physical therapy is often important to help maintain surgical site off-loading, facilitate gait training, and to help the patient with reconditioning.

Once the surgical site is healed, a prosthetist may provide a shoe or brace as necessary to accommodate an amputation or to help to off-load high-pressure areas that could lead to new wounds. For patients with a forefoot or midfoot amputation, accommodative padding may be incorporated with a shoe filler to decrease shear pressure. Some patients with Charcot neuroarthropathy do well with a rocker shoe and custom insole. In other patients with significant deformity that puts them at much higher risk for reulceration, a Charcot restraint orthotic walker (CROW) may be necessary (Fig. 49.52).

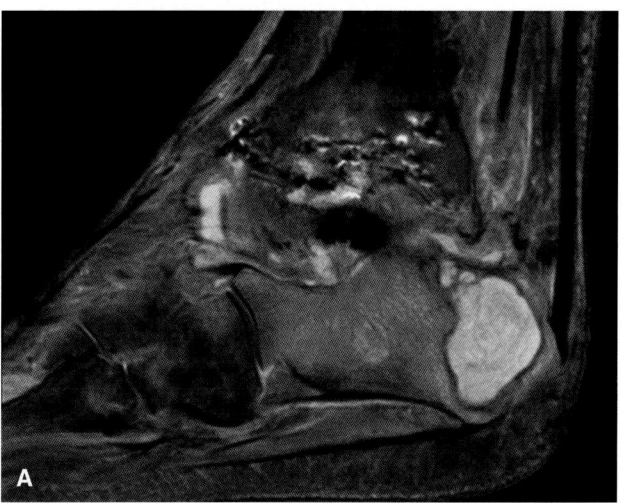

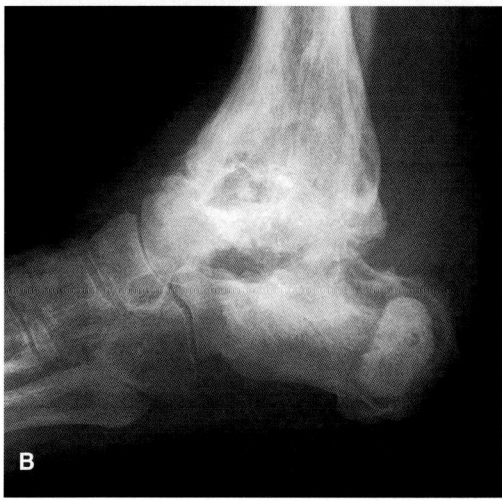

FIGURE 49.49 A. MRI STIR image depicts intraosseus calcaneal abscess and osteomyelitis. **B.** Postoperative radiograph following resection of infected bone and placement of antibiotic-loaded cement.

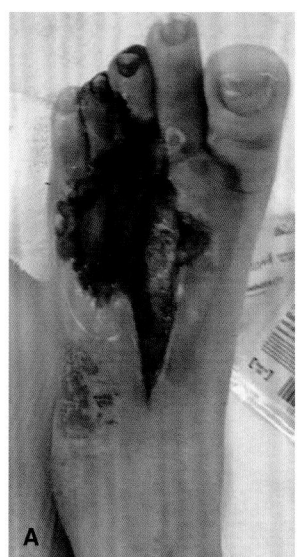
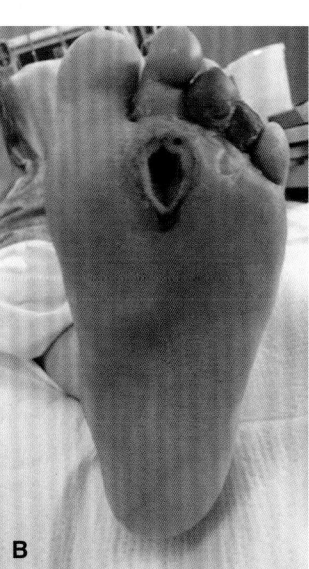
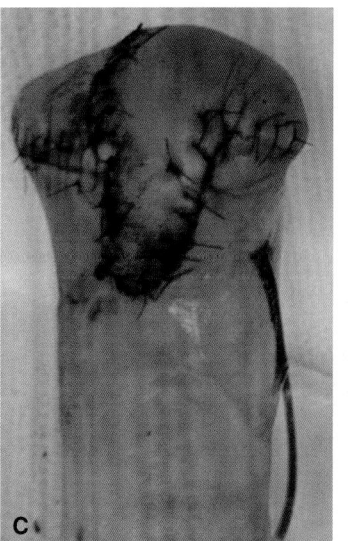
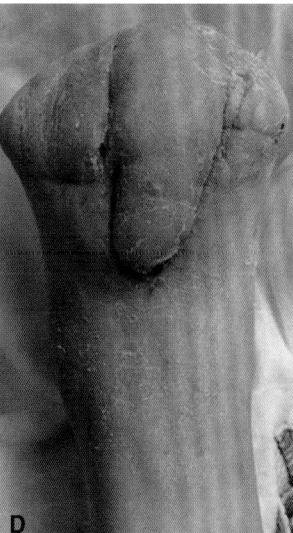

FIGURE 49.50 Clinical photographs **(A-D)** depicting healthy tissue from hallux and first ray mobilized to fill a large transmetatarsal amputation soft tissue defect following radical débridement of necrotic soft tissue and bone.

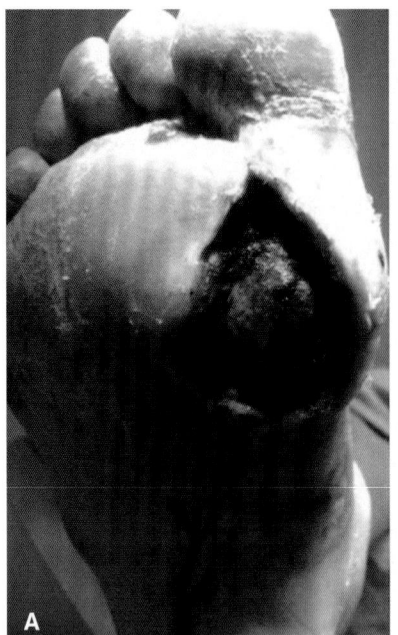

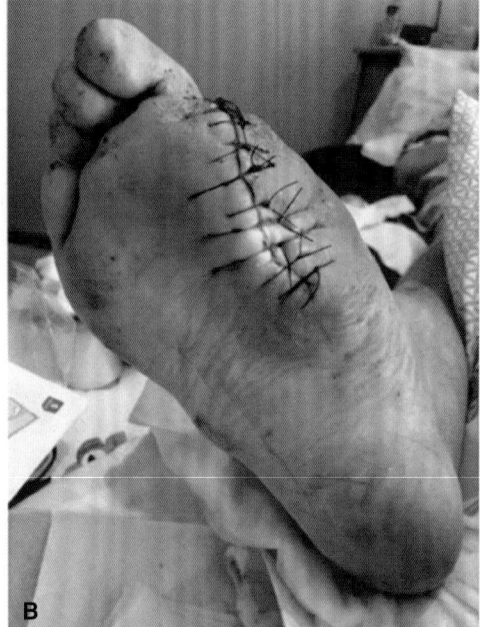

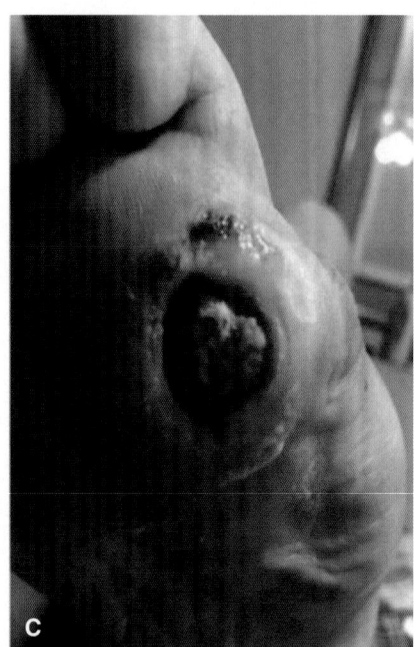

FIGURE 49.51 Bi-lobed flap for coverage of plantar medial wound in diabetic patient who refused transmetatarsal amputation. **A.** Photograph of plantar first metatarsal head wound with osteomyelitis. **B.** Partial first ray resection, which healed. **C.** Subsequent transfer ulcer developed plantar second metatarsal head. **D.** Partial second ray resection with large bi-lobed flap to cover plantar medial soft tissue defect. Flap débridement was necessary. **E.** Mature flap and ulcer-free foot at 2-year follow-up.

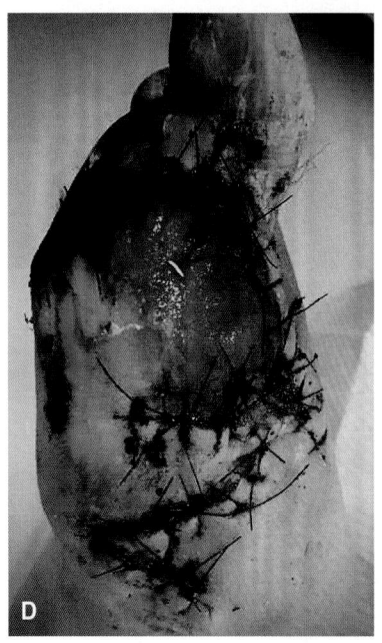

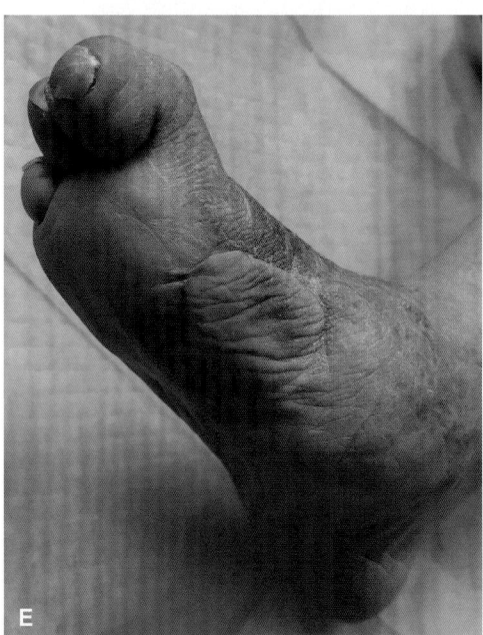

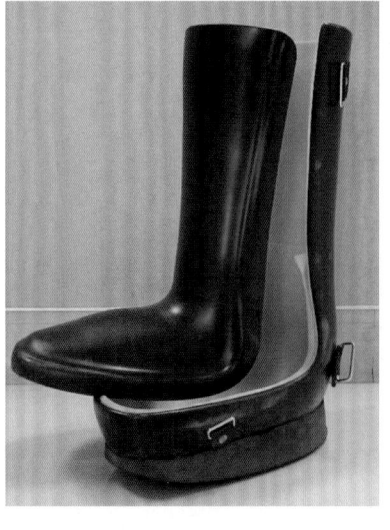

FIGURE 49.52 CROW boot.

REFERENCES

1. Fry DE, Polk HC. Infection in the surgical patient: prevention and treatment. *Drug Ther.* 1982;7:19-28.
2. Ki V, Rotstein C. Bacterial skin and soft tissue infections in adults: a review of their epidemiology, pathogenesis, diagnosis, and treatment and site of care. *Can J Infect Dis.* 2008;19:173-184.
3. Maharajan K, Patro DK, Menon J, et al. Serum procalcitonin is a sensitive and specific marker in the diagnosis of septic arthritis and acute osteomyelitis. *J Orthop Surg Res.* 2013;8:19.
4. Gedjerg N, LaRosa R, Hunter JG, et al. Anti-glucosaminidase IgG in sera as a biomarker of host immunity against Staphylococcus aureus in orthopedic surgery patients. *J Bone Joint Surg Am.* 2013;95:e171.
5. Blyme PJH, Lind T, Schantz K, et al. Ultrasonographic detection of foreign bodies in soft tissue: a human cadaver study. *Arch Orthop Trauma Surg.* 1990;110:24-25.
6. Boutin RD, Brossman J, Sartoris DJ, et al. Update on imaging of orthopedic infections. *Orthop Clin North Am.* 1998;29:41-66.
7. Kuhns LR, Borlaza GS, Seigel RS, et al. An in vitro comparison of computed tomography, xeroradiography, and radiography in the detection of soft-tissue foreign bodies. *Radiology.* 1979;132:218-219.
8. Sherertz RJ, Bassetti S, Bassetti-Wyss B. "Cloud" health-care workers. *Emerg Infect Dis.* 2001;7:241-243.
9. Davis N, Curry A, Gambhir AK, et al. Intra-operative bacterial contamination in operations for joint replacement. *J Bone Joint Surg Br.* 1999;81:886-889.
10. Isenberg HD, ed. *Clinical Microbiology Procedures Handbook.* 2nd ed. Washington, DC: ASM Press; 2004.
11. Garcia LS. *Updates to the Clinical Microbiology Procedures Handbook.* 2nd ed. Washington, DC: ASM Press; 2007.
12. Murray RP, Baron EJ, Jorgensen JH, et al., eds. *Manual of Clinical Microbiology.* 9th ed. Washington, DC: ASM Press; 2007.
13. Trampuz A, Piper KE, Jacobson MJ, et al. Sonication of removed hip and knee prosthesis for diagnosis of infection. *N Engl J Med.* 2007;357:654-663.
14. Moojen DJ, Spijkers SN, Schot CS, et al. Identification of orthopedic infections using broad-range polymerase chain reaction and reverse line blot hybridization. *J Bone Joint Surg Am.* 2007;89:1298-1305.
15. Nunez LV, Buttaro MA, Morandi A, et al. Frozen sections of samples taken intraoperatively for diagnosis of infection in revision hip surgery. *Acta Orthop.* 2007;78:226-230.
16. Heitmann C, Patzakis MJ, Tetsworth KD, Levin LS. Musculoskeletal sepsis: principles of treatment. *Instr Course Lect.* 2003;52:733-744.
17. Stevens DL, Bisno AL, Chambers HF, et al. Practice guidelines for the diagnosis and management of skin and soft tissue infections: 2014 update by the Infectious Diseases Society of America. *Clin Infect Dis.* 2014;59:e10-e52.
18. Roukis TS. Bacterial skin contamination before and after surgical preparation of the foot, ankle, and lower leg in patients with diabetes and intact skin verses patients with diabetes and ulceration: a prospective controlled therapeutic study. *J Foot Ankle Surg.* 2010;49:348-356.
19. Sayner LR, Rosenblum BI, Giurini JM. Elective surgery of the diabetic foot. *Clin Podiatr Med Surg.* 2003;20:783-792.
20. Somerville DA. The effect of age on the normal bacterial flora of the skin. *Br J Dermatol.* 1969;81:14.
21. Swartz MN. Cellulitis. *N Engl J Med.* 2004;350:904-912.
22. McNamara DR, Tleyjeh IM, Berbari EF, et al. Incidence of lower-extremity cellulitis: a population-based study in Olmsted county, Minnesota. *Mayo Clin Proc.* 2007;82:817-821.
23. Hirschmann JV, Raugi GJ. Lower limb cellulitis and its mimics: Part I. Lower limb cellulitis. *J Am Acad Dermatol.* 2012;67:163.e1-163.e12.
24. Bisno AL, Stevens DL. Streptococcal infections of the skin and subcutaneous tissues. *N Engl J Med.* 1996;334:240-245.
25. Chartier C, Grosshans E. Erysipelas. *Int J Dermatol.* 1996;29:459-467.
26. Dupuy A, Benchikhi H, Roujeu JC, et al. Risk factors for erysipelas of the leg (cellulitis): case-control study. *BMJ.* 1999;318(7198):1591-1594.
27. Field LA, Adams BB. Tinea pedis in athletes. *Int J Dermatol.* 2008;47:485-492.
28. Semel JD, Goldin H. Association of athlete's foot with cellulitis of the lower extremities: diagnostic value of bacterial cultures of ipsilateral interdigital space samples. *Clin Infect Dis.* 1996 23:1162-1164.
29. Day MR, Day RD, Harkless LB. Cellulitis secondary to web space dermatophytosis. *Clin Podiatr Med Surg.* 1996;13:759-766.
30. Pecci M, Comeau D, Chawla V. Skin conditions in the athlete. *Am J Sports Med.* 2009;37:406-418.
31. Tlougen BE, Mancini AJ, Mandel JA, et al. Skin conditions in figure-skaters, ice-hokey players and speed skaters: Part II. Cold-induced, infectious and inflammatory dermatoses. *Sports Med.* 2011;41:967-984.
32. Crawford F, Hollis S. Topical treatments for fungal infections of the skin and nails of the foot. *Cochrane Database Syst Rev.* 2007;(3):CD001434.
33. DeLauro NM, DeLauro NM Onychocryptosis. *Clin Podiatr Med Surg.* 2004;21:617-630.
34. Heidelbaugh JJ, Lee H. Management of the ingrown toenail. *Am Fam Physician.* 2009;79:303-308.
35. Reyzelman AM, Trombello KA, Vayser DJ, et al. Are antibiotics necessary in the treatment of locally infected ingrown toenails? *Arch Fam Med.* 2000;9:930-932.
36. Tosti, A, Piraccini BM, Ghetti E, et al. Topical steroids verses systemic antifungals in the treatment of chronic paronychia: an open, randomized double-blind and double dummy study. *J Am Acad Dermatol.* 2002;47:73-76.
37. Adams BB. Skin infections in athletes. *Dermatol Nurs.* 2008;20:39-44.
38. Raz R, Miron D, Colodner R, et al. 1-Year trial of nasal mupirocin in the prevention of recurrent staphylococcal nasal colonization and skin infections. *Arch Intern Med.* 1996;56:1009-1112.
39. Perez C, Huttner A, Assal M, et al. Infectious olecranon and patellar bursitis: short-course adjuvant antibiotic therapy is not a risk factor for recurrence in adult hospitalized patients. *J Antimicrob Chemother.* 2010;65:1008-1014.
40. Lawson KS, Schwarian JS, Awbrey BJ. Septic bursitis of the foot: diagnosis, management, and end-result. *J Foot Surg.* 1990;29:379-384.
41. Valeriano-Marcet J, Carter JD, Vasey FB. Soft tissue disease. *Rheum Dis Clin North Am.* 2003;29:77-88.
42. Beltran J. MR imaging of soft tissue infection. *Magn Reson Imaging Clin N Am.* 1995;3:743-751.
43. Stell IM, Gransden WR. Simple tests for septic bursitis: comparative study. *BMJ.* 1998;316:1877.
44. Baumbach SF, Lobo CM, Badyine I, et al. Prepatellar and olecranon bursitis: literature review and development of a treatment algorithm. *Arch Orthop Trauma Surg.* 2014;134:359-370.
45. Dellinger EP, Caplan ES, Weaver LD, et al. Duration of preventive antibiotic administration for open extremities fractures. *Arch Surg.* 1988;123:333-339.
46. Lee J. Efficacy of cultures in the management of open fractures. *Clin Orthop Relat Res.* 1997;339:71-75.
47. Higham M. Infections in a puncture wound after it has "healed." *Hosp Pract.* 1983;4:47-54.
48. Patzakis MJ, Wilkins J, Brien WW, et al. Wound site as a predictor of complications following deep nail punctures to the foot. *West J Med.* 1989;150:545-547.
49. Weber E. Plantar puncture wounds: a survey to determine the incidence of infection. *J Accid Emerg Med.* 1996;13:274-277.
50. Schwab RA, Powers RD. Conservative therapy of plantar puncture wounds. *J Emerg Med.* 1995;13:291-295.
51. Fitzgerald RH, Cowan JDE. Puncture wounds of the foot. *Orthop Clin North Am.* 1975;6:965-972.
52. Eidelman M, Bialik V, Miller Y, et al. Plantar puncture wounds in children: analysis of 80 hospitalized patients and late sequela. *Isr Med Assoc J.* 2003;5:268-271.
53. Haverstock BD, Grossman JP. Puncture wounds of the foot. Evaluation and treatment. *Clin Podiatr Med Surg.* 1999;16:583-596.
54. Centers for Disease Control. Recommendations of the Immunization Practices Advisory Committee: diphtheria, tetanus, and pertussis: guidelines for vaccine prophylaxis and other preventative measures. *Ann Intern Med.* 1985;103:869-905.
55. Griego RD, Rosen T, Orengo IF, Wolf JE. Dog, cat, and human bites: a review. *J Am Acad Dermatol.* 1995;33:1019-1029.
56. Fleisher GR. The management of bite wound. *N Engl J Med.* 1999;340:138-140.
57. Donate G, Emerick Salas R, Naidu D, et al. Nonvenomous bite injuries of the foot: case reports and review of the literature. *Int J Low Extrem Wounds.* 2008;7:41-44.
58. Patrick GR, O'Rourke KM. Dog and cat bites: epidemiological analyses suggest different prevention strategies. *Public Health Rep.* 1998;113:252-257.
59. Anderson CR. Animal bites. *Postgrad Med.* 1992;92:134-146.
60. Goldstein EJ. Bite wounds and infection. *Clin Infect Dis.* 1992;14:633-638.
61. Dire DJ. Emergency management of dog and cat bite wounds. *Emerg Med Clin North Am.* 1992;10:719-736.
62. Weber DJ, Wolfson JS, Swartz MN, Hooper DC. Pasteurella multicoda infections: report of 34 cases and review of the literature. *Medicine.* 1984;63:133-157.
63. Muguti GI, Dixon MS. Tetanus following human bite. *Br J Plast Surg.* 1992;45:614-615.
64. Richman KM, Rickman LS. The potential for transmission of human immunodeficiency virus through human bites. *J Acquir Immune Defic Syndr.* 1993;6:402-406.
65. Gold BS, Barish RA, Dart RC. North American snake envenomation: diagnosis, treatment, and management. *Emerg Med Clin North Am.* 2004;22:423-443.
66. Sakalkale R, Mansell C, Whalley D, et al. Rat-bite fever: a cautionary tale. *N Z Med J.* 2007;120:U2545.
67. Horseman MA, Surni S. A comprehensive review of *Vibrio vulnificus*: and important cause of severe sepsis and skin and soft-tissue infection. *Int J Infect Dis.* 2011;15:e157-e166.
68. Wiggins ME, Akelman E, Weiss APC. The management of dog bites and dog infections to the hand. *Orthopedics.* 1994;17:617-623.
69. Rea WJ, Wyrick WJ Jr. Necrotizing fasciitis. *Ann Surg.* 1970;172:957-964.
70. Angoules AG, Kontakis G, Drakoulakis E, et al. Necrotising fasciitis of upper and lower limb: a systematic review. *Injury.* 2007;38(suppl 5):S19-S26.
71. Mulla ZD. Treatment options in the management of necrotising fasciitis caused by Group A Streptococcus. *Expert Opin Pharmacother.* 2004;5(8):1695-1700.
72. Simonart T. Group A beta-haemolytic streptococcal necrotising fasciitis: early diagnosis and clinical features. *Dermatology.* 2004;208:5-9.
73. Wong CH, Chang HC, Pasupathy S et al. Necrotizing fasciitis: clinical presentation, microbiology, and determinants of mortality. *J Bone Joint Surg Am.* 2003;85-A:1454-1460.
74. Bellapianta JM, Ljungquist K, Tobin E, et al. Necrotizing fasciitis. *J Am Acad Orthop Surg.* 2009;17:174-182.
75. Young MH, Aronoff DM, Engleberg NC. Necrotizing fasciitis: pathogenesis and treatment. *Exp Rev Anti-Infect Ther.* 2005;3:279-294.
76. Edlich RF, Cross CL, Dahlstrom JJ, et al. Modern concepts of the diagnosis and treatment of necrotizing fasciitis. *J Emerg Med.* 2010;39:261-265.
77. Massey PR, Sakran JV, Mills AM, et al. Hyberbaric oxygen therapy in necrotizing soft tissue infections. *J Surg Res.* 2012;177:146-151.
78. Mathews CJ, Weston VC, Jones A, et al. Bacterial septic arthritis in adults. *Lancet.* 2010;375:846-855.

79. Esterhai JL Jr, Gleb I. Adult septic arthritis. *Orthop Clin North Am.* 1991;22:503-514.
80. Kang SN, Sanghera T, Mangwani J, et al. The management of septic arthritis in children. *J Bone Joint Surg Br.* 2009;91-B:1127-1133.
81. Goldenberg DL, Reed JI. Bacterial arthritis. *N Engl J Med.* 1985;312:764-771.
82. Rao N. Septic arthritis. *Curr Treat Options Infect Dis.* 2002;4:279-287.
83. Gupta MN, Sturrock RD, Field M. A prospective 2-year study of 75 patients with adult-onset septic arthritis. *Rheumatology (Oxford).* 2001;40:24-30.
84. Weston VC, Jones AC, Bradbuy N, et al. Clinical features and outcome of septic arthritis in a single UK Health District 1982-1991. *Ann Rheum Dis.* 1999;58:214-219.
85. Kaandorp CJ, Dinant HJ, van de Laar MA, et al. Incidence and sources of native and prosthetic joint infection: a community based prospective survey. *Ann Rheum Dis.* 1997;56:470-475.
86. Kaandorp CJ, Van Schaardenburg D, Krijnen P, et al. Risk factors for septic arthritis in patients with joint disease. A prospective study. *Arthritis Rheum.* 1995;38:1819-1825.
87. Edwards CJ, Cooper C, Fisher D, et al. The importance of the disease process and disease-modifying anti-rheumatic drug treatment in the development of septic arthritis in patients with rheumatoid arthritis. *Arthritis Rheum.* 2007;57;1151-1157.
88. Garcia-De La Torre I. Advances in the management of septic arthritis. *Rheum Dis Clin North Am.* 2003;29:61-75.
89. Gavet F, Tournadre A, Soubrier M, et al. Septric arthritis in patients aged 80 and older: a comparison with younger adults. *J Am Geriatr Soc.* 2005;53:1210-1213.
90. Bauer T, Boisrenoult P, Jenny JY. Post-arthroscopy septic arthritis: current data and practical recommendations. *Orthop Traumatol Surg Res.* 2015;101:S347-S350.
91. Geirsson AJ, Statkevicius S, Vikingsson A. Septic arthritic in Iceland 1990-2002: increasing incidence due to iatrogenic infections. *Ann Rheum Dis.* 2008;67:638-643.
92. Armstrong RW, Bolding F, Joseph R. Septic arthritis following arthroscopy: clinical syndromes and analysis of risk factors. *Arthroscopy.* 1992;8:213-223.
93. Ross JJ. Septic arthritis of native joints. *Infect Dis Clin North Am.* 2017;31:203-218.
94. Newman JH. Review of septic arthritis throughout the antibiotic era. *Ann Rheum Dis.* 1976;35:198-205.
95. Bohl DD, Frank RM, Lee S. Sensitivity of the saline load test for traumatic arthrotomy of the ankle with ankle arthroscopy simulation. *Foot Ankle Int.* 2018;39:736-740.
96. McCarthy JJ, Noonan KJ. Toxic synovitis. *Skeletal Radiol.* 2008;37:963-965.
97. Goldenberg DL. Septic arthritis. *Lancet.* 1998;351:197-202.
98. Smith JW, Chalupa P, Shabaz Hasan M. Infectious arthritis: clinical features, laboratory findings, and treatment. *Clin Microbiol Infect.* 2006;12:309-314.
99. Garcia-Arias M, Balsa A, Mola EM. Septic arthritis. *Best Pract Res Clin Rheumatol.* 2011;25:407-421.
100. Li SF, Henderson J, Dickman E, et al. Laboratory tests in adults with monoarticular arthritis: can they rule out a septic joint? *Acad Emerg Med.* 2004;11:276-280.
101. Soderquist B, Jones I, Fredlund H. Bacterial or crystal-associated arthritis? Discriminating ability of serum inflammatory markers. *Scand J Infect Dis.* 1998;30:591-596.
102. Margaretten ME, Kohlwes J, Moore D, et al. Does this adult patient have septic arthritis? *JAMA.* 2007;297:1478-1488.
103. Hughes JG, Vetter EA, Patel R, et al. Culture with BACTEC Peds Plus/F bottle compared with conventional methods for detection of bacteria in synovial fluid. *J Clin Microbiol.* 2001;39:4468-4471.
104. Hunter JG, Gross JM, Dahl JD, et al. Risk factors for failure of a single surgical debridement in adults with acute septic arthritis. *J Bone Joint Surg Am.* 2015;97:558-564.
105. Holtom PD, Borges L, Zalavras CG. Hematogenous septic ankle arthritis. *Clin Orthop Relat Res.* 2008;466:1388-1391.
106. Louie JS, Liebling MR. The polymerase chain reaction in infectious and post-infectious arthritis. A review. *Rheum Dis Clin North Am.* 1998;24:227-236.
107. Rye SY, Greenwood-Quintance KE, Hanssen AD, et al. Low sensitivity of periprosthetic tissue PCR for prosthetic knee infection diagnosis. *Diagn Microbiol Infect Dis.* 2014;79:448-453.
108. Mariaux S, Tafin UF, Borens O. Diagnosis of persistent infection in prosthetic two-stage exchange: PCR analysis of sonication fluid from bone cement spacers. *J Bone Jt Infect.* 2017;2:218-223.
109. Tarabichi M, Shohat N, Goswami K, et al. Can next generation sequencing play a role in detecting pathogens in synovial fluid? *Bone Joint J.* 2018;100:127-133.
110. Wilkinson VH, Rowbotham EL, Grainger AJ. Imaging in foot and ankle arthritis. *Semin Musculoskelet Radiol.* 2016;20:167-174.
111. Jaramillo D, Treves ST, Kasser JR. Osteomyelitis and septic arthritis in children: appropriate use of imaging to guide treatment. *AJR Am J Roentgenol.* 1995;165:399-403.
112. Vanquickenborne B, Maes A, Nuyts J, et al. The value of (18)FDG-PET for the detection of infected hip prosthesis. *Eur J Nucl Med Mol Imaging.* 2003;30:705-715.
113. Termatt MF, Raijmakers PG, Scholten HJ, et al. The accuracy of diagnostic imaging for the assessment of chronic osteomyelitis: a systematic review and meta-analysis. *J Bone Joint Surg Am.* 2005;87:2464-2471.
114. Smith RL, Schurman DJ, Kajiyama G. The effect of antibiotics on the destruction of cartilage in experimental infectious arthritis. *J Bone Joint Surg Am.* 1987;69-A:1063-1069.
115. Goldenberg DL, Brandt KD, Cohen AS, et al. Treatment of septic arthritis: comparison of needle aspiration and surgery as initial modes of joint drainage. *Arthritis Rheum.* 1975;18:83-90.
116. Parisien JS, Shaffer B. Arthoscopic management of pyoarthrosis. *Clin Orthop Relat Res.* 1992;275:243-247.
117. Mankovecky MR, Roukis TS. Arthroscopic synovectomy, irrigation, and debridement for treatment of septic ankle arthrosis: a systemic review and case series. *J Foot Ankle Surg.* 2014;53:615-619.
118. Aïm F, Delambre J, Bauer T. Efficacy of arthroscopic treatment for resolving infection in septic arthritis of native joints. *Orthop Traumatol Surg Res.* 2015;101:61-64.
119. van Huyssteen AL, Bracey DJ. Chlorhexidine and chondrolysis in the knee. *J Bone Joint Surg Br.* 1999;81:995-996.
120. Vispo Seara JL, Barthel T, Schmitz H, et al. Arthroscopic treatment of septic joints: prognostic factors. *Arch Orthop Trauma Surg.* 2002;122:204-211.
121. Böhler C, Dragana M, Puchner S, et al. Treatment of septic arthritis of the knee: a comparison between arthroscopy and arthrotomy. *Knee Surg Sports Traumatol Arthrosc.* 2016;24:3147-3154.
122. Peres LS, Marchitto RO, Pereira GS, et al. Arthrotomy vs arthroscopy in the treatment of septic arthritis in the knee in adults: a randomized clinical trial. *Knee Surg Sports Traumatol Arthrosc.* 2016;24:3155-3162.
123. Stutz G, Kuster MS, Kleinstuck F, et al. Arthroscopic management of septic arthritis: stages of infection and results. *Knee Surg Sports Traumatol Arthrosc.* 2000;8:270-274.
124. Lauper N, Davat M, Gjika E. Native septic arthritis is not an immediate surgical emergency. *J Infect.* 2018;77:47-53.
125. Peltola H, Pääkkönen M, Kallio P. Osteomyelitis-Septic Arthritis (OM-SA) Study Group. Prospective, randomized trial of 10 days versus 30 days of antimicrobial treatment, including a short-term course of parenteral therapy, for childhood septic arthritis. *Clin Infect Dis.* 2009;48:1201-1210.
126. Peltola H, Pääkkönen M. Management of a child with suspected acute septic arthritis. *Arch Dis Child.* 2012;97:287-292.
127. Jagodzinski NA, Kanwar R, Graham K. Prospective evaluation of a shortened regimen of treatment for acute osteomyelitis and septic arthritis in children. *J Pediatr Orthop.* 2009;29:518-525.
128. Liu C, Bayer A, Cosgrove SE, et al. Clinical practice guidelines by the Infectious Diseases Society of America for the treatment of methicillin-resistant *Staphylococcus aureus* infections in adults and children. *Clin Infect Dis.* 2011;52:e18-e55.
129. Arnold JC, Cannavino CR, Ross MK. Acute bacterial osteoarticular infections: eight-year analysis of C-reactive protein for oral step-down therapy. *Pediatrics.* 2012;130:e821-e828.
130. Thompson RM, Gourineni P. Arthroscopic treatment of septic arthritis in very young children. *J Pediatr Orthop.* 2017;37:e53-e57.
131. Nelaton A. *Elements de Pathologie Chirurgicale.* Paris, France: Germer-Bailliere; 1844-1859.
132. Kremers HM, Nwojo ME, Ransom JE, et al. Trends in the epidemiology of osteomyelitis: a population-based study. 1969 to 2009. *J Bone Joint Surg Am.* 2015;97:837-845.
133. Zuluaga AF, Galvis W, Saldarriaga JG, et al. Etiologic diagnosis of chronic osteomyelitis: a prospective study. *Arch Intern Med.* 2006;166:95-100.
134. Patzakis MJ, Rao S, Wilkins J. Analysis of 61 cases of vertebral osteomyelitis. *Clin Orthop Relat Res.* 1991;264:178-183.
135. Cierny G III, Mader JT, Pennick JJ. A clinical staging system for adult osteomyelitis. *Clin Orthop Relat Res.* 2003;414:7-24.
136. Varoga D, Wruck CJ, Tohidnezhad M, et al. Osteoclasts participate in the innate immunity of the bone by producing human beta defensin-3. *Histochem Cell Biol.* 2009;131:207-218.
137. O'Keefe RJ, Teot LA, Singh D, et al. Osteoclasts constitutively express regulators of bone resorption: an immunohistochemical and in situ hybridization study. *Lab Invest.* 1997;76:457-465.
138. Puzas JE, Hicks DG, Reynolds SD, et al. Regulation of osteoclastic activity in infection. *Methods Enzymol.* 1994;236:47-58.
139. Tkaczyk C, Hamilton MM, Datta V, et al. Staphylococcus aureus alpha toxin suppresses effective innate and adaptive immune responses in a murine dermonecrosis model. *PLoS One.* 2013;8:e75103.
140. Herman M, Vaudaux D, Pittet D, et al. Fibronectin, fibrinogen, and laminin act as mediators of adherence in clinical staphylococcal isolates to foreign material. *J Infect Dis.* 1988;158:693-701.
141. Ryden C, Tung HS, Nikolaev V, et al. Staphylococcus aureus causing osteomyelitis binds to a nonapeptide sequence in bone sialoprotein. *Biochem J.* 1997;327:825-829.
142. Nishitani K, Sutipornpalangkul W, de Mesy Bentley KL, et al. Quantifying the natural history of biofilm formation in vivo during the establishment of chronic implant-associated Staphylococcus aureus osteomyelitis in mice to identify critical pathogen and host factors. *J Orthop Res.* 2015;33:1311-1319.
143. Hudson MC, Ramp WK, Nicholson AS, et al. Internalization of *Staphylococcus aureus* by cultured osteoblasts. *Microb Pathog.* 1995;19:409-419.
144. Hoiby N, Bjarnsholt T, Givskov M, et al. Antibiotic resistance of bacterial biofilms. *Int J Antimicrob Agents.* 2010;35:322-332.
145. Ciampolini J, Harding KG. Pathophysiology of chronic bacterial osteomyelitis. Why do antibiotics fail so often? *Postgrad Med J.* 2000;76:479-483.
146. Inzana JA, Schwarz EM, Kates SL, et al. A novel murine model of established Staphylococcal bone infection in the presence of a fracture fixation plate to study therapies utilizing antibiotic-laden spacers after revision surgery. *Bone.* 2015;72:128-136.
147. Khalil H, Williams R, Stenbeck G, et al. Invasion of bone cells by *Staphylococcus epidermidis.* *Microbes Infect.* 2007;9:460-465.
148. Nelson JP. Musculoskeletal infection. *Surg Clin North Am.* 1980;60:213-222.
149. Costerton JW, Stewart PS, Greenberg EP. Bacterial biofilms: a common cause of persistent infections. *Science.* 1999;284:1318-1322.
150. Conlon BP. Staphylococcus aureus chronic and relapsing infections: evidence of a role for persister cells: an investigation of persister cells, their formation and their role in *S aureus* disease. *Bioessays.* 2014;36:991-996.
151. Otto M. Staphylococcal infections: mechanisms of biofilm maturation and detachment as critical determinants of pathogenicity. *Annu Rev Med.* 2013;64:175-188.
152. Boles BR, Horswill AR. Staphylococcal biofilm disassembly. *Trends Microbiol.* 2011;19:449-455.
153. Costerton JW. Cystic fibrosis pathogenesis and the role of biofilms in persistent infection. *Trends Microbiol.* 2001;9:50-52.
154. van den Kieboom J, Bosch P, Plate JDJ, et al. Diagnostic accuracy of serum inflammatory markers in late fracture-related infection: a systemic review and meta-analysis. *Bone Joint J.* 2018;100-B:1542-1550.

155. Stucken C, Olszewski DC, Creevy WR, et al. Preoperative diagnosis of infection in patients with nonunions. *J Bone Joint Surg Am.* 2013;95:1409-1412.
156. Ryan EC, Ahn J, Wukich DK, et al. Diagnostic utility of erythrocyte sedimentation rate and C-reactive protein in osteomyelitis of the foot in persons without diabetes. *J Foot Ankle Surg.* 2019;58:484-488.
157. Corved S, Portillo ME, Pasticci BM, et al. Epidemiology and new developments in the diagnosis of prosthetic joint infection. *Int J Artif Organs.* 2012;35:923-934.
158. Atkins BL, Athanasou N, Deeks JJ, et al. Prospective evaluation of criteria for microbiological diagnosis of prosthetic-joint infection at revision arthroplasty. The OSIRIS Collaborative Study Group. *J Clin Microbiol.* 1998;36:2932-2939.
159. Costerson JW. *The Biofilm Primer.* New York, NY: Springer; 2007.
160. Palmer MP, Altman DT, Altman GT, et al. Can we trust intraoperative culture results in nonunions? *J Orthop Trauma.* 2014;28:384-390.
161. Achermann Y, Vogt M, Leunig M, et al. Improved diagnosis of periprosthetic joint infection by multiplex PCR of sonication fluid from removed implants. *J Clin Microbiol.* 2010;48:1208-1214.
162. Tarabichi M, Shohat N, Goswami K, et al. Diagnosis of periprosthetic joint infection: the potential of next-generation sequencing. *J Bone Joint Surg Am.* 2018;100:147-154.
163. Tani S, Lepetsos P, Stylianakis A, et al. Superiority of the sonication method against conventional periprosthetic tissue cultures for diagnosis of prosthetic joint infections. *Eur J Orthop Surg Traumatol.* 2018;28:51-67.
164. Rosai J. *Rosai and Ackerman's Surgical Pathology.* 9th ed. St. Louis, MO: Mosby; 2004.
165. Costeron JW. Biofilm theory can guide the treatment of device-related orthopedic infections. *Clin Orthop Relat Res.* 2005;437:7-11.
166. Wu JS, Gorbachova T, Morrison WB, et al. Imaging-guided bone biopsy for osteomyelitis: are there factors associated with positive or negative cultures? *Am J Roentgenol.* 2007;188:1529-1534.
167. Ardran GM. Bone destruction not demonstrable by radiography. *Br J Radiol.* 1951;278:107-109.
168. Chandnani VP, Beltran J, Morris SN, et al. Acute experimental osteomyelitis and abscesses: detection with MR imaging versus CT. *Radiology.* 1990;174:233-236.
169. Govaert GA, IJpma FFA, McNally, M, et al. Accuracy of diagnostic imaging modalities for peripheral post-traumatic osteomyelitis—a systematic review of the recent literature. *Eur J Nucl Med Mol Imaging.* 2017;44:1393-1407.
170. Horger M, Eschmann SM, Pfannenberg C. The value of SPET/CT in chronic osteomyelitis. *Eur J Nucl Med Mol Imaging.* 2003;30:1665-1673.
171. Przybylski MM, Holloway S, Vyce SD, et al. Diagnosing osteomyelitis in the diabetic foot: a pilot study to examine the sensitivity and specificity of Tc(99m) white blood cell-labelled single photon emission computed tomography/computed tomography. *Int Wound J.* 2016;13:382-389.
172. Restrepo S, Vargas D, Riascos R, et al. Musculoskeletal infection imaging: past, present, and future. *Curr Infect Dis Rep.* 2005:7:365-372.
173. Gold RH, Hawkins RA, Katz RD. Bacterial osteomyelitis: findings on plain radiography, CT, MR, and scintigraphy. *AJR Am J Roentgenol.* 1991;157:365-370.
174. Erdman WA, Tamburro F, Jason HT, et al. Osteomyelitis: characteristic and pitfalls of diagnosis with MR imaging. *Radiology.* 1991;180:533-539.
175. Lee YJ, Sadigh S, Mankad K, et al. The imaging of osteomyelitis. *Quant Imaging Med Surg.* 2016;6:184-198.
176. Hargreaves BA, Worters PW, Pauly KB, et al. Metal-induces artifacts in MRI. *AJR Am J Roentgenol.* 2011;117:85-95.
177. Hayter CL, Koff MF, Shah P. MRI after arthroplasty: comparison of MAVRIC and conventional fast spi-echo techniques. *AJR Am J Roentgenol.* 2011;197:W405-W411.
178. Merkel K, Fitzgerald RJ, Brown M. Scintigraphic evaluation in musculoskeletal sepsis. *Orthop Clin North Am.* 1984;15:401-416.
179. Schauwecker DS. The scintigraphic diagnosis of osteomyelitis. *AJR Am J Roentgenol.* 1992;158:9-18.
180. Palestro CJ, Love C, Schneider R. The evolution of nuclear medicine and the musculoskeletal system. *Radiol Clin North Am.* 2009;47:505-532.
181. Waldvogel FA, Medoff G, Swartz MN. Osteomyelitis: a review of clinical features, therapeutic considerations, and unusual aspects. *N Engl J Med.* 1970;282:198-316.
182. Cierny G III, Mader JT. The surgical treatment of adult osteomyelitis. In: Evarts C, McCollister MD, ed. *Surgery of the Musculoskeletal System.* New York, NY: Churchill Livingstone; 1983:4814-4834.
183. Cierny G III, DiPasquale D. Treatment of chronic infection. *J Am Acad Orthop Surg.* 2006;14:S105-S110.
184. Cierny G III. Chronic osteomyelitis: results of treatment. *Instr Course Lect.* 1990;39:495-508.
185. Clawson DK, Dunn AW. Management of common bacterial infections of bones and joints. *J Bone Joint Surg Am.* 1967;49:164-182.
186. Kelly PJ, Martin WJ, Coventry MB. Chronic osteomyelitis: II. Treatment with closed irrigation and suction. *JAMA.* 1970;213:1843-1848.
187. Murray BE. The life and times of the Enterococcus. *Clin Microbiol Rev.* 1990;3:46-65.
188. Cetinkaya Y, Falk P, Mayhall CG. Vancomycin-resistant enterococci. *Clin Microbiol Rev.* 2000;13:686-707.
189. Ellington JK, Reilly SS, Ramp WK, et al. Mechanisms of *Staphylococcus aureus* invasion of cultured osteoblasts. *Microb Pathog.* 1999;26:317-323.
190. Proctor RA, von Eiff C, Kahl BC, et al. Small colony variants: a pathogenic form of bacteria that facilitates persistent and recurrent infections. *Nat Rev Microbiol.* 2006;4:295-305.
191. Kania RE, Lamers GE, Vonk MJ, et al. Demonstration of bacterial cells and glycocalyx in biofilms on human tonsils. *Arch Otolaryngol Head Neck Surg.* 2007;133:115-121.
192. Horst SA, Hoerr V, Beineke A, et al. A novel mouse model of Staphylococcus aureus chronic osteomyelitis that closely mimics the human infection: an integrated view of disease pathogenesis. *Am J Pathol.* 2012;181:1206-1214.
193. Giron KP, Gross ME, Musher DM, et al. In vitro antimicrobial effect against *Streptococcus pneumoniae* of adding rifampin to penicillin, ceftriaxone, or 1-ofloxacin. *Antimicrob Agents Chemother.* 1995;39:2798-2800.
194. Pankey G, Ashcraft D, Patel N. In vitro synergy of daptomycin plus rifampin against Enterococcus faecium resistant to both linezolid and vancomycin. *Antimicrob Agents Chemother.* 2005;49:5166-5168.
195. Baldoni D, Haschke M, Rajacic Z, et al. Linezolid alone or combined with rifampin against methicillin-resistant *Staphylococcus aureus* in experimental foreign-body infection. *Antimicrob Agents Chemother.* 2009;54:1142-1148.
196. Trampuz A, Widmer AF. Infections associated with orthopedic implants. *Curr Opin Infect Dis.* 2006;4:349-356.
197. Mohamed W, Sommer U, Sethi S, et al. Intracellular proliferation of *S. aureus* in osteoblasts and effects of rifampin and gentamicin on *S. aureus* intracellular proliferation and survival. *Eur Cell Mater.* 2014;28:258-268.
198. Mathes SJ, Alpert BS, Chang N. Use of the muscle flap in chronic osteomyelitis: experimental and clinical correlation. *Plast Reconstr Surg.* 1982;69:815-829.
199. McCoy WF, Bryers JD, Robbins J, et al. Observations of fouling biofilm formation. *Can J Microbiol.* 1981;27:910-917.
200. Selan L, Passariello L, Rizzo L, et al. Diagnosis of vascular graft infections with antibodies against staphylococcal slime antigens. *Lancet.* 2002;359:2166-2168.
201. Kobayashi M, Bauer TW, Tuohy MJ, et al. Brief ultrasonication improves detection of biofilm-formation bacteria around metal implants. *Clin Orthop Relat Res.* 2007;457:210-213.
202. Greer S, Kasabian A, Thorne C, et al. The use of a subatmospheric pressure dressing to salvage a Gustilo grade IIIB open tibial fracture with concomitant osteomyelitis to avert a free flap. *Ann Plast Surg.* 1998;41:687.
203. Ilizarov GA. The tension-stress effect on the genesis and growth of tissues: Part I. The influence of stability of fixation and soft tissue preservation. *Clin Orthop Relat Res.* 1989;238:249-281.
204. Ilizarov GA. The tension-stress effect on the genesis and growth of tissues: Part II. The influence of the rate and frequency of distraction. *Clin Orthop Relat Res.* 1989;239:263-285.
205. Taylor GI, Miller GD, Ham FJ. The free vascularized bone graft: a clinical extension of microvascular techniques. *Plast Reconstr Surg.* 1975;55:526-531.
206. Ger R. Muscle transposition for treatment and prevention of chronic posttraumatic osteomyelitis of the tibia. *J Bone Joint Surg Am.* 1977;59:784-791.
207. Wahlig H, Dingeldein E, Bergmann R, et al. The release of gentamicin from polymethylmethacrylate beads: an experimental and pharmacokinetic study. *J Bone Joint Surg Br.* 1978;60:270-275.
208. Argenta LC, Morykwas MJ, Marks MW. Vacuum-assisted closure: state of clinic art. *Plast Reconstr Surg.* 2006;117(suppl):127S-142S.
209. Datiashvili RO, Knox KR. Negative pressure dressings: an alternative to free tissue transfers? *Wounds.* 2005;17:206-212.
210. Hanssen AD. Local antibiotic delivery vehicles in the treatment of musculoskeletal infection. *Clin Orthop Relat Res.* 2005;437:91-96.
211. Ostermann PA, Seligson D, Henry SL. Local antibiotic therapy for severe open fractures: a review of 1085 consecutive cases. *J Bone Joint Surg Br.* 1995;77:93-97.
212. Enneking WF, Spanier SS, Goodman MA. A system for the surgical staging of musculoskeletal sarcoma. *Clin Orthop Relat Res.* 1982;170:62-75.
213. Salvati EA, Chekofsky KM, Brause BD, et al. Reimplantation in infection: a 12-year experience. *Clin Orthop Relat Res.* 1982;170:62-75.
214. Cierny G III. Infected tibial nonunions (1981-1995): the evolution of change. *Clin Orthop Relat Res.* 1999;360:97-105.
215. Bucholz H, Engelbrecht H. Depot effects of various antibiotics mixed with Palacos resins. *Chiurg.* 1970;41:511-515.
216. Seldes RM, Winiarsky R, Jordan LC, et al. Liquid gentamicin in bone cement: a laboratory study of a potentially more cost-effective cement spacer. *J Bone Joint Surg Am.* 2005;87:268-272.
217. Adams K, Couch L, Cierny G, et al. In vitro and in vivo evaluation of antibiotic diffusion from antibiotic-impregnated polymethylmethacrylate beads. *Clin Orthop Relat Res.* 1992;2778:244-252.
218. Torholm C, Lidgren L, Lindberg L, et al. Total hip joint arthroplasty with gentamicin-impregnated cement. A clinical study of gentamicin excretion kinetics. *Clin Orthop.* 1983;181:99-106.
219. Rasyid HN, van der Mei HC, Frijlink HW, et al. Concepts for increasing gentamicin release from handmade bone cement beads. *Acta Orthop.* 2009;80:508-513.
220. Diefenbeck M, Mückley T, Hofmann GO. Prophylaxis and treatment of implant-related infections by local application of antibiotics. *Injury.* 2006;37(suppl 2):S95-S104.
221. Holton PD, Warren CA, Greene NW. Relation of surface area to in vitro elution characteristics of vancomycin-impregnated polymethylmethacrylate spacers. *Am J Orthop.* 1998;27:207-210.
222. McKee MD, Wild LM, Schemitch EH, et al. The use of antibiotic-impregnated, osteoconductive, bioabsorbable bone substitute in the treatment of infected long bone defects: early results of a prospective trial. *J Orthop Trauma.* 2002;16:622-627.
223. Inzana JA, Trombetta RP, Schwarz EM, et al. 3D printed bioceramics for dual antibiotic delivery to treat implant-associated bone infection. *Eur Cell Mater.* 2015;30:232-247.
224. Arkudas A, Balzer A, Buehrer G, et al. Evaluation of angiogenesis of bioactive glass in the arteriovenous loop model. *Tissue Eng Part C Methods.* 2013;19:117-119.
225. Hus S, Chang J, Liu M, et al. Study on antibacterial effect of 45S5 Biogalss. *J Mater Sci Mater Med.* 2009:20:281-286.
226. Munukka E, Leppäranta O, Korkeamäki M, et al. Bactericidal effects of bioactive glasses on clinically important aerobic bacteria. *J Mater Sci Mater Med.* 2008;19:27-32.
227. Drago L, Romanò D, De Vecchi E, et al. Bioactive glass BAG-S53P4 for the adjunctive treatment of chronic osteomyelitis of the long bones: an in vitro and prospective clinical study. *BMC Infect Dis.* 2013;13:584-592.

228. Ferrao P, Myerson MS, Schuberth JM, et al. Cement spacer as definitive management for postoperative ankle infection. *Foot Ankle Int.* 2012;33:173-178.
229. Masquelet AC, Fitoussi F, Begue T, et al. Reconstruction des os longs par membrane induite et autogreffe spongieuse. [Reconstruction of the long bones by the induced membrane and spongy autograft]. *Ann Chir Plast Esthet.* 2000;45:346-353.
230. Aho OM, Lehenkari P, Ristiniemi J, et al. The mechanism of action of induced membranes in bone repair. *J Bone Joint Surg Am.* 2013;95:597-604.
231. Morelli I, Drago L, George DA, et al. Masquelet technique: myth or reality? A systematic review and meta-analysis. *Injury.* 2016;47(suppl 6):S68-S76.
232. Perry W. The effect of methylmethacrylate in chemotaxis of polymorphonuclear leukocytes. *J Bone Joint Surg Am.* 1978;60:492-498.
233. Ehanire I, Tucci M, Franklin L, et al. The effects of tobramycin on MG63 cell viability and function. *Biomed Sci Instrum.* 2007;43:182-187.
234. Patel R, Osmon DR, Hanssen AD. The diagnosis of prosthetic joint infection. *Clin Orthop Relat Res.* 2005;437:55-58.
235. Patrick BN, Rivey MP, Allington DR. Acute renal failure associated with vancomycin- and tobramycin-laden cement in total hip arthroplasty. *Ann Pharmacother.* 2006;40:2037-2042.
236. Kim JW, Cuellar DO, Hao J. Custom-made antibiotic cement nails: a comparative study of different fabrication techniques. *Injury.* 2014;45:1179-1184.
237. Scolaro JA, Mehta S. Stabilisation of infected peri-articular nonunions with antibiotic impregnated cement coated locking plate: technique and indications. *Injury.* 2016;47:1353-1356.
238. Sachs BL, Shaffer JW. A staged Papineau protocol for chronic osteomyelitis. *Clin Orthop Relat Res.* 1984;184:256-263.
239. Dahl LB, Hoyland AL, Dramsdahl H, et al. Acute hematogenous osteomyelitis in children: a population-based retrospective study 1965-1994. *Scand J Infect Dis.* 1998;30:573-577.
240. Song KM, Sloboda JF. Acute hematogenous osteomyelitis in children. *J Am Acad Orthop Surg.* 2001;9:166-175.
241. Lew DP, Waldvogel FA. Osteomyelitis. *Lancet.* 2004;364:369-379.
242. Stone B, Street M, Leigh W, et al. Pediatric tibial osteomyelitis. *J Pediatr Orthop.* 2016;36:534-540.
243. Mooney ML, Haidet K, Liu J, et al. Hematogenous calcaneal osteomyelitis in children: a systematic review of the literature. *Foot Ankle Spec.* 2017;10:63-68.
244. Perlman MH, Patzakis MJ, Kumar PJ. The incidence of joint involvement with adjacent osteomyelitis in pediatric patients. *J Pediatr Orthop.* 2000;20:40-43.
245. Arnold JC, Bradley JS. Osteoarticular infections in children. *Infect Dis Clin North Am.* 2015;29:557-574.
246. Funk SS, Copley LA. Acute hematogenous osteomyelitis in children: pathogenesis, diagnosis, and treatment. *Orthop Clin North Am.* 2017;48:199-208.
247. Li M, An Diep B, Villaruz AE, et al. Evolution of virulence in epidemic community-associated methicillin-resistant *Staphylococcus aureus. Proc Natl Acad Sci U S A.* 2009;29:55-58.
248. Staheli LT. Infections. In: Staheli LT, ed. *Practice of Pediatric Orthopedics.* 2nd ed. Philadelphia, PA: Lippincott Williams & Wilkins; 2006:345-364.
249. Scott RJ, Christofersen MR, Robertson WW Jr, et al. Acute osteomyelitis in children: a review of 116 cases. *J Pediatr Orthop.* 1990;10:649-652.
250. Labbe JL, Peres O, Leclair O, et al. Acute osteomyelitis in children: the pathogenesis revisited? *Orthop Traumatol Surg Res.* 2010;96:268-275.
251. Herring JA, Tachdjian MO. *Tachdjian's Pediatric Orthopedics: From the Texas Scottish Rite Hospital for Children*; 2014. http://www.clinicalkey.com/dura/browse/bookChapter/3-s.20-C2009159017X
252. McCarthy JJ, Dormans JP, Kozin SH, et al. Musculoskeletal infections in children. Basic treatment principles and recent advancements. *J Bone Joint Surg Am.* 2004;86:850-863.
253. Kahn DS, Pritzker KP. The pathophysiology of bone infection. *Clin Orthop.* 1973;96:12-19.
254. Bouchoucha S, Drissi G, Trifa M, et al. Epidemiology of acute hematogenous osteomyelitis in children: a prospective study over a 32 month period. *Tunis Med.* 2012;90:473-478.
255. Sreenivas T, Nataraj A, Menon J, et al. Acute multifocal hematogenous osteomyelitis in children. *J Child Orthop.* 2011;5:231-235.
256. Unkila-Kallio L, Kallio MJ, Eskola J, et al. Serum C-reactive protein, erythrocyte sedimentation rate, and white blood cell count in acute hematogenous osteomyelitis of children. *Pediatrics.* 1994;93:59-62.
257. Lazzarini L, Mader JG, Calhoun JH. Osteomyelitis in long bones. *J Bone Joint Surg Am.* 2004;86:2305-2318.
258. Chau CLF, Griffith JF. Musculoskeletal infections: ultrasound appearances. *Clin Radiol.* 2005;60:149-159.
259. Rosenfeld S, Bernstein DT, Daram S, et al. Predicting the presence of adjacent infections in septic arthritis in children. *J Pediatr Orthop.* 2016;36:70-74.
260. Hald J, Sudmann E. Acute hematogenous osteomyelitis: early diagnosis with computed tomography. *Acta Radiol Diagn.* 1982;23:55-58.
261. Crim JR, Seeger LL. Imaging evaluation of osteomyelitis. *Crit Rev Diagn Imaging.* 1994;35:201-256.
262. Floyed RL, Steele RW. Culture-negative osteomyelitis. *Pediatr Infect Dis J.* 2003;22:731-736.
263. Martinez-Aguilar G, Hammerman WA, Mason EO, et al. Clindamycin treatment of invasive infections caused by community-acquired, methicillin-resistant and methicillin-susceptible *Staphylococcus aureus* in children. *Pediatr Infect Dis J.* 2003;22:593-598.
264. Harik NS, Meltzer MS. Management of acute hematogenous osteomyelitis in children. *Expert Rev Anti-Infect Ther.* 2010;8:175-181.
265. Le Saux N, Howeard A, Barrowman NJ, et al. Shorter courses of parenteral antibiotic therapy do not appear to influence response rates for children with acute hematogenous osteomyelitis: a systematic review. *BMC Infect Dis.* 2002;2:16.
266. Giannestras NJ. Infections in the foot. In: Giannestras NJ, ed. *Foot Disorders, Medical and Surgical Management.* 2nd ed. Philadelphia, PA: Lea and Febiger; 1973:631-641.
267. Mollan RAB, Piggot J. Acute osteomyelitis in children. *J Bone Joint Surg Br.* 1977;59:2-7.
268. Street H, Puna R, Huang M, et al. Pediatric acute hematogenous osteomyelitis. *J Pediatr Orthop.* 2015;35:634-639.
269. Hung NN. Cortical bone fenestrations with continuous antibiotic irrigation to mediate hematogenous tibial osteomyelitis in children. *J Pediatr Orthop B.* 2010;19:497-506.
270. Le Saux N, Howeard A, Barrowman NJ, et al. Shorter courses of parenteral antibiotic therapy do not appear to influence response rates for children with acute hematogenous osteomyelitis: a systematic review. *BMC Infect Dis.* 2002;2:16.
271. Copley LA, Baron T, Garcia C, et al. A proposed scoring system for assessment of severity of illness in pediatric acute hematogenous osteomyelitis using objective clinical and laboratory findings. *Pediatr Infect Dis J.* 2014;33:35-41.
272. Hollmig ST. Deep vein thrombosis associated with osteomyelitis in children. *J Bone Joint Surg Am.* 2007;89:1517.
273. Guiterrez K. Bone and joint infections in children. *Pediatr Clin North Am.* 2005;52:779-794.
274. Ramos OM. Chronic osteomyelitis in children. *Pediatr Infect Dis J.* 2002;21:431-432.
275. Belthur MV, Birchansky SB, Verdugo AA, et al. Pathologic fractures in children with acute *Staphylococcus aureus* osteomyelitis. *J Bone Joint Surg Am.* 2012;94:34-42.
276. Peters W, Irving J, Letts M. Long-term effects of neonatal bone and joint infection on adjacent growth plates. *J Pediatr Orthop.* 1992;12:806-810.
277. Armstrong DG, Boulton AJM, Bus SA. Diabetic foot ulcers and their recurrence. *N Engl J Med.* 2017;376:2367-2375.
278. Singh N, Armstrong DG, Lipsky BA. Preventing foot ulcers in patients with diabetes. *JAMA.* 2005;293:217-228.
279. http://diabetes.org/diabetes-basics/statistics/
280. Frykberg RG, Wittmayer B, Zgonis T. Surgical management of diabetic foot infections and osteomyelitis. *Clin Podiatr Med Surg.* 2007;24:460-482.
281. Fincke BG, Miller DR, Turpin R. A classification of diabetic foot infections using ICD-9-CM codes: application to a large computerized medical database. *BMC Health Serv Res.* 2010;10:192.
282. Yang W, Dall TM, Halder R, et al. Economic costs of diabetes in the U.S. in 2012. *Diabetes Care.* 2013;36:1033-1046.
283. Lipsky BA. Diabetic foot infections: current treatment and delaying the 'post-antibiotic era.' *Diabetes Metab Res Rev.* 2016;32:246-253.
284. Oyibo SO, Jude EB, Tarawneh I, et al. A comparison of two diabetic foot ulcer classification systems: the Wagner and the University of Texas wound classifications systems. *Diabetes Care.* 2001;24:84-88.
285. Lipsky BA, Aragon Sanchez J, Diggle M, et al. IWGDY guidance on the diagnosis and management of foot infections in persons with diabetes. *Diabetes Metab Res Rev.* 2016;32:45-74.
286. Causey MW, Ahmed A, Wu B, et al. Society for Vascular Surgery limb stage and patient risk correlate with outcomes in an amputation prevention program. *J Vasc Surg.* 2016;63:1563-1573.
287. Beropoulis E, Stavroulakis K, Schwindt A, et al. Validation of the Wound, Ischemia, foot Infection (WIfI) classification system in nondiabetic patients treated by endovascular means for critical limb ischemia. *J Vasc Surg.* 2016;64:95-103.
288. Mills JL, Conte MS, Armstrong DG, et al. The Society for vascular surgery lower extremity threatened limb classification system: risk stratification based on wound, ischemia, and foot infection (WIfI). *J Vasc Surg.* 2014;59:220-234.
289. Prompers L, Huijberts M, Apelqvist J. High prevalence of ischaemia, infection, and serious comorbidity in patients with diabetic foot disease in Europe. Baseline results from Eurodiale study. *Diabetologia.* 2007;50:18-25.
290. Cutting KF, White R. Defined and refined: criteria for identifying wound infection revisited. *Br J Community Nurs.* 2004;9:6-15.
291. Hobizal KB, Wukich DK. Diabetic foot infections: current concept review. *Diabet Foot Ankle.* 2012;3:1-8.
292. Lavery LA, Armstrong DG, Peters EJ, et al. Probe-to-bone test for diagnosing diabetic foot osteomyelitis: reliable or relic? *Diabetes Care.* 2007;30:270-274.
293. Lavery LA, Armstrong DG, Wunderlich RP, et al. Risk factors for foot infections in individuals with diabetes. *Diabetes Care.* 2006;29:1288-1293.
294. Grayson ML, Gibbons GW, Balogh K, et al. Probing to bone in infected pedal ulcers. A clinical sign of underlying osteomyelitis in diabetic patients. *JAMA.* 1995;273:721-723.
295. Butalia S, Palda VA, Sargeant RJ, et al. Does this patient with diabetes have osteomyelitis of the lower extremity? *JAMA.* 2008;299:806-813.
296. Dinh MT, Abad CL, Safdar N. Diagnostic accuracy of the physical examination and imaging tests for osteomyelitis underlying diabetic foot ulcers: meta-analysis. *Clin Infect Dis.* 2008;47:519-527.
297. Domek N, Dux K, Pinzur M, et al. Association between hemoglobin A1c and surgical morbidity in elective foot and ankle surgery. *J Foot Ankle Surg.* 2016;55:939-943.
298. Joseph WS, LeFrock JL. The pathogenesis of diabetic foot infections—immunopathy, angiopathy, and neuropathy. *J Foot Surg.* 1987;26:7-11.
299. Lipsky BA, Berendt AR, Cornia PB, et al. Infectious Diseases Society of America clinical practice guideline for the diagnosis and treatment of diabetic foot infections. *Clin Infect Dis.* 2012;54:132-173.
300. Peters EJ, Lipsky BA, Berendt AR, et al. A systematic review of the effectiveness of interventions in the management of infection in the diabetic foot. *Diabetes Metab Res Rev.* 2012;28:142-162.
301. Marangos MN, Skoutelis AT, Nightingale CH, et al. Absorption of ciprofloxacin in patients with diabetic gastroparesis. *Antimicrob Agents Chemother.* 1995;39:2161-2163.
302. Costantini TW, Acosta JA, Hoyt DB, et al. Surgical resident and attending physician attitudes toward glucose control in the surgical patient. *Am Surg.* 2008;74:993-996.
303. Farrokhi F, Smiley D, Umpierrez GE. Glycemic control in non-diabetic critically ill patients. *Best Pract Res Clin Endocrinol Metab.* 2011;25:813-824.
304. Stryker LS, Abdel MP, Morrey ME, et al. Elevated postoperative blood glucose and preoperative hemoglobin A1C are associated with increased wound complications following total joint arthroplasty. *J Bone Surg Am.* 2013;95:808-812.
305. Karunaker MA, Staples KS. Does stress-induced hyperglycemia increase the risk of preoperative infectious complications in orthopedic trauma patients? *J Orthop Trauma.* 2010;24:752-756.

306. Hwang JS, Kim SJ, Bamne AB, et al. Do glycemic markers predict occurrence of complications after total knee arthroplasty in patients with diabetes? *Clin Orthop Relat Res.* 2015;473:1726-1731.

307. Goldstein DT, Durinka JB, Martino N, et al. Effect of preoperative hemoglobin A(1c) level on acute postoperative complications of total joint arthroplasty. *Am J Orthop (Belle Mead NJ).* 2013;42:88-90.

308. Chastil J, Anderson MB, Stevens V, et al. Is hemoglobin A1c or perioperative hyperglycemia predictive of periprosthetic joint infection or death following primary total joint arthroplasty? *J Arthroplasty.* 2015;30:1197-1202.

309. Wukich DK, Joseph A, Ryan M, et al. Outcomes of ankle fractures in patients with uncomplicated versus complicated diabetes. *Foot Ankle Int.* 2011;32:120-130.

310. Shohat N, Tarabichi M, Tischler EH, et al. Serum fructosamine: a simple and inexpensive test for assessing preoperative glycemic control. *J Bone Joint Surg Am.* 2017;99:1900-1907.

311. Akinci B, Yener S, Yesil S, et al. Acute phase reactants predict the risk of amputation in diabetic foot infection. *J Am Podiatr Med Assoc.* 2011;101:1-6.

312. Hinchliffe RJ, Brownrigg JR, Apelqvist J, et al. IWGDF guidance on the diagnosis, prognosis and management of peripheral artery disease in patients with foot ulcers in diabetes. *Diabetes Metab Res Rev.* 2016;32:37-44.

313. Ramsey DE, Manke DA, Sumner DS. Toe blood pressure. A valuable adjunct to ankle pressure measurement for assessing peripheral arterial disease. *J Cardiovasc Surg (Torino).* 1983;24:43-48.

314. Bakker K, Apelqvist J, Lipsky BA, et al. The 2015 IWGDF guidance on the prevention and management of foot problems in diabetes. *Int Wound J.* 2016;13:1072.

315. Carrington AL, Shaw JE, Van Schie CH, et al. Can motor nerve conduction velocity predict foot problems in diabetic subjects over a 6-year outcome period? *Diabetes Care.* 2002;25:2010-2015.

316. Gazzaruso C, Coppola A, Falcone C, et al. Transcutaneous oxygen tension as a potential predictor of cardiovascular events in type 2 diabetes: comparison with ankle–brachial index. *Diabetes Care.* 2013;36:1720-1725.

317. Adams BE, Edlinger JP, Ritterman Weintraub ML, et al. Three-year morbidity and mortality rates after nontraumatic transmetatarsal amputation. *J Foot Ankle Surg.* 2018;57:967-971.

318. Reekers J, Lammer J. Diabetic foot and PAD: the endovascular approach. *Diabetes Metab Res Rev.* 2012;28:36-39.

319. Zil-E-Ali A, Shfi S, Ali MH. Think before chopping a diabetic foot: insight to vascular intervention. *Cureus.* 2017;9:1194.

320. Lipsky BA. Osteomyelitis of the foot in diabetic patients. *Clin Infect Dis.* 1997;25:1318-1326.

321. Malone M, Bowling FL, Gannass A, et al. Deep wound cultures correlate well with bone biopsy culture in diabetic foot osteomyelitis. *Diabetes Metab Res Rev.* 2013;29:546-550.

322. Mijuskovic B, Kuehl R, Widmer AF. Culture of bone biopsy specimens overestimates rate of residual osteomyelitis after toe or forefoot amputation. *J Bone Joint Surg Am.* 2018;5;100:1448-1454.

323. Lavery LA, Sariaya M, Ashry H, et al. Microbiology of osteomyelitis in diabetic foot infections. *J Foot Ankle Surg.* 1995;34:61-64.

324. Senneville E, Melliez H, Beltrand E, et al. Culture of percutaneous bone biopsy specimens for diagnosis of diabetic foot osteomyelitis: concordance with ulcer swab cultures. *Clin Infect Dis.* 2006;42:57-62.

325. Ertugrul BM, Lipsky BA, Savk O. Osteomyelitis or Charcot neuro-osteoarthropathy? Differentiating these disorders in diabetic patients with a foot problem. *Diabet Foot Ankle.* 2013;5:4.

326. Ertuğrul MB, Baktıroğlu S. Diyabetik Ayak ve Osteomiyeliti [Diabetic foot and osteomyelitis]. *J Klinik.* 2005;18:8-13.

327. Toledano TR, Fatone EA, Weis A, et al. MRI evaluation of bone marrow changes in the diabetic foot: a practical approach. *Semin Musculoskelet Radiol.* 2011;15:257-268.

328. Knight D, Gray HW, McKillop JH, et al. Imaging for infection: caution required in the Charcot joint. *Eur J Nucl Med.* 1988;10:523-526.

329. Capriotti G, Chianelli M, Signore A. Nuclear medicine imaging of diabetic foot infection: results of meta-analysis. *Nucl Med Commun.* 2006;27:757-764.

330. Palestro CJ, Mehta HH, Patel M, et al. Marrow versus infection in the Charcot joint: indium-111 leukocyte and technetium-99m sulfur colloid scintigraphy. *J Nucl Med.* 1998;39:346-350.

331. Joseph, WS, Axler DA. Microbiology and antimicrobial therapy of diabetic foot infections. *Clin Podiatr Med Surg.* 1990;7:467-481.

332. Ertugrul MB, Baktiroglu S, Salman S, et al. The diagnosis of osteomyelitis of the foot in diabetes: microbiological examination vs. magnetic resonance imaging and labeled leukocyte scanning. *Diabet Med.* 2006;23:649-653.

333. Sheehy SH, Atkins BA, Bejon P, et al. The microbiology of chronic osteomyelitis: prevalence of resistance to common empirical anti-microbial regimens. *J Infect.* 2010;60:338-343.

334. King CM, Castellucci-Garza FM, Lyon L. Microorganisms associated with osteomyelitis of the foot and ankle. *J Foot Ankle Surg.* 2020;59:491-494.

335. Acree ME, Morgan E, David MZ. *S. aureus* infections in Chicago, 2006-2014: increase in CA MSSA and decrease in MRSA incidence. *Infect Control Hosp Epidemiol.* 2017;38:1226-1234.

336. Raff MJ, Melo JC. Anaerobic osteomyelitis. *Medicine (Baltimore).* 1978;57:83-103.

337. Lipsky BA, Berendt AR, Deery HG, et al. Diagnosis and treatment of diabetic foot infections. Infectious Diseases Society of America. *Clin Infect Dis.* 2004;39:885-910.

338. Tan JS, Friedman NM, Hazelton-Miller C, et al. Can aggressive treatment of diabetic foot infections reduce the need for above-ankle amputation? *Clin Infect Dis.* 1996;23:286-291.

339. Melamed EA, Peled E. Antibiotic impregnated cement spacer for salvage of diabetic osteomyelitis. *Foot Ankle Int.* 2012;33:213-219.

340. Krause FG, DeVries G, Meakin C, et al. Outcome of transmetatarsal amputations in diabetics using antibiotic beads. *Foot Ankle Int.* 2009;30:486-493.

341. Liu S, He CZ, Cai YT, et al. Evaluation of negative-pressure wound therapy for patients with diabetic foot ulcers: systematic review and meta-analysis. *Ther Clin Risk Manag.* 2017;13:533-544.

Cartilage Replacement Techniques

Alan Ng and Nilin M. Rao

DEFINITION

Cartilage damage is commonly seen throughout the body and frequently seen in the femoral condyle, humeral head, talus, capitellum of the humerus and metatarsal heads, with the most common sites being the ankle and the knee. Foot and ankle surgeons most commonly see cartilage damage in the talus and metatarsal heads, which lead to pain and decreased motion in the joints. The following chapter will discuss cartilage restoration techniques as they pertain to the ankle; however, these principles and techniques can be applied to many other areas of the foot as well.

Unlike other load-bearing joints, the ankle joint is commonly described as a nearly flawless joint. It is rare to see osteoarthritis development in the ankle joint, unless the joint has undergone some level of prior trauma. It has been shown that primary, nontrauma induced osteoarthritis of the ankle (OA) only accounts for 7%-9% of ankle arthritis, leaving about 78% of OA cases seen in the ankle to be secondary to prior trauma.[1] Posttraumatic arthritis in the ankle joint can be extremely painful and often times debilitating, leading to significant difficulties with ambulation and eliciting negative changes in lifestyle. The specialized nature of the ankle joint cartilage and its innate inability to regenerate causes brisk degeneration of the ankle joint, leading to significant pain and eventual problems with ambulation. Cartilage repair and regenerative techniques have been developed and implemented in an attempt to beat the body's natural ability for bony adaptation, preventing arthritic changes that subsequently occur following trauma. These techniques have been shown to alleviate pain, increase joint mobility, and allow patients to avoid larger, more incapacitating end stage surgery, such as total ankle arthroplasty or ankle arthrodesis. The fundamental purpose of replacing damaged cartilage is to preserve and restore the biomechanical, structural, and functional properties of the innate articular cartilage. Accomplishing this goal should lead to subsequent improvement in the clinical symptoms and overall function of the joint.[2]

The ankle joint is a synovial hinge joint, with three articulating bones. The ankle joint complex consists of the tibia, fibula, and the most common ankle joint bone to undergo cartilage injury, the talus. The talus is a uniquely shaped bone that can be divided into three separate anatomic regions: the talar body, neck, and head. The body, or talar dome, articulates with the tibia on its superior and medial side, and the fibula on its lateral surface to form the ankle joint. The transverse diameter of the talar body is greater anteriorly than posteriorly, causing increased joint stability with dorsiflexion. The talus is the second largest of the tarsal bones, has no muscular or tendinous attachments, and is one of the bones in the human body with over 60% of its surface area covered by articular cartilage.[3]

Cartilage is a resilient and smooth elastic tissue that covers and protects the ends of long bones at the joints. Cartilage matrix is composed of glycosaminoglycans, proteoglycans, collagen fibers, and, sometimes, elastin. Cartilage does not contain blood vessels or nerves, making it avascular and aneural. Chondrocytes obtain their nutrition from the synovial fluid by diffusion. The compression of the articular cartilage generates fluid flow, which assists diffusion of nutrients to the chondrocytes. Compared to other connective tissues, cartilage has a very slow turnover of its extracellular matrix (ECM) and does not regenerate. There are three different types of cartilage: elastic, hyaline, and fibrous. Hyaline cartilage is the native cartilage found on the joint surfaces of human long bones. Hyaline cartilage has fewer cells than elastic and fibrous cartilage and more intercellular space. The function of the articular cartilage is dependent on the molecular composition of the ECM. The ECM consists mainly of proteoglycan and type II collagen. The main proteoglycan is aggrecan, which forms large aggregates with hyaluronan. These negatively charged aggregates hold water in the tissue. The type II collagen constrains the proteoglycans, and the ECM responds to tensile and compressive forces experienced by the cartilage. The mechanical properties of articular cartilage in load-bearing joints have been extensively studied. These properties include the response of cartilage in frictional, compressive, shear, and tensile loading. Cartilage is resilient and displays viscoelastic properties. The layers of articular cartilage include hyaline cartilage, tidemark, calcified cartilage, and subchondral bone.

Cartilage has limited repair capabilities because chondrocytes are bound in lacunae and are unable to migrate to damaged areas. This causes a lot of difficulty in healing of any cartilage damage. Deposition of new matrix is slow because hyaline cartilage does not have a blood supply. Damaged hyaline cartilage is usually replaced by fibrocartilage scar tissue. Hyaline cartilage in the talus is different than cartilage seen anywhere else in the human body. The cells and ECM components are identical, but it behaves differently with less thickness than cartilage in the knee, response to injury, and susceptibility to injury.[4] Mean ankle joint articular cartilage thickness ranges from 1.0 to 1.7 mm thick, compared to the articular cartilage in the knee that ranges from 1.5 to 6.0 mm in thickness depending on location.[5,6] One study found the mean maximum

cartilage thickness to be 2.38 mm with the thickest articular cartilage occurring over the talar shoulders, where osteochondral lesions commonly occur, and not in the center of the talar dome as commonly believed.[6]

An osteochondral defect (OCD) is a focal area of damage involving injury to both the cartilage and the adjacent subchondral bone.[7] OCDs can be caused by acute trauma, microtrauma, avascular necrosis, osteochondritis dissecans, or intraoperatively.[8] The etiology of osteochondral lesions of the talus is frequently attributed to ankle trauma, but these lesions can also stem from alcohol abuse, chronic steroid use, endocrine abnormalities, or genetics.[9,10] The literature has reported an occurrence of up to 73% in ankle fracture cases and 42% in people with lateral ankle instability.[11] Osteochondral injuries are graded according to the stability, severity, and location of the fragment, as well as presence of secondary degenerative changes seen.[12]

When evaluating talar dome lesions and selecting the proper treatment method, it is important to be able to correctly identify the etiology behind the lesion. The literature tends to use the terms osteochondritis dissecans, chondral lesions, and OCD interchangeably; however, these terms are separate defects with clear pathological differences. Acute chondral lesions on the articular surface do not penetrate subchondral bone; with damage occurring to chondrocytes and the ECM, requiring no inflammatory healing response. Acute OCDs not only damage articular cartilage but also penetrate subchondral bone, causing an inflammatory healing response. Both of these terms refer to acute traumatic lesions. Osteochondritis dissecans is a more chronic pathology, occurring over several months, and involves the development of avascular necrosis to the bone underlying the defect. The avascular fragment separates from a normal, vascular bony bed beneath a sclerotic rim. The larger wedge segment of bone can lose its blood supply, causing the osteochondral surface to become avascular, leading to osteochondral surface breaks into multiple fragments and separation from an avascular bed. This extension can lead to necrotic bone under the subchondral bone, causing subchondral fracture and bone surface collapse.

Talar dome OCDs can be classified as constrained or unconstrained, depending on whether the defect extends to breach the subchondral plate at either the medial or lateral shoulder of the talar dome.[13] Constrained lesions have an intact margin of healthy bone and cartilage after debridement, whereas, unconstrained lesions tend to lack distinct margins, such as a shoulder lesion that extends into the gutter of the ankle or a lesion with an underlying cyst.[13]

Talar dome OCDs can also be classified as laminated or delaminated. Chondral delamination is the separation of the articular cartilage from the underlying subchondral bone at the tidemark.[14] Eighty percent of OCDs in the ankle are not delaminated and involve articular cartilage and subchondral bone.[15] These injuries have been reported as the result of shearing stress that is concentrated at the junction of noncalcified and calcified cartilage.[14,16-18] The delamination line runs parallel to the joint surface, but the overlying articular cartilage remains initially intact. The mechanism of injury associated with delamination injuries, acute shear forces, has been shown to produce painful lesions. Cartilage delamination injuries can occur as an isolated chondral injury or in association with a second cartilage injury. Early identification of these injuries is important, as they have a poor prognosis when unrecognized or untreated. Identification of these lesions preoperatively can alert the surgeon of the

extent of the cartilage injury; therefore, the extent of debridement necessary to treat the lesion. Advanced imaging is necessary for detection of chondral delamination injuries. On magnetic resonance imaging (MRI), chondral delamination injuries show linear T2-weighted signal near the intensity of joint fluid at the interface of the articular cartilage and subchondral bone.[16]

A long-standing debate among foot and ankle surgeons is why osteochondral lesions are so painful when cartilage lacks nerve innervation. It is theorized that pain is caused by synovial fluid forced underneath cartilage, into subchondral bone, leading to subchondral cyst formation and increased pressure within the talus.[19]

The outcome after an acute talar dome osteochondral impaction injury is variable. The chondral surface may remain intact and there may be resolution of the subchondral bone marrow edema, without complication. On the other hand, the relatively poor, retrograde blood supply of the talar dome predisposes to incomplete healing and the development of focal areas of ischemic and devascularized subchondral bone in which there may be resorption of subchondral trabeculae, replacement with fibrotic tissue, and successive development of cystic changes. In addition, any fissuring or break in the chondral surface and subchondral plate can lead to synovial fluid inflow into the subchondral bone.

Bone marrow edema is usually evident within hours of injury and will generally persist for several months. Microfissures or microfractures of the subchondral bone, hemorrhage, and edema have been seen as histologic correlates in areas of post-traumatic bone marrow edema in animal studies.[20,21] Bone marrow lesions are thought to be affiliated with pain because they denote a recovery response to underlying traumatic insult and trabecular injury.[22] Cystic change almost invariably develops at sites of preexisting bone marrow edema signal. The cystic change associated with talar dome osteochondral lesions may vary from a predominately fibrotic to predominantly fluid-filled content.[13]

There has been much controversy in the cartilage regeneration community regarding the efficacy of microfracture over the recent years. The original theory behind microfracture has always been that subchondral penetration causes bone marrow stimulation, leading to the formation of fibrocartilage. Fibrocartilage is not as durable and effective as the original hyaline cartilage; however, the literature shows its short-term efficacy in serving as a temporary solution for pain caused by acute OCDs. Recent literature has shown the lack of long-term efficacy surrounding microfracture, leading to a newer theory behind approaching acute lesions. It does not make sense to damage subchondral bone and cancellous bone, and the body does not have the ability to heal bone that is insufficient. True microfracture can only be used on delaminated cartilage lesions. Many cases of ankle osteochondral lesions involve "failed" subchondral bone or bone cysts. Microfracture allows for fluid penetration below subchondral bone, which leads to increased interosseous pressure. Bone is "soft," so putting more holes into it makes it softer, and the body cannot recover this injury, leading to failure of this treatment protocol.

A study by Solheim et al.[23] investigated the survival of cartilage repair in the knee by microfracture ($n = 119$) or mosaicplasty/osteochondral autograft transplantation (OAT) ($n = 84$) and found only 60% survival of microfracture at 3 years. They concluded that microfracture articular cartilage repairs failed more often and earlier than the OAT repairs, both in the whole cohort and in a subgroup of patients matched for age and size of treated lesions, indicating that the OAT repair is more durable.[23]

ADVANCED IMAGING AND CLASSIFICATIONS

The most common classification systems used by foot and ankle surgeons for the grading of OCDs in the talus are the Berndt and Harty radiographic classification system, Ferkel and Sgaglione computerized tomography (CT) staging system, and the Hepple MRI staging system (Fig. 50.1). These grading systems are used by foot and ankle surgeons to assist with determination of severity and stability of the lesion, as well as plan management. The Berndt and Harty radiographic staging system for the acute injury has been widely adopted as a radiographic and arthroscopic classification. However, its clinical use is limited, as there is no demonstrated correlation with prognosis and it does not guide management. In addition, it does not take into account the status of the articular surface, the presence of subchondral cystic change or bone marrow edema. A number of different CT, MRI, and arthroscopic staging systems have been advocated; however, their clinical use and prognostic significance are not yet established, limiting their clinical application (Fig. 50.2).

The ultimate goal of imaging chondral and osteochondral lesions in the ankle is primarily their detection, demonstration of their position and extent, including status of the chondral surface, demonstration of any associated chondral delamination, assessment of the integrity of the subchondral plate, and assessment of the cancellous subchondral bone for bone marrow edema like signal, sclerosis, cystic change, and for presence of an unstable osteochondral fragment. Plain film radiographs, CT, and bone scan may be helpful in detection and characterization of these lesions; however, MRI is the only imaging modality that will provide a comprehensive assessment of all these pathologies and has become the gold standard for assessment of OCDs.[13]

> ### PEARLS
> The author cautions that MRI can often overestimate the extent of the lesion and the only true way to assess the lesion is through direct visualization.

Plain film radiography is of limited sensitivity in the demonstration of chondral and osteochondral pathology in the ankle.[24] Weight-bearing radiographs should be performed in order to obtain a more accurate assessment of the alignment. A routine ankle series should include anteroposterior (AP), lateral, and mortise views. In the setting of acute trauma, plain radiographs may demonstrate an acute osteochondral fracture. In the chronic setting, central osteophyte formation may occur at the site of an overlying chondral defect. Plain radiographs may also demonstrate the development of subchondral cystic change in a chronic osteochondral lesion. Unstable osteochondral fragments and displaced osteochondral loose bodies may also be demonstrable on plain radiography.

Modern multislice helical CT involves acquisition of a thin slice volume data set in the transverse plane that can be reconstructed in any plane and also reconstructed into three dimensional images. CT arthrography will provide detailed assessment of the chondral surfaces and may be used as an alternative means of assessment when MRI is contraindicated.[25] The major disadvantage of CT arthrography compared with MRI lies in its invasive nature and its use of ionizing radiation. In the acute setting, CT can provide an assessment for fractures in cases where plain radiographs are equivocal or demonstrate a complex fracture. In the setting of chronic osteochondral lesions, CT will demonstrate the presence of subchondral sclerosis and cystic change, central osteophytes, and *in situ* and displaced ossific loose bodies. CT is superior to MRI in demonstrating small cracks in the subchondral plate associated with cystic change, which may allow propulsion of synovial fluid into the cyst. CT will not demonstrate the chondral surfaces and will not demonstrate bone marrow edema, making MRI the preferred advanced imaging modality for the assessment of ankle joint chondral and osteochondral lesions.

MRI provides a noninvasive assessment of the chondral surfaces, subchondral plate, subchondral bone, joint fluid, capsule, and ligaments. MRI is currently the best single imaging modality for assessment of ankle joint chondral and osteochondral lesions. MRI reportedly has a sensitivity of 0.96 and a specificity of 0.96 in the diagnosis of these lesions.[26]

FIGURE 50.1 The Berndt and Harty radiographic classification system, the Ferkel and Sgaglione CT staging system, and the Hepple MRI staging system. (Data From Hepple S, Winson IG, Glew D. Osteochondral lesions of the talus: a revised classification. *Foot Ankle Int.* 1999;20(12):789–793; Berndt AL, Harty M. Transchondral fractures (osteochondritis dissecans) of the talus. *J Bone Joint Surg Am.* 1959;41-A:988–1020; and Ferkel RD, Sgaglione NA. Arthroscopic treatment of osteochondral lesions of the talus: long term results. *Orthop Trans.* 1993-1994;17:1011.)

Berndt and Harty Radiographic Classification	
Stage 1	• Small area of subchondral compression
Stage 2	• Partial fragment detachment
Stage 3	• Complete fragment detachment but not displaced
Stage 4	• Displaced fragment

Ferkel and Sgaglione CT Staging System	
Stage 1	• Cystic lesion within dome of talus with an intact roof on all view
Stage 2a	• Cystic lesion communication to talar dome surface
Stage 2b	• Open articular surface lesion with the overlying nondisplaced fragment
Stage 3	• Nondisplaced lesion with lucency
Stage 4	• Displaced fragment

Hepple MRI Staging System	
Stage 1	• Articular cartilage edema
Stage 2a	• Cartilage injury with underlying fracture and surrounding bony edema
Stage 2b	• Stage 2a without surrounding bone edema
Stage 3	• Detached but nondisplaced fragment
Stage 4	• Displaced fragment
Stage 5	• Subchondral cyst formation

Outerbridge Arthroscopic Grading System	
Grade 0	Normal cartilage
Grade I	Softening and swelling
Grade II	Superficial fissures
Grade III	Deep fissures, without exposed bone
Grade IV	Exposed subchondral bone

ICRS (International Cartilage Repair Society) Grading System	
Grade 0	Normal cartilage
Grade 1	Nearly normal (superficial lesions)
Grade 2	Abnormal (lesions extend <50% of cartilage depth)
Grade 3	Severely abnormal (>50% of cartilage depth)
Grade 4	Severely abnormal (through the subchondral bone)

FIGURE 50.2 Outerbridge arthroscopic grading system and the ICRS (International Cartilage Repair Society) grading system. (Data from Outerbridge RE. The etiology of chondromalacia patellae. *J Bone Joint Surg Br.* 1961;43:752–757. ICRS: From https://cartilage.org/society/publications/icrs-score/)

Recent developments in MRI assessment of articular cartilage include quantitative T2 mapping, T1Q mapping, diffusion imaging, and delayed gadolinium-enhanced MRI of cartilage. These techniques can provide some assessment of water and proteoglycan content and integrity of the collagen matrix in articular cartilage before the onset of macrostructural changes.[27-30] These techniques remain largely a research tool not widely used in clinical practice.

Diagnostic joint injection is another important tool in the evaluation of osteochondral lesions of the talus. Pain relief is usually short term (days and not weeks) and not specific, but a positive response to injection confirms that the pain source is intra-articular. Re-examination of the ankle 5-10 minutes after injection helps to document a positive response. Preinjection pain on palpation at the anterior joint line is usually no longer present and the patient usually reports pain relief when walking in the office. One can also utilize joint injection prior to weight-bearing stress inversion imaging.[31]

TREATMENT OPTIONS AND TECHNIQUES

Early diagnosis of osteochondral lesions of the talus is imperative and has been shown to lead to better patient outcomes.[32] Clinically, patients with osteochondral lesions of the talus tend to present with low-grade aching ankle pain months after an ankle sprain or other ankle trauma. Patients typically describe an aching, deep pain and express ankle instability, catching, or locking. Physical exam findings tend to include reduced or painful ankle joint range of motion and mild nonpitting edema. Tenderness or pain may be elicited with palpation either medially or laterally on the ankle joint as well. Treatment depends on the location and size of the defect as well as presence of secondary degenerative changes. At earlier stages, nonsurgical, conservative treatment options should be initiated, including non–weight bearing and immobilization in a controlled ankle movement (CAM) boot or short leg cast, corticosteroid injections, and/or physical therapy. Conservative treatment options should be exhausted prior to surgical intervention; however, nonsurgical treatment options of osteochondral lesions of the talus have been reported to have success in only 45% of cases.[26,33] Berndt and Harty found that 75% of nonoperatively managed lesions had poor results.[33]

Cartilage repair in the ankle joint can be approached arthroscopically or through an open or mini-arthrotomy (Fig. 50.3). There are several advantages to the arthroscopic approach over the open approach. Arthroscopy is less invasive, requiring only two small stab incisions for portal access. This allows the surgeon and patient to avoid open arthrotomies and risky malleolar osteotomies. Barg et al.[34] reviewed 342 patients who underwent medial malleolar osteotomy and found a 2.3% complication rate. Complications included delayed union, nonunion, broken or painful screws, and nonspecific pain.[34] The arthroscopic approach can improve patient outcomes by allowing outpatient treatment, decreasing postoperative morbidity, and permitting faster and more functional rehabilitation.[35] This major disadvantage to the arthroscopic technique is the large learning curve that comes with the technique. In some rare cases, with hard to reach osteochondral lesions, the open approach is necessary. The open approach provides full joint access, direct visualization of the ankle joint and is good for surgeons lacking confidence and/or experience in arthroscopy. Disadvantages to this approach include increased risk of infection and wound dehiscence, the possibility for increased surgical time, increased risk of neurovascular compromise, and longer recovery time.

PERILS and PITFALLS

- Proper padding is important to avoid traction neuropraxia to the foot.
- Three to four layers of cast padding is sufficient.
- Be sure to place the heel ~6 in away from the end of the table to allow for proper ankle joint distraction.

Several surgical treatment options are available for treatment of cartilaginous lesions, including excision and debridement, marrow stimulation techniques, osteochondral autografts, and osteochondral allografts. Excision and debridement or curettage of osteochondral fracture fragments should be considered for small osteochondral lesions of the talus that are <1.5 cm². This procedure is typically performed arthroscopically through standard anteromedial and anterolateral portals or with an open ankle arthrotomy. Another popular treatment option indicated for smaller OCDs of the talus <1.5 cm² is subchondral bone drilling or microfracture. Marrow stimulation techniques are typically used as first line treatment options due to their relative ease, quicker recovery time, and ability to perform arthroscopically. This technique has been falling out of favor in recent literature due to the concept of bone marrow stimulation causing irreversible damage to the subchondral bone, leading to continued pain and procedural

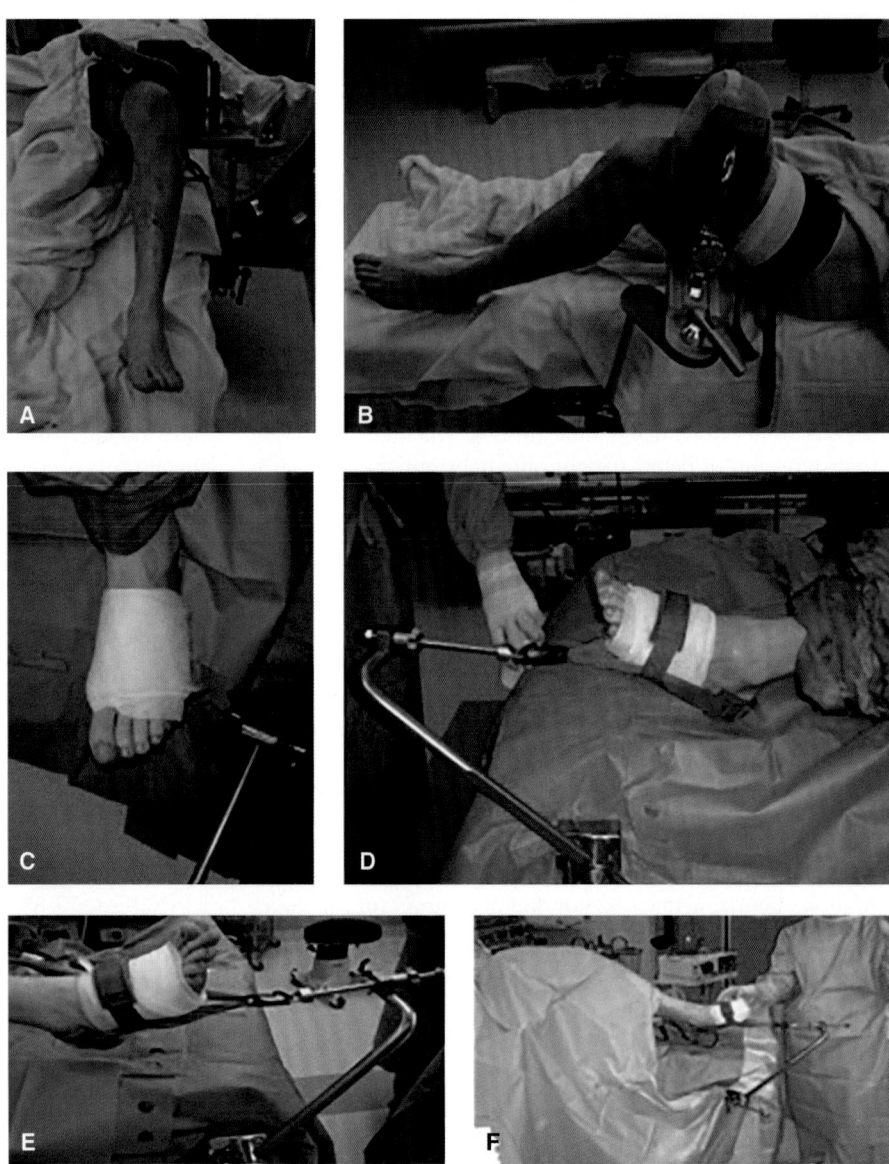

FIGURE 50.3 A-F. The authors preferred arthroscopic positioning with an ankle distractor.

failure. Seow et al.[36] reviewed 17 animal studies with 520 chondral lesions with the purpose of clarifying the morphology of subchondral bone following bone marrow stimulation, in preclinical, translational animal models. Their results demonstrated that the morphology of subchondral bone did not recover following bone marrow stimulation. Compared with untreated chondral defects, bone marrow stimulation resulted in superior morphology of superficial subchondral bone and cartilage but inferior morphology, specifically bone density, of the deep subchondral bone.[36]

The current indications for microfracture include lesions <1.5 cm in diameter or 150 mm² in surface area, noncystic lesions, and relative indications of <50 years of age and body mass index under 30. True microfracture should only be used on delaminated cartilage lesions, which is difficult in the ankle since 80% involve the subchondral plate.[15] The procedure is contraindicated in patients with large cystic lesions, failure of multiple surgeries, and acute lesions that have not undergone and exhausted conservative treatment.

Retrospective studies looking at the success rates of microfracture show good to excellent results in 39%-96% of cases.[37]

This large variation in success has sparked a lot of debate in the foot and ankle community regarding the efficacy of microfracture as a standard treatment option for cartilage repair. The technique is performed after excision and debridement of the OCD and can be performed arthroscopically or open as well. When performed with an open approach, a K-wire or Steinman pin is used to drill holes into the subchondral bone, resulting in bone marrow stimulation. This technique is frequently performed in conjunction with diagnostic arthroscopy in which surgeons insert an awl through the arthroscopic portals and perform microfracture with multiple perforations perpendicular to the joint surface, into the subchondral bone, for bone marrow stimulation.

Microfracture involves drilling through the subchondral bone, allowing bone marrow substrates to leave the subchondral bone and fill the defect. This process leads to angiogenesis and the production of a clot primarily composed of fibrocartilage, which provides high tensile strength and support. Fibrocartilage contains both type I and type II collagen, compared to hyaline cartilage which is primarily type II collagen. Although microfracture can be effective in alleviating the pain caused by

OCDs, it is important to remember that fibrocartilage is much less durable and has less proteoglycan than hyaline cartilage. Fibrocartilage also lacks the intrinsic biochemical and viscoelastic properties, as well as the shock absorption and force distribution capabilities of hyaline cartilage, and therefore may be insufficient for larger defects. Marrow stimulation procedures do not promote the excretion of growth factors or ECM proteins necessary for repair and regeneration of healthy hyaline cartilage, making it a short-term solution.[38] Considerations of growth factors and ECM protein supplementation had been discussed recently and show promise in cartilage regeneration. The goal is to allow for formation of type 2 collagen/hyaline cartilage regrowth. Recent literature has shown long-term failure in patients who have undergone microfracture, with recurrence of pain and joint stiffness. The literature shows the progression of better patient outcomes initially for microfracture with poor outcomes during long-term follow-up. Hunt et al.[39] found 54% of patients had fair or poor results after arthroscopy and microfracture at 66 weeks.[39]

Microfracture is a relatively simple, economical, single-stage procedure with appreciable short to mid-term pain relief. Incomplete regeneration, high interindividual variability, and poor repair outcome, especially in older individuals and larger defects, are just some of the shortcomings. There are many theories in recent literature trying to understand why microfracture fails in patients. One study reviewed 42 patients who underwent microfracture for osteochondral lesions of the talus. Serial MRIs were taken up until 8 years postoperatively. They found that patients demonstrated long-term subchondral bone edema following microfracture as well as subchondral cyst deterioration, theorizing that subchondral plate never fully recovers following microfracture perforations, leading to recurrent pain. They concluded that the lasting morphological changes in the subchondral bone may be indicative of long-term failure of the microfracture procedure.[40] According to the most recent literature on microfracture in the knee joint, multiple studies have shown microfracture long-term results to be inferior to other treatment options in lesions >2.5 cm² and in older individuals.

A study by Salzmann et al.[41] retrospectively looked at a large cohort of 454 patients with a mean defect size of 2.97 cm² treated by microfracture in the knee. In the study, index microfracture surgery was considered "failure" in patients that had revision surgery at the knee joint with pain related to the initial surgical site. They found a failure rate of 27.1% (123 patients), and the mean time between initial microfracture and the follow-up revision surgery was 1.6 years. Failure subjects had significantly smaller total defect dimensions and a smaller dimension of the largest lesion of the knee joint.[41]

Steadman et al.[42] targeted patients younger than 19 years old and evaluated 26 patients with a mean defect size of 1.77 cm² treated with microfracture. They were able to follow-up with 22/26 patients at an average of 5.8 years. They reported 3 patients, two who underwent microfracture of the patella and one who underwent microfracture of the trochlear groove, which had Lysholm scores of <80 at a minimum of 2 years after microfracture surgery and determined these to be a failure of the index procedure.[42]

Gobbi et al.[43] evaluated 53 athletes who had undergone microfracture procedures in the knee between 1991 and 2001 with at least a 10-year follow-up. At 10-15 years of follow-up, investigators found that patients who underwent microfracture to treat full-thickness chondral defects >3 cm² in size tended to fail within 1 year and required additional surgery. They also found that patients who underwent microfracture procedures for lesions smaller than 2.5 cm² demonstrated functional improvements for the first 5 years postoperatively, followed by gradual deterioration of results with reduced activity levels.[43]

Bae et al.[44] evaluated the survival of microfracture in patients with degenerative osteoarthritis in their knees (Fig. 50.4). They reviewed 134 knees in 124 patients in whom microfracture was performed with a mean follow-up of 11.2 years. They found a survival rate of 88.8% at 5 years and 67.9% at 10 years, with 51 patients going on to total knee arthroplasty at a mean of 6.8 years after the index microfracture procedure. Six of the knees were categorized as clinical failures.[44]

> ### PERILS and PITFALLS
> These intraoperative pictures (Fig. 50.5) are an arthroscopic presentation of fibrocartilage regrowth, note the fibrillated appearance of the fibrocartilage.

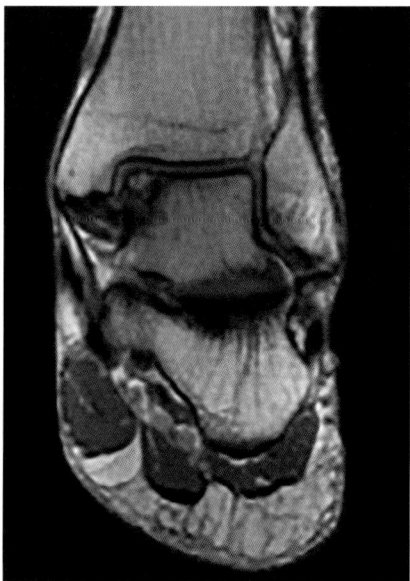
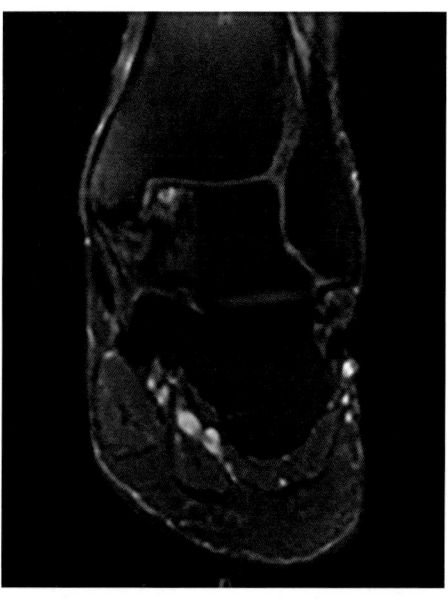

FIGURE 50.4 MRI of insufficient bone.

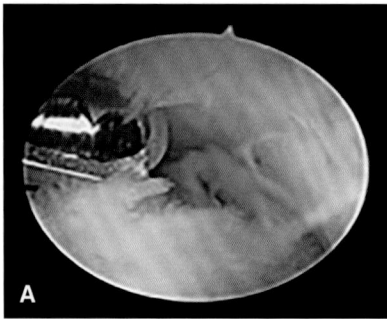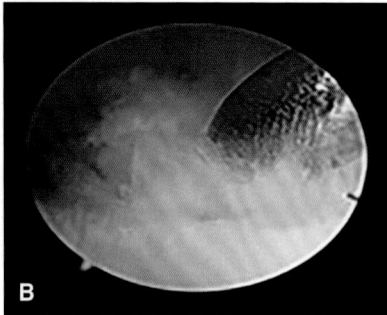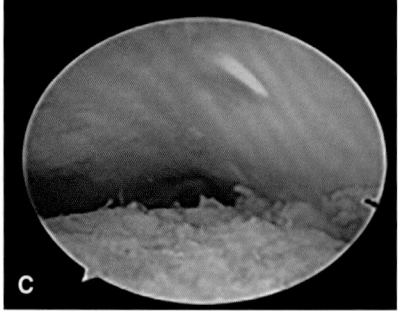

FIGURE 50.5 **A.** Photograph of repeat arthroscopic debridement prior to allograft placement. **B.** Microfracture performed when patient was 16 years old. **C.** Photograph of arthroscopic microfracture postdebridement 7 years later.

Abrasion chondroplasty is a similar first line technique that has been gaining a lot of traction in the literature recently. The procedure begins with arthroscopic excision of loose chondral or osteochondral fragments. The procedure can be performed with a curette, hand burr, or motorized arthroscopic shaver. The surface is abraded until underlying subchondral bone bleeds with debridement of the calcified layer. The edges of the defect are debrided with the same instruments, leaving edges perpendicular to the bone surface. Debridement during arthroscopy should not be too aggressive, maintaining as much subchondral bone as possible to keep the bone plate and overlying cartilage repair tissue contoured to the normal congruency of the opposing joint surface. A mechanical shaver is then used to trim down damaged cartilage with the goal of creating a stable, articular surface. A study by Gobbi et al.[45] compared microfracture, abrasion chondroplasty, and OAT in 33 patients with a mean follow-up of 53 months. They concluded that there were no differences between final outcomes between the three procedures; however, there was significantly improved pain immediately postoperatively with abrasion chondroplasty and microfracture compared to the OAT procedure. Their results also showed that abrasion chondroplasty had the least number of patients with persistent pain and poor final outcomes following the procedures.[45]

With much controversy in the literature surrounding the efficacy of microfracture, abrasion chondroplasty has become a viable option as an effective replacement procedure. Abrasion chondroplasty allows for marrow stimulation without destroying the subchondral bone under the osteochondral lesion. Findings from studies conducted on abrasion chondroplasty confirm the spontaneous repair response originates from the bone marrow spaces and results in the formation of a fibrous type of cartilage tissue. Although this contains most of the matrix components found in hyaline cartilage, significant quantities of fibrous constituents are also present.[46] One of the first relevant clinical trials evaluated patients suffering from OA and painful knee conditions that were subjected either to concomitant abrasion chondroplasty and osteotomy or to osteotomy alone. Individuals treated by the combined approach manifested a significantly higher proportion of hyalinelike cartilage repair tissue and had a lower incidence of tissue degeneration 12 months after surgery than did those who received only an osteotomy. However, no difference in the clinical outcome was observed after 2 (and up to 9) years.[47]

Abrasion chondroplasty with growth factors implantation has shown benefit in the literature. A study by Gobbi et al.[48] investigated the medium-term clinical outcomes of cartilage repair using abrasion chondroplasty followed by a hyaluronic acid-based scaffold with activated bone marrow aspirate concentrate (HA-BMAC) and compared their results with those treated by microfracture. They evaluated 50 patients with mean age of 45 years old, grade IV cartilage injury and lesion size of 1.5-24 cm^2. Patients were observed prospectively for 5 years. Their results showed that 64% of the microfracture group were classified as normal or nearly normal at 2 years, compared to 100% that were classified as normal at 2 years in the HA-BMAC group. Normal or nearly normal objective assessments in the microfracture group declined significantly after 5 years to 28% of patients, whereas, all the patients with HA-BMAC maintained improvements at 5 years.[48]

Another study by Gobbi et al.[49] evaluated the long-term clinical outcomes of 23 patients that were treated with abrasion chondroplasty in conjunction with hyaluronic acid-based scaffolds embedded with mesenchymal stem cells (MSCs) sourced from bone marrow aspirate concentrate (Fig. 50.6). Patients with a mean age of 48.5, who had median cartilage lesion size of 6.5 cm^2, were prospectively followed for an average of 8 years. They concluded that repair of full-thickness chondral lesions in the knee with HA-BMAC provides good to excellent clinical outcomes at long-term follow-up in the treatment of small to large lesions.[49]

PEARLS

Utilization of a 2.5- to 3.5-mm shaver is adequate to remove the calcified layer.

In many cases, marrow stimulation procedures may not be adequate, leaving the patient with continued pain and requiring more advanced cartilage restoration techniques. There are multiple options for cartilage restoration including cartilage replacements, biological cartilage scaffolds, and pluripotent cells.

Cartilage replacement allografts provide donor allografts for repair of OCDs and allow the ability for hyaline cartilage regeneration in a single staged procedure. In addition, osteochondral allografts have increased healing potential since they are more metabolically active, have a denser concentration of chondrocytes, and initiate less of an immune response.[37,50,51] Osteochondral allografts provide the advantage of abundant supply as well as the avoidance of donor site morbidity that comes with autografting. They also provide the advantage of allowing the surgeon to perform the repair in a single procedure.

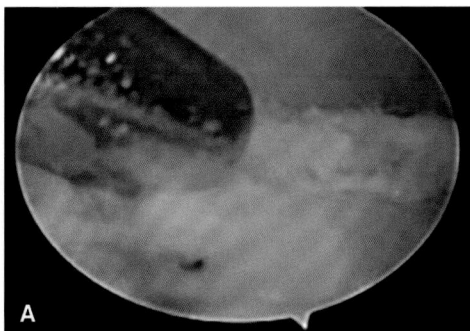 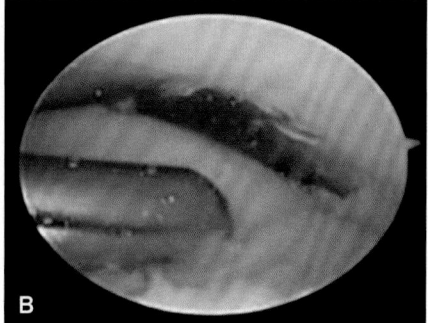

FIGURE 50.6 A, B. Intraoperative demonstration of arthroscopic abrasion chondroplasty performed for debridement of an osteochondral lesion in the ankle joint.

Disadvantages to ostcochondral allografts include the possibility for graft rejection and extended recovery time.[52]

Traditionally, osteochondral allografts have been reserved for lesions that are difficult to treat with other methods. These tend to present as large cystic lesions or unconstrained talar shoulder lesions. This technique was first described in 2001, using fresh, cadaver allografts for treatment of osteochondral lesions. Osteochondral allografts provide the advantage of allowing for the repair of any lesion, regardless of the size or shape.

In recent years, allograft cartilage has progressed significantly and become far more available for surgeons. Donor, cartilage allografts are now available in various sizes for direct repair of OCDs.

One type of allograft cartilage used for cartilage restoration includes adult cartilage cells, under the age of 35. This graft contains cartilage cells combined with cartilage allograft matrix to make a biologically active cartilage scaffold. This allograft provides functioning, viable chondrocytes and an ECM that contains the necessary chondrogenic growth factors for cartilage repair. These include type II collagen, proteoglycans, and endogenous growth factors. The advantage of this graft is the unique puttylike handling properties that easily conform to OCDs of various shapes and sizes. The graft is indicated for lesions up to 5 cm², which can be filled with one graft. Surgical application of this graft can be applied either through an open arthrotomy or arthroscopically in a similar fashion as application of particulated juvenile allograft cartilage (PJAC).[53]

After induction of anesthesia and obtaining a sterile field in the usual aseptic manner, a noninvasive ankle distractor is applied and the standard anteromedial and anterolateral arthroscopic portals are obtained. The osteochondral lesion of the talus is identified and debrided down to healthy subchondral bone using arthroscopic shavers and curettes, with care taken to ensure a sharp line of transition of healthy cartilage around the lesion. In cases in which the subchondral bone is not intact, the first layer of fibrin glue applied prevents the concern of bleeding of the cancellous bone, allowing the implant to take. The ankle joint is prepared for implantation by drying the joint with an abdominal insufflator and normal arthroscopic suction until the affected surface is dry. Direct drying of the osteochondral bed is accomplished with cotton tip applicators prior to glue placement. Once the subchondral bone of the osteochondral lesion of the talus is dry, the cartilage graft is inserted through a 10-gauge catheter in either anterior portal onto a layer of fibrin glue. A second layer of fibrin glue is then applied over the cartilage to fill the remaining defect.

The insufflator is again used to ensure that the fibrin glue is dry to the touch before closing the arthroscopic portals.[50]

Another allograft cartilage commonly used among foot and ankle surgeons is PJAC, which is the authors preferred technique. PJAC is comprised of morselized cartilage fragments from cadaveric donors under the age of 13 years old, since higher levels of type II collagen and proteoglycan production are typically seen in cartilage donors from this age group compared with adults.[54] The juvenile allograft cartilage is chondroinductive, chondroconductive, and chondrogenic making it an ideal graft option for cartilage regeneration. Juvenile chondrocytes have the ability to migrate from the ECM and proliferate to form neocartilage that integrates with surrounding native articular cartilage.[53,55-58] PJAC undergoes minimal amounts of manipulation and processing, thereby increasing the risk of disease transmission that comes with its use.[56]

In the past, PJAC was indicated for patients with symptomatic osteochondral lesions of the talus larger than 1.5 cm in diameter, revision OCD repair, and lesions involving the shoulder of the talus.[59] The current literature shows that PJAC can be used effectively on both large and small osteochondral lesions and as an index procedure to treat the lesion.[60] Contraindications for the use of PJAC include degenerative arthritic changes, a history of infection, and large cystic lesions. Large cystic lesions are often treated with cancellous chips, structural bone graft, or flowable calcium phosphate injections, followed by placement of PJAC over the top of the cartilage defect.[61]

> **PEARLS**
>
> Large cystic lesions are no longer a contraindication if the cyst is addressed intraoperatively.

The technique used for PJAC placement was first described in the literature in 2010 and performed with an open ankle joint arthrotomy.[62] In 2012, a more efficient and noninvasive technique for performing the PJAC technique arthroscopically was published by the author, which he had been performing since 2008.[50]

After induction of anesthesia and obtaining a sterile field in the usual aseptic manner, a noninvasive ankle distractor is applied and the standard anteromedial and anterolateral arthroscopic portals are obtained. The osteochondral lesion of the talus is identified and debrided down to healthy subchondral bone using arthroscopic shavers and curettes, with care

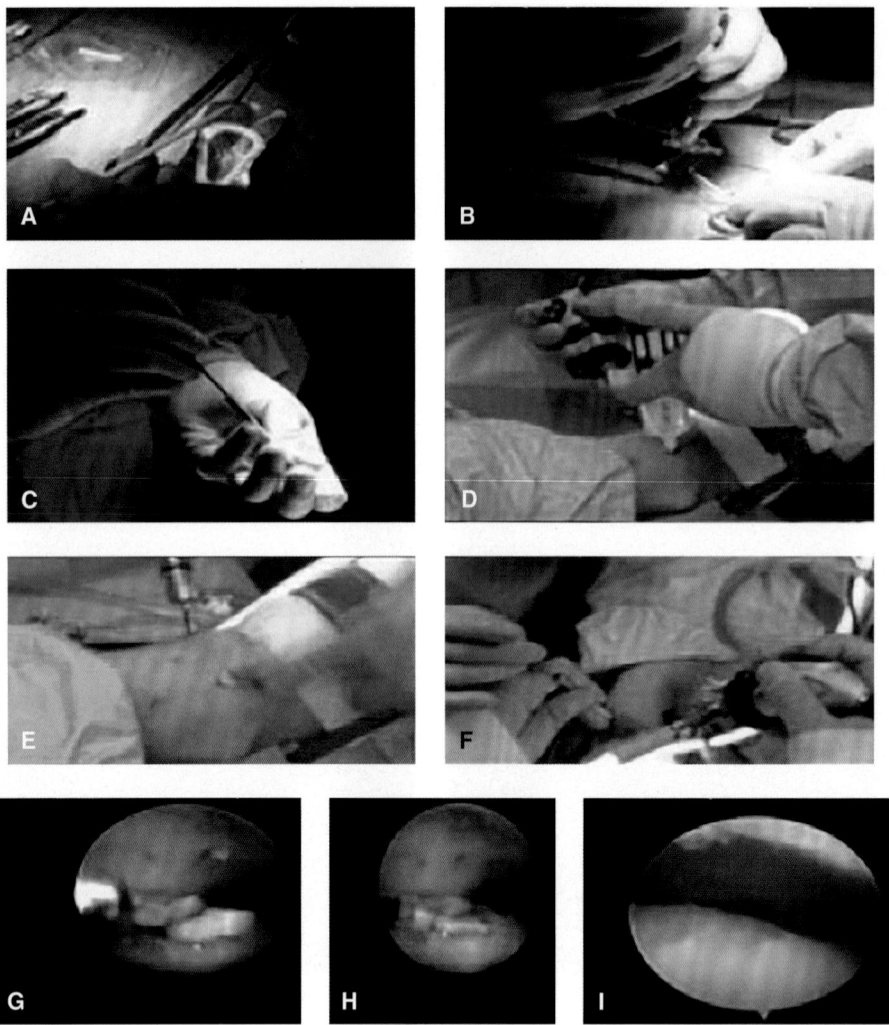

FIGURE 50.7 **A-C.** An 18-g needle is inserted into the PJAC packet and the fluid is pulled out with a syringe, isolating the PJAC particles. The packet is carefully opened and the PJAC particles are pushed into a 10-g angiocath with a freer elevator. **D.** Fibrin glue is inserted onto the OCD through an anterior portal. **E, F.** The PJAC is then placed into the portal and placed into the OCD, followed by another layer of fibrin glue. **G, H.** Shows pictures of the PJAC placed into the OCD. **I.** Demonstrates an arthroscopic second look of the healed OCD at a later date.

taken to ensure a sharp line of transition of healthy cartilage around the lesion. In cases in which the subchondral bone is not intact, the first layer of fibrin glue applied prevents the concern of bleeding of the cancellous bone, allowing the implant to adhere to the adhesive surface. The ankle joint is prepared for implantation by drying the joint with an abdominal insufflator and normal arthroscopic suction to create a dry environment. Utilizing the insufflator allows for maintaining of joint distension and prevents the joint from overheating. Direct drying of the osteochondral bed is accomplished with cotton tip applicators prior to glue placement. Once the subchondral bone of the osteochondral lesion of the talus is dry, the cartilage graft is inserted through a 10-gauge catheter in the anteromedial portal onto a layer of fibrin glue (Fig. 50.7). A second layer of fibrin glue is then applied over the cartilage to fill the remaining defect. The insufflator is again used to ensure that the fibrin glue is dry to the touch before closing the arthroscopic portals (Fig. 50.8).[50] Studies have shown that chondrocytes have the ability to migrate through fibrin glue within 2 weeks.[63,64]

PERILS and PITFALLS

- Abdominal insufflator is set to 20-30 mm Hg of continuous flow to distend and dry out the joint.
- Be sure to turn off the flow before inserting the graft.
- Once the graft is in place and sealed, turn the insufflation back on to distend and dry the joint and set the glue.

PEARLS

Use an 18-gauge blunt tip needle to insert the fibrin glue, this will allow accurate placement of the glue.

PEARLS

If the lesion is nonconstrained, contour the graft along the nonconstrained area and carefully seal the area with fibrin glue.

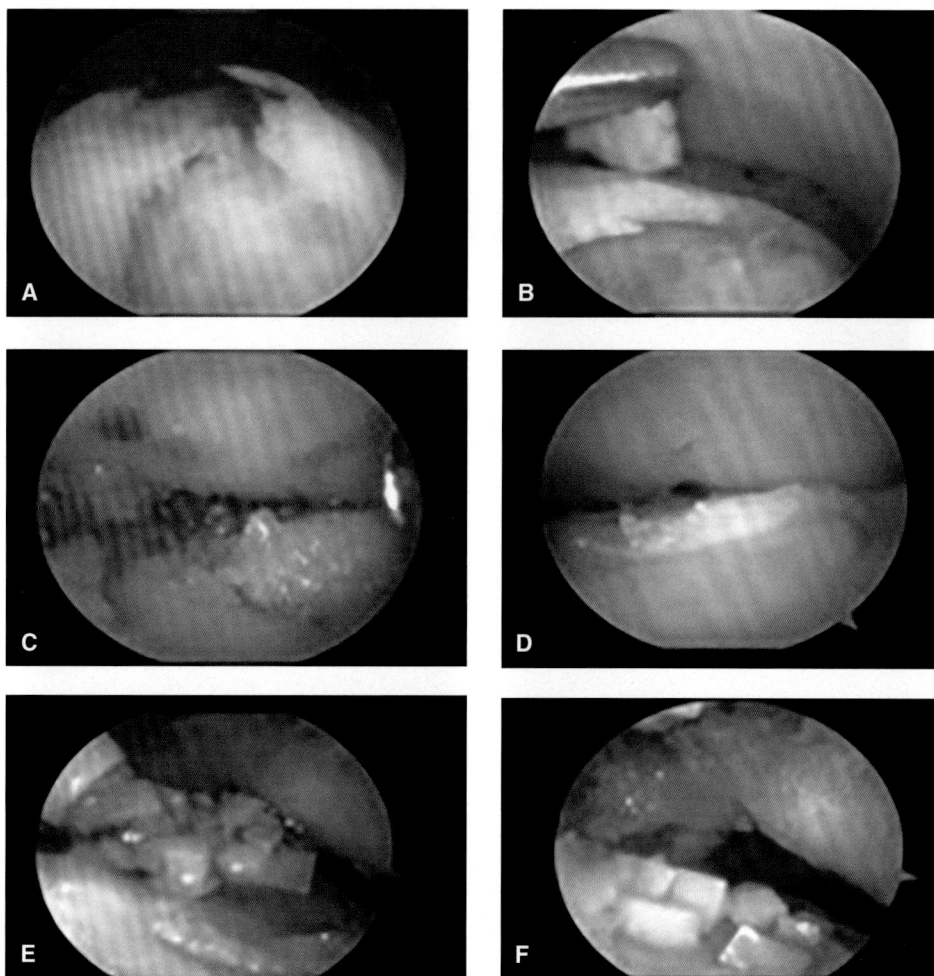

FIGURE 50.8 A, B. Removal of the talar osteochondral defect with debridement to firm edges. **C, D.** After drying out the ankle joint with the abdominal insufflator, fibrin glue is placed on the base of the lesion under dry scope. **E, F.** Arthroscopic PJAC placement on top of fibrin glue base under dry scope.

Kruse et al.[50] presented a case of arthroscopic repair of an osteochondral lesion of the talus using PJAC in a 30-year-old woman. The full-thickness lesion was located posteromedially on the talus and measured 7 × 5 mm. At 2-year follow-up, the patient presented pain free and had returned to full activity with no restrictions.[50]

A retrospective review by Chopra et al.[65] reviewed clinical outcomes utilizing the validated FAOS scoring system in patients who were treated with an arthroscopic implantation of PJAC between 2008 and 2016. They evaluated 32 patients with mean age of 40.7 years and mean follow-up time of 24 months. Their results demonstrated that all but four, 26/32 (82%), patients scored a good or excellent result in activities of daily living. They found that 26/32 (82%) patients had at least good results in both pain and symptoms, and 25/32 (78%) had at least a fair result for functional sports and quality of life. They concluded that although the use of PJAC implantation for repair of OCDs exists as a fairly new line of treatment, their study results provide strong evidence of the potential effectiveness of this procedure.[65]

The use of juvenile cartilage increases the number of immature chondrocytes, which are more metabolically active and capable of spontaneous repair.[66] This increased activity among the juvenile chondrocytes gives them the ability to differentiate into hyalinelike cartilage instead of fibrocartilage, which is seen in other OCD repair techniques.[50] The benefits of juvenile chondrocytes over adult chondrocytes have been widely demonstrated in many *in vitro* studies. Cartilage gene expression transforms with age, and the gene expression of juvenile cartilage is more favorable for cartilage regeneration than that of adult chondrocytes. The genes that direct cartilage growth and expansion are up-regulated, whereas in adult cartilage, genes that control structural integrity of cartilage are up-regulated.[55,57,67,68] The ability of juvenile chondrocytes to produce and maintain matrix is increased through increased metabolic activity, cell density, proliferation rate, and outgrowth.[55,69,70] Moreover, juvenile chondrocytes have been shown to be immune privileged, making it possible to utilize them as an allogeneic source for cartilage repair.

A study by Lanham et al.[71] compared outcomes of particulated juvenile articular cartilage and bone marrow aspirate concentrate for articular cartilage lesions of the talus. They evaluated 12 patients, 6 from each treatment group that underwent surgery between 2010 and 2013. Lesion size was 2.0 ± 1.1 cm²

for the BMAC group and 1.9 ± 0.9 cm² for the PJAC group with a mean follow-up of 25.7 months. They concluded that PJAC yielded better clinical outcomes at 2 years when compared with BMAC for articular lesions of the talus that were on average >1.5 cm² in size.[71]

A retrospective case-control study by Dekker et al.[72] looked at 15 patients who underwent particulated juvenile cartilage allograft transplant for treatment of OLTs with an average of 34.6-month follow-up. They defined failure of the procedure as no change or worsening of symptoms and/or the need for a subsequent cartilage restoration procedure. Their results showed a failure rate of 40% (6/15) in this series. They concluded that patients with lesions >125 mm² area had a significantly increased risk of clinical failure.[72]

Tan et al.[73] performed a histological and gross evaluation through second-look arthroscopy of osteochondral lesions of the talus after failed treatment with PJAC in four patients. They found no obvious patients or surgical factors associated with poor outcomes.[73]

A study by Karnovsky et al.[74] compared juvenile articular allograft cartilage and bone marrow aspirate concentrate vs microfracture with and without bone marrow aspirate concentrate in the arthroscopic treatment of talar osteochondral lesions. They looked at 30 patients who underwent microfracture and 20 patients who received PJAC-BMAC treatment between 2006 and 2014. Additionally, 17 microfracture patients received supplemental BMAC treatment. Average follow-up for functional outcomes was 30.9 months. They found that PJAC-BMAC and microfracture resulted in improved functional outcomes; however, while the majority of patients improved, functional outcomes and quality of repair tissue were still not normal. They concluded that lesions repaired with PJAC still appeared fibrocartilaginous on MRI and did not result in significant functional gains as compared to microfracture.[74]

Wang et al.[75] analyzed the functional outcomes of 27 patients treated with PJAC for symptomatic articular cartilage lesions in the patellofemoral joint with a mean follow-up of 3.84 years. They found significantly improved pain and function in patients treated with PJAC for symptomatic patellofemoral articular cartilage defects. No patients required reoperation for graft-related issues. Postoperative MRI results showed majority lesion fill in more than 69% of patients, but persistent morphologic differences between graft site and normal adjacent cartilage remain.[75]

Laboratory studies have proven the increased efficacy of juvenile cartilage over adult cartilage. A study by Adkisson et al.[68] took cartilage samples from juvenile (<13 years old) and adult (>13 years old) donors. The chondrogenic activity of the freshly isolated human articular chondrocytes and of expanded cells after monolayer culture was measured by proteoglycan assay, gene expression analysis, and histology. They found that proteoglycan content in neocartilage produced by juvenile chondrocytes was 100-fold higher than in neocartilage produced by adult cells. They also found that collagen type II and type IX mRNA in fresh juvenile chondrocytes were 100 to 700-fold higher, respectively, than in adult chondrocytes. The distributions of collagens II and IX were similar in native juvenile cartilage and in neocartilage made by juvenile cells. Juvenile cells grew significantly faster in monolayer cultures than adult cells, and proteoglycan levels produced in agarose culture were significantly higher in juvenile cells than in adult cells

after multiple passages. Lastly, they found that juvenile chondrocytes did not stimulate lymphocyte proliferation.[68]

Micronized cartilage matrix (MCM) was recently introduced to the cartilage restoration space, consisting of dehydrated allogeneic cartilage chips that act as a scaffold or matrix for hyaline cartilage formation following microfracture and debridement of osteochondral lesions of the talus. MCM contains proteoglycans and type II collagen, consistent with the components necessary for hyaline cartilage formation. The surgical technique also requires the use of platelet-rich plasma (PRP) to provide chondrogenic precursors and help influence differentiation.[76]

The indications for this procedure are very similar to microfracture, including lesions <1.5 cm in diameter or 150 mm² in surface area, noncystic lesions, and relative indications of <50 years of age and body mass index under 30. The procedure is contraindicated in patients with large cystic lesions, failure of multiple surgeries, and acute lesions that have not undergone and exhausted conservative treatment.

The surgical technique for application of MCM begins with standard debridement of the OLT, arthroscopically, with shavers and curettes to the level of healthy subchondral bone and cartilage. Microfracture is then performed in a standard fashion with arthroscopic awls and the ankle joint is then evacuated and dried out using an abdominal insufflator and normal arthroscopic suction for at least 5 minutes. Any small cysts should be packed with harvested bone marrow aspirate, cancellous chips, or flowable calcium phosphate. The MCM and the bone marrow aspirate or PRP are mixed in a 1:1 ratio and applied to the OLT by injection through the arthroscopic portal. The remainder of the defect is coated with fibrin glue and allowed to dry for 5 minutes, with care taken to ensure that the deficit is filled adequately and the cartilage is smooth. If the OLT cannot be adequately visualized or prepared arthroscopically, this procedure can also be performed through open ankle arthrotomy; however, it is important to still apply the MCM dry and take special care to maintain an even level with the surrounding cartilage.[77]

A proof of concept *in vitro* study, by Shieh et al.,[78] combined MCM with MSCs and concluded that MCM can serve as a scaffold for the growth of cartilage tissue for the treatment of osteochondral lesions.[78] A case report by Desai et al.[79] outlined the successful treatment of a talar OCD with debridement, marrow stimulation, and MCM through an arthroscopic approach.[79]

Human amniotic allografts have been in widespread use in a variety of applications including burn care, dentistry, ophthalmic, ear, nose and throat, and spine surgery since the early 20th century.[80-87] The pluripotent cells present in human amniotic allograft tissue are considered multipotent, meaning they can differentiate into various tissue types including muscle, tendon, bone, or cartilage.[88] They are also thought to have some level of immunogenicity. Amniotic tissues are composed of multiple types of collagen, hyaluronan, proteoglycans, morphogenetic proteins, and glycosaminoglycan. They are thought to be a reservoir for growth factors and house no antigenicity due to the amnion extraction process from the placental tissue.[88] Advances in technology have delivered a safe and consistent application for amniotic allograft over the last several years and clinicians are beginning to learn the potential benefits that the undifferentiated tissues can have on the healing process.

Human amniotic allograft is indicated for talar dome lesions <2 cm² as an adjunctive measure to marrow stimulating techniques. The surgical technique for application of amniotic

grafts begins with induction of anesthesia and obtaining a sterile field in the usual aseptic manner. A noninvasive ankle distractor is applied and the standard anteromedial and anterolateral arthroscopic portals are obtained. Standard circumferential debridement of the OCD is performed arthroscopically with shavers and curettes to the level of healthy subchondral bone. Marrow stimulation techniques are then implemented in a standard fashion. The ankle joint is then evacuated and dried out using an abdominal insufflator and normal arthroscopic suction for ~5 minutes. Human amniotic allograft is then used and applied directly to the lesion via needle technique and under direct visualization.

Studies show that human amniotic membrane contains pluripotent MSCs that can be influenced to produce chondrocytes. A study conducted in 2014 evaluated the use of hypothermically stored human amniotic membrane for cartilage repair in adult sheep. The study showed that the defects that successfully retained the graft had evidence of diffuse chondrocyte cell proliferation and showed a stromal matrix similar to hyaline cartilage.[89]

A new prospective study conducted recently by Tabet et al.[90] evaluated the effectiveness of hypothermically stored amniotic membrane (HSAM) for articular cartilage repair in 10 patients with at least International Cartilage Repair Society (ICRS) grade III lesions in the knee. Their MRI MOCART scoring demonstrated at least some degree of defect fill in 100% of patients, indicating increased proteoglycan content. They concluded that HSAM-treated patients show decreases in pain scores, along with increases in overall knee assessment scores up to 12 months postsurgery. Their evidence suggests that HSAM may be a viable treatment option for cartilage defects.[90]

Osteochondral autograft transplantation surgery (OATS), also called mosaicplasty, is a reconstructive bone grafting technique that uses one or more cylindrical osteochondral grafts from an area of low impact or allograft source and transplants them into a prepared defect site on the talus (Figs. 50.9 and 50.10). The goal of the OAT procedure is to reproduce the mechanical, structural, and biochemical properties of the original hyaline articular cartilage.[91]

The OAT procedure is indicated in patients with larger, >1 cm^2, isolated lesions and subchondral cystic lesions of the talus.[92] This procedure is also indicated in smaller defects where primary treatment (excision, debridement, and bone marrow stimulation) fails to resolve the symptoms.[91] Osteochondral lesions of the talus can occur secondary to avascular necrosis. These lesions have been shown to be at higher risk for failure due to the decreased vascularity in the talus and resulting in poor graft incorporation.[93]

Treating defects >4 cm^2 is not recommended with autograft transplantation due to donor site morbidity.[94] Surgeons are encouraged to use allograft for transplantation instead. Contraindications to this procedure include infection, inflammatory arthropathy, neuropathy, vascular disease, degenerative joint disease of the ankle joint, uncorrectable malalignment, lesions of the talar shoulder and ligamentous instability.[95]

For a successful procedure, perpendicular access must be available for both the plug harvest and transfer. An oblique distal fibular osteotomy can be utilized for lateral talar dome lesions that are otherwise difficult to access. Medial talar dome lesions that prove to be difficult to access can be approached in the same manner, with a medial malleolar osteotomy.

PEARLS

Predrilling for osteotomy fixation, prior to the osteotomy, is crucial to ensuring anatomic reduction of the osteotomy.

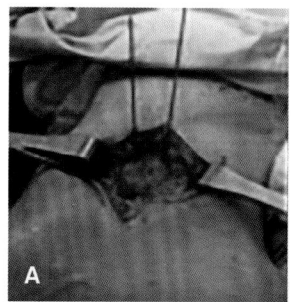
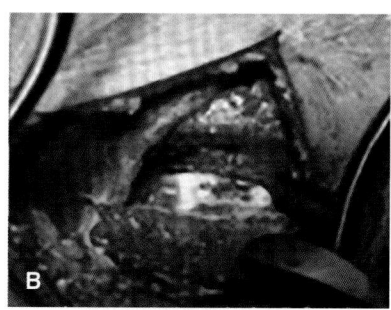
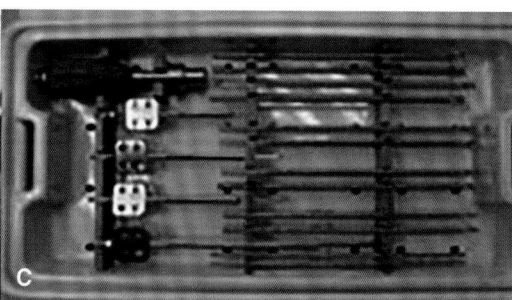
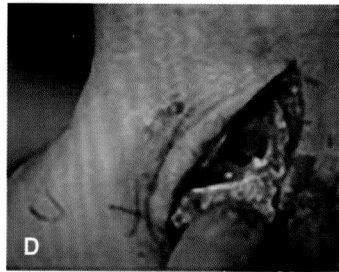
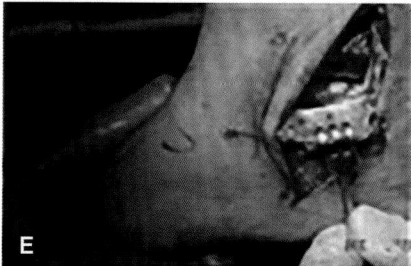
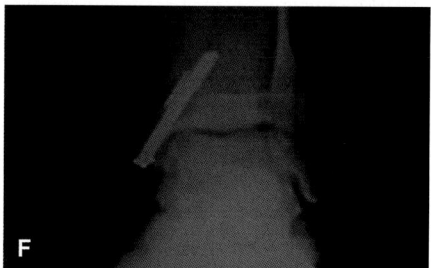

FIGURE 50.9 Osteochondral allograft transplant surgery (OATS). **A.** K-wire guide to ensure proper osteotomy placement, **(B)** the OCD is accessed and measured, **(C)** the recipient site is drilled out with reamers, **(D)** prepared recipient site, **(E)** plug seated into recipient site, and **(F)** postoperative radiographs following OATS procedure.

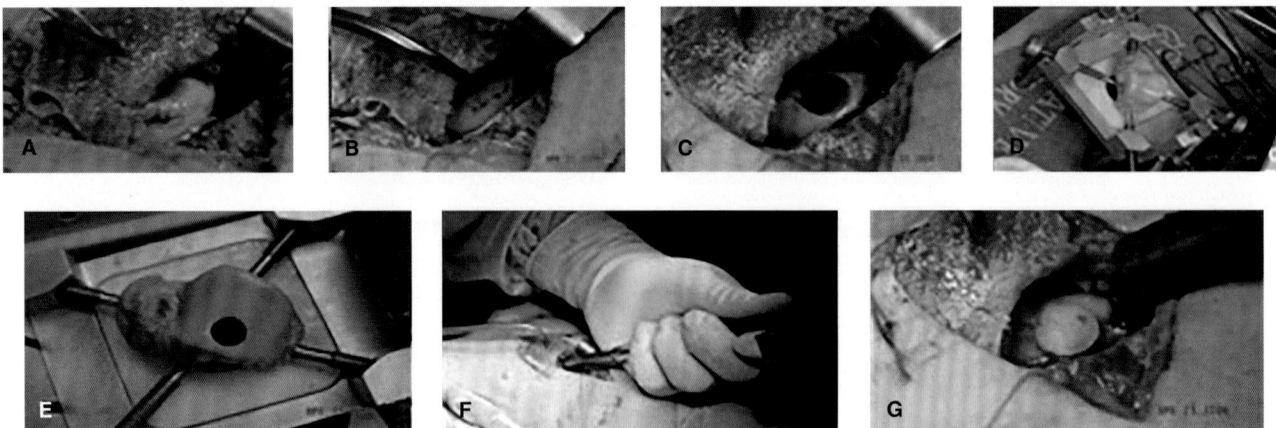

FIGURE 50.10 Osteochondral allograft transplant surgery (OATS). **A-C.** OCD is located and site is prepared for allograft plug, **(D, E)** plug is measured and matched on the allograft talus, and **(F, G)** allograft plug is sized, dilated, and inserted into recipient site.

For autologous harvest, sites should be located at non–weight-bearing portions such as the intercondylar notch and medial or lateral femoral condyles of the knee. The plantar and medial aspect of the talar head is another option for foot and ankle surgeons. Autologous harvest provides the advantage of increased chances of graft incorporation and reduced risk of disease transmission. The major disadvantage to this procedure is donor site morbidity. Although osteochondral allograft eliminates donor site complications, there remains a low risk of disease transmission, which patients should be aware of.

Arthroscopy can be performed first utilizing standard anteromedial and anterolateral portals to assess the size and location of the lesion. If arthroscopy is not an option, an open ankle arthrotomy can be used in order to visualize and gain access to the ankle joint. After inspecting the ankle joint for any other significant pathology, the osteochondral lesion is identified and a probe is used to inspect the surrounding cartilage for any other pathologic lesions. Excision and debridement is done to prepare the recipient site by establishing a healthy, stable articular rim around the defect and for accurate measurement of the lesion. Next, it is important to proceed with autograft or allograft donor harvest, prior to drilling the recipient site. If using autograft, the donor graft harvest site should be easily accessible with minimal morbidity. With the cylindrical harvester seated to the articular cartilage firmly, a manual technique should be used to reduce the risk of thermal necrosis and adverse effects on the viable chondrocytes. Access to the osteochondral lesion is then performed through malleolar arthrotomy or plafondplasty. The osteotomy is planned with a Kirschner wire and visualized under fluoroscopy to ensure that the osteotomy is placed in the proper orientation. Preplacement of screws is accomplished prior to the osteotomy to ensure anatomic reduction. The recipient site is then drilled to the same depth and diameter as that of the harvested plug, ensuring that the base has a stable vascularized zone in order to both potentiate vascular ingrowth for incorporation of the graft and to promote healing of fibrocartilage between plugs when used with mosaicplasty. The graft should be pressed fit with digital pressure. When utilizing multiple plugs, many surgeons have found beginning with the peripheral plugs and working centrally to be the most optimal way of approaching insertion.[96,97]

Fresh osteochondral allografts are currently used to treat a broad spectrum of osteoarticular lesions. Partial or total talar block replacement is another procedure commonly used to treat patients with OCDs (Fig. 50.11). It is used as a primary treatment option for large OCDs (>2 cm², 6-10 mm deep) and, in particular, for poor talar shoulder lesions. It is also used as a secondary procedure following failure of other regenerative techniques.

Different surgical techniques for both partial and total allograft transplantation procedures have been described, with differences between different techniques focusing primarily on the use of specifically developed instrumentations, the use of jigs from the ankle prosthesis instrumentation, and the use of an external fixation to assist with intraoperative joint distraction.

Regarding partial grafts, the dimension and shape of the portion of the talus being replaced should be evaluated, sized, and measured allowing for adequate reproduction onto the corresponding location of the donor fresh graft (Fig. 50.12). The graft is then shaped to fit the defect. Once the donor site is prepared, the osteochondral graft is positioned to replace the portion of the talus that was resected. Fixation can be achieved by using bioabsorbable poly-L-lactic acid osteochondral darts or headless titanium compression screws. Allograft transplantation may be performed from a medial or lateral transmalleolar approach or from an anterior approach. An external fixation device may be applied for intraoperative distraction of the ankle joint. Custom-made or total ankle replacement cutting jigs may be used to help both the recipient site preparation and the cut of the osteochondral allograft, in order to obtain a fit as close to perfect as possible. Using an oscillating saw, the talar dome and distal tibia are resected, being careful to avoid injuring the neurovascular bundle at the posteromedial corner of the ankle joint and the fibula posterolaterally (Fig. 50.13). The allograft surfaces are then to be positioned in the host ankle and fixed with screws, taking care to avoid the weight-bearing areas. Finally, congruency, range of motion, and stability of the ankle are checked from dorsiflexion to plantar flexion.[98]

PERILS and PITFALLS

Always cut the donor graft to the exact size or greater than the recipient size. You can always trim down the graft, but you cannot add more volume to the cut graft.

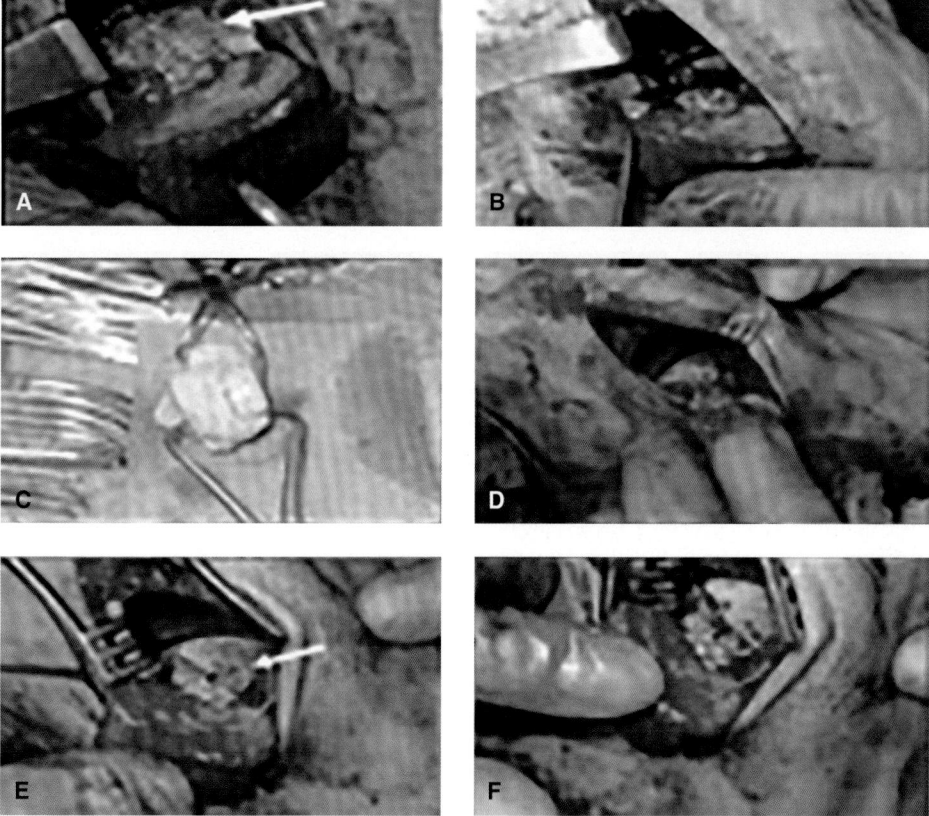

FIGURE 50.11 Talar allograft block replacement. **A.** Exposure of the deficit, **(B)** border of the talus, **(C)** talar allograft, **(D)** placement of the graft, **(E)** chondral dart fixation, and **(F)** testing of range of motion.

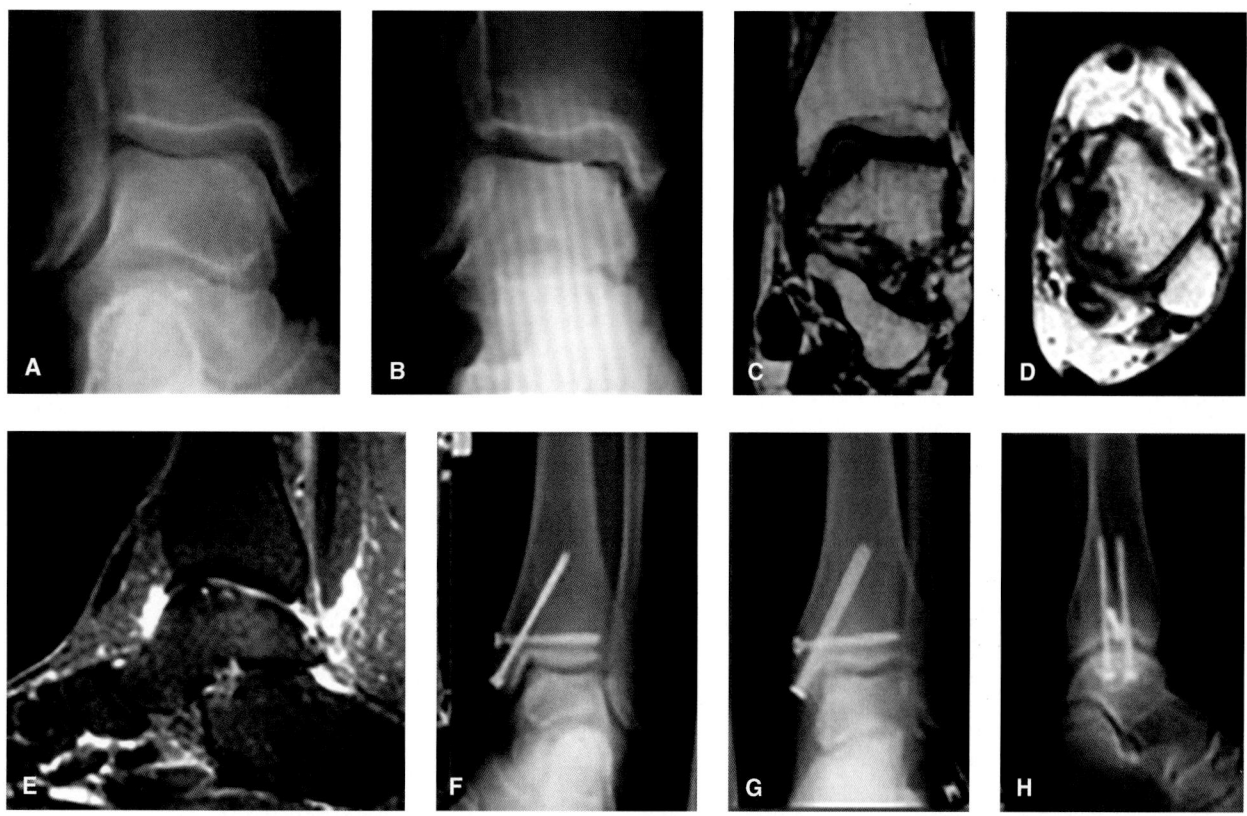

FIGURE 50.12 A 48-year-old female with severe ankle pain. **A, B.** Preop radiographs of osteochondral shoulder lesion of the talus. **C-E.** Preop MRI of osteochondral shoulder lesion of the talus. **F-H.** Postop radiographs following talar block allograft replacement in the talus.

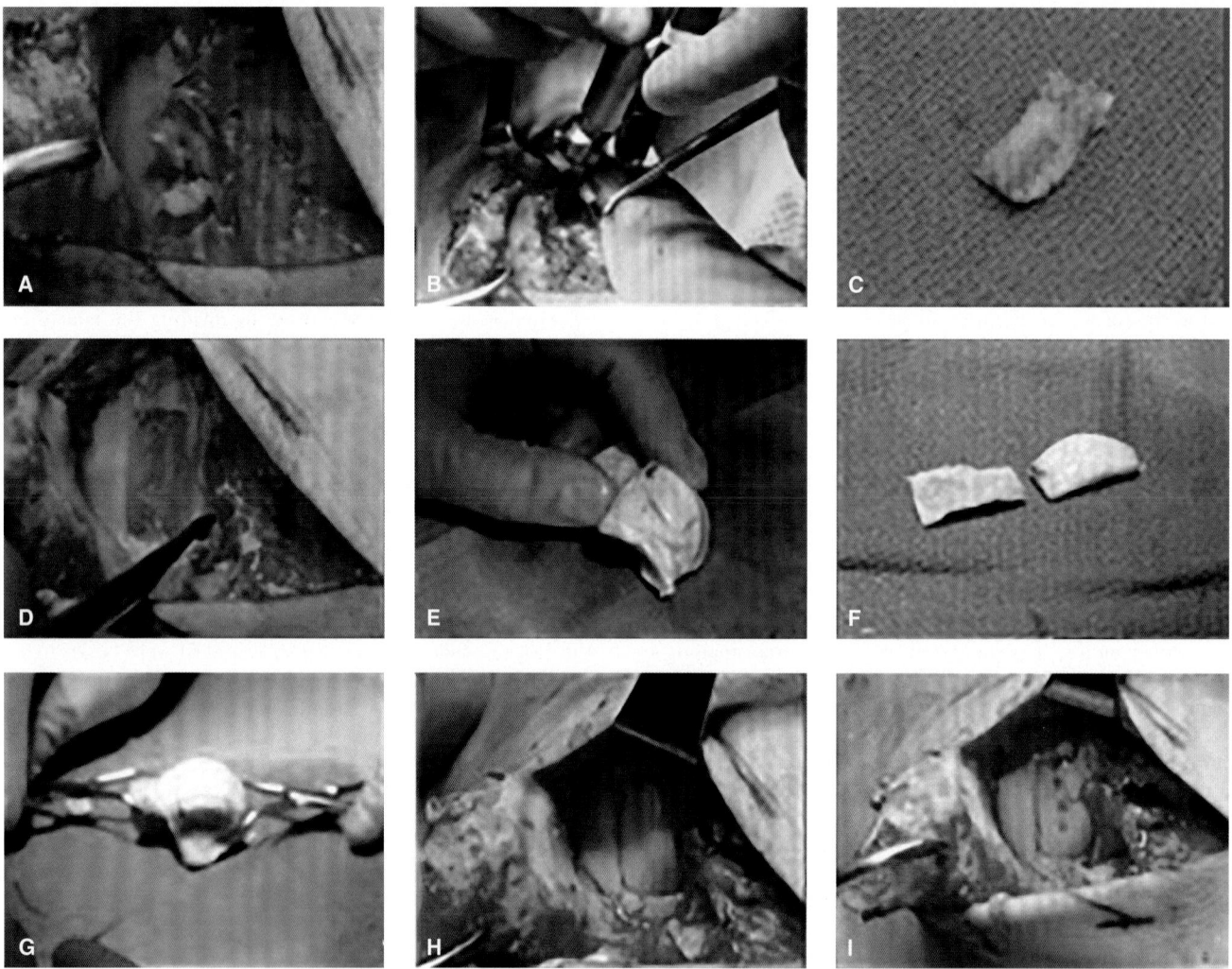

FIGURE 50.13 A-D. The location and resection of degenerated talus. **E-G.** The degenerated,resected portion of the talus is measured and matched to the talar allograft block, marked and cut to size. **H, I.** The viable talar allograft block is press fit into place, replacing the resected, degenerated portion of the talus.

PERILS and PITFALLS
- The more vertical the osteotomy is, the more unstable it becomes.
- Utilize a transverse screw or a buttress plate to avoid superior translation of the osteotomy.

POSTOPERATIVE COURSE

This chapter has detailed several different treatment options for cartilage repair and regeneration. Correct, pathology specific, procedural selection is imperative for providing the best chance of repair; however, it is just as important to choose the appropriate postoperative protocol following these advanced procedures. This section outlines typical postoperative protocols for the procedures described in this chapter, providing a framework for the reader.

Marrow stimulation procedures such as excision and debridement, microfracture, and abrasion chondroplasty all have a similar typical postoperative course. This includes immobilization in a fracture boot for 4 weeks. Some physicians choose to keep their patients non–weight bearing for 4-6 weeks; however, this comes with the risk of arthrofibrosis and disuse muscle atrophy. The author's postoperative protocol includes immediate weight bearing in a fracture boot with early range of motion at 2 weeks, followed by physical therapy at 4 weeks. The author's typical postoperative protocol involves having patients remain in the fracture boot for 4 weeks followed by transition into an ankle brace and continued physical therapy. Full return to activity without restrictions is expected around 3 months. If pain should persist at 6 months, the author recommends a MRI to evaluate for failure of subchondral bone and failure to heal the marrow stimulation site.

The postoperative course following PJAC includes non–weight bearing for 4 weeks in a fracture boot with range of motion starting at 2 weeks. These range of motion exercises should include dorsiflexion and plantarflexion without inversion or inversion range of motion. Patients should start physical therapy with no axial loading to the ankle and no single leg exercises at 4 weeks. At 8 weeks, patients are able to begin non-impact exercises, that is biking, swimming, rowing, with no axial

impact exercises, that is running, stairs, hopping, for 4 months. The author advises against obtaining an MRI too early in the postoperative course since the PJAC graft will be hydrophilic for up to 18 months. This could lead to MRI reports stating that the OCD is still present. After second looks at months 4, 6, 12, and 18, stable cartilage is seen at month 4, with full incorporation of cartilage at ~18 months. If pain and stiffness persist at 4-6 months postoperatively, the author recommends considering repeat arthroscopy to clean out arthrofibrosis, which is seen with overgrowth of the repair site.

Postoperative course for cartilage replacement depends on the type of replacement cartilage. If using a free graft, one should consider non–weight bearing in a fracture boot for 6 weeks, due to the large segment of single cartilage graft. Most of the literature suggests 6 weeks of non–weight bearing immediately after surgery with immobilization in a splint or short leg cast. At 6 weeks, a below the knee CAM boot is applied and active, assisted range of motion of the ankle is permitted outside of the boot. Weight bearing as tolerated is usually initiated between 6 and 8 weeks postoperatively, and patients are fully weight bearing by 12 weeks. A physical therapy program focusing on joint range of motion and mobility, balance, and strength should be started around 8 weeks. When using cartilage replacements, it is suggested to obtain serial imaging in the form of plain film radiographs, MRI, and/or CT scans to ensure union and incorporation of the graft.

Platelet-rich plasma, bone marrow aspirate concentrate, and other replacement cells are typically used in conjunction with marrow stimulation procedures. The typical postoperative course for these procedures includes weight bearing in a fracture boot for 4-6 weeks. Physical therapy is recommended at weeks 4-6 with limited activity for 3 months.

Scaffolds used in solitude, without replacement cells or marrow stimulation, should be treated in the same manner as marrow stimulation. Typical protocol includes weight bearing in a fracture boot for 4 weeks followed by initiation of physical therapy at 4-6 weeks.

OATS typically involves a medial or lateral osteotomy to gain access to the talus. Postoperative protocol should include 6-8 weeks of immobilization and non–weight bearing pending osteotomy healing, followed by 3-4 weeks in a fracture boot after the commencement of weight bearing. Physical therapy should be initiated at 6-8 weeks postsurgery, once the osteotomy has been healed.

The postoperative protocol for talar block replacement should also be approached in a similar manner to the postoperative course for OATS procedure, due to the medial or lateral malleolar osteotomy necessary for access to the talus. This protocol includes 6-8 weeks of non–weight bearing until the medial/lateral osteotomy is healed, followed by weight bearing in a fracture boot for 3-4 weeks, and introduction of physical therapy at 6-8 weeks postsurgery, depending on osteotomy healing. The author recommends getting a CT scan postoperatively to evaluate talar block allograft incorporation and suggests extending the non–weight-bearing period if necessary, pending interoperative observation.

THEORY AND NEW TREATMENTS ON THE HORIZON

The talar dome is a common location for OCDs (osteochondral defects/lesions), exceeded in frequency only by the knee and possibly the elbow. However, the etiology and morphology of these lesions have been controversial. Traditionally, talar dome lesions have been described as being most commonly located in the posteromedial or anterolateral region (aka: DIAL a PIMP mechanism of injury; although this may be correct in some instances, more recent literature shows that this is not always true) with the former location being deeper and cup shaped in morphology and the latter being more shallow and wafer shaped. However, this description of morphology has been highly controversial over the years.

A study by Elias et al.[99] established a novel, nine-zone anatomical grid system on the talar dome for an accurate depiction of lesion location. This was done by dividing the talar dome articular surface in an equal 3 × 3 grid configuration, with zone 1 being most anteromedial and zone 9 being most posterolateral (Fig. 50.14). The surface area of each of the 9 zones of the articular talar dome was identical. Two observers retrospectively reviewed MRI examinations of 428 ankles in 424 patients (211 males and 213 females; mean age 43 years) with reported osteochondral talar lesions. The frequency of involvement and size of lesion for each zone were recorded.[99]

Lesions in the medial third of the talar dome were significantly larger in surface area involvement and deeper than those at the lateral talar dome. Lesions in the transverse center third of the talar dome (zones 2, 5, and 8) were larger in surface area than either medial or lateral zones. Most importantly, the medial central talar dome (zone 4) was most frequently involved individual zone with 227 of the 428 (53.0%) lesions located there.[99]

Malleolar osteotomies allow for access to the ankle joint when an open approach is required (Fig. 50.15). A cadaveric study by Muir et al.[100] evaluated 9 cadaveric ankles dissected in

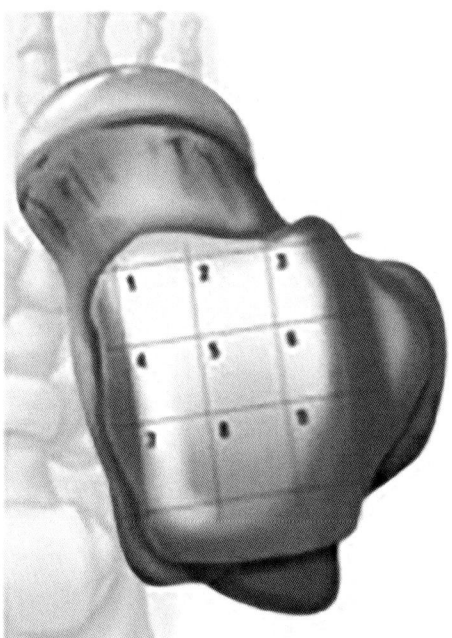

FIGURE 50.14 Anatomical nine-zone grid scheme on the talar dome. Diagram shows the 9 equal surface area zones, with zones 1, 4, and 7 positioned on the medial talus and zones 1, 2, and 3 positioned anteriorly. (Reproduced from Elias I, Zoga AC, Morrison WB, Besser MP, Schweitzer ME, Raikin SM. Osteochondral lesions of the talus: localization and morphologic data from 424 patients using a novel anatomical grid scheme. *Foot Ankle Int.* 2007;28(2):154-161.)

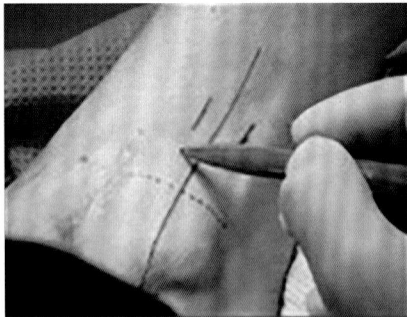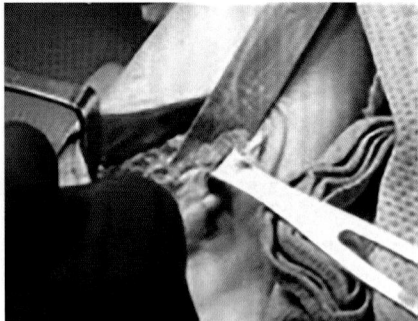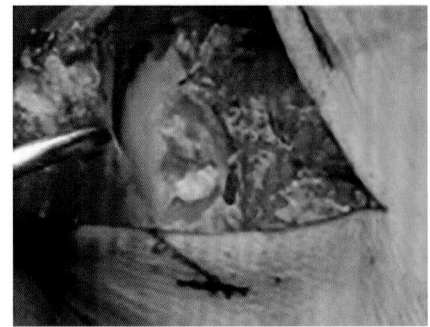

FIGURE 50.15 Lateral malleolar osteotomy performed for access to talar dome lesion.

a standard fashion to expose the talar dome. Seven approaches were used, including 4 arthrotomies (anteromedial, antero-lateral, posteromedial, and posterolateral) and 3 osteotomies (anterolateral, distal fibula, and medial malleolar). Their results showed that on average, 17% of the medial talar dome and 20% of the lateral talar dome could not be accessed without an osteotomy. On the lateral aspect of the superior talar dome, an anterolateral osteotomy added a mean of 22% sagittal plane exposure. They concluded that malleolar osteotomies provide access to the entire medial and lateral sides; however, there remains a mean residual 15% of the central talar dome that cannot be accessed in a perpendicular manner with any approach.[100]

Malleolar osteotomies can be performed on the distal tibia or fibula for medial or lateral joint access. Osteotomy techniques were first described by Ray and Coughlin in 1947, describing a transverse osteotomy.[101] Other techniques have been described since then including oblique, crescentic, step-cut, modified step-cut, invert U, and bi-plane chevron osteotomies.[102] When performing malleolar osteotomies, it is important to predrill your fixation screw holes to allow for proper apposition and alignment when replacing the medial or lateral malleolus at the conclusion of the procedure. Malleolar osteotomies allow for perpendicular access; however, an osteotomy displacement can

result in local ankle arthritis. Gaulrapp et al.[103] demonstrated in their series of oblique osteotomies that they commonly led to osteoarthritis. Their study evaluated 22 patients who underwent oblique osteotomies and reported up to 50% of ankles developed arthritic changes within 5 years of the operation.[103] The main risk associated with malleolar osteotomies is postfixation displacement, leading to delayed healing or malunion (Fig. 50.16). Van Bergen et al.[104] reported that a screw angle mismatch leads to excessive shear stress across the osteotomy site that can result in postoperative displacement.[104] A study by Bull et al.[102] reviewed 50 biplane medial malleolar chevron osteotomies fixated with 2 lag screws. Their results showed a 30% nonunion rate with an average of 2 mm of incongruence seen on radiographs. They suggested the use of a medial buttress plate in addition to two parallel screws to reduce postoperative osteotomy displacement.[102]

PEARLS

The author rarely utilizes malleolar osteotomies these days since almost all osteochondral defects can be accessed through standard anterior portals if proper noninvasive distraction is performed.

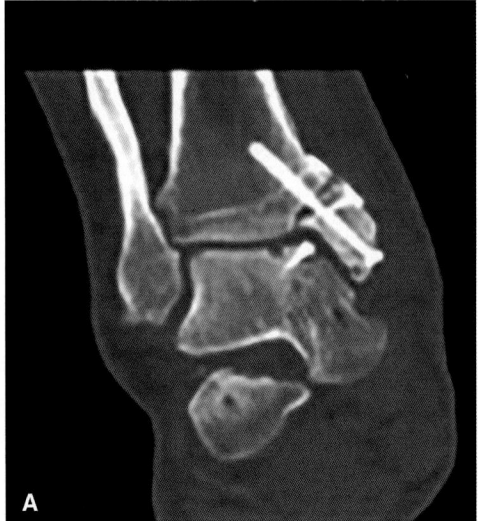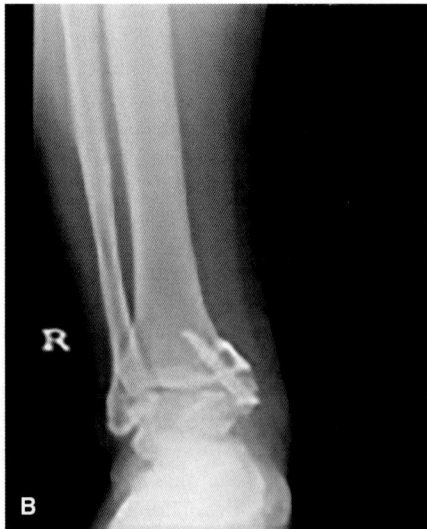

FIGURE 50.16 CT image **(A)** and plain film radiograph **(B)** of failed medial malleolar osteotomy performed for talar access.

There is much debate in the literature surrounding the question of why some osteochondral lesions are painful and others are not. One new ideology reevaluates the theory that pain is caused by the chondral lesion itself and redirects the source to be initiated by underlying bone marrow edema. It is believed that intra-articular pressure forces synovial fluid through micro fissures in the subchondral plate, causing subchondral cysts and the formation of bone marrow lesions.

A new technique involves injecting flowable synthetic calcium phosphate directly into the bone marrow lesion. This technique buttresses the internal architecture of the bone marrow lesion, providing stability and allowing healing with internal support.

The technique involves standard arthroscopic technique followed by identification and visualization of the osteochondral lesion to identify the location of the defect to assist in triangulation to make sure placement is accurate. The injectable synthetic calcium phosphate is then placed directly into the bone marrow lesion under fluoroscopic and/or arthroscopic guidance. Using fluoroscopy and the original MRI as reference, a cannula is inserted into the area of the bone marrow lesion with care taken to correlate and triangulate positioning on true AP and lateral views. Injection is done under thumb pressure only, in order to flow into the area of insufficient bone. Leakage into the joint often will occur and is easily removed with an arthroscopic shaver. The leakage into the joint may be a sign of accurate placement. Another indication of proper placement includes the extrusion of fat bubbles from the osteochondral lesion.

New indications for this procedure are being tested and developed constantly. It has the ability to stabilize insufficient or necrotic bone seen with failed microfracture and holds much promise for the future.

A relatively new technique using the flapped chondral fragment as an autograft has emerged called lift, drill, fill, and fix (LDFF). This approach is limited to lesions in which the chondral fragment remains intact. The approach is contraindicated when the flap is loose and floating. The procedure requires subchondral drilling of the defect, followed by fixation of the overlying cartilage flap with a recessed absorbable compressive screw. The procedure can be performed either open or arthroscopically. There is not much literature to support the technique; however, the results from the limited studies do seem promising.[105] One study looked at 9 subjects with a 4-year follow-up period and their results showed 78% good results and 22% fair results when using the Berndt-Harty clinical outcomes scale.[106] Another study looked at 7 patients who underwent arthroscopic LDFF for large, painful osteochondral lesions of the talus present for more than 1 year. Their results demonstrated improvement in the AOFAS score to 99 and pain numeric rating scale improvement to 0.1.[107] Although results do seem promising, more large, long-term prospective studies are needed to know the long-term benefits of LDFF.

Pluripotent cell injections have become a hot topic in recent years. Studies show that pluripotent MSCs can be influenced to produce chondrocytes. A study by Tabet et al.[89] conducted in 2014 evaluated the use of hypothermically stored human amniotic membrane for cartilage repair in adult sheep. The study showed that the defects that successfully retained the graft had evidence of diffuse chondrocyte cell proliferation and showed a stromal matrix similar to hyaline cartilage.[89] Unfortunately, there is not much in the literature on this technique currently;

however, we can expect to see many more studies in the near future on this emerging topic.

The treatment of OCD repair is evolving and there are many options for cartilage repair. It is the physician/surgeon's duty to review the literature and make an educated decision on the best way to approach each individual lesion. The author's preferred technique for OCDs of all sizes includes ankle arthroscopic debridement and OCD visualization. This is followed by excision of loose chondral or osteochondral fragments, and abrasion chondroplasty with an arthroscopic shaver, leaving the edges of the defect perpendicular to the bone surfaces. In cases where bone marrow lesions lie under the OCD, injectable synthetic calcium phosphate is placed directly into the bone marrow lesion under fluoroscopic and/or arthroscopic guidance. The purpose of the flowable synthetic calcium phosphate is to buttress the internal architecture of the bone marrow lesion, providing stability and allowing healing with internal support. The authors then perform the arthroscopic PJAC technique previously described to fill the OCD.[50]

New studies are ongoing to show long-term efficacy of various techniques and will hopefully help to guide treatment algorithms in the future. Other techniques are constantly being explored and performed arthroscopically. Utilization of adult cartilage cells and scaffolds, use of pluripotent amnion membrane, and using a biologic stimulant such as BMAC to enhance the regrowth of hyaline or hyalinelike cartilage are being performed. Treatment of OCDs of the talus has historically followed treatment guidelines that have been established in the knee. We have seen the rise and fall of techniques such as microfracture and the change in thought process that we use to guide our treatments. In the future, we will see new techniques and technologies to assist us in improving patient outcomes. The primary goal of all OCD treatment is the restoration of the articular cartilage to most closely resemble its native state, consisting of type 2 collagen.

REFERENCES

1. Valderrabano V, Horisberger M, Russell I, et al. Etiology of ankle arthritis. *Clin Orthop Relat Res*. 2009;467(7):1800-1806.
2. Hayes DW Jr, Averett RK. Articular cartilage transplantation. Current and future limitations and solutions. *Clin Podiatr Med Surg*. 2001;18:161-176.
3. Steele JR, Dekker TJ, Federer AE, Liles JL, Adams SB, Easley ME. Osteochondral lesions of the talus: current concepts in diagnosis and treatment. *Foot Ankle Orthop*. 2018;3(3).
4. Anderson DD, Chubinskaya S, Guilak F, et al. Peculiarities in ankle cartilage. *Cartilage*. 2017;8(1):12-18.
5. Shepherd DE, Seedhom BB. Thickness of human articular cartilage in joints of the lower limb. *Ann Rheum Dis*. 1999;58:27-34.
6. Millington SA, Grabner M, Wozelka Mag R, et al. Quantification of ankle articular cartilage topography and thickness using a high resolution stereophotography system. *Osteoarthritis Cartilage*. 2007;15:205-211.
7. Weiss JM, Shea AG, Jacobs Jr, et al. Incidence of osteochondritis dissecans in adults. *Am J Sports Med*. 2018;46(7):1592-1595.
8. Kravitz AB. Osteochondral autogenous transplantation for an osteochondral defect of the first metatarsal head: a case report. *J Foot Ankle Surg*. 2005;44:152-155.
9. Kessler JI, Weiss JM, Nikizad H, et al. Osteochondritis dissecans of the ankle in children and adolescents: demographics and epidemiology. *Am J Sports Med*. 2014;42(9):2165-2171.
10. Barnes CJ, Ferkel RD. Arthroscopic debridement and drilling of osteochondral lesions of the talus. *Foot Ankle Clin*. 2003;8(2):243-257.
11. Siegel SJ, Mount AC. Step-cut medial malleolar osteotomy: literature review and case studies. *J Foot Ankle Surg*. 2012;51(2):226-233.
12. Bohndorf K, Imhof H, Schibany N. Diagnostic imaging of acute and chronic osteochondral lesions of the talus. *Orthopade*. 2001;30(1):9-12.
13. Linklater JM. Imaging of talar dome chondral and osteochondral lesions. *Tech Foot Ankle Surg*. 2008;7:140-151.
14. Levy AS, Lohnes J, Sculley S, LeCroy M, Garrett W. Chondral delamination of the knee in soccer players. *Am J Sports Med*. 1996;24:634-639.
15. Steadman JR, Rodkey WG, Rodrigo JJ. Microfracture: surgical technique and rehabilitation to treat chondral defects. *Clin Orthop Relat Res*. 2001;(391 suppl):S362-S369.

16. Kendell SD, Helms CA, Rampton JW, Garrett WE, Higgins LD. MRI appearance of chondral delamination injuries of the knee. *Am J Roentgenol.* 2005;184:1486-1489.

17. Hopkinson WJ, Mitchell WA, Curl WW. Chondral fractures of the knee: cause for confusion. *Am J Sports Med.* 1985;13:309-312.

18. Ateshian GA, Lai WM, Zhu WB, et al. An asymptomatic solution for the contact of two biphasic cartilage layers. *J Biomech.* 1994;27:1347-1360.

19. Van Dijk CN, Reilingh ML, Zengerink M, et al. Osteochondral defects in the ankle: why painful? *Knee Surg Sports Traumatol Arthrosc.* 2010;18:570-580.

20. Rangger C, Kathrein A, Freund MC, et al. Bone bruise of the knee: histology and cryosections in 5 cases. *Acta Orthop Scand.* 1998;69:291-294.

21. Ryu KN, Jin W, Ko YT, et al. Bone bruises: MR characteristics and histological correlation in the young pig. *Clin Imaging.* 2000;24:371-380.

22. Eriksen EF, Ringe JD. Bone marrow lesions: a universal bone response to injury? *Rheumatol Int.* 2012;32(3):575-584.

23. Solheim E, Hegna J, Inderhaug E. Long-term survival after microfracture and mosaicplasty for knee articular cartilage repair: a comparative study between two treatments cohorts. *Cartilage.* 2018;11:71-76.

24. Loomer R, Fisher C, Lloyd-Smith R, et al. Osteochondral lesions of the talus. *Am J Sports Med.* 1993;21:13-19.

25. Schmid MR, Pfirrmann CW, Hodler J, et al. Cartilage lesions in the ankle joint: comparison of MR arthrography and CT arthrography. *Skeletal Radiol.* 2003;32:259-265.

26. Badekas T, Takvorian M, Souras N. Treatment principles for osteochondral lesions in the foot and ankle. *Int Orthoped.* 2013;37(9):1697-1706.

27. Young AA, Stanwell P, Williams A, et al. Glycosaminoglycan content of knee cartilage following posterior cruciate ligament rupture demonstrated by delayed gadolinium-enhanced magnetic resonance imaging of cartilage (dGEMRIC). A case report. *J Bone Joint Surg Am.* 2005;87:2763-2767.

28. Hannila I, Nieminen MT, Rauvala E, et al. Patellar cartilage lesions: comparison of magnetic resonance imaging and T2 relaxation-time mapping. *Acta Radiol.* 2007;48:444-448.

29. Li X, Benjamin Ma C, Link TM, et al. In vivo T(1rho) and T(2) mapping of articular cartilage in osteoarthritis of the knee using 3 T MRI. *Osteoarthritis Cartilage.* 2007;15:789-797.

30. Mamisch TC, Menzel MI, Welsch GH, et al. Steady-state diffusion imaging for MR in-vivo evaluation of reparative cartilage after matrix-associated autologous chondrocyte transplantation at 3 tesla—preliminary results. *Eur J Radiol.* 2008;65:72-79.

31. Prado MP, Kennedy JG, Raduan F, Nery C. Diagnosis and treatment of osteochondral lesions of the ankle: current concepts. *Rev Bras Ortop.* 2016;51(5):489-500.

32. Pettine KA, Morrey BF. Osteochondral fractures of the talus. *J Bone Joint Surg.* 1987;69(1):89-92.

33. Berndt AL, Harty M. Transchondral fractures (osteochondritis dissecans) of the talus. *J Bone Joint Surg.* 1959;41-A:988-1020.

34. Barg A, Pagenstert G, Leumann A, et al. Malleolar osteotomy-osteotomy as approach. *Orthopade.* 2013;42(5):309-321.

35. Van Dijk CN, van Bergen CJ. Advancements in ankle arthroscopy. *J Am Acad Orthop Surg.* 2008;16:635-646.

36. Seow D, Yasui Y, Hutchinson ID, Hurley ET, Shimozono Y, Kennedy JG. The subchondral bone is affected by bone marrow stimulation: a systematic review of preclinical animal studies. *Cartilage.* 2019;10(1):70-81.

37. McGahan PJ, Pinney SJ. Current concept review: osteochondral lesions of the talus. *Foot Ankle Int.* 2010;31:90-98.

38. O'Driscoll SW. The healing and regeneration of articular cartilage. *J Bone Joint Surg Am.* 1998;80:1795-1812.

39. Hunt SA, Sherman O. Arthroscopic treatment of osteochondral lesions of the talus with correlation of outcome systems. *Arthroscopy.* 2003;19(4):360-367.

40. Shimozono Y, Coale M, Yasui Y, O'Halloran A, Deyer TW, Kennedy JG. Subchondral bone degradation after microfracture for osteochondral lesions of the talus: an MRI analysis. *Am J Sports Med.* 2018;46(3):642-648.

41. Salzmann GM, Sah B, Südkamp NP, Niemeyer P. Reoperative characteristics after microfracture of knee cartilage lesions in 454 patients. *Knee Surg Sports Traumatol Arthrosc.* 2013;21(2):365-371.

42. Steadman JR, Briggs KK, Matheny LM, Guillet A, Hanson CM, Willimon SC. Outcomes following microfracture of full-thickness articular cartilage lesions of the knee in adolescent patients. *J Knee Surg.* 2015;28(2):145-150.

43. Gobbi A, Kumar A, Karnatzikos G. Microfracture treatment in athletes with knee grade IV chondral lesions: a 10-year follow up. Paper #16.3.5. Presented at the International Cartilage Repair Society World Congress 2012. May 12–15. Montreal.

44. Bae DK, Song SJ, Yoon KH, Heo DB, Kim TJ. Survival analysis of microfracture in the osteoarthritic knee-minimum 10-year follow-up. *Arthroscopy.* 2013;29(2):244-250.

45. Gobbi A, Francisco RA, Lubowitz JH, Allegra F, Canata G. Osteochondral lesions of the talus: randomized controlled trial comparing chondroplasty, microfracture, and osteochondral autograft transplantation. *Arthroscopy.* 2006;22(10):1085-1092.

46. Furukawa T, Eyre DR, Koide S, Glimcher MJ. Biochemical studies on repair cartilage resurfacing experimental defects in the rabbit knee. *J Bone Joint Surg Am.* 1980;62:79-89.

47. Akizuki S, Yasukawa Y, Takizawa T. Does arthroscopic abrasion arthroplasty promote cartilage regeneration in osteoarthritic knees with eburnation? A prospective study of high tibial osteotomy with abrasion arthroplasty versus high tibial osteotomy alone. *Arthroscopy.* 1997;13:9-17.

48. Gobbi A, Whyte GP. One-stage cartilage repair using a hyaluronic acid-based scaffold with activated bone marrow-derived mesenchymal stem cells compared with microfracture: five-year follow-up. *Am J Sports Med.* 2016;44:2846-2854.

49. Gobbi A, Whyte GP. Long-term clinical outcomes of one-stage cartilage repair in the knee with hyaluronic acid-based scaffold embedded with mesenchymal stem cells sourced from bone marrow aspirate concentrate. *Am J Sports Med.* 2019;47(7):1621-1628.

50. Kruse DL, Ng A, Paden M, Stone PA. Arthroscopic de novo NT® juvenile allograft cartilage implantation in the talus: a case presentation. *J Foot Ankle Surg.* 2012;51:218-221.

51. Bartlett W, Skinner JA, Gooding CR, et al. Autologous chondrocyte implantation versus matrix-induced autologous chondrocyte implantation for osteochondral defects of the knee: a prospective, randomized study. *J Bone Joint Surg Br.* 2005;87:640-645.

52. Malinin T, Temple HT, Buck BE. Transplantation of osteochondral allografts after cold storage. *J Bone Joint Surg Am.* 2006;88:762-770.

53. Lu Y, Dhanaraj S, Wang Z, et al. Minced cartilage without cell culture serves as an effective intraoperative cell source for cartilage repair. *J Orthop Res.* 2006;24:1261-1270.

54. Farr J. Allograft particulate cartilage transplantation: DeNovo natural tissue (NT) graft. In: Brittberg M, Gersoff W, eds. *Cartilage Surgery: An Operative Manual.* Philadelphia, PA: WB Saunders; 2010: 175-180.

55. Yanke AB, Tilton AK, Wetters NG, Merkow DB, Cole BJ. DeNovo NT particulated juvenile cartilage implant. *Sports Med Arthrosc Rev.* 2015;23(3):125-129.

56. Harris JD, Frank RM, McCormick FM, et al. Minced cartilage techniques. *Oper Tech Orthop.* 2014;24:27-34.

57. Farr J, Cole BJ, Sherman S, et al. Particulated articular cartilage: CAIS and DeNovo NT. *J Knee Surg.* 2012;25:23-29.

58. Farr J, Tabet SK, Margerrison E, et al. Clinical, radiographic, and histological outcomes after cartilage repair with particulated juvenile articular cartilage: a 2-year prospective study. *Am J Sports Med.* 2014;42:1417-1425.

59. Adams SB, Yao JQ, Schon LC. Particulated juvenile articular cartilage allograft transplantation for osteochondral lesions of the talus. *Tech Foot Ankle Surg.* 2011;10(2):92-98.

60. Saltzman BM, Lin J, Lee S. Particulated juvenile articular cartilage allograft transplantation for osteochondral talar lesions. *Cartilage.* 2017;8(1):61-72.

61. Ng A, Bernhard A, Bernhard K. Advances in ankle cartilage repair. *Clin Podiatr Med Surg.* 2017;34(4):471-485.

62. Hatic SO, Berlet GC. Particulated juvenile articular cartilage graft (DeNovo NT Graft) for treatment of osteochondral lesions of the talus. *Foot Ankle Spec.* 2010;3(6):361-364.

63. Willers C, Wood DJ, Zheng MH. A current review of the biology and treatment of articular cartilage defects. *J Musculoskeletal Res.* 2003;7:157-181.

64. Visna P, Pasa L, Cizmar I, et al. Treatment of deep cartilage defects of the knee using autologous chondrograft transplantation and by abrasive techniques: a randomized controlled study. *Acta Chir Belg.* 2004;104:709-714.

65. Chopra V, Chang D, Ng A, Kruse DL, Stone PA. Arthroscopic Treatment of Osteochondral Lesions of the Talus Utilizing Juvenile Particulated Cartilage Allograft: A Case Series. *J Foot Ankle Surg.* 2020;59(2):436-439.

66. Namba RS, Meuli M, Sullivan KM, Le AX, Adzick NS. Spontaneous repair of superficial defects in articular cartilage in a fetal lamb model. *J Bone Joint Surg Am.* 1998;80:4-10.

67. Lui PPY. Identity of tendon stem cells—how much do we know? *J Cell Mol Med.* 2013;17:55-64.

68. Adkisson HD, Martin JA, Amendola RL, et al. The potential of human allogeneic juvenile chondrocytes for restoration of articular cartilage. *Am J Sports Med.* 2010;38(7):1324-1333.

69. Adkisson HD, Gillis MP, Davis EC, et al. In vitro generation of scaffold independent neocartilage. *Clin Orthop Relat Res.* 2001;391:S280-S294.

70. Bonasia DE, Martin JA, Marmotti A, et al. Cocultures of adult and juvenile chondrocytes compared with adult and juvenile chondral fragments in vitro matrix production. *Am J Sports Med.* 2011;39:2355-2361.

71. Lanham NS, Carroll JJ, Cooper MT, Perumal V, Park JS. A comparison of outcomes of particulated juvenile articular cartilage and bone marrow aspirate concentrate for articular cartilage lesions of the talus. *Foot Ankle Spec.* 2017;10(4):315-321.

72. Dekker TJ, Steele JR, Federer AE, Easley ME, Hamid KS, Adams SB. Efficacy of particulated juvenile cartilage allograft transplantation for osteochondral lesions of the talus. *Foot Ankle Int.* 2018;39(3):278-283.

73. Tan EW, Finney FT, Maccario C, Talusan PG, Zhang Z, Schon LC. Histological and gross evaluation through second-look arthroscopy of osteochondral lesions of the talus after failed treatment with particulated juvenile cartilage: a case series. *J Orthop Case Rep.* 2018;8(2):69-73.

74. Karnovsky SC, DeSandis B, Haleem AM, Sofka CM, O'Malley M, Drakos MC. Comparison of juvenile allogenous articular cartilage and bone marrow aspirate concentrate versus microfracture with and without bone marrow aspirate concentrate in arthroscopic treatment of talar osteochondral lesions. *Foot Ankle Int.* 2018;39(4):393-405.

75. Wang T, Belkin NS, Burge AJ, et al. Patellofemoral cartilage lesions treated with particulated juvenile allograft cartilage: a prospective study with minimum 2-year clinical and magnetic resonance imaging outcomes. *Arthroscopy.* 2018;34(5):1498-1505.

76. Adams GD, Mall NA, Fortier LA, et al. BioCartilage: background and operative technique. *Oper Tech Sports Med.* 2013;21:116-124.

77. Mascarenhas R., Saltzman B.M., Fortier L.A., Cole B.J. BioCartilage: New frontiers in cartilage restoration. In: *Cartilage e-book.* CIC Edizioni Internazionali; Rome. 2015:183-193.

78. Shieh AK, Singh SG, Nathe C, et al. Effects of micronized cartilage matrix on cartilage repair in osteochondral lesions of the talus. *Cartilage.* 2018;11:316-322.

79. Desai S. Surgical treatment of a tibial osteochondral defect with debridement, marrow stimulation, and micronized allograft cartilage matrix: report of an all-arthroscopic technique. *J Foot Ankle Surg.* 2016;55(2):279-282.

80. Hatch EL. Burns and bravery. In: Hatch EL, Médico E, eds. *My Life as a Country Doctor in Mexico;* 1999:193-195.

81. Gwei-Djen L, Needham J. Medieval preparations of urinary steroid hormones. *Int J Hist Med.* 1964;8:101-121.

82. Davis S. Skin transplantation: with a review of 550 cases at the Johns Hopkins Hospital. *Johns Hosp Med J.* 1910;15:307-396.

83. Sabella N. Use of the fetal membranes in skin grafting. *Med Reconcil NY.* 1913;83:478-480.

84. Stern M. The grafting of preserved amniotic membrane to burned and ulcerated surfaces. Substituting skin grafts. *J Am Med Assoc.* 1913;60:973-974.

85. Douglas B. Homografts of fetal membranes as a covering for large wounds—especially those from burns: an experimental and clinical study (preliminary report). *J Tenn Med Assoc.* 1952;45:230-235.

86. DeRotth A. Plastic repair of conjunctival defects with fetal membranes. *Arch Ophthal.* 1940;23:522-525.

87. Shimberg M. The use of amniotic fluid concentrates in orthopaedic conditions. *J Bone Joint Surg.* 1938;20:167-177.

88. Sachs BP, Stern CM. Activity and characterization of a low molecular fraction present in human amniotic fluid with broad spectrum antibacterial activity. *Br J Obstet Gynaecol.* 1979;86:81-86.

89. Tabet SK, Clark AL, Chapman EB, Thal D. The use of hypothermically stored amniotic membrane cartilage repair: a sheep study. *Stem Cell Discov.* 2015;5(4):62-71.

90. Tabet SK, Kimmerling KA, Mowry KC, Munson NR. Implantation of Fresh Amniotic Membrane for the Treatment of Cartilage Defects. 2019 ISAKOS Biennial Congress ePoster #316. 2019.

91. Zengerink M, Struijs P, Tol J, et al. Treatment of osteochondral lesions of the talus: a systemic review. *Knee Surg Sports Traumatol Arthrosc.* 2010;18(2):238-246.

92. Laffenetre O. Osteochondral lesions of the talus: current concept. *Orthop Traumatol Surg Res.* 2010;96(5):554-566.

93. Gautier E, Kolker D, Jacob R. Treatment of cartilage defects of the talus by autologous osteochondral grafts. *Bone Joint J.* 2002;84(2):237-244.

94. Hangody L, Fules P. Autologous osteochondral mosaicplasty for the treatment of full-thickness defects of weight-bearing joints: ten years of experimental and clinical experience. *J Bone Joint Surg Am.* 2003;85a(suppl 2):25-32.

95. Berlet G, Hyer C, Philbin T, et al. Does fresh osteochondral allograft transplantation of talar osteochondral defects improve function? *Clin Orthop Relat Res.* 2011;469(8):2356-2366.

96. Richter DL, Tanksley JA, Miller MD. Osteochondral autograft transplantation: a review of the surgical technique and outcomes. *Sports Med Arthrosc Rev.* 2016;24(2):74-78.

97. Bisicchia S, Rosso F, Amendola A. Osteochondral allograft of the talus. *Iowa Orthop J.* 2014;34:30-37.

98. Vannini F, Buda R, Pagliazzi G, Ruffilli A, Cavallo M, Giannini S. Osteochondral allografts in the ankle joint: state of the art. *Cartilage.* 2013;4(3):204-213.

99. Elias I, Zoga AC, Morrison WB, Besser MP, Schweitzer ME, Raikin SM. Osteochondral lesions of the talus: localization and morphologic data from 424 patients using a novel anatomical grid scheme. *Foot Ankle Int.* 2007;28(2):154-161.

100. Muir D, Saltzman CL, Tochigi Y, Amendola N. Talar dome access for osteochondral lesions. *Am J Sports Med.* 2006;34(9):1457-1463.

101. Ray RB, Coughlin EJ Jr. Osteochondral dissecans of the talus. *J Bone Joint Surg Am.* 1947;29(3):697-706.

102. Bull PE, Berlet GC, Canini C, Hyer CF. Rate of malunion following bi-plane chevron medial malleolar osteotomy. *Foot Ankle Int.* 2016;37(6):620-626.

103. Gaulrapp H, Hagena FW, Wasmer G. Postoperative evaluation of osteochondrosis dissecans of the talus with special reference to medial malleolar osteotomy [in German]. *Zeitschrift fur Orthopadie und ihre Grenzgebiete.* 1996;134(4):346-353.

104. van Bergen CJ, Tuijthof GJ, Sierevelt IN, van Dijk CN. Direction of the oblique medial malleolar osteotomy for exposure of the talus. *Arch Orthop Trauma Surg.* 2011;131(7):893-901.

105. Reilingh ML, Kerkhoffs GMMJ. Lift, drill, fill and fix (LDFF): a cartilage preservation technique in osteochondral talar defects. In: *Cartilage Lesions of the Ankle.* Berlin: Springer; 2015.

106. Reilingh ML, Kerhoffs GM, Telkamp CJ, et al. Treatment of osteochondral defects of the talus in children. *Knee Surg Sports Traumatol Arthrosc.* 2014;22(9):2243-2249.

107. Kerhoffs GMMJ, Reilingh ML, Gerards RM, et al. Lift, drill, fill and fix (LDFF): a new arthroscopic treatment for talar osteochondral defects. *Knee Surg Sports Traumatol Arthrosc.* 2016;24(4):1265-1271.

Acquired Peripheral Nerve Pathologies

D. Scot Malay, Andreas C. Kaikis, and William Brownell

Acquired peripheral nerve pathologies are common in the lower extremities, and all of the nerves in the foot, ankle, and leg are susceptible to injury by entrapment, compression, traction, laceration, intraneural tumor formation, or incarceration in scar. Although the term *nerve entrapment* can be used to describe any type of localized, acquired peripheral nerve trunk lesion due to external influences, Kopell and Thompson[1] classically described entrapment neuropathy as "a region of localized injury and inflammation in a peripheral nerve that is caused by mechanical irritation from some impinging anatomical neighbor." In practice, acquired peripheral neuropathy has many local causes, and clinical signs and symptoms vary according to the extent of nerve damage and the specific nerve trunk involved. Although the biomedical literature is replete with reviews of nerve entrapment syndromes,[2,3] much still remains to be learned about the diagnosis and treatment of the wide variety of painful and disabling acquired neuropathies that affect the lower extremities. Peripheral nerve pain and paresthesia can also develop secondary to the presence of an intraneural lesion, such as nerve sheath tumor, a lipoma, or a ganglion cyst.[4] The evaluation and management of acquired peripheral nerve pathologies, whether due to an extra- or intraneural lesion, involves fundamental methods that apply to any peripheral nerve lesion, as well as specialized methods used to address specific types of lesions.

Anatomically speaking, all peripheral nerve trunks are mixed nerves containing sensory, motor, and autonomic fibers. Approximately 50% of the peripheral nerve trunk is made up of connective tissue[5] (Fig. 51.1). It is this intraneural connective tissue that, when appropriately stimulated, may proliferate and disrupt the internal continuity of the peripheral nerve trunk. Resultant intraneural fibrosis, alone or in combination with extraneural scarring, can cause symptomatic neuritis. Diagnosis of such a nerve lesion requires a thorough knowledge of both the segmental (*dermatomal*) distribution and the specific cutaneous distribution (*anatomical nerve trunk*) supplying the lower extremities (Fig. 51.2). Furthermore, an understanding of the motor innervation to the lower extremity aids in diagnosis when an abnormal deep tendon reflex or muscle weakness is present (Table 51.1).

ETIOLOGY OF LOCALIZED ACQUIRED PERIPHERAL NEUROPATHY

Localized, acquired peripheral neuropathy may develop after acute gross *trauma* or recurrent microtrauma, induced by either endogenous or exogenous sources, when inflammation infiltrates the nerve trunk and surrounding tissues. Severe pain in the peripheral nervous system can be attributed to three pathophysiologic conditions: end-neuroma (stump neuroma), neuroma-in-continuity, and nerves that are impinged upon by an adjacent anatomic or pathologic structure, such as scar tissue, or by an intraneural lesion, such as a tumor. Usually, the gross continuity of the nerve trunk is maintained, and the nerve may swell proximal to the point of injury or compression.[6] In cases of nerve entrapment, a fusiform or eccentric neuroma-in-continuity usually develops at the point of impingement. Intraneural fibrosis subsequently proceeds to disrupt the nerve fiber's myelin sheath and alters impulse conduction causing neuritis. Intraneural fibrosis also inhibits axonal remyelination.[7] If the pathologic influence is allowed to continue, or if acute sectioning or compression or traction injury occurs, then various degrees of nerve trunk disruption can occur. Blunt injuries that disrupt the myelin sheath of the nerve fibers can result in neuropraxia, which can last anywhere from hours to weeks, as the myelin sheath regenerates and a full or nearly full recovery ensues. More forceful compression, or traction, or even chemical or thermal injury, can damage the myelin sheath as well as axons, resulting in axonotmesis and more symptoms that require longer to heal, with a reduced likelihood of full recovery. Still further, partial- and full-thickness lacerations, avulsions, and crush injuries can disrupt even the epineural sheath and the gross structural integrity of the nerve trunk, resulting in neurotmesis, and almost guaranteeing a long and incomplete recovery, even when surgical intervention is employed to restore gross structural continuity. When axons are disrupted, distal wallerian degeneration will ensue, and actual myxoid degeneration of intraneural connective tissue with multifocal ganglion formation can develop.[8-11] Extraneural scarring and adhesion (perineural fibrosis) aggravate neuritis, and as extraneural fibrosis and resultant compression progresses, occlusion of the vasa nervorum ensues. Nerve ischemia leads to further degeneration, decreased impulse conduction, and increased symptoms. When the connective tissue framework of the nerve is altered, there is a heightened inflammatory response around the nerve. An excessive deposition of collagen interacts with regenerating nerve fibers causing a haphazard pattern known as a neuroma.[12] The neuroma then alters signal conduction through the affected nerve and causing hyperexcitability by abnormal accumulation of potassium and sodium ion channels on the axons in the neuroma, characterized as *ectopic neuralgia*.[13] Ectopic neuralgia facilitates the spontaneous pain that patients feel that causes discharges without any noxious impetus.

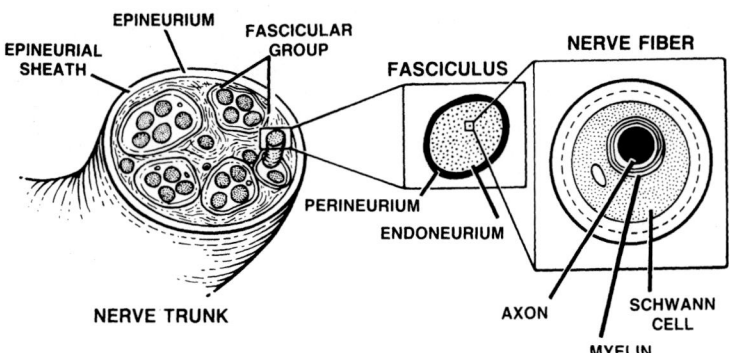

FIGURE 51.1 Peripheral nerve trunk functional and structural anatomy.

The natural history of untreated localized acquired peripheral neuropathy is unpredictable. Symptoms may spontaneously worsen, resolve to a degree, or resolve only to recur on an intermittent basis. When nerve injury has resulted in regional denervation, reinnervation from collateral sprouting of adjacent donor nerves can occur, either spontaneously or by means of surgical neurotization with adjacent nerve. A wide variety of mechanisms, ranging from repetitive microtrauma to acute injury, compression and traction and sectioning injuries, damage secondary to medications and toxins, can cause localized, acquired peripheral neuropathy. It should also be noted that entrapment neuropathy is very common in patients with

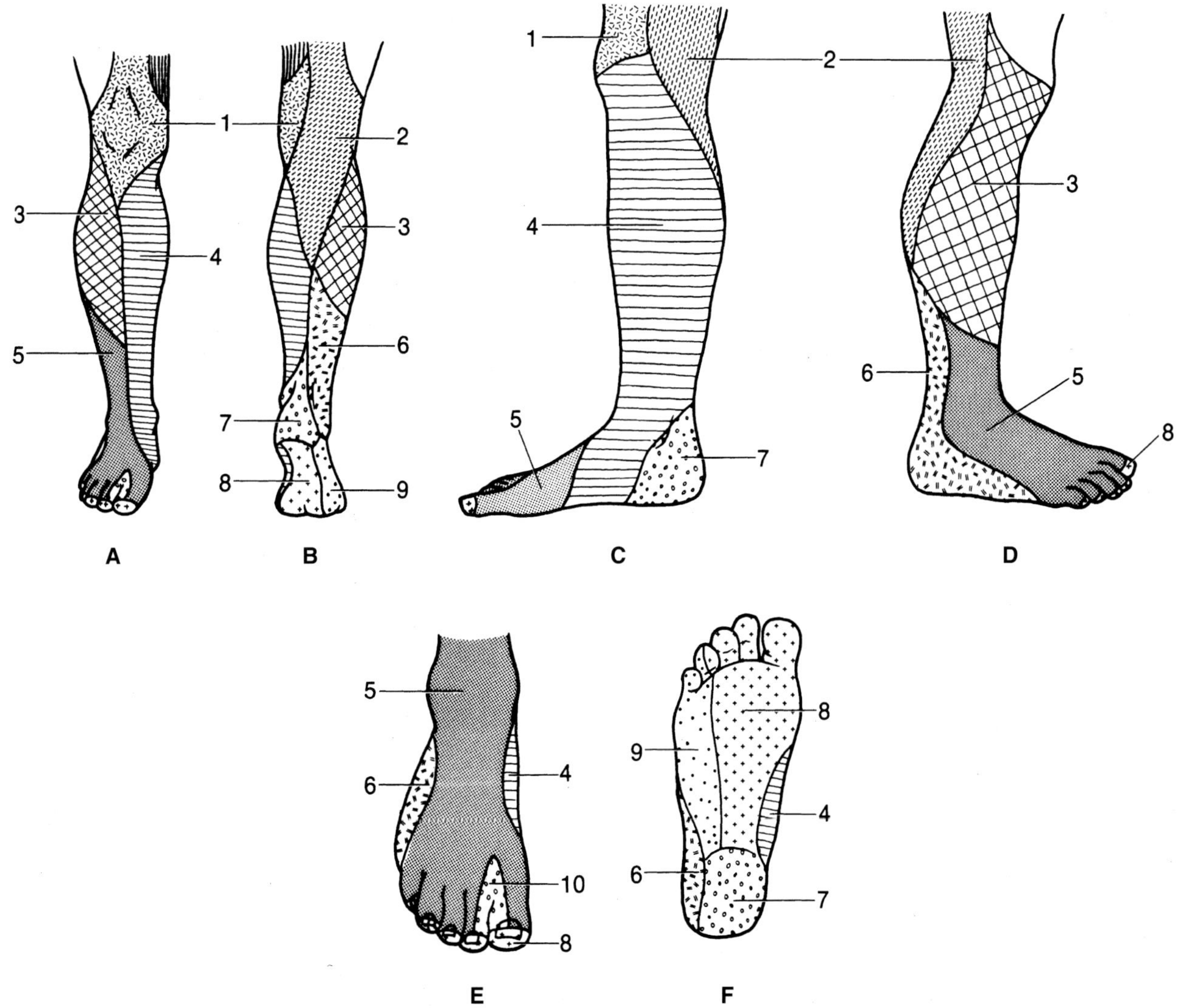

FIGURE 51.2 Peripheral nerve distribution. **A.** Anterior. **B.** Posterior. **C.** Medial. **D.** Lateral. **E.** Dorsal. **F.** Plantar. *1*, medial and intermediate femoral cutaneous nerves (L2-L3); *2*, posterior femoral cutaneous nerve (S1-S3); *3*, lateral sural cutaneous nerve (L5, S1-S2); *4*, saphenous nerve (L3-L4); *5*, superficial peroneal nerve (L4-L5, S1); *6*, sural nerve (L5, S1-S2); *7*, medial calcaneal branch of tibial nerve (S1-S2); *8*, medial plantar nerve (L4-L5); *9*, lateral plantar nerve (S1-S2); *10*, deep peroneal nerve (L4-L5).

TABLE 51.1 Motor Innervation to the Leg and Foot

Anatomic Location	Muscle(s)	Peripheral Nerve	Spinal Level(s)
Anterior leg	Tibialis anterior	Deep peroneal	L4-L5
	Extensor digitorum longus	Deep peroneal	L4-L5
	Extensor hallucis longus	Deep peroneal	L4-L5
	Peroneus tertius	Deep peroneal	L4-L5
Lateral (peroneal) leg	Peroneus longus	Superficial peroneal	L5, S1-S2
	Peroneus brevis	Superficial peroneal	L5, S1-S2
Superficial posterior leg	Gastrocnemius	Tibial	S1-S2
	Plantaris	Tibial	L5, S1-S2
	Soleus	Tibial	S1-S2
Deep posterior leg	Popliteus	Tibial	L4-L5, S1
	Tibialis posterior	Tibial	L4-L5
	Flexor digitorum longus	Tibial	S2-S3
	Flexor hallucis longus	Tibial	S2-S3
Dorsal pedal	Extensor digitorum brevis	Deep peroneal	L5, S1-S2
First plantar layer	Abductor hallucis	Medial plantar	S2-S3
	Flexor digitorum brevis	Medial plantar	S2-S3
	Abductor digiti minimi	Lateral plantar	S2-S3
Second plantar layer	Quadratus plantae	Lateral plantar	S2-S3
	First lumbrical	Medial plantar	S2-S3
	Second, third, and fourth lumbricals	Lateral plantar	S2-S3
Third plantar layer	Flexor hallucis brevis	Medial plantar	S2-S3
	Oblique and transverse heads of adductor hallucis	Lateral plantar	S2-S3
	Flexor digiti minimi brevis	Lateral plantar	S2-S3
Fourth plantar layer	Plantar interossei	Lateral plantar	S2-S3
	First and second dorsal interossei	Deep peroneal, lateral plantar	S1-S3
	Third and fourth dorsal interossei	Lateral plantar	S2-S3

diabetes mellitus, and isolated median or tibial nerve entrapment might precede the development of systemic polyneuritis, although it is often found in association with generalized polyneuropathy.[14]

Endogenous or spontaneous peripheral nerve entrapments are common. These develop after neighboring anatomical structures have repeatedly microtraumatized an adjacent nerve trunk by means of direct pressure and inhibition of normal peripheral nerve mobility. Neighboring anatomical structures include muscle bellies and fibrous bands, osseous surfaces, and combinations of soft tissue and bone. Congenital anatomical relationships may become a source of nerve compression because of developmental anomalies or abnormal circumstances, such as conditions of overuse that surpass the nerve's ability to adapt to changes in the local environment. This concept has been referred to as the *stress anatomy* of a particular nerve trunk and pertains to conditions of excessive tension or compression on a nerve associated with movement of the extremity.[1]

Other endogenous mechanisms of localized acquired peripheral neuropathy include *neoplastic disorders*, such as metastatic infiltration,[15] neurilemoma (schwannoma),[4,16-23] ganglion cyst,[9-11,24] varix, and lipoma, to name a few. Moreover,

microvascular dysfunction and subcutaneous atrophy complicating such metabolic diseases as rheumatoid arthritis and other connective tissue disorders,[25] diabetes mellitus,[14] peripheral vascular disease,[24] hyperlipidemia,[26] and hypothyroidism may underlie endogenous forms of peripheral nerve entrapment. Moreover, peripheral nerves in patients with diabetes are more prone to injury than those of persons who do not have diabetes.[27,28] Still further, the recognized *double-crush hypothesis* of peripheral nerve dysfunction proposes that a proximal nerve lesion along an axon, or the presence of concomitant metabolically induced peripheral neuropathy (as observed in diabetes mellitus), predisposes the nerve to injury at a more distal site along its course because of impaired axoplasmic flow.[29-35] The double-crush syndrome may also predispose a patient to persistent symptoms despite appropriate nonsurgical or surgical management of a peripheral nerve lesion.[36]

Exogenous causes of localized acquired peripheral neuropathy are also numerous. Gross traumatic events, including nerve trunk laceration,[37-39] blunt trauma, compartment syndrome,[40-42] fracture or dislocation, injection injury,[5,43-48] and excessive traction with resultant intraneural hematoma, have been implicated.[49-51] Nerve entrapment also has many iatrogenic causes

including tourniquet compression,[52-55] pressure related to positioning of the anesthetized patient during surgery, bandage or cast pressure,[56,57] and surgical misadventure.[52,58-61] Postoperative scarring secondary to normal wound healing may also create acquired neuropathy, even after proper incision planning, layer dissection, hemostasis, nerve manipulation, and wound closure. Scar incarcerated nerves are usually very difficult presentations for the foot and ankle surgeon to identify and treat successfully. Finally, local infection and hematoma causing postinflammatory fibrosis may also affect peripheral entrapment neuropathy.

DIFFERENTIAL DIAGNOSIS

In general, the distribution of pain proximal to the point of nerve damage may make an accurate diagnosis of localized acquired peripheral neuropathy difficult. Localized symptoms may be attributed to surgical scar, bony irregularities, stump neuroma, infection, or foreign object reaction. One case reported a retained Penrose drain in a below-knee amputation that mimicked nerve entrapment and neuroma pain.[62] In all cases, one must distinguish lower extremity nerve entrapment from lumbosacral radiculopathy. In fact, a major diagnostic dilemma exists in the case of suspected nerve entrapment associated with unrelated lumbosacral arthritis or intervertebral disk disease.[63] Furthermore, autonomic overtones with vasoconstriction, decreased skin temperature, distal cyanosis, and development of causalgialike pain (complex regional pain syndrome [CRPS] type 2) or reflex sympathetic dystrophy syndrome (CRPS type 1) can cloud the clinical diagnosis.[64-67] Whenever a CRPS is suspected, appropriate consultation with a pain specialist is advisable, since the treatment of these conditions often requires specialized treatment methods. Chronic compartment syndrome should also be considered in the differential diagnosis.[68] Similarly, chronic tenosynovitis or a smoldering infection (abscess or osteomyelitis) may mimic the pain of localized nerve entrapment. Patients who may stand to gain secondarily from ongoing symptoms can also create diagnostic difficulties, and consultation may be helpful. Finally, peripheral polyneuropathy associated with metabolic, toxic, or infectious processes must also be included in the differential diagnosis.

SIGNS, SYMPTOMS, AND DIAGNOSIS

The key diagnostic criterion associated with localized acquired peripheral neuropathy is *pain* created by irritation of the involved nerve. The pathologic condition may affect the entire nerve trunk, or it may asymmetrically involve only a portion of its diameter. Sensory abnormalities tend to predominate over motor dysfunction, especially in the early phases of entrapment. Pain is usually well localized over the sensory distribution of the involved nerve and typically has the nature of a sharp or burning sensation. Dysesthesia, hypesthesia, hyperpathia, hyperesthesia, and allodynia may also be present.

Pain associated with an entrapped motor component of the nerve is typically less well defined in terms of its distribution. Motor nerve pain takes the form of a dull, aching sensation associated with the muscle and joint innervated by the involved nerve. In the advanced case, severe muscle tenderness may result in disuse atrophy, weakness, dystonia, guarding of the painful extremity, and postural abnormality. Pain caused

by peripheral nerve entrapment is usually aggravated by limb motion and patient activity, and it may be severely debilitating. Spontaneous pain is usually characterized by patients. This pain is reported by patients to be a continuous ache with spiking instances of pain and is often associated with reflex motor activity that may cause jerking of the limb[69] or dystonia. Rest pain is a less frequent finding, and it may mimic peripheral vascular disease without the signs of ischemia.

The actual diagnosis of localized acquired peripheral neuropathy is made after a history and physical examination. The patient may not recall a specific traumatic event to which the onset of signs and symptoms may be attributable, particularly in the presence of underlying metabolic disease. Objective evaluation centers on the sensorimotor examination.[70] An altered one- and two-point static and moving touch-pressure threshold distinction over the sensory distribution of the involved nerve is an early finding.[71-73] Usually, if the nerve trunk is not too deeply situated, palpation or percussion of the nerve at the suspected point of irritation can elicit pain and paresthesia. Distal tingling on percussion with or without radiation of pain and paresthesia along the sensory distribution of the nerve, or *Tinel sign*, is usually present from the early stages of localized acquired neuropathy. *Valleix sign*, or proximal radiation of pain and paresthesia along the neuraxis on percussion at the point of nerve injury, may also be present. Moreover, active or passive manipulation of the extremity may exacerbate symptoms. Manual muscle strength testing is usually not helpful unless the neuropathy is advanced and muscle pain and atrophy are present. In difficult cases, nerve conduction velocity (NCV) and electromyographic measurements may be helpful. Conduction velocity is decreased in most cases of nerve entrapment, whereas electromyography (EMG) is of little use unless nearly complete conduction blockade is present.[65] Electrodiagnostic findings should not override one's clinical assessment, because both NCV and EMG vary with the patient's age, skin temperature, and other conditions that may lead to false-negative values. Finally, diagnostic local steroid injection, combined with a local anesthetic agent, may be used as part of the evaluation. The local anesthetic rapidly inhibits impulse conduction, whereas the glucocorticosteroid alleviates both perineural and intraneural inflammation and fibrosis when it is infiltrated around the nerve trunk. Immediate and dramatic resolution of symptoms indicates accurate localization of the nerve trunk lesion. Dramatic relief of symptoms is usually associated with a decrease in the local inflammatory process. Dramatic relief followed by recurrence of symptoms after a period of time points toward deep, diffuse scarring or a permanent anatomical structure as the cause of nerve entrapment.

PROGNOSIS, TREATMENT, AND COMPLICATIONS

Because a significant proportion of the anatomical continuity of the involved nerve trunk is usually preserved, the prognosis after nonsurgical treatment of localized acquired peripheral neuropathy is often relatively good.[37] Prognosis varies with the patient's age, the cause and extent of the nerve defect, and the location and duration of the lesion. The younger the patient, the more distal the site of injury, and the shorter the duration of symptoms, the better the prognosis will be. In general, after 6-8 weeks, the risk of peripheral nerve changes secondary to ongoing degeneration outweighs the risks associated with corrective surgical intervention.[5,74,75] However, entrapment neuropathies

can be severely debilitating and patients with the condition could become dependent on opioid analgesic medications, so it is imperative to understand how to diagnose and treat the pathology. Prevention of centralization of pain is important for the patient's long-term well-being.

Conservative measures may initially include removal of any direct external compression or tension that could be aggravating nerve function, along with the use of nonsteroidal anti-inflammatory drugs (NSAIDs). Interestingly, changes in ankle position have been shown to alter the dimensions of the fibro-osseous canals of the tarsal tunnel, with ankle dorsiflexion being associated with a significant decrease in the dimension of the tunnel and potentially associated with entrapment of the tibial nerve.[76] Abnormal mechanical stress may be alleviated with orthoses, careful casting or splinting, or application of a desensitizing shield as indicated. Immobilization for 7-10 days to eliminate motion that may be perpetuating local inflammation, and hence nerve irritation, can also be useful, as long as CRPS is not present. Local infiltration of steroid combined with a local anesthetic at the site of entrapment is a mainstay of conservative therapy.[59,77] Perineural infiltration of glucocorticosteroid decreases both intraneural and extraneural inflammation and fibrosis and allows axonal reorganization and remyelination within the nerve trunk. The addition of hyaluronidase to the injected solution can further enhance breakdown of perineural fibrosis, especially in cases involving hypertrophic scars.[78] Furthermore, therapeutic ultrasound or friction massage may aid in resolution of perineural fibrosis and may thereby diminish symptoms of nerve entrapment. Electroacupuncture has also been reported to be of use in the treatment of pain resulting from recalcitrant stump neuroma.[79]

Radiofrequency ablation (RFA) and cryoablation are two modalities that destroy nerve tissue, thereby inhibiting impulse conduction. Cryoneurolysis initially demonstrated severe, reversible damage to nerves with scar or neuroma formation. Cryoablation was introduced in 1917 by Trendelenburg, who demonstrated that freezing tissues caused severe but temporary nerve damage that could regenerate without scar or neuroma formation.[80] This concept of severe, reversible damage to nerves without neuroma formation was formally termed "cryoanalgesia" in 1976.[81] The physical basis for cryoanalgesia is founded on the Joule-Thompson principle (also known as the Kelvin effect), which states that gas under pressure escaping through a small orifice expands and rapidly cools. The endothermic rapid cooling process absorbs energy, in the form of heat, from the surrounding environment. When applied in a high-frequency cyclic fashion to tissues containing peripheral nerve, the resultant freeze-thaw cycle causes axonotmesis. Although contraindicated in the presence of infection, coagulopathy, and pain of unknown origin, cryoanalgesia has shown some efficacy for the treatment of interdigital neuroma, peripheral neuropathy, CRPS, as well as periungual warts and myxoid cysts.[82-85]

RFA is a method that can be used to diminish symptoms related to nerve pain. RFA is founded on the controlled disruption of local tissues due to the production of heat that is formed as radio energy, as a function of current per unit area, produces heat as the radio waves pass through the aqueous environment of the tissues. When precisely applied to peripheral nerve, the radio energy causes ionic agitation that alters neural architecture, thereby impeding impulse conduction and nociception.[86] In an effort to minimize the likelihood of neuroma formation that has been observed with application of continuous radiofrequency energy, pulsed RFA has been shown to be favorable as it produces less of an inflammatory response within the treated nerve trunk.[87] RFA has been used for the treatment not only of painful peripheral neuroma[88-90] but also of certain bone tumors,[91] plantar fasciitis,[92,93] and muscle hypertrophy.[94] Nerve tissue treated with RF can regenerate to a degree over time, and it may be necessary in the future to treat the nerve again with RF if symptoms, such as spasticity, recur.

ADJUNCT MEDICATIONS

Pharmacologic adjuncts to the management of nerve-related pain span a wide range of agents. These include selective serotonin and norepinephrine reuptake inhibitors (such as duloxetine)[95,96]; topical capsaicin[97]; tricyclic antidepressants[98-100]; anticonvulsants (carbamazepine, phenytoin, gabapentin, pregabalin)[101-103]; local anesthetics (orally administered mexiletine, or intravenous and topical lidocaine)[101,104]; adrenergic agonists (clonidine transdermal patch)[105]; aldose reductase inhibitors (sorbinil, tolrestat, epalrestat), particularly for diabetic neuropathy[106-109]; prostaglandin E_1[110,111]; transdermal nitric oxide[112]; and, traditionally, B-complex vitamins.

When denervation is severe, range-of-motion exercises and electrical nerve stimulation may be used to maintain joint function and muscle tone. Generally, after neuroma formation (from acute or chronic injury, such as entrapment, crush or contusion, partial laceration, or previous nerve suture), axon regeneration distalward through the area of injury takes about 7-14 days. Thereafter, nerve regenerates at the rate of ~1 mm/day or roughly 1 in per month, calculated by measuring the distance from the point of injury to the muscle belly or end organ being tested.[113] Conservative therapy is continued if pain is alleviated, adequate sensorium returns, and conduction velocity improves.

If the pain of nerve entrapment is disabling and fails to respond to conservative treatment, if the clinical picture worsens with advancing sensory loss that threatens position sense or weight-bearing sensation, or if motor weakness and atrophy develop, then surgical intervention should be considered. At this point, the risk of permanent nerve damage exceeds the risks of surgical intervention.[5] It is important to inform the patient that symptoms may recur, or worsen, or that disturbing anesthesia may result after surgery. The primary surgical goal is pain relief, and there is no single technique that has become the "gold standard" for the treatment of neuroma.[114] The aim, however, is to inhibit chaotic axonal sprouting and to direct regeneration into an unscarred terminal field while minimizing perineural fibrosis.[115] Surgical intervention by the authors is typically undertaken with the use of general anesthesia, and without the use of muscle relaxants, peripheral nerve blocks, and tourniquet hemostasis, as these interventions can alter the functional evaluation of the target nerve, particularly if a mixed sensorimotor nerve trunk is the target structure and intraoperative nerve monitoring (IONM) is part of the surgical plan.

NONBIODEGRADABLE INDWELLING CATHETER FOR TEMPORARY DELIVERY OF LOCAL ANESTHETIC

When dealing with a painful peripheral mononeuritis, a common method of diagnosis and, albeit short-lived, therapy is the use of local anesthetic blockade of the involved nerve trunk just proximal to the suspected lesion. This can be undertaken in the office or hospital setting and could potentially yield up to a few

hours of pain relief, depending upon the local anesthetic agent used. In some cases, it might be worthwhile to include a mixture of soluble and perhaps crystalline corticosteroid, depending upon the particular patient's systemic and local conditions.

In some cases, it might behoove the surgeon to surgically place a nonbiodegradable indwelling catheter into the tissues with the terminal portion of the catheter positioned immediately adjacent to, or proximal to, the specific nerve defect or point of entrapment in order to deliver a set volume of local anesthetic at a specified rate over a period of several days, during which time the patient can be as ambulatory as possible. In this way, rather than affording the patient just a few hours during which they could experience how they would feel if the involved nerve was not conducting impulses, they could have

several days, typically a 3-to-5-day period, to more fully appreciate how it would be with the specific nerve lesion blocked. Placement of the indwelling catheter can be done using a variety of anesthetic approaches, with the patient positioned supine. The local anesthetic ropivacaine can be particularly useful in this regard. When positioning the catheter, the involved nerve trunk is first isolated via a small extensile exposure at or just proximal to the lesion, after which a second skin entry is made with a scalpel ~10 cm proximal to the distal lesion, and the indwelling catheter path is created from proximal to distal using a tunneling device lined with a sheath designed to tear when the two halves of the sheath are separated from proximal to distal (Fig. 51.3). Once the tunneler-sheath complex is properly positioned, the metal tunneler is pulled from the

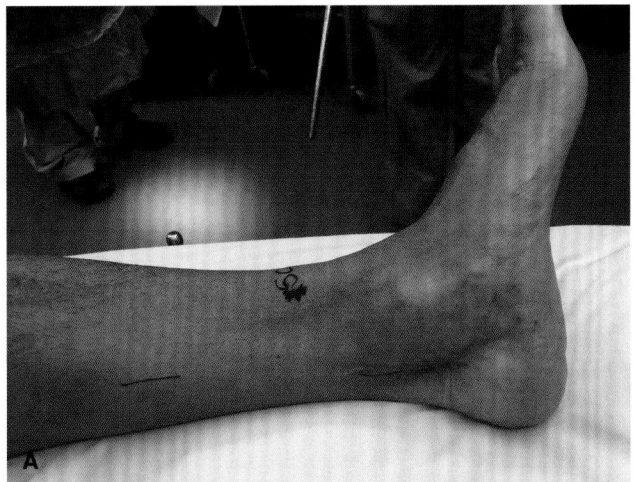
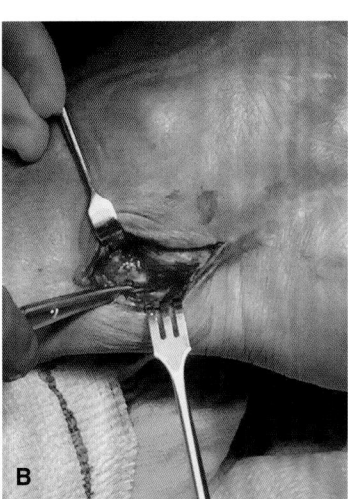
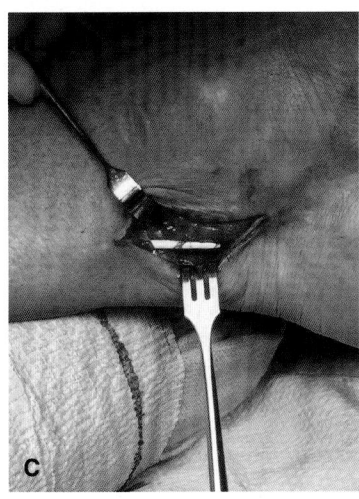
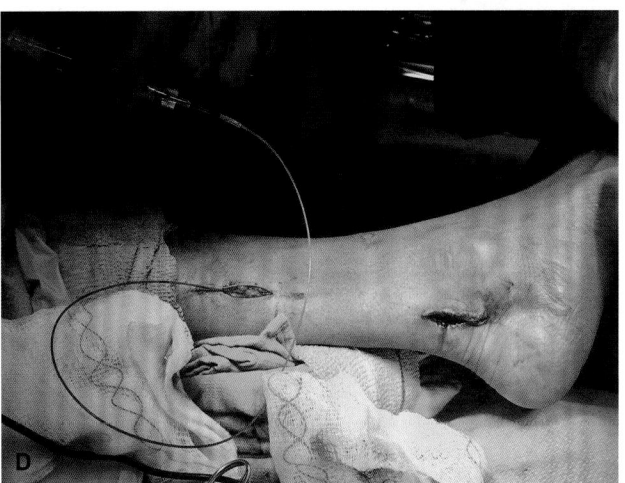

FIGURE 51.3 Placement of a temporary nonbiodegradable indwelling catheter for delivery of local anesthetic over a period of 3-5 days, to ascertain clinical function and pain relief in order to guide therapeutic decision making following a trial course of several days during which the target nerve's function is temporarily blocked. **A.** Left lower extremity in patient following previous failed tarsal tunnel external neurolysis. **B.** Small incision used to isolate the tibial nerve at proximal margin of the laciniate ligament. **C.** Fenestrated distal tip of catheter tunneler sheath, through which the indwelling catheter will be introduced from an entry portal 7-10 cm more proximal in the leg, after which the tunneler sheath will be split and pulled from the subcutaneous tunnel. **D.** Temporary nonbiodegradable indwelling catheter positioned in the leg, as local anesthetic is forced through the catheter and distal release of the agent observed to bathe the tibial nerve in the distal wound, prior to closing the wounds, securing the catheter, and connecting the proximal terminal of the catheter to a portable elastomeric bulb reservoir with an inline flow gauge to control the rate of local anesthetic delivery over the subsequent 3-5 days.

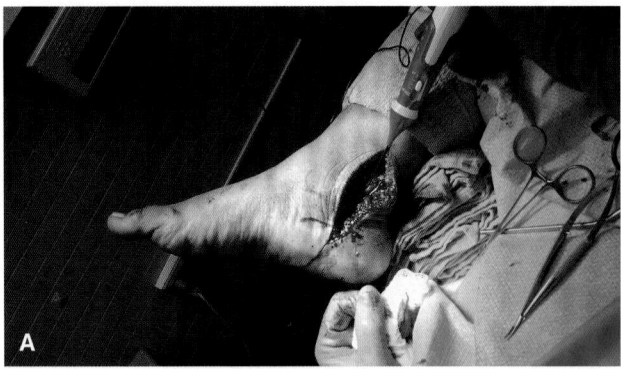 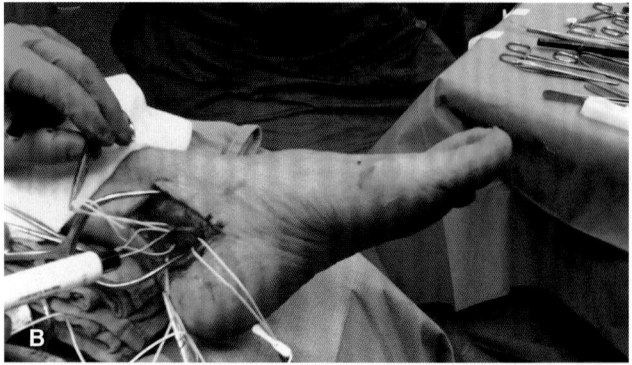

FIGURE 51.4 Direct current nerve stimulator used to assess stimulated function. **A.** Direct current stimulation of the right tibial nerve and its branches in the tarsal tunnel. **B.** Direct current–stimulated function assessment of the tibial nerve and its branches, in a case of left medial plantar muscular branch intraneural ganglion cyst.

sheath, which is left in place so that the indwelling catheter can be passed through the sheath to the target nerve lesion, after which the two halves of the sheath are separated and removed by pulling the proximal tabs of the sheath apart, leaving the catheter in place. It is important to maintain a substantial amount of intact subcutaneous fat and superficial fascia about the catheter, and some catheters are coated with silver to minimize the risk of infection. Once the catheter is properly positioned, the surgeon should test fluid flow by injecting either saline or local anesthetic with a syringe connected to the catheter's proximal Luer lock coupling, thereby assuring that the distal fenestrations in the catheter will adequately bathe the target nerve. Once the flow is assured, the catheter is connected to an elastomeric bulb pump filled with a specified amount of the desired local anesthetic solution, and the bulb reservoir set to deliver the desired volume and rate of local anesthetic over the ensuing 3-to-5 days. For nerve trunks about the ankle and distal leg, a setting of 4 cc per hour, with a bulb containing 440 cc of local anesthetic, can provide ~4.5 days of nerve blockade, after which the patient's clinical response can be discussed, and, if pronounced relief was experienced, then neurectomy might be indicated if subsequent operative assessments support that course of action. Use of the temporary indwelling catheter to deliver local anesthetic over a period of several days can provide the patient and surgeon with a great deal of useful information that can be considered in regard to the long-term management of the patient.

EXTERNAL NEUROLYSIS

Surgical management of localized acquired peripheral neuropathy centers primarily on external neurolysis, which is the fundamental maneuver upon which all surgical manipulations of the peripheral nerve are based. External neurolysis and all subsequent peripheral nerve manipulations are significantly enhanced with the use of either loupe magnification or the operative microscope, as well as use of fine-tipped microsurgical instrumentation and bipolar radiofrequency electrocoagulation. It is important to localize normal nerve trunk proximal and distal to the target lesion, such as a region of scar entrapment or a nerve sheath tumor, in order to expedite and make adequate external neurolysis possible. After exposure of the

involved nerve trunk, and before complete external neurolysis is performed, intraoperative electrical nerve stimulation, using either a direct current (DC), handheld, battery-powered device (Fig. 51.4) or a more sophisticated device powered by alternating current (AC) that can be used to measure electrical activity in the nerve when connected to straight or hooked probes (electrodes) that are applied to the nerve both proximal and distal to the nerve trunk lesion or point of entrapment (Fig. 51.5). The more sophisticated AC device enables the surgeon, with the help of a nerve monitor, to measure and display the electrical activity within the nerve and innervated muscle (EMG) and can be used to produce distal motor activity and thereby aid in identifying the nerve lesion and evaluating the degree of conduction blockade if the particular nerve in question innervates skeletal muscle; if the particular nerve trunk in question does not innervate skeletal muscle, action potentials can still be measured as they course through the nerve.

External neurolysis entails freeing the entrapped nerve from any impinging local structures, incising any adjacent fibrous bands, and, when present, dissecting and mobilizing the nerve trunk from surrounding scar tissue. Gross and magnified inspection of the nerve consists of visual examination and palpation, and may also include intraoperative electroneurodiagnostic measurements of the nerve's electrical activity, as briefly mentioned above and in greater detail below (see Intraoperative Nerve Monitoring, below). Typically, as a result of injury, either acute or in response to repetitive microtrauma, some form of indurated neuroma-in-continuity exists, and is the cause of the patient's pain and paresthesia, dystonia, and disability. A terminal bulb neuroma (amputation or stump neuroma) may also be present, especially when small branching sensory fibers are entangled in diffuse scar after previous surgery or trauma. This condition is often associated with recurrent intermetatarsal neuroma following previous intervention to remove a Morton neuroma by means of traction excision of the common intermetatarsal nerve trunk. Less commonly, the nerve trunk appears completely normal to gross visual inspection; however, palpation and magnified visual inspection, or intraoperative electroneurodiagnostic measurements, indicate the presence of pathologic intraneural fibrosis.

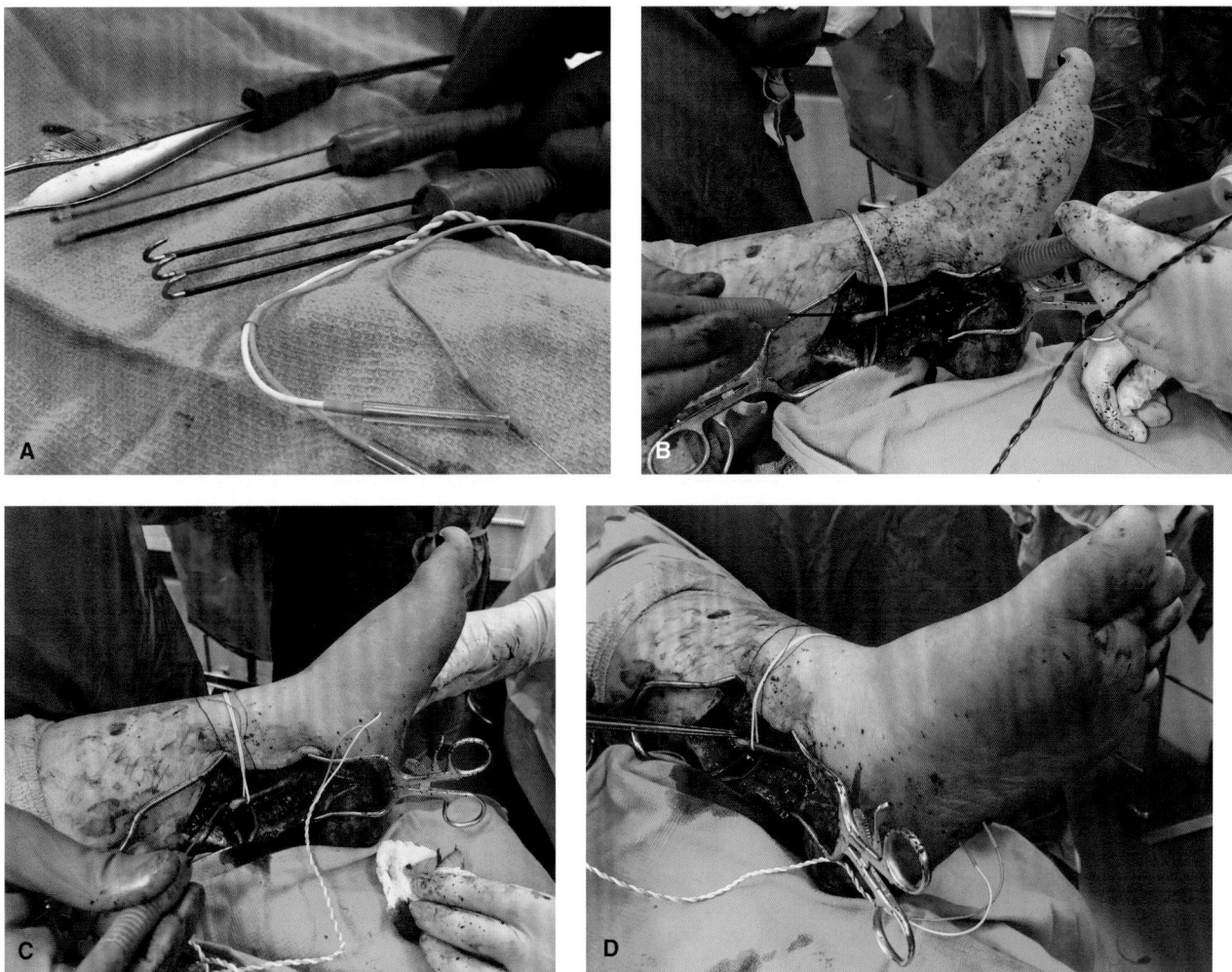

FIGURE 51.5 Intraoperative nerve monitoring left tibial nerve and its branches.
A. Bipolar radio energy forceps, 2- and 3-prong curved electrodes, and electromyograph needles.
B. Intraoperative nerve stimulation and functional measurement, 2-prong electrode proximal, and
3-prong distal. **C.** Abductor hallucis electromyography. **D.** Abductor digiti minimi electromyography.

Following amputation of a portion of the lower extremity, an amputation stump neuroma may develop and cause pain. In such cases, it is important to understand that amputation stump pain can be due to intrinsic or extrinsic factors.[116] Extrinsic amputation stump pain can result from an ill-fitting prosthesis that does not properly distribute load, thereby producing focal pressure that may result in ulceration, bursitis, soft tissue inflammation, contusion, or stress fracture, often with associated nerve stump irritation. Intrinsic stump pain may be associated with an aggressive bone edge or heterotopic ossification from denuded and reactive periosteum, also with associated nerve stump irritation. Following amputation, or nerve sectioning after trauma, a suspected stump neuroma may be visualized by ultrasound (US) or magnetic resonance imaging (MRI) scans, and prior studies have shown that intraoperative US can be used to localize a neuroma and may reduce the extent of surgical dissection.[117,118] Sonographic guidance of local anesthetic, corticosteroid, and alcohol injections for the treatment of painful nerve conditions has also been

described,[119] and this can increase the precision with which the injected preparation is localized, and reduce the required volume and the effect on surrounding, nontargeted tissues. A DC nerve stimulator can also be used to identify nerve that is incarcerated in scar tissue.

More often than not we are dealing with in-continuity nerve lesions due to localized entrapment or intraneural tumor formation in the foot, ankle, or distal leg. Once an in-continuity nerve lesion is isolated, intraoperative direct nerve stimulation or evoked nerve action potentials (NAPs) can be recorded in major nerve trunk lesions. Investigators have shown that in-continuity nerve lesions with complete loss of gross nerve function might display intraoperative NAPs indicative of axonotmesis in the process of regeneration.[120] IONM, which is described in greater detail below, can also be helpful in making surgical decisions related to prognosis and the extent of surgical manipulation needed for any particular nerve lesion. These tests are useful during external neurolysis of the tibial nerve in the leg or tarsal tunnel, the medial and lateral plantar nerves in the foot,

the common peroneal nerve (CPN) at the fibular neck, and the superficial and deep peroneal nerves (DPN) and branches thereof in the leg, anterior tarsal tunnel, and foot. As mentioned above, direct nerve stimulation may be performed with a DC stimulator grounded in adjacent soft tissues, or with a more sophisticated AC unit capable of stimulating the nerve and measuring the resultant electrical activity in the nerve trunk and in muscle innervated by the nerve in question. Intraoperative nerve stimulation requires that attention be paid to tourniquet-induced nerve trunk ischemia because this condition may inhibit impulse conduction, usually within 20 minutes after exsanguination, and may result in spurious measurements.[121] Moreover, to be effective, the surgeon must avoid the influence of local or regional anesthesia on the nerve trunk being tested. Gross visualization of distal skeletal muscle contraction on direct nerve stimulation proximal to the lesion (eg, pedal intrinsic musculature contraction on stimulation of the posterior tibial nerve or its branches in the tarsal tunnel) indicates axonal regeneration and the need only for external neurolysis, in most cases. In the absence of stimulated distal motor function, or when one is testing nerves that do not innervate skeletal muscle, evoked NAPs conducted through the lesion may be recorded, the presence of which indicates a regenerating lesion in continuity.[122] Measurement of evoked NAPs requires electrodiagnostic equipment that is more advanced than a simple DC, handheld nerve stimulator, and such equipment is readily available for use in the operating room of most hospitals. Identification of evoked NAPs traversing the lesion indicates that axonal regeneration is in progress and only external neurolysis is needed. Absence of both stimulated muscle function and evoked NAPs indicates the absence of axonal regeneration and suggests the need for more than simple external neurolysis. Operative electrodiagnostic information is used to supplement direct nerve inspection and palpation. A normal nerve trunk should feel soft and supple to palpation, and it should display a pink to white coloration with evidence of an intact vasa nervorum.

INTRAOPERATIVE NERVE MONITORING

IONM can be used to electrically assess nerve function in the operating room[123] and may be useful in regard to intraoperative decision making as it pertains to how far to go in regard to neurolysis, external vs internal, and whether or not excision may be indicated. IONM is useful when it comes to trying to determine functional changes associated with our surgical manipulations, since it can be used to measure nerve function in response to surgical ischemia, traction, and direct compression associated with manipulation, as well as changes in the values associated with surgical intervention. The practice of IONM has been commonplace since the 1930s and has advanced a great deal since the 1980s as the electronic equipment used to measure nerve function has improved and surgeons and technicians have gained experience with the techniques involved. IONM has traditionally been used for central nervous system operations involving the brain and spine, as well as thyroid surgery,[124,125] acoustic neuroma dissection,[126] and during nerve sheath tumor excision.[127] More recently, the use of IONM to assess peripheral nerve responses has extended to surgery localized to the brachial plexus,[128,129] rotator cuff,[130] hip,[131] as well as the carpal[132] and tarsal (Fig. 51.6)[133] tunnels.

IONM enables the surgeon to measure a number of physiologic functions of nerve and muscle, including motor evoked potentials (MEP), somatosensory evoked potentials (SSEP), and EMG; these measurements can be used to calculate NCV and response latency.[134] To be effective, the surgeon and the monitor should discuss the planned intervention, and how IONM will be used to accomplish the aims of the intervention, prior to the surgery. MEPs are electrical activity measured in skeletal muscle in response to direct stimulation of exposed motor cortex, indirect transcranial magnetic stimulation of the motor cortex, or direct stimulation of a peripheral nerve that innervates a muscle of interest. SSEPs are electrical activity measured in the brain as a result of touch-pressure stimulation in the periphery, and this particular modality is not generally used

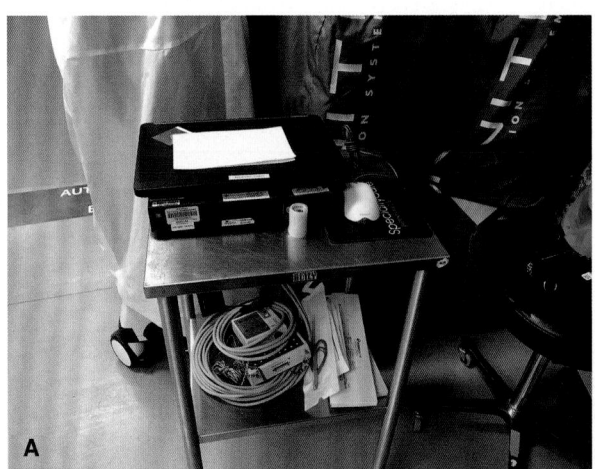
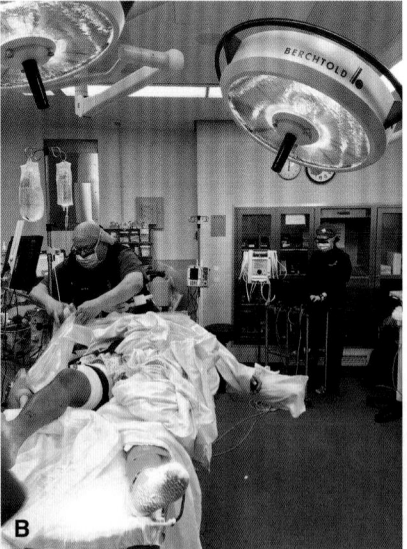

FIGURE 51.6 Intraoperative nerve monitoring used to assess stimulated function and to electronically measure and record conduction velocity, latency, and electromyography. **A.** Nerve monitoring equipment. **B.** The intraoperative nerve monitor (in the background).

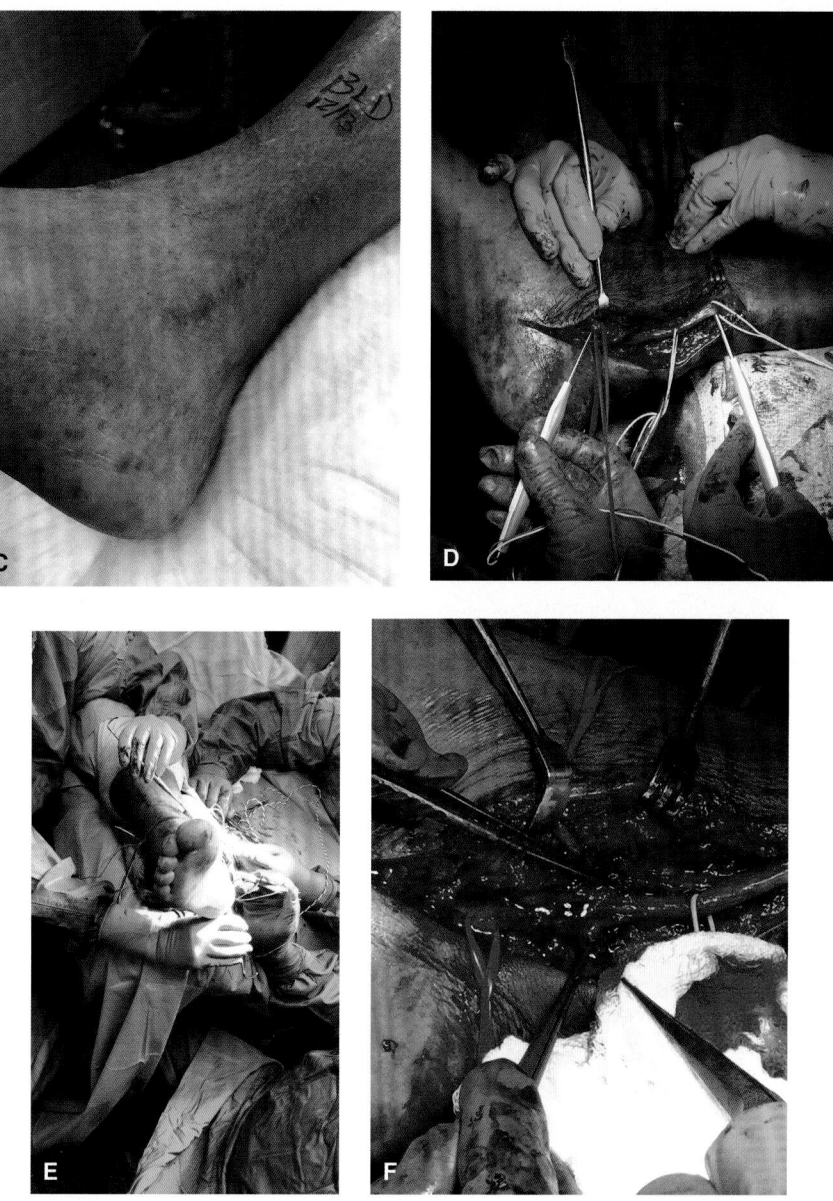

FIGURE 51.6 (*Continued*) **C.** Preoperative clinical view of target tarsal tunnel, right lower extremity. **D.** Intraoperative view of external neurolysis of tibial nerve with monitoring curved electrodes in position along the tibial nerve trunk. **E.** Stimulated function of the tibial nerve and its branches in the tarsal tunnel. **F.** View of tibial nerve intraneural fasciculi exposed and free following endoneurolysis.

in peripheral nerve surgery. When performing peripheral nerve surgery, stimulated EMG can be used in the operating room to assess motor NCV, as well as latency, and these assessments are performed by electrically stimulating the nerve in question and recording the resultant compound muscle action potentials in the corresponding innervated muscle. Stimulated EMG can be used to inform the surgeon of anatomical variations in the orientation of fibers and fasciculi in a named, anatomic motor nerve, and to quantify the influence of an impinging anatomic structure, scar tissue, or hardware on the nerve in question.

In addition to the neurophysiologist monitoring nerve function, the peripheral nerve surgeon should also discuss the

planned surgery with the anesthesiologist, since halogenated inhalant anesthetics, muscle relaxants, and local anesthetics can influence impulse conduction. As a rule, general anesthesia is used, whereas paralytic agents, local anesthetics in the surgical field, and tourniquet-induced ischemia are avoided when IONM is employed. If a tourniquet is used to aid hemostasis during part of the dissection, it is deflated for at least long enough to reperfuse the extremity prior to measuring nerve function. In the operating room, the surgeon will expose the peripheral nerve lesion and use double- and triple-hook nerve probes to stimulate and record impulse conduction in the nerve trunk. Hooked electrodes are positioned in various locations along the course of the nerve trunk of interest, typi-

TABLE 51.2 Electroneurodiagnostic Measurement Guidelines*a*

Peripheral Nerve	Minimum Amplitude (μV)	Minimum Conduction Velocity (m/s)	Maximum Latency (ms)
Tibial	2	41	6.1
Peroneal	3	41	6.1
Sural	6	>40	4.2

*a*Values are derived from clinical measurements[135] and are debatable in regard to intraoperative norms, where measurements vary with temperature, length of exposed nerve, and other operative variables.

cally proximal and distal to the level of injury, entrapment, or intraneural lesion, and typically a minimum of 7-10 centimeters (cm) apart, and the monitor needs to know the distance in order to calculate conduction velocities and latencies. Needle electrodes are also used to record electromyographic responses in selected skeletal muscle bellies. The neurophysiologist that serves as the nerve monitor is an individual certified to set up and use the monitoring equipment in the operating room. The monitor informs the surgeon of the measurements that are obtained and produces a report of the operative findings. The nerve monitor may be employed by the hospital, or by a company that the hospital hires for this purpose.

Guidelines for electroneurodiagnostic measurements can be found in a number of publications, including the University of Michigan Nerve Conduction Manual,[135] and although the values for amplitude, conduction velocity, and latency are well established for patients in the clinical setting, where the nerves remain protected and secure *in situ*, precise normal values remain debatable in the operating room, where the involved peripheral nerve is exposed to the ambient room environment, anesthetic agents, altered vascular perfusion, and direct manipulation by surgical instrumentation. With this in mind, surgeons are advised to use published values as a guideline (Table 51.2) and to compare the measurements that they obtain prior to, and then after, complete external neurolysis and, if indicated, surgical excision of scar tissue, tumor, or any extra- or intraneural pathology that may be suspected to be the cause of the patient's symptomatology. In general, with intraoperative EMG and conduction velocity monitoring, we aim to see increased velocity and decreased latency due to improved nerve fiber function, and greater amplitude as more axons conduct the stimulated impulses. In addition to the quantitative electromyographic and conduction velocity measurements, we also want to observe gross skeletal muscle function in the distribution of the motor nerve being stimulated (the same as if a DC nerve stimulator were being used). If the nerve trunk involved does not innervate skeletal muscle (even though visceral motor innervation to sweat glands, vascular smooth muscle, and arrector pili exists), such as when dealing with the sural nerve about the ankle, then gross visualization of stimulated muscle function cannot be used as a guide to treatment, and IONM is the only way to try to quantify impulse conduction. Some improvement in the quantitative intraoperative measurements might be observed immediately in the operating room, but clinical improvement in terms of pain reduction and improved function more often

than not requires days to weeks to become clinically evident, since restoration of damaged myelin sheaths and axon bud formation and growth progresses over time following surgical decompression of the nerve trunk. Immediately in the operating room, at the least, we do not want to see worsening of the measurements, and we hope to see improvement, even if it is subtle. The closer the intraoperative measurements are to normal, the more likely it is that external neurolysis, with or without endoneurolysis and/or transposition, will be considered sufficient in the operating room, and the less likely it is that surgical excision or ablation of the nerve trunk will be required. In other words, if, after external neurolysis and whatever other surgical manipulations are deemed indicated in the operating room, the electroneurodiagnostic measurements are near normal, or if they improve, then it is unlikely that excision of the nerve will be necessary, and it is indicated to give the nerve time to further recover (improve axon and nerve fiber architecture and function) in the postoperative setting. If, however, the measurements are markedly worse than what would be expected under normal conditions, and gross stimulated function of skeletal muscle is not evident if a motor nerve is being assessed, and if the patient's symptoms include severe pain and, perhaps, prior surgical attempts to decompress the nerve trunk, then excision of the nerve may be indicated. Excision of a mixed sensory and motor nerve, such as the tibial nerve or its major branches, or even the superficial peroneal nerve (SPN) and/or its major branches, is a very serious undertaking, and appropriate preoperative discussion of the expected outcomes, potential risks and complications, as well as the potential benefits and expectations, has to have taken place and been documented.

NERVE TRANSPOSITION, WRAPPING, AND CAPPING

When external neurolysis of an in-continuity lesion is deemed adequate, it may be of further benefit to transpose the freed nerve trunk to a nearby protected, well-vascularized, soft tissue bed, preferably between or within intact skeletal muscle bellies, fascia, or robust subcutaneous fat, or to an area where the nerve will be less vulnerable to traction or manipulation associated with joint flexion and extension, and the remaining nerve should not be subject to substantial contact or weight-bearing forces.[136-138] Transposition is particularly important when the nerve is predisposed to re-entrapment in scar tissue secondary to wound healing.

Wrapping the exposed or transposed nerve in a free flap consisting of fascia, subcutaneous fat, vein, muscle, or vascularized soft tissue has been shown to decrease the likelihood of recurrent pain,[139-141] and so too has transplantation of the nerve stump into a vein.[142] Entubulation with a 0.007- to 0.02-in-thick silicone elastomer sheet has not been shown to be beneficial in preventing reentrapment of a major nerve trunk, such as the posterior tibial nerve in the tarsal tunnel,[143] and it has been used experimentally to induce nerve injury to model nerve pathology in laboratory animals.[144,145] Although our experience with silicone sheath entubulation in the distant past yielded poor results because of profound intraneural edema, fibrosis, and dysvascularity (Figs. 51.7 and 51.8), experimental entubulation with carbohydrate polymer gel resulted in decreased incidence of perineural adhesion.[146,147] Furthermore, absorbable nerve guide implants in

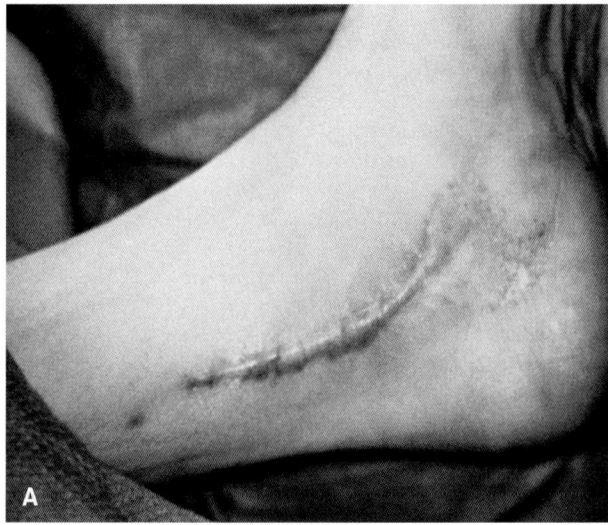

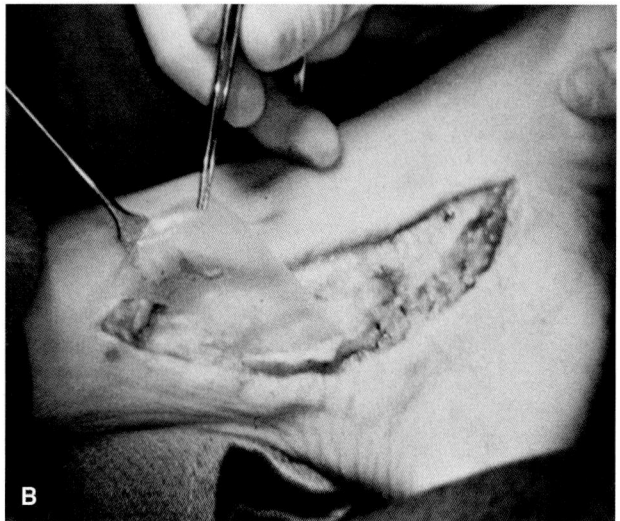

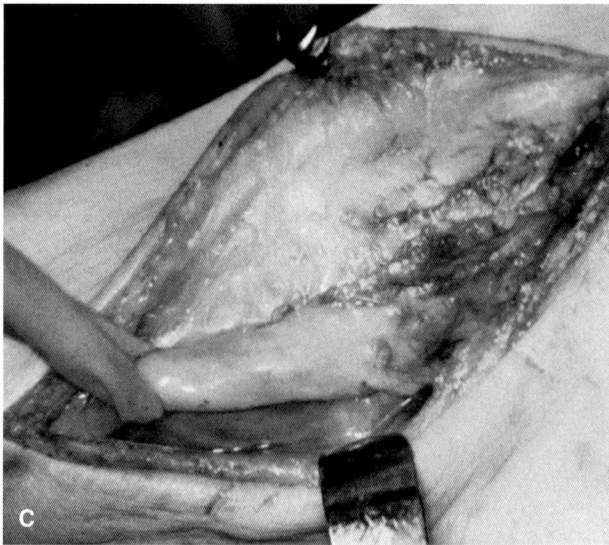

FIGURE 51.7 Silicone entubulation was used for treatment of recalcitrant left tarsal tunnel syndrome in a 53-year-old woman with a diagnosis of complex regional pain syndrome type 1 (formerly reflex sympathetic dystrophy) and yielded only two symptom-free months before recurrence of pain. The silicone sheath was removed 8 months after implantation. Before entubulation, treatment had included five previous tarsal tunnel decompressions, steroid injections, transcutaneous electrical nerve stimulation, epidural blocks, carbamazepine, and narcotic analgesics, as well as numerous hospitalizations for treatment of chronic pain. Approximately 1 year after removal of the silicone sheath, the patient continued to suffer and was considering posterior tibial neurectomy. **A.** Hypertrophic scar and dermatitis 8 months after silicone entubulation of the posterior tibial nerve. **B.** Hypertrophic scar excised and silicone sheath removed. **C.** Gross hypertrophy of the nerve trunk after 8 months of entubulation.

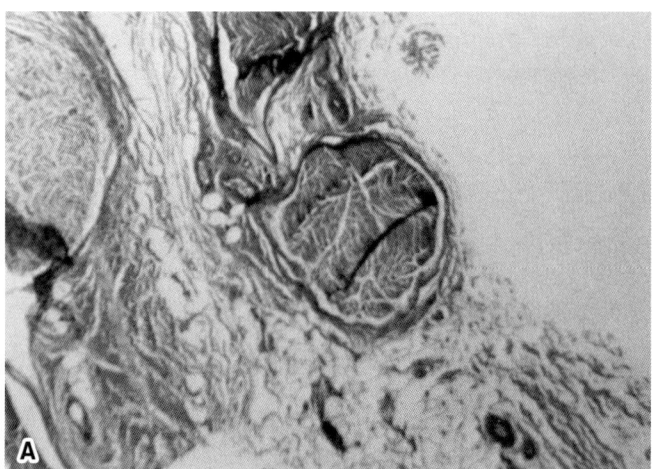

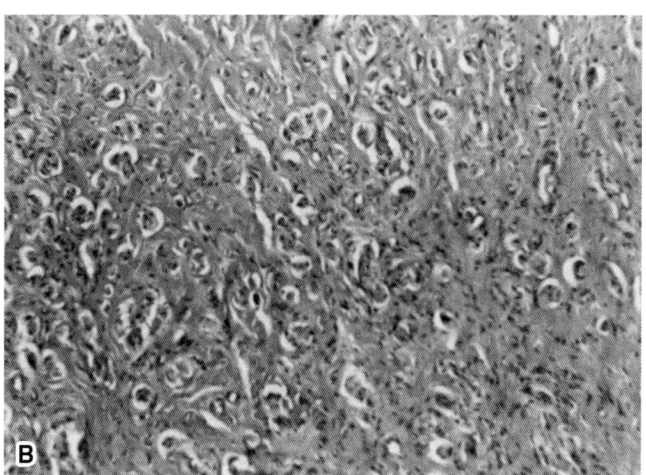

FIGURE 51.8 Histological appearance of a hypertrophic posterior tibial nerve after 1 year of silicone sheath entubulation for the treatment of recalcitrant tarsal tunnel syndrome (not the same patient as in Fig. 51.3). **A.** Hyperplastic epineural sheath fibrosis and perineural fibrofatty tissue (×60). **B.** Intraneural fibrosis and vessel hypoplasia (×160).

the shape of tubelike conduits (Fig. 51.9F), caps, and wraps (Fig. 51.9G), derived from bovine deep flexor tendons[148-151] or porcine small intestine submucosa,[152,153] have been used to connect nerve trunks with other nerves as well as segmental allogeneic nerve grafts (Fig. 51.9D and E), cover sectioned nerve stumps, and shield in-continuity lesions while promoting repair with growth factor migration and aiding the development of pliable incorporation with surrounding adventitia.

In more recent investigations, the use of amnion-derived adhesion barriers to wrap exposed nerve has shown some benefit in regard to minimizing perineural scar formation and indicates a need for ongoing evaluation of this approach.[154-156] Still further, stem cell therapies continue to be investigated in regard to their effectiveness in promoting functional repair when used as an adjunct to surgical manipulation of a peripheral nerve trunk.[157-159]

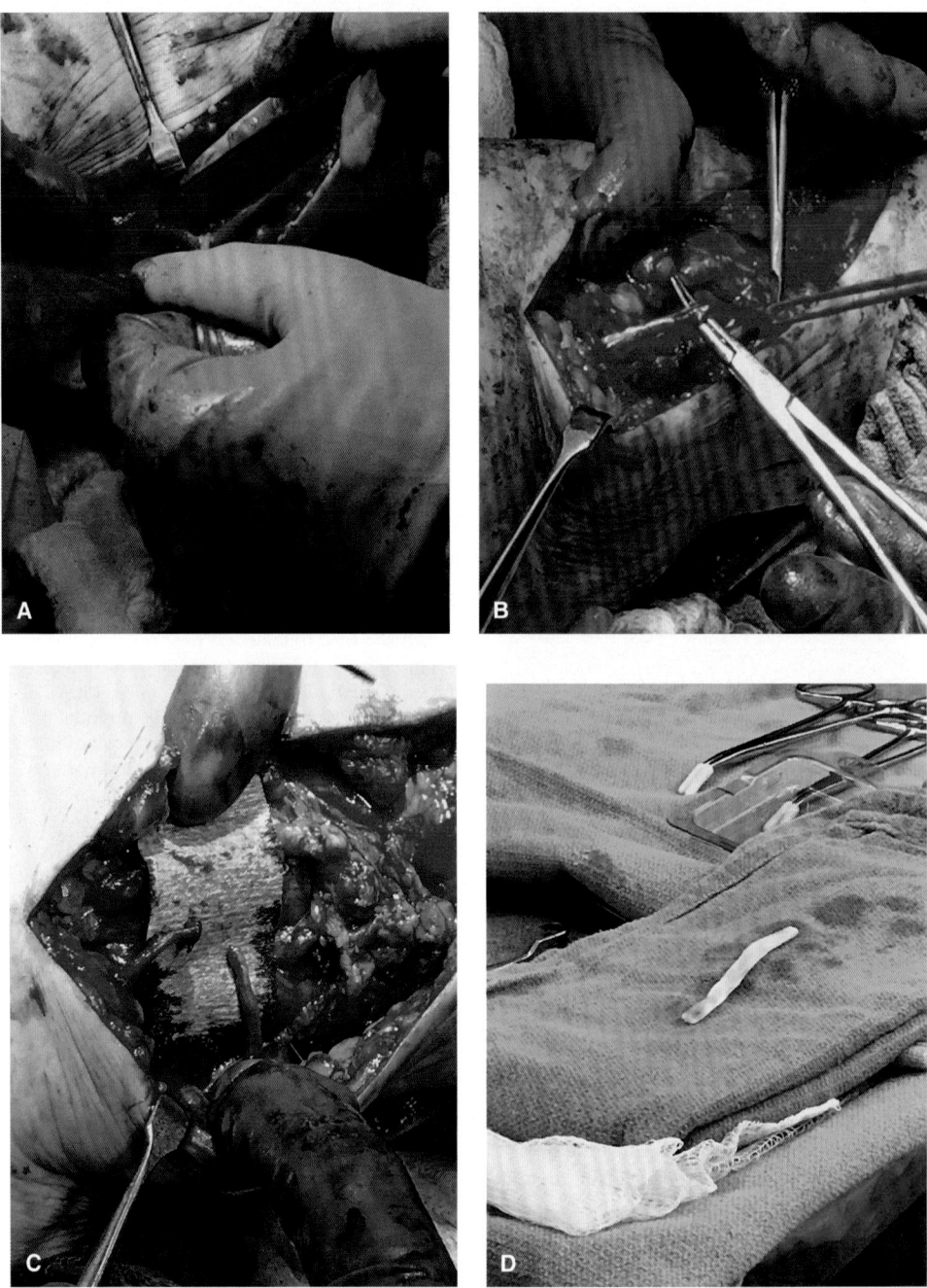

FIGURE 51.9 Nerve-to-nerve transposition for treatment of painful sural neuroma in a 57-year-old female 2 years status post sural nerve entrapment following peroneal tendon surgical repair and then failed sural neuroma excision and stump preparation and transfer into the deep surface of peroneus brevis muscle belly, thereafter successfully treated with sural-to-superficial peroneal nerve-to-nerve transposition with interposed allogeneic nerve graft. **A.** Procurement of sural nerve stump. **B.** Procurement of superficial peroneal nerve distal to muscle branches. **C.** Prepared superficial peroneal and sural nerve stumps in anterior leg compartment. **D.** Allogeneic nerve graft.

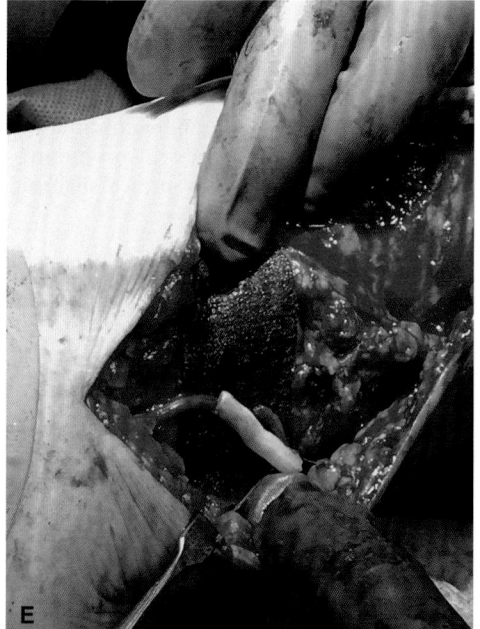

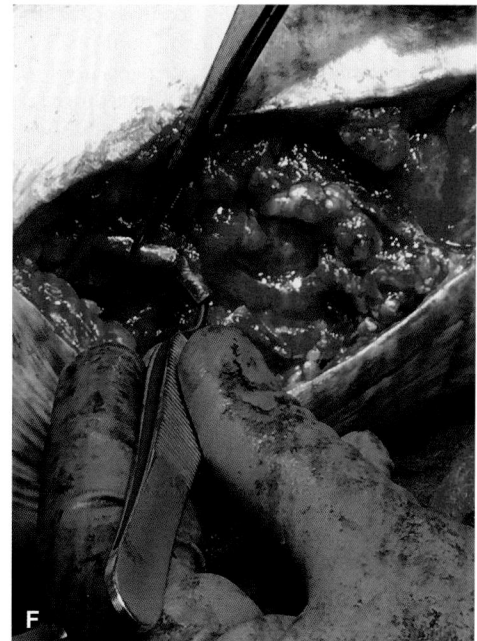

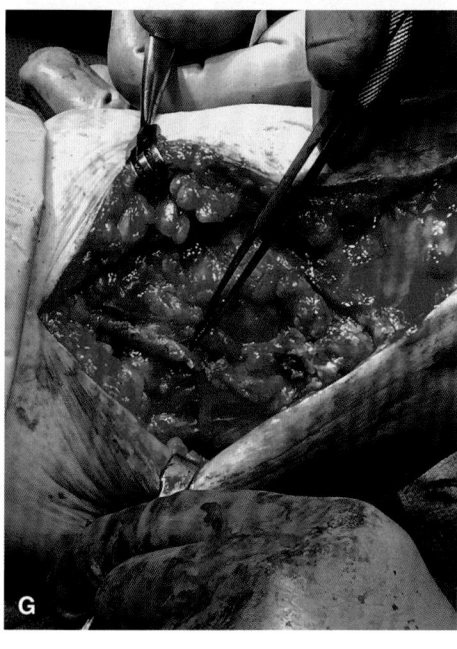

FIGURE 51.9 (*Continued*) **E.** Interposition of allogeneic nerve graft between superficial peroneal and sural nerve terminals. **F.** Superficial peroneal nerve stump and proximal-medial terminal of the allogeneic nerve graft already positioned in 2-3 mm proximity within xenograft collagen conduit, and sural nerve stump and distal-lateral terminal of the allogeneic nerve graft about to be positioned in proximity within a second xenograft collagen conduit. **G.** Final superficial peroneal to sural nerve transposition with interposition of an allogeneic nerve graft with the host-to-allograft interface positioned within xenograft collagen conduits at the proximal-medial and distal-lateral connections, wrapped in xenograft collagen securement localized deep to robust superficial fascia and subcutaneous fat layer.

ENDONEUROLYSIS (INTERNAL NEUROLYSIS)

When external neurolysis reveals a palpable neuroma-in-continuity of a major peripheral nerve trunk, endoneurolysis (internal neurolysis) should be considered.[5,160,161] Endoneurolysis is rarely indicated in the small nerve trunks distal to the metatarsus, although indications are prevalent in regard to the nerves in the hindfoot, ankle, and leg. This technique creates the potential for iatrogenic intraneural damage; however, it may be helpful when skeletal muscle function or plantar or contact area sensation is at risk or in extremely debilitated patients or those with recalcitrant symptoms that outweigh the potential risks. Internal neurolysis entails release of interfascicular fibrosis and scarring (Figs. 51.10 and 51.11) and requires the use of magnification and fine-tipped instruments. After external neurolysis, the nerve trunk is gingerly manipulated with

0.25-in Penrose drains or vessel loops, and the intraneural lesion is isolated. IONM is then performed, and electroneurodiagnostic measurements are made. It may then be helpful to inject a small amount of normal saline solution just under the epineurium in an effort to inflate the epineural sheath and to allow easier identification of intraneural adherence between the perineurium and epineurium, although this maneuver is not always necessary. The saline solution is used as an adjunct to internal neurolysis and does not itself effect neurolysis.[5] Under loupe magnification, the epineural sheath is incised at the point of adherence, and may be excised, and the individual fascicles defined by perineurium are gently teased apart with microsurgical instrumentation.

After opening the epineurium and addressing intraneural fibrosis and freeing the nerve fascicles, intraoperative stimulated distal motor function or evoked NAPs may then be

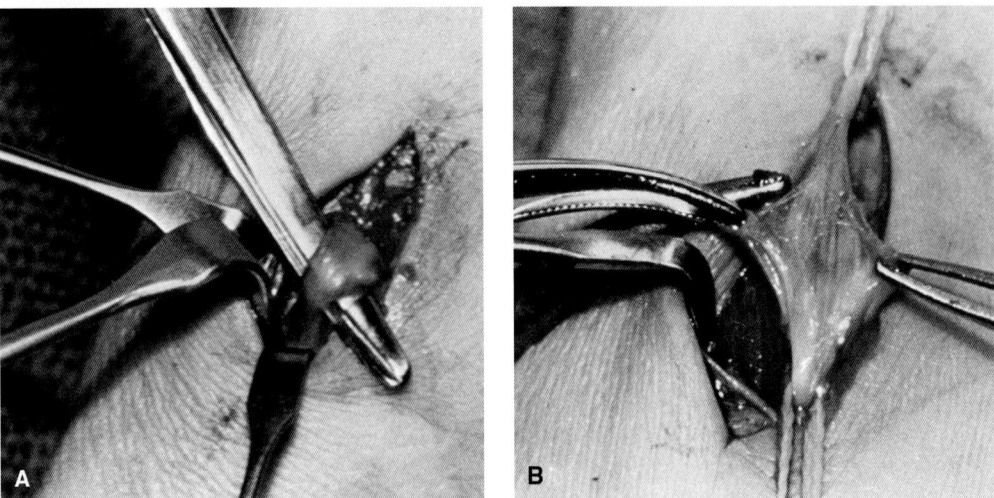

FIGURE 51.10 Internal neurolysis of deep peroneal neuroma-in-continuity in a 14-year-old boy who had suffered contusion of anterior tarsal tunnel 11 months earlier. After endoneurolysis, the patient experienced 95% symptomatic relief for only 12 weeks. Deep peroneal neurectomy was performed 5 months later, because symptoms worsened in spite of aggressive conservative management. **A.** Identification of deep peroneal neuroma-in-continuity. **B.** Epineural sheath retracted and fascicular separation completed.

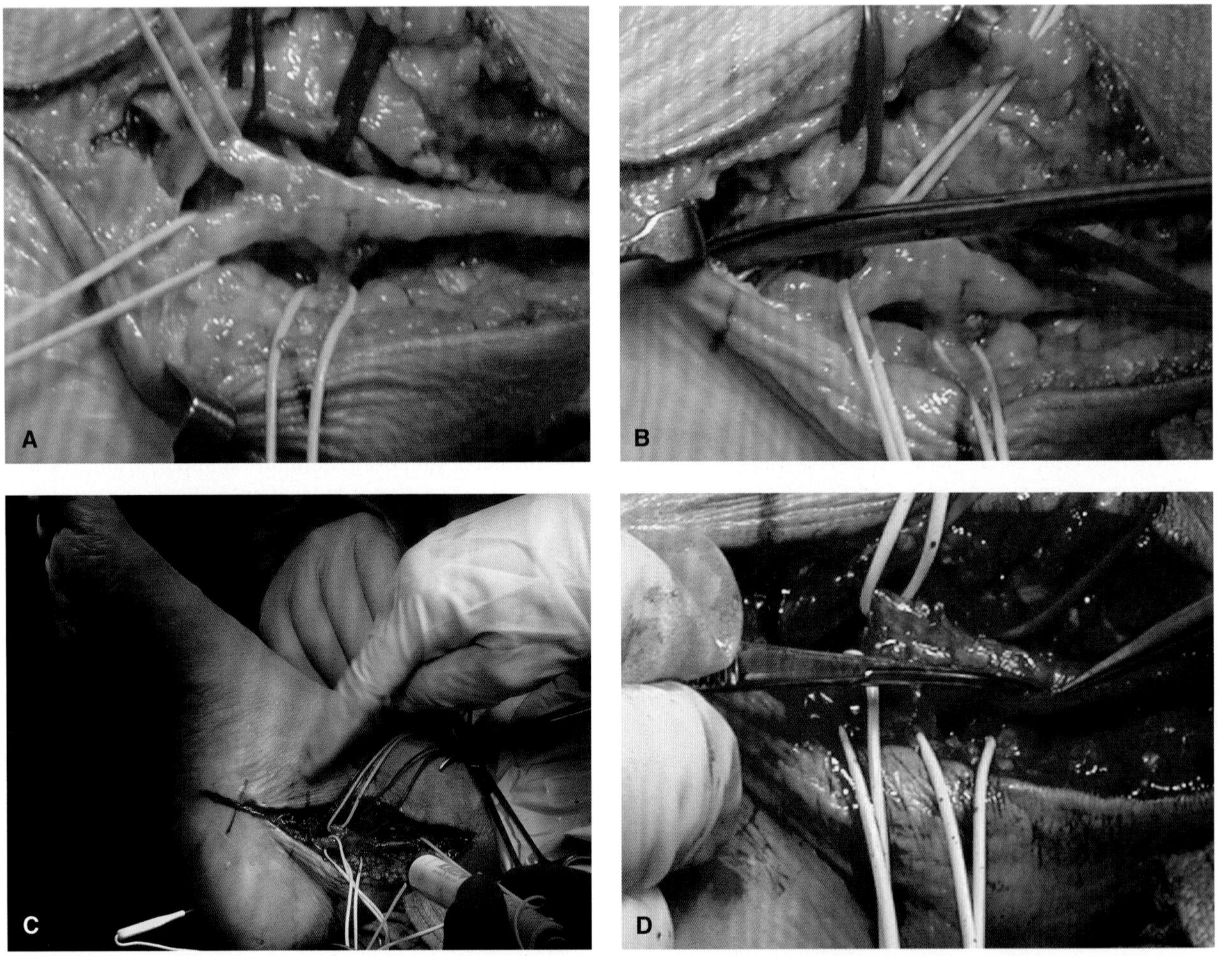

FIGURE 51.11 Internal neurolysis (endoneurolysis) of tibial neuroma-in-continuity following open reduction and internal fixation of a medial malleolus fracture in a middle-aged female. **A.** Distal bifurcation of the right tibial nerve in the tarsal tunnel (proximal, right side of image, distal, left side of image), with anterior venae comitans in *red* vessel loops, and medial plantar, lateral plantar, and medial calcaneal nerve branches isolated in *yellow* vessel loops. **B.** Initiation of dilation of the porta pedis. **C.** Direct current stimulated function of tibial nerve and branches, note ground electrode in heel pad. **D.** Excision of epineurium with fine-tipped forceps and scissors under loupe magnification.

measured once again, and compared to the pre-endoneurolysis measurements. If stimulated function or evoked NAPs are registered, in particular if they have improved, then endoneurolysis can be considered to have been effective and further functional improvement can be anticipated. If axonal conduction is not measurable at the time of surgery, it may still be beneficial to allow additional time for axon and nerve fiber regeneration and rehabilitation of the extremity after the operation, especially if permanent loss of the nerve trunk would create a serious functional deficit, such as skeletal muscle paralysis and/or plantar sensory denervation. After endoneurolysis, the epineural sheath is left open and a portion of it may be submitted for pathological inspection, an amnion-derived fibrosis barrier may or may not be used to shield the open nerve trunk, and the overlying tissues are reapproximated.

NEURECTOMY

In patients with severe in-continuity nerve trunk damage involving a distal sensory nerve, or even when a sensorimotor nerve that innervates skeletal muscle is the cause of a patient's severe pain, perhaps with a history of recurrent symptoms after previous neurolysis, excision of the involved portion of the nerve may be the preferred method of treatment.[162-165] Revision neurectomy may also be preferred when treating a symptomatic stump neuroma following trauma or previous surgery. Sectioning a peripheral nerve trunk results in Wallerian degeneration of the distal nerve fibers, whereas the proximal axons and cell bodies convert to a repair mode with distal propagation that is governed by a group of peptides known as neurotrophic factors (NTFs). NTFs can be found in nerve tissues in both the central and peripheral nervous systems, and also in end-organs that guide budding neurite and newly formed axons (neurotropism).[166] Combined neurotrophism and neurotropism promote and guide regeneration of nerve following sectioning, either as the result of traumatic or surgical injury, and the presence of distal endoneural tubes, or some semblance of scaffolding, can guide regeneration and limit the risk of chaotic, bulbous stump neuroma formation.[167-169] Chronic hyperglycemia can impede neurotrophism.[170]

Neurectomy of an in-continuity lesion involves retracting the nerve trunk from surrounding tissues, then sharply sectioning it proximally and distally and allowing the cleanly sectioned stump to retract back into adjacent, protective soft tissues, preferably amidst intact skeletal muscle bellies, and importantly not in close proximity to overlying denervated skin or moving joint structures or gliding tendons. This method is known as traction neurectomy, and it is the simplest form of neurectomy, and the one most commonly associated with subsequent development of a symptomatic stump. In an effort to minimize the likelihood of development of a symptomatic nerve stump following neurectomy, a number of options are available to the surgeon, and these will be discussed in greater detail below.

Neurectomy produces proximal and distal stumps that could potentially become recurrently symptomatic, and special attention to minimizing the risk of development of a symptomatic stump is worthwhile. A distal stump could potentially become symptomatic if it is not a terminal branch and if another nerve trunk communicates with the distal stump near the level of sectioning (for instance, after excision of the third common metatarsal nerve off of the medial plantar nerve, or the lateral plantar nerve, proximal to the communicating branch between the medial and lateral plantar nerves). In regard to the distal stump, it is best to section the nerve as far distal as is possible,

and the residual distal stump can be electrocoagulated with bipolar radiofrequency energy. As for the proximal portion of the excised nerve, it is dissected proximally until grossly normal nerve trunk is identified, followed by sharp transection and procurement of the distal portion for histopathologic inspection, then preparation of the fresh proximal nerve stump in order to prevent subsequent development of a symptomatic stump.

PREVENTION OF STUMP NEUROMA FORMATION: EPINEURAL CLOSURE, NEUROMYODESIS, NEURO-OSTEODESIS, AND NERVE-TO-NERVE ANASTOMOSIS

Before a sectioned nerve stump is allowed to retract into a well-vascularized and protected soft tissue bed, it may behoove the surgeon to prepare the fresh nerve stump in order to diminish the likelihood that a symptomatic stump will develop, as mentioned above. Epineural closure with 7-0 or 8-0 nylon sutures can be helpful in the prevention of formation of a symptomatic stump neuroma,[171-173] although budding neurites may still escape the reapproximated nerve terminal in search of distal endoneural tubes that are no longer present. Use of a purse string suture or even application of a vascular clip to close epineurium distal to the fascicular bundles within the nerve can also be helpful at limiting escape of budding neurites from the proximal terminal of the nerve. It may also be helpful to use the bipolar electrocoagulator to denature the proteinaceous tissues at the nerve terminal, in an effort to block budding neurite proliferation and subsequent development of a symptomatic stump neuroma. In the past, experimental use of tissue glues such as cyanoacrylate and fibrin adhesive were used to try to prevent the development of a painful stump neuroma secondary to excess neurite budding[174-176]; however, the clinical efficacy of these methods, as well as epineural sheath closure, remains to be proven on a large scale. Collagen conduits (Fig. 51.9F) and caps, made of type I bovine or porcine collagen, have also been used to prevent the budding neurite proliferation post neurectomy, and these are resorbable, kink resistant up to 60 degrees, impede intraluminal neuroma formation,[114,177,178] and they have been shown to stabilize the nerve stump and minimize stump neuroma formation.[179]

Other techniques that have been shown to be useful in the prevention of formation of a symptomatic amputation neuroma include transposition of the free nerve stump into innervated skeletal muscle (neuromyodesis) or into nearby bone (neuro-osteodesis) (Figs. 51.12-51.14). Bipolar electrocoagulation and/or purse string suture closure of the epineurium can also be performed in addition to transposition into muscle or bone. Neuromyodesis and neuro-osteodesis both satisfy the requirements for a well-vascularized and protected location necessary for unremarkable healing of a freshly sectioned nerve trunk. The premise of translocating the affected nerve to muscle or bone is to provide an area that is not superficial where the nerve can be irritated by adjacent anatomic, or extracorporeal, contact or pressure, and where it is not in close proximity to overlying denervated skin. Neuromyodesis varies slightly from simple traction neurectomy where the nerve stump retracts into an area where it is surrounded by intact skeletal muscle bellies, whereas with neuromyodesis, the epimysium is sectioned and the muscle fasciculi gently teased apart and the stump inserted, and then the epineurium is anchored to the muscle belly with 7-0 or 8-0 nylon suture. When the nerve stump is transposed into bone, the periosteum is incised and reflected after which the cortex is opened with a trephine or drill, just large enough to implant the sectioned nerve terminal into the medullary cavity,

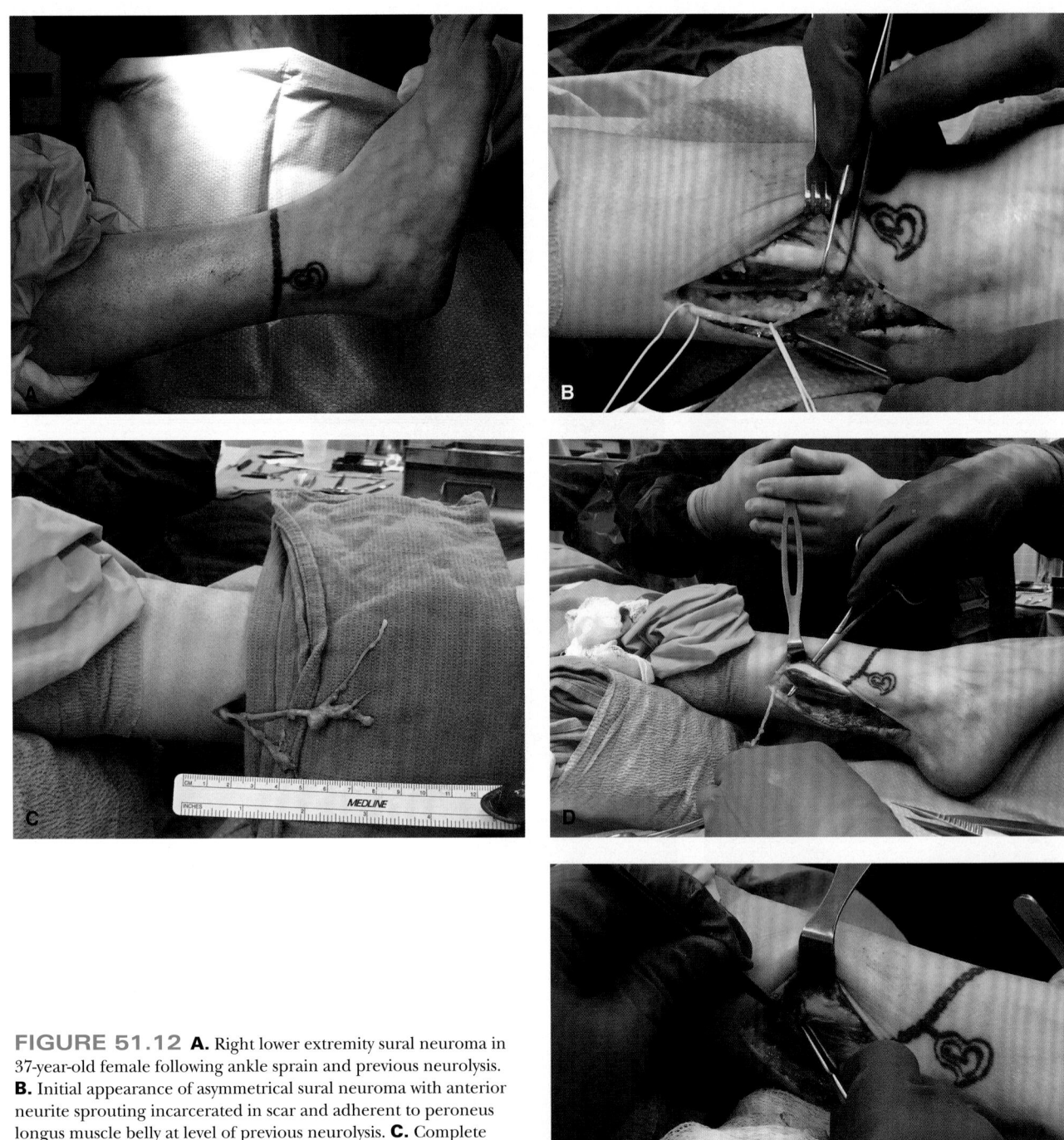

FIGURE 51.12 A. Right lower extremity sural neuroma in 37-year-old female following ankle sprain and previous neurolysis. **B.** Initial appearance of asymmetrical sural neuroma with anterior neurite sprouting incarcerated in scar and adherent to peroneus longus muscle belly at level of previous neurolysis. **C.** Complete microsurgical (loupe magnification) neurolysis of plexiform stump neuroma. **D.** Freshened sural stump transposed deep to peroneus longus and brevis enroute to implantation into the shaft of the fibula. **E.** Neuro-osteodesis of sural terminal into the diaphysis of the fibula, deep to muscle.

and the nerve stump positioned into the bone. With the nerve stump secured within the skeletal muscle belly, or in the medullary cavity of a bone, it is unlikely that it will adhere to a moving tendon or joint structure, and it is well protected from extrinsic forces.[114] Regardless of the location of the transposition of the stump, the residual nerve trunk must be redirected such that its final position is without excessive tension on the transplanted nerve. To this end, the knee and ankle, and even the subtalar and metatarsophalangeal joints if distal enough in the foot, should be positioned such that the transposed nerve remains under relaxed tension throughout the range of motion of the involved joints.

A proximal nerve stump can also be repositioned into a nearby nerve trunk, preferably one that is large enough and distal to any branches that innervate skeletal muscle (Fig. 51.9). Centrocentral anastomosis was first described in hand surgery literature in 1984 and aims to unite two nerves of similar origin together within a single epineurium via epineural repair with fine suture.[180] Histologically, centrocentral anastomosis promotes organized, regular nerve formation with a balance

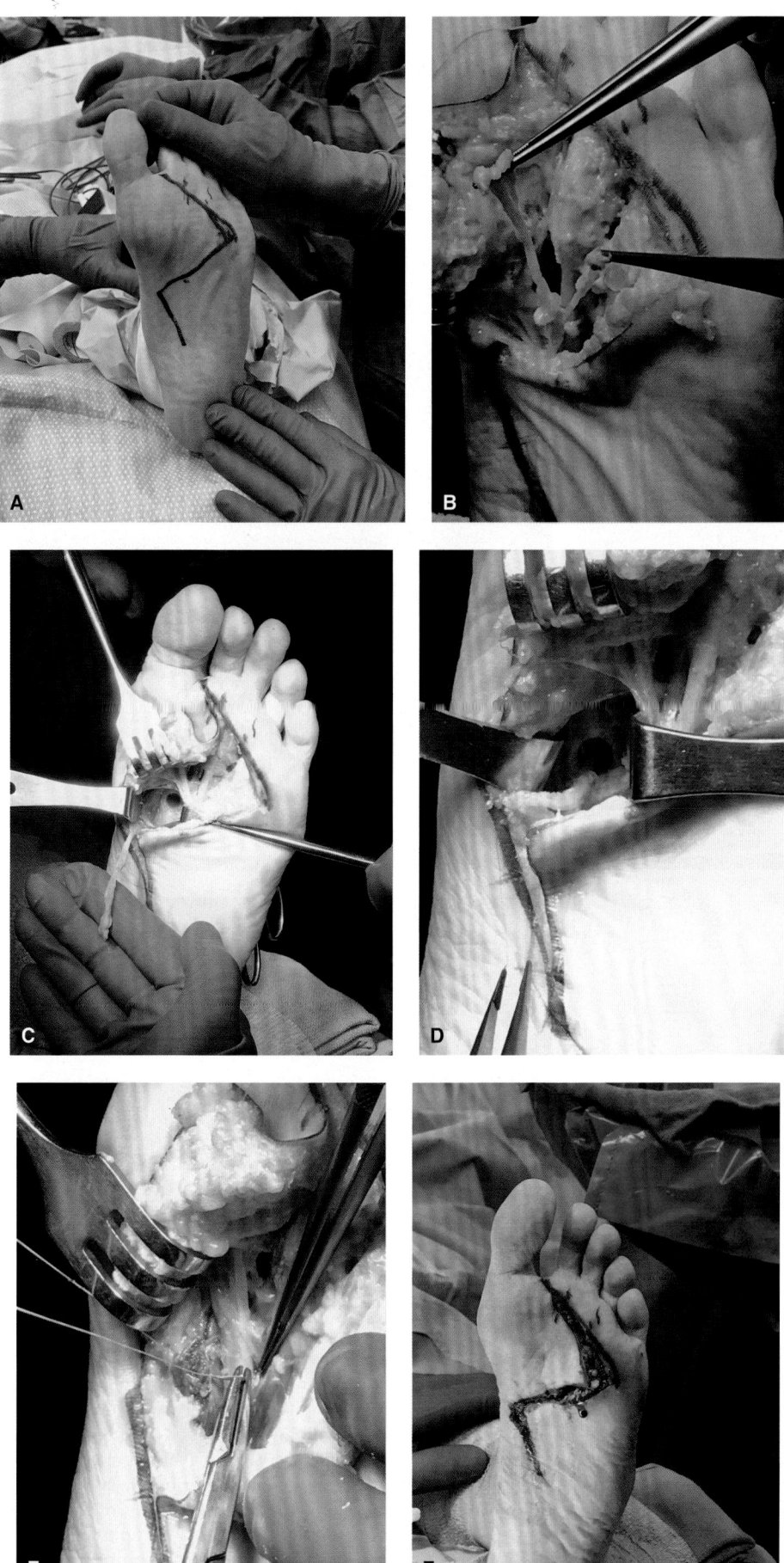

FIGURE 51.13 A. Plantar view of planned zigzag incision to expose suspected stump neuroma in the left foot of a young adult female following previous 2nd intermetatarsal plantar neuroma excision by means of traction neurectomy via a dorsal approach. **B.** Isolation of the stump neuroma of the common digital nerve in the second intermetatarsal space with a lateral articular branch excised from the 3rd metatarsophalangeal joint. **C.** Isolation of the lateral (third) branch of the medial plantar nerve, proximal to the communicating branch with the lateral plantar nerve, prepared for implantation into a trephine bone channel in the plantar aspect of the base of the first metatarsal. **D.** The freshly prepared nerve stump inserted into the hole in the bone, which is then lightly packed with loose preparation demineralized bone matrix putty and then the epineurium is anchored to adjacent periosteum. **E.** Reapproximation of intrinsic skeletal muscles superficial to the neuro-osteodesis. **F.** Reapproximation of the superficial fascia-subcutaneous fat layer prior to skin closure.

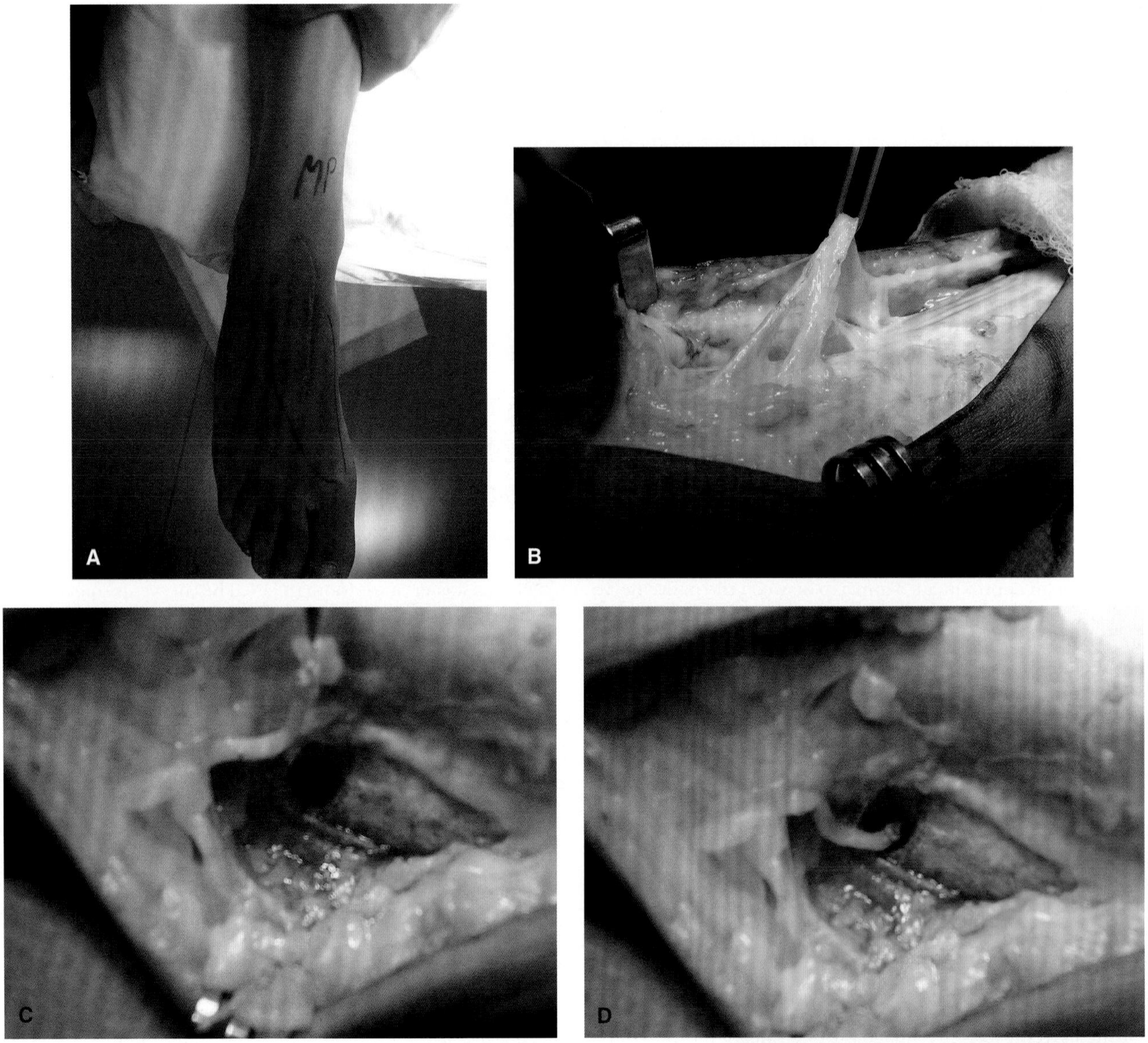

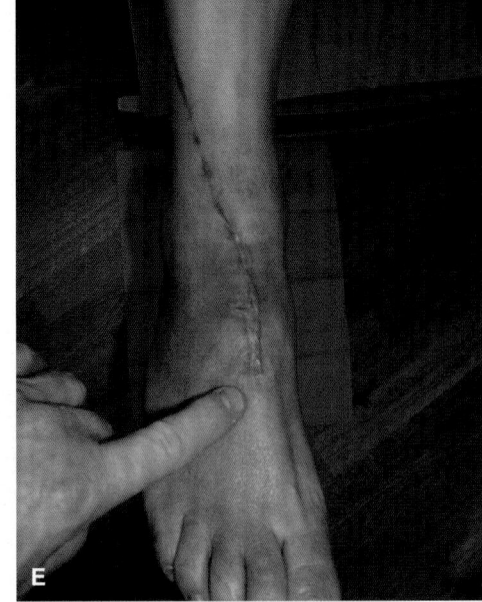

FIGURE 51.14 Medial dorsal cutaneous neuroma following previous dorsal tarsal surgery. **A.** Dorsal scar and planned curvilinear incision. **B.** View of expansive budding neuritic proliferation from proper digital branch of medial dorsal cutaneous nerve (distal medial perspective). **C.** Trephine hole in dorsal aspect 2nd metatarsal base. **D.** Fresh nerve stump implanted into bone. **E.** Well-healed incision and tolerance to direct, deep palpation at the site of neuro-osteodesis.

between myelinated and unmyelinated fibers.[114] Placement of a collagen conduit about the anastomosis can minimize neurite budding into surrounding adventitia, and an amnion-derived barrier could impede perineural fibrosis.[181] Recurrent forefoot stump neuromas treated with centrocentral anastomosis and a concomitant nerve conduit illustrates the necessity to conduct interventions that will limit nerve disarray during regeneration. The concept of embedding the terminal nerve into an appropriate area devoid of possible pressure or traction that could reignite symptomatology is important. Our preference is to augment centrocentral anastomosis with the adjunct use of a surrounding collagen allograft conduit. The use of the conduit and anastomosis may provide an environment that decreases inflammation and pain-generating substances. At the cellular level and tissue levels, it guides axon propagation with neural cell adhesion molecules that limit perineural fibrosis.

Bibbo and colleagues[182,183] have described nerve-to-nerve transfer with an entubulated intercalary nerve allograft for the treatment of lower extremity neuroma-in-continuity, as well as stump neuroma. The intercalary graft consists of an allograft nerve trunk and a surrounding allograft collagen tube (conduit or wrap), into which the fresh nerve stump is, or stumps are, sutured with an approximate 3-mm gap between the native nerve and the allograft, following excision of the painful neuroma (Fig. 51.9). The premise of this approach is to allow for rapid nerve regeneration owing to the natural nerve skeleton framework, thus providing a satisfactory substitute for harvested autograft nerve. The resected end of the stump neuroma incorporates into a secondary peripheral nerve and allows the nerve end to take advantage of the "cytoskeletal architecture" of the recipient nerve to prevent aberrant electrical transmission. Similarly, for in-continuity lesions, the intercalary graft is positioned between the fresh nerve stump created by excision of the painful neuroma and the recipient nerve trunk, preferably distal to any motor branches (innervating skeletal muscle) of the recipient nerve trunk.

Occasionally, sharp resection of a neuroma-in-continuity followed by primary neurorrhaphy or cable grafting is indicated for recalcitrant lesions that affect the posterior tibial or CPNs or their skeletal muscle branches. This may be considered in cases involving extreme axonal damage with significant motor paralysis or plantar sensory deficit. Release of nerve trunk tension and appropriate splinting of the extremity are crucial to the successful completion of neurorrhaphy.

After neurolysis, either external only or external and internal combined, perhaps including transposition or resection, a small amount of soluble steroid infiltrated about the remaining nerve trunk or stump may be helpful. Placement of a percutaneous perineural indwelling catheter (local anesthetic pain pump) (Fig. 51.3), or maintenance of an epidural block, can be useful in the immediate postoperative phase and can be continued for several days or weeks if the clinical situation warrants continued pharmacologic therapy. Periodic administration of local anesthetic or soluble steroid agent about the epineurium is sometimes necessary to effect sustained pain relief, especially in patients with a previous diagnosis of causalgia or chronic pain. Wound closure is performed in anatomical layers; typically leaving the fascia open or only partially closed if it is likely to impinge on the healing nerve. It is preferable to relocate the involved nerve trunk away from the vicinity of primarily closed deep fascia. Meticulous hemostasis is mandatory.

As long as the anatomical continuity of the nerve is maintained, and preoperative nonsurgical measures were exhausted before deciding to take the patient to the operating room,

postoperative prognosis is generally good. Usually, the patient is allowed to move the extremity freely as tolerated. The patient may experience profound improvement in sensorimotor function almost immediately after neurolysis. Axonal conduction may further improve over the next few weeks to months as regeneration progresses. After transposition with epineural anchoring in a new location, postoperative splinting for 2 weeks is recommended. After neurorrhaphy at or distal to the ankle, splinting for at least 3 weeks is recommended. Appropriate joint positioning may be helpful in reducing tension on the nerve trunk after relocation or neurorrhaphy. Follow-up physical therapy may be used as indicated, and repeat conduction velocity or quantitative sensory test measurements may be necessary to monitor regeneration if clinical improvement is less well marked.

LOCALIZED ACQUIRED NEUROPATHIES OF THE LOWER EXTREMITY

SAPHENOUS NERVE

Acquired neuropathy of the saphenous nerve (L3-L4) caused by direct trauma is uncommon, except in certain contact sports such as soccer and football.[1,184] The nerve is mechanically vulnerable to injury where it emerges through the fascia inferior to the sartorius muscle (Fig. 51.15). Spontaneous entrapment may develop secondary to chronic compression associated with genu valgum and medial tibial positioning. In a recent cohort of treatment outcomes for sural neuromas, 90% of symptomatic sural neuromas develop as a result of previous lower extremity surgery.[185] Postoperative scarring with subsequent entrapment after arthroscopy and arthrotomy of the knee may also occur. The saphenous nerve is also vulnerable to injury during ankle surgery.[186-190] We have also encountered entrapment of the nerve at the dorsomedial aspect of the first metatarsal base more frequently than elsewhere, although on occasion, we have treated patients for neuropathy involving the nerve at the anterior aspect of the medial malleolus.

Saphenous nerve entrapment can also affect obese, middle-aged patients and has been associated with the condition known as *adiposa dolorosa*. Complaints of pain and altered sensorium inferior and medial to the patella and along the medial aspect of the leg and foot indicate saphenous nerve compression. Focal

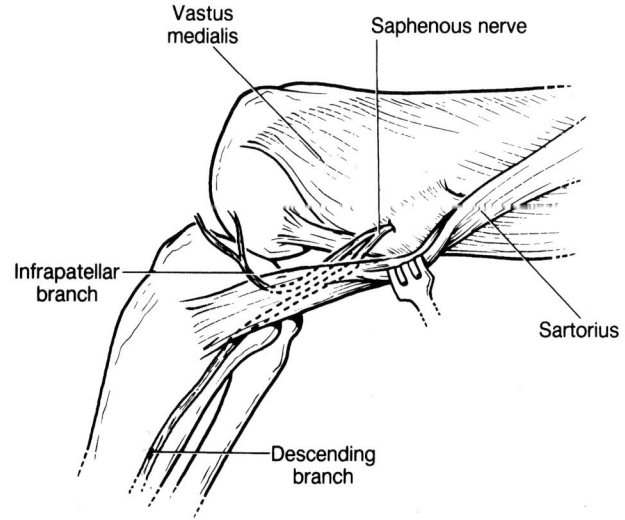

FIGURE 51.15 Course of the saphenous nerve.

nerve trunk tenderness at the point of emergence through the subsartorial fascia may be present, and palpation here may elicit both Tinel and Valleix signs. Local anesthetic and steroid infiltration at this location may prove both diagnostic and therapeutic. Differential diagnoses include compensatory knee changes secondary to faulty foot biomechanics and well as actual internal derangements of the knee itself. At the level of the medial malleolus, the differential diagnosis is facilitated by the superficial position of the nerve and by its immediate identification with the saphenous vein, and the patient may have a history of previous malleolar fracture or severe deltoid ligament sprain. When entrapment is present at the malleolar level, palpation readily produces pain or paresthesia. Entrapment medial to the base of the first metatarsal bone produces more of a diagnostic challenge. One must rule out synovitis, ligamentous strain, and degenerative disease of the first metatarsocuneiform joint, as well as acute tendinitis of the tibialis anterior tendon. The key diagnostic finding is pain on palpation, with the pain or paresthesia following a linear pattern along the course of the saphenous nerve. The nerve is usually acutely tender to palpation.

Conservative treatment consists of rest, as well as oral administration of NSAIDs. Local steroid infiltration is also recommended. When entrapment occurs at the base of the first metatarsal bone, a steroid injection may be combined with soft padding of the tongue and throat of the shoe. Surgical repair entails external neurolysis at the point of entrapment. Exposure is achieved by means of a longitudinal medial curvilinear incision centered over the point of entrapment. Surgery should usually be done with the use of a tourniquet, and dissection should be as atraumatic as possible along anatomical planes. When the nerve shows substantial thickening and whitish hyalinization, we have had better success with local neurectomy. Neurectomy with neuromyodesis or neuro-osteodesis has proved to be a beneficial procedure for the relief of chronic saphenous neuritis. There is usually little difficulty with loss of sensation related to neurectomy of the saphenous nerve at or distal to the ankle. Most of the saphenous neurectomies that we have performed have been at the level of the first metatarsal base in association with chronic neuritis secondary to prominent metatarsocuneiform exostosis.

COMMON PERONEAL NERVE

Localized *traumatic common peroneal (L4-L5, S1) neuropathy* is prevalent because the nerve trunk is vulnerable to injury, given that it lies against fibular periosteum while it courses through a narrow fibrous hiatus in the origin of the peroneus longus (Fig. 51.16).[39,191] Compression secondary to cast pressure,[56] sitting for long periods with one's legs crossed, improper positioning on the operating room table,[192] or decubitus pressure affecting the bedridden patient[193] are possible etiologic factors. Moreover, popliteal cysts[194] osseous tumors of the fibula, prominent bone associated with fibular melorheostosis,[195] traumatic ganglia at the fibular head,[10,11] intraneural ganglion cysts,[4] an enlarged fabella,[196] bilateral CPN entrapment associated with excessive weight loss in an adult,[197] lepromatous infection, or changes associated with diabetes mellitus and rheumatoid arthritis have been associated with CPN entrapment.

The CPN is the most common nerve to be injured when the lower extremity is traumatized, and patients who require surgical treatment respond best when direct primary suture is used as compared to use of an interposed graft.[198] The CPN is particularly vulnerable to injury when the ankle is sprained,[199] and traction secondary to sudden ankle supination or adduction of the leg

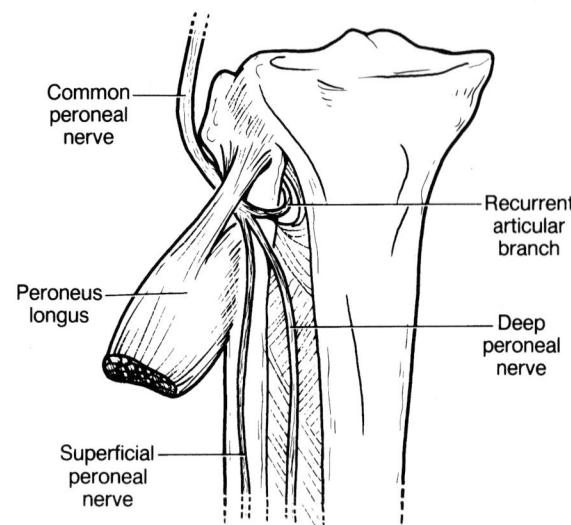

FIGURE 51.16 Course of the common peroneal nerve and its branches.

commonly injures the CPN at the fibular neck. In such cases, the entrapment has been attributed to intraneural hemorrhage caused by rupture of the vasa nervorum with resultant hematoma-induced nerve compression.[50,51] High fibular fractures (Maisonneuve) associated with pronation-eversion ankle injuries can directly traumatize the CPN and its branches. In fact, such fractures are typically not treated with open reduction because of the risk of damage to the peroneal nerve during surgery.

Pain and altered sensation over the lateral aspect of the leg and dorsum of the foot are major complaints associated with CPN entrapment. Weakness of ankle dorsiflexion and foot eversion may develop after long-standing nerve compression or after acute trauma about the neck of the fibula. Almost immediate drop foot deformity may ensue. Percussion or rolling of the nerve trunk along the posterior aspect of the fibular neck may elicit Tinel sign, or proximal radiation of pain and paresthesia may propagate along the sciatic neuraxis. We have observed profound dropfoot simply as a result of habitual sitting with one leg crossed over the other while at work, a position that causes compression of the CPN against the neck of the fibula. It has also been shown that the repetitive ankle plantar flexion test has diagnostic sensitivity and accuracy of 94.4%, each; the positive and the negative predictive values of the test are 89.5% and 94.1%, respectively, as an indicator of CPN entrapment neuropathy.[200]

In the presence of weak or absent ankle dorsiflexion, one must distinguish between CPN entrapment and lumbosacral radiculopathy and plexopathy. This is done by extending the knee to test the quadriceps femoris (L2-L3, L4), by abducting and adducting the hip to test the gluteals (L5, S1) and thigh adductors (L2-L4), by inverting the foot to test the tibialis posterior (L4-L5), and by plantar flexing the toes to test the flexor digitorum longus (S2-S3). A serious CPN entrapment causes weak ankle dorsiflexion and foot eversion while sparing the quadriceps femoris, hip abductors and adductors, foot inversion, and digital plantar flexion.[192] Other considerations in the differential diagnosis include peroneal tenosynovitis, anterior crural compartment syndrome with resultant drop foot deformity, and ruptured plantaris or partial tear of the lateral head of the gastrocnemius. One should also consider CPN entrapment when dealing with chronic lateral ankle instability, a situation in which ankle stress radiographs may be helpful in ruling out entrapment neuropathy. A partial sciatic neuritis or sciatic

nerve entrapment at the sciatic notch may also create signs and symptoms similar to those caused by CPN entrapment, and electrodiagnostic testing is often helpful in isolating the locus of injury.

In regard to imaging, in most instances when the target structure of interest is a peripheral nerve trunk, including the CPN, specific MRI neural sequences with complete nerve coverage is more worthwhile than are standard orthopedic pulse sequences,[201] and high-resolution contrast multiplanar reconstructions of these 3D sequences allow good depiction of peripheral nerves.[202]

Conservative therapy focuses on decreasing local inflammation and reducing traction or pressure on the nerve trunk as it rounds the fibular neck and courses through the fibro-osseous hiatus in the origin of peroneus longus. NSAIDs combined with orthoses to alleviate heel varus stress are often useful in patients with chronic cases. In patients with an acute case, careful casting or splinting with the ankle neutral or in slight dorsiflexion and the knee gently flexed can be used to alleviate tension on the nerve while it recovers. A spring brace or modified ankle-foot orthosis to prevent drop foot deformity, and physical therapies to augment muscle rehabilitation are useful therapeutic adjuncts.

Operative neurolysis of the CPN involves a posterolateral curvilinear approach about the fibular neck, to allow adequate visualization of the nerve proximally in the popliteal fossa, as well as distally beyond its trifurcation. It is usually necessary to incise the fascia at the inferior margin of the peroneus longus origin to obtain adequate freedom of the nerve trunk as it branches and changes direction to run distally in the leg. The CPN is decompressed by division of both edges of the fibular fibrous arch.

SUPERFICIAL PERONEAL NERVE

Localized acquired *neuropathy of the superficial peroneal nerve* (L4-L5, S1) was previously thought to be relatively uncommon,[203-205] although its branches—the medial and intermediate (Lemont nerve)[206] dorsal cutaneous nerves—are vulnerable to a variety of injuries because of their subcutaneous location.[207,208] The SPN may be subjected to traction injury caused by severe ankle supination. Specific sites of entrapment are superior at the fibular neck or distal where the nerve or its branches emerge through the deep crural fascia (Fig. 51.17). Entrapment at this location is typically related to athletic activity, particularly running and jumping.[209,210] Biomechanically speaking, compression neuropathy of the SPN or its terminal branches has been associated with a rigid forefoot valgus with a plantar flexed first ray.[211] We have noted entrapment of the medial dorsal cutaneous nerve at the anterior ankle and, more frequently, at the base of the first metatarsal related to bony prominence and direct shoe irritation of the nerve.

Contusions to the front of the leg or dorsum of the foot (commonly seen in soccer players) or simply pressure from tight shoes, especially in elderly patients with subcutaneous atrophy complicating peripheral vascular disease, diabetes mellitus, or rheumatoid arthritis, frequently result in localized acquired neuropathy of the SPN or its terminal branches (Fig. 51.18). Furthermore, postoperative nerve entrapment may affect Lemont nerve just anterior to the lateral malleolus or on the dorsum of the foot, as well as the medial dorsal cutaneous nerve on the dorsum of the foot and at the medial aspect of the first metatarsophalangeal joint.[58,59]

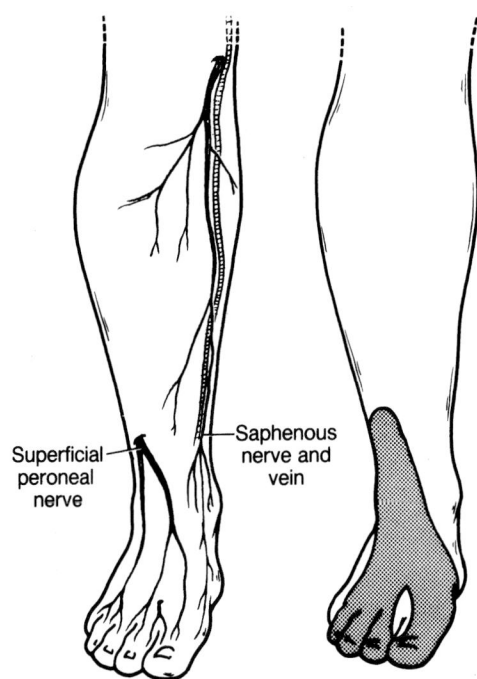

FIGURE 51.17 Emergence of the superficial peroneal nerve and its distribution. Note the course of the saphenous nerve and vein.

SPN mononeuritis has also been attributed to the presence of neural fibrolipoma,[212] as well as schwannoma,[213] anterior compartment muscle herniation through the deep fascia has also been associated with SPN entrapment neuropathy,[214] and so too has incarceration of the nerve between fibular fracture fragments following closed reduction of a fibula fracture.[215]

The SPN has been associated with iatrogenic postsurgical injury, and this may be related to variations in its course and distribution in the leg. Interestingly, an ultrasound and dissection cadaver study showed that the SPN divided prior to emergence through the deep fascia from the muscle compartment to the subcutaneous layer in 46.88% (15 of 32).[216] Surgeons are reminded to recall that the accessory DPN has been

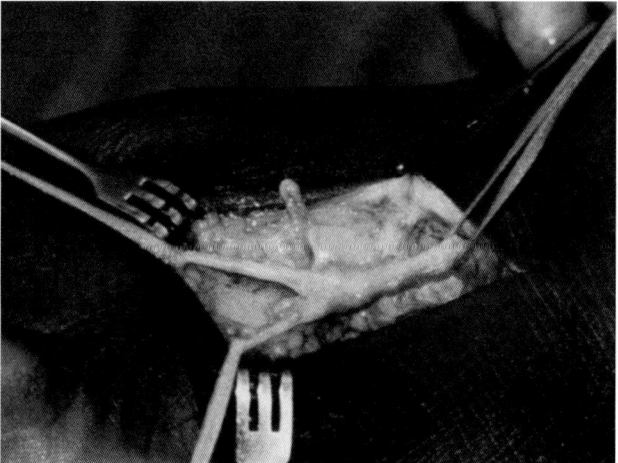

FIGURE 51.18 Posttraumatic asymmetric neuroma-in-continuity involving the common digital branch of the intermediate dorsal cutaneous nerve, in the left foot.

shown to be present in ~19% of clinical reports that looked for its presence, and it courses posterior to the peroneal musculature and the lateral malleolus to innervate extensor digitorum brevis muscle, and it can be vulnerable to injury when operating about the fibula.[217] Unfortunately, injury to the SPN is not uncommonly associated with prior leg surgery,[182,218] including ankle arthroscopy,[219-221] ankle arthrodesis,[183] and total ankle replacement, which has been shown to put the branches of the SPN at particular risk.[222] Attempts to identify the course of the SPN when performing ankle arthroscopy by means of the transillumination test has been shown to be of little to no value,[223] so surgeons are advised to pay attention when preparing portals for ankle arthroscopy, and the use of ultrasound can also be helpful in this regard.

Although injury to the SPN is rare when semi-blind fasciotomy is performed for the treatment of chronic exertional compartment syndrome, up to 8% of patients who underwent the procedure report sensory deficits suggestive of iatrogenic injury to the nerve,[224] and nerve allograft has been used successfully to treat this injury.[225] Because of the vulnerability of the SPN to injury when anterior compartment fasciotomy is undertaken, it may be advisable to identify the course of the nerve with ultrasound prior to dissection.[226] Similarly, injury to the SPN and its branches in association with placement of the anterolateral portal for ankle arthroscopy has prompted some surgeons to employ ultrasound to identify the SPN and its branches prior to creating the anterolateral ankle portal.[227]

Symptoms of entrapment of the SPN or its branches usually consist of sharp, burning pain and decreased sensory perception over the nerve's distribution. Tinel sign may be elicited on percussion of the nerve trunk as it pierces the deep fascia about 7-10 cm superior to the ankle. Retrograde pain along the peroneal neuraxis is common, and lumbar radiculopathy as well as compartment syndrome must be considered in the differential diagnosis.

Conservative treatment focuses on alleviation of abnormal traction or pressure on the nerve trunk. Orthoses to balance rigid forefoot valgus or heel varus deformities can be used to decrease inversion stress and the resultant nerve traction. In the acute case, splinting or immobilization with the foot slightly everted is appropriate. Local infiltration of a soluble steroid is usually beneficial and may be of diagnostic and therapeutic value. Symptoms are typically alleviated or are considerably reduced after two or three injections.

In recalcitrant cases, external neurolysis at the point where the nerve and its branches emerge through the deep crural fascia may be indicated (Fig. 51.19). A longitudinal anterolateral approach is used, and a 4- to 6-cm longitudinal fasciotomy is usually adequate. The superficial fascia and skin are closed, and the deep fascia is not reapproximated in an effort to avoid re-entrapment. Nerve trunk translocation and partial or complete deep fascial closure may be necessary if muscle herniation poses a potential problem. Gentle range-of-motion exercise is started immediately in an effort to avoid any reincarceration. All efforts should be made to prevent the need to resect the entrapped nerve trunk or its branches proximal to the ankle, because this produces extensive anesthesia over the dorsum of the foot. When debilitating neuritis is localized to either of the terminal branches of the SPN, surgical neurolysis or neurectomy may be necessary to alleviate pain (Figs. 51.20 and 51.21). Chiodo and Miller demonstrated that translocation

of the superficial peroneal neuromas into the fibula had better outcomes compared to translocation into the peroneus brevis.[228] Centrocentral anastomosis has also been reported in the literature for painful neuromas of the SPN with the use of an allograft intercalary nerve technique.[183] The repair was then fastened to the mid leg where the anastomosis was free to glide without tension and fastened in a cushion of muscle.

DEEP PERONEAL NERVE

Entrapment neuropathy of the deep peroneal nerve (L4-L5, S1), also known as the anterior tibial nerve, typically occurs at or just distal to the ankle. The nerve is situated in intimate proximity to the long extensor tendons and their binding retinacula, as well as the extensor digitorum brevis and its muscular slips, at the anterior aspect of the ankle and tarsus (Fig. 51.22). The resultant symptom complex has been termed the *anterior tarsal tunnel* or *anterior tarsal syndrome*.[211,229-232] Acute injuries in the form of direct trauma, as well as chronic biomechanically induced microtrauma related to cavus foot deformity aggravated by tight shoes, are also frequent etiologic factors. Severe ankle supination can place excessive traction on the DPN, either at its origin near the fibular neck or, more commonly, deep to the cruciate crural ligament (anterior tarsal tunnel). Osteophytosis of the talonavicular, navicular-cuneiform, or tarsal-metatarsal joints may cause entrapment at the midfoot. The DPN and its branches may become entrapped in resultant scar after surgery using the anterior ankle incisions from total ankle arthroplasty or fusion and more distally from first ray procedures. As previously noted, the accessory DPN has a prevalence of ~19%, and it courses posterior to the peroneal musculature and the lateral malleolus to innervate extensor digitorum brevis muscle, and it can be vulnerable to injury when operating about the fibula.[217] Reports of symptomatology following tibial osteotomy,[233] Lapidus arthrodesis,[234] and minimum incision or percutaneous first metatarsal osteotomy[235] have been described; injury to the DPN has been described following talonavicular joint arthroscopy,[236] and also in association with trauma including Lisfranc joint injury,[237] rupture of the peroneus longus muscle,[238] and posttraumatic intraneural ganglion cyst formation following trauma.[239]

DPN entrapment produces first interspace pain, sensory deficit, and paresthesia. Prolonged entrapment at or distal to the ankle may cause extensor digitorum brevis and interosseous atrophy with resultant weakness. Entrapment near the origin of the DPN can weaken the anterior compartment musculature and can cause dropfoot deformity. EMG and weight-bearing radiographs may be useful in localizing the level of entrapment. Differential diagnosis includes exertional anterior compartment syndrome as well as sinus tarsitis.

Conservative treatment entails removal of any external aggravating factors, the use of NSAIDs, and local infiltration of steroid at the point of entrapment. Immobilization of the ankle is frequently necessary in the case of acute injury of the DPN. Often, conservative management of anterior tarsal tendinitis alleviates the symptoms of deep peroneal neuritis when the neuropathy is caused by impingement resulting from edematous anterior tendon sheaths. If conservative efforts fail, external neurolysis should be performed (Fig. 51.23). Visualization of the nerve proximal to the cruciate crural ligament is recommended, and care should

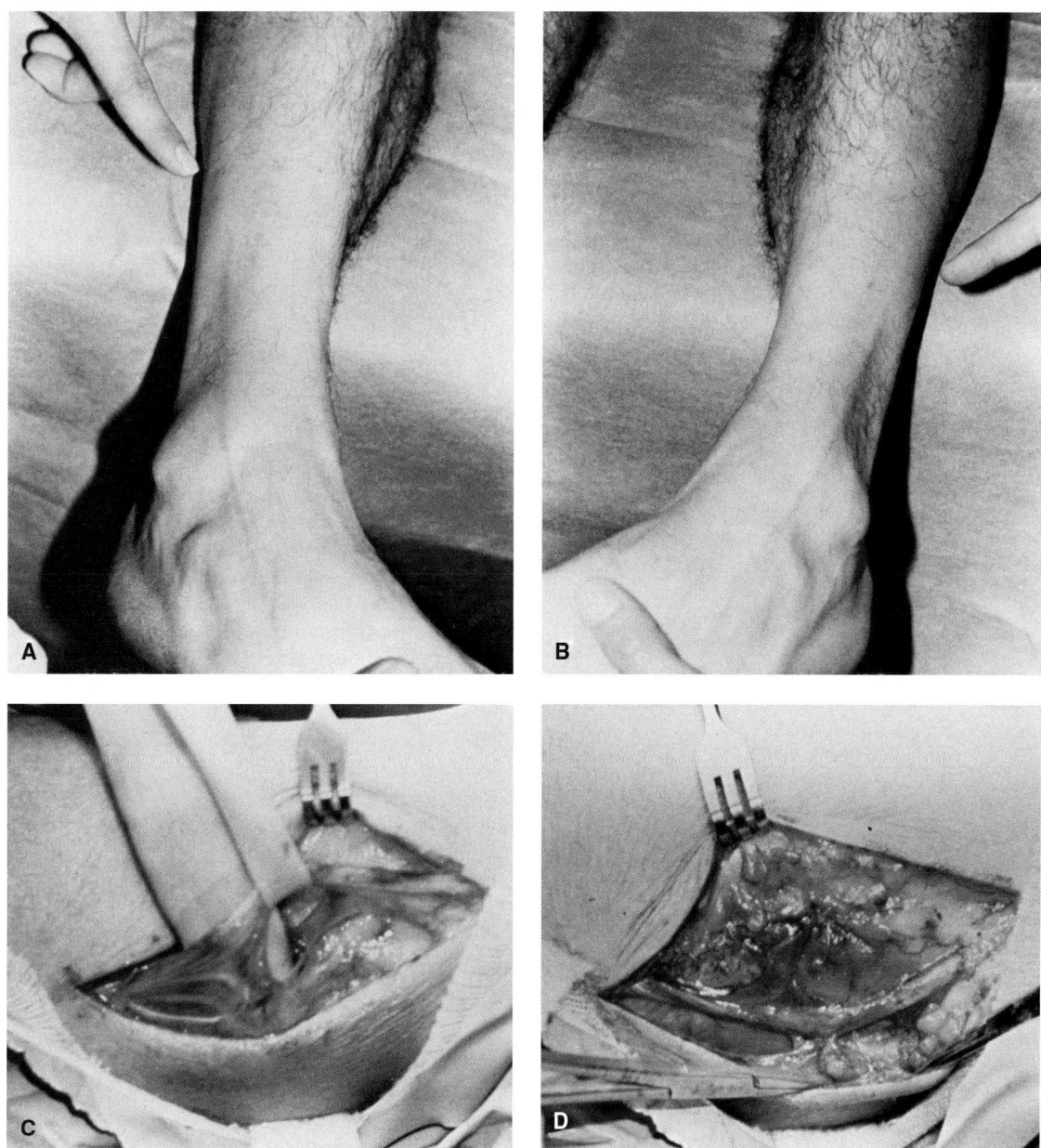

FIGURE 51.19 Superficial peroneal entrapment neuropathy associated with muscle herniation in a 58-year-old man. This patient had bilateral chronic burning pain and paresthesia, as well as a "lump" on the front of each leg, which had begun after he became a paratrooper more than 35 years earlier. Symptoms were immediately alleviated bilaterally after external neurolysis, nerve relocation, and herniorrhaphy, and there had been no recurrence of symptoms 18 months postoperatively. **A.** Clinical appearance of the right leg. **B.** Clinical appearance of the left leg. **C.** Superficial peroneal external neurolysis and identification of deep fascial defect. Peroneal musculature is being manually repositioned deep to the crural fascia. **D.** Deep crural fascia has been reapproximated, thereby containing the underlying muscles. The superficial peroneal nerve has been relocated posteriorly away from deep fascial wound and has been anchored with absorbable epineurial suture to the deep surface of the subcutaneous fat layer before wound closure.

be taken to identify the intermediate (Lemont) and medial dorsal cutaneous nerves superficially. If the decision is made to section the DPN, it should be incised proximal to the cruciate crural ligament to avoid predisposing the patient to symptomatic stump neuroma irritation from the neighboring tendons in the anterior tarsal tunnel.

SURAL NERVE

The sural nerve (L5, S1-S2) and its distal extension, the lateral dorsal cutaneous nerve, as well as the communicating branch between the sural nerve and Lemont (intermediate dorsal cutaneous) nerve, traverse the subcutaneous tissues in close proximity to the Achilles tendon, the lateral malleolus and

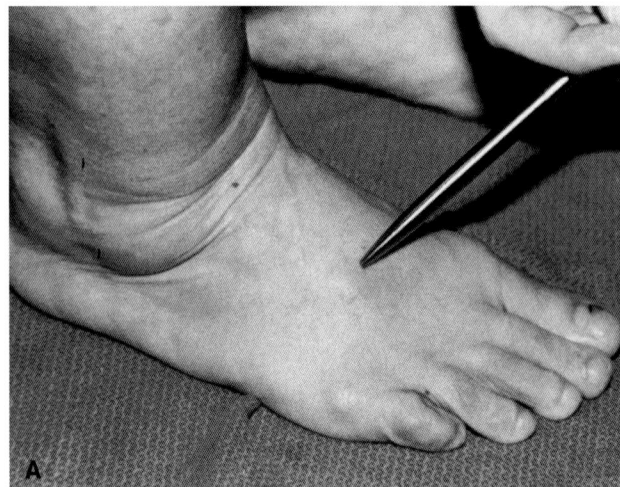
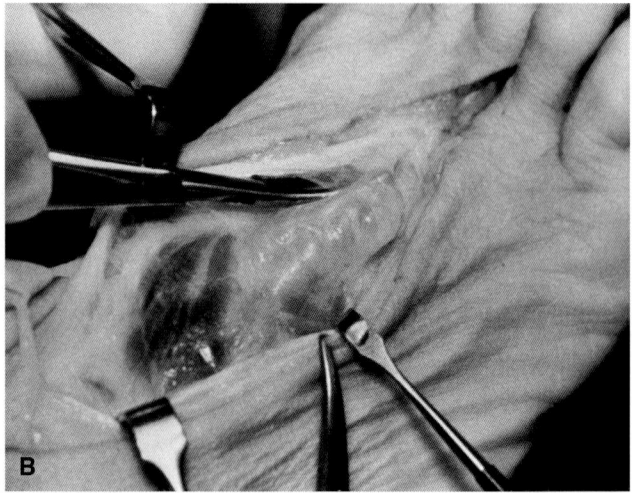
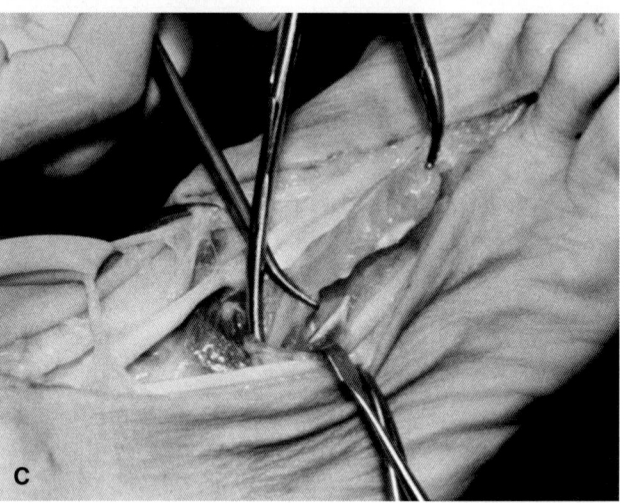

FIGURE 51.20 Chronic pain affecting the dorsum of the right foot in a 55-year-old woman. Burning and paresthesia, as well as a "binding" sensation and the development of a "lump" in her foot, began 2 years earlier after a severe inversion sprain of the right ankle. She subsequently could not work and suffered pain in her entire forefoot. Chronic lateral ligamentous instability persisted, and stress radiography indicated a ruptured anterior talofibular ligament. External neurolysis of the intermediate dorsal cutaneous nerve and ganglion cyst excision, as well as delayed primary repair of the anterior talofibular ligament, produced immediate and complete relief. The freed intermediate dorsal cutaneous nerve was relocated with an epineural anchor suture into robust subcutaneous fat, and an indwelling catheter was used to maintain neural blockade for the first 3 postoperative days. At 2 years postoperatively, a new ganglion developed, and symptoms partially recurred. Subsequent ganglion excision yielded total alleviation of symptoms. **A.** Exquisitely tender, indurated, linear subcutaneous bulge situated over the dorsolateral aspect of the lesser tarsus. Palpation-induced pain extending from the anterolateral aspect of the ankle to the forefoot. **B.** Ganglion cyst identified and noted to engulf the intermediate dorsal cutaneous nerve distally. **C.** Before excision, the stalk of the ganglion cyst is traced to the lateral margin of the talonavicular joint. The cyst probably resulted from rupture of joint capsule at the time of the severe sprain.

fibular collateral ligaments, and the lateral aspect of the hindfoot and metatarsus (Fig. 51.24). *Entrapment of the sural nerve* or its branches usually follows direct trauma and, unfortunately, is commonly related to surgical intervention and postsurgical scarring about the Achilles tendon, the lateral malleolus, and the lateral aspect of the hindfoot (Fig. 51.25). The sural nerve is vulnerable to injury when the Achilles tendon is surgically addressed for lengthening or repair following rupture, and this is particularly concerning when a minimal incision or percutaneous approach is employed[240,241]; some surgeons have explored

methods to minimize the risk of damaging the sural nerve when the sinus tarsi approach is used to gain access for open reduction and internal fixation of displaced calcaneal fractures.[242] A displaced fifth metatarsal base fractures can tent the sural nerve (Fig. 51.26), thus causing posttraumatic entrapment, and the nerve is vulnerable to scar incarceration after surgical manipulation of fifth metatarsal fractures. Peroneal tendon sheath and calcaneocuboid joint capsular degeneration with ganglion formation have also been implicated as causes of sural nerve compression neuropathy.[243] Sural compression neuropathy

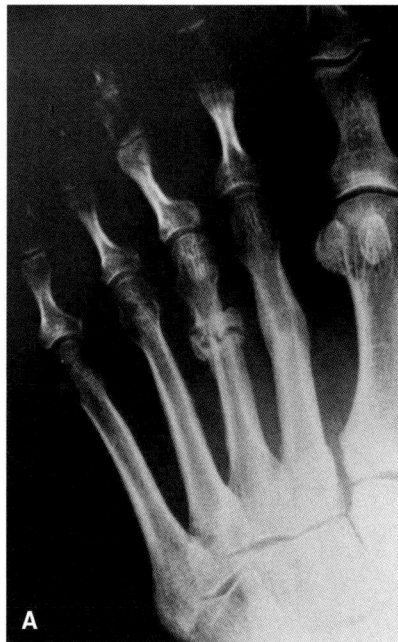
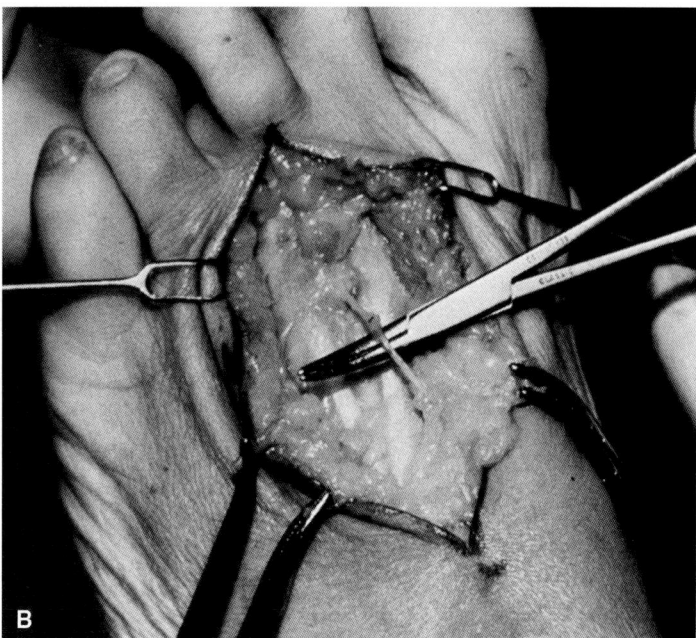
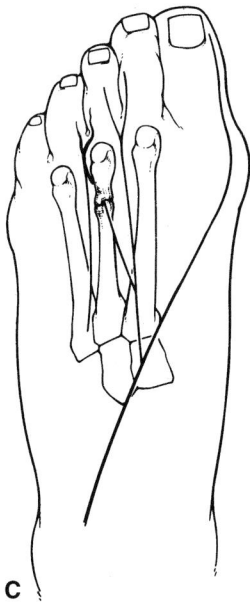

FIGURE 51.21 Postsurgical incarceration of the second metatarsal branch of the medial dorsal cutaneous nerve effecting reflex sympathetic dystrophy in a 52-year-old woman 1 year after minimal-incision surgical second and third metatarsal osteotomies. The patient had failed to respond to long-term pain therapy in two pain clinics, transcutaneous electrical nerve stimulation, and numerous epidural blocks. Although she complained of constant burning pain affecting the entire foot, examination revealed focal tenderness at the third metatarsal, and a field block infiltrated at the base of the metatarsal provided dramatic relief within minutes. Surgery revealed incarceration of the sensory nerve in bone callus and metatarsal nonunion. Proximal neurectomy and resection of the nonunion with plate fixation yielded significant partial relief of symptoms. Complete relief of symptoms coincided with settlement of a pending lawsuit. **A.** Radiograph showing healed osteotomy of second and hypertrophic nonunion of third metatarsal. **B.** Surgical exploration reveals sensory nerve incarcerated in bone callus. **C.** Schematic representation of nerve incarcerated in bone callus.

may also be acquired secondary to long-term chronic tendinitis of the Achilles or peroneal tendons and related induration of the peritendinous connective tissue. We have seen several cases in which enlargement of the peroneal tubercle or a large os peroneum on the lateral aspect of the calcaneus caused severe compression neuropathy.

Signs and symptoms include sensory alteration along the distribution of the sural nerve. Tinel sign may be elicited on percussion at the point of entrapment. Conservative care entails the use of systemic anti-inflammatory medications and local steroid infiltration combined with gentle range-of-motion physical therapy. Because of the subcutaneous location of the nerve, phonophoresis of dexamethasone-lidocaine ointment has also proved to be a useful treatment modality, especially when injection therapy is not desirable.

Surgical intervention is frequently necessary when dense subcutaneous scarring incarcerates the sural nerve or its branches or when a bony prominence is responsible for direct compression. External neurolysis through a curvilinear skin incision over the point of entrapment may yield a good result; however, sharp nerve resection is commonly necessary to alleviate pain caused by sural nerve entrapment. When external neurolysis is performed, the incidence of re-entrapment appears to be directly related to the quality of the soft tissues in which the freed nerve can be relocated. When the soft tissue bed is of poor quality, neurolysis appears to have little value as the sole operative manipulation. In such cases, neurectomy usually provides relief of pain, but the procedure should be performed far enough proximally to place the stump of the remaining nerve trunk in a good-quality bed. Placement of the sural nerve stump into the protective and well-vascularized confines of the medullary canal of the fibula is a useful option, especially in patients with recurrent sural entrapment or extensive subcutaneous scarring. Whenever sural neurolysis is performed, care must be

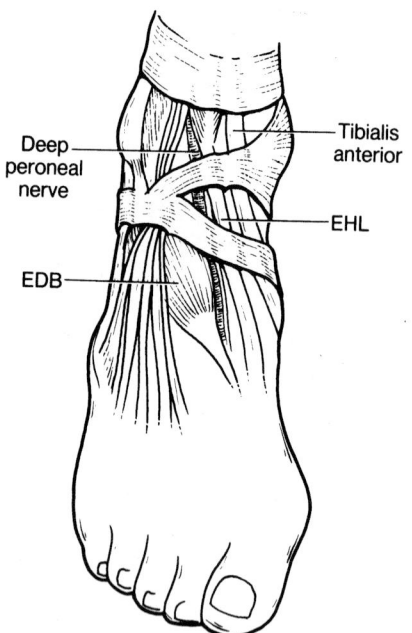

FIGURE 51.22 Course of the deep peroneal nerve. EHL, extensor hallucis longus; EDB, extensor digitorum brevis.

taken to ligate any damaged branches of the lesser saphenous vein because even a small hematoma may provide the mechanism for re-entrapment of the nerve.

TIBIAL NERVE

Proximal entrapment along the tibial neuraxis may occur anywhere from the posterior aspect of the lower thigh distally into the leg and is often the result of direct penetrating trauma. Most frequently, tibial nerve (L4-L5, S1-S3) entrapment occurs in the fibro-osseous tarsal tunnel, where the nerve runs deep to the flexor retinaculum, which is also known as the *laciniate ligament.* Compression neuropathy in this region produces a symptom complex commonly known as the *tarsal tunnel syndrome.*[244-257]

Posterior Tarsal Tunnel Syndrome

(We acknowledge the work that Michael S. Downey, DPM, FACFAS, and Dean L. Sorrento, DPM, FACFAS, did in the previous edition of this textbook in regard to their presentation focusing on tarsal tunnel syndrome, much of which we have included and expanded upon in this edition.)

Entrapment of the tibial nerve can occur at any point along the course of the nerve; however, when the entrapment occurs where the tibial nerve course posterior to the medial malleolus in the tarsal tunnel, the condition is referred to as posterior

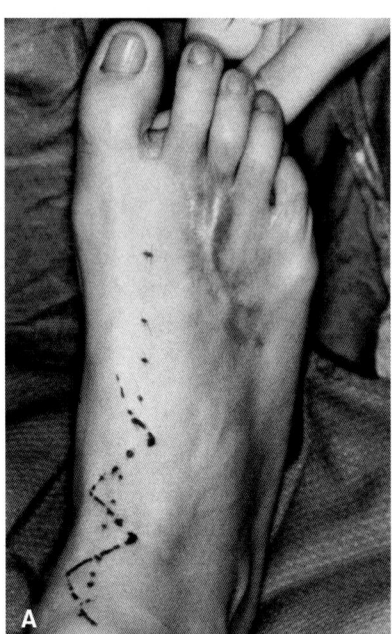
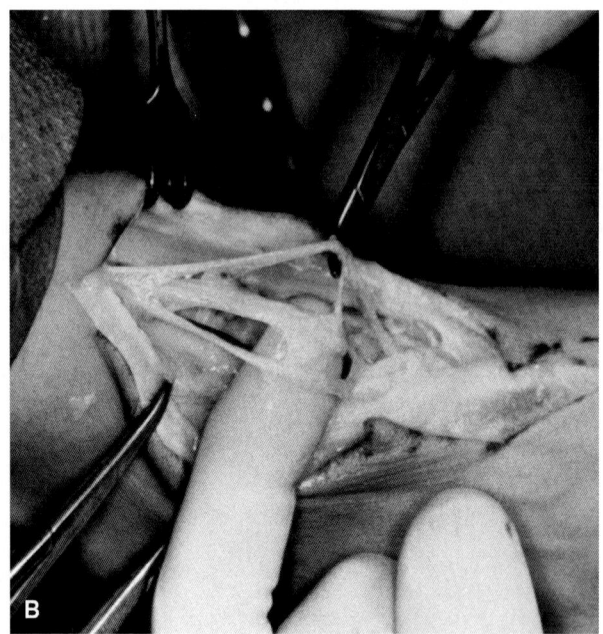

FIGURE 51.23 Chronic pain related to anterior tarsal tunnel syndrome in a 31-year-old woman who suffered a severe contusion to the dorsum of the foot and anterior ankle 13 months earlier. Reflex sympathetic dystrophy had been previously diagnosed, and more than 20 local anesthetic or steroid injections, transcutaneous electrical nerve stimulation, narcotic analgesics, and a 2-month course of weekly epidural blocks failed to alleviate her constant burning pain. Examination indicated deep peroneal neuritis, and a local anesthetic block of this nerve yielded major although incomplete relief. External neurolysis yielded complete relief that lasted only 2 months before symptoms gradually recurred and once again failed to respond to aggressive physical therapy and neurolytic injections. Nine months after external neurolysis, the patient returned to surgery, and a deep peroneal neurectomy was performed. Relief was prompt and complete, and the patient returned to full activities with no recurrence of symptoms at 1-year follow-up. **A.** First operation: the course of the deep peroneal nerve and the proposed Z incision line are marked. **B.** External neurolysis of the deep peroneal nerve.

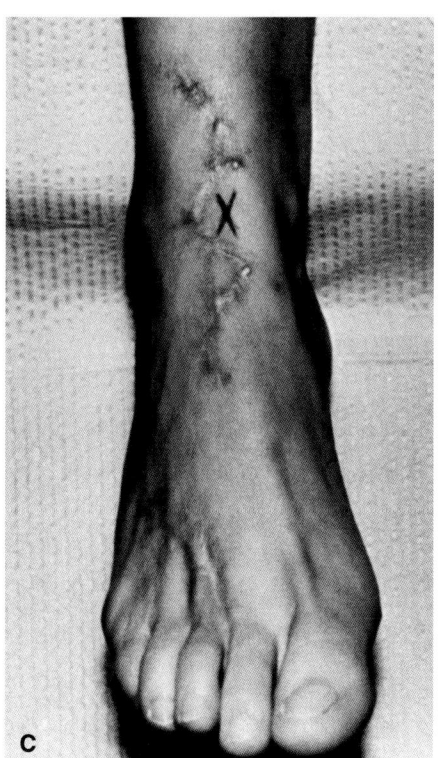 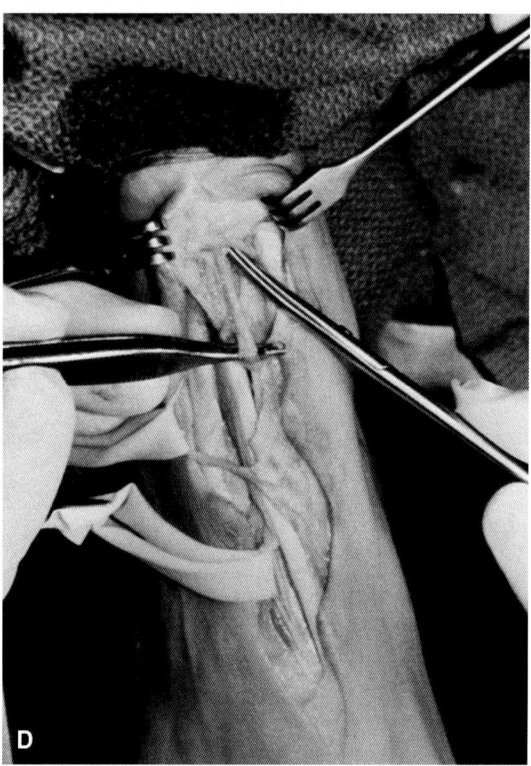

FIGURE 51.23 (*Continued*) **C.** Nine months after external neurolysis, *X* marks nidus of maximum pain that extends throughout the entire foot and ankle. **D.** Second operation: neurectomy of the deep peroneal nerve from above ankle to the metatarsus.

tarsal tunnel syndrome (PTTS). Kopell and Thompson described entrapment of the tibial nerve in their 1960 report,[2] and Keck[244] and Lam[258] separately introduced the term *tarsal tunnel syndrome* to describe the condition created by compression

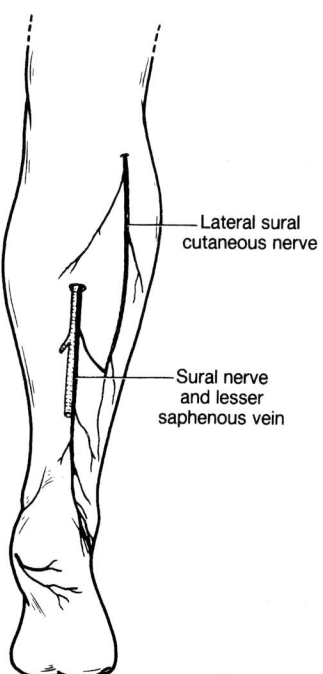

Lateral sural cutaneous nerve

Sural nerve and lesser saphenous vein

FIGURE 51.24 Emergence of the sural nerve and the lesser saphenous vein.

of the tibial nerve within the fibro-osseous tunnel posterior to the medial malleolus. PTTS is an entrapment neuropathy of the tibial nerve or any of its branches.[259] Keep in mind, when the tibial nerve is involved the syndrome is specifically the posterior TTS; this differs from the anterior tarsal tunnel syndrome, which involves the DPN (as previously described in this text). Although the condition can occur bilaterally,[260-263] it most commonly presents as a unilateral malady. Clinical manifestations of posterior TTS typically include burning, cold sensation,[264] aching, radiating, sharp, electric-type pain along the distribution of the involved nerves.[244,258,259,265] Several causes are possible, and this may complicate confirmation of the diagnosis.[260] Although objective tests, such as electrodiagnostic studies, quantitative sensory testing (QST), and MRI, provide helpful information, they do not replace the history and clinical examination in making the diagnosis.[266] Treatment options range from conservative to surgical and depend on the origin, severity, and duration of the nerve entrapment.[267]

Anatomy of the Posterior Tarsal Tunnel

The distal extent of the deep posterior compartment of the leg forms the tarsal tunnel. Located posterior to the medial malleolus, it is a fibro-osseous space formed inferiorly by the medial talar surface, the sustentaculum tali, and the medial calcaneal wall. The flexor retinaculum (laciniate ligament) is a specialized continuation of the deep fascia of the leg, and it covers and forms the roof of the tarsal tunnel.[268] The flexor retinaculum originates from the medial malleolus and inserts into the posterior inferior aspect of the calcaneal tuberosity. Specifically, it can be found roughly 2 cm on either side of a line drawn

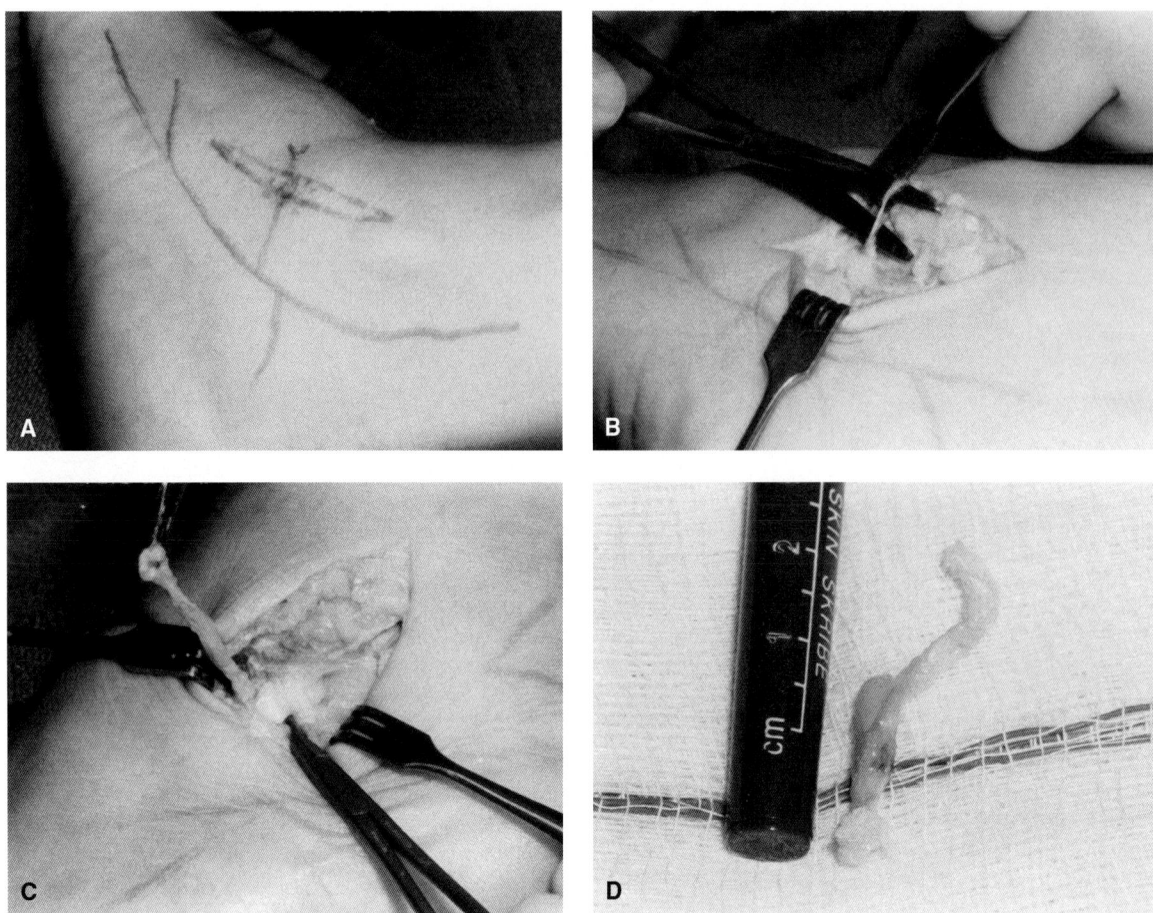

FIGURE 51.25 Posttraumatic neuroma-in-continuity of a communicating branch of the sural nerve. **A.** Dorsolateral aspect of the left foot and ankle marking the course of the sural nerve and area of paresthesia, and the point of a positive Tinel sign, along the course of communicating branch between sural nerve and intermediate dorsal cutaneous nerve. **B.** Communicating branch isolated, with the neuroma-in-continuity coming into view. **C.** Sharp resection of a large neuroma-in-continuity. **D.** Posttraumatic neuroma after resection.

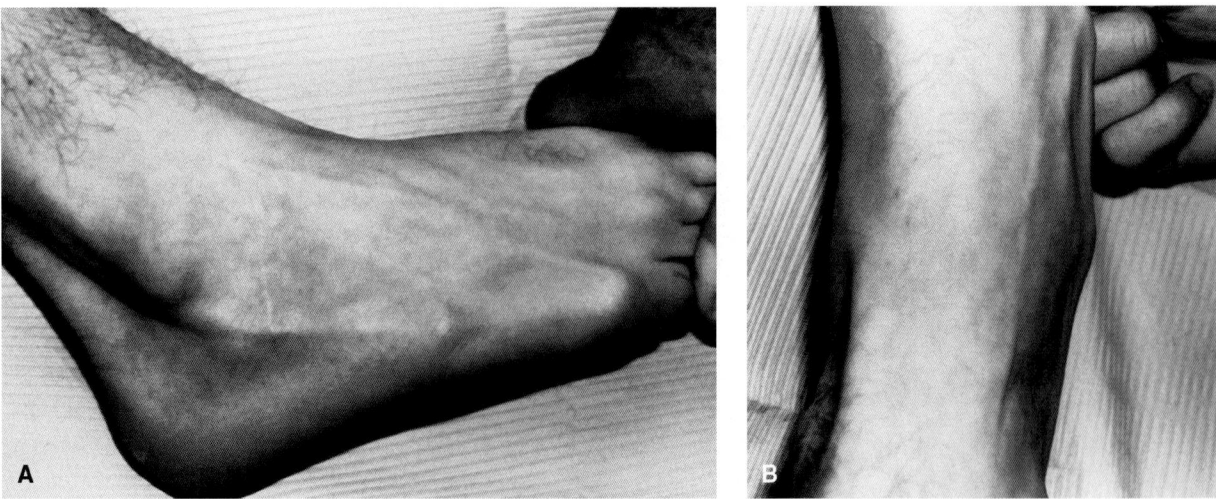

FIGURE 51.26 Tenting of the sural nerve after hypertrophic bone callus formation at the site of a fifth metatarsal base fracture. **A.** Lateral view of the passively supinated right foot reveals a tented sural nerve trunk. **B.** Dorsoplantar view shows a tented sural nerve at the base of a hypertrophic fifth metatarsal.

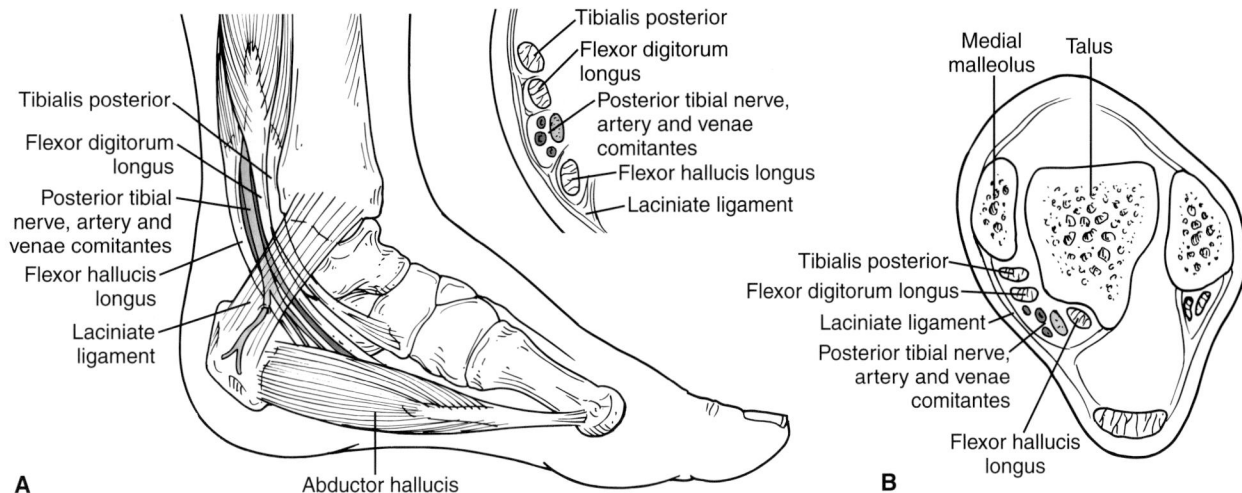

FIGURE 51.27 Schematic sagittal and coronal views of the tarsal tunnel. **A.** The course of the tibial nerve deep to the flexor retinaculum (laciniate ligament), with the medial calcaneal branch emerging through the retinaculum. From anteromedial to posterolateral the contents of the posterior tarsal tunnel include the tibialis posterior tendon (A), the flexor digitorum longus tendon (B), the tibial nerve, artery, and venae comitans (C), and the flexor hallucis longus tendon (D), with the overlying laciniate ligament (E). **B.** Transverse plane cross section of the tarsal tunnel depicts the talus (A), medial malleolus (B), tibialis posterior (C), flexor digitorum longus (D), flexor retinaculum (E), posterior tibial artery, nerve, and venae comitans (F), and flexor hallucis longus (G).

from the center of the medial malleolus to the center of the calcaneal tuberosity. The proximal and distal aspects of the tarsal tunnel are key landmarks for surgical decompression.[269-271] Located within the confines of the tarsal tunnel are the tibialis posterior, flexor digitorum longus, and flexor hallucis longus tendons. These tendons are contained in separate fibrous compartments formed by projections from the undersurface of the flexor retinaculum (Fig. 51.27).

Surgically, it is important to understand the course and relationship of the tibial nerve to the surrounding muscles in the leg. In the upper two-thirds of the leg, the nerve is located in the deep posterior compartment between the tibialis posterior muscle and the flexor digitorum longus muscle anteriorly. As it courses to the inferior one-third of the leg, the flexor hallucis longus muscle is situated lateral to the nerve, and the flexor digitorum longus muscle is anteromedial. The nerve remains lateral and slightly posterior to the posterior tibial artery.[268] As the tibial nerve courses distally, it divides into the medial and lateral plantar nerves, as well as the medial calcaneal nerve to the medial and plantar-medial aspects of the heel. The level of branching of these nerves is highly variable.[269,272] In a cadaver study,[269] the tibial nerve was noted to bifurcate within the tarsal tunnel in 95% of the specimens. The medial and lateral plantar nerves course through the distal tarsal tunnel to the porta pedis, where the nerves are separated by a fibrous septum that runs from the deep surface of the abductor hallucis to the medial wall of the calcaneus inferior to the sustentaculum tali (Fig. 51.28), dividing the porta pedis into anterior and posterior

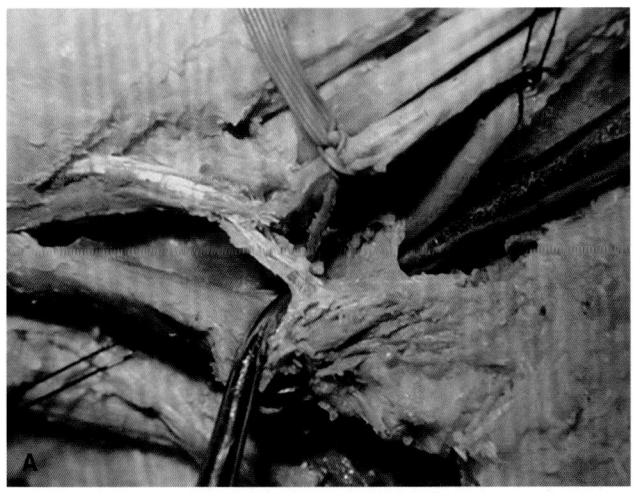
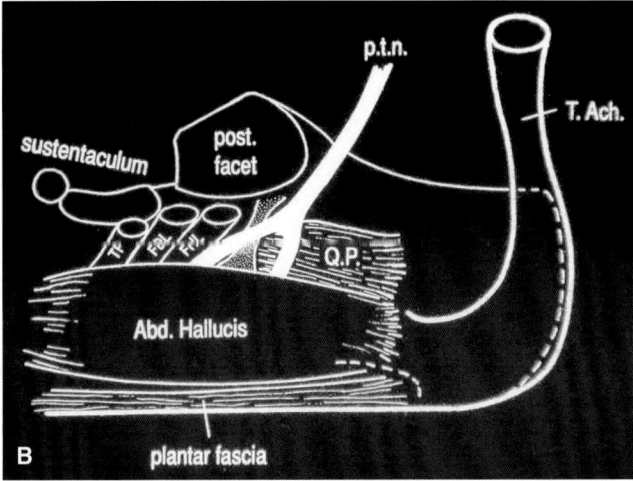

FIGURE 51.28 The tarsal tunnel and porta pedis. **A.** Cadaver dissection right tarsal tunnel and porta pedis showing fibrous septum deep to abductor hallucis and separating the anterior and posterior calcaneal canals, through which course the medial and lateral plantar nerves and their branches, respectively. **B.** Schematic representation of the tarsal tunnel and porta pedis.

calcaneal tunnels. The medial plantar nerve is larger and initially passes superior to the abductor hallucis and is bound by the plantar calcaneonavicular ligament. As it courses through the porta pedis into the plantar vault of the foot, the medial plantar nerve sends motor branches to the abductor hallucis, flexor hallucis brevis, flexor digitorum brevis, and first lumbrical and provides sensory innervation to the medial plantar foot and medial three and one-half toes. The lateral plantar nerve is smaller and passes through a fibrous arch formed by the fascia of the abductor hallucis muscle inferiorly and the fascia of the flexor digitorum longus and quadratus plantae superiorly. Distally, it emerges between the flexor digitorum brevis and abductor digiti minimi muscles and sends its first branch to the latter. It then continues to innervate the other intrinsic muscles, except the extensor digitorum brevis, and it provides sensation to the lateral plantar foot and lateral one and one-half toes. Edwards et al. pointed out that the lateral plantar nerve is vulnerable because of its more proximal passage through the fibrous opening of the abductor hallucis.[64] Additionally, the lateral plantar nerve was found to be supplied by a vessel derived from the medial plantar artery in 65% of cases.[273] This vessel runs between the flexor digitorum brevis and the quadratus plantae and thus is rendered susceptible to compression. The third branch of the tibial nerve, namely the medial calcaneal nerve, arises from the main trunk of the tibial nerve in 69%-90% of specimens, whereas the remainder of the time, it arises from the lateral plantar nerve. The branching pattern of the nerve is variable, with the most frequent pattern being a single medial calcaneal nerve off the posterior tibial nerve that travels below the flexor retinaculum or pierces it. Havel et al. found a single medial calcaneal nerve branch in 79% of their specimens and multiple branches in 21%.[272] The medial calcaneal nerve innervates the plantar and medial aspects of the heel.

Etiology of Posterior Tarsal Tunnel Syndrome

The most common cause of PTTS is idiopathic, occurring in 21%-36% of cases.[271] In ~60%-80% of cases, a specific cause of PTTS can be identified.[245,274-276] When the cause is known, trauma accounts for the majority of cases and ranges in incidence from 17%[245] to 87.5%[277] (Fig. 51.11). In their 87 cases, Grumbine and associates found a traumatic cause in 34.5% of their patients, followed by systemic disease (33.3%), biomechanical causes (17.2%), and idiopathic causes (14.9%).[278] In another review of 186 cases, female patients had a higher predilection (56%), the average patient age was 47 years; the most common causes included trauma (17%), varicosities (13%), heel varus (11%), fibrosis (9%), and heel valgus (8%).[271]

The posterior tibial nerve is particularly vulnerable to compression after traumatic injuries of the hindfoot and ankle.[279] Myerson and Berger reported a case of a fractured sustentaculum tali fragment that migrated into the tarsal tunnel and created compression.[255] Similarly, a fractured medial tubercle of the posterior process of the talus has been shown to compress the tibial nerve.[280] In one larger series, distal tibia and ankle trauma accounted for 49 of 56 cases of PTTS.[21] Sports-related injuries have also been a documented cause.[281-283]

Oh and Meyer found that 13% of traumatic injuries were associated with jogging and aerobic exercise.[284] PTTS has also been attributed to traction injury associated with total ankle replacement,[285] lateralizing calcaneal osteotomy,[286] and limb lengthening procedures.[287]

In addition to trauma, space-occupying lesions also cause compression on the tibial nerve.[288] The most common type of space-occupying lesion is varicosity.[289] Other lesions include ganglion (Fig. 51.4),[24,290] lipoma,[291-293] neurilemoma (Fig. 51.29),[20,21,294-297] thickened flexor retinaculum,[271] heterotopic calcification,[298] and accessory muscle.[249,299-302] While not a specific lesion, PTTS has been associated with chronic venous insufficiency.[303] Although most lesions are benign, a case of synovial sarcoma causing PTTS has been documented.[304] Proliferative synovitis secondary to inflammatory arthropathies and metabolic disorders can cause compression in the tarsal tunnel and needs to be excluded.[305] Finally, bony abnormalities such as tarsal coalition[306] and talar exostosis[307] have been described as causative factors in PTTS.

PTTS has been found to be associated with systemic disease.[308,309] Park and Del Toro, in a study of 49 patients, found that 34.4% of the patients had systemic disease, most commonly diabetes and inflammatory arthritis.[310] Oloff and coworkers reported similar results in an analysis of 73 cases.[308] Systemic diseases were encountered in 34.7% of patients, with diabetes (20.4%) and inflammatory arthritis (12.2%) constituting the majority. Rheumatoid arthritis,[311] hypothyroidism,[312] seronegative arthropathy,[313,314] hyperlipidemia,[26] lymphoma,[315] and leukemia[316] have also been linked to PTTS.

Foot deformities have also been correlated with PTTS. Radin found that two-thirds of patients had varus deformity of the heel with a pronated forefoot.[245] He believed that compensatory pronation contracts the abductor hallucis and compresses the distal tarsal tunnel. Pes planovalgus deformity can contribute to PTTS by increasing tension on the posterior tibial nerve. Daniels et al., in a cadaver study, demonstrated that surgically created pes valgus feet increased posterior tibial nerve tension through ankle joint dorsiflexion, hindfoot eversion, and combined ankle joint dorsiflexion-hindfoot eversion.[317] In a follow-up laboratory study, surgical reconstruction of pes valgus deformity decreased tension on the posterior tibial nerve.[318] Although these investigators did not advocate surgery, they did recommend the use of an ankle-foot orthosis to control the pes valgus deformity. The stress of prolonged stretch or tension on a nerve has been shown to have physical consequences. Lundborg and Rydevik found that elongation of a nerve by 15% resulted in complete intraneural vascular occlusion.[319]

In addition to tension, foot position can cause increased pressure within the tarsal tunnel. Trepman and associates measured tarsal tunnel pressures of cadaver specimens in neutral and maximum eversion and inversion.[320] These investigators found a significant increase in pressure with maximum inversion and eversion compared with neutral. Hence, foot deformity may be a contributing factor in the pathogenesis of PTTS. This, too, is supported by the clinical onset of PTTS following some cases of total ankle replacement,[285] lateralizing calcaneal osteotomy,[286] and limb lengthening procedures.[287]

Clinical Presentation of Posterior Tarsal Tunnel Syndrome

The symptoms of PTTS can often be diffuse with variable physical findings.[276] The history and physical examination can be essential to making the diagnosis. Patients with PTTS may relate a history of previous trauma that precipitated the pain. Most frequently, symptoms are unilateral with an insidious onset, but they have been found to occur bilaterally.[260,289,290]

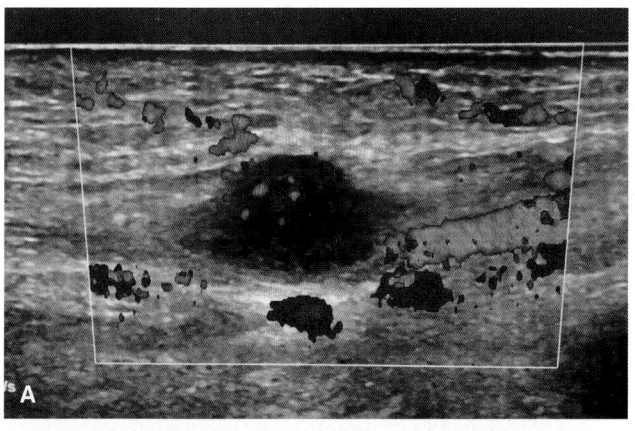
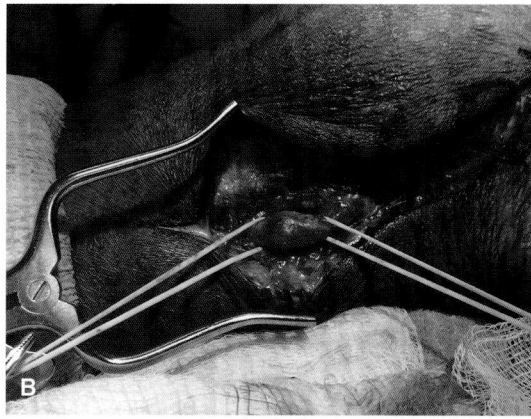
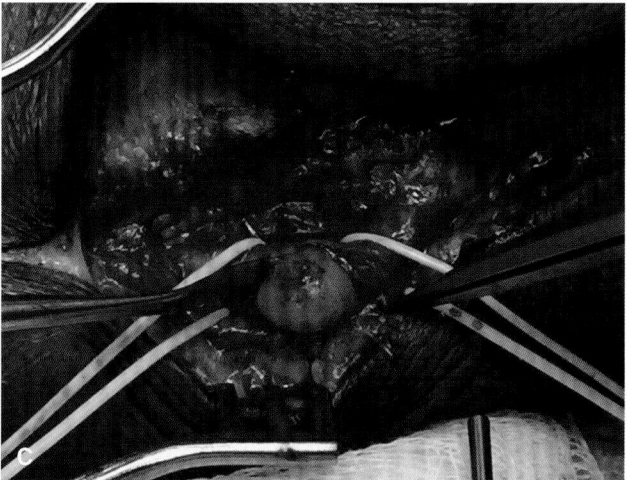
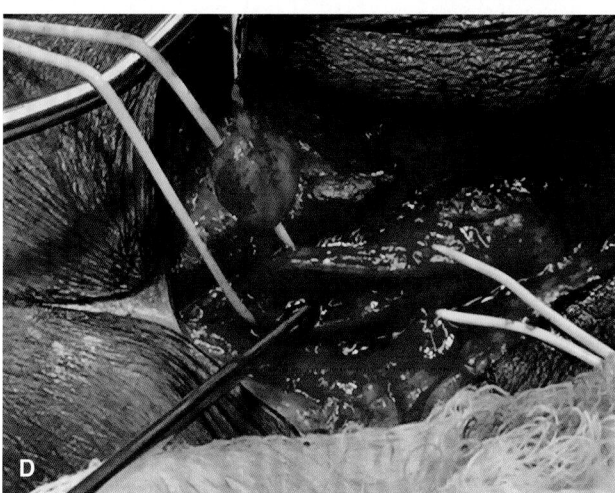
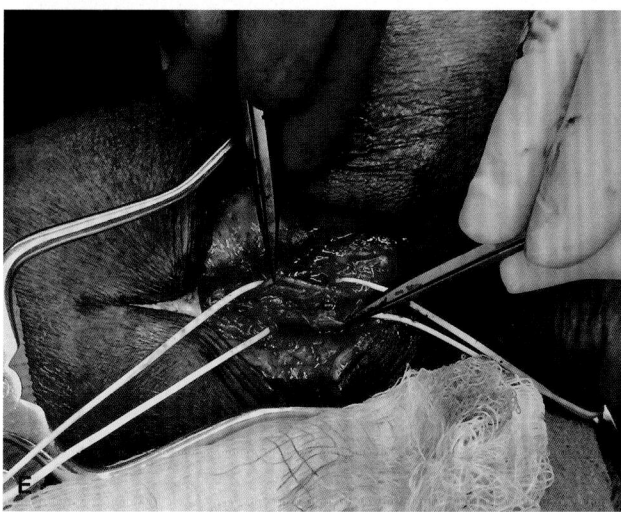

FIGURE 51.29 A. Color flow Doppler ultrasound shows hypoechoic lesion and arterial (*red*) and venous (*blue*) flow in tarsal tunnel, corresponding to clinically evident nodule associated with pain and paresthesia in an adult male. **B.** Isolation of fusiform enlargement of tibial nerve, indicative of intraneural soft tissue mass, prior to intraoperative assessment of stimulated electrical activity and muscle function. **C.** Epineurotomy reveals lamellar soft tissue nodule suggestive of schwannoma. **D.** Intraneural lesion separated from intact nerve fibers and fasciculi, effecting complete excision with preservation of functional nerve elements. **E.** After excision of the neurilemoma, which was subsequently microscopically identified as schwannoma, residual functional nerve elements are again assessed for stimulated function and the results compared with pre-excision values.

Common clinical features seen in most patients include burning, tingling, and numbness over the distribution of the involved nerve or nerves.[245,272,274,277,321] With plantar nerve involvement, symptoms are localized to the toes and distal sole of the foot. When the medial calcaneal branch is involved, symptoms are localized to the heel.[284]

Classically, these symptoms are aggravated by multiple activities such as prolonged standing or walking and are relieved by rest, elevation, and removal of shoes.[266,322] Nocturnal aggravation of symptoms is a common finding. Mosimann found that

42% of patients had nocturnal paresthesia.[277] When advanced, this paresthesia may radiate proximally to the calf and leg (ie, Valleix phenomenon).[64,244,244,245]

Positive *Tinel sign* and *sensory impairment* of the involved plantar nerves are two of the most common findings in PTTS.[284] Tinel sign is elicited by percussion of the tibial nerve over the tarsal tunnel. When the sign is positive, an electrical sensation or tingling sensation radiates distally into the sole of the foot or digits.[323] A positive sign is present in 50%-90% of cases.[321,324] Sensory impairment has been reported in more than two of

three patients and is most simply evaluated by pinprick and two-point discrimination.[321]

Tenderness with direct palpation over the tarsal tunnel is another common clinical finding.[267] Motor symptoms, such as weakness or muscle atrophy, are relatively rare and present only in advanced cases. Oh and Meyer found weakness of toe flexion the only reliable motor function test, a finding present in 19% of their cases.[284]

Diagnosis of Posterior Tarsal Tunnel Syndrome

The key to making the diagnosis of PTTS is the history and physical examination with neurologic evaluation. As already described, the two most helpful tests are positive Tinel sign and sensory loss in the distribution of the involved branches. Despite these tests, PTTS can be a challenging diagnosis.[325]

Oh and Meyer[284] pointed out that two neurologic conditions that can be confused with PTTS are L5 or S1 radiculopathy and sensory polyneuropathy. Clinical and objective findings help to distinguish among these conditions. Objective findings favoring radiculopathy include a positive straight leg raise test, calf muscle atrophy, radiating pain to the lower back, sensory abnormalities on the dorsum of the foot, and absent or negative Tinel sign. Clinical signs suggestive of polyneuropathy consist of a bilateral presentation, a stocking-glove distribution of sensory loss, and absent or negative Tinel sign. Painful conditions in the heel, medial ankle, or low back regions should be included in the differential diagnosis of PTTS.[325-327] It is important to rule out more proximal sites of nerve entrapment because PTTS has been reported to occur with additional nerve lesions in the same limb.[328]

The history and physical examination serve as guides for other tests, to narrow the differential diagnosis further. For example, radiographs may be used to determine foot deformity, fracture, or accessory ossicles. Injections of local anesthetic or corticosteroid can aid in the diagnosis and can provide

temporary relief. Laboratory studies may be indicated to rule out metabolic disorders such as hypothyroidism, rheumatoid arthritis, or diabetes mellitus. *Perthes tourniquet test* may be of value if varicosities are the suspected cause.[299] This test consists of inflating a cuff around the lower calf of the affected side from 30 to 50 mm Hg, which causes occlusion of the superficial venous system but not the deep venous system or arterial system. If the deep venous system of the tarsal tunnel is incompetent (eg, valvular damage or insufficiency), the posterior tibial venae comitans in the tarsal tunnel will engorge and will reproduce the symptoms.

Magnetic Resonance Imaging in Posterior Tarsal Tunnel Syndrome

MRI has been a valuable tool in the diagnosis of PTTS primarily because of its ability to demonstrate space-occupying soft tissue lesions.[305,329,330] Erickson et al., using MRI, were able to identify neurilemomas, tenosynovitis, ganglion cysts, posttraumatic fibrosis, and posttraumatic neuromas causing PTTS.[305] Kerr and Frey found lesions in 82% of their cases, with the most common causes being a focal mass lesion and varicose veins.[306] Another study by the same authors used MRI to study 40 symptomatic feet.[331] Electrodiagnostic studies confirmed the diagnosis in 20 ft. Seventeen of these 20 (85%) had positive MRI findings, with the most common being flexor hallucis tenosynovitis. Surgery was required in 21 ft and confirmed MRI findings in 19 of the 21. MRI may also be helpful in patients in whom revisional surgery is considered because it has been able to show incomplete release of the flexor retinaculum.[332] Downey also described the combined use of the Perthes test and MRI to confirm venous insufficiency of the venae comitans as a cause of PTTS[330] (Fig. 51.30).

Electrodiagnostic Studies in Posterior Tarsal Tunnel Syndrome

Clinical electrodiagnostic tests serve to objectively confirm the diagnosis of PTTS. Keep in mind that electrodiagnostic nerve

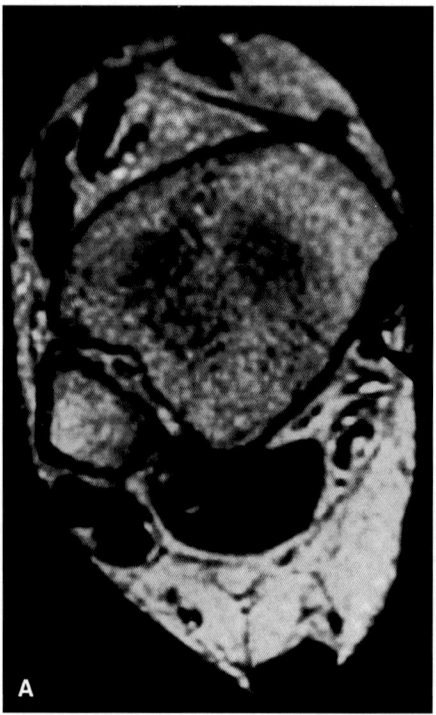 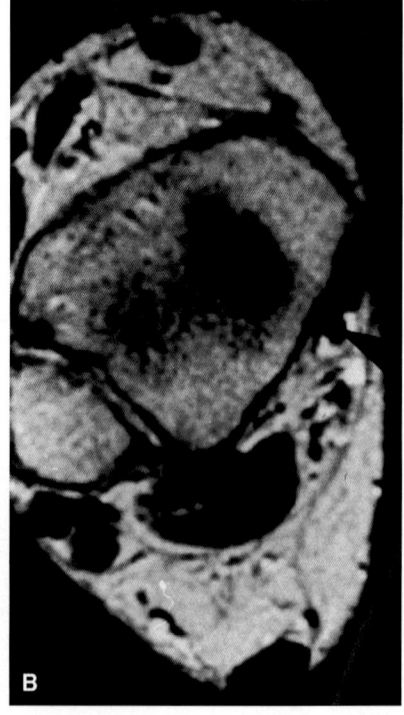

FIGURE 51.30 T2-weighted transverse plane axial magnetic resonance images at a level just proximal to the ankle, in a patient with suspected tarsal tunnel syndrome with venous insufficiency and varicosities evident in the lower extremities. **A.** Prior to tourniquet inflation, the posterior tibial artery is noted as a low-intensity (*black*) structure due to signal void, and the venae comitans are hardly evident even though they are usually noted as high-intensity structures resulting from flow enhancement. **B.** After inflation of a midcalf tourniquet to 50-mm Hg pressure, enough to occlude the superficial venous return, the venae comitans become more noticeable on either side of the artery, suggesting venous insufficiency as a cause of the patient's tarsal tunnel syndrome, and subsequent surgical dissection revealed varicosities of the venae comitans. (Courtesy of Michael S. Downey, DPM, FACFAS; Philadelphia, PA.)

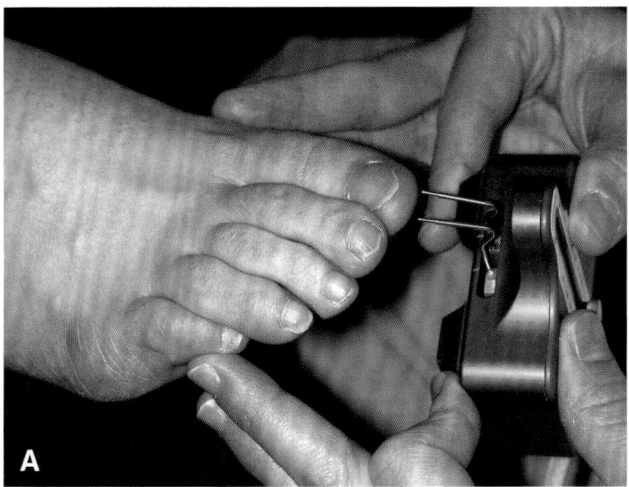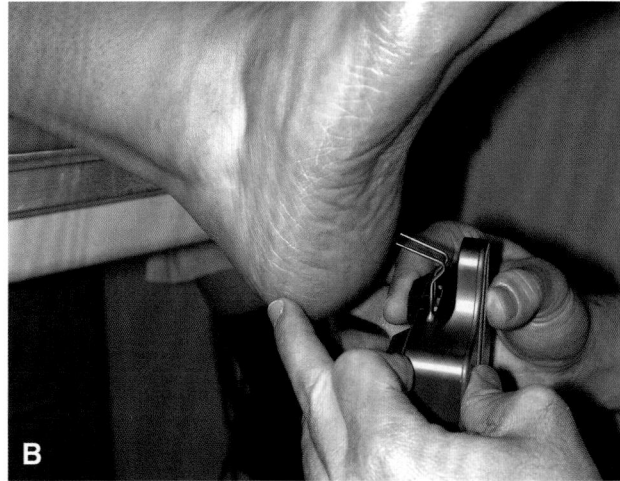

FIGURE 51.31 Quantitative sensory testing. Assessing sensibility to two-point pressure in the distribution of the medial plantar nerve **(A)**, and the medial calcaneal nerve **(B)**.

testing can also be performed in the operating room (see Intraoperative Nerve Monitoring, above), and preoperative test results can be used as a reference for intraoperative findings. Electrodiagnostic nerve tests can be divided into three categories: motor, sensory, and mixed nerve conduction velocities. Overall, these tests have a diagnostic accuracy of up to 90%.[333] Typically, these tests are performed with the patient in a supine position. Comparison studies with the patient in a weight-bearing position have failed to demonstrate a significant difference.[334] Results of motor conduction tests in PTTS are variable. Historically, a prolonged distal motor latency was used as a diagnostic criterion for PTTS, but later reports demonstrated a low sensitivity with prolonged latencies in 17%-52% of cases.[274] Terminal latency sensitivity has been reported to be 47% overall.[284] Thus, normal distal motor latencies alone are inadequate to rule out PTTS. Sensory nerve conduction velocities, conversely, have been superior in confirming the diagnosis of PTTS.[333] Pathologic sensory nerve conduction can be expressed by the absence of compound NAPs or slow NCV.[274] Despite higher sensitivity, false-positive results for sensory nerve conduction have been reported in up to 8% of cases.[333] Mixed NCV of the medial and lateral plantar nerves was described by Saeed and Gatens.[335] The purpose of this test was to increase the sensory conduction by recording a larger amplitude of signal and to improve on the poor sensitivity of motor conduction studies. Abnormalities using these tests were reported in 12 of 14 cases. The use of needle EMG can demonstrate denervation of the involved intrinsic foot muscles, but it is of limited value when nerve conduction studies localize the lesion to the tarsal tunnel.[284]

Quantitative Sensory Testing in Posterior Tarsal Tunnel Syndrome

Clinical electrodiagnostic studies are sometimes negative and often are not sensitive enough to identify early clinical problems of nerve entrapment. As a result, Dellon popularized the use of *QST techniques* for peripheral nerve entrapment syndromes.[336] Specifically, these techniques quantify perception thresholds for pressure and vibration, a function of large myelinated fibers. In cases of peripheral nerve compression, these fibers are typically affected first. The particular method for testing these fibers makes use of a pressure-specified

sensory device that permits measurement of the cutaneous pressure threshold for one- and two-point static or moving discrimination (Fig. 51.31).[71] In patients with PTTS, it has been found to be more sensitive, but less specific, than electrodiagnostic studies. In a report of 26 cases of PTTS, all patients were found to have abnormal pressure-specified sensory device tests compared with age-matched normal subjects, whereas only 17 had abnormal electrodiagnostic studies.[73] Indications for QST in the lower extremity have included heel pain, Morton neuroma, PTTS, DPN entrapment, sural nerve entrapment, and diabetic neuropathy. Advantages of this technique in the management of peripheral nerve entrapments are ease of interpretation of the results, ease of test performance with less pain to the patient, and earlier recognition and diagnosis of nerve compression or entrapment, particularly if smaller nerves are involved.[336] Interestingly, patients with medial plantar heel pain have been shown to display abnormal sensibility, even early in the clinical course of their heel pain, within the branches of the posterior tibial nerve, and specifically, within the distribution of the medial calcaneal nerve and the medial plantar nerve.[337]

The diagnosis of PTTS is first and foremost a clinical one, and hence when strong clinical findings suggesting PTTS are present, the diagnosis should not be reversed in the face of negative electrodiagnostic, MRI, or QST findings because these tests serve to support rather than make the diagnosis. These studies can be helpful at times, especially when trying to evaluate other potential causes of nerve pain, such as a space-occupying lesion, peripheral neuropathy, or lumbar radiculopathy.[338]

Conservative Treatment of Posterior Tarsal Tunnel Syndrome

Once a diagnosis of PTTS has been made, conservative therapy should generally be attempted before surgical intervention. Treatment options vary and should focus on the cause, if it can be determined. In some instances of severe nerve entrapment or compression, or when a space-occupying mass is diagnosed, immediate surgical intervention may be considered appropriate. One of the first lines of therapy in the conservative management of PTTS consists of controlling the inflammation around the posterior tibial nerve. The use of NSAIDs and of

corticosteroid injections has proven effective, especially in the presence of inflammatory arthropathy with associated tenosynovitis.[245]

Orthoses have been beneficial in cases of foot deformity. Medial longitudinal arch supports and medial heel wedges have been successful for flexible valgus deformities.[282,339] Rask suggested that orthotics may decrease tension across the posterior tibial nerve by counteracting hyperpronatory forces.[340] Other conservative measures include physical therapy to enhance mobilization of the posterior tibial nerve and to decrease tension. Iontophoresis may eradicate local symptoms of tenosynovitis.[340,341] If edema secondary to venous stasis is a contributing factor, compressive stockings may be beneficial.[21] Occasionally, a trial of immobilization in a short leg cast or an ankle-foot orthosis may be beneficial.[338] Should conservative methods of treatment fail, or when conservative measures are unlikely to alleviate the nerve compression, then surgical intervention is indicated.

Surgical Treatment of Posterior Tarsal Tunnel Syndrome

Surgical decompression of the tarsal tunnel varies based on the origin of the nerve entrapment. Regardless of cause, a detailed inspection of the tarsal tunnel and its contents is recommended.[342] Obviously, any space-occupying lesion or bone mass must be evaluated carefully and appropriately excised if possible. Although specific procedures and techniques vary, perhaps the most common approach was outlined by Lam.[258] He described three components to decompress the tarsal tunnel adequately. The first consists of release of the flexor retinaculum overlying the tarsal tunnel without deep suture closure. The second is to release the abductor fascia in the porta pedis. The third is to release the posterior tibial nerve and associated plantar branches from any surrounding entrapment. Traditionally, the procedure has been performed through a standard open incision posterior to the medial malleolus. Minimal incisions with endoscopic release of the retinaculum have been described, but further studies are needed to validate this technique.[343,344]

Other strategies often employed include use of a tourniquet to improve visualization, intraoperative nerve stimulation to assess nerve function, and a postoperative drain. Typically, postoperative care has consisted of early mobilization usually combined with non–weight bearing for 1-4 weeks, followed by physical therapy. A removable splint or bivalved below-knee cast may be used to encourage early mobilization to reduce fibrosis.[345]

The incidence of surgical success varies in the literature from 44% to 95%.[245,271,346,347] Takakura and associates reported that patients with space-occupying lesions and coalitions did much better than those with traumatic and idiopathic causes.[348] These investigators also found poorer results with a longer interval between onset of symptoms and operation.

Turan and associates examined the results of surgery in 18 patients with long-standing (median, 60 months) PTTS.[349] At an average clinical follow-up of 18 months, 61% of patients had an excellent outcome (ie, no remaining symptoms). Varicose veins were the most consistent pathoanatomical finding. Three patients (17%) had symptoms similar to those experienced before surgery, and they were considered to have had a failed result. All three patients had previous trauma, with two of the three having the longest duration of symptoms.

Mahan et al. reported that 71.1% of patients demonstrated improvement postoperatively.[248] Trauma accounted for 40% of the cases. These investigators also provided technical recommendations, including the following: atraumatic technique, use of surgical loupes, adequate hemostasis, use of a closed-suction drain postoperatively, and a comprehensive release including the abductor fascia. Similarly, Stern and Joyce found very good or excellent results in 11 of 15 surgical procedures of PTTS.[350] In an attempt to correlate patient satisfaction with cause of the disorder, their study revealed that a traumatic origin yielded the best results.

Bailie and Kelikian analyzed 34 patients after tarsal tunnel surgery.[351] Subjectively, patients described a satisfactory outcome in 72% of cases. Seventy-six percent had a traumatic cause, whereas 24% of these conditions were nontraumatic. Functional outcome was assessed using the functional foot score, which considered functional disability and performance of activities of daily living. Postoperative functional foot scores were significantly worse for the patients with traumatic cases than for those with atraumatic disorders. This finding correlated with patient satisfaction because 14% of the patients in the nontraumatic group were not satisfied with the surgical outcome, whereas 34% of those in the traumatic group were not satisfied. Although most other cases consisted of a proximal entrapment of the medial and lateral plantar nerves, these investigators did note an association between atraumatic origin and distal impingement at the abductor hallucis fascia. Hence, they emphasized release of the deep lamina of the abductor hallucis fascia to the level of the plantar fascia in all cases, regardless of cause.

Pfeiffer and Cracchiolo questioned the long-term benefits of surgical intervention.[346] They reviewed clinical results after tarsal tunnel release in 32 ft with an average follow-up of 31 months. Only 44% had a good or excellent result (benefited markedly from the operative procedure), and 38% had a poor result (patients dissatisfied with no long-term relief of pain). Of the 5 ft with an excellent result, three had a space-occupying lesion near the tarsal tunnel that was treated at the same time. These investigators concluded that "unless there is an associated lesion near or within the tarsal tunnel preoperatively, decompression of the posterior tibial nerve should be considered with caution."

Most authors agree that surgical results are improved under the following conditions: (1) young patients, (2) short history of symptoms, (3) early diagnosis, and (4) an identifiable lesion.[346,348,350] Complications of tarsal tunnel surgery, reported in ~13% of cases, include wound infection, hematoma, suture abscess, and hypertrophic scar.[349,351]

Recurrent Posterior Tarsal Tunnel Syndrome

Recurrent PTTS is a difficult entity to treat, and the results are less predictable. Factors that have been associated with failure of tarsal tunnel release include older patients,[258,348] double-crush syndrome,[352] idiopathic cases,[346] incorrect initial diagnosis, and inadequate release.[270] Zahari and Ly reported two cases of recurrence related to postoperative ankle injuries.[353] These investigators rereleased the retinaculum and injected steroid to retard scar formation.

Initial surgical treatment often simply focuses on releasing the flexor retinaculum without addressing the plantar branches. MRI has been shown to be effective in evaluating

incomplete release of the flexor retinaculum.[332] In fact, inadequate decompression has been reported as the most common indication for revisional surgery.[257,270] Skalley and associates analyzed clinical results after revisional tarsal tunnel release.[270] Revisional surgery was performed a mean of 3.5 years after initial release. These investigators identified three groups of patients based on intraoperative findings and clinical outcome. The first group (4 ft), which did poorly, revealed posterior tibial nerve scarring and inadequate distal release at the initial surgery. The second group (5 ft) overall noted an improvement, had scarring of the nerve, and had an adequate distal release. The third and final group (4 ft), which did well, had no posterior tibial nerve scarring but inadequate distal release. These workers concluded that the results of epineurolysis from scarring of the posterior tibial nerve are less predictable, and they would not recommend surgical exploration after previous tarsal tunnel surgery with an adequate distal release. Their technique did note the use of intraoperative nerve stimulation to identify the nerve encased in scar tissue.

Other methods have been described to abate the scarring process in revisional surgical treatment. Barrier techniques designed to insulate the posterior tibial nerve from recurrent scar tissue incarceration (ie, adhesive neuralgia) have been tried. One such method is silicone entubulation or ensheathment, which has been used for treating nerve entrapments (Figs. 51.7 and 51.8).[354] This method, however, was found to cause a fibrous capsule around the nerve and ultimately to lead to re-entrapment. In two patients with a recurrent PTTS, Novotny and associates reported excellent results using a radial forearm free flap.[257] These investigators found this technique to be effective in limiting scar formation. Instead of using a silicone barrier, the use of amnion-derived barrier materials[154-156] and stem cell therapies[157-159] have been shown to be of some benefit in minimizing exuberant scar formation and aid nerve regeneration.

The use of autogenous saphenous vein graft wrapping has been advocated as a barrier technique for recurrent nerve entrapments. Sotereanos et al. described the procedure for recurrent entrapment of the median nerve in the upper extremity secondary to scar formation.[355] Under loupe magnification, the greater saphenous vein is wrapped around the nerve with its endothelial surface against the nerve. Theoretically, the autogenous vein is believed to provide an external barrier against scarring of the nerve and the surrounding tissues that allows improvement in the vascular supply to the nerve. These investigators also suggested that the vein acts as a gliding conduit for the nerve and the vascular endothelium prevents internal scar formation.

The use of this technique for recurrent PTTS has been examined in several clinical series.[356-358] Gould reported wrapping a total of 65 nerves in the lower extremity, including the posterior tibial, superficial peroneal, common and deep peroneal, sural, and intermetatarsal. He reported 63% good or excellent results (ie, no pain or occasional pain with exertion) and 37% fair to poor results. Seventy-five percent of the patients were gratified with the results. The best outcomes were noted in patients with external adhesions, and those with internal scarring did not do as well; histology inspection at 17 months postsurgery demonstrated viable vein graft with satisfactory vascularity evidenced by patent adventitial lumens, and there was no evidence of vein graft degeneration.[338] Although internal scar within the nerve was not detected, no obvious gliding surface between the nerve and vein graft was identified, a finding suggesting this to be a less likely mechanism. Easley and Schon reviewed their series of vein wrapping procedures used for adhesive neuralgia in 25 patients.[358] They used the saphenous vein in 19 cases and a fetal umbilical vein in 6 cases. Twenty-one of their 25 cases were entrapment neuropathies of the posterior tibial nerve. Seventeen of the 25 patients (68%) were satisfied with the procedure (with or without reservations), whereas 8 patients (32%) gained minimal or no relief of their symptoms. The indications for vein wrapping in this series were (1) intractable neurogenic pain, (2) failure of the nonoperative management protocol, (3) temporary relief of symptoms after previous neurolysis with subsequent recurrence, and (4) clinical findings consistent with adhesive neuralgia. Long-term studies are needed to assess the benefits of this technique for PTTS accurately.

Preferred Surgical Technique for Posterior Tarsal Tunnel Syndrome

Tarsal tunnel decompression is performed with or without the use of a midthigh pneumatic tourniquet. When a tourniquet is used, certain factors must be remembered: (1) the tourniquet creates an ischemic state, possibly making the posterior tibial nerve unresponsive to an intraoperative nerve stimulator; (2) intraoperative nerve monitoring measurements are affected by ischemia; (3) the pulse of the posterior tibial artery is not palpable, making entrance to the third compartment slightly more hazardous; and (4) the tourniquet is usually deflated before wound closure to ensure hemostasis. Still further, in regard to IONM and nerve stimulation, local anesthetic and muscle paralyzing agents cannot generally be used, and certain general anesthetics also influence functional measurements of the nerve. Furthermore, loupe magnification and fine-tipped instrumentation are used.

The approach is through a 10- to 15-cm, retromalleolar, curvilinear incision extending from ~3 cm superior to the flexor retinaculum, gently curving distal to the inferior margin of the abductor hallucis muscle, and onto the plantar skin if necessary. The incision is deepened through the subcutaneous layer with meticulous hemostasis obtained. This dissection is done bluntly to avoid damage to the medial calcaneal nerve branch, which may present in the wound, and requires identification and protection. When the flexor retinaculum is reached, the subcutaneous layer is bluntly reflected.

Once the flexor retinaculum is exposed, care is taken to identify the third canal of the tarsal tunnel, with the aim of achieving external neurolysis of the tibial nerve and its branches (see External Neurolysis, above). The posterior tibial artery may be palpated if a tourniquet is not used. If a tourniquet is used, the tibialis posterior, flexor digitorum longus, and flexor hallucis longus tendons will be palpated with the third canal lying between the flexor longus tendons. Passive manipulation of the foot, lesser digits, and hallux aids in the identification of these tendinous structures. Alternatively, the venae comitans can usually be visualized through the flexor retinaculum. Occasionally, a perforating vein that pierces the flexor retinaculum can be used to identify the third canal because it is presumed to communicate with the venae comitans of the posterior tibial artery. If the third canal cannot be located by these methods, as often occurs in revisional tarsal tunnel surgical procedures, the posterior tibial nerve may be identified proximal to the tarsal tunnel and followed distally. Once the third canal of the

flexor retinaculum has been identified, the roof is incised in its entirety from proximal to distal, to allow access to its contents.

The posterior tibial nerve is isolated and is freed of any constricting connective tissue or scarring. A vessel loop or a Penrose drain is placed around the nerve trunk to aid in operative retraction and manipulation. Once the posterior tibial nerve is isolated, the dissection is carried distally until all the branches have been isolated. Generally, the medial calcaneal nerve branches first, followed by the medial plantar and lateral plantar branches. Vessel loops or Penrose drains are similarly placed around the branches to aid in operative retraction and manipulation. An intraoperative nerve stimulator may be used to aid in the identification of the nerve or its branches and to assess their function, and IONM can provide useful electrical information to guide surgical decision making in the operating room (Fig. 51.6) (see Intraoperative Nerve Monitoring, above).

The dissection is then carried distally to the abductor canal, where the plantar nerves enter the plantar vault via the porta pedis. Dilation of the abductor canal and of the channels for the medial and lateral plantar nerves is then performed. This may be accomplished bluntly with the surgeon's finger or sharply by excising the septum between the plantar nerves, which runs from the deep surface of abductor hallucis to the medial cortex of the calcaneus plantar to the sustentaculum tali. To incise the septum between the medial and lateral plantar nerves, the deep fascia overlying the abductor hallucis muscle is incised (Figs. 51.11 and 51.28), and the muscle is retracted inferiorly. The underlying fascial origin of the muscle is then exposed. This forms the medial plantar roof of the distal tarsal tunnel, which is the porta pedis. This fascia is incised, to expose the underlying medial and lateral nerve branches. The fascial septum between the medial and lateral plantar nerves can then be released or excised, thus completing the external neurolysis of the posterior tibial nerve.

If a local neoplasm (Fig. 51.29), bony prominence, or other compressive problem is observed, it is excised. Sectioning and ligation of varicosities of the venae comitans can be performed when these lesions contribute to the neural compression. If an aneurysmal defect of the posterior tibial artery is identified, it may be repaired, but this should be done only by a surgeon well oriented in this vascular technique. Attention is then returned to the proximal end of the tarsal tunnel, where blunt dilation is again performed with the surgeon's finger or similar instrumentation.

After complete external neurolysis, the nerve is assessed. If necessary, internal neurolysis is then performed (see Description of Internal Neurolysis [Endoneurolysis], above). Furthermore, depending on the patient's specific history and needs, nerve transposition, wrapping, excision, and stump relocation can then be performed (see explanation of these surgical maneuvers, above). The wound is then flushed with copious amounts of sterile isotonic saline. After complete release, the flexor retinaculum is left open to reduce the chances of postoperative fibrosis and re-entrapment. If a tourniquet has been used, it is usually deflated, and hemostasis is achieved. A closed-suction drain may be used. A small amount of short-acting phosphate-type steroid may be infiltrated. The subcutaneous layer is then reapproximated using 3-0 or 4-0 absorbable suture. The skin is then closed with 5-0 or 6-0 absorbable or 4-0 or 5-0 nonabsorbable suture. Saline-moistened sponges and a dry sterile dressing are then applied, followed by application of a soft dressing that will allow the patient to flex the knee, ankle, and

metatarsophalangeal joints early in the postoperative phase. Venous thromboprophylaxis is employed, in keeping with the patient's specific needs.

A dressing change is usually performed the first postoperative week, and the patient's wound inspected, and motion of the ankle and foot assessed. The patient is kept non–weight bearing for the first 10-21 days, depending on the extent of the incision onto the plantar skin. Active dorsiflexion-plantar flexion exercises are employed to encourage free movement between the nerve and adjacent tissues. Prolonged immobilization has been found to allow a greater chance of reincarceration of the nerve. At 4 weeks, the patient is allowed to begin partial weight bearing, with full ambulation allowed after about 6-8 weeks. Scar massage, ultrasonography or iontophoresis, and other rehabilitative modalities are begun based on the patient's specific indications and needs.

PLANTAR NERVES

Direct trauma affecting the plantar medial arch, fractures, or dislocations involving the calcaneus, or surgery performed on the hindfoot may damage nerve trunks and surrounding connective tissues and may thus produce *plantar nerve entrapment*. Similarly, space-occupying lesions, including ganglion cyst[359] or schwannoma,[360] or a fibrolipoma (Fig. 51.32), in the plantar vault may obliterate normal anatomy and lead to plantar nerve compression. Distally, branches of the plantar medial and lateral nerves can become entrapped after plantar fasciectomy, and those of the medial plantar nerve can be injured during first metatarsophalangeal sesamoidectomy and/or bunionectomy, where injury to the medial plantar nerve can result in formation of Joplin neuroma, a lesion that can be successfully managed with excision of the neuroma and implantation of the proximal stump into the medial arch.[361]

Symptoms associated with plantar nerve entrapment may be similar to those encountered with PTTS, Morton neuroma, and even lumbosacral radiculopathy, and the clinician must distinguish between these conditions. The cutaneous distribution over the sole of the foot, however, does not include the plantar medial aspect of the heel, which receives its innervation from the medial calcaneal nerve. Complaints of sharp or burning pain, numbness, and paresthesia, along with plantar sensory deficit, are common with intermetatarsal plantar neuroma of nerve entrapment.

Recalcitrant cases of plantar nerve entrapment often require surgical neurolysis, and the surgeon should aim to minimize intrinsic skeletal muscle function and try to maintain plantar sensation. If the entrapment site is located proximally in the plantar vault, the surgical approach is similar to that used for tarsal tunnel decompression, with a curvilinear incision that extends from the tunnel onto the plantar aspect of the foot over the belly of abductor hallucis then onto the plantar skin in a fashion that does not compromise vascularity while affording access to the target nerve/s. When the entrapment is located distally, the approach may vary depending on the specific location of the nerve incarceration. A plantar Z incision can be used to expose the entire plantar vault and readily allows exposure distally to the plantar digital sulcus (Figs. 51.13 and 51.33). The basic maneuvers of external neurolysis, IONM, endoneurolysis, nerve and stump transposition, and neurectomy (all described above) are used in the surgical management of plantar nerve lesions. When neurectomy

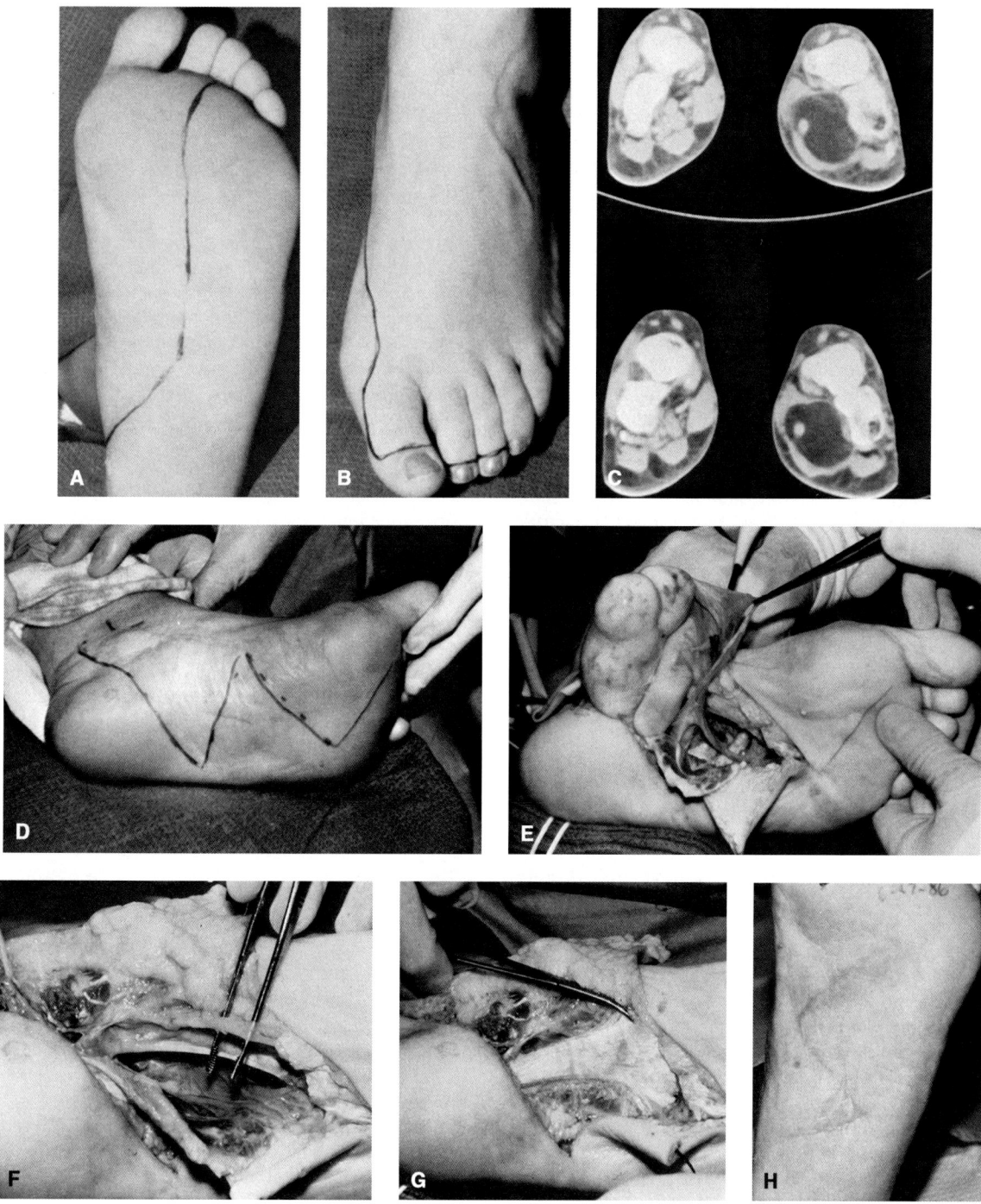

FIGURE 51.32 Rapidly progressing tarsal tunnel syndrome and suspected plantar mass in a 32-year-old woman with pain, paresthesia, and numbness of the plantar medial aspect of the left foot. She related that her arch had enlarged over the previous 18 months. Examination revealed moderate enlargement of the left foot relative to the right. The entire medial arch and the tips of the first, second, and third toes were essentially anesthetic. Ankle dorsiflexion–induced radiation of pain into the medial arch and first three toes, and Tinel sign was evident at the left tarsal tunnel. A computed tomography scan displayed a fibrous mass extending from the tarsal tunnel to the first intermetatarsal space, and lesion calcification raised suspicion of malignant tumor. A diagnosis of tarsal tunnel syndrome with tumor of the plantar vault was made, and, after oncology consultation, excisional biopsy through a plantar Z incision was performed. A fibrolipoma was excised, and obliteration of the plantar intrinsic musculature and compression of the medial plantar nerve were observed. The wound was primarily closed and healed unremarkably after 6 weeks of no weight bearing. The patient related 80% restoration of plantar sensation, with relief of pain 24 hours postoperatively, and nearly complete recovery 4½ months postoperatively. She related no recurrence of symptoms at 4 years postoperatively. **A.** Plantar area of primarily anesthesia with paresthesia, as outlined by the patient. **B.** Dorsal view of symptomatic area as outlined by the patient. The area is consistent with the medial plantar nerve distribution. **C.** Computed tomography scan displays a large mass in the plantar vault with fibrous tissue density and an area of calcification. **D.** Zigzag incision approximates relaxed skin tension lines to minimize scarring and to maximize exposure. **E.** Large mass (13 × 5 cm) histologically designated as a fibrolipoma. **F.** Apparently viable medial plantar nerve identified along the margin of the lesion along with atrophied muscle. **G.** Plantar fascia reapproximated and large void required the use of two closed-suction drains. **H.** Four and one-half months postoperatively, a fine-line scar is nontender, nearly full restoration of plantar sensorium has returned, and paresthesia is absent.

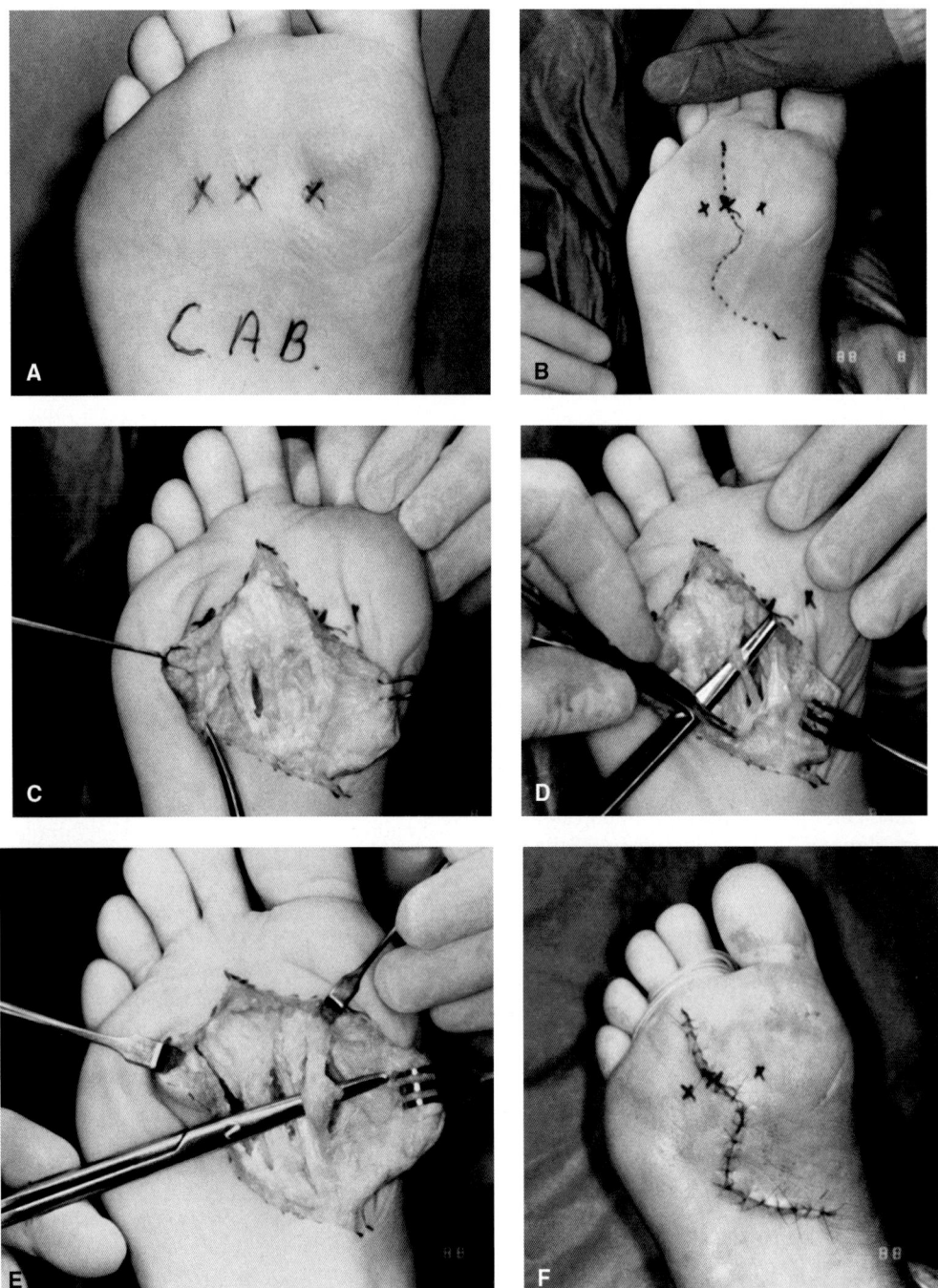

FIGURE 51.33 Recurrent intermetatarsal stump neuromas in a 25-year-old woman after two previous neuroma operations in the second and third interspaces. The patient also related a history of hallux valgus repair followed by neuroma pain in the first interspace. Neuritis redeveloped within 8 weeks after each previous surgical procedure and was more severe each time. All previous operations were performed through dorsal approaches. Examination revealed pain on digital and ankle dorsiflexion and was most severe in the first, second, and third intermetatarsal spaces. Pain radiated plantarly to the retro-medial malleolar area. Surgical neurolysis was performed through a modified plantar zigzag incision, and incarcerated stump neuromas were resected from the first, second, and third intermetatarsal spaces. Intraoperative digital dorsiflexion displayed nerve trunk tethering. The residual freshly sectioned nerve trunk was allowed to retract proximally into the plantar vault. Pain relief was prompt and complete, and weight bearing was resumed at 6 weeks postoperatively. Twenty-two months postoperatively, the patient had no reported recurrence of symptoms. **A.** *Xs* identify points of maximum tenderness. **B.** Incision designed to access three interspaces and allow identification of normal anatomy proximal to the region of scar tissue before the exploration of distal cicatrix. Moreover, the incision accounts for relaxed skin tension in an effort to minimize scar formation. **C.** Deep fascial layer obtained before medial, lateral, and distal undermining is performed. **D.** Intermetatarsal nerves are identified by separation of the digitations of the plantar fascia just proximal to the normal bifurcation. **E.** After identification of the normal nerve proximally, the nerve trunk is traced distally into scar. Here, the nerve is scarred to the flexor plate and tendon on the lateral plantar aspect of the joint. **F.** A thin plantar scar may be expected after primary closure, compression bandaging, closed-suction drainage, and 5-6 weeks of no weight bearing.

is performed in the plantar foot, whether it be in the inter-metatarsal space, or proximal to the common metatarsal nerve trunk, innervated muscle tissue or bone is typically easily accessed for implantation of the nerve end. Methods to impede symptomatic stump neuroma are also employed, since recurrent symptomatic nerve stump can occur in any patient following simple traction neurectomy (see Neurectomy and Prevention of Stump Neuroma Formation, above).

Articular Theory of Intraneural Ganglion Formation

The plantar nerves and their branches can also develop intra-neural ganglion formation[362,363]; surgeons are encouraged to consider the articular theory of intraneural ganglion formation,[363-368] a condition that has been shown to affect the articular branches of the tibial nerve and its branches to the ankle and subtalar joints.[368,369] It has even been recommended that the small articular branches, when associated with intraneural ganglion formation, be sectioned and excised in order to prevent recurrence.[369,370]

Neurogenic Heel

Neurogenic heel pain, often a condition that becomes evident after implementation of treatment for plantar fasciitis, only to have the plantar-medial heel pain persist and, ultimately, the conclusion made that entrapment of a branch of the tibial nerve, most often the lateral plantar nerve, and in particular, the first branch of the lateral plantar nerve, is often causative. In 1981, Przylucki and Jones described entrapment of the first branch of the lateral plantar nerve as a cause of persistent plantar heel pain associated with plantar fasciitis.[370] Then, in 1984, Baxter and Thigpen described good results in 32 (94.1%) of 34 patients following external neurolysis of the first branch of the lateral plantar nerve for relief of recalcitrant plantar fasciitis.[371] Since these early reports, clinical and MRI has been described as revealing atrophy of the abductor digiti quinti in cases of recalcitrant plantar fasciitis, indicative of entrapment of the lateral plantar nerve, in particular the first branch.[372] In 2003, Rose et al. showed that plantar-medial heel pain was associated with abnormal sensibility in the medial plantar and medial calcaneal nerves.[337] Ultrasound-guided radiofrequency denervation of the medial plantar nerve in runners for relief of refractory plantar medial heel pain.[373] Moreover, surgeons are advised to dissect carefully when performing calcaneal osteotomy, since it has been shown that there may be no named, anatomic "safe zone," where the nerves about the heel are not vulnerable to iatrogenic injury.[374]

Morton Intermetatarsal Neuroma

Mechanical impingement of the plantar intermetatarsal nerve (common plantar digital nerve), where the nerve engages the distal margin of the overlying (dorsally situated) deep transverse intermetatarsal ligament, can lead to in-continuity neuroma formation with intraneural fibrosis,[375-378] which is often painful enough to impede stance and gait. Although the precise prevalence of Morton neuroma remains unknown, it is generally considered a condition that occurs more commonly in females than in males,[379] and this could be related to shoe gear.

The diagnosis of Morton plantar intermetatarsal neuroma, much like the tarsal tunnel syndrome, is primarily a clinical diagnosis. A strong indicator of the presence of an intermetatarsal neuroma is Mulder sign, which is a palpable click that is elicited with simultaneous medial-to-lateral compression of the metatarsus at the level of the symptomatic intermetatarsal space, combined with alternating dorsally elevating and plantarly lowering the medial and lateral aspects of the metatarsus about the symptomatic intermetatarsal space. The Mulder's click is elicited if the symptomatic intermetatarsal nerve is large enough. It has been shown that the clinical findings of focal pain to deep palpation, pain that is aggravated by weight-bearing activity and alleviated with rest, and the presence of Mulder's click convey a diagnostic sensitivity of 98%.[380] Accurate clinical electroneurodiagnostic measurements of the function of the plantar nerves can be difficult to obtain,[402] and functional entrapment may cause severe symptoms despite normal nerve conduction velocities. Moreover, a study of the ultrasonic measurement of the intermetatarsal nerve in asymptomatic, healthy subjects, it was shown that enlargement was prevalent, leading the investigators to conclude that ultrasound is an unreliable method for diagnosing intermetatarsal neuroma, and that the clinical examination remains the gold standard for diagnosis.[381] Magnetic resonance images that reveal the intermetatarsal nerve to be >5 mm in transverse diameter and correlated with clinical symptoms, whereas the intermetatarsal bursal fluid collections of ≤3 mm are considered normal.[382]

A wide range of nonsurgical treatments have been described for the treatment of symptomatic Morton plantar intermetatarsal neuroma.[383,384] The conservative treatment of plantar nerve entrapment can be gratifying, especially when abnormal subtalar joint pronation is the causative factor. The use of a soft insole pad, a flexible sole, and a low-heeled shoe may also be helpful. For Morton metatarsalgia, a simple metatarsal projection pad positioned just proximal to the metatarsal heads can be very helpful and should be employed for a reasonable period of time prior to determining that nonsurgical care has not been adequate. Orthoses combined with NSAIDs, as well as local infiltration of corticosteroid[385-387] at the point of entrapment, in some cases, resolves the symptoms. In fact, local infiltration of corticosteroid, usually a mixture of short- and long-acting agents, combined with a metatarsal pad, is generally the most effective nonsurgical intervention, although the risk of plantar fat pad atrophy secondary to multiple corticosteroid injections should be balanced with the potential benefits. Alcohol injection,[388,389] cryotherapy,[390] radiofrequency denervation,[391-393] extracorporeal shockwave therapy,[394] and chemical denervation using botulinum toxin.[395]

The surgical management of recalcitrant Morton plantar intermetatarsal neuroma continues to hinge on excision, an intervention that is generally known to be effective in 85%-90% of cases when simple traction neurectomy is performed. A review of 41 patients, average age 44 (range 25-69) years and average follow-up of 7.4 (range 5-12) years, showed that traction neurectomy via a dorsal intermetatarsal approach for Morton neuroma resulted in clinically and statistically significant improvements in the AOFAS and VAS pain scores overall; however, 7% of the patients subjectively reported poor outcomes.[396] Dorsal and plantar incision approaches both yield satisfactory results, and a randomized controlled trial comparing the incision approaches did not make a difference in terms of satisfactory outcomes, although the types of complications varied,

with more scar issues associated with the plantar approach.[397] Dissection of the plantar intermetatarsal neuroma and the distal proper digital nerves is enhanced with the use of loupe magnification and fine-tipped instruments, and this is important for two main reasons: (1) the common and proper digital nerves often produce numerous small unnamed branches that propagate to the adjacent soft tissues, which could predispose to recurrent symptoms if left intact[398] and (2) preservation of the plantar soft tissues of the intermetatarsal space, in particular the intermetatarsal fat body, is crucial to avoiding the development of weight-bearing pain related to diminishing the function of the plantar fat pad in the ball of the foot. External neurolysis, including sectioning of the deep transverse intermetatarsal ligament, or translocation of the plantar nerve so that it courses dorsal to the transverse ligament after first sectioning it and then reapproximating it with suture. In addition to accurate dissection and preservation of the plantar intermetatarsal fat body, it is also important to section the proper digital branches, and any other unnamed branches, as far distal as possible, and the proximal common trunk well proximal to any grossly abnormal nerve, and proximal to the proximal margin of the deep transverse intermetatarsal ligament, after which the new proximal nerve stump is prepared in a fashion to diminish chaotic, bulbous budding neurites from becoming a symptomatic stump neuroma with recurrent pain (see Preventing Stump Neuroma, above). Our preferred method is to employ a plantar approach, sectioning the nerve proximal to the transverse ligament, purse string closure of the epineurium of the proximal nerve stump and bipolar electrocoagulation of redundant epineural tissue distal to the purse string suture, after which the freshly prepared nerve stump is transposed and sutured to the deep surface of an adjacent intrinsic skeletal muscle, or into nearby metatarsal bone (method described above). Adjacent interspaces can be approached using a plantar zigzag incision. The plantar approach also makes proximal nerve stump preparation and relocation easier than does the dorsal approach, which is limited from the dorsal aspect as it gets difficult to separate adjacent metatarsals and visualize the common plantar nerve proximal to the distal third of the metatarsus. After manipulating the nerve, a soft dressing is applied and the patient uses crutches to remain non–weight bearing on the operated foot for ~21 days in order to allow the plantar incision to heal. Metatarsophalangeal and ankle dorsiflexion and plantar flexion exercises are conducted daily, and venous thromboprophylaxis is conducted as deemed fit for the particular patient. The excised neuroma is submitted for pathological inspection.

Symptomatic stump neuroma occurring at the level of, and proximal to, the deep transverse intermetatarsal ligament may develop secondary to nerve stump incarceration or tethering after surgical excision of the plantar nerve in the treatment of Morton neuroma,[399-401] and implementation of methods to minimize symptomatic stump formation (as previously described) is advisable when the intermetatarsal neuroma is initially excised. If a symptomatic stump neuroma develops, and fails to resolve with nonsurgical supportive measures, then revision surgery may be indicated. The surgical management of a symptomatic stump in the plantar metatarsus is approached from the plantar surface, typically with a zigzag incision, and neuro-osteodesis or nerve-to-nerve transposition are our favored methods, assuming nonsurgical methods have failed.

REFERENCES

1. Kopell HP, Thompson WAL. *Peripheral Entrapment Neuropathies.* 2nd ed. Huntington, NY: Robert E. Krieger; 1976:1-88.
2. Kopell HP, Thompson WAL. Peripheral entrapment neuropathies of the lower extremity. *N Engl J Med.* 1960;262:56-60.
3. Carrel JM, Davidson DM. Nerve compression syndromes of the foot and ankle: a comprehensive review of symptoms, etiology, and diagnosis using nerve conduction testing. *J Am Podiatry Assoc.* 1975;65:322-341.
4. Pendleton C, Broski S, Spinner R. Concurrent Schwannoma and intraneural ganglion cyst involving branches of the common peroneal nerve. *World Neurosurg.* 2020;135:171-172.
5. Brown BA. Internal neurolysis in traumatic peripheral nerve lesions in continuity. *Surg Clin North Am.* 1972;52:1167-1175.
6. Duncan D. Alterations in the structure of nerves caused by restricting their growth with ligatures. *J Neuropathol Exp Neurol.* 1948;7:261-273.
7. Birch R, St. Clair Strange FG. A new type of peripheral nerve lesion. *J Bone Joint Surg Br.* 1990;72:312-313.
8. Brooks DM. Nerve compression by simple ganglia. *J Bone Joint Surg Br.* 1952;34:391-400.
9. Ellis VH. Two cases of ganglia in the sheath of the peroneal nerve. *Br J Surg.* 1937;24:141-142.
10. Wadstein T. Two cases of ganglia in the sheath of the peroneal nerve. *Acta Orthop Scand.* 1932;2:221-231.
11. Jacobs RR, Maxwell JA, Kepes J. Ganglia of the nerve: presentation of two unusual cases, a review of the literature, and a discussion of pathogenesis. *Clin Orthop.* 1975;113:135-144.
12. Wagner E, Ortiz C. The painful neuroma and the use of conduits. *Foot Ankle Clin.* 2011;16:295-304.
13. Vernadakis A, Koch H, Mackinnon S. Management of neuromas. *Clin Plast Surg.* 2003;30:247-268.
14. Rota E, Morelli N. Entrapment neuropathies in diabetes mellitus. *World J Diabetes.* 2016;7(17):342-353. doi: 10.4239/wjd.v7.i17.342.
15. Wilson RL. Management of pain following peripheral nerve injuries. *Orthop Clin North Am.* 1972;12:343-359.
16. Davidson MR. Heel neuroma: identification and removal. *J Am Podiatry Assoc.* 1977;67:431-435.
17. Davidson MR, Liston H, Jacoby RP, et al. Heel neuroma. *J Am Podiatry Assoc.* 1977;67:589-594.
18. Altman MI, Hinkes MP. Heel neuroma: a case history. *J Am Podiatry Assoc.* 1982;72:517-519.
19. Brietstein RJ. Compression neuropathy secondary to neurilemmoma. *J Am Podiatry Assoc.* 1985;75:160-161.
20. Dowling GL, Skaggs RE. Neurilemmoma (Schwannoma) as a cause of tarsal tunnel syndrome. *J Am Podiatry Assoc.* 1982;72:45-48.
21. Menon A, Dorfman HD, Renbaum J, et al. Tarsal tunnel syndrome secondary to neurilemmoma of the medial plantar nerve. *J Bone Joint Surg Am.* 1980;62:301-303.
22. Levin AS, Titchnal WO, Clark J. Tarsal tunnel syndrome secondary to neurilemmoma. *J Am Podiatry Assoc.* 1977;67:429-431.
23. Sasaki H, Nagano S, Yokouchi M, et al. Utility of intraoperative monitoring with motor-evoked potential during the surgical enucleation of peripheral nerve schwannoma. *Oncol Lett.* 2018;15(6):9327-9332. doi: 10.3892/ol.2018.8456.
24. Kenzora JE, Lenet MD, Sherman M. Synovial cyst of the ankle joint as a cause of tarsal tunnel syndrome. *Foot Ankle.* 1982;63:181-183.
25. Mondelli M, Romano C, Della Pota PD, et al. Electrophysiological evidence of "nerve entrapment syndromes" and subclinical peripheral neuropathy in progressive systemic sclerosis (scleroderma). *J Neurol.* 1995;242:185-194.
26. Ruderman MI, Palmer RH, Olarte MR, et al. Tarsal tunnel syndrome caused by hyperlipidemia. *Arch Neurol.* 1983;40:124-125.
27. Wieman TJ, Patel VG. Treatment of hyperesthetic neuropathic pain in diabetics: decompression of the tarsal tunnel. *Ann Surg.* 1995;221:660-664.
28. Tassler PL, Dellon AJ, Scheffler NM. Computer assisted measurement in diabetic patients with and without foot ulceration. *J Am Podiatr Med Assoc.* 1995;85:679-684.
29. Upton AR, McComas AJ. The double crush in nerve entrapment syndromes. *Lancet.* 1973;2(7825):359-362.
30. Osterman AL. The double crush syndrome. *Orthop Clin North Am.* 1988;19(1):147-155.
31. Morgan G, Wilbourn AJ. Cervical radiculopathy and coexisting distal entrapment neuropathies: double crush syndromes? *Neurology.* 1998;50:78-83.
32. Chaudhry V, Clawson LL. Entrapment of motor nerves in motor neuron disease: does double crush occur? *J Neurol Neurosurg Psychiatry.* 1997;62:71-76.
33. Wilbourn AJ, Gilliatt RW. Double crush syndrome: a critical analysis. *Neurology.* 1997;49:21-29.
34. Lundborg G, Dahlin LB. Anatomy, function, and pathophysiology of peripheral nerves and nerve compression. *Hand Clin.* 1996;12:185-193.
35. Simpson RL, Fern SA. Multiple compression neuropathies and the double crush syndrome. *Orthop Clin North Am.* 1996;27:381-388.
36. Idler RS. Persistence of symptoms after surgical release of compressive neuropathies and subsequent management. *Orthop Clin North Am.* 1996;27:409-416.
37. Simeone FA. Acute and delayed traumatic peripheral entrapment neuropathies. *Surg Clin North Am.* 1972;52:1329-1337.
38. Seddon HJ. Three types of nerve injury. *Brain.* 1943;66:238-288.
39. Mathews GJ, Osterholm JL. Painful traumatic neuromas. *Surg Clin North Am.* 1972;51:1313-1324.
40. Subotnick SI. Compartment syndromes in the lower extremities. *J Am Podiatry Assoc.* 1975;65:342-348.

41. Matsen FA, Clawson DK. Compartment syndromes (symposium). *Clin Orthop.* 1975;113:2-110.
42. Mthethwa J, Chikate A. A review of the management of tibial plateau fractures. *Musculoskelet Surg.* 2018;102(2):119-127. doi: 10.1007/s12306-017-0514-8.
43. Schut L. Nerve injuries in children. *Surg Clin North Am.* 1972;52:1307-1312.
44. Bigos SJ, Coleman S. Foot deformities secondary to gluteal injection in infancy. *J Pediatr Orthop.* 1984;4:560-563.
45. Matsen DD. Early neurolysis in treatment of injury of peripheral nerves due to faulty injection of antibiotics. *N Engl J Med.* 1950;242:973-975.
46. Clark WK. Surgery for injection injury of peripheral nerves. *Surg Clin North Am.* 1972;52:1325-1328.
47. Preston D, Logigian E. Iatrogenic needle induced peroneal neuropathy in the foot. *Ann Intern Med.* 1988;108:921-922.
48. Kim DH, Murovic JA, Tiel R, Kline DG. Management and outcomes in 353 surgically treated sciatic nerve lesions. *J Neurosurg.* 2004;101(1):8-17.
49. Highet WB, Holmes W. Traction injuries to the lateral popliteal nerve and traction injuries to peripheral nerves after suture. *Br J Surg.* 1942;30:212-233.
50. Nobel W. Peroneal palsy due to hematoma in the common peroneal nerve sheath after distal torsional fractures and inversion ankle sprains: report of two cases. *J Bone Joint Surg Am.* 1966;48:1484-1495.
51. Mansoor IA. Delayed incomplete traction palsy of the lateral popliteal nerve. *Clin Orthop.* 1969;66:183-187.
52. Seddon HJ. A classification of nerve injuries. *BMJ.* 1942;2:237-239.
53. Denny Brown D, Brenner C. Paralysis of nerve induced by direct pressure and by tourniquet. *Arch Neurol Psychiatry.* 1944;51:1-26.
54. Younger AS, Kalla TP, McEwen JA, Inkpen K. Survey of tourniquet use in orthopaedic foot and ankle surgery. *Foot Ankle Int.* 2005;26(3):208-217.
55. Li YS, Chen CY, Lin KC, Tarng YW, Hsu CJ, Chang WN. Open reduction and internal fixation of ankle fracture using wide-awake local anaesthesia no tourniquet technique. *Injury.* 2019;50(4):990-994. doi: 10.1016/j.injury.2019.03.011.
56. Gordon SL, Dunn EJ. Peroneal nerve palsy as a complication of clubfoot treatment. *Clin Orthop.* 1977;101:229-231.
57. Redfern DJ, Sauvé PS, Sakellariou A. Investigation of incidence of superficial peroneal nerve injury following ankle fracture. *Foot Ankle Int.* 2003;24(10):771-774.
58. Joplin RJ. The proper digital nerve, vitallium stem arthroplasty, and some thoughts about foot surgery in general. *Clin Orthop.* 1971;76:199-212.
59. Kenzora JE. Symptomatic incisional neuromas on the dorsum of the foot. *Foot Ankle.* 1984;5;2-15,
60. de Cesar Netto C, Johannesmeyer D, Cone B, et al. Neurovascular structures at risk with curved retrograde TTC fusion nails. *Foot Ankle Int.* 2017;38(10):1139-1145. doi: 10.1177/1071100717715909.
61. Talusan PG, Cata E, Tan EW, Parks BG, Guyton GP. Safe zone for neural structures in medial displacement calcaneal osteotomy: a cadaveric and radiographic investigation. *Foot Ankle Int.* 2015;36(12):1493-1498. doi: 10.1177/1071100715595696.
62. Liu K, Huang K, et al. A neglected retained Penrose drain mimicking an amputation stump neuroma. *J Trauma.* 2007;62(4):1051-1052.
63. Banerjee T, Koons DD. Superficial peroneal nerve entrapment: report of two cases. *J Neurosurg.* 1981;55:991-992.
64. Edwards WG, Lincoln CR, Bassett FH, et al. The tarsal tunnel syndrome: diagnosis and treatment. *JAMA.* 1969;207:716-720.
65. Kopell HP, Goodgold J. Clinical and electrodiagnostic features of carpal tunnel syndrome. *Arch Phys Med Rehabil.* 1968;49:371-375.
66. Thimineur MA, Aberski L. Complex regional pain syndrome type I (RSD) or peripheral mononeuropathy? A discussion of three cases. *Clin J Pain.* 1996;12:145-150.
67. Trevino SG, Panchbhavi VK, Castro-Aragon O, Rowell M, Jo J. The "kick-off" position: a new sign for early diagnosis of complex regional pain syndrome in the leg. *Foot Ankle Int.* 2007;28(1):92-95. Erratum in: *Foot Ankle Int.* 2007;28(3):vi.
68. Shepsis AA, Lynch G. Exertional compartment syndromes of the lower extremity. *Curr Opin Radiol.* 1996;8:143-147.
69. Mitchell SW. *Injuries of Nerves and Their Consequences.* Philadelphia, PA: Lippincott; 1872.
70. Omer GE. Physical diagnosis of peripheral nerve injuries. *Orthop Clin North Am.* 1981;12:207-228.
71. Tassler PL, Dellon AL. Correlation of measurements of pressure perception using the pressure specified sensory device with electrodiagnostic testing. *J Occup Environ Med.* 1995;37:862-866.
72. Dellon ES, Keller KM, Dellon AE. Validation of cutaneous pressure threshold measurements for the evaluation of hand function. *Ann Plast Surg.* 1997;38:485-492.
73. Tassler PL, Dellon AL. Pressure perception in the normal lower extremity and in the tarsal tunnel syndrome. *Muscle Nerve.* 1996;19:285-289.
74. Mont MA, Dellon AL, Chen F, et al. The operative treatment of peroneal nerve palsy. *J Bone Joint Surg Am.* 1996;78:863-869.
75. Nahabedian MY, Dellon AL. Meralgia paresthetica: etiology, diagnosis, and outcome of surgical decompression. *Ann Plast Surg.* 1995;35:590-594.
76. Bueno-Gracia E, Salcedo-Gadea J, López-de-Celis C, Salcedo-Gadea E, Pérez-Bellmunt A, Estébanez-de-Miguel E. Dimensional changes of the tibial nerve and tarsal tunnel in different ankle joint positions in asymptomatic subjects. *J Foot Ankle Surg.* 2019;58(6):1129-1133. doi: 10.1053/j.jfas.2019.03.005.
77. Smith JR, Nery HG. Local injection therapy of neuromata of the hand with triamcinolone acetonide. *J Bone Joint Surg Am.* 1970;52:71-83.
78. Grumbine NA, Radovic PA. Volume injection adhesiotomy. *J Am Podiatr Med Assoc.* 1989;79:121-123.
79. Sidlow CJ, Frankel SL, Chioros PG, et al. Electroacupuncture therapy for stump neuroma pain. *J Am Podiatr Med Assoc.* 1989;79:31-33.
80. Trendelenberg W. Uber landauende nerveausschaltung mit siche regenerationsfahigkeit. *Z Gesamte Exp Med.* 1917;5:371-374.
81. Lloyd J, Barnard J, Glynn C. Cryoanalgesia: a new approach to pain relief. *Lancet.* 1976;2:932-934.
82. Trescot A. Cryoanalgesia in interventional pain management. *Pain Physician.* 2003;6:345-360.
83. Hodor L, Barkal K, Hatch-Fox LD. Cryogenic denervation of the intermetatarsal space neuroma. *J Foot Ankle Surg.* 1997;36(4):311-314.
84. Caporusso EF, Fallat LM, Savoy-Moore R. Cryogenic neuroablation for treatment of lower extremity neuromas. *J Foot Ankle Surg.* 2002;41(5):286-290.
85. Margic K, Pirc J. Treatment of complex regional pain syndrome (CRPS) involving upper extremity continuous sensory analgesia. *Eur J Pain.* 2003;7(1):43-47.
86. Markman JD, Philip A. Interventional approaches to pain management. *Anesthesiol Clin.* 2007;25:883-898.
87. Cahana A, Zunder J, et al. Pulsed radiofrequency: current clinical and biological literature available. *Pain Med.* 2006;7(5):411-423.
88. Cione JA, Cozzarelli J, Mullin CJ. A retrospective study of radiofrequency thermal lesioning for the treatment of neuritis of the medial calcaneal nerve and its terminal branches in chronic heel pain. *J Foot Ankle Surg.* 2009;48(2):142-147.
89. Moore JL, Rosen R, Cohen J, Rosen B. Radiofrequency thermoneurolysis for the treatment of Morton's neuroma. *J Foot Ankle Surg.* 2011;51(1):20-22.
90. Arslan A, Koca TT, Utkan A, Sevimli R, Akel I. Treatment of chronic plantar heel pain with radiofrequency neural ablation of the first branch of the lateral plantar nerve and medial calcaneal nerve branches. *J Foot Ankle Surg.* 2016;55(4):767-771.
91. Migues A, Velan O, et al. Osetoid osteoma of the calcaneus: percutaneous radiofrequency ablation. *J Foot Ankle Surg.* 2005;44(6):469-472.
92. Sollitto RJ, Plotkin EL, et al. Early clinical results of the use of radiofrequency lesioning in the treatment of plantar fasciitis. *J Foot Ankle Surg.* 1997;36(3):215-219.
93. Hormozi J, Lee S, Hong DK. Minimal invasive percutaneous bipolar radiofrequency for plantar fasciotomy: a retrospective study. *J Foot Ankle Surg.* 2011;50(3):283-286.
94. Park Y, Jo Y, Bang S, et al. Radiofrequency volume reduction of gastrocnemius muscle hypertrophy for cosmetic purposes. *Aesthetic Plast Surg.* 2007;31:53-61.
95. Wernicke JF, Wang F, et al. An open label 52-week clinical extension comparing duloxetine with routine care in patients with diabetic peripheral neuropathic pain. *Pain Med.* 2007;8(6):503-513.
96. Kajdasz DK, Iyengar S, et al. Duloxetine for the management of diabetic peripheral neuropathic pain: evidence based findings from post hoc analysis of three mulitcenter, randomized, double-blind, placebo-controlled, parallel-group studies. *Clin Ther.* 2007;20:2536-2546.
97. Fusco BM, Giocovazzo M. Peppers and pain: the promise of capsaicin. *Drugs.* 1997;53:909-913.
98. Sindrup SH, Gram LF, Brosen K. The selective serotonin reuptake inhibitor paroxetine is effective in the treatment of diabetic neuropathy symptoms. *Pain.* 1990;42:135-141.
99. Max MB, Lynch SA, Muir J, et al. Effects of desipramine, amitriptyline, and fluoxetine on pain in diabetic neuropathy symptoms. *N Engl J Med.* 1992;326:1250-1256.
100. Gomez Perez FJ, Choza R, Rios M, et al. Nortriptyline fluphenazine versus carbamazepine in the symptomatic treatment of diabetic neuropathy. *Arch Med Res.* 1996;27:525-528.
101. Page JC, Chen EY. Management of painful diabetic neuropathy: a treatment algorithm. *J Am Podiatr Med Assoc.* 1997;87:370-374.
102. Backonja M, Beydoun A, et al. Gabapentin for the symptomatic treatment of painful neuropathy in patients with diabetes mellitus: a randomized controlled trial. *J Am Med Assoc.* 1998;280(21):1831-1837.
103. Wright ME, Rizzolo D. An update on the pharmacologic management and treatment of neuropathic pain. *JAAPA.* 2017;30(3):13-17. doi: 10.1097/01.JAA.0000512228.23432.f7.
104. Ho KY, Huh BK, White WD, et al. Topical amitriptyline versus lidocaine in treatment of neuropathic pain. *Clin J Pain.* 2008;24(1):51-55.
105. Byas Smith MG, Max MB, Muir J, et al. Transdermal clonidine compared to placebo in painful diabetic neuropathy using a two stage "enriched enrollment" design. *Pain.* 1995;60:267-270.
106. Aida K, Tawata M, Shindo H, et al. Isoliquiritigenin: a new aldose reductase inhibitor from glycyrrhizae radix. *Planta Med.* 1990;56:254-256.
107. Masson EA, Boulton AJ. Aldose reductase inhibitors in the treatment of diabetic neuropathy: a review of the rational and clinical evidence. *Drugs.* 1990;39:190-197.
108. Hotta N, Sakamoto N, Shigata Y, et al. Clinical investigation of epalrestat, an aldose reductase inhibitor, on diabetic neuropathy in Japan. *J Diabetes Complications.* 1996;10:168-171.
109. Snyder MJ, Gibbs LM, Lindsay TJ. Treating painful diabetic peripheral neuropathy: an update. *Am Fam Physician.* 2016;94(3):227-234.
110. Shindo H, Tawata M, Inoue M, et al. The effect of prastaglandin E1 alpha CD on vibratory threshold determined with SMV 5 vibrometer in patients with diabetic neuropathy. *Diabetes Res Clin Pract.* 1994;24:173-176.
111. Toyota T, Hirata Y, Ikeda Y, et al. Lipo PGE1, a new lipoencapsulated preparation of prostaglandin E1: placebo and prostaglandin E1 controlled multicenter trials in patients with diabetic neuropathy and leg ulcers. *Prostaglandins.* 1993;46:453-457.
112. Walton DM, Minton SD, Cook AD. The potential of transdermal nitric oxide treatment for diabetic peripheral neuropathy and diabetic foot ulcers. *Diabetes Metab Syndr.* 2019;13(5):3053-3056. doi: 10.1016/j.dsx.2018.07.003.
113. Kline DG. Early evaluation of peripheral nerve lesions in continuity with a note on nerve recording. *Am Surg.* 1968;34:77-81.
114. Gould J, Naranje S, McGwin G Jr, et al. Use of collagen conduits is management of painful neuromas of the foot and ankle. *Foot Ankle Int.* 2013;34:932-940.
115. Siegfried J and Zimmermann M Samii M. Centocentral anastomosis of peripheral nerves: a neurosurgical treatment of amputation neuromas. In: *Phantom and Stump Pain.* Springer-Verlag: Berlin Heidelberg, NY 1981:123-125.
116. Henrot P, Stines J, Walter F, et al. Imaging of the painful lower limb stump. *Radiographics.* 2000;20:s219-s235.
117. Thomas A, Bull M, et al. Perioperative ultrasound guided needle localization of amputation stump neuroma. *Injury.* 1999;30(10):689-691.
118. Provost N, Bonaldi V, et al. Amputation stump neuroma: ultrasound features. *J Clin Ultrasound.* 1997;25:85-90.

119. Gruber H, Kovacs P, et al. Sonographically guided phenol injection in painful stump neuroma. *Am J Roentgenol.* 2004;182(4):952-954.
120. Oberle JW, Antoniadis G, Rath SA, et al. Value of nerve action potentials in the surgical management of traumatic nerve lesions. *Neurosurgery.* 1997;41:1337-1342.
121. Parry GJ, Cornblath DR, Brown MJ. Transient conduction block following acute peripheral nerve ischemia. *Muscle Nerve.* 1985;8(5):409-412.
122. Kline DG, Nulsen FE. The neuroma in continuity: its preoperative and operative assessment. *Surg Clin North Am.* 1972;52:1189-1209.
123. Kim SM, Kim SH, Seo DW, Lee KW. Intraoperative neurophysiologic monitoring: basic principles and recent update. *J Korean Med Sci.* 2013;28(9):1261-1269.
124. Luginbuhl A, Schwartz DM, Sestokas AK, Cognetti D, Pribitkin E. Detection of evolving injury to the brachial plexus during transaxillary robotic thyroidectomy. *Laryngoscope.* 2012;122(1):110-115. doi: 10.1002/lary.22429.
125. Pisanu A, Porceddu G, Podda M, Cois A, Uccheddu A. Systematic review with meta-analysis of studies comparing intraoperative neuromonitoring of recurrent laryngeal nerves versus visualization alone during thyroidectomy. *J Surg Res.* 2014;188(1):152-161. doi: 10.1016/j.jss.2013.12.022.
126. Oh T, Nagasawa DT, Fong BM, et al. Intraoperative neuromonitoring techniques in the surgical management of acoustic neuromas. *Neurosurg Focus.* 2012;33(3):E6. doi: 10.3171/2012.6.FOCUS12194.
127. Sasaki H, Nagano S, Yokouchi M, et al. Utility of intraoperative monitoring with motor-evoked potential during the surgical enucleation of peripheral nerve schwannoma. *Oncol Lett.* 2018;15(6):9327-9332. doi: 10.3892/ol.2018.8456.
128. Kwok K, Davis B, Kliot M. Resection of a benign brachial plexus nerve sheath tumor using intraoperative electrophysiological monitoring. *Neurosurgery.* 2007;60:316-320.
129. Huang S, Garstka ME, Murcy MA, et al. Somatosensory evoked potential: preventing brachial plexus injury in transaxillary robotic surgery. *Laryngoscope.* 2019;129(11):2663-2668. doi: 10.1002/lary.27611.
130. Shinagawa S, Shitara H, Yamamoto A, et al. Intraoperative neuromonitoring during reverse shoulder arthroplasty. *J Shoulder Elbow Surg.* 2019;28(8):1617-1625. doi: 10.1016/j.jse.2019.01.007.
131. Overzet K, Kazewych M, Jahangiri FR. Multimodality intraoperative neurophysiological monitoring (IONM) in anterior hip arthroscopic repair surgeries. *Cureus.* 2018;10(9):e3346. doi: 10.7759/cureus.3346.
132. Timpson WL, Kong X, Hamlet WP, Gross P, Gozani SN. Time-dependent changes in median nerve sensory amplitude after local anesthetic administration and tourniquet application. *Am J Orthop (Belle Mead NJ).* 2006;35(11):515-519.
133. Still GP, Pfau ZJ, Cordoba A, Jupiter DC. Intraoperative nerve monitoring for tarsal tunnel decompression: a surgical technique to improve outcomes. *J Foot Ankle Surg.* 2019;58(6):1203-1209. doi: 10.1053/j.jfas.2019.04.009.
134. Grundy BL, Jannetta PJ, Procopio PT, Lina A, Boston JR, Doyle E. Intraoperative monitoring of brain-stem auditory evoked potentials. *J Neurosurg.* 1982;57:674-681.
135. Albers JW. *Nerve Conduction Manual.* Ann Arbor, MI: Electroneuromyography Laboratory, Department of Physical Medicine and Rehabilitation, University of Michigan Hospital. https://www.google.com/search?q=University+of+Michigan+tibial+nerve+electroneurodiagnostic+measures&rlz=1C5CHFA_enUS848US848&oq=University+of+Michigan+tibial+nerve+electroneurodiagnostic+measures&aqs=chrome.69i57.60215j1j8&sourceid=chrome&ie=UTF-8. Accessed January 19, 2020.
136. Madden JW, Peacock EE. Some thoughts on repair of peripheral nerves. *South Med J.* 1971;64:17-21.
137. Mackinnon SE, Dellon AL, Hudson AR, et al. Nerve regeneration through a pseudosynovial sheath in a primate model. *Plast Reconstr Surg.* 1985;75:833-837.
138. Lindsey JT, Bryan WW, Robinson JB Jr, et al. The effect of a muscle wrap on nerve healing in a rat model. *J Reconstr Microsurg.* 1996;12:475-478.
139. Jones NF, Shaw WW, Katz G, et al. Circumferential wrapping of a flap around a scarred peripheral nerve for salvage of end stage traction neuritis. *J Hand Surg Am.* 1997;22:527-535.
140. Koch H, Haas F, et al. Treatment of painful neuromas by resection and nerve stump transplantation into a vein. *Ann Plast Surg.* 2003;51(1):45-50.
141. Krishnan K, Pinzer T, Schackert G. Coverage of painful peripheral nerve neuromas with vascularized soft tissue: method and results. *Neurosurgery.* 2005;56(2 suppl):369-378.
142. Koch H, Hubmer M, et al. Treatment of painful neuroma of the lower extremity by resection and nerve stump transplantation into a vein. *Foot Ankle Int.* 2004;25(7):476-481.
143. Malay DS. Update: peripheral entrapment neuropathy. In: McGlamry ED, ed. *Reconstructive Surgery of the Foot and Leg: Update '88.* Tucker, GA: Podiatry Institute; 1988:153-154.
144. Le Beau JM. Growth factor expression in normal and diabetic rats during peripheral nerve regeneration through silicone tubes. *Adv Exp Med Biol.* 1992;321:37-44.
145. Tu Y, Chen Z, Hu J, et al. Chronic nerve compression accelerates the progression of diabetic peripheral neuropathy in a rat model: a study of gene expression profiling. *J Reconstr Microsurg.* 2018;34(7):537-548. doi: 10.1055/s-0038-1642023.
146. Petersen J, Russell L, Andrus K, et al. Reduction of extraneural scarring by ADCON T/N after surgical intervention. *Neurosurgery.* 1996;38:976-983.
147. Palatinsky EA, Maier KH, Touhalisky DK, et al. ADCON T/N reduces in vivo perineural adhesions in a rat sciatic nerve reoperation model. *J Hand Surg Br.* 1997;22:331-335.
148. Archibald SJ, Shefner J, Krarup C, Madison RD. Monkey median nerve repaired by nerve graft or collagen nerve guide tube. *J Neurosci.* 1995;15(5):4109-4123.
149. Archibald SJ, Krarup C, Li ST, Madison RD. A collagen-based nerve guide conduit for peripheral nerve repair: an electrophysiological study of nerve regeneration in rodents and nonhuman primates. *J Comp Neurol.* 1991;307:1-12.
150. Li ST, Archibald SJ, Krarup C, Madison R. Peripheral nerve repair with collagen conduits. *Clin Mater.* 1992;9:195-200.
151. Mackinnon SE, Dellon AL, Hudson AR, Hunter DA. A primate model for chronic nerve compression. *J Reconstr Microsurg.* 1985;1:185-194.
152. Hodde J, et al. Vascular endothelial growth factor in porcine-derived extracellular matrix. *Endothelium.* 2004;8(1):11-24.
153. Brooks DN, et al. Processed nerve allografts for peripheral nerve reconstruction: a multicenter study of utilization and outcomes in sensory, mixed and motor nerve reconstructions. *Microsurgery.* 2012;32:1-85.
154. Fairbairn NG, Randolph MA, Redmond RW. The clinical applications of human amnion in plastic surgery. *J Plast Reconstr Aesthet Surg.* 2014;67(5):662-675. doi: 10.1016/j.bjps.2014.01.031.
155. Gaspar MP, Kane PM, Vosbikian MM, Ketonis C, Rekant MS. Neurolysis with amniotic membrane nerve wrapping for treatment of secondary Wartenberg syndrome: a preliminary report. *J Hand Surg Asian Pac Vol.* 2017;22(2):222-228. doi: 10.1142/S0218810417200015.
156. Dy CJ, Aunins B, Brogan DM. Barriers to epineural scarring: role in treatment of traumatic nerve injury and chronic compressive neuropathy. *J Hand Surg Am.* 2018;43(4):360-367. doi: 10.1016/j.jhsa.2018.01.013.
157. Fairbairn NG, Meppelink AM, Ng-Glazier J, Randolph MA, Winograd JM. Augmenting peripheral nerve regeneration using stem cells: a review of current opinion. *World J Stem Cells.* 2015;7(1):11-26. doi: 10.4252/wjsc.v7.i1.11.
158. Kubiak CA, Grochmal J, Kung TA, Cederna PS, Midha R, Kemp SWP. Stem-cell-based therapies to enhance peripheral nerve regeneration. *Muscle Nerve.* 2020;61(4):449-459. doi: 10.1002/mus.26760.
159. Pisciotta A, Bertoni L, Vallarola A, Bertani G, Mecugni D, Carnevale G. Neural crest derived stem cells from dental pulp and tooth-associated stem cells for peripheral nerve regeneration. *Neural Regen Res.* 2020;15(3):373-381. doi: 10.4103/1673-5374.266043.
160. Grabb WC. Management of nerve injuries in the forearm and hand. *Orthop Clin North Am.* 1970;1:419-431.
161. Gould N, Trevino S. Sural nerve entrapment by avulsion of the base of the 5th metatarsal bone. *Foot Ankle.* 1981;2:153-155.
162. Dellon AL, Mont MA, Mullick T, et al. Partial denervation for persistent neuroma pain around the knee. *Clin Orthop.* 1996;329:216-222.
163. Dellon AL, Mont MA, Krackow KA, et al. Partial denervation for persistent neuroma pain after total knee arthroplasty. *Clin Orthop.* 1995;316:145-150.
164. Nahabedian MY, Dellon AL. Outcome of operative management of nerve injuries in the ilioinguinal region. *J Am Coll Surg.* 1997;184:265-268.
165. Antoniadis G, Richter HP. Pain after surgery for ulnar neuropathy at the elbow: a continuing challenge. *Neurosurgery.* 1997;41:585-589.
166. Deister C, Schmidt CE. Optimizing neurotrophic factor combinations for neurite outgrowth. *J Neural Eng.* 2006;3(2):172-179.
167. Srour RK, Crikelair GF, Moss ML. Neurotrophism in relation to muscle and nerve grafts in rats. *Surg Forum.* 1974;25(0):508-511.
168. Mackinnon SE. New directions in peripheral nerve surgery. *Ann Plast Surg.* 1989;22(3):257-273.
169. Brushart TM. Neurotropism and neurotrophism. *J Hand Surg Am.* 1987;12(5 Pt 1):808-809.
170. Dobrowsky RT, Rouen S, Yu C. Altered neurotrophism in diabetic neuropathy: spelunking the caves of peripheral nerve. *J Pharmacol Exp Ther.* 2005;313(2):485-491.
171. Aszman OC, Muse V, Dellon AL. Evidence in support of collateral sprouting after sensory nerve resection. *Ann Plast Surg.* 1996;37:520-525.
172. Mucci SJ, Dellon AL. Restoration of lower lip sensation: neurotization of the mental nerve with the supraclavicular nerve. *J Reconstr Microsurg.* 1997;13:151-155.
173. Ress AM, Babovic S, Angel MF, et al. Free radical damage in acute nerve compression. *Ann Plast Surg.* 1995;34:388-395.
174. Martini A, Fromm B. A new operation for the prevention and treatment of amputation neuromas. *J Bone Joint Surg Br.* 1989;71:379-382.
175. Moss ALH. Ideas and innovations: the preparation of divided nerve ends. *Br J Plast Surg.* 1990;43:247-249.
176. Narakas A. The use of fibrin glue in the repair of peripheral nerves. *Orthop Clin North Am.* 1988;19:187-199.
177. Waitayawinyu T Parisi DM, Miller B, et al. A comparison of polyglycolic acid versus type I collagen bioabsorbable nerve conduits in a rat model: an alternative to autografting. *J Hand Surg Am.* 2007;32:1521-1529.
178. Weber RA, Breidenbach WC, Brown RE, et al. A randomized prospective study of polyglycolic acid conduits for digital nerve reconstruction in humans. *Plast Reconstr Surg.* 2001;106:1036-1045.
179. O'Reilly MA, et al. Neuromas as the cause of pain in the residual limbs of amputees: an ultrasound study. *Clin Radiol.* 2016;71(10):1068.e1-1068.e6.
180. Gorkisch K, Boese-Landgraft J, Vaubel E. Treatment and prevention of amputation neuromas in hand surgery. *Plast Reconstr Surg.* 1984;73:293-296.
181. Lidor C, et al. Centrocentral anastomosis with autologous nerve graft treatment of foot and ankle neuromas. *Foot Ankle Int.* 1996;17:85-88.
182. Bibbo C, Rodrigues-Colazzo E. Nerve transfer with entubulated nerve allograft transfers to treat recalcitrant lower extremity neuromas. *J Foot Ankle Surg.* 2017;56:82-86.
183. Bibbo C, Rodrigues-Colazzo E, Finzen AG. Superficial peroneal to deep peroneal nerve transfer with allograft conduit for neuroma in continuity. *J Foot Ankle Surg.* 2018;57:514-517.
184. Kopell HP, Thompson WAL. Knee pain due to saphenous nerve entrapment. *N Engl J Med.* 1960;263:351-353.
185. Lans J, Gamo L, DiGiovanni C, et al. Etiology and treatment outcomes for Sural neuroma. *Foot Ankle Int.* 2019;40:545-552.
186. Nakasa T, Ikuta Y, Tsuyuguchi Y, Ota Y, Kanemitsu M, Adachi N. Application of a peripheral vein illumination device to reduce saphenous structure injury caused by screw insertion during arthroscopic ankle arthrodesis. *J Orthop Sci.* 2019;24(4):697-701. doi: 10.1016/j.jos.2018.12.007.
187. Yammine K, Assi C. Neurovascular and tendon injuries due to ankle arthroscopy portals: a meta-analysis of interventional cadaveric studies. *Surg Radiol Anat.* 2018;40(5):489-497. doi: 10.1007/s00276-018-2013-5.
188. Tonogai I, Hayashi F, Tsuruo Y, Sairyo K. Anatomic study of anterior and posterior ankle portal sites for ankle arthroscopy in plantarflexion and dorsiflexion: a cadaveric

study in the Japanese population. *J Foot Ankle Surg.* 2018;57(3):537-542. doi: 10.1053/j.jfas.2017.11.029.
189. Kaplan N, Fowler X, Maqsoodi N, DiGiovanni B, Oh I. Operative anatomy of the medial gastrocnemius recession vs the proximal medial gastrocnemius recession. *Foot Ankle Int.* 2017;38(4):424-429. doi: 10.1177/1071100716682993.
190. Eglitis N, Horn JL, Benninger B, Nelsen S. The importance of the saphenous nerve in ankle surgery. *Anesth Analg.* 2016;122(5):1704-1706. doi: 10.1213/ANE.0000000000001168.
191. Fisher MA, Gorelick PB. Entrapment neuropathies: differential diagnosis and management. *Postgrad Med.* 1985;77:160-174.
192. Pickett JB. Localizing peroneal nerve lesions. *Am Fam Physician.* 1985;31:189-196.
193. Cozen L. Management of footdrop in adults after permanent peroneal nerve loss. *Clin Orthop.* 1969;167:151-158.
194. Zeng X, Xie L, Qiu Z, Sun K. Compression neuropathy of common peroneal nerve caused by a popliteal cyst: a case report. *Medicine (Baltimore).* 2018;97(16):e9922. doi: 10.1097/MD.0000000000009922.
195. Puffer RC, Sabbag OD, Logli AL, Spinner RJ, Rose PS. Melorheostosis causing compression of common peroneal nerve at fibular tunnel. *World Neurosurg.* 2019;128:1-3. doi: 10.1016/j.wneu.2019.04.208.
196. Mangierri JV. Peroneal nerve injury from an enlarged fabella: a case report. *J Bone Joint Surg Am.* 1973;55:395-397.
197. Margulis M, Ben Zvi L, Bernfeld B. Bilateral common peroneal nerve entrapment after excessive weight loss: case report and review of the literature. *J Foot Ankle Surg.* 2018;57(3):632-634. doi: 10.1053/j.jfas.2017.10.035.
198. Horteur C, Forli A, Corcella D, Pailhé R, Lateur G, Saragaglia D. Short- and long-term results of common peroneal nerve injuries treated by neurolysis, direct suture or nerve graft. *Eur J Orthop Surg Traumatol.* 2019;29(4):893-898. doi: 10.1007/s00590-018-2354-0.
199. Le Hanneur M, Amrami KK, Spinner RJ. Explaining peroneal neuropathy after ankle sprain. *Eur J Orthop Surg Traumatol.* 2017;27(7):1025-1026. doi: 10.1007/s00590-017-1967-z.
200. Iwamoto N, Kim K, Isu T, Chiba Y, Morimoto D, Isobe M. Repetitive plantar flexion test as an adjunct tool for the diagnosis of common peroneal nerve entrapment neuropathy. *World Neurosurg.* 2016;86:484-489. doi: 10.1016/j.wneu.2015.09.080.
201. Tran TMA, Lim BG, Sheehy R, Robertson PL. Magnetic resonance imaging for common peroneal nerve injury in trauma patients: are routine knee sequences adequate for prediction of outcome? *J Med Imaging Radiat Oncol.* 2019;63(1):54-60. doi: 10.1111/1754-9485.12840.
202. Thawait SK, Chaundhry V, Thawait GK, et al. High-resolution MR neurography of diffuse peripheral nerve lesions. *AJNR Am J Neuroradiol.* 2011;32:1365-1372.
203. Lowdon IMR. Superficial peroneal nerve entrapment: a case report. *J Bone Joint Surg Br.* 1985;67:58-59.
204. Kernohan J, Levack B, Wilson JN. Entrapment of superficial peroneal nerve: three case reports. *J Bone Joint Surg Br.* 1985;67:60-61.
205. McAuliffe TB, Fiddian NJ, Browett JP. Entrapment neuropathy of the superficial peroneal nerve: a bilateral case. *J Bone Joint Surg Br.* 1985;67:62-63.
206. Lemont H. The branches of the superficial peroneal nerve and their clinical significance. *J Am Podiatry Assoc.* 1975;65:310-314.
207. Fabre T, Piton C, Andre D, et al. Peroneal nerve entrapment. *J Bone Joint Surg Am.* 1998;80:47-53.
208. Daghino W, Pasquali M, Faletti C. Superficial peroneal nerve entrapment in a young athlete: the diagnostic contribution of magnetic resonance imaging. *J Foot Ankle Surg.* 1997;36:170-172.
209. Mitra A, Stern JD, Perrotta VJ, et al. Peroneal nerve entrapment in athletes. *Ann Plast Surg.* 1995;35:366-368.
210. Piza Katzer H, Pilz E. Compression syndrome of the superficial fibular nerve [German]. *Handchir Mikrochir Plast Chir.* 1997;29:124-126.
211. Cangialosi CP, Schnall SJ. The biomechanical aspects of anterior tarsal tunnel syndrome. *J Am Podiatry Assoc.* 1980;70:291-292.
212. Nodelman LO, Silverman TJ, Theodoulou MH. Neural fibrolipoma of the ankle: a case report and review of the literature. *J Foot Ankle Surg.* 2016;55(5):1063-1066. doi: 10.1053/j.jfas.2015.12.012.
213. Maselli F, Testa M. Superficial peroneal nerve schwannoma presenting as lumbar radicular syndrome in a non-competitive runner. *J Back Musculoskelet Rehabil.* 2019;32(2):361-365. doi: 10.3233/BMR-181164.
214. Paolasso I, Cambise C, Coraci D, et al. Tibialis anterior muscle herniation with superficial peroneal nerve involvement: Ultrasound role for diagnosis and treatment. *Clin Neurol Neurosurg.* 2016;151:6-8. doi: 10.1016/j.clineuro.2016.09.019.
215. Corey RM, Salazar DH. Entrapment of the superficial peroneal nerve following a distal fibula fracture. *Foot Ankle Spec.* 2017;10(1):69-71. doi: 10.1177/1938640016640887.
216. Bowness J, Turnbull K, Taylor A, et al. Identifying the emergence of the superficial peroneal nerve through deep fascia on ultrasound and by dissection: implications for regional anesthesia in foot and ankle surgery. *Clin Anat.* 2019;32(3):390-395. doi: 10.1002/ca.23323.
217. Tomaszewski KA, Roy J, Vikse J, Pękala PA, Kopacz P, Henry BM. Prevalence of the accessory deep peroneal nerve: a cadaveric study and meta-analysis. *Clin Neurol Neurosurg.* 2016;144:105-111. doi: 10.1016/j.clineuro.2016.03.026.
218. Kang J, Yang P, Zang Q, He X. Traumatic neuroma of the superficial peroneal nerve in a patient: a case report and review of the literature. *World J Surg Oncol.* 2016;14(1):242. doi: 10.1186/s12957-016-0990-6.
219. Zekry M, Shahban SA, El Gamal T, Platt S. A literature review of the complications following anterior and posterior ankle arthroscopy. *Foot Ankle Surg.* 2019;25(5):553-558. doi: 10.1016/j.fas.2018.06.007.
220. Blázquez Martín T, Iglesias Durán E, San Miguel Campos M. Complications after ankle and hindfoot arthroscopy. *Rev Esp Cir Ortop Traumatol.* 2016;60(6):387-393. doi: 10.1016/j.recot.2016.04.005.
221. Darland AM, Kadakia AR, Zeller JL. Branching patterns of the superficial peroneal nerve: implications for ankle arthroscopy and for anterolateral surgical approaches to the ankle. *J Foot Ankle Surg.* 2015;54(3):332-337. doi: 10.1053/j.jfas.2014.07.002.
222. McAlister JE, DeMill SL, Hyer CF, Berlet GC. Anterior approach total ankle arthroplasty: superficial peroneal nerve branches at risk. *J Foot Ankle Surg.* 2016;55(3):476-479. doi: 10.1053/j.jfas.2015.12.013.
223. Harnroongroj T, Chuckpaiwong B. Is the arthroscopic transillumination test effective in localizing the superficial peroneal nerve? *Arthroscopy.* 2017;33(3):647-650. doi: 10.1016/j.arthro.2016.10.011.
224. de Bruijn JA, van Zantvoort APM, Hundscheid HPH, Hoogeveen AR, Teijink JAW, Scheltinga MR. Superficial peroneal nerve injury risk during a semiblind fasciotomy for anterior chronic exertional compartment syndrome of the leg: an anatomical and clinical study. *Foot Ankle Int.* 2019;40(3):343-351. doi: 10.1177/1071100718811632.
225. Ogrodnik J. Superficial peroneal nerve injured during fasciotomy: a successful repair with cadaveric nerve allograft. *Am Surg.* 2018;84(2):e59-e60.
226. Balius R, Bong DA, Ardèvol J, Pedret C, Codina D, Dalmau A. Ultrasound-guided fasciotomy for anterior chronic exertional compartment syndrome of the leg. *J Ultrasound Med.* 2016;35(4):823-829. doi: 10.7863/ultra.15.04058.
227. Poggio D, Claret G, López AM, Medrano C, Tornero E, Asunción J. Correlation between visual inspection and ultrasonography to identify the distal branches of the superficial peroneal nerve: a Cadaveric study. *J Foot Ankle Surg.* 2016;55(3):492-495. doi: 10.1053/j.jfas.2016.01.014.
228. Chiodo CP, Miller SD. Surgical treatment of superficial peroneal neuroma. *Foot Ankle Int.* 2004;25:689-694.
229. Adelman KA, Wilson G, Wolf JA. Anterior tarsal tunnel syndrome. *J Foot Surg.* 1988;27:299-302.
230. Gessini L, Jandolo B, Pietrangeli A. The anterior tarsal syndrome. *J Bone Joint Surg Am.* 1984;66:786-787.
231. Kanabe K, Kubota H, Shirakura K, et al. Entrapment neuropathy of the deep peroneal nerve associated with the extensor hallucis brevis. *J Foot Ankle Surg.* 1995;34:560-562.
232. Reed SC, Wright CS. Compression of the deep branch of the peroneal nerve by the extensor hallucis brevis muscle: a variation of the anterior tarsal tunnel syndrome. *Can J Surg.* 1995;38:545-546.
233. Jeong JH, Chang MC, Lee SA. Deep peroneal nerve palsy after opening wedge high tibial osteotomy: a case report. *Medicine (Baltimore).* 2019;98(27):e16253. doi: 10.1097/MD.0000000000016253.
234. So E, Van Dyke B, McGann MR, Brandao R, Larson D, Hyer CF. Structures at risk from an intermetatarsal screw for Lapidus bunionectomy: a cadaveric study. *J Foot Ankle Surg.* 2019;58(1):62-65. doi: 10.1053/j.jfas.2018.08.010.
235. Kaipel M, Reissig L, Albrecht L, Quadlbauer S, Klikovics J, Weninger WJ. Risk of damaging anatomical structures during minimally invasive hallux valgus correction (Bösch technique): an anatomical study. *Foot Ankle Int.* 2018;39(11):1355-1359. doi: 10.1177/1071100718786883.
236. Xavier G, Oliva XM, Rotinen M, Monzo M. Talonavicular joint arthroscopic portals: a cadaveric study of feasibility and safety. *Foot Ankle Surg.* 2016;22(3):205-209. doi: 10.1016/j.fas.2015.08.005.
237. Deol RS, Roche A, Calder JD. Return to training and playing after acute Lisfranc injuries in elite professional soccer and rugby players. *Am J Sports Med.* 2016;44(1):166-170. doi: 10.1177/0363546515616814.
238. Hiramatsu K, Yonetani Y, Kinugasa K, et al. Deep peroneal nerve palsy with isolated lateral compartment syndrome secondary to peroneus longus tear: a report of two cases and a review of the literature. *J Orthop Traumatol.* 2016;17(2):181-185. doi: 10.1007/s10195-015-0373-8.
239. Lu H, Chen L, Jiang S, Shen H. A rapidly progressive foot drop caused by the posttraumatic Intraneural ganglion cyst of the deep peroneal nerve. *BMC Musculoskelet Disord.* 2018;19(1):298. doi: 10.1186/s12891-018-2229-x.
240. Patel MS, Kadakia AR. Minimally invasive treatments of acute Achilles tendon ruptures. *Foot Ankle Clin.* 2019;24(3):399-424. doi: 10.1016/j.fcl.2019.05.002.
241. Manegold S, Tsitsilonis S, Schumann J, et al. Functional outcome and complication rate after percutaneous suture of fresh Achilles tendon ruptures with the Dresden instrument. *J Orthop Traumatol.* 2018;19(1):19. doi: 10.1186/s10195-018-0511-1.
242. Park JH, Chun DI, Park KR, et al. Can sural nerve injury be avoided in the sinus tarsi approach for calcaneal fracture?: A cadaveric study. *Medicine (Baltimore).* 2019;98(42):e17611. doi: 10.1097/MD.0000000000017611.
243. Pringle RM, Protheroe K, Mukherjee SK. Entrapment neuropathy of the sural nerve. *J Bone Joint Surg Br.* 1974;56:465-468.
244. Keck C. The tarsal tunnel syndrome. *J Bone Joint Surg Am.* 1962;44:180-182.
245. Radin EL. Tarsal tunnel syndrome. *Clin Orthop.* 1983;181:167-170.
246. Gathier JC, Bruyn GW, Van Der Meer WK. The medial tarsal tunnel syndrome. *J Neurol Neurosurg Psychiatry.* 1970;73:87-96.
247. Nobel W, Marks SC, Kubik T, et al: The anatomical basis for femoral nerve palsy following iliacus hematoma. *J Neurosurg.* 52:533, 1980
248. Mahan KT, Rock JJ, Hillstrom HJ. Tarsal tunnel syndrome: a retrospective study. *J Am Podiatr Med Assoc.* 1996;86:81-91.
249. Canter DE, Siesel KJ. Flexor digitorum accessorius longus muscle: an etiology of tarsal tunnel syndrome? *J Foot Ankle Surg.* 1997;36:226-229.
250. Mellado JM, Rosenberg ZS, Beltran J, et al. The peroneocalcaneus internus muscle: MR imaging features. *AJR Am J Roentgenol.* 1997;169:585-588.
251. Peterson DA, Stinson W, Lairimore JR. The long accessory flexor muscle: an anatomical study. *Foot Ankle Int.* 1995;16:637-640.
252. Pla ME, Dillingham TR, Spellman NT, et al. Painful legs and moving toes associated with tarsal tunnel syndrome and accessory soleus muscle. *Mov Disord.* 1996;11:82-86.
253. Boyer MI, Hochban T, Bowen V. Tarsal tunnel syndrome: an unusual case resulting from an intraneural degenerative cyst. *Can J Surg.* 1995;38:371-373.

254. Jaffe KA, Wade JD, Chivers FS, et al. Extraskeletal osteosarcoma: an unusual presentation as tarsal tunnel syndrome. *Foot Ankle Int.* 1995;16:796-799.

255. Myerson MS, Berger BI. Nonunion of a fracture of the sustentaculum tali causing tarsal tunnel syndrome: a case report. *Foot Ankle Int.* 1995;16:740-742.

256. Baba H, Wada M, Annen S, et al. The tarsal tunnel syndrome: evaluation of surgical results using multivariate analysis. *Int Orthop.* 1997;21:67-71.

257. Novotny DA, Kay DB, Parker MG. Recurrent tarsal tunnel syndrome and the radial forearm free flap. *Foot Ankle Int.* 1996;17:641-643.

258. Lam SJ. A tarsal-tunnel syndrome. *Lancet.* 1962;2:1354-1355.

259. Galinski AW. Tarsal tunnel syndrome: a case report. *J Am Podiatry Assoc.* 1970;60:169-170.

260. Goodman CR, Kehr LE. Bilateral tarsal tunnel syndrome: a correlative perspective. *J Am Podiatr Med Assoc.* 1988;78:292-294.

261. Komagamine J. Bilateral tarsal tunnel syndrome. *Am J Med.* 2018;131(7):e319. doi: 10.1016/j.amjmed.2017.10.028.

262. Bhat AK, Madi S, Mane PP, Acharya A. Bilateral tarsal tunnel syndrome attributed to bilateral fibrous tarsal coalition and symmetrical hypertrophy of the sustentaculum tali. *BMJ Case Rep.* 2017;2017. pii: bcr-2017-220087. doi: 10.1136/bcr-2017-220087.

263. Morinaga K, Shimizu T. Diagnosing bilateral tarsal tunnel syndrome. *Am J Med.* 2017;130(10):e437-e438. doi: 10.1016/j.amjmed.2017.05.009.

264. Kokubo R, Kim K, Isu T, et al. The impact of tarsal tunnel syndrome on cold sensation in the pedal extremities. *World Neurosurg.* 2016;92:249-254. doi: 10.1016/j.wneu.2016.04.095.

265. Troy TV. Tarsal tunnel syndrome: a case report. *J Am Podiatry Assoc.* 1972;62:399.

266. Kuritz HM, Sokoloff TH. Tarsal tunnel syndrome. *J Am Podiatry Assoc.* 1975;65:825-840.

267. Mann RA. Tarsal tunnel syndrome. *Orthop Clin North Am.* 1974;5:109-115.

268. Saraffian S. Neurology. In: Saraffian S, ed. *Anatomy of the Foot And Ankle: Descriptive, Topographic, Functional.* 2nd ed. Philadelphia, PA: JB Lippincott; 1993.

269. Dellon AL, MacKinnon SE. Tibial nerve branching in the tarsal tunnel. *Arch Neurol.* 1984;41:645-646.

270. Skalley TC, Schon LC, Hinton RY, et al. Clinical results following revision tibial nerve release. *Foot Ankle Int.* 1994;15:360-367.

271. Cimino WR. Tarsal tunnel syndrome: review of the literature. *Foot Ankle.* 1990;11:47-52.

272. Havel PE, Ebraheim NA, Clark SE, et al. Tibial nerve branching in the tarsal tunnel. *Foot Ankle.* 1988;9:117-119.

273. Flanigan DC, Cassell M, Saltzman CL. Vascular supply of nerves in the tarsal tunnel. *Foot Ankle Int.* 1997;18:288-292.

274. Oh SJ, Sarala PK, Kuba T, et al. Tarsal tunnel syndrome: electrophysiological study. *Ann Neurol.* 1979;5:327-330.

275. Kaplan PE, Kernahan WT Jr. Tarsal tunnel syndrome: an electrodiagnostic and surgical correlation. *J Bone Joint Surg Am.* 1981;63:96-99.

276. DeLisa JA, Saeed MA. The tarsal tunnel syndrome. *Muscle Nerve.* 1983;6:664-670.

277. Mosimann W. The tarsal tunnel syndrome [author's translation]. *Ther Umsch.* 1975;32:428-434.

278. Grumbine NA, Radovic PA, Parsons R, et al. Tarsal tunnel syndrome: comprehensive review of 87 cases. *J Am Podiatr Med Assoc.* 1990;80:457-461.

279. Naito J, Takebe K. Postoperative tarsal tunnel syndrome: case presentation and discussion. *J Foot Surg.* 1980;19:85-87.

280. Stefko RM, Lauerman WC, Heckman JD. Tarsal tunnel syndrome caused by an unrecognized fracture of the posterior process of the talus (Cedell fracture): a case report. *J Bone Joint Surg Am.* 1994;76:116-118.

281. Zuckerman SL, Kerr ZY, Pierpoint L, Kirby P, Than KD, Wilson TJ. An 11-year analysis of peripheral nerve injuries in high school sports. *Phys Sportsmed.* 2019;47(2):167-173. doi: 10.1080/00913847.2018.1544453.

282. Jackson DL, Haglund B. Tarsal tunnel syndrome in athletes: case reports and literature review. *Am J Sports Med.* 1991;19:61-65.

283. Yamamoto S, Tominaga Y, Yura S, et al. Tarsal tunnel syndrome with double causes (ganglion, tarsal coalition) evoked by ski boots: case report. *J Sports Med Phys Fitness.* 1995;35:143-145.

284. Oh SJ, Meyer RD. Entrapment neuropathies of the tibial (posterior tibial) nerve. *Neurol Clin.* 1999;17:593-615.

285. Primadi A, Kim BS, Lee KB. Tarsal tunnel syndrome after total ankle replacement—a report of 3 cases. *Acta Orthop.* 2016;87(2):205-206. doi: 10.3109/17453674.2015.1132196.

286. Walls RJ, Chan JY, Ellis SJ. A case of acute tarsal tunnel syndrome following lateralizing calcaneal osteotomy. *Foot Ankle Surg.* 2015;21(1):e1-e5. doi: 10.1016/j.fas.2014.07.006.

287. Lamm BM, Paley D, Testani M, Herzenberg JE. Tarsal tunnel decompression in leg lengthening and deformity correction of the foot and ankle. *J Foot Ankle Surg.* 2007;46(3):201-206.

288. Boc SF, Hatef J. Space occupying lesions as a cause of tarsal tunnel syndrome [Letter]. *J Am Podiatr Med Assoc.* 1995;85:713-715.

289. Gould N, Alvarez R. Bilateral tarsal tunnel syndrome caused by varicosities. *Foot Ankle.* 1983;3:290-292.

290. Kawakatsu M, Ishiko T, Sumiya M. Tarsal tunnel syndrome due to three different types of Ganglion during a 12-year period: a case report. *J Foot Ankle Surg.* 2017;56(2):379-384. doi: 10.1053/j.jfas.2016.11.005.

291. Krzywosinski TB, Bingham AL, Fallat LM. Intraneural lipoma of the tibial nerve: a case report. *J Foot Ankle Surg.* 2017;56(1):125-128. doi: 10.1053/j.jfas.2016.07.002.

292. O'Malley GM, Lambdin CS, McCleary GS. Tarsal tunnel syndrome: a case report and review of the literature. *Orthopedics.* 1985;8:758-760.

293. Myerson M, Soffer S. Lipoma as an etiology of tarsal tunnel syndrome: a report of two cases. *Foot Ankle.* 1989;10:176-179.

294. Belding RH. Neurilemmoma of the lateral plantar nerve producing tarsal tunnel syndrome: a case report. *Foot Ankle.* 1993;14:289-291.

295. Aydin AT, Karaveli S, Tuzuner S. Tarsal tunnel syndrome secondary to neurilemmoma of the medial plantar nerve. *J Foot Surg.* 1991;30:114-116.

296. Watanabe K, Fukuzawa T, Mitsui K. Tarsal tunnel syndrome caused by a Schwannoma of the posterior tibial nerve. *Acta Med Okayama.* 2018;72(1):77-80. doi: 10.18926/AMO/55667.

297. Albert P, Patel J, Badawy K, et al. Peripheral nerve schwannoma: a review of varying clinical presentations and imaging findings. *J Foot Ankle Surg.* 2017;56(3):632-637. doi: 10.1053/j.jfas.2016.12.003.

298. Willis AR, Samad AA, Prado GT, Gabisan GG. Heterotopic ossification and entrapment of the tibial nerve within the tarsal tunnel: a case report. *J Foot Ankle Surg.* 2016;55(5):1106-1109. doi: 10.1053/j.jfas.2016.01.032.

299. DiStefano V, Sack JT, Whittaker R, et al. Tarsal tunnel syndrome: review of the literature and two case reports. *Clin Orthop.* 1972;88:76-79.

300. Sammarco GJ, Conti SF. Tarsal tunnel syndrome caused by an anomalous muscle. *J Bone Joint Surg Am.* 1994;76:1308-1314.

301. Cheung Y. Normal variants: accessory muscles about the ankle. *Magn Reson Imaging Clin N Am.* 2017;25(1):11-26. doi: 10.1016/j.mric.2016.08.002.

302. Carrington SC, Stone P, Kruse D. Accessory soleus: a case report of exertional compartment and tarsal tunnel syndrome associated with an accessory soleus muscle. *J Foot Ankle Surg.* 2016;55(5):1076-1078. doi: 10.1053/j.jfas.2015.07.011.

303. Orozco-Villaseñor S, Martin-Oliva X, Elgueta-Grillo J, et al. Tarsal tunnel syndrome secondary to venous insufficiency. *Acta Ortop Mex.* 2015;29(3):186-190.

304. Southerland CC Jr, Spinner SM. Synovial sarcoma presenting as tarsal tunnel syndrome. *J Am Podiatr Med Assoc.* 1987;77:70-72. Erratum appears in *J Am Podiatr Med Assoc.* 1987;77:222.

305. Erickson SJ, Quinn SF, Kneeland JB, et al. MR imaging of the tarsal tunnel and related spaces: normal and abnormal findings with anatomic correlation. *AJR Am J Roentgenol.* 1990;155:323-328.

306. Takakura Y, Kumai T, Takaoka T, et al. Tarsal tunnel syndrome caused by coalition associated with a ganglion. *J Bone Joint Surg Br.* 1998;80:130-133.

307. Puleo DM, Knudsen HA, Sharon SM. Talar exostosis as a cause of tarsal tunnel syndrome. *J Am Podiatr Med Assoc.* 1987;77:147-149.

308. Oloff LM, Jacobs AM, Jaffe S. Tarsal tunnel syndrome: a manifestation of systemic disease. *J Foot Surg.* 1983;22:302-307.

309. Rinkel WD, Castro Cabezas M, van Neck JW, Birnie E, Hovius SER, Coert JH. Validity of the Tinel sign and prevalence of tibial nerve entrapment at the tarsal tunnel in both diabetic and nondiabetic subjects: a cross-sectional study. *Plast Reconstr Surg.* 2018;142(5):1258-1266. doi: 10.1097/PRS.0000000000004839.

310. Park TA, Del Toro DR. The medial calcaneal nerve. Anatomy and nerve conduction technique. *Muscle Nerve.* 1995;18:32-38.

311. Grabois M, Puentes J, Lidsky M. Tarsl tunnel syndrome in rheumatoid arthritis. *Arch Phys Med Rehabil.* 1981;62:401-403.

312. Schwartz MS, Mackworth Young CG, McKeran RO. The tarsal tunnel syndrome in hypothyroidism. *J Neurol Neurosurg Psychiatry.* 1983;46:440-442.

313. Olivieri I, Gemignani G, Siciliano G, et al. Tarsal tunnel syndrome in seronegative spondyloarthropathy. *Br J Rheumatol.* 1989;28:537-539.

314. Kucukdeveci AA, Kutlay S, Seckin B, et al. Tarsal tunnel syndrome in ankylosing spondylitis [Letter]. *Br J Rheumatol.* 1995;34:488-489.

315. Aynardi M, Raikin SM. Recurrence of extranodal natural killer/T-cell lymphoma presenting as tarsal tunnel syndrome. *Am J Orthop (Belle Mead NJ).* 2018;47(5). doi: 10.12788/ajo.2018.0025.

316. Obayashi O, Obata H, Naito K, et al. Recurrence of acute myelogenous leukemia with granulocytic sarcoma-associated tarsal tunnel syndrome in an elderly patient. *J Orthop Sci.* 2018;23(3):596-599. doi: 10.1016/j.jos.2016.06.009.

317. Daniels T, Lau J, Hearn T. The effect of foot position and load on tibial nerve tension. *Foot Ankle Int.* 1998;19:73-78.

318. Lau JT, Daniels TR. Effects of tarsal tunnel release and stabilization procedures on tibial nerve tension in a surgically created pes planus foot. *Foot Ankle Int.* 1998;19:770-777.

319. Lundborg G, Rydevik B. Effects of stretching the tibial nerve of the rabbit. *J Bone Joint Surg Br.* 1973;55:390-401.

320. Trepman E, Kadel NJ, Chisholm K, et al. Effect of foot and ankle position on tarsal tunnel compartment pressure. *Foot Ankle Int.* 1999;20:721-726.

321. Oh SJ, Kim HS, Ahmad BK. The near nerve sensory nerve conduction in tarsal tunnel syndrome. *J Neurol Neurosurg Psychiatry.* 1985;48:999-1003.

322. Lau JT, Daniels TR. Tarsal tunnel syndrome: a review of the literature. *Foot Ankle Int.* 1999;20:201-209.

323. Tinel J. The sign of "tingling" in lesions of the peripheral nerves. *Arch Neurol.* 1971;24:574-576.

324. Linscheid RL, Burton RC, Fredericks EJ. Tarsal tunnel syndrome. *South Med J.* 1970;63:1313-1323.

325. Julsrud ME. An unusual cause of tarsal tunnel syndrome. *J Foot Ankle Surg.* 1995;34:289-293.

326. Havens RT, Kaloogian H, Thul JR, et al. A correlation between os trigonum syndrome and tarsal tunnel syndrome. *J Am Podiatr Med Assoc.* 1986;76:450-454.

327. Romansky NM, Fried LC, Frugh A. Relief of low back pain from treatment of tarsal tunnel syndrome. *J Foot Surg.* 1986;25:327-329.

328. Sammarco GJ, Chalk DE, Feibel JH. Tarsal tunnel syndrome and additional nerve lesions in the same limb. *Foot Ankle.* 1993;14:71-77.

329. Zeiss J, Ebraheim N, Rusin J. Magnetic resonance imaging in the diagnosis of tarsal tunnel syndrome: case report. *Clin Imaging.* 1990;14:123-126.

330. Downey MS. MRI of tarsal tunnel pathology. In: Ruch JA, Vickers NS, eds. *Reconstructive Surgery of the Foot and Leg: Update '92.* Tucker, GA: The Podiatry Institute; 1992:104-110.

331. Kerr R, Frey C. MR imaging in tarsal tunnel syndrome. *J Comput Assist Tomogr.* 1991;15:280-286.

332. Zeiss J, Fenton P, Ebraheim N, et al. Magnetic resonance imaging for ineffectual tarsal tunnel surgical treatment. *Clin Orthop.* 1991;264:264-266.

333. Galardi G, Amadio S, Maderna L, et al. Electrophysiologic studies in tarsal tunnel syndrome: diagnostic reliability of motor distal latency, mixed nerve and sensory nerve conduction studies. *Am J Phys Med Rehabil.* 1994;73:193-198.
334. DiGiacomo MA, Bernstein AL, Scurran BL, et al. Electrodiagnosis of the tarsal tunnel syndrome. *J Am Podiatry Assoc.* 1980;70:94-96.
335. Saeed MA, Gatens PF. Compound nerve action potentials of the medial and lateral plantar nerves through the tarsal tunnel. *Arch Phys Med Rehabil.* 1982;63:304-307.
336. Dellon AL. Management of peripheral nerve problems in the upper and lower extremity using quantitative sensory testing. *Hand Clin.* 1999;15:697-715.
337. Rose JD, Malay DS, Sorrento DL. Neurosensory testing of the medial calcaneal and medial plantar nerves in patients with plantar heel pain. *J Foot Ankle Surg.* 2003;42(4):173-177.
338. DiGiovanni BF, Gould JS. Tarsal tunnel syndrome and related entities. *Foot Ankle Clin.* 1998;3:405-426.
339. Jackson DL, Haglund BL. Tarsal tunnel syndrome in runners. *Sports Med.* 1992;13:146-149.
340. Rask M. Medial plantar neuropraxia (Jogger's foot). *Clin Orthop.* 1978;134:193-195.
341. Francis H, March L, Terenty T, et al. Benign joint hypermobility with neuropathy: documentation and mechanism of tarsal tunnel syndrome. *J Rheumatol.* 1987;14:577-581.
342. Mendicino SS, Mendicino RW. The tarsal tunnel syndrome and its surgical decompression. *Clin Podiatr Med Surg.* 1991;8:501-512.
343. Day FN III, Naples JJ. Tarsal tunnel syndrome: an endoscopic approach with 4 to 28 month follow up. *J Foot Ankle Surg.* 1994;33:244-248.
344. Day FN III, Naples JJ. Endoscopic tarsal tunnel release: update 96. *J Foot Ankle Surg.* 1996;35:225-229.
345. Downey MS. Surgical management of peripheral nerve entrapment syndromes. In: Oloff LM, ed. *Musculoskeletal Disorders of the Lower Extremity.* Philadelphia, PA: WB Saunders; 1994:685-717.
346. Pfeiffer WH, Cracchiolo A III. Clinical results after tarsal tunnel decompression [see comments]. *J Bone Joint Surg Am.* 1994;76:1222-1230.
347. Carrel JM, Davidson DM, Goldstein KT. Observations on 200 surgical cases of tarsal tunnel syndrome. *Clin Podiatr Med Surg.* 1994;11:609-616.
348. Takakura Y, Kitada C, Sugimoto K, et al. Tarsal tunnel syndrome: causes and results of operative treatment. *J Bone Joint Surg Br.* 1991;73:125-128.
349. Turan I, Rivero-Melian C, Guntner P, et al. Tarsal tunnel syndrome: outcome of surgery in longstanding cases. *Clin Orthop.* 1997;343:151-156.
350. Stern DS, Joyce MT. Tarsal tunnel syndrome: a review of 15 surgical procedures. *J Foot Surg.* 1989;28:290-294.
351. Bailie DS, Kelikian AS. Tarsal tunnel syndrome: diagnosis, surgical technique, and functional outcome. *Foot Ankle Int.* 1998;19:65-72.
352. Golovchinsky V. Double crush syndrome in lower extremities. *Electromyogr Clin Neurophysiol.* 1998;38:115-120.
353. Zahari DT, Ly P. Recurrent tarsal tunnel syndrome. *J Foot Surg.* 1992;31:385-387.
354. Merle M, Dellon AL, Campbell JN, et al. Complications of silicon polymer intubulation of nerves. *Microsurgery.* 1989;10:130-133.
355. Sotereanos DG, Giannakopoulos P, Mitsionis GI, et al. Vein graft wrapping for the treatment of recurrent compression of the median nerve. *Microsurgery.* 1995;16:752-756.
356. Gould JS. Autogenous vein wrapping for painful nerves in continuity. *Foot Ankle Clin.* 1998;3:527-536.
357. Campbell JT, Schon LC, Burkhardt LD. Histopathologic findings in autogenous saphenous vein graft wrapping for recurrent tarsal tunnel syndrome: a case report. *Foot Ankle Int.* 1998;19:766-769.
358. Easley ME, Schon LC. Peripheral nerve vein wrapping for intractable lower extremity pain. *Foot Ankle Int.* 2000;21:492-500.
359. Chang KV, Wu WT, Özçakar L. Extra-tunnel compression mimicking tarsal tunnel syndrome: ultrasound imaging for a plantar ganglion cyst. *Med Ultrason.* 2018;20(4):540-541. doi: 10.11152/mu-1788.
360. Carter J, Ben-Ghashir N, Chandrasekar CR. Giant schwannoma of the medial plantar nerve. *Foot (Edinb).* 2016;26:4-6. doi: 10.1016/j.foot.2015.10.002.
361. Melendez MM, Patel A, Dellon AL. The diagnosis and treatment of Joplin's neuroma. *J Foot Ankle Surg.* 2016;55(2):320-323. doi: 10.1053/j.jfas.2014.09.045.
362. Kuran B, Aydoğ T, Erçalık C, et al. Medial calcaneal neuropathy: a rare cause of prolonged heel pain. *Agri.* 2017;29(1):43-46. doi: 10.5505/agri.2015.13540.
363. Spinner RJ. Letter to the editor. *J Foot Ankle Surg.* 2005;44(1):74-75.
364. Dellon AL, Rosson GD, Anderson SR, Amrami KK. Tibial intraneural ganglia in the tarsal tunnel: is there a joint connection? *J Foot Ankle Surg.* 2007;46(1):27-31.
365. Blitz NM, Prestridge J, Amrami KK, Spinner RJ. A posttraumatic, joint-connected sural intraneural ganglion cyst—with a new mechanism of intraneural recurrence: a case report. *J Foot Ankle Surg.* 2008;47(3):199-205.
366. Blitz NM, Amrami KK, Spinner RJ. Magnetic resonance imaging of a deep peroneal intraneural ganglion cyst originating from the second metatarsophalangeal joint: a pattern of propagation supporting the unified articular (synovial) theory for the formation of intraneural ganglia. *J Foot Ankle Surg.* 2009;48(1):80-84.
367. Spinner RJ, Amrami KK. Commentary: superficial peroneal intraneural ganglion cyst originating from the inferior tibiofibular joint: the latest chapter in the book. *J Foot Ankle Surg.* 2010;49:575-578.
368. Prasad N, Amrami KK, Yangi K, Spinner RJ. Occult isolated articular branch cyst of the lateral plantar nerve. *J Foot Ankle Surg.* 2017;56(1):78-81. doi: 10.1053/j.jfas.2016.09.008.
369. Laumonerie P, Lapègue F, Reina N, et al. Degenerative subtalar joints complicated by medial plantar intraneural cysts: cutting the cystic articular branch prevents recurrence. *Bone Joint J.* 2018;100-B(2):183-189. doi:10.1302/0301-620X.100B2.BJJ-2017-0990.R1.
370. Przylucki H, Jones CL. Entrapment neuropathy of muscle branch of lateral plantar nerve: a cause of heel pain. *J Am Podiatry Assoc.* 1981;71(3):119-124.
371. Baxter DE, Thigpen CM. Heel pain—operative results. *Foot Ankle.* 1984;5(1):16-25.
372. Jaring MRF, Khan AZ, Livingstone JA, Chakraverty J. A case of bilateral Baxter's neuropathy secondary to plantar fasciitis. *J Foot Ankle Surg.* 2019;58(4):771-774. doi: 10.1053/j.jfas.2018.11.010.
373. Counsel PD, Davenport M, Brown A, et al. Ultrasound-guided radiofrequency denervation of the medial calcaneal nerve. *Clin J Sport Med.* 2016;26(6):465-470.
374. Wills B, Lee SR, Hudson PW, et al. Calcaneal osteotomy safe zone to prevent neurological damage: fact or fiction? *Foot Ankle Spec.* 2019;12(1):34-38. doi: 10.1177/1938640018762556.
375. Baker LD, Kuhn HH. Morton's metatarsalgia: localized degenerative fibrosis with neuromatous proliferation of the fourth plantar nerve. *South Med J.* 1944;37:123-127.
376. Goldman F. Intermetatarsal neuromas-light and electron microscopic observations. *J Am Podiatry Assoc.* 1980;70:265-278.
377. Wu KK. Morton's interdigital neuroma: a clinical review of its etiology, treatment, and results. *J Foot Ankle Surg.* 1996;35(2):112-119.
378. Giannini S, Bacchini P, Ceccarelli F, Vannini F. Interdigital neuroma: clinical examination and histopathologic results in 63 cases treated with excision. *Foot Ankle Int.* 2004;25(2):79-84.
379. LiMarzi GM, Scherer KF, Richardson ML, et al. CT and MR imaging of the postoperative ankle and foot. *Radiographics.* 2016;36(6):1828-1848.
380. Pastides P, El-Sallakh S, Charalambides C. Morton's neuroma: a clinical versus radiological diagnosis. *Foot Ankle Surg.* 2012;18(1):22-24. doi: 10.1016/j.fas.2011.01.007.
381. Symeonidis PD, Iselin LD, Simmons N, Fowler S, Dracopoulos G, Stavrou P. Prevalence of interdigital nerve enlargements in an asymptomatic population. *Foot Ankle Int.* 2012;33(7):543-547. doi: 10.3113/FAI.2012.0543.
382. Zanetti M, Strehle JK, Zollinger H, Hodler J. Morton neuroma and fluid in the intermetatarsal bursae on MR images of 70 asymptomatic volunteers. *Radiology.* 1997;203(2):516-520.
383. Thomson L, Aujla RS, Divall P, Bhatia M. Non-surgical treatments for Morton's neuroma: a systematic review. *Foot Ankle Surg.* 2020;26(7):736-743. doi: 10.1016/j.fas.2019.09.009.
384. Matthews BG, Hurn SE, Harding MP, Henry RA, Ware RS. The effectiveness of non-surgical interventions for common plantar digital compressive neuropathy (Morton's neuroma): a systematic review and meta-analysis. *J Foot Ankle Res.* 2019;12:12. doi: 10.1186/s13047-019-0320-7.
385. Jain S, Mannan K. The diagnosis and management of Morton's neuroma: a literature review. *Foot Ankle Spec.* 2013;6(4):307-317. doi: 10.1177/1938640013493464.
386. Ruiz Santiago F, Prados Olleta N, Tomás Muñoz P, Guzmán Álvarez L, Martínez Martínez A. Short term comparison between blind and ultrasound guided injection in Morton neuroma. *Eur Radiol.* 2019;29(2):620-627. doi: 10.1007/s00330-018-5670-1.
387. Mahadevan D, Attwal M, Bhatt R, Bhatia M. Corticosteroid injection for Morton's neuroma with or without ultrasound guidance: a randomised controlled trial. *Bone Joint J.* 2016;98-B(4):498-503. doi: 10.1302/0301-620X.98B4.36880.
388. Santos D, Morrison G, Coda A. Sclerosing alcohol injections for the management of intermetatarsal neuromas: a systematic review. *Foot (Edinb).* 2018;35:36-47. doi: 10.1016/j.foot.2017.12.003.
389. Perini L, Perini C, Tagliapietra M, et al. Percutaneous alcohol injection under sonographic guidance in Morton's neuroma: follow-up in 220 treated lesions. *Radiol Med.* 2016;121(7):597-604. doi: 10.1007/s11547-016-0622-9.
390. Cazzato RL, Garnon J, Ramamurthy N, et al. Percutaneous MR-guided cryoablation of Morton's neuroma: rationale and technical details after the first 20 patients. *Cardiovasc Intervent Radiol.* 2016;39(10):1491-1498. doi: 10.1007/s00270-016-1365-7.
391. Masala S, Cuzzolino A, Morini M, Raguso M, Fiori R. Ultrasound-guided percutaneous radiofrequency for the treatment of Morton's neuroma. *Cardiovasc Intervent Radiol.* 2018;41(1):137-144. doi: 10.1007/s00270-017-1786-y.
392. Brooks D, Parr A, Bryceson W. Three cycles of radiofrequency ablation are more efficacious than two in the management of Morton's neuroma. *Foot Ankle Spec.* 2018;11(2):107-111. doi: 10.1177/1938640017709905.
393. Moore JL, Rosen R, Cohen J, Rosen B. Radiofrequency thermoneurolysis for the treatment of Morton's neuroma. *J Foot Ankle Surg.* 2012;51(1):20-22. doi: 10.1053/j.jfas.2011.10.007.
394. Seok H, Kim SH, Lee SY, Park SW. Extracorporeal shockwave therapy in patients with Morton's neuroma a randomized, placebo-controlled trial. *J Am Podiatr Med Assoc.* 2016;106(2):93-99. doi: 10.7547/14-131.
395. Climent JM, Mondéjar-Gómez F, Rodríguez-Ruiz C, Díaz-Llopis I, Gómez-Gallego D, Martín-Medina P. Treatment of Morton neuroma with botulinum toxin A: a pilot study. *Clin Drug Investig.* 2013;33(7):497-503. doi: 10.1007/s40261-013-0090-0.
396. Reichert P, Zimmer K, Witkowski J, Wnukiewicz W, Kuliński S, Gosk J. Long-term results of neurectomy through a dorsal approach in the treatment of Morton's neuroma. *Adv Clin Exp Med.* 2016;25(2):295-302. doi: 10.17219/acem/60249.
397. Akermark C, Crone H, Skoog A, Weidenhielm L. A prospective randomized controlled trial of plantar versus dorsal incisions for operative treatment of primary Morton's neuroma. *Foot Ankle Int.* 2013;34(9):1198-1204. doi: 10.1177/1071100713484300.
398. Amis JA, Siverhus SW, Liwnicz BH. An anatomic basis for recurrence after Morton's neuroma excision. *Foot Ankle.* 1992;13(3):153-156.
399. Johnson JE, Johnson KA, Unni KK. Persistent pain after excision of an interdigital neuroma. *J Bone Joint Surg Am.* 1988;70:651-657.
400. Malay DS. Recurrent intermetatarsal neuroma. In: McGlamry ED, ed. *Reconstructive Surgery of the Foot and Leg: Update '89.* Tucker, GA: Podiatry Institute; 1989:321-324.
401. Beskin JL, Baxter DE. Recurrent pain following interdigital neurectomy: a plantar approach. *Foot Ankle.* 1988;9:34-39.
402. David WS, Doyle JJ. Segmental near nerve sensory conduction studies of the medial and lateral plantar nerve. *Electromyogr Clin Neurophysiol.* 1996;36:411-417.

Pediatric Surgery

Juvenile and Adolescent Hallux Valgus

Kieran T. Mahan and Caitlin Mahan Madden

DEFINITION

Juvenile hallux valgus typically refers to patients who present with hallux valgus deformity before age 20.[1] The deformity in these patients has specific characteristics that differ from the adult. There is a high incidence of metatarsus adductus, a high hallux abductus angle (HAA), as well as a high proximal articular set angle (PASA). As a result, addressing the deformity surgically requires specifically addressing each of the components. Because hallux valgus is most often a disorder of adults, when it occurs at a younger age, special attention should be paid to the characteristics.

Another group with the same characteristics of deformity is the adolescent-onset patients. These are patients who may not present until adulthood but developed the deformity at an early age. These patients should be addressed with the same consideration as juvenile hallux valgus patients.

CLASSIFICATION

Juvenile hallux valgus can be classified as either a juvenile or adult presentation (both with juvenile onset).

The deformity can be further classified as with or without metatarsus adductus (Fig. 52.1). This is an important distinction because with metatarsus adductus the disorder is more frequent and the severity is worse. Those without metatarsus adductus usually have a rectus foot with a moderate to severe intermetatarsal angle (IMA). They are less likely to have a high HAA or high PASA. The patients with metatarsus adductus may have a more moderate IMA but because of the adductus foot, high HAA, and high PASA, the deformity is more severe and more frequent (Fig. 52.2).

ETIOLOGY

Shoes are an extrinsic factor in the development of juvenile hallux abducto valgus (HAV). They do not appear to have a determinative effect on causing the deformity but may be an aggravating factor. Intrinsic factors can include heredity, obesity, pes valgus, ankle equinus, metatarsus adductus etc. In most patients, the etiology is multifactorial.[2,3]

A particular dilemma is the role of pes valgus.[2] Hohman stated that "Hallux valgus is always combined with pes planus, and pes planus is always the predisposing factor in hallux valgus." Coughlin and Mann did not see the presence of pes planus as frequently unless a neurologic disorder was involved.[4] They concluded, however, that the presence of pes planus accelerated the development of hallux valgus.

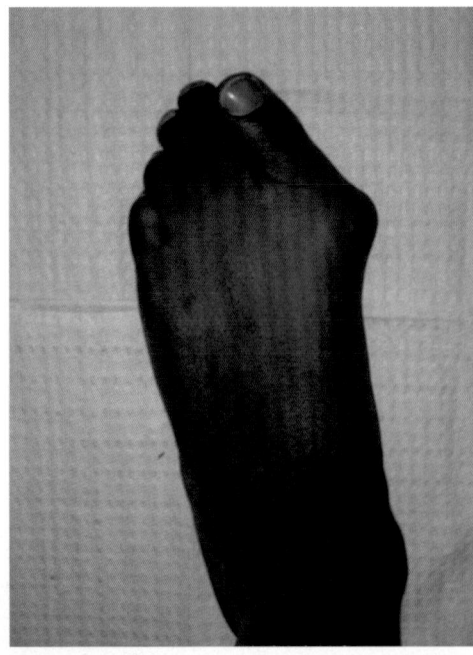

FIGURE 52.2 Photograph of left foot in an adolescent with juvenile hallux abducto valgus.

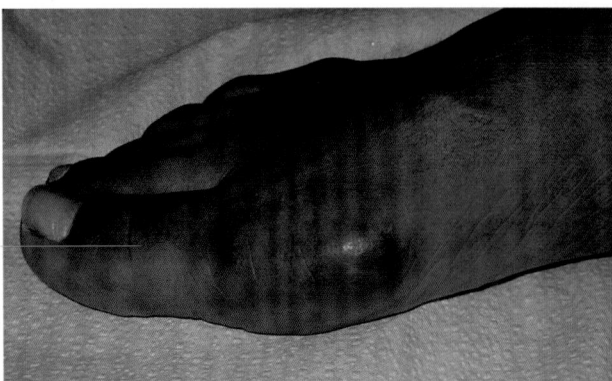

FIGURE 52.1 Photograph of a painful medial eminence from juvenile hallux abducto valgus.

INDICATIONS AND PITFALLS

As with most surgeries that we perform, pain is the most certain of the indications. Attempts to alleviate the pain may include topical creams, larger shoes, short course of anti-inflammatories, etc. Patients who have metatarsus adductus as a component may have significant hallux abductus. This can create impingement or overlapping with the second toe. Severe deformity that creates problems with gait or the likelihood of creating a second toe and metatarsophalangeal joint deformity is also an indication for surgery.

The timing of surgery is also important with respect to bone growth. Girls complete bone growth before boys on average, both within the 12-16 year time frame. If the deformity is stable, with controllable deforming forces, and little pain, then the surgical correction can be deferred until after bone growth is completed. If the foot type is rectus, with more moderate deformity, then deferring surgery can again be the best option. If the deformity is the more severe type with metatarsus adductus, or with uncontrolled deforming forces, or more severe pain and deformity, then correction before closure of the physeal plate should be attempted. Another advantage of doing the procedure early is that it allows for the possibility of epiphysiodesis.

Most commonly, there is an IMA of 15 or above or an elevated metatarsus adductus angle (MAA) as an indication for surgery.

Pitfalls largely include failure to address each of the components of the deformity, particularly PASA and metatarsus primus varus (Fig. 52.3). If either of those components is not addressed, the chance of recurrence is high. Having a high index of suspicion for metatarsus adductus is critical and measuring the MAA using Sgarlato technique appears to be the most accurate method.

> **PERILS and PITFALLS**
> - Failure to address multiple components
>   - PASA
>   - Metatarsus primus varus
> - Not measuring MAA with Sgarlato technique
> - Failure to consider age and bone growth when choosing procedure

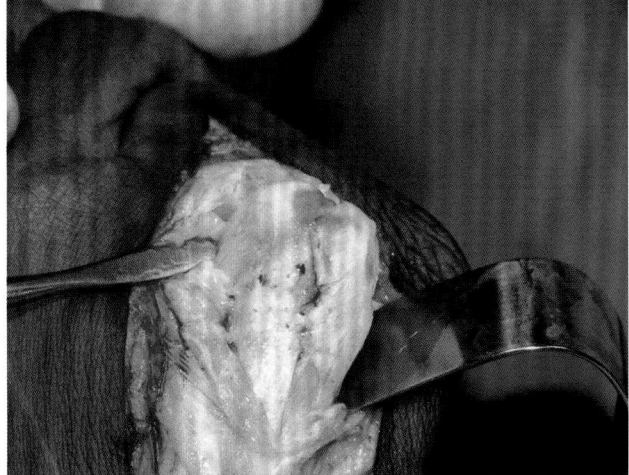

FIGURE 52.3 Intraoperative view of high PASA, often found to exceed preoperative measurements.

ANATOMY

The PASA is one of the defining aspects of juvenile HAV. It has been demonstrated that preoperative x-ray measurement is not reliable. Amarnek et al. (1985) demonstrated that the intraoperative measurement exceeded the preoperative x-ray measurement of PASA by 7 degrees.[5] It significantly underestimates the actual value as measured intraoperatively. As a result, it is critical to evaluate the PASA intraoperatively. In addition, it is best to prepare the patient and parents that there may need to be a procedure done to correct PASA during the surgery.

Another aspect of PASA correction is the tangential articular set angle. First described by Schechter and Doll in 1985, this angle is formed by the slope of the articular cartilage of the first metatarsal head and the perpendicular line to the long axis of the second metatarsal.[6] This angle changes after correction of the IMA and the metatarsus primus varus, creating an exaggeration of the PASA. Therefore, it is important to not only evaluate the PASA intraoperatively but to do that evaluation after the correction of the IMA and MPV. Coughlin (1995) stated that "The success of surgical correction of juvenile hallux valgus deformity is intimately associated with the magnitude of the distal metatarsal articular angle (DMAA)" (authors' note DMAA = PASA).[7]

One defining aspect of juvenile HAV is metatarsus adductus. Pontious et al.[8] demonstrated an incidence of metatarsus adductus of 75% in a group of juvenile HAV patients, and Banks et al.[9] showed an incidence of 67% in their group of juvenile HAV patients. In a study of adult patients, there was an incidence of 35% in the hallux valgus patients compared to 13% in controls. Whatever the exact number, there is clearly an increased incidence of metatarsus adductus in this juvenile HAV population. The significance of this is due to the effect of the MAA on the IMA. The "true IMA" is calculated by taking the measured MAA and subtracting 15 (the normal angle). The result is added to the IMA to come up with the "true IMA." The effect means that the greater the MAA, the greater the effect on the deformity and the greater likelihood of the need for proximal correction. In an unpublished study of 154 total juvenile patients with 82 juvenile hallux valgus patients, the senior author demonstrated by linear regression analysis and analysis of variance techniques that with metatarsus adductus the deformity is more frequent and more severe.

As it turns out, how the MAA is measured matters. Engel's angle is not accurate for purposes of this measurement.[10] It tends to significantly underestimate the effect on the true IMA. Consequently, the standard technique by Sgarlato is what should be used to calculate the MAA. McConnell, Cardenas, Mahan, and Meyr studied 140 preoperative hallux valgus feet, measuring both the standard MAA and Engel's angle.[11] The "true" IMA was 16.37 for the standard MAA and only 10.39 for Engel's angle. They concluded that the standard MAA was more sensitive than Engel's angle. Crawford and Green similarly found that Engel's angle is less reliable than the Sgarlato angle.[12] Dawoodi and Perera in 2012 reviewed five methods of measuring MAA and found that there is indeed sensitivity in the incidence of HAV by different measurement techniques.[10]

Yu and DiNapoli in 1989 wrote about the relationship between the radiographic angles in hallux valgus: with an increased MAA, as the hallux abductus increases, so too does the PASA, while the IMA tends to be smaller.[13] This paper in the Podiatry Institute seminar text was a thorough description of

what happens in juvenile hallux valgus. In these patients, even though the IMA may not be high, the effect of the MAA means that proximal correction is more likely to be necessary. Griffiths and Paladino in 1992 reported the same relationships.[14]

The conclusion is that metatarsus adductus is much more common in juvenile and adolescent hallux valgus patients and results in more severe hallux abductus and an increased PASA.[15] As a result, proximal correction and PASA correction are frequently necessary in these patients, as distinct from the adult hallux valgus patient. Failure to address one or both components when present will most likely lead to recurrence.

PHYSICAL EXAMINATION

A thorough physical examination allows the clinician to determine the severity of the hallux valgus deformity and to identify any concomitant biomechanical issues. A thorough review of the patient's history and family history is also critical. Parents of pediatric and adolescent patients should be questioned to help round out the examination. They can help identify time of onset (both of appearance of the bunion and start of symptoms) and can provide insight into the patient's ability (or willingness) to adhere to treatment, especially postoperatively. Children may be brought in by parents who are concerned about the appearance of their child's foot, even in the absence of pain. Adolescents may focus on difficulties with shoes in addition to cosmetic concerns. They may be more seriously involved in athletics, and a discussion of this can help determine the effect the hallux valgus deformity has on function, in addition to guiding timing for surgery if indicated. Evaluation of cleats, dance shoes, or other specialized athletic footwear is also helpful.

A key task for the clinician is to determine the amount of pain the hallux valgus deformity is causing the patient. In the absence of pain, it may be possible to delay surgery even for a moderate to severe deformity, whereas a milder deformity that is painful and affecting normal function may necessitate surgery at an earlier stage. Observing the patient's gait can be very helpful in this regard. A painful deformity may cause a limp, which may lead to other compensatory changes. In toeing, out toeing, genu valgum or varum, and equinus may also be seen during gait.

Examined in static weight bearing, the juvenile hallux valgus does differ from the adult hallux valgus. Transverse plane deformity is more common and typically more severe, whereas frontal plane valgus rotation is less common in juvenile patients. Inflammation at the medial aspect of the first metatarsal head may present as a "bump" of red or tender skin, possibly with a bursa lying beneath but rarely with the palpable degenerative osseous changes that are seen with adult HAV. In the juvenile deformity, signs of a hypermobile flatfoot may be evident. The rearfoot should be examined from the back to determine the degree of rearfoot valgus. In a hypermobile foot that is flat in weight bearing, one sees a medial arch appear upon heel raise. Limb length discrepancy, internal malleolar torsion, pronation, and signs of ligamentous laxity should all be kept in mind when examining the juvenile hallux valgus patient.

A non–weight-bearing examination, typically with the patient sitting in an examination chair, allows for evaluation of joint mobility. The first MTPJ should be assessed in dorsiflexion and plantarflexion, and horizontal (or transverse) motion should be attempted. A "tracking" or "track bound" joint indicates deviation of the first MTPJ axis, which is often seen with

an increase in PASA.[16] Hypermobility at the midfoot or rearfoot may indicate a more generalized ligamentous laxity. Spasticity or equinus at the ankle can be a sign of an underlying neurological condition, such as cerebral palsy. Thorough examination of the first MCJ should also be performed. If a more general ligamentous or neuromuscular condition is suspected, the other lower extremity joints should be evaluated bilaterally, and more specific blood work or imaging done as needed.

Additional deformities should also be noted. Crossover or underlapping second toe is less common in juvenile HAV but may indicate a more progressive deformity. Metatarsus adductus and pes plano valgus are frequently seen with juvenile HAV, and the severity of these must be taken into account when planning treatment.

IMAGING AND DIAGNOSTIC STUDIES

Radiographic evaluation of the juvenile hallux valgus should start with a full set of weight-bearing radiographs, similar to an adult evaluation. Standard angles and measurements should be taken. X-ray views, in particular the dorsal-plantar (DP) and lateral, should be taken in the patient's usual angle and base of gait. A sesamoid axial view is useful for evaluating the rotational aspect of the deformity. The age of the patient should be kept in mind, and any open or partially open epiphysis must be carefully noted. Typically, closure of the epiphysis at the base of the first metatarsal occurs between 14 and 16 years of age.

There are several radiographic angles that are utilized to evaluate hallux valgus deformities. The IMA between the first and second metatarsals is normally <9 degrees, with a measurement >15 degrees indicating a severe deformity. The HAA and hallux abductus interphalangeal angle can also be measured (Fig. 52.4). Tibial sesamoid position is evaluated on a DP view, and the length of the first metatarsal is determined

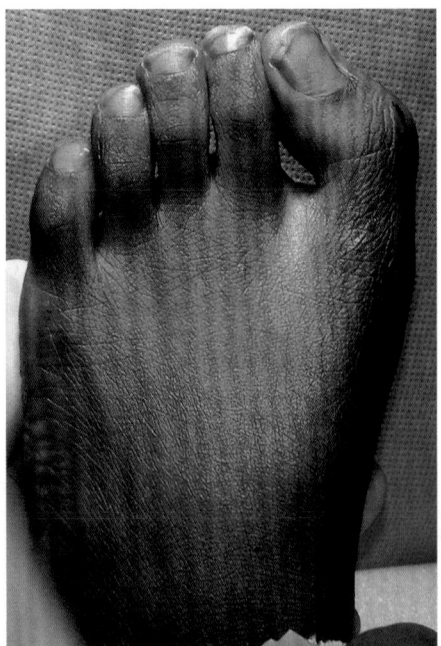

FIGURE 52.4 Photograph demonstrating high hallux interphalangeus.

by checking the first metatarsal protrusion distance. Lateral views can identify medial arch alignment and first metatarsal elevatus.

Measurement of the PASA and the MAA are of particular importance in the juvenile hallux valgus patient. To more accurately capture metatarsus adductus, a weight-bearing DP radiograph should be taken with the subtalar joint in neutral position.

Several ways of then measuring the MAA have been proposed. Dawoodi and Perera[10] confirmed previous findings by Griffiths and Palladino, demonstrating a correlation between MAA and hallux valgus. Out of five methods for measuring MAA, they found that Sgarlato method was the only one with significant correlation to hallux valgus. They also found it to have a high inter- and intraobserver reliability. It utilizes the bisection of the second metatarsal and a line perpendicular to the longitudinal bisection of the lesser tarsus. Specifically, the lesser tarsus bisection is taken from the line between the most lateral aspects of the fourth metatarsal-cuboid joint and the calcaneal-cuboid joint, and the line between the most medial aspects of the talonavicular joint and the first metatarsal-medial cuneiform joint. Engel's angle, while reliably reproducible, was found to underestimate the correlation of metatarsus adductus and HAV. An accurate MAA measurement also allows calculation of the true IMA. The true IMA is defined by the formula IMA + (MAA − 15) = true IMA.[13] Thus, it is important to use care in both taking and measuring radiographs.

PASA is defined as the angle between the line perpendicular to the long axis bisection of the first metatarsal and the orientation of the proximal aspect of the articular cartilage at the first metatarsal head. This is sometimes referred to as the DMAA in the literature. Due to the inherent difficulty in assessing cartilage on a plain radiograph, the PASA should be evaluated intraoperatively. On x-ray, the accepted normal range is 0-8 degrees. A high PASA can indicate adaptive changes at the first metatarsal head, and this should be considered when discussing treatment options.[8]

TREATMENT

Conservative treatment is limited for juvenile hallux valgus. Although it is possible that in some instances orthotics may serve to slow down the development of hallux valgus, this would be most likely in circumstances where the underlying flatfoot is a frontal plane deformity. Overall, there is no significant evidence that orthotics alter the long-term outcome of juvenile hallux valgus.[17]

Modifications of shoe gear, injections or short courses of nonsteroidal anti inflammatories for bursitis, and splints or padding have all been mentioned in the literature. Usually, conservative vs surgical treatment is more a question of whether the pain and/or the deformity rise to the level of warranting surgical care.

PERIOPERATIVE CARE

Adolescents require direct participation and explanation in order to make the surgery successful. They are at the age range where questions come naturally. It is important to involve the patient in his/her own care. It is important for them to understand that a scar will be left and also for them to understand all of the possible complications of the surgery.[18]

Pain control is understandably important.[19] Intraoperative popliteal blocks after the patient is asleep can be very effective. Acetaminophen with codeine is not effective for pain relief. It is a precursor drug that must be metabolized in the liver to morphine and a similar metabolite.[20] Varying metabolism rates can result in either ineffective pain management and/or excessive respiratory suppression. Tramadol may be an option in some patients. Oxycodone is as well. All of the narcotics can be problematic so a reliance on NSAIDs, where possible, is desirable.

Preoperative crutch training should be performed so that it is not necessary immediately after surgery when the patient may be groggy and/or nauseous.

SOFT TISSUE AND CAPITAL PROCEDURES

The concept of the lateral release has become more controversial lately with some authors arguing that it is not necessary. If the adductor tendon is shortened due to a high HAA, then it makes sense to us to release the lateral compartment and rebalance the soft tissues around the joint. This can, and should, be done without disrupting significant blood supply. Ruch has described the technique well in previous editions of McGlamry, but essentially the maneuver consists of

1. Dissection down onto the floor of the first interspace where the conjoined extensor expansions cross.
2. Utilizing the Metzenbaum, one arm is placed above and one below the expansion. The area beneath is spread to keep the neurovascular bundle away from the overlying structures. One cut is made through the expansions to expose the adductor tendon (Fig. 52.5).

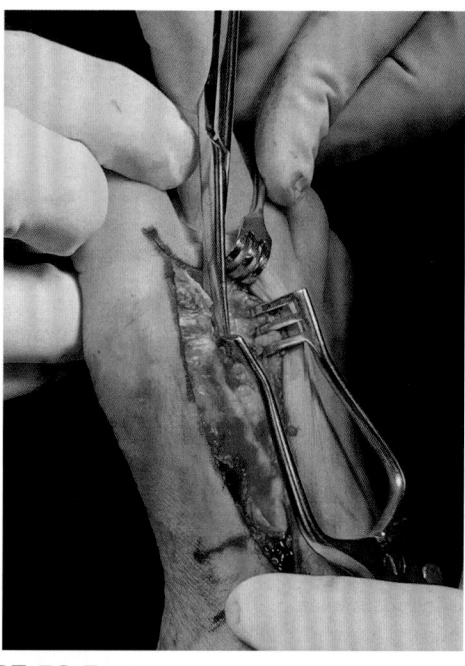

FIGURE 52.5 Standard interspace dissection as part of juvenile hallux abducto valgus repair.

3. With a no. 15 blade, a line is drawn along the dorsal side of the tendon. The tendon is detached distally, cutting in toward bone. A straight hemostat is tagged onto the tendon distally and the tendon is dissected proximally. The tendon can either be saved for later transfer, or more commonly, a piece is resected.

4. A freer elevator can be used to *lightly* press down on the fibular sesamoid, putting it under tension. The ligament is then incised and released.

5. If further release is necessary, then the lateral head of the flexor hallucis brevis can be released. This must be done carefully to avoid lacerating the flexor hallucis longus tendon. The procedure is also the functional equivalent of a sesamoid excision and so carries an increased risk of hallux varus. Sesamoid excision or release of the lateral head of the brevis is uncommon in juvenile hallux valgus.

6. The extensor hallucis brevis may also be released if it is contracted.

The medial eminence is not typically very enlarged. The sagittal groove is not typically very pronounced. Nonetheless, we typically take a small piece off of the medial eminence, angling the cut so that it is mostly dorsal medial.

HEAD OSTEOTOMIES

Although the emphasis in juvenile hallux valgus patients is on proximal correction because of the frequency of metatarsus adductus, capital osteotomies have a legitimate place for a subset of these patients.[21,22]

The Austin, Kalish, or Offset-V can be performed in those patients with a rectus foot and moderate IMA. These procedures can also be combined with epiphysiodesis or with the proximal correction of an opening wedge osteotomy of the medial cuneiform.

Although occasionally there may be a distal physis, usually a secondary physis is not an issue, which makes these procedures attractive. They can be performed without the need for casting or non–weight bearing. Bone is typically stable and healthy in these young patients and internal fixation is tolerated well. Two 2.7-mm screws give good fixation. In the rectus foot type, there is less chance of an elevated PASA. If the PASA is indeed elevated, it must be corrected. Wedging the cut for bicorrection and rotating the distal fragment to correct for the PASA are two techniques that can create correction.

Our own preference is not to use the Akin osteotomy to create a "cheater" amount of correction for the PASA. We do use the Akin for correction of an increased distal articular set angle (DASA). Using the Akin in lieu of PASA correction may lead to recurrence over time secondary to the remaining angulation of the cartilage. If an Akin is necessary, either for DASA correction or to fine-tune the overall correction, it can be done with an oblique cut with screw fixation (typically one 2.7-mm screw) or with a transverse cut and staple fixation.

The Green-Reverdin osteotomy is not used as a primary procedure but is frequently combined with a more proximal osteotomy to correct the PASA. Green has described the technique. The top cuts are made with one parallel to the PASA and one perpendicular to the long axis of the first metatarsal. This is for the PASA correction. The bottom cut is angled so that it will exit above and proximal to the sesamoids, to avoid sesamoid damage. The lateral cortex on the dorsal cut is preserved and closed gently in the wedge to preserve osteotomy stability. The plantar cut is through and through. Fixation can be done with a variety of techniques but most often we use a buried K-wire, which is simple and inexpensive.

SHAFT OSTEOTOMIES

Shaft osteotomies such as the scarf or z-osteotomy can gain a significant amount of IMA reduction.[23] Although the head can be swiveled to some degree to achieve PASA correction, there is a risk of troughing, which can create shortening of the metatarsal. These types of osteotomies are better used in adolescent hallux valgus without metatarsus adductus, PASA, or severe deformity.

BASE OSTEOTOMIES

Proximal correction is required more commonly in juvenile hallux valgus because of the influence of metatarsus adductus. The type of correction can vary, but a proximal closing base wedge osteotomy provides excellent correction of the IMA and metatarsus primus varus. An IMA of >15, or less in the adductus foot type, is an indication for the closing base wedge osteotomy or other proximal correction such as the crescentic osteotomy, Lapidus fusion, or opening base wedge osteotomy.

The crescentic osteotomy provides correction in multiple planes with less metatarsal shortening. Fixation and achieving sufficient stability are more difficult than a wedge osteotomy where there is an intact hinge that provides an inherent amount of stability. The opening base wedge osteotomy provides correction and usually requires plate fixation. Either graft material (autogenous or allogeneic) or specialized plates that allow for a specific amount of correction with metallic wedging are utilized to achieve the correction. The additional length can create jamming of the first MPJ, particularly if the first metatarsal is already long or if there is an adductus foot. This makes it less useful for juvenile hallux valgus correction. If the first metatarsal is short, the procedure is more useful. Al-Nammari et al. described a double osteotomy consisting of an opening wedge osteotomy of the base of the first metatarsal and an Akin osteotomy.[24]

The oblique closing base wedge is highly technique dependent. John Ruch developed, popularized, and refined the modern oblique base wedge osteotomy. The location of the hinge determines where the head of the metatarsal will end up. Most commonly, the hinge is located perpendicular to the weight-bearing surface, which results in transverse plane motion. The objective is to keep the first metatarsal even with the second and to prevent dorsiflexion. Both improper hinge location and premature weight bearing can result in dorsiflexion. Dorsiflexion results in metatarsalgia.

For juvenile hallux valgus, the physis may be open and it should be avoided. It can usually be identified as a somewhat darker line along the base of the metatarsal. If there is a question, an intraoperative x-ray can be used to confirm the location. The hinge is located just distal to the physis on the medial side.

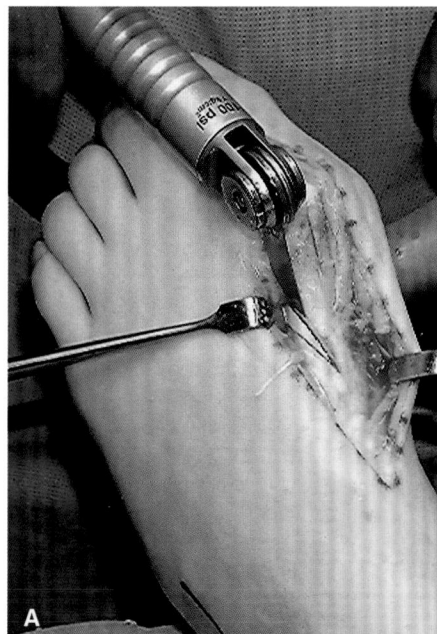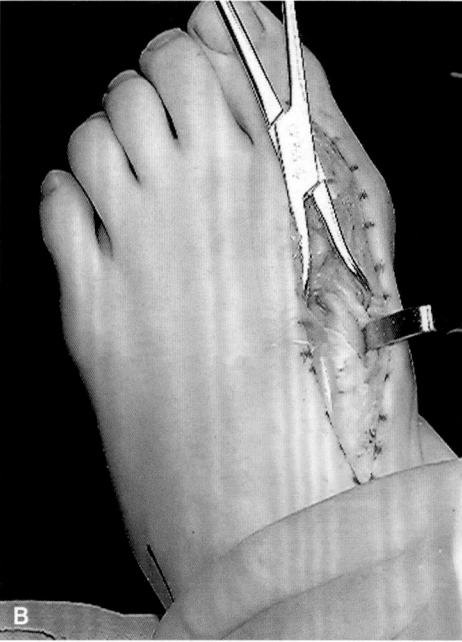

FIGURE 52.6 A. CBWO for the foot with metatarsus adductus and juvenile hallux abducto valgus. **B.** Temporary fixation is used to check the correction with fluoroscopy and stabilize during application of permanent fixation.

The technique itself is performed after resection of the medial eminence and interspace work when those are necessary, as is typical. The extensor hallucis longus tendon sheath is incised and retracted laterally. The periosteal incision is made in line with the osteotomy and minimal reflection is performed. A subperiosteal pocket is formed on the lateral side of the metatarsal. The vein end of a Senn retractor can be placed in this pocket to protect the neurovascular bundle. This also separates the periosteum from the part of the osteotomy that will be removed. The osteotomy cut must be oblique enough for the fixation (Fig. 52.6A). The more transverse the osteotomy, the more difficult screw fixation becomes and the more tension that is placed on the hinge. The osteotomy can be drawn out with a skin marker and/or scored with the saw. The distal cut can be made first to preserve stability of the proximal cut. It is critical to ensure that the proximal cut ends up being ~45 degrees to the long axis of the metatarsal. The cuts are made so that they converge just proximal to the hinge. The saw is used to score the dorsal cortex, to penetrate it, and then to saw down the lateral side. It is worked proximally back to the desired spot. The second cut is made in a similar fashion. The wedge can then be removed with a dental pick. The osteotomy can be tested for closure (Fig. 52.6B). If it does not bend easily, the hinge can be feathered slightly. It is important to make sure that the plantar and dorsal cortices have been cut and that only the medial hinge is intact. Once the osteotomy can be closed, a bone clamp is used to maintain the closure. It is now important to be sure that adequate correction has been obtained. If a small amount of additional correction is necessary, the osteotomy can be closed and "feathered." A larger amount of correction requires a thin sliver off the proximal portion of the bone.

Stability requires at least two points of fixation. An intact hinge is one point of stability. Loss of the hinge can cause the osteotomy to rotate around a solitary screw and then shift proximally. This can be a devastating complication requiring surgical correction. In order to prevent this complication, two screws are most commonly used. The proximal or anchor screw is used to prevent proximal shifting. We typically use a 2.7-mm cortical screw for this. The interfragmental compression screw is perpendicular to the osteotomy in order to achieve maximal compression and stability. The compression screw can be a 2.7- or 3.5-mm cortical screw placed with interfragmental technique or a partially threaded 4.0-mm cancellous screw. The screws are stacked vertically in order to avoid collision. The anchor screw is more dorsal and the compression screw is more plantar. Intraoperative x-rays can be taken after screw placement to confirm correction and fixation.

LAPIDUS

Lapidus described the metatarsocuneiform fusion in 1934 for the juvenile hallux valgus deformity with metatarsus primus varus.[25] The procedure includes a first metatarsocuneiform joint arthrodesis along with medial eminence resection and soft tissue realignment at the first metatarsophalangeal joint. In 1987, Clark et al. performed the Lapidus arthrodesis on adolescent patients with a HAV deformity with a hypermobile first ray.[26] The authors found 91% of the patients to have excellent or good results with only one recurrence of the deformity. The Lapidus procedure may best be used when there is instability of the first ray and a long first metatarsal as the fusion results in significant shortening of the ray. Other indications to perform a Lapidus on a juvenile hallux valgus deformity include a large IMA >25 degrees, any underlying neuromuscular diseases, or genetic conditions such as Down syndrome.[27] Corticocancellous grafting may be utilized to compensate for

the shortening resulting from the Lapidus fusion.[28] Fixation may be accomplished with screws or K-wires if crossing an open growth plate.

METATARSUS ADDUCTUS AND JUVENILE HALLUX VALGUS

As described above, metatarsus adductus is significantly intertwined with juvenile hallux valgus. For the most part, the significance of this is that proximal correction is required in these patients. Sometimes, however, the metatarsus adductus must be addressed. It is infrequent that all five metatarsals need to be corrected. More commonly, only the medial three metatarsals may be adducted. The need to address all five metatarsals complicates the repair significantly. Performing all five metatarsal osteotomies can be difficult in terms of dissection, perfecting alignment and fixation. It is beyond the scope of this chapter to address this repair, but it is important that there are alternatives to a full repair. A medial opening wedge osteotomy can address both metatarsus primus varus and the medial component of metatarsus adductus. The procedure was described in a paper by Lynch utilizing a technique by the late James Ganley DPM.[29] Through a dorsal medial incision, the tibialis anterior is identified and protected. The osteotomy is made anterior to the mid portion of the medial cuneiform with the lateral hinge intact. An osteotome is used to pry open the osteotomy until the desired amount of correction is obtained. The defect is measured and an optimal bone graft is shaped. Allogeneic bone bank bone is ideal in these circumstances. The medial cuneiform heals well and autogenous bone is usually not necessary. A graft with strong cortical walls is necessary to maintain correction. Precut wedges are available from some banks or allogeneic iliac crest or patella can be fashioned for use. Grafts measuring 4-6 mm are usually sufficient for correction.

Another approach to take if the adductus involves more of the forefoot is to combine the opening wedge cuneiform osteotomy with a closing wedge osteotomy of the cuboid. This technique is limited by the small size of the lateral aspect of the cuboid. There is not enough room to allow for much fixation, but a Steinmann pin is more than adequate because of the vascularity of the cuboid. The approach does not as directly correct all five metatarsals but it provides sufficient correction in most instances.

As patients age, the high hallux abductus will also create abductus of the lesser digits with deformity at the metatarsophalangeal joints. The lesser toes must be corrected in order to maintain permanent correction in these circumstances. Release of the MPJ with pinning across the joint may be helpful in maintaining this correction.

EPIPHYSIODESIS

Epiphysiodesis is a unique approach for correction of juvenile HAV. By arresting the lateral physis of the first metatarsal base and allowing the medial physis to continue to grow, the first metatarsal will adduct closing down the IMA as the child grows.[30-32] Epiphyseal stapling uses the body's growth potential to aid in the reduction of the IMA. There is less surgery and less postoperative disability, as immediate postoperative weight bearing can be accomplished.

Phemister was the first to report a case of epiphysiodesis to inhibit bone growth in 1933. He took a bone graft from the epiphyseal plate and reversed it to create an epiphysiodesis. This was done at the distal femur and proximal tibia to correct a limb length discrepancy.[33] Blount, Clark, and Zeier used staples in the distal femur or proximal tibia to correct angular deformities in bones in 1949 and 1952.[34,35]

Ellis in 1951 was the first surgeon to use the principles of epiphysiodesis for the correction of metatarsus primus adductus.[36] He used two to three staples to cross the lateral physis of the first metatarsal base. He performed this procedure on 20 feet with good results. However, his longest follow-up was only 14 months.

Fox and Smith in 1983 described using a trephine plug taken from the calcaneus to place in the lateral physis of the first metatarsal base.[37] They reviewed four children with 6 feet with a 10-year follow-up. The key for them was that appropriate timing was necessary as this was an irreversible physeal arrest.

In 1994, Seiberg, Green, and Green reported on the lateral stapling at the base of the first metatarsal in 15 feet and 9 children.[38] They reported good results with this potentially reversible technique. They indicated that it was a low risk, well-tolerated procedure, which is usually performed in association with an ancillary bunion procedure.

In 2006, Dickmore et al. reported on 21 patients and 38 feet on lateral physeal stapling technique for juvenile HAV in conjunction with a modified McBride bunionectomy.[39] All patients were reviewed radiographically. Group 1 included 12 patients, 22 feet that had their physeal plates closed at the last radiographic evaluation. For one patient, 2 feet, the preoperative radiographs could not be located. Group 2 consisted of six patients, 10 feet that still had their growth plates open. Three patients, 5 feet, were excluded as no long-term x-rays were available and these patients could not be contacted.

They reported good reduction of the IMA. An average IMA of 13.1 degrees preoperatively reduced about 7 degrees, to 6.2 degrees in group 1. In group 2, the IMA averaged 13.5 degrees preoperatively and reduced about 5 degrees, to 8.5 degrees. The physeal plates in group 2 were not completely closed, and they had the potential for further reduction.

The HAA was likewise significantly reduced. In group 1, the average preoperative 25.6 HAA reduced approximately 14 degrees, to 11.5 degrees. Group 2 with a 22.7 preoperative HAA reduced approximately 9 degrees, to 13.5 degrees. There is a potential further decrease since their physeal plates were not closed. There was no sign of metatarsus primus elevatus noted in their cases. The authors stressed the need for good control of pronatory forces postoperatively to prevent recurrence of HAV.

Timing is the most important consideration regarding epiphyseal stapling. There is a small window of opportunity during the adolescent growth spurt to be able to utilize this effective technique. Adequate ossification of the epiphysis is necessary to hold the staple in the epiphysis and metaphysis. Consequently, most patients are at least 9 years of age. The golden period for surgery is between 9 and 14 years of age. Females mature earlier than males and surgery is often between the ages of 10 and 12 for females and between the ages of 11 and 14 for males. The radiographic age is more important than the chronologic age. The radiographic age can be determined by comparing a patient's foot and ankle x-rays to a radiographic atlas such as Hoerr's *Radiographic Atlas of Skeletal Development of the Foot and Ankle*.[40] In the atlas, many examples will be labeled as a skeletal

age of a younger female and an older male for the same x-ray (eg, female 10 years old; male 13 years old) because of the different ages of maturity.

Once the radiographic age has been determined, it is necessary to determine how much potential growth there is in the first metatarsal. Nelson in 1981 found that the adolescent growth spurt occurred earlier in females.[41] The growth spurt averages between 9 and 14 years for females, as opposed to males, 12-15 years of age. Females grew on an average of 10 mm or 15% of their entire first metatarsal length during this period. Males grew on an average of 12 mm, which equated to 17% of their entire first metatarsal length during this period. Because of the variability of the size of feet and specifically the first metatarsals, the percentage of growth is utilized to determine the potential growth once the skeletal age has been determined. Nelson's growth chart is useful in estimating this percentage of potential growth.[35,41]

Finally, the amount of growth necessary to obtain correction needs to be determined. Tracing the first metatarsal relative to the second metatarsal and cutting the medial physis of the tracing can move the first metatarsal into a corrected position. The amount of the gap medially for the opening wedge osteotomy would equal the amount of medial growth needed to gain correction (Fig. 52.7). When the potential growth is close to the determined necessary growth, the timing of the surgery can be estimated. If using the staple technique, surgery should be performed earlier rather than later as it does take some months for the staple to actually arrest the lateral physis.

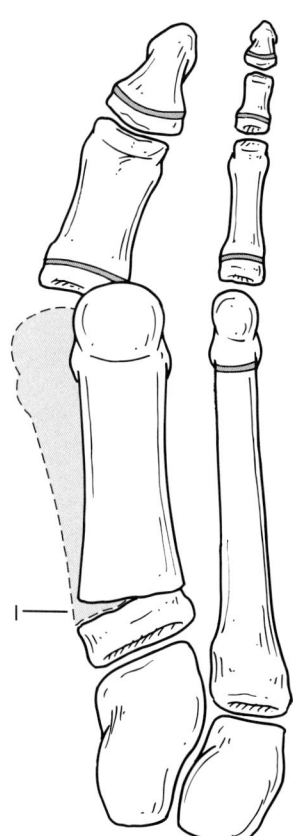

FIGURE 52.7 Template showing the desired medial growth of 3 mm to obtain angular correction.

Some authors prefer the stapling technique as growth can be potentially restored to the lateral physis by removing the staple if necessary. This also precludes the need for bone graft. The staple should penetrate the plantar cortex to avoid the potential of metatarsus primus elevatus. The staple should be placed dorsal to plantar in the lateral 25% of the metatarsal base across the physis.

A "Johnson staple" can be fashioned by bending a 0.062 smooth K-wire to 15 degrees to allow it to sit flush on the dorsal surface of the first metatarsal. The width of the staple is usually ~1.5 cm. The arms of the staple should be excessively long to be cut to an appropriate length intraoperatively.

The procedure is usually done in conjunction with a McBride bunionectomy. Following the McBride bunionectomy, the proximal base of the first metatarsal is identified laterally. The extensor tendon is reflected. A linear incision through the periosteum is reflected exposing the first metatarsocuneiform joint, the epiphysis, the physis (which is a whiter color), and the metaphysis (Fig. 52.8A). A 0.062 smooth K-wire is driven from dorsal to plantar in the epiphysis parallel to the first metatarsocuneiform joint. This is the key maneuver of the procedure. Intraoperative radiographic evaluation of the K-wire location is used to confirm that the K-wire is not in the joint, has not crossed the physis, and has penetrated the plantar cortex (Fig. 52.8B).

A guide is used to measure the length of the staple and to drive a parallel 0.062 smooth K-wire distally into the metaphysis bone from dorsal to plantar (Fig. 52.8C). Radiographic evaluation is used to confirm that the K-wire has penetrated the plantar cortex. As the K-wires are removed, the appropriate length of the arms of the staple can be measured by locking the K-wire in your K-wire removal. These can be cut to the appropriate length prior to insertion. The appropriate lengths can be confirmed with an AO depth gauge if necessary. The staple is slipped into the predrilled holes and lightly tapped in place. The staple location is confirmed radiographically.

The periosteum is closed over the staple and the wound is closed in layers. Postoperatively, the patient is treated as one would for a McBride bunionectomy since no osteotomy was performed. Night splints for the HAV to hold the toes straight are recommended until the physis is closed. Orthotic control of any pronatory forces is also recommended.

The epiphysiodesis procedure has proven quite successful if utilized in the window of opportunity of the adolescent growth spurt. The simplicity and potential reversibility of this procedure avoid the additional recovery necessitated by elective osteotomies.

COMPLICATIONS

Bone healing complications are uncommon in young patients. Nonetheless, delayed or nonunions may occur. Serial x-rays and having a high index of suspicion should lead to prompt treatment. Continued immobilization and bone stimulation are options if the bone is in good position. If the bone is in an unacceptable position, then surgical intervention will be required. In those circumstances, use of some degree of autogenous bone may help to augment healing. Calcaneal bone is excellent for this indication. When surgical repair is necessary, the fixation must be rigid, particularly if a graft is used. Although

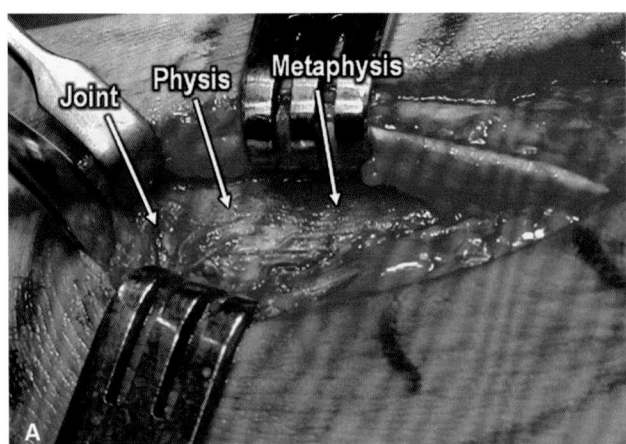

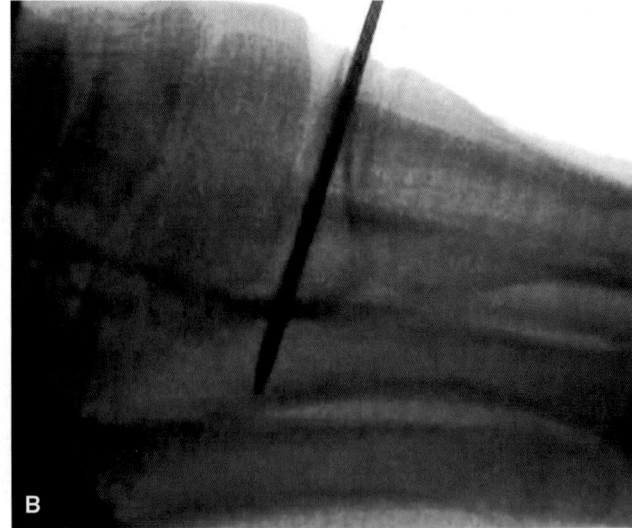

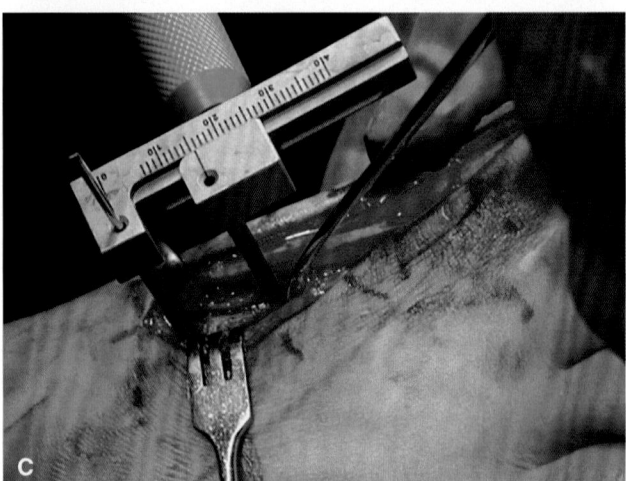

FIGURE 52.8 A. The joint, the physis, and the metaphysis are identified. **B.** After placement of K-wire, placement is visualized by fluoroscopy. Placement is key, with the K-wire parallel to the first met cuneiform joint and in the epiphysis. **C.** A guide is used for placement of the second K-wire parallel to the first and at the exact distance of the prefabricated staple.

allogeneic bone has been successfully used in these indications, autogenous bone is our preference.

Under or overcorrection are difficult problems to address. A hallux varus generally requires some type of surgical repair. Prevention is the best way to treat hallux varus. Avoiding negative IMA correction, overcorrecting the PASA, fibular sesamoidectomy, or releasing the lateral head of the flexor hallucis brevis are all part of the broad strategy to prevent hallux varus. Although it may be possible to get away with one of those mistakes, performing two of those mistakes will generally result in hallux varus. If hallux varus does occur early intervention is key so that muscle tendon balance can be restored without having to resort to fusion of the first MPJ.

Double osteotomies such as a closing base wedge and Reverdin or Green-Reverdin result in a greater likelihood of stiffness in the first metatarsophalangeal joint.[42] The prolonged immobilization can be a factor as well as the amount of dissection around the joint. Careful dissection around the joint is critical. Preserving as much of the dorsal synovial fold as possible can help to prevent this stiffness and maintain vascularity to the head. Early mobilization of the joint is also important and that requires secure fixation of both osteotomies. We generally use a cast for 2-3 weeks, followed by a removable casting device so that range of motion exercises can begin.

AUTHORS' PREFERRED TECHNIQUE

An adolescent with hallux valgus and a rectus foot without other deformities such as pes valgus, metatarsus adductus, and equinus can be adequately treated with a head or shaft osteotomy if the IMA is moderate.

Most of the adolescent hallux valgus patients may have some degree of metatarsus adductus. In those patients with high IMA and/or metatarsus adductus, our preferred technique is to perform proximal correction with a closing base wedge osteotomy and PASA correction with a Green-Reverdin as needed. The bone quality is ideal for a closing base wedge osteotomy, and this may tempt one to use a single screw. However, in order to prevent hinge fracture and shortening and/or dorsiflexion, the anchor screw is most useful and should accompany the compression screw. Make the cut long enough, usually at a 45-degree angle to the long axis of the shaft. If the cut is too transverse, there is too much tension on the hinge, which is subject to fracture and displacement. Pontious et al. found that there was an almost 5-degree increase in IMA reduction for a base osteotomy vs a head osteotomy in juvenile hallux valgus.[8]

The Green-Reverdin is performed if there is an increased PASA after the proximal correction is performed. The lower cut is aimed proximal to the sesamoids to avoid their injury. The

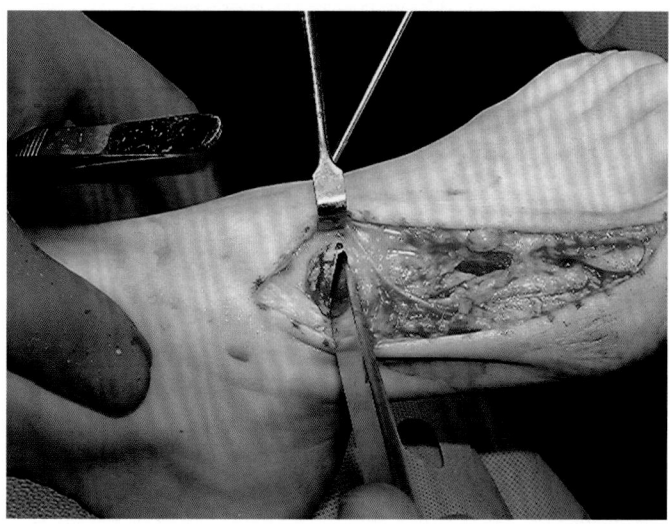

FIGURE 52.9 Opening wedge type Fowler osteotomy in the medial cuneiform to abduct the forefoot.

upper cuts are made perpendicular to the long axis of the first metatarsal and parallel to the first metatarsal head cartilage. The resulting wedge should correct the PASA down to zero. Because this cut is within the joint, stiffness can occur and early mobilization of the joint is important. Consequently, the fixation of both osteotomies must be secure enough to allow for that motion. Although the Green-Reverdin can be fixated in numerous ways, our preference is to use a single buried k-wire.

If the MAA is high, an approach that we use is to combine an opening wedge Fowler osteotomy with a closing wedge cuboid osteotomy to address the adductus foot (Figs. 52.9-52.11). A modified McBride and closing base wedge osteotomy can be performed and a Green-Reverdin if the PASA is sufficiently elevated to warrant correction. A Lapidus fusion is indicated for those patients with more significant hypermobility at the first metatarsal cuneiform joint (Fig. 52.12A and B).

PEARLS

- Indications for procedure must be stringently reviewed.
- Adequate correction of the intermetatarsal angle and PASA must be achieved.
- Deforming forces such as pes plano valgus and equinus must be addressed.
- It is important to begin early range of motion exercises, ~3 weeks postoperatively, following the double osteotomy.
- If metatarsus primus varus is present, an additional procedure such as the Fowler may be indicated.
- Aggressive treatment and recognition of metatarsus adductus is necessary to prevent recurrence.

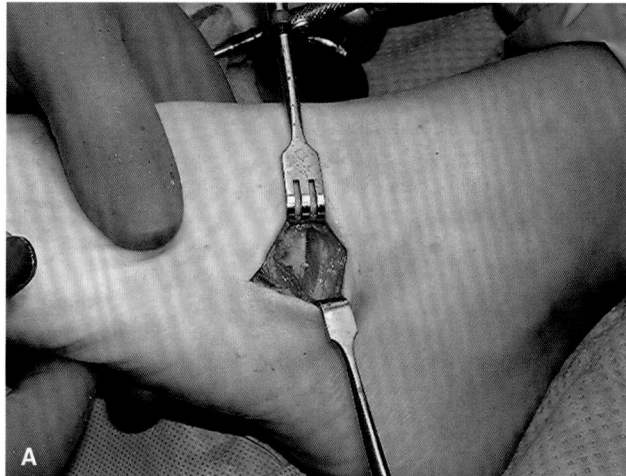
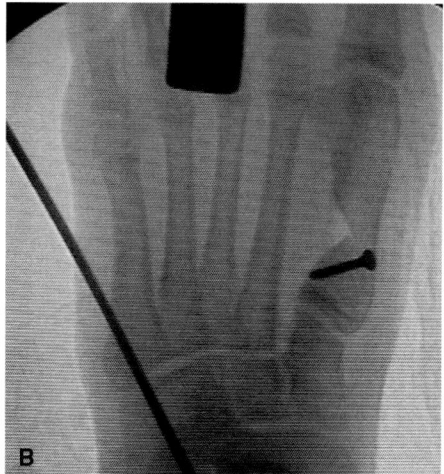

FIGURE 52.10 **A.** Closing wedge osteotomy of the cuboid to increase forefoot abduction in the juvenile hallux valgus patient with metatarsus adductus. **B.** Intraoperative radiograph demonstrating correction of the deformity.

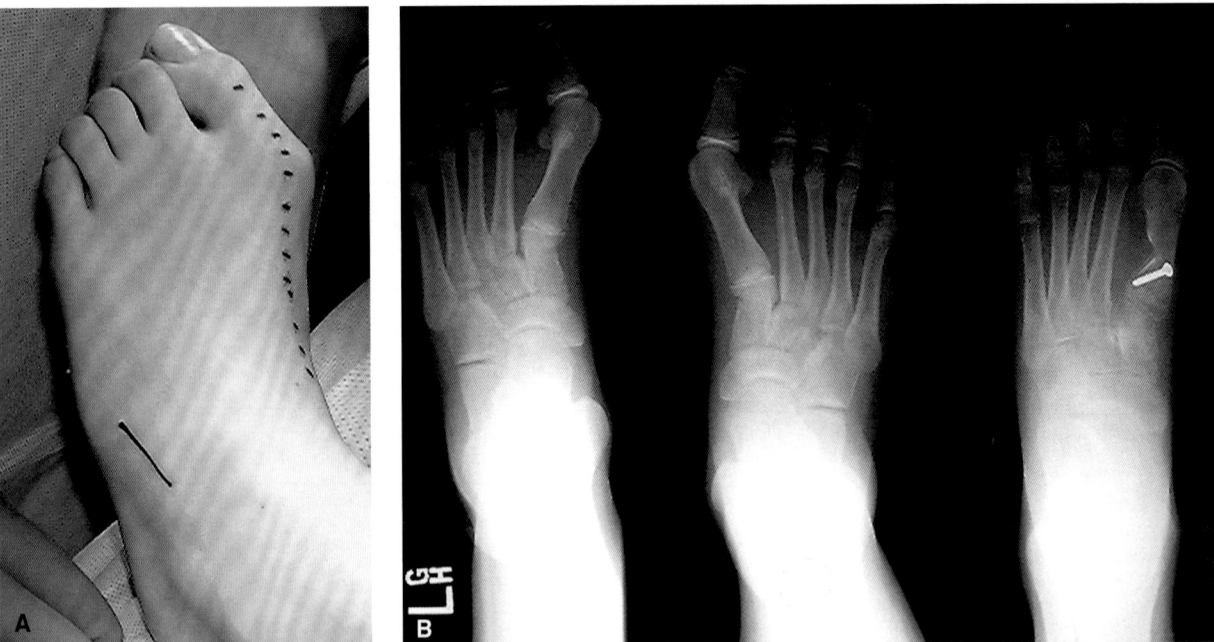

FIGURE 52.11 **A.** Preoperative clinical photograph. Note C-shaped deformity of foot. **B.** Side-by-side radiographs of bilateral preop and left postop views after closing base wedge, modified McBride, Fowler and closing cuboid osteotomy.

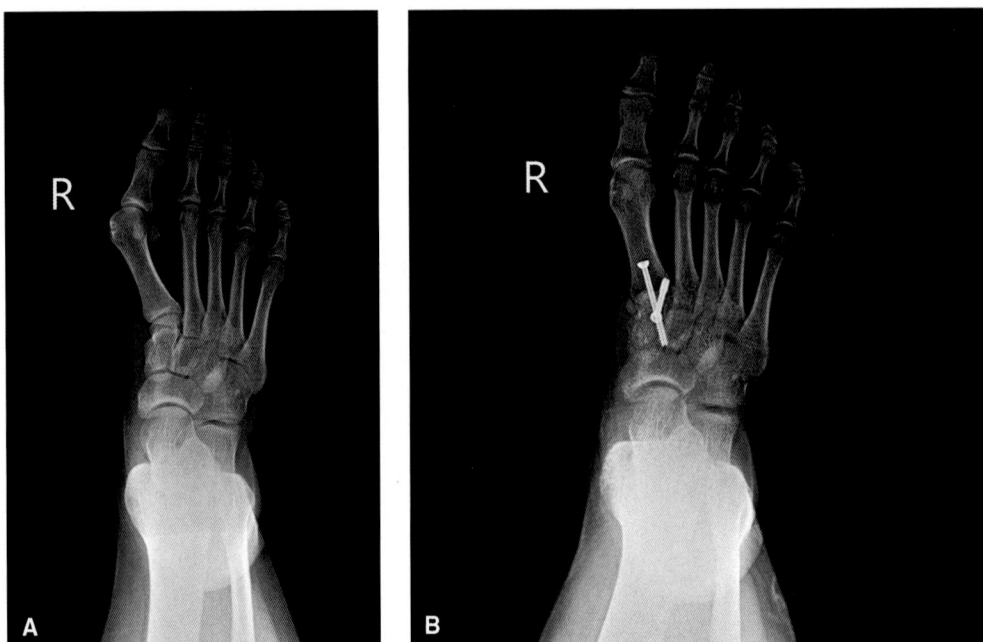

FIGURE 52.12 **A.** Preoperative radiograph of adolescent hallux abducto valgus. **B.** Four months postoperative view after Lapidus bunionectomy.

REFERENCES

1. Yu G, Landers P, Lo K, Shook J. Juvenile and adolescent hallux abducto valgus deformity. In: DeValentine S, ed. *Foot and Ankle Disorders in Children.* New York, NY: Churchill Livingstone; 1992:369-404.
2. Kilmartin TE, Wallace WA. The significance of pes planus in juvenile hallux valgus. *Foot Ankle.* 1992;13(2):53-56.
3. Vyas S, Conduah A, Vyas N, Otsuka NY. The role of the first metatarsocuneiform joint in juvenile hallux valgus. *J Pediatr Orthop B.* 2010;19(5):399-402.
4. Coughlin MJ, Mann RA. The pathophysiology of the juvenile bunion. *Instr Course Lect.* 1987;36:123-136.
5. Amarnek DL, Jacobs AM, Oloff LM. Adolescent hallux valgus: its etiology and surgical management. *J Foot Surg.* 1985;24(1):54-61.
6. Schecter A, Doll P. Tangential angle to the second axis. A new angle with implications in bunion surgery. *J Am Podiatr Med Assoc.* 1985;75(10):505-512.
7. Coughlin MJ. Roger A. Mann Award. Juvenile hallux valgus: etiology and treatment. *Foot Ankle Int.* 1995;16(11):682-697.
8. Pontious J, Mahan KT, Carter S. Characteristics of adolescent hallux abducto valgus. A retrospective review. *J Am Podiatr Med Assoc.* 1994;84(5):208-218.
9. Banks AS, Hsu YS, Mariash S, Zirm R. Juvenile hallux abducto valgus association with metatarsus adductus. *J Am Podiatr Med Assoc.* 1994;84(5):219-224.
10. Dawoodi AI, Perera A. Reliability of metatarsus adductus angle and correlation with hallux valgus. *Foot Ankle Surg.* 2012;18(3):180-186.
11. McConnell W, Cardenas V, Mahan K, Meyr A. *Calculation of the True First Intermetatarsal Angle Based on the Metatarsus Adductus Angle and Engel's Angle.* Proceedings of the Podiatry Institute. Tucker, GA: The Podiatry Institute; 2018:7-10.
12. Crawford M, Green D. *Metatarsus Adductus: Radiographic and Pathomechanical Analysis.* Proceedings of the Podiatry Institute. Tucker, GA: The Podiatry Institute; 2014:25-30.
13. Yu G, DiNapoli R. *Surgical Management of Hallux Abducto Valgus with Concomitant Metatarsus Adductus.* Proceedings of the Podiatry Institute. Tucker, GA: The Podiatry Institute; 1989:262-268.
14. Griffiths TA, Palladino SJ. Metatarsus adductus and selected radiographic measurements of the first ray in normal feet. *J Am Podiatr Med Assoc.* 1992;82(12):616-622.
15. Mahan KT, Jacko J. Juvenile hallux valgus with compensated metatarsus adductus. Case report. *J Am Podiatr Med Assoc.* 1991;81(10):525-530.
16. Guidera KJ, Drennan JC. Foot and ankle deformities in arthrogryposis multiplex congenita. *Clin Orthop Relat Res.* 1985;(194):93-98.
17. Kilmartin TE, Barrington RL, Wallace WA. A controlled prospective trial of a foot orthosis for juvenile hallux valgus. *J Bone Joint Surg Br.* 1994;76(2):210-214.
18. Mahan CC, Mahan KT. Patient preparation in pediatric surgery. *Clin Podiatr Med Surg.* 1987;4(1):1-9.
19. Mahan KT, Strelecky DC. Recent concepts in understanding a child's pain. *J Am Podiatr Med Assoc.* 1991;81(5):231-242.
20. Tobias JD, Green TP, Coté CJ, AAP section on anesthesiology and pain medicine, AAP committee on drugs. Codeine: Time To Say "No". *Pediatrics.* 2016;138(4):e20162396.
21. Selner AJ, Selner MD, Tucker RA, Eirich G. Tricorrectional bunionectomy for surgical repair of juvenile hallux valgus. *J Am Podiatr Med Assoc.* 1992;82(1):21-24.
22. Pittman SR, Burns DE. The Wilson bunion procedure modified for improved clinical results. *J Foot Surg.* 1984;23(4):314-320.
23. Agrawal Y, Bajaj SK, Flowers MJ. Scarf-Akin osteotomy for hallux valgus in juvenile and adolescent patients. *J Pediatr Orthop B.* 2015;24(6):535-540.
24. Al-Nammari SS, Christofi T, Clark C. Double first metatarsal and akin osteotomy for severe hallux valgus. *Foot Ankle Int.* 2015;36(10):1215-1222.
25. Grace D, Delmonte R, Catanzariti AR, Hofbauer M. Modified Lapidus arthrodesis for adolescent hallux abducto valgus. *J Foot Ankle Surg.* 1999;38(1):8-13.
26. Clark H, Veith R, Hansen S. Adolescent bunions treated by the modified Lapidus procedure. *Bull Hosp Jt Dis Orthop Inst.* 1987;47:109-122.
27. Mahan KT, Diamond E, Brown D. Podiatric profile of the Down's syndrome individual. *J Am Podiatry Assoc.* 1983;73(4):173-179.
28. Mahan KT. Calcaneal donor bone grafts. *J Am Podiatry Assoc.* 1994;84(1):1-9.
29. Lynch FR. Applications of the opening wedge cuneiform osteotomy in the surgical repair of juvenile hallux abducto valgus. *J Foot Ankle Surg.* 1995;34(2):103-123.
30. Wertheimer SJ. Role of epiphysiodesis in the management of deformities of the foot and ankle. *J Foot Surg.* 1990;29(5):459-462.
31. Ribotsky BM, Nazarian S, Scheuller HC. Epiphysiodesis of the first metatarsal with cancellous allograft. *J Am Podiatr Med Assoc.* 1993;83(5):263-266.
32. Sheridan LE. Correction of juvenile hallux valgus deformity associated with metatarsus primus adductus using epiphysiodesis technique. *Clin Podiatr Med Surg.* 1987;4(1):63-74.
33. Phemister DB. Operative arrest of longitudinal bones in the treatment of deformities. *J Bone Joint Surg Am* 1993;15:1.
34. Blount WP, Clark GR. Control of bone growth by physeal stapling. *J Bone Joint Surg Br* 1949;31A:464.
35. Blount WP, Zeier F. Control of bone growth. *JAMA* 1952;148:451.
36. Ellis VH. A method of correcting metatarsus primus varus. *J Bone Joint Surg Br* 1951;33B:415.
37. Fox IM, Smith SD. Juvenile bunion correction by epiphysiodesis of the first metatarsal. *J Am Podiatry Assoc.* 1983;73(9):448-455.
38. Seiberg M, Green R, Green D. Epiphysiodesis in juvenile hallux abducto valgus. A preliminary retrospective study. *J Am Podiatr Med Assoc.* 1994;84(5):225-236.
39. Dickemore C, et al. Epiphyseal stapling for juvenile hallux valgus. Podiatry Institute Update 2006. Dekalb, GA: Podiatry Institute Publishing, 2006.
40. Hoerr NL, Pyle SI, Francis CC. Radiographic atlas of skeletal development of the foot and ankle. Springfield, IL: Thomas, 1962.
41. Nelson JP. Mechanical arrest of bone growth for the correction of pedal deformities. *J Foot Surg* 1981;20:14.
42. Loretz L, DeValentine S, Yamaguchi K. The first metatarsal bicorrectional head osteotomy (distal "L"/Reverdin-Laird procedure) for correction of hallux abducto valgus: a retrospective study. *J Foot Ankle Surg.* 1993;32(6):554-568.

CHAPTER **53**

Clubfoot

Mitzi L. Williams, Matthew D. Doyle, and Matthew B. Dobbs

DEFINITION

Congenital clubfoot (talipes equinovarus) is a complex multiplanar deformity involving cavus, adductus, varus, and equinus (Fig. 53.1). While a variety of deformities can present in infancy, clubfoot is truly defined by its hindfoot varus deformity in association with equinus. The condition affects 1 out of every 1000 live births with a male-to-female ratio of 2:1.[1] It remains one of the most common birth defects, which can be isolated or of neurologic influence. While many are isolated birth defects, 20% are linked to neuromuscular and/or genetic conditions. Specifically, mutations in the PITX1-TBX4-HOXC transcriptional pathway have been noted to cause familial clubfoot and vertical talus in a small number of families.[2] In children, 50% present bilaterally. Hawaiians and Maoris have been reported to have the greatest prevalence at 7 per 1000 live births.[1,3]

HISTORY

Clubfoot treatment has undergone transformation over the last three decades. Kite was the first in the United States to have his nonoperative treatment protocol accepted, with a series of manipulation and casting.[4] However, many cases of clubfeet were still treated operatively. While Kite encouraged a noninvasive manipulation, his method was faulty. Counterpressure on the calcaneocuboid joint blocked the migration of the calcaneus from being able to move from a varus position to a more valgus position beneath the talus. Over the last few decades, there has been a paradigmatic shift in treatment of clubfoot, due to the work of Dr. Ignacio Ponseti.[5,6]

As the son of a watchmaker, Dr. Ignacio Ponseti was accustomed to working with delicate small components. He was further given the opportunity as a physician to perform retrospective reviews of children who had undergone posteromedial releases

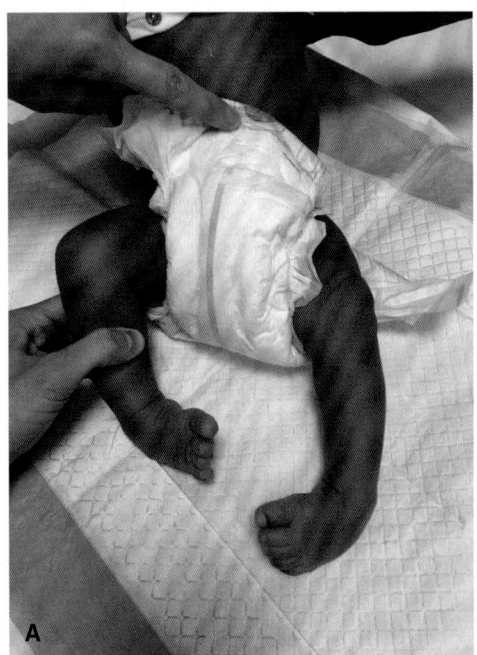
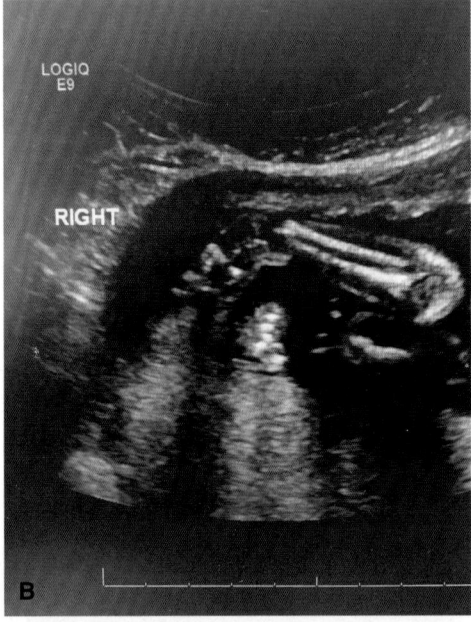

FIGURE 53.1 A. Clubfoot deformity demonstrating cavus, adductus, varus, and equinus. **B.** Suspected clubfoot on ultrasound *in utero.*

and surgical reconstructions at an early age. He concluded that these young children had developed stiff, undercorrected, and often painful feet. Likewise, their function was compromised.[7–9] Not only did he study these children from a functional standpoint but he also studied them on a cellular level.

From a histopathologic standpoint, he concluded that many children with clubfoot, when operated on especially under the age of 1, had developed an abundance of scar tissue, an increase in collagen fibrils, and retracting fibrosis, which led to recurrence of the deformity.[10] These microscopic and macroscopic findings led him to the development of a less invasive approach. He developed the Ponseti approach for management of clubfoot and confirmed its success by long-term follow-up studies.[5,11]

The Ponseti method is now the first line of treatment for the management of both idiopathic/isolated clubfoot, while it is also the accepted first line of treatment for the syndromic/nonisolated clubfoot.[12] Numerous studies demonstrate the effectiveness of the Ponseti method and need for subsequent bracing compliance until the age of 4.[5,11] Poor bracing compliance is the greatest reason for recurrence.[13] Following the Ponseti method, boots and an abduction bar brace must be utilized as recurrent equinus, inversion, and/or adduction can occur. Upon recurrence, the Ponseti method is still valuable in reducing deformity, while 40% of the clubfoot population will require some form of surgery for management of clubfoot in their lifetime.[2,14]

Still, the Ponseti method can minimize how grandiose of a procedure may be required to obtain a plantigrade foot.

CLASSIFICATION

Today, two common classification systems are used to quantify the degree of deformity and estimate treatment success—Pirani and Dimeglio (Fig. 53.2).[15,16] The Pirani classification examines six clinical signs involving contracture of the hindfoot and midfoot. When unilateral, the affected side is then compared to the contralateral, unaffected foot. Dimeglio examined the reducibility and motion of each of the four deformities present as well as additional aggravating factors. This was then translated into a grading system: grade I being mild, grade II significantly reducible, grade III partially reducible, and grade IV teratologic. Both classifications have

been found to have good interobserver reliability.[17,18] Other systems exist but have not been widely used.

PIRANI CLASSIFICATION[15]

- Hindfoot score 0-3
  - ▶ Posterior crease 0, 0.5, 1
  - ▶ Empty heel 0, 0.5, 1
  - ▶ Rigid equinus 0, 0.5, 1
- Midfoot score 0-3
  - ▶ Curvature of the lateral border 0, 0.5, 1
  - ▶ Medial crease 0, 0.5, 1
  - ▶ Talar head reducibility 0, 0.5, 1
- Total score 0-6

DIMEGLIO CLASSIFICATION[16]

- Reducibility
  - ▶ Heel equinus in sagittal plane = 0-4 points
  - ▶ Heel varus in frontal plane = 0-4 points
  - ▶ Internal rotation/supination = 0-4 points
  - ▶ Forefoot adduction in transverse plane = 0-4 points
- Aggravating elements
  - ▶ Posterior crease = 1 point
  - ▶ Medial crease = 1 point
  - ▶ Cavus = 1 point
  - ▶ Fibrous musculature = 1 point
- Total score = 0-20

ANATOMIC FEATURES

Anatomically, this complex deformity involves the ankle, subtalar, and midfoot joints. The anatomy of these joints is distorted and remains the focus during correction. Both osseous and soft tissue components contribute to the deformity. The talus and calcaneus are both positioned in equinus. The hindfoot is positioned in varus due to subtalar joint inversion as well as internal rotation and adduction. The talus is smaller than normal, and the body is laterally rotated within the mortise while the head and neck are medially and

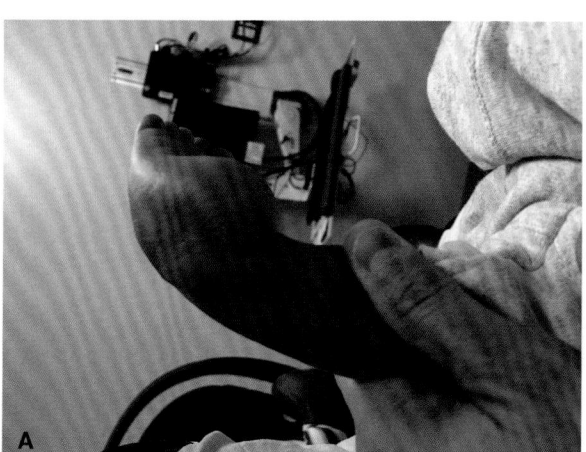
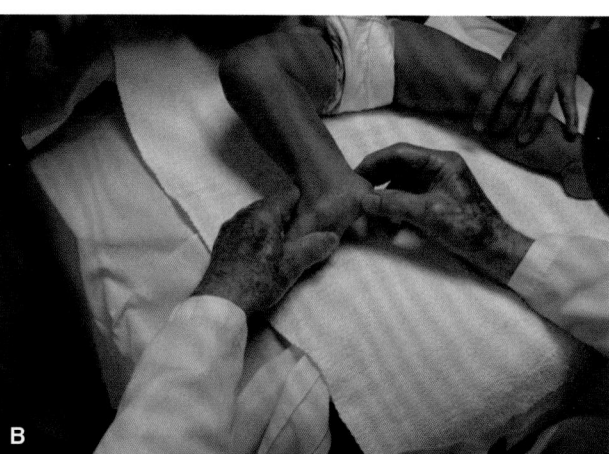

FIGURE 53.2 **A.** Posterior crease. **B.** Emptiness of heel.

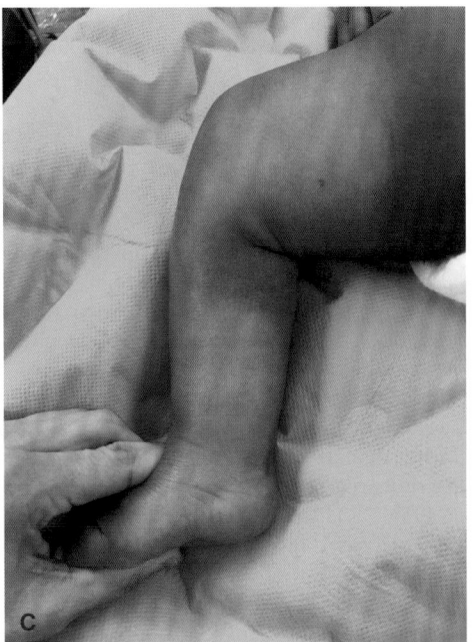
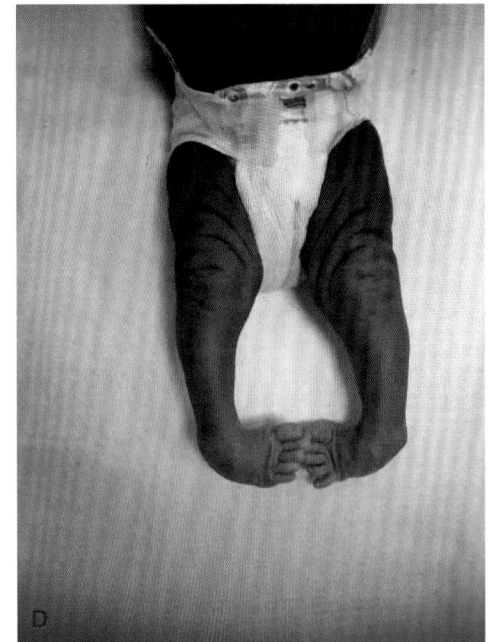
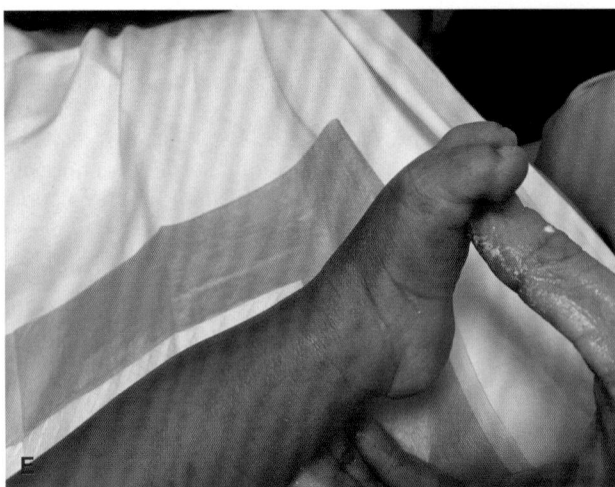
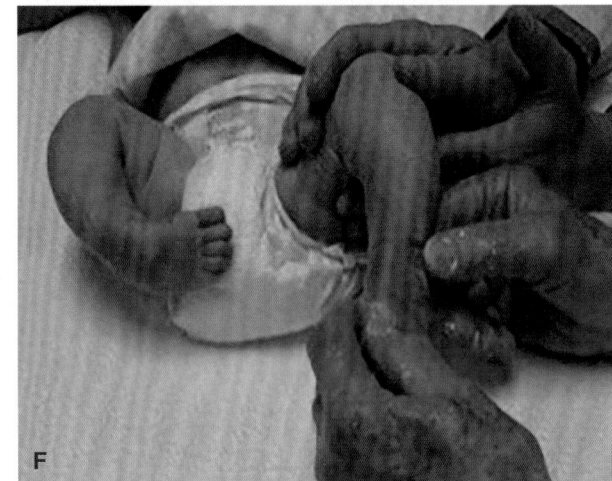

FIGURE 53.2 (*Continued*) **C.** Rigid equinus. **D.** Curvature of lateral border. **E.** Medial crease. **F.** Talar head reducibility.

plantarly deviated. Adding to the hindfoot complexity, the calcaneus is internally rotated below the head and neck of the talus and in an equinus position. Along the transverse tarsal joint, the navicular is rotated medially around the talar head so much that it may contact the medial malleolus. The cuboid is translated medially in relation to the calcaneus. Instead of these joints being parallel to each other, they lie on top of one another. The midfoot and forefoot are adducted and plantar flexed on the hindfoot, creating a cavus. The forefoot is not as inverted as the hindfoot. Occasionally, internal tibial torsion or bowing of the tibia is present (Fig. 53.3).

Fibrous hyperplasia of the posterior and medial structures has been described as myofibroblastlike cells and changes in muscle fibers, although this has been disputed.[19–26] Contractures of the posteromedial structures and leg atrophy have been described including contractures of the gastroc-soleus complex, tibialis posterior, flexor digitorum longus, flexor hallucis longus, ankle, subtalar and talonavicular joint capsules, and deltoid ligament.[7,27–29]

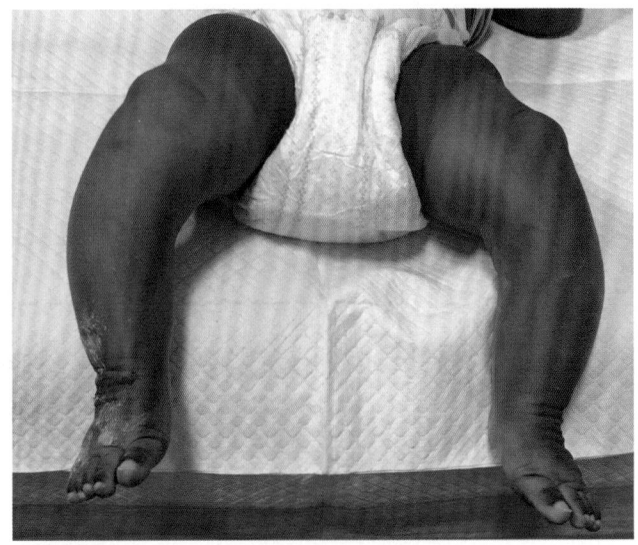

FIGURE 53.3 Bowing of the tibia.

ANATOMY OF CLUBFOOT

Untreated clubfoot has profound effects on gait and function. The goal of treatment is to obtain a stable, plantigrade foot with mobility (Fig. 53.4). If untreated, the deformity becomes much more difficult to treat conservatively and worsens over time. Patients may have little or even no pain during ambulation but will undoubtedly develop abnormal, thickened skin and bursae on the dorsolateral foot. Children with neglected clubfeet are often unable to wear shoe gear. Weakness of the lower extremity and a smaller calf size may decrease the ability to participate in sports and activity. Since the talus and calcaneus are notably plantar flexed, there is an equinus gait and compensation that occurs with knee hyperextension and hip external rotation. There is also an increase in knee and hip joint moments and decrease in ankle moments, likely due to a weak calf and plantarflexors. A weak posterior muscle group can lead to decreased push-off strength. Complete footdrop may also occur.

Conservative treatment using the Ponseti technique has provided a functional, plantigrade foot in 85%-95% of patients.[6,10,11,30–32] It has been reported that even after treatment, there is decreased ankle range of motion when compared to unaffected children, but overall, there is increased ankle range of motion and strength as well as less pain after casting.[33] This is accompanied by decreased peak pressures over the medial forefoot and hindfoot as well as increased pressure over the lateral midfoot. Residual intoeing is seen in up to 33% of children with moderate clubfoot using the Dimeglio scoring system.[34] Normal ankle sagittal plane motion may be obtained using casting or physical therapy in children with severe clubfoot, and almost two-thirds of patients have normal kinematic ankle motion if treated properly.[34,35]

PATHOGENESIS

Clubfoot may be associated with multiple other congenital disorders such as myelomeningocele, myelodysplasia, and arthrogryposis, most of which are neurologic.[36] While the true pathogenesis has not been elucidated, the origin is multifactorial, and many note that clubfoot has a partial genetic factor.[2,36–39] Since most cases are idiopathic and not associated with an additional congenital condition, it has been suggested that clubfoot is associated with a more complex trait, rather than a single gene. Current literature has examined the presence of mutations and deletions of transcription factor PITX.[2,40,41] The incidence among different races ranges from 0.39 to 7 per 1000.[21,42] Chinese populations have been reported to have the lowest incidence. This adds to the notion that genetics plays a role in its development. The male-to-female ratio is as high as 2.5:1.[35,38] Twenty-four percent of cases have a positive family history, and siblings have a 30-fold increased risk of congenital clubfoot. More recently, transcription factors have been tied to the etiology.[2] A recent study demonstrated a single dominant gene with 33% penetrance in Pacific and Maori populations.[43]

Additionally, environmental factors, such as smoking, as well as abnormal muscle fiber ratio and nerve abnormalities, abnormal soft tissue and bone formation, and even vascular

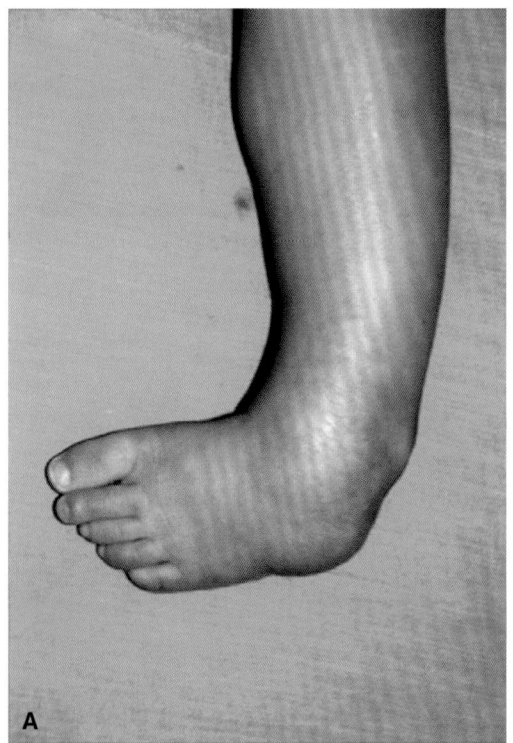
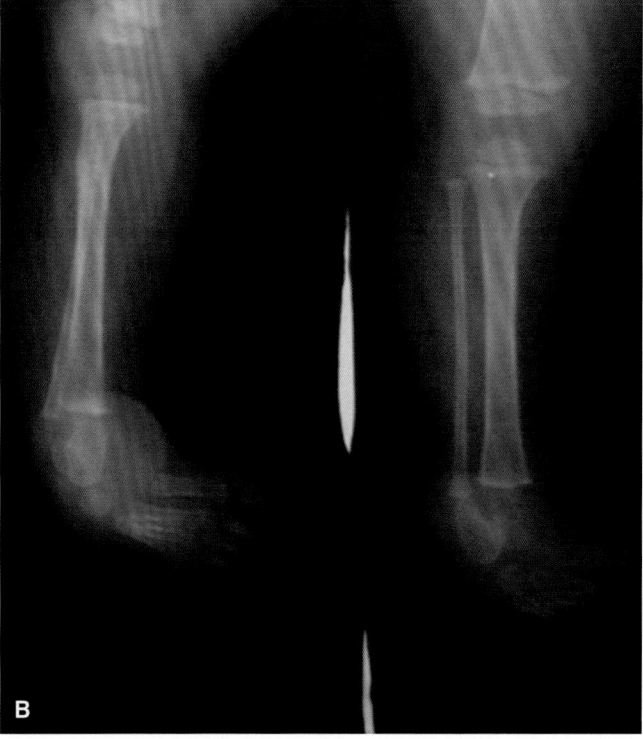

FIGURE 53.4 Untreated clubfoot: **(A)** One notes the enlarged bursa along the lateral aspect of the foot which is loaded in ambulation. The head of the talus is laterally deviated and in malalignment within the ankle mortise. The hindfoot remains in varus and equinus. The calcaneus never migrated beneath the talus out of varus. **B.** X-rays of untreated clubfoot.

malformations have been described.[44-47] Cigarette smoke has an odds ratio of 1.34 for clubfoot.[44] Family history has an odds ratio of 6.52. The combined odds ratio is 20.30.

PHYSICAL EXAMINATION

It is critical to perform a thorough physical examination on all clubfoot patients, which includes an examination of the hips, all four extremities, the neck, and spine to rule out other associated anomalies. Assessing for a sacral dimple is important to rule out spinal cord issues, such as a tethered cord, sacral agenesis, or spina bifida. In terms of the feet, the treating physician must ensure an accurate diagnosis of clubfoot as well as rule out associated nerve or muscle problems indicative of atypical clubfoot. While all clubfeet share the same general characteristics, they are quite heterogeneous in etiology. Isolated clubfoot, those clubfeet that occur without other associated diagnoses are the most common type, but this number is getting smaller. This is due to more careful physical examinations uncovering nerve and muscle abnormalities in many clubfoot children that were not diagnosed as babies in the past. In order to diagnose these nerve and muscle problems, a few simple examination techniques are required. Simply stimulating the bottom of the babies' foot should elicit strong dorsiflexion and plantarflexion of the toes (Fig. 53.5). If the infant cannot do this or does it weakly in any of the toes, this should raise the suspicion of underlying congenital nerve problem or muscle weakness. Similarly, stimulation of the plantar lateral aspect of the foot should elicit firing of the peroneus brevis. This examination tactic should be done at each cast change to get a clear picture of motor ability in the foot. This is important as those children with weak/absent dorsiflexion and/or eversion have a more difficult treatment course with high relapse risk. This needs to be explained to the parents. Clubfoot is a heterogeneous disorder that despite what its name implies, is not an isolated foot problem. Instead, it is a developmental limb defect, and the amount of involvement of the soft tissue structures of the lower limb can be highly variable between patients. The ability to perform a more careful physical examination will lead

the treating physician and patient into the era of personalized medicine where risk of relapse will be able to be better predicted based on specific physical examination findings.

IMAGING AND DIAGNOSTIC STUDIES

Imaging

- Imaging including x-rays, MRIs, or CT scans is not routinely used for evaluation of clubfoot in an infant.
- If the foot is not improving as expected with the Ponseti method, then plain film x-rays may be performed.
- With rigid, recurrent, or neglected clubfoot, one may utilize x-rays and/or advanced imaging given the probable need for surgical procedures.

TREATMENT

The Ponseti method has proven to be successful in the treatment of both isolated and nonisolated clubfoot (Fig. 53.6). The method should be executed prior to any pediatric invasive procedures and likewise may be attempted with any pediatric recurrence.[14] Quite often, the method provides a stretch and can improve overall foot position minimizing procedures needed to obtain a plantigrade foot. Still, it is important to recognize that without proper bracing following serial casting, recurrence is likely.[13] Despite the methods' effectiveness, 40% of children will require some form of surgical intervention in their lifetime.[2,14] Proper use of the method can minimize the extent of procedures required or eliminate the need for surgery.

The Ponseti Method

- A full musculoskeletal examination is performed prior to treatment.
- The Magic Move (first step): A dorsiflexory force is applied beneath the first metatarsal head with counterpressure applied to the lateral talar head. This maneuver reduces the cavus and medial crease. This is performed, as the forefoot is not as inverted as compared to the hindfoot.
- Do not touch the calcaneus or cuboid.
- Upon resolution of the medial crease, the forefoot is abducted with counterpressure applied to the lateral talar head. Upon reduction of the adduction, inversion, and cavus, one can proceed with correction of the equinus.
- A complete Achilles tenotomy is performed to reduce equinus if <10 degrees of dorsiflexion is noted at the level of the ankle joint. A final cast is applied and left intact for 2.5-3 weeks.
- Abduction bar bracing is utilized until age 4 at minimum. The affected foot is externally rotated at 50-70 degrees to the lower leg and an unaffected foot is positioned to 30-40 degrees to the lower limb.

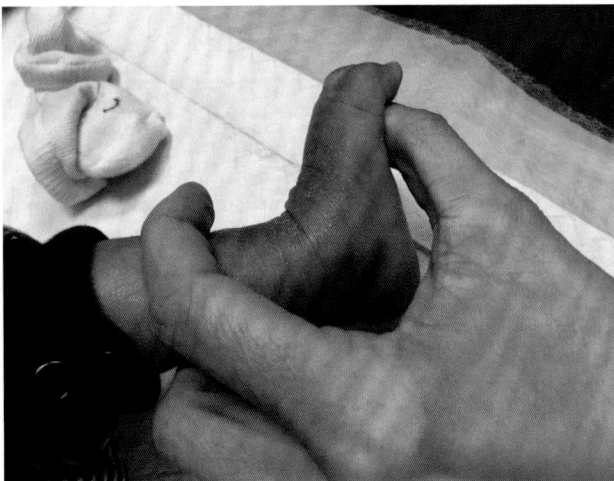

FIGURE 53.5 Stimulating bottom of the infant's foot should elicit strong plantar flexion and dorsiflexion of digits.

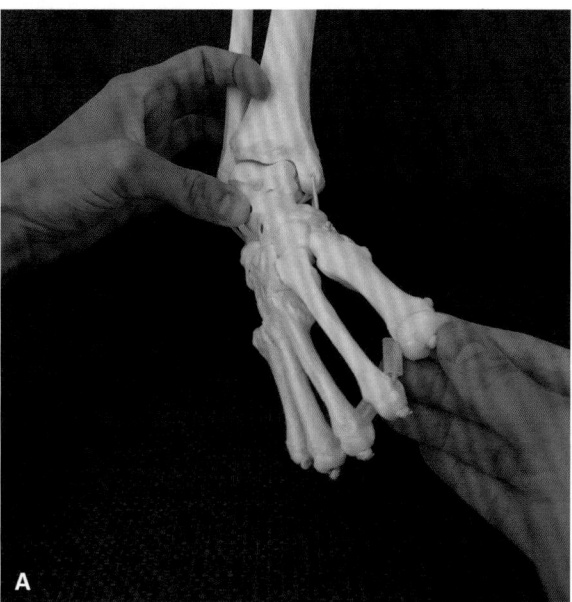 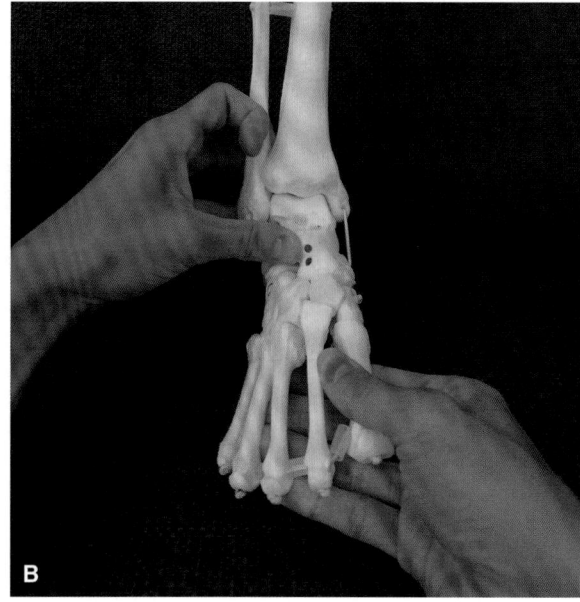

FIGURE 53.6 The Ponseti method: **(A)** Dorsiflexory force beneath the first metatarsal head and **(B)** abduction of the forefoot with counterpressure on the lateral talar head.

PEARLS

CASTING (Fig. 53.7)
- A thin layer of Webril or cast padding is utilized from the toes up to the groin.
- A well-molded plaster cast is utilized and secured from the toes to just below the knee. Once completed, plaster is continued above the knee while maintaining 90-110 degrees of knee flexion to minimize cast slippage.
- Excess plaster is removed to expose the toes.
- Semirigid casting material may be utilized in place of plaster while proper manipulation is key.
- Often with recurrences, a well-molded plaster cast is fashioned below the knee, and fiberglass is applied over the plaster and extends above the knee.
- It is essential to apply long leg casts, as below the knee casts will lead to slippage and/or lack of correction.
- Soothing techniques: bottle-feeds, sound machines, toys.
- Casts are changed weekly leading to Achilles tenotomy.

PERILS and PITFALLS

CASTING
- Improper manipulation and/or forceful manipulation in casts
- Inappropriate pressure applied to calcaneus
- Counterpressure to the calcaneocuboid joint
- Excessive cast padding
- Removal of casts prior to appointment
- Cast slippage

The Complex Clubfoot[48]
- May present with deep plantar crease initially and extreme cavus. Hyperabduction may lead to tightening of the quadratus plantae and pulling of the flexors. This leads to worsening cavus.
- Resistant to classic Ponseti method.
- Often identified around the time of the second cast.
- This condition can also be the result of improper manipulation and casting. Cast slippage can be associated with the complex subset.
- The 4-finger technique is utilized: Pushing upward beneath the first and fifth metatarsals while applying a dorsiflexory force on the posterior superior aspect of the calcaneus.

Atypical Clubfoot
- Noted at birth.
- Weak or absent active dorsiflexion of the toes and ankle as well as weak active eversion of the foot.
- Associated with neurologic and/or motor deficits.
- Deep plantar crease initially and extreme cavus. Hyperabduction may lead to tightening of the quadratus plantae and pulling of the flexors. This leads to worsening cavus.
- Resistant to classic Ponseti method.
- The 4-finger technique is utilized: Pushing upward beneath the first and fifth metatarsals while applying a dorsiflexory force on the posterior superior aspect of the calcaneus.
- Higher risks of relapse given motor strength deficit.

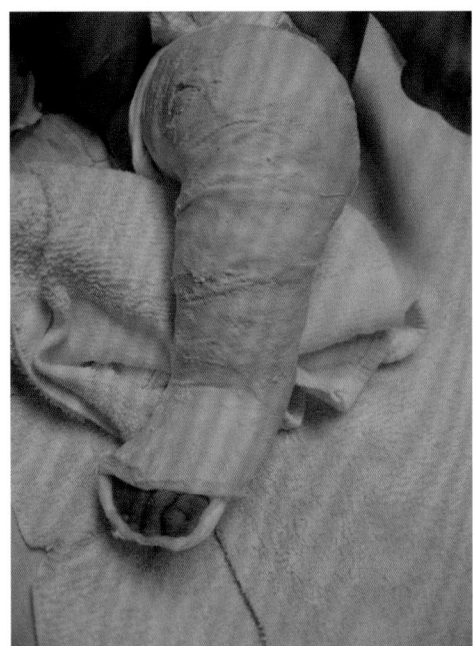

FIGURE 53.7 Ponseti casting for clubfoot.

COMPLEX CLUBFOOT

Complex clubfoot is used to describe a type of clubfoot that is more resistant to standard casting technique and develops a distinct phenotype during the casting process (Fig. 53.8). This type of clubfoot is usually not recognized at birth as being different. Often, correction ceases to occur in the middle of the casting series and the foot becomes short and fat, with a retracted first ray. Cast slipping is common, and if it occurs, a deep plantar crease is evident indicating entire midfoot cavus. Fortunately, Ponseti recognized this entity and developed modified casting technique to correct that is extremely effective. The emphasis is on dorsiflexing the first and fifth ray to stretch the plantar crease. Serial casts result in achieving 30-40 degrees of external rotation. At that time, a tenotomy is done and the foot casted in 50 degrees of external rotation and 10 degrees of dorsiflexion. Trying to externally rotate the foot further results in a midfoot breach laterally. Hyperflexion of the knee up to 110 degrees is helpful to prevent

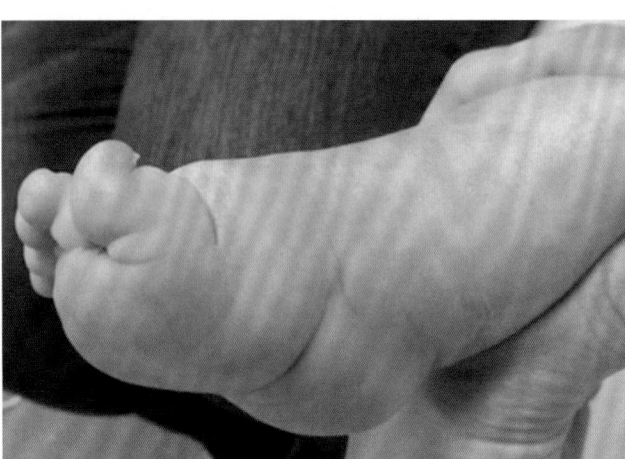

FIGURE 53.8 Complex clubfoot.

slipping. Care should be taken to use posterior plaster slab for lower leg and dorsal slab for the knee to minimize the amount of plaster rolls. This technique leads to better molding. Foot abduction bracing is used after the casting, but care should be taken to set the feet at 50 degrees of external rotation and not greater.

ATYPICAL CLUBFOOT

Atypical clubfoot, which is mistakenly used synonymously with complex clubfoot, is a different entity though the casting treatment is the same as it is for complex clubfoot. Atypical clubfeet share many of the same clinical features as complex clubfoot, but these are identifiable at birth with a good physical examination. Patients with atypical clubfeet have weak or absent active dorsiflexion of the toes and ankle as well as weak active eversion of the foot. This subset is associated with neurological and/or motor deficits. Casting is done as for complex clubfoot, but these patients are at higher risk of relapse due to lack of motor strength.

BRACING PERIOD

In many ways, the bracing period can be much more challenging for parents and families as compared to casting. There is always a feeling of accomplishment and relief among parents upon completion of casts. The break in period for braces can come as a surprise. It is important to educate all caregivers on the importance of bracing and the high risks for recurrence of clubfoot without proper bracing compliance. Immediately following the casting period, the child transitions to boots attached to an abduction bar (Fig. 53.9). It is important to educate caregivers that while the braces do not cause pain, they are a change especially for an infant.

Parents should attempt to soothe their child as compared to removing the braces while the child is crying. Demonstrating how the child can use the legs attached to the bar is often helpful as well. Boots should be snug while not too tight. Sores can

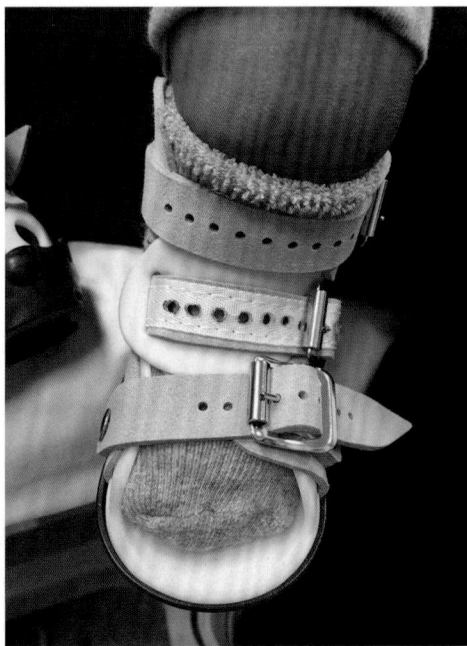

FIGURE 53.9 Ponseti Mitchell braces. It is important to remember that the boots should be snug to minimize motion and slippage.

develop if straps are too tight. If sores do arise, various products such as moleskin, Molefoam, Mepilex, lamb's wool, athletic tape, etc., may be utilized. If ulcerations or tissue necrosis occurs, a bracing vacation may be needed with expectation of return to casting. The feet and ankles are stretched daily, and ankle dorsiflexion is performed prior to brace application. The braces do not correct for any deformities. The braces simply maintain correction obtained from casting or surgery.

Weaning of Braces

- 23 hours per day for 3 months followed by
- 18 hours per day for 3 months followed by
- 16 hours per day for 3 months followed by
- Naptime and nighttime use until age 4

Authors Preferred Bracing Approach

- Ponseti Mitchell boots attached to the abduction bar: D bar enterprises until 6 months of age (Fig. 53.10).
- Transfer child to Dobbs articulated abduction bar at 6 months of age (strong kicking).
- Children are followed closely after the weaning process as some children need supramalleolar orthoses (SMOs), ankle foot orthoses (AFOs), knee ankle foot orthoses (KAFOs), or hip knee ankle foot orthoses (HKAFOs).
- Motion and physical therapy is often utilized until ambulation and can be dependent on coexisting conditions.

SURGICAL MANAGEMENT

EVALUATION

Up to 40% of patients with clubfoot treated successfully by the Ponseti method do experience recurrence of deformity.[2,14] Hence, it has become important not only to adhere to the strict details of the Ponseti method during the casting period while also promoting bracing compliance until 4 years of age. Some children, especially in the presence of neurologic influence, require not only nighttime bracing but also daytime ankle-foot orthoses in conjunction with nighttime abduction bar bracing. Still, despite successful execution of the method and bracing compliance, the deformity can still reoccur. The authors have studied symptomatic recurrence. Possible causes for recurrence include the intrinsic contractile nature of the soft tissues in clubfoot deformity,[49]

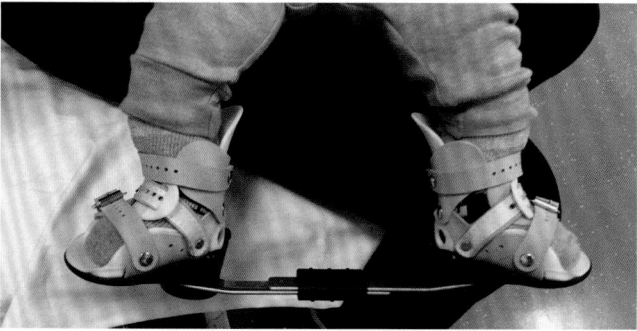

FIGURE 53.10 Ponseti Mitchell boots abduction bar.

genetic and neuromuscular factors, casting techniques,[50] different designs of braces,[50] and variable brace wear time due to parental nonadherence.[13]

While the syndromic foot or nonisolated clubfoot has an increased risk for symptomatic recurrence along with an earlier age in which recurrence is noted, the isolated clubfoot can still reoccur. It is essential to follow this pediatric population after the age of 5 to minimize the severity of recurrence if possible. In a study by van Praag et al., recurrence was seen in 19% (71) of 382 children who were eligible for the study who were typically discharged after the age of 5 years from their clinic. This alludes to the importance of continued follow-up until after that age.[14] Treatment with casting for the recurrence was successful in many patients and may be a reasonable choice for recurrent idiopathic clubfeet.[14]

Achilles Tenotomy

The majority of children with clubfoot will require an Achilles tenotomy to reduce the equinus deformity (Fig. 53.11). A topical anesthetic is utilized on the skin in the posterior ankle region. EMLA or lidocaine plain is most typically utilized under occlusion. The authors do not inject any further local anesthesia prior to the procedure as this can obscure the margins of the Achilles tendon. An assistant holds the leg with the foot in dorsiflexion. A Beaver Blade is introduced by the surgeon through the skin onto the medial edge of the tendoachilles about 1 cm proximal to its calcaneal insertion. The tendon is felt with the tip of the knife. The knife is introduced in front of the tendon and then rotated 45 degrees. The angle of dorsiflexion of the ankle will suddenly increase about 10-15 degrees.[51]

Advancing the blade too far laterally can place the peroneal artery or lesser saphenous vein at risk of being severed. After the tenotomy is performed and temporary dressing is applied, the child is monitored for good skin perfusion and digital refill over several minutes. The temporary dressing is removed and gauze is applied. Local anesthesia may be utilized at this time. A well-molded long-leg plaster cast is then applied, maintaining the foot in maximum dorsiflexion and in about 70 degrees of external rotation to the lower leg. The final cast is left intact for about 3 weeks to allow for tendon healing.

Using a more rounded Beaver Blade may reduce the risk of vascular injury. This makes palpation of the tendon edge easier. If the Achilles is easily palpable, the procedure may be performed in clinic without anesthesia. If serial Achilles tenotomies are performed for recurrence, the authors are more likely to perform a small open procedure in the operating room. Likewise, if patient's comorbidities or disposition make it unsafe to perform in clinic, the authors will perform the procedure in the operating room under general anesthesia. Majority of children under 12 months of age can undergo Achilles tenotomies in the office provided the borders of the Achilles are easily palpable.

A thorough lower extremity vascular examination is recommended prior to performing a percutaneous Achilles tenotomy. This should include palpation of the dorsalis pedis and posterior tibial pulses. Doppler ultrasound may be considered in those patients with an absent dorsalis pedis or posterior tibial pulse.[51] If both are absent or diminished on Doppler, then consideration should be given to performing an arteriogram to assess whether the peroneal artery is the dominant supply to the foot.[51] If the peroneal artery is dominant, then consideration should be given to performing an open Achilles tenotomy.

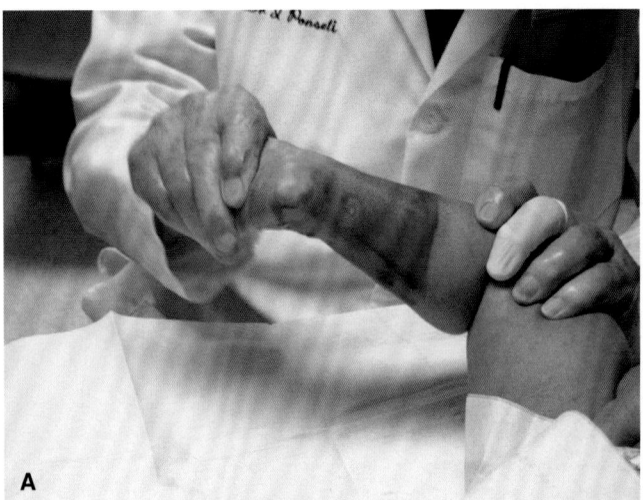

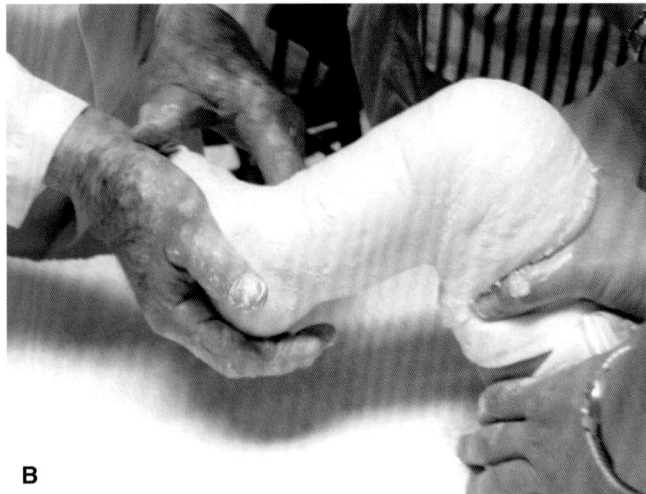

FIGURE 53.11 A. Achilles tenotomy. **B.** Long leg plaster casting with emphasis on dorsiflexion at the level of the ankle following Achilles tenotomy.

Anterior Tibialis Tendon Transfer

Some children of walking age demonstrate supination during swing and stance phase of gait. While often not complaining of pain, one may see callus formation as result of abnormal pressure and lateral column overload. This muscle imbalance is common among children with clubfoot given overactivity of supinating muscles and underactivity of everting muscles. While not every child born with clubfoot will require this procedure, it remains quite common and has been considered part of the formal method.

Prior to the procedure, if the foot is not fully corrected, it is essential to proceed with serial Ponseti casting to obtain a well-corrected foot prior to tendon transfer. Casts at this time are still well-molded plaster casts with a fiberglass cast overlay above the knee. The knee is flexed to minimize slippage and rotation. Many children at this time are 3 years of age or older and continue to attempt ambulation in bilateral casts. It is important to educate caregivers on cast care to minimize blisters, skin breakdown, or infections that may delay this procedure.

Casting should be done prior to tendon transfer in all patients. On average, three casts are needed to fully achieve correction. The tendon transfer itself will only maintain correction—it cannot be used to achieve correction. The preoperative casts are long leg bent 30 degrees to allow full weight bearing. After surgery, a long leg plaster cast is used with knee bent to 90 degrees to prevent weight bearing for 4 weeks. At that time, the tendon button is removed and a short leg weight-bearing cast is used for an additional 2 weeks. Following cast removal, AFO bracing is helpful for 6 weeks along with nighttime stretching splint and physical therapy.

Surgical Technique: Anterior Tibial Tendon Transfer

- Medial incision is fashioned over the first metatarsal cuneiform joint.
- The anterior tibial tendon is released from its insertion site.
- The tendon is reflected, and a whip stitch is performed to the anterior tibial tendon.

- The tendon is directed beneath retinacular tissue and transferred to the lateral cuneiform.
- A Bio-Tenodesis screw is utilized to improve pull out strength while the suture is pulled through plantar skin. A suture button can be utilized. Care is taken to not over tighten as maceration, ulceration, and skin necrosis can occur.
- An Achilles lengthening procedure often is performed in conjunction with any persistent equinus.
- A long leg cast is applied with the knee flexed to 90 degrees.
- It often takes 6 weeks for the tendon to incorporate into bone.

Postoperative Protocol

- Long leg split plaster cast with knee bent 90 degrees to prevent weight bearing for 4 weeks
- Short leg weight-bearing cast for 2 weeks
- AFO bracing for 6 weeks and formal physical therapy to work on strengthening, gait, and range of motion
- Nighttime dorsiflexion AFOs for 6 months

Posteromedial Release

Historically, the posterior medial release was the treatment of choice prior to the Ponseti technique. Many young children underwent grandiose incisions releasing tendons, joint capsules, and ligamentous structures of the posterior and medial compartments in attempt to reduce the talonavicular and subtalar joints. From review of these cases, surgeons noted outcomes to not be as favorable. Children had stiff feet with often-recurrent deformities that led to overall poorer functional outcome scores. While a smaller percentage of children need this procedure to date, the majority of children do not require such releases.

A posteromedial release is performed upon failure of Ponseti casting or the presence of resistant recurrent deformity. The critical aspects of the deformity must be understood in order to distinguish which structures require release. A surgeon

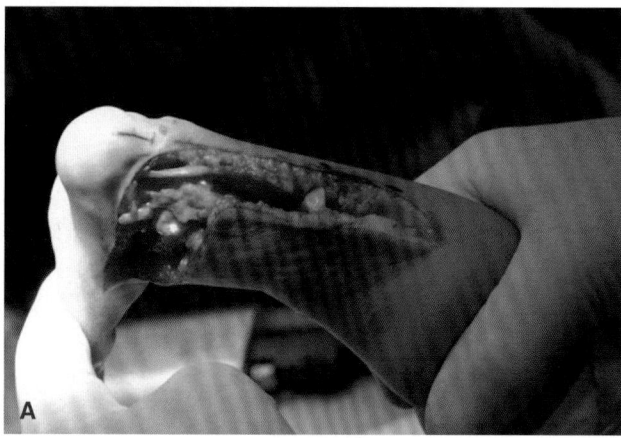
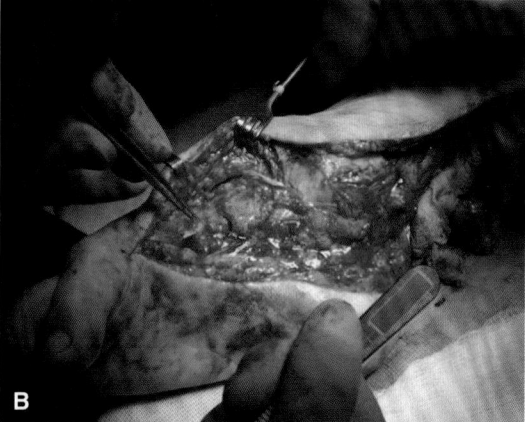

FIGURE 53.12 A. Posteromedial release. **B.** Scar tissue following previous posteromedial release. Notice obliteration of tissue planes and extreme scarring.

appreciates that the navicular is medially subluxed upon the talar head in close proximity to the medial malleolus. The calcaneus is supinated, and often equinus persists. A deep plantar crease is indicative of a cavus deformity.

A complete posteromedial release requires extensive dissection of the posterior ankle and subtalar joints along with the medial, lateral, and plantar aspects of the foot (Fig. 53.12). A medial incision is fashioned extending along the medial arch transcending posteriorly across the posterior aspect of the ankle to expose both the ankle and subtalar joints. This posterior arm of the incision may be a vertical or a transverse continuum from the medial incision. Care is taken to preserve neurovascular structures. A vessel loop is utilized to identify medial structures for retraction and protection. The medial plantar nerve is followed and protected while the abductor hallucis muscle is mobilized from the calcaneus and further released at the musculotendinous junction. The Achilles is lengthened or completely released based on age of the patient. The posterior tibial, flexor digitorum longus, and flexor hallucis longus tendons are lengthened proximal to the medial malleolus. Lengthening proximal to the porta pedis or proximal to the tarsal tunnel region may minimize adhesions. The talonavicular joint capsule, subtalar joint capsule, and calcaneocuboid capsules can then be released. Finally, the posterior ankle capsule is released to allow for the talus to rotate posteriorly into the ankle mortise when the ankle is dorsiflexed.

A plantar release is fashioned posterior to the neurovascular bundle. A plane is created between the subcutaneous tissue and plantar aponeurosis. Division of the aponeurosis allows for further correction of the cavus deformity. Following sequential soft tissue release, the talonavicular and subtalar joints are pinned to maintain alignment. One may utilize a 2-3 K-wire construct as needed for stability. A 0.062 smooth K-wire is antegraded from the posterior talus into the talar head to transcend the reduced talonavicular joint. The base of the first metatarsal is slightly abducted and held. A subsequent K-wire may be utilized across the subtalar joint. A third K-wire may be utilized from the lateral column into the calcaneus. If a tourniquet is utilized, it is important to deflate prior to closure to assess for appropriate perfusion.

A splint or bivalved cast is applied to reduce motion while also minimize edema postoperatively. Immobilization is advised for a minimum of 4-6 weeks. Often, the initial splint is left intact

for 7-14 days based on the extent of the release followed by subsequent above the knee casting for the remaining period of time. Children with increased risks for skin necrosis such as loss of protective sensation are seen in shorter intervals. It remains important to monitor all children undergoing such releases given the risks of edema, tissue necrosis, vascular compromise, bleeding problems, and dehiscence.

A full posterior, medial, and lateral release can often be avoided if recurrence is casted early in life prior to osseous adaptive changes. Often, casting can be utilized to correct for the medial soft tissue contracture, and if equinus and stiffness remains, a posterior release may be executed in resistant clubfeet. Wires may or may not be utilized. Following releases, a child is casted for 4 weeks in long leg plaster casts bivalved and non–weight bearing. This may be extended as needed.

Posterior Clubfoot Release

- Achilles tendon lengthening
- Posterior ankle and subtalar joint release
- Peroneal retinaculum release
- Flexor digitorum longus and flexor hallucis longus lengthening

Medial Clubfoot Release

- Posterior tibial tendon lengthening
- Flexor hallucis longus and flexor digitorum longus release
- Talonavicular joint capsulotomy
- Abductor hallucis tendon release
- Medial and plantar calcaneocuboid joint release
- Interosseous subtalar joint release

Lateral Clubfoot Release

- Lateral subtalar joint release
- Calcaneofibular ligament release
- Calcaneocuboid complete release

Plantar Clubfoot Release

- Plantar fascia release
- Flexor digitorum brevis release
- Abductor digiti minimi release
- Long plantar ligament release

Fixation Following Soft Tissue Release

- Pinning of subtalar joint
- Pinning of talonavicular joint
- Possible pinning of lateral column

OSSEOUS PROCEDURES

Osseous Procedures

- Opening cuneiform and closing cuboid osteotomies: Reduces adduction.
- Calcaneal osteotomies: Lateral closing osteotomy to reduce heel varus.
- Triple arthrodesis: Multiplanar deformity with pain/often-degenerative changes with unstable foot. Procedure is performed in attempt at recreating a stable tripod.
- Midfoot osteotomy: through and through osteotomy performed to correct for cavus. Can be dorsiflexory while also correct for any residual adduction.
- Supramalleolar osteotomies: Multiplanar correction for varus deformity. May be utilized in setting of flat top talus.
- Talectomy: removal of the talus often performed in children with deformities that are rigid, recurrent, and resistant to treatment. Most children have some form of neurologic or motor deficit.

CLUBFOOT AND SPINA BIFIDA

Despite the successful outcome of the Ponseti method with respect to management of clubfoot, recurrence rates remain higher among patients with neuromuscular imbalance. The method may be executed perfectly, while without proper daytime and nighttime bracing in spina bifida patients, the deformity generally reoccurs to varying degrees. The muscular imbalance is a driving force in impending deformity without static control postcorrection. The majority of spina bifida patients will have a foot deformity manifest within their lifetime.[52] Often if congenital, the deformity is clubfoot.

Challenges with bracing are common. These children present with loss of sensation and sensitive skin. This combination often leads to skin breakdown, blisters, or ulcerations. If the child is given time outside of the braces for the healing of skin lesions, recurrence of the deformity can occur and subsequently braces will not fit. This becomes a challenging cycle, one of which requires subsequent casting to correct for any recurrent deformities. With 30%-50% of patients with spina bifida presenting with clubfoot, Arkin et al. noted the Ponseti method lead to reliable initial correction and confirmed the approach to be useful at reducing the need for extensive soft tissue release.[12] Arkin further noted that midterm evaluation of the Ponseti method for clubfoot in spina bifida shows a successful outcome

in 42.3%.[12] An open excision of the Achilles was advised. Given complexity of this neuromuscular imbalance, families should be counseled about high risk of recurrence and potential need for surgical intervention.

Foot and ankle deformities in spina bifida may result from congenital, developmental, or iatrogenic causes. Clubfoot and vertical talus are classic examples of congenital deformities. Developmental deformities are associated with the level of neurologic involvement.[53] Despite function, the goal is a plantigrade, supple, braceable foot to minimize ulceration. Often, hindfoot varus and equinus tend to be recurrent deformities in spina bifida. These children if unsuccessful with subsequent casting may require posterior releases. The surgeon should use weight bearing to assist with maintenance of correction with braces.

COMPLICATIONS

Not only can complications arise from surgery but also from the casting process. Often, complications are linked to subsequent deformities resulting from poor casting technique. It remains key to not evert the forefoot and focus on supination of the forefoot initially. One should not solely abduct until the medial crease or essentially the cavus deformity is reduced. By pushing up under the first metatarsal head, one reduces the cavus and realigns the forefoot to the rearfoot. At times, the 4-finger technique may be utilized to further address the cavus. Please refer to the alternative maneuver for both atypical and complex clubfoot within this chapter.

One of the easiest means of minimizing complications is to never apply counterpressure to the calcaneocuboid joint. Despite many recognizing the faultiness with Kite's maneuver, it is quite easy to block the calcaneus from moving beneath the talus if one's thumb is on the prominent anterior process. Blockage of the calcaneus will leave the heel inverted and in varus. This may also lead to a posteriorly deviated fibula or inability for the talus to move within the ankle joint. Forceful manipulation can in essence also lead to an eventual flat top talus later in life or immediate distal tibial fractures. While reasons for development of a flat top talus are multifaceted and may be a clubfoot developmental finding, one must be gentle with manipulations. The flat top talus remains a challenging often-surgical problem. The ability to restore normal morphology of the talus does not exist. Hence, the surgeon attempts to realign around a disfigured talus. Many attempt supramalleolar osteotomies, calcaneal osteotomies, or midfoot osteotomies with inconsistent results.

The atypical and complex clubfoot types are of utmost importance for any physician to recognize. Failure to identify these specific groups may lead to further edema, disfigurement, rigidity, and progressive challenging deformities. There is still controversy over the etiology of the atypical clubfoot. A child presenting with a significant deep plantar crease or neurologic influence needs to closely be monitored as this atypical presentation is noted at birth. The complex subset may arise during the casting process. Hyperabduction with these groups will lead to the quadratus plantae pulling the flexors and worsening cavus deformity.

Improper casting technique may also lead to a complex clubfoot or mixed deformity. It is important if a complex foot deformity arises to adjust one's technique and approach to casting. Often the 4 finger technique is utilized.[48]

Likewise, surgical complications can arise. Often, this healthy young population will heal, while with any surgery, they are at risk of dehiscence, wound healing problems, infection, inability to close surgical sites, nerve problems, stiffness, pain, hardware problems, and unfortunate recurrence. Parents and caregivers should be educated on these potential outcomes well prior to surgery. Infections, wounds, and unfortunate limb loss are all outcomes of clubfoot treatment that should be discussed with parents and caretakers. Children with coexisting syndromes carry increased risks with higher likelihood for poorer outcomes.

AUTHORS' PREFERRED TREATMENT

CLUBFOOT

- The Ponseti method is performed as first-line treatment for the isolated and nonisolated/syndromic clubfoot.
- If <10 degrees of dorsiflexion is noted, then an Achilles tenotomy is performed. A final cast is applied immediately thereafter and left intact for 3 weeks.
- Children utilize the abduction bar braces until age of 4.
- The Ponseti method is utilized for recurrences.
- Surgical intervention may be needed for various symptomatic deformities that are not alleviated by casting: surgery is specific to the deformity while the most common procedures have been discussed in this chapter. Surgical procedures are primarily dictated by age of the patient and rigidity of the deformity.

REFERENCES

1. Chung CS, Nemechek RW, Larsen IJ, Ching GH. Genetic and epidemiological studies of clubfoot in Hawaii. General and medical considerations. *Hum Hered.* 1969;19:321-342.
2. Dobbs MB, Gurnett CA. The 2017 ABJS Nicolas Andry Award: advancing personalized medicine for clubfoot through translational research. *Clin Orthop Relat Res.* 2017;475:1716-1725.
3. Beals RK. Club foot in the Maori: a genetic study of 50 kindres. *N Z Med J.* 1978;88:144-146.
4. Kite JH. *The Clubfoot.* New York, NY: Grune & Stratton; 1964.
5. Cooper DM, Dietz FR. Treatment of idiopathic clubfoot. A thirty-year follow-up note. *J Bone Joint Surg Am.* 1995;77:1477-1489.
6. Ponseti IV. Treatment of congenital clubfoot. *J Bone Joint Surg Am.* 1992;74(3):448-454.
7. Ippolito E. Update on pathological anatomy of clubfoot. *J Pediatr Orthop.* 1995;4:17-24.
8. Ippolito E, Ponseti IV. Congenital clubfoot in the human fetus. A histological study. *J Bone Joint Surg Am.* 1980;62:8-22.
9. Dobbs MB, Nunley R, Schoenecker PL. Long-term follow up of patients with clubfoot treated with extensive soft tissue release. *J Bone Joint Surg Am.* 2006;88:986-996.
10. Ponseti IV. *Congenital Clubfoot: Fundamentals of Treatment.* Oxford University Press, Oxford Medical Publications; 1996.
11. Laaveg SJ, Ponseti IV. Long-term results of treatment of congenital clubfoot. *J Bone Joint Surg Am.* 1980;62(1):23-31.
12. Arkin, C, Ihnow S, Dias L, Swaroop VT. Midterm results of the Ponseti method for treatment of clubfoot in patients with spina bifida. *J Pediatr Orthop.* 2018;38(10):e588-e592.
13. Dobbs MB, Rudzki JR, Purcell DB, Walton T, Porter K, Gurnett CA. Factors predictive of outcome after use of the Ponseti methods for the treatment of idiopathic clubfoot. *J Bone Joint Surg.* 2004;86-A(1):22-27.
14. van Praag VM, Lysenko M, Harvey B, Yankanah R, Wright JG. Casting is effective for recurrence following Ponseti treatment of clubfoot. *J Bone Joint Surg Am.* 2018;100:1001-1008.
15. Pirani S, Outerbridge H, Moran M, Sawatsky BJ. *A Method of Evaluating the Virgin Clubfoot with Substantial Interobserver Reliability, vol 71,* Miami, FL: POSNA; 1995.
16. Dimeglio A, Bensahel H, Souchet P, et al. Classification of clubfoot. *J Pediatr Orthop.* 1995;4:129-136.
17. Flynn JM, Donohoe MPT, Mackenzie WG. An independent assessment of two clubfoot-classification systems. *J Pediatr Orthop.* 1998;18:323-327.
18. Cosma D, Vasilescu DE. A clinical evaluation of the Pirani and Dimeglio idiopathic clubfoot classifications. *J Foot Ankle Surg.* 2015;54:582-585.
19. Fried A. Recurrent congenital clubfoot: the role of the *m. tibialis* posterior in etiology and treatment. *J Bone Joint Surg Am.* 1959;41:243-252.
20. Hersch A. The role of surgery in the treatment of clubfeet. *J Bone Joint Surg Am.* 1967;49:1684-1696.
21. Turco VJ. Surgical correction of the resistant club foot: one-stage posteromedial release with internal fixation. *J Bone Joint Surg Am.* 1971;53:477-497.
22. Fukuhara K, Schollmeier G, Uhthoff HK. The pathogenesis of clubfoot: a histomorphometric and immunohistochemical study of fetuses. *J Bone Joint Surg Br.* 1994;76:350-357.
23. Gray DH, Katz JM. A histochemical study of muscle in club foot. *J Bone Joint Surg Br.* 1989;63:417-423.
24. Ionasescu V, Maynard JA, Ponseti IV, Zellweger H. The role of collagen in the pathogenesis of idiopathic clubfoot. *Helv Pediatr Acta.* 1995;29:305-314.
25. Isaccs H, Handelsman JE, Badenhorst M, Pickering A. The muscles in clubfoot: a histological, histochemical, and electron microscopic study. *J Bone Joint Surg Br.* 1977;59:465-472.
26. Khan AM, Ryan MG, Gruber MM, et al. Connective tissue structures in clubfoot: a morphologic study. *J Pediatr Orthop.* 2001;21:708-712.
27. Howard CB, Benson MK. Clubfoot: its pathological anatomy. *J Pediatr Orthop.* 1993;13:654-659.
28. Irani RN, Sherman MS. The pathological anatomy of idiopathic clubfoot. *Clin Orthop.* 1972;84:14-20.
29. Ippolito E, De Maio F, Mancini F, et al. Leg muscle atrophy in idiopathic clubfoot congenital clubfoot: is it primitive or acquired? *J Child Orthop.* 2009;3:171-178.
30. Abdelgawad AA, Lehman WB, van Bosse HJ, et al. Treatment of idiopathic clubfoot using the Ponseti method: minimum 2-year follow-up. *J Pediatr Orthop B.* 2007;16(2):98-105.
31. Bor N, Coplan JA, Herzenberg JE. Ponseti treatment for idiopathic clubfoot: minimum 5-year followup. *Clin Orthop Relat Res.* 2008;467(5):1263-1270.
32. Banskota B, Yadav P, Rajbhandari T, et al. Outcomes of the Ponseti method for untreated clubfeet in Nepalese patients seen between the ages of one and five years and followed for at least 10 years. *J Bone Joint Surg Am.* 2018;100:2004-2014.
33. Sinclair MF, Bosch K, Rosenbaum D, Bohm S. Pedobarographic analysis following Ponseti treatment for congenital clubfoot. *Clin Orthop Relat Res.* 2009;467:1223-1230.
34. Gottschalk HP, Karol LA, Jeans KA. Gait analysis of children treated for moderate clubfoot with physical therapy versus the Ponseti cast technique. *J Pediatr Orthop.* 2010;30:235-239.
35. El-Hawary R, Karol LA, Jeans KA, Richards BS. Gait analysis of children treated for clubfoot with physical therapy or the Ponseti cast technique. *J Bone Joint Surg Am.* 2008;90:1508-1516.
36. Wynne-Davies R. Family studies and the cause of congenital club foot, talipes equinovarus, talipes calcaneo-valgus and metatarsus varus. *J Bone Joint Surg Br.* 1964;46:445-463.
37. Wynne-Davies R. Genetic and environmental factor is in the etiology of talipes equinovarus. *Clin Orthop Relat Res.* 1972;84:9-13.
38. Lochmiller C, Johnston D, Scott A, et al. Genetic epidemiology study of idiopathic talipes equinovarus. *Am J Med Genet.* 1998;79:90-96.
39. Dietz F. The genetics of idiopathic clubfoot. *Clin Orthop Relat Res.* 2002;401:39-48.
40. Alvarado DM, McCall K, Aferol H. Pitx1 haploinsufficiency causes clubfoot in humans and a clubfoot-like phenotype in mice. *Hum Mol Genet.* 2011;20:3943-3952.
41. Alvarado DM, Buchan JG, Frick SL, et al. Copy number analysis of 413 isolated talipes equinovarus patients suggest role for transcriptional regulators of early limb development. *Eur J Hum Genet.* 2012;21:373-380.
42. Shimizu N, Hamada S, Mitta M, et al. Etiological considerations of congenital clubfoot deformity. In: Tachdjian MO, Simons G, eds. *The Clubfoot: The Present and A View of the Future.* New York, NY: Springer; 1993:31-38.
43. Chapman C, Stott NS, Port RV, Nicol RO. Genetics of club foot in Maori and Pacific people. *J Med Genet.* 2000;37:680-683.
44. Honein MA, Paulozzi LJ, Moore CA. Family history, maternal smoking, and clubfoot: an indication of a gene-environment interaction. *Am J Epidemiol.* 2000;152(7):658-665.
45. Dickinson KC, Meyer RE, Kotch J. Maternal smoking and the risk for clubfoot in infants. *Birth Defects Res A Clin Mol Teratol.* 2008;82(2):86-91.
46. Hootnick DR, Levinsohn EM, Crider RJ, et al. Congenital arterial malformations associated with clubfoot. A report of two cases. *Clin Orthop Relat Res.* 1982;167:160-163.
47. Levinsohn EM, Hootnick DR, Packard DS Jr. Consistent arterial abnormalities associated with a variety of congenital malformations of the human lower limb. *Invest Radiol.* 1991;26(4):364-373.
48. Ponseti IV, Zhivkov M, Davis N, Sinclair M, Dobbs MB, Morcuende J. Treatment of the complex idiopathic clubfoot. *Clin Orthop Relat Res.* 2006;451:171-176.
49. Colburn M, Williams M. Evaluation of the treatment of idiopathic clubfoot by using the Ponseti method. *J Foot Ankle Surg.* 2003;42(5):259-267.
50. Zhao D, Li H, Zhao L, Liu J, Wu Z, Jin F. Results of clubfoot management using the Ponseti method: do the details matter? A systematic review. *Clin Orthop Relat Res.* 2014;472(4):1329-1336.
51. Dobbs MB, Gordon JE, Walton T, Schoenecker PL. Bleeding complications following percutaneous tendoachilles tenotomy in the treatment of clubfoot deformity. *J Pediatr Orthop.* 2004;24(4):353-357.
52. Swaroop VT, Dias L. Orthopaedic management of spina bifida-part II: foot and ankle deformities. *J Child Orthop.* 2011;5:403-414.
53. Guille JT, Sarwark JF, Sherk HH, Kumar SJ. Congenital and developmental deformities of the spine in children with myelomeningocele. *J Am Acad Orthop Surg.* 2006;14:294-302.

Pediatric Deformities

Mitzi L. Williams and Matthew B. Dobbs

INTRODUCTION

This chapter will review some of the more common congenital foot and ankle deformities among children. Many of these deformities have a genetic influence while others may arise secondary to a failure in differentiation *in utero*. A complete pediatric history and physical examination is key in excluding any neurologic component.

ANATOMIC FEATURES AND FUNCTIONAL ANALYSIS

Foot deformity in infants is one of the most common congenital musculoskeletal conditions. Diagnosis and treatment requires sound knowledge of normal physiologic development, neurology, histology, and radiologic interpretation. While many pediatric conditions can be attributed to genetics and in fact assist with diagnosis of various syndromes, others are a direct product of trauma or overuse. One must appreciate the delicate nature of these anatomic structures and the variation in which they present. With experience, and a firm understanding of normal pediatric lower extremity anatomy, one can delineate abnormal structural conditions in hopes of early treatment modalities. Early intervention for many diagnoses leads to improved functional outcomes.

Many congenital foot deformities will be noted *in utero* via ultrasound and furthermore reviewed with detailed ultrasounds and amniocentesis. One may find the foot deformity to be a component of a syndrome identified via amniocentesis. Still both formal diagnosis and rigidity of conditions such as talipes equinovarus (clubfoot), congenital vertical talus, calcaneovalgus, and other deformities associated with syndromes will be verified by clinical examination. An amniocentesis may be advised with high-risk pregnancies or if noninvasive testing reveals concerning results. If performed, the fluid from the sac surrounding the fetus is aspirated and sent for evaluation between the 15th and 20th week of pregnancy.

Amniocentesis does not detect all birth defects, and this is important when counseling families. It can be used to detect Down syndrome, sickle cell, cystic fibrosis, muscular dystrophy, and Tay-Sachs, for example. With respect to foot deformities that may be associated with various syndromes, an amniocentesis can be helpful in assessing for any connection to neural tube defects such as spina bifida and/or chromosomal abnormalities. At the same time, one generally undergoes a detailed ultrasound that compliments the amniocentesis in detecting any structural abnormalities such as heart defects or cleft palate (Table 54.1).

Given the ossification pattern of the foot, x-rays in an infant may not be required unless difficulties with treatment exist, diagnosis is unclear, or postoperative alignment is reviewed often with respect to the talus. X-rays, for example, are rarely indicated in the treatment of clubfoot unless there is difficulty with reduction. As for vertical talus, a stress plantar flexion lateral x-ray is utilized to either confirm or exclude the diagnosis as noted in Figure 54.1.

OSSIFICATION

Ossific development of the foot begins *in utero*.[1,2] At birth, the talus, calcaneus, cuboid, metatarsals, and phalanges are ossified, while the navicular and cuneiforms are cartilaginous. Hence, when excluding the diagnosis of vertical talus, one is attempting to realign the talus with the first metatarsal on lateral plain film radiographs and not the navicular in infants. The lateral cuneiform ossifies at 6 months, intermediate cuneiform at 12 months, and medial cuneiform at 18 months (Fig. 54.2). The navicular does not ossify until 2.5-5 years of age. Fusion of secondary growth centers with respect to the calcaneus and

TABLE 54.1	Amniotic Fluid Is Tested at 15-20 Weeks' Gestation for Hundreds of Chromosomal Abnormalities, Genetic Disorders, and Neural Tube Defects	
Amniocentesis Identifies	**Examples**
Chromosomal abnormalities	Down syndrome, Edward syndrome, Patau syndrome
Genetic disorders	Cystic fibrosis, Tay-Sachs, sickle cell disease
Neural tube defects	Spina bifida
Severity of fetal anemia	Infants with Rh disease
Paternity testing	

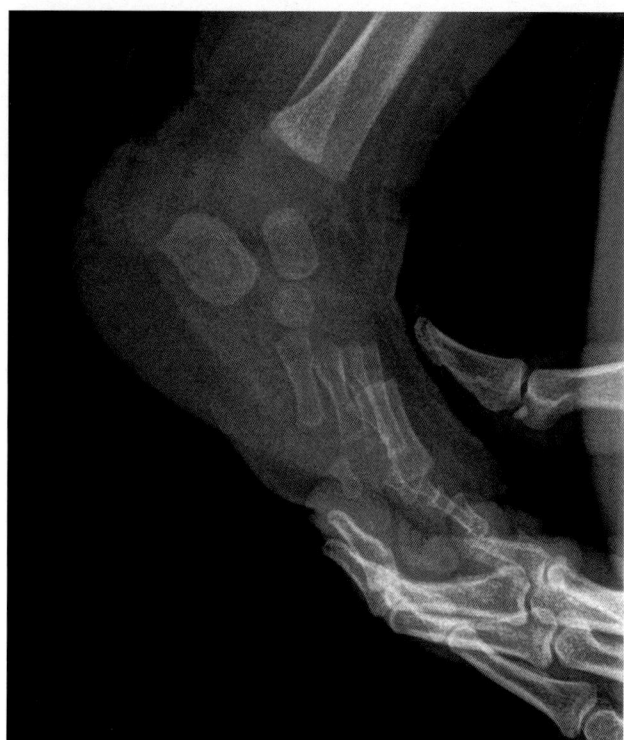

FIGURE 54.1 Stress plantar flexion view excluding vertical talus.

fifth metatarsal base occurs near 15 years of age. These ossification patterns (Table 54.2) are helpful in interpreting images and excluding fractures as compared to normal anatomy, while an awareness of the time frame for physeal closure assists with surgical procedure selection.

Bone growth can be influenced by systemic and local factors. Systemic factors include genetics, hormones, overall nutrition, and infection. Nutritional deficits may be linked to diet while may also be secondary to conditions associated to prematurity or systemic illnesses. Advances in neonatal care have significantly increased infant survival rates especially among very low birth weight infants. These children should be followed closely as these nutritional deficiencies can be multifactorial. Likewise, any unusual growth disturbance can have a grave impact on limb length and/or lead to angular deformities.

Local factors influencing growth of a single epiphysis often include trauma, vascular insult, or osteomyelitis. Trauma can include obvious fractures or mechanical injuries, while radiation may locally impact bone growth or lead to a growth hormone deficiency. Infections can also cause long-term harm with respect to bone growth. Caution should be taken with infection management and proper peripheral and central line care among infants as line infections may lead to bone infections. Hence, the premature closure of an isolated physis is a possibility. Saphenous peripheral lines, for example, are in close proximity to the distal tibia and can lead to angular deformities in the years to come if osseous infection ensues.

PHYSICAL EXAMINATION AND DEVELOPMENT

Parents quite often have worries with respect to their child's growth, development, and/or gait. Intoeing remains one of the most common reasons for referral and concern. Intoeing is rarely secondary to surgical pathology and is often attributed to metatarsus adductus, internal tibial torsion (in toddlers), and femoral anteversion (among children younger than 10). Other conditions such as clubfoot must be excluded by focusing on the hindfoot. Given the need for early clubfoot manipulation and poorer outcomes associated with its neglected form, one must recognize its presence from metatarsus adductus and initiate Ponseti manipulation and casting early in life. One must also distinguish complex clubfoot for its significant plantar crease and excessively plantarflexed metatarsals. For hyperabduction in this complex clubfoot, subset will lead to a worsening cavus deformity. It is important to identify the segment responsible for intoeing and hence determine if intervention is necessary (Table 54.3; Figs. 54.3 and 54.4).

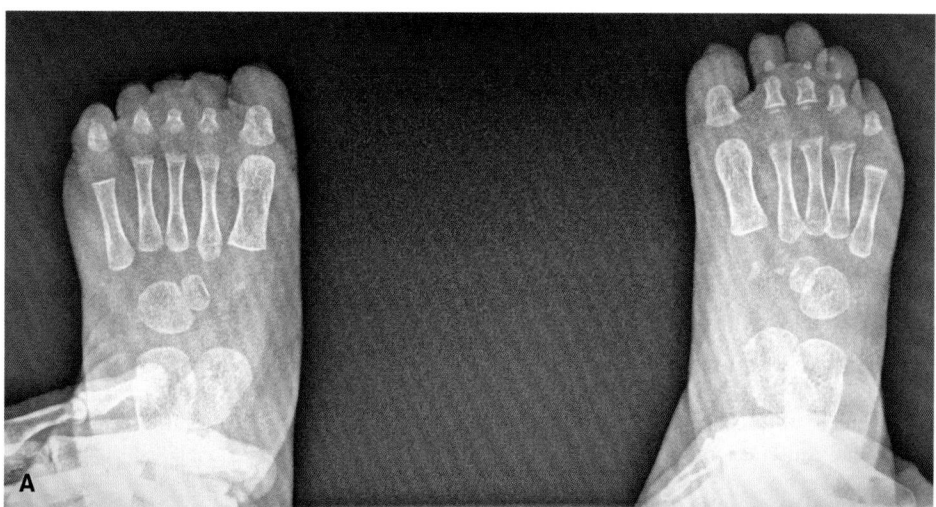
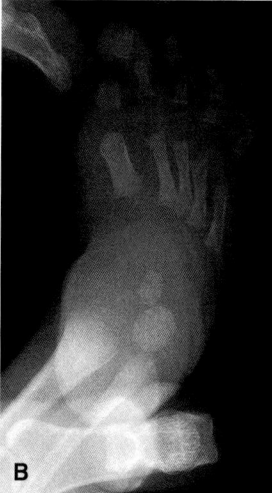

FIGURE 54.2 A. AP view of an 18-month-old female with toe deformities. **B.** AP view of infant's clubfoot.

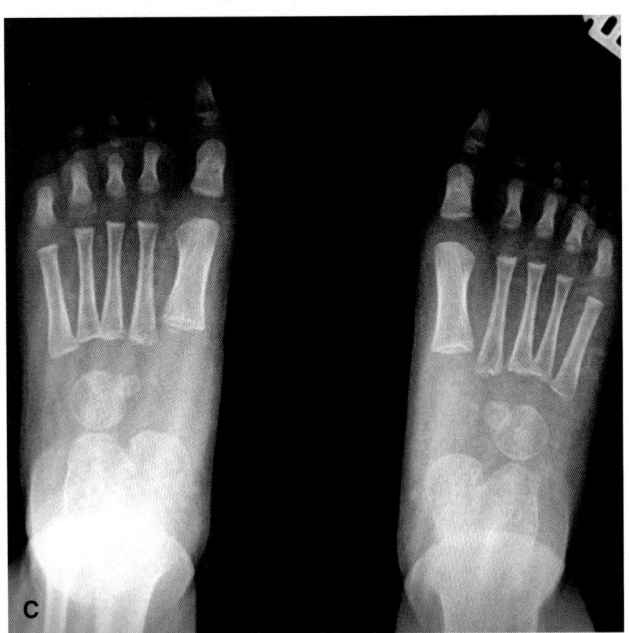

FIGURE 54.2 (*Continued*) **C.** AP weight-bearing foot x-rays of a 3-year-old healthy male.

Physicians must also educate parents that it is normal for the infant foot to be flat. With age, the arch develops and the osseous structures and intrinsic musculature matures. Hence, it is normal for a young toddler or child to have flatfeet. The arch continues to develop with growth. It is not until age 6 that the arch further develops. It is important to exclude neurologic conditions associated with intoeing, cavus feet, and varus position. Equally, it is essential to understand how ligamentous laxity, connective tissue disorders, Down syndrome, coalitions, and autism can influence flatfeet. Excluding underlying neurologic driving forces and recognizing pathologic biomechanical influences is key (Figs. 54.5 and 54.6).

TABLE 54.2	Ossification Chart: Variation Can Exist	
Bone	**Primary Center of Ossification Appearance**	**Secondary Center of Ossification Appearance**
Calcaneus	3- to 4-mo fetus	4-10 y
Talus	3- to 4-mo fetus	8-9 y
Cuboid	9-mo fetus	
Lateral cuneiform	6 mo of age	
Intermediate cuneiform	12 mo of age	
Medial cuneiform	18 mo of age	
Navicular	2.5-5 y of age	10 y
First metatarsal	3-mo fetus (shaft)	3 y (base)
Second to fifth metatarsal	3-mo fetus	3 y (head)
Phalanges	3- to 4-mo fetus	6 mo-2 y (head)
Sesamoids	7-8 y	

TABLE 54.3	Intoeing Etiology	
Intoeing	**Signs**	
Metatarsus adductus (often infants)	• Medial deviation of forefoot from plantar aspect • C-shaped foot	• Bleck method: heel bisector line from heel to forefoot
Internal tibial torsion (often toddlers)	• Patella centered in frontal plane • Foot points inward due to tibial rotation	• Internally rotated thigh-foot angle • Negative foot progression angle
Femoral anteversion (often school-aged children)	• Medially deviated patellae • Clumsy gait with speed	• Increased internal hip rotation (60-90 degrees) • Decreased external hip rotation (10-15 degrees)

PATHOGENESIS

CONDITIONS

Curly Toe

Curly toe is a common congenital digital deformity that presents as a flexion deformity often involving the third, fourth, or fifth toes.[4] One or multiple toes may be affected. The affected toe is essentially plantarflexed, medially deviated, and in varus rotation with the apex of the deformity involving the distal interphalangeal (DIP, or both DIP and proximal interphalangeal (PIP) joints. This condition can be hereditary, with a positive family history and autosomal dominant pattern of inheritance.[5] Still, despite the genetic influence for some, the etiology of the deformity is not completely understood. Children with excessive pronation or metatarsus adductus have presented more frequently with these flexion contractures,[6] which may suggest that the flexor stabilization mechanism is an important driving force in this deformity (Fig. 54.7).

Curly toes are often noticed early in infancy and can be an early source of parental anxiety. At this stage, they are rarely symptomatic. Parental reassurance, education, and evaluation for any other neurologic manifestations are the main goals of that initial visit. Spontaneous self-correction of the deformity before the age of 6 occurs in up to 24% of the patients.[7] Hence, the remaining percentage of curly toes may persist. Therefore, delaying surgical intervention until the age of 6 is generally recommended. In the presence of skin problems secondary to pressure and/or infections, one could proceed with surgery prior to age 6. Likewise, children undergoing surgery under the age of 6 for other reasons may elect for surgical correction of the toe(s) to minimize future episodes of anesthesia. Finally, if the condition is becoming more semirigid and there is concern that one's window to perform a tendon release will be lost, then one may proceed sooner.

Treatment

Toe strapping is one of the available nonoperative treatment modalities, which can be attempted at any age.[7] Its effectiveness, however, is controversial. In a study by Turner, toe strapping

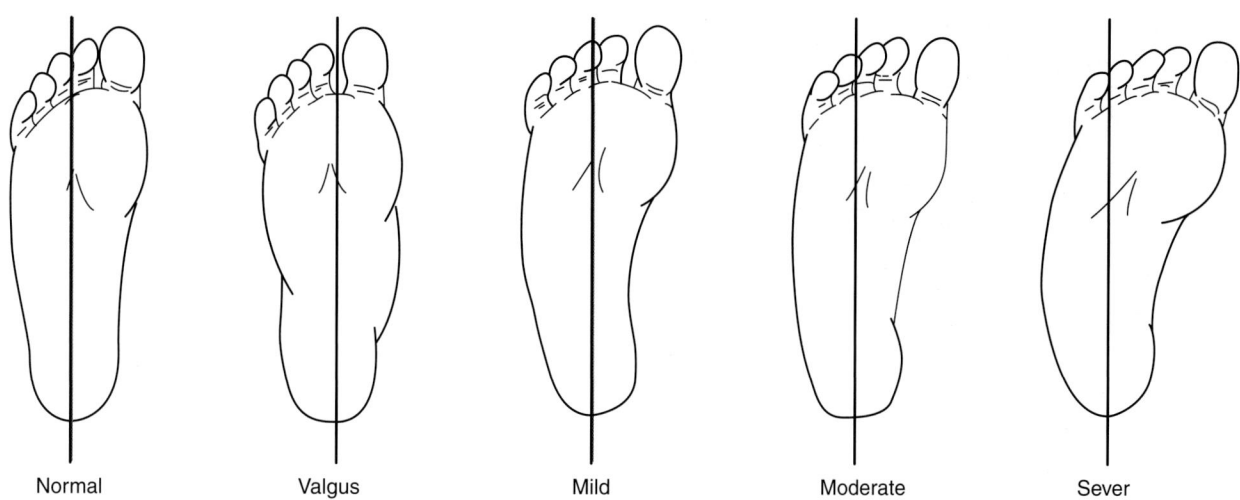

| Normal | Valgus | Mild | Moderate | Sever |

FIGURE 54.3 Bleck method for evaluation of metatarsus adductus. (Reprinted with permission from Bleck EE, Minaire P. Persistent medial deviation of the neck of the talus: a common cause of in-toing in children. *J Pediatr Orthop.* 1983;3:149 Ref.[3])

was performed daily on 28 children over 5 months of age for an average of 13 months.[8] No statistically significant difference was noted in the improvement rates between the study group versus a control group, consisting of children, who received no treatment. In another study, Smith and colleagues performed daily toe strapping for 3 months on 68 children with underlapping and overlapping toes, all of whom were no older than 10 days.[7] The authors observed a 94% improvement rate, which led them to suggest that toe strapping may be more successful in younger children. It is important to recognize that children in time may improve without treatment. The authors do not advocate for routine strapping and/or taping of curly toes in infancy.

Surgical treatment ultimately is reserved for patients with persistent deformity and symptomatic deformities. Patients may present with blisters or calluses at the tip of the underlapping toe or the plantar aspect of the adjacent toe. Others may present with nail deformities or pain in shoes.[9] Waiting until the child is at least 6 years old to assess if a toe will self-correct is appropriate provided the deformity is flexible. If the deformity is progressively becoming stiffer, from the ages of 2-6, one could proceed with surgery sooner to minimize the risk of an osseous procedure. Hence, tendon transfers and flexor tenotomies are performed. Arthroplasties, arthrodesis procedures, and phalangectomies are reserved for patients with semirigid or rigid contractures.

Girdlestone and Taylor have popularized flexor-to-extensor tendon transfer for treatment of claw toes in 1951.[10] The procedure allows recreating the dynamic pull of the intrinsic muscles and provides triplanar correction.[11] This procedure

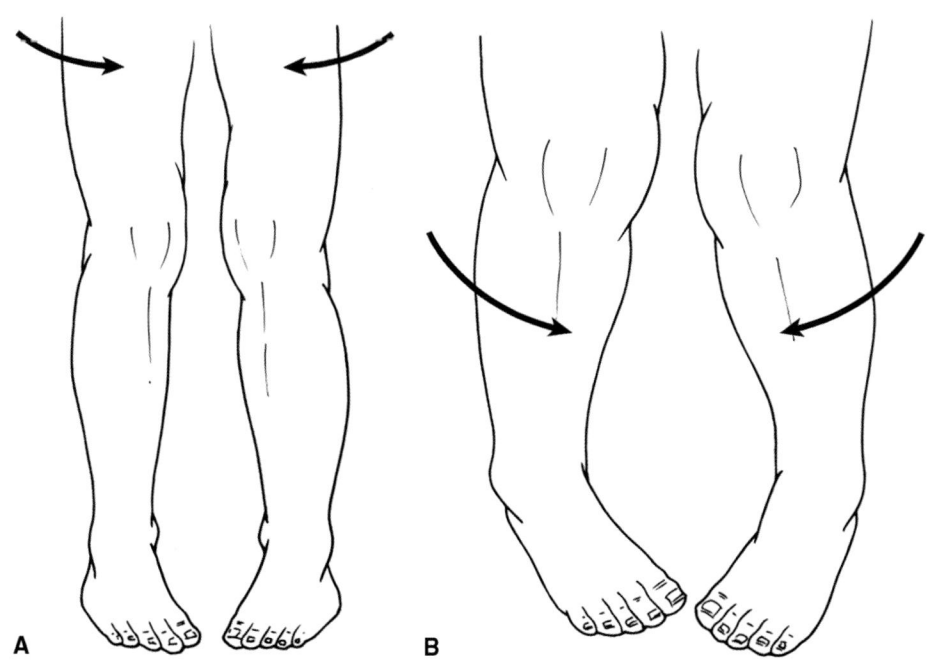

A   B

FIGURE 54.4 A. The knees are noted to be medially deviated hence not centered in the frontal plane in the presence of femoral anteversion. **B.** The knees will be centered with internal tibial torsion.

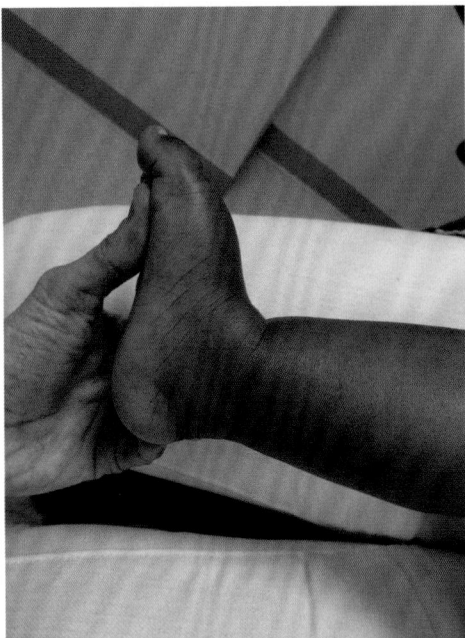

FIGURE 54.5 Undeveloped arch at 2 years of age.

was shown to be effective for correction of central curly toes 2, 3, and 4. The procedure is performed through a dorsolateral incision made over the extensor expansion. The long flexor is divided close to its insertion and transferred dorsolaterally, slightly distal to the extensor expansion, where it is attached under tension. Toe stiffness is a side effect following this procedure.[4]

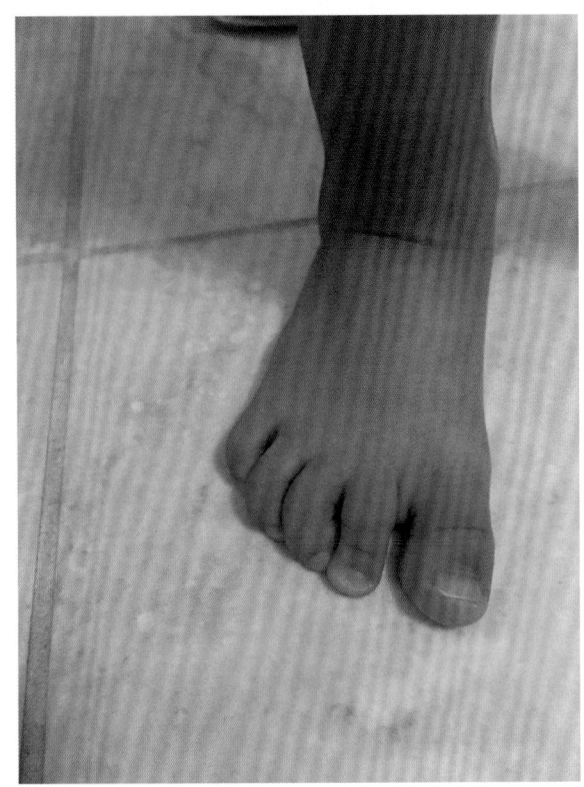

FIGURE 54.7 Reducible curly toes in a 3-year-old patient.

A flexor tenotomy is preferred to flexor to extensor tendon transfer to avoid postoperative toe stiffness. The procedure is performed through a small transverse stab incision on the plantar aspect of the toe.[12] The long and short flexor tendons

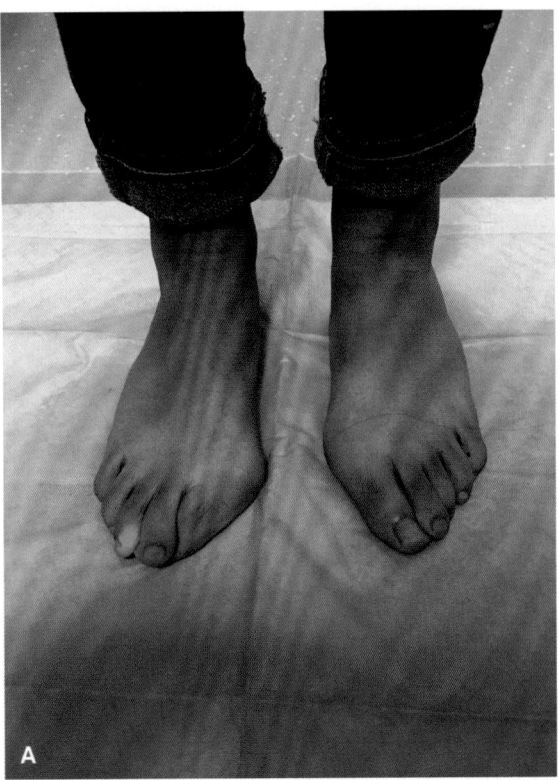

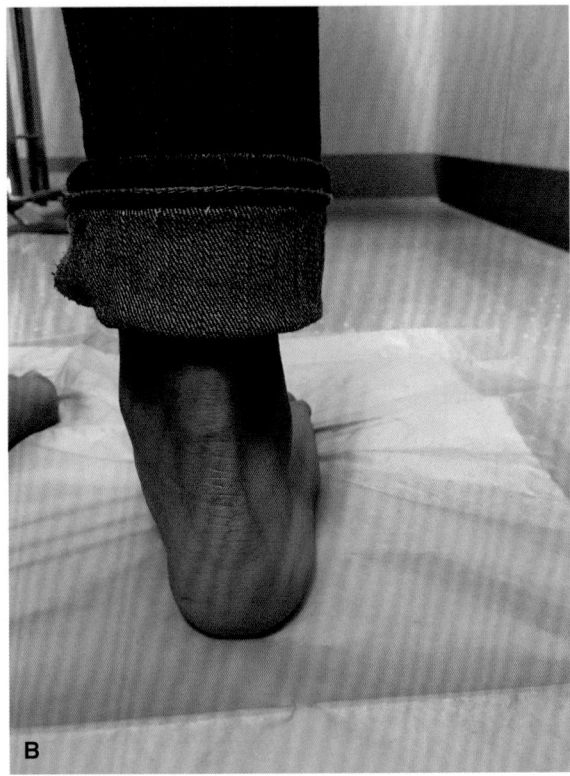

FIGURE 54.6 **A, B.** Pathologic flatfoot associated with middle facet coalition.

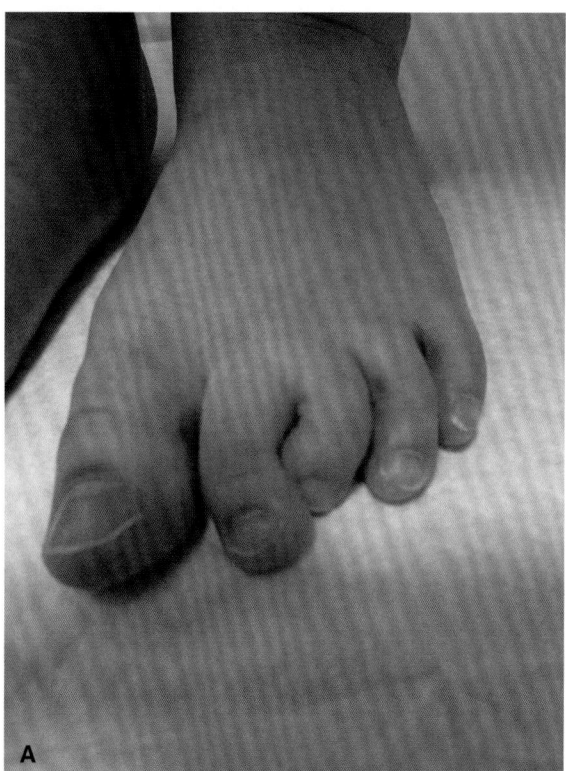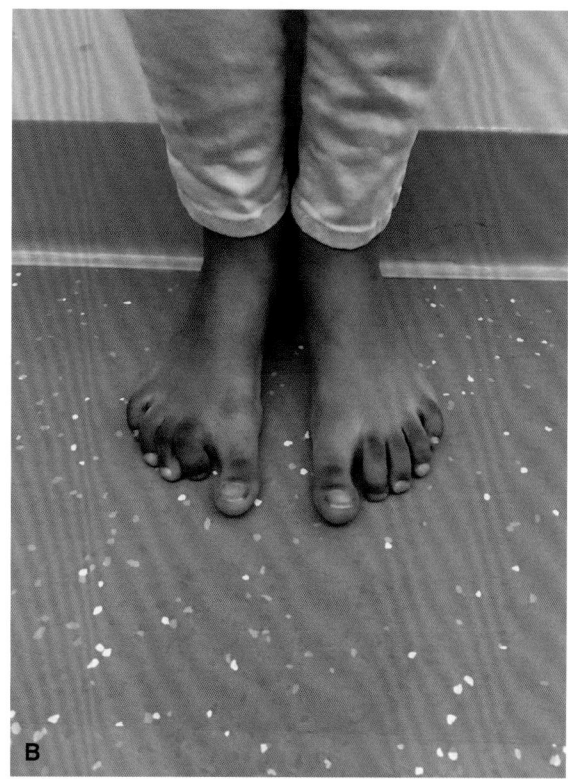

FIGURE 54.8 **A.** Flexible curly toe. **B.** Rigid curly toe.

are released. No sutures are needed with this type of small incision. Studies comparing flexor-to-extensor transfer and flexor tenotomy procedures suggest similar success rates with both procedures, with patient satisfaction being higher with flexor tenotomy.[4,13] A flexor tenotomy is also preferred for treatment of the underlapping fifth toe, for which flexor-to-extensor tendon transfer is not indicated[9] (Fig. 54.8).

Treatment of a rigid or semirigid overlapping toe involves PIP joint arthroplasty or fusion with concomitant flexor tenotomy or transfer.[9] Dorsolateral closing wedge arthroplasty may be performed to shorten and derotate the digit.[14] The procedure may be supplemented with capsular releases and phalangeal osteotomies for corrections of severe deformities. Postoperatively, the toe is usually held reduced with a K-wire for 6 weeks to prevent loss of correction. A skin plasty may also be performed. Treatment of a rigid underlapping fifth toe still represents a surgical challenge.

CURLY TOE PEARLS

- Reducible deformity: flexor tenotomy of long flexor or both short and long flexor tendons performed via plantar transverse stab incision.
- Rigid deformity: osseous procedures with K-wire pinning.
- Twenty-four percent of curly toes among the pediatric population will improve without treatment by age 6.[15]
- No sutures are needed following flexor tenotomy. On average, it takes about 14 days for skin healing.
- Following procedure, a short leg walking cast with toe plate may be utilized to keep the toes stretched for 10-14 days.

CURLY TOE PITFALLS

- Release of the long and short flexor tendons to reduce the deformity at PIP may lead to lack of purchase of toes for some children. Likewise, the authors have seen overcompensation for this lack of purchase by increased flexion of adjacent lesser toes that did not undergo a flexor tenotomy in the nonsyndromic foot under the age of 4. Further studies reviewing the long flexor release alone verse combined short and long flexor release may be indicated.

Polydactyly

Polydactyly is a congenital digital malformation characterized by formation of supernumerary digits (Fig. 54.9). It can be classified as preaxial: extra hallux; postaxial (most common): extra fifth toe; and central (rarest): middle three toes involved.[16] While it is a common congenital deformity of the hand and foot, with incidence in the foot of ~1 per 1000 live births,[17] the preaxial and central manifestations remain rare. Bilateral involvement is seen in 25%-50% of patients.[18] No gender predilection is observed.

In addition to duplication of phalanges, there may be a duplication of metatarsals. X-rays are important in assessing the extranumerary bones while also assessing if the growth and position of such bones will cause problems to the remainder of the foot. These x-rays are often obtained at a time in which the patient is of surgical age. Treatment must be individualized in accordance with the needs of the patient.[19]

The authors have met asymptomatic parents who did not undergo excision of simple extranumerary postaxial digits for example. Therefore, not every child must undergo surgical

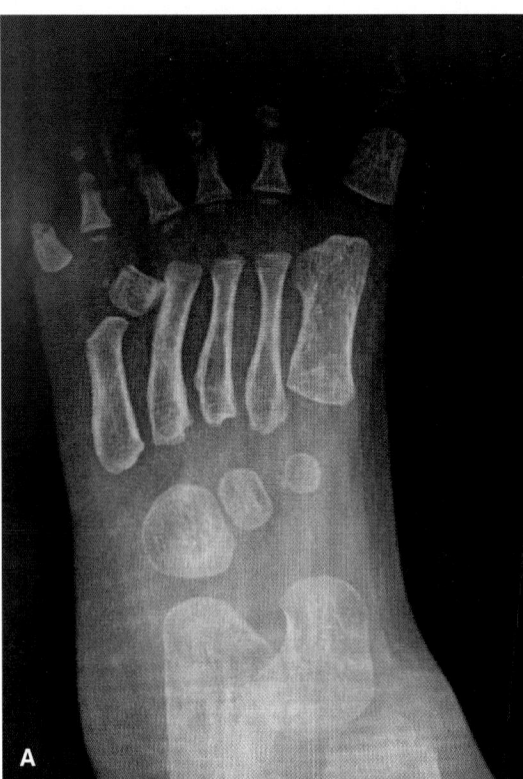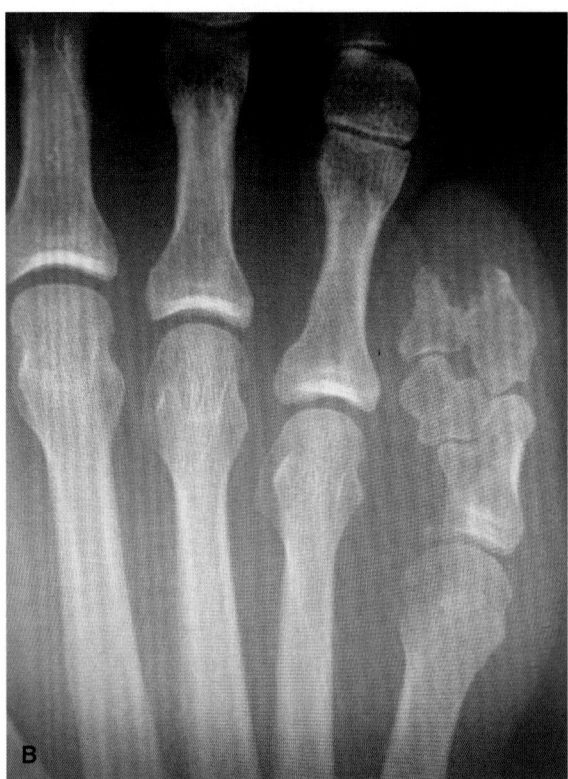

FIGURE 54.9 A. AP foot x-ray of a 2-year-old male with polydactyly. Risks of angular deformity exist with growth. **B.** AP foot x-ray of child's asymptomatic biological father demonstrating no history of surgical amputation.

excision. Unfortunately, the duplication of metatarsals and rays do pose additional risk of angular growth deformities if not resected. Many find the extranumerary toe to eventually cause shoe irritation.

POLYDACTYLY PEARLS

- Most incisions can be elliptical in nature around the toe and carried out dorsally to remove any duplicated metatarsal.
- It is important to obtain hemostasis in the operating room as any void secondary to ray resections or toe amputations may lead to hematomas.
- Surgery is not advised in children <12 months of age given anesthesia and recurrence risks. If the soft cartilaginous structures are left behind and growth continues, it may lead to a subsequent surgery.
- Radiographic evaluation is key in determining which digit or portion of ray should be removed. Often, one attempts to preserve the most normal-appearing toe. The most normal-appearing toe is not always the most lateral or medial toe. In these situations, the incision is not elliptical since a more central ray is excised.

Syndactyly

Syndactyly of toes is a common inherited condition in which there is cutaneous webbing. The webbing may be complete or incomplete in nature. Quite often the second and third toes

are conjoined. While this condition often causes parental anxiety and a consultation, the child often remains asymptomatic. For this reason, the authors do not advise desyndactylization unless pain and/or functional deficits exist secondary to syndactyly of the digits.

Syndactyly can be classified into two types (Fig. 54.10). Type 1 (zygosyndactyly) is a cutaneous webbing only. This condition is likely to not cause any shoe fitting problems or functional deficits. As for type 2 (polysyndactyly), this may cause some symptoms in children. Polysyndactyly is a more complex sequel of failure of differentiation of the apical ectodermal ridge during the first trimester.[19] The fourth and fifth toes are often conjoined with a postaxial duplicated fifth toe. The child often has a duplicated nail plate as well. With growth, some children do experience pain with shoe gear secondary to the increased width of the foot. The duplicated nail plate (synonychia) can also become inflamed causing pain or infections in young children. With symptomatic polysyndactyly, the duplicated toe and/or ray is removed. It is important to educate parents that it is often not the simple webbing that causes problems with development.

SYNDACTYLY PEARLS

- Syndactyly in the absence of polydactyly often remains asymptomatic.
- Desyndactylization carries risk including skin necrosis, loss of toe, and infection.

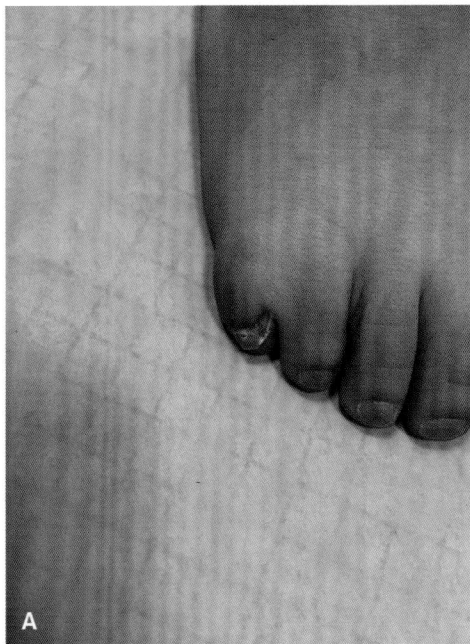

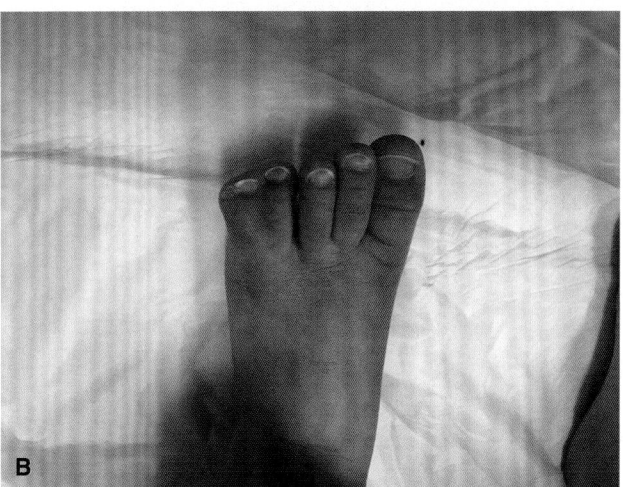

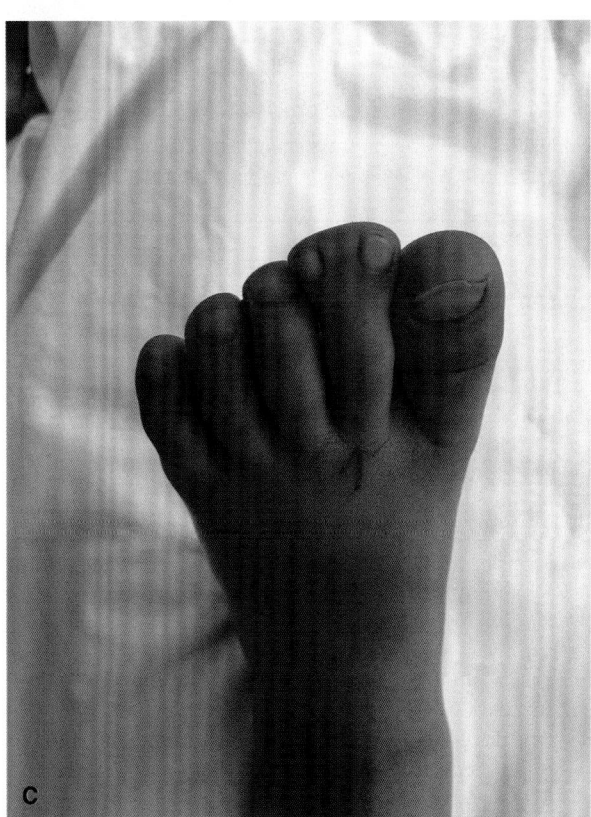

FIGURE 54.10 Syndactyly of toes. **A.** Zygosyndactyly or simple webbing. **B.** Polysyndactyly. **C.** Duplicated distal portion of the second toe.

Macrodactyly

Macrodactyly is a rare congenital deformity of the hands and feet characterized by the enlargement of soft tissue and osseous elements of the digit (Fig. 54.11).[20] The condition may occur as a part of a syndrome, such as Klippel-Trenaunay-Weber, *Proteus*, neurofibromatosis, or as an isolated phenomenon.[21] The etiology of the deformity is unknown, though some studies implicate hyperinduction of a neurotrophic mechanism responsible for normal pedal growth.[22] Slight male predilection has been noted.[23] Second and third digits are affected most often.[23] The enlargement of the bony phalanges and accumulation of the fibrofatty tissue defines the deformity.

Two forms of the deformity exist. In the first, the toes are enlarged in proportion to a hypertrophied foot, while the other presents with toes enlarged as compared to the rest of the foot. The amount of soft tissue involvement may be monitored via the metatarsal spread angle. The axes of the first and fifth metatarsals on an anteroposterior (AP) x-ray form this angle.[24] This angle may be compared to the contralateral foot. Shoe gear fitting problems can exist for both forms of macrodactyly and unfortunately obtaining a cosmetically acceptable foot is very challenging. Quite often this cannot be obtained.

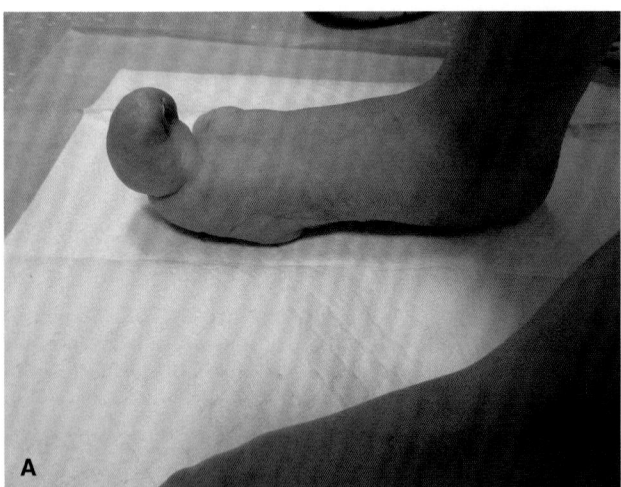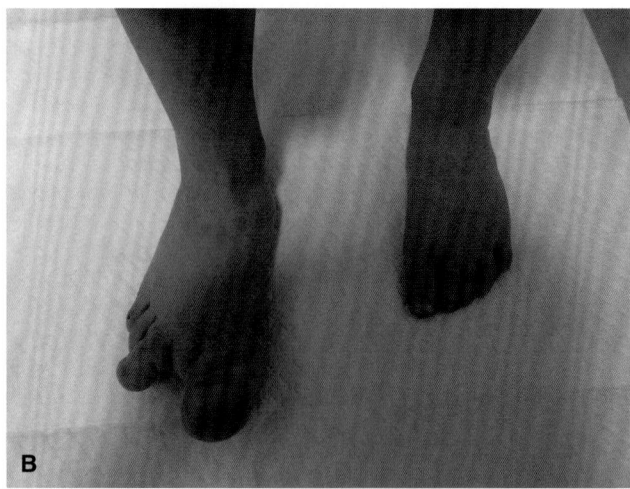

FIGURE 54.11 **A, B.** A 5-year-old male with macrodactyly.

Surgical options are utilized to promote improved function and to reduce pain. Reconstruction can be achieved by epiphysiodesis, amputation, resection of phalanges, or partial ray resections.[25] Debulking procedures may be used in conjunction with the above while is often not helpful when executed alone. Parents must be educated that many of these procedures rely on the child's available growth for the unaffected toes and structures to obtain further length and size. While length may be affected with epiphysiodesis, the girth of the toe will likely remain enlarged. As one can imagine, the cosmetic appearance of the foot is a continuous complaint.

MACRODACTYLY PEARLS

- Indications for digit-sparing procedures, however, may be limited to mild cases of static macrodactyly.
- A functional amputation remains the most definitive procedure.
- Ray resections may be recommended when one toe is grossly enlarged.

MACRODACTYLY PITFALLS

- Macrodactyly of the first ray remains a perplexing surgical problem.
- Hypertrophic tissue can regenerate after debulking.
- Delayed wound healing and bleeding from surgical site is common.
- In patients with Klippel-Trenaunay-Weber syndrome, local gigantism, hemangiomas, and venous varicosities surgery places child at increased risks for infection, wound healing problems, bleeding, and poor cosmesis.

Varus Fifth Toe

A varus fifth toe is present a birth and likely attributed to genetics. The fifth toe is noted to be overlapping the fourth toe in a dorsiflexed and adducted manner (Fig. 54.12). The toenail itself is more laterally deviated and remains a source of irritation in shoes. The authors find this deformity to be often bilateral in presentation and one in which treatment is surgical.[26,27]

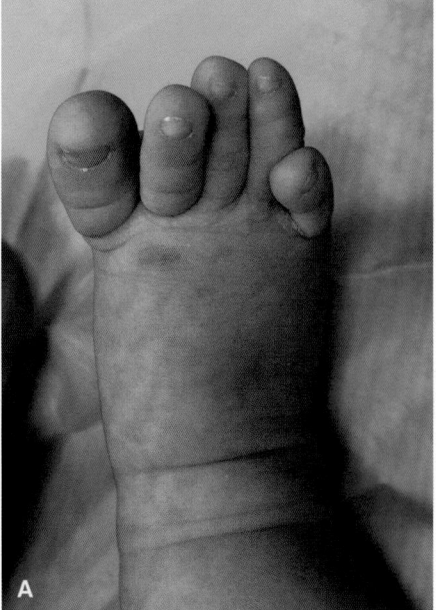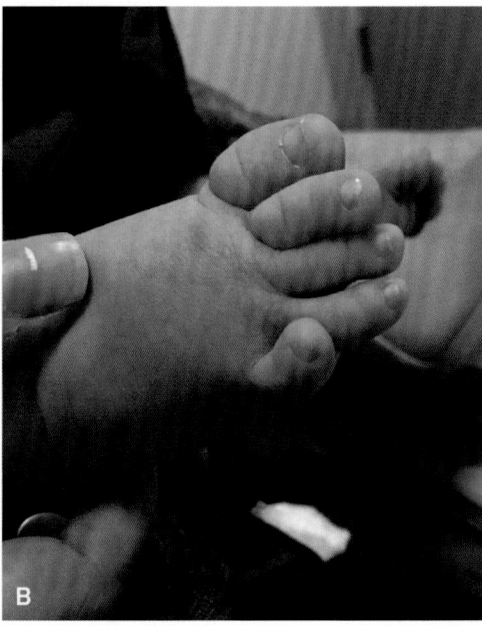

FIGURE 54.12 **A, B.** Varus overlapping fifth toe in a 3-month-old male.

For children under the age of 2, manipulation and gentle stretching may be utilized while has not proven to be successful at long-term deformity reduction. The authors have used casting to reduce this deformity in infants with good success. Plaster is used and must be molded correctly to stretch the toe. Children over the age of 2 who have pain or shoe gear complaints associated with deformity may progress toward surgery. Many children do require surgery given the challenges of shoe gear with such deformity. The Butler procedure is most typically utilized. A racquet-shaped incision is fashioned to allow for circumferential release. The extensor tendon and entire dorsal capsule is released. One is often concerned at the end of this procedure, as the fifth toe remains white for a while. This does take time for the color of the toe to improve over 24 hours. Cooling techniques should be avoided postoperatively.

Figure Butler Procedure

VARUS FIFTH TOE PEARLS

- Treatment is surgical.
- Butler procedure: release of dorsal MPJ capsule, tenotomy of extensor digitorum longus tendon, circumferential incision around the base of the fifth MPJ, dorsal and plantar longitudinal extensions.[28-30]
- McFarland procedure: extensor tenotomy, dorsal and medial capsulotomy of the fifth MPJ, proximal phalangectomy, and syndactylization of the fourth and fifth toes.[31]

VARUS FIFTH TOE PITFALLS

- Recurrence after soft tissue release may occur. A proximal phalangectomy may be indicated at this time.
- Vascular compromise, necrosis of tissue, and loss of digit can arise.

Longitudinal Epiphyseal Bracket

A longitudinal epiphyseal bracket is a congenital condition in which the epiphysis is continuous from distal to proximal along the medial aspect of the phalanx or first metatarsal. Historically, this condition was termed a delta phalanx for its U configuration and abnormal growth.[32] Growth of the abnormal epiphysis leads to a shortened, wide, and often triangular or trapezoidal bone. Etiology is not completely understood yet thought to be a failure of proper fetal formation of the primary ossification centers from the apical ectodermal ridge.[33,34] Many children present with coexisting deformities such as polydactyly, syndactyly, or coalitions. Others may present with Apert syndrome. An MRI is most helpful at diagnosis of a longitudinal epiphyseal bracket (Fig. 54.13).

LONGITUDINAL EPIPHYSEAL BRACKET PEARLS

- Treatment is surgical often between 6 and 24 months of age.
- In infants, the deformity may not be seen on x-rays, but it will be visible on MRI.[35]
- Surgery: resection of the abnormal longitudinal section of the epiphysis, preserve the transverse extensions of the epiphysis proximally and distally, possible interposition of polymethylmethacrylate or fat, osteotomy with bone graft of the affected bone to assist with length and angular deformity. Pinning of the first ray is often performed with removal at 6 weeks.
- Mubarak et al. demonstrated improved longitudinal growth in the first metatarsal after surgery.[35]

LONGITUDINAL EPIPHYSEAL BRACKET PITFALLS

- Inappropriate graft positioning may lead to deformity often in the form of a plantarflexed or dorsiflexed metatarsal.
- Angular deformity of the metatarsal phalangeal joint can arise.
- Look for coexisting deformities such as polydactyly, syndactyly, and tarsal coalitions.

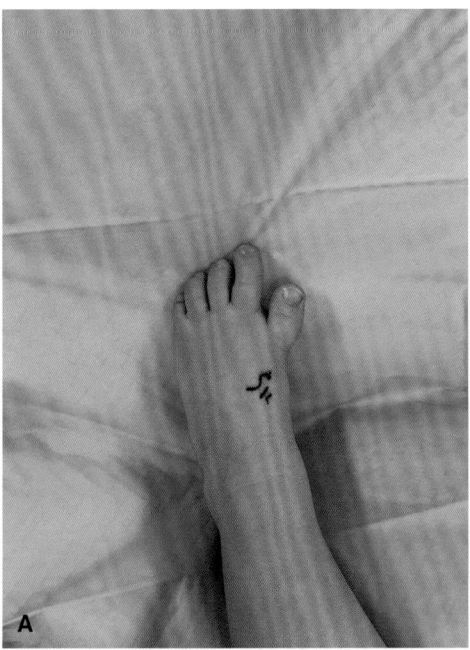

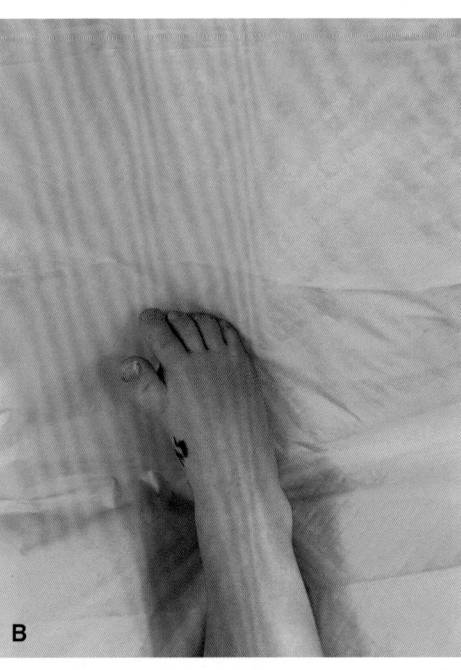

FIGURE 54.13 Surgical resection of longitudinal epiphyseal bracket and application of graft. **A, B.** Preoperative clinical photos.

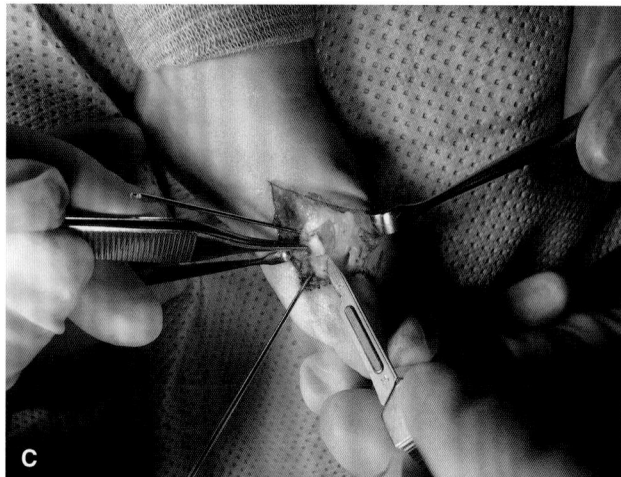

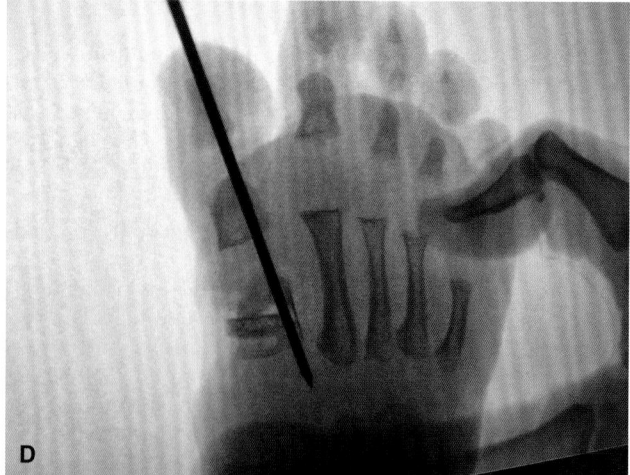

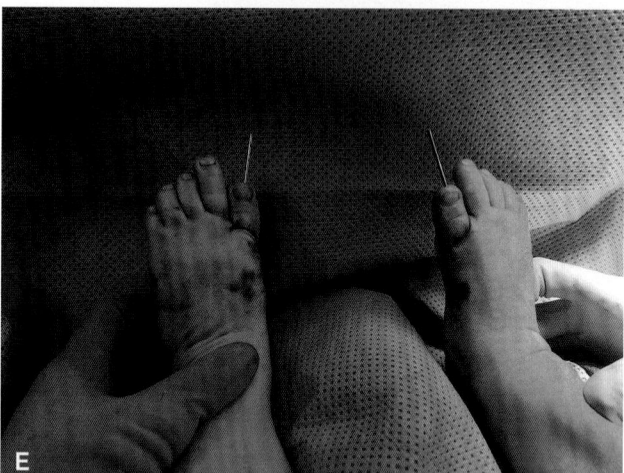

FIGURE 54.13 (*Continued*) **C.** Surgical excision of longitudinal epiphyseal bracket. **D, E.** Pinning following osseous graft application.

Subungual Exostosis

Subungual exostosis is a benign bone growth deep to the nail, which causes pain and toenail dystrophy (Fig. 54.14). At times, the nail becomes so traumatized by the bone growth that it falls off and the bone growth becomes visually apparent. Bone growth tends to involve the dorsomedial aspect of the distal phalanx with the hallux most typically affected.[36]

Symptoms often include pain and toenail irritation leading to surgical excision. As this condition progresses, one may lose complete soft tissue or nail bed coverage of the exostosis, which makes surgical coverage of the distal phalanx difficult in nature. In some instances, the child must heal secondarily and granulate over the phalanx. Treatment is toenail removal with excision of the abnormal bone growth and repair of available nail bed. Recurrence risks are higher if the exostosis is not fully resected initially.

> ## SUBUNGUAL EXOSTOSIS PEARLS
> - Exostosis is trabecular bone capped by fibrocartilage.
> - An osteochondroma is capped with hyaline cartilage.[37]
> - Osteochondromas are the most common bone tumor of the foot.[37]
> - Saucerization: use of a high-speed burr to saucerize the cancellous bone following excision of the abnormal bone growth is advised.

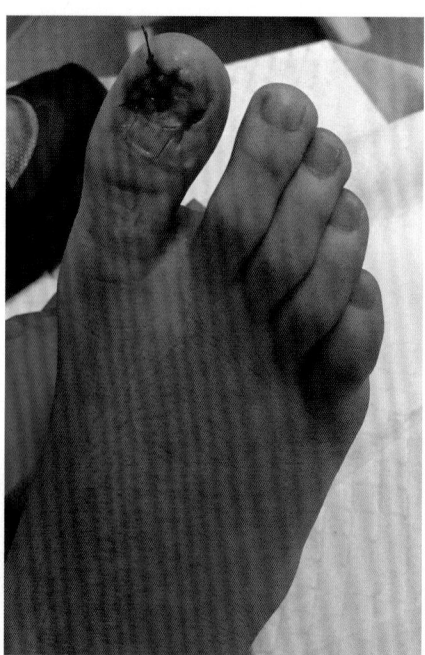

FIGURE 54.14 Subungual exostosis. Status postexcision demonstrating a lack of tissue available to close.

Metatarsus Adductus

Any deformity that is associated with intoeing tends to cause concern and fear among parents. Many parents note a visual deformity of the foot at birth yet quite often flexible metatarsus adductus is overlooked. Upon inspection, metatarsus adductus produces medial deviation of metatarsals at the level of the tarsometatarsal joint. The infant's foot may appear to have a slightly higher arch with a valgus rearfoot and medially deviated metatarsals. Equinus is not present.

In a screening of 2401 neonates, Widhe and associates noted foot abnormalities in 4% of infants, with 1% having metatarsus adductus.[38] 0.7% of infants had calcaneovalgus. Wynne-Davies found an incidence of metatarsus adductus of 1 in 1000 births and reported that if 1 child were affected, the risk of deformity in a second child in the same family was 1 in 20.[39] This alludes to a genetic component, while etiology is not completely understood.

It is important to distinguish metatarsus adductus from clubfoot. Equinus and varus of the heel does not exist with metatarsus adductus. Whereas Ponseti casting is employed for clubfoot despite degree of stiffness, one must closely evaluate degree of flexibility of metatarsus adductus to determine treatment. If the deformity is flexible hence easily reducible, one may closely monitor. This flexible type may reduce when the foot is stimulated into active eversion. Often, these deformities will resolve gradually. Parents may be reassured and educated on how to gently stretch the foot.

There is debate over the semirigid metatarsus adductus foot deformity. Many physicians do not advocate for casting this group, while others will cast to reduce the deformity. Braces utilized at night often follow casting. If the foot type is rigid and the deformity cannot be reduced, then casting is advised to assist with serial correction over time. Still this diagnosis always sparks debate over treatment with many questioning how much metatarsus adductus is pathologic as an adult.

In a 7-year follow-up of 130 untreated feet, Rushforth found that 10% had moderate deformity but were asymptomatic and that only 4% had residual deformity and stiffness.[40] Long-term research would be beneficial in furthering our knowledge on this deformity and its effects into adulthood.

Proper manipulation of the deformity is key in creating a supple rectus foot. One holds the heel in neutral position while the forefoot is abducted. Counter pressure is applied to the cuboid, so the abduction occurs at the level of the tarsometatarsal complex. This is the same gentle stretch that parents may perform at home. The authors often encourage stretching with diaper changes if advised. For the flexible and easily reducible deformity, one does not have to cast as this often improves with time. With semirigid and rigid metatarsus adductus, the authors recommend casting to gently manipulate the foot into a more rectus position (Fig. 54.15). Care should be taken to not evert the forefoot when casting. For a child under 6 months, a short leg cast with soft/nonrigid casting material may be used while plaster if utilized provides for an improved mold. One may alternatively prefer a long leg cast with a bent knee. In older children between 6 months and 3 years of age, one may also utilize casting to minimize the deformity.

If the foot is resistant to casting and the deformity remains severe, then surgical intervention is advised. Often, this rigid foot type has a significant medial crease and overactive abductor hallucis. Hence, surgical intervention includes release of the abductor hallucis, capsulotomy of the first tarsometatarsal joint, and serial cast correction.[41] The authors find these soft tissue procedures to be more typically executed between 2.5 and 4 years of age. Osseous procedures are often reserved for children 8 years of age or older. This often includes either midfoot osteotomies or metatarsal osteotomies with or without soft tissue release. Surgery is dependent on both severity and stiffness of deformity.

Authors' Preferred Method for Casting

- Long leg casting as described by Dr. Ponseti for metatarsus adductus.
- After casting, a shoe and bar brace is worn at nighttime until 2 years of age.

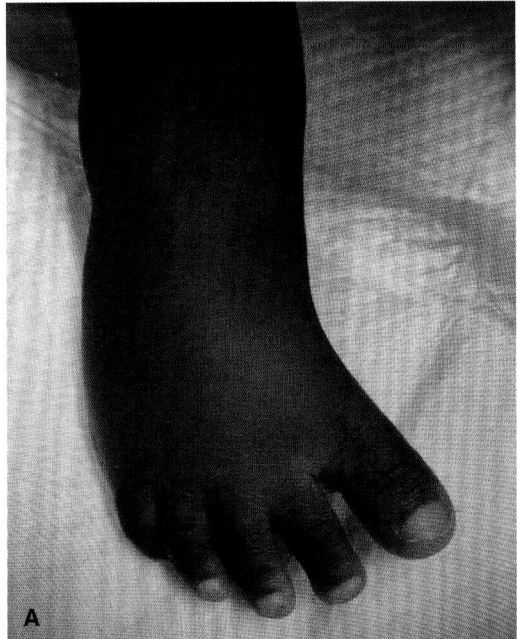 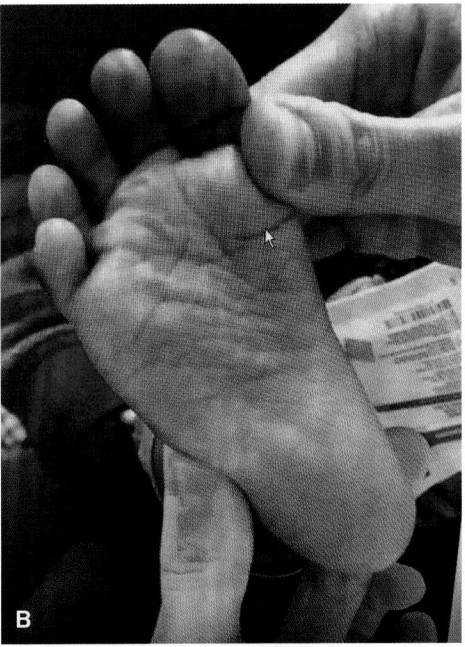

FIGURE 54.15 Metatarsus adductus semirigid presentation undergoing serial casting. **A.** Clinical presentation before casting. **B.** Reducible with force.

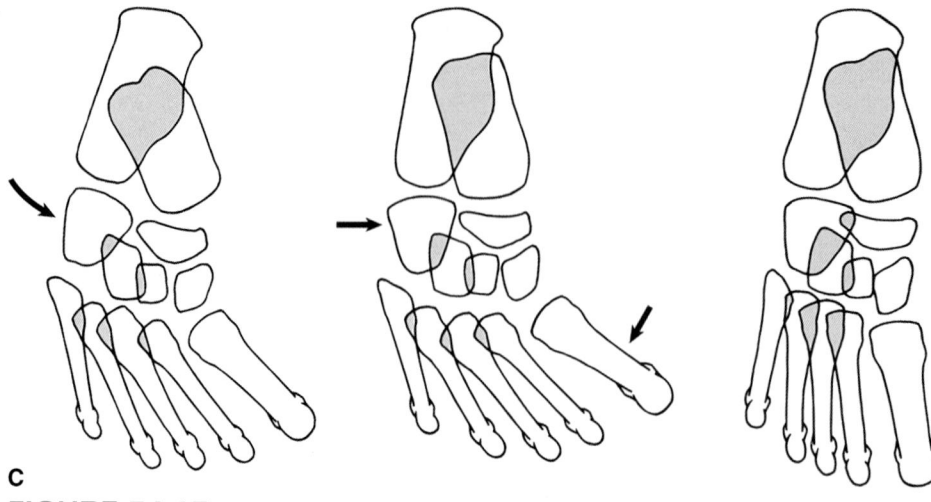

C

FIGURE 54.15 (*Continued*) **C.** Manipulation for metatarsus adductus.

METATARSUS ADDUCTUS PEARLS

- Flexible deformity: monitor and instruct parents on stretching maneuvers.
- Rigid deformity: serial casting advised followed by shoe and bar brace for sleep.
- May use soft casting material for serial casting. Benefits include fewer risks of wound development and greater parent satisfaction. Plaster provides an improved mold.
- Maneuver: hold the heel in neutral, apply counter pressure to the cuboid, and abduct the forefoot.
- 2.5- to 4-year-old children who fail casting: consider abductor hallucis release, capsulotomy of the first tarsometatarsal joint, and subsequent casting.
- Older children: may consider Heyman-Herndon release, metatarsal osteotomies, or opening wedge osteotomy of the medial cuneiform/closing osteotomy of cuboid.
- It is important to perform a hip examination and confirm no dislocatable or dislocated hip is present. In the presence of metatarsus adductus and breech position, a hip ultrasound can be helpful in excluding infant hip pathology.

METATARSUS ADDUCTUS PITFALLS

- Eversion of the forefoot can cause unwanted deformity. Care should be taken to use the cuboid or CC joint as the fulcrum. If the talus is used, this also results in excessive hindfoot valgus.
- It is important to differentiate from congenital skewfoot.
- We do not fully understand how much metatarsus adductus is pathologic in adulthood.

Brachymetatarsia

Brachymetatarsia can be defined by the presence of an unusually shortened metatarsal. This is a congenital deformity, which does not always manifest in pain. Many patients present with complaints of poor cosmesis. It is important that the clinician discern which patient truly has pain or lesser metatarsalgia as compared to others with asymptomatic cosmetic complaints. This is important as the surgical intervention for correction carries risk of necrosis, tissue loss, digital loss, and need for amputation.

Pathologic brachymetatarsia often presents as pain plantar to the adjacent metatarsal heads as compared to the plantar aspect of the shortened metatarsal itself. The fourth metatarsal is often the shortened metatarsal with pain beneath the third and/or fifth metatarsal heads. One may note a subluxation of the metatarsal phalangeal joint hence a floating toe. Of surgical note, the length of the shortened metatarsal needed to restore a more normal parabola must be assessed.

Conservative care includes rigid supportive shoes complimented by custom orthoses to off-load the metatarsal heads. Beyond this, there is not a plethora of options outside of surgical intervention. Surgery is dependent on the length of the metatarsal needed to restore the metatarsal parabola. Compliance also plays a special role with these surgical candidates especially when external fixation is considered.

When 1-1.5 cm of length is needed, one may consider a one-stage procedure in which an osteotomy of the metatarsal is fashioned and a graft is inserted. Stable internal fixation is utilized to secure the graft in place. Care is taken to not compress the graft. One should gradually distract the osteotomy prior to graft placement in the operating room with a deflated tourniquet. The patient is nonweight bearing for a minimum of 6-8 weeks. When more length is desired, callus distraction and use of external fixation is executed. The patient must be compliant and understand the directions with callus distraction or else the results can be catastrophic.

The principles of callus distraction are key. Two pins are inserted on either side of the osteotomy. A pin guide and/or the external fixator frame may be utilized. The osteotomy is performed in the proximal metaphysis of the shortened metatarsal. If the osteotomy is performed in the proximal metaphysis, distraction is typically started at ~7 days by use of a monorail. The rate and amount of distraction has been debated. Still the rate of 0.25 mm every 6 hours for a total of 1 mm a day has shown to produce more predictable bone remodeling. Histologic repair is ongoing and should not be stopped despite the radiographic lucency that often appears. One should continue with callus distraction until the desired length is achieved. The external fixator is left intact until osseous consolidation, which may be the time equivalent it took to obtain length. Hence, if it took 4 weeks to obtain length, the external fixator may be needed for a total length of 8 weeks. The authors find the external fixator frame is needed for a minimum of 4 weeks following desirable length.

BRACHYMETATARSIA PEARLS

- Callus distraction facilitates gradual lengthening of bone and provides sufficient time for the soft tissue to adapt.
- Place pins prior to osteotomy. Pins should be bicortical and parallel to one another. Use the external fixator as a guide for proper placement to avoid angulation. The latent period is generally 7 days prior to distraction.
- Turn 0.25 mm every 6 hours per day to equal 1 mm/day.
- Smaller frequent turning intervals result in efficient osteogenesis.
- The osteotomy should be perpendicular to the metatarsal.
- Pins attached to the external fixator or a K-wire may be utilized in the digit itself to alter alignment.

BRACHYMETATARSIA PITFALLS

- Overlengthening of the metatarsal results in dislocation of the metatarsal phalangeal joint.
- Necrosis, ulceration, vasospasm, ischemic changes, loss of toe remain risks of surgery.
- Angular deformities may occur secondary to poor pin placement or osteotomy.
- Patients may be displeased with surgical outcome, as the phalanx may still appear short despite surgical lengthening of the metatarsal. It is important to address expectations of the patient prior to any surgical intervention.

Talipes Equinovarus (Clubfoot)

Please refer to Chapter 53 Talipes Equinovarus by same authors.

Congenital Vertical Talus (Congenital Convex Pes Valgus)

In infancy, this rare deformity often resembles calcaneovalgus or a severe planovalgus foot type. Although the exact incidence of vertical talus is unknown, the estimated prevalence is 1 in 10 000 live births.[42] Due to the hindfoot valgus, equinus, and fixed dorsal dislocation of the navicular on the talus, many have referred to this deformity as a rocker-bottom flatfoot. Despite these findings, it is the rigidity of the deformity and true equinus that distinguishes itself from others such as positional calcaneovalgus or an oblique talus. A true congenital vertical talus cannot be easily reduced nor passively corrected. The condition is defined by its inability to reduce, or in essence rigidity, along with equinus. In fact, it is recommended that an oblique talus in the setting of equinus be treated as a vertical talus. Recognition of this deformity is key as without treatment vertical talus can lead to significant disability.[43]

Unfortunately, the condition is often not recognized in newborns because of the difficulty in differentiating it from other, more common benign positional foot anomalies. Without treatment, vertical talus can lead to pain and disability that hampers daily activities and leads to a more sedentary lifestyle. Traditional surgical management for vertical talus is invasive and fraught with both short-term and long-term complications. These complications include both undercorrection and overcorrection of the deformity, scaring, neurovascular injury, infection, wound dehiscence, and the need for multiple surgical procedures during growth. The scar tissue created with extensive soft tissue releases in a child's foot can lead to stiffness and pain over time, which has been shown to be true for both

vertical talus and clubfoot. A minimally invasive alternative has proved successful in providing correction while avoiding the need for extensive soft tissue release procedures.

In most cases, the etiology of vertical talus deformity remains unknown. Approximately one-half of cases of vertical talus occur in conjunction with neurologic disorders[44] or genetic defects and/or syndromes.[45] The remaining children present with further congenital anomalies and are considered idiopathic or isolated cases.[43] The most common neurologic disorders associated with vertical talus are distal arthrogryposis and myelomeningocele.[44] The most common genetic defects include aneuploidy of chromosomes 13, 15, and 18.[46] New insight is gained into pathogenesis from the discovery that mutations in the PITX1-TBX4-HOXC transcriptional pathways cause familial clubfoot and vertical talus in a small number of families.[47] Syndromes associated with vertical talus include De Barsy, Costello, and Rasmussen syndromes.[48] Finally, of the 50% of cases of vertical talus that are isolated, almost 20% have a positive family history of vertical talus.

In most of the isolated cases, the condition is inherited in an autosomal dominant fashion. This supports a significant number of isolated cases have a genetic etiology.[49] Still, while no one single gene defect has been held accountable of all cases of vertical talus, its etiology is heterogeneous. For example, in patients with myelomeningocele, a weak posterior tibialis muscle with strong ankle dorsiflexors could contribute to the deformity. Weakness of the foot intrinsics may play a role for other children with neurologic influence. Children with abnormal muscle biopsies such as arthrogryposis may be prone to vertical talus given skeletal muscle abnormalities.[45] Congenital vascular insufficiency of the lower extremities has also been proposed as a potential cause of vertical talus based on magnetic resonance angiography findings that demonstrated congenital arterial deficiencies of the lower extremity in a group of patients with vertical talus.[50] Beyond its etiology, early detection is helpful in reduction of deformity and overall outcomes.

Pathoanatomy

The hindfoot is in equinus and valgus as a result of contracture of the Achilles tendon and the posterolateral ankle and subtalar joint capsules. The midfoot and forefoot are dorsiflexed and abducted secondary to contractures of the tibialis anterior, extensor digitorum longus, extensor hallucis brevis, peroneus tertius and brevis, and extensor hallucis longus tendons as well as the dorsolateral aspect of the talonavicular capsule. The navicular is dorsally and laterally dislocated on the head of the talus, resulting in the development of a hypoplastic and wedge-shaped navicular. Both the talar head and neck are abnormal in shape and orientation. The position of the talus stretches vertically and weakens the plantar soft tissues, including the spring ligament, giving the foot a rocker-bottom appearance. The rigid equinus in the hindfoot is often accompanied by either dorsolateral subluxation or frank dorsal dislocation of the calcaneocuboid joint. The posterior tibial tendon and the peroneus longus and brevis are commonly subluxated anteriorly over the medial and lateral malleolus, respectively; the subluxated tendons then function as ankle dorsiflexors rather than plantar flexors.

Clinical Features

Hindfoot equinus, hindfoot valgus, forefoot abduction, and forefoot dorsiflexion are present in all patients with vertical talus. The rigidity of the deformities is the key to differentiating vertical talus from the more common and less severe conditions, such as calcaneovalgus foot, posteromedial bowing of

the tibia, and oblique talus (without an equinus contracture). A quick and easy clinical examination finding is testing for tendo Achilles contracture. This must be done with subtalar joint inverted. If ankle dorsiflexion is not limited, then the deformity is not vertical talus and is likely positional in nature. Because of the frequency of neuromuscular and genetic abnormalities associated with vertical talus, it is important to perform a complete and careful physical examination of the entire patient. The clinician should look for facial dysmorphic features that require a referral to a clinical geneticist or abnormalities suggestive of a neuromuscular etiology, which would require MRI evaluation of the neuroaxis and referral to a pediatric neurologist. The presence of a sacral dimple, in particular, should alert the examiner to possible central nervous system anomalies.

It is of upmost importance for the examiner to document the ability of the child to dorsiflex and plantar flex the toes. This is done by stimulating the plantar and dorsal aspects of the foot. This should be done on multiple occasions during the early treatment stage because the examination can be difficult, and results from serial examinations are more accurate. The presence of dorsiflexion and plantar flexion of the toes is recorded as absent, slight, or definitive. This should be recorded for the great toe alone as well as the lesser toes as a separate group. In our experience, slight or absent ability to move the toes with stimulation correlates with a vertical talus deformity that is more rigid and less responsive to treatment. It may also be indicative of a congenital neurologic or muscular anomaly.

Clinically, a congenital vertical talus foot has a convex plantar surface that results in a rocker-bottom appearance. The skin on the dorsum of the foot has a crease secondary to forefoot and midfoot dorsiflexion. The extreme dorsiflexion of the forefoot creates a gap dorsally where the navicular and talar head would articulate in a normal foot. If the gap reduces with plantar flexion of the forefoot, then the deformity has a degree of flexibility and may fall on the spectrum of oblique talus. This is important to assess because even if the talonavicular reduces in plantar flexion indicating an oblique talus, this does not mean that treatment is not needed. In this situation, the examiner must then assess for contracture of the Achilles tendon with the subtalar joint inverted. In our experience, oblique tali that have a contracture of the Achilles tendon need treatment just like true vertical tali.

Imaging
While x-rays are not indicated routinely in the management of clubfoot, they are useful in the diagnosis of vertical talus. The obliquity of the talus is apparent on x-rays and is almost in line with the longitudinal axis of the tibia in the sagittal plane. A stress plantar flexion lateral radiograph demonstrates that the navicular remains dorsally dislocated upon the talar head in vertical talus. It is important to remember that the navicular does not ossify until 2.5-5 years of age. Hence, in a vertical talus, the longitudinal axis of the talus fails to align with the longitudinal axis of the first metatarsal in a lateral radiograph when manually plantar flexed. The talus remains vertical as compared to the first metatarsal. On the lateral view of the foot in plantar flexion, the lateral talar axis-first metatarsal base angle (TAMBA) can be used as one criterion to help distinguish vertical talus from oblique talus. Values >35 degrees have been considered diagnostic for vertical talus.[51] However, vertical talus cannot be ruled out with values <35 degrees. In such cases, the presence of or absence of hindfoot equinus must be documented to distinguish between vertical talus and oblique talus. It can be difficult to differentiate those oblique tali that need

treatment from those that do not based on radiographs alone. In oblique tali, the talonavicular joint reduces in plantar flexion, but this does not necessarily mean treatment is not needed. In these situations, a careful clinical examination must be done to test for the presence or absence of hindfoot equinus by dorsiflexing the ankle with the subtalar joint inverted. If equinus is present, then the deformity is rigid and warrants treatment in the same manner as vertical talus. Left alone the oblique tali with tight tendo Achilles often present in adolescence as painful flatfeet with short Achilles tendon.

Classification
Current classification systems for vertical talus are purely descriptive and not prognostic in nature. The problem with this is that it does not have a dynamic component to account for motor strength in the lower legs. In our experience, weak or absent motor function in the lower leg musculature is predictive of not only poor response to initial treatment but also a risk of relapse. The child's ability to dorsiflex and plantar flex the toes can be evaluated by lightly stimulating the dorsal and plantar aspects of the foot. Movement can be graded as definitive, slight, or absent. This simple examination can be repeated at each clinical visit to improve accuracy. A new classification system that takes this into account is needed because the ability to better predict the response to treatment will allow for the development of an individualized treatment program for patients.

It should also be noted that current classification systems have attempted to define oblique talus as a milder form of vertical talus based on radiographic and clinical examination criteria. However, these attempts at classification have not translated into consistent treatment recommendations because some oblique tali do require treatment despite being milder in nature. In our experience, oblique tali that have an associated Achilles tendon contracture are at risk of becoming symptomatic with time. For this reason, we consider oblique tali and vertical tali to be related entities that occur along a spectrum of severity.

Vertical Talus Imaging
- *Stress plantar flexion x-ray (standard of care):* in vertical talus, the talus fails to align with the first metatarsal. The talus remains vertical when compared to the first metatarsal. In infancy, the navicular is not visible. One focuses on the talus with respect to the first metatarsal. An oblique talus or calcaneovalgus will realign or essentially reduce.
- *Neutral lateral x-ray:* in vertical talus, the long axis of the talus is vertical when compared to the first metatarsal. The calcaneus is in equinus.
- *Stress dorsiflexion x-ray:* persistent rigid hindfoot equinus is noted with vertical talus.

While vertical talus is nonreducible requiring serial casting to manipulate the foot into an improved position, calcaneovalgus remains flexible in nature (Fig. 54.16). Goals of relocating the talonavicular joint and alleviating equinus are key. Over the years, many methods of surgical treatment have been discussed, while the basic principles of reduction remain the same. The talonavicular dislocation must be reduced and stabilized. The hindfoot equinus must be alleviated to restore a normal talocalcaneal relationship. Lastly, the forefoot that is everted and in calcaneus should be corrected and stabilized upon a corrected hindfoot.

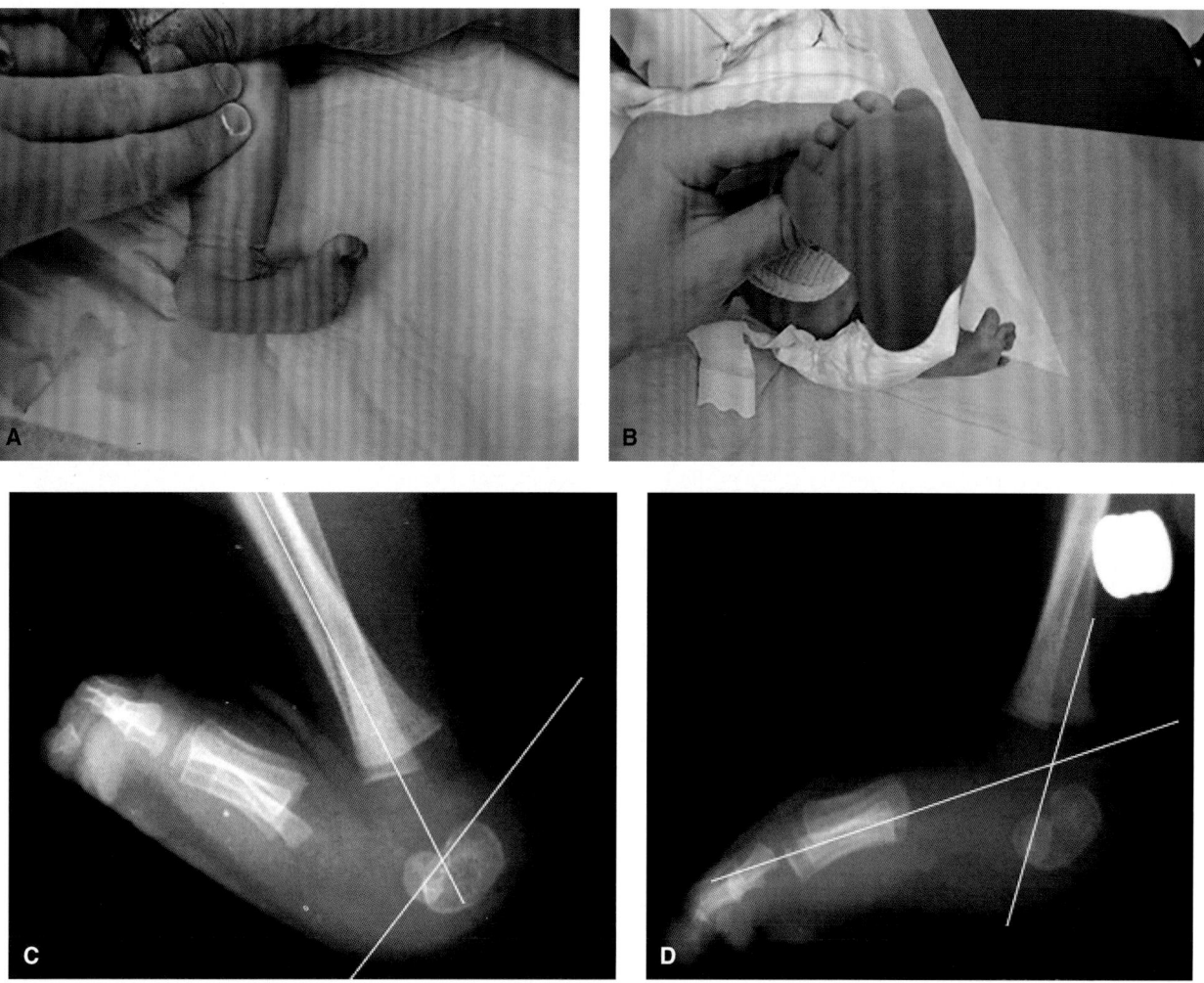

FIGURE 54.16 **A, B.** Vertical talus clinical photos. **C.** Lateral x-ray demonstrating vertical talus. **D.** Stress lateral plantar flexion x-ray demonstrating vertical talus.

As Ignacio Ponseti, MD, pioneered the method for serial casting and deformity correction for clubfoot without aggressive surgical releases, Matthew B Dobbs, MD, has essentially done the same for the treatment of vertical talus. Historically, large releases for this deformity were performed with persistent risks of stiffness, diminished function, and pain. The Dobbs method is a minimally invasive approach that relies on serial manipulation and casting. Achieving correction without extensive surgery leads to more functional and flexible feet.[43] With the retracting fibrosis and abundance of collagen that forms, it is advantageous to avoid large releases at an early age and approach reduction from a less invasive standpoint. While the majority of deformity correction is the result of manipulation and casting, the child does undergo at least an Achilles tenotomy and talonavicular joint pinning upon reduction.

Following tenotomy and talonavicular pinning, the foot is casted and monitored closely over the next 6 weeks following surgery. The wire is then removed in the operating room or office and the child transitions to a shoe and bar brace. The foot is held in a straight position. Shoe and bar braces are utilized until the child is 2 years of age. The authors use the abduction bar, designed by Dr. Dobbs, as there is no

dorsiflexion bend in it unlike the Ponseti bar. It is important not to brace in dorsiflexion, as the feet are most tight dorsolateral. Since the introduction of the Dobbs method in 2006,[52,53] many subsequent studies have demonstrated its efficacy in achieving initial correction in patients with isolated or nonisolated vertical talus.[54-62]

Traditional management involved lengthening the contracted dorsolateral tendons, dorsolateral capsular contractures, and reducing both the talonavicular joint and subtalar joint. Lengthening both the Achilles and peroneals along with performing a posterolateral capsulotomy followed.[63] Many performed all procedures in a single-stage approach.[64-69] Extensive surgical release is not necessary for most cases of vertical talus, as good results have been achieved with a minimally invasive approach that emphasizes serial manipulation and casting.[43]

To perform this manipulation, the treating provider must have knowledge of the subtalar joint and experience in treating clubfoot with manipulation and casting. The ability to accurately locate the talar head is essential. All components of the deformity are corrected simultaneously except for the hindfoot equinus, which is corrected with release of the Achilles.

Dobbs Method for Manipulation and Casting[43,52]

- Manipulations are gentle and consist of stretching the foot into plantar flexion with one hand, while counterpressure is applied as the thumb of the opposite hand gently pushes the talus dorsally and laterally (from the medial side of the foot).
- Do not touch the calcaneus. The calcaneus needs to glide smoothly beneath the talus from its valgus position.
- After 1-2 minutes of manipulation, a long leg plaster cast is applied to hold the foot into this manipulated position. The cast is applied in two sections, with the short leg portion applied first. This allows for an appropriate mold of the foot.
- The foot should be held in position achieved by stretching while an assistant rolls the plaster.
- Mold carefully around the talar head, malleoli, and above the calcaneus posteriorly.
- Remove excess plaster dorsally to expose the toes.
- The cast is then extended above the knee with knee in 90 degrees of flexion.
- Weekly casting is advised. An average of five casts is utilized to reduce the deformity. Hindfoot equinus still persists. In the final cast, the foot resembles a clubfoot. This position is critical to maximally stretch the dorsolateral soft tissues so you should achieve maximal equinovarus. This is analogous to achieving 70 degrees of external rotation in final clubfoot cast.
- When reduction of the talonavicular and calcaneocuboid joints is achieved, the child is scheduled for surgery.

Authors' Preferred Method[43,52]: Vertical Talus

- Serial manipulation and casting to improve the talonavicular and hindfoot alignment as described in the Dobbs method for manipulation and casting.
- When reduction is achieved, a small dorsal medial incision is fashioned over the talonavicular joint. The surgeon confirms reduction of talonavicular joint.
- If the joint is not completely reduced, a small capsulotomy is made in the anterior subtalar joint region to allow an elevator to be placed. This assists with talonavicular reduction.
- A K-wire is placed in retrograde fashion across the talonavicular joint.
- We recommend burying the wire to minimize migration of hardware especially in the child young.
- Rarely, the peroneus brevis, tibialis anterior, and/or dorsal extensor tendons are contracted after manipulation/casting. In severe nonisolated vertical talus, the tendons may still be contracted and lengthening is advised.
- Upon stabilization of the talonavicular joint, an Achilles tenotomy is performed.
- A long leg cast is applied with the ankle and foot in neutral position.
- The cast is changed 2 weeks postsurgery to manipulate the ankle to 10 degrees of dorsiflexion.

- The K-wire is removed in the operating room at 6 weeks postsurgery. A final cast is applied for 1 week followed by boot and bar brace system 24 hours per day for 2 months. The child then wears the boot and bar system at night for 2 years. The boots are pointed straight ahead. Do not place a dorsiflexion bend in the bar.
- It is important to stretch the foot into plantar flexion and adduction.
- The authors use an abduction bar designed by Dr Dobbs (https://www.dobbsbrace.com). Some research has been performed with other bars.[70]

VERTICAL TALUS PITFALLS

- Given a newborns foot, one may be fooled into thinking the calcaneus is the medial talar head. Pressure on the calcaneus will block reduction of the deformity.
- A common error is not achieving maximal equinovarus positioning in the last cast before K-wire placement. This may lead to relapse.
- Poor compliance with bracing increases risks for relapse.

Calcaneovalgus

Severe calcaneovalgus foot deformity is a deformity in which the foot is hyperdorsiflexed and often abutting the anterior aspect of the tibia. The forefoot is abducted with marked heel valgus. Plantar flexion is often restricted and limited to a neutral position. While parents may be very concerned about the appearance of this deformity, it often improves on its own. Most calcaneovalgus deformities will improve by 3-6 months of age without intervention. Caregivers can assist with gentle manipulations emphasizing plantar flexion at the level of the ankle. Gentle inversion and adduction can also be helpful based on the deformity.

While calcaneovalgus most typically improves on its own, it is more important to exclude deformities associated with abnormal packing *in utero* such as hip dysplasia or posteromedial bowing of the tibia. It is important to recognize that the initial infant's hip examination may be normal while there is a greater association of hip dysplasia in children who have calcaneovalgus on one foot and metatarsus adductus on the contralateral foot. Advanced imaging in the form of ultrasound or x-rays, based on the child's age, can be helpful in excluding a silent hip dysplasia.

PEARLS IN EVALUATING FOR HIP DYSPLASIA

- Document clinical hip examination and any unusual neurologic findings (tone, unusual spasticity for age).
- Ortolani maneuver: posterior dislocation of the hip is reducible.
- Barlow maneuver: by adducting the hip and applying pressure on the knee with force directed posteriorly, one can dislocate the hip.
- Ultrasound: often utilized to exclude a dislocated hip.

The incidence for calcaneovalgus is 1 in 1000 live births (Fig. 54.17). With intrauterine crowding or packing deformities, the first child was found to be more at risk. Such is found to be the case for hip dysplasia as well.

Of importance, one must exclude congenital vertical talus from calcaneovalgus. This is essential as congenital vertical talus foot deformities if left untreated can lead to gross rocker bottom foot deformities with either inability to ambulate without pain or functional deficits. One will note the calcaneus to be in equinus in vertical talus, whereas the heel is easily palpable, void of equinus, and in a dorsiflexed position with calcaneovalgus. Stress plantar flexion radiographs are most helpful in distinguishing between the two deformities. In congenital vertical talus, the talus will not align with the first metatarsal while the deformity will reduce with calcaneovalgus.

Generally, this deformity will improve by 3-6 months. Still given the small number of children who have persistent valgus deformities beyond this age group, casting can be utilized to assist with reduction of the deformity during the time frame in which a child is not ambulatory. Bracing and manipulations for the more severe cases can follow serial casting. The authors have noted some children with persistent deformities in the absence of neurologic conditions hence the role of casting in the infant. There is definite variation among clinicians as to casting, treatment modalities, and plan of care. Some clinicians may not advise casting in this group of infants with a reducible deformity. For residual calcaneovalgus deformities that persist beyond 12 months, it is prudent to exclude any neurologic influence.

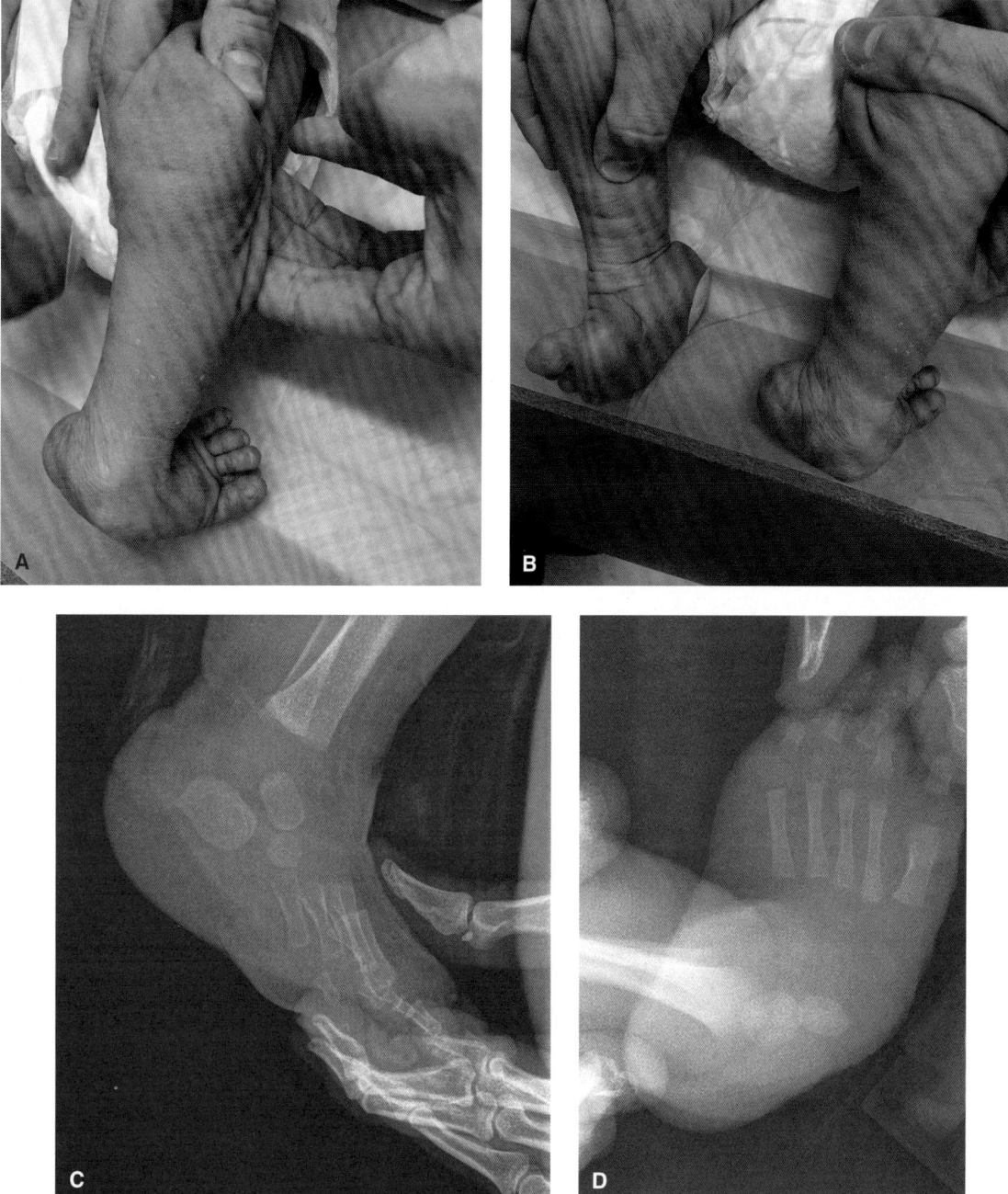

FIGURE 54.17 **A.** Calcaneovalgus in a 1-week-old male. **B.** Clubfoot right and calcaneovalgus left. **C.** Stress plantar flexion radiograph demonstrating aligned talus and first metatarsal. **D.** AP x-ray of calcaneovalgus.

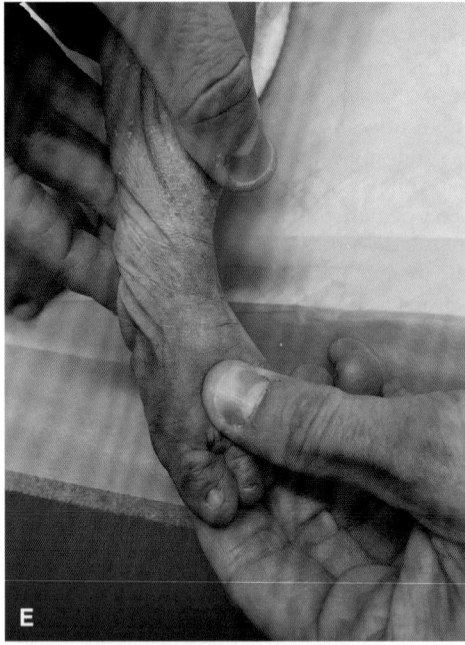
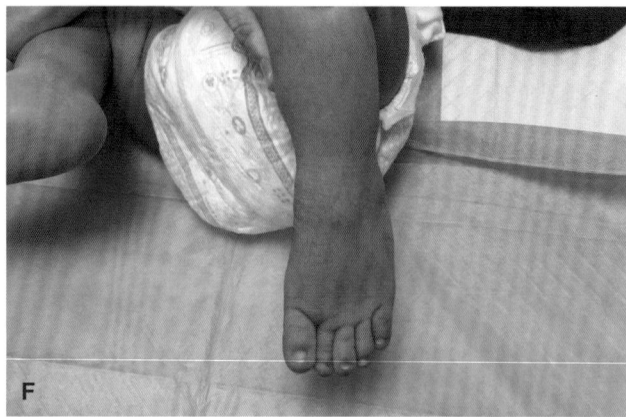
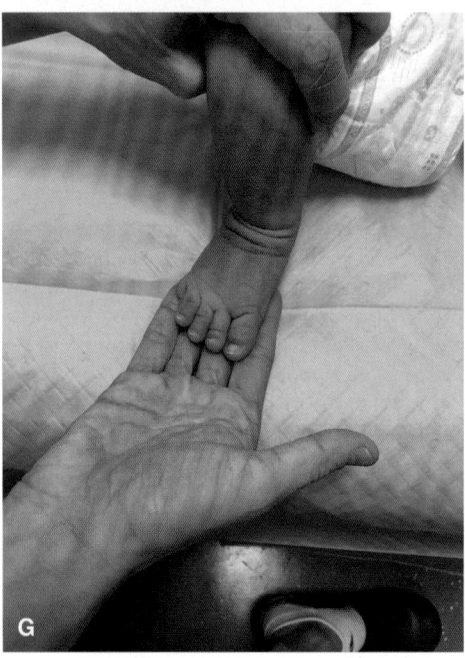
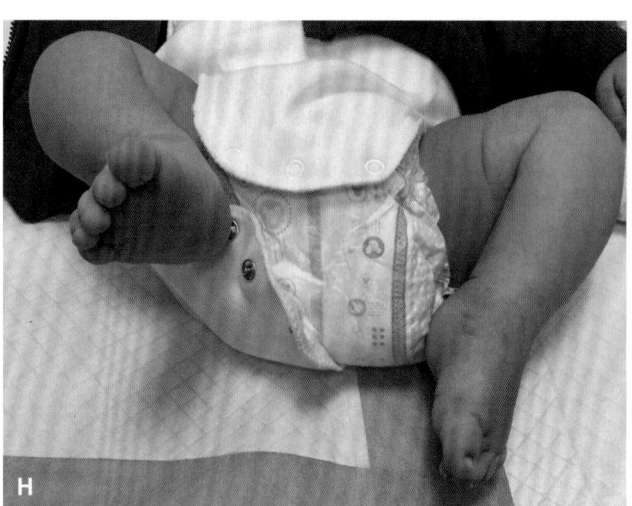

FIGURE 54.17 (*Continued*) **E.** Clinical manipulation of deformity. **F.** After serial casting for calcaneovalgus. **G.** After Ponseti serial casting. **H.** Postserial casting.

CALCANEOVALGUS PEARLS

- Educate parents that the majority of children with calcaneovalgus deformities will improve without care.
- Severe cases may benefit from serial casting to improve alignment and minimize risks of valgus pediatric foot deformities.[71] This can be complimented by manipulations and ankle-foot orthoses for additional months to assist with alignment.
- Exclude vertical talus by ordering stress plantar flexion x-rays.
- Exclude hip dysplasia.

Tarsal Coalitions and Flatfoot Deformities

Despite the prevalence of tarsal coalitions being 1%-2%, they appear frequently in high-volume pediatric foot and ankle clinics. Quite often, this condition can be found among young patients presenting with pediatric pes valgus while are not limited to this foot type alone. Likewise, many patients, prior to diagnosis, present with injuries, pain, stiffness, or flatfeet. Coalitions are essentially unusual unions between bones that can restrict motion and cause adaptive arthritic changes to surrounding joints. The condition is due to a failure of segmentation of the primitive mesenchyme during development.[72]

It is important to recognize that children may have more than one coalition present even in the same foot given this developmental reason for occurrence. The authors have treated children who have both a middle facet coalition and calcaneonavicular coalition in the same isolated foot. Hence, it is important to review all of the imaging. While coalitions can affect any joint, the most common tarsal coalitions of the foot include calcaneonavicular coalitions, middle facet talocalcaneal coalitions, and talonavicular coalitions in that order. Bilaterality has been reported in 50% of patients with talocalcaneal coalitions.

TARSAL COALITION PEARLS

- Talonavicular coalition: 1% of all coalitions, autosomal recessive disease, often bilateral, usually associated with orthopedic anomalies such as clinodactyly, symphalangism, ball and socket ankle, may be an incidental finding on x-rays
- Calcaneonavicular coalition: often presents at 8-12 years of age, most common coalition, embryologic failure of tarsal segmentation
- Talocalcaneal coalition: often presents between 12 and 15 years of age, autosomal dominance with variable penetrance, second most common tarsal coalition

Physical Examination

Pediatric patients can present with various positional deformities in association with coalitions yet the pronated flatfoot tends to be most common. Often when compared to an unaffected side, the foot will feel more stiff with limited subtalar joint motion. The patient often describes this stiffness as a "locked up" sensation when participating in pivoting activities. In the presence of a flatfoot, the deformity is often not reducible as compared to a pediatric pes planovalgus foot void of a coalition. Pain often exists along the dorsal lateral aspect of the foot in the presence of calcaneonavicular coalition. A double medial malleolus sign or prominence inferior to the medial malleolus is typically present with talocalcaneal coalitions. Again, timing of these symptoms tends to correspond with ossification of the tarsal bones.[73]

Imaging and Diagnostic Studies

These images are utilized on patients with stiffness and/or pain of the foot when evaluating for tarsal coalitions. Bilateral x-rays are often helpful for comparison.

1. Weight-bearing AP bilateral foot x-rays.
2. Weight-bearing lateral bilateral foot x-rays.
3. 45-degree internal oblique x-ray bilateral (detects calcaneonavicular coalitions)
4. Harris and Beath bilateral x-rays (detects talocalcaneal coalitions)
5. Hindfoot alignment x-rays bilateral

There are several radiographic signs often associated with coalitions while are not specific to coalitions. Moraleda and Mubarak reviewed the prevalence of the C sign on lateral weight-bearing x-rays and its association to talocalcaneal coalitions. In this study, a complete C sign was noted in 15% of talocalcaneal coalitions.[74] An interrupted C sign was present in 77% of talocalcaneal coalitions while also present in 45% of flexible pediatric flatfeet without a coalition.[74] Talar beaking may also be noted on the lateral radiograph with talocalcaneal coalitions while is not exclusive to such deformity. As for calcaneonavicular coalitions, an anteater sign or elongated anterior process is often visualized on the lateral radiograph.

A CT scan is most helpful in evaluating coalitions and joint involvement. Rozansky and colleagues described a radiologic classification of talocalcaneal coalitions (Fig. 54.18). This classification was based on the CT 3D reconstruction and remains very helpful in both the anatomic assessment of talocalcaneal coalitions and surgical planning. Long-term studies on prognosis are needed specifically following the middle facet coalition as compared to a more posteriorly deviated subtalar joint coalition.

There is little controversy over the diagnosis of a tarsal coalition while treatment modalities due vary especially with respect to talocalcaneal coalitions. The debate and/or variation of surgical options lie in the decision to resect alone vs resection in association with realignment procedures. There is debate over arthrodesis guidelines as well. In 1994, Wilde and colleagues reviewed their results from treating talocalcaneal coalitions and found unsatisfactory results in feet with a CT scan showing a relative coalition area >50%.[76] In this study, patients had more than 16 degrees of heel valgus, narrowing of the posterior talocalcaneal joint, and impingement of the lateral talar process on the calcaneus. Talar beaking was noted to be more of a traction spur and present in 33% of feet with a relative coalition size >50% and in 70% of feet with smaller coalitions. They recommended arthrodesis as a result for patients in which the talocalcaneal coalition involved more than 50% of the joint.[76]

Luhmann and Schoenecker reviewed results from 25 symptomatic talocalcaneal coalitions.[77] They recommended that all pediatric symptomatic talocalcaneal coalitions that failed nonoperative treatment and did not have an arthritic hindfoot be treated with resection as opposed to arthrodesis. They further concluded satisfactory results in patients with >50% joint involvement and >21 degrees of hindfoot valgus yet the valgus was addressed. The valgus of the heel was addressed postresection with an orthotic or surgical calcaneal osteotomy or lateral column lengthening procedure.[77] Arthrodesis was reserved for patients who failed the above and/or developed an arthritic hindfoot.

Mosca and colleagues reviewed 13 symptomatic talocalcaneal coalitions and concluded that a calcaneal lengthening osteotomy is a good alternative to triple arthrodesis for a painful foot with significant hindfoot valgus and an unresectable solid talocalcaneal tarsal coalition.[78] Gantsoudes and colleagues found that excision of the coalition to improve motion is the best solution to minimize impending pathology and alleviate pain. They also determined that correction of the preoperative valgus deformity could be necessary as a secondary procedure with good results in pain reduction.[79]

As noted, there is variation to the surgical management of talocalcaneal coalitions. Literature supports multiple treatment pathways from a resection vs arthrodesis standpoint. Likewise, there is support from a staged resection standpoint followed by orthoses vs resection of coalition with realignment procedures. One should think of the coalition and valgus position as two separate deformities. In the younger population, restoring some motion can be helpful as the child develops. Evaluating the child for excessive hindfoot valgus and/or peritalar subluxation should assist the surgeon in offering realignment procedures. In the presence of degenerative joint changes, arthrodesis should be considered.

Authors' Preferred Treatment

1. Resection of calcaneonavicular coalitions with or without fat graft interposition.
2. Resection of talocalcaneal coalitions with fat graft interposition in skeletally immature patients with no severe valgus deformity. This is complimented with orthoses if there is a mild valgus deformity.

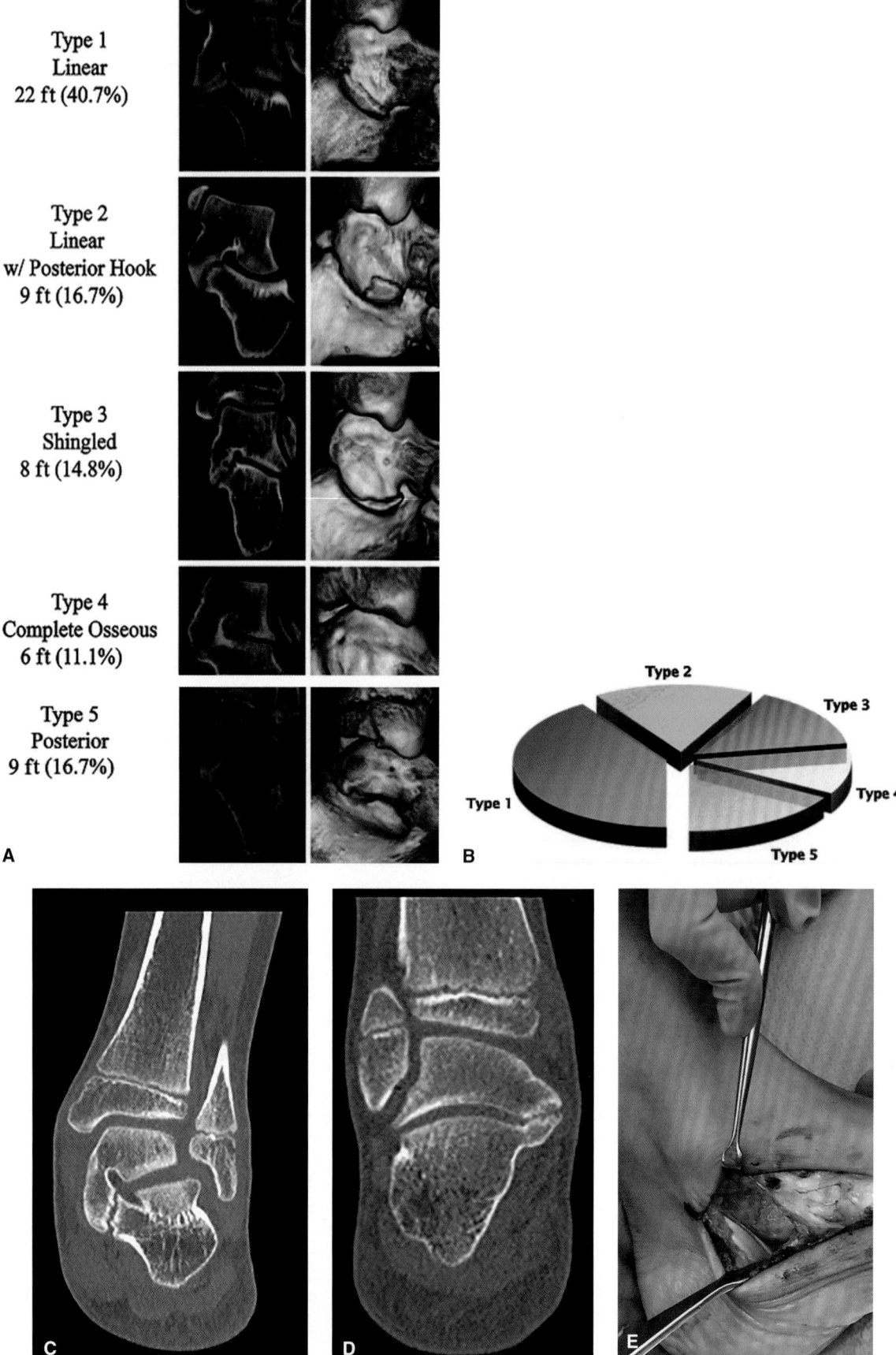

Type 1
Linear
22 ft (40.7%)

Type 2
Linear
w/ Posterior Hook
9 ft (16.7%)

Type 3
Shingled
8 ft (14.8%)

Type 4
Complete Osseous
6 ft (11.1%)

Type 5
Posterior
9 ft (16.7%)

A

Type 2

Type 3

Type 1

Type 4

Type 5

B

C

D

E

FIGURE 54.18 **A.** Talocalcaneal coalition classification scheme. **B.** Distribution by type of coalition. **C.** CT scan showing middle facet coalition with hindfoot valgus. **D.** CT scan showing middle facet coalition fairly rectus. **E.** Intraoperative talocalcaneal middle facet coalition. (Permission to reprint both **A** and **B** from Rozansky A, Varley E, Moor M, Wenger D, Mubarak S. A radiologic classification of talocalcaneal coalitions based on 3D reconstruction. *J Child Orthop.* 2010;4:129-135 Ref.[75])

3. Patients with a significant valgus deformity and/or peritalar subluxation undergo talocalcaneal coalition resection with fat graft interposition. In the absence of severe degenerative joint changes, realignment procedures are often staged to promote motion and minimize recurrence of coalition. In 6-12 months, children are offered realignment procedures based on the deformity and skeletal age. Often, procedures include a gastrocnemius recession, calcaneal lengthening osteotomy, and possible medial cuneiform osteotomy. Some children do undergo both resection and realignment in one stage if the valgus is grossly pathologic. The authors pay close attention to peritalar subluxation, hindfoot valgus, and the role of equinus.

4. Arthrodesis procedures are offered to older patients with degenerative joint changes or patients who have failed resection with or without realignment procedures.

5. All coalition patients are educated on the risks of requiring an arthrodesis at some point in their lifetime. Likewise, coalitions occupying over 50% of the joint are educated that they are at increased risk for need for arthrodesis in their lifetime.

Surgical Technique: Talocalcaneal Coalition Resection

1. Patient is positioned in the supine position.
2. Thigh tourniquet may be utilized.
3. The leg is prepped and draped with the ability to move the foot for intraoperative imaging. Buttocks region prepped for fat graft harvest.
4. A medial utility incision is fashioned from the medial malleolus along the medial subtalar joint transcending to the level of the talonavicular joint region. Care is taken to not fashion this incision too dorsal or plantar. This incision may be elongated posteriorly for type 5 talocalcaneal coalitions.
5. The posterior tibial tendon is often retracted superior, while the FDL is retracted inferior. The FHL and bundle will need to be retracted with stage 5 talocalcaneal coalitions.
6. A series of osteotomes can then be utilized to resect the coalition. This is continued until there is normal-appearing cartilage. One may complement this resection by using a rongeur or burr.
7. Intraoperative motion is then assessed. Intraoperative CT scans can confirm adequate resection.
8. Fat graft is then placed into the site of coalition resection.
9. Tendon sheaths are repaired.
10. Tourniquet is deflated prior to closure if utilized.
11. Bulky Jones splint applied for 2 weeks, followed by weight bearing in removable boot for 2-4 weeks prior to supportive shoes. Early range of motion is key once skin is healed.
12. The addition of realignment procedures requires 6 weeks nonweight bearing with immobilization.

Surgical Technique: Calcaneonavicular Coalition Resection

1. Oblique incision fashioned along the dorsal lateral aspect of the foot from the anterior process of the calcaneus to the navicular. Incision stops at the level of the extensors dorsally.
2. Extensor digitorum brevis is reflected.
3. A series of osteotomes are utilized to resect the entire coalition and most plantar bar.
4. Tourniquet is deflated prior to closure. Hemostasis is achieved prior to closure.
5. Fat graft may be inserted into the area of resection. The authors do not pack this void with any muscle belly.
6. Layer closure.

TARSAL COALITION PEARLS

- The CT scan and weight-bearing alignment x-rays should assist in surgical planning.
- Staged resection and realignment procedures may be best for the young pediatric patient.
- A full coalition resection is key to minimize recurrence or unsatisfactory results.
- A 3D CT scan defines size of coalition, location, and orientation of the talocalcaneal coalition. Intraoperative CT scans can be helpful to confirm adequate resection.
- MRI may be helpful in very young children with high suspicion for immature coalitions.
- Early range of motion once skin healing achieved can minimize recurrence.

TARSAL COALITION PITFALLS

- Inadequate resection of any coalition will lead to persistent pain or inability to reduce deformity.
- Inadequate hemostasis in the operating room can lead to hematomas, infection, and/or subsequent dehiscence.
- Failure to rebalance a foot with pathologic pronation in the form of peritalar subluxation and/ or hindfoot valgus can lead to pain.

Accessory Navicular

An accessory navicular is thought to be a normal variant that may become symptomatic following trauma or arises from biomechanical overuse. Quite often this accessory bone presents bilaterally and is visibly apparent. Parents often question the prominence noted. Prevalence of accessory navicular bones is between 14% and 26%.[80-82]

Three types of accessory navicular bones exist.[83,84] Type 1, otherwise known as os tibiale externum, is a small ossicle within the substance of the posterior tibialis tendon. Type 2 is an 8- to 12-mm ossicle. There is a medial and plantar extension of the navicular, which is connected to the navicular by a cartilaginous bridge. Type 3, known as the cornuate or gorilliform navicular, is a rare morphological entity.

Children often present with symptomatic accessory naviculars secondary to an acute injury. One may complain of a rotational injury, fall, or direct blow that causes tenderness overlying the accessory navicular. Contrary to this, others may present with tenderness to the prominence due to an overuse or biomechanical strain from a pronated flatfoot. It is extremely important to understand the biomechanical influence that the foot has on prognosis. For this reason, one cannot simply remove a symptomatic accessory navicular alone in a child with a pronated flatfoot as the faulty mechanics will continue to cause the posterior tibial tendon to work excessively hard.

Hence, it is important to recognize the foot type presenting with an accessory navicular (Fig. 54.19). Controversy exists regarding how often these accessory bones are painful. Still it is important to attempt conservative care as many children will improve without surgery. Conservative care includes off-loading via a cast or off-loading boot followed by rigid supportive shoes.[80] An orthotic is also utilized in the presence of pronation or deformity.

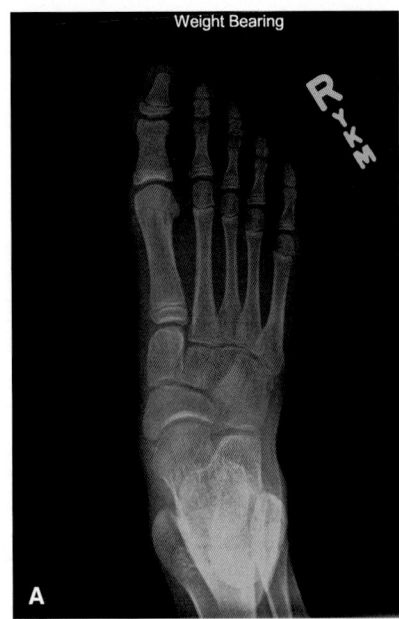

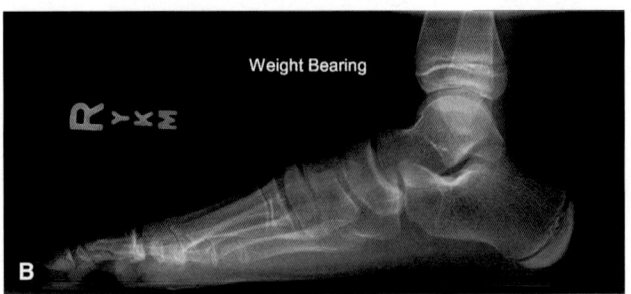

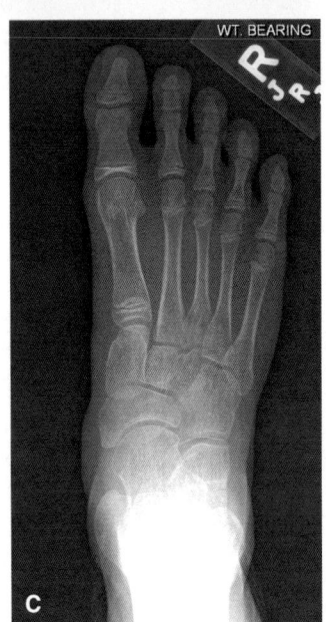

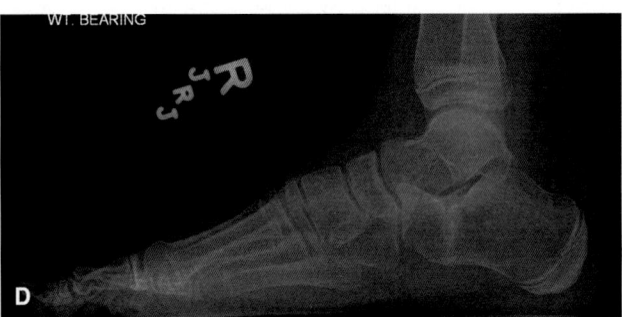

FIGURE 54.19 Accessory navicular.
A. Preoperative AP x-ray. **B.** Lateral x-ray.
C. Postoperative AP. **D.** Lateral radiographs
addressing the valgus deformity in
association with symptomatic accessory
navicular. **E.** MRI demonstrating accessory
navicular.

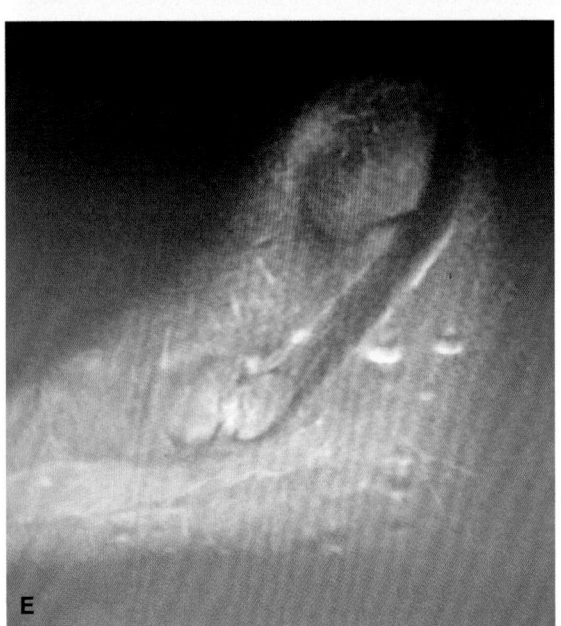

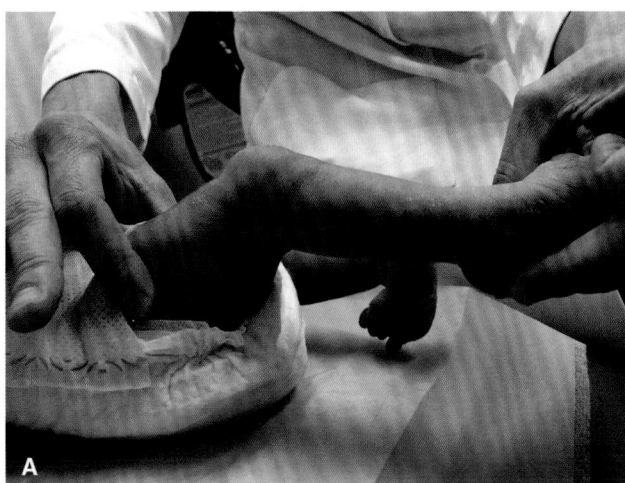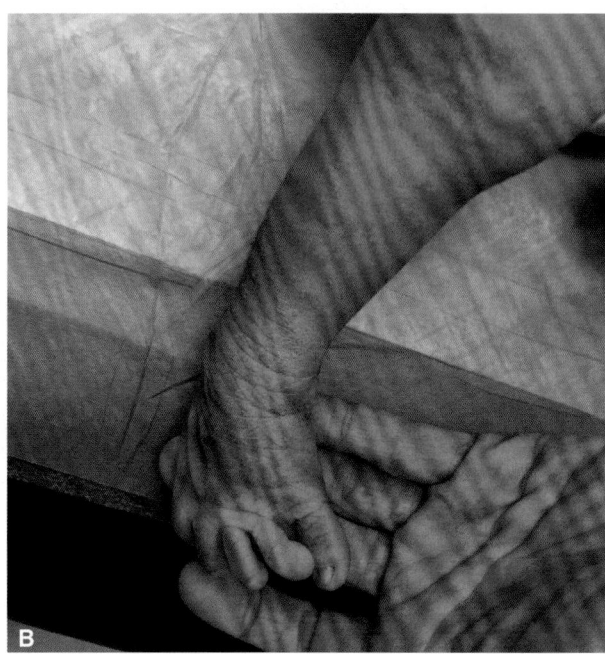

FIGURE 54.20 Arthrogryposis. **A.** Flexion of the knees. **B.** Equinovarus right foot.

Surgical intervention is offered for children who fail conservative care. Excision of the accessory navicular is performed by shelling the ossicle out of the posterior tibial tendon. The tendon is then repaired.[85] The attachments of the posterior tibial tendon are not disrupted. In the presence of a pronated flatfoot, the authors suggest rebalancing the foot. Hence, if the faulty mechanics are not addressed, the medial column can continue to be a source of pain. In the presence of excessive pronation and/or a valgus deformity, the Kidner procedure[86] is generally performed and complimented with various realignment procedures. In the presence of open growth plates, the authors often utilize a gastrocnemius recession, a calcaneal lengthening procedure, and possible opening medial cuneiform osteotomy. If growth plates are closed, then one may substitute the medial cuneiform osteotomy for a medial column fusion procedure for first ray purchase if needed. A pediatric pronated flatfoot should be evaluated on an individual basis, as not every child needs the same procedures.

ACCESSORY NAVICULAR PEARLS

- Symptomatic accessory naviculars may require a minimum 6-8 weeks of off-loading for pain to improve.
- Recurrent pain is common if the child has a pronated flatfoot and is not controlled in supportive rigid soled shoes with orthoses. Failure of these conservative modalities may lead to surgery.

Arthrogryposis

Arthrogryposis is a challenging congenital deformity in which multiple joint contractures exist. These contractures are debilitating if not treated early. Despite all conservative and surgical modalities centered on maintaining function and minimizing joint deformities, this condition remains quite difficult to obtain and maintain correction. Arthrogryposis occurs in ~1 of every 3000 live births.[87] Treatment methods should be centered on maintaining flexibility. One often notes a posture of elbow extension, wrist flexion, ulnar deviation, knee extension or flexion, and equinovarus foot deformities. At times, vertical talus or an equinovarus deformity may be appreciated.

Arthrogryposis multiplex congenital, or arthrogryposis, is not a diagnosis of itself, but in essence describes more than 400 conditions (Fig. 54.20).[87] These conditions share the presentation of an infant born with two or more joint contractures in multiple body areas.[87,88] Generally, all four extremities are involved while at times involvement may be limited to the upper or lower extremities. Prenatal diagnosis has been made as early as 19 weeks' gestation, based on absent fetal movement and contractures.[89]

Clubfeet are the most common foot deformities associated with arthrogryposis with an incidence of 78%-90% as compared to congenital vertical talus, which has a much lower incidence of 3%-10%.[88,90] Often the deformity is rigid in nature.[90-94] In the past, these children primarily underwent surgical releases and talectomies. Now there is research to support Ponseti serial casting for this subset of patients.[95,96] While these children may require longer periods of casting and manipulation, their risks of requiring major releases has been reduced. Hip motion is often preserved while the knees are stiff in flexion or extension. Still these children are more at risk of requiring a surgical procedure within their lifetime.

ARTHROGRYPOSIS PEARLS

- Arthrogrypotic clubfeet: Ponseti casting is initiated early in infancy. Relapses are common despite treatment and are generally casted again. In children who do not kick normally, one may consider an AFO molded to correct heel varus and forefoot adductus with the anterior ankle strap starting inside laterally to roll the ankle into valgus.[97]

- Equinovarus: a plantar crease will traverse the bottom of the foot medial to lateral. The appearance of this foot mimics an atypical clubfoot.[96] A 4-finger technique is utilized to provide dorsiflexion of the metatarsals with both thumbs, while the calcaneus is dorsiflexed. The Achilles tenotomy is performed once the cavus has been corrected.
- Congenital vertical talus: Dobbs method is very effective.[52,53] This maneuver relies on using the medial head of the talus as a fulcrum to reduce the talonavicular joint while bringing the foot into plantar flexion and adduction. It is key to apply both dorsal and lateral force on the talus. One must correct for the talus deformity in the sagittal and coronal planes. The Achilles is released after the talonavicular joint is reduced. The talonavicular joint undergoes pinning after improved alignment from serial casting.

Spina Bifida

Spina bifida is a birth defect in which there is incomplete development of the fetus' spine during the first month of pregnancy. While the incidence has decreased with proper prenatal care and the recommendation of folic acid, it still remains a large cause for disability within the United States. Spina bifida affects more infants each year as compared to muscular dystrophy or cystic fibrosis. Approximately 1500 pregnancies per year are affected.[98] Seventy-five percent of patients with spina bifida will have foot deformities. The three main types of spina bifida include spina bifida occulta, meningocele, and myelomeningocele.

Rarely, spina bifida occulta will cause any problems as a child develops. In fact, it has been estimated that 10%-20% of the population is unaware they have it. If symptoms present, one often experiences weakness and/or numbness of the legs. One may also experience bladder infections and incontinence.

Meningocele is the least common type of spina bifida. With this, the meninges protrude through the opening of the spine resulting in a sac on the back. The spinal cord has developed normally, and hence, the child has no neurological deficits. Surgery is performed in infancy to close the opening.

Myelomeningocele remains the most severe form of spina bifida. Infants with this condition are born with a portion of the undeveloped spinal cord protruding through the back. This sac contains cerebral spinal fluid and blood vessels surrounding the cord, which is not protected. Infants born with myelomeningocele are at risk for neurologic deficits. These deficits are dependent on the location and level of the spinal cord lesion. Many children will have weakness or even paralysis below the level of the spinal lesions. Some also experience hydrocephalus, loss of bladder or bowel function, scoliosis, and deformities of the feet.

Almost all patients with spina bifida will experience problems with foot deformity. Similar to arthrogryposis, children may present with clubfoot, vertical talus, equinovarus, or valgus deformities. These positional deformities are often complicated by a loss of protective sensation, weakness, or paralysis. Hence, risks of skin necrosis, ulceration, infections, and limb loss exists in this patient population. The skin in these very young patients tends to be sensitive and a source of breakdown in braces. This breakdown forces many families to discontinue the braces

for a period of time increasing the risk for recurrence of any corrected deformity.

In a patient who has the potential to ambulate the goals of casting, serial manipulation, and/or surgery are to create a plantigrade foot, which is supple with preserved motion. The foot must be braceable. This can be challenging when denervated muscles react spastically or the joint is severely unbalanced. The nonambulatory patient equally requires a plantigrade foot, which can be braced to minimize decubitus ulcerations. Early intervention especially in treating clubfoot or vertical talus can minimize rigid osseous deformities. Bracing is essential for this population to maintain position. Most require daytime and nighttime bracing throughout their life to minimize deformities. Multispecialty clinics are helpful for these children given multiple complex medical concerns.

SPINA BIFIDA PEARLS

- Thoracic or high lumbar (L1, L2): flail foot without deformity or equinus.[44,99-101] Caution should be taken to not cause a calcaneus deformity.
- Midlumbar (L3-L4): clubfoot,[44,102-104] possible valgus ankle or pes planovalgus.[105,106]
- Low level (L5, sacral): calcaneus deformity, neurologically normal-appearing[44,99,101,107] valgus ankle or pes planovalgus, vertical talus.[44]
- Procedures that make the foot rigid should be avoided.
- Most deformities upon correction do require lifelong bracing. Feet without deformity should be braced to minimize deformity.

SPINA BIFIDA BRACING PEARLS

- Thoracic, upper lumbar lesions: hip-knee-ankle-foot orthoses (HKAFOs), often wheelchair bound, with some quadriceps function and strong adductors a knee-ankle-foot Orthotic (KAFOs) may be considered.
- Lower lumbar, sacral lesions: good quadriceps function KAFOs and eventual AFOs.
- Sacral lesions: AFOs.
- Ground reaction AFOs prevent ankle sag into dorsiflexion.

Cerebral Palsy

Foot and ankle deformities are common in patients with cerebral palsy (Fig. 54.21). Children may present with equinovarus deformities or equinus contractures most typically. The degree of spasticity drives various deformities. While hemiplegia more often leads to an equinovarus deformity, equinovalgus deformity is seen more commonly in children with spastic diplegia and quadriplegia.[108]

Articulating ankle-foot orthoses can be quite helpful in the presence of mild equinus. As equinus becomes more rigid, botulinum toxin injections and/or serial casting become useful. Surgical intervention is reserved for fixed equinus or deformities that do not respond to conservative modalities such as stretching and casting. Goals are to obtain a plantigrade braceable foot.

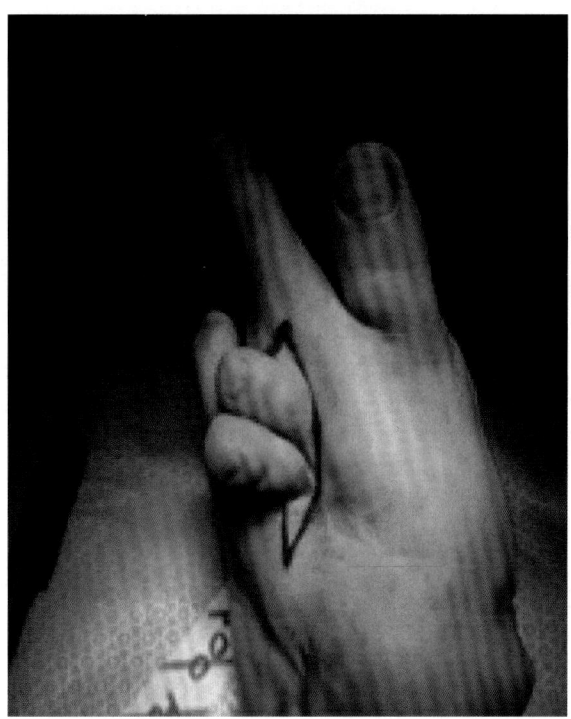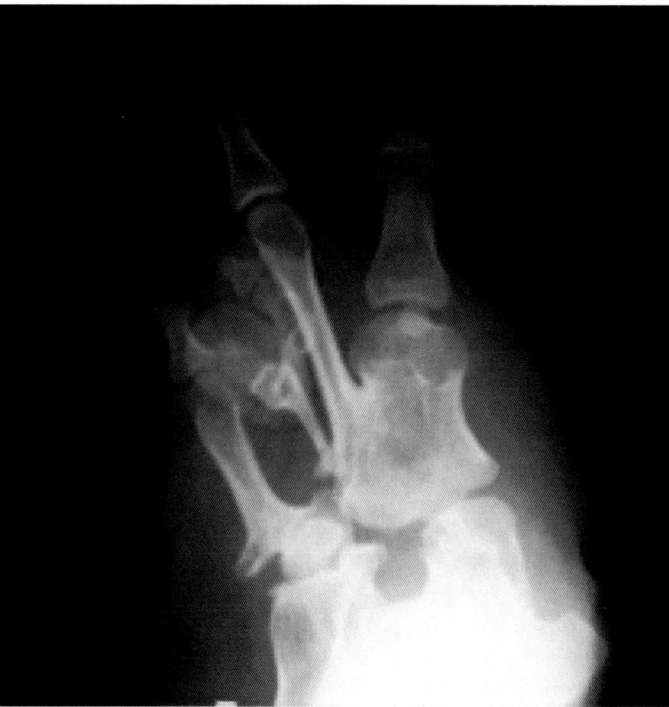

FIGURE 54.21 A 15-year-old female with Apert syndrome and cerebral palsy.

Down Syndrome

Musculoskeletal disorders occur in 20%-27% of patients with Down syndrome.[109,110] Foot and ankle deformities comprise 30% of all reported orthopedic complaints.[111] Many children present with increased body mass index, hypotonia, ligamentous laxity, and ankle instability. These traits often lead to pes planovalgus and progressive ankle valgus deformities, which in return place additional stress on one's knees, hips, and back. It is important to provide these children with conservative support given the ligamentous laxity that often exists. Orthoses and/or supramalleolar orthoses are often utilized early in childhood based on the deformity. Surgical intervention depends on the individual deformity and is reserved upon failure of conservative care. If the impending deformity is greatly at risk of causing harm to surrounding joints, then realignment procedures are discussed early in life.

REFERENCES

1. Gardner E, Gray DJ, O'Rahilly R. The prenatal development of the skeleton and joints of the human foot. *J Bone Joint Surg Am.* 1959;41:847.
2. O'Rahilly R, Gardner E, Gray DJ. The skeletal development of the foot. *Clin Orthop Relat Res.* 1960;16:7.
3. Bleck EE, Minaire P. Persistent medial deviation of the neck of the talus: a common cause of in-toing in children. *J Pediatr Orthop.* 1983;3:149.
4. Pollard JP, Morrison PJ. Flexor tenotomy in the treatment of curly toes. *Proc R Soc Med.* 1975;68(8):480-481.
5. Wagreich C. Congenital deformities. In: Banks A, Downey MS, Martin DE, Miller SJ, eds. McGlamry's Forefoot Surgery, 1st ed. Baltimore, MD: Williams & Wilkins; 2001.
6. Downey M, et al. Common pediatric digital deformities. In: DeValentine S, ed. *Foot and Ankle Disorders in Children.* St. Louis, MO: Mosby; 1992.
7. Smith WG, Seki J, Smith RW. Prospective study of a noninvasive treatment for two common congenital toe abnormalities (curly/varus/underlapping toes and overlapping toes). *Paediatr Child Health.* 2007;12(9):755-759.
8. Turner PL. Strapping of curly toes in children. *Aust N Z J Surg.* 1987;57(7):467-470.
9. Talusan PG, Milewski MD, Reach JS Jr. Fifth toe deformities: overlapping and underlapping toe. *Foot Ankle Spec.* 2013;6(2):145-149.
10. Taylor RG. The treatment of claw toes by multiple transfers of flexor into extensor tendons. *J Bone Joint Surg.* 1951;33-B(4):539-542.
11. Biyani A, Jones DA, Murray JM. Flexor to extensor tendon transfer for curly toes. 43 children reviewed after 8 (1-25) years. *Acta Orthop Scand.* 1992;63(4):451-454.
12. Ross ER, Menelaus MB. Open flexor tenotomy for hammer toes and curly toes in childhood. *J Bone Joint Surg.* 1984;66(5):770-771.
13. Hamer AJ, Stanley D, Smith TW. Surgery for curly toe deformity: a double-blind, randomised, prospective trial. *J Bone Joint Surg.* 1993;75(4):662-663.
14. Choi JY, Park HJ, Suh JS. Operative treatment for fourth curly toe deformity in adults. *Foot Ankle Int.* 2015;36(9):1089-1094.
15. Sweetnam R. Congenital curly toes; an investigation into the value of treatment. *Lancet.* 1958;2:398.
16. Burger E, Baas M, Hovius S, Hoogeboom J, Nieuwenhoven C. Preaxial polydactyly of the foot. *Acta Orthop.* 2018;89(1):113-118.
17. Phelps DA, Grogan DP. Polydactyly of the foot. *J Pediatr Orthop.* 1985;5(4):446-451.
18. Fahim R, Thomas Z, DiDomenico LA. Pediatric forefoot pathology. *Clin Podiatr Med Surg.* 2013;30(4):479-490.
19. McCarty J, Drennan J, eds. *Drennan's the Child's Foot and Ankle.* 2nd ed. Williams & Wilkins; 2009.
20. Hop MJ, van der Biezen JJ. Ray reduction of the foot in the treatment of macrodactyly and review of the literature. *J Foot Ankle Surg.* 2011;50(4):434-438.
21. Barsky AJ. Macrodactyly. *J Bone Joint Surg Am.* 1967;49(7):1255-1266.
22. Inglis K. Local gigantism (a manifestation of neurofibromatosis): its relation to general gigantism and to acromegaly; illustrating the influence of intrinsic factors in disease when development of the body is abnormal. *Am J Pathol.* 1950;26(6):1059-1083.
23. Kalen V, Burwell DS, Omer GE. Macrodactyly of the hands and feet. *J Pediatr Orthop.* 1988;8(3):311-315.
24. Chang CH, Kumar SJ, Riddle EC, et al. Macrodactyly of the foot. *J Bone Joint Surg Am.* 2002;84:1189.
25. Grogan DP, Bernstein RM, Habal MB, et al. Congenital lipofibromatosis associated with macrodactyly of the foot. *Foot Ankle.* 1991;12:40.
26. Morris EW, Scullion JE, Mann TS. Varus fifth toe. *J Bone Joint Surg Br.* 1982;64:99.
27. Paton RW. V-Y for correction of varus fifth toe. *J Pediatr Orthop.* 1990;10:248.
28. Black GB, Grogan DP, Bobechko WP. Butler arthroplasty for correction of the adducted fifth toe: a retrospective study of 36 operations between 1968 and 1982. *J Pediatr Orthop.* 1985;5:439.
29. Cockin J. Butler's operation for an over-riding fifth toe. *J Bone Joint Surg Br.* 1968;50:78.
30. Thompson GH. Bunions and deformities of the toes in children and adolescents. *Instr Course Lect.* 1996;45:355.
31. Tachdijian M. *Pediatric Orthopedics.* 2nd ed. Philadelphia, PA: WB Saunders; 1990.
32. Jones GB. Delta phalanx. *J Bone Joint Surg Br.* 1964;46:226.
33. Light TR, Ogden JA. The longitudinal epiphyseal bracket: implications for surgical correction. *J Pediatr Orthop.* 1981;1:299.
34. Stevens P. Toe deformities. In: Drennan J, ed. *The Child's Foot and Ankle.* New York, NY: Raven Press; 1992:183.
35. Mubarak SJ, O'Brien TJ, Davids JR. Metatarsal epiphyseal bracket: treatment by central physiolysis. *J Pediatr Orthop.* 1993;13:5.
36. Landon GC, Johnson KA, Dahlin DC. Subungual exostoses. *J Bone Joint Surg Am.* 1979;61:256.

37. Franklin TP, Miguel MQ, Félix MR, Leydi MQ, Herbert PC. Subungual osteochondroma: review of the Literature. *MOJ Orthop Rheumatol.* 2017;8(5):00327. doi: 10.15406/mojor.2017.08.00327.

38. Widhe T, Aaro S, Elmstedt E. Foot deformities in the newborn—incidence and prognosis. *Acta Orthop Scand.* 1988;59:176.

39. Wynne-Davies R. Family studies and the cause of congenital clubfoot, talipes equinovarus, talipes calcaneovalgus and metatarsus varus. *J Bone Joint Surg Br.* 1964;46:445.

40. Rushforth GF. The natural history of hooked forefoot. *J Bone Joint Surg Br.* 1978;60:530.

41. Thomson AM. Hallux varus and metatarsus varus: a five-year study (1954-1958). *Clin Orthop Relat Res.* 1960;16:109.

42. Jacobsen ST, Crawford AH. Congenital vertical talus. *J Pediatr Orthop.* 1983;3(3):306-310.

43. Miller M, Dobbs MB. Congenital vertical talus: etiology and management. *J Am Acad Orthop Surg.* 2015;23:604-611.

44. Sharrard WJ, Grosfield I. The management of deformity and paralysis of the foot in myelomeningocele. *J Bone Joint Surg Br.* 1968;50(3):456-465.

45. Merrill LJ, Gurnett CA, Connolly AM, Pestronik A, Dobbs MB. Skeletal muscle abnormalities and genetic factors related to vertical talus. *Clin Orthop Relat Res.* 2011;469(4):1167-1174.

46. Townes PL, Manning JA, Dehart GK Jr. Trisomy 18 (16-18) associated with congenital glaucoma and optic atrophy. *J Pediatr.* 1962;61:755-758.

47. Dobbs MB, Gurnett CA. The 2017 ABJS Nicolas Andry Award: advancing personalized medicine for clubfoot through translational research. *Clin Orthop Relat Res.* 2017;475:1716-1725.

48. Julia S, Pedespan JM, Boudard P, et al. Association of external auditory canal atresia, vertical talus, and hypertelorism: confirmation of Rasmussen syndrome. *Am J Med Genet.* 2002;110(2):179-181.

49. Dobbs MB, Gurnett CA, Pierce B, et al. HOXD10 M319K mutation in a family with isolated congenital vertical talus. *J Orthop Res.* 2006;24(3):448-453.

50. Kruse L, Gurnett CA, Hootnick D, Dobbs MB. Magnetic resonance angiography in clubfoot and vertical talus: a feasibility study. *Clin Orthop Relat Res.* 2009;467(5):1250-1255.

51. Hamanishi C. Congenital vertical talus: classification with 69 cases and new measurement system. *J Pediatr Orthop.* 1984;4(3):318-326.

52. Dobbs MB, Purcell DB, Nunley R, Morcuende JA. Early results of a new method of treatment for idiopathic congenital vertical talus. *J Bone Joint Surg Am.* 2006;88(6):1192-1200.

53. Dobbs MB, Purcell DB, Nunley R, et al. Early results of a new method of treatment for idiopathic congenital vertical talus. Surgical technique. *J Bone Joint Surg Am.* 2007;89(suppl 2Pt.1):111-121.

54. Bhaskar A. Congenital vertical talus: preatment by the reverse Ponseti technique. *Indian J Orthop.* 2008;42(3):347-350.

55. Aydin A, Atmaca H, Muezzinoglu US. Bilateral congenital vertical talus with severe lower extremity external rotational deformity: treated by reverse Ponseti technique. *Foot (Edinb).* 2012;22(3):252-254.

56. Khader A, Huntley JS. Congenital vertical talus in Cri du Chat ayndrome: a case report. *BMC Res Notes.* 2013;6:270.

57. Eberhardt O, Fernandez FF, Wirth T. The talar axis-first metatarsal base angle in CVT treatment: a comparison of idiopathic and non-idiopathic cases treated with the Dobbs method. *J Child Orthop.* 2012;6(6):491-496.

58. Eberhardt O, Wirth T, Fernandez FF. Minimally invasive treatment of congenital foot abnormalities in infants: new findings and midterm-results (German). *Orthopade.* 2013;42(12):1001-1007.

59. Aslani H, Sadigi A, Tabrizi A, Bazavar M, Mousavi M. Primary outcomes of the congenital vertical talus correction using the Dobbs method of serial casting and limited surgery. *J Child Orthop.* 2012;6(4):307-311.

60. Chalayon O, Adams A, Dobbs MB. Minimally invasive approach for the treatment of non-isolated congenital vertical talus. *J Bone Joint Surg Am.* 2012;94(11):e73.

61. Alaee F, Boehm S, Dobbs MB. A new approach to treatment of congenital vertical talus. *J Child Orthop.* 2007;1(3):165-174.

62. Eberhardt O, Fernandez FF, Wirth T. Treatment of vertical talus with the Dobbs method (German). *Z Orthop Unfall.* 2011;149(2):219-224.

63. Walker AP, Ghali NN, Silk FF. Congenital vertical talus: the results of staged operative reduction. *J Bone Joint Surg Br.* 1985;67(1):117-121.

64. Seimon LP. Surgical correction of congenital vertical talus under the age of 2 years. *J Pediatr Orthop.* 1987;7(4):405-411.

65. Stricker SJ, Rosen E. Early one-stage reconstruction of congenital vertical talus. *Foot Ankle Int.* 1997;18(9):535-543.

66. Duncan RD, Fixsen JA. Congenital convex pes valgus. *J Bone Joint Surg Br.* 1999;81(2):250-254.

67. Kodros SA, Dias LS. Single stage surgical correction vertical talus. *J Pediatr Orthop.* 1999;19(1):42-48.

68. Oppenheim W, Smith C, Christie W. Congenital vertical talus. *Foot Ankle.* 1985;5(4):198-204.

69. Mazzocca AD, Thompson JD, Deluca PA, Romness MJ. Comparison of the posterior approach versus the dorsal approach in the treatment of congenital vertical talus. *J Pediatr Orthop.* 2001;21(2):212-217.

70. Garg S, Porter K. Improved bracing compliance in children with clubfeet using a dynamic orthosis. *J Child Orthop.* 2009;3(4):271-276.

71. Giannestras NJ. Recognition and treatment of flatfeet in infancy. *Clin Orthop Relat Res.* 1970;70:10.

72. Vincent KA. Tarsal coalition and painful flatfoot. *J Am Acad Orthop Surg.* 1998;6:274-281.

73. Olney BW. Tarsal coalition. In: McCarthy JJ, Drennan JC, eds. *Drennan's the Child's Foot and Ankle.* New York, NY: Wolters Kluwer/Lippincott Williams& Wilkins; 2010:160-173.

74. Moraleda L, Gantsoudes GD, Mubarak SJ. C sign: talocalcaneal coalition of flatfoot deformity? *J Pediatr Orthop.* 2014;34:814-819.

75. Rozansky A, Varley E, Mubarak SJ, et al. A radiologic classification of talocalcaneal coalitions based on 3D reconstruction. *J Child Orthop.* 2010;4:129-135.

76. Wilde PH, Torode IP, Dickens DR, et al. Resection for symptomatic talocalcaneal coalition. *J Bone Joint Surg Br.* 1994;76:797-801.

77. Luhmann SJ, Schoenecker PL. Symptomatic talocalcaneal resection: indications and results. *J Pediatr Orthop.* 1998;18:748-754.

78. Mosca VS, Bevan WP. Talocalcaneal tarsal coalitions and the calcaneal lengthening osteotomy: the role of deformity correction. *J Bone Joint Surg Am.* 2012;94:1584-1594.

79. Gantsoudes GD, Roocroft JH, Mubarak SJ. Treatment of talocalcaneal coalitions. *J Pediatr Orthop.* 2012;32:301-307.

80. Grogan DP, Gasser SI, Ogden JA. The painful accessory navicular: a clinical and histopathological study. *Foot Ankle.* 1989;10:618.

81. Kruse RW, Chen J. Accessory bones of the foot: clinical significance. *Mil Med.* 1995;160:464.

82. Shands AR Jr, Wentz IJ. Congenital anomalies, accessory bones, and osteochondritis in the feet of 850 children. *Surg Clin North Am.* 1953;97:1643.

83. Ray S, Goldberg VM. Surgical treatment of the accessory navicular. *Clin Orthop Relat Res.* 1983;177:61.

84. Sella EJ, Lawson JP, Ogden JA. The accessory navicular synchondrosis. *Clin Orthop Relat Res.* 1986;209:280.

85. Kopp FJ, Marcus RE. Clinical outcome of surgical treatment of the symptomatic accessory navicular. *Foot Ankle Int.* 2004;25:27.

86. Kidner F. The prehallux (accessory scaphoid) in its relation to flatfoot. *J Bone Joint Surg.* 1929;11:831.

87. Hall JG. Arthrogryposis multiplex congenital: etiology, genetics, classification, diagnostic approach, and general aspects. *J Pediatr Orthop B.* 1997;6(3):159-166.

88. Bevan WP, Hall JG, Bamshad M, et al. Arthrogryposis multiplex congenital (amyoplasia): an orthopaedic perspective. *J Pediatr Orthop.* 2007;27(5):594-600.

89. Sepulveda W, Stagiannis KD, Cox PM, et al. Prenatal findings in generalized amyoplasia. *Prenat Diagn.* 1995;15:660.

90. Zimber S, Craig CL. The arthrogrypotic foot plan of management and results of treatment. *Foot Ankle.* 1983;3(4):211-219.

91. Menelaus MB. Talectomy for equinovarus deformity in arthrogryposis and spina bifida. *J Bone Joint Surg Br.* 1971;53(3):468-473.

92. Carlson WO, Speck GJ, Vicari V, et al. Arthrogryposis multiplex congenital. A long-term follow up study. *Clin Orthop Relat Res.* 1985;(194):115-123.

93. Drummond DS, Cruess RL. The management of the foot and ankle in arthrogryposis multiplex congenital. *J Bone Joint Surg Br.* 1978;60(1):96-99.

94. Hall JG, Reed SD, Driscoll EP. Part 1. Amyoplasia: a common, sporadic condition with congenital contractures. *Am J Med Genet.* 1983;15(4):571-590.

95. Morcuende JA, Dobbs MB, Frick SL. Results of the Ponseti method in patients with clubfoot associated with arthrogryposis. *Iowa Orthop J.* 2008;28:22-26.

96. Ponseti IV, Zhivkov M, Davis N, et al. Treatment of the complex idiopathic clubfoot. *Clin Orthop Relat Res.* 2006;451:171-176.

97. van Bosse, HJ. Syndromic feet, arthrogryposis and myelomeningocele. *Foot Ankle Clin.* 2015;20:619-644.

98. Parker SE, Mai CT, Canfield MA, et al. Updated National Birth Prevalence estimates for selected birth defects in the United States, 2004-2006. *Birth Defects Res A Clin Mol Teratol.* 2010;88(12):1008-1016.

99. Frischhut B, Stöckl B, Landauer F, et al. Foot deformities in adolescents and young adults with spina bifida. *J Pediatr Orthop B.* 2000;9(3):161-169.

100. Broughton NS, Graham G, Menelaus MB. The high incidence of foot deformity in patients with high level spina bifida. *J Bone Joint Surg Br.* 1994;76(4):548-550.

101. Frawley PA, Broughton NS, Menelaus MB. Incidence and type of hindfoot deformities in patients with low level spina bifida. *J Pediatr Orthop.* 1998;18(3):312-313.

102. Akbar M, Bresch B, Seylar TM, et al. Management of orthopaedic sequelae of congenital spinal cord disorders. *J Bone Joint Surg Am.* 2009;91(suppl 6):87-100.

103. de Carvalho Neto J, Dias LS, Gabrieli AP. Congenital talipes equinovarus in spina bifida: treatment and results. *J Pediatr Orthop.* 1996;16(6):782-785.

104. Flynn JM, Herrera-Soto JA, Ramirez NF, et al. Clubfoot release in myelodysplasia. *J Pediatr Orthop B.* 2004;13(4):259-262.

105. Abraham E, Lubicky JP, Songer MN, et al. Supramalleolar osteotomy of the ankle valgus in myelomeningocele. *J Pediatr Orthop.* 1996;16(6):774-781.

106. Burkus JK, Moore DW, Raycroft JF. Valgus deformity of the ankle in myelodysplastic patients. Correction by stapling of the medial part of the distal tibial physis. *J Bone Joint Surg Am.* 1983;65(8):1157-1162.

107. Fraser RK, Hoffman EB. Calcaneus deformity in the ambulant patient with myelomeningocele. *J Bone Joint Surg Br.* 1991;73(6):994-997.

108. Bennet GC, Rang M, Jones D. Varus and valgus deformities of the foot in cerebral palsy. *Dev Med Child Neurol.* 1982;24:499-503.

109. Mik G, Gholve PA, Scher DM, Wildmann RF, Green DW. Down syndrome: orthopedic issues. *Curr Opin Pediatr.* 2008;20:30-36.

110. Diamond LS, Lynne D, Sigman B. Orthopedic disorders in patients with Down's syndrome. *Orthop Clin North Am.* 1981;12:57-71.

111. Merrick J, Ezra E, Josef B, et al. Musculoskeletal problems in Down syndrome European Orthopaedic Society Survey: the Israeli sample. *J Pediatr Orthop B.* 2000;9:185-192.

Pediatric Foot and Ankle Fractures

David W. Gray and Jason M. Kennedy

DEFINING "PEDIATRIC" INJURIES

Musculoskeletal injuries to the foot and ankle are common complaints in children and adolescents. Pediatric fractures of the foot and ankle represent up to 13% of all fractures in the pediatric population. Physeal or "growth plate" fractures occur only in the growing skeleton. "Growth plate" fractures account for 18%-30% of all childhood and early adolescent fractures.

The peak incidence of physeal fractures occurs between the ages of 11 and 12 years in females. In males, the peak incidence is slightly older at 14 years of age.[1-4] Males reach skeletal maturity on average 2 years later than females.[1-4]

Classifying patients as "pediatric" by chronologic age alone is too simplistic. The definition of a pediatric fracture pattern should be reserved for those patients with bone growth remaining. Children mature at different chronologic ages. A better way of approaching "pediatric fractures" is by skeletal maturity. Patients near skeletal maturity have less growth potential, less potential for remodeling of a displaced fracture, and should be treated as skeletally mature.

When caring for pediatric patients, the surgeon must be able to estimate the skeletal maturity of the individual. For example, a girl that is chronologically 12 years of age with an ankle fracture may have a "bone age" of 14 years. A bone age is a reflection of the different rates of maturation of the skeleton seen across the population as a whole. Using a standardized radiograph of the left hand and wrist is one method of assessing the "age" or stage of bone maturation (Fig. 55.1).[5] A bone age of 14 for girls, and a bone age of 16 for boys, is considered mature. Patients within the last 1-2 years of skeletal growth should be treated within the context of adult guidelines for acceptable amounts of fracture displacement.

ANATOMY OF THE IMMATURE SKELETON

The "growth plate" in the bone of children is the primary method of longitudinal bone growth. The terms "physis," "epiphyseal plate," and "physeal" denote the region of the "growth plate." The major areas of the long bone in children are the epiphysis, the physis, the metaphysis, and the diaphysis.

Long bones and the bones of the foot and ankle are formed through a cartilaginous anlage. With the process of appendicular skeleton growth, the cartilage anlage (template) is replaced through endochondral ossification creating the adult skeleton.

The primary ossification center forms in the diaphysis of the long bones, and this ossification spreads toward the metaphysis ultimately arriving at the area of the physis. In the tarsal bones, the primary ossification center forms within the mid-portion of the cartilage anlage expanding peripherally in the bone.

The secondary ossification centers in long bones form in the epiphysis. The epiphysis is located at the end of the long bone supporting the hyaline articular joint surface. The physis is a cartilage region (growth plate) that is positioned between the epiphysis and the metaphysis. The physeal area is organized with germinal layer of cells nearest the epiphysis. From the germinal layer, new chondrocytes develop. These chondrocytes produce cartilage matrix creating longitudinal growth. Over time the chondrocytes hypertrophy, produce less cartilage matrix, and die. As new vasculature grows in from the metaphyseal side, the cartilage matrix produced by the chondrocytes from the physis undergoes provisional calcification. With time, the vascular ingrowth from the metaphysis allows osteoblasts and osteoclasts

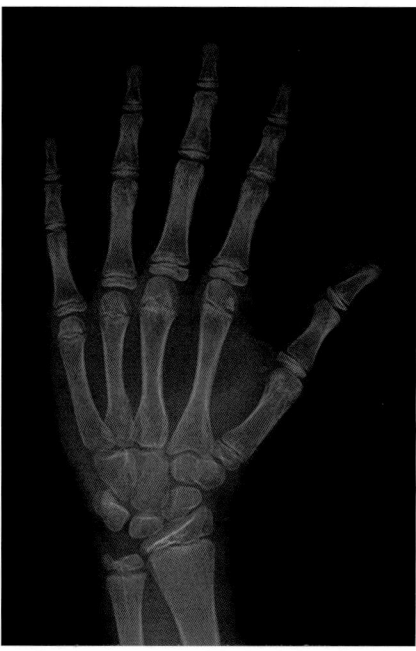

FIGURE 55.1 AP radiograph of left hand and wrist for bone age in 11-year + 6-month chronologic age girl. In this patient the Bone age correlates with chronologic age.

to populate the area. Calcified cartilage is removed, and the osteoblasts produce osteoid, which undergoes ossification. Bone formation is dynamic and undergoes constant process of turnover throughout life.[6-9]

Appositional growth of the bone along the diaphysis occurs with the aid of the periosteum. The periosteum is thicker in children than in adults. The periosteum is located along the diaphysis and metaphysis of the bone.

The perichondrium is a fibrous layer that covers the nonarticular portions of the epiphysis. The perichondrium blends with the periosteum in the region of the physis. At the physis, the perichondrium forms the fibrous perichondrial ring of La Croix. The zone of Ranvier is an area of fibroblasts, chondroblasts, and osteoblasts, providing peripheral growth of

the physis. Both the perichondrial ring of La Croix and zone of Ranvier provide additional stability to the region of the metaphysis and epiphysis (Fig. 55.2).[8,10,11]

THE IMMATURE SKELETON—CHARACTERISTICS, REMODELING, AND GROWTH ARREST

In the immature skeleton, there are unique opportunities and unique challenges. The surgeon, if well informed, will take advantage of continued growth in treatment decisions. This may allow closed treatment options not available in adults. At other times, surgical intervention will be required in an effort to preserve growth.

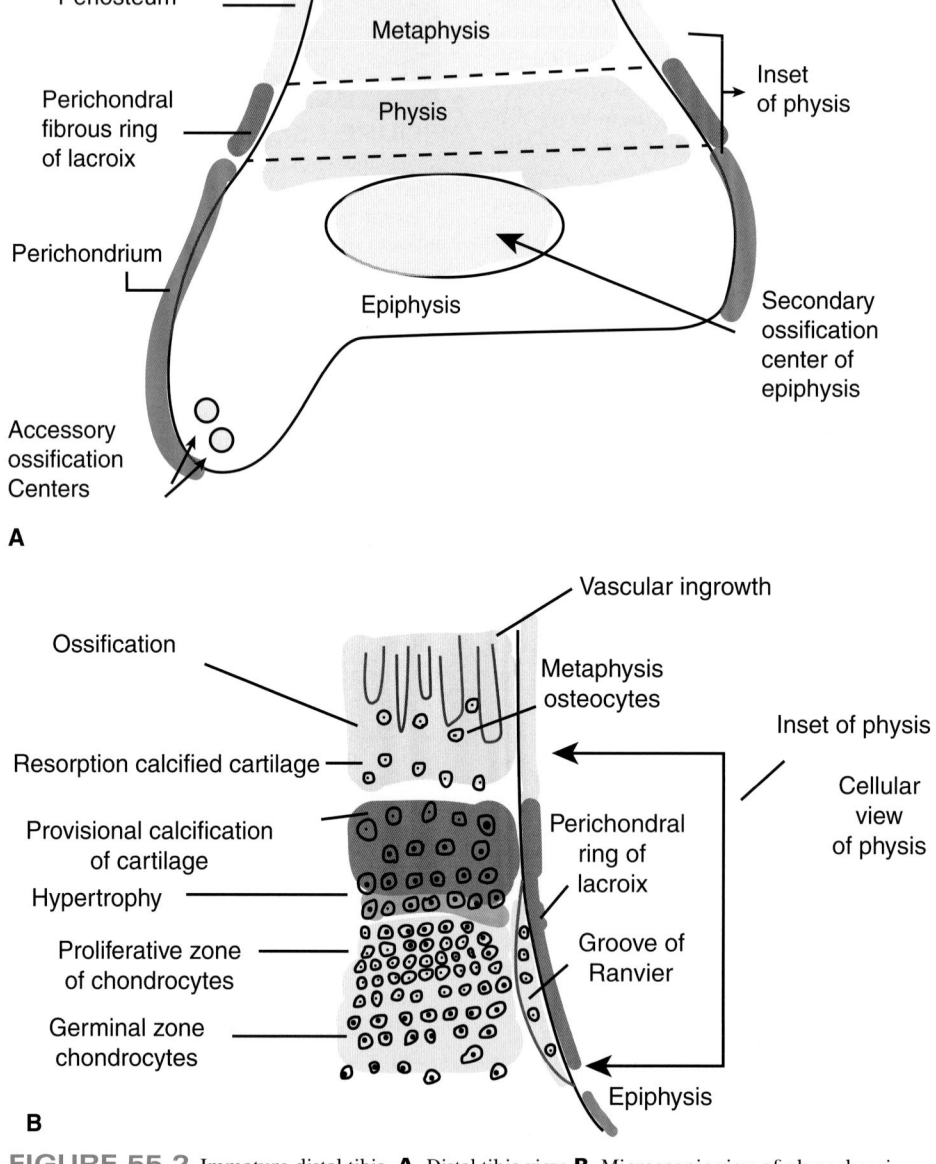

FIGURE 55.2 Immature distal tibia. **A.** Distal tibia view. **B.** Microscopic view of physeal region. Physis consists of cartilage matrix with cellular zones of metabolic activity. The germinal layer of the physis is adjacent to the epiphysis. The area of provisional calcification of the cartilage is at the physeal metaphyseal junction. The provisional zone of calcification undergoes calcification and resorption with vascular ingrowth. With vascular ingrowth, osteoblasts, osteocytes, and osteoclasts arrive.

The mechanical properties of the immature skeleton allow plastic deformation of bone, buckle (torus) fractures, and greenstick fractures. Bone in children is more elastic than adults. The decrease in stiffness allows the bone to absorb more energy prior to complete failure. Thus, explaining the ability of skeletally immature bone to show plastic deformation with injury.[12]

Immature bone can also fail within the physis. Early literature postulated that physeal fracture lines occurred in the area of hypertrophic chondrocytes and zone of provisional calcification. Multiple studies have found that fracture propagation can occur through any zone of the physis.[8,13–15]

Fracture remodeling is more predictable in children than adults because of ongoing bone growth. The growing skeleton is capable of correcting translation of displaced fracture ends, creating overgrowth (increased length) of a bone after an injury, and correcting angular deformity. Remodeling potential of a bone is related to the skeletal maturity of the patient, the proximity of the fracture to a rapidly growing physis, the preservation of cellular function of the physis, and the orientation of the deformity in relationship to the plane of joint motion.[16,17]

The remodeling process occurs through physeal growth and appositional growth. The periosteum creates new bone formation on the concavity (compression side) of the deformity. Resorption of bone occurs along the convexity (tension side) of the deformity. While translational, and angular deformities have the potential to remodel, there is a limit to how much can be spontaneously corrected. Rotational deformities and intra-articular displacement have little capacity to remodel.

While remodeling is commonly seen in children, the possibility of growth arrest represents the other end of the spectrum of physeal fractures. The cells of the physis are at risk with fracture, infection, soft tissue injury with disruption at the physeal area, vascular insult, and pin fixation across the physis. Pins crossing the physis that are >7%-9% of the cross-sectional area of the physeal region have the potential to create a growth arrest.[18,19]

Complete growth arrest may lead to limb length inequality depending on the patient's skeletal maturity. Partial growth arrest is capable of producing angular deformity in the coronal plane, sagittal plane, or both. Angular deformity leads to mechanical axis deviations with changes in stress across the joint. With radiographic follow-up after injury, the presence of Harris lines on the radiographs gives the surgeon an opportunity to observe either the presence of symmetric growth or the absence of symmetric growth after an injury (Fig. 55.3).

SALTER-HARRIS CLASSIFICATION SYSTEM OF PHYSEAL FRACTURES IN CHILDREN

Classification systems have evolved to describe growth plate fractures of the appendicular skeleton. The Salter-Harris classification was adopted after 1963 (Fig. 55.4).[15]

It is applied to all physeal fractures of long bones, metacarpals, metatarsals, and phalanges. The Salter-Harris classification is not applicable to the talus, calcaneus, navicular, cuneiforms, and cuboid.

The Salter-Harris V Pattern is unique in the classification as it is "retrospective" in nature. The existence of a separate Salter-Harris V fracture vs a "missed" known Salter-Harris pattern has been debated in the literature. Unexplained episodes

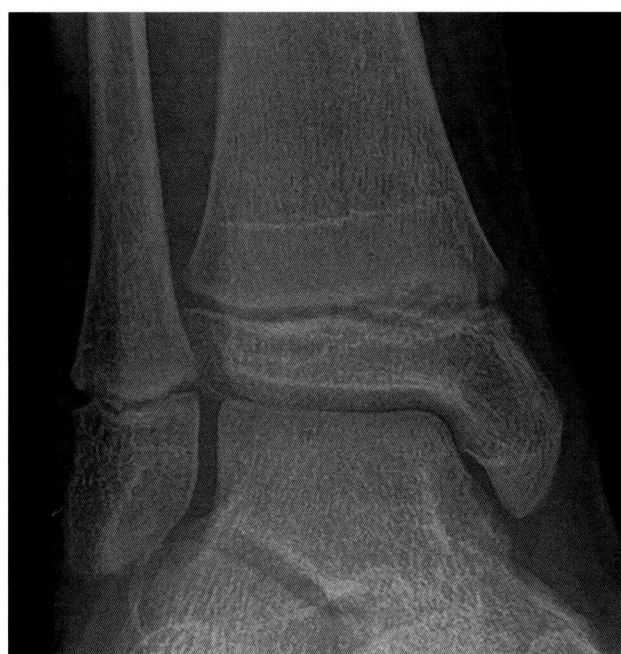

FIGURE 55.3 Harris line. There is an ossification line across the metaphysis of the tibia proximal to the physis. The line represents an area of increased ossification at the time of fracture healing. As growth resumes, the near symmetric line across the metaphysis indicates symmetric growth of the distal tibia has occurred 1 year after a Salter-Harris III fracture of the medial malleolus. There is a faint Harris line visible on the fibula as well.

of physeal growth arrest after trauma are reported supporting the Salter-Harris V concept.[20–22] It is presumed to be a compression injury, or vascular insult after an injury, with no identifiable previous Salter-Harris I-IV fracture pattern. Treatment is aimed at addressing limb length inequality or angular deformity if a Salter-Harris V injury is present. So even with the literature debate, the type V fracture pattern remains part of the Salter-Harris classification.

Authors have proposed modifications and additions to the Salter-Harris classification.[8,13,22–26] The increased complexity with the additional proposed types of fractures has not allowed widespread adoption of their use. Today, the 1963 Salter-Harris classification system of I through V remains the most widely used in clinical practice.[27]

HISTORY AND PHYSICAL EXAMINATION OF THE FOOT AND ANKLE IN CHILDREN

The history and physical examination is straightforward. Clearly understanding the mechanism of injury is a key component. In young children, accurate details may be lacking. A limping child is not always a musculoskeletal injury. The differential diagnosis includes infection, tumor, childhood arthritis, and nonaccidental trauma.

If the trauma is witnessed, the patient immediately refused to bear weight, or had immediate onset of an antalgic gait, then it is most likely a musculoskeletal injury. If the injury is not witnessed, or the mechanism is not clear, then the history becomes even more important. Details about presumed place of injury and the individuals overseeing the child at the time need to

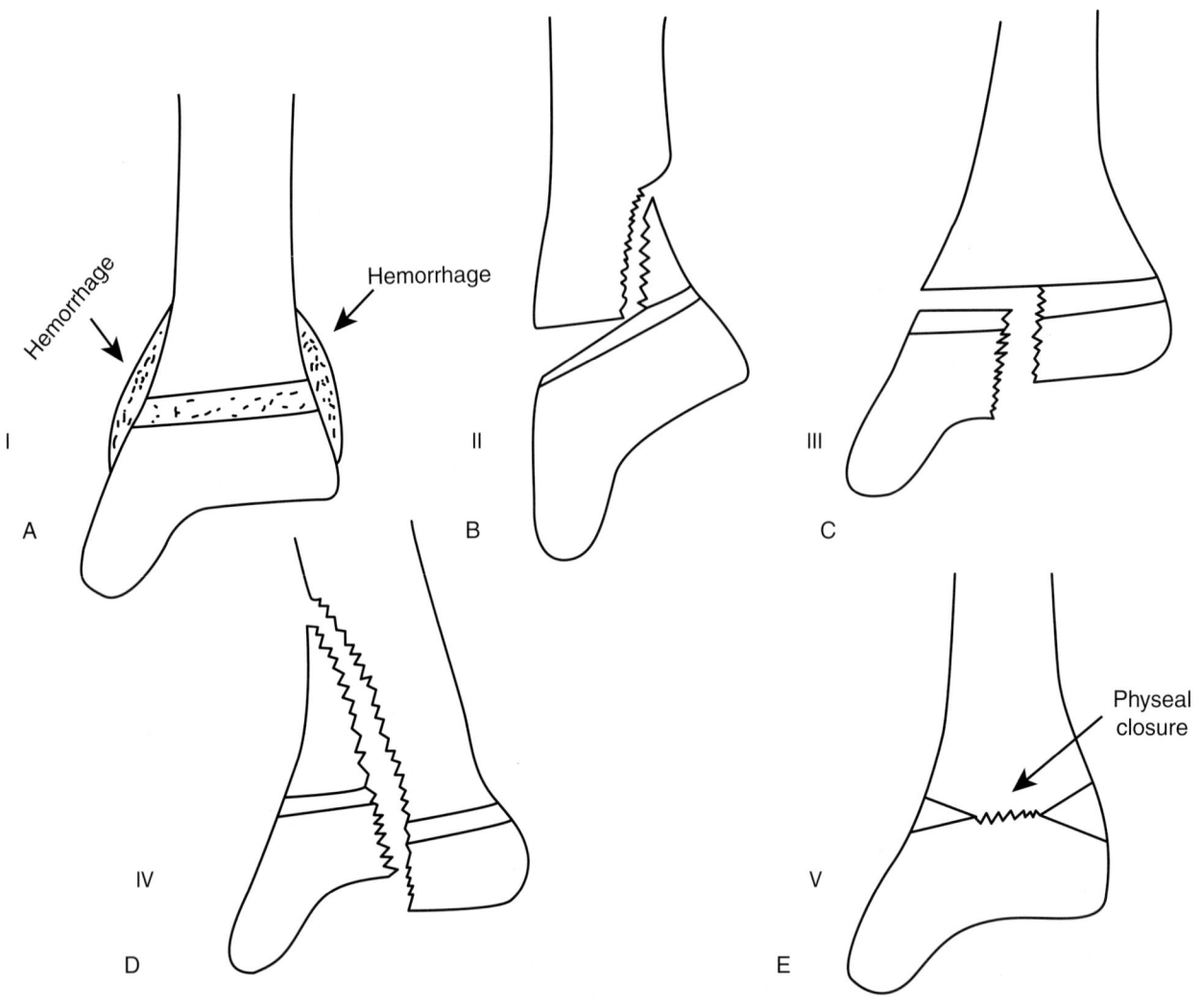

SALTER-HARRIS CLASSIFICATION

FIGURE 55.4 Salter-Harris classification of physeal injuries. **A.** Type I—fracture of physis. **B.** Type II—fracture of physis with metaphyseal involvement. **C.** Type III—fracture of physis with epiphyseal involvement. **D.** Type IV—physeal, epiphyseal, and metaphyseal involvement. **E.** Type V—represents a previous injury with no known prior Salter-Harris I-IV pattern presenting with late physeal arrest. (Redrawn with permission from Salter R, Harris R. Injuries involving the epiphyseal plate. *J Bone Joint Surg Am.* 1963;45-A(3):587-622.)

be clarified. Questions regarding swelling, redness, duration of symptoms, recent illnesses, fevers, constitutional symptoms, and night pain are critical.

The surgeon should be patient and calm. Point tenderness over the bone vs the muscle or ligaments must be noted. The joints above and below the areas of concern should be included in the examination. Hypersensitivity should be noted. Regional pain syndromes are seen in children and adolescence. Gait pattern should be examined. Is the child able to bear weight? For example, if the child will crawl bearing weight on the knee, but refuses to bear weight on the foot, then the etiology is likely in the lower leg, ankle, or foot. In younger children, the examination may take a few minutes of gaining the patient's confidence. It is not unusual to have to repeat the palpation of the extremity several times to delineate the area of maximal tenderness.

When the potential differential diagnoses include the possibilities of musculoskeletal infection, tumor, nonaccidental

PEARLS

Young children may respond more favorably sitting on a parent's lap for the examination. In the anxious child, distraction with a book, toy, or video may allow the examiner the opportunity to palpate the extremity looking for tenderness.

trauma, or juvenile arthritis, the examination needs to include the whole child. The surgeon should look for skin rashes, signs of trauma, bruises, scratches, burns, joint effusions, and restriction of joint motion. Laboratories for complete blood count with white blood cell differential, renal panel, liver panel, erythrocyte sedimentation rate, and C-reactive protein may provide further guidance for the surgeon. Advanced imaging also may play a role in the workup of the patient.

ANKLE INJURIES

INCIDENCE

Fractures of the distal tibia and fibula constitute about 5% of all pediatric fractures. Injury to the physis of the distal tibia and fibula accounts for about 15%-18% of all the growth plate fractures seen in children and early adolescents. To put this in to context, the literature states the most common physeal injuries are seen in the phalanges of the fingers at 37% of all physeal fractures. Physeal fractures of the distal tibia and distal fibula are almost equal to the percentage of physeal fractures seen at the wrist.[2–4,28]

ANATOMY OF THE DISTAL TIBIA AND FIBULA IN CHILDREN

The distal tibial ossification center appears between 6 months and 2 years of age. The medial malleolus ossification typically forms as the continuation of the main secondary ossific nucleus of the distal tibia (Fig. 55.5). The medial malleolus may also have accessory ossification center(s). The literature also discusses a separate ossicle, the os subtibiale. Whether previous references were truly a separate ossicle or instead accessory ossification centers creating variations in ossification within the epiphysis is unclear. With potential variations in the ossification pattern of the medial

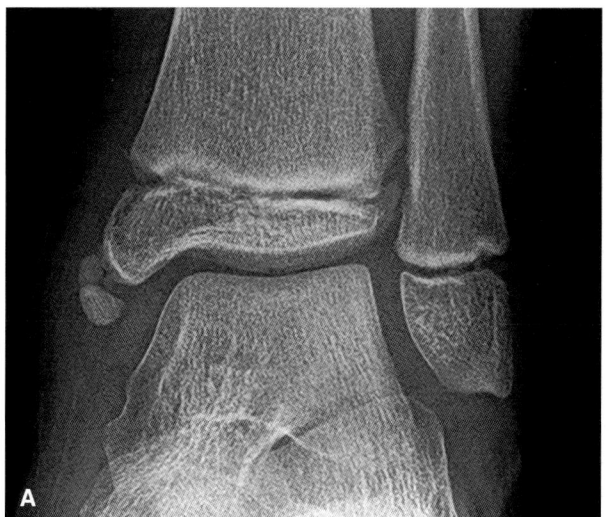
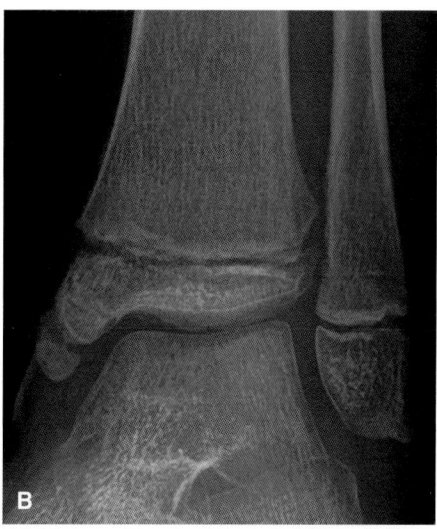
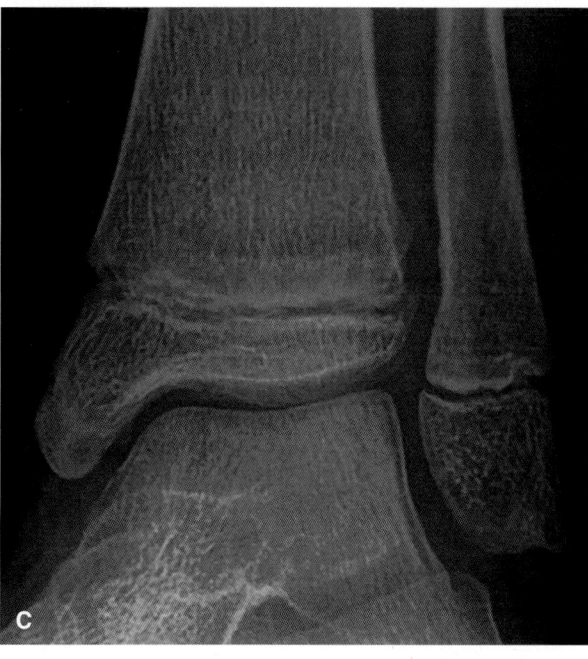

FIGURE 55.5 Medial malleolus ossification. **A.** Injury film showing a minimally displaced Salter-Harris III fracture of the medial malleolus in a boy of 7 years. The injury film report described the accessory ossification centers of the medial malleolus as multiple avulsion fractures. The area of the ossification centers has smooth edges on radiographs. **B.** At Three months, the area of the medial malleolus fracture line is healed. The accessory ossification centers are coalescing. **C.** At 9 months, the accessory ossification centers of the medial malleolus and the secondary ossification center have coalesced. The Harris line is also visible in the metaphysis of the distal tibia and fibula.

malleolus, these accessory ossification centers may be confused with avulsion fractures.[29–31]

The distal fibula ossification center appears between 9-24 months of age. The physis of the fibula in children is at the level of the ankle joint. Closure of the distal fibula physis occurs 12-24 months following distal tibial closure.[30,32] The os subfibulare has been postulated to be an accessory ossification center.[30] Os subfibulare has also been reported as the result of trauma.[33] Both postulates for an os subfibulare may be correct. Some radiographic findings may be related to variation in epiphyseal ossification, others related to avulsions, or periosteal sleeve avulsions of epiphyseal cartilage that later ossify.

In the skeletally immature skeleton, the deltoid ligament, anterior talofibular ligament, calcaneofibular ligament, and posterior talofibular ligament originate distal to the physis on the epiphysis. The teaching has been that since the ligaments originate on the epiphysis at the ankle, children are more likely to have physeal injuries not sprains. While in practice there are many physeal fractures, ultrasound has shown that children and adolescents can have ligamentous injury of the ankle.[34] The surgeon must note whether the location of the maximal area of tenderness is directly on the bony anatomy or over the soft tissue structures.

LONGITUDINAL GROWTH OF THE DISTAL TIBIA IN CHILDREN

The growth of the distal tibia accounts for about 40% of the growth of the tibia after the age of 5 years. Distal tibial growth ranges from 4 to 6 mm a year in the literature. Less growth occurs in the last 12-18 months prior to skeletal maturity.[35–40] In adolescence, the growth of the distal tibia physis begins closure centrally and extends medially first over a 12-18-month period. The anterolateral corner of the physis is the area last to close explaining the Tillaux fracture pattern.[41] This information about expectations of continued growth allows for counseling of a patient and family about risks of potential limb length inequality after injury.

CLASSIFICATION OF ANKLE FRACTURES

Salter-Harris and Dias-Tachdjian

The Salter-Harris classification system is the most commonly used to describe the ankle fracture patterns at the specific location of injury. Dias and Tachdjian modified the Lauge-Hansen classification to describe the mechanism of injury for fracture patterns seen in children and adolescents.[42,43] The Dias system consists of four descriptions of mechanism of injury producing many of the fracture patterns that are seen. The first word in the classification indicates the position of the foot. The second term describes the direction of force producing the injury. So, while most surgeons record the Salter-Harris classification of the fracture, understanding the direction of injury forces as delineated by Dias-Tachdjian is necessary for fracture reduction maneuvers (Fig. 55.6).

Dias-Tachdjian Supination-External Rotation (see Fig. 55.6A)

Grade I—This produces a Salter II fracture of the distal tibia. The tibial fracture line is usually from the physis distally on the lateral side and extends obliquely in a cephalad and medial direction.

Grade II—If the supination-external rotation force continues, the fibula will fracture in a spiral pattern.

Dias-Tachdjian Pronation-Eversion-External Rotation (see Fig. 55.6B)

The distal tibia fracture is usually a Salter I or a Salter II with lateral displacement of tibial fracture. This is accompanied by a transverse or short oblique fracture of the fibula. The most common fracture pattern is with the distal tibia metaphyseal spike is on the lateral side.

Dias-Tachdjian Supination-Inversion (see Fig. 55.6C)

Grade I—The inversion force separates the distal fibular epiphysis typically creating a Salter I or Salter II fracture of the distal fibula.

Grade II—With increasing inversion, the distal tibia is fractured. The distal tibia fracture often is a Salter-Harris III or IV injury of the medial malleolus. Occasionally, a Salter-Harris I or II fracture of the distal tibia can occur.

Dias-Tachdjian Supination-Plantarflexion (see Fig. 55.6D)

A plantarflexion force produces a distal tibia injury with posterior displacement of the epiphysis, plantarflexion of the distal tibia fragment, or a fracture of the epiphysis posteriorly. With plain radiography, this injury is often best identified on the lateral radiographs. Salter I or Salter II fracture patterns of the distal tibia are most common.

Transitional Fractures

As children enter adolescence, the distal tibia physis begins to close creating different fracture patterns then seen in younger children. These have been termed "transitional fractures." The juvenile Tillaux fracture and the triplane fracture are two transitional fractures occurring near or in adolescence. The original Dias-Tachdjian classification did not address these injuries. Dias in a follow-up article discussed external rotation as a primary mechanism for Tillaux and triplane injuries.[44]

Both the juvenile Tillaux fracture and triplane fracture patterns are intra-articular fractures of the distal tibia. The juvenile Tillaux is a Salter-Harris III fracture of the anterolateral epiphysis of the distal tibia (Fig. 55.7). The triplane consists of an intra-articular fracture line through the epiphysis extending through the physis into the metaphysis. The fracture line runs in sagittal, transverse (axial), and frontal (coronal) planes. The triplane fracture is a Salter-Harris IV injury to the distal tibia.[45,46] The triplane fractures may be two-part, three-part, or four-part injuries (Figs. 55.8-55.10).[47,48]

IMAGING OF THE PEDIATRIC ANKLE

Ottawa rules have been reviewed in children. Indication for radiographs in pediatric patient is refusal to bear weight and bone tenderness to palpation.[49,50] Anteroposterior, lateral, and mortise views are recommended. While most surgeons prefer three views, if only two views are obtained, the mortise, and the lateral radiographs approach the accuracy of three views in skeletally mature patients.[51]

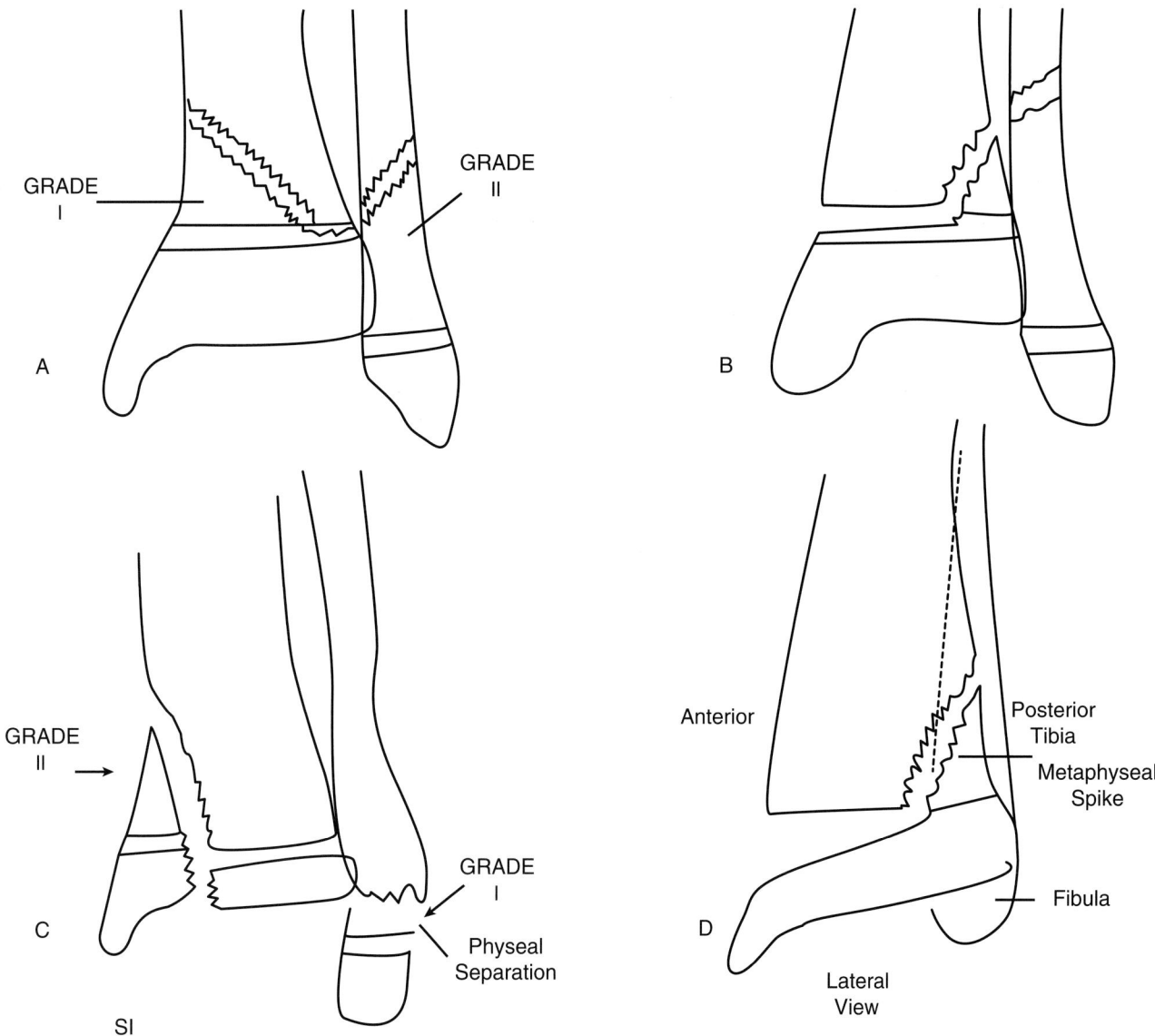

FIGURE 55.6 Dias-Tachdjian classification. (Redrawn with permission from Dias LS, Tachdjian MO. Physeal injuries of the ankle in children: classification. *Clin Orthop Relat Res.* 1978(136):230-233.) **A.** Supination-external rotation. Grade I and grade II. **B.** Pronation-eversion-external rotation. **C.** Supination-inversion. Grade I and grade II. **D.** Supination-plantarflexion.

While two views with mortise and lateral radiographs may be satisfactory in adults, the growing skeleton does not have the same relationships as mature skeleton (Fig. 55.11). The mean age at which tibia and fibula overlap on the AP view of the ankle is 5 years.[52] The tibiofibular overlap on the mortise radiograph occurs later. The mean age for overlap on the mortise view in females is 10 years. The tibiofibular overlap on the mortise radiographs for males is later with a mean age of 16 years.[52]

Comparison radiographs of the uninvolved ankle are useful when evaluating the syndesmosis, potential accessory ossification centers, avulsion injuries, and occult fractures. Ankle stress views are infrequently used in children. Manipulating a young child's ankle in the office is an unpleasant experience for the child and the child's family.

Advanced imaging is useful in complex fracture patterns. Ultrasonography can be used for evaluating potential nondisplaced physeal injuries vs ligamentous sprains.[34,53]

Computed tomography (CT) scans assist with defining intra-articular fragments, the amount of fracture displacement, and preoperative planning. Magnetic resonance imaging (MRI) allows soft tissue visualization and articular cartilage definition. The MRI may be helpful in evaluating the extent of injury, ligamentous injuries, injury to the non-ossified areas of the epiphysis, and occult fractures.[54] In evaluating a potential accessory ossicle, the MRI may be helpful delineating an area of injury vs a variation in ossification of the epiphysis.

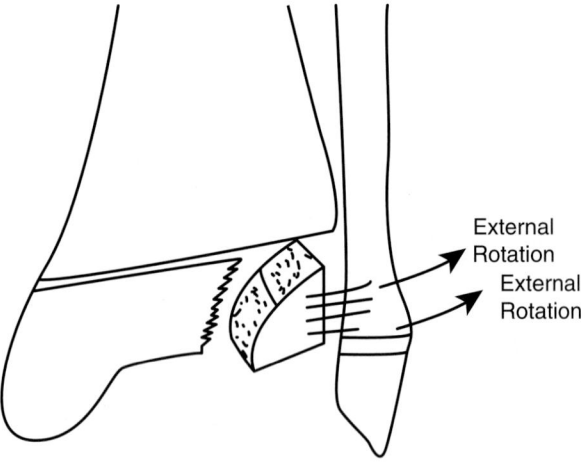

JUNENILE TILLAUX FRACTURE

FIGURE 55.7 Juvenile Tillaux fracture. External rotation mechanism with Salter-Harris III fracture of the epiphysis.

TREATMENT OF DISTAL TIBIA AND FIBULA ANKLE FRACTURES

Treatment of Salter-Harris Type I and Type II Distal Tibia Fractures

Salter-Harris type I and II fractures may or may not have displacement on the radiographs. The radiograph may have a normal appearance other than soft tissue swelling or slight widening of the physis. A nondisplaced Salter-Harris II fracture is often easier to recognize on radiographs because of the metaphyseal fracture line. Comparison view of the opposite ankle may be

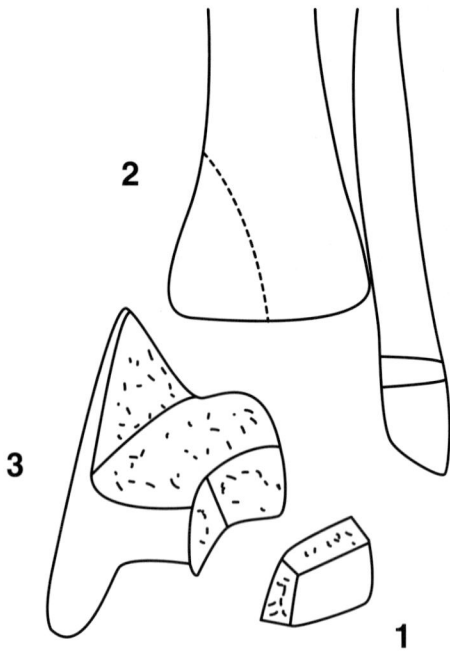

FIGURE 55.9 Three-part triplane fracture. Salter-Harris IV fracture distal tibia. (*1*) The epiphyseal fragment, anterolateral; (*2*) Main portion of tibia proximally; (*3*) Fracture fragment with components of distal epiphysis, physis, and metaphyseal spike posteriorly.

helpful for Salter-Harris I fractures. If there is no displacement on radiographs, the patient is tender over the physis, and there is a clear history of trauma, then immobilization should be used with follow-up radiographs at 7 and 14 days.

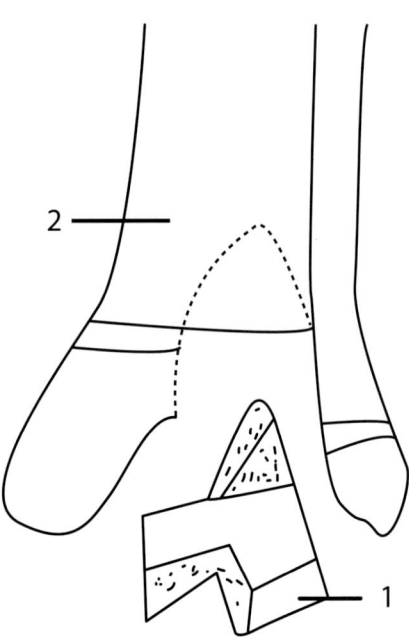

FIGURE 55.8 Two-part triplane fracture. A Salter-Harris IV fracture distal tibia. (*1*) The distal fragment with metaphyseal, physeal, and epiphyseal components. (*2*) The proximal tibia also with metaphyseal, physeal, and epiphyseal components.

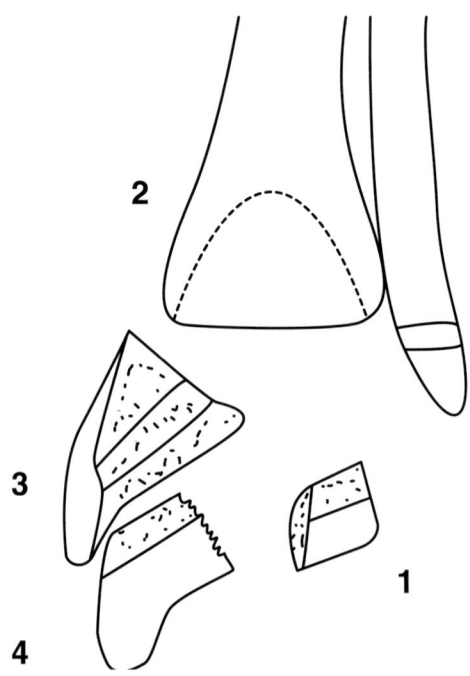

FIGURE 55.10 Four-part triplane fracture. Salter-Harris IV fracture of the distal tibia. (*1*) The epiphyseal fragment, anterolateral; (*2*) Main portion of tibia proximally; (*3*) Fracture fragment with components of distal epiphysis, physis, and metaphyseal spike posteriorly; (*4*) Epiphyseal fragment anteromedially at the medial malleolus.

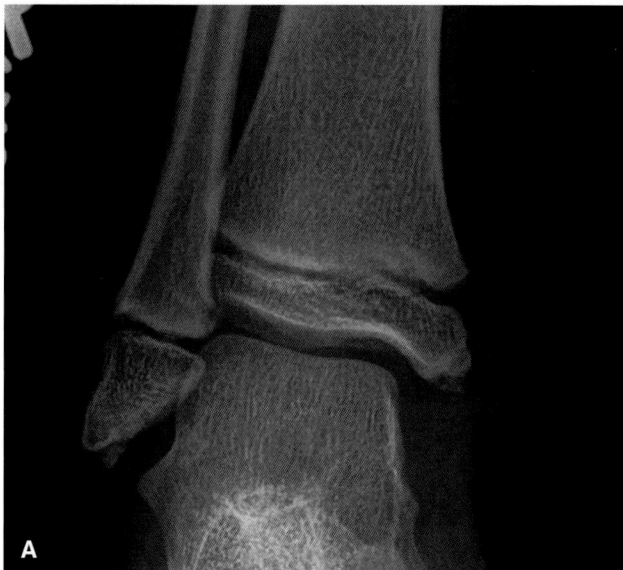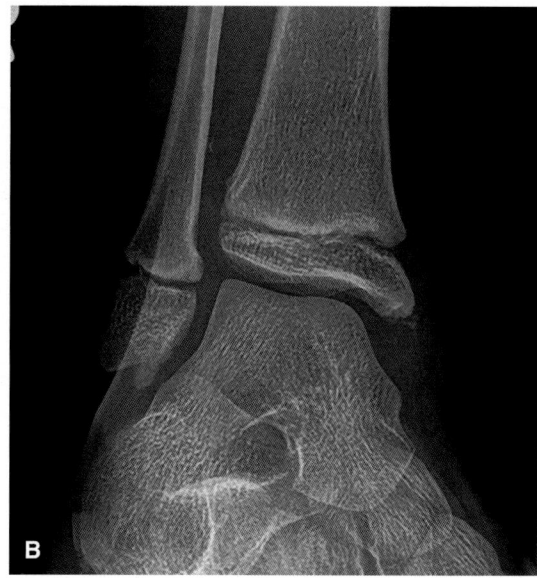

FIGURE 55.11 Radiographic anatomy of the immature ankle. Seven-year-old girl. **A.** AP view. **B.** Mortise. The accessory ossification areas within the cartilaginous epiphysis on the medial malleolus, and distal fibular epiphysis may be misinterpreted as avulsion fractures. The incisura at the distal tibia-fibula articulation is not quite visible on radiographs. There is overlap of the tibia and fibula on the AP but not on the Mortise, which is normal for this age. (From Bozic KJ, Jaramillo D, DiCanzio J, et al. Radiographic appearance of the normal distal tibiofibular syndesmosis in children. *J Pediatr Orthop.* 1999;19(1):14-21.)

Displaced Salter-Harris I and II fractures may require manipulation depending on the amount of displacement. If there is >3 mm of physeal displacement on the injury film, there is a 70% increase risk of growth arrest over nondisplaced injuries.[55] In displaced fractures, up to 12 degrees of distal tibia varus or valgus tilt correcting spontaneously in younger patients has been reported in older literature.[56] Conversely, Spiegel et al. reported growth arrest with Salter-Harris II fractures.[57] Reliance on fracture remodeling alone may lead to a deformity that cannot remodel if a growth arrest occurs. The goal of reduction should be <5 degrees of varus, or valgus alignment, and minimal physeal displacement (<3 mm).[55–57]

Authors' Preferred Treatment Nondisplaced Distal Tibia Salter-Harris I and II Fractures

Nondisplaced Salter-Harris I and II fractures are treated in an above knee cast. If there is any question about displacement, or the fracture pattern, a CT scan is done. A delayed reduction past 10-14 days involves forceful manipulation, or an open reduction, with risk to the physis. In patients with >2 years of anticipated growth remaining, it is preferable to avoid late reductions maneuvers after 10-14 days. Late manipulations have the potential of creating a physeal arrest. Early follow-up radiographs are advisable within 5-7 days of the injury to monitor for displacement so prompt changes in the treatment plan can be undertaken.

Patients are non–weight bearing for 6 weeks. At 4 weeks, the cast is often changed to a below knee cast. At 6 weeks, fractures of the distal tibia are typically changed to a fracture boot, allowed to weight bear, and rehabilitation begins. Return to activity occurs at 12-16 weeks. Follow-up is suggested for 18-24 months for potential premature growth arrest.

PEARLS

An above knee cast may aid in maintaining a non–weight-bearing status, and it allows rotational control assisting in the prevention of fracture displacement. An above knee cast may also increase comfort by minimizing tibial rotation through the knee joint minimizing fracture motion in the first few weeks.

Authors' Preferred Treatment Displaced Distal Tibia Salter-Harris I and II Fractures

Manipulation of displaced fractures involves reversing the mechanism of injury as described in Dias-Tachdjian classification. Anesthesia is used to avoid unnecessary additional trauma on the physis with repeated reduction attempts. Data in the literature suggest that multiple reduction attempts may be related to premature physeal closure. The severity of the mechanism of injury and the initial displacement seem to be significant predictors of growth arrest after a physeal injury.[55,56]

Displaced Salter-Harris I and II fractures have fracture reductions performed for displacement of more than 3 mm, varus/valgus tilt of more than 5 degrees, or more than 5 degrees of plantarflexion/dorsiflexion tilt. While remodeling may occur with angulations of 10 degrees or more, it seems advisable to minimize the angulation. Achieving fracture alignment acutely is easier than a late osteotomy to correct deformity.

Once satisfactory alignment is achieved, displaced Salter-Harris I fractures may be treated with immobilization in an above knee cast alone. If there are concerns about stability, 1.6-, 2.0-, or 2.4-mm smooth cross pins are used depending on patient size. To decrease the chance of infection, percutaneous smooth pins are removed by 4 weeks. The pins are by necessity,

either juxta-articular or intra-articular. Buried pins may be used, but this requires a second trip to the operating room for pin removal prior to weight bearing. After pin removal, a below knee cast is used until healing allows weight bearing at 6-8 weeks.

> ### PEARLS
>
> Caution with pins is advised. Larger pins have a risk of growth arrest if greater in size than 7%-9% of the cross-sectional area of the physis.[18,19] Smaller pins carry the risk of pin breakage.

After fracture reduction of a displaced Salter-Harris II fracture, percutaneous cannulated 4.0- or 4.5-mm screw(s) are placed using a lag technique within the metaphysis above the physis. If an open reduction is required, the incision should be made to allow either access to the metaphyseal spike or the ability to access the persistent area of physeal gap depending on the location of soft tissue interposition. If the metaphyseal fragment is large enough to allow adequate screw fixation, a non–weight bearing below knee cast can be used. If there are worries about stability, then an above knee cast is used for the first few weeks.

In displaced distal tibia fractures, weight bearing is typically allowed by 6 weeks. Rehabilitation follows with return to activity by 12-16 weeks. Follow-up care is provided for 18-24 months for potential premature growth arrest.

Treatment of Medial Malleolus Salter-Harris Type III and IV Fractures

The medial malleolus fracture is typically a grade II supination-inversion injury creating either a Salter-Harris III or IV fracture. The articular cartilage and the physis must be anatomically reduced. Nondisplaced fractures may be treated in an above

knee cast non–weight bearing. These fractures need careful follow-up when treated with immobilization alone. The use of a CT scan after cast placement may be warranted to accurately judge the displacement.

While these can be treated with immobilization alone, the trend is operative fixation. The medial malleolus fractures tend to be unstable patterns. The medial malleolus may also have a delayed union, nonunion, and physeal growth arrest with the development of a bony bridge across the physis.[58–60]

Physeal injuries to the ankle have been shown to have an 11% risk of arthritis at skeletal maturity.[61] Anatomic preservation of the joint surface is the goal. The recommendation is to treat any displacement >1-2 mm with a goal of restoring the articular surface and anatomic alignment of the physis.[58–60,62] While it is clear that a bridging bone will form across a mismatched, displaced physis, growth arrest does occur even with anatomic reduction.[58] With a risk of physeal growth arrest, and delayed union, a 1 mm step-off is an indication for operative treatment of medial malleolus physeal fractures.[60]

With a displaced medial malleolus injury, a medial approach using the anterior incision at the medial malleolus is used. The approach allows joint visualization, fracture reduction, and screw placement.[63] Indirect techniques and arthroscopic assist techniques have been described in pediatric ankle fractures.[64,65]

Authors' Preferred Treatment Medial Malleolus Salter-Harris III and IV Fractures

Nondisplaced Salter-Harris III and IV medial malleolus fractures are treated with one to two percutaneous 4.0-mm cannulated screws parallel to the physis if the fracture pattern allows (Fig. 55.12). There is a strong recommendation in the literature for treating fractures with as little as 1 mm of stepoff.[60] Fracture fixation, even in nondisplaced medial malleolus fractures, in

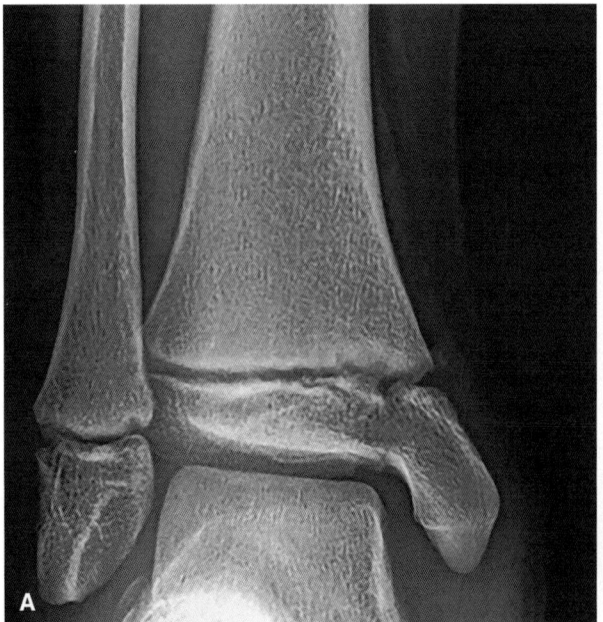
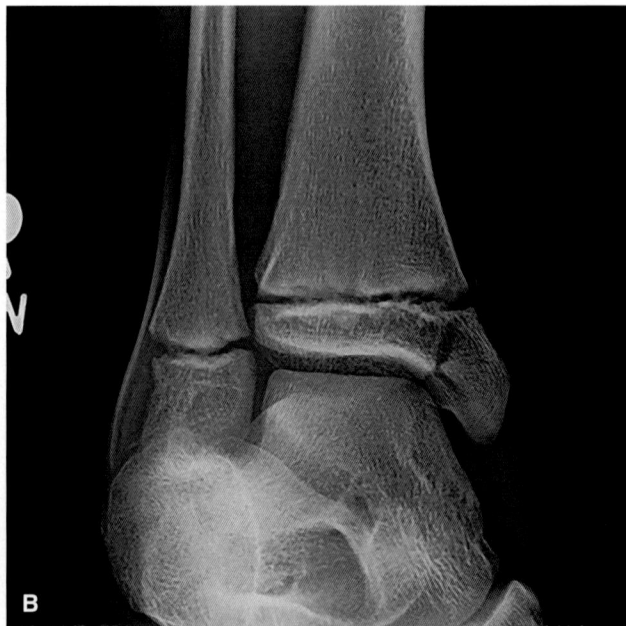

FIGURE 55.12 Medial malleolus Salter-Harris III fracture. **A.** Ten-year-old boy with an AP view. **B.** Mortise view. Note there is overlap of tibia and fibula on AP view but no overlap on the Mortise view. This is normal for this age.[52] The area of the incisura is beginning to show on the radiographs.

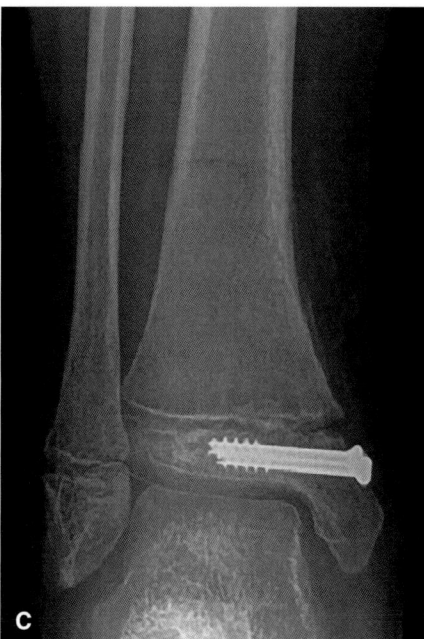

FIGURE 55.12 (*Continued*) **C.** Treated with open reduction and cannulated screw fixation parallel to the physis.

the authors' opinion, is a more predictable outcome with the benefit of preventing loss of alignment.

Displaced Salter-Harris III and IV medial malleolus fractures are approached through an anterior medial approach. Screw fixation is in the epiphysis parallel to the physis when the fracture pattern allows. Arthroscopy has not been required.

A below knee cast is acceptable if the patient is able to remain strictly non–weight bearing. Weight bearing is delayed until fracture healing is convincing on the radiographs. This may take 6 weeks. Once healing has occurred, progressive

weight bearing with rehabilitation is begun. Return to activity occurs at 12-16 weeks. Follow-up is provided for 18-24 months for potential premature growth arrest.

In patients with a low transverse medial malleolus fracture, internal fixation with smooth pins across the physis, tension band technique, or short 3.5- or 4.0-mm screws perpendicular to the fracture stopping short of the physis may be used. These fixation methods required in low transverse fractures may benefit from an above knee cast to "back-up" the internal fixation (Fig. 55.13). These are smaller fracture fragments subject to loss of fixation with rotation of the tibia.

Treatment of Juvenile Tillaux Fracture

This is a Salter-Harris III fracture of the anterior lateral epiphysis of the tibia due to an external rotation force.[44] The anterior inferior tibiofibular ligament pulls the anterolateral epiphyseal fragment away from the distal tibia (Fig. 55.14). The anterolateral epiphysis is the last area of the physis of the distal tibia to close near skeletal maturity.

If the fracture is nondisplaced, it may be treated in an above knee cast strictly with no weight bearing. A CT scan is often done to verify there is no displacement. If there is >2 mm of displacement, reduction and internal fixation with screws should be performed.[66,67] The anterolateral approach to the ankle is used. The incision is often smaller (2.5-3 cm) than described for extensile approaches.[63]

PEARLS

Percutaneous screw fixation of the Tillaux fracture involves an anterolateral trajectory. The superficial peroneal nerve is at risk with the anterolateral approach. With a percutaneous technique, the nerve may be injured with a drill, tap, or screw.

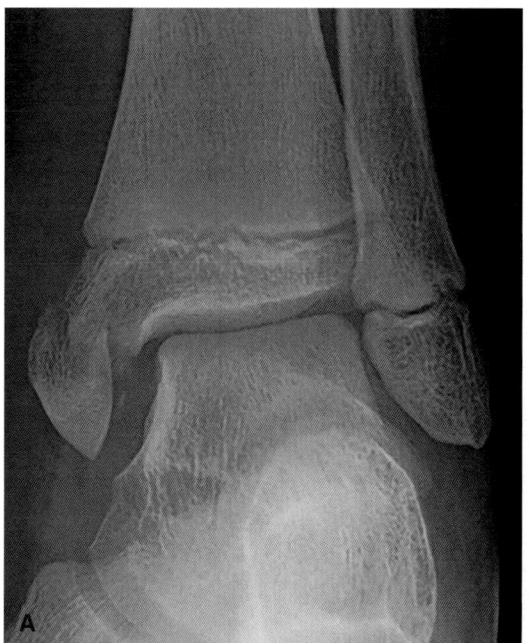
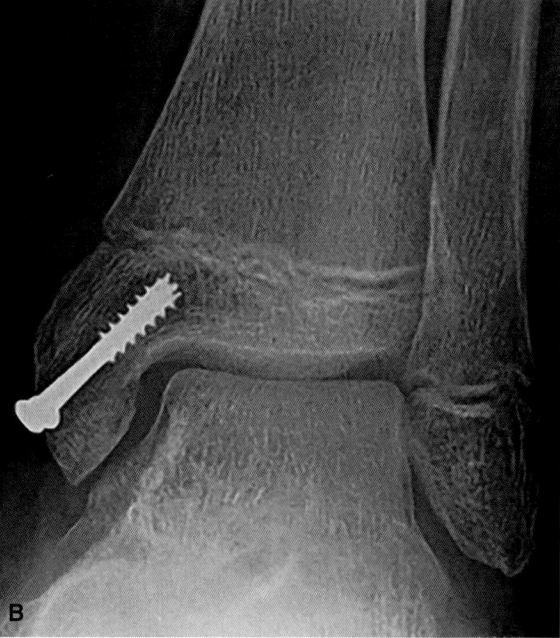

FIGURE 55.13 Low medial malleolus fracture. **A.** Low medial malleolus fracture within epiphysis. **B.** Open reduction with screw fixation in a 12-year-old girl avoiding the medial physis.

Treatment of Triplane Fracture of the Distal Tibia and Fibula

The triplane fracture pattern consists of an intra-articular fracture line through the epiphysis extending through the physis into the metaphysis. The fracture line runs in sagittal, transverse (axial), and frontal (coronal) planes. It is a Salter-Harris IV injury to the distal tibia.[45–48] The fractures can be two-part, three-part, or four-part injuries (see Fig. 55.8-55.10). Understanding the definition and patterns is key to treatment. A total of 48% of triplane fractures may have associated fibula fractures, and 8.5% may have ipsilateral tibial shaft fractures.[68]

Nondisplaced fractures can be treated with immobilization. The mechanism of injury involves rotational forces, so the preference is for above knee immobilization when no internal fixation is used. While nondisplaced fractures do occur, most of these fractures are displaced. A CT scan is useful in determining displacement, defining the anatomy, and in preoperative planning. If there is displacement >2 mm, reduction of the fracture with internal fixation should be planned.

Authors' Preferred Treatment Displaced Salter-Harris III and IV Fractures—Juvenile Tillaux And Triplane Fractures

The majority of the Tillaux and triplane fractures are best treated with reduction and internal fixation. Nondisplaced Salter-Harris III Tillaux or Salter-Harris IV triplane fractures may be treated with above knee cast treatment. CT scan is done to verify the displacement is <2 mm.

The displaced Tillaux fracture is internally rotated to achieve reduction. Direct compression or the use of a tenaculum closes the fracture allowing placement of cannulated 4.0-mm screws parallel to the physis in the epiphysis for skeletally immature patients (Fig. 55.14). Two screws are typically used.

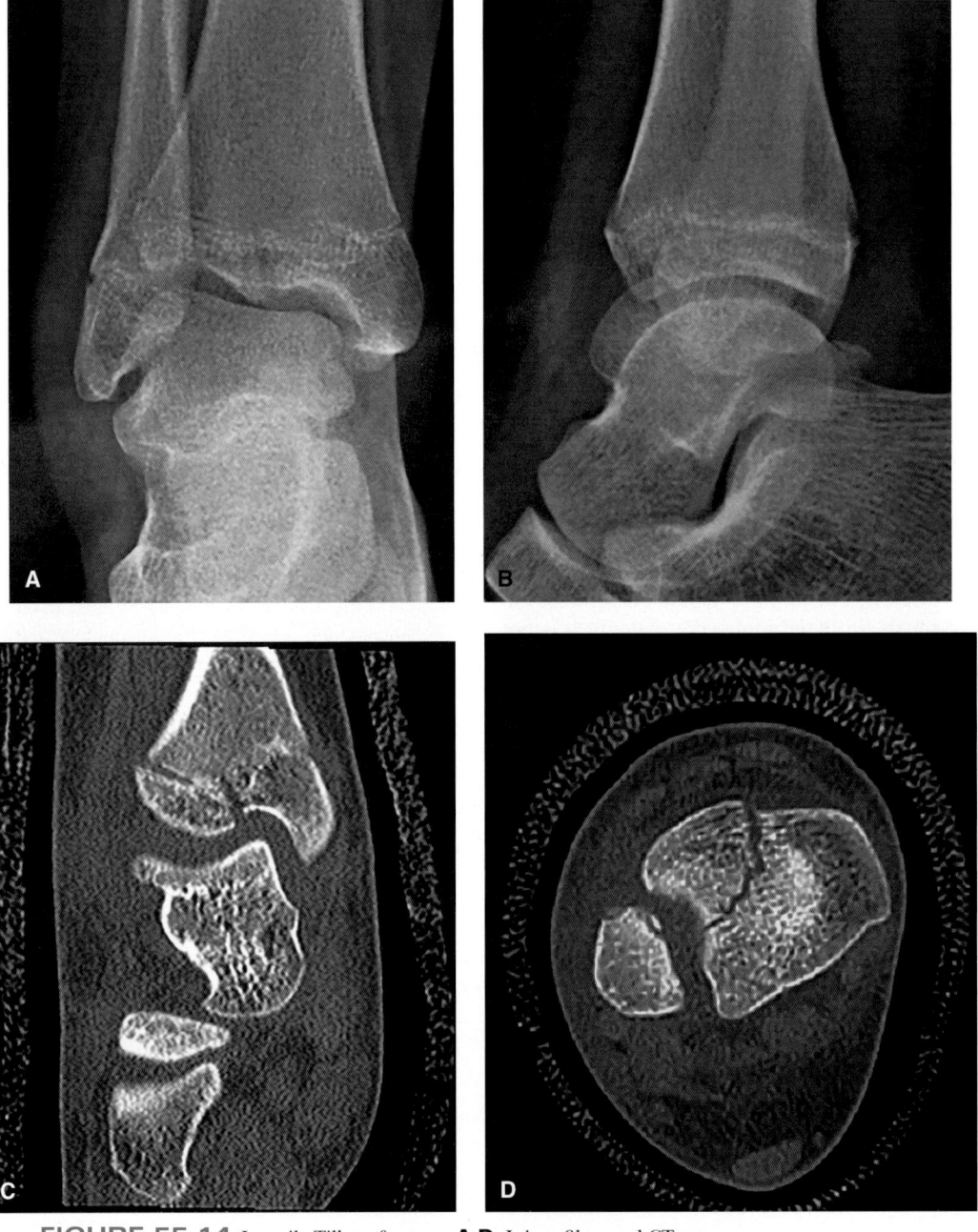

FIGURE 55.14 Juvenile Tillaux fracture. **A-D.** Injury films and CT scan.

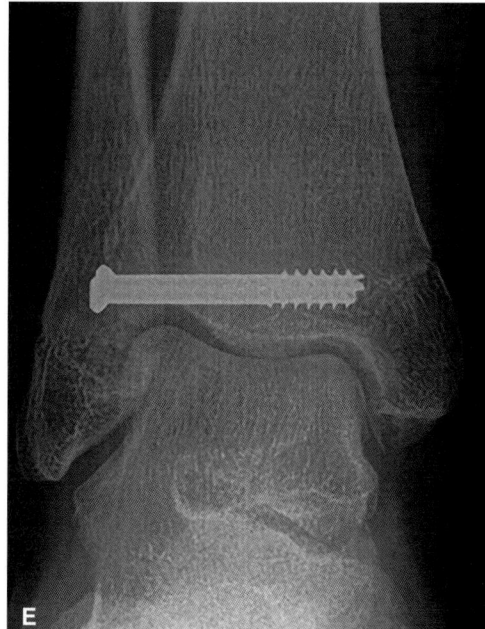
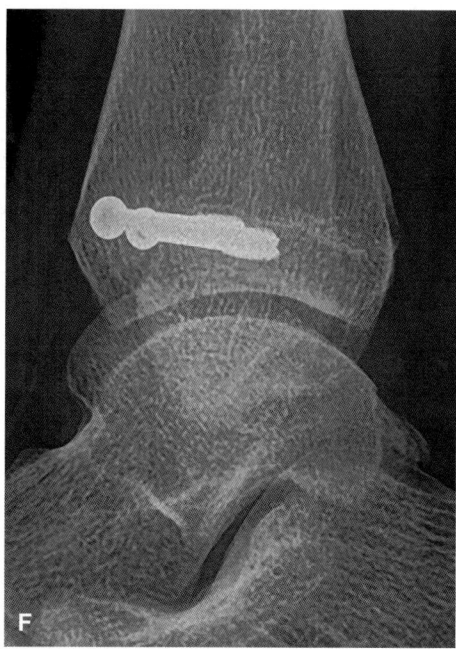

FIGURE 55.14 (*Continued*) **E, F.** Six months postoperatively after open reduction with internal fixation. The physes are closed. On the injury films, the physis is clearly closing on the distal tibia, so screws are allowed to enter the physeal scar on the medial side of the distal tibia further from subchondral bone. In younger patients with a completely open physis, screws should be parallel to the physis contained within the epiphysis below the physis.

Percutaneous screw fixation with reduction is used by some surgeons, but accurate reduction is required. Care must be taken to not injure the superficial peroneal nerve, so the use of a small 2.5-3 cm anterolateral approach is common.[63]

Displaced triplane fractures are imaged with a CT scan to determine displacement and for planning screw placement. Closed manipulation and percutaneous screw fixation may be possible; however, the surgeon should be prepared to use open reduction through any of the common ankle approaches. Anteromedial, posterormedial, anterolateral, and posterolateral approaches are used.[63] In younger patients, screw fixation should avoid the physis. In older adolescent patients, it is not as necessary to avoid the physis if the patient is within a year of skeletal maturity.

A closed reduction attempt is the first step in the operating room. An internal rotation maneuver is done for lateral displacement, while abduction is the primary manipulation for medial displacement. If the closed reduction is successful, percutaneous cannulated 4.0- or 4.5-mm screws can be used. If a closed reduction is not satisfactory, then open reduction is performed.

Open reduction of a two-part triplane fracture that is medially displaced is through an anteromedial incision.[63] A two-part triplane fracture that is laterally displaced is treated through an anterolateral incision.[63] Three-part and four-part triplane fractures (Fig. 55.15) may require more than one incision.

Postoperative care, when treated with internal fixation, is in a below knee cast non–weight bearing for 4-6 weeks. If there is a displaced fibula fracture that reduces with the triplane reduction, concerns regarding internal fixation stability, or concerns about the patient maintaining a non–weight bearing status, then an above knee cast is used. At 6 weeks, once healing is present, a fracture boot with progressive weight bearing and rehabilitation can begin. Return to activity may be achieved by 12-16 weeks. Follow-up until skeletal maturity is provided for potential risk of premature growth arrest.

PEARLS

In the treatment of a triplane injury, the fracture fragment containing the metaphyseal spike is often addressed first. This fragment can, at times, be secured with screws across the metaphysis above the physis following a closed manipulation. Then the separate epiphyseal fractures are addressed as needed with open reduction and internal fixation.

Treatment of Metaphyseal Distal Tibia Fractures

Metaphyseal distal tibia fractures range from incomplete injuries to injuries with near 100% displacement. If the fibula remains intact, the fibular length may protect against excessive valgus angulation of the distal tibia. Buckle (torus) fractures of the distal tibia in younger patients are treated with cast immobilization with no manipulation.

Guidelines for acceptable angulation are extrapolated from tibial shaft fracture treatment guidelines. Recurvatum, or apex posterior, deformity in tibial shaft fractures remodels poorly. Valgus angulation has also been shown to incompletely remodel in tibial shaft fractures.[69–71] Remodeling of a tibial shaft fracture is more reliable under the age of 10 years. Even so the spontaneous correction of the deformity over 12-18 months is not always complete.[72]

Authors' Preferred Treatment of Distal Tibia Fractures

While the expectation is that the distal tibia metaphysis should remodel more than the tibial diaphysis, it is prudent to minimize the angulation of a complete metaphyseal distal tibia fracture to 10 degrees or less in patients under 10 years of age. In patients over 10-11 years of age, there is less remodeling for tibial shaft fractures with less tolerance for residual angulation.

Initial cast treatment is most often with an above knee cast that is flexed at the knee. This cast helps avoid the cast sliding off the foot, controls rotation, and dissuades weight bearing. Weight bearing by 4-6 weeks is possible.

PEARLS

Dorsiflexion of the ankle to neutral for cast application may create apex posterior angulation (recurvatum) of a tibia fracture. Plantarflexion in the cast is acceptable to achieve satisfactory fracture alignment. After several weeks, the foot and ankle are dorsiflexed as the fracture healing allows.

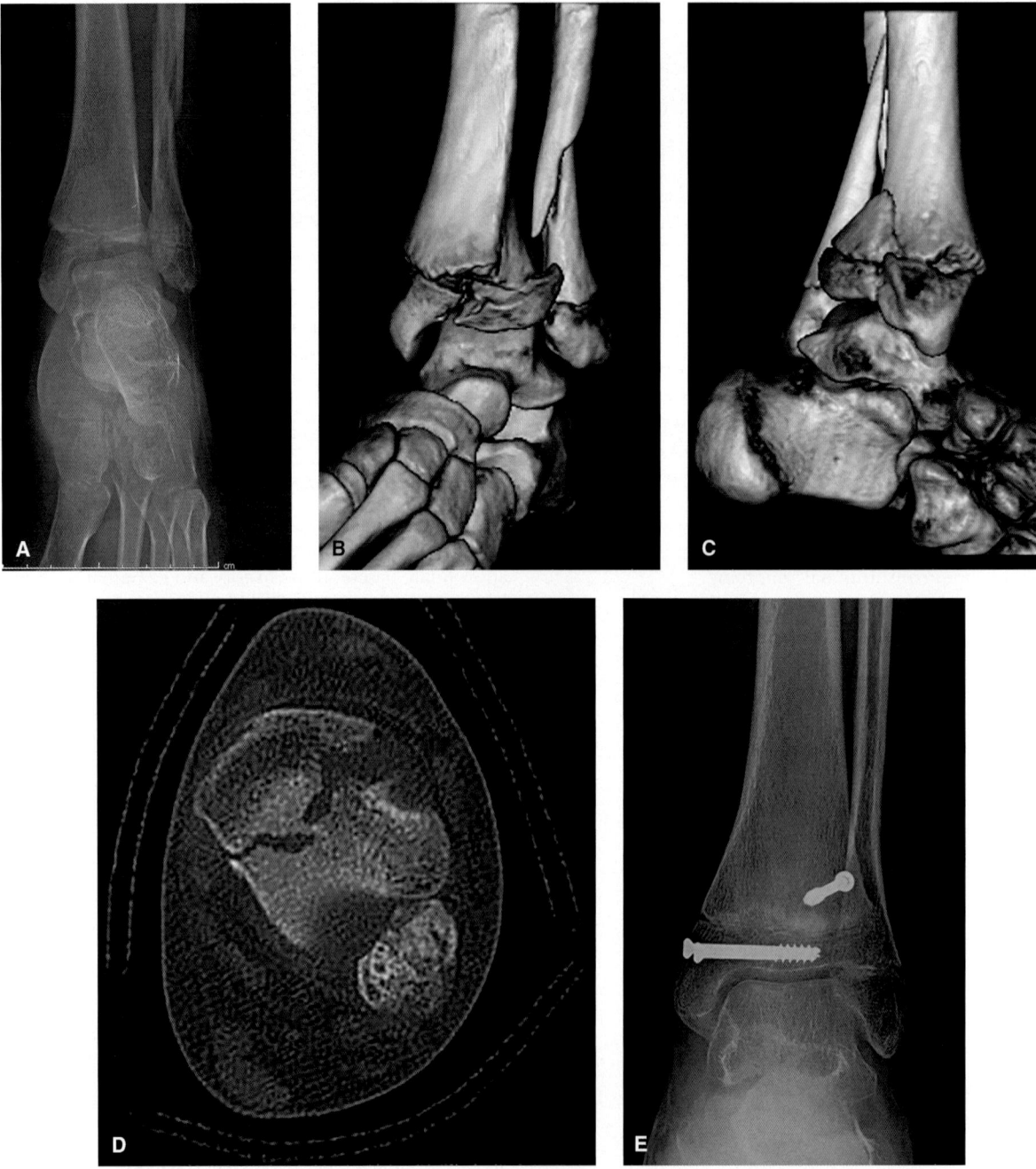

FIGURE 55.15 Four-part triplane fracture in a 13-year-old girl injured in soccer. **A-D.** The medial side of the epiphysis has a coronal split between the medial malleolus and the posterior epiphysis, which is attached to the metaphyseal spike. The anterolateral epiphysis is a separate fragment as well. **E-G.** Internal fixation. The fibula reduction occurred with reduction of the tibia.

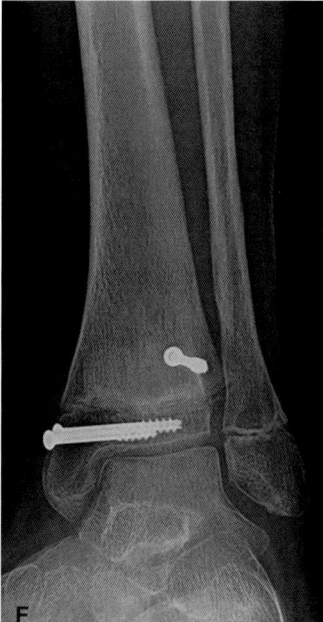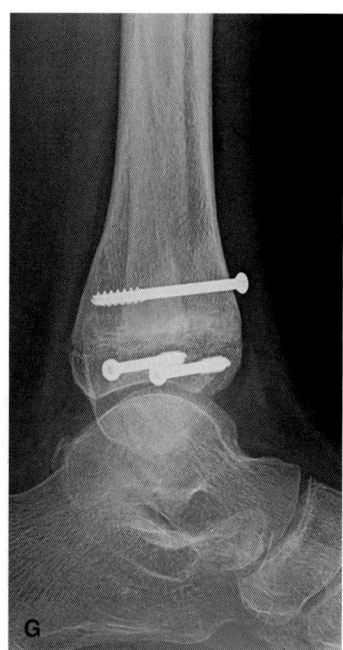

FIGURE 55.15 (*Continued*)

Toddler's Fracture of the Tibia

This is a nondisplaced or minimally displaced tibia fracture in the setting of an intact fibula (Fig. 55.16). It is typically seen in children under the age of 3-4 years.[73] The tibia has a spiral/oblique fracture occurring in the distal metaphysis or diaphysis. Twisting injuries while standing, jumping off of furniture, or coming down a slide are common mechanisms. The injury may not be witnessed. Patients may present with a limp or with refusal to bear weight. On examination, gentle rotation of the tibia often reproduces discomfort. It is imperative to take a history asking about constitutional symptoms.

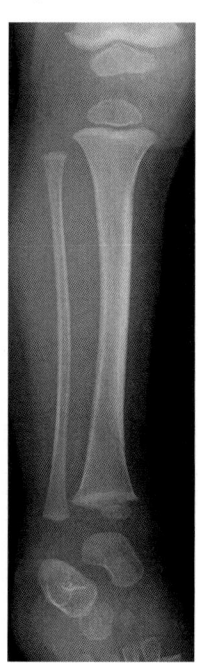

FIGURE 55.16 Toddler fracture in the distal tibial metaphysis.

The fracture line can be difficult to discern on radiographs. AP, lateral, and oblique views of the tibia are helpful. Follow-up radiographs at 10-14 days may show the fracture line or periosteal new bone formation if not visible initially. Treatment of a toddler's fracture is cast immobilization for 4-6 weeks until radiographic healing is assured.

Authors' Preferred Treatment of Toddler's Fracture of the Tibia

In patients with no constitutional symptoms, and a normal radiograph, a presumptive diagnosis of toddler's fracture is appropriate based on the history and examination.[74] An above knee cast is often used. Early follow-up in the first 2 weeks is required with a presumptive diagnosis.

In a presumptive toddler's fracture, if the patient is not improving during the first 7-14 days, or there is new onset of constitutional symptoms, then the cast is removed for reassessment with radiographs out of cast. The potential differential diagnosis includes musculoskeletal infection, tumor, nonaccidental trauma, or juvenile arthritis. Laboratory blood work and advanced imaging may be necessary. While this evaluation is ongoing, immobilization is maintained.

> **PEARLS**
>
> Subsequent completion (displacement) of a toddler's tibia fracture with weight bearing can occur when treated with a below knee cast or fracture boot. The immobilization must extend past the proximal extent of the tibia fracture, and it should ideally provide rotational control at the fracture site. An above knee cast is preferable.

Treatment of Adolescent Tibial Pilon Fractures

These injuries are small in number in the literature. The average age in one study was 15 years and 10 months of age.[75] This is an adult injury pattern. Treatment principles follow adult guidelines.

Treatment of Syndesmosis Injuries of the Distal Tibia and Fibula

Isolated syndesmotic injuries are very rare in the pediatric age group.[76] This injury is more likely to be seen in older adolescent patients near the end of skeletal growth.[77]

The majority of syndesmotic injuries reported are associated with fractures of the distal fibula or tibia. Syndesmotic injuries have been reported in triplane fractures.[78] Imaging in younger patients may lead to confusion. Comparison views of the uninjured ankle can be of help. The mean age at which tibia fibula overlap on the AP view of the ankle is 5 years. The tibiofibular overlap on the mortise radiograph occurs around the age of 10 years for females, and as late 16 years for males.[52] Treatment guidelines follow adult principles.

Treatment of the Distal Fibula Fracture

Salter-Harris I and II fractures of the distal fibula are often minimally displaced and treated with immobilization alone. A below knee cast, fracture boot, or ankle brace is used for patient comfort.[79,80] The literature does show that ultrasound or MRI can be used if there is a need to discern a Salter-Harris I fracture from another etiology.[34,81] Weight bearing is typically allowed as the patient becomes comfortable.

Isolated displaced Salter-Harris I and II displaced fractures of the fibula are uncommon but encountered.[82] If translated significantly, the concern is the relationship of the mortise and associated ligamentous structures. These may require open treatment.

Displaced fractures of the fibula or lateral malleolus are also associated with displaced Salter-Harris III and IV fractures of distal tibia. These will often reduce with reduction of the tibial fracture. The fibula does not necessarily require internal fixation. If the syndesmosis is a concern, or the fibula fracture is not reduced satisfactorily, then open reduction and internal

fixation is performed. Occasionally, internal fixation of the distal fibula fracture provides stability to prevent lateral or valgus angulation of a distal tibia fracture

Authors' Preferred Treatment of Distal Fibula Fractures

Most Salter-Harris I fractures of the distal fibula are nondisplaced and can be treated with a below knee cast or fracture boot depending on patient. Displaced fractures of the fibula are often associated with displaced Salter-Harris III and IV fractures of distal tibia (Figs. 55.17 and 55.18). The fibula may reduce with treatment of the tibia fracture (see Fig. 55.15).

Isolated displaced epiphyseal fractures of the distal fibula may require open reduction and internal fixation. When translation of 30% or more through the fibular physis persists after manipulation, open reduction and internal fixation techniques with a smooth pin may be used. Low fractures (avulsions) through the fibular epiphysis involving >30% of the epiphysis may also benefit from pin, small screw, or suture fixation provided the fibular fracture fragment is not comminuted.

Treatment of Ankle Sprains

In younger patients, it is more typical to see pain with tenderness over the lateral malleolus at the physis. These represent nondisplaced Salter-Harris I fractures. If the tenderness is over the ligaments, and not the bone, then this may represent an ankle sprain.[81]

Sprains can be treated with ankle brace, fracture boot, or cast depending on patient's comfort, and ability to bear weight.[79,80] After 3-4 weeks of immobilization, rehabilitation with gradual return to activity over the next 4-6 weeks is the typical course. Adolescent patients with severe sprains or sprains involving the syndesmosis are treated as adults.

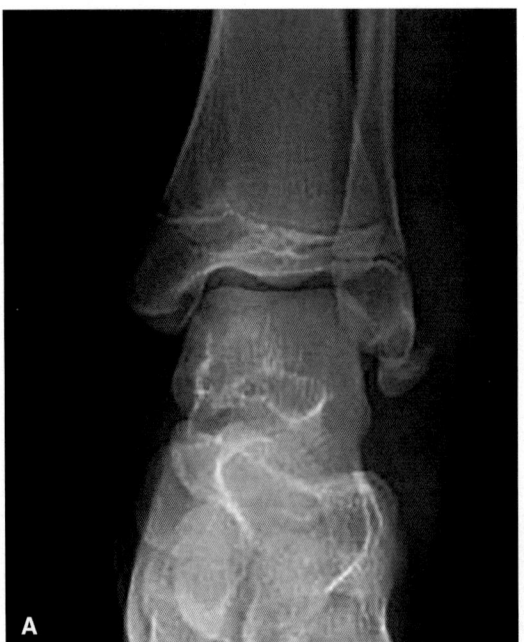
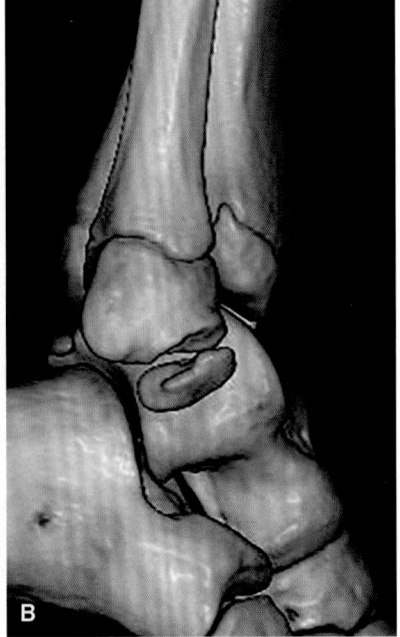

FIGURE 55.17 Low epiphyseal fibula fracture 13-year-old girl after soccer injury. **A, B.** Injury film and CT reconstruction lateral view. Axial, coronal, and sagittal CT verified fragment size at 15 mm in anteroposterior plane and 10 mm in depth.

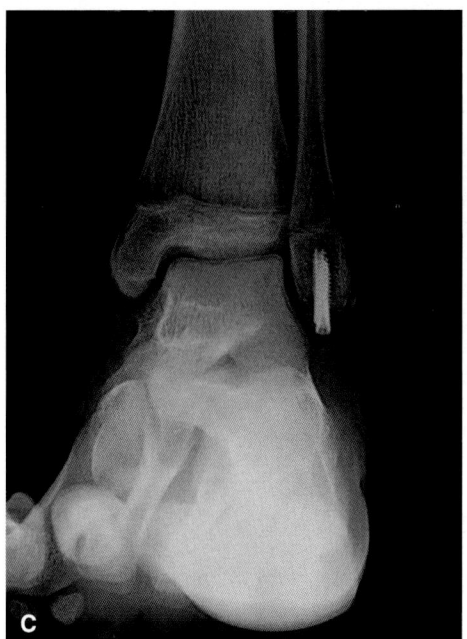
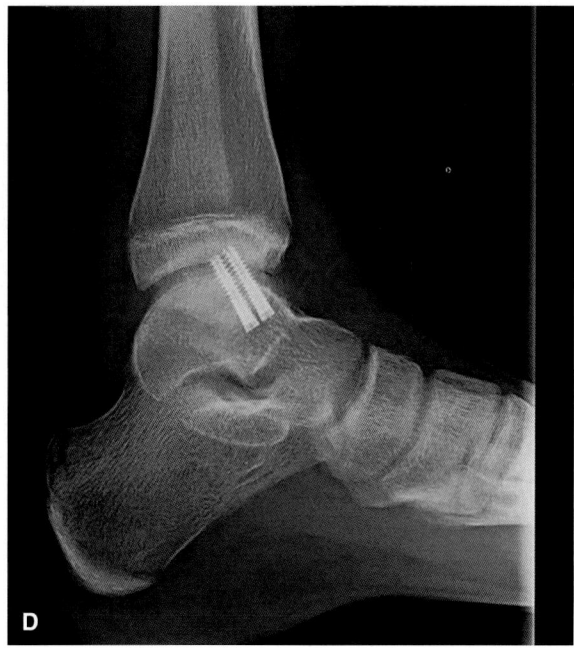

FIGURE 55.17 (*Continued*) **C, D.** Open reduction and internal fixation with headless compression screws.

PEARLS

Recurrent ankle sprains in older children and adolescent patients may be seen in tarsal coalitions.

Treatment of Accessory Ossicle—Os Subtibiale and Os Subfibulare

Differentiating whether an "avulsion fragment" seen at the tip of the fibula or medial malleolus is a fracture or it is a variation of normal epiphyseal ossification can be difficult. The literature does support that there are variations in the epiphyseal ossification pattern.[29,30]

The os subfibulare as a nonunion related to an avulsion fracture from the anterotalofibular ligament is also seen in the literature.[33]

Comparison radiographs of the opposite ankle are valuable. If the area of the ossicle is tender, then immobilization in a cast or fracture boot may help alleviate symptoms. If a patient remains symptomatic, or there is confusion, MRI may be of benefit.[54]

FIGURE 55.18 Displaced distal fibula Salter-Harris I fracture. Thirteen-year-old boy presents 2 weeks after injury. **A.** Note the mismatch of the width of the metaphysis and epiphysis. **B.** Lateral view the fibular epiphysis is posterior to the fibular metaphysis.

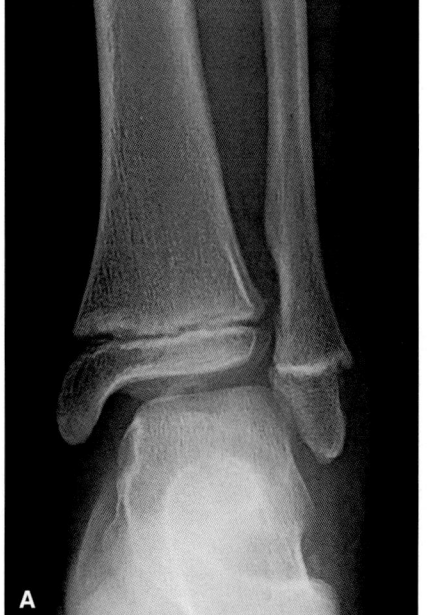
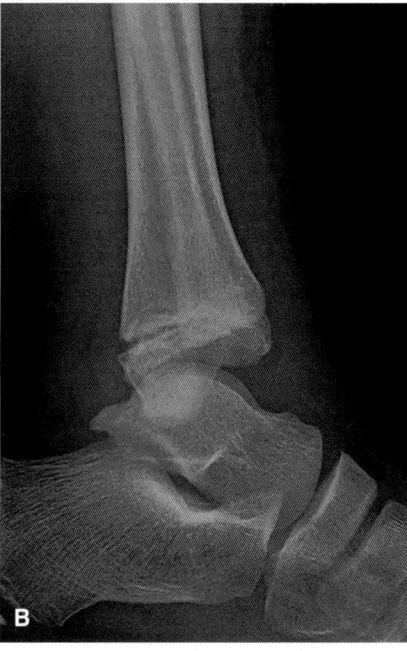

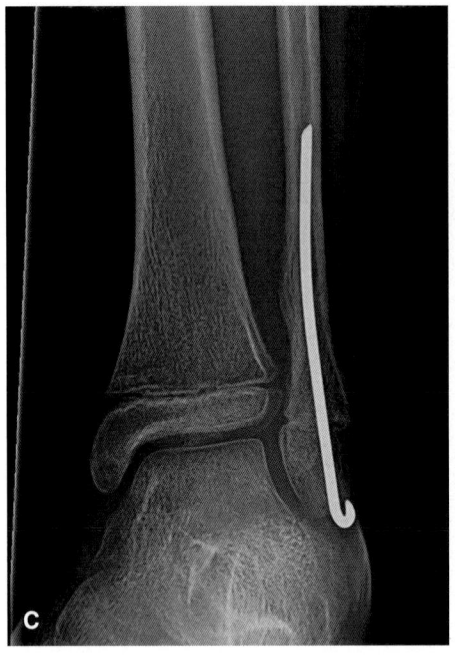

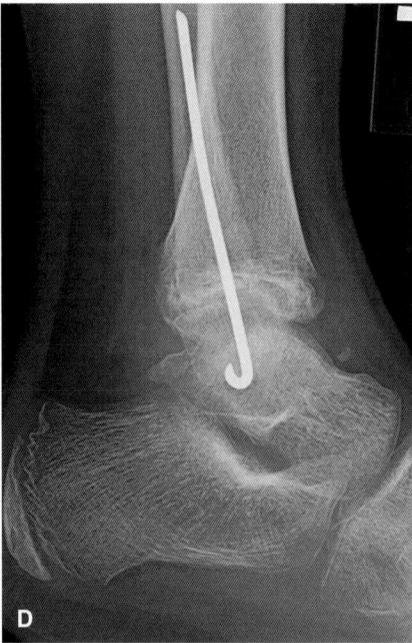

FIGURE 55.18 (*Continued*) **C, D.** Required open reduction and a smooth rod. On the mortise view **(C)** the fibula and tibia do not overlap. The incisura is beginning to appear on the radiograph. The lack of overlap is normal up to the age of 16 years for males. (Reproduced with permission from Bozic KJ, Jaramillo D, DiCanzio J, et al. Radiographic appearance of the normal distal tibiofibular syndesmosis in children. *J Pediatr Orthop.* 1999;19(1):14-21.)

COMPLICATIONS UNIQUE TO PEDIATRIC PATIENTS

Splint and Cast Application Complications

Complications related to splints and casts are under reported. Young patients have difficulty with verbalizing complaints. Pressure sores with skin breakdown may easily occur (Fig. 55.19). These injuries are often unrecognized until the cast or splint is removed.

Prefabricated fiberglass splints with no additional circumferential soft wrap on the skin prior to splint application are often applied. Skin breakdown from the elastic wrap rubbing directly on the skin occurs in children. In commonly applied posterior splints to the lower extremity, the foot is able to plantar flex sliding cephalad. This creates skin pressure over the heel from the splint and the dorsum of the foot from the elastic wrap.

> ### PEARLS
>
> The use of circumferential soft padding with plaster, fiberglass, or commercially available splints aids in the protection of the skin from pressure and elastic wraps. Given the concerns for heel pressure sores, avoiding posterior splints for lower extremity injuries in pediatric and adolescent age groups seem advisable.

Complications of Limb Length Discrepancy and Angular Deformity after Ankle Injuries

The literature is clear that the severity of the mechanism of injury and the initial displacement seem to be significant predictors of growth arrest after a physeal injury.[55,56,83] Delayed union, malunion, nonunion, stiffness, pain, and arthritis are potential sequelae of ankle injuries in all age groups. In follow-up, an 11% risk of arthritis in skeletal maturity has been reported in patients with fractures during childhood and adolescence.[61,82] Changes in distal tibial angulation produce changes in the contact areas of the tibiotalar joint.[84]

If a physeal arrest occurs, it may create an angular deformity, limb length inequality, or prevent satisfactory remodeling of a displaced fracture. Physeal distal tibial growth ranges from 4 to 6 mm/y allowing estimations on the loss of longitudinal growth possible. It should be remembered that there is less than the anticipated growth remaining in the 12-18 months prior to complete physiologic physeal closure.[35–40] Limb length discrepancy can be managed with epiphysiodesis, acute shortening osteotomy, limb lengthening, or physeal bar resection.

Distal tibia or distal fibula growth arrest can affect the ankle mortise due to asymmetric growth and alterations in the

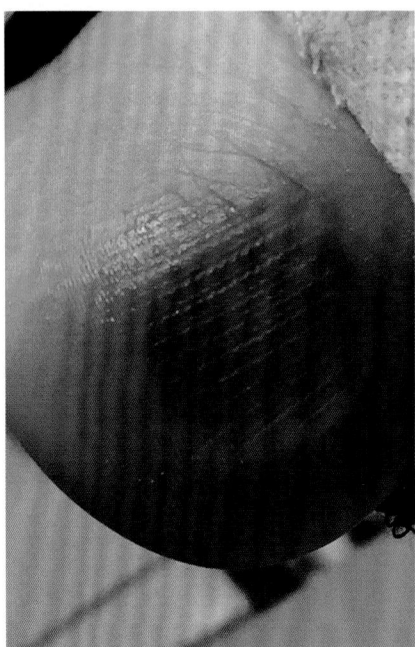

FIGURE 55.19 Pressure sore heel. Skin breakdown with pressure sore in a 4-year-old patient after 36 hours in posterior fiberglass splint. This unnecessarily complicates treatment of a minimally displaced tibia fracture.

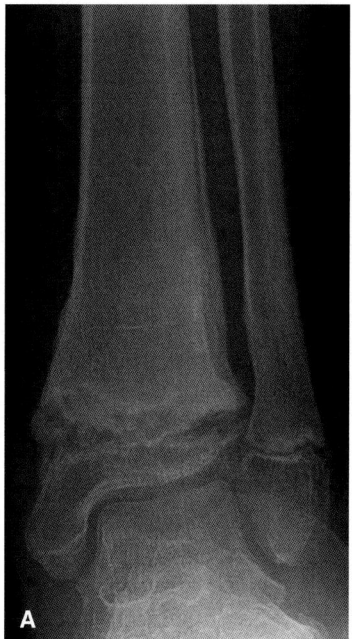 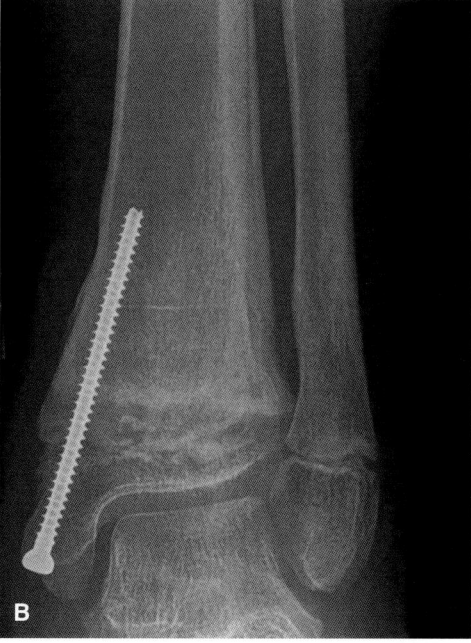 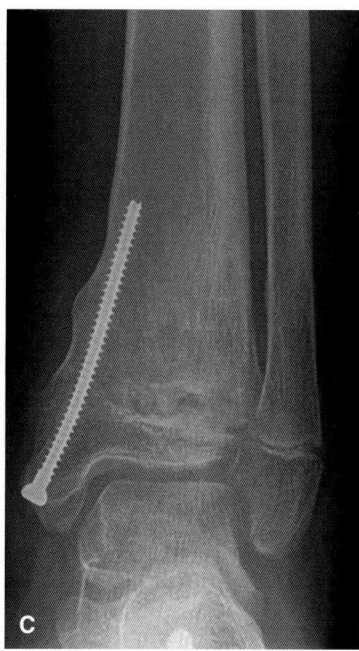

FIGURE 55.20 Guided growth with hemiepiphysiodesis. Thirteen-year-old ambulatory boy with a low lumbar myelomeningocele presented at 8 weeks after a displaced Salter-Harris I fracture of the distal tibia for which he had no active treatment. **A.** Injury displacement through the distal tibia epiphysis with partial healing, and long standing shortened fibula predating the injury. **B.** Medial screw hemiepiphysiodesis. **C.** Eighteen months later, the distal tibia alignment has corrected. Bending of implants with an epiphysiodesis is well documented. Note the asymmetry of the physeal line on the tibia after correction. The fibular station remains short with the fibular physis proximal to the level of the tibial plafond. This is often seen in myelomeningocele.

relationship between the tibia and fibula.[32] Angular deformity or mechanical axis deviation may be treated with an osteotomy, with guided growth, or physeal bar resection (Fig. 55.20). A bar resection may be considered when <35% of the physis is involved in patients with a bone age <10-12 years.[39]

FOOT INJURIES

INCIDENCE AND OVERVIEW

Pediatric foot fractures may represent up to 8% of all pediatric fractures and ankle fractures in children.[2-4] The majority of the pediatric foot fractures are treated with immobilization and do not require surgical intervention. In younger pediatric patients, the large areas of cartilage in the skeletally immature foot are more elastic with different injury patterns in children than adults.[8,12] As patients enter adolescence, foot fracture guidelines follow adult treatment plans. The classification systems for children's fractures of the foot are a combination of adult and pediatric methodology.

ANATOMY OF THE FOOT IN CHILDREN

The bones of the hindfoot and midfoot form as a cartilaginous anlage. The calcaneus and talus have an apparent ossification center by the 8th month of gestation. Both the calcaneus and talus ossification centers are visible on newborn radiographs. The calcaneus begins ossification prior to the talus. Of all the tarsal bones, the calcaneus has a predictable secondary ossification center, the calcaneal apophysis at the posterior edge.

The secondary ossification center of the calcaneal apophysis appears by 10 years of age. The cuboid ossification center develops around the 9th month of gestation while the navicular does not show evidence of ossification until about 3 years of age.[85-87]

The talus has three major anatomic regions consisting of the body, the neck, and the head. Ossification begins in the head and neck area and spreads toward the body of the talus.

Posteriorly, a secondary ossification center, the os trigonum, may develop from the area of the posterior talar tubercles.[88]

The majority of the talus is covered by articular cartilage and no tendons attach to the talus.[89] The artery of the tarsal canal provides the main blood supply to the talar body. The artery of the tarsal sinus and the deltoid artery are the other main arterial supplies to the talus. Within the talus are numerous interosseous anastomoses that are important in the survival of the talus with displaced fractures.[90]

The metatarsals and phalanges have a physis producing endochondral growth. In the second through fifth metatarsals, the physis is distal located at the junction of the head and neck of the metatarsal. The first metatarsal has the physis proximally at the base. The phalanges of the toes have the physis located on the proximal end of the phalanx.

GROWTH OF THE FOOT IN CHILDREN

The foot grows more slowly after the age of 5 adding only about 0.9 cm/y. In general, by the chronologic age of 12, girls have achieved 96% and boys 88% of the adult length of the foot.[91,92] This is helpful in estimating the growth remaining and the ability for a displaced injury to remodel.

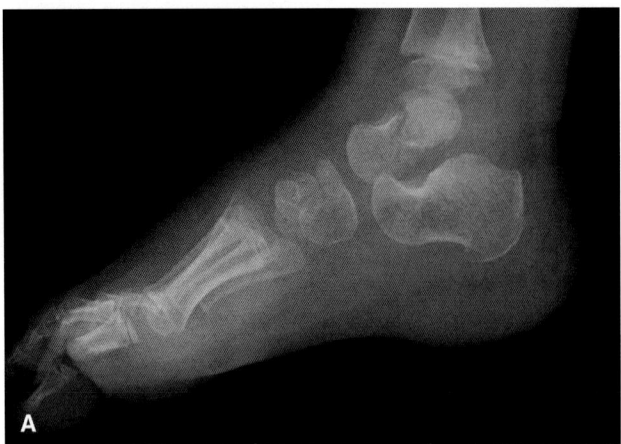
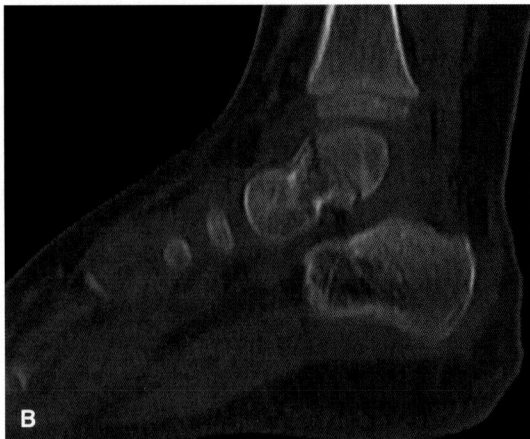

FIGURE 55.21 Talar Body Fracture. 3-year-old patient climbing on a motorcycle when the motorcycle fell onto his lower leg and foot. **A.** Injury Lateral. **B.** CT sagittal view. Note the fracture line extends posterior to the Lateral Talar Process. Examined in the operating room. The fracture was stable with range of motion. Patient was treated in an above knee cast.

TALUS FRACTURES

Incidence and Overview

Less than 1% of all pediatric fractures occur in the talus.[2] Fractures of the talus may occur in the talar neck, head, or body (Fig. 55.21). They may also present as avulsion fractures and as osteochondral fractures.[93] Higher acuity fractures of the talus with associated increasing rates of complications are seen more frequently in older children.[94]

A common mechanism of injury for talar neck fractures is a fall from a height with dorsiflexion of foot. The talus is injured as it contacts the anterior distal tibia.[93] Talar neck fractures in children require a great deal of energy to produce a fracture compared to the other bones in the foot.[95] Associated injuries should be assessed as well. As is the case with calcaneal fractures, fractures of the spine or other extremity injuries may be present.

Talar Neck Fractures Classification

The Hawkins classification is used for children and adolescent patients.[96,97]

The type IV classification was added by Canale and Kelly.[98] It is a type III injury with a talonavicular joint dislocation.

Imaging of Pediatric Talar Neck Fractures

Radiographs of the foot, AP, lateral, and oblique are standard views. Canale and Kelly proposed a pronated oblique view to evaluate the talar neck displacement and angulation. The foot is pronated about 15 degrees from the AP view with the beam of the radiograph at 75 degrees to the plate.[98] CT is valuable in assessing the fracture lines and displacement. A subchondral lucent line, the Hawkins sign, is interpreted as a radiographic indicator of satisfactory vascularization of the talar body after fracture.[96] The appearance of the Hawkins sign on a radiograph is variable. It may appear as early as 6 to 8 weeks after injury, or it may be delayed for months.

Treatment Talar Neck Fractures

Talar Neck Type I Fracture

A total of 5 mm or less of displacement and 5 degrees or less of angulation are considered nondisplaced.[96–98] Talar neck type I fractures are deemed acceptable to treat without surgical intervention.[98] A CT scan may help confirm that the fracture is nondisplaced.

Talar Neck Type II, III, and IV Fractures

These are displaced injuries that require reduction. CT scan preoperatively helps with the fracture assessment. In a type IV talar neck fracture, the talonavicular joint may be unstable requiring pinning after the talus has been treated.

Neurovascular compromise may be present necessitating urgent reduction. If there is no neurovascular compromise, and no imminent skin necrosis from a displaced fracture, Lindvall et al. showed there was no change in the outcome with early surgery vs surgery 24 hours later.[99] Up to 50% of type III fractures may be open injuries leading to deep infection rates in adults as high 38%.[100]

Open reduction and internal fixation may make use of more than one approach to the talus. As in adults, the most common approaches are posterolateral, anterolateral, and anteromedial. Open approaches to the talus do have the potential to interfere with the tenuous blood supply to a displaced talus.

Authors' Preferred Treatment of Talar Neck Fractures

The type I nondisplaced talar neck fracture is managed in a cast non–weight bearing for 6-8 weeks. A CT scan verifies the alignment is acceptable. Progressive weight bearing can be allowed if evidence of healing is visible on radiographs, but activity is restricted until the Hawkins sign is visible. Patients are followed for 18-24 months because of the risk of avascular necrosis.

In a displaced type II talar neck fracture, plantarflexion with pronation is a typical maneuver to realign the fracture. The calcaneus is manipulated to allow reduction of the subtalar joint. Prompt reduction helps with soft tissue compromise. If the reduction is felt to be satisfactory, then the foot may be immobilized in plantarflexion for 4 weeks. This is followed by gradual dorsiflexion to neutral with cast change. Follow-up radiographs are necessary to follow for loss of alignment as the swelling subsides in the cast. Rotational malalignment negatively impacts the subtalar joint.[101] CT scan after initial reduction is useful to confirm alignment after initial reduction.

After a closed reduction of a type II talar neck fracture, smooth wires or screws may be placed thru a small incision medial to the extensor hallucis tendon avoiding the anterior neurovascular bundle across the talar neck fracture. While closed reduction and immobilization is described in the literature, rotational alignment of the neck is difficult to assess. Open reduction with internal fixation is used for type II fractures when the quality of the reduction is in doubt.

Displaced type II, III and IV talar neck fractures are rare in children. They are more frequently seen in adolescent patients. Guidelines, surgical approaches, and screw fixation for talar neck fracture treatment follow the adult literature. Talar neck fractures should be followed for 18-24 months because of the risks associated with these injuries.

Complications of Talar Neck Fractures

In the pediatric and adolescent age groups, complications do occur. Nonunion rates of 14%, avascular necrosis rates of 16%, and arthrosis in 57% of patients have been reported.[97,102,103] With increasing fracture displacement, the incidence of complications increases. While displacement does increase the risk of avascular necrosis of the talus, avascular necrosis does occur in nondisplaced fractures.[98,103]

Revascularization of the talus is a slow process. Collapse of the talar dome can occur even with prolonged restriction of weight bearing.[96] MRI is often used to assess for avascular necrosis, but false negative reports of avascular necrosis do occur on MRI.[104]

Talar Body Fractures

Classification of Talar Body Fractures

Talar body fractures also include injuries to other areas of the talar body. These include fractures of the talar dome, the talar processes, and posterior tubercles. Sneppen suggested five types of talar body fractures (Table 55.1).[105] Fortin suggested a talar body classification consisting of three groups (Table 55.2).[89]

Treatment of Talar Body Proper (Cleavage) Fractures

Fractures through the talar body proper are also infrequent in children.[93] The location of the inferior fracture line in relationship to the lateral process of the talus has been suggested as the method to differentiate a talar body fracture from talar neck fracture (Fig. 55.21). If the inferior fracture line extends posterior to the lateral process of the talus, it should be classified as a talar body fracture.[106] Talar body shear fractures or cleavage fractures may be treated with a cast if nondisplaced.

TABLE 55.1	Sneppen Classification of Talar Body Fractures
Sneppen Grade	
1	Transchondral/osteochondral fracture
2	Shear fracture of the main body—coronal, sagittal, or horizontal planes
3	Posterior tubercle fracture
4	Lateral process fracture
5	Crush fracture

Data from Sneppen O, Christensen SB, Krogsoe O, et al. Fracture of the body of the talus. *Acta Orthop Scand.* 1977;48(3):317-324.

TABLE 55.2	Fortin Groups of Talar Body Fracture Classification
Fortin Group	**Description**
Group I	Cleavage fracture of talar body proper
Group II	Talar process or tubercle fractures
Group III	Compression/impaction fractures

Data from Fortin PT, Balazsy JE. Talus fractures: evaluation and treatment. *J Amer Academy Ortho Surgeon.* 2001;9(2):114-127.

Reduction and internal fixation are recommended for displacement in a manner similar to talar neck fractures for adults.

Treatment of Fractures of the Lateral Process of the Talus

The lateral process articulates with the fibula and the subtalar joint. It is covered by articular cartilage. These injuries are thought to be related to inversion with forced dorsiflexion.[107] Lateral process fractures garnered more attention with the increase in snowboarding activity.[108]

The fracture can be missed on radiographs. The fracture may best be seen on the mortise view and the lateral views of the ankle. CT scan is helpful in assessing the fracture pattern and size of the fragment.

If nondisplaced, the lateral process fracture can be treated non–weight bearing in a cast for up to 6 weeks. Open reduction with 2.7- or 3.5-mm screw fixation can be used if displaced more than 2-3 mm provided the fracture fragment is large enough. Comminuted fractures of the lateral process are not amenable to open reduction. Comminuted fractures can remain symptomatic after immobilization and rehabilitation. If symptomatic, the fragments can be later excised.[108–110]

Osteochondral Fractures of the Talus

Overview

The presentation of patients with osteochondral fractures of the talus is varied. Patients may have an ankle sprain with the osteochondral injury seen on initial radiographs. Some patients have had ongoing pain in the ankle after a remote history of trauma. Others have no known history of trauma.

Given the variability of the initial presentation, there is confusion in the literature with the terms *osteochondritis dissecans* and *osteochondral fractures of the talus*. Konig used the term *"osteochondritis dissecans"* in 1888 referring to "loose" bodies in a joint.[111] The postulate was that these "loose" bodies of bone were secondary to an inflammatory process with necrosis of the bone. The literature since that time has frequently used the terminology osteochondritis dissecans. Much of the attention in the literature has been directed at the knee.

Berndt and Harty in 1959 suggested that the term should instead be *"osteochondral fractures of the talus"* rather than *"osteochondritis dissecans".*[112] The Berndt and Harty study presented evidence that the medial, and lateral lesions of the talus can be caused by trauma.

This disputed the idea that the medial talar lesion is not related to trauma, while the lateral talar lesion is related to trauma. Anatomical specimens showed that the lateral talus impacts the fibula with dorsiflexion and inversion, while the posteromedial talus is injured with plantar flexion and inversion.

Other authors have agreed with trauma as an etiology for the majority of these radiographic findings both on the medial and lateral side of the talus.[113–117] While the literature reports many of the radiographic findings are likely secondary to injury, the concept of osteochondritis dissecans as an etiology remains, especially on the medial side of the talus. The percentage of talar lesions that literature attributes to trauma varies.

Classification of Osteochondral Fractures of the Talus

In the article by Anderson et al., the Berndt and Harty classification of osteochondral fractures was modified (Table 55.3).[113] MRI studies and radiographs were used. The resulting Anderson modification of the Berndt-Harty classification allows for findings not seen on plain radiography (Fig. 55.22).

Treatment of Osteochondral Fractures of the Talus

Treatment algorithms are difficult to discern in children and adolescents. The literature is varied on etiology of the lesions. The literature is inconsistent on outcomes. Some articles place patients with no symptoms, but with radiographic findings, in the good result category. Others question whether the patient should be listed as a good result if the radiograph is abnormal.

TABLE 55.3	Anderson Modification of Berndt and Harty Classification of Osteochondral Fractures of the Talus
Stage	**Fracture Type**
Stage I	Compression and subchondral bruising from compression—seen on MRI. Not visible on initial radiograph
Stage II	Incomplete separation of fragment
Stage IIA	Incomplete separation of fragment with subchondral cyst
Stage III	Fragment has complete separation but remains within the bed nondisplaced
Stage IV	Detached fragment that is displaced

Data from Berndt AL, Harty M. Transchondral fractures (osteochondritis dissecans) of the talus. *J Bone Joint Surg Am.* 1959;41-A:988-1020; Anderson IF, Crichton KJ, Grattan-Smith T, et al. Osteochondral fractures of the dome of the talus. *J Bone and Joint Surg Am.* 1989;71(8):1143-1152.

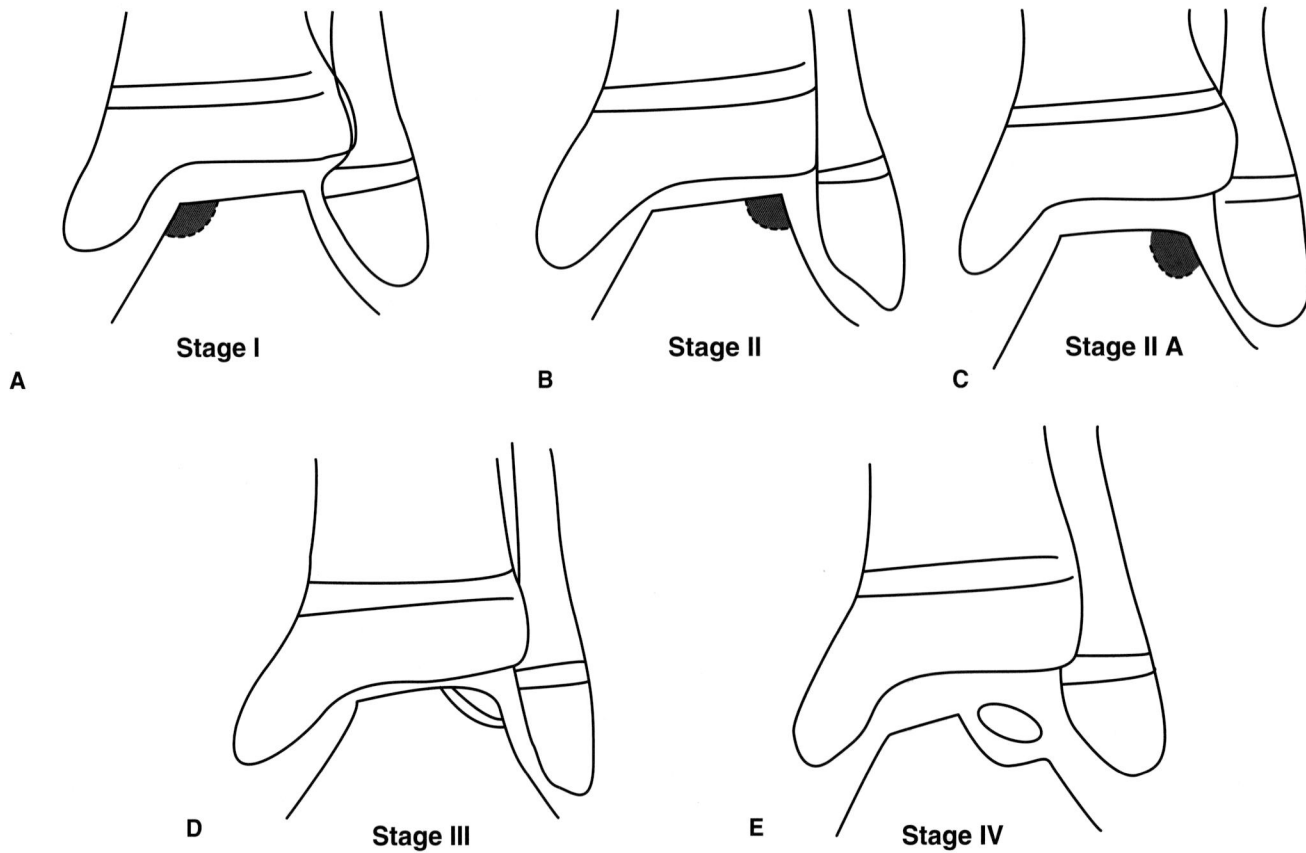

FIGURE 55.22 Anderson modification of Berndt Harty classification for talar dome osteochondral fractures. **A.** Stage I - area of subchondral edema related to compression or bruising seen on MRI. **B.** Stage II - incomplete lesion. **C.** Stage II A - incomplete lesion with subchondral cyst. **D.** Stage III - complete lesion but not displaced. **E.** Stage IV - displaced lesion. (Redrawn with permission from Berndt AL, Harty M. Transchondral fractures (osteochondritis dissecans) of the talus. *J Bone Joint Surg Am.* 1959;41-A:988-1020; Anderson IF, Crichton KJ, Grattan-Smith T, et al. Osteochondral fractures of the dome of the talus. *J Bone and Joint Surg Am.* 1989;71(8):1143-1152.)

What is clear is that results based solely on symptoms do not correlate with radiographic findings. Higuera et al. reported 94% of children, and adolescent patients had good to excellent clinical ratings based on symptoms.[115] In this same study, only 68% had good to excellent results based on radiographic healing.

Perumal et al. in a group of 31 skeletally immature patients showed that after 6 months only 16% had complete clinical and radiographic healing.[118] In the group that had persistent radiographic findings, 42% underwent surgery after an additional 6 months of nonoperative care based on continued pain with persistent radiographic findings. A total of 46% of patients had radiographic findings after a year of nonoperative treatment although they had no clinical symptoms. In the surgical group of 13 patients, radiographs showed complete healing in 54% within 16 weeks and in 30% by 1 year. A total of 15% of the surgical patients had no clinical symptoms but maintained persistent radiographic findings.

Patients under the age of 16 seem to have better outcomes than adults.[119] Others have found that patients under the age of 12 seem to have more favorable outcomes than older patients.[115,116] A group of 30 patients with 30 years of follow-up showed only two with arthritis of the ankle.[120] All of these varying statistics and outcome measures make the discussion confusing for patients and their families. The resolution of symptoms does not necessarily imply a normal radiograph in the literature.

Treatment of Stage I, II, and IIA Osteochondral Fractures of the Talus

Initial treatment is nonoperative immobilization with the use of a cast or fracture boot for 6-8 weeks followed by activity modifications (Fig. 55.23). Anderson et al. felt that the stage IIA lesions should be considered for earlier surgical intervention because of the subchondral cyst.[113] Pediatric literature, however, supports a trial of fracture boot, ankle brace, and activity modifications for type IIA lesions as long as the clinical symptoms are subsiding.[115–118] Those patients with continued symptoms and an abnormal radiograph beyond 6 months are candidates for arthroscopy with options for drilling, microfracture, bone grafting, or fixation of the lesion.[115,116,118]

Treatment of Stage III Osteochondral Fractures of the Talus

Literature in children and younger adolescent patients also supports an initial trial of a cast or fracture boot for 6-8 weeks.[115–118] If acutely painful, then non–weight bearing is advised. Weight bearing with activity restrictions is allowed once comfortable. If patients are improving, they may be followed for as long as 6 months prior to surgical treatment. Surgical treatment options with arthroscopy include drilling, microfracture, bone graft, or internal fixation of the lesion.[121]

Treatment of Stage IV Osteochondral Fractures of the Talus

These are displaced and surgery is recommended. Fragment removal with microfracture techniques is commonly employed. Occasionally, the fragment can be repaired with trimming to allow reduction and securing with bioabsorbable internal fixation.

Authors' Preferred Treatment of Osteochondral Fractures of the Talus

Osteochondral talar dome fractures, stages I, II, IIA, and III, are initially treated with cast or fracture boot immobilization. MRI is done if the symptoms are not improving in the first 4-6 weeks of immobilization. If there are mechanical symptoms such as "catching" or "locking," the MRI is done at initial presentation.

For type I, type II, and IIA lesions, a trial of a fracture boot or cast treatment with non–weight bearing is employed. If there is clinical improvement, radiographs are followed at 4-6-week intervals. If at 3 months, there is no pain, and a normal radiograph, full activity may be resumed after rehabilitation.

Activity modification is attempted for 6 months to 1 year in type I, type II, and type IIA lesions in skeletally immature, asymptomatic patients with continued radiographic findings. The fracture boot is generally discontinued at 3 months. Asymptomatic patients with continued radiographic findings are followed for 6-12 months before serious surgical discussions are entertained in the skeletally immature population.

Type I, type II, and IIA lesions with persistent clinical symptoms, surgical options are discussed earlier in the treatment

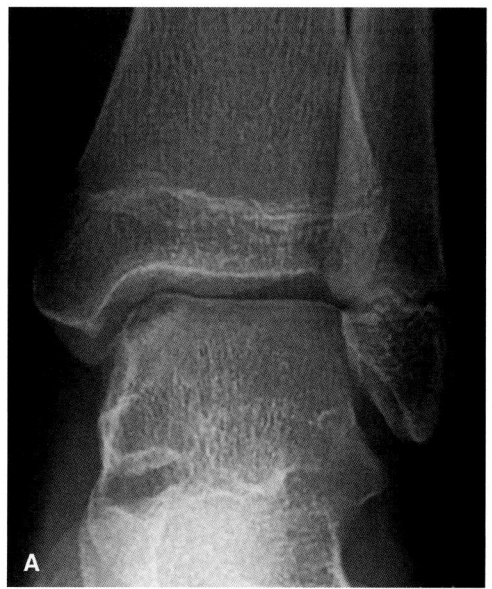
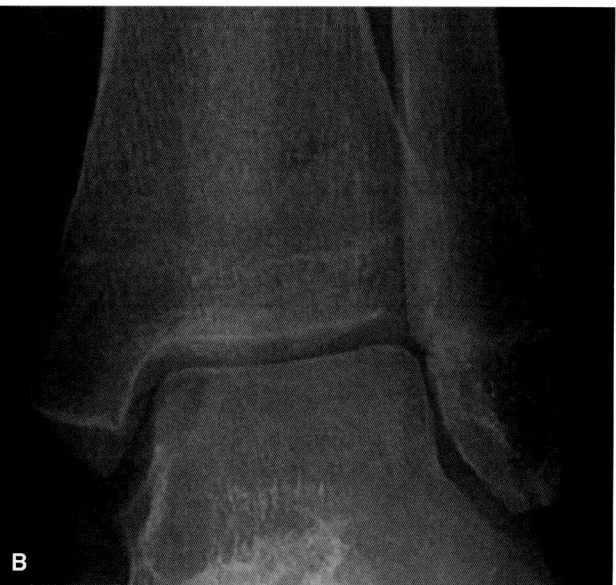

FIGURE 55.23 Osteochondral injury talar dome. Radiographs of 13-year-old girl with ankle pain and history of recurrent ankle sprains. **A.** Berndt-Harty type IIA. Treated with restricted activity for 4 months. **B.** Improvement at 4 months. Patient asymptomatic.

course. Patients that have persistent severe symptoms after 6-8 weeks may be candidates for surgery. This is seen infrequently in the pediatric literature. The majority of patients have some improvement in symptoms with immobilization initially.

A trial of fracture boot with activity modification is given for type III lesions, most frequently in those under 12 years of age. Patients with improving symptoms in the first 6 weeks may continue nonoperative treatment for up to 6 months. This allows for the possibility of radiographic healing to occur. If the symptoms are not improving in the first 6 weeks, surgical treatment is considered.[115,116,118] If symptoms persist, or patients are not willing to continue with activity modification, then surgery is discussed.[118] Details in the history such as mechanical symptom and severity of symptoms may move the discussion to surgery more quickly. In skeletally mature patients, surgical intervention is considered earlier in the treatment process.

The type IV lesions are offered surgery with arthroscopic methods. Arthroscopic debridement and microfracture can be augmented with bone marrow aspirate and allogeneic cartilage matrix scaffold. Allogeneic cartilage matrix graft has shown favorable results in small case series studies in lesion sizes 1.5 cm^2.[122] Open treatment as a backup for very large lesions is discussed. Surgical intervention consists most often of arthroscopic removal of the free fragment. Few are amenable to repair.

CALCANEAL FRACTURE

Incidence and Overview

Fractures of the calcaneus are rare in children. The series in the literature are small.[123–126] The low rates of calcaneal fractures may be related to the number of incomplete or nondisplaced fractures that are missed. Rates of missed calcaneal fractures reported on the patient's first examination range from 27% to 55%.[125–128]

The most common mechanism of injury is a fall from a height in both children and adolescent patients. In younger children under the age of 10 years, the injuries can be from a fall or jump from a height as little as 2-4 ft high. Over the age of 10, the calcaneal fractures are more commonly associated higher energy such as falls of 10 ft or more or motor

vehicle accidents.[126,128,129] Associated injuries of the spine and extremities were found in 20% of children under 12 and 50% in patients 13 years or older.[128]

Extra-articular fractures are more common in children. A total of 60% of the calcaneal fractures in patients <14 years are extra-articular. Under the age of 7 years, the percentage of extra-articular calcaneal fractures approaches 90% of the calcaneal fractures.[127,128]

As patients reach the age of 14 years, the percentage of extra-articular fractures drops below 40% with the majority of calcaneal fractures having intra-articular involvement.[125,129] The hypothesis in the literature has been that the larger cartilaginous component with increased elasticity of the immature calcaneus is protective in the younger age groups. In children, and adolescents, the intra-articular calcaneal fracture patterns that occur tend to have less comminution compared to adults.[125,129]

Classification of Calcaneus Fractures

Schmidt and Weiner modified components from existing classification systems including the Essex-Lopresti classification and Chapman and Galway study to create a classification for children.[128,130,131] For adolescent age patients, the CT-based Sanders classification is more typically used.[132] The fracture patterns in children 14 years and older are more likely to resemble adult fracture patterns.[129]

The Schmidt and Weiner fracture patterns that do not violate the posterior facet of the subtalar joint are types 1, type 2, and type 3 (Table 55.4). The type 4 is a fracture line entering the posterior facet of the subtalar joint, but no associated compression injury. Type 5A is a compression of the posterior facet with a tongue-type injury. Type 5B is a joint depression injury of the posterior facet. The type 6 in the Schmidt-Weiner classification denotes significant bone loss, soft tissue loss, and includes the loss of the Achilles insertion.

Imaging of the Pediatric Calcaneus

Standard foot radiographs consist of AP, lateral, and axial views of the calcaneus. On radiographs, Bohler angle and the angle of Gissane may have more variability in younger children due

TABLE 55.4 Schmidt and Weiner Calcaneal Fracture Patterns in Children		
Type	**Subtype**	**Description**
Type 1	1A Tuberosity or apophysis 1B Sustentaculum 1C Anterior process 1D Distal anterolateral at calcaneus—cuboid joint 1E Avulsion off body	Fractures not entering the posterior facet of subtalar joint
Type 2	2A Posterior beak 2B Avulsion of Achilles insertion	2A Beak fracture of tuberosity not involving Achilles insertion 2B Avulsion fracture at Achilles insertion
Type 3	No subtype	Linear fracture that does not involve the subtalar joint
Type 4	No subtype	Fracture line into posterior facet of subtalar joint
Type 5	5A Tongue type 5B Joint depression	Compression fractures involving posterior facet of subtalar joint 5A Tongue type 5B Joint depression
Type 6	No subtype	Bone loss and loss of Achilles insertion

With permission from Schmidt TL, Weiner DS. Calcaneal fractures in children. An evaluation of the nature of the injury in 56 children. *Clin Orthop Relat Res.* 1982;(171):150-155.

to the asymmetric ossification of the calcaneus.[85] In Boyle et al., 763 radiographs on patients 1-14 years of age were examined.[133] The average Bohler angle was 35 degrees and average angle of Gissane was 111 degrees. The angle of Gissane was highest in the 0-2-year age group at 119 degrees. The Bohler angle was highest at age 3-8 years at 40 degrees. Comparison view of the noninjured foot is useful. If both feet are injured, then the Boyle study provides some guidelines. When an intra-articular fracture is suspected, a CT scan should be ordered.

Treatment of Calcaneal Fractures

Historically, extra-articular and intra-articular fractures in children have been treated nonoperatively. Multiple articles have been published suggesting that children with nondisplaced and minimally displaced intra-articular fractures have favorable results when treated without surgery.[125–127,134,135] Most of the follow-up has been short in the pediatric literature. Brunet's article had on average 16 years of follow-up on 18 fractures with all patients, except for two individuals, under the age of 11 years at the time of injury.[134] Brunet's series was unique in that follow-up contained fractures with more than 5-mm intra-articular displacement and loss of Bohler angle of up to 8 degrees at the time of injury. With all initial injury patterns included, the average American Academy of Foot and Ankle Score was 96 at follow-up. The good functional scores were seen despite radiographs showing evidence of arthrosis, calcaneal widening, and loss of Bohler angle in some patients. Some studies have suggested that younger children may be able to remodel intra-articular fractures in the calcaneus.[134,136] Other nonoperative series have shorter follow-up. Good function was reported, but restriction of subtalar motion and radiographic changes consistent with arthritis were noted in studies.[125,126]

Even with some indication in the literature that intra-articular displacement may be able to remodel, there are no guidelines on how much remodeling can occur. Since there are concerns about the long-term prognosis in nonoperative treatment, the literature has articles supporting operative treatment in children and adolescent patients.[129,137,138] The operative treatment studies have shown satisfactory reductions, improved alignment, and fewer wound complications than adults. The functional outcome scores, as of present, are small in numbers with short-term follow-up. As with nonoperative treatment, the long-term concerns of loss of subtalar motion and arthrosis remain in the surgically treated patients.

Extra-articular Calcaneus Treatment

Extra-articular fractures of calcaneus in children are usually treated in a cast. At 4 weeks, patients can often begin to weight bear as tolerated for another 2-3 weeks. At 6 weeks, healing is usually adequate to begin progressive rehabilitation.

Tongue Fractures and Intra-articular Calcaneus Treatment

Nondisplaced intra-articular fractures can be treated with nonoperative treatment. CT scan is advised to look for intra-articular displacement. Immobilization with strict non–weight bearing is utilized for 6-8 weeks. Depending on the fracture healing seen on radiographs, protected weight bearing at 6-8 weeks is allowed. Most patients are full weight bearing and can participate in rehabilitation by 3 months.

The tongue fracture may create shortening of the Achilles or skin pressure concerns from fracture fragment displacement.

If there is concern regarding soft tissue compromise, then the fracture should be addressed. If the posterior facet is displaced in a tongue fracture, reduction and internal fixation is performed.

Displaced intra-articular fractures are moving toward surgery in the pediatric groups.[127,129,137–139] Articular gaps or step-offs measuring 2 mm are being used as indications for open reduction and internal fixation. The surgical approaches are based on "L"-shaped incision with "no touch" skin techniques.[140,141] Minimally invasive approaches allowing Kirschner wires and screw fixation have been described for children and adolescents.[139,142,143] Care should be taken though in minimally invasive techniques. There is no plate fixation to create a buttress of the lateral wall with a potential for loss of fixation.[137,144,145] After surgery, patients are non–weight bearing for 6-8 weeks. At 8 weeks, most surgeons allow partial weight bearing and full weight bearing by 3 months. Return to activity is at 4-6 months.

Authors' Preferred Treatment of Calcaneus Fractures

There seems to be consensus on the use of anatomic reductions with adult guidelines for operative treatment of tongue fractures and intra-articular fractures of the calcaneus in patients over the age of 10 years. In patients under 10 years of age, there are surgeons and literature that will advocate for nonoperative care with reliance on remodeling. When looking at overall fracture care in children, intra-articular displacement is not accepted in the other major joints of the lower extremity. The literature is moving toward operative treatment of displaced intra-articular injuries in younger patients if technically feasible. Anatomic reduction for displaced intra-articular displacement of >2 mm is now considered in patients under the age of 10 years.

Complications of Calcaneus Fractures

Wound complications in the pediatric literature are lower than in the adult literature.[137] Some patients do require removal of the lateral-based internal fixation.[129]

Long-term follow-up is lacking in the operative pediatric age groups. The outcomes of late arthritis, pain, and subtalar stiffness remain a concern across all treatment modalities.

MIDTARSAL INJURIES

Isolated injuries of the cuboid, navicular, and cuneiforms are sparse in the literature. Fractures and dislocations of the midtarsal foot more often occur in association with other injuries of the foot. It is likely these injuries have been under reported accounting for the lack of available literature in children.

Cuboid Fractures

Isolated cuboid fractures have been described in younger children under the age of 4 years (Fig. 55.24).[146] There may or may not be a history of trauma. Questions about fever, recent illness, and constitutional symptoms must be posed. A cuboid fracture may be a source of limping in preschool children. If lateral foot pain is elicited with the examiner holding the heel, and abducting the forefoot, this may be a sign of an occult cuboid fracture.[147]

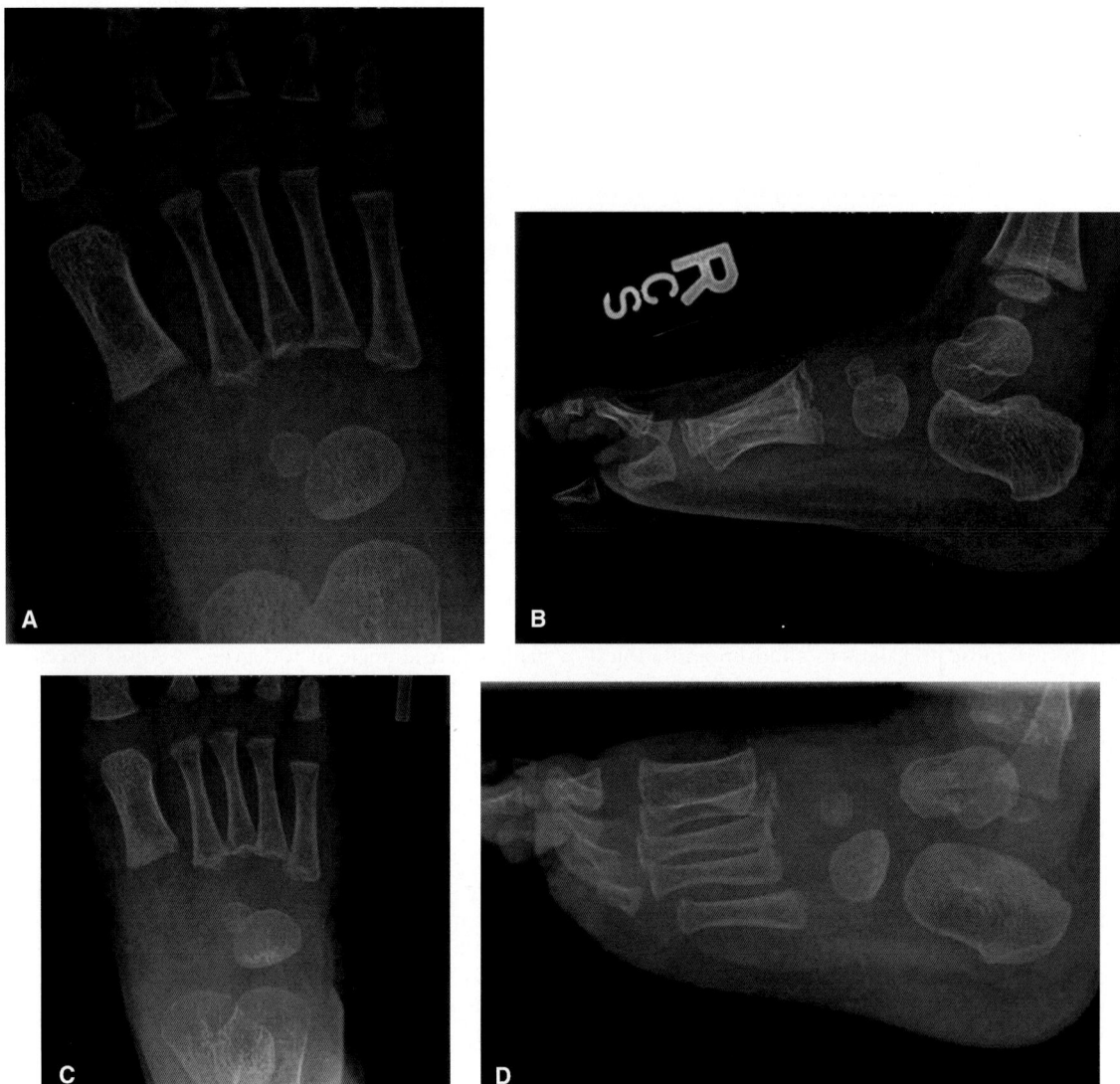

FIGURE 55.24 Cuboid fracture in 3-year-old patient limping after a trampoline birthday party. **A, B.** AP and lateral radiograph at 1 week. **C, D.** At 3 weeks, there is evidence of fracture healing with increased density in the proximal cuboid.

Initial AP, lateral, and oblique radiographs may be normal. Follow-up radiographs may show evidence of new bone formation within the cuboid indicating a healing fracture. Treatment is cast or fracture boot immobilization with weight bearing as tolerated for 3 weeks. Most patients are asymptomatic at this time, but some patients may need additional protection for 2-3 weeks to avoid re-injury.

Midtarsal Dislocations

Midtarsal dislocations involving the calcaneocuboid and talonavicular joints have been described in the pediatric age group in a small series described by Hosking et al.[148] The displacement can be identified on the lateral radiograph with subluxation at the calcaneocuboid joint.[148] Forefoot supination is thought to be the mechanism of injury.[149,150] Imaging is AP, lateral, and oblique radiographs. CT scan of the foot is advisable to clearly identify the injury. A midtarsal subluxation/dislocation can be seen with other injuries to the foot. Treatment is closed or open

reduction with smooth pin fixation. A non–weight-bearing cast is used for 6 weeks. Midtarsal dislocations are rare injuries in children. The importance of this dislocation pattern is the knowledge that these can be missed on radiographs if the surgeon is unaware of this entity.

Lisfranc Injuries

Incidence and Overview
The anatomy of the Lisfranc complex has been well described in the literature. Lisfranc injuries in children <10 years of age are rare.[151] In a 12-year retrospective review, 56 Lisfranc injuries in children and teenagers were identified from 3563 metatarsal fracture patients.[152] In this retrospective review, all of the 56 Lisfranc injuries occurred in patients over 11 years of age.

Lisfranc injuries can be related to a direct force to the foot or an indirect force that is applied longitudinally to a plantarflexed foot.[151,153] Varying positions of the patient and foot at

the time of injury have been described. Sport activity is a common source for Lisfranc injuries in adolescents.[152]

Classification of Lisfranc Injuries

Hardcastle et al. in 1982 published a classification system.[154] In 1986, Myerson et al. published a study modifying the classification system and discussed the Lisfranc complex.[155] The article by Myerson et al. used the word "complex" to include the cuneiforms, metatarsals, cuboid, and tarsal bones.

In adults, Myerson et al. found 14 of 76 patients had medial displacement injury patterns. This supported the literature view that the medial complex and base of second metatarsal are more resistant to displacement than the lateral side.[155] In children, and young adolescent patients, the displacement patterns appear to be different. A total of 52% of patients with open physes had a Myerson B1 pattern with medial displacement.[152] A total of 56% of patients with a closed physes had a Myerson B2 with lateral displacement.[152] As adolescents finish their growth, the injury patterns move to the lateral displacement injury patterns as seen in adults. This seems to indicate that the immature foot is more vulnerable to medial displacement. In the literature, partial incongruity (Myerson type B) patterns are most prevalent in children and adolescents.[151,152,156]

Imaging of Lisfranc Joint in Children

In 2018, Knijneberg et al. published data on the radiographic appearance of the Lisfranc joint in children using non–weight-bearing radiographs.[157] In children under the age of 6 years, the distance between the first metatarsal and second metatarsal is 3 mm or less. In patients <6 years of age, there is more variability in the second metatarsal base to medial cuneiform base with measurements of 3-7.5 mm. This is a radiographic appearance due to the normal expansion of the ossification front from more centrally in the bone to the periphery that occurs with skeletal maturation. By the age of 6 years, the values for both the first metatarsal to second metatarsal distance and the second metatarsal base to medial cuneiform distance approach adult values of 2 mm or less.[157]

Anteroposterior, oblique, and lateral radiographs of the foot are standard. Look for "fleck" injuries in the region of the base of the second metatarsal. Recognize that in young patients under the age of 6 years, the distances between the first and second metatarsal and second metatarsal and medial cuneiform may be >2 mm. Comparison radiographs of the foot can be very helpful. If patients are able to bear weight, standing radiographs as stress views are advised. CT scan is helpful for treatment planning.[158] An MRI may at times be of benefit in suspected ligamentous injuries with normal radiographs.[159]

Treatment of Lisfranc Injuries

In the pediatric literature, older patients are more likely to have open reduction and internal fixation (Fig. 55.25). Hill et al. found that 67% of patients with closed physes underwent open reduction and internal fixation.[152] Myerson et al. reported patients with good results had an average first metatarsal second metatarsal base distance of 2.9 mm and an average lateral talometatarsal angle of 5 degrees.[155] Adult recommendations are that patients with a >2 mm gap at the base of the second metatarsal to have a reduction of the injury performed. The talometatarsal angle of 15 degrees or more was associated with poor outcomes by Myerson et al., so a talometatarsal angles >5 degrees should be evaluated for intervention.

Authors' Preferred Treatment of Lisfranc Injuries

Nondisplaced injuries are treated in a non–weight-bearing cast. Follow-up weight-bearing films are done once the patient is comfortable to stand for the radiograph. At 8 weeks, patients are allowed to bear weight in a cast or fracture boot if the patients are free of pain. Restriction of activity is continued for up to 12 weeks.

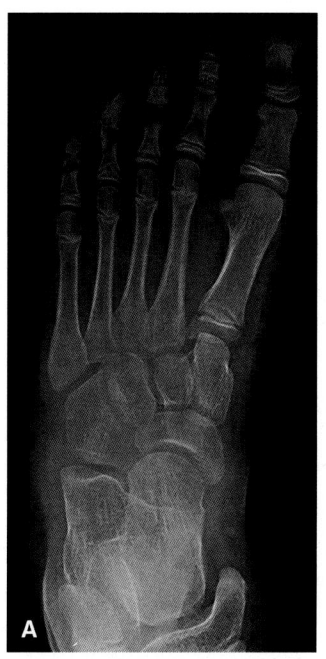
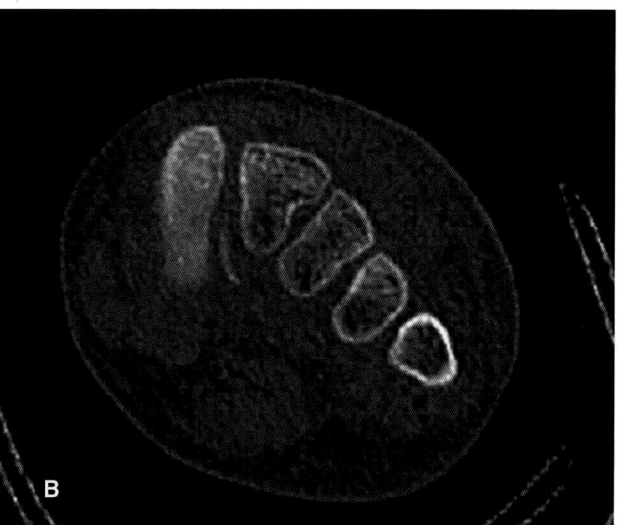

FIGURE 55.25 Lisfranc injury in a 10-year-old boy during soccer. **A.** Injury. **B.** CT scan.

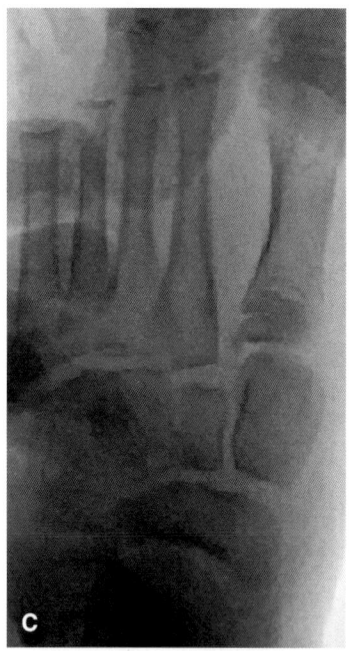

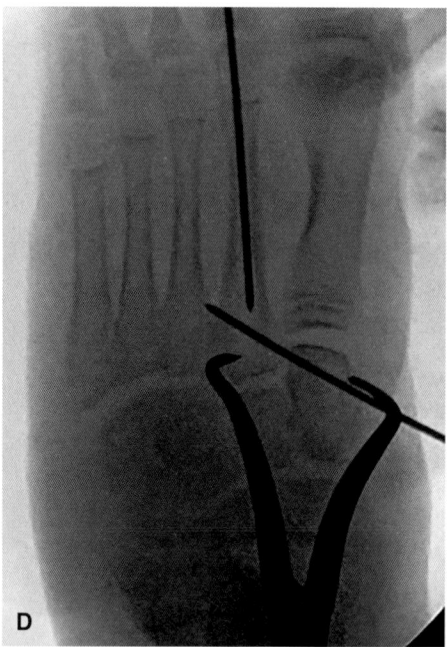

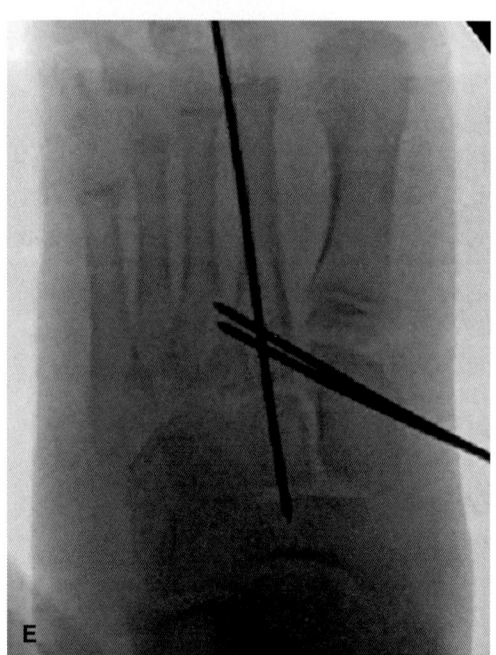

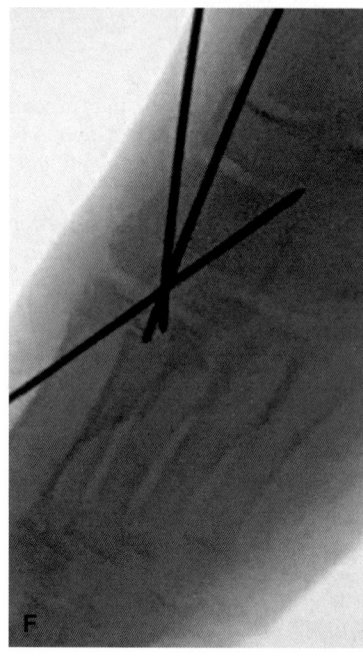

FIGURE 55.25 (*Continued*) **C.** Stress view in the operating room with gap between medial cuneiform and second metatarsal. **D-F.** Percutaneous reduction with tenaculum of second metatarsal to medial cuneiform. Smooth pin fixation to avoid base of first metatarsal physis. Reduction of second metatarsal base to medial cuneiform using crossing pins, and stabilization of second metatarsal to middle cuneiform.

If the injury is displaced, then closed reduction with longitudinal traction or tenaculum can be used initially. The sequence of events is to assess the medial side and move laterally.[160] Occasionally, a cast alone has been reported in the literature if the reduction is stable, but the literature supports internal fixation after reduction.[155] Smooth wire construct or screw fixation is used. If the closed reduction is not adequate, then open reduction is done. Dorsomedial and dorsolateral incisions are used depending on the need.[154,156,161,162]

Smooth pins are used in younger children, while in older patients screw fixation may be used. If the base of the first metatarsal has an open physis requiring internal fixation, and there is more than 1 year of anticipated growth remaining, a smooth pin is placed across the physis at the base of the first metatarsal instead of a screw. Pin fixation is typically removed at 6 weeks as long as there are no earlier signs of infection. Non–weight bearing is continued for another 6 weeks. Screw fixation removal is considered around 12 weeks prior to beginning unrestricted weight bearing.

PEARLS

Screw fixation across an open physis base of the first metatarsal may lead to growth arrest and a short first ray.

Complications of Lisfranc Injuries

Midtarsal injuries have the same concerns as in adults. Long-term concerns about function, pain, and arthritis. Acutely, swelling and compartment syndrome must be evaluated. Displaced late injuries have poor outcomes in adults.[154]

METATARSAL FRACTURES

Incidence and Overview

Up to 73% of all metatarsal fractures and tarsal fractures occur in the first metatarsal in children <5 years.[163] Metatarsal physeal fractures represent 1%-2% of all physeal fractures in children.[2,3,28] Most of the metatarsal fractures in the pediatric age group are either first or fifth metatarsal fractures.[163,164]

First metatarsals fractures are more common in children <5 years of age. These are often buckle fractures of the base of the first metatarsal. In the younger child under the age of five, the mechanism of injury is typically a fall.

Over the age of 10 years, the most common fracture of the metatarsals involves the fifth metatarsal.[163,164] Fifth metatarsal fractures in this older age group are more likely to occur with a fall from a level surface or in sporting activity. Fractures of the second, third, and fourth metatarsals are seen in isolation but usually occur with another metatarsal fracture.[163,164]

Metatarsal Classification of Fractures

Metatarsal fractures are described by the anatomic location. The fractures may involve the base, the diaphysis, the neck, or the head. If the anatomic location involves the physeal region, the Salter-Harris classification is used. There are two classifications useful for treatment of fifth metatarsal fractures in pediatric populations. These are discussed under treatment.

Treatment of Metatarsal Fractures

Studies providing recommendations on the criteria for the amount of displacement for metatarsal fractures in children and adolescents are lacking. Consideration for reduction of metatarsal fractures in adults is suggested for 4 mm of displacement of the metatarsal fracture and >10 degrees of angulation in the sagittal plane.[165,166]

Since 100% displaced fractures in younger children are capable of remodeling without surgical intervention, it is difficult to define strict guidelines in the pediatric population.[163,164,167]

First Metatarsal Fracture Treatment

First metatarsal fractures are frequently seen in younger patients under the age of 6 years. They are typically torus fractures that are minimally displaced. A buckle fracture of the base of the first metatarsal may be one of the many etiologies of a limping child without clear witnessed trauma by adult caregivers (Fig. 55.26). Manipulation of a buckle fracture is not required. Treatment can be a below knee cast or small pediatric fracture boot for 3 weeks. Return to activity is allowed as tolerated after 4-6 weeks.

Fifth Metatarsal Fracture Classification and Treatment

The majority of fifth metatarsal fractures do well with nonoperative treatment, but the time to healing can be considerably longer than expected. The apophysis of the fifth metatarsal base appears around age of 8 years. The apophysis fuses at ~12 years in girls and 15 years of age in boys.[168]

Herrera-Soto et al. proposed a classification for fractures of the fifth metatarsal for children and adolescents based on a review of 103 patients (Fig. 55.27).[169] A type I/fleck fracture is an apophyseal injury of the fifth metatarsal base. A type II/

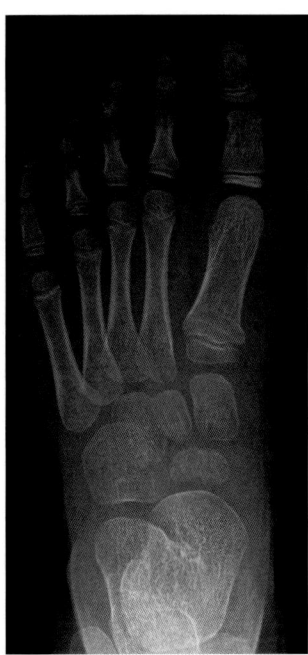

FIGURE 55.26 Buckle fracture tibial side of the base of first metatarsal in a 6-year-old patient.

intra-articular fracture involves the fifth metatarsal and cuboid articulation. A type III/Jones fracture is a proximal diaphyseal injury of the fifth metatarsal that is consistent with the adult Jones fracture.

Type I Herrera-Soto fractures were treated with a cast and weight bearing for 3-6 weeks as tolerated regardless of displacement. Two of thirty apophyseal fractures did not have evidence of healing on radiographs, but they were asymptomatic. All patients with a type I fracture had satisfactory clinical outcome.[169]

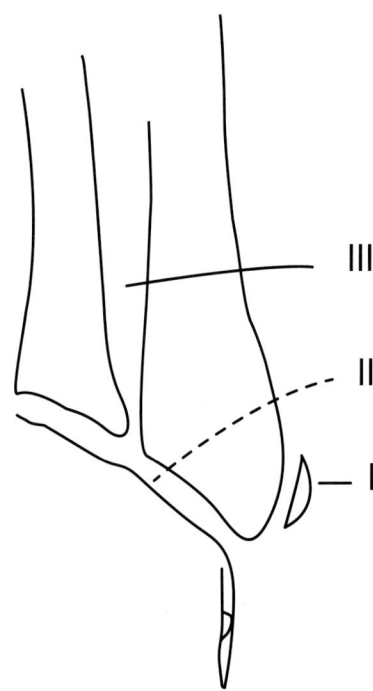

FIGURE 55.27 Illustration of Herrera-Soto fifth metatarsal classification. Herrera-Soto JA, Scherb M, Duffy MF, et al. Fractures of the fifth metatarsal in children and adolescents. *J Pediatr Orthop.* 2007;27(4):427-431.

The type II Herrera-Soto intra-articular fractures were troublesome when treated with early weight bearing. These type II group showed longer times to healing with an average of 6 weeks to healing. A total of 25% of the intra-articular fractures were treated longer than 8 weeks in a cast. With more than 3 mm of displacement, longer healing times were noted. A large proportion of these intra-articular fractures were delayed in healing or showed progressive displacement. The Herrera-Soto recommendation, after review, was that the type II intra-articular fractures of the fifth metatarsal should be treated initially with non–weight-bearing ambulation in a cast.[169]

The type III/Jones fractures had both nonoperative and operative management. If nonoperative management is used, the patients should be advised to remain non–weight bearing on the involved foot until fracture healing is visible. Repeat fractures do occur. In an active adolescent patient, internal fixation of the type III Herrera-Soto (Jones) fracture may allow faster return to activity.[169]

Mahan et al. proposed a different classification with fifth metatarsal fractures grouped using the distance from the tip of the fifth metatarsal base tuberosity.[170] Three groups were identified. The fracture grouping consisted of <20 mm from the tip of the tuberosity, 20-40 mm from the tuberosity, and >40 mm from the tip of the fifth metatarsal tuberosity. A total of 238 fifth metatarsal fractures in patients under the age of 18 years were reviewed. Fifteen patients were treated with surgery. Mahan et al. concluded that fractures <20 mm from the tip of the tuberosity are generally best treated initially with immobilization. The three complications of surgery all occurred in the <20 mm zone from the tip of the tuberosity. Fracture fixation is a concern with this smaller proximal fragment, and as expected two of the three complications were loss of fixation in this group. The other complication was an infection. The 20-40 mm zone represented the "at risk" group that corresponds to the adult Jones fracture. This 20-40 mm zone was the most common group to have operative intervention.[170]

Authors' Preferred Treatment of Fifth Metatarsal Fractures

Herrera-Soto type I avulsions of the apophysis are treated with a below knee cast or fracture boot depending on comfort. Weight bearing is often delayed for 2-3 weeks, but once comfortable, weight bearing is allowed. After 3-4 weeks, patients are changed to a fracture boot if they are in a cast. Rehabilitation begins around 8 weeks and anticipated return to activity occurs at 12 weeks.

Type II Herrera-Soto fractures are treated non–weight bearing in a cast until healing is visualized. These are slow to heal, and resorption of bone across the fracture site is common. Progressive displacement does occur (Fig. 55.28). It may take longer than 8 weeks to heal and up to 3 months to achieve adequate union for return to activity.[169]

The displaced Herrera-Soto type II fractures within 20 mm of the tip of the tuberosity have marginal fixation with a screw. If operative screw fixation is performed for a fracture within 20 mm of the tuberosity (Herrera-Soto type II), the postoperative treatment is non–weight bearing. Weight bearing is delayed until fracture healing occurs to avoid loss of fixation. In those patients with >3-5 mm of displacement, surgery is discussed if there is a possibility of adequate screw fixation. A surgical failure with loss of fixation is difficult to address. Attentive postoperative patience regarding weight bearing is a must.

For patients with Herrera-Soto type III fracture (the Jones fracture), surgery with screw fixation is discussed. In active patients, this is often chosen. If patients choose nonoperative treatment, non–weight-bearing immobilization is used until evidence of healing is seen.

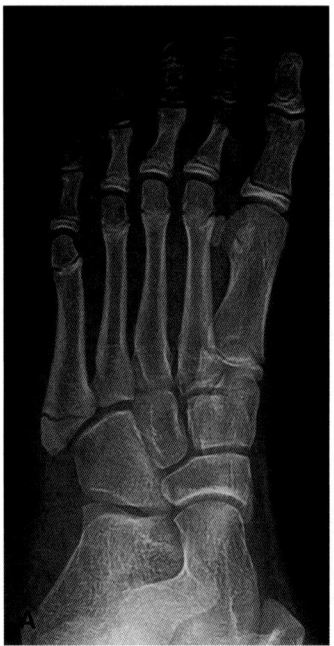 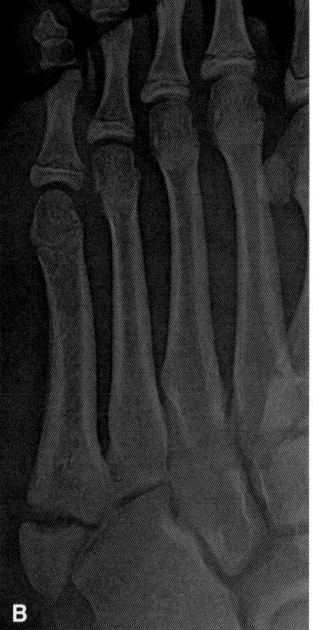 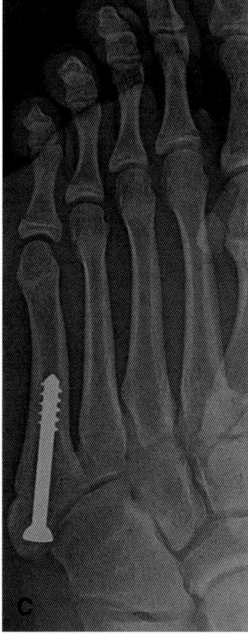

FIGURE 55.28 Fifth metatarsal base Herrera-Soto type II intra-articular fracture. **A.** Initial radiograph. **B.** Displaced at 3 weeks after full weight bearing. **C, D.** Healed fracture after screw fixation after reduction.

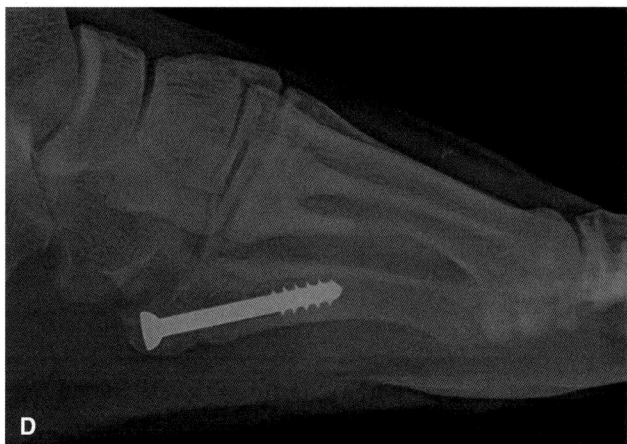

FIGURE 55.28 (*Continued*)

Multiple Metatarsal Fracture Treatment

These are not common in the pediatric age groups. A retrospective study of 1110 patients with metatarsal fractures was undertaken at Boston Children's Hospital.[171] A total of 98 patients under the age of 19 years were identified with more than one metatarsal fracture. Thirteen of these ninety-eight patients had surgery. In the nonsurgical group, the average age was younger at 9.1 vs 14.2 years of age in the surgical group. The suggestion from this retrospective study is that younger patients with <75% displacement should be considered for nonoperative care.[171] Robertson et al. retrospectively found that the surgical treatment was more likely to occur with displaced fractures showing an average translation of 84%, multiple metatarsal fractures, and an age over 12 years.[167]

The majority of metatarsal fractures are satisfactorily treated with immobilization alone. There is greater potential for correction of angular deformity in children under the age of 10; however, sagittal plane deformity should likely be <10 degrees.[172] With sagittal plane deformity, reduction and maintenance of reduction are the treatment goals.

Authors' Preferred Treatment of Multiple Metatarsal Fractures

Many of the multiple metatarsal fractures involve metatarsals 2 through 4. Shortening is often controlled by the interosseous soft tissues, and sagittal plane deformities may be small enough that a below knee cast can be used. Non–weight bearing for comfort for 2-3 weeks can be used. When comfortable, patients are allowed to bear weight often eliminating any mild plantar flexion.

Closed or open reduction is more often considered as patients' approach 11-12 years of age, with shortening of more than 4-5 mm, or sagittal plane deformity approaching 10 degrees. Smooth pin fixation is commonly used as the internal fixation choice. Pins are removed at 4 weeks.

PHALANGEAL FRACTURES

Incidence and Overview

Phalangeal fractures of the toes represent 3%-7% of all physeal fractures in children.[2,3,28] Common mechanisms of injuries include axial compression or a direct blow by a falling object. Fractures involving bare feet or crush injuries may have accompanying soft tissue compromise or injury. Distal tuft fractures and Salter-Harris I or II fractures of the distal phalanx of the toe may be associated with nail bed injury. Intra-articular fractures with small fragments are challenging to treat. Shaft fractures of the phalanx may be associated with tendon injury. Devastating injuries have been reported with escalator and lawn mower trauma.[173]

Classification of Phalangeal Fractures

Phalangeal fractures are described by the anatomic location. The Salter-Harris classification system is added for those fractures involving the physeal region. The physis is located proximally on each of the phalanges.

Treatment of Phalangeal Fractures

Phalangeal Shaft Fractures and Closed Salter-Harris I and II Fractures

Phalangeal shaft fractures and closed Salter-Harris I and II fractures of the phalanges are primarily treated with nonoperative treatment. This consists of buddy taping, hard-soled shoe, or symptomatic treatment. Displaced angulated diaphyseal fractures or closed Salter-Harris I and II fractures may benefit from a closed reduction. If the angular deformity of the toe would create shoe wear issues, or pressure on the adjacent toe(s), then a reduction maneuver to achieve parallel alignment of the toes is warranted.

Manipulation can be performed with a regional toe block.[174] After manipulation, buddy taping is used. Occasionally, a percutaneous pin may be necessary if the fracture cannot be maintained in a parallel alignment with the other toes.

> **PEARLS**
>
> Toe blocks in pediatric patients under the age of 10 years can be difficult to perform. Sedation with the aid of anesthesia may be helpful.

Salter-Harris III and IV Phalangeal Fractures, Intra-articular Fractures Involving the Phalangeal Condyles, and Phalangeal Neck Fractures

Physeal phalangeal Salter-Harris III and IV fractures and intra-articular fractures of the condyles of the phalanx may require percutaneous pinning or open reduction procedures. Nondisplaced fractures may be treated with buddy tape and protected weight bearing. Follow-up with radiographs during the first 3 weeks observing for displacement are necessary when nonoperative means are chosen.

Percutaneous methods of fixation with smooth pins may be used for fractures with concern about loss of alignment. Involvement of 25% or more of the joint surface or 2 mm of displacement are indications for operative intervention.[162,175–177] Fixation of these intra-articular fractures includes smooth pins, mini-fragment screws, and headless compression screws. The surgeon's enthusiasm for treatment should be tempered by literature that suggests 60% complication rates in these fracture patterns with treatment.[176]

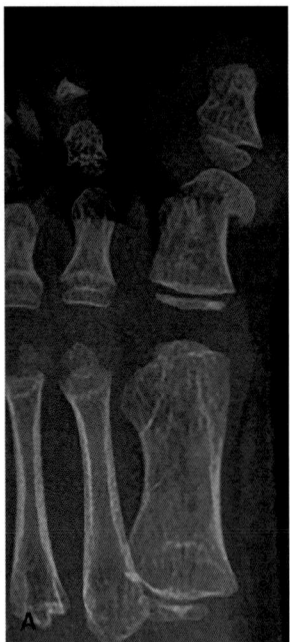
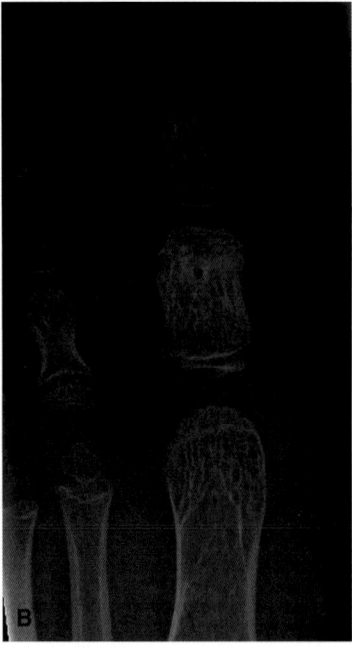
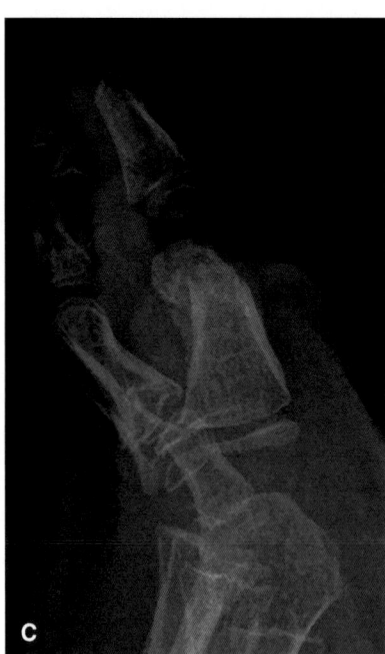

FIGURE 55.29 Great toe phalangeal neck fracture. 3-year-old patient. **A.** Injury film. Treated with closed manipulation under sedation and local block. Taping and above knee cast to prevent weight bearing. **B, C.** Five weeks after injury.

Phalangeal neck fractures may be treated with closed manipulation when displaced (Fig. 55.29). Follow-up radiographs during the first 3 weeks is advisable because of the risk of displacement and rotation of the fragment. Percutaneous smooth wire fixation may be employed for neck fractures that are prone to displacement with loss of rotational alignment.[177]

Closed manipulation, often with pinning, is used for displaced phalangeal neck fractures that if left untreated would create an angular deformity or rotational deformity.

Authors' Preferred Treatment of Salter-Harris III and IV Phalangeal Fractures, Intra-articular Fractures Involving the Phalangeal Condyles, and Phalangeal Neck Fractures

Great toe intra-articular fractures of the condyles, and Salter-Harris III and IV fractures at the proximal end of the phalanges, with 25% or more joint involvement, or 2 mm of displacement are considered for operative treatment. If the fracture fragment appears amenable to fixation, smooth wires or mini-fragment screws may be used. In minimally displaced Salter-Harris III and IV fractures, and with condylar fractures of the great toe that are not displaced, percutaneous pin fixation is considered to prevent further displacement. If nonoperative treatment is chosen for nondisplaced injuries, the patients are followed weekly for the first several weeks looking for early displacement.

Lesser toe intra-articular fractures, closed Salter-Harris III and IV fractures, or phalangeal neck fractures are more frequently treated by closed methods. Either simple immobilization or manipulation for angular deformity and immobilization are primarily used for toes 2 through 5. Achieving stable fixation of an intra articular fracture of a lesser toe is difficult without the risk of splitting the fracture fragment. Additionally, pin fixation across the smaller physis may lead to premature physeal closure. Fractures creating joint instability with angular deformity will require more active treatment on a case by case basis.

Open Salter-Harris I and II Fractures of the Great Toe

Salter-Harris I and II fractures of the great toe proximal phalanx are important to recognize as potentially open injuries. The eponym in the finger for an open fracture at the base of the distal phalanx with a nail bed injury is the "Seymour" fracture. In clinical practice, this fracture may present to the surgeon a few days later with early infection or several weeks later with established osteomyelitis. The initial radiograph may be unimpressive. The nail does not have to be grossly displaced to be an open injury. The patient will have bleeding at the base of the nail or in the area of the eponychial fold. The fracture is through the physis of the distal phalanx, and the displaced fracture tears through the soft tissue disrupting the germinal matrix and nail bed creating an open injury.

Open Salter-Harris I and II fractures of the base of the proximal phalanx require irrigation, debridement, and repair of the nail bed and matrix (Fig. 55.30). Removal of any foreign debris from the physis is performed, and the fracture reduction is done. Smooth pin fixation of the fracture may be indicated to ensure stable reduction and to protect the soft tissue repair. Thorough inspection and irrigation are required. Antibiotic treatment in the literature varies on length of treatment. The literature, which includes hand literature for the similar Seymour fracture, reports a dose of parenteral antibiotics at the time of debridement, which is followed by 7-14 days of oral treatment.[178–182]

PEARLS

Pinning across the DIP joint with an open fracture of distal phalanx, while increasing fracture stability, does present a risk of DIP joint sepsis in the face of an open fracture with potential microscopic contamination.

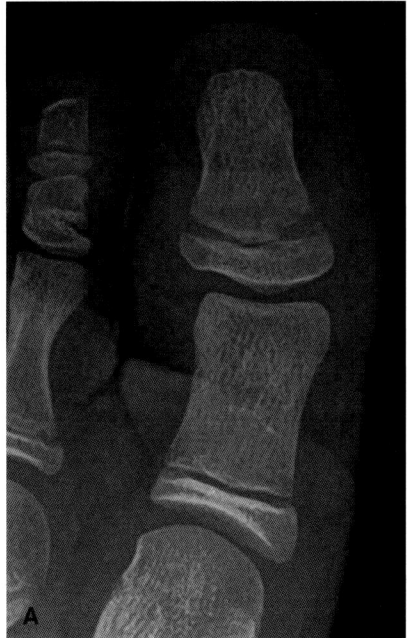
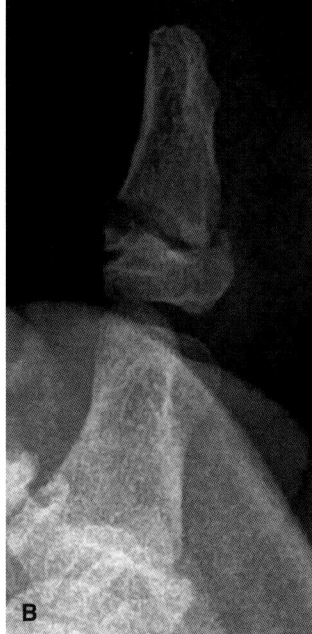
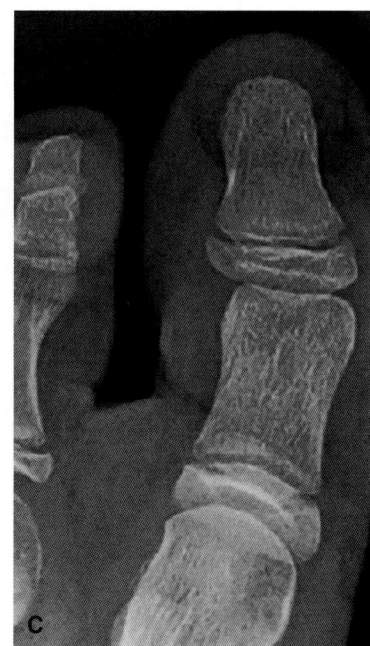
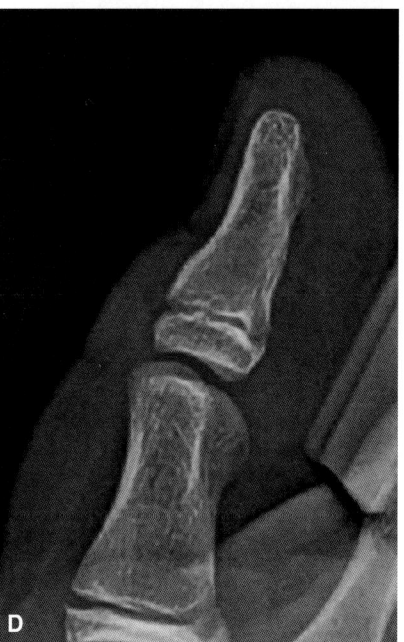

FIGURE 55.30 Open Salter-Harris II fracture great toe. **A, B.** Injury films. **C, D.** Radiographs 1 year after injury. Symmetric Harris line visible at proximal physis just distal to physis indicating growth after injury.

Authors' Preferred Treatment of Open Salter-Harris I and II Fracture of the Great Toe

An Open Salter-Harris I and II fracture of the great toe distal phalanx is treated acutely with a dose of parenteral antibiotics, irrigation, debridement, and nail bed repair. This is followed by 7-14 days of oral antibiotics. Nail bed repair, suture of the nail to the eponychial fold, and toe spica wrap may provide adequate fracture stability. When smooth pin fixation is performed, the pin is stopped in the epiphysis, if possible, to not violate the interphalangeal joint. If it is necessary to cross the interphalangeal joint with a pin, the surgeon must monitor closely for joint sepsis. Consider pin removal at 2 weeks and move to a toe spica wrap.

There is no clear guidance in the literature on treating delayed presentations of open fractures. If a patient presents late with signs of infection, the presumption is one of osteomyelitis. Treatment is with operative irrigation, debridement, and appropriate antibiotic therapy depending on the chronicity. Cultures are taken at the time of debridement to guide antibiotic therapy. In the case of established infection, treatment with antibiotics may range from 4 to 6 weeks.

Complications

Pediatric intra-articular phalangeal fractures are difficult to address. Physeal closure, joint stiffness, and pain are described in the literature.[172] Intra-articular fractures treated with surgery have shown loss of fixation, pin migration, and nonunion with the complication rates in the great toe approaching 60%.[176] Osteomyelitis may be the presenting problems for previously unrecognized open Salter-Harris I and II fractures of the distal phalanx of the great toe.

STRESS FRACTURES OF THE FOOT

Stress fractures are relatively rare in children but are seen in the tarsals and metatarsals. These are usually the result of repetitive activity such as endurance sports or high-level competitive activities. Exacerbation is seen in children competing in simultaneous or year-round sports or multiple competitive teams in the same sport. There is emerging evidence on serum vitamin-D relationship to fracture risk and healing.[183,184] Supplementation appears to be an important adjunct to the traditional activity modification and restrictions with cast, fracture boot, and non–weight bearing.

REHABILITATION OF FOOT AND ANKLE FRACTURES IN CHILDREN

Rehabilitation can be self-directed at home with simple instructions, or formal therapy can be prescribed. Young children often improve without formal therapy because of their unrestrained activity levels. Conversely, formal therapy is a challenge in young children as they are more interested in play then regimented exercise routines. Older children, adolescent patients, and patients trying to return to sports quickly do benefit from a more structured program. Strength, balance, and proprioceptive function are important prerequisites for return to physical activity.

PEARLS

Parents should be warned that many children will walk with a limp and an external rotation gait related to atrophy of the gastrocnemius and soleus muscles after immobilization or activity restriction. This may take 6 weeks or more to resolve.

REFERENCES

1. Mann DC, Rajmaira S. Distribution of physeal and nonphyseal fractures in 2,650 long-bone fractures in children aged 0-16 years. *J Pediatr Orthop.* 1990;10(6):713-716.
2. Mizuta T, Benson WM, Foster BK, et al. Statistical analysis of the incidence of physeal injuries. *J Pediatr Orthop.* 1987;7(5):518-523.
3. Peterson HA, Madhok R, Benson JT, et al. Physeal fractures: Part 1. Epidemiology in Olmsted County, Minnesota, 1979-1988. *J Pediatr Orthop.* 1994;14(4):423-430.
4. Worlock P, Stower M. Fracture patterns in Nottingham children. *J Pediatr Orthop.* 1986;6(6):656-660.
5. Greulich WW, Pyle SI. *Radiographic Atlas of Skeletal Development of the Hand and Wrist.* 2nd ed. Stanford, CA: Stanford University Press; 1959:xvi, 256.
6. Ballock RT, O'Keefe RJ. The biology of the growth plate. *J Bone Joint Surg Am.* 2003;85-A(4):715-726.
7. Ballock RT, O'Keefe RJ. Physiology and pathophysiology of the growth plate. *Birth Defects Res C Embryo Today.* 2003;69(2):123-143.
8. Ogden, John A. *Skeletal Injury in the Child.* 3rd ed. ed. New York; London: Springer, 2000.
9. O'Keefe RJ, Jacobs J, Chu C, Einhorn T, eds. *Orthopaedic Basic Science: Foundations of Clinical Practice.* 4th ed. Rosemont, IL: American Academy of Orthopaedic Surgeons; 2013:xv, 544.
10. Burkus JK, Ogden JA. Development of the distal femoral epiphysis: a microscopic morphological investigation of the zone of Ranvier. *J Pediatr Orthop.* 1984;4(6):661-668.
11. Shapiro F, Holtrop ME, Glimcher, MJ. Organization and cellular biology of the perichondrial ossification groove of Ranvier: a morphological study in rabbits. *J Bone Joint Surg Am.* 1977;59(6):703-723.
12. Currey JD, Butler G. The mechanical properties of bone tissue in children. *J Bone Joint Surg Am.* 1975;57(6):810-814.
13. Bright RW, Burstein AH, Elmore SM. Epiphyseal-plate cartilage. A biomechanical and histological analysis of failure modes. *J Bone Joint Surg Am.* 1974;56(4):688-703.
14. Ogden JA, Ganey T, Light TR, et al. *The pathology of acute chondro-osseous injury in the child. Yale J Biol Med.* 1993;66(3):219-233.
15. Salter R, Harris R. Injuries involving the epiphyseal plate. 1963;45-A(3):587-622.
16. Ryöppy S, Karaharju EO. Alteration of epiphyseal growth by an experimentally produced angular deformity. *Acta Orthop Scand.* 1974;45(4):490-498.
17. Wilkins KE. Principles of fracture remodeling in children. *Injury.* 2005;36(suppl 1):A3-A11.
18. Dahl WJ, Silva S, Vanderhave KL. Distal femoral physeal fixation: are smooth pins really safe? *J Pediatr Orthop.* 2014; 34(2):134-138.
19. Janarv PM, Wikström B, Hirsch G. The influence of transphyseal drilling and tendon grafting on bone growth: an experimental study in the rabbit. *J Pediatr Orthop.* 1998;18(2):149-154.
20. Bowler JR, Mubarak SJ, Wenger DR. Tibial physeal closure and genu recurvatum after femoral fracture: occurrence without a tibial traction pin. *J Pediatr Orthop.* 1990;10(5):653-657.
21. Hresko MT, Kasser JR. Physeal arrest about the knee associated with non-physeal fractures in the lower extremity. *J Bone Joint Surg Am.* 1989;71(5):698-703.
22. Peterson HA, Burkhart SS. Compression injury of the epiphyseal growth plate: fact or fiction? *J Pediatr Orthop.* 1981;1(4):377-384.
23. Moen CT, Pelker RR. Biomechanical and histological correlations in growth plate failure. *J Pediatr Orthop.* 1984;4(2):180-184.
24. Peterson HA. Physeal fractures: Part 2. Two previously unclassified types. *J Pediatr Orthop.* 1994;14(4):431-438.
25. Peterson HA. Physeal fractures: Part 3. Classification. *J Pediatr Orthop.* 1994;14(4):439-448.
26. Rang, Mercer, University of the West Indies (Mona Jamaica), and Lascelles Community Fund. *The Growth Plate and Its Disorders.* Edinburgh, London,: E. & S. Livingstone, 1969.
27. Cepela DJ, Tartaglione JP, Dooley TP, et al. Classifications in brief: Salter-Harris classification of pediatric physeal fractures. *Clin Orthop Relat Res.* 2016;474(11):2531-2537.
28. Peterson CA, Peterson HA. Analysis of the incidence of injuries to the epiphyseal growth plate. *J Trauma.* 1972;12(4):275-281.
29. LaMont L, Ladenhauf HN, Edobor-Osula F, et al. Secondary ossification centers in the development of the medial malleolus. *J Pediatr Orthop.* 2015;35(3):314-317.
30. Ogden JA, Lee J. Accessory ossification patterns and injuries of the malleoli. *J Pediatr Orthop.* 1990;10(3):306-316.
31. Powell H. Extra centre of ossification for the medial malleolus in children. *J Bone Joint Surg Br.* 1961;43B(1):107-113.
32. Karrholm J, Hansson LI, Selvik G. Changes in tibiofibular relationships due to growth disturbances after ankle fractures in children. *J Bone Joint Surg Am.* 1984;66(8):1198-1210.
33. Berg EE. The symptomatic os subfibulare. Avulsion fracture of the fibula associated with recurrent instability of the ankle. *J Bone Joint Surg Am.* 1991;73(8):1251-1254.
34. Farley FA, Kuhns L, Jacobson JA, et al. Ultrasound examination of ankle injuries in children. *J Pediatr Orthop.* 2001;21(5):604-607.
35. Anderson M, Green WT, Messner MB. Growth and predictions of growth in the lower extremities. *J Bone Joint Surg Am.* 1963;45-A:1-14.
36. Anderson M, Messner MB, Green WT. Distribution of lengths of the normal femur and tibia in children from one to eighteen years of age. *J Bone Joint Surg Am.* 1964;46:1197-1202.
37. Anderson M, Green WT. Lengths of the femur and the tibia; norms derived from ortho-roentgenograms of children from 5 years of age until epiphysial closure. *Am J Dis Child.* 1948;75(3):279-290.
38. Kelly PM, Dimeglio A. Lower-limb growth: how predictable are predictions? *J Child Orthop.* 2008;2(6):407-415.
39. Lalonde KA, Letts M. Traumatic growth arrest of the distal tibia: a clinical and radiographic review. *Can J Surg.* 2005;48(2):143-147.
40. Pritchett JW. Longitudinal growth and growth-plate activity in the lower extremity. *Clin Orthop Relat Res.* 1992(275):274-279.
41. Ogden JA, McCarthy SM. Radiology of postnatal skeletal development. VIII. Distal tibia and fibula. *Skeletal Radiol.* 1983;10(4):209-220.
42. Dias LS, Tachdjian MO. Physeal injuries of the ankle in children: classification. *Clin Orthop Relat Res.* 1978(136):230-233.
43. Lauge-Hansen N. Fractures of the ankle. II. Combined experimental-surgical and experimental-roentgenologic investigations. *Arch Surg.* 1950;60(5):957-985.
44. Dias LS, Giegerich CT. Fractures of the distal tibial epiphysis in adolescence. *J Bone Joint Surg Am.* 1983;65(4):438-444.
45. Lynn MD. The triplane distal tibial epiphyseal fracture. *Clin Orthop Relat Res.* 1972;86:187-190.
46. Marmor L. An unusual fracture of the tibial epiphysis. *Clin Orthop Relat Res.* 1970;73:132-135.
47. Cooperman DR, Spiegel PG, Laros GS. Tibial fractures involving the ankle in children. The so-called triplane epiphyseal fracture. *J Bone Joint Surg Am.* 1978;60(8):1040-1046.
48. Karrholm J, Hansson LI, Laurin S. Computed tomography of intraarticular supination–eversion fractures of the ankle in adolescents. *J Pediatr Orthop.* 1981;1(2):181-187.
49. Chande VT. Decision rules for roentgenography of children with acute ankle injuries. *Arch Pediatr Adolesc Med.* 1995;149(3):255-258.
50. Dowling S, Spooner CH, Liang Y, et al. Accuracy of Ottawa Ankle Rules to exclude fractures of the ankle and midfoot in children: a meta-analysis. *Acad Emerg Med.* 2009;16(4):277-287.
51. Vangsness CT Jr, Carter V, Hunt T, et al. Radiographic diagnosis of ankle fractures: are three views necessary? *Foot Ankle Int.* 1994;15(4):172-174.
52. Bozic KJ, Jaramillo D, DiCanzio J, et al. Radiographic appearance of the normal distal tibiofibular syndesmosis in children. *J Pediatr Orthop.* 1999;19(1):14-21.
53. Diaz MJ, Hedlund GL. Sonographic diagnosis of traumatic separation of the proximal femoral epiphysis in the neonate. *Pediatr Radiol.* 1991;21(3):238-240.
54. Smith BG, Rand F, Jaramillo D, et al. Early MR imaging of lower-extremity physeal fracture-separations: a preliminary report. *J Pediatr Orthop.* 1994;14(4):526-533.
55. Barmada A, Gaynor T, Mubarak SJ. Premature physeal closure following distal tibia physeal fractures: a new radiographic predictor. *J Pediatr Orthop.* 2003;23(6):733-739.
56. Carothers CO, Crenshaw AH. Clinical significance of a classification of epiphyseal injuries at the ankle. *Am J Surg.* 1955;89(4):879-889.
57. Spiegel PG, Cooperman DR, Laros G. Epiphyseal fractures of the distal ends of the tibia and fibula. A retrospective study of two hundred and thirty-seven cases in children. *J Bone Joint Surg Am.* 1978;60(8):1046-1050.

58. Kay RM, Matthys GA. Pediatric ankle fractures: evaluation and treatment. *J Am Acad Orthop Surg.* 2001;9(4):268-278.

59. Kling TF Jr, Bright RW, Hensinger RN. Distal tibial physeal fractures in children that may require open reduction. *J Bone Joint Surg Am.* 1984;66(5):647-657.

60. Luhmann SJ, Oda JE, O'Donnell J, et al. An analysis of suboptimal outcomes of medial malleolus fractures in skeletally immature children. *Am J Orthop.* 2012;41(3):113-116.

61. Caterini R, Farsetti P, Ippolito E. Long-term followup of physeal injury to the ankle. *Foot Ankle.* 1991;11(6):372-383.

62. Blackburn EW, Aronsson DD, Rubright JH, et al. Ankle fractures in children. *J Bone Joint Surg.* 2012;94(13):1234-1244.

63. Hoppenfeld S, De Boer PG, Hutton R. *Surgical Exposures in Orthopaedics: The Anatomic Approach.* 2nd ed. Philadelphia, PA: J.B. Lippincott Co.; 1994:xviii, 604.

64. Lintecum N, Blasier RD. Direct reduction with indirect fixation of distal tibial physeal fractures: a report of a technique. *J Pediatr Orthop.* 1996;16(1):107-112.

65. McGillion S, Jackson M, Lahoti O. Arthroscopically assisted percutaneous fixation of triplane fracture of the distal tibia. *J Pediatr Orthop B.* 2007;16(5):313-316.

66. Crawford AH. Triplane and Tillaux fractures: is a 2 mm residual gap acceptable? *J Pediatr Orthop.* 2012;32(suppl 1):S69-S73.

67. Kaya A, Altay T, Ozturk H, et al. Open reduction and internal fixation in displaced juvenile Tillaux fractures. *Injury.* 2007;38(2):201-205.

68. Rapariz JM, Ocete G, Gonzalez-Herranz P, et al. Distal tibial triplane fractures: long-term follow-up. *J Pediatr Orthop.* 1996;16(1):113-118.

69. Bennek J, Steinert V. Bone development after abnormal healing of lower leg shaft fractures in children. *Zentralbl Chir.* 1966;91(17):633-639.

70. Hansen BA, Greiff J, Bergmann F. Fractures of the tibia in children. *Acta Orthop Scand.* 1976;47(4):448-453.

71. Shannak AO. Tibial fractures in children: follow-up study. *J Pediatr Orthop.* 1988;8(3):306-310.

72. Swaan JW, Oppers VM. Crural fractures in children. A study of the incidence of changes of the axial position and of enhanced longitudinal growth of the tibia after the healing of crural fractures. *Arch Chir Neerl.* 1971;23(4):259-272.

73. Dunbar JS, Owen HS, Nogrady MB, et al. Obscure tibial fracture of infants—the toddler's fracture. *J Can Assoc Radiol.* 1964;15:136-144.

74. Halsey MF, Finzel KC, Carrion WV, et al. *Toddler's fracture: presumptive diagnosis and treatment. J Pediatr Orthop.* 2001;21(2):152-156.

75. Letts M, Davidson D, McCaffrey M. The adolescent pilon fracture: management and outcome. *J Pediatr Orthop.* 2001;21(1):20-26.

76. Pesl T, Havranek P. Rare injuries to the distal tibiofibular joint in children. *Eur J Pediatr Surg.* 2006;16(4):255-259.

77. Kramer DE, Cleary MX, Miller PE, et al. Syndesmosis injuries in the pediatric and adolescent athlete: an analysis of risk factors related to operative intervention. *J Child Orthop.* 2017;11(1):57-63.

78. Cummings RJ. Triplane ankle fracture with deltoid ligament tear and syndesmotic disruption. *J Child Orthop.* 2008;2(1):11-14.

79. Barnett PL, Lee MH, Oh L, et al. Functional outcome after air-stirrup ankle brace or fiberglass backslab for pediatric low-risk ankle fractures: a randomized observer-blinded controlled trial. *Pediatr Emerg Care.* 2012;28(8):745-749.

80. Boutis K, Willan AR, Babyn P, et al. A randomized, controlled trial of a removable brace versus casting in children with low-risk ankle fractures. *Pediatrics.* 2007;119(6):e1256-e1263.

81. Boutis K, Narayanan UG, Dong FF, et al. Magnetic resonance imaging of clinically suspected Salter-Harris I fracture of the distal fibula. *Injury.* 2010;41(8):852-856.

82. Korsh J, Adolfsen S. Displaced Salter-Harris type I distal fibula fractures: two case reports and a review of the literature. *J Foot Ankle Surg.* 2017;(56):845-850.

83. Leary JT, Handling M, Talerico M, et al. Physeal fractures of the distal tibia: predictive factors of premature physeal closure and growth arrest. *J Pediatr Orthop.* 2009;29(4):356-361.

84. Tarr RR, Resnick CT, Wagner KS, et al. Changes in tibiotalar joint contact areas following experimentally induced tibial angular deformities. *Clin Orthop Relat Res.* 1985;(199):72-80.

85. Howard CB, Benson MK. The ossific nuclei and the cartilage anlage of the talus and calcaneum. *J Bone Joint Surg Br.* 1992;74(4):620-623.

86. Hoerr NL. *Radiographic Atlas of Skeletal Development of the Foot and Ankle, A Standard of Reference.* Springfield, IL: Thomas; 1962:163.

87. Kuhns LR, Finnstrom O. *New standards of ossification of the newborn. Radiology.* 1976;119(3):655-660.

88. Grogan DP, Walling AK, Ogden JA. Anatomy of the os trigonum. *J Pediatr Orthop.* 1990;10(5):618-622.

89. Fortin PT, Balazsy JE. Talus fractures: evaluation and treatment. *J Am Acad Orthop Surg.* 2001;9(2):114-127.

90. Mulfinger GL, Trueta J. The blood supply of the talus. *J Bone Joint Surg Br.* 1970;52(1):160-167.

91. Anderson M, Blais M, Green WT. Growth of the normal foot during childhood and adolescence; length of the foot and interrelations of foot, stature, and lower extremity as seen in serial records of children between 1-18 years of age. *Am J Phys Anthropol.* 1956;14(2):287-308.

92. Anderson M, Blais M, Green WT. Lengths of the growing foot. *J Bone Joint Surg Am.* 1956;38-A(5):998-1000.

93. Jensen LB, Wester JU, Rasmussen F, et al. Prognosis of fracture of the talus in children. 21 (7-34)-year follow-up of 14 cases. *Acta Orthop Scand.* 1994;65(4):398-400.

94. Smith JT, Curtis TA, Spencer S, et al. Complications of talus fractures in children. *J Pediatr Orthop.* 2010;30(8):779-784.

95. Peterson L, Romanus B, Dahlberg E. Fracture of the collum tali—an experimental study. *J Biomech.* 1976;9(4):277-279.

96. Hawkins LG, Fractures of the neck of the talus. *J Bone Joint Surg Am.* 1970;52(5):991-1002.

97. Letts RM, Gibeault D. Fractures of the neck of the talus in children. *Foot Ankle.* 1980;1(2):74-77.

98. Canale ST, Kelly FB Jr. Fractures of the neck of the talus. Long-term evaluation of seventy-one cases. *J Bone Joint Surg Am.* 1978;60(2):143-156.

99. Lindvall E, Haidukewych G, DiPasquale T, et al. Open reduction and stable fixation of isolated, displaced talar neck and body fractures. *J Bone Joint Surg Am.* 2004;86(10):2229-2234.

100. Marsh JL, Saltzman CL, Iverson M, et al. Major open injuries of the talus. *J Orthop Trauma.* 1995;9(5):371-376.

101. Sangeorzan BJ, Wagner UA, Harrington RM, et al. Contact characteristics of the subtalar joint: the effect of talar neck misalignment. *J Orthop Res.* 1992;10(4):544-551.

102. Kruppa C, Snoap T, Sietsema DL, et al. Is the midterm progress of pediatric and adolescent talus fractures stratified by age? *J Foot Ankle Surg.* 2018;57(3):471-477.

103. Rammelt S, Zwipp H, Gavlik JM. Avascular necrosis after minimally displaced talus fracture in a child. *Foot Ankle Int.* 2000;21(12):1030-1036.

104. Henderson RC. Posttraumatic necrosis of the talus: the Hawkins sign versus magnetic resonance imaging. *J Orthop Trauma.* 1991;5(1):96-99.

105. Sneppen O, Christensen SB, Krogsoe O, et al. Fracture of the body of the talus. *Acta Orthop Scand.* 1977;48(3):317-324.

106. Inokuchi S, Ogawa K, Usami N. Classification of fractures of the talus: clear differentiation between neck and body fractures. *Foot Ankle Int.* 1996;17(12):748-750.

107. Hawkins LG. Fracture of the lateral process of the talus. *J Bone Joint Surg Am.* 1965;47:1170-1175.

108. Kirkpatrick DP, Hunter RE, Janes PC, et al. The snowboarder's foot and ankle. *Am J Sports Med.* 1998;26(2):271-277.

109. Heckman JD, McLean MR. Fractures of the lateral process of the talus. *Clin Orthop Relat Res.* 1985;(199):108-113.

110. Leibner ED, Simanovsky N, Abu-Sneinah K, et al. Fractures of the lateral process of the talus in children. *J Pediatr Orthop B.* 2001;10(1):68-72.

111. Konig. Ueber freie Korper in den Gelenken. *Deutsche Zeitschr Chir.* 1888;27:90-109.

112. Berndt AL, Harty M. Transchondral fractures (osteochondritis dissecans) of the talus. *J Bone Joint Surg Am.* 1959;41-A:988-1020.

113. Anderson IF, Crichton KJ, Grattan-Smith T, et al. Osteochondral fractures of the dome of the talus. *J Bone Joint Surg Am.*1989;71(8):1143-1152.

114. Canale ST, Belding RH. Osteochondral lesions of the talus. *J Bone Joint Surg Am.* 1980;62(1):97-102.

115. Higuera J, Laguna R, Peral M, et al. Osteochondritis dissecans of the talus during childhood and adolescence. *J Pediatr Orthop.* 1998;18(3):328-332.

116. Letts M, Davidson D, Ahmer A. Osteochondritis dissecans of the talus in children. *J Pediatr Orthop.* 2003;23(5):617-625.

117. Wester JU, Jensen IE, Rasmussen F, et al. Osteochondral lesions of the talar dome in children. A 24 (7-36) year follow-up of 13 cases. *Acta Orthop Scand.* 1994;65(1):110-112.

118. Perumal V, Wall E, Babekir N. Juvenile osteochondritis dissecans of the talus. *J Pediatr Orthop.* 2007;27(7):821-825.

119. Bruns J, Rosenbach B. Osteochondrosis dissecans of the talus. Comparison of results of surgical treatment in adolescents and adults. *Arch Orthop Trauma Surg.* 1992;112(1):23-27.

120. Bauer M, Jonsson K.Linden B. Osteochondritis dissecans of the ankle. A 20-year follow-up study. *J Bone Joint Surg Br.* 1987;69(1):93-96.

121. Lahm A, Erggelet C, Steinwachs M, et al. Arthroscopic management of osteochondral lesions of the talus: results of drilling and usefulness of magnetic resonance imaging before and after treatment. *Arthroscopy.* 2000;16(3):299-304.

122. Ahmad J, Maltenfort M. Arthroscopic treatment of osteochondral lesions of the talus with allograft cartilage matrix. *Foot Ankle Int.* 2017;38(8):855-862.

123. Jonasch E. Calcaneus fractures in children. *Hefte Unfallheilkd.* 1979;134:170.

124. Landin LA. Fracture patterns in children. Analysis of 8,682 fractures with special reference to incidence, etiology and secular changes in a Swedish urban population 1950-1979. *Acta Orthop Scand Suppl.* 1983;202:1-109.

125. Schantz K, Rasmussen F. Calcaneus fracture in the child. *Acta Orthop Scand.* 1987;58(5):507-509.

126. Wiley JJ, Profitt A. Fractures of the os calcis in children. *Clin Orthop Relat Res.* 1984;(188):131-138.

127. Inokuchi S, Usami N, Hiraishi E, et al. Calcaneal fractures in children. *J Pediatr Orthop.* 1998;18(4):469-474.

128. Schmidt TL, Weiner DS. Calcaneal fractures in children. An evaluation of the nature of the injury in 56 children. *Clin Orthop Relat Res.* 1982;(171):150-155.

129. Buckingham R, Jackson M, Atkins R. Calcaneal fractures in adolescents. CT Classification and results of operative treatment. *Injury.* 2003;34(6):454-459.

130. Chapman HG, Galway HR. Os Calcis fractures in children. *J Bone Joint Surg Br.* 1977;59B:510.

131. Essex-Lopresti P. The mechanism, reduction technique, and results in fractures of the os calcis. *Br J Surg.* 1952;39(157):395-419.

132. Sanders R, Fortin P, DiPasquale T, et al. Operative treatment in 120 displaced intraarticular calcaneal fractures. Results using a prognostic computed tomography scan classification. *Clin Orthop Relat Res.* 1993;(290):87-95.

133. Boyle MJ, Walker CG, Crawford HA. The paediatric Bohler's angle and crucial angle of Gissane: a case series. *J Orthop Surg Res.* 2011;6:2.

134. Brunet JA, Calcaneal fractures in children. Long-term results of treatment. *J Bone Joint Surg Br.* 2000;82(2):211-216.

135. Mora S, Thordorson DB, Zionts LE, et al. Pediatric calcaneal fractures. *Foot Ankle Int.* 2001;22(6):471-477.

136. Thomas HM. Calcaneal fracture in childhood. *Br J Surg.* 1969;56(9):664-666.

137. Petit CJ, Lee BM, Kasser JR, et al. Operative treatment of intraarticular calcaneal fractures in the pediatric population. *J Pediatr Orthop.* 2007;27(8):856-862.

138. Pickle A, Benaroch TE, Guy P, et al. Clinical outcome of pediatric calcaneal fractures treated with open reduction and internal fixation. *J Pediatr Orthop.* 2004;24(2):178-180.

139. Dudda M, Kruppa, C, Geßmann J, et al. Pediatric and adolescent intra-articular fractures of the calcaneus. *Orthop Rev (Pavia).* 2013;5(2):82-85.

140. Benirschke SK, Sangeorzan BJ, Extensive intraarticular fractures of the foot. Surgical management of calcaneal fractures. *Clin Orthop Relat Res.* 1993;(292):128-134.

141. Letournel E. Open treatment of acute calcaneal fractures. *Clin Orthop Relat Res.* 1993;(290):60-67.

142. Abdelgawad AA, Kanlic E. Minimally invasive (sinus tarsi) approach for open reduction and internal fixation of intra-articular calcaneus fractures in children: surgical technique and case report of two patients. *J Foot Ankle Surg.* 2015;54(1):135-139.

143. Tong L, Li M, Li F, et al. A minimally invasive (sinus tarsi) approach with percutaneous K-wires fixation for intra-articular calcaneal fractures in children. *J Pediatr Orthop B.* 2018;27(6):556-562.

144. Sanders R, Gregory P. Operative treatment of intra-articular fractures of the calcaneus. *Orthop Clin North Am.* 1995;26(2):203-214.

145. Sanders R. Intra-articular fractures of the calcaneus: present state of the art. *J Orthop Trauma.* 1992;6(2):252-265.

146. Simonian PT, Vahey JW, Rosenbaum DM, et al. Fracture of the cuboid in children. A source of leg symptoms. *J Bone Joint Surg Br.* 1995;77(1):104-106.

147. Senaran H, Mason D, De Pellegrin M. Cuboid fractures in preschool children. *J Pediatr Orthop.* 2006;26(6):741-744.

148. Hosking KV, Hoffman EB, Midtarsal dislocations in children. *J Pediatr Orthop.* 1999;19(5):592-595.

149. Elftman H, The transverse tarsal joint and its control. *Clin Orthop.* 1960;16:41-46.

150. Main BJ, Jowett RL. Injuries of the midtarsal joint. *J Bone Joint Surg Br.* 1975;57(1):89-97.

151. Wiley JJ. Tarso-metatarsal joint injuries in children. *J Pediatr Orthop.* 1981;1(3):255-260.

152. Hill JF, Heyworth BE, Lierhaus A, et al. Lisfranc injuries in children and adolescents. *J Pediatr Orthop B.* 2017;26(2):159-163.

153. Wiley JJ. The mechanism of tarso-metatarsal joint injuries. *J Bone Joint Surg Br.* 1971;53(3):474-482.

154. Hardcastle PH, Reschauer R, Kutscha-Lissberg E, et al. Injuries to the tarsometatarsal joint. Incidence, classification and treatment. *J Bone Joint Surg Br.* 1982;64(3):349-356.

155. Myerson MS, Fisher RT, Burgess AR, et al. Fracture dislocations of the tarsometatarsal joints: end results correlated with pathology and treatment. *Foot Ankle.* 1986;6(5):225-242.

156. Buoncristiani AM, Manos RE, Mills WJ. Plantar-flexion tarsometatarsal joint injuries in children. *J Pediatr Orthop.* 2001;21(3):324-327.

157. Knijneberg L, Dingemans S, Terra M, et al. Radiographic anatomy of the pediatric Lisfranc joint. *J Pediatr Orthop.* 2018;38(10):510-513.

158. Leenen LP, van der Werken C. Fracture-dislocations of the tarsometatarsal joint, a combined anatomical and computed tomographic study. *Injury.* 1992;23(1):51-55.

159. Potter HG, Eland JT, Gusmer PB, et al. Magnetic resonance imaging of the Lisfranc ligament of the foot. *Foot Ankle Int.* 1998;19(7):438-446.

160. Trevino SG, Kodros S. Controversies in tarsometatarsal injuries. *Orthop Clin North Am.* 1995;26(2):229-238.

161. Schenck RCJ, Heckman JD. Fractures and dislocations of the forefoot: operative and nonoperative treatment. *J Am Acad Orthop Surg.* 1995;3(2):70-78.

162. Kay RM, Tang CW. Pediatric foot fractures: evaluation and treatment. *J Am Acad Orthop Surg.* 2001;9(5):308-319.

163. Owen RJ, Hickey FG, Finlay DB. A study of metatarsal fractures in children. *Injury.* 1995;26(8):537-538.

164. Singer G, Cichocki M, Schalamon J, et al. A study of metatarsal fractures in children. *J Bone Joint Surg Am.* 2008;90(4):772-776.

165. Shereff MJ. Fractures of the forefoot. *Instr Course Lect.* 1990;39:133-140.

166. Buddecke, DE, Polk MA, Barp EA. Metatarsal fractures. *Clin Podiatr Med Surg.* 2010;27(4):601-624.

167. Robertson NB, Roocroft JH, Edmonds EW. Childhood metatarsal shaft fractures: treatment outcomes and relative indications for surgical intervention. *J Child Orthop.* 2012;6(2):125-129.

168. Dameron TB Jr. Fractures and anatomical variations of the proximal portion of the fifth metatarsal. *J Bone Joint Surg Am.* 1975;57(6):788-792.

169. Herrera-Soto JA, Scherb M, Duffy MF, et al. Fractures of the fifth metatarsal in children and adolescents. *J Pediatr Orthop.* 2007;27(4):427-431.

170. Mahan ST, Hoellwarth JS, Spencer SA, et al. Likelihood of surgery in isolated pediatric fifth metatarsal fractures. *J Pediatr Orthop.* 2015;35(3):296-302.

171. Mahan ST, Lierhaus AM, Spencer SA, et al. Treatment dilemma in multiple metatarsal fractures: when to operate? *J Pediatr Orthop B.* 2016;25(4):354-360.

172. Devalentine SJ. Epiphyseal injuries of the foot and ankle. *Clin Podiatr Med Surg.* 1987;4(1):279-310.

173. Lim KB, TEy IK, Lokino ES, et al. Escalators, rubber clogs, and severe foot injuries in children. *J Pediatr Orthop.* 2010;30(5):414-419.

174. Hatch RL, Hacking S. Evaluation and management of toe fractures. *Am Fam Physician.* 2003;68(12):2413-2418.

175. Buch BD, Myerson MS. Salter-Harris type IV epiphyseal fracture of the proximal phalanx of the great toe: a case report. *Foot Ankle Int.* 1995;16(4):216-219.

176. Kramer DE, Mahan ST, Hresko MT. Displaced intra-articular fractures of the great toe in children: intervene with caution! *J Pediatr Orthop.* 2014;34(2):144-149.

177. Mayr J, Peicha G, Grechenig W, et al. Fractures and dislocations of the foot in children. *Clin Podiatr Med Surg.* 2006;23(1):167-189.

178. Engber WD, Clancy WG. Traumatic avulsion of the finger nail associated with injury to the phalangeal epiphyseal plate. *J Bone Joint Surg Am.* 1978;60(5):713-714.

179. Kensinger DR, Guille JT, Horn BD, et al. The stubbed great toe: importance of early recognition and treatment of open fractures of the distal phalanx. *J Pediatr Orthop.* 2001;21(1):31-34.

180. Lin JS, Popp JE, Balch Samora J. Treatment of acute Seymour fractures. *J Pediatr Orthop.* 2019;39(1):e23-e27.

181. Pinckney LE, Currarino G, Kennedy LA. The stubbed great toe: a cause of occult compound fracture and infection. *Radiology.* 1981;138(2):375-377.

182. Reyes BA, Ho CA. The high risk of infection with delayed treatment of open Seymour fractures: Salter-Harris I/II or Juxta-epiphyseal fractures of the distal phalanx with associated nailbed laceration. *J Pediatr Orthop.* 2017;37(4):247-253.

183. Minkowitz B, Cerame B, Poletick E, et al. Low vitamin D levels are associated with need for surgical correction of pediatric fractures. *J Pediatr Orthop.* 2017;37(1):23-29.

184. Sonneville KR, Gordon CM, Kocher MS, et al. Vitamin D, calcium, and dairy intakes and stress fractures among female adolescents. *Arch Pediatr Adolesc Med.* 2012;166(7):595-600.

Soft Tissue Surgery

Tendon Transfers

Emily A. Cook, Jeremy J. Cook, Michael L. Sganga, and N. Jake Summers

Tendon transfers play a vital role in the reconstructive arsenal of any foot and ankle surgeon. Tendon transfers involve the knowledge of how to redistribute forces acting on and around foot and ankle joints. Understanding fundamental principles of tendon transfers, anatomy, and biomechanics is essential in order to establish a plantigrade and balanced foot.

Muscular function involves both acceleration (motor, push-off strength) and deceleration (braking) through a spring effect. There are 10 extrinsic muscles that provide extension, flexion, pronation, and supination about the foot and ankle. When there is an imbalance between the acceleration and deceleration, tendon transfers may become necessary. In this chapter, the authors will provide the surgeon with options that restore balance and counteract flexible deformities in the foot and ankle. A functional approach is utilized to classify common tendon transfers. Each technique is described in terms of indications, outcomes, and postoperative management. The indications for tendon transfers are extensive and dependent upon the specific pathology and deformity. Some common deformities/pathologies where a tendon transfer may be considered include the following:

INDICATIONS

- Tibialis posterior dysfunction (flexible flatfoot)
- Cavus, cavovarus, equinovarus deformities
- Digital imbalances: Hammertoes, hallux malleus
- Hallux varus/valgus
- Dropfoot
- Clubfoot
- Cerebral palsy
- Charcot-Marie-Tooth (CMT) disease
- Poliomyelitis
- Multiple sclerosis
- Nerve palsies (peroneus, sciatic)
- Neglected Achilles
- Amputations

ANATOMY

The role of tendons in the body is to serve as a bridge between muscle and bone. They are composed of collagen protein organized into bundles of fibrils, which in turn are part of larger collections of fascicles of collagen. Each fascicle is surrounded by a thin layer of connective tissue known as an endotenon.

Neurovascular elements are present between these fascicles within this layer. Several fascicles grouped together form a tendon. Tendons are surrounded by an epitenon, which also contains neurovascular elements in addition to lymphatic vessels. Immediately superficial to this layer is the paratenon, which serves as an additional supportive tissue that varies in composition and function. Depending on location, tendons associated with a synovial sheath have an inner layer that is lined with synovial cells, which blends with the epitenon to form a connective tissue bridge termed the mesotendon. The mesotendon provides neurovascular elements from outside the tendon via an attachment point on the epitenon called the hilum. In areas where the mesotendon is absent, tissue is supplied instead by plicae or vinculae, which are simply redundant connective tissue from the tendon sheath. Typically, a synovial sheath is present only if the course of the tendon requires that it pass deep to a ligament or if it radically changes direction.[1-4]

VASCULAR SUPPLY

Each tendon receives its blood supply from three sources:

1. Myotendinous junction
2. Osteotendinous junction
3. Paratenon, mesotendon, and vincula/plicae

Periosteal vessels communicate with vascular elements of the endotenon at the insertion site. At the myotendinous junction, vessels within the muscle are contiguous with the vessels of the endotenon. The majority of blood is provided by the paratenon. Those tendons without a synovial sheath receive external vascular supply throughout its course via connection to plicae and vincula. When the sheath is present, direct connection via the vincula is compromised and the synovial lining provides most of the nutrients. Most of the tendons of the lower extremity lack a sheath and therefore rely primarily on direct vascular perfusion.[1,5]

PRINCIPLES

PREOPERATIVE ASSESSMENT

Whether or not a patient is a surgical candidate and the mental and physical ability to properly rehabilitate from a tendon transfer are important but are beyond the scope of this chapter. A thorough history is vital when assessing for functional deformity imbalances. Ascertaining the primary problems and

overall patient goals play an important part in whether surgical intervention should be considered over alternative treatments.

A thorough non–weight-bearing and weight-bearing examination including gait analysis should be performed on every patient. The musculoskeletal examination should determine the overall foot type and assess for possible proximal deformities from the spine down as well as possible limb length discrepancies. Relevant stress testing is important to rule out possible ligamentous instability that can influence the deformity and overall success of a tendon transfer.

A major limitation of any tendon transfer procedure is its dependency on structural stability. These procedures are unable to correct deformities that are fixed or rigid. Joint range of motion (ROM) and assessment of the rigidity of the deformity must be determined. If there are semirigid or rigid structural deformities, these cannot be addressed through tendon transfers alone. Procedures such as realignment arthrodesis and osteotomies should be performed before the actual tendon transfer. Tendon transfers are adjunctive procedures in this setting and are not the primary procedure if the deformity is fixed. Identification of soft tissue and joint contractures is important as these may require releases or lengthening. The surrounding soft tissue needs to be supple without severe scarring to allow tendons to move freely.

When considering a transfer, one must evaluate the structure and function of the tendon and muscle to be transferred and assess if the muscle is spastic or flaccid. One of the most important considerations is of muscle strength, including cyclic muscle strength during rest and throughout gait evaluation. For the sake of completeness, we advise that each muscle be positioned at the end of ROM and that the examiner applies a counterforce to the foot while the patient exerts resistance. The examiner then labels the resistance according to a scale that is set between 0 and 5 (Table 56.1).[6] Manual muscle testing of individual muscles and muscle compartments should be performed. Muscle testing should be compared to the contralateral side and should be retested to confirm the testing accuracy

of assigned strength grade and for monitoring of progressive diseases on subsequent visits.

Literature supports the idea that a tendon transfer typically results in the loss of at least one muscle grade. When selecting the muscle for transfer, a muscle is considered appropriate if it has a grade of four or higher. This grading becomes less relevant when the transfer is intended to be used as a static rather than a dynamic structure.[3,7-9]

In order to ascertain the function of a muscle, additional testing or consultations may be needed. Electromyography (EMG) and nerve conduction velocity (NCV) studies may be helpful in the selection process. Radiographic images can further evaluate alignment, osseous, and joint pathology. CT may be helpful to provide anatomic details to rule out arthritic joint changes. MRI may be needed to evaluate for soft tissue pathology and the tendon(s) being considered for transfer.

The consequences of transferring a tendon must also be considered as to how this may influence function and compensation. Some tendons have natural connections distally to a transfer such as the flexor digitorum longus (FDL) connection to the flexor hallucis longus (FHL) via the knot of Henry, which compensate well. Other transfers may lead to unintended consequences, such as a progressive flatfoot deformity following a tibialis posterior transfer, and these can be avoided by performing ancillary simultaneous procedures.

TIMING

Preoperative assessment must also consider the status of the underlying functional deficit. Optimal timing for a tendon transfer requires an understanding of the pathology and reason for the functional imbalance. The potential for further recovery or deterioration of the structures must be clear before proceeding with any tendon transfer. Determining whether the functional status is static or dynamic will guide the procedural timing. For progressive deformities, it is sometimes ideal to proceed with the tendon transfer to help prevent contractures from worsening. Although it may be ideal to wait for pediatric patients to become mature enough to follow rehabilitation instructions, this may not be in the patient's best interest to avoid progression of deformity. Once deformities become fixed or rigid, tendon transfers in isolation are no longer effective. For degenerative tendons, it is better to address them in the tendinosis stage before tendons degenerate into a hypoperfusion state that eventually leads to rupture.

Conversely, bone stock must be adequate in order to achieve strong tendon to bone fixation without disrupting growth plates in pediatric patients or experiencing fractures in osteopenic bone. In cases of nerve injuries, it is best to wait for 1-2 years from the time of injury to allow as much recovery as possible. During this time, the foot and ankle surgeon should continue to perform repeat muscle testing and may consider obtaining an EMG just before surgery for planning. Consultation with specialists treating a patient's specific disease can further aid in determining the best time to proceed with a tendon transfer.

FACTORS THAT INFLUENCE TENDON TRANSFER STRENGTH

Detailed knowledge of anatomy and function of the foot and ankle is imperative but is beyond the scope of this chapter. Skeletal muscle architecture is predictive of functional capacity, and research on the lower extremity has been scarce. Much

TABLE 56.1	Grading and Evaluation of Muscle Strength
5	Normal power
4+	Full ROM; overcomes gravity and near-full resistance
4	Full ROM; overcomes gravity and moderate resistance
4−	Full ROM; overcomes gravity and mild resistance
3+	Full ROM; overcomes gravity and slight resistance
3	Full ROM; overcomes gravity only
3−	Full ROM; overcomes partial gravity only
2+	Partial ROM against gravity or full ROM with gravity eliminated
2	Full ROM with gravity eliminated
2−	Partial ROM with gravity eliminated
1	No visible motion; palpable contraction
0	No motor activity

ROM, range of motion.

Data from Kendall FP, McCreary EK, Provance PF, et al. Fundamental concepts. In: Lappies P, ed. *Muscles: Testing and Function, with Posture and Pain.* 5th ed. Baltimore, MD: Lippincott Williams & Wilkins; 2005:1-48.

of the early data were drawn from small samples of cadavers of variable age and gender, which makes the reliability of their data less certain. Furthermore, the measurement techniques were poorly described, which adds to the wide variation in data points. Ward and colleagues performed a landmark study designed to accurately measure muscle architecture for the lower extremities, including the largest force-generating and excursion capacity muscle groups at each joint.[10]

The tendon being considered for transfer must have adequate strength as most transfers typically lose one muscle grade of strength. In the vast majority of cases, the muscle strength for the tendon being transferred should be a minimum of 4/5. As mentioned earlier, in the rare case that a static tendon transfer is planned instead of a dynamic tendon transfer, muscle strength is less of a concern.[3,7-9]

Functional muscle strength is dependent on more than simply gross power. Several biomechanical and anatomic features augment or diminish muscle strength. For instance, a tendon transfer that passes beneath a retinaculum prevents bowstringing but at the cost of weakening the tendon's power. Another modifier of strength is where the tendon transfer will lie in relation to the joint axis. A centrally aligned tendon relative to the axis of a joint exerts little influence at that joint. The further the tendon is from the joint axis, the greater the influence the tendon transfer exerts as this lengthens the lever arm. It is also ideal to plan a tendon transfer to exert its pull as direct as possible. Acute angulations cause weakening of the force vector, which is something that occurs, for example, when transferring a posterior tibialis tendon through the interosseous membrane.

Another key concept is that the relative muscle strength of the tendon(s) transfer should be similar to the deficit it is replacing. Sarrafian and colleagues eloquently describe ankle-foot motors where the position of a tendon relative to the axis of a joint influences the action. Within the ankle joint, tendons that lie posterior to the ankle joint axis exert a plantar flexion force across the ankle. Tendons that lie anterior to the axis of ankle joint motion exert a dorsiflexory force. The relative muscle strength of plantar flexion generates four times more energy than dorsiflexion in a rectus foot. And within plantar flexion, the triceps surae generates almost 90% of the plantar flexion energy by itself. Within the foot, the axis of motion of the talocalcaneonavicular joint (TCNJ) and midtarsal joint are fairly similar. Tendons that lie medial to the TCNJ are invertors, and tendons that lie lateral to the TCNJ are evertors. Inversion strength generates two times more energy than eversion energy in a rectus foot type. Within the toes, all tendons passing dorsal to the metatarsophalangeal joint (MTPJ) axis of motion are extensors while those plantar function as flexors. Tendons passing through the vertical axis of a metatarsal head either medially or laterally will exert a varus or valgus force, respectfully (Table 56.2).[11]

An additional modifier of tendon transfer strength is synergism. Synergistic or in-phase muscle transfers are more ideal because this decreases the degree of reeducation needed for posttransfer rehabilitation and better preserves strength. The foot and ankle surgeon should avoid nonphasic tendon transfers when possible.

PRINCIPLES OF TENDON EXCURSION IN TENDON TRANSFERS

Another important consideration for matching compatible muscles is excursion. Excursion is the ability of a muscle to change length, and it is ideal if the relative excursions of the

TABLE 56.2	Ankle-Foot Motors of the Ankle and Talocalcaneonavicular Joints				
Ankle Joint					
Plantar flexion	Triceps surae	16.4	Dorsiflexion	TA	2.5
	FHL	0.9		EDL	0.8
	FDL	0.4		EHL	0.4
	TP	0.4		P. tertius	0.5
	PL	0.4			
	PB	0.3			
Total		**18.8**	**Total**		**4.2**
Talocalcaneonavicular Joint					
Inversion	Triceps surae	4.8	Eversion	PL	1.7
	TP	1.8		PB	1.3
	FDL	0.8		EDL	0.8
	FHL	0.8		P. tertius	0.5
	TA	1.0		EHL	0.1
				TA	0.3
Total		**8.2**	**Total**		**4.8**

Measurements reflect the work capacity related to the joint axis expressed in meter kilograms.

FHL, flexor hallucis longus; FDL, flexor digitorum longus; TP, tibialis posterior; PL, peroneus longus; PB, peroneus brevis; TA, tibialis anterior; EDL, extensor digitorum longus; EHL, extensor hallucis longus; P. tertius, peroneus tertius.

Data from Sarrafian Shahan K, Kelikian Armen S. Functional anatomy of the foot and ankle. In: *Sarrafian's Anatomy of the Foot and Ankle*. 3rd ed. Philadelphia, PA: Lippincott Williams & Wilkins; 2011:507-643.

tendon(s) being transferred are similar. Ward and colleagues calculated the estimated excursion for each extrinsic lower extremity muscle in order to aid surgeons in selecting the appropriate donor muscle for a tendon transfer surgery. These measurements have been previously performed and found to be useful in matching donor and host muscle architectures in the upper extremity, leading to better functional outcomes.[10]

For each muscle, Ward and colleagues calculated the normalized muscle fiber length, which is an index of a muscle's excursion. Their technique permitted comparison regardless of the fact that muscles may be fixed in various degrees of tension and position. The results of their work can be seen in Table 56.3. They also accounted for differences in muscle design using the fiber length–to–muscle length ratio (Lf/Lm ratio). This ratio indicates a muscle's excursion design. "For example, if a muscle contains fibers that span the entire muscle length (Lf/Lm ratio = 1), it is designed more for excursion compared with a muscle that has fibers spanning only half of the muscle length (Lf/Lm ratio = 0.5)." This ratio allows for excursion design comparisons beyond normalized fiber length alone.[10]

They determined that among the ankle muscle groups, fiber length was exceptionally similar within muscle groups. The outlier was the tibialis posterior, which has the shortest fibers associated with the ankle, and the authors linked this to the high frequency of tendinopathy. This is relevant because a dystrophic tendon may not behave predictably regardless of anatomic baseline. It should also be noted that excursion can be adversely impacted if there is excessive scarring or fibrosis

TABLE 56.3 **Comparison of the Muscle Excursion (Lf/Lm ratio) and Maximum Force-Producing Capacity (PCSA) of Extrinsic Lower Extremity Muscles**

Muscle[a]	Fiber Length (cm)	Lf/Lm Ratio	PCSA (cm²)
Tibialis anterior	6.83 ± 0.79	0.27 ± 0.05	10.9 ± 3.0
Extensor hallucis longus	7.48 ± 1.13	0.31 ± 0.06	2.7 ± 1.5
Extensor digitorum longus	6.93 ± 1.14	0.24 ± 0.04	5.6 ± 1.7
Peroneus longus	5.08 ± 0.63	0.19 ± 0.03	10.4 ± 3.8
Peroneus brevis	4.54 ± 0.65	0.19 ± 0.03	4.9 ± 2.0
Gastrocnemius medial head	5.10 ± 0.98	0.19 ± 0.03	21.1 ± 5.7
Gastrocnemius lateral head	5.88 ± 0.95	0.27 ± 0.03	9.7 ± 3.3
Soleus	4.40 ± 0.99	0.11 ± 0.02	51.8 ± 14.9
Flexor hallucis longus	5.27 ± 1.29	0.20 ± 0.05	6.9 ± 2.7
Flexor digitorum longus	4.46 ± 1.06	0.16 ± 0.09	4.4 ± 2.0
Tibialis posterior	3.78 ± 0.49	0.12 ± 0.02	14.4 ± 4.9

[a]Values are expressed as mean ± standard deviation. Lf = fiber length (excursion), Lm = muscle length, Lf/Lm ratio (muscle excursion design), PSCA = physiologic cross-sectional area (maximum force-producing capacity).

Data from Ward SR, Eng CM, Smallwood LH, Lieber RL. Are current measurements of lower extremity muscle architecture accurate? *Clin Orthop Relat Res.* 2009;467(4):1074-1082.

from trauma. In cases of prior injury, surgery, or trauma, there may be insufficient excursion of the tendon to be transferred. Each muscle-tendon excursion unit can also be influenced by age, gender, and other factors.

Ward and colleagues also measured the physiologic cross-sectional area (PCSA) of each extrinsic lower extremity muscle. PCSA functions as an estimate of strength proportional to a muscle's maximum force-producing capacity. They calculated that ankle plantarflexors as a functional unit had more than six times greater force-producing capacity relative to the dorsiflexors.[10] These concepts do not operate in a vacuum and are influenced by position relative to a single or multiple joints. The moment arm can either augment or diminish the functional ranges of these muscles as detailed in the prior section.

TENDON ANCHORING PRINCIPLES

Determining the tension of the tendon transfer when anchoring is a vital component to the overall success. The authors prefer to place tendons under more tension than relaxation as the tendons will almost always stretch out but rarely regain muscle strength if anchored too loose.

There are many techniques for anchoring tendons to bones and tendons to tendons that are beyond the scope of this chapter. The authors prefer a tendon-to-bone interface using an interference screw when possible. This provides a strong repair and often decreases the length of tendon needed for the transfer. The goal is to establish a strong interface for the tendon transfer insertion site so that the patient can start rehabilitation as soon as possible.

TENDON HEALING AND POSTOPERATIVE COURSE

Tendons heal in a manner that is very similar to wound healing. There are four stages that span a period beginning just hours after the injury and ending 8-12 weeks later. Initially, an inflammatory reaction occurs within 72 hours of the insult and will

last as long as 7 days. Infiltration of cells from the endotenon, epitenon, and peritenon forms a stabilizing fibroblastic callus while the local inflammatory cascade is active. The next phase is marked by proliferation of endotenon cells and increased production of disorganized collagen fibers. During this phase, which lasts between 7 and 14 days, the tendon is still quite weak and requires protection in the form of a cast or splint. The third stage of tendon healing involves further collagen production but in a more organized manner. Alignment of the fibers with the long axis of the tendon begins and is enhanced by passive ROM activity. Finally, the maturation phase will begin after ~5 weeks postinjury. At this point, collagen production is greatly reduced, and remodeling of the site becomes the primary activity.[1,4]

Postoperative care varies based on the tendon transfer(s) being performed, concomitant procedures, patient comorbidities, bone quality, and method of tendon insertion fixation. But in general, an initial period of immobilization is necessary to protect the tendon transfer as it is still very weak. Passive isometric motion should be initiated as soon as possible. The authors' goal is to begin protected passive ROM in 3 weeks. The patient is advanced based on the procedures performed, but the goal is to begin rehabilitation with progressive strengthening exercises once the cast is discontinued. Reeducation of the tendon transfer can take time, and if the transfer was out of phase, intense rehabilitation is usually necessary. Table 56.4 is an adaptation from van Dijk and colleagues with additional information in order to provide a helpful overview of the anticipated postoperative course for the majority of foot and ankle tendon transfers.[12] This can be modified as necessary dependent upon the specific procedures performed and other variants, which may impact the projected postoperative course.

PHASES OF GAIT

When transferring tendons or performing tenotomies, it is important to consider the concept of phasic activity. Broadly, each extrinsic muscle is classified as either a stance-phase

TABLE 56.4 Typical Postoperative Course Following Tendon Transfers of the Foot and Ankle		0-2 Weeks	2-4 Weeks	6-8 Weeks	8-12 Weeks	12-24 Weeks	>24 Weeks
Weight bearing status	Non–weight bearing	X					
	Partial weight bearing		X	X			
	Full weight bearing				X	X	X
Immobilization status	Immobilization in splint/cast	X	X				
	Immobilization in protective boot		X				
Range of motion	Passive range of motion		X	X	X		
	Active range of motion			X	X	X	
Nonimpact activity	Strengthening			X	X	X	X
	Proprioceptive training			X	X	X	X
	Eccentric/concentric exercises				X	X	X
	Isotonic exercises				X	X	X
High-impact activity	Running					X	X
	Sport-specific training						X

van Dijk PAD, Lubberts B, Verheul C. Rehabilitation after surgical treatment of peroneal tendon tears and ruptures. *Knee Surg Sports Traumatol Arthrosc.* 2016;24:1165.

or swing-phase muscle. Muscles active in the swing-phase are located within the anterior compartment. Unlike their counterparts within the stance-phase; swing-phase muscles are also active, albeit briefly, during the opposing phase of gait. Exclusively stance-phase muscles within the leg include the posterior and lateral muscle groups. The specific muscles and their dominant gait phase are illustrated in Table 56.5.[11]

When circumstances permit, tendon transfers that augment muscle activity in the same gait phase as the harvested tendon generally result in a simpler postoperative course. This is most apparent in cases where extensive physical therapy is required following a tendon transfer. Homophasic transfers tend to recover function much more rapidly, with some reporting full recovery in as little as 7-8 weeks.[3] Out-of-phase transfers are less predictable and may have a far more protracted course. Although phase conversion is a frequent goal, many of these procedures remain beneficial without phase conversion by providing biologic splintage.[3,13,14]

FUNCTIONAL CLASSIFICATION FOR SELECTING TENDON TRANSFER(S)

The sheer volume of information covering the versatility of every tendon transfer, indications, and outcomes is prohibitive in terms of presentation. Almost as expansive as the procedures themselves are the ways by which they can be classified.

In order to consolidate the deluge of available information, we have classified the procedures into categories according to the action they seek to enhance. By identifying the muscles and/or muscle compartments that are imbalanced, the goal is to then determine which procedures would best reestablish function. The actions include the goal of reestablishing flexion, extension, supination, and pronation. These categories have been further subdivided into the following anatomic locations: ankle joint, TCNJ, or coxa pedis within the foot and MTPJ. These procedures and categories are presented in tabular form for easy reference in Table 56.6.

Tendon transfers marked with an asterisk in Table 56.6 are reviewed in greater detail in the following sections as it is beyond the scope of this chapter to review every possible tendon transfer of the foot and ankle. Rather it is more important

TABLE 56.5 Primary Active Extrinsic Lower Extremity Muscles During Normal Phases of Gait via Electromyography			
Gait Phase	**Foot Position**	**Primary Muscle Activity**	**Percent of Cycle**
Stance phase	Heel strike	TA EDL EHL	0%-15%
	Midstance/ forefoot loading	Gastrocnemius Soleus TP	15%-30%
	Heel off/ propulsion	FDL FHL Peroneus longus Peroneus brevis	30%-62%
Swing phase	Toe off	TA EDL EHL	62%-100%

TA, tibialis anterior; EDL, extensor digitorum longus; EHL, extensor hallucis longus; TP, tibialis posterior; FDL, flexor digitorum longus; FHL, flexor hallucis longus.

TABLE 56.6	Functional Classification of Tendon Transfers Organized by Their Primary Method of Restoring Function to the Ankle or Foot	
To reestablish extension		
Ankle joint	TP into intermediate cuneiform (via IOM) +/− PL transfer (Bridle)*	
	PB into intermediate cuneiform	
	EDL/EHL into intermediate cuneiform	
	EDL into intermediate or lateral cuneiform or peroneus tertius (modified Hibbs tenosuspension)*	
TCNJ	EHL into first metatarsal (Jones tenosuspension)*	
To reestablish flexion		
Ankle Joint	FHL to Achilles/calcaneus*	
	PL/PB to Achilles/calcaneus	
	FDL to Achilles/calcaneus	
	TA to Achilles/calcaneus	
TMTJ	FHL into first metatarsal	
MTPJ	FDL/FHL into respective phalanx*	
To reestablish pronation		
TCNJ	STATT or TA into lateral cuneiform*	
	PL to PB transfer*	
	FHL to PB transfer	
To reestablish supination		
TCNJ	FDL transfer into navicular or medial cuneiform*	
	PB to PL transfer	
	Young suspension (rerouting TA around navicular)	

*Reviewed in detail in subsequent sections of this chapter.

TP, tibialis posterior; IOM, interosseous membrane; PL, peroneus longus; PB, peroneus brevis; EDL, extensor digitorum longus; EHL, extensor hallucis longus; FHL, flexor hallucis longus; FDL, flexor digitorum longus; TA, tibialis anterior; STATT, split tibialis anterior tendon transfer; TCNJ, talocalcaneonavicular joint; MTPJ, metatarsophalangeal joint.

Data from van Dijk PAD, Lubberts B, Verheul C. Rehabilitation after surgical treatment of peroneal tendon tears and ruptures. *Knee Surg Sports Traumatol Arthrosc.* 2016;24:1165.

for the surgeon to understand tendon and mechanical principles alongside unique deformity and patient characteristics to determine the best tendon transfer.

INTEROSSEOUS POSTERIOR TIBIAL TENDON TRANSFER

DEFINITION

Posterior tibial tendon (PTT) transfers are typically performed for treatment of footdrop, as a result of a broad spectrum of disorders of motor function deficits, resulting in loss of ankle dorsiflexion or dorsiflexory strength. They may also be performed in some cases of foot imbalance or flexible foot deformities to reduce the advantage of the invertors and restore balance and strength to the evertors.

Loss of ankle dorsiflexion and hindfoot eversion may result from a variety of conditions including cerebrovascular accident, common peroneal nerve palsy, common peroneal nerve injury, or L5 radiculopathy. A broad spectrum of motor or nerve functional deficits and associated deformities may lead to the need for this tendon transfer. It is essential that the function of the PTT is retained.[15]

INDICATIONS

PTT transfers may be indicated in cases of loss of ankle dorsiflexion and hindfoot eversion, while posterior muscle compartment and PTT function remains intact. This may include loss of peroneal nerve function, loss or imbalance of evertors such as the peroneus brevis and peroneus longus (PL) tendons, and equinus contractures.

In some cases, nerve injuries may recover with time, and footdrop or weakness may recover. Appropriate time and therapy should be allowed prior to proceeding with a PTT transfer. A minimum of 12-18 months should be allowed in order to confirm that nerve function is not likely to recover.

Flaccid paralysis with complete loss of tibial and common peroneal nerve function causes loss of motor function distal to the knee, causing loss of all major muscle antagonists in the lower leg. In these cases, tendon transfer may not be necessary as an imbalance may not necessarily exist or lead to contractures, and as all function is lost, a tendon transfer would provide no new advantage. These conditions remain relatively stable over time.

ANATOMIC FEATURES AND FUNCTIONAL ANALYSIS

POSTERIOR TIBIALIS TENDON

The PTT originates from the posterior tibia, interosseous membrane, and the fibula, coursing through the deep posterior leg compartment, curving posterior to the medial malleolus, and inserting on to the navicular tuberosity, spring ligament, and plantar midtarsal bones.

INTEROSSEOUS MEMBRANE

The interosseous membrane forms the ligamentous stabilizer between the tibia and fibula and forms the fibular syndesmosis, maintaining an anatomic ankle joint mortise. The membrane is wider proximally and narrows as it courses distally toward the ankle joint.

SCIATIC NERVE

The sciatic nerve branches into the tibial and common peroneal nerves just proximal to the popliteal fossa, with the common peroneal nerve moving from posterior to anterior

at the lateral leg at the fibular neck, supplying innervation to the anterior and lateral compartments of the lower leg and to the main dorsiflexors of the ankle via the superficial peroneal nerve. The common peroneal nerve is often affected with neuropathies or trauma, compromising the dorsiflexory functions. The tibial nerve is typically spared in these cases and provides innervation and function to the deep posterior compartment, including the PTT, and must be functional for the PTT to be functional and for a successful tendon transfer.

EXTENSOR RETINACULUM

The extensor retinaculum is the thick fibrous retinacular layer located on the dorsum of the foot and ankle, superficial to the course of the extensor tendons, creating a fulcrum point and preventing bowstringing of the extensors at the ankle joint. The decision to transfer a tendon deep vs superficial to the extensor retinaculum is important in surgical decision-making, as harvested tendon strength, tendon length, and desired location of new insertion are key factors in determining the new course of the transferred PTT.

PHYSICAL EXAMINATION

Physical examination findings will typically consist of gait abnormality and dorsiflexory weakness. "Slap foot gait" with dragging of the foot during swing phase may be seen. This may also lead to a high steppage gate with exaggerated flexion of the knee and hip during swing phase. Loss of great toe flexion after push off accompanied by intrinsic lesser toe extensor compensation during swing phase if often seen. Patients will often have difficulty walking on their heels.

The hindfoot will invert during swing phase with heel strike occurring more laterally on the calcaneus. A Coleman block test can be used to aid in determining if hindfoot is flexible or rigid.[15] Rigid deformities will require osseous correction via arthrodesis or osteotomy either prior to or in conjunction with tendon transfer.

Manual muscle strength testing reveals the inability to dorsiflex the ankle and the great toe, with notable weakness. The strength of the peroneal tendons and other ankle evertors should be thoroughly evaluated to ensure normal function and strength. Note the presence of spastic antagonist muscles.

Nerve palsies and other disease conditions may lead to varus hindfoot and equinus contractures as well as lesser toe digital claw toe contracture deformities due to chronic compensation. Loss of anterior compartment strength will lead to flexor advantage and plantar flexion contractures over time. Digital contractures may be masked during physical examination by the plantar flexed position of the foot. Dorsiflexing the ankle during physical examination will aid in revealing any claw toe deformities or equinus contracture deformities that are present. This is important in determining necessary adjunctive procedures when considering a tendon transfer.

Nerve dysfunction may also lead to loss of or diminished sensation to the dorsum of the foot.

PATHOGENESIS

NEUROMUSCULAR

Conditions including cerebral palsy, cerebrovascular accident, CMT, lumbar disc disease, Duchenne muscular dystrophy, and polio may lead to loss of dorsiflexory strength.

TRAUMA

Injury to the common peroneal nerve may lead to loss of dorsiflexory function. Tibialis anterior (TA) tendon ruptures may be extensive enough that repair is not possible or not successful. Neglected ruptures with severe contracture or atrophy may require a tendon transfer.

CONGENITAL

Congenital cavovarus foot or clubfoot deformities that are flexible and reducible, may benefit from a posterior tibialis tendon transfer in certain cases.

Other conditions in which a posterior tibialis tendon transfer may be considered include the following[16-18]:

- Tibialis anterior tendon rupture (trauma)
- Cerebrovascular accident
- Lumbar spine radiculopathy
- Hereditary sensorimotor neuropathy
- Common peroneal nerve injury (trauma)
- Charcot-Marie-Tooth
- Leprosy
- Poliomyelitis
- Spastic cerebral palsy

IMAGING AND DIAGNOSTICS

Standard weight-bearing AP, oblique, and lateral radiographs are typically sufficient to evaluate the weight-bearing contractures and deformities and any rigid bone or joint contractures due to long-standing conditions. An MRI may be helpful in evaluating the condition of the PTT health or identifying any mass or space-occupying lesions that may have contributed to a nerve palsy. It may also be helpful to confirm that weakness is not due to a TA tendon rupture rather than a neuromuscular dysfunction. Neurologic workup may include EMG or NCV studies.[19,20]

TREATMENT

The goal of treatment is to restore the balance between the invertors and evertors of the foot and to achieve a plantar grade foot without footdrop during the swing phase of gait. The ideal goal of surgical treatment being to achieve a functional gait without the need for an ankle-foot orthosis (AFO), or other stabilizing brace.[21] An out-of-phase transfer may restore dorsiflexory function or may only act as a static restraint of the plantar flexion deformity.[19,20,22]

It is recommended that a neurology consultation and a complete neurological workup, including any electrodiagnostic studies, be performed prior to proceeding with tendon transfer.

This may also be helpful in assessing the baseline function of the PTT to determine most likely posttransfer tendon function and strength.[15,19-21]

NONOPERATIVE

Nonoperative treatment may consist of AFO bracing techniques with a dorsiflex assist and plantar flexion stop modification. Physical therapy focusing on joint mobilization, contracture releases, and stretching may be beneficial. Botulinum toxin injections may be indicated in some cases as well. Flexible deformities tend to respond better to bracing and stretching options compared to more rigid or spastic contractures. Bracing can be extremely difficult in rigid or fixed deformities.[23]

SURGICAL PROCEDURE AND TECHNIQUE

- An Achilles tendon or gastrocnemius lengthening should be performed in most cases, although not always necessary. This can be performed percutaneously, open, or endoscopically depending on surgeon preference and patient indications.
- A 3- to 4-cm incision is made over the medial aspect of the navicular tuberosity at the insertion of the PTT. Blunt dissection is carried down to the tendon sheath, which is incised, exposing the posterior tibialis tendon (Fig. 56.1).
- The tendon may be sharply released from the insertion, maintaining as much distal tendon fibers as possible. Care should be taken to avoid the medial plantar nerve and vein during release and isolation of the distal tendon fibers (Fig. 56.2).
- Alternatively, a saw or osteotome may be used to resect and elevate bone from the insertion of the navicular tuberosity and increase harvest length or be used for bone-to-bone implantation after transfer.

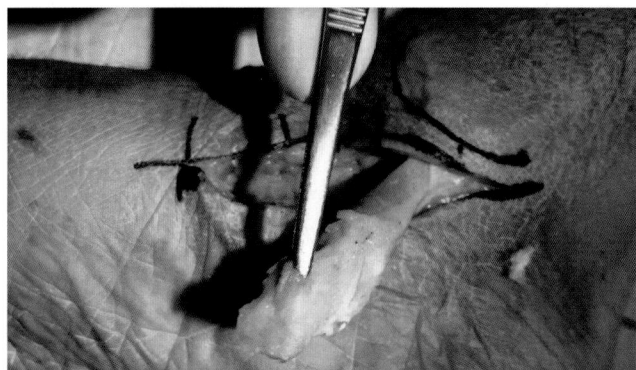

FIGURE 56.2 The posterior tibialis tendon is sharply released from the navicular tuberosity, maintaining as much length as possible.

- A second 3-cm incision is made on the posterior medial aspect of the calf at the myotendinous junction of the PTT. The incision is typically in line with and 1 cm posterior to the posteromedial border of the tibia. Blunt dissection is carried down to the first visible muscle belly. The FDL muscle is usually encountered first. Deep to the FDL, directly on the posterior medial surface of the tibia, the PTT and muscle can be identified (Fig. 56.3).
- A blunt retractor can be used to circumferentially isolate and elevate the PTT through this incision.
- Mobilize the distal PTT within the tendon sheath with a blunt scissor or probe, alternating tension on the tendon proximally and distally until the tendon can be pulled through the proximal incision. In some instances, the flexor retinaculum may need to be released in order to facilitate proximal passage (Fig. 56.4). Once the tendon has been brought into the second incision, keep the tendon covered with a moist sponge.
- A third incision 4-5 cm in length is made on the anterior aspect of the lower leg at the intersection of the middle and distal third of the fibula, 1 cm lateral to the tibial crest or on the medial surface of the fibula and just distal to the second incision.

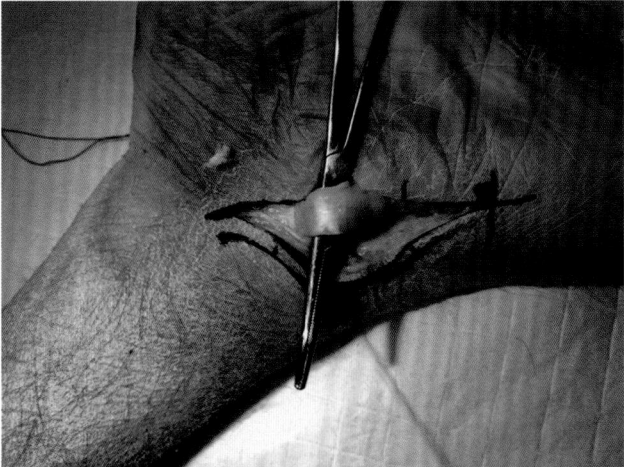

FIGURE 56.1 Incision #1 extends along the medial foot ending at the navicular tuberosity, and the posterior tibialis tendon is exposed.

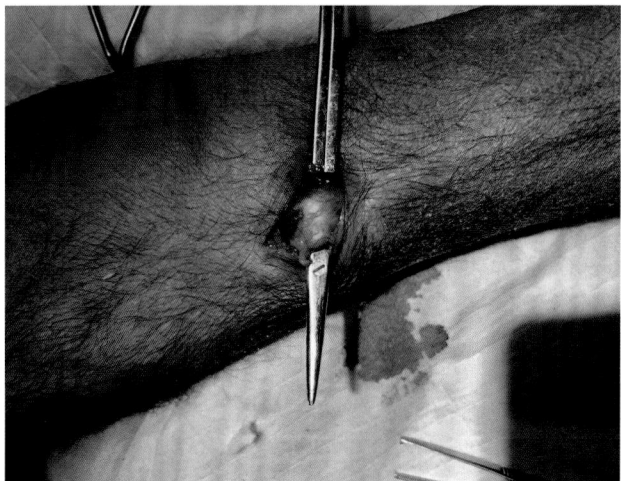

FIGURE 56.3 Incision #2 is on the posterior medial calf at the level of the posterior tibialis myotendinous junction. The posterior tibial tendon is deep to the FDL.

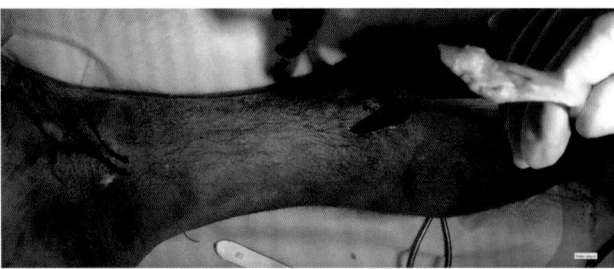

FIGURE 56.4 The posterior tibialis tendon is passed from incision #1 through incision #2.

- Blunt dissection is carried down along the medial face of the fibula or lateral face of the tibia until the interosseous membrane is identified. This decision is usually based upon the neurovascular bundle's position seen on the preoperative MRI. Careful medial retraction of the tibial anterior muscle and neurovascular structures may be necessary.
- Through the second incision, blunt dissection is performed with a large right angle hemostat along the posterior tibia, angle toward the third incision, and used to penetrate the interosseous membrane from posterior to anterior, thus protecting and preventing injury to the neurovascular bundle. The window in the membrane can then be enlarged to ~4 cm.
- The PTT is then passed from the second incision along the posterior tibia, staying in contact with the bone, through the interosseous membrane window, and delivered into the third incision laterally (Fig. 56.5).

- At this point, the tendon is whip stitched at its distal end with a large fiber absorbable suture.
- Using intraoperative fluoroscopy, the desired insertion of the tendon is identified, typically the lateral cuneiform.
- A fourth incision is made over the lateral cuneiform 3 cm in length, with blunt dissection down to the cuneiform, where the periosteum is elevated and the bone exposed.
- A tendon passer or long aortic clamp or forceps is then passed from the distal dorsal foot incision proximally in a retrograde fashion to the lateral leg incision. The tunnel is widened and mobilized, and the tendon is then passed from proximal to distal and delivered to the dorsum of the foot (blunt dissection from distal to proximal may be performed either superficial or deep to the extensor retinaculum, depending on surgeon preference and desired muscle strength) (Fig. 56.6).
- The tendon may then be fixed to the insertion point on the intermediate or lateral cuneiform, or cuboid, with the surgeon's preferred method of fixation through a bone tunnel or bone anchor (Tenodesis screw, EndoButton, Corkscrew anchor).
- Alternatively, the tendon may be tenodesed to the extensor tendons to act as a static restraint rather than an active dorsiflexor.[19,20]

positioning PEARLS

The patient should be placed in a supine position with an ipsilateral hip bump to orient the foot and toes upward and prevent excessive external rotation and aid in exposure if peroneal tendons need accessed for adjunctive procedures.

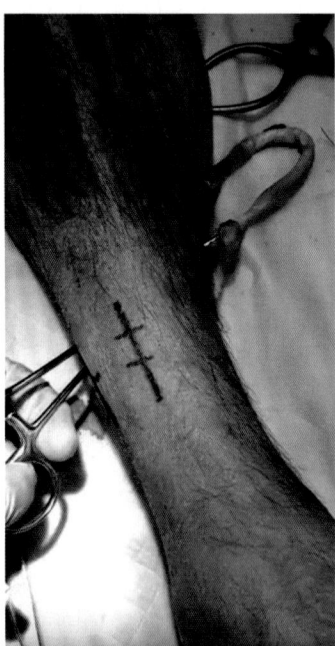

FIGURE 56.5 Incision #3 is along the anterior lower leg, 1 cm lateral to the tibial crest and just distal to incision #2. A 4-cm window is carefully made in the interosseous membrane through incision #2 using a right-angle hemostat. The posterior tibial tendon is then passed through the interosseous window into incision #3.

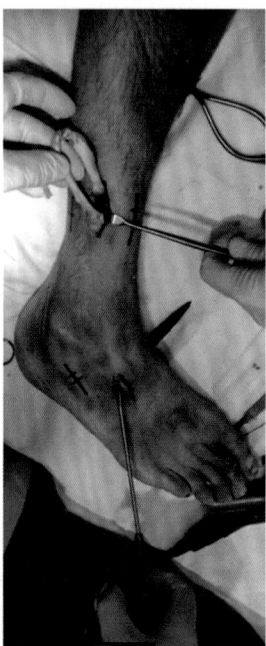

FIGURE 56.6 Incision #4 is made directly over the lateral cuneiform, location confirmed with fluoroscopy. The posterior tibial tendon is then whip stitched and passed from incision #3 to incision #4 with the aid of a long tendon passer.

EXPOSURE PEARLS

Longitudinal incisions are preferred, and care should be taken with transverse or oblique incisions, as they will place neurovascular structures at greater risk. Multiple relatively small incisions are utilized, but having adequate exposure at the distal PTT harvest site will aid in obtaining as much tendon length as possible and prevent complications associated with lack of sufficient tendon length for transfer. A larger incision at the transferred tendon insertion site may also aid in ease of anchor placement and fixation. Ideal position of the proximal tendon harvest incision can provide maximum length.[24]

AUTHORS' PREFERRED TREATMENT

The authors prefer a four-incision technique for tendon transfer with a distal sharp release of the PTT fibers and with the second incision located 7 cm above the medial malleolus in male patients and 6.5 cm above the medial malleolus in female patients in order to maximize harvested tendon length.[24]

An interosseous transfer is preferred due to the increased ankle dorsiflexion and ROM as well as improved tendon gliding compared to circumferential PTT transfers.[25,26] We prefer an interosseous membrane window size of ~5 cm or 2.5 times the size of the oblique tendon diameter in order to reduce the risk of tendon entrapment.[26] Ensuring that a portion of the muscle belly is present at the window is also preferred. An oblique angle between the second and third incisions is key in obtaining maximum tendon length and preserving muscle strength.

A tendon transfer deep to the extensor retinaculum is preferred, as it shows comparable strength and gliding of the tendon compared to above the retinaculum and prevents bowstringing of the tendon.[26]

An absorbable Bio-Tenodesis screw and bone tunnel fixation is preferred for fixation vs either bone anchors or Pulvertaft weave, as Tenodesis tends to have more variability and less reliability in tendon displacement and load to failure.[27]

PERILS and PITFALLS

- Proper preoperative assessment and planning is key to having a successful outcome. Full knowledge of the PTT function is vital. Appropriate patient education and rehab expectations in a reverse-phase tendon transfer such as the PTT transfer is important for successful outcomes.[28,29]
- Appropriate tensioning of the transferred PTT is important in achieving adequate ankle dorsiflexion. Overtensioning the transferred tendon is recommended, as some stretching will naturally occur over time. Ensuring that the tendon is stretched and pulled tightly through the interosseous membrane prior to anchoring will aid in appropriate tensioning. The ankle should be placed in 5-10 degrees of ankle joint dorsiflexion, and the PTT should be tensioned to ~90%-100% of elongation when anchoring the tendon.

- Have a low threshold for performing an Achilles lengthening or a gastrocnemius recession to prevent any residual contractures and to weaken the antagonist flexor advantage.
- The PTT transfer through the interosseous membrane at the appropriate level and with an adequately sized window will prevent constriction of the tendon and prevent weakness or loss of function after the transfer.
- Appropriate understanding of the advantages and disadvantages of transferring either deep or superficial to the extensor retinaculum is important.
- Do not begin ankle joint ROM exercises until the surgical incisions are healed. This will aid in prevention of infection and wound dehiscence. Allowing adequate time for the tendon insertion site to heal appropriately before beginning ROM and strengthening exercises will usually allow sufficient time for the wounds to heal.

POSTOPERATIVE CARE

The patient is placed non–weight bearing (NWB) in a well-padded posterior splint or short leg cast in the operating room in order to protect the transferred tendon until the anchor point is sufficiently healed. Sutures are typically removed at weeks 2-3 postoperatively. Care should be taken to maintain ankle in a dorsiflexed position during all postoperative visits and cast exchanges.

Partial weight bearing or touchdown weight bearing may begin at week 3; however, full protected weight bearing in a cast or protective tall walking boot should not be initiated until at least week 6 postoperatively.

Full weight bearing and protected ambulation in an AFO or protective tall walking boot is begun at 8-10 weeks postoperatively along with initiating physical therapy. No plantar flexion stretching should be performed during physical therapy at this time, and focus should be placed on posterior muscle group stretching and dorsiflexion and eversion strengthening.

The patient should be educated that a protective AFO will likely be needed for ~4-6 months postoperatively.[12]

BRIDLE PROCEDURE

DEFINITION

The Bridle procedure is essentially a PTT transfer that is augmented with a peroneal longus and TA tenodesis. As described previously, these are broadly indicated for the treatment of dropfoot and steppage gait. While the PTT transfer is largely concerned with dorsiflexion, the Bridle allows for greater frontal plane stability in the setting of more severe muscular imbalance. The anastomosis of these three tendons creates an evenly distributed pull for the PTT that maintains a more neutrally

positioned foot. The procedure aims to restore extension primarily and control the coronal secondarily.

INDICATIONS

Particularly in the setting of posttraumatic neurologic compromise, nerve function may gradually return over the course of 12-18 months. If recovery becomes evident, it may take several months of targeted physical therapy to restore muscle strength after nerve function is restored. Allow for adequate recovery prior to initiating a Bridle procedure.

Loss of ankle dorsiflexion and hindfoot frontal plane deformities may result from a variety of conditions including cerebrovascular accident, common peroneal nerve palsy, common peroneal nerve injury, or L5 radiculopathy. A broad spectrum of motor or nerve functional deficits and associated deformities may lead to the need for this tendon transfer. A functional PTT is an absolute requirement for this procedure.[15]

A footdrop in the setting of significant nonrigid frontal plane deformities is usually the best indication for the Bridle procedure. For example, a patient with baseline flatfoot deformity may find that after an isolated PTT transfer, the valgus may become worsened, particularly if the peroneal tendons remain functional or spastic. Conversely, a patient with flexible hindfoot varus due to concomitant peroneal compromise is also a better candidate for the Bridle over the isolated PTT transfer.

Flaccid paralysis with complete loss of tibial and common peroneal nerve function causes loss of motor function distal to the knee, which results in loss of all major muscle antagonists in the lower leg. In the setting of complete paralysis, with a foot that is braceable in a plantigrade position, a tendon transfer may not be necessary as an imbalance may not necessarily exist or necessarily lead to contractures. Under these conditions, a tendon transfer would provide no significant advantage.

Unlike the previously mentioned PTT transfer, a ruptured TA tendon is less conducive to the success of this procedure. A hypertrophic peroneal longus is not contraindicated for use since it acts as a tenodesis, but a thin, degenerated peroneal longus should be used with caution.

ANATOMIC FEATURES AND FUNCTIONAL ANALYSIS

Key anatomic structures such as the posterior tibialis tendon, interosseous membrane, sciatic nerve, and extensor retinaculum are covered in the posterior tibialis tendon transfer section.

ANTERIOR TIBIALIS

The anterior tibialis arises from the lateral condyle, interosseous membrane, and upper half of the lateral tibia. Within the anterior muscle compartment, it becomes tendinous at the transition between the middle and distal third of the tibia. It is contained within a synovial sheath from its myotendinous

junction to the distal insertion on the medial cuneiform and first metatarsal base. Prior to emerging onto the dorsal foot, it passes deep to the extensor retinaculum.

PERONEAL LONGUS

The PL origin is a composite of the lateral surfaces of the head and superior two-thirds of the fibula. Within the lateral compartment, it becomes tendinous proximal to the ankle. The tendon courses distally in tandem with the peroneus brevis within a common synovial sheath. At the level of the posterior ankle, the tendon lies posterior and lateral to the brevis tendon within an anatomic tunnel composed of a retrofibular sulcus that is usually concave and covered by the superior peroneal retinaculum (SPR). The SPR acts as the primary restraint that maintains the relative position of the peroneal tendons within the retrofibular groove. Beyond the fibula, the peroneal tendons turn anteriorly and emerge along the lateral calcaneus.

PHYSICAL EXAMINATION

Please refer to the posterior tibialis tendon transfer section.

PATHOGENESIS

Pathogenesis is similar to what is seen with conditions where a posterior tibialis tendon transfer may be beneficial. These include but are not limited to congenital deformities, neuromuscular conditions, and traumatic events. Direct injury to the common peroneal nerve may lead to loss of function. Injury to the knee, fractures, dislocations, and ligament repairs have been associated with both direct compression and indirect traction insults to the common peroneal nerve. Indirect traction following knee or hip replacement has also been reported.[16-18]

IMAGING AND DIAGNOSTICS

Similar to the imaging and diagnostics to a posterior tibialis tendon transfer, radiographs, MRI, and neurologic workup including EMG and NCV are important considerations.[19,20] Special attention should be paid to the fibular head and common peroneal nerve region. MRI may also be helpful in further assessing integrity of the posterior tibialis, anterior tibialis, and PL tendons.

TREATMENT

The goal of treatment is to restore the balance between the invertors and evertors of the foot and to achieve a plantar grade foot without footdrop during the swing phase of gait. The addition of the TA and PL tendon transfers, in addition to the posterior tibialis tendon transfer, are sometimes necessary in order to achieve this goal. This is an out-of-phase transfer, and depending on each situation, the goal may be to restore dorsiflexion or to only act as a static restraint from a plantar flexion deformity.[19,20,22]

NONOPERATIVE

Nonoperative treatment may consist of AFO bracing techniques with a dorsiflex assist and plantar flexion stop modification. Physical therapy focusing on joint mobilization, contracture releases, and stretching may be beneficial. Botulinum toxin injections may be indicated in some cases exacerbated by spasticity. Flexible deformities tend to respond better to bracing and stretching options compared to more rigid or spastic contractures. Bracing can be extremely difficult in rigid or fixed deformities.[23]

SURGICAL PROCEDURE AND TECHNIQUE

The procedural steps for the posterior tibialis tendon transfer are performed as described above. After the posterior tibialis tendon is passed through the interosseous membrane window and delivered into the third anterolateral incision and whip stitched, the whip-stitched tendon is set aside and wrapped in moist gauze.

A fourth incision is made ~5-8 cm above the distal tip of the fibula and centered over the peroneal tendons in the posterolateral distal leg. The PL tendon is then transected ~6 cm from the distal fibular tip. The distal tendon is whip stitched. The decision to tenodese the proximal peroneal longus stump to the peroneal brevis is usually determined by the presence of a functional lateral compartment. No tenodesis is necessary if the longus is nonfunctional.[30]

A fifth incision is made 1 cm proximal to the base of the fifth metatarsal and centered over the peroneal brevis. The brevis is retracted, and the distal segment of the PL tendon is identified deep and inferior to the brevis tendon. The peroneal longus is then pulled distally into this incision. With a hemostat gripping the whip stitch, the transected distal segment of the PL tendon is passed subcutaneously anterior to the fibula and deep to the extensor retinaculum toward the third incision anterior to the ankle.

Using intraoperative fluoroscopy, the desired insertion of the tendon transfer is identified, typically the lateral or intermediate cuneiform.

A sixth incision is made between the intermediate and the lateral cuneiforms ~3 cm in length. The neurovascular structures are retracted medially followed by blunt dissection down to the dorsal surface of the cuneiforms, where the periosteum is elevated and the bone exposed. The decision to secure into the intermediate or lateral cuneiform is discussed in greater detail below but is dependent on preoperative coronal deformities.

If not done previously, the PTT distal stump is debulked to match the diameter of the proximal nonpathologic tendon. With the foot placed in slight dorsiflexion, the overlap of the tibialis posterior, TA and PL are identified.

Next a longitudinal incision is made within the TA, and the posterior tibialis tendon is passed through this slit from deep to superficial. Then, a longitudinal incision is made through the peroneal longus as it passes superficial to the TA. The tibialis posterior is passed deep to superficial through the peroneal tendon opening.

A tendon passer or long aortic clamp or forceps is then passed from the distal dorsal foot (sixth) incision proximally in a retrograde fashion to the anterolateral leg (third) incision. The tunnel is widened and mobilized, and the tendon is then passed from proximal to distal and delivered to the dorsum of the foot. Blunt dissection from distal to proximal may

be performed either superficial or deep to the extensor retinaculum, depending on surgeon preference and desired muscle strength. If the posterior tibial strength is borderline or tendon length is potentially inadequate, then a subcutaneous passage is preferred. Otherwise, passing the PTT deep to the extensor retinaculum is preferred.

With the foot placed in 5-10 degrees of ankle joint dorsiflexion, the PTT is tensioned to ~90%-100% of elongation. The PTT may then be fixed to the insertion point with the surgeon's preferred method of fixation through a bone tunnel or bone anchor (interference screw, EndoButton, Corkscrew anchor, etc.).

With the PTT distal insertion secured, the frontal plane alignment is balanced by pulling the TA and PL tendons proximally. Nonabsorbable 2-0 suture secures the tritendon anastomosis to maintain the frontal plane balance. Nonabsorbable simple interrupted sutures are placed at the proximal and distal apices of the slits in the TA and peroneal longus tendons to prevent propagation of the splits once the patient becomes ambulatory.

POSITIONING PEARLS

The patient should be placed in a supine position with an ipsilateral hip bump to orient the foot and toes upward and prevent excessive external rotation and to aid in access of the peroneal tendons.

EXPOSURE PEARLS

Longitudinal incisions are preferred, and care should be taken with transverse or oblique incisions, as they will place neurovascular structures at greater risk. Multiple relatively small incisions are utilized, but having adequate exposure at the distal PTT harvest site will aid in obtaining as much tendon length as possible and prevent complications associated with lack of sufficient tendon length for transfer. A larger incision at the transferred tendon insertion site may also aid in ease of anchor placement and fixation. Ideal position of the proximal tendon harvest incision can provide maximum length.[24]

AUTHORS' PREFERRED TREATMENT

- Some descriptions of the technique do not incorporate the "fifth" incision over the lateral foot.[31] The author has found that this incision significantly expedites the case and makes passing the distal peroneal tendon to the anterior ankle incision far easier with a more controlled dissection.

- Most typically, a six-incision technique with a distal sharp release of the PTT fibers provides the greatest exposure to obtain adequate tendon length. Research suggests that the second incision should be located 7 cm above the medial malleolus in male patients and 6.5 cm above the medial malleolus in female patients in order to maximize the harvested tendon length.[25] The lateral leg (fourth) incision placement is more variable than the others. This is due to the range of low-lying muscle belly commonly associated with the peroneals.

- An interosseous transfer is preferred due to the increased ankle dorsiflexion and ROM as well as improved tendon gliding compared to circumferential PTT transfers.[26] The author prefers an interosseous membrane window size of ~5 cm or 2.5 times the size of the oblique tendon diameter in order to reduce the risk of tendon entrapment.[25] Adhesions are far more likely if the posterior tibial muscle belly is not partially transferred through the interosseous aperture. An oblique angle between the second and third incisions is key in obtaining maximum tendon length and preserving muscle strength.
- A tendon transfer deep to the extensor retinaculum is preferred, as it shows comparable strength and gliding of the tendon compared to above the retinaculum, and prevents bowstringing of the tendon in PTT transfers.[26]
- The decision to place the PTT in either the intermediate or lateral cuneiform is largely dependent on surgeon preference. For patients with a significant nonrigid valgus deformity, we prefer to insert into the intermediate cuneiform. Otherwise, we will primarily select the lateral cuneiform for securing the PTT transfer.
- An interference screw and bone tunnel fixation is preferred for fixation vs either bone anchors or Pulvertaft weave, as tenodesis tends to have more variability and less reliability in tendon displacement and load to failure.[27]

POSTOPERATIVE CARE

The postoperative care for a Bridle procedure is similar to the recovery for a posterior tibialis tendon transfer as described above.

HIBBS TENOSUSPENSION

DEFINITION

The Hibbs tenosuspension is a tendon transfer of the extensor digitorum longus (EDL) tendons to the dorsal midfoot. The term "clawfoot" was first described by Hibbs in 1919 as a high-arch foot, plantar calluses, and prominent metatarsal heads secondary to digital deformities.[32]

Although the Hibbs tenosuspension fell out of favor due to complications for many years, advances in patient selection, surgical technique, instrumentation, and anchoring have allowed significant improvements resulting in an increase in the modified Hibbs procedure being performed. This procedure and its modifications have been extensively described by DiDomenico and colleagues, which the authors have since adopted as detailed below.[33]

INDICATIONS

A Hibbs tenosuspension may be considered whenever there is retrograde buckling involving all lesser MTPJs. A flexible forefoot equinus is often associated with this deformity as well.

There are several associated conditions such as neuromuscular disease,[33] rheumatoid, and diabetic patients as well as those with muscular imbalances such as cavus and flatfoot conditions where "clawfoot" can be observed.[34,35]

PERILS and PITFALLS

- Proper preoperative assessment and planning is key to having a successful outcome. Full knowledge of the posterior tibial, anterior tibialis, and PL tendons function is vital. Clinical examination is adequate, but EMG gives greater detail. Appropriate patient education and rehabilitation expectations in a reverse-phase tendon transfer such as the PTT transfer is important for successful outcomes.[28,29]
- The traditional description of the Bridle procedure incorporates an Achilles tendon lengthening, usually because of the chronic equinus contracture. Our preference is to assess the equinus under anesthesia with a Silfverskiöld test. This guides us to perform either a gastrocnemius recession or the Achilles tendon lengthening.[30] This is typically performed prior to the Bridle procedure to allow for better tendon balancing and minimize strain to the Bridle anastomosis.
- Appropriate tensioning of the transferred PTT is important in achieving adequate ankle dorsiflexion. Overtensioning the transferred tendon is recommended, as some stretching will naturally occur over time. Ensuring that the tendon is stretched and pulled tightly through the interosseous membrane prior to anchoring will aid in appropriate tensioning. The ankle should be placed in 5-10 degrees of ankle joint dorsiflexion, and the PTT should be tensioned to ~90%-100% of elongation when anchoring the tendon.
- The PTT transfer through the interosseous membrane at the appropriate level and with an adequately sized window will prevent in constriction of the tendon and prevent weakness or loss of function after the transfer.
- Appropriate understanding of the advantages and disadvantages of transferring either deep or superficial to the extensor retinaculum is important.
- Do not begin ankle joint ROM exercises until the surgical incisions are healed. This will aid in prevention of infection and wound dehiscence. Allowing adequate time for the tendon insertion site to heal appropriately before beginning ROM and strengthening exercises will usually allow sufficient time for the wounds to heal.

INDICATIONS

- Reducible extensor digital contractures: claw toes or hammertoes digits 2-5
- Cavus foot
- Extensor substitution/recruitment
- Clawfoot
- Neuromuscular diseases

ANATOMIC FEATURES

A detailed understanding of the anatomy of the distal interphalangeal joint (DIPJ), proximal interphalangeal joint (PIPJ), MTPJ, and dorsal midfoot is especially important for the surgical success of a Hibbs procedure. The EDL originates from the lateral condyle of the tibia, travels along the anterolateral leg,

becomes tendinous, and passes deep to the extensor retinaculum at the ankle joint. The EDL divides into four tendon slips that travel distally to each of the four lesser toes. At the level of the MTPJ, the EDL has membranous extensions into the extensor expansion and plate. The EDL trifurcates with the central slip attaching to the middle phalanx and medial and lateral terminal slips inserting into the distal phalanx.[36]

There are many other anatomic structures, which influence the MTPJ that is beyond the scope of this section. But, it is important to understand that the collateral ligaments stabilize in the transverse plane while the plantar plate provides sagittal stability.[37,38] Furthermore, the EDL functions as a dorsiflexor of the ankle through the swing phase of gait. It also extends the PIPJ, DIPJ, and MTPJ of the four lesser toes.[39]

FUNCTIONAL ANALYSIS OF THE ANATOMY

There is often a biomechanical imbalance resulting in digital contractures most commonly from extensor substitution. Extensor substitution occurs during swing phase whenever the EDL gains a mechanical advantage over the lumbricals. Digital deformities can develop as a result of the MTPJ extension and IPJ plantar flexion from the flexors. When extensor substitution is exhibited, there can be a neurologic component leading to atrophy of the intrinsic musculature. This allows the EDL to become a deforming force on the MTPJ and easily overpower the lumbricals. This creates unopposed pull of the EDL and FDL tendons leading to claw toes[39] (Fig. 56.7).

PHYSICAL EXAMINATION

Physical examination should focus on the deforming forces and flexibility. Biomechanical analysis in both weight bearing and NWB should be performed. Most importantly, the digits and foot should be reducible. A Kelikian push-up test at the MTPJ level is very useful in determining how readily reducible and flexible the deformity is.[40] A neurology consult can help to determine a neurogenic etiology if the source of the contractures is unclear.[41] Evaluate the digits at DIPJ, PIPJ, and MTPJ level to ensure that reduction is possible. If there is hindfoot or

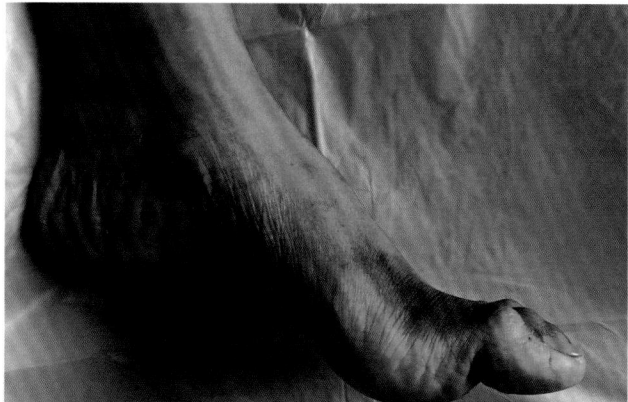

FIGURE 56.7 Preoperative clinical images showing claw toes and extensor substitution.

midfoot involvement, evaluate for flexibility and possible concomitant procedures.

One should always include a thorough vascular workup. If there is concern, consider vascular consultation or additional tests such as noninvasive arterial studies including pulse volume recordings, Doppler, ankle-brachial indices, toe-brachial indices, and digital pressures if available at your local vascular lab.

PATHOGENESIS

In the cavus foot with an overpowering and tight posterior muscle group or Achilles tendon and often a weak TA, extensor substitution can develop as the EDL is now recruited to aid with dorsiflexion. This leads to retrograde buckling at the MTPJ and development of metatarsalgia and hammertoes. Essentially, the EDL overpowers the intrinsic musculature and the lumbricals, eventually becoming a deforming force at the MTPJ. This leads to dorsal subluxation at the MTPJ and increased plantar pressure. This can occur in cases of CMT, postpolio, or with other neurologic causes.[39-42]

IMAGING AND DIAGNOSTIC STUDIES

Appropriate imaging consists initially of plain film weight-bearing X-rays of the foot in AP, medial oblique and lateral projections. A calcaneal axial image is also very useful. (Fig. 56.8A and B). A good AP projection is helpful in assessing transverse and sagittal plane deformity,[37] while the lateral view is critical to assess the sagittal plane. As noted previously, neurologic workup with EMG/NCV to assess muscle function can be helpful.

TREATMENT

NONOPERATIVE

Nonoperative treatment can include taping, toe crest pads, strapping of the toes, Budin or other splints, orthotics, or shoe modifications. Typically, patients having pain, callus buildup, or ulceration will proceed with surgical correction unless they are poor surgical candidates.

SURGICAL PROCEDURE AND TECHNIQUE

A thigh tourniquet is preferred, although performing the procedure without tourniquet and meticulous dissection is also acceptable. The incision courses from the proximal fourth metatarsal base to the second metatarsal neck obliquely (Fig. 56.3). A minimally invasive approach has been described; however, the authors prefer this oblique approach in order to clearly visualize and avoid neurovascular structures.[11] A primary structure at risk for this procedure is the intermediate dorsal cutaneous nerve, which runs longitudinal through this approach (Fig. 56.9). Gentle retraction with double skin hooks helps protect the soft tissues and the superficial location of the intermediate dorsal cutaneous nerve branches while still aiding in visualization.

The EDL and EBD tendons are subsequently encountered and are carefully exposed longitudinally taking care to avoid disruption of any other soft tissue structures. The four tendon

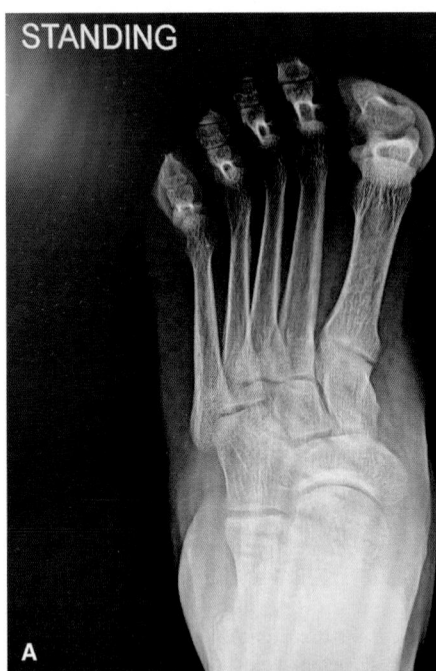

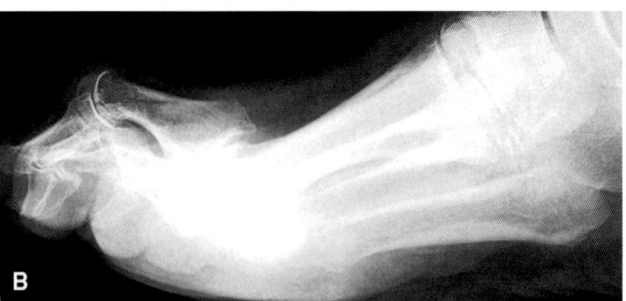

FIGURE 56.8 A. Preoperative AP radiograph demonstrate digital contractures of one to five. **B.** Preoperative lateral radiograph further demonstrates severity of digital contractures involving all five digits.

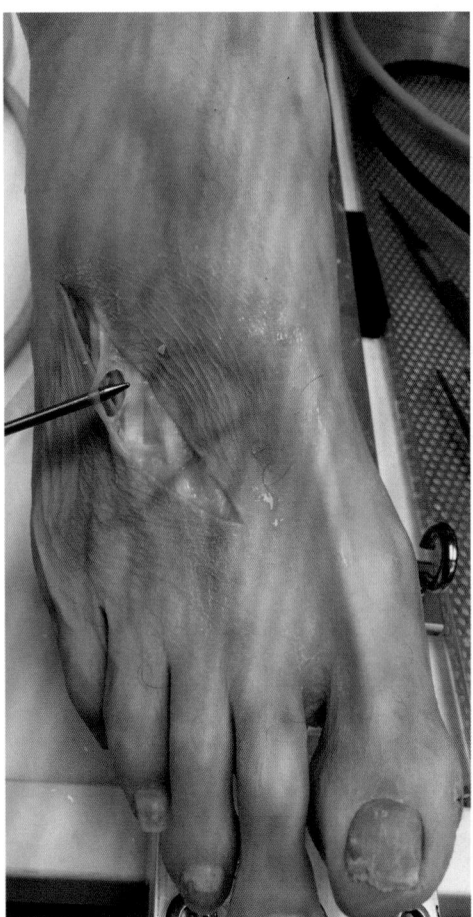

FIGURE 56.9 The incision for a Hibbs tenosuspension begins at the proximal fourth metatarsal base and extends to the second metatarsal neck obliquely. Note the superficial nature and longitudinal course of the extensors beneath the intermediate dorsal cutaneous nerve and its associated branches.

slips of the EDL are now exposed and freed from the surrounding soft tissues. All four EDL tendon slips are then transected at different levels as proximally as the incision allows within the dorsal midfoot. The surgeon may elect to lengthen the tendon slip to the fifth digit in lieu of transecting it. By transecting the EDL tendon slips at different levels, this helps minimize tendon bulk.[43]

The distal EDL will be transferred to the extensor digitorum brevis (EDB) and the proximal EDL tendon slips will be transferred into either the peroneus tertius or midfoot. DiDomenico and colleagues describe an elegant method through the use of Allis clamps and small mosquito hemostats to maintain organization of multiple tendon slips as described here[33]:

- Tag each proximal EDL tendon slip stump with a mosquito hemostat.
- The proximal EDL tendon slip stumps are then retracted proximally with ends pulled medially (second and third) and laterally (fourth and possibly fifth).
- Tag each distal EDL tendon slip stump with an Allis clamp.
- The distal EDL tendon slip stumps are then freed as distally as possible and retracted out of the way within their respective web spaces for later repair to the EDB.

Organizing the clamps in this way assists with easy identification as Allis clamps attached to the distal EDL signifies the tendon slips to be transferred to the distal EDB. The mosquito clamps to the proximal EDL signifies the tendon slips to be transferred into the peroneus tertius or midfoot.

Next, a tenolysis frees the EDB tendon slips to digits 2, 3, and 4, and these are released and transected as far distally as possible. The proximal EDB tendon slip stumps are then each tagged with an Allis clamp and retracted as proximal as possible.[33]

Additional soft tissue and/or osseous work can now be easily completed as each unique deformity dictates. This may include but is not limited to PIPJ arthrodeses; MTPJ releases, repair, or rebalancing; FDL tendon transfers; and metatarsal osteotomies.

At this point, the digits should sit in a relatively neutral alignment without residual contracture.

Attention is redirected to the distal EDL tendon stumps (tagged with Allis clamps lying in the web spaces) where tendon slips 2-4 are each tenodesed under physiologic tension to the respective proximal EDB tendon stumps 2-4 (tagged with Allis clamps lying proximally). This results in a distal longus stump to proximal brevis stump transfer proximal to the level of each MTPJ. The fifth EDL tendon is either left intact with a Z-lengthening or transected and transferred to the fourth EDB (both the fourth and fifth EDL distal tendon slips are tenodesed to the fourth digit's EDB proximal tendon).[33]

The proximal EDL tendon slips (tagged with mosquito hemostats) are then transferred into the peroneus tertius and/or midfoot (intermediate or lateral cuneiform). This decision is made through a combination of surgeon preference guided by the underlying foot deformity. As long as the transfer is secure, and the pull is relatively direct and the deforming force is reduced without too much bulk, it does not matter and is surgeon preference. One option is to tenodese the 2-4 EDL proximal tendon slips (or 2-5 EDL tendon slips) together with suture into a single confluent unit. They can then be transferred as a single unit into either the peroneus tertius or intermediate cuneiform as appropriate. To reduce bulk, EDL tendon slips 2-4 can be trimmed so they are different lengths and form a more tapered structure. Another variation is to separately transfer the lateral EDL tendons into the peroneus tertius or lateral cuneiform. Other variants are possible depending on the deformity and surgeon preference. As mentioned earlier, the EDL fifth tendon slip is either kept intact and lengthened or tenodesed to the peroneus tertius.[33,43]

If opting to transfer EDL tendon slips into the intermediate or lateral cuneiform as a single unit, this requires identification of the cuneiform and cautious dissection onto the dorsal surface. Once this is achieved, a guidewire with a tendon-passing loop is drilled from dorsal to plantar centered within the selected cuneiform as confirmed on intraoperative fluoroscopy. A bone tunnel is then drilled with a cannulated drill according to the measured size of the tendons for application of tenodesis screw fixation. The tendons as a group are then transferred from dorsal to plantar within the target cuneiform pulling the suture ends out of the bottom of the foot. The tendons are placed under tension and neutral alignment of the foot, with the ankle dorsiflexed. An interference screw is then inserted from dorsal to plantar within the selected cuneiform to fixate the tendons into bone. A common size for this interference screw is 4 × 10 mm.

This modification to the Hibbs procedure as described above serves to weaken the overall strength of the extensors, remove its deformity force on the digits, and transfer the power of the EDL proximally and laterally (Fig. 56.10A and B).

Wound closure is performed in layers per surgeon preference generally using 4-0 absorbable suture for deep subcutaneous tissue and 3-0 or 4-0 nonabsorbable suture for the skin. A cast or splint is applied while the patient is still under anesthesia on the operative table with the ankle in neutral to slightly dorsiflexed position to minimize early stress on the repair. The cast can be bivalved to accommodate for swelling.

---

positioning PEARLS

- Supine with the patients heel slightly off the end of the bed.
- Always bump the ipsilateral hip and ensure complete access to the surgical sites without difficulty.
- A thigh tourniquet is preferred to decrease tension on tendons about the ankle.

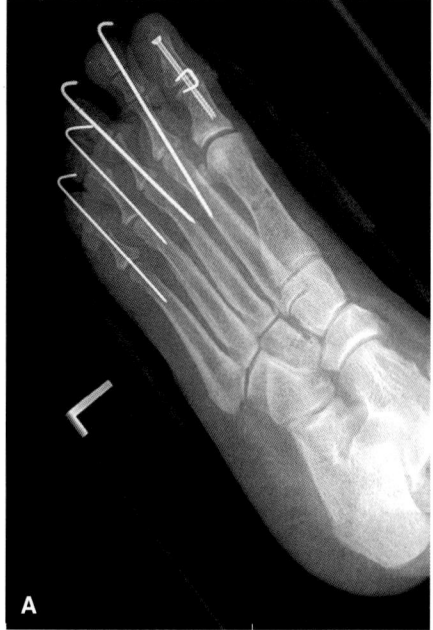
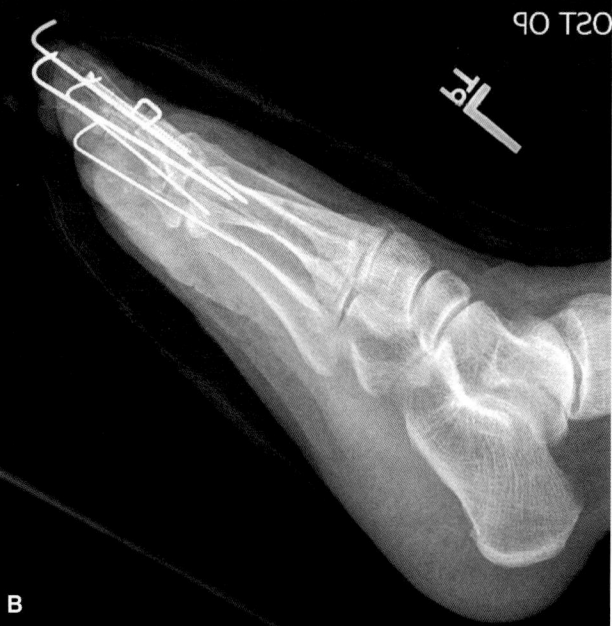

FIGURE 56.10 Postoperative appearance of the foot after Modified Hibbs, arthrodesis PIPJ 1-5, and Jones tenosuspension. **A.** AP radiograph of postoperative correction. **B.** Lateral radiograph of postoperative correction.

PEARLS

EXPOSURE AND DISSECTION

- Surgical exposure is oblique lateral dorsal midfoot starting at the fourth metatarsal base and coursing toward the second metatarsal neck.
- Care must be taken with the thin skin envelope and to avoid all neurovascular structures as they run longitudinally.
- The intermediate dorsal cutaneous nerve and associated branches are known structures at risk for this procedure.
- All four extensor tendons are transected at midmetatarsal level. Consider transecting the tendons at different lengths to minimize bulk and scarring during eventual transfer.
- The lateral tendons should be a direct line of pull to the peroneus tertius or lateral cuneiform, if not further tenolysis of the tendon sheath is needed.

SURGICAL PEARLS

- The deformity must be flexible and reducible. If a Hibbs is performed alone, the deformity must be completely reducible.
- Appropriate selection of concomitant procedures is of paramount importance in order to reduce the deformity.
- The soft tissue envelope is very thin on the dorsal foot, and gentle retraction and meticulous tendon handling and management are crucial to a proper repair.
- Careful suture and tendon management simplifies the procedure.
- Allis clamp and small mosquito hemostat is preferred for atraumatic grasping of the tendons and to maintain organization of the tendon slips.
- Harvest and prepare all tendons prior to any digital bony work or arthrodesis to preserve tension.
- Once the tendons are harvested, all digital and MTPJ work may be performed prior to final transfer.
- The foot should be in a roughly neutral and plantigrade alignment prior to tenodesing the EDL stumps to the EDB to simulate weight-bearing tension.
- All distal stumps of EDL are transferred to the EDB proximal tendons stumps at a level proximal to the MTPJ.
- When tenodesing the proximal EDL tendon slips together, 0 Vicryl is a suitable choice.
- Peroneus tertius must be of adequate bulk for the transfer. If it appears too small, be prepared to transfer into the cuneiform.
- Ensure that the ankle is in slight dorsiflexion during final tensioning of the repair.
- Care must be taken with closure to ensure no overlap and minimize scaring.

AUTHORS' PREFERRED TREATMENT

- The authors prefer the oblique incisional approach given the care needed to avoid neurovascular structures such as the superficial intermediate nerve.
- Our preference is to perform all proximal dissection and tendon harvesting first and then address the digits prior to final tensioning of the proximal tendon transfer.
- Tenodesis is performed with a tendon weave and whip stitch using 2-0 Vicryl.

- Our preference is to transfer into the cuneiform with an interference screw system.
- Layered closure preference is 4-0 running Vicryl and an overlying 3-0 nylon mattress for the skin.

PERILS and PITFALLS

- Injury to superficial nerves
- Excessive tension from retraction, which can lead to incision healing or scarring complications
- Under tensioning the tendon repair
- Not correcting digital or MTPJ deformities or addressing other deforming forces
- Transferring a weak or nonfunctional EDL
- Performing a modified Hibbs procedure in a rigid deformity

POSTOPERATIVE CARE

Anticipated postoperative care for an isolated Hibbs tenosuspension involves an initial period of NWB with immobilization for 2-4 weeks with the goal of initiating passive ROM at week 3. Progressive rehabilitation begins with ROM exercises and nonimpact activity including strengthening, proprioceptive training, and eccentric and isotonic exercises. By weeks 6-8, the patient is transitioned to a supportive sneaker. High impact activity is typically avoided until weeks 12 or later (Table 56.4).

Other procedures will dictate the postoperative course. A concomitant Jones tenosuspension and HIPJ fusion are often performed. There may be additional cavus reconstructive procedures such as calcaneal, midfoot, or first metatarsal osteotomies. The recovery will be dictated by those procedures, but early ROM is encouraged to avoid binding of the tendons. Even in cases where tendons scar and have limited excursion, the results are often favorable as the deforming force has been properly addressed (Fig. 56.11A and B).

REHABILITATION

Physical therapy is helpful and is usually initiated after week 4. Physical therapy can aid in reduction of scar tissue formation, edema control, and provides assistance with maintenance of protected weight bearing and progression without overuse or stress to the repair.

JONES TENOSUSPENSION WITH HALLUX INTERPHALANGEAL JOINT FUSION

DEFINITION

The Jones tenosuspension was first described by Sir Robert Jones in 1916[44] as the transfer of the extensor hallucis longus (EHL) from its insertion in the hallux to a drill-hole through the neck of the first metatarsal and tied onto itself. It is a tendon transfer that also functions as a tenosuspension as it is designed to support and elevate the first ray in a flexible deformity. This procedure was indicated for clawfoot with a clawed hallux or when the extensor tendons overpowered the digits with retrograde MTPJ buckling leading to deformity.[33] The description

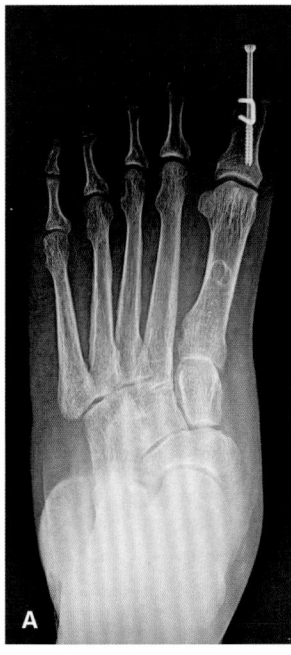
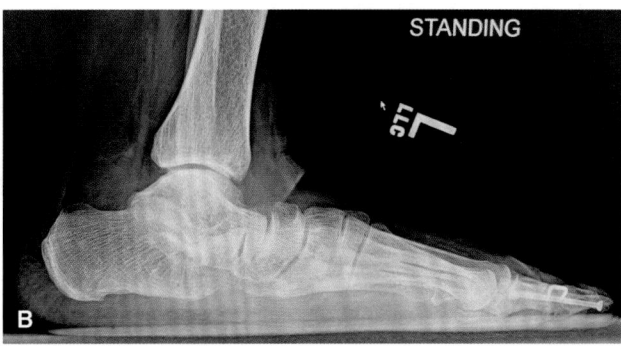

FIGURE 56.11 Final radiographic outcome at 2 years post-op following K-wire removal at 6 weeks. **A.** AP weight-bearing radiograph demonstrated maintenance of correction 2 years following a modified Hibbs, arthrodesis PIPJ 1-5, and Jones tenosuspension in a severely contracted flexible forefoot deformity. **B.** Lateral weight-bearing radiograph 2 years postoperatively showing good alignment of digits in the sagittal plane.

of clawfoot pertinent to this procedure included contracture of the plantar fascia, Achilles tendon (equinus), and hallux. The original procedure described a long central incision with wide dissection to transfer the EHL and adjunctive release of the plantar fascia.[44]

There have been many iterations of the Jones tenosuspension over the past century, but the most contemporary version is supplemented with a HIPJ arthrodesis. Other modifications could be as minor as different dissection and anchoring methods, while others applied the same concept lesser digits. This procedure is frequently combined with other adjunct procedures aimed at cavus correction.

This section describes the modified Jones tenosuspension with HIPJ arthrodesis that includes reduction of the incision and dissection with a contemporary interference anchoring technique.

INDICATIONS

A Jones tenosuspension with fusion of the HIPJ may be considered in cases where there is clawing of the hallux (concomitant hyperextension of the MTPJ and flexion of the HIPJ) creating retrograde buckling at the MTPJ or flexible plantar flexed first metatarsal (Fig. 56.12).

INDICATIONS

- Hallux malleus
- Cavus foot
- Flexible plantar flexed first ray
- HIPJ ulcerations
- Plantar first metatarsal head ulceration
- Clawfoot and clawed hallux
- Hallux varus resulting in hallux claw toe
- Prophylaxis after removal of tibial and fibular sesamoids

ANATOMIC FEATURES

Hallux malleus or claw toe is currently defined as the extension of the first MTPJ and flexion of the IPJ. The etiology is believed to be muscular imbalances among the FHL, EHL, and the PL.[45]

FUNCTIONAL ANALYSIS OF THE ANATOMY

Deformity can be driven by a variety of muscular imbalances involving the EHL, FHL, TA, and PL. This is further deformed by the FHL causing HIPJ flexion, the EHL being overpowered,

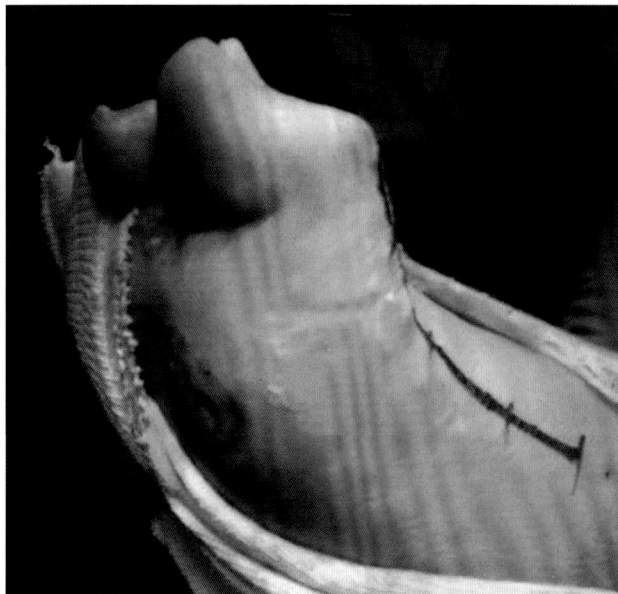

FIGURE 56.12 Preoperative photograph of hallux malleus with planned Jones tenosuspension. Notice the retrograde buckling causing an ulceration plantar to the first metatarsal head.

and the PL causing plantar flexion of the first ray leading to extension at the MTPJ.

PHYSICAL EXAMINATION

Sensate patients will exhibit pain under the first metatarsal head and extension at the MTPJ with weakness in the EHL. There may be relative weakness in the TA compared to the PL as seen with peroneal overdrive syndrome. A semireducible HIPJ flexion contracture is typically present as well. Preulcerative lesions and hyperkeratotic lesions can also be present at the plantar first metatarsal head or dorsal HIPJ. Shoe fit and difficulty with walking and activity are also common. Ensuring that the first ray is flexible and able to be reduced (Fig. 56.13) is paramount. A rigid deformity requires further osseous work, and these cases should be approached with caution and a knowledge of the limited ability to correct with soft tissue procedures alone.

Other features are seen in the cavus foot type, including tight plantar fascia, ankle equinus, hammertoes or claw toes of the lesser digits, and hindfoot cavus or varus. A neurologic evaluation and possible consultation is often recommended.

PATHOGENESIS

The most accepted theory is in the setting of a weakened TA, which results in a plantar flexed first ray due to the antagonistic overpowering of the PL. Furthermore, a weakened TA leads to recruitment of the EHL and EDL to act as ankle dorsiflexors that leads to the clawing of the hallux.[46] Although it may appear that the EHL and FHL are the obvious deforming forces, they may not be the primary etiology of the hallux claw toe.[46] Another commonly encountered example is a hallux malleus often seen in long-standing hallux varus deformity.[47] There are several other conditions and deformities that may culminate with an MTPJ contracture, but it is beyond the scope of this chapter to discuss them all. An efficient and widely accepted approach is to categorize them into either idiopathic or neurologic etiology,

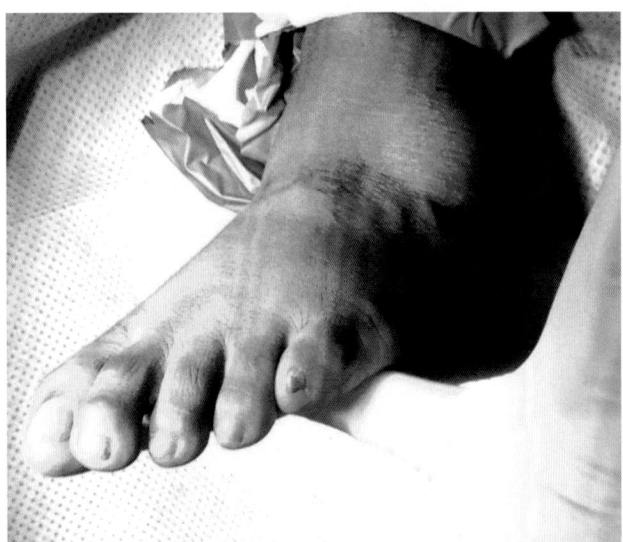

FIGURE 56.13 Kelikian push-up test showing reducibility of the MTPJ.

with a subdivision of upper and lower motor neuron disorders. The most common lower motor neurologic causes that are also associated with cavus foot type are CMT, Poliomyelitis, Roussy-Levy syndrome, and Friedrich ataxia. These medical conditions often are associated with foot and ankle deformities including hallux malleus where a Jones tenosuspension may be considered.[48] This is an important consideration as a progressive muscle imbalance may lead to recurrence. Specifically, in CMT disease, the long extensors progressively weaken.[49] Similar to the challenges with a Hibbs in CMT, the transfer could eventually become ineffective as the EHL weakens. This would allow the flexors to overpower the remaining EHB at the level of the MTPJ. The resultant flexion deformity could cause chronic tripping or stubbing injuries to the hallux. Therefore, osseous procedures are often preferred over tendon rebalancing procedures to dorsiflex the first ray in cases of CMT.

IMAGING AND DIAGNOSTIC STUDIES

Plain film weight-bearing radiographs consisting of foot AP, medial oblique, and lateral and weight-bearing sesamoid axial can help assess for arthritic changes within the joint (Fig. 56.14A and B). Neurologic workup with EMG/NCV to assess muscle function can also be helpful in some cases.

TREATMENT

NONOPERATIVE

Nonoperative treatment options include off-loading the first metatarsal head/hallux IPJ, orthotics, padding, shoe modifications, and physical therapy.

SURGICAL PROCEDURE AND TECHNIQUES: STEP-BY-STEP

The procedure consists of harvesting the EHL tendon and transferring it to the first metatarsal by a variety of means. Classically, this was described as side-to-side drill tunnel with tying of the tendon over itself.[44] The authors' preferred technique is a dorsal-to-plantar interference screw to anchor the EHL to the first metatarsal.

Various approaches and incisional techniques have been presented in the literature. We use a two-incision minimally invasive approach in order to avoid excessive dissection. The first incision is a semielliptical transverse incision centered over the HIPJ with which the surgeon can excise an ulcer, callus, or lesion and dorsiflex at the HIPJ with removal of the skin wedge. The second incision is made longitudinally over the first metatarsal neck and head.

Within the first incision (transverse HIPJ), dissection is carried down to the EHL tendon that is harvested as distal as possible. A complete release of the extensor hood and freeing the tendon as proximal as possible is carried out bluntly along the tendon sheath. A whip stitch with 2-0 or larger suture is performed in the tendon, and an Allis clamp can be used to grasp the tendon (Fig. 56.15).

The second incision is approximately a 2- to 3-cm longitudinal incision, parallel to the EHL and centered dorsally over the planned transfer site within the first metatarsal. The tendon is then passed to this incision and delivered out of the incision for

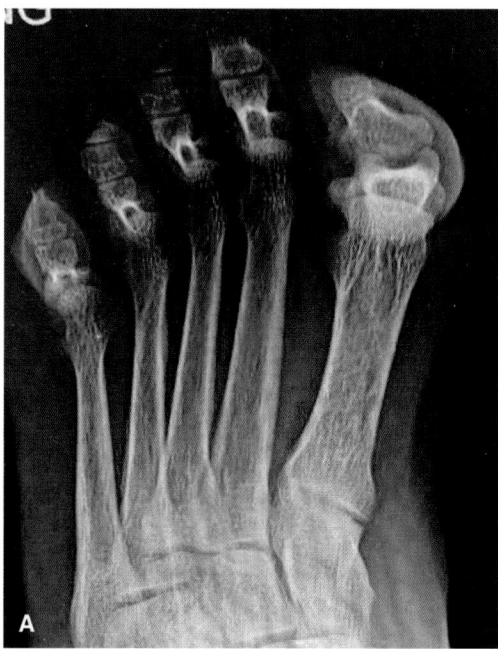

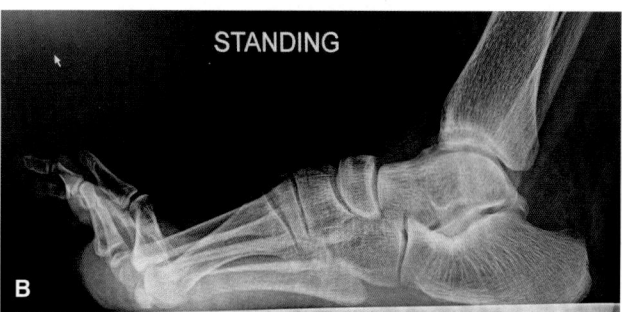

FIGURE 56.14 A. Preoperative AP radiograph with severely contracted hallux. **B.** Preoperative lateral radiograph with plantar flexed first ray and hallux contracture.

transfer. A periosteal elevator is used to make a subperiosteal dissection centrally at the first metatarsal for a dorsal-to-plantar drill hole.

The hallux IPJ joint is then prepared for arthrodesis. Utilizing a sagittal saw, a transverse osteotomy is performed to remove the necessary portion of the proximal phalanx head. The base of the distal phalanx is then prepped with a rongeur or curette until all cartilage is denuded. After thorough irrigation, the adjacent surfaces are fish-scaled with a small osteotome and then drilled with a small drill to fenestrate both sides of the joint. The fusion is then fixated by surgeon choice. For fixation, we prefer a single-headed central screw introduced through a third percutaneous incision at the distal tip of the hallux, with the screw passed from distal to proximal. We will frequently supplement this with an additional dorsal compression staple

typically sized 8 × 8 or 10 × 10 to counteract any rotational stress (Fig. 56.16).

Once the HIPJ fusion has been completed, the EHL is transferred into the first metatarsal utilizing manufacturer guidelines for the interference screw of choice. This generally includes sizing the tendon for drilling and selecting the appropriately sized interference screw (Fig. 56.17). An appropriate sized drill hole is then made centrally within the first metatarsal (Fig. 56.18). The typical interference screw size is ~4 × 10 mm. After drilling, the whip-stitched tendon is passed from dorsal to

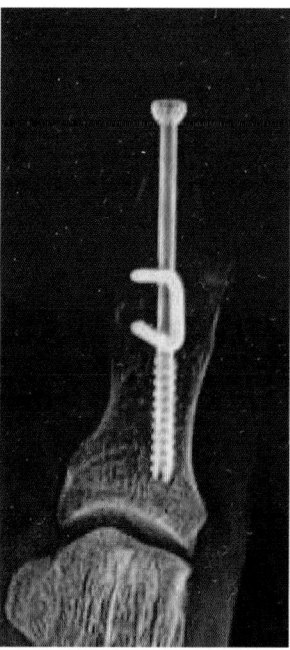

FIGURE 56.16 AP radiograph showing HIPJ fixation utilizing a single headed screw from distal to proximal and dorsal compression staple to counteract rotational force.

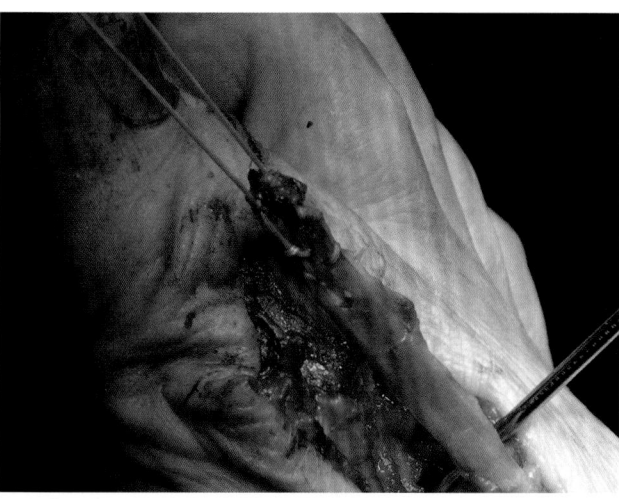

FIGURE 56.15 The EHL tendon is whip stitched in order to prepare for the transfer.

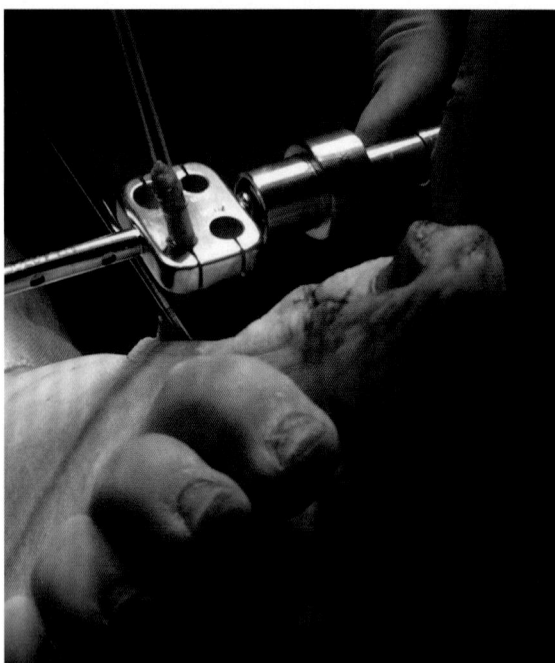

FIGURE 56.17 The EHL whip-stitched tendon is measured to determine the appropriate size drill tunnel and interference screw needed.

plantar through the drill hole, and the suture tail is pulled out through the plantar aspect of the foot. The transferred EHL is tensioned with the foot and ankle in neutral to slightly dorsiflexed position to allow for proper repair. Of note, we do recommend overtensioning as the tendon transfer will stretch out over time. The interference screw is then inserted from dorsal to plantar within the drill hole alongside the transferred EHL tendon.

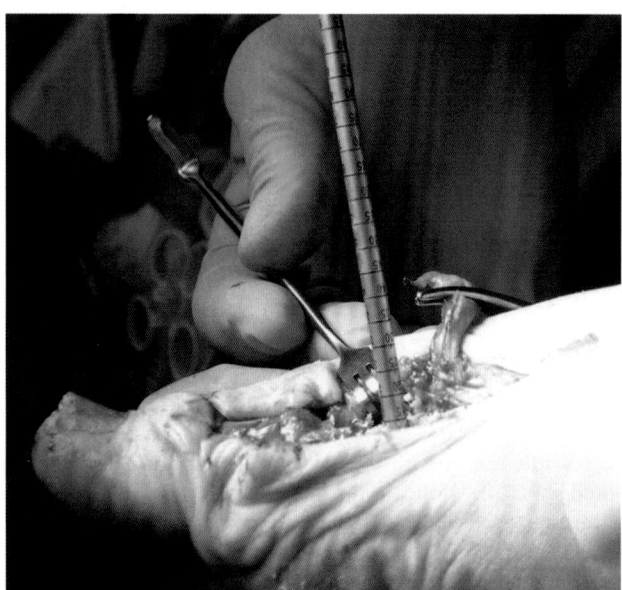

FIGURE 56.18 A drill tunnel is then created centrally within the first metatarsal from dorsal to plantar.

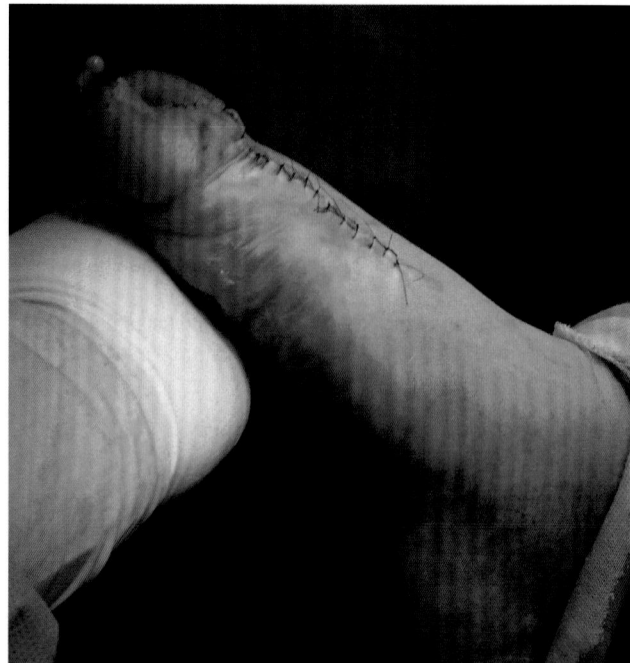

FIGURE 56.19 Evaluation of final correction after a Jones tenosuspension with HIPJ fusion was confirmed by loading the foot intraoperatively and visualizing the reduction of hallux contracture. Note that this patient pre-dates the authors' switch to a two incisional approach. A separate transverse semielliptical skin plasty centered over the HIPJ would have provided additional correction without excess tissue dorsally.

Strength of the repair is checked, and incisions are irrigated. Final postoperative appearance should have minimal residual deformity and should be checked for any contracture or malalignment that may need to be addressed (Fig. 56.19). Closure per surgeon preference is in layers. Typically, patients are placed into a neutral non–weight-bearing cast on the operative table and can be bivalved for swelling as needed.

positioning PEARLS
- Supine with a bump under the ipsilateral hip.
- Ensure that fluoroscopy is available and positioned on the operative side for ease of use.

PEARLS
EXPOSURE
- Two-incision approach preferred
  - Incision #1: elliptical transverse skin wedge excised at dorsal HIPJ; allows for excision of ulcer or lesion if needed and aids in IPJ correction.
  - Release EHL at distal incision, use an Allis clamp to grasp and a Kelly clamp to release all adhered structures from distal to proximal into the incision over the first metatarsal neck.
  - Incision #2: dorsal first metatarsal along EHL roughly 2-3 cm long centered over planned transfer site.
  - Dissect down to bone and use a Freer to expose the metatarsal.

AUTHORS' PREFERRED TREATMENT

We prefer to transfer with an interference screw to the first metatarsal neck via two incisions as described above along with a HIPJ fusion.

PERILS and PITFALLS
- Avoid larger than needed interference screw.
- Drill centrally in first metatarsal to avoid a stress riser.
- Stable fixation for HIPJ fusion.
- Avoid overzealous handling of EHL to prevent damage.
- Consider first MTPJ fusion instead if there is an arthritic or pathologic joint.
- Not protecting the tendon transfer long enough postoperatively.

POSTOPERATIVE CARE

Anticipated postoperative care for an isolated Jones tenosuspension involves an initial period of NWB with immobilization for 2-4 weeks with the goal of initiating passive ROM at week 3. Progressive rehabilitation begins with ROM exercises and nonimpact activity including strengthening, proprioceptive training, and eccentric and isotonic exercises. By weeks 6-8, the patient is transitioned to a supportive sneaker. High impact activity is typically avoided until weeks 12 or later (Table 56.4). Other procedures such as calcaneal or midfoot osteotomies, patient comorbidities, and bone stock may take precedent in recovery course.

REHABILITATION

Physical therapy is helpful and is usually initiated after week 4. Physical therapy can aid in reduction of scar tissue formation, edema control, and provides assistance with maintenance of protected weight bearing and progression without overuse or stress to the repair.

FHL TENDON TRANSFER WITH V-Y ADVANCEMENT FOR CHRONIC ACHILLES TENDON RUPTURES

DEFINITION

A chronic or neglected Achilles rupture occurs when rupture of the Achilles tendon is missed or delayed, when nonoperative

treatment of acute ruptures yields suboptimal results, or if there is a rerupture of the Achilles tendon. In general, if an Achilles rupture is not appropriately treated within 8 weeks, it is usually considered a chronic or neglected Achilles tendon rupture.

Depending on the severity of the chronic Achilles rupture, the repair may require excision of the diseased segment of the tendon along with lengthening of the tendon to achieve an end-to-end repair. Further supplementation with a tendon transfer may also be considered. This section describes the repair of a chronic Achilles tendon rupture requiring a V-Y advancement coupled with an FHL tendon transfer.

INDICATIONS

INDICATIONS
- To reestablish ankle joint plantar flexion
- Chronic Achilles tendinosis involving >50% of the tendon (midsubstance or insertional)
- Achilles rupture with >3 cm gap

ANATOMIC FEATURES

The entire gastrocnemius-soleus-Achilles is also called the triceps surae complex and crosses the knee, ankle, and subtalar joints (STJs). The gastrocnemius muscle originates from the distal femoral condyles above the knee. It has a medial and lateral muscle belly that crosses the knee joint to join the soleus muscle. The gastrocnemius and soleus combine to form the Achilles tendon, which inserts broadly into the posterosuperior calcaneal tuberosity.

The Achilles tendon is loosely covered by paratenon. The vascularity of the Achilles tendon is from the paratenon, the proximal muscle belly, and calcaneal insertion, which leaves a watershed area within the tendon of poor vascularity. The watershed area occurs in a zone that occurs ~2-6 cm proximal from the insertion into the calcaneus.[50]

FUNCTIONAL ANALYSIS OF THE ANATOMY

The Achilles tendon is the strongest and largest tendon in the body. Its primary function is ankle joint plantar flexion. The rupture most commonly occurs within the watershed region of the Achilles tendon. The proximal gastrocnemius-soleus complex retracts proximally with resultant diastasis between the ruptured tendon ends. A pseudotendon of nonfunctional scar tissue often forms within the tendon gap over time.

There are many tendons, including the PL, PB, and FDL, which are candidates for augmenting a weakened triceps surae but less ideal because they only provide mechanical support. As noted above, a significant portion of Achilles pathology occurs within the relatively dysvascular watershed area of the tendon. An FHL transfer can provide both functional support and vascular augmentation due to its relatively low lying muscle belly. Unlike many other examples given in this chapter, the FHL transfer functions partially as a musculotendinous flap that is utilized to strengthen plantar flexion but also treat a region of hypoperfusion.[29,50-53]

PHYSICAL EXAMINATION

HISTORY

If the patient can recall the details surrounding an Achilles rupture event, it is often described as being hit on the back of the heel or leg. More commonly, the inciting event is reported as being benign with some transient pain that quickly resolves. They may have been diagnosed or self-diagnosed with an ankle sprain and have had chronic weakness since the injury. The patient may relate difficulty in walking or balance. Inclines, stairs, and ladders are often difficult. They may not have pain given the chronicity of the problem.

It is also possible that the Achilles pathology was not traumatic in nature but rather a chronic progressive degeneration from a hindfoot varus, equinus, Haglund deformity, retrocalcaneal bursitis, age, weight, or comorbidity related or a combination of these factors. In these cases, the pain usually progressively worsens as the tendon slowly degenerates.

EXAMINATION

If there is a palpable gap at the chronic Achilles rupture site, then the diagnosis is more easily determined. The ability to detect the gap may be diminished by excessive edema, particularly in obese patients, or if pseudotendon or scar tissue has formed. The Thompson test will either be positive or more commonly exhibit less plantar flexion than the contralateral side. There may be less plantar flexion at rest, which is best seen with the patient in the prone position (Fig. 56.20).

With muscle strength testing, there is often plantar flexion weakness at the ankle joint. But there is often some plantar flexion strength due to residual function of the posterior tibialis tendon, FHL, FDL, and peroneals and plantaris. Ambulation is still possible, but patients are typically unable to perform a single leg heel rise or walk on their toes (Fig. 56.21).

With ROM testing, there is increased ankle joint dorsiflexion when compared to the contralateral side (Fig. 56.22). In more severe cases, the patient may present with a calcaneal gait

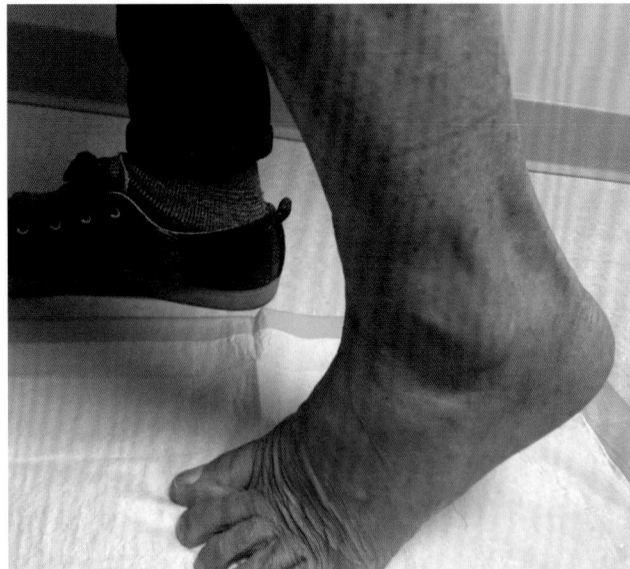

FIGURE 56.21 Subtle chronic gastrocnemius-soleus tear within the muscle belly resulting in the patient unable to heel rise without assistance from the contralateral leg.

and fat pad atrophy, which can even lead to skin breakdown and wounds (Fig. 56.23).

PATHOGENESIS

Achilles ruptures can occur from forceful dorsiflexion of the ankle and are most commonly associated with sporting activities. Achilles ruptures are most commonly seen in males, 30-40 years old. Spontaneous silent ruptures are also possible, particularly in the setting of steroid use or systemic inflammatory diseases.

Chronic breakdown of the Achilles can occur from repeated mechanical stress, which leads to degeneration and scarring. With aging, the capacity to heal is diminished, and in the setting of repetitive injury, eventually the tendon becomes dysvascular and hypertrophic.[52-57]

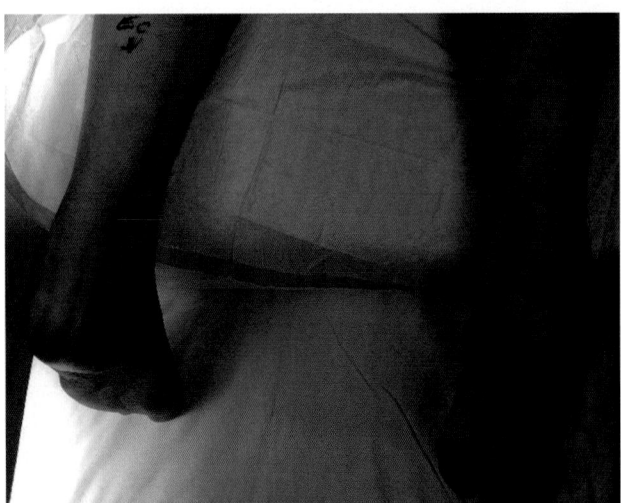

FIGURE 56.20 This patient had less plantar flexion at rest on the left side supporting a chronic Achilles rupture.

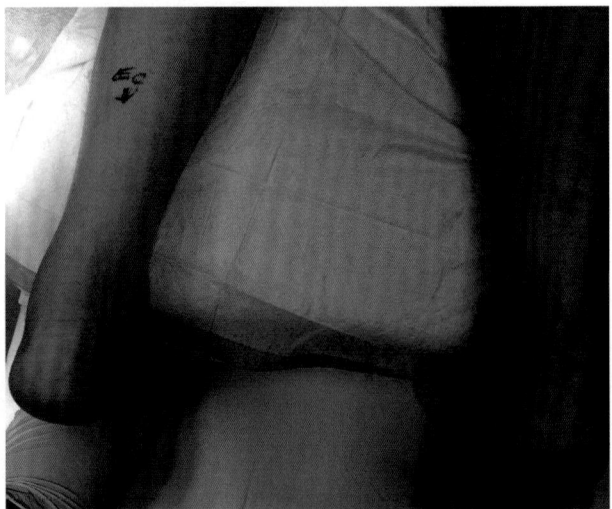

FIGURE 56.22 The left side has significantly more dorsiflexion than the right consistent with a chronic Achilles rupture.

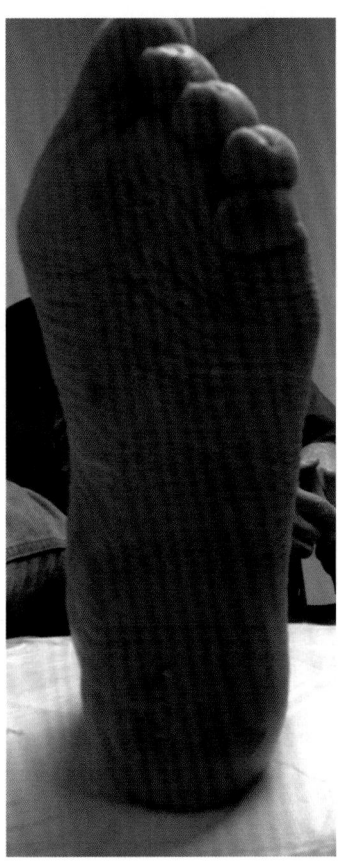

FIGURE 56.23 This patient has severe fat pad atrophy and preulcerations secondary to a calcaneal gait from a chronic Achilles tendon rupture.

IMAGING AND DIAGNOSTIC STUDIES

Frequently a chronic or neglected Achilles tendon rupture can be diagnosed clinically. Radiographs may be obtained to rule out an avulsion fracture. An MRI or ultrasound may be performed if the diagnosis is unclear, to assess the gap, to assess for other pathology, and to confirm the integrity of tendon transfer candidates. An MRI will provide more information than an ultrasound and allows quantification of the gap, which can help guide the recommended treatments and prognosis. If there is a large gap, an allograft may need to be secured in advance for the planned surgical date (Fig. 56.24A and B).

TREATMENT

NONOPERATIVE

If the patient is not a surgical candidate, permanent bracing is an option. Either a custom molded locked or spring-loaded AFO will provide the most support. Other supportive care may include heel lifts, activity modification, physical therapy, and nonsteroidal anti-inflammatory drugs. Patients who are more active do not tolerate permanent bracing or basic supportive care well.

GASTROCNEMIUS SOLEUS V-TO-Y LENGTHENING

An inverted V is made completely within the aponeurosis or myotendinous zone (apex proximal with medial and lateral arms exiting the distal medial and lateral borders). The arms should be at least two times the length of the true gap in order to achieve enough length. Using a #15 or #10 blade, the V is made only within the aponeurosis or tendinous portion, leaving the underlying muscle belly intact (Fig. 56.28).

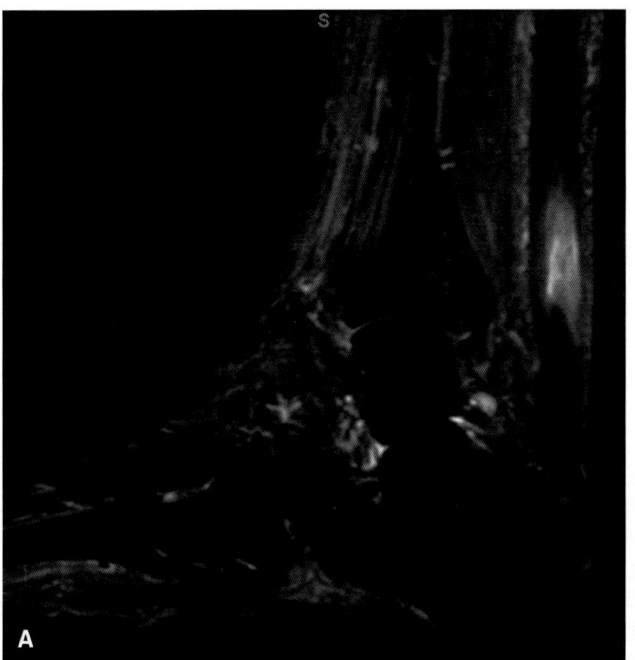

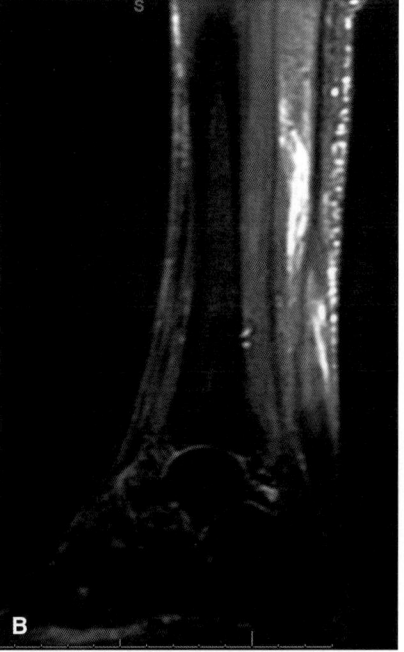

FIGURE 56.24 **A.** MRI demonstrating chronic Achilles rupture within the watershed region with formation of pseudotendon and scar tissue. **B.** MRI can be helpful to assess severity as in this case where there was chronic tendinosis and thickening extending into the gastrocnemius-soleus region.

positioning PEARLS

- A thigh tourniquet is necessary as a calf tourniquet will prevent mobilization of the gastrocnemius soleus muscle.
- A prone position is necessary.
- It is easier to apply the thigh tourniquet while the patient is still in the supine position.
- Ensure the tourniquet connection and tubing lies laterally or posterolateral.
- Either general or spinal anesthesia is necessary.
- If using general anesthesia, have chest rolls ready and positioned before flipping patient prone.
- Prepare padding for the brachial plexus and ulnar nerves at the elbow; protect the genitalia.
- Prepping and draping both limbs to above the knee allows comparison of the tension between the repaired side to the uninjured contralateral side.
- Haystack the sheets to allow the ankles to hang off the end (Fig. 56.25).
- When covering the toes with sterile adhesive, keep the hallux separately wrapped from the lesser toes to aid in confirming the FHL harvest later in the case.

PEARLS

- The incision is centered midline over the pathologic Achilles tendon.
- Distally, the incision placement should curve medially to avoid injury to the sural nerve, which lies ~5 mm lateral to the Achilles; this also avoids a painful posterior heel scar from shoe irritation and improves access to the FHL (Fig. 56.26A and B).
- The proximal incision can be midline with the overall length determined by potential concomitant procedures such as a V-to-Y lengthening, turndown, or allograft replacement of the Achilles (Fig. 56.26B).
- If the proximal incision must be extended up to or proximal to the myotendinous junction, the sural nerve must be identified and protected; remember that the sural nerve crosses from lateral to central at the myotendinous junction and then dives beneath the medial head of the gastrocnemius muscle belly.
- The lesser saphenous vein runs with the sural nerve, which can help in identifying the nerve more proximally.
- Distal exposure should be full thickness to the level of paratenon; avoid any unnecessary dissection.
- Paratenon: incise longitudinally and tag to allow maximum repair at the end of the case.
- Paratenon: it is common that there is inadequate paratenon over the ruptured site but preserve as much as possible to optimize the vascularity of the repair (Fig. 56.27).

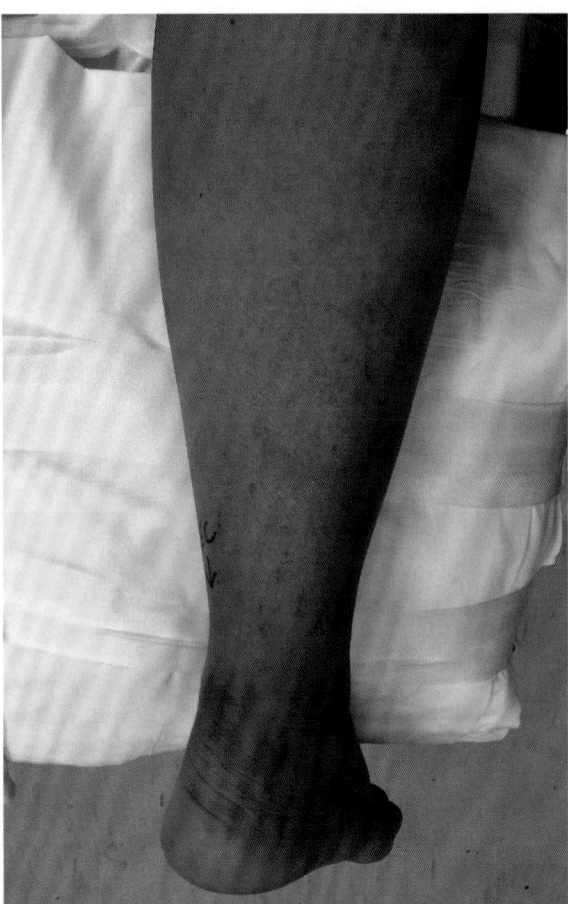

FIGURE 56.25 Patient positioning for repair of a chronic Achilles tendon rupture with FHL transfer includes placing the patient in the prone position, thigh tourniquet, and hay stacking sheets to allow both ankles to hang off of the end of the table.

Correct Measurement of the Achilles Gap

- Expose the ruptured Achilles. In chronic cases, there is usually a nonviable pseudotendon present within the ruptured area. Sharply resect this along with the nonviable ends of the Achilles tendon.
- Measure the true tendon gap after resecting the nonviable portions. In order to match the contralateral Achilles resting tension, ensure that both extremities have ~30 degrees of knee flexion and ~20 degrees of ankle joint plantar flexion.
- <1 cm gap: typically end-to-end repair is possible.
- 1-3 cm gap: often end-to-end repair is possible after placing longitudinal traction of the Achilles tendon for 5-10 minutes.
- 3-8 cm gap: often V-to-Y lengthening with FHL tendon transfer to augment the repair is possible (depends on length of aponeurosis) and is described below.
- >8 cm gap: consider an Achilles turndown (depends on length of remaining tendinous tissue) or allograft.[58,59]

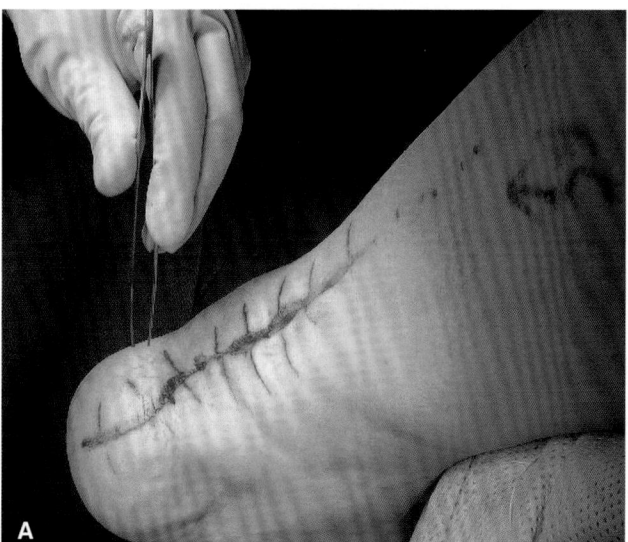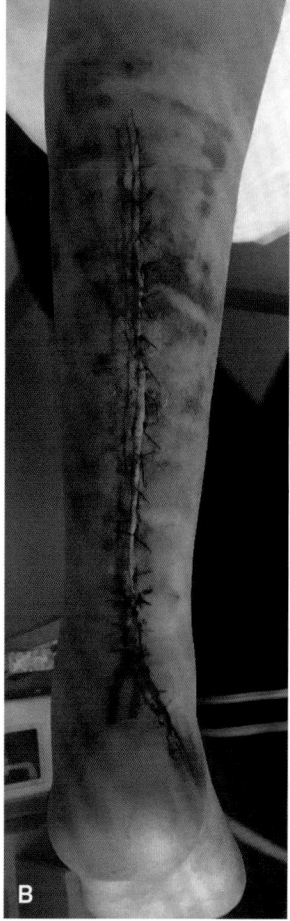

FIGURE 56.26 The incision may vary depending on the underlying pathology. **A,B.** The primary pathology here is insertional Achilles pathology with a Haglund deformity, which was very inferior on the calcaneus. Achilles tendon repair with FHL tendon transfer was performed with an incision midline to the Achilles proximally but curved slightly medial and ended at the inferior calcaneus. The primary pathology here is chronic midsubstance Achilles rupture with a 7-cm gap. Achilles tendon repair with FHL tendon transfer was performed with an incision midline to the Achilles proximally but curved medially to aid in the FHL transfer. Given the more proximal pathology, the incision did not need to be extended as distal. The proximal incision was extended superiorly to allow for a V-Y Achilles lengthening due to the large gap.

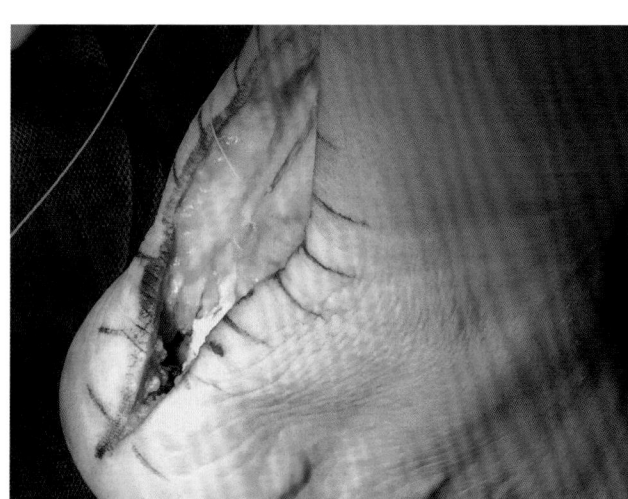

FIGURE 56.27 The paratenon is preserved and sutured over the final Achilles repair to optimize vascularity.

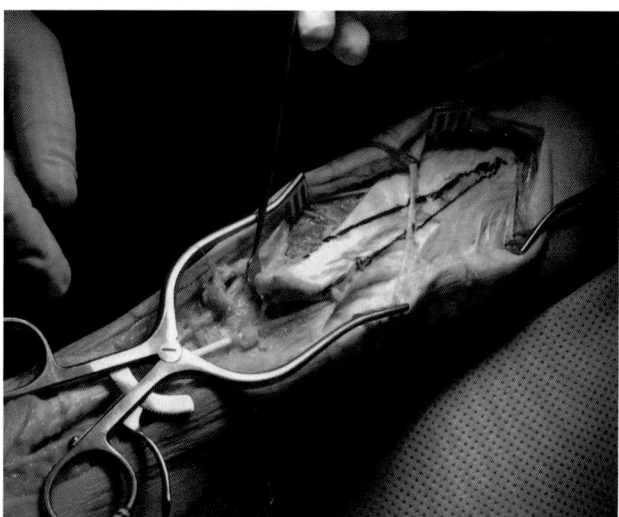

FIGURE 56.28 A gastrocnemius soleus V-Y lengthening was required due to a 7-cm gap. The arms of the V should be at least two times the length of the true gap. The base of the V is advanced distally to allow for an end-to-end repair of the Achilles.

The base of the V is advanced distally until enough length is achieved to perform an end-to-end repair of the Achilles gap. Advance the base by utilizing strong nonabsorbable suture on each end of the Achilles tendon in preparation for the end-to-end repair (surgeon's choice on suture type, size, and suturing technique; our technique is described under the section "Authors' Preferred Treatment").

Apply strong continuous traction to the tendon using a weight if needed. Release small portions of the tendon from the muscle along the V incision while continuously applying firm traction to the tendon end. Continue releasing additional portions of the tendon from the muscle, but ensure that there is always some muscle belly still attached to the tendon. The muscle fibers will slide and stretch over time. Rather than release too much tendon, it is better to take additional time allowing the muscle fibers to stretch. Continue this process until the gap is closed with the two tendon ends reapproximated under similar resting tension and position to the contralateral side.

The inverted V has now been converted to a Y with the long arm of the Y the same length of the closed gap. The newly converted Y is repaired after completing the FHL tendon transfer.

FHL TENDON HARVEST (ONE-INCISION APPROACH)

The FHL lies immediately deep to the posterior compartment fascia deep to the Achilles tendon. Begin the dissection along the medial border of the Achilles tendon and reflect the Achilles laterally if still intact or reflect the ends inferiorly and superiorly if not intact. Alternatively, a split Achilles tendon approach may be utilized during a Haglund resection with Achilles tendon repair and also allows access for an FHL tendon transfer[56] (Fig. 56.29). Cautiously penetrate only the posterior

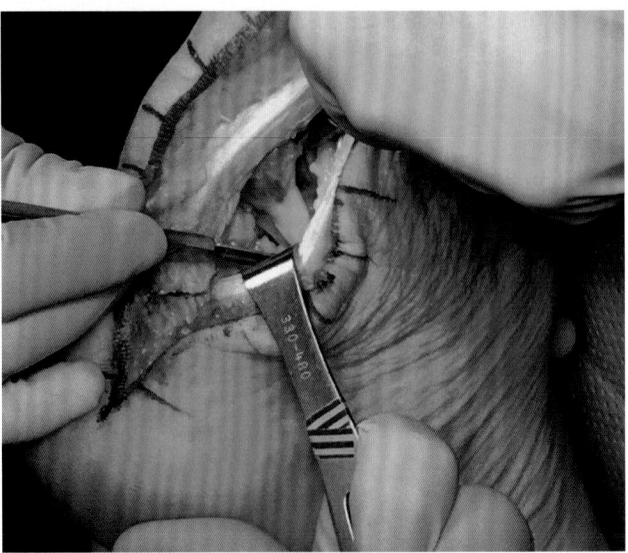

FIGURE 56.30 If utilizing an interference screw for the FHL transfer, sufficient tendon length can be obtained by bluntly dissecting while plantar flexing and inverting the foot.

compartment fascia with a longitudinal incision as the posterior tibial artery and tibial nerve are just medial to the FHL tendon. Once through the posterior compartment fascia, the FHL muscle is readily identified without much additional dissection as it often extends to the level of the ankle joint. Exposure of the FHL muscle and tendon can be achieved with careful, blunt dissection. Dissect along the lateral aspect of the FHL to avoid the neurovascular bundle medially and release the FHL tendon sheath once posterior to the medial malleolus. The FHL tendon can now be further mobilized away from the neurovascular bundle. To obtain as much tendon length as possible, plantar flex the hallux and ankle while simultaneously applying proximal traction to the FHL tendon (Fig. 56.30). Cautiously transect the FHL tendon staying away from the neurovascular bundle immediately adjacent to the FHL. Typically, when combined with an interference screw for the transfer fixation, there is adequate tendon length through this single-incision approach.[60]

FHL TENDON HARVEST (ALTERNATIVE TWO-INCISION APPROACH)

If using other forms of fixation, greater length of the FHL tendon will be required. This necessitates a separate incision along the medial foot to expose the FHL tendon at the master knot of Henry. This separate incision is made from the inferior portion of the talonavicular (TN) joint to the medial first metatarsal shaft. There is often an extensive venous plexus within the Knot of Henry region that can lead to hematoma, prolonged swelling, and pain as well as additional scar tissue, surgical time, and dissection. Identify the abductor hallucis and flexor hallucis brevis and retract dorsally. The FHL and FDL along with the master knot of Henry are beneath and can be identified by visualizing tendon excursion when separately flexing and extending the hallux (FHL) and lesser toes (FDL). Resect the appropriate length of FHL tendon being cautious of the venous plexus and medial plantar nerve. The remaining distal stump of the FHL may be tenodesed to the FDL if desired, but given the multiple connections that exist between

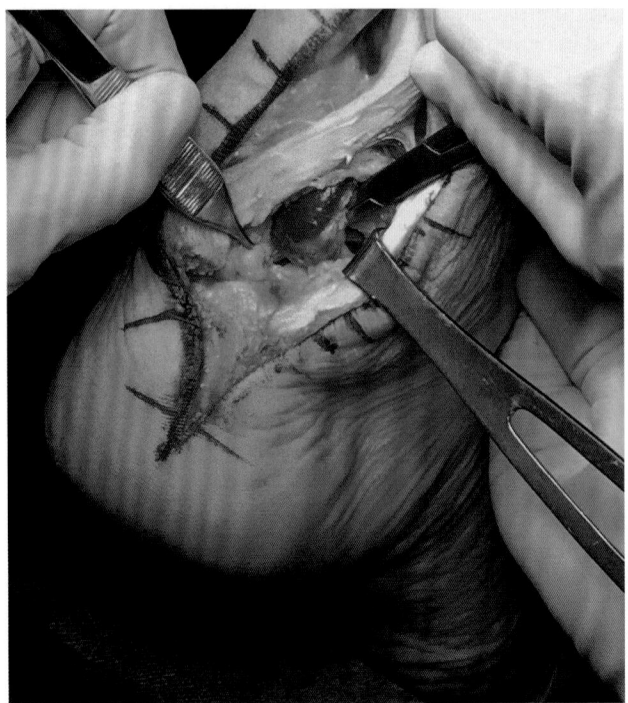

FIGURE 56.29 The FHL muscle belly lies immediately deep to the posterior compartment fascia, which is accessed in this example via a split Achilles tendon approach for a concomitant Haglund resection.

the FHL and FDL in the setting of the venous plexus and adjacent medial plantar nerve, one can usually avoid performing this tenodesis.

FHL TENDON HARVEST (ONE-INCISION APPROACH CONTINUED)

Once adequate tendon length has been obtained, whip stitch the distal stump of the FHL tendon (Fig. 56.31). Measure the FHL tendon diameter to determine the appropriate-sized interference screw (Fig. 56.32) and then follow manufacturer guidelines for preparing the drill tunnel prior to securing the FHL tendon into the calcaneus. Regardless of the specific implant, the transfer site should be oriented such that the guidewire for the drill is in line with the pull of the Achilles tendon (Fig. 56.33). This tunnel should be placed just anterior to the Achilles tendon insertion (Fig. 56.34). A through and through drill tunnel technique allows one to pull the suture attached to the FHL through the plantar heel, which makes proper tensioning of the FHL easier (Fig. 56.35). To determine the ideal FHL tension, ensure that both ankles are ~20 degrees plantar flexed and use the resting tension of the contralateral ankle as a guide. The interference screw is inserted while maintaining the FHL under the desired tension (Fig. 56.36A and B). After fixating the FHL into the calcaneus, test the strength of the interference screw by pulling on the FHL.

Achilles Tendon Repair

- When performing the end-to-end repair, match the contralateral resting tension with the knee extended and foot plantar flexed ~20 degrees to avoid making the repair too loose.
- Reapproximate the ends by placing traction on the sutures (Fig. 56.37A and B).
- Hand tie the opposite side with intratendinous knots.
- Confirm there is similar tension to the contralateral limb. Then, hand tie the other side of the repair with intratendinous knots.
- Test the strength of the repair by gently dorsiflexing the foot to ensure that there is no gapping at the repair site and that the FHL fixation remains seated within the calcaneus.
- After completing the Achilles tendon repair, the FHL muscle belly can be sutured to the anterior Achilles using absorbable suture to increase the vascularity of the diseased Achilles tendon.
- The tagged paratenon is then reapproximated with absorbable suture over the repaired area as best as possible.
- The wound is closed in layers.
- A strong and padded below-knee posterior splint is applied with the ankle held in neutral to a slight plantar flexed position.

ACHILLES TENDON REPAIR

The last part of the case is directed to repairing the Achilles tendon. When performing the end-to-end repair, match the contralateral resting tension with the knee extended and foot plantar flexed ~20 degrees to avoid making the repair too loose. Reapproximate the ends by placing traction on the sutures

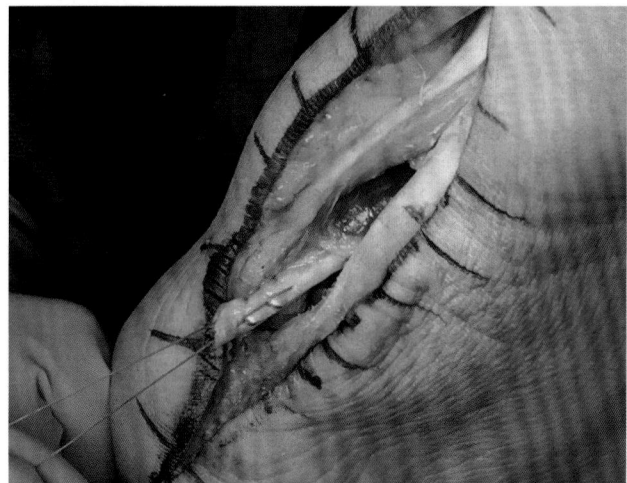

FIGURE 56.31 The FHL tendon is whip stitched with a nonabsorbable 2-0 suture using a modified Krakow technique. Avoid inadvertently compromising the suture by selecting suture that is easily visible in the event the tendon stump requires debulking during the transfer.

(Fig. 56.37A and B). The goal is that there should be similar tension such that both feet should have equivalent position.

Prior to closure, test the strength of the repair by gently dorsiflexing the foot to ensure that there is no gapping at the repair site and that the FHL fixation remains seated within the calcaneus. After completing the Achilles tendon repair, the FHL muscle belly can be sutured to the anterior Achilles using absorbable suture to increase the vascularity of the diseased Achilles tendon. The tagged paratenon is then reapproximated with absorbable suture over the tendon repair with as little suture as possible. Close the incision in layers.

A strong and padded below-knee posterior splint is applied while the patient is still on the operative table with the ankle held in neutral to a slight plantar flexed position.

AUTHORS' PREFERRED TREATMENT

- We prefer an end-to-end anastomosis for a neglected Achilles rupture when possible. But direct repair is usually not possible. A V-Y lengthening of the Achilles with

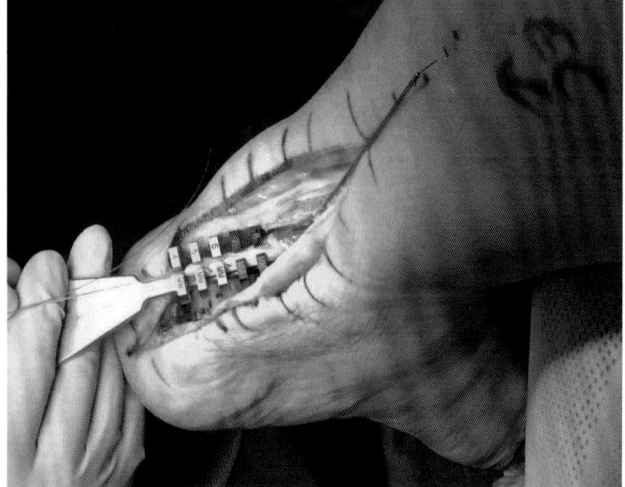

FIGURE 56.32 The whip-stitched FHL tendon is usually either a size 4 or 5 mm.

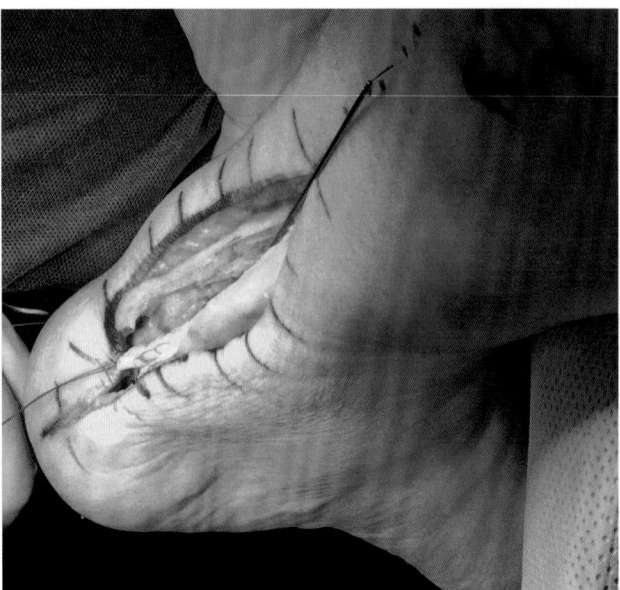

FIGURE 56.33 A guidewire with an attached tendon passer is oriented in line with the pull of the Achilles tendon.

FHL tendon transfer is usually necessary. Sometimes, an FHL tendon transfer will also be included with an end-to-end repair if additional strength is needed.

- Do not perform an FHL tendon transfer in isolation as it will have insufficient strength
- We avoid an Achilles turndown when at all possible to avoid excessive bulk. Patients often find the bulkiness at the turndown level uncomfortable. Allograft is also avoided when possible. Although rare, tissue rejection and/or infection of the allograft has devastating consequences.
- We recommend placing weighted traction on the gastrocnemius-soleus as soon as the pseudotendon is excised. This will allow the muscle to start stretching while performing

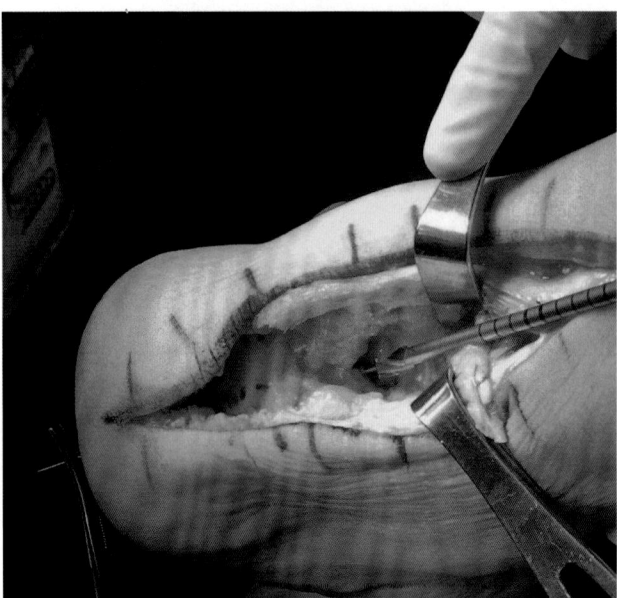

FIGURE 56.34 The drill tunnel starts just anterior to the Achilles tendon insertion and exits inferiorly.

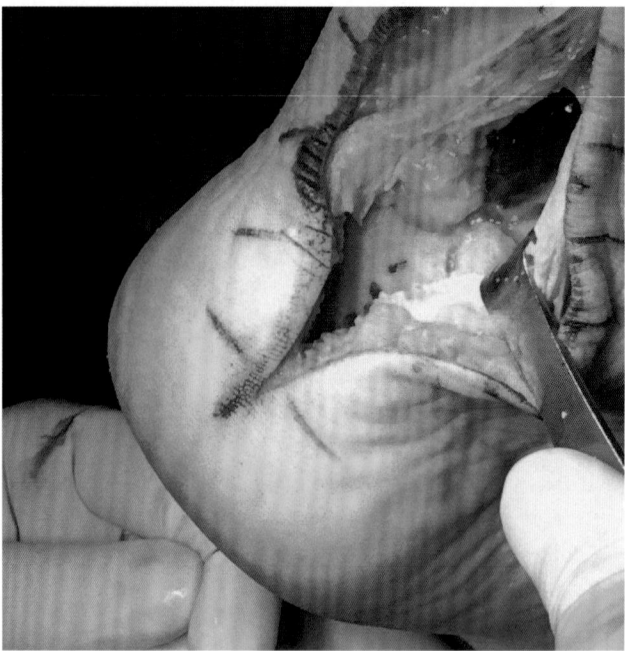

FIGURE 56.35 The FHL tendon is pulled into the tunnel with the suture exiting through the plantar heel. This allows for precise tensioning of the FHL tendon transfer.

the FHL tendon transfer and V-Y lengthening. We use a locking Krakow stitch within the remaining tendon end as described below. The suture ends can then be attached to a weight while performing additional procedure steps.

- By fixating the FHL tendon transfer with an interference anchor, less tendon is required allowing the procedure to be performed through a single incision that ends at the level of the medial malleolus.
- While there are many techniques available to perform an end-to-end repair of the Achilles gap, the authors prefer a locking Krakow stitch with a single suture for each tendon end (one suture for the proximal Achilles tendon; one suture for the distal Achilles tendon). We often utilize suture tape because it is flat and does not pull through the tendon as easily as traditional suture. Frequently, we place three to five locked loops on each side of the tendon. This is repeated for the opposite tendon end and hand tied together.
- Locking Krakow: Start within the medial or lateral end of the tendon exiting out the respective side. Leave just enough suture to hand tie later. Advance up the tendon with three to five locked loops. Only suture one-third of the tendon on each side to avoid strangulation. Once three to five locked loops are completed, pass the suture tape to the opposite side within the substance of the tendon. Complete another three to five locked loops down the other side of the tendon, exiting at the end. If performed correctly, there will be two suture tails exiting out the distal medial and lateral tendon end.
- We often supplement the repair with amniotic tissue as we have found this to help reduce tendon adhesions and scarring, which is commonly encountered with this procedure.
- We use as little suture as possible as using too much suture can impair tendon healing, increase scarring, and increase risk for suture reactions.
- Unless contraindicated, we place patients on DVT prophylaxis following this surgery.

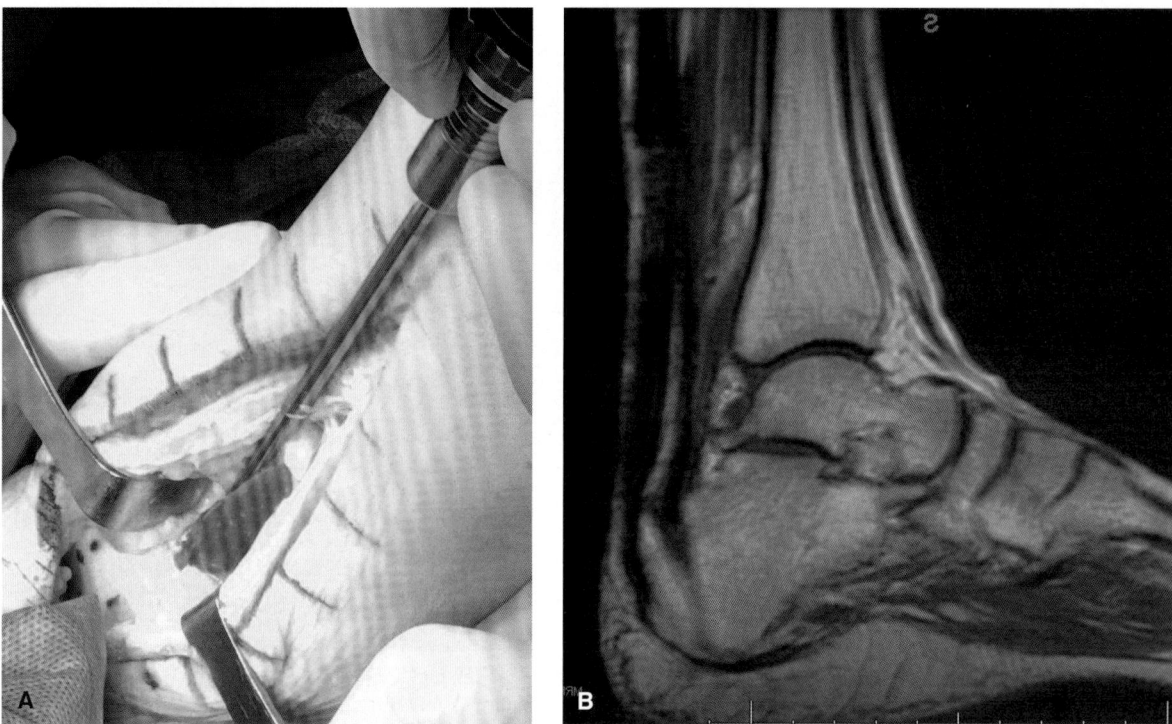

FIGURE 56.36 **A.** While holding the desired tension with the foot and leg in the proper position, the interference anchor is inserted into the calcaneus alongside the FHL tendon. **B.** MRI demonstrating trajectory and final position of the interference screw with FHL tendon transfer.

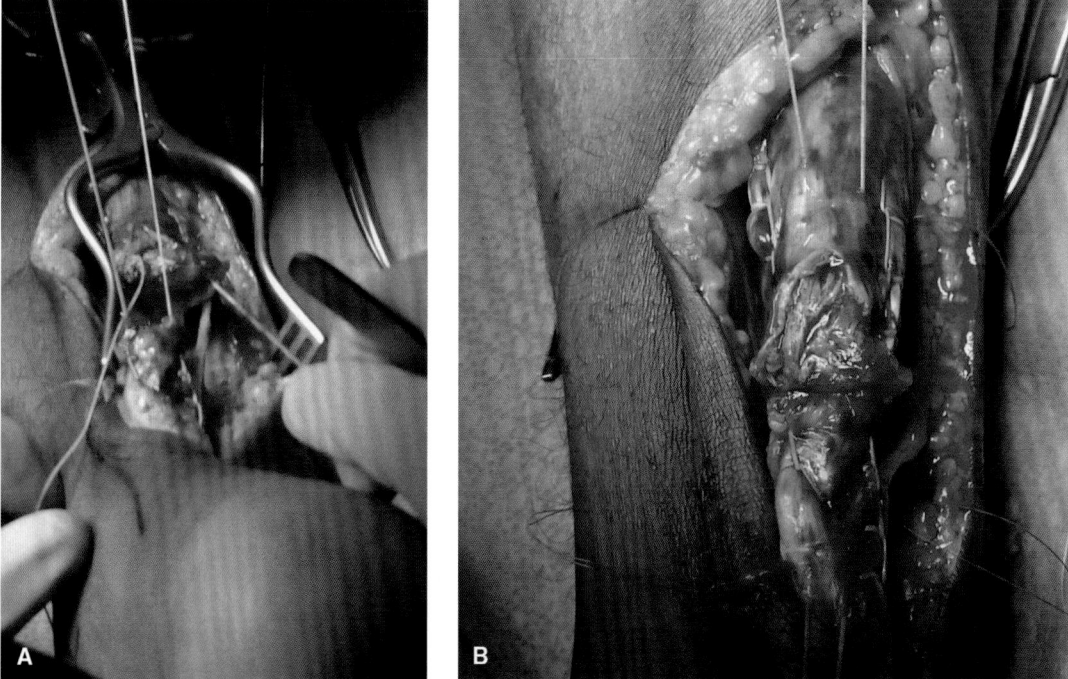

FIGURE 56.37 **A.** A modified Krakow suture was placed in the proximal Achilles tendon stump and another modified Krakow suture was placed in the distal Achilles tendon stump. **B.** The modified Krakow sutures in the distal Achilles stump are pulled proximally, and the modified Krakow sutures in the proximal Achilles tendon stump are pulled distally in order to reapproximate the end-to-end repair.

Our preferred order of surgical management is as follows:

1. Resect pseudotendon and measure true gap; decide if performing end-to-end repair, V-Y, FHL tendon transfer, etc.
2. Place locking Krakow sutures within both ends of the Achilles tendon.
3. Place continuous weighted traction to the gastrocnemius-soleus via the locked Krakow sutures (keep in traction until Achilles repair at the end).
4. Perform V-Y lengthening within the gastrocnemius-soleus aponeurosis/myotendinous region.
5. Perform FHL tendon transfer and fixate into calcaneus with an interference screw.
6. Perform Achilles tendon repair.
7. Repair as much paratenon as possible using the least amount of absorbable suture as possible. Supplement repair with amniotic tissue if needed and close.

PERILS and PITFALLS

- The FHL tendon transfer is an adjunctive procedure and should not be performed in isolation of a chronic Achilles tendon rupture.
- Dissection: Be cautious of the sural nerve as distally is it ~5 mm adjacent to the lateral Achilles tendon. It may be entrapped within the rupture site as well. Proximally, the sural nerve crosses from lateral to central at the myotendinous junction and then dives beneath the medial head of the gastrocnemius muscle belly.
- FHL tendon transfer: The neurovascular bundle is immediately medial to the FHL tendon. When harvesting the FHL, it is important to dissect along the lateral FHL and to release the tendon sheath allowing mobilization of the tendon further away from the neurovascular bundle when transecting it.
- FHL tendon transfer: Plantar flex and invert the foot, ankle, and hallux in order to achieve adequate length for the tendon transfer via an interference anchor.
- FHL tendon transfer: The calcaneal cancellous bone often easily compresses when inserting the interference screw and tendon, and therefore, underdrilling or increasing the size of the interference screw is often necessary especially if there is any osteopenia.
- V-Y lengthening: Sliding the tendon often requires a good amount of force and patience, but be careful to always keep some muscle belly attached to the tendon to avoid devascularizing the repair.
- It is important to avoid under- and overtightening the repair. Add some additional tension as the muscle always stretches out some. This is achieved by comparing the resting tension to the contralateral limb.
- Setting patient expectations is important. They should expect a prolonged recovery and understand that outcomes of neglected Achilles tendon ruptures are inferior to acute Achilles ruptures.

POSTOPERATIVE CARE

For weeks 0-2, the patient is strict NWB in a posterior splint in neutral position. At week 2, if incisions are healed, then sutures

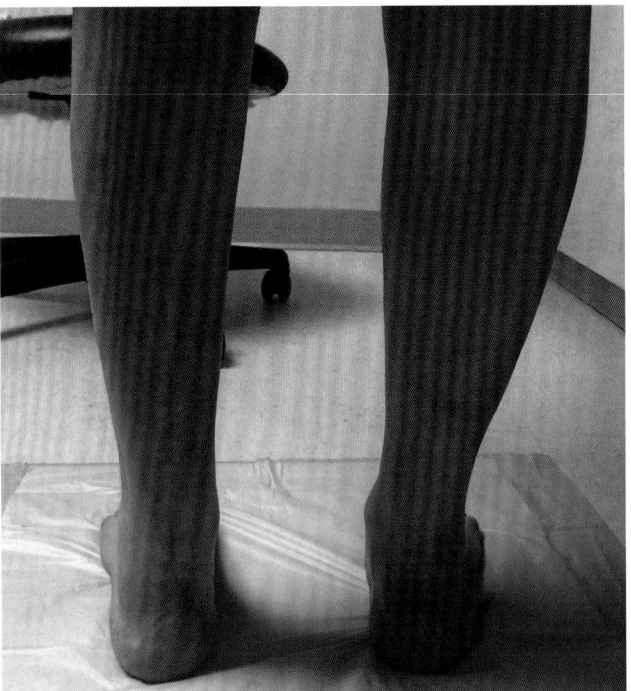

FIGURE 56.38 The patient is 1 year postoperative from a V-Y Achilles lengthening and end-to-end repair with FHL tendon transfer. The patient has been progressively improving, but there is still apparent muscle atrophy within the left calf.

are removed. The patient is then transitioned to either a neutral cast or below-knee immobilization boot and may partial weight bear with crutch assist as tolerated. If more than two-thirds of the Achilles was excised, then the non–weight-bearing period is extended for a total of 4 weeks. Gentle passive ROM exercises are typically initiated at week 4, and active ROM with progressive strengthening exercises are initiated between weeks 6-8. The boot is typically discontinued between weeks 10 and 12 as tolerated. The patient should be educated that they will experience calf atrophy and will have a prolonged course of calf weakness[61] (Fig. 56.38).

REHABILITATION

Start physical therapy at between weeks 6 and 12, 2-3 times per week: performed with boot removed, start with passive Achilles stretching, then a graduated Achilles strengthening program that includes gait training. High-impact activities such as running, jumping, or cutting should be avoided for at least 6 months from the date of surgery.

DIGITAL FLEXOR TENDON TRANSFER

DEFINITION

A hammertoe deformity is a specific flexion deformity present at the PIPJ; however, it is also commonly accompanied by a flexion contracture at the DIPJ and, often, an extension contracture at the MTPJ. There may also be a transverse plane deformity of varying severity ranging from mild to severe, such as those seen

with crossover toe deformities.[62] Hammertoe, claw toe, and mallet toe deformities are often described interchangeably; however, a true hammertoe is defined by the sagittal plane flexion contracture at the PIPJ, though all are associated with a biomechanical imbalance of the intrinsic and extrinsic musculature to the toes.

CLASSIFICATION

FLEXOR STABILIZATION DEFORMITY

Typically occurs in a pronated foot type, which leads to early activation of the FDL tendon, creating a mechanical advantage over the intrinsic muscles and leading to an adductovarus contracture deformity.[35,63]

FLEXOR SUBSTITUTION DEFORMITY

Typically occurs due to weakness at the triceps surae, leading to deep posterior leg muscle compensation and overpowering of the interossei by the extrinsic flexors.[63]

EXTENSOR SUBSTITUTION DEFORMITY

Occurs during the swing phase of the gait cycle, with hyperactivity of the extrinsic extensors leading to an overpowering of the lumbricals and a bowstring type contracture at the MTPJ.[35,63] Digital deformities can be further classified as flexible, semi-rigid, or rigid/fixed.[37]

INDICATIONS

Surgical correction is indicated for hammertoes, claw toes, mallet toes, extensor contractures, MTPJ instability, plantar plate insufficiency, and crossover toes when conservative options have failed and patients continue to have pain and disability. Dorsal callus or ulceration at the PIPJ, or distal tip callus or ulceration of the toe without signs of infection are common indications requiring surgical correction when conservative treatment has been unsuccessful.

The presence of plantar metatarsal head callus or porokeratosis causing pain, or chronic plantar metatarsalgia and retrograde buckling pressure may also indicate the need for surgical intervention.[64] Neuropathic patients may require earlier intervention in order to prevent ulcerations and infection. Soft tissue rebalancing and tendon transfers are typically most beneficial in flexible deformities, but combined with adjunctive procedures, can also be indicated in rigid contractures.

ANATOMIC FEATURES AND FUNCTIONAL ANALYSIS

DYNAMIC STABILIZERS

EDL tendon extends from the lower leg deep to the retinaculum at the ankle to each of the lesser toes, forming the primary extensor of the lesser toes at the MTPJs. The EDB extends from its origin at the lateral foot to each of the four medial toes, excluding the fifth toe, forming the lone intrinsic dorsal muscle of the foot. The extensor hood maintains the orientation and directional force of the extensor tendons to the toes, consisting of the proximal extensor sling and distal extensor wing. The interossei muscles insert into the extensor sling, while the lumbricals insert into the extensor wing, creating an intricate balance that allows the extensors to work in concert with the intrinsic flexors to extend at the MTPJ, PIPJ, and DIPJ.

The flexor digitorum brevis tendons (FDB) and the FDL tendons work in concert to provide extrinsic flexion at the PIPJ and DIPJ, respectively, and minimally at the MTPJ. The interossei and lumbricals provide the major flexion forces at the MTPJs, as well as working in concert with the extensors to extend the PIPJ and DIPJ.

STATIC STABILIZERS

The plantar plate extends from its origin at the shaft of the metatarsals as an extension of the plantar fascia and inserts into the deep transverse intermetatarsal ligaments, and onto the base of the proximal phalanx, providing insertion points for collateral ligaments, and functions as the primary static stabilizing force of the MTPJ and PIPJ. The plantar plate is often contiguous with the flexor tendon sheath and joint capsule plantarly at the MTPJ.

The medial and lateral collateral ligaments along with the plantar plate provide the main stabilizers for the MTPJ.[65]

PHYSICAL EXAMINATION

Obtaining a detailed family history and any history of high-arch foot types and neuropathic symptoms or conditions can be important in determining the pathology of the digital deformities and aid in determining the appropriate treatment. Any history of trauma, injury, gait problems, or weakness should also be evaluated. Patients will often complain of rubbing and pressure in shoe gear, callus to dorsal or distal tufts of the toes, pain and metatarsalgia to the ball of the foot, or painful corns. Both weight-bearing and non–weight-bearing examinations should be completed, including a gait evaluation. Evaluating posterior muscle group contractures or weakness is also important. Evaluation of the foot type and extent of the digital deformities should include determination of sagittal, transverse, and frontal plane malalignment and contracture, reducibility/rigidity of deformities. A Kelikian push-up test is often employed to assess flexibility of the contractures.[40] A dorsal drawer test, Lachman vertical stress test, or a positive Thompson and Hamilton sign may also be employed to assess the stability and functionality of the plantar plate.[66-68] A thorough neurovascular examination should be completed, as correction of severe digital deformities, especially those long-standing in nature, can compromise the neurovascular structures.

PATHOGENESIS

Due to the intricate balance between the static and dynamic stabilizers and the intrinsic and extrinsic muscles, any disruption of this balance can lead to digital contracture deformity.[68] Any change to the axis of rotation of the MTPJ will change the vector of pull for both extrinsic and intrinsic musculature and lead

to deformity. Loss or weakening of the intrinsic flexors will lead to MTPJ extension by the extensor tendons, creating a chain reaction that extends at the MTPJ and contracts at the PIPJ, further weakening the ability of the already weak intrinsic musculature to flex at the MTPJ and extend at the PIPJ and DIPJ.

CONGENITAL

Cavovarus foot, clubfoot, pronation deformities are a few causes that may lead to digital deformities. Pronated foot types can cause loss of normal quadratus plantae force vector and lead to adductovarus frontal and sagittal plane deformities, often seen in the pronated foot type. Severe cavovarus foot types can increase the normal force vector angle of the long flexors, leading to similar frontal and sagittal plane deformities.[69]

IATROGENIC

Imbalances may be created as a result of surgery. Over-dorsiflexion or over-plantar flexion of a metatarsal after osteotomy can disrupt the tendon-ligamentous balance. Lengthening, shortening, or overtensioning of tendons proximally may disrupt the balance and lead to deformities.

INFLAMMATION

Systemic conditions such as rheumatoid arthritis may lead to chronic inflammation and weakening of the static stabilizers including the joint capsule, collateral ligaments, and plantar plate.

NEUROMUSCULAR

Conditions including cerebral palsy, cerebrovascular accident, CMT, lumbar disc disease, muscular dystrophies, multiple sclerosis, Friedreich ataxia, spinal dysraphism, and polio may lead to imbalance and deformity. Many other causes of neuromuscular dysfunction can contribute.

TRAUMA

Injury and scarring to the extrinsic muscles of the lower leg including nerve injury, compartment syndrome, fractures, and lacerations can create weakness and lead to a distal imbalance and resultant digital deformity. Chronic trauma to the joint stabilizers including the plantar plate may lead to injury, attenuation, and deformity.

OTHER

Chronic external deforming forces such as small shoes, compact toe box, and repetitive motions may lead to buckling of the digits over time. Age-related attenuation and weakening of muscles, tendons, and ligaments may also contribute to deformity developing over time.

IMAGING AND DIAGNOSTICS

Weight-bearing AP, oblique, and lateral radiographs are typically sufficient for evaluation of the deformities and to evaluate the involvement of any long-standing arthritides,

inflammatory conditions, periarticular erosions, subluxation, and multiplane deformities. An MRI may be utilized to assess the viability of the plantar plate if suspicion of attenuation or insufficiency is present. Dorsiflexion at the MTPJ during MRI may be helpful, but often, clinical testing can be more reliable than MRI. Ankle-brachial index (ABI), toe pressures (toe-brachial index [TBI]), and TcPO2 studies may also be utilized if vascular status is in question. Neurologic workup may include EMG or NCV studies in the setting of neurologic pathology.

TREATMENT

The goal of treatment is to restore the balance between the static and dynamic stabilizers and intrinsic and extrinsic musculature. Weakening the overpowering tendon and restoring tension to the weaker tendon should ideally restore appropriate anatomic balance. Repair of any compromised static stabilizers such as the collateral ligaments and plantar plate may also be employed. The end result should reestablish a neutral anatomically positioned digit that is stable in all planes.

NONOPERATIVE

Conservative treatment tends to be most appropriate with reducible flexible deformities and should be employed prior to surgical intervention. Stretching and strengthening exercises may provide some benefit, although this tends to have little effect on reestablishing a balanced digit. Accommodating deformity and managing symptoms is often the extent of nonoperative treatment. This can be employed via shoe gear modification (wider, deeper, flexible) or via padding and cushioning such as metatarsal pads, toe separators, gel toe sleeves, foam, Lamb's wool, and digital toe strapping and splints. The long-term benefits of these options will vary greatly from patient to patient.

SURGICAL PROCEDURE AND TECHNIQUE

Digital flexor tendon transfers are rarely performed as a stand-alone procedure. It is commonly accompanied by a variety of other soft tissue and osseous procedures, performed as a whole to attempt to restore normal biomechanical function and balance to the MTPJ. The plantar plate should be assessed and any attenuation or rupture may indicate a need for repair. Elongated or plantarly prominent metatarsals may require shortening or dorsiflexory osteotomies. Repair of collateral ligaments and transpositional osteotomies may be necessary to correct transverse plane deformities. Interphalangeal joint procedures such as arthroplasty, arthrodesis, intramedullary implants, or soft tissue releases may also be needed.

Progressive skin, tendon, capsule, and ligamentous releases may need to be performed in order to reduce the deformity and the digit to a neutral and rectus position. These should be performed prior to tendon transfer as deemed necessary.

Metatarsal osteotomies should be considered, particularly in the setting of an MTPJ extension contracture. After soft tissue releases are completed, and assessment of the reducibility of the joint should be performed.

FDL to Extensor Transfer

A single-incision approach has been described for FDL to extensor transfers and is most easily performed through the PIPJ when adjunctive PIPJ procedures are necessary; however, a multi-incision approach will be described here.

A longitudinal incision is made over the dorsal aspect of the MTPJ from proximal to distal and extended over the base of the proximal phalanx. This allows for exposure of the MTPJ as needed for appropriate soft tissue releases or metatarsal osteotomies. A curvilinear incision may be preferred to aid in prevention of skin and scar contracture postoperatively. The incision can be extended distally over the PIPJ in cases of more rigid contractures, when adjunctive PIPJ procedures are necessary. Any hyperkeratotic skin, callus, or corn to the dorsal PIPJ may be excised if needed.

A second incision is made in either a longitudinal or transverse fashion to the plantar aspect of the toe at the proximal skin crease. Blunt dissection is carried down subcutaneously where the flexor tendon sheath can be identified and incised sharply, exposing the long and short flexor tendons. The FDL tendon is identified between the two slips of the FDB tendon and is elevated and isolated with a hemostat or Freer (Fig. 56.39).

A third small stab incision is made at the plantar aspect of the distal skin crease at the DIPJ, where dissection can be carried down to the FDL tendon, or a percutaneous release and tenotomy of the FDL tendon can be performed (Fig. 56.40).

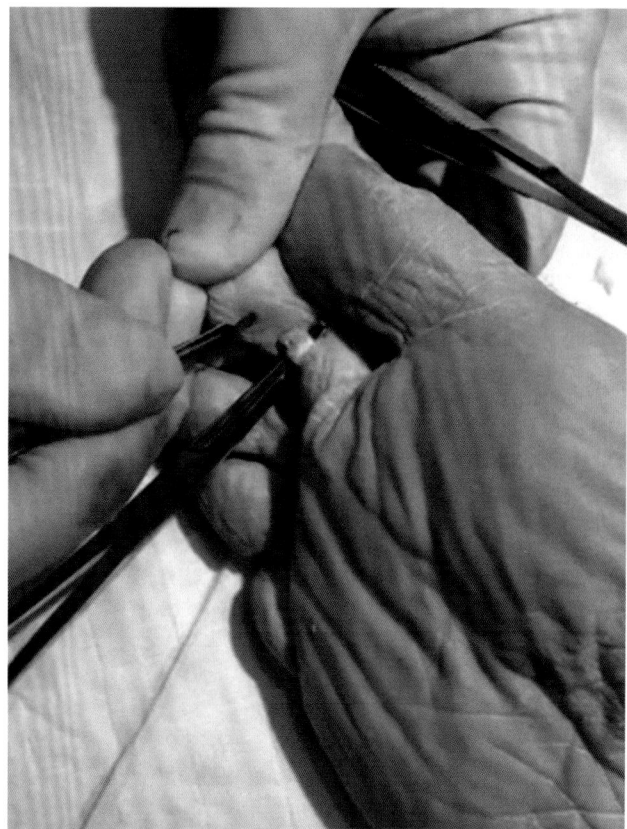

FIGURE 56.40 After making a small incision in the DIPJ, a tenotomy is performed to release the insertion of the FDL tendon.

Care should be taken with percutaneous tenotomy to avoid the joint capsule and ligaments of the DIPJ. An open incision vs a percutaneous release may allow for more distal dissection for increased tendon length if desired.

The previously placed hemostat or Freer is now used to pull the FDL tendon through the proximal plantar incision for complete visualization (Fig. 56.41). The FDL tendon is then split into equal halves longitudinally, creating a medial and lateral slip along its midline. This can be performed with a sharp blade or a nylon suture.

Attention is redirected to the dorsal incision, where blunt dissection is used to identify the extensor tendons. The extensor tendon and sheath are then sharply incised longitudinally along its midline overlying the proximal phalanx. Blunt dissection is then carried down medially and laterally directly on the bone of the proximal phalanx through this incision down to the proximal plantar incision directly below. Care should be taken to stay subperiosteal to protect the neurovascular structures.

A small hemostat is passed from dorsal to plantar on the medial side of the phalanx, where the medial slip of the now split FDL tendon is grasped and passed from plantar to dorsal. This is repeated for the lateral side (Fig. 56.42).

Once both slips of the FDL tendon have been passed to the dorsum of the proximal phalanx, the entire foot and ankle and the toe should be held in a neutral position, with slight plantar flexion of 10-20 degrees of the toe at the MTPJ. Both slips of the FDL tendon are then sutured into the extensor tendon with a 4-0 absorbable suture.

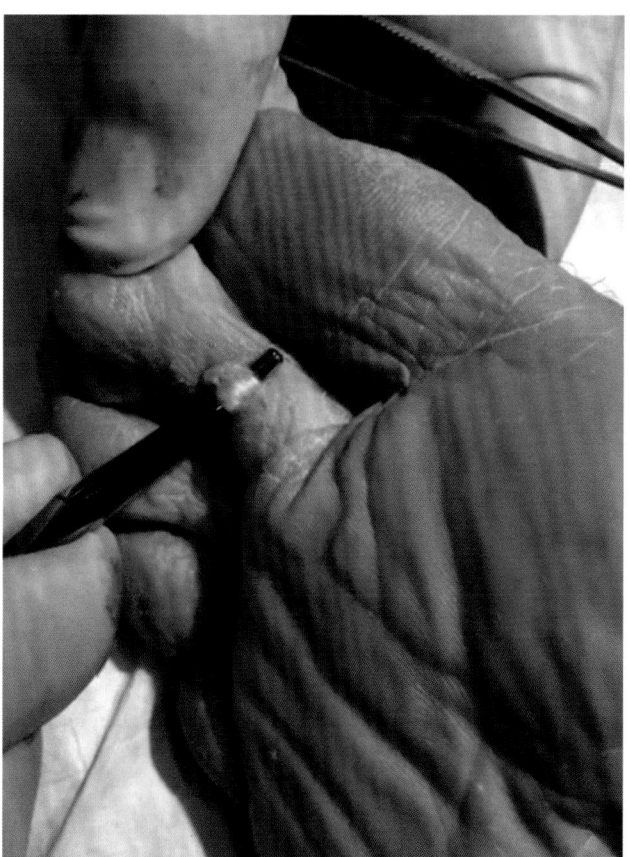

FIGURE 56.39 The FDL tendon is identified within a plantar incision at the proximal skin crease of the toe.

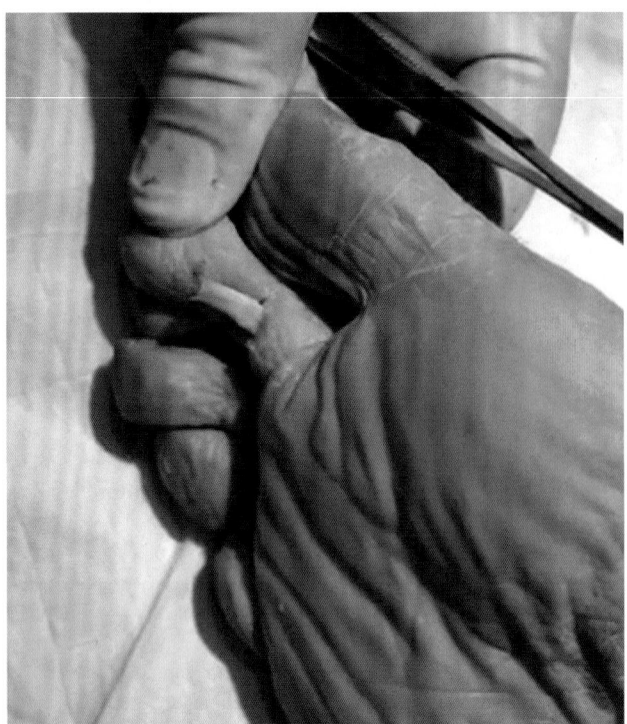

FIGURE 56.41 The FDL tendon is passed into the proximal plantar incision. It will be subsequently split in half longitudinally.

Evaluate the position of the toe and correction of the deformity, including any residual contractures. The toe should maintain the previously describe slightly plantar flexed position at the MTPJ. The incisions are then all irrigated and closed with absorbable sutures deeply and a nonabsorbable suture to the skin. A Kirschner wire (K-wire) may be placed across the PIPJ and MTPJ to maintain correction and protect the repair if desired.

Any tourniquet used should be deflated to evaluate appropriate revascularization to the toe, and the dressings and

appropriate splint should be applied in order to maintain the plantar flexed position of the toe.

FDL Transfer via Drill Tunnel

The previous surgical technique is followed until the FDL tendon is released and pulled through the proximal planar incision and the dorsal incision is carried down through the extensor tendon.

Dissection is carried down through the longitudinal incision of the extensor tendon, where a guidewire is placed from dorsal to plantar perpendicular to the long axis of the proximal phalanx. A 2.0-mm drill is then used to place a drill hole through the shaft of the proximal phalanx from dorsal to plantar (Fig. 56.43). The hole should be large enough to pass the FDL tendon through the tunnel. The size of the FDL tendon and the size of the phalanx may dictate the size of the drill tunnel. You should try to avoid making a drill tunnel larger than ⅓-½ the diameter of the phalanx. The FDL tendon is whip stitched at the end of the tendon plantarly, and a suture passer is used to pass the suture and the FDL tendon between the FDB slips from plantar to dorsal through the drill tunnel (Fig. 56.44).

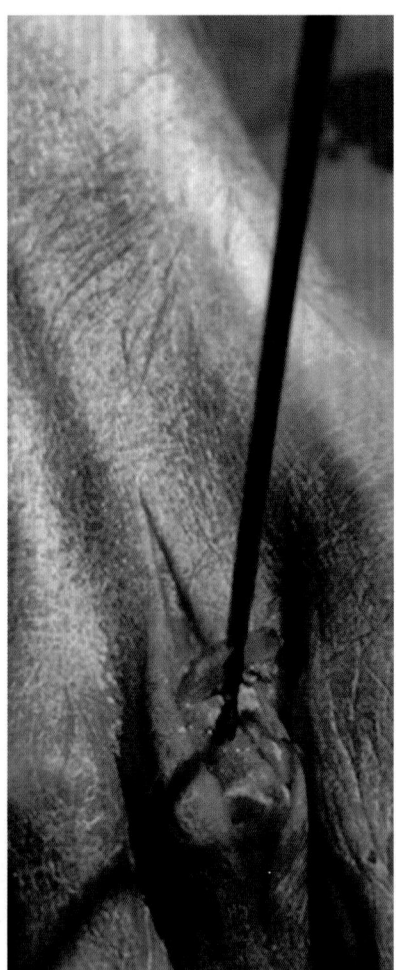

FIGURE 56.43 A 2.0-mm drill tunnel is created from dorsal to plantar within the proximal phalanx shaft.

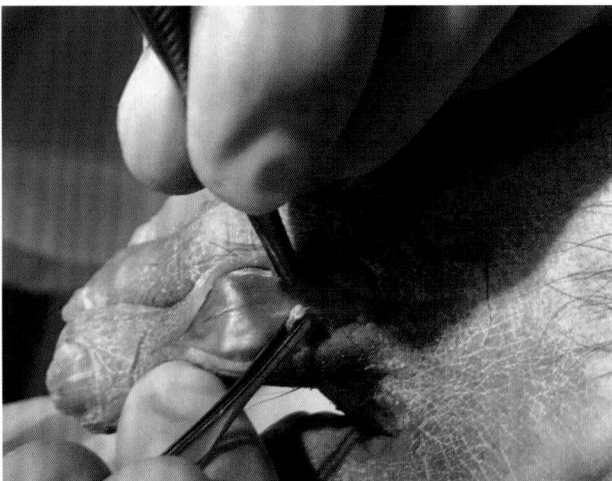

FIGURE 56.42 The medial and lateral FDL tendon slips are passed from plantar to dorsal around the phalanx. These slips are sutured together dorsally with the toe held in the corrected position.

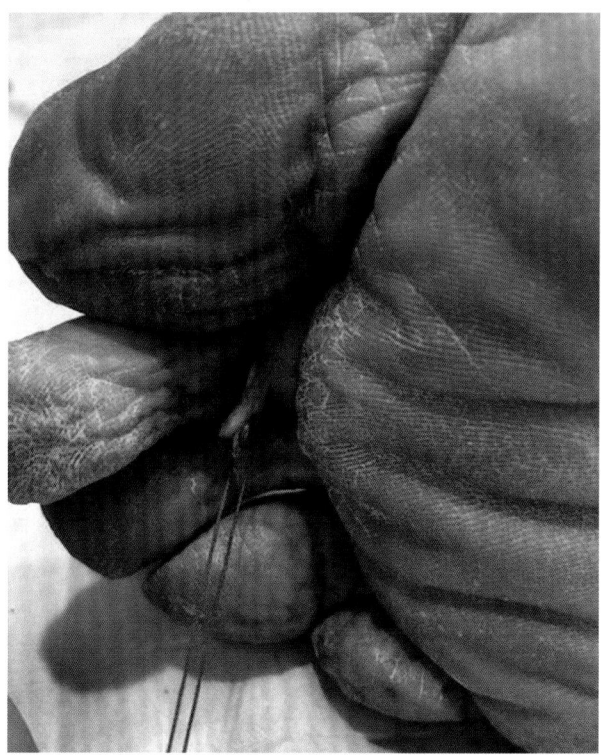

FIGURE 56.44 The FDL tendon is whip stitched and passed from plantar to dorsal through the drill tunnel utilizing a suture passer.

Position the foot as describe above, with the described plantar flexion of the toe at the MTPJ, and secure the FDL tendon to the EDB tendon with a 4-0 absorbable suture or with a small bioabsorbable interference screw. Closure, dressings, and splinting remain the same as described above.

positioning PEARLS

- The patient should be placed in a supine position with an ipsilateral hip bump to orient the foot and toes upward and prevent excessive external rotation.
- As a dorsal and plantar approach are both necessary, the patient should be positioned according to surgeon preference toward the end of the table to allow for visualization of both approaches.

EXPOSURE PEARLS

- Longitudinal incisions both dorsally and plantarly may allow for better exposure and visualization of the tendons and joints. An MTPJ exposure is almost always necessary for appropriate treatment. Care should be taken with transverse or oblique incisions as they will place neurovascular structures at greater risk.

AUTHORS' PREFERRED TREATMENT

- The author prefers a longitudinal curvilinear dorsal approach with a transverse proximal plantar incision and percutaneous stab incision to distal plantar incision.

- A metatarsal osteotomy is performed in some cases, in a standard dorsal distal-to-plantar proximal fashion, angled parallel to the weight-bearing surface of the foot. A small 1- to 2-mm wafer of bone is usually removed with the metatarsal osteotomy to aid in maintaining the anatomic axis of rotation around the metatarsal head after shortening and to avoid any plantar prominence as the metatarsal head is translated proximally.
- An absorbable interference screw is preferred for fixation with transfer through a drill tunnel, as less tendon is required and there is less stiffness and better anatomic width and thickness of the digit, resulting in a more pleasing appearance of the toe with less sausagelike appearance that can occur when tendons are transferred medially and laterally.
- When hammertoe implants are used at the PIPJ, either a bone tunnel cannot be used or the appropriate implant should be selected that will allow for bone tunnel drilling through the implant if desired.

PERILS and PITFALLS

- Proper preoperative assessment of any underlying bony etiology or associated ligamentous instability or attenuation is key to achieving a successful outcome.
- Proper postoperative protection of the soft tissue repairs is also important in a good long-term outcome and prevention of common complications and patient complaints.
- Overcorrection of the deformity in plantar flexion tends to be less of a problem than undercorrection or failure of soft tissue repairs. Being more aggressive toward at least 20 degrees of plantar flexion when fixating the tendon transfer appears to reduce the risk of these complications and preventing the most common patient complaints. The normal biomechanical stress to the toe and the joint during ambulation allow for stretching of an overtightened tendon and tends to be more forgiving.
- An obliquely angled drill tunnel either medially or laterally may also aid in correction of transverse plane deformities.
- Swelling and numbness are some of the most common complications inherent to digital surgery. Overaggressive dissection, poor neurovascular status, suture reactions, anchor placement, tendon size, and improper postoperative care may lead to prolonged swelling and numbness. Wire or pin placement may contribute and may need to be removed early.
- MTPJ and PIPJ stiffness: Early ROM exercises may be beneficial, but care should be taken to protect the repaired soft tissues as well. Appropriate patient expectations are important. Patients should understand that some stiffness will reduce the risk of recurrence of the deformity.
- Recurrence: Recurrence can be a common problem, and the complex biomechanical relationships at the MTPJ makes this a difficult problem to treat. Recurrence may be due to improper procedure selection, undercorrection, inappropriate tensioning, undiagnosed neurologic issues, scar contracture, or failure of fixation.
- Floating toe, lack of toe purchase, angular deformity: Care should be taken to perform the needed adjunctive procedures to reduce risks associated with residual deformity. Appropriate positioning, tensioning, and postoperative splinting may aid in prevention of floating toe or loss of purchase.

POSTOPERATIVE CARE

The patient is placed partial weight bearing (PWB) with crutches in a stiff-soled postoperative shoe with a compression dressing left in place for 1 week postoperatively. The toe is strapped and splinted via both the dressings and the use of ¼ inch silk tape to splint the toe in a neutral and slightly plantar flexed position. Dressings are changed at week 1 and week 2 postoperatively. Sutures are typically removed at week 2 postoperatively depending on approximation and healing of the incisions.

Once sutures are removed, continued daily strapping vs prefabricated digital loop splints are used to maintain the position and protect the soft tissue repairs and tendon transfer, continuing to maintain slight plantar flexion of the digit.

Patients are usually progressed to weight bearing as tolerated (WBAT) in a supportive sneaker at week 6 postoperatively, depending on pain and swelling to the area and any adjunctive procedures that were performed.

REHABILITATION

Some surgeons advocate for early ROM exercises to the MTPJ at weeks 2-3 postoperatively; however, as failure of the soft tissue repairs and tendon transfers tends to lead toward more patient dissatisfaction than does stiffness of the joint, aggressive ROM exercises are not begun until week 6 postoperatively. Stiffness can be increased with this delay but over time improves. Therefore, gentle ROM exercises are often initiated at weeks 2-3 because of the stiffness commonly associated with this procedure.

SPLIT TIBIALIS ANTERIOR TENDON TRANSFER (STATT) OR SPLIT ANTERIOR TIBIALIS TRANSFER (SPLATT)

DEFINITION

This is a modification of the complete TA tendon transfer, where the TA tendon is split distally at the insertion, transferring the lateral portion to a new insertion, typically on either the lateral cuneiform or the cuboid.

INDICATIONS

TA tendon transfers and split TA tendon transfers were initially indicated for use in the treatment of idiopathic clubfoot in children via the Ponseti method[70]; however, after the introduction of the STATT procedure by Hoffer et al.,[71] indications have expanded to include treatment of a broad range of flexible equinovarus deformities in both children and adults, including many progressive neurologic disorders including[3,72-80]:

- Primary pediatric clubfoot
- Recurrent/residual clubfoot
- Dynamic forefoot supinatus
- Flexible cavovarus
- Spastic equinovarus

- Progressive neurologic disorders
- Nerve injury
- Tarsometatarsal joint amputations

Flexible deformities with an imbalance between the invertors (anterior and PTTs) and the evertors (peroneal tendons) are the primary indications, regardless the original etiology of the imbalance, as long as the TA tendon retains its muscle strength. The presence of dynamic supination during gait with confirmed imbalance between inversion and eversion strength is prime indication for a split TA tendon transfer.[77] There have even been some indications presented for STATT procedure in cases of total ankle replacements in varus ankle deformities, with good to excellent results[78]; however, this is not well studied.

ANATOMIC FEATURES AND FUNCTIONAL ANALYSIS

The STATT procedure allows the force and pull of the TA muscle to be transferred laterally to compensate for weak evertors that have created an unopposed supinatory pull by the anterior and PTTs and a resulting dynamic supination of the forefoot.[72,75] This tendon transfer allows a rebalancing of the inverters and evertors and restores the natural talo-first metatarsal angle.[73] TA tendons with a muscle strength of <4+ or 5 should be considered a contraindication for an STATT procedure (Table 56.1).[6,81] Rigid deformities should also be considered a contraindication for an STATT procedure. The anatomic ROM at the ankle joint and the dynamic flexibility of the TA tendon should be evaluated prior to surgical intervention, in order to allow for enough tendon length to successfully transfer the lateral portion of the tendon to its new insertion point laterally. Any accompanying structural or osseous deformities should be assessed, as they may require correction at the time of the TA tendon transfer, which is rarely performed in isolation without other adjunctive procedures. Any osseous procedures and corrections should be performed prior to tendon rebalancing.

PHYSICAL EXAMINATION

A thorough preoperative workup and evaluation of the deformities, its pathogenesis, flexibility, and reducibility should always be performed, including an assessment of the muscle strength grade of the TA tendon itself. The strength and function of the peroneal tendons should also be assessed, as this will aid in determining the best point of insertion for the split TA tendon laterally. More severe deformities may require greater correction and more lateral insertion of the transferred tendon. Some have advocated that the STATT procedure should be transferred to the cuboid in most cases; however, a thorough evaluation of the function and deformity as well as the available length of TA tendon may dictate a more medial insertion point in the lateral cuneiform.[28]

The physical examination should include both a static evaluation of the position and flexibility of the deformity as well as a dynamic gait evaluation and biomechanical examination. A supinated foot during the swing phase of gait, with initial foot strike occurring to the lateral border of the foot, is typically

observed during gait analysis. A more flexible deformity lends itself to a better result when performing an STATT procedure.[73] A Coleman block testing may also be necessary to assess the reducibility of a varus deformity. Gastrocnemius and Achilles equinus contractures should be assessed and a Silfverskiöld test should be performed, as a posterior heel cord lengthening is almost always necessary.

PATHOGENESIS

Equinovarus deformities may occur for a variety of reasons and are commonly seen in pediatric clubfoot but may also occur due to a variety of other causes. Trauma resulting in nerve or spinal cord injury and dysfunction may lead to deformity. Traumatic brain injury or cerebrovascular events may lead to this deformity. Progressive neurological conditions such as CMT, poliomyelitis, syringomyelia, spinal dysraphism, cerebral palsy, and multiple sclerosis may also lead to spastic equinovarus deformities.

IMAGING AND DIAGNOSTICS

Weight-bearing plain film AP and lateral radiographs of both the foot and ankle and a weight-bearing calcaneal axial radiograph should be considered. In cases of severe deformities, an appropriate MRI or CT may be necessary, with an MRI being most valuable to assess the condition of the distal TA tendon. These imaging studies are important to assess underlying deformities that may require concomitant correction at the time of the tendon transfer. Some have advocated for EMG or foot and ankle motion analysis to aid in appropriate tendon and procedure selection.[82]

TREATMENT

SURGICAL PROCEDURE AND TECHNIQUE

A three-incision technique is employed for harvesting, transfer, and anchoring of the split TA tendon.

The initial incision is made over the dorsomedial foot at the insertion of the TA tendon on the medial aspect of the medial cuneiform and first metatarsal base. The incision can be performed proximal-to-distal, oblique along the course of the tendon, or in a curvilinear fashion if preferred. Intraoperative fluoroscopy may be helpful in locating the desired medial aspect of the first tarsometatarsal joint and minimizing dissection.

The second incision is made on the anterior medial lower leg just proximal to the ankle and the extensor retinaculum directly overlying the course of the TA tendon from proximal to distal.

The third incision is made dorsolaterally on the foot overlying the lateral cuneiform or the cuboid depending on the planned point of insertions. Intraoperative fluoroscopy should be used to locate the desired point of insertion and plan the incision.

The anterior tibialis tendon sheath is carefully incised at the insertion, identifying the tendon and directly visualizing the tendon just proximal to the insertion. The tendon sheath

should then be incised and the tendon exposed at the second proximal anterior lower leg incision. A sharp incision should be made through the center of the tendon at the lower leg, where a long strand of umbilical tape or large nylon suture is then inserted through the incised tendon and passed from proximal to distal through the tendon sheath with a suture passer, exiting the medial foot incision at the insertion of the TA tendon. The two ends of the umbilical tape or suture are then used to split the tendon longitudinally from proximal to distal by pulling the tape or suture distally to the insertion. The lateral portion of the split tendon is then dissected away from the insertion, maintaining as much of the distal fibers and insertion as possible. Once released, the lateral portion of the tendon is then pulled proximally through the second incision at the anterior lower leg.

A tendon passer or a closed loop wire such as a Luque wire should be passed from distal to proximal from the lateral incision to the anterior leg incision, taking care to ensure it remains deep to the extensor retinaculum and within the extensor tendon sheath. Some advocate for passing the tendon subcutaneously in order to preserve muscle strength. The end of the lateral portion of the split tendon should be tagged with a whip-stitched suture, and the tendon passer is then used to pass the suture and the split TA tendon from proximal to distal exiting the lateral incision on the foot at the new desired anchor point.

The split TA tendon is finally anchored into the bone at the lateral incision either to the cuboid or the lateral cuneiform via a tendon anchor or an interference screw. The foot should be held in a neutral dorsiflexed and slightly everted position while the transferred tendon is anchored under appropriate physiologic tension. In cases of insufficient tendon, the split tendon may be tenodesed into the peroneus tertius tendon; however, this will decrease the strength of the pull and correction of deformity, and the presence of the peroneus tertius tendon should be confirmed prior to surgery.

positioning PEARLS

- Patient positioning should allow for adequate access to both the medial and lateral foot as well as the anterior lower leg and ankle.
- A supine position with appropriate ipsilateral hip or leg bump to achieve the desired position is preferred, tending to overbump into an internally rotated position for better view of the lateral foot, as the foot and ankle will more easily be adjusted intraoperatively with external rotation or a frog-leg position to aid in medial exposure as needed.

AUTHORS' PREFERRED TREATMENT

The authors' preferred technique consists of an initial tendoachilles lengthening or gastrocnemius lengthening, determined preoperatively. This is almost always accomplished percutaneously for both procedures. Once the lateral TA tendon is passed to the lateral foot, the tendon is then anchored via an interference screw to the cuboid.[83] The drill tunnel is angled slightly dorsolateral to medial plantar. Bioabsorbable interference screws have been shown to have more secure fixation and

less complications related to failure of fixation and rupture of the transferred tendon.[28,84,85]

Claw toe deformities are common before surgery in spastic equinovarus deformities and will often occur postoperatively in patients even when it was not initially present prior to surgery. Therefore, the author will typically perform a complete tenotomy of the long and short toe flexors along with the STATT procedure and heel cord lengthening.[86]

PERILS AND PITFALLS

Common complications can range from minor to major, with minor complications being more common.[3,74,76,87] Complications may include infection, tendon rupture of either one or both portion of the split tendon, neurovascular injury, tendonitis and tenosynovitis, hallux extensus, undercorrection, and overcorrection. Many complications may be avoided with appropriate surgical technique and preoperative decision-making. Transferring the tendon too far laterally and over- or undertensioning the tendon should be avoided. It is always recommended to over tighten some as the tendon loosens up some. Determining whether a split tendon transfer is sufficient or if a complete tendon transfer will be necessary can also affect outcomes. Appropriate selection of adjunctive procedures is also key in limiting complications particularly those stemming from over- or undercorrection.

Inappropriate positioning of the foot during tendon tensioning and anchoring is a common pitfall. Care should be taken with spastic cerebral palsy patients to not transfer too laterally or overtension, as this patient group is more prone to overcorrection into valgus.[28,88]

POSTOPERATIVE CARE

Patients are placed NWB in a well-padded compression dressing and posterior splint or cast with the foot in a dorsiflexed and slightly everted position. Patients are typically kept strictly NWB for 6-8 weeks. Dressings are changed at week 1, and sutures are removed at week 2 or 3 according to wound healing and postoperative edema. Patients are transferred to protected weight bearing in an appropriate immobilization boot and progressed from partial to full weight bearing with the assistance of physical therapy (Table 56.4).

REHABILITATION

Appropriate physical therapy is begun at 6-8 weeks postoperatively when protected weight bearing is begun. Adjunctive surgical soft tissue and bone procedures may drive the postoperative course of weight bearing; however, physical therapy should begin at 6-8 weeks postoperatively, and active ROM and strengthening exercises should begin prior to weight bearing if a more lengthy period of NWB is necessary. Physical therapy and rehabilitation should focus on strengthening and re-training of the TA muscle, balance, proprioception, and gait training. Progressive strengthening and progressive weight bearing are advanced concomitantly as strength and function improve. Recovery should be relatively rapid, as this

is an in-phase transfer of the TA tendon. Physical therapy is continued for ~3 months as the patient returns to regular shoe gear.

PERONEAL LONGUS TO BREVIS TENDON TRANSFER

DEFINITION

The peroneal longus to brevis transfer is most commonly applied to decrease deforming plantarflexory force on the first ray and augment eversion associated with a weak peroneal brevis.[31,89,90]

INDICATIONS

A variety of circumstances can lead to weakness of the pronators of the foot. Most commonly, these are neurogenic, traumatic, chronic degenerative, or iatrogenic in etiology. Regardless of the cause, weak eversion can result in overload of the lateral column, which increases the risk of pain and ulceration.

ANATOMIC FEATURES AND FUNCTIONAL ANALYSIS

PERONEAL LONGUS

The PL origin is a composite of the lateral surfaces of the head and superior two-thirds of the fibula. Within the lateral compartment, it becomes tendinous proximal to the ankle. The tendon courses distally in tandem with the peroneus brevis within a common synovial sheath. At the level of the posterior ankle, the tendon lies posterior and lateral to the brevis tendon within an anatomic tunnel composed of a retrofibular sulcus that is usually concave and covered by the SPR. The SPR acts as the primary restraint that maintains the relative position of the peroneal tendons within the retrofibular groove. Beyond the fibula, the peroneal tendons turn anteriorly and emerge along the lateral calcaneus. At the level of the peroneal tubercle, the common tendinous sheath becomes divided by a septum from the inferior peroneal retinaculum. The peroneal longus resides within the inferior sheath and courses distally. It then passes beneath the cuboid groove anteromedially toward its insertion on the plantar lateral aspect of the medial cuneiform and the first metatarsal base. The PL is antagonistic to the TA tendon. It plantar flexes the first ray and is a weak evertor of the foot relative to the peroneal brevis.[11,91]

PERONEAL BREVIS

The peroneus brevis originates along the posterior surface of the middle one-third of the fibula and partially from the intermuscular septum. It becomes tendinous proximal to the ankle and enters the retrofibular groove described above. Beyond the fibula, the peroneal tendons turn anteriorly and emerge along the lateral calcaneus. At the level of the peroneal tubercle, the common tendinous sheath becomes divided by a septum from the inferior peroneal retinaculum. The peroneal brevis resides within the superior sheath and courses distally where it inserts onto the base of the styloid process of the fifth metatarsal.

The peroneus brevis opposes the tibialis posterior and primarily acts as the primary evertor of the foot.[11,91]

PHYSICAL EXAMINATION

Physical examination findings will typically consist of weak eversion against resistance. The patient may relate a history of frequent ankle inversion sprains. This may be correlated clinically with the presence of a positive anterior drawer or inversion stress test compared to the nonpathologic limb. The presence of a cavovarus foot type and evidence of peroneal overdrive are potential findings seen with this pathology.[92,93] In an NWB environment, the foot will often assume an inverted position (Fig. 56.45). During the stance phase of gait, the patient may demonstrate a limited eversion of the hindfoot.[93] It is important to assess the strength of the peroneal longus prior to transfer.

PATHOGENESIS

The etiology of weakness of the peroneal brevis is highly variable. This includes neurologic conditions such as CMT. Other more common conditions include untreated chronic peroneal brevis tendon ruptures and even severe avulsion fractures. Chronic lateral ankle instability and hindfoot varus deformities increase stress on the peroneal tendon causing a slow tendinopathy over time. Iatrogenic mediated consequences of a lateral ankle stabilization procedure and complete or partial fifth ray resection for infection can diminish this eversion strength.[90,92,93]

IMAGING AND DIAGNOSTICS

Standard weight-bearing AP, oblique, and lateral radiographs are typically sufficient to evaluate the weight-bearing contractures and deformities and any rigid bone or joint contractures due to long-standing conditions.[89,91,92] An MRI may be helpful in evaluating the condition of the peroneal tendons and may also identify an accessory bone within either tendon. This imaging also helps to confirm that the weakness is not due to peroneal brevis tendon rupture or loss of insertion attachment (Fig. 56.46). Electrodiagnostic studies, including EMG or NCV studies, may be helpful in determining a functional peroneal longus.[89,90,92,93]

TREATMENT

Reestablishment of frontal plane function is the primary objective. Although the peroneal longus is a weak evertor relative to the peroneal brevis, this transfer is highly effective restoring

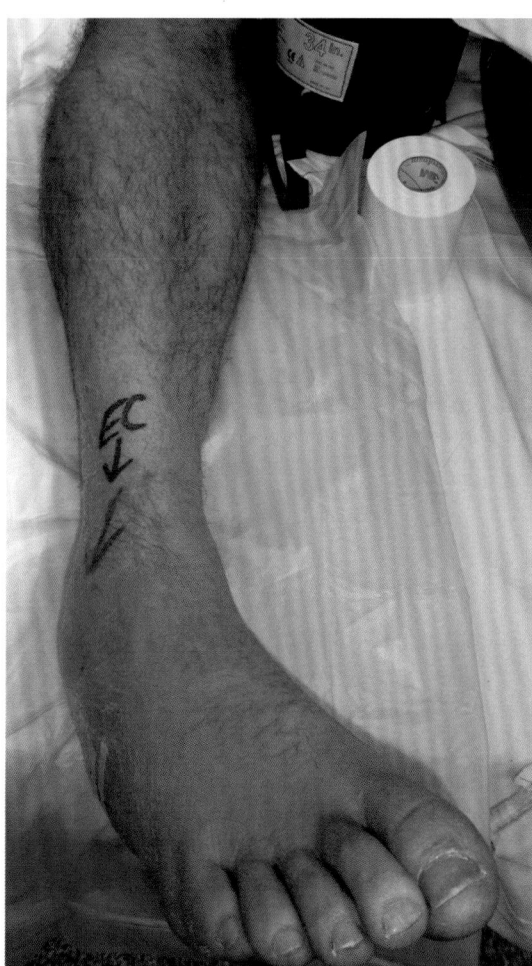

FIGURE 56.45 Without a functional peroneal brevis, the tibialis anterior and posterior overpower the modest eversion force of the peroneal longus.

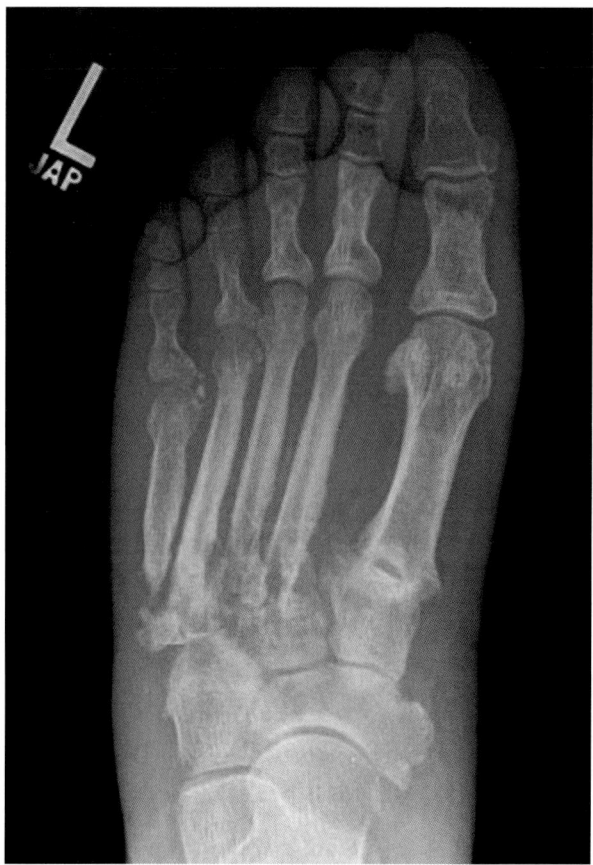

FIGURE 56.46 AP radiograph of frontal plane changes following resection of osteomyelitis of the fifth metatarsal base.

midtarsal joint pronation. In the setting of a flexible first ray, this procedure can alleviate force under the first MTPJ.

NONOPERATIVE

As long as the patient has a flexible deformity that permits a stable plantigrade foot, then bracing is a viable alternative. If, however, bracing fails to prevent ulceration or more normal ambulation, then these nonsurgical options may not be possible on a long-term basis.[89]

SURGICAL PROCEDURE AND TECHNIQUE

- An ~4- to 5-cm linear incision is made over the course of the peroneal tendons and should be centered over the calcaneal-cuboid joint (Fig. 56.47).
- This is a relatively safe zone, where the only structures at risk during dissection are the sural nerve and the peroneus brevis tendon itself. At this level, the peroneus brevis is superior and just lateral to the PL tendons. Once through the peroneal sheath, each tendon can be easily identified. Follow the path of the PL as it dives inferior to the cuboid and then confirm its action on the first ray by applying tension to it (Fig. 56.48).
- With the foot in slightly inverted to neutral position, transect the PL tendon ~1-1.5 cm proximal to its course immediately plantar to the cuboid. 2-0 nonabsorbable suture is then used to tag each end.
- With the foot still in neutral position, mark the peroneus brevis tendon ~1 cm proximal to its insertion. Align the tendons in the desired position. Prior to performing the side-to-side suturing technique, use a scalpel blade to roughen up the tendon surfaces that will be in contact. A 4-0 or 3-0 nonabsorbable suture is used to secure the proximal peroneal tendon stump to the intact peroneus brevis together (Fig. 56.49).
- Management of the distal peroneal longus stump is largely dependent on surgeon preference. With rare exception, the distal PL tendon stump should be attached to the cuboid. For simplicity, this can be achieved by direct suturing to the cuboid periosteum or with a small

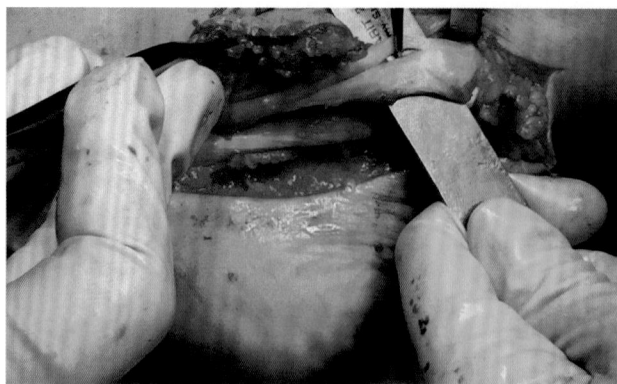

FIGURE 56.48 Evaluate and debride any pathologic peroneal brevis so that the transfer is secured to a robust substrate.

bone anchor. First ray alignment is achieved with careful tensioning such that it is maintained in a static and supported position. If a secondary goal of the procedure was to alleviate pressures beneath the first ray, then objective can be addressed at this time.

> ### *positioning* PEARLS
>
> The lateral decubitus position provides the surgeon with the best exposure, but a supine position with an ipsilateral hip bump will permit access to the medial column should a reverse Cotton also be necessary.

EXPOSURE PEARLS

If the transfer is to be performed concomitantly with a calcaneal osteotomy, then the incision placement can be altered to reflect that choice. The incision is made in a hockey stick orientation centered over the course of the peroneals. This starts ~2 cm proximal to the lateral malleolus and extends ~3 cm distal to the lateral malleolus. The same structures at risk apply and the same technique previously described applies, but the attachment site to the brevis is now more proximal. The only variation is that in some instances, the SPR may be visibly attenuated.

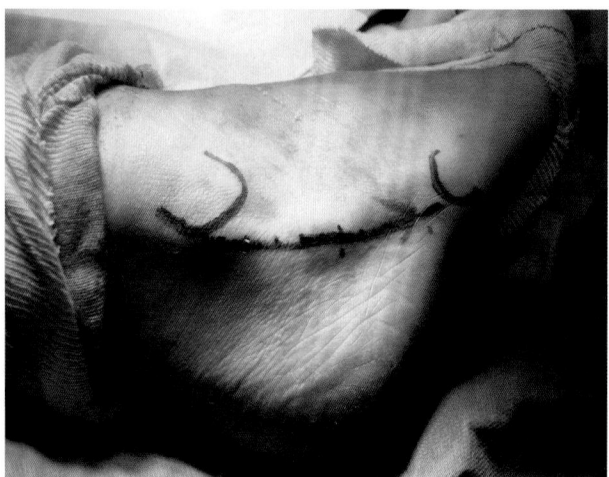

FIGURE 56.47 Incision placement for tendon transfer only without ancillary procedures.

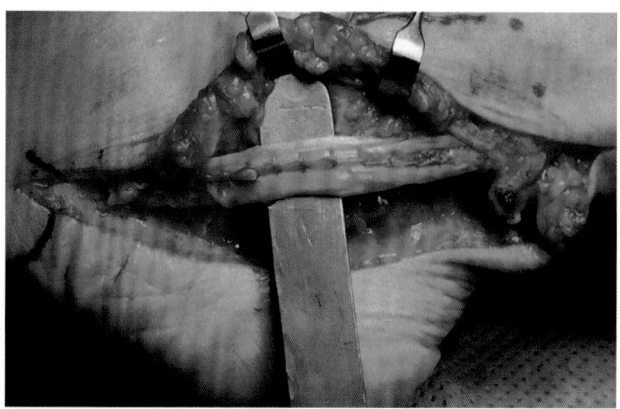

FIGURE 56.49 A locking suture technique is used to facilitate the transfer.

In those instances, the SPR can be reflected off the posterior fibula and tightened during final closure to secure the peroneal tendons into anatomic position.

AUTHORS' PREFERRED TREATMENT

- A thigh tourniquet is necessary for hemostasis.
- A side-by-side tendon transfer is our preferred technique because it is efficient and fairly robust. Some individuals may desire a Pulvertaft tendon weave for transfer. This requires a sturdy brevis and adequate length of the longus. Within the peroneal brevis, the scalpel blade should be passed longitudinally through the midsubstance of the tendon. Although the ultimate length of the incision is dictated by the diameter of the proximal PL stump, the typical incision is ~1 cm in length and care is taken to avoid transecting the tendon. A total of 2-3 longitudinal is usually applied, with each split at least 2 cm apart. The proximal PL tendon stump is then weaved through the longitudinal incisions within the peroneus brevis.

PERILS and PITFALLS

- Understanding the specific pathology is critical for optimizing outcomes. This procedure will not correct a rigid deformity; likewise, a nonfunctional peroneal longus is also ineffective.
- An MRI is helpful in evaluating the health of the peroneal tendons preoperatively. In some cases, significant tendon pathology may be present, which may direct you toward the most optimal transfer site.
- If the "weak" peroneal brevis is due to a fifth base excision or a complete rupture of the brevis, then distal attachment points must be identified. In cases where a peroneal brevis rupture occurred proximal to the fifth metatarsal insertion, the peroneal longus proximal stump can be attached to the remaining peroneal brevis stump. It is strongly recommended to back up this attachment with a small anchor into the fifth metatarsal. In some instances, a biologic sheet is used to augment the transfer site (Fig. 56.50). If an accessory bone is present, then the peroneal longus transection should occur proximal to it.
- All soft tissue releases and osseous procedures, including calcaneal osteotomy and dorsiflexory osteotomy of the medial cuneiform, should be performed prior to final balancing and transfer of the peroneal longus tendon.

POSTOPERATIVE CARE

If the peroneal longus to peroneal brevis transfer is performed with osseous procedures, then those procedures dictate postoperative care. Otherwise, immediately post-op, a well-padded posterior splint or short leg cast is applied. The foot is placed into a slightly plantar flexed and everted position in order to protect the transferred tendon. Sutures are removed per protocol ~2-3 weeks postoperatively. Educate the patient and staff to avoid foot inversion during cast and dressing changes.

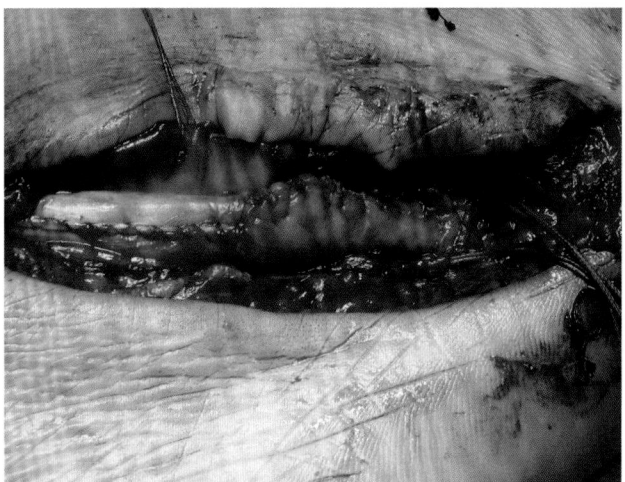

FIGURE 56.50 A soft tissue anchor is used to supplement the peroneal tendons attachment to the fifth metatarsal with a biological sheet surrounding the transfer junction.

By week 3, the patient is transferred into a removable pneumatic boot and they are permitted to begin touch-down or partial weight bearing. NWB passive ROM exercises may begin at the end of week 3 under the supervision of physical therapy.[12,29] Inversion should be avoided during these sessions.

Full weight bearing in the pneumatic boot starts at week 6 along with gradual active strengthening protocols. Final protected ambulation in sturdy high-tide boot, ankle brace, or AFO begins 8-10 weeks postoperatively (Table 56.4).

In patients in whom the tendon condition is less robust or significant pathology was evident intraoperatively, the cast is maintained for an additional week and the subsequent milestones are delayed by that week.

FLEXOR DIGITORUM LONGUS TENDON TRANSFER FOR FLATFOOT

DEFINITION

This technique involves transfer of the FDL tendon into the navicular to replace a pathologic posterior tibialis and as an adjunct for correction of flatfoot deformity. First described by Goldner and colleagues at Duke University[94] in 1974, the FDL transfer was utilized in talipes equinovalgus treatment. They reported an FDL transfer with imbrication of the spring ligament alongside lengthening of the Achilles tendon.[94] As we have gained a better understanding of the progressive stages of this condition, the surgical approach has similarly matured. Soft tissue repairs for flatfoot and flexible adult acquired flatfoot deformity (AAFD) or posterior tibial tendon dysfunction (PTTD) have gained an increased role in reconstruction alongside osseous procedures over time.

Flatfoot is a complex and dynamic deformity with a progressive nature and multiple symptoms. With better understanding of the pathomechanics and progressive imbalances leading to a flatfoot, reconstructive surgeons have advanced their approaches to correction.

CLASSIFICATION

CLASSIFICATION	
Classification for AAFD/PTTD[96,99]	
Stage	**Clinical Findings**
I *Pain along PTT without deformity or minimal deformity*	Intact medial longitudinal arch Able to single-limb heel rise with inverting calcaneus
II *Attenuation of PTT with flexible deformity*	Loss of medial longitudinal arch Forefoot abduction Forefoot supination Hindfoot can be reduced to neutral Unable to single-limb heel rise
III *Rigid hindfoot valgus*	Loss of medial longitudinal arch Unable to single-limb heel rise Hindfoot cannot be reduced to neutral
IV *Ankle valgus with flatfoot deformity*	Valgus tilting of the talus in the ankle joint on standing radiographs Stage II or III with valgus at the ankle caused by deltoid insufficiency

Originally, Johnson and Strom proposed three stages of AAFD.[95] Stage I is described as posterior tibial tendonitis alone without hindfoot valgus. Stage II encompassed flexible flatfoot and PTT elongation. This was later subdivided into stages IIa and IIb in an effort to guide surgical decision-making more effectively.[96-99] Stage IIa has less AP radiograph changes with minimal foot abduction and <30% TN joint uncovering. Stage IIb can be differentiated by a more abducted foot and a TN joint uncovering >30%.[97,98] This distinction improves osseous procedure selection by more accurately defining the deformities planar dominance. Stage III describes complete disruption of the PTT and a more rigid deformity with fixed hindfoot valgus as well as some degenerative changes. Typically, stage III will have sinus tarsi pain or subfibular impingement symptoms. As this is a progressive deformity, Myerson added a stage IV to describe the progressive changes that occur within the ankle joint. This includes valgus angulation of the talus, arthritic changes, and deltoid ligamentous complex insufficiency.[99]

INDICATIONS

INDICATIONS
■ Adult acquired flatfoot deformity
■ Reducible/flexible pes planus
■ Progressive hindfoot valgus, forefoot abduction, and forefoot varus most commonly caused by PTTD
■ PTTD stage I or II
■ Stage IIb: FDL transfer alone not adequate
■ Failed conservative management

Early stages of flatfoot (stages I and II) are traditionally treated with a modified Kidner procedure, soft tissue and sometimes bony work accompanied by an FDL transfer.[100] There remains

significant debate regarding the "best treatment" for flexible stage II deformities. More recent approaches include the FDL transfer as a component of the overall correction with trends toward joint preservation and are far less likely to be used as a stand-alone procedure. One such contemporary combination of osseous and soft tissue procedures was described by Pomeroy et al. in the "All-American" approach in 1997. This approach utilizes an FDL transfer to the medial cuneiform to improve the lever arm, a double calcaneal osteotomy with lateral column lengthening, and a medial displacement osteotomy (MDCO) as well as an Achilles or gastrocnemius lengthening as indicated.[101] To counter this, other authors have described bony approaches without tendon transfers. DiDomenico et al. discussed the need to correct the structural abnormalities of the hindfoot with extra-articular osteotomies and medial column fusion without FDL transfer and presented successful outcomes in 34 patients.[102,103]

ANATOMIC FEATURES

POSTERIOR TIBIALIS

The posterior tibial muscle originates from the posterior tibia, interosseous membrane, and the fibula, coursing through the deep posterior leg compartment, curving posterior to the medial malleolus, and inserting on to the navicular tuberosity, spring ligament, and plantar midtarsal bones.

FLEXOR DIGITORUM LONGUS

The FDL arises from the posterior aspect of the tibia and the fascia of the tibialis posterior. It becomes tendinous proximal to the ankle joint and enters the second tunnel within the tarsal tunnel. At this level, it is adjacent to the PTT and courses behind the medial malleolus. This relationship is maintained until it exits the tarsal tunnel moving laterally toward its insertion on the proximal phalanges.

MASTER KNOT OF HENRY

As the FDL and FHL emerge from their calcaneal tunnels, they share a common sheath without a separating septum. This structure begins plantar-laterally relative to the navicular tuberosity.

FUNCTIONAL ANALYSIS OF THE ANATOMY

Flexible AAFD will present with loss of arch height and weakened push-off. An imbalance facilitated by attenuation of the PTT. The PTT has a limited 1-2 cm excursion, and any fault whether major or minor will have a negative impact on the ability of the tendon to do its job.[104]

The FDL is an excellent option for replacing PTT compromise, when indicated. The FDL is in phase with the PTT and has a similar line of pull. The FDL has been shown to have similar strength to the peroneus brevis, which is the PTT's antagonist.[14] Wacker et al. described MRI findings of the PTT and FDL in patients with AAFD. They found that fatty infiltrate and complete rupture correlated with nonfunctional PTT and PTT without complete rupture showed atrophy. This study also identified hypertrophy of the FDL in these cases.[105] Following an FDL transfer, functional deficiencies are minimal. This is due to the presence of the master knot of Henry within the midfoot, which maintains the distal FDL attachment and remains

functional alongside the FHL and is further augmented by action of the FDB. Although the FDL meets many of the criteria for an optimal tendon transfer, it does not replace the PTT trajectory of its extensive distal attachments.

PHYSICAL EXAMINATION

Examination in the NWB and weight-bearing state is imperative. A relaxed stance position, heel rise, and a gait analysis are also strongly encouraged.

- The forefoot may appear abducted in relation to the rearfoot.
- There is often posteromedial hindfoot pain below the medial malleolus.
- Patients will relate a widening of the foot or a "fallen arch" over time and change in position or shape of the foot. Lateral pain at the sinus tarsi or subfibular region is also a common finding from impingement of the lateral malleolus on the calcaneus.[106]
- Gait abnormalities are commonly observed as well. These may consist of early heel-off, abductory twist, push-off weakness, or an apropulsive gait pattern.
- Typically, heel inversion is limited or absent on heel rise as well as limited ability to run or participate in sporting activity.

PATHOGENESIS

AAFD is a progressive hindfoot valgus, forefoot abduction, and forefoot varus. PTTD is the most common etiology. The PTT itself is a powerful supinator of the STJ and adductor of the midfoot. The PTT contracts in early stance to unlock the TN and calcaneocuboid (CC) joints and in toe-off to supinate the hindfoot and locking the TN and CC joints. This helps create a rigid level for propulsion by way of gastrocnemius soleus contraction.

As hindfoot valgus progresses into PTTD, the PTT attenuates and the spring ligament is left unsupported. The peroneus brevis overpowers the weakened PTT and leads to forefoot abduction. Gradual loss of arch height can be noted over time and as PTTD progresses from stage I to stage II.[107] As the hindfoot valgus and forefoot abduction progress, this leads to insufficiency of the medial column and first metatarsal elevatus or forefoot varus; initially, this will be flexible but can become rigid.[108]

IMAGING AND DIAGNOSTIC STUDIES

Plain film weight-bearing radiographs consisting of three views of the foot and ankle should be obtained. It is important in long-standing cases to assess for ankle pathology as well. Calcaneal axial and long-leg alignment views are helpful in assessing the hindfoot to leg relationship. MRI is frequently utilized to evaluate overall condition of the PTT as well as the status of the spring ligament. It also helps to ascertain if the FDL is structurally suitable for transfer.

TREATMENT

NONOPERATIVE

Symptomatic management is the mainstay of conservative care. This includes nonsteroidal anti-inflammatory medications,

physical therapy, and immobilization in a cast or pneumatic boot, shoe modifications, custom orthosis, Richie or Arizona type braces.

SURGICAL INTERVENTION

All other osteotomies and osseous procedures should be performed prior to the tendon transfer. Under thigh tourniquet control with the ipsilateral hip bumped, a posterior medial curvilinear incision from just posterior to the medial malleolus along the course of the PTT to the naviculocuneiform joint is created (Fig. 56.51). The flexor retinaculum is encountered, and all attempts to keep this structure intact at the medial malleolus should be made. Dissection continues bluntly proximal and posterior to the medial malleolus allowing for isolation of the PTT sheath. This is encountered at the level of the medial malleolus and incised down toward the navicular to release the tendon. The PTT is then inspected for tears and degeneration. Careful attention must be paid to the undersurface of the tendon, where the majority of pathology is found in earlier stages. Degenerative tendon will appear yellowed, thickened, frayed, torn or firm, and bulbous (Fig. 56.52). At this point, the decision is made as to whether or not the PTT can be debrided, repaired, augmented with a side-to-side transfer of the FDL or excised or bypassed with an FDL transfer. The spring ligament should be evaluated and built into the repair or primarily repaired with a figure-of-8 nonabsorbable stitch if amenable.

The FDL tendon is harvested through the same single medial incision. The easiest way to find the tendon and isolate it is starting proximally at the medial malleolus and isolating the tendon sheath of the FDL directly behind and below the PTT sheath (Fig. 56.53). The lesser digits can be flexed and extended to assist. At this level, the FDL tendon sheath is directly posterior and lateral to the PTT sheath. Once the tendon is isolated, the appropriate tendon should be further confirmed by applying traction on the tendon and evaluating the digital movement. With the FDL, the lesser toes will move with force while the hallux will only move slightly. In order to obtain adequate tendon length, carry the dissection more distally. Inferior to the

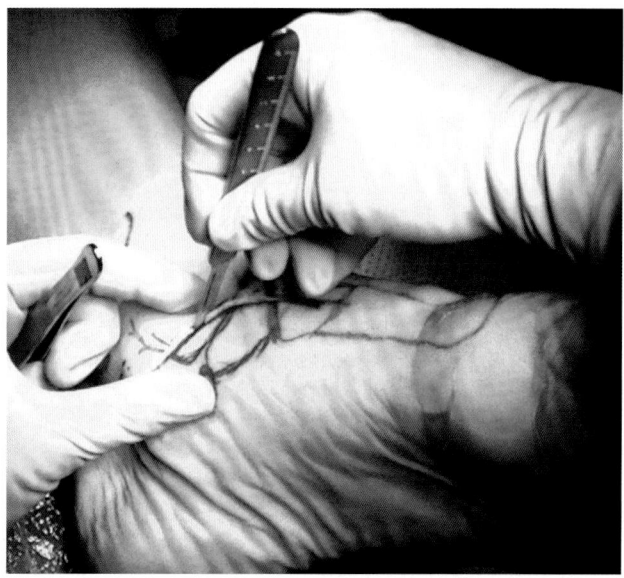

FIGURE 56.51 A medially oriented curvilinear incision permits access to both the posterior tibial tendon and the flexor digitorum longus.

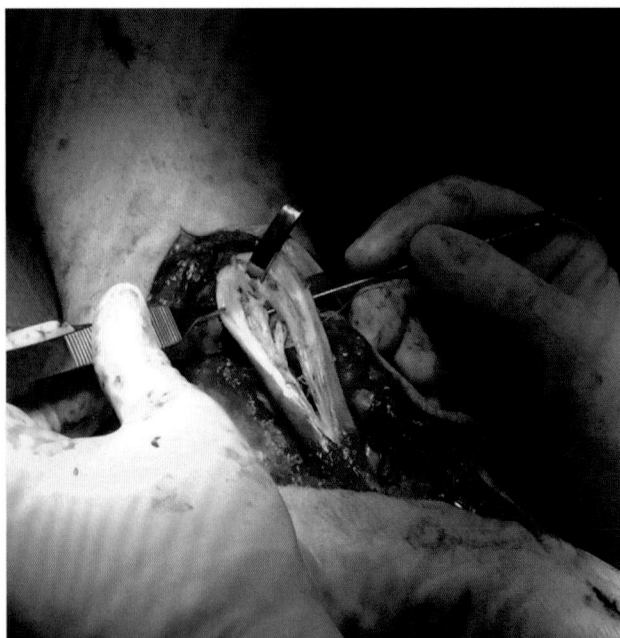

FIGURE 56.52 The tibialis posterior tendon may appear simply hypertrophic or severely diseased.

navicular, near the knot of Henry, a venous plexus is frequently encountered that can be difficult to maintain hemostasis (Fig. 56.54). Deliberate dissection and judicious use of cautery can minimize this issue. Trace the FDL as far distal as possible without disrupting the knot of Henry. It is important to avoid the medial planter branch of the tibial nerve in this area. Plantar flex the ankle, flex the digits, and invert the foot to maximize tendon length. Then, incise the tendon distally with a #15 blade. There is usually no need to secure the distal segment of the FDL, since the attachments to the FHL via the master knot of Henry are often adequate.

A whip stitch is applied to the FDL proximal stump with absorbable or nonabsorbable 0 suture (Fig. 56.55). At this point, a decision needs to be made as to where the FDL tendon will be transferred. Several options have been described such as anastomosis to the PTT, anchoring to the navicular tuberosity

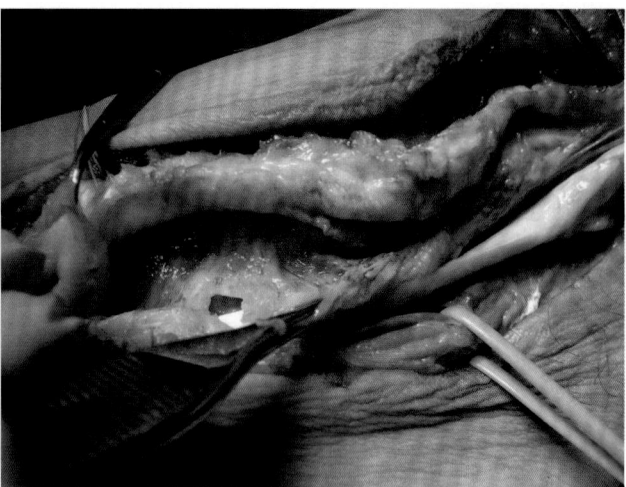

FIGURE 56.54 Careful dissection can identify the subnavicular venous plexus; vessel loops can be used to retract the veins while further dissection is performed.

or rarely to the medial cuneiform. The authors prefer to use a bone tunnel through the navicular and an interference screw. It is also the authors' preference to preserve as much of the PTT as possible. If the PTT is significantly dystrophic, then it can be sacrificed and the PTT distal stump should be preserved. Attention is brought to the navicular tuberosity, and a drill tunnel is created passing from plantar to dorsal through the navicular tuberosity and exiting in the navicular body dorsally. This allows for a more plantar transfer of the tendon into the bone.

Utilizing the interference screw system of your choice, the guidewire is drilled from the plantar medial navicular tuberosity into the dorsal body with care to avoid joint surfaces, and it exits percutaneously dorsal on the foot. The tendon is measured and a proper reamer is selected to over drill the guidewire for creation of the tendon transfer tunnel. The foot is positioned in maximal inversion and then the tendon is passed through the tunnel, and the guidewire is pulled out of the top of the foot percutaneously. There is no standardized tensioning technique; however, in the authors' experience, a more tensioned transfer is better than attempting to attain a physiologic tension since these tend to gradually stretch out over time particularly in obese patients. Tensioning this repair is usually the

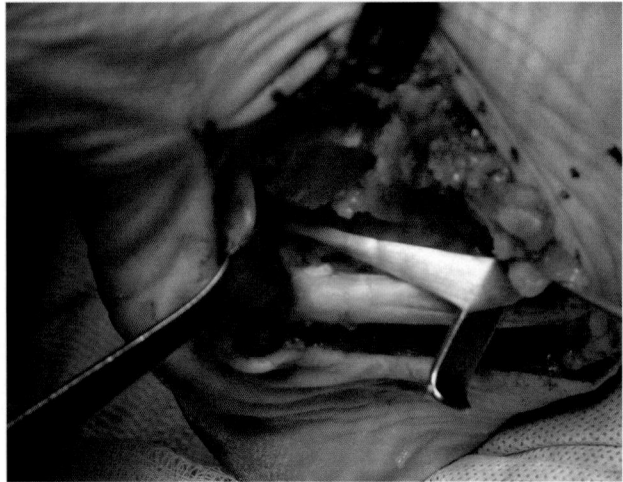

FIGURE 56.53 The FDL identified directly behind and below the PTT sheath.

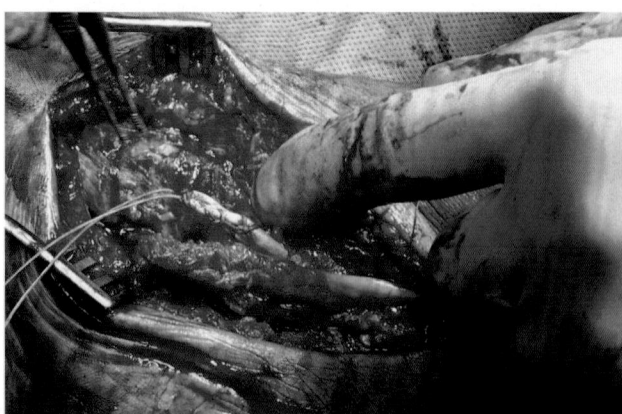

FIGURE 56.55 The FDL tendon has been whip stitched to maintain control of the tendon during insertion.

last step of the flatfoot reconstruction and will need to be protected from stress once anchored. The remaining tendon can be sutured back onto itself if there is enough length or sutured onto the distal PTT stump for additional support if it remains.

For the sake of completeness, there are traditionally four types of transfers that can be performed.

1. The first method is a side-by-side tenodesis or on lay of the FDL into the PTT.
2. One can employ an interweave technique such as Pulvertaft with the FDL weaved into the PTT.
3. Anchoring to bone or through a tunnel using a tendon anchor or interference screw technique as described above with the tenodesis or interference screw of surgeon choice.
   a. We prefer to use a nonmetallic interference screw.
4. Lastly, one can use a classic drill hole through the navicular with the FDL being sewn back upon itself and the periosteum to hold fixation of the tendon.

What to do with the PTT:

Some authors excise the PTT with the theory that it is a pain generator and will not function in the future, while others keep it intact or debride and repair it.[14,19] Aronow discussed the bulky nature of a hypertrophied PTT with the repair and tight flexor retinaculum closure relating increased scar tissue and pain postoperative in these cases.[19] There is no definitive evidence to suggest one over the other at this time. The authors will always intraoperatively evaluate the tendon; however, in cases of degeneration and substantial dysfunction, we will excise the PTT. If there is viable tendon remaining, it can be left intact or a tenodesis side-by-side to the FDL can be performed at the same time. We suggest that MRI and intraoperative findings guide these decisions on a case-by-case basis. Interestingly, a study by Rosenfeld et al. looked at patients who underwent an FDL transfer and medial displacement calcaneal osteotomy (MDCO) for stage II AAFD. They compared contralateral sides by MRI and found a mean 23% atrophy of the PTT and mean 27% hypertrophy of the FDL. They further found when the PTT was maintained, the FDL was hypertrophied 11% at 14 months. While in the PTT excision group, the FDL was hypertrophied 44% suggesting that excising the PTT is a more functional tendon transfer.[109]

positioning **PEARLS**

- Supine with the patient's heel slightly off the end of the bed.
- Use of a bump is largely dependent on the concomitant procedures.
- A thigh tourniquet is preferred to decrease tension on tendon for transfer.
- Ensure that fluoroscopy is available and positioned on the operative side for ease of use.

AUTHORS' PREFERRED TREATMENT

The authors prefer to perform an FDL transfer I to the navicular with a PEEK interference screw. The tunnel is drilled plantar to dorsal through and through from the navicular tuberosity to the dorsal body ensuring not to violate the adjacent joints. This provides a strong anchoring point within the body of the navicular reducing the risk for fracture. These procedures are usually complemented with osseous procedures such as an MDCO and/or lateral column lengthening as clinically indicated. Most commonly, we prefer a Cotton medial cuneiform osteotomy or other medial column procedure to address forefoot varus or insufficiency. If the patient has an existing hallux valgus deformity, then a Lapidus procedure is preferred in place of a Cotton osteotomy. We always address any equinus present whether gastrocnemius, soleus, or a combination.

EXPOSURE AND SURGICAL PERILS AND PITFALLS

- Be sure that the surgical plan addresses equinus, hindfoot, and forefoot osseous pathology; if not addressed, the FDL will likely suffer a similar fate as the PTT.
- Evaluate for coalition, rigidity, or peroneal spasm; these can change your surgical approach.
- Avoid transferring a dystrophic, weak, or nonfunctional FDL.
- Avoid applying a draping barrier over toes 1-5 as a unit. Instead, isolate the hallux from the lesser digits to help differentiate FHL and FDL.
- Avoid over dissecting the master knot of Henry, too much leads to loss of the connection with the FHL. This can be left intact as less tendon is required if anchoring with an interference screw.
- If the FDL is significantly hypertrophic, be sure to taper it to a caliber that the navicular can tolerate, taper at least the length of the implant being used.
- Overtensioning, although these authors will over tension knowing the repair with stretch.
- Overzealous drilling can lead to navicular fracture.
- Failure to address forefoot varus or medial column insufficiency.

POSTOPERATIVE CARE AND REHABILITATION

The authors will utilize a supinated cast applied in the operating room to hold the repair and off-load stress on the FDL transfer. These casts can be bivalved as needed to allow for edema. For an FDL transfer and gastrocnemius lengthening alone, which is less common, the patient will be NWB for 2-4 weeks with the goal of initiating passive ROM at week 3. Progressive rehabilitation begins with ROM exercises and nonimpact activity including strengthening, proprioceptive training, and eccentric and isotonic exercises. By weeks 6-8, the patient is transitioned to a supportive sneaker with orthotic. High-impact activity is typically avoided until weeks 12 or later (Table 56.4).

The FDL tendon transfer is rarely performed as a standalone procedure, and other procedures will often take precedent for weight bearing and advancement into physical therapy. Rehab typically will start early, 4 weeks if possible. This will aid in edema control, improve ROM, decrease scar tissue formation, assist with weight-bearing transition, retrain tendon function, and build strength.

REFERENCES

1. Platt MA. Tendon repair and healing. *Clin Podiatr Med Surg.* 2005;22:553-560.
2. Benjamin M, Ralphs J. Tendons and ligaments—an overview. *Histol Histopathol.* 1997;12:1135-1144.
3. Miller S, Groves MJ. Principles of muscle-tendon surgery and tendon transfers. In: McGlamry ED, ed. *Comprehensive Textbook of Foot Surgery*, vol. 2. Philadelphia, PA: Lippincott Williams & Wilkins; 2001:1523-1566.
4. Armagan O, Shereff M. Tendon injury and repair. In: Myerson M, ed. *Foot and Ankle Disorders*, vol. 2. Philadelphia, PA: WB Saunders; 2000:942-971.
5. Fenwick S, Hazleman B, Riley G. The vasculature and its role in the damaged and healing, tendon. *Arthritis Res.* 2002;4:252-260.
6. Kendall FP, McCreary EK, Provance PF, et al. Fundamental concepts. In: Lappies P, ed. *Muscles: Testing and Function, With Posture and Pain*. 5th ed. Baltimore, MD: Lippincott Williams & Wilkins; 2005:1-48.
7. Daniels L, Worthingham K. Techniques of manual examination. In: *Muscle Testing*. 7th ed. Philadelphia, PA: WB Saunders Co.; 2002.
8. Martin EG, Lovett RW. A method of testing muscular strength in infantile paralysis. *JAMA.* 1915;LXV(18):1512-1513.
9. Samilson RL, Dillin W. Cavus, cavovarus, and calcaneovarus: an update. *Clin Orthop.* 1983;177:125-132.
10. Ward SR, Eng CM, Smallwood LH, Lieber RL. Are current measurements of lower extremity muscle architecture accurate? *Clin Orthop Relat Res.* 2009;467(4):1074-1082.
11. Sarrafian Shahan K, Kelikian Armen S. Functional anatomy of the foot and ankle. In: *Sarrafian's Anatomy of the Foot and Ankle*. 2nd ed. Philadelphia, PA: Lippincott Williams & Wilkins; 2011:507-643.
12. van Dijk PAD, Lubberts B, Verheul C. Rehabilitation after surgical treatment of peroneal tendon tears and ruptures. *Knee Surg Sports Traumatol Arthrosc.* 2016;24:1165.
13. Clark G, Lui E, Cook K. Tendon balancing in pedal amputations. *Clin Podiatr Med Surg.* 2005;22:447-467.
14. Silver RL, De La Garza J, Rang M. The myth of muscle balance: a study of relative muscle strengths and excursions of normal muscles about the foot and ankle. *J Bone Joint Surg Br.* 1985;67:432-437.

Interosseous Posterior Tibial Tendon Transfer

15. Shane AM, Reeves CL, Cameron JD, Vazales R. Posterior tibial tendon transfer. *Clin Podiatr Med Surg.* 2016;33:29-40.
16. Watkins M, Jones JB, Ryder CT, et al. Transplantation of the posterior tibial tendon. *J Bone Joint Surg Am.* 1954;36:1181-1189.
17. Root L, Miller S, Kirz P. Posterior tibial tendon transfer in patients with cerebral palsy. *J Bone Joint Surg Am.* 1987;69:1133-1139.
18. Pinzur M, Kett N, Trilla M. Combined anteroposterior tibial tendon transfer in post-traumatic peroneal palsy. *Foot Ankle.* 1988;8:271-275.
19. Aronow MS. Tendon transfer options in managing the adult flexible flatfoot. *Foot Ankle Clin N Am.* 2012;17:205-226.
20. Mann RA. Tendon transfers and electromyography. *Clin Orthop Relat Res.* 1972;85:64-66.
21. Waters R, Frazier J, Garland D. Electromyographic gait analysis before and after operative treatment for hemiplegic equinus and equinovarus deformity. *J Bone Joint Surg Am.* 1982;64:284-288.
22. Dreher T, Wolf SI, Heitzmann D, et al. Tibialis posterior tendon transfer corrects the foot drop component of cavovarus foot deformity in Charcot-Marie-Tooth disease. *J Bone Joint Surg Am.* 2014;96:456-462.
23. Easley ME, Scott AT. Tendon transfer for foot drop. In: Easley ME, ed. *Operative Techniques in Foot and Ankle Surgery*. Philadelphia, PA: Lippincott Williams & Wilkins; 2011.
24. Thamphongsri K, Harnroongroj T, Jarusriwanna A, Chuckpaiwong B. How to harvest the greatest length of tibialis posterior tendon for tendon transfer: a cadaveric study. *Clin Anat.* 2017;30:1083-1086.
25. Wagner P, Ortiz C, Vela O, et al. Interosseous membrane window size for tibialis posterior tendon transfer—geometrical and MRI analysis. *Foot Ankle Surg.* 2016;22:196-199.
26. Wagner E, Wagner P, Zanolli D, et al. Biomechanical evaluation of circumtibial and transmembranous routes for posterior tibial tendon transfer for dropfoot. *Foot Ankle Int.* 2018;39:843-849.
27. Marsland D, Stephen JM, Calder T, et al. Strength of interference screw fixation to cuboid vs Pulvertaft weave to peroneus brevis for tibialis posterior tendon transfer for foot drop. *Foot Ankle Int.* 2018;39:858-864.
28. Kuo KN, Wu KW, Krzak JJ, Smith PA. Tendon transfers around the foot: when and where. *Foot Ankle Clin N Am.* 2015;20:601-617.
29. Landsman A, Cook E, Cook J. Tenotomy and tendon transfer about the forefoot, midfoot, and hindfoot. *Clin Podiatr Med Surg.* 2008;25:547-569.

Bridle Procedure

30. Johnson JE, Paxton ES, Lippe J, et al. Outcomes of the Bridle procedure for the treatment of foot drop. *Foot Ankle Int.* 2015;36:1287-1296.
31. Myerson MS, Kadakia AR. *Reconstructive Foot and Ankle Surgery: Management of Complications.* 3rd ed. Philadelphia, PA: Elsevier; 2018.

Hibbs Tenosuspension

32. Hibbs RA. An operation for "clawfoot". *JAMA.* 1919;73:1583-1585.
33. DiDomenico LA, Luckino FAIII, Butto DN. Tendon transfers for digital deformities and hammertoes. In: Cook EA, Cook JJ, eds. *Hammertoes.* Switzerland: Springer Nature Switzerland AG; 2019:209-239.

34. Hansen S Jr. Transfer of the extensor digitorum communis to the midfoot. In: *Functional Reconstruction of the Foot and Ankle.* Philadelphia, PA: Lippincott; 2000:451.
35. Boberg J, Eilts C. Lesser digital deformities: etiology, procedure selection, and arthroplasty. In: Southerland JT, et al., eds. *McGlamry's Comprehensive Textbook of Foot and Ankle Surgery.* Philadelphia, PA: Lippincott; 2013:117-123.
36. Richardson BA, Knabel M, Swenson E. Anatomy of the intermetatarsal, lesser metatarsophalangeal and lesser interphalangeal joints. In: Cook EA, Cook JJ, eds. *Hammertoes.* Switzerland: Springer Nature Switzerland AG; 2019:1-19.
37. Boberg JS. Surgical decision making in hammertoe surgery. In: Vickers NS, et al., eds. *Reconstructive Surgery of the Foot and Leg: Update 1997.* Tucker, GA: Podiatry Institute; 1997:3-6.
38. Cook EA, Cook JJ, Cook R. Lesser MTPJ reconstruction. In: Cook EA, Cook JJ, eds. Hammertoes. Switzerland: Springer Nature Switzerland AG; 2019:265-286.
39. Schwend RM, Drennan JC. Cavus foot deformity in children. *J Am Acad Orthop Surg.* 2003;11:201-211.
40. Bouchard JL, Castellano BD. Clawtoe deformities and contractures of the forefoot. In: Camasta CA, Vickers NS, Ruch JA, eds. *Reconstructive Surgery of the Foot and Leg, Update 1988.* Tucker, GA: Podiatry Institute Publishing; 1998:14-21.
41. Piazza S, Ricci G, Ineco EC, et al. Pes cavus and hereditary neuropathies: when a relationship should be suspected. *J Orthop Traumatol.* 2010;11:195-201.
42. Boffeli TJ, Tabatt JA. Minimally invasive early operative treatment of progressive foot and ankle deformity associated with Charcot-Marie-Tooth Disease. *J Foot Ankle Surg.* 2015;54:701-708.
43. Grambart ST. Hibbs Tenosuspension. *Clin Podiatr Med Surg.* 2016;33:63-69.

Jones Tenosuspension

44. Jones R. The soldier's foot and the treatment of common deformities of the foot, part II. *Br Med J.* 1916;1:749-753.
45. Abousayed M, Kwon JY. Hallux claw toe. *Foot Ankle Clin.* 2014;19(1):59-63.
46. Giannini S, Girolammi M, Ceccarelli F, et al. Modified Jones operation in the treatment of pes cavovarus. *Ital J Orthop Traumatol.* 1985;11:165-170.
47. Wood WA. Acquired hallux varus: a new corrective procedure. *J Foot Surg.* 1981;20:194-197.
48. Faraj A. A modified Jones procedure for post-polio claw hallux deformity. *J Foot Ankle Surg.* 1997;36(5):356-359.
49. Pareyson D, Scaioli V, Laura M. Clinical and electrophysiological aspects of Charcot-Marie-Tooth disease. *Neuromolecular Med.* 2006;8:3-22.

FHL Tendon Transfer

50. Lagergren C, Lindholm A. Vascular distribution in the Achilles tendon; an angiographic and microangiographic study. *Acta Chir Scand.* 1959;116:491-495.
51. Marks RM. Achilles tendinopathy, peritendinitis, pantendinitis, and insertional disorders. *Foot Ankle Clin.* 1999;4:789-810.
52. Jozsa L, Kvist M, Balint BJ. The role of recreational sport activity in Achilles tendon rupture: a clinical, pathoanatomical and sociological study of 292 cases. *Am J Sport Med.* 1989;17:338-343.
53. Wong M, Ng S. Modified flexor hallucis longus transfer for Achilles insertional rupture in elderly patients. *Clin Orthop.* 2005;431:201-206.
54. Maffulli N, Ajis A, Longo UG, et al. Chronic rupture of the tendon Achilles. *Foot Ankle Clin.* 2007;12(4):583-596.
55. Wapner KL, Pavlock GS, Hecht PJ, et al. Repair of chronic Achilles tendon rupture with flexor hallucis longus tendon transfer. *Foot Ankle Int.* 1993;14:443-449.
56. McGarvey WC, Palumbo RC, Baxter DE, et al. Insertional Achilles tendinosis. Surgical treatment through a central tendon splitting approach. *Foot Ankle Int.* 2002;23:19-25.
57. Sebastian H, Datta B, Maffulli N, et al. Mechanical properties of reconstructed Achilles tendon with transfer of peroneus brevis or flexor hallucis longus tendon. *J Foot Ankle Surg.* 2007;46(6):424-428.
58. Raikin SM, Elias I, Bessler MP, et al. Reconstruction of retracted Achilles tendon rupture with V-Y lengthening and FHL tendon. *Foot Ankle Int.* 2007;28:1238-1248.
59. Raikin SM. Chronic Achilles tendon ruptures using V-Y advancement and FHL transfer. In: Easley ME, Wiesel SW, eds. *Operative Techniques in Foot and Ankle Surgery*. Philadelphia, PA: Lippincott Williams & Wilkins; 2011.
60. DeCarbo WT, Hyer CF. Interference screw fixation for flexor hallucis longus tendon transfer for chronic Achilles tendinopathy. *J Foot Ankle Surg.* 2008;47(1):69-72.
61. Martin RL, Manning DM, Carcia CR, et al. An outcome study of chronic Achilles tendinosis after excision of the Achilles tendon and flexor hallucis longus tendon transfer. *Foot Ankle Clin.* 2007;12(4):583-596.

Digital FDL Tendon Transfer

62. Coughlin M, Dorris J, Polk E. Operative repair of the fixed hammertoe deformity. *Foot Ankle Int.* 2000;21:94-104.
63. Didomenico L, Rollandini J. A closer look at tendon transfers for crossover hammertoe. *Podiatry Today.* 2014;27:44-51.
64. Bus SA, Maas M, de Lange A, Michels RP, et al. Elevated plantar pressures in neuropathic diabetic patients with claw/hammer toe deformity. *J Biomech.* 2005;38:1918-1925.
65. Bhatia D, Myerson MS, Curtis MJ. Anatomical restraints to dislocation of the second metatarsophalangeal joint and assessment of repair technique. *J Bone Joint Surg Am.* 1994;75:1371.
66. Ford L, Collins K, Christensen J. Stabilization of the subluxed second metatarsophalangeal joint: flexor tendon transfer versus primary repair of the plantar plate. *J Foot Ankle Surg.* 1998;37:217-222.
67. Thompson F, Hamilton W. Problem of the second metatarsophalangeal joint. *Orthopedics.* 1987;10:83-89.

68. Butterworth M. Tendon transfers for management of digital and lesser metatarsophalangeal joint deformities. *Clin Podiatr Med Surg*. 2016;33:71-84.
69. Niklas B. Surgical management of digital deformities. In: *Hallux Valgus and Forefoot Surgery*. New York: Churchill; 1994:359-357.

STATT

70. Ponseti IV, Campos J. The classic: observations on pathogenesis and treatment of congenital clubfoot. *Clin Orthop Relat Res*. 2009;467:1124-1132.
71. Hoffer MM, Reiswig JA, Garrett AM, et al. The split anterior tibial tendon transfer in the treatment of spastic varus hindfoot of childhood. *Orthop Clin North Am*. 1974;5:31-38.
72. Hoffer MM, Barakat G, Koffman M. 10-year follow-up of split anterior tibial tendon transfer in cerebral palsied patients with spastic equinovarus deformity. *J Pediatr Orthop*. 1985;5:432-434.
73. Lampasi M, Bettuzzi C, Palmonari M, et al. Transfer of the tendon of tibialis anterior in relapsed congenital clubfoot: long-term results in 38 feet. *J Bone Joint Surg Br*. 2010;92:277-283.
74. Mulhern JL, Protzman NM, Brigido SA. Tibialis anterior tendon transfer. *Clin Podiatr Med Surg*. 2016;33:41-53.
75. Thompson GH, Hoyen HA, Barthel T. Tibialis anterior tendon transfer after clubfoot surgery. *Clin Orthop Relat Res*. 2009;467:1306-1313.
76. Johnson CH. Tendon transfers. In: Chang TJ, ed. *Master Techniques in Podiatric Surgery: The Foot and Ankle*. Philadelphia, PA: Lippincott Williams & Wilkins; 2004:249-263.
77. Kuo KN, Hennigan SP, Hastings ME. Anterior tibial tendon transfer in residual dynamic clubfoot deformity. *J Pediatr Orthop*. 2001;21:35-41.
78. Hamel J. Early results after tibialis anterior tendon transfer for severe varus in total ankle replacement. *Foot Ankle Int*. 2012;33:553-559.
79. Dreher T, Wenz W. Tendon transfers for the balancing of hind and mid-foot deformities in adults and children. *Tech Foot Ankle Surg*. 2009;8:178-189.
80. Ortiz C, Wagner E. Tendon transfers in cavovarus foot. *Foot Ankle Clin N Am*. 2014;19:49-58.
81. Atesalp S, Bek D, Demiralp B, et al. Correction of residual dynamic varus deformity using the tibialis anterior tendon. *J Bone Joint Surg Br*. 2006;88:23-24.
82. Krzak JJ, Corcos DM, Graf A, et al. Effect of fine wire electrode insertion on gait patterns in children with hemiplegic cerebral palsy. *Gait Posture*. 2013;37:251-257.
83. Hosalkar H, Goebel J, Reddy S, et al. Fixation techniques for split anterior tibialis transfer in spastic equinovarus feet. *Clin Orthop Relat Res*. 2008;466:2500-2506.
84. Drakos MC, Gott M, Karnovsky SC, et al. Biomechanical analysis of suture anchor vs tenodesis screw for FHL transfer. *Foot Ankle Int*. 2017;38:797-801.
85. Wu KW, Huang SC, Kuo KN, et al. The use of bio-absorbable screw in a split anterior tibial tendon transfer: a preliminary result. *J Pediatr Orthop B*. 2009;18:69-72.
86. Vogt JC, Bach G, Cantini B, Perrin S. Split anterior tibial tendon transfer for varus equinus spastic foot deformity Initial clinical findings correlate with functional results: a series of 132 operated feet. *Foot Ankle Surg*. 2011;17:178-181.
87. Radler C, Gourdine-Shaw MC, Herzenberg JE. Nerve structures at risk in the plantar side of the foot during anterior tibial tendon transfer: a cadaver study. *J Bone Joint Surg Am*. 2012;94:349-355.
88. Chang CH, Albarracin JP, Lipton GE, et al. Long-term follow-up of surgery for equinovarus foot deformity in children with cerebropalsy. *J Pediatr Orthop*. 2002;22:792-799.

PL to PB Tendon Transfer

89. Coughlin J. Disorders of tendons. In: Hurley R, ed. *Surgery of the Foot and Ankle*. 7th ed. vol. 2. St. Louis, MO: Mosby; 1999:786-861.
90. Hamilton GA, Ford LA, Perez H, et al. Salvage of the neuropathic foot by using bone resection and tendon balancing: a retrospective review of 10 patients. *J Foot Ankle Surg*. 2005;44:37-44.
91. Matthews J. The developmental anatomy of the foot. *Foot*. 1998;8(1):17-25.
92. Manoli A II, Graham B. The subtle cavus foot, "the underpronator". *Foot Ankle Int*. 2005;26(3):256-263.
93. Deben SE, Pomeroy GC. Subtle cavus foot: diagnosis and management. *J Am Acad Orthop Surg*. 2014;22:512-520.

FDL Transfer for Flatfoot

94. Goldner JL, Keats PK, Bassett FH III, et al. Progressive talipes equinovalgus due to trauma or degeneration of the posterior tibial tendon and medial plantar ligaments. *Orthop Clin North Am*. 1974;5:39-51.
95. Johnson KA, Strom DE. Tibialis posterior tendon dysfunction. *Clin Orthop*. 1989;239:196-206.
96. Deland JT. Adult acquired flatfoot deformity. *J Am Acad Orthop Surg*. 2008;16(7):399-406.
97. Deland JT, Page A, Sung IH, et al. Posterior tibial tendon insufficiency results at different stages. *HSS J*. 2006;2:157-160.
98. Vora AM, Tien TR, Parks BG, et al. Correction of moderate and severe acquired flexible flatfoot with medializing calcaneal displacement osteotomy and flexor digitorum longus tendon transfer. *J Bone Joint Surg Am*. 2006;88(8):1726-1734.
99. Myerson MS. Adult acquired flatfoot deformity. *J Bone Joint Surg Am*. 1996;78(5):780-792.
100. Maskill JT, Pomeroy GC. Flexor digitorum longus tendon transfer and modified Kidner technique in posterior tibial tendon dysfunction. *Clin Podiatr Med Surg*. 2016;33:15-20.
101. Pomeroy GC, Manoli A II. A new operative approach for flatfoot secondary to posterior tibial tendon insufficiency: a preliminary report. *Foot Ankle Int*. 1997;18(4):206-212.
102. Didomenico LA, Thomas ZM, Fahim R. Addressing stage II posterior tibial tendon dysfunction: biomechanically repairing the osseous structures without the need of performing the flexor digitorum longus transfer. *Clin Podiatr Med Surg*. 2014;31:391-404.
103. Didomenico LA, Stein DY, Wargo-Dorsey M. Treatment of posterior tibial tendon dysfunction without flexor digitorum tendon transfer: a retrospective study of 34 patients. *J Foot Ankle Surg*. 2011;50:293-298.
104. Haddad SL, Mann RA. Flatfoot in adults. In: Coughlin MJ, Mann RA, Saltzman C, eds. *Surgery of the Foot and Ankle*. 8th ed. St Louis, MO: Mosby; 2011:1007-1086.
105. Wacker JT, Calder JD, Engstrom CM, et al. MR morphometry of posterior tibialis muscle in adult acquired flatfoot. *Foot Ankle Int*. 2003;24(4):354-357.
106. Malicky ES, Crary JL, Houghton MJ, et al. Talocalcaneal and subfibular impingement in symptomatic flatfoot in adults. *J Bone Joint Surg Am*. 2002;84:2005-2009.
107. Gazdag AR, Cracchiolo A III. Rupture of the posterior tibial tendon: evaluation of injury of the spring ligament and clinical assessment of tendon transfer and ligament repair. *J Bone Joint Surg Am*. 1997;79:675-681.
108. Cohen BE, Ogden F. Medial column procedures in the acquired flatfoot deformity. *Foot Ankle Clin*. 2007;12:287-299, Vi.
109. Rosenfeld PF, Dick J, Saxby TS. The response of the flexor digitorum longus and posterior tibial muscles to tendon transfer and calcaneal osteotomy for stage II posterior tibial tendon dysfunction. *Foot Ankle Int*. 2005;26:671-674.

Tendon Tears/Lacerations

John T. Marcoux and Sara Shirazi

Tendon trauma results from exogenous and/or endogenous insult to the tendon. Although the mechanism of injury can differ, evaluation and treatment principles between acute and chronic tendon injuries are similar. Exogenous tendon trauma often results from acute laceration or crush injuries. Endogenous tendon injuries are usually attritional in nature and develop from repetitive stress applied to the tendon leading to reactive tendinopathy, tendon disrepair, and degenerative tendinopathy. In some instances, an acute on chronic tendon injury occurs when a specific high-intensity event leads to an acute rupture in an underlying pathologic tendon.[1]

Tears and lacerations about the foot and ankle are encountered fairly routinely by foot and ankle surgeons. Acute tendon lacerations may not always be readily appreciated by the patient or by emergency room/urgent care providers. It is imperative that as the foot and ankle specialist, you have a high index of suspicion any time a laceration penetrates through the deep fascia about the foot and ankle. Appropriate management of lower extremity tendon injuries requires a thorough understanding of the mechanism of injury as well as an accurate and thorough examination in order to deliver a timely diagnosis. An advanced understanding of anatomy and imaging modalities and knowledge of available treatment options will help to achieve recovery of tendon strength and excursion. Failure to diagnose a tendon laceration can lead to long-term functional consequences and disability. Neglected or inadequate repair may also lead to an imbalance between the tendon and its antagonist, which results in biomechanical deformity, compensation, or predisposition to adverse sequelae such as arthrosis or ulceration in some patients. It is also important to recognize that these conditions not only impact quality of life but result in both a direct and indirect economic burden to the patient and health care system.[2-4]

This chapter will serve to expand on the general knowledge of the management of common acute and chronic tendon lacerations and ruptures about the foot and ankle with the exception of Achilles tendon disorders/tears, which is discussed in Chapter 58. It will discuss tendon anatomy, current models on tendon pathology, and healing as well as the general principles including pearls and pitfalls of the physical examination, diagnostic imaging modalities, and surgical options.

ANATOMY AND FUNCTION

Tendons primary functional responsibility is to translate the load of muscular contractions to joint movement. The principal role of the tendon is to resist tension; however, they must allow for a certain degree of compliance within musculoskeletal biomechanics. A tendon is stronger per unit area than muscle and has a tensile strength approximately equal to bone but with additional flexibility, elasticity, and extensibility. The parallel arrangement of collagen fibers acts to resist tension so that contractile energy is not lost during load transmission. The loads encountered in everyday activities are typically well below the tissues ultimate tensile strength; however, in quick eccentric contraction that can occur with rapid deceleration, more significant stresses can be observed, which can result in tendon injury.[5,6]

Tendons are living connective tissue, which consist of dense yet flexible type I collagen fibrils oriented in a parallel fashion embedded in a hydrated proteoglycan matrix. The structure is maintained by tenocytes, which are primarily responsible for maintaining the extracellular matrix in response to its environment. The smallest structural unit is the collagen fibril. Each fibril is built from soluble tropocollagen molecules forming cross-links to create insoluble collagen molecules, which then aggregate progressively into microfibrils, fibrils, and finally fibers. Bundles of fibers are bound together by thin layers of loose connective tissue known as the epi- and endotenon, which allow the fiber groups to glide on each other in an almost frictionless manner. They also carry blood vessels, nerves, and lymphatics to the deeper portions of the tendon. The paratenon in tendons with a straight course or the synovial sheath in tendons with an angle course supports the entire tendon and is composed of a loose, fatty, areolar tissue, or synovial sheath (Fig. 57.1).[7] This three-dimensional structure provides the tendon with high tensile force and resilience while preventing separation of the fibers under mechanical stress.

In the past, it was generally believed that tendons were avascular with low metabolic activity. We now understand that the tendon derives its blood supply from several main sources. An understanding of this vascular supply is necessary in order to ensure that healing can be observed after either acute injury or surgical repair. Tendons obtain their blood supply from muscular branches at the myotendinous junction, vessels from the mesotenon or paratenon, and lastly vessels at the tendo-osseous junction. The branches from the myotendinous junction only supply the distal or proximal one-third of the tendon, and the mesotenon provides circulation to the entirety of the tendon. There are some areas of compromised vasculature, which is believed to lead to predictably weak areas predisposed to rupture.[8]

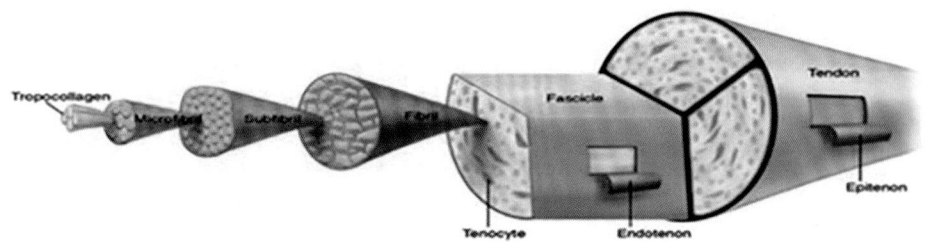

FIGURE 57.1 Schematic diagram showing the organization of the components of a collagen fiber.

TENDON INJURY/TENDINOPATHY

PATHOGENESIS

Controversy surrounds the pathogenesis of tendinopathy as it is not fully understood at the current time. There is a multitude of extrinsic and intrinsic factors that may influence the development of tendinopathy.[9] Extrinsic factors include occupation, sporting activities, local environmental conditions, posture, and biomechanical factors. Intrinsic factors include age, gender, body weight, anatomic variation, and systemic diseases such as diabetes mellitus.[10,11]

It is extremely rare for a healthy tendon to develop a spontaneous intrasubstance tendon rupture following rapid, strong tensile loading of the tendon. These individuals are more likely to develop an avulsion fracture at the tendon insertion site or myofascial injury. Tendons in the foot such as the tibialis posterior, peroneal tendons, and Achilles tendon are much more likely to develop attritional tears based upon the biomechanical stresses applied to them. Repetitive eccentric loading of these tendons is implicated as a major etiology in the development of progressive tendinopathy and subsequent rupture. Characteristic changes occur in tendon structure that results in a tendon being incapable of sustaining repeated tensile loads. Acute overload within the tendon is sensed by the tenocyte, which results in a cascade of cell-based reactive physiologic responses.[12]

Several models regarding the etiology for tendon pathology have been proposed. These have been divided in three main categories:

1. Collagen disruption/tearing
2. Inflammation
3. Tendon cell response

Cook and Purdam in 2009 proposed a model of tendon pathology based around a continuum model, which incorporates clinical, histological, and imaging information. Their model describes the early stages of reactive tendon pathology as a noninflammatory, proliferative tissue reaction, usually in response to acute overload or compression.[13] The tendon thickens due to the up-regulation of large proteoglycans and an increase in bound water, with minimal collagen damage or separation. Tendon dysrepair is characterized by greater tissue matrix breakdown, with collagen separation, proliferation of abnormal tenocytes, and some increase in tendon neovascularity. These two stages are considered to have some degree of reversibility if provided an appropriate healing environment. The final stage is degenerative tendinopathy, an essentially irreversible stage, which sees further disruption of collagen, widespread cell death, and extensive ingrowth of neovessels and nerves into the tendon substance. This model of tendinopathy development attempts to provide a framework describing what treatments might be best aligned with the stage of tendinopathy, along with descriptions of the clinical presentation of each stage.[12,14,15,58]

TENDON HEALING

The stages of tendon healing have been studied primarily from experimentally induced tendon damage in animal models. There are three main phases of tendon healing each with its own particular cellular and molecular cascades (Table 57.1). The phases of healing overlap, and their duration is dependent on the location and severity of the tendon damage. The initial phase is an *inflammatory stage* that begins in the first 48-72 hours after injury. The blood vessels within the tendon sheath create the formation of a hematoma. The resulting clot releases

TABLE 57.1	The Three Phases of Tendon Healing	
Stages of Tendon Healing		
Inflammatory	The blood vessels within the tendon sheath create the formation of a hematoma. The resulting clot releases various chemotactic factors, which attract inflammatory cells.	48-72 h
Repair/proliferative	Recruitment of various growth factors to provide a vascular network responsible for the survival of newly forming fibrous tissue at the injury site.	Begins day 3 to 6 wk
Remodeling	Consolidation—characterized by a decrease in cellularity and matrix production. Replacement of type III collagen by type I collagen. The collagen fibers structure is organized along the longitudinal axis of the tendon, which helps to restore tendon stiffness and tensile strength.	Begins 6-8 wk postinjury
	Maturation—increase in collagen fiber cross-linking and the formation of more mature tendon tissue.	Begins 10 wk postinjury

Data from Docheva D, Muller SA, et al. Biologics for tendon repair. *Adv Drug Deliv Rev*. 2015;84:222–239 and Lin TW, Cardenas L, Soslowsky LJ. Biomechanics of tendon injury and repair. *J. Biomech*. 2004;37:865–877.

various chemotactic factors, which attract inflammatory cells to the injured area. This is followed by the *reparative* or *proliferative stage*, which starts ~72 hours after the injury and lasts for ~6 weeks. It involves the recruitment of various growth factors to provide a vascular network responsible for the survival of newly forming fibrous tissue at the injury site. Fibroblasts are continuously recruited, and proteoglycans, collagens, and other components of the extracellular matrix are synthesized and then arranged randomly within the matrix. The tendon in this stage appears scarlike and has an extensive blood vessel network. The *remodeling stage* is the last phase of tendon healing and is divided into a consolidation and maturation component. The consolidation component of the remodeling stage begins ~6-8 weeks following the injury and is characterized by a decrease in cellularity and matrix production as the tissue becomes more fibrous through the replacement of type III collagen by type I collagen. The collagen fiber structure is organized along the longitudinal axis of the tendon, which helps to restore tendon stiffness and tensile strength. After ~10 weeks following the injury, the maturation stage begins, which includes an increase in collagen fiber cross-linking and the formation of more mature tendon tissue.[6,16-18] Unfortunately, the repaired tendon does not achieve the same characteristics of a normal, noninjured tendon.

In order to provide structural support during tendon healing, the appropriate sized suture, material, and technique should be chosen based upon the size of the tendon to prevent gapping, relieve tension on the suture ends, and avoid suture failure. Typically, a nonabsorbable suture of 2 to 2-0 is utilized in larger tendon repairs and 2-0 in smaller tendinous structures. A taper needle is preferred to prevent further damage to the injured tendon. Many grasping or locking suture techniques such as a Bunnell, Krackow, Mason-Allen, and Kessler constructs can be utilized for tendon reapproximation (Fig. 57.2).

Studies show that the optimal distance between where the suture is placed and the cut end of the tendon is 0.7 and 1.0 cm. This provides improved repair strength with less chance of suture pull out.[19] For most tendons, four core suture strands crossing the tendon ends leads to an increase in resistance of gap formation and avoidance of failure during cyclical loading. A two-strand suture construct is insufficient; however, greater than four-strand sutures may lead to bulkiness, damage, or strangulation to the tendon end. Addition of tension to the four-strand sutures is beneficial in withstanding the pull of muscles after surgery and reduced the risk of gapping during early tendon motion.[59] A study by Wu and Tang in 2014 showed that 10% of tendon shortening markedly increased the gap resistance forces without any obvious increase in tendon bulkiness. If using a suture material with relatively poor knot holding ability, it is recommended that four to five knots are utilized

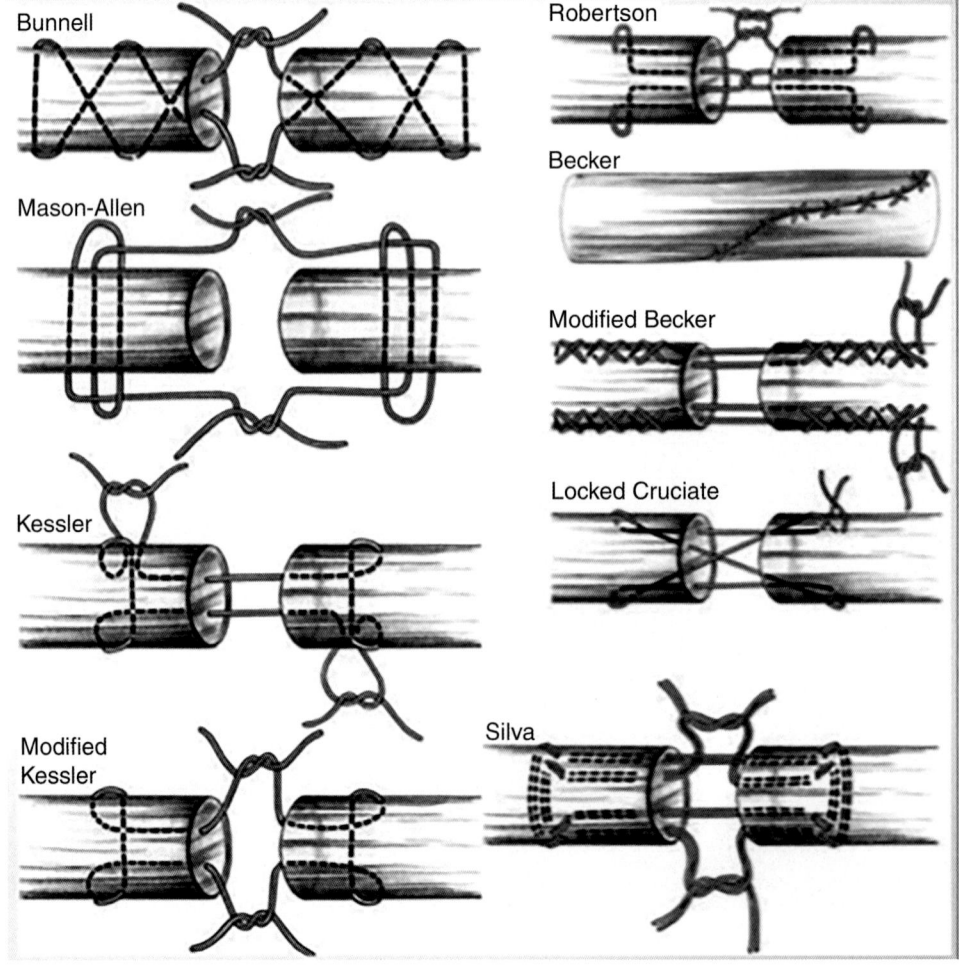

FIGURE 57.2 Various suture techniques for tendon repair.

to prevent slippage.[20] Repair of the tendon sheath should be carefully performed to avoid inadvertent suturing of the tendon that would result in adhesions and restrict tendon gliding.

IMAGING AND DIAGNOSTIC STUDIES

The diagnosis of acute and chronic tendon injury is made following a history and clinical examination, and imaging studies can be used as an adjunct to provide more information regarding the extent of injury as well as providing a basis for potential surgical repair.

RADIOGRAPHS

Radiographs are a common medical imaging study, which are often obtained as a baseline study following foot and ankle trauma. Although radiographs provide no direct information on tendon pathology, they are helpful in assessing for osseous pathology or dislocation in the acute trauma setting (Fig. 57.3A and B).

Weight-bearing radiographs of the foot and ankle are beneficial to obtain in patients with chronic tendinopathy such as tibialis posterior tendon dysfunction to assess for osseous malalignment and arthrosis.

COMPUTED TOMOGRAPHY SCANS

A computed tomography (CT) scan is a useful three-dimensional imaging tool, which allows the physician to visualize osseous and soft tissue pathology following a traumatic injury. Similar to radiographs, the density of the tissue determines the brightness and contrast of the images. Bone, which has a much higher attenuation coefficient over soft tissue structures, is more easily visualized and with greater detail than soft tissue structures. Therefore, a CT scan is not the imaging of choice unless a concomitant osseous injury is suspected or needs to be assessed further.

On CT scan, tendons appear homogeneous, oval or round, and well demarcated. A partial tendon rupture appears to have an increase in girth or radiolucent areas within the tendon substance itself. A complete rupture is visualized as a void either filled with fluid or fat, or simply the absence of a portion of the tendon. A concern associated with CT scans is the dosage of ionizing radiation.[21]

MAGNETIC RESONANCE IMAGING

Magnetic resonance imaging (MRI) is another three-dimensional imaging modality that has long been considered the gold standard for diagnostic imaging of tendon pathology. MRI provides excellent contrast of anatomic structures in multiple planes while avoiding radiation exposure to the patient. Normal tendons appear with low signal intensity on all conventional imaging sequences. When visualizing an abnormal tendon on MRI, one will see changes in signal intensity within the tendon or peritendinous structures (Fig. 57.4). Tendinopathy can result in changes such as focal thickening, thinning, longitudinal splits, contour irregularity, or complete tendon discontinuity. Fluid within the tendon sheath is often pathologic; however, it is important to note that a small amount of fluid within a tendon sheath such as the flexor hallucis longus (FHL) may be physiologic.

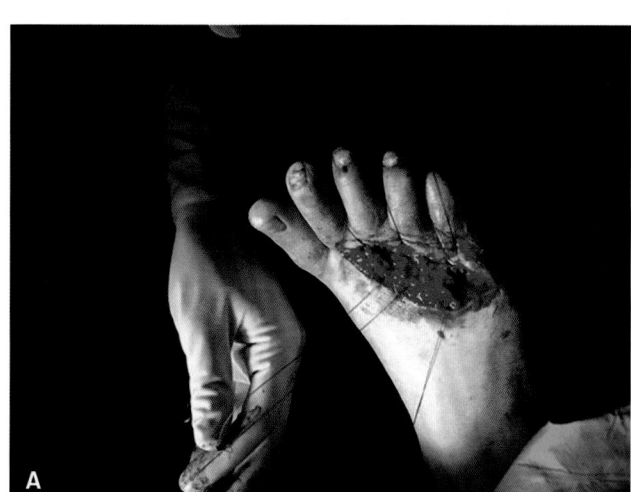

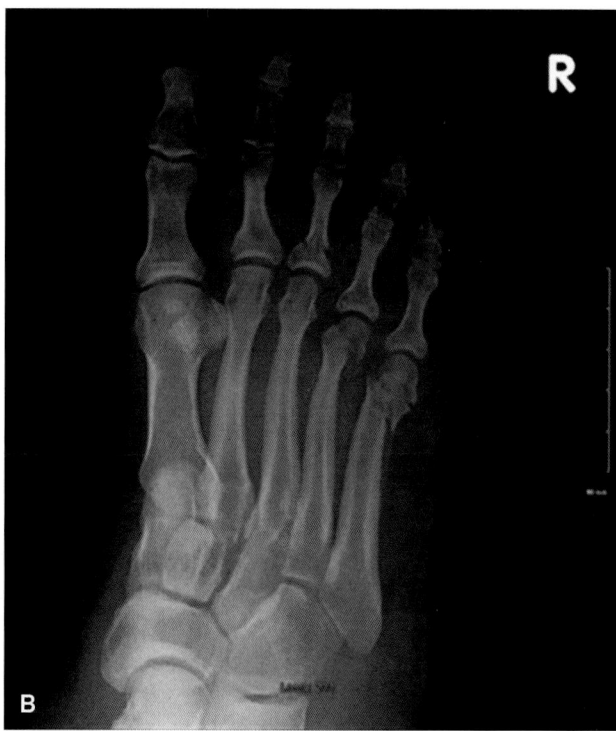

FIGURE 57.3 A. Large dorsal foot laceration with multiple tendon lacerations and underlying open fractures. **B.** Plain radiograph demonstrating multiple open fractures.

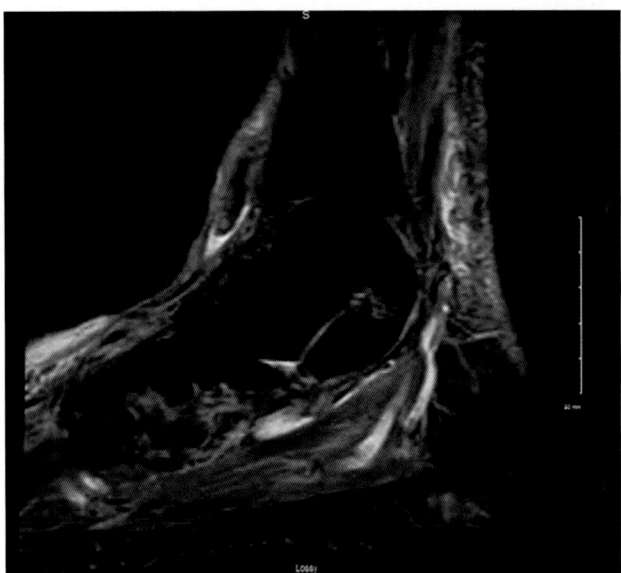

FIGURE 57.4 Sagittal STIR MRI of tibialis anterior tendon rupture with proximal retraction.

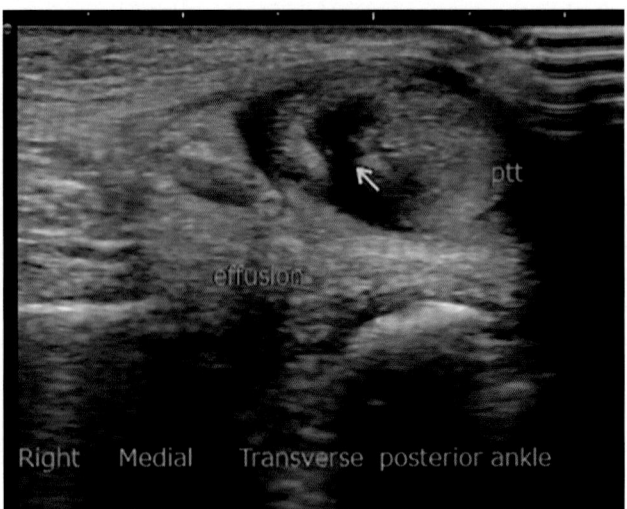

FIGURE 57.5 Transverse ultrasonography imaging of posterior tibial tendinopathy at the level of the posteromedial ankle. The *arrow* signifies effusion. The hyperechoic/*white area* at the bottom is the medial malleolus.

The "magic angle phenomenon" occurs if the tendon is oriented 55 degrees to the magnetic field and, depending on the type of sequence and the echo time of the study, may result in images that demonstrate a higher signal intensity within the tendon. To reduce the concern of false-positive tendinopathy findings, the clinician should request plantar flexed ankle views when imaging for potential tendon pathology for the peroneal and long flexor tendons as they course around the malleoli.[22]

ULTRASONOGRAPHY

Ultrasonography use for musculoskeletal imaging has increased significantly over the last several years. It provides a cost-effective, noninvasive, dynamic, real-time imaging that can be extremely helpful in evaluating tendon pathology. Other benefits of ultrasonography include a lack of ionizing radiation and no difficulty in imaging patients with local orthopedic hardware or implanted medical devices such as cardiac pacemakers.[23] A combination of longitudinal and transverse imaging can be performed to evaluate the tendon with the use of a high-frequency transducer probe. On ultrasound, the fascicular structure is seen as multiple, closely spaced echogenic parallel lines on longitudinal scanning, whereas in the transverse plane, multiple echogenic dots or lines are visible.[24] Tendons exhibit anisotropy on ultrasound owing to their regular, uniform structure. The brightly reflective fascicles within the tendon are best seen when the ultrasound beam is perpendicular to the orientation of the fascicles. If the beam is not perpendicular, which can occur when examining tendons that change direction around the ankle, the echogenic appearance is lost and can mimic tendinopathy. Assessment of acute tendon lacerations or tears under ultrasonography reveals discontinuity of fibers and anechoic fluid visible within the tear.[25,26] As fresh hematoma organizes at the rupture, its echogenicity increases, and it may be difficult to differentiate the tear from the adjacent tendon, which can result in false-negative sonogram results. Dynamic imaging during muscle contraction or passive movement is often helpful to

further assess the tendon integrity. Ultrasound of tendinopathy typically shows loss of the normal fibrillar structure with increased spacing of the hyperechoic fibrillar lines and generally reduced echogenicity and tendon thickening (Fig. 57.5).[27]

The major limitation associated with the use of ultrasonography in the evaluation of tendon pathology is that the quality of the study is significantly user dependent. Lack of familiarity with the equipment or with musculoskeletal ultrasound imaging and interpretation can limit the diagnostic accuracy of the study.[28]

ACUTE TENDON LACERATIONS

Traumatic skin lacerations about the foot and ankle may result in acute tendon disruptions, which are most common over the dorsal aspect of the foot and ankle. The long flexor tendons in the foot are relatively well protected except in the distal forefoot where they become more superficial. Acute tendon lacerations can easily be missed if a complete musculoskeletal assessment is not performed, especially in minor skin lacerations. Occasionally during foot and ankle reconstructive surgery, failure to adequately protect or identify anatomic structures can lead to iatrogenic tendon laceration.[29,30]

In the emergency room or urgent care setting, information should be obtained from the patient to determine the mechanism of injury, tetanus status, and time when the laceration occurred. Physical examination of the laceration should assess the cleanliness of the soft tissues, neurovascular status, and musculoskeletal strength of the tendons in the area of concern. It is often easy to assess if a long extensor tendon has been lacerated by confirming the presence of an extensor lag due to loss of physiologic tension within the tendon (Fig. 57.6A). It is also helpful to try and palpate to determine where the lacerated tendon ends are located. Depending on the position of the foot and degree of muscle contraction at the time of injury, these could either be proximal or distal to the skin laceration site.[4,31]

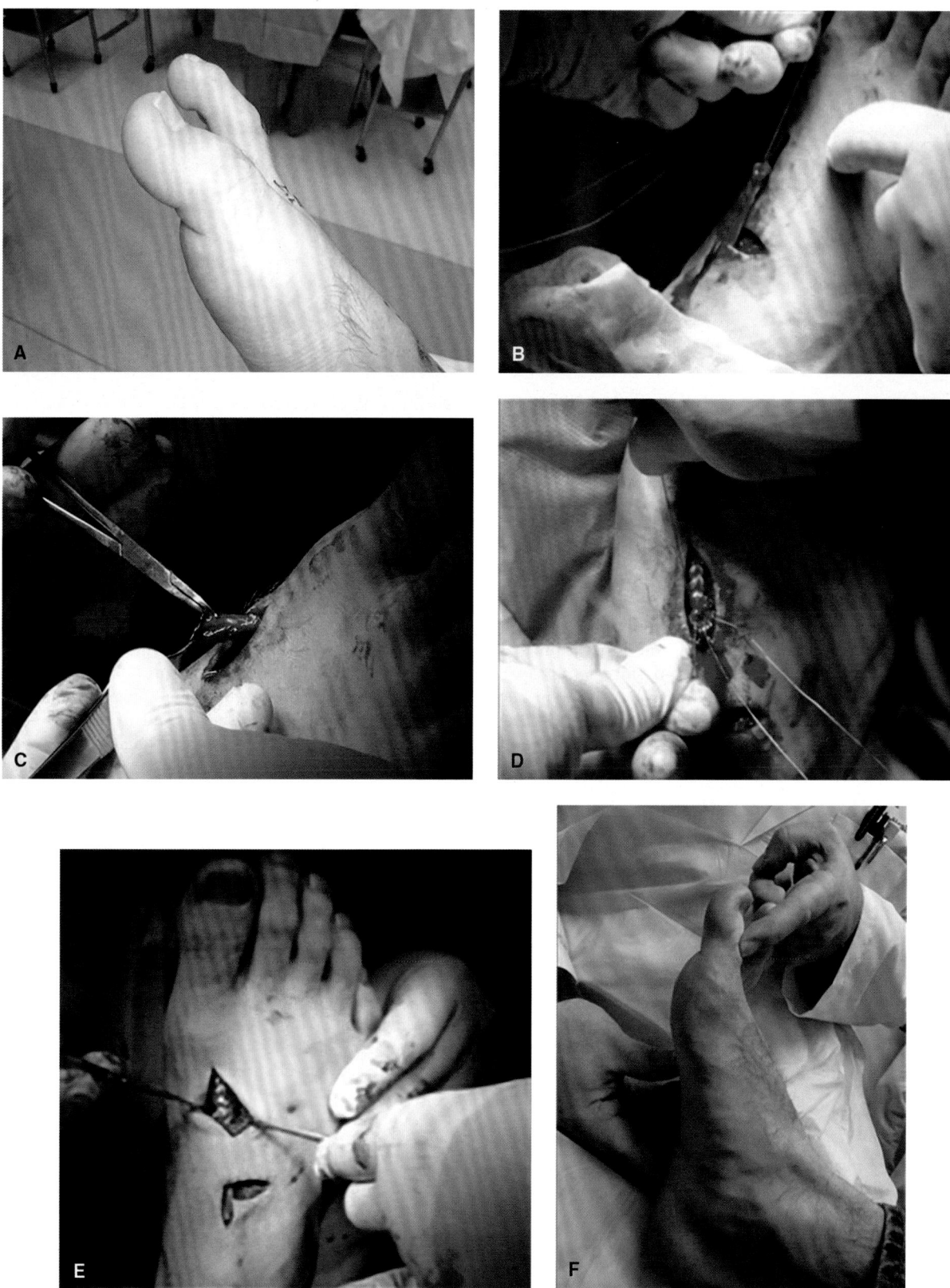

FIGURE 57.6 A. Extensor lag resulting from EHL tendon laceration. **B.** Following retrieval and suturing of the proximal EHL tendonwas pulled distally to determine the appropriate location to incise skin and retrieve the distal stump. Unlike most tendon lacerations, due to maximal dorsiflexion of hallux and ankle at the time of this injury, the proximal tendon stump is not retracted proximally. **C.** Distal EHL tendon is retrieved through secondary incision followed by débridement of hematoma and suturing. **D.** EHL tendon reapproximation at physiologic tension with four-strand technique. **E.** Final repair prior to tendon sheath closure. **F.** Return of functional strength and excursion of EHL tendon following repair.

Surgical repair is usually employed for open lacerations of tendons followed by postoperative splinting to protect the tendon during the early phases of healing. Radiographs should be obtained if there is a concern for possible foreign body or concomitant fracture. Musculoskeletal ultrasound or MRI studies are often not cost-effective or necessary to confirm the diagnosis; however, if musculoskeletal ultrasound is easily available, it can be utilized as an adjunct to establish the location of the tendon ends.[19]

Acute tendon lacerations distal to the metatarsophalangeal joint do not result in proximal retraction of the tendon due to the extensor expansion apparatus. If clean, these may be treated with tendon and skin reapproximation or even managed conservatively with splinting.[32] For most acute tendon lacerations, if surgical intervention is not able to proceed emergently, the laceration should be flushed and skin closed with a nonabsorbable suture. A posterior splint should be applied in an effort to avoid retraction of the tendon.[32,33]

The primary repair of acute tendon lacerations is typically straightforward and the techniques applicable to all tendons. Retrieval of the tendon ends often necessitates a secondary incision rather than extending the original skin laceration to any significant extent. Careful handling of the skin and peritendinous structures prevents further embarrassment to the traumatized tissues. After the tendon ends are located, they should be débrided of hematoma and nonviable tissue. Nonabsorbable suture should be passed up and down each tendon segment, resulting in repair of both the medial and lateral halves of the tendon. Tapered suture needles are always preferred over cutting needles to prevent further tearing of the tendon. During the course of the repair, the tendon should be kept well moistened in order to prevent desiccation of the tendon. The tendon can then be passed down the sheath by means of a suture lasso or tendon passer. Prior to tying the sutures, the foot and ankle is typically placed into a position to maintain optimal length-tension relationship. Typically, four core strands of suture are utilized to tie the surgical knots at the laceration interface. This technique permits dispersion of force equally on both sides of the tendon, resulting in an increase in strength and resistance to gap formation at the repair site. Additional nonabsorbable suture can be used at the level of the laceration to augment the primary repair in larger tendons. The foot and ankle should be held in neutral position during soft tissue closure. Effort should be made to cover the tendon repair with the vascular tendon sheath to minimize the development of fibrosis and adhesion (Fig. 57.6B-F and Video 57.1).[34]

Occasionally, acute tendon lacerations are unable to be repaired in a timely fashion. Reasons for the delay vary but examples include a delay in proper diagnosis, poor soft tissue envelope or contamination of the wound, or concomitant medical issues that delay safe surgical intervention. This delay can make primary repair of the tendon with end-to-end anastomosis unattainable. In these instances where there is insufficient tendon length to provide apposition, secondary repair of the tendon is recommended. There are multiple techniques available to the surgeon to provide the necessary length to regain function of the tendon. These include V to Y lengthening, turndown onlay grafting, or the use of autogenous or allogeneic tissue grafts to span the length between the proximal and distal tendon stumps (Fig. 57.7).[61]

Commercially available biologic tissue scaffolds should not be utilized to span the tendon deficit as an alternative to an

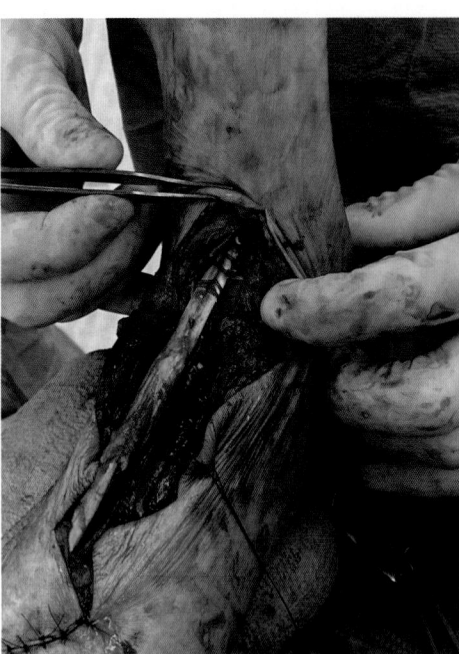

FIGURE 57.7 Delayed repair of tibialis anterior tendon with posterior tibial allograft tendon.

anatomic graft but may be considered an onlay adjunct to augment the repair.

SPECIFIC TENDON RUPTURES

TIBIALIS ANTERIOR

The tibialis anterior is active in the stance and swing phases of the gait cycle. It functions to decelerate the foot via eccentric loading at heel strike and provides dorsiflexion of the foot via concentric contraction in the swing phase. The tibialis anterior muscle originates from the proximal two-thirds of the lateral tibial shaft and interosseous membrane. It becomes tendinous at the distal tibial metaphysis and is covered in a synovial sheath. It courses beneath the superior and inferior extensor retinaculum to insert at the medial and plantar surface of the first cuneiform and base of the first metatarsal.[30] It demonstrates a 45- to 67-mm area of hypovascularity on the anterior aspect of the tendon in the area of the retinaculum, 5-30 mm from the insertion, and corresponds to the most common site of rupture.[34,35] Another study on anterior tendon abnormalities on MRI scans did not support these theories. It demonstrated that signal intensity abnormalities were most commonly found either in the posterior portion (39%) of the tendon—close to the bone—or in a diffuse distribution (54%). Only 7% of abnormalities were found in the anterior portion of the tendon. They associated these pathologic findings to mechanical irritation of the tendon by local osteophytes.[22]

Tibialis anterior tendon ruptures are not very common. Acute open lacerations usually affect younger patients, while spontaneous rupture usually affects middle-aged and older patients due to degeneration of the tendon underneath the extensor retinaculum. Spontaneous tears are typically insidi-

ous in nature, and aside from age, patients with a history of gout, uncontrolled diabetes mellitus, inflammatory arthropathy, or postcorticosteroid injection are also at higher risk for causing microdamage and subsequently rupture to the tendon.[36,37,60]

The clinical presentation and therefore the diagnosis of spontaneous ruptures of the tibialis anterior tendon in the elderly are often delayed and underreported. These injuries are often not painful and are in low-demand patients who are able to compensate for the weakness.[38] Although ankle dorsiflexion may be significantly weakened, substitution of the extensor digitorum longus (EDL) and extensor hallucis longus (EHL) may allow the tear can go unrecognized initially.[39] Patients with chronic tendon rupture may develop clawing of the toes due to extensor substitution.

Physical examination should include static and dynamic assessment of the patient using the contralateral limb for comparison.

Clinical findings include a loss of the normally visualized and prominent tendon at the anterior medial ankle (Fig. 57.8). Manual muscle testing reveals weakness and decreased range of motion to ankle dorsiflexion with recruitment of the EHL and extensor digitorum. This results in the production of eversion rather than inversion with dorsiflexion (Video 57.2). There may also be a palpable and visible defect or palpable mass (pseudotumor) present at the anterior ankle from retraction of the ruptured tendon end. The proximal aspect of the tendon typically retracts between 2 and 10 cm and becomes entrapped in the superior extensor retinaculum.[30]

A neurologic examination should be performed to insure that the weakness is not due to other potential causes such as an L4 radiculopathy or peroneal neuropathy. Assessment of overall foot structure, degree of equinus, joint quality, and circulation also need to be determined if surgical intervention may be required. During the gait examination, compensatory gait patterns may be seen such as toe dragging, steppage, circumduction, or foot slap at heel strike. These may become more apparent with prolonged activity as the substituting muscles begin to fatigue.

The diagnosis is made primarily based on the clinical examination; however, ultrasonography and MRI are both excellent imaging modalities if further assessment of the tendon is desired. Ultrasonography provides a dynamic assessment of the tendon and demonstrates disorganization of the regular fibrillar pattern with hypoechoic or anechoic findings

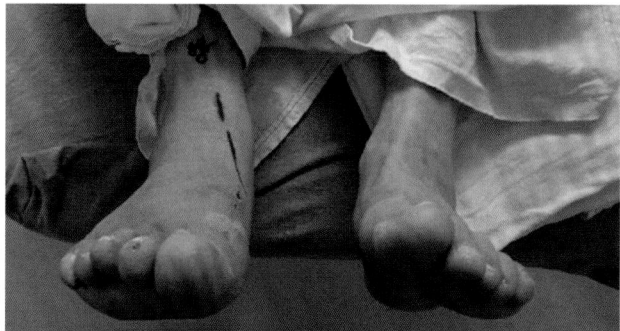

FIGURE 57.8 Clinical appearance of an anterior tibialis tendon rupture next to the contralateral nonpathological extremity.

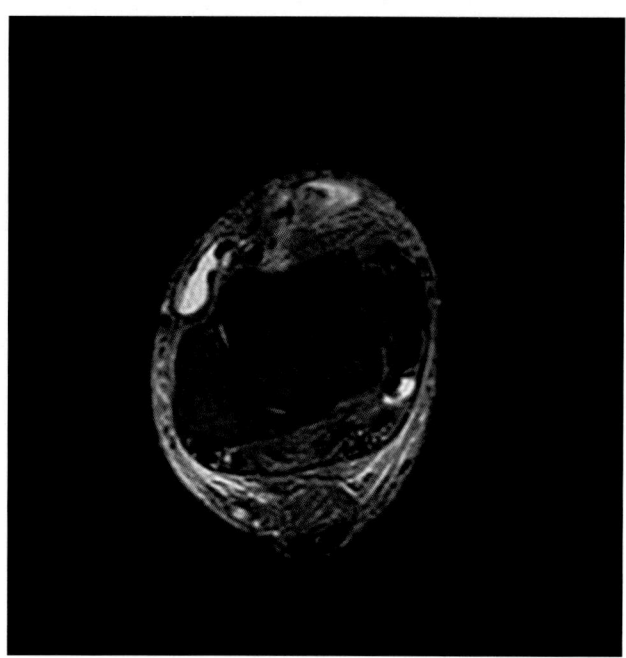

FIGURE 57.9 Axial MIR sequence MRI demonstrating anterior tibial tendon rupture.

corresponding to the rupture site. MRI findings of the rupture demonstrate tendon discontinuity as well as surrounding focal high signal intensity corresponding to local edema (Fig. 57.9).[21]

Treatment of spontaneous tibialis anterior tendon rupture needs to be individualized to the patient based on age, functional capacity, and medical comorbidities. Elderly individuals with low functional demands, chronic ruptures, or extensive medical comorbidities may be successfully managed conservatively with the use of a dorsiflexion assist molded ankle-foot orthosis.[38] The purpose of the brace is to counteract the unopposed pull of the peroneus longus tendon and reduce the need for substitution by the long extensor tendons. Conservative therapy without the use of an appropriate brace places the patient at greater risk for falls and potential injury due to gait compensation.

Surgical management of tibialis anterior tendon ruptures is recommended in younger individuals with higher functional demands or in patients who have failed conservative treatment. Primary repair of the tendon can be performed if the injury is recent and with adequate tendon length, quality, and mobility. The procedure is performed with the patient in the supine position. A thigh tourniquet can be placed for hemostasis if desired. Incision is made from approximately the medial cuneiform to the superior extensor retinaculum. To avoid linear scar contracture over the anterior ankle, multiple "Z" skin incisions may be considered. Anatomic dissection is carried down to the tibialis anterior tendon, and the tendon is débrided. Options for repair include end-to-end anastomosis with the use of a Krackow, Bunnell, or modified Kessler technique with a nonabsorbable suture of the surgeon's choice.

A secondary repair option available if end-to-end anastomosis is not possible is the use of the turn down onlay flap or sliding graft utilizing half of the proximal tibialis anterior stump to fill the gap. Nonanatomic repair can be performed

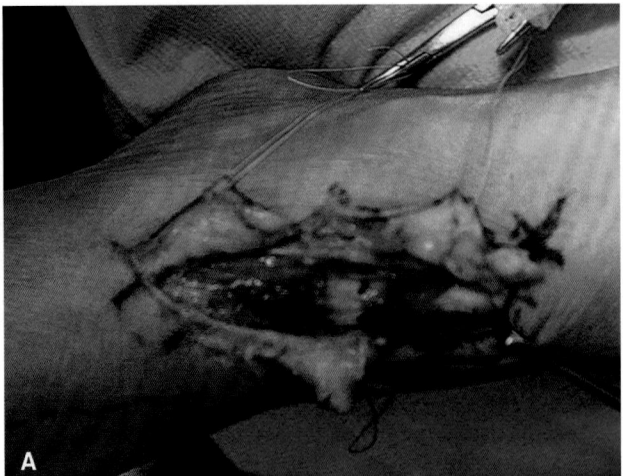

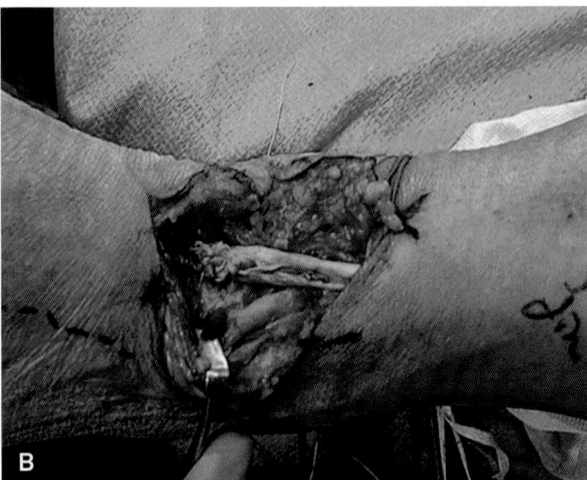

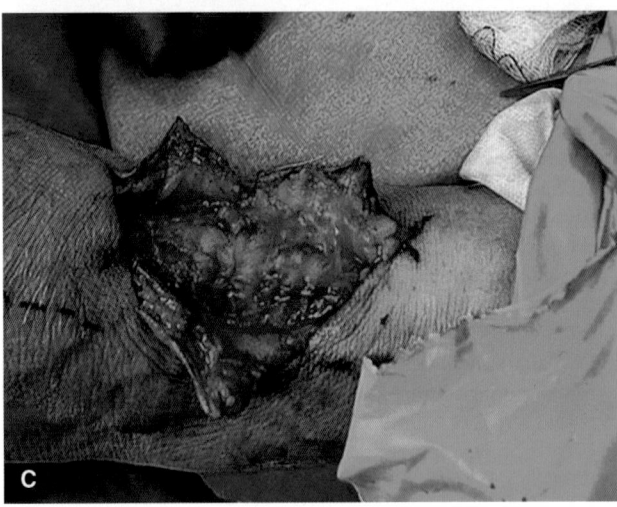

FIGURE 57.10 A. Multiple Z-skin incisions to repair rupture of anterior tibialis tendon to avoid linear scar contracture. **B.** Nonanatomic repair of anterior tibialis tendon rupture utilizing bone anchor for tendon reattachment. **C.** Tendon sheath closure overlying repair to avoid fibrosis and tendon adhesions.

by means of a tendon anchor placed within the medial cuneiform or navicular but perpendicular to the pull of the tendon to avoid pullout of the device. Traditional and knotless tendon anchor devices are available to provide secure fixation to bone (Fig. 57.10A-C).

Adjacent tendon transfer and free autograft or allograft are other potential reconstruction options. Several tendon options for repair have been described in the literature including the use of EHL, EDL, peroneus brevis, and posterior tibial tendon transfer. The most common procedure is the use of the EHL tendon. The EHL tendon can be detached at the metatarsophalangeal joint and the remaining distal aspect sutured to the EHB tendon. The proximal aspect of the EHL is anastomosed to the proximal stump of the ruptured tibialis anterior tendon in a side-to-side fashion. The EHL is then transferred through a bone tunnel in the medial cuneiform and held in place with an interference screw or sutured back onto itself.

To try and provide normal physiologic tension, the ankle should be held in slight dorsiflexion during reapproximation or anastomosis for all of these repairs. This position should be maintained and protected throughout the remainder of the procedure. Layered closure of the tendon sheath, retinaculum, subcutaneous tissue, and skin is then performed. Per surgeon preference, use of collagen matrix or amniotic graft can be considered to augment repair and prevent

adhesions.[62] A short leg cast should be applied following the procedure with the ankle held in slight dorsiflexion to protect the repair.

For chronic, neglected ruptures, it is important to assess for underlying gastrocnemius equinus. A gastrocnemius recession or Achilles tendon lengthening may be necessary to help restore the balance between dorsiflexion and plantar flexion in order to protect the surgical repair.

TIBIALIS POSTERIOR

The tibialis posterior muscle is the most central muscle in the leg, which is located in the deep posterior compartment. The tendon originates at the upper third of the leg posteriorly at the tibia, fibula, and interosseous membrane. The tendon develops in the distal third of the leg and then passes posterior to the medial malleolus where it takes an acute turn. The tendon sits in a shallow groove in the posteromedial aspect of the distal tibia and is tethered by the flexor retinaculum, which functions as a seat belt, to keep the tendon in the groove and prevent dislocation. The tendon primarily inserts into the navicular tuberosity but sends slips to the cuneiforms, cuboid, and metatarsal bases of 2, 3, and 4. Just distal to the medial malleolus is an area that is relatively hypovascular and is thought to contribute to degeneration of the tendon. The tibialis pos-

terior tendon is approximately twice the size of the FHL and flexor digitorum longus (FDL) tendons, and slightly smaller than the anterior tibialis tendon.[39] The location of the TP tendon relative to the axes of the subtalar and ankle joints facilitates inversion and plantar flexion, respectively. During the gait cycle, the tibialis posterior tendon functions as a dynamic stabilizer of the arch with the assistance of static stabilizers such as the spring ligament, deltoid ligament, and talonavicular joint capsule. It functions during the midstance phase of the gait cycle to support the arch by controlling the midtarsal joint and aids in inversion of the foot and plantar flexion of the ankle. Electromyography research has revealed that individuals with a low arched foot and tibialis posterior tendon dysfunction are associated with greater tibialis posterior muscle activity during stance phase, compared to normal or healthy subjects.[40]

The clinical presentation of tibialis posterior tendon pathology is variable depending on the degree of tendinopathy and whether progressive deformity has developed. Acute lacerations rarely occur in this tendon; however, progressive tendinopathy is extremely common in clinical practice. Patients with progressive tibialis posterior tendinopathy often present with acute on chronic complaints of pain and swelling around the area of the medial malleolus and navicular with weight-bearing activities. It is most commonly seen in females older than age 50 and is often associated with underlying disorders such as a preexisting flatfoot, obesity, change in activity, injury, diabetes mellitus, or previous treatment such as corticosteroid injections.[41] Examination should include non–weight-bearing and weight-bearing assessment of both lower extremities looking for structural and biomechanical pathology. Non–weight-bearing examination should include palpation of the rearfoot to assess tenderness and swelling along the tendon or impingement laterally. The range of motion and quality of joint motion should be assessed to determine the flexibility of the deformity and whether adequate ankle dorsiflexion is available. Neurovascular status should always be fully assessed. Weight-bearing examination should assess overall lower extremity alignment. The classically described "too many toes sign" can be seen when viewing the patient from behind and reveals increased forefoot abduction and valgus of the heel. The flexibility of the foot can then be assessed by performing

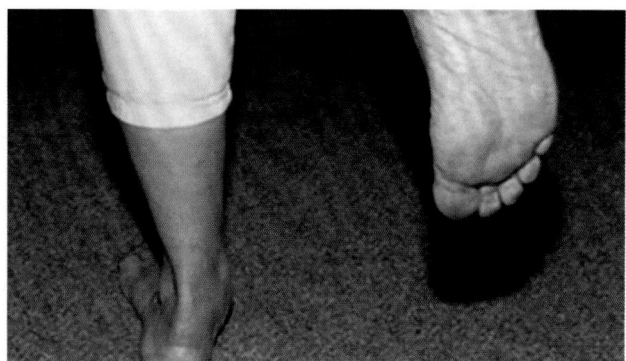

FIGURE 57.11 Clinical photo of posterior tibial tendon dysfunction here while patient performs single heel raise test.

the Hubscher maneuver. The single heel raise test historically has been performed to evaluate for the supinatory strength of the tendon (Fig. 57.11). The single heel raise test requires the patient to lift the unaffected foot off the ground and then attempt to raise the heel off the ground by elevating onto the toes of the affected foot. If the tibialis posterior is intact, the heel will invert as the patient lifts off the ground. This often results in complaints of pain and decreased strength when compared to the contralateral side. However, patients may be able to bypass the pathologic tibialis posterior tendon by recruiting other muscles to help raise onto their toes, or they may raise up on both tiptoes and then balance on the pathologic foot. This occurs by means of the plantar fascia plantar flexing the metatarsal heads.[42]

Gait analysis should also be performed looking for structural malalignment and pathologic compensation. Typical findings reveal rearfoot valgus with abduction of the forefoot and a lack of resupination in midstance with an early heel off. Weight-bearing radiographs of the foot and ankle should be evaluated to assess structural alignment and degree of arthrosis. A comprehensive classification system was developed by Johnson and Strom in 1989 and revised based on the clinical experience of Myerson in 2007. This classification system takes into account the clinical and radiographic findings and offers treatment suggestions based on the stage of deformity (Table 57.2).

TABLE 57.2	Classification System for Tibialis Posterior Tendon Dysfunction as Described by Johnson and Strom With Myerson Modification		
Stage	**Deformity**	**Findings**	**Treatment**
I	No deformity PT synovitis (+) single leg raise	(+) positive single leg raise	Conservative treatment (taping, firm shoes, physical therapy, rest)
II	**Flatfoot deformity** Flexible hindfoot Normal forefoot (−) single leg raise	**(−) single leg raise** Mild sinus tarsi pain (+) too many toes sign **Arch collapse**	AFO Tendon reconstruction Calcaneal osteotomy
III	Flatfoot deformity **Rigid hindfoot** Rigid forefoot abduction	(−) single leg raise (+) too many toes sign **Severe sinus tarsi pain** **STJ arthritis**	STJ fusion Triple arthrodesis
IV	Flatfoot deformity Rigid hindfoot valgus (talar tilt on x-ray) Rigid forefoot abduction **Deltoid ligament compromise**	(−) single leg raise (+) too many toes sign Severe sinus tarsi pain **Ankle pain** **Talar tilt in ankle mortise**	Pantalar arthrodesis Triple arthrodesis with TAR Triple arthrodesis with supramalleolar osteotomy

Data from Bluman EM, Title CI, Myerson MS. Posterior tibial tendon rupture: a refined classification system. *Foot Ankle Clin.* 2007;12(2):233–249 and Johnson KA, Strom DE. Tibialis posterior tendon dysfunction. *Clin Orthop.* 1989;239:196–206.

CLASSIFICATION

MRI evaluation may be utilized to confirm the clinical diagnosis or assist in surgical planning. MRI findings vary depending on the degree of tendinopathy present and involvement of the static stabilizers such as the spring ligament.[43]

Nonoperative treatment may be considered in the early stages with immobilization followed by physical therapy, orthotic management, and weight loss if necessary. In later stages, nonoperative treatment is considered in patients with low functional demands or those with medical comorbidities that do not allow surgical reconstruction. In these individuals, the use of an ankle-foot orthosis such as an Arizona or Richie brace is often attempted. The goal of these conservative modalities is not to correct the underlying pathology but to provide symptomatic relief and improve function. However, there is no clear consensus on which interventions are most effective and at which stage of progression.[44]

Surgical treatment is often necessary in patients with progressive tibialis posterior tendon dysfunction. It is imperative that the surgeon assess and plan to not only address the pathologic tendon but the biomechanical/structural deformities that are present. Failure to do so will result in further compromise of the repair over time. It is out of the scope of this chapter to review all ancillary procedures that may be required in addressing chronic tibialis posterior tendon ruptures. Procedures may include calcaneal osteotomies, limited fusions, and gastrocnemius recession or Achilles tendon lengthening. Tibialis posterior tenosynovectomy and tendon débridement/tubularization are occasionally performed in early-stage pathology. The primary procedure for a flexible deformity involves an FDL tendon transfer with possible repair/augmentation of the spring ligament. The procedure is performed with the patient in the supine position. A thigh tourniquet can be placed for hemostasis if desired. The skin incision is made from the posterior aspect of the medial malleolus and continued down to the medial cuneiform along the medial aspect of the foot. The saphenous nerve and medial marginal vein are retracted superiorly after the venous tributaries are ligated. The tendon sheath of the tibialis posterior tendon is entered, and the tendon is detached and débrided if salvageable. The FDL tendon is located in the tendon sheath posteriorly adjacent to the tibialis posterior and is easily entered. Although the FDL tendon can be anastomosed in side-to-side fashion to provide increased supinatory strength, it is often released distally and transferred to the navicular. To ensure adequate tendon length, the FDL tendon should be followed distally to the master knot of Henry where it crosses with the FHL tendon. The FDL tendon should be released as far distal and the distal aspect whipstitched. A drill hole of acceptable size based upon the cross-sectional area of the FDL tendon can be performed either medial to lateral or superior to inferior in the navicular tuberosity, based on surgeon preference. Care should be taken to avoid violation of the talonavicular joint or fracture of the navicular tuberosity. The foot should be held in a slightly plantar flexed and inverted position to allow for appropriate tension of the FDL tendon. Once this is established, an appropriate sized interference screw should be inserted while holding the position and ensuring stability of the transfer (Fig. 57.12A-C). If the spring ligament is found to be attenuated, this may be augmented or repaired with a suture tape construct. Layered closure of the tendon sheath, retinaculum, subcutaneous tissue, and skin is then performed with the foot stabilized to protect the transfer.

The postoperative course varies depending on the procedures performed. If only soft tissue procedures are performed, a non–weight-bearing splint for 6 weeks followed by 2 weeks weight bearing in a removable boot is sufficient. In cases where concomitant fusions or osteotomies are performed, the patient should remain non–weight-bearing for 6-8 weeks before gradually transitioning to full weight bearing in a removable boot for an additional 2 weeks.[45]

PERONEAL TENDONS

DEFINITION

The peroneus longus muscle takes origin from the upper two-thirds of the lateral fibula and begins to become tendinous in the midtibial region. It is fully tendinous ~4 cm from lateral malleolus. The peroneus brevis takes origin from the lower two-thirds of the lateral fibula and often continues to receive muscular fibers into the posterior lateral malleolar surface. The peroneus brevis lies against the posterior surface of the fibula with the peroneus longus directly posterior to the brevis. As the tendons course around the lateral malleolus, they are tethered down by the superior peroneal retinaculum in a groove created by the posterior fibula and a fibrocartilaginous ridge. The ridge effectively deepens the groove and contributes to stability of the tendons behind the fibula as they turn anterior and slightly plantarly into the lateral foot. The peroneal tendons are contained within a synovial sheath that courses behind the retromalleolar groove and splits at the level of the peroneal tubercle where the inferior peroneal retinaculum attaches. The peroneus brevis is contained in superior sheath above the peroneal tubercle with the peroneus longus in the inferior sheath along the lateral aspect of the calcaneus. The peroneus brevis continues on to insert at the styloid process of the fifth metatarsal base. The peroneus longus tendon courses within the sheath and turns distal medially at the peroneal groove and into the cuboid tunnel on the lateral and inferior surface of the cuboid before inserting into the plantar surface of the first metatarsal base and medial cuneiform.

The peroneal tendons both function together as strong evertors of the foot and provide weak plantar flexion of the ankle. The peroneus longus also stabilizes the first ray during midstance and propulsion, while decelerating ankle dorsiflexion in the propulsive phase of gait. The peroneus brevis in particular is the strongest evertor of the foot and antagonist to muscles that supinate the foot. It also stabilizes the fifth ray during midstance and early propulsion.[46]

Peroneal tendinopathy is an often overlooked and underdiagnosed cause of lateral ankle pain and disability. While peroneal tendinopathy is relatively uncommon in young, healthy patients, traumatic injuries that result in ankle instability or laxity in the superior peroneal retinaculum may facilitate peroneal subluxation and subsequent tears. This is especially true if there is underlying anatomic susceptibility such as patients with a peroneus quartus, low-lying muscle belly, or insufficient retromalleolar groove. Diagnosis of peroneal tendon tears and subluxation requires a high level of suspicion and accurate clinical evaluation. The evaluation of patients with

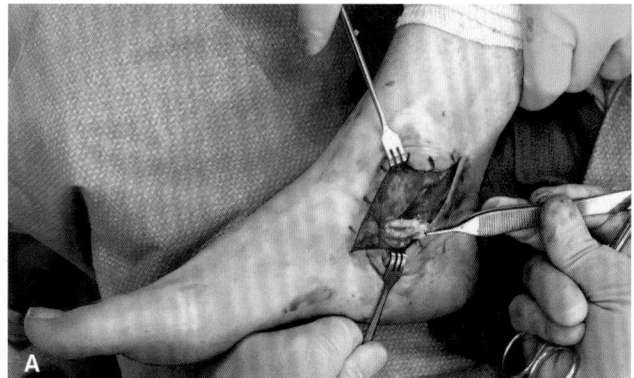

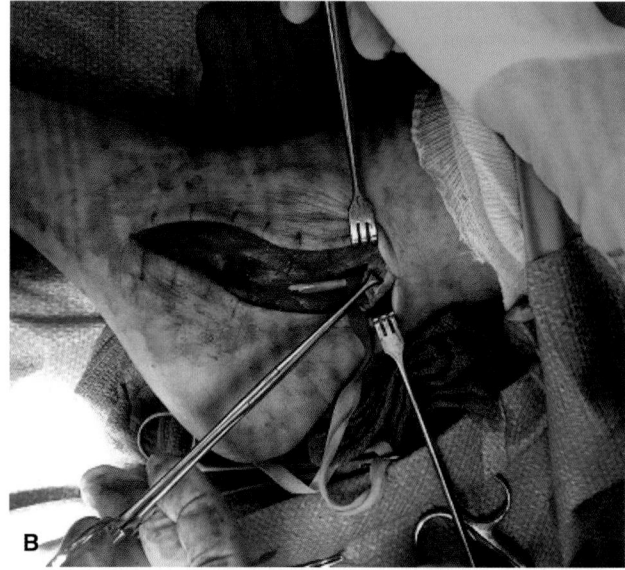

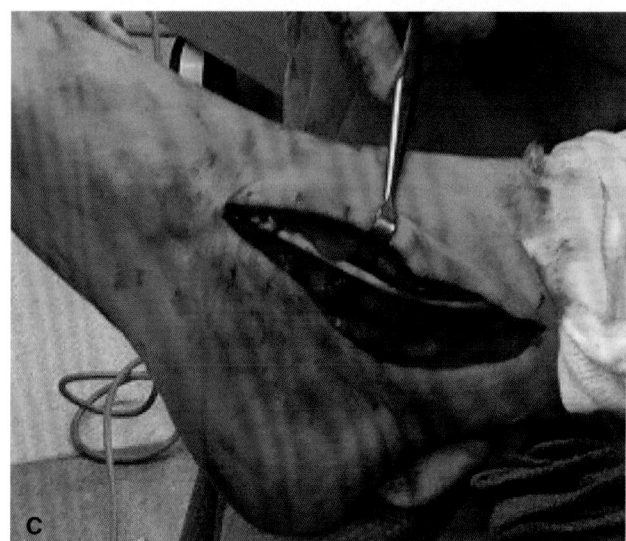

FIGURE 57.12 A. Distal extent of tibialis posterior tendon rupture following corticosteroid injections prior to excision. **B.** Proximal extent of tendon rupture (in Alice clamp) with FDL tendon exposed prior to distal release and transfer. **C.** FDL tendon transfer to navicular for TP tendon rupture.

long-standing lateral ankle pain requires determination of a possible mechanism of injury, concomitant symptoms such as snapping or subluxation of the tendons, and lateral ankle instability. Attritional tears of the peroneus brevis tendon due to progressive degeneration are fairly common in middle-aged to elderly patients behind the distal fibula. Tears of the peroneus longus tendon occur less frequently than peroneus brevis tears and are more commonly seen in patients with a cavus foot, ankle instability, enlarged peroneal tubercle, or os peroneum. Peroneus longus tears are more likely to result in further rearfoot imbalance into inversion as compared to isolated peroneus brevis pathology.[47,48]

Peroneal muscle strength and the location of pain are important to distinguish as well as retromalleolar edema or associated deformities such as a pes cavus deformity (Fig. 57.13A).

If pes cavus is a contributing etiologic factor, then a Coleman block test should be performed to determine if the osseous deformity is from a varus deformity in the rearfoot, plantar flexed first ray, or a combination of both. Provocative maneuvers such as a peroneal compression test to assess for peroneal subluxation should be performed. This is performed by having the patient flex their knee to 90 degrees and the ankle in

relaxed plantar flexion. The clinician places either their thumb or index and middle fingers from the superior peroneal retinaculum on the posterior-distal fibula to the lateral calcaneus and pushes down on the peroneal tendons. The patient then forcefully everts and dorsiflexes their foot and ankle against resistance. The test is considered positive if the patient complains of pain and accompanied subluxation or snapping of the tendons (Fig. 57.13B).[49,50]

Medical imaging studies can be used to assist in developing a diagnosis. In the presence of an acute inversion ankle injury, plain radiographs of the ankle can assess for avulsion fractures of the posterior/distal fibula, peroneal tubercle, or os peroneum. Stress radiographs can be utilized to determine if any underlying ankle instability is present. Although advanced imaging is not always required, an MRI may be obtained to correlate with clinical findings or to help with surgical planning. The peroneus brevis tendon often appears flat or crescentic on axial views. The tendon is susceptible to longitudinal splits, resulting in increased signal intensity on MRI, irregularity, and a "C"-shaped configuration from compression of the peroneus longus.[51] The ability for ultrasound to dynamically visualize tendons in real time makes ultrasonography a preferred imaging

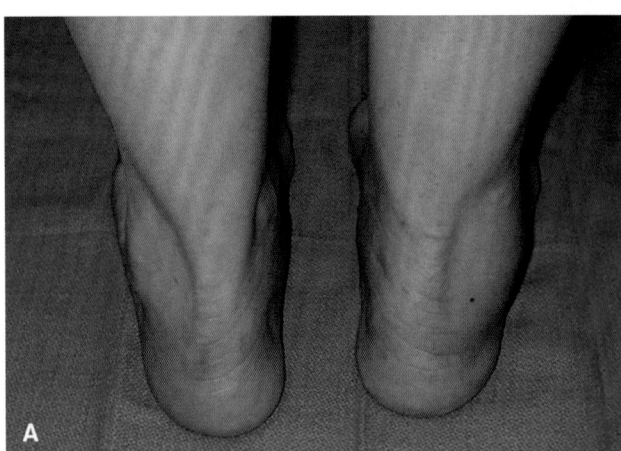 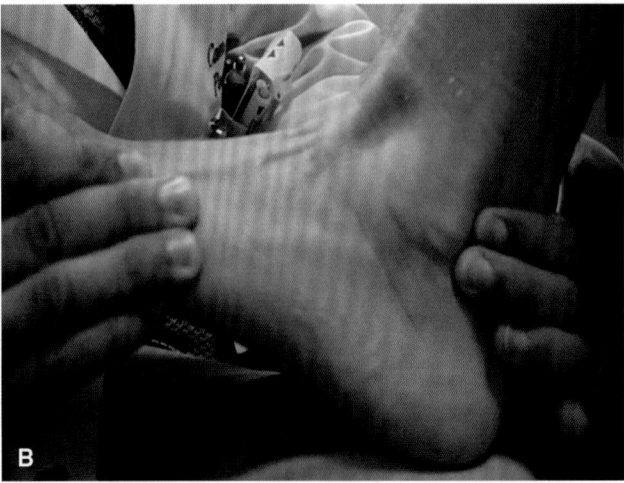

FIGURE 57.13 A. Retromalleolar edema seen in a patient with chronic peroneal tendinopathy.
B. Peroneal compression test for peroneal subluxation.

modality compared with MRI in order to visualize and detect peroneal tendon subluxation.[52] Risk factors for peroneal tendon dysfunction such as a low-lying muscle belly, peroneus quartus, or peroneal tendon dislocation may also be demonstrated. The surgeon must remember that the extent of tendon pathology is often not definitive until intraoperative assessment can be made.

Conservative management of chronic peroneal tendinopathy/peroneal subluxation has not been found to be effective.[53] Surgical management is often warranted, and it is extremely important that the surgeon reassess intraoperatively and be prepared to address all contributing etiologic factors at the time of surgery and avoid recurrence of pathology.[54] The surgical plan for management of peroneal tendon pathology should follow a continuum. Osseous pathology such as a varus deformity in the calcaneus or shallow fibular groove should be addressed first with a Dwyer calcaneal osteotomy with or without lateral displacement calcaneal osteotomy or fibular groove deepening procedure. Once osseous realignment has been performed, the peroneal tendon pathology should be addressed as these remain mobile after repair. The next structures to address are the lateral ankle ligaments as these are immobile and require neutral ankle position after repair. Finally, the superior peroneal retinaculum should be tightened and repaired to the posterior-distal fibula with the elimination of any pseudopocket if peroneal subluxation was present.

At the time of surgery, the patient should be in a lateral position with the aid of a bean bag with pillows between the legs and padding to avoid nerve palsy or pressure from osseous prominences. A thigh tourniquet can be used for hemostasis if desired. Incisional approaches are based on the pathology; if not completely sure of the degree of ankle instability, then stress radiographs of the ankle should be performed once the patient is anesthetized.

The standard approach to peroneal tendon pathology and subluxation repair involves an incision overlying the peroneal tendons from posterior to the fibula and follows the course of the tendons toward the peroneal tubercle and distally as necessary. The sural nerve should be posterior to the incision but is often encountered if the tendon repair is combined with a calcaneal osteotomy for varus correction. The communicating branch of the sural nerve can often be encountered as it travels to the dorsal foot and merges with the intermediate dorsal cutaneous

nerve. Dissection should continue down to the tendon sheath and retinaculum. The tendon sheath is opened, and the tendons are inspected for tenosynovitis and longitudinal tears. The surgeon should assess for presence of space-occupying structures in the fibro-osseous tunnel such as low-lying peroneal muscle belly, peroneus quartus as well as the extent of the fibular groove and fibrocartilaginous rim of the distal fibula. Distally where the sheath splits, one should assess for a hypertrophic peroneal tubercle, which could lead to deterioration of the tendon.

Although there is little evidence-based support for this in the literature, the "50% rule" has often been used to guide management decisions when tendon pathology is encountered. The surgeon estimates the percentage of cross-sectional tendon involvement to determine if the tendon can be débrided and tubularized or if a tenodesis procedure is necessary.[55]

If <50% of the tendon is involved, the tendon can be débrided in a longitudinal fashion and an appropriately sized, nonabsorbable monofilament suture with a taper needle. The knot should be buried within the tendon by starting internally and then proceeding with tubularization of the tendon with a running baseball suture technique (Fig. 57.14A-D).

If >50% of the cross-sectional area is ruptured, a side-to-side tenodesis procedure is appropriate if the viability and excursion of the corresponding muscle are still adequate. Distally, the peroneus longus tendon is sectioned distally and anchored to the cuboid to maintain a static effect on the first ray. An everted position is maintained by placing a towel bump under the medial foot. The epitenon of the peroneus brevis and longus tendon should be roughened at the area of the tenodesis to encourage a fibrous union. The side-to-side anastomosis is performed utilizing nonabsorbable sutures, which may be reinforced with absorbable sutures as needed.[56] Once the side-to-side anastomosis is completed, the diseased portion of the tendon is then excised (Fig. 57.15A and B). Tendon sheath and superior retinaculum as well as subcutaneous layers should be closed in careful fashion to prevent fibrosis and adhesions. A short-leg non–weight-bearing cast should be applied postoperatively.

COMPLICATIONS

General complications with any of these repairs include hematoma, wound dehiscence, neuritis and tendon

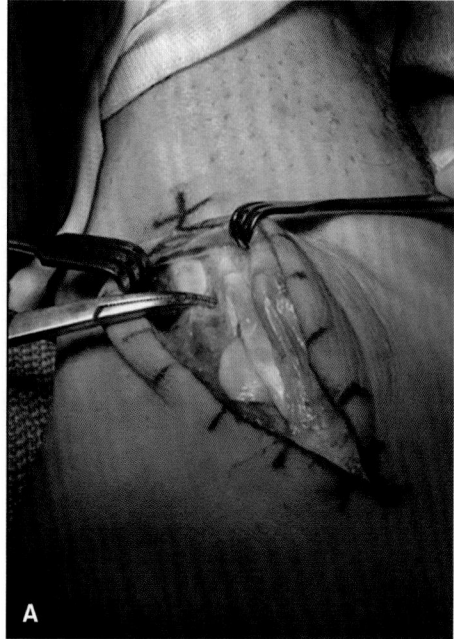
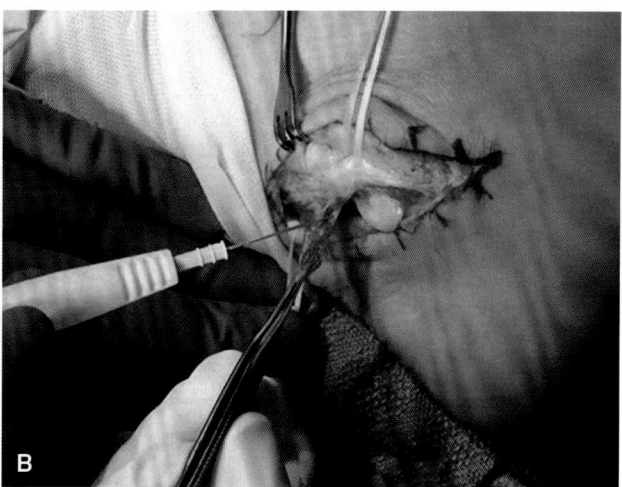
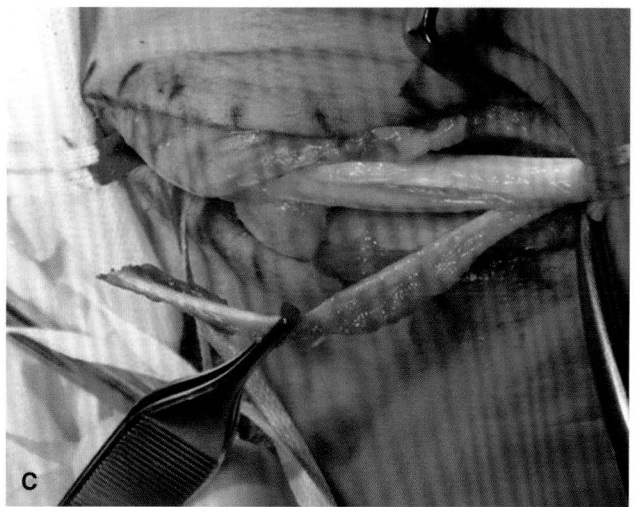
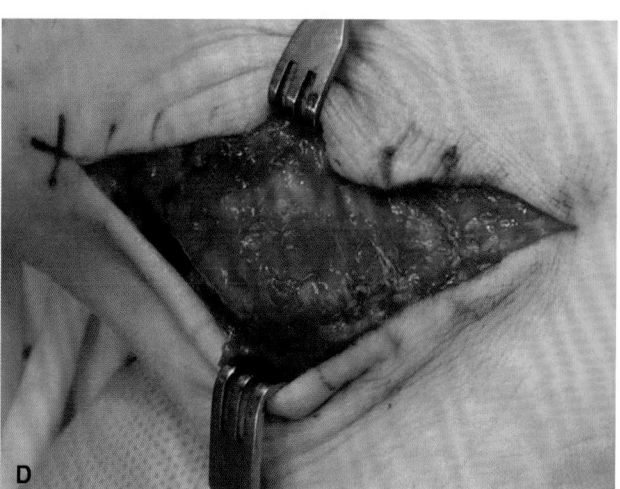

FIGURE 57.14 A. Bucket handle peroneus brevis split tear with subluxation over distal fibula.
B. Resection of low-lying peroneus brevis muscle belly. **C.** Débridement followed by retubularization
of the longitudinal tear, which encompasses <50% of the cross-sectional diameter of the tendon.
D. Peroneal retinaculum and tendon sheath repair.

adhesions/fibrosis, and postoperative infection. Negative
sequelae can be diminished with the use of thoughtful incision placement to avoid neurovascular structures as well as
meticulous surgical technique, which includes anatomic
dissection, gentle tissue handling, and anatomic closure of
the tendon sheath.

If postoperative neuritis does occur, it is often successfully
managed with corticosteroid injections and physical therapy
modalities. If the neuritis or nerve entrapment persists, external neurolysis or neurectomy with implantation into muscle
more proximally can be considered. The use of amniotic membrane grafts overlying the tendon repair has been reported to
reduce inflammation and tendon adhesions.[57] Early protected

range of motion is also helpful to mobilize tendons and reduce
fibrosis and adhesions. If adhesions are problematic, they can
be managed with either open or tenoscopic lysis of adhesions
with subsequent early range of motion. Rerupture of the tendon may occur if the deforming forces are not resolved, and the
foot is not adequately stabilized. This is not generally a short-
term complication, but rather a complication that occurs over
time, particularly when the choice of procedures has not been
adequate to give the foot enough long-term support. Examples
of this may include not addressing a plantar flexed first ray
or rearfoot varus in a patient with peroneal tendinopathy or
rearfoot valgus and equinus in a patient with tibialis posterior
tendon dysfunction.

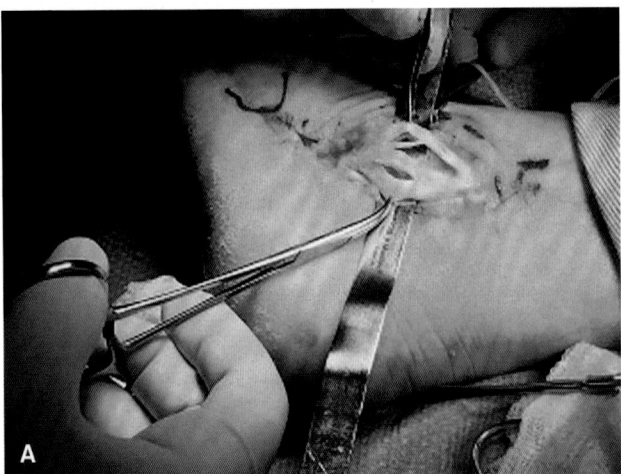
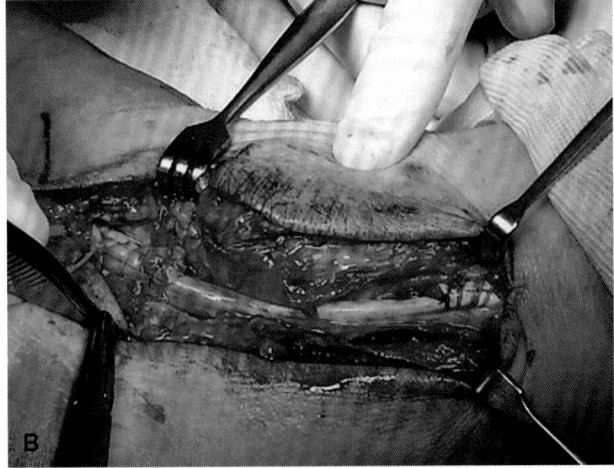

FIGURE 57.15 **A.** Intraoperative finding of multiple longitudinal tears within the peroneus brevis tendon, which could not be repaired. **B.** Side-to-side tenodesis performed as tenodesis of peroneus brevis was not viable due to extensive tears.

POSTOPERATIVE CARE

Following surgical repair of the tendon, patients should be non–weight bearing in a postoperative lower leg splint or short-leg cast for 2-4 weeks. Patients may be allowed to bear weight in a protected fashion in a walking boot or cast at 4 weeks depending on surgeon preference, type of repair performed, and concomitant procedures performed. Physical therapy typically starts at 6 weeks postoperatively with the initial goal to restore range of motion and strength. Passive and active assisted range of motion exercises in combination with gentle scar massage are helpful to prevent the development of scar tissue and maintain the gliding of the tendon within the sheath. Strengthening exercises start with isometric exercises in pain-free range and electrical stimulation of the involved muscle tendon unit. Proprioception and balance activities can be initiated in a seated or partial weight-bearing attitude. The use of aquatherapy and equipment such as a stationary bike can be a helpful adjunct in providing limited weight bearing while still providing excursion of the tendon to prevent fibrosis and reactive tendinitis. At ~8 weeks postoperatively, proprioceptive exercises are gradually expanded from protected weight bearing to full weight bearing to tolerance. Eccentric, concentric, and isotonic progressive resistive exercises are initiated with the use of a TheraBand and other modalities as available. As the strength and proprioception improve, gait training is initiated in a controlled fashion without the protection of the walking boot. Running and sport-specific rehabilitation activities should not be initiated until at least 12 weeks from the repair and not until range of motion, strength, proprioception, and gait training have returned to functional levels. It is important to emphasize that the progression through rehabilitation following tendon repair is variable. The general tendon rehabilitation protocol as described above should be used as a guide. A specific rehabilitation protocol should be tailored according to individual patient needs based upon discussions between the surgeon, physical therapist, and patient. It should be dependent upon the exact nature of tendon injury repair as well as the functional demands and expectations of the patient.[46]

PEARLS and PITFALLS

- Clinical evaluation of resting tension and function should be performed for any laceration penetrating the deep fascia.
- Lacerations distal to the MPJ may not need to be repaired if the extensor expansion remains viable.
- MRI and ultrasonography are the best imaging modalities to assess for tendon pathology. MRI allows for greater visualization of surrounding structures; however, ultrasound allows for real-time, dynamic assessment of the tendon.
- Grasping or locking suture constructs with 4-strand core sutures provide increased strength and resistance to gap formation while avoiding excessive bulk.
- Taper suture needles should be utilized to prevent further tendon trauma.
- During tendon reapproximation/repair, the foot should be placed in physiological tension and protected throughout remainder of procedure and postoperatively.
- Closure of the tendon sheath and use of an amniotic membrane may help prevent fibrosis and adhesions.

Chronic Ruptures

- Assessment of underlying structural deformities need to be considered and appropriately managed to avoid recurrence/rerupture.
- Intraoperative assessment and sequence of repair should follow a continuum. Correct osseous deformities followed by tendon and ligament repair.
- If greater than or less than 50% of the cross-sectional diameter of the tendon is ruptured, this helps determine débridement and repair vs tenodesis/tendon grafting.
- Tenodesis is appropriate only if the viability and excursion of the muscle are adequate.
- If tendon reapproximation is not possible, an adjacent tendon graft, tendon transfer, or nonanatomic repair may be considered.

REFERENCES

1. Abate M, et al. Pathogenesis of tendinopathies: inflammation or degeneration? *Arthritis Res Ther.* 2009;11(3):235. doi: 10.1186/ar2723.
2. Tan J, Wang B, Xu Y, Tang JB. Effects of direction of tendon lacerations on strength of tendon repairs. *J Hand Surg Am.* 2003;28:237-242.
3. Floyd DW, Heckman JD, Rockwood CA. Tendon lacerations in the foot. *Foot Ankle.* 1983;4:8-14.
4. Bell W, Schon L. Tendon lacerations in the toes and foot. *Foot Ankle Clin.* 1996;1:355-372.
5. James R, Kesturu G, et al. Tendon: biology, biomechanics, repair, growth factors, and evolving treatment options. *J Hand Surg Am.* 2008;33:102-112.
6. Lin TW, Cardenas L, Soslowsky LJ. Biomechanics of tendon injury and repair. *J Biomech.* 2004;37(6):865-877.
7. Gagliano N, et al. Tendon structure and extracellular matrix components are affected by spasticity in cerebral palsy patients. *Muscles Ligaments Tendons J.* 2013;3(1):42-50. doi: 10.11138/mltj/2013.3.1.042.
8. Fenwick SA, et al. The vasculature and its role in the damaged and healing tendon. *Arthritis Res.* 2002;4(4):252-260. doi: 10.1186/ar416.
9. Lewis JS. Rotator cuff tendinopathy: a model for the continuum of pathology and related management. *Br J Sports Med.* 2010;44:918-923.
10. DeOliveira RR, Lemos A, et al. Alterations of tendons in patients with diabetes mellitus: a systematic review. *Diabet Med.* 2011;28:886-895.
11. Gaida JE, Alfredson H, et al. Asymptomatic Achilles tendon pathology associated with a central fat distribution in men and peripheral fat distribution in women: a cross-sectional study of 298 individuals. *BMC Musculoskelet Disord.* 2010;11:41. doi: 10.1186/1471-2474-11-41.
12. Cook JL, Rio E, Purdam CR, et al. Revisiting the continuum model of tendon pathology: what is its merit in clinical practice and research? *Br J Sports Med.* 2016;50:1187-1191.
13. Cook JL, Purdam CR. Is tendon pathology a continuum? A pathology model to explain the clinical presentation of load-induced tendinopathy. *Br J Sports Med.* 2009;43(6):409-416.
14. McCreesh K, Lewis J. Continuum model of tendon pathology-where are we now? *Int J Exp Pathol.* 2013;94:242-247.
15. Shepherd JH, Screen HR Fatigue loading of a tendon. *Int J Exp Pathol.* 2013;94:260-270.
16. Docheva D, Muller SA, et al. Biologics for tendon repair. *Adv Drug Deliv Rev.* 2015;84:222-239.
17. Yang, G, et al. Tendon and ligament regeneration and repair: clinical relevance and developmental paradigm. *Birth Defects Res C Embryo Today.* 2013;99(3):203-222. doi: 10.1002/bdrc.21041.
18. Galloway MT, et al. The role of mechanical loading in tendon development, maintenance, injury, and repair. *J Bone Joint Surg Am.* 2013;95(17):1620-1628. doi: 10.2106/JBJS.L.01004.
19. Tang JB, et al. Core suture purchase affects strength of tendon repairs. *J Hand Surg Am.* 2005;30(6):1262-1266.
20. Wu YF, Tang JB. Recent developments in flexor tendon repair techniques and factors influencing strength of the tendon repair. *J Hand Surg Eur Vol.* 2014;39:6-19.
21. Cheung Y. Rosenberg ZS, Magee T, et al. Normal anatomy and pathological conditions of ankle tendons: current imaging techniques. *Radiographics.* 1992;12:429.
22. Mengiardi B, Pfirrmann CWA, Schöttle PB, et al. Magic angle effect in MR imaging of ankle tendons: influence of foot positioning on prevalence and site in asymptomatic subjects and cadaveric tendons. *Eur Radiol.* 2006;16(10):2197-2206.
23. Kaleho P, Allenmark C, Peterson L, et al. Diagnostic value of ultrasound. *Sports Med.* 1992;20:378-381.
24. Hodgson RJ, O'Connor PJ, Grainger AJ. Tendon and ligament imaging. *Br J Radiol.* 2012;85:1157-1172.
25. Pathria MN, Zlatkin M, Sartoris DJ, et al. Ultrasonography of the popliteal fossa and lower extremities. *Radiol Clin North Am.* 1988;1:77-85.
26. Waitches GM, Rockets M, Brage M, et al. Ultrasonographic-surgical correlation of ankle tendon tears. *J Ultrasound Med.* 1998;17:249-256.
27. Vincent LM. Ultrasound of soft tissue abnormalities of the extremities. *Radiol Clin North Am.* 1988;26(1):131-144.
28. Martinoli C, Cittachini G Jr, Pastorino C, et al. High resolution ultrasound of tendon echostructure: normal findings and pathologic changes. *Radiology.* 1992;185(suppl):144.
29. Gillott E, Ray PS. Repair of iatrogenic rupture of the flexor hallucis longus tendon following an akin osteotomy: a case report and review of literature. *FAOJ.* 2012;5(5):1.
30. Harkin E, et al. Treatment of acute and chronic tibialis anterior tendon rupture and tendinopathy. *Foot Ankle Clin.* 2017;22(4):819-831.
31. Simonet WT, Sim L. Boot-top tendon lacerations in ice hockey. *J Trauma.* 1995;38:30.
32. Kass JC, Palumbo F, Mehl S, Camarinos N. Extensor hallucis longus tendon injury: an in-depth analysis and treatment protocol. *J Foot Ankle Surg.* 1997;36:24-27.
33. Joseph RM, Barhorst J. Surgical reconstruction and mobilization therapy for a retracted extensor hallucis longus laceration and tendon defect repaired by split extensor hallucis longus tendon lengthening and dermal scaffold augmentation. *J Foot Ankle Surg.* 2012;51:509-516.
34. Peterson W, Stein V, Tillman B. Blood supply of the tibialis anterior tendon. *Arch Orthop Trauma Surg.* 1999;119:371-375.
35. Al-Qattan MM. Surgical treatment and results in 17 cases of open lacerations of the extensor hallucis longus tendon. *J Plast Reconstr Aesthet Surg.* 2007;60:360-367.
36. Beischer AD, Beamond BM, Jowett AJ, O'Sullivan R. Distal tendinosis of the tibialis anterior tendon. *Foot Ankle Int.* 2009;30:1053-1059.
37. Patten A, Pun WK. Spontaneous rupture of tibialis anterior tendon: a case report and literature review. *Foot Ankle Int.* 2000;21(8):697-700.
38. Markarian GG, Kelikian AS, Brage M, et al. Anterior tibialis tendon ruptures: an outcome analysis of operative versus nonoperative treatment. *Foot Ankle Int.* 1998;19(12):792-802.
39. Bluman EM, et al. Posterior tibial tendon rupture: a refined classification system. *Foot Ankle Clin.* 2007;12(2):233-249.
40. Semple R, Murley GS, et al. Tibialis posterior in health and disease: a review of structure and function with specific reference to electromyographic studies. *J Foot Ankle Res.* 2009;2:24.
41. Bubra PS, et al. Posterior tibial tendon dysfunction: an overlooked cause of foot deformity. *J Family Med Prim Care.* 2015;4(1):26-29. doi: 10.4103/2249-4863.152245.
42. Walters JL, Mendicino SS. The flexible adult flatfoot. Anatomy and pathomechanics. *Clin Podiatr Med Surg.* 2014;31(3):329-336.
43. Hsu TC, Wang TO, Hsieh FL. Ultrasonographic examination of the posterior tibial tendon. *Foot Ankle Int.* 1997;18:34-38.
44. Bowring B, Chockalingam N. Conservative treatment of tibialis posterior tendon dysfunction—a review. *Foot (Edinb).* 2010;20(1):18-26.
45. Gluck GS, et al. Tendon disorders of the foot and ankle, part 3: the posterior tibial tendon. *Am J Sports Med.* 2010;38(10):2133-2144. doi: 10.1177/0363546509359492.
46. Van Dijk P, et al. Rehabilitation after surgical treatment of peroneal tendon tears and ruptures. *Knee Surg Sports Traumatol Arthrosc.* 2016;24(4):1165-1174.
47. Sammarco GJ, DiRaimondo CV. Chronic peroneus brevis tendon tears. *Foot Ankle.* 1989;9:163-170.
48. Sammarco GJ. Peroneal tendon injuries. *Orthop Clin North Am.* 1994;25:135-145.
49. Sobel M, Bohne WHO, Levy ME. Longitudinal attrition of the peroneal brevis tendon in the fibula groove: an anatomic study. *Foot Ankle.* 1990;11:124-128.
50. Saxena A, Pham B. Longitudinal peroneal tears. *J Foot Ankle Surg.* 1997;36(3):173-179.
51. Rademaker J, et al. Alterations in the distal extension of the musculus peroneus brevis with foot movement. *Am J Roentgenol.* 1997;168(3):787-789.
52. Grant TH, Kelikian AS. Ultrasound diagnosis of peroneal tendon tears. *J Bone Joint Surg Am.* 2005;87:1788-1794.
53. Squires N, Myerson MS, Gamba C. Surgical treatment of peroneal tendon tears. *Foot Ankle Clin.* 2007;12(4):675-695.
54. Jaffe D, et al. Functional outcomes of peroneal reconstruction with peroneal tendon transfer. *Foot Ankle Orthop.* 2017;2(3). doi: 10.1177/2473011417S000219.
55. Pedowitz RA, Higashigawa K, et al. The "50%" rule in arthroscopic and orthopaedic surgery. *Arthroscopy.* 2011;27(12):1602-1603.
56. Rawson S, et al. Suture techniques for tendon repair; a comparative review. *Muscles Ligaments Tendons J.* 2013;3(3):220-228.
57. Demirkan F, Colakoglu N, Herek O, et al. The use of amniotic membrane in flexor tendon repair: an experimental model. *Arch Orthop Trauma Surg.* 2002;122:396.
58. Cook, JL, Purdam CR. Is compressive load a factor in the development of tendinopathy? *Br J Sports Med.* 2012;46(3):163-168.
59. Lawrence TM, Davis TR. A biomechanical analysis of suture materials and their influence on a four-strand flexor tendon repair. *J Hand Surg Am.* 2005;30:836-841.
60. Dooley BJ, Kudelka P, Menelaus MB. Subcutaneous rupture of the tendon of tibialis anterior. *J Bone Joint Surg Br.* 1980;62-B:471-472.
61. Wong JC, Daniel JN, Raikin SM. Repair of acute extensor hallucis longus tendon injuries: a retrospective review. *Foot Ankle Spec.* 2014;7:45-51.
62. DiDomenico LA, Blasko GA, Cane L, Cross DJ. Repair of lacerated anterior tibial tendon with acellular tissue graft augmentation. *J Foot Ankle Surg.* 2012;51(5):642-644.

Achilles Tendon Disorders

Alfred J. Phillips, Gina H. Nalbandian, and David J. Caldarella

DEFINITION

Achilles tendon disorders comprise diseases associated with the Achilles tendon and its insertion into the calcaneal tuberosity. These disorders include Achilles insertional tendonitis/tendinosis, retrocalcaneal bursitis, Haglund deformity, noninsertional Achilles tendinosis, peritendinitis, Achilles tendon ruptures, and neglected Achilles ruptures. These disorders will be described in three sections: insertional Achilles tendon disorders, noninsertional Achilles tendinitis/tendinosis, and Achilles tendon ruptures.

CLASSIFICATION

Achilles tendinopathy (Puddu et al., 1976)
1. Peritendinitis
2. Peritendinitis and tendinosis
3. Tendinosis
   2 and 3 can lead to rupture

ANATOMIC FEATURES

The Achilles tendon and its insertion into the posterior aspect of the calcaneus is a complex anatomical system that stabilizes the posterior aspect of the ankle, plantar flexes the foot on the ankle, and aids in the propulsion of the lower extremity through the gait cycle (Fig. 58.1A and B). This biomechanical mechanism translates the leg over the foot through the ankle joint during gait. There are three muscles that contribute to the Achilles tendon complex: the soleus muscle, the gastrocnemius muscle (medial and lateral head), and the plantaris muscle. The gastrocnemius muscle originates from muscle bellies each arising from opposite condyles of the femur. The medial belly is larger and longer than the lateral. The gastrocnemius muscle fibers are fast twitch type 1. The gastrocnemius muscle belly stabilizes the knee posteriorly but also assists as a plantar flexor and a posterior stabilizer of the ankle joint. The Soleus muscle belly originates inferior to the knee joint from the proximal tibia and is wider and flatter than either gastrocnemius muscle bellies. It is a true plantar flexor of the ankle. The muscle is a slow twitch type 1 and primarily has a postural function. The plantaris muscle is small and arises from the medial aspect of the lateral condyle of the femur. It is absent in 6%-8% of the population.[1] The tendon crosses the knee joint and courses distally between the gastrocnemius and soleus muscle bellies. The tendon distally courses along the medial aspect of the Achilles tendon. The plantaris inserts into the anteromedial border of the Achilles tendon. It seldom inserts into the flexor retinaculum. Pathologically, it has been linked to medial pain of the noninsertional Achilles tendinosis. Due to its lack of significant function, it has been used as a tendon graft in repair of Achilles tendon ruptures both acute and neglected. The tendons associated with these muscles constitute the conjoined tendon known as the Achilles tendon.

The tendon fibers twist in orientation during descent. *Edama et al.* described 3 types of twisting after dissection of 132 legs from 78 cadavers.[2] Type I contains the least amount of twist, type II moderate, and type III extreme. Eighty-seven percent of the Achilles tendons dissected met the criteria of the type II (moderate) group. During descent, the fibers of the Achilles tendon course in a counterclockwise direction on a right lower extremity and a clockwise direction on the left lower extremity. The twist begins just proximal to the myotendinous junction and ends at the insertion into the midsection of the posterior calcaneal tuberosity. The intensity of the twisting appears between 2 and 5 cm proximal to the Achilles tendon insertion in the area typical for noninsertional Achilles tendinosis. The majority of the fibers originating from the medial head of the gastrocnemius insert into the posterior aspect of the Achilles tendon insertion, whereas the fibers originating from the lateral head and the soleal muscle body insert into the anterior portion of the Achilles tendon insertion. Some studies have also indicated that fibers from the Achilles tendon insertion continue to course around the posterior inferior aspect of the calcaneus and continue within the plantar fascia. This is especially noted in younger individuals.[3]

The posterior calcaneal tuberosity is divided into three sections; the superior facet, middle facet, and inferior facet (Fig. 58.2). The Achilles tendon inserts primarily into the middle facet below the posterosuperior aspect of the calcaneal tuberosity, essentially two centimeters distal to the posterior superior aspect of the calcaneal tuberosity.[2] The normal tendon at its insertion is ~5-6 mm in depth from anterior to posterior.[4] The middle facet is trapezoidal in shape and has many linear grooves marking the site of insertion. Ballal described the area of insertion as a footprint. The mean width of the footprint is 28.3 mm and the length 7.8 mm.[5] Pathologically, this is the area where the retrocalcaneal exostosis originates. Interestingly, the majority of fibers inserting into the anterior aspect of the

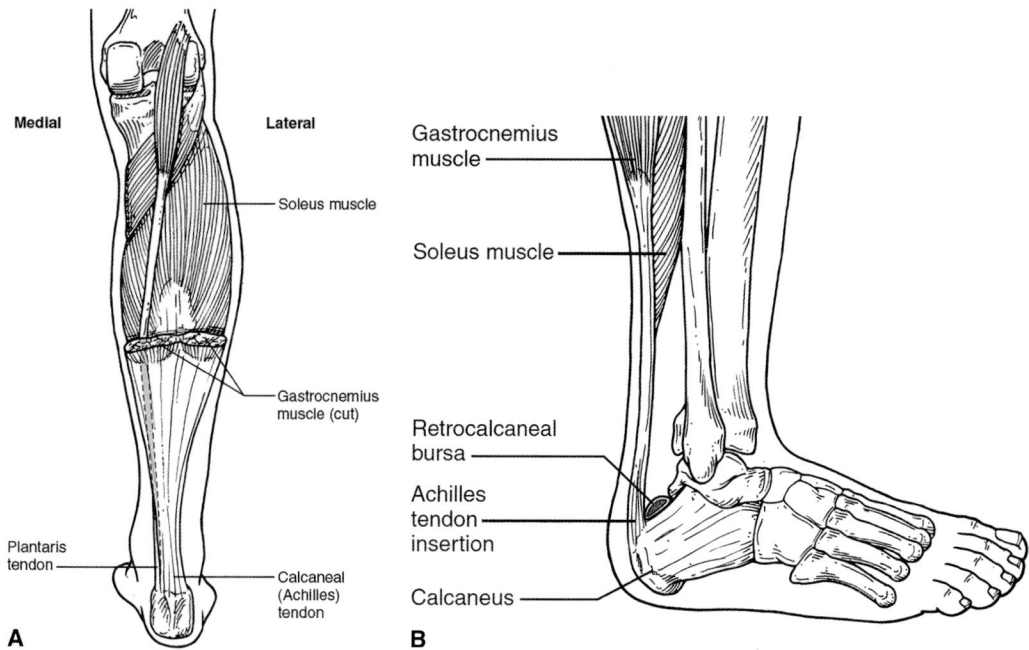

FIGURE 58.1 **A, B.** Lateral and posterior view of the anatomic depiction of the Achilles tendon complex: the soleus muscle is clearly seen deep to the gastrocnemius muscle (medial and lateral heads). The plantaris muscle is found crossing the knee joint and seen coursing along the anteromedial aspect of the Achilles tendon.

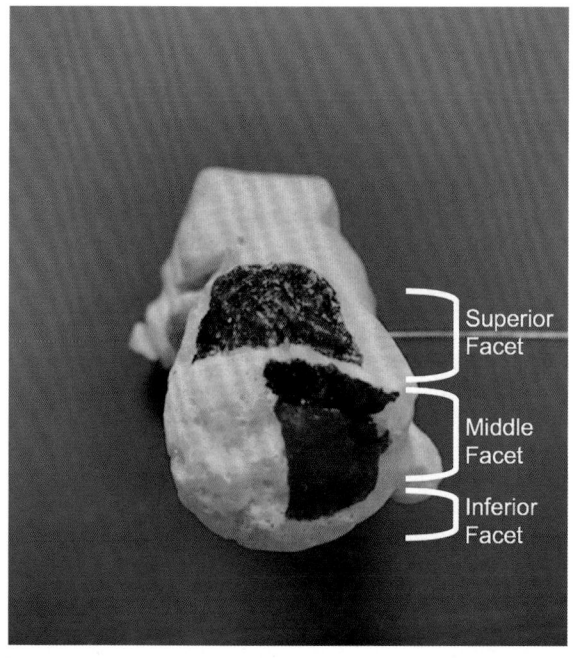

FIGURE 58.2 Site of attachment of the Achilles tendon to the calcaneal tuberosity. Right calcaneal tuberosity, posterior view. The calcaneal tuberosity was divided into three parts: superior facet, middle facet, and inferior facet. *Green,* superior facet site of the retrocalcaneal bursa; *blue,* fibers from the lateral head of the gastrocnemius; *red,* fibers from the medial head of the gastrocnemius; *yellow,* fibers from the soleus muscle. (With permission from Edama M, et al. Structure of the Achilles tendon at the insertion on the calcaneal tuberosity. *J Anat.* 2016;229(5):610-614.)

calcaneal tuberosity from the soleal muscle is where the majority of the degenerative process in Achilles tendinosis occurs.

The Achilles insertion is crescent shaped from medial to lateral taking on the shape of posterior aspect of calcaneus. There are also medial and lateral bands of the Achilles that insert into the medial and lateral aspect of the calcaneus, respectively.[6] The tendon fibers are smooth and tightly woven. Tendon fibers are arranged in individual fascicles covered by endotenon, while the tendon itself is covered with an epitenon. The Achilles tendon is covered with a loose visceral layer of tissue called the paratenon, which is present throughout the course of the conjoined tendon that carries the neurovascular supply to the tendon.

The Achilles tendon vascular supply occurs with the perimysial vessels at the myotendinous junction, along the course of the Achilles tendon through the paratenon, and at the insertion of the Achilles tendon. The primary vascular system is along the Achilles tendon via the paratenon and a capillary vascular loop. The least amount of blood supply occurs 2-6 cm proximal to the Achilles insertion and is frequently referred to as the watershed area. The vascular density of blood vessels in the midportion of the Achilles tendon is approximately half of what it is at the myotendinous junction and the Achilles tendon insertion.[7]

The nerve supply to the Achilles tendon is provided by musculature surrounding the tendon and its periphery as well as cutaneous nerves in the area including branches from the sural nerve. The cutaneous and deep nerve fibers penetrate the paratenon accompanying blood vessels, some of which continue into the tendon themselves. Overall there is a minimal nerve supply to the tendon itself, and the number of nerve endings in the paratenon is relatively low.[8]

A retrocalcaneal bursa is present at the junction between the anterior aspect of the Achilles tendon and the posterior

superior aspect of the calcaneal tuberosity. It is present at birth and protects the Achilles tendon from fraying on the posterior superior aspect of the calcaneal tuberosity. The posterior aspect of the bursa lies on the cartilaginous portion of the anterior aspect of the Achilles tendon, while the anterior aspect of the bursa lies on the superior calcaneal facet. The bursa aids in helping to maintain a constant distance between the Achilles tendon and the ankle joint axis of rotation during dorsiflexion and plantar flexion.

FUNCTIONAL ANATOMICAL CONSIDERATIONS

Foot structure and biomechanics of the lower extremity have an effect on the Achilles tendon. The two extremes of foot structure are the pes cavus and pes valgus foot type. Each of these foot types positions the calcaneus in a way that shortens the combined Achilles tendon structure creating equinus. Pes cavus foot shortens the tendon due to the varus position of the calcaneus. The pes valgus shortens the tendon by the declination of the calcaneal longitudinal axis with the midfoot collapse. Each of these scenarios results in equinus. The forefoot and rearfoot motion contribute to the amount of ankle dorsiflexion and could contribute to the pathology of IAT as well.[9] The increased physical tension caused by the equinus creates pathological changes to the Achilles tendon.

PATHOGENESIS OF TENDINOSIS

Histologically, the tendon is an organized network of primarily tenocytes and tenoblasts at the cellular level and connective tissue consisting of collagen type I and elastin at the noncellular level. Pathologically, this organized network degenerates and as a result drastically changes the histological structure of the tendon. The glistening white structure of the tendon becomes gray and fatty in the gross appearance, and microscopically the collagen and elastin become disorganized and degenerate. Collagen I turns into weak collagen III.[8] During the reparative process, sensory nerves develop and grow with the evolving vascular supply in response to repetitive loading and response to injury. Levels of the P substance within the degenerating portion of the tendon increase due to this neurovascular ingrowth. This creates pain at the site of degeneration, which is present with both insertional and noninsertional Achilles tendinosis.[7,10]

INSERTIONAL ACHILLES DISORDERS

INSERTIONAL ACHILLES TENDINITIS/TENDINOSIS AND RETROCALCANEAL EXOSTOSIS

The terms tendinitis and tendinosis can sometimes be used interchangeably when discussing Achilles tendon disorders. Tendinitis is an acute inflammatory reaction that is painful but generally short-term if treated aggressively. Tendinosis is a degenerative process where the tendon fibers deteriorate and collapse creating long-term effects. Both tendinitis and tendinosis are primarily caused by physical stress and strain on the tendon.

Insertional Achilles tendinosis presents as pain at the insertion of the Achilles tendon into the posterior aspect of the calcaneus. Typically, those with Achilles tendinosis present when a patient has been treated at home with rest or anti-inflammatory

medication for acute Achilles tendinitis and does not improve. Insertional Achilles tendinosis is generally more challenging to treat. It is common in athletes and those playing recreational sports but also in obese and elderly patients. Achilles tendinosis accounts for 10% of all running injuries.[11] There is also a genetic predilection that can increase Achilles tendinosis dramatically.[12] Systemic etiologies include diabetes, seronegative spondyloarthropathies, gout, and rheumatoid arthritis.

Biomechanically, Achilles tendinosis can occur in situations in which there is relatively high physical stress placed on the insertion of the Achilles tendon such as gastrocsoleus or gastrocnemius equinus. This physical stress creates microtears within the tendinous insertion creating an inflammatory disorder (tendinitis) that eventually develops into a degenerative process (tendinosis) if not treated. Some studies have reported the presence of small amounts of inflammatory cells from specimens taken from surgical débridement.[13,21] This indicates a combination of acute and chronic histologic findings. This is generally caused by physical strain at the insertion from either equinus, the shape of the calcaneus, or either a cavus or valgus foot type. This creates tension on the more superficial (posterior) fibers and compression on the deeper (anterior) fibers, which leads to the development of a degenerative process in the anterior aspect of the Achilles tendon. The anterior portion of the Achilles tendon undergoes endochondral ossification at its insertion due to the physical stress and degenerative process. This ossification results in the enthesis or retrocalcaneal exostosis.[14] The enthesopathy known as retrocalcaneal exostosis is thus a development due to the physical stress as well. Benjamin et al. described the exostosis developing due to endochondral ossification as a way for the bone to have greater surface area on the tendon.[15] Exostoses are as common on the asymptomatic side as they are on the symptomatic side.[13-16] There is a correlation between a large exostosis being symptomatic and a small exostosis in the contralateral limb being asymptomatic.[16,13] There are also nonmechanical etiologies such as steroid use, use of estrogen, fluoroquinolones, and inflammatory arthritides, which also can result in the degradation of the insertion of the Achilles tendon.

PHYSICAL EXAMINATION

On examination, patient presents with a painful posterior prominence, localized edema, and occasional erythema at the Achilles tendon insertion. The tendon insertion appears thicker than a normal tendon insertion. Pain is either upon palpation of the prominence or at the Achilles insertion or just superior to this. Frequently, there is pain upon palpation in both areas. There is occasionally pain upon forced dorsiflexion of the foot on the lower leg. Typically, patients have an ankle equinus condition, and it is recommended that a Silfverskiold test be performed to differentiate between the soleus equinus and gastrocnemius equinus. Local numbness or paresthesias can be noted around the area due to nerve compression or traction. Inability to perform a single limb heel raise and weakness of the gastro-soleal complex are commonly seen in the clinical physical examination. Gait evaluation reveals an early heel off and a quick lateral lumbar shift to the contralateral limb.

IMAGING AND DIAGNOSTIC STUDIES

Lateral and calcaneal axial radiographs are typically performed of the foot. Irregularities are frequently noted at the insertion

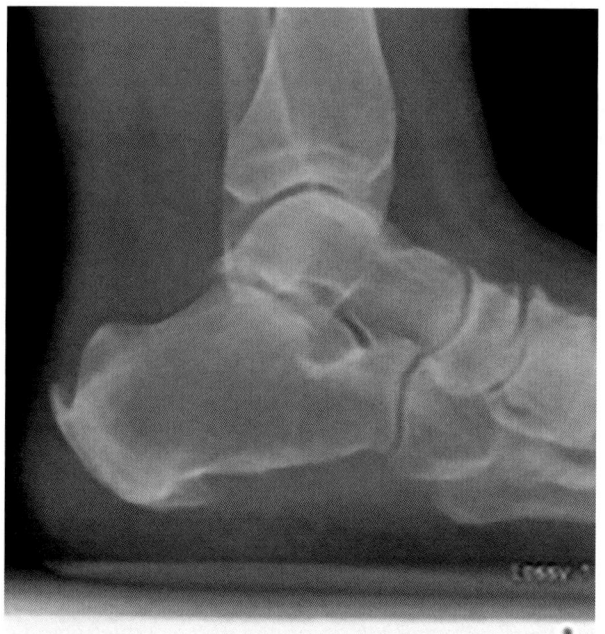

FIGURE 58.3 Lateral radiograph revealing moderate retrocalcaneal spur.

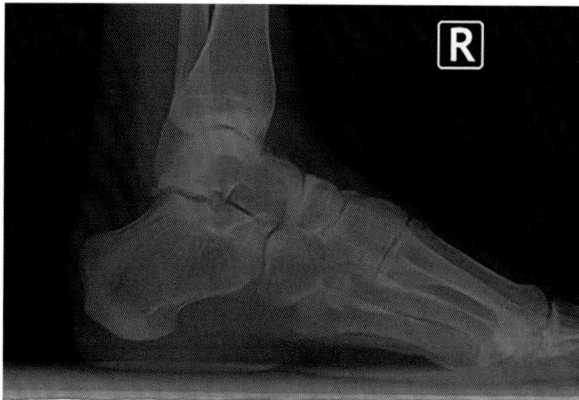

FIGURE 58.4 Hypoechogenicity (lower on the *gray* scale) on ultrasound reveals disorganized composition of the microstructure of the tendon indicating insertional Achilles tendinitis.

of the Achilles tendon. These consist of small or large bone spurring (ossification) (Fig. 58.3). Kager triangle can be evaluated from a lateral view. Obscurity of the Kager triangle would indicate the probability of retrocalcaneal bursitis.[17] An increase in the calcaneal inclination angle has been linked to insertional tendinosis; however, Shibuya et al. refuted this assumption stating that there is no statistical difference in the calcaneal inclination angle in those that have exostoses and those that do not.[18] The calcaneal axial view will help to determine the presence of calcaneal varus and the positioning of the exostosis if present.

Diagnostic ultrasound is an effective tool in diagnosing Achilles tendon pathology. The ultrasound can measure cross-sectional area, thickness from anterior to posterior. Hypoechoic (lower on the gray scale) areas indicate pathology of the tendon as well as determine the thickness of the paratenon. This helps to identify paratendinitis. It is also helpful in evaluating and measuring the size of a retrocalcaneal exostosis[13] (Fig. 58.4). Hypoechoic signals can also measure the integrity of the tendon insertion and can reveal disorganized composition of the micro structure of the tendon. In 2014, Chimenti RL reported increased vascularity on color or power Doppler supporting these histological findings.[19] MRI obtains similar information. Nicholson et al. developed a classification system based on MRI findings to aid in treatment. The classification was based on sagittal cuts on a STIR image.[20]

Type I revealed 6- to 8-mm thickness with nonuniform splits in the tendon or punctate areas of degeneration. Type II revealed thickness >8 mm and uniform degeneration of the intrasubstance of the tendon involving <50% of the width of the tendon. Type III revealed thickening of the tendon >8 mm with uniform degeneration involving more than 50% of the width of the tendon. Treatment recommendations based on this classification supported nonoperative treatment for type I and operative treatment for type II and III.

Nicholson demonstrated that the majority of patients with type I involvement responded to nonoperative treatment, whereas those with type II and III degeneration required surgical intervention (Fig. 58.5).[20]

NONOPERATIVE TREATMENT

Three to six months of nonoperative treatment is recommended for insertional Achilles tendinosis. Casting and immobilization of the Achilles tendon via a CAM walker or fiberglass cast is a viable option in the acute setting of Achilles tendinitis. Change of activity and heel lifts can also reduce symptoms initially. After reduction of acute pain, an aggressive physical therapy program is recommended. Physical therapy will consist of eccentric and concentric muscle strengthening. Studies have reported a 67% success rate in reduction of pain with physical therapy with eccentric muscle strengthening that did not allow dorsiflexion beyond perpendicular.[21]

Extracorporeal shockwave therapy (ESWT) is a "mechanico-therapy" using a physical force via high energy acoustic waves to change the biology in the local area.[19] ESWT affects the area by inducing angiogenesis to promote tissue regeneration and provide pain relief. The devices can deliver focused and radial therapy options to treat Achilles tendinopathy. High- and low-energy ESWT has been used for the treatment of Achilles tendinopathy. The literature has been unequivocal in supporting ESWT therapy. Studies have indicated that it is effective in both noninsertional and insertional tendinopathy.[22–24] Rompe and colleagues found that ESWT had better patient satisfaction and relief of pain than eccentric muscle strengthening. Many practitioners consider this a safe and reliable alternative to surgical intervention when other conservative efforts have failed. However, a recent systematic review of ESWT as treatment for tendinosis for common tendons of the lower limb gave a low level of evidence.[25]

Cortisone injections are not recommended for treatment of insertional Achilles tendinosis. Numerous studies have revealed increased risk of rupture due to the injection.[26] It is an accepted practice to inject into a retrocalcaneal bursa as treatment for bursitis; however, care should be given not to

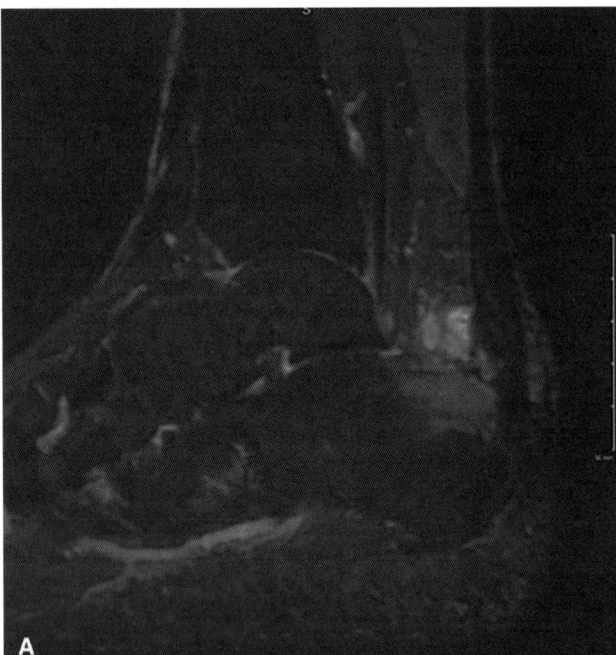 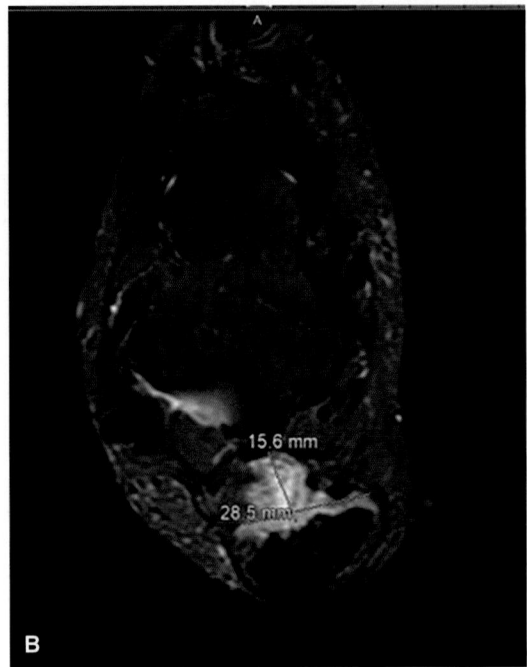

FIGURE 58.5 A. Sagittal and **B.** Axial T2 MRI images reveal a thickened achilles tendon with hypoechoic changes typical of a type III degeneration.

inject the tendon. The injection should be given just posterior to the posterior superior aspect of the calcaneal tuberosity, and there should be no tension when pressing the plunger. Tension would indicate that the needle is in the tendon. Alternatively, the use of an ultrasound is beneficial in prevention of an intratendinous injection.

SURGICAL TREATMENT

Surgical treatment for insertional Achilles tendinosis can be performed by minimally invasive as well as an open surgical procedure. Minimally invasive procedures include ultrasound-guided radiofrequency procedures and minimally open tenotomies or débridements to remove degenerated tendinous tissue. Successful excision of bone spurs performed through endoscopy with an open flexor hallucis longus (FHL) tendon transfer has been noted in the literature.[27] The authors have not had any significant experience with endoscopic excision of bone spurs in a patient with and insertional Achilles tendinosis.

Recent systematic reviews conclude that minimally invasive procedures and open procedures have similar patient satisfaction, but there are more potential complications with open procedures.[13] Open procedure complications include nerve entrapment, wound dehiscence, etc. Generally, however, the minimally invasive procedures are performed on patients with less tendinosis than those with open procedures. Also, a minimally invasive procedure might be chosen when the patient is medically unable to undergo an open procedure and is looking for some relief. Ultrasound can be used in minimally invasive surgery such as ultrasonic débridement with radiofrequency.[28]

Open procedures are done from a prone position. There are a variety of incisions available depending on the location of the retrocalcaneal spur or area of diseased tendon. The approach can be lateral, medial, or split through the tendon. Ettinger reported the ability to visualize all the pathology through a trans-tendinous incision.[29] It is also felt that the central splitting incision is less likely to disrupt the vasculature as well as less of a risk of cutting nerves. The goals of the surgical dissection are to identify the diseased tendon that requires débridement and to identify the retrocalcaneal exostosis that will be resected (if present). It is important to remember during the dissection to only reflect what is necessary. The retrocalcaneal exostosis can vary in size from a spur less than a half centimeter in length and width to one that encompasses the entire calcaneal tuberosity. This will help prevent an intraoperative or postoperative rupture of the Achilles, which can be challenging to repair. It is important to appreciate the fact that the Achilles tendon insertion does fan out medially and laterally around the posterior aspect of the calcaneal tuber. In the author's experience, it is quite simple to reflect the posterior calcaneal exostosis without transecting the entire Achilles tendon insertion.

If there is no retrocalcaneal exostosis, the damaged Achilles tendon, which is typically on the anterior aspect of the tendinous insertion, is excised. Débridement is performed on whatever side the damage is noted from ultrasound or MRI imaging. If the damage is centrally located, then usually a split tendon technique is utilized. It has been suggested that if <50% of the tendon is reflected it is not necessary to utilize a tendon anchor or perform an FHL tendon transfer. It is the author's preference to utilize the FHL tendon transfer when there is significant degeneration of the Achilles tendon and/or >50% of the insertion requires reflection. The dissection for the FHL transfer will be covered in the noninsertional section.

When a retrocalcaneal exostosis is noted and dissected, it can be excised with hand instruments such as an osteotome

and mallet or power instrumentation. The osseous resection should be planned beforehand utilizing preoperative radiographs and confirmed intraoperatively with fluoroscopy. It is the author's preference to use a sagittal saw to perform the majority of these resections. Care must be given not to remove excess amounts of bone. Once the spur is resected, osteotomes are used to mobilize the spur and a 15 blade is utilized to carefully perform any additional dissection to remove the spur. The reciprocating rasp or hand rasp can be used to smooth all edges. If the amount of reflection of the tendon is minimal, the wound is closed, but if the reflection is deemed significant, it is the author's opinion that bone anchors are indicated. At this time the surgeon's choice for bone anchors can be utilized. The goal of the reattachment is to apply and reattach healthy tendon to the footprint of the Achilles tendon on the middle facet of the calcaneal tuberosity. Before beginning the anchoring process, it is important to assess whether the tendon length is enough to reach the insertion point at the calcaneal tuberosity. If not, there should be some consideration of performing a gastrocnemius recession via a Strayer or a proximal gastrocnemius medial release (PGMR) in order to obtain some length. There are data supporting both two- and four-anchor constructs. Ettinger's study supported the use of single- or double-row anchor constructs vs a single anchor.[29] Literature does not identify that four anchors are better than two, but if the surgeon feels that they can obtain better apposition of the tendon on the footprint with four anchors then this is recommended. The author's suturing technique is illustrated in the figures (Fig. 58.6).

Once the anchors have been locked in place and the sutures tightened, closure can begin. It is important to close the peritenon layer since it contains the vascular supply of the tendon. This layer is generally repaired with the deep fascial layer at the same time utilizing a 3-0 absorbable suture. The subcutaneous tissues and skin are then reapproximated with 4-0 absorbable and 4 nonabsorbable sutures, respectively. Care should be given to perform a delicate closure in order to prevent wound dehiscence. Dehiscence is a common complication in open Achilles tendon repairs.

HAGLUND DEFORMITY

Haglund deformity is a separate entity compared to insertional Achilles tendinosis and/or retrocalcaneal exostosis. It is typically a large prominence located in the posterior lateral superior aspect of the calcaneal tuberosity. Patrick Haglund described this deformity in 1928.[30] The deformity is also referred to as a "pump bump" or "winter heel".[31] It can be an abnormally large prominence on the posterior superior aspect of the calcaneal tuberosity. It can also be a result of the orientation of the heel exposing the posterior lateral superior process as in a calcaneal varus deformity. Pressure from shoe gear on the prominence creates a subcutaneous bursa, erythema, and edema. This is generally seen in younger middle-aged active patients. Haglund deformity also can create pressure within the retrocalcaneal space creating bursitis. Similar physical stress that affected the Achilles tendon itself places pressure between the Haglund deformity and the tendon causing the bursitis pain. Inflammation in this area can lead to pathology when there is the presence of a Haglund deformity.

It is very important to distinguish between a Haglund deformity and a retrocalcaneal exostosis. These terms have been used interchangeably within the literature. The authors of this chapter identified the Haglund deformity as the prominence of the posterior superolateral aspect of the calcaneal tuberosity. A retrocalcaneal exostosis is the calcification at the insertion of the Achilles tendon into the calcaneus.

Physical examination of a patient with Haglund deformity presents with a prominent posterior lateral calcaneal tuberosity. Typically it is a heel that is in slight varus. There is pain upon palpation of the prominence. At times there is pain to palpation at the site of the retrocalcaneal bursa. There is also usually a palpable subcutaneous bursa between the prominence and

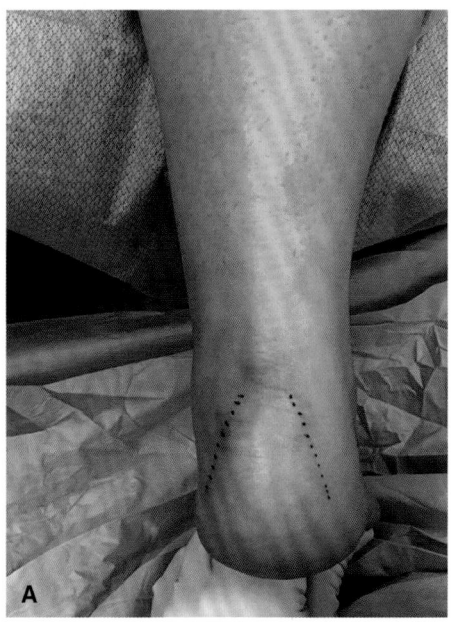
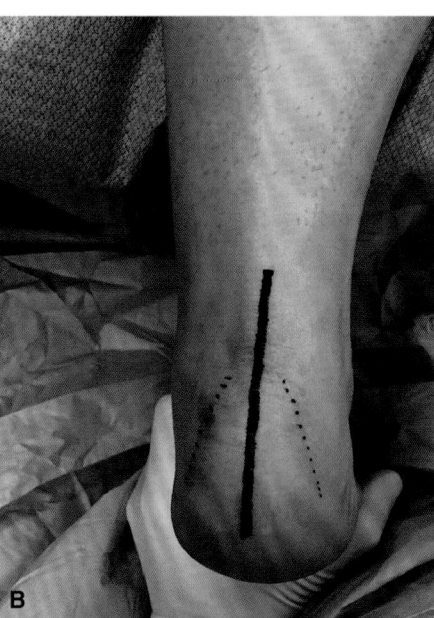

FIGURE 58.6 A. Patient is placed in the prone position. The *dotted lines* represent the lateral and medial flare and broad insertional fibers of the Achilles tendon. **B.** A central linear posterior incision is generally utilized. Alternatively, a medially biased linear incision can provide adequate access including the lateral aspect of the distal Achilles tendon insertional area.

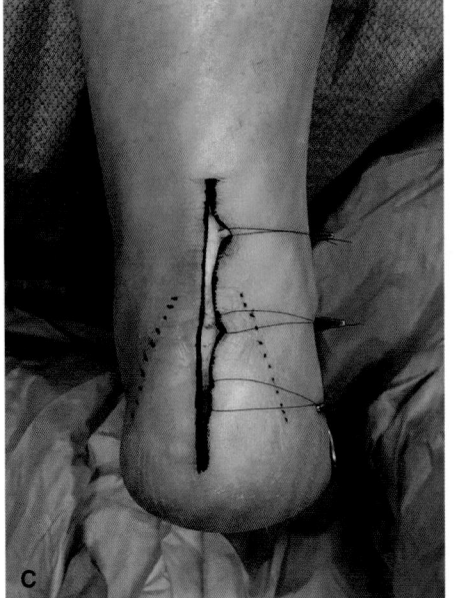

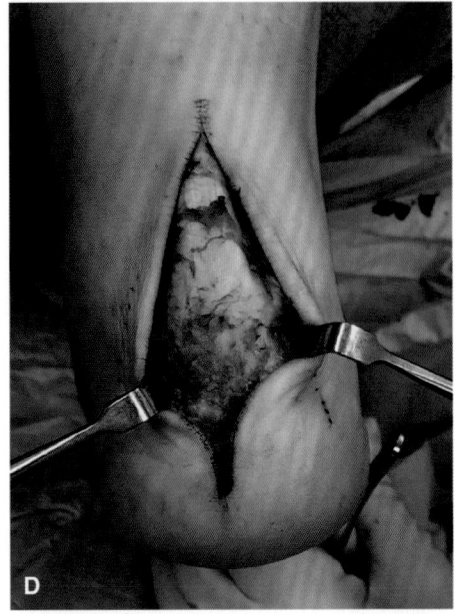

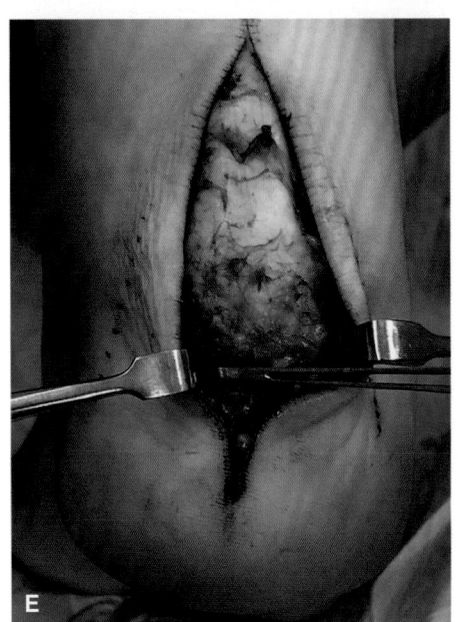

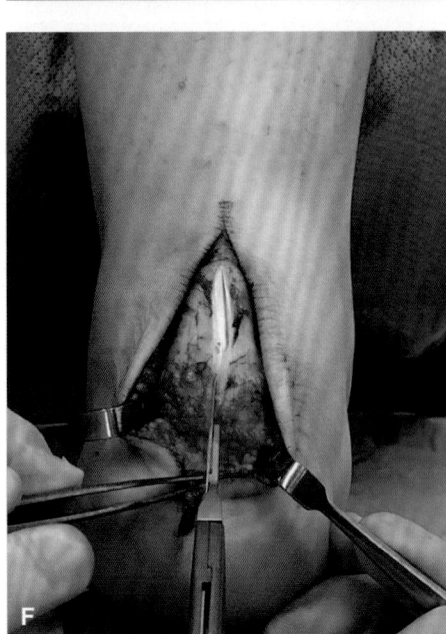

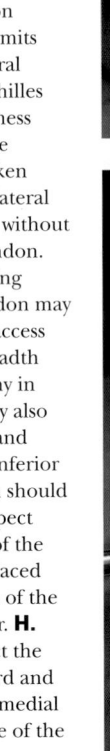

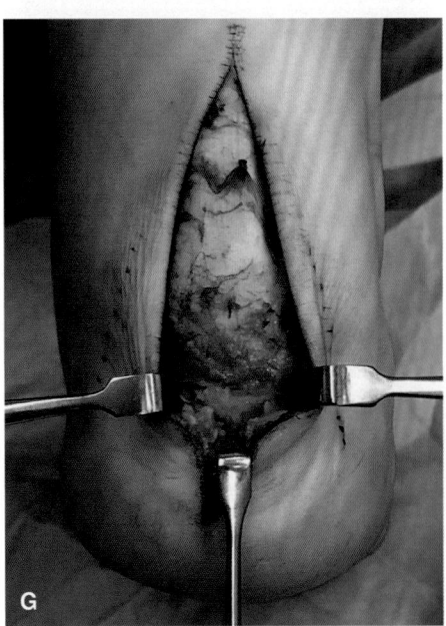

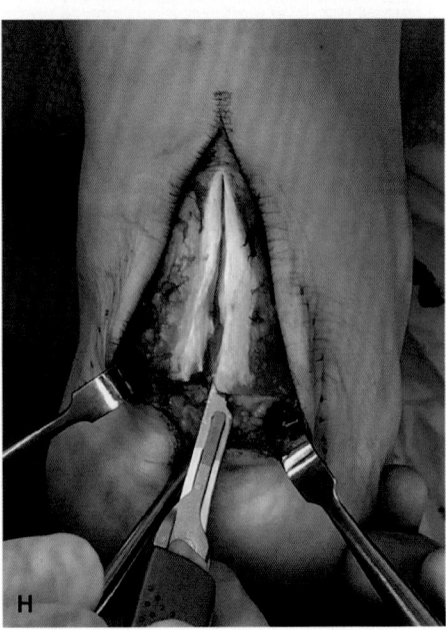

FIGURE 58.6 (*Continued*) **C.** Care is taken to limit anatomic dissection with "no-touch" provisional suture retraction. Absorbable stay sutures are placed as noted to avoid excessive handling and lessen potential for wound healing in this vulnerable area of the posterior heel. **D.** Anatomic dissection completed to the level of the deep fascia overlying the distal Achilles tendon footprint. Adequate exposure permits access to the broad medial to lateral extent of the distal insertional Achilles tendon. **E.** A transverse full-thickness incision is planned as noted by the position of the forceps. Care is taken to preserve the most medial and lateral insertional Achilles tendon fibers without transecting the entire Achilles tendon. **F.** A proximal-based central splitting incision through the Achilles tendon may be executed to provide optional access to the entire medial to lateral breadth of insertional calcific tendinopathy in select patients. This approach may also aid in retaining the most medial and lateral expansion fibers. **G.** The inferior location of the transverse incision should approximate the most inferior aspect of the primary insertional fibers of the Achilles tendon. The inferiorly placed retractor is placed at the junction of the posterior/inferior calcaneal tuber. **H.** A no. 15 blade is utilized to reflect the distal insertional fibers medialward and lateralward without "exiting" the medial or lateral expansion fibers or flare of the Achilles tendon as possible.

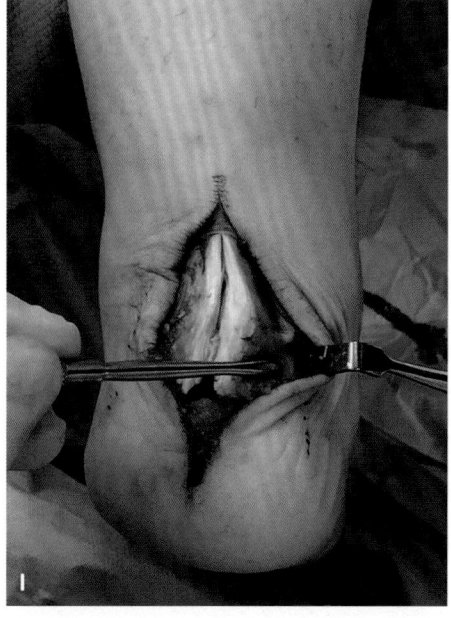

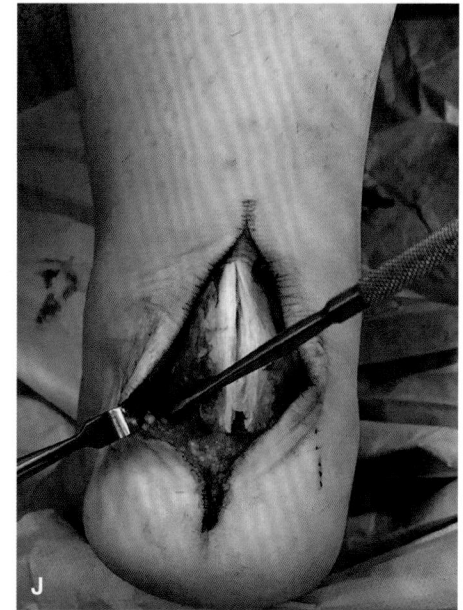

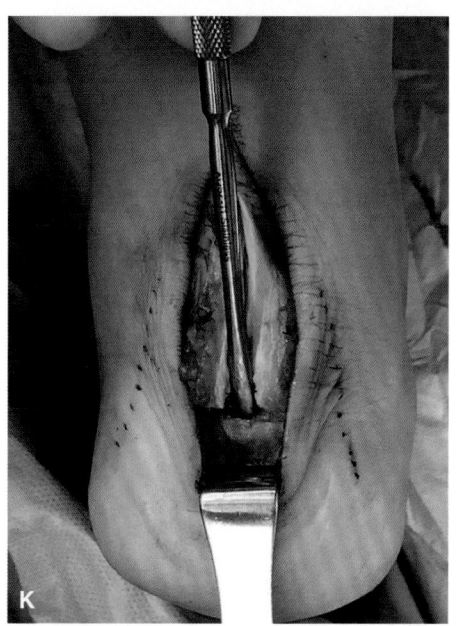

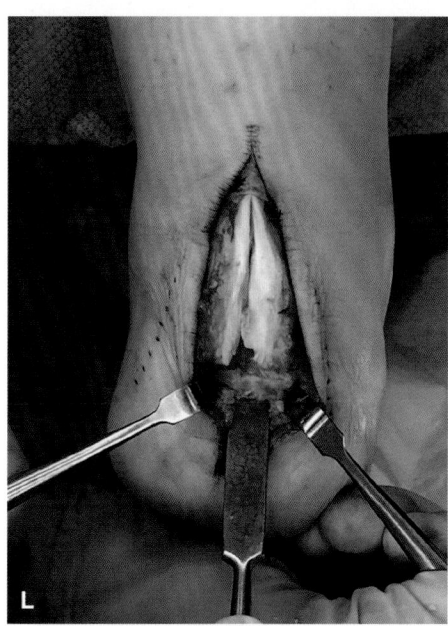

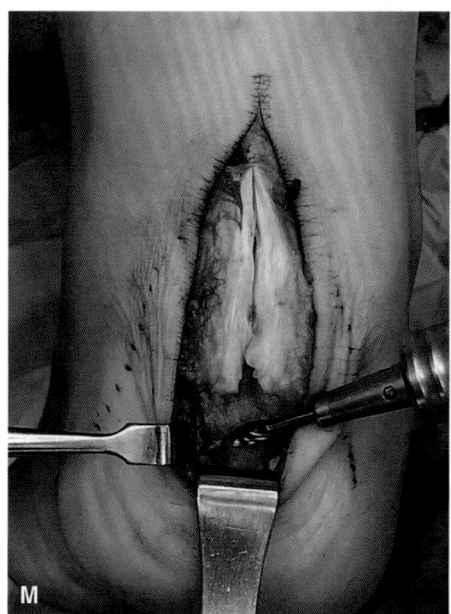

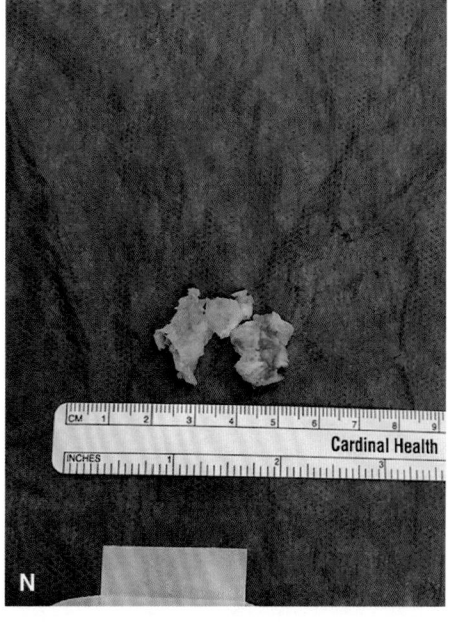

FIGURE 58.6 (*Continued*)
I. Preservation of the underlying medial flair of the Achilles tendon insertional fibers is noted. **J.** Preservation of the underlying lateral flair of the Achilles tendon insertional fibers similarly is noted by the position of the Freer elevator. **K.** The Freer elevator denotes the position and relationship of the distal extent of the insertional fibers centrally following transverse reflection at the zone of calcific changes. The large retractor is positioned to demonstrate where the central Achilles distal insertion thins out onward to the plantar calcaneus. **L.** Once the central distal fibers of the Achilles tendon are reflected as demonstrated, the primary zone of insertional Achilles calcific tendinopathy (IACT) is evident. Débridement and resection of all nonviable fibrous/calcific tendinopathy is critical. **M.** Adequate débridement of all insertional diseased Achilles tendon is accomplished with power instrumentation. A remodeled posterior calcaneal tuber is prepared towards a satisfactory cancellous substrate. **N.** Débridement of all calcified and nonviable fibrous tissue can be proportionately performed centrally, medially, and/or laterally within the zone(s) of involvement.

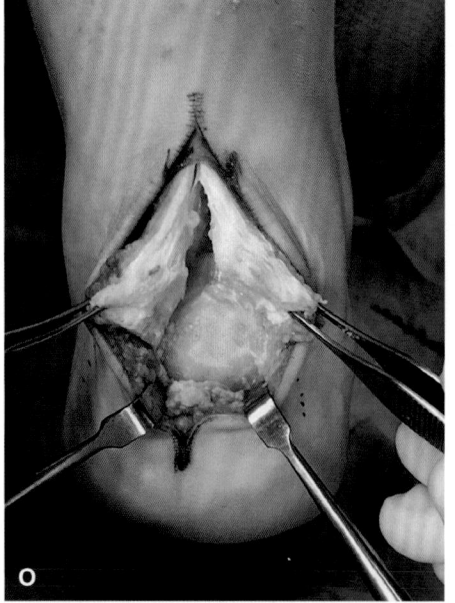

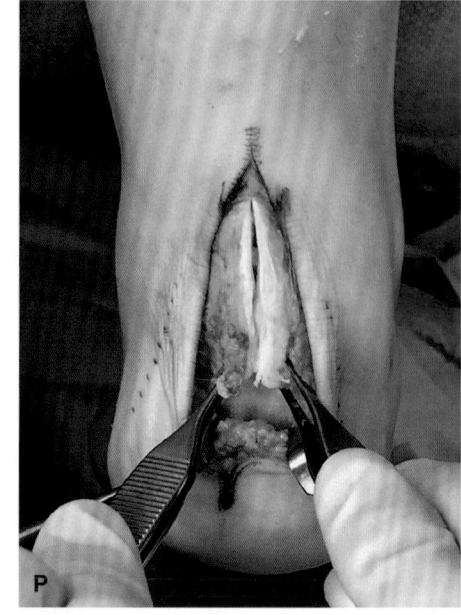

FIGURE 58.6 (*Continued*)
O. Intraoperative view illustrating adequate débridement and resection and a well-remodeled posterior calcaneal tuber. **P.** The forceps demonstrate the planned reapproximation of the distal Achilles tendon. Following final débridement of the calcific changes at the level of the posterior tuber, further anterior-based debulking of diseased fibrous thickening of the distal insertional Achilles tendon may be required. **Q.** Cross-sectional anatomy demonstrating the primary zone of the Achilles tendon insertion centrally noted. Note that the proximal third surface of the calcaneal tuber has no direct insertional attachment. Inferiorly, note the thinning of the Achilles tendon insertion at the distal third of the calcaneal tuber. **R.** Note that the proximal third of the posterior calcaneus is generally preserved as a region of physiologic dissipation of force and "off-loading" of insertional repair of the distal Achilles tendon. Concurrent adventitious bursa may be noted and excised. Note the prepared cancellous substrate as the primary "target" for reattachment. **S.** The proximal row of planned reattachment of the retained insertional Achilles fibers is created first; aligned and prepared to reapproximate the Achilles tendon at its near anatomic position as possible. **T.** Note that the orientation and relationship of the prepared bone tunnels of the proximal row is aligned with anticipated reattachment point within the target site of the primary reinsertion of the distal Achilles tendon.

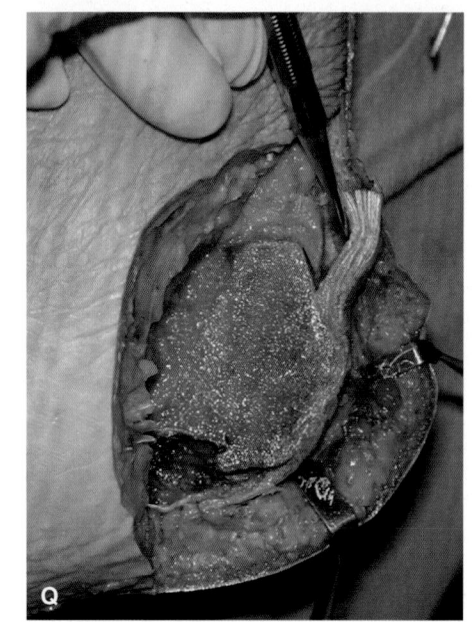

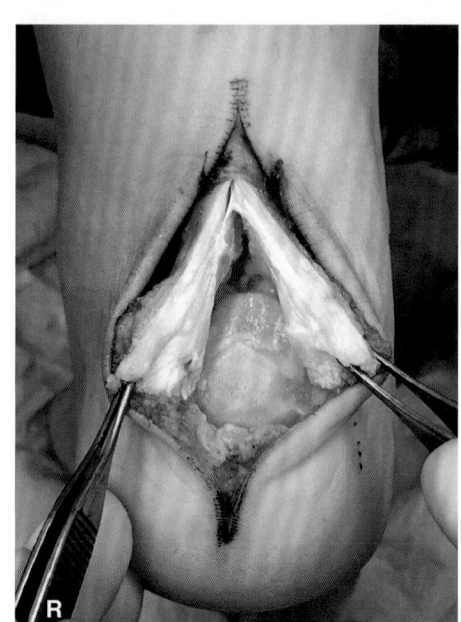

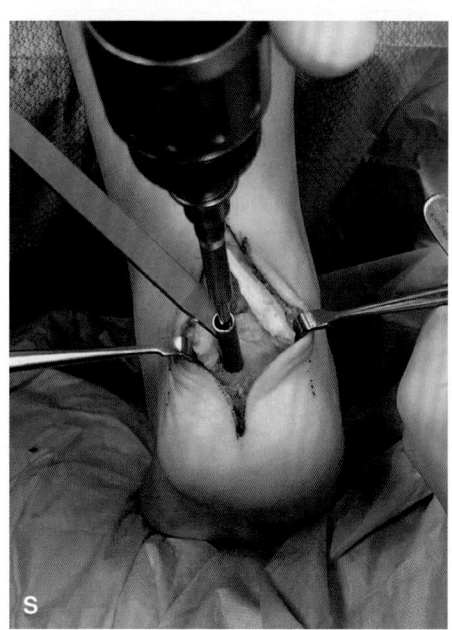

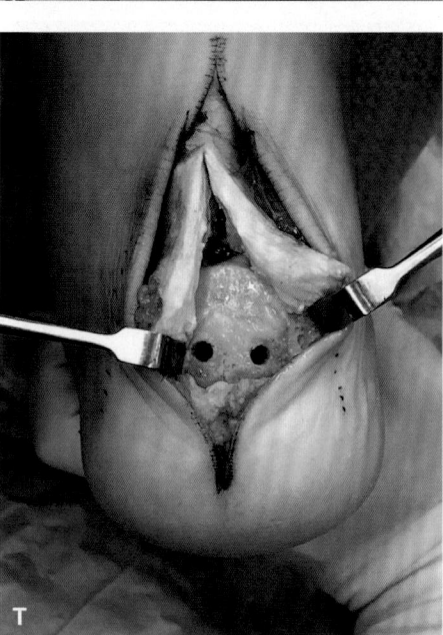

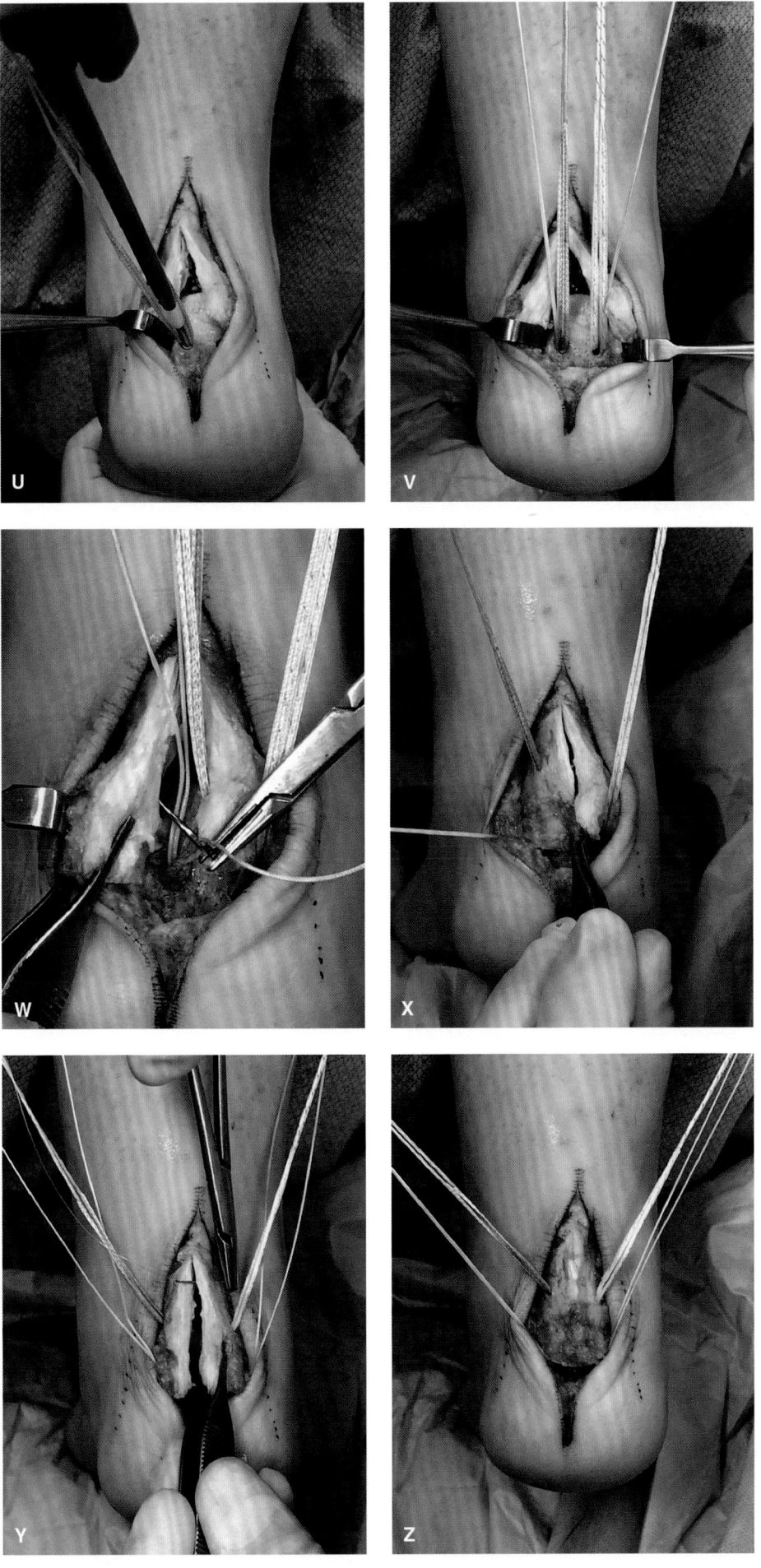

FIGURE 58.6 (*Continued*) **U.** The posterior lateral and medial soft tissue interference screws are all oriented to approximate the "Dead Man's Angle," which optimizes the stability and hold strength of the closed bone tunnel anchor. **V.** The proximal row posterior lateral and medial interference screws each securing two primary strands of polyblend suture tape and one "rescue" strand of polyblend suture. **W.** Next the polyblend suture tape is "transferred" from a deep to superficial position within the distal Achilles tendon substrate both lateralward and medialward. **X.** The *blue* polyblend suture tape strands (medially) shown exiting out from an anterior to posterior position within the distal Achilles tendon insertion. **Y.** The medial and lateral polyblend suture tape strands are now exited from deep to superficial in preparation to reapproximate the distal Achilles tendon footprint to the posterior calcaneus. **Z.** The distal rescue polyblend suture strands inferiorly are preserved for possible augmentation or reinforcement. These additional strands can be helpful in further augmentation of the primary repair or may be discarded following confirmation of a solid reapproximation with the primary polyblend tape.

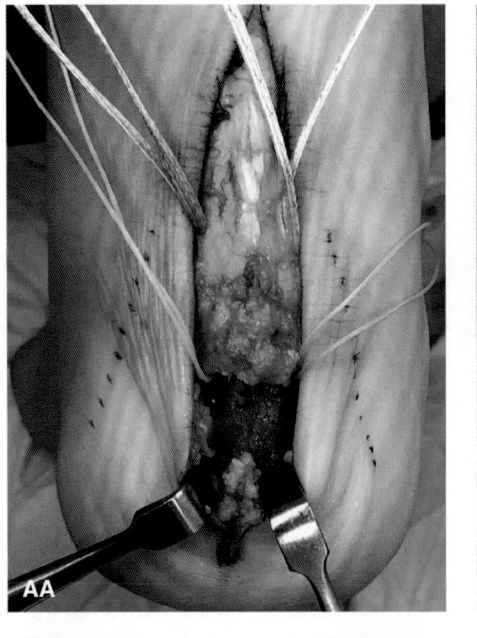

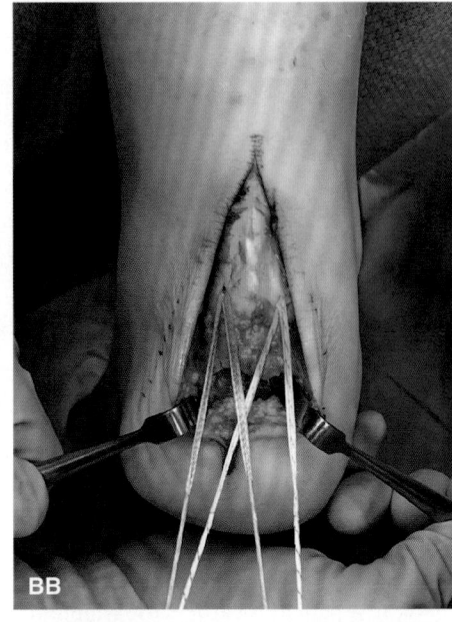

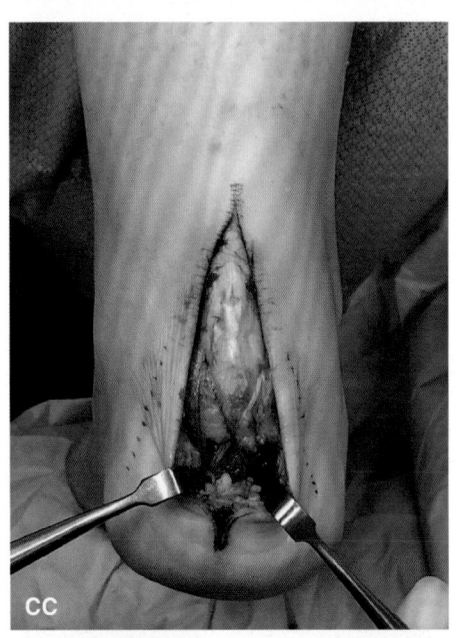

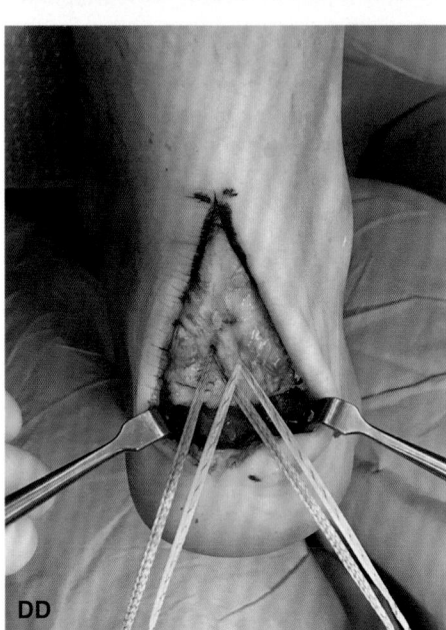

FIGURE 58.6 (*Continued*)
AA. Next, the distal row of closed bone tunnels posterolateral and posteromedial are positioned, drilled, and tapped. Note the position and orientation of the distal row placement within the inferior zone of the prepared posterior calcaneal tuber. **BB.** Provisional orientation of the intended crossing configuration to secure "reattachment" of the distal Achilles tendon footprint. The linear Achilles central splitting incision is first reapproximated with an absorbable suture material. **CC.** Stable reattachment of the crossing suture tape construct. The distal retractors are noted at the posterior plantar junction of the calcaneal tuber. **DD.** An example of the same crossing suture tape via a single transverse incisional approach. No linear central Achilles tendon splitting incision is made; as such the proximal and distal bone tunnel placement remains similarly placed. **EE.** Final reapproximation completing the distal reattachment of the insertion of the Achilles tendon within the appropriate "central zone" and anatomic footprint. **FF.** Final closure with interrupted nonabsorbable mattress suture centrally and simple sutures at the proximal and distal pole of the incision.

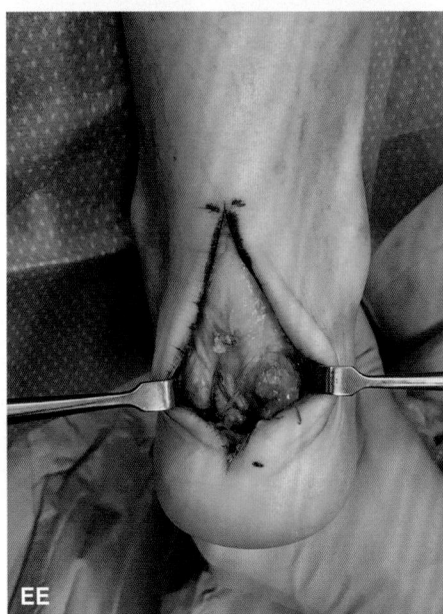

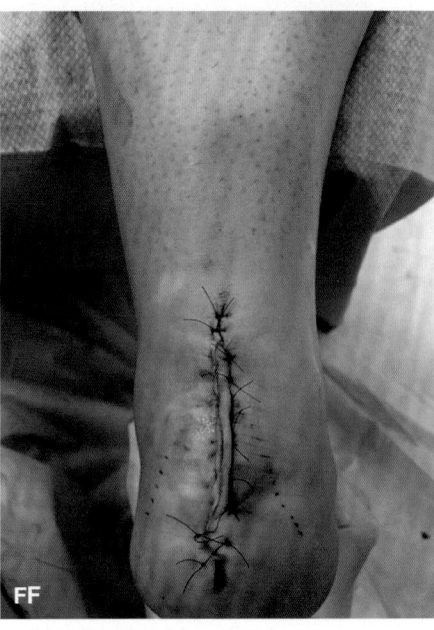

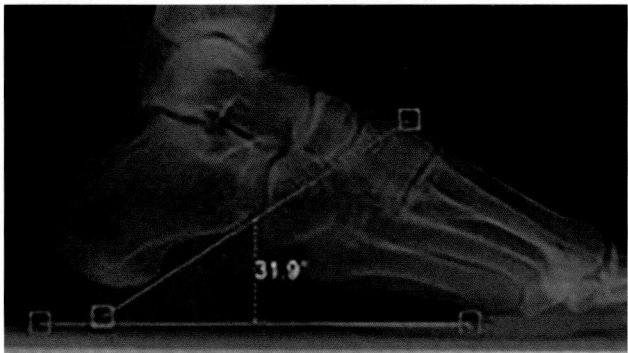

FIGURE 58.7 The calcaneal inclination angle/calcaneal pitch angle measures the angle between the line from the inferior aspect of the calcaneal tuberosity to the anterior tubercle and aligned from the inferior calcaneal tuberosity and the weight-bearing surface.

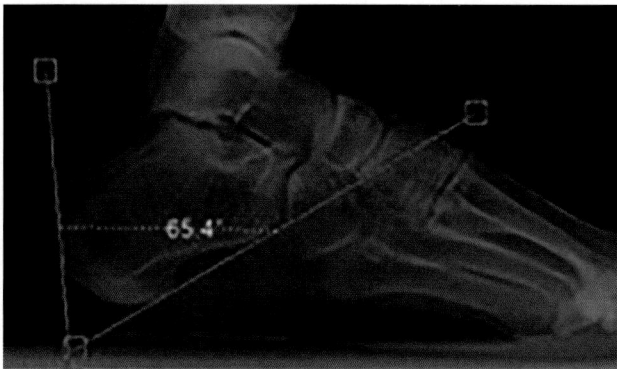

FIGURE 58.8 The Fowler Philip angle is the angle between the inferior aspect of the calcaneal tuberosity to the anterior tubercle with the line of the superior posterior aspect of the calcaneus.

the skin. A patient is particularly symptomatic at the end of the day or after wearing a shoe with a heel counter at the same height of the prominence. In these situations, the Haglund area is erythematous and edematous.

Imaging of the Haglund deformity is generally performed through a weight-bearing lateral calcaneal radiograph. At first inspection evaluation of the outline on the Kager triangle is important. The absence of radiolucency in the posterior inferior aspect is indicative of a chronic bursitis secondary to the effects of the Haglund deformity.[32] Calcaneal inclination angle, Fowler Philip angle and parallel pitch lines have been historically implemented to evaluate Haglund deformity by radiographs. The calcaneal inclination angle/calcaneal pitch angle measures the angle between the line from the inferior aspect of the calcaneal tuberosity to the anterior tubercle and aligned from the inferior calcaneal tuberosity and the weight-bearing surface and is normally 17 to 32 degrees. The Fowler Philip angle is the angle between the

inferior aspect of the calcaneal tuberosity to the anterior tubercle with the line of the superior posterior aspect of the calcaneus and is normally between 45 and 70 degrees. Bulstra et al. measured the calcaneal inclination angle and the Fowler Philip angle in both patients with a Haglund deformity and those without a Haglund deformity. The study revealed that only the calcaneal inclination angle had a correlation with a Haglund deformity and this occurred only in women.[33] Another radiographic parameter is the parallel pitch lines. The parallel pitch lines are determined by a line that begins at the superior posterior aspect of the posterior facet and courses posteriorly parallel to a line from the inferior aspect of the calcaneal tuberosity to the anterior tubercle. If the superior line exposes the superior portion of the calcaneal tuberosity superiorly, that is evidence of a Haglund deformity. The authors have also found that if the prominence is truly posterior superolateral, an oblique ankle view can be helpful in visualizing the prominence (Figs. 58.7-58.10).

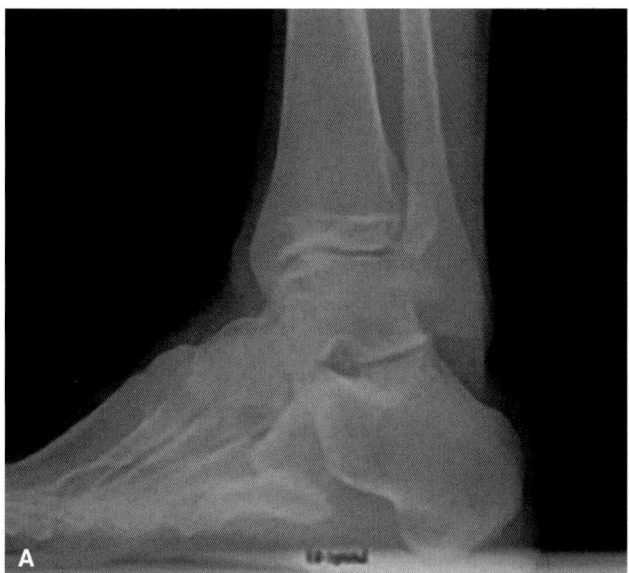

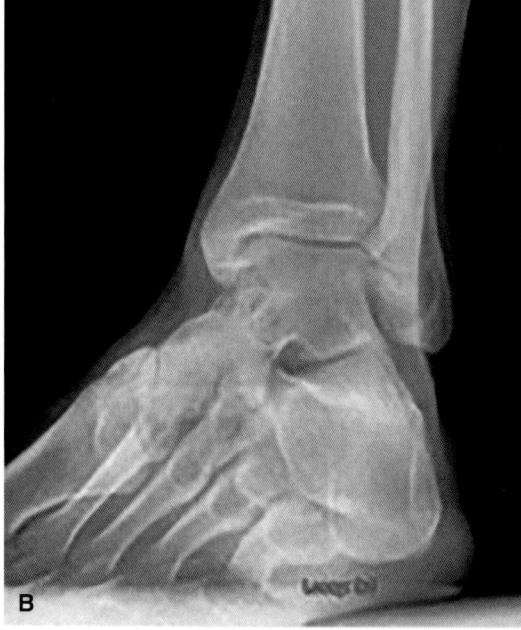

FIGURE 58.9 A, B. If the superior portion of the calcaneal tuberosity prominence is truly posterior superolateral, an oblique ankle view can also be helpful in visualizing the prominence as shown here. This provides a better angle that can be missed on a lateral view.

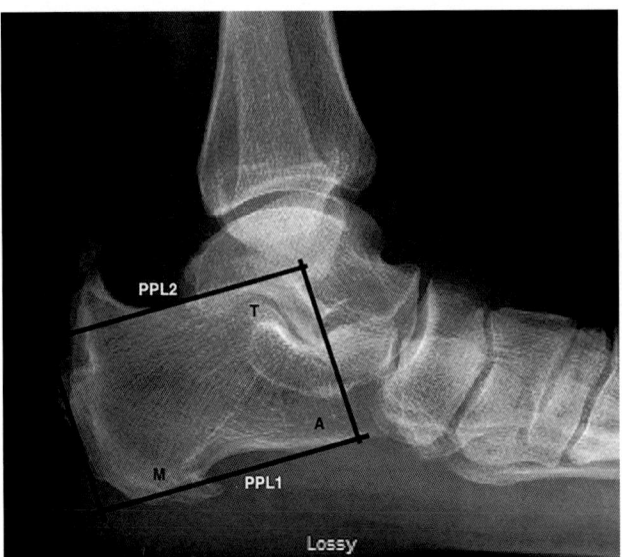

FIGURE 58.10 The parallel pitch line is defined by the baseline tangent to the anterior tubercle (*A*) and the medial tuberosity (*M*) creating (*PPL1*) and a parallel line (*PPL2*) from the talar articular facet (*T*). It is pathologic if the bursal projection of the tuberosity extends beyond the PPL2.

TREATMENT

Nonoperative Treatment

Nonoperative treatment consists of essentially directing pressure away from the Haglund deformity. The first-line of defense is addressing pressure from shoegear. Avoidance of high-heeled shoes with a mid-level heel counter is helpful. Generally wearing a shoe with an open heel or a shoe that has a heel counter that does not rub against the prominence can relieve the pain.

Various padding techniques via silicone or felt can also help in off-loading the deformity. Anti-inflammatory medication does have a role in reducing this inflammation of an acutely symptomatic Haglund deformity.

Surgical Treatment

The patient is placed in a prone or lateral position. The prominence is noted at the posterior superior aspect of the lateral calcaneal tuberosity. Generally a J-type incision is made over the prominence. The incision is deepened through the subcutaneous tissue. During dissection, a superficial bursa is frequently encountered with a synovial lining. This can be meticulously dissected and removed from the wound. During this dissection, the surgeon should be aware of a terminal branch from the sural nerve that typically runs across this area. Frequently when this is identified, it is noted that it is thickened and yellow in color. If this occurs, the author recommends excision of this cutaneous branch. At this time, an incision is then made through the deep fascial peritenon layer to bone. It is best at this time to reflect the tendinous insertion from proximal to distal on both sides of the wound. Once the desired area for resection is identified, the prominence can be resected with either hand instruments via an osteotome and mallet or an oscillating or sagittal saw. The area can then be smoothed with a reciprocating rasp. Bone wax can be applied to the exposed bone to help prevent excessive bleeding/hematoma from developing. Dissection can be made posteriorly to the calcaneal tuberosity to identify the retrocalcaneal bursa and excised if inflamed. After copious lavage of saline, the wound can then be closed in layers. Generally, a 3-0 absorbable suture can be utilized to close the paratenon and deep fascial layer and subcutaneous and skin closure performed with 4-0 absorbable and 4-0 nonabsorbable suture, respectively (Fig. 58.11).

An alternative to a Haglund resection for a young active person who has a prominent Haglund's that extends the entire

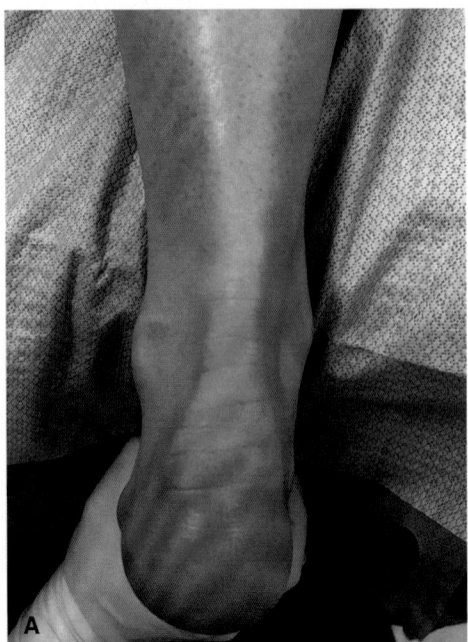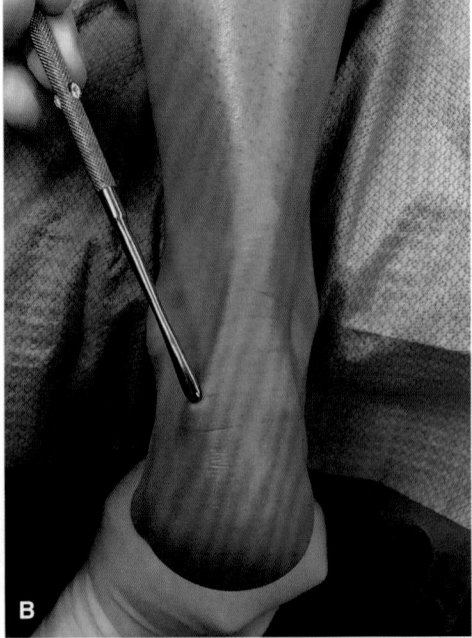

FIGURE 58.11 **A.** Haglund deformity as noted presents as posterolateral superior calcaneal prominence without insertional Achilles tendinopathy. **B.** Freer elevator identifying apex of Haglund deformity and basis of the nidus of mechanical pain.

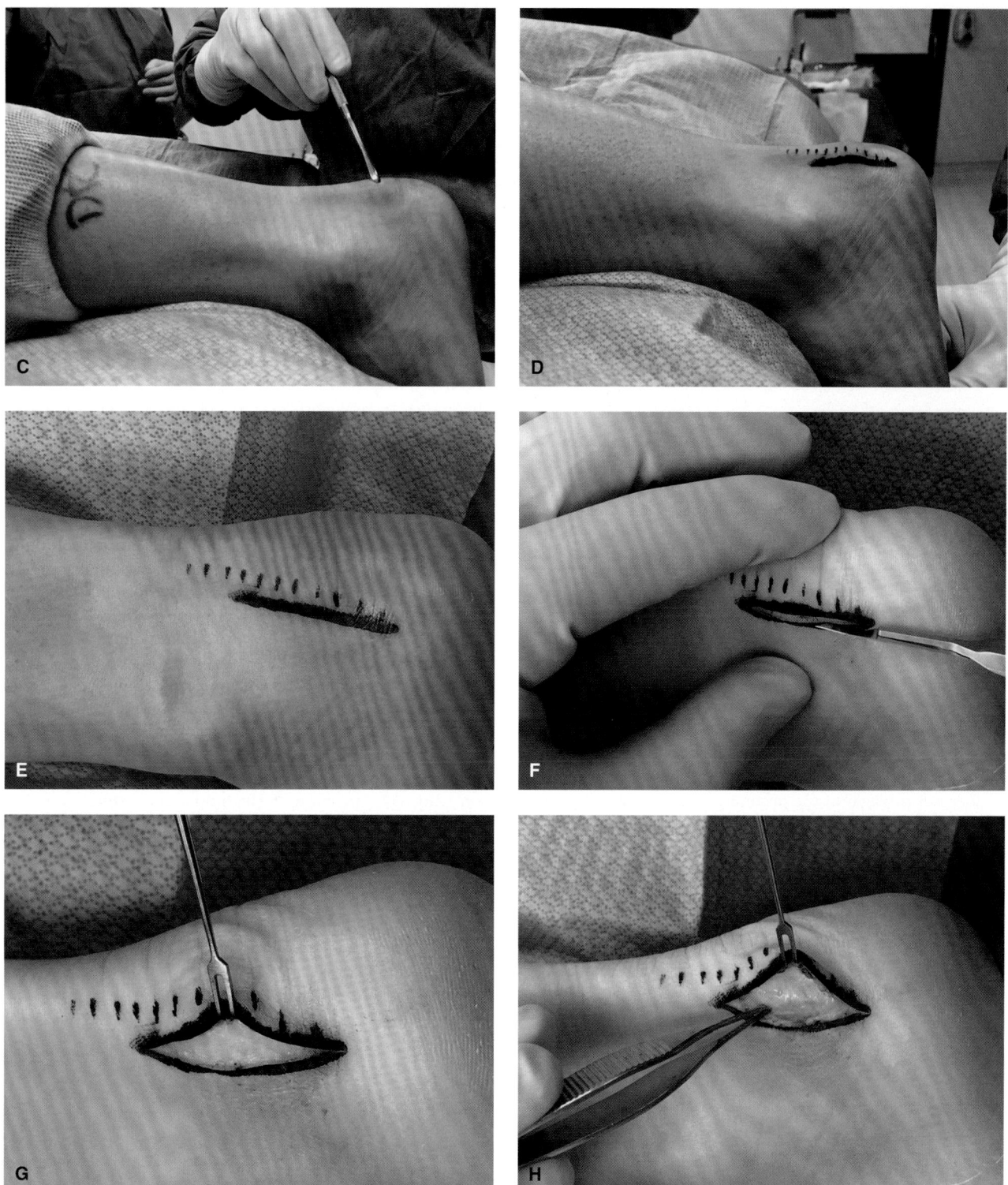

FIGURE 58.11 (*Continued*) **C.** Lateral perspective of posterior superolateral osseous projection and apex of true Haglund deformity ("Pump bump"). No involvement of distal insertional Achilles tendinopathy. **D.** *Dotted line* represents distal lateral extent and lateral border of the Achilles tendon. *Solid line* represents the standard surgical incision plan for access to Haglund deformity. **E.** Surgical incision anterior and parallel to lateral border of distal Achilles tendon fibers. Surgical incision posterior and parallel to primary sural nerve course. **F.** Skin incision is made perpendicular to the overlying posterolateral anatomy. **G.** Anatomic dissection is atraumatically noted to the overlying subcutaneous tissue plane. **H.** Forceps demonstrating the overlying deep fascia at the lateral extent and border of the distal lateral Achilles tendon.

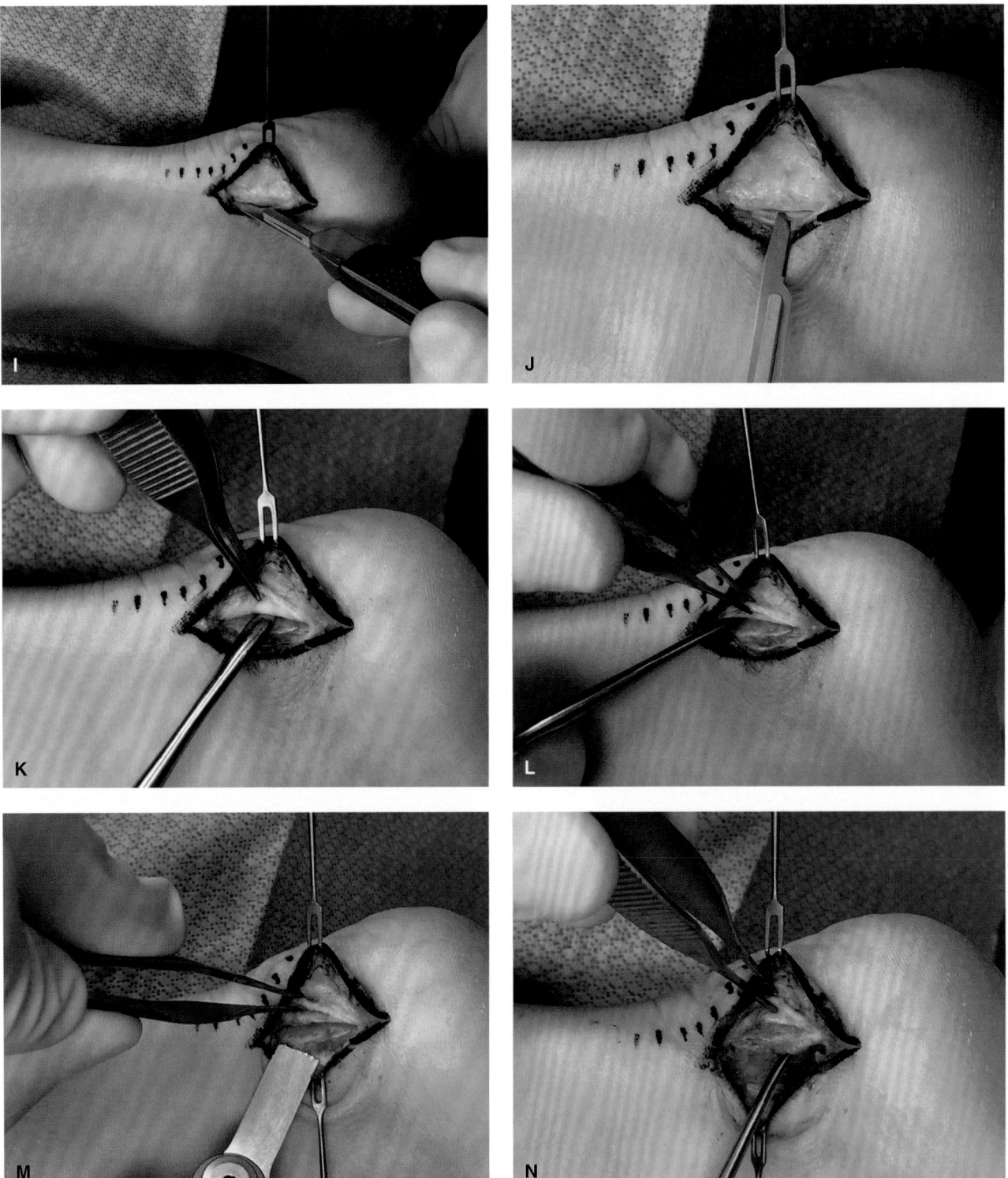

FIGURE 58.11 (*Continued*) **I.** Deep fascia and periosteal linear incision is begun proximally and is made parallel and lateral to the lateral distal fibers of the Achilles tendon. **J.** Number 15 blade demonstrating linear incision completed overlying the superior posterolateral calcaneal tuber. **K.** Freer elevator accessing entrance to the Haglund deformity while preserving the distal lateral insertional fibers of the Achilles tendon. **L.** Freer elevator demonstrating subperiosteal exposure to the prominent apex of the underlying Haglund deformity. **M.** Sagittal saw blade being introduced to resect the prominent apex of the Haglund deformity. **N.** Deep fascia and periosteum being held in forceps. Resected osseous prominence at apex of Haglund deformity being lifted by Freer elevator.

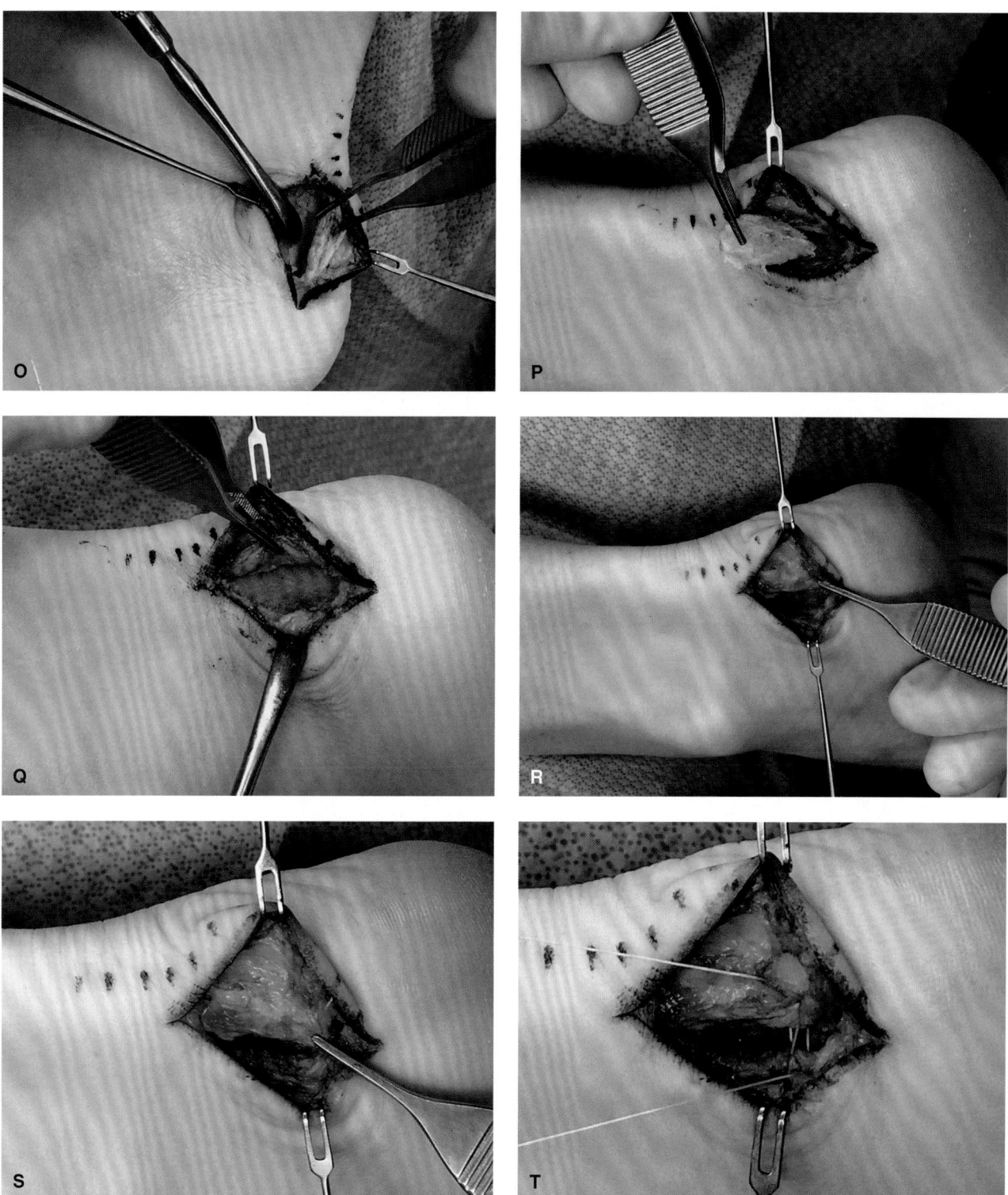

FIGURE 58.11 (*Continued*) **O.** Superior posterolateral calcaneal tuber following initial resection. **P.** Removal of primary Haglund deformity prominence. **Q.** Final appearance of resected Haglund deformity with further remodeling of the posterior superolateral prominence noted. **R.** Forceps demonstrating deep fascia layer overlying the resected and completed Haglund deformity correction. **S.** Reapproximation of the deep fascia lateralward with no involvement or disruption of the lateral border of the distal extent of the Achilles tendon insertion. **T.** Absorbable "over and over" interrupted deep fascial closure.

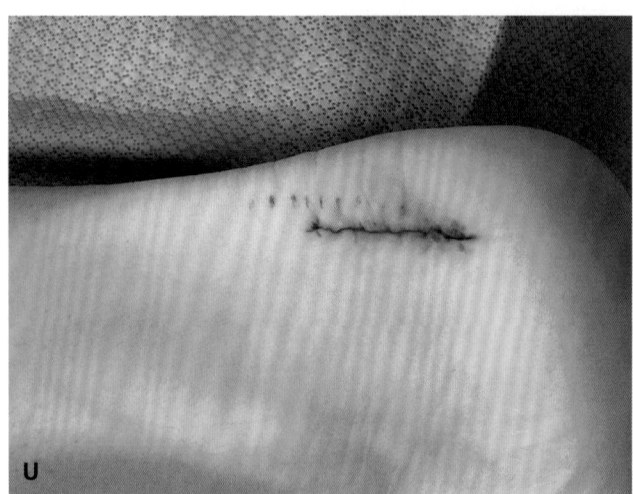

FIGURE 58.11 (*Continued*) **U.** Final appearance and resection of Haglund deformity with running absorbable intradermal skin closure.

posterior superior aspect of the calcaneal tuberosity is a Zadek osteotomy.[34] This is an oblique dorsal wedge osteotomy of the calcaneal tuberosity that essentially decompresses the area between the calcaneal tuberosity and the distal end of the Achilles tendon. It removes pressure from the retrocalcaneal bursa and thus can reduce inflammation. Performance of the osteotomy prevents aggressive excision of the superior prominence, which in itself can potentially create pain from scarring within this retrocalcaneal area. The osteotomy can provide a long-term result (Figs. 58.12 and 58.13).

NONINSERTIONAL ACHILLES TENDINITIS AND ASSOCIATED DISORDERS

Noninsertional Achilles tendinosis is defined as tendinosis between 2 and 6 cm proximal to the insertion of the Achilles tendon into the calcaneus (Fig. 58.14). Noninsertional Achilles tendinosis occurs in athletes, particularly runners, including weekend warrior's. Lyshom and Wiklander reported 7%-9% incidence in runners from running clubs.[35] There is a lower incidence in patients with comorbid diseases such as diabetes, obesity, etc. Noninsertional Achilles tendinopathy accounts for 55%-65% of all Achilles tendinopathy.[36] It is generally referred

to throughout the literature as an overuse injury or as a failed healing response.[37] It also occurs in the elderly and has been linked closely to quinolone use.[38]

Etiology of noninsertional Achilles tendinosis is multifaceted. This portion of the Achilles tendon is highly vulnerable to disease. The diameter of the tendon is the lowest in this area making it weaker. It is well documented that there is decreased intratendinous vascularity in this area with an increase of neovascular growth superficially. The twisting of the Achilles tendon fibers is the greatest in this area creating intratendinous tension. The biomechanical etiology is associated with lower limb length discrepancy, limited ankle dorsiflexion, training errors, and lack of flexibility.[39] Valgus and the cavus foot deformities are contributing factors resulting in altered rotational forces on the Achilles tendon. The distribution of pressure from a cavus or a valgus foot type translated through the subtalar joint to the Achilles tendon creates tension among the tendon fibers. Twisting of the Achilles tendon fibers combined with abnormal biomechanics, decreased vascularity, and physical stress risk the integrity of this portion of the Achilles tendon. The Achilles tendon loses its normal elasticity, and its tensile strength diminishes. Repetitive loading leads to tendon

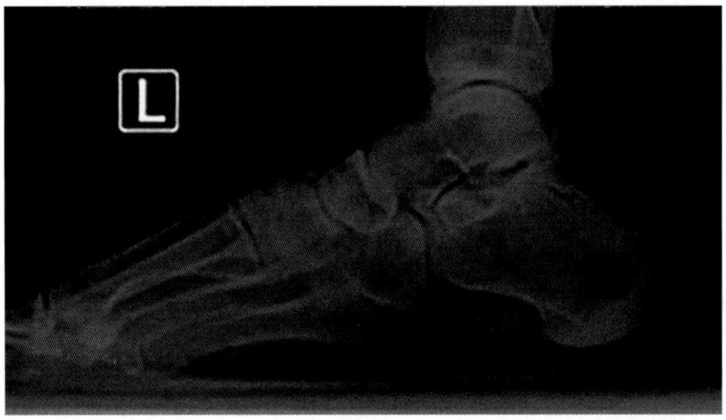

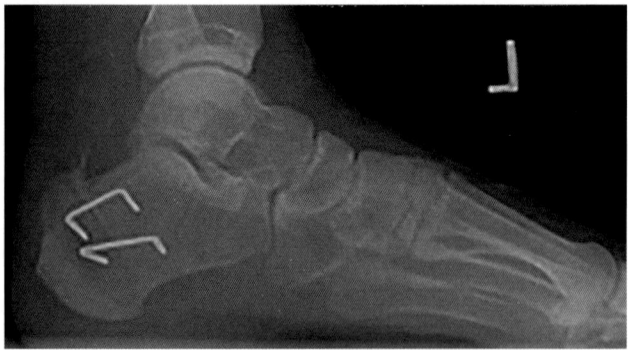

FIGURE 58.12 Lateral radiograph of prominent Haglund deformity. Lateral view of preoperative radiograph of a haglund deformity before Zadek Osteotomy.

FIGURE 58.13 Lateral view of postoperative radiograph depicting a Zadek osteotomy. This osteotomy extends the entire posterior superior aspect of the calcaneal tuberosity and consists of an oblique dorsal wedge osteotomy of the calcaneal tuberosity, which decompresses the area between the calcaneal tuberosity and the distal end of the Achilles tendon.

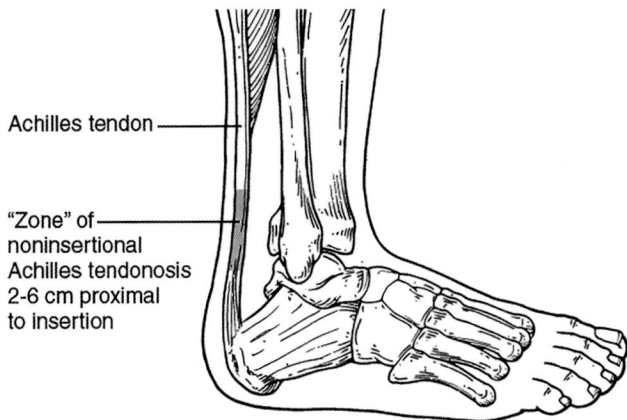

FIGURE 58.14 Anatomic description of insertion of the Achilles tendon. Noninsertional Achilles tendinosis is defined as tendinosis between 2 and 6 cm proximal to the insertion of the Achilles tendon, as depicted here.

degeneration, manifested as loss of normal collagen patterns and replacement of normal tissue with a disorganized array of collagen and proliferative extracellular matrix. The tendon becomes infiltrated with mucoid material, fibrocartilage, calcification, and lipid droplets.

Vascularity appears to increase at the site of the tendinopathy as part of the reparative process. Neovascularization occurs in 50%-88% of symptomatic tendons. This is visualized as thick walls, a tortuous appearance, and small lumens on the anterior/ventral side of the Achilles tendon within the paratenon, which is not seen in asymptomatic tendons. The healthy Achilles tendon is superficially innervated by the paratenon, but does not have a rich nervous supply itself. It is normally aneuronal; conversely, chronic painful tendons have been shown to exhibit new ingrowth of nerve fibers accompanying the peritendinous neovascularization from the paratenon into the tendon proper. Sensory nerve ingrowth has been observed as a reaction to repetitive loading and also as a response to injury. In theory, an increase in nerve fibers in the area creates a type of nerve entrapment or neuropathy that results in pain.[6]

CLINICAL PRESENTATION

The typical patient would present with a history of insidious onset of pain in the Achilles tendon above the insertion. Pain occurs first thing in the morning or after rest; however, it can also occur during strenuous activity. The pain generally prevents patients from participating in sporting activities and even long walks. Uncommonly, a patient presents with a history of an injury three or four weeks before they develop a thickening of the tendon. This could be a sign of a partial Achilles rupture, which should be differentiated from chronic Achilles tendinosis because the treatment protocol would be different.

PHYSICAL EXAMINATION

Clinical evaluation of the Achilles tendon reveals focal edema at the mid substance area of the Achilles tendon. This is typically anteromedially but can appear to be the periphery of the entire tendon. This is generally between 2 and 6 cm proximal

to the Achilles tendon insertion. There is pain upon palpation of the area, and the tendon appears thickened. There is usually a painful arc sign, which is pain at the site during active ankle joint range of motion. A sign of Achilles tendinosis is when the ankle joint is put through range of motion and the focal edematous area moves with it. In contrast to this, paritonitis is when the focal edematous area does not move. There is frequently pain upon passive and active range of motion at the site of the localized edema. There is a negative Thompson sign. Frequently, the plantaris tendon can be palpated at or just distal to the site of pain as the plantaris tendon courses parallel to the conjoined tendon. This can indicate a pathologic relationship and frequently is resistant to conservative therapy.

IMAGING

Ultrasound and MRI are the best imaging modalities for noninsertional Achilles tendinopathy. The ultrasound image will reveal hypoechoic areas of damaged tendons and also reveal areas of inflammation of the paratenon. This helps in differentiating between tendinopathy and peritendinitis. Color Doppler ultrasound will identify the neovascularization of the anterior portion of the tendon and help identify the site of treatment. This is generally quick and inexpensive. An MRI will provide a more specific look at the Achilles tendon and quantifies the amount of Achilles tendon damage by identifying both normal and abnormal tissue. It also has the ability to provide a 3D image, which can help for better visualization of the pathology. MRIs can help direct the treatment regimen and also help predict success rates. The ultrasound and the MRI can be utilized to identify pathological tendinous changes as well as to measure the length, width and depth of the Achilles tendon.

TREATMENT

Conservative Treatment

Noninvasive treatment can be successful in ~75% of patients with noninsertional Achilles tendinosis. Initial treatment depends on the acuity of the symptoms. A patient with acute pain is immobilized in a neutral or slightly plantar flexed ankle position within a CAM walker and provided a prescription for a nonsteroidal anti-inflammatory medication. After symptoms dissipate, physical therapy is initiated. Cessation from all athletic activities is advised and prevents early recurrence or failure of initial treatment.

Eccentric muscle strengthening is the mainstay of physical therapy for noninsertional Achilles tendinosis. Eccentric muscle exercises aid in reducing pain in the Achilles tendon by strengthening the gastrocnemius and soleal muscle bellies and stretching out the myotendinous unit. This reduces the neovascularization occurring in the damaged tendon by reducing the number of P receptors at the injury site. Recent studies have revealed improved results with partial ankle range of motion strengthening rather than total range of motion. Alfredson and colleagues compared the effectiveness between eccentric and concentric muscle strengthening. After 12 weeks, 82% of all participants improved with eccentric muscle strengthening and 36% improved with concentric muscle strengthening. The authors reported that this was sustained for 12 months.[36]

Platelet-rich plasma (PRP) injections have been utilized to aid in the reparative process in insertional and noninsertional Achilles tendinosis. There have been multiple studies on its efficacy indicating mixed response.[40] PRP acts to promote migration of cells in tendon repair. At the early stage of tendon repair, paratenon-derived cells (PDCs) are thought to play a more important role than tendon proper–derived cells (TDCs). In one study, the PRP group demonstrated a significantly higher migration rate than the control group in both TDCs and PDCs.[42] These results suggested that PRP promoted the proliferation of PDCs as well as TDCs, further suggesting that treatment with PRP may enhance the healing properties at the initial stage of tendon repair. The use of PRP in Achilles pathology, chronic plantar fasciitis, osteochondral lesions of the talus, ankle osteoarthritis, and diabetic foot ulcers has shown some clinical benefit.[41,42] However, a large systematic meta-analysis did not reveal promising results.[43] Anecdotally many physicians report good results with PRP injections and perform it commonly. However, given the abundance of conflicting and poor-quality evidence, no clear indications for the use of PRP currently exist. The lack of standardization in the PRP preparation and delivery method has contributed to the inconsistent results. Better studies need to be done to further investigate this theory as most systematic meta-analysis studies report poor results.[41,42]

The use of shockwave therapy in noninsertional Achilles tendinosis is similar to the role that it has with insertional Achilles tendinosis. Proponents of shockwave therapy favor it for both noninsertional and insertional Achilles tendinosis. Dry needling, hydrodissection, and polidocanol (sclerosing agent) have also been reported as therapies.[44] These and other injections are performed to disrupt the neovascularization at the rupture site to relieve pain.

Surgical Treatment

Surgical/invasive treatment of noninsertional Achilles disorders consist of both minimally invasive and open surgical procedures. Percutaneous tenotomy through a probe delivering radiofrequency coblation has increased in popularity. Radiofrequency coblation increases the neovascularization but reduces the number of nerve fibers thus reducing pain in the tendon. Débridement of pathological tissue is performed through a vibrating plastic probe admitting radiofrequency cooled by a saline pump. A 25-28 kHz frequency delivered by the probe is specific for débriding diseased tissue.[45] Many authors have reported successful outcomes using this modality.[46,47] However, there is a need for randomized control studies to document its efficacy (Fig. 58.15).

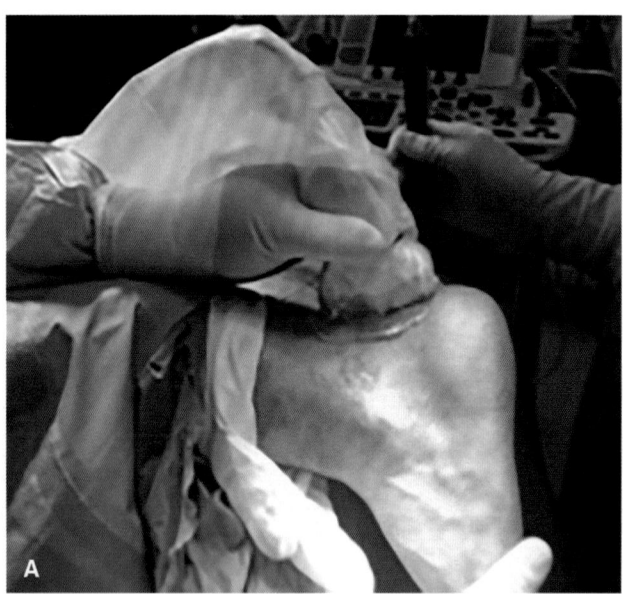

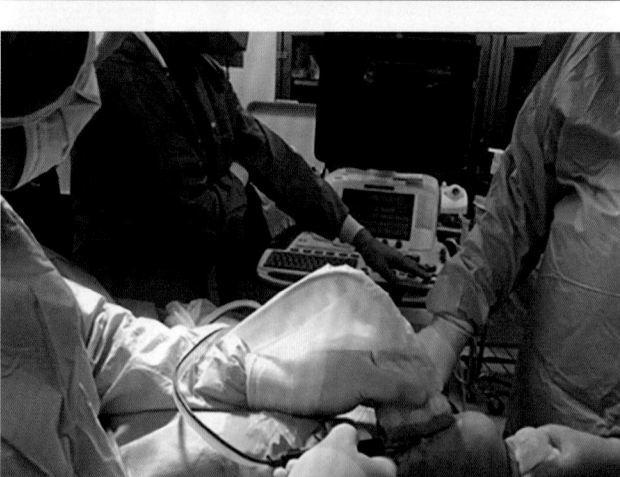

FIGURE 58.15 A-C. Percutaneous tenotomy depicted here. Débridement of pathological tissue is performed through a vibrating plastic probe admitting radiofrequency cooled by a saline pump; 25-28 kHz frequency delivered by the probe is specific for débriding diseased tissue.

The authors have utilized this modality with successful reduction of symptoms of both noninsertional and insertional Achilles tendinosis. The procedure can be performed in the office setting, in a hospital procedure room, or in the OR. The patient is placed in a prone position. An ultrasound is utilized to identify the Achilles tendon. Two stab incisions are performed (one lateral and one medial) ~1 cm proximal to the point of tenderness. A hemostat is utilized to dissect to the tendon. The probe delivering the radiofrequency treatment is then inserted through the Achilles tendon as parallel as possible to the longitudinal tendon fibers. Care is required to avoid transversely crossing the Achilles tendon in that this could lead to partial or total rupture.[48] The probe needs to be moved quickly through the tissue to prevent burning the tissue. The procedure generally takes up to 3 minutes. Suture or Steri-Strips are applied to the incisions for reapproximation. A light dressing and Ace wrap are placed over the wounds. The patient is immobilized in an appropriately oriented CAM walker for 4-6 weeks to allow for proper healing. When there is decreased pain and edema, the patient is allowed to return to normal shoe gear.

Open procedures are generally chosen in more severe cases of degeneration. These procedures include localized débridement of degenerated tendon and an FHL tendon transfer. An FHL tendon transfer is performed similarly to that for the insertional Achilles tendinosis; however, more attention is given to mobilizing the FHL muscle belly.

The procedure is performed in a prone position. The area of thickened tendon is identified and a curvilinear incision is made encompassing this area and extending to the posterior calcaneus. Dissection is then made down to the deep fascia separating the deep fascia and superficial fascia along the wound margins. A linear deep fascial incision is made through the deep fascia and the paratenon exposing the diseased tendon. Frequently, the paratenon is adherent to the underlying tendon

and requires meticulous dissection to reflect it. The diseased tendon is then débrided and removed from the wound.

Once the débridement of the degenerated Achilles tendon has been performed, attention is directed anteriorly into the retrocalcaneal space. Dissection is made into the intracompartmental septum between the deep and superficial compartments. Care should be taken during this dissection to avoid the neurovascular bundle, which courses just medial to where the intracompartmental septum will be incised. Identifying the FHL can be performed intraoperatively before the septum is incised by deep palpation while flexing and extending the hallux with the foot in a dorsiflexed position. The septum is then incised with iris or tenotomy scissors creating a 3-4 cm opening. The muscle belly of the FHL is then easily visualized and a hemostat is used to wrap umbilical tape around the FHL tendon/muscle belly. The foot and the hallux are then maximally plantar flexed. The FHL is pulled proximally, and care is taken to transect the tendon as distal as possible in order to gain maximum length. Once the tendon is transected and the end is visualized, a whipstitch is performed to prepare the tendon for transfer into the calcaneus. The tendon can be weaved through the Achilles tendon or sewn side to side. It is the author's preference to drill a hole in the calcaneus and utilize an interference screw to fixate the tendon in place with the appropriate resting tension. The author's preference is to insert the tendon into either the medial posterior or the posterior aspect of the calcaneal tuberosity. The muscle belly of the FHL is then sutured to the midsubstance of the Achilles tendon in an effort to bring vascularity to the tendon (Fig. 58.16). The FHL tendon is then sutured side to side to the achilles tendon. Paratenon and deep closure performed with a 3-0 absorbable stitch. Subcutaneous and skin closure is performed with 4-0 absorbable sutrue and 4-0 nonabsorbable suture respectively. While in a prone position, the patient is casted in gravity equinus with a fiberglass cast.

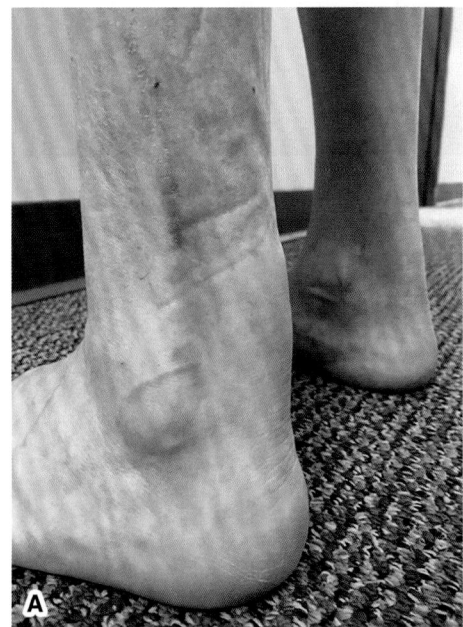
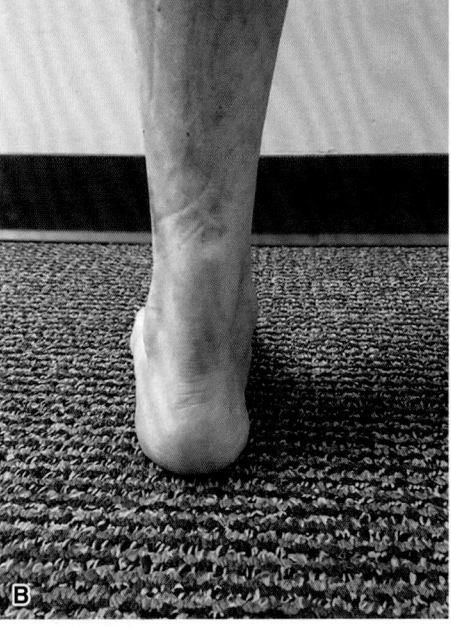
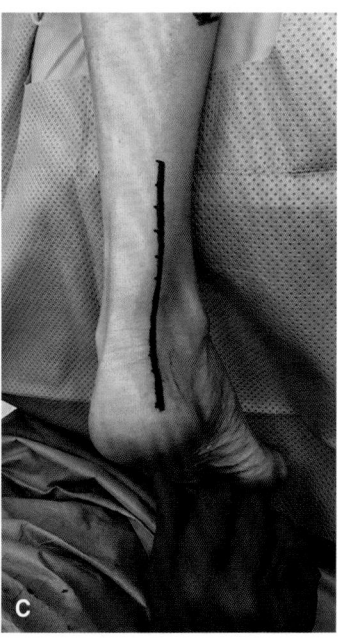

FIGURE 58.16 **A.** Patient with recalcitrant pain and functional weakness secondary to chronic midsubstance Achilles degenerative tendinopathy. Chronic fusiform edema with bulbous thickening of the midsubstance Achilles tendon is noted. **B.** Note the marked chronic thickening broadly within the entire midsubstance of the Achilles tendon. **C.** Achilles tendon midsubstance débridement and FHL tendon transfer is reserved for recalcitrant cases that fail meaningful conservative treatment. A medially biased longitudinal incision is planned and placed to reduce risk of wound complications and access to the FHL muscle/tendon unit via a single incision approach.

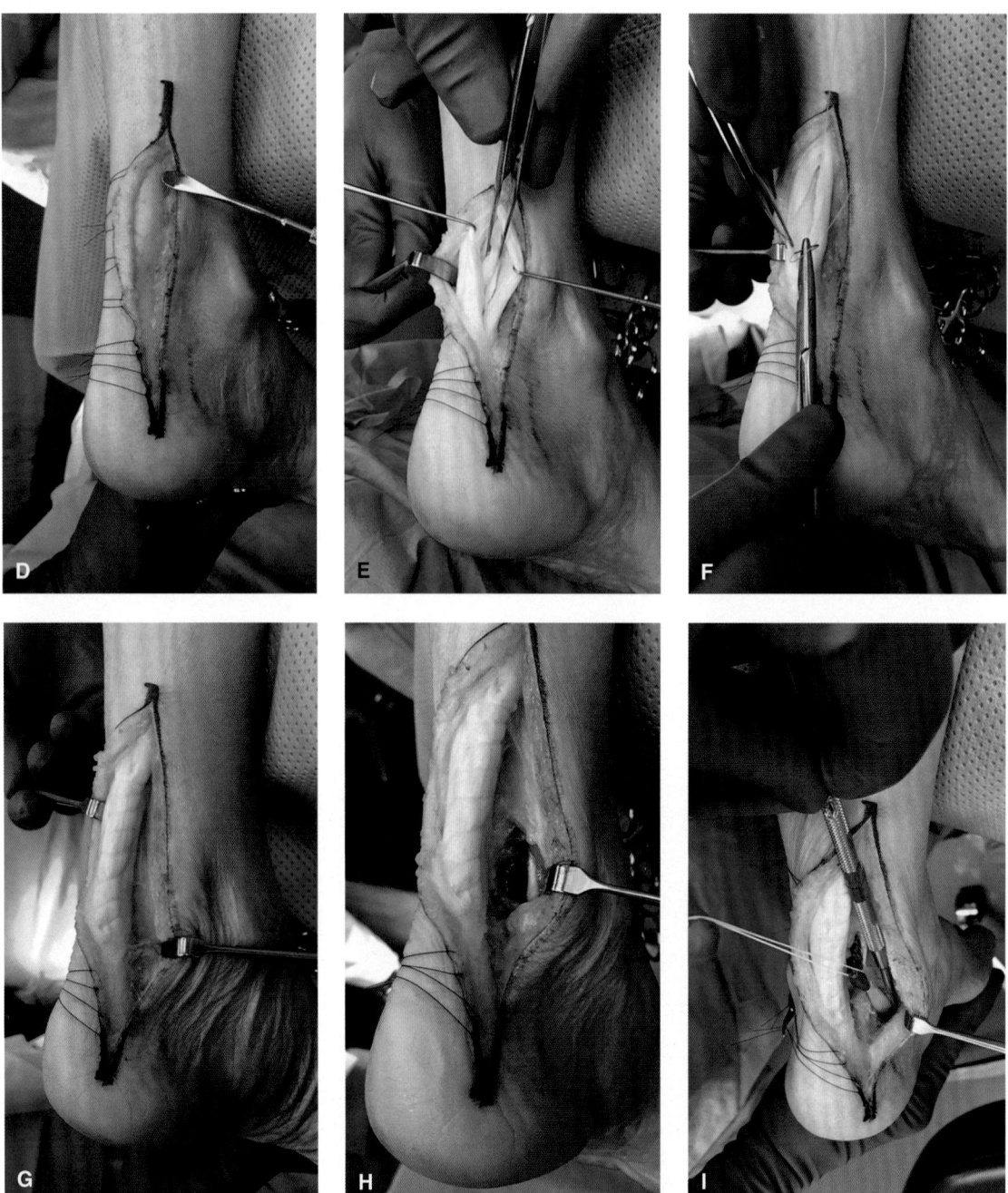

FIGURE 58.16 (*Continued*) **D.** Note the skin stay sutures are placed as a "no-touch" atraumatic technique to avoid excessive handling of the skin and soft tissues. The bulbous zone of degenerative midsubstance Achilles tendinopathy is identified with the Freer elevator. **E.** The midsubstance Achilles tendinopathy is débrided sharply of its mucoid/myxoid degenerative substrate. Generally, (and even in cases less than) 50% degenerative involvement of the cross section of the Achilles tendon being noted, a relatively low threshold is considered to adjunctively perform an FHL tendon transfer. **F.** Following débridement of the degenerative midsubstance Achilles tendinopathy, an absorbable suture is utilized to retuberalize the Achilles tendon. **G.** Note the completion of the Achilles "retuberalization." The FHL muscle/tendon unit is easily found deep to the Achilles tendon at its midsubstance below the underlying deep fascia at this level. **H.** A small incision is made overlying the deep fascia at the level of the FHL muscle belly/proximal tendon to recruit the FHL muscle/tendon unit. **I.** Anatomic dissection is carefully performed distalward and to the course of the FHL tendon near its relationship to the middle facet and sustentaculum tali. The Freer elevator identifies the site of planned transection of the FHL tendon to ensure adequate tendon length is recruited.

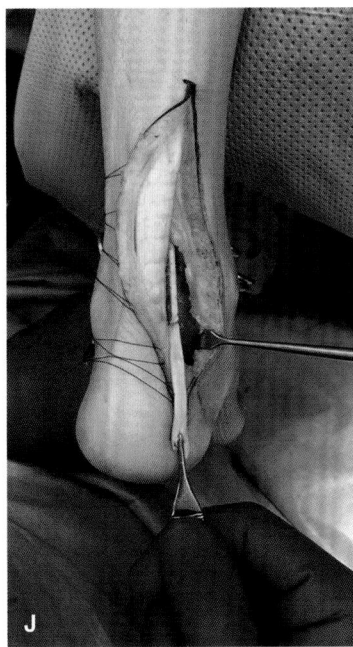
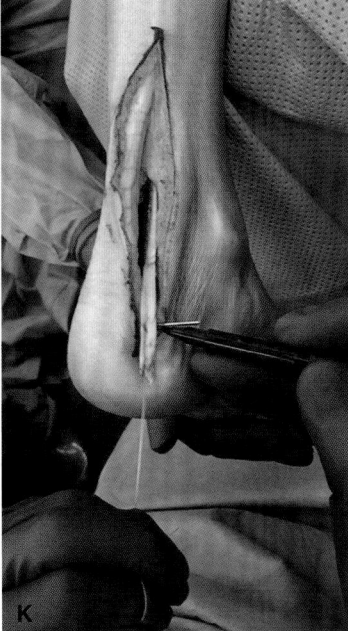
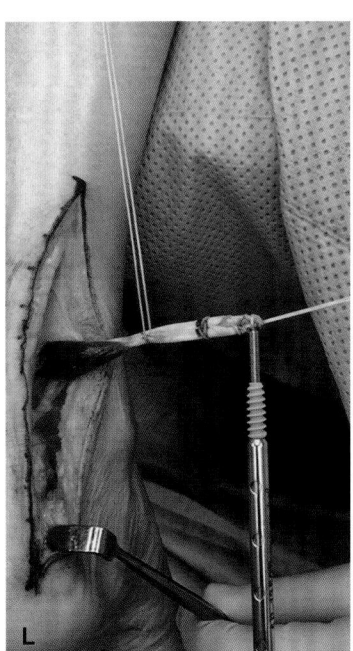

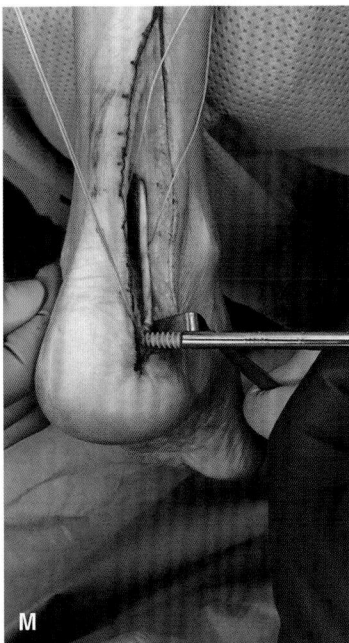
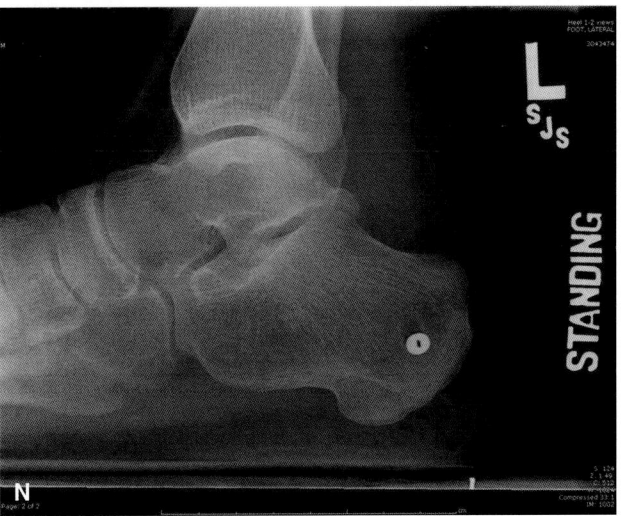

FIGURE 58.16 (*Continued*) **J.** Once the FHL is harvested and transected, adequate length is noted to ensure a solid osseous primary tenodesis of the FHL tendon to the calcaneus. The FHL tendon transfer location is placed directly anterior to the primary insertion zone of the native Achilles tendon. **K.** A K-wire is placed medially 1 cm anterior to the Achilles tendon insertion as a guide toward preparation of a closed bone tunnel. Note the position of the FHL muscle belly, which will be anastomosed to the zone of the débrided and retuberalized Achilles tendon. **L.** A nonabsorbable looped polyblend suture is positioned to ultimately perform a side-to-side anastomosis of the FHL muscle to the region of the lateral and anterior Achilles tendon. **M.** A biocomposite interference screw is utilized to secure the FHL tendon transfer to the medial calcaneus, which "sets" the physiologic tension of this tendon transfer. Note the position of the FHL muscle/tendon unit. **N.** A first-generation metallic interference screw is shown in this case simply to denote the position of the bone tunnel in relation to the primary insertion site of the native Achilles tendon.

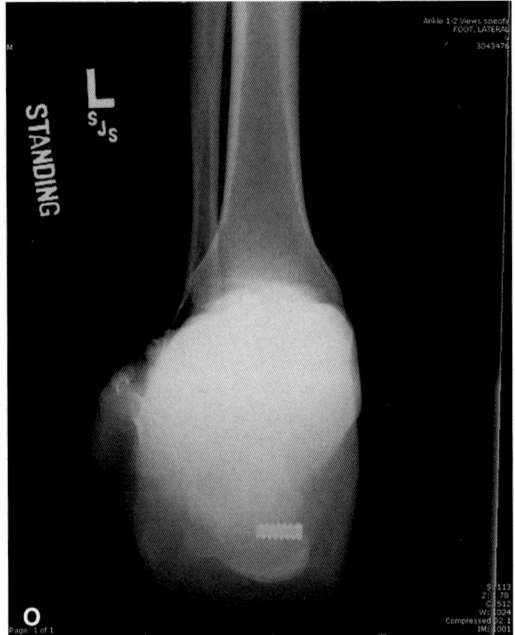
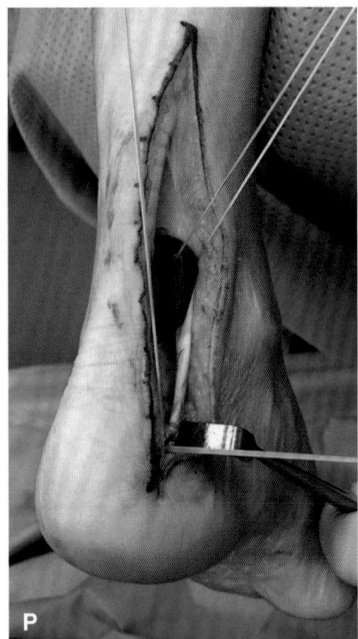
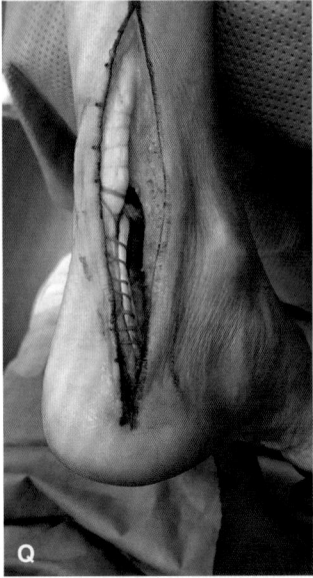
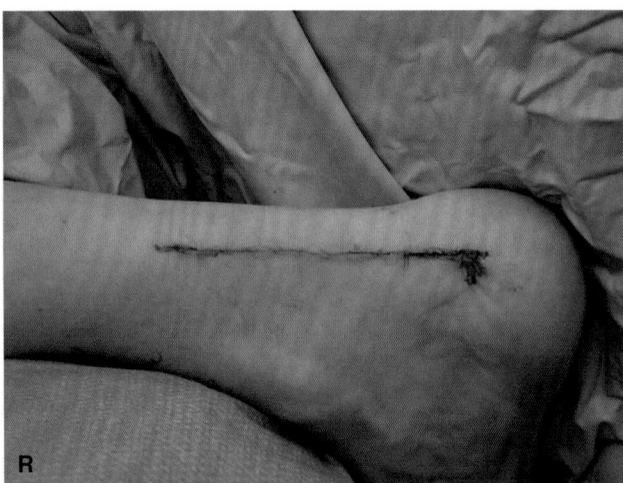

FIGURE 58.16 (*Continued*) **O.** A postoperative modified hindfoot alignment/axial view demonstrating the position and placement of the calcaneal bone tunnel. **P.** Once the FHL tendon is secured via interference fit within the calcaneal bone tunnel, the FHL tendon and muscle are anastomosed from a distal to proximal direction sequentially. The FHL muscle/tendon unit effectively becomes further "positioned" in line with the contractile axis of the Achilles tendon. **Q.** Final anastomosis completed. The conjoined "alignment" of the Achilles / FHL anastomosis is co-linear, therefore negating any medial overpowering or resultant varus heel position. The FHL muscle tendon unit is optimally positioned in this technique functionally, physiologically, and mechanically. **R.** Final closure.

ACHILLES TENDON RUPTURES

ETIOLOGY

An Achilles tendon rupture can be a devastating injury. It most frequently occurs in people while participating in athletic events. Both seasoned athletes as well as weekend warriors are affected by this injury. There are a reported 31 Achilles ruptures per 100,000 people annually. Achilles tendon ruptures most frequently occur in the 37- to 44-year-old age group. It is theorized that this is due to the aging population staying active in athletic activities.[49]

Most commonly, Achilles tendon ruptures occur indirectly from a forced dorsiflexion of the foot with a contracted gastroc-soleus complex.[50] The ruptures generally occur in the midsubstance of the achilles tendon within the watershed area. This is typically where the injury occurs during athletics and usually occurs in patients who have had no previous Achilles tendon pain or pathology. Achilles ruptures can also occur at the myotendinous junction as well as the insertion of the Achilles. Achilles tendon ruptures occurring at the insertion tend to have a history of chronic Achilles tendinosis.[51] Current evidence has suggested that multiple secondary risk factors can predispose one to the

risk of Achilles tendon rupture including tendon degeneration, poor tendon vascularity, corticosteroid use, fluoroquinolone use, and previous rupture on the contralateral side.[52]

KUWADA CLASSIFICATION OF ACHILLES TENDON RUPTURES		
Type I	Partial tear <50%: posterior fibers torn first	Typically treated with conservative management
Type II	Complete tear <3 cm defect	Typically treated with end-to-end anastomosis
Type III	Complete tear 3-6 cm defect	Often requires tendon/synthetic graft
Type IV	Complete tear >6 cm defect	Often requires tendon/synthetic graft and gastrocnemius recession

CLINICAL PRESENTATION AND PHYSICAL EXAMINATION

Commonly patients present with a history of an athletic injury. They relate a twist of the leg on the ankle and a pop or "give" at the back of the ankle. Achilles tendon ruptures in basketball and tennis are quite common. Patients relate that they feel like someone kicked them in the back of the heel. Initially, most patients are not certain they have a serious injury.

Upon examination, there is edema and ecchymosis noted in the posterior lower leg. The patient is then placed in a prone position with the feet off the end of the table. Inspection of both lower legs is performed. Examination of a noninjured limb will reveal an intact Achilles tendon coursing from the posterior calf to the posterior aspect of the calcaneus with normal tension and the foot slightly plantar flexed. Examination of the injured limb will reveal the foot perpendicular to the leg (Figs. 58.17 and 58.18 A&B). There will be edema at the Achilles tendon preventing visualization of the tendon. Careful palpation is then performed from the gastrocsoleus complex distally to the calcaneal tuberosity. Palpation is performed to identify any delves or thickening of the tendon and to localize any specific sites

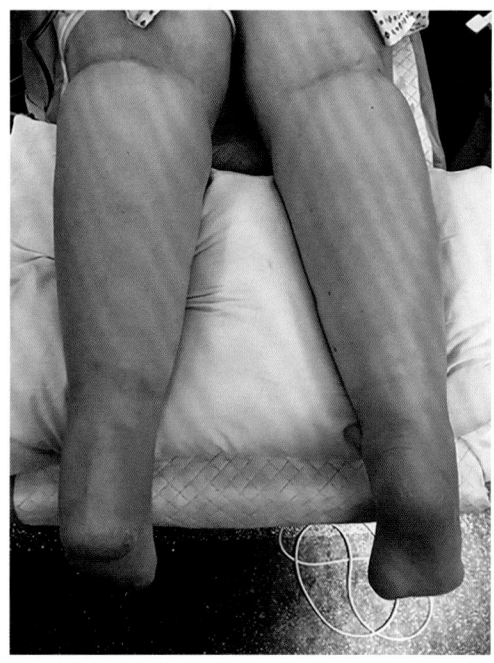

FIGURE 58.17 A discrepancy is evident between the ruptured Achilles (*left*) and intact Achilles (*right*). The *right* has resting plantar flexion, indicating a functional and intact Achilles tendon, while the *left* is in dorsiflexion and unable to plantar flex.

of pain. A Thompson test is then performed. The test is positive if by squeezing the posterior calf the foot does not plantar flex. Passive range of motion of the ankle will generally reveal excessive dorsiflexion and instability or "floppiness" of the retrocalcaneal area. During stance, the patient will be unable to perform a single or double limb heel raise.

At this time, it is important to obtain imaging to identify the specific site of the rupture along the tendon and the length of the rupture. The ruptures can occur at the insertion, along the course of the tendon, or at the musculotendon junction. Imaging will help identify the specific site of injury. Both ultrasound and MRI can be utilized for this evaluation. MRI is more

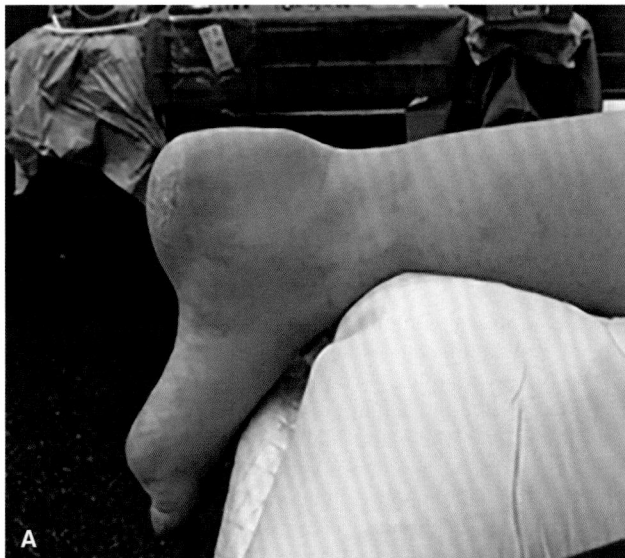

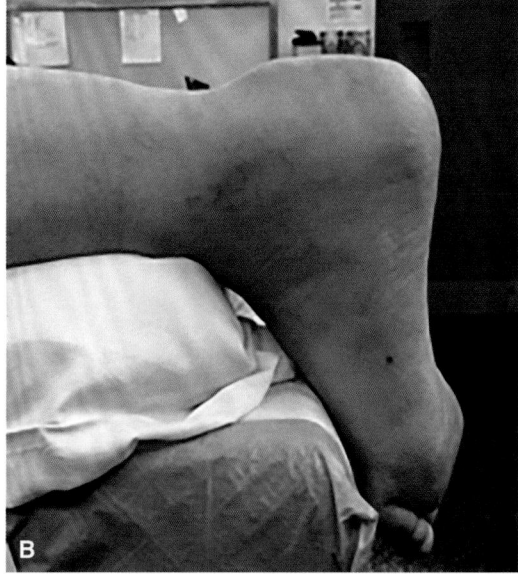

FIGURE 58.18 A, B. A dell may be visible with an Achilles rupture.

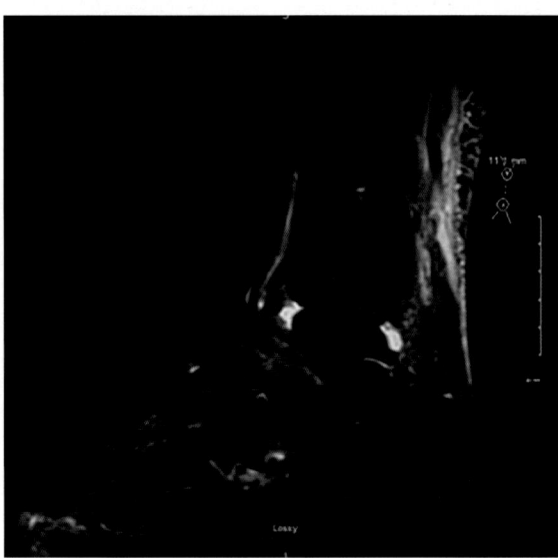

FIGURE 58.19 Acute Achilles tendon rupture on T2 MRI with an 11.1-mm defect.

commonly used and identifies the gap quite readily. This will aid in determining the type of repair (Fig. 58.19).

OPERATIVE VS NONOPERATIVE TREATMENT

There has been much debate on whether to surgically repair the Achilles tendon rupture or to treat this injury with immobilization. Surgical treatment involves repair of the Achilles tendon either through an open incision or through a minimally invasive technique. Nonoperative treatment via non–weight-bearing cast involves the application of a plantar flexed cast for 2 weeks followed by gradual dorsiflexion of the cast every 2 weeks. The patient is allowed to weight-bear from 6 to 8 weeks post injury and begin an aggressive physical therapy program.

Operative treatment is associated with a significant reduction in rerupture rate compared with nonoperative treatment. However, operative treatment results in a significantly higher rate of other complications. Approximately 1 in 9 patients undergoing operative repair of an acute Achilles tendon rupture develops a postoperative complication, with the three most common adverse events being wound problems (5.2%), venous thromboembolic events (3.6%), and sural nerve injury (2.0%). Advanced aging and active tobacco use are independent risk factors for developing such complications.[53] General incidence of major complications for acute Achilles tendon rupture is as high as 9.13% and the overall incidence rates of rerupture are 5%. Achilles tendon ruptures treated nonoperatively combined with early mobilization had a high risk of complications when compared with open treatment and minimal incision treatment.[54] This has been supported by recent systematic reviews, which have concluded that surgical treatment can effectively reduce the incidence of rerupture. However, inherent to surgical repair, there is an increased risk of wound dehiscence and infection.[55] According to recent literature, surgical repair leads to lower rerupture rates, superior functional results, and a shorter time to return to activity.[49,56,57] Nonoperative treatment obviously has no surgical complications but can have similar functional results. There have been no statistically significant differences found in the functional outcomes between surgical and nonsurgical groups for DVT, number of patients returning

to sport, or amount of ankle joint range of motion (dorsiflexion/plantar flexion).[58] It still remains a controversial topic.

OPEN VS MINIMALLY INVASIVE

Minimally invasive repair of Achilles tendon ruptures has gained increased popularity, and its use is evolving.[58] A percutaneous surgical approach, or minimally invasive surgery, reduces surgical exposure in order to minimize the risk of wound complications. However, this can be technically more demanding to perform with a steep learning curve, due to the limited direct visualization. This makes it more difficult to approximate the stump, as well as increases the risk of sural nerve injury. There have been studies comparing minimal and open surgical repair. Wu and his colleagues reviewing the treatment of 2060 patients in a meta-analysis concluded that minimal incision surgery with aggressive physical therapy and rehabilitation had the least amount of complications compared to other treatment and rehabilitation regimens.[54] In another meta-analysis, Grassi et al reported less complications and increased patient satisfaction when comparing minimally invasive and open surgical repair of the Achilles tendon.[58]

OPEN ACHILLES TENDON REPAIR

Open repair is performed with the patient in a prone position with both feet at the end of the table. Once the patient has been placed into the prone position, appropriate padding should be utilized to protect areas of pressure such as the patella.

The author generally uses a long lazy S–type incision, which begins approximately about 3-4 cm proximal medial to the suspected rupture to avoid the sural nerve. The incision ends 3-4 cm distal to the rupture lateral to the Achilles. The incision is deepened through subcutaneous tissue to the deep fascial area. At this stage, the hematoma of the rupture should be visualized. The deep fascia and underlying paratenon are usually intact. A linear incision is made through the deep fascia and the paratenon. Care should be taken in dissection of the paratenon, which will be engorged with blood and easily identifiable. At this time any residual hematoma between the two ends of the tendon is removed with copious lavage and use of a curette. At this time a Krackow-type stitch is placed in both the proximal and distal ends of the tendon rupture with an 0 nonabsorbable suture material. The foot is then held in a plantar flexed position. The ruptured tendon is reapproximated and the suture tied. If the plantaris tendon is available, it can be weaved on either side of the tendon to augment the repair. The wound is then closed in layers. Careful attention is made to reapproximate the paratenon layer over the ruptured tendon due to the fact that the paratenon layer holds the vascular supply to the tendon. The deep fascial layer and the paratenon are generally closed in the same layer. A closed drain is typically used if there is concern with bleeding or the possibility of hemorrhagic pooling in areas around the repair. Subcutaneous closure is performed with a continuous 4-0 absorbable suture. Skin closure is then performed with a combination of simple interrupted and mattress sutures with a nonabsorbable nylon or Prolene. A compression dressing is then applied to the foot and lower leg with the foot in a plantar flexed position. During the application of the dressing and the cast, it is important to have an assistant holding the foot in the desired position. A below-knee fiberglass cast is then applied and bivalved for edema (Fig. 58.20).

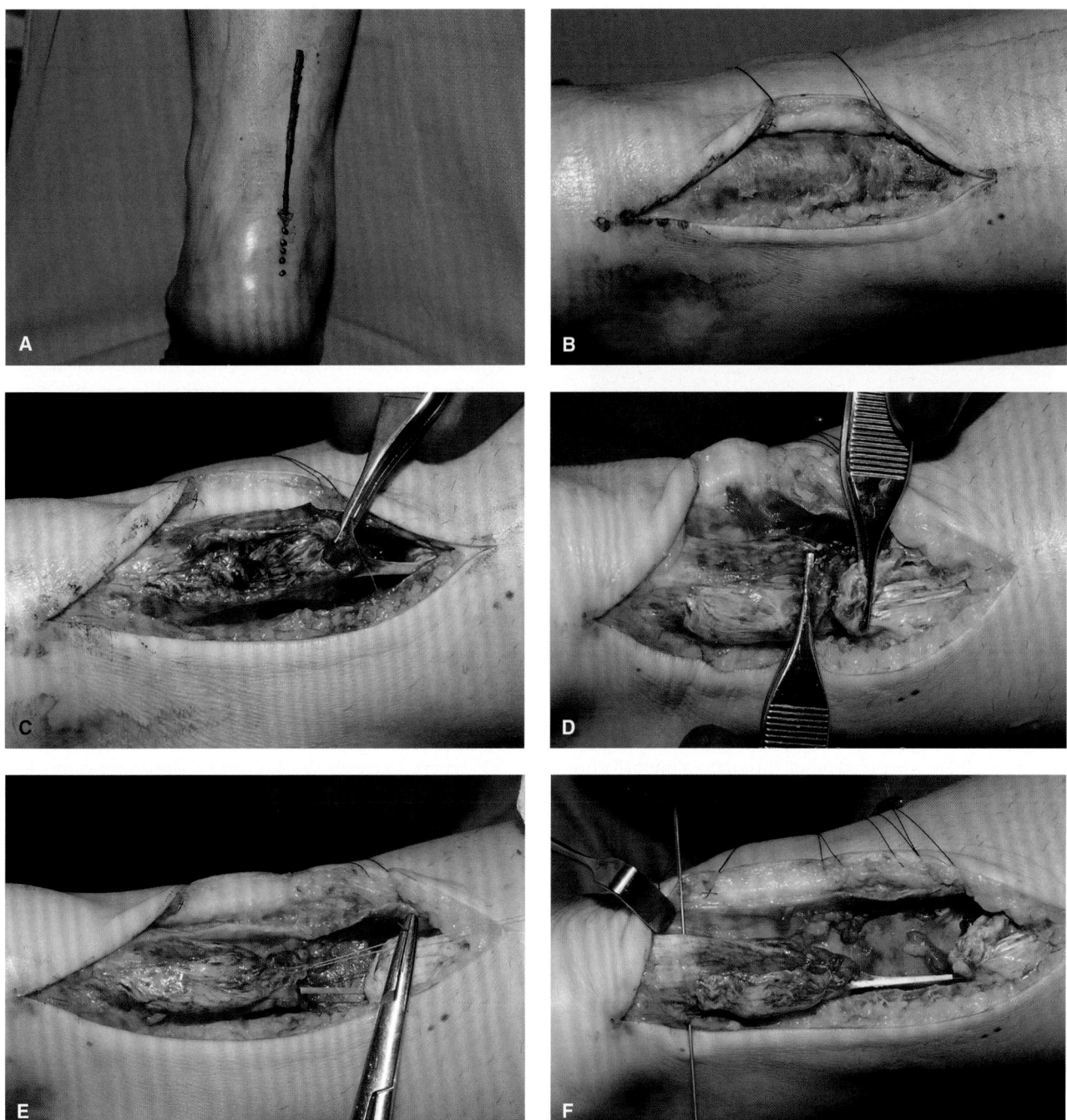

FIGURE 58.20 **A.** A medially biased linear incision plan is shown for an open repair of a subacute midsubstance Achilles tendon rupture. A medially biased incision provides adequate access for an open repair and may reduce the potential for wound healing complications. **B.** Stay sutures are utilized as shown to aid in atraumatic handling of the skin and soft tissues throughout the procedure. Note the hemorrhagic paratenon and deep fascia layer, which is identified and preserved for reapproximation following open repair of a midsubstance Achilles tendon rupture. **C.** The forceps are shown grasping the proximal segment of the Achilles tendon rupture site. Note the plantaris tendon course adjacent to the midsubstance Achilles tendon rupture site. **D.** The proximal and distal margins at the zone of the midsubstance Achilles tendon rupture site are evaluated and approximated. Débridement of the proximal and distal "ends" is limited to only nonviable fibrous tissue interposition and is generally not required in acute and/or subacute Achilles tendon ruptures. **E.** Initially, a nonabsorbable suture is utilized as a provisional stitch to "gather" the proximal fibers of the midsubstance Achilles tendon rupture site toward reapproximation of the primary repair. **F.** A Keith needle is shown in this example as a starting point for either a modified Bunnell or modified Krackow suture technique.

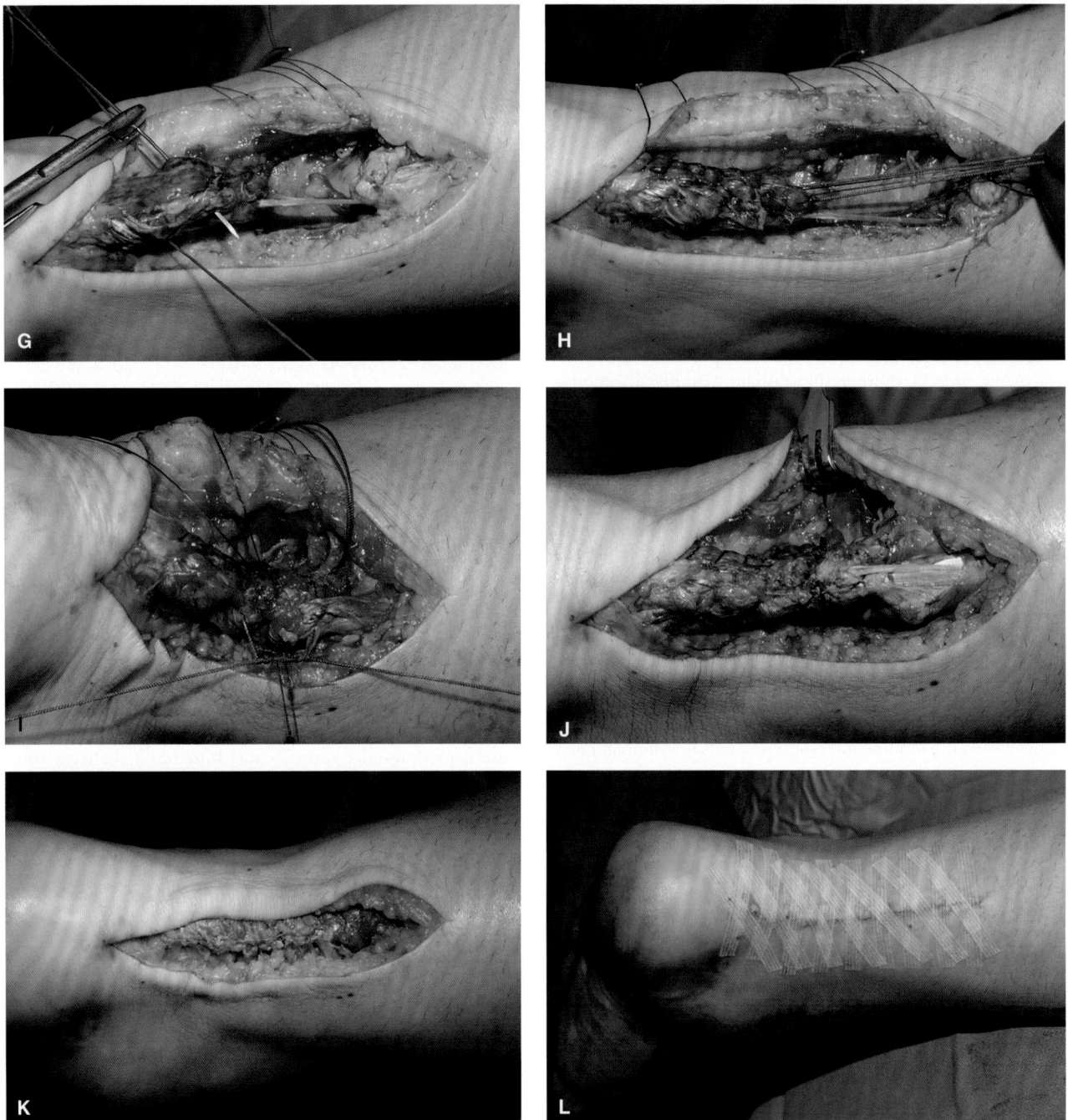

FIGURE 58.20 (*Continued*) **G.** A nonabsorbable polyblend suture material is generally utilized to maintain integrity throughout the proximal and distal Achilles tendon segments. Care is taken to limit suture volume as the tensile strength of polyblend suture is proportionately quite strong. **H.** The proximal segment is shown utilizing a two-strand technique. A modified Bunnell stitch is placed more anteriorward. A modified Krackow stitch technique is also shown utilizing an absorbable strand of PDS. **I.** Care is taken to pass each given strand (regardless of the stitch pattern) across the Achilles rupture site laterally in a modified "gift box" surgical technique. The lateral suture strands are shown with the surgical knots tied away from the primary end to end. Placing the suture knots distal and proximal to the rupture site and within native Achilles tendon substrate may enhance the strength of the repair and limit gap healing attenuation at the repair site. The medial suture strand (in comparison) is shown with the surgical knot to be completed near to the primary end to end repair site. **J.** The final "reapproximation" of the midsubstance Achilles tendon rupture site with focused attention to restoring and securing return to physiologic tension. The contralateral extremity can be used as a template to further gauge appropriate tension is restored to the injured side. The benefits of utilizing static compression hose and/or sequential compression devices on the contralateral extremity aimed at optimizing DVT prophylaxis should be thoughtfully considered at the time of surgery. **K.** The paratenon and deep fascia is closed in layers to restore the vascular, nutritional and gliding function of the Achilles tendon. Care is taken meticulously with a non-absorbable suture to restore the paratenon and deep fascial layers over the entire Achilles tendon. **L.** Final closure demonstrating a running intradermal suture technique, reinforced with standard steri-strips. The foot is generally held and splinted in a gravity equinus position in open primary repair of midsubstance Achilles tendon ruptures.

MINIMALLY INVASIVE ACHILLES TENDON REPAIR

Regarding minimally invasive Achilles tendon repair, it is recommended to use a well-padded thigh pneumatic tourniquet. The foot and leg are then scrubbed, prepped, and draped in the usual aseptic manner.

It is imperative to assess for plantar flexion of operative and contralateral legs with calf squeeze and to note a palpable dell to mark out incision prior to surgery. Using a no. 15 blade, an ~3-cm longitudinal incision is made just medial to the midsection of the Achilles tendon along the rupture site. The incision is deepened to the level of the subcutaneous tissue with care taken to protect all vital neurovascular structures. All crossing bleeders are subsequently cauterized by Bovie as appropriate. Careful dissection is then taken down to the level of the paratenon, taking care to avoid the sural nerve. Skin flaps are carefully handled. A longitudinal incision is then made in the peritenon and opened up exposing the ruptured tendon. Evacuation of the hematoma is performed at this time, if needed. Frayed tendon edges are débrided with a no. 15 blade and curette at this stage. Wound is copiously irrigated. It is then imperative to note whether there is sufficient tendon to perform a primary repair. The proximal stump of the Achilles tendon is then grasped with an Allis clamp (one positioned medially, and one laterally), taking precaution to not grasp the surrounding paratenon. This would allow for proper placement of the percutaneous Achilles repair system jig and excursion of the proximal tendon stump. The jig is placed in the incision and advanced proximally between the tendon and paratenon. Advancing the device between the tendon and paratenon aids in avoiding injury to the sural nerve. The device is opened just enough to ensure that the proximal tendon is between the two arms of the jig, taking care to pull on the tendon with Allis clamps for stability. Digital palpation is used to confirm that the tendon stump is captured.

A variety of sutures are thrown percutaneously in the jig creating a locking stitch, 4-5 cm proximally. Each construct is individually tested to be sure that it captures the tendon and will not pull out. The device is then slowly removed from the leg, pulling the suture through the incision site and within the paratenon, avoiding the sural nerve.

Attention is then turned to the distal portion of the Achilles tendon. One medial and one lateral stab incision is made over the calcaneus just proximal to the Achilles insertion and overlying the superior facet of the calcaneus. A 3.5-mm drill with drill guide is used to drill holes at an angle converging toward the midline within these stab incisions. The tunnels are angled so they do not intersect. A 4.75-mm tap is then used to prepare the drill holes. A suture lasso is then passed through the distal Achilles tendon stump to retrieve the proximal nonabsorbable suture and tape strands. The strands are then passed through the distal Achilles stump with an Allis clamp holding tension on the distal stump. The strands are then secured into the calcaneus on the medial and lateral sides with a 4.75-mm interference screw on each side, whereas the foot is held in appropriate plantar flexion. When fastening these strands, attention is paid to the contralateral foot to ensure that appropriate tension is applied. Proper repair of the tendon should be noted. Plantar flexion at the ankle joint should be noted with calf squeeze.

Copious irrigation is then performed with normal saline. The paratenon is closed using 4-0 Monocryl. Deep closure is then performed with 4-0 Vicryl followed by skin closure with interrupted simple, vertical, and horizontal mattress sutures with 4-0 Prolene. Tourniquet is deflated. The foot is then dressed with 4 × 4 gauze, 4 in. Kerlix, and 4 in. Ace. The patient is placed in a posterior splint in gravity equinus (Fig. 58.21).

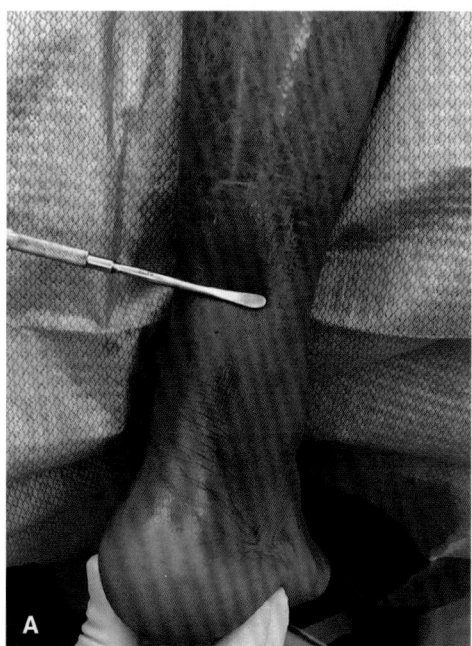 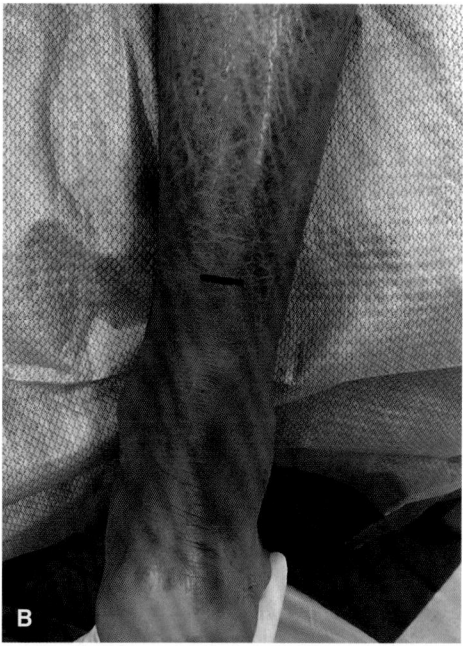

FIGURE 58.21 **A.** Patient is placed in the prone position. Identification of the exact level of the midsubstance Achilles tendon rupture site. **B.** A limited transverse incision is made ~1.0 cm proximal to the midsubstance Achilles tendon rupture site. Alternatively, a small longitudinal incision may be made overlying the medial aspect of the Achilles tendon rupture site and extended as necessary.

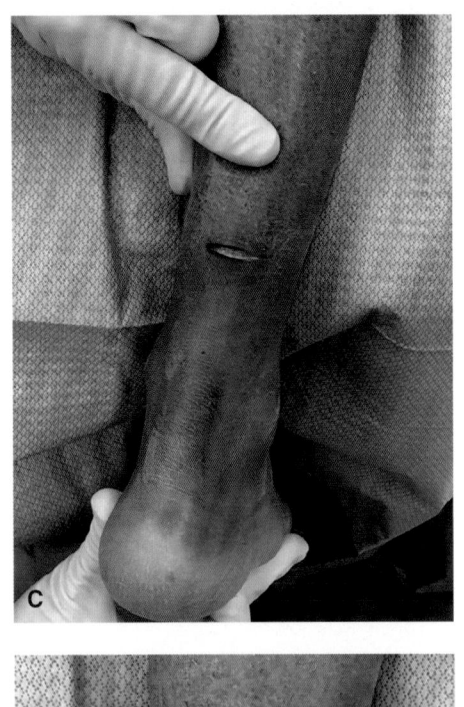
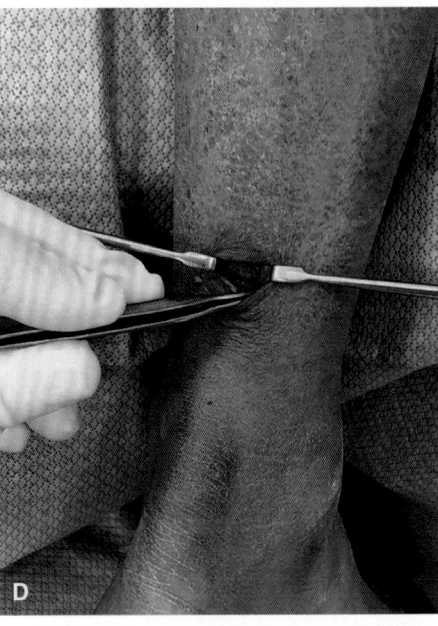
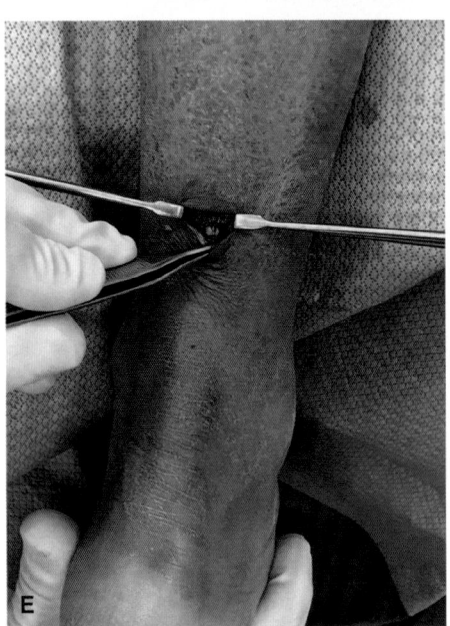
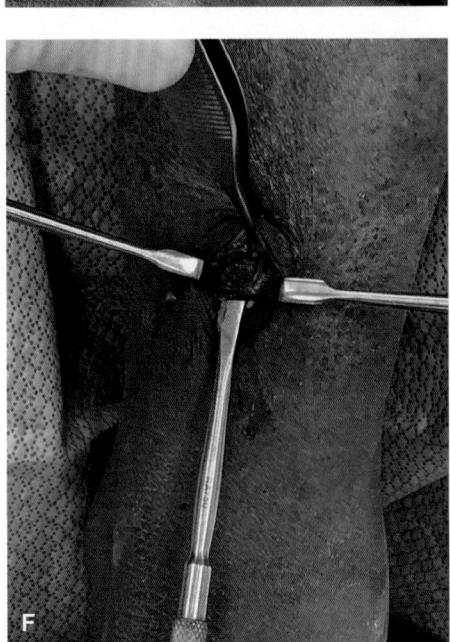
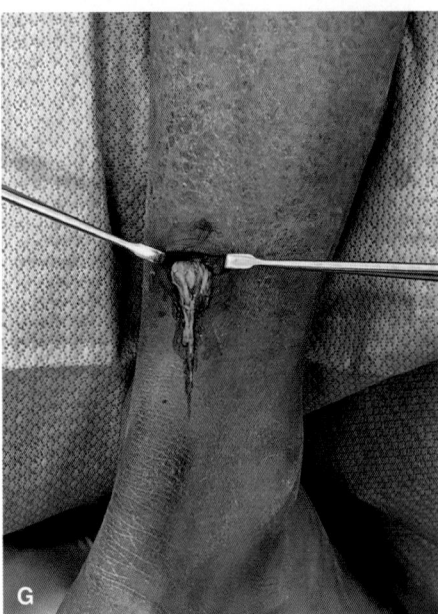
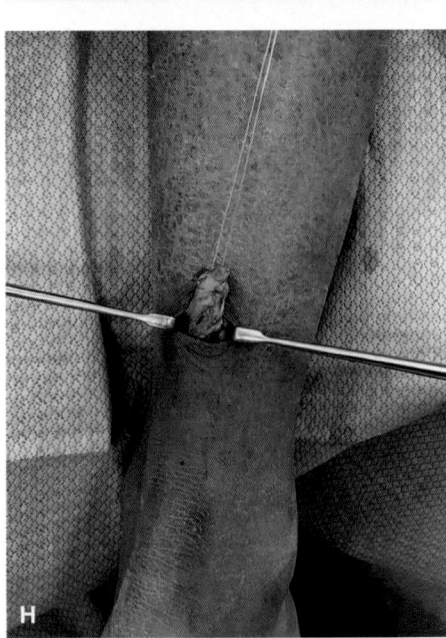

FIGURE 58.21 (*Continued*)
C. The transverse incision is controlled to the level of the deep fascia. **D.** Care is taken to anatomically dissect and identify and preserve the paratenon as shown. **E.** A small transverse incision is then made overlying the paratenon exposing the midsubstance Achilles tendon rupture site. **F.** A Freer elevator is utilized to free any adhesions involving the midsubstance Achilles tendon rupture site; this maneuver aids in restoring full gliding function and physiologic tension at the Achilles tendon rupture site and preserves the paratenon. **G.** Midsubstance proximal Achilles tendon rupture fibers shown in relation to the placement of the transverse incision. **H.** A provisional absorbable suture is used to gain control of the proximal stump of the Achilles tendon.

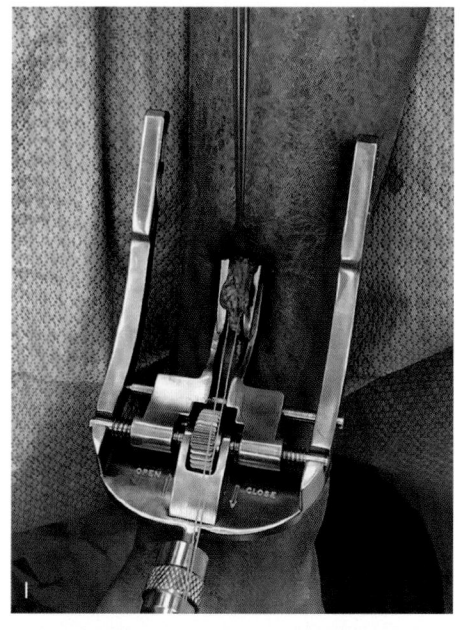

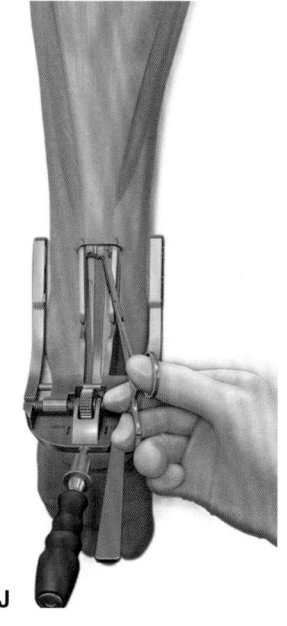

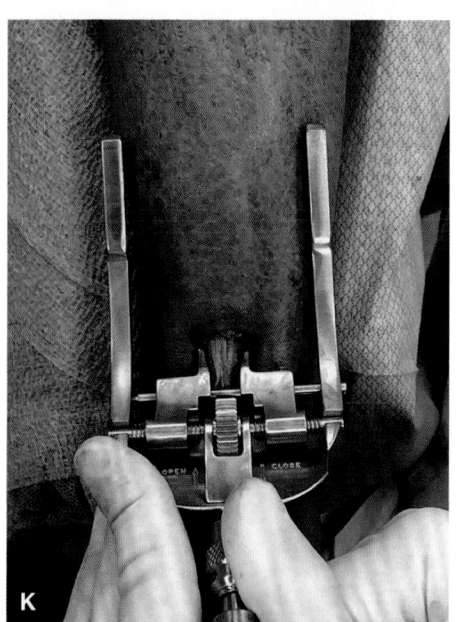

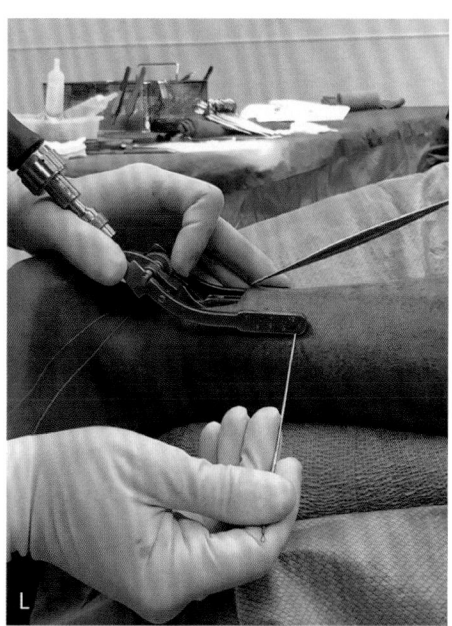

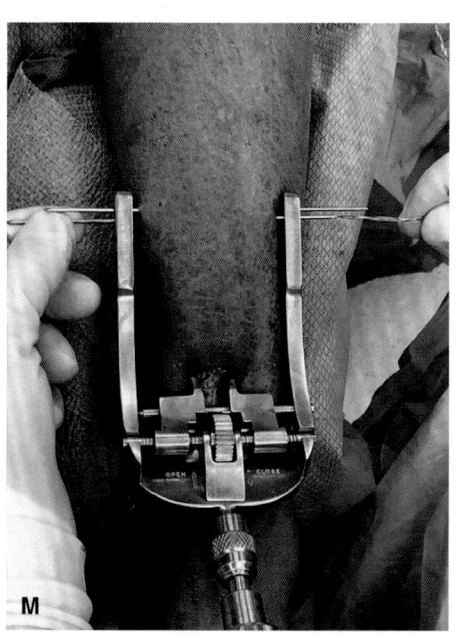

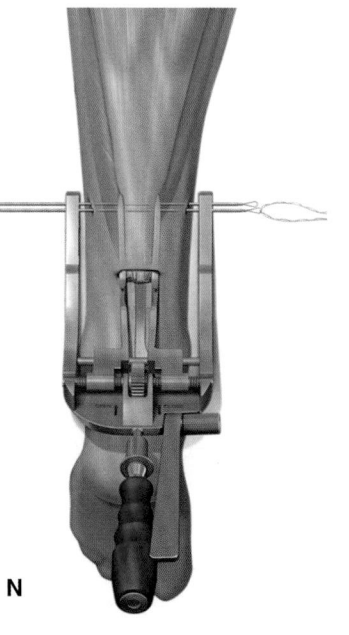

FIGURE 58.21 (*Continued*)
I. The PARS jig is guided into the Achilles tendon rupture site within the paratenon; while distal traction is placed on the controlling provisional suture as shown. **J.** Illustration demonstrating placement of the PARS jig while controlling the proximal Achilles tendon rupture segment. **K.** The PARS jig internal arms are then dialed in to securely engage the proximal Achilles tendon segment. **L.** Care is made to ensure the proximal Achilles tendon segment is anatomically well aligned and positioned with respect to the PARS jig targeted no. 1–7 dedicated hole sequences as shown. **M.** An initial Keith needle may be inserted in the most proximal PARS jig hole to provisionally secure and position the proximal Achilles tendon segment within the PARS jig. The remaining percutaneous sutures are placed in stepwise fashion. **N.** Illustration demonstrating proximal hole securing proximal Achilles tendon segment.

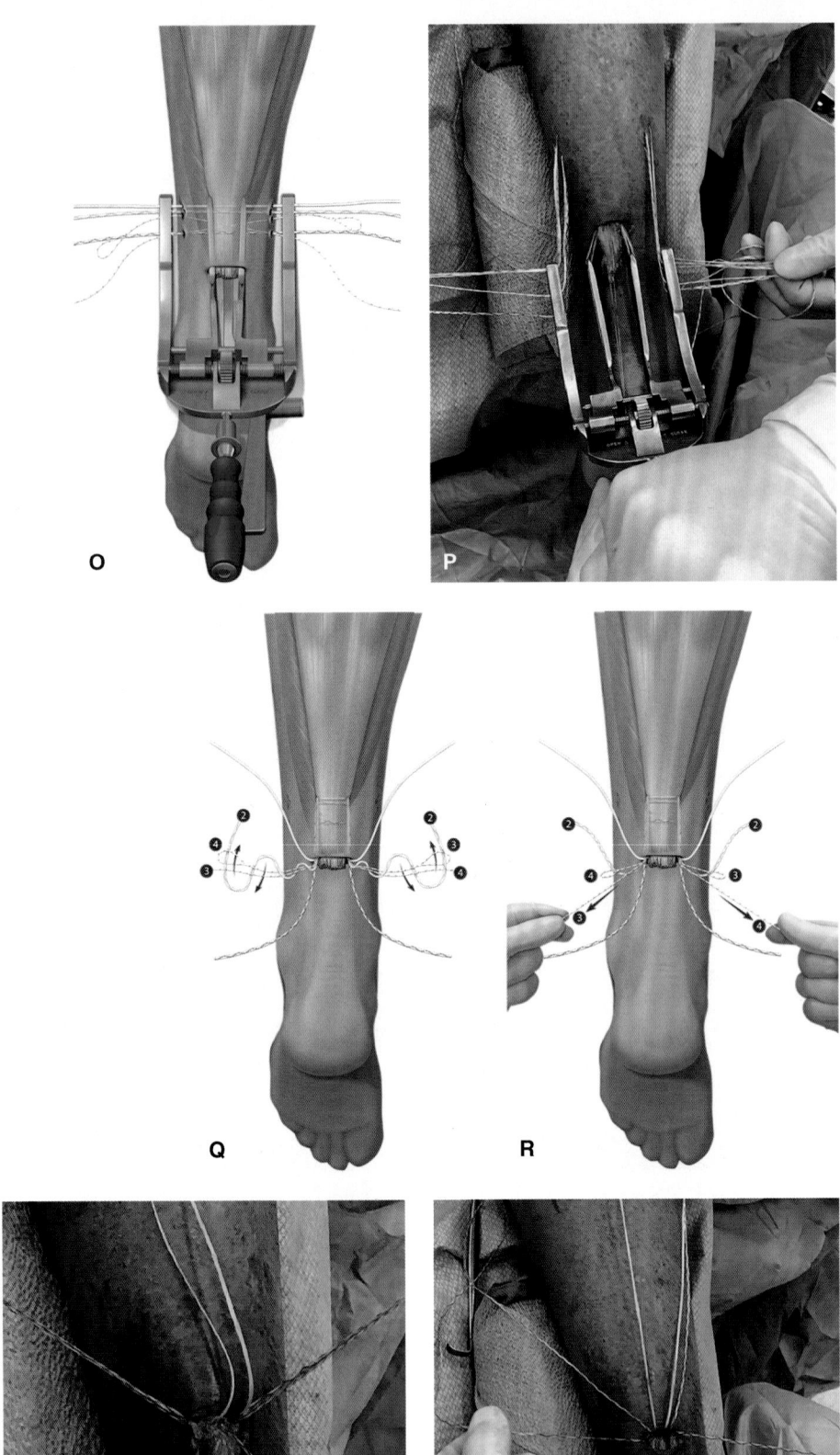

FIGURE 58.21 (*Continued*)
O. Illustration demonstrating final placement and position of all proximal Achilles tendon suture strands before removing the PARS jig. **P.** Once all percutaneous sutures have been passed sequentially, the PARS jig is removed as shown. **Q.** Illustration demonstrating the no. 2 suture strand being wrapped around the no. 3 and 4 suture tape and back through the looped ends positioned both medially and laterally. **R.** Illustration demonstrating the looped suture (no. 3/4) being pulled through creating the locked suture construct medially and laterally. **S.** Once completed three matched polyblend suture strands remain medially and laterally securing the proximal Achilles tendon. Two locked suture tape. One free suture strand. **T.** The final proximal construct demonstrating two locked and one gliding nonabsorbable polyblend suture as shown.

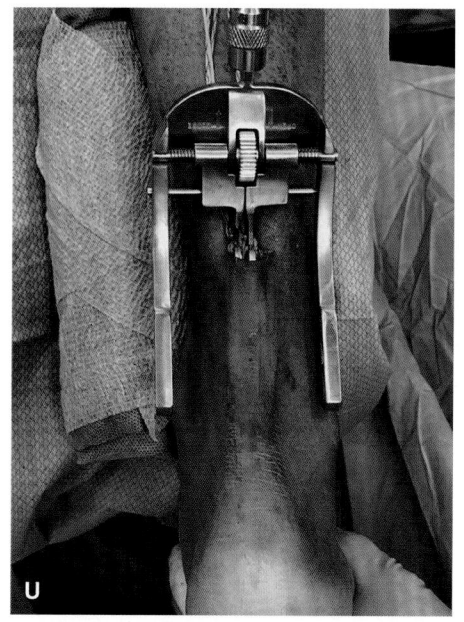

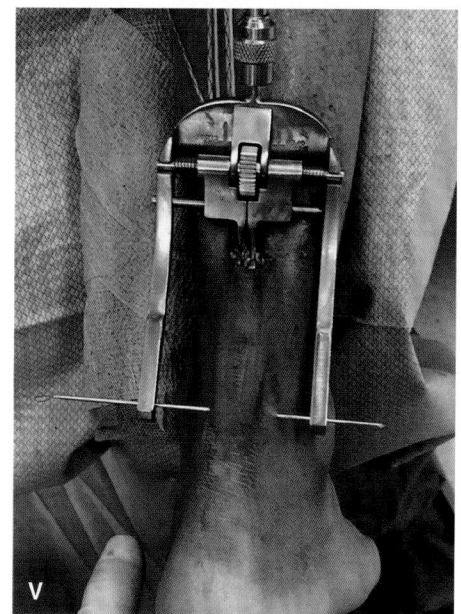

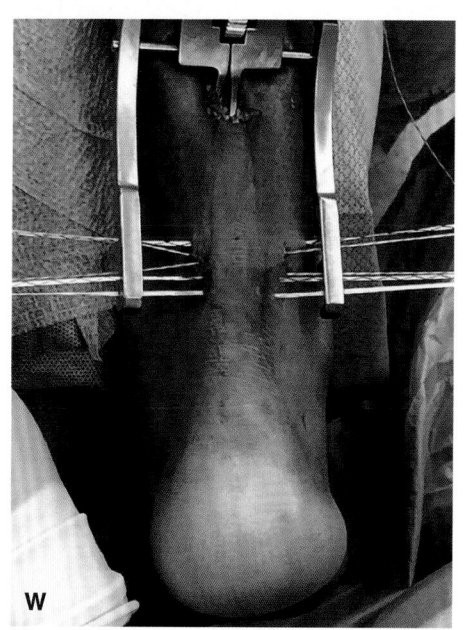

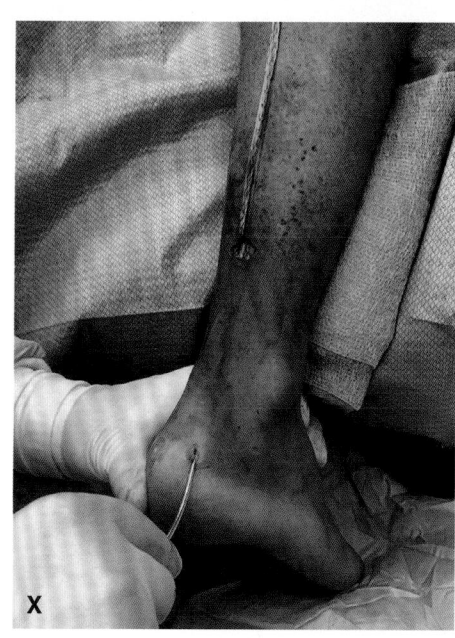

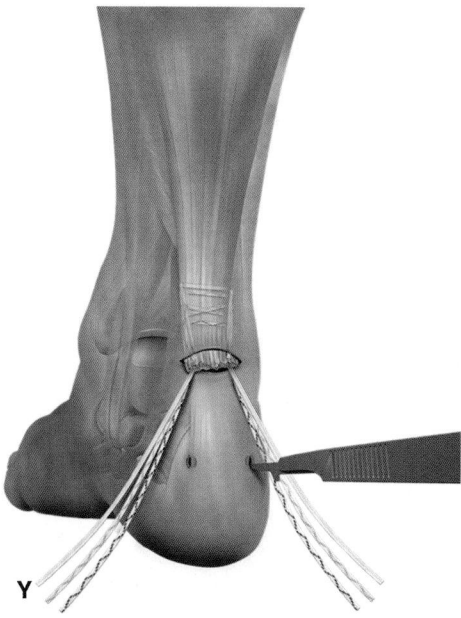

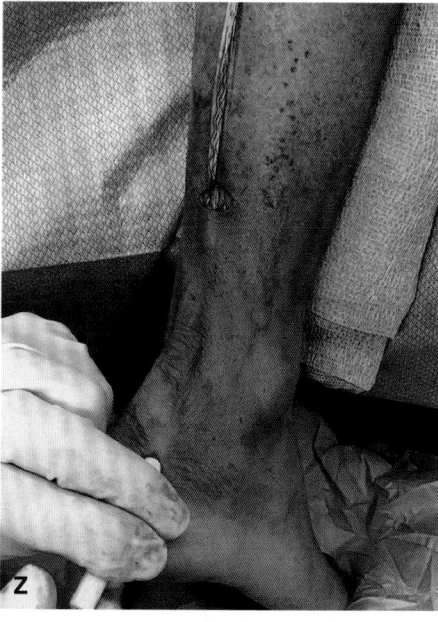

FIGURE 58.21 (*Continued*)
U. The PARS jig can then be reversed and inserted distally in similar fashion to secure the distal Achilles tendon segment. **V.** The percutaneous sutures are then placed and completed via stepwise fashion to the distal Achilles tendon segment as previously shown. **W.** The completed distal Achilles tendon suture construct as shown in a direct repair via a "PARS to PARS" surgical technique. **X.** Alternatively, the proximal Achilles tendon segment can be directly secured distally within the posterior calcaneal tuber via stable interference screw fixation. **Y.** Illustration demonstrating completion of proximal suture construct; and posterolateral and posteromedial sites for distal tensioned interference screw fixation placement. **Z.** An anatomically designed suture passer is placed within a stab incision within the distal extent of the Achilles tendon. The suture passer is controlled within the substance of the distal Achilles tendon fibers and advanced to the zone of midsubstance Achilles tendon rupture site.

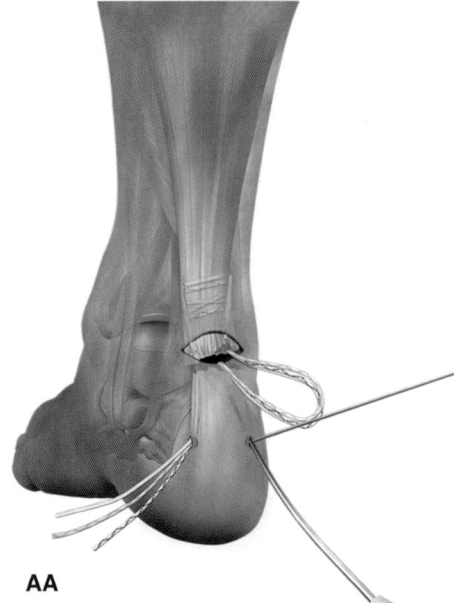

AA

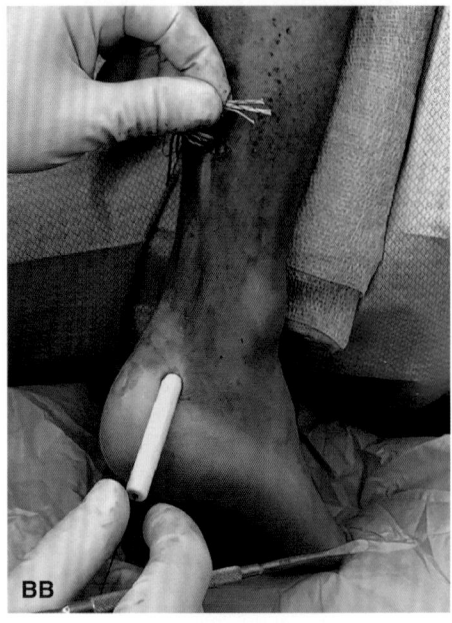

BB

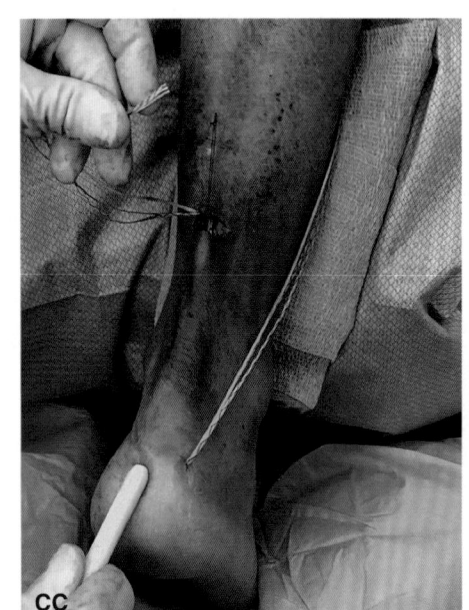

CC

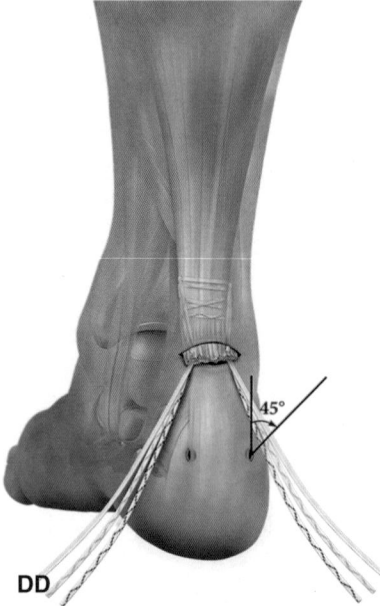

DD

FIGURE 58.21 (*Continued*)
AA. Illustration demonstrating advancement of the distally inserted suture passer to retrieve the proximal suture tape construct. **BB.** A suture passing lasso is then advanced distally to proximally to the level of the proximal lateral Achilles tendon suture construct as shown. **CC.** A suture passing lasso is shown advancing distally to proximally to the level of the proximal medial Achilles tendon suture construct. The proximal lateral suture construct is now shown shuttled distally through the distal Achilles tendon segment to the posterolateral calcaneal tuber. **DD.** Illustration demonstrating the direction of the distal calcaneal medial and lateral bone tunnels. **EE.** Schematic drawing illustrating the placement site and appropriate drill angle of the closed bone tunnels. These bone tunnels are placed slightly medially and laterally and just proximal to the primary insertional footprint of the Achilles' tendon. **FF.** Once completed, the foot is secured in a plantar flexed position and the proximal lateral and proximal medial suture constructs are appropriately tensioned and affixed into closed calcaneal bone tunnels via interference screw fixation.

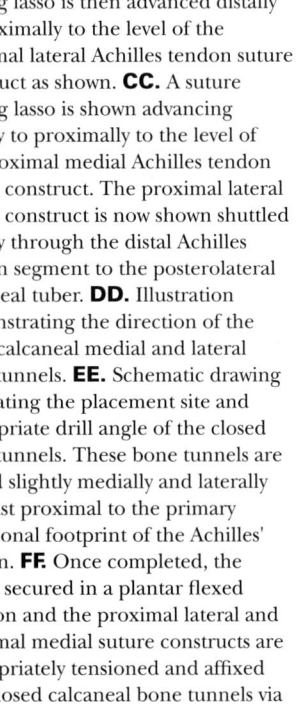

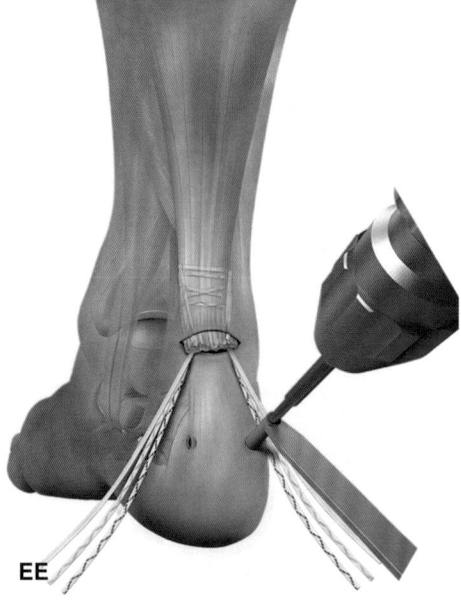

EE

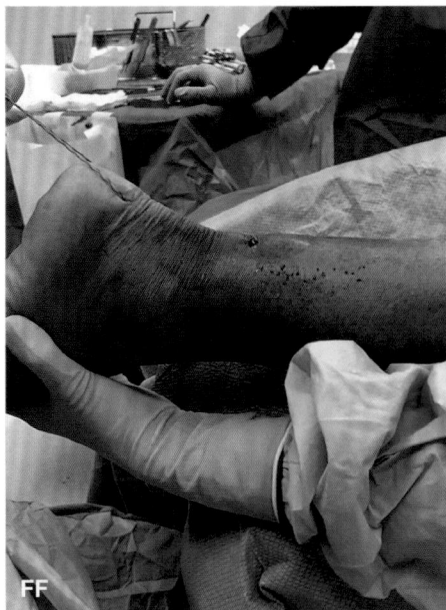

FF

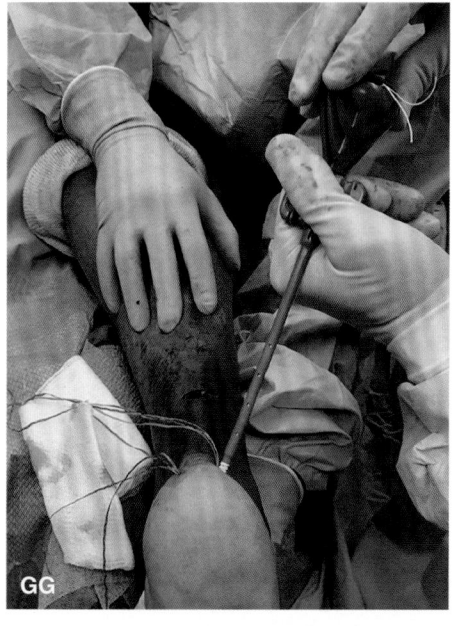

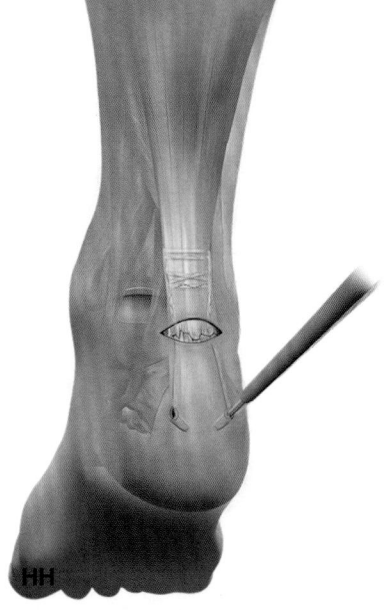

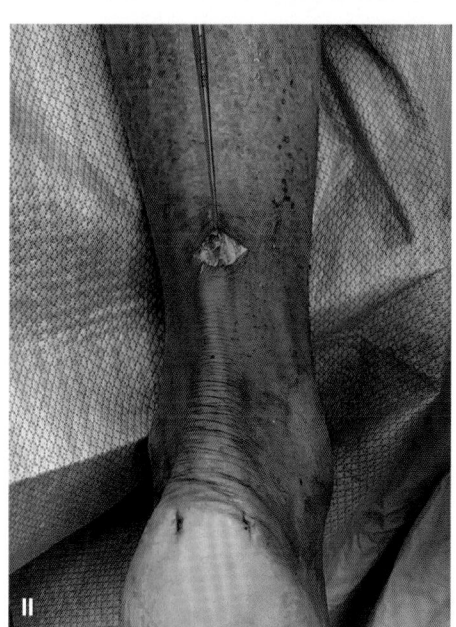

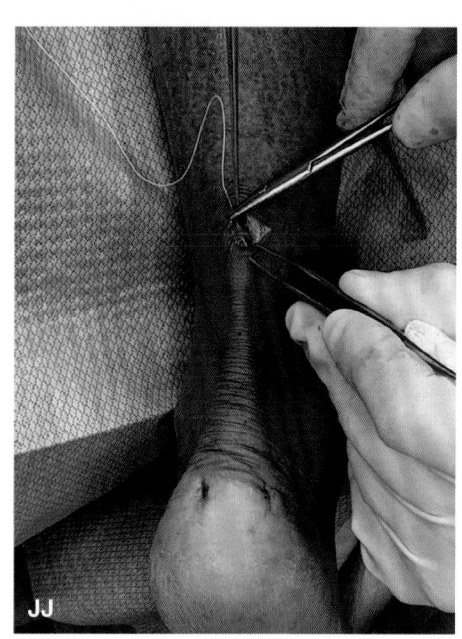

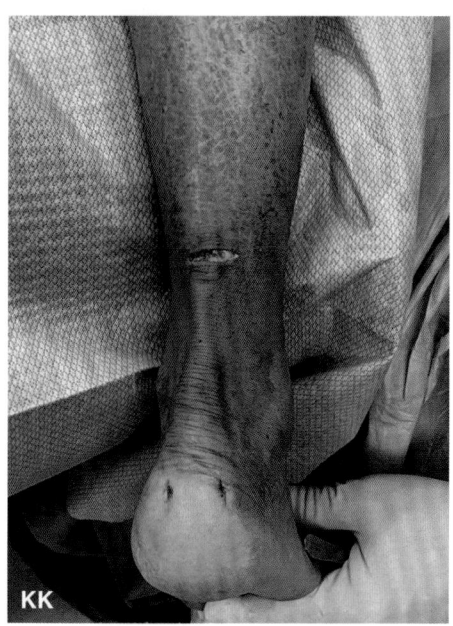

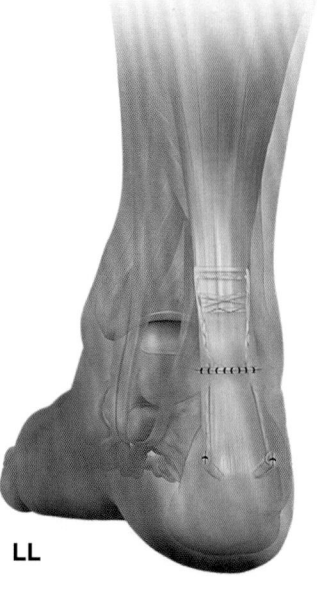

FIGURE 58.21 (*Continued*) **GG.** Interference screw fixation being placed to secure the suture tape strands within the distal medial and distal lateral bone tunnels. **HH.** Illustration demonstrating the angle, position and relationship of the distal medial and lateral calcaneal interference screw placement. **II.** Completion of the minimally invasive midsubstance Achilles tendon rupture via a dual distal interference fixation construct. **JJ.** Repair of the paratenon layer in preserving its gliding function. **KK.** Final view demonstrating restoration of physiologic tension of the midsubstance Achilles tendon rupture site. **LL.** Illustration demonstrating final proximal locked suture construct secured via distal interference screw fixation.

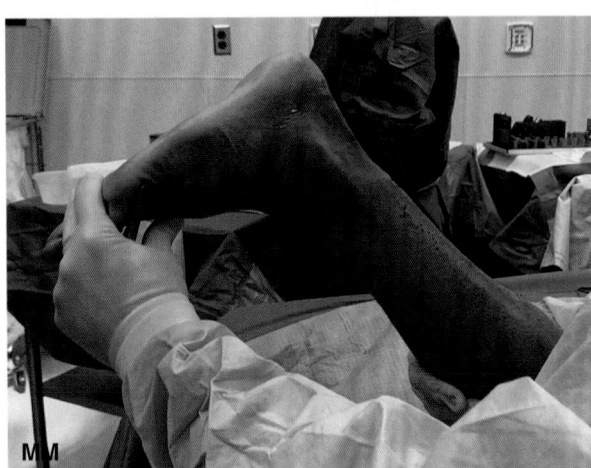
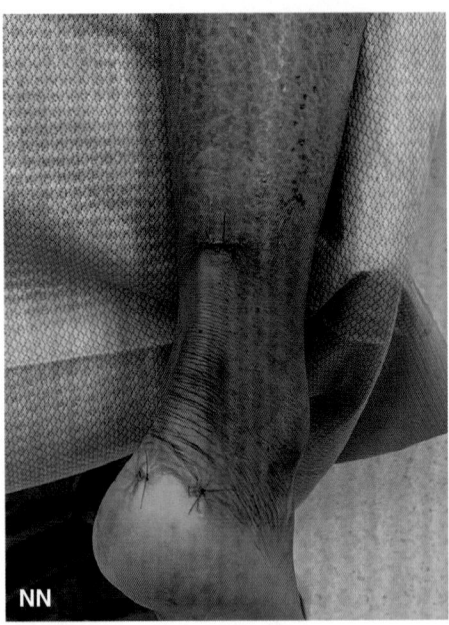

FIGURE 58.21 (*Continued*) **MM.** Lateral view demonstrating restoration of physiologic tension. **NN.** Final closure of the minimally invasive midsubstance Achilles tendon rupture with nonabsorbable suture.

NEGLECTED ACHILLES TENDON RUPTURES

Neglected Achilles tendon ruptures can be a challenge to treat. A chronic or neglected Achilles tendon rupture is defined as rupture that has not been treated in 6 weeks or more from the injury. The rupture gap can typically be 2-10 cm in length. The patient usually presents with a limp due to loss of function of the gastrosoleal complex. There is decreased tone in the gastrocnemius muscle bellies. The gap can sometimes be difficult to palpate due to scar tissue. The Thompson test and the knee flexion test can be performed to help make the diagnosis. An MRI or ultrasound testing will confirm the diagnosis to develop a surgical plan.

Treatment of neglected Achilles tendon ruptures is typically surgical intervention. The Achilles tendon is overlengthened and thus poorly functional, and surgical correction is the only way to correct the deformity. If surgical intervention is not possible, bracing in a ground reactive force ankle foot orthosis would be the best option. There is no standard procedure for surgical intervention of the neglected Achilles tendon ruptures. The procedure chosen is determined by the deficit.

Guidelines popularized by Myerson can be helpful in preoperative planning. These guidelines are determined by the gap size, which is determined by MRI or ultrasound (Fig. 58.22). This is due to the fact that the gap of the rupture can vary. A gap size of 1-2 cm can be treated with an end-to-end anastomosis and a posterior ankle compartment fasciotomy. A gap size between 2 and 5 cm requires a V-Y tendon lengthening augmented with a tendon transfer, if needed. A gap size >5 cm requires a tendon transfer alone or in combination with a V-Y advancement or a turn down.[59,60] A preoperative plan can be implemented, but it is not uncommon that the gap intraoperatively is greater than noted preoperatively, secondary to nonviable/scar tissue.

The author has had success with gastrocnemius recession/Strayer fasciotomy as an alternative to the V-Y advancement in order to bring the proximal end of the tendon distally to perform an end-to-end anastomosis of the tendon ends. An FHL tendon transfer has been also successfully utilized by the author to augment the repair.

Autogenous grafting has been described using FHL, peroneus brevis, or plantaris tendons.[61] In these cases, the tendon is either woven through the two ends of the Achilles to bridge the gap or, in the case of the FHL, laid across the gap with the muscle bridging the deficit. Allogeneic grafting techniques have been utilized via quadriceps tendon, semitendinosus tendon, Achilles tendon, etc.[62] Care is taken to suture the grafts with normal physiologic tension at the rupture site, with the foot in slight plantar flexion (Fig. 58.23).

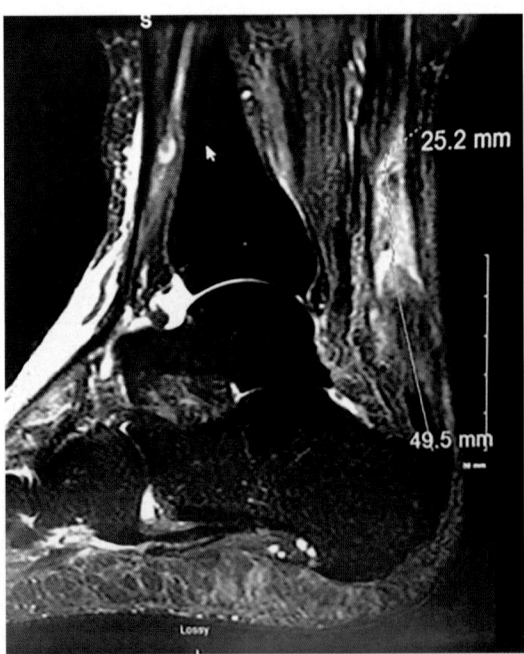

FIGURE 58.22 T2 MRI depicting a neglected Achilles tendon rupture with a defect of 24.3 mm.

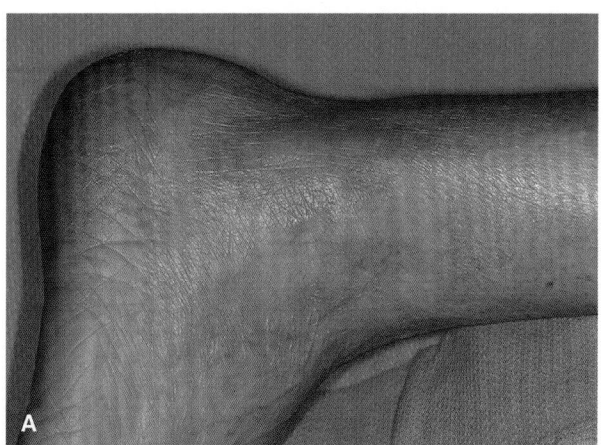

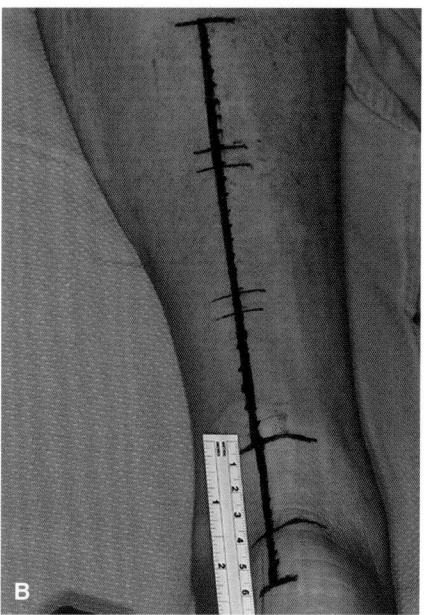

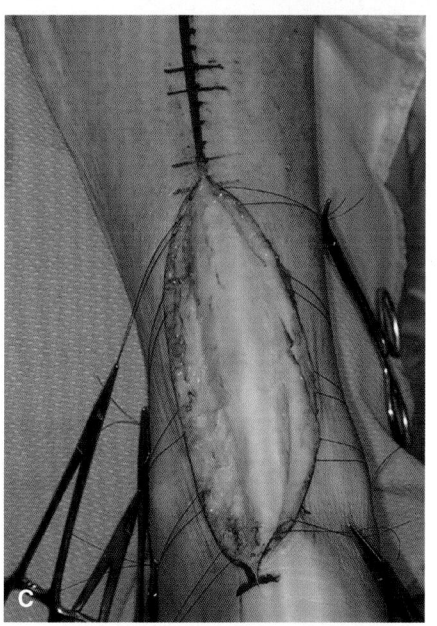

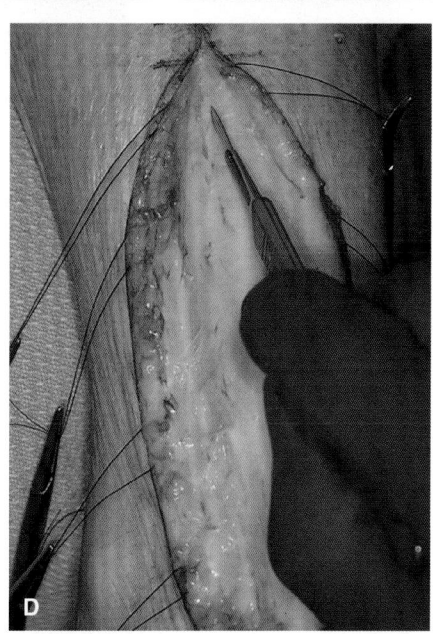

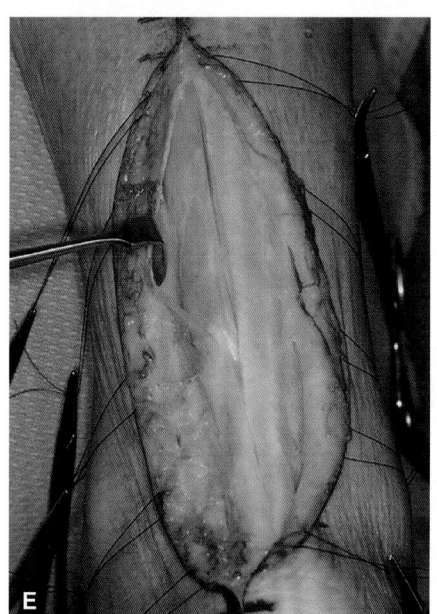

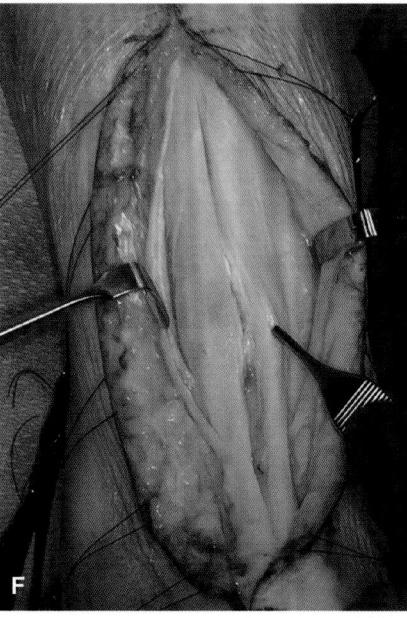

FIGURE 58.23 A. Note the obvious concavity and palpable "dell" at the level of the chronic midsubstance Achilles rupture site. The gap distance approximates 4.5 cm with a relatively preserved insertional Achilles tendon. **B.** A medially biased longitudinal incision is planned toward a delayed primary repair and adjunctive FHL tendon transfer. Proximal extension of the incision is planned should the gap distance be unable to be coapted and a proximally based gastrocnemius "turndown" procedure also be required. **C.** The incision is carried to the level of the deep fascia overlying the site of the neglected midsubstance Achilles tendon chronic rupture. Stay sutures are utilized to protect the skin and soft tissues from excessive handling and to reduce potential of wound healing delay or complication. **D.** The deep fascia and paratenon is incised beginning proximally overlying the proximal Achilles tendon fibers. **E.** Care is taken to reflect and preserve the deep fascia as possible overlying the entire length and zone of the chronic midsubstance Achilles tendon rupture site. **F.** Note the fibrous interposition at the level of the identified chronic midsubstance Achilles tendon rupture site. The forceps identifies the proximal extent of the rupture site.

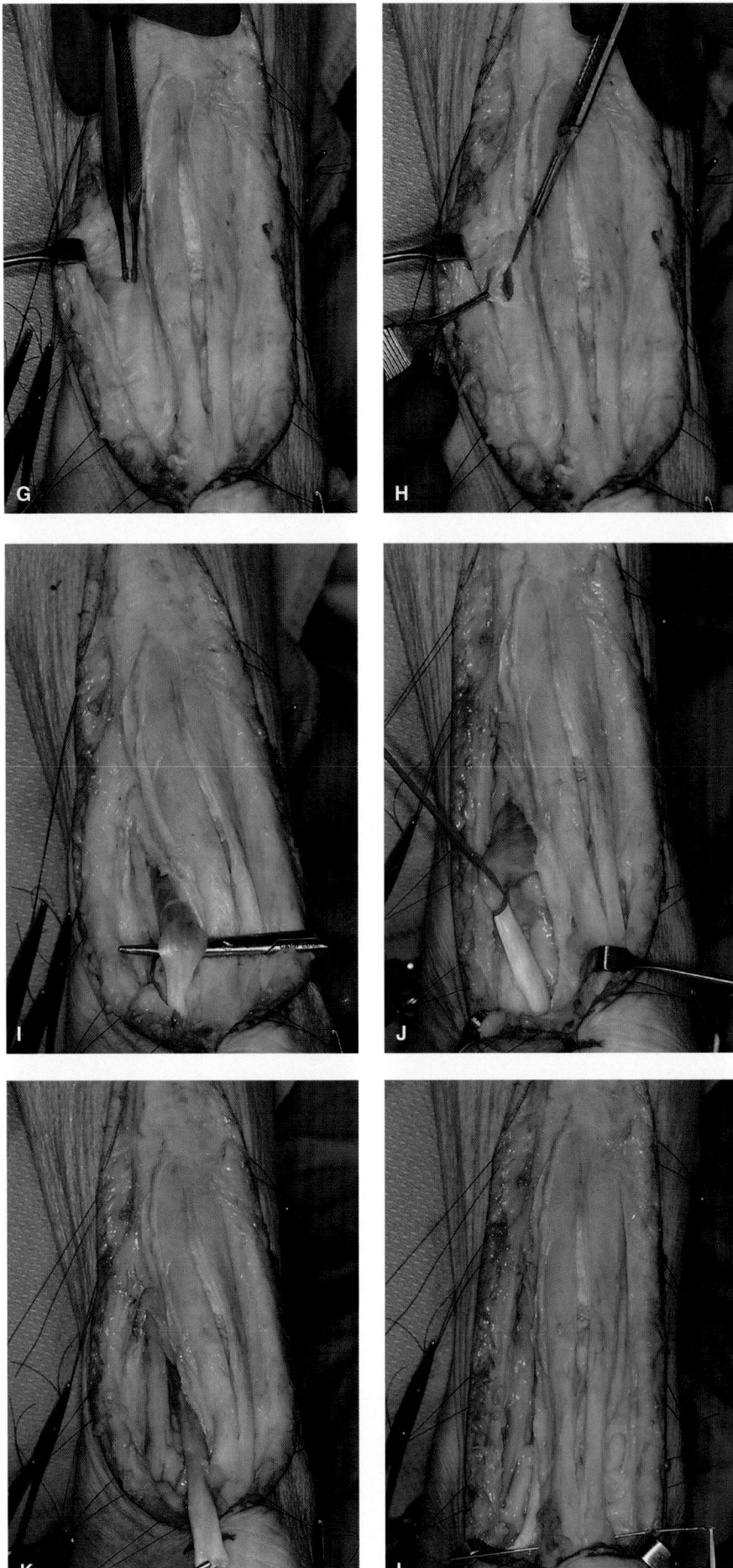

FIGURE 58.23 (*Continued*) **G.** The proximal extent of the rupture site is identified within the confines of the linear incision through the thickened deep fascia/paratenon layer. The forcep medially identifies the position and deep fascia overlying the FHL muscle/tendon unit. **H.** A small linear incision is made overlying the deep fascia to identify the muscle/tendon unit of the Flexor Hallucis Longus. The muscle belly will be utilized to support the "end to end" reconstruction of the débrided neglected chronic midsubstance Achilles tendon repair site. **I.** The FHL myotendinous junction in view as dissection is carried out distally to recruit the FHL tendon. **J.** A vessel loop as shown can effectively be used to manipulate and control the FHL tendon towards distal dissection and recruitment of adequate FHL harvest length. Care is made to resect the FHL via the primary incision distally at or near the level of the sustentaculum. **K.** The forcep identifying the FHL towards a planned "side to side" anastomosis adjunct to the delayed primary repair of the neglected midsubstance Achilles tendon rupture. **L.** A modified Bunnell type suture technique is employed distally via a "Keith" needle with a non-absorbable polyblend suture to secure the distal Achilles tendon.

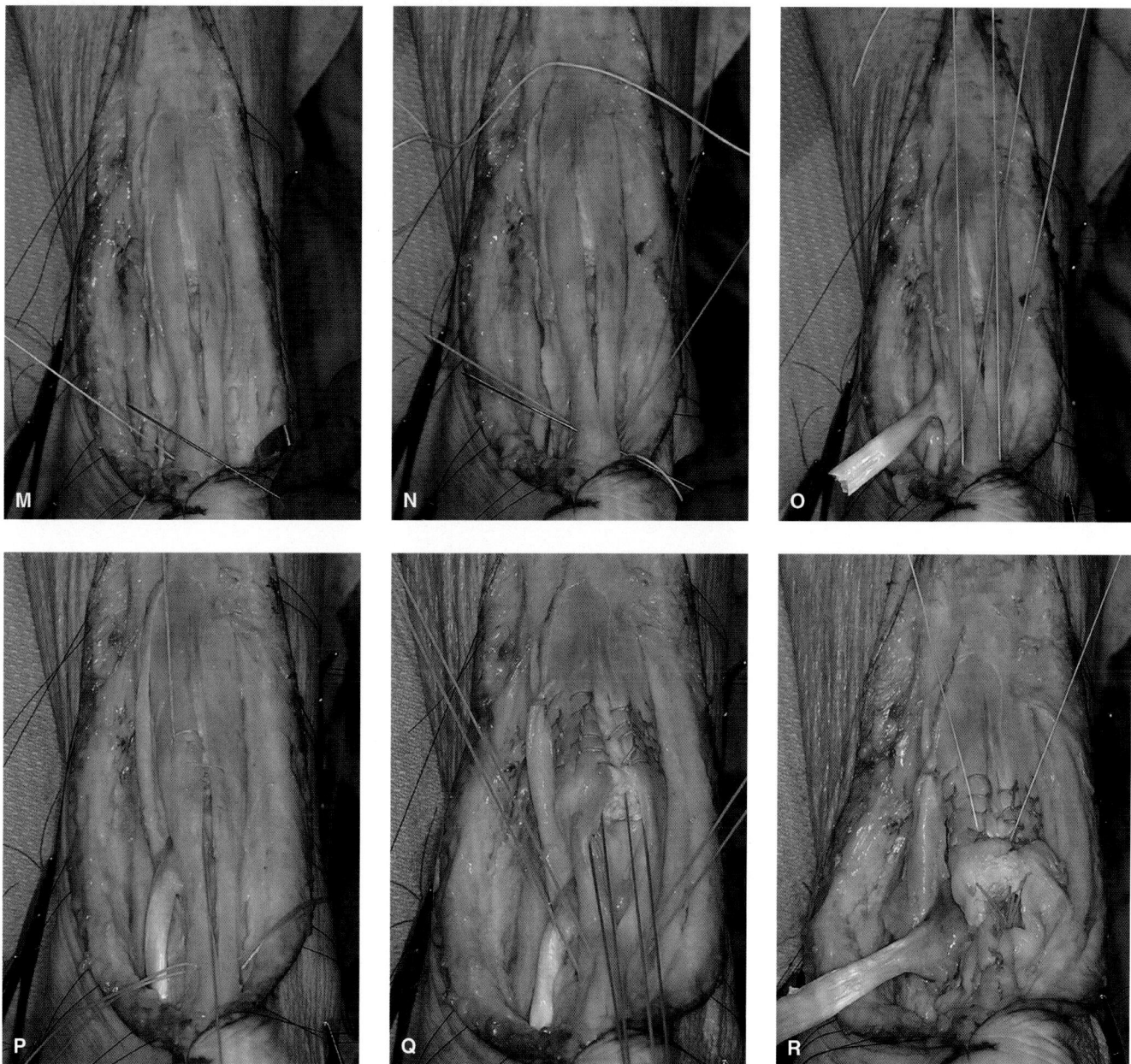

FIGURE 58.23 (*Continued*) **M.** A single strand is passed and biased posteriorly throughout the distal Achilles tendon segment to level of the recognized gap of the neglected Achilles midsubstance rupture site. **N.** An additional strand is then completed in similar fashion and biased anteriorly as shown. **O.** Effectively, two strands of polyblend suture are positioned as shown; one strand more posteriorly placed and one strand more anteriorly placed. Both strands will be utilized in reinforcing the distal Achilles tendon segment at the "end to end" repair site. **P.** A modified "Krackow" technique is utilized to create control over the proximal Achilles tendon. Two strands are created in like kind to the distal Achilles strands to serve to reapproximate the gap distance at the chronic Achilles tendon rupture site. **Q.** Final suture strand positions shown. The two proximal strands via a modified Krackow suture application. The two distal strands via a modified Bunnell suture application. **R.** An additional single strand of absorbable suture is utilized to aid in approximating the rupture site while the nonabsorbable polyblend is passed to the respective opposite sides of Achilles tendon.

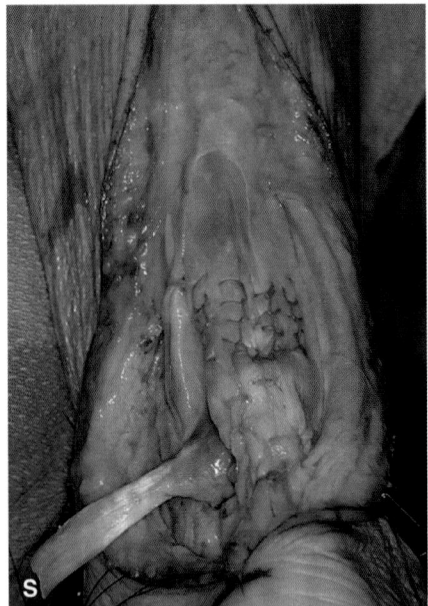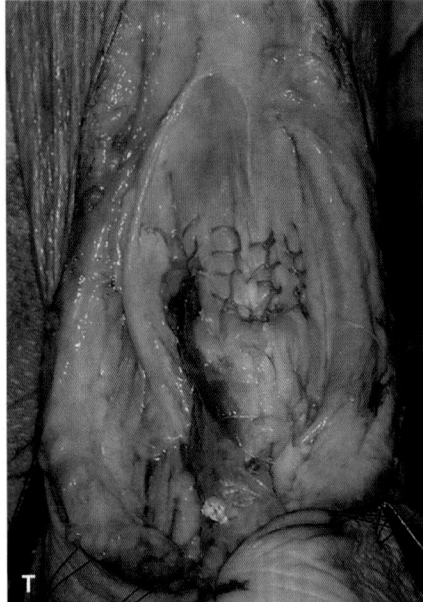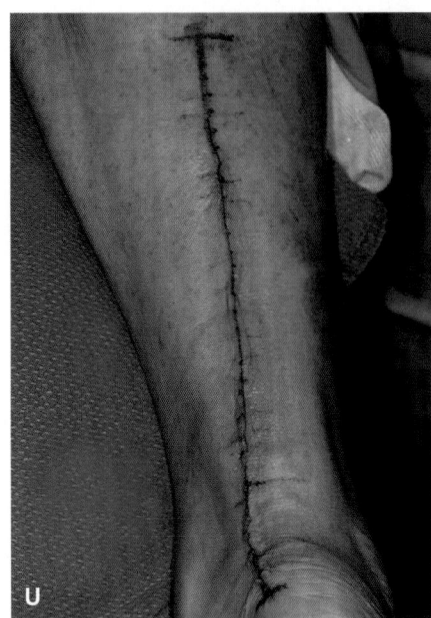

FIGURE 58.23 (*Continued*) **S.** The two distal polyblend nonabsorbable strands are passed through unto the proximal Achilles tendon. The two proximal polyblend nonabsorbable strands are passed through unto the distal Achilles tendon. The neglected rupture site now reapproximated at physiologic tension. **T.** The FHL muscle is shown anastomosed "side to side" to the level of the reconstructed "end to end" Achilles tendon repair site. The FHL tendon distally has been first secured via a medially based closed bone tunnel via interference screw fixation. **U.** Final closure.

PEARLS

- Situate patient in prone position with both limbs evident to evaluate for Achilles tendon rupture.
- Affected side will be dorsiflexed.

PERILS and PITFALLS

- Be cautious of the sural nerve and lesser saphenous vein when dissecting.

PERILS and PITFALLS

- Be cautious of the neurovascular bundle when dissecting for the FHL tendon in the prone position.
- Plantar flex the hallux to be sure the correct tendon is being transferred.

ACKNOWLEDGMENT

The authors wish to acknowledge Leo Caldarella for his work in editing and preparation of the clinical and intraoperative photographs that illustrate the surgical techniques provided throughout this Chapter. The authors additionally express their gratitude to Leo Caldarella for his work in editing and preparation of the surgical case illustration video segments throughout this Chapter. The authors also acknowledge his work in proof reading of the captions and legends accompanying the surgical case illustrations in both the print and video formats found throughout this Chapter.

REFERENCES

1. O'Brien M. The anatomy of the Achilles tendon. *Foot Ankle Clin.* 2005;10:225-238.
2. Edama M, et al. Structure of the Achilles tendon at the insertion on the calcaneal tuberosity. *J Anat.* 2016;229(5):610-614.
3. Kim PJ, et al. The variability of the Achilles tendon insertion: a cadaveric examination. *J Foot Ankle Surg.* 2010;49(5):417-420.
4. Chimenti RL, et al. Altered tendon characteristics and mechanical properties associated with insertional Achilles tendinopathy. *J Orthop Sports Phys Ther.* 2014;44(9):680-689.
5. Ballal MS, Walker CR, Molloy AP. The anatomical footprint of the Achilles tendon: a cadaveric study. *Bone Joint J.* 2014;96-B(10):1344-1348.
6. Lohrer H, et al. The Achilles tendon insertion is crescent shaped—an in vitro anatomic investigation. *Clin Orthop Relat Res.* 2008;466:2230-2237.
7. Van Sterkenburg MN, Van Dijk CN. Mid-portion Achilles tendinopathy: why painful? an evidence-based philosophy. *Knee Surg Sports Traumatol Arthrosc.* 2011;19(8):1367-1375.
8. Milz S, et al. Three-dimensional reconstructions of the Achilles tendon insertion in man. *J Anat.* 2002;200(Pt 2):145-152. doi: 10.1046/j.0021-8782.2001.00016.x.
9. Chimenti R, et al. Forefoot and rearfoot contributions to the lunge position in individuals with and without insertional Achilles tendinopathy. *Clin Biomech.* 2016;36:44-45.
10. Bjur D, et al. The innervation pattern of the human Achilles tendon: studies of the normal and tendinosis tendon with markers for general and sensory innervation. *Cell Tissue Res.* 2005;320(1):201-206.
11. Francis P, et al. The proportion of lower limb running injuries by gender, anatomical location and specific pathology: a systematic Review. *J Sports Sci Med.* 2019;18(1):21-31.
12. Kraemer R, et al. Analysis of hereditary and medical risk factors in Achilles tendinopathy and Achilles tendon ruptures: a matched pair analysis. *Arch Orthop Trauma Surg.* 2012;132(6):847-853.
13. Chimenti RL, et al. Current concepts review update: insertional Achilles tendinopathy. *Foot Ankle Int.* 2017;38(10):1160-1169.
14. Rufai A, et al. Structure and histopathology of the insertional region of the human Achilles tendon. *J Orthop Res.* 1995;13(4):585-593.
15. Benjamin M, et al. The mechanism of formation of bony spurs (enthesophytes) in the Achilles tendon. *Arthritis Rheum.* 2000;43(3):576-583.
16. Chimenti RL, et al. Insertional Achilles tendinopathy associated with altered transverse compressive and axial tensile strain during ankle dorsiflexion. *J Orthop Res.* 2017;35(4):910-915.
17. Van Sterkenburg MN, et al. Appearance of the weight-bearing lateral radiograph in retrocalcaneal bursitis. *Acta Orthop.* 2010;81(3):387-390.
18. Shibuya N, et al. Is calcaneal inclination higher in patients with insertional Achilles tendinosis? A case-controlled, cross-sectional study. *J Foot Ankle Surg.* 2012;51(6):757-761.
19. Taylor J, et al. Extracorporeal Shockwave Therapy (ESWT) for refractory Achilles tendinopathy: a prospective audit with 2-year follow up. *Foot (Edinb)* 2016;26:23-29.

20. Nicholson CW, et al. Prediction of the success of nonoperative treatment of insertional Achilles tendinosis based on MRI. *Foot Ankle Int.* 2007;28(4):472-477.
21. Shakked RJ, Raikin SM. Insertional tendinopathy of the Achilles: debridement, primary repair, and when to augment: debridement, primary repair, and when to augment. *Foot Ankle Clin.* 2017;22(4):761-780.
22. Rompe JD, et al. Eccentric loading versus eccentric loading plus shock-wave treatment for midportion Achilles tendinopathy: a randomized controlled trial. *Am J Sports Med.* 2009;37(3):463-470.
23. Saxena A, et al. Extra-corporeal Pulsed-Activated Therapy ('EPAT' sound wave) for Achilles tendinopathy: a prospective study. *J Foot Ankle Surg.* 2011;50(3):315-319.
24. Al-Abbad H, Varghese Simon J. The effectiveness of extracorporeal shock wave therapy on chronic Achilles tendinopathy: a systematic review. *Foot Ankle Int.* 2013;34(1):33-41.
25. Korakakis V, et al. The effectiveness of extracorporeal shockwave therapy in common lower limb conditions: a systematic review including quantification of patient-rated pain reduction. *Br J Sports Med.* 2018;52(6):387-407.
26. Hart L. Corticosteroid and other injections in the management of tendinopathies: a review. *Clin J Sport Med.* 2011;21(6):540-541.
27. Li H-Y, Hua Y-H. Achilles tendinopathy: current concepts about the basic science and clinical treatments. *Biomed Res Int.* 2016;2016:9.
28. Burke CJ, Adler RS. Ultrasound-guided percutaneous tendon treatments. *Am J Roentgenol.* 2016;207(3):495-506.
29. Ettinger S, et al. Operative treatment of the insertional Achilles tendinopathy through a transtendinous approach. *Foot Ankle Int.* 2016;37(3):288-293.
30. Vaishya R, et al. Haglund's syndrome: a commonly seen mysterious condition. *Cureus.* 2016;8(10):e820.
31. Syed TA, Perera A. A proposed staging classification for minimally invasive management of haglund's syndrome with percutaneous and endoscopic surgery. *Foot Ankle Clin.* 2016;21(3):641-664.
32. Van Sterkenberg MN, et al. Appearance of the weight-bearing lateral radiograph in retrocalcaneal bursitis. *Acta Orthop.* 2010;81(3):387-390.
33. Bulstra GH, et al. Can we measure the heel bump? Radiographic evaluation of haglund's deformity. *J Foot Ankle Surg.* 2015;54(3):338-340.
34. Zadek I. An operation for the cure of achillobursitis. *Am J Surg.* 1939;43(2):542-546.
35. Lysholm J, Wiklander J. Injuries in runners. *Am J Sports Med.* 1987;15:168-171.
36. Alfredson H, Spang C. Clinical presentation and surgical management of chronic Achilles tendon disorders—A retrospective observation on a set of consecutive patients being operated by the same orthopedic surgeon. *Foot Ankle Surg.* 2018;24:490-494.
37. Decarbo WT, Bullock MJ. Midsubstance tendinopathy, surgical management. *Clin Podiatr Med Surg.* 2017;34(2):175.
38. Khaliq Y, et al. Fluoroquinolone-associated tendinopathy: a critical review of the literature. *Clin Infect Dis.* 2003;36(11):1404-1410.
39. Pearce CJ, Carmichael J, Calder JD. Achilles tendinoscopy and plantaris tendon release and division in the treatment of non-insertional Achilles tendinopathy. *Foot Ankle Surg.* 2012;18:124-127.
40. Moraes VY, et al. Platelet-rich therapies for musculoskeletal soft tissue injuries. *Cochrane Database Syst Rev.* 2014;2014(4):CD010071.
41. Henning PR, Grear BJ. Platelet-rich plasma in the foot and ankle. *Curr Rev Musculoskelet Med.* 2018;11(4):616-623.
42. Imai S, et al. Platelet-rich plasma promotes migration, proliferation, and the gene expression of scleraxis and vascular endothelial growth factor in paratenon-derived cells in vitro. *Sports Health.* 2019;11(2):142-148.
43. Filardo G, et al. Platelet -rich plasma in tendon-related disorders: results and indications. *Knee Surg Sports Traumatol Arthrosc.* 2018;26:1984-1999.
44. Singh A, et al. Noninsertional tendinopathy of the Achilles. *Foot Ankle Clin.* 2017;22(4):745-760.
45. Nunley, James A. The Achilles Tendon : Treatment and Rehabilitation. Springer, 2009.
46. Yeap EJ, et al. Radiofrequency coblation for chronic foot and ankle tendinosis. *J Orthop Surg.* 2009;17(3):325-330.
47. Shibuya N, et al. Is percutaneous radiofrequency coblation for treatment of Achilles tendinosis safe and effective? *J Foot Ankle Surg.* 2012;51(6):767-771.
48. Sanchez PJ, et al. Percutaneous ultrasonic tenotomy for Achilles tendinopathy is a surgical procedure with similar complications. *J Foot Ankle Surg.* 2017;56(5):982-984.
49. Ochen Y, et al. Operative treatment versus nonoperative treatment of Achilles tendon ruptures: systematic review and meta-analysis. *BMJ.* 2019;364:k5120.
50. Schipper O, Cohen B. The acute injury of the Achilles. *Foot Ankle Clin.* 2017;22:689-714.
51. Egger AC, Berkowitz MJ. Achilles tendon Injuries. *Curr Rev Musculoskelet Med.* 2017;10:72-78.
52. Godoy-Santos AL, et al. Fluoroquinolones and the risk of Achilles tendon disorders: update on a neglected complication. *J Urol.* 2018;113:20-25.
53. Stavenuiter XJR, et al. Postoperative complications following repair of acute Achilles tendon rupture. *Foot Ankle Int.* 2019;40:679-686. doi: 10.1177/1071100719831371.
54. Wu Y, et al. Complications in the management of acute Achilles tendon rupture: a systematic review and network meta-analysis of 2060 patients. *Am J Sports Med.* 2019;47:2251-2260.
55. Holm C, et al. Achilles tendon rupture—Treatment and complications: a systematic review. *Scand J Med Sci Sports.* 2015;25(1):e1-e10.
56. Zhou K, et al. Surgical versus non-surgical methods for acute Achilles tendon rupture: a meta-analysis of randomized controlled trials. *J Foot Ankle Surg.* 2018;57(6):1191-1199.
57. Deng S, et al. Surgical treatment versus conservative management for acute Achilles tendon rupture: a systematic review and meta-analysis of randomized controlled trials. *J Foot Ankle Surg.* 2017;56(6):1236-1243.
58. Grassi A, et al. Minimally invasive versus open repair for acute Achilles tendon rupture: meta-analysis showing reduced complications, with similar outcomes, after minimally invasive surgery. *J Bone Joint Surg.* 2018;100(22):1969-1981.
59. Myerson MS. Achilles tendon ruptures. *Instr Course Lect.* 1999;48:219-230.
60. Kraeutler M, Purcell J, Hunt K. Chronic Achilles ruptures. *Foot Ankle Int.* 2017;38(8):921-929.
61. Maffulli N, et al. Chronic Achilles tendon rupture. *Open Orthop J.* 2017;11:660-669.
62. Song Y-J, Hua Y-H. Tendon allograft for the treatment of chronic Achilles tendon rupture: a systematic review. *Foot Ankle Surg.* 2019;25:252-257.

SUGGESTED READINGS

Abate M, et al. Platelet rich plasma compared to dry needling in the treatment of non-insertional Achilles tendinopathy. *Phys Sportsmed.* 2019;47:232-237.

Alfredson H. Midportion Achilles tendinosis and the plantaris tendon. *Br J Sports Med.* 2011;45(13):1023-1025.

Alfredson H. Where to now with Achilles tendon treatment? *Br J Sports Med.* 2011;45(5):386-386.

Alfredson H. Clinical commentary of the evolution of the treatment for chronic painful midportion Achilles tendinopathy. *Br J Phys Ther.* 2015;19(5):429-432.

ÅStrõm M, et al. Imaging in chronic Achilles tendinopathy: a comparison of ultrasonography, magnetic resonance imaging and surgical findings in 27 histologically verified cases. *Skeletal Radiol.* 1996;25(7):615-620.

Bisaccia DR, Aicale R, Tarantino T, Peretti GM, Maffulli N. Biological and chemical changes in fluoroquinolone-associated tendinopathies: a systematic review. *Br Med Bull.* 2019;130:39-49.

Bullock MJ, et al. Achilles impingement tendinopathy on magnetic resonance imaging. *J Foot Ankle Surg.* 2017;56(3):555-563.

Catanzariti AR, Hentges M. Combined tendon and bone allograft transplantation for chronic Achilles tendon ruptures. *Clin Podiatr Med Surg.* 2016;33(1):125-137.

Caudell GM. Insertional Achilles Tendinopathy. *Clin Podiatr Med Surg.* 2017;34(2):195-205.

Chen X, et al. The efficacy of platelet-rich plasma on tendon and ligament healing: a systematic review and meta-analysis with bias assessment. *Am J Sports Med.* 2018;46(8):2020-2032.

Chimenti RL, et al. Utility of ultrasound for imaging osteophytes in patients with insertional Achilles tendinopathy. *Arch Phys Med Rehabili.* 2016;97(7):1206-1209.

Chimenti RL, et al. Percutaneous ultrasonic tenotomy reduces insertional Achilles tendinopathy pain with high patient satisfaction and a low complication rate. *J Ultrasound Med.* 2019;38:1629-1635.

d'Agostino MC, et al. Shock wave as biological therapeutic tool: from mechanical stimulation to recovery and healing, through mechanotransduction. *Int J Surg.* 2015;24(Pt B):147-153.

Ficek K, et al. Calcaneal CT is a useful tool for identifying Achilles tendon disorders: a pilot study. *J Orthop Surg Res.* 2017;12(1):1-8.

Gillis CT, Lin JS. Use of a central splitting approach and near complete detachment for insertional calcific Achilles tendinopathy repaired with an Achilles bridging suture. *J Foot Ankle Surg.* 2016;55(2):235-239.

Greenhagen RM, et al. Intermediate and long-term outcomes of the suture bridge technique for the management of insertional Achilles tendinopathy. *Foot Ankle Spec.* 2013;6(3):185-190.

Guelfi M, et al. Long-term beneficial effects of platelet-rich plasma for non-insertional Achilles tendinopathy. *Foot Ankle Surg.* 2015;21:178-181.

Habets B, et al. Return to sport in athletes with midportion Achilles tendinopathy: a qualitative systematic review regarding definitions and criteria. *Sports Med (Auckland, N.Z.).* 2018;48(3):705-723.

Hahn F, et al. Changes in plantar pressure distribution after Achilles tendon augmentation with flexor hallucis longus transfer. *Clin Biomech.* 2008;23(1):109-116.

Hardy A, et al. Functional outcomes and return to sports after surgical treatment of insertional Achilles tendinopathy: surgical approach tailored to the degree of tendon involvement. *Orthop Traumatol Surg Res.* 2018;104(5):719-723.

Heckman DS, et al. Tendon disorders of the foot and ankle, part 2: Achilles tendon disorders. *Am J Sports Med.* 2009;37(6):1223-1234.

Hickey B, et al. It is possible to release the plantaris tendon under ultrasound guidance: a technical description of ultrasound guided plantaris tendon release (UPTR) in the treatment of non-insertional Achilles tendinopathy. *Knee Surg Sports Traumatol Arthrosc.* 2019;27:2858-2862.

Howell MA, et al. Calcific insertional Achilles tendinopathy-Achilles repair with flexor hallucis longus tendon transfer: case series and surgical technique. *J Foot Ankle Surg.* 2019;58(2):236-242.

Huh J, et al. Characterization and surgical management of Achilles tendon sleeve avulsions. *Foot Ankle Int.* 2016;37(6):596-604.

Hunt KJ, et al. Surgical treatment of insertional Achilles tendinopathy with or without flexor hallucis longus tendon transfer: a prospective, randomized study. *Foot Ankle Int.* 2015;36(9):998-1005.

Irwin TA. Current concepts review: insertional Achilles tendinopathy. *Foot Ankle Int.* 2010;31(10):933-939.

Jerosch J. Endoscopic calcaneoplasty. *Foot Ankle Clin.* 2015;20(1):149-165.

Johannsen F, et al. 10-year follow-up after standardised treatment for Achilles tendinopathy. *BMJ Open Sport Exerc Med.* 2018;4(1):e000415.

Johansson K, et al. Macroscopic anomalies and pathological findings in and around the Achilles tendon: observations from 1661 operations during a 40-year period. *Orthop J Sports Med.* 2014;2(12):2325967114562371.

Johnston E, et al. Chronic disorders of the Achilles tendon: results of conservative and surgical treatments. *Foot Ankle Int.* 1997;18(9):570-574.

Kang S, et al. Insertional Achilles tendonitis and haglund's deformity. *Foot Ankle Int.* 2012;33(6):487-491.

Kedia M, et al. The effects of conventional physical therapy and eccentric strengthening for insertional Achilles tendinopathy. *Int J Sports Phys Ther.* 2014;9(4):488-497.

Khan WS, et al. Analysing the outcome of surgery for chronic Achilles tendinopathy over the last 50 years. *World J Orthop.* 2015;6(6):491-497.

Khan KM, Maffulli N. Tendinopathy: an Achilles' heel for athletes and clinicians. *Clin J Sport Med.* 1998;8(3):151-154.

Leppilahti J, et al. Ruptures of the Achilles tendon: relationship to inequality in length of legs and to patterns in the foot and ankle. *Foot Ankle Int.* 1998;19(10):683-687.

Lin Y-J, et al. V-Y tendon plasty for reconstruction of chronic Achilles tendon rupture: a medium-term and long-term follow-up. *Orthop Surg.* 2019;11(1):109-116.

Lohrer H, et al. Surgical treatment for Achilles tendinopathy—a systematic review. *BMC Musculoskelet Disord.* 2016;17(207):207.

Maffulli N, et al. Chronic Achilles tendon disorders. *Clin Sports Med.* 2015;34(4):607-624.

Mansur NSB, et al. Shockwave therapy associated with eccentric strengthening for Achilles insertional tendinopathy: a prospective study. *Foot Ankle Spec.* 2019;12:540-545. doi: 10.1177/1938640019826673.

Masci L, et al. How to diagnose plantaris tendon involvement in midportion Achilles tendinopathy—clinical and imaging findings. *BMC Musculoskelet Disord.* 2016;17(99):97.

Mcalister JE, Hyer CF. Safety of Achilles detachment and reattachment using a standard midline approach to insertional enthesophytes. *J Foot Ankle Surg.* 2015;54(2):214-219.

Mcbeth ZL, et al. Proximal to distal exostectomy for the treatment of insertional Achilles tendinopathy. *Foot Ankle Spec.* 2018;11(4):362-364.

McShane JM, et al. Noninsertional Achilles tendinopathy: pathology and management. *Curr Sports Med Rep.* 2007;6(5):288-292.

Meulenkamp B, et al. Protocol for treatment of Achilles tendon ruptures; a systematic review with network meta-analysis. *Syst Rev.* 2018;7(1):1-7.

Miao XD, et al. Treatment of calcified insertional Achilles tendinopathy by the posterior midline approach. *J Foot Ankle Surg.* 2016;55(3):529-534.

Molyneux P, et al. Ultrasound characteristics of the mid-portion of the Achilles tendon in runners: a systematic review protocol. *Syst Rev.* 2017;6(1):1-4.

Monto RR. Platelet rich plasma treatment for chronic Achilles tendinosis. *Foot Ankle Int.* 2012;33(5):379-385.

Moraes VY, et al. Platelet-rich therapies for musculoskeletal soft tissue injuries. *Cochrane Database Syst Rev.* 2013;2013(12):CD010071.

Morath O, et al. The effect of sclerotherapy and prolotherapy on chronic painful Achilles tendinopathy—a systematic review including meta-analysis. *Scand J Med Sci Sports.* 2018;28(1):4-15.

Murawski CD, et al. A single platelet-rich plasma injection for chronic midsubstance Achilles tendinopathy: a retrospective preliminary analysis. *Foot Ankle Spec.* 2014;7(5):372-376.

Natarajan S, Narayanan VL. Haglund deformity—surgical resection by the lateral approach. *Malays Orthop J.* 2015;9(1):1-3.

Nesse E, Finsen V. Poor results after resection for haglund's heel: analysis of 35 heels in 23 patients after 3 years. *Acta Orthopaedica.* 1994;65(1):107-109.

Ortmann FW, Mcbryde AM. Endoscopic bony and soft-tissue decompression of the retrocalcaneal space for the treatment of haglund deformity and retrocalcaneal bursitis. *Foot Ankle Int.* 2007;28(2):149-153.

Oshri Y, et al. Chronic insertional Achilles tendinopathy: surgical outcomes. *Muscles Ligaments Tendons J.* 2012;2(2):91-5.

Pearce CJ, Tan A. Non-insertional Achilles tendinopathy. *EFORT Open Rev.* 2017;1(11):383-390.

Peek AC, et al. The Achilles tendon. *Orthop Trauma.* 2016;30(1):1-7.

Pfeffer G, et al. Achilles pullout strength after open calcaneoplasty for haglund's syndrome. *Foot Ankle Int.* 2018;39(8):966-969.

Pilson H, et al. Single-row versus double-row repair of the distal Achilles tendon: a biomechanical comparison. *J Foot Ankle Surg.* 2012;51(6):762-766.

Puddu G, et al. A classification of Achilles tendon disease. *Am J Sports Med.* 1976;4(4):145-150.

Rigby RB, et al. Early weightbearing using Achilles suture bridge technique for insertional Achilles tendinosis: a review of 43 patients. *J Foot Ankle Surg.* 2013;52(5):575-579.

Rompe JD, Furia J, Maffulli N. Eccentric loading compared with shock wave treatment for chronic insertional Achilles tendinopathy. A randomized, controlled trial. *J Bone Joint Surg.* 2008;90(1):52-61.

Ruergård A, et al. Results of minimally invasive Achilles tendon scraping and plantaris tendon removal in patients with chronic midportion Achilles tendinopathy: a longer-term follow-up study. *SAGE Open Med.* 2019;7:2050312118822642.

Santamato A, et al. Power doppler ultrasound findings before and after focused extracorporeal shock wave therapy for Achilles tendinopathy: a pilot study on pain reduction and neovascularization effect. *Ultrasound Med Biol.* 2019;45:1316-1323.

Schlussel MM, et al. Platelet-rich plasma in Achilles tendon healing 2 (PATH-2) trial: statistical analysis plan for a multicentre, double-blinded, parallel-group, placebo-controlled randomised clinical trial. *Trials.* 2018;19(1):1-10.

Schon LC, et al. Flexor hallucis longus tendon transfer in treatment of Achilles tendinosis. *J Bone Joint Surg.* 2013;95(1):54-60.

Singh D. Cholesterol level in non-insertional Achilles tendinopathy. *Foot.* 2015;25(4):228-231.

Staggers J, et al. Reconstruction for chronic Achilles tendinopathy: comparison of flexor hallucis longus (FHL) transfer versus V-Y advancement. *Int Orthop.* 2018;42(4):829-834.

Stenson JF, et al. Predicting failure of nonoperative treatment for insertional Achilles tendinosis. *Foot Ankle Spec.* 2018;11(3):252-255.

Trofa DP, et al. Professional athletes' return to play and performance after operative repair of an Achilles tendon rupture. *Am J Sports Med.* 2017;45(12):2864-2871.

Vega J, et al. Endoscopic Achilles tendon augmentation with suture anchors after calcaneal exostectomy in haglund syndrome. *Foot Ankle Int.* 2018;39(5):551-559.

Wagner E, et al. Technique and results of Achilles tendon detachment and reconstruction for insertional Achilles tendinosis. *Foot Ankle Int.* 2006;27(9):677-684.

Waldecker U, et al. Epidemiologic investigation of 1394 feet: coincidence of hindfoot malalignment and Achilles tendon disorders. *Foot Ankle Surg.* 2012;18(2):119-123.

Wang C-C, et al. Ultrasound-guided minimally invasive surgery for Achilles tendon rupture: preliminary results. *Foot Ankle Int.* 2012;33(7):582-590.

Wei M, et al. Recent research from Chinese people's liberation army general hospital highlight findings in tendinopathy. *Health Med Week.* 2017:1920.

Weinstabl R, et al. Classifying calcaneal tendon injury according to MRI findings. *J Bone Joint Surg Br.* 1991;73(4):683-685.

Wilson F, et al. Exercise, orthoses and splinting for treating Achilles tendinopathy: a systematic review with meta-analysis. *Br J Sports Med.* 2018;52(24):1564-1574.

Xia Z, et al. Surgical correction of haglund's triad using a central tendon-splitting approach: a retrospective outcomes study. *J Foot Ankle Surg.* 2017;56(6):1132-1138.

Yammine K, Assi C. Efficacy of repair techniques of the Achilles tendon: a meta-analysis of human cadaveric biomechanical studies. *Foot (Edinb).* 2017;30:13-20.

Zhang Q, et al. Sonoelastography shows that Achilles tendons with insertional tendinopathy are harder than asymptomatic tendons. *Knee Surg Sports Traumatol Arthrosc.* 2017;25(6):1839-1848.

Ankle Ligament Repair

Ryan B. Rigby

ANATOMIC FEATURES

Three separate segments of ligament tissue constitute the lateral ankle ligament complex. The anterior talofibular ligament (ATFL) is the most commonly injured and a primary ankle stabilizer.[1] Most commonly, this is a bifurcate ligament consisting of two bands (Fig. 59.1) and less commonly, it contains a third band, all together constituting the ATFL.[2] Originating ~10 mm anterior and superior to the tip of the lateral malleolus the ATFL inserts upon the lateral talar body just distal to the lateral wall articular surface. The ATFL is most taut in plantar flexion and inversion and is roughly 20 mm in length.[2-8]

The calcaneofibular ligament (CFL) is commonly involved in lateral ankle injuries, but to a lesser degree than the ATFL. The CFL lies deep to the peroneal tendons and demonstrates a more cylindrical morphological appearance. Average dimensions are found to be around 3-5 mm in thickness and 4-8 mm in width. The CFL forms an angle of 10-45 degrees posterior to the axis of the fibula by originating on the anterior tip and extending to the lateral wall of the calcaneus. Because of this, the CFL is most taut with the ankle in dorsiflexion and inversion.[3-9] Isolated CFL injuries may occur but are rare.[10,11]

The posterior talofibular ligament (PTFL) is rarely injured and is under maximum tensile force during maximum dorsiflexion.[3,4,8] With an average diameter of 6.5 mm, the PTFL is considered the strongest band. The PTFL is disrupted in only 5% of lateral ankle injuries and seldom requires surgical repair.[7]

INDICATIONS

Patients often present complaining of a "weak ankle." Upon further discussion, several scenarios may be encountered. Typically, patients recall an initial ankle injury whether a fracture or sprain. Although less common, one incident may be enough to result in chronic ankle instability. Patients often describe difficulty with uneven terrain, side to side motion, and/or a lack of confidence in the ankle during sporting activities. A minimum of 6 months of conservative treatment is traditionally regarded as the time allotted for ligament healing to occur. Conservative treatment has been reported to be successful in the majority of patients.[12-17] Typically, 80%-85% of acute ankle sprains heal with conservative modalities. Acute lateral ligament repair is uncommon and typically only considered in the setting of high-level athletes, or in conjunction with other pathologies acutely requiring

surgery. acute or subacute setting. However, in the situation of an "acute on chronic" scenario, reconstruction may be elected without waiting the typical minimum of 6 months.

INDICATIONS FOR LATERAL ANKLE LIGAMENT SURGICAL REPAIR

- Chronic ankle instability and/or pain refractory to conservative treatment
- Difficulty with uneven ground or terrain
- History of significant ankle sprain or multiple sprains
- Chronic ATFL and/or CFL tear
- Chronic functional or mechanical ankle instability
- See Table 59.1 for acute ligament repair indications

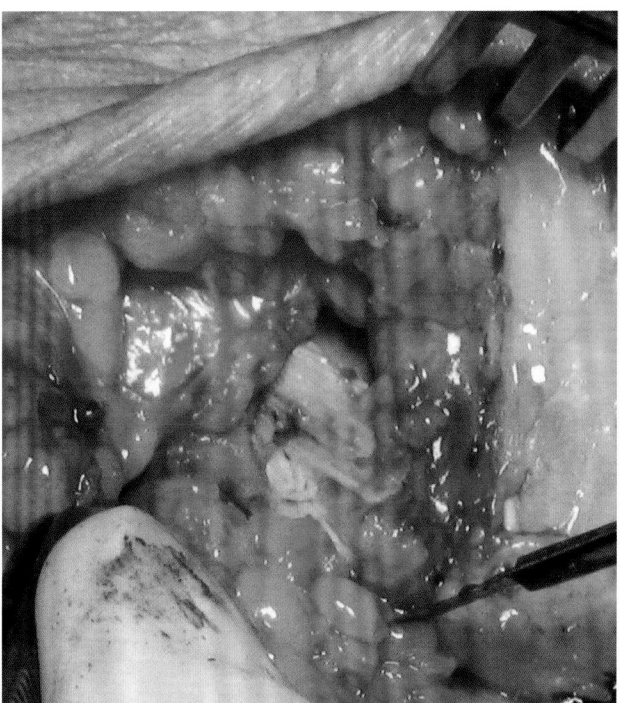

FIGURE 59.1 Intraoperative photo of the anterior talofibular ligament in bifurcate form.

TABLE 59.1	Scenarios to Consider Primary Repair of Acute Disrupted Lateral Ankle Ligaments

1. "Acute on chronic" ligament injury
2. Acute subluxed peroneal tendons requiring repair with associated ligament injury
3. Acute unstable OCD requiring surgical repair with associated ligament injury
4. Acute syndesmosis repair with associated lateral collateral ligament injury
5. High-level/high-demand athlete with grade III injury

PHYSICAL EXAMINATION/FUNCTIONAL ANALYSIS OF THE ANATOMY

Initial examination should include resting stance position. It is imperative to identify any structural frontal plane malalignment, as such findings may be the underlying etiology, and if neglected, contribute to recurrent instability. A discussion should take place with patients who present with frontal plane deformity, especially those with cavus or hindfoot varus, as these patients may require additional procedures to realign the foot.[9,18] Planus foot structure has also been found to increase the chance of ankle injury.[19] Depending upon the severity of deformity, foot orthosis or surgical reconstruction of the malalignment should be considered concomitantly with the ligament repair.

Evaluation of the lateral collateral ligaments should include direct palpation to the ATFL, and the CFL. Patients may or may not have pain with palpation to the chronically insufficient ligaments. Pain is not always a presenting complaint, nor a requirement to necessitate reconstruction.

Stress maneuvers are mandatory in order to adequately feel and assess the degree of instability.[20-22] The anterior drawer maneuver should be performed with the patient sitting with the knee relaxed in a flexed position. One hand is placed cupping. Pulling anteriorly on the heel, with resistance on the tibia posteriorly, elicits excursion of the talus from the ankle mortise. Positive findings include pain with this maneuver, a feeling of "clunking" of the talus in and out of the mortise, and excessive talus excursion anteriorly. Comparison to the contralateral limb may be helpful; however, patients often present with some degree of instability bilaterally. The "pucker" sign is seen when the ATFL is entirely insufficient and negative pressure within the ankle joint creates a vacuum, pulling the lateral skin in toward the joint where a healthy, intact ATFL would normally resist such forces. Additionally, the inversion stress test is performed with a stabilizing hand again upon the distal tibia while the other hand provides an inversion maneuver of the hindfoot. It is helpful to position the inverting hand with the fingers feeling the lateral process of the talus to determine whether the instability occurs between the tibia and talus or alternatively, inferior at the level of the subtalar joint. A positive test may result in pain, or obvious excessive inversion again with comparison to the contralateral limb.

Palpation of the peroneal tendons should occur during the examination. Frequent lateral ankle ligament injuries often result in concomitant peroneal pathology. It is possible that the pain patients often experience is entirely related to peroneal pathology.

The syndesmosis should be evaluated especially in the "acute on chronic" setting as frequent injuries to the lateral ankle may precipitate chronic attenuation of the syndesmosis. Patients may present with complaints consistent with classic lateral ankle instability; however, an underlying subtle syndesmotic instability may additionally be present. Subtle syndesmotic instability is difficult to assess clinically, while an magnetic resonance imaging (MRI) and/or arthroscopic assessment provides valuable diagnostic information in this regard.

Patients with ankle instability often develop intra-articular pathology (Figs. 59.2 and 59.3). Pain may be found with palpation to the tibiotalar joint line, especially the medial and lateral gutters. Pain in these areas support the role for arthroscopic débridement at the time of stabilization. Pain at the joint line

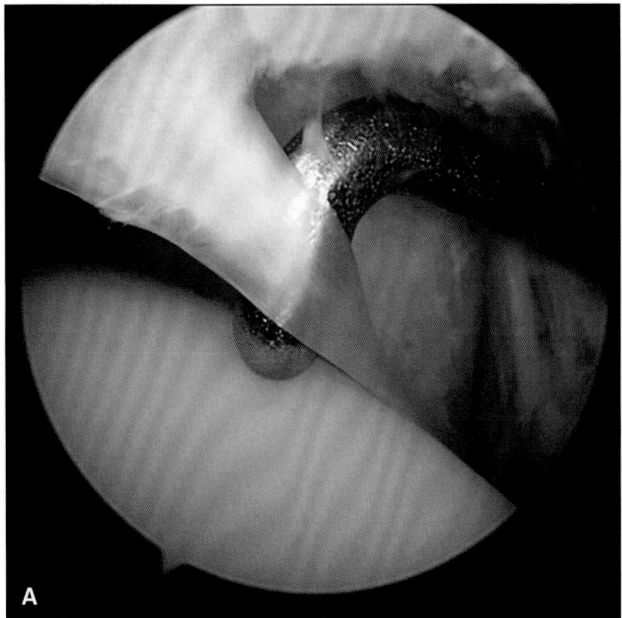

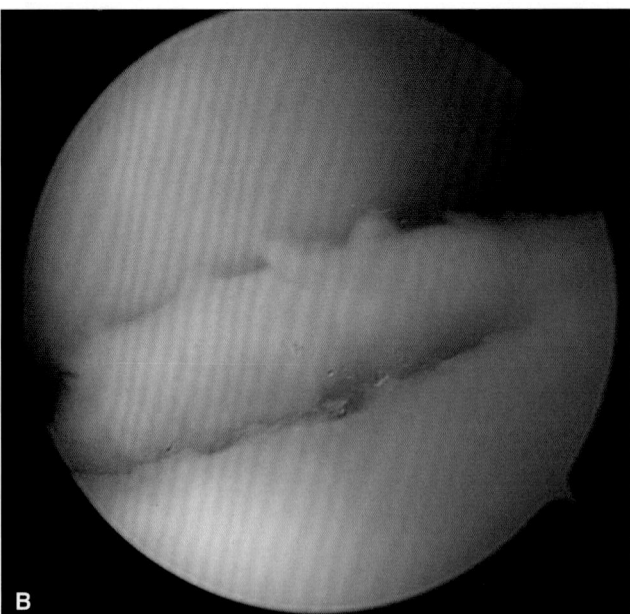

FIGURE 59.2 **A.** Intra-articular fibrous band visualized arthroscopically. **B.** Osteochondral defect of the talus visualized arthroscopically.

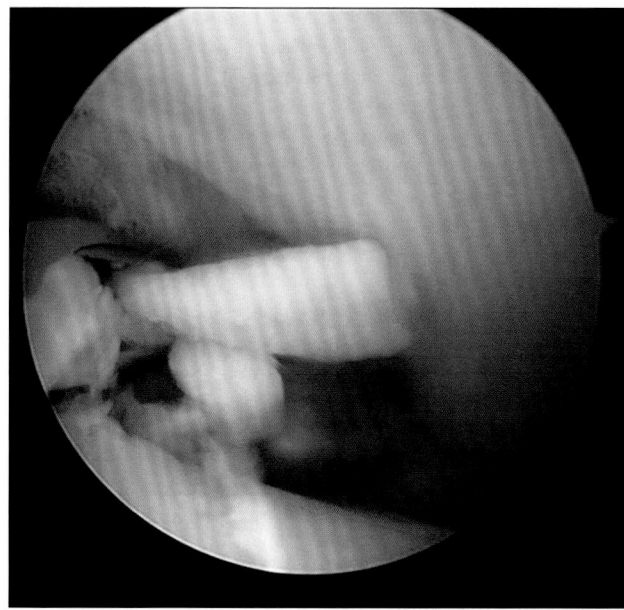

FIGURE 59.3 Intra-articular loose bodies visualized arthroscopically in a patient with chronic lateral ankle instability.

may also raise suspicion for symptomatic osteochondral lesion of the talus (OLT).

Subtle medial ankle instability is more difficult to appreciate clinically. Patients with medial instability often continue to have pain over the anterior deltoid region, and this is better assessed with MRI and arthroscopic examination.

PATHOGENESIS

Lateral ankle instability may develop following a one-time insult to the ligamentous structures. Even though pain and swelling eventually dissipates, ligament attenuation or laxity may persist. This may result in less control or stability during lateral ankle movements. Such changes may predispose further incidents, ultimately leading to chronic instability. Cavus patients with hindfoot varus deformity are more susceptible to lateral ankle injury. Ground reactive forces in these patients shift the subtalar and ankle joint into a lateral movement, decreasing the threshold for these joints to shift beyond their intrinsic anatomic position.

Patients who have sustained ankle or hindfoot fractures often have associated soft tissue injuries. As a result, despite fracture treatment, residual ligament damage may persist resulting in instability.

IMAGING

RADIOGRAPHS

Plain film radiographs are mandatory. Radiographs should include both standard three views of the ankle as well as three views of the foot and should be weight bearing. The tibiotalar joint should be carefully inspected as long-term instability may result in degenerative changes. Furthermore, periarticular structures often show signs of chronic instability such as osteophyte formation, or avulsion fragments from the tip of the medial or lateral malleolus (Fig. 59.4). Radiographs should further be assessed for frontal plane tilting, which typically results once complete insufficiency of the collateral ligaments has taken place. Once incongruent tilting occurs, degeneration of the articular surface is accelerated (Fig. 59.5A-C). Mild tilting without severe joint destruction may be amenable to ligament reconstruction with or without supramalleolar osteotomy. Advanced destruction, however, typically requires joint destructive procedures, such as ankle arthrodesis or total ankle arthroplasty.[23]

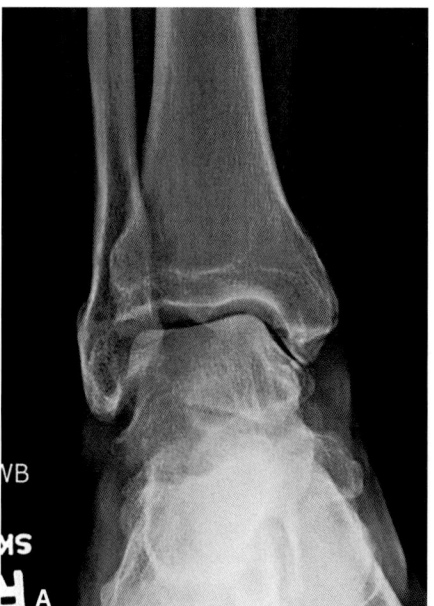
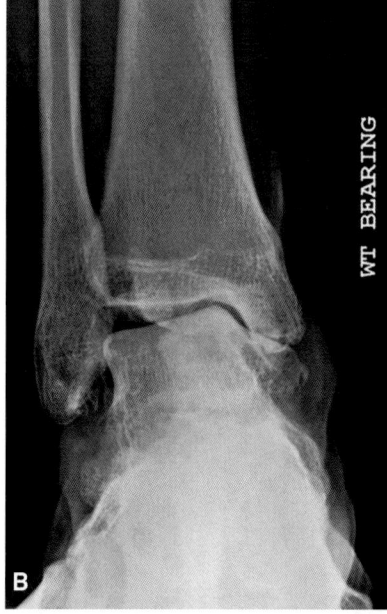
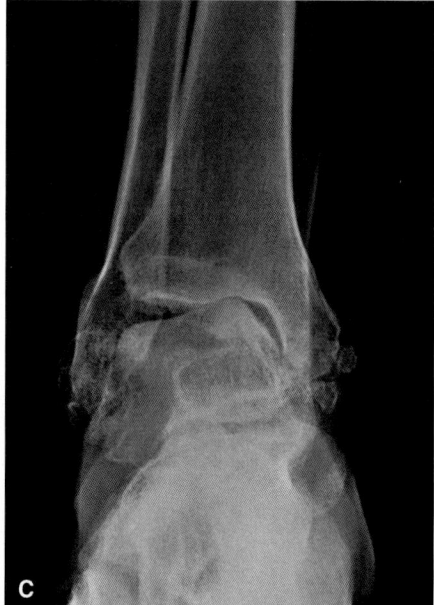

FIGURE 59.4 A. Early varus incongruent tilting secondary to chronic insufficiency of the lateral collateral ligaments. **B.** Moderate varus incongruent tilting with joint space narrowing starting to occur. **C.** Late presentation of severe varus incongruent tilting with the development of advanced joint arthrosis.

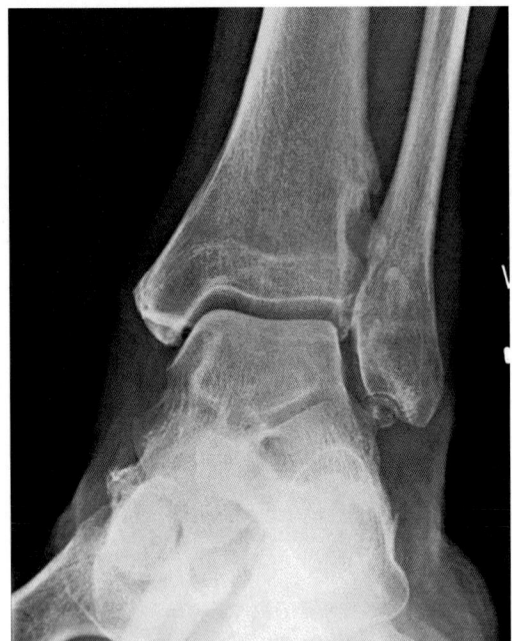

FIGURE 59.5 Chronic distal fibular avulsion fragment indicating prior lateral collateral ligament injury.

STRESS RADIOGRAPHS

The decision for surgery is based upon patient history, clinical examination, radiographs, and MRI. Stress radiographs are not always necessary to confirm instability; however, valuable information is obtained from dynamic live testing. Such information is helpful for surgical planning. For example, subtalar instability can be very difficult to diagnose based upon history, examination, standard radiographs, and MRI; however, upon live stress fluoroscopic examination, a combination of tibiotalar and subtalar or isolated subtalar instability may be discovered.

If live fluoroscopy is unavailable in the clinical setting, this can be performed in the operating room before the surgery has begun. At minimum, anterior drawer and talar tilt maneuvers are performed (Fig. 59.6A-D). It is important to assess the subtalar joint under live stress as well for tilting, along with excessive medial to lateral shifting of the joint indicating instability.

MRI

MRI, when possible, is a very valuable imaging modality.[24] As discussed, many other associated etiologies may be contributing to the patient's pain and/or instability. MRI is extremely helpful in identifying these pathologies and may suggest the need for peroneal exploration along with arthroscopy, at the time of reconstruction. The following structures should be scrutinized when viewing the MRI images preoperatively for surgical planning: ATFL, CFL, syndesmosis, peroneal tendons, medial deltoid integrity, and the articular surfaces. One should keep in mind that MRI may show the ATFL to be intact; however, chronic tearing may present on MRI as attenuation or thickening of the ATFL as longterm instability affects the integrity of these ligament fibers (Fig. 59.7A-I).[25]

CT

As ankle ligament insufficiency is typically a soft tissue pathology, CT is rarely employed. However, in cases of ankle malalignment, CT may help to determine the extent of degeneration present and assist in surgical decision making.

ULTRASOUND

Ultrasound may evaluate the ATFL, but is more helpful for peroneal tendon evaluation. Ultrasounds diagnostic ability is limited in providing information about the syndesmosis, and intra-articular pathology.

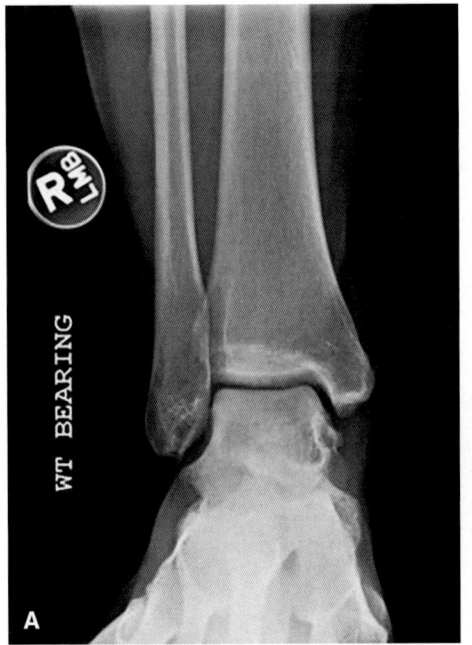
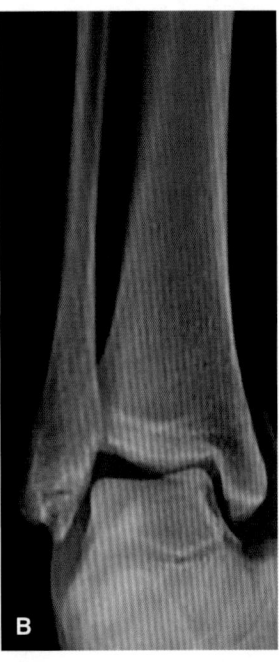

FIGURE 59.6 **A.** Nonstress weight bearing preoperative AP radiograph. **B.** Inversion stress examination demonstrating varus tilting indicating instability.

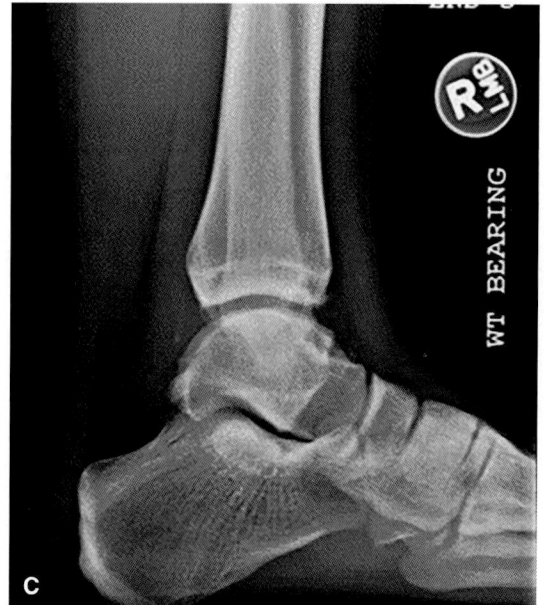
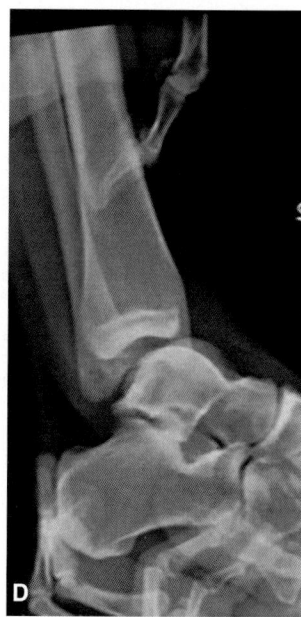

FIGURE 59.6 (*Continued*) **C.** Nonstress weight bearing preoperative lateral radiograph. **D.** Anterior drawer stress examination demonstrating instability.

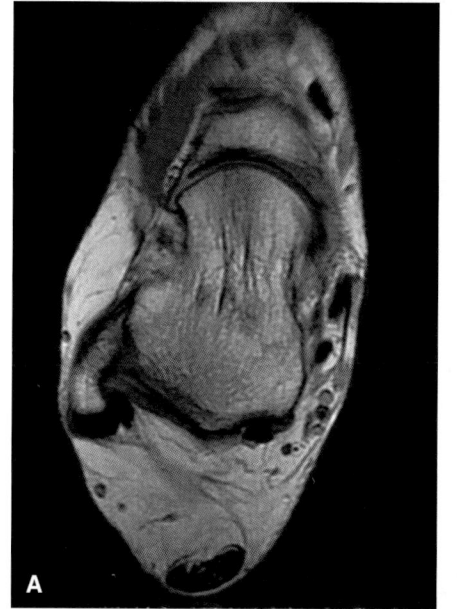
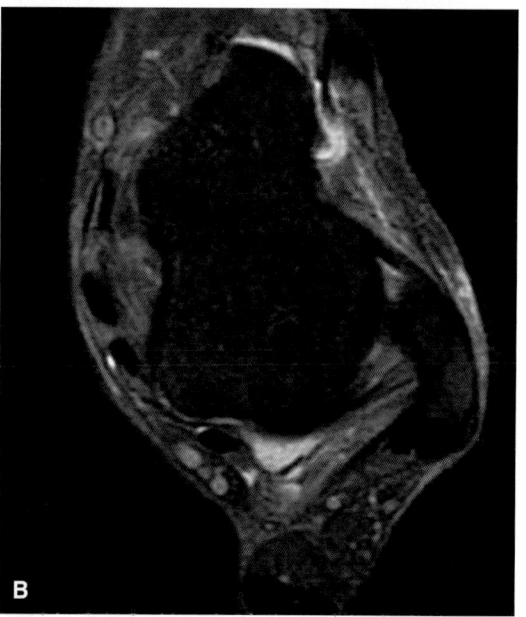
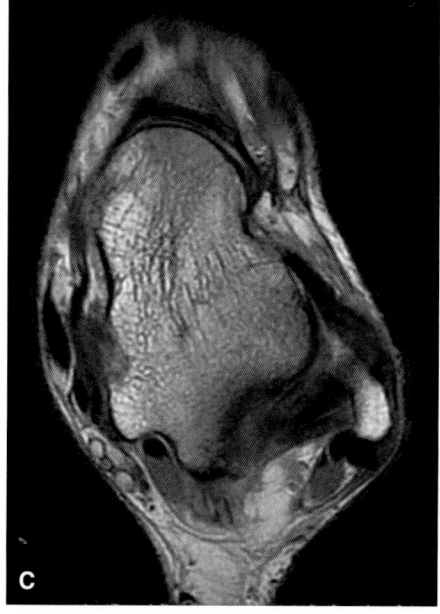
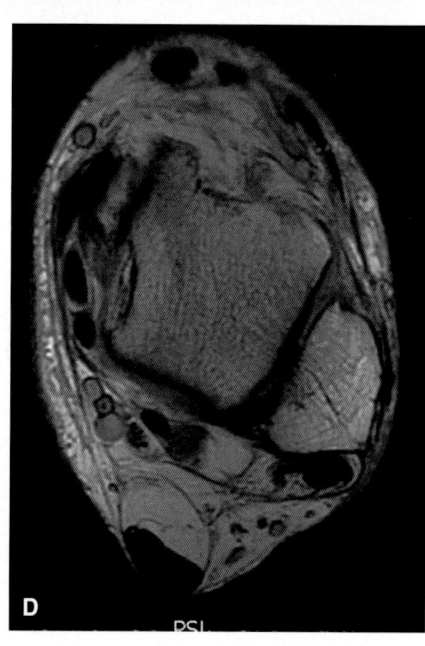

FIGURE 59.7 **A.** MRI example of a normal ATFL on T1 image. **B.** MRI example of a normal ATFL on T2 image. **C.** MRI example of abnormal ATFL with chronic thickening on T1 image. **D.** MRI example of abnormal ATFL with chronic thinning on T1 image.

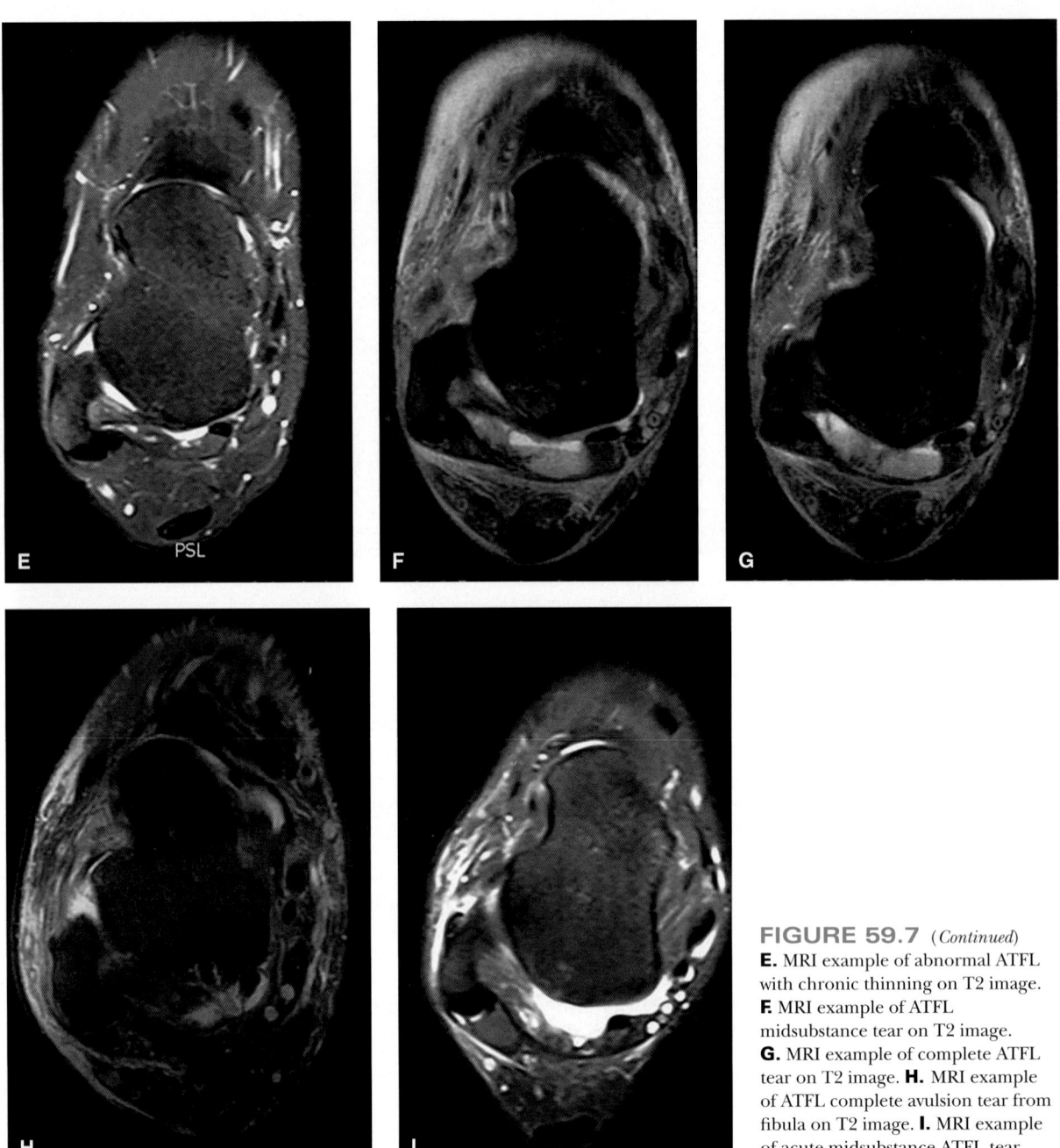

FIGURE 59.7 (*Continued*)
E. MRI example of abnormal ATFL with chronic thinning on T2 image.
F. MRI example of ATFL midsubstance tear on T2 image.
G. MRI example of complete ATFL tear on T2 image. **H.** MRI example of ATFL complete avulsion tear from fibula on T2 image. **I.** MRI example of acute midsubstance ATFL tear.

ROLE OF ARTHROSCOPY

Ankle instability often results in or presents with intra-articular pathology. For this reason, many authors advocate for the utilization of arthroscopy when performing ankle ligament repair.[26-30] Excessive motion within the tibiotalar joint often leads to hypertrophic synovitis, osteochondral defects, loose bodies, periarticular spur formation along with accelerated articular surface thinning (Fig. 59.8A and B). MRI may provide valuable diagnostic information for intra-articular pathology, but arthroscopy brings a true visual experience and allows simultaneous treatment of encountered pathology. For example, chronic ATFL or deltoid tears may be visualized and assessed arthroscopically. The decision to perform arthroscopy should be made based upon imaging, history, and clinical examination. Patients with

chronic ankle instability, who undergo only ligament stabilization without arthroscopy, may result in a sufficiently stable ankle that remains painful.

LATERAL ANKLE SURGICAL REPAIR

ACUTE

In general, acute ankle sprains heal without long term sequelae the majority of the time, with appropriate functional rehabilitation.[12-16,31] It has been reported that conservative treatment is effective 80% of the time whereas 20% of patients with acute lateral ankle injuries will develop chronic instability.[31] Acute surgical repair is typically not warranted. There are a few unique exceptions to this rule. One exception is the "acute on chronic"

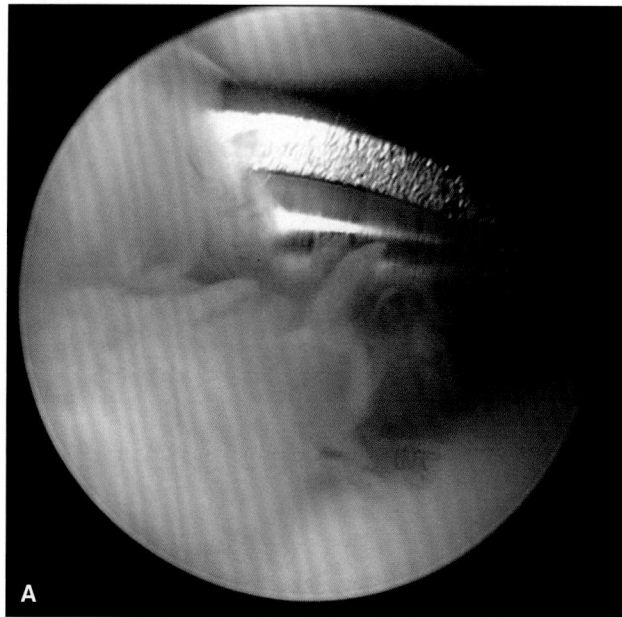 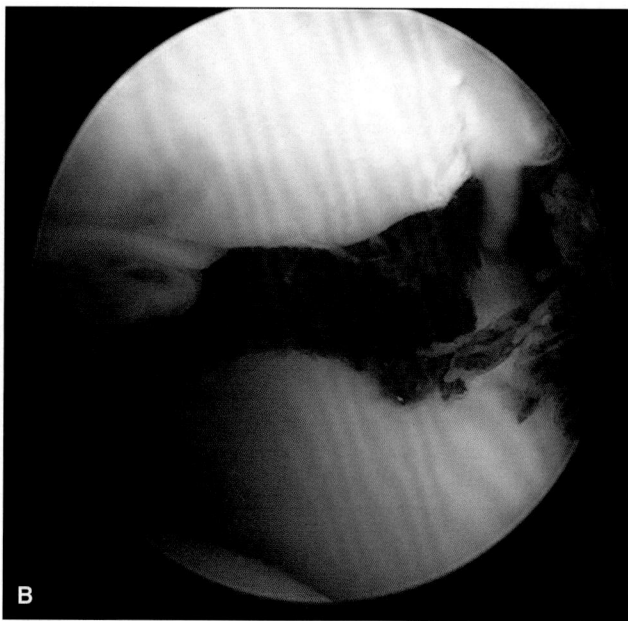

FIGURE 59.8 A. Arthroscopic shaver débridement of hypertrophic synovitis often found in association with chronic lateral ankle instability. **B.** Hypertrophic synovitis identified arthroscopically in the anterolateral ankle in a patient with chronic lateral ankle instability.

scenario. In this situation, a patient presents complaining of a recent injury to the ankle. Upon further discussion, if the patient reports this is not a "first time" ankle sprain, a discussion should ensue determining how many prior sprains have occurred and how frequently does the ankle "give out." A decision is made between the patient and surgeon whether this is occurring frequently enough to warrant surgical repair. Does instability prevent the patient from participating in the desired activities? If such discussion determines that significant chronic instability exists, a repair in the acute setting is appropriate.

Acute repair may also be considered when other concomitant injuries require surgical intervention such as acute peroneal subluxation, unstable osteochondral defects, and syndesmotic disruption. In these cases, if MRI demonstrates significant injury to the ATFL or CFL, a primary repair may be considered at time of surgical repair for these other ankle injuries. Doing so may be beneficial in protecting such structures as the syndesmosis or a repaired OLT, as undue strain may be placed upon these structures if ankle instability develops or persists.

Some debate exists regarding high-level athletes whereupon early high demand is often placed upon the ankle. Some authors advocate primary repair of acute ligament disruption for grade III injuries in high-level athletes.[32-36] For such patients, many factors are considered, such as timing of season play, future play, and specific sport and positional demands.

CHRONIC REPAIR

Arthroscopic Brostrom Technique

The patient is positioned on the operating room table in the supine position, and a general anesthesia is administered. A well-padded thigh tourniquet is placed. A noninvasive ankle joint distractor is used with a padded thigh holder. It is imperative to use a surgical marker and outline the superior border

of the peroneal tendons, the distal fibula, and the superficial peroneal nerve. This creates a safe zone in which to perform the repair (Fig. 59.9). Standard anteromedial and anterolateral ankle joint portals are created with care to avoid the anterior neurovascular and tendinous structures. Inspection of the joint is performed along with débridement as needed. Chronic disruption of the ATFL may be noted via arthroscopic visualization. Any other procedures are then completed for any associated intra-articular pathologies. Specific attention should be made to perform adequate intra-articular débridement using a shaver and/or an ablator to the anterolateral ankle joint removing any hypertrophic synovitis, which may create an impingement if not adequately débrided as the repair is tensioned. The anterior face of the distal fibula is débrided creating a raw bone surface to facilitate adhesion of the repaired ligamentous and

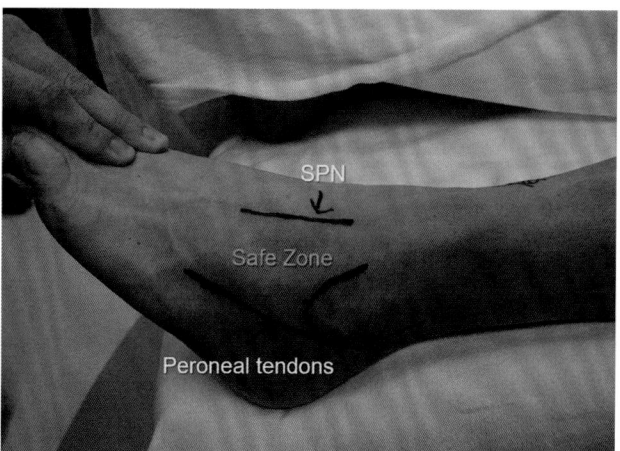

FIGURE 59.9 Preoperative outline of anatomic structures creating a "safe zone" to perform the arthroscopic Brostrom procedure.

capsular tissues. Before placing bone anchors, the borders of the medial, lateral, and distal fibula should be identified. The anterolateral portal becomes the access point to the distal anterior fibula for anchor placement. Each step is visualized with the 30-degree arthroscope inserted through the anteromedial portal. Preparation for the first of two bioabsorbable bone anchors is made by inserting the drill guide through the anterolateral portal and held into position directly midline and ~1 cm superior to the distal tip of the fibula. Avoid angling the guide inferiorly as this may shear off the distal tip of the fibula; instead, angle the guide superior into the midbody of the distal fibula. It is also imperative to direct this guide to avoid disruption of the medial and lateral cortical margins of the fibula with the drill bit. The drill is then fully seated and removed without moving the guide from its position upon the fibula facilitating anchor placement. The first anchor is inserted through the drill guide under arthroscopic visualization. This is usually a 2.4- or 3.0-mm biocomposite bone anchor. The handle and drill guide are removed, and the sutures now exit the anterolateral portal. In order to bring the sutures through the residual ATFL, ankle capsule, and inferior extensor retinaculum (IER), a sharp suture passer is used. As two anchors are typically used, the first two suture arms are now passed to the first of four locations, making sure to stay within the safe zone between the peroneal tendons and superficial peroneal nerve. The first suture arm from the inferior bone anchor is typically passed and exits the skin just superior to the peroneal tendons and is ~1.5-2 cm anterior and inferior to the distal fibula. The suture passer percutaneously pierces the skin angling toward the anterolateral portal and should course deep enough to capture the capsule and any residual ATFL along with the IER. A looped nitinol wire is then advanced through the suture passer device and captures only one strand from the bone anchor, which is then pulled down through the tissue and out the skin at location no. 1 (Fig. 59.10). A second pass is made in a similar manner to pull the second suture strand through the tissues into location no. 2.

A second bone anchor is then placed superior to the first anchor into the midline of the fibula using the same technique and ideally is positioned level with the dome of the talus with as much of a bone bridge between anchors as possible. Again, these sutures exit the lateral portal and the suture passer captures each individual strand ultimately pulled through the tissues and exits the skin for location no. 3 and no. 4. Ultimately, this creates a four-strand construct each exiting the skin with about 1 cm between each suture arm along the course of the retinaculum in the safe zone.

At this juncture, any other concomitant procedures are performed after which a small accessory portal is made between the two sets of suture (between location no. 2 and no. 3). Only the skin is incised, and an angled probe is inserted to subcutaneously gather all four sutures into this accessory incision; however, it is important that the sutures are separated back to their corresponding bone anchor. Use an instrument to clear any subcutaneous adipose tissue that could prevent the sutures from lying directly on the retinaculum. Any distraction device being utilized is then removed and the foot is held in an everted position with neutral dorsiflexion/plantar flexion. Surgical knots are then tensioned for each suture set correlating to their respective anchors within the fibula advancing the residual ATFL and IER further upon the anterior face of the distal fibula. The arthroscope may be left in the medial portal to visualize this step and observe the tissue advancement to the anterior face of the fibula, which also helps confirm and avoid any iatrogenic impingement of tissue into the lateral gutter. The arthroscope may be left in the medial portal to visualize this step and observe the tissue advancement to the anterior face of the fibula, which also helps confirm and avoid any iatrogenic impingement of tissue into the lateral gutter. The authors have not seen this occur, but still recommend visual confirmation that this area is clear of any possible impinging tissue.

If insufficient stability has been achieved, one option is to shuttle all four suture arms subcutaneously to the proximal lateral fibula making a small accessory incision and using a knotless suture anchor to secure all four sutures into the fibula. This has been demonstrated to provide increased mechanical stability.[37] Alternatively, conversion to an open procedure can also be performed.

Patients are placed into a CAM walker immobilization boot and allowed to weight bear at 3 days postoperatively. Physical therapy and transition to a stabilizing ankle brace typically is initiated between 4 and 6 weeks postoperatively. Postoperative protocols vary based upon individual patient factors and morbidities.

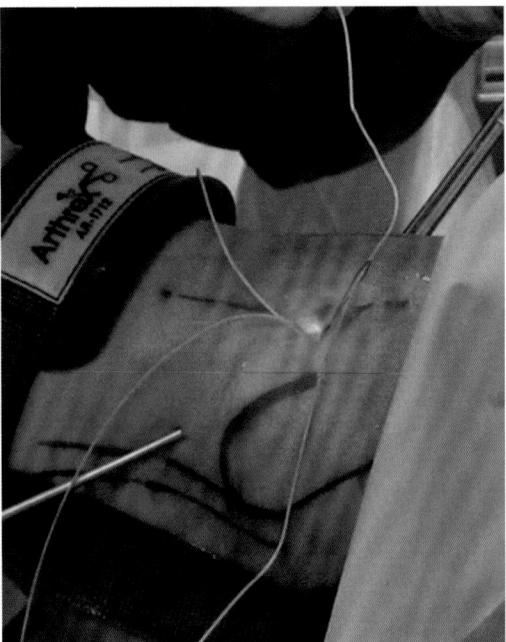

FIGURE 59.10 Suture passer at position no. 1 capturing first suture arm from the portal.

ARTHROSCOPIC BROSTROM—POSITIONING PEARLS

- Patient positioned supine
- Thigh holder elevates leg off the table with knee flexed
- Noninvasive ankle joint distractor is utilized

ARTHROSCOPIC BROSTROM—TECHNICAL PEARLS

- Outline important anatomic structures creating a "safe zone" to work within.
- Perform adequate arthroscopic lateral ankle joint débridement to prevent postoperative impingement.
- Maintain as much space between fibular anchors as possible.
- If further stability is desired after knot tie, shuttle suture arms subcutaneously to the lateral fibula and further tension with an additional anchor.

Open Brostrom procedure With Open Fibular Physis or Without Tape

On the rare occasion that instability develops in the adolescent, stabilization should be achieved without the use of bone anchors in the fibula to spare the open physis. The following technique may also be utilized for patients in whom tape augmentation will not be employed. The patient is brought to the operating room and after general anesthesia is positioned into a lateral decubitus position using a bean bag and an axillary roll and padding any bony prominences. Arthroscopy is recommended as an adjunct procedure for lateral ankle stabilization; however, in the author's experience for this age group, typically little intra-articular pathology is identified, but this should be determined on a case-by-case basis. The leg is prepped and draped, and a well-padded thigh tourniquet is utilized. A longitudinal utility incision is made overlying the distal anterior fibula. Care should be made to keep this incision within the safe zone between the superficial peroneal nerve and the peroneal tendons. Initial dissection should avoid disruption of the IER, which may be incorporated later into the repair. An arthrotomy into the lateral tibiotalar joint is performed. The arthrotomy should be carefully created from superior to inferior directly in front of the anterior face of the distal fibula. As the arthrotomy is carried inferiorly towards the distal tip of the fibula one should take care to avoid damaging the peroneal tendons, which are coursing in this area. Furthermore, the arthrotomy is typically shifted slightly distal as transection of the residual ATFL and the capsule will occur. Doing so leaves sufficient ligamentous tissue attached to the fibula for repair. Anatomic structures are assessed including the residual ATFL, IER, and distal fibula. Suture repair is then performed in a pants over vest fashion to restore tension to the ligament tissue. When doing so, it is imperative to place a bump under the distal tibia lifting the heel off the table, avoiding anterior excursion of the talus. The foot is held in an everted and dorsiflexed manner while tensioning occurs. Avoid cutting the repair sutures at this time. If possible, the sutures are then passed further posterior through a fibular flap from deep to superficial in four locations and then passed in the same fashion, from deep to superficial in four separate locations along the course of the IER fibers from lateral to medial. This creates a pants over vest repair of the periosteal flap with the IER providing inversion stability by advancing the IER further upon the distal fibula. Stability is then analyzed by performing gentle anterior drawer and inversion stress maneuvers. Forceful maneuvers should be avoided as compromise of the suture/tissue interface may occur. If satisfactory stability has been achieved, the wound is irrigated and closed in layered fashion. A dressing is applied while the tourniquet is released.

If other simultaneous procedures allow, patients are placed into a CAM walker immobilization boot and allowed to weight bear at 3 days postoperatively. Physical therapy and transition to a stabilizing ankle brace typically is initiated between 4 and 6 weeks postoperatively. Postoperative protocols vary based upon individual patient factors and morbidities.

Open Brostrom Augmentation Using Tape

The patient is brought to the operating room and following general anesthesia is positioned into a lateral decubitus position using a bean bag, an axillary roll is placed, and padding is applied to any bony prominences. The leg is prepped and draped, and a well-padded thigh tourniquet is utilized. The leg may be externally rotated and placed into a noninvasive ankle joint distractor. The standard anterior lateral and anterior medial ankle joint portals are created using a "nick and spread" technique avoiding the anterior neurovascular and tendinous structures. A thorough inspection of the joint is performed, and any intra-articular pathology is addressed. The arthroscopy instrumentation is removed, and the portals are closed. The thigh holder may be removed from under the drapes by operating room personnel, and the leg is allowed to rest in a lateral position allowing excellent exposure to the lateral aspect of the ankle. The author prefers a longitudinal utility incision overlying the distal anterior fibula extending along the course of the ATFL. This incision is ideal as it may be shifted slightly inferior, if needed, to address peroneal pathology. Care should be made to keep this incision within the safe zone between the superficial peroneal nerve and the peroneal tendons. Initial dissection should avoid disruption of the IER, which may be incorporated later into the repair. An arthrotomy into the lateral tibiotalar joint is performed, at which time evacuation of residual arthroscopic fluid typically occurs. The arthrotomy

should be carefully created from superior to inferior directly before the anterior face of the distal fibula. As the arthrotomy is carried inferiorly towards the distal tip of the fibula, one should take care to avoid damaging the peroneal tendons, which are coursing in this area. Starting within the arthrotomy, a periosteal flap is created and lifted in a posterior direction about 5 mm. There is no reason to continue this flap too far posterior as the periosteum typically thins on the most lateral fibula especially in elderly individuals and the structural ability of the flap may be compromised. The capsule and residual remnants of the ATFL are identified distal to the arthrotomy. The quality of this tissue widely varies from individual to individual. The ATFL may be chronically thickened from repetitive injuries or alternatively attenuated from long-term insulting incidents to this ligamentous structure. It is helpful to establish a plane between the capsule and the IER that is the ideal location for the tape augmentation to lie. Gentle retraction distally of the capsule and residual ligament allow exposure to the lateral wall of the talus including the insertion point of the ATFL just distal to the articular surface of the lateral talus (Fig. 59.11). This is the ideal location to place the first anchor of the tape augmentation. Various anchor sizes may be utilized, the most common of which is a 4.75-mm biocomposite anchor that has been loaded with the tape. The drill for this anchor should be angled 45 degrees back into the body of the talus, and care should be taken to avoid angling too far superior breaching the articular surface. Alternatively, placement of this anchor too inferior may result in placing the anchor into the sinus tarsi. This anchor can be easily and safely placed if care is taken to drill at the insertion point of the ATFL fibers, which furthermore allows the tape to be placed directly over top the ATFL repair, in alignment with the fibers, providing ideal biomechanical augmentation for the ATFL. It is imperative to tap for this anchor to avoid breakage of the anchor during insertion. The anchor should be secured well within the body of the talus with two arms of tape intact

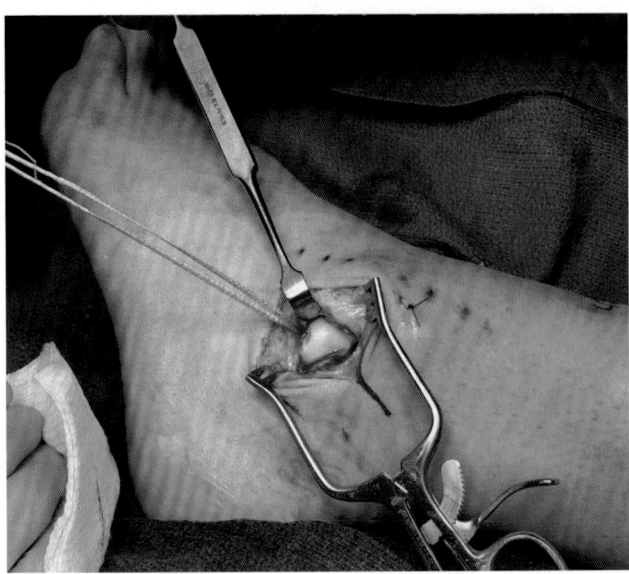

FIGURE 59.12 Intraoperative photo showing first anchor placement into the talus for tape augmentation.

(Fig. 59.12). Avoid leaving the anchor proud in this area to avoid impingement within the lateral gutter with dorsiflexion. Using a free needle, pass both arms of the tape through the ATFL/capsule lying directly over the anchor. If possible, retract the IER distally to avoid capturing this structure with the free needle. The free end of the tape is then set aside while two anchors are placed into the anterior face of the distal fibula. A variety of anchors may be used in this area depending upon fibula size and bone quality. The author prefers to use an all-suture type anchor to minimize bone loss. Using the origin of the ATFL fibers as a reference point, which will be the second anchor location for securing the tape augmentation, one suture anchor is placed above this point and one below keeping as much of a bone bridge between these areas as possible. The superior anchor is often level with the dome of the talus and the inferior anchor near the anterior tip of the fibula. Care should be taken to avoid plunging these anchors too deep, as a posterior cortical breach may cause peroneal irritation. Furthermore, these anchors should be centered within the midbody of the fibula and directed to avoid disrupting both the articular surface medially and the cortex laterally. The anchors are typically preloaded with sutures that are then passed from intra-articular out through the residual ATFL/capsule in four separate locations and hand tied to advance the ligament. When doing so, it is imperative to place a bump under the distal tibia lifting the heel off the table, avoiding anterior excursion of the talus. The foot is held in an everted and dorsiflexed manner while tensioning occurs. Avoid cutting the repair sutures at this time. The free arms of the tape are then placed over top the repaired ligament, and a second anchor secures the tape at the origin of the ATFL between the two fibular anchors in a blind tunnel fashion. The tape runs along the course of the ATFL fibers and is tensioned with the foot held in a neutral inversion/eversion position. However, the author prefers to place the tape with the foot in 30 degrees plantar flexion, as this is when the ATFL fibers should be near max tension. If the tape is tensioned securely in 30 degrees plantar flexion, as the foot is dorsiflexed to neutral the tape should lessen enough to

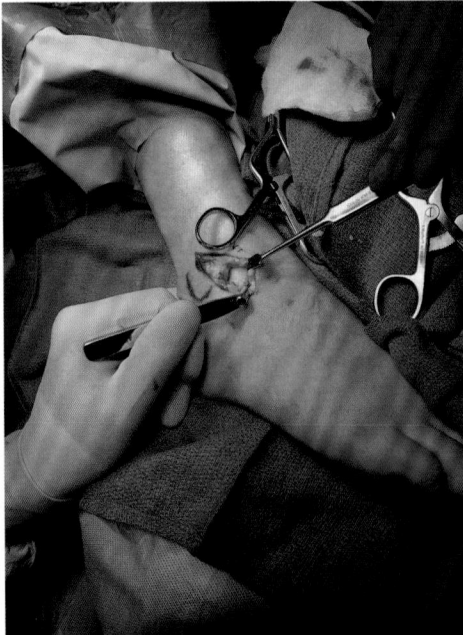

FIGURE 59.11 Intraoperative photo demonstrating location for tape augmentation first anchor placement. Soft tissue guide is angled at ~45 degrees into the body of the talus.

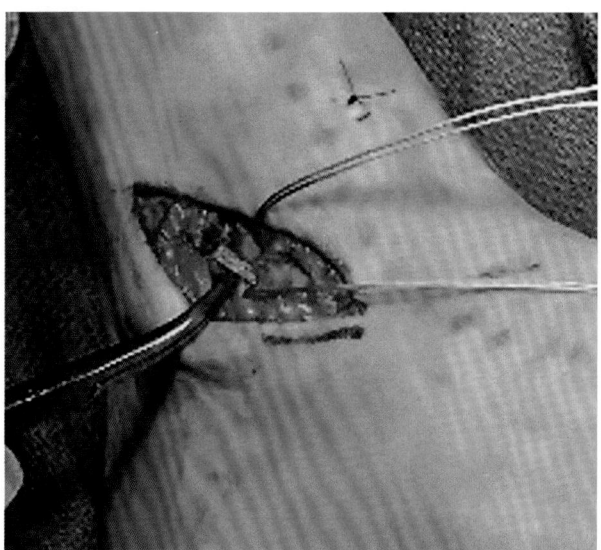

FIGURE 59.13 Tape augmentation placed over top Brostrom repair with hemostat testing tension.

OPEN BROSTROM WITH TAPE AUGMENTATION—TECHNICAL PEARLS

- Place a bump under distal tibia to avoid anterior excursion of the talus within the mortise.
- Incorporate IER in a pants over vest fashion using a periosteal flap.
- Tape anchors should be placed at fibular origin and talus insertion.
- Tape should be kept extra-articular and overtop the ATFL repair, but under the IER/periosteal pant over vest repair.

OPEN BROSTROM WITH TAPE AUGMENTATION—PERILS AND PITFALLS

- Avoid placing talus tape anchor into the sinus tarsi.
- Avoid overtensioning tape; hemostat should be able to insert under tape at neutral position.
- Angle fibula Tape anchor proximal to help avoid plunging the anchor through the posterior cortex.

slip an instrument such as a curved hemostat under the tape confirming the overtensioning has been avoided (Fig. 59.13). Range of motion of the ankle is assessed to confirm overtensioning has not occurred. The excess tape is then cut sharply flush with the bone. The bone anchor sutures are then passed further posterior through the fibular flap from deep to superficial in four locations and then passed in the same fashion, from deep to superficial in four separate locations along the course of the IER fibers from lateral to medial. This creates a pants over vest repair of the periosteal flap with the IER providing inversion stability by advancing the IER further upon the distal fibula. Stability is then analyzed by performing gentle anterior drawer and inversion stress maneuvers and compared to preoperative analysis. Forceful maneuvers should be avoided as compromise of the suture/tissue interface may occur. If satisfactory stability has been achieved the wound is irrigated and closed in layered fashion. A dressing is applied while the tourniquet is released.

If other simultaneous procedures allow, patients are placed into a CAM walker immobilization boot and allowed to weight bear at 3 days postoperatively. Physical therapy and transition to a stabilizing ankle brace typically is initiated between 3 and 4 weeks postoperatively. Postoperative protocols vary based upon individual patient factors and morbidities.

OPEN BROSTROM WITH TAPE AUGMENTATION—POSITIONING PEARLS

- Patient is positioned in lateral decubitus using a bean bag.
- Axillary roll is placed, and any bony prominences are well padded.
- Surgical limb is externally rotated with thigh holder for arthroscopy.
- Noninvasive ankle joint distractor is utilized.
- After arthroscopy is completed, the thigh holder and distractor are removed by operative room personnel and the leg is allowed to rest in a lateral position.

Allograft Repair

The patient is brought to the operating room and following general anesthesia is positioned into a lateral decubitus position using a bean bag, an axillary roll is placed, and padding is applied to any bony prominences. The leg is prepped and draped, and a well-padded thigh tourniquet is positioned. Autografts may be utilized but discouraged, because of donor site morbidities. Alternatively, an allograft is prepared. The author prefers a frozen semitendinosus allograft ~140-155 mm in length. The graft is soaked in warm saline and, once thawing has occurred, is whip-stitched on both ends and placed onto a tensioner device while the initial portion of the procedure occurs. The leg may be externally rotated and placed into noninvasive ankle joint distractor if arthroscopy is to be performed. Following arthroscopy, a curvilinear incision is made overlying the distal fibula extending within the safe zone between the superficial peroneal nerve and peroneal tendons. The insertion point for the distal ATFL fibers is cleared just distal to the talus articular surface. Using blind tunnel techniques, a guide pin is placed from lateral to medial at the insertion point of the ATFL. The graft is then sized, and the appropriate reamer is then employed to the desired depth based upon tenodesis screw lengths. One end of the graft is then secured using a tenodesis screw. The origin of the ATFL is then identified upon the anterior face of the distal fibula and a guidewire is driven from anterior to posterior within the midbody of the fibula. A retractor should be placed posterior to the fibula protecting the peroneal tendons as the guidewire exits the posterior fibular cortex. Again, a reamer is chosen based upon tendon diameter and a through and through bone tunnel is created from anterior to posterior. The guidewire is then introduced from the posterior fibula inferior to the newly created bone tunnel and angled anterior and inferior with the guidewire attempting to exit at the origin of the CFL. Again, the peroneal tendons should be protected as the guidewire and the reamer exit the fibula. Care should be taken when planning these bone tunnels to avoid sheering off the distal fibula during reaming. It is helpful to start the first bone tunnel at the ATFL origin but angle the guidewire slightly proximal creating adequate posterior fibula cortex as it exits this area. This

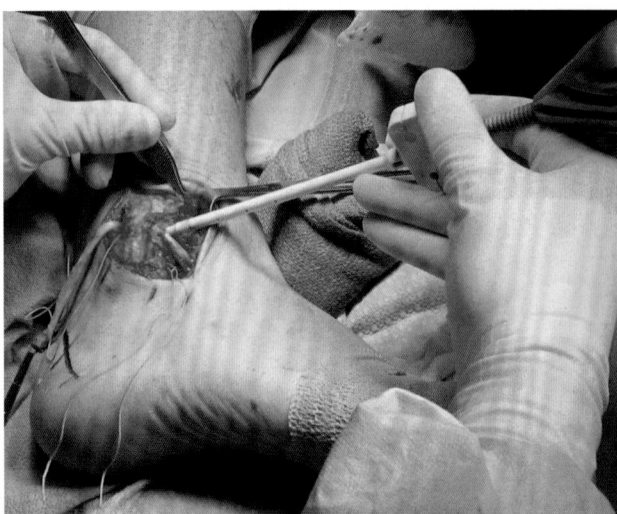

FIGURE 59.14 Semitendinosus allograft for nonanatomic lateral ankle reconstruction. Anchor is being placed into the fibula securing the ATFL portion of the graft.

ALLOGRAFT—TECHNICAL PEARLS

- Allograft should be secured using tenodesis anchors, at the origin and insertion points of the ATFL and CFL.
- Tension ATFL portion of the graft first and independently of the CFL portion.
- First reamer in fibula should be angled slightly proximal to maintain as much distal fibula as possible for second reamer pass.

ALLOGRAFT—PERILS AND PITFALLS

- Protect peroneal tendons using an instrument when reaming fibula from anterior to posterior.
- Excess graft should be resected to avoid bottom out inside medial calcaneal wall.
- Talus and calcaneus anchors secured on both ends of the graft are mandatory; a third anchor in the fibula prevents detrimental excursion of the graft within the fibula.

allows ample bone below for the second bone tunnel. The final bone tunnel is created by retracting the peroneal tendons inferiorly and placing a guidewire at the insertion of the CFL upon the calcaneus. The guidewire should be angled inferior so as to avoid violating the subtalar joint. Again, reaming occurs over the guidewire. A blind tunnel within the calcaneus may be created; alternatively, a through and through tunnel with the reamer exiting the calcaneus medially provides easier tensioning of the graft. However, care should be taken to avoid the medial neurovascular bundle if this technique is employed. Using a passer, the graft is pulled from anterior to posterior through the fibular bone tunnel. With the foot in a neutral dorsiflexion/plantar flexion and avoiding excessive eversion, the allograft is secured within the fibula using a tenodesis screw (Fig. 59.14). The graft is then passed again through the next bone tunnel from posterior exiting at the origin of the CFL, following which, the graft is then secured into the calcaneus. The author prefers the through and through tunnel for which the slotted guidewire is advanced through the plantar medial calcaneus and is used to pull the whip-stitch sutures externally on the plantar medial heel. Final tensioning then occurs with the foot in a neutral dorsiflex/plantar flexed position and very little eversion while a final tenodesis screw secures the graft within the calcaneus. The sutures exiting the medial side are pulled and cut flush with the skin. Range of motion is assessed for residual instability or overconstrainment. The wound is irrigated and closed in standard layered fashion. The tourniquet is released, and a well-padded below-the-knee splint is applied with the foot in slight eversion. The patient remains non–weight bearing for 6 weeks following which an immobilization boot is used for 4-6 weeks. An ankle brace and physical therapy begin around 8-12 weeks postoperatively.

ALLOGRAFT—POSITIONING PEARLS

- Patient is positioned in lateral decubitus using a bean bag.
- Axillary roll is placed, and any bony prominences are well padded.
- Ankle is placed on several folded towels or blankets bringing the lateral ankle towards the ceiling.

DECISION MAKING

Many procedures have been described to restore ankle stability. The Brostrom or Brostrom-Gould procedure has become a popular anatomic procedure.[21,38-44] Furthermore, the Brostrom procedure has been described to be a safe procedure for adolescent patients.[45] Controversy exists regarding whether the CFL requires direct repair. Authors have reported good outcomes without repairing the CFL.[40] As described in the techniques in this chapter, the author has not found it necessary to directly repair the CFL.

The addition of tape to augment the procedure has also been reported with favorable outcomes.[46,47] Procedure selection is multifactorial. Ultimately, for traditional lateral ankle stabilization, the open Brostrom with augmentation tape is the author's most commonly performed procedure. The arthroscopic Brostrom procedure has been described with outcomes comparable to those of other procedures[37,40,48-54] In the author's opinion, the arthroscopic Brostrom is ideal when the majority of the pathology is intra-articular and MRI reveals ATFL partial or complete disruption. For example, a patient with symptomatic OLT in which MRI reports ATFL pathology is benefitted by stabilization, as subtle instability may place undue sheer or strain upon the newly repaired OLT. These patients may not present with severe or gross instability with stress maneuvers; however, subtle instability is not conducive to cartilage healing and may decrease the success of the OLT repair. If the peroneal tendons are the primary concern, and an MRI additionally reports ATFL/CFL pathology, a minimally invasive brostrom repair may ensure critical lateral ankle stability for long term peroneal repair success. The question remains, if an open incision is already created to repair the peroneal tendons why not complete the stabilization via open incision? Arguably, this is a reasonable option; however, the dissection anteriorly to perform an open Brostrom procedure requires a larger incision and more dissection and ultimately leads to increased swelling, operative time, and pain, whereas a smaller peroneal incision in combination with an arthroscopic Brostrom repair has the potential to decrease complications.

In the setting of revision lateral ankle instability repair, using an allograft has been and continues to be a viable option.[55-57]

As anatomic repairs can be performed using a small incision and high patient satisfaction, performing a primary repair using autograft or allograft is typically viewed as unnecessary. Some authors have described percutaneous techniques for allograft repair in attempts to decrease incision size and the potential for complications.[58] Allograft often requires 4-6 weeks of crutches, results in increased swelling and stiffness, and requires a larger incision. The incorporation of tape augmentation to an anatomic repair, in the author's experience, has decreased the incidence of allograft reconstruction. Patients who have undergone traditional open Brostrom stabilization without tape augmentation may choose to undergo revision Brostrom with tape augmentation prior to allograft repair. Ultimately, a conversation should take place between surgeon and patient in choosing which procedure is ideal, on a case-by-case basis.

MEDIAL ANKLE LIGAMENTS

ANATOMIC FEATURES

The medial ligament complex is most commonly described as a multilayer, multiband structure. The deltoid links the ankle, subtalar, and talonavicular joints by spanning the medial malleolus, talus, calcaneus, and navicular bones. Typically, the medial ligament complex is broken down into two main segments, the superficial and deep ligaments. Each of these are composed of separate bands. The superficial component resists eversional forces of both the ankle and subtalar joints, whereas the deep portion resists external rotation along with lateral translation of the talus.[59-61] The superficial deltoid is composed of the tibionavicular, the tibiospring, the tibiocalcaneal, and the superficial posterior tibiotalar bands. The deep layer consists of the anterior tibiotalar and posterior tibiotalar bands with the posterior being the larger of the two.

SURGICAL REPAIR

ACUTE

Indications, Imaging, and Decision Making

Isolated deltoid injuries requiring primary surgical repair are infrequent, but do occur under certain circumstances, most commonly in high-level athletes. In the setting of an acute injury to the medial ankle ligaments, the decision on whether to treat conservatively or surgically is typically based upon three questions (Table 59.2). First, is the deltoid tear a partial or complete rupture, as declared via advanced imaging? Second, has the injury created gross instability of the medial ankle? This is usually assessed via weight-bearing radiographs, gravity or manual static stress radiographs, and live fluoroscopic assessment. And thirdly, is the patient a high-level athlete for whom primary repair may assist in quicker return to sports or decrease the likelihood of long-term sequelae? A partial deltoid tear most often can be treated conservatively, as the ankle typically remains stable. If a complete tear has been identified via MRI, the patient is brought under live fluoroscopy or analyzed under static stress radiographs. If gross instability has developed, and the patient is active or athletic, a primary repair should be discussed and considered. Debate

TABLE 59.2	Decision Making for the Treatment of Acute Deltoid Injury Is Based Upon Three Questions
	1. Is the deltoid tear a partial or complete rupture? (determined via advanced imaging)
	2. Has the injury created gross instability of the medial ankle?
	3. Is the patient a high-level athlete?

remains as to whether an acute deltoid, occurring in association with ankle fracture, should be primarily repaired as discussed in the "Ankle Fracture" chapter.

Arthroscopic Deltoid Repair Technique

The patient is brought to the operating room and following general anesthesia is positioned supine. The leg is prepped and draped, and a well-padded thigh tourniquet is positioned. The ankle is placed into a noninvasive joint distractor. The standard anterior lateral and anterior medial ankle joint portals are created using a "nick and spread" technique avoiding the anterior neurovascular and tendinous structures. A thorough inspection of the joint is performed, and any intra-articular pathology is addressed. The deltoid is assessed arthroscopically for disruption along with instability. The distractor is removed, and the ankle is then stressed under fluoroscopic stress examination. A decision is made to perform surgical stabilization based upon preoperative imaging, along with intraoperative arthroscopic and fluoroscopic findings. Although some variation may occur, most commonly, the deltoid has avulsed off the tip of the medial malleolus. Primary repair is performed by placing one or two bone anchors arthroscopically (Fig. 59.15). The sutures then exit the anteromedial portal (Fig. 59.16). A suture passer is used to percutaneously pass both suture arms separately capturing the deltoid complex and exiting the skin below the

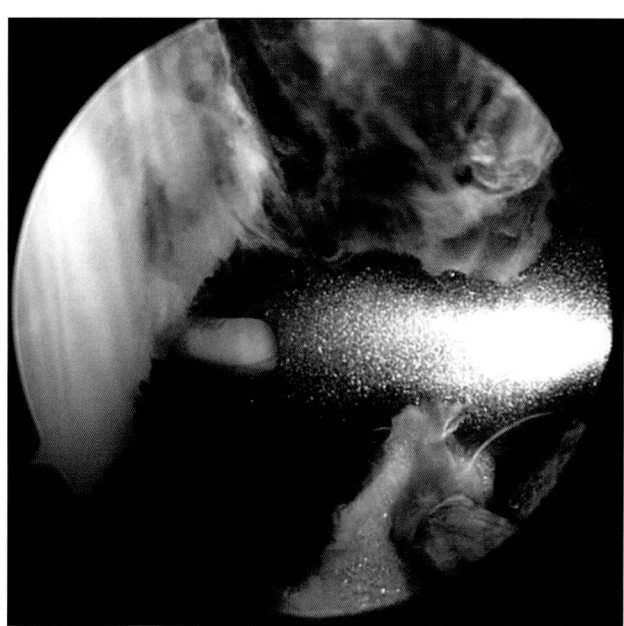

FIGURE 59.15 Arthroscopic photo demonstrating bone anchor placement within the medial malleolus for acute primary deltoid repair.

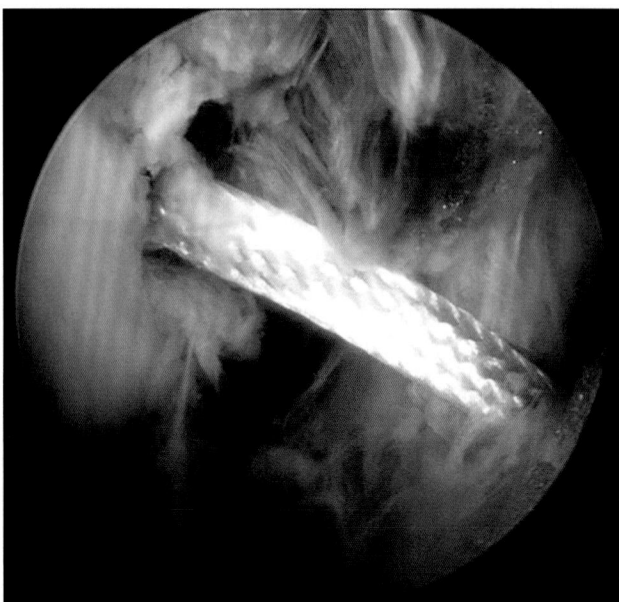

FIGURE 59.16 Arthroscopic photo of suture used for arthroscopic repair of acute deltoid tear.

closed in standard fashion. The tourniquet is released, and a well-padded below-the-knee splint is applied with the foot in slight inversion. The patient remains non–weight bearing for 6 weeks following which an immobilization boot is used for 4-6 weeks. An ankle brace and physical therapy begin around 8-12 weeks postoperatively.

ARTHROSCOPIC DELTOID REPAIR— POSITIONING PEARLS

- Patient is positioned supine.
- Thigh holder elevates leg off the table with knee flexed.
- Noninvasive ankle joint distractor is utilized.

ARTHROSCOPIC DELTOID REPAIR— TECHNICAL PEARLS

- Shifting anteromedial portal slightly inferior and medial assists with anchor placement.
- Perform adequate arthroscopic débridement of the medial gutter.
- Visualize via arthroscopy the suture passer capturing ligament tissue.
- Remove any distraction device prior to tensioning repair.

ARTHROSCOPIC DELTOID REPAIR— PERILS AND PITFALLS

- Significant deltoid instability should be repaired via open approach.
- Avoid passing sutures through posterior tibial tendon.

medial malleolus (Fig. 59.17A-C). A second anchor may be placed in the same fashion if desired. A small accessory incision is created between the suture arms to confirm that the sutures have not captured the posterior tibial tendon. The foot is held in an inverted position and the sutures are tensioned restoring stability to the deltoid complex (Fig. 59.18). Fluoroscopic stress examinations are repeated confirming that adequate stability has been restored to the medial ankle. If recurrent stability persists, an open repair should then be performed. Once stability has been achieved, the incisions are irrigated and

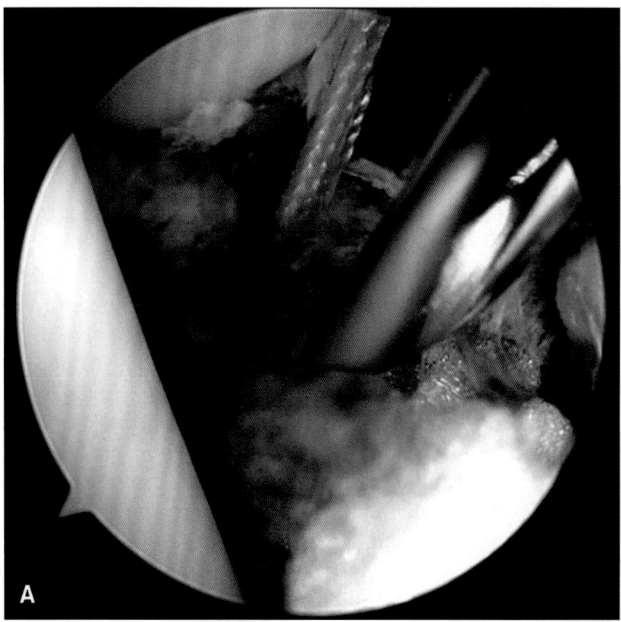
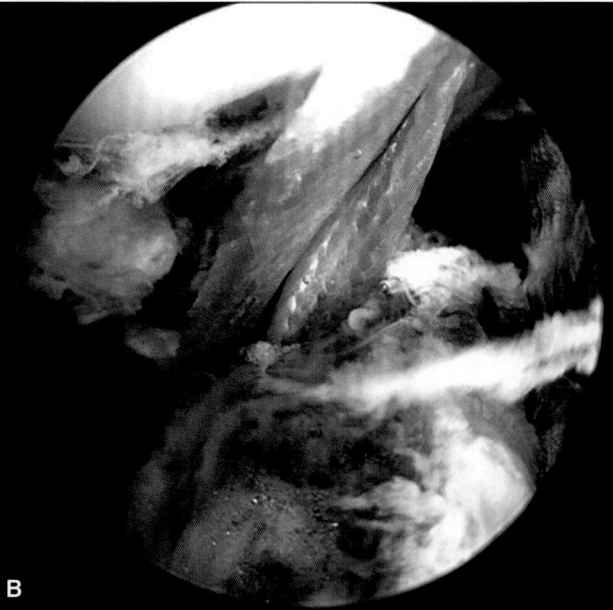

FIGURE 59.17 **A.** Arthroscopic visualization showing suture passer capturing deltoid for repair. **B.** Sutures secured into the torn deltoid before repair is tensioned and completed.

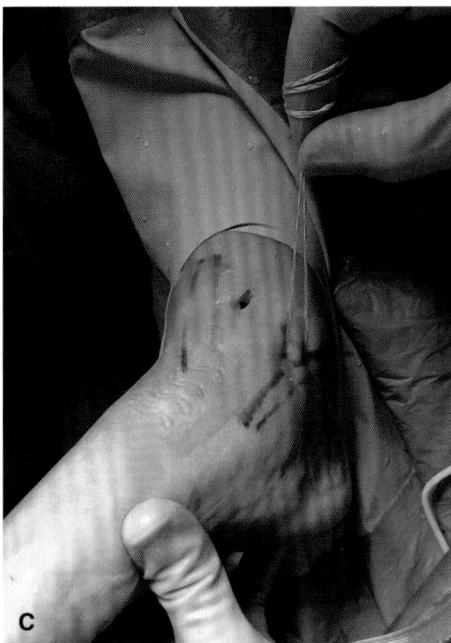

FIGURE 59.17 (*Continued*) **C.** Arthroscopic deltoid repair suture placement.

CHRONIC

Indications, Imaging, and Decision Making

In the chronic setting, deltoid insufficiency is most often divided into two groups. The first is referred to as "subtle" while the other is identified as "obvious" deltoid insufficiency. Subtle deltoid insufficiency may present with normal radiographic findings. The medial clear space and ankle mortise appear within normal limits on static routine radiographs. However,

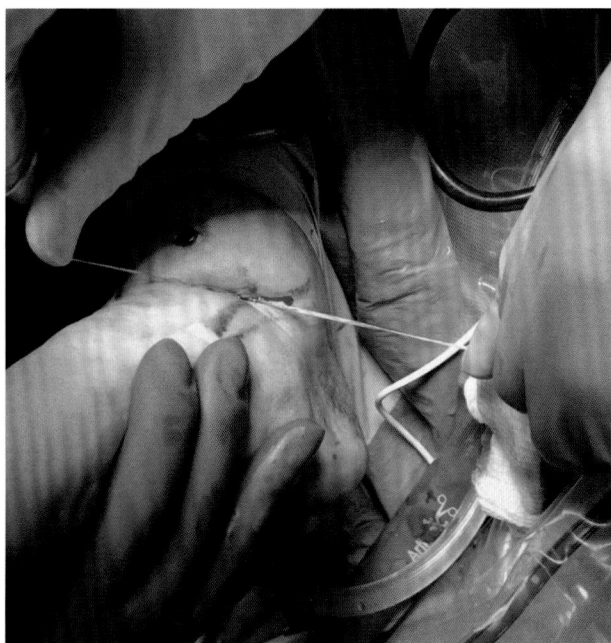

FIGURE 59.18 Hand tie completion of arthroscopic deltoid repair with foot held in slight inversion.

when incongruent valgus tilting of the tibiotalar joint is visualized radiographically, obvious disruption of the medial deltoid complex has taken place and can be deemed insufficient. An exception to this rule is posttraumatic erosion of the lateral tibiotalar joint creating valgus incongruence in the setting of a preserved deltoid complex. If the underlying etiology is truly deltoid insufficiency and valgus incongruence of the joint has occurred, the decision on joint sparing vs joint destruction procedures is based upon the extent of the articular surface erosion. This is determined using radiographs, MRI, and/or CT scans along with arthroscopic assessment. In the setting of significant joint degeneration, restoring congruency via deltoid reconstruction may be less successful, and joint destructive procedures should be considered. However, in the context of total ankle replacement, a deltoid reconstruction is often necessary to provide sufficient soft tissue balancing. If caught early, valgus incongruence may be corrected via deltoid reconstruction. One should keep in mind the importance of foot position and realize how influential foot deformity may be upon the success or failure of deltoid reconstruction. For example, in stage 4 posterior tibial tendon dysfunction, whereupon ankle valgus has developed in association with planovalgus foot structure, an isolated deltoid reconstruction alone will fail. It is imperative that a well balanced, plantar grade foot has been achieved in order for deltoid reconstruction to be successful long term.

Subtle Chronic Medial Instability Diagnosis and Repair

Patient history provides the first clue to this condition as they often describe a feeling of "giving way."[60,61] Subtle chronic medial instability is often found in association with chronic lateral ankle instability. Stress radiographs for lateral ankle instability may be of some assistance as severe anterior drawer excursion is not possible without some degree of concomitant medial instability. With live stress fluoroscopy, it is not always possible to identify subtle medial instability. Arthroscopy, however, provides very helpful diagnostic information. Arthroscopic evaluation of the medial ankle gutter may reveal chronic avulsion of the deltoid from the medial malleolus. Another means of analyzing the deltoid arthroscopically is the so-called drive through sign. A 4.0-mm shaver or instrument is inserted through the medial portal and should not be able to enter the medial gutter. If the instrument can easily pass between the medial talus and the medial malleolus, instability likely is present. A portion of patients complaining of "ankle instability" have both lateral and medial instability, and a repair of both collateral ligaments may be necessary to achieve satisfactory stability.[60,61]

If subtle medial instability has been identified, an incision is made overlying the medial malleolus. Care is taken to center this and avoid disrupting the posterior tibial tendon and the saphenous nerve and vein. It is difficult and not necessary to directly repair the deep deltoid when only subtle instability is present. For this reason, focus is made to the superficial deltoid. The posterior tibial tendon is retracted inferiorly, and a cuff of tissue is created from off the anterior and distal portion of the medial malleolus. The tip of the medial malleolus is roughened using a rasp or curette to facilitate soft tissue adhesion. Two bone anchors are placed into the medial malleolus usually into the anterior and posterior colliculus. If enough tissue is present, a periosteal flap of tissue can be created from inferior to superior to assist in the repair. The superficial deltoid is advanced further upon the medial malleolus.

After suture knots are secured, instead of cutting the suture arms pass them superior through the periosteal flap before tying. Arthroscopy can be repeated with stress testing to confirm that stability has been restored to the medial ankle. Lateral ankle instability procedures may then be performed if needed. Closure is completed and the patient is kept non–weight bearing for 4 weeks, followed by 4 weeks in a CAM walker boot. At 6-8 weeks, physical therapy begins and the patient is transitioned into an ankle brace and shoe gear. Side to side activity is limited until 12 weeks postoperative.

Obvious Deltoid Instability Repair

The patient is brought to the operating room and following general anesthesia is positioned into a supine position. The leg is prepped and draped, and a well-padded thigh tourniquet is positioned and inflated. The author prefers a frozen semitendinosus allograft ~155 mm in length (Fig. 59.19). The graft is soaked in warm saline and, once thawing has occurred, is whip-stitched on both ends and placed onto a tensioner device while the initial portion of the procedure occurs. An incision is made on the medial ankle starting along the posterior border of the tibia above the ankle joint and extending over the medial malleolus distally. The posterior tibial tendon sheath is opened, and the tendon is retracted inferiorly (Fig. 59.20). Remnants of deltoid tissue are of poor tissue quality and may be resected or retracted inferiorly as a cuff of tissue off the distal tip of the medial malleolus. A guidewire is placed at the insertion of the deep deltoid fibers on the medial talus wall (Fig. 59.21). The tendon is sized and the appropriate reamer is used, and one end of the graft is inserted using a "blind tunnel" method. A spade-tip guidewire is placed at the inferior pole of the medial

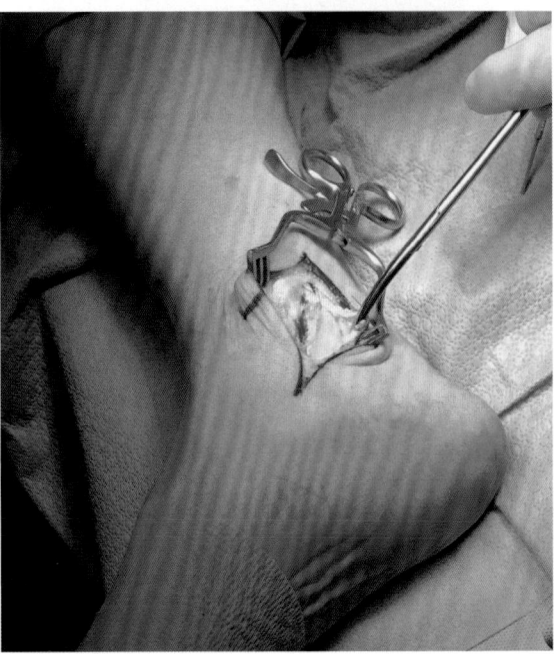

FIGURE 59.20 Incision placement for chronic deltoid reconstruction. Posterior tibial tendon sheath has been incised to allow inferior retraction.

malleolus within the intercollicular groove (Fig. 59.22A and B). This guidewire is advanced toward the anterior lateral distal tibia (Fig. 59.23). It is vital that a small anterolateral incision be made before the spade tip exits the cortex in order to retract the soft tissues in this area, especially the neurovascular bundle as this instrument is very aggressive and may cause injury (Fig. 59.24). A 6.0-mm reamer is then advanced started at the medial malleolus about 40 mm into the distal tibia (Fig. 59.25). The spade-tip guidewire is used as a knotless ACL button is looped around the graft (Fig. 59.26). The button is pulled out the anterolateral tibial cortex and the loop brings the midportion of the graft into the distal tibia at least 15 mm; however, care is taken to avoid pulling the graft into the full 40 mm of reamed tunnel

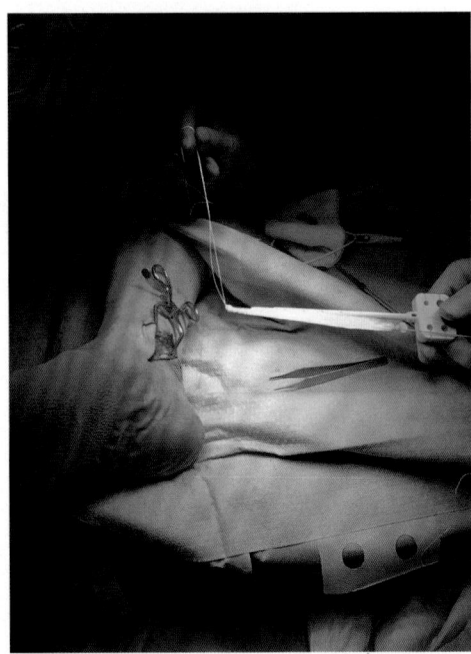

FIGURE 59.19 Semitendinosus allograft with whipstitch ends ready for insertion into medial wall of talus using a blind tunnel technique.

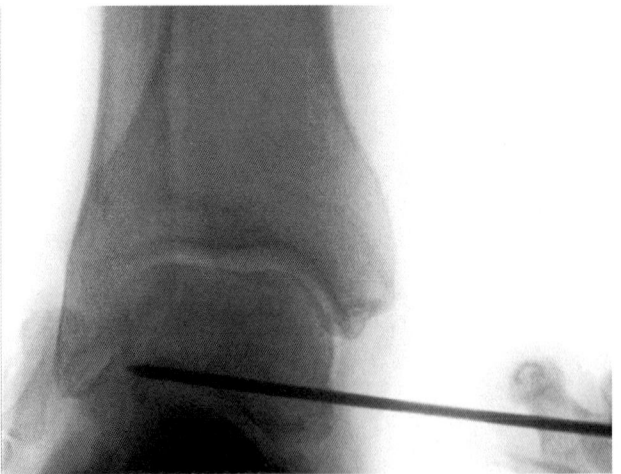

FIGURE 59.21 Intraoperative fluoroscopy AP view showing guidewire placement for reaming and allograft implantation.

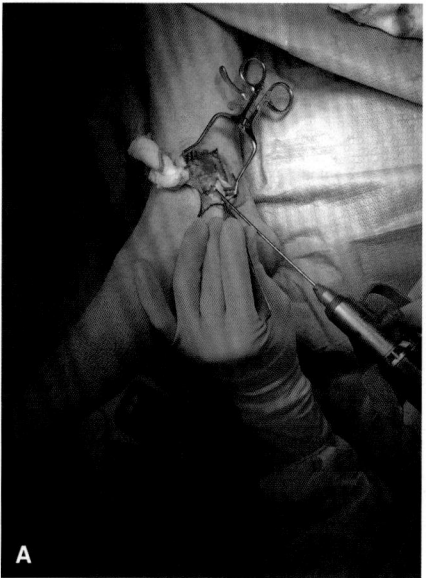

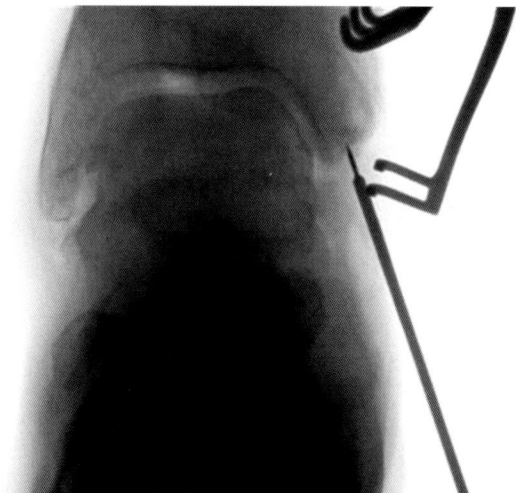

FIGURE 59.22 A. Intraoperative photo showing guidewire starting point and angle. **B.** Intraoperative fluoroscopy AP view showing guidewire starting point and angle. Note how the guidewire is carefully centered within the medial malleolus.

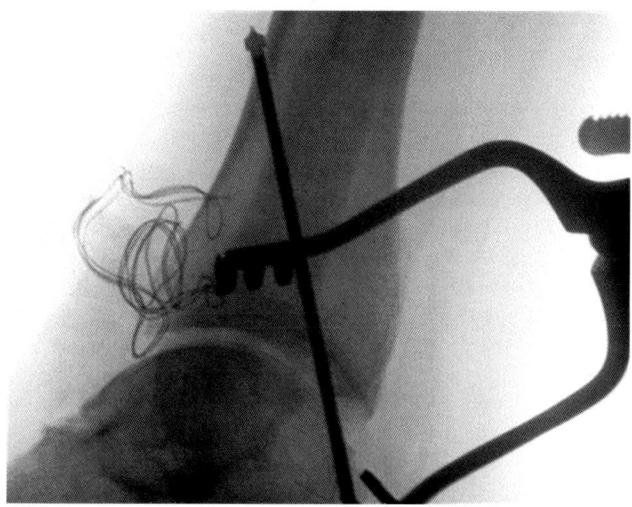

FIGURE 59.23 Intraoperative fluoroscopy lateral view demonstrating placement of guidewire before reaming.

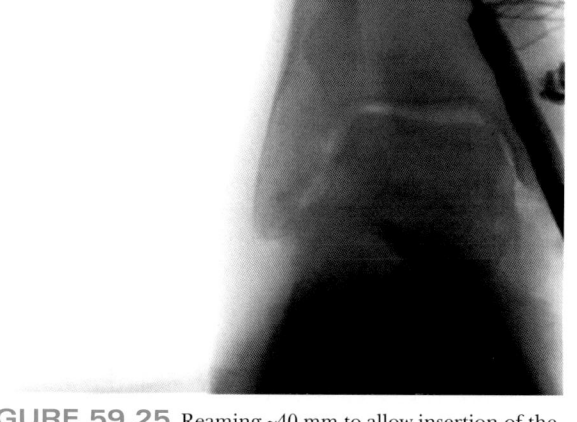

FIGURE 59.25 Reaming ~40 mm to allow insertion of the allograft within the distal tibia.

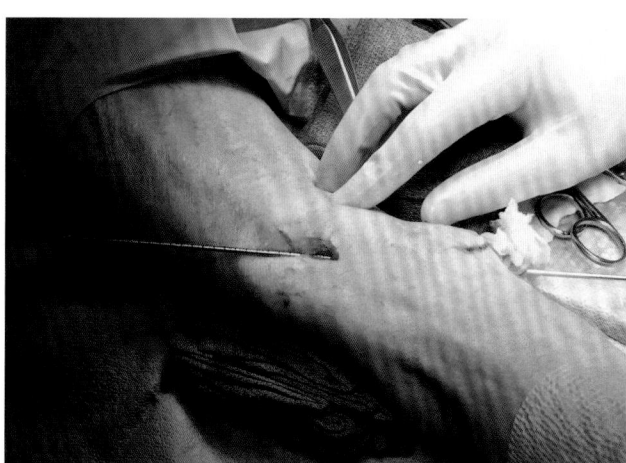

FIGURE 59.24 Small accessory incision is created to gently retract and protect the neurovascular bundle before the guidewire exits the anterolateral tibial cortex.

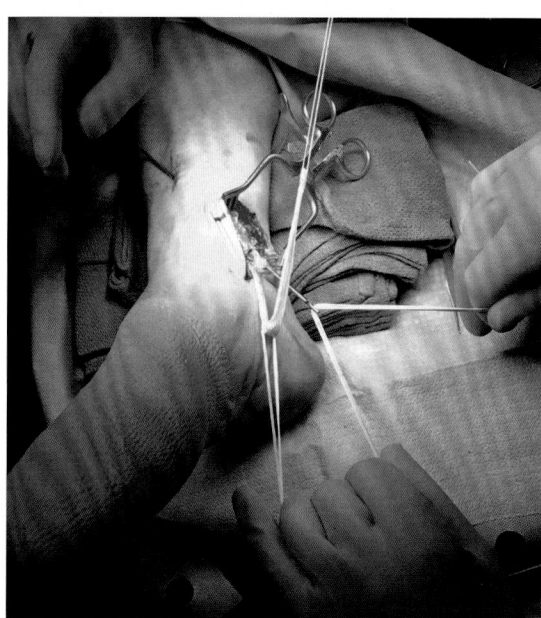

FIGURE 59.26 The looped button captures the graft in the middle and pulls the midportion of the graft into the distal tibia.

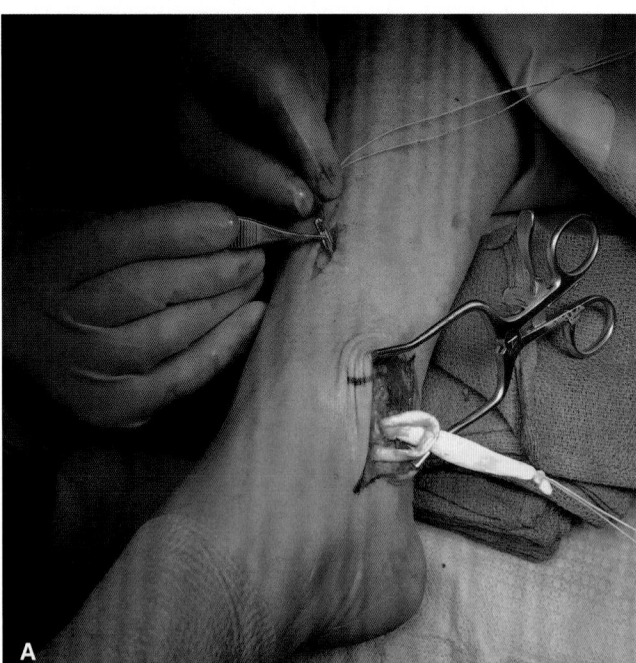

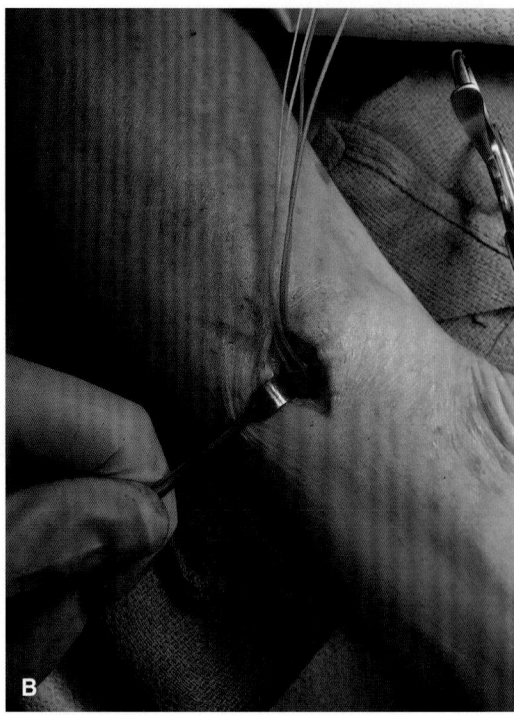

FIGURE 59.27 **A.** Suture button passed through the distal tibia and into the accessory incision. The allograft is then pulled into the distal tibia. **B.** Button placement along the anterior cortex of the tibia.

(Fig. 59.27A and B). At this juncture, one arm of the graft is secured into the talus, and the midportion of the graft is within the medial malleolus. A guidewire is then placed into the sustentaculum tali and angled slightly inferior to avoid breaching the subtalar joint (Fig. 59.28A and B). Again using the appropriate reamer for the graft, a through and through tunnel is made exit-

ing the lateral cortex. The length of the graft is then measured preserving at minimum 15-20 mm to enter the calcaneus, and the excess graft is sharply removed. Using a suture passer that exits from the lateral heel the graft is pulled into the body of the calcaneus. The ankle is held in a neutral dorsiflexion/plantar flexion position; however, inversion may be necessary to correct

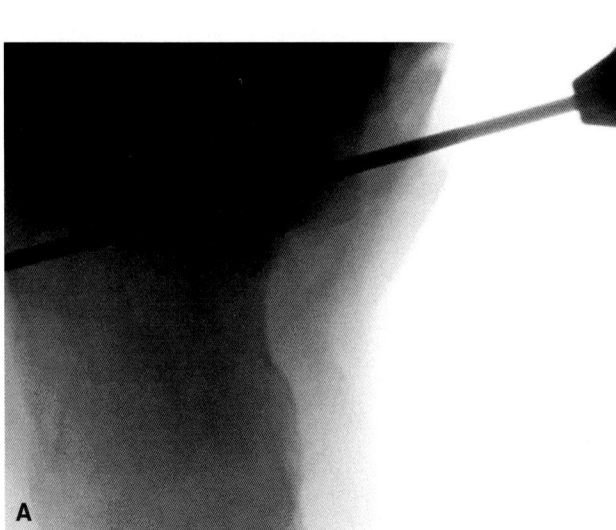

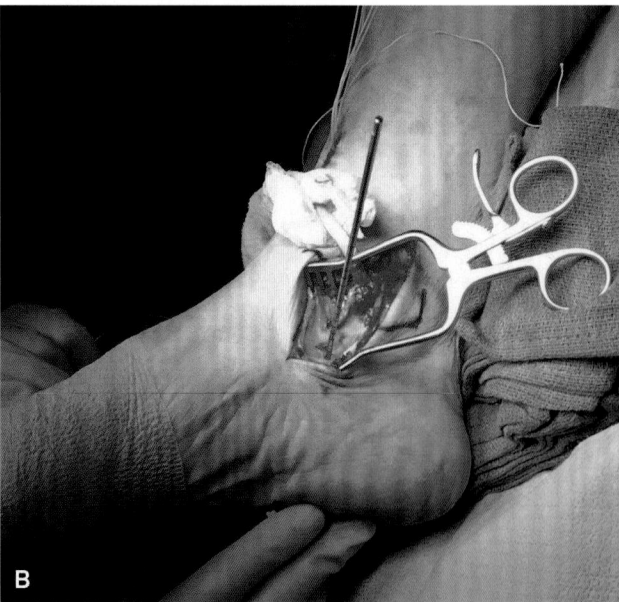

FIGURE 59.28 **A.** Intraoperative fluoroscopy calcaneal axial view showing guidewire placement into the sustentaculum tali. **B.** Intraoperative photograph showing guidewire placement into the sustentaculum tali.

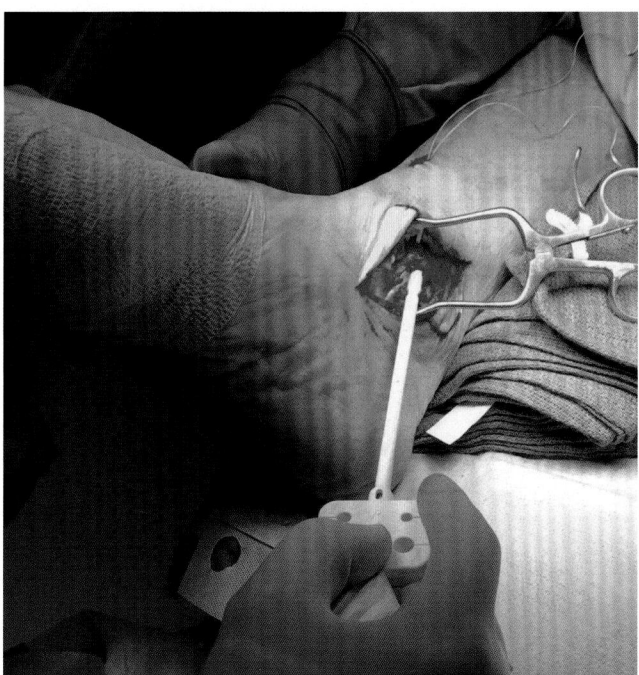

FIGURE 59.29 Final anchor placed into the medial malleolus securing the overall tension of both arms of the graft.

the valgus position. Fluoroscopy is helpful in avoiding overtensioning or creating a varus ankle. After tensioning the graft, a tenodesis screw is inserted into the calcaneus securing this arm of the graft. Stability is then assessed via stress maneuvers and range of motion observed under fluoroscopy. The button may then provide further tension if desired, further pulling the graft into the distal tibia. Once final tensioning has occurred, a third tenodesis screw is inserted into the medial malleolus securing the midbody of the graft into position (Fig. 59.29). The graft has now reconstructed the deep and superficial deltoid complex. Intraoperative stress fluoroscopic images confirm joint congruity and stability. The cuff of tissue created initially may be used over the graft and sutured to a periosteal flap off the medial malleolus, or smaller anchors may be placed to repair this tissue. However, this should only take place with caution as additional anchors in the medial malleolus increase the chance of stress riser and this tissue is often of poor quality. The wound is irrigated and closed in standard layered fashion. The tourniquet is released, and a well-padded below-the-knee splint is applied with the foot in slight inversion. The patient remains non–weight bearing for 6 weeks following which an immobilization boot is used for 4-6 weeks. An ankle brace and physical therapy begin around 8-12 weeks postoperatively (Fig. 59.30A-D).

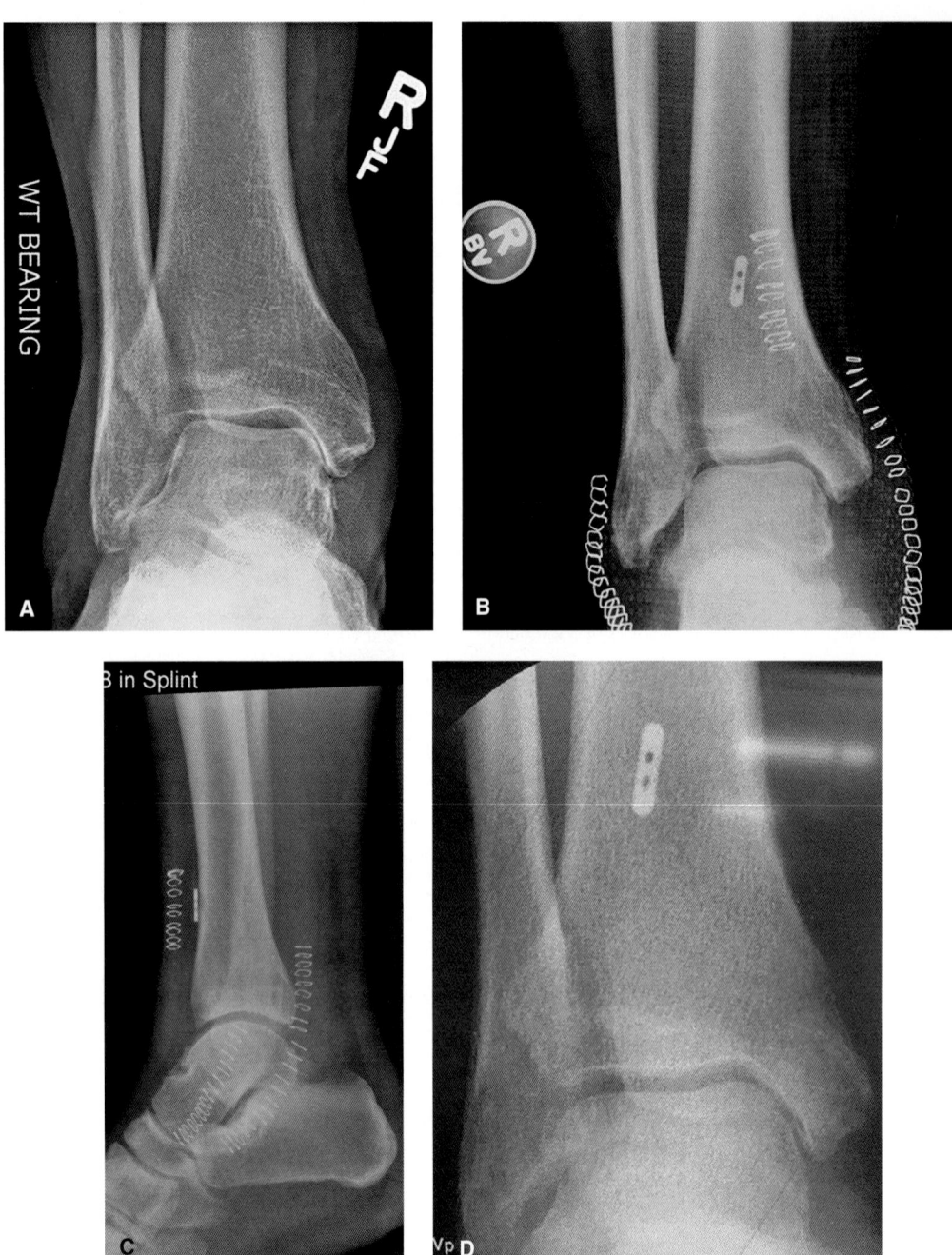

FIGURE 59.30 **A.** Preoperative AP radiograph showing valgus ankle tilting indicating deltoid insufficiency. **B.** Initial postoperative AP radiograph showing suture button placement; the tunnel in the medial malleolus to house the allograft can be visualized as well. Overall reduction of the valgus deformity has been reduced. **C.** Initial postoperative lateral radiograph showing suture button placement on the anterior tibial cortex. **D.** Final 6-month follow-up AP radiograph demonstrating maintenance of the tibiotalar joint congruency.

REFERENCES

1. Johnson E, Markolf K. The contribution of the anterior talofibular ligament to ankle laxity. *J Bone Joint Surg Am.* 1983;65(1):81-88.
2. Khawaji B, Soames R. The anterior talofibular ligament: a detailed morphological study. *Foot (Edinb).* 2015;25(3):141-147.
3. Ozeki S, Yasuda K, Kaneda K, Yamakoshi K, Yamanoi T. Simultaneous strain measurement with determination of a zero strain reference for the medial and lateral ligaments of the ankle. *Foot Ankle Int.* 2002;23(9):825-832.
4. Ozeki S, Kitaoka H, Uchiyama E, Luo ZP, Kaufman K, An KN. Ankle ligament tensile forces at the end points of passive circumferential rotating motion of the ankle and subtalar joint complex. *Foot Ankle Int.* 2006;27(11):965-969.
5. de Asla RJ, Kozánek M, Wan L, Rubash HE, Li G. Function of anterior talofibular and calcaneofibular ligaments during in-vivo motion of the ankle joint complex. *J Orthop Surg Res.* 2009;4:7.
6. Bahr R, Pena F, Shine J, Lew WD, Engebretsen L. Ligament force and joint motion in the intact ankle: a cadaveric study. *Knee Surg Sports Traumatol Arthrosc.* 1998;6(2):115-121.
7. Zwipp H, Rammelt S, Grass R. Ligamentous injuries about the ankle and subtalar joints. *Clin Podiatr Med Surg.* 2002;19(2):195-229, v.
8. Renstrom P, Wertz M, Incavo S, et al. Strain in the lateral ligaments of the ankle. *Foot Ankle.* 1988;9(2):59-63.
9. Colville MR. Surgical treatment of the unstable ankle. *J Am Acad Orthop Surg.* 1998;6(6):368-377.
10. Rigby R, Cottom JM, Rozin R. Isolated calcaneofibular ligament injury: a report of two cases. *J Foot Ankle Surg.* 2015;54(3):487-489.

11. Puffer JC. The sprained ankle. *Clin Cornerstone*. 2001;3(5):38-49.
12. Ajis A, Maffulli N. Conservative management of chronic ankle instability. *Foot Ankle Clin*. 2006;11(3):531-537.
13. Hubbard TJ, Kramer LC, Denegar CR, Hertel J. Contributing factors to chronic ankle instability. *Foot Ankle Int*. 2007;28(3):343-354.
14. Tochigi Y. Effect of arch supports on ankle-subtalar complex instability: a biomechanical experimental study. *Foot Ankle Int*. 2003;24(8):634-639.
15. Petersen W, Rembitzki IV, Koppenburg AG, et al. Treatment of acute ankle ligament injuries: a systematic review. *Arch Orthop Trauma Surg*. 2013;133(8):1129-1141.
16. Lynch SA, Renström PA. Treatment of acute lateral ankle ligament rupture in the athlete. Conservative versus surgical treatment. *Sports Med*. 1999;27(1):61-71.
17. Karlsson J, Bergsten T, Lansinger O, Peterson L. Reconstruction of the lateral ligaments of the ankle for chronic lateral instability. *J Bone Joint Surg Am*. 1988;70(4):581-588.
18. Espinosa N, Smerek J, Kadakia AR, Myerson MS. Operative management of ankle instability: reconstruction with open and percutaneous methods. *Foot Ankle Clin*. 2006;11(3):547-565.
19. Mei-Dan O, Kahn G, Zeev A, et al. The medial longitudinal arch as a possible risk factor for ankle sprains: a prospective study in 83 female infantry recruits. *Foot Ankle Int*. 2005;26(2):180-183.
20. Trevino SG, Davis P, Hecht PJ. Management of acute and chronic lateral ligament injuries of the ankle. *Orthop Clin North Am*. 1994;25(1):1-16.
21. Brostrom L. Sprained ankles. VI. Surgical treatment of "chronic" ligament ruptures. *Acta Chir Scand*. 1966;132(5):551-565.
22. Griffith JF, Brockwell J. Diagnosis and imaging of ankle instability. *Foot Ankle Clin*. 2006;11(3):475-496.
23. McBride DJ, Ramamurthy C. Chronic ankle instability: management of chronic lateral ligamentous dysfunction and the varus tibiotalar joint. *Foot Ankle Clin*. 2006;11(3):607-623.
24. Park HJ, Cha SD, Kim SS, et al. Accuracy of MRI findings in chronic lateral ankle ligament injury: comparison with surgical findings. *Clin Radiol*. 2012;67(4):313-318.
25. Kanamoto T, Shiozaki Y, Tanaka Y, Yonetani Y, Horibe S. The use of MRI in pre-operative evaluation of anterior talofibular ligament in chronic ankle instability. *Bone Joint Res*. 2014;3(8):241-245.
26. Henderson I, La Valette D. Ankle impingement: combined anterior and posterior impingement syndrome of the ankle. *Foot Ankle Int*. 2004;25(9):632-638.
27. Ferkel RD, Chams RN. Chronic lateral instability: arthroscopic findings and long-term results. *Foot Ankle Int*. 2007;28(1):24-31.
28. Hintermann B, Boss A, Schäfer D. Arthroscopic findings in patients with chronic ankle instability. *Am J Sports Med*. 2002;30(3):402-409.
29. Maiotti M, Massoni C, Tarantino U. The use of arthroscopic thermal shrinkage to treat chronic lateral ankle instability in young athletes. *Arthroscopy*. 2005;21(6):751-757.
30. Berlet GC, Saar WE, Ryan A, Lee TH. Thermal-assisted capsular modification for functional ankle instability. *Foot Ankle Clin*. 2002;7(3):567-576, ix.
31. Chan KW, Ding BC, Mroczek KJ. Acute and chronic lateral ankle instability in the athlete. *Bull NYU Hosp Jt Dis*. 2011;69(1):17-26.
32. Kerkhoffs GM, Van Dijk CN. Acute lateral ankle ligament ruptures in the athlete: the role of surgery. *Foot Ankle Clin*. 2013;18(2):215-218.
33. Takao M, Miyamoto W, Matsui K, Sasahara J, Matsushita T. Functional treatment after surgical repair for acute lateral ligament disruption of the ankle in athletes. *Am J Sports Med*. 2012;40(2):447-451.
34. van den Bekerom MP, Kerkhoffs GM, McCollum GA, Calder JD, van Dijk CN. Management of acute lateral ankle ligament injury in the athlete. *Knee Surg Sports Traumatol Arthrosc*. 2013;21(6):1390-1395.
35. Pihlajamäki H, Hietaniemi K, Paavola M, Visuri T, Mattila VM. Surgical versus functional treatment for acute ruptures of the lateral ligament complex of the ankle in young men: a randomized controlled trial. *J Bone Joint Surg Am*. 2010;92(14):2367-2374.
36. White WJ, McCollum GA, Calder JD. Return to sport following acute lateral ligament repair of the ankle in professional athletes. *Knee Surg Sports Traumatol Arthrosc*. 2016;24(4):1124-1129.
37. Cottom JM, Baker JS, Richardson PE, Maker JM. A biomechanical comparison of 3 different arthroscopic lateral ankle stabilization techniques in 36 cadaveric ankles. *J Foot Ankle Surg*. 2016;55(6):1229-1233.
38. Ajis A, Younger AS, Maffulli N. Anatomic repair for chronic lateral ankle instability. *Foot Ankle Clin*. 2006;11(3):539-545.
39. Krips R, van Dijk CN, Halasi PT, et al. Long-term outcome of anatomical reconstruction versus tenodesis for the treatment of chronic anterolateral instability of the ankle joint: a multicenter study. *Foot Ankle Int*. 2001;22(5):415-421.
40. Lee KT, Park YU, Kim JS, Kim JB, Kim KC, Kang SK. Long-term results after modified Brostrom procedure without calcaneofibular ligament reconstruction. *Foot Ankle Int*. 2011;32(2):153-157.
41. Molloy AP, Ajis A, Kazi H. The modified Broström-Gould procedure–early results using a newly described surgical technique. *Foot Ankle Surg*. 2014;20(3):224-228
42. Hennrikus WL, Mapes RC, Lyons PM, Lapoint JM. Outcomes of the Chrisman-Snook and modified-Broström procedures for chronic lateral ankle instability. A prospective, randomized comparison. *Am J Sports Med*. 1996;24(4):400-404.
43. Schmidt R, Cordier E, Bertsch C, et al. Reconstruction of the lateral ligaments: do the anatomical procedures restore physiologic ankle kinematics? *Foot Ankle Int*. 2004;25(1):31-36.
44. Bell SJ, Mologne TS, Sitler DF, Cox JS. Twenty-six-year results after Broström procedure for chronic lateral ankle instability. *Am J Sports Med*. 2006;34(6):975-978.
45. Kocher MS, Fabricant PD, Nasreddine AY, Stenquist N, Kramer DE, Lee JT. Efficacy of the modified Broström procedure for adolescent patients with chronic lateral ankle instability. *J Pediatr Orthop*. 2017;37(8):537-542.
46. Coetzee JC, Ellington JK, Ronan JA, Stone RM. Functional results of open Broström ankle ligament repair augmented with a suture tape. *Foot Ankle Int*. 2018;39(3):304-310.
47. DeVries JG, Scharer BM, Romdenne TA. Ankle stabilization with arthroscopic versus open with suture tape augmentation techniques. *J Foot Ankle Surg*. 2019;58(1):57-61.
48. Cottom JM, Baker JS, Richardson PE. The "all-inside" arthroscopic Broström procedure with additional suture anchor augmentation: a prospective study of 45 consecutive patients. *J Foot Ankle Surg*. 2016;55(6):1223-1228.
49. Prissel MA, Roukis TS. All-inside, anatomical lateral ankle stabilization for revision and complex primary lateral ankle stabilization: a technique guide. *Foot Ankle Spec*. 2014;7(6):484-491
50. Giza E, Shin EC, Wong SE, et al. Arthroscopic suture anchor repair of the lateral ligament ankle complex: a cadaveric study. *Am J Sports Med*. 2013;41(11):2567-2572.
51. Drakos MC, Behrens SB, Paller D, Murphy C, DiGiovanni CW. Biomechanical comparison of an open vs arthroscopic approach for lateral ankle instability. *Foot Ankle Int*. 2014;35(8):809-815.
52. Yeo ED, Lee KT, Sung IH, Lee SG, Lee YK. Comparison of all-inside arthroscopic and open techniques for the modified Broström procedure for ankle instability. *Foot Ankle Int*. 2016;37(10):1037-1045.
53. Cottom JM, Rigby RB. The "all inside" arthroscopic Broström procedure: a prospective study of 40 consecutive patients. *J Foot Ankle Surg*. 2013;52(5):568-574.
54. Rigby RB, Cottom JM. A comparison of the "all-inside" arthroscopic Broström procedure with the traditional open modified Broström-Gould technique: a review of 62 patients. *Foot Ankle Surg*. 2019;25(1):31-36.
55. Coughlin MJ, Schenck RC Jr, Grebing BR, Treme G. Comprehensive reconstruction of the lateral ankle for chronic instability using a free gracilis graft. *Foot Ankle Int*. 2004;25(4):231-241.
56. Xu X, Hu M, Liu J, Zhu Y, Wang B. Minimally invasive reconstruction of the lateral ankle ligaments using semitendinosus autograft or tendon allograft. *Foot Ankle Int*. 2014;35(10):1015-1021.
57. Caprio A, Oliva F, Treia F, Maffulli N. Reconstruction of the lateral ankle ligaments with allograft in patients with chronic ankle instability. *Foot Ankle Clin*. 2006;11(3):597-605.
58. Klammer G, Schlewitz G, Stauffer C, Vich M, Espinosa N. Percutaneous lateral ankle stabilization: an anatomical investigation. *Foot Ankle Int*. 2011;32(1):66-70.
59. Campbell KJ, Michalski MP, Wilson KJ, et al. The ligament anatomy of the deltoid complex of the ankle: a qualitative and quantitative anatomical study. *J Bone Joint Surg Am*. 2014;96(8):e62.
60. Hintermann B. Medial ankle instability. *Foot Ankle Clin*. 2003;8(4):723-738.
61. Hintermann B, Knupp M, Pagenstert GI. Deltoid ligament injuries: diagnosis and management. *Foot Ankle Clin*. 2006;11(3):625-637.

Wounds and Flaps

John S. Steinberg, Christopher E. Attinger, and Jayson N. Atves

INTRODUCTION

The modern understanding and management of lower extremity wounds has truly undergone a renaissance in the new millennium. A combination of advances in technology and the evolution of evidence-based understanding have led to significant progressions in the assessment and treatment of chronic nonhealing lower extremity wounds. The application of these practices has produced more efficient utilization of patient-specific treatments and a better appreciation of the nonhealing foot and ankle wound environment. Despite this vigor, the complex foot and ankle wound continues to bear significant burden on the health care system at large and on the well-being of those patients suffering from these complex wounds.

When compared to acute wounds, which can often be treated outright with standard therapies, chronic wounds demand more advanced treatment modalities and consideration overall. We anticipate the wound of a healthy patient to heal through primary or secondary intention within roughly 2 weeks with continued remodeling thereafter. This process is predictable and consistent in acute wounds with little deviations based in age, gender, location, or etiology. The chronic wound, though, stagnates and does not improve in size or character secondary to factors that inhibit the wound healing cascade.

There are numerous factors that may contribute to an acute wound's degeneration into a chronic state. Some of the most common causes found in the lower extremity include ischemia, infection, neuropathy, deformity, or any combination thereof. Diabetes mellitus, for example, bears an assortment of local and systemic complications that affect a myriad of tissue types and organ systems, all of which may deleteriously effect wound healing. In fact, it is well known and established that diabetes can wreak havoc on the tissues requisite for healing and in those most pertinent for preventing wound formation. In these ways, diabetes truly represents the personification of complex and nonhealing wounds. In both the United States and many other nations, the prevalence of diabetes mellitus has reached epidemic proportions. The annual incidence of foot and ankle wounds in diabetics is about 2% in most Western countries, though rates have been reported as high as 6%.[1] Recent data also suggest that the lifetime risk of diabetic foot and ankle wounds may be as high as 34%.[1] For these reasons and numerous others, early assessment and appropriate intervention is vital when confronted with the complex nonhealing wound, regardless of its exact etiology.

It is important, however, to consider that although a great number of complicated and nonhealing wounds emanate from the diabetic population, diabetes as a pathology in and of itself is an insufficient scapegoat for classifying the etiology of a wound. Further investigation must be undertaken to define the causal relationship for wound formation and chronicity. With this in mind, the terms "diabetic wound," "diabetic ulceration," or "diabetic foot" are classic misnomers that lead us to assume the etiological basis for a wound is diabetes or its complications. While the complications associated with diabetes may in fact be the reason(s) for a wound's chronicity, it should not be assumed without a proper assessment and these fairly antiquated terms should only be used as grossly generalized descriptors. Rather, the terms should be replaced by more accurate and nonleading descriptors like "complex wound," "complicated wound," "chronic wound," or "nonhealing wound." In nondiabetic patients, for instance, the burden of etiological proof placed upon the physician and team is just the same as it is for a diabetic patient.

Certainly, the nonhealing foot and ankle wound is a complex structure and environment that is undeniably disadvantaged due to an assortment of potential local and/or systemic complications that may hinder wound healing. Therefore, proper assessment and treatment of chronic wounds is of the utmost importance. With this in mind, it is imperative that clinicians be vigilant and attentive to this dynamic patient population, modify wound healing strategies appropriately, and engage in aggressive and perhaps varied treatment practices when warranted. In this chapter, we review the principles in the evaluation and treatment of nonhealing wounds of the foot and ankle and offer an assortment of strategies aimed at their prevention, eradication, and suppression.

ANATOMIC AND PHYSIOLOGIC FEATURES

ANATOMY

A basic knowledge of the anatomy of skin and its adjacent tissues is necessary in evaluating and treating chronic wounds. Five anatomic layers should be considered: (1) skin (epidermis and dermis); (2) superficial fascia; (3) deep fascia; (4) periosteum; and (5) bone (Fig. 60.1). The epidermis is the most superficial layer of skin, the majority of which has no direct vascular supply but rather is incumbent upon the processes of osmotic vascular flow. The dermis is often regarded as the most important skin component to wound healing due to the

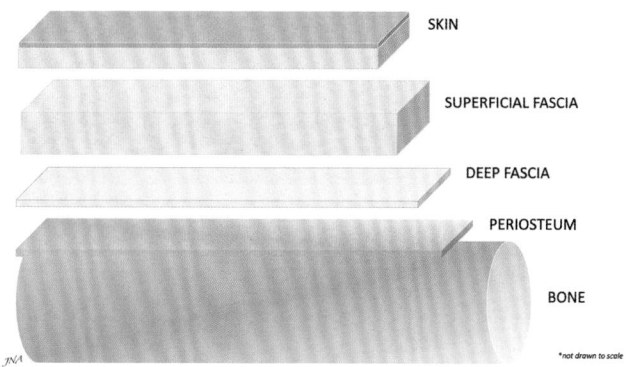

FIGURE 60.1 The five anatomic layers of dissection: (1) skin; (2) superficial fascia; (3) deep fascia; (4) periosteum; and (5) bone.

fact that granulation tissue is seen at this level. The superficial fascia contains superficial adipose tissue, cutaneous nerves, and superficial veins. The deep fascia is a thin but strong continuous layer separating superficial structures from deep structures, including deep vessels and nerves, muscle, tendon, and bone. The periosteal layer includes the contiguous structures of periosteum, capsule, and ligamentous structures. The bone layer consists of bone and all its varied structures. One should bear in mind that these tissue layers have an intimate working knowledge of their micro- and macro-architecture and anatomic variation when managing a chronic wound so that appropriate treatment modalities can be identified and implemented as necessary, be it surgically or otherwise.

PRINCIPLES OF WOUND HEALING

A review of the normal wound healing cascade is necessary to more clearly understand the chronic nonhealing wound. Wound healing is a natural physiological reaction to tissue injury. However, this is not a simple phenomenon but rather involves a complex interplay between numerous cell types, cytokines, mediators, and the vascular system. The traditional cascade of wound healing is described as the sequential and overlapping progression through three phases: inflammation, proliferation, and remodeling[2] (Fig. 60.2). The initial vasoconstriction of blood vessels and platelet aggregation is designed to stop bleeding. This is followed by an influx of a variety of inflammatory cells, starting with the neutrophils. These inflammatory cells, in turn, release a variety of mediators and cytokines to promote angiogenesis, thrombosis, and reepithelialization. The fibroblasts, in turn, lay down extracellular components, which will serve as scaffolding for ultimate wound healing and closure.

The inflammatory phase begins with hemostasis at the initial insult after platelets have collected and adhered at the site of injury to form a hemostatic plug. In this phase, the body activates the clotting cascade and forms a clot to stop continued bleeding. During this process, platelets that have traveled to the site of injury come into contact with collagen, resulting in their activation and aggregation. Thrombin initiates the formation of a fibrin plug, which strengthens the platelet clumps into a stable clot. Additionally, platelets contain intracellular structures including alpha-granules that contain growth factors, clotting factors, and other proteins involved in wound healing. Transforming growth factor (TGF-beta) and platelet-derived angiogenesis factor (PDAF) play roles in wound matrix production by promoting collagen production and new capillary formation. Platelet-derived growth factor (PDGF) is one of the key components of wound healing, which recruits and activates proinflammatory cells such as fibroblasts, macrophages, monocytes, and neutrophils. These cells, in turn, secrete growth factors such as TGF-beta, fibroblast growth factor (FGF), endothelial growth factor (EGF), and vascular endothelial growth factor (VEGF). These cellular interactions and communications are critical elements in the wound healing cascade. This phase normally lasts a matter of days after the initial insult.

The proliferation or epithelialization phase begins with the proliferation and migration of epidermal cells. Epidermal cells will form linkages with one another and initiate deposition of basement membrane components and degrade the extracellular matrix. Neovascularization occurs at the wound bed causing the formation of granulation tissues, which infiltrates the temporary matrix. Fibroblast plays a crucial role in orchestrating the reorganization of the extracellular matrix into a collagenous matrix through the use of proteases and other enzymes. Growth factors such as VEGF contribute to the stimulation of angiogenesis to support wound healing. This phase of wound healing can normally last days to weeks in duration.

The remodeling or maturation phase involves slow advances in new tissue strength and flexibility with wound contraction facilitated by fibroblasts that have converted to myofibroblasts stimulated by growth factors. Collagen is continually remodeled through enzymatic degradation by matrix metalloproteinases (MMPs) until final collagen deposition and wound reepithelialization have occurred. This phase's duration can vary greatly lasting for weeks to years.

PHYSICAL EXAMINATION

Proper and timely physical examination is critical in healing a nonhealing wound. The first step in wound evaluation is to assess the vascularity of the wound site both locally and systemically. The next step is to establish the level of contamination or infection present. Further evaluation of any gross foot or ankle deformity should be conducted with a musculoskeletal examination. Finally, a thorough evaluation of the quality and character of the wound itself is vitally important during a dermatological examination. All portions of the examination should include a subjective assessment via patient or family inquiry for symptoms associated with advanced or underlying pathology or wound progression.

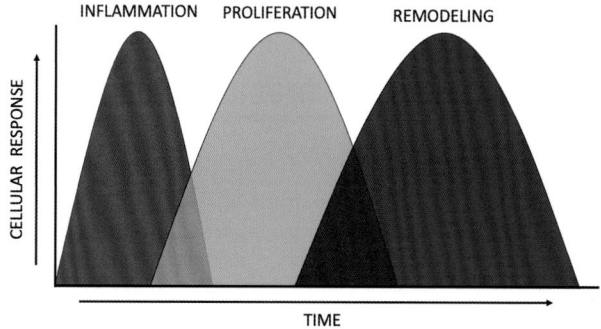

FIGURE 60.2 The traditional wound healing cascade is described as three overlapping phases: inflammation, proliferation, and remodeling.

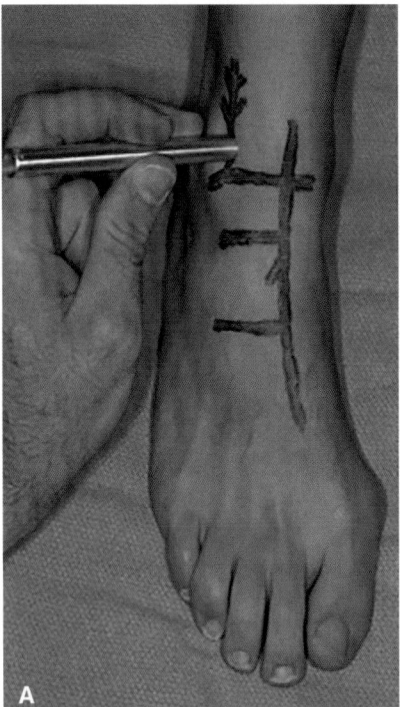 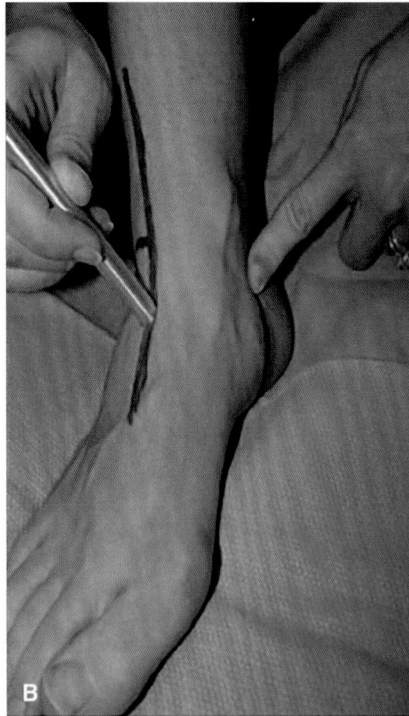 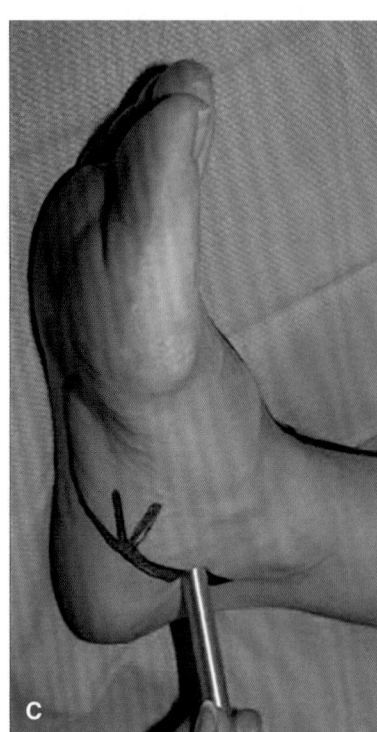

FIGURE 60.3 Audible Doppler vascular examination will provide much in the way of determining vascular flow by way of the **(A)** perforating peroneal artery, **(B)** anterior tibial and dorsalis pedis arteries, and **(C)** posterior tibial artery.

VASCULAR EXAMINATION

Oxygenation and nutrition delivery are requisites for the healing of any wound. The vascular patency can be assessed at the wound site through both noninvasive and invasive methods. Initial evaluation of skin color (pallor), hair distribution (absence or presence), atrophy of skin and nail, and temperature gradients to the affected limb can raise the clinical suspicion for ischemia. The capillary fill time and any form of edema should also be evaluated.

Palpation of pulses is a sensitive measure of blood flow about a wound site; however, it is not completely predictive of vascular patency. The dorsalis pedis (DP) artery, posterior tibial (PT) artery, and the perforating peroneal artery are the three large vessels that feed the foot. Regardless of the absence or presence of palpable arterial pulses, in a nonhealing wound further investigation with a handheld Doppler is warranted (Fig. 60.3).

Utilizing a Doppler will provide much in the way of determining sufficient or insufficient vascular flow by way of the main three arteries to the foot. One should be able to discern between triphasic, biphasic, and monophasic pulse signals at each artery individually. Anything less than triphasic signal should be considered abnormal and warrants further vascular investigation. Of note, one should implement measures to ensure that retrograde flow is not present within a single source artery by manually compressing the other main arteries while listening for changes in the audible Doppler examination flow (Fig. 60.4).

An ankle brachial index (ABI) is a measure of systolic pressure differences between the ankle artery pressure divided by the brachial artery pressure. Although there is no absolute threshold that predicts successful wound healing, some general guidelines can be helpful. An ABI of 0.90 or less is considered abnormal, 0.71-0.90 indicating mild PAD, 0.41-0.70 indicating moderate PAD, and 0.40 or less indicating severe PAD.[3] It is important to note that noncompressible or calcific vessels will falsely elevate the ABI measure due to noncompliance of the vessel walls.[3] In the chronic wound environment, patients are more likely to require an amputation with an ABI of <0.50.[4]

More advanced and invasive imaging techniques may be necessary for further evaluation, including arterial duplex ultrasound, angiogram, and magnetic resonance arteriogram. Subjective questioning for symptoms associated with vasculopathies includes inquiries of cramping pains to the feet, legs, or thighs either when walking that is relieved by rest or when lying recumbently that is relieved by dependency and/or walking.

Infection Assessment

As all open wounds will be colonized with microorganisms, we define infection by the presence of the classic signs of inflammation, including rubor (redness), tumor (swelling), dolor (pain), calor (heat), and function laesa (loss of function). As these findings may be altered in patients with peripheral neuropathy or PAD, some clinicians accept secondary signs, such as friable granulation tissue or wound undermining, lymphadenopathy, and superficial thrombophlebitis (Fig. 60.5) as evidence of a fulminant infection. The assessment of superficial infection or cellulitis should include observation for responses to elevation and dependency and monitoring by drawing a line of demarcation as a reference to advancing or receding infection (Fig. 60.6). Wound depth should be probed utilizing a sterile instrument as this will enable the clinician to fully examine the extent of the wound and may aid in the diagnosis of bone infection.[5,6]

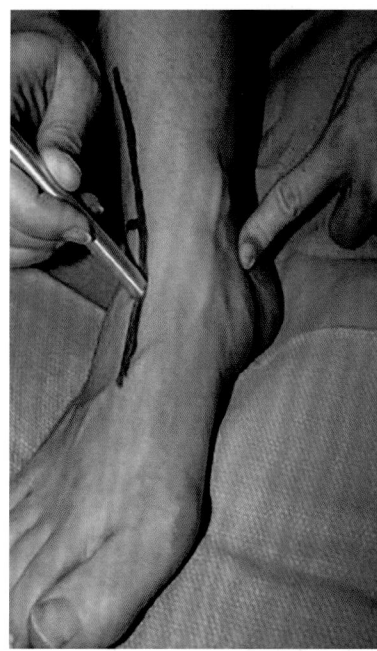
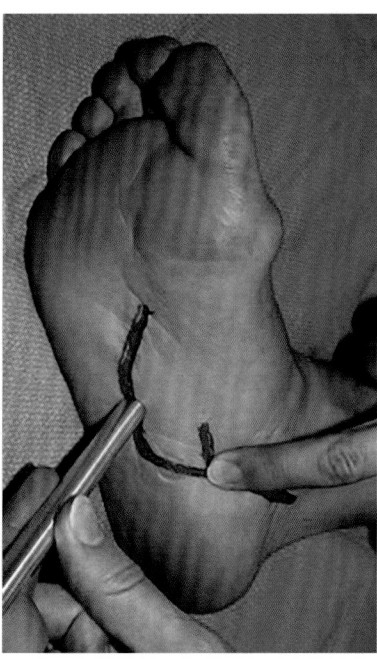

FIGURE 60.4 One should implement measures to ensure that retrograde flow is not present within a single source artery by manually compressing the other main arteries while listening for changes in the audible Doppler examination flow.

Subjective questioning for constitutional symptoms associated with infection includes inquiries of nausea, fever, diarrhea, constipation, cough, chills, cramps, and malaise. However, in many immunocompromised patients, these systemic factors present with a lesser frequency and severity as the patient may be unable to mount a sufficient immune response to infection. Patients should also be questioned about recent illness, hospitalization, or visit to the emergency room or urgent care, as these types of information can go undetected if not pursued. Baseline vital signs should always be evaluated including fever or hypothermia, tachycardia (heart rate,

> 100 beats/min), and hypotension (systolic blood pressure < 90 or 20 mm Hg below baseline).[7]

MUSCULOSKELETAL EXAMINATION

A careful examination and palpation of any bony prominences with a perceptible decrease in soft tissue overlay is an important component of the musculoskeletal examination. Soft tissue changes can predispose the lower extremity to ulceration and should be given consideration. Further, diabetic patients experience collagen glycosylation, which is demonstrated to decrease the mobility of joints as well as tendons resulting in stiffening of the tissues themselves or "cheiroarthropathy."[8-14] Individual joint range of motion and manual muscle testing with, ideally, gait analysis should be performed. The clinician should give consideration to all joints of the foot and ankle regardless of their proximity to the wound and note where joint and/or tendon contractures exist. Gait analysis offers a unique manner in which to observe the patient in a dynamic and functional manner and may clue the clinician in to a biomechanical fault not easily observed without this observation. Obviously, these examinations can may be limited depending on the exact environment or patient limitations, but the importance of a thorough musculoskeletal examination nonetheless remains.

DERMATOLOGICAL EXAMINATION

A thorough assessment of the wound itself and regional tissue of the extremity should always be made and is often paired with the infection assessment. The visual character of the wound base should be made with objective measurements of size, shape, and location as well as subjective estimations of depth according to tissues layers making sure to note any specific exposed deep tissues (tendon, muscle, capsule, bone, etc.). Wound appearance conveys much information, especially when compared to previous wound observations and the differentiation and quantification between granular, fibrotic, and eschar tissues is paramount and can lead treatment decision-making. The edges

FIGURE 60.5 Patient displaying signs tracking rubor, indication of superficial thrombophlebitis of the great saphenous vein with a concomitant soft tissue infection of the foot.

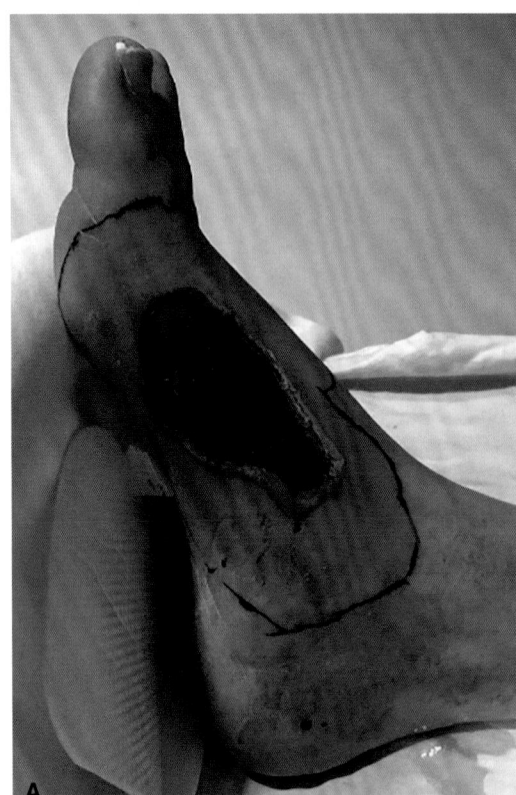 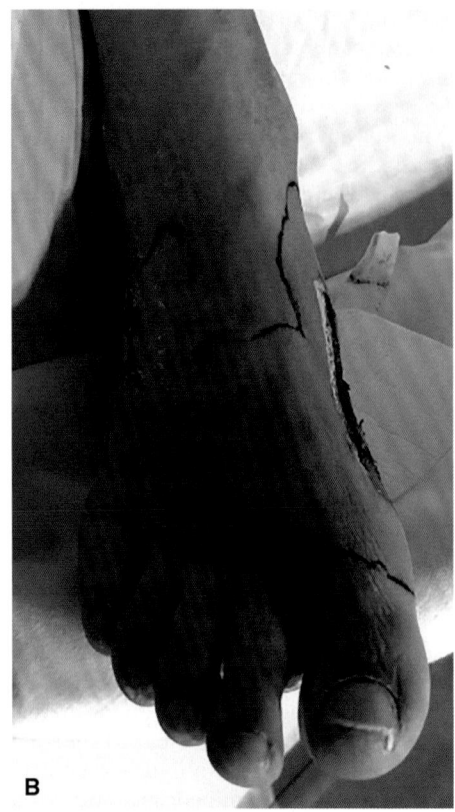

FIGURE 60.6 A, B. Cellulitis should include monitoring by outlining a line of demarcation as a reference to advancing or receding infection.

of the wound should be characterized and inspected for under-mining or probing and any odor and drainage emanating from a wound should also be noted and described.

PATHOGENESIS

Determination of chronic wound etiology is of the utmost importance in order to guide the most appropriate course of wound optimization. That said, it is imperative to understand that wound character may evolve over time, especially in the complex or comorbid patient population. Consequently, a thoughtful understanding and careful consideration of the patient, wound, and treatment types is vital to a successful out-come.[15] Additionally, the fact that many nonhealing wounds may have a combination of multifactorial etiology should not escape the physician. In this light, we present the most common etiological factors associated with complex nonhealing wounds of the foot and ankle.

ISCHEMIA

Vascular compromise plays a major role in the chronicity of nonhealing wounds. It is important to remember that a chronic wound is not always ischemic; however, due to the vascular pathology associated with diseases like diabetes mellitus, wounds may progress in this direction and never return. Vasculopathy associated with diabetes mellitus has two major components: macrovascular and microvascular processes. Systemic macro-vascular pathologic processes include cerebrovascular, car-diovascular, and, perhaps most pertinent to this discussion,

peripheral vascular/arterial disease (PVD/PAD). Microvascular dysfunction revolves around issues with the microcirculation at the level of arterioles and capillaries and is more of a dysfunc-tion in physiology than anatomy.

PAD is one of the most devastating sequelae of diabetes.[16] Diabetic patients with PAD have a higher risk of lower extrem-ity amputations.[17] The hallmark atherosclerotic process is fibro-fatty plaque deposition initiated by an inflammatory process within the vessel walls. The plaques may progress to a point at which complete occlusion may occur. Wound care specialists are often the first to identify systemic ischemic disease as mani-fested by the symptoms of a nonhealing wound. The ischemia discovered will often persist much further systemically and in fact is a common marker for carotid and cardiac vessel disease. "Critical limb ischemia" is a term used to describe the point at which, without intervention, limb amputation is strongly pre-dictive.[18] Revascularization can be conducted through open or endovascular approaches. Open technique may include the harvesting of superficial veins including the greater and lesser saphenous veins to be used as the vessel that bypasses the area of obstruction. Endovascular techniques utilize a vari-ety of ablative techniques and technologies to remove focal plaques through a minimally invasive technique.[19] Prior to lower extremity revascularization, an arteriogram or magnetic resonance angiography should be performed to identify and localize the exact areas of occlusion.

The microvascular environment is also altered in patients with pathology such as diabetes.[20-22] Generally speaking, there are two components in the diabetic microvascular system that are in an altered state. First, there is increased vascular permeability. Sec-ond, there is an impairment in the regulation of vascular tone

and local blood flow.[23] This, in part, has to do with a thickening of the capillary basement membrane and a decrease in capillary diameter.[24,25] Suffice to say, though, there are numerous factors at play in the pathological microvascular environment that predispose patients to insufficient ability to provide adequate vascular flow to the tissues of the foot and ankle.

The proper assessment and treatment of vascular disease must be addressed prior to or in conjunction with wound care modalities. If blood flow is compromised to the affected extremity, the wound will not heal or will at least be severely retarded in healing. The wound is entirely dependent upon adequate nutrition and oxygenation. Thus, vascular evaluation and possibly consultation is necessary in the treatment of a chronic wound (Fig. 60.7).

INFECTION

Infection is an obvious impediment to wound healing and as such must be addressed early and aggressively. However, with the rise of antibiotic resistance, it is unrealistic, irresponsible, and often unacceptable to treat all bacterial infections of the lower extremity with a single large spectrum antibiotic. The appropriate and judicious use of antibiotics specifically targeting the offending organism is necessary to slow the growing concerns of bacterial resistance.[26-29] Although the antibiotic choices available appear to be plentiful, a cautious and systematic evaluation of the infectious process with the isolation of the offending organism(s) is necessary to impede growing bacterial resistance. Selective antibiotic use is essential for the appropriate treatment of infections. This is of particular importance given the number of years that it takes for new drug research and development. Appropriate consultation with an infectious disease will help ensure the best possible practices are implemented and at the same time will help to ensure antibiotic efficacy into the future.

NEUROPATHY

Peripheral neuropathy has been cited as a pivotal process that contributes to the chronicity of foot and ankle wounds and can affect up to 66% of patients with diabetes.[30-33] Peripheral neuropathy can be generally defined as a progressive loss of peripheral nerve fibers. In the diabetic patient, for instance, this typically presents in a symmetrical fashion and involves sensory, motor, and autonomic neuropathy or a combination thereof. The etiology of peripheral neuropathy is most attributable to hyperglycemia.[34] Hyperglycemia contributes to metabolism disturbances that negatively impact nerve function. Other contributing factors include focal areas of nerve entrapment, which can lead to degeneration of the nerve fibers. Nerve entrapment may benefit from surgical decompression.[35]

Sensory neuropathy can often present as a painful process with patients reporting symptoms of "pins and needles" or "burning" type sensation in earlier stages. Peripheral neuropathy may progress to a point in which complete loss of sensation occurs. The typical insensate process begins distally at the toes and fingers and progresses proximally in a "stocking and glove" distribution. The most critical aspect of peripheral neuropathy is that patients are unaware of focal areas of trauma, which may lead to the development of a wound.[32] This wound continues to be traumatized and inadequately treated and thus degenerates into a chronic wound.

Motor and autonomic neuropathies may also contribute to the chronicity of a nonhealing wound. Motor neuropathy can lead to an imbalance of the muscles or muscle atrophy in the lower extremities. This process may lead to areas of increased pressure that can subsequently lead to tissue breakdown. Autonomic neuropathy involves the denervation of the sympathetic nervous system, leading to the shunting of arterial blood flow away from the nutrient capillaries. This arterial to venous shunting diverts the nutrients and oxygen away from the underlying

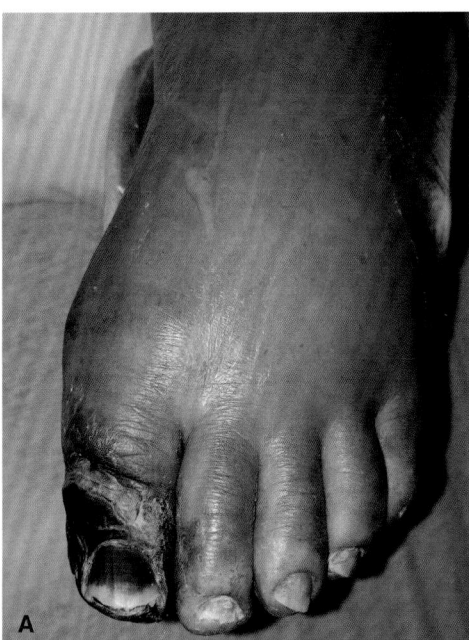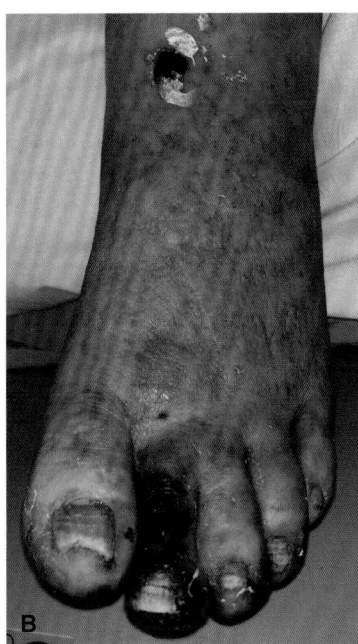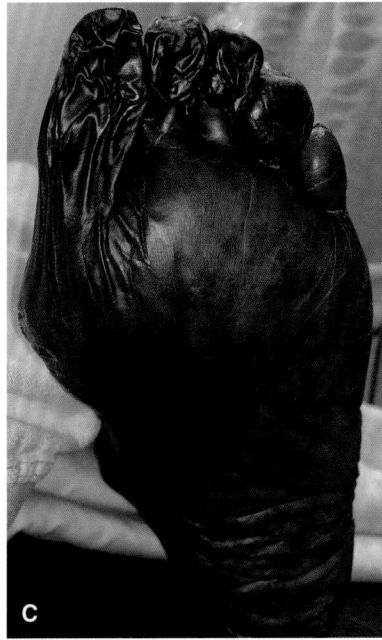

FIGURE 60.7 A-C. Vascular disease may be subtle or, as in these cases, more distinct. Ischemic changes to the distal extremity may progress slowly or rapidly depending on the oxygenation and nutritional demands of the tissues.

soft tissues. Therefore, the tissues become less tolerant to stresses leading to tissue breakdown. It is hypothesized that this process may explain loss of sweat production in the lower extremities and fat pad atrophy of the plantar foot.

Peripheral neuropathy is a significant contributing factor in the development and chronicity of chronic foot and ankle wounds.[36] Proper management consists of early detection, strict glucose control, and oral medications that target symptomatic relief including tricyclics, selective serotonin reuptake inhibitors, anticonvulsants, antiarrhythmics, narcotics, and nonsteroidal anti-inflammatories.[37] Although there is no cure for this progressive disease, management can blunt its progression that can ultimately lead to an insensate foot and ankle.

DEFORMITY

Any foot or ankle deformity, ranging from the subtle to the obvious, may play a causal role in wound development and chronicity, be it directly or indirectly[36,38] (Fig. 60.8). Hallux limitus, hammertoes, equinus, bony prominence, and Charcot collapse are some of the most common deformities that will potentiate wound development and chronicity; however, countless other deformities may exist secondary to acute or progressive pathology.[38-40] Areas of erythema and/or callous formation may indicate an underlying bony deformity. Radiographic evaluation is a must when a wound is identified, particularly if the wound is located on a weight-bearing surface, as a bony irritation elsewhere on the foot or ankle can potentiate wound formation or support chronicity. It is useful to place a metallic or vitamin marker or otherwise in the area of irritation in order to correlate with a bony prominence. An underlying bony deformity can also be identified utilizing a plantar pressure measuring device that can isolate areas of increased peak plantar pressures, where available. A foot or ankle deformity in and of itself may not directly produce a wound; however, in conjunction with the processes such as peripheral neuropathy and PVD, it places the foot and ankle at an increased risk of wound formation.

Additionally, soft tissue changes can predispose the lower extremity to ulceration or wound formation and should always

be assessed. The limitation of joint mobility at the ankle caused by contracture of the Achilles tendon has been defined as an equinus deformity. Equinus has been implicated as a major deforming force in the development and chronicity of plantar wound formations as well as midfoot Charcot collapse.[41-48] Measuring of the maximal passive dorsiflexion available at the ankle with the subtalar joint locked and the knee extended and then flexed accomplishes this task. Distinction between gastrocnemius or isolated equinus vs gastrocnemius-soleus or combined equinus is significant when considering the surgical lengthening of equinus via gastrocnemius-soleus recession (GSR) vs tendo-Achilles lengthening (TAL), respectively. Other tendinous imbalances may be seen in nearly any of the muscles and tendons of the foot and ankle including the digits. Chronic changes to multiple tissue types and architecture of the foot and ankle may cause progressive digital contracture. Although innocuous appearing, digital contractures in higher risk patients, especially those with either PVD and/or peripheral neuropathy, can result in the accelerated progression of preulcerative and ultimately chronic wound formation. A simple in-office flexor tenotomy at the level of the contracted digital joint or as supplementation of other procedure types can remedy this deformity in a proportion of patients and provide for lasting prophylactic relief. Regardless, careful consideration for the patient's surgical history and a thorough musculoskeletal assessment must be made in the formulation of appropriate supplemental or primary procedure selection for the correction or accommodation of biomechanical or anatomic deformity.

IMAGING AND DIAGNOSTICS STUDIES

RADIOGRAPHS

Plain film radiographs in multiple views are a standard to rule in or rule out the presence of foreign bodies, tissue emphysema, or bony prominence or deformity and may be particularly helpful in the diagnosis of infection as well as give preliminary signs of underlying vascular disease (Fig. 60.9). Some radiographic

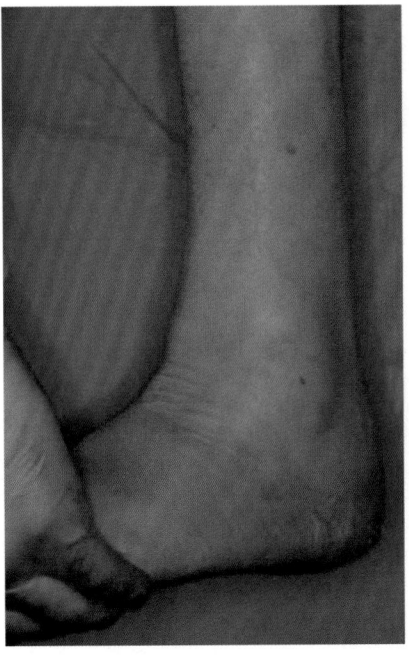 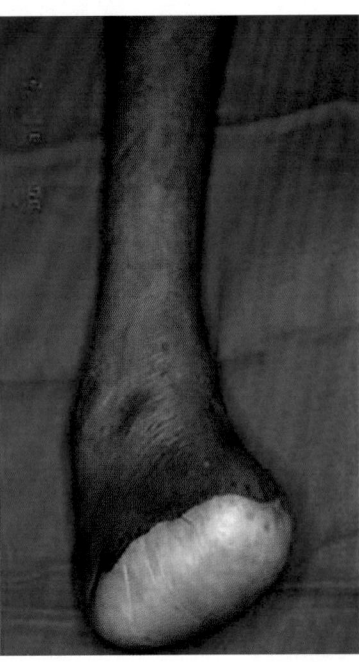

FIGURE 60.8 Clinical deformity is a precursor to excessive pressure distribution and subsequent wound/ulcer formation.

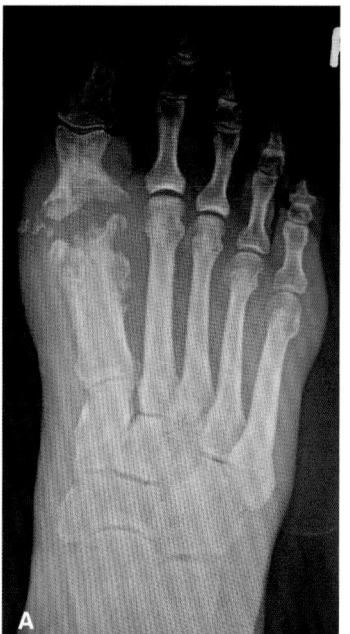
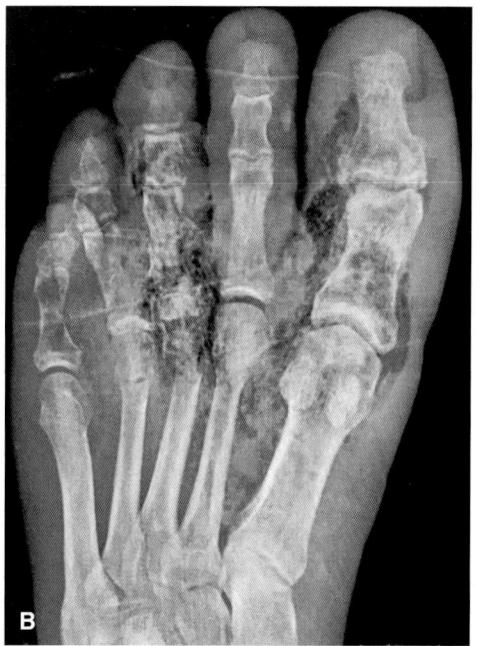
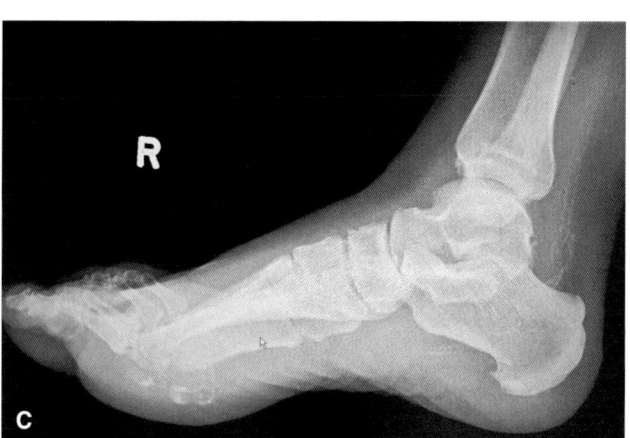
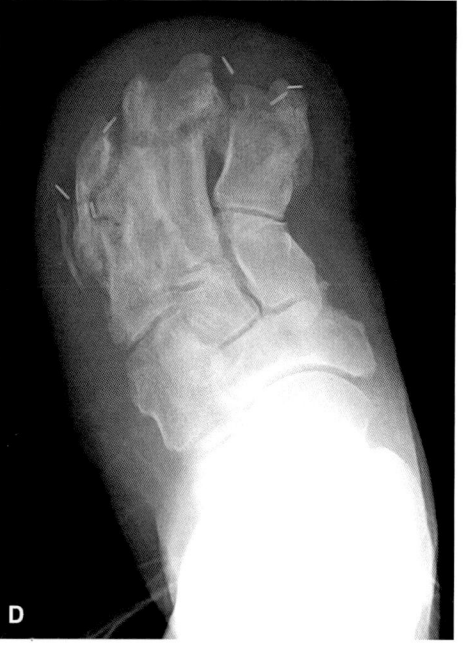

FIGURE 60.9 Radiographs can provide important imaging for determining location and extent of infection, integrity and orientation of osseous structures, and potentially an insight into possible vascular disease. **A.** Chronic osteomyelitis of the first MTPJ. **B.** Acute soft tissue emphysema of the forefoot. **C.** Vascular calcification of the posterior tibial artery. **D.** Diffuse metatarsal heterotopic ossification following transmetatarsal amputation.

markers of bone infection include periosteal reaction, cortical erosions, bone sequestrum, and involucrum. However, there may be a radiographic delay of up to 14-21 days in these findings and thus repeat radiographs over several weeks may be helpful.

ADVANCED IMAGING

Advanced imaging techniques such as magnetic resonance imaging (MRI), computed tomography (CT), or radiolabeled scintigraphy/nuclear scans may be appropriate for some patients in whom initial evaluations suggest osteomyelitis

(OM).[49] MRI may be useful to image the deeper layers of the foot and ankle. CT may be used to visualize changes in the cortical bone due to infection or for anatomical contour, position, and alignment. Nuclear medicine bone scans reflect changes in metabolic activity of bone, and these modalities are very sensitive but fairly nonspecific for bone infection. Indium-111 WBC-labeled and technetium-99 WBC-labeled (HMPAO-hexamethylpropyleneamine) scans are considered more specific for infection. When late images are utilized, these scans have reported comparable levels of sensitivity and specificity as histopathologic evaluations of bone for the diagnosis of OM.[50]

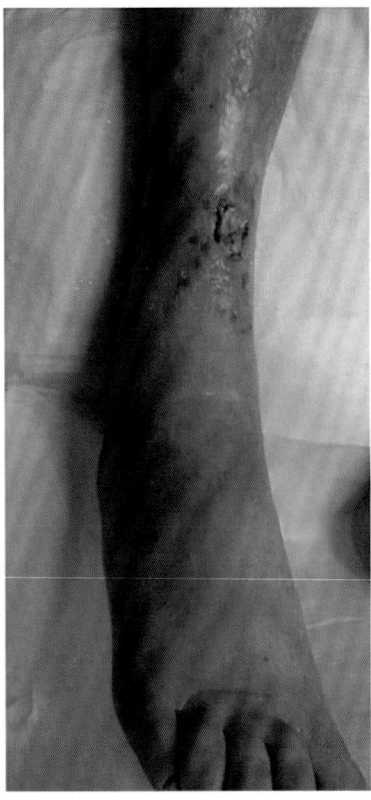 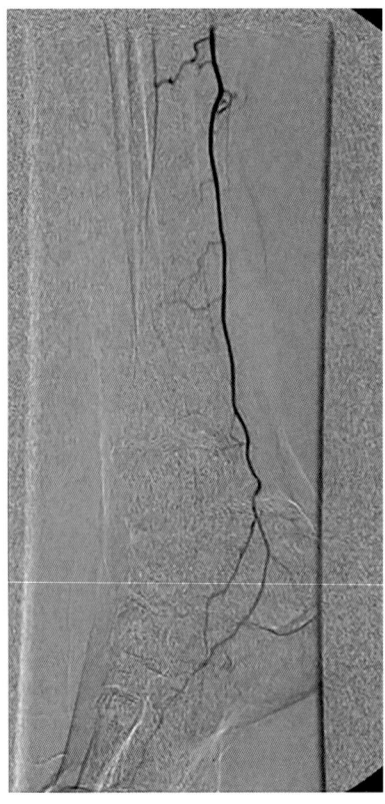

FIGURE 60.10 Clinical wound appearance with corresponding angiography showing insufficient flow of the anterior tibial artery.

LABORATORY TESTING

One should obtain a baseline of laboratory work for all except the most mild of infections. Laboratory tests are of particular importance in patients with soft tissue infections that show signs and symptoms of systemic toxicity. These laboratory tests include blood cultures, complete blood cell count with differential, creatinine, bicarbonate, creatine phosphokinase, and C-reactive protein (CRP) levels.[51] An elevated white blood cell (WBC) count can indicate an aggressive infectious process. Immature polymorphonuclear leukocyte (PMN) bands may also be an important indicator of infection. An increase in bands occurs with acute infections when the production of mature WBCs cannot sustain with the demands of the body to ward off infection. This process is referred to as a "left shift."

CULTURES

Definitively diagnosing bone infection requires collecting a bone specimen that has a positive culture or histological evidence of inflammation and necrosis, and preferably both.

Gram stain and culture and sensitivity are valued tools to aid in the diagnosis and treatment of infection. If a culture is warranted, both aerobic and anaerobic cultures should be taken. Culture and sensitivity reports will guide the clinician to prescribe appropriate antibiotics as well as guide appropriate timing for definitive closure. Deep tissue and bone cultures are best taken in the operating room with swab cultures of drainage, purulence, or open wound surfaces. The selective use of cultures is of key importance as superficial swab cultures often grow normal skin flora and nonpathogenic contaminants. Patients who are immunocompromised are often more likely to have infections, which are polymicrobial in natures or contain atypical pathogens.

ANGIOGRAPHY

Although a proper discussion of the intricacies of angiography is certainly warranted, its shear length precludes a proper discussion within this chapter. Angiography, though, is considered the gold standard in diagnostic evaluation of peripheral vascular patency. The lumen of peripheral vessels can be visualized directly with remarkable clarity, detail, and accuracy with a catheterization of selective vessels and at a low risk to most patients. Additionally, progresses in the interventional aspect of angiography have advanced to where specific wall lesions can provide greater patency with amazing increases to overall vascularity. In the face of uncertainty of the exact vascular status of a complex nonhealing wound, or when noninvasive testing has revealed vascular pathology, one should not hesitate to advocate for angiography for its immensely beneficial diagnostic and potentially therapeutic benefits (Fig. 60.10).

TREATMENT

The fundamental tenants in the management of most lower extremity wounds include eradication of infection, optimization of tissue perfusion and adequate offloading with correction, accommodation, or stabilization of static or dynamic deformity. Chronic wound formation in particular requires adherence to a multifactorial algorithm, which affords the greatest healing potential while mitigating costs and minimizing recidivism. A variety of management factors are essential to obtaining and preserving a healthy wound bed, which includes, but is not limited to, patient comorbidities, nutrition, glucose control, smoking status, ambulatory status, wound etiology, availability of resources, adherence, and perhaps the most important being wound location and topography. Outside of the modifiable patient-centered factors as a means of

ameliorating the chronicity of complex wounds, the local establishment and maintenance of a healthy wound bed remains central in chronic wound treatment. This is made possible with the judicious use of debridement and offloading, with supplementation by topical formulations, dressings, bioengineered alternative tissues (BATs), negative pressure wound therapy (NPWT), and hyperbaric oxygen (HBO) therapy.

Given the complexity of this patient population, the management of the chronic foot and ankle wound environment is best suited for a multidisciplinary or team approach. This aspect of treatment cannot be overstated; however, it is often underappreciated and certainly underutilized. This is perhaps due to a myriad of a reason, but most obvious may be due to an absence of resources and a lack of appropriate edification on part of the surgeon or a combination thereof. To be fair, the culmination of well-equipped podiatric surgery, plastic surgery, and vascular surgery teams is an increasingly elusive constellation in both the private and hospital settings. Many practices, hospitals, or systems simply lack the available infrastructure and/or physician expertise or enthusiasm to adequately support the demands of this type of pathology. However, the consortium offered by a multidisciplinary approach including specialized evaluation, intervention, and perhaps most importantly interspecialty collaboration may truly be considered the ideal foundation for the management of the complex foot and ankle wound environment.

DEBRIDEMENT

The word debridement derives from the French *débridement*, which translates to "to remove a constraint." This term was first used by Henri LeDran (1685-1770) in the context of an incision of skin and fascia to release swelling associated with injury.[52] However, during 18th and 19th century wartime, this definition was refined to include removal of all materials incompatible with healing in order to prevent gangrene and it is this definition that still guides practitioners today.[53] Presently, debridement is the excision of dead, damaged, or infected tissues in order to optimize healing potential of the remaining presumably healthy and viable tissues (Fig. 60.11). This is performed

in an assortment of individual or combined methods and settings in preparation of a wound bed for closure.[54] However, it is important to remember that debridement is merely one, albeit vital, factor in modern wound bed preparation.

Mechanical debridement is perhaps the oldest form of debridement and utilizes a procession of moist or wet flushes or dressings, which are subsequently removed after drying. This causes nonselective debridement of loose tissues and slough. Examples include direct wound irrigation with saline or the like, wet-to-dry dressings, NPWT with instillation and hydrotherapy including bath and whirlpool. This is best suited to wounds with large amounts of loose tissue and is relatively cost-effective given the simple and ubiquitous nature of simple dressing materials like saline and gauze. Additionally, dressing changes are quite simple so changes can be taught to be performed independently in many cases. However, mechanical debridement is considered nonselective in nature and thus may remove or damage healthy tissues if not performed meticulously. This process may be time-consuming as dressings must be changed often and may be painful in the non-neuropathic patient. Additionally, bath and whirlpool therapies can create an unwanted risk of bacterial exposure, can damage fragile tissue, and may risk complications.

Enzymatic debridement utilizes chemical agents to debride necrotic wound tissue. Chemical enzymes are fast-acting products that slough necrotic tissue, some of which are selective, while others are not. Collectively, these enzymes are derived from microorganisms like *Clostridium histolyticum* or from plants, including collagenase, varidase, papain, and bromelain. This method is most useful for debridement of wounds with a large amount of necrotic tissue with little risk to healthy tissues. However, enzymatic debridement is a relatively slow process and a prescription is often required that may be fairly expensive depending on insurance coverage or resource availability. A secondary dressing may be required to absorb exudate, and this may be a painful process to the non-neuropathic patient.

Autolytic debridement utilizes the body's own enzymatic processes to debride necrotic tissues and slough. This process

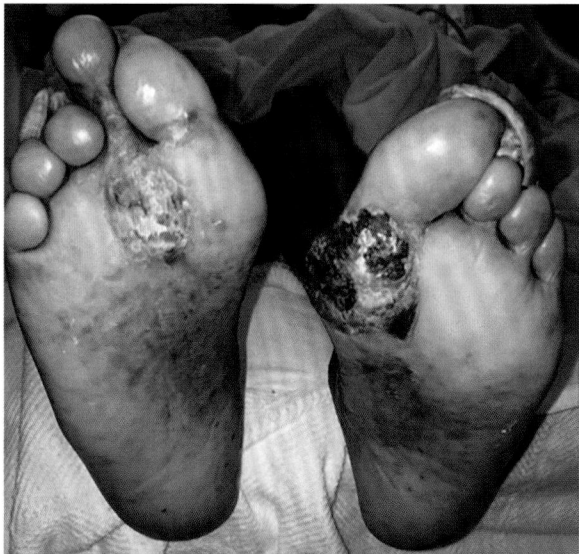
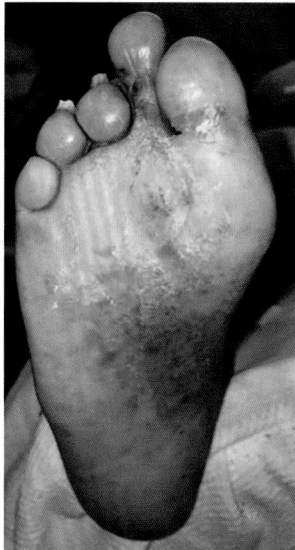
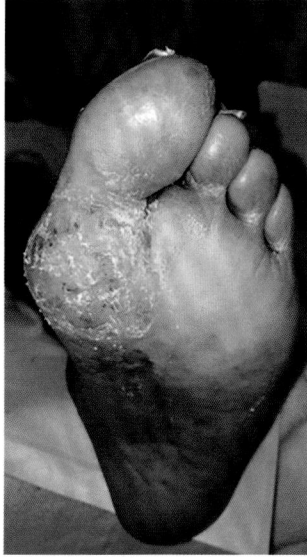

FIGURE 60.11 Sharp debridement of eschar is often utilized in office to prevent wound/ulcer formation, especially in patients who are unable to undergo surgical deformity correction.

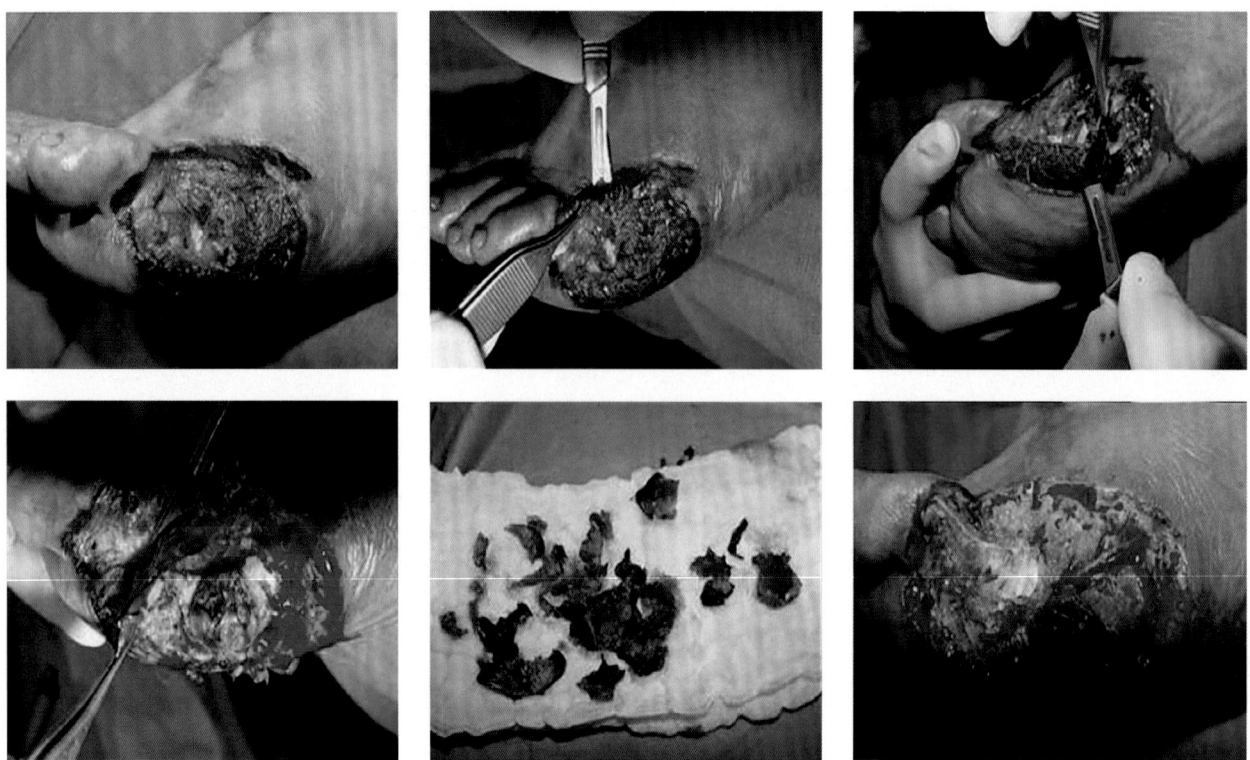

FIGURE 60.12 Debridement is the excision of dead, damaged, or infected tissues in order to optimize healing potential of the remaining healthy and viable tissues.

interrupts dead and devitalized tissue over time by allowing wound fluids to maintain constant contact in the wound bed in order to hydrate, soften, and liquefy necrotic tissue and eschar. This method is achieved with the use of occlusive or semiocclusive dressings with or without the supplementation of hydrocolloids, hydrogels, and transparent films and is suitable for wounds where the amount of dead tissue is not extensive and where no infection exists. Autolytic debridement is selective for necrotic tissues, is easy to perform, and is virtually painless to the patient. However, this is by far the slowest type of debridement and the wound must be rigorously monitored for signs of infection. For these reasons, this method is most times reserved for patients with no resource availability or those requiring holiday from other debridement types.

Biologic debridement employs medical maggots that have been grown in a sterile environment. Several young larvae of the green bottle fly (*Lucilia sericata*) are introduced into a wound bed and secured with a specialized nonocclusive dressing or "maggot house." The maggots nourish selectively on necrotic tissue of the "host" without injuring healthy living tissue and can quite effectively debride a wound in a matter of just a few days. The larvae derive nutrients by secreting a broad spectrum of enzymes that liquefy necrotic tissue for consumption. In an optimum environment, maggots molt twice, increasing in overall size and leaving a clean wound free of necrotic tissue when they are removed. This method has gained popularity over time, but some patients can find the method painful and a patient's aversion to maggots being placed onto the body may impede its use. This debridement method has the advantage of being nonsurgical in nature and works faster than autolytic and enzymatic debridement with little risk to healthy

tissues and as such can be considered a feasible alternative in the treatment of chronic wounds.[55]

Surgical debridement is arguably the most common and varied type of debridement. A myriad of instrumentation and adjuncts are utilized to physically excise nonviable tissue from the wound bed, either at bedside, in clinic, or in an operating room (Fig. 60.11). The surgeon will debride tissue to viability, as determined by tissue character and the presence of vascularity in healthy tissues using any combination of instruments including rongeur, curette, blade, scissors, forceps, and the like (Fig. 60.12). Adjuncts like the micro water jet device have been developed for an even more meticulous and selective debridement. A novel method used by the authors to ensure sufficient debridement of wounds, especially those pending definitive closure, is to completely paint the wound with methylene blue immediately prior to debridement (Fig. 60.13). This provides a clear delineation between more superficially exposed tissues that may harbor bioburden and the healthy tissues immediately deep to this color. Surgical debridement on the whole is best suited for progressive or recalcitrant wounds, larger sized wounds or those in abnormal/precarious locations, grossly infected wounds, and wounds considered of an unknown etiology, which necessitate surgical biopsy or resection. This is easily considered the fastest method of debridement as it is very selective, limited only by the skill and experience of the surgeon. Overall, surgical debridement affords superior control over what and how much tissue is removed, is the fastest way to achieve a clean wound bed, and can speed the healing process in nearly every patient. Although surgical debridement may not be considered as cost-effective given the resources required, it has the benefit of providing relatively expedient wound bed preparation and subsequent closure of a majority of wound types, regardless of etiology.

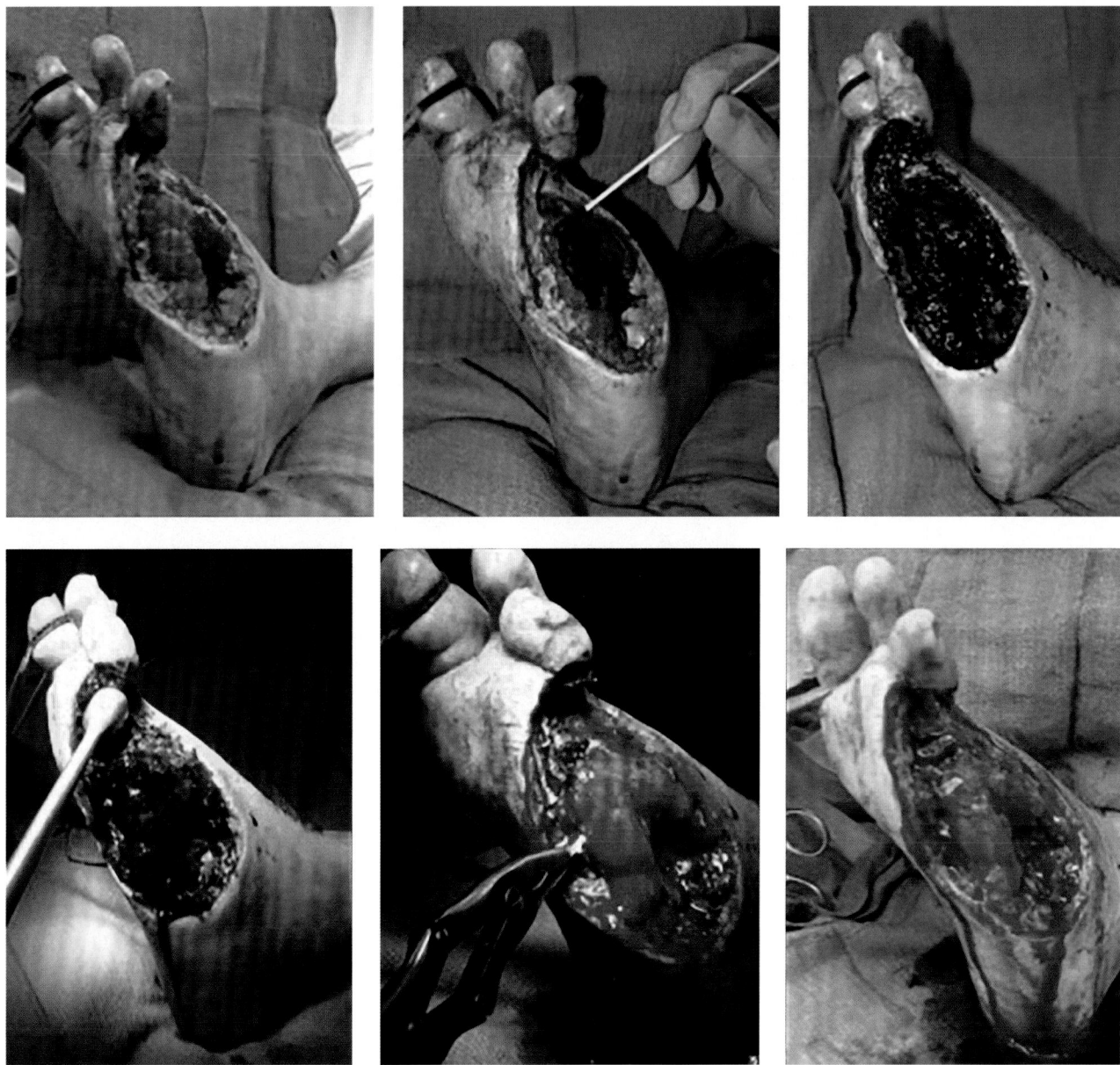

FIGURE 60.13 A method to ensure that sufficient debridement is to completely paint the wound with methylene blue immediately prior to debridement.

OFFLOADING

Vertical and horizontal forces play a deleterious role in the development and chronicity of complex wounds on the plantar aspect of the foot. Vertical forces have been measured to be elevated in areas of ulceration and joint breakdown.[41,47,48,56] The role of horizontal or shear forces have not been as well elucidated.[43,57-59] Regardless, these forces are profound in the environment of a foot that is insensate, is lacking normal mobility, has decreased soft tissue density, and has a potentially compromised blood supply. Ideally, prevention of wound development through the use of functional and accommodative devices and/or extradepth shoes and multidensity insoles is the end goal. However, delayed recognition of an at-risk foot and ankle may result in a nonhealing wound.

There are many modalities available for offloading. The goal is complete non–weight bearing with crutch, walker, knee walker or knee scooter ambulation, or wheel chair use. However, this goal is impractical or even unrealistic for the majority of patients with nonhealing wounds. Some of the more commonly used offloading devices include total contact casting (TCC), removable cast walkers (RCWs), half or wedge shoes, extradepth shoes, and aperture padding. However, these modalities do not equally nor completely offload a wound site.[60,61] It is important to think about the forces not only at the wound site but around the wound periphery as well. For example, a donut-shaped pad with a central aperture would seem to sufficiently offload a small plantar wound. In reality, the forces are transferred to the periphery of the wound and with that increased stress about the wound periphery can inhibit wound closure. This "edge effect" may inhibit wound closure.[62,63] Furthermore,

it is important to evaluate the degree of mobility or rather immobility about the surrounding joints, which will affect the forces experienced at the wound site. The goal of offloading is to redistribute forces evenly throughout the plantar surface of the foot not only at the wound site. This tact will ensure that new ulcerations at different sites do not form as a sequelae of focal stress reduction.

Total Contact Casts

Total contact casts (TCCs) have been the gold standard for offloading of lower extremity wounds and have been validated through randomized controlled trials.[64,65] Although reported complications of TCCs are relatively low, there are some potential drawbacks.[66] First, the TCC technique is time-consuming and labor intensive. The application alone takes a level of skill, technique, and understanding, which makes it difficult for anyone who only occasionally applies it. Improper application can lead to aggravation of current wounds or worse off, the formation new wounds. Furthermore, accommodation for swelling is certainly limited just as it would be in a traditional circumferential cast. Second, inspection of the wound site is impaired and an infection manifested by ascending erythema or increased drainage cannot be adequately visualized or identified due to coverage of the dressing. Third, a TCC can be unwieldy due to its size and weight. This may cause the patient to become unbalanced and at an increased risk for fall as well as at risk for. Despite these potential pitfalls, the TCC has been used successfully in an assortment of environments that employ experienced personnel and who also provide proper education to the patient.

Removable Walking Casts

There are several offloading devices that fall into the category of removable walking cast (RWC). Pressure relief walker (ie, DH Pressure Relie Walker, Royce Medical/Center Orthopedics, Camerillo, CA) and pneumatic walkers (ie, XP Diabetic Walker, Aircast, Summit, NJ) are two more common types. In general, RCWs are similar to CAM walkers in that they extend distally past the toes and come proximally to the midcalf. The outer structural components are generally made of a hard plastic or metal composite with padding along the interior. The plantar surface most often has a rocker bottom sole and is held in place upon the lower extremity with Velcro strapping. RCWs not only redistribute pressure but limit range of motion of the foot and ankle, thus stabilizing joint motion surrounding the wound itself. The pressure relief walker contains a multidensity insert with removable pegs that attempt to offload locally, also available for use in a shoe, allowing for ankle joint motion when appropriate. The pneumatic walker contains adjustable airbladders within the shell to maximize fit and reduce foot motion or "pistoning" within the device. Both types of RCWs have shown to effectively reduce pressures at a plantar wound site.[60-68] RCWs are off-the-shelf products that are easy to apply but come in limiting sizes and standard contours. The convenience of these products makes them a prevalent offloading choice. However, it should be noted that since RCWs can be easily removed, the patient may elect to remove the device outside of prescribed instances, rendering the device useless. Strategies to prevent nonadherence in this fashion include applying a layer of fiberglass casting material or Coban dressing around the RCW, effectively making the RCW function at an "instant TCC."[69]

Other Offloading Strategies

Many other strategies and techniques for offloading exist, including half or wedge shoes and accommodative devices. Half shoes or wedge shoes provide a platform of decreased weight bearing. The design is similar to a surgical shoe except that an elevated heel or forefoot is incorporated. This allows for the weight to be shifted either to the rearfoot or the forefoot depending on wound location. These have shown to effectively but partially offload, just not to the degree of a TCC or RCW.[67,68,70] Many patients report difficulty with balance and nonadherence with these devices.

Accommodative devices such as felted foam and aperture pads are also used to offload wounds. Accommodative devices are typically made by layering different materials of different durometers. For example, felted foam pads have been shown to reduce peak plantar pressures.[67] The use of felted foam pad involves the removal of a portion of the felted foam that corresponds to the wound site but incorporates the entirety of the plantar aspect of the foot. An accurate fit is essential to the success of this device both around the wound site and within the shoe itself. A donut-shaped pad should be used with caution due to the "edge effect" as previously described. Further, anchoring such a device may be difficult as it may migrate from the wound site or cause adhesive reaction to the surrounding tissues.

External Fixators

The use of external fixation is a viable alternative to the aforementioned offloading strategies, especially when strict offloading or additional structural stability is absolutely necessary. An external fixator may be applied either immediately following a definitive reconstructive closure attempt or during an interim period where an open surgical site requires offloading or structural support. Patients with tenuous or fragile grafts or flaps or other procedures like joint arthroplasty or fusion, osteotomy, and hardware removal/exchange may benefit from the weight relief and/or structural support provided by an external fixator (Fig. 60.14). A wire or pin frame may be applied in innumerable construct fashions and a number of manufacturers provide circular or "Ilizarov" frames, principally aimed at offloading or providing immobilization of a particular area about the foot and ankle. The primary shortcoming to this type of offloading is the morbidity associated with such a construct. Well-known potential complications associated with external fixation frames include pin or wire site irritation and/or infection, pin or wire failure, pin or wire-associated fracture, as well as external fixator associated psychosis or "cage rage." Certainly, not every patient is considered a candidate for this type of offloading, and those under consideration should be properly counseled about the realistic expectations, the benefits of such a construct, and the potential for complication.

ADJUVANTS

Topical Formulations

There exist a plethora of topical solutions utilized in conjunction with debridement for the conservative management of wounds in the form of pastes, ointments, and gels. These include debriding agents, antibiotics, and prograntulation formulations. The ease of application and noninvasive nature make these products make these products a simple but effective adjunct to wound care.

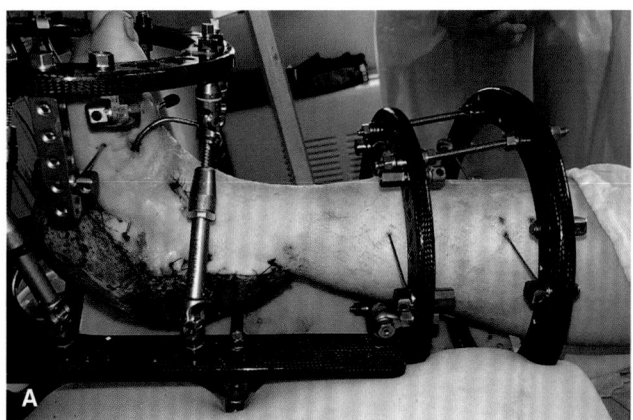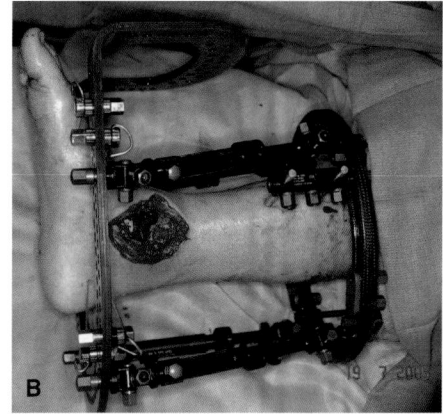

FIGURE 60.14 A, B. External fixation is an excellent solution for offloading or providing structural stability to patients with tenuous or fragile grafts or flaps, joint arthroplasty, fusion, osteotomy, and hardware removal/exchange.

Commonly utilized topical antibiotics include triple antibiotic, mupirocin, gentamicin, silver sulfadiazine, and cadexomer iodine. Triple antibiotic is a formulation of bacitracin zinc, neomycin sulfate, and polymyxin B sulfate. Topical antibiotics have been shown to be effective against uncomplicated soft tissue infection and have a place in the management of mild non-healing wound infections.[71,72] Bacitracin zinc is effective against gram-positive bacteria, including *Staphylococcus*. Neomycin sulfate belongs in the class of the aminoglycosides and hence has activity against gram-negative bacteria with some gram-positive coverage. Polymyxin B sulfate is effective against gram-negative bacilli like *Pseudomonas*. Mupirocin primarily has activity against *Staphylococcal* and *Streptococcal* species. Further, mupirocin has been demonstrated to be effective against methicillin-resistant *Staphylococcus aureus* (MRSA).[73,74] Gentamicin belongs to the aminoglycoside class of antibiotics, with broad-spectrum activity, which includes *Pseudomonas*. On a whole, topical antibiotics should be reserved for mild superficial infections. Topical antibiotics can be used in combination with oral antibiotics for infection control. The authors do not recommend prolonged use of topical antibiotics due to the potential development of drug resistance. Daily application for the management of mild infection associated with chronic wound or in patients who cannot tolerate oral or parental antibiotics are examples of judicious use of this type of therapy.

Two other commonly used antibacterial topicals include silver sulfadiazine (Silvadene, King Pharmaceuticals Inc., Bristol, TN) and cadexomer iodine (Iodosorb/Iodoflex, Smith & Nephew, Largo, FL). Silver sulfadiazine is a commonly used topical cream with broad-spectrum activity including both gram-positive and gram-negative bacteria. Caution should be used, however, for patients with sensitivities or allergies to sulfamides. Cadexomer iodine ointment consists of a starch polymer bead infused with 0.9% iodine. Exudate is absorbed by the starch polymer with the subsequent release of the iodine, which acts as an antibacterial in the wound. Although this product has been primarily used for venous stasis ulcerations, it has a significant role in the exudative nonhealing wounds.[75] Silver sulfadiazine and cadexomer iodine can be used to decrease the likelihood of infection in an uninfected wound site. Hence, these products can be used for a sustained duration without deleterious effects.

There are also topical products that promote granulation at a wound site. We will focus our discussion on the two more commonly utilized products: becaplermin and hydrogels. Becaplermin (Regranex Gel, Systagenix, New Brunswick, NJ) consists of recombinant human platelet-derived growth factor (rhPDGF). Becaplermin should be applied daily to the wound site and covered by a saline-moistened gauze dressing with debridement performed at each office visit. Of note, this product does require refrigeration between applications. Literatures have demonstrated that becaplermin is a safe product that promotes wound healing at a faster rate vs a placebo gel.[76-78] Hydrogels (AmericGel Wound Dressing, Amerx Health Care Crop, Clearwater, FL and Curasol Gel Wound Dressing, Healthpoint Ltd., Fort Worth, TX) have been shown effective, relatively inexpensive products used to promote wound healing.[79] Hydrogels will create a sustained moist environment with daily applications. Hydrogels will consist of polymers (ie, polyethylene glycol), water, humectant (promotor of moisture retention), and other added ingredients, which come in a variety of forms, including gels and sheets. These added ingredients may include antibacterial components and debriding agents. This product should be reserved for smaller, superficial, and minimally exudative wounds.

Dressings

Dressing materials represent a great diversity of function in the approach to wound healing, including the promotion of granulation tissue formation by actively preventing infection and filling potential space where fluid may otherwise collect, while simultaneously drawing exudate away from the wound bed and protecting the wound from pressure and shear. An understanding of the different dressing categories and uses allows for a better patient-specific dressing selection.[15,80]

Twice-daily normal saline-moistened gauze dressing changes have historically been a fundamental treatment regimen for wounds of any kind. A moist environment promotes wound healing and the ease of application allows for frequent direct inspection. Further, the gauze dressing acts as a physical barrier to bacterial contamination. The clinician must be careful not to oversaturate the gauze, which may iatrogenically cause maceration of the surrounding tissues and worsening of the

primary wound character. Further, undersaturation will transform the moistened gauze into a wet-to-dry dressing, which may damage healthy tissues during its removal. Some of the more common solutions include diluted acetic acid (vinegar) and diluted sodium hypochlorite (Dakin solution). Daily or twice-daily dressing changes with gauze moistened with diluted acetic acid may be utilized for wounds that are questionably or mildly infected and specifically has been shown to be effective in the treatment multibacterial infected wounds including *Pseudomonal* infections.[81,82] Diluted sodium hypochlorite can been used as part of daily or twice daily dressing changes in wounds that are grossly infected; however, use of even diluted sodium hypochlorite should be used for no more than 3-4 days consecutively due to the potential caustic effects on healthy surrounding tissues and cells involved in wound healing (ie, fibroblasts, keratinocytes, neutrophils, endothelial cells).[83,84] It is important to note that topical dressing solutions should not be used in isolation when an infection is suspected. Oral or parenteral antibiotics should be utilized in conjunction with the dressing solutions along with appropriate debridement and offloading.

Silver-impregnated dressings are frequently applied to wound sites as silver ions have demonstrated to have antimicrobial activity.[85-87] Silver-impregnated dressing materials have reported to have positive effects on wound healing, although there are very few robust studies specifically examining its efficacy in the nonhealing wound.[88-90] These dressing materials contain a reservoir of silver that is released when contacted with fluid within the wound. Silver is also added as a component with other dressing materials, including hydrocolloids, alginates, foams, and polyesters. Due to their antibacterial properties, these dressing materials can be left in place for 3-7 days before requiring replacement, depending on the amount of exudate produced. Further, these products can be used in combination with other wound adjuncts including NPWT.

There are other large categories of dressing materials used on chronic wounds, the more commonly utilized categories being absorptive wound fillers, foams, hydrocolloids, and collagens. Absorptive wound fillers include alginates and starch copolymers. This encompasses a large group of dressing materials that come in a wide variety of forms including sheets, ropes, strands, powders, and pastes. These dressing materials are used in exudative wounds and function by drawing fluid away from the wound surface. Depending on the amount of exudate, the dressing should be changed every 1-3 days. Of note, care should be taken with excessively packing the absorptive wound filler because this can become a nidus for infection if not removed in total, especially in deeper or tracking wounds. Foams are most often constructed from polyurethane (polymer), which provide for a moist environment allowing for autolytic debridement. These also come in a variety of forms and should be changed every 1-7 days. Hydrocolloids will also create an environment for autolytic debridement by interacting with the wound bed, creating an occlusive or semiocclusive gel. Consistent with most dressing materials, this product comes in a variety of forms. However, hydrocolloids have a limited capacity to absorb fluid and thus should not be used for more exudative wounds.

Topical collagens are typically combined with other materials including alginates or hydrogels. Collagen has the ability to absorb significant volumes of exudate and dissolves at the wound site. Promogran (Systagenix, New Brunswick, NJ) is composed of collagen and oxidized regenerative cellulose. Promogran's mechanism of action involves its interaction with

MMPs and TIMPs in the wound bed,[91,92] thereby stimulating wound healing. In a dry wound, this product should be moistened with sterile saline prior to application in order to change the product into a gel.

Contact dressings in and of themselves do not have any wound healing properties. They are, however, often used in conjunction with other wound care products. Contact dressings can be applied directly on the wound surface or over other products. Some examples include Adaptic (Systagenix, New Brunswick, NJ) and Mepitel (Molnlycke, Goteborg, Sweden). Adaptic is a cellulose fabric mesh coated with a light oil emulsion that is often used at surgical incision sites. Mepitel is a semitransparent polyamide coated with silicone. Generally, contact dressings are porous, allowing exudate to leave the wound site. Further, these dressings are low adherent or nonadherent to the wound surface, which minimizes pain and irritation during dressing removal.

Bioengineered Alternative Tissue

Living cell-based bioengineered alternative tissue (BAT) products stimulate the wound healing process in the wound bed or can serve to deliver growth factors when applied to the wound. Importantly, BAT products promote the conversion of a stagnant wound to an acute wound and are used in different wound types and at different stages than autogenous skin grafting. Some BATs contain living fibroblast and keratinocytes in addition to growth factors. When selecting a specific BAT product, it is important to bear in mind the different layers of tissue and their architecture. In some cases, a specific product choice can be made to match the wound depth and nature. When BAT products are used incorrectly, though, the results have a lesser degree of predictable success. Whereas proper selection increases the likelihood of successful wound closure.

Each BAT product has been specifically designed to interact with the wound environment in a unique manner. As such, not all BATs are the same, in terms of structure and function. "Dermoinductive" BATs are derived from living cell cultures, which contain human living keratinocytes and/or fibroblasts imbedded within the product. These cells actively participate in the recruitment and activation of the wound tissues. Generally, these are utilized for superficial wounds. "Dermoconductive" BATs serve as a scaffolding matrix, which allows for an organized infiltration of cells from the surrounding tissue. Generally, these are utilized for deeper wounds, which allow for the wound to "build up."

Numerous companies produce an array of different BATs, which may be used in the same degree. The decision for use should be based on the percent decrease in wound dimensions and/or degree of granulation tissue noted in the wound bed. Prior to application, and regardless of the specific BAT used, the wound should be free of infection and adequate tissue vascularity should be established. Each product will have its own specifics for application; however, a general protocol should be adhered to. Application should begin with thorough wound debridement. Depending on the fenestration requirements, the products are then applied to the wound and should be "tacked down" utilizing sutures or staples. The authors prefer absorbable sutures or staples depending on wound size, location, and topography. A nonadherent dressing is then applied atop, and the wound is evaluated weekly for the possibility of infection. Most BAT products will integrate within 3-4 weeks.

The BAT products can promote complete epithelialization of a wound; however, a split-thickness skin graft may be more effective and efficient in achieving final closure. In contrast, the BAT products may require sequential application of different products or repeated applications of the same product to ultimately achieve closure.

Negative-Pressure Wound Therapy

NPWT has become ubiquitous in the treatment of both acute and chronic wounds. Whether it is used as a supplement to primary wound closure, as a precursor to delayed closure, or for preparation of the wound bed for additional therapies, NPWT plays an important role in all processes of wound closure.

Since its inception, NPWT has been reported with successful outcomes in the medical and surgical literature for the treatment of an assortment of wound types.[93-101] NPWT will promote granulation by decreasing bacterial bioburden and increasing capillary budding at the wound base. Additionally, its superiority over more "standard" wound care modalities has been well established and its variability of use via adjustable settings and formations makes it an excellent adjunct to wound treatment.

Standard NPWT protocol includes the setting of −125 mm Hg of negative pressure with options between continuous and intermittent suction. A common example of a portable NPWT device is the vacuum-assisted closure (VAC) (Kinetic Concepts International, San Antonio, TX). This apparatus essentially contains a motorized suction unit connected to plastic tubing, which is then inserted into an open-cell foam that is cut to the shape of the wound and placed directly onto the wound bed. Multiple wounds can be linked and serviced by a single unit and semiadherent or nonadherent dressings may be placed into the wound base in order to prevent adhesion of new granulation tissues into the foam. The foam is covered by a transparent occlusive "drape" dressing and negative pressure is set at a continuous or intermittent pattern with easy adjustability. A new foam and dressing is reapplied every 3-7 days.

As NPWT has become increasingly prevalent, various adjunctive techniques and modifications have been adopted. The use of NPWT atop the application of split-thickness skin grafts and BATs provides a more predictable and uniform antishear dressing vs historical gauze "bolster" dressings.[102-107]

Hyperbaric Oxygen Therapy

HBO therapy has been demonstrated to be effective as an adjunctive therapy in some chronic wound management.[108-110] This wound care modality should be used as a supplement in conjunction with other wound care modalities and specifically may be beneficial in patients with microvascular disease causing local wound ischemia. Transcutaneous oximetry may be beneficial in assessing local tissue perfusion prior to utilizing HBO. HBO involves the administration of 100% oxygen inhaled while in a compression chamber. The compression chamber is set at an ambient pressure of >1 atmosphere absolute (typically 2.0-2.5 atmosphere absolutes). Each treatment session or "dive" lasts 60-120 minutes and is generally conducted 1-2 times daily for a total of 15-30 treatments. HBO therapy essentially attempts to increase oxygenation at wound sites by increasing the partial pressure of oxygen in the arterial circulation, which, in turn, increases the diffusion of oxygen into those tissues. This increased level of oxygenation at wound sites has been

purported to have positive effects including enhancement of antibacterial components, increasing fibroblast activation, upregulation of growth factors, promotion of collagen synthesis, and angiogenesis.[110-115]

Important considerations for HBO, as with all wound care modalities, are that PVD must be considered and addressed. Regardless of the physiology of HBO, oxygenation will not reach the wound tissues if peripheral vascular occlusion exists. Particularly, large vessel disease will limit oxygenated blood from reaching the target tissues.

Adverse effects of HBO include barotrauma to the tympanic membrane and sinuses and transient myopia. Further, elevated levels of oxygen can be toxic to brain and lung tissues. HBO is an expensive wound care modality and is time-consuming and not without potential complications. Therefore, a careful assessment of the cost-benefit ratio should be conducted prior to use and only ever in a state-sanctioned HBO facility with properly licensed HBO specialists.

PLASTIC AND RECONSTRUCTIVE LADDER

CONSIDERATIONS

Following the eradication of infection and the optimization of local and systemic healing factors, a wound is said to be prepared or "primed" for closure. At this juncture, an assortment of options exists on the plastic and reconstructive ladder (Fig. 60.15) for definitive closure including (1) primary closure and delayed primary closure; (2) secondary closure; (3) skin grafting; (4) intrinsic tissue flaps; (5) extrinsic tissue flaps; and (6) free tissue transfers.[116] It is incumbent upon the surgeon

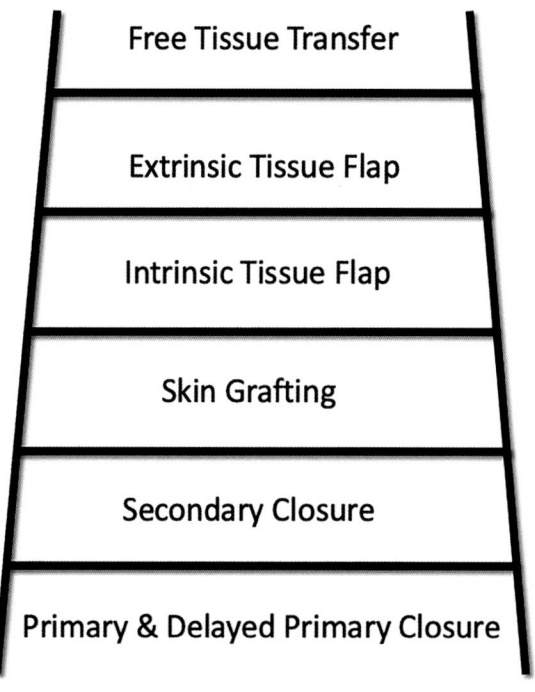

FIGURE 60.15 Modern plastic and reconstructive ladder for definitive closure includes (1) primary closure and delayed primary closure; (2) secondary closure; (3) skin grafting; (4) intrinsic tissue flaps; (5) extrinsic tissue flaps; and (6) free tissue transfers.

to choose the most appropriate method(s) of reconstruction based on the availability of resources, logistical feasibility for both the patient and surgeon, wound characteristics including location and topography, and concomitant factors, which may either advance or retard wound healing. In general, a greater majority of chronic wounds will ascribe to a more simplistic nature of closure via primary, delayed primary, or secondary closure and skin grafting, where warranted. A minority of complex wounds will require definitive closure via tissue flap reconstruction, and in these cases, it is only when necessary to cover vital structures like bone, tendon, or capsule. It is dependent upon the surgeon to discern when and where to implement or supplement with each of these methods of reconstruction in order to provide the most expedient and longest lasting, if not conclusive result for the patient.

Of note, Mathes and Nahai[117] used the metaphor of the reconstructive ladder to integrate flap procedures with the standard procedures of the time (Fig. 60.16). The original goal of the "ladder" was to allow the surgeon to consider options for wound closure in a systematic way with the steps of the ladder arranged from simple to complex in ascending order, and the surgeon figuratively climbed as far as necessary to bring the goal of wound closure to fruition. This framework presumably increased the reliability of outcomes and decreased morbidity by identifying the simplest procedure suitable for a problem while eliminating unnecessarily complicated strategies. However, the term "ladder" carries with it the connotation that one must progress from one level to the next in succession, and perhaps this undertone has perpetuated over the years. This tact could not be more untrue, however. In actuality, one may move to any level or level(s) on the plastic and reconstructive ladder as long as appropriate. In this way, it is important to consider that the reconstructive ladder is merely a useful metaphor, where one can progress from any level to any other without the necessity to stop at each level along the way.

Maximizing lower extremity function, though, is a significant consideration for any wound and for every patient. Regardless of confounding factors associated with the successful closure or reconstruction of a nonhealing wound, the ability to maximize a patient's function is of dire consequence. Poor consideration for a patient's functional demands and limitations can perpetuate a cascade of events that ultimately results in failure or

recurrence. Supplementary procedures to afford a preservation or increase in functional limb capacity may include soft tissue procedures like tendon lengthening or tendon transfer or bony procedures such as exostectomy, amputation, or joint arthroplasty or fusion. Notably, considerations for functional limb preservation can afford patients a more expedited recovery, greater likelihood for avoidance of recurrence, and a superior quality of life. For these reasons, limb function should always be a consideration prior to definitive procedure selection on the plastic and reconstructive ladder.

TISSUE HANDLING

Regardless of the precise method of closure selected, proper tissue handling is paramount and may quite literally "make or break" an attempted wound closure. Bunnell[118] first coined the term "atraumatic technique" to describe how soft tissues should be handled during surgery. An atraumatic technique should be implemented at all times in order to preserve vascularity to the existing tissues and maximize the potential for healing. One should minimize excessive traction and manipulation of the tissues. This is best accomplished with strictly intent motions and manipulations and blunt retraction only when necessary for proper visualization. Proper instrumentation selection is key to preserving an atraumatic technique. A thorough understanding and knowledge of the available instrumentation and more importantly how well a particular surgical task can be accomplished in one's hands is crucial. For example, the authors often prefer to forego the use of forceps for tissue handling unless absolutely necessary, especially during suturing as this may cause repeated trauma to the microvasculature of the wound periphery. Rather, the use of strategically positioned and oriented sutures is best utilized for transposition, rotation, and overall manipulation of tissues during a definitive closure. Ideally, when utilizing suture material, one should use a nonabsorbable monofilament. The authors prefer a vertical mattress technique when reapproximating skin layers directly and absorbable monofilament when affixing grafts and supplementing with staples where warranted.

PRIMARY CLOSURE (PRIMARY INTENTION)

Primary closure, also known as healing by primary intention, is the direct and normally uncomplicated healing of smaller and clean soft tissue defects, often surgical incisions. These wounds require new blood vessels and keratinocytes to migrate only a small distance and as such typically do not succumb to chronicity unless plagued by mitigating local or systemic factors. The phases of the wound healing cascade are respected without interruption. Small cutaneous wounds like paper cuts usually heal by primary intention as the skin edges are closely approximated and results in dermal coaptation for definitive closure.

SECONDARY CLOSURE (SECONDARY INTENTION)

Secondary closure, also known as healing by secondary intention, is the indirect healing of unapproximated dermal layers. This is accomplished via the gradual filling of a soft tissue deficit with the formation of a granulation tissue matrix and epithelialization atop. Intuitively, this type of closure requires more time, energy, and observation relative to primary closure, however, may be the preferred method of definitive closure based on its

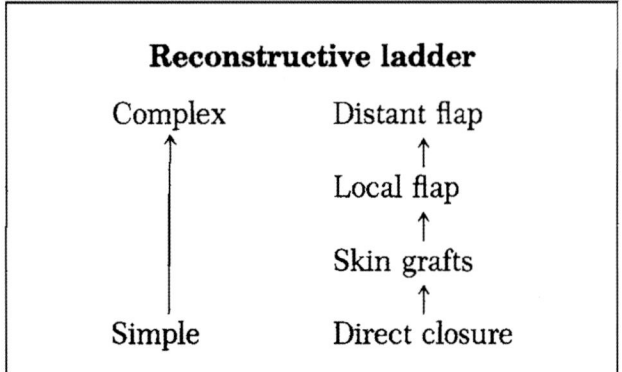

FIGURE 60.16 Original plastic and reconstructive ladder as delineated by Mathes and Nahai. (Reprinted with permission from Mathes S, Nahai F. *Clinical Application for Muscle and Musculocutaneous Flaps.* St Louis, MO: Mosby; 1982:3.)

simplicity. Still, this closure places the wound at a greater likelihood of infection secondary to its maintenance in an "open" state and must be carefully monitored during its progression through the healing cascade.

DELAYED PRIMARY CLOSURE (TERTIARY INTENTION)

Delayed primary closure, or healing by tertiary intension, is a variation of primary closure but with the caveat that the wound undergoes a period of purposeful observation prior to definitive closure. This period of observation permits sufficient time for the eradication of infection and devitalized tissues as well as for the maximization of tissue perfusion and systemic factors for healing. Local eradication of infection and devitalized tissues is best achieved by serial debridement with an array of adjuvants, as mentioned earlier in this chapter. Advances in technology, such as NPWT, have provided an array of options for facilitating delayed primary closure. As part of closure by tertiary intention, free flaps and rotational flaps are used to provide soft tissue coverage, along with the innovation of secondary intention wound granulation with NPWT-assisted dressings and hemostatic bandages.[119]

GRAFTS

Grafting involves transferring of a portion of tissue, devoid of its blood supply, from one part of the body to another. A skin graft specifically provides coverage of a wound and reduces the complications and disability associated with prolonged healing. Skin grafts have low complication rates compared with more invasive procedures, such as cutaneous flaps or the like. The donor site may be left to heal secondarily from the remaining dermal structures and wound margins or may be closed primarily with excision of the exposed dermal tissues and approximation of the remaining tissue edges. Skin grafts, in general, can be classified as *autografts* (from the same individual), *allografts* (from the same species), or *xenografts* (from different species).[120] Xenografts are used only as temporary biologic dressings as they will not show the discrete signs of healing.[121] Advances in cultured epithelia may provide new alternatives in skin graft coverage.[122] Cultured epithelial cells for grafting can expand up to 10 000 times the original surface area and can provide a significant amount of skin graft coverage in the severely burned patients.[123] Autogenous skin grafts are divided into two general types: full-thickness skin grafts (FTSGs) and split-thickness skin grafts (STSGs), with distinction based on the thickness of dermis within the graft.

Split-Thickness Skin Grafts

As the name suggests, STSGs include the epidermis and a portion of the dermis. STSGs vary in the amount of dermis that is included, and they are generally classified as thin (0.008-0.012 in), intermediate (0.013-0.016 in), and thick (0.017-0.02 in)[124] (Fig. 60.17). The thinner the graft, the more likely a graft is to "take." The reason may be the increased number of small vessels located in the superficial dermis that are transected during the harvesting process. These transected vessels aid in the revascularization process. Thinner grafts also have less tissue to support with the available blood supply. The higher initial success rate is the main advantage to using a thin graft over thicker grafts. However, a thinner graft undergoes a greater degree of contraction because of the smaller amount of dermis that is

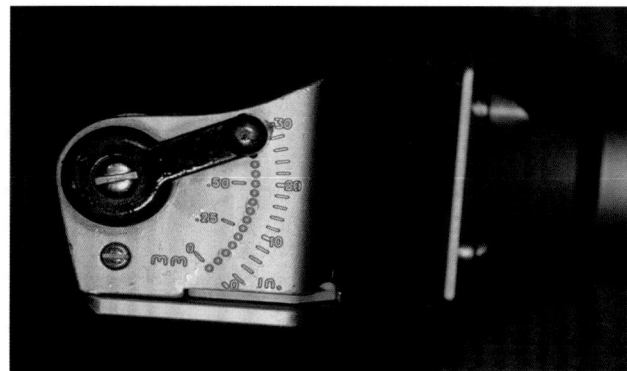

FIGURE 60.17 Skin graft thickness may be set directly at the dermatome device.

present. Thicker grafts retain more of the dermal appendages, a feature that makes them more durable and provides a better cosmetic appearance. One must balance these considerations with the anticipated stress that will be applied to the area once it is healed. STSGs should only be used in areas of adequate vascularity with a healthy wound base and are not to be used to cover vital or relatively avascular structures such as tendon, cartilage, or bone.[125] However, a tendon that is covered by paratenon or bone that is covered by periosteum may support an STSG. Furthermore, an STSG may be used to cover small avascular regions, <0.5 cm in diameter, by a process known as "bridging."[126] When harvesting a skin graft, the donor site should be prepared with saline or mineral oil to allow the dermatome to slide smoothly across the skin surface and prevent binding or bunching of the skin that can lead to uneven graft thickness harvesting. The dermatome is held at ~45 degrees relative to the skin with firm and constant pressure applied as the dermatome is advanced. An assistant can help to guide the graft as it presents itself in the dermatome. When enough graft has been harvested, the dermatome is lifted from the surface in a scooping action and should be kept running until it leaves the skin surface. This allows the graft to be separated cleanly from the donor site. Adequate graft should be taken to cover the wound. If extra graft is harvested, it may be replaced on the donor site and will aid in reepithelization at this level. Frequently, the STSG is meshed to allow the graft to expand and to cover more surface area and to permit drainage, either with a mechanical mesher or manually with a scalpel blade via a "pie crusting" technique (Fig. 60.18).

Full-Thickness Skin Grafts

FTSGs include the epidermis, dermis, and most of the dermal appendages. These types of skin grafts are more durable because of the overall thickness and the retention of sebaceous glands. Moreover, hair follicles remain in the graft; therefore, an appropriate donor site should be chosen for the desired cosmetic result. Because there is more tissue to be supported while the blood supply is being reestablished, this graft has a higher failure rate. The flexor creases, such as the popliteal fossa, the inguinal area, and the gluteal fold, are common donor sites. Small grafts, sometimes referred to as "pinch grafts," can also be taken from the sinus tarsi area. Harvesting the graft in line with the flexor crease results in formation of a scar parallel to the RSTLs and facilitates primary closure of the donor site. Harvesting of the graft begins by drawing the outline of the incisions on the skin. An elliptic incision in a 3:1 length allows

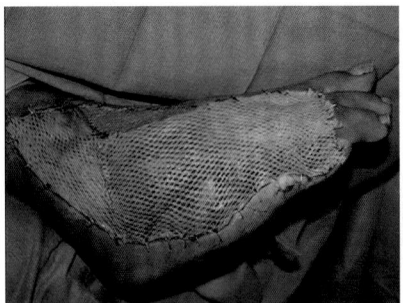 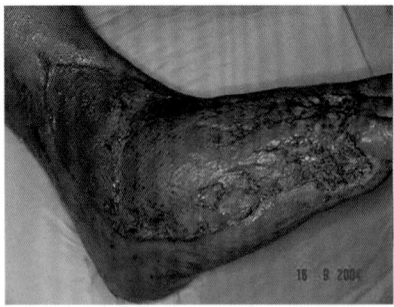 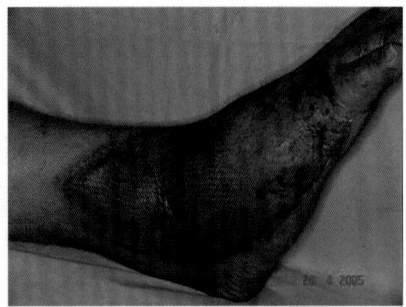

FIGURE 60.18 Split-thickness skin grafts (STSGs) are an excellent choice for definitive closure of a "primed" wound bed.

primary closure with minimal tension. Adequate graft should be harvested to allow for minimal tension across the graft when it is sutured to the recipient site. The graft is excised from the donor area by dissecting through the dermis and taking as little adipose tissue as possible with the skin. The donor site is then closed primarily. All remaining adipose tissue should be removed by stretching the graft. FTSGs are not meshed, but pie crusting may be used to promote drainage if a potential hematoma or seroma is of great concern. More sutures are often required with a FTSG to stretch the tissue back to its original size. As with STSG, the graft must be in complete contact with the recipient bed. The postoperative course is also similar to that of patients with an STSG. Seroma, hematoma, infection, and shear forces are the greatest threats to graft survival. Once healing has taken place, a FTSG provides a more cosmetically pleasing and durable result than an STSG.

FLAPS

The term "flap" is defined as a segment of tissue that is transferred or rotated to restore a tissue defect.[127] Unlike grafts, though, flaps will retain in some capacity, their own vascular supply, and sensorium in many instances. The base of the flap, which retains vascularity, is referred to as the *pedicle*. The pedicle may include a portion of skin, subcutaneous tissue, and the vascular supply, or it may be limited to the vascular structures, such as an island flap or free flap, as is later discussed.

Classification

It is important to understand that although there exists a multitude of methods in which to classify flaps, there is no system that perfectly classifies all flaps types,[128] especially since the nomenclature for many types of flaps cannot be standardized. However, for purposes of this chapter, we offer two well-known and well-accepted methods by which to simplistically categorize flaps. Flaps may be classified by either the motion the flap undergoes or by its vascularity. Flaps classified according to motion may take place from a local or a distant donor site. Flaps categorized by vascularity may be categorized into random and axial patterns.

Classification by Motion
Local Flaps
Local flaps encompass a wide array of flap types. Most simplistically, these flaps are created in the soft tissues in close proximity to the defect and may be further subdivided as advancement, rotational, transpositional, and interpolational flaps.[129] Advancement flaps have fixed points that are stretched as the donor tissue is

pulled into the recipient bed. Examples of advancement flaps include bipedicle flaps and V to Y advancement flaps. Rotational flaps are semicircular and are rotated about a pivot point (Fig. 60.19). Transpositional flaps are also rotated about a point, however, are composed of linear dimensions such as squares or rectangles, not circular or semicircular. Interpolational flaps are also rotated about a pivot point; however, they differ from rotational and transpositional flaps as the flap will pass over or under intact tissue between donor and recipient sites.[129]

Distant Flaps
Distant flaps are those that are transferred from another region of the body, such as a free flap or cross-extremity flap. These flaps are often used for larger defects of the foot and ankle region. Distant flaps require more advanced technical expertise including such specialized techniques as microsurgery and are most often performed by an experienced plastic surgeon trained in free tissue transfer techniques.

Classification by Vascularity Grabb and Myers[130] were the first to classify cutaneous flaps according to the source of vascularity. This classification is particularly useful because the vessels supplying the flap are the chief factor, which limits their motion. Flaps classified on their vascular supply fall into two categories: random-pattern flaps and axial-pattern flaps.

Random Flaps
A random flap is vascularized by the cutaneous dermal-subdermal plexus. These flaps lack a primary artery and vein and rely on the perfusion of the dermal-subdermal vessels from the pedicle of the flap. The ability of the pedicle to provide adequate blood to the tissues limits a random flap's length. A length-to-base ratio of 1:1 is generally accepted to provide adequate vascular perfusion to the distal end of the flap.[131] Thus, the base must remain wide, a feature that can greatly limit flap mobility and rotation. Some have reported success with a 2:1 ratio; however, a 1.5:1 ratio provides consistently successful outcomes and anecdotally the most practical in foot and ankle surgery.

Axial Flaps
Axial flaps contain a primary artery and vein that are incorporated into the pedicle of the flap. Therefore, perfusion depends on the axial artery rather than the width of the pedicle and cutaneous perfusion. Any portion of the flap distal to the direct supply of the axial artery is effectively a random flap and is perfused by the dermal-subdermal plexus. As a result, this portion of the flap is subject to the length-to-base ratio at the distal end to maintain a good vascular supply.

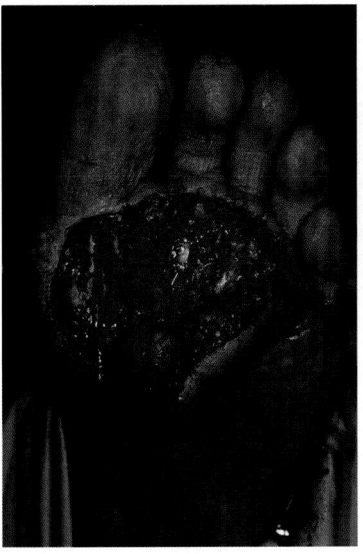
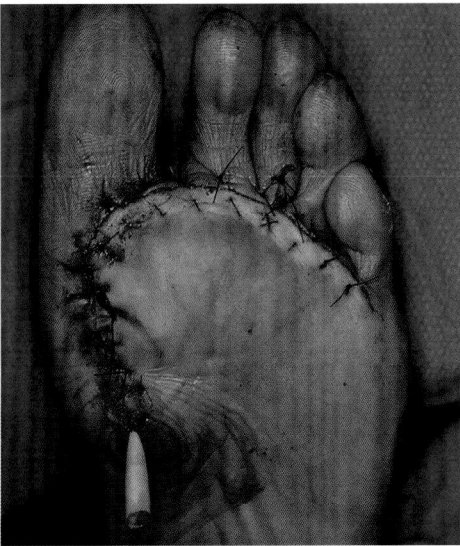
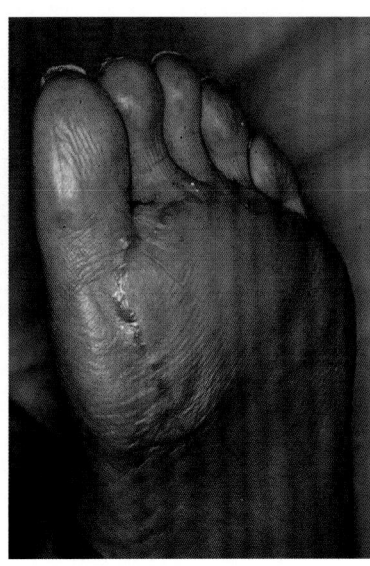

FIGURE 60.19 Clinical appearance of a semicircular rotational flap, rotated about a single pivot point.

Local Flaps

Random Flaps

V to Y and Y to V Flap

The V to Y skin flap is advancement flaps that are useful in lengthening scar contractures or in reducing contracted digits[132] (Fig. 60.20). Because this is a random pattern flap, the apex may be placed either proximally or distally. Generally,

the wider the base of the flap, the greater the blood supply to the distal segment, thereby reducing the risk of flap necrosis. The full thickness of the tissues should be undermined minimally before advancement to release any existing tension limiting the flap's mobility. The flap is advanced in the direction opposite the apex to create the lengthening desired with the conversion of a V-shaped incision to a Y-shaped incision.

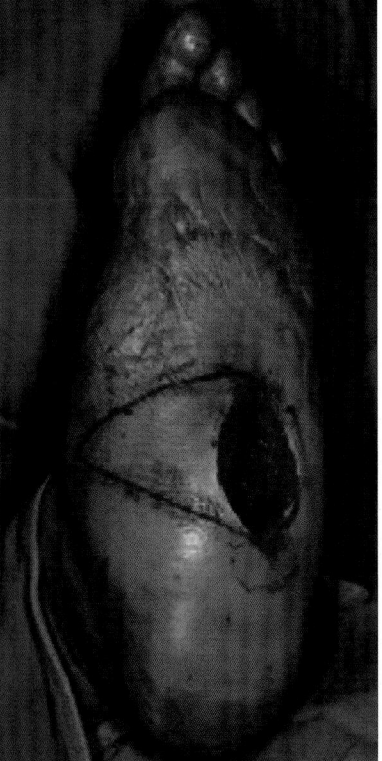
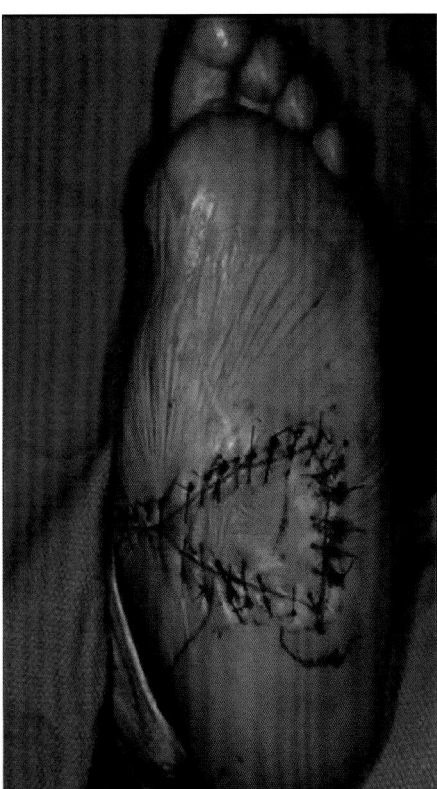
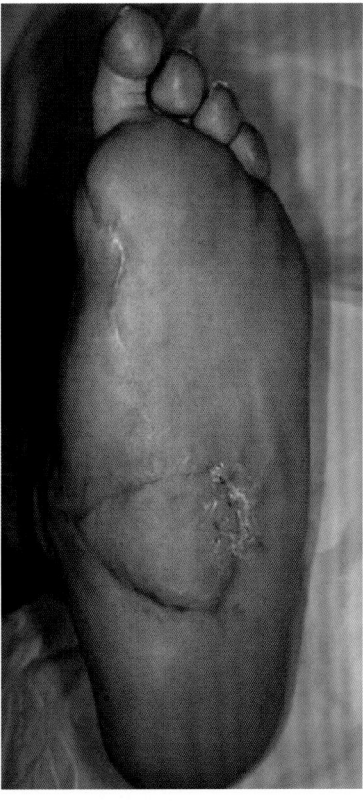

FIGURE 60.20 Clinical appearance of a V to Y flap, advanced in the direction opposite the apex to create the tissue transposition desired with the conversion of a V-shaped incision to a Y-shaped incision.

The Y to V approach can also be used to create length, but with this technique, the lengthening occurs perpendicular to the stem of the Y, because the flap is advanced in the direction of the apex.[133] More commonly, the Y to V approach is used to cover defects or to create shortening in line with the direction of advancement.

A variation of the V to Y skin plasty is an advancement flap used to cover small defects on the plantar surface of the foot.[134] The base of the V is oriented next to the wound defect. The wound is excised full thickness, including the plantar fascia and a complete triangular V flap is incised and advanced into the defect. As all of the vascularity comes from the underlying perforating vessels within the V, there is very little undermining performed in this instance. Once the V flap is advanced, the donor defect is closed producing the stem of the Y. For still larger defects, two opposing flaps, or a double V to Y flaps, may be used and advanced toward each other in order to provide definitive closure.[135]

Z-Plasty Flap

The Z-plasty flap consists of two small, random-pattern flaps that are transposed on each other to create length along one central axis and shortening in the perpendicular axis[136] (Fig. 60.21). Although this technique is relatively simple, the procedure requires careful planning and is best utilized for treating scars and linear contractures found over the lesser metatarsophalangeal joints. A central concept of the Z-plasty flap is that the desired gain in length is created at the expense of shortening in the transverse axis.[137,138] Because the skin in the foot is less mobile, the transverse shortening can present distinct problems, which may be addressed by using multiple smaller Z-plasties that allow the same overall gain in length but limit shortening in the transverse axis. The physician must determine the amount of lengthening required during their surgical planning. Limiting factors are based on local skin properties,

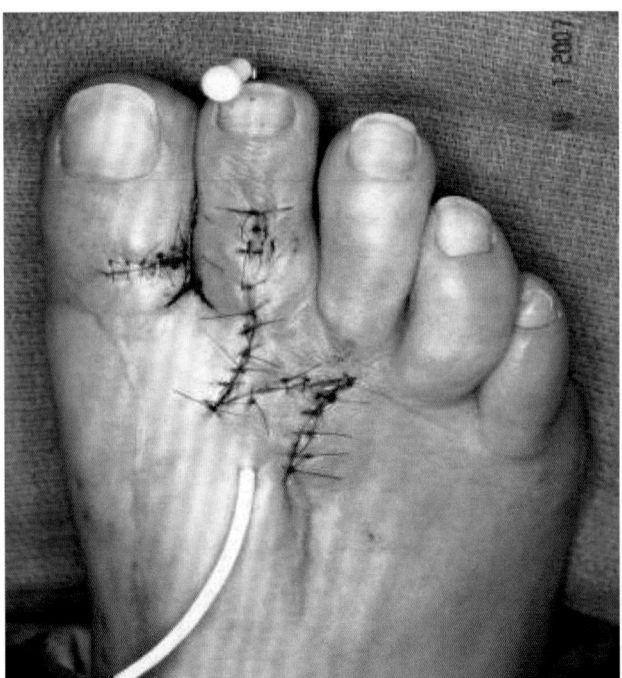

FIGURE 60.21 Clinical appearance of a Z-plasty flap overlying the second MTPJ. This flap consists of two small, random pattern flaps that are transposed on each other to create length along one central axis and shortening in the perpendicular axis.

including skin elasticity. However, theoretically, the increase in length is determined by the angle of the two lateral arms in relation to the central arm. Angles from 30 to 75 degrees have been used, with greater lengthening achieved with the larger angles.[139] Unfortunately, as the angle increases, a corresponding increase in the difficulty of rotating the flaps occurs. In the foot, an angle of 60 degrees is most commonly used and theoretically provides a 75% increase in length along the central arm.[139] Once the appropriate angle has been determined, the flap should be drawn on the skin with a marker. The central arm is drawn along the line of contracture. The two remaining arms are then drawn in opposite directions at the desired angle to the central arm, creating the "Z." It is imperative that all three arms are of equal length to ensure proper alignment of the flaps following transposition. Once elevated, the flaps are transposed into place. The physician should verify that the central arm has changed direction and that the flaps have been transposed properly. Suturing should be performed on a bias, so each stitch aides in the advancement of the flap into the defect and to reduce the tension at the apex of the flap.

Unilobed Flap

Schrudde and Petrovici[140] popularized the unilobed rotation flap as a random pattern flap that may be used when a simple 3:1 ratio is important. As the flap is rotated into place, the donor site begins to close. Ideally, the final linear scar created at the donor site should be designed to be parallel to the relaxed skin tension lines (RSTLs). Three variations of the unilobed flap are described depending on the shape of the defect where differences in the design were shown for defects varying from round, oval, or semicircular. Schrudde and Petrovici[140] reported their experience with the unilobed flap in 1308 flaps; however, only 0.6% of these were on the plantar aspect of the foot.

Bilobed Flap

Esser[141] first described the use of the bilobed flap for closure of soft tissue defects (Fig. 60.22). The bilobed flap is an interpolational flap. The technique has since been used for closure of defects on a wide range of anatomic locations with variations including cutaneous, fasciocutaneous, and myocutaneous flaps.[135,142–145] The flap is similar to the unilobed flap, but a second flap is created to reduce the tension required to close the donor site. This is accomplished by sequentially reducing the size of the flaps, with the first flap being 75% of the size of the defect and the second flap being 50% of the size of the original defect. In addition, the large surface area of the flap tends to reduce tension and the possibility of wound dehiscence. The bilobed flap is indicated for moderate-sized plantar defects or lesions that are too large to be closed adequately with a unilobed flap. Relative contraindications include poor vascular status, atrophic skin, mechanical lesions, infection, and adjacent scarring that would limit the flap's mobility.

The design of the bilobed flap resembles that of the unilobed flap where the first lobe begins at the halfway mark of the defect and is 75% of the size of the deficit. The second lobe is created at an angle 90 degrees to the first lobe and is ~50% the size of the original defect. A 60-degree angle between the two flaps is sufficient to maintain viability.[141,144,145] The flaps are raised from the deep fascial junction, so the flap contains skin and subcutaneous fascia. The surrounding tissue should be undermined at this same level to reduce tension on the flaps. Care should be taken to avoid grasping the flap with forceps to avoid compression injury and flap necrosis. A skin hook may be used to facilitate tissue

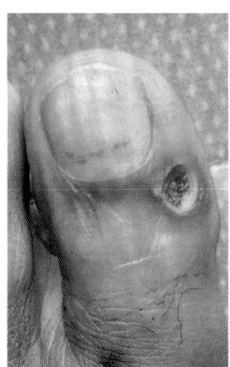 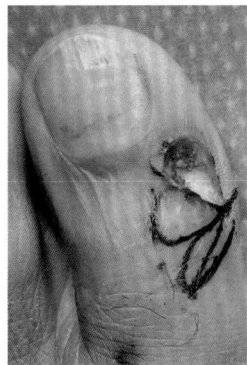 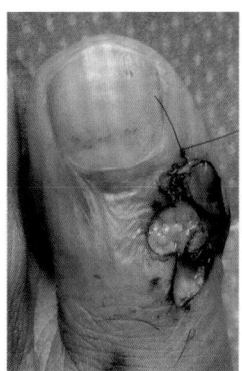 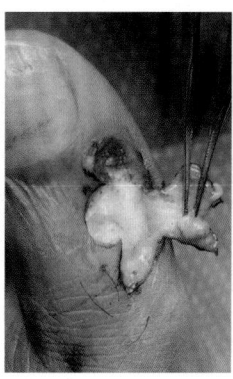 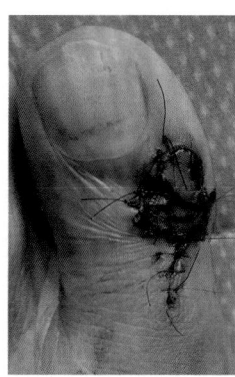

FIGURE 60.22 The bilobed flap is similar to the unilobed flap, but where a second flap is created to reduce the tension required to close the donor site.

elevation. The flaps are rotated into place simultaneously with the first segment filling the wound defect and the second filling the donor site of the first flap. The donor site of the second flap should close as the tissue is rotated. As with the unilobed flap, the flaps should be oriented with the final linear incision of the second donor site parallel to the RSTLs. Sanchez-Conejo-Mir et al.[145] reported on the use of 17 bilobed flaps for repair of defects on the sole of the foot. The bilobed flap was used to close defects ranging in size from 1.5 to 3.0 cm. The authors discouraged use of the bilobed flap for lesions >3.0 cm due to the tension created across the pedicle of the flap with rotation.[145]

Limberg/Rhombic Flap

Limberg[146] first described a local randomized flap in the shape of a rhombus for coverage of skin defects, but the Limberg or rhombic flap was popularized in clinical practice by Borges.[147] The primary advantage of this flap is that it preserves a large amount of the normal skin adjacent to the deficit that would otherwise have been excised with a standard elliptic or fusiform closure. This is a random pattern, transpositional flap with many potential applications, particularly where ulceration may recur easily and when the mobility of the skin may be better in one direction than another. The first step is to excise the wound in the shape of a rhombus, which is an equilateral parallelogram, all sides being equivalent in length. Two of the opposing angles created will measure 120 degrees, whereas the remaining two angles will measure 60 degrees. The RSTLs should be parallel to a line bisecting the two 120-degree angles. The flap is then created by making a vertical line off one of the 120-degree angles. This relationship must serve as the basis for the initial line or orientation. In this manner, the flap rotates around one of the 60-degree angles. The line must be of equal length to the sides of the rhombus. A second line is then made at a 60-degree angle to the first and parallel to one of the sides of the defect. This line must also be of equal length and creates an adjacent mirror image of the excised central deficit. The flap is then elevated full thickness and is rotated into the defect. If properly designed, the flap fills the defect and the donor site is closed. The linear incision that results when the donor site is closed should be parallel to the RSTLs. A major disadvantage of the Limberg/rhombic procedure is that the skin must be mobile to prevent excessive tension across the flap and to obtain closure of the donor site. A flap designed in the proper orientation to the RSTLs takes full advantage of the line of maximum extensibility, to allow the donor site to close with minimal tension. A Limberg/rhombic

flap retains more of the normal skin tissue as compared with the amount required for an elliptic excision.

Double Z Rhombic Flap

The double Z rhombic flap was originally described by Cuono[148] for repair of defects with a potential for increased tension on the wound or in conjunction with joint contracture. In the foot, this flap is useful when excising lesions from digits in which a long elliptic excision would create a greater risk of creating residual contracture by crossing more than one joint. The double Z rhombic flap consists of two Z-plasties that, when transposed, advance tissue from opposite sides to fill the wound or lesion. Excision of the lesion in the shape of a rhombus with angles of 60 and 120 degrees is performed with an imaginary line drawn between the two 60-degree angles oriented parallel to the RSTLs. This technique ensures that once the flaps are transposed, three of the five incision lines, including the longer central arm, will be parallel to the RSTLs, reducing the risk of contracture. The first arm of the "Z" is made by continuing one of the sides of the rhombus at the 120-degree angle a distance equal to the sides of the defect. The second arm is then made at an angle of 60 degrees to the first and of equal length. The procedure is then repeated at the other 120-degree angle, in the opposite direction.

Fillet of Toe Flap

The fillet of toe flap was popularized by Snyder and Edgerton[149]; however, the idea of utilizing locally retained tissues following amputation for adjacent coverage has evolved to include larger portions of the surrounding areas of the foot (Fig. 60.23). The main advantage of the fillet flap lies in the fact that the tissues of the flap are similar characteristics to the area being covered. It is ideal for lesions in the forefoot and midfoot, especially over bony prominences or areas. The procedure is performed in conjunction with digital or ray amputation or disarticulation. The phalanges are carefully dissected free of all surrounding soft tissue and are excised, including the nail and matrix. Care must be taken to avoid the medial and lateral neurovascular bundles. Excision of the long and short tendons as well as the plantar plate will make the flap more pliable and easier to rotate toward the deformity. Redundant tissue should be removed with great care in order to avoid compromising the neurovascular bundles. Excising redundant tissue also prevents involutions and skin depressions that can lead to further complications. The advantage of using this approach to cover smaller defects is that one of the flaps can be deepithelialized and rotated over the most prominent area and then covered with the second flap.[150]

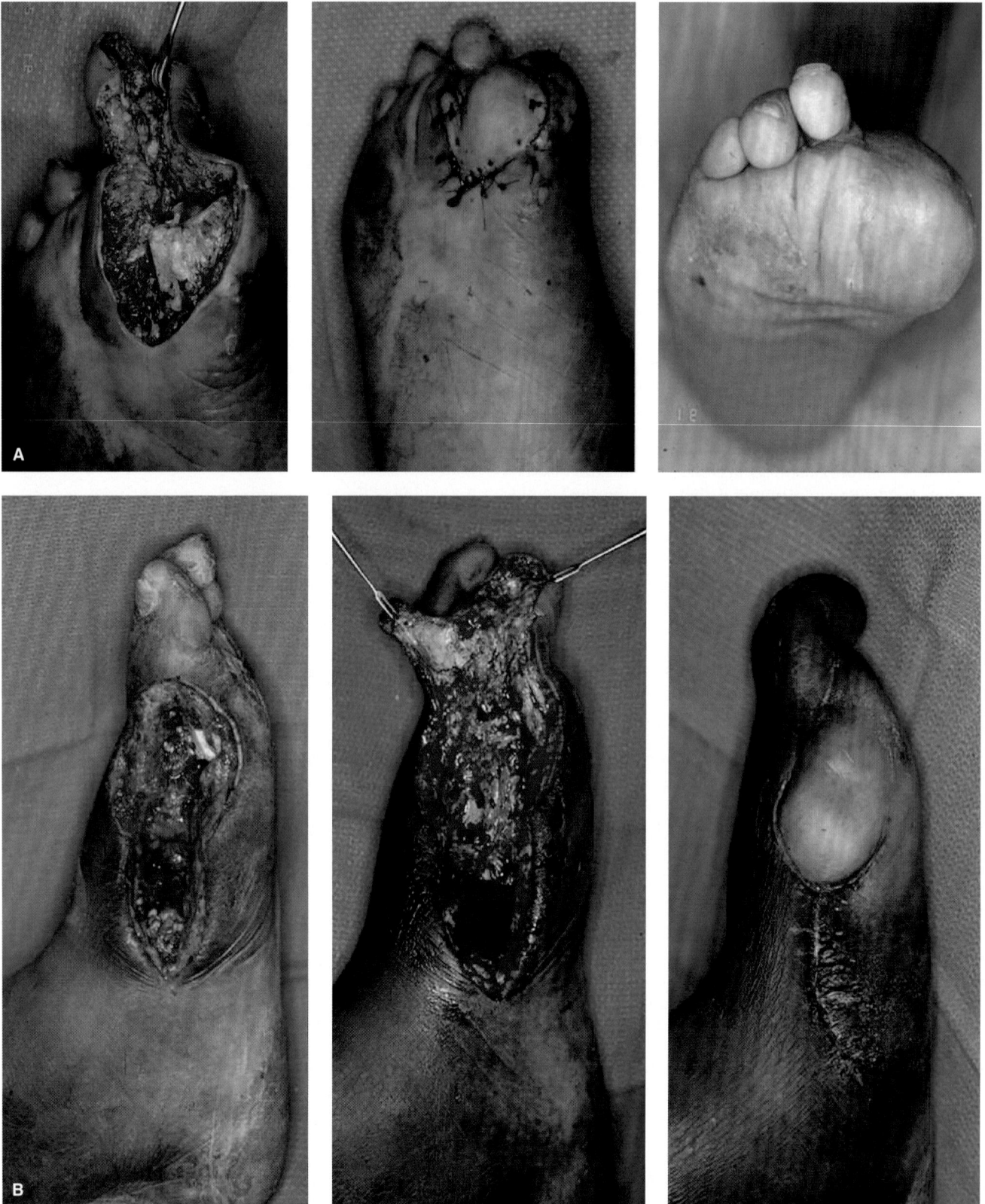

FIGURE 60.23 A, B. The fillet flap utilizes tissues similar to the area being covered and has evolved to include larger portions of the surrounding areas of the foot performed in conjunction with digital, ray, or even partial foot amputation or disarticulation.

Web Space Flap

The web space flap has been used successfully to cover a variety of forefoot defects that are usually distal and relatively small.[151,152] The flap may be based on the dorsal or plantar vasculature of the toe. The plantar-based flap alleviates the need to transect the deep transverse intermetatarsal ligament to maintain its structural integrity.[152] The major advantage of this procedure is that the donor site is in an inconspicuous non–weight-bearing area providing for a more pleasing cosmetic result. Adequate blood flow to the digit is essential when one contemplates this procedure. Once the vascular pedicle has been identified by Doppler examination, a template is used to determine the size of the flap to be elevated. The medial aspect of the second toe is commonly employed because of the reliable pattern of the vasculature.[152] Other reports support the use of the lateral aspect of the great toe.[153] The flap is then incised circumferentially through the skin and is elevated, beginning distally with care to keep the subcutaneous fat and the neurovascular bundle intact with the flap. Maintaining the fat around the neurovascular bundle helps to prevent damage to these structures.[152] The pedicle is then freed of surrounding soft tissue as far proximally as necessary to gain the desired rotation. A subcutaneous tunnel is then made to the wound site, and the flap is pulled through this tunnel and sutured into place. A skin graft is often required to cover the donor site defect. This technique has been described for coverage of plantar defects overlying the metatarsal heads.[152]

Axial Flaps

Cutaneous Flaps of the Foot

Cutaneous axial flaps within the foot have been extensively described. These flaps have the benefit of a reliable and robust vascular pedicle and thus provide for durable coverage about deficits in the foot and ankle. Their use, as evidenced by their location upon the plastic and reconstructive ladder, should be considered advanced and their undertaking should be of the most judicious manner for pre-, intra-, and postoperative considerations. The authors recommend a thorough and intimate understanding of the anatomy and mechanics of flap motion in order to anticipate any manner of success with these flaps.

Dorsalis Pedis Artery Flap

The DP artery flap has been used for both local and distant coverage of tissue defects with primary indications for use with wounds of the medial or lateral foot and ankle and anterior ankle.[154] This flap provides substantial coverage of either malleoli and may also be used to cover defects of the heel or over the Achilles tendon area. Additionally, the flap has also been used to cover distal forefoot wounds by rotating the flap distally.[155] Advantages of this approach include the ability to maintain sensorium to the flap and its relatively large size. A disadvantage is that the dissection may be quite challenging, and the DP artery and its numerous cutaneous branches are easily disrupted.[156] The donor site may become problematic because sensation is lost to this area. STSGs overexposed tendons on the dorsum of the foot may limit the take of the graft and may create additional problems with healing. Elevation of the flap should begin at the distal medial corner where the first dorsal metatarsal artery may be identified and ligated. The tissue is then elevated in a proximal direction just beneath the deep fascia that overlies the extensor tendons. Care must be taken to leave the paratenon of the extensor tendons intact.

As the dissection continues, the deep plantar artery is identified and is ligated between the base of the first and second metatarsals. The extensor hallucis brevis tendon should be identified and either transected or elevated with the flap because the DP artery passes deep to this tendon. As elevation of the flap continues, the DP artery, veins, and the deep peroneal nerve are carefully elevated from the tarsal bones. Care is taken to leave all soft tissue dorsal to the artery intact because the small arterioles supplying these tissues are tenuous. At the proximal most aspect of the flap, the neurovascular bundle may be dissected even further proximally to allow for a vascular pedicle of greater length. The donor site is covered using an STSG.

Reverse Dorsalis Pedis Artery Flap

The reverse DP flap has been described to close forefoot defects.[155,157] This flap is based on the proximal communicating branch of the DP artery. In one report, the DP neurovascular flap was passed posteriorly through the intraosseous membrane between the tibia and fibula to provide coverage of heel defects.[158]

Dorsal Metatarsal Artery Flap

A variation of the DP cutaneous flap is the first dorsal metatarsal artery flap.[159] This flap is more distally based and originates from the first dorsal metatarsal artery. Although the artery is always present, its origin varies between the DP artery (90.6%) and the lateral tarsal artery (9.4%).[160] Hayashi and Maruyama[161] reported 11 cases of reverse first dorsal metatarsal artery flaps with satisfactory results in all patients. This flap has been reported several times for coverage of defects surrounding the first metatarsophalangeal joint and hallux.[162-164]

Medial Plantar Artery Flap

Historically, perhaps the most versatile arterial flap within the foot is the medial plantar artery flap (Fig. 60.24). It may be utilized for coverage of defects both distally and proximally in the foot, heel, ankle, and distal leg.[165,166] This flap has many advantages, including glabrous tissue, a consistent reliable blood supply, a donor site in a relatively non–weight-bearing location, a significant amount of tissue for coverage, and the ability to maintain sensation to the flap. Additionally, this flap works well for covering large defects in the plantar midfoot, often times associated with Charcot foot collapse. The flap is based on the smaller of the two terminal branches of the PT artery. As such, attempts should be made to map the course of the medial plantar artery with a Doppler ultrasound examination preoperatively. Excellent results have been reported in patients with either plantar or posterior heel wounds who were managed with medial plantar artery flaps.[167]

Dissection begins distally, proximal to the metatarsal heads in the non–weight-bearing instep. The incision is carried to the plantar fascia that is elevated with the flap. The medial plantar artery can be found consistently in the cleft between the abductor hallucis muscle and the flexor digitorum brevis muscle. The artery is ligated distally and is elevated with the flap. Once the flap has been mobilized on three sides, it can be rotated into place, leaving the proximal base intact. Carefully planning the arc of rotation ensures that enough tissue will be present to cover the defect without creating excessive dog ears or tension. If the wound recurs, a free flap may be required for coverage because an island flap can rarely be re-rotated.

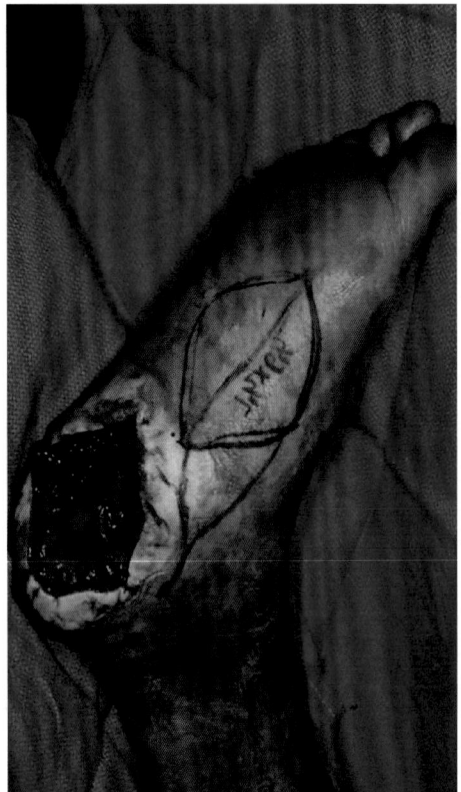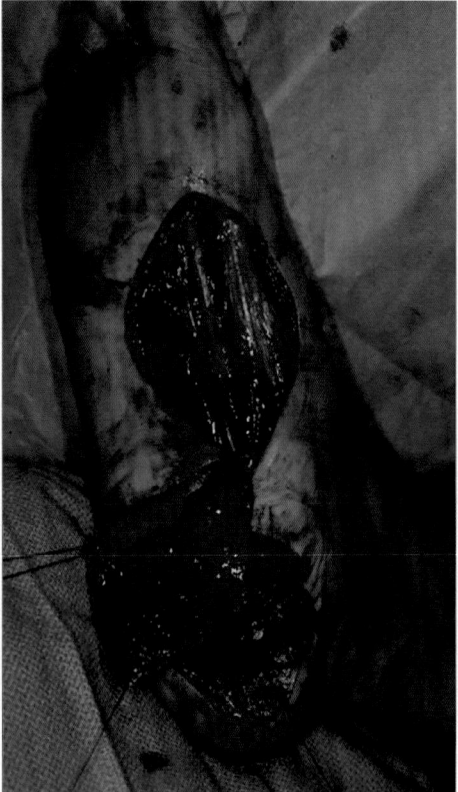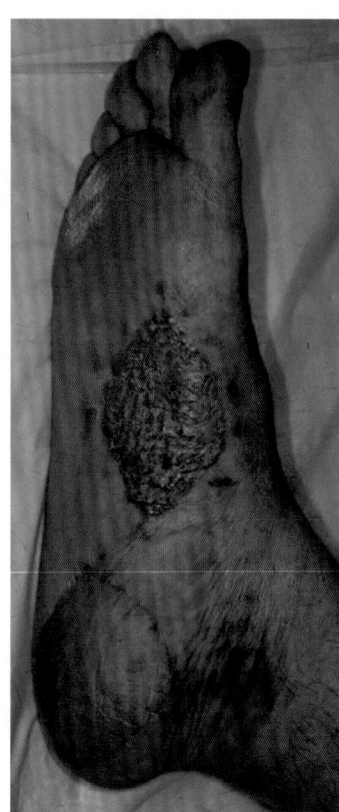

FIGURE 60.24 Clinical appearance of a medial plantar artery flap, which works well for covering large defects in the plantar midfoot and rearfoot.

Lateral Plantar Artery Flap

The lateral plantar artery flap is similar to the medial plantar artery flap but is used less frequently. The flap utilizes the plantar glabrous skin, but the tissue available for rotation is from a primarily weight-bearing surface and is considered more durable for this characteristic. This procedure may be useful for wounds plantar to the base of the fifth metatarsal or lateral aspect of the forefoot. Few reports have described the use of this flap solely as a fasciocutaneous flap. More often, the lateral plantar artery flap has been described in conjunction with a flexor digitorum brevis muscle flap.[168,169]

Lateral Calcaneal Artery Flap

The lateral calcaneal artery flap was originally described by Grabb and Argenta[170] and is a relatively simple axial pattern artery flap that may be used to provide sensate soft tissue coverage at the posterior heel region[171] (Fig. 60.25). The procedure may also be used to provide plantar heel coverage by extending the flap distally toward the fifth metatarsal base. However, with this additional length, the distal aspect of the tissue may not be as well perfused from the artery and may act more like a random pattern flap. Therefore, in longer flaps, this more distal area of coverage may not be as reliable.[172]

The flap includes the lateral calcaneal artery, the lesser saphenous vein, and the sural nerve. The lateral calcaneal artery is located within the subcutaneous tissues until it dives deep forming many tributaries to supply the plantar heel. The lateral calcaneal artery is most often the terminal branch of the peroneal artery, but on occasion, it may be derived from the PT artery. The sural nerve and lesser saphenous vein lie just

anterior to the lateral calcaneal artery as it passes posterior to the lateral malleolus.

Several considerations exist regarding the use of this type of procedure; however, one must ensure that at least one other vessel is adequately perfusing the foot before the lateral calcaneal artery is sacrificed. Investigators have suggested that antegrade flow of the lateral calcaneal artery should be confirmed with the use of Doppler ultrasound examination and manual occlusion of the posterior and anterior tibial vessels.[172]

Initially, the course of the lateral calcaneal artery and of the lesser saphenous vein is marked on the skin. The rotation and size of the flap are then determined by using a template from the wound defect to the pedicle and then transposing it to lie over the mapped artery. The axial pattern can provide vasculature for as much as an 8-cm flap, with an additional 6 cm of tissue available for transfer, but through a random pattern vascular supply as the flap angles distally toward the fifth metatarsal base.[170] The flap should be centered directly over the artery, and a proximal base of at least 4 cm is preferred.[172]

Dissection begins distally and is carried to the level of the calcaneal periosteum. Mobilization of the flap progresses in a retrograde manner, and one should pay particular attention to leave the calcaneal periosteum and the peroneal tendon sheaths intact. The neurovascular structures should not be visualized because dissection is at a deeper level. Once the flap is mobilized, it is rotated into position and is secured using skin closure. The foot and ankle should be splinted to limit ankle dorsiflexion and any tension on the pedicle. The donor site defect is often closed using an STSG. A depression on the lateral

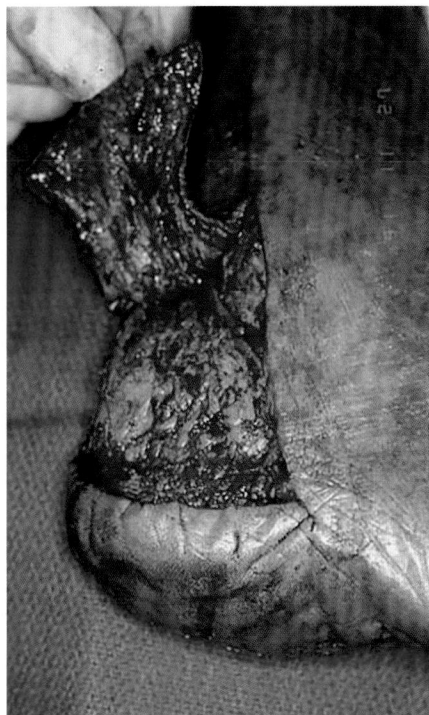
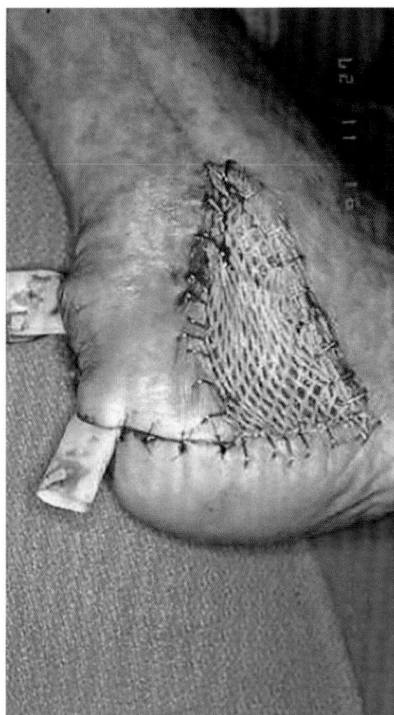
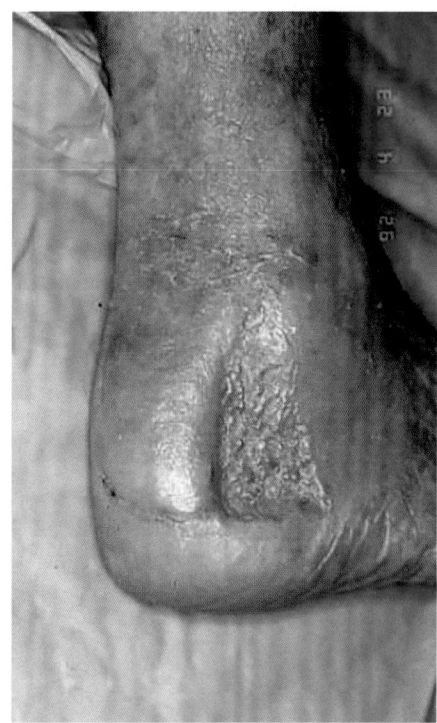

FIGURE 60.25 Clinical appearance of a lateral calcaneal artery flap, which is an axial pattern flap that may be used to provide sensate soft tissue coverage at the posterior heel.

aspect of the hindfoot remains, but it has been well tolerated. Disruption of the sural nerve is a significant disadvantage of this procedure.[173]

Hovius et al.[174] reported good results after performing seven lateral calcaneal artery neurovascular flaps for chronic heel and lateral malleolar ulcers. Similar results with the lateral calcaneal artery flap for heel and lateral malleolar lesions have been reported by other authors.[170,173,175] Additionally, the flap can provide good coverage of exposed distally Achilles tendon lesions.[171]

Muscle Flaps of the Foot The first documented local muscle flap was described in 1906 in which a pectoralis minor muscle flap was used for breast reconstruction; however, local muscle flaps have also been described extensively in the lower extremity. In the 1960s, Ralph Ger pioneered soft tissue reconstruction in the lower extremity for posttraumatic and venous stasis wounds using pedicled soleus and flexor digitorum longus muscle flaps.[176] Historically speaking, advances in anesthesia, antibiotics, and wound healing gradually popularized the use of these types of flaps and in doing so improved postoperative outcomes. Local muscle flaps improve the blood supply to the recipient region, which may also enhance antibiotic delivery, and promote wound healing, including to underlying bone.[177] Additionally, muscle flaps provide for bulk and padding to areas necessitating more robust defect coverage.

Abductor Hallucis Muscle Flap The abductor hallucis muscle may be used to cover defects of the medial malleolus and medial heel[178] (Fig. 60.26). The medial plantar artery supplies the muscle, and the nutrient branch can be identified, entering the lateral aspect of the muscle belly approximately two to three finger-breadths proximal to the navicular tuberosity. The approach is through a medial incision, just above Brinton line. The tendon is transected distally, and the muscle belly is elevated. Release of the origin provides greater rotation distally if needed.

Abductor Digiti Minimi Muscle Flap The abductor digiti minimi (ADM) muscle is located in the first layer of the lateral foot between the flexor digitorum brevis (FDB) medially and the 5th metatarsal and cuboid laterally. It takes its origin from the medial and lateral calcaneal tubercles and its adjacent intermuscular septum and inserts onto the lateral aspect of the base of the fifth proximal phalanx. The main vascular supply is the proximal branch of the lateral plantar artery, which is its dominant pedicle inserting medial to the muscle's origin on the calcaneus[179] with one or more minor pedicles also supplying it. When raised, the muscle survives based on the single dominant vessel supply. The ADM is useful for small coverage of plantar and lateral defects of the foot and lateral distal and plantar calcaneus[180] (Fig. 60.27).

Flexor Digitorum Brevis Muscle Flap Bostwick[181] described a technique using the flexor digitorum brevis with a skin graft (Fig. 60.28). The FDB is supplied predominantly by the lateral plantar artery and, to a lesser extent, by the medial plantar artery.[182] The approach is through a midline plantar incision, and the plantar fascia is dissected from the muscle. The four tendons distally are transected, and the muscle is rotated back on itself. Care must be taken not to injure the lateral plantar nerve during dissection. If more rotation is needed, the muscle belly may be dissected from its origin off the calcaneus as well.[183] Graziano et al.[184,185] successfully used the FDB muscle belly in the management of osteomyelitis of the heel and for plantar

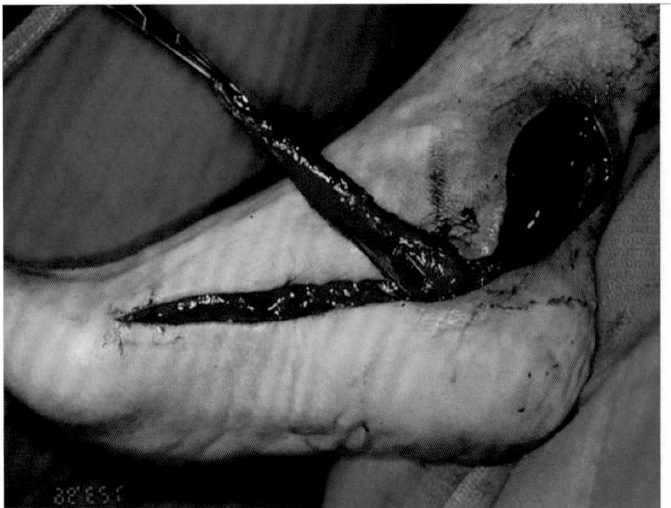
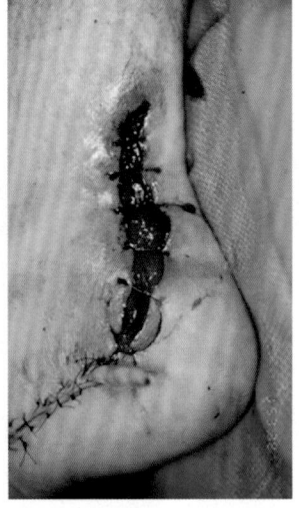
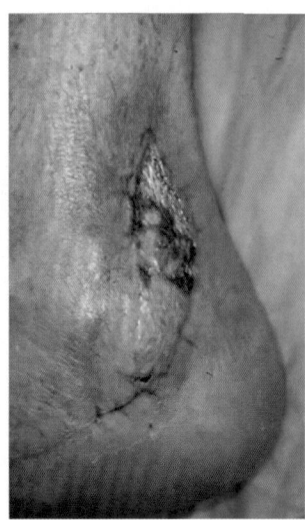

FIGURE 60.26 Clinical appearance of an abductor hallucis muscle flap, which may be used to cover defects of the medial malleolus and medial heel.

ulcerations. In a different report, the FDB was used to close a heel defect after wide excision in seven patients with malignant lesions.[186]

Extensor Digiti Minimi Muscle Flap The extensor digitorum brevis (EDB) may be used to cover defects of the lateral malleolus, anterior ankle, and forefoot[187] (Fig. 60.29). The vascular supply to the muscle is from the lateral tarsal artery, a branch of the DP. The muscle takes origin from the calcaneus in the floor of the sinus tarsi. The muscle may be rotated proximally after severing the four tendons and rotating it back on itself. Alternatively, the EDB may be freed from its origin and rotated distally as an island muscle flap with the lateral tarsal artery attached as the pedicle. The EDB muscle belly has been used for soft tissue defects of the lateral malleolus, the medial malleolus, dorsal foot wounds, distal tibial wounds, and coverage of Achilles tendon defects.[188-191]

Cutaneous Flaps of the Leg Cutaneous flaps of the leg have also been described for coverage for foot and ankle and leg defects and may be adipofascial, myocutaneous, or fasciocutaneous. In most cases, the flaps are based on reverse-flow axial arteries, most often perforator branches from the anterior tibial, PT, or peroneal arteries. Perforator artery flap reconstruction began in 1989, with the utilization of the inferior epigastric artery cutaneous flap without the need for a rectus abdominis muscle for reconstruction of the floor of the mouth and groin.[192] In the appropriate situation, though, the utilization of cutaneous perforator flaps of the leg may obviate the need for a free tissue transfer, sparing the patient a more complicated primary surgery and protracted recovery and rehabilitation, as well as providing more aesthetically pleasing coverage without the need for secondary procedures for recontouring and less donor site morbidity. Of note, in a comparative study of anterior tibial, PT, and peroneal artery flaps, Satoh et al.[193] concluded that the

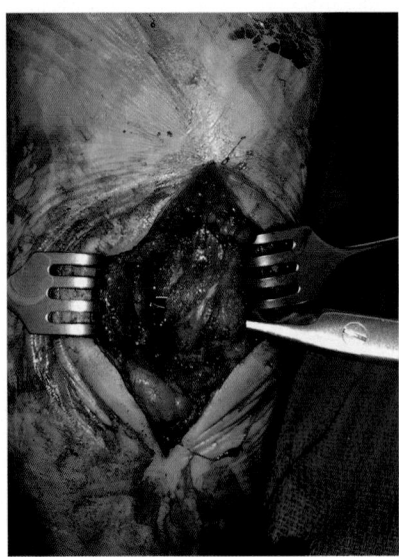
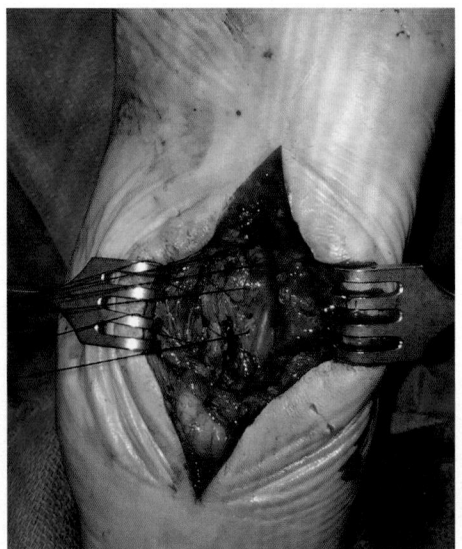
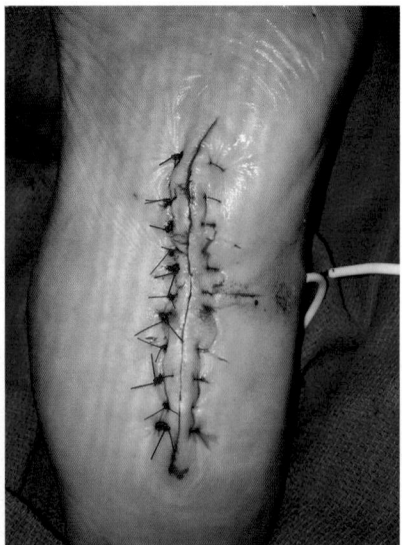

FIGURE 60.27 Clinical appearance of a plantar abductor digiti minimi muscle flap, which is useful for small coverage of plantar and lateral defects of the foot and ankle.

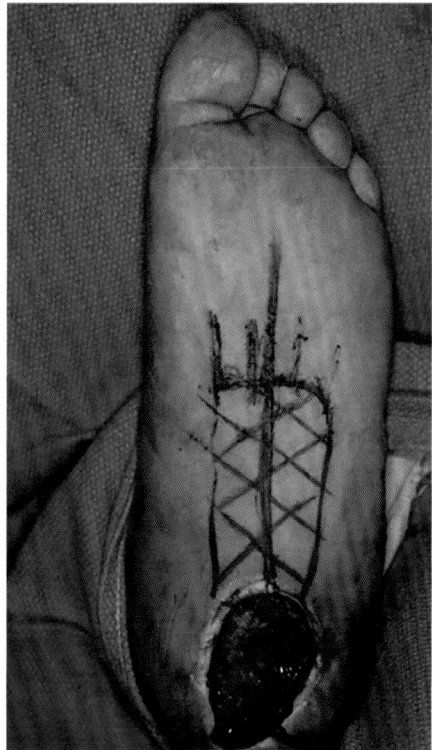
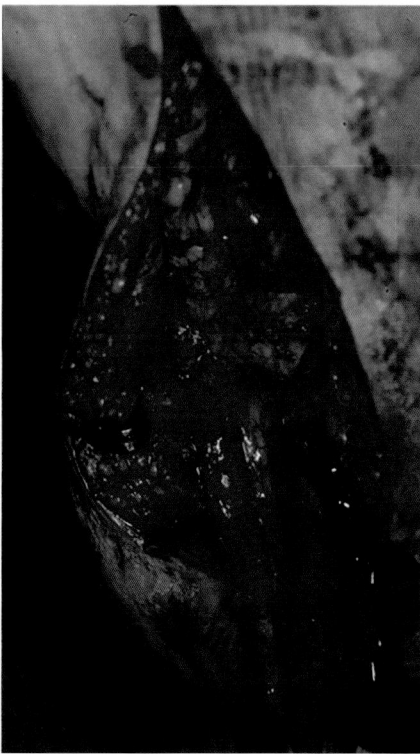
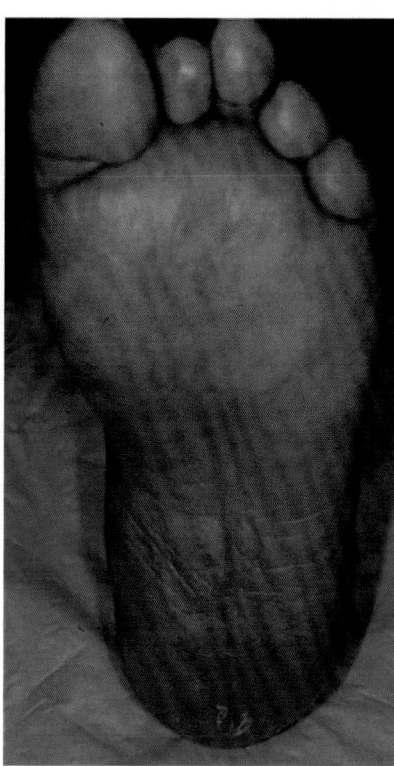

FIGURE 60.28 Clinical appearance of a flexor digitorum brevis muscle flap, which is useful for small coverage of the heel and plantar ulcerations.

anterior tibial reverse-flow flaps were more likely to become congested or necrose.

Peroneal Artery Perforator Flap A fasciocutaneous flap of the anterolateral distal leg described by Masquelet et al.[194] is based distally from the perforating branch of the peroneal artery. This flap may be used for coverage of wounds over the lateral malleolus, posterior heel, and distal leg. Identification of the perforating branch of the peroneal artery can be confirmed by Doppler examination or angiography preoperatively. The arterial branch should be mapped on the anterolateral aspect of the lower leg. Dissection is initiated proximally, and the pedicle of the flap is most often based distally. This flap may be used as an island flap to provide greater rotation or excursion of transfer. Yoshimura et al.[195] reported on 14 cases of peroneal island flaps for wound coverage in the lower extremities, all of

which healed without necrosis. Cheng et al.[196] saw unanimous peroneal artery perforator flap survival in 55 patients with chronic lower limb wounds, citing low postoperative morbidity, good daily functions, and relatively satisfactory aesthetic results, without sacrificing any major vessels or nerves.

Reverse Sural Artery Perforator Flap The reverse sural artery flap was described by Ponten[197] in 1981 and later developed by several other cohorts[198,199] (Fig. 60.30). The flap is based in the perforators of the peroneal artery system and is effective for deficits about the distal leg and ankle. A significant advantage of this flap is its constant vascular supply that does not require sacrifice or manipulation of a major artery. Although, a growing consensus is that impaired venous drainage is one of the preeminent factors that may contribute to flap necrosis in the early postoperative period.[200] Akhtar and Hameed[201] saw 66 of

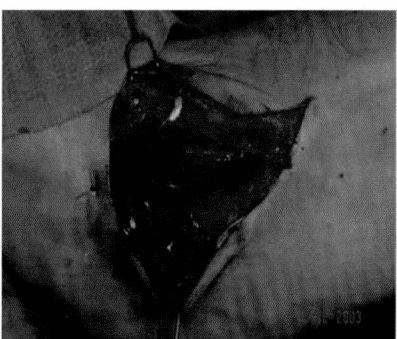
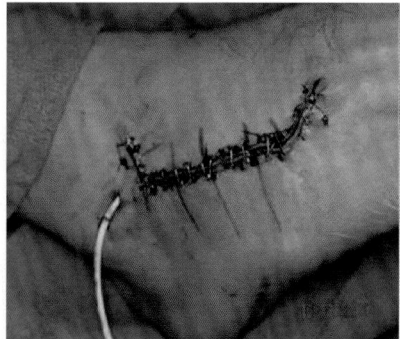
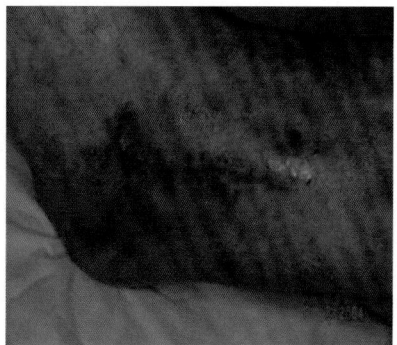

FIGURE 60.29 Clinical appearance of an extensor digitorum brevis muscle flap, which may be used to cover defects of the lateral malleolus, anterior ankle, or forefoot.

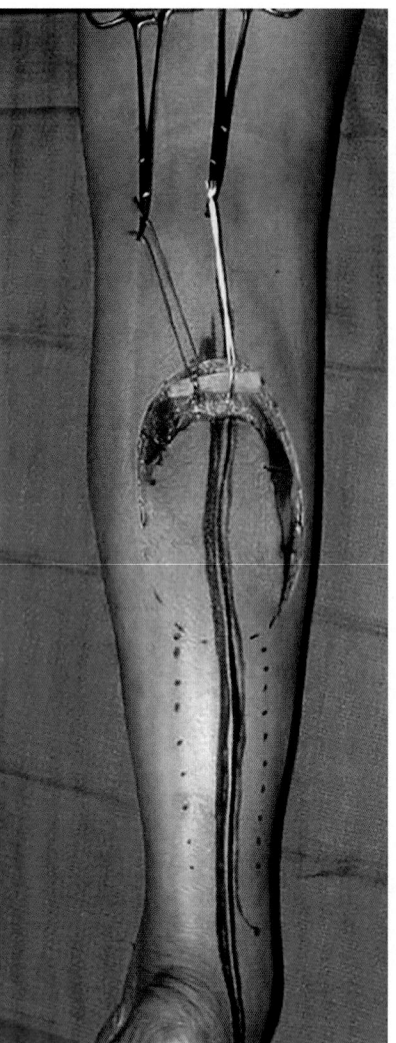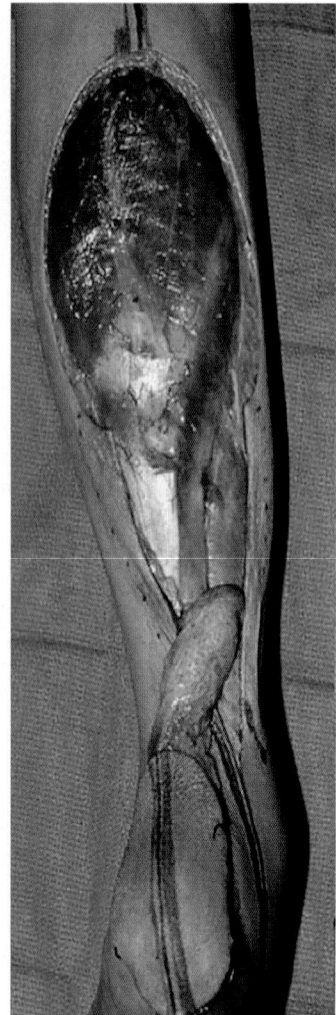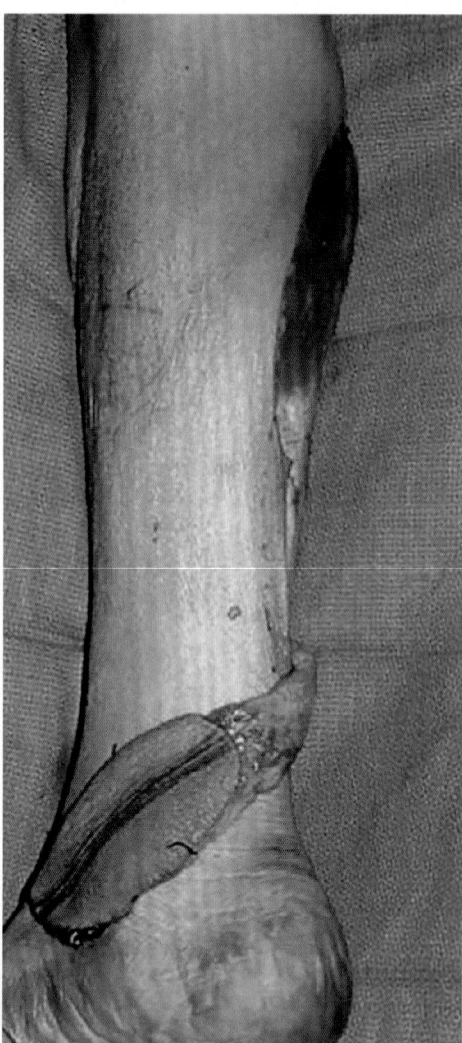

FIGURE 60.30 The reverse sural artery flap provides a constant vascular supply that does not require sacrifice or manipulation of a major artery.

84 patients with complete flap survival, no considerable donor site morbidity, and all with satisfactory functional outcomes. Jeng et al.[202] related good results with a modified superficial sural island flap.

Posterior Tibial Artery Perforator Flap In 1986, Amarante et al.[203] described a flap based from the perforators of the PT artery (Fig. 60.31). The PT artery is the direct continuation of the popliteal artery and primarily the dominant vessel of the tri-furcation.[204] It is accompanied by two venae comitantes and through its course in the leg supplies normally four perforators, at constant levels at 4.0, 6.5, 8.0, and 10.0 cm above the medial malleolus.[203,205] Yang et al.[206] described complete flap survival with utilization of the PT artery perforator flap for 23 of 28 patients with chronic wounds about the lower limb, citing it as a feasible option for the management of small- to medium-sized defects about the malleoli, calcaneus, or Achilles.

Anterior Tibial Artery Perforator Flap Wee[207] described the use of the anterior tibial artery flap and its perforators for foot and ankle defects. However, this flap is rarely used in the distal third of the leg and ankle due to the variable origin, course, and small dimension of its perforator vessels, making it considerably more likely to undergo flap congestion, if not necrosis.[193,208]

Saphenous Artery Perforator Flap The saphenous artery per-forator (SAP) flap is historically used for coverage of soft tis-sue defects about the knee and proximal leg. The SAP flap (Fig. 60.32), based from the descending genicular artery, pro-vides robust circulation and generous coverage to the recipient region. The saphenous artery arises as one of three branches of the descending genicular artery. In this area of the lower extremity, the vascular supply is robust and orients in pre-dictable branching patterns. Three types of branching occur, depending on whether all three branches shared a common origin (60%); one of the branches has an isolated origin (30%); or all three branches have isolated origins (10%).[209] Nenad et al.[210] retrospectively analyzed 50 patients for a mean of 4 years following distally based saphenous neurofasciocutane-ous perforator flaps and found a 70% success rate.

Ad Hoc Perforator Flaps
The concept of the "ad hoc" perforator flap was first suggested by Quaba in 1990.[211] By definition, the ad hoc flap can be

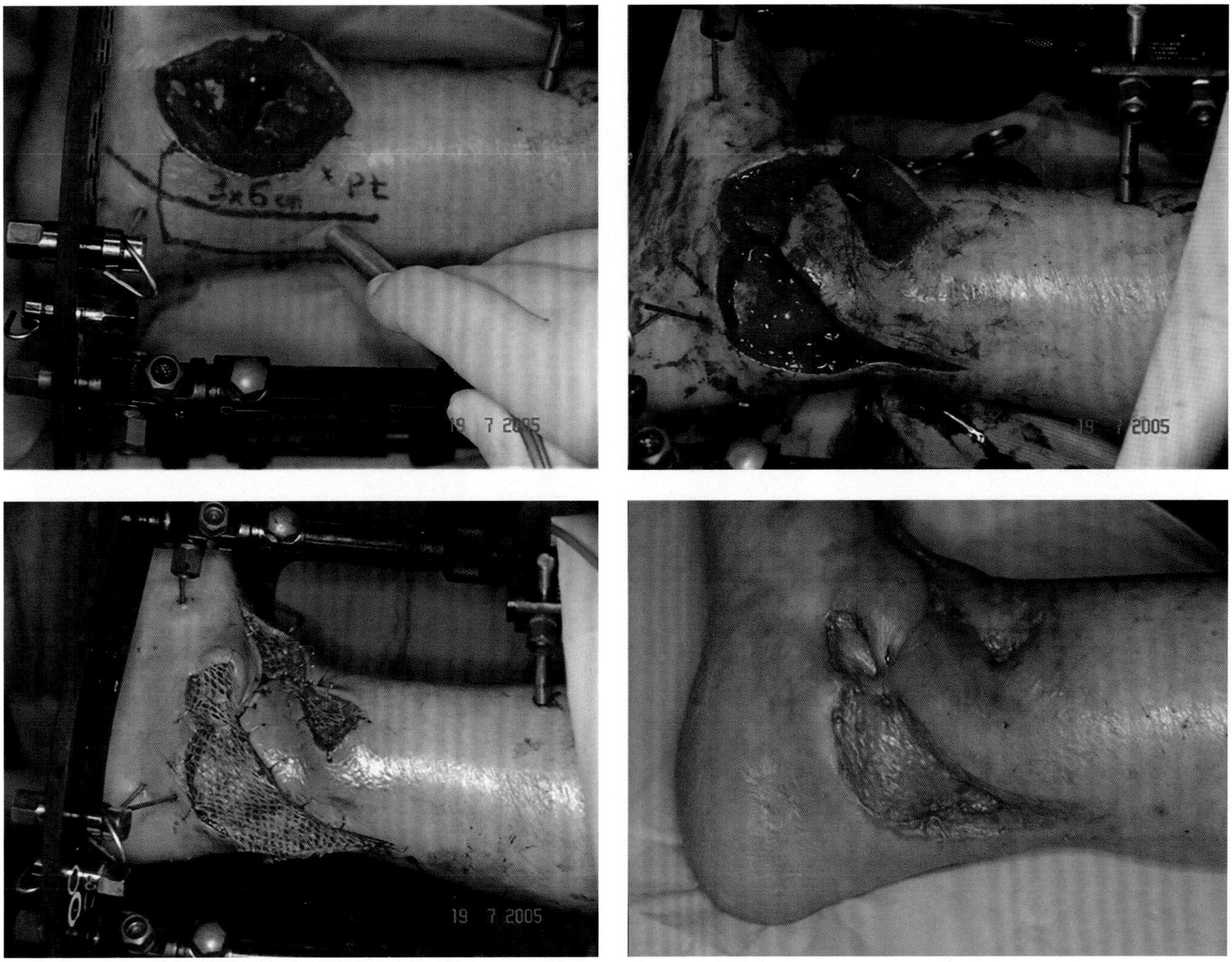

FIGURE 60.31 Clinical appearance of a posterior tibial artery perforator flap for coverage about the exposed medial ankle joint.

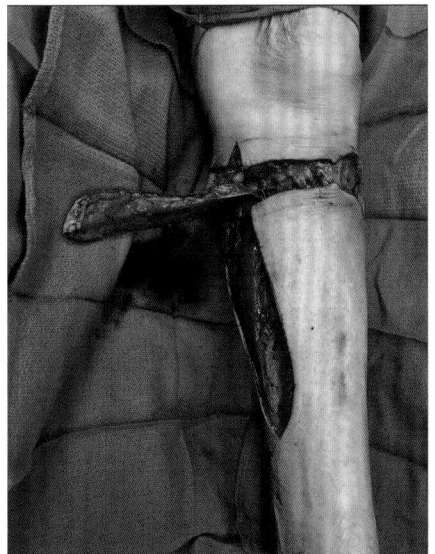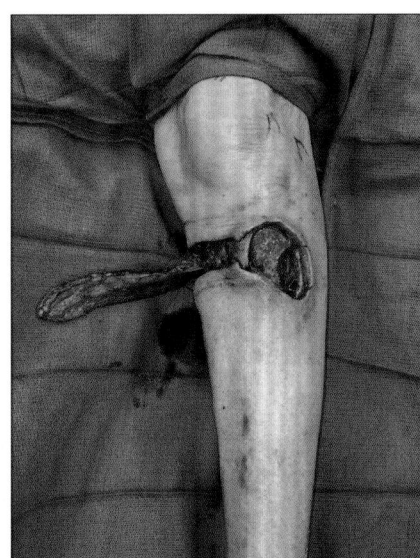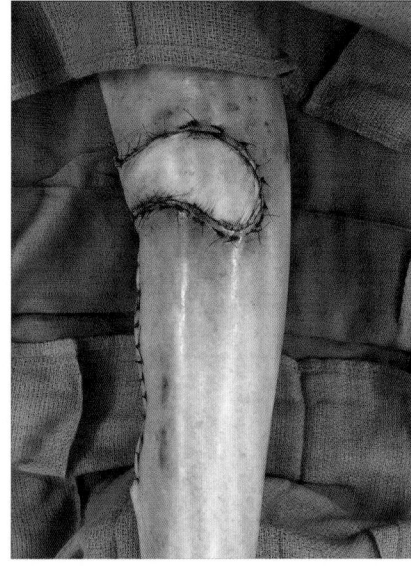

FIGURE 60.32 The saphenous artery perforator flap is based from the descending genicular artery and provides robust circulation and generous coverage to the recipient region.

based on any perforator vessel rather than its discrete source artery. This has been described as analogous to the "free-style free flap" concept popularized by Wei and Mardini.[212] It diverts the knowledge and importance of any flap source vessel to the suprafascial location of any of the major perforator arteries, as mapped by Taylor and Palmer.[213] The presence of a positive audible Doppler signal in a donor territory adjacent to the defect allows execution of the flap. In this way, sufficient understanding of the cutaneous circulation, a working knowledge of the regional vascular anatomy, and experience in raising local skin flaps, the reconstructive surgeon can be liberated from the limitations of molding the defect to a previously described local flap.[214] One must confirm both the direction of course and the area of potential vascular territory of the perforator vessel in order to assure successful retention of the flap.

It should be noted that comorbid individuals may pose a particular difficulty in the design, evaluation, and execution of this flap type due to pathological changes in the vascular and soft tissue anatomy, which can potentially alter the micro- and macrostructure of perforator vessels and their surrounding soft tissues. Patients with diabetes mellitus, in particular, may prove to be a relative contraindication due to these pathological anatomic variations and abnormalities, which may hinder flap design, execution, and longevity.

Muscle Flaps of the Leg As with muscle flaps of the foot, muscular flaps of the leg provide for increased vascularity, enhanced bulk, padding, and robust coverage about deficits in the leg and ankle. Gastrocnemius, soleus, and peroneus brevis muscle flaps have historically met the unique needs of significant tissue deficits in the leg and ankle and additionally are subject to myocutaneous utilization where warranted. However, the potential for substantial compromise to the overall stability and function of the extremity cannot be denied with these muscular flaps and as such their use should be respected and judicious consideration should be exercised.

Gastrocnemius Muscle Flap
Medial and lateral gastrocnemius muscle flaps have a versatility of uses and may be used with a wide arc of rotation for coverage spanning the thigh, knee, and proximal to middle leg.[215] Each head of the gastrocnemius muscle is supplied by an individual sural artery branching from the popliteal artery and entering the muscle belly ~3 cm proximal to the knee joint line. There are also several direct fasciocutaneous and septocutaneous vessels arising from the popliteal artery and its trifurcation, respectively. The medial and lateral gastrocnemius head muscle flaps may be harvested individually or simultaneously.[216] This muscle flap has been utilized in cases with significant bone tumor resection in the proximal tibia with good results, owing to its versatility of use.[217] A review of 218 medial gastrocnemius muscle flaps revealed good results with 76.2% strength in maximal plantarflexion force and 87% not significantly limited in walking.[218]

Soleus Muscle Flap The soleus muscle flap is considered a reliable local flap option, both by itself or in conjunction with other local flaps, to reconstruct less extensive wounds in the middle to distal third of the leg.[219] Kauffman et al.[220] saw nine of twelve patients achieve a healed and stable wound after a soleus muscle flap. They attributed their failures to comorbid conditions like PVD, smoking, and planned radiation and concluded that these factors should be considered relative contraindications for the

soleus muscle flap use. Additionally, a myocutaneous version of the soleus flap has also been reported that incorporates the medial portion of the soleus muscle into the flap.[221]

Peroneus Brevis Muscle Flap
The peroneus brevis muscle flap is an interesting option for soft tissue coverage in the distal leg and ankle. Although infrequently utilized for defect coverage about the distal leg and ankle, the donor site can always be closed primarily and the anatomy is relatively constant. Its arc of rotation allows coverage of more anterior defects of the ankle, the Achilles tendon, the heel as well as of lateral and medial malleoli. It is simple to harvest and is transposed into the wound without advanced dissection. As long as the peroneus longus is maintained, ankle function should not be adversely affected.[222] Ensat et al.[223] saw great success in ten patients undergoing distally based peroneus brevis muscle flaps. And a review of literature saw an overall complication rate of 41.6% in this muscle flap in 192 patients, comparable to alternatives in this region like the distally based sural fasciocutaneous flap.[223]

Distant Flaps

Free Tissue Flaps A free tissue transfer or free flap is a portion of tissue that is transferred with its vascular pedicle from one part of the body to another (Fig. 60.33). This requires that the flap's artery and vein be reanastomosed to vessels at or near the recipient site via microsurgical techniques by a skilled plastic surgeon. The tissue may be skin, fascia, adipose, muscle, bone, or a combination thereof. Free flaps are indicated when a defect exists and a local flap or skin graft is inappropriate because of the defect's size, location, or vascular supply. When skin and fascia are combined, this technique provides a more durable result than a skin graft and can be applied over tendon, bone, or joints because it does not rely on the underlying tissue for its blood supply.

As with all flaps, multiple classifications exist for the categorization of free flaps. These are often based in tissue composition, vascular anatomy, and harvest technique. However, for purposes of simplicity, a classification according to structural components is most frequently employed. Muscle flaps are commonly used in reconstruction of three-dimensional defects where significant bulk is required to fill a large negative space and/or coverage over bone or joint or hardware. Muscle flaps, though, may also provide a thin, pliable, and well-contoured coverage based on the amount of muscle initially dissected with the flap. The initial bulky appearance of muscle flaps is often diminished over time due to atrophy.[224] In such a case, appropriately sized muscle flaps may actually lead to a well-contoured flap; however, debulking can be performed at a later time if necessary. Just as with local muscle flaps, free muscle flaps offer enhanced vascularity that is capable of suppressing bacteria by aiding in the delivery of neutrophils and antibiotics to the site.[225-227] Therefore, muscle flaps are often employed for largely contaminated wounds and chronically infected wounds with large amounts of negative space.

Fasciocutaneous free flaps are ideal for wound resurfacing and are capable of restoring contour and facilitating adequate tendon glide along the flap-native wound interface.[228] These flaps are also useful for staged reconstruction of underlying tissue components, as they can be rapidly reevaluated. Fasciocutaneous free flaps are susceptible to large amounts of subcutaneous adipose tissue at the donor site and in this

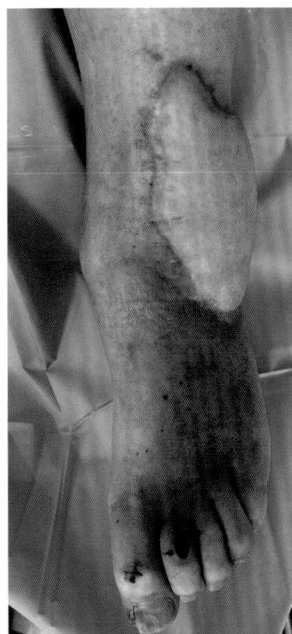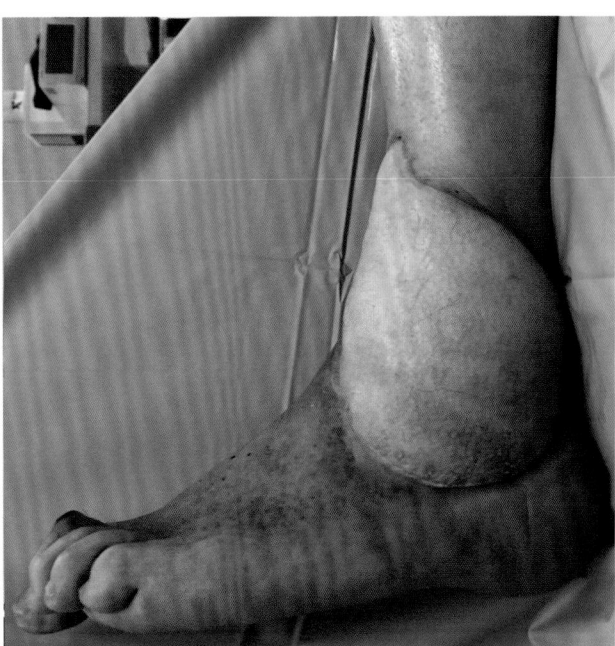

FIGURE 60.33 Clinical appearance of a well-healed anterolateral thigh-free tissue flap status post attempted ankle fusion with subsequent infection, explantation of hardware with significant soft tissue deficit.

way may be relatively bulky. Surgical debulking procedures and liposuction may be required at a later time to improve contour.

Perforator free flaps are flaps that receive their blood supply from branches of named vessels that "perforate" through the muscle or fascial septum to supply the overlying skin and subcutaneous tissues. Unlike fasciocutaneous free flaps, however, these flaps are harvested above the level of deep fascia using retrograde "ad hoc" perforator dissection techniques until adequate pedicle length is achieved. This technique facilitates wound resurfacing with ultrathin adipocutaneous flaps, enhances the freedom of flap design, and minimizes the need for secondary debulking.[229] With knowledge of perforator anatomy and flow characteristics, nearly any perforator in the body can be utilized as a source of vascular supply for a free tissue flap. Primary disadvantages of perforator-free flap harvest include high variability in perforator size and location from one patient to the next, greater complexity of dissection, and a higher risk of fat necrosis and flap loss due to their more tenuous vascular supply.[230-232] For these reasons, perforator flaps are ideal for coverage of moderately sized defects and require detailed preoperative planning to enhance the safety and efficiency of flap harvest.

Common donor sites for free tissue transfers to the foot and ankle include the anterolateral thigh (ALT), vastus lateralis (VL), Thoracodorsal Artery Perforator (TDAP),[233] rectus abdominis,[234] gracilis,[235] and the radial forearm (RF).[236] Flap selection, though, is dependent on the wound dimensions, required pedicle length, presence of infection and/or exposed vital structures, aesthetic and functional demands of the donor and recipient site, potential to restore sensation, patient positioning in the operating room, and the patient's body habitus.[228]

When assessing candidacy for a free flap, there are multiple factors and considerations that should be addressed. Central to this, as is much of the aforementioned chapter, is addressing wound etiology and comorbidities, wound optimization and infection control, evaluation and/or establishment of adequate blood flow, proper nutrition, and lifestyle modifications. Considerations must be made for comorbidities that may influence wound healing such as cardiac disease, renal disease, infection, vasculopathy, diabetes mellitus, neuropathy, venous hypertension, lymphatic obstruction, immunological deficiency, hypercoagulability, connective tissue disease, malnutrition, autoimmune disease, vasospasm, neoplasm, and psychiatric illness.[237]

Timing of free flap reconstruction is dependent on the establishment of a healthy, vascularized wound bed with clinical signs of healing. Many authors agree that reconstruction should be attempted as early as possible following an adequate debridement and recipient-site optimization. However, this course may also vary depending on wound etiology as some wounds require adjunctive measures, such as revascularization procedures, or other medical management to optimize healing potential at the recipient site prior to free tissue transfer. There is wide agreement for immediate flap coverage in the setting of exposed vital structures or the need to salvage a disvascular limb.

Advances in microsurgical technique have contributed to significantly reduced rates of postoperative complications and ultimately free flap failure at high-volume centers. Flap loss, though, can be due to intrinsic factors that compromise blood supply or extrinsic factors such as infection, hypotension, compression, and/or the use of vasoconstricting agents.[238] Other complications include functional limitations, sensory impairment, donor-site scar, and the need for revision/debulking. Lakhiani et al.[238] described donor-site morbidities from commonly utilized thigh-based flaps and proposed that flap selection is highly individualized, and the implications of aesthetic, perioperative, and/or functional morbidities should not be underestimated. Patients should be counseled on potential risks specific to each flap type in order to optimize outcomes and overall satisfaction.

In the appropriate setting, free tissue transfer has proven to be an effective primary solution for complex wound reconstruction. Advances in knowledge of vascular anatomy, surgical technique, and postoperative patient care have enabled substantial improvements in microvascular success rates. As data have shown, vigilance in all stages of selection, planning, execution, and rehabilitation is essential to optimize outcomes for this population.

CONCLUSION

With the myriad of local and systemic complications seen in this patient population, treating the complex foot and ankle wound can be a monumental undertaking for both the patient and physician, alike. Multiple factors and considerations are at play and must be given attention, respect, and careful consideration in both their assessment and management. A fundamental understanding and working knowledge of the complex interactions between the numerous and varying physiologic components involved in wound healing is paramount. It is unrealistic to assume that we will ever discover or develop a single element or modality that will prevent, heal, or prophylax against all complex wounds. However, advances and innovations in technology will continue to occur and our understanding and the ability to efficaciously treat this pathology will continue to evolve. Our thought processes and decision-making skills must be rooted in the culmination of evidence-based medicine, not merely isolated research. This tact should be supported by our individual and collective clinical prowess and experience. The surgeon must adapt to the wound as it presents and evolves and cater treatment modalities to the patient and the environment in which they are treated. Regardless of the exact setting, the multidisciplinary approach must be pursued and utilized to the maximum extent. This consortium of disciplines and patient-specific treatment modalities is paramount in order to prevent, heal, and suppress the nonhealing wounds of the foot and ankle in order to ultimately provide the patient with the most expedient and functional outcome possible.

REFERENCES

1. Armstrong DG, Boulton AJM, Bus SA. Diabetic foot ulcers and their recurrence. *N Engl J Med.* 2017;376:2367-2375.
2. Broughton G, Janis JE, Attinger CE. The basic science of wound healing. *Plast Reconstr Surg.* 2006;117(7 suppl):12S-34S.
3. Khan NA, Rahim SA, Annad SS, et al. Does the clinical examination predict lower extremity peripheral arterial disease? *J Am Med Assoc.* 2006;295(5):536-546.
4. Marston WA, Davies SW, Armstrong B, et al. Natural history of limbs with arterial insufficiency and chronic ulceration treated without revascularization. *J Vasc Surg.* 2006;44(1):108-114.
5. Grayson MI, Gibbons GW, Balogh K, et al. Probing to bone in infected pedal ulcers: a clinical sign of underlying osteomyelitis in diabetic patients. *JAMA.* 1995;273:721-725.
6. Lavery LA, Armstrong DG, Peters EJG, et al. Probe-to-bone test for diagnosing diabetic foot osteomyelitis: Reliable or relic. *Diabetes Care.* 2007;30(2):270-274.
7. Stevens DL, Bisno AL, Chambers HF, et al. Infections Disease Society of America: practice guidelines for the diagnosis and management of skin and soft-tissue infections. *Clin Infect Dis.* 2005;41:1373-1406.
8. Campbell RR, Hawkins SJ, Maddison PJ, et al. Limited joint mobility in diabetes mellitus. *Ann Rheum Dis.* 1985;44:93-97.
9. Mueller MJ, Diamond JE, Delitro A, et al. Insensitivity, limit mobility and plantar ulcers in patients with diabetes mellitus. *Phy Ther.* 1989;69(6):453-462.
10. Arkkila PET, Kantoa IM, Vilkari JSA. Limited joint mobility in type 1 diabetic patients: correlation to other diabetic complications. *J Intern Med.* 1994;236:215-223.
11. Grant WP, Sullivan R, Sonenshine DK, et al. Electron microscopic investigation of the effect of diabetes mellitus on the Achilles tendon. *J Foot Ankle Surg.* 1997;36(4):272-278.
12. Reddy CK. Cross-linking in collagen by nonenzymatic glycation increases the matrix stiffness in rabbit Achilles tendon. *Exp Diabesity Res.* 2004;5(2):143-153.
13. Couppe C, et al. Human Achilles tendon glycation and function in diabetes. *J Appl Physiol.* 2016;120:130-137.
14. Ahmed A, et al. Expressional changes in growth and inflammatory mediators during Achilles tendon repair in diabetic rats: new insights into a possible basis for compromised healing. *Cell Tissue Res.* 2014;357:109-117.
15. Attinger CE, Janis JE, Steinberg JS, et al. Clinical approach to wounds: debridement and wound bed preparation including the use of dressings and wound-healing adjuvants. *Plast Reconstr Surg.* 2006;117(7 suppl):72S-109S.
16. Donahue RP, Orchard TJ. Diabetes mellitus and macrovascular complications. *Diabetes Care.* 1992;15:1141-1155.
17. Jude EB, Oylbo SO, Chalmers N, et al. Peripheral arterial disease in diabetic and non-diabetic patients: a comparison of severity and outcome. *Diabetes Care.* 2001;24:1433-1437.
18. Trans Atlantic Inter-Society Consensus Working Group (TASG). Management of peripheral arterial disease (PAD). *J Vasc Surg.* 2000;51(1 pt 2):S1-S296.
19. Dashioghi HH, O'Brien-Irr MS, Lukan J, et al. Does preferential use of endovascular interventions by vascular surgeons improve limb salvage, control symptoms and survival of patients with critical limb ischemia? *Am J Surg.* 2006;192:572-576.
20. Jorneskog G, Brismar K, Fagrell B. Skin capillary circulation is more impaired in the toes of the diabetic than non-diabetic patients with peripheral vascular disease. *Diabet Med.* 1995;12(1):36-41.
21. Jorneskog G, Brismar K, Fagrell B. Skin capillary circulation severely impaired in toes of patients with IDDM, with and without late diabetic complications. *Diabetologia.* 1995;38(4):474-480.
22. Jorneskog G, Brismar K, Fagrell B. Pronounced skin capillary ischemia in the foot of diabetic patients with bad metabolic control. *Diabetologia.* 1998;41(4):410-415.
23. Schramm JC, Dinh T, Veves A. Microvascular changes in the diabetic foot. *Int J Low Extrem Wounds.* 2006;5(3):149-159.
24. Rayman G, Malik RA, Sharma AK, et al. Microvascular response to tissue injury and capillary ultrastructure in the foot skin of type I diabetic patients. *Clin Sci.* 1995;89:467-474.
25. Jaap AJ, Shore AC, Stockman AJ, et al. Skin capillary density in subjects with impaired glucose tolerance and patients with type 2 diabetes. *Diabet Med.* 1996;13:160-164.
26. Chambers HF. The changing epidemiology of *Staphylococcus aureus? Emerg Infect Dis.* 2001;7:178-182.
27. Barret TW, Moran GJ. Update on emerging infections: news from the centers for disease control and prevention [commentary]. *Ann Emerg Med.* 2004;43:45-47.
28. Cohen PR, Kurzrock R. Community-acquired methicillin-resistant *Staphylococcus aureus* skin infection: an emerging clinical problem. *J Am Acad Dermatol.* 2004;50:277-280.
29. Moran GJ, Krishnadasan A, Gorwitz RJ, et al.; EMERGEncy ID Net Study Group. Methicillin-resistant *S. aureus* infections among patients in the emergency department. *N Engl J Med.* 2006;355(7):666-674.
30. Dyck PJ, Kratz KM, Karnes JL, et al. The prevalence by staged severity of various types of diabetic neuropathy, retinopathy, and nephropathy in a population-based cohort: The Rochester Diabetic Neuropathy Study. *Neurology.* 1993;43(4):817-824.
31. Young MJ, Boulton AJ, MacLeod AF, et al. A multicenter study of the prevalence of diabetic peripheral neuropathy in the United Kingdom hospital clinic population. *Diabetologia.* 1993;36(2):150-154.
32. Kumar S, Ashe HA, Parnell LN, et al. The prevalence of foot ulceration and its correlates in type 2 diabetic patients: a population-based study. *Diabet Med.* 1994;11(5):480-484.
33. Cabezas-Cerrato J. The prevalence of clinical diabetic polyneuropathy in Spain: a study in primary care and hospital clinic groups. Neuropathy Spanish Study Group of the Spanish Diabetes Society (SDS). *Diabetologia.* 1998;41(11):1265-1269.
34. Diabetes Control and complications Trial Research Group. The effect of intensive treatment of diabetes on the development and progression of long-term complications in insulin-dependent diabetes mellitus. *N Engl J Med.* 1993;329(14):977-986.
35. Slemienow M, Alghoul M, Molski M, et al. Clinical outcome of peripheral nerve decompression in diabetic and non-diabetic peripheral neuropathy. *Ann Plast Surg.* 2006;54(4):385-390.
36. Relber GE, Vileikyte L, Boyko EJ, et al. Causal pathways for incident lower-extremity ulcers in patients with diabetes from two settings. *Diabetes Care.* 1999;22(1):157-162.
37. Rathur HM, Boulton AJM. Recent advances in the diagnosis and management of diabetic neuropathy. *J Bone Joint Surg Br.* 2005;87-B(12):1605-1610.
38. Boyko EJ, Ahroni J, Stensel V, et al. A prospective study of risk factors for diabetic foot ulcers. The Seattle Diabetic Foot Study. *Diabetes Care.* 1999;22(7):1036-1042.
39. Larsen K, Fabrin J, Holstein PE. Incidence and management of ulcers in diabetic Charcot feet. *J Wound Care.* 2001;10(8):323-328.
40. Ledoux WR, Shafer JB, Smith DG. Relationship between foot type, foot deformity, and ulcer occurrence in the high-risk diabetic foot. *J Rehabil Res Dev.* 2005;42(5):665-672.
41. Boulton AJM, Hardisty CA, Betts RP, et al. Dynamic foot pressure and other studies as diagnostic and management aid in diabetic neuropathy. *Diabetes Care.* 1983;(61):26-33.
42. Barry DC, Sabacinski KA, Habershaw GM, et al. Tendo Achilles procedures for chronic ulcerations in diabetic patients with transmetatarsal amputations. *J Am Podiatric Med Assoc.* 1993;83(2):96-100.
43. Armstrong DG, Peters EJ, Athanasion KA, et al. Is there a critical level of plantar foot pressure to identify patients at risk for neuropathic foot ulceration? *J Foot Ankle Surg.* 1998;37:303-307.
44. Armstrong DG, Sacpoole-Shea S, Nguyen H, et al. Lengthening of the Achilles tendon in diabetic patients who are at high risk for ulceration of the foot. *J Bone Joint Surg Am.* 1999;81(4):535-538.
45. Lin Ss, Lee TH, Wapner KL. Plantar forefoot ulceration with equinus deformity of the ankle in diabetic patients: the effect of tendon-Achilles lengthening and total contact casting. *Orthopedics.* 1996;19(5):465-475.
46. Lavery LA, Armstrong DG, Boulton AJM. Ankle equinus deformity and its relationship to high plantar pressure in a large population with diabetes mellitus. *J Am Podiatr Med Assoc.* 2002;92(9):479-482.
47. Holstein P, Lohmann M, Bitsch M, et al. Achilles tendon lengthening, the panacea for planar forefoot ulceration? *Diabetes Metab Res Rev.* 2004;20(suppl 1):S37-S40.

48. Orendurff MS, Rohr ES, Sangeorzan BJ, et al. An equinus deformity of the ankle accounts for only a small amount of the increased forefoot plantar pressure in patients with diabetes. *J Bone Joint Surg Br.* 2006;88(1):65-68.
49. Lauri C, Tamminga M, Glaudemans WJM, et al. Detection of osteomyelitis in the diabetic foot by imaging techniques: a systematic review and meta-analysis comparing MRI, white blood cell scintigraphy, and FDG-PET. *Diabetes Care.* 2017;40:1111-1120.
50. Erngrul MB, Bakdroglu S, Salman S, et al. The diagnosis of osteomyelitis of the foot in diabetes: microbiological examination vs. magnetic resonance imaging and labeled leukocyte scanning. *Diabet Med.* 2006;23(6):649-653.
51. Pecoraro RE, Reiber GE, Burgess EM. Pathways to diabetic limb amputation: basis for prevention. *Diabetes Care.* 1990;12:513-521.
52. Kamolz LP, Wild, T. Wound bed preparation: the impact of debridement and wound cleansing. *Wound Med.* 2013;1:44-50.
53. Cornell RS, Meyr AJ, Steinberg JS, Attinger CE. Debridement of the noninfected wound. *J Vasc Surg.* 2010;52(3 suppl):31S-36S.
54. Guthrie HC, Clasper JC. Historical origins and current concepts of wound debridement. *J R Army Med Corps.* 2011;157(2):130-132.
55. Sun X, Jiang K, Chen J, et al. A systematic review of maggot debridement therapy for chronically infected wounds and ulcers. *Int J Infect Dis.* 2014;25:32-37.
56. Ahroni JH, Boyko EJ, Forsberg R. Reliability of F-scan in-shoe measurements of plantar pressure. *Foot Ankle Int.* 1998;19(10):668-673.
57. Pollard JP, Le Quesene LP, Tappin JW. Forces under the foot. *J Biomech Eng.* 1989;5:37-40.
58. Delbridge L, Ctercteko G, Fowler C, et al. The aetiology of diabetic neuropathic ulceration of the foot. *Br J Surg.* 1985;72:1-6.
59. Perry JE, Hall JO, Davis BL. Simultaneous measurement of plantar pressure and shear forces in diabetic individuals. *Gait Posture.* 2002;15:101-107.
60. Lavery LA, Vela SA, Lavery DC, et al. Reducing dynamic foot pressures in high risk diabetic subjects with foot ulcerations: a comparison of treatments. *Diabetes Care.* 1996;19(8):818-821.
61. Lavery LA, Vela SA, Fleischill JG, et al. Reducing plantar pressure in the neuropathic foot: a comparison of footwear. *Diabetes Care.* 1997;20(11):1706-1710.
62. Armstrong DG, Losmond PJ, Todd WF. Potential risks of accommodative padding in the treatment of neuropathic ulcerations. *Ostomy Wound Manage.* 1995;41(7):44-46, 48-49.
63. Armstrong DG, Athanasion KA. The edge effect: how and why wounds grow in size and depth. *Clin Podiatr Med Surg.* 1998;15(1):105-108.
64. Mueller MJ, Diamond JK, Sinacore DR, et al. Total contact casting in treatment of diabetic plantar ulcers. Controlled clinical trial. *Diabetes Care.* 1989;12(6):384-388.
65. Armstrong DG, Nguyen HC, Lavery LA, et al. Off-loading the diabetic foot wound: a randomized clinical trial. *Diabetes Care.* 2001;24(8):1019-1022.
66. Wukich DK, Motko J. Safety of total contact casting in high-risk patients with neuropathic foot ulcers. *Foot Ankle Int.* 2004;25(8):556-560.
67. Fleischill JG, Lavery LA, Vela SA, et al. Comparison of strategies for reducing pressure at the site of neuropathic ulcers. *J Am Podiatr Med Assoc.* 1997;87(10):466-472.
68. Armstrong DG, Stacpoole-Shea S. Total contact casts and removable cast walkers. *J Am Podiatr Med Assoc.* 1999;89(10):50-53.
69. Armstrong DG, Short B, Espensen EH, Abu-Rumman PL. Technique for fabrication of an "Instant Total-Contact Cast" for treatment of neuropathic diabetic foot ulcers. *J Am Podiatr Med Assoc.* 2002;92(7):405-408.
70. Chantelau E, Breuer U, Leisch AC, et al. Outpatient treatment of unilateral diabetic foot ulcers with 'half shoes'. *Diabet Med.* 1993;10(3):267-270.
71. Hood R, Shermock KM, Emerman C. A prospective, randomized pilot evaluation of topical triple antibiotic versus mupirocin for the prevention of uncomplicated soft tissues wound infection. *Am J Emerg Med.* 2004;22(1):1-2.
72. Lipsky BA, Berendt AR, Deery HG, et al. Diagnosis and treatment of diabetic foot infections. *Plast Reconstr Surg.* 2006;117(7 suppl):212S-238S.
73. Strock LL, Lee MM, Rutars RL, et al. Topical Bactroban (mupirocin): efficacy in treating burn wounds infected with methicillin-resistant staphylococci. *J Burn Care Rehabil.* 1990;11(5):454-459.
74. Smoot EC III, Kucan JO, Graham DR, et al. Susceptibility testing of topical antibacterials against methicillin-resistant *Staphylococcus aureus*. *J Burn Care Rehabil.* 1992;13(2 pt 1):198-202.
75. Apelqvist J, Ragnarson TG. Cavity foot ulcers in diabetic patients: a comparative study of cadexomer iodine ointment and standard treatment. An economic analysis alongside a clinical trial. *Acta Derm Venereol.* 1996;76(3):231-237.
76. Steed DL; Diabetic Ulcer study Group. Clinical evaluation of recombinant human platelet-derived growth factor the treatment of lower extremity diabetic ulcers. *J Vasc Surg.* 1995;21(1):71-78.
77. Wieman, TJ, Smiell JM, Su Y. Efficacy and safety of a topical gel formulation of recombinant human platelet-derived growth factor-BB (Becaplermin) in patients with chronic neuropathic diabetic ulcers. *Diabetes Care.* 1998;21(5):822-827.
78. Steed DL. Clinical evaluation of recombinant human platelet-derived growth factor for the treatment of lower extremity ulcers. *Plast Reconstr Surg.* 2006;117(78):143S-149S.
79. Jensen JL, Seeley J, Gillin B. Diabetic foot ulcerations. A controlled, randomized comparison of two moist wound healing protocols Carrasyn hydrogel wound dressing and wet-to-moist saline gauze. *Adv Wound Care.* 1998;11(7 suppl):2-4.
80. Seaman S. Dressing selection in chronic wound management. *J Am Podiatr Med Assoc.* 2002;92(1):24-33.
81. Phillips I, Lobo AZ, Fernandes R, et al. Acetic acid treatment of superficial wounds infected by *Pseudomonas aeruginosa*. *Lancet.* 1968;1(7532):11-14.
82. Milner SM. Acetic acid to treat *Pseudomonas aeruginosa* in superficial wounds and burns. *Lancet.* 1992;340:61.
83. Kozol RA, Gillies C, Elgebaly SA. Effects of sodium hypochlorite (Dakin's Solution) on cells of the wound module. *Arch Surg.* 1988;123:420-423.
84. Wilson JR, Mills JG, Prather ID, et al. A toxicity index of skin and wound cleansers used on in vitro fibroblasts and keratinocytes. *Adv Skin Wound Care.* 2005;18(7):373-378.
85. Russell AD, Hugo WB. Antimicrobial activity and action of silver. *Prog Med Chem.* 1994;31:351-370.
86. Tredget EE, Shankowsky HA, Groeneveld A, et al. A matched-pair, randomized study evaluating the efficacy and safety of Acticoat silver-coated dressing for the treatment of burn wounds. *J Burn Care Rehabil.* 1998;19(6):531-537.
87. Ip M, Liu SL, Poon VKM, et al. Antimicrobial activities of silver dressings: an in vitro comparison. *J Med Microbiol.* 2006;55:59-65.
88. Jorgensen B, Price P, Anderson KE, et al. The silver-releasing foam dressing, Contrees Foam, promotes faster healing of critically colonized venous leg ulcers: a randomized, controlled trial. *Int Wound J.* 2005;2(1):64-73.
89. Mesume S, Vallet D, Morere MN, et al. Evaluation of a silver-release hydroalginate dressing in chronic wounds with signs of local infection. *J Wound Care.* 2005;14(9):411-419.
90. Munter KC, Beele H, Russell L, et al. Effect of a sustained silver-releasing dressing on ulcers with delayed healing: the CONTOP study. *J Wound Care.* 2006;15(5):199-206.
91. Cullen B, Smith R, McCullock E, et al. Mechanism of action of PROMOGRAN, a protease modulating matrix, for the treatment of diabetic foot ulcers. *Wound Repair Regen.* 2002;10(1):16-25.
92. Lobmann R, Zemlin C, Motzkau M, et al. Expression of matrix metalloproteinases and growth factors in diabetic foot wounds treated with a protease absorbent dressing. *J Diabetes Complications.* 2006;20(5):329-335.
93. Fleischmann W, Strecker W, Bombelli M. Vacuum sealing as treatment of soft tissue damage in open fractures. *Unfallchirurg.* 1993;96(9):488-492.
94. Fleishcmann W, Lange E, Kinsel L. Vacuum assisted wound closure after dermatofasciotomy of the lower extremity. *Unfallchirurg.* 1996;99(4):283-287.
95. Fleischmann W, Lang E, Russ M. Treatment of infection by vacuum sealing. *Unfallchirurg.* 1997;100(4):301-304.
96. Morykwas MJ, Argenta LC, Shelton-Brown EI, et al. Vacuum-assisted closure: a new method for wound control and treatment: animal studies and basic foundation. *Ann Plast Surg.* 1997;38(6):553-562.
97. Argenta LC, Morykwas MJ. Vacuum-assisted closure: a new method for wound control and treatment: clinical experience. *Ann Plast Surg.* 1997;38(6):565-576.
98. Joseph E, Mamort CA, Bergman S, et al. A prospective randomized trial of vacuum-assisted closure versus standard therapy of chronic non-healing wounds. *Wounds.* 2000;12:60-67.
99. McCallon SK, Knoight CA, Vallules JP, et al. Vacuum-assisted closure versus saline-moistened gauze in the healing of postoperative diabetic foot wounds. *Ostomy Wound Manage.* 2000;46:28-32, 34.
100. Eginton MT, Brown KR, Seabrook GR, et al. A prospective randomized evaluation of negative-pressure wound dressings for diabetic foot wounds. *Ann Vasc Surg.* 2003;17(6): 645-649.
101. Armstrong DG, Lavery LA. Negative pressure wound therapy after atrial diabetic foot amputation: a multicenter randomized controlled trial. *Lancet.* 2005;366:1704-1710.
102. Molnar JA, DeFranzo AJ, Hadaegh A, et al. Acceleration of Integra incorporation in complex tissue defects with subatmospheric pressure. *Plast Reconstr Surg.* 2004;113(5): 1339-1346.
103. Molnar JA, DeFranzo AJ, Marks MW. Sing-staged approach to skin grafting the exposed skull. *Plast Reconstr Surg.* 2000;105(1):174-177.
104. Espensen EH, Nixon BP, Lavery LA, et al. Use of subatmospheric (VAC) therapy to improve bioengineered tissue grafting in diabetic foot wounds. *J Am Podiatr Med Assoc.* 2002;92(7):395-397.
105. Scherer LA, Shiver S, Chang M, et al. The vacuum assisted closure device: a method of securing skin grafts and improving graft survival. *Arch Surg.* 2002;137(8):930-935.
106. Isago T, Nozaki M, Kikuchi Y, et al. Skin graft fixation with negative-pressure dressing. *J Dermatol.* 2003;30(9):673-678.
107. Moisidis E, Heath T, Boorer C, et al. A prospective, blinded, randomized, controlled clinical trial of topical negative pressure use in the skin graft. *Plast Reconstr Surg.* 2004;114(4):917-922.
108. Coctor N, Pandya S, Supe A. Hyperbaric oxygen therapy in diabetic foot. *J Postgrad Med.* 1992;38(3):112-114, 111.
109. Fagia E, Favales F, Aldeghi A, et al. Adjunctive systemic hyperbaric oxygen therapy in treatment of severe prevalently ischemic diabetic foot ulcer. A randomized study. *Diabetes Care.* 1996;19(12):1338-1348.
110. Abidia A, Laden G, Kuthan G, et al. The role of hyperbaric oxygen therapy in ischemic diabetic lower extremity ulcers: a double-blinded randomized-controlled trial. *Eur J Vasc Surg.* 2003;25(6):513-518.
111. Hunt TK, Pal MP. The effect of varying ambient oxygen tensions on wound metabolism and collagen synthesis. *Surg Gynecol Obstet.* 1972;135(4):561-567.
112. Ellis ME, Mandel BK. Hyperbaric oxygen treatment: 10 years' experience of a regional infectious disease unit. *J Infect.* 1983;6(1):17-28.
113. Zhao LL, Davidson JD, Wee SC, et al. Effect of hyperbaric oxygen and growth factors on rabbit ear ischemic ulcers. *Arch Surg.* 1994;129(10):1045-1049.
114. Sheikh AY, Gibson JJ, Rollins MD, et al. Effect of hypoxia on vascular endothelial growth factor levels in a wound model. *Arch Surg.* 2000;135(11):1293-1297.
115. Kang TS, Corti GK, Quan SY, et al. Effect of hyperbaric oxygen on growth factor profile of fibroblasts. *Arch Facial Plast Surg.* 2004;6(1):31-35.
116. Attinger CE, Clemens MW, Ducic I, Levin MM, Zelen C. Chapter 23: the use of local muscle flaps in foot and ankle reconstruction. In: Dockery GD, ed. *Lower Extremity Soft Tissue & Cutaneous Plastic Surgery.* 2nd ed. Kidlington, England: Elsevier Science; 2011.
117. Mathes S, Nahai F. *Clinical Application for Muscle and Musculocutaneous Flaps.* St Louis, MO: Mosby; 1982:3.
118. Bunnell S. An essential in reconstructive surgery: atraumatic technique. *Cal State J Med.* 1921;19:204.
119. Manring MM, Hawk A, Calhoun JH, Andersen RC. Treatment of war wounds: a historical review. *Clin Orthop Relat Res.* 2009;467:2168-2191.
120. Snell GD. The terminology of tissue transplantation. *Transplantation.* 1964;2:655-657.

121. Salisbury R, Caines R, McCarthy LR. Comparison of the bacterial cleaning effects of different biologic dressings on granulating wounds following thermal injury. *Plast Reconstr Surg.* 1980;66:596-598.
122. Kumagai N, Nishina H, Tanabe H, et al. Clinical application of autologous cultured epithelia for the treatment of bum wounds and bum scars. *Plast Reconstr Surg.* 1988;82:99-108.
123. Latarjet J, Gangolphe M, Hezez G, et al. The grafting of burns with cultured epidermis as autografts in man. *Scand J Plast Reconstr Surg.* 1987;21:241.
124. Rothstein AS. Skin grafting techniques. *J Am Podiatry Assoc.* 1983;73:79-85.
125. Vistnes LM. Grafting of skin. *Surg Clin North Am.* 1977;57:939-959.
126. McGregor I. *Fundamental Techniques of Plastic Surgery and Their Applications.* 7th ed. New York, NY: Churchill-Livingstone; 1980:55-99.
127. Barsky ED. *Principles of Plastic Surgery.* 2nd ed. New York, NY: McGraw-Hill; 1964:65.
128. Hallock GG. The complete classification of flaps. *Microsurgery.* 2004;24:157-161.
129. Fleetwood J, Barrett S, Day S. Skin flaps: the Burow advancement flap for closure of plantar defects. *J Am Podiatr Med Assoc.* 1987;77:246-249.
130. Grabb WC, Meyers MB. *Skin Flaps.* Boston, MA: Little, Brown; 1975.
131. Marcinko DE. Plastic surgery in podiatry (simplified illustrated technique). *J Am Podiatr Med Assoc.* 1988;27:103-110.
132. Dockery GL. Principles of forefoot plastic surgery. In: Butterworth RF, Dockery GL, eds. *Color Atlas and Text of Forefoot Surgery.* Chicago, IL: Mosby-Year Book; 1992.
133. Shaw DT, Li CS. Multiple Y-V plasty. *Ann Plast Surg.* 1979;2:436-440.
134. Colen LB, Replogle SL, Mathes SJ. The V-Y plantar flap for reconstruction of the forefoot. *Plast Reconstr Surg.* 1988;81:220-227.
135. Zimany A. The bilobed flap. *Plast Reconstr Surg.* 1953;11:424-454.
136. McGregor IA. The Z-plasty. *Br J Plast Surg.* 1966;19:82-87.
137. McGregor IA. The Z-plasty in hand surgery. *J Bone Joint Surg Br.* 1967;49:448-457.
138. Woolf RM, Broadbent TR. The four-flap Z-plasty. *Plast Reconstr Surg.* 1972;49:448-457.
139. Crawford ME, Docker GL. Use of Z-skin plasty in scar revisions and skin contractures of the lower extremity. *J Am Podiatr Med Assoc.* 1995;85:28-35.
140. Schrudde J, Petrovici V. The use of slide-swing plasty in closing skin defects: a clinical study based on 1,308 cases. *Plast Reconstr Surg.* 1981;67:467-481.
141. Esser JFS. Gestielte lokale Nasenplastik mit zweizipfligen Lappen, Deckung des sekunderen Defektes vom ersten Zipfel durch den Zweiten. *Dtsch Z Chir.* 1918;143:385.
142. Morgan BL, Samilan MR. Advantage of the bilobed flap for closure of small defects of the face. *Plast Reconstr Surg.* 1973;52:35-37.
143. McGregor JC, Soutar DS. A critical assessment of the bilobed flap. *Br J Plast Surg.* 1981;34:197-205.
144. Miller SJ. The bilobed skin flap rotation. *Clin Podiatr Med Surg.* 1986;3:253-258.
145. Sanchez-Conejo-Mir J, Bueno MJ, Moreno G, et al. The bilobed flap in sole surgery. *J Dermatol Surg Oncol.* 1985;11:913-917.
146. Limberg AA. Design of local flaps. In: Gibson T, ed. *Modern Trends in Plastic Surgery.* 2nd ed. London, UK: Butterworth; 1966:38-61.
147. Borges AF. The rhombic flap. *Plast Reconstr Surg.* 1981;67:458-465.
148. Cuono C. Double Z-rhombic repair of both large and small defects of the upper extremity. *J Hand Surg Am.* 1984;9:197-202.
149. Snyder GB, Edgerton MT. The principle of the island neurovascular flap in the management of ulcerated anesthetic weight-bearing areas of the lower extremity. *Plast Reconstr Surg.* 1965;36:518-528.
150. Attinger CE. Use of soft tissue techniques for salvage of the diabetic foot. In: Kominsky S, ed. *Medical and Surgical Management of the Diabetic Foot.* St. Louis, MO: Mosby-Year Book; 1994:323-366.
151. Banchke HJ, Colen LB. An island flap from the first web space of the foot to cover plantar ulcers. *Br J Plast Surg.* 1980;33:242-244.
152. Granick MS, Newton ED, Fistrell JW, et al. The plantar digital web space island flap for reconstruction of the distal sole. *Ann Plast Surg.* 1987;19:68-74.
153. Colen LB, Buncke HJ. Neurovascular island flaps from the plantar vessels and nerves for foot reconstruction. *Ann Plast Surg.* 1984;12:327-332.
154. Furlow LT. The dorsalis pedis flap. In: Strauch B, Vasconer LO, Hall-Findlay EJ, eds. *Grabb's Encyclopedia of Flaps.* Boston, MA: Little, Brown; 1990:1654-1660.
155. Ishikawa K, Isshiki N, Suzucki S, et al. Distally based dorsalis pedis flap from the first web of the foot in hand reconstruction. *J Hand Surg Am.* 1977;2:387-395.
156. Man D, Acland RD. The microarterial anatomy of the dorsalis pedis flap and its clinical applications. *Plast Reconstr Surg.* 1980;65:419-423.
157. Smith AA, Aarons JA, Reyes R, et al. Distal foot coverage with a reverse dorsalis pedis flap. *Ann Plast Surg.* 1995;34:191-200.
158. Gajhwala KJ, Mehta IM, Mahalusmuivala SM, et al. A new approach to heel ulcers: dorsalis pedis neurovascular trans-interosseous island flap. *Br J Plast Surg.* 1987;40:241-245.
159. Early MJ, Milner RH. A distally based first web flap in the foot. *Br J Plast Surg.* 1989;42:507-511.
160. Lee JH, Dauber W. Anatomic study of the dorsalis pedis-first dorsal metatarsal artery. *Ann Plast Surg.* 1997;38:50-55.
161. Hayashi A, Maruyama Y. Reverse first dorsal metatarsal artery flap for reconstruction of the distal foot. *Ann Plast Surg.* 1993;31:117-122.
162. Senyuva C, Yucel A, Fassio E. Reverse first dorsal metatarsal artery adipofascial flap. *Ann Plast Surg.* 1996;36:158-161.
163. Saki S. A distally based island first dorsal metatarsal artery flap for coverage of a distal plantar defect. *Br J Plast Surg.* 1993;46:480-482.
164. Satoh K, Kaieda K. Resurfacing the distal part of the foot with a dorsal foot skin island flap pedicled on the plantar vasculature. *Plast Reconstr Surg.* 1995;95:176-180.
165. Shanahan RE. The medial plantar flap. In: Strauch B, Vasconez LO, Hall-Findlay EJ, eds. *Grabb's Encyclopedia of Flaps.* Boston, MA: Little, Brown, 1990:1638-1640.
166. Shaw WW, Hidalgo DA. Anatomic basis of plantar flap design: clinical applications. *Plast Reconstr Surg.* 1986;78:637-649.
167. Leung PC, Hung LK, Leung KS. Use of the medial plantar flap in soft tissue replacement around the heel region. *Foot Ankle.* 1988;8:327-330.
168. Saki S, Soeda S, Kanou T. Distally based lateral plantar artery island flap. *Ann Plast Surg.* 1988;21:165-169.
169. Suzuki S, Nose K, Ogawa Y, et al. The "reverse flow" flexor digitorum brevis myocutaneous flap for reconstruction of chronic ulcer on the metatarsal pad. *Jpn J Plast Reconstr Surg.* 1985;28:562.
170. Grabb WC, Argenta LC. The lateral calcaneal artery skin flap (the lateral calcaneal artery, lesser saphenous vein, and sural nerve skin flap). *Plast Reconstr Surg.* 1981;68:723-730.
171. Maha KT. Lateral calcaneal artery skin flap for posterior heel coverage. *Clin Podiatr Med Surg.* 1986;3:277-287.
172. Argenta LC. Reconstruction of soft-tissue defects of the posterior heel with a lateral calcaneal artery island flap (Discussion). *Plast Reconstr Surg.* 1987;79:420-421.
173. Yanal A, Park S, Iwao T, et al. Reconstruction of a skin defect of the posterior heel by a lateral calcaneal flap. *Plast Reconstr Surg.* 1985;75:642-646.
174. Hovius SER, Hofman A, Meulen JC. Experiences with the lateral calcaneal artery flap. *Ann Plast Surg.* 1988;21:532-535.
175. Lin SD, Lai CS, Chiu YT, et al. The lateral calcaneal artery adipofascial flap. *Br J Plast Surg.* 1996;49:52-57.
176. Attinger CE, Ducic I, Zelen C. The use of local muscle flaps in foot and ankle reconstruction. *Clin Podiatr Med Surg.* 2000;17(4):681-711.
177. D'Avila F, Franco D, D'Avila B, Arnaut M Jr. Use of local muscle flaps to cover leg bone exposures. *Rev Col Bras Cir.* 2014;41(6):434-439.
178. Ger R. Abductor hallucis brevis muscle flap. In: Strauch B, Vasconez LO, Hall-Findlay EJ, eds. *Grabb's encyclopedia of flaps.* Boston, MA: Little, Brown; 1990:1666-1668.
179. Ger R. The technique of muscle transposition and the operative treatment of traumatic and ulcerative lesions of the leg. *J Trauma.* 1971;11:502-510.
180. Mathes SJ, Nahai F. *Reconstructive Surgery: Principles, Anatomy and Technique.* New York, NY: Churchill Livingstone and Quality Medical Publishing, Inc.; 1997.
181. Bostwick J III. Reconstruction of the heel pad by muscle transposition and split-skin graft. *Surg Gynecol Obstet.* 1976;143:973-974.
182. Ger R. Flexor digitorum brevis muscle flap. In: Strauch B, Vasconez LO, Hall-Findlay EJ, eds. *Grabb's Encyclopedia of Flaps.* Boston, MA: Little, Brown; 1990:1669-1670.
183. Scheflan M, Hanai F. Foot: reconstruction. In: Mathes SJ, Nahal F, eds. *Clinical Applications for Muscle and Musculocutaneous Flaps.* St. Louis, MO: CV Mosby; 1982:594.
184. Graziano TA, Baratta JB, Menditto L, et al. A surgical alternative in the management of chronic neurotropic ulcerations of the foot. *J Foot Ankle Surg.* 1993;32:295-298.
185. Graziano T, Giampapa V. Muscle transposition in the management of chronic osteomyelitis and ulceration of the heel. *J Foot Surg.* 1989;28:68-71.
186. Furukawa M, Nakagawa K, Hamada T. Long-term complications of reconstruction of the heel using a digitorum brevis muscle flap. *Ann Plast Surg.* 1993;30:345-358.
187. Landi A, Soragni O, Monteleone M. The extensor digitorum brevis muscle island flap for soft-tissue loss around the ankle. *Plast Reconstr Surg.* 1985;75:892-897.
188. Leitner D, Gordon L, Buncke H. The extensor digitorum brevis as a muscle island flap. *Plast Reconstr Surg.* 1985;76:777-780.
189. Hing DN, Buncke HJ, Alpert BS. Applications of the extensor digitorum brevis muscle for soft tissue coverage. *Ann Plast Surg.* 1987;19:530-537.
190. Gibstein LA, Abrasson DL, Sampson CE, et al. Musculofascial flaps based on the dorsalis pedis vascular pedicle for coverage of the foot and ankle. *Ann Plast Surg.* 1996;37:152-157.
191. Giordano P, Argensen G, Pequignot JP. Extensor digitorum brevis as an island flap in the reconstruction of soft-tissue defects in the lower limb. *Plast Reconstr Surg.* 1989;83:100-109.
192. Saint-Cyr M, Schaverien M. Perforator flaps: history, controversies, physiology, anatomy, and use in reconstruction. *Plast Reconstr Surg.* 2009;123:132-145.
193. Satoh K, Aoyama R, Onizuka T. Comparative study of reverse flow island flaps in the lower extremities: peroneal, anterior tibial, and posterior tibial island flaps in 25 patients. *Ann Plast Surg.* 1993;30:48-56.
194. Masquelet AC, Beveridge J, Romana C, et al. The lateral supramalleolar flap. *Plast Reconstr Surg.* 1988;81:74-81.
195. Yoshimura M, Shimada T, Imura S, et al. Peroneal island flap for skin defects in the lower extremity. *J Bone Joint Surg Am.* 1985;67:935-941.
196. Cheng L, Yang X, Chen T, Li Z. Peroneal artery perforator flap for the treatment of chronic lower extremity wounds. *J Orthop Surg Res.* 2017;12:170.
197. Ponten B. The fasciocutaneous flap: its use in soft tissue defects of the lower leg. *Br J Plast Surg.* 1981;34:215-220.
198. Donski PK, Fogdestam I. Distally based fasciocutaneous flap from the sural region. *Scand J Plast Reconstr Surg.* 1983;17:191-196.
199. Masquelet AC, Gilbert A. *An Atlas of Flaps of the Musculoskeletal System. Transfers from the Lower Limb.* 1st ed. Essex: CRC Press; 2010;186-187.
200. Sugg KB, Schaub TA, Concannon MJ, et al. The reverse superficial sural artery flap revisited for complex lower extremity and foot reconstruction. *Plast Reconstr Surg Glob Open.* 2015;3(9):e519.
201. Akhtar S, Hameed A. Versatility of the sural fasciocutaneous flap in the coverage of lower third leg and hind foot defects. *J Plast Reconstr Aesthet Surg.* 2006;59(8):839-845.
202. Jeng SF, Wei FC. Distally based sural island flap for foot and ankle reconstruction. *Plast Reconstr Surg.* 1997;99:744-750.
203. Amarante J, Costa H, Reis J, et al. A new distally based fasciocutaneous flap of the leg. *Br J Plast Surg.* 1986;39:338-340.
204. Blondeel PN, Morris SF, Hallock GG, Neligan PC, eds. Anatomy of the integument of the lower extremity. In: *Perforator flaps, Anatomy, Technique and Clinical Applications.* Baltimore, MD: Quality Medical Publishing (QMP); 2006:542-577.
205. Jones EB, Cronwright K, Lalbahadur A. Anatomical studies and five years clinical experience with the distally based medial fasciocutaneous flap of the lower leg. *Br J Plast Surg.* 1993;46:639-643.
206. Yang X, Chen G, Zeng H, et al. Distal posterior tibial artery perforator flaps for the treatment of chronic lower extremity wounds. *Int J Clin Exp Med.* 2016;9(10):19553-19560.
207. Wee JTK. Reconstruction of the lower leg and foot with the reverse pedicled anterior tibial flap: a preliminary report of a new fasciocutaneous flap. *Br J Plast Surg.* 1986;39:327-337.

208. Georgescu AV. Propeller perforator flaps in the distal lower leg: evolution and clinical applications. *Arch Plast Surg.* 2012;39:94-105.
209. Garcia-Pumarino R, Franco JM. Anatomical variability of descending genicular artery. *Ann Plast Surg.* 2014;73(5):607-611.
210. Nenad T, Reiner W, Schlageter M, Hoffmann R, et al. Saphenous perforator flap for reconstructive surgery in the lower leg and the foot: a clinical study of 50 patients with posttraumatic osteomyelitis. *J Trauma.* 2010;68(5);1200-1207.
211. Quaba AA, Davison PM. The distally-based dorsal hand flap. *Br J Plast Surg.* 1990;43:28-39.
212. Wei F, Mardini S. Free-style free flaps. *Plast Reconstr Surg.* 2004;114:910-916.
213. Taylor GI, Palmer JH. The vascular territories (angiosomes) of the body: experimental study and clinical applications. *Br J Plast Surg.* 1987;40:113-141.
214. Quaba O, Quaba A. Pedicled perforator flaps for the lower limb. *Semin Plast Surg.* 2006;20(2):103-111.
215. Ger R, Efron G. New operative approach in the treatment of chronic osteomyelitis of the tibial diaphysis. A preliminary report. *Clin Orthop Relat Res.* 1970;70:165-169.
216. Dibbell DG, Edstrom LE. The gastrocnemius myocutaneous flap. *Clin Plast Surg.* 1980;7:45-50.
217. Buchner M, Zeifang F, Bernd L. Medial gastrocnemius muscle flap in limb-sparing surgery of malignant bone tumors of the proximal tibia: mid-term results in 25 patients. *Ann Plast Surg.* 2003;51:266-272.
218. Daigeler A, Drücke D, Tatar K, et al. The pedicled gastrocnemius muscle flap: a review of 218 cases. *Plast Reconstr Surg.* 2009;123(1):250-257.
219. Song P, Pu LLQ. The soleus muscle flap: an overview of its clinical applications for lower extremity reconstruction. *Ann Plast Surg.* 2018;81(6 suppl 1):S109-S116.
220. Kauffman CA, Lahoda LU, Cederna PS, Kuzon WM. Use of soleus muscle flaps for coverage of distal third tibial defects. *J Reconstr Microsurg.* 2004;20(8):593-597.
221. Costa H, Malheiro E, Silva A, et al. The distally based posterior tibial myofasciocutaneous island flap in foot reconstruction. *Br J Plast Surg.* 1996;49:111-114.
222. Lorenzetti F, Lazzeri D, Bonini L, et al. Distally based peroneus brevis muscle flap in reconstructive surgery of the lower leg: postoperative ankle function and stability evaluation. *J Plast Reconstr Aesthet Surg.* 2010;63(9):1523-1533.
223. Ensat F, Hladik M, Larcher L, et al. The distally based peroneus brevis muscle flap-clinical series and review of the literature. *Microsurgery.* 2014;34(3):203-208.
224. Lakhiani C, Evans KK, Attinger CE, Chapter 16: Free Flap Reconstruction for Soft Tissue Coverage of the Diabetic Lower Extremity. In: Zgonis T, ed. *Surgical Reconstruction of the Diabetic Foot.* 2nd ed. Philiadelphia, PA: Lippincott Williams & Wilkins. 2017.
225. Heller L, Kronowitz SJ. Lower extremity reconstruction. *J Surg Oncol.* 2006;94:479-489.
226. Mathes SJ, Alpert BS, Chang N. Use of the muscle flap in chronic osteomyelitis: experimental and clinical correlation. *Plast Reconstr Surg.* 1982;69:815-829.
227. Mathes SJ, Feng LG, Hunt TK. Coverage of the infected wound. *Ann Surg.* 1983;198:420-429.
228. Saint-Cyr M, Wong C, Buchel EW, Colohan S, Pederson WC. Free tissue transfers and replantation. *Plast Reconstr Surg.* 2012;130(6):858e-878e.
229. Hansen SL, Young DM, Lang P, Sbitany H. *Plastic Surgery: Principles,* volume 1. 3rd ed. London: Elsevier Health Sciences; 2013. Chapter 24, Flap classification and applications.
230. Hallock GG. Anatomic basis of the gastrocnemius perforator-based flap. *Ann Plast Surg.* 2001;47:517.
231. Blondeel N, Vanderstraeten GG, Monstrey SJ, et al. The donor site morbidity of free DIEP flaps and free TRAM flaps for breast reconstruction. *Br J Plast Surg.* 1997;50:322-330.
232. Kimura N. A microdissected thin tensor fasciae latae perforator flap. *Plast Reconstr Surg.* 2002;109:69.
233. Blemer E, Stock W. Total thumb reconstruction: a one-stage reconstruction using an osteocutaneous forearm flap. *Br J Plast Surg.* 1985;36:52-55.
234. Gulmbertaeau JC, Panconi B. Recalcitrant non-union of the scaphoid treated with a vascularized bone graft based on the ulnar artery. *J Bone Joint Surg Am.* 1990;72:88-97.
235. Storm T, Cohen J, Newton ED. Free vascularized bone graft. *J Foot Ankle Surg.* 1996;35:436-439.
236. Morrison WA, O'Brien B, MacLeod A. Clinical experiences in free flap transfer. *Clin Orthop.* 1978;133:132-139.
237. DeFazio MV, Han KD, Attinger CE, Volume 4: Chapter 8: Foot Reconstruction. In: Neligan PC. ed. Plastic Surgery. 4th ed. Atlanta, GA: Elsevier. 2018;184-218.
238. Lakhiani C, DeFazio MV, Han K, Falola R, Evans KK. Donor-site morbidity following free tissue harvest from the thigh: a systemic review and pooled analysis of complications. *J Reconstr Microsurg.* 2016;32(05):342-357.

Complex Soft Tissue Injuries

Peter A. Blume, Trusha Jariwala, and Laura P. Rowe

DEFINITION

Complex soft tissue injuries represent one of the most difficult families of traumatic injuries for the foot and ankle surgeon to treat. They consist of a heterogeneous family of injuries caused by high-energy mechanisms, which include falls, motor vehicle crashes, auto vs pedestrian or cyclist accidents, industrial or farm accidents, gunshot wounds, crush injuries, and degloving injuries. These high-energy mechanisms lead to significant soft tissue damage, necrosis, and contamination with potential infection. The great majority of patients who present with severe soft tissue injuries have concomitant osseous injuries (fractures or dislocations), often open, and may have injuries to other sites requiring more complex, coordinated care.

Complex soft tissue injuries can belong to a number of subtypes, though due to their diverse nature a single injury may belong to various subtypes. Among the most common types of complex injuries in high-energy trauma are degloving, avulsion, crush, and mangling. Degloving refers to the separation of skin and subcutaneous layers from underlying tissues. The skin may be fully detached during the injury, or it may retain its attachment along one aspect. Soft tissue avulsion resembles degloving but involves the detachment of deeper tissue layers such as muscle or fascia. Arteries, veins, and nerves may be involved in the tissue that has been avulsed. The survival of the avulsed soft tissue depends on the blood supply that it retains, as well as that which can be established after injury. Crush injuries result from massive force on a part of the body and are common in industrial accidents. The damage to skin may appear less significant than the damage to internal tissue as seen during debridement. Mangling injuries involve the highest energy forces and manifest with involvement of all soft tissue layers and bone, often with traumatic amputations and vascular injury. However, it should be noted that all injuries are unique and can belong to more than a single of these subtypes.

Recently, there has been a new approach to dealing with complex osseous and soft tissue injuries called the combined orthoplastic approach. According to recent research, when these severe limb-threatening injuries occur, multiple specialties (particularly orthopedic and plastic surgery) have to combine efforts in coordinating patient care. This orthoplastics approach is set forth in "Standards for the management of the open fractures of the lower limbs."[1] In a multicenter prospective cohort study, the combined orthoplastic approach provided statistically improved outcomes compare to single specialty approach in severe limb injuries.[2] As foot and ankle surgeons, trained in orthopedic trauma and various plastic and reconstructive techniques, we are vital members of the team attempting to salvage and heal complex foot and ankle trauma.

CLASSIFICATION

There are no specific classifications for complex soft tissue injuries of the lower extremity. However, due to the high-energy mechanism of action in these injuries that usually leads to concomitant osseous injury, the most significant classification to mention here is the Gustilo-Anderson classification for open fractures. The Gustilo-Anderson classification was first proposed in 1976, based on both retrospective and prospective data, to describe patterns of open fractures and effects of early vs delayed closure, use of internal fixation, and an antibiotic use algorithm with infection rate.[3] They categorized open fractures (and by extension their soft tissue injuries) in three grades based on wound size, level of contamination, and fracture pattern.

The three categories and their descriptions are as follows[3]:

- Type I: an open fracture with a clean wound <1 cm long.
- Type II: an open fracture with a laceration >1 cm long without extensive soft tissue damage, flaps, or avulsions.
- Type III: either an open segmental fracture, an open fracture with extensive soft tissue damage, or a traumatic amputation.

Initially, Gustilo et al. concluded that the infection rate can be reduced 84.4% in type I and type II injuries with primary closure with internal fixation and use of prophylactic antibiotics.[3] However, they appreciated that the type III injuries varied widely in their severity, infection rate, and prognosis. Thus, they later proposed the division of type III fractures, based on additional retrospective study, into subtypes A, B, and C as follows[4]:

- Type IIIA: open fractures with adequate soft tissue coverage of a fractured bone despite extensive soft tissue laceration or flaps, or high-energy trauma regardless of the size of the wound.
- Type IIIB: open fractures with extensive soft tissue loss with periosteal stripping and bone exposure. This usually is associated with massive contamination.
- Type IIIC: open fractures associated with arterial injury requiring repair.

GUSTILO-ANDERSON CLASSIFICATION, WITH MODIFICATIONS

Gustilo Type	I	II	IIIA	IIIB	IIIC
Energy	Low	Moderate	High	High	High
Wound size and contamination	<1 cm Clean	1-10 cm Moderate	>10 cm Extensive	>10 cm Extensive	>10 cm Extensive
Soft tissue Damage	Minimal	Moderate	Extensive	Extensive	Extensive
Skin coverage	Local	Local	Local	Free/rotational graft	Flap coverage
Vascular injury	Normal	Normal	Normal	Normal	Arterial damage requiring repair

Adapted from Gustilo RB, Mendoza RM, Williams DN. Problems in the management of type III (severe) open fractures: a new classification of type III open fractures. *J Trauma.* 1984;24(8):742-746.

Type III fractures are generally likely to correspond with complex soft tissue injuries. These injuries have both bone and soft tissue involvement, in which both musculoskeletal and soft tissue injuries must be addressed: the bone stabilized to allow for soft tissue healing, and the soft tissue maintained to be able to cover the bone and avoid infection or necrosis.

Tscherne and Oestern described a classification for closed and open fractures in 1982. The open fracture classification also described the severity of the soft tissue damage with the predicted rate of infection.[5] This classification is based on the rate of kinetic energy mechanism of action affecting the soft tissue and physiologic consequences of the trauma on the overlying soft tissue envelope. The soft tissue damage spanned from minor skin laceration to extensive damage with neurovascular compromise. Per Tscherne and Oestern recommendation, grade 1 and 2 injuries are reasonable for primary fixation with closure of soft tissue. However, staged fracture care resulted in decreased rate of soft tissue complication.[6] In a recent study comparing Gustilo-Anderson and Tscherne's classifications for open fractures, Tscherne's classification showed higher specificity as a predictor of infection rate.[7]

In 1985, Byrd, Spicer, and Cierney proposed a classification of open tibial fractures,[8] which is shown in the classification box. Like the Gustilo-Anderson classification, it relates only to open fractures and ultimately relies on subjective criteria; however, unlike other classifications, it focuses on soft tissue coverage and viability for staged local or free flap coverage. The initial paper focuses on type III and IV fractures, of which they report 98% limb salvage for type III and 82% limb salvage for type IV injuries.

BYRD-SPICER CLASSIFICATION OF OPEN TIBIAL FRACTURES, ORIENTED TOWARD SOFT TISSUE RECONSTRUCTABILITY

Type I	Low-energy forces causing spiral or oblique fracture with skin lacerations <2 cm and relatively clean wound
Type II	Moderate-energy forces causing a comminuted or displaced fracture with moderate adjacent skin and muscle contusion but without devitalized muscle
Type III	High-energy forces causing significantly displaced fracture with severe comminution, segmental fracture, or bone defect; with extensive associated skin loss and devitalized muscle
Type IV	Fracture pattern as in III but with extreme-energy forces (eg, high-velocity gunshot, shotgun, crush, or degloving) or associated vascular injury requiring repair

Adapted from Byrd HS, Spicer TE, Cierney G III. Management of open tibial fractures. *Plast Reconstr Surg.* 1985;76(5):719-730.

TSCHERNE CLASSIFICATION FOR OPEN FRACTURES

Grade	Typical Fracture Pattern/ Injuries	Typical Soft Tissue Damage
01	Fracture resulting from indirect trauma (AO A1-A2)	Skin laceration; none to minimal
02	Fracture resulting from direct trauma (AO A3, B, C)	Skin laceration; circumferential contusions; moderate contamination
03	Comminuted fractures; farming injuries; high-velocity gunshot wounds	Extensive; major vascular and/or nerve damage; compartment syndrome
04	Subtotal and complete amputation	Extensive; major vascular and/or nerve damage

Data from Oestern HJ, Tscherne H. 148. Klassifizierung der Frakturen mit Weichteilschaden. *Langenbecks Arch Chiv.* 1982;358:483.

The concept of a scoring system for mangled extremities was introduced in 1985, with a comprehensive scoring system taking into account severity of injury to the extremity's skin, nerves, arteries, veins, and bone, as well as overall injury severity, preexisting health, shock, and time to treatment.[9] In 1990, the simpler mangled extremity severity score (MESS) was proposed for lower extremity injuries, which scores the patient's age and degree of hypotension, as well as the energy of the injury and the extent and duration of ischemia to the limb.[10,11] The authors proposed that a MESS greater than seven conferred poor prognosis to the limb and might guide a surgeon to propose primary amputation rather than extended and possible fruitless limb salvage. More recent research has suggested

that MESS is not the only prognostic factor, and that surgical techniques have advanced, so that less than half of patients in a recent study with MESS of eight underwent amputation.[12]

MANGLED EXTREMITY SEVERITY SCORE		
Category	Description	Score
Age (y)	<30	0
	30-50	1
	>50	2
Extremity injury type	Low energy (simple fracture, stab)	1
	Medium energy (dislocation, comminuted fracture)	2
	High energy (crush, MVA, military gunshot)	3
	High energy as above, with gross contamination or soft tissue avulsion	4
Ischemia (score doubled if ischemic time >6 h)	Reduced pulse, normal perfusion	1
	No pulse, poor capillary refill, paresthesias	2
	Cool numb extremity	3
Shock	Normotensive	0
	Transient hypotension (systolic pressure <90 mm Hg)	1
	Persistent hypotension (systolic pressure <90 mm Hg)	2

Total score is tallied from the four individual scoring categories. MESS greater than seven is considered prognostic of limb amputation.

Adapted from Helfet DL, Howey T, Sanders R, et al. Limb salvage versus amputation. Preliminary results of the mangled extremity severity score. *Clin Orthop Relat Res.* 1990;(256):80-86.

There are many classification systems for various types and mechanisms of severe and high-energy injuries; none is specific for complex lower extremity soft tissue injuries. Each classification has some degree of subjectivity in its application, so that intraobserver variability can occur when applying the classification to a specific patient.[13] Some classifications can be prognostic—such as the MESS, Gustilo-Anderson score, or Tscherne-Oestern classification. Others steer treatment—such as the Gustilo-Anderson or Byrd-Spicer classifications. In a clinical situation, classifications may guide treatment, but treatment should ultimately be determined by clinician judgment and experience as well as the patient's clinical condition.

ANATOMIC FEATURES

As mentioned earlier, complex soft tissue injuries often leave major soft tissue defects for the surgeon to heal. There are many factors that need to be considered when determining the best means of closure. Sir Harold Delf Gillies, a pioneer of modern plastic surgery, stated, "The next best skin is the nearest skin".[14]

When planning a wound closure, the nearby skin and muscle should be evaluated for its viability and its potential uses in covering deep defects. Coverage is particularly important, and particularly problematic, on the weight-bearing surfaces of the foot as many wound coverage options will not provide durable long-term solutions. Other factors that need to be considered prior to definitive coverage include infection control, perfusion rate, and local friction or stress.[15]

The reconstructive ladder is a widely used concept in wound closure.[16] This ladder lists options for wound coverage or closure in order of their complexity. The ladder rungs, from simplest to most complex, are

- Secondary intention
- Primary closure
- Delayed primary closure
- Split-thickness skin graft (STSG)
- Full-thickness skin graft
- Local random flap
- Rotational flap
- Free flap

In theory, a surgeon should start at the simplest possible rung and move upward as needed, though in practice a higher complexity procedure may be chosen to obtain early definitive closure. Certain rungs may not be available or feasible for a given wound. For example, STSG, which is excellent for most non–weight-bearing surfaces (Fig. 61.1), is relatively contraindicated on a weight-bearing surface as it will not have the durability to withstand the pressure and shear forces of walking and standing. Similarly, local rotational flaps, which are excellent when nearby tissue is viable as in Figure 61.2, are not a good option when the nearby tissues are compromised by the initial injury.

PHYSICAL EXAMINATION

Patients who sustain complex soft tissue injuries usually present to an emergency department for stabilization and evaluation after their injury. For any patient presenting after a trauma, the initial examination and stabilization/resuscitation follows the ABCDE (airway, breathing, circulation, disability, exposure) pathway. After these vital elements are addressed, the secondary examination consists of a quick but detailed examination of the entire body, with care taken to assess pain, deformity, circulation, and motor and sensation to each extremity.

For the foot and ankle surgeon consulted to examine a patient with high-energy trauma leading to soft tissue injury, the examination must assess the vascular inflow to the extremity. Pulses may be difficult to palpate, in which case a handheld Doppler should be used to assess for arterial patency. Sensation and motor should be tested if the patient is conscious.

Any open or closed wounds should be examined for extent; loss of skin and subcutaneous tissue; exposure of underlying tissue including muscle, tendon, bone, or neurovascular structures; and contamination. Common contaminants in complex foot and ankle injuries include shoe material, road debris, and dirt or plant material. Skin should also be examined for regions that are closed but threatened, such as skin tenting from displaced fracture fragments, or fracture blisters. While the initial assessment is important, the extent of soft tissue devascularization and death will only become evident over subsequent examinations and debridements.

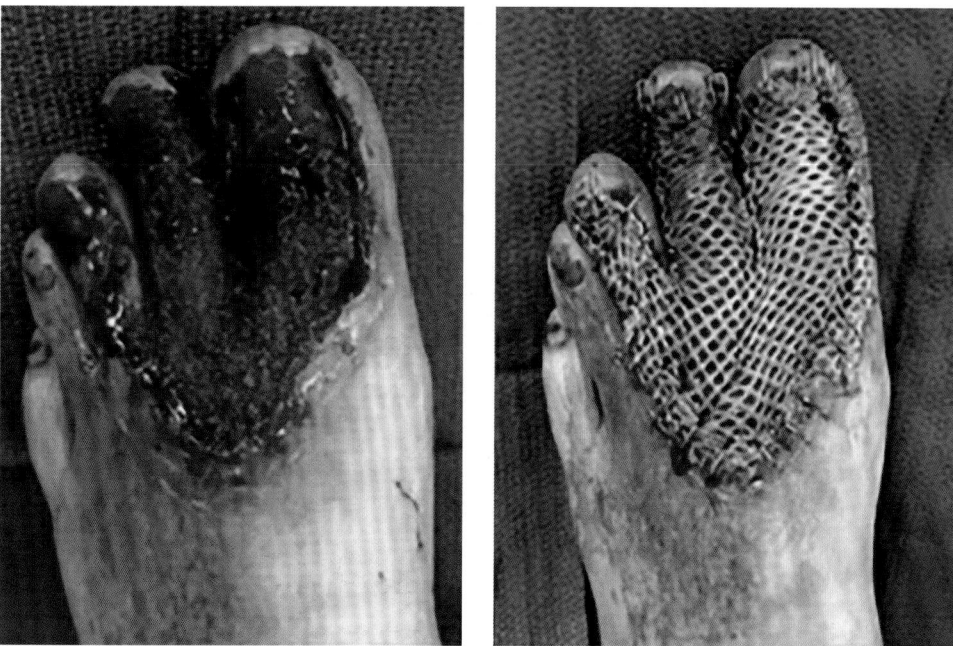

FIGURE 61.1 STSG applied to uninfected, granular wound bed on non–weight-bearing surface.

At the time of initial evaluation, if the patient is responsive, a brief history should be obtained. A useful mnemonic for abbreviated history taking in urgent trauma situations is AMPLE: Allergies, Medications, Pertinent medical history, Last oral intake, and Events leading to injury. Tetanus immunization status should also be ascertained. Learning the time of injury, either from the patient or emergency medical technician, also guides treatment, as timing of antibiotic administration and debridement can affect the patient's prognosis.

IMAGING AND DIAGNOSTIC STUDIES

The initial evaluation of any complex soft tissue injury in the foot and ankle must at minimum include radiographs. Initial radiographs may be sufficient to provide initial treatment with stabilization. If significant bone comminution is involved, it is prudent to obtain the better three-dimensional resolution afforded by computed tomography (CT) to plan more definitive treatment.[17] There is generally no immediate indication for

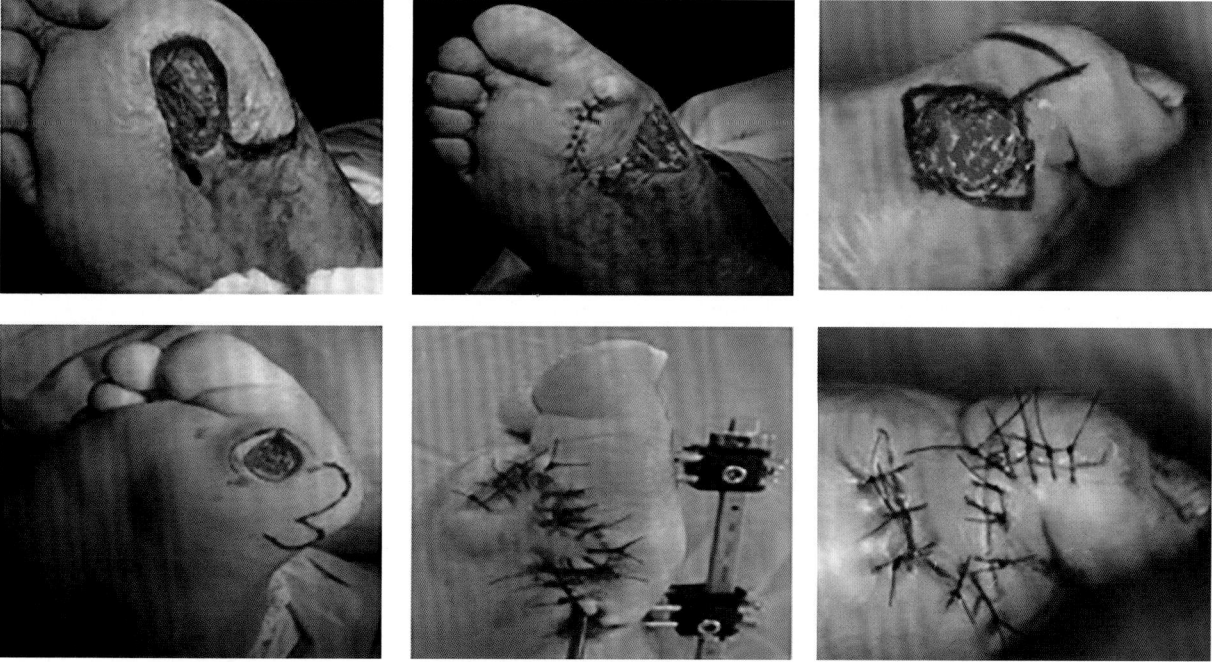

FIGURE 61.2 Examples of local random flaps: unilobed (**upper left and center**), bilobed (**lower left and center**), and rhomboid (**upper right and lower right**).

magnetic resonance imaging (MRI) or ultrasound, though the postoperative course may require these modalities to assess for fluid collections or deep tissue infection.

Complex soft tissue injuries involving potential vascular injury may also require immediate computed tomography arteriogram (CTA) or angiogram to further assess for vascular patency. Intraoperatively, intravenous (IV) fluorescein can be administered, and fluorescence imaging can be used to assess perfusion of questionable tissues.

TREATMENT

The standard of care for complex soft tissue injuries is urgent or emergent surgery for irrigation with debridement of contaminants and nonviable tissue. The "golden hour" period of 6-8 hours after the injury was long held to be the ideal period for debridement, but recent studies have generally shown that moderate surgical delay (ie, 8-24 hours after injury) has little effect on complication rates.[18,19] Severely mangled, crushed, or ischemic extremities may require primary amputation. Nonoperative treatment of severe soft tissue injuries is *not* recommended unless the patient is so critically ill that they are not considered a candidate for limb-salvaging surgery.

During the foot and ankle surgeon's initial history and examination on presentation to the emergency department, a bedside irrigation and closed reduction of any deformity can be performed if the patient is able to tolerate it. A regional or peripheral nerve block with local anesthesia may be beneficial to allow examination and treatment. Early reduction and stabilization of the deformity confers an improved chance of survival on soft tissues, as it reduces tension and may also increase blood flow if it had been previously compromised by deformity.[20] During this period, tetanus prophylaxis should be administered: none if the patient has known tetanus vaccination within 10 years, or else both tetanus toxoid immunization and 250-500 units of tetanus immunoglobulin if tetanus immunization status is unknown or over 10 years.[21] Intravenous (IV) antibiotics should be initiated as soon as possible; studies have shown increased infection if antibiotics are administered over 3 hours after injury or even after 66 minutes from time of injury.[22-24]

After the patient is brought to the operating room, the first step is to perform a thorough debridement of contaminated and devitalized tissue. There are many ways of performing tissue debridement, including mechanical, hydrosurgical, ultrasonic, and enzymatic.

Mechanical debridement can be performed with standard surgical instruments, including scalpels, curettes, or rongeurs. Mechanical debridement has the advantage of being simple to set up and readily available at any site that can perform surgeries (including in small or resource-poor settings), but its disadvantages include the propensity to damage viable tissue while removing nonviable tissue.

In recent years, hydrosurgical and ultrasound debridement have gained increased use among foot and ankle surgeons due to their ability to remove devitalized and contaminated tissue more selectively, with less damage to underlying healthy tissue. The hydrosurgery system available in the United States is the Versajet (Smith & Nephew, Largo, Florida). This hydrosurgery

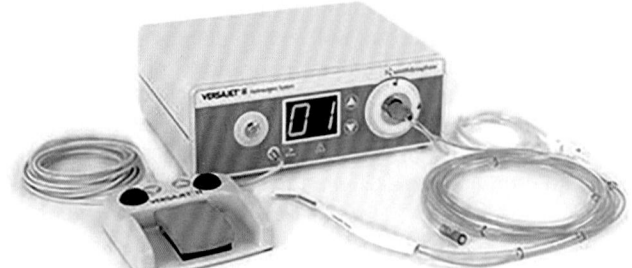

FIGURE 61.3 Versajet hydrosurgery system (Smith & Nephew, Largo, Florida).

device uses water dissection, which works using high pressure jet of sterile saline emitted by the handpiece that creates a Venturi effect and allows for selective debridement.[25] Versajet hydrosurgery aids in preservation of viable tissue, reduces healing time, reduces bacterial load, and aids in creating a smooth bed for grafts (Fig. 61.3).[26]

Low-frequency contact ultrasound debridement (LFCUD) is another novel debridement method that helps to preserve healthy structures while debriding, reduces blood loss, and improves wound bed preparation.[27] Currently, the only LFCUD device on the market in the United States is the SonicOne O.R. (Misonix, Farmingdale, New York) (Fig. 61.4). With ultrasonic debridement, the surgeon can selectively remove devitalized tissue layer by layer. Fluid irrigation running via the handpiece allows the surgeon to irrigate the field and capture the debris from the wound bed while debriding.

Both of these newer wound debridement technologies have tremendously improved wound healing time and the preservation of viable tissue, especially with complex soft tissue injuries.[25-27] The goal of debridement is to eliminate contamination, to prepare the wound bed for incorporation of potential grafts, and to expedite wound healing.

Irrigation of the wound is also a critical component of the initial operative management of severe soft tissue injuries. Irrigation dislodges and removes contaminating debris and bacteria from the wound. Many studies have been done, mostly

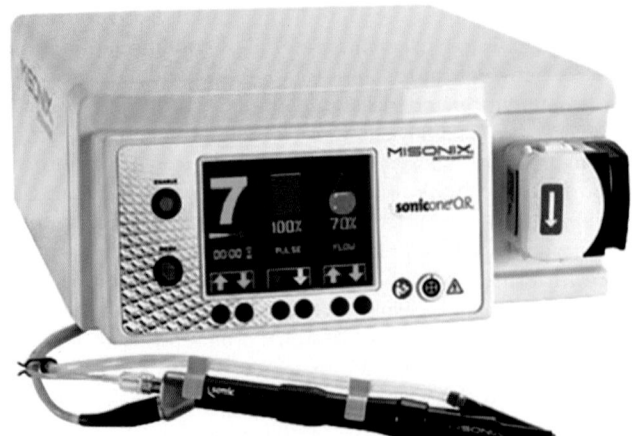

FIGURE 61.4 SonicOne O.R. ultrasonic debridement system (Misonix, Farmingdale, New York).

on open fractures, to elucidate the ideal type and quantity of fluid, as well as pressure of delivery, to decrease rate of infection and repeat surgeries. The theoretical appeal of adding antiseptic or soap to irrigation solution is self-evident, though they also have the potential to irritate tissues or inhibit their healing.[28] High-pressure (35-70 psi) pulsatile lavage has been shown to dislodge more bacteria from a wound[29] but also theorized to seed some of the bacteria deeper and to damage the soft tissue relative to low-pressure lavage.[30,31] Gravity irrigation delivers the irrigating solution with less pressure but has the advantage of being low cost and available at virtually any hospital.

Studies have indicated that castile soap solution led to lower wound complication rates than bacitracin solution,[32] that normal saline led to fewer reoperations than castile soap solutions,[33] and that distilled water led to comparable infection rates compared to normal saline.[34] A large, randomized, prospective trial demonstrated no difference in infection or reoperation rates between high-pressure pulse lavage, low-pressure pulse lavage, or very-low pressure irrigation (ie, gravity irrigation).[33] Amount of irrigation for open fractures has traditionally been recommended as 3 L times the Gustilo grade of the fracture,[33,34] though there is little evidence cited for this recommendation. Routinely culturing acute soft tissue injuries, which are considered contaminated, is not recommended, as initial cultures have only poor correlation with later cultures if infection does develop.[24]

Depending on the orthopedic injuries, proper reduction and stabilization are crucial to achieve for appropriate healing. The chief purpose of fixation is to achieve stabilization, either temporary or definitive, of the bone and soft tissue. There are two main forms of fixation: internal and external. Internal fixation, though used less commonly, is an option for stabilization for open fractures, especially with clean wound appearance, major displacement and dislocation, or injuries with negative wound culture from the initial debridement and irrigation and no subsequent signs of infection. There are many articles that report the infection rate after open reduction and internal fixation for open fractures is usually very low, citing many other risk factors that can lead to infection.[1,35,36]

Each patient with a complex soft tissue injury needs to be evaluated individually, as wound infection depends on many factors including degree and material of contamination, time elapsed between injury and treatment, patient comorbidities, treatment-related risks, and injury severity.[37] According to a recent meta-analysis, there is no significant difference in infection rate between internal and external fixation for open fractures.[37] Literature suggests that internal fixation is safe after proper wound debridement has been performed in open fractures with soft tissue defects.[1] It is important to note that with using internal fixation as the initial mode of stabilization, patients are usually kept on antibiotics for a longer period of time.[38] The type of internal fixation used depends on the injury pattern, soft tissue coverage, and surgeon's preference; the most common types of internal fixation are Kirschner wires, screws, plates, and intramedullary rods. Hardware with antibiotic coating is available; however, there is no definitive research that shows a significant difference from

uncoated hardware.[24] The overall success of internal fixation varies based on the type injury.

External fixation is commonly used in orthopedic injuries with concomitant soft tissue injury; it can be applied in one, two, or three planes. Without going into too much historical detail, external fixators have been classified into generations one through five. Generation one is a rigid A-frame with little flexibility; generation two is the unilateral frame with biplanar stabilization; generation three is the Ilizarov circular device with angular and rotational stability, axial micromotion, and multiplanar fixation; generation four is a mobile unilateral device that has the versatility of circular frames and ease of being unilateral; and generation five is multiplanar and multiaxial fixation with circular frames.[39]

The components of the external fixation methods commonly used for initial trauma stabilization are pins, bars, and clamps. The concept of pin-to-bar allows independent pin fixation based on the deformity and soft tissue healing simultaneously.[39,40] It is usually utilized as a temporary fixation system; however, with portable traction, it can also be used as definitive fixation. When utilizing external fixation for complex soft tissue injuries, premade frames may be impossible to use due to significant soft tissue defects or bone comminution. Placing the pins first in unaffected bone allows the surgeon to achieve the best fixation in any injury scenario. Triangular "delta" frames, widely used on complex ankle and hindfoot injuries, are an example of the pin-to-bar approach. Antibiotic-coated pins are available; however, as with internal fixation there is not much research evidence on the superiority of those hardware. The type of frame used also depends on the surgeon's training and preference. The final goal, as with internal fixation, is to achieve appropriate stabilization for healing.

After reduction and stabilization of the underlying bone trauma, and proper wound debridement and irrigation, the final step is to initiate wound management. If there is adequate skin and the wound is relatively clean, the goal is to perform primary closure or set up for delayed primary closure at a second surgery. Generally with complex soft tissue injuries, there is not enough skin available for primary closure. In these scenarios, the goal is delayed wound closure expedited with aids such as negative pressure wound therapy (NPWT), excellent local wound care, and application of biologic coverings. Depending on the wound bed, wound location, and local soft tissue, final coverage may be possible via skin graft, local flap, or distant (free) flap.

NPWT in the past two decades becomes a vital component of managing many complex wounds. It was first mentioned by Morykwas et al. in 1997, when they demonstrated that NPWT on pig wounds with pressure of 125 mm Hg helped healing tremendously by improving blood flow to the area and decreasing bacterial load.[41,42] Later, more advanced versions of NPWT with easier application techniques came to the market; but the basic principle remained the same. NPWT helps to remove fluid, induce wound contraction, and promote angiogenesis at microscopic level.[43] NPWT can be utilized either temporarily after the initial surgery or as the definitive treatment.

There are many wound care modalities and products, whose application depends on the nature of the wound

itself. The most common dressing solutions used for complex injuries with large soft tissue defects are normal saline, Dakin solution (diluted sodium hypochlorite), povidone-iodine, silver sulfadiazine, hydrogel, hydrocolloids, petrolatum gauze, polymeric membrane dressing, hydrofiber, foam, and others.[44] These products have specific characteristics that make them more efficient at treating some wounds over others. Proper knowledge of these characteristics is important to efficiently treat patients, but it is not the topic of this chapter.

STSGs are often an excellent option for final wound closure with soft tissue defects, though they are generally considered too fragile for the stresses faced by plantar weight-bearing skin. STSG contains epidermis and some layers of dermis and can be classified as thin (0.008-0.012 in), intermediate (0.012-0.016 in), and thick (0.016-0.020 in) depending on the amount of dermis harvested.[15] The author prefers fenestrating the skin graft either via mesher or scalpel to avoid seroma or hematoma formation under the graft. The author uses NPWT as the postoperative dressing after application of STSG for 5 days immediately postoperatively.

A major advantage of STSG is that patients are the donor themselves; no additional resources are needed. However, for STSG to incorporate in the wound, the wound bed has to be healthy and without any drainage, edema, or erythema.[45] STSG cannot be applied over infection or exposed bone.

At times even during a repeat operative procedure, the wound bed is not ready for STSG. In those cases, other bioengineered grafts can be utilized. Bioengineered grafts have become more popular in the past decade for initial wound coverage prior to final skin grafts or flap closure. These graft products have various different wound healing properties that expedite the preparation of the wound bed for more definitive closure. Some of these products are Integra Bilayer Matrix (Integra Life Sciences, Plainsboro, New Jersey), Graftjacket Regenerative Tissue Matrix (Wright Medical, Memphis, Tennessee), Stravix (Osiris Therapeutic, Columbia, Maryland), and many more.

Integra Bilayer Matrix is a cross-linked bovine tendon collagen and glycosaminoglycan, which acts as a scaffold for the fibroblast.[46] When this graft was used in a clinical setting with degloving soft tissue injuries, it showed great wound healing properties even with exposed bone or tendon in the wound.[47] Integra can be used even when bone is exposed in the wound bed, which increases its value in complex soft tissue injuries.[47] Graftjacket regenerative tissue matrix is collagen-based graft that is made from donated human skin; since it is derived from human skin, it has almost all acellular components of human skin and acts as a scaffold for deposition of new cells.[48] Stravix is a cryopreserved human placental tissue that has tensile strength ten times greater than dehydrated amniotic membrane and which provides durability and elasticity to the wounds.[49] Previously, when these modern graft technologies were unavailable, human or animal dermal allografts, such as cadaveric or porcine skin, were utilized for wound coverage and preparation for definitive coverage. Overall, modern bioengineered graft products provide another component in the armamentarium for initial wound coverage, while accelerating healing and preparing for definitive coverage.

PEARLS

- Atraumatic technique and preservation of tissue: soft tissue for coverage and bone for length and function. Leave all possible tissue intact to act as a biologic barrier even if there is limited perfusion in the region; retention sutures are useful to obtain coverage.
- Adequate debridement: limited utilization of ultrasonic debridement or hydrosurgery, followed by pulse lavage. It is vital to protect neurovascular bundles and apply advanced moist wound therapy during the immediate postoperative period.
- Stabilization: to reduce motion of soft tissue and tendons and to reduce shearing forces on the degloved tissue or open fracture. External fixation can play a major role in protecting the soft tissue, especially at the level of an articulation.
- Temporary coverage with biologic tissue, for example, biologic grafts or cadaveric or porcine skin graft, to protect underlying tendon, bone, and soft tissue, is paramount to preservation of traumatized soft tissue and bone.
- NPWT plays a major role in aiding production of granulation tissue over tendon and bone as an interim step toward flap or skin graft reconstruction.

CASE STUDIES AND AUTHORS' PREFERRED TREATMENT

As every complex soft tissue injury is complex in its own way, the best way to describe the authors' preferred treatment, as well as pitfalls that can be encountered along the way, seemed to be the presentation of several case studies.

CASE 1—CRUSH INJURY

A 24-year-old male was brought to the emergency room after a work injury in which his foot was crushed between a forklift and the wall. A complete initial trauma workup was performed by the emergency medicine team. Upon physical examination of the extremity, the patient had a laceration in the dorsal first interspace with exposed tendon and muscle actively bleeding; severe plantar transverse degloving extended from first to fourth interspaces with exposed flexor tendons and surrounding muscles. These two lacerations communicated (Fig. 61.5) is capillary refill time was delayed and sensation was decreased to all digits, however, he had palpable dorsalis pedis and posterior tibial arteries as well as intact range of motion of the involved digits. Plain radiographs showed comminuted fracture of distal first metatarsal, intra-articular second metatarsal base fracture, and Lisfranc injury involving widening between first and second metatarsal and fracture of medial cuneiform (Fig. 61.6).

He was emergently taken to the operating room within 30 minutes of podiatric surgical evaluation. The initial procedure included irrigation via pulse lavage and debridement, with stabilization of fractures via circular Ilizarov external fixation. Due to the high risk of desiccation from the plantar degloving injury, the plantar flap was reapproximated

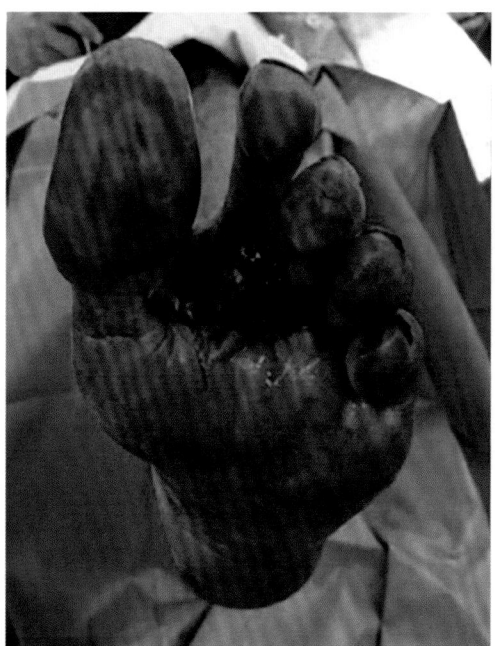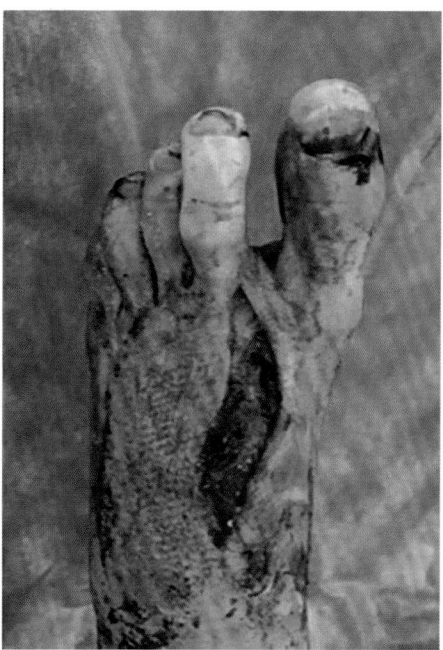

FIGURE 61.5 A severe crush injury in a 24-year-old male in which the foot was crushed between the wall and a forklift, showing large dorsal and plantar lacerations.

and closed primarily, leaving the dorsal laceration packed open (Fig. 61.7). As there was adequate initial reduction of the fractures by radiograph, no further imaging was obtained (Fig. 61.8). During the hospital stay, the fourth and fifth digits began to necrose; further surgery was postponed until demarcation became complete.

Over the next 3 weeks, digits 4 and 5 became completely necrotic, with distal tuft necrosis of digits 1, 2, and 3, along with mild necrosis of the plantar degloved flap along the plantar first and second interspaces (Fig. 61.9). About a month after the initial injury, the patient was taken back to

surgery for partial amputations of digits 1-3 and complete amputation of digits 4 and 5, along with wound debridement with LFCUD (Fig. 61.10). Placental (Stravix) graft was applied to the dorsal and plantar wounds, and NPWT was initiated to expedite wound healing. Monthly radiographs were obtained to evaluate for the fracture healing. About 10 weeks after the original injury and stabilization, all the fractures healed and the external fixator was removed; daily wound care continued at the graft sites. At 3 months after the injury, all wounds were closed including the external fixator pin sites (Fig. 61.11).

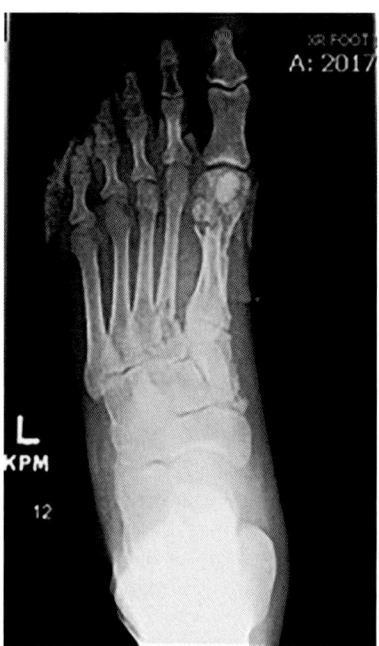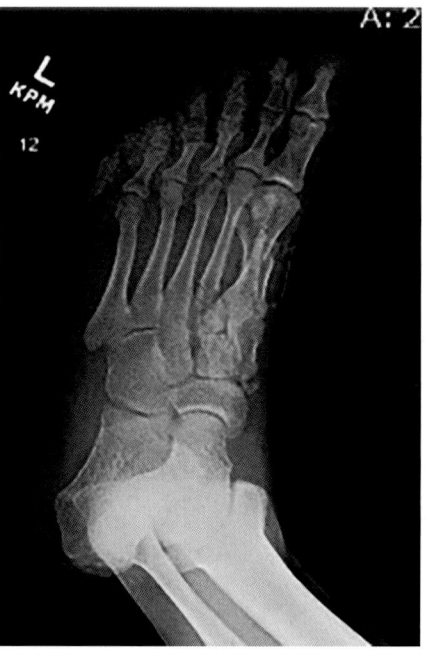

FIGURE 61.6 AP and medial oblique radiographs showed comminuted fracture of the distal first metatarsal, intra-articular fracture of the base of the second metatarsal, and injury to Lisfranc ligament.

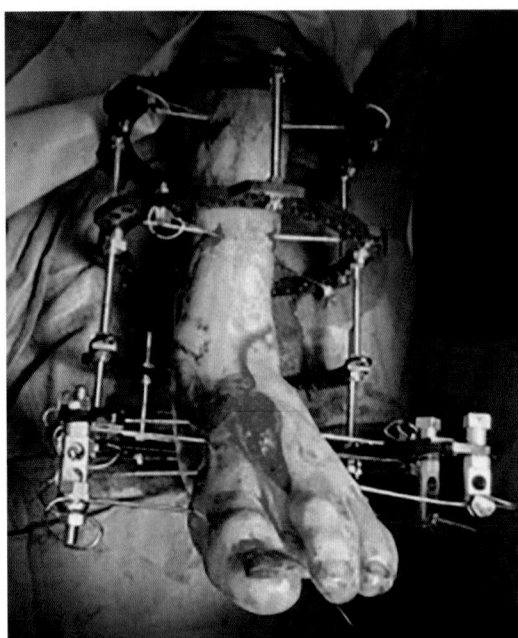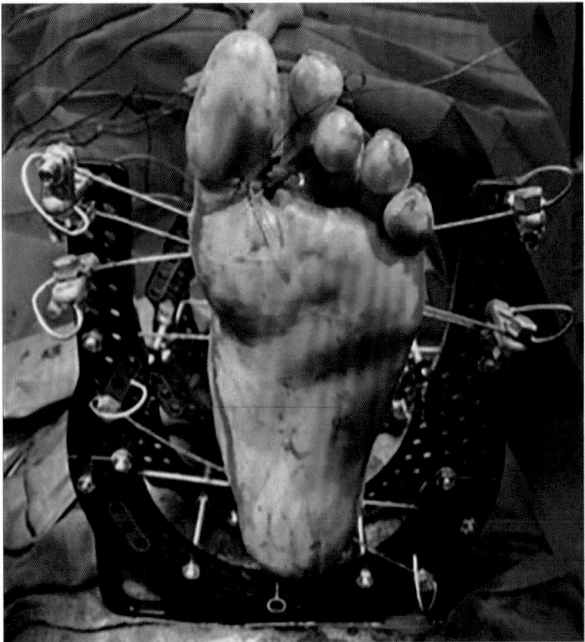

FIGURE 61.7 After debridement and irrigation, primary closure of the plantar laceration was performed while dorsal soft tissue defect was left open for drainage.

CASE 2—DEGLOVING INJURY

A 46-year-old male presented to the emergency room after motor vehicle accident with severe degloving injury to his forefoot. An initial trauma evaluation was performed in the emergency room. On physical examination of the affected limb, the first digit was partially amputated and degloved with a dorsal skin bridge and delayed capillary refill time, the second digit was completely amputated at the level of metatarsophalangeal joint (MTPJ), the third digit was unstable at the MTPJ level, and the fourth and fifth digits were intact but with sluggish capillary refill. The entire plantar, dorsal, and medial aspect of forefoot displayed full-thickness degloving with exposed tendons and metatarsals 1 and 2 (Figs. 61.12 and 61.13). Dorsalis pedis and posterior tibial arteries were palpable, and there was no active bleeding.

The patient was emergently taken to the operating room for debridement and stabilization. Reduction of the hallux

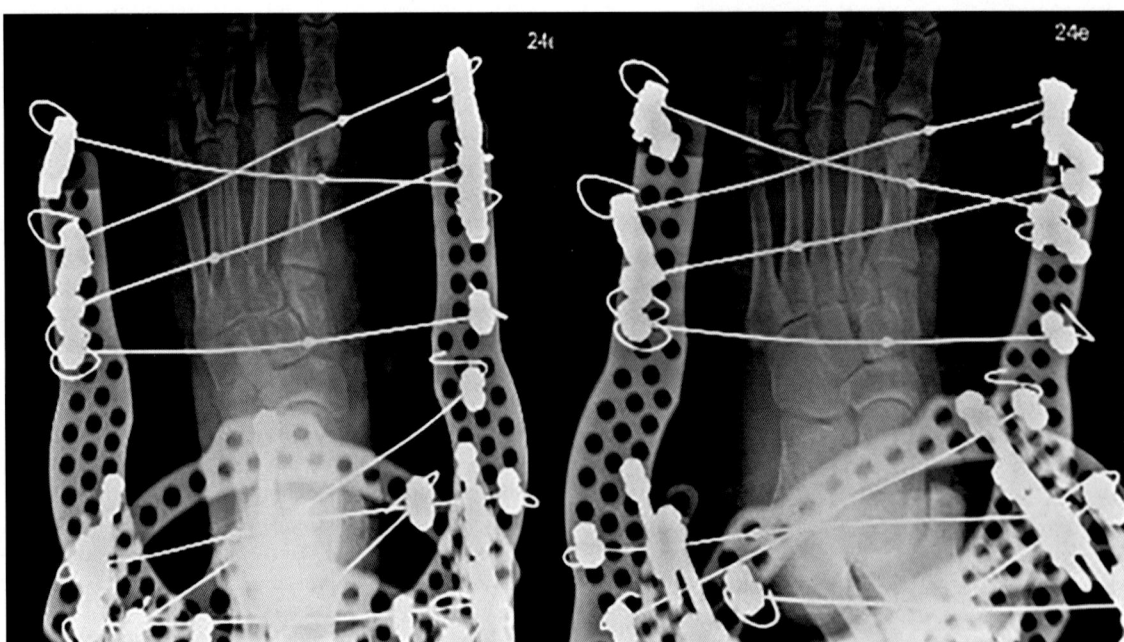

FIGURE 61.8 Postoperative AP and oblique radiographs demonstrating initial stabilization of the fractures with Ilizarov external fixator, reduction of the fractures/dislocations.

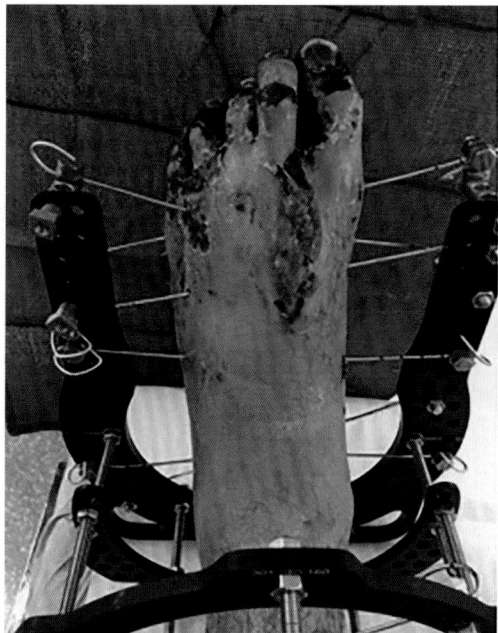
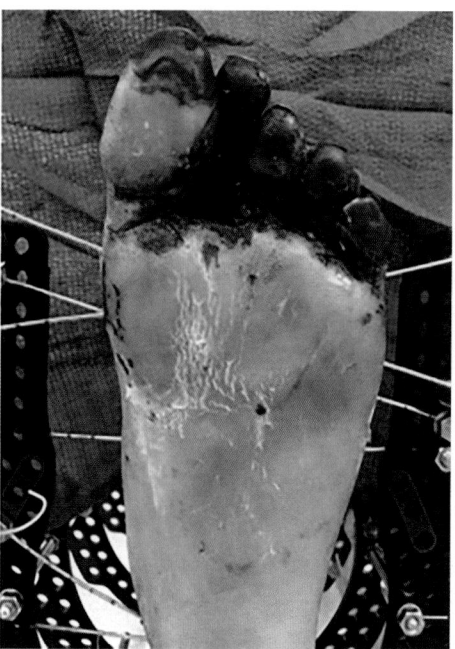

FIGURE 61.9 Necrosis developed to the entire fourth and fifth digits as well as partially to the digits 1-3.

was attempted, but it became dusky and required amputation. Digits 3-5 were reduced to an acceptable position and stabilized using K-wires (Fig. 61.14). Using pulsatile lavage, the surgical site was irrigated with 4 L of normal saline. Soft tissue coverage was obtained using local plantar advancement muscle flap and skin plasties, leaving about a 3 × 3-cm area of the medial forefoot open for drainage (Fig. 61.15). He was started on cefazolin upon admission to the hospital.

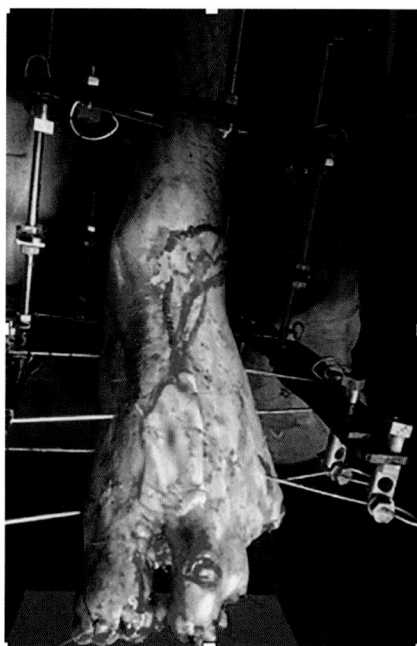

FIGURE 61.10 Subsequent partial amputation of digits 1-3 and complete amputation of digits 4-5 were performed, along with biological graft application to the dorsal wound.

Daily dressing changes with flap checks for viability were performed postoperatively.

About 3 weeks after initial surgery, the patient developed a hematoma on the plantar aspect, which was evacuated in the office and managed with continued local wound care. At about 8 weeks postoperatively, the K-wires were removed, and he was transitioned to partial weight bearing in pneumatic walker. At this time, the distal third digit started to become cyanotic (Fig. 61.16). At about the 12-week mark after injury, he underwent partial third digit amputation with wound debridement. He was also made full weight bearing at this time. Fifteen weeks from the initial injury, the patient had healed all the flaps with viable partial third digit and complete fourth and fifth digits (Fig. 61.17).

CASE 3—OPEN FRACTURE-DISLOCATION

A healthy 42-year-old male construction worker was transferred from an outside hospital for a left foot injury sustained when an excavator load fell on his foot. He did not sustain any other injuries. The outside hospital gave tetanus prophylaxis as well as intravenous cefazolin and gentamicin prior to transfer. On initial examination, he was found to have a curvilinear laceration ~15 cm long, with partial degloving distally, over the dorsal medial midfoot, with exposed extensor hallucis longus (EHL) tendon and first and second metatarsal (Fig. 61.18). Sensation was absent to the hallux and diminished to other digits; capillary refill was intact to all digits. Radiographs (Fig. 61.18) revealed lateral dislocation of the hallux on the first metatarsal and laterally dislocated transverse fractures of metatarsals 2-4.

He was taken to the operating room the same day for irrigation, debridement, open reduction of the fractures and dislocation, internal fixation of metatarsals 2 and 3, and external fixation of the first MTPJ (see Fig. 61.18).

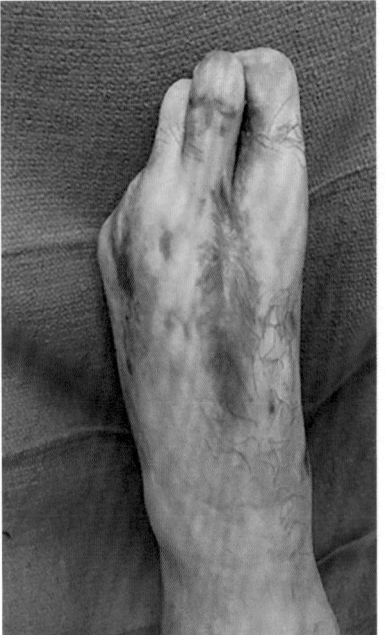 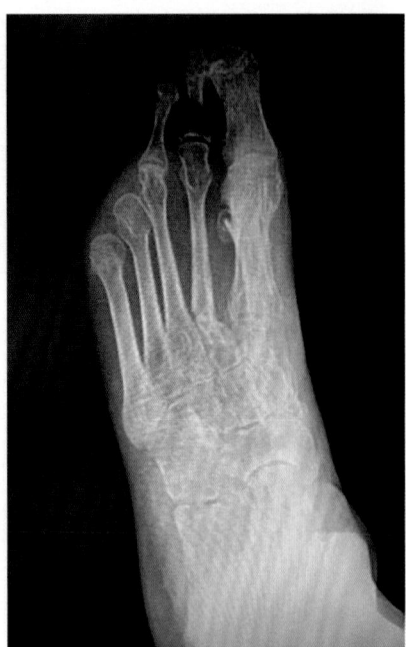

FIGURE 61.11 About 3 months after the initial injury, all the wounds and fractures healed with a stable foot for ambulation as showed in the AP radiograph.

The lateral portion of the flap was sutured down for coverage, though its vascular supply during the case was observed to be marginal. He was started on cefazolin for coverage while wounds were open.

Daily wound checks revealed gradual necrosis of most of the degloved skin flap, seen in Figure 61.19. He was taken back to surgery for debridement of necrotic tissue and hematoma with ultrasound debridement. There were no signs of infection, though EHL and abductor tendons were exposed in the wound. Placental biologic graft was placed over the debrided wound, and NPWT was initiated the following day. He was

maintained on NPWT for 4 weeks, after which time he had graft incorporation with granular tissue and almost total coverage of EHL and EDL tendons (Fig. 61.19). He was taken to surgery again for wound debridement and STSG placement.

Subsequent follow-up showed radiographic healing of the metatarsal fractures, so he underwent uneventful external fixation removal 9 weeks after the initial injury. At 6 months postinjury, he had complete take and healing of the graft as well as radiographic healing of fractures and dislocation (Fig. 61.20). He did have residual stiffness of the MTPJs for which he was referred to physical therapy.

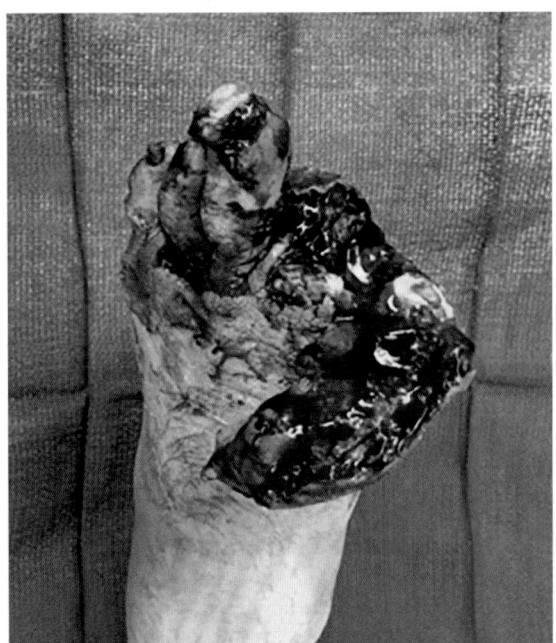 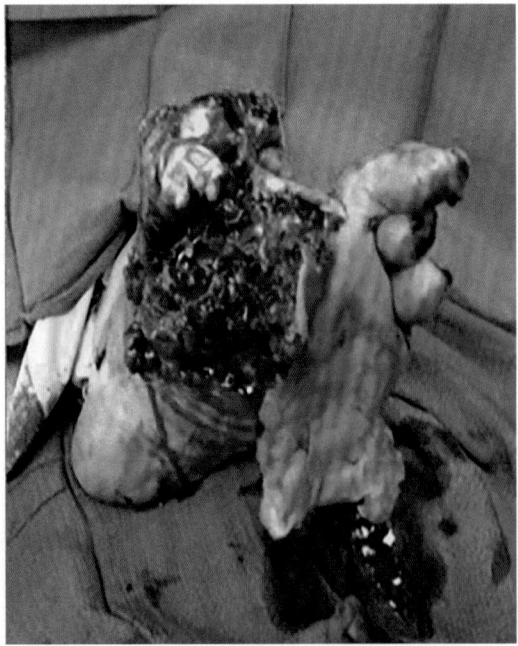

FIGURE 61.12 A 46-year-old male developed a severe degloving injury in a motor vehicle accident, with mangled forefoot with sluggish blood flow to the forefoot.

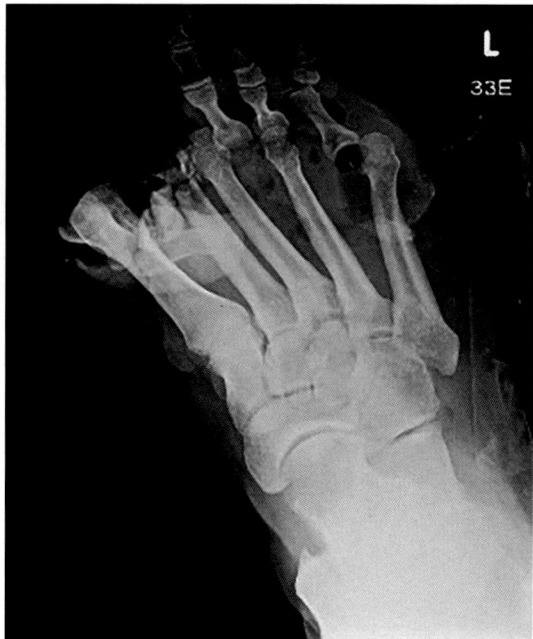
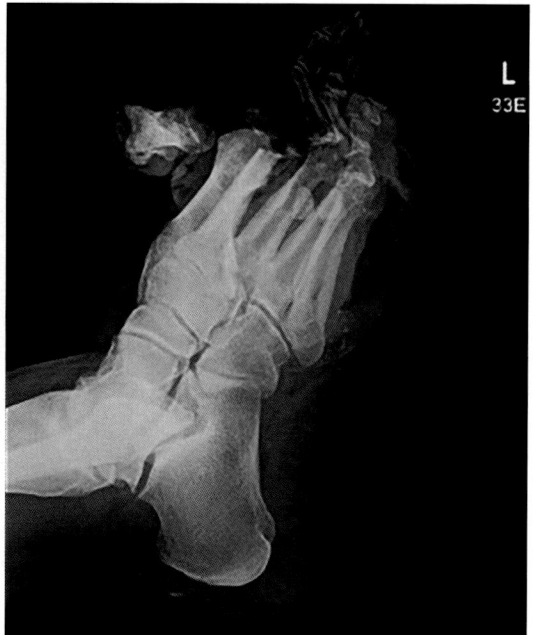

FIGURE 61.13 As demonstrated in the AP and lateral non–weight-bearing radiographs, injuries included traumatic amputation of the second digit, dislocated and degloved first digit, and dislocated MTP joints 3-5.

PERILS and PITFALLS

- Lack of appropriate evaluation of vascular status, lack of preservation of venous and arterial flow leading to tissue necrosis, bone loss, and bone infection
- Incomplete debridement
- Inadequate stabilization, which can lead to hematoma, seroma, and extensive tissue necrosis
- Lack of temporary tissue coverage, which can lead to desiccation, necrosis, and tissue loss with infection.
- Infection, often polymicrobial, and potentially osteomyelitis

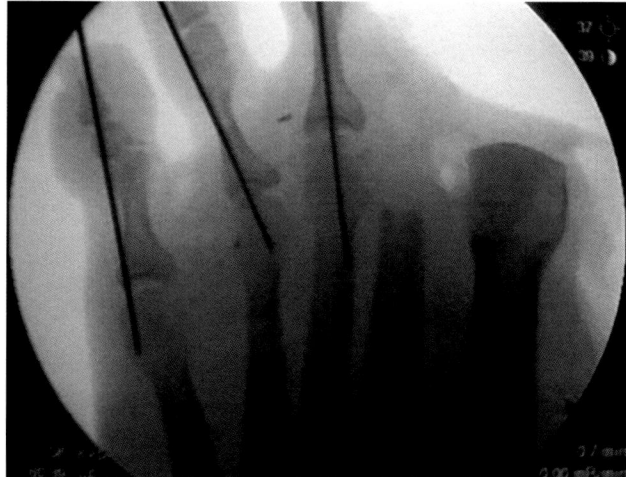

FIGURE 61.14 Intraoperative fluoroscopic images demonstrate fracture stabilization with pins.

POSTOPERATIVE CARE AND REHABILITATION

Postoperative care of the patient with complex soft tissue injuries of the foot and ankle is centered on excellent wound management, addressing the systemic factors that may affect wound healing, and preventing major causes of morbidity and mortality in the hospitalized trauma patient. For most complex soft tissue injuries, postoperative care starts with the expectation of one or more second-look operations for additional debridement and irrigation, generally within 48-72 hours, as well as wound closure when the wound bed is adequately prepared.

Management of the wound necessitates dressing changes.[50] Dressing changes can remove fluid and allow an opportunity for additional debridement (mechanical or excisional) at bedside. Dressings should be chosen that provide a good wound healing environment; antibiotic-impregnated dressings or antiseptics (eg, povidone-iodine) should generally be avoided as they inhibit cell growth within the wound.[24] Dressing changes moreover allow the surgical team to monitor the affected skin and soft tissues for viability and signs of necrosis or infection. Signs of necrosis include dusky, cool, or black skin with delayed capillary refill. Signs of infection may be obvious, such as frank purulence or erythema with lymphangitic extension, or may be more subtle, such as increased malodor or increased pain at the site. The wound check is thus one of the most important activities for the surgical team, as it informs both the timing and extent of repeat operations.

Postoperative care also includes management of any chronic or acute medical conditions that may inhibit wound healing. Uncontrolled diabetes mellitus, malnutrition, and peripheral vascular disease (PVD) are all known to delay and diminish wound healing potential.

Diabetes mellitus, particularly when poorly controlled, is well known to cause delayed wound healing and an increase in

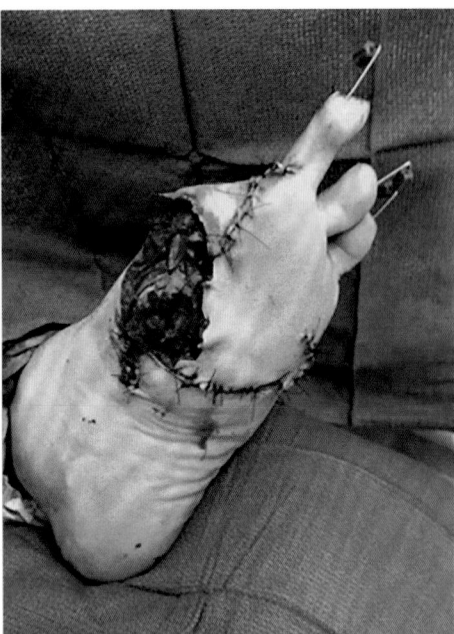 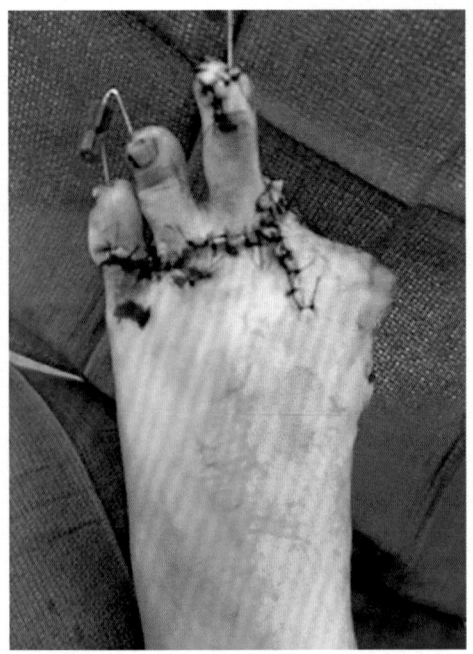

FIGURE 61.15 Initial surgical procedure included amputation of the first digit and K-wire stabilization of MTP joints 3-5 as well as debridement and irrigation. The medial soft tissue defect was left open.

surgical complications.[51] It does this via the direct mechanism of hyperglycemia inhibiting cellular activities, as well as by indirect routes of peripheral and autonomic neuropathy, PVD, and impaired immune function. Appropriate glycemic control in the inpatient and critical care setting has been shown to decrease diabetes-associated morbidity and mortality.[52,53]

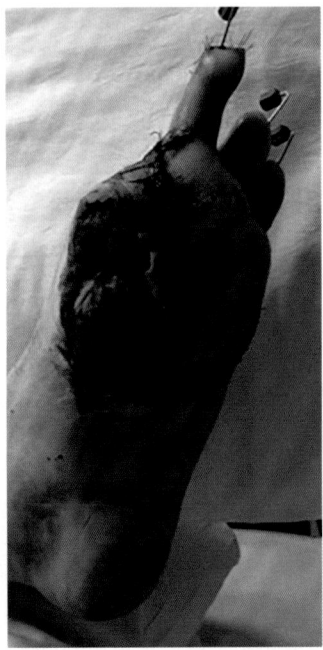

FIGURE 61.16 Subsequent cyanosis of the third digit developed with K-wire removal around 8 weeks after initial surgery. The patient required subsequent partial amputation of the third digit.

PVD is as important a factor for healing acute traumatic wounds as it is for healing chronic pressure, neuropathic, or vascular ulcers. Without adequate arterial blood supply, cells within wounds do not have enough oxygen or nutrients to perform their reparative work. Fewer inflammatory and immune cells are able to migrate to the wound. Patients with complex injuries may have known PVD, with a history of claudication or nonhealing wounds, but they may also have undiagnosed or occult PVD. A surgical team should have a low index of suspicion for patients with poorly healing soft tissue injuries and any risk factors for PVD. Risk factors include diabetes, tobacco use, hypertension, hyperlipidemia, obesity, coronary artery disease, and history of cerebrovascular disease. If there is suspicion for PVD, appropriate testing should be performed and consults made to vascular surgeons or interventionalists as indicated.

Malnutrition is another modifiable factor, which can delay wound healing. Malnutrition can be present in patients with normal or elevated body mass, as a person can easily consume excessive calories from nutritionally poor food sources. Serum albumin is a lab test that has long been used as a marker of nutritional status, with a value under 3.5 mg/dL regarded as a sign of malnutrition.[54-56] However, multiple other disease states can lower serum albumin, including chronic liver or kidney disease and chronic inflammation. Albumin also has a relatively long half-life of 20 days, making it a poor marker for monitoring acute response to dietary therapy. Serum prealbumin has a shorter half-life and is more sensitive as a marker of nutritional status.[57] Prealbumin levels under 15-20 mg/dL are markers of poor nutrition and should be monitored serially to evaluate response to nutrition therapy. However, isolated undernourishment without other disease states does not necessarily decrease albumin or prealbumin levels significantly, so lab values should be used in conjunction with the patient's clinical status.[58]

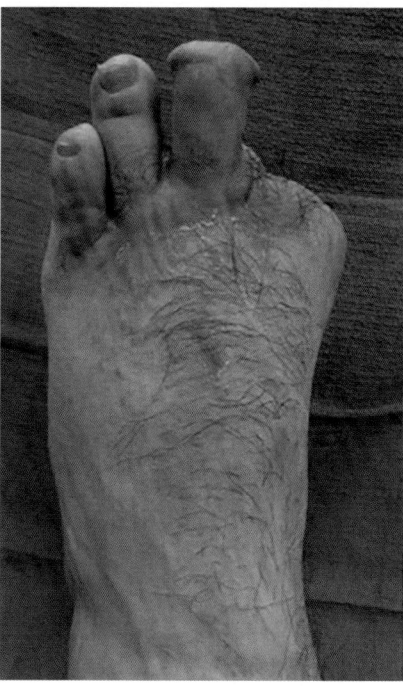
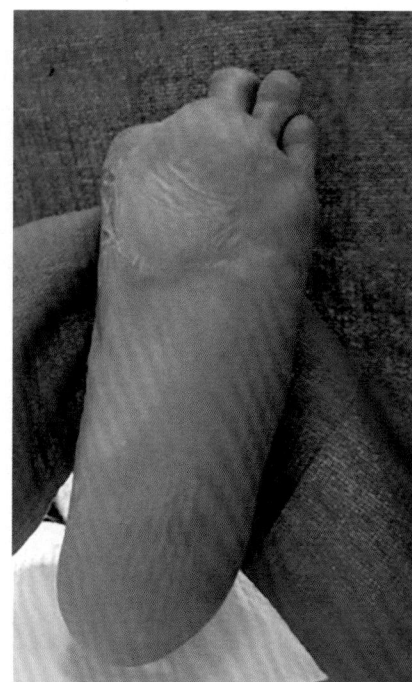
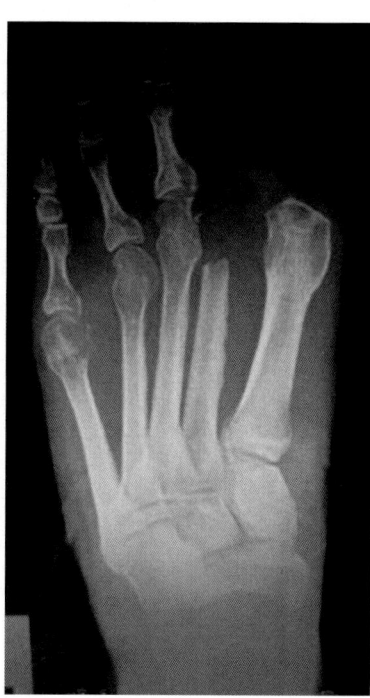

FIGURE 61.17 At 15 weeks after the initial injury, all the incisions and tissue defects healed. AP radiograph shows evidence of well-aligned MTP joints 3-5.

Vitamins A, C, and D are considered valuable for healing, as well as zinc if it is deficient; supplementing with these may benefit wound healing.[59] Registered dieticians are a vital member of the team whenever there is any concern about nutritional status.

Deep vein thrombosis (DVT) prevention is another critical aspect of postoperative management of patients with complex lower extremity injuries. Such patients are at elevated risk of DVT due to their recent trauma and surgery with subsequent immobility. While DVT has its own morbidity, it is also a potential cause of mortality by leading to pulmonary embolism (PE). Additional risk factors for DVT and PE, which include

malignancy, oral contraceptives, congestive heart failure, advanced age, or personal or family history of DVT, should be ascertained. Unless there are contraindications such as allergy or active bleeding, all patients should be started on medical DVT prophylaxis after their initial debridement surgery. Low molecular weight heparin is generally easier to administer and more effective in prevention of DVT and PE than unfractionated heparin.[60,61]

Physical therapy is also of value even in the early postoperative stages before definitive wound closure. While the soft tissue and osseous injuries will likely limit motion at the

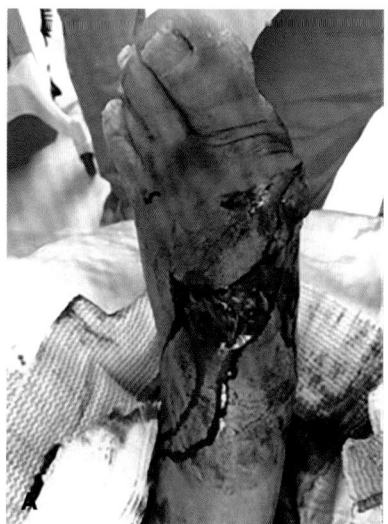
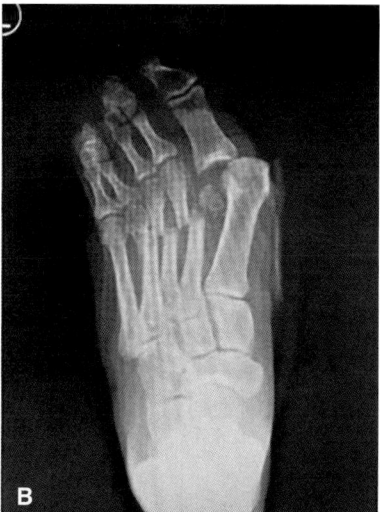
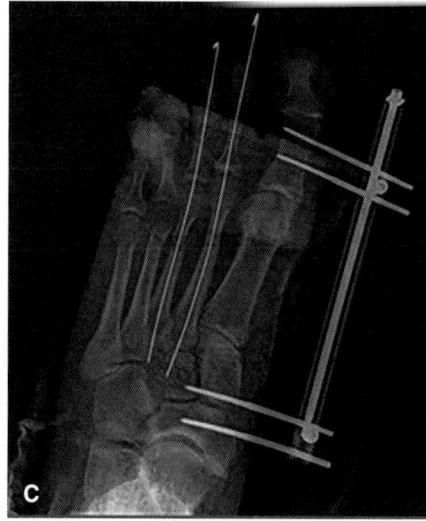

FIGURE 61.18 A 42-year-old man sustained open fracture-dislocation with degloving injury when an excavator load fell on his foot. First and second metatarsals are exposed under the degloved skin **(A)**. AP radiographs show dislocation of first MTP joint and fracture of metatarsals 2-4, before **(B)** and after **(C)** reduction.

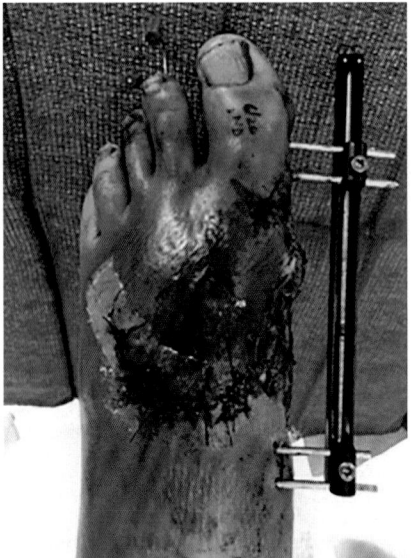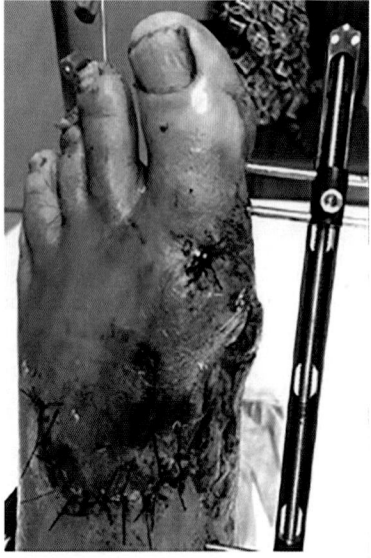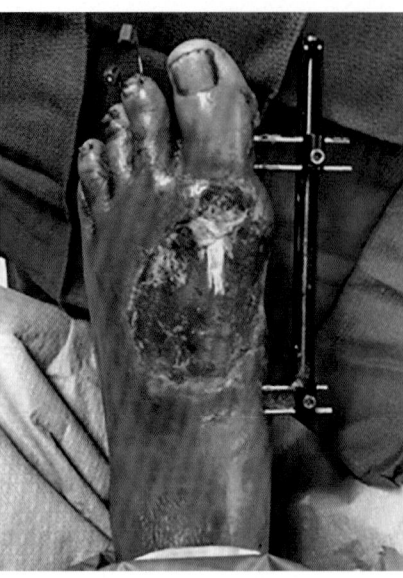

FIGURE 61.19 The degloved skin flap developed subsequent necrosis, requiring debridement (not pictured), biologic graft application, and NPWT. After 4 weeks of NPWT, the wound had adequate granulation tissue for definitive STSG placement.

affected limb, attempts should be made to mobilize adjacent uninjured joints, as well as the contralateral limb if it is unaffected. This will provide mechanical prevention of DVT, help to prevent edema and deconditioning, prepare the patient for an extended recovery, and give the patient the ability to participate actively in their recovery. After definitive treatment, physical therapy at the site of the injury may be initiated as allowed by osseous and soft tissue healing and should include range of motion as soon as possible to prevent joint stiffness or contractures.[62]

For some patients, postoperative complications such as infection or tissue necrosis may necessitate amputation to remove all infected or devitalized tissue. For others, the initial injury may be of such severity that primary or delayed amputation has the best likelihood of providing a functional limb. Factors that may influence a surgical team and patient toward a secondary amputation include infection, insensate limb, substantial plantar skin loss, substantial bone loss or deformity, and the patient's preoperative functional status. Insensate foot at presentation is no longer considered a primary indication for amputation.[63]

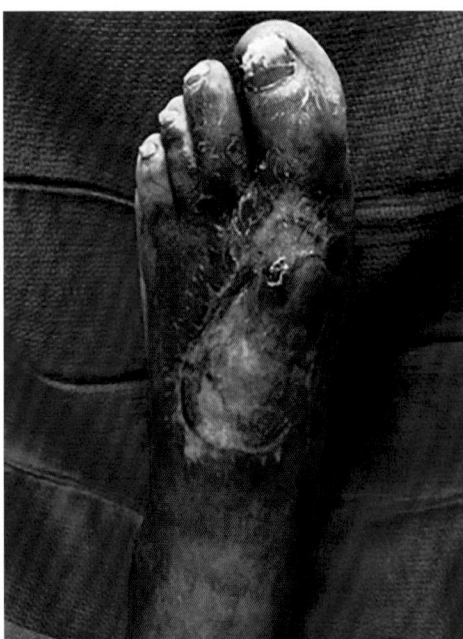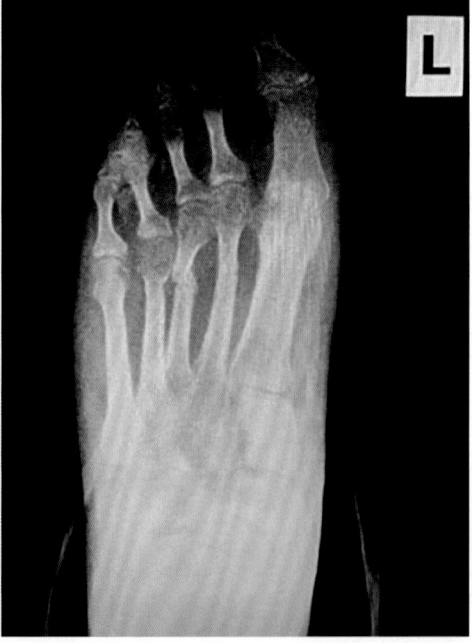

FIGURE 61.20 At 6 months after the injury, healed skin graft with restored metatarsal parabola, although a delayed union of the third metatarsal is evident on the AP radiograph. Patient had residual stiffness and edema of the medial MTP joints.

Patients who undergo primary or early amputation for severe, complex lower extremity injuries may suffer more depression and stump complications[64] but have a shorter hospital stay and possibly easier transition to prosthesis use than those who undergo delayed amputation.[65]

CONCLUSION

Complex soft tissue injuries of the foot and ankle can be limb threatening and life changing. Appropriate treatment of them involves rapid evaluation, early antibiotic administration, appropriate medical resuscitation and stabilization prompt and thorough debridement with irrigation and stabilization of concomitant osseous injuries, good local wound care, management of medical comorbidities, likely repeat debridements, and definitive wound closure planning as soon as possible. The goal of treatment is a functional limb and return to an acceptable activity level, and the surgeon should focus on function rather than on limb salvage at all costs; for some patients, this may mean recommending early amputation rather than subjecting them to protracted hospital stays and repeated painful surgeries to salvage a nonfunctional foot. Treating these wounds requires a coordinated team approach, which may include trauma, vascular, and plastic reconstructive surgeons; internal medicine and infectious disease physicians; and dieticians and physical therapists in addition to the foot and ankle surgeon.

REFERENCES

1. Chummun S, Wright TC, Chapman TW, et al. Outcome of the management of open ankle fractures in an ortho-plastic specialist centre. *Injury.* 2015;46(6):1112-1115.
2. Boriani F, Ul Haq A, Baldini T, et al. Orthoplastic surgical collaboration is required to optimise the treatment of severe limb injuries: a multi-centre, prospective cohort study. *J Plast Reconstr Aesthet Surg.* 2017;70(6):715-722.
3. Gustilo RB, Anderson JT. Prevention of infection in the treatment of one thousand and twenty-five open fractures of long bones: retrospective and prospective analyses. *J Bone Joint Surg Am.* 1976;58(4):453-458.
4. Gustilo RB, Mendoza RM, Williams DN. Problems in the management of type III (severe) open fractures: a new classification of type III open fractures. *J Trauma.* 1984;24(8):742-746.
5. Tscherne H, Oestern HJ. [A new classification of soft-tissue damage in open and closed fractures (author's transl)]. *Unfallheilkunde.* 1982;85(3):111-115.
6. Ibrahim DA, Swenson A, Sassoon A, et al. Classifications in brief: the Tscherne classification of soft tissue injury. *Clin Orthop Relat Res.* 2017;475(2):560-564.
7. Oliveira RV, Cruz LP, Matos MA. Comparative accuracy assessment of the Gustilo and Tscherne classification systems as predictors of infection in open fractures. *Rev Bras Ortop (Sao Paulo).* 2018;53(3):314-318.
8. Byrd HS, Spicer TE, Cierney G III. Management of open tibial fractures. *Plast Reconstr Surg.* 1985;76(5):719-730.
9. Gregory RT, Gould RJ, Peclet M, et al. The mangled extremity syndrome (M.E.S.): a severity grading system for multisystem injury of the extremity. *J Trauma.* 1985;25(12):1147-1150.
10. Helfet DL, Howey T, Sanders R, et al. Limb salvage versus amputation. Preliminary results of the mangled extremity severity score. *Clin Orthop Relat Res.* 1990;(256):80-86.
11. Johansen K, Daines M, Howey T, et al. Objective criteria accurately predict amputation following lower extremity trauma. *J Trauma.* 1990;30(5):568-572; discussion 572-563.
12. Loja MN, Sammann A, DuBose J, et al. The mangled extremity score and amputation: Time for a revision. *J Trauma Acute Care Surg.* 2017;82(3):518-523.
13. Durrant CA, Mackey SP. Orthoplastic classification systems: the good, the bad, and the ungainly. *Ann Plast Surg.* 2011;66(1):9-12.
14. Gillies HD, Millard DR. *The Principles and Art of Plastic Surgery.* Boston, MA: Little, Brown; 1957.
15. Blume PA, Donegan R, Schmidt BM. The role of plastic surgery for soft tissue coverage of the diabetic foot and ankle. *Clin Podiatr Med Surg.* 2014;31(1):127-150.
16. Capobianco CM, Zgonis T. Soft tissue reconstruction pyramid for the diabetic Charcot foot. *Clin Podiatr Med Surg.* 2017;34(1):69-76.
17. Schepers T, Rammelt S. Complex foot injury: Early and definite management. *Foot Ankle Clin.* 2017;22(1):193-213.
18. Srour M, Inaba K, Okoye O, et al. Prospective evaluation of treatment of open fractures: Effect of time to irrigation and debridement. *JAMA Surg.* 2015;150(4):332-336.
19. Malhotra AK, Goldberg S, Graham J, et al. Open extremity fractures: Impact of delay in operative debridement and irrigation. *J Trauma Acute Care Surg.* 2014;76(5):1201-1207.
20. Rittmann WW, Schibli M, Matter P, et al. Open fractures. Long-term results in 200 consecutive cases. *Clin Orthop Relat Res.* 1979(138):132-140.
21. Rhee P, Nunley MK, Demetriades D, et al. Tetanus and trauma: a review and recommendations. *J Trauma.* 2005;58(5):1082-1088.
22. Patzakis MJ, Wilkins J. Factors influencing infection rate in open fracture wounds. *Clin Orthop Relat Res.* 1989;(243):36-40.
23. Lack WD, Karunakar MA, Angerame MR, et al. Type III open tibia fractures: Immediate antibiotic prophylaxis minimizes infection. *J Orthop Trauma.* 2015;29(1):1-6.
24. Zalavras CG. Prevention of infection in open fractures. *Infect Dis Clin North Am.* 2017;31(2):339-352.
25. Vanwijck R, Kaba L, Boland S, et al. Immediate skin grafting of sub-acute and chronic wounds debrided by hydrosurgery. *J Plast Reconstr Aesthet Surg.* 2010;63(3):544-549.
26. Gurunluoglu R. Experiences with waterjet hydrosurgery system in wound debridement. *World J Emerg Surg.* 2007;2:10.
27. Murphy CA. The effect of 22.5 kHz low-frequency contact ultrasound debridement (LFCUD) on lower extremity wound healing for a vascular surgery population: a randomised controlled trial. *Int Wound J.* 2018;15(3):460-472.
28. Cheng Q, Zhang XF, Di DH, et al. Efficacy of different irrigation solutions on the early debridement of open fracture in rats. *Exp Ther Med.* 2015;9(5):1589-1592.
29. Brown LL, Shelton HT, Bornside GH, et al. Evaluation of wound irrigation by pulsatile jet and conventional methods. *Ann Surg.* 1978;187(2):170-173.
30. Boyd JI III, Wongworawat MD. High-pressure pulsatile lavage causes soft tissue damage. *Clin Orthop Relat Res.* 2004;(427):13-17.
31. Hassinger SM, Harding G, Wongworawat MD. High-pressure pulsatile lavage propagates bacteria into soft tissue. *Clin Orthop Relat Res.* 2005;439:27-31.
32. Anglen JO. Comparison of soap and antibiotic solutions for irrigation of lower-limb open fracture wounds. A prospective, randomized study. *J Bone Joint Surg Am.* 2005;87(7):1415-1422.
33. Bhandari M, Jeray KJ, Petrisor BA, et al. A trial of wound irrigation in the initial management of open fracture wounds. *N Engl J Med.* 2015;373(27):2629-2641.
34. Olufemi OT, Adeyeye AI. Irrigation solutions in open fractures of the lower extremities: evaluation of isotonic saline and distilled water. *SICOT J.* 2017;3:7.
35. Franklin JL, Johnson KD, Hansen ST Jr. Immediate internal fixation of open ankle fractures. Report of thirty-eight cases treated with a standard protocol. *J Bone Joint Surg Am.* 1984;66(9):1349-1356.
36. Wiss DA, Gilbert P, Merritt PO, et al. Immediate internal fixation of open ankle fractures. *J Orthop Trauma.* 1988;2(4):265-271.
37. Kortram K, Bezstarosti H, Metsemakers WJ, et al. Risk factors for infectious complications after open fractures; a systematic review and meta-analysis. *Int Orthop.* 2017;41(10):1965-1982.
38. Doshi P, Gopalan H, Sprague S, et al. Incidence of infection following internal fixation of open and closed tibia fractures in India (Infiniti): A multi-centre observational cohort study. *BMC Musculoskelet Disord.* 2017;18(1):156.
39. Kemper DD, Lowenberg DW, Ong A, et al. *Principles of External Fixation.* 2014 [cited January 7, 2019]. https://ota.org/sites/files/2018-06/G11-Principles%20of%20External%20 Fixation.pdf.
40. Moss DP, Tejwani NC. Biomechanics of external fixation. *Bull NYU Hosp Jt Dis.* 2007;65(4):294-299.
41. Argenta LC, Morykwas MJ. Vacuum-assisted closure: a new method for wound control and treatment: clinical experience. *Ann Plast Surg.* 1997;38(6):563-576; discussion 577.
42. Morykwas MJ, Argenta LC, Shelton-Brown EI, et al. Vacuum-assisted closure: a new method for wound control and treatment: animal studies and basic foundation. *Ann Plast Surg.* 1997;38(6):553-562.
43. Maurya S, Bhandari PS. Negative pressure wound therapy in the management of combat wounds: A critical review. *Adv Wound Care (New Rochelle).* 2016;5(9):379-389.
44. Dabiri G, Damstetter E, Phillips T. Choosing a wound dressing based on common wound characteristics. *Adv Wound Care (New Rochelle).* 2016;5(1):32-41.
45. Zgonis T, Stapleton JJ, Roukis TS. Advanced plastic surgery techniques for soft tissue coverage of the diabetic foot. *Clin Podiatr Med Surg.* 2007;24(3):547-568, x.
46. Moiemen NS, Staiano JJ, Ojeh NO, et al. Reconstructive surgery with a dermal regeneration template: Clinical and histologic study. *Plast Reconstr Surg.* 2001;108(1):93-103.
47. Graham GP, Helmer SD, Haan JM, et al. The use of Integra® dermal regeneration template in the reconstruction of traumatic degloving injuries. *J Burn Care Res.* 2013;34(2):261-266.
48. Brigido SA, Boc SF, Lopez RC. Effective management of major lower extremity wounds using an acellular regenerative tissue matrix: a pilot study. *Orthopedics.* 2004;27(1 suppl):s145-s149.
49. Cooke M, Tan EK, Mandrycky C, et al. Comparison of cryopreserved amniotic membrane and umbilical cord tissue with dehydrated amniotic membrane/chorion tissue. *J Wound Care.* 2014;23(10):465-474, 476.
50. Schultz GS, Sibbald RG, Falanga V, et al. Wound bed preparation: a systematic approach to wound management. *Wound Repair Regen.* 2003;11(suppl 1):S1-S28.
51. Jehan F, Khan M, Sakran JV, et al. Perioperative glycemic control and postoperative complications in patients undergoing emergency general surgery: what is the role of plasma hemoglobin A1c? *J Trauma Acute Care Surg.* 2018;84(1):112-117.
52. Greenhalgh DG. Wound healing and diabetes mellitus. *Clin Plast Surg.* 2003;30(1):37-45.
53. van den Berghe G, Wouters P, Weekers F, et al. Intensive insulin therapy in critically ill patients. *N Engl J Med.* 2001;345(19):1359-1367.
54. Ingenbleek Y, Van Den Schrieck HG, De Nayer P, et al. Albumin, transferrin and the thyroxine-binding prealbumin/retinol-binding protein (TBPA-RBP) complex in assessment of malnutrition. *Clin Chim Acta.* 1975;63(1):61-67.

55. Molnar JA, Vlad LG, Gumus T. Nutrition and chronic wounds: improving clinical outcomes. *Plast Reconstr Surg.* 2016;138(3 suppl):71S-81S.

56. Pinzur MS, Stuck RM, Sage R, et al. Syme ankle disarticulation in patients with diabetes. *J Bone Joint Surg Am.* 2003;85-A(9):1667-1672.

57. Delliere S, Cynober L. Is transthyretin a good marker of nutritional status? *Clin Nutr.* 2017;36(2):364-370.

58. Lee JL, Oh ES, Lee RW, et al. Serum albumin and prealbumin in calorically restricted, nondiseased individuals: a systematic review. *Am J Med.* 2015;128(9):1023.e1021-1022.

59. Quain AM, Khardori NM. Nutrition in wound care management: a comprehensive overview. *Wounds.* 2015;27(12):327-335.

60. Knudson MM, Morabito D, Paiement GD, et al. Use of low molecular weight heparin in preventing thromboembolism in trauma patients. *J Trauma.* 1996;41(3):446-459.

61. Lassen MR, Borris LC, Nakov RL. Use of the low-molecular-weight heparin reviparin to prevent deep-vein thrombosis after leg injury requiring immobilization. *N Engl J Med.* 2002;347(10):726-730.

62. Hsu JR, Owens JG, DeSanto J, et al. Patient response to an integrated orthotic and rehabilitation initiative for traumatic injuries: the PRIORITI-MTF study. *J Orthop Trauma.* 2017;31(suppl 1):S56-S62.

63. Bosse MJ, McCarthy ML, Jones AL, et al. The insensate foot following severe lower extremity trauma: An indication for amputation? *J Bone Joint Surg Am.* 2005;87(12):2601-2608.

64. Demiralp B, Ege T, Kose O, et al. Amputation versus functional reconstruction in the management of complex hind foot injuries caused by land-mine explosions: a long-term retrospective comparison. *Eur J Orthop Surg Traumatol.* 2014;24(4):621-626.

65. Williams ZF, Bools LM, Adams A, et al. Early versus delayed amputation in the setting of severe lower extremity trauma. *Am Surg.* 2015;81(6):564-568.

Gastroc Recession

Troy J. Boffeli and Samantha A. Luer

DEFINITION

Equinus deformity of the ankle has been historically described as a limitation of passive ankle joint dorsiflexion to <90 degrees angle of the foot to the leg. The Silfverskiold test is widely used in practice to differentiate between gastrocnemius equinus and combined gastrocnemius-soleus equinus.[1] A positive Silfverskiold sign is defined as ankle equinus that is present when the knee is extended but that disappears when the knee is flexed, which indicates gastrocnemius equinus.[1] Combined gastrocnemius-soleus equinus does not improve with flexion of the knee.[1] DiGiovanni defined gastrocnemius equinus as <5 degrees dorsiflexion with the knee extended and gastrocnemius-soleus equinus as <10 degrees dorsiflexion with the knee flexed.[2]

INDICATIONS

INDICATIONS FOR GASTROCNEMIUS RECESSION

- Isolated gastrocnemius equinus
- An adjunctive procedure to address gastrocnemius equinus with associated foot/ankle pathologies
  - Diabetic foot ulcers
  - Neuromuscular diseases
  - Flatfoot or cavus deformity
  - Plantar fasciitis
  - Achilles tendinitis/tendinopathy
  - Hallux valgus
  - Metatarsalgia
  - Ankle DJD/total ankle replacement

Indications for surgical lengthening in patients with gastrocnemius equinus include gastrocnemius equinus present with or without an associated lower extremity disorder that has not responded to conservative care.[3] There are patients who present with symptomatic isolated gastrocnemius contracture, but more commonly the contracture is a primary or secondary condition noted in conjunction with other pathologic conditions of the foot and ankle. Common conditions that have been linked to gastrocnemius equinus include adult-acquired flatfoot, metatarsalgia, diabetic forefoot ulceration, plantar fasciitis, Achilles tendinitis/tendinosis, Charcot neuropathic arthropathy, recurrent ankle sprains, hallux valgus, neuromuscular diseases, and many others.[4] Gastrocnemius equinus is therefore most commonly corrected as an adjunctive procedure as part of a bigger operation which has implications regarding patient positioning and postoperative ambulatory status.

The etiology and severity of gastrocnemius equinus contracture should be considered when surgical management is recommended. Specific procedures are indicated for a more aggressive lengthening verses a less aggressive lengthening which can be applied to both spastic and nonspastic equinus. For spastic equinus associated with neuromuscular diseases and longstanding contracture, gastrocnemius lengthening alone is generally not aggressive enough. Historically, isolated neurectomy and/or proximal resection of the heads of the gastrocnemius muscle have been performed especially in cases of fixed knee flexion and muscular ankle joint equinus associated with spastic gastrocnemius.[5] Tendo-Achilles lengthening (TAL) procedures (Chapter 58) are more commonly indicated as they allow more aggressive correction of combined gastrocnemius-soleus equinus and spastic equinus contracture. For nonspastic equinus, the desired degree of lengthening is important which is often determined by patient specific factors as well as the severity of contracture. Factors to consider for an individual patient include age, desired activity level, underlying medical conditions, risk profile of various surgical techniques, scar concerns, and the potential need to wear a rigid ankle brace postoperatively due to weakness.

ANATOMIC FEATURES

The gastrocnemius and soleus muscles make up the triceps surae also known as the gastrocnemius-soleus complex of the superficial posterior compartment of the leg. The gastrocnemius muscle is the most superficial muscle of the posterior compartment, and its heads originate on the posterior aspect of the femoral condyles just proximal to the knee joint.[6,7] The medial head of the gastrocnemius muscle is broader and thicker while the lateral head occasionally contains a sesamoid bone (flabella). The gastrocnemius remains separate from the soleus for the length of the muscle belly and only connects into the soleus aponeurosis distally after the gastrocnemius aponeurosis becomes tendinous. The soleus muscle is deep to the gastrocnemius and is broad, flat, and pennate. It originates from the upper third of the tibia, fibula, and interosseous membrane.[6,7] The Achilles tendon is the convergence of

these muscles and inserts on the midportion of the posterior calcaneal tuberosity. The paratenon, a thick elastic sleeve of dense connective tissue, surrounds the Achilles tendon to permit gliding and separate the tendon from the deep fascia of the leg.[7] An additional muscle in the superficial group of the superficial posterior leg compartment is the plantaris, absent in 7% of individuals.[6] The plantaris muscle belly is small, flat, and fusiform. It usually originates with the lateral head of the gastrocnemius then the thin tendon passes obliquely between the gastrocnemius and soleus muscles and inserts along the medial edge of the Achilles tendon.[7]

FUNCTIONAL ANALYSIS OF THE ANATOMY

The main function of the gastrocnemius muscle is propulsion of the body forward during gait, while the soleus is a postural muscle that also functions as a peripheral vascular pump.[6] The gastrocnemius and plantaris muscles cross the knee, ankle, and subtalar joints, while the soleus crosses only the ankle and subtalar joints. This concept that the gastrocnemius and plantaris are three-joint muscles while the soleus is a two-joint muscle is clinically very important and is the basis of the Silfverskiold test described above and in the next section.[5] Both heads of the gastrocnemius are subject to contracture and functional shortening, although research has demonstrated that the medial head of the gastrocnemius is typically tighter.[6] Surgical release should therefore focus on complete release of the medial aspect of the gastrocnemius for improved lengthening. The soleus muscle in comparison is rarely associated with functional shortening.[6] When there is a limitation in ankle joint dorsiflexion with the knee extended, but not with the knee flexed, this is directly caused by gastrocnemius and plantaris tightness. The plantaris is a rudimentary muscle and often forgotten, but it does function much like the gastrocnemius and must be addressed during surgical procedures for equinus.[5]

Neurovascular structures of importance which can be at risk during dissection are different depending on the level of the procedure along the posterior muscle complex. The tibial nerve, the larger component of the sciatic nerve (anterior divisions L4-S3), innervates all muscles of the superficial posterior compartment of the leg.[7] Proximally, the popliteal artery and vein as well as the tibial nerve lie lateral to the medial head of the gastrocnemius. Inferior to the popliteus muscle, the tibial nerve disappears between the heads of the gastrocnemius and deep to the soleus, eventually lying medial to the Achilles tendon. The tibial nerve divides into the medial and lateral plantar nerves at the flexor retinaculum. The posterior leg compartment muscles receive vascular supply from the posterior tibial artery, which is the larger of the two terminal branches of the popliteal artery. The posterior tibial artery begins at the inferior border of the popliteus muscle and courses deep to the soleus muscle in an inferomedial direction. Additional important structures are the saphenous nerve and sural nerve. The saphenous nerve is the longest branch of the femoral nerve and runs with the great saphenous vein along the medial side of the leg outside the posterior fascia along the soleus muscle belly. At the level of the ankle, the saphenous nerve and great saphenous vein are anterior to the medial malleolus. The sural nerve is formed by union of a branch of the tibial nerve (medial sural cutaneous nerve) and a branch of the common peroneal nerve

(lateral sural cutaneous nerve); because of an inconstant union site, it can have a variable origin. The sural nerve courses with the small saphenous vein superficial to the deep fascia of the posterolateral leg. At the level of the ankle joint, the sural nerve is lateral to the Achilles tendon and posterior to the lateral malleolus. The sural nerve is the main contributor to the Achilles tendon and paratenon structures, and because of its proximity to the tendon and aponeurosis posteriorly, it is often at risk during gastrocnemius recession.[7]

PHYSICAL EXAMINATION

The diagnosis of gastrocnemius equinus is determined clinically by physical examination. At least 23 different methods have been described in the literature to measure ankle joint dorsiflexion.[8] The Silfverskiold test has historically been used to differentiate between gastrocnemius equinus and combined gastrocnemius-soleus equinus.[1] It is performed with the patient seated comfortably in an examination chair with their knee fully extended. The patient's ankle is dorsiflexed with the knee extended and then with the knee flexed. A positive Silfverskiold sign is defined as ankle equinus that is present when the knee is extended but that disappears when the knee is flexed which indicates gastrocnemius equinus.[1] Combined gastrocnemius-soleus equinus does not improve with flexion of the knee.[1] Traditionally the foot position while performing a Silfverskiold test was in a "neutral position." The neutral position of the foot is hard to reproduce and can be a potential source of error. Dayton et al. recommend a supinated foot position as a more reliable position for measuring clinical ankle joint range of motion.[9] During clinical testing, it is also important to note that the motion should be passive. If active motion is evaluated, the anterior muscles fire to actively dorsiflex the foot and the resting tone of the gastrocnemius is turned off, demonstrating improved dorsiflexion.[4] However, the desired measurement is the dorsiflexion achieved in a simulated stance, where the anterior muscles are not active and the gastrocnemius tone is pertinent.

Compensatory signs of ankle equinus include knee recurvatum, hip flexion, lumbar hyperlordosis, and forefoot overload.[1,5] These signs should be observed for during resting stance and gait evaluation.

Lastly, a complete physical examination prior to surgical intervention should be performed including a thorough neurologic, dermatologic, and vascular evaluation. Neurological examination is important to rule out spasticity. The patient's skin quality including appearance, texture, turgor, and edema can suggest underlying comorbidities. Poor skin quality, arterial supply, or chronic edema can also predict delayed incision healing. Skin condition, edema, and vascular supply should be optimized preoperatively when possible, and the surgeon should give consideration to less invasive procedures if wound healing concerns cannot be reversed.

PATHOGENESIS

Spastic equinus contracture of the gastrocnemius-soleus complex is well documented in the literature for patients with systemic neurologic or spastic imbalance. Common neurologic conditions associated with spastic ankle equinus include

cerebral palsy, Charcot-Marie-Tooth (CMT), traumatic brain injuries, and cerebrovascular accident (CVA). Spastic contracture typically involves both the gastrocnemius and soleus muscle bellies.[6] Patients with spastic equinus frequently require aggressive lengthening due to severity of contracture and are more often treated with TAL rather than gastrocnemius recession. These conditions often require ongoing foot and ankle bracing, which decreases the concern for over-lengthening as compared to elective lengthening in nonneurogenic equinus.

Nonspastic equinus contracture in comparison is a result of functional shortening of the gastrocnemius-soleus complex, often an isolated contracture of the gastrocnemius muscle.[6] This functional shortening can cause increased pressure on the foot in otherwise healthy individuals. Increased pressure on the foot occurs because the posterior calcaneus is tethered due to a short gastrocnemius-soleus complex, placing a plantar flexion force on the arch and increasing the plantar pressures on the forefoot as well as causing early heel rise during the stance phase of gait.[6] The tight posterior complex can also accentuate hindfoot valgus through the subtalar joint. Eventually this leads to failure of the medial column of the foot, producing a flatfoot deformity because the subtalar joint is forced into an everted position and can no longer invert during the stance phase of gait; compensation through pronation of the foot.[7] Throughout the literature, authors believe that these abnormal forces caused by a functionally shortened gastrocnemius leads to multiple forefoot and midfoot pathologies, as discussed previously.

IMAGING AND DIAGNOSTIC STUDIES

A weight-bearing lateral radiograph of the ankle is commonly obtained to rule out bony equinus, especially in gastrocnemius-soleus and fixed equinus. Anterior ankle impingement associated with bones spurs and ankle degenerative joint disease can create a bony block that limits the ankle from adequate dorsiflexion.

TREATMENT

NONOPERATIVE MANAGEMENT

Posterior muscle group stretching is the main nonoperative treatment that is recommended to address gastrocnemius equinus. Both static and eccentric stretching programs have been published in the literature. The goal is to attempt to increase ankle dorsiflexion and reduce symptoms. Radford et al. found in a systematic review that static calf muscle stretches provide a small but statistically significant increase in ankle dorsiflexion, particularly after 5-30 minutes of stretching.[10] There was also a trend that the longer the stretch, the greater the increase in ankle dorsiflexion.[10] However, the increase in ankle dorsiflexion with static stretching although statistically significant was not substantial (increase of 2.1-3.0 degrees after 5-60 minutes of stretching when compared with no stretching). Therefore, Radford et al. recommended that calf muscle stretching may only be beneficial when a small increase in ankle range of motion is needed. Other nonoperative treatment modalities may be incorporated to treat associated pathologies including night splints, orthoses, physical therapy, padding, rigid/supportive shoe gear, and bracing.

SURGICAL PROCEDURES AND TECHNIQUES

Intramuscular Aponeurotic Gastrocnemius Recession (Baumann)

The Baumann procedure, first described by Baumann and Koch, is very conducive to being performed in the supine position with an incision at the medial midsubstance of the gastrocnemius muscle belly.[11] The medial incision provides a less visible scar high on the inside of the calf, which may be preferred by patients who would like to avoid a visible scar on the back of the calf. The proximal location of this procedure makes it a true gastrocnemius only lengthening, which provides less aggressive lengthening.[11,12] This conservative lengthening may not be enough for some conditions, but benefits of the procedure include optimal preservation of muscle mass and strength, which is important for pediatric and athletic patients.[12]

> *positioning* PEARLS
>
> - Procedure performed in a supine position. Natural external rotation of the leg provides good visibility when performing supine procedures like flatfoot reconstruction.[12]

1. Longitudinal, 3-5 cm incision performed at the medial midsubstance of the gastrocnemius muscle belly, which is proximal compared to a traditional Strayer gastrocnemius recession (Fig. 62.1A and B). Incision deepened bluntly to the deep crural fascia without raising flaps or undermining the subcutaneous layer off the fascia (Fig. 62.1C-E). Watch for the great saphenous vein and saphenous nerve during dissection and be sure to retract if seen.
2. Crural fascia is divided to expose the soleus and gastrocnemius muscles (Fig. 62.1F and G). Look for the white aponeurosis on the anterior aspect of the gastrocnemius muscle, which is in contact with the white aponeurosis on the posterior aspect of the soleus muscle (Fig. 62.1H). The interval between the soleus and gastrocnemius muscles can then be separated with a probing finger.
3. The gastrocnemius muscle is retracted posteriorly, and the plantaris tendon as well as the aponeurotic surface of the gastrocnemius muscle can be visualized on the anterior aspect of the muscle.
4. A long, narrow blade retractor or speculum is inserted to provide exposure and flatten the muscle belly in preparation for recession (Fig. 62.1I).
5. Plantaris tendon is sharply divided.
6. The foot is dorsiflexed while the surgeon performs a transverse gastrocnemius recession with a scalpel. Multiple transverse cuts at various levels of the retinaculum increase the amount of dorsiflexion achieved and should be performed in a parallel fashion at least 1 cm apart. Cuts are made until normal ankle dorsiflexion is achieved.
7. Surgical site irrigated. Layered closure performed. Dorsiflexion of the foot during closure of the deep crural fascia prevents the underlying muscle bellies from bulging out (Fig. 62.1J).

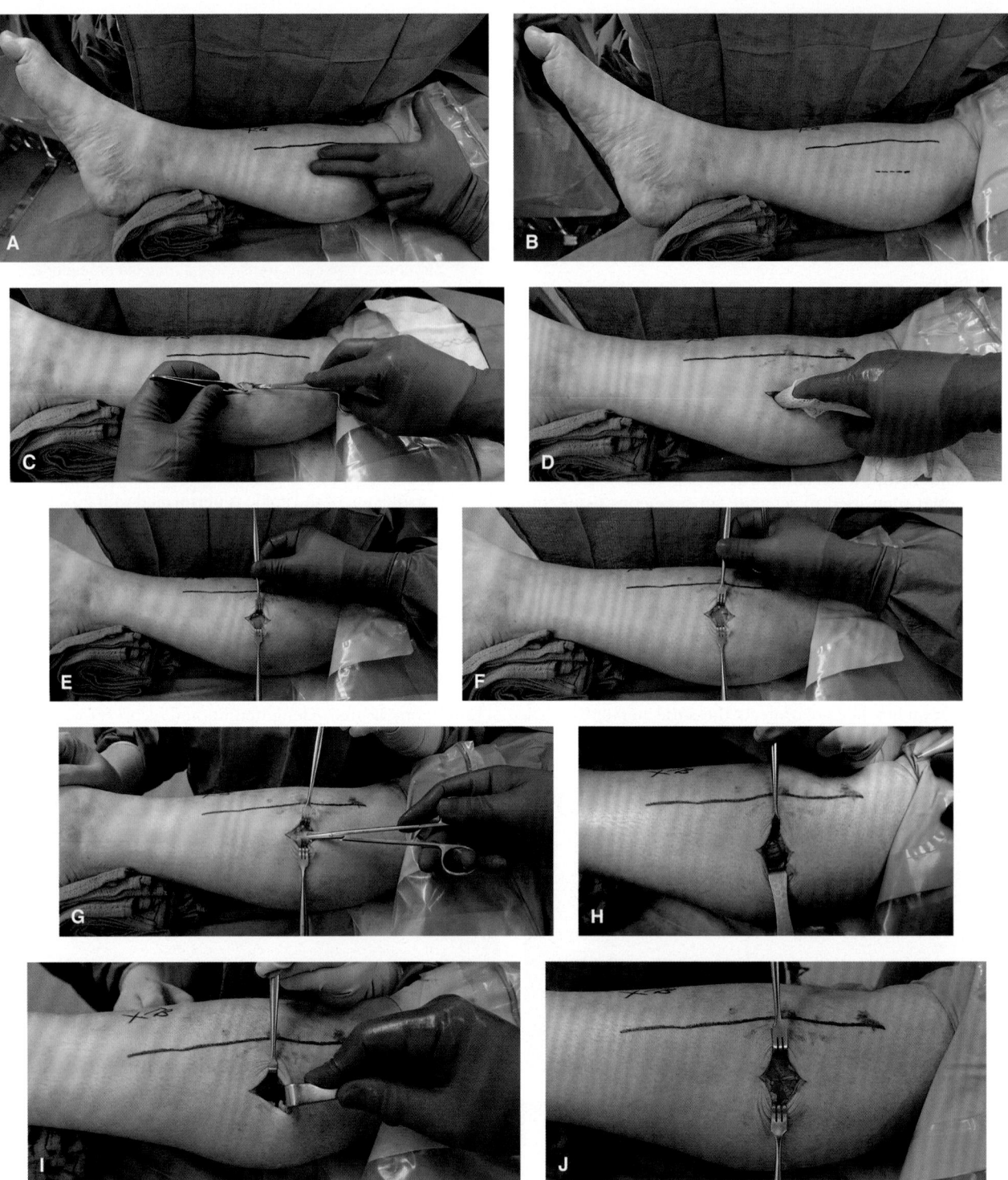

FIGURE 62.1 The Bowman intramuscular gastrocnemius recession is performed through an incision on the medial side of the calf.
A. The *straight line* on the anterior shin indicates the palpable medial aspect of the tibia. Proper location of the incision from anterior to posterior is beneficial in order to find the interval between the gastrocnemius and soleus muscle bellies. The appropriate distance from the palpable medial aspect of the tibia can be determined generally by two finger widths. **B.** Incision location is identified with *hash marks*. This high medial calf incision is generally less visible as compared to a posterior midline incision so there are cosmetic advantages to this approach. Incision deepened bluntly to the deep crural fascia without raising flaps or undermining the subcutaneous layer off the fascia. **C.** Mosquito shown as blunt instrumentation. **D.** However, a wet sponge with the surgeon's index figure is also utilized as dissecting tool to expose the deep fascia. Care must be taken to watch for the great saphenous vein and saphenous nerve during separation of the subcutaneous tissues. **E.** Deep crural fascia is exposed. **F, G.** A small midline incision is then made with a No. 15 blade and finished with a dissecting scissors to protect the underlying muscles and avoid risk to neurovascular structures. **H.** Deep retractors are placed anterior and posterior along the incision to expose the underlying soleus and gastrocnemius muscles. The interval between the soleus and gastrocnemius muscles can then be separated with a probing finger. Soleus muscle is retracted, and the plantaris tendon as well as the posterior aponeurotic surface of the gastrocnemius muscle can be visualized. The plantaris tendon is transected. **I.** A deep angled retractor is shown here for exposure and to flatten the muscle surface to improve cutting efficiency. Long narrow speculums are helpful, and proprietary cutting jigs are available for this purpose. **J.** The deep crural fascia is reapproximated with absorbable suture. Dorsiflexion of the foot during closure of the fascia prevents the underlying muscle bellies from bulging out. Closure of this layer helps prevent scar tissue adhesions between the skin and muscle which can lead to an unsightly puckered scar.

Distal Gastrocnemius Recession (Strayer)

The Strayer gastrocnemius recession is the workhorse of equinus surgery since it is highly conducive to supine surgery, provides adequate lengthening, and is relatively friendly to the sural nerve provided the surgical exposure is deep to the peritenon level.[13] It is possible to perform gastrocnemius only Strayer lengthening but only if exposure is above the conjoined tendon just below the gastrocnemius muscle belly.[13]

1. Patient in supine position and operative leg is often manipulated in a frog-leg manner or elevated on a bump of towels. Procedure can be performed wet or with a thigh tourniquet inflated.
2. The Strayer gastrocnemius recession is performed just below the muscle belly of the gastrocnemius. The longitudinal incision is performed along the medial edge of the palpable tendon and is ~3-5 cm in length (Fig. 62.2A).
3. Hemostat then used to separate subcutaneous tissue and identify crossing veins. Care taken to avoid disruption of the veins as this can obscure the operative field. Further subcutaneous adipose tissue is dissected utilizing a moist sponge and the surgeon's index finger. Retractors placed and deep fascia is visualized (Fig. 62.2B).
4. No. 15 blade is used to incise the deep fascia and paratenon in line with the skin incision. Blunt dissection below the level of the paratenon exposes the underlying gastrocnemius aponeurosis and protects the sural nerve, which is superficial to this deep layer.

5. A small speculum or deep retractors are placed under the deep fascia and paratenon to further visualize the entire gastrocnemius aponeurosis from medial to lateral (Fig. 62.2C).

> ### PEARLS
> - It is important to be sure the speculum/deep retractor is at the appropriate level. This protects vital neurovascular structures from being transected during the procedure.

6. No. 15 blade with long handle is then used to cut the gastrocnemius aponeurosis entirely from lateral to medial. Cut should be down to the underlying muscle belly, but avoid cutting into the muscle itself to decrease risk of hematoma. The plantaris tendon is easily visualized along the medial edge of the gastrocnemius aponeurosis and should also be transected.
7. Dorsiflexion of the ankle is performed with goal of getting the foot at a >90-degree angle to the lower leg.
8. Surgical site irrigated. Layered closure performed. Approximation of the deep fascia with absorbable sutures is important to avoid adhesion of the skin to the underlying muscle tissues. Such adhesions can create an unsightly dell at the incision site.

Endoscopic Gastrocnemius Recession

Indications, degree of lengthening, and recovery for endoscopic gastrocnemius recession is similar to the Strayer technique with

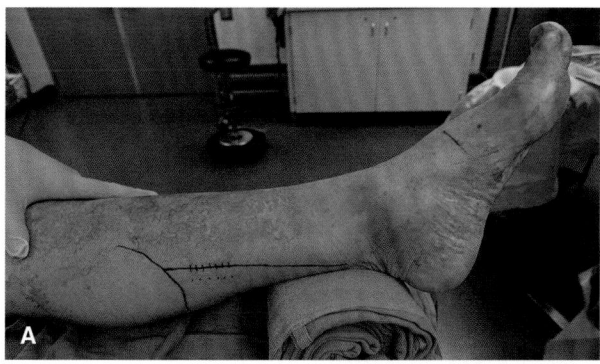
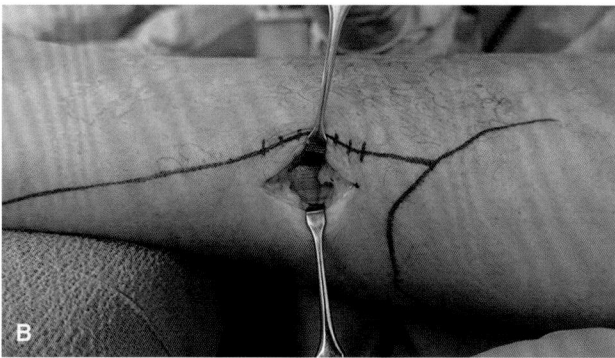
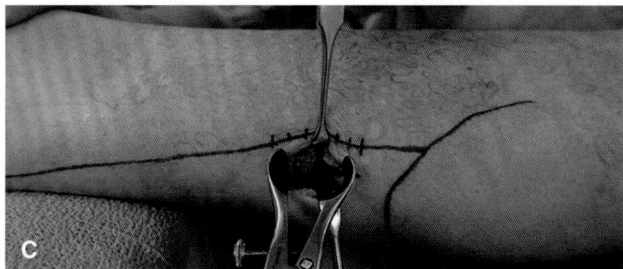

FIGURE 62.2 A. The traditional medial Strayer incision is shown here in *hash marks* along the medial aspect of the gastrocnemius retinaculum. The authors prefer to adjust the incision slightly posterior as pictured with dots to facilitate better access laterally when performing the recession. Also pictured, a bump of towels can be placed under the operative ankle to assist with positioning and exposure. **B.** The gastrocnemius aponeurosis is visualized after incising the deep crural fascia. **C.** Incision of the aponeurosis from lateral to medial at a depth which exposes the soleus muscle accomplishes gastrocnemius lengthening combined with conservative soleus lengthening. Incising the aponeurosis from lateral to medial also minimizes the underlying muscle from bulging into the operative field. A narrow, long speculum can be used to fully visualize the lateral aponeurosis and assist with retraction of the paratenon and deep fascia.

procedure selection largely based on surgeon preference. Risk profile regarding injury to the surrounding tissue is technique and experience dependent. A skilled surgeon could potentially have less nerve complications or bleeding due to better visibility although the procedure is technology dependent, which can add time, cost, and frustration. The endoscopic approach is minimally invasive creating only a small medial scar.[14,15]

1. When patient is placed in a supine position, a stack of towels under the operative ankle can be used to facilitate passage of instrumentation under the calf. A tourniquet is utilized for this procedure (thigh or high calf), as bleeding during the procedure will obscure visualization through the endoscope.

2. Incision is placed in a similar location as the distal gastrocnemius recession (Strayer), just below the gastrocnemius muscle belly along the medial edge of the palpable tendon. However, only 1 cm in length of the incision is required to pass the endoscope. This small incision is important for patients with cosmetic concerns.

3. A No. 15 blade is used to incise the skin then a hemostat as well as a wet sponge is utilized to dissect the subcutaneous tissue and fat. No. 15 blade again is used to incise the deep fascia and paratenon of the gastrocnemius aponeurosis in line with the incision.

4. Then the blunt end of the scalpel or other blunt instrument is used to sweep the paratenon from the underlying gastrocnemius aponeurosis. The fascial elevator is then introduced through the incision across the aponeurosis from medial to lateral.

5. After the fascial elevator is removed, it is replaced by the cannula/obturator. Obturator then removed and the 4 mm, 30-degree endoscope is inserted into the cannula (size and angle of the scope is variable based on surgeon preference). The gastrocnemius aponeurosis can then be visualized.

PEARLS

- It is important to be sure to rotate the endoscope 180 degrees to verify the saphenous vein and sural nerve are protected behind the paratenon/deep fascia.

6. Endoscope then removed from the cannula in order to lock the cutting instrument onto the scope.

7. Endoscope with cutting instrument then reintroduced through the incision. Care is taken to identify the lateral edge of the gastrocnemius aponeurosis and adjacent subcutaneous tissue.

8. Active dorsiflexion of the operative ankle is performed as blade of the cutting instrument is deployed. From watching the monitor, the surgeon can indirectly visualize a lateral to medial gastrocnemius aponeurosis recession. Active ankle dorsiflexion during the cut is vital because it avoids overlengthening.

9. Surgical site irrigated. Layered closure performed.

Open Tongue and Groove Gastrocnemius Recession (Baker)

The tongue and groove procedure, first described by Baker in 1956 as a modification of the Vulpius procedure, is generally performed in the prone position which creates added burden with many reconstructive procedures. The midline posterior

incision also creates a more visible scar. Complete gastrocnemius and partial soleus lengthening is achieved due to the procedure being performed below the conjoined tendon. The central incision allows direct visualization and retraction of the sural nerve, but even a well protected nerve can become problematic due to scar tissue. The open nature of the procedure allows direct suture repair to avoid both over lengthening and recurrence associated with tendon retraction.

1. Patient placed in prone position. Operative leg should hang off table or bump to allow for dorsiflexion during the procedure. Procedure can be performed wet or with a thigh tourniquet inflated. Alternatively, the procedure can be performed supine, which has added challenges related to holding the leg off the table or turning the leg for visualization.

2. Incision located midline on the posterior calf below the gastrocnemius muscle belly at the level of the conjoined gastrocnemius and soleus tendons (Fig. 62.3A). The sural nerve often will run from proximal medial to distal lateral, crossing the incision (Fig. 62.3B). This is conducive to identification and retraction of the nerve but also predisposes to scar tissue around the nerve postoperatively. Incision performed with a No. 15 blade.

3. A hemostat and a wet sponge are utilized to dissect the subcutaneous tissue and fat.

4. Deep fascia is cut longitudinally first with a No. 15 blade and then finished with a dissecting scissors taking care to avoid the sural nerve which lies below.

5. The nerve is then located and retracted to one side to allow safe incision of the paratenon, which is then bluntly swept away from the underlying gastrocnemius aponeurosis (Fig. 62.3C).

6. The central one-third of the aponeurosis is incised transversely at the most proximally aspect of the incision (Fig. 62.3D). The authors prefer this approach as the aponeurosis is wide and difficult to expose at the most medial and lateral aspects at this high level just below the muscle belly. An inverted central tongue is created by cutting the medial and lateral one-third portions of the aponeurosis at the distal aspect of the incision (Fig. 62.3E).

7. The ankle is dorsiflexed with the knee extended to obtain the desired amount of slide lengthening (Fig. 62.3F). The lengthened tendon is then sutured along both sides in the desired position with a braided nonabsorbable suture.

8. Surgical site irrigated. The paratenon and deep fascia are then repaired using absorbable suture, taking great care to avoid the exposed sural nerve (Fig. 62.3G). Skin closure performed with nonabsorbable suture (Fig. 62.3H).

AUTHORS PREFERRED TREATMENT

Procedure selection among the various approaches to address gastrocnemius equinus can be viewed as either an opportunity or a challenge. While all approaches work, guidelines are lacking to assist the surgeon with ideal procedure selection based on an individual patient's operative needs. The majority of the literature involving equinus procedure selection is level three or four evidence.[16] We believe that there are a multitude of factors that contribute to ideal procedure selection including positioning for adjunctive procedures (supine or prone), site of incision which has implications regarding scar visibility,

postoperative weight bearing status related to adjunctive procedures, risk of injury to the sural nerve, potential over-lengthening or incomplete lengthening, and degree of lengthening desired. Our approach is to incorporate these factors along with patient specific indications for optimal procedure selection. Table 62.1 highlights multiple procedure selection considerations incorporated into the decision-making process for the various gastrocnemius recession procedures. The authors would like to acknowledge that there is always more than one appropriate procedure for a given patient and that this approach is intended to raise awareness of factors that are worthy of consideration when performing ankle equinus surgery.

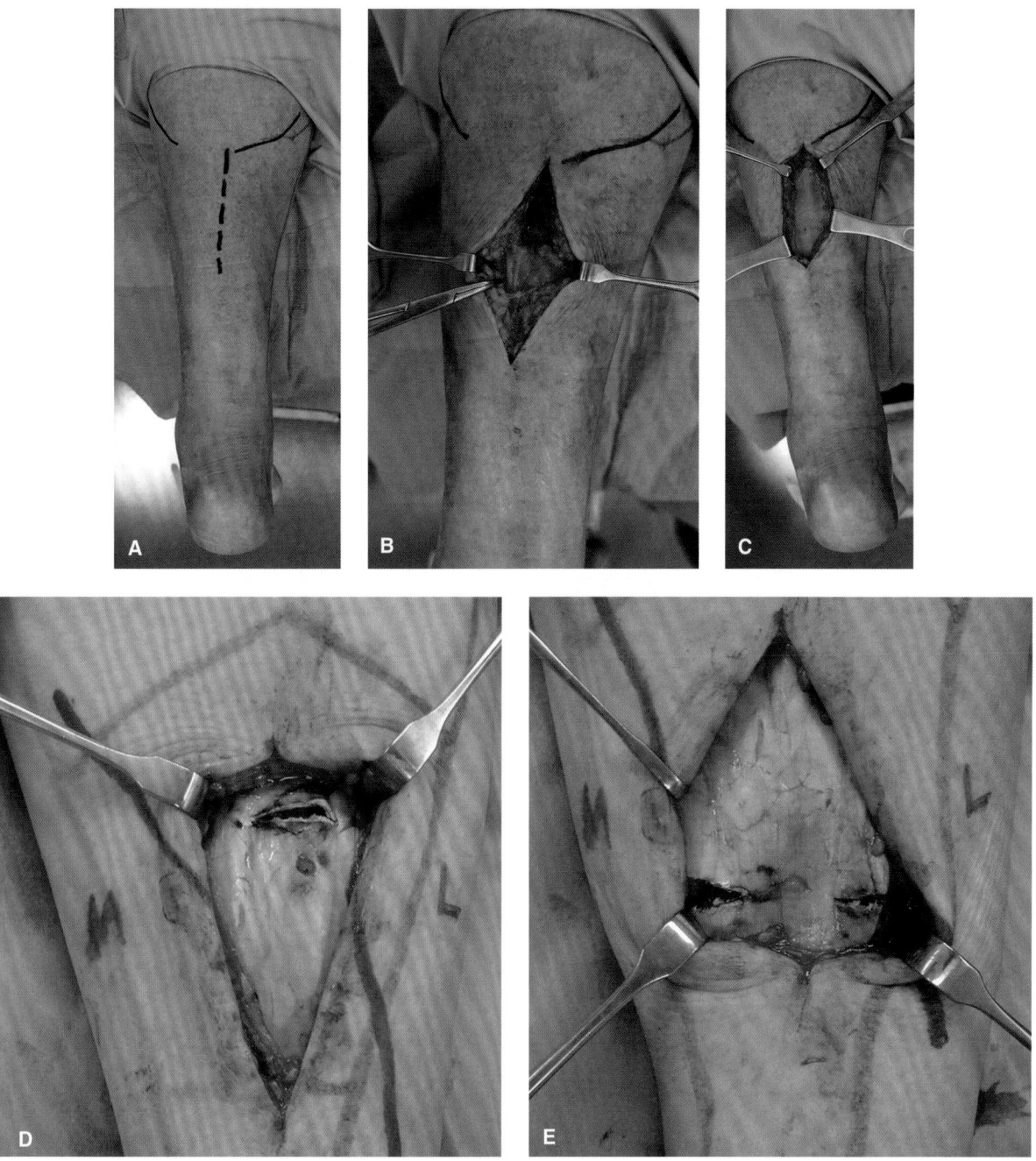

FIGURE 62.3 **A.** Incision planning for tongue and groove gastrocnemius recession is shown here. The *dotted lines* represent a midline posterior incision in the region of proposed tongue and groove recession. This is below the level of the gastrocnemius muscle belly and usually below the level of the conjoined tendon. **B.** The sural nerve is almost always identified during blunt dissection after incising the deep fascia. The nerve runs from proximal medial to distal lateral crossing the incision which is conducive to nerve identification and retraction but also predisposes to scar tissue around the nerve. **C.** It is important to maintain the nerve in the native tissue yet still mobilize and retract the nerve prior to incising the paratenon. **D.** The central one-third of the aponeurosis is incised proximally between the medial and lateral heads of the gastrocnemius muscle bellies. **E.** An inverted central tongue is created by medial and lateral one-third aponeurosis incisions at the distal aspect of the incision.

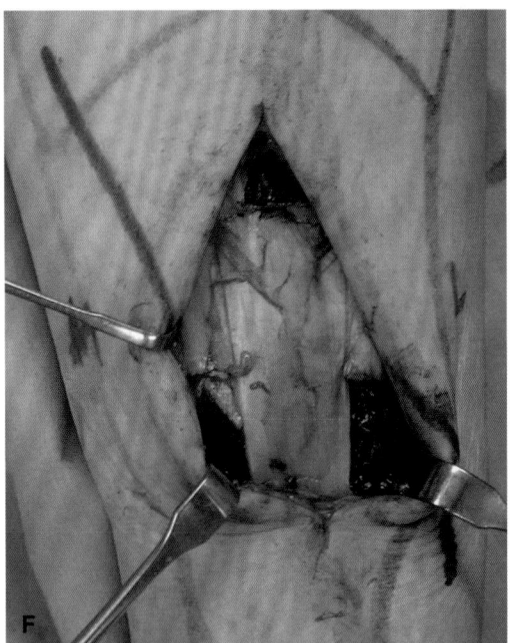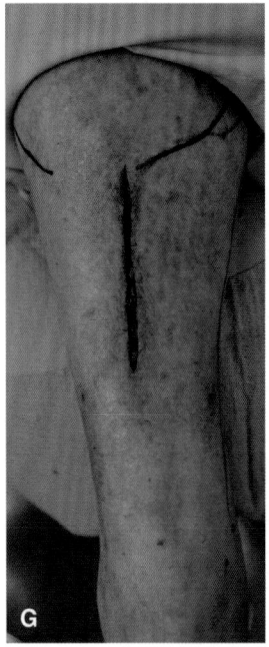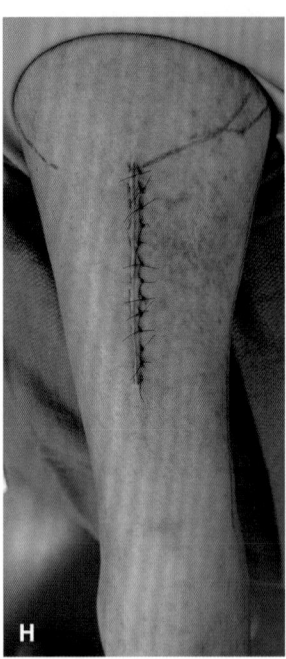

FIGURE 62.3 (*Continued*) **F.** Ankle is then dorsiflexed, and slide lengthening is performed. The amount of lengthening is easily visualized with open procedure. The authors commonly place 3 sutures along each side of the lengthened tendon in an effort to maintain this stretched position. Layered closure is performed. **G.** Paratenon is closed to limit adhesions followed by closure of the deep crural fascia which is reapproximated with absorbable suture. Care must be taken to avoid injury or compression on the sural nerve during closure. **H.** Skin closed with nonabsorbable interrupted suture or a running suture for improved cosmetic appearance.

TABLE 62.1 Gastrocnemius Recession Procedure Selection Considerations				
Criteria	Intramuscular Gastroc Recession (Baumann)	Endoscopic Gastroc Recession	Distal Gastroc (Strayer)	Open Tongue & Groove (Baker)
Position	Supine	Supine	Supine	Prone
Incision/scar	High on medial calf, less visible scar	Minimally invasive, smallest scar	Medial with risk of skin puckering	Midline on posterior calf, most visible scar
Zone	True, isolated gastroc	Gastroc or Gastro-soleal	Gastroc or Gastro-soleal	Gastro-soleal
Weight bearing status	WB helps maintain stretch	WB with below knee fracture boot	WB with below knee fracture boot	WB with below knee fracture boot
PROS	1. Hidden scar 2. Conservative lengthening 3. Preserves muscle mass	1. Small incision 2. Good visualization for complete release	1. Quick procedure 2. Supine when performing adjunctive procedures	1. Suture at desired length to avoid retraction or overlengthening 2. Best visualization
CONS	1. Wide tendon 2. Muscle bleeding 3. Least aggressive 4. Need proper incision placement	1. Time to setup 2. Added cost 3. Special training 4. Nerve risk 5. Equipment dependent	1. Visibility on lateral side challenging 2. Need to maintain stretch if NWB	1. Added time and hassle of prone position 2. Visible scar 3. Sural nerve risk
Typical patient selection	Positive Silfverskiold in younger, athletic patients	Patients who desire cosmetic scar	Patients undergoing multiple supine procedures (Flatfoot reconstruction)	Isolated equinus procedure or multiple prone procedures

Multiple factors should be considered when selecting the ideal approach to gastrocnemius equinus correction including the underlying condition being treated, individual patient circumstances, and influence of adjunctive procedures.

POSTOPERATIVE CARE

Postoperatively it is important to maintain the ankle in a dorsiflexed position following gastrocnemius recession. This can be achieved utilizing a variety of methods. The authors typically apply either a below the knee fracture boot or a short leg posterior splint postoperatively depending on the adjunctive proceidures performed. Patients are educated to keep the boot/splint on at all times to maintain length of the gastrocnemius. A night splint can be used while sleeping once the sutures are removed, provided adjunctive procedures allow removal of the boot or posterior splint. The night splint is less bulky than the below knee fracture boot and also prevents the relaxed plantarflexion position of the foot/ankle while sleeping. Some surgeons recommend that patients wear a night splint or other brace for at least 3 months status post gastrocnemius recession.

Immediate weight bearing in a below the knee fracture boot is generally tolerated and frequently desired following gastrocnemius recession unless adjunctive procedures were performed that necessitate nonweight bearing. Postoperative weight bearing can help maintain stretch of the gastrocnemius and aid in prevention of venous thromboembolism.

REHABILITATION

Physical therapy is not routinely prescribed status post gastrocnemius recession. If patients are having trouble or are delayed in returning to their preoperative activity level, physical therapy is ordered.

REFERENCES

1. Barouk P, Barouk L. Clinical diagnosis of gastrocnemius tightness. *Foot Ankle Clin.* 2014;19(9):659-667.
2. DiGiovanni CW, Kuo R, Tejwani N, et al. Isolated gastrocnemius tightness. *J Bone Joint Surg Am.* 2002;84A(6):962-970.
3. Deheer PA. Equinus and lengthening techniques. *Clin Podiatr Med Surg.* 2017;34(2):207-227.
4. Chen L, Greisberg J. Achilles lengthening procedures. *Foot Ankle Clin.* 2009;14: 627-637.
5. Downey MS, Schwartz JM. Ankle equinus. In: Southerland JT, ed. *McGlamry's Comprehensive Textbook of Foot and Ankle Surgery.* 4th ed. Philadelphia, PA: Lippincott Williams & Wilkins; 2013:541-583.
6. Cohen JC. Anatomy and biomechanical aspects of the gastrocsoleus complex. *Foot Ankle Clin.* 2009;14:617-626.
7. Dayton P. Anatomic, vascular and mechanical overview of the achilles tendon. *Clin Podiatr Med Surg.* 2017;34(2):107-113.
8. Gatt A, De Giorgio S, Chockalingam N, Formosa C. A pilot investigation into the relationship between static diagnosis of ankle equinus and dynamic ankle and foot dorsiflexion during stance phase of gait: time to revisit theory? *Foot (Edinb).* 2017;30:47-52.
9. Dayton P, Feilmeier M, Parker K, et al. Experimental comparison of the clinical measurement of ankle joint dorsiflexion and radiographic tibiotalar position. *J Foot Ankle Surg.* 2017;56:1036-1040.
10. Radford JA, Burns J, Buchbinder R, Landorf KB, Cook C. Does stretching increase ankle dorsiflexion range of motion? A systematic review. *Br J Sports Med.* 2006;40: 870-875.
11. Baumann JU, Koch HG. Ventrale aponeurotische verlangerung des musculus gastrocnemius. *Oper Orthop Traumatol.* 1989;1:254-258.
12. Rong K, Ge W, Li X, Xu X. Mid-term results of intramuscular lengthening of gastrocnemius and/or soleus to correct equinus deformity in flatfoot. *Foot Ankle Int.* 2015;36(10):1223-1228.
13. Pinney SJ, Sangeorzan BJ, Hansen ST. Surgical anatomy of the gastrocnemius recession (strayer procedure). *Foot Ankle Int.* 2004;25(4):247-250.
14. Harris RC III, Strannigan KL, Piraino J. Comparison of the complication incidence in open versus endoscopic gastrocnemius recession: a retrospective medical record review. *J Foot Ankle Surg.* 2018;57:747-752.
15. Schweinberger MH, Roukis TS. Surgical correction of soft-tissue ankle equinus contracture. *Clin Podiatr Med Surg.* 2008;25:571-585.
16. Cychosz CC, Phisitkul P, Belatti DA, Glazebrook MA, DiGiovanni CW. Gastrocnemius recession for foot and ankle conditions in adults: Evidence-based recommendations. *Foot Ankle Surg.* 2015;21(2):77-85.

Special Surgery

3D Printing

Selene G. Parekh

MIDSHAFT DEROTATIONAL METATARSAL OSTEOTOMY WITH CUSTOM 3D PRINTED PLATE FOR CORONAL CORRECTION OF HALLUX VALGUS

DEFINITION

- Hallux valgus is a common deformity affecting 23% of people ages 18-65 and 36% of people over the age of 65.[1,2] The deformity involves subluxation of the first metatarsophalangeal joint with subsequent lateral deviation of the hallux and medial deviation of the first metatarsal.[3] It is speculated that modern footwear is the primary culprit for the deformity, most notably a narrow toebox and heel height.[3-14] Various correction modalities have been proposed, with simple bunionectomy and joint hemiresection falling out of favor in the last two decades.[15] Additionally, rates of dissatisfaction have been found in up to 10.6%, rates of recurrent deformity in up to 4.9%, and hardware removal in up to 16% in the early term.[15] Longer-term studies have reported rates of recurrent deformity in up to 50% of patients.[16-19] Specific risk factors have been attributed to this unsatisfactory rate including intermetatarsal angle, hallux valgus angle, metatarsus adductus, age, and hyperlaxity.[20-23] An often missed risk factor is metatarsal pronation.[24] This pronation deformity has been found in up to 87% of hallux valgus patients.[25] A tarsometatarsal joint–sparing rotational osteotomy has been used to correct this rotational deformity, though the intraoperative correction is restricted to fluoroscopic guidance.[26] The incorporation of a custom 3D printed plate allows for the integration of more exact surgery. A more exact rotational correction can be performed, and 3D radiographic reconstructions more precisely plan the most appropriate anatomical location for the sesamoids.

CLASSIFICATION

Radiographic Hallux Valgus Severity
- Mild   Hallux valgus angle <30 degrees
                           Intermetatarsal angle <13 degrees
- Moderate   Hallux valgus angle 30-40 degrees
                           Intermetatarsal angle 13-20 degrees
- Severe   Hallux valgus angle 40 degrees+
                           Intermetatarsal angle 20 degrees+

INDICATIONS

CT scans must be obtained to evaluate pronation deformity, sesamoid dislocation, and approximate rotation >15 degrees. Sesamoid dislocation is defined as the alignment of the sesamoids with the intersesamoidal ridge. Dislocation occurs as the sesamoids cross under the ridge. Rotational deformity can be approximated by a Cobb angle with one ray perpendicular to the ground and the second ray coming down to the vertex through the Z-axis of the first metatarsal head (coronal view). The Z-axis may be approximated by drawing a superior line along the X-axis that bisects the medial and lateral corners of the upper first metatarsal head. A second line is then drawn inferiorly that bisects the medial and lateral lower corners (sulci). Connecting the midpoints of these two lines yields the Z-axis of the first metatarsal. Severe hallux valgus approaching the upper limits of deformity may be poor candidates for this procedure.

ANATOMIC FEATURES

The significant muscular attachments are located around the first metatarsophalangeal joint. The extensor hallucis brevis inserts superiorly onto the proximal phalanx. The extensor hallucis longus inserts superiorly onto the distal phalanx. With respect to the fibular sesamoid, the adductor hallucis inserts laterally (also inserts into the base of the proximal phalanx), and the lateral head of the flexor hallucis brevis muscle inserts inferiorly. Similarly, the tibial sesamoid has an inferior insertion to the medial head of the flexor hallucis brevis muscle and a medial insertion by the abductor hallucis muscle. The abductor hallucis muscle also inserts into the lateral aspect of the proximal phalanx. The ligamentous structures of the sesamoids are also important as the sesamoids connect to the proximal phalanx distally through phalangeal-sesamoid ligaments and superiorly through the metatarsal-sesamoid ligaments (two sets of each medially and laterally). Significant nervous structures are the medial branch of the superficial peroneal nerve, located along the mid to distal first metatarsal shaft, and the saphenous nerve is located proximally. The dorsalis pedis is located at the most proximal junction between the first and second metatarsals, before it bifurcates into deep and superficial branches. The superficial branch continues distally between the two metatarsals.

FUNCTIONAL ANALYSIS OF THE ANATOMY

Hallux valgus is characterized by a valgus deviation of the phalanx and a varus deviation of the first metatarsal. As the metatarsal head deviates, the sesamoids remain with the insertion points of the flexor hallucis brevis insertion points and are connected to the valgus deviating phalanx by the sesamoid-phalangeal ligament. As the deformity increases, the adductor hallucis becomes the major force of deformity, as well as the extensor hallucis longus.

PHYSICAL EXAMINATION

The extent of deformity can often be visualized by the presence of a medial eminence, as well as any resting deformity present at the first MTPJ. Pronation should be recognized in particular. Care should be taken in examining the range of motion of the first MTPJ. Additionally, mobility of the first tarsometatarsal joint must also be determined and any discomfort noted. Inferiorly, the sesamoids should be palpated for discomfort and signs of dislocation recognized (this can be examined upon dorsiflexion and plantar flexion of the first MTP). Callous formation must also be recognized, as well as concomitant deformity about the lesser toes.

PATHOGENESIS

The pathogenesis of hallux valgus was previously described, with adductor hallucis becoming a major driver of deformity. Of significance is also the driving force of pronation. As the hallux valgus deformity increases, the major contributors to pronation become more clear. As the sesamoids dislocate into the first intermetatarsal space, they maintain their ligamentous attachment to the proximal phalanx. However, in the coronal plane, the lateral and medial ligaments that attach to the first metatarsal will cause pronation to occur.[27] Another driving force is the extensor hallucis longus, with its distal insertion at the distal phalanx. As the hallux valgus deformity increases, the EHL will begin to cause pronation and plantar flexion at the proximal phalanx. This may further exacerbate the coronal deformity at the first metatarsal head and cause asymmetric wear of the first MTPJ's articular surface.

IMAGING AND DIAGNOSTIC STUDIES

Radiographs are sufficient for the diagnosis of hallux valgus, and in the settings of pronation, a CT scan is helpful. Additionally, a CT scan is required for construction of the custom implant.

TREATMENT

The patient is positioned prone, followed by prep and draping in the normal fashion. Once anesthesia is induced, a tourniquet may be applied. An incision is made at the medial aspect of the first metatarsal. The incision should follow the approximate axis of the first ray. The abductor hallucis muscle must be retracted plantar-medially to adequately visualize the first metatarsal

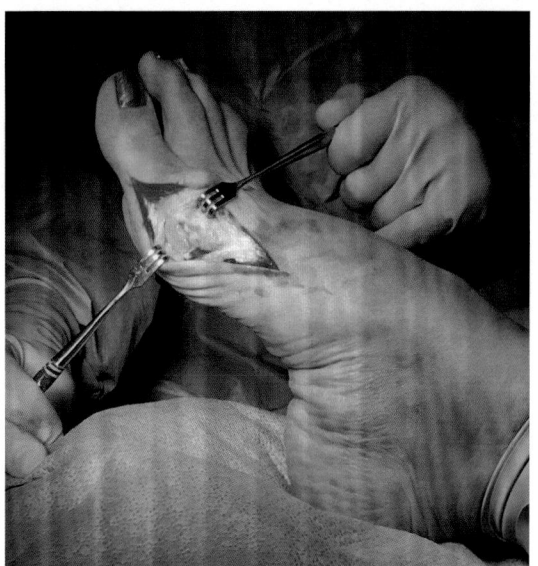

FIGURE 63.1 Hallux valgus exposure. A medial incision is made along the axis of the first metatarsal, and the extensor hallucis longus is retracted plantar-medially.

(Fig. 63.1). A custom drill guide is then placed along the midshaft of the first metatarsal (Fig. 63.2). The custom guide will fit onto the metatarsal in a specific location as its ventral surface mirrors the topography around the osteotomy site. Two Kirschner wires (K-wires) are placed into the proximal component of the guide, followed by the placement of two K-wires into the distal component. A 1.1-mm drill bit is then used to make the oblique osteotomy within the guide holes of the custom guide. There are typically eight sites used to make the osteotomy (Fig. 63.2). Once the osteotomy has been completed, the drill guide may be removed, while the anchoring K-wires stay in place. The proximal portion must then be removed in

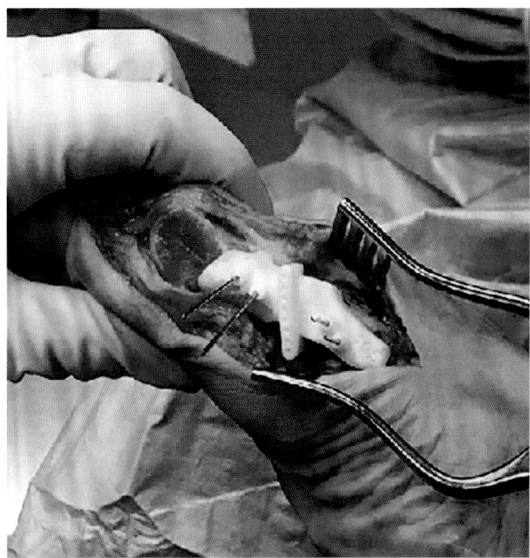

FIGURE 63.2 Custom midshaft derotational osteotomy guide. The contours of the custom guide will fit onto a preplanned location on the first metatarsal. Subsequent placement of proximal and distal Kirschner wires anchors the guide and allows for the osteotomy to be performed along the guide's midpoint.

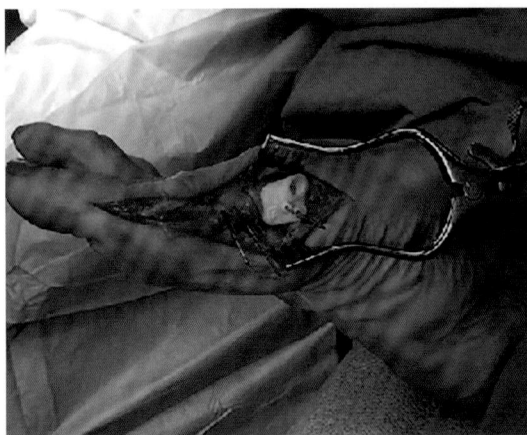

FIGURE 63.3 Second guide plate. A proximal guide is now placed onto the first metatarsal and a transfixiant bump made using a 6-mm drill bit; the perforation must only be 2 mm.

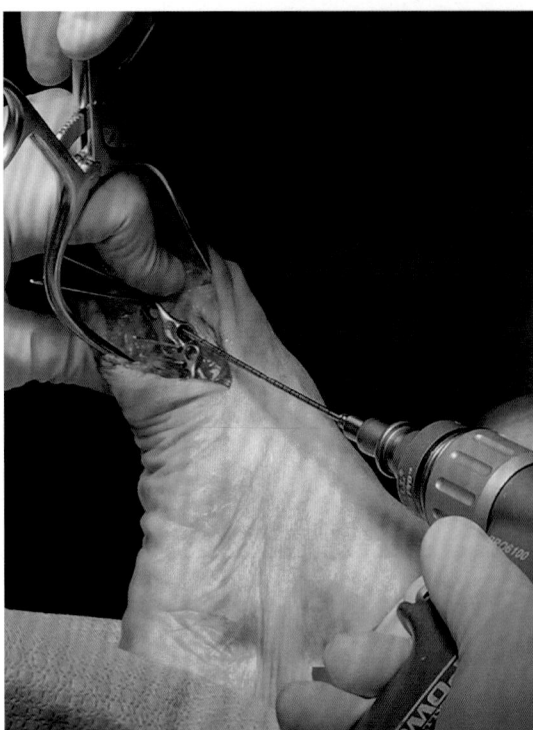

FIGURE 63.4 Custom plate placement and transfixiant screw. The custom plate may now be placed onto the first metatarsal and the distal segment rotated to allow for the distal Kirschner wires to fit into the plate. The entrypoint for the transfixiant screw may now be prepared with a fluoroscopically guided guidewire and subsequent reaming.

the same fashion. A second smaller drill bit guide is then placed on the proximal K-wires. A transfixiant screw hole is then created with the guide; a 6-mm drill bit is used and advanced 2 mm (Fig. 63.3). The smaller drill bit guide may now be removed and a final cut guide placed onto the proximal K-wires. A custom cut guide is then used to remove the medial eminence. The cut guide is then removed, and the custom plate is placed (Fig. 63.4). The distal metatarsal segment must be rotated until the anchoring K-wires line up with the plate. Once adequately placed, the proximal screw holes of the plate are drilled and the three nonlocking screws are placed. Subsequently, the distal screw holes are then reamed and three additional nonlocking screws are placed (Fig. 63.5). The transfixiant screw hole may now be reamed and a final screw placed. Positioning of the plate is fluoroscopically inspected in three planes. Once adequate placement has been confirmed, the surgical tourniquet is then deflated and the incision site is closed.

PEARLS

The cutting guide for the medial eminence is an optional guide for this procedure. It is helpful in the management of moderate to severe hallux valgus in the presence of pronation deformity.

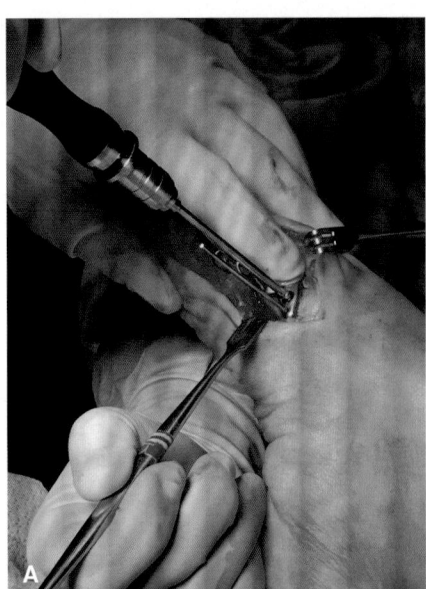
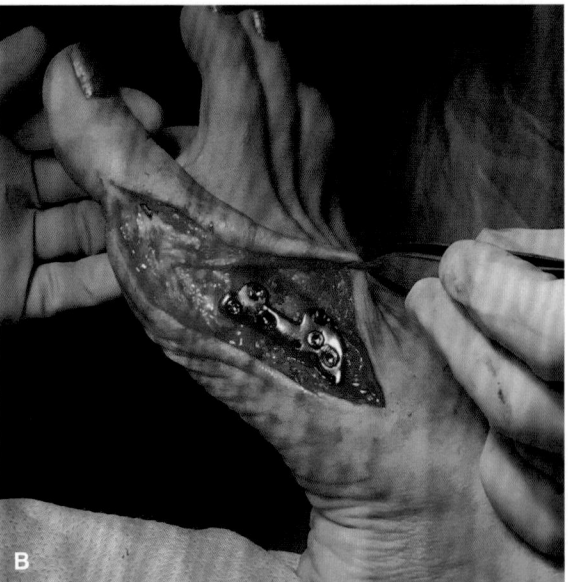

FIGURE 63.5 Final plate fixation. **A.** The proximal and distal screw holes within the plate are reamed and the screws placed one by one, with the transfixiant screw being the last to be placed. **B.** The fixation construct should fit as preoperatively planned; final fluoroscopic inspection will precede closure.

AUTHORS' PREFERRED TREATMENT

The custom plate used for pronation deformity in hallux valgus is a reliable bunion correcting construct when the first TMT joint is nonarthritic in moderate to severe hallux valgus. The preoperative planning helps to better align dislocated sesamoids into a more anatomic position. The custom medial eminence cutting guide is most often used in these settings.

PERILS and PITFALLS

- The midshaft derotational osteotomy may be inadequate in treating severe hallux valgus.
- Initial placement of the drill bit guide must be correlated with preoperative planning images regardless of fit.
- Transfer metatarsalgia, as well as any other concomitant deformities, must be addressed. Hallux valgus interphalangeus is common.

POSTOPERATIVE CARE

The patient is placed in a three-sided splint, and radiographs are performed the day after surgery. For the initial 2 weeks, the patient is to remain non–weight bearing. At the 2-week mark, the incision may be inspected and the sutures removed if adequate healing has taken place. If the healing is satisfactory, the patient may then be placed into a circumferential cast for an additional 8 weeks. At the end of this term, additional radiographs are ordered. If there is sufficient evidence of early union of the osteotomy site, the patient may be placed in a CAM boot. Crutches will be initially used, before transition into partial and then full weight bearing. Four to six weeks afterward, the patient may begin transitioning out of the walking boot in the absence of residual symptoms.

REHABILITATION

Rehabilitation must not take place until the osteotomy site has healed. Once the patient transitions into the walking boot, early mobility work may begin for the first MTP joint, with more strenuous movements occurring until transition out of the walking boot. Once out of the walking boot, early weight-bearing exercise may begin in a transitional period, leading into low-impact exercise.

3D PRINTED TOTAL NAVICULAR REPLACEMENT

DEFINITION

Avascular necrosis of the navicular is a less common injury, with a number of presentations.[28-31] It has a central watershed area predisposing it to AVN and can occur in the settings of trauma, sickle cell disease, corticosteroid use, excessive alcohol use, and Gaucher disease.[28,29] Some of the more unique occurrences happen due to the navicular being one of the last bones to ossify, and it may remain suboptimally ossified into adulthood. Because of this, the navicular is prone to compression between the tarsal bones, restricting the periosteal blood supply and driving osteonecrosis in the central watershed area.[28-31] In the adolescent, the osteochondroses counterpart has been termed Koehler disease.[32] The suboptimal ossification-related injury occurring in the adult, particularly females, is called Mueller-Weiss disease.[31] Mueller-Weiss staging is appropriate in determining navicular AVN progression in traumatic settings. Core decompression and vascular bone grafts are less effective in the later stages of the disease, necessitating salvage arthrodesis. When enough viable navicular remains talonavicular arthrodesis, talonavicular-cuneiform, double, and triple arthrodesis may be used depending on the surrounding joint pathology.[33,34] In stage 5 of the disease, a bone block arthrodesis must be undertaken. These are associated with unsatisfactory clinical outcomes and low rates of arthrodesis.[33] Using a 3D printed custom construct, optimal anatomic surface area is generated along with submicron structure to drive bone ingrowth. The custom contouring with built in plates allows for an anatomic fit and appropriate medial column length. These factors help maximize outcomes in midfoot salvage and are useful in concomitant deformity.

CLASSIFICATION

Mueller-Weiss Radiographic Classification
- Stage 1   Subtle talar varus deformity
- Stage 2   Dorsolateral displacement of the talus and associated cavovarus and dorsal angulation of the Meary-Tomeno line
- Stage 3   Compression or splitting of the navicular, resulting in a lowered longitudinal arch and neutral Meary-Tomeno line
- Stage 4   Navicular compression leading to hindfoot equinus, loss of longitudinal arch, and plantar angulation of the Meary-Tomeno line
- Stage 5   Talocuneiform neoarticulation and navicular remnant extrusion

---

INDICATIONS

- At stage 5, 3D printed navicular replacement is an option for medial column lengthening and midfoot arthrodesis.
- The custom implant may be considered in stage 3 or 4 of the disease if the bone is nonsalvageable or if there are concerns for a successful arthrodesis.

ANATOMIC FEATURES

The navicular articulates with the talus, all three cuneiforms, and the calcaneus. It also serves as the attachment point for the tibialis posterior as well as the spring ligament. The dorsal blood supply originates from the dorsalis pedis, and the plantar supply from the medial branch of the posterior tibial artery.[35]

FUNCTIONAL ANALYSIS OF THE ANATOMY

The central body of the navicular is predisposed to avascular necrosis because of its watershed area.[35,36] Due to its anatomic location and attachment points for the posterior tibial tendon and spring ligament, progressive necrosis drives deformity.

The Meary-Tomeno line is a radiographic demarcation made between the axis of the first metatarsal and the axis of the talus. In early stages of the disease, it deviates dorsally before deviating plantarly as deformity progresses. Early navicular changes result in talar varus and eventual cavovarus; as the navicular further degrades, the midfoot collapses, along with the longitudinal arch.[33]

PHYSICAL EXAMINATION

The initial examination should focus on an adequate range of motion present about the talus. Any varus misalignment of the talus will reduce the arc range of motion of the subtalar joint, and potentially inhibit eversion. Progressive deformity will demonstrate cavus, before equinus and pes planus deformities. End-stage pathology will have midfoot collapse and residual dorsal fragments of the navicular. Dorsiflexion changes can also be noted in the midfoot due to the new pseudoarticulation.

PATHOGENESIS

Obstruction of the navicular blood supply drives osteonecrotic changes in the central body of the navicular.[35,36] Obstruction may occur due to fracture, although typically, this occurs only in the subtypes of displaced body and stress fractures.[37] The Mueller-Weiss variant, often occurring in adult females, is due to suboptimal ossification of the navicular. Compressive changes due to surrounding articular forces drive vascular obstruction and spontaneous avascular necrosis.[31]

IMAGING AND DIAGNOSTIC STUDIES

Initial staging of navicular avascular necrosis may be done with radiographs, with MRI being useful in suspected cases. Due to accumulating deformity about the navicular, radiographs are adequate in later stages of the disease. A bilateral CT scan is required for optimal planning of the custom navicular implant.

TREATMENT

The patient is positioned prone, followed by prep and draping in the normal fashion. Once anesthesia is induced, a tourniquet may be applied. Two incisions will be used; one dorsal and one slightly medial. The medial incision is made between the tibialis anterior and posterior. The incision should allow for adequate exposure of the talonavicular as well as navicular-cuneiform joints. The tibialis anterior may be retracted medially and dorsally and must be protected for the remainder of the procedure. The dorsal incision must expose both the talonavicular as well as the navicular-cuneiform joints. A skin bridge ~2 cm wide will separate the two incisions.[33] The necrotic navicular must now be thoroughly removed from the joint cavity utilizing both exposure sites. Additionally, the anterior talonavicular and dorsal cuneonavicular ligaments may need to be released, as well as the spring ligament and posterior tibial tendon attachment. The adjacent joint needs to then be prepared for pseudoarthrodesis. The talar head and neighboring cuneiforms must be debrided symmetrically down to cancellous bone.

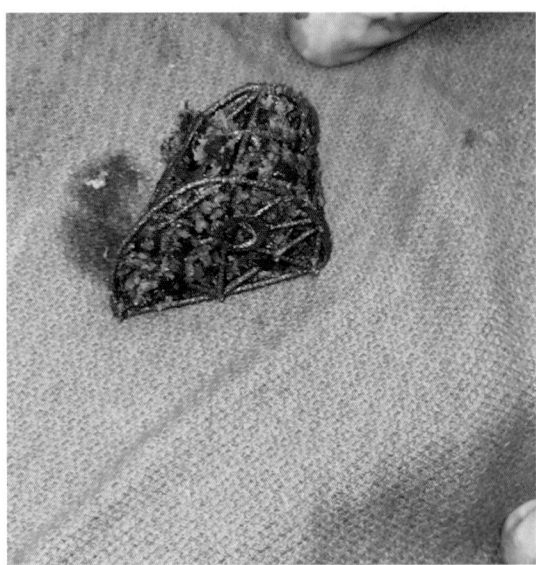

FIGURE 63.6 Bone graft placement within custom construct. The custom implant is impregnated with allograft or autograft, along with additional adjuvant at the surgeon's discretion.

The tourniquet is then deflated to ensure that bleeding cancellous bone has been exposed.[33] Next bone grafting needs to be prepared. Both autograft and allograft constructs may be used. The implant must be impregnated and the neighboring joint surfaces well covered (Fig. 63.6). The implant is then introduced into the joint space, and any asymmetrical defects in the surrounding joints must be corrected (Fig. 63.7). The implant

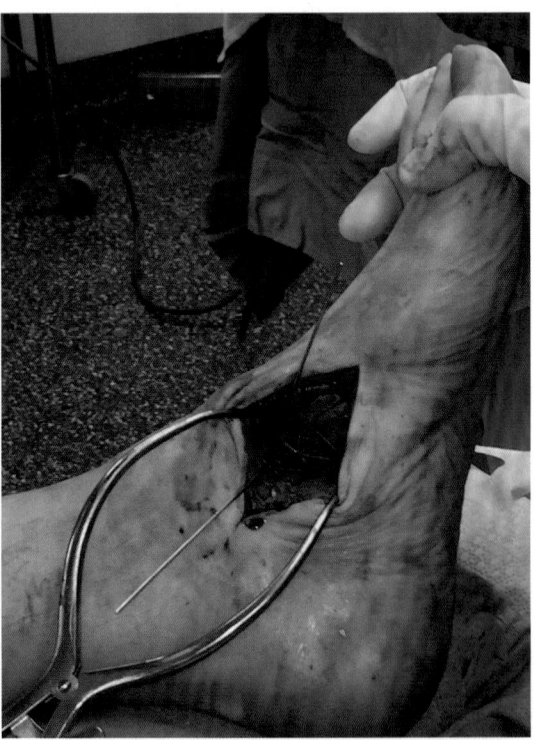

FIGURE 63.7 Placement of the custom construct. Once the surrounding joints have been prepared, the bone graft impregnated custom construct may then be placed along with fluoroscopically guided guidewires.

will have built in pores for talar and cuneiform fixation. Fluoroscopy must be used to appropriately place guidewires. The placement of fixation may vary from implant to implant depending on customization (Fig. 63.7). Following adequate guidewire placement, reaming and screw placement will follow. Depending on the construct, compression screws may also be used. The stage of deformity will dictate whether subtalar as well as the navicular-cuneiform joints need arthrodesis. These should be fluoroscopically identified as well as the articulations about the medial column construct. After additional joint inspection or arthrodesis, both exposure sites may be closed following thorough irrigation.

PEARLS

- Deformity stages between 2 and 4 will have varying amounts of viable bone, with defects often present laterally. The adequacy of this construct may be helpful as the viability is reduced, more comorbidities are present, and in the presence of severe deformity.
- In stages 4 and 5, relative stability is the goal, and the subtalar and cuneonavicular joints may require arthrodesis.

AUTHORS' PREFERRED TREATMENT

Patients undergoing revisions of midfoot arthrodesis for nonunions and infected nonunions are prime candidates for this procedure due to the high rate of bone ingrowth for custom constructs. Late-stage avascular cases demonstrate satisfactory results when performing this procedure, and in the presence of comorbidities, this procedure may be a consideration. All stage 5 Mueller-Weiss cases are recommended for this procedure as the fusion rate is unsatisfactory for traditional bone block arthrodesis.

PERILS and PITFALLS

- The custom 3D printed navicular replacement is a powerful tool in managing segmental defects of the medial column. However, in advanced deformity, the subtalar and cuneonavicular joints may also require arthrodesis.
- Long-term posterior tendon and spring ligament insufficiency will drive additional forces through the medial column fusion construct. Dissipation of these forces through the cuneiform-metatarsal joints and spared hindfoot joints may predispose to arthritis in the long term.

POSTOPERATIVE CARE

The patient is kept exclusively non–weight bearing for 8 weeks. In the early postoperative period, a three-sided splint is used, with subsequent radiography occurring the day after surgery. At 2 weeks, the splint is removed and the exposure sites carefully examined. If adequate healing has taken place, the sutures may be removed and a circumferential cast may be placed. At 8 weeks, additional radiographs should be taken to evaluate for a solid pseudofusion. The midfoot should additionally be stiff and cool to the touch. If a stable construct is present, the patient may be transitioned into CAM walking boot. CT scans are advised to definitively confirm bone ingrowth. Four to six weeks after CAM boot transition, the patient may be weaned out of the boot into full weight bearing. The use of orthotics is suggested.

REHABILITATION

Rehabilitation must be avoided until a solid fusion construct is in place. If present at 8 weeks, minimal low-impact therapy may begin. Significant increases in rehabilitative volume should not occur until the patient has begun to transition out of the CAM boot.

3D PRINTED TOTAL TALUS REPLACEMENT

DEFINITION

Avascular necrosis of the talus is a debilitating disease when large segments are involved, often warranting bone block tibiotalocalcaneal arthrodesis. Successful arthrodesis is typically achieved in only 66% of these patients.[38-42] Total talus replacement has demonstrated viability as a joint-sparing alternative to arthrodesis.[43-48] The first generation of the implant incorporated a synthetic talar body with a notch fitting into the talar head. In a 1997 study, follow-up ranged from 10 to 36 years, and patients demonstrated satisfactory outcomes.[43] In another study published in 2015, a third-generation implant replacing the entire talus with a synthetic alumina ceramic talus demonstrated satisfactory outcomes at an average of 4.4 years postoperatively.[48] There have been two recent publications demonstrating the use of 3D printed total talar replacements and their benefit with respect to early clinical outcomes and restoration of talar height.[49,50] This operative modality is helpful in ensuring a more optimal "fit" and addressing concomitant deformity (cavus or pes planus).[49] Further, a number of case series have been reported combining total talus replacement with the tibial component of ankle arthroplasty, and a two component total talus has also been developed that allows for screws to be placed into the calcaneus resulting in a pseudoarthrodesis.[51]

INDICATIONS

- Advanced stage avascular necrosis of the talus, and talus extrusion injuries; in the setting of nonarthritic tibiotalar, subtalar, and talonavicular joints.
- There are a number of case series adapting the total talus to ankle arthroplasty revisions, as well as a two component system for pseudoarthrodesis of the subtalar joint. Further studies are needed.

ANATOMIC FEATURES

A knowledge of ankle arthroplasty is helpful in the approach to total talus implantation as the exposure is similar with the interval between the extensor hallucis longus and extensor digitorum longus muscles. A strong understanding of the talar

ligaments is paramount in releasing the diseased talus. Just inferior to the lateral gutter lies the anterior talofibular ligament, and inferior to the medial gutter lies the superficial deltoid ligament. Inferior to the talus lies the plantar interosseous talocalcaneal ligament, and plantar-medially just behind the talar head is the cervical ligament. The cervical ligament can be troublesome to release. At the anterior aspect of the talus resides the anterior talonavicular ligament. Posteriorly, there are four ligaments of importance; the two superior ligaments are the posterior talofibular ligament and the posterior tibiotalar segment of the deltoid. Inferiorly, the two ligaments are the posterior talocalcaneal ligament and the median talocalcaneal ligament.

FUNCTIONAL ANALYSIS OF THE ANATOMY

Given the loss of the talar ligaments, there is a loss of stability; however, the remaining deltoid imparts significant stability medially as does the calcaneofibular complex laterally. Posteriorly, the tibiocalcaneal component of the deltoid as well as the posterior calcaneofibular ligaments remain intact. Additionally, the contractile tissue about the hindfoot and midfoot impart stability. The only concern is with anterior displacement between the synthetic talus and the navicular; the connective tissues of the superior midfoot impart enough stability that activities of daily living are well tolerated. However, more strenuous activities should only be performed in supportive footwear encapsulating the entire foot.

PHYSICAL EXAMINATION

Distal pulses must be examined followed by inspection for superficial inflammatory changes such as temperature or redness. Mobility about the ankle, subtalar, and talonavicular joints must now be examined. Appropriate articulations may be examined through ankle flexion, extension, inversion, and eversion; followed by locking the hindfoot and ankle with one hand and then stabilizing the midfoot at the plane just posterior to the metatarsal heads - minimal flexion and extension should be present. Stiffness, pain, and any crepitus should be noted. Any indications of lost height between the ankle and hindfoot should also be noted.

PATHOGENESIS

Due to the multiple articular surfaces of talus, there is a very limited blood supply, which is prone to injury and subsequent avascular necrosis.[54] The anterior talus is supplied by the anterior tibial artery, the talar body is supplied by the posterior tibial artery, and the perforating peroneal artery supplies the lateral aspect of the talus as well as the area of the talus inferior to the talar head. There is also an anastomosis known as the sinus tarsi artery between the anterior and posterior tibial arteries. In settings of fracture, the talus is often salvageable as long as some collateral blood supply remains in each of the segments; however, the incidences of avascular necrosis greatly increase with crush and extrusion injuries.[52-54]

IMAGING AND DIAGNOSTIC STUDIES

Radiographs are reliable in assessing avascular necrosis of the talus with observable changes in bone quality and collapse. When AVN is not obvious and suspected, MRI is helpful and more sensitive in detecting osteonecrotic changes. A subsequent CT must be ordered for planning and manufacturing of the synthetic total talus.

TREATMENT

The patient is positioned prone, draped in the normal fashion, and anesthesia is induced. A tourniquet may be applied and is encouraged. An incision is made between the extensor hallucis longus (EHL) and extensor digitorum longus, ~4 cm proximal to the tibiotalar joint and extending 2 cm distal to the talonavicular joint. The EHL sheath is opened and the tendon retracted laterally. The superficial peroneal nerve must be protected, and the anterior neurovascular bundle also retracted laterally. Dissection should be carried down into the plane exposing the tibiotalar joint (Fig. 63.8). A dorsal closing wedge osteotomy is then performed at the level of the talar neck using an oscillating saw. The plantar interosseous ligaments must be severed, but care must be taken in not damaging the subtalar joint (Fig. 63.9). The wedge is then removed with a rongeur. The anterior talonavicular ligament may now be released. A Cobb elevator is then placed in the talonavicular joint and worked medial to lateral;

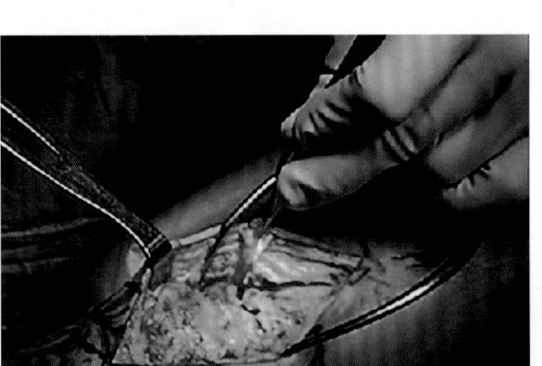

FIGURE 63.8 Incision and exposure. **A.** An incision is made between the extensor hallucis longus (EHL) and extensor digitorum longus. **B.** Dissection is carried down into the plane exposing the tibiotalar joint.

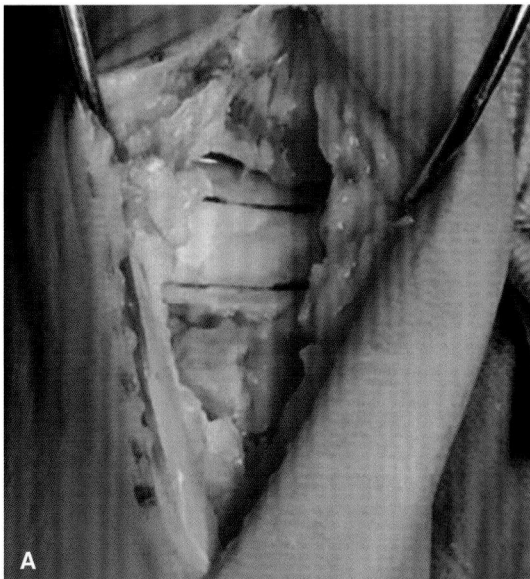
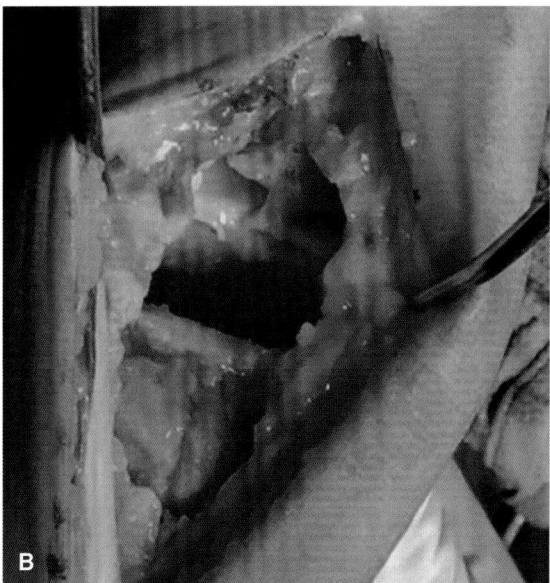

FIGURE 63.9 Dorsal wedge closing osteotomy. **A.** A dorsal closing wedge osteotomy is performed at the level of the talar neck using an oscillating saw. **B.** Removal of the wedge segment and visualization of the remaining posterior segment.

particular attention must be made medially where the cervical ligament must be removed. Prior to talar head removal, the medial superficial deltoid and lateral talofibular ligament must be transected. The talar head may now be removed. A twisting "alligator roll" may be applied in order to free the talar segment from its connective tissue. Articular surfaces must be protected during the removal of this segment (Fig. 63.10). Three parallel vertical osteotomies are now performed on the talar body and dome, again with care not to disturb the surrounding structures. There may be additional attachments from the plantar interosseous ligament that must be additionally freed from its attachment to the talus. The three segments of the talar body may now be explanted utilizing a rongeur. Plantar-medially the spring ligament is an important structure that must be protected. Additionally, the deltoid ligament must be preserved

as much as possible. It should be noted that the two superior ligaments, the posterior tibiotalar ligament (deltoid), and posterior talofibular ligament are attached, as well as the two inferior ligaments, the median talocalcaneal and posterior talocalcaneal ligaments (Fig. 63.11). Once removed, the talar cavity must be carefully inspected for bony fragments or connective tissue that may cause impingement. Two plastic trials are provided by the manufacturer, and both must be trialed into the cavity and approximate anatomic articulation demonstrated (Fig. 63.12). Preoperative assessment of the contralateral ankle and hindfoot range of motion may be helpful. Once the appropriate trial is selected, the cavity is thoroughly irrigated and the implant placed. The surgical window is then closed and a sterile dressing placed. In the acute postoperative period, the patient is placed in an immobilizing brace (Fig. 63.13).

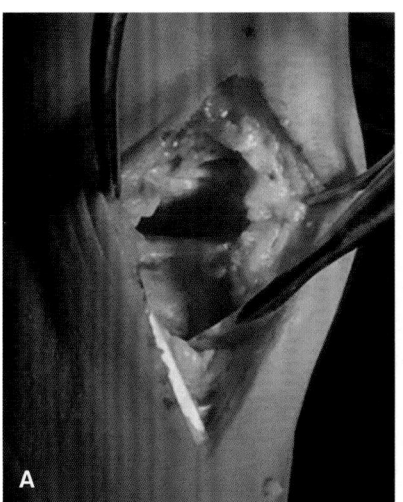
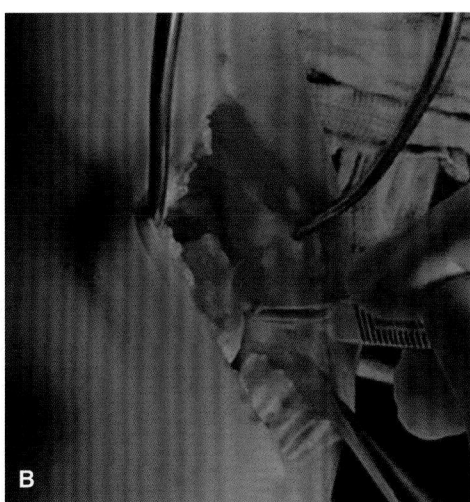
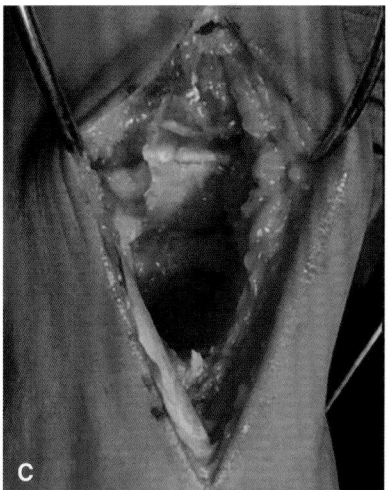

FIGURE 63.10 Anterior talar segment. **A.** Release of the anterior talonavicular ligament. **B.** Removal of ligamentous structures within the talonavicular joint, particular attention is made medially where the cervical ligament is located. **C.** Anterior void after talar segment explantation.

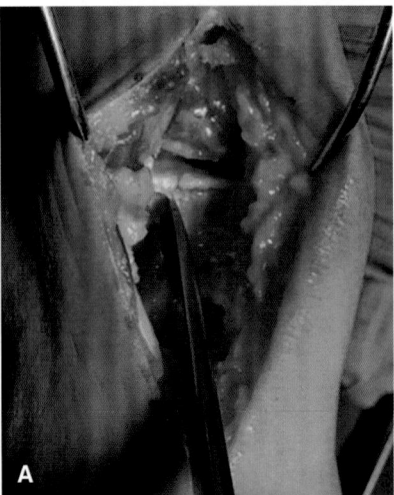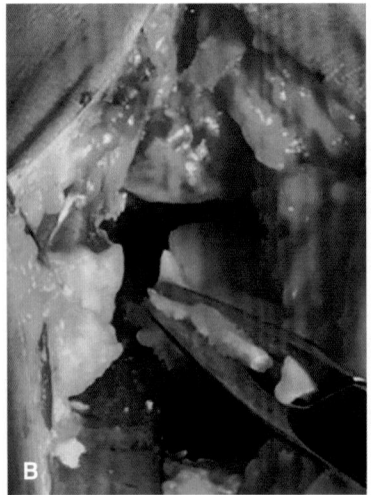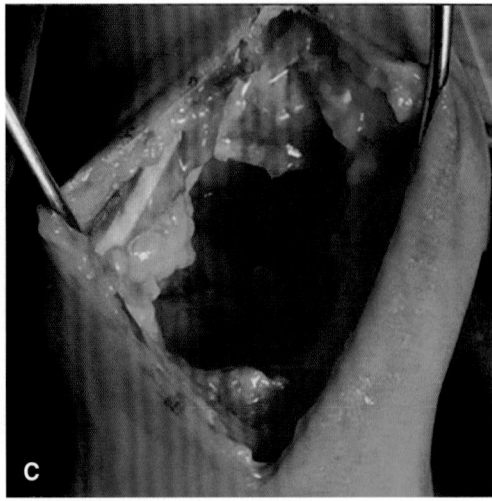

FIGURE 63.11 Posterior talar segment. **A.** Three parallel vertical osteotomies are performed on the talar body and dome. **B.** The three segments of the talar body being explanted; the rongeur can be used. **C.** Complete explantation of the talus and visualization of the remaining soft tissues.

PEARLS

- The dorsal closing wedge osteotomy should encompass the talar neck.
- Make sure to release the ligamentous structures distal to the medial and lateral gutters before removal of the talar body. Also remember that there may be residual attachment of the plantar interosseous ligament at each stage of talar segment explantation.

AUTHORS' PREFERRED TREATMENT

In large segments of avascular necrosis, core decompression and vascular bone defects are much less effective. Total talus replacement is a novel technique in salvage while preserving neighboring joint articulation. In scenarios of neighboring arthritis, additional interventions may be used in conjunction with the total talus implant. Combinations with the tibial component of ankle arthroplasty and/or with the two component

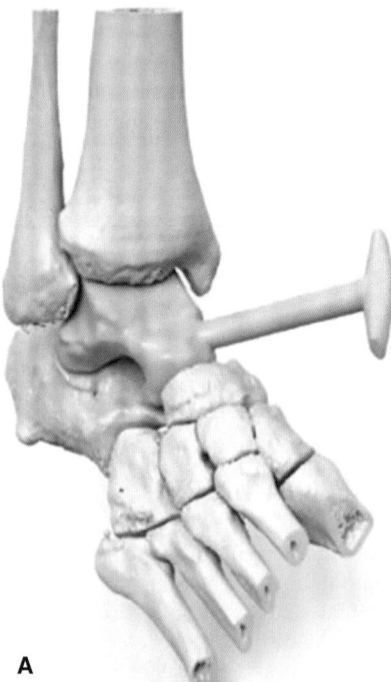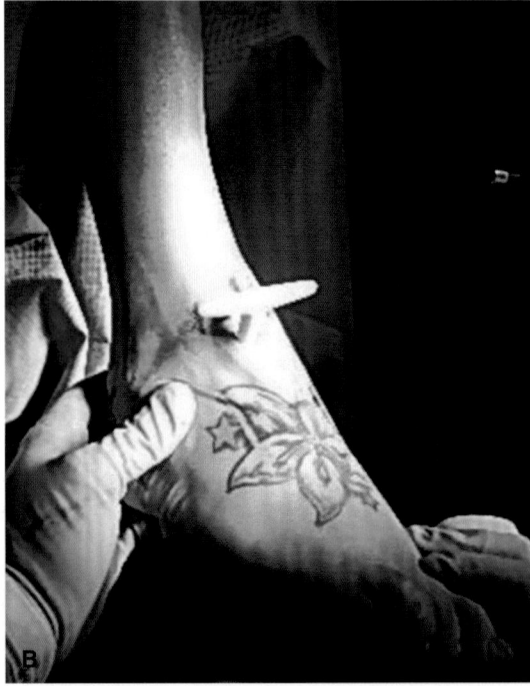

FIGURE 63.12 Trial implant. **A.** Preoperative digital rendering of the trial implant and predicted surrounding joint articulations. **B.** Implanted trial talus and articulation inspection. An audible "thump" will be heard when the appropriate trial has been placed.

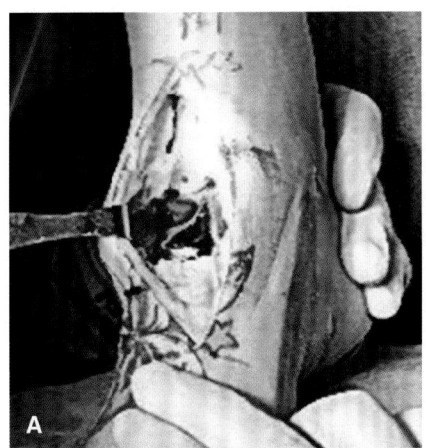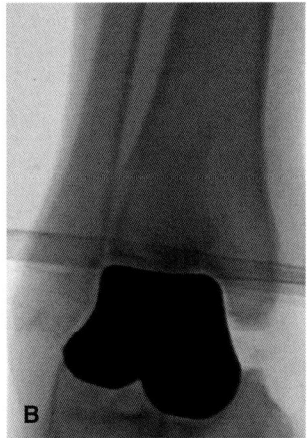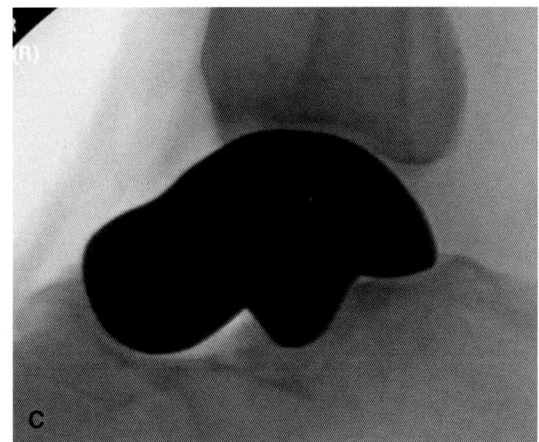

FIGURE 63.13 3D printed total talus implant. **A.** Implanted custom total talus replacement. **B.** A/P postoperative radiograph. **C.** Sagittal postoperative radiograph.

subtalar screw implant have demonstrated satisfactory clinical results in the acute postoperative period. Additional studies will be needed to investigate the longevity of these implants.

POSTOPERATIVE CARE

Patients should remain non–weight bearing for the initial 3 weeks. At this point, the sutures are removed if appropriate, radiographs obtained, and the patient transitioned into a CAM walking boot. Showering is allowed, but foot submersions should not occur for another 2 months. The patient may transition to weight bearing as tolerated, beginning with crutches. By 6 weeks, the patient should be weight bearing. Transition to non-CAM boot wear should begin with 2 hours of free wear, with subsequent increases of 2 hours each day.

REHABILITATION

Early range of motion exercises may begin once the patient has transitioned to the CAM walking boot; this should occur three times per day along with making the motions of the alphabet with their big toe. At 6 weeks, physical therapy may begin. High-impact exercise is restricted to minimize any sclerotic development between the bone-metal interfaces; low-impact exercise is encouraged.

3D PRINTED SALVAGE CONSTRUCTS FOR TIBIOTALOCALCANEAL PSEUDOARTHRODESIS: INCORPORATING THE DEATH STAR

DEFINITION

Segmental defects of the tibial shaft were previously discussed, except for those that extend into the hindfoot. These large

defects are most commonly caused by extensive trauma, non-unions, osteomyelitis, and neurofibromatosis, though smaller defects can arise from failed ankle arthroplasty.[55-58] These cases become substantially more difficult depending on the tibial void that is present. Bone transport techniques may be used along the entire void length, though there are many complications. The duration of the therapy is also extensive with each centimeter of osteogenesis taking a month, and the final arthrodesis taking 6 months, and remaining in external fixation for a year or more is not well tolerated.[59,60] Large bulk allografts are another option, though the rate of arthrodesis is unsatisfactory.[38] The incorporation of 3D printed custom constructs with structural enhancements has substantial promise in these cases. The osteogenic characteristics of the implants help drive the formation of a stable fusion construct, and the custom designs help restore as much anatomic alignment as is possible. In certain cases, the tibial shaft construct may be extended distally into the calcaneus, and in others, a rounded talar body construct, the "death star," may be used to better recapitulate a fusion mass resembling the body of the native talus.[59,60]

ANATOMIC FEATURES

As these cases are typical in the setting of salvage, the pertinent anatomy may be missing. These can extend superiorly up the tibial shaft or distally through the talus and calcaneus. Additionally, anterior defects extending into the midfoot and medial and lateral columns may be attempted. A knowledge of the native anatomy is important, specifically maintaining height, width, and rotation. The development of a well-aligned stable construct is paramount, and when done correctly, can be well tolerated when considering the patient's gait.

FUNCTIONAL ANALYSIS OF THE ANATOMY

As previously discussed in the segmental defects of the tibial shaft chapter, a cortically aligned tibial cage will better distribute load distally and mitigate potential stress shielding around the implant. Voids encompassing the talus have varying characteristics. The goals of distal salvage are to create a fusion construct that recapitulates the talar declination angle and distributes dynamic loads through the hindfoot and forefoot. With a pseudoarthrodesis encompassing the subtalar joint, native talar height and a Bohler angle between 20 and 40 degrees must be recapitulated to as close as anatomically possible. As these constructs most often have a tibial intramedullary nail incorporated into the construct, an interlocking nail going through the talar body component (or tibial segment extension) should form a relatively normal Meary's angle between the forefoot and the fusion construct. Though difficult, a pseudoarthrodesis that best mirrors normal anatomic alignment will better preserve surrounding joint articulations; however, accelerated articular wear is impossible to fully mitigate.

PHYSICAL EXAMINATION

Distal pulses and sensations should be clinically examined along with skin quality. Depending on the setting, additional clinical examinations may be needed. Any limb length discrepancies should be examined, as well as normal articulation within the knee and ankle. The range of motion about the talus should be done carefully and any crepitus present noted. Any lack of resistance in the articulations should also be taken into account. Due to talar collapse, pes planus may be present and should be examined for rigidity. Movement of the midfoot should also be examined, and any abnormal articulations or length discrepancies in the medial and lateral columns should be carefully noted.

PATHOGENESIS

These large segment defects can happen for a number of reasons including trauma, damaging the tibial segment and the talus. Another reason could be obstruction of the talar blood supply, leading to AVN. Failed ankle arthroplasty or osteomyelitis are yet more possible reasons. Understanding the nature of the deformity is more important in these cases, and specifically how much bone is salvageable.

IMAGING AND DIAGNOSTIC STUDIES

- Diagnostic radiographic imaging should be the initial imaging modality; however, CT studies must be undertaken to better understand the deformity present (Fig. 63.14). Additionally, MRI is helpful in understanding any soft tissue pathology that is present. A preoperative CT is mandatory for design of the custom implant.

TREATMENT

Since bone ingrowth of the distal segment is of concern, it is recommended that this procedure be carried out in two stages, allowing for the subsequent use of the Masquelet induced membrane technique[61,62] (Fig. 63.15).

The patient is placed in a supine position, followed by induction of general anesthesia along with standard prepping and draping. Debridement must be carried out in settings of trauma or osteomyelitis as previously outlined in the chapter on segmental defects of the tibial shaft. This must also be extended into the hindfoot and any other regions encompassed by the void. The ankle and subtalar joints should now be prepared for pseudoarthrodesis. Upon the final debridement, an intercalary bone segment is placed approximating the length of the contralateral limb. If using the induced membrane technique in a stable setting, a craniomedial exposure may be used, exposing the tibial defect for intercalary cement placement. A dorsal exposure may be used between the extensor digitorum longus and extensor hallucis longus for the placement of cement within the talar void. The talus must be explanted using the technique outlined in the total talus replacement chapter. The soft tissue may then be closed, and the induced membrane will be fully formed in 6-8 weeks.

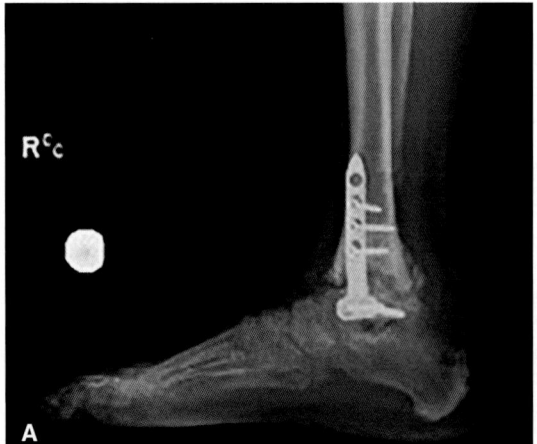
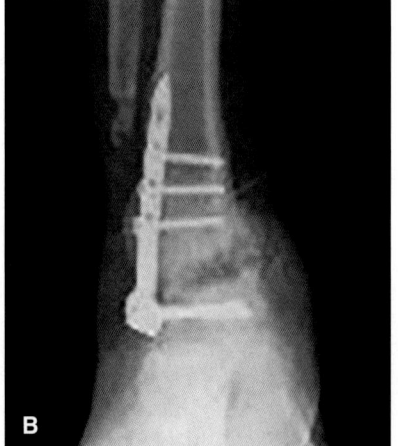
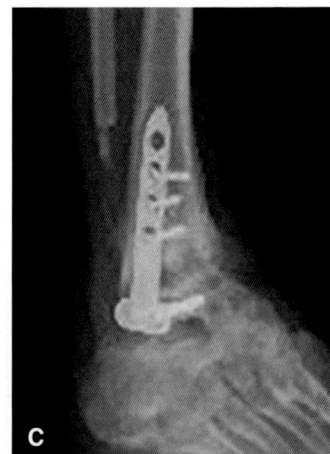

FIGURE 63.14 Preoperative assessment of talar salvage with failed ankle arthrodesis. **A–C.** Sagittal, A/P, and oblique radiographic views of ankle arthrodesis nonunion, with talar collapse, and evidence of surrounding joint involvement.

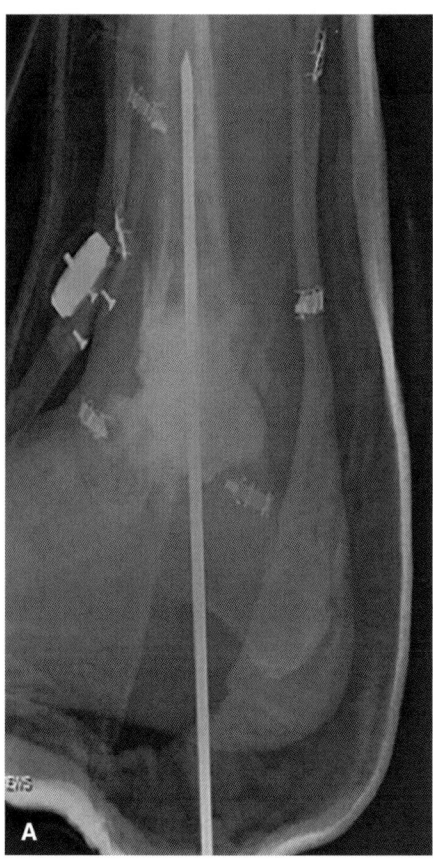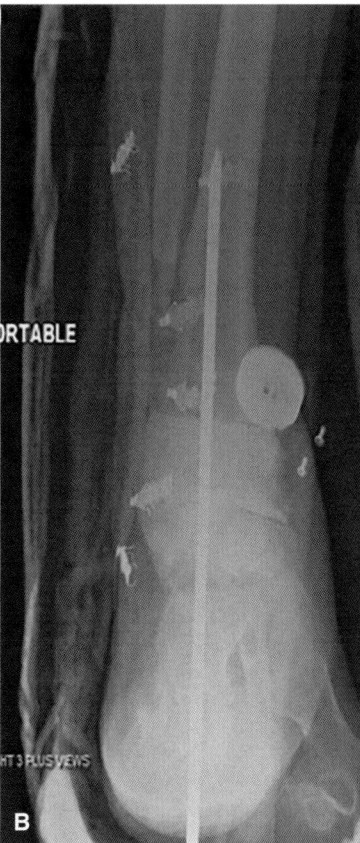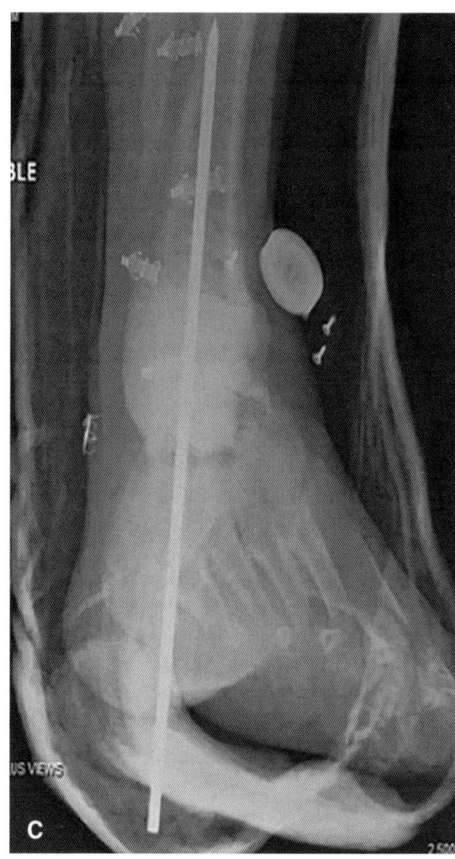

FIGURE 63.15 External fixation staging. **A–C.** Sagittal, A/P, and oblique radiographic views of external fixation using a tibiotalocalcaneal Kirschner wire and circumferential cast. Antibiotic impregnated intercalary cement was used to fill the defect to adequate length and staging scheduled for induction of membrane formation.

There are three specific construct modalities for the TTC pseudoarthrodesis: a tibial shaft cage extending into the hindfoot, a tibial shaft cage combined with the death star, and a death star used by itself (used for the figures in this chapter). The death star is advantageous in optimizing the surface area for bone ingrowth at the level of the calcaneus and the navicular (also at the level of the tibiotalar joint in the absence of larger tibial defects).

A craniomedial exposure is used to access the tibial shaft for placement of the tibial cage. Distraction may be used for an appropriate fit. If using the induced membrane technique, the cage may be placed inside the membrane after the cement is removed. Distally, another incision is made or remade between the EHL and EDL. Previously used cement must be removed, and an induced membrane may be used to envelop the custom implant. Depending on the construct used, the surrounding joints must now be prepared for pseudoarthrodesis. This may include the calcaneus and navicular, as well as the tibiotalar joint depending on the chosen construct. Once prepared, bleeding cancellous bone should be visible, and the implant may be placed.

For tibial cages extending into the hindfoot, the calcaneus and talar neck/navicular must be prepared prior to placement of the cage (may be membrane enveloped). As previously mentioned, tibial cages can be combined with the death star to optimize the surface area for bone growth at the level of the calcaneus and the midfoot structures. When using this construct, lining up the proximal to distal pores is important, as is ensuring the alignment of any anterior to posterior pores in

the death star needed for an interlocking screw to be placed through an intramedullary nail. Additionally, the final construct of using just the death star should follow the same guidelines as previously mentioned. Pore orientation should be as close to preoperative planning as possible to ease the placement of the intramedullary nail and interlocking screws.

Once the chosen construct has been placed, fluoroscopic guidance can be used to ensure adequate positioning of the pores. A stab incision is made at the proximal tibia and a guidewire slowly advanced distally. Fluoroscopic guidance through the implant pores is a necessity and may prove difficult in combined cage and death star constructs. Once the pores have been appropriately aligned with the guidewire, a reamer is used to prepare the canal for nail placement. The tibial nail must be advanced slowly, as to minimize as much translation as possible. Fluoroscopic guidance is advised for adequate placement of the nail within the implant pores. Once the tibial nail is adequately placed, a supplemental interlocking screw may then be advanced through the nail. Depending on the deformity, the interlocking screw may be placed at a number of locations along the posterior distal lower extremity. The neurovascular tissue must be protected as much as possible, as well as any salvageable connective tissue. A guidewire and subsequent reamer must be fluoroscopically advanced through the construct pore and intramedullary nail. Once appropriately placed, alignment of the distal extremity may be checked, and adequate compression across the construct further inspected. Once the construct has been placed to the surgeon's discretion, the surgical field may be closed (Fig. 63.16).

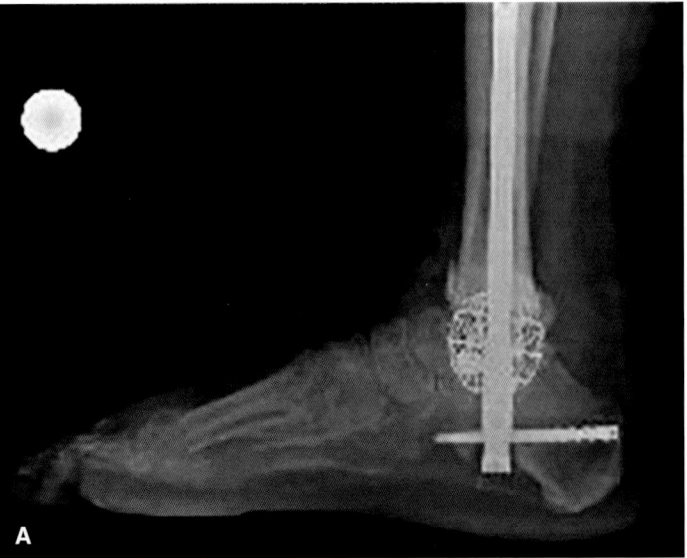
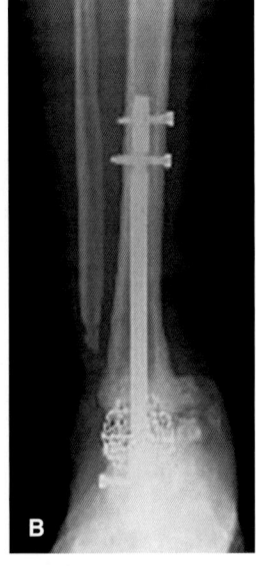
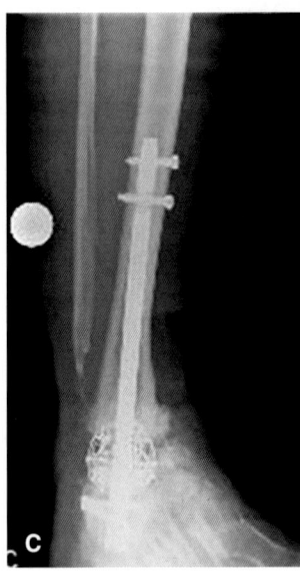

FIGURE 63.16 Postoperative assessment of TTC "death star." **A–C.** Sagittal, A/P, and oblique views of TTC pseudoarthrodesis. Placement of the custom implant must be inspected for proper placement especially as translation is common when placing intramedullary fixation through the custom construct's pore.

PEARLS

- The death star may be used when the talar neck and head are salvageable and will increase the surface area for bone ingrowth. It is particularly useful in the salvage of failed ankle arthroplasty.
- Tibial cages may be combined with the death star or extended into the hindfoot.

AUTHORS' PREFERRED TREATMENT

In recreating an anatomical construct, the use of an extended cage into the hindfoot is generally avoided. Using the rounded death star allows for a much more anatomic alignment around the calcaneus and distal forefoot. This is readily apparent radiographically by both Meary's and Bohler angles. In a limited case series, this procedure has also been invaluable in multirevision osteomyelitis cases spanning significant positions of the distal tibia and hindfoot.

PERILS and PITFALLS

- Even with the osteogenic potential of these implants, there is still a significant risk for inadequate bone ingrowth. Adequate compression is very important as is optimizing the surface area for bone ingrowth whenever possible. The use of the Masquelet induced membrane technique is advised.
- When placing the intramedullary nail and interlocking screw, some degree of translation is impossible to avoid. The internal fixation must be advanced slowly, and care used as the surrounding bone's quality may be suspect.

POSTOPERATIVE CARE

The postoperative period is similar to that for the tibial cage but with an extended period of non–weight bearing. In the early postoperative period, a three-sided cast is placed with subsequent radiographs taken. Patients must remain non–weight bearing during the initial 10-12 weeks. At the 2-week period, the cast may be removed and the wound inspected. Subsequent suture removal may occur if adequate healing has taken place, and the patient may now be placed in a circumferential cast. At 10 weeks, additional radiographs, including a CT scan, may be ordered. If evidence of bone ingrowth exists, the patient can be transitioned into a CAM walking boot for the next 6-8 weeks.[56,58] At this time, radiographs should be ordered. If there is continuing bone ingrowth, transition into weight bearing is allowed. Full transition into activities of daily living should be slowly introduced as tolerated. High-impact exercise is restricted and low-impact exercise encouraged.

REHABILITATION

Rehabilitation is restricted until evidence of bone ingrowth is present. Once present, early rehabilitation should emphasis maintenance of lower extremity mobility and short durations of weight bearing. Transition to more advanced physical therapy should occur through the duration of CAM boot wear. Additional rehabilitation modalities may be indicated in patients with neurovascular defects relating to debridement or trauma.

3D PRINTED CAGES FOR SEGMENTAL DEFECTS OF THE TIBIAL SHAFT

DEFINITION

Segmental defects of the tibial shaft are clinically challenging to manage. Voids are caused by osteomyelitis, neoplasm,

trauma, or hardware explantation.[63] The clinical algorithm has evolved significantly over the last century with the development of advanced hardware and biologic implantation.[64-67] Tibiofibular synostosis was an early attempt at salvage that proved to be unsatisfactory, followed by bone grafting, which is ideal in constructs spanning defects that are between 0.3 and 3 cm.[64,66,68-70] However, nonunions, refracture, and poor function are common complications.[64,70] Bone transport distraction osteogenesis is another option for larger defects spanning up to 10 cm; however, there is a long treatment duration associated with complications.[64,71-74] Single stage titanium cages were first implemented in the early 2000's and have demonstrated optimal bone ingrowth, but there have been high rates of limb length discrepancies and in some cases angular deformities.[75-78] With the implementation of custom cages, rates of limb length discrepancy may be further reduced while taking advantage of the osteogenic potential of additive manufacturing.[49,50,59,60]

CLASSIFICATION

- ■ Void size
  - ▶ Under 2 mm—acute limb shortening (immediate healing, soft tissue tension relieved in the short term, and primary closure may be obtained; poorly tolerated with larger defects)
  - ▶ 0.3-3 cm—autologous nonvascularized cancellous bone graft (osteoconductive material well suited for moderate deformity; associated with nonunion, refracture, and poor function)
  - ▶ 2-10 cm—bone transport distraction osteogenesis (well suited to large defects and in the management of associated soft tissue defects; long treatment duration with associated complications)
  - ▶ 2 cm+—single stage titanium cage (high degree of bone integration; restricted to specific lengths with high rate of postoperative limb length discrepancy)
  - ▶ 2 cm+—3D printed custom cage (highest degree of bone integration well suited for salvage cases with high-risk comorbidities, no associated complications; high cost)

INDICATIONS

- ■ Traumatic bone defects >2 cm, nonunions, revisions.
- ■ 3D printed custom cages are particularly useful in the setting of advanced multirevision cases, patients with advanced comorbidities, and in large defects where distraction osteogenesis would be poorly tolerated.

ANATOMIC FEATURES

Depending on the location and size of the defect, a custom cage can be designed with similar contouring to that of the missing bone. This is particularly important in defects encompassing the metaphysis. Custom implants should only be attempted in stable settings, and in cases of advanced trauma or osteomyelitis, staging must be considered. Other pertinent anatomic variables affecting staging include the health of the surrounding soft tissues and neurovascular structures.

FUNCTIONAL ANALYSIS OF THE ANATOMY

Mitigating limb length discrepancies are paramount in using custom cages to correct a tibial defect. CT reconstructions accurately reconstruct the missing defect, and an intramedullary nail is then used to lock it in place under adequate compression. Distal interlocking screws may also be incorporated into the intramedullary nail. Optimizing modulus properties of the tibial cage involve adequate placement of the cage within the defect and controlling any translation that may occur during the placement of the intramedullary nail. Congruency of the implant with the surrounding tibial cortex ensures proper load distribution and accounts for any possible angular deformity. Long-term success of the implant is highly dependent on reducing any angular deformity and not allowing any residual stress shielding to occur along the bone-metal interfaces of the custom implant. However, custom constructs accurately predict areas of stress shielding, and this may be relatively controlled.

PHYSICAL EXAMINATION

Distal pulses and sensations should be clinically examined along with skin quality. Depending on the setting (trauma, osteomyelitis, or neoplasm), additional clinical examinations may be needed. Any limb length discrepancies should be examined, as well as normal articulation within the knee and ankle. Additional deformity within either joints must also be incorporated into the surgical algorithm to better compliment the management of the segmental defect.

PATHOGENESIS

Segmental defects of the tibial shaft are most often encountered in advanced trauma. Severe comminution encountered in motor vehicle accidents can create segments of nonviable diaphyseal bone. Osteomyelitis is another major contributor that can occur in the setting of compound fractures or due to seeding from a distant site. Concomitant comorbidity significantly increases the chance for osteomyelitis to occur. There are a number of orthopedic neoplasms requiring bone resection that could lead to segmental defects. Additionally, the explantation of hardware may be another cause, in settings of discomfort, osteomyelitis, and residual deformity.

IMAGING AND DIAGNOSTIC STUDIES

A CT scan is needed to plan for the printed construct; x-rays should be used in the initial diagnosis.

TREATMENT

The patient is placed in a supine position, followed by induction of general anesthesia along with standard prepping and draping. Given the need to plan and construct the custom implant, staging is used in the setting of trauma or osteomyelitis. When debriding in acute settings, it is helpful to abstain from tourniquet use.

Trauma or osteomyelitis preparation: Incisions should be advanced proximally and distally from an open fracture site in order to properly debride the surgical site. In cases of closed comminuted fracture, a smaller incision may be used. Debridement of all nonviable tissue should be undertaken. The guidelines of color, consistency, contractility, and capacity should be exercised during muscle debridement, and extra care should be taken to avoid viable tissue as much as possible. Any cortical fragments that can be removed with minimal force using forceps should be discarded. The exception is when free fragments within the metaphysis are still viable. Ideal exposure, however, should be considered when retaining these fragments. All articular fragments are usually preserved. Once the debridement is completed, the tourniquet if used should be deflated to inspect for additional nonviable/nonbleeding tissue. Following thorough debridement, the surgical site should be flushed with saline and an external fixation device placed. The residual void is then filled with antibiotic impregnated cement beads, typically containing tobramycin and vancomycin. Subsequent debridements are then performed every 24-96 hours until the soft tissue envelope is viable for closure. In each subsequent debridement, the same technique is used, except that an intercalary cement spacer is used prior to the final closure. Additionally, more extensive soft tissue reconstructions may be required in higher-grade Gustilo fractures.[79] A CT scan is then undertaken and the custom implant manufactured.

In the setting of stable void defects (neoplasm or hardware explantation), a CT scan is performed during the first consultation with the delay in custom cage implantation only being as long as the manufacturing process. In staged settings (trauma and osteomyelitis), the antibiotic spacer should be placed for a minimum of 4-6 weeks (Fig. 63.17). Prior to the second stage procedure, comprehensive clinical testing, including WBC, sedimentation rate, and C-reactive protein, and radiographs should be undertaken to rule out infection. This time period also provides an interval for the development of a pseudomembrane around the antibiotic spacer. This membrane is used concomitantly with the custom cage (Masquelet technique) contributing additional

osteoinductive effects.[61,62,80] Multiple implants will be provided with slightly different lengths. The implants may be trialed and fluoroscopically inspected for optimal fit (Fig. 63.18). Prior to implantation, the selected custom implant must be seeded with bone graft. This can be autologous or cadaveric, and additional biologics may be incorporated at the surgeon's discretion. The implant is then placed within the induced membrane. Distraction may be used to adequately place the membrane enclosed custom implant within the void defect (Fig. 63.19). Once adequately stable, fluoroscopy confirms appropriate positioning. The hip should then be flexed and the knee also flexed into the preferred position for intramedullary nail implantation. The guidewire must be fluoroscopically guided for ideal positioning within the intramedullary canal as well as proper positioning through a pore within the custom implant. Once appropriately positioned, subsequent reaming and nail implantation may begin. The nail must be advanced carefully through the cage pore while mitigating as much translation as possible. Once sufficiently advanced, interlocking distal locking screws may be placed. Prior to closure, positioning and alignment should be checked under fluoroscopy (Fig. 63.20).

positioning PEARLS

- Distraction can be used in the implantation of the custom cage.
- Plan on an extra set of hands to help mitigate translation while maneuvering the intramedullary nail through the cage pore.

PEARLS

In staged procedures, make sure that the final intercalary concrete block restores limb length to the approximate contralateral side. This ensures that the induced membrane will approximately cover the entire custom cage.

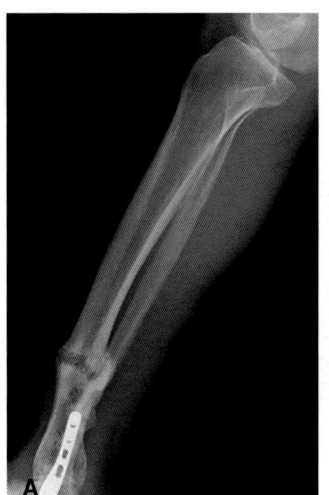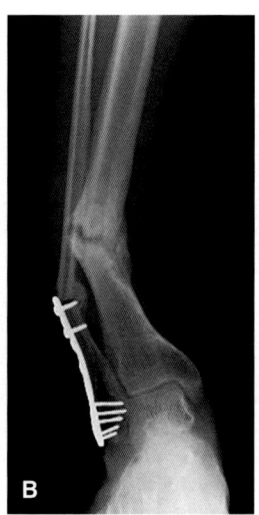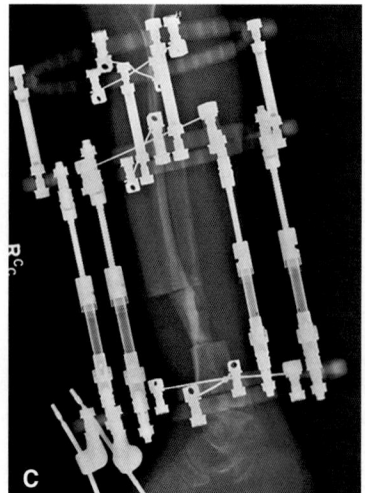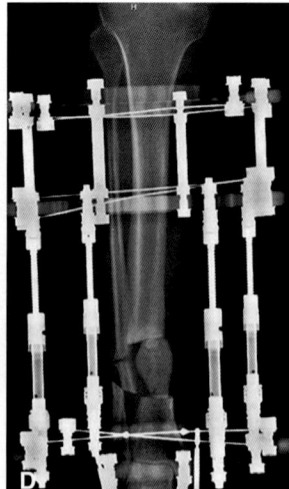

FIGURE 63.17 Angular deformity and external fixation staging. **A, B.** Sagittal and A/P views of preoperative angular deformity. **C, D.** Sagittal and A/P views of external fixation staging with the placement of an intercalary antibiotic impregnated cement spacer to induce membrane formation.

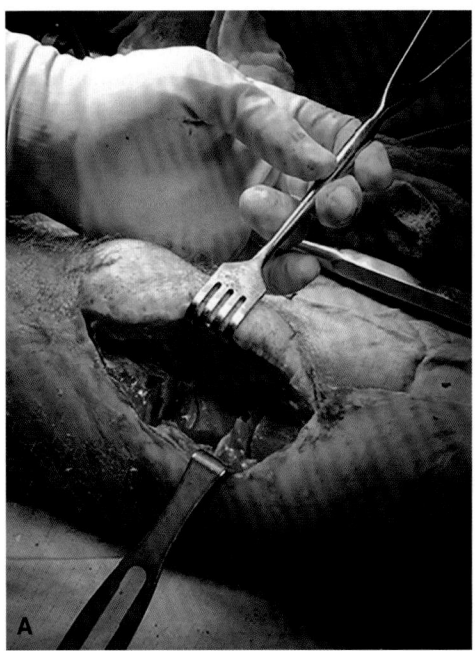
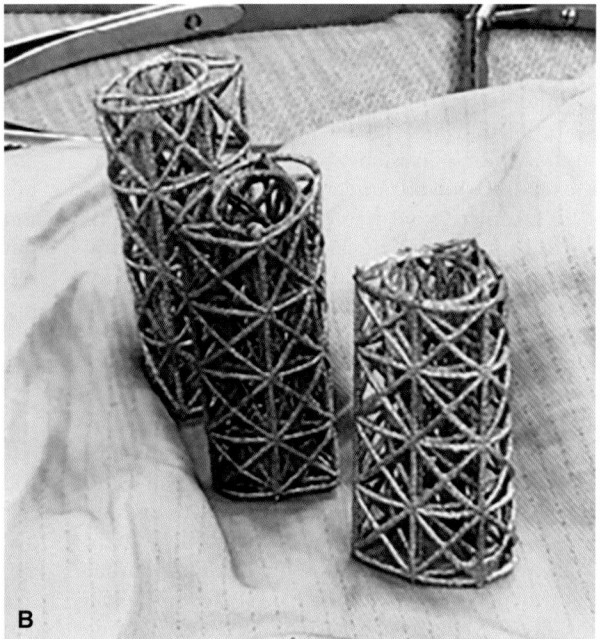

FIGURE 63.18 Void exposure and implant sizing. **A.** Careful exposure of the void must be carried out with attention made toward the viability of the surrounding tissue. **B.** The custom 3D printed implant will come in three sizes to ensure optimal fit; once an appropriate trial has been selected, fluoroscopic inspection must follow.

AUTHORS' PREFERRED TREATMENT

Custom cage implantation has been successful in salvage procedures encompassing >2 cm of void defect. In settings of multirevision trauma and osteomyelitis, custom cage implantation along with the Masquelet induced membrane technique have resulted in 100% bone integration and no reported residual limb length discrepancies.

PERILS and PITFALLS

- CT planned custom cages are accurate; however, surgeon guided clinical judgment is paramount in optimizing clinical outcomes.
- Translation of the custom cage is nearly impossible to avoid when placing the intramedullary nail. Optimize clinical alignment and length as it is the most important factor.

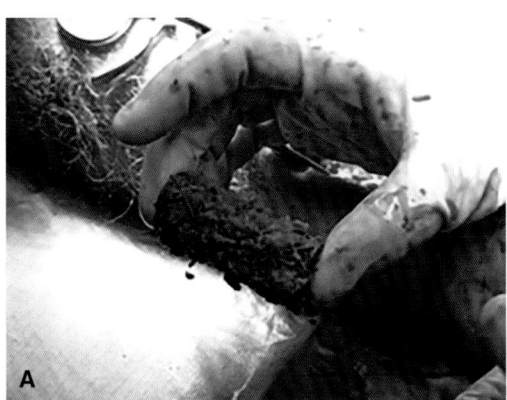
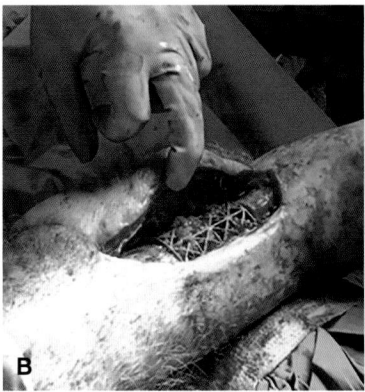
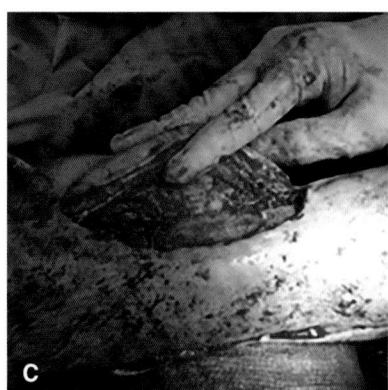

FIGURE 63.19 Implantation of the bone graft infused construct using the Masquelet induced membrane technique. **A.** Allograft or autograft may be used to fill the custom construct; additional augment may also be chosen. **B.** The bone infused implant is then placed within the void and the cortices aligned. **C.** The induced membrane is then placed around the implant, with subsequent placement of the intramedullary nail.

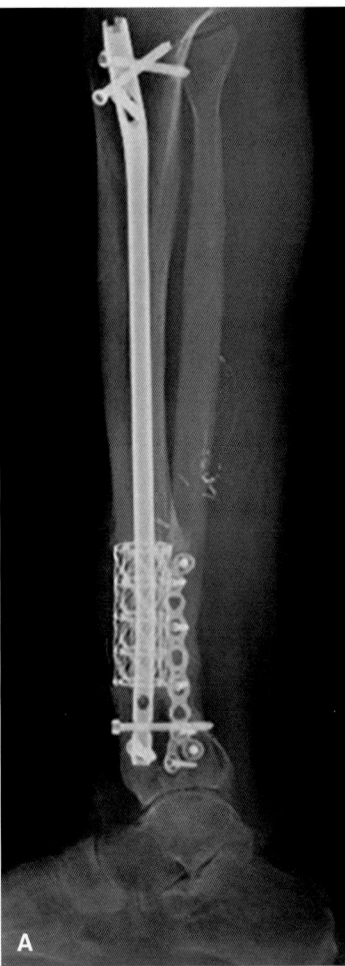
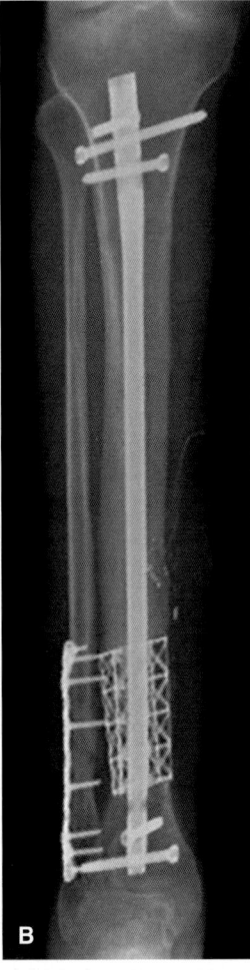

FIGURE 63.20 Postoperative implant assessment.
A, B. Sagittal and A/P views of the postoperative placement of the custom implant; alignment must be inspected along the cortices of the implant. Radiographic findings of translation may not necessarily rule in suboptimal placement of the implant if the patient is found to be clinically aligned.

POSTOPERATIVE CARE

Depending on risk factors and the setting of the surgery, some patients may need to be treated with an aggressive course of postoperative antibiotics and lifelong antibiotic therapy thereafter. Ideally, postoperative care is patient specific given the variables necessitating limb salvage. In the early postoperative period, a three-sided cast is placed with subsequent radiographs taken. Patients must remain non–weight bearing during the initial 8 weeks. At the 2-week period, the cast may be removed and the wound inspected. Subsequent suture removal may occur if adequate healing has taken place; then, the patient may now be placed in a circumferential cast. At 8 weeks, additional radiographs, including a CT scan, may be ordered. If evidence of bone ingrowth exists, the patient can be transitioned into a CAM walking boot for the next 6-8 weeks.[80] At this time, radiographs should then be ordered. If there is evidence of continuing bone ingrowth, the patient may be transitioned into weight bearing. Full transition into activities of daily living should be slowly introduced as tolerated. High-impact exercise is restricted and low-impact exercise encouraged.

REHABILITATION

Rehabilitation is restricted until evidence of bone ingrowth is present. Once present, early rehabilitation should emphasize maintenance of lower extremity mobility and short durations of weight bearing. Transition to more advanced physical therapy should occur through the duration of CAM boot wear. Additional rehabilitation modalities may be indicated in patients with neurovascular defects relating to debridement or trauma.

REFERENCES

1. Munteanu SE, Menz HB, Wark JD, et al. Hallux valgus, by nature or nurture? A twin study. *Arthritis Care Res (Hoboken).* 2017;69(9):1421-1428.
2. Nix S, Smith M, Vicenzino B. Prevalence of hallux valgus in the general population: a systematic review and meta-analysis. *J Foot Ankle Res.* 2010;3:21.
3. Thomas S, Barrington R. Hallux valgus. *Curr Orthop.* 2003;17:299-307.
4. Thompson FM, Coughlin MJ. The high price of high-fashion footwear. *J Bone Joint Surg Am.* 1994;76-A:1586-1593.
5. Menz HB. *Foot Problems in Older People: Assessment and Management.* Edinburgh, UK: Churchill Livingstone Elsevier; 2008.
6. Nix SE, Vicenzino BT, Collins NJ, Smith MD. Characteristics of foot structure and footwear associated with hallux valgus: a systematic review. *Osteoarthr Cartil.* 2012;20:1059-1074.
7. Perera AM, Mason L, Stephens MM. The pathogenesis of hallux valgus. *J Bone Joint Surg Am.* 2011;93:1650-1661.
8. Coughlin MJ. Hallux valgus. *J Bone Joint Surg Am.* 1996;78-A:932-966.
9. Frey C. Foot health and shoewear for women. *Clin Orthop Relat Res.* 2000;372:32-44.
10. Dawson J, Thorogood M, Marks SA, et al. The prevalence of foot problems in older women: a cause for concern. *J Public Health.* 2002;24:77-84.
11. Al-Abdulwahab SS, Al-Dosry R. Hallux valgus and preferred shoe types amongst young healthy Saudi Arabian women. *Ann Saudi Med.* 2000;20:319-321.
12. Menz HB, Morris ME. Determinants of disabling foot pain in retirement village residents. *J Am Podiatr Med Assoc.* 2005;95:573-579.
13. Nguyen US, Hillstrom HJ, Li W, et al. Factors associated with hallux valgus in a population-based study of older women and men: the MOBILIZE Boston Study. *Osteoarthr Cartil.* 2010;18:41-46.
14. Dufour AB, Casey VA, Golightly YM, Hannan MT. Characteristics associated with hallux valgus in a population-based foot study of older adults. *Arthritis Care Res (Hoboken).* 2014;66:1880-1886.
15. Barg A, Harmer JR, Presson AP, Zhang C, Lackey M, Saltzman CL. Unfavorable outcomes following surgical treatment of hallux valgus deformity: a systematic literature review. *J Bone Joint Surg Am.* 2018;100(18):1563-1573. doi: 10.2106/JBJS.17.00975.
16. Choi GW, Choi WJ, Yoon HS, et al. Additional surgical factors affecting the recurrence of hallux valgus after Ludloff osteotomy. *Bone Joint J.* 2013;95-B:803-808.
17. Choi GW, Kim HJ, Kim TS, et al. Comparison of the modified McBride procedure and the distal chevron osteotomy for mild to moderate hallux valgus. *J Foot Ankle Surg.* 2016;55:808-811.
18. Crespo Romero E, PeñuelaCandel R, Gómez Gómez S, et al. Percutaneous forefoot surgery for treatment of hallux valgus deformity: an intermediate prospective study. *Musculoskelet Surg.* 2017;101:167-172.
19. Fakoor M, Sarafan N, Mohammadhoseini P, et al. Comparison of clinical outcomes of scarf and chevron osteotomies and the McBride procedure in the treatment of hallux valgus deformity. *Arch Bone Jt Surg.* 2014;2:31-36.
20. Okuda R, Kinoshita M, Yasuda T, et al. Hallux valgus angle as a predictor of recurrence following proximal metatarsal osteotomy. *J Orthop Sci.* 2011;16:760-764.
21. Aiyer A, Shub J, Shariff R, et al. Radiographic recurrence of deformity after hallux valgus surgery in patients with metatarsus adductus. *Foot Ankle Int.* 2016;37:165-171.
22. Shibuya N, Jupiter DC, Plemmons BS, et al. Correction of hallux valgus deformity in association with underlying metatarsus adductus deformity. *Foot Ankle Spec.* 2017;10:538-542.
23. Agrawal Y, Bajaj SK, Flowers MJ. Scarf-Akin osteotomy for hallux valgus in juvenile and adolescent patients. *J Pediatr Orthop B.* 2015;24:535-540.
24. Okuda R, Kinoshita M, Yasuda T, et al. Postoperative incomplete reduction of the sesamoids as a risk factor for recurrence of hallux valgus. *J Bone Joint Surg Am.* 2009;91:1637-1645.
25. Kim Y, Kim JS, Young KW, et al. A new measure of tibial sesamoid position in hallux valgus in relation to the coronal rotation of the first metatarsal in CT scans. *Foot Ankle Int.* 2015;36:944-952.
26. Wagner P, Ortiz C, Wagner E. Rotational osteotomy for hallux valgus. A new technique for primary and revision cases. *Tech Foot Ankle Surg.* 2017;16:3-10.
27. Mortier JP, Bernard JL, Maestro M. Axial rotation of the first metatarsal head in a normal population and hallux valgus patients. *Orthop Traumatol Surg Res.* 2012;98:677-683.
28. Maceira E, Rochera R. Müller-Weiss disease: clinical and biomechanical features. *Foot Ankle Clin.* 2004;9(1):105-125.
29. Lui TH. Arthroscopic triple arthrodesis in patients with Müller Weiss disease. *Foot Ankle Surg.* 2009;15(3):119-122.
30. Reade B, Atlas G, Distazio J, Kruljac S. Mueller-Weiss syndrome: an uncommon cause of midfoot pain. *J Foot Ankle Surg.* 1998;37(6):535-539.
31. Haller J, Sartoris DJ, Resnick D, et al. Spontaneous osteonecrosis of the tarsal navicular in adults: imaging findings. *Am J Roentgenol.* 1988;151(2):355-358.

32. McCauley RG, Kahn PC. Osteochondritis of the tarsal navicula: radioisotopic appearances. *Radiology.* 1977;123(3):705-706.

33. Mayich DJ. The treatment of Mueller-Weiss disease: a systematic approach. *Tech Foot Ankle Surg.* 2016;15(2):59-73.

34. Zhang H, Li J, Qiao Y, et al. Open triple fusion versus TNC arthrodesis in the treatment of Mueller-Weiss disease. *J Orthop Surg Res.* 2017;12(1):13.

35. Prathapamchandra V, Ravichandran P, Shanmugasundaram J, Jayaraman A, Salem RS. Vascular foramina of navicular bone: a morphometric study. *Anat Cell Biol.* 2017;50(2):93-98.

36. Golano P, Fariñas O, Sáenz I. The anatomy of the navicular and periarticular structures. *Foot Ankle Clin.* 2004;9:1-23.

37. Saxena A, Fullem B, Hannaford D. Results of treatment of 22 navicular stress fractures and a new proposed radiographic classification system. *J Foot Ankle Surg.* 2000;39:96-103.

38. Jeng CL, Campbell JT, Tang EY, Cerrato RA, Myerson MS. Tibiotalocalcaneal arthrodesis with bulk femoral head allograft for salvage of large defects in the ankle. *Foot Ankle Int.* 2013;34(9):1256-1266.

39. Adelaar RS, Madrian JR. Avascular necrosis of the talus. *Orthop Clin North Am.* 2004;35(3):383-395, xi.

40. Delanois RE, Mont MA, Yoon TR, Mizell M, Hungerford DS. Atraumatic osteonecrosis of the talus. *J Bone Joint Surg Am.* 1998;80:529-536.

41. Hawkins LG. Fractures of the neck of the talus. *J Bone Joint Surg Am.* 1970;52(5):991-1002.

42. Vallier HA, Nork SE, Barei DP, Benirschke SK, Sangeorzan BJ. Talar neck fractures: results and outcomes. *J Bone Joint Surg Am.* 2004;86(8):1616-1624.

43. Harnroongroj T, Vandurongwan V. The talar body prosthesis. *J Bone Joint Surg Am.* 1997;79(9):1313-1322.

44. Taniguchi A, Takakura Y, Sugimoto K, et al. The use of a ceramic talar body prosthesis in patients with aseptic necrosis of the talus. *J Bone Joint Surg Br.* 2012;94:1529-1533.

45. Tsukamoto S, Tanaka Y, Maegawa N, et al. Total talar replacement following collapse of the talar body as a complication of total ankle arthroplasty: a case report. *J Bone Joint Surg Am.* 2010;92:2115-2120.

46. Angthong C. Anatomic total talar prosthesis replacement surgery and ankle arthroplasty: an early case series in Thailand. *Orthop Rev.* 2014;6(3):5486.

47. Ando Y, Yasui T, Isawa K, Tanaka S, Tanaka Y, Takakura Y. Total talar replacement for idiopathic necrosis of the talus: a case report. *J Foot Ankle Surg.* 2015;55(6):1292-1296.

48. Taniguchi A, Takakura Y, Tanaka Y, et al. An alumina ceramic total talar prosthesis for osteonecrosis of the talus. *J Bone Joint Surg Am.* 2015;97:1348-1353.

49. Tracey J, Arora D, Gross CE, Parekh SG. Custom 3D-printed total talar prostheses restore normal joint anatomy throughout the hindfoot. *Foot Ankle Spec.* 2019;12(1): 39-481938640018762567.

50. Scott D, Parekh S. Outcomes following 3D printed total talus arthroplasty. *Foot Ankle Orthop.* 2018;3(3):2473011418S00419.

51. Regauer M, Lange M, Soldan K, et al. Development of an internally braced prosthesis for total talus replacement. *World J Orthop.* 2017;8:221-228.

52. Gelberman RH, Mortensen WW. The arterial anatomy of the talus. *Foot Ankle Int.* 1983;2:64-72.

53. Mulfinger GL, Trueta J. The blood supply of the talus. *J Bone Joint Surg Br.* 1970;52(1): 160-167.

54. Haliburton RA, Sullivan CR, Kelly PJ, Peterson LF. The extra-osseous and intra-osseous blood supply of the talus. *J Bone Joint Surg Am.* 1958;40(5):1115-1120.

55. Carrier DA, Harris CM. Ankle arthrodesis with vertical Steinmann's pins in rheumatoid arthritis. *Clin Orthop Relat Res.* 1991;268:10-14.

56. Barrett GR, Meyer LC, Bray EW III, Taylor RG Jr, Kolb FJ. Pantalar arthrodesis: a long-term follow-up. *Foot Ankle.* 1981;1:279-283.

57. Kitaoka HB, Romness DW. Arthrodesis for failed ankle arthroplasty. *J Arthroplasty.* 1992;7:277-284.

58. Russotti GM, Johnson KA, Cass JR. Tibiotalocalcaneal arthrodesis for arthritis and deformity of the hind part of the foot. *J Bone Joint Surg Am.* 1988;70:1304-1307.

59. Hamid KS, Parekh SG, Adams SB. Salvage of severe foot and ankle trauma with a 3D printed scaffold. *Foot Ankle Int.* 2016;37(4):433-439.

60. Dekker TJ, Steele JR, Federer AE, Hamid KS, Adams SB Jr. Use of patient-specific 3D-printed titanium implants for complex foot and ankle limb salvage, deformity correction, and arthrodesis procedures. *Foot Ankle Int.* 2018;39(8):916-921.

61. Masquelet AC, Fitoussi F, Begue T, Muller GP. Reconstruction of the long bones by the induced membrane and spongy autograft. *Ann Chir Plast Esthet.* 2000;45:346-353.

62. Masquelet AC, Begue T. The concept of induced membrane for reconstruction of long bone defects. *Orthop Clin North Am.* 2010;41:27-37.

63. Clements JR, Carpenter BB, Pourciau JK. Treating segmental bone defects: a new technique. *J Foot Ankle Surg.* 2008;47(4):350-356.

64. DeCoster TA, Gehlert RJ, Mikola EA, Pirela-Cruz MA. Management of posttraumatic segmental bone defects. *J Am Acad Orthop Surg.* 2004;12(1):28-38.

65. Weinberg H, Roth VG, Robin GC, Floman Y. Early fibular bypass procedures (tibiofibular synostosis) for massive bone loss in war injuries. *J Trauma.* 1979;19(3):177-181.

66. Watson JT, Anders M, Moed BR. Management strategies for bone loss in tibial shaft fractures. *Clin Orthop Relat Res.* 1995;(315):138-152.

67. Huntington TW. VI. Case of bone transference: use of a segment of fibula to supply a defect in the tibia. *Ann Surg.* 1905;41(2):249.

68. Agiza AR. Treatment of tibial osteomyelitic defects and infected pseudarthroses by the Huntington fibular transference operation. *J Bone Joint Surg Am.* 1981;63(5):814-819.

69. Goldstrohm GL, Mears DC, Swartz WM. The results of 39 fractures complicated by major segmental bone loss and/or leg length discrepancy. *J Trauma.* 1984;24(1):50-58.

70. Christian EP, Bosse MJ, Robb G. Reconstruction of large diaphyseal defects, without free fibular transfer, in Grade-IIIB tibial fractures. *J Bone Joint Surg Am.* 1989;71(7):994-1004.

71. Green SA, Jackson JM, Wall DM, Marinow H, Ishkanian J. Management of segmental defects by the Ilizarov intercalary bone transport method. *Clin Orthop Relat Res.* 1992;(280):136-142.

72. Ilizarov GA, Ledyaev VI. The replacement of long tubular bone defects by lengthening distraction osteotomy of one of the fragments. *Clin Orthop Relat Res.* 1992;280:7-10.

73. DeCoster TA, Simpson AH, Wood M, Li G, Kenwright J. Biologic model of bone transport distraction osteogenesis and vascular response. *J Orthop Res.* 1999;17(2):238-245.

74. Polyzois D, Papachristou G, Kotsiopoulos K, Plessas S. Treatment of tibial and femoral bone loss by distraction osteogenesis: experience in 28 infected and 14 clean cases. *Acta Orthop Scand.* 1997;68(suppl 275):84-88.

75. Betz AM, Hierner R, Baumgart R, et al. Primary shortening—secondary lengthening. A new treatment concept for reconstruction of extensive soft tissue and bone injuries after 3rd degree open fracture and amputation of the lower leg. *Handchir Mikrochir Plast Chir.* 1998;30(1):30-39.

76. Meffert RH, Inoue N, Tis JE, Brug E, Chao EY. Distraction osteogenesis after acute limb-shortening for segmental tibial defects: comparison of a monofocal and a bifocal technique in rabbits. *J Bone Joint Surg.* 2000;82(6):799-808.

77. Green SA. Skeletal defects. A comparison of bone grafting and bone transport for segmental skeletal defects. *Clin Orthop Relat Res.* 1994;(301):111-117.

78. Marsh JL, Prokuski L, Biermann JS. Chronic infected tibial nonunions with bone loss. Conventional techniques versus bone transport. *Clin Orthop Relat Res.* 1994;(301): 139-146.

79. Southam BR, Archdeacon MT. "Iatrogenic" segmental defect: how I debride high-energy open tibial fractures. *J Orthop Trauma.* 2017;31:S9-S15.

80. Gupta G, Ahmad S, Zahid M, Khan AH, Sherwani MK, Khan AQ. Management of traumatic tibial diaphyseal bone defect by "induced-membrane technique". *Indian J Orthop.* 2016;50(3):290.

Compartment Syndrome of the Lower Extremity and Foot

Michael H. Theodoulou and Jennifer Buchanan

Compartment syndrome is an identified condition seen in the acute (ACS) and chronic (CECS) setting. Acutely, it is appreciated in the trauma patient who has sustained significant injury with closed myofascial compartments that will allow for increased intracompartmental pressure to promote progressive ischemic pain in the extremity. Frequently, this increased pressure is resulting from acute local hemorrhage. In the chronic condition, this results from a constant exertional activity that promotes demand for increased blood flow in an idiopathic or congenitally constrained compartment. The exact mechanism for chronic exertional compartment syndrome is not known. The acute presentation does demand immediate surgical intervention to reduce the risk of long-term injury. The chronic form often time impacts athletes or individuals who participate in high demand activities such as in the military that will not permit the individual to participate appropriately. Chronic cases of compartment syndrome are also managed surgically but most frequently done through more minimally invasive techniques. Clinically, the diagnosis is often made due to the severity of pain. Compartment pressures have been the quantitative examination of choice in establishing a diagnosis of compartment syndrome. Generally accepted findings of intracompartmental pressures <30 mm Hg difference with diastolic pressure can promote the clinical presentation of compartment syndrome or an absolute measured compartment pressure >30-40 mm Hg. This chapter will be devoted to the discussion of the anatomy of the lower leg and its compartments as well as those proposed for the foot. We will appreciate the pathophysiology of compartment syndrome, its clinical and procedural identification, recommended treatments, and sequelae of compartment syndrome.

ANATOMY

There are defined compartments of the lower leg. Consistently, these have been appreciated as anterior, lateral, superficial posterior, and deep posterior (Fig. 64.1). Compartments of the foot are somewhat more controversial with regard to presentation and actual existence.

Within the contents of the anterior compartment reside the muscles of tibialis anterior, extensor hallucis longus, the extensor digitorum longus, and peroneus tertius. Vessels identified include the anterior tibial artery and vein. The deep peroneal nerve provides innervation to this area. Structural definition of the borders consists of the anterior tibia, anteromedial fibula, the interosseous membrane, and the anterior intermuscular septum (Fig. 64.2). Within the lateral compartment resides the peroneus longus and brevis muscles. Vascular support to this region is from the fibular and posterior tibial arteries. The common peroneal nerve innervates this region. Structurally, it is bound by the posterolateral margin of the fibula and the anterolateral and posterolateral intermuscular septa (Fig. 64.3). Within the superficial posterior compartment lies

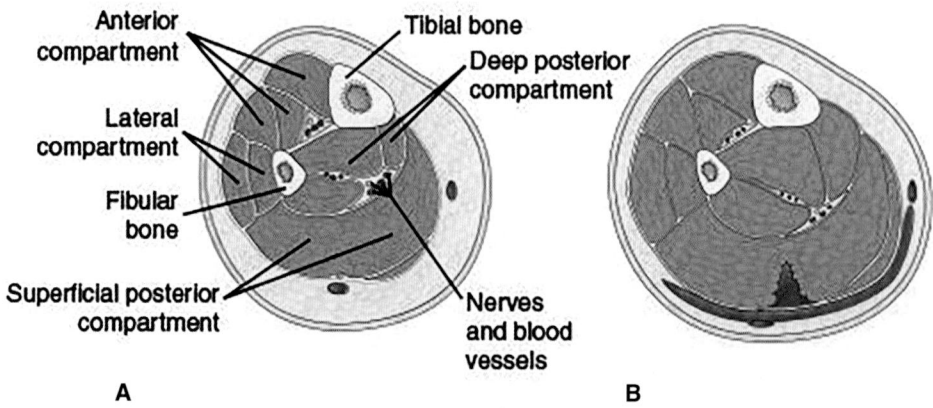

FIGURE 64.1 A, B. Compartments of the leg. (Reproduced with permission from *Lippincott's Nursing Advisor*. Philadelphia, PA: Lippincott Williams & Wilkins; 2014.)

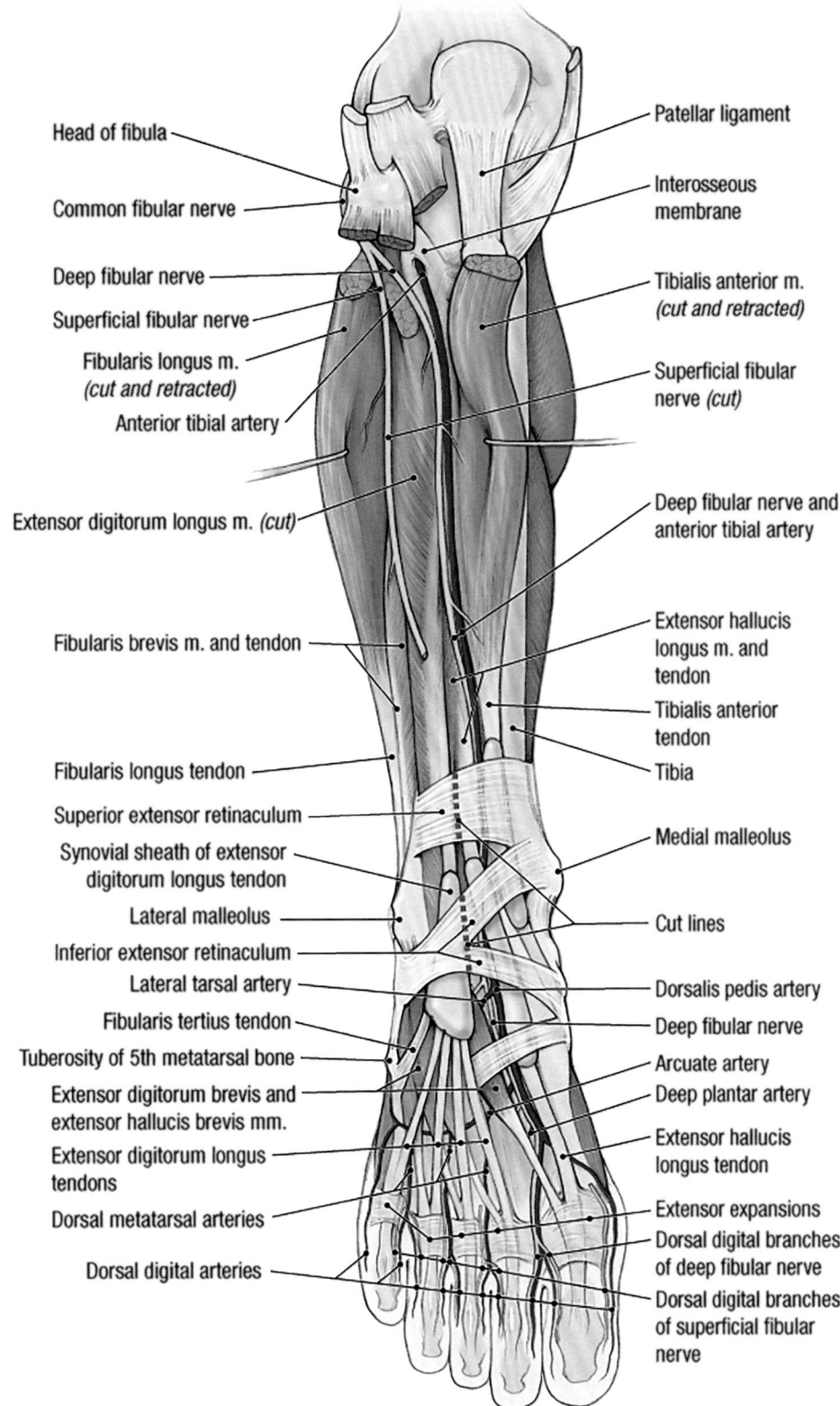

Head of fibula

Common fibular nerve

Deep fibular nerve

Superficial fibular nerve

Fibularis longus m.
(cut and retracted)

Anterior tibial artery

Extensor digitorum longus m. *(cut)*

Fibularis brevis m. and tendon

Fibularis longus tendon

Superior extensor retinaculum

Synovial sheath of extensor
digitorum longus tendon

Lateral malleolus

Inferior extensor retinaculum

Lateral tarsal artery

Fibularis tertius tendon

Tuberosity of 5th metatarsal bone

Extensor digitorum brevis and
extensor hallucis brevis mm.

Extensor digitorum longus
tendons

Dorsal metatarsal arteries

Dorsal digital arteries

Patellar ligament

Interosseous
membrane

Tibialis anterior m.
(cut and retracted)

Superficial fibular
nerve *(cut)*

Deep fibular nerve and
anterior tibial artery

Extensor hallucis
longus m. and
tendon

Tibialis anterior
tendon

Tibia

Medial malleolus

Cut lines

Dorsalis pedis artery

Deep fibular nerve

Arcuate artery

Deep plantar artery

Extensor hallucis
longus tendon

Extensor expansions

Dorsal digital branches
of deep fibular nerve

Dorsal digital branches
of superficial fibular
nerve

FIGURE 64.2 Anterior leg compartment anatomy. (Reproduced with permission from Tank P. *Grant's Dissector*. Philadelphia, PA: Lippincott Williams & Wilkins; 2013.)

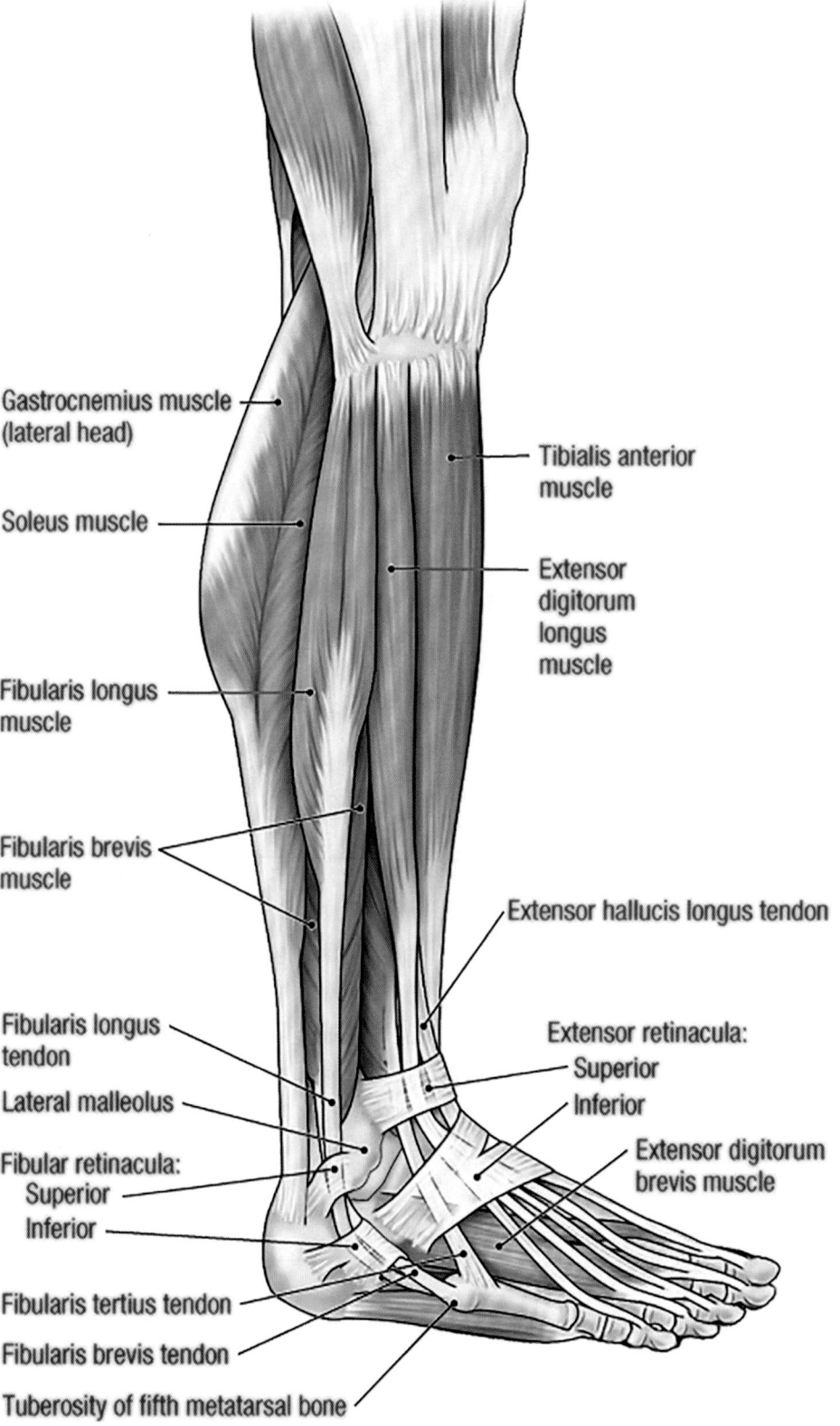

Gastrocnemius muscle
(lateral head)

Soleus muscle

Fibularis longus
muscle

Fibularis brevis
muscle

Fibularis longus
tendon

Lateral malleolus

Fibular retinacula:
 Superior
 Inferior

Fibularis tertius tendon

Fibularis brevis tendon

Tuberosity of fifth metatarsal bone

Tibialis anterior
muscle

Extensor
digitorum
longus
muscle

Extensor hallucis longus tendon

Extensor retinacula:
 Superior
 Inferior

Extensor digitorum
brevis muscle

FIGURE 64.3 Lateral leg compartment. (Reproduced with permission from Tank P. *Grant's Dissector*. Philadelphia, PA: Lippincott Williams & Wilkins; 2013.)

the gastrocnemius, soleus, and plantaris muscles. It is anteriorly bounded by the intermuscular septa with the deep posterior muscles, superiorly by the posterior tibia and fibula. The tibial nerve innervates this region with blood supply supporting the muscles to include sural branches of the popliteal artery, the sural, posterior tibial, and peroneal arteries (Fig. 64.4). Finally, the deep posterior muscle group presents the muscles of tibialis posterior, flexor digitorum longus, and flexor hallucis longus. The posterior aspect of the tibia, intramuscular septae

of the lateral and superficial posterior muscle compartments serve as borders. It is innervated by the tibial nerve with arterial supply emanating from the posterior tibial and peroneal arteries (Fig. 64.5).

Compartments of the foot continue to remain controversial and whether their existence may contribute to a syndrome of ischemia resulting from increased intracompartmental pressure. The allocation of muscles within specific compartments and whether communication exists remains uncertain. Early study

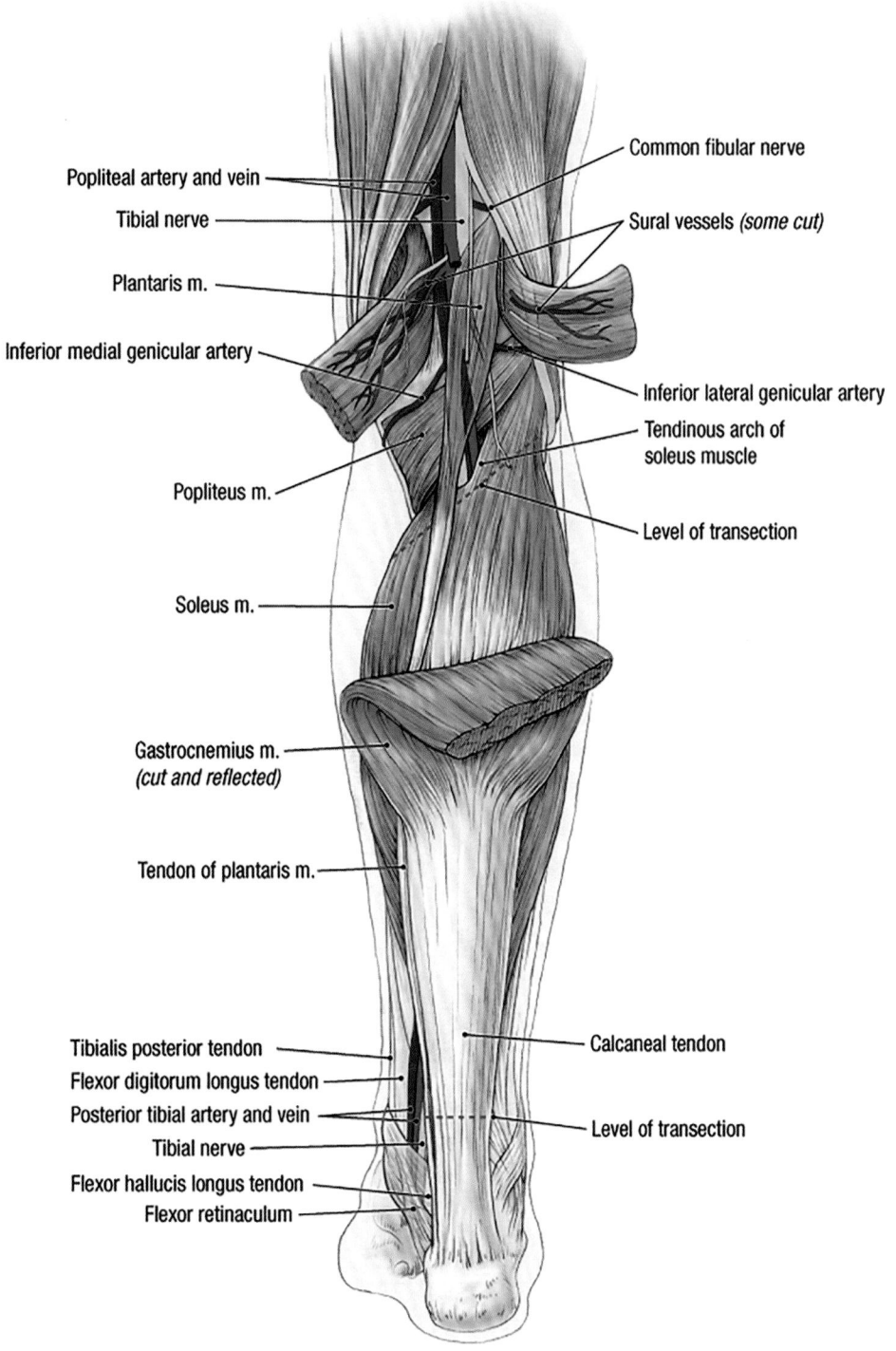

FIGURE 64.4 Superficial posterior leg compartment. (Reproduced with permission from Tank P. *Grant's Dissector*. Philadelphia, PA: Lippincott Williams & Wilkins; 2013.)

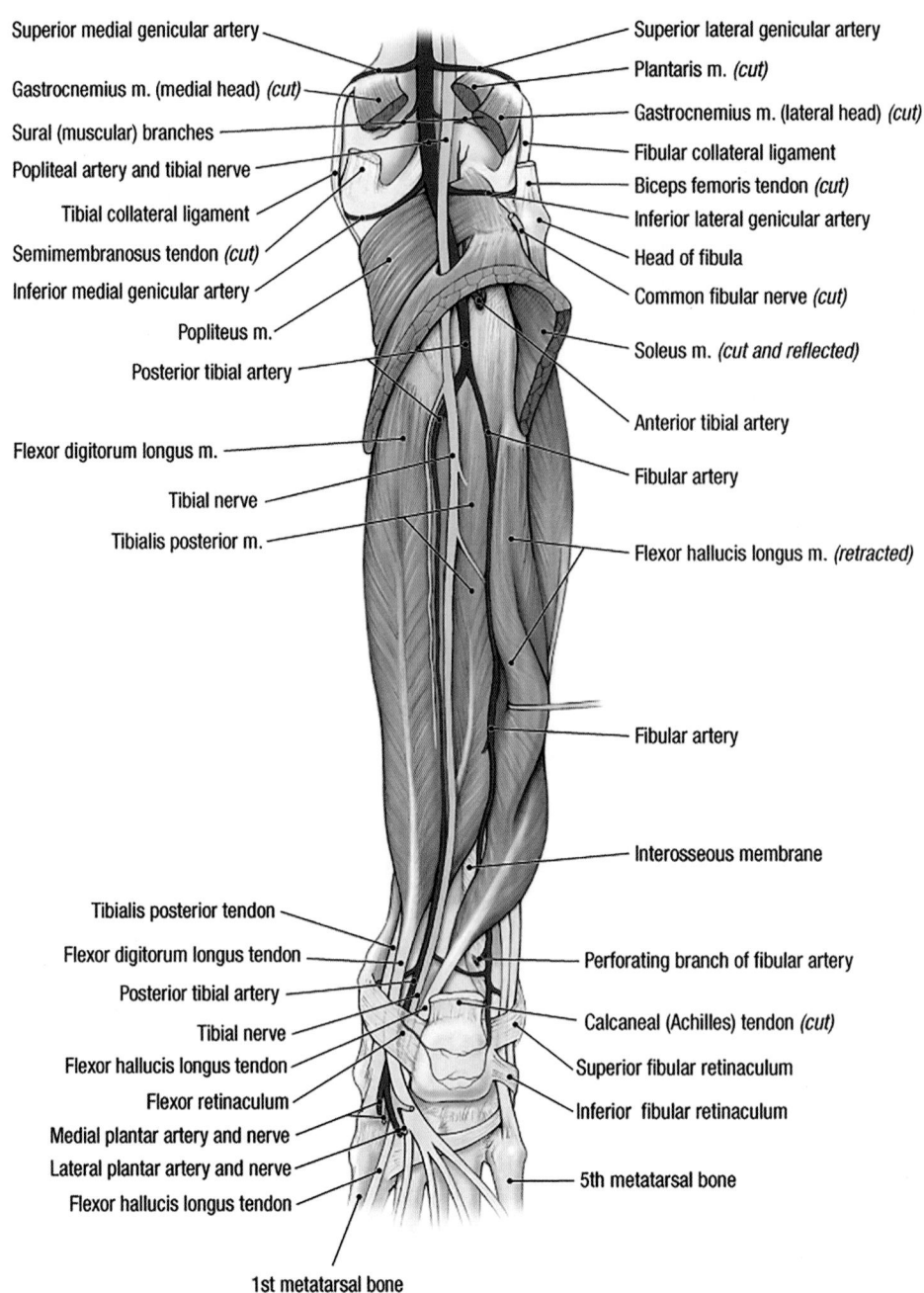

Superior medial genicular artery

Gastrocnemius m. (medial head) *(cut)*

Sural (muscular) branches

Popliteal artery and tibial nerve

Tibial collateral ligament

Semimembranosus tendon *(cut)*

Inferior medial genicular artery

Popliteus m.

Posterior tibial artery

Flexor digitorum longus m.

Tibial nerve

Tibialis posterior m.

Tibialis posterior tendon

Flexor digitorum longus tendon

Posterior tibial artery

Tibial nerve

Flexor hallucis longus tendon

Flexor retinaculum

Medial plantar artery and nerve

Lateral plantar artery and nerve

Flexor hallucis longus tendon

1st metatarsal bone

Superior lateral genicular artery

Plantaris m. *(cut)*

Gastrocnemius m. (lateral head) *(cut)*

Fibular collateral ligament

Biceps femoris tendon *(cut)*

Inferior lateral genicular artery

Head of fibula

Common fibular nerve *(cut)*

Soleus m. *(cut and reflected)*

Anterior tibial artery

Fibular artery

Flexor hallucis longus m. *(retracted)*

Fibular artery

Interosseous membrane

Perforating branch of fibular artery

Calcaneal (Achilles) tendon *(cut)*

Superior fibular retinaculum

Inferior fibular retinaculum

5th metatarsal bone

FIGURE 64.5 Deep posterior leg compartment. (Reproduced with permission from Tank P. *Grant's Dissector.* Philadelphia, PA: Lippincott Williams & Wilkins; 2013.)

and literature suggested four compartments of the foot to include a medial, lateral, central, and interosseous. Manoli and Weber performed infusion studies suggesting nine domains to the foot through infusion technique and separated the central compartment into a superficial and deep as well as dividing the four interosseous spaces and adding a separate chamber for the adductor hallucis muscle[1] (Fig. 64.6). Utilizing MRI, Reach et al. defined a tenth compartment that includes the extensor digitorum and hallucis brevis muscles.[2] Ling and Kumar did not identify an inelastic medial compartment as it was bound by the skin and subcutaneous tissue medially. They appreciated closed compartments medially and laterally to the hindfoot with

a suggestion that only a plantar incision is required to decompress this space. They recognized that within the intermediate chamber one could cause ischemia with sequelae as the vital structures of the medial and lateral plantar arteries to pass in this zone as well as the branches of the tibial nerve.[3] Faymonville et al. analyzed topographic anatomy by injecting epoxy-resin into 32 cadaveric specimens. They identified six compartments including dorsal, medial, lateral, superficial central, deep forefoot, and deep hindfoot. There was appreciated communication between deep hindfoot, deep forefoot, and superficial central.[4]

Further, vital neurovascular structures were found to pass between the medial and deep hindfoot chambers. In the

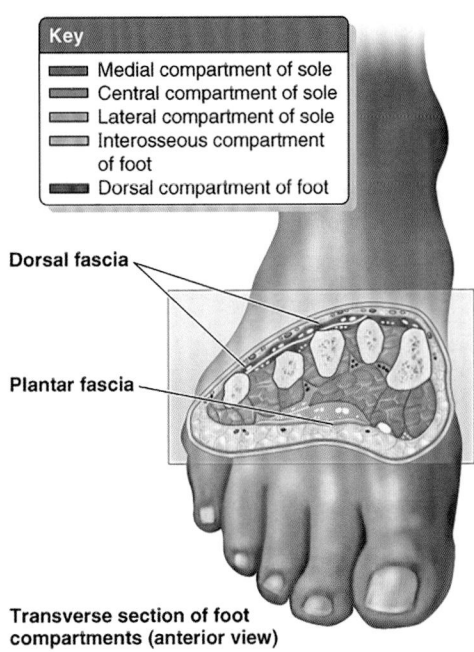

Transverse section of foot compartments (anterior view)

FIGURE 64.6 Proposed foot compartments. (Reproduced with permission from Moore K, Agur A, Dalley A II. *Essential Clinical Anatomy*. Philadelphia, PA: Wolters Kluwer; 2015.)

forefoot, these structures passed through the deep compartment. Finally, it was recognized that the quadratus plantae might be effected in cases of calcaneal fracture with increased compartmental pressure as it resides in the deep central hindfoot. This may explain the sequelae of a calcaneal fracture–induced compartment syndrome of claw toes that will be discussed later in the chapter.

CLINICAL AND DIAGNOSTIC OBSERVATIONS

Nudel et al., utilizing a mathematical model, reported on the challenges of establishing compartment syndrome. Their model quantitatively demonstrated the highly nonuniform build up of intracompartmental pressure based on anatomic location and time.[5] Their work identifies the general observation that the clinical findings of pain, paralysis, and even compartment pressure measurement do not demonstrate reproducible diagnosis of compartment ischemia. With that said, the failure to identify and appropriately manage the condition can result in neurologic impairment, devitalized tissue, loss of function, amputation, and death.

Having a high level of suspicion for the presentation, particularly in the acute presentation, is often prompted by the appreciation of the mechanism of injury to the extremity. Brink et al. performed a retrospective study at a level I trauma center identifying cases of acute compartment syndrome of the foot and described associated mechanisms of injury. Over a 7-year analysis, they identified 31 patients and 33 feet. The majority of cases were identified with high-energy trauma as those seen in vehicular motor accidents, but they did find a 20% incidence associated with low-energy mechanism. In all but one of their cases, foot fracture was noted. There was one case of open

fracture. Interestingly, there seemed to be an equal prevalence of single and multiple injury diagnoses, with 17 and 14 being identified respectively. The majority of fractures associated with acute compartment syndrome involved tarsal bones.[6] Ojike et al., in 2009, performed a systematic review of the literature and found only level IV case series. Within that series, 39 cases of foot compartment syndrome were identified with the most common cause resulting from crush injury.[7] Calcaneal fractures are notable in literature to suffer from this sequelae. Park et al. retrospectively reviewed 303 patients with calcaneal fractures. Logistic regression analysis was used to assess association prediction. The only strongly associated factor was Sanders type IV fracture.[8] Myerson and Manoli suggest a 10% incidence of compartment syndrome in calcaneal fractures. With identified sequelae of claw toe and other deformities in more than half of these patients.[9] These may support the validity of the deep hindfoot chamber as noted by Faymonville et al.

However, there are multiple case reports identified in writing that would not immediately raise the suspicion for acute compartment syndrome. Brandao et al. present a case of bilateral foot compartment syndrome associated with frostbite. Their patient was admitted with thermal ischemia of hallux due to cold exposure and identified gangrene. Increasing rhabdomyolysis without explanation prompted measurement of compartments with the medial demonstrating absolute pressure of >100 mm Hg and dorsally 50 mm Hg.[10] Patil et al. present a case of compartment syndrome of the foot that developed following infection resulting from hydrocortisone injection for plantar fasciitis. It was appreciated that suppurative infection in the deep myofascial compartment prompted pressure-induced ischemia that responded to fasciotomy.[11] For those practitioners intimately involved in the management of the diabetic foot, the concept of infection producing ischemia may not seem foreign, and the performance of urgent/emergent incision and drainage of deep abscesses for tissue preservation is identified. Maharaj et al., speak to this in their publication identifying anatomic compartments of the diabetic foot. They appreciate increased compartment pressures resulting from infection producing rapid necrosis and the need for the scalpel to reduce the risk of sepsis and proximal amputation.[12]

Given the established challenges that do not allow the condition of compartment syndrome to be fitted into a clean model of identification, the clinician must have some parameters that will help formulate an expedient diagnosis as timely treatment is of the essence in acute cases. The hallmark clinical description of the five P's to include pain, paresthesias, poikilothermia (skin temperature change), paralysis, and pulselessness have been appreciated. The pain of passive stretch of muscles within a given compartment is generally accepted as the most sensitive diagnostic finding for the process. Pain is found to be diffuse to the extremity or foot and progressive requiring advancing analgesic agents. Tense swelling of the extremity has been reported by several authors to be a predictor, particularly in foot compartment syndrome (Figs. 64.7 and 64.8). Myerson appreciated this with calcaneal fractures, and Fakouhri and Manoli reported this finding in a small case series of 12 patients. Sensory changes have been found to be nonspecific for the condition with the most specific being loss of two-point discrimination. Motor weakness and the presence or absence

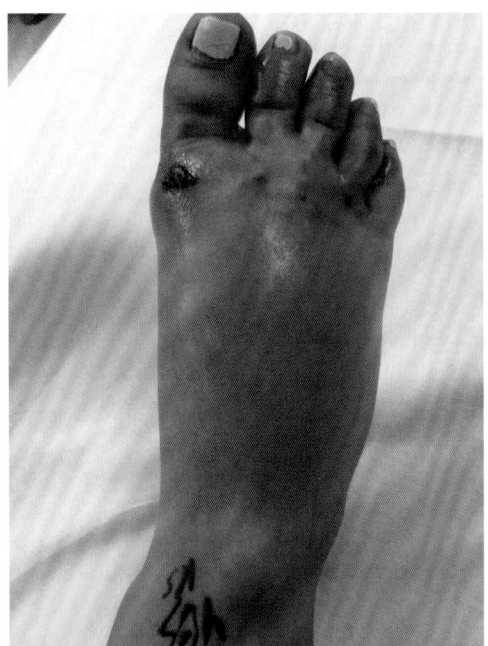

FIGURE 64.7 Preoperative foot compartment syndrome. (Picture courtesy Harry Schneider, DPM.)

of palpable pulses have demonstrated limited predictive value. A serial examination is critical to document any developing changes.

With the difficulty of physical examination alone to identify acute compartment syndrome, most clinicians and authors agree that compartment pressure monitoring is the most reliable and objective measure for the disorder. The threshold of absolute pressure of >30 mm Hg warranting emergent fasciotomy is well established. But is this accurate? This number was based on many uncontrolled studies in the 1970s when the use of a wick catheter was employed to identify intermuscular pressure. This value did come into question as subsequent studies did suggest high false positive with this technique. In the mid-1990s, the Whiteside technique of

subtracting compartment pressure from patient's diastolic pressure became more widely accepted. The thought was the ability of diastolic flow to overcome localized compartment pressure. A value was established again of 30 mm Hg of pressure exceeding or within the patients mean arterial pressure within the compartment would warrant fasciotomy. This would represent perfusion pressure. Nelson in 2013 suggested a false positive rate varying from 18% to 84% using pressure perfusion for tibial fractures.[13]

Commonly used devices for compartment pressure measurements include the Stryker intracompartmental pressure monitor system (Fig. 64.9), arterial line manometer, and the Whiteside apparatus. In a study by Boody and Wongworawat, in 2005, they looked at these devices to determine accuracy. They also looked at variations of catheters and needles employed. They appreciated that side port needles and slit catheters were more accurate than straight needles. They also acknowledged that arterial manometer was most accurate but found appropriate efficacy of the Stryker unit. They presented a concern with the Whiteside apparatus suggesting it lacked precision with two of the three needle configurations overestimating pressure and overall had the highest standards of error.[14]

Besides concerns for the accuracy of the device in establishing a diagnosis of compartment syndrome, there has been a study regarding the introduction of the needles into the appropriate compartments. In a study by Finnoff et al., they looked at two techniques for placement of the catheter into the medial compartment of the foot and relationship to neurovascular structures. In literature, two methods for deployment have been described. The Reach technique uses a side port needle placed medial 6 cm distal to the most prominent portion of the medial malleolus. It is inserted parallel to the plantar surface and advanced 1 cm from medial to lateral. The Mollica technique enters the needle just inferior to medial cuneiform parallel to the plantar surface and again advanced 1 cm from medial to lateral. Looking at 10 cadaver specimens, the authors identified that both approaches entered the medial compartment; however, using the Reach method may be safer as it is further away from the neurovascular bundle.[15]

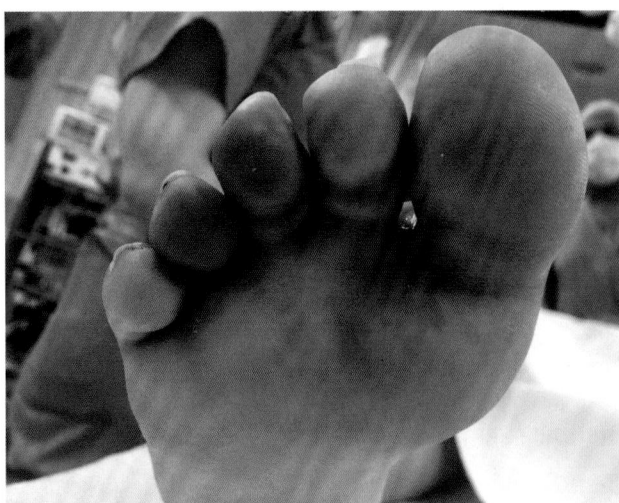

FIGURE 64.8 Cyanosis and progressive ischemia of digits in ACS. (Image courtesy of Harry Schneider, DPM.)

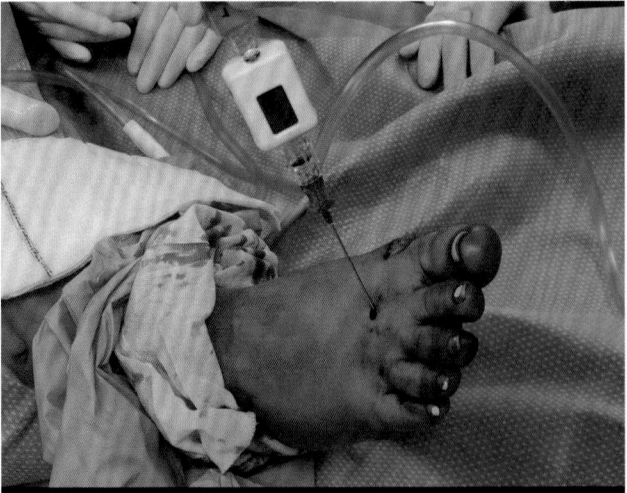

FIGURE 64.9 Use of compartment pressure monitoring device. (Image courtesy of Harry Schneider, DPM.)

In the diagnosis and management of chronic exertional compartment syndrome (CECS), the approach is not dissimilar to the acute. The difference is in the etiology. In chronic cases, its identification must be established by generating similar demand on the muscular compartment.

Methods of Measuring Intracompartmental Pressure

- Catheters of varying type to include commercially available self-contained Stryker device, catheter attached to arterial line attached to manometer, and Whiteside apparatus.
- Absolute pressure of >30 mm Hg warrants emergent fasciotomy.
- Whiteside technique of subtracting compartment pressure from diastolic with concept of ability for diastolic flow to overcome pressure.

With reproducible pain and defining with compartment pressure measuring technique. The real challenge is determining the pain is resulting from increased compartment pressures as the differential diagnosis is varied and is one often of exclusion with advanced negative testing such as imaging, electrophysiologic examinations to rule out other musculoskeletal and neurologic disorders.

Intracompartmental manometry is performed to all four compartments before exercise and at 1 and 5 minutes postactivity. In a report by Pedowitz et al., they retrospectively reviewed 131 patients with 45 having a definition of CECS and 75 being ruled out by intracompartmental pressures. It was appreciated that in the clinical setting of this disorder, the final compartment pressure findings were appreciated: (1) preexercise pressure measurements of ≥15 mm Hg; (2) a 1-minute postexercise pressure of ≥30 mm Hg; and (3) a postexercise pressure after 5 minutes of ≥20 mm Hg.[16] More recently, a systematic review and meta-analysis were performed by Aweid et al. that subjects and controls demonstrated similar elevation of compartment pressures during activity, but there was no overlap at 1-minute postexercise with subjects showing pressures notably more elevated as controls returned to normal. This would suggest that the 5-minute measurement is not necessary to support the diagnosis.[17]

Are there other available tests to assess chronic exertional compartment syndrome? There is a single report utilizing neurosensory testing for recurrent deep posterior compartment syndrome. In this sample of one subject, Williams et al. demonstrated incomplete release of this compartment due to an anatomic variant that was appreciated using noninvasive neurosensory testing. They were able to identify improvement using this examination following repeat release of the compartment before and after treadmill running. They suggest that this study is readily performed without pain to the patient and is sensitive for assessing compartment syndrome when other tests have failed.[18]

In conclusion, the diagnosis of compartment syndrome both acute and chronic relies on high clinical suspicion by the clinician through identification of history, injury mechanism, or in chronic cases documented reproduction of pain, physical examination, and supported use of intracompartment pressure measurement. The failure to identify and appropriately manage this disorder can have significant sequelae in the function of the limb.

PATHOPHYSIOLOGY OF COMPARTMENT SYNDROME

ACUTE COMPARTMENT SYNDROME

Common causes of ACS described by Donaldson include fracture, crush injury, injection injury, penetrating trauma, constrictive dressings, casts, burns, infections, bleeding disorders, arterial injury, reperfusion, and extravasation of drugs.[19]

ACS is defined as a critical pressure increase within a confined compartment space resulting in reduced perfusion pressure to the tissues in the compartment. Tissue perfusion is proportional to the difference between capillary perfusion pressure (CPP) and the interstitial fluid pressure (IFP).[19] Normal CPP is 25-30 mm Hg, and the IFP in resting muscle is 4-8 mm Hg.[20] When fluids enter the compartment, the tissue and venous pressure increases and when this becomes greater than the CPP, the capillaries collapse. This results in reduced oxygenation and builds up of metabolic by-products from the tissue creating ischemia and further edema. This creates a self-perpetuating cycle of edema and ischemia. Any oxygen that is present has to diffuse a further distance through the edema within the tissue to reach cells resulting in further ischemia. Muscles and nerves within the compartment will die after 4-6 hours of anoxia if the complete cessation of blood flow occurs. Therefore, surgical decompression at this point is critical to reducing the risk of tissue damage. Weakness, paralysis, paresthesias, and anesthesia occur with prolonged anoxia, and the sequelae are discussed later in this chapter. In a classic article by Rorabeck, it was noted that almost complete recovery of limb function was achieved if fasciotomy is performed within 6 hours of the injury.[21]

A systemic effect of compartment syndrome is rhabdomyolysis, which occurs as a result of muscle breakdown and release of intracellular molecules including potassium, calcium, phosphate, uric acid, and creatinine kinase (CK). Metabolic acidosis is common, and an increased anion gap may be present. Biomarkers that can be measured include both blood CK levels and urine myoglobin levels in addition to electrolyte measurements. Myoglobin spills into the urine staining it red or brown, and the patient may complain of myalgias and weakness.[22] Long et al. have recently published a review of this process for emergency physicians.[23] It is typically diagnosed with a CK greater than five times the upper limit of normal or >5000 units/L though should be considered in combination with the clinical presentation as there is not an absolute cutoff. In severe cases, this can result in renal failure, electrolyte imbalances, liver injury, and disseminated intravascular coagulation. Acute kidney injury can occur in up to 50%, but the risk is lower if CK is <15-20 000 units/L.[24] Restoring electrolyte balance and fluid support is critical in preventing renal failure in these patients and should be addressed along with surgical decompression of the affected compartments.

CHRONIC EXERTIONAL COMPARTMENT SYNDROME

This form of compartment syndrome is related to overuse in individuals who engage in repetitive physical activities such as running but is not entirely understood. It primarily occurs in the lower extremities and therefore is of interest to this text.

The most commonly affected compartments in the left are anterior > deep posterior > lateral and rarely the superficial posterior compartment. As in ACS, there is an elevation of intramuscular pressure to the point where the compartment becomes tight and painful. This typically resolves with rest. There are some theories that this is due to tighter or thicker fascia, but this remains unclear. Many studies have demonstrated decreased blood flow and oxygenation in the legs of symptomatic patients.[25] Exercise substantially increases blood flow to active muscles. During contractions, intramuscular pressure can exceed 500 mm Hg. Perfusion occurs when the muscle relaxes. If relaxation does not allow for a large enough arterial-venous gradient of at least 30 mm Hg, then perfusion to the compartment is compromised.[26] Initially, there is no permanent damage; however, repetitive incidents can cause ischemia of the involved muscles. If there is significant tissue damage, an inflammatory cascade results in further swelling, which may prevent normalization of pressure and then CECS can become a more emergent syndrome.

Interestingly, there are reports of athletes who develop rhabdomyolysis and subsequently develop compartment syndrome. In a case report, a 22-year-old college football player presented to the ED after a typical leg workout and was found to have rhabdomyolysis but despite systemic supportive therapy, developed worsening thigh pain. Compartmental pressures were tested, and due to an elevation above 30 mm Hg, he was taken to the OR for emergent fasciotomies.[27]

MANAGEMENT OF COMPARTMENT SYNDROME

Immediate treatment of ACS, once identified, involves an emergent release of the involved compartments as soon as possible. Any restrictive dressings should be released immediately. Supportive systemic therapy should be initiated as well including fluid management and maintenance of systemic pressure. The limb should be kept at the level of the heart to prevent further decrease in arterial flow.[28]

According to Donaldson, the principles of performing a fasciotomy include

1. Adequate and extensile incision
2. Complete release of all involved compartments
3. Preservation of vital structures
4. Thorough debridement
5. Skin coverage at a later date within 2 weeks

RELEASE OF LEG COMPARTMENT

A two-incision technique includes a long (20-25 cm) anterolateral incision placed halfway between the tibial crest and the shaft of the fibula over the anterior intermuscular septum. Care must be taken to avoid the superficial peroneal nerve just posterior to the intermuscular septum when making an incision between the two compartments transversely. A medial incision is made 2 cm posterior to the medial tibial border. It must be placed anterior to the posterior tibial artery to avoid injury to the perforating vessels that supply the skin. A skin bridge of >5 cm should be kept between the incisions (Figs. 64.10-64.12). A transverse incision can then be made between the deep and superficial compartments. The soleus may also need to be released from the posterior tibia as well.[29] A single lateral

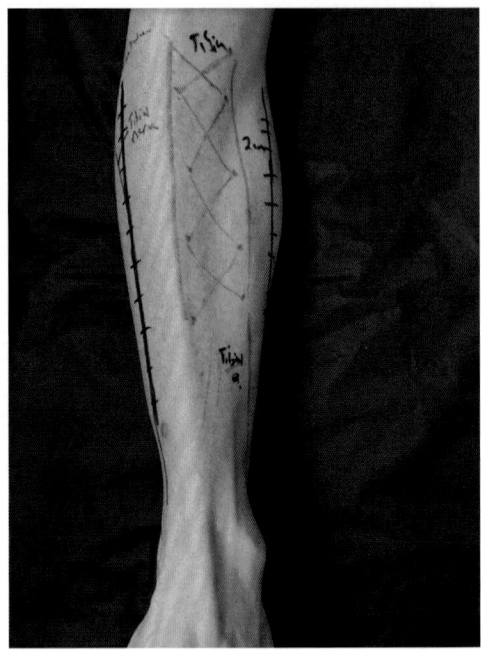

FIGURE 64.10 Dual incision approach for compartments of leg.

incision overlying the fibula has also been described. This can be useful with tibial fractures to help maintain soft tissue stability and provide for a better cosmetic outcome.[30] From this incision, the septum between the anterior and lateral compartments is identified and released taking care to avoid the superficial peroneal nerve. The lateral compartment muscles are elevated from the posterior intramuscular septum to enter the superficial posterior compartment. The deep posterior compartment can be difficult to access and decompress. This involves dividing the origin of the soleus muscle from the fibula to access the deep compartment. Regardless of the method, it is important to make the incisions long enough as the inadequate compartmental release has been well documented with smaller incisions.[31]

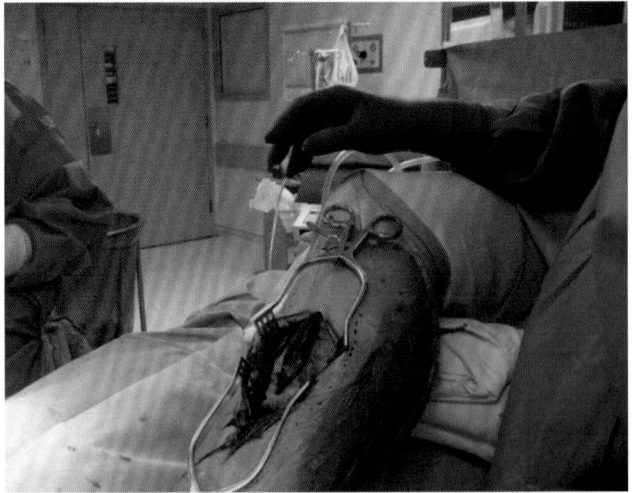

FIGURE 64.11 Exposure to anterior compartment with fasciotomy.

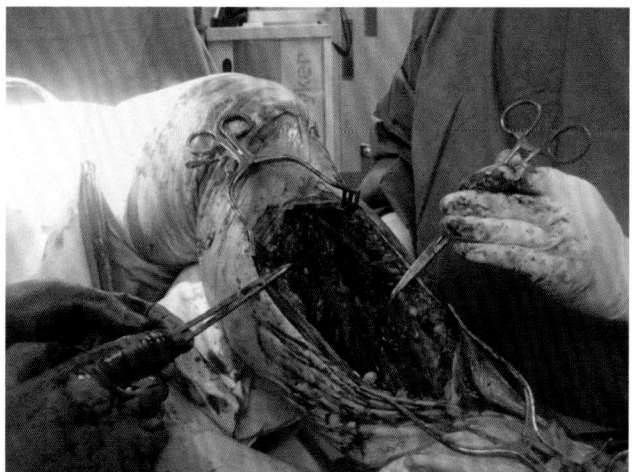

FIGURE 64.12 Posterior compartment approach demonstrating developing myonecrosis of the deep posterior musculature.

RELEASE OF FOOT COMPARTMENTS

Myerson has described a three incision approach, which is commonly used for surgical decompression of the foot[32] (Fig. 64.13). This is based on the nine compartment model by Manoli and Weber. Two dorsal incisions are created overlying the medial aspect of the 2nd metatarsal and the other over the lateral aspect of the 4th metatarsal, maintaining an adequate skin bridge. Superficial fascia is divided, and the interosseous and adductor compartments are released. A medial incision is made starting 4 cm from the posterior aspect of the heel and 3 cm superior to the plantar surface of the foot and is carried distally 6 cm. Following the incision, the fascia of the abductor hallucis muscle is visible and should be split. The abductor muscle is then detached from the fascia and retracted superiorly exposing a fascial layer. Upon incision of this fascia entry and release of the superficial compartment is obtained and the flexor digitorum brevis is retracted inferiorly, and the medial fascia of the lateral compartment is identified. The fascia is then released exposing the abductor digiti quinti and flexor digiti minimi.[1,33] The calcaneal compartment communicates with the deep posterior compartment of the lower leg, and therefore injuries of the calcaneus and tibial fractures may require more proximal decompression in the leg as described above.[9] Also, it may demand a release of the distal tarsal tunnel proximally.[34] An alternative method described by Dunbar et al. is a "pie-crusting" technique where multiple stab incisions are made over the intermetatarsal spaces followed by blunt dissection. This is done to reduce the need for skin grafting, which is often needed following extensive incisions.[35] Stabilization of forefoot or midfoot fractures should be performed at the time of decompression; however, calcaneal fracture management should be delayed until soft tissue swelling has receded.

Wound closure is typically delayed and often requires some type of skin grafting techniques. Dermatotraction using skin staples and elastic cords such as vessel loops is used to gently bring the edges together as the swelling resolves and once the skin margins are within 1 cm delayed primary closure can be performed[36] (Fig. 64.14). Vacuum-assisted wound closure is also used widely and can even be performed from the time of initial decompression and can aid in the reduction of soft tissue edema.[37] Split-thickness skin grafting can then be used for any area they cannot be closed primarily.

In addition to surgical management, there is also a role for hyperbaric oxygen therapy (HBOT). The Undersea and Hyperbaric Medical Society (UHMS) approve the use of HBOT in cases continued edema or ischemic tissue, the unclear demarcation between viable and nonviable tissue, residual neuropathy, or prolonged ischemia time. A total of 1-2 daily HBOT treatments are recommended for up to 7-10 days postfasciotomy.

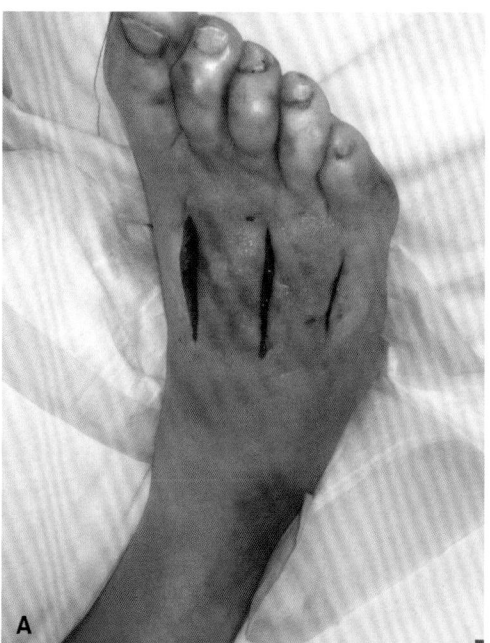
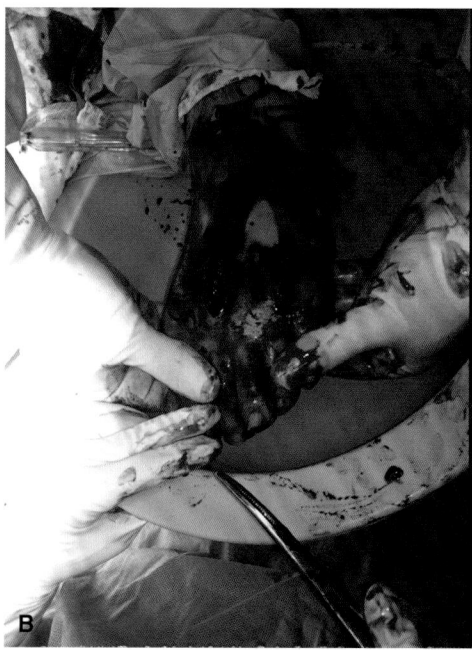

FIGURE 64.13 A, B. Three dorsal incision approach to interosseous compartments of the foot.

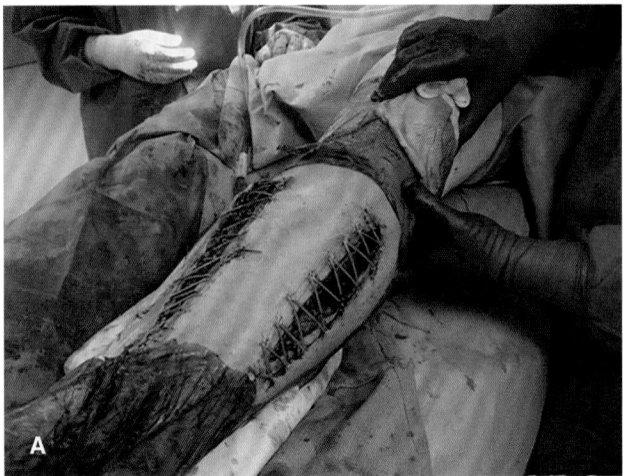
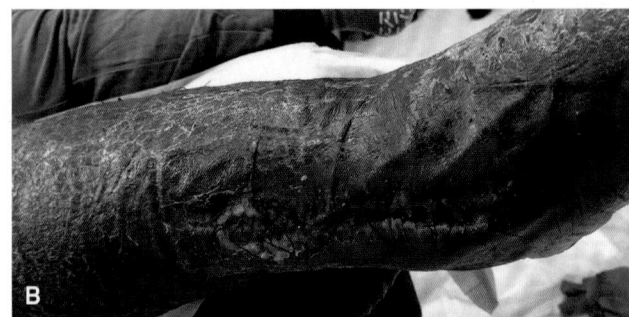

FIGURE 64.14 A, B. Use of vessel loop for early approximation of wounds and return to OR for delayed primary closure.

It increases arterial oxygen pressure increasing perfusion to anoxic tissues. This stimulates angiogenesis and activates fibroblasts and macrophages to aid in wound healing. It also reduces reactive oxygen species in the tissues locally to reduce reperfusion injury.[38]

PERILS and PITFALLS

ANTERIOR COMPARTMENT FASCIOTOMY
- Anterior compartment is one of the most commonly missed during lower extremity fasciotomy.
- Incision is placed either directly on or posterior to the fibula.
- Lateral incision should be made one finger width anterior to the fibular edge to be directly over the septum between the lateral and anterior compartments.

MANAGEMENT OF CHRONIC EXERTIONAL COMPARTMENT SYNDROME

Nonoperative measures in CECS are generally regarded with poor success. Changing activities to reduce the strain of muscles in the compartment can be helpful but generally not well received by the competitive athlete requiring treatment. Massage therapy can have a limited benefit. Blackman et al. studied seven patients with CECS who underwent a 5-week course of leg massage and stretching. Although the patients were able to increase the amount of activity before pain develop, their intracompartmental pressures were not affected and all but one experienced exercise-induced pain.[39] Functional manual therapy has been described in a case study with a triathlete to have success in returning to the desired level of activity without pain, which was maintained 3 years post-treatment.[40]

If a patient wishes to pursue the same level of activity that results in increased compartmental pressure, then surgical intervention can be warranted. Many different techniques are described in the literature to release the involved compartments in CECS. Smaller incisions are typically used over those that are used in the acute setting. Mouhsine et al. describe

an open minimal double incision surgical approach to treat leg CECS in a series of 18 athletes. Two vertical skin incisions are made over the anterior compartment, 15 cm apart. Blunt dissection is performed subcutaneously down to the fascia (Fig. 64.15). The superficial peroneal nerve is identified in the lower incision 10-12 cm proximal to the lateral malleolus. Once this is safely identified and retracted, the anterior and lateral fascial compartments are released with a scissor (Figs. 64.16 and 64.17). The use of an endoscope can also aid in this procedure to allow for smaller skin incisions. A third incision can be used in patients with long extremities. After skin closure, a compression bandage should be applied, and the extremity elevated for 24 hours. Compression should be used for the first 2-3 days following the release and patients are encouraged to begin early range of motion exercises and weight bearing to prevent scarring and adhesions. Physical therapy may also be helpful to improve mobilization. Patients can typically return to sports a mean 25 days after surgery.[41]

Surgical treatment of CECS is generally successful for anterior and lateral compartment releases. Detmer et al. demonstrated 90% improvement following fasciotomy,[42] and Styf and Korner had 95% good results after anterior compartment fasciotomy.[43] Schepsis et al. had excellent results in 96% of patients with anterior compartment release; however, 35% of patients had unsatisfactory results after fasciotomy for deep posterior compartment syndrome.[44] A retrospective review of military personnel who underwent surgical release for CECS by Waterman et al. in 2013 found that 44.7% of the patients suffered from a recurrence of their symptoms.[45] Complications from the surgical release can include infection, nerve injury, wound dehiscence, and development of seroma or hematoma, scar tissue, and recurrence; therefore, proceeding with surgical intervention should be well thought out and discussed at length with the patient before proceeding.

SEQUELAE OF COMPARTMENT SYNDROME

A variety of clinical presentations may develop resulting from ischemic contracture of the lower extremities. Deformity and functional impact are determined by compartments impacted and degree of nerve injury. Follow-up care is established in an

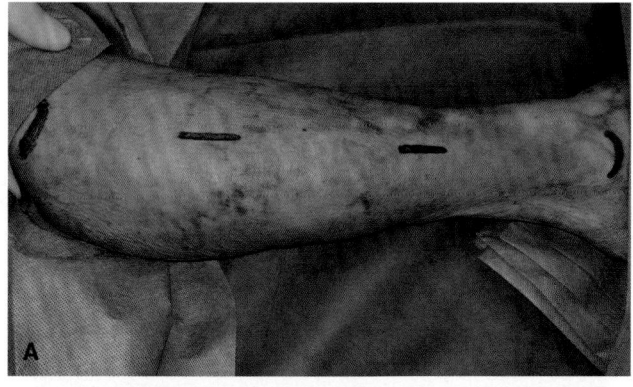

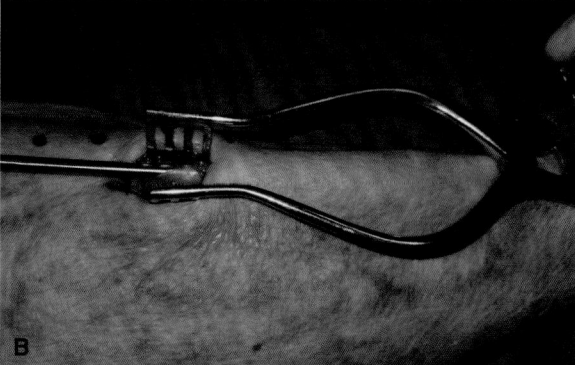

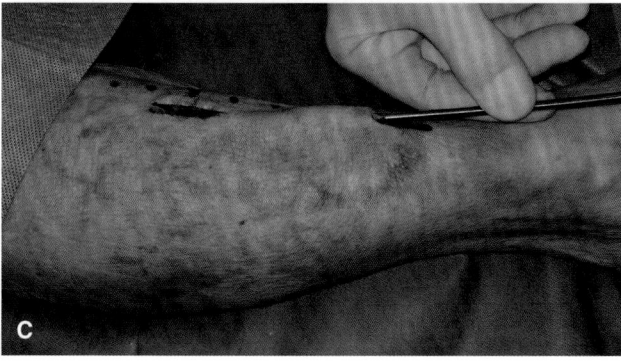

FIGURE 64.15 A-C. Two incision approach. (Pictures courtesy of Ron Ray, DPM.)

algorithmic fashion to include the performance of any necessary nerve releases or decompression, soft tissue releases, and osseous procedures for more rigid consequences to include reconstructive osteotomy and arthrodesis. In severe refractory cases, amputation of the limb is an available option.

In 2009, Kashuk et al. published a prospective review of lower extremity compartment syndrome. This was conducted at an academic level 1 trauma center. Over 7 years, variables to include demographics, injury mechanism, tissue death, amputation, and mortality were considered. The authors hypothesized that delayed diagnosis leading to limb loss was a preventable event. In their sample of 83 patients, 7 patients were to have had a late diagnosis, without the performance of compartment measures, resulting in muscle necrosis requiring multiple surgical debridements, wound closure issues, and long-term disability.[46] In the United Kingdom, the trauma society of the British Orthopaedic Association

established national guidelines for ACS in 2014. Attempting to assess the efficacy of this guideline, Bodansky et al. retrospectively looked at data from four major trauma centers over 5 years. Seventy-five patients were identified. Unfortunately, the guidelines did not improve time to surgery, time to the second visit, or identifying clinical findings. Twenty-one patients had severe complications that included one death and four amputations. Complications also included nine individuals with chronic pain to include six permanent nerve injuries and three chronic regional pain syndromes.[47] In 2016, Glass et al. performed a systematic review of controlled trials. They identified nine studies that met criteria. Fifty-seven patients and 64 limbs were investigated. Overall study quality was considered "very low" with one study considered "low." It was appreciated that delayed compartment decompression, more than 6 hours to time of surgery, yielded outcomes of 19 limb amputations, two deaths, and most surviving limbs having functional

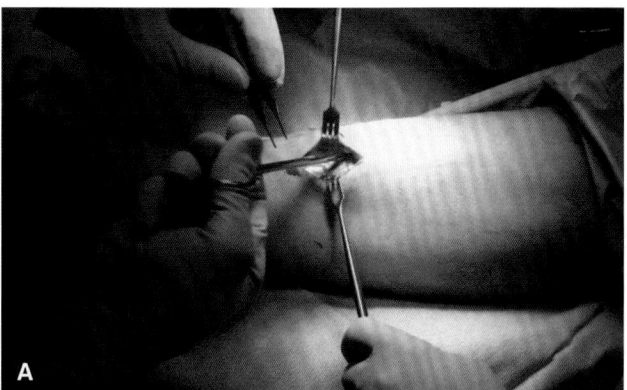

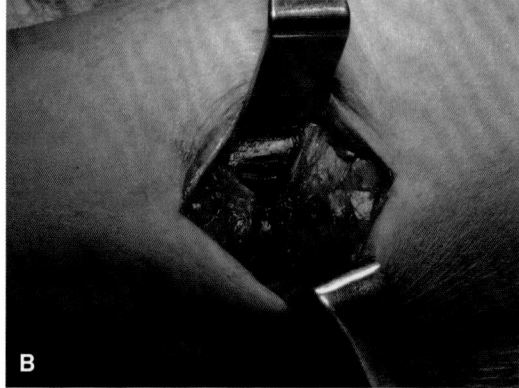

FIGURE 64.16 A, B. Small anterolateral incision with septal separation of the anterior and lateral muscle groups.

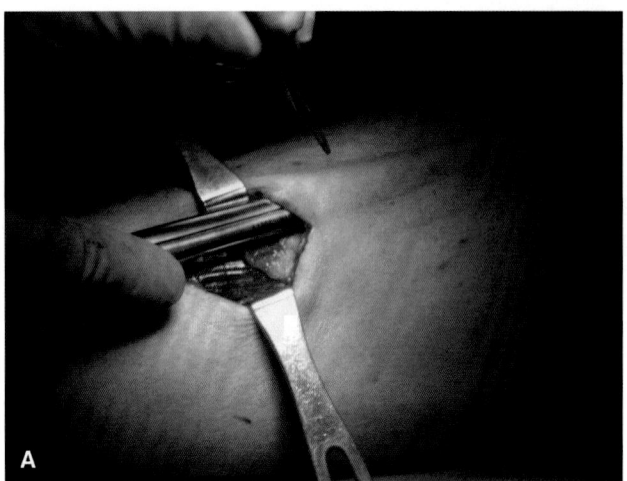 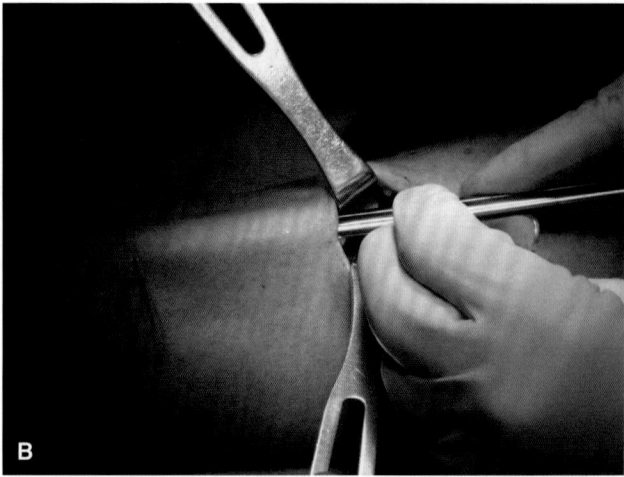

FIGURE 64.17 A, B. Incising with scissors cephalad and caudal to ensure full release of the compartment.

deficits.[48] Lollo and Grabinsky also appreciated risk for kidney injury in their sample of 124 patients. They identified its mean peak serum CK levels of 58 600 units/mL. Their study produced a limb amputation rate of 12.9%, foot numbness in 20.5%, and drop foot in 18.2%. Long-term follow-up confirmed patients with moderate residual lower extremity pain of 10.2% and only 69.2% returned to work.[49]

In a prospective study looking at outcomes and quality of life following foot fasciotomy for acute presentation, Han et al. reviewed 14 patients over an average of 24 months. Two patients developed claw toe deformities, three patients had residual sensory deficits, and four required orthoses or shoe modification to ambulate comfortably. In a report managing long-term sequelae to lower extremity compartment syndrome, Lintz et al. reviewed a 25-year period identifying 151 patients. Of these, 10 required subsequent foot and ankle surgery to relieve acquired deformities. It was appreciated that most developed an acquired equinus with the need for posterior release to include soft tissue lengthening and three necessitated significant hindfoot fusion.[50]

Chronic exertional compartment syndrome is more challenging to define identified sequelae other than the inability to resume desired activity athletic or work. Clearly, lifestyle modification may achieve relief of this process, but this may not be desirable or acceptable to the individual. There is an adequate amount of literature generated from the military community looking at exertional compartment syndrome of the lower extremity and foot. It is appreciated the demand on the lower extremities in the performance of their duties and the relatively high frequency of leg pain attributed to this disorder. A large sample of 611 patients with 754 surgical procedures was reported by Waterman et al. in a military population. They demonstrated that more than three-quarters of the surgeries were executed on the anterior and lateral compartments of the leg. Symptom recurrence was identified in 44.7% of the patients, and 27.7% were unable to return to full duty.[45] Packer et al. hypothesized in their report that higher preoperative compartment measures would generate improved outcomes of satisfaction with fasciotomy. In their cohort, a nonoperative sample of 27 patients and an operative sample of 73 patients were presented. The mean follow-up was 5.6 and 5.2 years, respectively. The operative

group demonstrated higher success and satisfaction rates. They could not identify the correlation of compartment pressures. The authors did appreciate a higher failure rate when both anterior and lateral compartments were released.[51] The efficacy for decompression of the deep posterior compartment remains challenged in available literature and outcomes suggested. In 2014, Winkes et al. performed a systematic review. They identified seven studies of level III evidence and 131 patients meeting criteria. Only four studies met intracompartmental pressure requirements. Multiple surgical procedures were entertained with no one method demonstrating superiority. Success rates were modest from 30% to 65% with higher ICP proving a greater success. Factors that would influence outcome particularly failure were not identified.[52] Finally, the entity of acute on chronic exertional compartment syndrome is suggested by a case report written by Popovic et al. in 2011. The authors present a recreational soccer player with sequelae of foot drop necessitating peroneal longus tendon transfer.[53]

Both acute and chronic compartment syndrome require a high level of suspicion by the treating physician supported by well-established history, physical findings, and supported by quantitative measuring of intracompartment pressures. Given the devastating consequences associated with failure to identify this injury process, it is imperative that timely identification and emergent decompression in the acute setting is performed.

REFERENCES

1. Manoli A II, Weber TG. Fasciotomy of the foot: an anatomical study with special reference to release of the calcaneal compartment. *Foot Ankle.* 1990;10(5):267-275.
2. Reach JS Jr, Amrami KK, Felmlee JP, Stanley DW, Alcorn JM, Turner NS. The compartments of the foot: a 3-tesla magnetic resonance imaging study with clinical correlates for needle pressure testing. *Foot Ankle Int.* 2007;28(5):584-594.
3. Ling ZX, Kumar VP. The myofascial compartments of the foot: a cadaver study. *J Bone Joint Surg Br.* 2008;90(8):1114-1118.
4. Faymonville C, Andermahr J, Seidel U, et al. Compartments of the foot: topographic anatomy. *Surg Radiol Anat.* 2012;34(10):929-933.
5. Nudel I, Dorfmann L, deBotton G. The compartment syndrome: is the intra-compartment pressure a reliable indicator for early diagnosis? *Math Med Biol.* 2017;34(4):547-558.
6. Brink F, Bachmann S, Lechler P, Frink M. Mechanism of injury and treatment of trauma-associated acute compartment syndrome of the foot. *Eur J Trauma Emerg Surg.* 2014;40(5):529-533.
7. Ojike NI, Roberts CS, Giannoudis PV. Foot compartment syndrome: a systematic review of the literature. *Acta Orthop Belg.* 2009;75(5):573-580.

8. Park YH, Lee JW, Hong JY, Choi GW, Kim HJ. Predictors of compartment syndrome of the foot after fracture of the calcaneus. *Bone Joint J.* 2018;100-b(3):303-308.

9. Myerson M, Manoli A. Compartment syndromes of the foot after calcaneal fractures. *Clin Orthop Relat Res.* 1993;(290):142-150.

10. Brandao RA, St John JM, Langan TM, Schneekloth BJ, Burns PR. Acute compartment syndrome of the foot due to frostbite: literature review and case report. *J Foot Ankle Surg.* 2018;57(2):382-387.

11. Patil SD, Patil VD, Abane S, Luthra R, Ranaware A. Acute compartment syndrome of the foot due to infection after local hydrocortisone injection: a case report. *J Foot Ankle Surg.* 2015;54(4):692-696.

12. Maharaj D, Bahadursingh S, Shah D, Chang BB, Darling RC III. Sepsis and the scalpel: anatomic compartments and the diabetic foot. *Vasc Endovascular Surg.* 2005;39(5):421-423.

13. Nelson JA. Compartment pressure measurements have poor specificity for compartment syndrome in the traumatized limb. *J Emerg Med.* 2013;44(5):1039-1044.

14. Boody AR, Wongworawat MD. Accuracy in the measurement of compartment pressures: a comparison of three commonly used devices. *J Bone Joint Surg Am.* 2005;87(11):2415-2422.

15. Finnoff JT, Henning PT, Cederholm SK, Hollman JH. Accuracy of medial foot compartment pressure testing: a comparison of two techniques. *Foot Ankle Int.* 2010;31(11):1001-1005.

16. Pedowitz RA, Hargens AR, Mubarak SJ, Gershuni DH. Modified criteria for the objective diagnosis of chronic compartment syndrome of the leg. *Am J Sports Med.* 1990;18(1):35-40.

17. Aweid O, Del Buono A, Malliaras P, et al. Systematic review and recommendations for intracompartmental pressure monitoring in diagnosing chronic exertional compartment syndrome of the leg. *Clin J Sport Med.* 2012;22(4):356-370.

18. Williams EH, Detmer DE, Guyton GP, Dellon AL. Non-invasive neurosensory testing used to diagnose and confirm successful surgical management of lower extremity deep distal posterior compartment syndrome. *J Brachial Plex Peripher Nerve Inj.* 2009;4:4.

19. Donaldson J, Haddad B, Khan WS. The pathophysiology, diagnosis, and current management of acute compartment syndrome. *Open Orthop J.* 2014;(M8):185-193.

20. Wattel F, Mathieu D, Neviere R, Bocquillon N. Acute peripheral ischaemia and compartment syndromes: a role for hyperbaric oxygenation. *Anaesthesia.* 1998;53(suppl 2):63-65.

21. Rorabeck CH, Clarke KM. The pathophysiology of the anterior tibial compartment syndrome: an experimental investigation. *J Trauma.* 1978;18(5):299-304.

22. Giannoglou GD, Chatzizisis YS, Misirli G. The syndrome of rhabdomyolysis: pathophysiology and diagnosis. *Eur J Intern Med.* 2007;18(2):90-100.

23. Long B, Koyfman A, Gottlieb M. An evidence-based narrative review of the emergency department evaluation and management of rhabdomyolysis. *Am J Emerg Med.* 2019;37(3):518-523.

24. Bosch X, Poch E, Grau JM. Rhabdomyolysis and acute kidney injury. *N Engl J Med.* 2009;361(1):62-72.

25. Mohler LR, Styf JR, Pedowitz RA, Hargens AR, Gershuni DH. Intramuscular deoxygenation during exercise in patients who have chronic anterior compartment syndrome of the leg. *J Bone Joint Surg Am.* 1997;79(6):844-849.

26. Dunn JC, Waterman BR. Chronic exertional compartment syndrome of the leg in the military. *Clin Sports Med.* 2014;33(4):693-705.

27. Bhalla MC, Dick-Perez R. Exercise induced rhabdomyolysis with compartment syndrome and renal failure. *Case Rep Emerg Med.* 2014;2014:735820.

28. Matsen FA III, Wyss CR, Krugmire RB Jr, Simmons CW, King RV. The effects of limb elevation and dependency on local arteriovenous gradients in normal human limbs with particular reference to limbs with increased tissue pressure. *Clin Orthop Relat Res.* 1980;(150):187-195.

29. Shadgan B, Menon M, Sanders D, et al. Current thinking about acute compartment syndrome of the lower extremity. *Can J Surg.* 2010;53(5):329-334.

30. DeLee JC, Stiehl JB. Open tibia fracture with compartment syndrome. *Clin Orthop Relat Res.* 1981;(160):175-184.

31. Jensen SL, Sandermann J. Compartment syndrome and fasciotomy in vascular surgery. A review of 57 cases. *Eur J Vasc Endovasc Surg.* 1997;13(1):48-53.

32. Myerson M. Diagnosis and treatment of compartment syndrome of the foot. *Orthopedics.* 1990;13(7):711-717.

33. Fulkerson E, Razi A, Tejwani N. Review: acute compartment syndrome of the foot. *Foot Ankle Int.* 2003;24(2):180-187.

34. Myerson MS. Management of compartment syndromes of the foot. *Clin Orthop Relat Res.* 1991;(271):239-248.

35. Dunbar RP, Taitsman LA, Sangeorzan BJ, Hansen ST Jr. Technique tip: use of "pie crusting" of the dorsal skin in severe foot injury. *Foot Ankle Int.* 2007;28(7):851-853.

36. Janzing HM, Broos PL. Dermatotraction: an effective technique for the closure of fasciotomy wounds: a preliminary report of fifteen patients. *J Orthop Trauma.* 2001;15(6):438-441.

37. Zannis J, Angobaldo J, Marks M, et al. Comparison of fasciotomy wound closures using traditional dressing changes and the vacuum-assisted closure device. *Ann Plast Surg.* 2009;62(4):407-409.

38. Strauss MB. The effect of hyperbaric oxygen in crush injuries and skeletal muscle-compartment syndromes. *Undersea Hyperb Med.* 2012;39(4):847-855.

39. Blackman PG, Simmons LR, Crossley KM. Treatment of chronic exertional anterior compartment syndrome with massage: a pilot study. *Clin J Sport Med.* 1998;8(1):14-17.

40. Collins CK, Gilden B. A non-operative approach to the management of chronic exertional compartment syndrome in a triathlete: a case report. *Int J Sports Phys Ther.* 2016;11(7):1160-1176.

41. Mouhsine E, Garofalo R, Moretti B, Gremion G, Akiki A. Two minimal incision fasciotomy for chronic exertional compartment syndrome of the lower leg. *Knee Surg Sports Traumatol Arthrosc.* 2006;14(2):193-197.

42. Detmer DE, Sharpe K, Sufit RL, Girdley FM. Chronic compartment syndrome: diagnosis, management, and outcomes. *Am J Sports Med.* 1985;13(3):162-170.

43. Styf JR, Korner LM. Chronic anterior-compartment syndrome of the leg. Results of treatment by fasciotomy. *J Bone Joint Surg Am.* 1986;68(9):1338-1347.

44. Schepsis AA, Martini D, Corbett M. Surgical management of exertional compartment syndrome of the lower leg. Long-term followup. *Am J Sports Med.* 1993;21(6):811-817; discussion 817.

45. Waterman BR, Laughlin M, Kilcoyne K, Cameron KL, Owens BD. Surgical treatment of chronic exertional compartment syndrome of the leg: failure rates and postoperative disability in an active patient population. *J Bone Joint Surg Am.* 2013;95(7):592-596.

46. Kashuk JL, Moore EE, Pinski S, et al. Lower extremity compartment syndrome in the acute care surgery paradigm: safety lessons learned. *Patient Saf Surg.* 2009;3(1):11.

47. Bodansky D, Doorgakant A, Alsousou J, et al. Acute compartment syndrome: do guidelines for diagnosis and management make a difference? *Injury.* 2018;49(9):1699-1702.

48. Glass GE, Staruch RM, Simmons J, et al. Managing missed lower extremity compartment syndrome in the physiologically stable patient: a systematic review and lessons from a Level I trauma center. *J Trauma Acute Care Surg.* 2016;81(2):380-387.

49. Lollo L, Grabinsky A. Clinical and functional outcomes of acute lower extremity compartment syndrome at a Major Trauma Hospital. *Int J Crit Illn Inj Sci.* 2016;6(3):133-142.

50. Han F, Daruwalla ZJ, Shen L, Kumar VP. A prospective study of surgical outcomes and quality of life in severe foot trauma and associated compartment syndrome after fasciotomy. *J Foot Ankle Surg.* 2015;54(3):417-423.

51. Packer JD, Day MS, Nguyen JT, Hobart SJ, Hannafin JA, Metzl JD. Functional outcomes and patient satisfaction after fasciotomy for chronic exertional compartment syndrome. *Am J Sports Med.* 2013;41(2):430-436.

52. Winkes MB, Hoogeveen AR, Scheltinga MR. Is surgery effective for deep posterior compartment syndrome of the leg? A systematic review. *Br J Sports Med.* 2014;48(22):1592-1598.

53. Popovic N, Bottoni C, Cassidy C. Unrecognized acute exertional compartment syndrome of the leg and treatment. *Acta Orthop Belg.* 2011;77(2):265-269.

SUGGESTED READINGS

Ascer E, Strauch B, Calligaro KD, Gupta SK, Veith FJ. Ankle and foot fasciotomy: an adjunctive technique to optimize limb salvage after revascularization for acute ischemia. *J Vasc Surg.* 1989;9(4):594-597.

Balius R, Bong DA, Ardevol J, Pedret C, Codina D, Dalmau A. Ultrasound-guided fasciotomy for anterior chronic exertional compartment syndrome of the leg. *J Ultrasound Med.* 2016;35(4):823-829. doi: 10.7863/ultra.15.04058.

Barshes NR, Pisimisis G, Kougias P. Compartment syndrome of the foot associated with a delayed presentation of acute limb ischemia. *J Vasc Surg.* 2016;63(3):819-822. doi: 10.1016/j.jvs.2015.01.043.

Bartolomei FJ, Colley JO III. Compartment syndrome. A dorsal pedal presentation. *J Am Podiatr Med Assoc.* 1989;79(3):139-141. doi: 10.7547/87507315-79-3-139.

Bedigrew KM, Stinner DJ, Kragh JF Jr, Potter BK, Shawen SB, Hsu JR. Effectiveness of foot fasciotomies in foot and ankle trauma. *J R Army Med Corps.* 2017;163(5):324-328. doi: 10.1136/jramc-2016-000734.

Blacklidge DK, Kurek JB, Soto AD, Kissel CG. Acute exertional compartment syndrome of the medial foot. *J Foot Ankle Surg.* 1996;35(1):19-22.

Bong MR, Polatsch DB, Jazrawi LM, Rokito AS. Chronic exertional compartment syndrome: diagnosis and management. *Bull Hosp Jt Dis.* 2005;62(3-4):77-84.

Botte MJ, Santi MD, Prestianni CA, Abrams RA. Ischemic contracture of the foot and ankle: principles of management and prevention. *Orthopedics.* 1996;19(3):235-244.

Brewer RB, Gregory AJ. Chronic lower leg pain in athletes: a guide for the differential diagnosis, evaluation, and treatment. *Sports Health.* (2012);4(2):121-127. doi: 10.1177/1941738111426115.

Brey JM, Castro MD. Salvage of compartment syndrome of the leg and foot. *Foot Ankle Clin.* 2008;13(4):767-772. doi: 10.1016/j.fcl.2008.08.003.

Burrus MT, Werner BC, Starman JS, et al. Chronic leg pain in athletes. *Am J Sports Med.* 2015;43(6):1538-1547. doi: 10.1177/0363546514545859.

Campano D, Robaina JA, Kusnezov N, Dunn JC, Waterman BR. Surgical management for chronic exertional compartment syndrome of the leg: a systematic review of the literature. *Arthroscopy.* 2016;32(7):1478-1486. doi: 10.1016/j.arthro.2016.01.069.

Cortina J, Amat C, Selga J, Corona PS. Isolated medial foot compartment syndrome after ankle sprain. *Foot Ankle Surg.* 2014;20(1):e1-e2. doi: 10.1016/j.fas.2013.08.006.

D'Abarno A, Bhimji SS. Anatomy, bony pelvis and lower limb, leg lateral compartment. In: *StatPearls.* Treasure Island, FL: StatPearls Publishing LLC; 2018.

Dayton P, Goldman FD, Barton E. Compartment pressure in the foot. Analysis of normal values and measurement technique. *J Am Podiatr Med Assoc.* 1990;80(10):521-525. doi: 10.7547/87507315-80-10-521.

Dodd A, Le I. Foot compartment syndrome: diagnosis and management. *J Am Acad Orthop Surg.* 2013;21(11):657-664. doi: 10.5435/jaaos-21-11-657.

Edwards PH Jr, Wright ML, Hartman JF. A practical approach for the differential diagnosis of chronic leg pain in the athlete. *Am J Sports Med.* 2005;33(8):1241-1249. doi: 10.1177/0363546505278305.

Fakhouri AJ, Manoli A II. Acute foot compartment syndromes. *J Orthop Trauma.* 1992;6(2):223-228.

Frink M, Klaus AK, Kuther G, et al. Long term results of compartment syndrome of the lower limb in polytraumatised patients. *Injury.* 2007;38(5):607-613. doi: 10.1016/j.injury.2006.12.021.

Fronek J, Mubarak SJ, Hargens AR, et al. Management of chronic exertional anterior compartment syndrome of the lower extremity. *Clin Orthop Relat Res.* 1987;(220):217-227.

Furulund OK, Hove LM. [Acute compartment syndrome—a clinical follow-up study]. *Tidsskr Nor Laegeforen.* 2000;120(28):3380-3382.

Gaines RJ, Randall CJ, Browne KL, Carr DR, Enad JG. Delayed presentation of compartment syndrome of the proximal lower extremity after low-energy trauma in patients taking warfarin. *Am J Orthop (Belle Mead NJ).* 2008;37(12):E201-E204.

Gajanan K, Kannan RY, Brotherston MT. Foot compartment syndrome. *J Trauma.* 2010;68(5):E117. doi: 10.1097/TA.0b013e31815eb17d.

Gerow G, Matthews B, Jahn W, Gerow R. Compartment syndrome and shin splints of the lower leg. *J Manipulative Physiol Ther.* 1993;16(4):245-252.

Gill CS, Halstead ME, Matava MJ. Chronic exertional compartment syndrome of the leg in athletes: evaluation and management. *Phys Sportsmed.* 2010;38(2):126-132. doi: 10.3810/psm.2010.06.1791.

Goldman FD, Dayton PD, Hanson CJ. Compartment syndrome of the foot. *J Foot Surg.* 1990;29(1):37-43.

Grewal SS, Amrami KK, Murthy NS, Spinner, RJ. The importance of normal pressures in the compartment of the leg. *Clin Anat.* 2017;30(8):1002-1004. doi: 10.1002/ca.22975.

Guyton GP, Shearman CM, Saltzman CL. The compartments of the foot revisited. Rethinking the validity of cadaver infusion experiments. *J Bone Joint Surg Br.* 2001;83(2):245-249.

Heckman JD, Champine MJ. New techniques in the management of foot trauma. *Clin Orthop Relat Res.* 1989;(240):105-114.

Hessmann MH, Ingelfinger P, Rommens PM. Compartment syndrome of the lower extremity. *Eur J Trauma Emerg Surg.* 2007;33(6):589-599. doi: 10.1007/s00068-007-7161-y.

Hill CE, Modi CS, Baraza N, Mosleh-Shirazi MS, Dhukaram V. Spontaneous compartment syndrome of the foot. *J Bone Joint Surg Br.* 2011;93(9):1282-1284. doi: 10.1302/0301-620x.93b9.27377.

Hutchinson MR, Ireland ML. Common compartment syndromes in athletes. Treatment and rehabilitation. *Sports Med.* 1994;17(3):200-208. doi: 10.2165/00007256-199417030-00006.

Kemp MA, Barnes JR, Thorpe PL, Williams JL. Avulsion of the perforating branch of the peroneal artery secondary to an ankle sprain: a cause of acute compartment syndrome in the leg. *J Foot Ankle Surg.* 2011;50(1):102-103. doi: 10.1053/j.jfas.2010.09.003.

Kiel J, Kaiser K. Tibial anterior compartment syndrome. In: *StatPearls.* Treasure Island, FL: StatPearls Publishing LLC; 2018.

Kinner B, Tietz S, Muller F, Prantl L, Nerlich M, Roll C. Outcome after complex trauma of the foot. *J Trauma.* 2011;70(1):159-168; discussion 168. doi: 10.1097/TA.0b013e3181fef5eb.

Knape JT. [Missed acute compartment syndrome of the lower leg]. *Ned Tijdschr Geneeskd.* 2005;149(5):268; author reply 268-269.

Krticka M, Ira D, Bilik A, Rotschein P, Svancara J. Fasciotomy closure using negative pressure wound therapy in lower leg compartment syndrome. *Bratisl Lek Listy.* 2016;117(12):710-714. doi: 10.4149/bll_2016_136.

Laframboise MA, Muir B. Acute compartment syndrome of the foot in a soccer player: a case report. *J Can Chiropr Assoc.* 2011;55(4):302-312.

Larsen MH, Nielsen HT, Wester JU. [Compartment syndrome of the lower part of the leg, exceptional trauma mechanism]. *Ugeskr Laeger.* 2003;165(27):2751-2752.

Lavery KP, Bernazzani M, McHale K, Rossy W, Oh L, Theodore G. Mini-open posterior compartment release for chronic exertional compartment syndrome of the leg. *Arthrosc Tech.* 2017;6(3):e649-e653. doi: 10.1016/j.eats.2017.01.010.

Lee BY, Guerra J, Civelek B. Compartment syndrome in the diabetic foot. *Adv Wound Care.* 1995;8(6):36, 38, 41-42 passim.

Lewis J, Mendicino RW, Mendicino SS. Compartment syndromes causing neuropathy. *Clin Podiatr Med Surg.* 1994;11(4):593-608.

Lintz F, Colombier JA, Letenneur J, Gouin F. Management of long-term sequelae of compartment syndrome involving the foot and ankle. *Foot Ankle Int.* 2009;30(9):847-853. doi: 10.3113/fai.2009.0847.

Lohrer H, Malliaropoulos N, Korakakis V, Padhiar N. Exercise-induced leg pain in athletes: diagnostic, assessment, and management strategies. *Phys Sportsmed.* 2019;47(1):47-59. doi: 10.1080/00913847.2018.1537861.

Lueders DR, Sellon JL, Smith J, Finnoff JT. Ultrasound-guided fasciotomy for chronic exertional compartment syndrome: a cadaveric investigation. *PM R.* 2017;9(7):683-690. doi: 10.1016/j.pmrj.2016.09.002.

Lui TH. Endoscopic fasciotomy of the superficial and deep posterior compartments of the leg. *Arthrosc Tech.* 2017;6(3):e711-e715. doi: 10.1016/j.eats.2017.01.019.

Mallik K, Diduch DR. Acute noncontact compartment syndrome. *J Orthop Trauma.* 2000;14(7):509-510.

Manista GC, Dennis A, Kaminsky M. Surgical management of compartment syndrome and the gradual closure of a fasciotomy wound using a DermaClose device. *Trauma Case Rep.* 2018;14:1-4. doi: 10.1016/j.tcr.2017.10.003.

Manoli A II. Compartment syndromes of the foot: current concepts. *Foot Ankle.* 1990;10(6):340-344.

Mar GJ, Barrington MJ, McGuirk BR. Acute compartment syndrome of the lower limb and the effect of postoperative analgesia on diagnosis. *Br J Anaesth.* 2009;102(1):3-11. doi: 10.1093/bja/aen330.

McKeag DB, Dolan C, Garrick JG. Overuse syndromes of the lower extremity. *Phys Sportsmed.* 1989;17(7):108-123. doi: 10.1080/00913847.1989.11709830.

Middleton S, Clasper J. Compartment syndrome of the foot—implications for military surgeons. *J R Army Med Corps.* 2010;156(4):241-244.

Mitchell IR, Meyer C, Krueger WA. Deep fascia of the foot. Anatomical and clinical considerations. *J Am Podiatr Med Assoc.* 1991;81(7):373-378. doi: 10.7547/87507315-81-7-373.

Mittlmeier T, Machler G, Lob G, Mutschler W, Bauer G, Vogl T. Compartment syndrome of the foot after intraarticular calcaneal fracture. *Clin Orthop Relat Res.* 1991;(269):241-248.

Moyer RA, Boden BP, Marchetto PA, Kleinbart F, Kelly JDt. Acute compartment syndrome of the lower extremity secondary to noncontact injury. *Foot Ankle.* 1993;14(9):534-537.

Murdock M, Murdoch MM. Compartment syndrome: a review of the literature. *Clin Podiatr Med Surg.* 2012;29(2):301-310, viii. doi: 10.1016/j.cpm.2012.02.001.

Myerson MS, Berger BI. Isolated medial compartment syndrome of the foot: a case report. *Foot Ankle Int.* 1996;17(3):183-185. doi: 10.1177/107110079601700313.

Owen C, Cavalcanti A, Molina V, Honore C. Decompressive fasciotomy for acute compartment syndrome of the leg. *J Visc Surg.* 2016;153(4):293-296. doi: 10.1016/j.jviscsurg.2016.05.013.

Perry MD, Manoli A II. Foot compartment syndrome. *Orthop Clin North Am.* 2001;32(1):103-111.

Raikin SM, Rapuri VR, Vitanzo P. Bilateral simultaneous fasciotomy for chronic exertional compartment syndrome. *Foot Ankle Int.* 2005;26(12):1007-1011. doi: 10.1177/107110070502601201.

Ramanujam CL, Wade J, Selbst B, Belczyk R, Zgonis T. Recurrent acute compartment syndrome of the foot following a calcaneal fracture repair. *Clin Podiatr Med Surg.* 2010;27(3):469-474. doi: 10.1016/j.cpm.2010.03.005.

Roberts CS, Gorczyca JT, Ring D, Pugh KJ. Diagnosis and treatment of less common compartment syndromes of the upper and lower extremities: current evidence and best practices. *Instr Course Lect.* 2011;60:43-50.

Schubert AG. Exertional compartment syndrome: review of the literature and proposed rehabilitation guidelines following surgical release. *Int J Sports Phys Ther.* 2011;6(2):126-141.

Sellei RM, Hildebrand F, Pape HC. [Acute extremity compartment syndrome: current concepts in diagnostics and therapy]. *Unfallchirurg.* 2014;117(7):633-649. doi: 10.1007/s00113-014-2610-7.

Sharma AK, Sharaf I, Ajay S. Compartment syndrome of the foot in a child. *Med J Malaysia.* 2001;56(suppl C):70-72.

Shaw CJ, Spencer JD. Late management of compartment syndromes. *Injury.* 1995;26(9):633-635.

Shuler FD, Dietz MJ. Physicians' ability to manually detect isolated elevations in leg intracompartmental pressure. *J Bone Joint Surg Am.* 2010;92(2):361-367. doi: 10.2106/jbjs.I.00411.

Silas SI, Herzenberg JE, Myerson MS, Sponseller PD. Compartment syndrome of the foot in children. *J Bone Joint Surg Am.* 1995;77(3):356-361.

Srikanth KN, Chong M, Porter K. Acute exertional compartment syndrome of the superficial posterior compartment of the leg. *Acta Orthop Belg.* 2006;72(4):507-510.

Tam JPH, Gibson AGF, Murray JRD, Hassaballa M. Fasciotomy for chronic exertional compartment syndrome of the leg: clinical outcome in a large retrospective cohort. *Eur J Orthop Surg Traumatol.* 2018;29(2):479-485. doi: 10.1007/s00590-018-2299-3.

Towater LJ, Heron S. Foot compartment syndrome: a rare presentation to the Emergency Department. *J Emerg Med.* 2013;44(2):e235-e238. doi: 10.1016/j.jemermed.2012.07.046.

Tremblay LN, Feliciano DV, Rozycki GS. Secondary extremity compartment syndrome. *J Trauma.* 2002;53(5):833-837. doi: 10.1097/01.Ta.0000031174.60867.Eb.

Uzel AP, Lebreton G, Socrier ML. Delay in diagnosis of acute on chronic exertional compartment syndrome of the leg. *Chir Organi Mov.* 2009;93(3):179-182. doi: 10.1007/s12306-009-0043-1.

Vajapey S, Miller TL. Evaluation, diagnosis, and treatment of chronic exertional compartment syndrome: a review of current literature. *Phys Sportsmed.* 2017;45(4):391-398. doi: 10.1080/00913847.2017.1384289.

van Zantvoort APM, de Bruijn JA, Hundscheid HPH, van der Cruijsen-Raaijmakers M, Teijink JAW, Scheltinga MR. Fasciotomy for lateral lower-leg chronic exertional compartment syndrome. *Int J Sports Med.* 2018;39(14):1081-1087. doi: 10.1055/a-0640-9104.

Vandergugten S, Zemmour L, Lengele B, Nyssen-Behets C. A cadaveric model of anterior compartment leg syndrome: subcutaneous minimally invasive fasciotomy versus open fasciotomy. *Orthop Traumatol Surg Res.* 2019;105(1):167-171. doi: 10.1016/j.otsr.2018.10.003.

Verleisdonk EJ, van der Werken C. [Missed acute compartment syndrome of the lower leg]. *Ned Tijdschr Geneeskd.* 2004;148(45):2205-2209.

Vora A, Myerson MS. Crush injuries of the foot in the industrial setting. *Foot Ankle Clin.* 2002;7(2):367-383.

Wallin K, Nguyen H, Russell L, Lee DK. Acute traumatic compartment syndrome in pediatric foot: a systematic review and case report. *J Foot Ankle Surg.* 2016;55(4):817-820. doi: 10.1053/j.jfas.2016.02.010.

Wesslen C, Wahlgren CM. Contemporary management and outcome after lower extremity fasciotomy in non-trauma-related vascular surgery. *Vasc Endovascular Surg.* 2018;52(7):493-497. doi: 10.1177/1538574418773503.

Wiger P, Zhang Q, Styf J. The effects of limb elevation and increased intramuscular pressure on nerve and muscle function in the human leg. *Eur J Appl Physiol.* 2000;83(1):84-88. doi: 10.1007/s004210000237.

Yang CC, Chang DS, Webb LX. Vacuum-assisted closure for fasciotomy wounds following compartment syndrome of the leg. *J Surg Orthop Adv.* 2006;15(1):19-23.

Ziv I, Mosheiff R, Zeligowski A, Liebergal M, Lowe J, Segal D. Crush injuries of the foot with compartment syndrome: immediate one-stage management. *Foot Ankle.* 1989;9(4):185-189.

Multiplanar External Fixation

Bradley M. Lamm and Jordan J. Ernst

HISTORICAL REVIEW

External fixation, at its essence, is a method of osseous and soft tissue stabilization by way of components that extend to, or are completely external to the limb, at a distance from the zone of injury or operative focus. Considering this, the first recorded use of external fixation was before the time of Christ, about 2400 years ago when Hippocrates fashioned bent wooden rods from a cornel tree between two taught leather cuffs.[1] This elementary device allowed for repositioning of the limb segments by way of distraction and angulation. Since that time, external fixation has taken on many forms and functions, being employed in a host of treatment paradigms for both trauma and reconstructive surgery. Advancement of external fixation has been the cumulative work of many pioneers. Malagaine, in 1840, first described transcutaneous components of external fixation when he employed a spike driven into the tibia connected to a strap to immobilize a tibia fracture.[2] The metamorphosis continued with the advent of unilateral type fixator devices about the turn of the 20th century, first by Parkhill and then Lambotte.[3,4] In the early 1900s, the concept of pin traction was introduced by both Codivilla and Steinmann.[5,6] Shortly after, Kirschner developed fine wire fixation.[7] Half pin fixation then followed. Stader, a veterinarian, developed a fixator that incorporated half pins and allowed for complete weight bearing in the device.[8] His device was utilized in treating wounded soldiers during World War II. Schanz and others then expounded on the biomechanical properties of half pins.[9] Hoffman, in 1938, refined the application of external fixation to where minimally invasive techniques were now possible.[10]

Perhaps the most recognizable name when discussing the history of external fixation is that of a Russian orthopedic surgeon, Gavril Abramovich Ilizarov.[11] In the 1950s, he developed the use of a modular circular fixator with transosseous tensioned wire fixation while working on assignment in Kurgan, in the Ural Mountains of Siberia. Here, he treated thousands of wounded veterans in Russia following World War II. He also developed a method of inducing bone growth with a minimally invasive corticotomy. He applied his techniques to the treatment of deformities, limb-length discrepancies, nonunions, osteomyelitis, fractures, and bone defects. Ilizarov worked in relative obscurity until 1967, when he treated an infected nonunion of the tibia and fibula sustained by Russian Olympic high jump champion, Valery Brumel, in a motor vehicle accident.

The injury resulted in a nonviable distal fibula, which was remediated by Ilizarov performing a corticotomy to restore fibular length via distraction osteogenesis. This treatment allowed Brumel to return to high-level competition.

An Italian professor, A. Bianchi Maiocchi, introduced Ilizarov's methods to the western world in 1981. Use of these techniques increased in North America in the mid-1980s due to the efforts of Drs. James Aronson, Victor Frankel, Stuart Green, and Dror Paley.

In 1994, Dr. J. Charles Taylor and his brother, engineer Harold Taylor, developed the Taylor Spatial Frame (TSF). The TSF, which modified the Ilizarov system, is an apparatus that uses a Stewart platform with a computer program to allow for precise gradual osseous and soft tissue correction in any plane.[12] The advantage of TSF over traditional Ilizarov devices is the ease of construct whereby no hinges, translation boxes, or rotational apparatuses are required. Instead, six adjustable struts connect two rings that span the deformity. This allows for simultaneous correction of multiplanar deformities with the same frame construction. The internet-based computer software utilizes deformity and mounting parameters that are entered into the program by the surgeon postoperatively. Deformity parameters define the malaligned position of the bony segments of the deformity, while mounting parameters define the position of the frame relative to the limb. With these inputs, a prescription of strut adjustments is created. These can be performed by the patient, caretaker, home health nurse, or surgeon. More recently, software utilizing the Center of Rotation of Angulation principle has been developed. This software touts point and click x-ray planning rather than the entering of deformity and mounting parameters. Collectively, these systems are often referred to as computer-assisted fixators. With these new technologies, the application of external fixation is truly limited only by the creativity and innovation of the surgeon.

As the technology of external fixation has advanced, so too have its indications. With this expansion of treatment options, several forms of external fixation have emerged, each with its own specific advantages and limitations. Circular fixation is typically preferred for static or dynamic correction of rearfoot and ankle deformities because of the versatility of its components, as well as its strength and stability, which allow for weight bearing (Figs. 65.1 and 65.2). Given the focus of this chapter, other types of fixators will be only briefly discussed and in relation to their features compared with circular fixation.

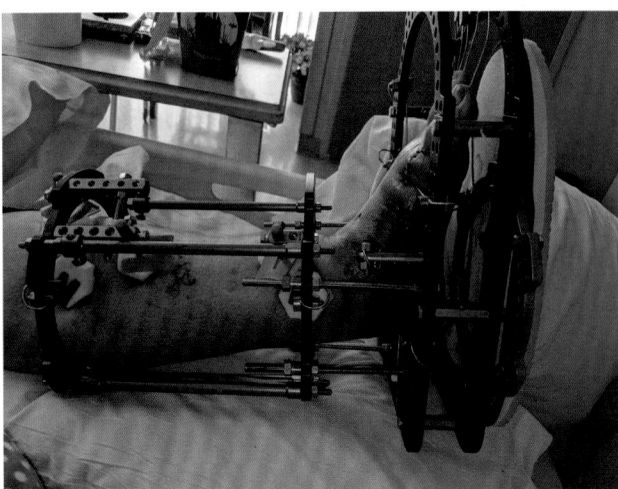

FIGURE 65.1 An example of a basic static frame configuration as described in the authors' preferred treatment. In this instance, the frame was utilized to augment internal fixation that was placed for Charcot deformity correction. The external fixator allowed her to remain ambulatory and expanded the area of fixation beyond the bone affected by the neuropathic process.

CLASSIFICATION

- Unilateral
- Pin to bar
- Hybrid
- Circular (ring)
  - Ilizarov
    - Static
    - Dynamic
  - Computer assisted

Unilateral frames, in contradistinction to circular frames, are placed only on one side of the limb or bone segment. There is less potential for interference with the contralateral limb. A less cumbersome design and more clothing options are additional benefits. These fixators are most suitable for deformities limited to a single plane. In the tibia, they are not suited for weight bearing as axial loading subjects the construct to cantilever bending and asymmetric loading.[13] On a smaller scale, a specialized application of this design is useful within the foot to treat brachymetatarsia via distraction osteogenesis.[14]

Pin to bar constructs utilize multiple light weight carbon fiber bars connected to transosseous pins. These are most often temporizing devices in the setting of acute trauma, meant to be in place for a short period of time until a more definitive method of fixation is appropriate. The pin to bar design allows for rapid application, which is ideal in damage control orthopedics where the patient is not medically optimized or has more serious injuries that must be dealt with. Half pins are placed independently and connected to one another via the carbon fiber rods until a closed construct is created.

Hybrid designs refer to a combination of ring fixation in addition to one of the other discussed fixator types. By combining the principles of circular fixation with more discrete configurations, a wide and versatile range of applications is possible. One example is where the fixator is tasked with spanning multiple major joints such as the ankle and knee. In this way, the circular frame can provide supreme rigidity to the leg, while the construct is spanned to areas where less rigidity is needed or a ring is impractical. An example is provided in Figure 65.3.

Circular fixators are composed of either full or partial rings. These rings are connected via threaded rods or struts. Full rings provide the most stability, but partial rings may be desired near joints where a full ring would prevent normal extremity function such as the shoulder and femur. With respect to the lower extremity, this is not typically an issue; however, a partial ring may be needed with an exceptionally

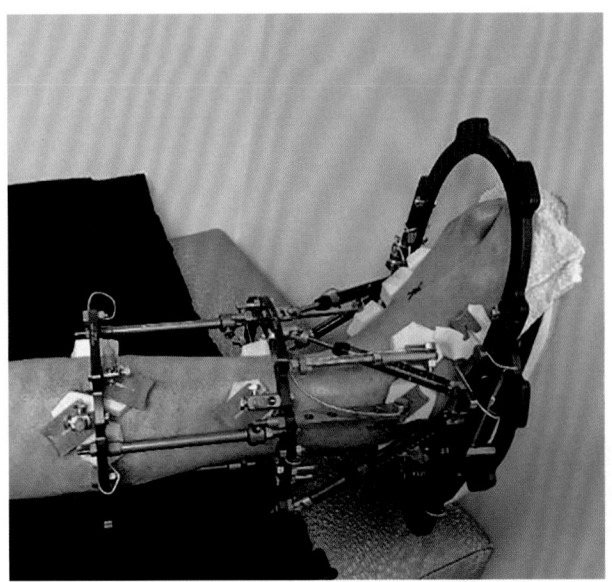

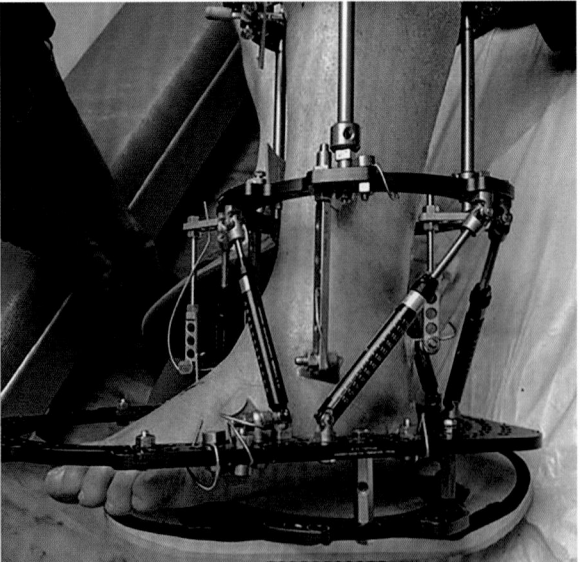

FIGURE 65.2 An example of a modification to our standard frame to allow for gradual Charcot deformity correction. In this case, the threaded rods connecting the distal tibial ring and foot block are replaced by struts that allow for the gradual correction.

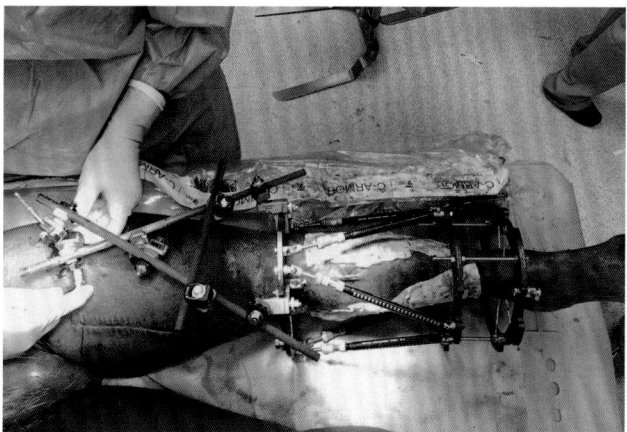

FIGURE 65.3 This polytrauma patient was involved in a motorcycle vs automobile accident. His injuries included a distal tibial fracture and distal femoral fracture. A hybrid construct was utilized to span the ankle as well as the knee. A circular fixator provided maximal stability to the tibial fracture while a pin to bar configuration extended from the proximal tibial ring to stabilize the femur until internal fixation could be placed at that location.

large limb. The circumferential nature of full rings prevents cantilever bending and allows for multiplanar fixation. Their modular nature allows easy adaptability not only to a variety of conditions but also the potential for adjustment and modification during the postoperative course as dictated by the surgical goals.

Circular frames may be further divided by function. With respect to the classic Ilizarov devices, static frames are utilized to maintain correction achieved at the time of the index operation, while dynamic fixators gradually correct deformity. Dynamic Ilizarov devices are best suited for simple uniplanar deformities while more complex scenarios are best left to computer-assisted fixators such as the TSF (Fig. 65.4).

Biomechanically, a fixator must be constructed in a way that provides the most stable exoskeleton for the deficient bone. This undertaking requires consideration of each segment and component of the fixator. With an appreciation for the various principles at each segment, these elements can be combined to provide the optimal construct. With respect to stability, this is not an absolute term, but rather a relative one, with various aspects of the application and construction contributing to the overall stability of the fixation.

When considering fixator rings, the smallest ring possible while still allowing for soft tissue edema postoperatively, in general at least 2 cm about the posterior and lateral compartments where the majority of the postoperative edema will reside, is desirable. The distance between the rings has an inverse relationship with stability. Longer gaps may require the use of telescopic rods with greater bending stiffness. An increased number of connections between the rings also increase stability.

Rings are affixed to the bone by both fine wires and pins, the diameters of which are directly proportional to rigidity. In general, half pins range from 4 to 6 mm and are stiffer than wires, which are typically 1.8 mm in adults and 1.5 mm in pediatric applications. Limitations such as the size of the bony segments and the surrounding anatomy dictate which implant is more appropriate at a given location.

After first considering the size of the rings and the type of implant, the next point of consideration is the position of these implants in relation to the bony segment of interests, their method of fixation to the ring, as well as their position relative to one another at each ring. The most stable construction of rings and connecting elements is wasted if this stability is not transferred to the bony segments through appropriate fixation.

Wires are attached to rings via slotted bolts and nuts. The inner hole of the ring should be utilized to maximize stability. When placing more than one wire at a given ring, maximal

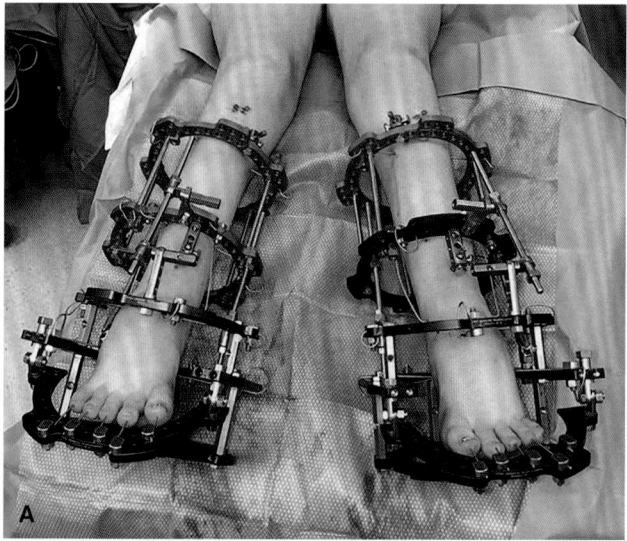
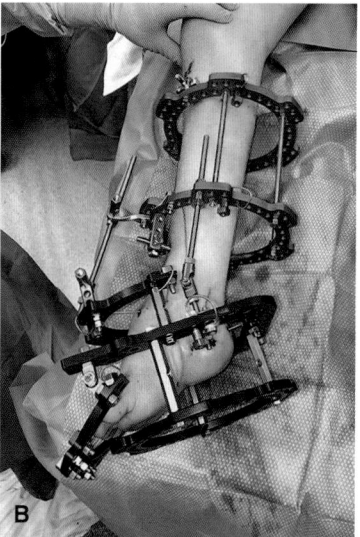

FIGURE 65.4 An example of a dynamic Ilizarov device used to correct a rigid congenital equinus deformity secondary to Zellweger syndrome. **A.** The anterior distraction rods are utilized to correct equinus by daily turns of the counting nut. **B.** The medial and lateral hinges allow for the gradual correction. Additionally, the threaded rods to which they are attached were utilized to achieve ankle joint distraction to avoid impingement during equinus correction.

divergence as allowed by the anatomic safe zones provides the most stability. A 90-degree crossing angle would provide maximal stability with regard to axial loading but is not possible given that one wire would have to traverse the posterior compartment. An angle <60 degrees allows for sliding of the bone segments. This can be mitigated with the use of olive wires. When placed in periarticular fashion, the wires should be placed with the joint in its end range of motion to avoid skin irritation.

Fine wires have a distinct advantage relative to half pins for small bone segments, osteopenic bone, periarticular bone segments, and pediatric patients. Wires impart no stability until tensioned. The greater the tension, the greater the stability. The desired amount of tension is dictated by the anatomical constraints and the amount of load bearing support needed. Fine wires can be retensioned during the postoperative course, another advantage relative to half pins. A specialized application of smooth wires is their ability to apply a directional force across a fracture or union site by inserting the wire straight and then bending the wire prior to fixation to the ring and applying tension. As the stored energy attempts to straighten the wire against the fixation bolts, compression is applied along the concave side and distraction along the convex side.

Half pins, given their diameter, tend to be stiffer than fine wires, providing better torsional control. As they do not traverse the entire limb, large crossing angles can be achieved without invading muscle compartments. Multiple variations exist from self-drilling to blunt tipped, cortical and cancellous thread patterns, as well as stainless steel or titanium. Coating with hydroxyapatite offers resistance to infection as well as greater bone fixation and extraction torque. This same extraction torque makes them ill suited for office removal.

Dimensional discrepancies in these two components account for their differential responses to weight bearing. This difference must be appreciated for proper implant selection. Half pins, given their attachment to the ring at only one point, are loaded in cantilever fashion, that is, loaded at one end. Conversely, wires are supported at both ends by the ring. The clinical relevance is that during weight bearing, the stress distribution across bone is more uniform with wires than with half pins.[15] The circumferential nature of ring fixators largely minimizes cantilever loading, but this can become an issue with an insufficient amount of connecting elements between rings.

Some surgeons prefer all wire frames, some rely on half pins. Our typical construct utilizes both wires and half pins at each tibial ring block. A wire is placed first, which facilitates orthogonal ring placement.

These variables in combination allow for the prerequisites of weight bearing, which are frame rigidity and fracture stability. The desired goal is axial compression without shear, bending, or torque. Cyclical micromotion is advantageous in an axial fashion. Shear forces are reduced by maximizing frame and fracture stability. Relating to fractures, maximizing contact, stabilization, as well as avoiding distraction, provides optimal stability.

This supreme control of the bone segments allows for comfortable ambulation. In those situations where bone healing is necessary, the ossification afforded by frame stability offloads the fixation points, further facilitating ambulation. Lack of stability causes undue transfer of axial loads through the pins and wires, effecting increased motion, discomfort, and possible infection. While this discomfort may de-incentivize a sensate

patient from weight bearing, these same issues may often go unrecognized in the neuropathic patient, which can be devastating if uncorrected. Truly, prevention is the best strategy, with careful attention to detail during frame design and application.

Within the pedal block, utilization of various connecting elements becomes necessary given that wires often do not lay flush against the ring, and that rings or partial ring configurations are placed in close proximity. Posts allow for fixation of wires at a distance from the ring, while plates allow for extension of connecting elements off of the ring, including to connect rings of different sizes. Hinges provide a means of various angled configurations to facilitate correction of malalignment as well as allow for range of motion. Commercially made options are available, but they can also be constructed from male posts connected by a bolt.

INDICATIONS

- Damage control orthopedics (see Fig. 65.3)
- Complex congenital deformities (see Fig. 65.4)
- Charcot neuroarthropathy (see Fig. 65.5)
- Nonunion (see Fig. 65.6)
- Open fractures (see Fig. 65.7)
- Malunion/neglected injuries (see Fig. 65.8)
- Complex deformity correction (see Fig. 65.9)
- Arthrodiastasis (see Fig. 65.10)
- Neurologic disorders (see Fig. 65.11)
- Bone transport/distraction osteogenesis/limb lengthening (see Figs. 65.12 and 65.13)
- Infected fracture/nonunion
- Closed fractures with severe soft tissue injury
- Arthrodesis
- Unstable/periarticular fractures
- Osteoporotic bone
- Failed internal fixation
- Augmentation of internal fixation
- Protection of flaps/grafts

With an understanding of the general principles of external fixation, the breadth of its indications is easily appreciated. During treatment with external fixation, soft tissue access is afforded, which allows for close surveillance. This is especially useful when the degree of soft tissue damage is evolving or expected to remain hostile. In the trauma setting, this may be done while awaiting a soft tissue envelope that is amenable to internal fixation, or even as the definitive mode of fixation. In situations that present chronic soft tissue defects, such as in Charcot deformity correction, the frame can allow for wound care to be easily performed while it is simultaneously offloaded (Fig. 65.5).

Patient factors that contribute to the complexity of the case may make external fixation a more suitable option. Those with neuropathy, obesity, upper extremity weakness, and inability to be non–weight bearing are situations where external fixation may confer a specific advantage over internal fixation. These same patients often exhibit poor healing potential and thus are precluded from extensile incisions to place internal fixation.

Conditions treated with external fixation are often complex including revision surgery, failed internal fixation, multiplanar deformities, a compromised soft tissue enveloped, and poor bone quality (Figs. 65.6 and 65.7).

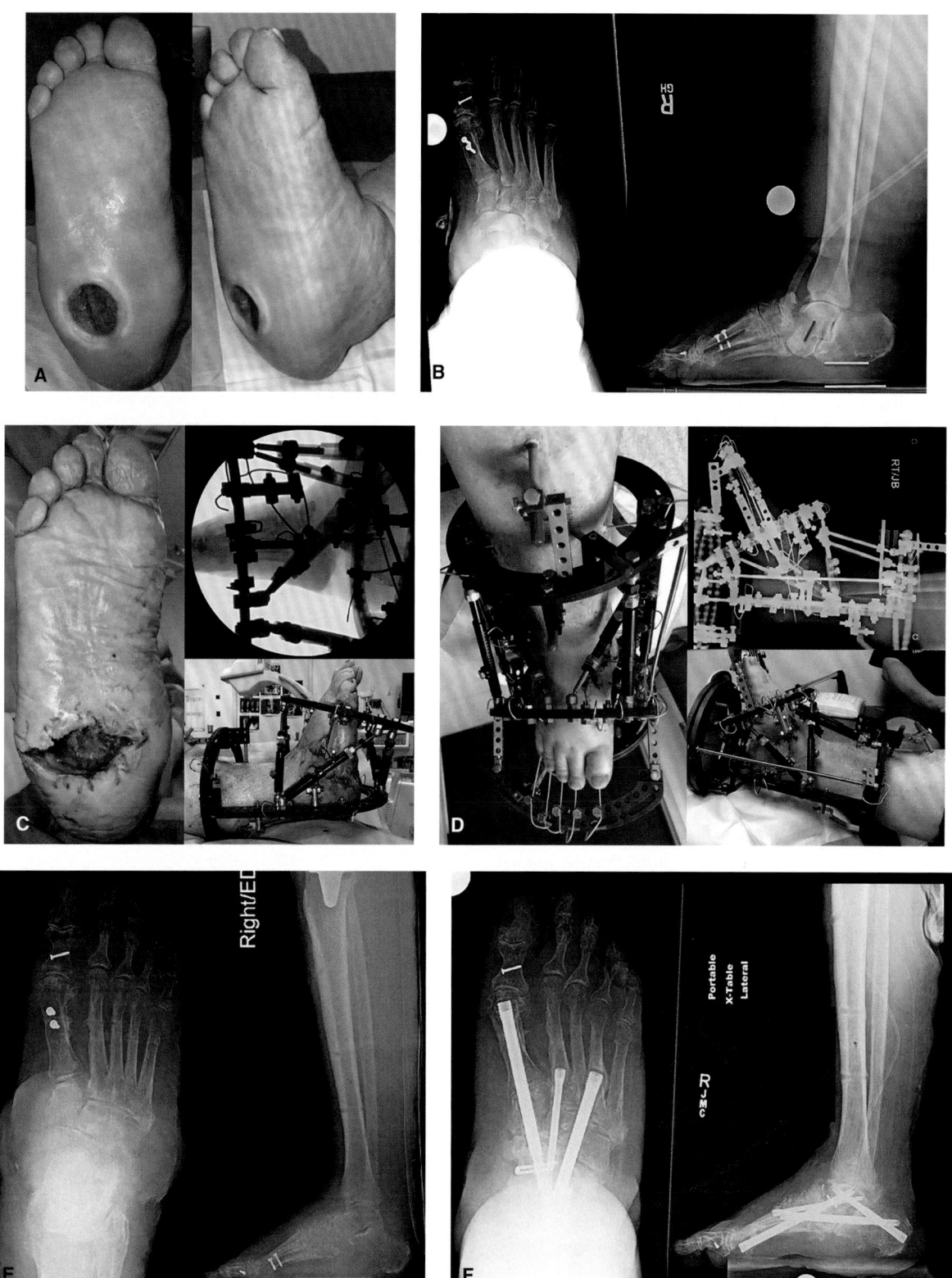

FIGURE 65.5 This patient presented with a long-standing ulceration due to a chronic Charcot midtarsal dislocation. **A.** The ulceration was plantar to the anterior calcaneus. **B.** Radiographs demonstrating the chronic midtarsal dislocation. **C.** The ulceration was excised in a full-thickness manner and a Butt frame configuration was applied for gradual correction. **D.** Clinical and radiographic images during her treatment course. **E.** Radiographs of obtained correction after fixator removal. **F.** Internal fixation was then applied to maintain correction.

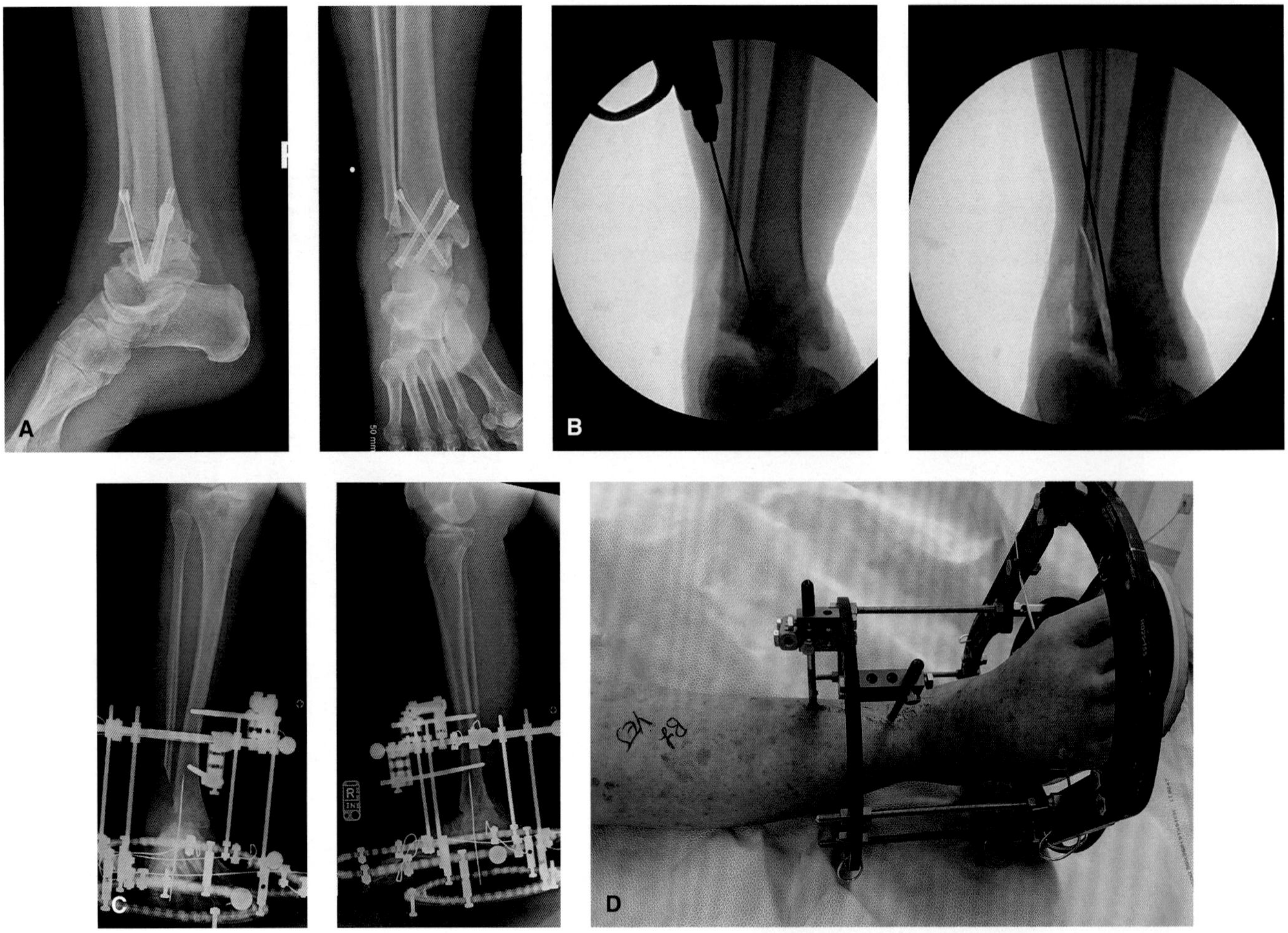

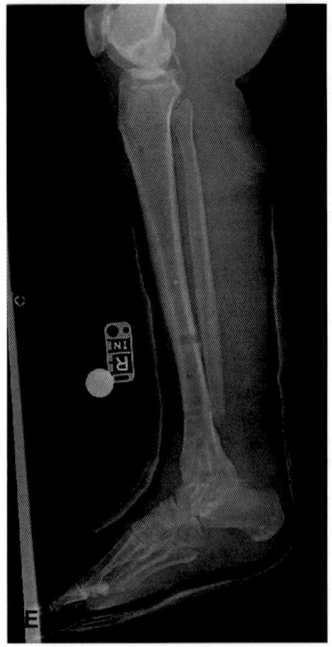
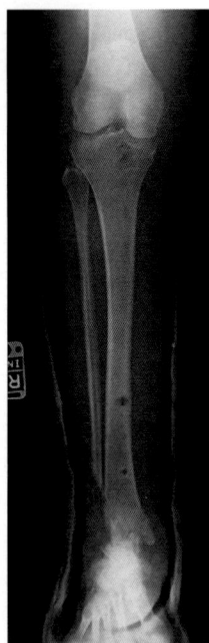

FIGURE 65.6 Example of a simple frame for an ankle nonunion.
A. Radiographs demonstrating an ankle nonunion with retained internal
fixation from an outside facility. **B.** Intraoperative fluoroscopic imaging
demonstrating the use of the distal tibia and remnant fibula for autogenous
grafting. **C.** Good alignment and compression was achieved. The subtalar
joint was also fused given symptomatic arthritis. **D.** A simple frame design
was sufficient. Threaded rods allowed for compression in the operating
room as well as the potential for additional compression postoperatively
if desired. **E.** Anterior-posterior and lateral radiographs after external
fixation removal demonstrating ankle and subtalar joint fusion in good
alignment. The patient was casted post removal for one month.

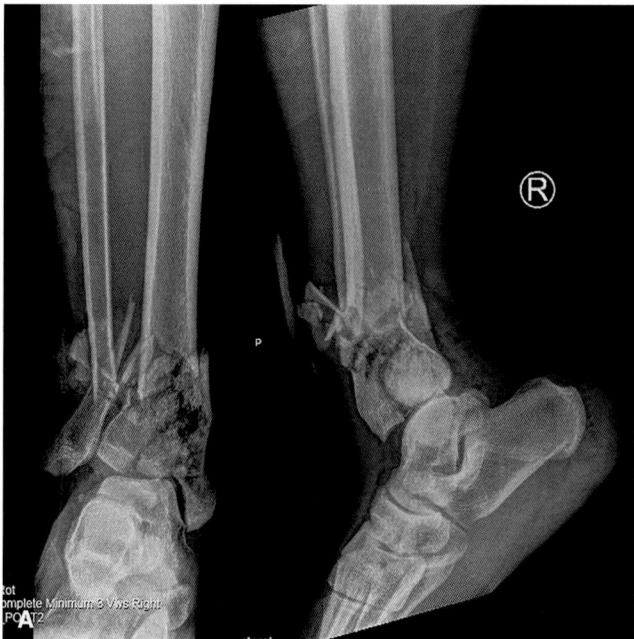
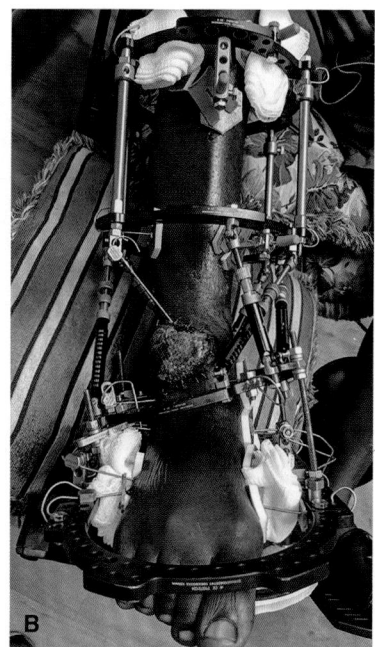
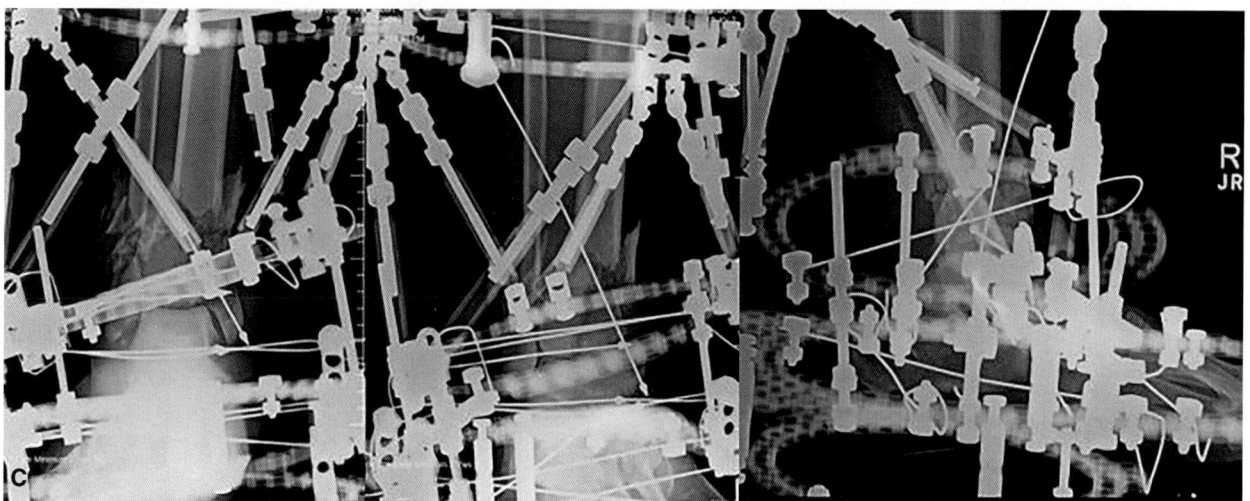

FIGURE 65.7 This patient sustained an open pilon fracture as the result of a forklift injury. He was initially treated with a pin to bar delta frame. Given the severity of the soft tissue injury, circular fixation was employed for a definitive method of treatment. Struts were utilized to allow for fine tuning of the reduction postoperatively. **A.** Date of injury radiographs. **B.** Circular fixation in place that affords stability while allowing easy wound access. **C.** Radiographs demonstrating acceptable reduction with the fixator in place.

With internal fixation, the precise deformity correction must be obtained at the time of the index surgery and cannot be altered during the postoperative period. With external fixation, adjustments can be performed during the treatment course to allow for optimal clinical and radiographic results (Fig. 65.8).

If there is an intact soft tissue envelope, external fixation allows for patients to shower, bathe, and even swim in a chlorinated pool.

The technical expertise required for its application, the frequency of follow-up visits necessary, as well as the labor intensive nature are some reasons that discourage surgeons from utilizing external fixation. With the appropriate training, however, the use of external fixation can create elegant solutions to correct otherwise debilitating conditions.

ANATOMICAL CONSIDERATIONS

In the application of external fixation, a sound working knowledge with cross-sectional and three-dimensional anatomy is crucial. Unlike internal fixation, external fixation is applied without direct visualization of the target structures. An appreciation of key surface landmarks of surface anatomy can be instrumental as well. Anatomic safe zones define the tissue corridors appropriate for placement of fixation.

The tibial shaft contains three borders: anterior, medial, and lateral, which define three surfaces. The anterior and medial borders define the medial surface, which is subcutaneous. The lateral surface is bordered by the anterior and lateral borders.

This surface is covered by anterior compartment musculature. The posterior surface is bound by the medial and lateral borders.

The tibial crest, or anterior border, should be palpated and identified. It may be more or less prominent depending on the body habitus of the individual. The medial border should be palpated as well. These two structures define the medial face or surface, which is an anatomic safe zone. It is smooth and convex, sloping from anterior and superficial to posterior and deep. This surface allows for safe insertion of smooth wires as well as half

pins as it is devoid of any overlying musculature or neurovascular structures. Our preferred technique places one half pin proximally, just medial to the crest, one in the mid-diaphysis, roughly perpendicular to the medial surface, and one distally at the tibial isthmus, which is the narrower medial face of the distal tibia.

Half pins and wires have different safe zones given their properties. As half pins do not extend into the soft tissue beyond the far cortex, they can be placed in an anterior to posterior fashion as the posterior neurovascular bundle is not in jeopardy.

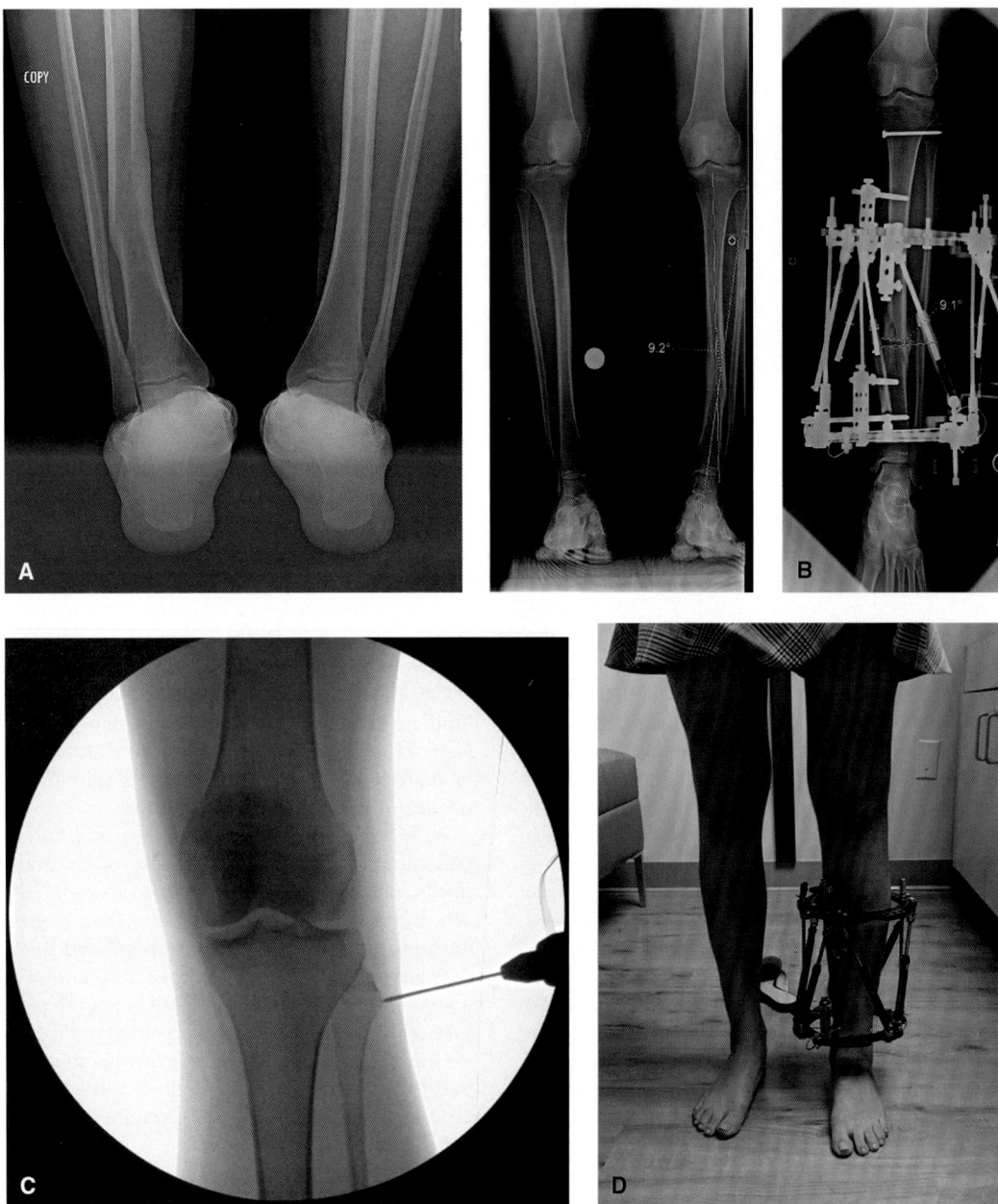

FIGURE 65.8 Example of a computer-assisted frame for uniplanar tibia deformity correction. Given the location of the fracture, a foot plate was not needed. **A.** Note the varus deformity of the tibia with a CORA in the mid-diaphysis. This was the result of a conservatively managed fracture after a motor vehicle accident. **B.** An osteotomy was performed at the CORA to allow for gradual correction. A proximal tibiofibular joint temporary arthrodesis screw was employed to prevent diastasis during correction. **C.** The guidewire for the screw is entered at the equator of the bone, also a useful reference for placing fixator wires. **D.** Clinical photograph with the deformity corrected and the fixator in place during the consolidation phase.

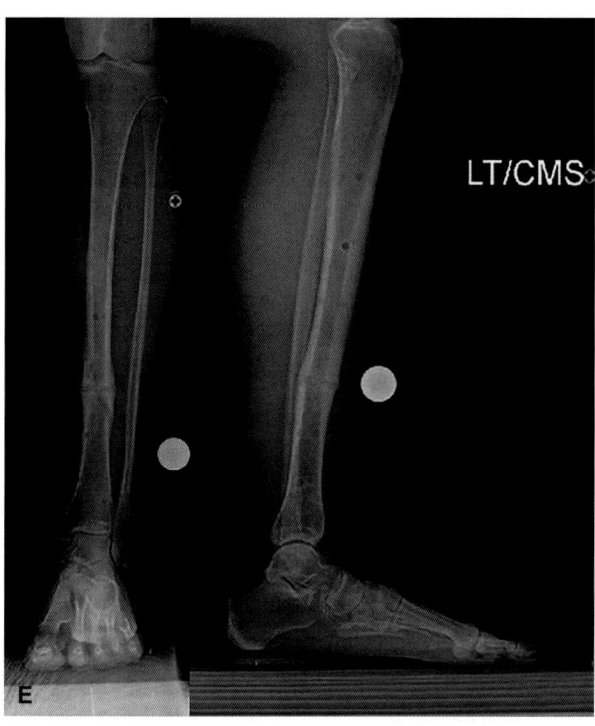

FIGURE 65.8 (*Continued*) **E.** Radiograph showing deformity correction and well-healed osteotomy.

Smooth wire placement is generally described as one of three configurations: axial, medial face, and fibular. Placement is largely based on surgeon preference and the number of wires desired at each ring. Axial wires are placed in a medial-lateral direction through the tibia, ensuring the wire is placed deep the anterior cortex. The medial face wire is placed parallel to the face from anterolateral to posteromedial. The fibular wire is placed from the medial face of the tibia and directed to the fibula posterolaterally.

When considering the path of the neurovascular structures along the leg, each is at more or less risk of injury depending on the cross-sectional level. Proximally, the common peroneal nerve branches at the fibular neck. At this level, therefore, placement of axial wires should be avoided at the neck and anterior to it where the common peroneal nerve branches course beneath the peroneal musculature. Throughout the length of the leg, the anterior neurovascular bundle runs along the anterior surface of the interosseous membrane. The axial wire should be placed anterior enough to avoid these structures. While the medial face wire does not pose a risk here, the fibular wire could do so.

The posterior neurovascular structures are easily avoided proximally given their position behind the tibia. Distally in the leg, these structures transition to a more medial location. Given this arrangement, wires are more safely placed from the medial to lateral direction when working distally. Also of importance is the distal tibiofibular recess, which extends 2 cm proximal to the ankle joint. In cases where the ankle is not fused, this should be kept in mind as wires placed in the zone pose a potential for joint sepsis.

Given its less exposed anatomy, talar wire fixation can be more difficult. Wires should pass through the talar body and are typically passed in a medial to lateral direction and from anteromedial to posterolateral. Talar wires are strategically employed when there is a reason to hold the position of the talus static while the pedal block is rotating around it as part of a deformity correction. One example is in the treatment of clubfoot or other varus deformities. Other situations include arthrodiastasis where the tibia and talus are being pulled in opposite directions. Certain scenarios can require the talar wires to be affixed to different ring levels depending on the component of the deformity being corrected. Correction of a subtalar inversion deformity would require holding the talus in static position to a tibial ring while the foot ring corrects the foot position. If residual equinus remained, the talar wires would then be attached to the foot plate to dorsiflex the foot at the ankle as one unit.

Calcaneal wires must avoid the posteromedial neurovascular bundle and are thus best placed medial to lateral, starting at the posterior tuber. Despite being the largest tarsal bone, the space for smooth wire or half pin fixation is quite limited. A posterior to anterior half pin is also an option.

With respect to the forefoot and midfoot, fixation at this level can add to the overall stability of the frame, even if the specific pathology does not demand fixation at this level. Typically, these wires are tensioned to a lesser degree and thus are more prone to failure given the increased micromotion. Two wires are typically placed, one medial to lateral and one lateral to medial. The wires are angulated along the plane of the transverse arch to capture at least two metatarsals each.

Given these angulations, various connecting elements are used to build the frame up to these wires. The first intermetatarsal space should be avoided given the location of the dorsalis pedis and deep plantar artery.

In certain instances, toe fixation can be performed as well. This not only adds overall stability to the fixator but prevents contractures that may develop as the result of lengthening or deformity correction that would put the flexor tendons on stretch.

PHYSICAL EXAMINATION

Paramount to the success of any operation is a thorough and detailed history and physical examination. A comprehensive

clinical examination including stance and gait analysis is imperative. Limb deformity principles are the foundation for proper surgical planning and correction. They provide accurate reference points and angles for producing predictable results.

With a comprehensive analysis, a customized treatment can be devised for the patient. This should include the goals of the patient with reasonable expectations set by the surgeon. The potential for complications should also be reviewed in detail.

A physical examination should include both static and dynamic components. The resting position of the limb should be observed for any contractures. Prior surgical scars should be documented and taken into consideration as well as any previous flaps or grafts. Gait analysis should be performed.

A full muscle inventory should be recorded and joint range of motion should be quantified. While radiographs provide an objective method of assessing limb position, they do not fully reveal function.

Cleary, neurovascular status should be assessed. Many times external fixation is employed in patients where these variables are compromised, as other methods of fixation would be overly prone to failure. These hosts may additionally present with acute or chronic infection. External fixation allows the surgeon to select the most ideal point of entry into the tissues, minimize soft tissue and blood flow reduction, and, is by virtue of its temporary nature, provide stability in the infected host where internal implants would tend to perpetuate infection.

Joint deformities should be categorized as either rigid or reducible. A deformity at one joint may be compensatory for a more proximal deformity. Over time, an initially supple scenario will become less so. A knowledge of this is essential, as correction of the more proximal deformity may unmask the more distal compensation. If the distal compensation has become rigid, correction of the more proximal deformity will now present a scenario where the distal compensatory position can no longer be reduced. An example would be a rigid subtalar joint inversion compensation for an ankle valgus deformity. The surgeon should appreciate that once the ankle is corrected, the heel will need to be realigned as well as it can no longer be everted back to neutral (Fig. 65.9).

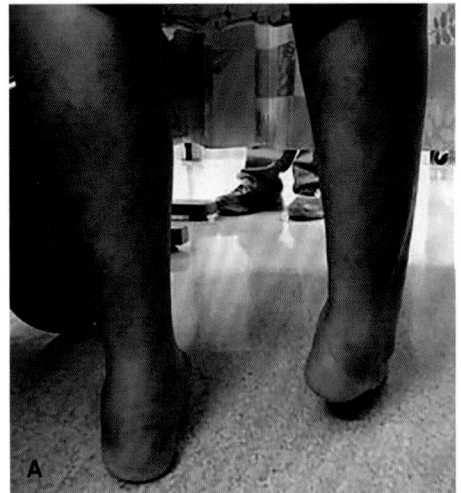
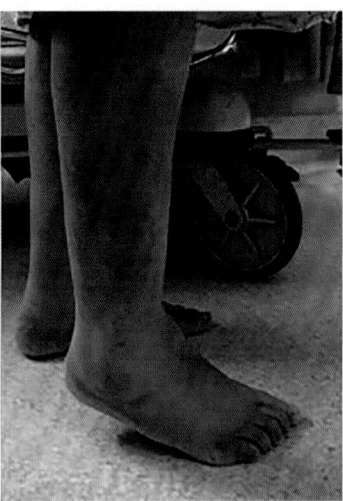
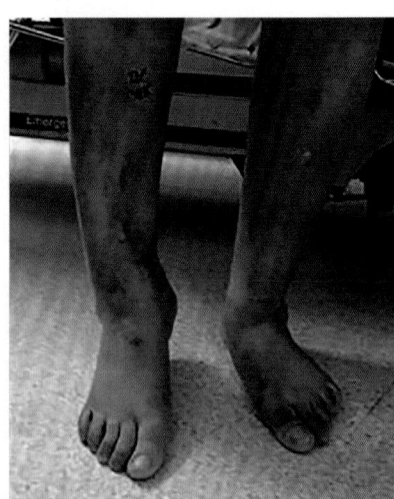
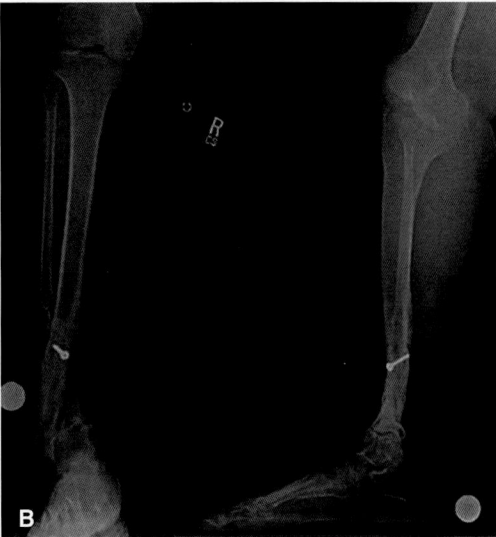
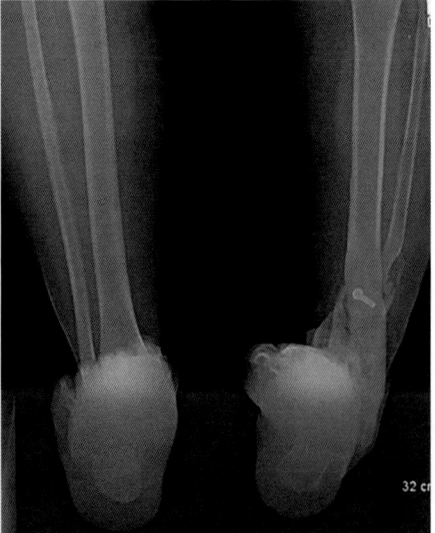

FIGURE 65.9 This patient sustained and open trauma as a child that resulted in a tibial deformity and ankle arthritis. She was minimally ambulatory given her deformity. Her correction was achieved with dynamic external fixation in a 2-stage fashion. **A.** Clinical images of her deformity. **B.** Radiographic images demonstrating her severe deformities.

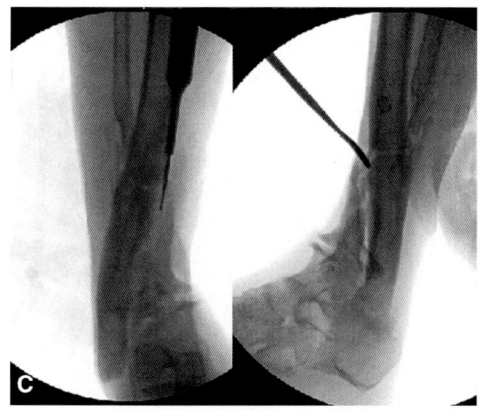
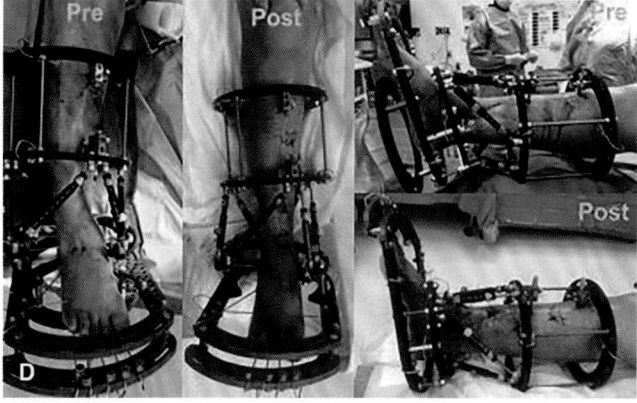

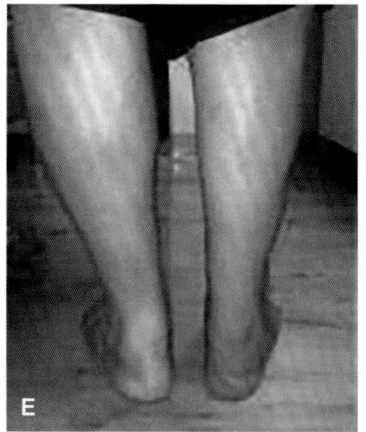
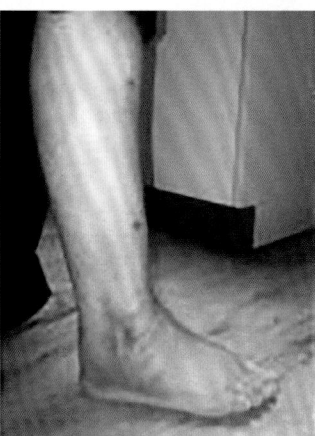
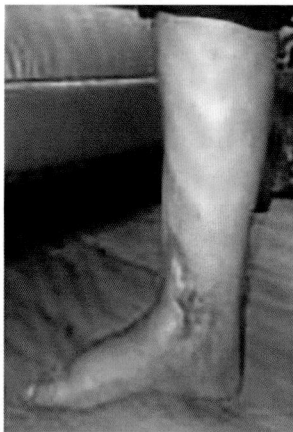
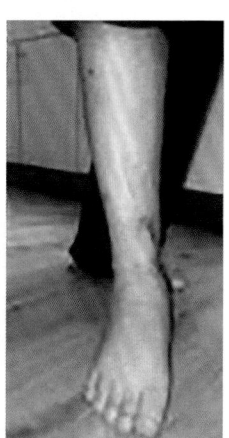

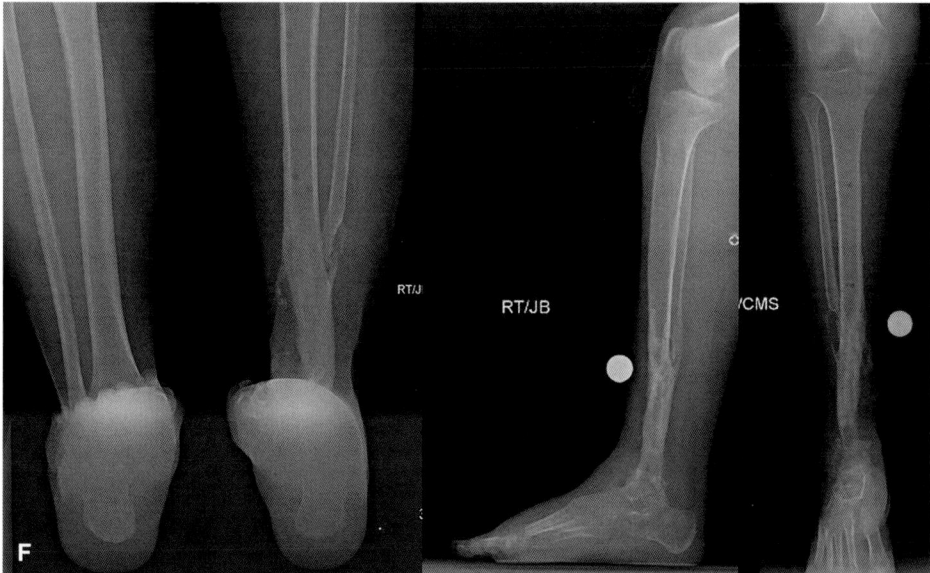

FIFURE 65.9 (*Continued*) **C.** In the first stage, a tibial osteotomy was performed through her nonunion to allow for gradual correction with the fixator. In the second stage, the ankle joint was prepared and then fused via compression through the fixator. **D.** Clinical images of the fixator pre- and postcorrection. **E.** Clinical images of the patient's markedly improved stance. **F.** Postcorrection radiographs.

PATHOGENESIS

The wide ranging utility and spectrum of pathology treated with external fixation likewise lends itself to a diverse patient population. Each subset requires careful consideration to understand how unique patient variables will affect the treatment course. These differences may ultimately play a role in determining the amount of time the patient is in the fixator, affect its construction, and even distinguish certain patients as more or less suited to undergo fixator application.

The cause and resultant effects of the deformity should be elicited, as this is essential to understanding the current condition. As external fixation is often employed in difficult revision cases, a full surgical history should be documented. A multiply operated limb imposes many potential challenges that demand attention if a successful outcome is to be attained. Among these are created and compensatory deformities, soft tissue envelope compromise, retained internal fixation, malunion/nonunion, contractures, osteopenia, avascular necrosis, infection, as well as chronic pain.

IMAGING

In deformity correction, radiographic analysis can elucidate the location and magnitude, as well as the planal components of the deformity. In addition to standard views of the foot and ankle, erect leg length films should be obtained to ascertain any limb length discrepancy that may influence the treatment plan. Further, calcaneal axial or Saltzman views should be obtained for full frontal plane assessment. Given that the calcaneus is the first point of contact during gait, its location relative to the tibia is crucial. If there is undue translation or angulation, frontal plane incongruity can compromise an otherwise well-aligned limb.

Stress views and real-time fluoroscopy can add additional dimensions to distinguish soft tissue deformities from osseous ones as well as quantify the amount of joint motion.

A normative angular range of radiographic parameters has been produced for the lower extremity.[16] While attaining normal values is not a guarantee of clinical success, a knowledge of what is normal is necessary to appreciate what is abnormal. In conjunction with an understanding of the principles of the center of rotation of angulation, a plan can be devised to accurately align the bony segments of the deformity into a functional position. The center of rotation of angulation defines the apex of the deformity.[17] A multiplanar deformity may have a unique CORA in each plane. The principles that govern effective application of the CORA to deformity correction should be understood. In this manner, an appropriate radiographic template can be used to assist with preoperative planning.

While not a surrogate for a formal bone density testing, the quality of the host bone can be preliminarily assessed. As fixed angle devices, external fixators are especially advantageous in osteoporotic bone.

Advanced imaging modalities can be acquired based on the specific pathology being addressed. Computed tomography is often times useful for evaluating the extent of nonunion. This modality also offers a more detailed assessment of bone quality. Magnetic resonance imaging can allow for an appreciation of additional soft tissue pathology that will be concomitantly addressed. This includes but is not limited to ligamentous injury, tendon damage, cartilaginous defects, as well as the presence and extent of infection.

---

positioning PEARLS

- The heel should rest a few centimeters proximal to the end of the table.
- The thigh is bumped to achieve a foot forward position.
- Draping includes the thigh to assess limb rotation and allow maneuverability of the limb for fluoroscopy.
- Large C-arm is placed on the contralateral side.
- Adequate space should be available on the table so the fixator does not injure the contralateral limb, or in some cases to allow for bilateral fixation.
- Folded towels should be available to assist with positioning the limb within the frame.
- Adequate sterile working space at the end for the operating table for multiplanar wire insertion should be available.

PEARLS

- Multiplanar and comprehensive deformity assessment.
- Ensure appropriate limb position within the frame.
- Respect the anatomic safe zones.
- Minimize soft tissue trauma.
- Employ and refine a systematic method of frame application.
- Apply sound biomechanical principles at each point of application to maximize frame stability.

AUTHORS' PREFERRED TREATMENT

Only when the surgeon possesses a true understanding of the principles and mechanics of external fixation can its true potential be unlocked. When looking at the completed external fixator construct, the task of its application can seem daunting, especially to the novice external fixation surgeon. However, through a systematic and detailed deconstruction of the individual steps, a reproducible and effective method of applying a mechanically sound external fixator can be learned. With a mastery of this algorithm and a sound working knowledge of external fixation and limb deformity principles, the approach can be modified and adapted to correct even the most severe deformities.

Critical to efficient frame application is the setup of the operative theater. Ample space should be available for maneuvering while inserting multiplanar fixation and obtaining fluoroscopic imaging. The most common fixation elements such as fixation bolts and nuts as well as tensiometers should be placed on a Mayo stand for rapid access. Other devices that should be readily available are threaded rods, wire cutters, wire benders, wrenches, drill sleeves, and power drivers.

The maintenance of general anesthesia should not include paralytics so as not to mask muscular contractions that would alert the surgeon to iatrogenic nerve insult.

Prior to application of the frame, open procedures are performed with a thigh tourniquet in place. Once the incisions are closed, the tourniquet is released. Bleeding during wire passage has a cooling effect that is thought to be protective to the tissues from thermal injury, which could potentiate infection and wire loosening. Some authors advocate the use of saline-soaked sponges while passing wires.

The limb is prepped proximally to the thigh to allow for assessment of patellar position and for manipulation of the limb under fluoroscopy. Bumps of folded blankets are instrumental in allowing for placement of rings as well as elevating the leg for lateral fluoroscopic imaging. A tibial block is assembled on the backfield consisting of two rings connected by four threaded rods. Bumps are placed under the knee and the tibial block is placed around the leg. A bump is then placed under the heel. In this, space is created about the tibia for application of the frame. Momentarily, the frame is held out of the way for placement of an axial fine wire medial to lateral in the mid tibia. The equator of the bone is sought with the wire tip, that is, the widest point of the bone. This will be represented radiographically as the tip appearing to rest directly on the cortical bone, neither above nor below. This ensures bicortical purchase. The wire is driven through the near cortex. Fluoroscopy is then taken to ensure an accurate trajectory. The driver is adjusted as necessary to facilitate wire placement perpendicular to the tibia, and the wire is then driven through the far cortex. The wire is then pulsed through the remaining soft tissues out of the other side of the limb until there is approximately an equal length of wire on each side. The wire is pulsed after penetration of the far cortex to allow the wire to push potential neurovascular structures aside rather than piercing them. This first wire sets the position of the tibial block, which is then brought to the wire. A wire fixation nut and bolt are used to secure the wire to the frame on either side. The wire is placed where it lies so to speak, that is, the hole nearest to the wire is used for fixation, utilizing the inner ring of holes as this affords the greatest stability. A transverse wire is then placed to the proximal ring in similar fashion. To complete the stability of the tibial block, half pins are added. Careful attention to detail during pin placement can avoid untoward consequences such as skiving off of the tibia or unicortical application. Posts are used as extensions from the circular rings to allow for placement of the half pins. The post is secured with a nut, which is not yet tightened, to allow for rotation of the post and proper pin placement. Starting proximally, the first pin is placed just medial to the tibial crest. A tissue sleeve is placed through post hole to make a small indentation in the tissues at the desired site of pin application. A stab incision is made with a no. 15 blade. The incision should only be made as long as the diameter of the pin. This will create the best skin seal about the pin and minimize the potential for pin tract infections. The drill is then placed though the drill sleeve, first visualizing the drill tip going through the incision, then placing the drill sleeve down to bone as well. Care is taken to avoid skiving of falling off of the medial face of the tibia into the soft tissues. The near cortex is drilled, fluoroscopy is then used to confirm the correct trajectory prior to breaching the far cortex. Once the far cortex is engaged, an image is taken perpendicular to the pin to allow for true assessment of bicortical purchase. Large C-arm fluoroscopy is instrumental in this task. If imaging is taken off axis, the pin may be driven too far and offend the soft tissues, or conversely, not far enough and be only unicortical, and thus unstable. The threaded portion of the pin should be entirely within bone, with the run out of the pin inserted just under the near cortex. The run out is the weakest part of the pin, thus, insertion within the near cortex provides a strengthening effect. Half pins are then placed in similar fashion along the medial tibial face off of the proximal ring and along the tibial isthmus at the distal ring. The nuts securing the half pin posts are then tightened. Additionally, short bolts are

placed in the appropriate holes of the posts to further secure the half pins. The tibial fine wires are tensioned to 130 mm Hg. The nuts are then tightened with a 10-mm wrench while the bolt is held static with a special slotted wrench with the tensiometer still applying tension. The tensiometers are then released. If multiple wires are utilized at a given ring, they should be tensioned in reciprocal fashion to avoid deformation of the ring. This entails tightening of the fixation nuts on the medial side of one wire and the lateral side of the other. The wires are then tensioned simultaneously on the opposite sides that are not yet tightened. While seemingly tedious at first, after several frame applications, these actions become second nature, and ultimately, reduce potential time-consuming complications from developing during the postoperative course.

The next phase consists of the application of the pedal block. An appropriately sized U-shaped foot ring is connected to the tibial block by way of additional threaded rods. The foot is secured by first placing the calcaneal wires. The foot is placed parallel to the frame with the ankle in neutral dorsiflexion. The first calcaneal wire is placed below the frame from medial to lateral, starting posterior to the neurovascular bundle. The next wire is placed from the posteromedial calcaneus and aimed laterally toward the fifth metatarsal base. This wire is placed above the frame as the intended target is the anterior calcaneal process, which is more superior than the calcaneal tuber. Crossing forefoot wires are placed, one starting medial and one lateral, capturing at least two metatarsals each. Given the trajectory of these wires, the frame often has to be built up to the wires utilizing plates and posts. Calcaneal wires are tension to 110 mm Hg while midfoot and forefoot wires are set to 90 mm Hg. The foot rings should always be closed. This is accomplished by using a full ring or by connecting the open ends of a partial ring with an arch or a threaded rod secured by posts. Failure to do so will result in ring deformation while the wires are tightened, analogous to goal posts bending toward each other.

The toes are then pinned in retrograde fashion if desired. These wires are not tensioned.

Finally, a walking ring is added to the foot plate via sockets. A postoperative shoe is attached to the walking ring by way of bolts and nylon threaded nuts to allow for traction during ambulation. The nylon threads prevent the nuts from backing off of the bolts. Pin sites are covered with slit sponges secured with plastic clips to prevent skin motion about the wires.

In the case of dynamic correction with computer software, precise fluoroscopic images are needed postoperatively. These images are taken with the x-ray beam shooting down the reference ring(s) to allow for accurate measurements that will be input into the deformity correction program. The fixator is overwrapped with an elastic bandage.

Although the exact fixator configuration will vary based on the specific deformities and pathology being addressed, an understanding of a basic static frame application will facilitate an appreciation of how more advanced constructs can be developed and adapted from this basic model. A clinical example of our standard static frame configuration as described above is provided in Figure 65.1. An adaptation of this is presented in Figure 65.2. In this frame, the distal tibial ring and foot plate are connected by struts instead of threaded rods to allow for gradual deformity correction. Note the talar wire connected to the distal tibial ring to hold the talus in place while the foot is rotated into a corrected position. The common fixator components are easily identified in each figure.

The surgeon should be familiar with the various fixator pieces to expedite assembly as well as allow for the most efficient and purposeful application, without excessive components or awkward configurations. The entire surgical team should be familiar with the various hardware trays, and a standard nomenclature should be adopted to allow communication between members and avoid operative delays.

Typically, surgical failures in external fixation cases relate to the application of the external fixator, which in large part stems from a lack of understanding of the device, not the type of fixator chosen. The stability and strength of external fixation, as with internal fixation, is largely dependent on its application.

The tibia's mechanical and anatomic axes are parallel, with the mechanical axis parallel and just medial to the anatomic axis. The calcaneus is aligned lateral to the tibia by 5-10 mm. When performing ankle or tibiotalocalcaneal arthrodesis, it is imperative to position the heel beneath the tibia so that the calcaneal bisection and mid-diaphyseal line of the tibia overlap. In the sagittal plane, the foot is placed at a right angle to the limb, and the tibial mid-diaphyseal line coincides with the lateral process of the talus. In the transverse plane, the foot is externally rotated to the limb for a 10-15 degree thigh foot axis.[18] These parameters should be kept in mind whether the position is obtained acutely such as in a single-stage arthrodesis or whether they will be achieved dynamically with the aid of deformity correction software.

As stated, the neuropathic patient presents a scenario for operative complications to be potentially devastating, both from their increased propensity for these complications as well as their tendency to be magnified in these patients. In these cases, more frequent office visits are required for close monitoring. External fixator stability is paramount. Issues typically do not interfere with the final surgical goal so long as they are swiftly remediated.

POSTOPERATIVE CARE

Complications can of course occur, with those universal to the management of lower extremity deformities as well as those unique to external fixation. Vigilance should be maintained for thromboembolic events; however, mobility assists with their prevention. Our standard protocol is a 1-month course of aspirin so long as there are no contraindications such as renal or gastrointestinal issues.

With respect to pin site care, a less is more attitude is generally employed. Crusts are left in place as a natural "seal" unless there is obvious accumulation of drainage beneath, or surrounding erythema. Pin site infections are not uncommon, but most are minor and can be addressed nonoperatively. A 10-day oral antibiotic regimen is usually sufficient, typically a first-generation cephalosporin. Culture-guided therapy can be implemented in the case of recurrent or persistent infection. The cause of the infection should be sought such as poor insertion technique, improper frame care, contamination such as animal dander, as well as excessive motion about the pin from a loss of tension. Limb edema that is repeatedly resolved with elevation creates a cycle where the skin is pistoning up and down the fixator pin, carrying contaminants on the wire or pin from superficial to deep, causing infection. Pin site necrosis can also occur from excessive tension about the skin, such as during gradual deformity correction or joint distraction. Major complications such as osteomyelitis, as well as nonunion and malunion can be encountered just as with internal fixation. If operative intervention is required, treatment can typically be continued while the issue is addressed (Fig. 65.10).

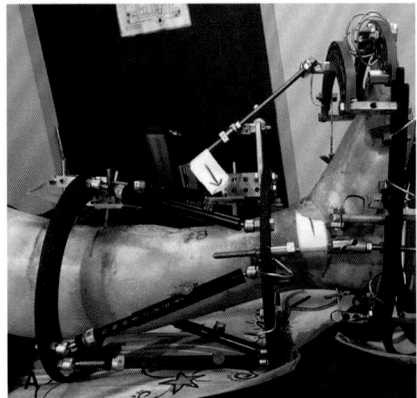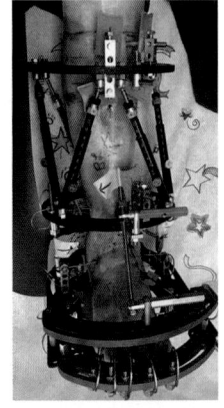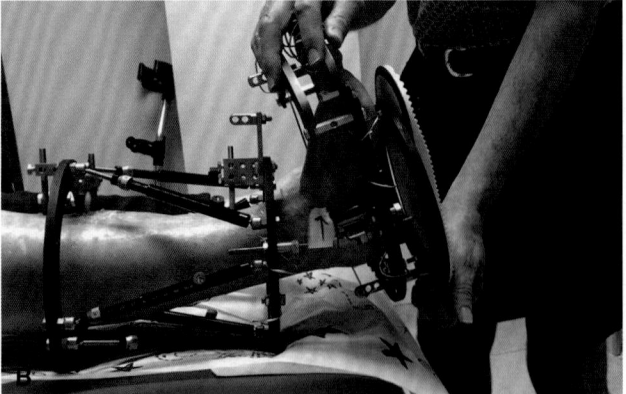

FIGURE 65.10 An example of a fixator construct for arthrodiastasis. **A.** Note the hinges that allow for range of motion exercise while in the fixator. Tape with arrows directs the patient on the proper method of turning the counting nuts for distraction. **B.** The patient undergoing active range of motion therapy with the anterior distraction rod removed.

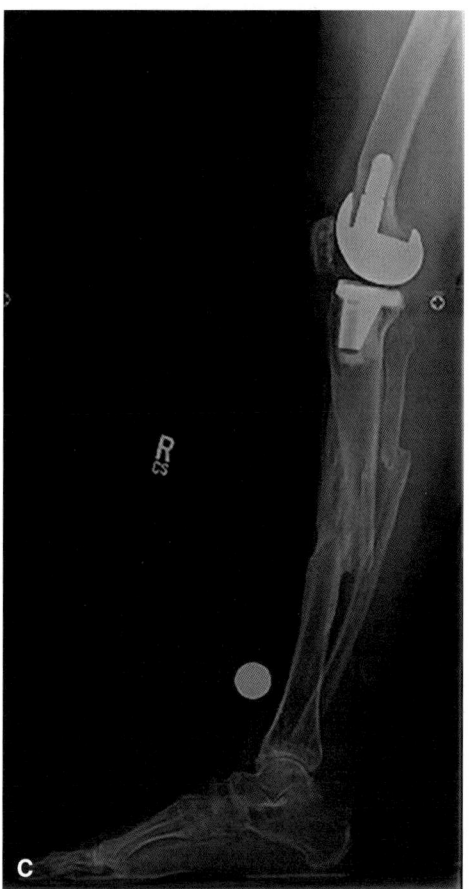
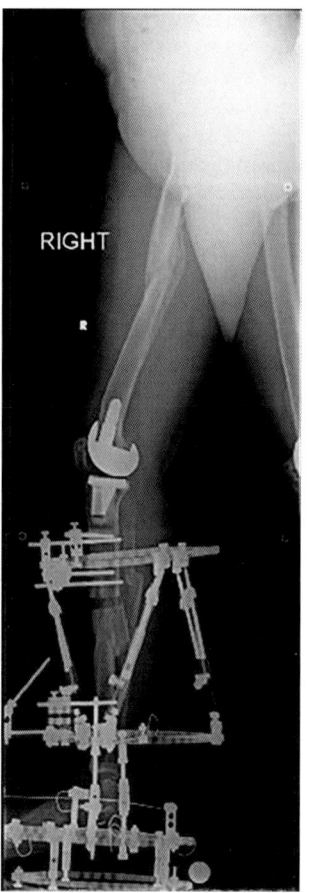
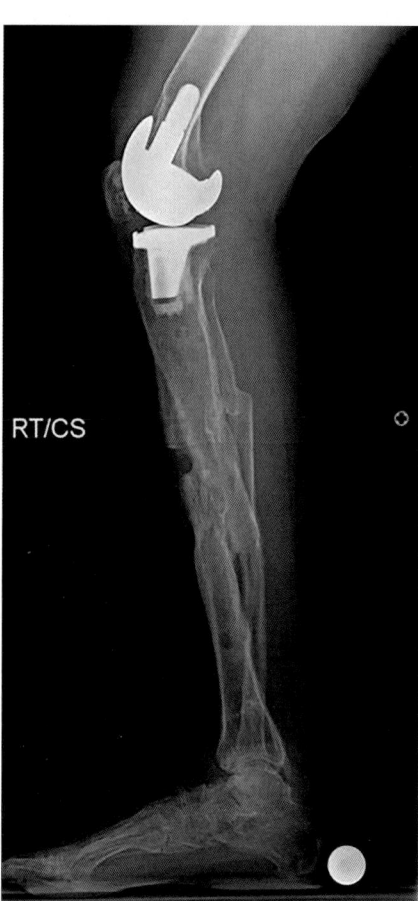

FIGURE 65.10 (*Continued*) **C.** Radiographs demonstrating the increased joint space. The fixator was also used to correct a proximal tibial deformity with tibial lengthening.

Other issues such as residual deformity, limb length inequality, as well as nerve complications are best mitigated with precise preoperative planning.

Nerve irritation or entrapment can occur with acute or gradual correction.[19] In general, the larger the degree of correction, the greater the likelihood of inducing tension or compression about the neurovasculature. While an exact amount of stretch or tension that will provoke symptoms cannot be quantified, it should be appreciated that even small degrees of correction can cause offense. This is especially true in the face of scar tissue from prior surgical intervention. Implants themselves can impinge or compress nerves during the treatment course. Early recognition and treatment by wither nerve decompression or removal of the offending implant is essential for recovery of nerve function. Prompt attention is required before permanent damage is incurred. While shortening does not place the tibial nerve on stretch, acute realignment of the rearfoot and ankle can produce stress as well as compression from osseous encroachment. We routinely perform concomitant tarsal tunnel decompression with deformity correction procedures. Common peroneal nerve decompression is also warranted with more proximal deformities, such as a proximal tibial valgus or external rotation correction (Fig. 65.11).

Wound issues can be mitigated with proper incision placement and planning. In the setting of acute shortening due to bone resection, transverse incisions should be considered. Vertical incisions are preferred otherwise and are mandatory with lengthening procedures where transverse incisions would be pulled apart. Careful planning is necessary in the presence of traumatized skin, flaps, and previous surgical incisions.

Fixation compromise can occur and at times requires revision surgery. Components can break with excessive loads. Smooth wires can fail from inadequate tension, while half pins tend to fail or cause stress fractures when part of an unstable construct.

REHABILITATION

The postoperative course after circular fixation is largely dependent upon the concomitant procedures performed. However, the authors routinely construct the fixator with the potential for weight bearing. In this way, one of the greatest benefits of external fixation over other forms of correction is utilized. Weight bearing limits disuse osteopenia, protects against deconditioning, and allows for maintenance of independence postoperatively. After admission, an assessment is performed by the physical therapy team to determine the patient's overall needs. Some patients ambulate quite naturally without any assistance in the fixator, while others are greatly aided by an assistive device such as a walker. In most instances, the patient can be discharged without the need for further therapy while

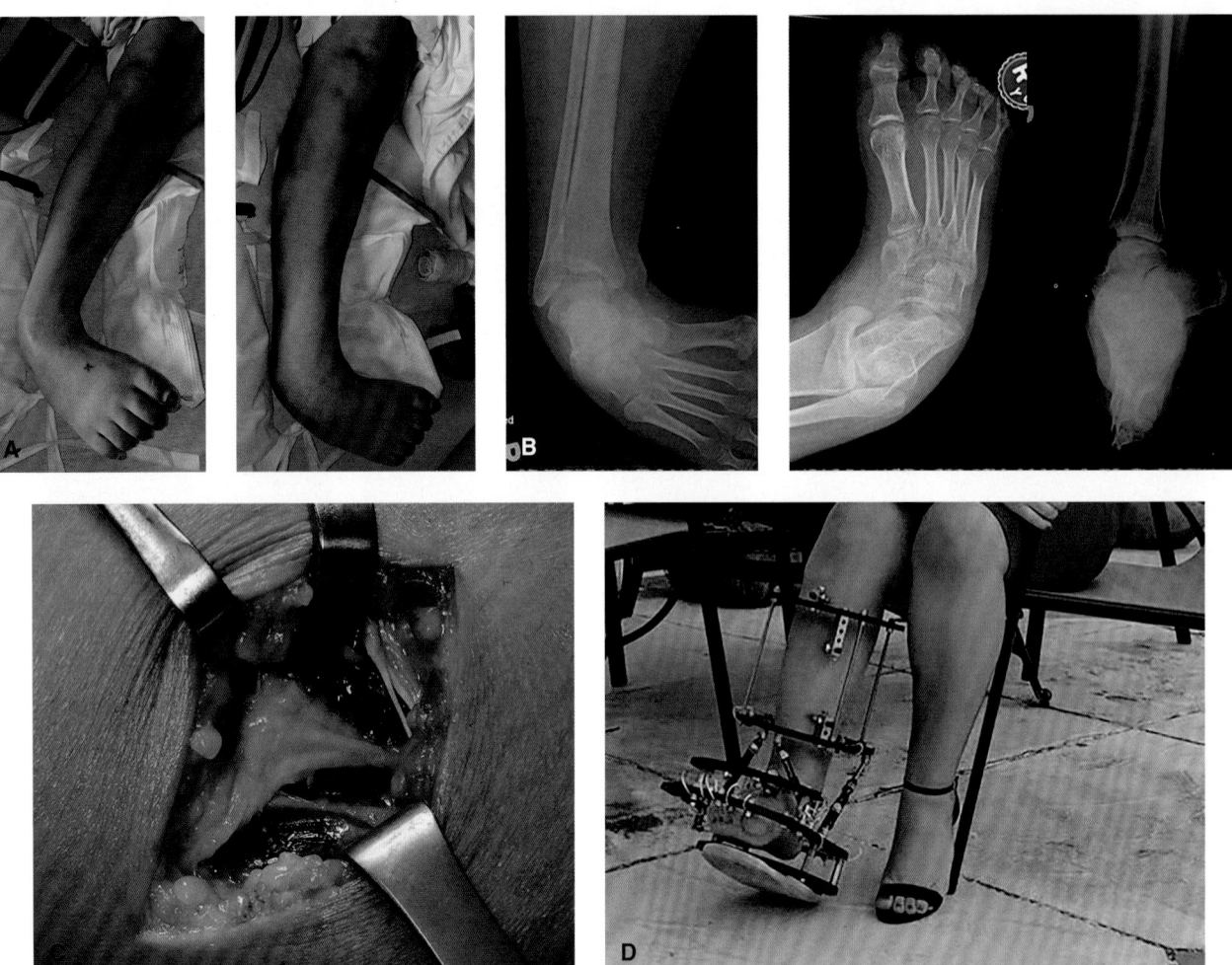

FIGURE 65.11 This patient incurred a recurrent midtarsal inversion deformity as the result of a fall. Despite casting as well as transarticular pinning at an outside location, her foot continued to reassume the deformed position. An extensive neurologic workup yielded diagnoses of focal dystonia and complex regional pain syndrome. **A.** Her deformity was that of equinovarus and was rigid. **B.** In addition to the midtarsal subluxation, the ankle was following into varus as well. **C.** Intraoperative image of the common peroneal nerve. Tarsal tunnel and common peroneal nerve decompressions were performed given the degree of correction and the neurologic etiology. **D.** The patient was quite active in the fixator.

the fixator is in place. If additional teaching is thought to be of benefit, such as negotiating stairs, home therapy can be ordered. More rigorous therapy is needed in the case of limb lengthening patients to prevent Achilles tendon and knee contractures. In these patients, a hinged fixator may be placed to allow for unobstructed ankle range of motion therapy. Contractures of the knee are best prevented by walking and standing, but should they develop, a knee cuff is a great tool to assist in remediation. This cuff is composed of circular fixator rings placed around a fiberglass thigh wrap. The rings are connected to the proximal tibial block in hinged fashion with a removable bar anteriorly. In this way, range of motion that is achieved during therapy can be captured.

Typically, the fixator is left in place for 2-4 months. When delayed union is encountered, the fixator can be modified in a noninvasive manner to encourage to promote bone healing.

This method is called dynamization. The technique is performed by systematically and sequentially destabilizing the construct. This can be accomplished by removing a strut, threaded rod, pin fixation cube, or even a segment of the external fixator. As the fixator is weakened, the bone is tasked with transferring more of the weight-bearing force placed on the limb. This increased stress prompts the bone to increase in cellularity and strength.

Upon fixator removal, 2-3 times/week gait training is utilized. Ambulation is first encouraged with a controlled ankle motion boot. In the case of arthrodesis, range of motion of the remaining essential joints is maximized. In arthrodiastasis cases, the preserved joint is aggressively rehabilitated to prevent any loss in the improved range of motion. Custom bracing is often utilized for at least 1 year postoperatively in the setting of arthrodesis procedures (Figs. 65.12 and 65.13).

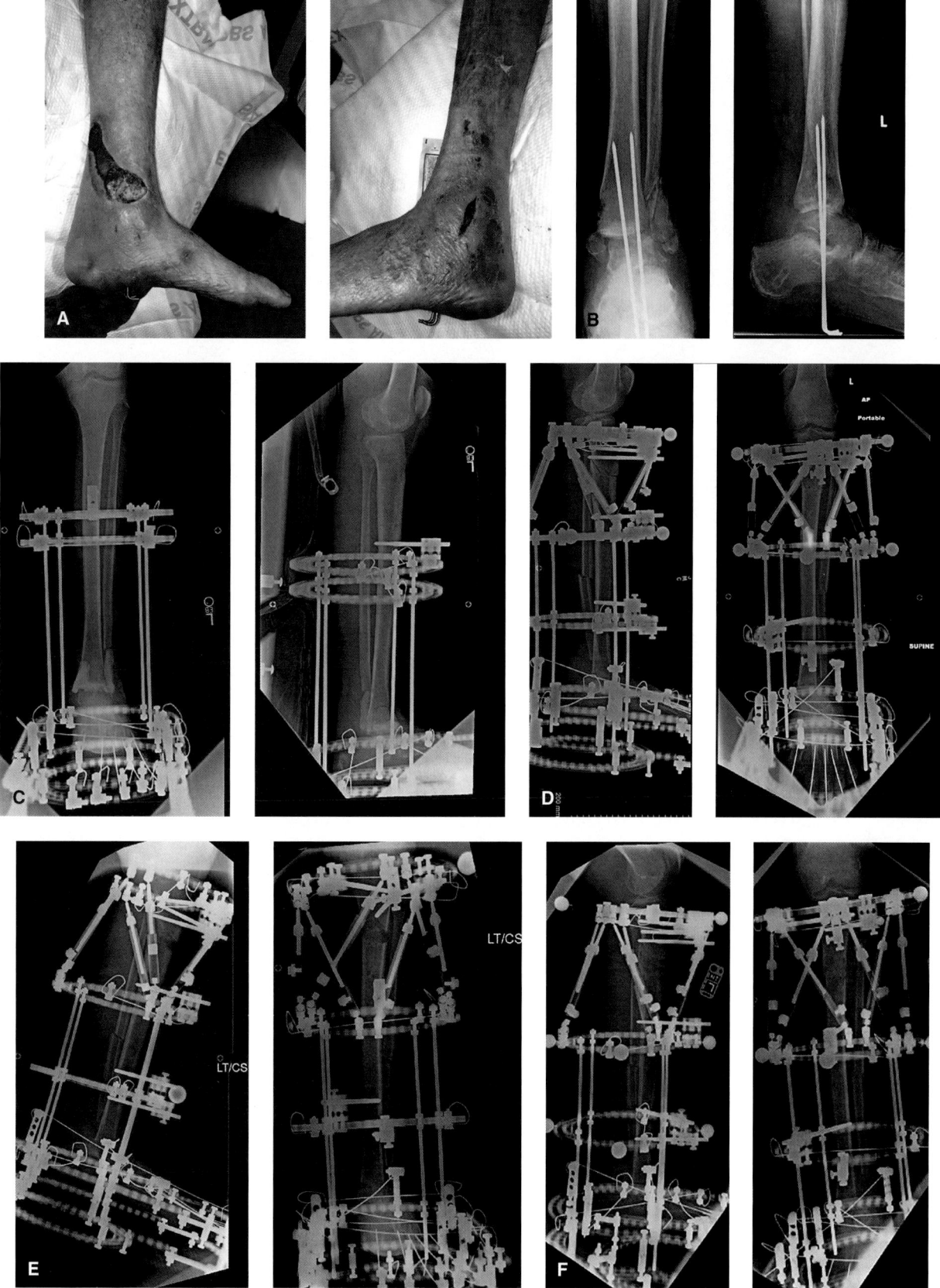

FIGURE 65.12 This patient sustained an open pilon fracture complicated by infection that necessitated substantial bone resection. Given the resulting limb length discrepancy, the fixator was utilized to both fuse the remnant talus to the resected distal tibia and lengthen the tibia proximally by distraction osteogenesis. **A.** Clinical photo on presentation to us after referral from the trauma surgeon. **B.** Initial radiographs. **C.** A simple static frame was employed to provide stability while an antibiotic spacer was in place to irradiate infection. **D.** A proximal tibial block was added with struts for gradual lengthening. The tibia and fibula were osteotomized. **E.** Imaging obtained during the lengthening phase. **F.** Restoration of limb length with robust regenerate formation to the tibial osteotomy.

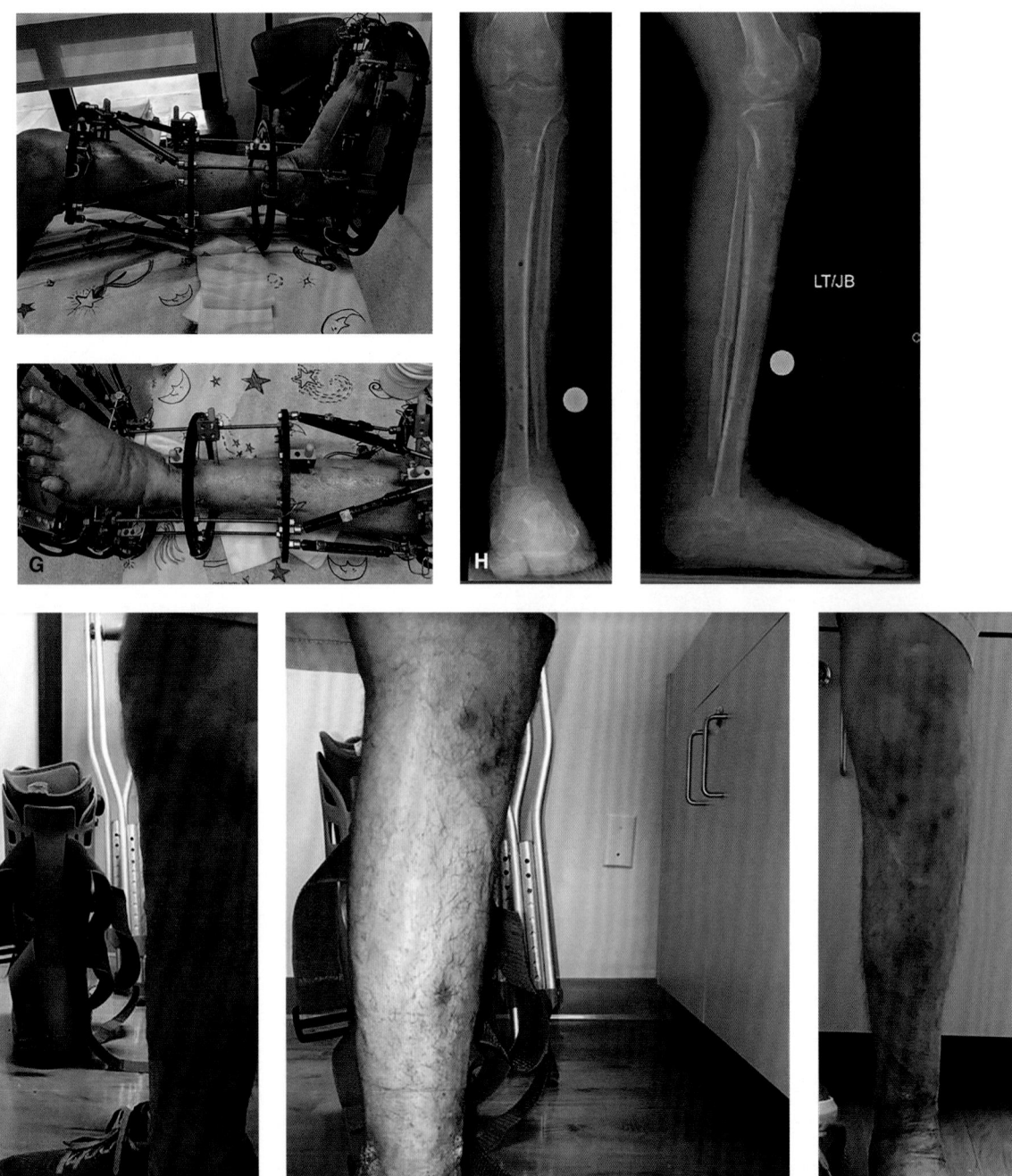

FIGURE 65.12 (*Continued*) **G.** Clinical images of the fixator in place. **H.** Radiographs obtained after fixator removal. **I.** Clinical result.

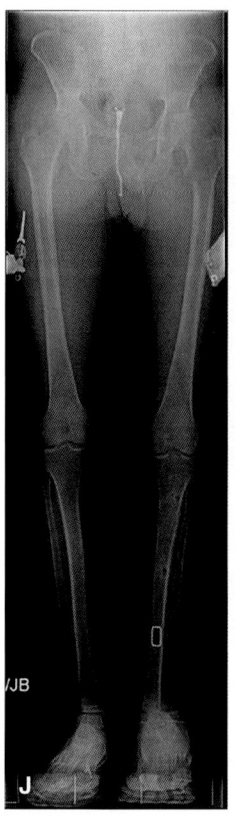
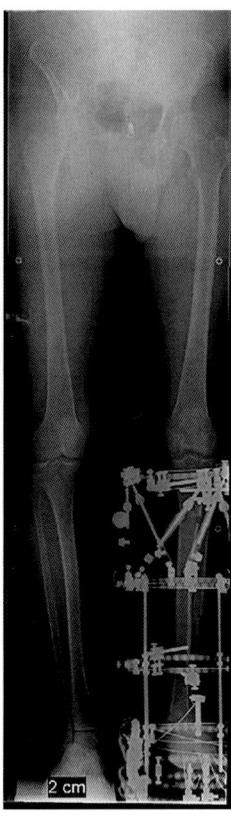

FIGURE 65.12 (*Continued*) **J.** Erect leg length films were used to assess limb length during the treatment course.

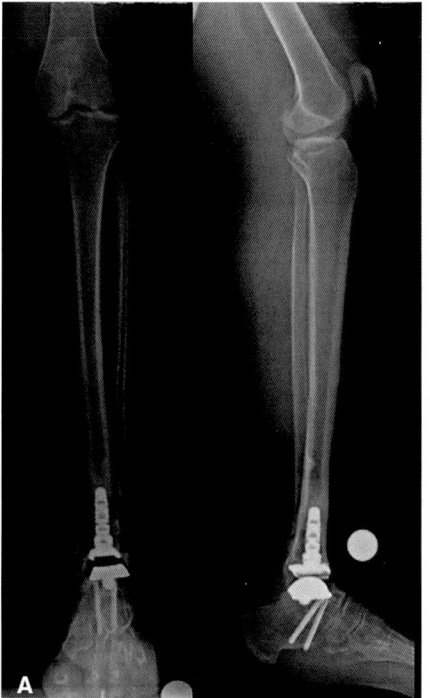
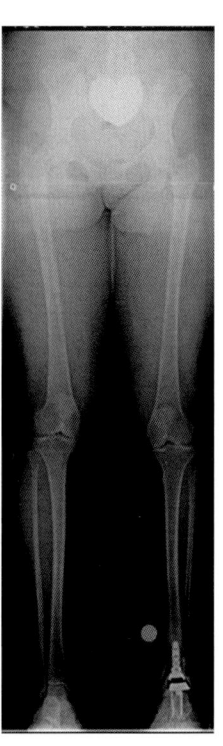
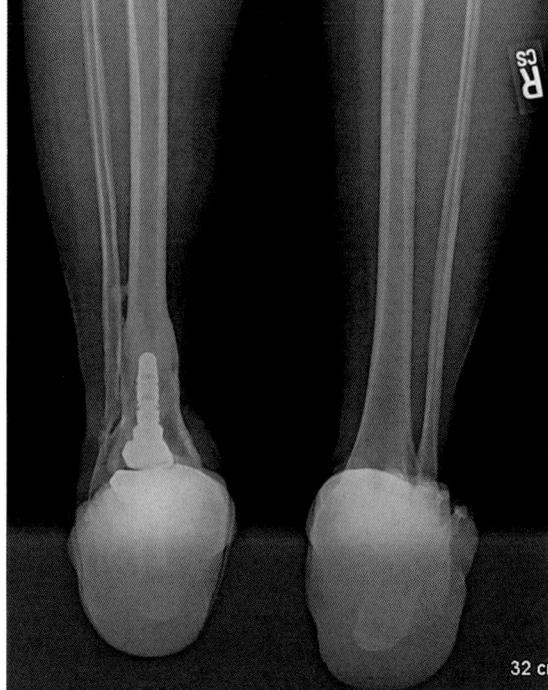

FIGURE 65.13 This patient sustained on open ankle fracture in her youth that resulted in ankle arthritis with equinus. A total ankle replacement was performed elsewhere. She presented to us with pain to her ankle as well as pain from a limb length discrepancy. **A.** Radiographs on presentation to our clinic. Note the differential knee levels given her limb length discrepancy.

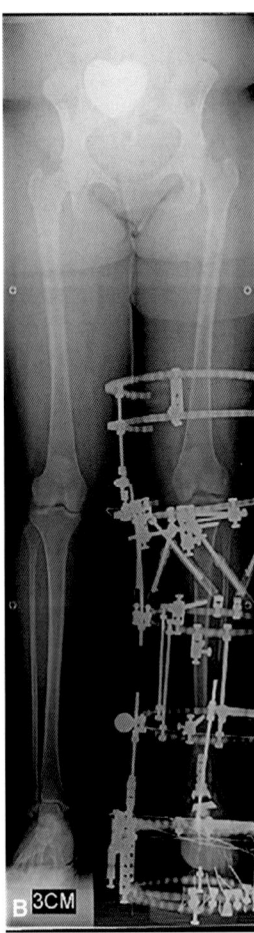
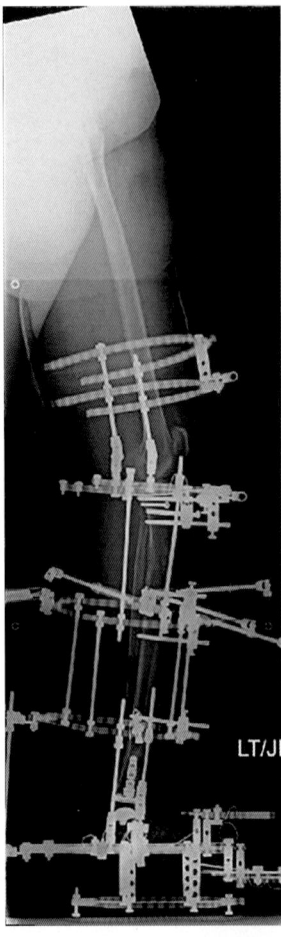
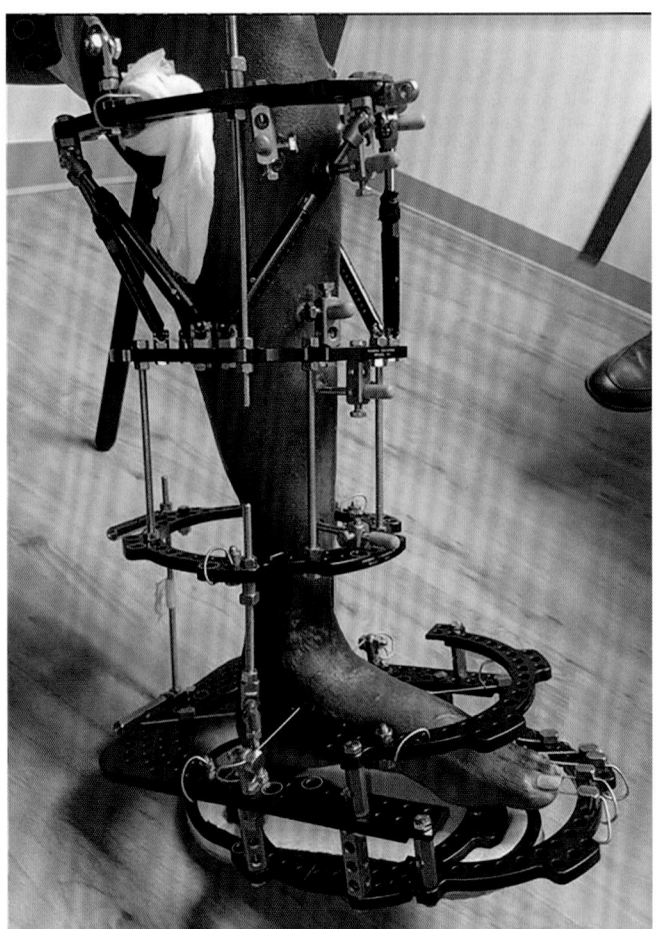
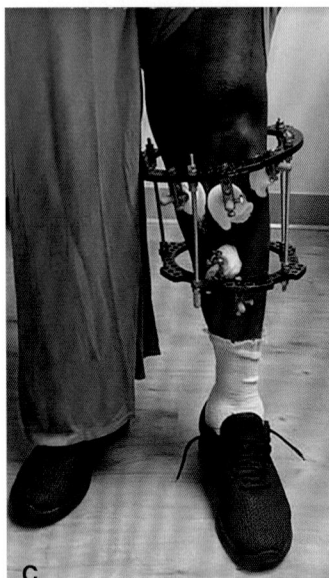
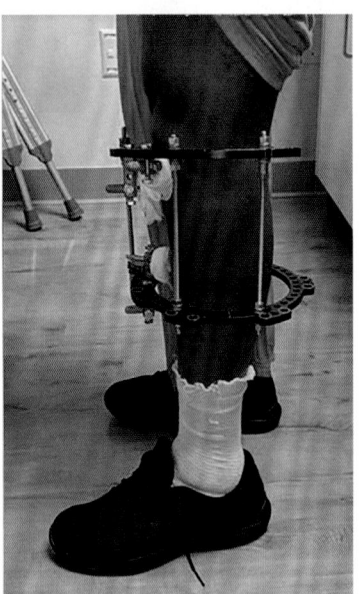
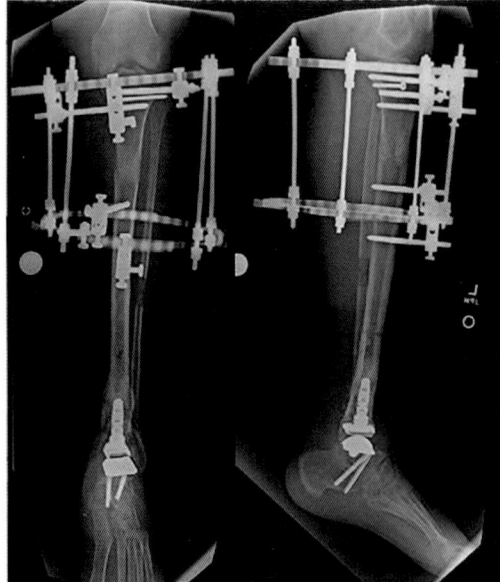

FIGURE 65.13 (*Continued*) **B.** A dynamic fixator was used to distract her ankle prosthesis as well as restore her limb length. A knee cuff was utilized for a knee contracture that developed during her course. This consists of rings extended on hinges and secured to the thigh by fiberglass. An anterior bar can be unlocked for range of motion and relocked to capture the gained range of motion. **C.** The fixator was dynamized by first removing the foot and distal tibial blocks. Note the marked increase in regenerate with the dynamization process.

REFERENCES

1. Hippocrates. *Works of Hippocrates.* Baltimore, MD: Williams & Wilkins; 1938.
2. Malgaigne JF. Pathologie externe. Considéracions cliniques sur les fractures de la rotule et leur traitment par les griffes. *J Conn Med Prat Pharmacol.* 1853;21:8-12.
3. The classic. A new apparatus for the fixation of bones after resection and in fractures with a tendency to displacement, with report of cases. By Clayton Parkhill. 1897. *Clin Orthop Relat Res.* 1983;(180):3-6.
4. Lambotte A. *Churugie Opératoire des Fractures.* Paris: Masson; 1913.
5. Codivilla A. The classic: on the means of lengthening, in the lower limbs, the muscles and tissues which are shortened through deformity. 1905. *Clin Orthop Relat Res.* 2008;466:2903-2909.
6. Romm S. Fritz Steinmann and the pin that bears his name. *Plast Reconstr Surg.* 1984;74:306-310.
7. Huber W. Historical remarks on Martin Kirschner and the development of the Kirschner (K)-wire. *Indian J Plastic Surg.* 2008;41:89-92.
8. Stader O. Treating fractures of long bones with the reduction splint. *North Am Vet.* 1934;20:62.
9. Schanz A. Handbuch der orthopädischen Technik für Ärzte und Bandagisten. Jena, Germany: Fischer; 1908.
10. Schwechter EM, Swan KG. Raoul Hoffmann and his external fixator. *J Bone Joint Surg Am.* 2007;89:672-678.
11. Golyakhovsky V. Gavriel A. Ilizarov: "The magician from Kurgan". *Bull Hosp Jt Dis.* 1988;48:12-16.
12. Chaudhary M. Taylor spatial frame-software-controlled fixator for deformity correction-the early Indian experience. *Indian J Orthop.* 2007;41:169-174.
13. Gasser B, Boman B, Wyder D, Schneider E. Stiffness characteristics of the circular Ilizarov device as opposed to conventional external fixators. *J Biomech Eng.* 1990;112:15-21.
14. Lamm BM. Percutaneous distraction osteogenesis for treatment of brachymetatarsia. *J Foot Ankle Surg.* 2010;49:197-204.
15. Pinzur MS. Simple solutions for difficult problems: a beginner's guide to ring fixation. *Foot Ankle Clin.* 2008;13:1-13, v.
16. Lamm BM, Stasko PA, Gesheff MG, Bhave A. Normal foot and ankle radiographic angles, measurements, and reference points. *J Foot Ankle Surg.* 2016;55:991-998.
17. Paley D. *Principles of Deformity Correction.* Berlin Heidelberg: Springer; 2002.
18. Paley D, Lamm BM, Katsenis D, Bhave A, Herzenberg JE. Treatment of malunion and nonunion at the site of an ankle fusion with the Ilizarov apparatus. Surgical technique. *J Bone Joint Surg Am.* 2006;88(suppl 1 Pt 1):119-134.
19. Lamm BM, Paley D, Testani M, Herzenberg JE. Tarsal tunnel decompression in leg lengthening and deformity correction of the foot and ankle. *J Foot Ankle Surg.* 2007;46:201-206.

SUGGESTED READINGS

Cherkashin AM, Samchukov ML, Birkholts F. Treatment strategies and frame configurations in the management of foot and ankle deformities. *Clin Podiatr Med Surg.* 2018;35:423-442.

Cooper P, Zgonis T, Polyzois VD. *External Fixators of the Foot and Ankle.* Philadelphia, PA: Lippincott Williams & Wilkins; 2013.

Fragomen AT, Rozbruch SR. The mechanics of external fixation. *HSS J.* 2007;3:13-29.

Lamm BM, Gottlieb HD, Paley D. A two-stage percutaneous approach to Charcot diabetic foot reconstruction. *J Foot Ankle Surg.* 2010;49:517-522.

Lamm BM, Mendicino RW, Catanzariti AR, Hillstrom HJ. Static rearfoot alignment: a comparison of clinical and radiographic measures. *J Am Podiatr Med Assoc.* 2005;95:26-33.

Paley D. Problems, obstacles, and complications of limb lengthening by the Ilizarov technique. *Clin Orthop Relat Res.* 1990;(250):81-104.

Paley D. The Ilizarov technology revolution: history of the discovery, dissemination, and technology transfer of the Ilizarov method. *J Limb Lengthen Reconstr.* 2018;4:115-128.

Paley D, Lamm BM, Purohit RM, Specht SC. Distraction arthroplasty of the ankle—how far can you stretch the indications? *Foot Ankle Clin.* 2008;13:471-484, ix.

Cages

Stephen A. Brigido and Dustin Constant

INTRODUCTION

Salvage of large segmental bone defects, nonunions, and angular deformities in the lower extremity can be difficult to treat for the most experienced of surgeons. While trauma is a common cause of large segmental bone defect, pathologies such as avascular necrosis, osteomyelitis, and Charcot neuroarthropathy are also common causes of large bone voids. As total ankle replacement continues to gain acceptance in the treatment of end-stage ankle arthritis, failed total ankle arthroplasty continues to be a challenge in the surgical setting when unable to revise.

While there are many techniques described as suitable treatment options for the above described foot and ankle pathologies, they all have significant limitations and associated comorbidities. Bone transport techniques have high union rates, but it requires external fixation to be in place upward of 1 year.[1] These technically demanding procedures are associated with pin tract infections, broken pins/fixators, and multiple fixator adjustments. Osteomyocutaneous flaps of the fibula,[2] allografts, and Masquelet techniques[3] have all been described in the setting of large boney defect and deformity; however, each of these procedures has a increased nonunion rate and often the need for multiple procedures. Tibiocalcaneal arthrodesis has demonstrated adequate fusion rate[4] but have a clear disadvantage in regard to limb length discrepancy and function.

Lessons learned from our colleagues in spinal surgery, as well as advances in titanium manufacturing and additive manufacturing, have given foot and ankle surgeons access to cage-type implants to fill large bone voids as an osteoconductive construct. Prefabricated cage implants come in predetermined shapes and sizes. Additive manufacturing, sometimes referred to as 3D printing, allows for lattice-type cages, spheres, and cylinders to be manufactured in an efficient and cost-friendly manner. These implants can be made in a multitude of shapes and sizes and also have the ability to be custom made to accurately fit the defect being treated.

HISTORY

The first mesh titanium cage was produced by Bohm, Harms, et. al in 1986.[5] The original intent was to act as a spacer where vertebral defects exist, but the design also allowed for harboring of bone graft. A novel technique for the use of titanium mesh cages to restore large boney defects in the lower extremity was first published by Cobos in 2000.[6] In the study, two successful cases were reported with excellent radiographic and clinical outcomes. Since then, many case studies have been published demonstrating successful utilization of titanium mesh cages in foot and ankle reconstruction.[7-9]

Adams[7] published an animal study in 2005 demonstrating that trabecular lattice structure of an implant allowed for early bone ingrowth and a substantial increase in implant strength over time. The evolution of trabecular metal implants designed for lower extremity reconstruction was described by Henricson in 2010.[10] This paper reported a series of 13 patients using a trabecular metal implant demonstrating good bone-to-implant interface. The positive outcomes were attributed to an implant design with porous structure and elasticity similar to that of native bone.

The largest study to date was published by Dekker in 2018.[8] This retrospective review of 15 consecutive cases utilizing patient-specific titanium cages demonstrated 87% success. Comorbidities included one infection and one nonunion that went on to below-knee amputation. In particular, this study demonstrated how a multitude of sizes and shapes of implants can be utilized to correct deformity, fill voids in traumatic high-energy injuries, and provide a viable option in the setting of failed total ankle arthroplasty.

MATERIALS

Cages used in foot and ankle surgery commonly come in two materials: titanium (typically titanium-aluminum-vanadium alloy [Ti6A14V]) and polyether ether ketone (PEEK). Titanium mesh cages were initially designed as fenestrated metal sheets used in cranio-maxillofacial surgery.[11] These titanium cages have evolved over time to be meshed, laser etched, and plasma coated to create a "trabecular" network of metal around the cage. Because osteoblast differentiation and osteogenic synthesis are stimulated by the roughened surface of titanium, implants made from traditional titanium can allow for good bone-to-implant contact and osteointegration.[12]

PEEK is a thermoplastic polymer that can be machined easily to form various shapes and sizes of orthopedic cages. PEEK is an inert platform that is used in various orthopedic, trauma, and spinal implants. PEEK differs from titanium in that it does not integrate well with surrounding bone and is thought to form a fibrous connective tissue interface.[13]

BENEFITS AND INDICATIONS

There are many benefits to using a cage in lower extremity reconstruction. One clear advantage is the ability to maintain appropriate limb length in cases that require repair of segmental bony defect or complete extrusion of the talus. There is also an inherit mechanical advantage with interference fit of the cage, which stabilizes the construct when combined with intramedullary fixation. The combination of cage and intramedullary fixation may reduce cantilever stress in both coronal and sagittal planes.[14] This creates an intraoperative stability about the surgical site that is often difficult to achieve.

Large harvest autogenous bone graft, fresh frozen allograft, and other allograft bone products can present several challenges in the operative setting. First, the bone scaffolds can be extremely difficult to fixate with hardware. These bone scaffolds are often fashioned to fit the defect manually, which is inaccurate. This can lead to graft fracture and poor native bone-to-graft apposition. Another significant challenge is graft resorption in the postoperative setting. As these grafts resorb and ultimately subside, additional stress is placed on the hardware. This can lead to broken hardware and nonunion.

The friction coefficient of trabecular metal cages is much higher than that of allograft bone and PEEK. The attraction of osteoblasts and increased formation of vascular supply around the fusion site further enhances the stability of the construct and reduces subsidence.[14]

The prevailing limitation of cage fixation lies within its cost. While nonadditive cages are more cost-effective, they are not as precise when restoring limb length and large segmental defects, nor are they as efficient as additive options when planning complex deformity correction. It has been reported that these implants can cost over $20 000 US.[8] The advantage of additive manufacturing is the seemingly endless customizable options in size, shape, and fixation.

> ## INDICATIONS
>
> Indications for the utilization of cages in foot and ankle reconstruction are as follows:
> - Revisional first MTP arthrodesis with significant bone loss or failed metatarsophalangeal joint implants
> - Flatfoot reconstruction, both extra- and intra-articular
> - Midfoot arthrodesis with significant bone loss
> - Primary hindfoot and ankle arthrodesis for treatment of avascular necrosis
> - Primary hindfoot and ankle arthrodesis for treatment of severe traumatic injury
> - Primary hindfoot and ankle arthrodesis for treatment of failed total ankle arthroplasty
> - Segmental defects of the limb secondary to tumor, osteomyelitis, and trauma

PREOPERATIVE PLANNING AND IMPLANT SELECTION

When considering the use of cages in the treatment of lower extremity pathology, one must consider a multitude of factors. Size and shape of the implant can only be determined after proper assessment of alignment and deformity. Appropriate

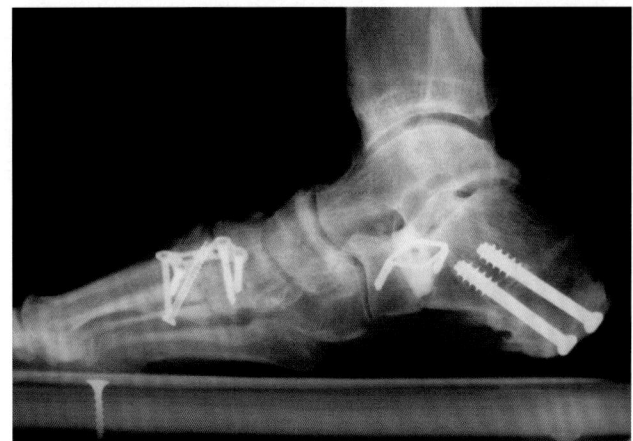

FIGURE 66.1 Lateral column calcaneal lengthening with titanium prefabricated cage in the shape of a wedge. (Radiograph courtesy of Christopher F. Hyer, DPM.)

radiographs are a necessity, and in the setting of limb deformity, full limb views must be obtained. Long leg views or computed tomography scanograms may be beneficial when addressing limb length for appropriate sizing of the implant. Magnetic resonance imagining and computed tomography may be beneficial to assess situations such as avascular necrosis, osteomyelitis, and prosthetic subsidence. In situations where additive manufacturing is preferred, protocol-specific computed tomography of the ipsilateral and in some instances bilateral limbs may be necessary.

Cages for the foot and ankle come in many sizes and shapes. The most commonly used prefabricated cage is in the form of a wedge. Wedges are constructed to offer uniplanar, biplanar, or event triplanar correction. These are beneficial in cases such as extra-articular osteotomies. Lateral column calcaneal lengthening, plantarflexory cuneiform osteotomies, and other bicorrectional osteotomies often benefit from wedge-shaped cages (Fig. 66.1). Other shapes include spherical, trapezoidal, circular (donut), and cylindrical. In a case with significant avascular necrosis and collapse of the talus, a spherical implant may offer the greatest ability to position foot in the most optimal position while maintaining the talonavicular articulation (Fig. 66.2). In the setting of failed ankle arthroplasty, the shape and size of the prosthetic will dictate the shape of the cage. For instance, a failed fixed bearing modular stem intramedullary total ankle implant may require a trapezoid shape cage due to the nature of the prosthetic footprint[15] (Fig. 66.3).

SURGICAL CONSIDERATIONS AND TECHNIQUE

FAILED FIRST METATARSOPHALANGEAL JOINT IMPLANT OR ARTHRODESIS

Failed first metatarsophalangeal arthrodesis or implants can leave a significant boney defect at the level of the joint. In some cases of failed arthrodesis, the revision surgery may allow for sufficient bone-on-bone apposition. In cases where direct bone-to-bone apposition is not an option, arthrodesis with cage fixation may be beneficial. Cage fixation is also beneficial in cases where silastic, metallic total and hemi-arthroplasty require explant due to failure. Cages can be utilized to not

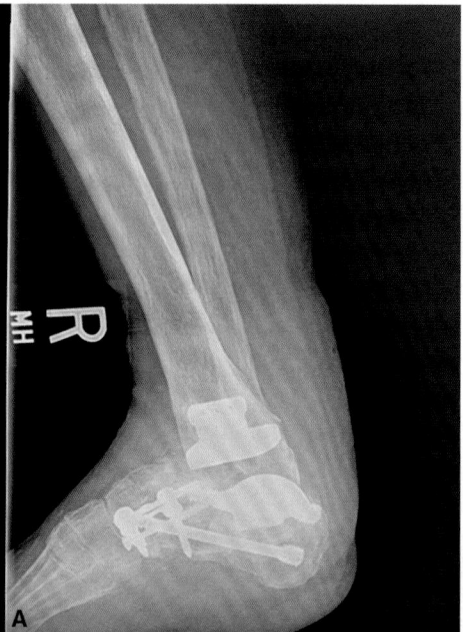
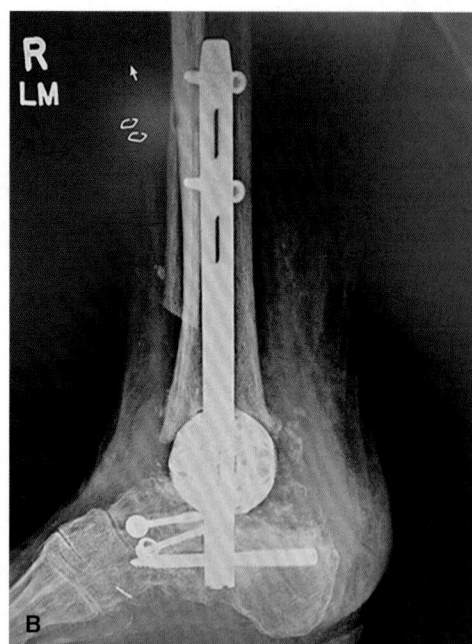

FIGURE 66.2 Preoperative **(A)** and postoperative **(B)** radiographs of a patient with a failed total ankle arthroplasty. Patient was treated with a spherical cage and intramedullary nail fixation.

only restore length of the first ray but also offer a stable, non-compressible construct, which can aid in early mobilization.[16] Historically, an autogenous iliac crest bone graft (ICBG) distraction arthrodesis was considered the gold standard for such cases; however, this is often associated with donor (harvest) site morbidity.[17] Donor site pain 6 months after surgery has been reported as high as 38% with 19% of those patients still experiencing pain 2 years postoperatively.[18] The clear advantage of autografts is the osteogenic properties, which are not offered with allografts. For this reason, calcaneal autograft, which has lower morbidity than iliac crest bone harvesting, combined with a cage may offer all the advantages of ICBG without the associated comorbidities.

SURGICAL PEARLS FOR FIRST METATARSOPHALANGEAL JOINT ARTHRODESIS WITH A CAGE

- Complete removal of failed implant or complete resection of nonunion in the case of failed fusion.
- Debridement of bone to healthy bleeding margins.
- Cage selection and shape should help assist in providing the appropriate position of the great toe for optimum ambulation.
- In selected cases, additive manufacturing may allow for the fusion plate to be incorporated into the cage (Fig. 66.4).

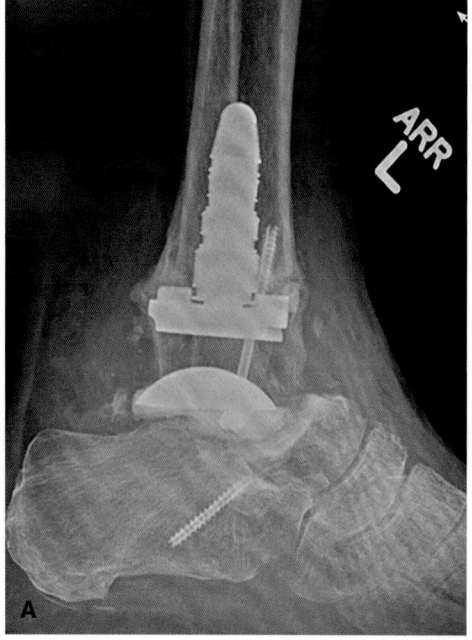
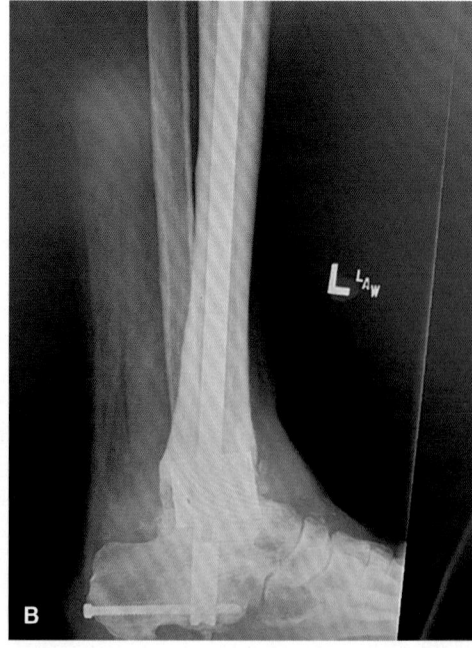

FIGURE 66.3 Preoperative **(A)** and postoperative **(B)** radiographs of a patient with a failed total ankle arthroplasty. Patient was treated with trapezoidal shaped cage and intramedullary nail fixation.

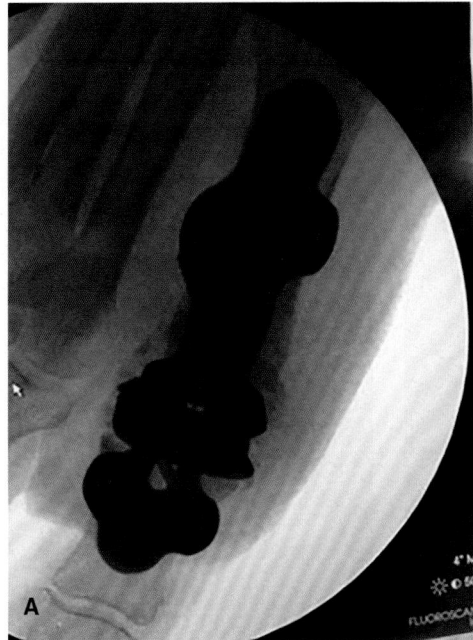

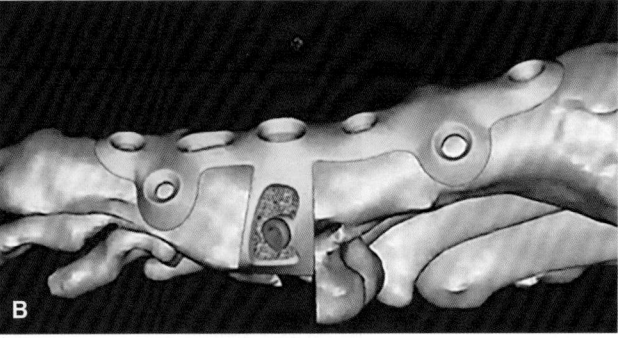

FIGURE 66.4 Preoperative planning image **(A)** with postoperative fluoroscopy of first metatarsophalangeal joint fusion **(B)** with additive manufactured cage and plate. (Photo courtesy of Additive Orthopedics.)

EXTRA-ARTICULAR OSTEOTOMY

In more recent years, the utilization of prefabricated wedged cages has drastically increased. Industry has now marketed cages toward extra-articular pes planus reconstruction. Wedges for plantarflexory cuneiform osteotomies and lateral column calcaneal lengthening are available with a large selection of sizes and shapes. The advantage of these wedges over the traditional allograft or autograft techniques is loss of correction due to graft resorption[19] (Fig. 66.5). As mentioned earlier, the open architecture and texture of the cage surface enhance bone ingrowth and osteoblast migration. When coupled with autograft or cancellous allograft packed within the cage, osteolysis around the osteotomy may be reduced.

SURGICAL PEARLS FOR EXTRA-ARTICULAR OSTEOTOMY

- Procedure performed no differently than standard surgical technique.
- Wedges may be used by themselves or may be used in conjunction with plates or staples for additional fixation.

HINDFOOT AND ANKLE FUSIONS WITH SUBSTANTIAL BONE LOSS

When addressing large segmental defects in the hindfoot and ankle, Berkowitz demonstrated that an isolated ankle fusion with bone-to-bone apposition was possible if the bone defect was <2 cm.[20] With the increased number of total ankle prosthetics available, a bone defect of this size can now often be addressed with a revision arthroplasty. Defects >2 cm create a mechanical disadvantage for all the muscles and tendons crossing the ankle joint and create abnormal stresses on the proximal joints of the lower extremity.[20] Cage fixation allows for the maintenance of length and ultimately helps preserve the biomechanics of the extremity to the best of the ability in the setting of salvage reconstruction. Early reports of cage and IM

nail fixation were used as a spacer and buttress, respectively. Newer technology allows for hardware fixation through the cage and, in some cases, may provide for added stability.

SURGICAL PEARLS FOR HINDFOOT AND ANKLE ARTHRODESIS WITH CAGES

- On the operating room table, position the patient on a stable platform in order to obtain all fluoroscopic views with ease. When considering a fibular takedown, it may be beneficial to place the patient in a slight lateral decubitus position with a beanbag or ipsilateral bump under the hip.
- After exposure of joints or removal of hardware, all bone margins should be adequately prepped to healthy bleeding bone.
- While placing the trial implants, the foot must be loaded in order to assess how well the implant fits. With a plantar flexed foot, one could easily oversize the implant leading to an equinus deformity.
- Autogenous or allograft bone can be used to pack the cage.

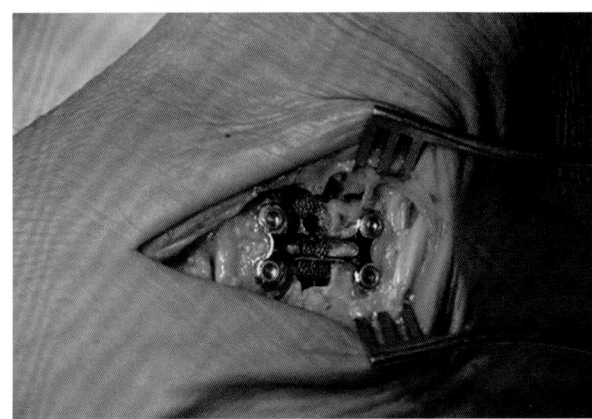

FIGURE 66.5 Picture of titanium cage used in calcaneal lateral column lengthening. Cage is fixation assisted via locking plate. (Photo courtesy of Christopher F. Hyer, DPM.)

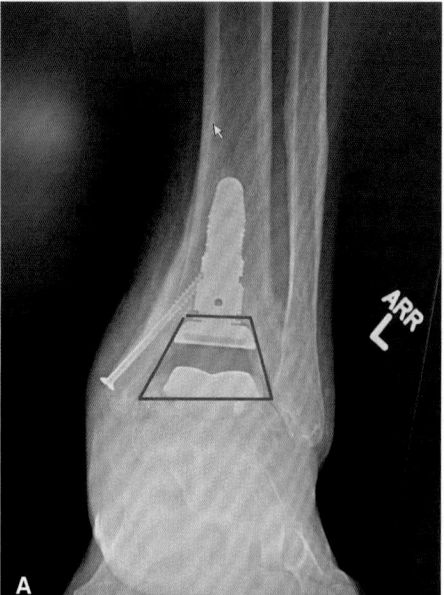
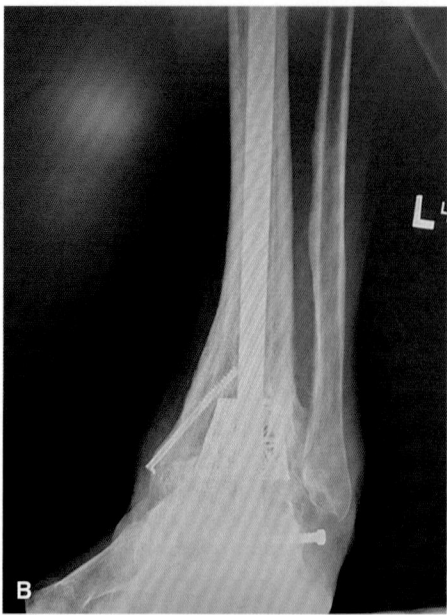

FIGURE 66.6 **A.** Preoperative planning using the "footprint" of the prosthetic to dictate size and shape of the cage. Notice *trapezoidal* shape that the failed total ankle replacement provides in the preoperative view and how well the construct fits the void in the **(B)** postoperative image.

SURGICAL PEARLS WHEN USING CAGES AFTER FAILED ANKLE ARTHROPLASTY

- Understanding the "footprint" of the failed ankle prosthetic will dictate the appropriate shape of cage used for repair (Fig. 66.6).
- Choices can range from trapezoid, square, rectangle, wedge, or spherical.
- Lateral approach with fibular takedown osteotomy often allows for access of prosthetic removal and increased visibility to ankle and subtalar joint.
- When using trapezoidal or square/rectangle-shaped cages, a sagittal saw may be best utilized for bone preparation. This will allow for good apposition between the bone and cage.
- When using spherical cages, an acetabular reamer may be used for bone preparation. This allows for progressive increase in reamer diameter, allowing the surgeon to obtain the optimum size of the implant for best fit (Fig. 66.7).
- When preparing the bone with an acetabular reamer, the foot must be positioned in the desired postoperative alignment. If the foot is plantar flexed while reaming, the radius of curvature of the tibia and calcaneus will not align.
- If using intramedullary nail fixation with the spherical cage, the guidewire and tibial reaming should be performed with the sizing template, not the final implant (Fig. 66.8).

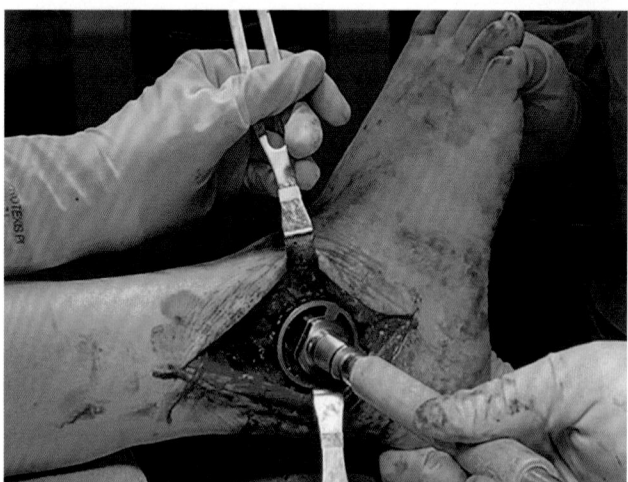

FIGURE 66.7 The use of an acetabular reamer to prepare the joint for arthrodesis with a cage.

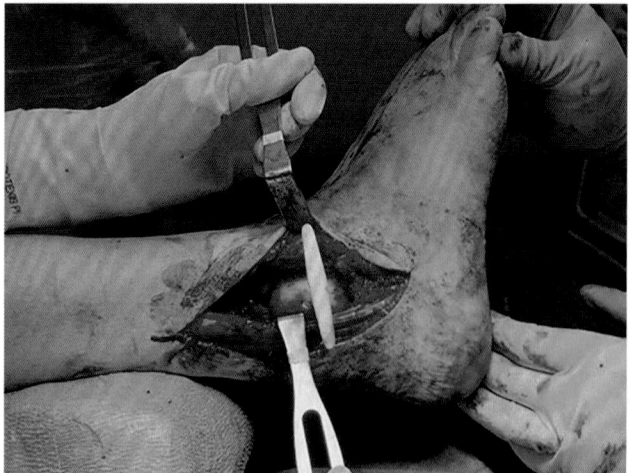

FIGURE 66.8 The use of the cage template to assist in positioning while fixating and reaming the tibia for nail insertion.

POSTOPERATIVE COURSE WHEN USING CAGES

The postoperative course when using a cage is very similar to that of a case using autograft or allograft bone. Patients are often placed in a multilayer compression dressing with posterior slab immediately after surgery. A non–weight-bearing period of 6-8 weeks is typically sufficient with serial radiographs dictating the exact course. Patients may be transitioned into a protective walking boot after non–weight bearing. Many surgeons will order computed tomography (CT scan) of the fusion site before the final transition into shoe gear and another at 12 months to ensure boney bridging.[8] While there are limited peer-reviewed data recommending the minimal amount of bone migration into the cage needed before weight bearing is initiated, it is generally accepted that 2 mm of bone penetrating each side of the cage is adequate for weight-bearing stability. Physical therapy may be beneficial in the addressing edema, strength deficits, gait abnormalities, as well as pelvic and lower extremity compensatory changes.

CONCLUSIONS

The use of cages, both prefabricated and additive, is another tool that foot and ankle surgeons may utilize to address the challenges of deformity correction, segmental bone loss, and allograft/autogenous bone grafting. Cage style implants eliminate the morbidity associated with harvesting large bone grafts from the iliac crest and lower extremity and decrease the healing time associated with bone transport in cases of segmental bone loss.

While this technology is promising and has become a tool with expanding indications for surgeons, there are several limitations. There is little known about the mechanical strength of these constructs and the effectiveness of how bone incorporates into the scaffold. There appears to be consensus among surgeons that the titanium alloy constructs are more effective than their PEEK counterpart. PEEK does not allow for boney incorporation and has been described as causing a fibrous interface between the cage and adjacent bone.

As with many new technologies, cost is a concern. A 2016 study demonstrated that these implants, when developed with additive manufacturing, can cost in excess of $20 000 US, excluding additional equipment such as intramedullary nails or plates. When including prefabricated cages, the average cost of a cage case was $11 700 US.[21] When compared to other types of salvage reconstruction (eg, spatial-based external fixation), these implants are still considered cost-effective. It is also reasonable to assume that as manufacturing for these implants continues to become more efficient, the cost of the product will decrease and become more readily available to surgeons.

In the setting of segmental bone loss, avascular necrosis, osteomyelitis, and deformity, reconstruction of the leg, ankle, and foot can be challenging for even the most experienced surgeon. Cages developed using prefabricated and additive techniques can provide surgeons an option that avoids the morbidity associated with large volume bone graft harvest and the complications associated with bone transport techniques or bone graft subsidence.

REFERENCES

1. Song HR, Cho SH, Koo KH, et al. Tibial bone defects treated by internal bone transport using the Ilizarov method. *Int Orthop.* 1998;22(5):293-297.
2. Chung YK, Chung S. Ipsilateral island fibula transfer for segmental tibial defects: integrate and retrograde fashion. *Plast Reconstr Surg.* 1998;101(2):375-382.
3. Wong TM, Lau TW, Li X, Fang C, Yeung K, Leung F. Masquelet technique for treatment of post traumatic bone defects. *Scientific World Journal.* 2014;2014:710302.
4. Myerson MS, Alvarez RG, Lam PW. Tibiocalcaneal arthrodesis for the management of severe ankle and hind foot deformities. *Foot Ankle Int.* 2000;21(8):643-650.
5. Bohm H, Harms J, Donk R, Zielke K. Correction and stabilization of angular kyphosis. *Clin Orthop Relat Res.* 1990;258: 56-61.
6. Cobos J, Lindsey R, Gugala Z. The cylindrical titanium mesh cage for treatment of a long bone segmental defect: description of a new technique and report of two cases. *J Orthop Trauma.* 2000;14:54-59.
7. Adams JE, Zobitz ME, Reach JS, An KN, Lewallen DG, Steinmann SP. Canine carpal joint fusion: a model for four-corner arthrodesis using a porous tantalum implant. *J Hand Surg Am.* 2005;30:1128-1135.
8. Dekker TJ, Steele JR, Federer AE, Hamid KS, Adams SB. Use of patient-specific 3D-printed titanium implants for complex foot and ankle limb salvage, deformity correction, and arthrodesis procedures. *Foot Ankle Int.* 2018;39(8):916-921.
9. Mulhern JL, Protzman NM, White AM, Brigido SA. Salvage of failed total ankle replacement using a custom titanium truss. *J Foot Ankle Surg.* 2016;55:868-873.
10. Henricson A, Rydholm U. Use of a trabecular metal implant in ankle arthrodesis after failed total ankle replacement. *Acta Orthop.* 2010;81:747-749.
11. Patel MF, Langdon JD. Titanium mesh (TiMesh) osteosynthesis: a fast and adaptable method of semi-rigid fixation. *Br J Oral Maxillofac Surg.* 1991;29(5):316-324.
12. Oliveres-Navarrete R, Hyzy SL, Gittens RA, et al. Rough titanium alloys regulate osteoblast production of angiogenic factors. *Spine J.* 2013;13(11):1563-1570.
13. Kurtz SM, Devine JN. PEEK biomaterials in trauma, orthopedic, and spinal implants. *Biomaterials.* 2007;28(32):4845-4869.
14. Zhang Y, Ahn PB, Fitzpatrick DC, Heiner AD, Poggie RA, Brown TD. Interfacial frictional behaviour: cancellous bone, cortical bone, and a novel porous tantalum biomaterial. *J Musculoskelet Res.* 1999;3:245-251.
15. Brigido SA, Didomenico LA. Primary zimmer trabecular metal total ankle replacement. Primary and revision total ankle replacement. In: Roukis T, et al., eds. *Primary and Revision Total Ankle Replacement.* Cham, Switzerland: Springer; 2016.
16. Coriaty N, Pettibone K, Todd N, Rush S, Carter R, Zdenek C. Titanium scaffolding for salvage of failed first ray procedures. *J Foot Ankle Surg.* 2018;57(3):593-599.
17. Brodsky JW, Ptaszek AJ, Morris SG. Salvage of first MTP arthrodesis utilizing ICBG clinical evaluation and outcome. *Foot Ankle Int.* 2000;21:290-296.
18. Goulet JA, Senunas LE, DeSilva GL, Greenfield ML. Autogenous iliac crest bone graft: complications and functional assessment. *Clin Orthop Relat Res.* 1997;339:76-81.
19. Lee IH, Chung CY, Lee KM, et al. Incidence and risk factors of allograft bone failure after calcaneal lengthening. *Clin Orthop Relat Res.* 2015;473:1765-1774.
20. Berkowitz MJ, Sanders RW, Walling AK. Salvage arthrodesis after failed ankle replacement: surgical decision making. *Foot Ankle Clin.* 2012;17:725-740.
21. Hamid KS, Parekh SG, Adams SB. Salvage of severe foot and ankle trauma with a 3D printed scaffold. *Foot Ankle Int.* 2013;34(12):1612-1618.

Interpositional Arthroplasty

Carl T. Hasselman and Alex J. Kline

Techniques for preservation of motion in arthritic joints using biological tissues has a long historical record with good success in many situations. Although arthrodesis has been the mainstay for many joints in the foot and ankle, the loss of motion in certain regions can limit normal function of the foot and alter gait function. Various techniques with mixed results have evolved over time in an attempt to alleviate pain and maximize function of the joint. This chapter will historically explore the various usage of biological tissues, the different techniques particular to a region in the lower extremity, and consider current and future roles that biological restoration of joint function play.

HISTORICAL OVERVIEW

The earliest reports of interposition arthroplasty were in the mid-1900s.[1] These authors discussed the use of porcine bladder or fascia lata to alleviate pain associated with degenerative arthritis of the hip. Since then, interpositional arthroplasty techniques have been described for many joints in the body to include the elbow,[2] shoulder,[3-8] hand,[9-20] knee,[21] and foot and ankle, which is the focus of this chapter. Over the years, biological materials used have included autograft tendons, allograft tendons, allograft meniscus, hematoma formations, and xenograft materials. Nonbiological materials, such as gold, carbon fiber, and ceramic materials, have been tried with poorer outcomes.[1,22] Current research into this area is focusing on stem cell technology, platelet-rich plasma, and newer biological materials as possible modifications on current techniques to improve outcomes.[23-25]

INDICATIONS

The indication for biological joint-preserving surgery is the younger patient with advanced arthritis that has failed conservative treatment, is limited in activities of daily living, and wishes to preserve function of the joint. A common question posed to patients by the author is "Which bothers you more, the loss of motion or the pain?" If the patient states both or just the loss of motion, then biological preservation of the joint is a better option. If the main complaint is pain and they do not mind the loss of motion, then arthrodesis is usually the better option with the understanding that the surrounding joints may become degenerative over following years.

A second indication may be the elderly patient with severe arthritis pain and significant medical comorbidities or any patient with limitations in function who could not tolerate the non–weight-bearing period needed for arthrodesis. In this situation, the early or immediate weight bearing offered by interpositional arthroplasty may allow a significant reduction in pain while not compromising the function of the patient.

These procedures are designed only to resurface the articular surface and do not correct deformities around the articular surface. If deformity is also present in conjunction with the arthritic condition, then procedures to correct the deformity must be combined with the joint-preserving surgery.

INDICATIONS

- Younger patient with advanced arthritis
- For patients wanting to maintain some motion
- Elderly patients with comorbidities that could not tolerate the postoperative requirements of an arthrodesis

ANKLE JOINT

Possible Joints for Interpositional Arthroplasty

- Ankle
- Subtalar
- Talonavicular
- Calcaneocuboid
- 4/5 Tarsometatarsal joints
- First metatarsophalangeal joint
- Lesser metatarsophalangeal joints
- Hammertoes
- Joints with persistent nonunion

The clinical presentation of ankle arthritis is variable and ranges from mild pain, stiffness, and swelling in early stages to disabling pain, significant loss of motion, and moderate to severe swelling in late stages. Radiographic changes noted as the arthritis progresses include joint space narrowing, osteophyte formation, subchondral sclerosis, and periarticular cystic formation. Ankle arthritis has been classified into four categories based on weight-bearing, plain radiograph of the ankle.[26] The classes were based on spur formation, sclerosis, joint narrowing, periarticular cysts, and ossicle formation. The

classifications are (1) doubtful, (2) minimal, (3) moderate, and (4) severe. Conservative measures include activity modification, bracing, nonsteroidal medications, and judicious use of corticosteroid injections.

Arthroscopic debridement and cheilectomy for symptomatic ankle arthritis is commonly used as a less invasive surgical treatment. The goal of this surgery is to remove loose bodies, excise anterior osteophytic spurs, and debride osteochondral lesions. Ankle arthroscopic debridement for the treatment of arthritis has recently undergone a thorough literature review regarding outcomes by the American Academy of Orthopedic Surgeons Ankle Arthritis Clinical Guideline Work Group.[27] These authors gave a grade B (fair evidence) treatment recommendation for the use of arthroscopic debridement of anterior bony osteophytes in patients with early stages of arthritis and spur formation (grades 1 and 2). They found that the evidence did not support the use of arthroscopic debridement for treatment of moderate and severe ankle arthritis (grades 3 and 4).

Prior to the introduction of interpositional arthroplasty, the only biological joint-sparing technique for moderate to severe arthritis was distraction arthroplasty using external fixation (arthrodiastasis).[28-31] This technique involves placing an external fixator that spans the ankle joint and distracts the ankle joint between 5 and 10 mm. The external fixator can be fixed, not allowing motion of the ankle, or articulated, allowing movement of the ankle. Patients are allowed to bear weight as tolerated for 8-14 weeks. At the time of distraction, the ankle joint may be surgically debrided open or arthroscopically and both have been described in the literature.[30,31] The mechanism of how joint distraction works is unclear, but theories have ranged from increased proteoglycans within the cartilage to decreases in subchondral sclerosis have been implied.[31] Unfortunately, the studies to date regarding outcomes of this technique are level IV (retrospective with small cohorts). The consensus statement by the American Academy of Orthopedic Surgeons is that distraction arthroplasty has shown efficacy in preliminary studies but the short- and long-term effectiveness of this technique is inconclusive based on current literature.[26] Regardless, this technique plays an important role for younger patients with moderate to severe arthritis who wish to maintain ankle motion. The development of degenerative arthritis in adjacent joints after ankle arthrodesis is significantly high in the younger patients,[32,33] and methods that can preserve ankle joint motion should be sought in this population.

Interpositional arthroplasty for the treatment of moderate to severe arthritis is a relatively newer technique and has been reported using allograft tendon,[34,35] allograft dermis,[36] and xenograft.[37] Although this technique has only a few published studies with small cohorts, the current results do show promise as a surgical intervention. With this technique, the concept is to place biological material between the talus and tibia in order to "cushion" the bones from contacting each other. Several approaches to the ankle have been described. Lee and Adams described using only an anterior approach and not securing the posterior graft.[34,35] Carpenter used an anterior incision combined with a posterior approach just lateral to the Achilles tendon.[36] Kline described smaller incisions at the anteromedial, anterolateral, posteromedial, and posterolateral borders of the ankle.[37] During the procedure, osteophytes are removed from the tibia, fibula, and talus to eliminate any impingement of the

ankle. The advantages to the two latter approaches are that the graft can be secured posteriorly as well as anteriorly and posterior osteophytes can be removed under direct visualization. The disadvantages are greater dissection of the soft tissues with increased chances of wound complications. The authors are currently working on arthroscopic techniques that will permit minimal soft tissue dissection; however, this technology is still being developed.

Once the ankle is exposed and all osteophytes are removed with an osteotome or burr, the joint is manually distracted with an external fixator,[35] femoral distractor,[36] or an osteotome/periosteal elevator.[34,37] With the ankle prepared and distracted, measurements are taken of the ankle surface area to be covered and the graft cut to the appropriate size (Fig. 67.1). In the case of Adams, the graft was one piece and stuffed posteriorly while attaching the graft anteriorly to the tibia and talus.[34] Lee placed separate grafts on the tibia and talus and used suture anchors on the joint surface to secure the graft anteriorly and midline.[35] Carpenter and Kline used separate grafts for the tibia and talus and secured the grafts at the four corners of the ankle joint[36,37] (Fig. 67.2). In the technique by Kline, the graft was pulled through the ankle joint by shuttling sutures attached to the graft through the four incisions around the ankle (Fig. 67.3). The graft was secured in each corner at both the distal tibia and talus using suture anchors (Fig. 67.4A). The postoperative course varied among authors with Adams allowing full weight bearing at 4 weeks and Carpenter and Kline beginning full weight at 3 weeks. Lee continued the external fixation during the postoperative state with fixator removal and full weight bearing between 3 and 6 weeks. With the exception of the case report by Adams,[34] the other three reports showed significant improvements in patient satisfaction and AOFAS scores (35-37 point improvements) with cohorts ranging from 4 to 20. Radiographic changes showed marked improvement in the joint space postoperatively when compared to the preoperative films (Fig. 67.5A-D). Although interposition arthroplasty for the ankle has only a 10-year history, the early studies show it is a viable option for younger patients with advanced arthritis

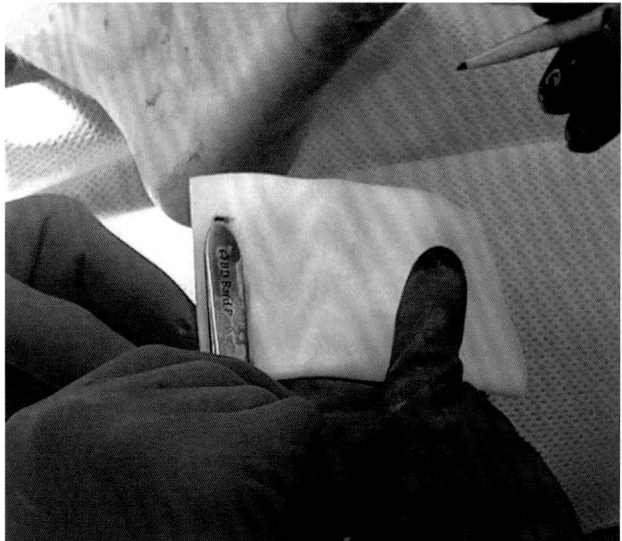

FIGURE 67.1 Xenograft material is measured and cut to cover the surface area of the distal tibia and talus. Bone marrow aspirate will be placed on the graft prior to insertion into the ankle.

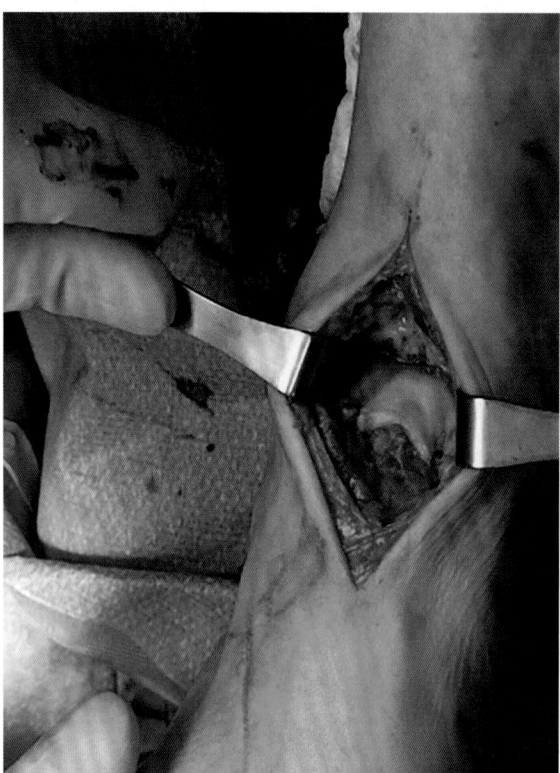

FIGURE 67.2 Anterior ankle exposed showing graft secured to distal tibia and talus with bone marrow aspirate in the graft. (Courtesy of Brian Carpenter.)

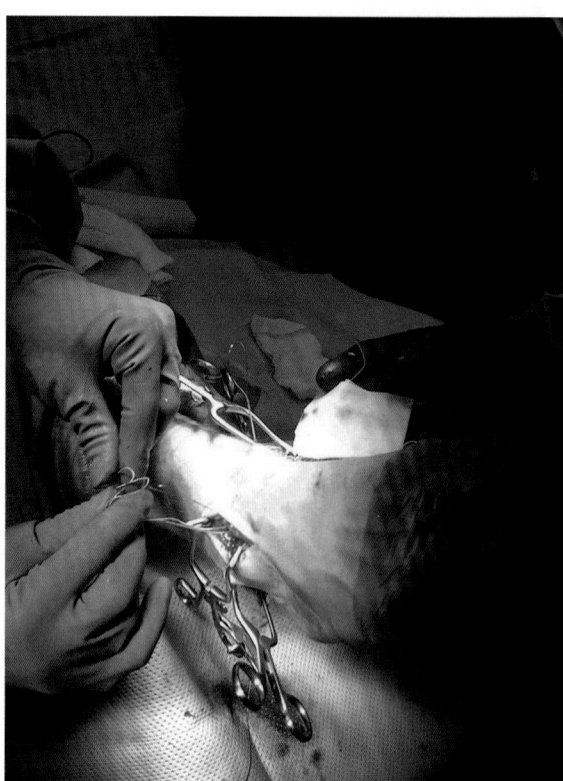

FIGURE 67.3 Intraoperative photo of graft being passed through the ankle using sutures as a shuttle to keep graft flat in the joint.

who wish to avoid arthrodesis and its subsequent complications. Further studies are needed to assess its long-term outcomes and overall efficacy as a surgical option.

Both arthrodiastasis and interpositional arthroplasty are techniques designed to biologically resurface the ankle joint, but they cannot correct deformities of the hindfoot. In the case of deformity at the ankle joint, procedures to correct the deformity such as supramalleolar osteotomies[38] should be done prior to or during the biological resurfacing procedure. In the case

of hindfoot deformity, procedures to realign the hindfoot[39] should be undertaken prior to or during the resurfacing procedure. It is the authors' preference that realignment procedures should be undertaken prior to any biological resurfacing procedure as often the realignment procedure may avoid the need for a second procedure. Only if the ankle and hindfoot are neutrally aligned and the younger patient persists with symptomatic arthritis should arthrodiastasis or interpositional arthroplasty be performed.

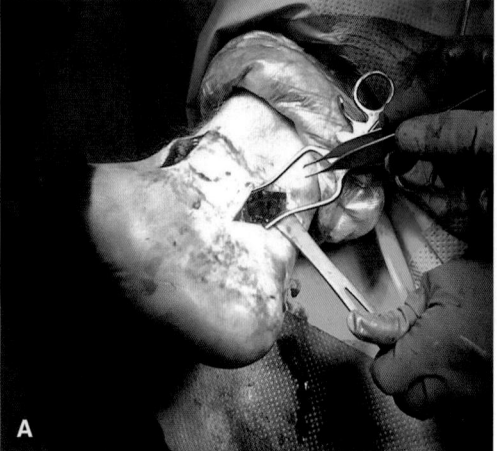
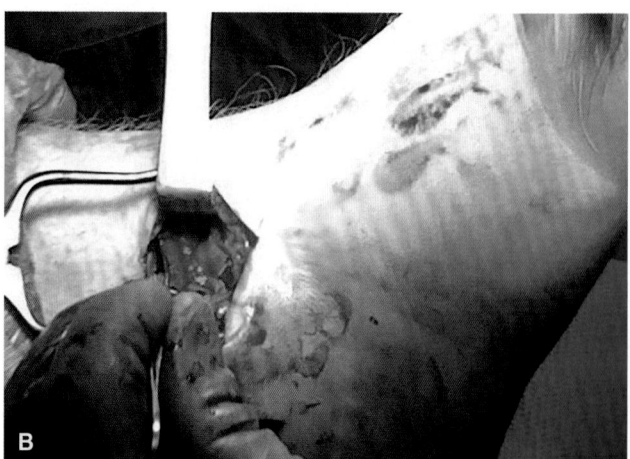

FIGURE 67.4 A. Posterior medial corner showing graft secured to distal tibia and talus.
B. Anterolateral corner of the ankle showing graft secured to distal tibia and talus.

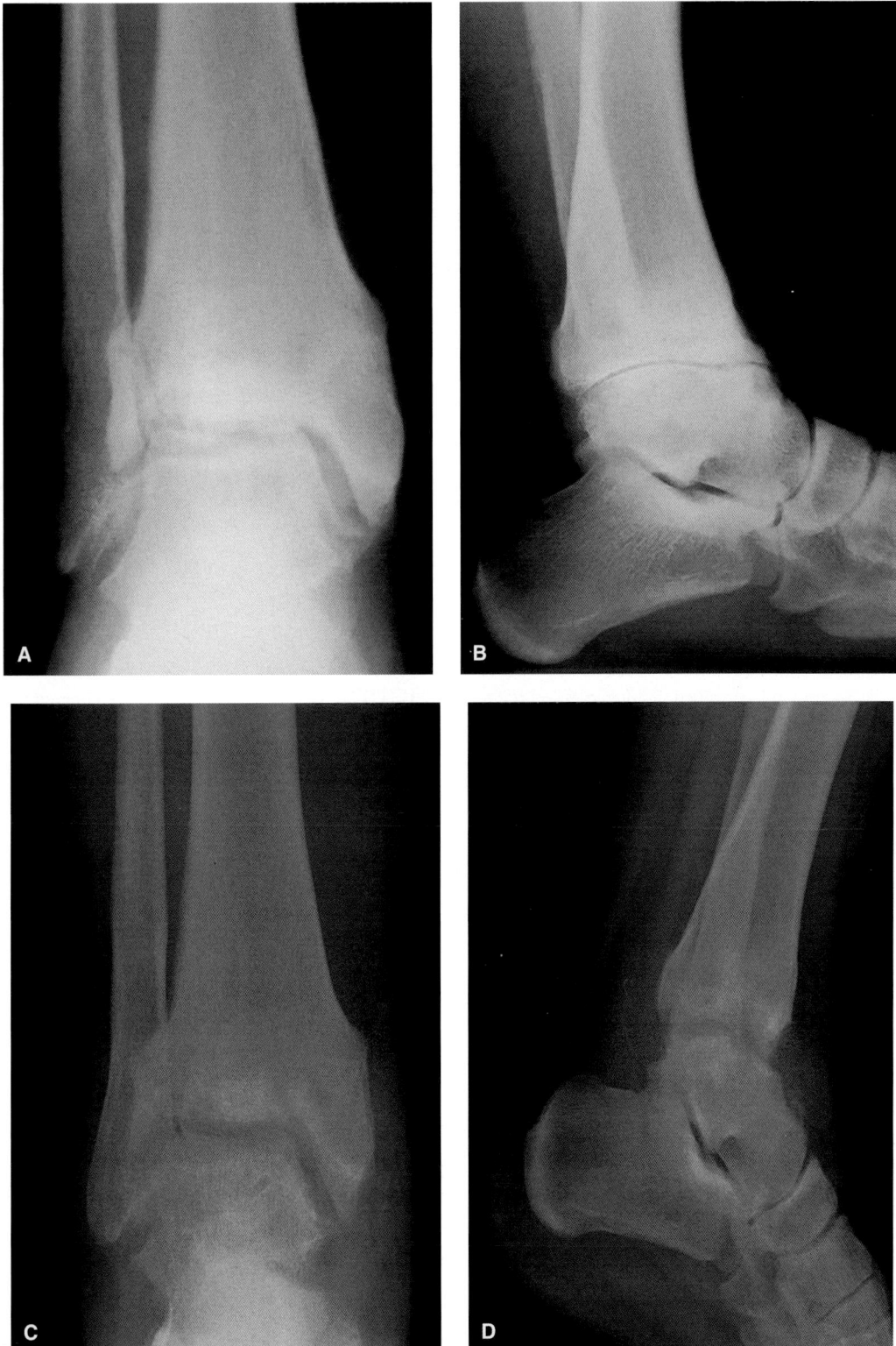

FIGURE 67.5 A, B. Preoperative AP and lateral radiographs of degenerative ankle.
C, D. Postoperative AP and lateral radiographs of same patient after interpositional arthroplasty and removal of arthritic spurs.

SUBTALAR JOINT

Interpositional arthroplasty as a treatment option for posttraumatic arthritis of the subtalar joint has been previously reported only once.[40] In this series of 22 patients with posttraumatic

subtalar arthritis, the average age was 39 years old. All had failed conservative treatment and were limited in activities of daily living. Either an extensile lateral approach or sinus tarsi approach was used to expose the joint. Tensor fascia lata autograft from the ipsilateral thigh or fat autograph from the posterior ankle

was harvested and sutured into place to resurface the posterior facet of the subtalar joint. Patients were not allowed to bear weight on the heel for 6 weeks. At 1-year follow-up, the authors reported a marked improvement in AOFAS scores, decrease in visual analogue pain score (VAS), and a poor result in only two patients. In the two patients with a poor result, arthrodesis was successful as a follow-up procedure. Although this is the only known report of interpositional arthroplasty for the subtalar joint, the results are promising and can be considered as a treatment option in the younger patient with posttraumatic subtalar arthritis. More recently, dermal allograft has been used as a biological material with promising results as well, and publications on this technique are forthcoming.[41]

TALONAVICULAR JOINT

Although arthrodesis of the talonavicular joint has been found to have good clinical outcomes, there have been two case reports of interpositional arthroplasty for this joint. In a report by Patel et al., an 89-year-old man with numerous cardiac and renal comorbidities underwent simultaneous bilateral interpositional arthoplasties of the talonavicular joints.[42] The patient had failed all conservative treatments, but an arthrodesis would prevent weight bearing and compromise his medical conditions. In their technique, a dorsomedial incision was made over the talonavicular joint and the distal 5 mm of talar head was resected. A fresh frozen Achilles allograft was folded over, shaped, and sutured into place where the talus was resected. The wound was closed and the patient allowed to bear weight immediately in a postoperative shoe. At 1-year postoperative follow-up, his pain continued to be markedly reduced. His AOFAS score and VAS score went from 16 and 9.5 preoperatively to 66 and 0.5 postoperative at 1 year. The second case report involved a 50-year-old female with posttraumatic arthritis of the talonavicular joint who had failed two attempts at arthrodesis.[43] In this case, the nonunion site at the talonavicular joint was resected and a piece of dermal allograft was sutured into the resected area. Postoperatively, the patient was allowed to bear weight in a walking boot. At 2-year postoperative follow-up, the AOFAS score had improved from 60 preoperative to 90 postoperative and she reported no pain with activities of daily living. Although these are just two case reports and there are no prospective or retrospective studies, these give the surgeon options in difficult situations such as these.

CALCANEOCUBOID JOINT

The use of interpositional arthroplasty to address calcaneocuboid nonunions has also been described.[44] In this case report, a 49-year-old female with rheumatoid arthritis had undergone a triple arthrodesis with failure to fuse of only the calcaneocuboid joint. Two more unsuccessful attempt at fusion were made. Because of her limited mobility, non–weight bearing was difficult to be compliant with. The authors went through a lateral incision and excised the fibrous nonunion of the calcaneocuboid joint. A piece of regenerative allograft tissue was sutured into the nonunion site. The patient was allowed full weight bearing in a leg brace for 1 month. At 1-year follow up, the patient had minimal pain with activities of daily living and radiographs showed graft survival in the region. Again, although this is just one case report

and there are no prospective or retrospective studies, this technique gives surgeons a possible salvage for difficult cases such as this. Further studies would be needed to compare calcaneocuboid arthrodesis to interpositional arthroplasty to determine its role in the treatment of symptomatic arthritis of this joint.

4/5 TARSOMETATARSAL JOINT

Historically, arthrodesis of the 4/5 tarsometatarsal (TMT) joints was the preferred method for surgical treatment of advanced arthritis of these lateral column joints.[45-47] However, biomechanical studies of gait and midfoot function subsequently showed the importance of motion at the lateral column for normal gait.[48-50] These studies show that most of the midfoot motion occurs through the lateral column. Furthermore, it was shown that during normal loading, most of the load is carried by the second and third TMT joints; however, as the load increases and foot position changes, the fourth and fifth TMT joints play an important role in load sharing.[49] It is the mobility of these joints that allow load distribution to occur. This mobility may explain why arthrodesis of the 4/5 TMT joints has been complicated by nonunions.[47,51-53] It is for these reasons that interposition arthroplasty for the 4/5 TMT joints has become more popular for the treatment of painful advanced arthritis.[54,55] In these reports, a dorsolateral incision was made over 4/5 TMT region and the articular surfaces of the cuboid and 4/5 metatarsal bases were resected. The ipsilateral peroneus brevis was split or the peroneus tertius harvested, and this autograph was sutured between the resected ends of the bones. Patients were made non–weight bearing for 6 weeks in a postoperative shoe. At 24-month follow-up, six out of the eight patients were markedly improved and said they would have the procedure again.[54] In the second series, all three patients were able to resume unrestricted activities without pain after 3 months.[55] Since these reports, many have used allograft tendon and dermal allograft as alternatives to autograph tendon with similar good results (Fig. 67.6A and B). The most important part of this technique is that an adequate resection is done to ensure that the bone ends do not make contact during weight bearing (Fig. 67.7). Interposition resection arthroplasty as a surgical treatment of symptomatic, advanced arthritis in the 4/5 TMT joints has become accepted as the primary treatment over arthrodesis.

FIRST METATARSOPHALANGEAL JOINT

Perhaps the most written about area in the lower extremity for interpositional arthroplasty is the first metatarsophalangeal joint (MTPJ). It has long been known as a treatment alternative for end-stage hallux rigidus when all conservative measures failed. There has been numerous studies reporting the use of autograph tissues as the interposition material. Regarding autologous tissue, areas where tissue were harvested include rib periosteum,[56] dorsal capsule of the first MTP,[57] medial capsule of the first MTP,[58] periosteum from the tibia,[59] extensor hallucis longus,[60] plantaris,[61] gracillus,[62] gastrocnemius,[60] and fascia lata.[63] Allograft materials have included meniscus,[64] amniotic membrane,[65] dermal tissue,[66] and regenerative matrix.[67] Although many different tissues have been identified for use, the basic technique involves making a dorsal or dorsomedial incision over the first MTP. The joint is debrided of all loose bodies and

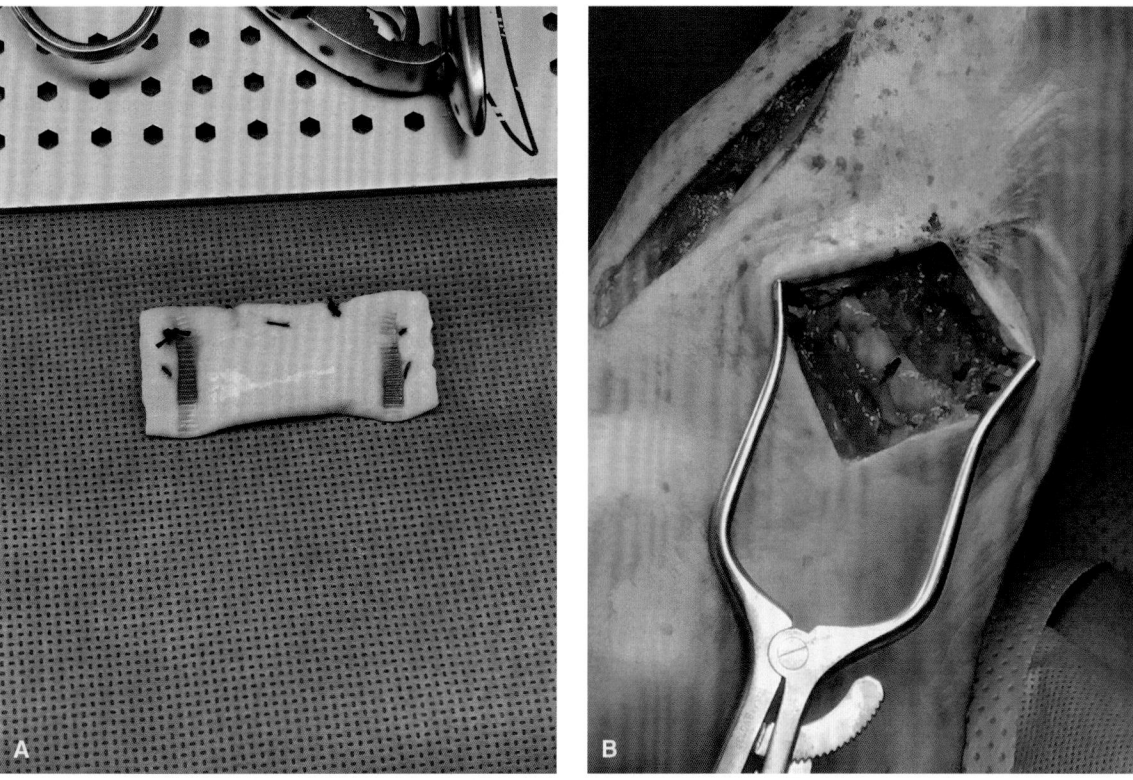

FIGURE 67.6 A. Dermal allograft material cut and rolled into the size of resected bone between the cuboid and 4/5 metatarsal. The graft is sutured into this shape. **B.** Intraoperative view of resected cuboid end with allograft tissue in place between the cuboid and 4/5 metatarsal bases. The space resected is filled with the graft.

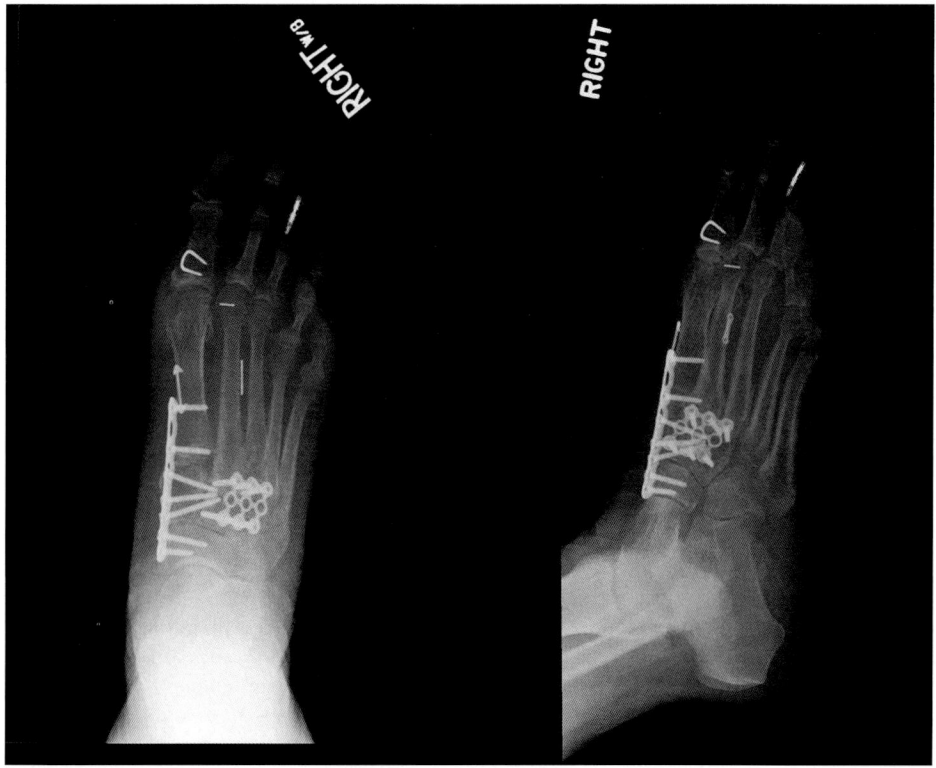

FIGURE 67.7 Oblique radiograph of the foot after resection arthroplasty. Note that the distal end of the cuboid does not contact the base of the 4/5 metatarsals.

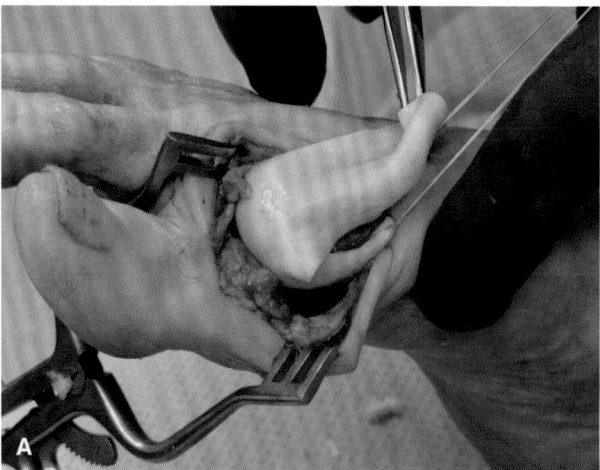
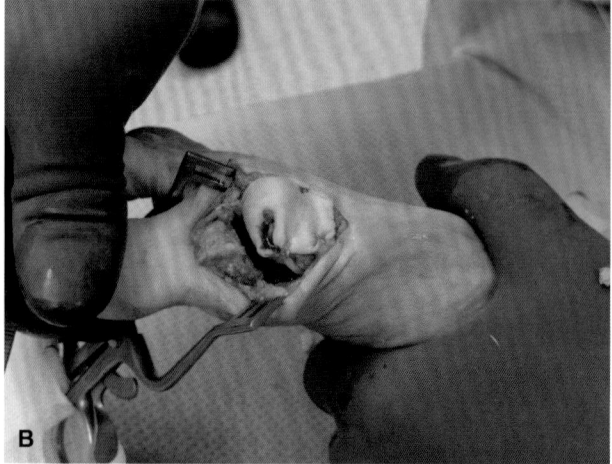

FIGURE 67.8 **A.** A piece of dermal allograft is wrapped around the metatarsal head after debridement of the joint. **B.** The dermal allograft is sutured at the sides and excess is trimmed so that the graft appears to make a boxing glove over the metatarsal head.

osteophytes. Any sesamoid osteophytes are removed as well. A dorsal cheilectomy of the metatarsal head is done, typically removing roughly the dorsal 25% of the metatarsal head. A portion of the base of the proximal phalanx is removed, and this is where many authors differ in their approach. Some remove only the dorsal 4 mm and angle to the plantar articular surface,[66] while others remove 4 mm of the entire phalangeal base, leaving a small rim of articular surface in the center.[68] Regardless, the graft is then placed between the metatarsal articular surface and the resected base of the phalanx. There are numerous variations on this technique with each report showing acceptable outcomes with their technique. Most reports have shown good to excellent results with 2- to 4-year follow-up. A review of the literature with autologous tissues showed good to excellent results at 2 years.[69] A variation of the above techniques using regenerative tissue has been described.[67] In this procedure, the regenerative matrix is wrapped around the metatarsal head and sutured into place like a boxing glove (Fig. 67.8A and B). The authors nicknamed the procedure "the boxing glove technique." A 5-year follow-up of this procedure showed that all six patients were satisfied and AOFAS scores improved from 38 to 66.

One of the most common concerns with interpositional arthroplasty is transfer metatarsalgia. Current interpositional arthroplasty techniques suggest minimal or no resection of the base of the proximal phalanx,[57-71] whereas previous techniques described resection of 25% of the base of the phalanx.[72,73] It appears that patients with an athletic lifestyle, a first metatarsal shorter than the second metatarsal, preexisting metatarsalgia, or greater resection of the phalangeal base have a higher incidence of transfer metatarsalgia after interpositional arthroplasty.[69] Transfer metatarsalgia did not seem to be a complication when minimal or no resection of the phalangeal base occurs during the procedure.[69]

More recently, the use of interpositional arthroplasty as a motion-preserving technique for failed implant arthroplasty has been recognized as an alternative to fusion with an intercalary graft.[74,75] The technique has been well described by Gene Curry, MD. In this technique, a dorsal incision is made over the first MTP joint and the joint exposed. Any prior implants are removed (Fig. 67.9) and the metatarsal head and phalangeal base are convexly reamed to create a spherical space between the metatarsal head and phalangeal base (Fig. 67.10).

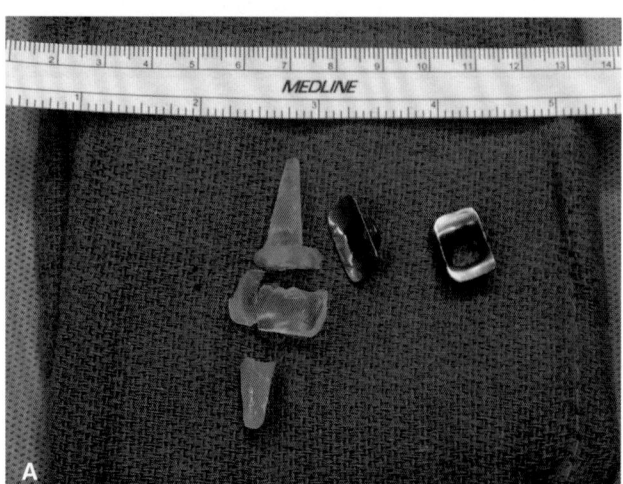
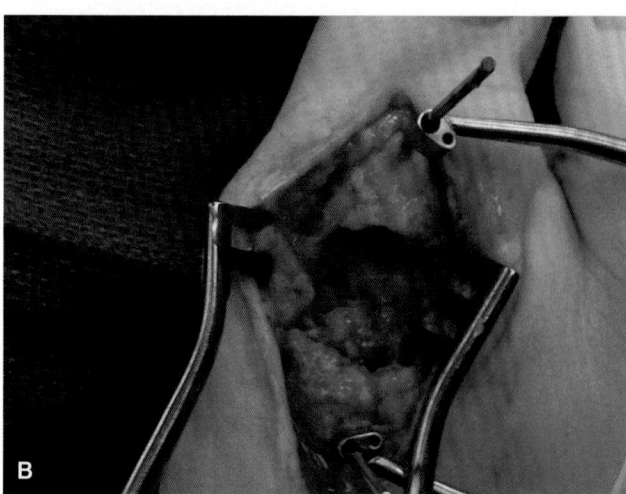

FIGURE 67.9 **A.** The removed failed implant from the MTP. **B.** The remaining joint distracted and nonviable tissue/synovitis removed from the area. (Courtesy of Gene Curry, MD.)

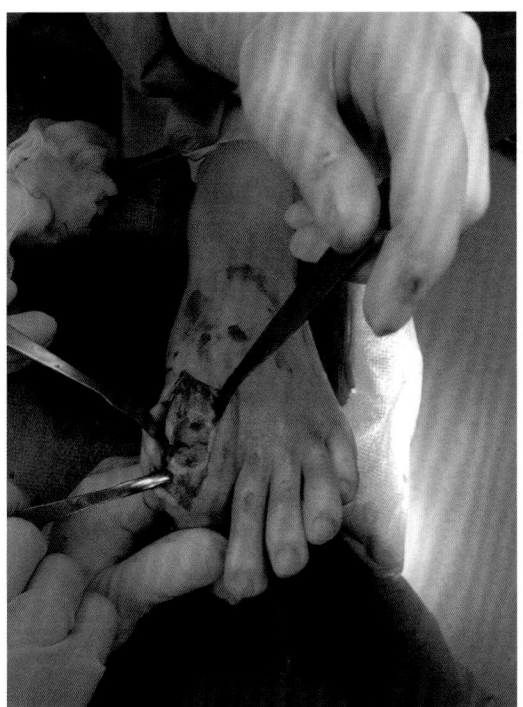

FIGURE 67.10 The metatarsal head and phalangeal base are conically reamed and drilled to prepare for the tendon allograft. (Courtesy of Gene Curry, MD.)

Semitendinosus allograft is sutured and shaped into a sphere that matches the defect created by reaming with care to ensure that the length of the first ray is maintained (Fig. 67.11A-C). The interposition graft is sutured into place (Fig. 67.12A and B). The wound is then closed in layers. The cited authors have immobilized the joint with a K-wire[74,75]; however, others allow immediate movement of the joint in a postoperative shoe. For those choosing K-wire placement, the patient is allowed to heel weight bear in a postoperative shoe for 6 weeks. At 6 weeks, the K-wire is removed and activities as tolerated may begin. These authors did feel that contraindications to this anchovy procedure include advanced hallux rigidus as a primary procedure, high demand athletes, severe sesamoidal arthritis, and patients with significant hallux valgus or varus deformities. These authors did report complications with this procedure to include angular deformity, transfer metatarsalgia, and decreased joint range of motion; however, it is an option for patients who wish to avoid the prolonged immobilization, protected weight bearing, alteration in shoe wear, and complications associated with intercalary bone block arthrodesis.

LESSER METATARSOPHALANGEAL JOINTS

Interpositional arthroplasty for the lesser MTPJs has been described as well for degenerative arthritis that has failed conservative treatment.[59,76-80] These reports specifically discussed end-stage Freiberg disease when the entire MTPJ was damaged

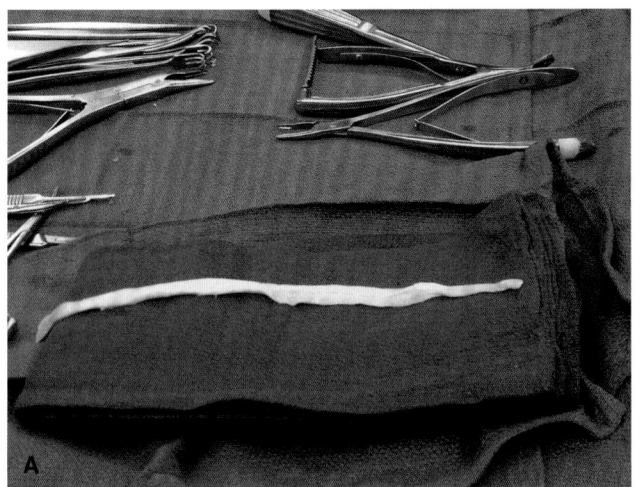

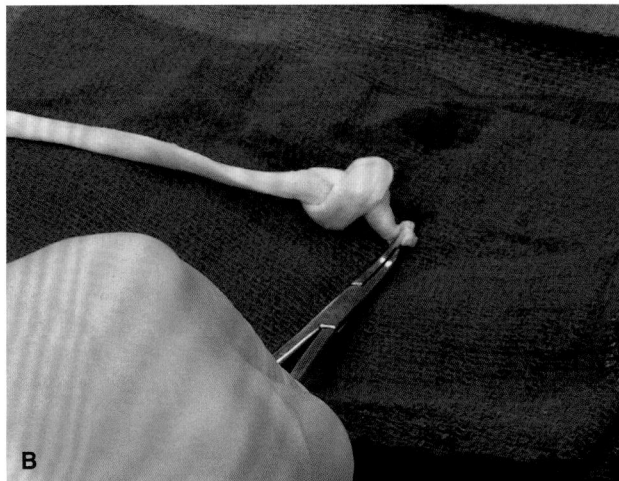

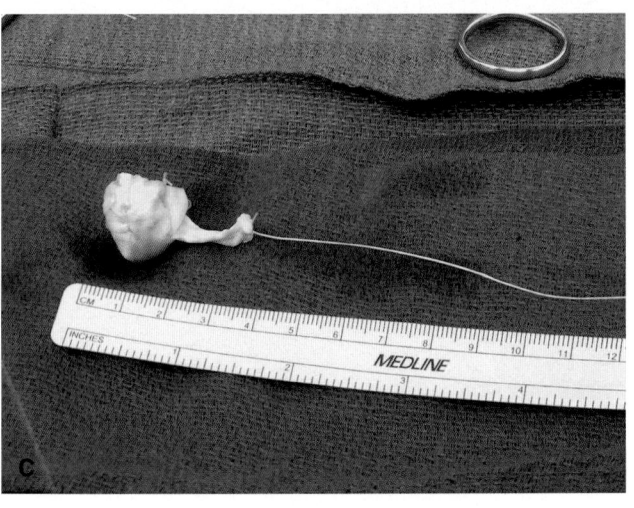

FIGURE 67.11 A-C. An allograft is wrapped in a ball large enough to fill the space created between the proximal phalanx and metatarsal head once the implant is removed and the bony surfaces debrided. It is knotted as shown with the final product shown in **(C)**. The tail end will be secured into the metatarsal head to prevent migration or dislocation of the graft. (Courtesy of Gene Curry, MD.)

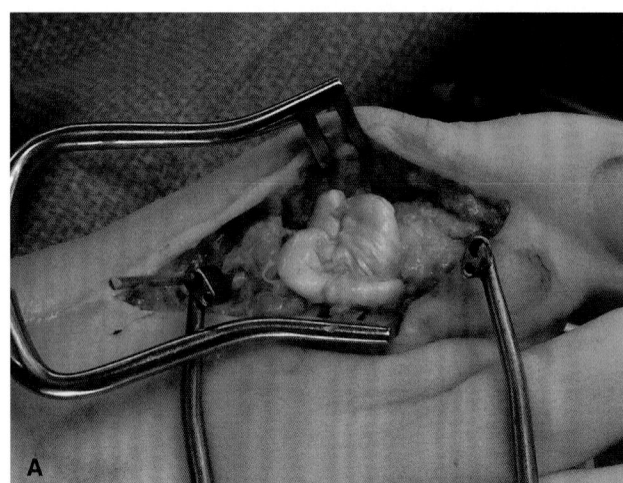
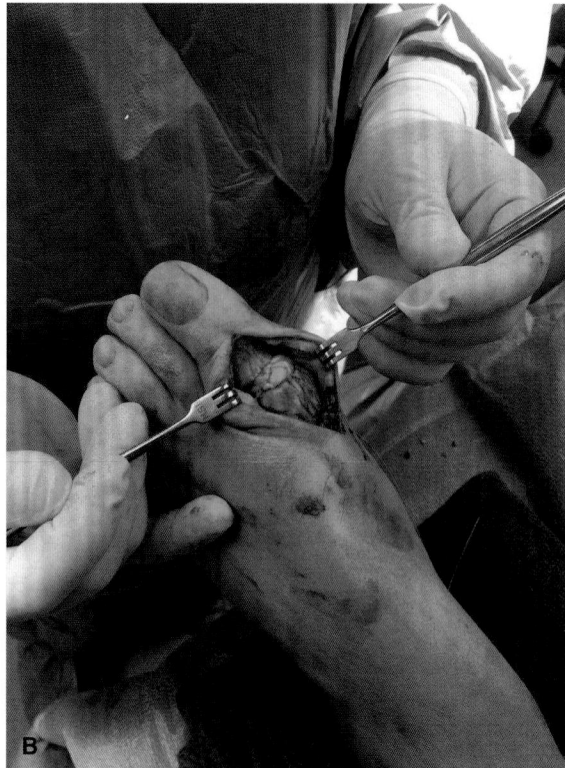

FIGURE 67.12 A, B. The tendon is in place and shaped to its final appearance in **(B)**. The wound is then closed in layers. (Courtesy of Gene Curry, MD.)

and lesser procedures such as osteotomies were not applicable. The interposition materials consisted of extensor digitorum longus,[76] extensor digitorum brevis,[77,78] palmaris longus,[79] semitendinosus allograft,[80] and local capsular tissue.[81] In all cases, the dorsal aspect of the metatarsal head was excised and the interpositional material secured to the plantar plate and/or metatarsal head with sutures. Postoperatively, the patient was allowed full weight bearing in a postoperative shoe with progression at 2 weeks to regular shoe wear. In a review and comparison of the reported techniques,[81] all studies showed a significant improvement in AOFAS scores and good to excellent patient satisfaction with the procedures. As fusion of the lesser MTP joints is not acceptable and metatarsal head resection leads to transfer metatarsalgia, interpositional arthroplasty is a very reasonable option for patients with advanced arthritis of these joints.

HAMMER TOES

Interpositional arthroplasty has also been described for hammer toe correction of fixed deformities.[82] Fixed hammer toe correction has traditionally been described as excisional arthroplasty[83] or arthrodesis[84] with good results in cosmesis, pain relief, and deformity correction. In the report of interpositional arthroplasty, the authors performed a resection of the head of the proximal phalanx and released the proximal portion of the extensor tendon. The extensor tendon was then sutured into the space created by the resection of the proximal phalangeal

head. The toes were taped together to prevent postoperative deformity. The authors followed 16 patients over a 2-year period. Although MOXFAQ scores improved postoperatively, most patients felt their pain was minimally if at all improved. This is the only known report of interpositional arthroplasty for hammer toe correction. Traditional methods of excisional arthroplasty and arthrodesis have shown superior results in this area.

SUMMARY

Interpositional arthroplasty is a valuable procedure in many areas of the foot and ankle when motion preservation is an important factor to consider. Many studies have shown the benefit of such procedures especially in the MTP joints and 4/5 TMT joints. In the ankle, this procedure could have a role in the treatment of advanced arthritis in younger patients who could not have implant arthroplasty and wish to preserve motion of the joint. This area is relatively new and optimal graft material, technique, and postoperative protocols are still unclear. In the hindfoot, it may play a role in persistent nonunions that have failed multiple attempts at arthrodesis or in the elderly where arthrodesis is not an option due to inability to tolerate long periods of immobilization or non–weight bearing. In the future, studies will focus on optimizing techniques, exploring the role of autologous plasma and stem cell therapy in graft incorporation and improving materials used for interposition.

REFERENCES

1. Gomez PF, Morcuende JA. Early attempts at hip arthroplasty. *Iowa Orthop J.* 2005;5:25-29.
2. Cheng SL, Morrey BF. Treatment of the mobile, painful arthritic elbow by distraction interposition arthroplasty. *J Bone Joint Surg Br.* 2000;82:233-238.
3. Strauss EJ, Verma NN, Salata MJ, et al. The high failure rate of biologic resurfacing of the glenoid in young patients with glenohumeral arthritis. *J Shoulder Elbow Surg.* 2014;23:409-419.
4. Muh SJ, Streit JJ, Shishani Y, et al. Biologic resurfacing of the glenoid with humeral head resurfacing for glenohumeral arthritis in the young patient. *J Shoulder Elbow Surg.* 2014;23:e185-e190.
5. Hammond J, Lin EC, Harwood DP, et al. Clinical outcomes of hemiarthroplasty and biological resurfacing in patients aged younger than 50 years. *J Shoulder Elbow Surg.* 2013;22:1345-1351.
6. Lollino N, Pellegrini A, Paladini P, et al. Gleno-humeral arthritis in young patients: clinical and radiographic analysis of humeral resurfacing prosthesis and meniscus interposition. *Musculoskelet Surg.* 2011;95(suppl 1):s59-s63.
7. Bois AJ, Whitney IJ, Somerson JS, et al. Humeral head arthroplasty and meniscal allograft resurfacing of the glenoid: a concise follow-up of a previous and survivorship analysis. *J Bone Joint Surg Am.* 2015;97:1571-1577.
8. Merolla G, Bianchi P, Lollino N, et al. Clinical and radiographic mid-term outcomes after shoulder resurfacing in patients aged 50 years old or younger. *Musculoskelet Surg.* 2013;97(suppl 1):s23-s29.
9. Gervis WH. Excision of the trapezium for osteoarthritis of the trapeziometacarpal joint. *J Bone Joint Surg Br.* 1949;31:537-539.
10. Froimson AI. Tendon arthroplasty of the trapeziometacarpal joint. *Clin Orthop Relat Res.* 1970;70:191-199.
11. Burton RI, Pellegrini VD. Surgical management of basal joint arthritis of the thumb: II. Ligament reconstruction with tendon interposition arthroplasty. *J Hand Surg Am.* 1986;11:324-332.
12. Tomaino MM, Pellegrini VD Jr, Burton RI. Arthroplasty of the basal joint of the thumb: long-term follow-up after ligament reconstruction with tendon interposition. *J Bone Joint Surg Am.* 1995;77:346-355.
13. Thompson JS. Suspensionplasty technique. In: *Atlas of the Hands Clinics.* Philadelphia, PA: WB Saunders; 1997:101-126.
14. Diao E. Trapezio-metacarpal arthritis: trapezium excision and ligament reconstruction not including the LRTI arthroplasty. *Hand Clin.* 2001;17:223-236.
15. Kuhns CA, Emerson ET, Meals RA. Hematoma and distraction arthroplasty for thumb basal joint osteoarthritis: a prospective, single-surgeon study including outcome measures. *J Hand Surg Am.* 2003;28:381-389.
16. Nusem I, Goodwin DR. Excision of the trapezium and interposition arthroplasty with gelfoam for the treatment of trapeziometacarpal osteoarthritis. *J Hand Surg Br.* 2003;28:242-245.
17. Gerwin M, Griffith A, Weiland AJ, et al. Ligament reconstruction basal joint arthroplasty without tendon interposition. *Clin Orthop Relat Res.* 1997;342:42-45.
18. Kriegs-Au G, Petie G, Fojtl E, et al. Ligament reconstruction with or without tendon interposition to treat primary thumb carpometacarpal osteoarthritis: a prospective randomized study. *J Bone Joint Surg Am.* 2004;86:209-218.
19. Martou G, Veltri K, Thoma A. Surgical treatment of osteoarthritis of the carpometacarpal joint of the thumb: a systematic review. *Plast Reconstr Surg.* 2004;114:421-432.
20. Wajon A, Ada L, Edmunds I. Surgery for thumb (trapeziometacarpal joint) osteoarthritis. *Cochrane Database Syst Rev.* 2005;4:CD004631.
21. Omori G, Koga Y, Kono S, et al. A case report of arthroscopic and histological long-term evaluation after resection interpositional knee arthroplasty with chromicized fascia lata (J-K membrane). *Acta Med Biol.* 1996;44:111-115.
22. Shawen SB, Anderson RB, Cohen BE, et al. Spherical ceramic interpositional arthroplasty for basal fourth and fifth metatarsal arthritis. *Foot Ankle Int.* 2007;28:896-901.
23. Koga H, Shimaya M, Muneta T, et al. Local adherent technique for transplanting mesenchymal stem cells as a potential treatment of cartilage defect. *Arthritis Res Ther.* 2008;10:R842575632.
24. Sekiya I, Muneta T, Horie M, et al. Arthroscopic transplantation of synovial stem cells improve outcomes in knees with cartilage defects. *Clin Orthop Relat Res.* 2015;473(7): 2316-2326.
25. Chu C, Rodeo S, Bhutani N, et al. Optimizing clinical use of biologics in orthopedic surgery: consensus recommendations from the 2018 AAOS/NIH U-13 conference. *J Am Acad Orthop Surg.* 2019;27(2):e50-e63.
26. Kellgren JH, Lawrence JS. Radiological assessment of osteoarthrosis. *Ann Rheum Dis.* 1957;16:494-502.
27. Labib SA, Raikin SM, Lau JT, et al. Joint preservation procedures for ankle arthritis. *Foot Ankle Int.* 2013;34(7):1040-1047.
28. Tellisi N, Fragomen AT, Kleinman D, et al. Joint preservation of the osteoarthritic ankle using distraction arthroplasty. *Foot Ankle Int.* 2009;30:318-325.
29. Ploegmakers JJ, van Roermund PM, van Melkebeek J, et al. Prolonged clinical benefit from joint distraction in the treatment of ankle osteoarthritis. *Osteoarthritis Cartilage.* 2005;13:582-588.
30. Paley D, Lamm BM, Purohit RM, et al. Distraction arthroplasty of the ankle—how far can you stretch the indications? *Foot Ankle Clin.* 2008;13:471-484.
31. Marijnissen AC, van Roermund PM, van Melkebeek J, et al. Clinical benefit of joint distraction in the treatment of ankle osteoarthritis. *Foot Ankle Clin.* 2003;8:335-346.
32. Fuchs S, Sandmann C, Skwara A, et al. Quality of life 20 years after arthrodesis of the ankle: a study of adjacent joints. *J Bone Joint Surg Br.* 2003;85:994-998.
33. Buchner M, Sabo D. Ankle fusion attributable to post traumatic arthrosis: a long term follow up of 48 patients. *Clin Orthop Relat Res.* 2003;406:155-164.
34. Adams HB, VanYperen JJ. Interposition ankle arthroplasty using Achilles tendon allograft ("the AAA procedure"): a case report. *J Foot Ankle Surg.* 2012;51:645-647.
35. Lee DK. Ankle arthroplasty alternatives with allograft and external fixation: preliminary clinical outcome. *J Foot Ankle Surg.* 2008;47:447-452.
36. Carpenter B, Duncan K, Ernst J, et al. Interposition ankle arthroplasty using acellular dermal matrix: a small series. *J Foot Ankle Surg.* 2017;56:894-897.
37. Kline AJ, Hasselman CT. Ankle interpositional xenograft arthroplasty. *Oper Tech Orthop.* 2010;20:195-200.
38. Stamatis ED, Cooper PS, Myerson MS. Supramalleolar osteotomy for the treatment of distal tibial angular deformities and arthritis of the ankle joint. *Foot Ankle Int.* 2003;24: 754-764.
39. Pagenstert GI, Hintermann B, Barg A, et al. Realignment surgery as an alternative treatment of varus and valgus ankle osteoarthritis. *Clin Orthop Relat Res.* 2007;462:156-168.
40. Kim G-L, Park JY, Hyun Y-S, et al. Treatment of traumatic subtalar arthritis with interpositional arthroplasty with tensor fascia lata or fat. *Eur J Orthop Surg Traumatol.* 2013;23:487-491.
41. Clanton TO. Personal communication. 2018.
42. Patel A, Eleftheriou KI, Anand A, et al. Bilateral excision arthroplasty and interpositional allograft for severe talonavicular osteoarthritis. *Foot Ankle Int.* 2013;34:1294-1298.
43. Kim DH, Berkowitz MJ. Allograft dermal matrix interpositional arthroplasty in the treatment of failed revision arthrodesis at the talonavicular joint. *Foot Ankle Int.* 2014;35: 619-622.
44. Kim DH, Berkowitz M, Pino E, et al. Interpositional arthroplasty of the calcaneocuboid joint using a regenerative tissue matrix to treat recurrent nonunion. *Orthopedics.* 2009;32:131.
45. Brunet JA, Wiley JJ. The late results of tarsometatarsal joint injuries. *J Bone Joint Surg Br.* 1987;69:437-440.
46. Hardcastle PH, Reschauer R, Kutscha-Lissberg E, et al. Injuries to the tarsometatarsal joint. Incidence, classification and treatment. *J Bone Joint Surg Br.* 1982;64:349-356.
47. Komenda GA, Myerson MS, Biddinger KR. Results of arthrodesis of the tarsometatarsal joints after traumatic injury. *J Bone Joint Surg Am.* 1996;78:1665-1676.
48. dePalma L, Santucci A, Sabetta SP, et al. Anatomy of the Lisfranc joint complex. *Foot Ankle Int.* 1997;18:356-364.
49. Lakin RC, Degnore LT, Pienkowski D. Contact mechanics of normal tarsometatarsal joints. *J Bone Joint Surg Am.* 2001;83:520-528.
50. Ouzounian TJ, Shereff MJ. In vitro determination of midfoot motion. *Foot Ankle Int.* 1989;10:140-146.
51. Hansen ST. *Functional Reconstruction of the Foot and Ankle.* Philadelphia, PA: Lippincott Williams & Wilkins; 2000:90-96.
52. Park DS, Schram AJ, Stone NM. Isolated lateral tarsometatarsal joint arthrodesis: a case report. *J Foot Ankle Surg.* 2000;39:239-243.
53. Mann RA. Biomechanics. In: *Disorders of the Foot.* Philadelphia, PA: WB Staunders; 1982:52-53.
54. Berlet GC, Anderson RB. Tendon arthroplasty for basal fourth and fifth metatarsal arthritis. *J Foot Ankle Surg.* 2002;23:440-446.
55. Mirmiran R, Hembree JL. Tendon interpositional arthroplasty of the fourth-fifth metatarsocuboid joint. *J Foot Ankle Surg.* 2002;41:173-177.
56. Engkvist O, Johansson SH. Perichondrial arthroplasty: a clinical study in twenty six patients. *Scand J Plast Reconstr Surg.* 1980;14:71-87.
57. Miller SD. Interposition resection arthroplasty for hallux rigidus. *Tech Foot Ankle Surg.* 2004;3:158-164.
58. Hahn MP, Gerhardt N, Thordarson DB. Medial capsular interpositional arthroplasty for severe hallux rigidus. *Foot Ankle Int.* 2009;30:494-499.
59. Ritsila V, Eskola A, Hoikka V, et al. Periosteal resurfacing of the metatarsal head in hallux rigidus and Freiberg's disease. *J Orthop Rheum.* 1992;5:78-84.
60. Cosentino GL. The Cosentino modification for tendon interpositional arthroplasty. *J Foot Ankle Surg.* 1995;34:501-508.
61. Barca F. Tendon arthroplasty of the first metatarsophalangeal joint in hallux rigidus: preliminary communication. *Foot Ankle Int.* 1997;18:222.
62. Miller D, Maffulli N. Free gracilis interposition arthroplasty for severe hallux rigidus. *Bull Hosp Jt Dis.* 2005;62:121-124.
63. Gould JS, Florence MN. Interpositional arthroplasty of the great toe metatarsophalangeal joint using autogenous fascia lata for advanced hallux rigidus. *Tech Foot Ankle Surg.* 2015;14:65-68.
64. DelaCruz EL, Johnson AR, Clair BL. First metatarsophalangeal joint interpositional arthroplasty using a meniscus allograft for the treatment of advanced hallux rigidus: surgical technique and short-term results. *Foot Ankle Spec.* 2011;4:157-164.
65. Garas DN, Holton JP. Interpositional arthroplasty technique for hallux rigidus using amniotic membrane and regenerative tissue matrix. *Tech Foot Ankle Surg.* 2016;15:197-201.
66. Aynardi MC, Atwater MD, Dein EJ, et al. Outcomes after interpositional arthroplasty of the first metatarsophalangeal joint. *Foot Ankle Int.* 2017;38:514-518.
67. Hyer CF, Granata JD, Berlet GC, et al. Interpositional arthroplasty of the first metatarsophalangeal joint using a regenerative tissue matrix for the treatment of advanced hallux rigidus: 5 year case series follow-up. *Foot Ankle Spec.* 2012;5:249-252.
68. Sanhudo JA, Gomes JE, Rodrigo MK. Surgical treatment of advanced hallux rigidus by interpositional arthroplasty. *Foot Ankle Int.* 2011;32:400-406.
69. Roukis TS. Outcome following autogenous soft tissue interpositional arthroplasty for end stage hallux rigidus: a systematic review. *J Foot Ankle Surg.* 2010;49:475-478.
70. Akgun RC, Sahin O, Demirors H, et al. Analysis of modified oblique Keller procedure for severe hallux rigidus. *Foot Ankle Int.* 2008;29:1203-1208.
71. Roukis TS, Landsman AS, Ringstrom JB, et al. Distally-based capsule-periosteum interpositional arthroplasty for hallux rigidus: indications, operative technique, and short-term follow-up. *J Am Podiatr Med Assoc.* 2003;93:349-366.
72. Lau JTC, Daniels TR. Outcomes following cheilectomy and interpositional arthroplasty in hallux rigidus. *Foot Ankle Int.* 2001;22:462-470.
73. Hamilton WG, O'Malley MJ, Thompson FM, et al. Capsular interposition arthroplasty for severe hallux rigidus. *Foot Ankle Int.* 1997;18(2):68-70.

74. Watson TS, Panicco J, Parekh A. Allograft tendon interposition arthroplasty of the hallux metatarsophalangeal joint: a technique and literature review. *Foot Ankle Int.* 2019;40:113-119.

75. Thomas D, Thordarson D. Rolled tendon allograft interpositional arthroplasty for salvage surgery of the hallux metatarsophalangeal joint. *Foot Ankle Int.* 2018;39:458-462.

76. El-Tayeby HM. Freiberg's infraction: a new surgical procedure. *J Foot Ankle Surg.* 1998;37:23-27.

77. Liao CY, Lin ACC, Lin CY, et al. Interpositional arthroplasty with palmaris longus tendon graft for osteonecrosis of the second metatarsal head: a case report. *J Foot Ankle Surg.* 2015;54:237-244.

78. Lui TH. Arthroscopic interpositional arthroplasty for Freiberg's disease. *Knee Surg Sports Traumatol Arthrosc.* 2007;15:555-559.

79. Ozkan Y, Ozturk A, Ozdemir R, et al. Interpositional arthroplasty with extensor digitorum brevis tendon in Freiberg's disease: a new surgical technique. *Foot Ankle Int.* 2005;29:448-492.

80. Stautberg E, Klein S, McCormick J, et al. Evaluation of outcomes following lesser toe metatarsophalangeal interpositional arthroplasty with semitendinosus allograft with description of anchovy technique. *Foot Ankle Orthop.* 2018;3:1.

81. Wahid A, Hickey B, Perera A. Functional outcomes of local pedicle graft interpositional arthroplasty in adults with severe Freiberg's disease. *Foot Ankle Int.* 2018;39:1290-1300.

82. Atinga M, Dodd L, Foote J, et al. Prospective review of medium term outcomes following interpositional arthroplasty for hammer toe deformity correction. *Foot Ankle Surg.* 2011;17:256-258.

83. O'Kane S, Pod FC, Kilmartin T. Review of proximal interphalangeal joint excisional arthroplasty for the correction of second hammer toe deformity in 100 cases. *Foot Ankle Int.* 2005;14:320-325.

84. Lehman DE, Smith RW. Treatment of symptomatic hammer toe with a proximal interphalangeal joint arthrodesis. *Foot Ankle Int.* 1995;16:535-541.

CHAPTER 68

Forefoot Revision Surgery

Thomas J. Chang

The topic of forefoot revision surgery can be very complex. These deformities can occur in all three planes and can also involve contributions from the hindfoot, ankle, and proximal areas as well. As with most cases in foot and ankle surgery, the long-term success of surgery is dependent on the biomechanical stability of the lower extremity. If biomechanical forces are not recognized and properly addressed, the outcome will likely be compromised long term.

Biomechanical imbalances are usually the predominant factor in a failed forefoot surgery. They need to be considered with any primary surgery and especially with revisional surgery. These revisional cases need to be addressed sequentially and logically for a successful revisional outcome. For the sake of this chapter on Forefoot Revision, we will accept that the areas of the hindfoot, ankle, and any proximal contributions are properly balanced and focus our attention to the forefoot area. This means imbalances of pes planus or pes cavus and even equinus are already addressed conservatively or surgically, and hindfoot balance has been created. We are now left with functional and alignment complications of the forefoot distal to the Lisfranc joint.

There are certain categories that may be considered when dealing with these complications. Initially, these can be due to poor procedural selection, noncompliance by the patient, and possibly other medical and physiological factors. Within the category of poor procedural selection, these might include adjacent nonfixated arthroplasties, digital and MPJ implants, minimal incision surgical approaches, and lesser metatarsal surgeries (Figs. 68.1-68.3). It is highly recommended to get the prior operative reports whenever possible. This will provide some clarity on what is currently left damaged and compromised from previous surgery, which will help guide your surgical planning for the revision surgery.

A logical algorithm for treating these forefoot revisions successfully is to consider basic principles of biomechanics in our reconstructive approach. If we can establish hindfoot and ankle stability, then the basis of building a successful platform for revision starts with the metatarsal parabola and forefoot loading Table 68.1. It is vital to establish a functional metatarsal parabola, and this will be the cornerstone and foundation for balancing the metatarsophalangeal joint (MPJ) as well as the digit for success. Once the metatarsal parabola is established, then the next level of focus is to establish a functional MPJ. When a functional MPJ is established, then the last building block is a stable digit. This will usually occur through arthrodesis of the PIPJ and/or coupled with a flexor tendon transfer to provide flexor power to a stable toe (Fig. 68.4).

A metatarsal parabola should be created where the second metatarsal is 1-2 mm longer than the adjacent first and third. Metatarsals 2 through 5 should appear with a descending length pattern on the AP radiograph. Short metatarsals can be lengthened and commonly long metatarsals are shortened (Fig. 68.5A-D). The length pattern of the metatarsal may also be part of the problem as soft tissue tension is vital to the balance of the MPJ. Shortening osteotomies of any type is often appropriate for adequate MPJ restoration. The most common is the Weil osteotomy, yet others have been described in an attempt to minimize the floating toe phenomena often seen and reported with the Weil. Treatment of a floating toe is difficult. The skin and soft tissues are often secondarily contracted and also need to be addressed. The standard approach is to perform a Z-plasty skin incision through the old MPJ scar, followed by a Z-plasty extensor tendon lengthening; release the MPJ capsule; and consider a plantar plate reefing to hold the toe down. If the metatarsal head is found to be structurally plantar flexed, then an elevational osteotomy should be performed.

As just discussed above, it is also vitally important that the metatarsals are balanced in the sagittal plane as well. A metatarsal primus elevatus will commonly cause overload of mechanical pressure to the central metatarsals and result in failure long term (Fig. 68.6). If the lesser metatarsals are malaligned in the sagittal plane, osteotomies to correct these are also recommended.

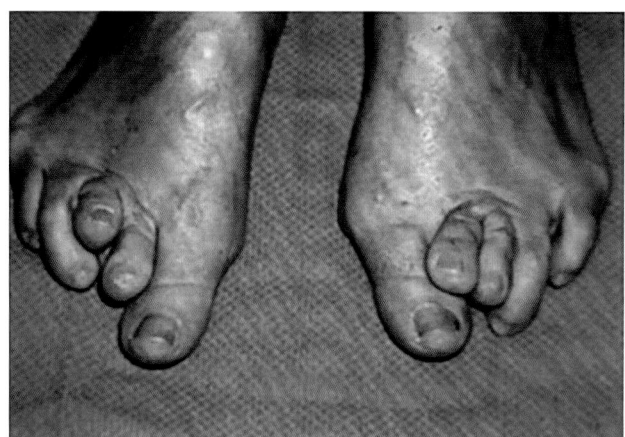

FIGURE 68.1 Forefoot deformity with deviated digits and multiple unstable rays.

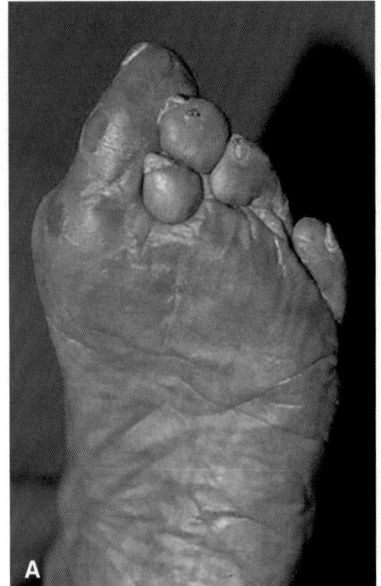
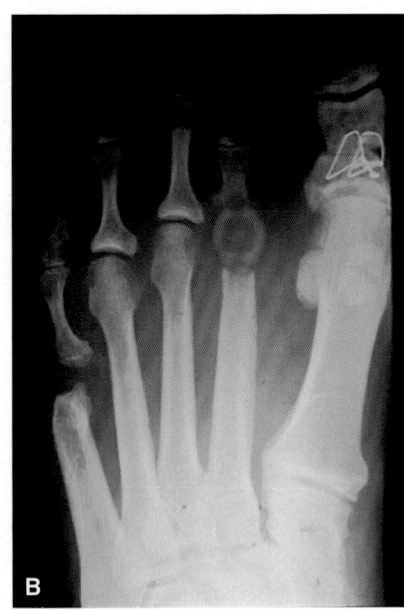

FIGURE 68.2 A. Shortened second ray and medial imbalance of lesser toes. **B.** Metatarsal head resections from 2 and 5 with MPJ implants.

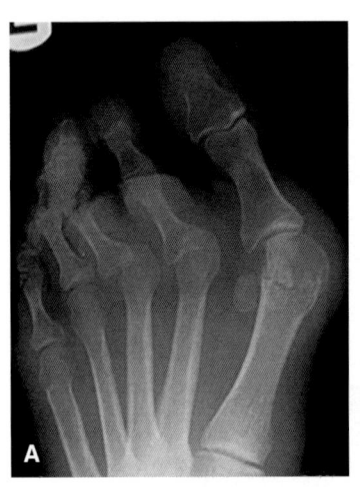
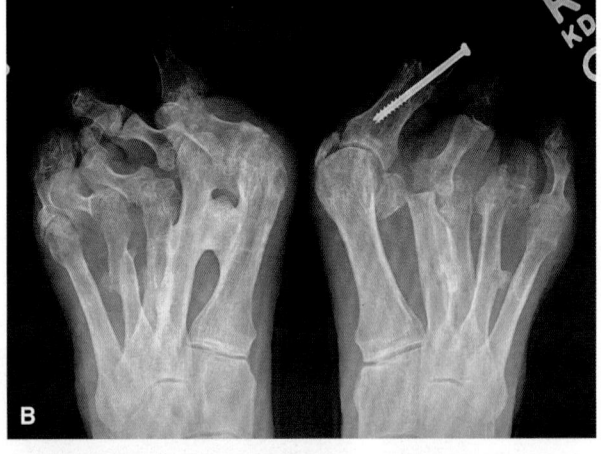
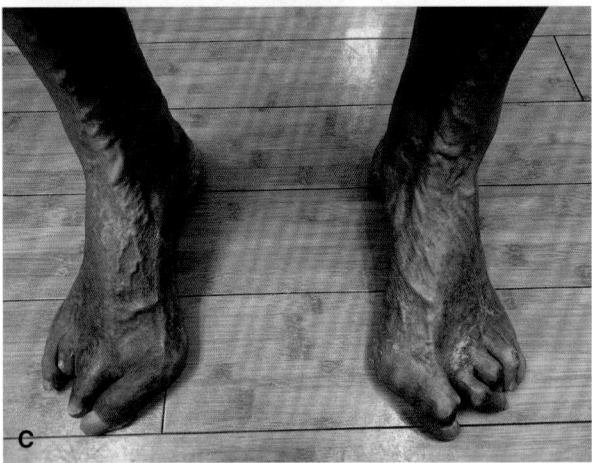

FIGURE 68.3 A. Forefoot derangement with more poorly aligned MPJs than those in an acceptable, rectus position. There is compromise and instability of the 1-3 MPJs. This illustrates a nonfunctioning metatarsal parabola, with dysfunctional MPJs and unstable digits. All three principles are compromised. **B.** Severe iatrogenic forefoot deformities after three failed surgeries. These are often debilitating with each step taken. **C.** Clinical appearance the x-ray in Figure B. Often the soft tissues are severely affected with chronic scar tissue and vascular insult.

TABLE **68.1** **Three Principles of Forefoot Reconstruction**
1) **Establish a balanced metatarsal parabola**
2) **Create a functional MPJ**
3) **Provide flexor stability to a stable digit**

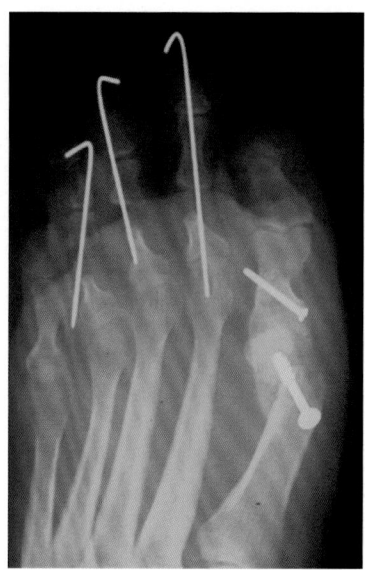

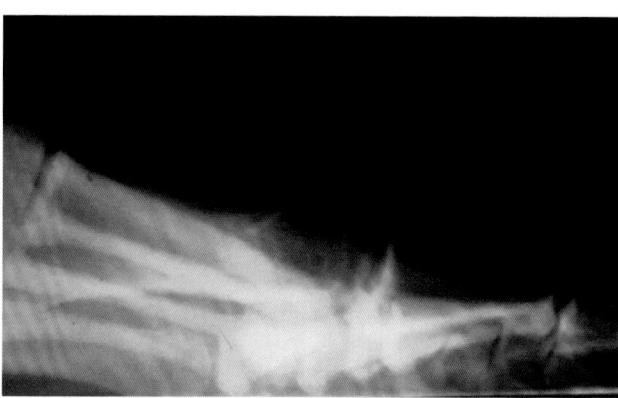

FIGURE 68.6 Intrinsic metatarsus primus elevatus with secondary central metatarsal overload. The deformity occurs within body of the first metatarsal.

FIGURE 68.4 Radiograph showing loss of the metatarsal parabola and nonfunctional MPJs and unstable digits. Reconstruction starts with the first principle of metatarsal parabola restoration.

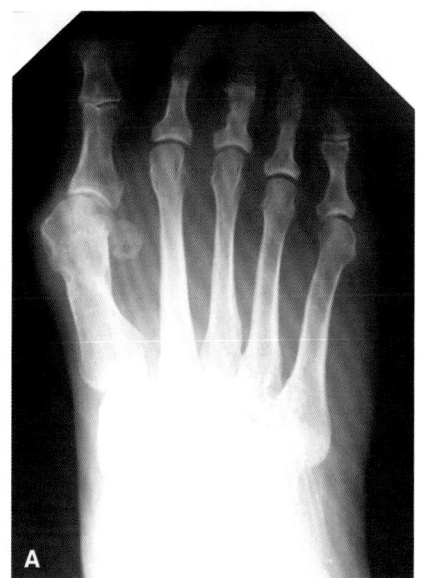

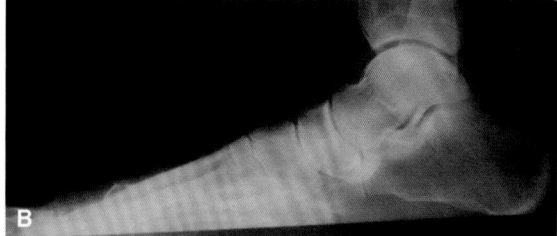

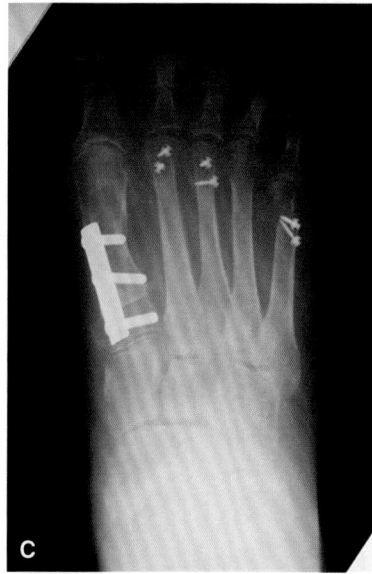

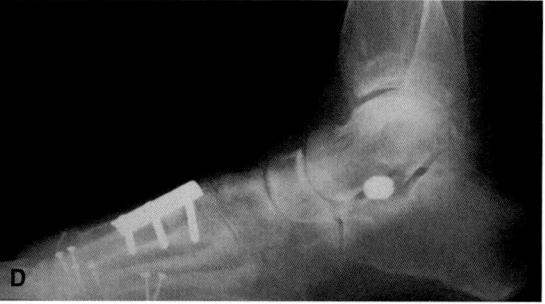

FIGURE 68.5 **A.** Iatrogenic shortening of the first ray and severe metatarsal overload of the central metatarsals. **B.** Note the collapse in the hindfoot with STJ pronation and medial column faulting. **C.** Attempt at reestablishing the metatarsal parabola and direct shortening from overload to the central metatarsals. *In situ* bone graft to the first and slight overshortening of the third metatarsal noted. **D.** Note the hindfoot balance addressed with subtalar arthroereisis. The forefoot sits in a rectus position now upon the stabilized rearfoot.

The first metatarsal clearly plays the dominant role in the stabilization of the whole forefoot, and care should be taken to provide positional stability in all planes along the first metatarsal in the first ray. This could include stabilization through a first metatarsal cuneiform joint arthrodesis or possibly sagittal plane manipulation through a sagittal scarf or other types of midshaft osteotomies. Camasta described the elevation to be one of intrinsic vs extrinsic elevatus of the first metatarsal.[1] In cases of extrinsic elevatus, a first metatarsal-cuneiform or even a naviculo-cuneiform arthrodesis might be best to establish alignment to the medial column. In cases of intrinsic elevatus, a metatarsal osteotomy, such as the sagittal scarf, can be considered for repair (Fig. 68.7A-F).

The first metatarsal length is also important to reestablish in certain situations, especially when the first MPJ is being salvaged. *In situ* bone grafts can be considered in cases where upward of 1.5-2 cm of bone length is required. It is difficult to get enough soft tissue stretching to adequately treat more than this in a single setting. The distal aspect of the toe should be carefully monitored to make sure the color does not look compromised. These cases should be done without the aid of a tourniquet to properly assess the vascularity to the toe. The appropriate bone graft can be used and usually secured with a locking plate construct. For cases requiring more than 1.5-2 cm, it is strongly recommended to utilize a mini distractor that will allow lengthening of the distal metatarsal in a linear controlled manner (Fig. 68.8A-F).

Once the parabola is balanced, then the next step can be focused on providing a functional MPJ. This means that the articular cartilage is facing in a straightforward direction, as well as dynamic balance of the intrinsic musculature around the joint. Within this, the extrinsic flexor and extensor tendons

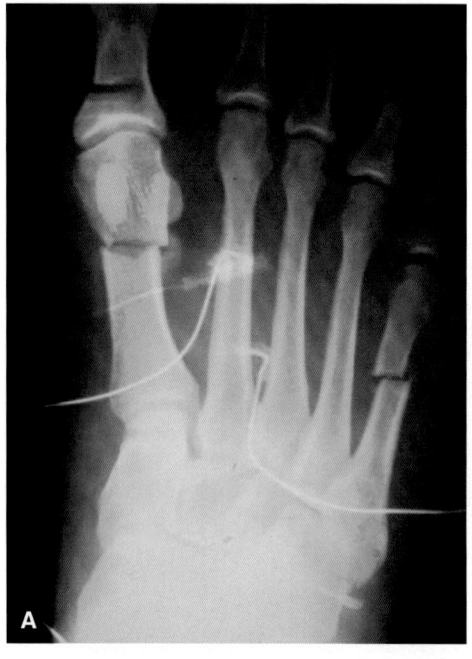

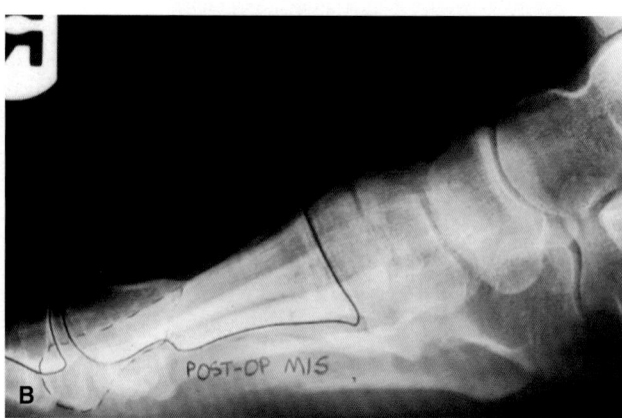

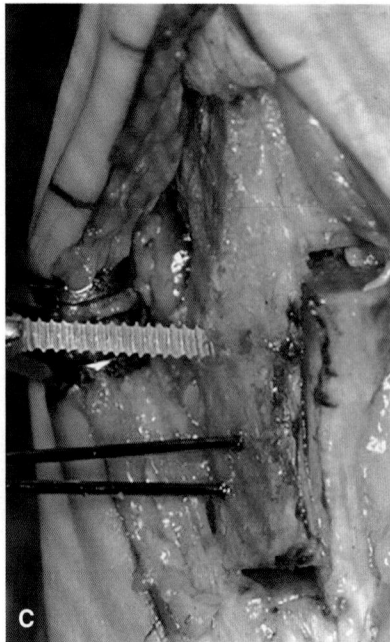

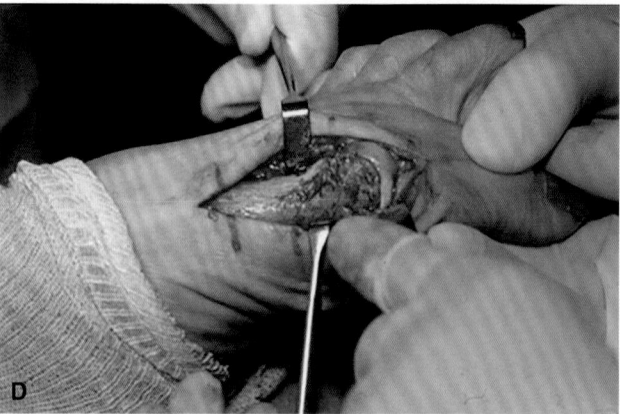

FIGURE 68.7 A. AP radiograph after MIS procedure to the first and fifth metatarsals. **B.** Clear metatarsus primus elevatus within the first metatarsal. **C.** Dorsal view of the sagittal scarf, rotation along the longitudinal arm allowing correction in the sagittal plane. The arms exit distal lateral and proximal medial. At least two screws are utilized from medial to lateral for stability. **D.** Intra-operative view of the intrinsic elevatus within the first metatarsal after failed osteotomy.

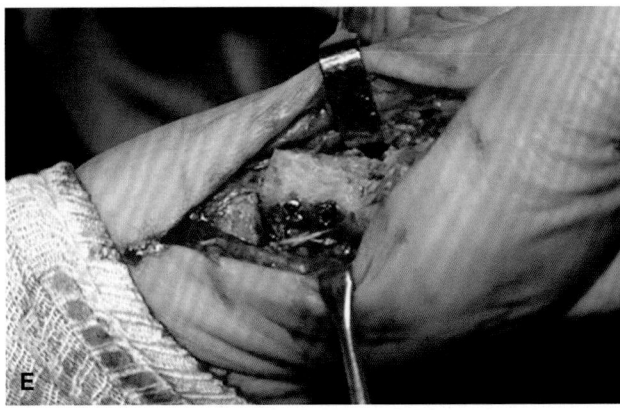

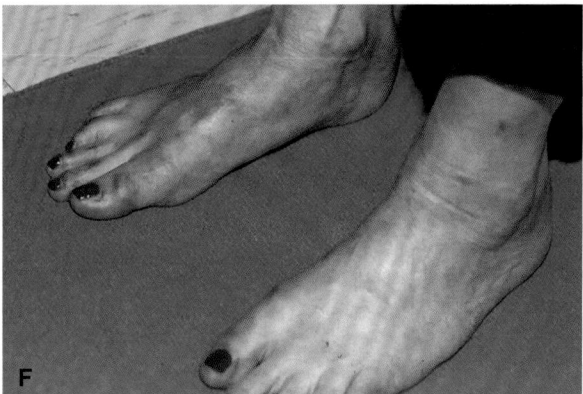

FIGURE 68.7 (*Continued*) **E.** Fixation of the sagittal scarf with two bicortical screws. Note the plantar flexion achieved with cortical overlap and stability provided to prevent troughing. **F.** 1 year post-op demonstrating the first metatarsal clinically back on the weight-bearing surface.

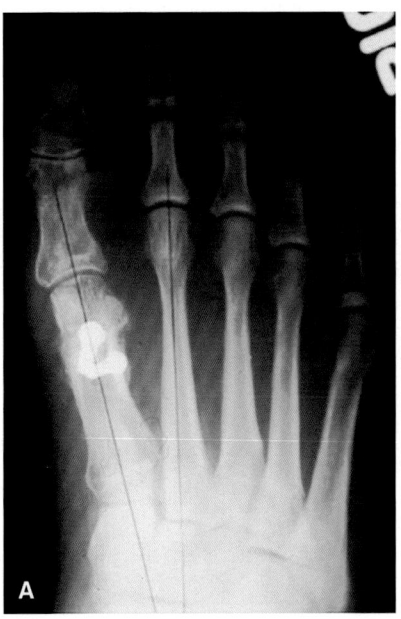

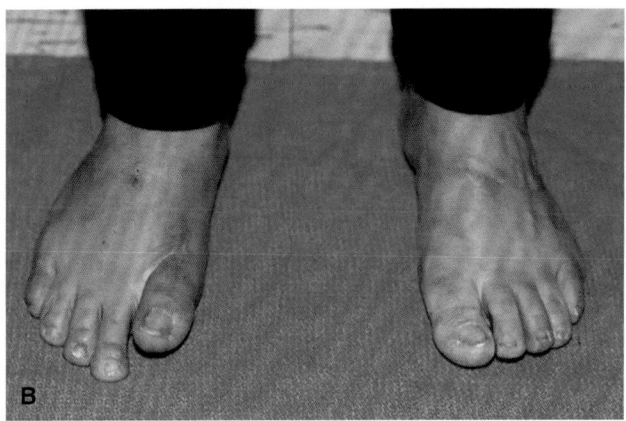

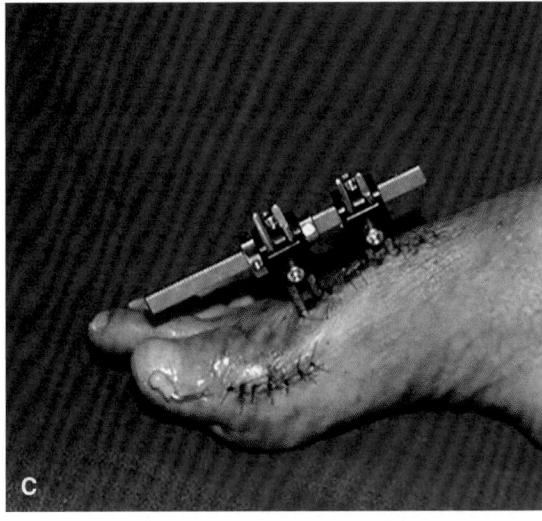

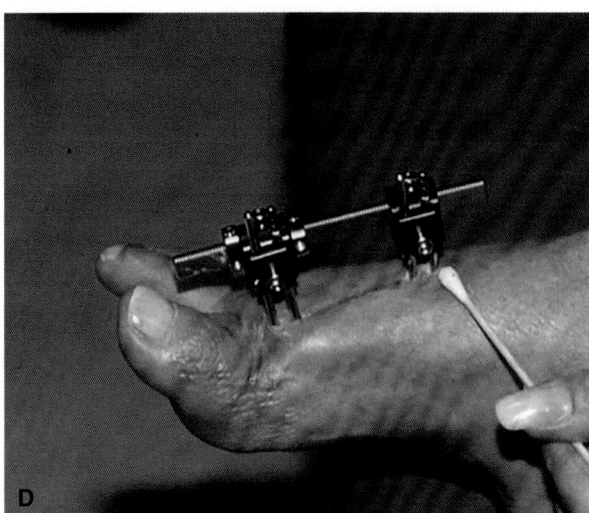

FIGURE 68.8 **A.** An inherently short first metatarsal after distal osteotomy. **B.** Clinical example of a cock-up hallux after excessive first ray shortening. **C.** Placement of a mini external fixator for gradual lengthening. Note the external pin across the first MPJ to stabilize this joint during proximal distraction. The corticotomy is usually made in the metaphyseal bone and lengthened roughly 1 mm/day. **D.** Distraction brought out to the desired length with daily pin care needed.

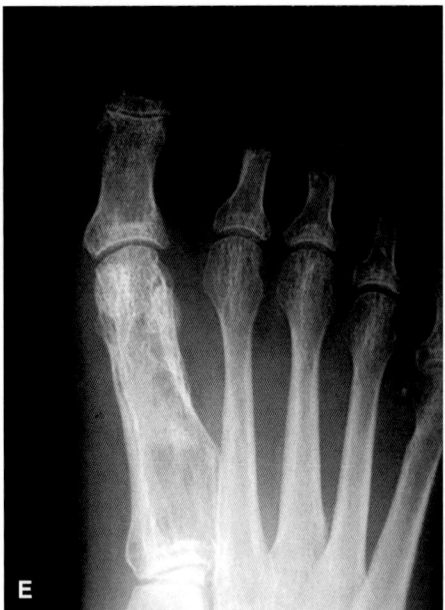
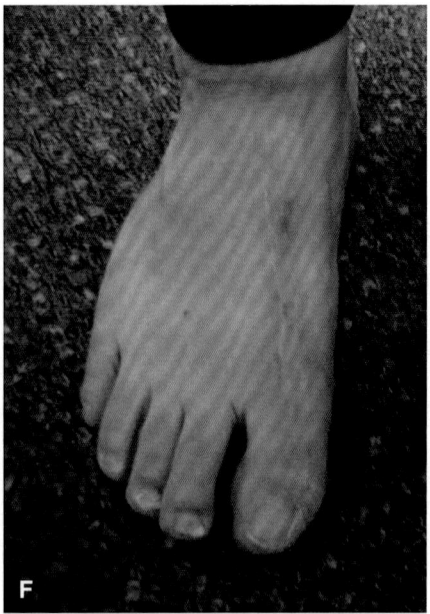

FIGURE 68.8 (*Continued*) **E.** Radiograph showing bone consolidation and fixator removed after obtaining the desired length. This may take 3-4 months for the bone to become dense enough for weight bearing. **F.** Final clinical picture of lengthened first ray and the ability to restore hallux purchase.

should also being balanced. The sequential release of the MPJ, well described by McGlamry in the past, is a good start to achieving this process. A dorsal, medial, and lateral MPJ capsulotomy is often performed initially, and then the reduction is evaluated with the Kelikian push-up test. If necessary, a flexor plate release with a McGlamry elevator will provide more relaxation to the planter MPJ musculature (Fig. 68.9).

With selected and adequate soft tissue releases at the MPJ, traditional methods of K-wires across the MPJ may still be used to hold the toe in a rectus alignment for 4-6 weeks. This is not always successful due to malalignment of the cartilage, as well as other soft tissues contributing to this deformity. The transverse plane

deviation may also be positional without any articular adaptation (Fig. 68.10A and B). Shortening osteotomies with a medial or lateral translation is often important to centralize the flexor tendon back beneath the metatarsal head (Fig. 68.11A and B). If there is a medial or lateral angulation to the articular surface, an angulation type of osteotomy behind the articular surface, such as a Reverdin, may be very helpful to reestablish the proper alignment of the cartilage in a functional direction (Fig. 68.12A-D).

When there is long-standing dorsal MPJ dislocation, the soft tissues are exceptionally challenging to balance properly. Surgical repair will require metatarsal shortening, often a flexor plate repair and possibly a flexor tendon transfer (Fig. 68.13A and B).

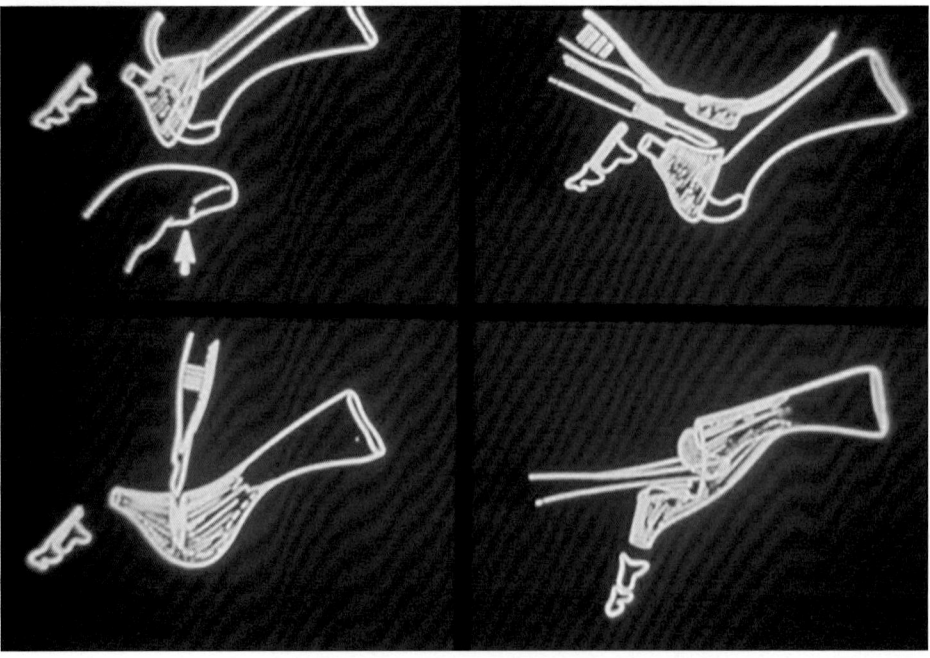

FIGURE 68.9 Schematic showing the Kelikian push-up test, extensor tendon release, MPJ capsulotomy, and flexor plate release. These are sequentially performed with the push-up test used between each step.

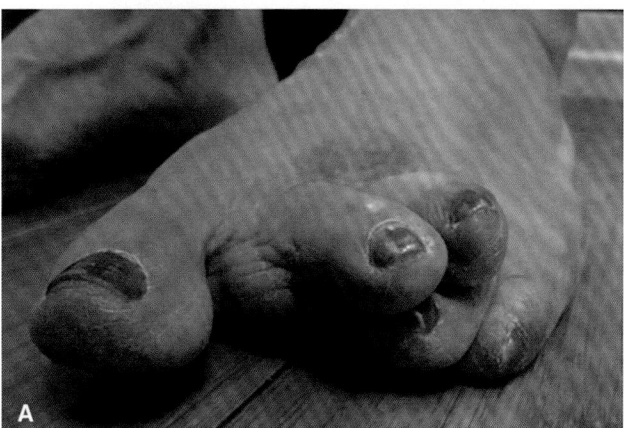

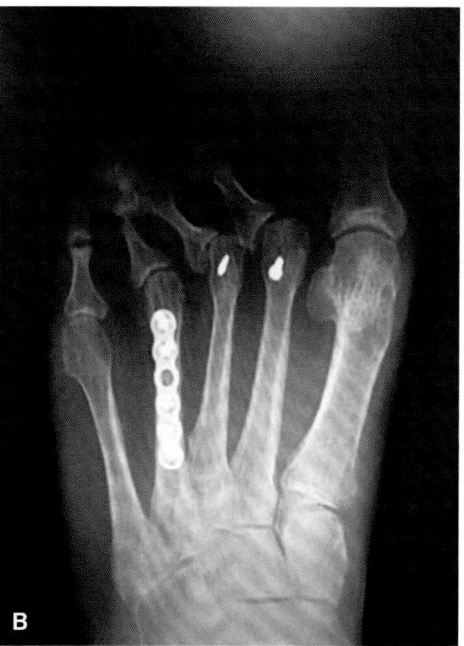

FIGURE 68.10 A. Clinical picture of severe transverse plane deviation with loss of soft tissue balancing. **B.** Radiograph with prior metatarsal osteotomies and loss of soft tissue balance. Note that the 2nd and 3rd joint spaces do not appear to be adapted yet.

One consideration is to perform a partial metatarsal head resection with external K-wire stabilization for 6 weeks (Fig. 68.14A-C). Care is taken to leave the partial metatarsal head resection at least the same length of the adjacent metatarsal or slightly longer. This joint destructive approach can also be utilized in rare cases of severe long-standing transverse plane contractions but is often more predictable when the MPJ dislocation is uniplanar (sagittal plane) rather than in multiple planes (dorsal and transverse). In significant transverse plane deformities at the MPJ, the long flexor tendon is also deviated within the interspace. This is often a recurrent deforming force which will return even after the K-wire is pulled after 6 weeks. Decompression of the metatarsal segment with the partial metatarsal head resection does help lessen the pull of the deviated flexor tendon but often this is persistent. Resection of the long flexor tendon with digital syndactyly has been suggested in extreme cases of flexor deviation. This case clearly shows the continued deforming force at the third MTPJ after partial head resection with K-wire fixation (Fig. 68.15A-C).

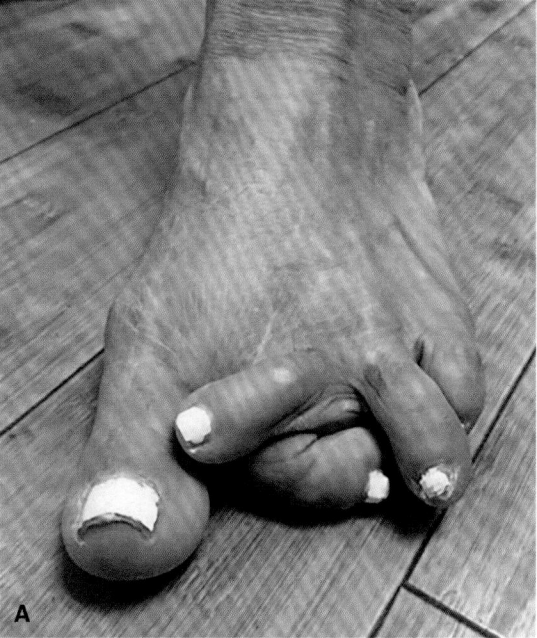

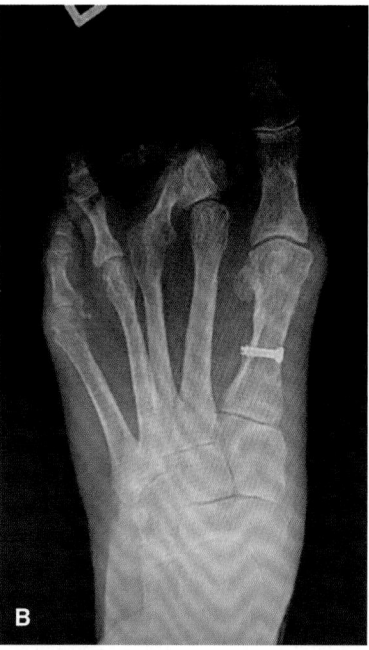

FIGURE 68.11 A. Severe MPJ instability after MPJ release, neuroma excision, and second toe arthroplasty. **B.** Radiograph depicting the MPJ imbalance above. The metatarsal parabola is also out of balance with the shortening along the first metatarsal.

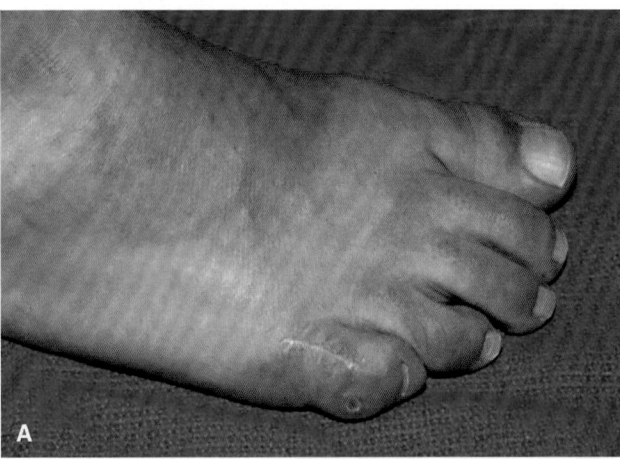
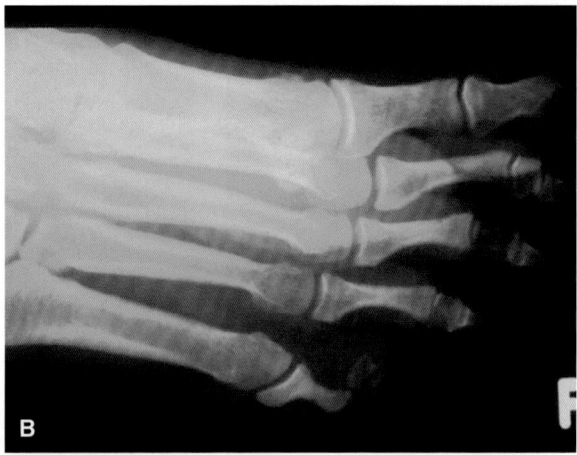
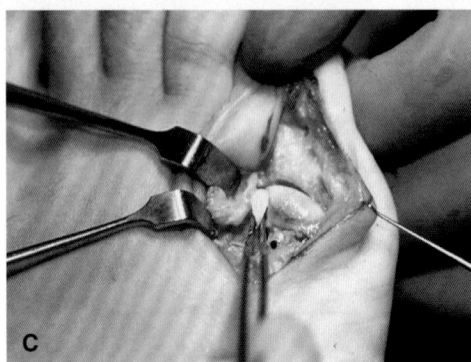
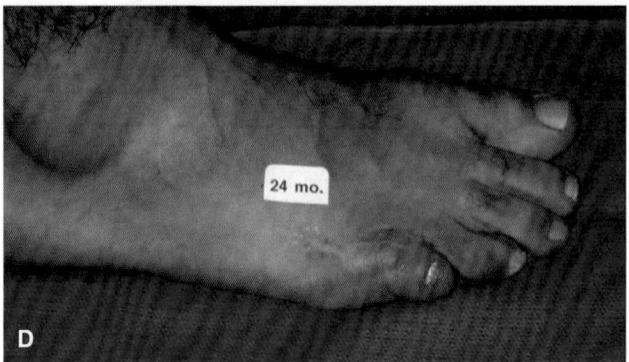

FIGURE 68.12 A. Malposition with a 90-degree rotation of the fifth toe. Note the continued recurrence of the PIPJ corn. **B.** Oblique radiograph illustrating the lateral plantar direction of the fifth MPJ. **C.** A Reverdin type of medial-based wedge performed to orient the cartilage in a rectus direction. Fixation is provided with a tapered absorbable pin. **D.** Two-year clinical follow-up with better alignment of the fifth toe. A partial syndactyly was also performed for long-term stability.

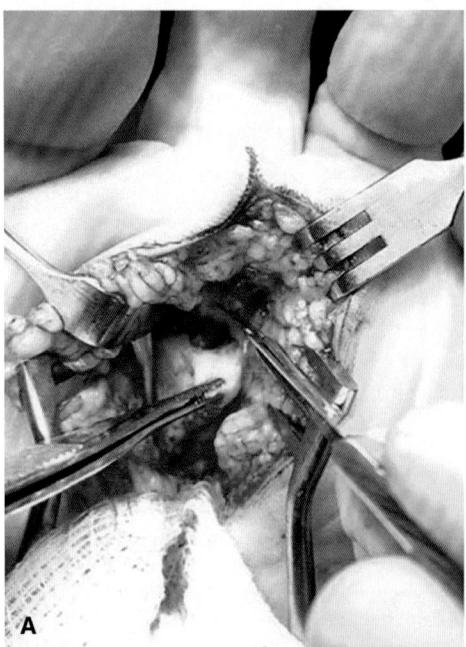
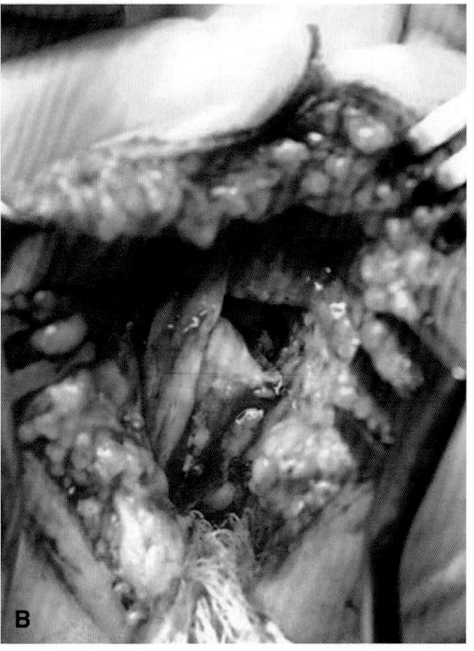

FIGURE 68.13 A. Plantar plate exposure from a direct plantar incision. This is performed centrally under the metatarsal head and carried down to the flexor tendon sheath. The rupture is usually directly under this flexor tendon sheath. **B.** A laterally based wedge taken from the flexor plate to align a medial deviated toe. Note the flexor tendon is sitting on the medial portion of the joint. Central relocation of the tendon is useful for long-term alignment of the toe.

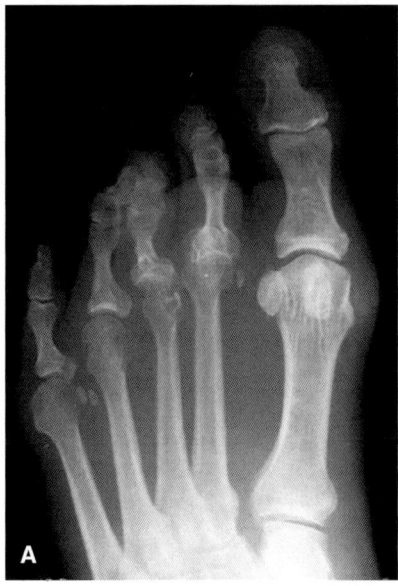
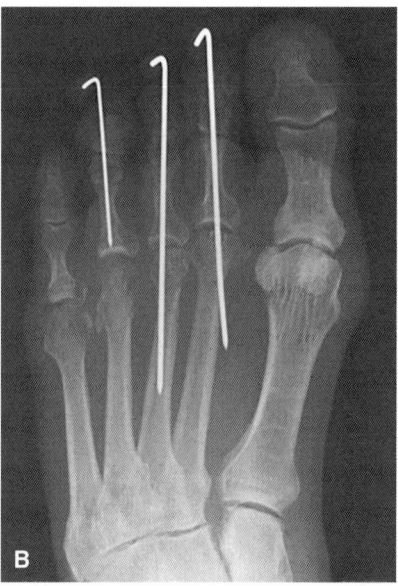
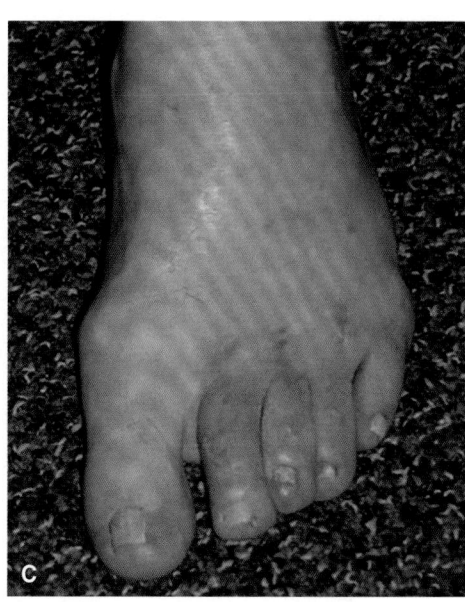

FIGURE 68.14 A. Radiograph depicting a dorsal dislocation of the second and third metatarsophalangeal joints. The parabola is out of balance here, and better balance is achieved with metatarsal shortening. **B.** Post-op radiograph showing partial metatarsal head resection and realignment stabilization of the second and third MPJs. K-wire stabilization of the MPJ is usually maintained for at least 6 weeks to provide soft tissue scarring and stability. **C.** Clinical picture at 8 months after pins were pulled at 8 weeks. Note the toes are slightly off the ground. This alignment is definitely improved in these cases, yet there may be some residual elevation in the sagittal plane.

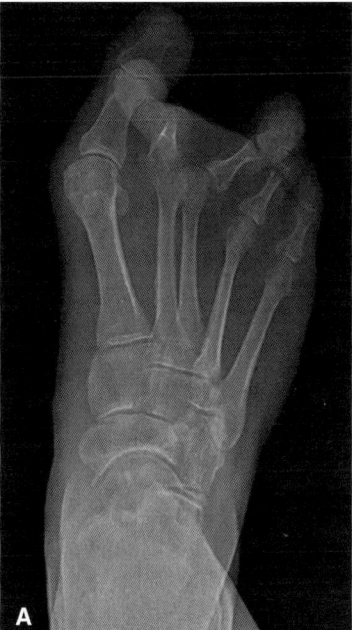
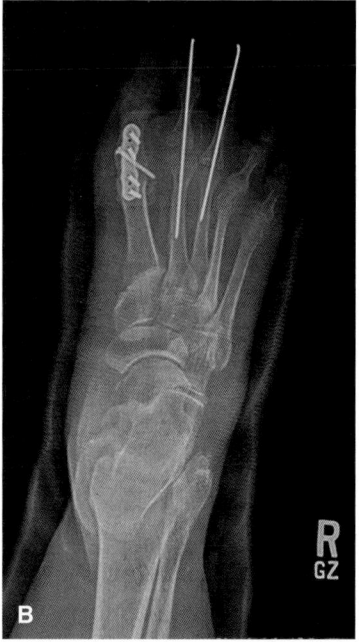
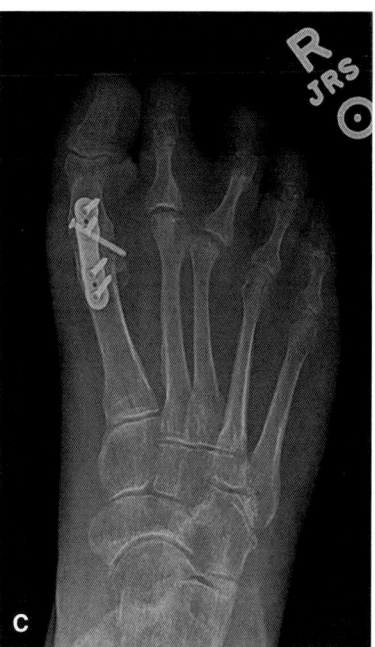

FIGURE 68.15 A. Example of second MTPJ dorsal dislocation and third MPJ transverse plane deviation. The transverse plane dislocations are more difficult to correct long term. **B.** Double partial metatarsal head resection with K-wire fixation utilized for severe MPJ deviation/subluxation. Note the stability provided by first MTPJ arthrodesis. Again, the K-wire stabilization is maintained for 6-8 weeks. **C.** Residual lateral malposition of the third MTPJ after pin is pulled. The toe is dramatically improved yet still mildly deviated. Transverse plane deviation is often complicated by the residual position of the flexor tendon and its role in recurrent deformity. A centrally placed flexor tendon transfer may be beneficial in some cases, or perhaps a slight overcorrected position during K-wire fixation may assist in more long-term transverse plane correction.

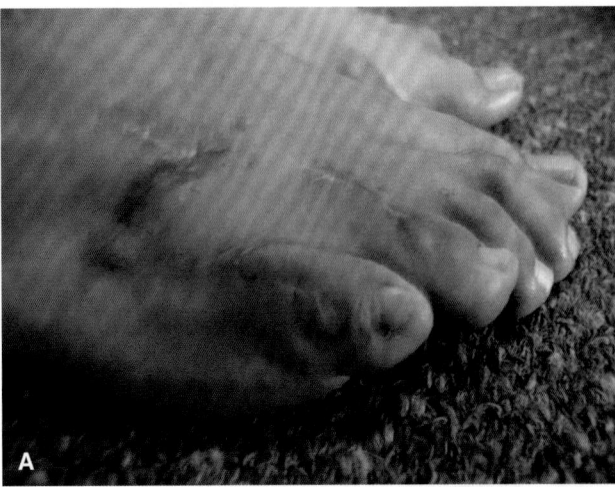
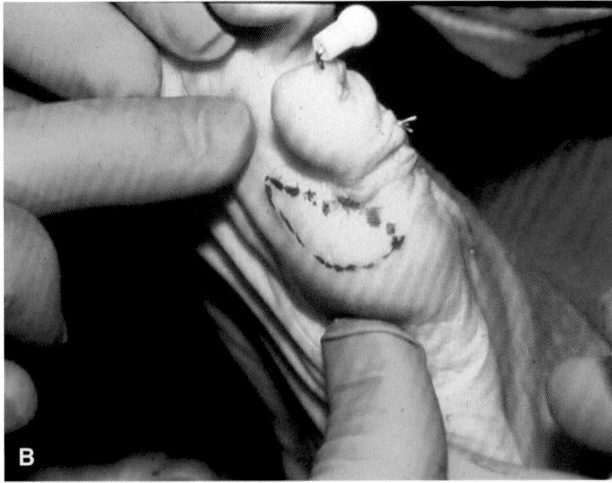

FIGURE 68.16 A. Dorsal migration of the fifth toe caused from residual plantar soft tissue left behind after digital surgery. The distal migration of the fat pad can be a deforming force during digital alignment. **B.** Removal of excessive plantar soft tissue seen after digital alignment will provide better soft tissue alignment to the final position of the digit in the sagittal plane.

There are even situations where significant dorsal MPJ contractures or long-standing contractures have resulted in a significant migration of the planter fat pad out distally. Dorsal dislocations may also be addressed with a partial metatarsal head resection with K-wire pinning in difficult long-standing cases. In these cases, after the MPJ is subsequently reduced in surgery, a plantar skin ellipse may be very helpful during closure to reduce the fullness of these distally migrated soft tissues. Failure to recognize this or remove this excess fullness plantarly during closure will leave a bulk of extra tissue, which might cause a recurrent dislocation of the MPJ during weight bearing (Fig. 68.16A and B).

In certain cases, the MPJ is destabilized from a phalangeal base resection (Fig. 68.17). This causes severe instability of the soft tissue support to the toe. Salvage approaches include placement of an MPJ implant, a partial syndactyly to an adjacent toe, and some authors have discussed a lesser MPJ arthrodesis (Fig. 68.18). An MPJ implant in some cases will provide length back to the lesser ray and provide tension to both the dorsal and plantar musculature to help bring the toe back to the weight-bearing surface. Appropriate soft tissue releases are required dorsally. The success of lesser MPJ implants is dramatically better when stability is noted in the first MTPJ (Fig. 68.19A-D).

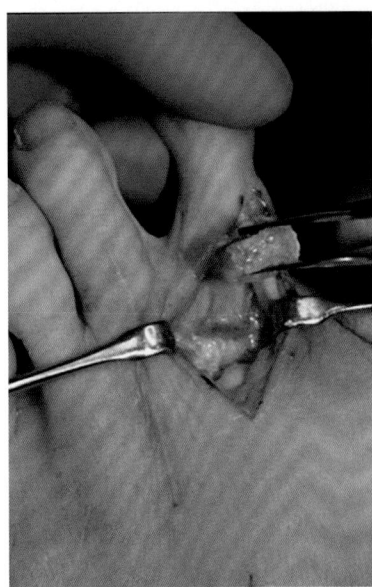

FIGURE 68.17 Significant instability to the MPJ and toe results after resection of the phalangeal base. This is difficult to salvage and should be avoided whenever possible.

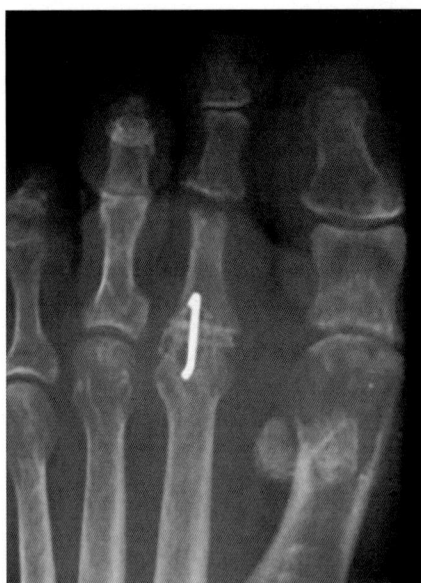

FIGURE 68.18 Second MPJ arthrodesis fusion has been described as a possible option for MPJ stability when considerable instability is present.

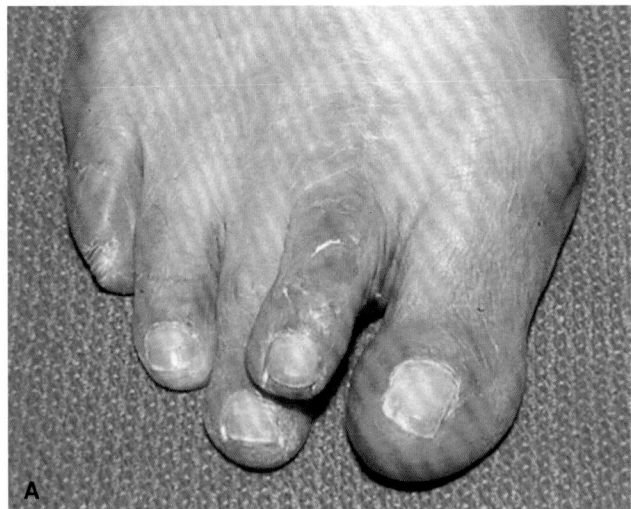
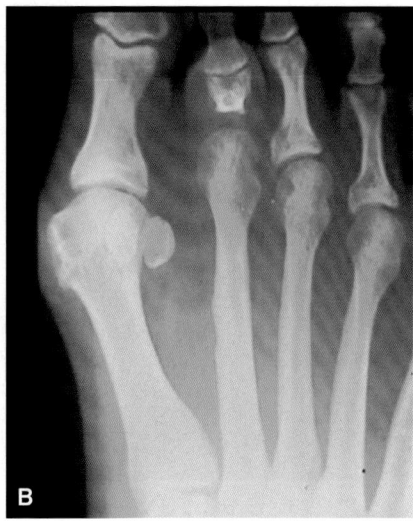
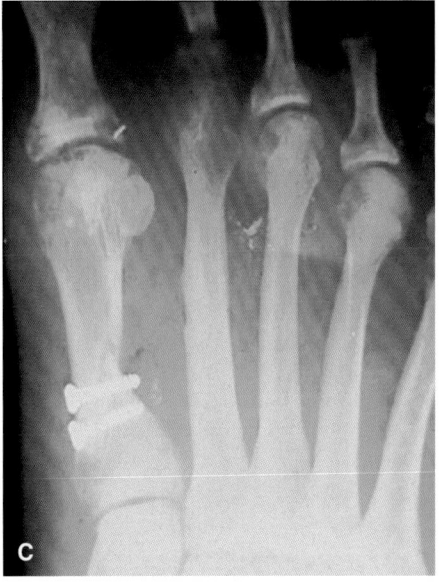
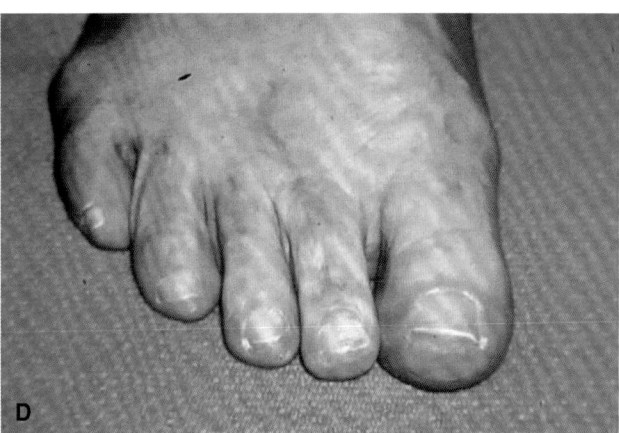

FIGURE 68.19 A. Clinical example showing loss of digital purchase and instability after phalangeal base resection. Note the contribution of the hallux valgus deformity to residual metatarsal imbalance. **B.** Radiograph of the above clinical example. Note the HAV deformity, which also needs to be considered for long-term correction. **C.** Correction of the hallux valgus and placement of a second MPJ implant to help restore length back to the second ray. The implant in this case can assist in restoring tension back to the flexor and extensor tendons. Stability restored to the first MPJ will play a vital role in the long-term success of central MPJ implants. **D.** Clinical follow-up of the case above with maintenance of hallux and second toe alignment.

Once the MPJ can be established to be functional, then it is time to provide stability to the toe (Fig. 68.20A and B). This is most easily achieved by arthrodesis of the PIPJ in many situations (Fig. 68.21A-F). There may be situations where an excess of bone has been removed, or there is just chronic instability due to loss of soft tissue support to the toe. A bone graft can be used to help reestablish the length of the toe and also the tension. This can be achieved using either allograft bone or autogenous bone from the calcaneus.

There will be situations where long-term stability to the toe is necessary through the utilization of the flexor tendon transfer. This will provide flexor power to a stable digit. This be achieved with the long or short flexor tendon and will take away the potential flexion of the distal phalanges upon the proximal phalanx, resulting in buckling of the PIPJ. Either the short or long flexor tendon can be directly anchored or transferred to the base of the proximal phalanx (Fig. 68.22A and B).

Excessive loss of bone will often result in a flail toe deformity (Fig. 68.23). These deformities are usually from an overaggressive arthroplasty technique which also results in loss of motor function. The surgery will require a structural bone graft, and this is usually taken from the lateral calcaneus. Once the graft is ready for implantation, a central K-wire stabilization across the bone graft is recommend as well as extending this proximal to the MPJ (Fig. 68.24A-E). It is important to cross the MPJ to

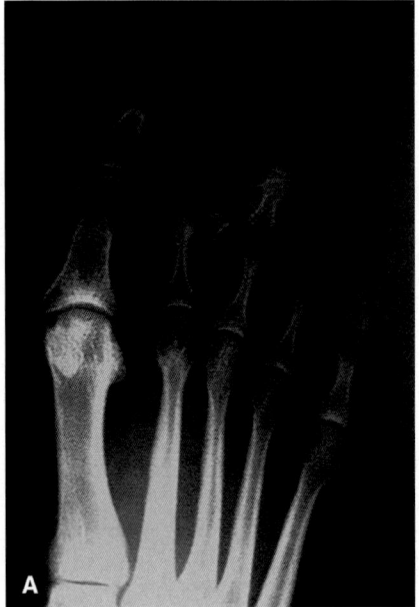
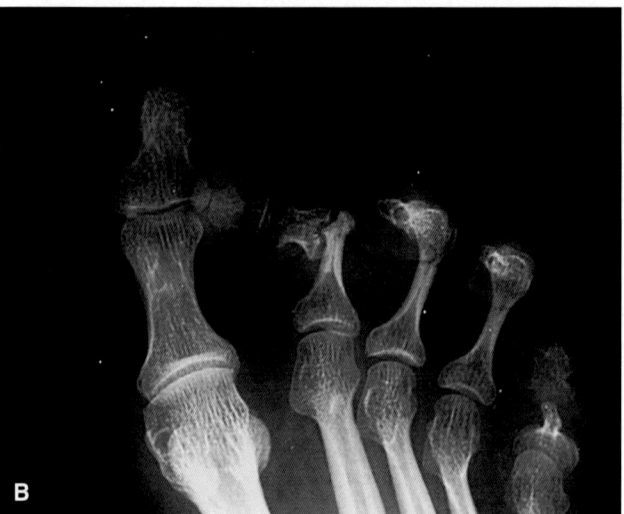

FIGURE 68.20 **A.** Example of lateral digital deviation and soft tissue imbalance after digital arthroplasty. **B.** Opposite deviation showing the power of the flexor tendon in exaggerating the instability after multiple adjacent nonfixated arthroplasties.

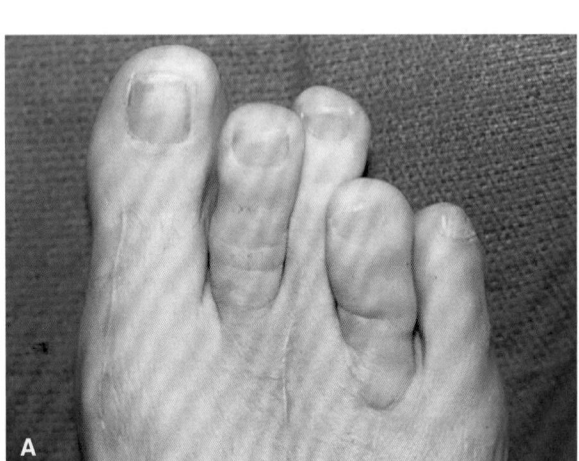
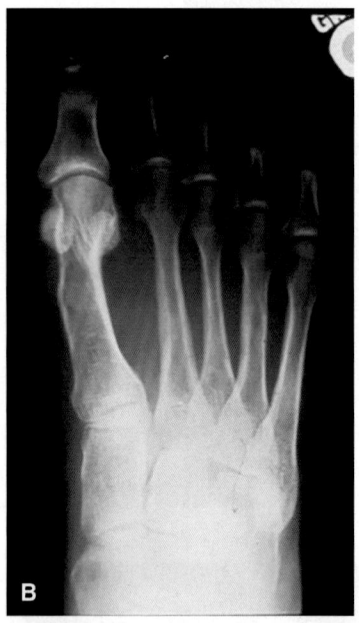
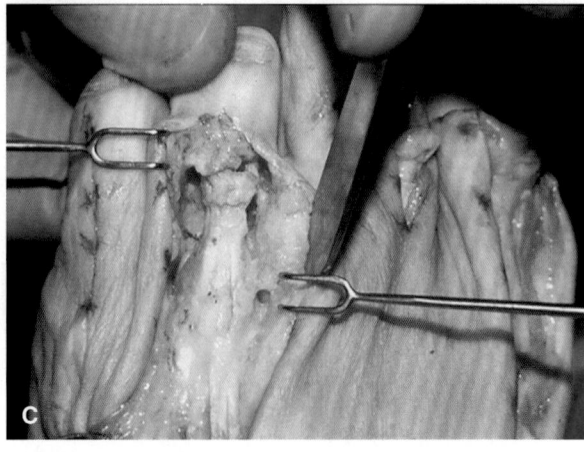

FIGURE 68.21 **A.** Clinical picture of multiple adjacent nonfixated arthroplasties. This is often the scenario for digital instability as soft tissues heal and contract randomly. This can be avoided or minimized by temporary stabilization across the PIPJ during the post-op course or even better prevented with PIPJ arthrodesis. **B.** Radiograph of the same patient. Note the arthroplasties from 2 to 5. **C.** Incisions should be made full thickness down to the deep fascia with minimal undermining. The prior arthroplasty sites are débrided and prepared for revisional fusion.

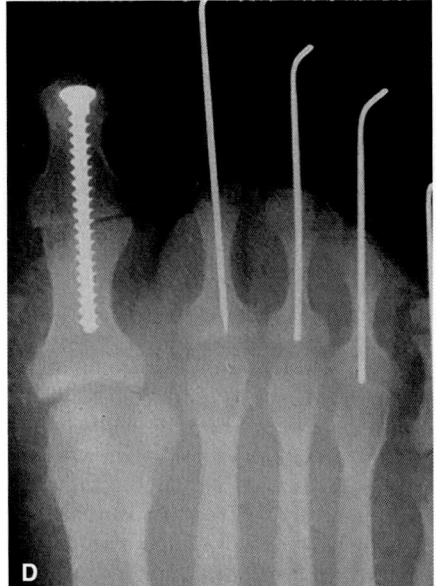

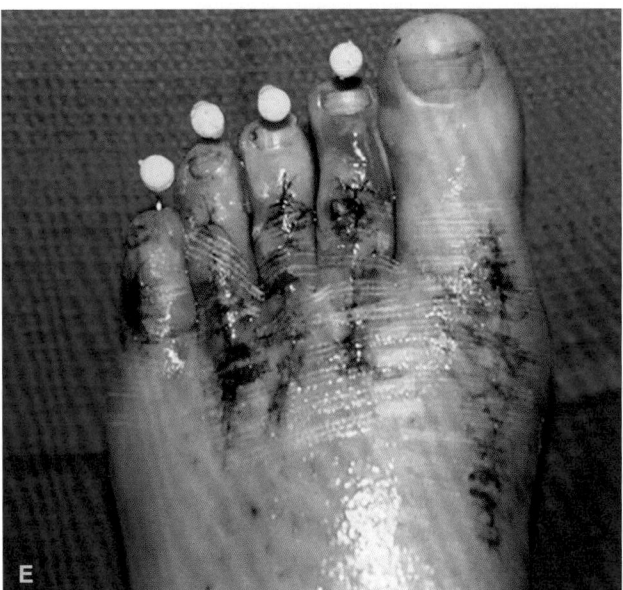

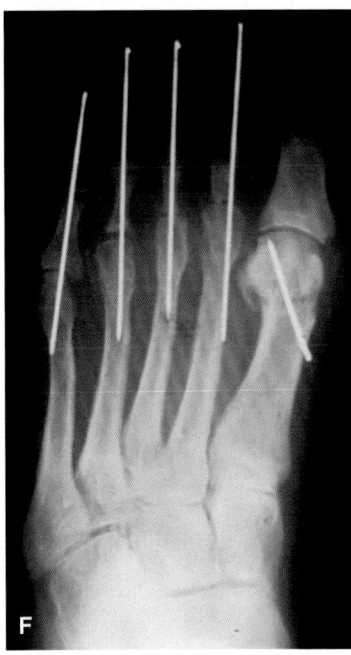

FIGURE 68.21 (*Continued*) **D.** Stabilization of toes 1-5 with an arthrodesis across the board. Slight shortening of the toes is routine after two procedures. **E.** Example of vascular injury not uncommonly seen after revision surgery on toes due to scar tissue and repeated soft tissue trauma. Aggressive dissection in revisional surgery can be unforgiving to the vascularity. **F.** Radiograph of the same patient with K-wires crossing the MPJ. Note the phalangeal bases were resected in this case. Salvage included a transfer of the long flexor tendons to the remaining bases of the proximal phalanx. It might be necessary to pull the K-wires out from the MPJs early to allow relaxation to the soft tissues and minimize vascular damage.

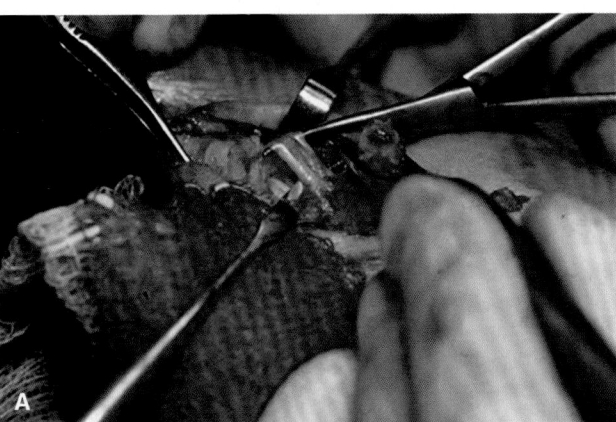

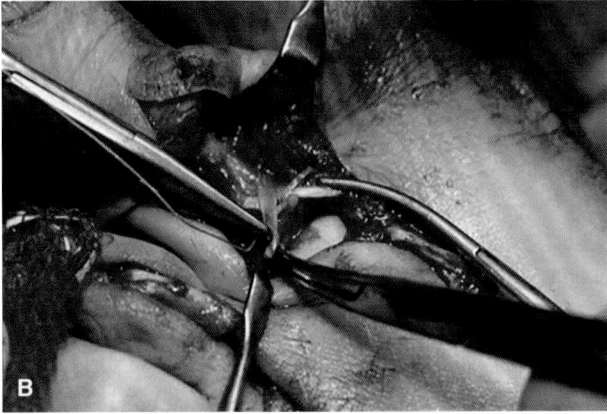

FIGURE 68.22 A. Dissection through the plantar capsule after PIPJ resection. The surgeon may choose either the FDL or FDB to assist in the flexor tendon transfer. **B.** Example of a central split in the FDB and then the tendon brought around the base of the phalanx and sutured together under proper tension.

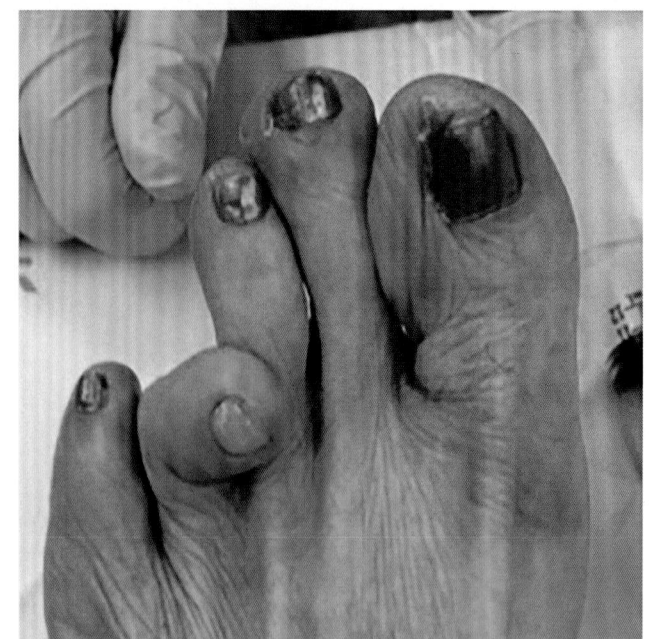

FIGURE 68.23 Example of a fourth flail toe, with significant loss of bone tissue and motor function.

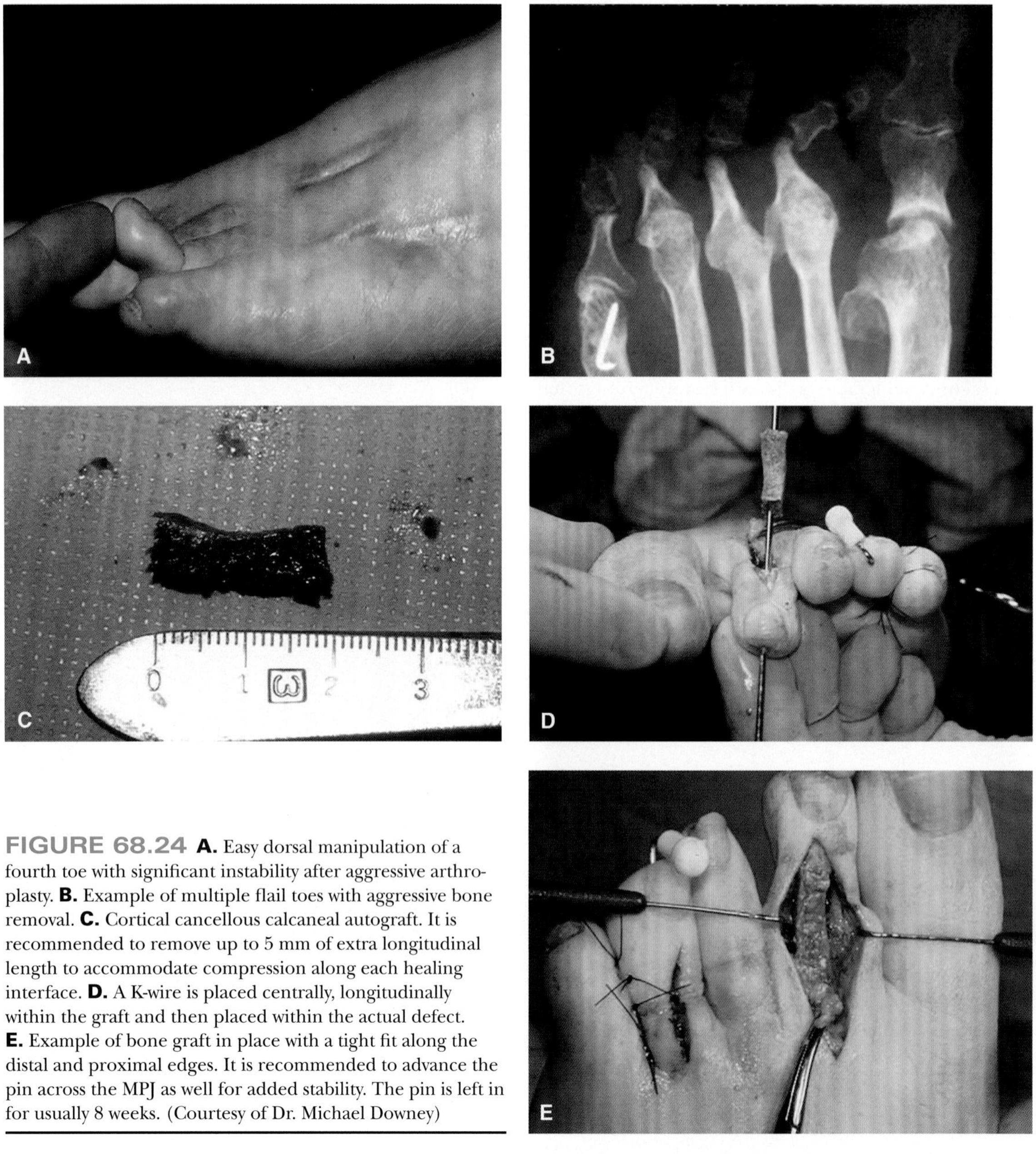

FIGURE 68.24 **A.** Easy dorsal manipulation of a fourth toe with significant instability after aggressive arthroplasty. **B.** Example of multiple flail toes with aggressive bone removal. **C.** Cortical cancellous calcaneal autograft. It is recommended to remove up to 5 mm of extra longitudinal length to accommodate compression along each healing interface. **D.** A K-wire is placed centrally, longitudinally within the graft and then placed within the actual defect. **E.** Example of bone graft in place with a tight fit along the distal and proximal edges. It is recommended to advance the pin across the MPJ as well for added stability. The pin is left in for usually 8 weeks. (Courtesy of Dr. Michael Downey)

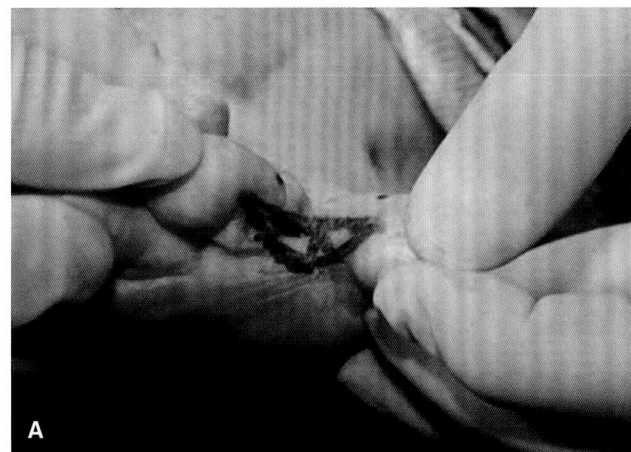

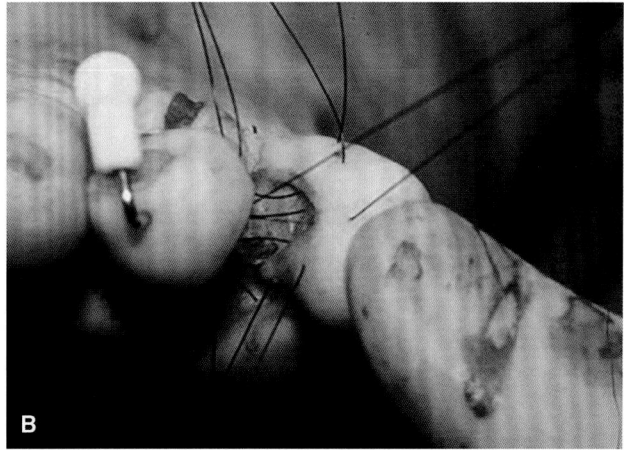

FIGURE 68.25 **A.** Planning of a syndactyly incision with marking one side of the interspace with a marker and squeezing the toes together. **B.** Picture demonstrating all the sutures should be ideally placed within the incision line before any of them are tied. This is much easier than placing one stitch at a time.

provide more needed stability to the graft during healing. The K-wire will often need to be maintained for upward of 8 weeks after surgery before being pulled out. Another option for providing digital stability in some cases is to consider syndactyly to a stable adjacent toe. This will also provide length back to some short unstable digits, and a partial syndactyly is also cosmetically acceptable (Fig. 68.25A and B).

In some unfortunate cases, there has been significant compromise to multiple segments of the metatarsal parabola (Fig. 68.26). If there are more poorly aligned MPJs than those in an acceptable, rectus position, which means that three or more may be involved, then it is often more reasonable to perform a pan metatarsal head resection (Fig. 68.27A and B). A pan metatarsal head resection follows the principles of reconstruction as resection of metatarsals 1-5 will restore a functional parabola back to the damaged forefoot. The first MPJ can be left with an arthroplasty, yet is more stable with a first MPJ arthrodesis. With the first MPJ, the strong recommendation is resection of all of the metatarsals to a normal parabola first, and then the proximal phalanx of the hallux is fused to the new first metatarsal length (Fig. 68.28). The first and second metatarsals

can be resected to equal lengths and then descending from the second through the fifth.

Many of the complications of forefoot surgery have been discussed. Each can present differently, clinically, and visually, yet can be broken down into certain general principles. As presented in this paper, the first step in rebuilding the foot requires a balanced metatarsal parabola. The next step would be to establish a functional MPJ. Finally, with the first two parameters stable, then we can provide flexor function to a stable digit. These biomechanical principles can be used to break down even the most difficult of deformities and provide an algorithm for successful revision in these cases.

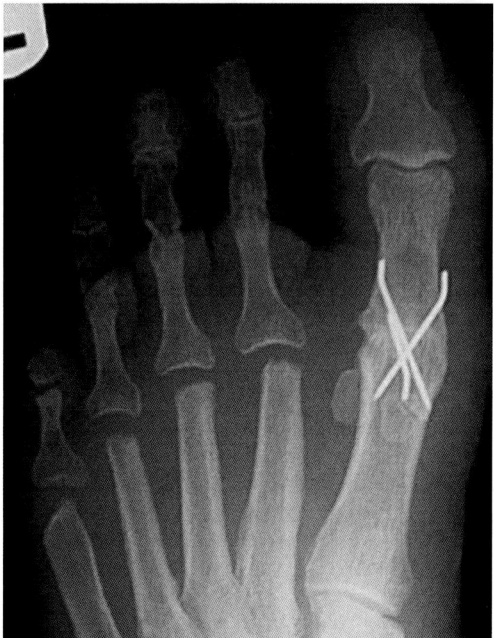

FIGURE 68.27 Pan metatarsal head resection approach for salvage of severe deformity with a first MPJ arthrodesis. For best long term results, all five metatarsals are resected to a proper parabola first before the first MTPJ fusion is performed.

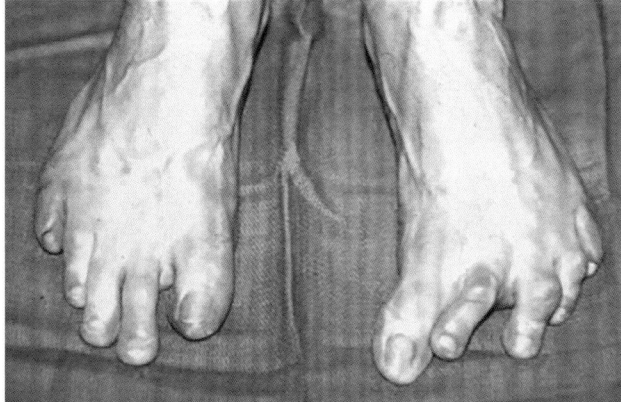

FIGURE 68.26 Clinical example of severe deformity. Hallux varus is present and the second toe is dislocated at the second MPJ, with loss of a functional parabola with unstable MPJs and digits.

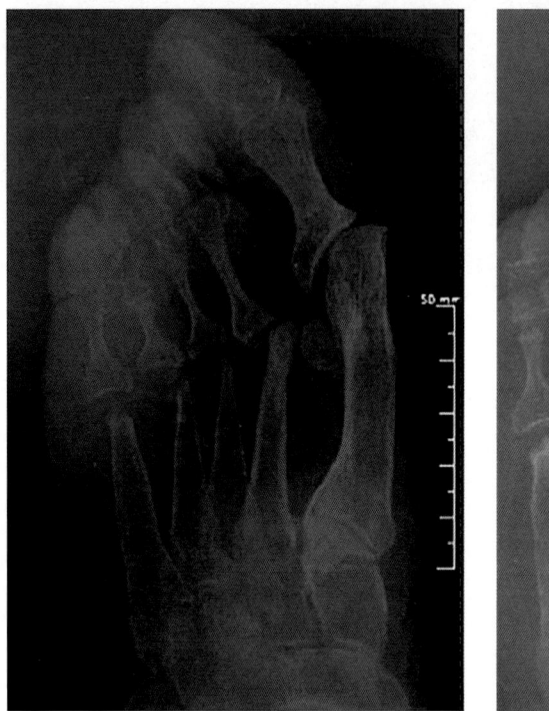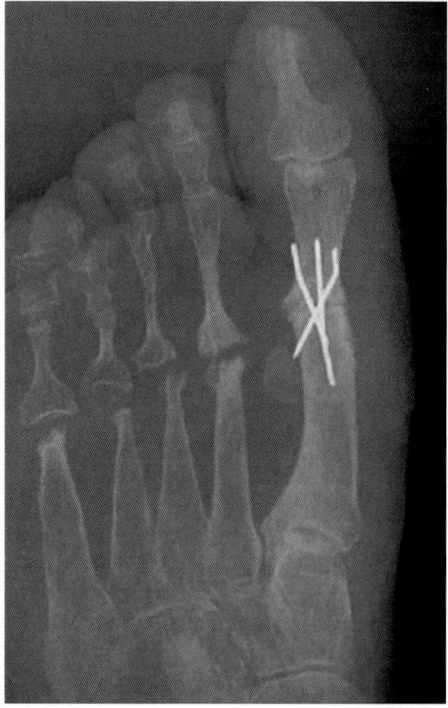

FIGURE 68.28 Example illustrating excessive length of the first metatarsal preserved. This will often lead to sub first metatarsal overload and painful calluses. This again stresses the need to resect all the five metatarsals to a functional metatarsal parabola first, before performing the first MPJ fusion.

REFERENCE

1. Camasta CA. Hallux limitus and hallux rigidus. Clinical examination, radiographic findings, and natural history. *Clin Podiatr Med Surg.* 1996;13(3):423-448.

CHAPTER 69

Rearfoot and Ankle Revision

Gage M. Caudell

INTRODUCTION

For years, hindfoot and ankle arthrodesis have been the procedures of choice for patients with end-stage rheumatological, primary and posttraumatic arthritis, avascular necrosis (AVN), flatfoot, cavovarus, congenital and neuromuscular deformities, failed ankle replacement, and Charcot.[1] Many of these patients will have also failed less aggressive procedures that resulted in them needing arthrodesis. Unfortunately, arthrodesis procedures themselves have their own risk including but not limited to adjacent joint arthritis, infection, malunion, and nonunion.[2] Fusion rates for hindfoot arthrodesis have been reported to be between 65% and 98%.[2-6] Revision arthrodesis of the hindfoot has also been found to have similar nonunion rates.[1,3,4,6,7] This chapter will go over potential causes of malunited and nonunited hindfoot and ankle arthrodesis and how we can hopefully rectify them.

CLINICAL FEATURES

Patients with hindfoot arthrodesis procedures most often will present with loss of range-of-motion, stiffness, and discomfort. These symptoms should be communicated with patients prior and after their surgery. Good communication between patient and physician can allow for patients to have a full understanding of what to expect.

When patients present weeks or months after surgery with swelling, increase warmth, pain out of proportion for what would be expected, and difficulty ambulating, considerations of complications from their surgery should be considered. Once deep vein thrombosis and infection have been rule out, malunited or nonunited arthrodesis should be considered.

Clinical examination should include evaluation of the area of discomfort, looking for a focal region of pain and discomfort. Evaluating the patient weight-bearing is crucial in determining if there is any malalignment that needs to be addressed.

Plain weightbearing radiographs including both foot and ankle images are necessary in allowing the surgeon to adequately evaluate the position of the arthrodesis and overall morphology. The internal fixation needs to be closely looked at for any failure including loosening and lucencies around the screws, breakage of the screw and/or plate, and positioning of the screws. On more than one occasion, I have witnessed a screw being too long and causing discomfort in the adjacent joint. Also, I have seen times with a subtalar joint arthrodesis was successful, but the screw from the posterior inferior heel was angled too far medially and exiting out of the calcaneus and entering the soft

tissue just inferior to the sustentaculum tali and resulting in impingement of the flexor hallucis longus tendon. Evaluation of the arthrodesis site on plain radiographs should show good trabeculation across the arthrodesis site. If no trabeculation is seen and there is a clear sclerotic line and potentially gapping at the arthrodesis site, one should suspect a nonunion.

Often times, computerized tomography (CT) scan will be necessary to either diagnose the nonunion or assist in further evaluating the malunion site (Fig. 69.1A-G). CTs arguably are the gold standard in determining if an arthrodesis site has successfully healed.

MALUNION CLINICAL FEATURES

The malunited arthrodesis can be very debilitating, causing the patient to alter their gate, put added stress to adjacent joints and muscles. Radiographically, it can sometimes be difficult to see that the patient's arthrodesis site is in a malunited position. Ankle arthrodesis may reveal a valgus or varus position on the anterior ankle radiograph. On the lateral radiography, one can see if the foot is 90 degrees to the leg or if the patient is in a recurvatum or procurvatum. Subtalar joint alignment is best viewed on a lateral radiograph, evaluating if the calcaneal inclination angle is sufficient and also the talar declination angle is within normal range. One must make sure that the talus is not too dorsiflexed within the ankle joint or you risk limiting ankle range-of-motion and increasing the stresses on the joint and lead to faster development of degenerative changes. Standing long leg calcaneal axial radiographs can assist in determining if the frontal plane alignment is appropriate. Last, talonavicular joint arthrodesis on both standing lateral and long leg calcaneal radiographs may show similar findings mentioned in regard to malunited subtalar joint arthrodesis. Standing anterior-posterior radiographs of the foot will also assist in determining if the talus is correctly lined up with the navicular and forefoot.

HINDFOOT NONUNION CLINICAL FEATURES

Patients that present with nonunion often times will complain of localized pain to the arthrodesis site. Patient likely will have significant swelling and sometimes warmth to the area of and around the nonunion site. If the surgeon has taken good notes in regard to their previous examinations of the patient, they may determine that the patient may have lost correction and

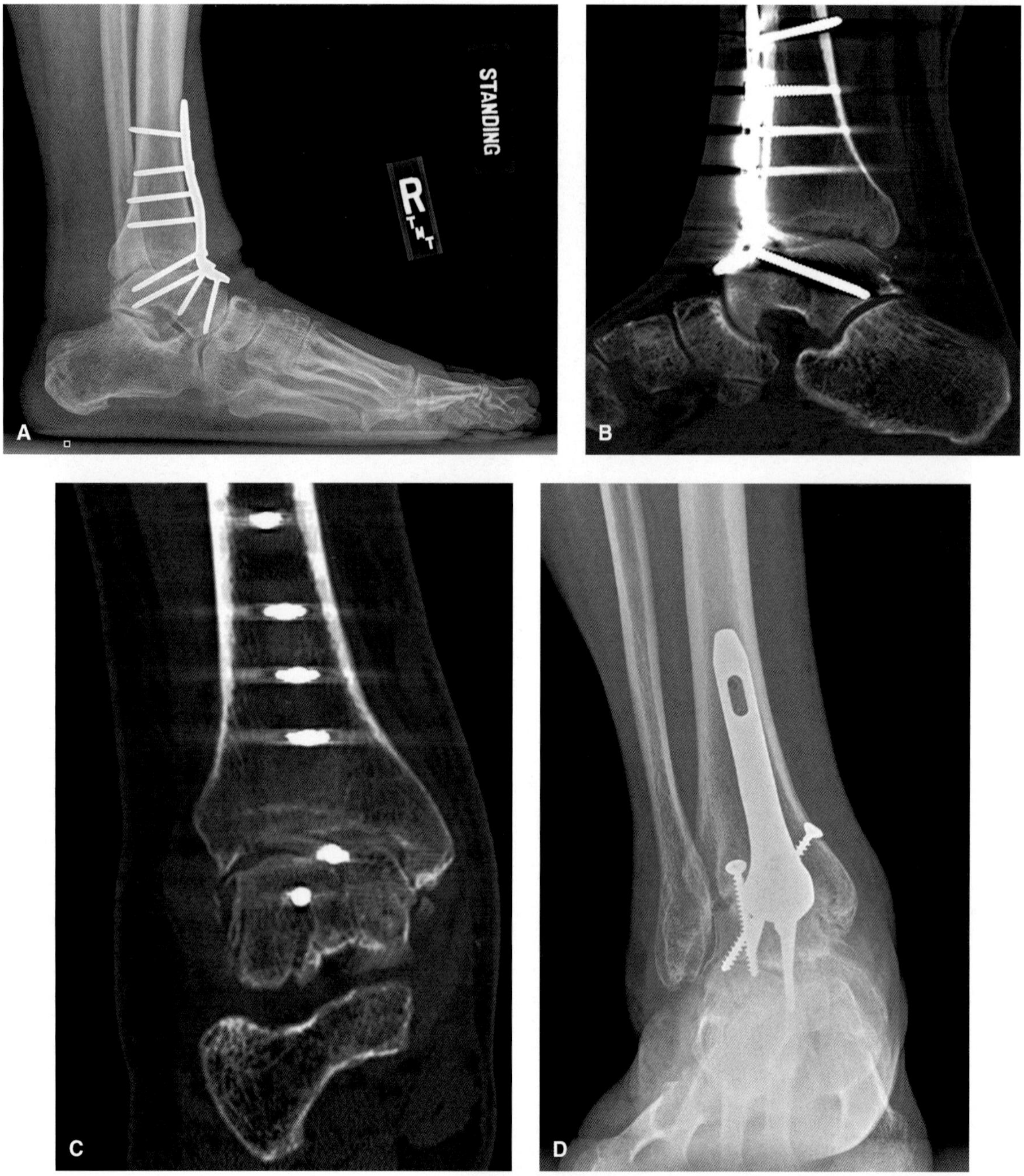

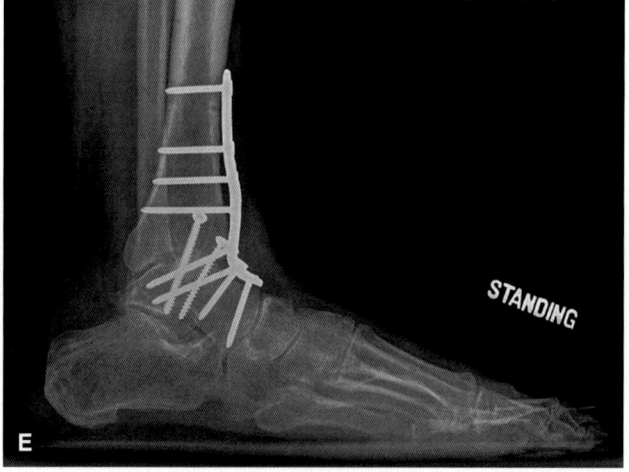

FIGURE 69.1 A. Patient underwent ankle arthrodesis for osteoarthritis. Six months postoperative you can see minimal consolidation at arthrodesis site. **B, C.** CT scan with metal suppression reveals no consolidation at arthrodesis site. **D, E.** 4 months status post revisional ankle arthrodesis with autogenous proximal tibia bone graft and addition of two interfragmentary screws placed using a compromised technique to add additional stability to construct.

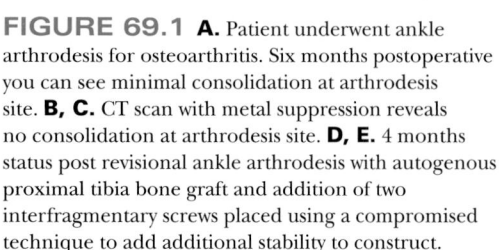

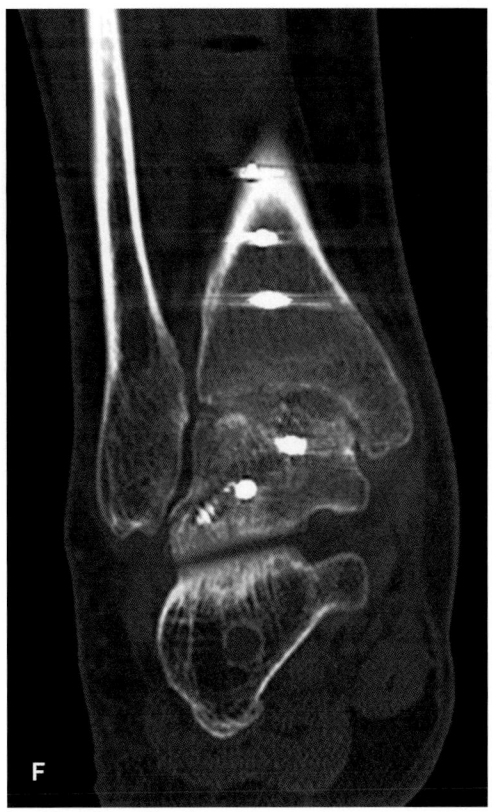

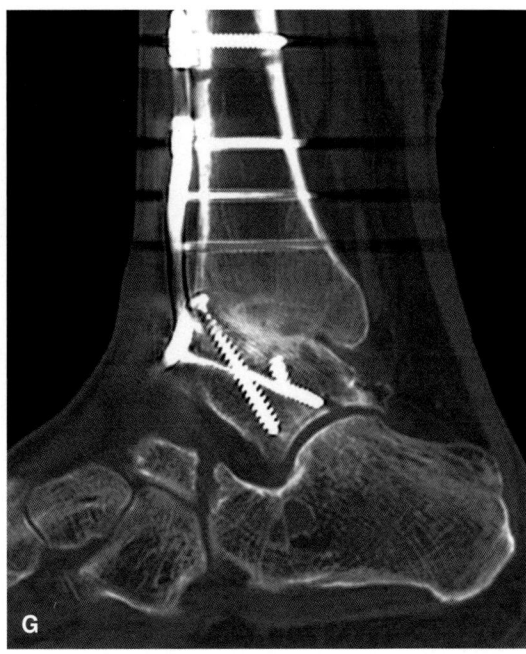

FIGURE 69.1 (*Continued*) **F, G.** CT scan 4 months status postrevisional ankle arthrodesis showing consolidation at arthrodesis site.

appear to have a malunion. Lastly, as already mentioned, plain radiographs and potentially CT scans will be beneficial in determining if the arthrodesis site did not heal.

PATHOGENESIS

The cause of a malunited or nonunited hindfoot arthrodesis can be multifactorial (Table 69.1). These factors can be broken down into patient and surgeon factors. Patient and surgeon factors can be further broken down into medical comorbidities and metabolic disorders, internal and external hardware selection and placement, postoperative planning, and patient compliance.

As a medical provider, one of our most challenging obligations is attempting to control patient compliance. It is in my opinion, we should try to the best of our abilities to educate and communicate with patients on what is expected of them before and after surgery. Educating patients on what their problem is and what is needed to achieve a successful outcome is imperative. When patients have a good understanding of their problem, they are more successful in following directions. Explaining in a generic way why biologically they have to be

non–weight-bearing for many weeks can help with compliance. When allowing a patient to come out of a rigid boot or splint for periods of time for showering and range-of-motion activities, they need to be instructed for how long and how to keep the extremity offloaded. Patients should receive a copy of instructions after surgery and after each office visit. This is provided to them so that there is no question of what was told and expected of them.

Patient compliant factors that may lead to malunion or nonunion include early weight-bearing and/or excessive motion due to not wearing the immobilization device that was given to them. These patients may present with increase pain and swelling. Serial plain radiographs are important to document if there is failure of the fracture or fusion site to heal. CT scan with metal suppression may also be useful. In instances of noncompliance, it is very important the surgeon documents this information and informs the patient that what they are doing may be a detriment to their ultimate outcome.

Many metabolic disorders have been associated with fracture healing. Even though this has not been researched in regard to arthrodesis, this information is important because the same type of bone healing applies in these patients. Common metabolic

TABLE 69.1	Patient Factors That Can Lead to Hindfoot Nonunions[5,8-17]			
Compliance	**Metabolic Disorders**	**Comorbidities**	**Substance Abuse**
Not wearing mobilization device	Vitamin D deficiency	Prior adjacent joint arthrodesis	Alcohol
Early weight bearing	Diabetes	Autoimmune disorders	Narcotics
	Hypogonadism	Neuropathy	Tobacco
	Calcium imbalance	Psychiatric disorders	NSAIDs
	Growth hormone deficiency	Pain disorders	
	PTH deficiency	Obesity	

disorders associated with impaired healing include vitamin D deficiency, diabetes, hypogonadism, and imbalances of calcium, growth hormone, and PTH.[8,18] A few of these disorders directly affect bone metabolism such as vitamin D, calcium, and PTH.[8]

Another patient nonunion factor that should be considered in patients undergoing arthrodesis is patients who have previously underwent adjacent joint arthrodesis or have severe arthritis to the effective joint and to the adjacent joints[1] (Fig. 69.2A-E). There

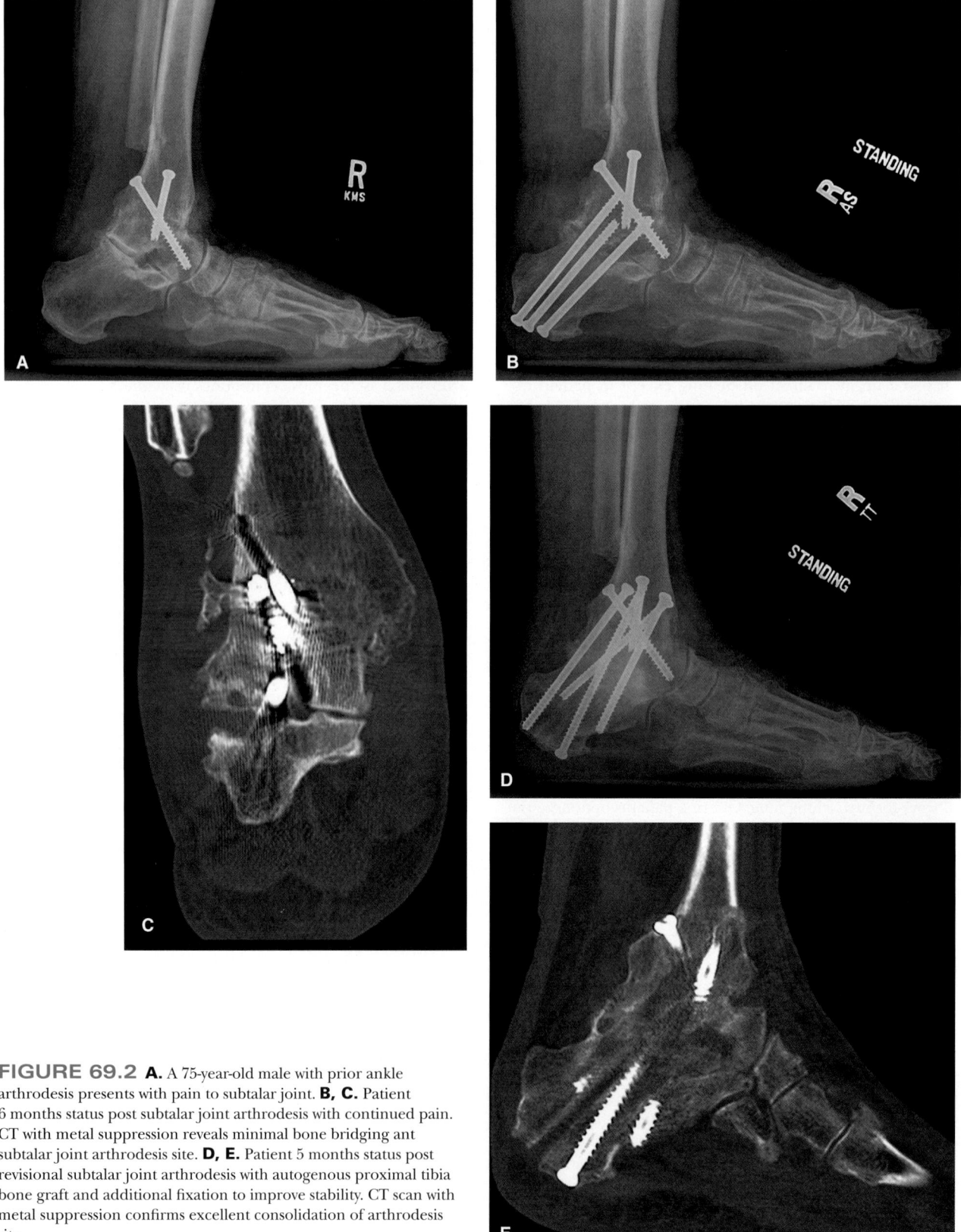

FIGURE 69.2 A. A 75-year-old male with prior ankle arthrodesis presents with pain to subtalar joint. **B, C.** Patient 6 months status post subtalar joint arthrodesis with continued pain. CT with metal suppression reveals minimal bone bridging ant subtalar joint arthrodesis site. **D, E.** Patient 5 months status post revisional subtalar joint arthrodesis with autogenous proximal tibia bone graft and additional fixation to improve stability. CT scan with metal suppression confirms excellent consolidation of arthrodesis site.

is evidence that positively correlates between delayed unions and nonunions with previous adjacent joint arthrodesis.[5,9]

As a surgeon, it is important for us to complete a game plan when managing our patients. We have to do a thorough preoperative history and physical, exhaust appropriate nonoperative treatment, create an appropriate surgical plan, and lastly, manage the patient after surgery in the most appropriate manner possible.

Understanding patients' comorbidities is crucial in attempting to prevent unnecessary complications. To explain this thoroughly, this topic would go well beyond what this chapter is designed to do. Mulligan et al. looked at preoperative risk factors for complications in elective foot and ankle reconstruction and found a strong correlation with alcohol, narcotic, tobacco use, mood or chronic pain disorders, obesity, and diabetes as significant risk factor complications after foot and ankle reconstructions.[10] Perlaman and Thordarson found a correlation with ankle nonunions in patients who used tobacco, consumed alcohol, had a psychiatric disorder, or used illegal drugs.[11] NSAID use has been strongly debated in orthopedics in regard to fracture and arthrodesis healing.[12,13] Dodwell et al. in 2010 looked at NSAID exposure and risk of nonunion and found no increase risk.[12] Wheetley et al. in 2019 meta-analysis looked at effects of NSAIDs on bone healing and concluded that it had a negative effect on healing except in pediatrics.[13] They also concluded that it may be dose or time dependent because studies looking at low-dose or short duration use did not affect union rates.[13] Other comorbidities such as diabetes and rheumatoid arthritis are known to increase risk of surgical complications.[14-16] O'Connor et al. published a level IV study finding an association with neuropathy as a significant risk factor of arthrodesis nonunion.[17]

Often times, we overlook patients economic and social living standards. It would be hard from a research standpoint to stratify the importance of these factors when managing patients surgically. Theoretically, patients with lower economic wellness may have less resources for having the proper equipment necessary for them to be compliant after surgery. They may also have a more difficult time staying off work because of financial restraints. A surgeon should never compromise the way they are going to appropriately manage the patient based on patients need to return to work but sometimes giving patients options that may allow them to return to work earlier and communicate with them reasons why they will be off work for such a long time. Offering patients options to purchase offloading devices at locations that will save them money can maximize compliance and healing and also provide the patient confidence that you are providing the best care.

When patients that have substandard living conditions, the surgeon should attempt to optimize this situation by having them have assistance from family members or friends. If needed, utilizing home health care and rehabilitation facilities should be considered. Communicating with the patient the reasoning behind these decisions are important so that the patients clearly understand you have their best interest at heart.

Surgical planning is instrumental in properly executing good rigid fixation and allowing for adequate bone healing (Table 69.2). Anatomic dissection and reducing excessive soft tissue stripping will help maintain the vascularity to the fusion site.[19] The use of external, internal fixation such as interfragmentary screws or plates have their advantages and disadvantages.

The ring external fixator was introduced by Dr. Gavril Ilizarov in the late 1950s. External fixation has advantages of preserving soft tissue and periosteum, does not disrupt fracture

TABLE 69.2	Surgical Factors That Can Lead to Hindfoot Nonunions[19-35]	
Dissection	**Joint Preparation**	**Fixation Failure**
Poor tissue handling	Inadequate cartilage removal	Improper hardware placement
Vascular compromise	Excision bone removal	Insufficient compression
		Insufficient stability

hematoma, and patients can be allowed to weight-bear early.[20] They can also have their disadvantages. Patient selection is important because some patients psychologically will have a difficult time with these devices. Pin track infections are the most common complications with external fixation.[20] Occurrences of pin track infections have been sited in the literature ranging from 1% to 100%.[21,22] Establishing safe zones before wire insertions is crucial in preventing neurovascular and muscle/tendon injury.[20] If the construct is too rigid, it may lead to bone healing problems and nonunion.[20]

Interfragmentary screw fixation for ankle and hindfoot arthrodesis is the most commonly used method in performing these procedures.[23] A two or three screw fixation technique using 6.5 mm or larger screws have been discussed often in the literature for ankle arthrodesis.[24] There is some evidence to support the use of two screws vs three screws due to the loss of contact joint surface.[25] If two or three screws enter the ankle joint in close proximity to one another and also cross at a very close proximity to one another, concerns of rotational instability should be considered. Clifford et al. in 2014 compared different internal fixation techniques for ankle arthrodesis and concluded that using a locking plate in an anterior or lateral configuration and the addition of a compression screw considerable increases primary bending stiffness of ankle arthrodesis compared to screw fixation.[24] Similar studies have also supported this.[23,26,27] Isolated talonavicular, subtalar, and calcaneocuboid joint arthrodesis when using screw fixation can have similar concerns.

The use of plate fixation in hindfoot arthrodesis is most commonly used for calcaneocuboid, tibiotalar, and tibiotalocalcaneal arthrodesis (TTCA). The use of locking plates has been found to be superior to conventional plates in regard to rigidity.[28] With exception of anterior ankle arthrodesis plating, we have to implant these devices on the compression side of the joint which can lead to distraction on the tension side and theoretically lead to potential nonunion (Fig. 69.3A-K). A good example is posterior plating for tibiotalar and or TTCA. In these instances, it is important for the surgeon to use interfragmentary screw fixation to the anterior portion of these joints to prevent distraction and potential nonunion.

Intramedullary rod fixation for TTCA for primary and revisional procedures has been discussed in the literature.[29-31] TTCA indications include severe osteoarthritis, AVN of the talus, and previous failed total ankle arthroplasty. Other conditions amenable for TTCA include severe rheumatoid arthritis, osteoarthritis of tibiocalcaneal and talocalcaneal joints, Charcot arthropathy, neuromuscular disease, trauma, severe deformity of clubfoot, congenital deformities, or pseudarthrosis.[30] Common complications using intramedullary fixation include neurovascular injury, infection, delayed and nonunion, and perioperative fracture.[30,31]

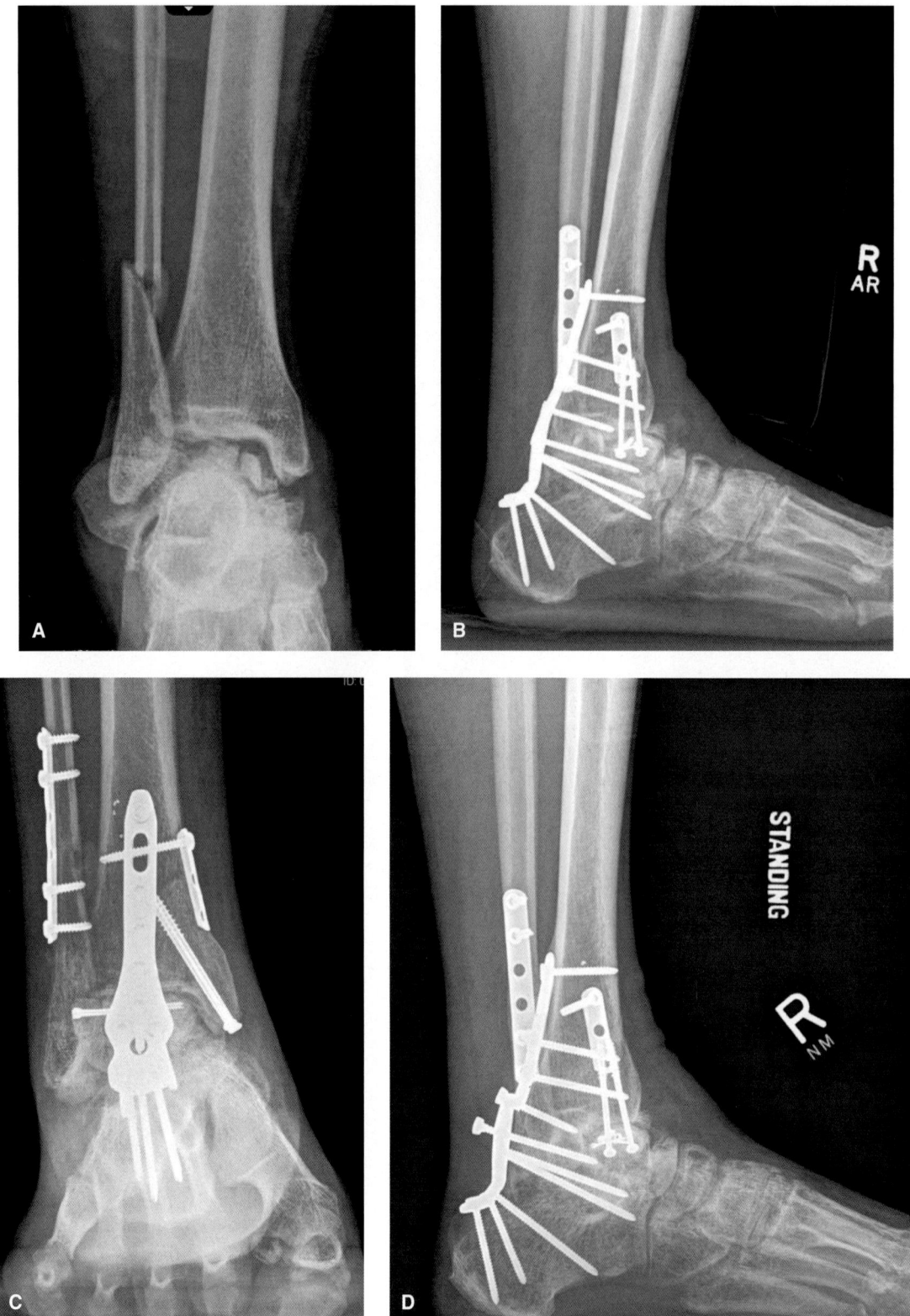

FIGURE 69.3 **A.** A 35-year-old male presents with severely comminuted talar body fracture and associated fibula fracture. **B, C.** Patient underwent primary tibiotalocalcaneal arthrodesis with autogenous iliac bone graft and 5 months postoperatively, hardware appears stable and patient complains of minimal pain. The plate was placed posteriorly due to the severe comminution of the talus and best visualization of the arthrodesis site. The fibula was left intact so that an ankle replacement surgery could be an option if necessary. **D, E.** Patient presents 8 months post-op TTC arthrodesis with failed hardware and severe pain to the ankle.

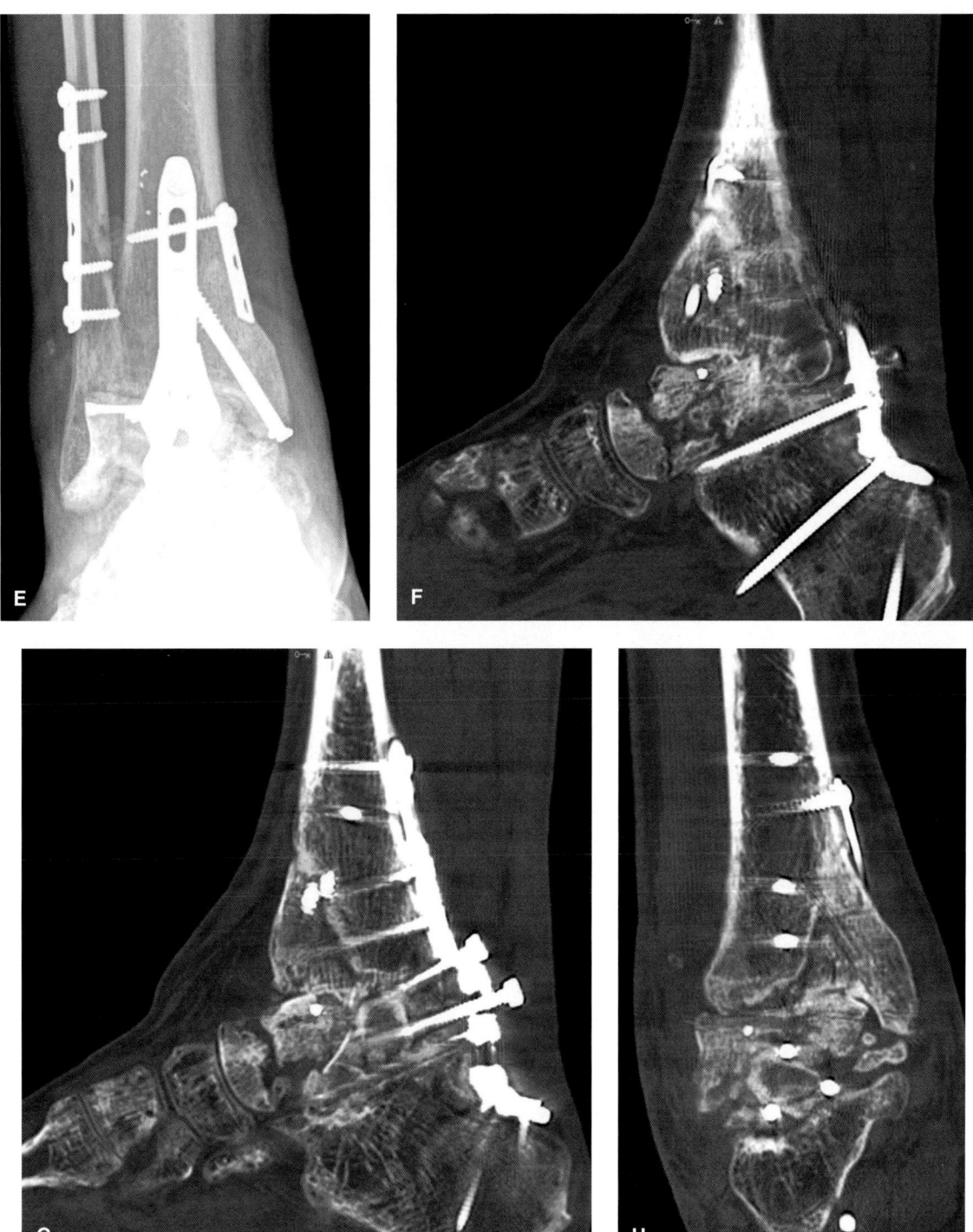

FIGURE 69.3 (*Continued*) **F, G.** Patients CT with metal suppression reveals minimal consolidation at tibiotalar and subtalar joint.

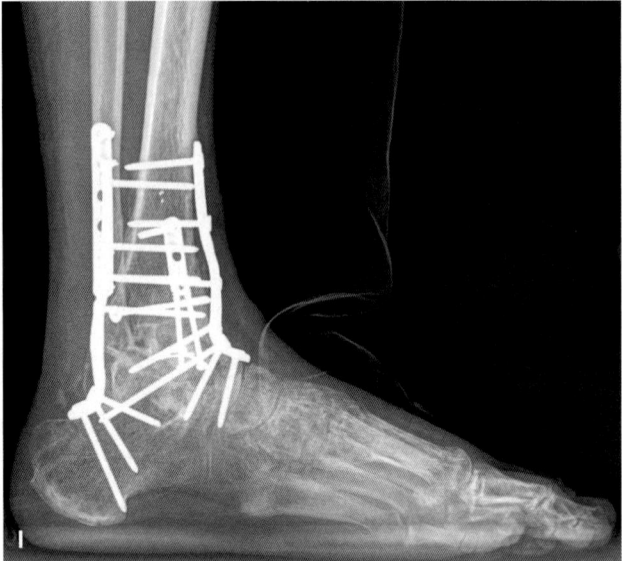

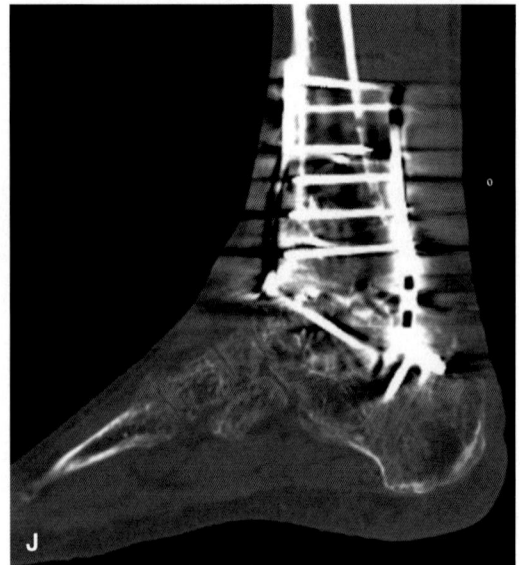

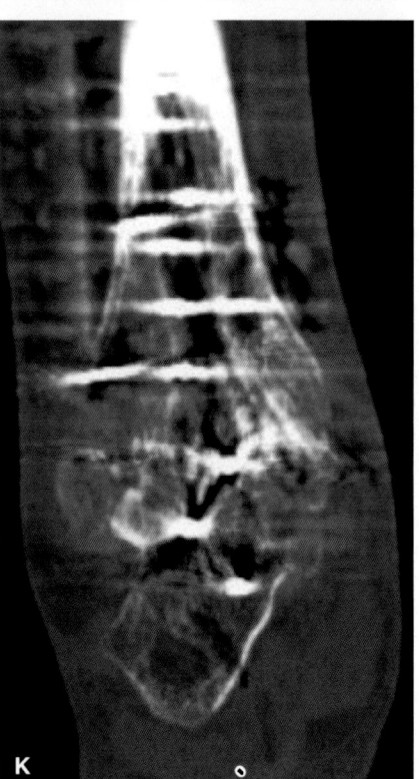

FIGURE 69.3 (*Continued*) **H-K.** Patient 5 months status post revisional TTC arthrodesis with autogenous iliac crest bone graft with evidence showing good consolidation of arthrodesis site.

Careful reaming is crucial to prevent fracture of the tibia during surgical insertion. Intraoperatively, it is crucial to determine proper length of the intramedullary rod to prevent postoperative stress on the tibia and prevent tibia stress fracture.[32] Evidence supports when using these implants, staying within the proximal or distal metaphysis of the tibia is advised.[32]

Intramedullary rod fixation should be considered in revisional surgery when there are concerns of loss of height due to bone resorption (in example AVN of the talus) and in cases of severe hindfoot deformity. A physician once said "you can easily cheat when using screws or plate fixation for hindfoot fusions, but you cannot with an intramedullary rod, the rod makes you get proper correction."

This philosophy is important and getting good anatomic position is critical for a good successful outcome.

TREATMENT

Once a malunion or nonunion has been diagnosed, the surgeon needs to determine appropriate management. Management of malunions may be just monitoring or prescribing custom fabricated orthotics or bracing. Nonunions unfortunately will not be tolerated long term and will need more aggressive treatment. Patients will often need to be immobilized for additional period of time and need adjunctive measures such

as bone stimulators and casting. In both situations of malunion and nonunion, additional surgical measures may be necessary.

NONUNION TREATMENT

Once an infection has been eliminated, resolved, or ruled out and/or nonoperative treatment has been exhausted, surgical management should be considered (Table 69.3). Prior to operative management, it is important for the surgeon to determine the potential cause of the nonunion so that it can best be avoided. The surgeon has to create a game plan that involves restoring healthy bleeding tissue to the arthrodesis site, good intra and postoperative stabilization, and an adjunctive treatment plan that includes bone stimulators and possible pharmacological drugs.

Nonunions of the hindfoot with no deformity should be managed in a very straightforward fashion. Most often you will use the same incisions that were used for the initial procedures. The surgeon should be cautious making additional incisions due to the risk of further damaging the blood supply to the arthrodesis site. If better internal stabilization can be obtained through new incisions, this would be an instance it should be considered. After dissecting to the arthrodesis site, any prior internal fixation that needs to be removed should be removed. You should always have a hardware removal set available so that if the screws are damaged, they can still be easily removed without causing further soft tissue harm and also reduce time in the operating room. Once the nonunion site is visualized, preparation of the joint is critical. Often, an osteotome or saw will be needed to initially break through the nonunion site. Once the nonunion site is free, a combination of curettes, osteotomes, rongeur, and round burr should be used. The most important job is to remove all fibrous nonviable tissue and to get to a level of good bleeding bone. A round burr when used appropriately can accomplish this. When using a burr, you will need to use saline often to prevent overheating and potential thermal necrosis.[33,34] Johnson et al. 2009 histological analysis study looked at curettage joint preparation technique and showed evidence that most surgeons likely do not remove enough calcified cartilage from the joint preparation site.[35] Curettage technique may prevent segmental shortening but you increase your risk of a nonunion. I routinely use a round burr exactly for this reason when performing both primary and revisional arthrodesis. Reducing the risk of segmental shortening is important, but removing the subchondral plate is more critical so that you can reduce the amount of cartilage present. Scaling/shingling the joint site to increase the amount of bone that is exposed may also help with healing.

TABLE 69.3	Tips for Successful Nonunion Repair[19-35]	
Patient Factors	**Surgical Factors**	**Postsurgical Factors**
Metabolic disorder management	Minimize vascular insult	Immobilization
Substance abuse monitoring	Joint preparation	Non–weight-bearing
	Bone graft utilization	Bone stimulator
	Stable internal/external fixation	

In my opinion, the use of orthobiologics is essential when managing hindfoot nonunions. I cannot recall any situation in which I did not use orthobiologics in revisional surgeries. Other authors have even suggested that this is standard of care.[5] One study found that 96% of foot surgeons almost always or always use bone grafting during nonunion surgery.[36] Autograft, allograft, and bone substitutes such as demineralized bone matrix (DBM), autologous platelet concentrate, and synthetic grafts have all been described in the literature.[1,37]

My preferred orthobiologic is combination of autogenous and allograft bone graft. I typically have the autogenous graft harvested from the proximal tibia or iliac crest. Evidence supports similar healing factors in proximal tibial bone graft when compared to iliac crest.[38] Proximal tibia bone graft has less donor site morbidity, and a larger quantity of cancellous bone can be harvested.[39] Allograft bone grafts I use are a combination of cancellous bone chips and bone morphogenic protein-2. By combining all three grafts, I have a good combination of osteogenic, osteoconductive, and osteoinductive properties.

The literature shows evidence that allograft incorporation is similar to autogenous incorporation. Muller et al. 2013 studied comparing autografts with allografts in hindfoot arthrodesis and osteotomies and found similar outcomes for both.[40] This systematic review looked at 928 hindfoot procedures. The authors did caution that the studies analyzed were of poor quality due to small sample sizes and compounding variables. Most of these studies are only looking at primary arthrodesis, instances where the blood supply to the surrounding bone should be rich. In revisional surgery, the blood supply may be compromised and using autogenous graft in my opinion may see better incorporation rates.

Bone stimulator use should be considered in both operative and nonoperative management of delayed hindfoot arthrodesis. Literature supports their use in hindfoot arthrodesis both in primary and delayed unions.[41,42] Pulse electromagnetic field therapy has been FDA approved for stimulation of bone growth for failed arthrodesis.[41] Routine use of bone stimulators for primary arthrodesis are most likely not needed, but for revisional arthrodesis, it is important consideration. Both implantable and external devices can be used. I routinely use low-intensity pulse ultrasound bone stimulation in my practice due to its support in the literature and its ease of use.[43]

MALUNION TREATMENT

The ideal position of an ankle arthrodesis is the foot 90 degrees to the leg, the heel in neutral to slight valgus (ie, 5 degrees), the foot displaced as much posteriorly on the leg as possible to allow for good contact between both joint surfaces, and it reduces the lever arm of the construct, and the foot rotated externally 10-15 degrees.[2,44] The patient may be able to tolerate mild variance of these positions. Often times they will be able to tolerate more of a variance of valgus or external rotation than compared to varus or internal rotation. If the foot is too dorsiflexed or plantarflexed in the sagittal plane, this will likely change the patients gait and put undo stress on contralateral joints, especially the knee and hip. The patient may have a slight limb shortening due to the surgical procedure, and this has not been shown to be detrimental and can facilitate toe clearance during swing phase of gait.[45]

Isolated and multi-joint malunited arthrodesis of the talonavicular, subtalar, calcaneal cuboid joints can present

with a forefoot varus or valgus, abduction or adduction, and sagittal plane malalignment do to a rocker bottom deformity or reduced ankle range-of-motion secondary to a talus dorsiflexed in the ankle mortise. The goal in each of these situations is to have the heel in a neutral to slight valgus position (ie, 5 degrees). If the talus is dorsiflexed in the ankle mortise, then the goal is to plantarflexed the talus so that the talar declination angle is ~21 degrees.

ANKLE MALUNION

The ankle malunion can be corrected with supramalleolar osteotomies, wedge cuts, straight cuts, or focal dome osteotomies.[1,46-48] Evaluation of appropriate radiographs should demonstrate the location of the deformity, the center of rotation of angulation (CORA). If uniplanar deformity correction is necessary, then a wedge osteotomy will likely be most appropriate. If the foot needs to be shifted anterior or posterior, then a straight cut will likely work well. If the patient has multiplanar deformity, a focal dome osteotomy may be needed.

Literature in regard to management of malunited ankle fractures is limited. Casillas and Allen in 2004 described wedge osteotomies, various fixation devices, and ancillary surgical procedures for ankle arthrodesis nonunions.[49] Cooper in 2001 and Raikin and Rampuri in 2008 also showed a similar algorithm.[44,50] Katsenis et al. in 2005 described a technique using Ilizarov external fixation that could simultaneously treat osteomyelitis, limb length discrepancy, and deformity.[51]

HINDFOOT MALUNION

When evaluating hindfoot malunions, the surgeon must evaluate for deformity in the hindfoot and midfoot. Common midfoot deformities that may occur after isolated hindfoot or triple arthrodesis would be forefoot supination or pronation and forefoot abduction or adduction. Correction of a forefoot deformity after an isolated talonavicular or subtalar joint arthrodesis may be correctable by performing a midfoot osteotomy or arthrodesis. In severe deformities, especially after a triple arthrodesis, a derotational osteotomy through the talonavicular and calcaneal cuboid joint may be necessary. In severe forefoot abduction or adduction deformities, closing or opening wedge osteotomies may be necessary.

Patients may develop a rocker bottom deformity, typically from a malunited calcaneal cuboid joint because the cuboid subluxed plantarly while performing a triple arthrodesis. A plantar closing wedge or a dorsal opening wedge osteotomy through the midtarsal joints may be considered.[52,53] This will allow for the talus to plantarflex and reduce stress on the ankle joint.

In patients with residual hindfoot varus or valgus after subtalar joint arthrodesis, a wedge cut through the joint or extraarticular osteotomy through the calcaneal tuberosity may be performed.[52] In severe valgus deformity or when patients have an increase in the talo-first metatarsal angle, a revisional bone block arthrodesis can be performed.

Patients may present with multiplanar deformities after triple arthrodesis. In situations like this, combination of derotational and wedge osteotomies may be considered. Figures 69.4-69.6

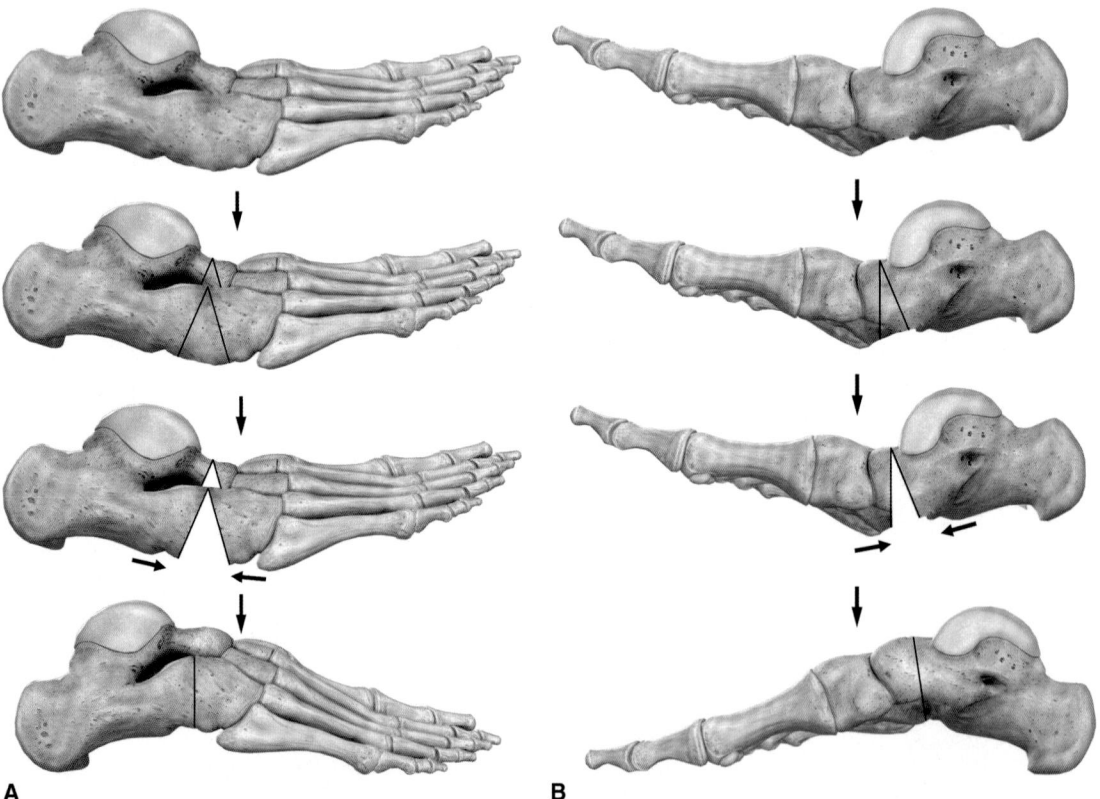

A   **B**

FIGURE 69.4 A, B. Illustration of a rocker bottom deformity. Closing wedge osteotomy with apex superiorly through the talonavicular and calcaneal cuboid arthrodesis site can correct this sagittal plane malalignment. Also, if there is frontal plane deformity to the forefoot, it can easily be rotated in the frontal plane to correct any residual varus or valgus. Adaptation from 3D4Medical Complete Anatomy. *(Reproduced with permission from 3D4 Medical Limited.)*

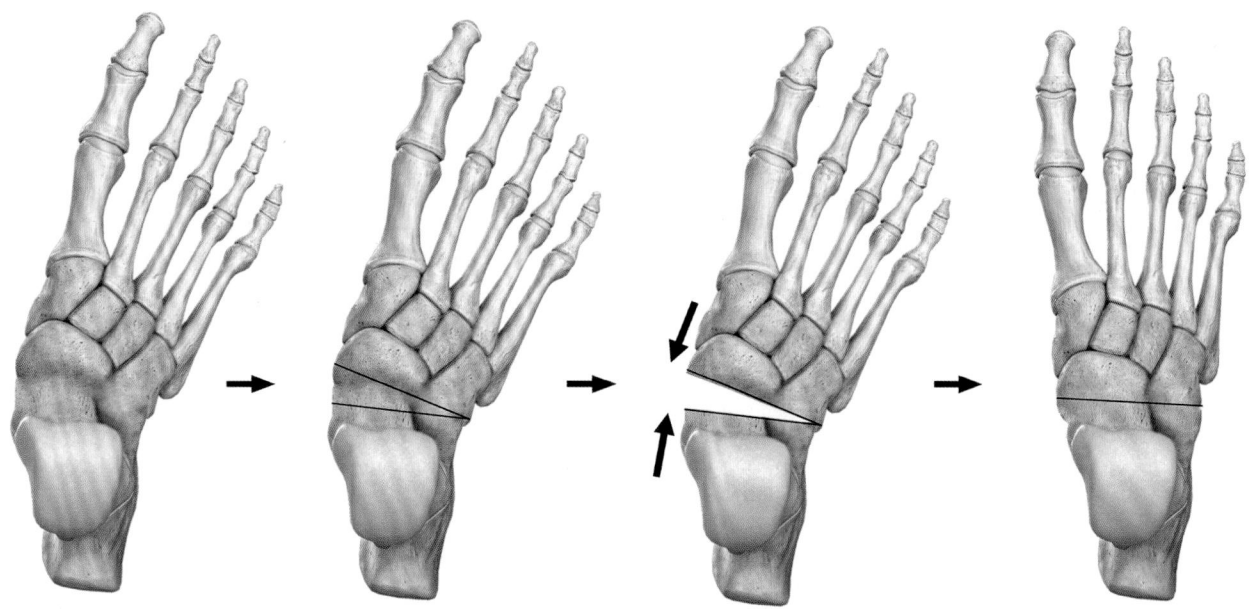

FIGURE 69.5 Illustration of an abducted forefoot after triple arthrodesis. This can be corrected with a closing wedge osteotomy with the apex laterally. Frontal plane correction can also be performed simultaneously through the osteotomy site. *(Reproduced with permission from 3D4 Medical Limited.)*

show both uniplanar and multiplanar derotational, opening, and closing wedge osteotomies that may be performed when correcting these deformities.

POSTOPERATIVE PROTOCOL

For patients undergoing revisional surgeries, postoperatively you will need to be more conservative, especially for non-unions. Postoperative management of malunions are managed similar to treatment used for primary arthrodesis procedures.

If utilizing bone graft or additional adjunctive procedure are necessary, consideration of longer immobilization and casting should be considered. Hindfoot arthrodesis procedures likely need to be non–weight-bearing for 10-12 weeks. For the first 2 weeks, the patient is immobilized in a Jones compression dressing with a posterior splint. The sutures are then removed and then the patient is casted. Around 6 weeks, the cast can be removed, and patients can be placed in a 3D Tall boot that is to be worn during the day and at night they are allowed to wear a splint that was prefabricated for them. Often times they will be allowed to perform hindfoot range-of-motion exercises

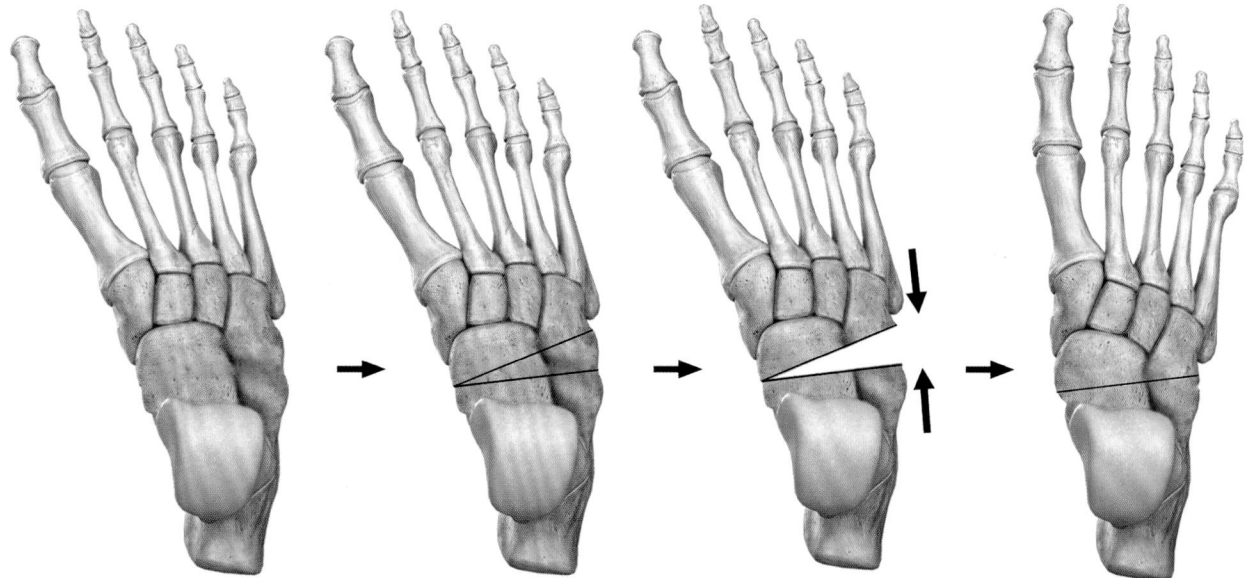

FIGURE 69.6 Illustration of an adducted forefoot after triple arthrodesis. This can be corrected with a closing wedge osteotomy with the apex medially. Frontal plane correction can also be performed simultaneously through the osteotomy site. *(Reproduced with permission from 3D4 Medical Limited.)*

with the exception of patients undergoing ankle arthrodesis. Weight-bearing at 10-12 weeks is gradual. For 2 weeks, instructions are given for a limited amount of steps and time needed between walking in a boot. The last 2 weeks, before returning to regular shoe, patient is allowed to walk without restrictions in the boot. Once the patient is allowed to return to regular shoe, they are placed in a lace-up ankle for support.

Physical therapy is often ordered after hindfoot arthrodesis procedures for 4-6 weeks. Obviously, we are not trying to regain motion to the joints that we fused but to regain strength, balance, and mental confidence.

Serial radiographs are taken at the time of surgery (intraoperative films), at their first postoperative visit (typically 2 weeks postsurgery), and then every 4 weeks. CT scan with metal suppression may need to be considered around 12-16 weeks postoperatively if there is suspicion of problems healing or in instances, the use of internal fixation makes it difficult to evaluate the fusion site. Most of these patients are then followed for 6-12 months with plain radiographs at each of their visits. Communicating with the patient routinely is important in determining how they are doing and what their expectations should be. Explaining, it will take 12 months to recover and that they most likely will always have some discomfort is important. The goal is not to make them pain free, it is to make their pain tolerable and to improve their quality of life.

NONUNION POSTOPERATIVE PROTOCOL

When treating patients undergoing revisional arthrodesis due to a nonunion, management is similar to all other hindfoot arthrodesis procedures with the exception they may be non–weight-bearing a few weeks longer, they may be casted longer, and they may utilize a bone stimulator. Most of these patients will be non–weight-bearing for 12-14 weeks and will be casted for at least 8 of those weeks.

Serial radiographs are taken in the same sequence as mentioned in patients undergoing revisional malunion surgery. Obtaining CT scan is more important in these patients to confirm the arthrodesis has healed. These patients are also followed for 6-12 months. Last, these patients need to have expectations that their recovery will be longer due to the duration of immobilization and because many of these patients have been in a compromised state many months before the original surgery. Thus, many have been immobilized for 6 months or greater.

SUMMARY

In summary, revisional hindfoot arthrodesis can be very challenging, especially when there is severe deformity or overlying comorbidities. Utilizing a systematic approach by first determining the cause of the malunion and nonunion, determining best surgical plan, and last, managing the patient postoperatively is crucial in allowing for a successful outcome.

REFERENCES

1. Murphy LJ, Mendicino RW, Catanzariti AR. Revisional hindfoot arthrodesis. *Clin Podiatr Med Surg.* 2009;26(1):59-78.
2. Yasui Y, et al. Ankle arthrodesis: a systematic approach and review of the literature. *World J Orthop.* 2016;7(11):700-708.
3. Klassen LJ, et al. Comparative nonunion rates in triple arthrodesis. *J Foot Ankle Surg.* 2018;57(6):1154-1156.
4. Neumann J, et al. Comparison of non-union and complication rates in primary versus revision tibiotalar arthrodesis. *Foot Ankle Orthop.* 2018;3(3):2473011418S00091.
5. Saxby T, Rosenfeld P. Triple arthrodesis: is bone grafting necessary? *J Bone Joint Surgery British* 2005;87-B(2):175-178.
6. Barg A, Saltzman C. Primary vs. revision ankle arthrodesis: comparison of fusion and complication rates. *Foot Ankle Surg.* 2017;23:47.
7. Easley ME, et al. Revision tibiotalar arthrodesis. *J Bone Joint Surg Am.* 2008;90(6):1212-1223.
8. Brinker MR, O'Connor DP. The biological basis for nonunions. *JBJS Rev.* 2016;4(6):01874474-201606000-00001.
9. Haskell A, Pfeiff C, Mann R. Subtalar joint arthrodesis using a single lag screw. *Foot Ankle Int.* 2004;25(11):774-777.
10. Mulligan RP, et al. Preoperative risk factors for complications in elective ankle and hindfoot reconstruction. *Foot Ankle Spec.* 2018;11(1):54-60.
11. Perlman MH, Thordarson DB. Ankle fusion in a high risk population: an assessment of nonunion risk factors. *Foot Ankle Int.* 1999;20(8):491-496.
12. Dodwell ER, et al. NSAID exposure and risk of nonunion: a meta-analysis of case–control and cohort studies. *Calcif Tissue Int.* 2010;87(3):193-202.
13. Wheatley BM, et al. Effect of NSAIDs on bone healing rates: a meta-analysis. *J Am Acad Orthop Surg.* 2019;27(7):e330-e336.
14. Tucker W, et al. Effect of type 1 and type 2 diabetes mellitus on complication and reoperation rates of ankle arthrodesis and total ankle arthroplasty. *Foot Ankle Orthop.* 2018;3(3):2473011418S00497.
15. Mäenpää H, Lehto MU, Belt EA. Why do ankle arthrodeses fail in patients with rheumatic disease? *Foot Ankle Int.* 2001;22(5):403-408.
16. Rabinovich RV, Haleem AM, Rozbruch SR. Complex ankle arthrodesis: review of the literature. *World J Orthop.* 2015;6(8):602.
17. O'Connor KM, et al. Clinical and operative factors related to successful revision arthrodesis in the foot and ankle. *Foot Ankle Int.* 2016;37(8):809-815.
18. Nauth A, et al. Principles of nonunion management: state of the art. *J Orthop Trauma.* 2018;32:S52-S57.
19. Harwood PJ, Ferguson DO. An update on fracture healing and non-union. *Orthop Trauma.* 2015;29(4):228-242.
20. Ali A, et al. Common complications of Ilizarov external fixator. *J Pak Orthop Assoc.* 2018;30(01):39-43.
21. Antoci V, et al. Pin-tract infection during limb lengthening using external fixation. *Am J Orthop (Belle Mead NJ).* 2008;37(9):E150-E1544.
22. Battle, J, Carmichael KD. Incidence of pin track infections in children's fractures treated with Kirschner wire fixation. *J Pediatr Orthop.* 2007;27(2):154-157.
23. Dohm MP, et al. A biomechanical evaluation of three forms of internal fixation used in ankle arthrodesis. *Foot Ankle Int.* 1994;15(6):297-300.
24. Clifford C, et al. A biomechanical comparison of internal fixation techniques for ankle arthrodesis. *J Foot Ankle Surg.* 2015;54(2):188-191.
25. So E, Brandão RA, Bull PE. A comparison of talar surface area occupied by 2- versus 3-screw fixation for ankle arthrodesis. *Foot Ankle Spec.* 2020;13(1):50-53.
26. Harris E, Moroney P, Tourné Y. Arthrodesis of the first metatarsophalangeal joint—A biomechanical comparison of four fixation techniques. *Foot Ankle Surg.* 2017;23(4):268-274.
27. Mueckley TM, et al. Biomechanical evaluation of primary stiffness of tibiotalar arthrodesis with an intramedullary compression nail and four other fixation devices. *Foot Ankle Int.* 2006;27(10):814-820.
28. Gautier E, Perren S, Cordey J. Strain distribution in plated and unplated sheep tibia an in vivo experiment. *Injury.* 2000;31:37-93.
29. Donnenwerth MP, Roukis TS. Tibio-talo-calcaneal arthrodesis with retrograde compression intramedullary nail fixation for salvage of failed total ankle replacement: a systematic review. *Clin Podiatr Med Surg.* 2013;30(2):199-206.
30. Franceschi F, et al. Tibiotalocalcaneal arthrodesis using an intramedullary nail: a systematic review. *Knee Surg Sports Traumatol Arthrosc.* 2016;24(4):1316-1325.
31. Roukis TS. Determining the insertion site for retrograde intramedullary nail fixation of tibiotalocalcaneal arthrodesis: a radiographic and intraoperative anatomical landmark analysis. *J Foot Ankle Surg.* 2006;45(4):227-234.
32. Noonan T, et al. Tibiotalocalcaneal arthrodesis with a retrograde intramedullary nail: a biomechanical analysis of the effect of nail length. *Foot Ankle Int.* 2005;26(4):304-308.
33. Tehemar SH. Factors affecting heat generation during implant site preparation: a review of biologic observations and future considerations. *Int J Oral Maxillofac Implants.* 1999;14(1):127-136.
34. Eriksson AR, Albrektsson T, Albrektsson B. Heat caused by drilling cortical bone: temperature measured in vivo in patients and animals. *Acta Orthop Scand.* 1984;55(6):629-631.
35. Johnson JT, et al. Joint curettage arthrodesis technique in the foot: a histological analysis. *J Foot Ankle Surg.* 2009;48(5):558-564.
36. Baumhauer JF, et al. Survey on the need for bone graft in foot and ankle fusion surgery. *Foot Ankle Int.* 2013;34(12):1629-1633.
37. Wee J, Thevendran G. The role of orthobiologics in foot and ankle surgery: allogenic bone grafts and bone graft substitutes. *EFORT Open Rev.* 2017;2(6):272-280.
38. Prall WC, et al. Proliferative and osteogenic differentiation capacity of mesenchymal stromal cells: influence of harvesting site and donor age. *Injury.* 2018;49(8):1504-1512.
39. Salawu O, et al. Comparative study of proximal tibia and iliac crest bone graft donor sites in treatment of orthopaedic pathologies. *Malays Orthop J.* 2017;11(2):15.
40. Müller MA, et al. Substitutes of structural and non-structural autologous bone grafts in hindfoot arthrodeses and osteotomies: a systematic review. *BMC Musculoskelet Disord.* 2013;14(1):59.
41. Saltzman C, Lightfoot A, Amendola A. PEMF as treatment for delayed healing of foot and ankle arthrodesis. *Foot Ankle Int.* 2004;25(11):771-773.
42. Dhawan SK, et al. The effect of pulsed electromagnetic fields on hindfoot arthrodesis: a prospective study. *J Foot Ankle Surg.* 2004;43(2):93-96.
43. Jones CP, Coughlin MJ, Shurnas PS. Prospective CT scan evaluation of hindfoot nonunions treated with revision surgery and low-intensity ultrasound stimulation. *Foot Ankle Int.* 2006;27(4):229-235.

44. Raikin SM, Rampuri V. An approach to the failed ankle arthrodesis. *Foot Ankle Clin.* 2008;13(3):401-416.

45. Thomas R, Daniels TR, Parker K. Gait analysis and functional outcomes following ankle arthrodesis for isolated ankle arthritis. *J Bone Joint Surg Am.* 2006;88(3):526-535.

46. Mendicino RW, Catanzariti AR, Reeves CL. Percutaneous supramalleolar osteotomy for distal tibial (near articular) ankle deformities. *J Am Podiatr Med Assoc.* 2005;95(1):72-84.

47. Sen C, et al. Correction of ankle and hindfoot deformities by supramalleolar osteotomy. *Foot Ankle Int.* 2003;24(1):22-28.

48. Lubicky JP, Altiok H. Transphyseal osteotomy of the distal tibia for correction of valgus/varus deformities of the ankle. *J Pediatr Orthop.* 2001;21(1):80-88.

49. Casillas MM, Allen M. Repair of malunions after ankle arthrodesis. *Clin Podiatr Med Surg.* 2004;21(3):371-383, vi.

50. Cooper PS. Complications of ankle and tibiotalocalcaneal arthrodesis. *Clin Orthop Relat Res.* 2001;391:33-44.

51. Katsenis D, et al. Treatment of malunion and nonunion at the site of an ankle fusion with the Ilizarov apparatus. *J Bone Joint Surg Am.* 2005;87(2):302-309.

52. Seybold JD. Management of the malunited triple arthrodesis. *Foot Ankle Clin.* 2017;22(3):625-636.

53. Toolan BC. Revision of failed triple arthrodesis with an opening-closing wedge osteotomy of the midfoot. *Foot Ankle Int.* 2004;25(7):456-461.

Free Flaps for Lower Extremity Trauma

Luke Bates, Peter Apel, and J. Randolph Clements

INTRODUCTION

Lower extremity salvage in the acute trauma setting remains a difficult reconstructive process. These efforts require a multi-specialty approach. High-energy soft tissue injuries of the distal leg and foot can be frequently encountered at trauma centers and are often associated with underlying fractures and bone loss. These complex soft tissue and bone defects often require free tissue transfers in conjunction with fracture fixation for definitive management.[1]

In 1968, Cobbett[2] performed the first toe-to-thumb transplant in a young woodworker after traumatic amputation by a circular saw. In 1973, O'Brien[3] performed the first successful free flap to the lower extremity, a free groin flap to the anterior ankle after gunshot wound to the anterior ankle. Since these pioneering procedures over a half a decade ago, there have been many advancements in free tissue transfer increasing successful limb salvage in patients with complex soft tissue and bone loss. This chapter will review the use of free flaps for lower extremity reconstruction.

VASCULAR ANATOMY, FLAP SELECTION, AND TIMING

VASCULAR ANATOMY

When considering soft tissue coverage options, it is important to understand soft tissue anatomy, cutaneous blood supply, flap location, incorporated tissue layers, and characteristics of ideal tissue for a lower extremity flap. In general, flaps can be described based on the blood supply to the flap, anatomic location of donor site, and the type of tissue that is being transferred. The skin is divided into three main layers: epidermis, dermis, and the subcutaneous. The arterial supply to the skin is divided into two networks; the deep network, also known as the subdermal plexus, lies between the dermis and the subcutaneous tissues, while the more superficial networks lies within the papillary layer of the dermis and supplies the epidermis by means of diffusion. These cutaneous networks are supplied by perforating arteries ("perforators") that bring blood from large vessels to the skin. These perforators start deep between layers of muscles and emerge via intermuscular septae to feed the skin as septocutaneous perforators, or through muscles, as musculocutaneous perforators. Fasciocutaneous flaps are generally based off known perforator anatomy.

FLAP SELECTION

Free flaps are the highest rung on the reconstructive ladder (Fig. 70.1). The reconstructive ladder describes the basic concept of soft tissue reconstruction by complexity. While the ladder has gradually evolved since in conception by incorporating negative pressure dressings and skin dermal matrix, the basic principles of escalating complexity remains the same. Flaps are distinguished from grafts by their blood supply; grafts rely on wound bed nourishment, while flaps bring their blood supply to the wound. Of the flaps, local flaps are the lowest in complexity and include advancement, rotational, and transposition flaps. Regional and distant flaps include an island that is elevated distant from the defect but remain attached to its blood supply via a pedicle. Free flaps are considered the most complex. The donor site of a free flap is not adjacent to the recipient site; therefore, the arterial and venous supply to the flap are detached from the donor site and reattached to donor vessels at the recipient site. These free flaps can include skin (cutaneous), fascia and skin (fasciocutaneous), muscle, muscle and skin (musculocutaneous), or bone and skin (osteocutaneous) based on tissue defect.

Free flaps are powerful reconstructive tools that can cover massive or infected wounds. Free flaps can cover exposed bone and implants in locations where no local flap is available. Lower extremity free flap selection is driven by three factors: (1) tissue type needed; (2) size and shape of the wound; and (3) surgeon experience. For soft tissue only wounds, the two main options are A) a single fasciocutaneous flap or B) a muscle flap paired with a split-thickness skin graft (Fig. 70.2A and B). The size of the wound is a major determinant of free flap selection. For example, radial forearm flaps (RFFs) and gracilis muscle flaps are suitable for smaller wounds, while anterolateral thigh flaps (ALTs) and latissimus muscle flaps are reserved for large wounds. Donor site morbidity is a lesser consideration for free flap selection, as most of the commonly used free flaps are well tolerated, especially when faced with a limb salvage vs amputation scenario. Lastly, surgeon experience is a major determinant of flap selection. Free flaps are technically demanding procedures and the importance of familiarity with the procedure should not be underestimated as the ideally planned but poorly executed free flap surgery is a still a failure.

TIMING

The "fix and flap" method described by Gopal et al.[4] in 2000 recommends immediate internal fixation and healthy soft

Free tissue transfer

Distance tissue transfer

Local tissue transfer

Tissue expansion

Autologous skin grafting 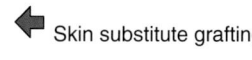 Skin substitute grafting

Direct wound closure

Healing by secondary intension

FIGURE 70.1 Reconstructive ladder.

tissue coverage within 72 hours. A delay in wound coverage >72 hours was associated with a significant increase in postoperative complications. Gopal et al.[4] reported a deep infection rate of 6% when reconstruction was performed within 72 hours and recommended the use of internal fixation over external

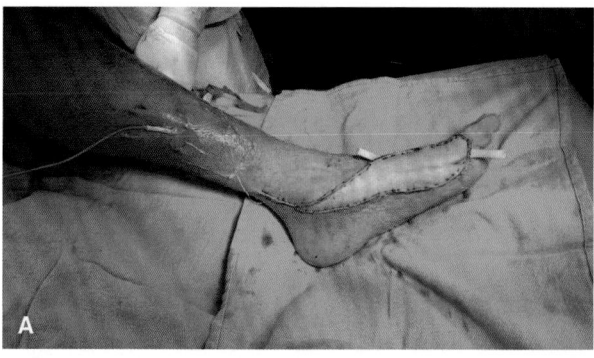

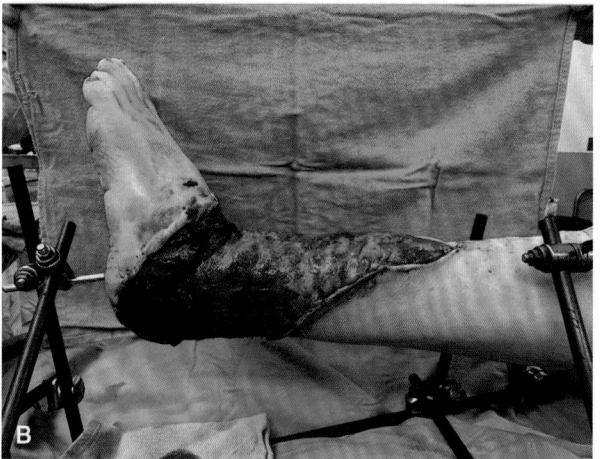

FIGURE 70.2 A. Fasciocutaneous radial forearm flap to the medial foot. **B.** Latissimus muscle flap to the anterior and posterolateral ankle.

fixation due to practical difficulties for flap reconstruction and chronic pin tract infections. Fischer et al.[5] showed that soft tissue coverage of open tibia fractures <10 days had lower infection rates compared to wounds covered after 10 days or wounds that were allowed to heal by secondary intention. While the literature remains inconclusive with regard to optimal timing for flap coverage, the orthopaedic and plastic surgery communities recommend coverage within the 72-hour time frame and not delayed longer than 10 days.

ADDITIONAL CONSIDERATIONS

Additional consideration should be given to protecting flaps from pressure postoperatively, especially for those placed posteriorly or laterally. The posterior aspect of the foot and ankle is obviously an area where pressure is applied with usual supine positioning, but the lateral ankle is also susceptible to pressure with the obligate external rotation of the hip that occurs during periods of prolonged bed rest. Wounds on the posterior lateral aspect of the ankle should be protected with an external fixator. External fixator pins can be placed in the tibia, and a kickstand or suspensory construct can be made. This prevents pressure on the flap. Failure to protect the flap can lead to venous congestion and flap loss.

COMMONLY USED FREE FLAPS FOR LOWER EXTREMITY RECONSTRUCTION

A full review of free flap options is beyond the scope of this chapter; thus, discussion is limited to the most used free flaps for lower extremity reconstruction due to their versatility, size, and familiarity.

FASCIOCUTANEOUS FLAPS

Anterolateral Thigh

The ALT flap is a perforator flap based on the descending branch of the lateral femoral circumflex artery. The ALT is commonly used and is familiar to most surgeons. It is a large flap and can be harvested up to 10 cm wide and up to 25 cm long with the donor site being able to be closed primarily. The pedicle is typically 8-10 cm, making the anastomosis out of the zone of injury for most wounds. The lateral femoral cutaneous nerve can be taken with the flap and neurotized to a lower extremity donor nerve to regain sensation in the flap. The sheer size of the ALT allows it to cover most large defects in the lower extremity. Unfortunately, this flap varies in thickness with body habitus and thus, the main drawback of the ALT flap is that in all but the thinnest patients, the subcutaneous fat layer of the thigh is a poor match for the thin skin of the foot and ankle. This thickness mismatch does not change with time as fasciocutaneous flaps do not atrophy like muscle flaps. Defatting can be performed at later time, but these necessitate further surgery. Despite this drawback, the ALT remains the workhorse large fasciocutaneous free flap due to its size, donor site tolerance, and familiarity.

Radial Forearm Flap

The RFF is medium-to-small sized longitudinally oriented fasciocutaneous flap, based on the radial artery and its associated vena comitantes. The cephalic vein and lateral antebrachial cutaneous nerve can optionally be included in the flap. The RFF

is harvested from the thin skin of the volar distal forearm and thus is well suited to medium-small wound of the foot because of its size, thickness, and contour. The vascular anatomy of the RFF is constant, and the perforators are abundant along the path of the radial artery, especially distally in the forearm. Pedicle lengths can be up to 18 cm and flap lengths can be 20 cm or more. The RFF can be customized to fit irregular defects. It can also be harvested as an osteocutaneous flap, as discussed below. There are drawbacks of the RFF, first the donor site morbidity as the forearm is easily visible and the donor site must be skin grafted. Secondly, the RFF is limited in width, which is unreliable beyond 10 cm. Nonetheless, it remains a favorite flap for lower extremity reconstruction because of its easy of harvest, familiarity, durability, and excellent contour match to the foot and ankle.

MUSCLE FLAPS

For lower extremity reconstruction, muscle flaps are usually taken as muscle only, with split-thickness skin grafts applied over top. Optionally, the muscle flaps can be taken with a skin paddle.

Latissimus Dorsi

The workhorse of the muscle flaps is the latissimus dorsi flap. This is a large thin flap, based on the thoracodorsal artery, and is widely used for reconstructive surgery thought the upper extremity, trunk, chest, and lower extremity. Its anatomy and harvest are familiar to most surgeons. The vessels are reliable, and the pedicle can be up to 15 cm. Vessels are 2-5 mm in diameter—large caliber for a microscopic anastomosis. In an adult male, the latissimus can be massive, up to 25 × 40 cm. It can cover nearly the entirety of the ankle and foot (see Fig. 70.2B) and is well suited to large defects. Drawbacks include workflow challenges with positioning as this flap is usually harvested in the lateral position and the patient must be repositioned for wound preparation and flap inset. Other drawbacks for use in the foot and ankle are the sheer size of the muscle flap as it can be quite bulky when applied to smaller wounds. Nonetheless, its widespread familiarity and durability make this a commonly used muscle flap.

Gracilis

The gracilis muscle flap is a medium-sized muscle flap, based off a gracilis branch which comes off the medial circumflex femoral artery. The pedicle is shorter than other flaps (6 cm), but the muscle is quite long, up to 30 cm. The gracilis is harvested from the medial thigh and can cover many defects in the lower extremity. The gracilis is an anatomically thin muscle but can easily be fanned out to cover larger defects, up to 10 cm wide. It is commonly used for medium-sized defects in the lower extremity (Fig. 70.3A and B).

BONE FLAPS

Fibula

Sources of free vascularized bone graft are limited throughout the human skeleton. The most common and largest bone free flap is the free fibula, which provides a long piece of bone

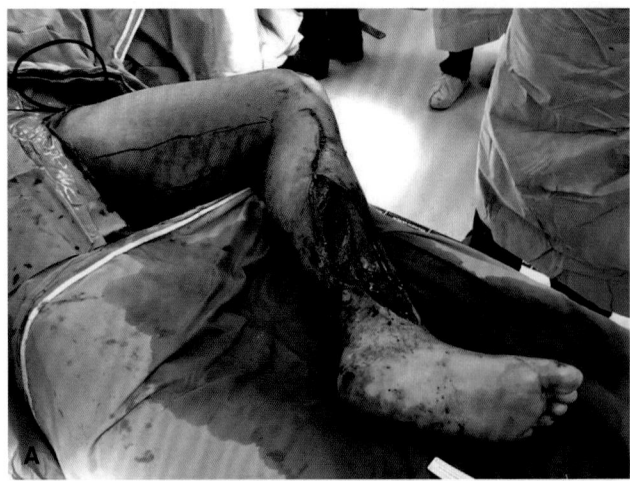

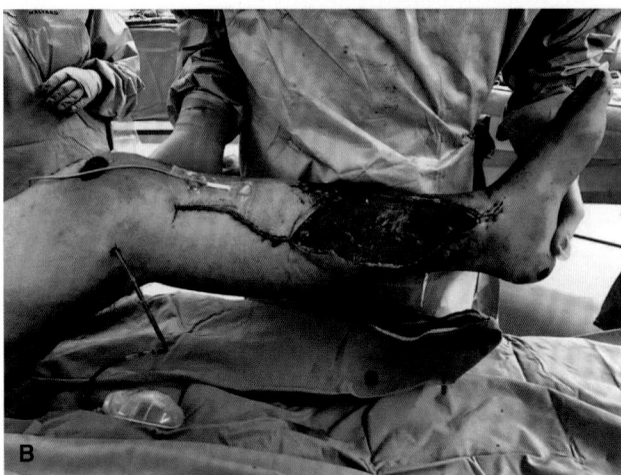

FIGURE 70.3 **A.** Soft tissue defect from grade 3B open distal 1/3 tibial fracture. **B.** Intraoperative clinical photo depicting gracilis muscle flap.

suitable for many large reconstructions. The free fibula flap is based off the peroneal artery and its donor site morbidity is generally well tolerated. The drawbacks of using the fibular free flap for foot and ankle defects are mainly related to its large size, up to 22 cm. Although it can be cut in half (double barreled), its size is often too much for the smaller bones of the foot and ankle. It is a difficult flap to take smaller than 12 cm as the perforator anatomy becomes less reliable as the size of the bone graft gets smaller. In addition, the free fibula is an all-cortical bone graft, which is advantageous for structural support applications but difficult to adapt to irregular boney defects or scenarios when cancellous graft is needed. Nonetheless, its familiarity and east of harvest make it a common choice for lower extremity reconstruction.

Free Iliac Crest Graft

Although less commonly used, the free iliac crest graft is an option for corticocancellous bone graft. The free iliac crest graft is based off the deep femoral circumflex artery and can provide a concave graft up to 5 × 15 cm in size. Although rarely used today, the free iliac crest graft provides a medium-sized piece of corticocancellous bone for foot reconstruction.

Medial Femoral Condyle

A more commonly used smaller free bone graft is the medial femoral condyle (MFC) from the distal femur. The MFC provides a medium-sized graft of corticocancellous bone (typically 5 × 5 cm) but can be harvested larger (up to 13 × 8 cm) or smaller (2.5 × 2.5 cm). This flap is based off the descending genicular artery, a branch of the superficial femoral artery. Its dissection is straightforward, and this graft can be reduced in size more easily than the free fibula to fit smaller defects. Its versatility in both upper extremity and lower extremity reconstruction makes it an attractive option for lower extremity reconstruction.

Osteocutaneous Flaps

Osteocutaneous grafts are chimeric grafts, which include skin, subcutaneous tissue, and bone. They are suitable for wounds of the foot that require reconstruction of skin, subcutaneous tissue, and bone.

Radial Forearm

The osteocutaneous radial forearm flap (OCRFF) is a flap that is well suited for use in the foot and ankle, given the thin skin of the forearm, and the small- to medium-sized bone that is provided. Unlike other bone flaps, the bone from the RFF is a unicortical block no wider than 1.5 cm. The donor site on the radius should be plated to avoid fracture (Fig. 70.4A and B). With prophylactic plating, the complication rates are very low.[6] One advantage of the radial forearm osteocutaneous flap is the long pedicle, which is often useful in getting the microvascular anastomosis out of the zone of injury. The main limitations of the OCRFF include the relative immobility of the bone-skin unit and difficulty with fixation of the bone to the recipient site.

Scapular/Parascapular

The scapular and parascapular flap can be harvested as a fasciocutaneous flap or as a chimeric flap, with skin, muscle, and bone from the lateral scapula. The muscle, bone, and skin can be harvested on separate branches, giving it the ability to fit complicated and diverse defects. Although advantageous in the amount of tissue provided, the parascapular flap is technically demanding to harvest and is limited due to the short pedicle (3-5 cm) making it less favorable for wounds with a large zone of injury.

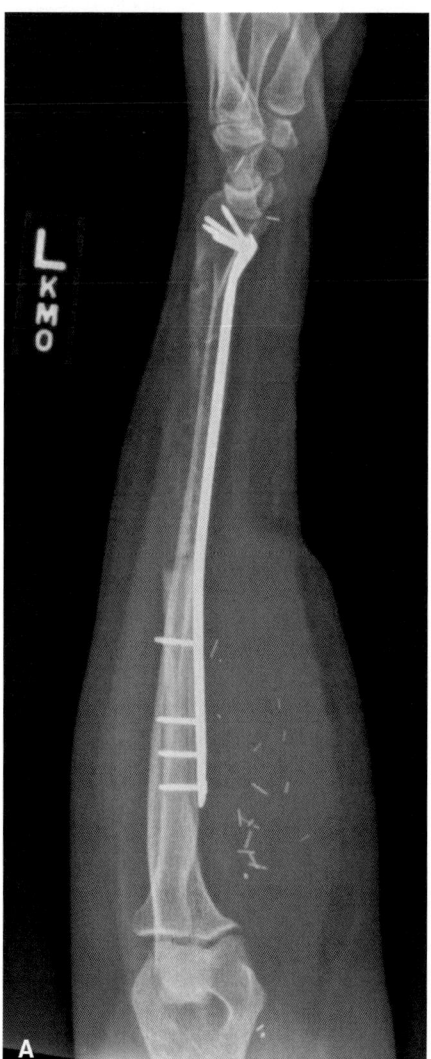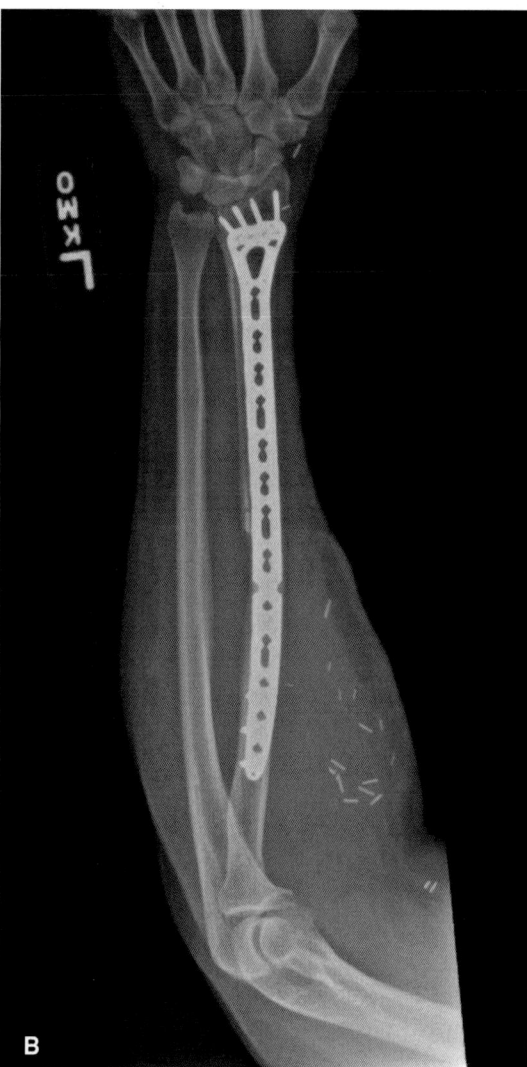

FIGURE 70.4 A. Lateral. **B.** Posteroanterior radiographs demonstrating prophylactic distal radius plating following harvest of an osteocutaneous radial forearm flap.

Arterial and Venous Anastomoses

Arterial and venous anastomoses ensure proper inflow and out-flow to free flap. Inadequate vascular anastomoses can lead to stoppage of flap perfusion or venous congestion, both of which usually lead to flap loss. The benefits of end-to-end (ETE) vs end-to-side (ETS) arterial anastomosis, one vs two venous anastomosis, and the use of venous couplers remain a subject of debate among microvascular surgeons. Advantages of an ETE anastomosis include technical ease and hemodynamic perfusion pattern[7,8] (Fig. 70.5A). Benefits to ETS anastomosis include vessel diameter discrepancies and need for preservation of arterial perfusion distal to anastomosis site[9,10] (Fig. 70.5B). Recent literature suggests there is no change in outcomes between ETE and ETS anastomoses but recommend ETS anastomosis when possible to preserve distal perfusion.[11] When considering venous anastomoses, two vessel venous anastomoses have historically been favored over single vessel anastomosis based on the hypothesis that increased venous output improved blood flow though the flap and reduced risk of venous thrombosis.[12] However, Hanasono et al.[13] recommended a single venous anastomosis as venous blood velocities are significantly greater when compared to double venous anastomoses, thus concluding a decreased risk for venous thrombosis and flap failure.

Venous couplers were described by Nakayama in 1962, who used an interlocking metal ring and pins to achieve patent venous anastomosis.[14] The Unilink coupler[15] was then later designed in the 1980s in Sweden and has since been refined. The purpose of the coupler was to provide intima to intima contact without intraluminal suture and which may promote

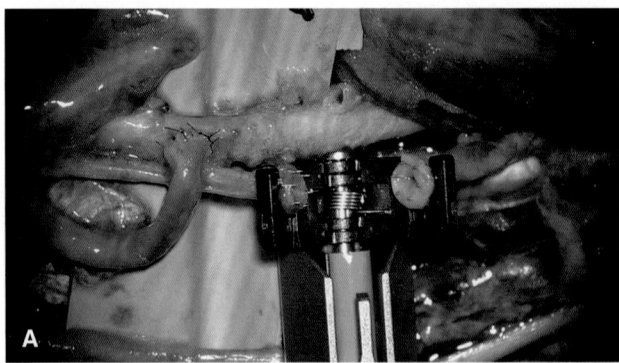

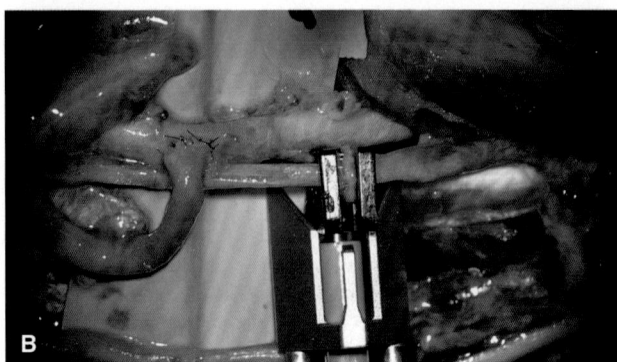

FIGURE 70.6 A. Venous coupler, prior to final coupling. **B.** Venous coupler, late stage of deployment.

thrombus formation. Recent literature suggests that these venous anastomotic couplers have an average patency rate of 98.5% and thrombus rate ranging from 0% to 3%[16] and reduce operating time, cost, and incidence of take-backs[17] (Fig. 70.6A and B).

COMPLICATIONS

Complications following free flaps are common. The most common complications include partial flap loss, reoperation, or reexploration. Oftentimes, major limb salvage efforts need additional procedures such as skin grafting, flap defatting, or revision of bony fixation. In experienced hands, catastrophic complications are rare. Free flap reexploration rates are reported between 6% and 14%[18] with complete flap failure <1% and partial flap loss <3% at many large microvascular centers.[19] Common complications include arterial or venous thrombus, hematoma, seroma, and surgical site infections. Bleeding disorders, albumin <3.5, diabetes, steroid usage, and operative time >510 minutes have all been associated with increased complications with lower extremity free flaps.[20]

LIMB SALVAGE VS PRIMARY AMPUTATION

Since the calling for objective guidelines for limb salvage vs primary amputation by Hansen in 1987, there have been multiple studies evaluating outcomes and predictive measures leading to amputation in the setting of lower extremity trauma. The

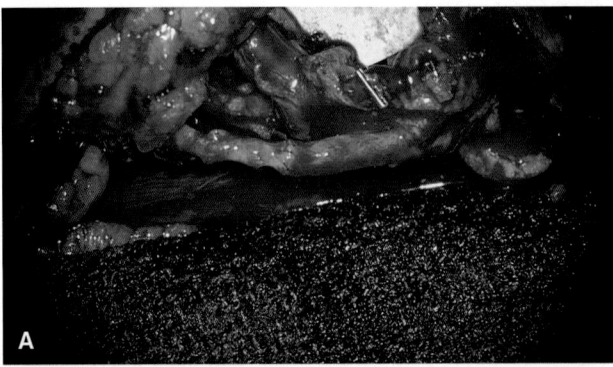

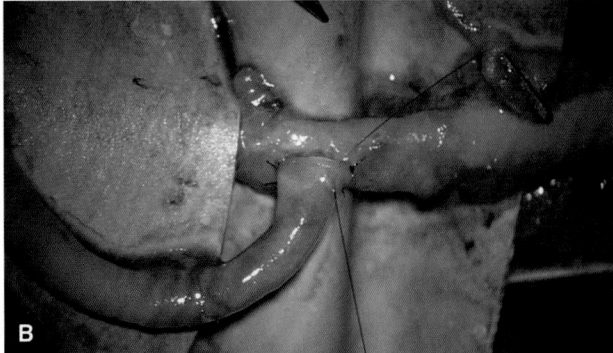

FIGURE 70.5 A. End-to-end anastomosis. Note the large venous anastomosis in the upper part of the picture. **B.** End-to-side anastomosis, with sutures being placed.

mangled extremity severity score (MESS), predicative salvage index (PSI), limb salvage index, and the nerve injury, ischemia, soft tissue injury, skeletal injury, shock, and age of patient (NISSSA) score have since been established to aid clinicians (Table 70.1). The most well-known, MESS study, evaluated four significant criteria, including severity of skeletal/soft tissue injury, limb ischemia, shock, and age, concluding that A MESS score >7 had a 100% predictive value for amputation.[21] Since 1990 when MESS was introduced, capabilities of managing extremity trauma have evolved. There have been considerable improvements in facture fixation, negative pressure wound therapy, and free tissue transfers, thus questioning the utility of the MESS.

Despite the above indices, clinicians continued to struggle deciding between primary amputation vs limb salvage. The Lower Extremity Assessment Project (LEAP)[22] set out to help

clinicians answer many of the questions surrounding when to amputate vs salvage the extremity. Overall, the LEAP trial found similar functional outcomes in patients in both amputation and reconstruction groups at 2 years.[22] Negative functional outcomes were associated with rehospitalization for major complication, lower educational level, nonwhite race, poverty, lack of private health insurance, poor social support, low self-efficacy, smoking, workers compensation, or patient seeking/receiving disability.[22] Using the data collected from the LEAP trial, Bosse et al.[23] sought to address the previous widespread notion that the absence of plantar sensation deemed the extremity unsalvageable. Bosse et al. found that while these patients had substantial impairment at follow-up, loss of plantar sensation did not adversely affect limb salvage.[23] Unfortunately, the LEAP study did not support the usefulness of any of the severity indices but suggests that patient's degree of self-efficacy as the single greatest factor at determining outcomes in patient with severe lower extremity trauma.[22]

TABLE 70.1	Predictive Indices for Primary Lower Extremity Amputation vs Limb Salvage in the Setting of Trauma		
MESI	Mangled Extremity Syndrome Index	▪ Injury Severity Score ▪ Tegmentum injury ▪ Vascular injury ▪ Fracture type ▪ Bone loss ▪ Wait time ▪ Age ▪ Comorbidities	>20 amputation
MESS	Mangled Extremity Severity Score	▪ Injury type ▪ Limb ischemia ▪ Shock ▪ Age ▪ Score ×2 for ischemia >6 hours	> 7 amputation
PSI	Predictive Salvage Index	▪ Level of arterial injury ▪ Degree of bone injury ▪ Degree of muscle injury ▪ Time to operating room	>8 amputation
LSI	Limb Salvage Index	▪ Arterial injury ▪ Nerve injury ▪ Bone injury ▪ Skin injury ▪ Muscle injury ▪ Deep venous injury ▪ Warm ischemia time	>6 likely amputation
NISSA	Nerve Injury, Ischemia, Soft tissue contamination, Skeletal injury, Shock, Age	▪ Nerve Injury ▪ Ischemia ▪ Soft tissue contamination ▪ Skeletal injury ▪ Shock ▪ Age	<7 salvage >11 amputation

CASE 1

A 22-year-old male sustained accidental gunshot wound to his left foot from large caliber hunting rifle. There was substantial bony and soft tissue loss with retained bullet fragments (Fig. 70.7A-C). He underwent irrigation and debridement with pinning of digits two and four, amputation of third digit, and wound VAC application on hospital day one followed by subsequent debridement, second digit amputation, amniotic tissue application, and wound VAC application on hospital day five (Fig. 70.8A and B). The fourth toe continued to decline, and patient subsequently returned to the operating room 2 weeks after initial injury for a repeat debridement and third toe amputation. A right ALT free flap was performed 1 month after initial injury followed by flap debulking 3 months later (Fig. 70.9A and B). He went on to heal uneventfully and able to ambulate on his operate extremity without difficulty (Fig. 70.9C).

CASE 2

A 57-year-old male presented to clinic with a chief complaint of a wound to his left foot. The patient described a remote 15-year-old crushing injury to his right foot that underwent open reduction with internal fixation. The patient also described a postoperative course that was complicated by delayed wound healing and osteomyelitis. He underwent hardware removal and a 6-week course of IV antibiotic therapy thereafter. The previous wound healed and had been without complication prior to his presentation to clinic. He was admitted to the hospital and underwent irrigation and debridement with bone biopsies the following day (Fig. 70.10A and B). Bone biopsies of the first metatarsal returned positive for chronic osteomyelitis. The patient returned to the operating room 4 days later for repeat debridement, partial resection of the first metatarsal to clean margin, antibiotic spacer placement, and wound VAC application. He returned to the operating room 1 month after his initial procedure for contralateral free radial forearm osteocutaneous flap with ETS vascular anastomosis, first

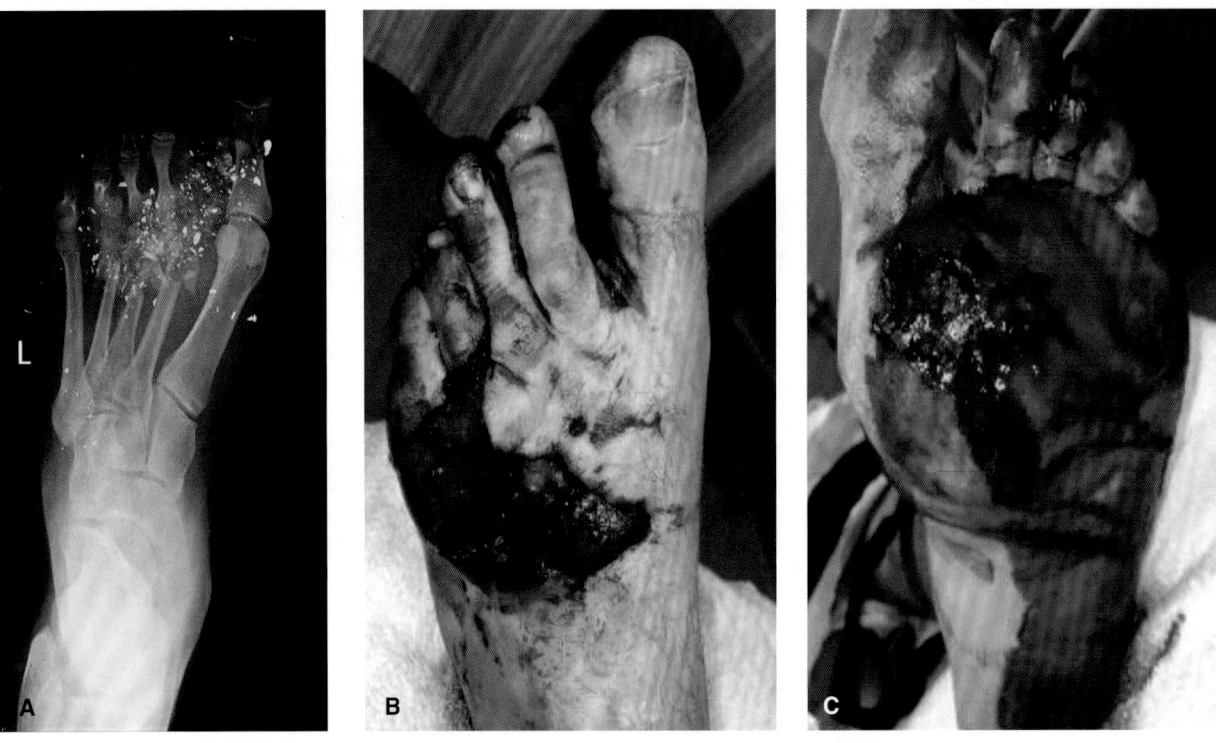

FIGURE 70.7 A. Anteroposterior radiograph with retained metallic fragments. **B, C.** Clinical photos from initial presentation. The patient underwent irrigation and debridement with pinning of digits two and four, amputation of third digit, and wound VAC application on hospital day one followed by subsequent debridement, second digit amputation, amniotic tissue application, and wound VAC application on hospital day five.

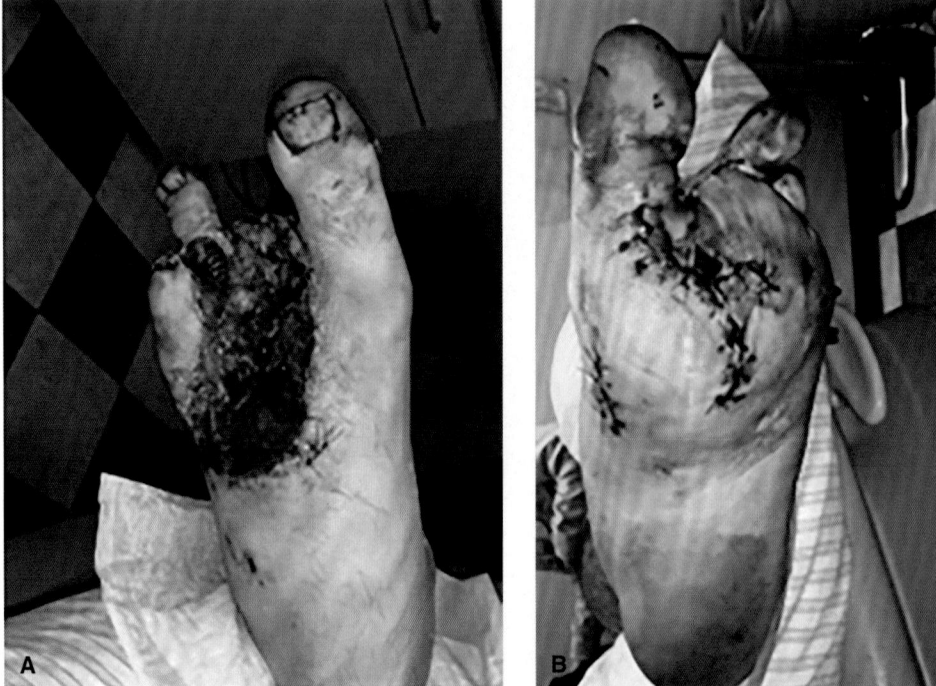

FIGURE 70.8 A. Clinical photos from hospital day five after two debridements and amniotic tissue application. The fourth toe continued to decline and the patient subsequently returned to the operating room 2 weeks after initial injury for a repeat debridement and third toe amputation. **B.** A right anterolateral thigh free flap was performed 1 month after initial injury followed by flap debulking 3 months later.

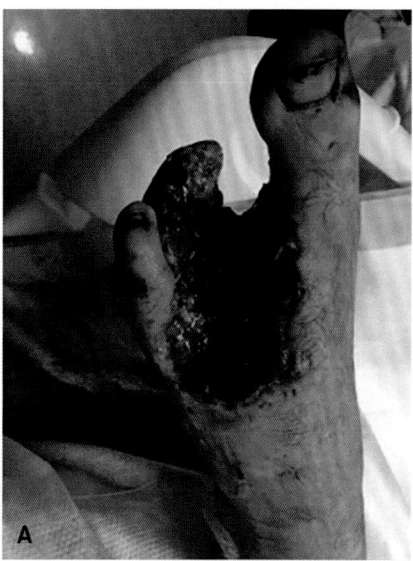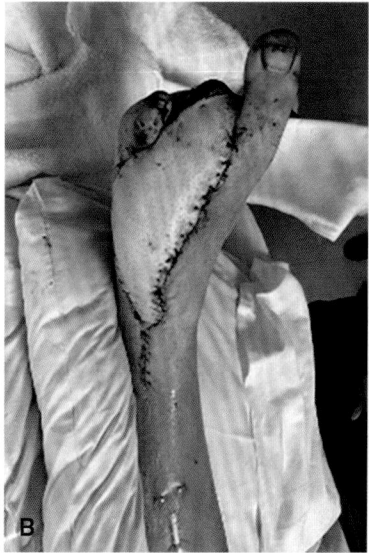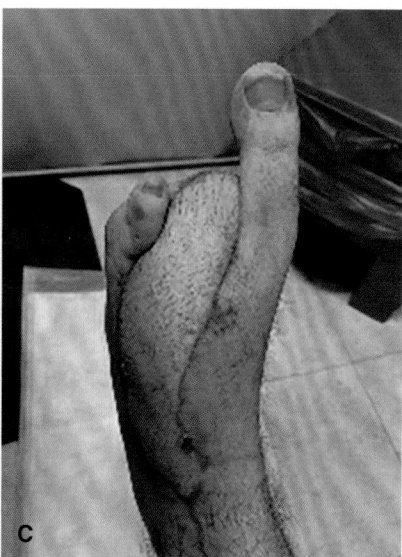

FIGURE 70.9 Clinical images of soft tissue defect **(A)** 4 weeks after in initial presentation, **(B)** immediate postop after anterolateral thigh flap, and **(C)** healed recipient site at 3 months after debulking. The patient went on to heal uneventfully and able to ambulate on their operate extremity without difficulty.

metatarsophalangeal joint, and first tarsometatarsal joint arthrodesis (Figs. 70.11A and B and 70.12A-D). On postoperative day zero, loss of signal to the implantable Doppler with delayed capillary fill was noted on postoperative examination. He returned emergently to the operating room for flap exploration with revision ETE arterial anastomosis. Five weeks

postoperatively, he underwent partial debridement with split-thickness skin grafting to remainder of harvest and donor site wounds. Three months postoperatively, he was noted excellent harvest and donor site healing with adequate bone healing across graft sites and transitioned to weight bearing as tolerated (Fig. 70.13A-C).

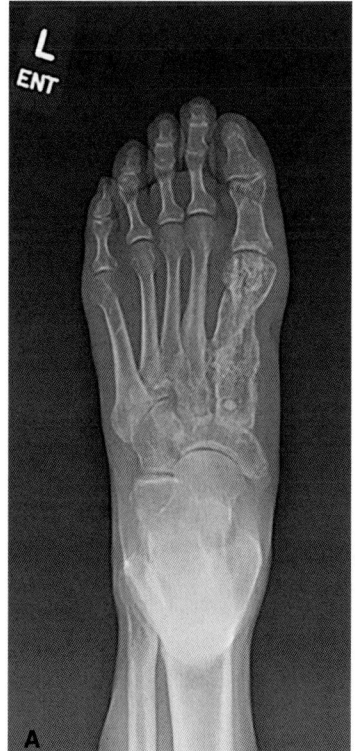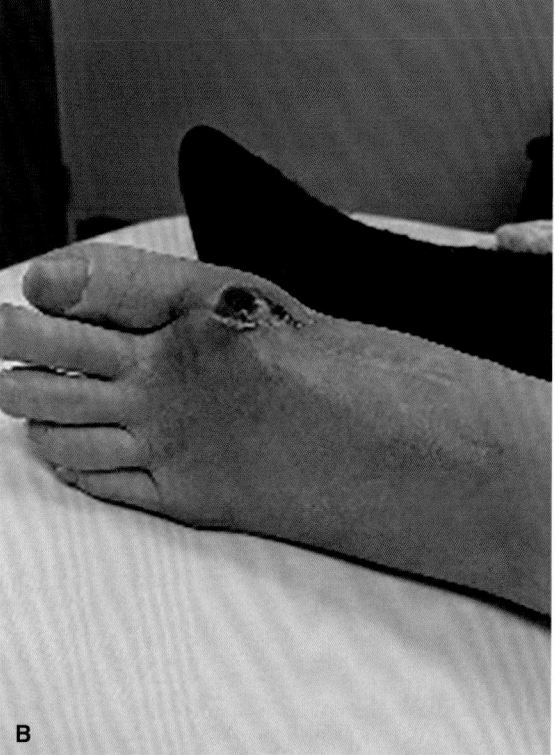

FIGURE 70.10 A. Anteroposterior radiograph of left foot with underlying osseous changes. **B.** Clinical photo from initial presentation with full-thickness ulceration and wound VAC application.

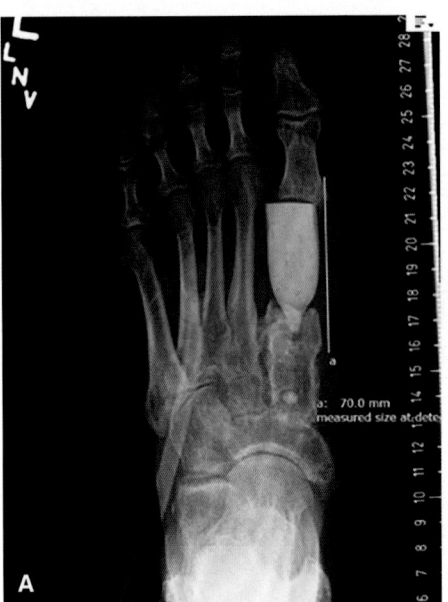
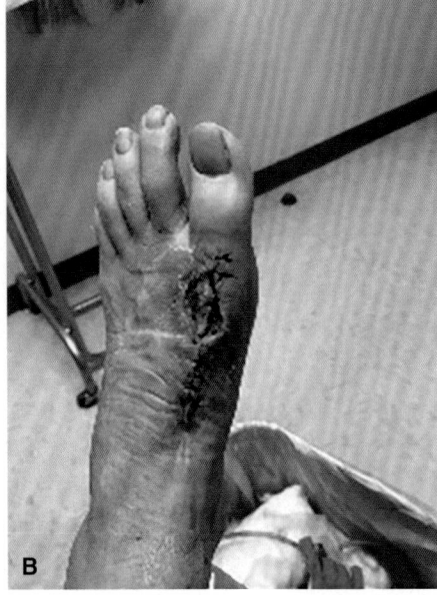

FIGURE 70.11 A. Intraoperative radiograph. **B.** Clinical photo after irrigation and debridement and subsequent antibiotic cement placement. The patient returned to the operating room 1 month after their initial procedure for contralateral free radial forearm osteocutaneous flap with end-to-side vascular anastomosis, first metatarsophalangeal joint, and first tarsometatarsal joint arthrodesis.

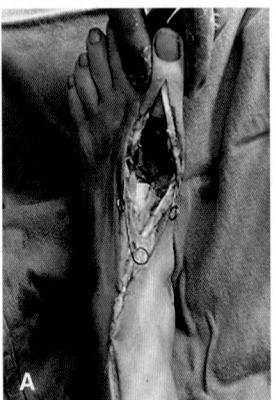
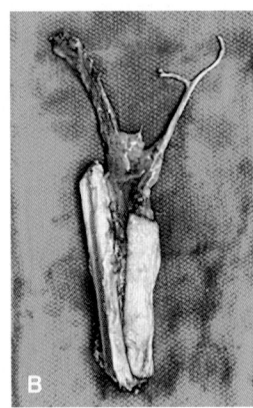
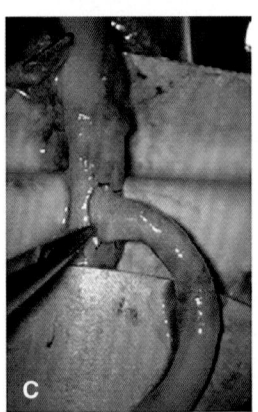
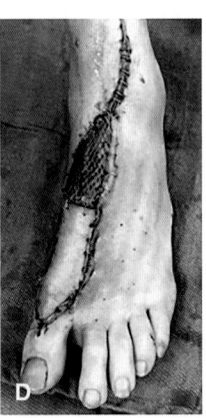

FIGURE 70.12 Intraoperative photographs of **(A)** bone and soft tissue defect, **(B)** harvested radial forearm osteocutaneous flap with donor vessels, **(C)** end-to-side arterial anastomosis, and **(D)** immediate postoperative photograph. On postoperative day zero, loss of signal to implantable Doppler with delayed capillary fill was noted on postoperative examination. The patient returned emergently to the operating room for flap exploration with revision end-to-end arterial anastomosis. Five weeks postoperatively, the patient underwent debridement with split-thickness skin grafting to remainder of harvest and donor site wounds. Three months postoperatively, excellent harvest and donor site healing was noted with adequate bone healing across graft sites and transitioned to weight bearing as tolerated.

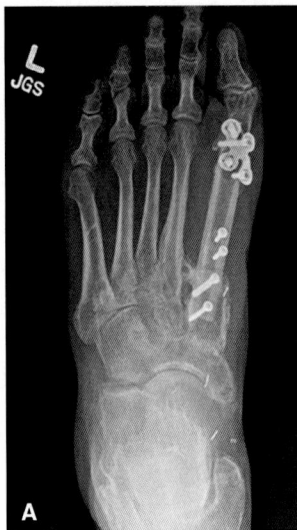
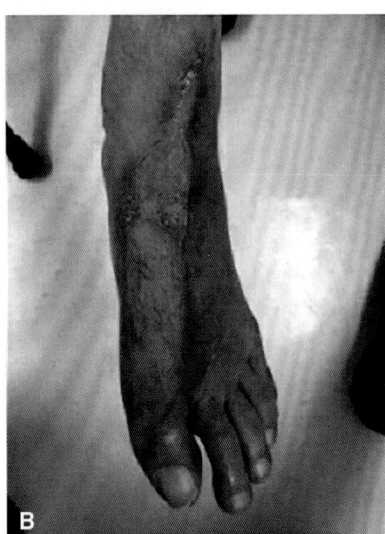
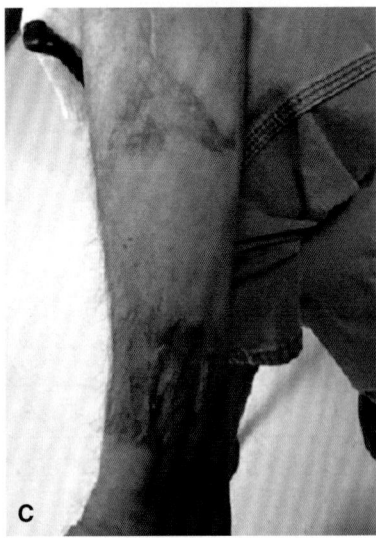

FIGURE 70.13 A. Anteroposterior radiograph. **B, C.** Clinical photographs at 3 months revealing osseous consolidation across the first tarsometatarsal joint and metatarsophalangeal joint and healed donor and recipient sites.

CASE 3

A 54-year-old male presented to the emergency department after accidental discharge of 20-gauge shotgun to the right foot (Figs. 70.14 and 70.15). Imaging was remarkable for comminuted fractures of metatarsals, multiple phalanx fractures, and numerous retained bullet fragments. Patient was taken to the operating room the following day for I&D, fasciotomies, and foreign body removal. Patient returned to the OR 3 days later for repeat debridement, antibiotic spacer placement to metatarsal two and three, fourth metatarsal pinning, and wound VAC application. The authors recommend using a 5cc syringe for 1st metatarsal spacer and a 3cc syringe for lesser metatarsals. These diameters match nicely, and the tapered tip of the syringe provides a nipple shape contact point. Patient was discharged home with close follow-up to discuss reconstruction options. Patient returned to OR 1 month after injury to begin two step reconstruction. Patient underwent repeat debridement, partial second ray amputation, first metatarsophalangeal arthrodesis, and antibiotic spacer exchange. He then returned 3 days later for contralateral free radial osteocutaneous flap with dorsalis pedis ETE anastomosis, Integra placement to right forearm, and split-thickness skin grafting to dorsal foot. He returned 3 weeks later for split-thickness skin grafting to harvest site. Patient healed uneventfully and was able to return to work 4 months postoperatively.

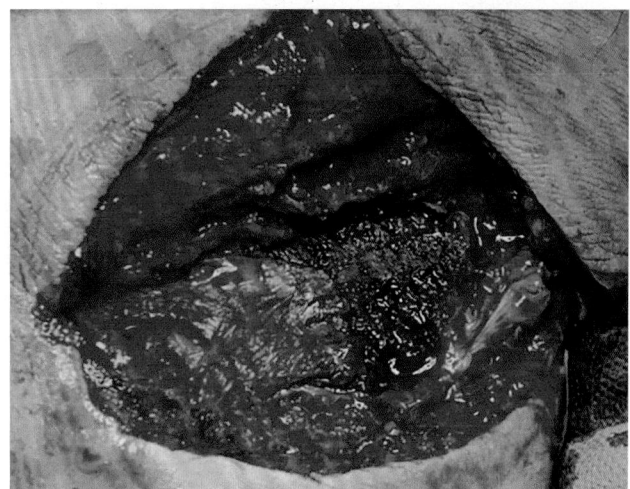

FIGURE 70.15 Exposed cancellous bone at the calcaneus at the base of the wound.

CASE 4

A 31-year-old male landscaper was injured by a commercial lawnmower with the epicenter of the injury to the left posterolateral heel. He was taken for an initial irrigation and debridement on the day of presentation where he was found to have exposed calcaneus. He returned to the operating room in 48 hours for a repeat irrigation and debridement, placement of a suspensory external fixator to the left leg, and a fasciocutaneous RFF (Fig. 70.16). Integra was placed on the RFF donor site. Allograft skin was placed over the pedicle of the free flap with plans for delayed skin grafting. His postoperative course

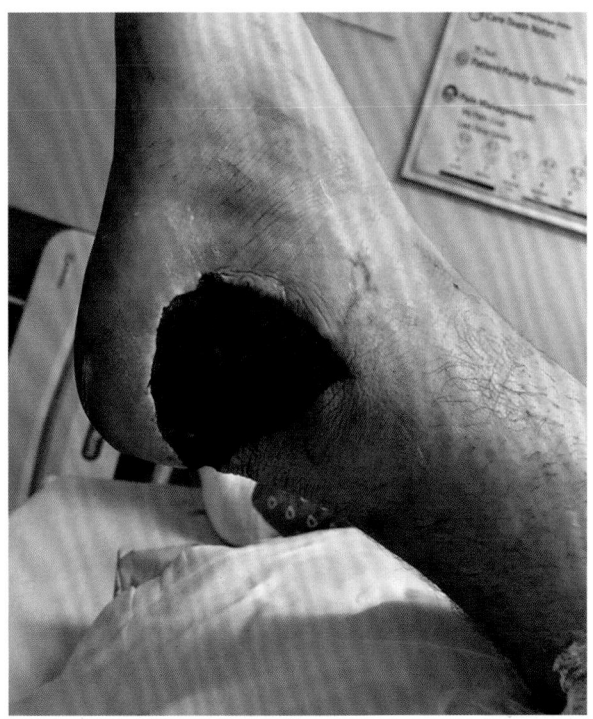

FIGURE 70.14 This is a posterolateral calcaneal wound.

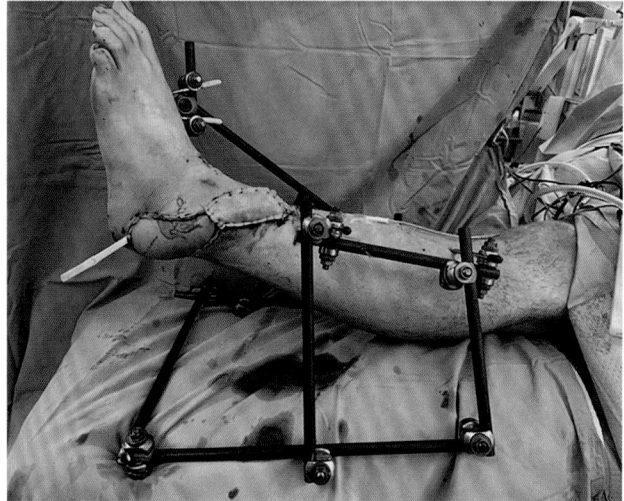

FIGURE 70.16 File placement of radial forearm flap with suspensory external fixation. Note the floating of the foot and elevation created by positioning of the frame. A Penrose drain has been placed under the flap. Allograft is placed in the proximal aspect of the pedicle flap.

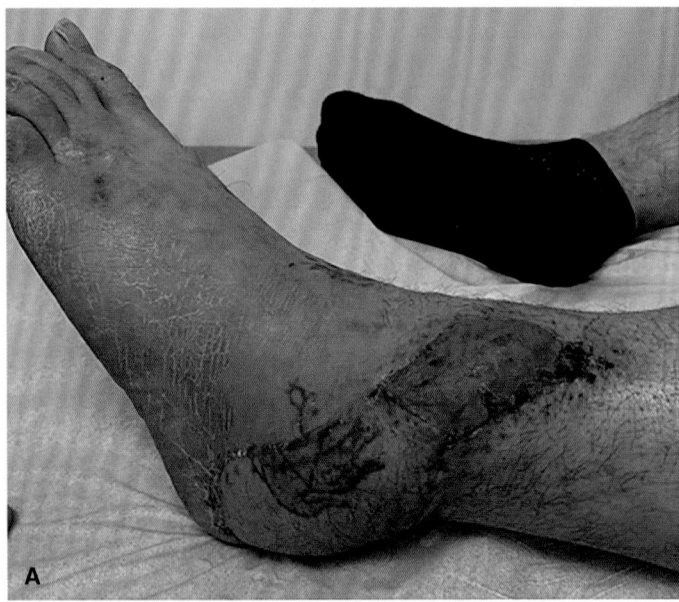
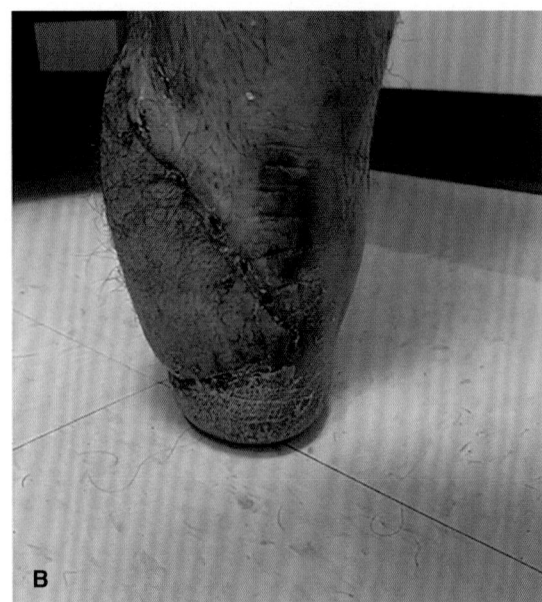

FIGURE 70.17 **A.** Final healed radial forearm flap after definitive autologous skin grafting on the proximal pedicle portion. **B.** Healed fasciocutaneous graft showing posterior distal Achilles tendon.

was unremarkable, and he returned to the operating room 3 weeks later for external fixator removal with skin grafting of the donor site and the pedicle of the flap. There was a partial loss of the skin graft on the arm and one of the tibial pin tracts had evidence of purulence. He returned to the operating room 3 days later for debridement of the tibial pin tract and re-skin grafting. He healed uneventfully and went on to full ambulation and returned to work 3 months after his initial injury (Figs. 70.17A and B and 70.18).

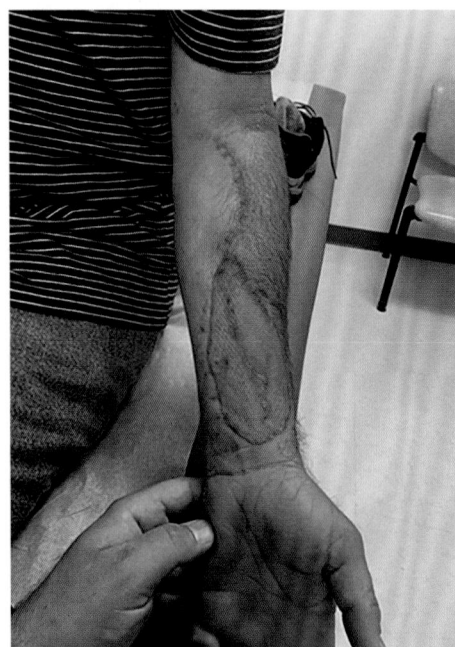

FIGURE 70.18 Donor site from radial forearm flap, after being covered by Integra and skin graft.

SUMMARY

In the absence of other reconstructive options, free flaps allow for limb reconstruction and limb salvage. Although dozens of different free flaps have been described, the reconstructive surgeon should have a small armamentarium of familiar flaps that can be performed efficiently and adapted to the clinical scenario. The above listed free flaps are appliable to a variety of wounds of the lower extremity. Flap selection should consider both patient and surgeon-related factors. Surgical planning ought to consider the tissue being reconstructed, the zone of injury, and the match of the donor and recipient tissue. Free flaps are technically demanding but can have high rates of success.

REFERENCES

1. Kaplan I, Ada S, Özerkan F, Bora A, Ademoglu Y. Reconstruction of soft tissue and bone defects in lower extremity with free flaps. *Microsurgery.* 1998;18(3):176-181. doi: 10.1002/(SICI)1098-2752.
2. Cobbett JR. Free digital transfer. Report of a case of transfer of a great toe to replace an amputated thumb. *J Bone Joint Surg Br.* 1969;51(4):677-679. doi: 10.1302/0301-620x.51b4.677.
3. O'Brien BMC, Morrison WA, Ishida H, MacLeod AM, Gilbert A. Free flap transfers with microvascular anastomoses. *Br J Plast Surg.* 1974;27(3):220-230. doi: 10.1016/S0007-1226(74)90079-4.
4. Gopal S, Majumder S, Batchelor AGB, Knight SL, De Boer P, Smith RM. Fix and flap: the radical orthopaedic and plastic treatment of severe open fractures of the tibia. *J Bone Joint Surg Br.* 2000;82(7):959-966. doi: 10.1302/0301-620X.82B7.10482.
5. Fischer MD, Gustilo RB, Varecka TF. The timing of flap coverage, bone-grafting, and intramedullary nailing in patients who have a fracture of the tibial shaft with extensive soft-tissue injury. *J Bone Jointt Surg Am.* 1991;73(9):1316-1322.
6. Satteson ES, Satteson AC, Waltonen JD, et al. Donor-site outcomes for the osteocutaneous radial forearm free flap. *J Reconstr Microsurg.* 2017;33(8):544–548. doi: 10.1055/s-0037-1602740.
7. Samaha FJ, Oliva A, Buncke GM, Buncke HJ, Siko PP. A clinical study of end-to-end versus end-to-side techniques for microvascular anastomosis. *Plast Reconstr Surg.* 1997;99(4):1109-1111. doi: 10.1097/00006534-199704000-00029.
8. Zhang L, Moskovitz M, Piscatelli S, Longaker MT, Siebert JW. Hemodynamic study of different angled end-to-side anastomoses. *Microsurgery.* 1995;16(2):114-117. doi: 10.1002/micr.1920160214.

9. Albertengo JB, Rodriguez A, Buncke HJ, Hall EJ. A comparative study of flap survival rates in end–to–end and end–to–side microvascular anastomosis. *Plast Reconstr Surg.* 1981;67(2):194-199. doi: 10.1097/00006534-198167020-00009.

10. Godina M. Preferential use of end–to–side arterial anastomoses in free flap transfers. *Plast Reconstr Surg.* 1999;64(5):673-682. doi: 10.1097/00006534-198006000-00028.

11. Heidekrueger PI, Ninkovic M, Heine-Geldern A, Herter F, Broer PN. End-to-end versus end-to-side anastomoses in free flap reconstruction: single centre experiences. *J Plast Surg Hand Surg.* 2017;51(5):362-365. doi: 10.1080/2000656X.2017.1283321.

12. Kroll SS, Schusterman MA, Reece GP, et al. Timing of pedicle thrombosis and flap loss after free-tissue transfer. *Plast Reconstr Surg.* 1996;98(7):1230-1233. doi: 10.1097/00006534-199612000-00017.

13. Hanasono MM, Kocak E, Ogunleye O, Hartley CJ, Miller MJ. One versus two venous anastomoses in microvascular free flap surgery. *Plast Reconstr Surg.* 2010;126(5):1548-1557. doi: 10.1097/PRS.0b013e3181ef8c9f.

14. Nakayama K, Tamiya T, Yamamoto K, Akimoto S. A simple new apparatus for small vessel anastomosis (free autograft of the sigmoid included). *Surgery.* 1962;52(6):918-931. doi: 10.5555/uri:pii:0039606062901459.

15. Ostrup LT, Berggren A. The UNILINK instrument system for fast and safe microvascular anastomosis. *Ann Plast Surg.* 1986;17(6):521-525. doi: 10.1097/00000637-198612000-00014.

16. Ardehali B, Morritt AN, Jain A. Systematic review: anastomotic microvascular device. *J Plast Reconstr Aesthet Surg.* 2014;67(6):752-755. doi: 10.1016/j.bjps.2014.01.038.

17. O'Connor EF, Rozen WM, Chowdhry M, et al. The microvascular anastomotic coupler for venous anastomoses in free flap breast reconstruction improves outcomes. *Gland Surg.* 2016;5(2):88-92. doi: 10.3978/j.issn.2227-684X.2015.05.14.

18. Kubo T, Yano K, Hosokawa K. Management of flaps with compromised venous outflow in head and neck microsurgical reconstruction. *Microsurgery.* 2002;22(8):391-395. doi: 10.1002/micr.10059.

19. Gill PS, Hunt JP, Guerra AB, et al. A 10-year retrospective review of 758 DIEP flaps for breast reconstruction. *Plast Reconstr Surg.* 2004;113(4):1153-1160. doi: 10.1097/01.PRS.0000110328.47206.50.

20. Veith J, Donato D, Holoyda K, Simpson A, Agarwal J. Variables associated with 30-day postoperative complications in lower extremity free flap reconstruction identified in the ACS-NSQIP database. *Microsurgery.* 2019;39(7):621-628. doi: 10.1002/micr.30502.

21. Helfet DL, Howey T, Sanders R, Johansen K. Limb salvage versus amputation. Preliminary results of the mangled extremity severity score. *Clin Orthop Relat Res.* 1990;(256):80-86. doi: 10.1097/00003086-199007000-00013.

22. Higgins TF, Klatt JB, Beals TC. Lower extremity assessment project (LEAP)—the best available evidence on limb-threatening lower extremity trauma. *Orthop Clin North Am.* 2010;41(2):233-239. doi: 10.1016/j.ocl.2009.12.006.

23. Bosse MJ, McCarthy ML, Jones AL, et al. The insensate foot following severe lower extremity trauma: an indication for amputation? *J Bone Jointt Surg Am.* 2005;87(12 I):2601-2608. doi: 10.2106/JBJS.C.00671.

Note: Page numbers followed by "*f*" refer to figures; page numbers followed by "*t*" refer to tables.

    879–880, 896–903
Talocalcaneal coalition resection, 1168
Talocalcaneonavicular joint (TCNJ), 1215, 1215*t*
Talocrural angle, supramalleolar osteotomy, 755
Talolisthesis, 631
Talonavicular arthrodesis, 945, 957*f*–958*f*
Talonavicular coalition, 37, 38*f*, 870, 872,
    903–905
Talonavicular coverage angle, 47
Talonavicular joint, 1463*b*, 1467
Talonavicular (TN) joint arthrodesis
    anatomic considerations, 541
    complications, 545, 545*f*
    definition, 541
    imaging, 542, 542*f*–543*f*
    indications, 541, 541*f*–542*f*
    nonunion of, 979*f*
    physical examination, 542
    postoperative care, 545
    surgical technique, 543–544, 543*f*, 544*f*
    treatment, 542–543
Talus, 1055
Talus fractures, 1193–1197
    incidence, 1193, 1193*f*
    lateral process of the talus, treatment of
        fractures of, 1194
    osteochondral fractures of talus, 1194–1197
    talar body fractures, 1194, 1194*t*
    talar neck fractures, 1193–1194
Talus-first metatarsal angle, 46
Tangential surfaces concept, 22, 22*t*
TAR. *See* Total ankle replacement (TAR)
Targeted antibiotic therapy
    for native ankle septic arthritis, 1018*t*
    for necrotizing soft tissue infections, 1015*t*
Targeted antimicrobial therapy, for adult
        osteomyelitis, 1028
Tarsal and carpal coalitions, 872
Tarsal coalition
    arthritic changes, 889
    articular involvement, 889
    associated abnormalities, 872–874
    classification, 874–875
    clinical findings, 875–878
    conservative therapy, 887–888
    definition, 870
    direct surgical treatment, 888–908
    etiology, 870–871
    incidence, 871–872
    invasive studies and evaluation, 885–887
    limitation of motion, 875
    limitation of subtalar and midtarsal joint
        motion, 876
    massive coalitions, 872–873
    metatarsal abnormalities, 872
    MRI signs, 885, 887*t*
    muscle spasm, 875
    pain, 875–876
    peroneal spastic flatfoot, 870
    radiographic and advanced imaging
        findings, 878–885
    symptomatic relief of, 888
    treatment, 887–908
    ultrasound evaluation, 885
Tarsal coalitions, 1165–1168, 1167*f*
    calcaneonavicular coalition resection, 1168
    imaging and diagnostic studies, 1166
    physical examination, 1166
    talocalcaneal coalition resection, 1168
    treatment for, 1166–1168
Tarsal tunnel syndrome, 429–430, 873,
    1101–1102
Tarsal-carpal coalition syndrome, 871
4/5 Tarsometatarsal joints, 1463*b*, 1467, 1468*f*
Tarsometatarsal (TMT) articulation, 492

Tarsometatarsal joint (TMTJ), 492
    arthrodesis, 455–464
    anatomic features, 455, 455*b*
    biomechanics, 455
    complications, 463–464
    etiology, 455–456, 455*b*, 456*f*
    indications for, 458*b*
    nonoperative management, 458
    physical examination, 456–457, 457*b*, 457*f*
    postoperative management, 463
    primary arthritis, 455
    radiographic evaluation, 457–458, 458*f*
    surgical planning and considerations,
        458–460, 459*f*–460*f*
    surgical technique
        countersinking axial screw placement,
            460–463, 463*f*
        deep peroneal nerve and dorsalis pedis
            artery, 460–463, 461*f*
        dorsal-central incision, 460–463, 461*f*
        fixation options, 460–463, 462*f*, 463*f*
        Freer elevator, 460–463, 461*f*
        intravenous sedation, 460
        medially based incision, 460–463,
            460*f*–463*f*
        patient positioning, 460
        soft tissue closure, 460–463
        two screw placement, 460–463
Taylor Spatial Frame (TSF), 764, 1436
Tc-99m sulfur colloid scanning, 1026
Techneitum-99m methylene diphosphonate
        (Tc-99m MDP) scan, 1017–1018,
        1026
    complex regional pain syndrome, 104, 105*f*
Technetium-99m hexamethyl-propyleneamine
        oxime (HMPAO)-labeled
        leukocyte scan (Ceretec), 1026
Temporary fixation of ankle fractures with
        external fixation, 719, 719*f*–720*f*
Tendinopathy
    acute tendon lacerations, 1265–1267, 1266*f*,
        1267*f*
    complications, 1273–1274
    imaging and diagnostic studies, 1264–1265
    pathogenesis, 1262
    postoperative care, 1275
    tendon healing, 1262–1264, 1262*t*, 1263*f*
Tendo Achilles lengthening (TAL), 442
    indications, 1392
Tendon anchoring principles, 1216
Tendon healing
    collagen fiber structure, 1262–1263
    grasping/locking suture techniques, 1263
    phases of, 1262–1263, 1262*t*
    remodeling stage, 1262–1263
    reparative/proliferative stage, 1262–1263
    stages of, 1262–1263, 1262*t*
    suture techniques, 1263, 1263*f*
Tendon proper–derived cells (TDCs),
        noninsertional Achilles
        tendinosis, 1295
Tendon sheath, giant cell tumor of, 916
Tendon transfers, 1213
    anatomic features and functional analysis,
        1218–1219
        extensor retinaculum, 1219
        interosseous membrane, 1218
        posterior tibialis tendon, 1218
        sciatic nerve, 1218–1219
    anatomy of, tendons, 1213
    Bridle procedure
        anatomic features and functional analysis,
            1223
        anterior tibialis, 1223
        definition of, 1222–1223
        exposure pearls, 1224

        imaging and diagnostics, 1223
        indications, 1223
        interosseous transfer, 1225
        nonoperative treatment, 1224
        pathogenesis, 1223
        peroneal longus, 1223
        physical examination, 1223
        positioning pearls, 1224
        postoperative care, 1225
        six-incision technique, 1224
        surgical procedure and technique, 1224
        treatment, 1223–1224
    digital flexor tendon transfer
        absorbable interference screw for, 1248
        anatomic features and functional analysis,
            1244
        chronic external deforming forces, 1245
        classification, 1244
        congenital, 1245
        definition of, 1243–1244
        dynamic stabilizers, 1244
        extensor substitution deformity, 1244
        FDL to extensor transfer, 1246–1247,
            1246*f*, 1247*f*
        FDL transfer via drill tunnel, 1247–1248,
            1247*f*–1248*f*
        flexor stabilization deformity, 1244
        flexor substitution deformity, 1244
        hammertoe implants for, 1248
        iatrogenic, 1245
        imaging and diagnostics, 1245
        indications, 1244
        inflammation, 1245
        neuromuscular, 1245
        nonoperative treatment of, 1245
        pathogenesis, 1244–1245
        physical examination, 1244
        postoperative care, 1249
        rehabilitation, 1249
        static stabilizers, 1244
        surgical procedure and technique,
            1245–1248
        trauma, 1245
        treatment of, 1245–1248
    exposure pearls, 1222
    FHL tendon transfer WITH V-Y
            advancement for chronic Achilles
            tendon ruptures, 1234, 1238*f*,
            1240–1243
        Achilles tendon repair, 1240
        anatomic features, 1234
        definition, 1234
        end-to-end anastomosis, 1240–1241
        FHL tendon harvest (alternative two-
            incision approach), 1239–1240
        FHL tendon harvest (one-incision
            approach), 1239–1240,
            1240*f*–1242*f*
        functional analysis of anatomy, 1234
        gastrocnemius soleus V-to-Y lengthening,
            1236–1239, 1238*f*
        imaging and diagnostic studies, 1236,
            1236*f*
        indications, 1234
        locking Krakow, 1241
        nonoperative treatment, 1236
        pathogenesis, 1235
        physical examination, 1235, 1235*f*–1236*f*
        postoperative care, 1243, 1243*f*
        rehabilitation, 1243
    flexor digitorum longus tendon transfer for
            flatfoot, 1254
        anatomic features, 1255
        classification, 1255
        cotton medial cuneiform osteotomy, 1258
        definition of, 1254